LIPPINCOTT®
Nursing
Procedures

NINTH EDITION

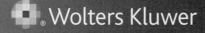
Wolters Kluwer

Philadelphia • Baltimore • New York • London
Buenos Aires • Hong Kong • Sydney • Tokyo

Chief Nurse: Anne Dabrow Woods, DNP, RN, CRNP, ANP-BC, AGACNP-BC
Director, Content Management: Jamie L. Blum
Acquisitions Editor: Susan M. Hartman
Editor-in-Chief: Collette Bishop Hendler, RN, MS, MA, CIC
Clinical Editor: Beverly Ann Tscheschlog, RN, MS
Senior Managing Editor: Diane Labus
Associate Editor: Ellen Sellers
Editor: Rosanne Hallowell
Editorial Assistant: Linda K. Ruhf
Graphic Arts and Design Manager: Stephen Druding
Image Coordinator: Joseph John Clark
Production Project Manager: Barton Dudlick
Manufacturing Coordinator: Beth Welsh
Marketing Manager: Amy Whitaker
Production Services: TNQ Technologies

10 8 9 7 6 5 4 3 2

Printed in Mexico

Library of Congress Cataloging-in-Publication Data

ISBN-13: 978-1-975178-58-1

Cataloging in Publication data available on request from publisher.

shop.LWW.com

Contents

Contributors and consultants

Amy Adkison, MSN, RN, RN-BC, NPD-BC
Clinical Education Specialist
Saint Luke's Health System
Kansas City, MO

Erin Alden, MN, ARNP-CNS, RN-BC, CMSRN, ACNS-BC
Acute Care Clinical Nurse Specialist/Stroke Coordinator
UW Medicine Valley Medical Center
Renton, WA

Jiji Andrews, MSN, RN, PCCN, CMSRN
Acute Care Clinical Education Specialist
Texas Health Resources University
Arlington, TX

Kristine Arcadi, MBA, MSN, RN, CMSRN
Unit Manager
Erie County Medical Center
Buffalo, NY

Patricia Barrella, MSN, RN, CHFN
Heart Failure Coordinator
Abington Memorial Hospital
Abington, PA

Donna Barto, DNP, RN, CCRN
Teaching Faculty
Rowan College Burlington County
Mt. Laurel, NJ

Claire Bethel, PhD, RN-BC
Magnet Program Coordinator
Banner Health
Tucson, AZ

Emerald Bilbrew, DNP, MSN, RN, CMSRN
Faculty
Fayetteville Technical Community College
Fayetteville, NC

Anndalos Bindra, MSN, RN-BC, CCRN-K, PHN
Magnet Program Manager, Nurse Manager
Valley Children's Healthcare
Madera, CA

Sarah Bixler, MSN, RN
Lecturer
Kent State University
Kent, OH

Sarah Bologna, MS, RN, CNS, ACNS-BC
Diabetes Clinical Nurse Specialist
Duke Health
Durham, NC

Donna Bond, DNP, RN, CCNS, AE-C, CTTS, FCNS
Pulmonary Clinical Nurse Specialist
Carilion Clinic
Roanoke, VA

Brianna Buzzuro, MSN, RN, CEN, TCRN, NPD-BC
Registered Nurse
Christiana Care Health System
Wilmington, DE

Amanda Cancelliere, BSN, RN, CPPS
Clinical Consultant
Chesterfield, NJ

Bridget Carey, MSN, RN, CWCN
Medical Education Manager
Smith & Nephew Advance Wound Management
Fort Worth, TX

Tiffany Carollo, RN, MS, CNS
Nurse Educator, Patient Education
Long Island Jewish Medical Center
New Hyde Park, NY

Tina Collins, MSN, RN, CCRN, CNS
Sepsis Coordinator, Critical Care Clinical Nurse Specialist
Henrico Doctors' Hospital
Richmond, VA

Melinda Constantine, RN, MSN, CMSRN, ONC
Director of Professional Development
New York Community Hospital
Brooklyn, NY

Laurie K. Donaghy, MSN, RN, CEN
Assistant Nurse Manager
Temple University Hospital
Philadelphia, PA

Taina Evans, MHA, BSN, RN
Director, Specialty Clinics—Clinic Administration
Boys Town National Research Hospital
Boys Town, NE

Ellie Z. Franges, DNP, ANP-BC, CRNP, CNRN
Nurse Educator
Ameritech College of Healthcare
Provo, UT

Anthodith Garganera, MSN/MHA, RN, CMSRN, CNL
Clinical Nurse Leader
Texas Health Presbyterian Hospital of Plano
Plano, TX

Theresa Garren-Grubbs, DNP, RN, CMSRN, CNL
Clinical Assistant Professor
South Dakota State University
Brookings, SD

Denise Giachetta-Ryan, MSN, MPH, RN, CNOR
Perioperative Specialist
Richmond University Medical Center
Staten Island, NY

Blaine Jumper, MSN, RN, CMSRN
Practical Nursing Instructor
Southwest Technology Center
Altus, OK

Chantel Knox, MSN, RN, CEN, TCRN
Clinical Registered Nurse IV
Saint Agnes Hospital
Baltimore, MD

Karen Krofft, DNP, RN-BC, OCN
Director of Nursing Support Services
Genesis Healthcare Systems
Zanesville, OH

Jennifer Lee, RN, MSN, FNP-C
Nurse Practitioner
Prisma Health Greenville Hospital
Greenville, SC

Lillian McAteer, MBA, BSN, BHA, RN, CPAN
Clinical Consultant
Wimberley, TX

Colleen McCracken, BSN, RN, CMSRN, CHPN, OCN
Staff Registered Nurse Educator
Froedtert Hospital
Milwaukee, WI

Kylene Mesaros, MSN, APRN, ACCNS-AG, CCRN
Critical Care Clinical Nurse Specialist
Summa Health System
Akron, OH

Amanda Murray, MSN, APRN, AGCNS-BC, CMSRN
Clinical Nurse Specialist
Norton Healthcare
Louisville, KY

Sheri Piper, RN, MSN, CCRN
Manager Nursing Patient Care
OSF Healthcare St. Joseph's Medical Center
Bloomington, IL

Michael Pulliam, BA, BSN, RN, CCRN, CEN, TCRN, CPAN
Staff, Charge Nurse
Cooper University Hospital
Camden, NJ

Noraliza Salazar, MSN, RN, CCRN-K, RN-BC, CNS
Cardiovascular Clinical Nurse Specialist
AHMC Seton Medical Center
Daly City, CA

Jere Shear, MSN, RN, CMSRN
Nurse Manager
Eastern Oklahoma VA Healthcare System
Muskogee, OK

Cheryl Sheffield, RN, PhD, CMSRN, OCN
Nursing Faculty
Lee College
Baytown, TX

Deirdre Smith, MSN, RN, CMSRN
Advanced Clinical Educator
Virtua Our Lady of Lourdes Hospital
Camden, NJ

Bridgette Smoot, MSN, RN, CMSRN
Staff Registered Nurse
Centra Lynchburg General Hospital
Lynchburg, VA

Theodore Urbano, MS, BSN, RN, CMSRN, CCP
Program Manager, Military Medical
   Treatment Facility Education & Training
   Plans & Policy
Defense Health Agency
Falls Church, VA

Jennifer Whitley, RN, MSN, MBA, CNOR, CST
Director, Surgical Technology Programs
Huntsville Hospital
Huntsville, AL

Kendra Wold, MSN, BS, RN, CNL
Clinical Consultant
Schertz, TX

Wendy Woodall, MSN, CMSRN, CNE
Deputy Chief, Department of Clinical
   Specialties
U.S. Army
Fort Sam Houston, TX

Demetra Zalman, MSN, CRNP
Acute Care Nurse Practitioner
Hospital of the University of Pennsylvania
Philadelphia, PA

Galen Ziegler, BSN, RN, CMSRN
Staff Registered Nurse
University of Maryland Upper Chesapeake
   Medical Center
Bel Air, MD

How to use this book

As a nurse, you're expected to know how to perform or assist with literally hundreds of procedures. From the most basic patient care, to complex treatments, to assisting with the most intricate surgical procedures, you need to be able to carry out nursing procedures with skill and confidence. But mastering so many procedures is a tall order.

Newly updated with the latest evidence-based research, this ninth edition of *Lippincott Nursing Procedures* provides step-by-step guidance on the most commonly performed nursing procedures you need to know, making it the ideal resource for providing the professional, hands-on care your patients deserve.

The A-to-Zs of organization

With over 400 procedures covered in detail, the current edition of *Lippincott Nursing Procedures* presents this wealth of information in the most efficient way possible. Many procedures books use such categories as fundamental procedures, body systems, and other types of procedures (such as psychiatric care) to organize the material. But with the proliferation in the number and types of procedures you need to understand, such an organization can become difficult to manage.

To address this, *Lippincott Nursing Procedures* organizes all procedures into an A-to-Z listing, making the book fast and easy to use. When you need to find a particular procedure quickly, you can simply look it up by name. No need to scan through the table of contents. No time lost turning to the index, looking for the name of the procedure you want, and then finding the right page in the book.

After you've found the entry for a particular procedure in the alphabetical listing, you'll find that each entry uses the same clear, straightforward structure. An introductory section appears first. After that, most or all of the following sections appear, depending on the particular procedure:

- The *Equipment* section lists all the equipment you'll need, including all the variations in equipment that might be needed. For instance, in the "electrical bone growth stimulation" entry, you'll see a general equipment list, which is followed by separate lists of the additional equipment you'll need for ultrasound stimulation and electromagnetic stimulation.
- As the name implies, the *Preparation of equipment* section guides you through preparing the equipment for the procedure.
- In the *Implementation* section—the heart of each entry—you'll find the step-by-step guide to performing the particular procedure.
- *Special considerations* alerts you to factors to keep in mind that can affect the procedure.
- *Patient teaching* covers procedure-related and home care information you need to teach to the patient and family.
- *Complications* details procedure-related complications to watch for.
- The *Documentation* section helps you keep track of everything you need to document related to the procedure.
- The expanded *References* section includes numbered citations keyed to the main text of each entry. These numbered citations serve as the clinical evidence that underpins the information and step-by-step procedures presented in the entry. (There'll be more on this in the next section of this "how to" guide.)

The continued use of the A-to-Z organization in the ninth edition and the clear structure of each entry make this book a powerful tool for finding and understanding the procedures you need to know.

Evidently speaking...

Lippincott Nursing Procedures strengthens its evidence-based approach to nursing care with an expanded numbered *References* section that appears in each entry. As mentioned earlier, the numbered citations are keyed to information that appears throughout each procedure.

As you read through an entry and come across a bullet describing a particular step in a procedure, you'll notice one or more red superscript numbers following the bullet. These numbers are citations for studies listed in the *References* section; the studies supply clinical evidence or detail "best practices" related to that bulleted step in the procedure. This is what is meant by *evidence-based practice*: a particular practice—say, performing hand hygiene—is supported by the clinical evidence. This evidence-based approach means the procedures you'll read about in *Lippincott Nursing Procedures* are best-practice procedures that rely on solid, authoritative evidence.

As you look at the numbered references in each entry, you may notice that many of them are followed by a level number. This level number appears in parentheses after the reference as the word "Level" followed by a Roman numeral that ranges from I to VII. These level numbers give you an indication of the strength of the particular reference, with Level I being the strongest and Level VII the weakest.

Here's how the rating system for this hierarchy of evidence works:
- *Level I:* Evidence comes from a systematic review or meta-analysis of all relevant randomized, controlled trials.
- *Level II:* Evidence comes from at least one well-designed randomized, controlled trial.
- *Level III:* Evidence comes from well-designed, controlled trials without randomization.
- *Level IV:* Evidence comes from well-designed case-control and cohort studies.
- *Level V:* Evidence comes from systematic reviews of descriptive and qualitative studies.
- *Level VI:* Evidence comes from a single descriptive or qualitative study.
- *Level VII:* Evidence comes from the opinion of authorities, reports of expert committees, or both.

In this book, the majority of cited references followed by a level are rated "Level I." These Level I references provide the strongest level of evidence to support a particular practice. You can use these levels to gauge the strength of supporting evidence for any particular practice or procedure.

Another important way *Lippincott Nursing Procedures* provides a more evidence-based approach is by offering rationales for many procedure steps. These rationales are set off from the main text in italics. For instance, you may see a bullet like this: "Explain the procedure to the patient and family (if appropriate) according to their individual communication and learning needs *to increase their understanding, allay their fears, and enhance cooperation.*" The second part of that bullet—the italicized portion—is the rationale, or reason, for performing the first part. The practice of answering the patient's questions is supported by the clinical evidence of the patient's decreased anxiety and increased cooperation.

Just the highlights, please

Lippincott Nursing Procedures, Ninth Edition, also benefits from other features that make it easy to use. Throughout, you'll find highlighting that greatly enhances the main text. Some examples:

- As mentioned earlier, footnotes appear in red for easier spotting.
- Colored letter tabs at the top of each page make finding a particular entry quick and easy.
- Full-color photos and diagrams highlight the main text, illustrating many of the step-by-step procedures in the *Implementation* section of each entry.
- Special alerts—with colorful, eye-catching logos—appear in many entries:

NURSING ALERT lets you know about potentially dangerous actions or clinically significant findings related to a procedure.

PEDIATRIC ALERT warns you of particular precautions to take concerning infants, young children, and adolescents.

ELDER ALERT cautions you about the special needs of this growing population.

HOSPITAL-ACQUIRED CONDITION ALERT warns you about conditions that the Centers for Medicare and Medicaid Services has identified as conditions that may occur as the result of hospitalization. Following various best practices can reasonably help to prevent such conditions; when these conditions do occur, they have payment implications for health care facilities.

- Short, boxed-off items appear throughout the book. These short pieces run the gamut, from explaining procedures in more detail, to highlighting equipment, to offering tips for clearer documentation, to name just a few. Several are set off with their own eye-catching icons and are enhanced with illustrations or full-color photos:

EQUIPMENT profiles an essential piece of equipment needed to perform the procedure.

TROUBLESHOOTING helps you to quickly identify problems and complications and isolate their probable cause, and guides you with step-by-step interventions.

PATIENT TEACHING provides helpful tips, reminders, and follow-up instructions to share with patients being discharged following their procedure.

Your go-to guide

Now that you know what the ninth edition of *Lippincott Nursing Procedures* has to offer—and have learned how to use it quickly and adeptly—you're ready to take on the task of performing a variety of nursing procedures. Whether you're a nursing student, a recent graduate, or an experienced practitioner, you're ready to provide all your patients with expert nursing care, with your go-to guide at your fingertips.

ABDOMINAL PARACENTESIS, ASSISTING

Paracentesis involves the aspiration of fluid from the peritoneal space through a needle, trocar, or angiocatheter inserted in the abdominal wall.[1] Used to diagnose and treat massive ascites resistant to other therapies, the procedure helps to determine the cause of ascites while relieving the resulting pressure.

Abdominal paracentesis may also precede other procedures, including radiography, peritoneal dialysis, and surgery; may detect intra-abdominal bleeding after a traumatic injury; and may be used to obtain a peritoneal fluid specimen for laboratory analysis. Contraindications include acute abdomen, which requires immediate surgery, and disseminated intravascular coagulation.[1] Relative contraindications include abdominal adhesions and other coagulopathies.[1] The procedure must be performed cautiously in patients who are pregnant and in those with bleeding tendencies, severely distended bowel, or infection at the intended insertion site.[1]

Equipment

Stethoscope ■ vital signs monitoring equipment ■ pulse oximeter and probe ■ scale ■ tape measure ■ marking pen ■ gloves ■ mask ■ gown ■ goggles ■ fluid-impermeable pads ■ specimen containers or laboratory tubes ■ labels ■ laboratory biohazard transport bag ■ antiseptic cleaning solution (povidone-iodine, chlorhexidine) ■ local anesthetic ■ sterile 4″ × 4″ (10-cm × 10-cm) gauze pads ■ tape ■ sterile paracentesis tray ■ sterile drapes ■ 5-mL syringe with 21G or 25G needle ■ disinfectant pad ■ Optional: sterile 50-mL syringe, drainage bag, suture materials, IV albumin, IV catheter insertion equipment, indwelling urinary catheter insertion equipment, laboratory request forms, prescribed analgesic.

If a preassembled tray isn't available, gather the following sterile supplies: trocar with stylet, 16G to 20G needle, or angiocatheter; 25G or 27G 1½″ (3.8 cm) needle; 20G or 22G spinal needle; scalpel; #11 knife blade; three-way stopcock.

Preparation of equipment

Inspect all equipment and supplies. If a product is expired, is defective, or has compromised integrity, remove it from patient use, label it as expired or defective, and report the expiration or defect as directed by your facility.

Implementation

■ Verify the practitioner's order.
■ Confirm that informed consent has been obtained and that the signed consent form is in the patient's medical record.[2,3,4,5]
■ Review the patient's history for hypersensitivity to latex or to the local anesthetic.
■ Conduct a preprocedural verification to make sure that all relevant documentation, related information, and equipment are available and correctly identified to the patient's identifiers.[6,7]
■ Verify that laboratory and imaging studies have been completed as ordered and that the results are in the patient's medical record. Notify the practitioner of any unexpected results.[6]
■ Gather and prepare the necessary equipment and supplies.
■ Perform hand hygiene.[8,9,10,11,12,13]
■ Confirm the patient's identity using at least two patient identifiers.[14]
■ Provide privacy.[15,16,17,18]
■ Reinforce the practitioner's explanation of the procedure according to the individual communication and learning needs *to increase understanding, allay fears, and enhance cooperation.*[19] Reassure the patient that the he or she should feel no pain but may feel a stinging sensation from the local anesthetic injection and pressure from the needle, trocar, or angiocatheter insertion. The patient may also sense pressure when the practitioner aspirates abdominal fluid.

■ Instruct the patient to void before the procedure. Alternatively, insert an indwelling urinary catheter, if ordered, *to minimize the risk of accidental bladder injury from insertion of the needle, trocar, or angiocatheter.*[1]
■ Obtain the patient's weight in kilograms.
■ Raise the patient's bed to waist level before performing patient care *to prevent caregiver back strain.*[20]
■ Perform hand hygiene.[8,9,10,11,12,13]
■ Obtain the patient's vital signs, oxygen saturation using pulse oximetry, and abdominal girth, and assess respiratory status *to serve as a baseline for comparison during and after the procedure.*[1] Use the tape measure to measure the patient's abdominal girth at the umbilical level. Use a felt-tipped marker to indicate the abdominal area measured.
■ Screen and assess for pain using facility-defined criteria that are consistent with the patient's age, condition, and ability to understand *to serve as a baseline for comparison during and after the procedure.*[1,21]
■ Treat the patient's pain, as needed and ordered, using nonpharmacologic, pharmacologic, or a combination of approaches. Base the treatment plan on evidence-based practices and the patient's clinical condition, past medical history, and pain management goals.[21]
■ Make sure the patient has a patent IV catheter in place, if ordered; insert a new IV catheter, *if necessary to provide access for administration of IV fluid and sedation, as needed.*
■ Position the patient in the supine position or on the side *to allow the fluid to pool in dependent areas.*[1]
■ Expose the patient's abdomen from diaphragm to pubis. Keep the rest of the patient covered *to avoid chilling.*
■ Make the patient as comfortable as possible, and place a fluid-impermeable pad under the patient *for protection from drainage.*
■ Remind the patient to stay as still as possible during the procedure *to prevent injury from the needle, trocar, or angiocatheter.*
■ Perform hand hygiene.[8,9,10,11,12,13]
■ Open the paracentesis tray using sterile no-touch technique *to ensure a sterile field.*
■ Put on a gown, a mask, goggles, and gloves *to comply with standard precautions.*[22,23,24]
■ Label all medications, medication containers, and other solutions on and off the sterile field.[25,26]
■ Assist the practitioner, as needed, with skin preparation and during the procedure.
■ Conduct a time-out immediately before starting the procedure *to perform a final assessment that the correct patient, site, positioning, and procedure are identified and, as applicable, that all relevant information and necessary equipment are available.*[27]
■ Using the scalpel, the practitioner may make a small incision before inserting the needle, trocar, or angiocatheter (usually 1″ to 2″ [2.5 to 5 cm] below the umbilicus). Listen for a popping sound, *which signifies that the needle, trocar, or angiocatheter has pierced the peritoneum.*
■ Assist the practitioner with collecting specimens in the proper containers. If the practitioner orders substantial drainage, connect the three-way stopcock and tubing to the needle, trocar, or angiocatheter. Run the other end of the tubing to the drainage bag. Alternatively, aspirate the fluid with a three-way stopcock and 50-mL syringe.
■ Label the specimen tubes in the presence of the patient *to prevent mislabeling,* and send them to the laboratory in a laboratory biohazard transport bag (with appropriate laboratory request forms if required by your facility).[14,24] If the patient is receiving antibiotics, note this information on the request form for consideration during the fluid analysis.
■ Gently turn the patient from side to side *to enhance drainage,* if necessary.[1]
■ As the fluid drains, monitor the patient's vital signs and oxygen saturation level frequently. Observe the patient closely for vertigo, faintness, diaphoresis, pallor, heightened anxiety, tachycardia, dyspnea, and hypotension, especially if more than 5 L of peritoneal fluid was aspirated at one time. In rare cases, *this loss may induce a fluid shift and hypovolemic shock.*[28] Immediately report signs of shock to the practitioner.
■ Administer IV albumin, as ordered, *to prevent hypovolemia and a decline in kidney function.*[21,28,29,30,31,32]
■ When the procedure ends and the practitioner removes the needle, trocar, or angiocatheter, apply pressure to the wound using sterile 4″ × 4″ (10-cm × 10-cm) gauze pads. If the wound still leaks after 5 minutes, the

practitioner may suture the incision.[1] Alternatively, if permitted in your facility, remove the paracentesis catheter, as directed (*some facilities permit a specially trained nurse to remove the catheter*).

■ Remove and discard your gloves,[22,24] perform hand hygiene,[8,9,10,11,12,13] and put on gloves.[22,24]

■ When drainage becomes minimal, remove and discard the pressure dressing; apply dry sterile gauze pads and tape them to the site.

NURSING ALERT If the patient has fragile skin, use dressings and tape specifically formulated for fragile skin *to prevent skin stripping during removal*.[33]

■ Help the patient assume a comfortable position.

■ Monitor the patient's vital signs, oxygen saturation level, and respiratory status at an interval determined by your facility *because no evidence-based research indicates best practice for the frequency of vital sign assessment after a procedure*.[34] Make sure that alarm limits are set properly for the patient's current condition and that alarms are turned on, functioning properly, and audible to staff.[35,36,37,38]

■ Check the dressing for drainage. Be sure to note drainage color, amount, and characteristics.

■ Reassess and respond to pain by evaluating the patient's response to treatment and progress toward pain management goals. Assess for adverse reactions and risk factors for adverse events that may result from treatment.[21]

■ Monitor the patient's intake and output at an interval determined by the patient's condition and your facility.[1]

■ Return the bed to the lowest position *to prevent falls and maintain patient safety*.[39]

■ Discard used supplies in the appropriate receptacles.[24]

■ Remove and discard your gloves and other personal protective equipment.[22,24]

■ Perform hand hygiene.[8,9,10,11,12,13]

■ Clean and disinfect your stethoscope using a disinfectant pad.[40,41]

■ Perform hand hygiene.[8,9,10,11,12,13]

■ Document the procedure.[42,43,44,45]

Special considerations

■ Throughout this procedure, help the patient remain still *to prevent accidental perforation of abdominal organs*.

■ If the patient shows signs of hypovolemic shock, reduce the vertical distance between the needle, trocar, or angiocatheter and the drainage collection container *to slow the drainage rate*. If necessary, stop the drainage.

■ If peritoneal fluid doesn't flow easily, try repositioning the patient *to facilitate drainage*.

■ After the procedure, observe for peritoneal fluid leakage. If this develops, notify the practitioner.[28]

■ Obtain the patient's weight (using the same scale) and abdominal girth daily. Compare these values with the baseline figures *to detect recurrent ascites*.

■ Ultrasound may be used to assist in locating the fluid and inserting the needle, trocar, or angiocatheter. Research suggests that ultrasound-guided paracentesis results in fewer adverse events that paracentesis performed without ultrasound guidance.[1,46]

■ Monitor for respiratory changes during the procedure, *because ascites may place pressure on the diaphragm, leading to respiratory distress*. Removal of ascitic fluid should help relieve this pressure and distress.[1,29]

■ The Joint Commission has issued a sentinel event alert concerning medical device alarm safety *because alarm-related events have been associated with permanent loss of function or death*. Among major contributing factors were improper alarm settings, alarm settings turned off inappropriately, and alarm signals that are inaudible to staff. Make sure that alarm limits are set properly and that alarms are turned on, functioning properly, and audible to staff. Follow facility guidelines for preventing alarm fatigue.[35]

Complications

Although rare, removing large amounts of fluid may cause hypotension, oliguria, and hyponatremia. Ascitic fluid may form again, drawing fluid from extracellular tissue throughout the body. Other possible procedural complications include fluid leakage from the puncture site after the procedure; perforation of abdominal organs, including the bowel or bladder, by the needle, trocar, or angiocatheter; wound infection; internal bleeding; cellulitis; and peritonitis.[28,29]

Documentation

Record the date and time of the procedure, the puncture site location, and whether the practitioner sutured the wound. Document the amount, color, viscosity, and odor of aspirated fluid in your notes as well as in the fluid intake and output record. Record the patient's vital signs, oxygen saturation level, weight (in kilograms), and abdominal girth measurements before and after the procedure. Also note the patient's tolerance of the procedure, vital signs, and any signs or symptoms of complications during the procedure. Note the number of specimens sent to the laboratory. Document teaching provided to the patient and family (if applicable), their understanding of that teaching, and any need for follow-up teaching.

REFERENCES

1 Wiegand, D. L. (2017). *AACN procedure manual for high acuity, progressive, and critical care* (7th ed.). St. Louis, MO: Elsevier.

2 The Joint Commission. (2021). Standard RI.01.03.01. *Comprehensive accreditation manual for hospitals*. Oakbrook Terrace, IL: The Joint Commission. (Level VII)

3 DNV GL-Healthcare USA, Inc. (2020). PR.2.SR.3. *NIAHO® accreditation requirements, interpretive guidelines and surveyor guidance—revision 20.0*. Milford, OH: DNV GL-Healthcare USA, Inc. (Level VII)

4 Centers for Medicare and Medicaid Services, Department of Health and Human Services. (2020). Condition of participation: Patient's rights. 42 C.F.R. § 482.13(b)(2).

5 Accreditation Association for Hospitals and Health Systems. (2020). Standard 15.01.11. *Healthcare Facilities Accreditation Program: Accreditation requirements for acute care hospitals*. Chicago, IL: Accreditation Association for Hospitals and Health Systems. (Level VII)

6 The Joint Commission. (2021). Standard UP.01.01.01. *Comprehensive accreditation manual for hospitals*. Oakbrook Terrace, IL: The Joint Commission. (Level VII)

7 Accreditation Association for Hospitals and Health Systems. (2020). Standard 30.00.14. *Healthcare Facilities Accreditation Program: Accreditation requirements for acute care hospitals*. Chicago, IL: Accreditation Association for Hospitals and Health Systems. (Level VII)

8 The Joint Commission. (2021). Standard NPSG.07.01.01. *Comprehensive accreditation manual for hospitals*. Oakbrook Terrace, IL: The Joint Commission. (Level VII)

9 Centers for Disease Control and Prevention. (2002). Guideline for hand hygiene in health-care settings: Recommendations of the Healthcare Infection Control Practices Advisory Committee and the HICPAC/SHEA/APIC/IDSA Hand Hygiene Task Force. *MMWR Recommendations and Reports, 51*(RR-16), 1–45. https://www.cdc.gov/mmwr/pdf/rr/rr5116.pdf (Level II)

10 World Health Organization. (2009). WHO guidelines on hand hygiene in health care: First global patient safety challenge, clean care is safer care. https://apps.who.int/iris/bitstream/handle/10665/44102/9789241597906_eng.pdf?sequence=1 (Level IV)

11 Centers for Medicare and Medicaid Services, Department of Health and Human Services. (2020). Condition of participation: Infection control. 42 C.F.R. § 482.42.

12 Accreditation Association for Hospitals and Health Systems. (2020). Standard 07.01.21. *Healthcare Facilities Accreditation Program: Accreditation requirements for acute care hospitals*. Chicago, IL: Accreditation Association for Hospitals and Health Systems. (Level VII)

13 DNV GL-Healthcare USA, Inc. (2020). IC.1.SR.1. *NIAHO® accreditation requirements, interpretive guidelines and surveyor guidelines – revision 20.0*. Milford, OH: DNV GL-Healthcare USA, Inc. (Level VII)

14 The Joint Commission. (2021). Standard NPSG.01.01.01. *Comprehensive accreditation manual for hospitals*. Oakbrook Terrace, IL: The Joint Commission. (Level VII)

15 The Joint Commission. (2021). Standard RI.01.01.01. *Comprehensive accreditation manual for hospitals*. Oakbrook Terrace, IL: The Joint Commission. (Level VII)

16 Centers for Medicare and Medicaid Services, Department of Health and Human Services. (2020). Condition of participation: Patient's rights. 42 C.F.R. § 482.13(c)(1).

17 Accreditation Association for Hospitals and Health Systems. (2020). Standard 15.01.16. *Healthcare Facilities Accreditation Program: Accreditation requirements for acute care hospitals.* Chicago, IL: Accreditation Association for Hospitals and Health Systems. (Level VII)

18 DNV GL-Healthcare USA, Inc. (2020). PR.2.SR.5. *NIAHO® accreditation requirements, interpretive guidelines and surveyor guidance—revision 20.0.* Milford, OH: DNV GL-Healthcare USA, Inc. (Level VII)

19 The Joint Commission. (2021). Standard PC.02.01.21. *Comprehensive accreditation manual for hospitals.* Oakbrook Terrace, IL: The Joint Commission. (Level VII)

20 Waters, T. R., et al. (2009). Safe patient handling training for schools of nursing. https://www.cdc.gov/niosh/docs/2009-127/pdfs/2009-127.pdf (Level VII)

21 The Joint Commission. (2021). Standard PC.01.02.07. *Comprehensive accreditation manual for hospitals.* Oakbrook Terrace, IL: The Joint Commission. (Level VII)

22 Siegel, J. D., et al. (2007, revised 2019). 2007 guideline for isolation precautions: Preventing transmission of infectious agents in healthcare settings. https://www.cdc.gov/infectioncontrol/pdf/guidelines/isolation-guidelines-H.pdf (Level II)

23 Accreditation Association for Hospitals and Health Systems. (2020). Standard 07.01.10. *Healthcare Facilities Accreditation Program: Accreditation requirements for acute care hospitals.* Chicago, IL: Accreditation Association for Hospitals and Health Systems. (Level VII)

24 Occupational Safety and Health Administration. (2012). Bloodborne pathogens, standard number 1910.1030. https://www.osha.gov/pls/oshaweb/owadisp.show_document?p_id=10051&p_table=STANDARDS (Level VII)

25 The Joint Commission. (2021). Standard NPSG.03.04.01. *Comprehensive accreditation manual for hospitals.* Oakbrook Terrace, IL: The Joint Commission. (Level VII)

26 Accreditation Association for Hospitals and Health Systems. (2020). Standard 25.01.27. *Healthcare Facilities Accreditation Program: Accreditation requirements for acute care hospitals.* Chicago, IL: Accreditation Association for Hospitals and Health Systems. (Level VII)

27 The Joint Commission. (2021). Standard UP.01.03.01. *Comprehensive accreditation manual for hospitals.* Oakbrook Terrace, IL: The Joint Commission. (Level VII)

28 Runyon, B. A. (2019). Diagnostic and therapeutic abdominal paracentesis. In: *UpToDate,* Chopra, S. (Ed.).

29 Phillip, V., et al. (2014). Effects of paracentesis on hemodynamic parameters and respiratory function in critically ill patients. *BMC Gastroenterology, 14,* 18. https://bmcgastroenterol.biomedcentral.com/track/pdf/10.1186/1471-230X-14-18 (Level VI)

30 Centers for Medicare and Medicaid Services, Department of Health and Human Services. (2020). Condition of participation: Nursing services. 42 C.F.R. § 482.23(c).

31 Accreditation Association for Hospitals and Health Systems. (2020). Standard 16.01.03. *Healthcare Facilities Accreditation Program: Accreditation requirements for acute care hospitals.* Chicago, IL: Accreditation Association for Hospitals and Health Systems. (Level VII)

32 The Joint Commission. (2021). Standard MM.06.01.01. *Comprehensive accreditation manual for hospitals.* Oakbrook Terrace, IL: The Joint Commission. (Level VII)

33 LeBlanc, K., et al. (2013). International skin tear advisory panel: A tool kit to aid in the prevention, assessment, and treatment of skin tears using a simplified classification system. *Advances in Skin & Wound Care, 26,* 459–476. (Level IV)

34 American Society of PeriAnesthesia Nurses. (2019). *2019–2020 perianesthesia nursing standards, practice recommendations and interpretative statements.* Cherry Hill, NJ: American Society of PeriAnesthesia Nurses. (Level VII)

35 The Joint Commission. (2013). Sentinel event alert 50: Medical device alarm safety in hospitals. Accessed May 2021 via the Web at https://www.jointcommission.org/assets/1/6/SEA_50_alarms_4_26_16.pdf (Level VII)

36 The Joint Commission. (2021). Standard NPSG.06.01.01. *Comprehensive accreditation manual for hospitals.* Oakbrook Terrace, IL: The Joint Commission. (Level VII)

37 Graham, K. C., & Cvach, M. (2010). Monitor alarm fatigue: Standardizing use of physiological monitors and decreasing nuisance alarms. *American Journal of Critical Care, 19,* 28–37.

38 American Association of Critical-Care Nurses. (2018). AACN practice alert: Managing alarms in acute care across the life span: Electrocardiography and pulse oximetry. https://www.aacn.org/clinical-resources/practice-alerts/managing-alarms-in-acute-care-across-the-life-span (Level VII)

39 Ganz, D. A., et al. (2013, reviewed 2021). *Preventing falls in hospitals: A toolkit for improving quality of care (AHRQ Publication No. 13-0015-EF).*

40 Rutala, W. A., et al. (2008, revised 2019). Guideline for disinfection and sterilization in healthcare facilities, 2008. https://www.cdc.gov/infection-control/pdf/guidelines/disinfection-guidelines-H.pdf (Level I)

41 Accreditation Association for Hospitals and Health Systems. (2020). Standard 07.02.03. *Healthcare Facilities Accreditation Program: Accreditation requirements for acute care hospitals.* Chicago, IL: Accreditation Association for Hospitals and Health Systems. (Level VII)

42 The Joint Commission. (2021). Standard RC.01.03.01. *Comprehensive accreditation manual for hospitals.* Oakbrook Terrace, IL: The Joint Commission. (Level VII)

43 Centers for Medicare and Medicaid Services, Department of Health and Human Services. (2020). Condition of participation: Medical record services. 42 C.F.R. § 482.24(b).

44 Accreditation Association for Hospitals and Health Systems. (2020). Standard 10.00.03. *Healthcare Facilities Accreditation Program: Accreditation requirements for acute care hospitals.* Chicago, IL: Accreditation Association for Hospitals and Health Systems. (Level VII)

45 DNV GL-Healthcare USA, Inc. (2020). MR.2.SR.1. *NIAHO® accreditation requirements, interpretive guidelines and surveyor guidance—revision 20.0.* Milford, OH: DNV GL-Healthcare USA, Inc. (Level VI)

46 Patel, P. A., et al. (2012). Evaluation of hospital complications and costs associated with using guidance during abdominal paracentesis procedures. *Journal of Medical Economics, 15,* 1–7. (Level IV)

ADMISSION

Admission to a nursing unit prepares a patient for a stay in a health care facility. Whether the admission is scheduled or follows emergency treatment, effective admission procedures should include certain steps to accomplish important goals. These steps include verifying the patient's identity using at least two patient identifiers,[1] assessing the clinical status, making the patient as comfortable as possible, introducing the patient to roommates (if possible) and staff, orienting the patient to the environment and routine, and providing supplies and special equipment needed for daily care.

The Joint Commission and DNV GL-Healthcare require that each patient undergo an admission assessment by a registered nurse within 24 hours after inpatient admission.[2,3,4] The *Healthcare Facilities Accreditation Program* requires that an initial assessment be performed by a registered nurse within the timeframe established by the individual facility.[5] During this assessment, the nurse should prioritize the patient's needs, always remaining aware of the patient's levels of fatigue and comfort, and should maintain the patient's privacy while obtaining the health history. According to the American Hospital Association's Patient Care Partnership (which replaced the Patient's Bill of Rights), the patient has the right to expect that examinations, consultations, and treatment will be conducted in a manner that protects the patient's privacy.[6]

Admission routines that are efficient and show appropriate concern for the patient can ease the patient's anxiety and promote cooperation and receptivity to treatment. Conversely, admission routines that the patient perceives as careless or excessively impersonal can heighten anxiety, reduce cooperation, impair the patient's response to treatment, and aggravate symptoms.

Equipment

Patient gown ■ vital signs monitoring equipment ■ stethoscope ■ disinfectant pad ■ patient scale with stadiometer ■ identification band ■ validated screening tool for unhealthy alcohol use ■ standardized fall risk assessment tool ■ standardized suicide screening tool ■ emergency equipment (code cart with cardiac medications, defibrillator, handheld resuscitation bag with mask, intubation equipment) ■ Optional: personal property form; gloves; oxygen delivery system; suction equipment; equipment for obtaining blood or urine specimens; patient care reminders; friction-reducing device or lateral transfer board (for a patient who weighs less than 200 lb [91 kg]) or ceiling lift with supine sling, mechanical transfer device, or air-assisted device (for a patient who weighs more than 200 lb [91 kg]);[7] tape measure; advance directive information; alert bracelets; tape; labels; chair or bed scale; facility-approved disinfectant; laboratory transport bag; laboratory request forms.

Preparation of equipment

Inspect all equipment and supplies. If a product is expired or defective, or has compromised integrity, remove it from patient use, label it as expired or defective, and report the expiration or defect as directed by your facility.

Adjust the lights, temperature, and ventilation in the room. Make sure that emergency equipment or special equipment, such as oxygen or suction equipment, is functioning properly and readily available, as needed.

Position the bed as the patient's condition requires. If the patient is ambulatory, place the bed in the low position; if the patient is arriving on a stretcher, place the bed in the high position. Fold down the top linens. Prepare emergency or special equipment, such as oxygen or suction, as needed.

Implementation

- Review the admission form and the practitioner's orders. Note the reason for admission, restrictions on activity and diet, and any orders for diagnostic tests requiring specimen collection.
- Gather and prepare the appropriate equipment.
- Perform hand hygiene.[8,9,10,11,12,13]
- Put on gloves, as needed, *to comply with standard precautions.*[14]
- Speaking slowly and clearly, greet the patient by the patient's proper name, and introduce yourself and any other staff members present.
- Confirm the patient's identity using at least two patient identifiers.[1] Apply an identification band, verifying that the identifiers are correct, including the patient's name and its spelling. Notify the admission office of any corrections.
- Escort the patient to the health care facility room and, if the patient isn't in distress, introduce the patient to the roommate (if present).
- If the patient is being admitted from the emergency department and arrives on a stretcher, summon the help of coworkers to transfer the patient from the stretcher to the bed using an appropriate transfer device.[7] Keep in mind that the patient may require immediate treatment depending on the patient's condition; *treatment takes priority over routine admission procedures.* (See *Managing emergency admissions.*)

Managing emergency admissions

After emergency department (ED) treatment, the patient is transported to the nursing unit. The patient arrives on the nursing unit with a temporary identification bracelet, the practitioner's orders, and a record of treatment. Provide privacy.[15,16,17,18] Read the record and receive hand-off communication from the person who was responsible for the patient's care in the ED. Ask questions, as necessary, *to avoid miscommunications that can cause patient care errors during transitions of care.*[19,20] Expect to receive the patient's weight in kilograms during the hand-off *to prevent medication errors.*[21] As part of the hand-off process, trace each tubing and catheter from the patient to the point of origin; use a standardized line reconciliation process.[22,23]

Tape the connections *to prevent accidental disconnection of the tubing.* If the patient has more than one connection to a port of entry into the body (e.g., if an IV catheter has more than one infusion infusing through it), label each tube near the insertion site. Label the infusion bag, ensuring that the label faces out *so it can be read easily.* Route tubing and catheters having different purposes in a standardized approach—for example, keeping IV lines routed toward the head and enteric lines routed toward the feet to prevent dangerous misconnections.[23] If different access sites are used, label each tubing at the distal end (near the patient connection) and proximal end (near the source container) *to distinguish the different tubing and prevent misconnections.*[23] If the patient has an electronic infusion device or other patient equipment with alarms, make sure that alarm limits are set according to the patient's current condition, and that alarms are turned on, functioning properly, and audible to staff.[24,25,26]

Obtain and record the patient's vital signs, and follow the practitioner's orders for treatment. If the patient is conscious and not in distress, explain any treatment orders. When the patient's condition allows, proceed with routine admission procedures.

- Provide privacy.[15,16,17,18]
- Help the patient change into a hospital gown or pajamas from home if appropriate.[27]
- Itemize all valuables, clothing, and prostheses in the medical record on the personal property form if your facility uses such a form. Encourage the patient to store valuables or money in the safe or, preferably, to send them home.
- Orient the patient to the room. Demonstrate how to use the equipment in the room, including the call system, bed controls, TV controls, telephone, and lights. Show an ambulatory patient where the bathroom and closets are located.
- Explain the admission procedure to the patient and family (if appropriate) according to their individual communication and learning needs *to increase their understanding, allay their fears, and enhance cooperation.*[28] Also explain the routine at your health care facility. Mention when to expect meals, vital signs assessments, and medications. Review visiting hours and any restrictions.
- Obtain and record the patient's vital signs.
- Measure the patient's height and weight (in kilograms). If the patient can't stand, use a chair or bed scale and ask the patient's height. *Knowing the patient's height and weight is important for planning treatments and diet and for calculating medication and anesthetic dosages.* Record the patient's weight in kilograms and document it prominently in the patient's medical record *to help prevent medication errors.*[21]
- Collect blood and urine specimens, if ordered. Label specimens in the presence of the patient *to prevent mislabeling*, place them in a laboratory biohazard transport bag with completed laboratory request forms (if needed), and send them to the laboratory immediately.[1]
- Notify the patient's practitioner of the patient's arrival. Report emergency or unexpected assessment findings.
- Obtain a complete patient history. Include all previous hospitalizations, illnesses, surgeries, and food and drug allergies.
- Screen the patient for influenza vaccination (as directed by your facility) and for tobacco and unhealthy alcohol use.[29] Use a validated screening tool to screen for unhealthy alcohol use.[29,30,31,32]
- Make sure that a complete list of the medications the patient was taking at home (including over-the-counter, supplements, and herbal preparations) is documented in the patient's medical record. Include doses, routes, and frequencies for all medications. Compare this list with the patient's current medications and reconcile and document any discrepancies (omissions, duplications, adjustments, deletions, or additions) in the patient's medical record *to reduce the risk of transition-related adverse drug events.*[33,34]
- Determine whether the patient has an advance directive and, if so, ask for a copy to place in the medical record. If the patient doesn't have one, provide information about advance directives to the patient.[35,36,37] (See the "Advance directives" procedure.)
- Review patient rights with the patient and family (if appropriate).[6,17]
- Perform an admission assessment. Ask the patient to tell you the reasons for coming to the facility. Record the answers (in the patient's own words) as the reason for seeking care. Follow up with a physical assessment, focusing on those reasons for seeking care. Record any marks, bruises, and discolorations on the nursing assessment form.
- Screen the patient for suicide ideation, using a brief, standardized, evidence-based screening tool.[38] If the patient is at risk for suicide, address the patient's immediate safety needs, and collaborate with the multidisciplinary team to determine the most appropriate setting for treatment.[38]
- Perform a structured pressure injury risk assessment as soon as possible after admission.[39,40,41]

HOSPITAL-ACQUIRED CONDITION ALERT Keep in mind that the Centers for Medicare and Medicaid Services considers a stage 3 or 4 pressure injury a hospital-acquired condition *because it can be reasonably prevented using a variety of best practices.* Make sure to follow pressure injury prevention practices (such as assessing skin integrity, encouraging mobility, and repositioning the patient, *to reduce the risk of pressure injuries.*[39,40]

- Determine the patient's risk of falling, using either a standardized fall risk assessment tool or one developed by your facility, and institute fall precautions.[41,42]

HOSPITAL-ACQUIRED CONDITION ALERT Keep in mind that the Centers for Medicare and Medicaid Services considers an injury from a fall a hospital-acquired condition *because it can be reasonably prevented using a variety of best practices.* Make sure to follow evidence-based fall prevention practices (such as performing a fall risk assessment and instituting fall precautions) *to reduce the risk of falls.*[41,43,44]

■ Screen and assess the patient's pain using facility-defined criteria that are consistent with the patient's age, condition, and ability to understand.[45]

■ If required by your facility, attach an alert bracelet to the patient's arm if the patient has a drug allergy, is at risk for falls, or has another condition that requires an alert bracelet; also place an alert in the patient's medical record.[46]

■ Assess and address the patient's safety needs.

■ After the assessment, inform the patient about any ordered tests and their scheduled times. Describe what the patient should expect for each test.

■ Develop an interdisciplinary care plan and review it with the patient.[47,48]

■ Before leaving the patient's room, make sure the patient is comfortable. Adjust the bed, and place the call light and other personal items within the patient's easy reach.

■ Post patient care reminders (concerning such topics as allergies and special needs) at the patient's bedside, as needed, *to notify coworkers.* (See *Using patient care reminders.*)

■ Remove and discard your gloves, if worn,[49] and perform hand hygiene.[8,9,10,11,12,13]

■ Clean and disinfect your stethoscope using a disinfectant pad.[50,51]

■ Perform hand hygiene.[8,9,10,11,12,13]

■ Put on gloves and, as needed, other personal protective equipment *to comply with standard precautions.*[49]

■ Clean and disinfect other reusable equipment (if used) according to the manufacturer's instructions *to prevent the spread of infection.*[50,51]

■ Remove and discard your gloves and, if worn, other personal protective equipment[49] and perform hand hygiene.[8,9,10,11,12,13]

■ Document the procedure.[52,53,54,55]

Special considerations

■ The Joint Commission issued a sentinel event alert concerning inadequate hand-off communication *because of the potential for patient harm*

Using patient care reminders

Patient care reminders are specially designed cards or signs or computer-generated alerts that are used to alert staff members of important information about a patient. These care reminders call attention to the patient's special needs and help ensure consistent care by communicating these needs to the facility's staff members, the patient's family, and other visitors. Examples of information that might be placed on a patient care reminder include:

■ allergies
■ aspiration risk
■ dietary restrictions
■ high risk of falls
■ fluid restrictions
■ specimen collection needs
■ transmission-based precautions
■ hearing impairments, including whether the patient is deaf or hearing impaired and the ear(s) affected
■ foreign language spoken.

Patient care reminders can also include:
■ mobility status
■ instructions to avoid performing venipuncture or taking blood pressure in a specific location
■ individualized turning schedule
■ nothing-by-mouth status.

Although patient care reminders serve as useful tools, health care providers should be careful not to violate a patient's privacy by posting the patient's name, diagnosis, details about surgery, or any other protected health information.

---

that can result when a receiver receives inaccurate, incomplete, untimely, misinterpreted, or otherwise inadequate information. To improve hand-off communication, standardize the critical information communicated by the sender. At a minimum, include the sender's contact information; illness assessment; patient summary, including events that led up to the illness or admission, hospital course, ongoing assessment, and plan of care; to-do action list; contingency plans; allergy list; code status; medication list; and dated laboratory test results and vital signs. Provide face-to-face communication whenever possible in an interruption-free location, using facility-approved, standardized tools and methods (for example, forms, templates, checklists, protocols, and mnemonics). Provide ample time and opportunity for questions, including the multidisciplinary team members and the patient and family when appropriate.[56]

■ If you're caring for a patient who brought medications from home, take an inventory and record this information on the nursing assessment form.[34] Instruct the patient not to take any medications unless authorized by the practitioner. Send authorized medications to the pharmacy for identification and relabeling.[57] Send other medications home with a responsible family member, or store them in the designated area outside the patient's room until discharge. *Use of unauthorized medications may interfere with treatment or cause an overdose.*

■ The Joint Commission issued a sentinel event alert concerning medical device alarm safety *because alarm-related events have been associated with permanent loss of function and death.* Among the major contributing factors were improper alarm settings, alarm settings turned off inappropriately, and alarm signals that are inaudible to staff. Make sure alarm limits are appropriately set and that alarms are turned on, functioning properly, and audible to staff. Follow facility guidelines for preventing alarm fatigue.[58]

■ Find out the patient's normal routine, and ask about any desired adjustments to the facility regimen; for instance, the patient may prefer to shower at night instead of in the morning. *Accommodating the patient with such adjustments, whenever possible, can ease anxiety and help the patient feel more in control of a potentially threatening situation.*

■ Place the patient who requires airborne precautions in an airborne infection isolation room *to reduce the risk of transmission.*[14]

■ Teach the patient and family about the importance of proper hand hygiene in preventing the spread of infection.[8,11] Encourage them to speak up if a health care worker fails to perform hand hygiene before having contact with the patient or the patient's environment.

■ Arrange for an interpreter, if necessary, *to ensure that the patient and family can communicate their concerns and understand information provided by the health care providers.*[59]

Documentation

After leaving the patient's room, document your assessment findings, including the patient's vital signs, height, weight, allergies, and drug and health history; a list of the patient's belongings and those sent home with family members; the results of your physical assessment; and a record of specimens collected for laboratory tests. Document teaching provided to the patient and family (if applicable), their understanding of the teaching, and any need for follow-up teaching.

REFERENCES

1 The Joint Commission. (2021). Standard NPSG.01.01.01. *Comprehensive accreditation manual for hospitals.* Oakbrook Terrace, IL: The Joint Commission. (Level VII)

2 The Joint Commission. (2021). Standard PC.01.02.03. *Comprehensive accreditation manual for hospitals.* Oakbrook Terrace, IL: The Joint Commission. (Level VII)

3 Centers for Medicare and Medicaid Services, Department of Health and Human Services. (2020). Condition of participation: Nursing services. 42 C.F.R. § 482.23(b)(3).

4 DNV GL-Healthcare USA, Inc. (2020). NS.3.SR.2. *NIAHO® accreditation requirements, interpretive guidelines and surveyor guidance—revision 20.0.* Milford, OH: DNV GL-Healthcare USA, Inc. (Level VII)

5 Accreditation Association for Hospitals and Health Systems. (2020). Standard 10.01.24. *Healthcare Facilities Accreditation Program: Accreditation requirements for acute care hospitals.* Chicago, IL: Accreditation Association for Hospitals and Health Systems. (Level VII)

6 American Hospital Association. (2003, revised 2019). The patient care partnership: Understanding expectation, rights and responsibilities. https://www.aha.org/system/files/2018-01/aha-patient-care-partnership.pdf

7 Waters, T. R., et al. (2009). Safe patient handling training for schools of nursing. https://www.cdc.gov/niosh/docs/2009-127/pdfs/2009-127.pdf (Level VII)

8 The Joint Commission. (2021). Standard NPSG.07.01.01. *Comprehensive accreditation manual for hospitals.* Oakbrook Terrace, IL: The Joint Commission. (Level VII)

9 Centers for Disease Control and Prevention. (2002). Guideline for hand hygiene in health-care settings: Recommendations of the Healthcare Infection Control Practices Advisory Committee and the HICPAC/SHEA/APIC/IDSA Hand Hygiene Task Force. *MMWR Recommendations and Reports, 51*(RR-16), 1–45. https://www.cdc.gov/mmwr/pdf/rr/rr5116.pdf (Level II)

10 World Health Organization. (2009). WHO guidelines on hand hygiene in health care: First global patient safety challenge, clean care is safer care. https://apps.who.int/iris/bitstream/handle/10665/44102/9789241597906_eng.pdf?sequence=1 (Level IV)

11 Centers for Medicare and Medicaid Services, Department of Health and Human Services. (2020). Condition of participation: Infection control. 42 C.F.R. § 482.42.

12 Accreditation Association for Hospitals and Health Systems. (2020). Standard 07.01.21. *Healthcare Facilities Accreditation Program: Accreditation requirements for acute care hospitals.* Chicago, IL: Accreditation Association for Hospitals and Health Systems. (Level VII)

13 DNV GL-Healthcare USA, Inc. (2020). IC.1.SR.1. *NIAHO® accreditation requirements, interpretive guidelines and surveyor guidance—revision 20.0.* Milford, OH: DNV GL-Healthcare USA, Inc. (Level VII)

14 Siegel, J. D., et al. (2007, revised 2019). 2007 guideline for isolation precautions: Preventing transmission of infectious agents in healthcare settings. https://www.cdc.gov/infectioncontrol/pdf/guidelines/isolation-guidelines-H.pdf (Level II)

15 Accreditation Association for Hospitals and Health Systems. (2020). Standard 15.01.16. *Healthcare Facilities Accreditation Program: Accreditation requirements for acute care hospitals.* Chicago, IL: Accreditation Association for Hospitals and Health Systems. (Level VII)

16 Centers for Medicare and Medicaid Services, Department of Health and Human Services. (2020). Condition of participation: Patient's rights. 42 C.F.R. § 482.13(c)(1).

17 The Joint Commission. (2021). Standard RI.01.01.01. *Comprehensive accreditation manual for hospitals.* Oakbrook Terrace, IL: The Joint Commission. (Level VII)

18 DNV GL-Healthcare USA, Inc. (2020). PR.2.SR.5. *NIAHO® accreditation requirements, interpretive guidelines and surveyor guidance—revision 20.0.* Milford, OH: DNV GL-Healthcare USA, Inc. (Level VII)

19 The Joint Commission. (2012). Hot topics in health care, transitions of care: The need for a more effective approach to continuing patient care. http://www.jointcommission.org/assets/1/18/Hot_Topics_Transitions_of_Care.pdf

20 The Joint Commission. (2021). Standard PC.02.02.01. *Comprehensive accreditation manual for hospitals.* Oakbrook Terrace, IL: The Joint Commission. (Level VII)

21 Emergency Nurses Association. (2016). Position statement: Weighing all patients in kilograms. https://www.ena.org/docs/default-source/resource-library/practice-resources/position-statements/weighingallpatientsinkilograms.pdf?sfvrsn=9c0709e_6 (Level VII)

22 U.S. Food and Drug Administration. (2017). Examples of medical device misconnections. https://www.fda.gov/medical-devices/medical-device-connectors/examples-medical-device-misconnections

23 The Joint Commission. (2014). Sentinel event alert 53: *Managing risk during transition to new ISO tubing connector standards.* http://www.jointcommission.org/assets/1/6/SEA_53_Connectors_8_19_14_final.pdf (Level VII)

24 American Association of Critical-Care Nurses. (2018). AACN practice alert: Managing alarms in acute care across the life span: Electrocardiography and pulse oximetry. https://www.aacn.org/clinical-resources/practice-alerts/managing-alarms-in-acute-care-across-the-life-span (Level VII)

25 Graham, K. C., & Cvach, M. (2010). Monitor alarm fatigue: Standardizing use of physiological monitors and decreasing nuisance alarms. *American Journal of Critical Care, 19,* 28–37.

26 The Joint Commission. (2021). Standard NPSG.06.01.01. *Comprehensive accreditation manual for hospitals.* Oakbrook Terrace, IL: The Joint Commission. (Level VII)

27 The Joint Commission. (2021). Standard RI.01.06.05. *Comprehensive accreditation manual for hospitals.* Oakbrook Terrace, IL: The Joint Commission. (Level VII)

28 The Joint Commission. (2021). Standard PC.02.01.21. *Comprehensive accreditation manual for hospitals.* Oakbrook Terrace, IL: The Joint Commission. (Level VII)

29 Centers for Medicare and Medicaid Services, & The Joint Commission. (2021). The specifications manual for national hospital inpatient quality measures (version 5.10). https://www.qualitynet.org/inpatient/specifications-manuals#tab1

30 National Institute on Alcohol Abuse and Alcoholism. (2003). Screening tests. https://pubs.niaaa.nih.gov/publications/arh28-2/78-79.htm

31 Ewing, J. A. (1984). Detecting alcoholism: The CAGE questionnaire. *Journal of the American Medical Association, 252*(14), 1905–1907.

32 Williams, N. (2014). The CAGE questionnaire. *Occupational Medicine, 64*(6), 473–474. https://academic.oup.com/occmed/article/64/6/473/1432970

33 The Joint Commission. (2021). Standard NPSG.03.06.01. *Comprehensive accreditation manual for hospitals.* Oakbrook Terrace, IL: The Joint Commission. (Level VII)

34 Accreditation Association for Hospitals and Health Systems. (2020). Standard 25.02.13. *Healthcare Facilities Accreditation Program: Accreditation requirements for acute care hospitals.* Chicago, IL: Accreditation Association for Hospitals and Health Systems. (Level VII)

35 Centers for Medicare and Medicaid Services, Department of Health and Human Services. (2020). Condition of participation: Patient's rights. 42 C.F.R. § 482.13(b)(3).

36 The Joint Commission. (2021). Standard RI.01.05.01. *Comprehensive accreditation manual for hospitals.* Oakbrook Terrace, IL: The Joint Commission. (Level VII)

37 DNV GL-Healthcare USA, Inc. (2020). PR.2.SR.1. *NIAHO® accreditation requirements, interpretive guidelines and surveyor guidance—revision 20.0.* Milford, OH: DNV GL-Healthcare USA, Inc. (Level VII)

38 The Joint Commission. (2021). Standard NPSG.15.01.01. *Comprehensive accreditation manual for hospitals.* Oakbrook Terrace, IL: The Joint Commission. (Level VII)

39 European Pressure Ulcer Advisory Panel, et al. (2019). Prevention and treatment of pressure ulcers/injuries: Quick reference guide. http://www.internationalguideline.com/static/pdfs/Quick_Reference_Guide-10Mar2019.pdf (Level VII)

40 Wound, Ostomy and Continence Nurses Society (WOCN). (2016). *Guideline for prevention and management of pressure ulcers (injuries): WOCN clinical practice guidelines series 2.* Mount Laurel, NJ: WOCN.

41 Accreditation Association for Hospitals and Health Systems. (2020). Standard 16.02.02. *Healthcare Facilities Accreditation Program: Accreditation requirements for acute care hospitals.* Chicago, IL: Accreditation Association for Hospitals and Health Systems. (Level VII)

42 Ganz, D. A., et al. (2013, reviewed 2021). *Preventing falls in hospitals: A toolkit for improving quality of care* (AHRQ Publication No. 13-0015-EF). Rockville, MD: Agency for Healthcare Research and Quality. https://www.ahrq.gov/professionals/systems/hospital/fallpxtoolkit/index.html (Level VII)

43 Jarrett, N., & Callaham, M. (2016). Evidence-based guidelines for selected hospital-acquired conditions: Final report. https://www.cms.gov/Medicare/Medicare-Fee-for-Service-Payment/HospitalAcqCond/Downloads/2016-HAC-Report.pdf

44 The Joint Commission. (2021). Standard PC.01.02.08. *Comprehensive accreditation manual for hospitals.* Oakbrook Terrace, IL: The Joint Commission. (Level VII)

45 The Joint Commission. (2021). Standard PC.01.02.07. *Comprehensive accreditation manual for hospitals.* Oakbrook Terrace, IL: The Joint Commission. (Level VII)

46 The Joint Commission. (2021). Standard RC.02.01.01. *Comprehensive accreditation manual for hospitals.* Oakbrook Terrace, IL: The Joint Commission. (Level VII)

47 The Joint Commission. (2021). Standard PC.01.02.05. *Comprehensive accreditation manual for hospitals.* Oakbrook Terrace, IL: The Joint Commission. (Level VII)

48 Centers for Medicare and Medicaid Services, Department of Health and Human Services. (2020). Condition of participation: Medical record services. 42 C.F.R. § 482.23(b)(4).

49 Occupational Safety and Health Administration. (2012). Bloodborne pathogens, standard number 1910.1030. https://www.osha.gov/pls/oshaweb/owadisp.show_document?p_id=10051&p_table=STANDARDS (Level VII)

50 Rutala, W. A., et al. (2008, revised 2019). Guideline for disinfection and sterilization in healthcare facilities, 2008. https://www.cdc.gov/infection-control/pdf/guidelines/disinfection-guidelines-H.pdf (Level I)

51 Accreditation Association for Hospitals and Health Systems. (2020). Standard 07.02.03. *Healthcare Facilities Accreditation Program: Accreditation requirements for acute care hospitals.* Chicago, IL: Accreditation Association for Hospitals and Health Systems. (Level VII)

52 The Joint Commission. (2021). Standard RC.01.03.01. *Comprehensive accreditation manual for hospitals.* Oakbrook Terrace, IL: The Joint Commission. (Level VII)

53 Centers for Medicare and Medicaid Services, Department of Health and Human Services. (2020). Condition of participation: Medical record services. 42 C.F.R. § 482.24(b).

54 Accreditation Association for Hospitals and Health Systems. (2020). Standard 10.00.03. *Healthcare Facilities Accreditation Program: Accreditation requirements for acute care hospitals.* Chicago, IL: Accreditation Association for Hospitals and Health Systems. (Level VII)

55 DNV GL-Healthcare USA, Inc. (2020). MR.2.SR.1. *NIAHO® accreditation requirements, interpretive guidelines and surveyor guidance—revision 20.0.* Milford, OH: DNV GL-Healthcare USA, Inc. (Level VII)

56 The Joint Commission. (2017). Sentinel event alert 58: Inadequate hand-off communication. https://www.jointcommission.org/assets/1/18/SEA_58_Hand_off_Comms_9_6_17_FINAL_(1).pdf (Level VII)

57 The Joint Commission. (2021). Standard MM.03.01.05. *Comprehensive accreditation manual for hospitals.* Oakbrook Terrace, IL: The Joint Commission. (Level VII)

58 The Joint Commission. (2013). Sentinel event alert 50: Medical device alarm safety in hospitals. https://www.jointcommission.org/assets/1/6/SEA_50_alarms_4_26_16.pdf (Level VII)

59 The Joint Commission. (2021). Standard RI.01.01.03. *Comprehensive accreditation manual for hospitals.* Oakbrook Terrace, IL: The Joint Commission. (Level VII)

ADMIXTURE OF DRUGS IN A SYRINGE

Combining two drugs in one syringe allows you to avoid the discomfort of two injections. Drugs can be mixed in a syringe using a multidose vial and ampule, two ampules, or two multidose vials. However, such combinations are contraindicated when the drugs aren't compatible and when the combined doses exceed the amount of solution that can be absorbed from a single injection site. Sterile no-touch technique must be followed during the procedure to prevent medication contamination and reduce the risk of infection.

The Association of Professionals in Infection Control and Epidemiology and the World Health Organization recommend using single-use or single-dose vials whenever possible. The risk of transmission posed by inappropriate handling of multidose vials has been clearly demonstrated, and mandates a practice of one vial per one patient whenever possible.[1,2] Infection transmission risk is reduced when multidose vials are dedicated to a single patient.[2,3,4] The Infusion Nurses Society also recommends that nurses administer pharmacy-prepared or commercially available products whenever possible.[3]

Equipment

Medication record ■ prescribed medications ■ alcohol pads ■ syringe ■ 5-micron filter needle or straw[3,5,6] ■ safety needle ■ Optional: gauze pad, ampule breaker, needless access transfer device, metal file, personal protective equipment.

The type and size of syringe and needle depend on the volume and viscosity of prescribed medications, the patient's body mass, and the injection site.

Preparation of equipment

Inspect all equipment and supplies. If a product is expired or defective, or has compromised integrity, remove it from patient use, label it as expired or defective, and report the expiration or defect as directed by your facility.

Before preparing the injection, make sure the preparation area is free from clutter, and clean the preparation surface with an alcohol pad.[1,2,7]

Implementation

■ Avoid distractions and interruptions when preparing medication *to prevent medication errors.*[8,9]

■ Review the practitioner's order to make sure that the prescribed medication, dose, rate, and administration route are appropriate for the patient's age and condition. Assess concerns about the order with the practitioner, pharmacist, or your supervisor, and if necessary the risk management department, or as directed by your facility.[10,11,12,13]

■ Reconcile the patient's medications when the practitioner prescribes new medication *to reduce the risk of medication errors, including omissions, duplications, dosing errors, and drug interactions.*[14,15]

■ Perform hand hygiene before assessing supplies and preparing medications *to prevent the transmission of infection.*[2]

■ Gather the medications and necessary equipment and supplies.

■ Compare the medication labels with the order in the patient's medical record.[10,11,12,13]

■ Verify the compatibility of the drugs to be combined.[16]

■ Check the patient's medical record for an allergy or a contraindication to the prescribed medications. If an allergy or a contraindication exists, don't administer the medications; notify the practitioner.[10,11,12,13]

■ Check the expiration date on each of the medications. If either of the medications is expired, return the expired medication to the pharmacy and obtain new medication.[10,11,12,13]

■ Visually inspect each solution for particles or discoloration or other loss of integrity; don't administer the medications if either has compromised integrity.[10,11,12,13]

■ Discuss any unresolved concerns about the medications with the patient's practitioner.[10,11,12,13]

■ Calculate the doses to be administered.

■ Have another nurse double-check your calculations if necessary.

NURSING ALERT Check if either of the prescribed medications is considered a high-alert medication, which can cause significant patient harm when used in error.[17] If required by your facility, have another nurse perform an independent double-check *to verify the patient's identity and to make sure that the correct medications are drawn up in the prescribed concentrations; the indications for both medications correspond with the patient's diagnosis; the dosage calculations are correct and the dosing formula used to derive the final dose is correct; the route of administration is safe and proper for the patient; and the prescribed time and frequency of administration are safe and proper for the patient.*[17]

■ Perform hand hygiene.[1,18,19,20,21,22,23]

NURSING ALERT If your facility's hazardous drug list contains either of the medications you're about to prepare, put on personal protective equipment as directed.[24] (See the "Hazardous drug preparation and handling" procedure.)

■ When preparing the medications, read the medication labels as you select the medications, as you draw each up, and after you have drawn each up *to verify the correct medication and dosage.*

Mixing drugs from a multidose vial and an ampule

■ Remove the medication vial's lid.

■ Disinfect the stopper with an alcohol pad.[2] Allow it to dry completely.[1,3]

■ Pull back the syringe plunger until the volume of air drawn into the syringe equals the volume to be withdrawn from the drug vial.

■ Insert the needle or needleless access device (attached to a syringe) into the top of the vial and inject the air. Then invert the vial and keep the needle's bevel tip below the level of the solution as you withdraw the prescribed dose.

■ Put the sterile needle cover over the needle or needleless access device.

■ Tap the stem of the ampule *to move any medication from the stem into the body of the ampule.*

■ Disinfect the neck of the ampule using the alcohol pad, and allow it to dry completely.[2,3]

■ If you're using an ampule that requires use of a metal file to open, draw the file carefully around the narrow part of the ampule *to weaken it.*[25]

■ Wrap a sterile gauze pad or an alcohol pad around the ampule's neck *to protect yourself from injury in case the glass splinters.*[1] Alternatively, insert the ampule's head into an ampule breaker.

- Break open the ampule, directing the force away from you.
- Change the needle or needleless access device to a 5-micron filter needle or straw *to filter out any glass splinters*.[3,5,26]
- Insert the needle or straw into the ampule. Don't touch the outside of the ampule with the needle or straw.
- Draw the correct dose into the syringe.
- When you have prepared the syringe, change the filter needle or straw to a safety needle *to administer the injection*.
- Discard the needles and the ampule in a puncture-resistant sharps container,[1] and discard all additional equipment appropriately.[1,27]

Mixing drugs from two multidose vials

- Remove the vial lid and disinfect the rubber stopper on the first drug vial with an alcohol pad and allow it to dry[1,2,3] *to decrease the risk of contaminating the medication as you insert the needle into the vial.*
- Pull back the syringe plunger until the volume of air drawn into the syringe equals the volume to be withdrawn from the drug vial.
- Without inverting the vial, insert the needle (or needleless access device) into the top of the vial, making sure that the needle's bevel tip doesn't touch the solution. Inject the air into the vial and withdraw the needle (or needleless access device). *This step replaces air in the vial, which prevents the creation of a partial vacuum when you withdraw the drug.*
- Repeat the steps above for the second vial. Then, after injecting the air into the second vial, invert the vial, withdraw the prescribed dose, and then withdraw the needle or needleless access device.
- Disinfect the rubber stopper of the first vial again, allow it to dry, and insert the needle (or needleless access device), taking care not to depress the plunger. Invert the vial, withdraw the prescribed dose, and then withdraw the needle (or needleless access device).
- Change the needle (or needleless access device) on the syringe, if indicated, to administer the injection.[3]
- Discard any needle (or needleless access device) in a puncture-resistant sharps container, and discard all additional equipment appropriately.[27]

Mixing drugs from two ampules

- Tap the stems of the ampules *to move any medication from the stems into the body of the ampules.*
- Disinfect the neck of each ampule with an alcohol pad and allow to dry completely.[2,3]
- If you're using an ampule that requires a metal filc to open it, draw the file carefully around the narrow part of the ampule *to weaken it*.[25]
- Open each ampule by wrapping a small gauze pad or alcohol pad around the neck of the ampule and quickly snapping off the top along the scored line at the neck.[1] Alternatively, insert the ampule's head into a ampule breaker. Snap the neck in the direction away from your body.
- Insert a syringe (with a filter needle or straw attached *to filter out any glass splinters*) into the first ampule without letting the needle to come into contact with the rim of the ampule. Make sure the needle or straw is in the solution.[2,3,4,26]
- Withdraw the amount ordered from the first ampule and remove the needle from the solution.
- Repeat the ampule preparation steps with the second ampule, changing the needle or straw before drawing up the medication from the ampule if possible.
- When you've prepared the syringe, change to a regular safety needle to administer the medication.[3]

Completing the procedure

- Discard all equipment in appropriate receptacles.[1,27]
- Perform hand hygiene.[1,18,19,20,21,22,23]
- Document the procedure.[28,29,30,31]

Special considerations

- When withdrawing the medication from an ampule, place the ampule upright on a flat surface, insert the needle into the solution, and then withdraw the ordered amount. Alternatively, after the needle is in the solution, you can invert the ampule, keeping the needle centered and in the solution to withdraw the ordered amount. *Surface tension holds the fluid in place when the ampule is inverted.*

- Never combine drugs if you're unsure of their compatibility, and never combine more than two drugs. *Although drug incompatibility usually causes a visible reaction, such as clouding, bubbling, or precipitation, some incompatible combinations produce no visible reaction, even though they alter the chemical nature and action of the drugs.* Check appropriate references and consult a pharmacist when you're unsure about specific compatibility. When in doubt, administer two separate injections.
- Some medications are compatible for only a brief time after being combined and should be administered within 10 minutes after mixing. *After this time, environmental factors, such as temperature, exposure to light, and humidity, may alter compatibility.*
- Always follow manufacturer's instructions for ampule storage and use.
- *To reduce the risk of contamination*, most facilities dispense parenteral medications in single-dose vials.
- Dedicate multidose medication vials to one patient whenever possible to reduce the risk of bloodborne pathogen transmission and infection. *Dedicating multidose vials to one patient reduces infection transmission risk.* If you must use multidose vials for more than one patient, you should keep the vials in, and access them from, a dedicated medication preparation area away from immediate patient treatment areas to prevent inadvertent contamination of the vials through direct or indirect contact with potentially contaminated surfaces or equipment, which could lead to infections in subsequent patients.[2,32,33] Label multidose vials with the date and time, your name and signature, and the patient's name and signature immediately upon piercing.[1,34]
- You should use vials labeled by the manufacturer as "single dose" or "single use" only for a single patient. *These medications may lack antimicrobial preservatives, and can become contaminated and serve as a source of infection if used inappropriately. Evidence shows that improper use of single-dose vials for multiple patients increases the risk of infection.*[35]
- Label a syringe after preparation, unless you've prepared it at the bedside for immediate administration.[6] If preparing several syringes at a time at the bedside or away from the bedside, label each after you prepare it and before preparing another syringe.[6]
- The Joint Commission issued a sentinel event alert concerning the transmission of pathogens related to the misuse of vials that caused viral and bacterial infections, including hepatitis B, hepatitis C, meningitis, and epidural abscesses. These infections were attributed to the reuse of single-dose vials that don't typically contain preservatives, re-entering multidose vials with used syringes and needles, and using multidose vials for multiple patients. To prevent these infections, follow evidence-based best practices, such as disinfecting the vial's rubber stopper before piercing; using single-dose vials only once and then discarding the vial; dedicating multidose vials to a single patient; and using a new syringe and needle when re-entering a multidose vial. Assign the appropriate "beyond-use" date when first entering a multidose vial, and store multidose vials as directed by your facility and according to the manufacturer's instructions.[33]

Complications

Infection may result from failure to follow such infection prevention techniques as performing hand hygiene, using sterile no-touch technique, dedicating multidose vials for single-patient use, and discarding solutions that have reached the beyond-use date.[1]

Documentation

Record the medication strength, dose, administration route, and date and time of administration. Record any adverse reactions to the prescribed medication, the date and time that you notified the practitioner, prescribed interventions, and the patient's response to those interventions.

References

1 World Health Organization. (2010). WHO best practices for injections and related procedures toolkit. https://apps.who.int/iris/bitstream/handle/10665/44298/9789241599252_eng.pdf;jsessionid=C4F0BA433E0D-467FFF3C6BBA8351F981?sequence=1 (Level IV)

2 Dolan, S. A., et al. (2016). APIC position paper: Safe injection, infusion, and medication vial practices in health care (2016). http://www.apic.org/Resource_/TinyMceFileManager/Position_Statements/2016APICSIPPositionPaper.pdf (Level VII)

3 Standard 20. Compounding and preparation of parenteral solutions and medications. Infusion therapy standards of practice (8th ed.). (2021). *Journal of Infusion Nursing, 44*, S59–S60. (Level VII)

4 Infusion Nurses Society. (2016). *Policies and procedures for infusion therapy* (5th ed.). Boston, MA: Infusion Nurses Society.

5 Hafez, M. A., & Al-Dars, A. M. (2012). Glass foreign bodies inside the knee joint following intra-articular injection. *The American Journal of Case Reports, 13*, 238–240. https://www.ncbi.nlm.nih.gov/pmc/articles/PMC3616057/

6 Institute for Safe Medication Practices. (2015). Safe practice guidelines for adult IV push medications. https://www.ismp.org/guidelines/iv-push (Level VII)

7 Accreditation Association for Hospitals and Health Systems. (2020). Standard 07.02.03. *Healthcare Facilities Accreditation Program: Accreditation requirements for acute care hospitals.*Chicago, IL: Accreditation Association for Hospitals and Health Systems. (Level VII)

8 Westbrook, J., et al. (2010). Association of interruptions with an increased risk and severity of medication administration errors. *Archives of Internal Medicine, 170*, 683–690. (Level IV)

9 Institute for Safe Medication Practices. (2012). Side tracks on the safety express: Interruptions lead to errors and unfinished...Wait, what was I doing? *Nurse Advise-ERR, 11*(2), 1–4. Web at https://www.ismp.org/resources/side-tracks-safety-express-interruptions-lead-errors-and-unfinished-wait-what-was-i-doing?id=37

10 The Joint Commission. (2021). Standard MM.06.01.01. *Comprehensive accreditation manual for hospitals.* Oakbrook Terrace, IL: The Joint Commission. (Level VII)

11 Accreditation Association for Hospitals and Health Systems. (2020). Standard 16.01.03. *Healthcare Facilities Accreditation Program: Accreditation requirements for acute care hospitals.* Chicago, IL: Accreditation Association for Hospitals and Health Systems. (Level VII)

12 Centers for Medicare and Medicaid Services, Department of Health and Human Services. (2020). Condition of participation: Nursing services. 42 C.F.R. § 482.23(c).

13 DNV GL-Healthcare USA, Inc. (2020). MM.1.SR.3. *NIAHO® accreditation requirements, interpretive guidelines and surveyor guidance—revision 20.0.* Milford, OH: DNV GL-Healthcare USA, Inc. (Level VII)

14 Institute for Healthcare Improvement. (2011). How-to guide: Prevent adverse drug events (medication reconciliation). http://app.ihi.org/LMS/Content/2cf9e482-3e91-4218-afe3-22f77b5025bc/Upload/HowtoGuidePreventADEs.pdf (Level VII)

15 Standard 13. Medication verification. Infusion therapy standards of practice (8th ed.). (2021). *Journal of Infusion Nursing, 44*, S46–S48. (Level VII)

16 Standard 59. Infusion medication and solution administration. Infusion therapy standards of practice. (8th ed.). (2021). *Journal of Infusion Nursing, 44*, S180–S182. (Level VII)

17 Institute for Safe Medication Practices. (2018). ISMP list of high-alert medications in acute care settings. https://www.ismp.org/sites/default/files/attachments/2018-08/highAlert2018-Acute-Final.pdf

18 The Joint Commission. (2021). Standard NPSG.07.01.01. *Comprehensive accreditation manual for hospitals.* Oakbrook Terrace, IL: The Joint Commission. (Level VII)

19 Centers for Disease Control and Prevention. (2002). Guideline for hand hygiene in health-care settings: Recommendations of the Healthcare Infection Control Practices Advisory Committee and the HICPAC/SHEA/APIC/IDSA Hand Hygiene Task Force. *MMWR Recommendations and Reports, 51*(RR-16), 1–45. https://www.cdc.gov/mmwr/pdf/rr/rr5116.pdf (Level II)

20 World Health Organization. (2009). WHO guidelines on hand hygiene in health care: First global patient safety challenge, clean care is safer care. https://apps.who.int/iris/bitstream/handle/10665/44102/9789241597906_eng.pdf?sequence=1 (Level IV)

21 Centers for Medicare and Medicaid Services, Department of Health and Human Services. (2020). Condition of participation: Infection control. 42 C.F.R. § 482.42.

22 Accreditation Association for Hospitals and Health Systems. (2020). Standard 07.01.21. *Healthcare Facilities Accreditation Program: Accreditation requirements for acute care hospitals.* Chicago, IL: Accreditation Association for Hospitals and Health Systems. (Level VII)

23 DNV GL-Healthcare USA, Inc. (2020). IC.1.SR.1. *NIAHO® accreditation requirements, interpretive guidelines and surveyor guidance - revision 20.0.* Milford, OH: DNV GL-Healthcare USA, Inc. (Level VII)

24 The United States Pharmacopeial Convention. (2019). USP general chapter <800> Hazardous drugs: Handling in healthcare settings. https://www.usp.org/compounding/general-chapter-hazardous-drugs-handling-healthcare (Level VII)

25 UNC Eshelman School of Pharmacy. (n.d.). Sterile compounding: Aseptically transferring drugs from a glass ampule. https://pharmlabs.unc.edu/labs/parenterals/ampule.htm

26 Standard 35. Filtration. Infusion therapy standards of practice (8th ed.). (2021). *Journal of Infusion Nursing, 44*, S102–S104. (Level VII)

27 Occupational Safety and Health Administration. (2012). Bloodborne pathogens, standard number 1910.1030. https://www.osha.gov/pls/oshaweb/owadisp.show_document?p_id=10051&p_table=STANDARDS (Level VII)

28 The Joint Commission. (2021). Standard RC.01.03.01. *Comprehensive accreditation manual for hospitals.* Oakbrook Terrace, IL: The Joint Commission. (Level VII)

29 Centers for Medicare and Medicaid Services, Department of Health and Human Services. (2020). Condition of participation: Medical record services. 42 C.F.R. § 482.24(b).

30 Accreditation Association for Hospitals and Health Systems. (2020). Standard 10.00.03. *Healthcare Facilities Accreditation Program: Accreditation requirements for acute care hospitals.* Chicago, IL: Accreditation Association for Hospitals and Health Systems. (Level VII)

31 DNV GL-Healthcare USA, Inc. (2020). MR.2.SR.1. *NIAHO® accreditation requirements, interpretive guidelines and surveyor guidance—revision 20.0.* Milford, OH: DNV GL-Healthcare USA, Inc. (Level VII)

32 Centers for Disease Control and Prevention. (2019). Frequently asked questions regarding safe practices for medical injections: Questions about multi-dose vials. https://www.cdc.gov/injectionsafety/providers/provider_faqs_multivials.html

33 The Joint Commission. (2014). Sentinel event alert 52: Preventing infection from the misuse of vials. https://www.jointcommission.org/-/media/deprecated-unorganized/imported-assets/tjc/system-folders/assetmanager/sea_52pdf.pdf?db=web&hash=45D132407D5F06D-35C75767A9087B176 (Level VII)

34 Accreditation Association for Hospitals and Health Systems. (2020). Standard 25.01.18. *Healthcare Facilities Accreditation Program: Accreditation requirements for acute care hospitals.* Chicago, IL: Accreditation Association for Hospitals and Health Systems. (Level VII)

35 Centers for Disease Control and Prevention. (2012). Single-dose/single-use vial position and messages. https://www.cdc.gov/injectionsafety/PDF/CDC-SDV-Position05022012.pdf

ADVANCE DIRECTIVES

The Patient Self-Determination Act of 1990 requires health care facilities to provide information to health care consumers about advance directives and their right to choose and refuse treatment.[1] An advance directive is a legal document used as a guideline for providing life-sustaining medical care to a patient with an advanced disease or disability who can no longer indicate his or her own wishes.[2] Advance directives include living wills and health care proxies.

A living will instructs health care providers about a patient's preferences for receiving life-sustaining treatment in the event that a patient becomes unable to communicate choices owing to such conditions as terminal illness, persistent vegetative state, or coma. In making a living will, a legally competent patient states which procedures the patient does or doesn't want carried out, such as intubation and mechanical ventilation, feeding tube insertion, parenteral or enteral nutrition and hydration, antibiotic therapy, dialysis, and cardiopulmonary resuscitation. The living will goes into effect when a patient can no longer communicate choices about medical care. (See *Understanding the living will*, page 10.)

With a health care proxy (also called *durable power of attorney for health care*), the patient designates another person to make decisions about medical care if the patient can't make decisions independently; this person is often referred to as a health care agent. (See *Understanding the health care proxy*, page 11.)

Equipment

Advance directive forms or a copy of the previously established advance directive ■ Optional: written on advance directives.

Understanding the Living Will

A living will is an advance care document that specifies a patient's wishes with regard to medical care should the patient become terminally ill, incompetent, or unable to communicate. A living will is commonly used with a health care agent.

All states and the District of Columbia have laws that outline the documentation requirements for living wills. The sample document below is from Ohio.

Living Will

If my attending doctor and one other practitioner who examines me determine, to a reasonable degree of medical certainty and in accordance with reasonable medical standards, that I am in a terminal condition or in a permanently unconscious state, and if my attending doctor determines that at that time I no longer am able to make informed decisions regarding the administration of life-sustaining treatment, and that, to a reasonable degree of medical certainty and in accordance with reasonable medical standards, there is no reasonable possibility that I will regain the capacity to make informed decisions regarding the administration of life-sustaining treatment, then I direct my attending doctor to withhold or withdraw medical procedures, treatment, interventions, or other measures that serve principally to prolong the process of my dying, rather than diminish my pain or discomfort.

I have used the term "terminal condition" in this declaration to mean an irreversible, incurable, and untreatable condition caused by disease, illness, or injury from which, to a reasonable degree of medical certainty as determined in accordance with reasonable medical standards of my attending doctor and one other practitioner who has examined me, both of the following apply:

1. There can be no recovery.
2. Death is likely to occur within a relatively short time if life-sustaining treatment is not administered.

I have used the term "permanently unconscious state" in this declaration to mean a state of permanent unconsciousness that, to a reasonable degree of medical certainty, is determined in accordance with reasonable medical standards by my attending doctor and one other practitioner who has examined me, as characterized by both of the following:

1. I am irreversibly unaware of myself and my environment.
2. There is a total loss of cerebral cortical functioning, resulting in my having no capacity to experience pain or suffering.

Nutrition and hydration

I hereby authorize my attending doctor to withhold or withdraw nutrition and hydration from me when I am in a permanent unconscious state if my attending doctor and at least one other practitioner who has examined me determine, to a reasonable degree of medical certainty and in accordance with reasonable medical standards, that nutrition or hydration will not or no longer will serve to provide comfort to me or alleviate my pain.

[Sign here for withdrawal of nutrition or hydration] _____

I hereby designate _____ as the person whom I wish my attending doctor to notify at any time that life-sustaining
[Print name of person to decide]
treatment is to be withdrawn or withheld pursuant to this Declaration.

_____   _____
[Sign your name here]   [Today's date]

Witnessed by: _____

[Living will person's name] voluntarily signed or directed another individual to sign this Living Will in the presence of the following who each attests that the Declarant appears to be of sound mind and not under or subject to duress, fraud, or undue influence.

_____   _____
[First witness signs here]   [Second witness signs here]

Adapted from Leading Age Ohio, et al. (2019). "Choices: Living well at the end of life; Advance directives packet (7th ed.)." [Online]. Accessed May 2021 via the Web at http://www.midwestcarealliance.org/aws/LAO/asset_manager/get_file/314696?ver=8392

Implementation

■ Perform hand hygiene.[3,4,5,6,7,8]
■ Confirm the patient's identity using at least two patient identifiers.[9]
■ Provide privacy.[10,11,12,13]
■ Assist with assessing the patient's level of capacity *to ensure that the patient can make care decisions.* This process may include evaluating the patient's ability to understand information, consider the alternatives, evaluate the alternatives, make decisions, and communicate choices. A doctor or advanced practice nurse may determine the patient's capacity for making decisions.[14]
■ Determine if the patient has an advance directive.[1]
■ Explain the procedure to the patient and family (if appropriate) according to their individual communication and learning needs *to increase their understanding, allay their fears, and enhance cooperation.*[15]

If the patient has an advance directive

■ Review the advance directive with the patient *to confirm that it still reflects the patient's wishes.*

■ Place a copy of the advance directive in a prominent location in the medical record *so that it's easily accessible to all health care providers.*[2,16,17,18,19]
■ Notify the practitioner and the rest of the health care team that the patient has an advance directive *so that it can be used to guide care.*[2,20]
■ Determine whether the patient's health care agent has a copy of the advance directive.
■ Encourage the patient to discuss the advance directive with family and health care agent *so that they understand the patient's wishes and can ask questions while the patient is competent and can explain the decision-making process.*[21]
■ Perform hand hygiene.[3,4,5,6,7,8]
■ Document the procedure and the presence of the patient's advance directive.[2,16,17,22,23,24,25]

If the patient doesn't have an advance directive

■ Provide the patient with verbal and written information about advance directives *so that the patient can make an informed decision about developing one.*[2,20,25]

Understanding the Health Care Proxy

The sample document below is an example of a health care proxy, which allows a competent patient to delegate to another person the authority to consent to or refuse health care treatment for the patient. This document helps ensure that the patient's wishes will be carried out if the patient should become incompetent.

Each state with a health care proxy law has specific requirements for executing the document. The sample form below is from Nebraska.

Power of attorney for health care

I appoint_____

whose address is_____

and whose telephone number is_____

as my attorney-in-fact for health care. _____

I appoint_____

whose address is_____

and whose telephone number is_____

as my successor attorney-in-fact for health care. _____

I authorize my attorney-in-fact appointed by this document to make health care decisions for me when I am determined to be incapable of making my own health care decisions. I have read the warning that accompanies this document and understand the consequences of executing a power of attorney for health care.

I direct that my attorney-in-fact comply with the following instructions or limitations (optional):_____

_____

I direct that my attorney-in-fact comply with the following instructions on life-sustaining treatment (optional):_____

_____

I direct that my attorney-in-fact comply with the following instructions on artificially administered nutrition and hydration (optional):

_____

I have read this power of attorney for health care. I understand that it allows another person to make life and death decisions for me if I am incapable of making such decisions. I also understand that I can revoke this power of attorney for health care at any time by notifying my attorney-in-fact, my physician, or the facility in which I am a patient or resident. I also understand that I can require in this power of attorney for health care that the fact of my incapacity in the future be confirmed by a second physician.

_____   _____
[signature of person making designation]   [date]

_____

Adapted from: Nebraska Supreme Court. (2016). "Nebraska power of attorney: Health care" [Online]. Accessed May 2021 via the Web at https://supreme-court.nebraska.gov/sites/default/files/DC-6-13-fillin16.pdf

■ Answer the patient's questions about advance directives or have a social worker or patient representative discuss advance directives with the patient *to provide accurate information*. Make sure the materials are in the patient's preferred language *to promote understanding*. Arrange for an interpreter, if necessary.[2,18,20,26,27]

■ Determine the patient's cognitive, developmental, and legal ability to participate in developing an advance directive. *Weight should be given to the patient's wishes regarding life-sustaining medical treatment.*

■ Assess the patient's religious and cultural beliefs that may affect life-sustaining medical treatments and end-of-life care decisions and practices.

■ Discuss the prognosis for treatment, treatment options, and potential outcomes with the patient and family, as needed.[26]

■ As needed, determine the need for a multidisciplinary conference to provide the patient and family with complete, comprehensive, and accurate information *to prevent them from receiving conflicting or confusing information from various health care providers*.

■ Encourage the patient to discuss developing an advance directive with the family.[21] If the patient would like to make an advance directive, assist the patient and family with coming to terms with the patient's decisions.

■ If indicated, have the patient sign the advance directive and obtain witness signatures as required by state law.

■ Perform hand hygiene.[3,4,5,6,7,8]

■ Document the procedure.[2,16,17,22,23,24,28]

Special considerations

■ Arrange for a translator, if necessary, *to ensure that the patient and family can communicate their concerns and understand health care providers' explanations*.[27,29]

■ If family members express opposition to the patient's advance directive, notify the patient's practitioner, the nursing supervisor, and the risk manager. Encourage family members to discuss their feelings with the patient and these individuals. A consult with the facility's ethics committee may be requested, as indicated.

■ The patient may revoke or change an advance directive at any time for any reason, which may include a change in clinical condition or simply a change of opinion.[20] The patient can revoke an advance directive either orally or in writing.

Documentation

Document the presence of an advance directive and that the practitioner was notified of its presence.[2,20] Include the name of the practitioner and the time of notification. Include the name, address, and telephone number of the health care agent. If the patient's wishes differ from those of the practitioner or family, note the discrepancies.

If the patient doesn't have an advance directive, document that the patient received written information about patient rights under state law to make health care decisions. If the patient refuses information on an advance directive, document this refusal using the patient's own words, in quotes, if possible. Record all conversations with the patient about decision making. Document that proof of capacity was obtained. Document teaching provided to the patient and family (if applicable), their understanding of that teaching, and any need for follow-up teaching.

REFERENCES

1 Congress.Gov. (1990). H.R.5067—Patient Self Determination Act of 1990. https://www.congress.gov/bill/101st-congress/house-bill/5067
2 Centers for Medicare and Medicaid Services, Department of Health and Human Services. (2020). Condition of participation: Patient's rights. 42 C.F.R. § 482.13(b)(3).
3 The Joint Commission. (2021). Standard NPSG.07.01.01. *Comprehensive accreditation manual for hospitals.* Oakbrook Terrace, IL: The Joint Commission. (Level VII)
4 Centers for Disease Control and Prevention. (2002). Guideline for hand hygiene in health-care settings: Recommendations of the Healthcare Infection Control Practices Advisory Committee and the HICPAC/SHEA/APIC/IDSA Hand Hygiene Task Force. *MMWR Recommendations and Reports, 51*(RR-16), 1–45. https://www.cdc.gov/mmwr/pdf/rr/rr5116.pdf (Level II)
5 World Health Organization. (2009). WHO guidelines on hand hygiene in health care: First global patient safety challenge, clean care is safer care. https://apps.who.int/iris/bitstream/handle/10665/44102/9789241597906_eng.pdf?sequence=1 (Level IV)
6 Centers for Medicare and Medicaid Services, Department of Health and Human Services. (2020). Condition of participation: Infection control. 42 C.F.R. § 482.42.
7 Accreditation Association for Hospitals and Health Systems. (2020). Standard 07.01.21. *Healthcare Facilities Accreditation Program: Accreditation requirements for acute care hospitals.* Chicago, IL: Accreditation Association for Hospitals and Health Systems. (Level VII)
8 DNV GL-Healthcare USA, Inc. (2020). IC.1.SR.1. *NIAHO® accreditation requirements, interpretive guidelines and surveyor guidance—revision 20.0.* Milford, OH: DNV GL-Healthcare USA, Inc. (Level VII)
9 The Joint Commission. (2021). Standard NPSG.01.01.01. *Comprehensive accreditation manual for hospitals.* Oakbrook Terrace, IL: The Joint Commission. (Level VII)
10 DNV GL-Healthcare USA, Inc. (2020). PR.2.SR.5. *NIAHO® accreditation requirements, interpretive guidelines and surveyor guidance—revision 20.0.* Milford, OH: DNV GL-Healthcare USA, Inc. (Level VII)
11 The Joint Commission. (2021). Standard RI.01.01.01. *Comprehensive accreditation manual for hospitals.* Oakbrook Terrace, IL: The Joint Commission. (Level VII)
12 Centers for Medicare and Medicaid Services, Department of Health and Human Services. (2020). Condition of participation: Patient's rights. 42 C.F.R. § 482.13(c)(1).
13 Accreditation Association for Hospitals and Health Systems. (2020). Standard 15.01.16. *Healthcare Facilities Accreditation Program: Accreditation requirements for acute care hospitals.* Chicago, IL: Accreditation Association for Hospitals and Health Systems. (Level VII)
14 Leo, R. J. (1999). Competency and the capacity to make treatment decisions: A primer for the primary care physicians. *The Primary Care Companion to the Journal of the Association of Medicine and Psychiatry, 1*(5), 131–141. (Level V)
15 The Joint Commission. (2021). Standard PC.02.01.21. *Comprehensive accreditation manual for hospitals.* Oakbrook Terrace, IL: The Joint Commission. (Level VII)
16 DNV GL-Healthcare USA, Inc. (2020). PR.3.SR.1a. *NIAHO® accreditation requirements, interpretive guidelines and surveyor guidance—revision 20.0.* Milford, OH: DNV GL-Healthcare USA, Inc. (Level VII)
17 The Joint Commission. (2021). Standard RC.02.01.01. *Comprehensive accreditation manual for hospitals.* Oakbrook Terrace, IL: The Joint Commission. (Level VII)
18 Accreditation Association for Hospitals and Health Systems. (2020). Standard 15.01.12. *Healthcare Facilities Accreditation Program: Accreditation requirements for acute care hospitals.* Chicago, IL: Accreditation Association for Hospitals and Health Systems. (Level VII)
19 Accreditation Association for Hospitals and Health Systems. (2020). Standard 15.01.10. *Healthcare Facilities Accreditation Program: Accreditation requirements for acute care hospitals.* Chicago, IL: Accreditation Association for Hospitals and Health Systems. (Level VII)
20 The Joint Commission. (2021). Standard RI.01.05.01. *Comprehensive accreditation manual for hospitals.* Oakbrook Terrace, IL: The Joint Commission. (Level VII)
21 National Institute on Aging & U.S. Department of Health and Human Services. (2018). Advance care planning: Healthcare directives. https://www.nia.nih.gov/health/advance-care-planning-healthcare-directives
22 The Joint Commission. (2021). Standard RC.01.03.01. *Comprehensive accreditation manual for hospitals.* Oakbrook Terrace, IL: The Joint Commission. (Level VII)
23 Centers for Medicare and Medicaid Services, Department of Health and Human Services. (2020). Condition of participation: Medical record services. 42 C.F.R. § 482.24(b).
24 Accreditation Association for Hospitals and Health Systems. (2020). Standard 10.00.03. *Healthcare Facilities Accreditation Program: Accreditation requirements for acute care hospitals.* Chicago, IL: Accreditation Association for Hospitals and Health Systems. (Level VII)
25 DNV GL-Healthcare USA, Inc. (2020). MR.2.SR.1. *NIAHO® accreditation requirements, interpretive guidelines and surveyor guidance—revision 20.0.* Milford, OH: DNV GL-Healthcare USA, Inc. (Level VII)
26 DNV GL-Healthcare USA, Inc. (2020). PR.3.SR.1. *NIAHO® accreditation requirements, interpretive guidelines and surveyor guidance—revision 20.0.*. Milford, OH: DNV GL-Healthcare USA, Inc. (Level VII)
27 Centers for Medicare and Medicaid Services, Department of Health and Human Services. (2020). Condition of participation: Patient's rights. 42 C.F.R. § 482.13(b)(2).
28 The Joint Commission. (2020). Standard RI.01.01.03. *Comprehensive accreditation manual for hospitals.* Oakbrook Terrace, IL: The Joint Commission. (Level VII)
29 DNV GL-Healthcare USA, Inc. (2020). PR.4.SR.1. *NIAHO® accreditation requirements, interpretive guidelines and surveyor guidance—revision 20.0.* Milford, OH: DNV GL-Healthcare USA, Inc. (Level VII)

AIRBORNE PRECAUTIONS

Airborne precautions, used in addition to standard precautions, prevent the spread of infectious droplet nuclei, which are small particles (less than 5 micrometers) suspended in the air and disperse over long distances by air currents. Susceptible individuals can inhale these suspended particles even without having face-to-face contact with the source of the particles (i.e., the infected individual).[1] (See *Conditions requiring airborne precautions.*)

NURSING ALERT For information on Coronavirus disease (COVID-19), please refer to the latest recommendations from the Centers for Disease Control and Prevention (CDC), located online at https://www.cdc.gov/coronavirus/2019-ncov/infection-control/control-recommendations.html?CDC_AA_refVal=https%3A%2F%2Fwww.cdc.gov%2Fcoronavirus%2F2019-ncov%2Fhcp%2Finfection-control.html, when caring for a patient with known or suspected Coronavirus disease.
NURSING ALERT Please refer to the latest recommendations from the CDC, located online at https://www.cdc.gov/vhf/ebola/hcp/index.html, when caring for a patient with known or suspected Ebola virus infection.

Effective airborne precautions require an airborne infection isolation room: a single-patient room that's equipped with monitored negative pressure (in relation to the surrounding area). An airborne infection isolation room should have 12 air exchanges/hour if the room has been newly constructed or renovated, or 6 air exchanges/hour if it's an existing room. The air is either vented directly to the outside of the building or filtered through high-efficiency particulate air (HEPA) filtration before recirculation.[1,5] According to the CDC, air pressure should be monitored daily, using visual indicators, while the room is in use.[5] The door to the room should be kept closed to maintain the proper air pressure balance between the isolation room and the adjoining hallway or corridor. An anteroom is preferred.

All people who enter an airborne infection isolation room must wear respiratory protection, provided by a disposable respirator (such as an N95 respirator or a HEPA respirator) or a reusable respirator (such as HEPA respirator or a powered air-purifying respirator [PAPR]) when

Conditions requiring airborne precautions

If a patient is known to have a condition requiring airborne precautions, the facility should follow the Centers for Disease Control and Prevention's (CDC's) isolation precautions *to prevent the spread of organisms spread by the airborne route.*[2] This table outlines some common conditions that require airborne precautions, including the required duration and any special considerations.[1]

CONDITION	PRECAUTIONARY PERIOD	SPECIAL CONSIDERATIONS (AS APPLICABLE)
Avian influenza	■ For 14 days after onset of signs and symptoms or until an alternate diagnosis is confirmed	■ N/A
Chickenpox (varicella)	■ Until lesions are crusted and no new lesions appear	■ Susceptible health care workers shouldn't enter the room if immune caregivers are available. ■ Contact precautions should be instituted.
Herpes zoster (disseminated disease [rash affects three or more dermatomes][3] in *any* patient or localized disease in *immunocompromised* patient until disseminated disease is ruled out)	■ Duration of illness	■ Susceptible health care workers shouldn't enter the room if immune caregivers are available. ■ Contact precautions should be instituted.
Measles (rubeola)	■ For 4 days after onset of rash ■ For duration of illness in immunocompromised patients	■ Susceptible health care workers shouldn't enter the room if immune caregivers are available.
Monkeypox	■ Until disease is confirmed and smallpox is excluded	■ Contact precautions should be instituted until lesions have crusted.
Severe acute respiratory syndrome	■ For duration of illness plus 10 days after resolution of fever	■ Eye protection (goggles or face shield) should be worn. ■ Contact precautions should be instituted. ■ Vigilant environmental disinfection should be performed.
Smallpox	■ For duration of illness until all scabs have crusted and separated (typically 3 to 4 weeks)	■ Contact precautions should be instituted. ■ Unvaccinated health care workers shouldn't provide care when immune health care workers are available.
Tuberculosis, extrapulmonary, draining lesion	■ Until patient improves clinically and drainage has ceased, or until three consecutive negative cultures of continued drainage are obtained[1]	■ Contact precautions should be instituted.
Tuberculosis, pulmonary or laryngeal disease, confirmed	■ Until patient improves clinically while on effective therapy (such as a decreased cough and fever or improved chest X-ray results) and has three consecutive sputum smears negative for acid-fast bacillus, collected on separate days[1]	■ N/A
Tuberculosis, pulmonary or laryngeal disease, suspected	■ Until active tuberculosis is deemed highly unlikely, and either another diagnosis explains the clinical findings or the results of three consecutive sputum smears for acid-fast bacillus, collected 8 to 24 hours apart, are negative[1,4]	■ At least one of the three sputum specimens should be collected in the morning.[1]

infectious pulmonary or laryngeal tuberculosis (TB) or smallpox is suspected or confirmed, and during procedures that cause aerosolization of viable organisms in patients with suspected or confirmed infectious TB skin lesions.[1,5] Regardless of the type or respiratory protection worn, ensure proper fit to the face each time a respirator is worn by performing a user seal check.[1,5] When using a PAPR, ensure proper functioning of the unit. The CDC has no recommendation for the type of personal protective equipment (for example, surgical mask or respiratory protection with an N95 or higher respirator) to be worn by susceptible health care personnel or those with presumed immunity who must have contact with patients with known or suspected measles, chickenpox, or disseminated herpes zoster.[1]

NURSING ALERT When a patient comes to your facility complaining of respiratory symptoms and an airborne infection is suspected, put a surgical mask on the patient's face (if tolerated) and immediately place the patient in a private room with the door closed until an airborne infection isolation room is available. If the patient can't tolerate a mask, place the patient in a private room with the door closed and wear a respirator when entering the room and caring for the patient.[1]

Equipment

Isolation sign ■ tissues ■ no-touch receptacle ■ Optional: respirators (either disposable N95 or HEPA respirators, or reusable HEPA respirators or PAPRs), surgical masks.

Preparation of equipment

Inspect all equipment and supplies. If a product is expired, is defective, or has compromised integrity, remove it from patient use, label it as expired or defective, and report the expiration or defect as directed by your facility. Keep all airborne precaution supplies outside the patient's room in a wall- or door-mounted cabinet, a cart, or an anteroom.

Implementation

■ Review the patient's medical record and verify the need for airborne precautions.
■ Gather and prepare the necessary equipment and supplies.
■ Perform hand hygiene.[6,7,8,9,10,11]
■ Confirm the patient's identify using at least two patient identifiers.[12]

EQUIPMENT

Respirator seal check

After you put on your respirator, perform a seal check by placing your hands over the face piece, as shown below, and then exhale gently. The seal is considered satisfactory if a slight positive pressure builds up inside the face piece without air leaking from the seal.[15] Air leaking is evidenced by the fogging of your glasses, a feeling of air trickling down your uncovered face, and lack of pressure buildup under the face piece.

If the respirator has an exhalation valve, cover the filter surface with your hands as much as possible and then inhale. The seal is considered satisfactory if the face piece collapses on your face and you don't feel air passing between your face and the face piece.

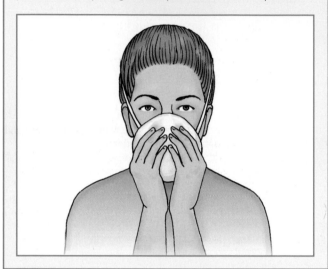

■ Situate the patient in a single-patient airborne infection isolation room with the door closed *to maintain negative pressure.*[1,13] If possible, the room should have an anteroom. Ensure that a private bathroom, if available, is also under negative air pressure. Monitor negative pressure according to regulations.

■ Explain isolation precautions to the patient and family (if appropriate) according to their individual communication and learning needs, *to increase their understanding, allay their fears, and enhance cooperation.*[14]

■ Keep the patient's door (and the anteroom door) closed at all times *to maintain negative pressure and contain the airborne pathogens.*[1] Put an AIRBORNE PRECAUTIONS sign on the door *to notify anyone entering the room of the situation.*

■ Before entering the room, if needed, put on a respirator according to the manufacturer's instructions.[1] Adjust the straps for a firm but comfortable fit. Check the seal. (See *Respirator seal check.*)

■ If you're using a PAPR, check for proper function, battery life, and air flow.

■ Perform hand hygiene.[6,7,8,9,10,11]

■ Enter the patient's room and remove the patient's mask, if the patient is wearing one.

■ Provide the patient with tissues, and instruct the patient to cover the nose and mouth with a tissue when coughing or sneezing. Place a sign in the patient's room as a reminder.[1]

■ Provide the patient with a no-touch receptacle for used-tissue disposal. Instruct the patient to dispose of tissues in the receptacle after use and to perform hand hygiene after contact with respiratory secretions and contaminated objects.[16]

■ Perform hand hygiene.[6,7,8,9,10,11]

■ If worn, remove your respirator after leaving the patient's room and closing the door. To remove your respirator, grasp the bottom and then the top elastic; avoid touching the front of the respirator, *because the front is considered contaminated.*[15]

■ As appropriate, discard the respirator in the appropriate receptacle, or store it for reuse. You may reuse an N95 respirator according to the manufacturer's recommendations if it's not damaged or soiled.[17]

■ Perform hand hygiene.[6,7,8,9,10,11]

■ Document the procedure.[18,19,20,21]

Special considerations

■ Fit testing is performed to confirm that the respirator adequately fits the user. It's performed initially and then periodically at a frequency determined by federal, state, and local regulations.[5,22] Fit testing should also be performed with changes in physical features that could affect the respirator (such as scarring, weight loss or gain, or dental changes).[22]

■ Teach visitors the proper way to wear respiratory protection, and make sure that they wear respiratory protection while in the patient's room.[5]

■ Limit the patient's movement from the airborne infection isolation room. If the patient must leave for essential procedures, make sure the patient wears a surgical mask that covers the nose and mouth.[1,5,13] Notify the receiving staff of the patient's isolation precautions *so that the precautions will be maintained and the patient will be promptly returned to the airborne infection isolation room.* If the patient has skin lesions from varicella, smallpox, or *M. tuberculosis*, the lesions should be covered *to decrease the risk of aerosolization during transport.*[1]

■ Depending on the type of respirator and recommendations from the manufacturer, discard your respirator or store it until the next use.[1] A reusable respirator should be stored by hanging it in a designated storage place or by placing it in a clean, breathable container such as a paper bag. Store respirators so they don't touch each other, and make sure that the respirator is clearly marked with the name of the person it belongs to *in order to minimize potential cross-contamination.*[17]

■ If a patient on airborne precautions requires surgery, schedule the procedure when a minimal number of health care workers and other patients are present. If possible, schedule it as the last case of the day *so that more time is available to clean and disinfect the operating room.* Use an operating room with an anteroom, if possible. Ensure that all health care workers involved in the surgery wear respiratory protection.[5,13]

■ After a patient with suspected or confirmed *M. tuberculosis* leaves an airborne infection isolation room, allow adequate time to elapse before allowing entry of another patient *to ensure removal of contaminated air from the room.* Consult with an infection preventionist about the appropriate length of time. The CDC recommends that a room with six air exchanges/hour be left empty for 69 minutes to effectively remove 99.9% of airborne contaminants.[5]

Complications

Social isolation is a complication of airborne precautions.

Documentation

Record the need for airborne precautions on the nursing care plan and as otherwise determined by your facility. Document initiation and maintenance of the precautions, and the patient's tolerance of the procedure. Document teaching provided to the patient or family (if applicable), their understanding of that teaching, and any need for follow-up teaching. Also document the date airborne precautions were discontinued.

REFERENCES

1 Siegel, J. D., et al. (2007, revised 2019). 2007 guideline for isolation precautions: Preventing transmission of infectious agents in healthcare settings. https://www.cdc.gov/infectioncontrol/pdf/guidelines/isolation-guidelines-H.pdf (Level II)

2 The Joint Commission. (2021). Standard IC.01.05.01. *Comprehensive accreditation manual for hospitals.* Oakbrook Terrace, IL: The Joint Commission. (Level VII)

3 Centers for Disease Control and Prevention. (2020). Shingles (herpes zoster): Clinical overview. https://www.cdc.gov/shingles/hcp/clinical-overview.html

4 Centers for Disease Control and Prevention. (2016). Tuberculosis (TB) fact sheet: Infection control in health-care settings. https://www.cdc.gov/tb/publications/factsheets/prevention/ichcs.htm

5 Centers for Disease Control and Prevention. (2005). Guidelines for preventing the transmission of *Mycobacterium tuberculosis* in health-care settings, 2005. *MMWR Recommendations and Reports, 54*(RR-17), 1–141. https://www.cdc.gov/mmwr/PDF/rr/rr5417.pdf (Level I)

6 Centers for Disease Control and Prevention. (2002). Guideline for hand hygiene in health-care settings: Recommendations of the Healthcare Infection Control Practices Advisory Committee and the HICPAC/SHEA/APIC/IDSA Hand Hygiene Task Force. *MMWR Recommendations and Reports, 51*(RR-16), 1–45. https://www.cdc.gov/mmwr/pdf/rr/rr5116.pdf (Level II)

7 The Joint Commission. (2021). Standard NPSG.07.01.01. *Comprehensive*

accreditation manual for hospitals. Oakbrook Terrace, IL: The Joint Commission. (Level VII)

8 World Health Organization. (2009). WHO guidelines on hand hygiene in health care: First global patient safety challenge, clean care is safer care. https://apps.who.int/iris/bitstream/handle/10665/44102/9789241597906_eng.pdf (Level IV)

9 Centers for Medicare and Medicaid Services, Department of Health and Human Services. (2020). Condition of participation: Infection control. 42 C.F.R. § 482.42.

10 Accreditation Association for Hospitals and Health Systems. (2020). Standard 07.01.21. *Healthcare Facilities Accreditation Program: Accreditation requirements for acute care hospitals.* Chicago, IL: Accreditation Association for Hospitals and Health Systems. (Level VII)

11 DNV GL-Healthcare USA, Inc. (2020). IC.1.SR.1. *NIAHO® accreditation requirements, interpretive guidelines and surveyor guidance—revision 20.0.* Milford, OH: DNV GL-Healthcare USA, Inc. (Level VII)

12 The Joint Commission. (2021). Standard NPSG.01.01.01. *Comprehensive accreditation manual for hospitals.* Oakbrook Terrace, IL: The Joint Commission. (Level VII)

13 Accreditation Association for Hospitals and Health Systems. (2020). Standard 07.01.10. *Healthcare Facilities Accreditation Program: Accreditation requirements for acute care hospitals.* Chicago, IL: Accreditation Association for Hospitals and Health Systems. (Level VII)

14 The Joint Commission. (2021). Standard PC.02.01.21. *Comprehensive accreditation manual for hospitals.* Oakbrook Terrace, IL: The Joint Commission. (Level VII)

15 Centers for Disease Control and Prevention. (n.d.). How to properly put on and take off a disposable respirator. https://www.cdc.gov/niosh/docs/2010-133/pdfs/2010-133.pdf

16 Centers for Disease Control and Prevention. (2009). Respiratory hygiene/cough etiquette in healthcare settings. https://www.cdc.gov/flu/professionals/infectioncontrol/resphygiene.htm

17 Centers for Disease Control and Prevention, The National Institute for Occupational Safety and Health (NIOSH). (2020). Pandemic planning: Recommended guidance for extended use and limited reuse of N95 filtered face-piece respirators in healthcare settings. https://www.cdc.gov/niosh/topics/hcwcontrols/recommendedguidanceextuse.html (Level VII)

18 The Joint Commission. (2021). Standard RC.01.03.01. *Comprehensive accreditation manual for hospitals.* Oakbrook Terrace, IL: The Joint Commission. (Level VII)

19 Centers for Medicare and Medicaid Services, Department of Health and Human Services. (2020). Condition of participation: Medical record services. 42 C.F.R. § 482.24.

20 Accreditation Association for Hospitals and Health Systems. (2020). Standard 10.00.03. *Healthcare Facilities Accreditation Program: Accreditation requirements for acute care hospitals.* Chicago, IL: Accreditation Association for Hospitals and Health Systems. (Level VII)

21 DNV GL-Healthcare USA, Inc. (2020). MR.2.SR.1. *NIAHO® accreditation requirements, interpretive guidelines and surveyor guidance—revision 20.0.* Milford, OH: DNV GL-Healthcare USA, Inc. (Level VII)

22 Occupational Safety and Health Administration. (2011). Respiratory protection, standard number 1910.134. https://www.osha.gov/laws-regs/regulations/standardnumber/1910/1910.134 (Level VII)

Air-fluidized therapy bed use

Originally designed for managing burns, the air-fluidized therapy bed is now used for patients with various debilities. By allowing harmless contact between the bed's surface and grafted sites, the bed promotes comfort and healing. The surface of the bed conforms to the patient's bony prominences as they are immersed into the bed's surface, which lowers the interface pressure by increasing the surface pressure distribution area.[1]

The traditional air-fluidized therapy bed is actually a large tub that supports the patient on a thick layer of silicone-coated microspheres of lime glass. Another version combines the air-fluidized section with a low-air-loss or cushioned section. (See *The air-fluidized therapy bed.*) A monofilament polyester filter sheet covers the microsphere-filled tub. Warmed air, propelled by a blower beneath the bed, passes through it. The resulting fluid-like surface reduces pressure on the skin to avoid obstructing capillary blood flow, which helps to prevent pressure injuries and to promote wound healing.[2,3] The air-fluidized bed's air temperature may be adjusted to help control hypothermia and hyperthermia. The microprocessor technology also allows manipulation of various sections of the unit

EQUIPMENT

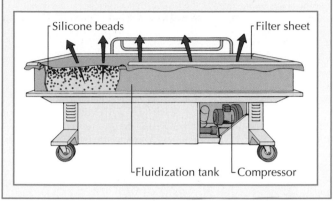

The air-fluidized therapy bed

The air-fluidized therapy bed is a large tub filled with microspheres that are suspended by air pressure and give the patient fluid-like support. The bed provides the advantages of flotation without the disadvantages of instability, patient positioning difficulties, and immobility.

Silicone beads   Filter sheet

Fluidization tank   Compressor

for optimum adjustment. Some models come with adjustable back and leg supports to promote optimal patient positioning.

An air-fluidized therapy bed may be indicated for patients with large Stage 3 or 4 pressure injuries or injuries on multiple turning surfaces.[4] An air-fluidized therapy bed may be contraindicated in a patient with an unstable spine. It also may be contraindicated in a patient who can't mobilize and expel pulmonary secretions, because the bed's lack of back support impairs productive coughing. Operation of an air-fluidized therapy bed is complex and requires special training.

Equipment

Air-fluidized therapy bed with microspheres ▪ filter sheet ▪ flat sheet or specialized sheet ▪ elastic cord ▪ friction-reducing device or lateral transfer board for a patient who weighs less than 200 lb (91 kg); ceiling lift with spine sling, mechanical transfer device, or air-assisted device (for a patient who weighs more than 200 lb [91 kg])[5] ▪ cushioning device or pillows[4] ▪ Optional: gloves, gown, mask with face shield, mask, goggles, breathable underpad.

Preparation of equipment

Inspect all equipment and supplies. If a product is expired, is defective, or has compromised integrity, remove it from patient use, label it as defective, and report the defect as directed by your facility.

A manufacturer's representative or a trained staff member usually prepares the bed for use. If you must help with the preparation, make sure the bed's microspheres reach to within ½″ (1.3 cm) of the top of the tub. Then position the filter sheet on the bed with its printed side facing up. Match the holes in the sheet to the holes in the edge of the bed's frame. If the bed has detachable aluminum rails, place them on the frame, with the studs in the proper holes. Depress the rails firmly, and then secure them by tightening the knurled knobs to seal the filter sheet. Place a flat sheet over the filter sheet or use the specialized sheet provided by the bed company, and secure it with the elastic cord. If using a flat sheet, place only one sheet *so that the patient is as close to the therapeutic surface as possible.*[6] If an underpad is necessary, don't use a reusable underpad; use only a breathable underpad *so that the permeability of the filter sheet is not altered.*[6] Turn on the air current *to activate the microspheres and to ensure that the bed is working properly;* then turn off the air current.

Implementation

▪ Consult with a wound, ostomy, and continence nurse or an educated skin care team member before using an air-fluidized bed *to make sure it's the best choice of support surface for the patient.*

▪ Gather and prepare the equipment and supplies and help prepare the air-fluidized therapy bed, if necessary.

- Perform hand hygiene[7,8,9,10,11,12]
- Confirm the patient's identity using at least two patient identifiers.[13]
- Provide privacy.[14,15,16,17]
- Explain the procedure to the patient and family (if appropriate) according to their individual communication and learning needs *to increase their understanding, allay their fears, and enhance cooperation.*[18] Demonstrate the operation of the air-fluidized therapy bed. Inform the patient the reason for its use, and explain that the patient will feel as though floating while on the bed.
- Raise the bed to waist level before transferring the patient *to prevent caregiver back strain.*[5]
- Perform hand hygiene[7,8,9,10,11,12]
- Put on gloves and, as needed, other personal protective equipment *to comply with standard precautions.*[19,20]
- With the help of three or more coworkers, transfer the patient to the bed using an appropriate patient transfer device.
- If the patient has an enteral feeding tube, elevate the head of the bed at least 30 degrees, unless contraindicated, *to help prevent aspiration.*[21]
- Place cushioning devices or pillows between the patient's legs, ankles, and other bony prominences *to help maintain alignment and prevent bony prominences from touching.*[4]
- Turn on the air current pressure *to activate the air-fluidized therapy bed.*
- Remove the patient transfer device.
- Monitor the patient's fluid and electrolyte status, *because an air-fluidized therapy bed increases evaporative water loss.*
- Reposition the patient at a frequency determined by the patient's condition and the support surface.[22] *Specialty beds don't eliminate the need for frequent assessment and position changes.*
- Adjust the bed's temperature for patient comfort according to the manufacturer's instructions. (The usual comfort range is 88° F [31° C] to 94° F [34.5° C]).[6]
- Return the bed to the lowest position *to prevent falls and maintain patient safety.*[23]
- Remove and discard your gloves and any other personal protective equipment, if worn.[24]
- Perform hand hygiene[7,8,9,10,11,12]
- Document the procedure.[25,26,27,28]

Special considerations

- *Because of the bed's drying effect,* always cover a patient's mesh graft for the first 2 to 8 days, as ordered. If the patient has excessive upper respiratory tract dryness, use a humidifier and mask, as ordered. Encourage coughing and deep breathing.
- To position a bedpan, roll the patient away from you; place the bedpan on the flat sheet and push it into the bed's microspheres, then reposition the patient and defluidize the bed if requested by the patient. To remove the bedpan, hold it steady and roll the patient away from you. If you have defluidized the bed, be sure to reactivate the air fluidization.
- If a filter sheet change is needed, notify the manufacturer for a replacement.[6]
- Note that the air-fluidized therapy bed has an emergency procedure to stop the action of the bed if the patient needs cardiopulmonary resuscitation. Follow the manufacturer's cardiopulmonary resuscitation (CPR) instructions to defluidize the bed and turn on maximum inflation.[6]
- If the patient has a flap or graft, make sure to keep the fluidization function on during patient transfers in and out of the bed *to prevent short-term pressure on the wound.*
- Perform a pressure injury risk assessment and skin assessment upon a patient's admission to the health care setting, and repeat the assessments on a regularly scheduled basis, or when there's a significant change in the patient's condition (e.g., surgery, a decline in health status).[4] Use a standardized pressure injury risk assessment tool.

HOSPITAL-ACQUIRED CONDITION ALERT Keep in mind that the Centers for Medicare and Medicaid Services considers a Stage 3 or 4 pressure injury to be a hospital-acquired condition, *because it may be prevented using a variety of best practices.* Make sure to follow pressure injury prevention practices (e.g., performing risk assessments, moisturizing the patient's skin, providing adequate hydration and nutrition, and using specialty support surfaces) *to reduce the risk of pressure injuries.*[29,30,31]

Documentation

Record the duration of therapy and the patient's response to it. Document the condition of the patient's skin and the existence of pressure injuries or other wounds. Document teaching provided to the patient and family (if applicable), their understanding of that teaching, and any need for follow-up teaching.

REFERENCES

1 Baranoski, S., & Ayello, E. A. (2020). *Wound care essentials: Practice principles* (5th ed.). Philadelphia, PA: Wolters Kluwer.

2 Haesler, E. (2018). Evidence summary: Pressure injuries: Active support surfaces for preventing and treating pressure injuries. *Wound Practice & Research: Journal of the Australian Wound Management Association, 26*(1), 50–51. (Level I)

3 Greenwood, C. E., et al. (2017). Pressure-relieving devices for preventing heel pressure ulcers. *Cochrane Database of Systematic Reviews, 2017*(5), CD011013. (Level I)

4 Wound Ostomy and Continence Nurses Society (WOCN). (2016). *Guideline for prevention and management of pressure ulcers (injuries): WOCN clinical practice guideline series 2.* Mount Laurel, NJ: WOCN.

5 Waters, T. R., et al. (2009). Safe patient handling training for schools of nursing. https://www.cdc.gov/niosh/docs/2009-127/pdfs/2009-127.pdf (Level VII)

6 Hill-Rom. (2005). Clinitron® Rite-Hite® air fluidized therapy unit: Quick reference guide. https://www.hill-rom.com/eLearningCourses/Clinitron/assets/pdf/Clinitron_Rite_Hite_Quick_Ref_Guide.pdf

7 The Joint Commission. (2021). Standard NPSG.07.01.01. *Comprehensive accreditation manual for hospitals.* Oakbrook Terrace, IL: The Joint Commission. (Level VII)

8 Centers for Disease Control and Prevention. (2002). Guideline for hand hygiene in health-care settings: Recommendations of the Healthcare Infection Control Practices Advisory Committee and the HICPAC/SHEA/APIC/IDSA Hand Hygiene Task Force. *MMWR Recommendations and Reports, 51*(RR-16), 1–45. https://www.cdc.gov/mmwr/pdf/rr/rr5116.pdf (Level II)

9 World Health Organization. (2009). WHO guidelines on hand hygiene in health care: First global patient safety challenge, clean care is safer care. https://apps.who.int/iris/bitstream/handle/10665/44102/9789241597906_eng.pdf?sequence=1 (Level IV)

10 Centers for Medicare and Medicaid Services, Department of Health and Human Services. (2020). Condition of participation: Infection control. 42 C.F.R. § 482.42.

11 Accreditation Association for Hospitals and Health Systems. (2020). Standard 07.01.21. *Healthcare Facilities Accreditation Program: Accreditation requirements for acute care hospitals.* Chicago, IL: Accreditation Association for Hospitals and Health Systems. (Level VII)

12 DNV GL-Healthcare USA, Inc. (2020). IC.1.SR.1. *NIAHO® accreditation requirements, interpretive guidelines and surveyor guidance—revision 20.0.* Milford, OH: DNV GL-Healthcare USA, Inc. (Level VII)

13 The Joint Commission. (2021). Standard NPSG.01.01.01. *Comprehensive accreditation manual for hospitals.* Oakbrook Terrace, IL: The Joint Commission. (Level VII)

14 The Joint Commission. (2021). Standard RI.01.01.01. *Comprehensive accreditation manual for hospitals.* Oakbrook Terrace, IL: The Joint Commission. (Level VII)

15 Centers for Medicare and Medicaid Services, Department of Health and Human Services. (2020). Condition of participation: Patient's rights. 42 C.F.R. § 482.13(c)(1).

16 Accreditation Association for Hospitals and Health Systems. (2020). Standard 15.01.16. *Healthcare Facilities Accreditation Program: Accreditation requirements for acute care hospitals.* Chicago, IL: Accreditation Association for Hospitals and Health Systems. (Level VII)

17 DNV GL-Healthcare USA, Inc. (2020). PR.2.SR.5. *NIAHO® accreditation requirements, interpretive guidelines and surveyor guidance—revision 20.0.* Milford, OH: DNV GL-Healthcare USA, Inc. (Level VII)

18 The Joint Commission. (2021). Standard PC.02.01.21. *Comprehensive accreditation manual for hospitals.* Oakbrook Terrace, IL: The Joint Commission. (Level VII)

19 Accreditation Association for Hospitals and Health Systems. (2020). Standard 07.01.10. *Healthcare Facilities Accreditation Program: Accreditation requirements for acute care hospitals.* Chicago, IL: Accreditation Association for Hospitals and Health Systems. (Level VII)

20 Siegel, J. D., et al. (2007, revised 2019). 2007 guideline for isolation precautions: Preventing transmission of infectious agents in healthcare

settings. https://www.cdc.gov/infectioncontrol/pdf/guidelines/isolation-guidelines-H.pdf (Level II)

21 Boullata, J. I., et al. (2017). ASPEN safe practices for enteral nutrition therapy. *Journal of Parenteral and Enteral Nutrition, 41*, 15–103. http://journals.sagepub.com/doi/full/10.1177/0148607116673053 (Level VII)

22 European Pressure Ulcer Advisory Panel, et al. (2019). Prevention and treatment of pressure ulcers/injuries: Quick reference guide. http://www.internationalguideline.com/static/pdfs/Quick_Reference_Guide-10Mar2019.pdf (Level VII)

23 Ganz, D. A., et al. (2013, reviewed 2021). *Preventing falls in hospitals: A toolkit for improving quality of care* (AHRQ Publication No. 13-0015-EF). Rockville, MD: Agency for Healthcare Research and Quality. https://www.ahrq.gov/professionals/systems/hospital/fallpxtoolkit/index.html (Level VII)

24 Occupational Safety and Health Administration. (2012). Bloodborne pathogens, standard number 1910.1030. https://www.osha.gov/pls/oshaweb/owadisp.show_document?p_id=10051&p_table=STANDARDS (Level VII)

25 The Joint Commission. (2021). Standard RC.01.03.01. *Comprehensive accreditation manual for hospitals.* Oakbrook Terrace, IL: The Joint Commission. (Level VII)

26 Centers for Medicare and Medicaid Services, Department of Health and Human Services. (2020). Condition of participation: Medical record services. 42 C.F.R. § 482.24(b).

27 Accreditation Association for Hospitals and Health Systems. (2020). Standard 10.00.03. *Healthcare Facilities Accreditation Program: Accreditation requirements for acute care hospitals.* Chicago, IL: Accreditation Association for Hospitals and Health Systems. (Level VII)

28 DNV GL-Healthcare USA, Inc. (2020). MR.2.SR.1. *NIAHO® accreditation requirements, interpretive guidelines and surveyor guidance—revision 20.0.* Milford, OH: DNV GL-Healthcare USA, Inc. (Level VII)

29 Jarrett, N., & Callaham, M. (2016). Evidence-based guidelines for selected hospital-acquired conditions: Final report. https://www.cms.gov/Medicare/Medicare-Fee-for-Service-Payment/HospitalAcqCond/Downloads/2016-HAC-Report.pdf

30 Accreditation Association for Hospitals and Health Systems. (2020). Standard 16.02.02. *Healthcare Facilities Accreditation Program: Accreditation requirements for acute care hospitals.* Chicago, IL: Accreditation Association for Hospitals and Health Systems. (Level VII)

31 Centers for Medicare and Medicaid Services, Department of Health and Human Services. (2021). Appendix I: Hospital-acquired conditions (HACS) list. https://www.cms.gov/Medicare/Medicare-Fee-for-Service-Payment/HospitalAcqCond/icd10_hacs

ALIGNMENT AND PRESSURE-REDUCING DEVICE APPLICATION

Various assistive devices can be used to maintain correct body positioning and to help prevent complications that commonly arise when a patient must be on prolonged bed rest. Alignment and pressure-reducing devices, or pressure-redistribution devices, include the cradle boot, abduction pillow, trochanter roll, hand roll, and wheelchair cushion. (See *Common alignment and pressure-reducing devices*, page 18.) Several of these devices—the cradle boot, trochanter roll, hand roll, and wheelchair cushion—are especially useful when caring for patients who have a loss of sensation, mobility, or consciousness.

Equipment

Heel suspension device ▪ heel suspension foam cushion ▪ abduction pillow ▪ trochanter rolls ▪ hand rolls ▪ wheelchair cushion ▪ pressure injury risk assessment tool ▪ Optional: washcloth, blanket or towel, roller gauze, hypoallergenic or adhesive tape, pillow.

Preparation of equipment

▪ Inspect all equipment and supplies. If a product is expired, is defective, or has compromised integrity, remove it from patient use, label it as expired or defective, and report the expiration or defect as directed by your facility.

Implementation

▪ Gather and prepare the appropriate equipment and supplies. If you're using a device that's available in different sizes, select the appropriate size for the patient.
▪ Perform hand hygiene.[5,6,7,8,9,10]
▪ Confirm the patient's identity using at least two patient identifiers.[11]

▪ Provide privacy.[12,13,14,15]
▪ Explain the procedure and the purpose of the alignment and pressure-reducing device to the patient and family (if appropriate) according to their individual communication and learning needs *to increase their understanding, allay their fears, and enhance cooperation.*[16]
▪ Assess the patient's skin and perform a structured pressure injury risk assessment, paying special attention to the location(s) where you'll be applying the device.[17] Note and record any areas of redness or swelling, and pay close attention to pressure points at the elbows, heels, trochanters, sacrum, coccyx, buttocks, and ischium, and beneath medical devices, *because these areas are more likely to develop pressure injuries.*[17]

HOSPITAL-ACQUIRED CONDITION ALERT Keep in mind that the Centers for Medicare and Medicaid Services consider a stage 3 or 4 pressure injury to be a hospital-acquired condition by the *because it can be reasonably prevented using a variety of best practices.* Make sure to follow evidence-based pressure injury prevention practices (such as assessing skin integrity, encouraging mobility, and repositioning the patient) *to reduce the risk of pressure injury.*[18,19]

Applying a heel suspension device
▪ Position the patient comfortable in either a sitting or supine position with the legs in a neutral position.
▪ Open the slit on the superior surface of the boot, place the patient's heel in the circular cutout area, then fasten the Velcro strap(s) according to the manufacturer's instructions. Check that you can insert two fingers beneath the strap(s) *to prevent a tight fit that might impair circulation.*
▪ Repeat the procedure with the patient's other foot, as needed.
▪ Position the patient's legs in a comfortable, neutral position *to prevent internal and external rotation.*
▪ Make sure that both knees are flexed 5 to 10 degrees *to prevent hyperextension of the knee and to decrease the risk of deep vein thrombosis.* Ensure that both heels are suspended off the bed, and that there isn't any pressure on the Achilles tendon.[1]

Applying a heel suspension foam cushion
▪ Place the patient in the supine position.
▪ Slide the cushion longitudinally under the patient's calves, avoiding the Achilles tendon.[1]
▪ Make sure the heels are suspended in the air.[1]
▪ Make sure that the patient's knees are flexed slightly *to avoid the risk of popliteal vein compression and deep knee thrombosis.*[3] Offload the heel *to distribute weight along the calf without placing pressure on the Achilles tendon.*[3]

Applying an abduction pillow
▪ Place the patient in the supine position, slide the pillow between the patient's legs, and gently arrange the straps beneath the patient's legs, making sure the straps are flat on the bed.
▪ Place the upper part of the patient's legs in the pillow's lateral indentations.
▪ Bring the straps around the patient's legs, securing them to the top of the pillow.
▪ Place the patient's legs in a neutral position *to prevent external hip rotation.*

Applying trochanter rolls
▪ Place the patient in a supine position.
▪ Position a trochanter roll, rolled towel, or blanket along the outside of the patient's thigh from the iliac crest to the mid-thigh. If you're using a rolled towel or blanket, tuck a few inches of material under the patient's hip and thigh *to hold the roll in place.*
▪ Place another roll along the other thigh.
▪ Make sure neither roll extends to the knee *to prevent peroneal nerve compression and palsy, which can lead to footdrop.*
▪ Place the patient's legs in a neutral position *to prevent external hip rotation.*

Applying hand rolls
▪ Place a hand roll or rolled washcloth in each of the patient's hands *to maintain a neutral position.*
▪ Secure the straps, if present, or apply roller gauze and secure with hypoallergenic or adhesive tape.

EQUIPMENT

Common alignment and pressure-reducing devices

Some common alignment and pressure-reducing devices include the cradle boot, abduction pillow, trochanter roll, hand roll, and wheelchair cushion.

Heel suspension device

A heel suspension device, such as a cradle boot (as shown below), elevates the heel and redistributes the weight of the leg along the calf without putting pressure on the Achilles tendon.[1,2,3] It helps to prevent footdrop, skin breakdown, internal and external rotation of the hip, strain on hip ligaments, and pressure on bony prominences.

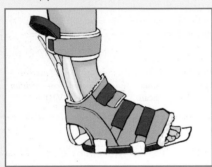

Heel suspension foam cushion

A specially designed foam cushion (as shown below) used under the full length of the calves helps keep the heels elevated for short-term use in alert, cooperative patients. Be sure to flex the patient's knees slightly to avoid the risk of popliteal vein compression and deep vein thrombosis.[3]

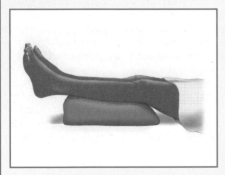

Abduction pillow

An abduction pillow (as shown below) is a wedge-shaped piece of sponge rubber with lateral indentations for the patient's thighs. Its straps wrap around the patient's thighs and maintain correct positioning by preventing internal rotation and adduction of the hip. Although a properly shaped bed pillow may temporarily substitute for a commercial abduction pillow, it's difficult to apply and fails to maintain proper lateral alignment.

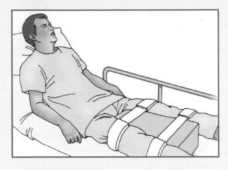

Trochanter roll

A trochanter roll is used to prevent hip external rotation by keeping the hip and thigh in a neutral position. A commercial trochanter roll is made of sponge rubber. You can also improvise a trochanter roll using a rolled blanket or towel if a commercial one is not available. To hold an improvised roll in place, gently tuck a few inches of the material beneath the patient's hip and thigh as he lies in a supine position, allowing his leg to rest against the rolled blanket or towel (as shown below).

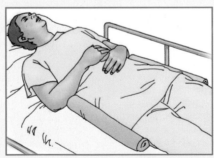

Hand roll

A hand roll, designed to prevent hand contractures, is available in hard and soft materials and is held in place by fixed or adjustable strap(s). You can improvise one from a rolled washcloth secured with roller gauze and adhesive tape if a commercial device is unavailable.

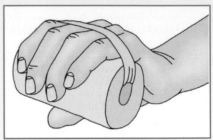

Wheelchair cushion

A wheelchair cushion is a pressure-reducing device filled with air, viscous fluid and foam, or gel and foam. When used with a properly fitted wheelchair, a pressure-reducing cushion can significantly reduce pressure injury formation at the sacrum and ischium in patients who need to use a wheelchair for 6 or more hours per day.[4] A convoluted foam cushion should be avoided because it doesn't protect the patient's skin from pressure injuries while seated.

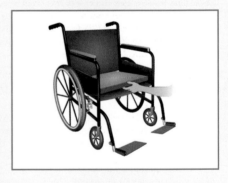

Applying a pressure-reducing wheelchair cushion
- Place the cushion into the wheelchair seat before the patient sits.
- Ensure the wheelchair width is adequate by checking that the patient's hips don't touch the sides of the wheelchair at their widest point.

Completing the procedure
- Reposition the patient periodically, at a frequency determined by the patient's condition and the support surface, *to reduce the duration and magnitude of pressure over affected body surfaces.*[17,20,21] If the patient can perform repositioning, explain how to make small, frequent position changes. Avoid positioning the patient on reddened areas.
- Perform structured pressure injury risk assessments at a frequency determined by the patient's condition.[17]
- Perform hand hygiene.[5,6,7,8,9,10]
- Document the procedure.[22,23,24,25]

Special considerations
- Remember that the use of assistive devices doesn't preclude regularly scheduled patient positioning, range-of-motion exercises, and skin care. Turn the patient at a frequency determined by the patient's tissue tolerance, level of activity and mobility, skin condition, medical condition, treatment goals, type of pressure redistribution support surface, and comfort. Remove the device as needed.[1]
- Monitor skin integrity underneath a strap.
- Consult a wound, ostomy, and continence nurse, as needed.

Patient teaching
Explain the use of appropriate devices to the patient and caregiver. Demonstrate the proper use of each device, emphasizing proper alignment of extremities, and have the patient or caregiver give a return demonstration *to check for proper technique.* Emphasize measures needed to prevent pressure injuries.

Complications

Contractures and pressure injuries can occur with the use of a hand roll and possibly other assistive devices. To avoid these problems, remove hand rolls every 2 hours.

Documentation

Record the use of alignment and pressure-reducing devices in the patient's medical record and in the nursing care plan, including the reason for the device. Include your assessment for complications. Document the findings of pressure injury risk assessments and skin assessments.[17] In addition, document teaching provided to the patient and family (if applicable), their understanding of that teaching, and any need for follow-up teaching. Document re-evaluation of patient care goals, as needed.

REFERENCES

1 Wound Ostomy and Continence Nurses Society (WOCN). (2016). *Guideline for prevention and management of pressure ulcers (injuries): WOCN clinical practice guideline series 2.* Mount Laurel, NJ: WOCN.

2 Rajpaul, K., & Acton, C. (2016). Using heel protectors for the prevention of hospital-acquired pressure ulcers. *British Journal of Nursing, 25*(Suppl. 6), S18–S26.

3 European Pressure Ulcer Advisory Panel (EPUAP), et al. (2019). Prevention and treatment of pressure ulcers/injuries: Clinical practice guideline (The International Guideline, 3rd ed.). Prague, Czech Republic: EPUAP, National Pressure Injury Advisory Panel, PanPacific Pressure Injury Alliance. (Level VII)

4 Brienza, D., et al. (2010). A randomized clinical trial on preventing pressure ulcers with wheelchair seat cushions. *Journal of the American Geriatrics Society, 58,* 2308–2314. (Level II)

5 The Joint Commission. (2021). Standard NPSG.07.01.01. *Comprehensive accreditation manual for hospitals.* Oakbrook Terrace, IL: The Joint Commission. (Level VII)

6 Centers for Disease Control and Prevention. (2002). Guideline for hand hygiene in health-care settings: Recommendations of the Healthcare Infection Control Practices Advisory Committee and the HICPAC/SHEA/APIC/IDSA Hand Hygiene Task Force. *MMWR Recommendations and Reports, 51*(RR-16), 1–45. https://www.cdc.gov/mmwr/pdf/rr/rr5116.pdf (Level II)

7 World Health Organization. (2009). WHO guidelines on hand hygiene in health care: First global patient safety challenge, clean care is safer care. https://apps.who.int/iris/bitstream/handle/10665/44102/9789241597906_eng.pdf?sequence=1 (Level IV)

8 Centers for Medicare and Medicaid Services, Department of Health and Human Services. (2020). Condition of participation: Infection control. 42 C.F.R. § 482.42.

9 Accreditation Association for Hospitals and Health Systems. (2020). Standard 07.01.21. *Healthcare Facilities Accreditation Program: Accreditation requirements for acute care hospitals.* Chicago, IL: Accreditation Association for Hospitals and Health Systems. (Level VII)

10 DNV GL-Healthcare USA, Inc. (2020). IC.1.SR.1. *NIAHO® accreditation requirements, interpretive guidelines and surveyor guidance—revision 20.0.* Milford, OH: DNV GL-Healthcare USA, Inc. (Level VII)

11 The Joint Commission. (2021). Standard NPSG.01.01.01. *Comprehensive accreditation manual for hospitals.* Oakbrook Terrace, IL: The Joint Commission. (Level VII)

12 Accreditation Association for Hospitals and Health Systems. (2020). Standard 15.01.16. *Healthcare Facilities Accreditation Program: Accreditation requirements for acute care hospitals.* Chicago, IL: Accreditation Association for Hospitals and Health Systems. (Level VII)

13 Centers for Medicare and Medicaid Services, Department of Health and Human Services. (2020). Condition of participation: Patient's rights. 42 C.F.R. § 482.13(c)(1).

14 The Joint Commission. (2021). Standard RI.01.01.01. *Comprehensive accreditation manual for hospitals.* Oakbrook Terrace, IL: The Joint Commission. (Level VII)

15 DNV GL-Healthcare USA, Inc. (2020). PR.2.SR.5. *NIAHO® accreditation requirements, interpretive guidelines and surveyor guidance—revision 20.0.* Milford, OH: DNV GL-Healthcare USA, Inc. (Level VII)

16 The Joint Commission. (2021). Standard PC.02.01.21. *Comprehensive accreditation manual for hospitals.* Oakbrook Terrace, IL: The Joint Commission. (Level VII)

17 European Pressure Ulcer Advisory Panel, et al. (2019). Prevention and treatment of pressure ulcers/injuries: Quick reference guide. http://www.internationalguideline.com/static/pdfs/Quick_Reference_Guide-10Mar2019.pdf (Level VII)

18 Jarrett, N., & Callaham, M. (2016). Evidence-based guidelines for selected hospital-acquired conditions: Final report. https://www.cms.gov/Medicare/Medicare-Fee-for-Service-Payment/HospitalAcqCond/Downloads/2016-HAC-Report.pdf

19 Accreditation Association for Hospitals and Health Systems. (2020). Standard 16.02.02. *Healthcare Facilities Accreditation Program: Accreditation requirements for acute care hospitals.* Chicago, IL: Accreditation Association for Hospitals and Health Systems. (Level VII)

20 Baranoski, S., & Ayello, E. A. (2020). *Wound care essentials: Practice principles* (5th ed.). Philadelphia, PA: Wolters Kluwer.

21 Greenwood, C. E., et al. (2017). Pressure-relieving devices for preventing heel pressure ulcers. *Cochrane Database of Systematic Reviews, 2017*(5), CD011013. (Level I)

22 The Joint Commission. (2021). Standard RC.01.03.01. *Comprehensive accreditation manual for hospitals.* Oakbrook Terrace, IL: The Joint Commission. (Level VII)

23 Centers for Medicare and Medicaid Services, Department of Health and Human Services. (2020). Condition of participation: Medical record services. 42 C.F.R. § 482.24.

24 Accreditation Association for Hospitals and Health Systems. (2020). Standard 10.00.03. *Healthcare Facilities Accreditation Program: Accreditation requirements for acute care hospitals.* Chicago, IL: Accreditation Association for Hospitals and Health Systems. (Level VII)

25 DNV GL-Healthcare USA, Inc. (2020). MR.2.SR.1. *NIAHO® accreditation requirements, interpretive guidelines and surveyor guidance—revision 20.0.* Milford, OH: DNV GL-Healthcare USA, Inc. (Level VII)

ANKLE-BRACHIAL INDEX CALCULATION

Calculating the ankle-brachial index helps diagnose peripheral artery disease (PAD). A common cause of impaired ambulation, PAD is the leading cause of lower extremity wounds and amputations. Risk factors associated with PAD include older age, smoking, hyperlipidemia, hypertension, obesity, diabetes mellitus, and atherosclerosis.[1,2] When a practitioner suspects PAD, the ankle-brachial index is considered the first-line noninvasive test for diagnosis.[3]

To calculate the ankle-brachial index, a handheld Doppler 8- to 10-MHz ultrasound probe is used to measure the systolic blood pressure from both of a patient's brachial arteries and the dorsalis pedis and posterior tibial arteries in both ankles. When measuring the systolic blood pressures of a patient's four extremities, each person in your facility should use a consistent sequence, such as this counterclockwise sequence: right brachial artery, right posterior tibial artery, right dorsalis pedis artery, left posterior tibial artery, left dorsalis pedis artery, and left brachial artery.

If the systolic blood pressure in a patient's right arm exceeds the systolic blood pressure in the left arm by 10 mm Hg or more, repeat the blood pressure measurement in the right arm and disregard the first measurement in that arm. Calculate the ankle-brachial index for each of the patient's legs by taking the higher of the two systolic blood pressures of the two arteries (posterior tibial or dorsalis pedis) in the ankle and dividing it by the higher of the two brachial artery systolic blood pressures (right arm or left arm). If repeat testing is needed, do so in a clockwise sequence, starting and ending with the left arm.[3]

Ankle-brachial index calculation is contraindicated in patients who can't remain supine during testing or who have an extremity injury that may worsen with application of a blood pressure cuff.[4]

Equipment

Sphygmomanometer with appropriately sized blood pressure cuff(s)[3] ▪ handheld Doppler ultrasound device with 8- to 10-MHz probe[3] ▪ conduction gel ▪ soft cloth ▪ calculator ▪ facility-approved disinfectant ▪ Optional: impermeable dressing, gloves.

Preparation of equipment

Inspect all equipment and supplies. If a product is expired, is defective, or has compromised integrity, remove it from patient use, label it as expired or defective, and report the expiration or defect as directed by your facility.

Implementation

▪ Review the medical record for the patient's history, including contraindications to the procedure.
▪ Gather and prepare the necessary equipment and supplies.

- Perform hand hygiene.[5,6,7,8,9,10]
- Confirm the patient's identity using at least two patient identifiers.[11]
- Provide privacy.[12,13,14,15]
- Explain the procedure to the patient and family (if appropriate) according to their individual communication and learning needs *to help increase their understanding, allay their fears, and enhance cooperation.*[16]
- Instruct the patient to remain still during blood pressure measurement. If the patient can't remain still because of tremors or some other condition, consider using another testing method, such as color duplex ultrasound imaging, computed tomography angiography, magnetic resonance angiography, or angiography.[3]
- Verify that the patient hasn't smoked or consumed caffeine for at least 2 hours before testing. *Smoking and caffeine consumption may alter test results.*[3]
- Ensure that the patient wears loose-fitting clothing *so that you can easily access the arms and legs for blood pressure measurement.*
- Have the patient rest quietly for 5 to 10 minutes in a supine position, with the head and heels supported.[2,3]
- Ensure a comfortable room temperature (66° to 72° F [18.9° to 22.2° C]).[3]
- Raise the patient's bed to waist level before providing care *to help prevent caregiver back strain.*[17]
- Perform hand hygiene.[5,6,7,8,9,10]
- Remain quiet during blood pressure measurement and instruct the patient to do the same, *because the systolic blood pressure increases with talking.*
- Assess the patient's extremities for blood pressure cuff placement. Avoid placing the cuff over a distal bypass *to help reduce the risk of bypass thrombosis.*[3] Don't apply a blood pressure cuff on an extremity with deep vein thrombosis, grafts, ischemic changes, an arteriovenous fistula, or an arteriovenous graft. Don't apply it over a peripherally inserted central catheter or midline catheter site. If the patient has lymphedema after undergoing a lumpectomy or mastectomy, don't use the affected arm.
- If a patient has an open lesion, cover it with an impermeable dressing to help reduce the risk of cross-contamination.[3]
- If you're using a counterclockwise sequence, begin by measuring the systolic blood pressure in the patient's right arm over the brachial artery. Position the blood pressure cuff about 1" (2.5 cm) above the antecubital fossa.[2] Apply conduction gel over the Doppler ultrasound probe sensor.[3] Turn on the Doppler ultrasound device.[3] Place the Doppler ultrasound probe sensor over the brachial artery at a 45- to 60-degree angle to the surface of the skin.[3] While listening to the brachial artery, inflate the blood pressure cuff at least 20 mm Hg above the point at which the audible Doppler signal disappears.[3] Don't inflate the cuff to more than 300 mm Hg; if you still detect blood flow, deflate the cuff rapidly to help avoid patient discomfort.[3] Slowly release the pressure in the blood pressure cuff until the pulse returns. Record the systolic blood pressure.[2,18]
- Measure the systolic blood pressure in the patient's lower extremities, continuing in a counterclockwise sequence, over the right posterior tibial artery, right dorsalis pedis artery, left posterior tibial artery, and left dorsalis pedis artery. Wrap the deflated blood pressure cuff around the patient's leg about 1" (2.5 cm) above the superior aspect of the medial malleolus.[2] Place the Doppler ultrasound probe sensor over the posterior tibial artery (as shown) at a 45- to 60-degree angle to the surface of the skin.[3]

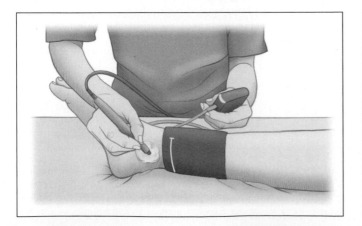

- While listening to the posterior tibial artery, inflate the blood pressure cuff at least 20 mm Hg above the point at which the audible Doppler signal disappears.[2] Slowly release the pressure in the blood pressure cuff until the pulse returns. Record the systolic blood pressure of the posterior tibial artery.[2,18] Repeat and record the systolic blood pressure measurement over the dorsalis pedis artery (as shown).[2] Repeat and record both systolic blood pressure measurement in the opposite leg.[3]

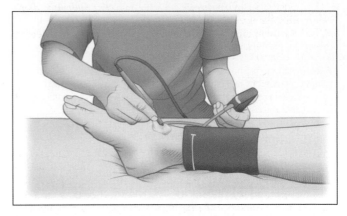

- Measure and record the systolic blood pressure in the patient's left arm over the brachial artery. Repeat the measurement in the patient's right arm over the brachial artery.[3]
- Turn off the Doppler ultrasound device.
- Wipe the conduction gel from the patient and the Doppler ultrasound probe using a soft cloth.[19]
- Return the patient's bed to the lowest position *to help prevent falls and maintain patient safety.*[20]
- Perform hand hygiene.[5,6,7,8,9,10]
- Average the two systolic blood pressure measurements from the right arm, unless the difference between the measurements exceeds 10 mm Hg, in which case use only the second right arm measurement.[3]
- Calculate and interpret the patient's ankle-brachial index. (See *Formulas for calculating ankle-brachial index.*)[3,18]
- Perform hand hygiene.[5,6,7,8,9,10]
- Put on gloves, if needed.[21,22]
- Clean and disinfect the Doppler ultrasound device, its probe, and other reusable equipment following the manufacturer's instructions, *to prevent the spread of infection.*[19,23,24]
- Remove and discard your gloves, if worn.[25]
- Perform hand hygiene.[5,6,7,8,9,10]
- Document the procedure.[26,27,28,29]

Formulas for calculating ankle-brachial index

To determine the patient's ankle-brachial index, use the following formulas:

Right ankle-brachial index = Higher systolic blood pressure over the right posterior tibial artery or the right dorsalis pedis artery ÷ Higher of the right or left arm systolic blood pressure

Left ankle-brachial index = Higher systolic blood pressure over the left posterior tibial artery or the left dorsalis pedis artery ÷ Higher of the right or left arm systolic blood pressure

Repeat the measurements if the initial ankle-brachial index is 0.8 to 1. Interpret the ankle-brachial index test results:
- An ankle-brachial index of 0.9 or lower confirms the diagnosis of lower extremity peripheral artery disease (PAD).[4,18]
- An ankle-brachial index of 0.91 to 1 is considered borderline for cardiovascular risk.

If the ankle-brachial index is 0.9 or lower or 1.4 or higher, the patient is considered at risk for cardiovascular events.[4]

Special considerations

■ Repeat the systolic blood pressure measurements after exercise if you strongly suspect PAD but the patient has a normal ankle-brachial index at rest.[2]

■ For a low or absent Doppler signal during measurements, check the equipment function, volume, and power level. Make sure that you have enough gel applied, and try changing the probe location or the choice of probe frequency. *Sound interference can occur from other equipment, debris in the speaker, and intermittent cable or battery contacts.*[19]

■ Vessel occlusion can occur from increased cuff pressure. Try releasing the pressure on the probe to correct this.

Complications

Improper technique for measuring the systolic blood pressure may result in inaccurate ankle-brachial index test results.

Documentation

Note the environmental temperature and any signs of the patient's inability to tolerate the supine position as well as the patient's ability to tolerate blood pressure readings. Document bilateral brachial and bilateral ankle blood pressure readings. Record your ankle-brachial index calculations and your interpretation of the calculation results. Document teaching provided to the patient and family (if applicable), their understanding of that teaching, and any need for follow-up teaching.

REFERENCES

1 Hayward, R. A. (2020). Screening for lower extremity peripheral artery disease. In: *UpToDate*, Elmore, J. G. (Ed.).

2 Kim, E. S., et al. (2012). Using the ankle-brachial index to diagnose peripheral artery disease and assess cardiovascular risk. *Cleveland Clinic Journal of Medicine, 79*, 651–661. (Level VII)

3 Aboyans, V., et al. (2012). Measurement and interpretation of the ankle-brachial index: A scientific statement from the American Heart Association. *Circulation, 126*, 2890–2909. https://www.ahajournals.org/doi/pdf/10.1161/cir.0b013e318276fbcb (Level VII)

4 Park, C. W. (2020). Ankle-brachial index measurement. http://emedicine.medscape.com/article/1839449-overview (Level VII)

5 Centers for Disease Control and Prevention. (2002). Guideline for hand hygiene in health-care settings: Recommendations of the Healthcare Infection Control Practices Advisory Committee and the HIPCAC/SHEA/APIC/IDSA Hand Hygiene Task Force. *MMWR Recommendations and Reports, 51*(RR-16), 1–45. https://www.cdc.gov/mmwr/pdf/rr/rr5116.pdf (Level II)

6 World Health Organization. (2009). WHO guidelines on hand hygiene in health care: First global patient safety challenge, clean care is safer care. https://apps.who.int/iris/bitstream/handle/10665/44102/9789241597906_eng.pdf?sequence=1 (Level IV)

7 The Joint Commission. (2021). Standard NPSG.07.01.01. *Comprehensive accreditation manual for hospitals.* Oakbrook Terrace, IL: The Joint Commission. (Level VII)

8 Accreditation Association for Hospitals and Health Systems. (2020). Standard 07.01.21. *Healthcare Facilities Accreditation Program: Accreditation requirements for acute care hospitals.* Chicago, IL: Accreditation Association for Hospitals and Health Systems. (Level VII)

9 Centers for Medicare and Medicaid Services, Department of Health and Human Services. (2020). Condition of participation: Infection control. 42 C.F.R. § 482.42.

10 DNV GL-Healthcare USA, Inc. (2020). IC.1.SR.1. *NIAHO® accreditation requirements, interpretive guidelines and surveyor guidance—revision 20.0.* Milford, OH: DNV GL-Healthcare USA, Inc. (Level VII)

11 The Joint Commission. (2021). Standard NPSG.01.01.01. *Comprehensive accreditation manual for hospitals.* Oakbrook Terrace, IL: The Joint Commission. (Level VII)

12 The Joint Commission. (2021). Standard RI.01.01.01. *Comprehensive accreditation manual for hospitals.* Oakbrook Terrace, IL: The Joint Commission. (Level VII)

13 Centers for Medicare and Medicaid Services, Department of Health and Human Services. (2020). Condition of participation: Patient's rights. 42 C.F.R. § 482.13(c)(1).

14 Accreditation Association for Hospitals and Health Systems. (2020). Standard 15.01.16. *Healthcare Facilities Accreditation Program: Accreditation requirements for acute care hospitals.* Chicago, IL: Accreditation Association for Hospitals and Health Systems. (Level VII)

15 DNV GL-Healthcare USA, Inc. (2020). PR.2.SR.5. *NIAHO® accreditation requirements, interpretive guidelines and surveyor guidance—revision 20.0.* Milford, OH: DNV GL-Healthcare USA, Inc. (Level VII)

16 The Joint Commission. (2020). Standard PC.02.01.21. *Comprehensive accreditation manual for hospitals.* Oakbrook Terrace, IL: The Joint Commission. (Level VII)

17 Waters, T. R., et al. (2009). Safe patient handling training for schools of nursing. https://www.cdc.gov/niosh/docs/2009-127/pdfs/2009-127.pdf (Level VII)

18 Mitchell, E. (2019). Noninvasive diagnosis of arterial disease. In: *UpToDate*, Eidt, J. F.,, & Mills, J. L. (Eds.).

19 Wallach Surgical Devices. (2013). User manual for the LifeDop® ABI handheld vascular system. https://www.coopersurgical.com/product-resources/bd7492df-958e-4d59-b10d-efb113a01ab4_man0007-dfu_reva.pdf

20 Ganz, D. A., et al. (2013, reviewed 2021). *Preventing falls in hospitals: A toolkit for improving quality of care* (AHRQ Publication No. 13-0015-EF). Rockville, MD: Agency for Healthcare Research and Quality. https://www.ahrq.gov/professionals/systems/hospital/fallpxtoolkit/index.html (Level VII)

21 Accreditation Association for Hospitals and Health Systems. (2020). Standard 07.01.10. *Healthcare Facilities Accreditation Program: Accreditation requirements for acute care hospitals.* Chicago, IL: Accreditation Association for Hospitals and Health Systems. (Level VII)

22 Siegel, J. D., et al. (2007, revised 2019). 2007 guideline for isolation precautions: Preventing transmission of infectious agents in healthcare settings. https://www.cdc.gov/infectioncontrol/pdf/guidelines/isolation-guidelines-H.pdf (Level II)

23 Rutala, W. A., et al. (2008, revised 2019). Guideline for disinfection and sterilization in healthcare facilities, 2008. https://www.cdc.gov/infection-control/pdf/guidelines/disinfection-guidelines-H.pdf (Level I)

24 Accreditation Association for Hospitals and Health Systems. (2020). Standard 07.02.03. *Healthcare Facilities Accreditation Program: Accreditation requirements for acute care hospitals.* Chicago, IL: Accreditation Association for Hospitals and Health Systems. (Level VII)

25 Occupational Safety and Health Administration. (2012). Bloodborne pathogens, standard number 1910.1030. https://www.osha.gov/pls/oshaweb/owadisp.show_document?p_id=10051&p_table=STANDARDS (Level VII)

26 Centers for Medicare and Medicaid Services, Department of Health and Human Services. (2020). Condition of participation: Medical record services. 42 C.F.R. § 482.24(b).

27 Accreditation Association for Hospitals and Health Systems. (2020). Standard 10.00.03. *Healthcare Facilities Accreditation Program: Accreditation requirements for acute care hospitals.* Chicago, IL: Accreditation Association for Hospitals and Health Systems. (Level VII)

28 The Joint Commission. (2021). Standard RC.01.03.01. *Comprehensive accreditation manual for hospitals.* Oakbrook Terrace, IL: The Joint Commission. (Level VII)

29 DNV GL-Healthcare USA, Inc. (2020). MR.2.SR.1. *NIAHO® accreditation requirements, interpretive guidelines and surveyor guidance—revision 20.0.* Milford, OH: DNV GL-Healthcare USA, Inc. (Level VII)

ANTIEMBOLISM STOCKING APPLICATION

Antiembolism stockings help prevent venous thromboembolism (VTE), a disorder that includes deep vein thrombosis (DVT) and pulmonary embolism.[1] They do so by compressing superficial leg veins, which in turn increases venous return by forcing blood into the deep venous system rather than allowing it to pool in the legs and form clots. Antiembolism stockings should provide graduated compression and produce a calf pressure of 14 to 15 mm Hg.[2,3,4,5]

HOSPITAL-ACQUIRED CONDITION ALERT Keep in mind that the Centers for Medicare and Medicaid Services considers VTE in patients who underwent total knee replacement or hip replacement to be a hospital-acquired condition *because it can be reasonably prevented using best practices.*[6,7] Be sure to follow evidence-based VTE prevention practices, such as using mechanical compression devices (including antiembolism stockings and an intermittent pneumatic compression device), early ambulation, and pharmacologic prophylaxis *to reduce the risk of VTE.*[8,9,10,11,12]

Patients who typically require antiembolism stockings include postoperative patients, older adult patients, and those who are bedridden, have varicose veins, or are otherwise at risk for DVT. Compression therapy has proven beneficial for the treatment of venous ulcers and chronic venous insufficiency, and therefore is considered a standard of care for patients with these conditions.[13] For patients with chronic venous problems, practitioners may order the use of intermittent pneumatic compression stockings for the duration of surgery and postoperatively. (See the "Sequential compression therapy" procedure.)

Guidelines caution against using antiembolism stockings in patients with dermatoses or open skin lesions, gangrene, severe arteriosclerosis or other ischemic vascular diseases, pulmonary edema or any massive edema, recent vein ligation, vascular or skin grafts, peripheral neuropathy or other causes of sensory impairment, an allergy to the material, or severe leg deformity.[3,4,14] Studies show that graduated compression stockings don't reduce the risk of DVT in stroke patients and may even increase the risk of skin complications in these patients.[15]

There's no evidence to support the use of one type of antiembolism stocking (knee-length, thigh-length, or waist-length) over another. Thus, patient compliance, ease of use, and cost will indicate the best choice of stocking type.[16]

Equipment

Tape measure ▪ antiembolism stockings of correct size.

Preparation of equipment

Obtain the correct size antiembolism stocking according to the manufacturer's specifications.[14] If the patient's measurements are outside the range indicated by the manufacturer, or if the patient's legs are deformed or edematous, ask the practitioner whether an order for custom-made antiembolism stockings is warranted.

▪ **Before applying a knee-length stocking:** Measure the patient using a tape measure to ensure a *proper fit*. (See *Measuring for antiembolism stockings*, on the right column.)

▪ **Before applying a thigh-length stocking:** Measure the upper thigh circumference at the gluteal fold, then the calf circumference at the greatest dimension, and lastly the leg length from the gluteal fold to the base of the heel.[1]

▪ **Before applying a waist-length stocking:** To measure for a waist-length stocking, first measure the upper thigh circumference at the gluteal fold.[1] Next, measure the calf circumference at the greatest dimension.[1] Last, measure the leg length by measuring from the gluteal fold to the base of the heel.[1] If the patient's thigh measurements are outside of the specified recommended range, consider knee-length stockings as another option.[1]

Implementation

▪ Verify the practitioner's order.
▪ Review the patient's medical record for any allergy to materials used by the manufacturer or contraindications to antiembolism stocking use.[4]
▪ Gather and prepare the necessary equipment and supplies.
▪ Perform hand hygiene.[17,18,19,20,21,22]
▪ Confirm the patient's identity using at least two patient identifiers.[23]
▪ Provide privacy.[24,25,26]
▪ Explain the procedure to the patient and family (if appropriate) according to their individual communication and learning needs *to increase their understanding, allay their fears, and enhance cooperation.*[27]
▪ Help the patient lie down if the patient isn't already doing so.
▪ Raise the bed to waist level when providing care *to prevent caregiver back strain.*[28]
▪ Perform hand hygiene.[17,18,19,20,21,22]
▪ Assess the condition of the patient's legs. Notify the practitioner before applying the stockings if you suspect arterial disease.[4]

Applying a knee-length stocking

▪ Following the manufacturer's instructions, insert your hand into the stocking from the top and grasp the heel pocket from the inside. Holding the heel, turn the stocking inside out. *This method allows easier application than gathering the entire stocking and working it up over the foot and ankle.*[3]
▪ Position the stocking over the foot and heel, making sure the heel is centered in the heel pocket.[3]
▪ Grasp a few inches (centimeters) of the stocking and begin pulling it up around the patient's ankle and calf,[3] as shown on the next page.

Measuring for antiembolism stockings

Measure the patient carefully **to ensure that the antiembolism stockings provide enough compression for adequate venous return.** Measure both legs, because if the right and left leg measure differently, you many need to order two different stocking sizes.[3]

To choose the correct knee-length antiembolism stocking, measure the circumference of the calf at its widest point[3,14] and the leg length from the popliteal fold (bend of the knee) to the base of the heel.[3,14]

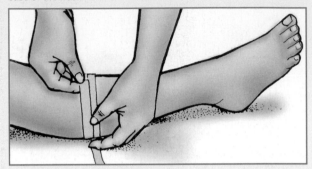

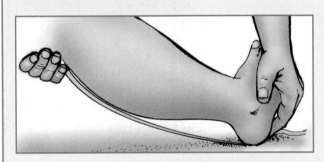

To choose the correct thigh-length stocking, measure the calf as for a knee-length stocking and the thigh at its widest point. Then measure leg length from the bottom of the heel to the gluteal fold (*bottom right*).[2]

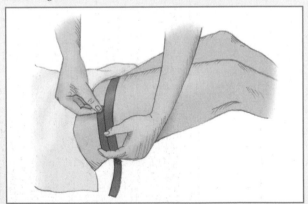

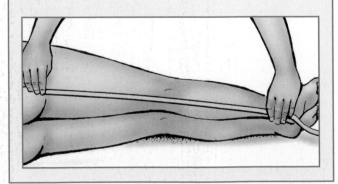

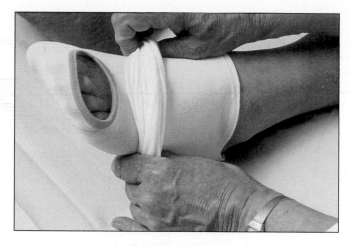

- Continue pulling the stocking up the patient's leg using short pulls, alternating front and back, as shown below. When you're finished pulling the stocking up the patient's leg, the bottom of the band (or change in the stocking's stitching) should fall 1″ to 2″ (2.5 to 5 cm) below the popliteal fold.[3]

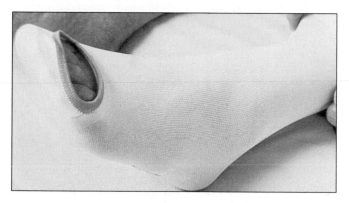

- Make sure the patient's toes are visible through the toe inspection area, if present; the patient's toes shouldn't stick out of the inspection area opening.[3]
- Repeat the procedure for the second stocking, if ordered.
- Return the bed to the lowest position *to prevent falls and maintain patient safety.*[29]
- Perform hand hygiene.[17,18,19,20,21,22]
- Document the procedure.[30,31,32,33]

Applying a thigh-length stocking
- Follow the procedure for applying a knee-length stocking, taking care to distribute the fabric evenly below the knee before continuing the procedure.
- As you apply the thigh portion of the stocking, start rotating the stocking inward so the panel (if present) is slightly toward the inside of the patient's leg, as shown below. When you've applied the stocking fully, the top band of the stocking should rest at the patient's gluteal fold.

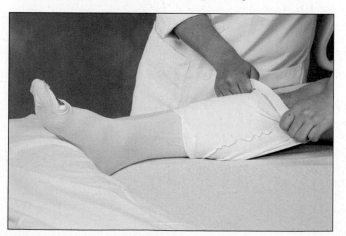

- Smooth out any wrinkles in the stocking fabric *to prevent skin breakdown.*[3,14]
- Make sure the patient's toes are visible through the toe inspection area, if present; the patient's toes shouldn't stick out of the inspection area opening.[3]
- Return the bed to the lowest position to prevent falls and maintain patient safety.[29]
- Repeat the procedure for the second stocking, if ordered.
- Perform hand hygiene.[17,18,19,20,21,22]
- Document the procedure.[30,31,32,33]

Applying a waist-length stocking with a waist belt
- Follow the procedure for applying a knee-length stocking, taking care to distribute the fabric evenly below the knee before continuing the procedure.
- When the stocking reaches the patient's knee, begin turning the stocking to position the side panel.
- Continue to apply the stocking until the stocking's upper thigh hem rests in the groin and at the gluteal fold. Make sure the seam is flat against the body and the side panel is at the hip bone.[1]
- Repeat the procedure for the second stocking.
- Unfold the waist belt and bring it around the patient's waist. The smooth side of the belt should rest against the patient's skin. Fasten the waist belt snaps to the stockings.[1]
- Fasten the waist belt snaps to the stockings.
- Connect the waist belt buckle, and adjust the waist belt so that it's tight enough to secure the stockings in place.
- Smooth out wrinkles in the stocking fabric *to prevent skin breakdown.*[1]
- Pull the toe area forward to smooth the ankle and instep area to promote toe comfort.[1] Make sure the patient's toes are visible through the toe inspection area, if present; the toes shouldn't stick out of the inspection area opening.[1]
- Return the bed to the lowest position *to prevent falls and maintain patient safety.*[29]
- Perform hand hygiene.[11,12,13,14,15,16]
- Document the procedure.[24,25,26,27]

Special considerations
- If the patient has a fluctuation in weight or develops edema or postoperative swelling, remeasure the patient and obtain stockings of the appropriate size.[1,2]
- Encourage the patient to wear the stockings day and night until the patient no longer has significantly reduced mobility.[2]
- Remove the stockings at least once daily *to bathe the skin and observe for irritation and breakdown.* Inspect the skin, provide skin care, and then reapply the stockings.[3,4,14]
- Inspect the skin (especially the ankles and heels) at least two to three times per day or per the manufacturer's recommendation, and be alert for an allergic reaction.[3,4] *Some patients can't tolerate the sizing in new antiembolism stockings.*
- Discontinue the use of antiembolism stockings if you note marking, blistering, or discoloration of the skin, especially over heels and bony prominences, or if the patient experiences pain or discomfort. Notify the practitioner, who may prescribe a sequential compression device as an alternative to antiembolism stockings.[4]
- Don't allow antiembolism stockings to roll or turn down at the top or toes *because the excess pressure could cause venous strangulation.*
- Have the patient wear the stockings in bed and during ambulation *to provide continuous protection against VTE.*
- Using warm water and mild soap, wash the antiembolism stockings when they become soiled.[3] Keep a second pair handy *so that the patient can wear them while the other pair is being laundered.*

Patient teaching
If the patient will require antiembolism stockings after discharge, teach the patient or a family member how to apply them correctly and explain why the patient needs to wear them *to adherence for maximal effectiveness of treatment.*[34] Instruct the patient and family member or caregiver to wash the stockings every 2 to 3 days, or more frequently if they become

visibly soiled.[3] Advise them to follow the manufacturer's washing instructions. Inform them that, with proper care, stockings commonly last for 2 to 3 months.

Complications

Complications from poorly fitting stockings include discomfort and tissue necrosis. Patients with impaired arterial blood flow may experience worsening ischemia, and patients who are allergic to the stocking material may develop contact dermatitis.[35]

Documentation

Record the date and time of antiembolism stocking application, stocking style and size, and the condition of the leg, foot, and toes before application.[3] Document teaching provided to the patient and family (if applicable), their understanding of the teaching, and any need for follow-up teaching.

REFERENCES

1 Sachdeva, A. et al. (2018). Graduated compression stockings for prevention of deep vein thrombosis. *Cochrane Database of Systematic Reviews, 11*, CD00f1484. https://www.ncbi.nlm.nih.gov/pmc/articles/PMC6477662/ (Level I)

2 CardinalHealth. (n.d.). T.E.D.™ anti-embolism stockings. https://www.cardinalhealth.com/en/product-solutions/medical/compression/t-e-d-anti-embolism-stockings.html

3 Covidien. (2014). T.E.D. anti-embolism stockings: Nursing procedure guide. https://docplayer.net/20753080-T-e-d-anti-embolism-stockings-nursing-procedure-guide-sizing-and-application-for-optimal-benefit.html (Level VII)

4 National Institute for Health and Care Excellence. (2018, updated 2019). Venous thromboembolism in over 16s: Reducing the risk of hospital-acquired deep vein thrombosis or pulmonary embolism. https://www.nice.org.uk/guidance/ng89 (Level VII)

5 Anderson, I. (2017). Treating patients with venous ulcers in the acute care setting: Part 1. *British Journal of Nursing, 26*, S32–S41. (Level VII)

6 Centers for Medicare and Medicaid Services, Department of Health and Human Services. (2021). Appendix I: Hospital-acquired conditions (HACS) list. https://www.cms.gov/Medicare/Medicare-Fee-for-Service-Payment/HospitalAcqCond/icd10_hacs

7 Centers for Medicare and Medicaid Services, & The Joint Commission. (2021). The specifications manual for national hospital inpatient quality measures (version 5.10.). https://www.qualitynet.org/inpatient/specifications-manuals#tab1

8 National Institute for Health and Care Excellence. (2010, revised 2018). *Guideline summary: Venous thromboembolism in adults admitted to hospital: Reducing the risk.* https://www.nice.org.uk/guidance/Qs3 (Level I)

9 Kearon, C., et al. (2016). Antithrombotic therapy for VTE disease. *Chest, 149*, 315–352. https://journal.chestnet.org/article/S0012-3692(15)00335-9/fulltext#sec7 (Level I)

10 Jarrett, N., & Callaham, M. (2016). Evidence-based guidelines for selected hospital-acquired conditions: Final report. https://www.cms.gov/Medicare/Medicare-Fee-for-Service-Payment/HospitalAcqCond/Downloads/2016-HAC-Report.pdf

11 Association of periOperative Registered Nurses. (2020). Venous thromboembolism. In *Guidelines for perioperative practice, 2020 edition.* Denver, CO: AORN, Inc. (Level VII)

12 Balk, E. M., et al. (2017). *Venous thromboembolism prophylaxis in major orthopedic surgery: Systematic review update* (AHRQ Publication No. 17-EHC021-EF). Rockville, MD: Agency for Healthcare Research and Quality. (Level VII)

13 Nelson, E. A., & Bell-Syer, S. E. M. (2014). Compression hosiery (stockings) for preventing venous leg ulcers returning. *Cochrane Database of Systematic Reviews, 2014*(9), CD002303. (Level VII)

14 Le, L. K. (2016). *Deep vein thrombosis prophylaxis.* Adelaide, Australia: Joanna Briggs Institute. (Level V)

15 Kappelle, L. J. (2011). Preventing deep vein thrombosis after stroke: Strategies and recommendations. *Current Treatment Options in Neurology, 13*, 629–635. https://www.ncbi.nlm.nih.gov/pmc/articles/PMC3207135/ (Level V)

16 Sajid, M. S., et al. (2012). Knee length versus thigh length graduated compression stockings for prevention of deep vein thrombosis in postoperative surgical patients. *Cochrane Database of Systematic Reviews, 2012*(5), CD007162. (Level II)

17 The Joint Commission. (2021). Standard NPSG.07.01.01. *Comprehensive accreditation manual for hospitals.* Oakbrook Terrace, IL: The Joint Commission. (Level VII)

18 Centers for Disease Control and Prevention. (2002). Guideline for hand hygiene in health-care settings: Recommendations of the Healthcare Infection Control Practices Advisory Committee and the HICPAC/SHEA/APIC/IDSA Hand Hygiene Task Force. *MMWR Recommendations and Reports, 51*(RR-16), 1–45. https://www.cdc.gov/mmwr/pdf/rr/rr5116.pdf (Level II)

19 World Health Organization. (2009). WHO guidelines on hand hygiene in health care: First global patient safety challenge, clean care is safer care. https://apps.who.int/iris/bitstream/handle/10665/44102/9789241597906_eng.pdf?sequence=1 (Level IV)

20 Centers for Medicare and Medicaid Services, Department of Health and Human Services. (2020). Condition of participation: Infection control. 42 C.F.R. § 482.42.

21 Accreditation Association for Hospitals and Health Systems. (2020). Standard 07.01.21. *Healthcare Facilities Accreditation Program: Accreditation requirements for acute care hospitals.* Chicago, IL: Accreditation Association for Hospitals and Health Systems. (Level VII)

22 DNV GL-Healthcare USA, Inc. (2020). IC.1.SR.1. *NIAHO® accreditation requirements, interpretive guidelines and surveyor guidance—revision 20.0.* Milford, OH: DNV GL-Healthcare USA, Inc. (Level VII)

23 The Joint Commission. (2021). Standard NPSG.01.01.01. *Comprehensive accreditation manual for hospitals.* Oakbrook Terrace, IL: The Joint Commission. (Level VII)

24 Centers for Medicare and Medicaid Services, Department of Health and Human Services. (2020). Condition of participation: Patient's rights. 42 C.F.R. § 482.13(c)(1).

25 Accreditation Association for Hospitals and Health Systems. (2020). Standard 15.01.16. *Healthcare Facilities Accreditation Program: Accreditation requirements for acute care hospitals.* Chicago, IL: Accreditation Association for Hospitals and Health Systems. (Level VII)

26 DNV GL-Healthcare USA, Inc. (2020). PR.2.SR.5. *NIAHO® accreditation requirements, interpretive guidelines and surveyor guidance—revision 20.0.* Milford, OH: DNV GL-Healthcare USA, Inc. (Level VII)

27 The Joint Commission. (2021). Standard PC.02.01.21. *Comprehensive accreditation manual for hospitals.* Oakbrook Terrace, IL: The Joint Commission. (Level VII)

28 Waters, T. R., et al. (2009). Safe patient handling training for schools of nursing. https://www.cdc.gov/niosh/docs/2009-127/pdfs/2009-127.pdf (Level VII)

29 Ganz, D. A., et al. (2013, reviewed 2021). *Preventing falls in hospitals: A toolkit for improving quality of care* (AHRQ Publication No. 13-0015-EF). Rockville, MD: Agency for Healthcare Research and Quality. https://www.ahrq.gov/professionals/systems/hospital/fallpxtoolkit/index.html (Level VII)

30 The Joint Commission. (2021). Standard RC.01.03.01. *Comprehensive accreditation manual for hospitals.* Oakbrook Terrace, IL: The Joint Commission. (Level VII)

31 Centers for Medicare and Medicaid Services, Department of Health and Human Services. (2020). Condition of participation: Medical record services. 42 C.F.R. § 482.24(b).

32 Accreditation Association for Hospitals and Health Systems. (2020). Standard 10.00.03. *Healthcare Facilities Accreditation Program: Accreditation requirements for acute care hospitals.* Chicago, IL: Accreditation Association for Hospitals and Health Systems. (Level VII)

33 DNV GL-Healthcare USA, Inc. (2020). MR.2.SR.1. *NIAHO® accreditation requirements, interpretive guidelines and surveyor guidance—revision 20.0* Milford, OH: DNV GL-Healthcare USA, Inc. (Level VII)

34 Kanaan, A. O., et al. (2012). Evaluating the role of compression stockings in preventing post thrombotic syndrome: A review of the literature. *Thrombosis, 2012*, 694851. https://www.hindawi.com/journals/thrombosis/2012/694851/ (Level I)

35 Lim, C. S., & Davies, A. H. (2014). Graduated compression stockings. *CMAJ, 186*, E391–E398. https://www.ncbi.nlm.nih.gov/pmc/articles/PMC4081237/

AQUAPHERESIS

Aquapheresis is a therapy that involves using ultrafiltration to remove fluid from the blood. It provides an alternative method for relieving congestion caused by fluid overload in patients with decompensated heart failure who are resistant to diuretics.[1]

Aquapheresis is provided using venovenous access and a device known as the Aquadex FlexFlow ultrafiltration system (shown below). This device mechanically withdraws blood through a catheter and passes it through a hemofilter, which removes excess sodium and water, restoring fluid balance. After the device filters the patient's blood, it returns it to the patient through the infusion port of the catheter. Sterile no-touch technique is followed during therapy.

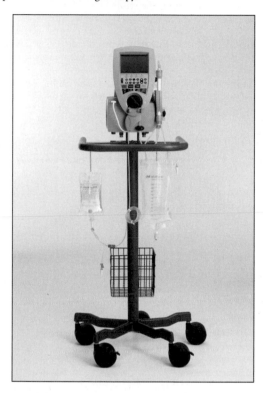

NURSING ALERT Only individuals who have received specialized training in administering aquapheresis therapy are permitted to administer the therapy.[2]

Equipment

Aquadex FlexFlow pump ▪ sterile, disposable, single-use extracorporeal blood circuit set ▪ scale ▪ electronic infusion device (preferably a smart pump with dose-error reduction software) ▪ antiseptic pads (chlorhexidine-based, povidone iodine, or alcohol) ▪ prescribed IV heparin bolus ▪ prescribed heparin infusion ▪ 500-mL bag of normal saline solution ▪ 10-mL prefilled syringes containing preservative-free normal saline solution ▪ graduated liquid waste receptacle ▪ gloves ▪ sterile end caps ▪ supplies for cleaning reusable equipment ▪ tape ▪ vital signs monitoring equipment ▪ stethoscope ▪ disinfectant pad ▪ appropriately sized venovenous access device (common sizes include #6 French dual-lumen extended-length peripheral catheter; #7 or #8 French dual-lumen central venous access catheter; and #8.5 French dual-lumen central venous access catheter [14G or 16G lumens]) [3] ▪ Optional: IV tubing labels, blood sampling equipment.

Preparation of equipment

Before therapy begins, the practitioner inserts a venovenous access device. The catheter must be able to accommodate a blood flow of 10 to 40 mL/minute.

Inspect all equipment and supplies. If a product is expired, is defective, or has compromised integrity, remove it from patient use, label it as expired or defective, and report the expiration or defect as directed by your facility. Follow the manufacturer's recommendations for use and care of the aquapheresis pump.

Implementation

▪ Verify the practitioner's order for aquapheresis in the patient's medical record, and ensure that diuretic and electrolyte replacement therapy has been discontinued before initiating therapy.
▪ Make sure that preprocedure laboratory test results are available and documented in the patient's medical record; report any abnormalities.
▪ Confirm that informed consent has been obtained and that the signed consent form is in the patient's medical record.[4,5,6,7,8]
▪ Gather and prepare the necessary equipment and supplies.
▪ Perform hand hygiene.[8,9,10,11,12,13]
▪ Confirm the patient's identity using at least two patient identifiers.[14]
▪ Provide privacy.[15,16,17,18]
▪ Reinforce the practitioner's explanation of the procedure, and answer the patient's questions.[4,5,6,7]
▪ Obtain the patient's weight in kilograms *to prevent medication dosing errors.*[19]
▪ Raise the bed to waist level during patient care *to prevent caregiver back strain.*[20]
▪ Perform hand hygiene.[8,9,10,11,12,13]
▪ Put on gloves *to comply with standard precautions.*[21,22,23]
▪ Perform a vigorous mechanical scrub of the access port for at least 5 seconds using an antiseptic pad and allow it to dry completely.[24,25]
▪ While maintaining sterility of the syringe tip, attach a prefilled syringe containing preservative-free normal saline solution to the access port. (Use a 10-mL syringe or a syringe specially designed to generate lower injection pressure.) Unclamp the catheter and slowly aspirate for a blood return that is the color and consistency of whole blood. If you don't obtain a blood return, take steps to locate an external cause of the obstruction.[26]
▪ If you obtain a blood return, slowly inject preservative-free normal saline solution into the catheter. Use a minimum volume of twice the internal volume of the catheter system. Don't forcibly flush the device; further evaluate the device if you meet resistance.[26]

Priming the blood circuit

▪ Plug the power cord into a grounded electrical outlet.
▪ Press the ON/OFF key on the front panel. (See *A look at the aquapheresis circuit,* page 26.)
▪ Place the blood pump cartridge into the blood pump on the machine console and snap it into place. Then turn the knob clockwise until you hear a beep.
▪ Insert the ultrafiltrate cartridge in the side of the console and snap it into place. Then turn the knob clockwise until you hear a beep.
▪ Insert the tubing into the blood leak and air sensors.
▪ Put the pressure sensor cables into their proper connectors, located on the console.
▪ Insert the data key provided with the blood circuit system into the reader on the front of the console; *this data key facilitates many of the system's functions.*[27]
▪ Hang the empty ultrafiltrate collection bag on the machine's weight scale hook, and close the drain valve located at the bottom of the bag.
▪ Remove the end caps from the infusion tubing of the circuit and the priming adapter on the ultrafiltrate drainage bag, and then attach the circuit infusion tubing to the priming adapter on the ultrafiltrate drainage bag.
▪ Remove the end caps from the withdrawal tubing and the priming spike adapter, and then attach the withdrawal tubing to the withdrawal priming spike adapter.
▪ Spike the 500-mL priming bag of normal saline solution with the priming spike, and then hang the bag on the priming hook, making sure that the ultrafiltrate bag hangs freely.
▪ Open the clamps on the withdrawal tubing, infusion tubing, and ultrafiltrate bag priming adapter.
▪ Press the PRIME key and follow the onscreen instructions; priming should be completed and the system should be free from air in about 4 minutes.

EQUIPMENT

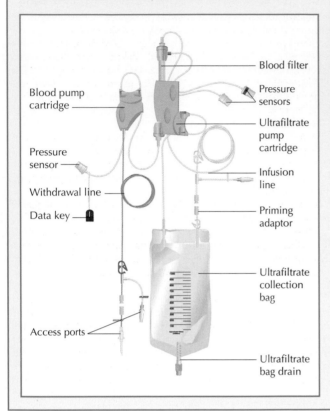

A look at the aquapheresis circuit

Aquapheresis requires a circuit such as the one below to filter fluid and sodium from the blood of patients with fluid overload.

Labels:
- Blood filter
- Pressure sensors
- Ultrafiltrate pump cartridge
- Blood pump cartridge
- Infusion line
- Pressure sensor
- Priming adaptor
- Withdrawal line
- Data key
- Ultrafiltrate collection bag
- Access ports
- Ultrafiltrate bag drain

■ Empty the priming solution from the fluid collection bag before starting therapy. *Priming solution drains into the collection bag; emptying the collection bag ensures accuracy of the patient's output measurement.*

■ Close the clamps on the blood circuit set, remove the end cap on the withdrawal catheter lumen, disconnect the withdrawal line from the IV spike, and connect the withdrawal line to the withdrawal catheter lumen.

■ Remove the end cap from the infusion catheter lumen, disconnect the infusion line from the ultrafiltrate priming adapter, and connect the infusion line to the infusion catheter lumen.

■ Trace each tube from the patient to the point of origin *to make sure that you've attached it to the proper catheter lumens.*[28,29]

■ Route tubing using a standardized approach if the patient has other tubing and catheters that have different purposes. Label the tubing at both the distal (near the patient connection) and proximal (near the source container) ends *to reduce the risk of misconnection if multiple IV lines will be used.*[30]

■ Put sterile end caps on the priming spike and the ultrafiltrate priming adapter.

Beginning anticoagulant therapy

■ Begin anticoagulant therapy at least 30 minutes before the procedure, as ordered, following safe medication administration practices.[27,31,32,33,34] Typically, an IV bolus dose of heparin is given, followed by a continuous heparin infusion *to reduce the risk of clot formation within the system.*

■ Avoid distractions and interruptions when preparing and administering medication *to prevent medication errors.*[35,36]

■ Compare the medication label with the order in the patient's medical record.[31,32,33,34]

■ Check the patient's medical record for an allergy or contraindication to the prescribed medication. If an allergy or contraindications exist, don't administer the medication and instead notify the practitioner.[31,32,33,34]

■ Check the expiration date on the medication. If the medication is expired, return it to the pharmacy and obtain new medication.[31,32,33,34]

■ Visually inspect the solution for particles or discoloration or other loss of integrity; don't administer the medication if integrity is compromised.[31,32,33,34]

■ Discuss any unresolved concerns about the medication with the patient's practitioner.[31,32,33,34]

■ If the patient is receiving the medication for the first time, teach him or her about potential adverse reactions, and discuss any other concerns related to the medication.[31,32,33,34]

■ Verify that the medication is being administered at the proper time, in the prescribed dose, and by the correct route *to reduce the risk of medication errors.*[31,32,33,34]

■ If your facility uses a barcode technology, scan your identification badge, the patient's identification bracelet, and the medication's bar code.[33]

NURSING ALERT Heparin, when administered IV, is considered a high-alert medication *because it can cause significant patient harm when used in error.*[37]

■ Before beginning the heparin infusion, have another nurse perform an independent double-check if required by your facility.[38] (See *Double-checking high-alert medications.*)

■ After comparing the results of the independent double-check (if required), begin infusing the heparin through the withdrawal port of the access device, if no discrepancies exist. If discrepancies exist, rectify them before beginning the infusion.[38]

■ Make sure that the infusion device alarm limits are set appropriately for the patient's condition, and that the alarms are turned on, functioning properly, and audible to staff.[39,40,41]

Beginning Aquapheresis therapy

■ Open the withdrawal and infusion tubing clamps.

■ Press the RUN key to begin therapy.[27]

■ If your unit has a hematocrit (HCT) monitor, make sure that the sensor clip is attached to the blood chamber on the blood circuit. Allow 5 to 10 minutes to elapse in the RUN mode *to complete the initial baseline measurement of the patient's HCT.* The text "Baselining" will appear; after baselining is complete, press the HCT key and then set the HCT limit, using the up and down arrows. *The HCT limit automatically restricts the fluid removal rate to help prevent excessive volume depletion.*[27] If the hematocrit sensor won't be used, leave the sensor clip on the dock on the back of the pump.[42]

■ Set the blood flow rate by pressing the BLOOD FLOW key. Use the arrow keys to adjust the value. For a central venous catheter, begin the flow rate at 40 mL/minute. For a peripheral dual-lumen extended-length catheter, begin the flow rate at 25 mL/minute.

■ After the blood flow rate is stable, increase the rate in increments of 10 mL/hour (or as prescribed) until the ordered rate is achieved. Use the

Double-checking high-alert medications

If required by your facility, have another nurse perform an independent double-check of your preparation of a high-alert medication such as heparin *to ensure safe administration.*[38] The second nurse must perform the following tasks:

■ Verify the patient's identity.

■ Ensure that the correct medication is being administered and is in the prescribed strength or concentration.

■ Ensure that the medication's indication corresponds with the patient's diagnosis.

■ Verify that the dosage calculations are correct and that the dosing formula used to derive the final dose is correct.

■ Verify that the route of administration is safe and appropriate for the patient.

■ Verify that the prescribed time and frequency of administration is safe and appropriate for the patient.[38]

■ Ensure that electronic infusion device settings are correct and that the infusion line is attached to the correct port.

arrow keys to adjust the rate. The average removal rate is 250 mL/hour.[3] Patients in volume-sensitive states, such as those with right-sided heart failure, hepatic disease, or cardiogenic shock, usually require lower rates (50 to 150 mL/hr).[3]

- Monitor the patient and the system for 10 minutes after beginning therapy. If after 10 minutes the system functions without alarming, secure the catheter.
- Monitor and record vital signs every 15 minutes during the first hour of treatment, and then hourly or more frequently as indicated by the patient's condition.[43]
- Record intake and output hourly; include the ultrafiltrate in the patient's output volume.[43]
- Monitor the system and respond to any alarms according to the manufacturer's guidelines. *The system has sensors to detect air bubbles in the blood circuit line, withdrawal line disconnect or occlusion, infusion line disconnect or occlusion, circuit life exceeded, circuit not primed, and a full ultrafiltrate bag.*[27] *For patient safety issues, the system will stop therapy and request assistance.*[27]
- Monitor the system for signs of clotting, such as frequent and unexpected infusion or withdrawal occlusions.[2]
- Maintain the patient's fluid restriction.
- Monitor the patient for signs of hypovolemia, such as tachycardia, hypotension, and diminished urinary output. Obtain blood samples for blood urea nitrogen and creatinine levels, as ordered, and monitor the results. (See the "Venipuncture" procedure.)
- Return the bed to the lowest level *to prevent falls and maintain patient safety.*[44]
- When the system alarms (indicating that the ultrafiltrate collection bag is full), empty the bag into a graduated liquid waste receptacle.

Discontinuing Aquapheresis therapy

- Press the STOP key *to stop the pumps.*[27]
- Trace each tubing from the patient to the point of origin before clamping *to make sure that you're clamping the correct tubing.*[28,29]
- Clamp the withdrawal catheter extension tubing.
- Disconnect the withdrawal blood circuit connection from the withdrawal catheter extension.
- Flush the withdrawal catheter IV access and cap with preservative-free normal saline solution.
- Clamp the infusion line.
- Disconnect the infusion line.
- Flush the infusion IV access and cap with preservative-free normal saline solution.
- Return the HCT sensor to its dock on the back of the console.
- Remove the blood circuit from the console by pressing the clips on the front and side cartridges and rotating the knobs while removing the tubing. Discard the system in an appropriate biohazard waste container.[22]
- Turn off the console by holding the ON/OFF key for 1 second.[27]
- Obtain the patient's weight in kilograms.[19]
- Discard used supplies in appropriate receptacles.[22]
- Remove and discard your gloves.[22]
- Perform hand hygiene.[8,9,10,11,12,13]
- Clean and disinfect your stethoscope using a disinfectant pad.[45,46]
- Perform hand hygiene.[8,9,10,11,12,13]
- Document the procedure.[47,48,49,50]

Cleaning the unit after each use

- Perform hand hygiene.[8,9,10,11,12,13]
- Put on clean gloves.[21,22,23]
- Clean and disinfect reusable equipment according to the manufacturer's instructions *to prevent the spread of infection.*[45,46]
- Remove and discard your gloves.[22]
- Perform hand hygiene.[8,9,10,11,12,13]

Special considerations

- When flushing the access catheter, consider using a pulsatile flushing technique; short boluses of 1 mL each interrupted by brief pauses may be more effective at removing deposits (such as fibrin, drug precipitate, and intraluminal bacteria) than a continuous low-flow technique.[26]
- Consider using the 10-in-10 test when assessing for venous access catheter patency. Using a 10-mL syringe attached to the access port, aspirate 10 mL of blood over 10 seconds. Assess for resistance, then infuse the 10 mL of blood over 10 seconds.[42]
- The Joint Commission issued a sentinel event alert concerning medical device alarm safety, *because alarm-related events have been associated with permanent loss of function or death.* Among the major contributing factors were improper alarm settings, alarm settings turned off inappropriately, and alarm signals that are inaudible to staff. Make sure alarm limits are set appropriately and that alarms are turned on, functioning properly, and audible to staff. Follow facility guidelines for preventing alarm fatigue.[51]
- Monitor partial thromboplastin time at specific intervals during therapy, as ordered; the recommended therapeutic range for therapy is 80 to 100 seconds.
- Patients receiving warfarin who have an International Normalized Ratio greater than 2 typically start on a continuous heparin infusion and don't receive an initial bolus of heparin. If heparin is contraindicated, the practitioner may prescribe argatroban. Low molecular weight heparin isn't recommended.[3]
- The average treatment time is 24 hours with a fluid removal goal of about 80% of the estimated weight over dry weight.[3]
- Adjust the ultrafiltration rates if the patient's blood pressure drops 10 mm Hg below baseline or if the patient's heart rate is greater than 130 beats/minute after two consecutive measurements within 5 minutes. Obtain orders to reduce the ultrafiltration rate or briefly stop ultrafiltration *to allow the patient time to recover.*
- The Joint Commission issued a sentinel event alert related to managing risk during transition to new International Organization for Standardization tubing standards that were designed to prevent dangerous tubing misconnections, which can lead to serious patient injury and death. During the transition, trace the tubing and catheter from the patient to the point of origin before connecting or reconnecting any device or infusion, at any care transition (such as a new setting or service), and as part of the hand-off process; route tubes and catheters having different purposes in different standardized directions; when there are different access sites or several bags hanging, label the tubing at the distal and proximal ends; use tubing and equipment only as intended; and store medications for different delivery routes in separate locations.[30]

Complications

Complications may include bleeding and infection.[52] An ultrafiltration alarm activates when ultrafiltrate pressure deviates from the usual range; this usually means clotting of the filter requiring that the filter be replaced. In this situation, first contact the practitioner to determine if treatment should be continued. Then, as applicable, follow the manufacturer's procedure for replacement of the circuit and filter, as outlined in the *Aquadex FlexFlow User's Guide.*[42]

Documentation

Record the date and time that therapy began; the reason for the therapy; the patient's weight before and after the treatment; vital signs and pressures (withdrawal, infusion, and ultrafiltrate pressures) throughout the treatment; patency and condition of catheter access sites; initial Aquadex FlexFlow settings, changes you made, and the reasons for such changes; the patient's intake and output; laboratory values; and the patient's tolerance of the procedure. Document teaching provided to the patient and family (if applicable), their understanding of that teaching, and any need for follow-up teaching.

REFERENCES

1 Costanzo, M. R. (2019). Ultrafiltration in acute heart failure. *Cardiac Failure Review, 5*(1), 9–18. https://www.ncbi.nlm.nih.gov/pmc/articles/PMC6396068/

2 CHF Solutions, Inc. (2017). Aquadex FlexFlow reference guide. https://www.nuwellis.com/wp-content/uploads/2021/04/16-05629-G_SmartFlow-Quick-Reference-Guide_MAY20.pdf

3 Nuwellis. (n.d.). Ultrafiltration with Aquadex Smartflow®. https://www.nuwellis.com/healthcare-professionals/ultrafiltration-with-aquadex-smartflow/

4 The Joint Commission. (2021). Standard RI.01.03.01. *Comprehensive accreditation manual for hospitals.* Oakbrook Terrace, IL: The Joint Commission. (Level VII)

5 Centers for Medicare and Medicaid Services, Department of Health and Human Services. (2020). Condition of participation: Patient's rights. 42 C.F.R. § 482.13(b)(2).

6 Accreditation Association for Hospitals and Health Systems. (2020). Standard 15.01.11. *Healthcare Facilities Accreditation Program: Accreditation requirements for acute care hospitals.* Chicago, IL: Accreditation Association for Hospitals and Health Systems. (Level VII)

7 DNV GL-Healthcare USA, Inc. (2020). PR.2.SR.3. *NIAHO® accreditation requirements, interpretive guidelines and surveyor guidance—revision 20.0.* Milford, OH: DNV GL-Healthcare USA, Inc. (Level VII)

8 The Joint Commission. (2021). Standard NPSG.07.01.01. *Comprehensive accreditation manual for hospitals.* Oakbrook Terrace, IL: The Joint Commission. (Level VII)

9 Centers for Disease Control and Prevention. (2002). Guideline for hand hygiene in health-care settings: Recommendations of the Healthcare Infection Control Practices Advisory Committee and the HICPAC/SHEA/APIC/IDSA Hand Hygiene Task Force. *MMWR Recommendations and Reports, 51*(RR-16), 1–45. https://www.cdc.gov/mmwr/pdf/rr/rr5116.pdf (Level II)

10 World Health Organization. (2009). WHO guidelines on hand hygiene in health care: First global patient safety challenge, clean care is safer care. https://apps.who.int/iris/bitstream/handle/10665/44102/9789241597906_eng.pdf?sequence=1 (Level IV)

11 Centers for Medicare and Medicaid Services, Department of Health and Human Services. (2020). Condition of participation: Infection control. 42 C.F.R. § 482.42.

12 Accreditation Association for Hospitals and Health Systems. (2020). Standard 07.01.21. *Healthcare facilities accreditation program: Accreditation requirements for acute care hospitals.* Chicago, IL: Accreditation Association for Hospitals and Health Systems. (Level VII)

13 DNV GL-Healthcare USA, Inc. (2020). IC.1.SR.1. *NIAHO® accreditation requirements, interpretive guidelines and surveyor guidance—revision 20.0.* Milford, OH: DNV GL-Healthcare USA, Inc. (Level VII)

14 The Joint Commission. (2021). Standard NPSG.01.01.01. *Comprehensive accreditation manual for hospitals.* Oakbrook Terrace, IL: The Joint Commission. (Level VII)

15 Accreditation Association for Hospitals and Health Systems. (2020). Standard 15.01.16. *Healthcare Facilities Accreditation Program: Accreditation requirements for acute care hospitals.* Chicago, IL: Accreditation Association for Hospitals and Health Systems. (Level VII)

16 Centers for Medicare and Medicaid Services, Department of Health and Human Services. (2020). Condition of participation: Patient's rights. 42 C.F.R. § 482.13(c)(1).

17 The Joint Commission. (2021). Standard RI.01.01.01. *Comprehensive accreditation manual for hospitals.* Oakbrook Terrace, IL: The Joint Commission. (Level VII)

18 DNV GL-Healthcare USA, Inc. (2020). PR.2.SR.5. *NIAHO® accreditation requirements, interpretive guidelines and surveyor guidance—revision 20.0.* Milford, OH: DNV GL-Healthcare USA, Inc. (Level VII)

19 Institute for Safe Medication Practices. (2020). 2020–2021 targeted medication safety best practices for hospitals. https://www.ismp.org/sites/default/files/attachments/2020-02/2020-2021%20TMSBP-%20FINAL_1.pdf

20 Waters, T. R., et al. (2009). Safe patient handling training for schools of nursing. https://www.cdc.gov/niosh/docs/2009-127/pdfs/2009-127.pdf (Level VII)

21 Siegel, J. D., et al. (2007, revised 2019). 2007 guideline for isolation precautions: Preventing transmission of infectious agents in healthcare settings. https://www.cdc.gov/infectioncontrol/pdf/guidelines/isolation-guidelines-H.pdf (Level II)

22 Occupational Safety and Health Administration. (2012). Bloodborne pathogens, standard number 1910.1030. https://www.osha.gov/pls/oshaweb/owadisp.show_document?p_id=10051&p_table=STANDARDS (Level VII)

23 Accreditation Association for Hospitals and Health Systems. (2020). Standard 07.01.10. *Healthcare facilities accreditation program: Accreditation requirements for acute care hospitals.* Chicago, IL: Accreditation Association for Hospitals and Health Systems. (Level VII)

24 Marschall, J., et al. (2014). SHEA/IDSA practice recommendation: Strategies to prevent central line-associated bloodstream infections in acute care hospitals. *Infection Control and Hospital Epidemiology, 35,* 753–771. https://www.jstor.org/stable/10.1086/676533#metadata_info_tab_contents (Level I)

25 Standard 36. Needleless connectors. Infusion therapy standards of practice (8th ed.). (2021). *Journal of Infusion Nursing, 44,* S104–S107. (Level VII)

26 Standard 41. Flushing and locking. Infusion therapy standards of practice (8th ed.). (2021). *Journal of Infusion Nursing, 44,* S113–S118. (Level VII)

27 Nuwellis. (n.d.). *Training and Education: Ultrafiltration training.* https://www.nuwellis.com/healthcare-professionals/training-and-education/

28 U.S. Food and Drug Administration. (2017). Examples of medical device misconnections. https://www.fda.gov/medical-devices/medical-device-connectors/examples-medical-device-misconnections

29 Standard 20. Compounding and preparation of parenteral solutions and medications. Infusion therapy standards of practice (8th ed.). (2021). *Journal of Infusion Nursing, 44,* S59–S60. (Level VII)

30 The Joint Commission. (2014). Sentinel event alert 53: Managing risk during transition to new ISO tubing connector standards. https://www.jointcommission.org/assets/1/6/SEA_53_Connectors_8_19_14_final.pdf (Level VII)

31 The Joint Commission. (2021). Standard MM.06.01.01. *Comprehensive accreditation manual for hospitals.* Oakbrook Terrace, IL: The Joint Commission. (Level VII)

32 Accreditation Association for Hospitals and Health Systems. (2020). Standard 16.01.03. *Healthcare facilities accreditation program: Accreditation requirements for acute care hospitals.* Chicago, IL: Accreditation Association for Hospitals and Health Systems. (Level VII)

33 Centers for Medicare and Medicaid Services, Department of Health and Human Services. (2020). Condition of participation: Nursing services. 42 C.F.R. § 482.23(c).

34 DNV GL-Healthcare USA, Inc. (2020). MM.1.SR.3. *NIAHO® accreditation requirements, interpretive guidelines and surveyor guidance—revision 20.0.* Milford, OH: DNV GL-Healthcare USA, Inc. (Level VII)

35 Westbrook, J., et al. (2010). Association of interruptions with an increased risk and severity of medication administration errors. *Archives of Internal Medicine,170,* 683–690. (Level IV)

36 Institute for Safe Medication Practices. (2012). Side tracks on the safety express: Interruptions lead to errors and unfinished…Wait, what was I doing? *Nurse Advise-ERR, 11*(2), 1–4. https://www.ismp.org/resources/side-tracks-safety-express-interruptions-lead-errors-and-unfinished-wait-what-was-i-doing?id=37

37 Institute for Safe Medication Practices. (2018). ISMP list of high-alert medications in acute care settings. https://www.ismp.org/sites/default/files/attachments/2018-08/highAlert2018-Acute-Final.pdf

38 Institute for Safe Medication Practices. (2013). Independent double checks: Undervalued and misused: Selective use of this strategy can play an important role in medication safety. at https://www.ismp.org/resources/independent-double-checks-undervalued-and-misused-selective-use-strategy-can-play (Level VII)

39 Graham, K. C., & Cvach, M. (2010). Monitor alarm fatigue: Standardizing use of physiological monitors and decreasing nuisance alarms. *American Journal of Critical Care, 19,* 28–37. http://ajcc.aacnjournals.org/content/19/1/28.full.pdf

40 American Association of Critical-Care Nurses. (2018). AACN practice alert: Managing alarms in acute care across the life span: Electrocardiography and pulse oximetry. https://www.aacn.org/clinical-resources/practice-alerts/managing-alarms-in-acute-care-across-the-life-span (Level VII)

41 The Joint Commission. (2021). Standard NPSG.06.01.01. *Comprehensive accreditation manual for hospitals.* Oakbrook Terrace, IL: The Joint Commission. (Level VII)

42 CHF Solutions, Inc. (2017). Aquadex Flexflow®: Reference guide. https://www.manualslib.com/manual/1350920/Chf-Solutions-Aquadex-Flexflow.html

43 The Joint Commission. (2021). Standard RC.02.01.01. *Comprehensive accreditation manual for hospitals.* Oakbrook Terrace, IL: The Joint Commission. (Level VII)

44 Ganz, D. A., et al. (2013-Reviewed 2021). Preventing falls in hospitals: A toolkit for improving quality of care (AHRQ Publication No.13-0015-EF). Rockville, MD: Agency for Healthcare Research and Quality. https://www.ahrq.gov/professionals/systems/hospital/fallpxtoolkit/index.html (Level VII)

45 Accreditation Association for Hospitals and Health Systems. (2020). Standard 07.02.03. *Healthcare Facilities Accreditation Program: Accreditation requirements for acute care hospitals.* Chicago, IL: Accreditation Association for Hospitals and Health Systems. (Level VII)

46 Rutala, W. A., et al. (2008, revised 2019). Guideline for disinfection and sterilization in healthcare facilities, 2008. https://www.cdc.gov/infection-control/pdf/guidelines/disinfection-guidelines-H.pdf (Level I)

47 The Joint Commission. (2021). Standard RC.01.03.01. *Comprehensive accreditation manual for hospitals.* Oakbrook Terrace, IL: The Joint Commission. (Level VII)

48 Centers for Medicare and Medicaid Services, Department of Health and Human Services. (2020). Condition of participation: Medical record services. 42 C.F.R. § 482.24(b).

49 Accreditation Association for Hospitals and Health Systems. (2020). Standard 10.00.03. *Healthcare facilities accreditation program: Accreditation requirements for acute care hospitals.* Chicago, IL: Accreditation Association for Hospitals and Health Systems. (Level VII)

50 DNV GL-Healthcare USA, Inc. (2020). MR.2.SR.1. *NIAHO® accreditation requirements, interpretive guidelines and surveyor guidance—revision 20.0.* Milford, OH: DNV GL-Healthcare USA, Inc. (Level VII)

51 The Joint Commission. (2013). Sentinel event alert 50: Medical device alarm safety in hospitals. https://www.jointcommission.org/assets/1/6/SEA_50_alarms_4_26_16.pdf (Level VII)

52 Kazory, A. (2016). Ultrafiltration therapy for heart failure: Balancing likely benefits against possible risks. *Clinical Journal of the American Society of Nephrology, 11*(8), 463–1471. https://www.ncbi.nlm.nih.gov/pmc/articles/PMC4974896/

ARTERIAL AND VENOUS SHEATH REMOVAL

Surgeons may place an arterial sheath, venous sheath, or both during endovascular procedures. Sheath removal can improve patient comfort and shorten the required time on bed rest, resulting in positive patient outcomes. Only those who have received special training should perform sheath removal because of its association with potentially life-threatening adverse events.

Methods used to control bleeding following sheath removal include manual compression (used alone or with a hemostasis pad), mechanical compression devices, collagen plug devices, staple- or clip-mediated closure devices, and percutaneous suture-mediated closure devices.[1] When using a plug-type device, staple- or clip-mediated closure device, or suture-mediated closure device, sheath removal can happen immediately after the procedure, regardless of the patient's coagulation status. Studies comparing methods used to control bleeding have not shown that any method is superior in terms of vascular complications.[1]

Equipment

Gloves ▪ gown ▪ mask and goggles or mask with face shield ▪ sterile gloves ▪ cardiac monitor ▪ blood pressure monitor ▪ permanent marker ▪ antiseptic solution (chlorhexidine-based or povidone-iodine) ▪ sterile gauze ▪ hypoallergenic tape ▪ fluid-impermeable pad ▪ prescribed analgesic ▪ emergency equipment (code cart with cardiac medications, defibrillator, handheld resuscitation bag with mask, intubation equipment ▪ Optional: suture removal kit, IV catheter insertion equipment, sterile normal saline solution, transparent dressing, mechanical compression device, noninvasive hemostasis pad, 10-mL syringe, prescribed local anesthetic (10 to 20 mL of 1% lidocaine).[2]

Preparation of equipment

Inspect all equipment and supplies. If a product is expired, is defective, or has compromised integrity, remove it from patient use, label it as expired or defective, and report the expiration or defect as directed by your facility. Make sure that emergency equipment is readily available and functioning properly. Administer an analgesic 20 to 30 minutes before the procedure[1], and assist with local anesthetic administration, as ordered, following safe medication administration practices *to promote patient comfort.*[2,3,4,5,6]

Implementation

▪ Verify the practitioner's order for sheath removal.
▪ Review the patient's medical record to assess for conditions that increase the patient's risk of bleeding, and check the patient's platelet count, prothrombin time, international normalized ratio, partial thromboplastin time, complete blood count, blood urea nitrogen and creatinine levels, and activated clotting time *to ensure that hemostasis can be achieved.*[1]

> **NURSING ALERT** Keep in mind that patients receiving potent oral and IV antiplatelet and antithrombin medications who have conditions such as hypertension and kidney dysfunction (defined as creatinine clearance of less than 60 mL/minute) are at increased risk for bleeding during percutaneous coronary intervention.[7]

▪ Gather and prepare the necessary equipment and supplies.
▪ Perform hand hygiene.[8,9,10,11,12,13,14,15]
▪ Confirm the patient's identity using at least two patient identifiers.[16]
▪ Provide privacy.[17,18,19,20]
▪ Explain the procedure to the patient and family (if appropriate) according to their individual communication and learning needs *to increase their understanding, allay their fears, and enhance cooperation.*[21] Include anticipated postprocedure activity restrictions, discomfort caused by pressure to the site, and signs and symptoms to report.
▪ Raise the bed to waist level before providing care *to prevent caregiver back strain.*[22]
▪ Perform hand hygiene.[8,9,10,11,12,13,14,15]
▪ Put on gloves as needed *to comply with standard precautions.*[23,24,25,26,27]
▪ Ensure the patient is connected to the cardiac monitor *to enable prompt recognition and treatment of complications that may occur during the procedure.* Also make sure that the patient is connected to a blood pressure monitor *to monitor blood pressure every 5 minutes until hemostasis is attained during arterial sheath removal.*[1] Make sure that alarm limits are set properly for the patient's current condition, and that the alarms are turned on, functioning, and audible to staff.[28,29,30,31]
▪ Obtain the patient's vital signs and assess the electrocardiogram (ECG) tracing on the cardiac monitor *to establish baselines for comparison.* Notify the practitioner if the patient's blood pressure is elevated, *because the practitioner may order medication to lower the patient's blood pressure before sheath removal, to decrease postprocedure bleeding.*[1,7]
▪ Assess neurovascular status in the extremity distal to the sheath insertion site *to establish a baseline for comparison.*[1]
▪ Mark the pulses distal to the sheath insertion site using a permanent marker *to facilitate finding the pulses for subsequent assessment.*[1]
▪ Confirm that a patent IV catheter is in place *in case the patient requires emergency IV fluids or medications.* If not, insert one.[1,2,32] (See the "IV catheter insertion and removal" procedure.)
▪ Position the patient with the head of the bed flat *to promote hemostasis.*[1]
▪ Place a fluid-impermeable pad under the affected extremity *to keep the bed linens clean and to provide a place to set the sheath after removal.*
▪ Remove and discard your gloves, if worn, in the appropriate receptacle.[23,26]
▪ Perform hand hygiene.[8,9,10,11,12,13,14,15]
▪ Put on gloves, a gown, and a mask and goggles or mask with face shield *to comply with standard precautions.*[23,24,25,26,27]
▪ If you're using a mechanical compression device, place it under the patient before sheath removal *to reduce patient movement and the risk of bleeding after sheath removal.*[1] If you're using a hemostasis pad, open it using sterile, no-touch technique, and open the sterile normal saline solution. (See the "Sterile technique, basic" procedure.)
▪ If the sheath is sutured in place, open a suture removal kit using sterile no-touch technique.
▪ Carefully remove the dressing covering the sheath insertion site.
▪ Inspect the insertion site for bruising, bleeding, and hematoma.
▪ Clean the insertion site with the antiseptic solution.[1]
▪ Attach a 10-mL syringe to the blood sampling port of the stopcock. Gently aspirate 5 to 10 mL of blood into the syringe *to ensure that the sheath is free of clots.*[1,34,35] Notify the practitioner if you can't aspirate blood through the sheath's sampling port.[1]
▪ Remove and discard your gloves in the appropriate receptacle.[23,26,33]
▪ Perform hand hygiene.[8,9,10,11,12,13,14,15]
▪ Put on sterile gloves.[1]
▪ Remove the sutures, if present. (See the "Suture removal" procedure.)

Arterial sheath removal using manual or mechanical compression

▪ Locate the femoral pulse proximal to the insertion site *so that you can properly position compression (manual or mechanical) 1 to 2 cm above the insertion site.*[1]

■ Hold the sheath with one hand while applying firm manual or mechanical pressure over the femoral artery with the other hand *to reduce bleeding.*

■ Remove the sheath slowly while the patient exhales *to prevent the patient from bearing down during removal, which can cause a vasovagal response.* Continue to apply pressure manually or with the mechanical device.[1]

NURSING ALERT If you meet resistance while withdrawing the sheath, stop the procedure and notify the practitioner.[1]

■ Apply continuous, firm pressure to the artery for approximately 20 minutes.[1] Ensure that the pressure is strong enough to stop the bleeding but not so strong that it obscures the pedal pulse. Continue to assess pulses distal to the insertion site (you might need a coworker to do this).

Arterial sheath removal using a noninvasive hemostasis pad with manual compression

■ Apply pressure 1 to 2 cm proximal to the insertion site.[1]

■ Place the hemostasis pad directly over the insertion site.

■ Remove the sheath slowly while the patient exhales *to prevent the patient from bearing down during removal, which can cause a vasovagal response.*

■ Momentarily reduce proximal pressure to let a small amount of blood from the insertion site moisten the noninvasive hemostasis pad *to activate the hemostasis mechanism,* and then reapply proximal pressure.[1]

■ After 3 to 4 minutes, slowly decrease pressure proximal to the insertion site while continuing to apply pressure to the insertion site for no less than 10 minutes. Continue to assess pulses distal to the insertion site (you might need a coworker to do this).[1]

■ Apply another sterile gauze pad over the hemostasis pad and cover the site with a transparent dressing *to reduce the risk of infection.*[1,36]

■ Leave the hemostasis pad in place for 24 hours.[1]

■ Remove manual pressure after hemostasis is achieved.

Venous sheath removal

■ Remove the venous sheath, if present, 5 to 10 minutes after removal of the arterial sheath, *because pressure at the arterial site must be maintained for a longer time.*[1]

■ Apply pressure over the venous and arterial sites for 10 more minutes or until the bleeding stops.[1]

■ If a hemostasis pad is used, momentarily reduce proximal pressure to let a small amount of blood from the insertion site moisten the noninvasive hemostasis pad *to activate the hemostasis mechanism* and then reapply proximal pressure.[1] After 3 to 4 minutes, slowly decrease pressure proximal to the insertion site while continuing to apply pressure to the insertion site for no less than 10 minutes. Then apply another sterile gauze pad over the hemostasis pad, cover the site with a transparent dressing, and leave it in place for 24 hours.

NURSING ALERT Avoid prolonged pressure on the femoral vein. *Prolonged venous occlusion, especially with pressure devices, may cause venous thrombosis.* Assess for neurovascular changes.[2]

Follow-up care

■ Apply sterile dressings to the arterial and venous insertion sites *to keep the areas clean and reduce the risk of infection.*[37] Use a sterile transparent dressing *to allow easier assessment of the puncture site.*[1]

■ Discard used supplies in appropriate receptacles.[23,26,33]

■ Return the bed to the lowest position to prevent falls and maintain patient safety.[37]

■ Remove and discard your gloves and other personal protective equipment.[23,26,33]

■ Perform hand hygiene.[8,9,10,11,12,13,14,15]

■ Screen for and assess the patient's pain using facility-defined criteria that are consistent with the patient's age, condition, and ability to understand.[38]

■ Treat the patient's pain as needed and ordered using nonpharmacologic, pharmacologic, or a combination of approaches. Base the treatment plan on evidence-based practices and the patient's clinical condition, medical history, and pain management goals. If you're administering pain medication, follow safe medication administration practices.[3,4,5,6]

■ Assess neurovascular status, vital signs, and the insertion site in the affected limb every 15 minutes for 1 hour, every 30 minutes for the next hour, and then every hour for 4 hours *to enable early detection of complications.*[1]

■ Tell the patient not to elevate the head of the bed greater than 30 degrees *to reduce the risk of disrupting homeostasis and relieve back discomfort.*

■ Instruct the patient to report any bleeding from the site, saturation of the dressing, or wetness or warmth on the groin or leg.

■ Tell the patient to report coolness, numbness, tingling, or pain in the affected extremity.

■ When applying mechanical or manual pressure after arterial sheath removal, keep the patient on bed rest for 1 to 6 hours, as directed by your facility. Note that bed rest time varies depending on the size of the sheath used; type of procedure; and use of bivalirudin, heparin, or antiplatelet medications during the procedure.[1,39]

■ Keep the patient on bed rest for 1 to 4 hours when achieving hemostasis through percutaneous suture-mediated closure and hemostasis pads, according to the manufacturer's instructions.[1]

■ Keep the patient on bed rest for no more than 4 hours after venous sheath removal; *venous sheath removal has a lower incidence of vascular complications than arterial sheath removal because the venous system is a lower-pressure system.*[1]

■ Reassess and respond to the patient's pain by evaluating the response to treatment and progress toward pain management goals. Assess for adverse reactions and risk factors for adverse events that may result from treatment.[38]

■ Perform hand hygiene.[8,9,10,11,13,14,15]

■ Document the procedure.[40,41,42,43,44]

Special considerations

■ Some practitioners prefer to use the radial artery for catheterization. *Because the radial artery is much smaller and located closer to the skin surface, accessing this artery eliminates internal bleeding and enables easy compression of any external bleeding.* After the catheter and sheath are removed from the radial artery, a compression device is placed around the wrist *to apply pressure.* Radial catheterization also eliminates the need for the patient to remain immobile. In general, patients find radial catheterization more comfortable than femoral catheterization *because they are able to sit up, walk, and eat immediately following removal.*[45]

■ In a patient with obesity, you may need a second person to assist in holding back skin and abdominal folds.[1]

■ In a patient with hypertension, you may need to apply pressure for a longer period of time *to ensure hemostasis.*[1]

■ Be sure to read the manufacturer's instructions for correct use of mechanical compression devices. *Tissue damage can occur with incorrect use of the devices.*

■ The compression time required to control bleeding depends on several factors, including the size of the sheath, administration of heparin and antiplatelet drugs, and blood coagulation levels.[1,2]

■ If you can't stop the bleeding following sheath removal, notify the practitioner.[1]

■ The Joint Commission issued a sentinel event alert concerning medical device alarm safety, *because alarm-related events have been associated with permanent loss of function or death.* Among the major contributing factors were improper alarm settings, alarm settings turned off inappropriately, and alarm signals not audible to staff. Make sure alarm limits are set appropriately and that alarms are turned on, functioning properly, and audible to staff. Follow facility guidelines for preventing alarm fatigue.[28]

Patient teaching

Provide the patient and family with written and oral discharge instructions. Tell the patient to avoid lifting anything heavier than 10 lb (4.5 kg) for 3 days and to avoid driving or operating machinery for 24 hours. Tell the patient that it's permissible to remove the dressing and shower after 24 hours, but that a tub bath or swimming is to be avoided until the skin is healed. After the initial 24 hours, the patient may clean the site with soap and water and apply a small adhesive bandage. Tell the patient to inspect the site daily and to notify the practitioner as soon as possible of any bleeding, redness, or discharge at the site or if a fever develops.

Complications

The most common complication following sheath removal is bleeding, which occurs most commonly at the femoral artery access site. Retroperitoneal bleeding may also occur. Vascular complications include hematoma, pseudoaneurysm, arteriovenous fistula, embolus, and thrombus formation.[46] Sensory or motor impairment may occur in the affected limb. Vasovagal complications may also occur.

Documentation

Record the date and time of sheath removal; note whether the sheath was intact.[1] Document whether you removed an arterial sheath, a venous sheath, or both, and note the location(s). Note the patient's pain assessment findings, any interventions you provided, and the patient's response to those interventions. Document the patient's laboratory values before sheath removal, and note that they were within normal limits. Record vital signs, neurovascular status, and heart rhythm before sheath removal. State whether you marked pulses distal to the sheath insertion site(s).

Note whether the patient has a patent IV line. Include that the patient was placed flat for sheath removal. Describe the condition of the sheath insertion site(s), noting redness, skin breakdown, drainage, bleeding, or hematoma formation. Note how many sutures you removed, if applicable. Explain any difficulties you encountered during sheath removal. Record the method of hemostasis you used and the time required for you to achieve hemostasis. Document your assessments, including neurovascular status, vital signs, and sheath insertion site. Note the patient's tolerance of the procedure.

Record any complications, the name of the practitioner you notified, the date and time of notification, any orders you received, your interventions, and the patient's response to those interventions. Include the patient's position after sheath removal and the duration of bed rest. Document teaching provided to the patient and family (if applicable), their understanding of that teaching, and any need for follow-up teaching.

REFERENCES

1 Wiegand, D. L. (2017). *AACN procedure manual for high acuity, progressive, and critical care* (7th ed.). St. Louis, MO: Elsevier.

2 Kern, M. J. (2017). *The interventional cardiac catheterization handbook* (4th ed.). Philadelphia, PA: Saunders.

3 Centers for Medicare and Medicaid Services, Department of Health and Human Services. (2020). Condition of participation: Nursing services. 42 C.F.R. § 482.23(c).

4 Accreditation Association for Hospitals and Health Systems. (2020). Standard 16.01.03. *Healthcare Facilities Accreditation Program: Accreditation requirements for acute care hospitals*. Chicago, IL: Accreditation Association for Hospitals and Health Systems. (Level VII)

5 The Joint Commission. (2021). Standard MM.06.01.01. *Comprehensive accreditation manual for hospitals*. Oakbrook Terrace, IL: The Joint Commission. (Level VII)

6 DNV GL-Healthcare USA, Inc. (2020). MM.1.SR.2. *NIAHO® accreditation requirements, interpretive guidelines and surveyor guidance—revision 20.0*. Milford, OH: DNV GL-Healthcare USA, Inc. (Level VII)

7 Merriweather, N., & Sulzbach-Hoke, L. M. (2012). Managing risk of complications at femoral vascular access sites in percutaneous coronary intervention. *Critical Care Nurse, 32*(5), 16–29. (Level VII)

8 Centers for Disease Control and Prevention. (2002). Guideline for hand hygiene in health-care settings: Recommendations of the Healthcare Infection Control Practices Advisory Committee and the HICPAC/SHEA/APIC/IDSA Hand Hygiene Task Force. *MMWR Recommendations and Reports, 51*(RR-16), 1–45. https://www.cdc.gov/mmwr/pdf/rr/rr5116.pdf (Level II)

9 World Health Organization. (2009). WHO guidelines on hand hygiene in health care: First global patient safety challenge, clean care is safer care. https://apps.who.int/iris/bitstream/handle/10665/44102/9789241597906_eng.pdf?sequence=1 (Level IV)

10 The Joint Commission. (2021). Standard NPSG.07.01.01. *Comprehensive accreditation manual for hospitals*. Oakbrook Terrace, IL: The Joint Commission. (Level VII)

11 Standard 16. Hand hygiene. Infusion therapy standards of practice (8th ed.). (2021). *Journal of Infusion Nursing, 44*, S53–S54. (Level VII)

12 Centers for Disease Control and Prevention. (2011, revised 2017). Guidelines for the prevention of intravascular catheter–related infections. https://www.cdc.gov/infectioncontrol/guidelines/bsi/recommendations.html (Level I)

13 Centers for Medicare and Medicaid Services, Department of Health and Human Services. (2020). Condition of participation: Infection control. 42 C.F.R. § 482.42.

14 Accreditation Association for Hospitals and Health Systems. (2020). Standard 07.01.21. *Healthcare Facilities Accreditation Program: Accreditation requirements for acute care hospitals*. Chicago, IL: Accreditation Association for Hospitals and Health Systems. (Level VII)

15 DNV GL-Healthcare USA, Inc. (2020). IC.1.SR.1. *NIAHO® accreditation requirements, interpretive guidelines and surveyor guidance—revision 20.0*. Milford, OH: DNV GL-Healthcare USA, Inc. (Level VII)

16 The Joint Commission. (2021). Standard NPSG.01.01.01. *Comprehensive accreditation manual for hospitals*. Oakbrook Terrace, IL: The Joint Commission. (Level VII)

17 The Joint Commission. (2021). Standard RI.01.01.01. *Comprehensive accreditation manual for hospitals*. Oakbrook Terrace, IL: The Joint Commission. (Level VII)

18 Centers for Medicare and Medicaid Services, Department of Health and Human Services. (2020). Condition of participation: Patient's rights. 42 C.F.R. § 482.13(c)(1).

19 Accreditation Association for Hospitals and Health Systems. (2020). Standard 15.01.16. *Healthcare Facilities Accreditation Program: Accreditation requirements for acute care hospitals*. Chicago, IL: Accreditation Association for Hospitals and Health Systems. (Level VII)

20 DNV GL-Healthcare USA, Inc. (2020). PR.2.SR.5. *NIAHO® accreditation requirements, interpretive guidelines and surveyor guidance—revision 20.0*. Milford, OH: DNV GL-Healthcare USA, Inc. (Level VII)

21 The Joint Commission. (2021). Standard PC.02.01.21. *Comprehensive accreditation manual for hospitals*. Oakbrook Terrace, IL: The Joint Commission. (Level VII)

22 Waters, T. R., et al. (2009). Safe patient handling training for schools of nursing. https://www.cdc.gov/niosh/docs/2009-127/pdfs/2009-127.pdf (Level VII)

23 Siegel, J. D., et al. (2007, revised 2019). 2007 guideline for isolation precautions: Preventing transmission of infectious agents in healthcare settings. https://www.cdc.gov/infectioncontrol/pdf/guidelines/isolation-guidelines-H.pdf (Level II)

24 Standard 17. Standard precautions. Infusion therapy standards of practice (8th ed.). (2021). *Journal of Infusion Nursing, 44*, S54–S58. (Level VII)

25 Accreditation Association for Hospitals and Health Systems. (2020). Standard 07.01.10. *Healthcare Facilities Accreditation Program: Accreditation requirements for acute care hospitals*. Chicago, IL: Accreditation Association for Hospitals and Health Systems. (Level VII)

26 Occupational Safety and Health Administration. (2012). Bloodborne pathogens, standard number 1910.1030. https://www.osha.gov/pls/oshaweb/owadisp.show_document?p_id=10051&p_table=STANDARDS (Level VII)

27 DNV GL-Healthcare USA, Inc. (2020). IC.1.SR.2. *NIAHO® accreditation requirements, interpretive guidelines and surveyor guidance—revision 20.0*. Milford, OH: DNV GL-Healthcare USA, Inc. (Level VII)

28 The Joint Commission. (2013). Sentinel event alert 50: Medical device alarm safety in hospitals. https://www.jointcommission.org/assets/1/6/SEA_50_alarms_4_26_16.pdf (Level VII)

29 The Joint Commission. (2021). Standard NPSG.06.01.01. *Comprehensive accreditation manual for hospitals*. Oakbrook Terrace, IL: The Joint Commission. (Level VII)

30 Graham, K. C., & Cvach, M. (2010). Monitor alarm fatigue: Standardizing use of physiological monitors and decreasing nuisance alarms. *American Journal of Critical Care, 19*, 28–37.

31 American Association of Critical-Care Nurses. (2018). AACN practice alert: Managing alarms in acute care across the life span: Electrocardiography and pulse oximetry. https://www.aacn.org/clinical-resources/practice-alerts/managing-alarms-in-acute-care-across-the-life-span (Level VII)

32 Standard 34. Vascular access device placement. Infusion therapy standards of practice (8th ed.). (2021). *Journal of Infusion Nursing, 44*, S97–S101. (Level VII)

33 Standard 21. Medical waste and sharps safety. Infusion therapy standards of practice (8th ed.). (2021). *Journal of Infusion Nursing, 44*, S60–S62. (Level VII)

34 Dressler, D. K., & Dressler, K. K. (2006). Caring for patients with femoral sheaths. *The American Journal of Nursing, 106*(5), 64A–64H. https://journals.lww.com/ajnonline/fulltext/2006/05000/caring_for_patients_with_femoral_sheaths__after.36.aspx?casa_token=tuNQayMhv7IAAAAA:S3Aug3Ek-1rB-ktXfZRDmPla8ZejJDzEfsi4OYbtGlHPceBd5Jh4aWbzxdPgsOmyEWG9GlTvEnSjioXJAirj0I2FX64#O4-36-2

35 Kern, M. (2013). Back to basics: Femoral artery access and hemostasis. *Cath Lab Digest, 21*(10). https://www.cathlabdigest.com/articles/Back-Basics-Femoral-Artery-Access-Hemostasis

36 Standard 42. Vascular access device (VAD) assessment, care and dressing changes. Infusion therapy standards of practice (8th ed.). (2021). *Journal of Infusion Nursing, 44,* S119–S123. (Level VII)

37 Ganz, D. A., et al. (2013, reviewed 2021). *Preventing falls in hospitals: A toolkit for improving quality of care* (AHRQ Publication No. 13-0015-EF). Rockville, MD: Agency for Healthcare Research and Quality. https://www.ahrq.gov/professionals/systems/hospital/fallpxtoolkit/index.html (Level VII)

38 The Joint Commission. (2021). Standard PC.01.02.07. *Comprehensive accreditation manual for hospitals.* Oakbrook Terrace, IL: The Joint Commission. (Level VII)

39 Walker, S., et al. (2008). Comparison of complications in percutaneous coronary intervention patients mobilized at 3, 4, and 6 hours after femoral arterial sheath removal. *Journal of Cardiovascular Nursing, 23*(5), 407–413. (Level II)

40 The Joint Commission. (2021). Standard RC.01.03.01. *Comprehensive accreditation manual for hospitals.* Oakbrook Terrace, IL: The Joint Commission. (Level VII)

41 Centers for Medicare and Medicaid Services, Department of Health and Human Services. (2020). *Condition of participation: Medical record services. 42 C.F. R. § 482.24(b).*

42 Accreditation Association for Hospitals and Health Systems. (2020). Standard 10.00.03. *Healthcare Facilities Accreditation Program: Accreditation requirements for acute care hospitals.* Chicago, IL: Accreditation Association for Hospitals and Health Systems. (Level VII)

43 DNV GL-Healthcare USA, Inc. (2020). MR.2.SR.1. *NIAHO® accreditation requirements, interpretive guidelines and surveyor guidance—revision 20.0.* Milford, OH: DNV GL-Healthcare USA, Inc. (Level VII)

44 Standard 10. Documentation in the health record. Infusion therapy standards of practice (8th ed.). (2021). *Journal of Infusion Nursing, 44,* S39–S42. (Level VII)

45 Balaji, N. R., & Shah, P. B. (2011). Radial artery catheterization. *Circulation, 124,* e407–e408. https://www.ahajournals.org/doi/pdf/10.1161/circulationaha.111.019802 (Level VII)

46 Sulzbach-Hoke, L. M., et al. (2010). Predictors of complications following sheath removal with percutaneous coronary intervention. *Journal of Cardiovascular Nursing, 25*(3), E1–E8. (Level IV)

ARTERIAL PRESSURE MONITORING

Arterial catheters provide direct arterial pressure monitoring, which permits continuous measurement of systolic, diastolic, and mean arterial pressures and allows for arterial blood sampling.[1] Because direct measurement reflects systemic vascular resistance (SVR) as well as blood flow, it's generally more accurate than indirect methods (such as palpation and auscultation of Korotkoff [audible pulse] sounds), which are based on blood flow. Direct monitoring is indicated when highly accurate or frequent blood pressure measurements are required, such as for patients with low cardiac output and high systemic vascular resistance. It can also be used for patients receiving titrated doses of vasoactive drugs and for those who require frequent blood sampling.

Arterial pressure monitoring is used in critical care settings. Catheter insertion, which can be performed at the beside under surgically sterile conditions, is performed by a practitioner. Guidelines recommend the radial, brachial, and dorsalis pedis sites over the femoral and axillary sites to reduce the risk of infection.[2,3] The catheter should be removed as soon as possible to decrease the risk of complications.[1,2,4]

HOSPITAL-ACQUIRED CONDITION ALERT Keep in mind that the Centers for Medicare and Medicaid Services considers vascular catheter–associated infection to be a hospital-acquired condition *because it can be reasonable prevented using a variety of best practices.* Make sure to follow infection prevention techniques, such as performing hand hygiene, maintaining sterile technique, limiting catheter manipulations, and removing the catheter as soon as it's no longer needed, *to reduce the risk of vascular catheter–associated infection.*[2,5,6]

A nurse caring for a patient undergoing arterial pressure monitoring must have an understanding of cardiac anatomy and physiology, the physiology of fluid and electrolyte balance, the pathophysiology of heart disease, and the hemodynamic alterations expected with cardiac

---

Understanding an arterial waveform

Normal arterial blood pressure produces a characteristic waveform, representing ventricular systole and diastole. The waveform has five distinct components: the anacrotic limb, the systolic peak, the dicrotic limb, the dicrotic notch, and end diastole.

The *anacrotic limb* marks the waveform's initial upstroke, which occurs as blood is rapidly ejected from the ventricle through the open aortic valve into the aorta. This rapid ejection causes a sharp rise in arterial pressure, which appears as the waveform's highest point, called the *systolic peak.*[1]

As blood continues into the peripheral vessels, arterial pressure falls, and the waveform begins a downward trend; this part is called the *dicrotic limb.* Arterial pressure usually will continue to fall until pressure in the ventricle is less than pressure in the aortic root. When this decrease occurs, the aortic valve closes. This event appears as a small notch (called the *dicrotic notch*) on the waveform's downside.[1] When the aortic valve closes, diastole begins, progressing until the aortic root pressure gradually descends to its lowest point. On the waveform, this point is known as *end diastole.*

Normal arterial waveform

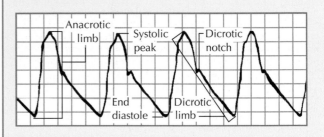

---

interventions and surgery. Competence in setting up and maintaining arterial monitoring equipment, evaluating waveforms, and making clinical decisions about changes in a patient's therapy are also crucial. (See *Understanding an arterial waveform.*)

Equipment

Disposable pressure transducer system ▪ bag of IV flush solution ▪ sterile nonvented or dead-end caps ▪ pressure tubing ▪ pressure infuser bag ▪ transducer holder on an IV pole ▪ monitoring system and equipment (module, bedside monitor, and cable) ▪ vital signs monitoring equipment ▪ labeling device ▪ Optional: single-patient-use joint stabilization device, indelible marker, arterial catheter, and insertion equipment.

Preparation of equipment

Inspect all equipment and supplies. If a product is expired, is defective, or has compromised integrity, remove it from patient use, label it as expired or defective, and report the expiration or defect as directed by your facility.[7]

If necessary, set up and prime the disposable pressure transducer system. (See the "Transducer system setup" procedure.) Make sure you keep all parts of the pressure monitoring system sterile.[2] When you've completed equipment preparation, turn on the bedside monitor and set the appropriate scale *to visualize the correct waveform.*[1]

Implementation

▪ Gather and prepare the necessary equipment and supplies.
▪ Perform hand hygiene.[2,8,9,10,11,12,13,14]
▪ Confirm the patient's identity using at least two patient identifiers.[15]
▪ Provide privacy.[16,17,18,19]
▪ Explain the procedure to the patient and family (if appropriate) according to their individual communication and learning needs *to increase their understanding, allay their fears, and enhance cooperation.*[20] Include the purpose of arterial pressure monitoring and the anticipated duration of catheter placement.

- Raise the bed to waist level before providing care *to prevent caregiver back strain.*[21]
- Perform hand hygiene.[2,8,9,10,11,12,13,14]
- Position the patient for easy access to the catheter insertion site.
- Obtain vital signs *to provide baseline date for comparison.*
- If the patient doesn't already have an arterial catheter in place, assist the practitioner, as needed, during catheter insertion.
- Immobilize the insertion site if necessary. Use a single-patient-use joint stabilization device with a radial or brachial site *to facilitate infusion delivery and maintain device patency.*[22]

NURSING ALERT Keep the catheter site visible at all times. Don't allow linens to cover the site. Arterial catheter dislodgement requires prompt recognition and intervention *to reduce the risk of exsanguination.*

Zeroing the transducer

- Position the patient and the transducer on the same level (usually with the patient supine and the head of the bed elevates 0 to 45 degrees).[1]
- Using the leveling device, level the zeroing stopcock of the transducer with the phlebostatic axis (fourth intercostal space, at the midpoint of the anterior-posterior diameter of the chest wall), which reflects central arterial pressure.[1,23]
- Mark the point of the phlebostatic axis with an indelible marker, if directed by your facility, *to ensure accuracy and consistency in leveling.*[1]
- Zero the system to atmospheric pressure *to negate the effects of atmospheric pressure and prepare the monitoring system for accurate arterial pressure monitoring.*[1] Zero the transducer system only with initial setup, if the transducer system is disconnected from the monitoring cable, if the monitoring cable is disconnected from the monitor, and when blood pressure values don't correspond with the patient's clinical status *to minimize the number of entries into the pressure monitoring system and subsequently reduce the risk of vascular catheter–associated infection.*[1,2]
- Observe the monitor for the arterial waveform and pressure reading. Perform a square wave test *to determine whether the system correctly reflects arterial pressure.* Note that the square wave test is affected by such system problems as air bubbles in the tubing, excessive tubing length, loose connections, and catheter patency.[1] (See *Performing a square-wave test.*)

Completing the procedure

- Make sure that alarms are set appropriately for the patient's current condition, and that alarms are turned on, functioning properly, and audible to staff.[24,25,26]
- Continuously observe the arterial waveform quality on the monitor and record variances *to ensure the accuracy of the waveform and detect changes in the patient's hemodynamic status.* A normal waveform has a peak systole, clear dicrotic notch, and end diastole.[1]
- Monitor the patient's vital signs and note trends in arterial pressure waveform readings at least every 2 hours. Correlate pressure readings with the patient's clinical condition and response to therapies.
- Monitor the insertion site for bleeding, hematoma formation, and such signs and symptoms of infection as pain, erythema, warmth, swelling, and purulent drainage.[1]
- Monitor the involved extremity for changes in temperature, pulse, color, sensation, capillary refill time, and movement *to detect neurovascular compromise that may occur in the affected extremity distal to the insertion site.*[1]
- Regularly evaluate the arterial pressure monitoring system for air bubble formation, which can lead to potentially lethal air emboli. Remove air bubbles by flushing them through a system stopcock.[1]
- Troubleshoot the arterial waveform, as needed.[1] Notify the practitioner, as appropriate. If the waveform suddenly becomes dampened, check the patient before attempting to determine its cause or fix the problem, *because a sudden hypotensive episode can look like a dampened waveform on the monitor and can be potentially life-threatening if not treated properly.* (See *Recognizing abnormal waveforms*, page 34.)
- Return the bed to the lowest position to prevent falls and maintain patient safety.[27]
- Perform hand hygiene.[2,8,9,10,11,12,13,14]
- Document the procedure.[28,29,30,31,32]

Performing a square-wave test

When using a pressure transducer system, you must ensure and document the system's accuracy. Along with leveling and zeroing the system to atmospheric pressure at the phlebostatic axis and interpreting waveforms, you can ensure accuracy by performing the square wave test (also called the dynamic response test). Perform the square wave test with initial system setup, at least once each shift, after opening the catheter system (such as for rezeroing or tubing changes), and when the arterial waveform appears to be dampened or distorted.[23]

To perform a square wave test, follow these steps:
- Activate the fast-flush device for 1 second and then release.
- Obtain a graphic printout.
- Observe for the desired response: The pressure wave rises rapidly, squares off, and is followed by one or two oscillations (as shown in the illustration below).
- Know that these oscillations should have an initial downstroke, which extends below the baseline and just one to two oscillations after the initial downstroke. Usually, but not always, the first upstroke is about one-third the height of the initial downstroke.
- Be aware that the intervals between oscillations should be no more than 0.12 second (three small boxes).
- Note that the arterial pressure waveform should also be clearly defined, with all the components of the waveform visible.[1]

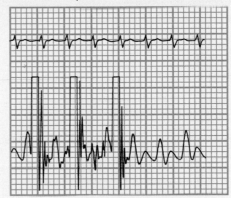

Underdamped square wave

If you observe extra oscillations after the initial downstroke or more than 0.08 second between oscillations, the waveform is underdamped (as shown in the illustration below). This effect can cause falsely high pressure readings and artifact in the waveforms. You can correct it by:
- using large-bore, shorter tubing
- removing air bubbles from the system
- using a damping device.[1]

After correcting the issue, repeat the square wave test and read the pressure waveform.

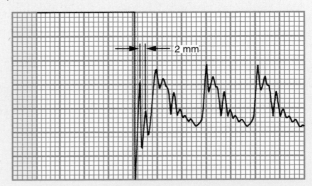

Overdamped square wave

If you observe a slurred upstroke at the beginning of the square wave and a loss of oscillations after the initial downstroke, the waveform is overdamped (as shown in the illustration page 34). This effect can cause falsely low pressure readings as well as lost sharpness of each

(Continued)

waveform peak and the dicrotic notch, which indicates pulmonic valve closure. You can correct this problem by:
- clearing the system of any blood or air
- checking to make sure the catheter has no kinks or obstructions
- using low-compliance, short monitoring tubing
- checking the bag of flush solution to make sure that fluid remains in the bag and the pressure is maintained at 300 mm Hg
- tightening any loose connections.[1]

After correcting the issue, repeat the square wave test and read the pressure waveform.

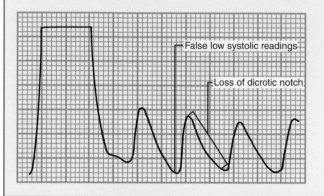

Special considerations

- Be aware that erroneous pressure readings can result from a catheter that's clotted or positional, loose connections, addition of extra stopcocks or extension tubing, inadvertent entry of air into the system, or improper calibrating, leveling, or zeroing of the monitoring system. If the catheter lumen clots, the flush system may be pressurized improperly. Regularly assess the amount of flush solution in the IV bag, and maintain 300 mm Hg of pressure in the pressure infuser bag.[1]
- Change disposable transducer systems, including flush device and flush solution used for invasive hemodynamic monitoring, every 96 hours, immediately upon suspected contamination, or when integrity of the system has been compromised. Limit the number of manipulations and entries to the system.[2,33]
- Change transparent semipermeable dressings at least every 7 days and gauze dressings at least every 2 days.[34]
- Perform hand hygiene before performing dressing changes, and use sterile technique and sterile gloves when redressing the site.[2,34] If signs or symptoms of infection are present or if the dressing becomes visibly soiled, loosened, or dislodged, immediately change the dressing and closely assess the site for redness. Note complaints of tenderness, and then clean and disinfect the site. Immediately notify the practitioner if you note such signs.[34]
- Don't routinely change arterial catheters *to reduce the risk of vascular catheter–associated infection.*[2]

Recognizing abnormal waveforms

Understanding a normal arterial waveform is relatively straightforward. However, an abnormal waveform is more difficult to decipher. Abnormal patterns and markings may provide important diagnostic clues to the patient's cardiovascular status, or they may simply signal trouble in the monitor. Use this chart to help you recognize and resolve waveform abnormalities.

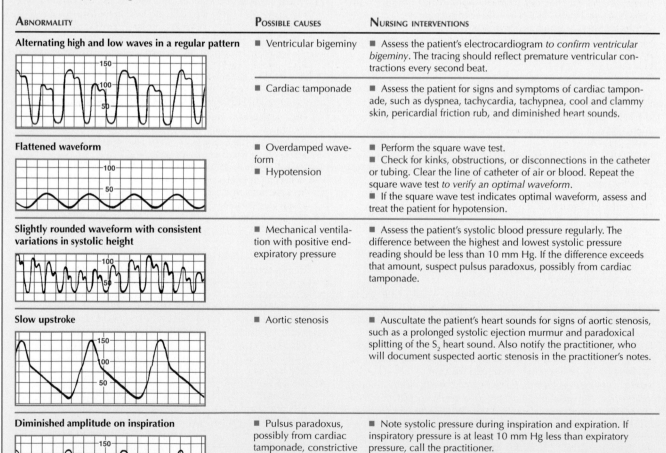

ABNORMALITY	POSSIBLE CAUSES	NURSING INTERVENTIONS
Alternating high and low waves in a regular pattern	■ Ventricular bigeminy	■ Assess the patient's electrocardiogram *to confirm ventricular bigeminy*. The tracing should reflect premature ventricular contractions every second beat.
	■ Cardiac tamponade	■ Assess the patient for signs and symptoms of cardiac tamponade, such as dyspnea, tachycardia, tachypnea, cool and clammy skin, pericardial friction rub, and diminished heart sounds.
Flattened waveform	■ Overdamped waveform ■ Hypotension	■ Perform the square wave test. ■ Check for kinks, obstructions, or disconnections in the catheter or tubing. Clear the line of catheter of air or blood. Repeat the square wave test *to verify an optimal waveform*. ■ If the square wave test indicates optimal waveform, assess and treat the patient for hypotension.
Slightly rounded waveform with consistent variations in systolic height	■ Mechanical ventilation with positive end-expiratory pressure	■ Assess the patient's systolic blood pressure regularly. The difference between the highest and lowest systolic pressure reading should be less than 10 mm Hg. If the difference exceeds that amount, suspect pulsus paradoxus, possibly from cardiac tamponade.
Slow upstroke	■ Aortic stenosis	■ Auscultate the patient's heart sounds for signs of aortic stenosis, such as a prolonged systolic ejection murmur and paradoxical splitting of the S_2 heart sound. Also notify the practitioner, who will document suspected aortic stenosis in the practitioner's notes.
Diminished amplitude on inspiration	■ Pulsus paradoxus, possibly from cardiac tamponade, constrictive pericarditis, or lung disease	■ Note systolic pressure during inspiration and expiration. If inspiratory pressure is at least 10 mm Hg less than expiratory pressure, call the practitioner. ■ If you're also monitoring pulmonary artery pressure, observe for a diastolic plateau. This abnormal waveform occurs when the mean central venous pressure (right atrial pressure), mean pulmonary artery pressure, and mean pulmonary artery occlusion pressure are within 5 mm Hg of one another.

■ The Joint Commission issued a sentinel event alert concerning medical device alarm safety, *because alarm-related events have been associated with permanent loss of function and death.* Among the major contributing factors were improper alarm settings, alarms turned off inappropriately, and alarm signals that are inaudible to staff. Make sure that alarm limits are set appropriately and that alarms are turned on, functioning properly, and audible to staff. Follow facility guidelines for preventing alarm fatigue.[24]

Complications

Arterial catheter insertion and pressure monitoring can cause such complications as arterial bleeding; infection at the insertion site, which can spread into the bloodstream; clot formation within the catheter, which can then be carried into the general circulation; catheter perforation of the vessel wall, which can be associated with excessive bleeding and extravasation of flush solution into the surrounding tissue; air embolism; arterial spasm; and impaired circulation to the extremity distal to the catheter insertion site, which, if not treated promptly, can lead to loss of tissue and, ultimately, loss of limb.[1]

Documentation

Document the color, warmth, sensation, and pulse strength of the extremity distal to the catheter insertion site at regular intervals determined by your facility. Note the alarm settings and confirmation that the alarms are turned on. Record the patient's vital signs. Document dressing, tubing, and flush solution changes, when appropriate. Document teaching provided to the patient and family (if applicable), their understanding of that teaching, and any need for follow-up teaching.

REFERENCES

1 Wiegand, D. L. (2017). *AACN procedure manual for high acuity, progressive, and critical care* (7th ed.). St. Louis, MO: Elsevier.

2 Centers for Disease Control and Prevention. (2011, revised 2017). Guidelines for the prevention of intravascular catheter–related infections. https://www.cdc.gov/infectioncontrol/guidelines/bsi/recommendations.html (Level I)

3 Standard 27. Site selection. Infusion therapy standards of practice (8th ed.). (2021). *Journal of Infusion Nursing, 44*, S81–S86. (Level VII)

4 Standard 45. Vascular access device removal. Infusion therapy standards of practice (8th ed.). (2021). *Journal of Infusion Nursing, 44*, S133–S137. (Level VII)

5 Jarrett, N., & Callaham, M. (2016). Evidence-based guidelines for selected hospital-acquired conditions: Final report. https://www.cms.gov/Medicare/Medicare-Fee-for-Service-Payment/HospitalAcqCond/Downloads/2016-HAC-Report.pdf

6 Marschall, J., et al. (2014). SHEA/IDSA practice recommendation: Strategies to prevent central line–associated bloodstream infections in acute care hospitals—2014 update. *Infection Control and Hospital Epidemiology, 35*(7), 753–771. http://www.jstor.org/stable/10.1086/676533 (Level I)

7 Standard 12. Product evaluation, integrity, and defect reporting. Infusion therapy standards of practice (8th ed.). (2021). *Journal of Infusion Nursing, 44*, S45–S46. (Level VII)

8 The Joint Commission. (2021). Standard NPSG.07.01.01. *Comprehensive accreditation manual for hospitals.* Oakbrook Terrace, IL: The Joint Commission. (Level VII)

9 Centers for Disease Control and Prevention. (2002). Guideline for hand hygiene in health-care settings: Recommendations of the Healthcare Infection Control Practices Advisory Committee and the HICPAC/SHEA/APIC/IDSA Hand Hygiene Task Force. *MMWR Recommendations and Reports, 51*(RR-16), 1–45. https://www.cdc.gov/mmwr/pdf/rr/rr5116.pdf (Level II)

10 World Health Organization. (2009). WHO guidelines on hand hygiene in health care: First global patient safety challenge, clean care is safer care. https://apps.who.int/iris/bitstream/handle/10665/44102/9789241597906_eng.pdf?sequence=1 (Level IV)

11 Centers for Medicare and Medicaid Services, Department of Health and Human Services. (2020). Condition of participation: Infection control. 42 C.F.R. § 482.42.

12 Accreditation Association for Hospitals and Health Systems. (2020). Standard 07.01.21. *Healthcare Facilities Accreditation Program: Accreditation requirements for acute care hospitals.* Chicago, IL: Accreditation Association for Hospitals and Health Systems. (Level VII)

13 Standard 16. Hand hygiene. Infusion therapy standards of practice (8th ed.). (2021). *Journal of Infusion Nursing, 44*, S53–S54. (Level VII)

14 DNV GL-Healthcare USA, Inc. (2020). IC.1.SR.1. *NIAHO® accreditation requirements, interpretive guidelines and surveyor guidance—revision 20.0.* Milford, OH: DNV GL-Healthcare USA, Inc. (Level VII)

15 The Joint Commission. (2021). Standard NPSG.01.01.01. *Comprehensive accreditation manual for hospitals.* Oakbrook Terrace, IL: The Joint Commission. (Level VII)

16 The Joint Commission. (2021). Standard RI.01.01.01. *Comprehensive accreditation manual for hospitals.* Oakbrook Terrace, IL: The Joint Commission. (Level VII)

17 Centers for Medicare and Medicaid Services, Department of Health and Human Services. (2020). Condition of participation: Patient's rights. 42 C.F.R. § 482.13(c)(1).

18 Accreditation Association for Hospitals and Health Systems. (2020). Standard 15.01.16. *Healthcare Facilities Accreditation Program: Accreditation requirements for acute care hospitals.* Chicago, IL: Accreditation Association for Hospitals and Health Systems. (Level VII)

19 DNV GL-Healthcare USA, Inc. (2020). PR.2.SR.5. *NIAHO® accreditation requirements, interpretive guidelines and surveyor guidance—revision 20.0.* Milford, OH: DNV GL-Healthcare USA, Inc. (Level VII)

20 The Joint Commission. (2021). Standard PC.02.01.21. *Comprehensive accreditation manual for hospitals.* Oakbrook Terrace, IL: The Joint Commission. (Level VII)

21 Waters, T. R., et al. (2009). Safe patient handling training for schools of nursing. https://www.cdc.gov/niosh/docs/2009-127/pdfs/2009-127.pdf (Level VII)

22 Standard 39. Joint stabilization. Infusion therapy standards of practice (8th ed.). (2021). *Journal of Infusion Nursing, 44*, S111–S112. (Level VII)

23 American Association of Critical-Care Nurses (AACN). (2016). AACN practice alert: PA/CVP monitoring in adults. https://www.aacn.org/clinical-resources/practice-alerts/pulmonary-artery-pressure-measurement (Level VII)

24 The Joint Commission. (2013). Sentinel event alert 50: Medical device alarm safety in hospitals. https://www.jointcommission.org/assets/1/6/SEA_50_alarms_4_26_16.pdf (Level VII)

25 The Joint Commission. (2021). Standard NPSG.06.01.01. *Comprehensive accreditation manual for hospitals.* Oakbrook Terrace, IL: The Joint Commission. (Level VII)

26 Graham, K. C., & Cvach, M. (2010). Monitor alarm fatigue: Standardizing use of physiological monitors and decreasing nuisance alarms. *American Journal of Critical Care, 19*, 28–37.

27 Ganz, D. A., et al. (2013, reviewed 2021). Preventing falls in hospitals: A toolkit for improving quality of care (AHRQ Publication No. 13-0015-EF). Rockville, MD: Agency for Healthcare Research and Quality. https://www.ahrq.gov/professionals/systems/hospital/fallpxtoolkit/index.html (Level VII)

28 The Joint Commission. (2021). Standard RC.01.03.01. *Comprehensive accreditation manual for hospitals.* Oakbrook Terrace, IL: The Joint Commission. (Level VII)

29 Centers for Medicare and Medicaid Services, Department of Health and Human Services. (2020). Condition of participation: Medical record services. 42 C.F.R. § 482.24(b).

30 Accreditation Association for Hospitals and Health Systems. (2020). Standard 10.00.03. *Healthcare Facilities Accreditation Program: Accreditation requirements for acute care hospitals.* Chicago, IL: Accreditation Association for Hospitals and Health Systems. (Level VII)

31 DNV GL-Healthcare USA, Inc. (2020). MR.2.SR.1. *NIAHO® accreditation requirements, interpretive guidelines and surveyor guidance—revision 20.0.* Milford, OH: DNV GL-Healthcare USA, Inc. (Level VII)

32 Standard 10. Documentation in the health record. Infusion therapy standards of practice (8th ed.). (2021). *Journal of Infusion Nursing, 44*, S39–S41. (Level VII)

33 Standard 43. Administration set management. Infusion therapy standards of practice (8th ed.). (2021). *Journal of Infusion Nursing, 44*, S123–S125. (Level VII)

34 Standard 42. Vascular access device assessment, care and dressing changes. Infusion therapy standards of practice (8th ed.). (2021). *Journal of Infusion Nursing, 44*, S119–S123. (Level VII)

ARTERIAL PUNCTURE FOR BLOOD GAS ANALYSIS

Arterial blood gas (ABG) analysis evaluates ventilation by measuring blood pH and the partial pressures of arterial oxygen (Pao_2) and carbon dioxide ($Paco_2$). Blood pH measurement reveals the blood's acid-base balance, Pao_2 indicates the amount of oxygen in the blood, and $Paco_2$ indicates the lungs' capacity to eliminate carbon dioxide. ABG samples can also be analyzed for total hemoglobin, oxygen saturation, saturation of dyshemoglobins, bicarbonate values, and base excess or deficit.[1] Obtaining an arterial blood sample requires percutaneous puncture of the brachial, radial, or femoral artery or withdrawal of a sample from an arterial line.

Typically, the practitioner orders ABG analysis when respiratory distress or failure is suspected. It's also performed during episodes of shock, after coronary artery bypass surgery, after resuscitation from cardiac arrest, after changes in respiratory therapy or status, during administration of oxygen or mechanical ventilation therapies, after acute kidney injury, and during prolonged anesthesia.[2]

Most ABG samples can be drawn by a respiratory therapist or specially trained nurse; however, collection from the femoral artery is usually performed by a practitioner. The radial artery is the preferred site because it is small and easy to stabilize.[2,3]

Equipment

Preheparinized ABG plastic Luer-lock syringe specially made for drawing blood for ABG analysis ■ 20G to 25G 1″ to 1½″ (2.5-cm to 3.8-cm) needle ■ gloves ■ antiseptic pad or swab (alcohol, chlorhexidine, or povidone-iodine)[3,4,5] ■ two 2″ × 2″ (5-cm × 5-cm) gauze pads ■ rubber cap for syringe hub ■ laboratory biohazard transport bag ■ label ■ small towel ■ adhesive bandage ■ Optional: mask and goggles or mask with face shield, gown, sterile gloves, 1% lidocaine solution without epinephrine or eutectic mixture of local anesthetics cream, 1-mL syringe with 22G needle, 1-mL ampule of aqueous heparin (1:1,000), plastic bag, crushed ice, Doppler ultrasound device, pulse oximeter, laboratory request form, soap, water, washcloth, towel.

Many health care facilities use a commercial ABG kit that contains some of the equipment listed above.

Preparation of equipment

If time allows, administer local anesthetic cream at least 1 hour before the procedure, *because it requires at least 1 hour to achieve its effect.*[6,7,8,9]

Inspect all equipment and supplies. If a product is expired, is defective, or has compromised integrity, remove it from patient use, label it as expired or defective, and report the expiration or defect, as directed by your facility.

Open the ABG kit and remove the sample label and the plastic bag. If the syringe isn't heparinized, you will have to heparinize it *to prevent the sample from clotting.* To do so, first attach the 22G needle to the syringe. Then open the ampule of heparin. Draw all the heparin into the syringe. Hold the syringe upright, and rotate the barrel while pulling the plunger back *to allow the heparin to coat the entire inside surface of the syringe.* Then slowly force the heparin toward the hub of the syringe, and expel all of the heparin.

ABG analysis should be performed within 10 minutes of obtaining the blood sample.[10,11] Fill a plastic bag with enough crushed ice to contain the syringe if you anticipate a delay in analysis.[10]

Implementation

■ Verify the practitioner's order.
■ Review the patient's medical record for current anticoagulation therapy, clotting disorders, and pertinent laboratory values *to determine the patient's risk of prolonged bleeding after the procedure.* Discuss any concerns with the patient's practitioner.
■ Review the patient's medical record for a history of allergies, such as to lidocaine, antiseptics, or tape.[2]

■ Confirm steady state conditions *to ensure accurate test results.* If the patient is receiving oxygen, make sure that this therapy has been underway for 20 to 30 minutes before collecting an arterial sample.[2] If the patient has received a nebulizer treatment, wait 20 minutes before collecting the sample. If the patient recently underwent suctioning or was placed on mechanical ventilation or the fraction of inspired oxygen (Fio_2) concentration has been changed, wait at least 15 minutes before collecting a blood sample.[4,10]
■ Gather and prepare the necessary equipment and supplies.
■ Perform hand hygiene.[7,8,9,10,11,12]

Performing the modified Allen test

The modified Allen test is a collateral circulation test performed to assess whether ulnar collateral blood flow is sufficient to allow for puncture of the radial artery. To perform the modified Allen test, position the patient with the wrist extended about 30 degrees. Place a rolled towel under the wrist to provide support. Instruct the patient to clench the fist. Occlude the radial and ulnar arteries with your index and middle fingers while the patient's fist remains clenched. Then ask the patient to slowly unclench the fist. The palm will be blanched from the lack of arterial blood flow, as shown below.

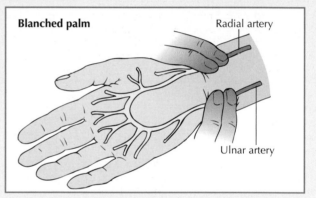

Blanched palm — Radial artery — Ulnar artery

Release the pressure on the patient's ulnar artery. If the patient's hand becomes immediately flushed, indicating that the arterial circulation has resumed, you can safely proceed with radial artery puncture at that site. If the hand doesn't appear flushed, the test is negative, indicating that circulation is inadequate; you'll need to select an alternative puncture site, such as the other radial artery or a brachial artery.[3] If you choose the other radial artery, you'll need to perform the modified Allen test before proceeding. If both radial sites are inadequate, consider using the femoral artery, if permitted by your facility.[3] If the patient is unable to cooperate with the modified Allen test, assess circulation manually with the help of an assistant.

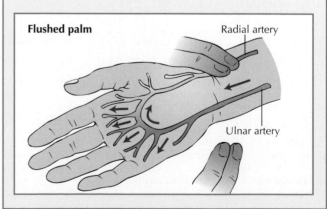

Flushed palm — Radial artery — Ulnar artery

- Confirm the patient's identity using at least two patient identifiers.[13]
- Provide privacy.[14,15,16,17]
- Explain the procedure to the patient and family (if appropriate) according to their individual communication and learning needs *to increase their understanding, allay their fears, and enhance cooperation.*[18] Tell the patient that the needle stick will cause some discomfort but that the patient must remain still during the procedure.
- Raise the bed to waist level before providing care *to prevent caregiver back strain.*[24]
- Perform hand hygiene.[12,13,14,15,16,17]
- Assess the radial pulse in both wrists *to determine the best site from which to draw the specimen.*
- Assess circulation to the patient's hand by assessing the radial and ulnar pulses or by performing the Allen test, pulse oximetry, or a Doppler flow study as directed by your facility.[2,25] Be aware that recent research questions the validity of performing a modified Allen test.[26,27,28] If the test is negative, do not use the radial artery; instead, select another site.[4] (See *Performing the modified Allen Test.*)
- Position the patient and place a rolled towel under the patient's wrist for support, if one is not already present. Once you have identified a site, note anatomic landmarks to be able to find the site again.[3]
- If visibly soiled, clean the intended puncture site with soap and water and then dry it with a towel.
- Perform hand hygiene.[12,13,14,15,16,17]
- Put on gloves and, as needed, a gown and a mask and goggles or a mask with face shield *to comply with standard precautions.*[3,29,30,31]
- If indicated and ordered, administer a local anesthetic, such as lidocaine, following safe medication administration practices.[6,7,8,9] Consider the use of lidocaine carefully *because the patient might be allergic to the drug.*[32] To administer lidocaine, draw up 0.5 mL of 1% lidocaine into a 1-mL syringe with a 25G needle. Disinfect the site with an antiseptic pad and then allow it to dry. Inject 0.2 to 0.3 mL intradermally around the artery. Wait for the anesthetic to take effect.
- Clean the intended puncture site with an antiseptic pad or swab [3,4,5] according to the manufacturer's recommendations and then allow it to dry completely.[2,5]
- Stabilize the artery with the index and middle fingers of your nondominant hand while holding the syringe over the puncture site with the other hand. If you need to palpate the site again, put on sterile gloves.[2,3,25]
- Hold the needle bevel up at a 30- to 60-degree angle (as shown below).[2]

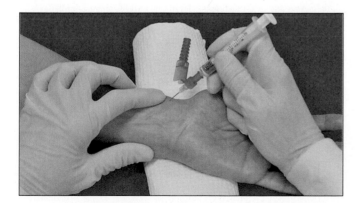

- Puncture the skin and the arterial wall in one motion, following the path of the artery.
- Watch for blood backflow in the syringe. Don't pull back on the plunger, *because arterial blood should enter the syringe automatically.* Obtain 1 mL of blood.
- Withdraw the needle while stabilizing the syringe.
- Press a gauze pad firmly over the puncture site for 5 minutes or until the bleeding stops. If the patient is receiving anticoagulant therapy or has a blood dyscrasia, apply pressure for 10 to 15 minutes; [2] if necessary, ask a coworker to hold the gauze pad in place while you prepare the sample for transport to the laboratory. Don't ask the patient to hold the pad *because failure to apply sufficient pressure can lead to formation of a painful hematoma, hindering future arterial punctures at that site.*
- Check the syringe for air bubbles. If any appear, remove them by holding the syringe upright and slowly ejecting some of the blood onto a 2″ × 2″ (5-cm × 5-cm) gauze pad *to prevent alteration of the test results.*[1]
- Use the syringe safety device to cover the needle, and then remove the needle and place a rubber cap directly on the syringe tip *to prevent the sample from leaking and to keep air out of the syringe.*
- Gently roll the syringe in your hands for 30 seconds *to mix the heparin, which prevents the sample from clotting.*[2]
- Label the syringe in the presence of the patient *to prevent mislabeling.*[18] The label should contain the patient's full name, another patient identifier (such as the patient's date of birth or medical record number), the date and time you collected the sample, and the measured FIO_2 or supplemental oxygen liter flow.[1]
- Put the labeled sample in the laboratory biohazard transport bag,[31] and attach a properly completed laboratory request form (if required by your facility), and immediately send the sample to the laboratory.[1,33] If the sample can't be sent to the laboratory immediately, put it on ice.[10,33]
- When the bleeding stops, apply a small adhesive bandage to the site.
- Monitor the patient for signs of circulatory impairment, such as swelling, discoloration, pain, numbness, and tingling in the arm or leg. Also watch for bleeding at the puncture site.
- Return the bed to the lowest position *to prevent falls and maintain patient safety.*[34]
- Discard used equipment in the appropriate receptacles.[31]
- Remove and discard your gloves and other personal protective equipment, if worn.
- Perform hand hygiene.[12,13,14,15,16,17]
- Document the procedure.[35,36,37,38]

Special considerations

- Chilling the sample extends the time to test the sample for up to 1 hour; if more than an hour has elapsed since collection, discard the sample.[4,10,33]
- Unless ordered, don't turn off existing oxygen therapy before collecting an arterial blood sample.
- Be sure to indicate on the laboratory request slip the amount and type of oxygen therapy the patient is receiving. If the patient isn't receiving oxygen, indicate that the patient is breathing room air.

Complications

If you use too much force when attempting to puncture an artery, the needle may touch the periosteum of the bone, causing the patient considerable pain. You may inadvertently advance the needle through the opposite wall of the artery. If this happens, slowly pull the needle back a short distance and check to see if you obtain blood return. If blood still fails to enter the syringe, withdraw the needle completely and attempt the puncture with a new needle and syringe. Don't make more than two attempts to withdraw blood from the same site. *Probing the artery may injure it and the radial nerve. Also, hemolysis will occur, altering test results.*

If arterial spasm occurs, blood won't flow into the syringe and you won't be able to collect the sample. If this happens, replace the needle with a smaller one and try the puncture again, *because a smaller-bore needle is less likely to cause arterial spasm.*

Documentation

Record the results of the modified Allen test, the time the sample was drawn, the patient's temperature, the site of the arterial puncture, the amount of time that pressure was applied to the site to control bleeding by you or a co-worker, and the type and amount of oxygen therapy the patient was receiving. Also document specific site preparation, the type and amount of local anesthetic administered (if used), the size of the needle used, and the number of attempts.[39] Document teaching you provided to the patient and family (if applicable), their understanding of that teaching, and any need for follow-up teaching.

REFERENCES

1 American Association for Respiratory Care (AARC). (2013). AARC clinical practice guideline: Blood gas analysis and hemoximetry 2013. *Respiratory Care, 58,* 1694–1703. http://rc.rcjournal.com/content/respcare/58/10/1694.full.pdf (Level VII)

2 Wiegand, D. L. (2017). *AACN procedure manual for high acuity, progressive, and critical care* (7th ed.). St. Louis, MO: Elsevier.

3 World Health Organization (2010). WHO guidelines on drawing blood: Best practices in phlebotomy. https://apps.who.int/iris/bitstream/handle/10665/44294/9789241599221_eng.pdf (Level IV)

4 Kacmarek, R. M., et al. (2021). *Egan's fundamentals of respiratory care* (12th ed.). St Louis, MO: Mosby.

5 Centers for Disease Control and Prevention. (2011, revised 2017). Guidelines for the prevention of intravascular catheter-related infections. https://www.cdc.gov/infectioncontrol/guidelines/bsi/recommendations.html (Level I)

6 The Joint Commission. (2021). Standard MM.06.01.01. *Comprehensive accreditation manual for hospitals.* Oakbrook Terrace, IL: The Joint Commission. (Level VII)

7 Centers for Medicare and Medicaid Services, Department of Health and Human Services. (2020). Condition of participation: Nursing services. 42 C.F.R. § 482.23(c).

8 Accreditation Association for Hospitals and Health Systems. (2020). Standard 16.01.03. *Healthcare Facilities Accreditation Program: Accreditation requirements for acute care hospitals.* Chicago, IL: Accreditation Association for Hospitals and Health Systems. (Level VII)

9 DNV GL-Healthcare USA, Inc. (2020). MM.1.SR.3. *NIAHO® accreditation requirements, interpretive guidelines and surveyor guidance—revision 20.0.* Milford, OH: DNV GL-Healthcare USA, Inc. (Level VII)

10 Fischbach, F., & Fischbach, M. A. (2018). *A manual of laboratory and diagnostic tests* (10th ed.). Philadelphia, PA: Wolters Kluwer.

11 Wan, X. Y., et al. (2018). Effects of time delay and body temperature on measurements of central venous oxygen saturation, venous-arterial blood carbon dioxide partial pressures difference, venous-arterial blood carbon dioxide partial pressures difference/arterial-venous oxygen difference ratio and lactate. *BMC Anesthesiology, 18,* 187. https://www.ncbi.nlm.nih.gov/pmc/articles/PMC6290537/(Level III)

12 Centers for Disease Control and Prevention. (2002). Guideline for hand hygiene in health-care settings: Recommendations of the Healthcare Infection Control Practices Advisory Committee and the HICPAC/SHEA/APIC/IDSA Hand Hygiene Task Force. *MMWR Recommendations and Reports, 51*(RR-16), 1–45. https://www.cdc.gov/mmwr/pdf/rr/rr5116.pdf (Level II)

13 The Joint Commission. (2021). Standard NPSG.07.01.01. *Comprehensive accreditation manual for hospitals.* Oakbrook Terrace, IL: The Joint Commission. (Level VII)

14 World Health Organization. (2009). WHO guidelines on hand hygiene in health care: First global patient safety challenge, clean care is safer care https://apps.who.int/iris/bitstream/handle/10665/44102/9789241597906_eng.pdf?sequence=1 (Level IV)

15 Centers for Medicare and Medicaid Services, Department of Health and Human Services. (2020). Condition of participation: Infection control. 42 C.F.R. § 482.42.

16 Accreditation Association for Hospitals and Health Systems. (2020). Standard 07.01.21. *Healthcare Facilities Accreditation Program: Accreditation requirements for acute care hospitals.* Chicago, IL: Accreditation Association for Hospitals and Health Systems. (Level VII)

17 DNV GL-Healthcare USA, Inc. (2020). IC.1.SR.1. *NIAHO® accreditation requirements, interpretive guidelines and surveyor guidance—revision 20.0.* Milford, OH: DNV GL-Healthcare USA, Inc. (Level VII)

18 The Joint Commission. (2021). Standard NPSG.01.01.01. *Comprehensive accreditation manual for hospitals.* Oakbrook Terrace, IL: The Joint Commission. (Level VII)

19 Accreditation Association for Hospitals and Health Systems. (2020). Standard 15.01.16. *Healthcare Facilities Accreditation Program: Accreditation requirements for acute care hospitals.* Chicago, IL: Accreditation Association for Hospitals and Health Systems. (Level VII)

20 Centers for Medicare and Medicaid Services, Department of Health and Human Services. (2020). Condition of participation: Patient's rights. 42 C.F.R. § 482.13(c)(1).

21 The Joint Commission. (2021). Standard RI.01.03.01. *Comprehensive accreditation manual for hospitals.* Oakbrook Terrace, IL: The Joint Commission. (Level VII)

22 DNV GL-Healthcare USA, Inc. (2020). PR.2.SR.5. *NIAHO® accreditation requirements, interpretive guidelines and surveyor guidance—revision 20.0.* Milford, OH: DNV GL-Healthcare USA, Inc. (Level VII)

23 The Joint Commission. (2021). Standard PC.02.01.21. *Comprehensive accreditation manual for hospitals.* Oakbrook Terrace, IL: The Joint Commission. (Level VII)

24 Waters, T. R., et al. (2009). Safe patient handling training for schools of nursing. https://www.cdc.gov/niosh/docs/2009-127/pdfs/2009-127.pdf (Level VII)

25 Standard 44. Blood sampling. Infusion therapy standards of practice (8th ed.). (2021). *Journal of Infusion Nursing, 44,* S125–S133. (Level VII)

26 Romeu-Bordas, Ó., & Ballesteros-Peña, S. (2017). Reliability and validity of the modified Allen test: A systematic review and meta-analysis. *Emergencias, 29,* 126–135. http://emergencias.portalsemes.org/descargar/validez-y-fiabilidad-del-test-modificado-de-allen-una-revisin-sistemtica-y-metanlisis/ (Level I)

27 Valgimigli, M. C. (2014). Transradial coronary catheterization and intervention across the whole spectrum of Allen test results. *Journal of the American College of Cardiology, 63,* 1833–1841. (Level VI)

28 Bertrand, O. F., et al. (2014). Allen or no Allen; That is the question! *Journal of American College of Cardiology, 63,* 1842–1844. (Level V)

29 Siegel, J. D., et al. (2007, revised 2019). 2007 guideline for isolation precautions: Preventing transmission of infectious agents in healthcare settings. https://www.cdc.gov/infectioncontrol/pdf/guidelines/isolation-guidelines-H.pdf (Level II)

30 Accreditation Association for Hospitals and Health Systems. (2020). Standard 07.01.10. *Healthcare Facilities Accreditation Program: Accreditation requirements for acute care hospitals.* Chicago, IL: Accreditation Association for Hospitals and Health Systems. (Level VII)

31 Occupational Safety and Health Administration. (2012). Bloodborne pathogens, standard number 1910.1030. https://www.osha.gov/pls/oshaweb/owadisp.show_document?p_id=10051&p_table=STANDARDS (Level VII)

32 Fresenius Kabi USA, LLC. (2018). Xylocaine (lidocaine HCl injection, USP) https://www.accessdata.fda.gov/drugsatfda_docs/label/2018/006488s097lbl.pdf

33 Mohammadhoseini, E., et al. (2015). Effect of sample storage temperature and time delay on blood gases, bicarbonate and pH in human arterial blood samples. *Iran Red Crescent Medical Journal, 17*(3), e13577. https://www.ncbi.nlm.nih.gov/pmc/articles/PMC4441774/ (Level V)

34 Ganz, D. A., et al. (2013, reviewed 2021). Preventing falls in hospitals: A toolkit for improving quality of care (AHRQ Publication No. 13-0015-EF). https://www.ahrq.gov/professionals/systems/hospital/fallpxtoolkit/index.html (Level VII)

35 The Joint Commission. (2021). Standard RC.01.03.01. *Comprehensive accreditation manual for hospitals.* Oakbrook Terrace, IL: The Joint Commission. (Level VII)

36 Centers for Medicare and Medicaid Services, Department of Health and Human Services. (2020). Condition of participation: Medical record services. 42 C.F.R. § 482.24.

37 Accreditation Association for Hospitals and Health Systems. (2020). Standard 10.00.03. *Healthcare Facilities Accreditation Program: Accreditation requirements for acute care hospitals.* Chicago, IL: Accreditation Association for Hospitals and Health Systems. (Level VII)

38 DNV GL-Healthcare USA, Inc. (2020). MR.2.SR.1. *NIAHO® accreditation requirements, interpretive guidelines and surveyor guidance—revision 20.0.* Milford, OH: DNV GL-Healthcare USA, Inc. (Level VII)

39 Standard 10. Documentation in the health record. Infusion therapy standards of practice (8th ed.). (2021). *Journal of Infusion Nursing, 44,* S39–S42. (Level VII)

Assessment techniques

A physical assessment involves four basic techniques: inspection, palpation, percussion, and auscultation.[1] Performing these techniques correctly helps elicit valuable information about a patient's condition.

Inspection requires the use of vision to observe the details of the patient's appearance, behavior, and movement.[2] Special lighting and various pieces of equipment—such as an otoscope, a tongue blade, and an ophthalmoscope—may be used to enhance vision or examine an otherwise hidden area. Inspection begins during the first patient contact and continues throughout the assessment.[1]

Palpation usually follows inspection, except when examining the abdomen or assessing infants and children.[1] Palpation involves touching the body to determine the size, shape, and position of structures; to detect and evaluate temperature, pulsations, and other movement; and to elicit tenderness.[1] The four palpation techniques include light palpation, deep palpation, light ballottement, and deep ballottement. Ballottement is used to evaluate a flowing or movable structure. It involves applying pressure against the structure you're assessing and then waiting to feel it rebound. This technique may be used, for example, to check the position of an organ or a fetus.

Percussion involves a quick, sharp tapping of the fingers or hands against body surfaces to produce sounds, detect tenderness, or assess reflexes.[1] Percussing for sound helps locate organ borders, identify organ shape and position, and determine whether an organ is solid or filled with fluid or gas. Organs and tissues produce sounds of varying loudness, pitch, and duration, depending on their density. For example, air-filled cavities such as the lungs produce markedly different sounds from those produced by the liver and other dense organs and tissues. Percussion techniques include indirect percussion, direct percussion, and blunt percussion.

Auscultation involves listening to various sounds of the body—particularly those produced by the heart, lungs, vessels, stomach, and intestines using a stethoscope. Most auscultated sounds result from the movement of air or fluid through these structures.[1]

Auscultation is usually performed after the other assessment techniques. When examining the abdomen, however, auscultation should occur after inspection but before percussion and palpation, which can alter bowel sounds. Auscultation is also best performed first on infants and young children, who may start to cry when palpated or percussed. Auscultation is most successful when performed in a quiet environment with a properly fitted stethoscope.[1]

Equipment

Flashlight or gooseneck lamp ▪ patient drape ▪ stethoscope ▪ disinfectant pad ▪ Optional: gloves.

Preparation of equipment

Inspect all equipment and supplies. If a product is expired, is defective, or has compromised integrity, remove it from patient use, label it as expired or defective, and report the expiration or defect as directed by your facility.

Implementation

▪ Gather all of the necessary equipment and supplies.
▪ Perform hand hygiene.[3,4,5,6,7,8]
▪ Confirm the patient's identity using at least two patient identifiers.[9]
▪ Provide privacy.[10,11,12,13]
▪ Explain all aspects of the procedure to the patient and family (if appropriate) according to their individual communication and learning needs *to increase their understanding, allay their fears, and enhance cooperation.*[14]
▪ Raise the bed to waist level before providing care *to prevent caregiver back strain.*[15]
▪ Ask the patient to undress, and then drape the patient appropriately.[1]
▪ Make sure the room is warm and adequately lit *to make the patient comfortable and aid visual inspection.*
▪ Warm your hands and the stethoscope.
▪ Perform hand hygiene.[3,4,5,6,7,8]
▪ Put on gloves if needed *to comply with standard precautions.*[16,17,18]

Inspection
▪ Use your eyes to observe the patient. Pay close attention to the details of the patient's appearance, behavior, and movement, such as facial expressions, mood, physique, and conditioning.[2] Focus on areas related to the patient's reason for seeking care.

▪ To inspect a specific body area, first make sure the area is sufficiently exposed. Survey the entire area, noting key landmarks and checking its overall condition. Focus on specifics—color, shape, texture, size, and movement. Note unusual findings as well as predictable ones.

Palpation
▪ Tell the patient what to expect, such as occasional discomfort as you apply pressure. Encourage the patient to relax, *because muscle tension and guarding can interfere with performance and results of palpation.*
▪ Provide just enough pressure to assess the tissue beneath one or both hands. Then release pressure and gently move to the next area, systematically covering the entire surface to be assessed. (See *Performing palpation,* page 40.)
▪ Use both hands (bimanual palpation) to trap a deep, underlying, hard-to-palpate organ (such as the kidney or spleen) or to fix or stabilize an organ (such as the uterus) with one hand while you palpate it with the other.

Percussion
▪ First, decide which of the percussion techniques best suits your assessment needs. Indirect percussion helps reveal the size and density of underlying thoracic and abdominal organs and tissues. Direct percussion helps assess an adult's sinuses for tenderness and elicits sounds in a child's thorax. Blunt percussion aims to elicit tenderness over organs, such as the kidneys, gallbladder, or liver. When percussing, note the characteristic sounds produced. (See *Identifying percussion sounds,* page 40.)
▪ To perform indirect percussion, place one hand on the patient and tap the middle finger with the middle finger of the other hand. (See *Performing indirect percussion,* page 41.)
▪ To perform direct percussion, tap your hand or fingertip directly against the body surface.
▪ To perform blunt percussion, strike the ulnar surface of your fist against the body surface. Alternatively, place the palm of one hand against the body, make a fist with the other hand, and strike the back of the first hand.

Auscultation
▪ First, determine whether to use the diaphragm or bell of the stethoscope. Use the diaphragm to detect high pitched sounds, such as breath and bowel sounds.[1] Keep in mind that bowel sounds shouldn't be described as absent until no sound is heard for 5 minutes.[20] Use the bell to detect lower-pitched sounds, such as heart and vascular sounds.[1]
▪ Place the diaphragm or bell of the stethoscope over the appropriate area of the patient's body and place the earpieces in your ears.
▪ Listen intently to individual sounds and try to identify their characteristics. Determine the intensity, pitch, and duration of each sound, and check the frequency of recurring sounds.

Completing the procedure
▪ Return the bed to the lowest position *to prevent falls and maintain the patient's safety.*[21]
▪ Remove and discard your gloves, if worn,[18] and perform hand hygiene.[3,4,5,6,7,8]
▪ Clean and disinfect your stethoscope using a disinfectant pad.[22,23]
▪ Perform hand hygiene.[3,4,5,6,7,8]
▪ Document the procedure.[24,25,26,27]

Special considerations
▪ Avoid palpating or percussing an area of the body known to be tender at the start of your examination. Instead, work around the area, and then gently palpate or percuss it at the end of the examination. *This progression minimizes the patient's discomfort and apprehension.*
▪ *To pinpoint an inflamed area deep within the patient's body,* perform a variation on deep palpation: Press firmly with one hand over the area you suspect is involved, and then lift your hand away quickly. If the patient reports that pain increases when you release the pressure, then you've identified rebound tenderness.[28]

Performing palpation

You should be familiar with four palpation techniques: light palpation, deep palpation, light ballottement, and deep ballottement. Remember to use the flattened finger pads for palpating tender tissues, feeling for crepitus (crackling) at the joints, and lightly probing the abdomen. Use the thumb and index finger for assessing hair texture, grasping tissues, and feeling for lymph node enlargement. Use the back, or dorsal, surface of the hand when feeling for warmth.

Light palpation

With the tips of two or three fingers held close together, depress the skin, indenting ½" (1.3 cm). Use the lightest touch possible, *because too much pressure blunts your sensitivity*.[19]

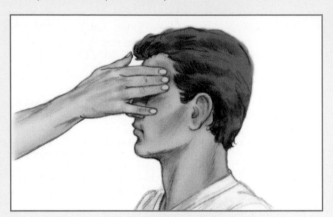

Deep palpation (bimanual palpation)

If the patient tolerates light palpation and you need to assess deeper structures, palpate deeply by increasing your fingertip pressure, indenting the skin about ¾" to 1½" (2 to 3.8 cm). Place your other hand on top of the palpating hand (as shown below), *to control and guide your movements*.[16]

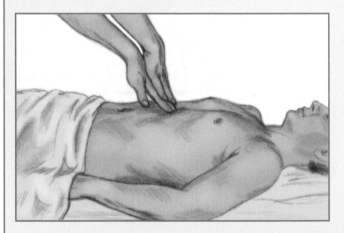

Light ballottement

Apply light, rapid pressure to the abdomen, moving from one quadrant to another. Keep your hand on the skin surface *to detect tissue rebound*.

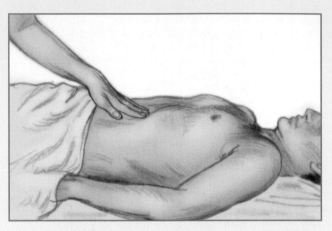

Deep ballottement

Apply abrupt, deep pressure on the patient's abdomen. Release the pressure completely, but maintain fingertip contact with the skin *to detect tissue rebound*.

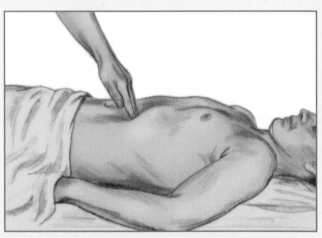

Identifying percussion sounds

Percussion produces sounds that vary according to the tissue being percussed. This chart lists important percussion sounds along with their characteristics and typical sources.

SOUND	INTENSITY	PITCH	DURATION	QUALITY	SOURCE
Resonance	Moderate to loud	Low	Long	Hollow	Normal lung
Tympany	Loud	High	Moderate	Drumlike	Gastric air bubble, intestinal air
Dullness	Soft to moderate	High	Moderate	Thudlike	Liver, full bladder, pregnant uterus
Hyperresonance	Very loud	Very low	Long	Booming	Hyperinflated lung (as in emphysema)
Flatness	Soft	High	Short	Flat	Muscle

Performing indirect percussion

To perform indirect percussion, place your nondominant hand firmly against the patient's body surface. With your wrist flexed loosely, use the middle finger of your dominant hand to tap the middle finger beneath the distal joint of your nondominant hand (as shown). Tap lightly and quickly, removing your dominant middle finger as soon as you deliver each tap. Move your nondominant hand and repeat the procedure, coving the entire area to be percussed.

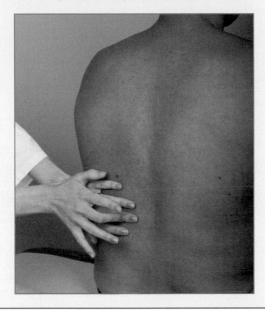

NURSING ALERT Suspect peritonitis if you elicit rebound tenderness when examining the abdomen.[28]

■ If you can't palpate because the patient fears pain, try distracting the patient with conversation. Then perform auscultation and gently press your stethoscope into the affected area *to try to elicit tenderness.*

Complications

Palpation may cause an enlarged spleen or infected appendix to rupture.

Documentation

Document your assessment findings and the technique used to elicit each finding—for example, "Right lower quadrant tenderness on deep palpation, no rebound tenderness." Indicate the practitioner notified of any abnormal findings and the time of the notification. Document interventions required to treat those findings as well as the patient's response to those interventions. Document teaching provided to the patient and family (if applicable), their understanding of that teaching, and any need for follow-up teaching.

REFERENCES

1 Craven, R. F., et al. (2021). *Fundamentals of nursing: Concepts and competencies for practice.* (9th ed.). Philadelphia, PA: Wolters Kluwer.

2 Bickley, L. et al. (2021). *Bates' guide to physical examination and health history taking* (13th ed.). Philadelphia, PA: Wolters Kluwer.

3 The Joint Commission. (2021). Standard NPSG.07.01.01. *Comprehensive accreditation manual for hospitals.* Oakbrook Terrace, IL: The Joint Commission. (Level VII)

4 Centers for Disease Control and Prevention. (2002). Guideline for hand hygiene in health-care settings: Recommendations of the Healthcare Infection Control Practices Advisory Committee and the HICPAC/SHEA/APIC/IDSA Hand Hygiene Task Force. *MMWR Recommendations and Reports, 51*(RR-16), 1–45. https://www.cdc.gov/mmwr/pdf/rr/rr5116.pdf (Level II)

5 World Health Organization. (2009). WHO guidelines on hand hygiene in health care: First global patient safety challenge, clean care is safer care. https://apps.who.int/iris/bitstream/handle/10665/44102/9789241597906_eng.pdf?sequence=1 (Level IV)

6 Centers for Medicare and Medicaid Services, Department of Health and Human Services. (2020). Condition of participation: Infection control. 42 C.F.R. § 482.42.

7 Accreditation Association for Hospitals and Health Systems. (2020). Standard 07.01.21. *Healthcare Facilities Accreditation Program: Accreditation requirements for acute care hospitals.* Chicago, IL: Accreditation Association for Hospitals and Health Systems. (Level VII)

8 DNV GL-Healthcare USA, Inc. (2020). IC.1.SR.1. *NIAHO® accreditation requirements, interpretive guidelines and surveyor guidance—revision 20.0.* Milford, OH: DNV GL-Healthcare USA, Inc. (Level VII)

9 The Joint Commission. (2021). Standard NPSG.01.01.01. *Comprehensive accreditation manual for hospitals.* Oakbrook Terrace, IL: The Joint Commission. (Level VII)

10 Centers for Medicare and Medicaid Services, Department of Health and Human Services. (2020). Condition of participation: Patient's rights. 42 C.F.R. § 482.13(c)(1).

11 Accreditation Association for Hospitals and Health Systems. (2020). Standard 15.01.16. *Healthcare Facilities Accreditation Program: Accreditation requirements for acute care hospitals.* Chicago, IL: Accreditation Association for Hospitals and Health Systems. (Level VII)

12 The Joint Commission. (2021). Standard RI.01.01.01. *Comprehensive accreditation manual for hospitals.* Oakbrook Terrace, IL: The Joint Commission. (Level VII)

13 DNV GL-Healthcare USA, Inc. (2020). PR.2.SR.5. *NIAHO® accreditation requirements, interpretive guidelines and surveyor guidance—revision 20.0.* Milford, OH: DNV GL-Healthcare USA, Inc. (Level VII)

14 The Joint Commission. (2021). Standard PC.02.01.21. *Comprehensive accreditation manual for hospitals.* Oakbrook Terrace, IL: The Joint Commission. (Level VII)

15 Waters, T. R., et al. (2009). Safe patient handling training for schools of nursing. Accessed June 2021 via the Web at https://www.cdc.gov/niosh/docs/2009-127/pdfs/2009-127.pdf (Level VII)

16 Siegel, J. D., et al. (2007, revised 2019). 2007 guideline for isolation precautions: Preventing transmission of infectious agents in healthcare settings. https://www.cdc.gov/infectioncontrol/pdf/guidelines/isolation-guidelines-H.pdf (Level II)

17 Accreditation Association for Hospitals and Health Systems. (2020). Standard 07.01.10. *Healthcare Facilities Accreditation Program: Accreditation requirements for acute care hospitals.* Chicago, IL: Accreditation Association for Hospitals and Health Systems. (Level VII)

18 Occupational Safety and Health Administration. (2012). Bloodborne pathogens, standard number 1910.1030. https://www.osha.gov/pls/oshaweb/owadisp.show_document?p_id=10051&p_table=STANDARDS (Level VII)

19 Jensen, S. (2019). *Nursing health assessment: A best practice approach,* (3rd ed.). Philadelphia, PA: Wolters Kluwer.

20 Craven, H. (Ed.). (2016). *Core curriculum for medical-surgical nursing* (5th ed.). Pitman, NJ: Academy of Medical-Surgical Nurses.

21 Ganz, D. A., et al. (2013, Reviewed 2021). Preventing falls in hospitals: A toolkit for improving quality of care (AHRQ Publication No. 13-0015-EF). Rockville, MD: Agency for Healthcare Research and Quality. https://www.ahrq.gov/professionals/systems/hospital/fallpxtoolkit/index.html (Level VII)

22 Rutala, W. A., et al. (2008, revised 2019). Guideline for disinfection and sterilization in healthcare facilities, 2008 https://www.cdc.gov/infection-control/pdf/guidelines/disinfection-guidelines-H.pdf (Level I)

23 Accreditation Association for Hospitals and Health Systems. (2020). Standard 07.02.03. *Healthcare Facilities Accreditation Program: Accreditation requirements for acute care hospitals.* Chicago, IL: Accreditation Association for Hospitals and Health Systems. (Level VII)

24 The Joint Commission. (2021). Standard RC.01.03.01. *Comprehensive accreditation manual for hospitals.* Oakbrook Terrace, IL: The Joint Commission. (Level VII)

25 Centers for Medicare and Medicaid Services, Department of Health and Human Services. (2020). Condition of participation: Medical record services. 42 C.F.R. § 482.24(b).

26 Accreditation Association for Hospitals and Health Systems. (2020). Standard 10.00.03. *Healthcare Facilities Accreditation Program: Accreditation requirements for acute care hospitals.* Chicago, IL: Accreditation Association for Hospitals and Health Systems. (Level VII)

27 DNV GL-Healthcare USA, Inc. (2020). MR.2.SR.1. *NIAHO® accreditation requirements, interpretive guidelines and surveyor guidance—revision 20.0.* Milford, OH: DNV GL-Healthcare USA, Inc. (Level VII)

28 Hinkle, J. L., & Cheever, K. H. (2018). *Brunner & Suddarth's textbook of medical-surgical nursing* (14th ed.). Philadelphia, PA: Wolters Kluwer.

AUTOLOGOUS BLOOD COLLECTION, PREOPERATIVE

Preoperative autologous blood collection is the collection, processing, and storage of the patient's own blood before a scheduled procedure that's likely to cause significant bleeding.[1]

Autologous blood transfusion has several advantages over transfusion of blood from a blood bank. First, it minimizes the risk of infectious disease transmission (with the exception of bacterial sepsis) and alloimmunization of red cell, platelet, and leukocyte antigens. It also provides a source of blood for individuals who have rare blood types or antibodies that make it difficult to find compatible blood. Last, some individuals who refuse blood from donors because of religious or other beliefs may be willing to accept a transfusion of their own blood.[1]

Despite the advantages, there may be rare adverse effects associated with autologous blood transfusion, including septic transfusion reactions that can occur if bacteria multiply during storage and nonhemolytic transfusion reactions that can result from white blood cell cytokine release during storage. In addition, if the recipient is misidentified before transfusion, a hemolytic reaction may occur or the patient may be exposed to a transfusion-transmitted disease.[1,2]

Sepsis or suspected bacteremia is a contraindication to autologous donation. The practitioner may also prefer not to use blood from a patient who has an infectious disease or active infection. There are no specific age requirements; children and older adult patients may participate. However, patients with certain medical conditions may not be acceptable candidates for preoperative donation. The hemoglobin level should be 11 g/dL or higher, or the hematocrit, if used, should be 33% or higher. If the patient weighs less than 110 lb (50 kg), it may be necessary to reduce the volume of blood obtained.[1]

Equipment

Gloves ■ vital signs monitoring equipment ■ 18G or 20G catheter and equipment for venipuncture and IV catheter insertion ■ blood collection bags with phlebotomy administration set ■ blood sample collection equipment ■ AUTOLOGOUS BLOOD label ■ laboratory biohazard transport bag ■ Optional: prescribed IV fluids, mask, protective eyewear or mask with face shield, gowns or aprons, blood scale.

Preparation of equipment

Inspect all IV equipment and supplies; if a product is expired, has compromised integrity, or is defective, remove it from patient use, label it as expired or defective, and report the expiration or defect as directed by your facility.[3]

Implementation

■ Verify the practitioner's order for autologous blood collection.[1]
■ Review the patient's medical record for factors that may affect peripheral vasculature, such as conditions that result in structural vessel changes (for example, diabetes and hypertension), history of frequent venipuncture or lengthy infusion therapy, skin variations, skin alterations (such as scars or tattoos), patient age, obesity, or fluid volume deficit *to determine the need for vascular visualization technology*.[4]
■ Verify that the patient's hemoglobin level is 11 g/dL or higher, and that hematocrit, if used, is 33% or higher.[1]
■ Confirm that informed consent has been obtained and that the consent form is in the patient's medical record.[1,5,6,7,8,9]
■ Perform hand hygiene.[10,11,12,13,14,15,16]
■ Confirm the patient's identity using at least two patient identifiers.[17]
■ Provide privacy.[18,19,20,21]
■ Explain the procedure to the patient and family (if appropriate) according to their individual communication and learning needs *to increase their understanding, allay their fears, and enhance cooperation*.[22,23] Make sure the patient understands that autologous blood may not be received exclusively if there's unexpected blood loss, if there's an emergency need for more units than collected, or if a less-than-desired number of units was collected. Also, make sure the patient understands that a risk of certain adverse effects still exists with autologous blood transfusion. Explain that all collections should be completed more than 72 hours before the anticipated surgery or transfusion.[1]

■ *To prevent hypovolemia*, encourage the patient to drink plenty of fluids before collection. Explain that the patient may feel light-headed during the collection but that the problem can be treated.[1]
■ Obtain and record vital signs before starting the collection *to provide a baseline for comparison*.[1]
■ Help the patient into a reclining supine position.
■ Raise the bed to waist level when providing care *to prevent caregiver back strain*.[24]
■ Perform hand hygiene.[10,11,12,13,14,15,16]
■ Prepare the collection bags according to the manufacturer's instructions.
■ Place the blood collection bag below the venipuncture site; close the clamp on the administration set.[25]
■ Prepare replacement IV fluids, if ordered.
■ Perform hand hygiene.[10,11,12,13,14,15,16]
■ Put on gloves and other personal protective equipment, as needed, *to comply with standard precautions*.[26,27,28,29,30]
■ Select an appropriate IV catheter insertion site.[31]
■ Prepare the patient's arm and IV catheter insertion site. Insert an 18G or 20G catheter.[32] (See the "IV catheter insertion and removal" procedure.)
■ Connect the collecting system to the IV catheter according to the manufacturer's instructions; slowly open the clamp to allow retrograde blood flow into the administration set and blood collection bag.[25]
■ Monitor the patient for adverse reactions.

NURSING ALERT Monitor the patient's vital signs closely for signs of hypotension during this process.

■ Administer replacement IV fluids, if ordered.
■ Monitor the volume or weight of the collected blood until the prescribed quantity is withdrawn.[25]
■ When blood collection is complete, reclamp the administration set tubing, remove the IV catheter, and perform site care.
■ Recheck the patient's vital signs *to evaluate the patient's response to the procedure*.[25]
■ Obtain a blood sample from the patient for a coagulation profile, hemoglobin, hematocrit, and calcium level, as ordered. Label the sample in the presence of the patient *to prevent mislabeling*.[2,17] Place the sample in a laboratory biohazard transport bag[26] and send it to the laboratory immediately.
■ Clearly label the blood collection bag with the patient's name, at least two patient identifiers, and an AUTOLOGOUS BLOOD label. Make sure there's a mechanism to clearly determine the date of collection and the identity of the person who collected the blood *to prevent blood administration errors*.[1,25]
■ Send the blood to the blood bank.
■ Return the bed to the lowest position *to prevent falls and maintain safety*.[33]
■ Discard all used supplies in appropriate receptacles.[26,27,34]
■ Remove and discard your gloves and any other personal protective equipment, if worn.[26,27,34]
■ Perform hand hygiene.[10,11,12,13,14,15,16]
■ Document the procedure.[35,36,37,38,39]

Special considerations

■ In the 4 to 6 weeks before surgery, the patient may be prescribed iron supplements *to improve preoperative hemoglobin levels*.[2]
■ Monitor the patient closely during and after the collection. Vasovagal reactions are usually mild and short in duration, but the patient may experience fatigue after the event.[40] Have the patient remain in a reclining supine position for at least 10 minutes after the collection, or have the patient sit in a forward-leaning position with the elbows or forearms on a table and feet flat on the floor. If the patient feels light-headed or dizzy, advise the patient to remain in a reclining supine position with the legs raised or to lie down with the head lower than the body until symptoms resolve.[41]
■ Instruct the patient to monitor the IV site for a few hours after the collection. Instruct the patient to apply firm pressure for 5 to 10 minutes if bleeding occurs and to notify the practitioner if bleeding continues.

■ The practitioner should discontinue anticoagulation drugs before elective or nonemergent surgery.[2]

Complications

Preoperative collection may cause vasovagal reactions, hypovolemia, nausea, vomiting, and such local reactions as bruising, hematoma, or sensory changes in the arm used for the donation.[41]

Documentation

Document the time the collection began and ended; the amount of blood collected; your assessments before and after the procedure, including vital signs; and the patient's tolerance of the procedure. Note the condition of the IV site and the dressing applied. Record that the blood sample was sent to the laboratory and that the blood was sent to the blood bank. Document teaching provided to the patient and family (if applicable), their understanding of that teaching, and any need for follow-up teaching.[25,36]

REFERENCES

1 AABB. (2018). *Primer of blood administration.* Bethesda, MD: AABB. (Level VII)

2 American Society of Anesthesiologists. (2015). Practice guidelines for perioperative blood management: An updated report by the American Society of Anesthesiologists Task Force on Perioperative Blood Management. *Anesthesiology, 122,* 241–275. https://pubs.asahq.org/anesthesiology/article/122/2/241/12287/Practice-Guidelines-for-Perioperative-Blood (Level VII)

3 Standard 12. Product evaluation, integrity, and defect reporting. Infusion therapy standards of practice (8th ed.). (2021). *Journal of Infusion Nursing, 44,* S45–S46. (Level VII)

4 Standard 22. Vascular visualization. Infusion therapy standards of practice (8th ed.). (2021). *Journal of Infusion Nursing, 44,* S63–S65. (Level VII)

5 DNV GL-Healthcare USA, Inc. (2020). PR.2.SR.3. *NIAHO® accreditation requirements, interpretive guidelines and surveyor guidance—revision 20.0.* Milford, OH: DNV GL-Healthcare USA, Inc. (Level VII)

6 The Joint Commission. (2021). Standard RI.01.03.01. *Comprehensive accreditation manual for hospitals.* Oakbrook Terrace, IL: The Joint Commission. (Level VII)

7 Centers for Medicare and Medicaid Services, Department of Health and Human Services. (2020). Condition of participation: Patient's rights. 42 C.F.R. § 482.13(b)(2).

8 Accreditation Association for Hospitals and Health Systems. (2020). Standard 15.01.11. *Healthcare Facilities Accreditation Program: Accreditation requirements for acute care hospitals.* Chicago, IL: Accreditation Association for Hospitals and Health Systems. (Level VII)

9 Standard 9. Informed consent. Infusion therapy standards of practice (8th ed.). (2021). *Journal of Infusion Nursing, 44,* S37–S39. (Level VII)

10 World Health Organization. (2009). WHO guidelines on hand hygiene in health care: First global patient safety challenge, clean care is safer care. https://apps.who.int/iris/bitstream/handle/10665/44102/9789241597906_eng.pdf?sequence=1 (Level IV)

11 The Joint Commission. (2021). Standard NPSG.07.01.01. *Comprehensive accreditation manual for hospitals.* Oakbrook Terrace, IL: The Joint Commission. (Level VII)

12 Centers for Disease Control and Prevention. (2002). Guideline for hand hygiene in health-care settings: Recommendations of the Healthcare Infection Control Practices Advisory Committee and the HICPAC/SHEA/APIC/IDSA Hand Hygiene Task Force. *MMWR Recommendations and Reports, 51*(RR-16), 1–45. https://www.cdc.gov/mmwr/pdf/rr/rr5116.pdf (Level II)

13 Standard 16. Hand hygiene. Infusion therapy standards of practice (8th ed.). (2021). *Journal of Infusion Nursing, 44,* S53–S54. (Level VII)

14 Centers for Medicare and Medicaid Services, Department of Health and Human Services. (2020). Condition of participation: Infection control. 42 C.F.R. § 482.42.

15 Accreditation Association for Hospitals and Health Systems. (2020). Standard 07.01.21. *Healthcare Facilities Accreditation Program: Accreditation requirements for acute care hospitals.* Chicago, IL: Accreditation Association for Hospitals and Health Systems. (Level VII)

16 DNV GL-Healthcare USA, Inc. (2020). IC.1.SR.1. *NIAHO® accreditation requirements, interpretive guidelines and surveyor guidance—revision 20.0.* Milford, OH: DNV GL-Healthcare USA, Inc. (Level VII)

17 The Joint Commission. (2021). Standard NPSG.01.01.01. *Comprehensive accreditation manual for hospitals.* Oakbrook Terrace, IL: The Joint Commission. (Level VII)

18 The Joint Commission. (2021). Standard RI.01.01.01. *Comprehensive accreditation manual for hospitals.* Oakbrook Terrace, IL: The Joint Commission. (Level VII)

19 DNV GL-Healthcare USA, Inc. (2020). PR.2.SR.5. *NIAHO® accreditation requirements, interpretive guidelines and surveyor guidance—revision 20.0.* Milford, OH: DNV GL-Healthcare USA, Inc. (Level VII)

20 Centers for Medicare and Medicaid Services, Department of Health and Human Services. (2020). Condition of participation: Patient's rights. 42 C.F.R. § 482.13(c)(1).

21 Accreditation Association for Hospitals and Health Systems. (2020). Standard 15.01.16. *Healthcare Facilities Accreditation Program: Accreditation requirements for acute care hospitals.* Chicago, IL: Accreditation Association for Hospitals and Health Systems. (Level VII)

22 The Joint Commission. (2021). Standard PC.02.01.21. *Comprehensive accreditation manual for hospitals.* Oakbrook Terrace, IL: The Joint Commission. (Level VII)

23 Standard 8. Patient education. Infusion therapy standards of practice (8th ed.). (2021). *Journal of Infusion Nursing, 44,* S35–S37. (Level VII)

24 Waters, T. R., et al. (2009). Safe patient handling training for schools of nursing. https://www.cdc.gov/niosh/docs/2009-127/pdfs/2009-127.pdf

25 Infusion Nurses Society. (2016). *Policies and procedures for infusion therapy* (5th ed.). Boston, MA: Infusion Nurses Society.

26 Occupational Safety and Health Administration. (2012). Bloodborne pathogens, standard number 1910.1030. https://www.osha.gov/pls/oshaweb/owadisp.show_document?p_id=10051&p_table=STANDARDS (Level VII)

27 Siegel, J. D., et al. (2007, revised 2019). 2007 guidelines for isolation precautions: Preventing transmission of infectious agents in healthcare settings. https://www.cdc.gov/infectioncontrol/pdf/guidelines/isolation-guidelines-H.pdf (Level II)

28 Standard 17. Standard precautions. Infusion therapy standards of practice (8th ed.). (2021). *Journal of Infusion Nursing, 44,* S54–S55. (Level VII)

29 Accreditation Association for Hospitals and Health Systems. (2020). Standard 07.01.10. *Healthcare Facilities Accreditation Program: Accreditation requirements for acute care hospitals.* Chicago, IL: Accreditation Association for Hospitals and Health Systems. (Level VII)

30 DNV GL-Healthcare USA, Inc. (2020). IC.1.SR.2. *NIAHO® accreditation requirements, interpretive guidelines and surveyor guidance—revision 20.0.* Milford, OH: DNV GL-Healthcare USA, Inc. (Level VII)

31 Standard 27. Site selection. Infusion therapy standards of practice (8th ed.). (2021). *Journal of Infusion Nursing, 44,* S81–S86. (Level VII)

32 Standard 66. Therapeutic phlebotomy. Infusion therapy standards of practice (8th ed.). (2021). *Journal of Infusion Nursing, 44,* S195–S196. (Level VII)

33 Ganz, D. A., et al. (2013-reviewed 2021). *Preventing falls in hospitals: A toolkit for improving quality of care* (AHRQ Publication No. 13-0015-EF). Rockville, MD: Agency for Healthcare Research and Quality. https://www.ahrq.gov/professionals/systems/hospital/fallpxtoolkit/index.html (Level VII)

34 Standard 21. Medical waste and sharps safety. Infusion therapy standards of practice (8th ed.). (2021). *Journal of Infusion Nursing, 44,* S60–S62 (Level VII)

35 The Joint Commission. (2021). Standard RC.01.03.01. *Comprehensive accreditation manual for hospitals.* Oakbrook Terrace, IL: The Joint Commission. (Level VII)

36 Standard 10. Documentation in the health record. Infusion therapy standards of practice (8th ed.). (2021). *Journal of Infusion Nursing, 44,* S39–S42. (Level VII)

37 Centers for Medicare and Medicaid Services, Department of Health and Human Services. (2020). Condition of participation: Medical record services. 42 C.F.R. § 482.24(b).

38 Accreditation Association for Hospitals and Health Systems. (2020). Standard 10.00.03. *Healthcare Facilities Accreditation Program: Accreditation requirements for acute care hospitals.* Chicago, IL: Accreditation Association for Hospitals and Health Systems. (Level VII)

39 DNV GL-Healthcare USA, Inc. (2020). MR.2.SR.1. *NIAHO® accreditation requirements, interpretive guidelines and surveyor guidance—revision 20.0.* Milford, OH: DNV GL-Healthcare USA, Inc. (Level VII)

40 Benditt, D. (2019). Reflex syncope in adults and adolescents: Clinical presentation and diagnostic evaluation. In: *UpToDate,* Kowey, P. (Ed.).

41 Kleinman, S. (2020). Blood donor screening: Procedures and processes to enhance safety for the blood recipient and the blood donor. In: *UpToDate,* Silvergleid, A. J. (Ed.).

AUTOLOGOUS BLOOD TRANSFUSION, PERIOPERATIVE

Perioperative autologous blood transfusion is the collection and transfusion of the patient's own blood collected intraoperatively from the operative site or from an extracorporeal circuit. One benefit of this procedure is that the patient can receive autologous blood, thereby, minimizing the need for allogenic blood transfusion.[1,2] It may be used during vascular or orthopedic surgery (because considerable bleeding can result from these surgeries) and during the treatment of traumatic injury. perioperative autologous blood transfusion is contraindicated when instances occur that increase the risk of blood contamination with bacteria, tumor cells, or other harmful substances.[1]

Various types of devices are available to retrieve blood from the operative site; apheresis devices are available to prepare the components intraoperatively. (See *Autologous blood recovery systems.*) Follow the manufacturer's instructions when collecting, storing, and transfusing the patient's blood using an autologous blood recovery system.[1,3]

Equipment

Gloves ▪ vital signs monitoring equipment ▪ antiseptic pad (chlorhexidine-based, povidone-iodine, or alcohol) ▪ 3-mL syringe ▪ 250-mL bag of normal saline solution ▪ blood administration set with microaggregate filter ▪ IV pole ▪ wall suction with pressure gauge ▪ autologous blood recovery system device with necessary supplies; for a Cell Saver® 5+ unit, suction tubing and collection kit (an autotransfusion drain usually has standalone functioning) ▪ AUTOLOGOUS BLOOD label ▪ Optional: mask with face shield or mask and goggles, gown, labels, 14G to 24G venous access catheter and insertion equipment.

Preparation of equipment

Inspect all IV equipment and supplies; if a product is expired, is defective, or has compromised integrity, remove it from patient use, label it as expired or defective, and report the expiration or defect as directed by your facility.[5]

Implementation

▪ Verify the practitioner's order for the rate of reinfusion and the amount of blood to be reinfused.
▪ Confirm that the informed consent has been obtained and that the signed consent form is in the patient's medical record.[6,7,8,9,10]
▪ Notify the perfusionist to set up the autologous blood recovery system device and connect the tubing to the setup following the manufacturer's instructions. (Note that the person responsible for this step may vary by facility. A perioperative nurse or anesthesia care provider may set up the device in some facilities.)

EQUIPMENT

Autologous blood recovery systems

Autologous blood recovery systems are used in surgical procedures to salvage red blood cells (RBCs) when there's rapid bleeding or high-volume blood loss. Shed blood is collected and stored in a reservoir, where waste is separated from the healthy RBCs. The waste collects into a separate bag; healthy RBCs are then returned to the patient. This process can be performed in 3 to 7 minutes. In emergencies, the autologous blood recovery system can process up to 800 mL of blood each minute.[4]

Advantages to autologous blood recovery systems include:
▪ up-to-date microprocessor and sensor technologies
▪ automated operation and manual operation options
▪ platelet sequestration
▪ RBC bags with integrated microaggregate filters
▪ features to ensure consistent processing and a high-quality blood product
▪ fast processing
▪ built-in safety features.

▪ Perform hand hygiene.[11,12,13,14,15,16,17,18]
▪ Confirm the patient's identity using at least two patient identifiers.[19]
▪ Perform hand hygiene.[11,12,13,14,15,16,17,18]
▪ Put on gloves and, as needed, other personal protective equipment *to comply with standard precautions.*[20,21,22,23,24,25]
▪ Make sure the collection chamber and the blood transfer bag are clearly marked with the patient's first and last name, identifying numbers, date and time of the collection initiation, and an AUTOLOGOUS BLOOD label. If applicable, include the time of, or condition for, expiration.[1,3,26]
▪ Obtain the patient's vital signs before the transfusion *to serve as a baseline for comparison.*[3]
▪ Ensure that the patient has adequate venous access, either peripheral or central, with an appropriate-size catheter (14G to 24G).[27] Verify patency by aspirating for a blood return. Insert an IV catheter if necessary. (See the "IV catheter insertion and removal" procedure.)
▪ Insert one spike of the standard Y-type blood administration set into the 250-mL bag of normal saline solution. Close all clamps and hang the blood administration set on an IV pole.
▪ The anesthesia care provider, perioperative nurse, or perfusionist will start blood collection according to the device manufacturer's instructions. (Some devices process and centrifuge the blood automatically.)
▪ Monitor the patient's vital signs closely during the blood collection for signs of hypotension. *Hypotension may occur as the result of hypovolemia.*
▪ Monitor the status of the blood collection.
▪ When sufficient blood has been collected, spike the blood transfer bag with the open port of the blood administration set, remove all air from the blood transfer bag, and hang the bag on the IV pole.
▪ Open the clamp from the normal saline solution and prime the filter and tubing *to remove all air from the tubing.* Close the clamp from the normal saline solution.
▪ Open the clamp from the blood transfer bag to the drip chamber of the blood administration set and prime the filter [3] and tubing with blood *to remove all air from the tubing.*
▪ If you're using a postprocedure transfusion device, follow the manufacturer's instructions *to properly connect the device to the patient.* (Staff members should receive training on all transfusion devices before use.)
▪ Perform a vigorous mechanical scrub of the needleless connector for at least 5 seconds using an antiseptic pad. Allow it to dry completely.[28,29]
▪ Attach the blood administration set to the venous access device and trace the tubing from the patient to its point of origin before beginning the transfusion *to make sure it's connected to the proper port.*[30] Route the tubing in a standardized direction if the patient has other tubing and catheters that have different purposes. Label the tubing at the distal (near the patient connection) and proximal (near the source container) ends *to reduce the risk of misconnection* if multiple IV lines will be used.[31]
▪ Begin the transfusion, as ordered.
▪ Monitor the patient throughout the procedure.[2]
▪ Obtain vital signs during the transfusion at an interval indicated by the patient's condition or at a frequency determined by your facility.[27]
▪ Make sure the transfusion is completed in the surgery suite or postanesthesia care unit within the time period defined by the system used[1] or within your facility's recommended time frame.
▪ Obtain the patient's vital signs after the transfusion is complete.[3]
▪ Disconnect the blood recovery system from the patient's drains, or have the anesthesia care provider, perioperative nurse, or perfusionist do so.
▪ Recheck the laboratory data for coagulation profile, hemoglobin, hematocrit, and calcium levels after the transfusion is complete, or as the practitioner orders. Notify the practitioner of critical test results within your facility's established time frame *so that the patient can be treated promptly.*[32]
▪ Discard used supplies in appropriate receptacles.[20,21,33]
▪ Remove and discard your personal protective equipment.[20,21,33]
▪ Perform hand hygiene.[11,12,13,14,15,16,17,18]
▪ Document the procedure.[34,35,36,37,38]

Managing problems of autologous blood transfusion

This chart describes the problems related to autologous blood transfusion, their possible causes, and interventions to manage them.

PROBLEM	POSSIBLE CAUSES	NURSING INTERVENTIONS
Citrate toxicity (rare, unpredictable)	■ Chelating effect on calcium of citrate in phosphate dextrose (CPD) ■ Predisposing factors, including hyperkalemia, hypocalcemia, acidosis, hypothermia, myocardial dysfunction, and liver or kidney problems	■ Watch for hypotension, arrhythmias, and myocardial contractility. ■ Prophylactic calcium chloride may be administered if more than 2,000 mL of CPD-anticoagulated blood is given over 20 minutes. ■ Stop infusing CPD and correct acidosis. Measure arterial blood gas values and serum calcium levels frequently *to assess for toxicity*.
Coagulation	■ Not enough anticoagulant ■ Blood not defibrinated in mediastinum	■ Add CPD or another regional anticoagulant at a ratio of 7 parts blood to 1 part anticoagulant. Keep blood and CPD mixed by shaking the collection bottle regularly. ■ Check for anticoagulant reversal. Strip chest tubes as needed.
Coagulopathies	■ Reduced platelet and fibrinogen levels ■ Platelets caught in filters ■ Enhanced levels of fibrin split products	■ Patients receiving autologous transfusions of more than 4,000 mL of blood may also need transfusion of fresh frozen plasma or platelet concentrate.
Emboli	■ Microaggregate debris ■ Air	■ Don't use equipment with roller pumps or pressure infusion systems. ■ Before transfusion, remove air from blood bags.[1] ■ Transfuse with a microaggregate filter.
Hemolysis	■ Trauma to blood caused by turbulence or roller pumps	■ Don't skim the operative field and don't use equipment with roller pumps. ■ When collecting blood from chest tubes, keep the vacuum below 30 mm Hg; when aspirating from a surgical site, keep the vacuum below 60 mm Hg.
Sepsis	■ Lack of sterile technique ■ Contaminated blood	■ Give broad-spectrum antibiotics, as prescribed.[1] ■ Use strict sterile technique. ■ Transfuse within 4 hours. ■ Don't infuse blood from infected areas or blood that contains feces, urine, or other contaminants.

Special considerations

■ If multiple units are to be transfused, change the blood administration set and filter after the completion of each unit or every 4 hours. If more than one unit can be infused within 4 hours, the administration set can be used for 4 hours.[27]

■ Be aware that you may need to replace clotting factors, fresh frozen plasma, or platelets if you're transfusing large volumes of blood.[1]

■ Certain religious groups refuse blood transfusions because of their beliefs. However, many of these groups permit autologous blood transfusion if it's kept in a continuous closed circuit.

■ The Joint Commission issued a sentinel event alert related to managing risk during transition to the new International Organization for Standardization tubing standards; the new standards were designed to prevent dangerous tubing misconnections, which can lead to serious patient injury and death. During the transition, be sure to trace the tubing and catheter from the patient to the point of origin before connecting or reconnecting any device or infusion, at any care transition (such as to a new setting or service), and as part of the hand-off process; route tubes and catheters having different purposes in different, standardized directions; label the tubing at both the distal and proximal ends (when there are different access sites or several bags hanging); use tubing and equipment only as intended; and store medications for different delivery routes in separate locations.[31]

Complications

More complications are associated with the reinfusion of filtered, unwashed blood than with the transfusion of filtered, washed blood. These complications include fever, hypotension, myocardial infarction, infections, particulate and air embolism, and thrombocytopenia. Complications are more pronounced when the time from salvage to transfusion is greater than 6 hours. (See *Managing problems of autologous blood transfusion*.)

Documentation

Document the time the collection began, the time the transfusion started and ended[3], and the venous access site used for the transfusion. Include the patient's vital signs before and after transfusion.[3] Note the amount of blood collected and transfused, the name of the person who administered the blood, and the system used.[1,3] Document any adverse reactions, the date and time the practitioner was notified, prescribed interventions, and the patient's response to those interventions.[1] Also document any post-transfusion laboratory studies obtained.[3] Document teaching provided to the patient and family (if applicable), their understanding of the teaching, and any need for follow-up teaching.[35]

REFERENCES

1 AABB. (2018). *Primer of blood administration*.Bethesda, MD: AABB. (Level VII)

2 American Society of Anesthesiologists. (2015). Practice guidelines for perioperative blood management: An updated report by the American Society of Anesthesiologists Task Force on Perioperative Blood Management. *Anesthesiology, 122*, 241–275. https://pubs.asahq.org/anesthesiology/article/122/2/241/12287/Practice-Guidelines-for-Perioperative-Blood (Level VII)

3 AABB. (2019). *Standards for perioperative autologous blood collection and administration* (8th ed.). Bethesda, MD: AABB. (Level VII)

4 Haemonetics Corporation. (2012). Cell Saver® 5+ standard of care in intraoperative autotransfusion. https://pdf.medicalexpo.com/pdf/haemonetics/cell-saver-5-standard-care-intraoperative-autotransfusion/78504-168063.html

5 Standard 12. Product evaluation, integrity, and defect reporting. Infusion therapy standards of practice (8th ed.). (2021). *Journal of Infusion Nursing, 344*, S45–S46. (Level VII)

6 The Joint Commission. (2021). Standard RI.01.03.01. *Comprehensive accreditation manual for hospitals*. Oakbrook Terrace, IL: The Joint Commission. (Level VII)

7 Centers for Medicare and Medicaid Services, Department of Health and Human Services. (2020). Condition of participation: Patient's rights. 42 C.F.R. § 482.13(b)(2).

8 Accreditation Association for Hospitals and Health Systems. (2020). Standard 15.01.11. *Healthcare Facilities Accreditation Program: Accreditation requirements for acute care hospitals.* Chicago, IL: Accreditation Association for Hospitals and Health Systems. (Level VII)

9 DNV GL-Healthcare USA, Inc. (2020). PR.2.SR.3. *NIAHO® accreditation requirements, interpretive guidelines and surveyor guidance—revision 20.0.* Milford, OH: DNV GL-Healthcare USA, Inc. (Level VII)

10 Standard 9. Informed consent. Infusion therapy standards of practice (8th ed.). (2021). *Journal of Infusion Nursing, 44,* S37–S39. (Level VII)

11 The Joint Commission. (2021). Standard NPSG.07.01.01. *Comprehensive accreditation manual for hospitals.* Oakbrook Terrace, IL: The Joint Commission. (Level VII)

12 Centers for Disease Control and Prevention. (2002). Guideline for hand hygiene in health-care settings: Recommendations of the Healthcare Infection Control Practices Advisory Committee and the HICPAC/SHEA/APIC/IDSA Hand Hygiene Task Force. *MMWR Recommendations and Reports, 51*(RR-16), 1–45. https://www.cdc.gov/mmwr/pdf/rr/rr5116.pdf (Level II)

13 World Health Organization. (2009). WHO guidelines on hand hygiene in health care: First global patient safety challenge, clean care is safer care. https://apps.who.int/iris/bitstream/handle/10665/44102/9789241597906_eng.pdf?sequence=1 (Level IV)

14 Guideline for hand hygiene. (2020). In Wood, A. (Ed.), *Guidelines for perioperative practice: 2020 edition.* Denver, CO: AORN, Inc. (Level VII)

15 Standard 16. Hand hygiene. Infusion therapy standards of practice (8th ed.). (2021). *Journal of Infusion Nursing, 44,* S53–S54. (Level VII)

16 Centers for Medicare and Medicaid Services, Department of Health and Human Services. (2020). Condition of participation: Infection control. 42 C.F.R. § 482.42.

17 Accreditation Association for Hospitals and Health Systems. (2020). Standard 07.01.21. *Healthcare Facilities Accreditation Program: Accreditation requirements for acute care hospitals.* Chicago, IL: Accreditation Association for Hospitals and Health Systems. (Level VII)

18 DNV GL-Healthcare USA, Inc. (2020). IC.1.SR.1. *NIAHO® accreditation requirements, interpretive guidelines and surveyor guidance—revision 20.0.* Milford, OH: DNV GL-Healthcare USA, Inc. (Level VII)

19 The Joint Commission. (2021). Standard NPSG.01.01.01. *Comprehensive accreditation manual for hospitals.* Oakbrook Terrace, IL: The Joint Commission. (Level VII)

20 Siegel, J. D., et al. (2007, revised 2019). 2007 guideline for isolation precautions: Preventing transmission of infectious agents in healthcare settings. https://www.cdc.gov/infectioncontrol/pdf/guidelines/isolation-guidclines-H.pdf (Level II)

21 Occupational Safety and Health Administration (2012). Bloodborne pathogens, standard number 1910.1030. https://www.osha.gov/pls/oshaweb/owadisp.show_document?p_id=10051&p_table=STANDARDS (Level VII)

22 Accreditation Association for Hospitals and Health Systems. (2020). Standard 07.01.10. *Healthcare Facilities Accreditation Program: Accreditation requirements for acute care hospitals.* Chicago, IL: Accreditation Association for Hospitals and Health Systems. (Level VII)

23 DNV GL-Healthcare USA, Inc. (2020). IC.1.SR.2. *NIAHO® accreditation requirements, interpretive guidelines and surveyor guidance—revision 20.0.* Milford, OH: DNV GL-Healthcare USA, Inc. (Level VII)

24 Guideline for transmission-based precautions. (2020). In Wood, A. (Ed.), *Guidelines for perioperative practice: 2020 edition.* Denver, CO: AORN, Inc. (Level VII)

25 Standard 17. Standard precautions. Infusion therapy standards of practice (8th ed.). (2021). *Journal of Infusion Nursing, 44,* S54–S55. (Level VII)

26 The Joint Commission. (2021). Standard NPSG.01.03.01. *Comprehensive accreditation manual for hospitals.* Oakbrook Terrace, IL: The Joint Commission. (Level VII)

27 Standard 64. Blood administration. Infusion therapy standards of practice (8th ed.). (2021). *Journal of Infusion Nursing, 44,* S135–S137. (Level VII)

28 Standard 36. Needleless connectors. Infusion therapy standards of practice (8th ed.). (2021). *Journal of Infusion Nursing, 44,* S68–S70. (Level VII)

29 Marschall, J., et al. (2014). SHEA/IDSA practice recommendation: Strategies to prevent central line–associated bloodstream infections in acute care hospitals: 2014 update. *Infection Control and Hospital Epidemiology, 35,* 753–771. https://www.jstor.org/stable/10.1086/676533#metadata_info_tab_contents (Level I)

30 U.S. Food and Drug Administration. (2017). Examples of medical device misconnections. https://www.fda.gov/medical-devices/medical-device-connectors/examples-medical-device-misconnections

31 The Joint Commission. (2014). Sentinel event alert 53: Managing risk during transition to new ISO tubing connector standards. http://www.jointcommission.org/assets/1/6/SEA_53_Connectors_8_19_14_final.pdf (Level VII)

32 The Joint Commission. (2021). Standard NPSG.02.03.01. *Comprehensive accreditation manual for hospitals.* Oakbrook Terrace, IL: The Joint Commission. (Level VII)

33 Standard 21. Medical waste and sharps safety. Infusion therapy standards of practice (8th ed.). (2021). *Journal of Infusion Nursing, 44,* S60–S62. (Level VII)

34 The Joint Commission. (2021). Standard RC.01.03.01. *Comprehensive accreditation manual for hospitals.* Oakbrook Terrace, IL: The Joint Commission. (Level VII)

35 Standard 10. Documentation in the health record. Infusion therapy standards of practice (8th ed.). (2021). *Journal of Infusion Nursing, 44,* S39–S42. (Level VII)

36 Centers for Medicare and Medicaid Services, Department of Health and Human Services. (2020). Condition of participation: Medical record services. 42 C.F.R. § 482.24(b).

37 Accreditation Association for Hospitals and Health Systems. (2020). Standard 10.00.03. *Healthcare Facilities Accreditation Program: Accreditation requirements for acute care hospitals.* Chicago, IL: Accreditation Association for Hospitals and Health Systems. (Level VII)

38 DNV GL-Healthcare USA, Inc. (2020). MR.2.SR.1. *NIAHO® accreditation requirements, interpretive guidelines and surveyor guidance—revision 20.0.* Milford, OH: DNV GL-Healthcare USA, Inc. (Level VII)

AUTOMATED EXTERNAL DEFIBRILLATION

Automated external defibrillators (AEDs) are commonly used to meet the need for early defibrillation, which is currently considered the most effective treatment for ventricular fibrillation (VF) and pulseless ventricular tachycardia. Some facilities now require every noncritical care unit to have an AED. These devices provide a means to facilitate early defibrillation in areas of a health care facility where staff members have no rhythm recognition skills and defibrillators aren't frequently used. When AEDs are used in health care facilities, first-responding staff should have training to use the AED and have a goal of delivering the first shock within 3 minutes of the patient's collapse.[1] AEDs are also commonly used in such public places as shopping malls, sports stadiums, and airplanes. Instruction in using an AED is required as part of both basic life support (BLS) and advanced cardiac life support (ACLS) training, pediatric advanced life support (PALS) training, and Heartsaver® AED courses.

AEDs provide early defibrillation even when no health care provider is present. The AED interprets the victim's cardiac rhythm and gives the operator step-by-step directions on how to proceed if defibrillation is indicated. (See *Understanding an AED.*)

The American Heart Association in its guidelines for cardiopulmonary resuscitation (CPR) and emergency cardiovascular care, recommends rapid integration of CPR with the use of an AED, as follows:[1,2]

■ For a witnessed adult cardiac arrest when an AED is immediately available, use the defibrillator as soon as possible. For adults with unmonitored cardiac arrest or for whom an AED isn't immediately available, initiate CPR, and then use the AED as soon as it is available.[1]

■ When two rescuers are available, one rescuer should begin CPR immediately while the second rescuer activates the emergency response system and obtains and prepares the defibrillator.[1]

■ CPR and defibrillation should be coordinated to minimize the time between stopping compressions and administering the shock.[1,3]

■ First responders should receive AED training with the goal of delivering the first shock for any spontaneous cardiac arrest within 3 minutes of collapse.[1,3]

■ For children ages 1 to 8, the use of a pediatric dose attenuator system along with an AED is preferable. If one isn't available, a standard AED is acceptable.[2]

■ If pediatric pads aren't available, the use of adult pads on a child is acceptable. Place the pads at least 1″ (2.5 cm) apart, or use an anterior-posterior pad position.[4]

■ For infants, the use of a manual defibrillator is preferred over an AED. However, if one isn't available, an AED with a pediatric dose attenuator system is acceptable. If neither defibrillator is available, an AED without a dose attenuator is acceptable as a last resort.[2]

EQUIPMENT

Understanding an AED

Each automated external defibrillator (AED) is equipped with a microcomputer that senses and analyzes a patient's heart rhythm at the push of a button. It then audibly or visually prompts the user to deliver a shock. AED models all have the same basic function, but each offers different operating options. For example, all AEDs communicate display directions via messages on a display screen or give voice commands, or both, but some AEDs simultaneously display a patient's heart rhythm as well.

All devices record the operator's interactions with the patient during defibrillation, in a solid-state memory module. Some AEDs have an integral printer for immediate event documentation. The patient's practitioner may review the documented events. Local and state regulations govern who is responsible for collecting AED case data for reporting purposes.

There are two types of automated defibrillators: one with monophasic waveforms and one with biphasic waveforms. Monophasic waveform defibrillators were introduced first, and some are still in use today. The energy level on this type of device is usually preset by the manufacturer. Most AEDs use biphasic waveforms. These devices are typically set to deliver escalating energy levels for the first three shocks and then, after the third shock, deliver subsequent shocks at the same energy as the third shock. Energy levels are commonly preconfigured at 120 to 200 joules. The optimal energy level for a biphasic waveform defibrillator hasn't been determined. The optimal dose for each device that has proven most effective in eliminating ventricular fibrillation should be noted on the device.

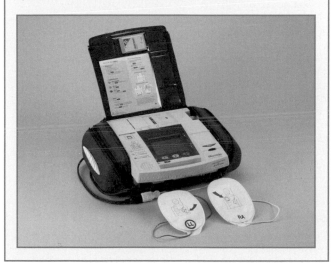

Equipment

AED ▪ two prepackaged, unopened AED electrodes ▪ facility-approved disinfectant ▪ Optional: gloves, vital signs monitoring equipment.

Preparation of equipment

Verify that the AED is charging when not in use. Examine cables, connectors, and accessories for tears, cuts, and exposed wires, and replace as needed. Verify that the electrode pads are in sealed packages and haven't expired; obtain new ones if the integrity of the packaging is compromised or if the electrodes have expired.

Implementation

- Perform hand hygiene.[5,6,7,8,9,10]
- Put on gloves, as needed, *to comply with standard precautions.*[11,12]
- After determining that the patient is unresponsive to questions and is apneic or only gasping, start CPR and follow BLS and ACLS protocols.[1,2]
- While you are performing CPR, ask a colleague to activate the emergency response system, bring the AED into the patient's room, and set it up as described below before the code team arrives.

- Turn on the AED and follow the visual or audible prompts.
- Open the foil packets containing the two AED electrode pads.
- Expose the patient's chest.
- Make sure the patient is in a dry environment and that the patient's chest is dry, *because if personnel or the patient's skin comes in contact with water, personnel may receive a shock and the patient may receive skin burns during defibrillation.* In addition, make sure that the areas where the electrodes will be applied are dry, *because moisture under the pads can decrease the effectiveness of contact with the skin.*[4]
- Remove any metal objects that the patient may be wearing, *because metal conducts electricity and could cause burns during defibrillation.*[4]
- Remove transdermal patches from the patient's chest (and back, if using anterior–posterior placement), *because the medication may interfere with current conduction and produce burns.*[4]
- Remove the plastic backing film from the AED electrodes.
- Place one electrode pad on the right side of the patient's bare, dry chest just below the clavicle. Place the second electrode pad on the left side of the patient's bare, dry chest to the left of the heart's apex.[4] Images showing proper placement are located on the anterior surface of the electrodes (depending on the manufacturer).

NURSING ALERT Don't interrupt CPR for electrode placement; *even a few seconds of interruption can decrease coronary blood flow.*[3]

NURSING ALERT Don't place the electrode pads directly over an implantable cardioverter-defibrillator or implanted pacemaker; *this placement may damage the device.* Keep the electrodes about 3″ (7.6 cm) from the device, as recommended.[4]

- Attach one AED electrode to each electrode cable (if not already attached), and then connect the cable to the AED.
- Now the machine is ready to analyze the patient's heart rhythm. Ask everyone to stand clear, and press the ANALYZE button when the machine prompts you to do so. Be careful not to touch or move the patient while the AED is in analysis mode, *because doing so may cause a delay in the AED's ability to analyze the rhythm.*[4] (If you get a CHECK ELECTRODES message, make sure the electrodes are correctly placed and the patient cable is securely attached; then press the ANALYZE button again.)
- Wait for the AED to analyze the patient's heart rhythm. When the patient needs a shock, the AED will prompt you with a STAND CLEAR message and emit a beep that changes into a steady tone as it's charging. If no shock is needed, the AED will display a NO SHOCK INDICATED message and prompt you to CHECK PATIENT.
- When the AED is fully charged and prompts you to deliver a shock, make sure no one is touching the patient or bed, and call out "Stand clear." Then press the SHOCK button on the AED. Most AEDs are ready to deliver a shock within 15 seconds. (Note that some fully automated AEDs automatically deliver a shock within 15 seconds after analyzing the patient's rhythm.)
- After the first shock, immediately continue CPR for about five cycles, beginning with chest compressions, for about 2 minutes. Don't delay compressions to recheck rhythm or pulse. After five cycles of CPR, the AED should analyze the rhythm again and deliver another shock, if indicated.[1]
- If a nonshockable heart rhythm is detected, the AED should instruct you to resume CPR. Then continue the algorithm sequence until the code leader arrives.
- If the patient regains a pulse, obtain vital signs and assess level of consciousness *to determine the patient's response to CPR and use of the AED.*[4]
- After the code, remove and transcribe the AED's computer memory module or tape, or prompt the AED to print a rhythm strip with code data. Analyze and store the code data as directed by your facility.
- Remove and discard your gloves.[13]
- Perform hand hygiene.[5,6,7,8,9,10]
- Put on gloves, as needed.[11,12]
- Clean, disinfect, and prepare the equipment for future use according to the manufacturer's instructions *to help prevent the spread of infection.*[14,15]
- Remove and discard your gloves, if worn.[13]
- Perform hand hygiene.[5,6,7,8,9,10]
- Document the procedure.[16,17,18,19]

Special considerations

- AEDs vary by manufacturer, so familiarize yourself with your facility's equipment.
- AED operation should be checked at an interval established by your facility, usually after each use and every 8 hours. Consider using a checklist to maintain the AED in a state of readiness.
- Acceptable alternative electrode placement includes bi-axillary positioning with pads placed on the right and left lateral chest walls, or placement of one pad in the standard apical position with the other pad on the right or left upper back.
- Excessive chest hair can interfere with optimal AED electrode adhesion and may need to be removed. Apply pressure to the pads to improve contact; if this is not working, rapidly remove the AED electrode and apply a new one.[4]
- Avoid placing the AED electrode pad on the sternum, *because bone blocks some of the energy and decreases effectiveness.*[4]
- After using an AED, give a synopsis to the code team leader that includes the patient's name, age, medical history, and chief complaint; time you found the patient in cardiac arrest, time you started CPR, and time you applied the AED; number of shocks the patient received; time the patient regained a pulse, if any; post-arrest care provided, if any; and physical assessment findings.

Complications

Defibrillation can cause accidental electric shock to those providing care and skin burns to the patient. Radiofrequency (RF) interference may result in improper device operation, a distorted electrocardiogram (ECG), or failure to detect a shockable rhythm. Avoid operation of the device near cauterizers, diathermy equipment, cellular phones, or other portable and mobile RF communication equipment.

Documentation

Document the procedure, including the patient's ECG rhythm before and after defibrillation; the number of times defibrillation was performed; the energy used with each attempt; whether a pulse returned; the dosage, route, and time of drug administration; whether CPR was performed; how the patient's airway was maintained; and the patient's outcome. Document teaching provided to the patient and family (if applicable), their understanding of that teaching, and any need for follow-up teaching.

REFERENCES

1 American Heart Association. (2020) Web-based integrated guidelines for cardiopulmonary resuscitation and emergency cardiovascular care—Part 5: Adult basic life support (BLS) and cardiopulmonary resuscitation (CPR) and quality. https://ECCguidelines.heart.org (Level II)

2 American Heart Association. (2020). Web-based integrated guidelines for cardiopulmonary resuscitation and emergency cardiovascular care—Part 11: Pediatric basic life support and cardiopulmonary resuscitation quality. https://ECCguidelines.heart.org (Level II)

3 American Heart Association. (2013). Strategies for improving survival after in-hospital cardiac arrest in the United States: 2013 consensus recommendations. *Circulation, 127*, 1538–1563. https://www.ahajournals.org/doi/pdf/10.1161/CIR.0b013e31828b2770 (Level VII)

4 Wiegand, D. L. (2017). *AACN procedure manual for high acuity, progressive, and critical care* (7th ed.). St. Louis, MO: Elsevier.

5 World Health Organization. (2009). WHO guidelines on hand hygiene in health care: First global patient safety challenge, clean care is safer care. https://apps.who.int/iris/bitstream/handle/10665/44102/9789241597906_eng.pdf?sequence=1 (Level IV)

6 The Joint Commission. (2021). Standard NPSG.07.01.01. *Comprehensive accreditation manual for hospitals.* Oakbrook Terrace, IL: The Joint Commission. (Level VII)

7 Centers for Disease Control and Prevention. (2002). Guideline for hand hygiene in health-care settings: Recommendations of the Healthcare Infection Control Practices Advisory Committee and the HICPAC/SHEA/APIC/IDSA Hand Hygiene Task Force. *MMWR Recommendations and Reports, 51*(RR-16), 1–45. https://www.cdc.gov/mmwr/pdf/rr/rr5116.pdf (Level II)

8 Centers for Medicare and Medicaid Services. (2020). Condition of participation: Infection control. 42 C.F.R. § 482.42.

9 Accreditation Association for Hospitals and Health Systems. (2020). Standard 07.01.21. *Healthcare Facilities Accreditation Program: Accreditation requirements for acute care hospitals.* Chicago, IL: Accreditation Association for Hospitals and Health Systems. (Level VII)

10 DNV GL-Healthcare USA, Inc. (2020). IC.1.SR.1. *NIAHO® accreditation requirements, interpretive guidelines and surveyor guidance—revision 20.0.* Milford, OH: DNV GL-Healthcare USA, Inc. (Level VII)

11 Siegel, J. D., et al. (2007, revised 2019). 2007 guideline for isolation precautions: Preventing transmission of infectious agents in healthcare settings. https://www.cdc.gov/infectioncontrol/pdf/guidelines/isolation-guidelines-H.pdf (Level II)

12 Accreditation Association for Hospitals and Health Systems. (2020). Standard 07.01.10. *Healthcare Facilities Accreditation Program: Accreditation requirements for acute care hospitals.* Chicago, IL: Accreditation Association for Hospitals and Health Systems. (Level VII)

13 Occupational Safety and Health Administration. (2012). Bloodborne pathogens, standard number 1910.1030. https://www.osha.gov/pls/oshaweb/owadisp.show_document?p_id=10051&p_table=STANDARDS (Level VII)

14 Rutala, W. A., et al. (2008, revised 2019). Guideline for disinfection and sterilization in healthcare facilities, 2008. https://www.cdc.gov/infectioncontrol/pdf/guidelines/disinfection-guidelines-H.pdf (Level I)

15 Accreditation Association for Hospitals and Health Systems. (2020). Standard 07.02.03. *Healthcare Facilities Accreditation Program: Accreditation requirements for acute care hospitals.* Chicago, IL: Accreditation Association for Hospitals and Health Systems. (Level VII)

16 The Joint Commission. (2021). Standard RC.01.03.01. *Comprehensive accreditation manual for hospitals.* Oakbrook Terrace, IL: The Joint Commission. (Level VII)

17 Centers for Medicare and Medicaid Services, Department of Health and Human Services. (2020). Condition of participation: Medical record services. 42 C.F.R. § 482.24(b).

18 Accreditation Association for Hospitals and Health Systems. (2020). Standard 10.00.03. *Healthcare Facilities Accreditation Program: Accreditation requirements for acute care hospitals.* Chicago, IL: Accreditation Association for Hospitals and Health Systems. (Level VII)

19 DNV GL-Healthcare USA, Inc. (2020). MR.2.SR.1. *NIAHO® accreditation requirements, interpretive guidelines and surveyor guidance—revision 20.0.* Milford, OH: DNV GL-Healthcare USA, Inc. (Level VII)

BALLOON VALVULOPLASTY CARE

Although surgery remains the treatment of choice for valvular heart disease, balloon valvuloplasty provides an alternative to valve replacement in patients with critical stenoses.[1] This technique enlarges the orifice of a heart valve that has been narrowed by a congenital defect, calcification, rheumatic fever, or aging. It evolved from percutaneous transluminal coronary angioplasty and uses the same balloon-tipped catheters for dilatation. Balloon valvuloplasty may be considered as a bridge to surgery or transcatheter aortic valve implantation.[1] It may be indicated for patients for whom surgery poses a high risk and for those who refuse surgery.

Balloon valvuloplasty is performed in a cardiac catheterization laboratory under local anesthesia, light sedation, moderate sedation, or general anesthesia.[2,3,4] The practitioner inserts a balloon-tipped catheter through the patient's femoral vein or artery using a sheath, threads it into the heart, and repeatedly inflates it against the leaflets of the diseased valve. This process increases the size of the orifice, improving valvular function and helping prevent complications from decreased cardiac output. (See *How balloon valvuloplasty works*, page 50.)

After balloon valvuloplasty, you should monitor the patient closely for complications, provide supportive care, and teach the patient and family about postprocedure care.

Equipment
Before and during balloon valvuloplasty
Antiseptic solution ▪ local anesthetic ▪ vital signs monitoring equipment ▪ gloves ▪ gown ▪ caps ▪ masks ▪ valvuloplasty or balloon-tipped catheter

■ sheath ■ IV catheter insertion supplies ■ prescribed IV solution and tubing ■ cardiac monitor and electrodes ■ oxygen source ■ oxygen delivery device ■ sterile label ■ prescribed sedative ■ emergency equipment (code cart with emergency medications, defibrillator, handheld resuscitation bag with mask, intubation equipment) ■ heparin (or other anticoagulant) for injection[5] ■ contrast medium ■ introducer kit for balloon catheter ■ introducer kit for balloon catheter ■ sterile gown ■ sterile gloves ■ sterile drapes ■ sterile dressings ■ pulse oximeter and probe ■ prescribed antiplatelet or antithrombotic medications ■ Optional: disposable head clippers, pulmonary artery (PA) catheter, Doppler ultrasound blood flow detector, sterile scissors, suture material.

After balloon valvuloplasty

Gloves ■ stethoscope ■ vital signs monitoring equipment ■ pulse oximeter and probe ■ prescribed IV solution ■ IV administration set ■ cardiac monitor and electrodes ■ pulmonary artery monitoring system ■ oxygen source ■ oxygen delivery device ■ Doppler ultrasound blood flow detector ■ disinfectant pad ■ facility-approved disinfectant ■ Optional: prescribed medications, electronic infusion device (preferably a smart pump with dose-error reduction software and interoperability with the electronic health record),[6] supplies for arterial blood gas (ABG) analysis, additional personal protective equipment (gown, mask with face shield or mask and goggles), prescribed analgesic, labels, bedpan.

Preparation of equipment

Inspect all equipment and supplies. If a product is expired, is defective, or has compromised integrity, remove it from patient use, label it as expired or defective, and report the expiration or defect as directed by your facility. Make sure that emergency equipment is readily available and functioning properly.

Implementation

Before balloon valvuloplasty

■ Verify the practitioner's orders.
■ Check the patient's medical record for allergies to the prescribed contrast medium, prescribed medications, local anesthetic, or latex, and for any other contraindications to the procedure.
■ If required by your facility, confirm that informed consent has been obtained and that the signed consent form is in the patient's medical record.[7,8,9,10]
■ Gather and prepare the necessary equipment and supplies.
■ Conduct a preprocedure verification *to make sure that all relevant documentation, related information, and equipment are available and matched correctly to the patient's identifiers.*[11,12]
■ Verify that the ordered laboratory and imaging studies have been completed and that the results are in the patient's medical record. Notify the practitioner of critical test results within your facility's established timeframe *so that the patient can be treated promptly.*[13] Ensure that results of coagulation studies, complete blood count, serum electrolyte studies, and blood typing and crossmatching are available.[11,12]
■ Review baseline hemodynamic parameters and patient medications *for contraindications to the procedure.*[14]
■ Perform hand hygiene.[15,16,17,18,19,20]
■ Confirm the patient's identity using at least two patient identifiers.[21]
■ Provide privacy.[22,23,24,25]
■ Reinforce the practitioner's explanation of the procedure, taking into account the patient's and family's (if appropriate) communication and learning needs, *to increase understanding, allay fears, and enhance cooperation.*[26] Include the procedure risks and alternatives, and answer the patient's questions.
■ Provide reassurance that, although awake during the procedure, the patient will receive a sedative and a local anesthetic beforehand *for comfort.*
■ Teach the patient what to expect *to ease anxiety and enhance cooperation.* For example, inform the patient that the hair in the groin area will be clipped and the skin cleaned with an antiseptic; a brief stinging sensation will be felt when the local anesthetic is injected; and there may be pressure as the catheter moves along the vessel. Describe the warm, flushed feeling that the patient will likely experience from injection of the contrast medium.

■ Explain that the procedure may last up to 4 hours, and that the patient may feel discomfort from lying on a hard table for that long.
■ If the procedure isn't an emergency, confirm the patient's nothing-by-mouth status before the procedure; minimum fasting recommendations are 2 hours for clear liquids, 6 or more hours for a light meal or nonhuman milk, and 8 or more hours for fried or fatty foods or meat.[27]
■ Have the patient void.
■ Raise the bed to waist level before providing care *to prevent caregiver back strain.*[28]
■ Perform hand hygiene.[15,16,17,18,19,20]
■ Obtain vital signs and oxygen saturation level using pulse oximetry *to serve as a baseline for comparison during and after the procedure.*
■ Perform a neurovascular assessment on all extremities. Assess the presence or absence and quality of all distal pulses. Assess faint or nonpalpable pulses using a Doppler ultrasound blood flow detector, as indicated. (See the "Doppler ultrasound device use" procedure.)[10]
■ Perform hand hygiene.[15,16,17,18,19,20]
■ Put on gloves *to comply with standard precautions.*[29,30,31]
■ Insert an IV catheter, as ordered, *to provide access for medications and to infuse prescribed IV fluid.* (See the "IV catheter insertion and removal" procedure.)
■ Clip hair from the insertion site, as needed; clean the site with antiseptic solution and allow it to dry completely.[32]
■ Administer an antiplatelet or antithrombotic agent, as ordered, following safe medication administration practices.[14,33,34,35,36]
NURSING ALERT Aspirin reduces the frequency of ischemic complications after percutaneous coronary intervention (PCI). Although the minimum effective aspirin dosage in the setting of PCI hasn't been established, it's recommended that 325 mg of aspirin be given at least 2 hours (preferably 24 hours) before PCI.[14]
■ Administer a sedative, as ordered, following safe medication administration practices.[33,34,35,36]
■ Remove and discard your gloves.[29]
■ Perform hand hygiene.[15,16,17,18,19,20]
■ Provide hand-off communication about the patient's history, condition, and care to the person who will assume responsibility for the patient's care during the procedure. Allow time for questions, as necessary, *to avoid miscommunications that can cause patient care errors during transitions of care.*[37]
■ Document the procedure.[30,39,40,41]

During balloon valvuloplasty

■ Receive hand-off communication from the person who was responsible for the patient's care. Ask questions, as necessary, *to avoid miscommunications that can cause patient care errors during transitions of care.*[37] As part of the hand-off process, trace each tubing and catheter from the patient to its point of origin using a standardized line recognition process.[37,42,43]
■ Perform hand hygiene.[15,16,17,18,19,20]
■ Confirm the patient's identity using at least two patient identifiers.[21]
■ Conduct a preprocedural verification *to make sure that all relevant documentation, related information, and equipment are available and correctly matched with the patient's identifiers.*[11,12]
■ Put on a cap and mask.
■ Perform hand hygiene.[15,16,17,18,19,20]
■ Put on a gown, and gloves *to comply with standard precautions.*[29,30,31]
■ Attach the patient to the cardiac monitoring equipment. Make sure that the alarm limits are set appropriately for the patient's current condition, and that the alarms are turned on, functioning properly, and audible to staff.[44,45,46,47]
■ Administer supplemental oxygen, as ordered.
■ The practitioner will put on a cap and mask, a sterile gown, and sterile gloves, and will then open the sterile supplies. Assist as necessary.
■ Confirm that the correct procedure has been identified for the correct patient at the correct site.[11,12]
■ Label all medications, medication containers, and other solutions on and off the sterile field.[48,49]
■ Using maximal barrier precautions, the practitioner will drape the patient and prepare and anesthetize the catheter insertion site (usually at

How balloon valvuloplasty works

In balloon valvuloplasty, the practitioner chooses an appropriate-sized balloon-tipped catheter using the following formula:

balloon size = patient's height (in cm) ÷ 10 + 10

Alternatively, the practitioner may directly measure the value diameter using two-dimensional echocardiography.[2] The practitioner then inserts the balloon-tipped catheter through the patient's femoral vein or artery using a sheath, threads it into the heart, and locates the stenotic valve.

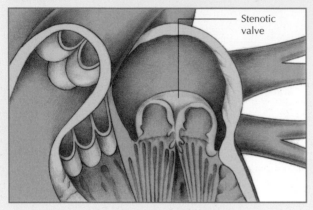

Stenotic valve

After locating the stenotic valve, the practitioner inflates the balloon, which increases the size of the valve opening.

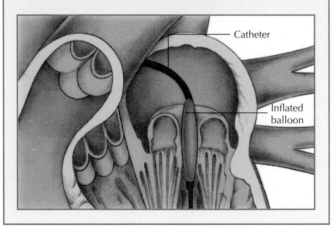

Catheter

Inflated balloon

the femoral artery). The practitioner may insert a PA catheter if one isn't already in place.[50]

■ Conduct a time-out immediately before starting the procedure *to ensure that the correct patient, site, positioning, and procedure are identified and, as applicable, that all relevant information and necessary equipment are available.*[51]

■ The practitioner will then insert a sheath into the site and thread a valvuloplasty or balloon-tipped catheter up into the heart.

■ The practitioner will inject a contrast medium *to visualize the heart valves and assess the stenosis*; the practitioner will also inject heparin or another anticoagulant[5] *to prevent the catheter from clotting.*[13,50]

■ Using low pressure, the practitioner will repeatedly inflate the balloon on the valvuloplasty catheter for a short time, usually 15 to 30 seconds, gradually increasing the time and pressure. If these actions don't reduce the stenosis, the practitioner may use a larger balloon.

■ Monitor the patient during the procedure. Assess the insertion site frequently for bleeding, and monitor International Normalized Ratio, prothrombin time, partial thromboplastin time, activated clotting time, and platelet count, as ordered.[5,50] Assess the patient's vital signs and oxygen saturation levels continually during the procedure, especially for aortic valvuloplasty.

NURSING ALERT During balloon inflation, the aortic outflow tract is completely obstructed, causing blood pressure to fall dangerously low. Ventricular ectopy also is common during balloon positioning and inflation. Start treatment for ectopy when signs or symptoms develop or when ventricular tachycardia is sustained. Carefully assess the patient's respiratory status; changes in rate and pattern can be the first sign of a complication such as an embolism.

■ After completion of valvuloplasty, a series of angiograms is taken *to evaluate the effectiveness of the treatment.* Assist as necessary.

■ The practitioner may then suture the sheath in place and cover the insertion site with a sterile dressing. The sutures typically remain in place until the effects of the anticoagulant have worn off.

■ Continue to closely monitor the patient.

■ Discard used supplies in appropriate receptacles.[52]

■ Remove and discard your gloves and other personal protective equipment.[52]

■ Perform hand hygiene.[15,16,17,18,19,20]

■ Document the procedure.[38,39,40,41]

After balloon valvuloplasty

■ Receive hand-off communication from the person who was responsible for the patient's care during the procedure. Ask questions as necessary *to avoid miscommunications that can cause patient care errors during transitions of care.*[37] As part of the hand-off process, trace each tubing and catheter from the patient to its point of origin using a standardized line reconciliation process.[37,42,43]

■ Verify the practitioner's orders.

■ Reconcile the patient's medications at the care transition *to reduce the risk for medication errors, including omissions, duplications, dosing errors, and drug interactions.*[53,54]

■ Gather and prepare the necessary equipment and supplies.

■ Perform hand hygiene.[15,16,17,18,19,20]

■ Confirm the patient's identity using at least two patient identifiers.[21]

■ Provide privacy.[22,23,24,25]

■ Explain the procedure to the patient and family (if appropriate) according to their communication and learning needs *to increase understanding, allay fears, and enhance cooperation.*[26]

■ Raise the patient's bed to waist level before providing care *to prevent caregiver back strain.*[28]

■ Put on gloves and other personal protective equipment as needed *to comply with standard precautions.*[29,30]

■ Attach the patient to a cardiac monitor and pulse oximeter. Make sure that the alarm limits are set appropriately for the patient's current condition and that the alarms are turned on, functioning properly, and audible to staff.[44,45,46,47]

■ Obtain the patient's vital signs *to serve as a baseline for comparison*, and continue to monitor them frequently at an interval determined by your facility and the patient's condition *to promptly recognize changes in the patient's condition.* Note that there's no evidence-based research to indicate best practice for the frequency of vital signs monitoring.[55]

■ Assess the sheath insertion site for bleeding, hematoma, and ecchymosis. If the sheath remains in place, refer to the "Arterial and venous sheath removal" procedure when removal is indicated. If the sheath was removed and a compression device remains in place over the insertion site, make sure that the device was applied properly.

■ Ensure that the patient is positioned properly; positioning will depend on the presence of a sheath or the time since sheath removal. Follow facility guidelines, the manufacturer's guidelines, or the practitioner's orders.[56]

■ If the patient is receiving IV heparin,[14] nitroglycerin, or another medicated infusion, administer the medication using an electronic infusion device[57] following safe medication administration practices *to prevent life-threatening dosing errors.*[33,34,35,58] Make sure that the electronic infusion device alarm limits are set appropriately and that the alarms are turned on, functioning properly, and audible to staff.[44,45,46] Trace the tubing from the patient to its point of origin *to make sure that it's connected to the proper port.*[43] Route the tubing in a standardized direction if the patient has other tubing and catheters that have different purposes. If multiple IV lines will be used, label the tubing at the distal end (near the patient connection) and proximal end (near the source container) *to reduce the risk of misconnection.*[44] If required by your facility, have another nurse perform an independent double-check *to verify the patient's identity and to ensure that the correct medication is hanging in the prescribed concentration, the medication's indication corresponds with the patient's diagnosis, the dosage calculations are correct and the dosing formula used to derive the final dose is correct, the route of administration is safe and proper for the patient, the pump settings are correct, and the infusion line is attached to the correct port.*[59,60] Compare the results of the independent double-check with the other nurse (if required) and, if no discrepancies exist, continue infusing the medication. If discrepancies exist, rectify them before continuing the infusion.[60]

■ Assess the patient's cardiac status; continue to monitor the patient's heart rate and rhythm, and auscultate regularly for murmurs, *which may indicate worsening valvular insufficiency*. Notify the practitioner if you detect a new or worsening murmur.

■ Administer oxygen, if ordered, as prescribed. Assess the patient's respiratory status, including oxygen saturation level using pulse oximetry; continue to monitor respiratory status for changes, *because changes in respiratory rate and pattern can be the first sign of a complication such as an embolism*. Monitor ABG results, as ordered.

■ Monitor the patient's arterial pressure, pulmonary artery pressure, and other hemodynamic parameters, as indicated.

■ Continue to monitor the insertion site for bleeding and to assess peripheral pulses distal to the insertion site as well as the color, sensation, temperature, and capillary refill time of the affected extremity. Use a Doppler ultrasound blood flow detector to assess pedal pulses *because they may be difficult to assess, especially if the sheath remains in place*. Compare findings bilaterally.

■ Administer IV fluids, as prescribed, *to help the kidneys excrete the contrast medium used during the procedure*. Closely monitor intake and output, and watch for signs of fluid overload, such as distended neck veins, atrial and ventricular gallops, dyspnea, pulmonary congestion, tachycardia, hypertension, and hypoxemia.

■ Assess for signs and symptoms of complications of the procedure, such as embolism (dyspnea, tachypnea, altered mental status, and tachycardia), hemorrhage (including retroperitoneal bleeding), myocardial ischemia (chest pain caused by obstruction of blood flow during valvuloplasty), and cardiac tamponade (decreased or absent peripheral pulses, pale or cyanotic skin, hypotension, and paradoxical pulse). Immediately report signs and symptoms of any of these complications.

■ Encourage the patient to perform deep-breathing exercises *to prevent atelectasis, which can occur with immobility*. Note that this step is especially important in older adult patients.

■ Screen for and assess the patient's pain using facility-defined criteria that are consistent with the patient's age, condition, and ability to understand. Treat the patient's pain as needed and ordered using nonpharmacologic, pharmacologic, or a combination of approaches. Base the treatment plan on evidence-based practices and the patient's clinical condition, past medical history, and pain management goals.[61]

■ Administer pain medications, as needed and prescribed, following safe medication administration practices.[33,34,35,58]

■ Assist the patient during meals, bedpan use, and position changes that are appropriate to the patient's activity limitations.

■ Reassess and respond to the patient's pain by evaluating the response to treatment and progress toward pain management goals. Assess for adverse reactions and risk factors for adverse events that may result from treatment.[61]

■ Return the patient's bed to the lowest position *to prevent falls and maintain patient safety*.[64]

■ Discard used supplies in appropriate receptacles.[52]

■ Remove and discard your gloves and any other personal protective equipment worn.[52]

■ Perform hand hygiene.[15,16,17,18,19,20]

■ Clean and disinfect your stethoscope using a disinfectant pad.[63,64]

■ Perform hand hygiene.[15,16,17,18,19,20]

■ Put on gloves and other personal protective equipment, as needed.[52]

■ Clean and disinfect reusable equipment according to the manufacturer's instructions *to prevent the spread of infection*.[63,64]

■ Remove and discard your gloves and other personal protective equipment.[52]

■ Perform hand hygiene.[15,16,17,18,19,20]

■ Document the procedure.[38,39,40,41]

Special considerations

■ Be aware that using heparin and a large-bore catheter can lead to arterial hemorrhage. Monitor the patient closely.

■ If the patient is receiving heparin, monitor partial thromboplastin time or activated clotting time and maintain the infusion according to your facility's protocol or the practitioner's order.[50,57] Notify the practitioner of critical test results within your facility's established time frame *so that the patient can receive prompt treatment*.[13]

■ The Joint Commission has issued a sentinel event alert concerning medical device alarm safety *because alarm-related events have been associated with permanent loss of function and death*. Among the major contributing factors were improper alarm settings, alarm settings turned off inappropriately, and alarm signals that are inaudible to staff. Make sure that alarm limits are set appropriately and that alarms are turned on, functioning properly, and audible. Follow facility guidelines for preventing alarm fatigue.[44]

■ The Joint Commission has issued a sentinel event alert related to managing risk during transition to the new International Organization for Standardization tubing standards that were designed to prevent dangerous tubing misconnections, *which can lead to serious patient injury and death*. During the transition, trace each tubing and catheter from the patient to its point of origin before connecting or reconnecting any device or infusion, at any care transition (such as a new setting or service), and as part of the hand-off process; route tubes and catheters serving different purposes in different standardized directions; label the tubing at both the distal and proximal ends (when there are different access sites or several bags hanging); use tubing and equipment only as intended; and store medications for different delivery routes in separate locations.[42]

■ The Joint Commission has issued a sentinel event alert concerning inadequate hand-off communication because of the potential for patient harm that can result when a receiver receives inaccurate, incomplete, untimely, misinterpreted, or otherwise inadequate information. To improve hand-off communication, standardize the critical information communicated by the sender. At a minimum, include the sender contact information; illness assessment; patient summary, including events leading up to the illness or admission, hospital course, ongoing assessment, and care plan; to-do action list; contingency plans; allergy list; code status; medication list; and dated laboratory test results and vital signs. Provide face-to-face communication whenever possible in an interruption-free location using facility-approved, standardized tools and methods (for example, forms, templates, checklists, protocols, and mnemonics). Provide ample time and opportunity for questions, and include the multidisciplinary team members and the patient and family when appropriate.[65]

Complications

Complications include bleeding and hematoma at the insertion site, vessel damage, arrhythmias, stroke, valvular rupture, ventricular rupture, valve regurgitation, infection, and an allergic reaction to the contrast medium.[66]

Documentation

Document the patient's vital signs and oxygen saturation levels before and during the procedure, assessment findings, diagnostic test results, complications and resulting interventions, and the patient's tolerance of the procedure. Record any teaching provided to the patient and family (if applicable), their understanding of that teaching, and any need for follow-up teaching.

REFERENCES

1 Baumgartner, H., et al. (2017). 2017 ESC/EACTS guidelines for the management of valvular heart disease. *European Heart Journal, 38*, 2739–2791. https://academic.oup.com/eurheartj/article/38/36/2739/4095039

2 Nobuyoshi, M., et al. (2009). Percutaneous balloon mitral valvuloplasty: A review. *Circulation, 119*, e211–e219. https://www.ahajournals.org/doi/pdf/10.1161/CIRCULATIONAHA.108.792952 (Level VII)

3 Assadi, R. (2020). Percutaneous mitral balloon valvuloplasty commissu-rotomy, valvotomy. https://emedicine.medscape.com/article/1839677-overview#a2

4 Keeble, T., et al. (2016). Percutaneous balloon aortic valvuloplasty in the era of transcatheter aortic valve implantation: A narrative review. *Open Heart, 3*, e000421. https://openheart.bmj.com/content/openhrt/3/2/e000421.full.pdf (Level VI)

5 Merriweather, N., & Sulzbach-Hoke, L. M. (2012). Managing risk of complications at femoral vascular access sites in percutaneous coronary intervention. *Critical Care Nurse, 32*(5), 16–29. (Level VII)

6 Standard 24. Flow-control devices. Infusion therapy standards of practice (8th ed.). (2021). *Journal of Infusion Nursing, 44*, S69–S73. (Level VII)

7 The Joint Commission. (2021). Standard RI.01.03.01. *Comprehensive accreditation manual for hospitals*. Oakbrook Terrace, IL: The Joint Commission. (Level VII)

8 Centers for Medicare and Medicaid Services, Department of Health and Human Services. (2020). Condition of participation: Patient's rights. 42 C.F.R. § 482.13(b)(2).

9 Accreditation Association for Hospitals and Health Systems. (2020). Standard 30.01.11. *Healthcare Facilities Accreditation Program: Accreditation requirements for acute care hospitals*. Chicago, IL: Accreditation Association for Hospitals and Health Systems. (Level VII)

10 DNV GL-Healthcare USA, Inc. (2020). PR.2.SR.3. *NIAHO® accreditation requirements, interpretive guidelines and surveyor guidance—revision 20.0*. Milford, OH: DNV GL-Healthcare USA, Inc. (Level VII)

11 The Joint Commission. (2021). Standard UP.01.01.01. *Comprehensive accreditation manual for hospitals*. Oakbrook Terrace, IL: The Joint Commission. (Level VII)

12 Accreditation Association for Hospitals and Health Systems. (2020). Standard 30.00.14. *Healthcare Facilities Accreditation Program: Accreditation requirements for acute care hospitals*. Chicago, IL: Accreditation Association for Hospitals and Health Systems. (Level VII)

13 The Joint Commission. (2021). Standard NPSG.02.03.01. *Comprehensive accreditation manual for hospitals*. Oakbrook Terrace, IL: The Joint Commission. (Level VII)

14 Dehmer, G. J., et al. (2014). SCAI/ACC/AHA expert consensus document: 2014 update on percutaneous coronary intervention without on-site surgical backup. *Circulation, 129*, 2610–2626. https://www.ahajournals.org/doi/pdf/10.1161/CIR.0000000000000037 (Level VII)

15 The Joint Commission. (2021). Standard NPSG.07.01.01. *Comprehensive accreditation manual for hospitals*. Oakbrook Terrace, IL: The Joint Commission. (Level VII)

16 Centers for Disease Control and Prevention. (2002). Guideline for hand hygiene in health-care settings: Recommendations of the Healthcare Infection Control Practices Advisory Committee and the HICPAC/SHEA/APIC/IDSA Hand Hygiene Task Force. *MMWR Recommendations and Reports, 51*(RR-16), 1–45. https://www.cdc.gov/mmwr/pdf/rr/rr5116.pdf (Level II)

17 World Health Organization. (2009). WHO guidelines on hand hygiene in health care: First global patient safety challenge, clean care is safer care. https://apps.who.int/iris/bitstream/handle/10665/44102/9789241597906_eng.pdf?sequence=1 (Level IV)

18 Centers for Medicare and Medicaid Services, Department of Health and Human Services. (2020). Condition of participation: Infection control. 42 C.F.R. § 482.42.

19 Accreditation Association for Hospitals and Health Systems. (2020). Standard 07.01.21. *Healthcare Facilities Accreditation Program: Accreditation requirements for acute care hospitals*. Chicago, IL: Accreditation Association for Hospitals and Health Systems. (Level VII)

20 DNV GL-Healthcare USA, Inc. (2020). IC.1.SR.1. *NIAHO® accreditation requirements, interpretive guidelines and surveyor guidance—revision 20.0*. Milford, OH: DNV GL-Healthcare USA, Inc. (Level VII)

21 The Joint Commission. (2021). Standard NPSG.01.01.01. *Comprehensive accreditation manual for hospitals*. Oakbrook Terrace, IL: The Joint Commission. (Level VII)

22 Accreditation Association for Hospitals and Health Systems. (2020). Standard 15.01.16. *Healthcare Facilities Accreditation Program: Accreditation requirements for acute care hospitals*. Chicago, IL: Accreditation Association for Hospitals and Health Systems. (Level VII)

23 Centers for Medicare and Medicaid Services, Department of Health and Human Services. (2020). Condition of participation: Patient's rights. 42 C.F.R. § 482.13 (c)(1).

24 DNV GL-Healthcare USA, Inc. (2020). PR.2.SR.5. *NIAHO® accreditation requirements, interpretive guidelines and surveyor guidance—revision 20.0*. Milford, OH: DNV GL-Healthcare USA, Inc. (Level VII)

25 The Joint Commission. (2021). Standard RI.01.01.01. *Comprehensive accreditation manual for hospitals*. Oakbrook Terrace, IL: The Joint Commission. (Level VII)

26 The Joint Commission. (2021). Standard PC.02.01.21. *Comprehensive accreditation manual for hospitals*. Oakbrook Terrace, IL: The Joint Commission. (Level VII)

27 American Society of Anesthesiologists. (2017). Practice guidelines for preoperative fasting and the use of pharmacologic agents to reduce the risk of pulmonary aspiration: Application to healthy patients undergoing elective procedures. *Anesthesiology, 126*, 376–393. (Level V)

28 Waters, T. R., et al. (2009). Safe patient handling training for schools of nursing. https://www.cdc.gov/niosh/docs/2009-127/pdfs/2009-127.pdf (Level VII)

29 Siegel, J. D., et al. (2007, revised 2019). 2007 guideline for isolation precautions: Preventing transmission of infectious agents in healthcare settings. https://www.cdc.gov/infectioncontrol/pdf/guidelines/isolation-guidelines-H.pdf (Level II)

30 Accreditation Association for Hospitals and Health Systems. (2020). Standard 07.01.10. *Healthcare Facilities Accreditation Program: Accreditation requirements for acute care hospitals*. Chicago, IL: Accreditation Association for Hospitals and Health Systems. (Level VII)

31 DNV GL-Healthcare USA, Inc. (2020). IC.1.SR.2. *NIAHO® accreditation requirements, interpretive guidelines and surveyor guidance—revision 20.0*. Milford, OH: DNV GL-Healthcare USA, Inc. (Level VII)

32 The Joint Commission. (2021). Standard NPSG.07.05.01. *Comprehensive accreditation manual for hospitals*. Oakbrook Terrace, IL: The Joint Commission. (Level VII)

33 Centers for Medicare and Medicaid Services, Department of Health and Human Services. (2020). Condition of participation: Nursing services. 42 C.F.R. § 482.23(c).

34 Accreditation Association for Hospitals and Health Systems. (2020). Standard 16.01.03. *Healthcare Facilities Accreditation Program: Accreditation requirements for acute care hospitals*. Chicago, IL: Accreditation Association for Hospitals and Health Systems. (Level VII)

35 The Joint Commission. (2021). Standard MM.06.01.01. *Comprehensive accreditation manual for hospitals*. Oakbrook Terrace, IL: The Joint Commission. (Level VII)

36 DNV GL-Healthcare USA, Inc. (2020). MM.1.SR.3. *NIAHO® accreditation requirements, interpretive guidelines and surveyor guidance—revision 20.0*. Milford, OH: DNV GL-Healthcare USA, Inc. (Level VII)

37 The Joint Commission. (2021). Standard PC.02.02.01. *Comprehensive accreditation manual for hospitals*. Oakbrook Terrace, IL: The Joint Commission. (Level VII)

38 The Joint Commission. (2021). Standard RC.01.03.01. *Comprehensive accreditation manual for hospitals*. Oakbrook Terrace, IL: The Joint Commission. (Level VII)

39 Centers for Medicare and Medicaid Services, Department of Health and Human Services. (2020). Condition of participation: Medical record services. 42 C.F.R. § 482.24(b).

40 Accreditation Association for Hospitals and Health Systems. (2020). Standard 10.00.03. *Healthcare Facilities Accreditation Program: Accreditation requirements for acute care hospitals*. Chicago, IL: Accreditation Association for Hospitals and Health Systems. (Level VII)

41 DNV GL-Healthcare USA, Inc. (2020). MR.2.SR.1. *NIAHO® accreditation requirements, interpretive guidelines and surveyor guidance—revision 20.0*. Milford, OH: DNV GL-Healthcare USA, Inc. (Level VII)

42 The Joint Commission. (2014). Sentinel event alert 53: Managing risk during transition to new ISO tubing connector standards. http://www.jointcommission.org/assets/1/6/SEA_53_Connectors_8_19_14_final.pdf (Level VII)

43 U.S. Food and Drug Administration. (2017). Examples of medical device misconnections. https://www.fda.gov/medical-devices/medical-device-connectors/examples-medical-device-misconnections

44 The Joint Commission. (2013). Sentinel event alert 50: Medical device alarm safety in hospitals. https://www.jointcommission.org/assets/1/6/SEA_50_alarms_4_26_16.pdf (Level VII)

45 The Joint Commission. (2021). Standard NPSG.06.01.01. *Comprehensive accreditation manual for hospitals*. Oakbrook Terrace, IL: The Joint Commission. (Level VII)

46 Graham, K. C., & Cvach, M. (2010). Monitor alarm fatigue: Standardizing use of physiological monitors and decreasing nuisance alarms. *American Journal of Critical Care, 19*, 28–37.

47 American Association of Critical-Care Nurses. (2018). AACN practice alert: Managing alarms in acute care across the life span – Electrocardiography

and pulse oximetry. https://www.aacn.org/clinical-resources/practice-alerts/managing-alarms-in-acute-care-across-the-life-span (Level VII)

48 The Joint Commission. (2021). Standard NPSG.03.04.01. *Comprehensive accreditation manual for hospitals*. Oakbrook Terrace, IL: The Joint Commission. (Level VII)

49 Accreditation Association for Hospitals and Health Systems. (2020). Standard 25.01.27. *Healthcare Facilities Accreditation Program: Accreditation requirements for acute care hospitals*. Chicago, IL: Accreditation Association for Hospitals and Health Systems. (Level VII)

50 Agu, N. C., & Rao, P. S. (2012). Balloon aortic valvuloplasty. *Pediatrics & Therapeutics, S5*, 004. https://www.longdom.org/open-access/balloon-aortic-valvuloplasty-2161-0665.S5-004.pdf (Level VII)

51 The Joint Commission. (2021). Standard UP.01.03.01. *Comprehensive accreditation manual for hospitals*. Oakbrook Terrace, IL: The Joint Commission. (Level VII)

52 Occupational Safety and Health Administration. (2012). Bloodborne pathogens, standard number 1910.1030. https://www.osha.gov/pls/oshaweb/owadisp.show_document?p_id=10051&p_table=STANDARDS (Level VII)

53 Standard 13. Medication verification. Infusion therapy standards of practice (8th ed.). (2021). *Journal of Infusion Nursing, 44*, S46–S49. (Level VII)

54 The Joint Commission. (2020). Standard NPSG.03.06.01. *Comprehensive accreditation manual for hospitals*. Oakbrook Terrace, IL: The Joint Commission. (Level VII)

55 American Society of PeriAnesthesia Nurses. (2019). *2019–2020 Perianesthesia nursing standards, practice recommendations and interpretive statements*. Cherry Hill, NJ: American Society of PeriAnesthesia Nurses. (Level VII)

56 Wiegand, D. L. (2017). *AACN procedure manual for high acuity, progressive, and critical care* (7th ed.). St. Louis, MO: Elsevier.

57 The Joint Commission. (2021). Standard NPSG.03.05.01. *Comprehensive accreditation manual for hospitals*. Oakbrook Terrace, IL: The Joint Commission. (Level VII)

58 DNV GL-Healthcare USA, Inc. (2020). MM.1.SR.2. *NIAHO® accreditation requirements, interpretive guidelines and surveyor guidance—revision 20.0*. Milford, OH: DNV GL-Healthcare USA, Inc. (Level VII)

59 Institute for Safe Medication Practices. (2018). ISMP list of high-alert medications in acute care settings. http://www.ismp.org/Tools/highalertmedications.pdf (Level VII)

60 Institute for Safe Medication Practices. (2014). Independent double-check: Undervalued and misused. https://www.ismp.org/resources/independent-double-checks-undervalued-and-misused-selective-use-strategy-can-play (Level VII)

61 The Joint Commission. (2021). Standard PC.01.02.07. *Comprehensive accreditation manual for hospitals*. Oakbrook Terrace, IL: The Joint Commission. (Level VII)

62 Ganz, D. A., et al. (2013, reviewed 2021). *Preventing falls in hospitals: A toolkit for improving quality of care* (AHRQ Publication No. 13-0015-EF). Rockville, MD: Agency for Healthcare Research and Quality. https://www.ahrq.gov/professionals/systems/hospital/fallpxtoolkit/index.html (Level VII)

63 Rutala, W. A., et al. (2008, revised 2019). Guideline for disinfection and sterilization in healthcare facilities, 2008. https://www.cdc.gov/infection-control/pdf/guidelines/disinfection-guidelines-H.pdf (Level I)

64 Accreditation Association for Hospitals and Health Systems. (2020). Standard 07.02.03. *Healthcare Facilities Accreditation Program: Accreditation requirements for acute care hospitals*. Chicago, IL: Accreditation Association for Hospitals and Health Systems. (Level VII)

65 The Joint Commission. (2017). Sentinel event alert 58: Inadequate hand-off communication. https://www.jointcommission.org/assets/1/18/SEA_58_Hand_off_Comms_9_6_17_FINAL_(1).pdf (Level VII)

66 Perez, O. A., et al. (2020). Balloon valvuloplasty. https://www.ncbi.nlm.nih.gov/books/NBK519532/

BARIATRIC BED USE

Obesity affects more than 42% of Americans.[1] A patient is considered to have obesity if the patient's body mass index (BMI) is 30 kg/m^2 or greater.[2] A typical hospital bed is designed to hold a patients who weighs up to 450 lb (204 kg) and who doesn't have a wide abdominal girth. A bariatric bed, a recent addition to hospital equipment, accommodates patients with obesity. Various types of bariatric beds are available, ranging from a simply larger versions of a standard bed to a bed with a low-air-loss mattress that provides pressure relief.

A bariatric bed provides more comfort for a patient with obesity than the standard-size bed. A bariatric bed also preserves self-esteem of a patient with obesity by fitting the patient's larger body size easily and providing special side rails that help the patient with turning and repositioning. A bariatric bed provides sufficient space that allows the caregiver to perform such routine care as boosting, turning, and transferring the patient in and out of bed with greater ease and less risk of injury. Most bariatric beds have a built-in scale that lets you weigh the patient more easily. Some types of bariatric beds convert easily to a cardiac chair.

Equipment

Bariatric bed ■ facility-approved pressure injury risk assessment tool ■ Optional: overhead trapeze, special sheets.

Preparation of equipment

Obtain a bariatric bed from central supply or contact the company representative to have a bed delivered. Inspect all equipment and supplies. If a product is expired, is defective, or has compromised integrity, remove it, label it expired or defective, and report the expiration or defect as direct by your facility.

Prepare the bed according to the manufacturer's guidelines. A manufacturer's representative may be involved in the patient assessment *to ensure that the appropriate type and size of bariatric bed are provided.* Choose the appropriate type of mattress to meet your patient's needs. Specialized sheets may be necessary. Attach an overhead trapeze, if indicated.

Implementation

■ Verify the practitioner's order for a bariatric bed.

■ Perform hand hygiene.[3,4,5,6,7,8]

■ Confirm the patient's identity using at least two patient identifiers.[9]

■ Provide privacy.[10,11,12,13]

■ Explain the procedure to the patient and family (if appropriate) according to their individual communication and learning needs *to increase their understanding, allay their fears, and enhance cooperation.*[14] Discuss the need for the use of a bariatric bed *so that the patient and family understand its benefits and therapeutic effects.*

■ Assess the condition of the patient's skin by performing a pressure injury risk assessment upon the patient's admission to the facility. Repeat the assessment regularly or when a significant change occurs in the patient's condition, such as surgery or a decline in the patient's condition, *to help determine the type of mattress that meets the patient's needs.*[15] (See the "Pressure injury prevention" procedure.)

HOSPITAL-ACQUIRED CONDITION ALERT Keep in mind that the Centers for Medicare and Medicaid Services considers a stage 3 or 4 pressure injury to be a hospital-acquired condition *because it can be reasonably prevented by using a variety of best practices.* Make sure to follow evidence-based pressure injury prevention practices (e.g., assessing skin integrity, encouraging mobility, and repositioning the patient) *to reduce the risk of pressure injury.*[16,17,18]

■ Consult with other health care team members, such as the practitioner, surgical team members, physical therapist, occupational therapist, wound care specialist, and respiratory therapist, *to discuss your assessment findings and choose the appropriate type of bariatric bed and mattress for the patient's needs.*

■ Prepare the equipment for the patient.

■ If the bariatric bed is a rental, ask the manufacturer's representative to conduct an in-service training program *to help all health care team members understand the bed's use and provide safe care.*

■ Make sure that written instructions come with the bariatric bed. Keep them at the patient's bedside.

■ Provide the patient with bariatric bed product information and ensure orientation to the bed's functions and controls *to help the patient understand its many features and how to use it safely.*

■ Perform hand hygiene.[3,4,5,6,7,8]

■ Document the procedure.[19,20,21,22]

Special considerations

■ Provide other bariatric equipment and supplies, as needed, such as hospital gowns, commodes, wheelchairs, lifts, scales, and stretchers, *to ensure patient comfort and safety.*
■ Obtain the assistance of the appropriate number of staff members to assist with repositioning, transferring, or transporting the patient *to ensure patient safety and prevent caregiver strain or injury.*[23]
■ When transferring the patient to another department, call first to ensure that the department can accommodate a larger bed and that staff members are familiar with its use.

Documentation

Document the type of bariatric bed ordered and the date and time of its delivery. Indicate that staff members were oriented to the bed's use by the manufacturer's representative. Also indicate that the patient was oriented to the safe use of the bed and that the patient completed a return demonstration. Note whether written product information was given to the patient or left at the patient's bedside. Also document any other bariatric equipment you provided, such as an overhead trapeze or specialized sheets. Note the type of mattress on the bariatric bed. Document the patient's skin condition when the patient is placed on the bed. Record the patient's response to the bariatric bed. Document teaching provided to the patient and family (if applicable), their understanding of that teaching, and any need for follow-up teaching.

References

1 Hayes, C. M., et al. (2017). Prevalence of obesity among adults and youth: United States, 2015–2016. *NCHS Data Brief, 288*, 1–8. https://www.cdc.gov/nchs/data/databriefs/db288.pdf

2 Centers for Disease Control and Prevention. (2021). Defining adult overweight and obesity. https://www.cdc.gov/obesity/adult/defining.html

3 The Joint Commission. (2021). Standard NPSG.07.01.01. *Comprehensive accreditation manual for hospitals.* Oakbrook Terrace, IL: The Joint Commission. (Level VII)

4 Centers for Disease Control and Prevention. (2002). Guideline for hand hygiene in health-care settings: Recommendations of the Healthcare Infection Control Practices Advisory Committee and the HICPAC/SHEA/APIC/IDSA Hand Hygiene Task Force. *MMWR Recommendations and Reports, 51*(RR-16), 1–45. https://www.cdc.gov/mmwr/pdf/rr/rr5116.pdf (Level II)

5 World Health Organization. (2009). WHO guidelines on hand hygiene in health care: First global patient safety challenge, clean care is safer care. https://apps.who.int/iris/bitstream/handle/10665/44102/9789241597906_eng.pdf?sequence=1 (Level IV)

6 Centers for Medicare and Medicaid Services, Department of Health and Human Services. (2020). Condition of participation: Infection control. 42 C.F.R. § 482.42.

7 Accreditation Association for Hospitals and Health Systems. (2020). Standard 07.01.21. *Healthcare Facilities Accreditation Program: Accreditation requirements for acute care hospitals.* Chicago, IL: Accreditation Association for Hospitals and Health Systems. (Level VII)

8 DNV GL-Healthcare USA, Inc. (2020). IC.1.SR.1. *NIAHO® accreditation requirements, interpretive guidelines and surveyor guidance—revision 20.0.* Milford, OH: DNV GL-Healthcare USA, Inc. (Level VII)

9 The Joint Commission. (2021). Standard NPSG.01.01.01. *Comprehensive accreditation manual for hospitals.* Oakbrook Terrace, IL: The Joint Commission. (Level VII)

10 The Joint Commission. (2020). Standard RI.01.01.01. *Comprehensive accreditation manual for hospitals.* Oakbrook Terrace, IL: The Joint Commission. (Level VII)

11 DNV GL-Healthcare USA, Inc. (2020). PR.2.SR.5. *NIAHO® accreditation requirements, interpretive guidelines and surveyor guidance—revision 20.0.* Milford, OH: DNV GL-Healthcare USA, Inc. (Level VII)

12 Centers for Medicare and Medicaid Services, Department of Health and Human Services. (2020). Condition of participation: Patient's rights. 42 C.F.R. § 482.13(c)(1).

13 Accreditation Association for Hospitals and Health Systems. (2020). Standard 15.01.16. *Healthcare Facilities Accreditation Program: Accreditation requirements for acute care hospitals.* Chicago, IL: Accreditation Association for Hospitals and Health Systems. (Level VII)

14 The Joint Commission. (2021). Standard PC.02.01.21. *Comprehensive accreditation manual for hospitals.* Oakbrook Terrace, IL: The Joint Commission. (Level VII)

15 Wound Ostomy and Continence Nurses Society (WOCN). (2016). *Guideline for prevention and management of pressure ulcers (injuries): WOCN clinical practice guideline series 2.* Mount Laurel, NJ: WOCN.

16 National Pressure Ulcer Advisory Panel, et al. (2014). Prevention and treatment of pressure ulcers: Quick reference guide. https://www.epuap.org/wp-content/uploads/2016/10/quick-reference-guide-digital-npuap-epuap-pppia-jan2016.pdf (Level VII)

17 Accreditation Association for Hospitals and Health Systems. (2020). Standard 16.02.02. *Healthcare Facilities Accreditation Program: Accreditation requirements for acute care hospitals.* Chicago, IL: Accreditation Association for Hospitals and Health Systems. (Level VII)

18 Jarrett, N., & Callaham, M. (2016). Evidence-based guidelines for selected hospital-acquired conditions: Final report. https://www.cms.gov/Medicare/Medicare-Fee-for-Service-Payment/HospitalAcqCond/Downloads/2016-HAC-Report.pdf

19 The Joint Commission. (2021). Standard RC.01.03.01. *Comprehensive accreditation manual for hospitals.* Oakbrook Terrace, IL: The Joint Commission. (Level VII)

20 Centers for Medicare and Medicaid Services, Department of Health and Human Services. (2020). Condition of participation: Medical record services. 42 C.F.R. § 482.24(b).

21 Accreditation Association for Hospitals and Health Systems. (2020). Standard 10.00.03. *Healthcare Facilities Accreditation Program: Accreditation requirements for acute care hospitals.* Chicago, IL: Accreditation Association for Hospitals and Health Systems. (Level VII)

22 DNV GL-Healthcare USA, Inc. (2020). MR.2.SR.1. *NIAHO® accreditation requirements, interpretive guidelines and surveyor guidance—revision 20.0.* Milford, OH: DNV GL-Healthcare USA, Inc. (Level VII)

23 Waters, T. R., et al. (2009). Safe patient handling training for schools of nursing. https://www.cdc.gov/niosh/docs/2009-127/pdfs/2009-127.pdf (Level VII)

Bed bath

Performing a bed bath not only cleans the patient's skin but also stimulates circulation, provides mild exercise, and promotes comfort. Bathing also allows assessment of skin condition, joint mobility, and muscle strength.

Studies have revealed that basins traditionally used for patient bathing are commonly contaminated with multidrug-resistant organisms, increasing the risk of hospital-acquired infections.[1,2] Moreover, soap-and-water bathing causes skin deterioration in patients who are hospitalized, which can lead to pressure injuries.[3] Hospital-acquired infections and pressure injuries are not only costly to the patient's health but also to the facility. Because the Centers for Medicare and Medicaid Services categorizes them as a hospital-acquired conditions, they can affect reimbursement.[3] Daily bathing with chlorhexidine-impregnated disposable cloths can help prevent such hospital-acquired infections as central line–associated bloodstream infection[4] and catheter-associated urinary tract infection. These no-rinse cloths produce a persistent antibacterial effect on the skin that reduces bacterial colonization. Additionally, use of premoistened disposable cloths that contain a no-rinse surfactant can be helpful for daily bathing for patients with contraindications to chlorhexidine or when bathing with chlorhexidine isn't preferable.

Chlorhexidine-impregnated disposable cloths are contraindicated for patients with known allergies to chlorhexidine gluconate or any other ingredients in the product.[5] Avoid using them in patients with lumbar puncture or in contact with the meninges.[5] Use with care in premature infants or infants under age 2 months because these products may cause skin irritation or chemical burns.[5]

Equipment

Gloves ■ patient gown ■ bath blanket or sheet ■ Optional: gown, mask with face shield or mask and goggles, shampoo cap, shampoo.

For bathing with commercially prepared disposable cloths

Commercially prepared disposable cloths (chlorhexidine-impregnated or other facility-approved, no-rinse cloth) ■ Optional: washcloth, moisturizer or chlorhexidine-compatible moisturizer.

For bathing with water, skin cleanser, and washcloth
Washcloths ▪ skin cleanser ▪ warm water ▪ towel ▪ Optional: deodorant, moisture barrier, skin protectant.

Preparation of equipment
Inspect all equipment and supplies. If a product is expired, is defective, or has compromised integrity, remove it from patient use, label it as expired or defective, and report the expiration or defect as directed by your facility. If the patient desires, warm the commercially-prepared disposable cloths following the manufacturer's instructions.[6] (Room-temperature cloths remain active; warming is for patient comfort and not required.[7]

Implementation
▪ Review the patient's medical record for a history of allergies to chlorhexidine-gluconate, other ingredients in the product, or other bathing products.[5]
▪ Gather and prepare the necessary equipment and supplies.
▪ Perform hand hygiene.[8,9,10,11,12,13]
▪ Confirm the patient's identity using at least two patient identifiers.[14]
▪ Provide privacy.[15,16,17,18]
▪ Explain the procedure to the patient and family (if appropriate) according to their individual communication and learning needs *to increase their understanding, allay their fears, and enhance cooperation.*[19]
▪ Adjust the temperature in the patient's room, and close any open doors and windows *to prevent drafts.*
▪ Perform hand hygiene.[8,9,10,11,12,13]
▪ Raise the bed to waist level before providing care *to prevent caregiver back strain.*[20]
▪ Perform hand hygiene.[8,9,10,11,12,13]
▪ Put on gloves and, as needed, other personal protective equipment *to comply with standard precautions.*[21,22,23]
▪ Inspect the patient's skin for contraindications to disposable cloth or skin cleanser use.
▪ Position the patient for comfort.
▪ Use a shampoo cap or wash the patient's hair with shampoo, if needed. Avoid contact between the shampoo and the rest of the body because shampoo can deactivate chlorhexidine.[7]
▪ Remove the patient's gown, and cover the patient with a bath blanket or sheet.

For bathing with commercially prepared disposable cloths
▪ If using chlorhexidine-impregnated cloths, wash the patient's face using a regular washcloth and warm water.[6] Begin with the eyes, and wash from the inner canthus to the outer canthus. Use a separate section of the washcloth to wash each eye *to avoid spreading ocular infection.* Alternatively, clean the patient's face using a premoistened disposable cloth that contains a no-rinse surfactant.
NURSING ALERT Don't use chlorhexidine-impregnated cloths above the jawline. Chlorhexidine may cause serious or permanent injury if it enters and remains in the eyes, ears, or mouth.[5]
▪ Remove and discard your gloves.[23]
▪ Perform hand hygiene.[8,9,10,11,12,13]
▪ Put on a new pair of gloves.[21,22,23]
▪ Open the package containing the commercially prepared disposable cloths. Check the temperature before use *to prevent burns or discomfort.* Keep in mind that gloves diminish the sense of heat.[7]
▪ Use the first cloth to clean the patient's neck, shoulders, and chest following the manufacturer's instructions for use. Clean the neck well, even if it isn't visibly soiled, *because the neck often accumulates debris and moisture.*[7]
▪ After cleaning each area of the patient's body, allow the skin to air-dry.[7] Don't rinse, wipe off, or dry the skin with a cloth *to maintain the antibacterial activity of chlorhexidine and the moisturizing effects of the disposable cloths.* If you're using chlorhexidine-impregnated cloths, after cleaning each body area, clean any tubing present at that site (for example, indwelling urinary catheter, chest drainage tube, gastrostomy tube, biliary drainage tube). Clean the area of the tubing that's located within 6" (15 cm) of the patient's body.[7] Use additional cloths, as needed.

▪ Use a second cloth to clean the patient's arms, hands, web spaces, and axillae.[7]
▪ Use a third cloth to clean the patient's abdomen and then the groin and perineum.[7] Ensure thorough cleaning with special attention to such commonly soiled areas as skinfolds and the perineum.[7] For an obese or incontinent patient, use additional cloths as needed.[7]
▪ After the patient's skin air-dries, cover the patient's chest, abdomen, and perineum with a bath blanket or sheet *to maintain modesty and promote comfort.*
▪ Remove and discard your gloves.[23]
▪ Perform hand hygiene.[8,9,10,11,12,13]
▪ Put on a new pair of gloves.[21,22,23]
▪ Use a fourth cloth to clean the patient's right leg, right foot, and web spaces.[7]
▪ Use a fifth cloth to clean the patient's left leg, left foot, and web spaces.[7]
▪ Use a sixth cloth to clean the back of the neck, back, and then buttocks.[7]
▪ Discard used cloths in an appropriate receptacle.
NURSING ALERT Discard each disposable cloth in an appropriate receptacle. Don't flush disposable cloths in the toilet.[7]
▪ Remove and discard your gloves.[23]
▪ Perform hand hygiene.[8,9,10,11,12,13]
▪ Put on a new pair of gloves.[21,22,23]
▪ If the patient's skin requires additional moisturizer, apply it as needed. If you bathed the patient with chlorhexidine, use a moisturizer with known compatibility with chlorhexidine, *because some products can neutralize the antibacterial effects of chlorhexidine.*[7]

For bathing with water, skin cleanser, and washcloth
▪ Wet the washcloth with warm water. Wash the patient's face. Begin with the eyes, and wash from the inner canthus to the outer canthus. Use a separate section of the washcloth to wash each eye *to avoid spreading ocular infection.*
▪ If the patient tolerates skin cleanser, apply some to the washcloth and then wash the rest of the face, ears, and neck using gentle strokes. Rinse thoroughly, *because residual cleanser may cause itching and dryness.*
▪ Dry the patient's skin with a towel. Allow the skin to remain damp but not wet *to prevent drying of the skin and subsequent skin breakdown.*[24]
▪ Wash, rinse, and dry the patient's neck, shoulders, and chest. Clean the neck well, even if it isn't visibly soiled. Wash skinfolds under the patient's breasts by lifting each breast. Cover the patient's chest with a sheet or bath blanket *to maintain modesty and comfort.*
▪ Wash, rinse, and dry the patient's arms, hands, web spaces, and axillae. If the patient tolerates and desires deodorant, apply it.
▪ Wash, rinse, and dry the patient's abdomen and then the groin and perineum. Ensure thorough cleaning, paying special attention to such commonly soiled areas as skinfolds and the perineum. Cover the patient with a sheet or bath blanket, as appropriate, *to maintain modesty and comfort.*
▪ Remove and discard your gloves.[23]
▪ Perform hand hygiene.[8,9,10,11,12,13]
▪ Put on a new pair of gloves.[21,22,23]
▪ If the patient tolerates cleanser, wet a clean washcloth with warm water and apply skin cleanser to the washcloth.
▪ Wash, rinse, and dry the patient's right leg, right foot, and web spaces.
▪ Wash, rinse, and dry the patient's left leg, left foot, and web spaces.
▪ Assist the patient to turn onto the side. Alternatively, turn the patient onto the side.
▪ If the patient experienced incontinence, use a disposable cloth to clean the soiled area. Remove and discard your gloves, perform hand hygiene, and put on a new pair of gloves.[8,9,10,11,12,13,21,22,23]
▪ Wash, rinse, and dry the back of the neck, back, and buttocks.
▪ Apply a moisture barrier and skin protectant to the patient's buttocks, if necessary.
▪ Assist the patient with putting on a clean gown. Alternatively, put a clean gown on the patient.
▪ Discard the used washcloth and towel in the appropriate receptacle.

Completing the procedure

- Return the bed to the lowest position *to prevent falls and maintain patient safety.*[25]
- Remove and discard your gloves and other personal protective equipment, if worn.[23]
- Perform hand hygiene.[8,9,10,11,12,13]
- Document the procedure.[26,27,28,29]

Special considerations

- Use absorbent underpads or briefs to wick incontinence-associated moisture away from the skin in a patient with incontinence, *because moisture trapped against the skin can cause skin maceration.*
- HOSPITAL-ACQUIRED CONDITION ALERT Keep in mind that the Centers for Medicare and Medicaid Services considers a stage 3 or 4 pressure injury a hospital-acquired condition because it can be reasonably prevented using a variety of best practices. Make sure to follow pressure injury prevention practices, such as assessing skin integrity, encouraging mobility, and repositioning the patient, *to reduce the risk of pressure injuries.*[30,31,32,33]
- Raise the side rails of the bed during a bed bath, as needed, *to aid in turning and repositioning.* Lower the side rails with care *to prevent any of the patient's body parts from getting caught between the rails or between the rails and the mattress.*[34]
- *To improve the patient's circulation, maintain joint mobility, and preserve muscle tone,* move the body joints through their full range of motion during the bed bath.
- When bathing an older adult with dementia, focus on getting to know the person rather than just the task of bathing *to help reduce discomfort and anxiety.*

Complications

Skin irritation, sensitization, or allergic reaction can occur.[5]

Documentation

Record the date and time of the bed bath. Note the patient's tolerance of the bath, range of motion, and self-care abilities, and document any unusual findings. Document teaching provided to the patient and family (if applicable), their understanding of that teaching, and any need for follow-up teaching.

REFERENCES

1 Marchaim, D., et al. (2012). Hospital bath basins are frequently contaminated with multidrug-resistant human pathogens. *American Journal of Infection Control, 40,* 562–564. (Level VI)

2 Hanrahan, K., et al. (2015). Sacred cow gone to pasture: A systematic evaluation and integration of evidence-based practice. *Worldviews on Evidence-based Nursing, 12,* 3–11.

3 Martin, E. T. (2017). Bathing hospitalized dependent patients with prepackaged disposable washcloths instead of traditional bath basins: A case-crossover study. *American Journal of Infection Control, 45,* 990–994. (Level IV)

4 Musuuza, J. S., et al. (2019) The impact of chlorhexidine bathing on hospital-acquired bloodstream infections: A systematic review and meta-analysis. *BMC Infectious Diseases, 19*(1), 416. https://www.ncbi.nlm.nih.gov/pmc/articles/PMC6518712/pdf/12879_2019_Article_4002.pdf

5 Sage Products. (n.d.). Sage 2% chlorhexidine gluconate (CHG) cloths: Drug facts. https://sageproducts.com/wp-content/uploads/CHG-Cloth-Drug-Facts.pdf

6 Sage Products. (n.d.). Comfort Bath® cleansing washcloths: Give a better bath by eliminating the basin—a CAUTI risk factor. https://sageproducts.com/comfort-bath-cleansing-washcloths/

7 Agency for Healthcare Research and Quality. (2013). Universal ICU decolonization: An enhanced protocol. https://www.ahrq.gov/professionals/systems/hospital/universal_icu_decolonization/universal-icu-apd.html

8 The Joint Commission. (2021). Standard NPSG.07.01.01. *Comprehensive accreditation manual for hospitals.* Oakbrook Terrace, IL: The Joint Commission. (Level VII)

9 Centers for Disease Control and Prevention. (2002). Guideline for hand hygiene in health-care settings: Recommendations of the Healthcare Infection Control Practices Advisory Committee and the HICPAC/SHEA/APIC/IDSA Hand Hygiene Task Force. *MMWR Recommendations and Reports, 51*(RR-16), 1–45. https://www.cdc.gov/mmwr/pdf/rr/rr5116.pdf (Level II)

10 World Health Organization. (2009). WHO guidelines on hand hygiene in health care: First global patient safety challenge, clean care is safer care. https://apps.who.int/iris/bitstream/handle/10665/44102/9789241597906_eng.pdf?sequence=1 (Level IV)

11 Centers for Medicare and Medicaid Services, Department of Health and Human Services. (2020). Condition of participation: Infection control. 42 C.F.R. § 482.42.

12 Accreditation Association for Hospitals and Health Systems. (2020). Standard 07.01.21. *Healthcare Facilities Accreditation Program: Accreditation requirements for acute care hospitals.* Chicago, IL: Accreditation Association for Hospitals and Health Systems. (Level VII)

13 DNV GL-Healthcare USA, Inc. (2020). IC.1.SR.1. *NIAHO® accreditation requirements, interpretive guidelines and surveyor guidance—revision 20.0.* Milford, OH: DNV GL-Healthcare USA, Inc. (Level VII)

14 The Joint Commission. (2021). Standard NPSG.01.01.01. *Comprehensive accreditation manual for hospitals.* Oakbrook Terrace, IL: The Joint Commission. (Level VII)

15 Accreditation Association for Hospitals and Health Systems. (2020). Standard 15.01.16. *Healthcare Facilities Accreditation Program: Accreditation requirements for acute care hospitals.* Chicago, IL: Accreditation Association for Hospitals and Health Systems. (Level VII)

16 Centers for Medicare and Medicaid Services, Department of Health and Human Services. (2020). Condition of participation: Patient's rights. 42 C.F.R. § 482.13(c)(1).

17 The Joint Commission. (2021). Standard RI.01.01.01. *Comprehensive accreditation manual for hospitals.* Oakbrook Terrace, IL: The Joint Commission. (Level VII)

18 DNV GL-Healthcare USA, Inc. (2020). PR.21.SR.5. *NIAHO® accreditation requirements, interpretive guidelines and surveyor guidance—revision 20.0.* Milford, OH: DNV GL-Healthcare USA, Inc. (Level VII)

19 The Joint Commission. (2021). Standard PC.02.01.21. *Comprehensive accreditation manual for hospitals.* Oakbrook Terrace, IL: The Joint Commission. (Level VII)

20 Waters, T. R., et al. (2009). Safe patient handling training for schools of nursing. https://www.cdc.gov/niosh/docs/2009-127/pdfs/2009-127.pdf (Level VII)

21 Siegel, J. D., et al. (2007, revised 2019). 2007 guideline for isolation precautions: Preventing transmission of infectious agents in healthcare settings. https://www.cdc.gov/infectioncontrol/pdf/guidelines/isolation-guidelines-H.pdf (Level II)

22 Accreditation Association for Hospitals and Health Systems. (2020). Standard 07.01.10. *Healthcare Facilities Accreditation Program: Accreditation requirements for acute care hospitals.* Chicago, IL: Accreditation Association for Hospitals and Health Systems. (Level VII)

23 Occupational Safety and Health Administration. (2012). Bloodborne pathogens, standard number 1910.1030. https://www.osha.gov/pls/oshaweb/owadisp.show_document?p_id=10051&p_table=STANDARDS (Level VII)

24 LeBlanc, K., et al. (2013). International skin tear advisory panel: A tool kit to aid in the prevention, assessment, and treatment of skin tears using a simplified classification system. *Advances in Skin & Wound Care, 26,* 459–476. (Level IV)

25 Ganz, D. A., et al. (2013, reviewed 2021). *Preventing falls in hospitals: A toolkit for improving quality of care* (AHRQ Publication No. 13-0015-EF). Rockville, MD: Agency for Healthcare Research and Quality. https://www.ahrq.gov/professionals/systems/hospital/fallpxtoolkit/index.html (Level VII)

26 The Joint Commission. (2021). Standard RC.01.03.01. *Comprehensive accreditation manual for hospitals.* Oakbrook Terrace, IL: The Joint Commission. (Level VII)

27 Centers for Medicare and Medicaid Services, Department of Health and Human Services. (2020). Condition of participation: Medical record services. 42 C.F.R. § 482.24(b).

28 Accreditation Association for Hospitals and Health Systems. (2020). Standard 10.00.03. *Healthcare Facilities Accreditation Program: Accreditation requirements for acute care hospitals.* Chicago, IL: Accreditation Association for Hospitals and Health Systems. (Level VII)

29 DNV GL-Healthcare USA, Inc. (2020). MR.2.SR.1. *NIAHO® accreditation requirements, interpretive guidelines and surveyor guidance—revision 20.0.* Milford, OH: DNV GL-Healthcare USA, Inc. (Level VII)

30 National Pressure Ulcer Advisory Panel, et al. (2014). Prevention and treatment of pressure ulcers: Quick reference guide. https://www.epuap.org/wp-content/uploads/2016/10/quick-reference-guide-digital-npuap-epuap-pppia-jan2016.pdf (Level VII)

31 Wound Ostomy and Continence Nurses Society (WOCN). (2016). *Guideline for prevention and management of pressure ulcers (injuries): WOCN clinical practice guideline series 2.* Mount Laurel, NJ: WOCN.

32 Jarrett, N., & Callaham, M. (2016). Evidence-based guidelines for selected hospital-acquired conditions: Final report. https://www.cms.gov/Medicare/Medicare-Fee-for-Service-Payment/HospitalAcqCond/Downloads/2016-HAC-Report.pdf

33 Accreditation Association for Hospitals and Health Systems. (2020). Standard 16.02.02. *Healthcare Facilities Accreditation Program: Accreditation requirements for acute care hospitals.* Chicago, IL: Accreditation Association for Hospitals and Health Systems. (Level VII)

34 U.S. Food and Drug Administration. (2010). A guide to bed safety—bed rails in hospitals, nursing homes and home health care: The facts. http://www.fda.gov/downloads/MedicalDevices/ProductsandMedicalProcedures/GeneralHospitalDevicesandSupplies/HospitalBeds/ucm125857.pdf

BED-MAKING, OCCUPIED

Bed linen changes promote comfort and help prevent skin breakdown and health care–associated infection for a bedridden patient. To help control health care–associated infections, the procedure must be preceded by hand hygiene, performed by using clean technique, and followed by proper handling and disposal of soiled linens. Bed linen changes for the bedridden patient necessitate the use of side rails to prevent the patient from rolling out of bed and, depending on the patient's condition, the use of a turning sheet to move the patient from side to side.

Making an occupied bed may require more than one person. It also entails loosening the bottom sheet on one side and fanfolding or rolling it to the center of the mattress instead of loosening the bottom sheet on both sides and removing it, as in an unoccupied bed. It calls also for making the foundation of the bed on both sides before applying the top sheet instead of making the foundation and applying the top sheet on one side and then the other.[1,2]

Equipment

Two sheets (one fitted, if available) ▪ pillowcase ▪ bedspread ▪ one or two bath blankets ▪ laundry bag ▪ Optional: fluid-impermeable pads, gloves, gown, mask and goggles or mask with face shield, overhead trapeze bar.

Implementation

▪ Gather and prepare the necessary equipment and supplies.
▪ Perform hand hygiene.[3,4,5,6,7,8]
▪ Provide privacy.[12,13,14,15]
▪ Confirm the patient's identity using at least two patient identifiers.[9]
▪ Explain the procedure to the patient and family (if applicable) according to their individual communication and learning needs *to increase their understanding, allay their fears, and enhance cooperation.*[10] Explain how the patient can help if able, and adjust the plan according to the patient's abilities and needs.
▪ Obtain the help of a coworker as needed *to prevent injuring yourself.*[11] Have the coworker stand on the opposite side of the bed from you.
▪ Move furniture away from the bed, if necessary, *to ensure ample working space.*
▪ Raise the side rail on the far side of the bed *to prevent falls.*[16]
▪ Raise the bed to waist level before performing patient care *to prevent caregiver back strain.*[11]
▪ If permitted, lower the head of the bed *to ensure tight-fitting, wrinkle-free linens.*
▪ Perform hand hygiene.[3,4,5,6,7,8]
▪ Put on gloves and other protective equipment, as needed, *to comply with standard precautions.*[17,18]
▪ When stripping the bed, watch for belongings that may have fallen among the linens.
▪ Cover the patient with a bath blanket *to avoid exposure and provide warmth and privacy.*
▪ Fanfold the top sheet and spread from beneath the bath blanket, and then bring them back over the blanket.
▪ Loosen the top linens at the foot of the bed and remove them separately. If reusing the top linens, fold each piece and hang each piece over the back of the chair. Otherwise, remove the top linens carefully and

place them in a laundry bag. *To avoid dispersing microorganisms*, don't fan the linens; hold them against your clothing, or place them on the floor.[2]
▪ If the mattress slid downward when the head of the bed was raised, have a coworker help push the mattress to the head of the bed before making the bed. *Adjusting the mattress after the bed is made loosens the linens.*
▪ Roll the patient to the far side of the bed, and turn the pillow lengthwise under the patient's head *to support the neck.* Ask the patient to help (if possible) by grasping the far side rail as the patient turns *so that the patient is positioned at the far side of the bed after turning.* Alternatively, have the patient use an overhead trapeze bar *to assist with repositioning.*[19]
▪ Loosen the soiled bottom linens on the side of the bed nearest you. Then roll the linens toward the patient's back in the middle of the bed (as shown below).

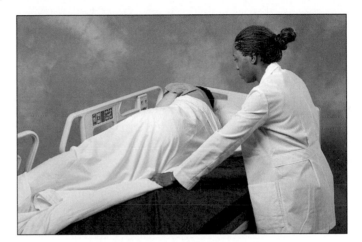

▪ Place a clean bottom sheet on the bed, with its center fold in the middle of the mattress. For a fitted sheet, secure the top and bottom corners over the side of the mattress nearest you. For a flat sheet, place its end even with the foot of the mattress. Miter the top corner as you would for an unoccupied bed *to keep linens firmly tucked under the mattress, preventing wrinkling.*
▪ Fanfold or roll the remaining clean bottom sheet toward the patient with its center fold in the middle of the mattress (as shown below).

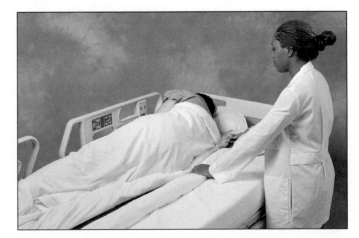

▪ If necessary, position a fluid-impermeable pad on the sheet *to absorb excretions or surgical drainage*, and fanfold or roll it toward the patient.
▪ Raise the other side rail, and roll the patient to the clean side of the bed.[16] Alternatively, have the patient use an overhead trapeze bar to assist with repositioning.
▪ Move to the unfinished side of the bed and lower the side rail nearest you. If a coworker is assisting, you can either remain on your side of the bed or switch sides with the coworker.
▪ Loosen and remove the soiled bottom linens separately and place them in the laundry bag.[20]

- Pull the clean bottom sheet taut. Secure the fitted sheet, or place the end of a flat sheet even with the foot of the bed, and miter the top corner. Unfold and smooth the fluid-impermeable pad, if used.
- Assist the patient to the supine position if the patient's condition permits.
- Remove the soiled pillowcase and place it in the laundry bag.[20]
- Slip the pillow into a clean pillowcase, tucking in the corners *to ensure a smooth fit*. Place the pillow beneath the patient's head, with its seam toward the top of the bed *to prevent it from rubbing against the patient's neck, causing irritation*. Place the pillow's open edge away from the door *to give the bed a finished appearance*.
- Unfold the clean top sheet over the patient with the rough side of the hem facing away from the bed *to avoid irritating the patient's skin*. Allow enough sheet to form a cuff over the bedspread.
- Remove the bath blanket from beneath the sheet and center the bedspread over the top sheet.
- Tuck the top sheet and bedspread under the foot of the bed, and miter the bottom corners. Fold the top sheet over the bedspread *to give the bed a finished appearance*.
- Loosen the top linens around the patient's feet *to allow room for the patient's feet and to prevent pressure that can cause discomfort, skin breakdown, and footdrop*.
- Return the bed to the lowest position *to prevent falls and maintain patient safety*.[21]
- Raise the head of the bed to a comfortable position.
- Raise side rails only if appropriate for the patient, and lock the bed's wheels *to ensure patient safety*.[22,23]
- Assess the patient's body alignment.
- Return the furniture to its proper place (if moved), and place the call light within the patient's reach.
- Remove the laundry bag from the room.
- Remove and discard your gloves and any other personal protective equipment if worn.[20]
- Perform hand hygiene.[3,4,5,6,7,8]
- Document the procedure.[24,25,26,27]

Special considerations

- Use a fitted bottom sheet when available, *because a flat sheet tends to loosen and become untucked easily, especially if the mattress is covered with plastic*.
- If the patient can't assist with repositioning, use a lift sheet or lift equipment for patient repositioning *to prevent friction injuries to the patient's skin*.[19]
- If the patient has a support surface, avoid or limit placing excess linens and fluid-impermeable pads on top of the support surface *because they can interfere with support surface functioning*.[19]
- *To prevent pressure injuries to the heels of an at-risk patient*, use heel suspension devices that elevate (float) and offload the heels completely and redistribute the weight of the leg along the calf without putting pressure on the Achilles tendon. Make sure that the patient's knees are flexed 5 to 10 degrees.[19,28]
- If the patient is being treated with traction, enlist the help of a coworker to make the bed. The patient may also assist by using an overhead trapeze bar during the bed-making procedure. (See *Making a traction bed*.)

Documentation

Although you wouldn't usually document a linen change, record the dates and times of linen changes for patients with incontinence, excessive wound drainage, pressure injuries, or diaphoresis. Document teaching provided to the patient and family (if applicable), their understanding of that teaching, and any need for follow-up teaching.

References

1   Pellatt, G. C. (2007). Clinical skills: Bed making and patient positioning. *British Journal of Nursing, 16*, 302–305.

2   Lynn, P. (2018). *Taylor's clinical nursing skills: A nursing process approach.* Philadelphia, PA: Wolters Kluwer.

3   The Joint Commission. (2021). Standard NPSG.07.01.01. *Comprehensive accreditation manual for hospitals.* Oakbrook Terrace, IL: The Joint Commission. (Level VII)

4   Centers for Disease Control and Prevention. (2002). Guideline for hand hygiene in health-care settings: Recommendations of the Healthcare Infection Control Practices Advisory *Recommendations and Reports, 51*(RR-16), 1–45. https://www.cdc.gov/mmwr/pdf/rr/rr5116.pdf (Level II)

5   World Health Organization. (2009). WHO guidelines on hand hygiene in health care: First global patient safety challenge, clean care is safer care. https://apps.who.int/iris/bitstream/handle/10665/44102/9789241597906_eng.pdf?sequence=1 (Level IV)

6   Centers for Medicare and Medicaid Services, Department of Health and Human Services. (2020). Condition of participation: Infection control. 42 C.F.R. § 482.42.

7   Accreditation Association for Hospitals and Health Systems. (2020). Standard 07.01.21. *Healthcare Facilities Accreditation Program: Accreditation requirements for acute care hospitals.* Chicago, IL: Accreditation Association for Hospitals and Health Systems. (Level VII)

8   DNV GL-Healthcare USA, Inc. (2020). IC.1.SR.1. *NIAHO® accreditation requirements, interpretive guidelines and surveyor guidance—revision 20.0.* Milford, OH: DNV GL-Healthcare USA, Inc. (Level VII)

9   The Joint Commission. (2021). Standard NPSG.01.01.01. *Comprehensive accreditation manual for hospitals.* Oakbrook Terrace, IL: The Joint Commission. (Level VII)

10   The Joint Commission. (2021). Standard PC.02.01.21. *Comprehensive accreditation manual for hospitals.* Oakbrook Terrace, IL: The Joint Commission. (Level VII)

11   Waters, T. R., et al. (2009). Safe patient handling training for schools of nursing. https://www.cdc.gov/niosh/docs/2009-127/pdfs/2009-127.pdf (Level VII)

12   Accreditation Association for Hospitals and Health Systems. (2020). Standard 15.01.16. *Healthcare Facilities Accreditation Program: Accreditation requirements for acute care hospitals.* Chicago, IL: Accreditation Association for Hospitals and Health Systems. (Level VII)

13   Centers for Medicare and Medicaid Services, Department of Health and Human Services. (2020). Condition of participation: Patient's rights. 42 C.F.R. § 482.13(c)(1).

14   The Joint Commission. (2021). Standard RI.01.01.01. *Comprehensive accreditation manual for hospitals.* Oakbrook Terrace, IL: The Joint Commission. (Level VII)

15   DNV GL-Healthcare USA, Inc. (2020). PR.2.SR.5. *NIAHO® accreditation requirements, interpretive guidelines and surveyor guidance - revision 20.0.* Milford, OH: DNV GL-Healthcare USA, Inc. (Level VII)

16   Morse, J. M., et al. (2015). The safety of hospital beds: Ingress, egress, and in-bed mobility. *Global Qualitative Nursing Research, 2*, 2333393615575321. https://www.ncbi.nlm.nih.gov/pmc/articles/PMC5371163/ (Level V)

17   Siegel, J. D., et al. (2007, revised 2019). 2007 guideline for isolation precautions: Preventing transmission of infectious agents in healthcare settings. https://www.cdc.gov/infectioncontrol/pdf/guidelines/isolation-guidelines-H.pdf (Level VII)

18   Accreditation Association for Hospitals and Health Systems. (2020). Standard 07.01.10. *Healthcare Facilities Accreditation Program: Accreditation requirements for acute care hospitals.* Chicago, IL: Accreditation Association for Hospitals and Health Systems. (Level VII)

19   Wound Ostomy and Continence Nurses Society. (2016). *Guideline for prevention and management of pressure ulcers (injuries): WOCN clinical practice guidelines series 2.* Mount Laurel, NJ: WOCN.

20   Occupational Safety and Health Administration. (2012). Bloodborne pathogens, standard number 1910.1030. https://www.osha.gov/pls/oshaweb/owadisp.show_document?p_id=10051&p_table=STANDARDS (Level VII)

21   Ganz, D. A., et al. (2013, reviewed 2021). *Preventing falls in hospitals: A toolkit for improving quality of care* (AHRQ Publication No. 13-0015-EF). Rockville, MD: Agency for Healthcare Research and Quality. https://www.ahrq.gov/professionals/systems/hospital/fallpxtoolkit/index.html (Level VII)

22   U.S. Food & Drug Administration. (2018). Recommendations for health care providers about bed rails. https://www.fda.gov/medical-devices/bed-rail-safety/recommendations-health-care-providers-about-bed-rails

23   U.S. Food and Drug Administration. (2010). A guide to bed safety: Bed rails in hospitals, nursing homes and home health care – The facts. https://www.fda.gov/media/75122/download

24   The Joint Commission. (2021). Standard RC.01.03.01. *Comprehensive accreditation manual for hospitals.* Oakbrook Terrace, IL: The Joint Commission. (Level VII)

25   Centers for Medicare and Medicaid Services, Department of Health and Human Services. (2019). Condition of participation: Medical record services. 42 C.F.R. § 482.24(b).

26   Accreditation Association for Hospitals and Health Systems. (2020). Standard 10.00.03. *Healthcare Facilities Accreditation Program: Accred-*

Making a traction bed

Making a traction bed requires specific measures for preparation and during the linen change. For a patient in traction, obtain help from a coworker. Work from head to toe *to minimize the risk of traction misalignment.* A patient in upper body traction won't be able to use an overhead trapeze bar; you'll need to support the extremity that the traction is applied to (the head for cervical traction or the arm for arm traction) when you're removing the pillows or sheets from under the patient's extremity, and you'll need to assist the patient with movement as needed.

Preparation

- Perform hand hygiene.[3,4,5,6,7,8]
- Bring clean linens and arrange them in the order of use on the bedside stand or a chair.
- Provide privacy.[12,13,14,15]
- Explain the procedure to the patient and family (if appropriate) according to their communication and learning needs *to increase understanding, allay their fears, and enhance cooperation.*[10]
- Obtain assistance from a coworker.
- Remove unnecessary furniture.
- Raise the bed to waist level before providing care *to prevent caregiver back strain.*[11]
- Perform hand hygiene.[3,4,5,6,7,8]
- Put on gloves and other protective equipment, as needed, *to comply with standard precautions.*[17,18]

Changing the linens

- Lower both side rails.
- Stand near the headboard, opposite your coworker.
- Pull the mattress gently to the head of the bed. Avoid sudden movements, *because they can misalign traction and cause patient discomfort.*
- Remove the pillow from the bed.
- Loosen the bottom linens and roll them from the headboard toward the patient's head.
- Remove the soiled pillowcase and replace it with a clean one.
- Fold a clean bottom sheet crosswise and place the sheet across the head of the bed. Tell the patient to raise the head and upper shoulders by grasping the overhead trapeze bar above the bed. With your coworker, fanfold or roll the bottom sheet quickly from the head of the bed under the patient's shoulders so that it meets the soiled linen. Tuck at least 12" (30.5 cm) of the bottom sheet under the head of the mattress. Miter the corners and tuck in the sides.
- Tell the patient to raise the buttocks by grasping the trapeze bar (as shown to the right). As a team, move toward the foot of the bed and, in one movement, roll the soiled linens and clean linens quickly and carefully under the patient.
- Instruct the patient to release the trapeze bar and to rest. Place a pillow under the patient's head for comfort.

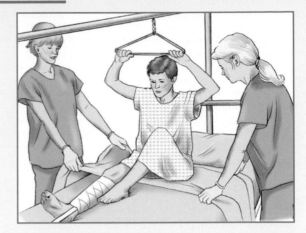

- If allowed, remove any pillows from under the patient's extremity. Otherwise, continue to move linens toward the foot of the bed and under the patient's legs and traction while your coworker lifts the pillows and supports the patient's extremity.
- Put soiled linens in a laundry bag.[20]
- Tuck the remaining loose linens securely under the mattress. *To ensure a tight-fitting bottom sheet,* have the patient raise off the bed by simultaneously grasping the trapeze bar and raising the buttocks while you pull the sheet tight. As needed, place a drawsheet or fluid-impermeable pad underneath the patient.
- If the bottom sheet doesn't cover the foot of the mattress, cover it with a drawsheet. Miter its corners and tuck in the sides.
- Replace the pillows under the patient's extremity, and then cover the patient with a clean top sheet. Fold over the top hem of the sheet approximately 8" (20.5 cm). If one or both of the patients legs are in traction, fit the lower end of the sheet loosely over the traction apparatus; don't press on the traction ropes. *To secure the sheet,* tuck in the corner opposite the traction under the foot of the bed and miter the corner. Neatly tuck in the lower corner of the sheet on the traction side *to expose the leg and foot.*
- If the traction apparatus exposes the patient's sides, cover the patient with a drawsheet—not a full sheet or spread.
- Return the bed to the lowest position *to prevent falls and ensure patient safety,* but don't allow the traction weights to touch the floor.[21]
- Raise the side rails only if appropriate for the patient, and lock the bed wheels *to ensure the patient's safety.*[22,23]
- Remove and discard your gloves and other personal protective equipment, if worn.[20]
- Perform hand hygiene.[3,4,5,6,7,8]

---

itation requirements for acute care hospitals.* Chicago, IL: Accreditation Association for Hospitals and Health Systems. (Level VII)

27 DNV GL-Healthcare USA, Inc. (2020). MR.2.SR.1. *NIAHO® accreditation requirements, interpretive guidelines and surveyor guidance - revision 20.0.* Milford, OH: DNV GL-Healthcare USA, Inc. (Level VII)

28 Haesler, E. (2017). Evidence summary: Pressure injuries – Preventing heel pressure injuries with positioning. *Wound Practice & Research, 25,* 212–214. https://pdfs.semanticscholar.org/897e/da1fa44e6e71d4585869f-b6093166447ac6e.pdf (Level V)

BED-MAKING, UNOCCUPIED

The daily changing and periodic straightening of bed linens is a routine procedure that promotes patient comfort and prevents skin breakdown. When preceded by hand hygiene, performed using clean technique, and followed by proper handling and disposal of soiled linens, this procedure also helps control health care–associated infections.

Equipment

Two sheets (one fitted, if available) ■ pillowcase ■ bedspread ■ laundry bag ■ Optional: gloves, gown, mask and goggles or mask with face shield, fluid-impermeable pads, drawsheet.

Implementation

- Gather the necessary equipment and supplies.
- Perform hand hygiene.[1,2,3,4,5,6]
- Explain the procedure to the patient and family (if appropriate) according to their communication and learning needs *to increase their understanding, allay their fears, and enhance cooperation.*[7] Help the patient to a chair if necessary.
- Move furniture away from the bed *to provide ample working space.*
- Lower the head of the bed and side rails *to make the mattress level and ensure tight-fitting, wrinkle-free linens.*
- Raise the bed to waist level *to prevent caregiver back strain.*[8]
- Perform hand hygiene.[1,2,3,4,5,6]
- Put on gloves and gown, mask and goggles, or mask with face shield, as needed, *to comply with standard precautions.*[9,10]
- When stripping the bed, watch for any belongings that may have fallen among the linens.
- Remove the pillowcase and place it in the laundry bag or in the middle of the bed. Set the pillow aside.
- Lift the mattress edge slightly and work around the bed, untucking the linens. If you plan to reuse the top linens, fold the top hem of the spread down to the bottom hem. Then pick up the hemmed corners, fold the

spread into quarters, and hang it over the back of the chair. Do the same for the top sheet. Otherwise, carefully remove and place the top linens in the laundry bag or pillowcase. *To avoid spreading microorganisms*, don't fan the linens, hold them against your clothing, or place them on the floor.[11,12]

■ Remove the soiled bottom linens and place them in the laundry bag.[11]

■ If the mattress has slid downward, push it to the head of the bed. *Adjusting it after the bed is made loosens the linens.*

■ Place the clean bottom sheet with its center fold in the middle of the mattress.

■ For a fitted sheet, secure the top and bottom corners over the mattress corners on the side of the bed nearest you. For a flat sheet, align the end of the sheet with the foot of the mattress and miter the top corner *to keep the sheet firmly tucked under the mattress*. To miter the corner, first tuck the top end of the sheet evenly under the mattress at the head of the bed. Then lift the side edge of the sheet about 12″ (30.5 cm) from the mattress corner and hold it at a right angle to the mattress. Tuck in the bottom edge of the sheet hanging below the mattress. Finally, drop the top edge and tuck it under the mattress. (See *Making a mitered corner*.)

■ After tucking under one side of the bottom sheet, place the drawsheet or fluid-impermeable pad (if needed) about 15″ (38 cm) from the top of the bed, with its center fold in the middle of the bed. Then tuck in the entire edge of the drawsheet on that side of the bed.

Making a mitered corner

To make a mitered corner, follow these instructions:

■ After placing the sheet on the bed, grasp the side edge of the sheet and lift it up to form a triangle (as shown below).

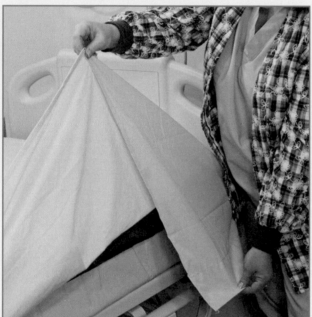

■ Then, place the sheet on the top of the bed, making a flat triangular fold (as shown below).

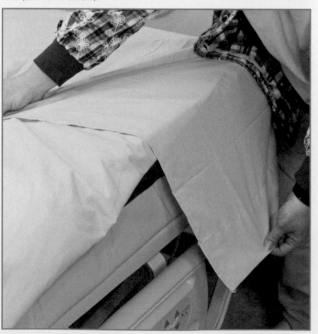

■ While holding the point of the triangle on the bed, tuck the sheet under the mattress (as shown below).

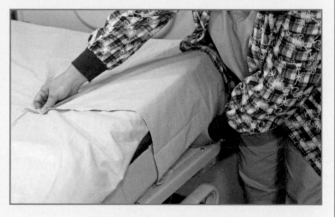

■ Take the triangular fold from the mattress and place it over the side of the mattress (as shown below).

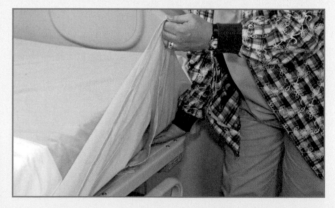

■ Tuck the remaining end of the triangular linen fold under the mattress (as shown below).

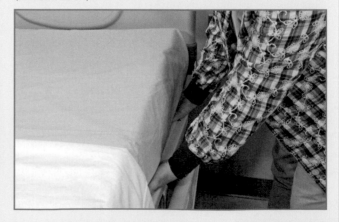

■ Place the top sheet with its center fold in the middle of the bed and its wide hem even with the top of the bed. Position the rough side of the hem face up *so that the smooth side shows when folded over the bedspread.* Allow enough sheet at the top of the bed to form a cuff over the bedspread.

■ Place the bedspread over the top sheet, with its center fold in the middle of the bed. (If the patient will be returning from surgery, use the alternative technique described in *Making a surgical bed*.)

■ Fit all remaining corners of the bottom sheet or tuck them under the mattress, and then pull the sheet at an angle from the head toward the foot of the bed. *Doing so tightens the linens, making the bottom sheet taut and wrinkle-free and promoting patient comfort.*

■ Tuck the top sheet and bedspread under the foot of the mattress. Then miter the bottom corners.

■ Fold the top sheet over the bedspread at the head of the bed *to form a cuff and to give the bed a finished appearance.* When making an open bed, fanfold the top linens to the foot of the bed.

■ Slip the pillow into a clean pillowcase, tucking in the corners. Then place the pillow on the bed with its seam toward the top of the bed *to prevent it from rubbing against the patient's neck, causing irritation,* and its open edge facing away from the door *to give the bed a finished appearance.*

■ Return the bed to the lowest position and lock its wheels *to prevent falls and maintain patient* safety.[13]

■ Return furniture to its proper place.

■ Assist the patient into bed and position the patient comfortably, as needed.

■ Place the call light within the patient's reach.

■ Remove the laundry bag from the room.[11]

■ Remove and discard your gloves and any other personal protective equipment if worn.

■ Perform hand hygiene.[1,2,3,4,5,6]

■ Document the procedure.[14,15,16,17]

Making a surgical bed

Preparation of a surgical bed permits easy patient transfer from surgery and promotes cleanliness and comfort. To make such a bed, take the following steps:

■ Perform hand hygiene.[1,2,3,4,5,6]

■ Assemble linens as you would for making an unoccupied bed, including two clean sheets (one fitted, if available), a drawsheet, a bath blanket, a spread or sheet, a pillowcase, facial tissues, an emesis basin, a plastic trash bag, fluid-impermeable pads, extra pillows, and other special equipment (such as an IV pole and suction apparatus) as needed.

■ Raise the bed to waist level *to prevent caregiver back strain.*[8]

■ Slip the pillow into a clean pillowcase and place it on a nearby table or chair.

■ Make the foundation of the bed using the bottom sheet and drawsheet.

■ Place an open bath blanket about 15″ (38 cm) from the head of the bed with its center fold positioned in the middle of the bed. *The blanket warms the patient and counteracts the decreased body temperature caused by anesthesia.*

■ Place a top sheet or bedspread on the bath blanket, and position it as you did the blanket. Then fold the bath blanket and top sheet or bedspread back from the top so that the blanket shows over the sheet. Similarly, fold the sheet or bedspread and bath blanket up from the bottom (as shown in illustration 1).

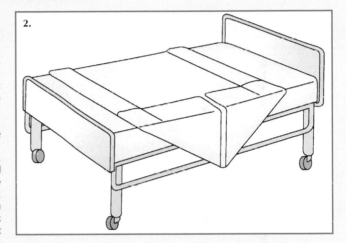

2.

■ *To make the patient comfortable and to prevent unnecessary movement and linen changes,* try to anticipate and be ready for any special needs. For nausea, keep an emesis basin, facial tissues, and fluid-impermeable pads at the bedside. Also, remove all liquids from the bedside. If you expect bleeding or discharge, place at least one fluid-impermeable pad on the bed.

■ Keep extra pillows handy *to elevate the patient's arms and legs, which promotes circulation, thereby preventing edema.* If necessary, have IV equipment, suction apparatus, a patient transfer device, or other special equipment ready.

■ Return the bed to the lowest position *to prevent falls and maintain the patient's safety.*[13]

■ Perform hand hygiene.[1,2,3,4,5,6]

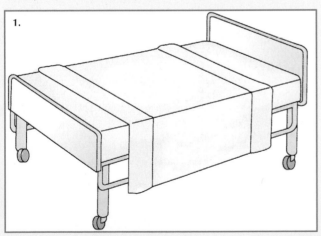

1.

■ On the side of the bed where you'll receive the patient, fold up the two outer corners of the sheet or bedspread and bath blanket so they meet in the middle of the bed (as shown in illustration 2).

■ Pick up the point hanging over this side of the bed and fanfold the linens back to the other side of the bed *so the linens won't interfere with patient transfer* (as shown in illustration 3).

■ Position the bed at hip level to transfer the patient, lock the wheels, and lower the side rails.[8] Ensure the side rails work properly.

■ Move the bedside stand and other objects out of the stretcher's path *to facilitate easy transfer when the patient arrives.*

■ After the patient is transferred to the bed, position the pillow for comfort and safety. Pull the top point of the top sheet or bedspread and blanket over the patient and open the folds. After covering the patient, tuck in the linens at the foot of the bed and miter the corners.

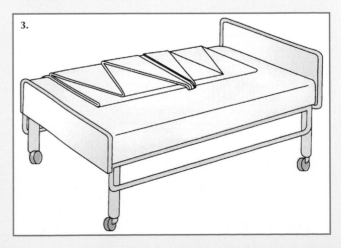

3.

Special considerations

▪ Because a hospital mattress is usually covered with plastic *to protect it and to facilitate cleaning between patients*, a flat-bottom sheet tends to loosen and become untucked. Use a fitted sheet, if available.[12]

Documentation

Although you wouldn't usually document a linen change, record the dates and times of linen changes for patients with incontinence, excessive wound drainage, or diaphoresis. Document teaching provided to the patient and family (if applicable), their understanding of that teaching, and any need for follow-up teaching.

REFERENCES

1 The Joint Commission. (2021). Standard NPSG.07.01.01. *Comprehensive accreditation manual for hospitals.* Oakbrook Terrace, IL: The Joint Commission. (Level VII)

2 Centers for Disease Control and Prevention. (2002). Guideline for hand hygiene in health-care settings: Recommendations of the Healthcare Infection Control Practices Advisory Committee and the HICPAC/SHEA/APIC/IDSA Hand Hygiene Task Force. *MMWR Recommendations and Reports, 51*(RR-16), 1–45. https://www.cdc.gov/mmwr/pdf/rr/rr5116.pdf (Level II)

3 World Health Organization. (2009). WHO guidelines on hand hygiene in health care: First global patient safety challenge, clean care is safer care. https://apps.who.int/iris/bitstream/handle/10665/44102/9789241597906_eng.pdf?sequence=1 (Level IV)

4 Centers for Medicare and Medicaid Services, Department of Health and Human Services. (2020). Condition of participation: Infection control. 42 C.F.R. § 482.42.

5 Accreditation Association for Hospitals and Health Systems. (2020). Standard 07.01.21. *Healthcare Facilities Accreditation Program: Accreditation requirements for acute care hospitals.* Chicago, IL: Accreditation Association for Hospitals and Health Systems. (Level VII)

6 DNV GL-Healthcare USA, Inc. (2020). IC.1.SR.1. *NIAHO® accreditation requirements interpretive guidelines and surveyor guidance - revision 20.0.* Milford, OH: DNV GL-Healthcare USA, Inc. (Level VII)

7 The Joint Commission. (2021). Standard PC.02.01.21. *Comprehensive accreditation manual for hospitals.* Oakbrook Terrace, IL: The Joint Commission. (Level VII)

8 Waters, T. R., et al. (2009). Safe patient handling training for schools of nursing. https://www.cdc.gov/niosh/docs/2009-127/pdfs/2009-127.pdf (Level VII)

9 Siegel, J. D., et al. (2007, revised 2019). 2007 guideline for isolation precautions: Preventing transmission of infectious agents in healthcare settings. https://www.cdc.gov/infectioncontrol/pdf/guidelines/isolation-guidelines-H.pdf (Level II)

10 Accreditation Association for Hospitals and Health Systems. (2020). Standard 07.01.10. *Healthcare Facilities Accreditation Program: Accreditation requirements for acute care hospitals.* Chicago, IL: Accreditation Association for Hospitals and Health Systems. (Level VII)

11 Occupational Safety and Health Administration. (2012). Bloodborne pathogens, standard number 1910.1030. https://www.osha.gov/pls/oshaweb/owadisp.show_document?p_id=10051&p_table=STANDARDS (Level VII)

12 Lynn, P. (2018). *Taylor's clinical nursing skills: A nursing process approach.* Philadelphia, PA: Wolters Kluwer.

13 Ganz, D. A., et al. (2013, reviewed 2021). *Preventing falls in hospitals: A toolkit for improving quality of care* (AHRQ Publication No. 13-0015-EF). Rockville, MD: Agency for Healthcare Research and Quality. https://www.ahrq.gov/professionals/systems/hospital/fallpxtoolkit/index.html (Level VII)

14 The Joint Commission. (2021). Standard RC.01.03.01. *Comprehensive accreditation manual for hospitals.* Oakbrook Terrace, IL: The Joint Commission. (Level VII)

15 Centers for Medicare and Medicaid Services, Department of Health and Human Services. (2020). Condition of participation: Medical record services. 42 C.F.R. § 482.24(b).

16 Accreditation Association for Hospitals and Health Systems. (2020). Standard 10.00.03. *Healthcare Facilities Accreditation Program: Accreditation requirements for acute care hospitals.* Chicago, IL: Accreditation Association for Hospitals and Health Systems. (Level VII)

17 DNV GL-Healthcare USA, Inc. (2020). MR.2.SR.1. *NIAHO® accreditation requirements, interpretive guidelines and surveyor guidance - revision 20.0.* Milford, OH: DNV GL-Healthcare USA, Inc. (Level VII)

BEDPAN AND URINAL USE

Bedpans and urinals permit patients who are bedridden to eliminate and allow you to observe and measure their urine and stool accurately. Female patients use bedpans for defecation and urination; male patients use bedpans for defecation and urinals for urination. After providing privacy, offer either device frequently, including before meals, visiting hours, morning and evening care, and treatments or procedures.

Equipment

Bedpan (either regular bedpan or fracture pan) or urinal with cover ▪ disposable cleaning wipes or washcloths, soap and water, and towel ▪ toilet tissue ▪ two pairs of gloves ▪ fluid-impermeable pads ▪ facility-approved disinfectant solution ▪ Optional: air freshener, pH balanced cleanser, bath blanket, small pillow, graduated cylinder, specimen container, bed linens.

Available in adult and pediatric sizes, a bedpan may be disposable or reusable (the latter can be sterilized). A fracture pan, a type of bedpan, is used when spinal injuries, body or leg casts, or other conditions prohibit or restrict turning the patient. Like a bedpan, the urinal may be disposable or reusable. Consider the use of disposable bedpans *to prevent the spread of* Clostridioides difficile *infection.*[1,2]

Preparation of equipment

Inspect all equipment and supplies. If a product is expired, is defective, or has compromised integrity, remove it from patient use, label it as expired or defective, and report the defect as directed by your facility. Inspect the bedpan or urinal, and make sure that it is clean before using.

Implementation

▪ Gather and prepare the necessary equipment and supplies.
▪ Perform hand hygiene.[3,4,5,6,7,8]
▪ Confirm the patient's identity using at least two patient identifiers.[9]
▪ Provide privacy.[10,11,12,13]
▪ Explain the procedure to the patient and family (if appropriate) according to their communication and learning needs *to increase their understanding, allay their fears, and enhance cooperation.*[14]

Placing a bedpan

▪ Raise the bed to waist level before providing care *to prevent caregiver back strain.*[15]
▪ If allowed, elevate the head of the bed slightly *to prevent hyperextension of the spine when the patient raises the buttocks.*
▪ Perform hand hygiene.[3,4,5,6,7,8]
▪ Put on gloves *to comply with standard precautions.*[16,17]
▪ Rest the bedpan on the edge of the bed. Then, turn down the corner of the top linens and draw up the patient's gown under the buttocks.
▪ Ask the patient to raise the buttocks by flexing the knees and pushing down on the heels. Place a fluid-impermeable pad under the patient's buttocks and then, while supporting the patient's lower back with one hand, center the curved, smooth edge of the bedpan beneath the buttocks.
▪ If the patient can't raise the buttocks, lower the head of the bed to horizontal and help the patient roll onto one side, with the buttocks toward you. Place a fluid-impermeable pad under the patient's buttocks, position the bedpan properly against the buttocks, and then help the patient roll back onto the bedpan.
▪ After positioning the bedpan, elevate the head of the bed further to 30 degrees or higher, if allowed, until the patient is sitting erect *to allow the patient to assume a normal elimination posture.* (See *Using a commode,* for information on another device that permits normal elimination posture.)
▪ If elevating the head of the bed is contraindicated, tuck a small pillow or folded bath blanket under the patient's back *to cushion the sacrum against the edge of the bedpan and support the lumbar region.*

■ If the patient can be left alone, place the bed in a low position and raise the side rails *to prevent falls and maintain the patient's safety*.[19] Place toilet tissue and the call light within the patient's reach, and instruct the patient to push the call light button after elimination. Don't leave a patient who is weak or disoriented alone.

■ Before removing the bedpan, raise the bed to waist level *to prevent caregiver back strain*.[15]

■ Lower the head of the bed slightly and ask the patient to raise the buttocks off the bed. Support the patient's lower back with one hand, and gently remove the bedpan with the other *to avoid skin injury caused by friction*.

■ If the patient can't raise the buttocks, ask the patient to roll to the opposite side so that the buttocks are toward you while you assist with one hand. Hold the pan firmly with the other hand to avoid spills.

■ Cover the bedpan with a fluid-impermeable pad, and place the bedpan on the chair.

■ Help clean the patient's anal and perineal area, as necessary, *to prevent irritation, infection, and skin breakdown*. As needed, turn the patient on the side; wipe carefully with toilet tissue; clean the area with a pH-balanced cleanser, disposable cleaning wipes, or soap and warm water; and dry well with a towel *to reduce the risk of pressure injury*.[20] Clean a female patient from front back *to avoid introducing rectal contaminants into the vaginal or urethral openings*.

HOSPITAL-ACQUIRED CONDITION ALERT Keep in mind that the Centers for Medicare and Medicaid Services considers a stage 3 or 4 pressure injury a hospital-acquired condition *because it can be reasonably prevented using a variety of best practices*. Make sure to follow evidence-based pressure injury prevention practices, such as keeping the skin clean and dry, assessing skin integrity, encouraging mobility, and repositioning the patient, *to reduce the risk of pressure injuries*.[21,22,23]

■ Remove and discard your gloves and perform hand hygiene.[3,4,5,6,7,8] Put on a new pair of gloves.[16,17]

Placing a urinal

■ Lift the corner of the top linens, hand the urinal to the patient, and allow the patient to position it.

■ If the patient can't position the urinal without help, spread the patient's legs slightly and hold the urinal in place *to prevent spills*.

■ After the patient voids, carefully withdraw the urinal and cover it or close the lid .

Completing the procedure after use of a bedpan or urinal

■ Give the patient disposable cleaning wipes (or a clean washcloth dampened with soap and warm water) and a towel *to wash and dry the hands*.[24] Check the bed linens for wetness or soiling, and straighten or change them, as needed.

■ Make the patient comfortable. Return the bed to the lowest position *to prevent falls and maintain the patient's safety*.[19]

■ Take the bedpan or urinal to the bathroom or utility room. Observe the color, odor, amount, and consistency of its contents.

■ If ordered, measure urine output or liquid stool in a graduated cylinder and place a specimen in a specimen container for laboratory analysis.[24] (See the "Urine specimen collection" procedure.)

■ Empty the contents of the bedpan or urinal into the toilet or designated waste area.[24]

■ Rinse the bedpan or urinal with water and clean it thoroughly using a facility-approved disinfectant solution *to prevent the spread of infection*.[25,26]

■ Dry, cover, and return the bedpan or urinal to the patient's bathroom for storage.

■ Remove and discard your gloves and perform hand hygiene.[3,4,5,6,7,8]

■ Use an air freshener, if necessary, *to eliminate offensive odors and minimize embarrassment*.

■ Document the procedure.[27,28,29,30]

Special considerations

■ Explain to the patient that drug treatment and changes in environment, diet, and activities may disrupt the patient's usual elimination schedule. Try to anticipate elimination needs, and offer the bedpan or urinal frequently *to help reduce embarrassment and minimize the risk of incontinence*.

Using a commode

An alternative to a bedpan, a commode is a portable chair made of plastic or metal with a large opening in the center of the seat. It may have a bedpan or bucket that slides underneath the opening, or it may slide directly over the toilet, adding height to the standard toilet seat. Unlike a bedpan, a commode allows the patient to assume a normal elimination posture, which aids in defecation. Consider the use of a disposable commode bucket *to prevent the spread of* Clostridioides difficile *infection*.[18]

Before the patient uses the commode, inspect its condition and make sure it's clean. Roll or carry the commode to the patient's room. Place it parallel and as close as possible to the patient's bed, and secure its brakes or wheel locks. If necessary, block its wheels with sandbags. Assist the patient onto the commode, provide toilet tissue, and place the call light within the patient's reach. Instruct the patient to push the call light when finished using the commode.

■ If necessary, assist the patient with cleaning, returning to bed, and getting comfortable. Offer the patient cleaning wipes or a clean washcloth dampened with soap and warm water and a towel *to wash and dry the hands*. Close the lid of the commode or cover the bucket. Roll the commode or carry the bucket to the bathroom. If ordered, observe and measure the contents before disposal. Rinse and clean the bucket, and then spray or wipe the bucket and commode seat with disinfectant. Use an air freshener, if appropriate, *to eliminate offensive odors and minimize embarrassment*.

■ Don't place a bedpan or urinal on top of the bedside stand or over-bed table *to avoid contaminating clean equipment and food trays*. Similarly, don't place it on the floor *to prevent the spread of microorganisms from the floor to the patient's bed linens when the patient uses the device*.

■ If the patient feels pain during turning or feels uncomfortable on a standard bedpan, use a fracture pan. Unlike the standard bedpan, you slip the fracture bedpan under the buttocks from the front rather than the side. *Because it's shallower than the standard bedpan*, you need only lift the patient slightly to position it. If the patient has obesity or is otherwise difficult to lift, ask a coworker to help you.

■ If the patient has an indwelling urinary catheter in place, carefully position and remove the bedpan *to avoid tension on the catheter, which could dislodge it or irritate the urethra*. After the patient defecates, wipe, clean, and dry the anal region, taking care to avoid catheter contamination. If necessary, clean the urinary meatus.

■ Don't leave the urinal, fracture pan, or regular bedpan in place for extended periods *to prevent skin breakdown*.[21,24]

■ For a thin patient, place a fluid-impermeable pad at the edge of the bedpan or use a fracture pan *to minimize pressure on the coccyx*.

Complications

Complications may include constipation, embarrassment, discomfort, and possible loss of dignity.

Documentation

Record the time, date, and type of elimination in the flowchart, and the amount of urine output or liquid stool on the intake and output record, as needed. In your notes, document the amount, color, clarity, and odor of the urine or stool and the presence of blood, pus, or other abnormal characteristics in urine or stool. Document the condition of the perineum. Document teaching provided to the patient and family (if applicable), their understanding of that teaching, and any need for follow-up teaching.

REFERENCES

1 Public Health Agency of Canada. (2013). *Clostridium difficile* infection: Infection prevention and control guidance for management in acute care settings. https://www.canada.ca/en/public-health/services/infectious-diseases/nosocomial-occupational-infections/clostridium-difficile-infection-prevention-control-guidance-management-acute-care-settings.html#tphp (Level VII)

2 Metcalf, D., et al. (2015). *Clostridium difficile* contamination of reprocessed hospital bedpans. *Canadian Journal of Infection Control, 30*, 33–36. (Level VI)

3 The Joint Commission. (2021). Standard NPSG.07.01.01. *Comprehensive accreditation manual for hospitals.* Oakbrook Terrace, IL: The Joint Commission. (Level VII)

4 Centers for Disease Control and Prevention. (2002). Guideline for hand hygiene in health-care settings: Recommendations of the Healthcare Infection Control Practices Advisory Committee and the HICPAC/SHEA/APIC/IDSA Hand Hygiene Task Force. *MMWR Recommendations and Reports, 51*(RR-16), 1–45. https://www.cdc.gov/mmwr/pdf/rr/rr5116.pdf (Level II)

5 World Health Organization. (2009). WHO guidelines on hand hygiene in health care: First global patient safety challenge, clean care is safer care. https://apps.who.int/iris/bitstream/handle/10665/44102/9789241597906_eng.pdf?sequence=1 (Level IV)

6 Centers for Medicare and Medicaid Services, Department of Health and Human Services. (2020). Condition of participation: Infection control. 42 C.F.R. § 482.42.

7 Accreditation Association for Hospitals and Health Systems. (2020). Standard 07.01.21. *Healthcare Facilities Accreditation Program: Accreditation requirements for acute care hospitals.* Chicago, IL: Accreditation Association for Hospitals and Health Systems. (Level VII)

8 DNV GL-Healthcare USA, Inc. (2020). IC.1.SR.1. *NIAHO® accreditation requirements, interpretive guidelines and surveyor guidance - revision 20.0.* Milford, OH: DNV GL-Healthcare USA, Inc. (Level VII)

9 The Joint Commission. (2021). Standard NPSG.01.01.01. *Comprehensive accreditation manual for hospitals.* Oakbrook Terrace, IL: The Joint Commission. (Level VII)

10 DNV GL-Healthcare USA, Inc. (2020). PR.2.SR.5. *NIAHO® accreditation requirements, interpretive guidelines and surveyor guidance—revision 20.0.* Milford, OH: DNV GL-Healthcare USA, Inc. (Level VII)

11 Accreditation Association for Hospitals and Health Systems. (2020). Standard 15.01.16. *Healthcare Facilities Accreditation Program: Accreditation requirements for acute care hospitals.* Chicago, IL: Accreditation Association for Hospitals and Health Systems. (Level VII)

12 Centers for Medicare and Medicaid Services, Department of Health and Human Services. (2020). Condition of participation: Patient's rights. 42 C.F.R. § 482.13(c)(1).

13 The Joint Commission. (2021). Standard RI.01.01.01. *Comprehensive accreditation manual for hospitals.* Oakbrook Terrace, IL: The Joint Commission. (Level VII)

14 The Joint Commission. (2021). Standard PC.02.01.21. *Comprehensive accreditation manual for hospitals.* Oakbrook Terrace, IL: The Joint Commission. (Level VII)

15 Waters, T. R., et al. (2009). Safe patient handling training for schools of nursing. https://www.cdc.gov/niosh/docs/2009-127/pdfs/2009-127.pdf (Level VII)

16 Siegel, J. D., et al. (2007, revised 2019). 2007 guideline for isolation precautions: Preventing transmission of infectious agents in healthcare settings. https://www.cdc.gov/infectioncontrol/pdf/guidelines/isolation-guidelines-H.pdf (Level II)

17 Accreditation Association for Hospitals and Health Systems. (2020). Standard 07.01.10. *Healthcare Facilities Accreditation Program: Accreditation requirements for acute care hospitals.* Chicago, IL: Accreditation Association for Hospitals and Health Systems. (Level VII)

18 Delaney, M. B. (2017). Kick the bucket: One hospital system's journey to reduce *Clostridium difficile. Journal of Emergency Nursing, 43,* 519–525. (Level VI)

19 Ganz, D. A., et al. (2013-reviewed 2021). *Preventing falls in hospitals: A toolkit for improving quality of care* (AHRQ Publication No. 13-0015-EF). Rockville, MD: Agency for Healthcare Research and Quality. https://www.ahrq.gov/professionals/systems/hospital/fallpxtoolkit/index.html (Level VII)

20 Wound Ostomy and Continence Nurses Society (WOCN). (2016). *Guideline for prevention and management of pressure ulcers (injuries): WOCN clinical practice guideline series 2.* Mount Laurel, NJ: WOCN.

21 National Pressure Ulcer Advisory Panel, et al. (2014). Prevention and treatment of pressure ulcers: Quick reference guide. https://www.epuap.org/wp-content/uploads/2016/10/quick-reference-guide-digital-npuap-epuap-pppia-jan2016.pdf (Level VII)

22 Accreditation Association for Hospitals and Health Systems. (2020). Standard 16.02.02. *Healthcare Facilities Accreditation Program: Accreditation requirements for acute care hospitals.* Chicago, IL: Accreditation Association for Hospitals and Health Systems. (Level VII)

23 Jarrett, N., & Callaham, M. (2016). Evidence-based guidelines for selected hospital-acquired conditions: Final report. https://www.cms.gov/Medicare/Medicare-Fee-for-Service-Payment/HospitalAcqCond/Downloads/2016-HAC-Report.pdf

24 Toney-Butler, T. J., & Gaston, G. (2020). Nursing bedpan management. https://www.ncbi.nlm.nih.gov/books/NBK499978/

25 Rutala, W. A., et al. (2008, revised 2019). Guideline for disinfection and sterilization in healthcare facilities, 2008. https://www.cdc.gov/infection-control/pdf/guidelines/disinfection-guidelines-H.pdf (Level I)

26 Accreditation Association for Hospitals and Health Systems. (2020). Standard 07.02.03. *Healthcare Facilities Accreditation Program: Accreditation requirements for acute care hospitals.* Chicago, IL: Accreditation Association for Hospitals and Health Systems. (Level VII)

27 The Joint Commission. (2021). Standard RC.01.03.01. *Comprehensive accreditation manual for hospitals.* Oakbrook Terrace, IL: The Joint Commission. (Level VII)

28 Centers for Medicare and Medicaid Services, Department of Health and Human Services. (2020). Condition of participation: Medical record services. 42 C.F.R. § 482.24(b).

29 Accreditation Association for Hospitals and Health Systems. (2020). Standard 10.00.03. *Healthcare Facilities Accreditation Program: Accreditation requirements for acute care hospitals.* Chicago, IL: Accreditation Association for Hospitals and Health Systems. (Level VII)

30 DNV GL-Healthcare USA, Inc. (2020). MR.2.SR.1. *NIAHO® accreditation requirements, interpretive guidelines and surveyor guidance - revision 20.0.* Milford, OH: DNV GL-Healthcare USA, Inc. (Level VII)

BEDSIDE SPIROMETRY

Bedside spirometry uses portable equipment to measure forced vital capacity (FVC) and forced expiratory volume (FEV). These measurements, in turn, allow for the calculation of other pulmonary function indexes, such as timed forced expiratory flow rate. Depending on the type of spirometer used, bedside spirometry can also allow direct measurement of vital capacity (VC) and tidal volume.

Bedside spirometry identifies the presence and severity of airflow obstruction. It's recommended for use in patients with respiratory signs and symptoms to determine whether their signs and symptoms result from respiratory disease or another condition.[1] Bedside spirometry can help diagnose chronic obstructive pulmonary disease by demonstrating obstructed airflow that isn't fully reversible.[1] It's also useful for evaluating a patient's preoperative anesthesia risk. Because the required breathing patterns can aggravate conditions such as bronchospasm, use of the bedside spirometer requires a review of the patient's history and close observation during testing. Forced expiration, which is required for measuring FVC and FEV, shouldn't be performed in a patient who's had recent abdominal, intracranial, or eye surgery or a patient with a pneumothorax, unstable angina, or a recent myocardial infarction.[2]

Performing bedside spirometry requires proper education and training in the procedure to ensure that test results are accurate.[3]

Equipment

Portable spirometer ▪ disposable mouthpiece ▪ stethoscope ▪ vital signs monitoring equipment ▪ disinfectant pad ▪ scale ▪ stadiometer ▪ Optional: gloves, gown, mask and goggles or mask with face shield, nose clip.

Preparation of equipment

Inspect all equipment and supplies. If a product is expired, is defective, or has compromised integrity, remove it from patient use, label it as expired or defective, and report the expiration or defect as directed by your facility. Review the manufacturer's instructions for assembly and use of the spirometer. If necessary, insert the breathing tube firmly to ensure a tight connection. If the unit comes with the tube preconnected, check the seals for tightness and the tubing for leaks. Insert the disposable mouthpiece and ensure that it's sealed tightly. Make sure that the unit has been calibrated according to the manufacturer's guidelines.

Implementation

▪ Verify the practitioner's orders, if required.

- Review the patient's medical record *to confirm that any inhaled long-acting beta-adrenergic agonist bronchodilator and oral beta-adrenergic agonist medications were withheld before spirometry testing, as ordered.*[3]

NURSING ALERT Oral and inhaled bronchodilators may be withheld from the patient before spirometry testing *to diagnose an underlying lung condition.* Be aware that the risk of bronchospasm increases if these medications are withheld. If spirometry testing is intended to evaluate bronchodilator response, bronchodilator medications are usually not withheld.[3]

- Gather and prepare the necessary equipment and supplies.
- Perform hand hygiene.[4,5,6,7,8,9]
- Confirm the patient's identity using at least two patient identifiers.[10]
- Provide privacy.[11,12,13,14]
- Explain the procedure to the patient and family (if appropriate) according to their communication and learning needs *to increase their understanding, allay their fears, and enhance cooperation.*[15] Emphasize that cooperation is essential *to ensure accurate results.*
- Instruct the patient to remove or loosen bras, belts, and other constricting clothing *to prevent alteration of test results from restricted thoracic expansion and abdominal mobility.*[3]
- Instruct the patient to void *to prevent abdominal discomfort.*
- Obtain the patient's weight (in kilograms) and height without shoes *to calculate predicted lung volumes.* Body mass index should be calculated as kg/m^2.[3] (See the "Height and weight measurement" procedure.)
- If the patient wears dentures that fit well, leave them in place *to promote a tight seal around the mouthpiece.*[3] However, if the dentures fit poorly, have the patient remove them *to prevent incomplete closure of the mouth around the mouthpiece, which could allow air to leak around the mouthpiece.*
- If the patient smokes, vapes, or uses a water pipe, confirm that the patient hasn't done so for at least 1 hour before the bedside spirometry procedure *to avoid acute bronchospasm due to smoke inhalation.*[3]
- Confirm that the patient hasn't performed vigorous exercise within 1 hour before testing *to avoid possible exercise-induced bronchoconstriction.*[3]
- Confirm the patient hasn't consumed intoxicants within 8 hours of testing *to avoid problems in coordination, comprehension, and physical ability.*[3]
- Perform hand hygiene.[4,5,6,7,8,9]
- Put on gloves and other personal protective equipment as needed *to comply with standard precautions.*[16,17]
- Enter the required information into the spirometer's computer system.
- Obtain the patient's blood pressure, pulse, and respiratory rate, and auscultate breath sounds *to serve as a baseline for comparison.*
- Ensure that the patient is either sitting straight in a chair with feet flat on the floor or standing with the chin slightly elevated.[3]
- If desired, allow the patient to practice the required breathing technique with the breathing tube unhooked. After practice, replace the tube and check the seal.
- Instruct the patient not to breathe through the nose. If the patient has difficulty complying, apply a nose clip.
- To measure VC, instruct the patient to inhale as deeply as possible, and then insert the mouthpiece so that the lips are sealed tightly around it *to prevent air leakage and to ensure an accurate digital readout or spirogram recording.*[3]
- Instruct the patient to exhale normally but completely, and then remove the mouthpiece *to avoid recording the next inspiration.*
- Repeat the maneuver at least three times, allowing adequate rest (more than 1 minute) between each maneuver. Typically, no more than four maneuvers are required to achieve acceptable repeatability. *Acceptable repeatability is achieved when the difference between the largest and the next-largest VC values for the maneuvers is 0.1 L or less.*[3]
- To measure FEV and FVC, adjust the spirometer settings to the appropriate mode according to the manufacturer's instructions.
- Repeat the procedure followed for VC measurement but instruct the patient to exhale as forcefully and completely as possible in one exhalation. Tell the patient when to start and activate the spirometer's recorder at the same time. Coach the patient throughout inspiration and exhalation.[3]
- Repeat the maneuver at least three times, allowing adequate rest (more than 1 minute) between each maneuver. Typically, no more than eight maneuvers are required to achieve acceptable repeatability for FVC and

FEV. *Acceptable repeatability is achieved when the difference between the largest and the next largest FVC and FEV values for the maneuvers is 0.1 L or less.*[3]
- Monitor the patient for increased shortness of breath, light-headedness, paroxysmal coughing, and chest pain.[3]
- Compare VC values between the maneuvers.

NURSING ALERT If a subsequent VC value is 20% lower than the original value and you're confident that there's no leak in the system, terminate the study, *because dangerous air trapping may result from forced exhalation.*

- After completing the procedure, generate a summary report from the spirometer's computer system.
- Obtain the patient's vital signs and assess respiratory status *to make sure the patient's condition is stable before leaving the bedside.* Notify the practitioner of any changes in the patient's condition.
- Discard the mouthpiece, and follow the manufacturer's instructions for cleaning and sterilizing the spirometer.[18,19]
- Remove and discard your gloves and any other personal protective equipment worn.[16,17]
- Perform hand hygiene.[4,5,6,7,8,9]
- Clean and disinfect your stethoscope using a disinfectant pad.[18,19]
- Perform hand hygiene.[4,5,6,7,8,9]
- Document the procedure.[20,21,22,23]

Special considerations

- Don't perform pulmonary function tests, including bedside spirometry, immediately after a large meal, *because the patient may experience abdominal discomfort.*
- Encourage the patient to perform maximally during the test; *doing so may help the patient to exhale more forcefully.*[3] If the patient coughs during expiration, wait until coughing subsides before repeating the measurement.
- Older adults patients with significant cognitive impairment and apraxia are less likely to perform spirometry correctly; however, advanced age alone shouldn't interfere with the ability to achieve accurate test results.
- Patients as young as age 2½ years may be able to perform spirometry maneuvers well enough to produce accurate results. Some spirometry software manufacturers offer developmentally appropriate visual incentives to enhance test performance in children.[3]
- Although FVC and VC are normally approximately equal, in patients with obstructive lung disease, FVC may be reduced but VC remains normal. In patients with restrictive lung disease, VC and FVC may be reduced.
- Although the reference data programmed in current spirometry software allow for automatic computation of predicted values, you shouldn't rely on the software alone when interpreting bedside spirometry results; they should be forwarded to the appropriate practitioner for interpretation. If software isn't available, a properly trained practitioner can calculate predicted values and compare patient results using a reference table of predicted normal values to aid diagnosis.

Complications

Forced exhalation can cause dizziness or light-headedness, precipitate or worsen bronchospasm, increase discomfort if the patient has inadequate pain control, rapidly increase exhaustion, cause hypoxia in a patient receiving oxygen therapy *because of the break in therapy,* and cause barotrauma in a patient with emphysema.[24] Forced expiration may cause increased pressure in the chest, abdomen, head, and eyes.[2]

Documentation

Record the date and time of the bedside spirometry; the patient's sex, age, height, and weight at the time of the testing; the patient's respiratory status before and after bedside spirometry; any complications that occurred; and the patient's tolerance of the procedure. If complications occurred, document the name of the practitioner notified, the date and time of notification, prescribed interventions, and the patient's response to those interventions. Document whether the patient was unable to complete the maneuvers. Record that the appropriate practitioner was notified of bedside spirometry results. Document teaching provided to the patient and family (if applicable), their understanding of that teaching, and any need for follow-up teaching.

REFERENCES

1 Qaseem, A., et al. (2011). Diagnosis and management of stable chronic obstructive pulmonary disease: A clinical practice guideline update from the American College of Physicians, American College of Chest Physicians, American Thoracic Society, and European Respiratory Society. *Annals of Internal Medicine, 155*, 179–191. https://annals.org/aim/fullarticle/479627/diagnosis-management-stable-chronic-obstructive-pulmonary-disease-clinical-practice-guideline (Level VII)

2 McCormack, M. C. (2020). Office spirometry. In: *UpToDate*, Stoller, J. K. (Ed.).

3 Graham, B. L., et al. (2019). Standardization of spirometry 2019 update. An official American Thoracic Society and European Respiratory Society technical statement. *American Journal of Respiratory and Critical Care Medicine, 200*(8), e70–e88. https://www.atsjournals.org/doi/pdf/10.1164/rccm.201908-1590ST (Level VII)

4 The Joint Commission. (2021). Standard NPSG.07.01.01. *Comprehensive accreditation manual for hospitals*. Oakbrook Terrace, IL: The Joint Commission. (Level VII)

5 Centers for Disease Control and Prevention. (2002). Guideline for hand hygiene in health-care settings: Recommendations of the Healthcare Infection Control Practices Advisory Committee and the HICPAC/SHEA/APIC/IDSA Hand Hygiene Task Force. *MMWR Recommendations and Reports, 51*(RR-16), 1–45. https://www.cdc.gov/mmwr/pdf/rr/rr5116.pdf (Level II)

6 World Health Organization. (2009). WHO guidelines on hand hygiene in health care: First global patient safety challenge, clean care is safer care. https://apps.who.int/iris/bitstream/handle/10665/44102/9789241597906_eng.pdf (Level IV)

7 Accreditation Association for Hospitals and Health Systems. (2020). Standard 07.01.21. *Healthcare Facilities Accreditation Program: Accreditation requirements for acute care hospitals*. Chicago, IL: Accreditation Association for Hospitals and Health Systems. (Level VII)

8 Centers for Medicare and Medicaid Services, Department of Health and Human Services. (2020). Condition of participation: Infection control. 42 C.F.R. § 482.42.

9 DNV GL-Healthcare USA, Inc. (2020). IC.1.SR.1. *NIAHO® accreditation requirements, interpretive guidelines and surveyor guidance—revision 20.0*. Milford, OH: DNV GL-Healthcare USA, Inc. (Level VII)

10 The Joint Commission. (2021). Standard NPSG.01.01.01. *Comprehensive accreditation manual for hospitals*. Oakbrook Terrace, IL: The Joint Commission. (Level VII)

11 Accreditation Association for Hospitals and Health Systems. (2020). Standard 15.01.16. *Healthcare Facilities Accreditation Program: Accreditation requirements for acute care hospitals*. Chicago, IL: Accreditation Association for Hospitals and Health Systems. (Level VII)

12 The Joint Commission. (2021). Standard RI.01.01.01. *Comprehensive accreditation manual for hospitals*. Oakbrook Terrace, IL: The Joint Commission. (Level VII)

13 Centers for Medicare and Medicaid Services, Department of Health and Human Services. (2020). Condition of participation: Patient's rights. 42 C.F.R. § 482.13(c)(1).

14 DNV GL-Healthcare USA, Inc. (2020). PR.2.SR.5. *NIAHO® accreditation requirements, interpretive guidelines and surveyor guidance—revision 20.0*. Milford, OH: DNV GL-Healthcare USA, Inc. (Level VII)

15 The Joint Commission. (2021). Standard PC.02.01.21. *Comprehensive accreditation manual for hospitals*. Oakbrook Terrace, IL: The Joint Commission. (Level VII)

16 Accreditation Association for Hospitals and Health Systems. (2020). Standard 07.01.10. *Healthcare Facilities Accreditation Program: Accreditation requirements for acute care hospitals*. Chicago, IL: Accreditation Association for Hospitals and Health Systems. (Level VII)

17 Siegel, J. D., et al. (2007, revised 2019). 2007 guideline for isolation precautions: Preventing transmission of infectious agents in healthcare settings. https://www.cdc.gov/infectioncontrol/pdf/guidelines/isolation-guidelines-H.pdf (Level II)

18 Rutala, W. A., et al. (2008, revised 2019). Guideline for disinfection and sterilization in healthcare facilities, 2008. https://www.cdc.gov/infection-control/pdf/guidelines/disinfection-guidelines-H.pdf (Level I)

19 Accreditation Association for Hospitals and Health Systems. (2020). Standard 07.02.03. *Healthcare Facilities Accreditation Program: Accreditation requirements for acute care hospitals*. Chicago, IL: Accreditation Association for Hospitals and Health Systems. (Level VII)

20 The Joint Commission. (2021). Standard RC.01.03.01. *Comprehensive accreditation manual for hospitals*. Oakbrook Terrace, IL: The Joint Commission. (Level VII)

21 Accreditation Association for Hospitals and Health Systems. (2020). Standard 10.00.03. *Healthcare Facilities Accreditation Program: Accreditation requirements for acute care hospitals*. Chicago, IL: Accreditation Association for Hospitals and Health Systems. (Level VII)

22 Centers for Medicare and Medicaid Services, Department of Health and Human Services. (2020). Condition of participation: Medical record services. 42 C.F.R. § 482.24(b).

23 DNV GL-Healthcare USA, Inc. (2020). MR.2.SR.1. *NIAHO® accreditation requirements, interpretive guidelines and surveyor guidance—revision 20.0*. Milford, OH: DNV GL-Healthcare USA, Inc. (Level VII)

24 Kacmarek, R. M., et al. (2021). *Egan's fundamentals of respiratory care* (12th ed.). St Louis, MO: Mosby.

BILIARY DRAINAGE CATHETER CARE

A biliary drainage catheter, also called a T-tube, facilitates biliary drainage in patients with obstruction of the biliary tree due to tumors, strictures, cholangitis, abscess, or choledocholithiasis (biliary stones) and after such surgical procedures as cholecystectomy, choledochostomy, or liver transplant.

A practitioner inserts a biliary drainage catheter into the common bile duct, anchors it to the abdominal wall, and connects it to a closed drainage system (as shown on the next page). Catheters can also drain internally into the small intestine. Placement of a biliary drainage catheter can occur in an interventional radiology suite using fluoroscopy, contrast dye, and a guidewire.

You should change a biliary drainage catheter dressing routinely, as needed and ordered, to prevent infection and skin excoriation from bile drainage. In preparation for catheter removal, the practitioner may request that you clamp the catheter to assess the patient's tolerance of the return of bile flow.

Equipment

Gloves ■ clamp or stopcock ■ vital signs monitoring equipment ■ graduated collection container ■ indelible marker ■ clean gauze pad ■ normal saline solution ■ prescribed antiseptic cleaning agent ■ two sterile basins ■ sterile precut drain dressings ■ hypoallergenic paper tape ■ Optional: prescribed pain medication, gown, protective eyewear, transparent dressing, skin protectant, biliary drainage catheter irrigation equipment, catheter securement device.

Preparation of equipment

Inspect all equipment and supplies. If a product is defective or has compromised integrity, remove it from patient use, label it as defective, and report the defect, as directed by your facility. Label all solution containers (with the patient's name and the date and time you opened it) using an indelible marker.

Implementation

■ Verify the practitioner's order.
■ Check the patient's medical recorder for a history of allergies.
■ Gather and prepare the necessary equipment and supplies.
■ Perform hand hygiene.[1,2,3,4,5,6]
■ Confirm the patient's identity using at least two patient identifiers.[7]
■ Provide privacy.[8,9,10,11]
■ Explain the procedure to the patient and family members (if appropriate) according to their communication and learning needs *to increase their understanding, allay their fears, and enhance cooperation.*[12]

Changing the dressing

■ Screen and assess the patient for pain using facility-defined criteria that are consistent with the patient's age, condition, and ability to understand.[13]

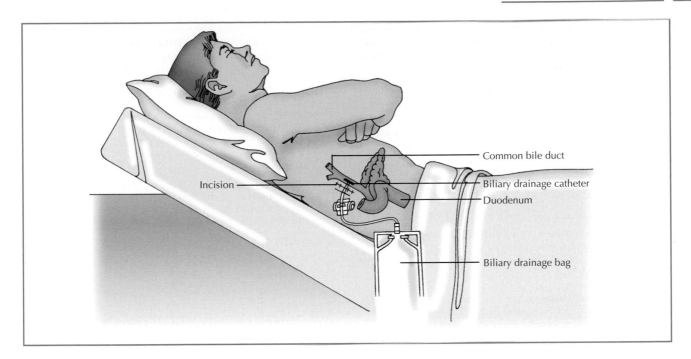

Common bile duct

Incision

Biliary drainage catheter

Duodenum

Biliary drainage bag

Before the dressing change, treat the patient's pain, as necessary and ordered, using nonpharmacologic, pharmacologic, or a combination of approaches.[13,14,15,16,17]

■ Raise the bed to hip level *to prevent caregiver back strain*. Position the patient to allow clear access to the dressing. Then raise the bed to waist level *to prevent caregiver back strain when providing care*.[18]

■ Perform hand hygiene.[1,2,3,4,5,6]

■ Put on gloves and, as necessary, other personal protective equipment *to comply with standard precautions*.[19,20,21]

■ Without dislodging the biliary drainage catheter, carefully remove the old dressing *to prevent skin stripping or tearing*.[22]

■ Inspect the dressing for drainage, and then dispose of it in an appropriate receptacle.[20]

■ Remove and discard your gloves.[19,20,21]

■ Perform hand hygiene.[1,2,3,4,5,6]

■ Open the sterile packages using sterile no-touch technique, and pour the prescribed antiseptic cleaning agent into a sterile basin and the normal saline solution into another sterile basin.

■ Perform hand hygiene.[1,2,3,4,5,6]

■ Put on gloves and follow sterile no-touch technique *to prevent contamination of the incision*.[19,20,21,23]

■ Inspect the incision and biliary drainage catheter insertion site for signs of infection, including redness, edema, warmth, tenderness, induration, and skin excoriation. Also assess the catheter and site for wound dehiscence or evisceration, if applicable.

■ Soak a sterile 4″ × 4″ (10-cm × 10-cm) gauze pad in the prescribed antiseptic cleaning agent and then use it to clean and remove dried matter and bile drainage from around the biliary drainage catheter. Starting always at the catheter insertion site, gently wiping outward in a continuous circular motion *to prevent recontamination of the catheter insertion site*.

■ Soak a new sterile 4″ × 4″ (10-cm × 10-cm) gauze pad in normal saline solution and use it to rinse the area. Dry the area with a sterile 4″ × 4″ (10-cm × 10-cm) gauze pad.

■ Lightly apply a skin protectant to the site, if necessary, *to protect the skin from injury caused by bile drainage*.

■ Apply sterile precut drain dressings, one extending from either side of the biliary drainage catheter, *to absorb bile drainage*.

■ Apply a sterile 4″ × 4″ (10-cm × 10-cm) gauze pad over the incision.

■ Apply a sterile 4″ × 4″ (10-cm × 10-cm) gauze pad or transparent dressing over the biliary drainage catheter and the incision dressings. *To avoid blocking bile drainage*, don't kink the tubing. Secure the dressings with hypoallergenic paper tape.

■ Reassess and respond to the patient's pain by evaluating the response to treatment and progress toward pain management goals. Assess for adverse reactions and risk factors for adverse events that may result from treatment.[13]

■ Return the patient's bed to the lowest position *to prevent falls and maintain patient safety*.[24,25]

■ Remove and discard your gloves.[19,20,21]

■ Perform hand hygiene.[1,2,3,4,5,6]

Emptying the drainage bag

■ Put on gloves *to comply with standard precautions*.[19,20,21]

■ Trace the biliary drainage catheter from the patient to its point of origin *to ensure you're emptying the correct drainage bag*.[26]

■ Place a graduated collection container under the outlet valve of the drainage bag.

■ Supporting the biliary drainage bag *to help prevent traction on the biliary drainage catheter and accidental removal*, open the outlet valve, empty the bag's contents completely into the container, and close the valve without contaminating the valve, tubing, or clamp (if used).[27]

■ Wipe the end of the outlet valve with a clean gauze pad *to remove residual bile drainage that may remain after the valve is closed*.

■ Measure carefully and record the character, color, and amount of drainage.

■ Discard the bile drainage, and rinse or discard the collection container appropriately.[19]

■ Check bile drainage amounts regularly *to ensure patient comfort and safety*.

■ Make sure that the biliary catheter drainage system is secured below the level of the catheter insertion site *to prevent backflow contamination*. Make sure that the catheter securement device is intact, or replace as necessary, *to prevent pulling and tension on the catheter*.[28]

■ Remove and discard your gloves.[19,20,21]

■ Perform hand hygiene.[1,2,3,4,5,6]

■ Obtain the patient's vital signs, monitor intake and output, and assess for any signs or symptoms of obstructed bile flow (such as chills, fever, tachycardia, nausea, right-upper-quadrant fullness and pain, jaundice, dark, foamy urine, and clay-colored stools. Report any signs or symptoms of such obstruction to the practitioner immediately.

Clamping the tube

■ Put on gloves *to comply with standard precautions*.[19,20,21]

■ Trace the biliary drainage catheter from the patient to its point of origin *to make sure you're clamping the correct catheter.*[26]

■ Occlude the biliary drainage catheter lightly with a clamp, or close the stopcock, if present. *Clamping the catheter 1 hour before and after meals diverts bile back to the duodenum to aid digestion.*

■ Monitor the patient's response to having the biliary drainage catheter clamped.

■ Supporting the biliary drainage bag *to help prevent traction on the biliary drainage catheter and accidental removal,* unclamp the biliary drainage catheter or open the stopcock, as ordered.[27]

■ Check bile drainage amounts regularly, and empty the biliary drainage bag into a graduated collection container for measurement, as necessary, *to ensure patient comfort and safety.*

Completing the procedure
■ Dispose of used equipment and materials appropriately.
■ Remove and discard your gloves[19,20,21] and perform hand hygiene.[1,2,3,4,5,6]
■ Document the procedure.[29,30,31,32]

Special considerations
■ The biliary drainage catheter usually drains from 300 to 500 mL of blood-tinged bile within the first 24 hours after surgery. Report drainage within that time period that exceeds 500 mL; if drainage is 50 mL or less, notify the practitioner, *because the tube may be obstructed.* (See *Managing biliary drainage catheter obstruction.*)

■ Bile drainage typically declines to 200 mL or less 4 days after surgery and the color changes to green-brown. Monitor the patient's fluid, electrolyte, and acid-base status carefully.

■ Secure the biliary drainage system below the level of the catheter insertion site *to prevent tension on the catheter.*[28]

■ Provide meticulous skin care and frequent dressing changes. Observe for bile leakage around the biliary drainage catheter, *which may indicate obstruction.*

■ Assess biliary drainage catheter patency and the catheter insertion site condition hourly for the first 8 hours postoperative and then every 4 hours until the practitioner removes the catheter.

■ If the patient has fragile skin, use dressings and tape specifically formulated for fragile skin *to prevent skin stripping and tearing during removal.*[22,23]

■ Monitor all the patient's urine and stool for color changes. Assess the patient for icteric skin and sclera, *which may indicate jaundice.*

■ If the practitioner orders it, follow these steps for flushing the biliary drainage catheter: (1) Perform hand hygiene.[1,2,3,4,5,6] (2) Put on gloves *to comply with standard precautions.*[19,20,21] (3) Turn the three-way stopcock off to the drainage bag. (4) Perform a vigorous mechanical scrub of the needleless connector on the flushing port of the stopcock using an antiseptic pad; allow it to dry completely. (5) While maintaining sterility of the syringe tip, attach a 10-mL prefilled syringe containing sterile, normal saline solution to the needleless connector. (6) Inject the prescribed volume (typically 3, 5, or 10 mL) of sterile, normal saline solution gently, as directed. (7) Remove and discard the syringe. (8) Turn the three-way stopcock off to the needleless connector on the flushing port of the stopcock. (9) Remove and discard your gloves [19,20,21] and perform hand hygiene.[1,2,3,4,5,6]

■ The Joint Commission has issued a sentinel event alert related to managing risk during transition to the new International Organization for Standardization tubing connector standards designed to prevent dangerous tubing misconnections, which can lead to serious patient injury and death. During the transition, be sure to trace the connection tubing and catheter from the patient to the point of origin before connecting or reconnecting any device or infusion, at any care transition (such as a new setting or service), and as part of the hand-off process. Route connection tubes and catheters with different purposes in different standardized directions. When different access sites exist or several bags are hanging, label the connection tubing at the distal and proximal ends. Use tubing and equipment only as intended. Store medications for different delivery routes in separate locations.[33]

> ## Managing biliary drainage catheter obstruction
>
> If the patient's biliary drainage catheter becomes obstructed after cholecystectomy, notify the practitioner and take these steps while you wait for the practitioner to arrive:
> ■ Unclamp the biliary drainage catheter (if it was clamped 1 hour before or after a meal), and connect the catheter to a closed gravity-drainage system.
> ■ Inspect the catheter carefully *to detect any kinks or obstructions.*
> ■ Prepare the patient for possible biliary drainage catheter irrigation or direct X-ray of the common bile duct (cholangiography). Describe these measures briefly to the patient *to reduce the patient's apprehension and promote cooperation.*
> ■ Provide encouragement and support to the patient.

Patient teaching
Inform the patient that loose bowel movements commonly occur in the first few weeks after surgery. Teach the patient how to care for the biliary drainage catheter at home, including providing meticulous skin care and dressing changes, *to prevent infection and skin breakdown.* Also instruct the patient how to flush the tube daily (or more frequently if ordered) with 3 to 10 mL of sterile normal saline or water, as ordered by the practitioner, *to prevent blockage.*[28,34,35] Also inform the patient about the signs and symptoms of catheter and biliary obstruction that the patient should report to the practitioner. Teach the patient how to manage the biliary drainage catheter when turning, walking, and performing activities of daily living. Caution the patient to avoid direct pulling or traction on the biliary drainage catheter,[27] and explain that bile stains clothing. Instruct the patient and family members to keep the drainage bag lower than the catheter insertion site *to help with drainage.*

Complications
Obstructed bile flow, skin excoriation or breakdown, biliary drainage catheter dislodgment, drainage reflux, and infection are the most common complications related to the use or clamping of a biliary drainage catheter.

Documentation
Document the date and time of the dressing change, the type of antiseptic cleaning agent you used, infection prevention and safety precautions you implemented, appearance of the insertion site and surrounding skin, and type of dressing you applied. Note whether drainage was present on the old dressing. Keep a precise record of the patient's bile drainage, color, character, and volume, patient temperature, and amount and frequency of urination and bowel movements. Document the patient's tolerance of the clamping procedure. Also document any patient report of pain during the procedure, resulting interventions, and the patient's response to those interventions. Document teaching you provided to the patient and family (if applicable), their understanding of that teaching, and any need for follow-up teaching.

REFERENCES
1 Centers for Disease Control and Prevention. (2002). Guideline for hand hygiene in health-care settings: Recommendations of the Healthcare Infection Control Practices Advisory Committee and the HICPAC/SHEA/APIC/IDSA Hand Hygiene Task Force. *MMWR Recommendations and Reports, 51*(RR-16), 1–45. https://www.cdc.gov/mmwr/pdf/rr/rr5116.pdf (Level II)

2 The Joint Commission. (2021). Standard NPSG.07.01.01. *Comprehensive accreditation manual for hospitals.* Oakbrook Terrace, IL: The Joint Commission. (Level VII)

3 World Health Organization. (2009). WHO guidelines on hand hygiene in health care: First global patient safety challenge, clean care is safer care. https://apps.who.int/iris/bitstream/handle/10665/44102/9789241597906_eng.pdf?sequence=1 (Level IV)

4 Accreditation Association for Hospitals and Health Systems. (2020). Standard 07.01.21. *Healthcare Facilities Accreditation Program: Accreditation requirements for acute care hospitals*. Chicago, IL: Accreditation Association for Hospitals and Health Systems. (Level VII)

5 Centers for Medicare and Medicaid Services, Department of Health and Human Services. (2020). Condition of participation: Infection control. 42 C.F.R. § 482.42.

6 DNV GL-Healthcare USA, Inc. (2020). IC.1.SR.1. *NIAHO® accreditation requirements, interpretive guidelines and surveyor guidance—revision 20.0*. Milford, OH: DNV GL-Healthcare USA, Inc. (Level VII)

7 The Joint Commission. (2021). Standard NPSG.01.01.01. *Comprehensive accreditation manual for hospitals*. Oakbrook Terrace, IL: The Joint Commission. (Level VII)

8 Accreditation Association for Hospitals and Health Systems. (2020). Standard 15.01.16. *Healthcare Facilities Accreditation Program: Accreditation requirements for acute care hospitals*. Chicago, IL: Accreditation Association for Hospitals and Health Systems. (Level VII)

9 Centers for Medicare and Medicaid Services, Department of Health and Human Services. (2020). Condition of participation: Patient's rights. 42 C.F.R. § 482.13(c)(1).

10 DNV GL-Healthcare USA, Inc. (2020). PR.2.SR.5. *NIAHO® accreditation requirements, interpretive guidelines and surveyor guidance—revision 20.0*. Milford, OH: DNV GL-Healthcare USA, Inc. (Level VII)

11 The Joint Commission. (2021). Standard RI.01.01.01. *Comprehensive accreditation manual for hospitals*. Oakbrook Terrace, IL: The Joint Commission. (Level VII)

12 The Joint Commission. (2021). Standard PC.02.01.21. *Comprehensive accreditation manual for hospitals*. Oakbrook Terrace, IL: The Joint Commission. (Level VII)

13 The Joint Commission. (2021). Standard PC.01.02.07. *Comprehensive accreditation manual for hospitals*. Oakbrook Terrace, IL: The Joint Commission. (Level VII)

14 The Joint Commission. (2021). Standard MM.06.01.01. *Comprehensive accreditation manual for hospitals*. Oakbrook Terrace, IL: The Joint Commission. (Level VII)

15 Accreditation Association for Hospitals and Health Systems. (2020). Standard 16.01.03. *Healthcare Facilities Accreditation Program: Accreditation requirements for acute care hospitals*. Chicago, IL: Accreditation Association for Hospitals and Health Systems. (Level VII)

16 Centers for Medicare and Medicaid Services, Department of Health and Human Services. (2020). Condition of participation: Nursing services. 42 C.F.R. § 482.23(c).

17 DNV GL-Healthcare USA, Inc. (2020). MM.1.SR.3. *NIAHO® accreditation requirements, interpretive guidelines and surveyor guidance—revision 20.0*. Milford, OH: DNV GL-Healthcare USA, Inc. (Level VII)

18 Waters, T. R., et al. (2009). Safe patient handling training for schools of nursing. https://www.cdc.gov/niosh/docs/2009-127/pdfs/2009-127.pdf (Level VII)

19 Siegel, J. D., et al. (2007, revised 2019). 2007 guideline for isolation precautions: Preventing transmission of infectious agents in healthcare settings. https://www.cdc.gov/infectioncontrol/pdf/guidelines/isolation-guidelines-H.pdf (Level II)

20 Occupational Safety and Health Administration. (2012). Bloodborne pathogens, standard number 1910.1030. https://www.osha.gov/pls/oshaweb/owadisp.show_document?p_id=10051&p_table=STANDARDS (Level VII)

21 Accreditation Association for Hospitals and Health Systems. (2020). Standard 07.01.10. *Healthcare Facilities Accreditation Program: Accreditation requirements for acute care hospitals*. Chicago, IL: Accreditation Association for Hospitals and Health Systems. (Level VII)

22 LeBlanc, K., et al. (2013). International skin tear advisory panel: A tool kit to aid in the prevention, assessment, and treatment of skin tears using a simplified classification system. *Advances in Skin and Wound Care, 26*, 459–476. (Level IV)

23 Accreditation Association for Hospitals and Health Systems. (2020). Standard 07.01.20. *Healthcare Facilities Accreditation Program: Accreditation requirements for acute care hospitals*. Chicago, IL: Accreditation Association for Hospitals and Health Systems. (Level VII)

24 Ganz, D. A., et al. (2013, reviewed 2021). Preventing falls in hospitals: A toolkit for improving quality of care (AHRQ publication no. 13-0015-EF). https://www.ahrq.gov/professionals/systems/hospital/fallpxtoolkit/index.html (Level VII)

25 Accreditation Association for Hospitals and Health Systems. (2020). Standard 16.02.02. *Healthcare Facilities Accreditation Program: Accreditation requirements for acute care hospitals*. Chicago, IL: Accreditation

Association for Hospitals and Health Systems. (Level VII)

26 U.S. Food and Drug Administration. (2017). Examples of medical device misconnections. https://www.fda.gov/medical-devices/medical-device-connectors/examples-of-medical-device-misconnections

27 Bauldoff, G., et al. (2019). *LeMone and Burke's medical-surgical nursing: Clinical reasoning in patient care* (7th ed.). Cranbury, NJ: Pearson Education.

28 Memorial Sloan Kettering Cancer Center. (2021). About your biliary drainage catheter. https://www.mskcc.org/cancer-care/patient-education/about-your-biliary-drainage-catheter

29 The Joint Commission. (2021). Standard RC.01.03.01. *Comprehensive accreditation manual for hospitals*. Oakbrook Terrace, IL: The Joint Commission. (Level VII)

30 Accreditation Association for Hospitals and Health Systems. (2020). Standard 10.00.03. *Healthcare Facilities Accreditation Program: Accreditation requirements for acute care hospitals*. Chicago, IL: Accreditation Association for Hospitals and Health Systems. (Level VII)

31 Centers for Medicare and Medicaid Services, Department of Health and Human Services. (2020). Condition of participation: Medical record services. 42 C.F.R. § 482.24(b).

32 DNV GL-Healthcare USA, Inc. (2020). MR.2.SR.1. *NIAHO® accreditation requirements, interpretive guidelines and surveyor guidance—revision 18.2*. Milford, OH: DNV GL-Healthcare USA, Inc. (Level VII)

33 The Joint Commission. (2014). Sentinel event alert 53: Managing risk during transition to new ISO tubing connector standards. http://www.jointcommission.org/assets/1/6/SEA_53_Connectors_8_19_14_final.pdf (Level VII)

34 Stanford Health Care. (2014). Interventional radiology patient discharge education biliary drain/stent placement or exchange. https://stanfordhealthcare.org/content/dam/SHC/clinics/interventional-radiology-clinic/docs/biliary-drain-patient-discharge-education.pdf

35 Dawood, A. (2020). Percutaneous biliary drainage. http://emedicine.medscape.com/article/1828052-overview#a1 (Level VII)

BIOHAZARDOUS WASTE HANDLING

Waste that contains blood or other potentially infectious body fluids is considered biohazardous waste (regulated medical waste).[1,2] You must handle such waste appropriately to prevent exposure to patients and other health care providers. Because of the increased risk of infection from exposure to blood or body fluids, proper handling of biohazardous waste is especially important in the operating room (OR).[1] (See *Types of biohazardous waste*, page 70.)

It's essential to separate biohazardous waste from other trash and store it in clearly labeled hazardous waste containers.[1,2] The assigned surgical team members responsible for handling waste should use personal protective equipment, as appropriate. A spill of potentially infectious waste requires immediate cleanup using a disinfectant registered with the Environmental Protection Agency (EPA), and disposal of all soiled materials in a biohazard bag.[3,4,5]

To prevent infection transmission, appropriately store, transport, and dispose of biohazardous waste according to the most stringent local, state, or federal regulations.[1] Dispose of sharps and pharmaceutical waste in appropriate, clearly labeled, puncture-proof containers.[1,5,6]

Equipment

Labeled, leakproof biohazardous waste container ▪ clear trash bags ▪ rigid containers with lids ▪ personal protective equipment (gloves, masks, eye protection, face shield, gown) ▪ puncture-proof containers ▪ Optional: solidifying equipment, EPA-registered disinfectant.

Preparation of equipment

Inspect all equipment and supplies. If a product is expired, is defective, or has compromised integrity, remove it from patient use, label it as expired or defective, and report the expiration or defect, as directed by your facility.

Implementation

▪ Put on gloves and other personal protective equipment, as appropriate, *to protect yourself from accidental exposure*.[2,4,5,6,7,8,9]

■ Place biohazardous waste in the appropriate biohazardous waste container at the point of use *to reduce the risk of exposure.* The container must be labeled clearly as biohazardous waste *so that it's easily identifiable and receives appropriate handling.*[1,5]

■ Separate regular trash from biohazardous waste, and place regular trash in clear trash bags *to enable proper disposal.*[1]

■ Store each type of biohazardous waste in an appropriate rigid container with a lid *to reduce the risk of infection transmission or exposure during storage and transportation.*[1]

■ Add a solidifying agent to a container that contains blood and other fluids, as indicated, *to solidify the contents to reduce exposure to biohazardous materials.*[7]

■ Notify the environmental services department that the containers are ready for disposal.

■ Clean spills immediately with an EPA-registered disinfectant, following the manufacturer's instructions for use, while wearing appropriate personal protective equipment *to avoid accidental exposure.*[3] Discard all soiled items in the biohazard bag.

■ Dispose of all sharps in puncture-proof containers specifically labeled for sharps or pharmaceutical waste.[2,5]

■ Remove and discard your gloves and any other personal protective equipment you wore.

■ Perform hand hygiene.[4,10,11,12,13,14,15]

Special considerations

■ All staff members should receive instruction on how to follow standard precautions and properly use personal protective equipment.[4]

■ Staff members should report any bloodborne pathogen exposure to a supervisor, as directed by the facility, including patient exposure or injury that occurs while handling biohazardous waste.[4]

■ Change sharps containers and trash bags when they're three-quarters full *to prevent injury to those handling them.*

Types of biohazardous waste

■ *Isolation waste* is any waste generated by a patient who's isolated because of a communicable disease.

■ *Cultures and stocks of infectious agents and associated biologicals* include specimen cultures from medical and pathology laboratories, cultures and stocks of infectious agents from research and industrial laboratories, waste resulting from the production of biologicals, discarded live and attenuated vaccines, and culture dishes and devices used to transfer, inoculate, and mix cultures.

■ *Human blood and blood products* include whole blood, serum, plasma, and other blood products.

■ *Pathologic waste* includes tissues, organs, body parts, and body fluids removed during surgery or autopsy.

■ *Contaminated sharps* include hypodermic needles, syringes, Pasteur pipettes, broken glass, and scalpel blades, all of which are considered infectious waste because of the possibility of contamination with bloodborne pathogens.

■ *Contaminated carcasses, body parts, and bedding* are materials from animals that have been intentionally exposed to pathogens during research, the production of biologicals, or in vivo testing of pharmaceuticals.

■ *Miscellaneous waste* includes waste that isn't designated as infectious but that's assumed to be and managed as infectious to protect the environment and the people handling such waste. Examples include:
   ■ waste from surgeries and autopsies, such as soiled dressings, sponges, drapes, lavage tubes, drainage sets, underpads, and surgical gloves
   ■ contaminated laboratory waste, such as specimen containers, slides and coverslips, disposable gloves, laboratory coats, and aprons
   ■ dialysis unit waste, such as contaminated disposable equipment and supplies, including tubing, filters, disposable sheets, towels, gloves, aprons, and laboratory coats
   ■ contaminated equipment, including discarded equipment and parts used in patient care, medical and industrial laboratories, research, and the production and testing of certain pharmaceuticals.

■ Manage waste generated during the care of patients requiring transmission-based precautions following the same methods used in other patient care areas.[4,7,9]

Complications

Patients or staff members may be exposed to bloodborne pathogens during handling of biohazardous waste in the OR. Improper disposal of waste, such as in an unapproved landfill, could also put others at risk for exposure.

Documentation

Although the handling of biohazardous waste doesn't require documentation, document any exposure, as required by your facility and according to Occupational Safety and Health Administration standards.[2]

REFERENCES

1 Guideline for perioperative practice: Safe environment of care. (2020). In Wood, A. (Ed.), *Guidelines for perioperative practice 2020 edition.* Denver, CO: AORN, Inc. (Level VII)

2 Occupational Safety and Health Administration. (2012). Bloodborne pathogens, standard number 1910.1030. https://www.osha.gov/pls/oshaweb/owadisp.show_document?p_id=10051&p_table=STANDARDS (Level VII)

3 Occupational Safety and Health Administration (OSHA) and the National Institute for Occupational Safety and Health (NIOSH). (2012). InfoSheet: Protecting workers who use cleaning chemicals. https://www.osha.gov/Publications/OSHA3512.pdf

4 Guideline for perioperative practice: Transmission based precautions. (2020). In Wood, A. (Ed.), *Guidelines for perioperative practice 2020 edition.* Denver, CO: AORN, Inc. (Level VII)

5 The Joint Commission. (2021). Standard EC.02.02.01. *Comprehensive accreditation manual for hospitals.* Oakbrook Terrace, IL: The Joint Commission. (Level VII)

6 Occupational Safety and Health Administration. (n.d.). OSHA technical manual: Hospital investigations—health hazards. https://www.osha.gov/dts/osta/otm/otm_vi/otm_vi_1.html (Level VII)

7 Guideline for perioperative practice: Environmental cleaning. (2020). In Wood, A. (Ed.), *Guidelines for perioperative practice 2020 edition.* Denver, CO: AORN, Inc. (Level VII)

8 Accreditation Association for Hospitals and Health Systems. (2020). Standard 07.01.10. *Healthcare Facilities Accreditation Program: Accreditation requirements for acute care hospitals.* Chicago, IL: Accreditation Association for Hospitals and Health Systems. (Level VII)

9 Siegel, J. D., et al. (2007, revised 2019). 2007 guideline for isolation precautions: Preventing transmission of infectious agents in healthcare settings. https://www.cdc.gov/infectioncontrol/pdf/guidelines/isolation-guidelines-H.pdf (Level II)

10 Accreditation Association for Hospitals and Health Systems. (2020). Standard 07.01.21. *Healthcare Facilities Accreditation Program: Accreditation requirements for acute care hospitals.* Chicago, IL: Accreditation Association for Hospitals and Health Systems. (Level VII)

11 World Health Organization. (2009). WHO guidelines on hand hygiene in health care: First global patient safety challenge, clean care is safer care. https://apps.who.int/iris/bitstream/handle/10665/44102/9789241597906_eng.pdf?sequence=1 (Level IV)

12 Centers for Disease Control and Prevention. (2002). Guideline for hand hygiene in health-care settings: Recommendations of the Healthcare Infection Control Practices Advisory Committee and the HICPAC/SHEA/APIC/IDSA Hand Hygiene Task Force. *MMWR Recommendations and Reports, 51*(RR-16), 1–45. https://www.cdc.gov/mmwr/pdf/rr/rr5116.pdf (Level II)

13 The Joint Commission. (2021). Standard NPSG.07.01.01. *Comprehensive accreditation manual for hospitals.* Oakbrook Terrace, IL: The Joint Commission. (Level VII)

14 Centers for Medicare and Medicaid Services, Department of Health and Human Services. (2020). Condition of participation: Infection control. 42 C.F.R. § 482.42.

15 DNV GL-Healthcare USA, Inc. (2020). IC.1.SR.1. *NIAHO® accreditation requirements, interpretive guidelines and surveyor guidance—revision 20.0.* Milford, OH: DNV GL-Healthcare USA, Inc. (Level VII)

BISPECTRAL INDEX MONITORING

Bispectral index monitoring involves the use of an electronic device that converts electroencephalogram (EEG) waves into a number. This number, statistically derived from raw EEG data, indicates the depth or level of a patient's sedation and provides a direct measure of the effects of sedatives and anesthetics on the patient's brain. Unlike reliance on subjective assessments and vital signs, bispectral index monitoring provides objective, reliable data the practitioner can use to make care decisions, minimizing the risks of oversedation and undersedation. When used appropriately, bispectral index monitoring can decrease the total amount of sedation needed to keep a patient adequately sedated.[1,2,3]

The bispectral index monitor is attached to a sensor applied to the patient's forehead. The sensor obtains information about the patient's electrical brain activity and then translates this information into a number from 0 (indicating no brain activity) to 100 (indicating a patient who's awake and alert). During general anesthesia, a target range between 40 and 60 is the area in which patients have a lower risk of experiencing intraoperative awareness on recall.[4] On a critical care unit and in an operating room, the use of bispectral index monitoring helps assess the level of sedation when the patient is receiving mechanical ventilation or neuromuscular blocking agents and during barbiturate coma therapy and bedside procedures.[5]

Equipment

Bispectral index monitor and interface cable ■ bispectral index sensor ■ washcloth ■ soap and water ■ Optional: gloves, alcohol pads, gauze.

Preparation of equipment

Inspect all equipment and supplies. If a product is expired, is defective, or has compromised integrity, remove it from patient use, label it as expired or defective, and report the expiration or defect, as directed by your facility. Place the bispectral index monitor close to the patient's bed, and plug the power cord into a wall outlet. Turn on the monitor, and allow it to initiate a self-test according to the manufacturer's instructions to ensure that the equipment is functioning properly.[6]

Implementation

- Verify the practitioner's orders if required.
- Gather and prepare the necessary equipment and supplies.
- Perform hand hygiene.[7,8,9,10,11,12]
- Confirm the patient's identity using at least two patient identifiers.[13]
- Provide privacy.[14,15,16,17]
- Explain the procedure to the patient and family (if appropriate) according to their communication and learning needs *to increase their understanding, allay their fears, and enhance cooperation.*[18] (See *Bispectral index monitoring.*)
- Raise the patient's bed to waist level before providing patient care *to prevent caregiver back strain.*[19]
- Perform hand hygiene.[7,8,9,10,11,12]
- Put on gloves as needed *to comply with standard precautions.*[20,21,22]
- Assess the patient's neurologic status, including level of sedation, responsiveness, and arousal, *to obtain baseline data for comparison.*[6]
- Identify the anatomical landmarks for accurate placement of the bispectral index sensor.[6]
- Clean the patient's forehead using a washcloth with soap and water and then allow it to dry. Alternatively, clean the intended sensor area with an alcohol pad and then dry it using a gauze pad *to remove debris and oily residue from the skin and optimize contact for sensor placement.*[6]
- Open the bispectral index sensor package and apply the sensor to the patient's forehead on the right or left side. Position the circle labeled "1" midline, approximately 2″ (about 5 cm) above the bridge of the patient's nose.[6]
- Position the circle labeled "3" on the right or left temple area, at the level of the outer canthus of the patient's eye, between the corner of the eye and the patient's hairline.[6]
- Position the circle labeled "4" above and parallel to the patient's eyebrow on the appropriate side.[6]
- Position the circle labeled "2" between the circles labeled "1" and "4" on the patient's forehead.[6]
- Apply gentle but firm pressure around the edges of the sensor, including the areas in between the numbered circles, *to ensure proper adhesion.*[6]
- Press firmly on each of the numbered circles for about 5 seconds *to ensure that the electrodes adhere to the skin.*[6]
- Connect the bispectral index sensor to the interface cable and bispectral index monitor.

Bispectral index monitoring

In bispectral index monitoring, the monitor is connected by an interface cable to a bispectral index sensor applied to the patient's forehead (as shown below).

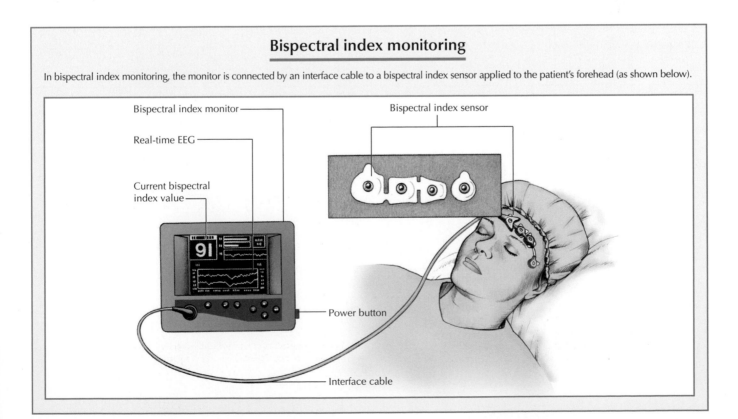

Bispectral index monitor

Real-time EEG

Current bispectral index value

Bispectral index sensor

Power button

Interface cable

■ Secure the digital signal converter near the patient's head, such as to a pillow or sheet, *to maximize the signal to the interface cable and reduce other electrical equipment interference.*[6]

■ Watch the bispectral index monitor for information related to impedance (electrical resistance) testing.

NURSING ALERT For the bispectral index monitor to display a reading, impedance values must be below a specified threshold. If they aren't, be ready to troubleshoot sensor problems. (See *Troubleshooting bispectral index sensor problems.*)

■ Select a smoothing rate (the time during which the monitor analyzes the data for calculation of the bispectral index; usually 15 or 30 seconds) using the ADVANCE SETUP button. Read and record the bispectral index value.

■ Read and record the bispectral index value.

■ Return the patient's bed to the lowest position *to prevent falls and maintain patient safety.*[23]

■ Check the bispectral index sensor site *to help ensure that the sensor didn't dislodge with patient repositioning.*

■ Assess the integrity of the patient's skin *to ensure the skin is intact,* and change the bispectral index sensor every 24 hours or more frequently, as needed, *to ensure adequate electrical contact.*[6]

■ Remove and discard your gloves, if worn.[20]

■ Perform hand hygiene.[7,8,9,10,11,12]

■ Document the procedure.[24,25,26,27]

Special considerations

■ Always evaluate the bispectral index value in conjunction with other patient assessment findings. Don't rely on the bispectral index value alone.[2] (See *Interpreting bispectral index values.*)

■ Keep in mind that patient movement may occur with low bispectral index values. Be alert for artifacts that could falsely elevate bispectral index values.

NURSING ALERT Bispectral index values may be elevated due to muscle shivering, tightening, or twitching; the use of electromechanical devices in close proximity to the patient; and problems with the bispectral index monitor or the sensor. Interpret the bispectral index value cautiously in these situations.[2]

■ Anticipate the need to adjust the dosage of sedation based on the patient's bispectral index value.[2]

■ Minimize patient position changes during bispectral index monitoring. *Studies have shown that changing a patient's position during monitoring can affect the bispectral values significantly.*

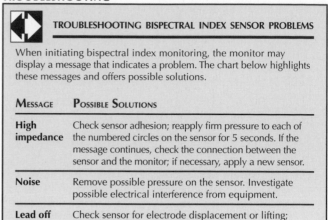

TROUBLESHOOTING BISPECTRAL INDEX SENSOR PROBLEMS

When initiating bispectral index monitoring, the monitor may display a message that indicates a problem. The chart below highlights these messages and offers possible solutions.

MESSAGE	POSSIBLE SOLUTIONS
High impedance	Check sensor adhesion; reapply firm pressure to each of the numbered circles on the sensor for 5 seconds. If the message continues, check the connection between the sensor and the monitor; if necessary, apply a new sensor.
Noise	Remove possible pressure on the sensor. Investigate possible electrical interference from equipment.
Lead off	Check sensor for electrode displacement or lifting; reapply with firm pressure or, if necessary, apply a new sensor.

NURSING ALERT Keep in mind that decreased stimulation, increased sedation, recent administration of a neuromuscular blocking agent or analgesia, or hypothermia may decrease the bispectral index value, thus indicating the need for a decrease in sedation or analgesia. Pain may cause an elevated bispectral index value, thus indicating a need for an increase in sedation or analgesia.[2,28]

Complications

The bispectral index sensors may cause skin irritation.[6]

Documentation

Document initiation of bispectral index monitoring, including the bispectral index sensor's location, the baseline bispectral index value, and baseline neurologic assessment findings. Record ongoing assessment findings and bispectral index values to provide a clear overall picture of the patient's condition. Note increases or decreases in bispectral index value, along with actions you took based on those values, including

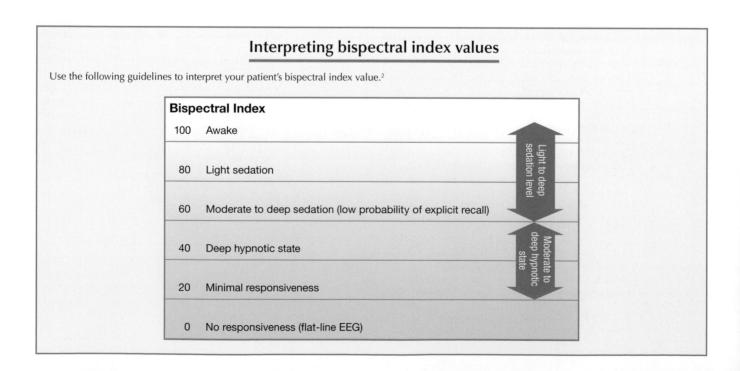

Interpreting bispectral index values

Use the following guidelines to interpret your patient's bispectral index value.[2]

Bispectral Index	
100	Awake
80	Light sedation
60	Moderate to deep sedation (low probability of explicit recall)
40	Deep hypnotic state
20	Minimal responsiveness
0	No responsiveness (flat-line EEG)

Light to deep sedation level

Moderate to deep hypnotic state

changes in sedative agent or analgesic administered. Document any teaching you provided to the patient and family members (if applicable), their understanding of that teaching, and any need for follow-up teaching.

REFERENCES

1 Shetty, R. M., et al. (2018). BIS monitoring versus clinical assessment for sedation in mechanically ventilated adults in the intensive care unit and its impact on clinical outcomes and resource utilization. *Cochrane Database of Systematic Reviews*, 2018(2), CD011240. https://www.ncbi.nlm.nih.gov/pmc/articles/PMC6353112/ (Level I)

2 Kelly, S. D. (2010). *Monitoring consciousness using the bispectral index™ (BIS™) during anesthesia: A pocket guide for clinicians* (2nd ed.). Boulder, CO: Covidien. http://wiki.med.uottawa.ca/download/attachments/7438404/BIS_PocketGuide.pdf

3 Jia, L., et al. (2020). Study of the rational dose of propofol in elderly patients under bispectral index monitoring during total intravenous anesthesia: A PRISMA-compliant systematic review. *Medicine (Baltimore), 99*(5), e19043. https://www.ncbi.nlm.nih.gov/pmc/articles/PMC7004673/ (Level IV)

4 Chang, B., et al. (2019). General anaesthesia tutorial 416: Bispectral index monitoring and intraoperative awareness. https://resources.wfsahq.org/wp-content/uploads/416_english.pdf

5 Goodwin, H., et al. (2012). "Cooperative sedation": Optimizing comfort while maximizing systemic and neurological function. *Critical Care, 16,*(2), 217. https://www.ncbi.nlm.nih.gov/pmc/articles/PMC3681362/pdf/cc11231.pdf (Level VII)

6 Wiegand, D. L. (2017). *AACN procedure manual for high acuity, progressive, and critical care* (7th ed.). St: Louis, MO: Elsevier.

7 Centers for Disease Control and Prevention. (2002). Guideline for hand hygiene in health-care settings: Recommendations of the Healthcare Infection Control Practices Advisory Committee and the HICPAC/SHEA/APIC/IDSA Hand Hygiene Task Force. *MMWR Recommendations and Reports, 51*(RR-16), 1–45. https://www.cdc.gov/mmwr/pdf/rr/rr5116.pdf (Level II)

8 World Health Organization. (2009). WHO guidelines on hand hygiene in health care: First global patient safety challenge, clean care is safer care. https://apps.who.int/iris/bitstream/handle/10665/44102/9789241597906_eng.pdf?sequence=1 (Level IV)

9 The Joint Commission. (2021). Standard NPSG.07.01.01. *Comprehensive accreditation manual for hospitals*. Oakbrook Terrace, IL: The Joint Commission. (Level VII)

10 Accreditation Association for Hospitals and Health Systems. (2020). Standard 07.01.21. *Healthcare Facilities Accreditation Program: Accreditation requirements for acute care hospitals*. Chicago, IL: Accreditation Association for Hospitals and Health Systems. (Level VII)

11 Centers for Medicare and Medicaid Services, Department of Health and Human Services. (2020). Condition of participation: Infection control. 42 C.F.R. § 482.24.

12 DNV GL-Healthcare USA, Inc. (2020). IC.1.SR.1. *NIAHO® accreditation requirements, interpretive guidelines and surveyor guidance—revision 20.0*. Milford, OH: DNV GL-Healthcare USA, Inc. (Level VII)

13 The Joint Commission. (2021). Standard NPSG.01.01.01. *Comprehensive accreditation manual for hospitals*. Oakbrook Terrace, IL: The Joint Commission. (Level VII)

14 Centers for Medicare and Medicaid Services, Department of Health and Human Services. (2020). Condition of participation: Patient's rights. 42 C.F.R. § 482.13(c)(1).

15 The Joint Commission. (2021). Standard RI.01.01.01. *Comprehensive accreditation manual for hospitals*. Oakbrook Terrace, IL: The Joint Commission. (Level VII)

16 Accreditation Association for Hospitals and Health Systems. (2020). Standard 15.01.16. *Healthcare Facilities Accreditation Program: Accreditation requirements for acute care hospitals*. Chicago, IL: Accreditation Association for Hospitals and Health Systems. (Level VII)

17 DNV GL-Healthcare USA, Inc. (2020). PR.2.SR.5. *NIAHO® accreditation requirements, interpretive guidelines and surveyor guidance—revision 20.0*. Milford, OH: DNV GL-Healthcare USA, Inc. (Level VII)

18 The Joint Commission. (2021). Standard PC.02.01.21. *Comprehensive accreditation manual for hospitals*. Oakbrook Terrace, IL: The Joint Commission. (Level VII)

19 Waters, T. R., et al. (2009). Safe patient handling training for schools of nursing. https://www.cdc.gov/niosh/docs/2009-127/pdfs/2009-127.pdf (Level VII)

20 Occupational Safety and Health Administration. (2012). Bloodborne pathogens, standard number 1910.1030. https://www.osha.gov/pls/oshaweb/owadisp.show_document?p_id=10051&p_table=STANDARDS (Level VII)

21 Siegel, J. D., et al. (2007, revised 2019). 2007 guideline for isolation precautions: Preventing transmission of infectious agents in healthcare settings. https://www.cdc.gov/infectioncontrol/pdf/guidelines/isolation-guidelines-H.pdf (Level II)

22 Accreditation Association for Hospitals and Health Systems. (2020). Standard 07.01.10. *Healthcare Facilities Accreditation Program: Accreditation requirements for acute care hospitals*. Chicago, IL: Accreditation Association for Hospitals and Health Systems. (Level VII)

23 Ganz, D. A., et al. (2013-reviewed 2021). Preventing falls in hospitals: A toolkit for improving quality of care (AHRQ publication no. 13-0015-EF). https://www.ahrq.gov/professionals/systems/hospital/fallpxtoolkit/index.html (Level VII)

24 The Joint Commission. (2021). Standard RC.01.03.01. *Comprehensive accreditation manual for hospitals*. Oakbrook Terrace, IL: The Joint Commission. (Level VII)

25 Centers for Medicare and Medicaid Services, Department of Health and Human Services. (2020). Condition of participation: Medical record services. 42 C.F.R. § 482.24(b).

26 Accreditation Association for Hospitals and Health Systems. (2020). Standard 10.00.03. *Healthcare Facilities Accreditation Program: Accreditation requirements for acute care hospitals*. Chicago, IL: Accreditation Association for Hospitals and Health Systems. (Level VII)

27 DNV GL-Healthcare USA, Inc. (2020). MR.2.SR.1. *NIAHO® accreditation requirements, interpretive guidelines and surveyor guidance—revision 20.0*. Milford, OH: DNV GL-Healthcare USA, Inc. (Level VII)

28 Coleman, R. M., et al. (2015). The use of the bispectral index in the detection of pain in mechanically ventilated adults in the intensive care unit: A review of the literature. *Pain Research and Management, 20,* e33–e37. https://www.ncbi.nlm.nih.gov/pmc/articles/PMC4325898/ (Level V)

BLADDER ULTRASONOGRAPHY

Urine retention, a potentially life-threatening condition, may result from neurologic or psychological disorders or obstruction of urine flow. It's also a common complication of some types of surgery.[1,2] Medications such as anticholinergics, antihistamines, antidepressants, opiates, and analgesics (especially spinal and epidural) can also cause urine retention. Traditionally, the amount of urine retained in the bladder was measured by urinary catheterization, which placed the patient at risk for catheter-associated urinary tract infection (CAUTI).

Bladder ultrasonography, also known as *bladder scanning*, is a noninvasive method of assessing bladder volume to monitor for urine retention and postvoid residual volume. Because bladder ultrasonography is a noninvasive means of measuring bladder volume, it reduces the risk of urinary tract infection by preventing unnecessary bladder catheterization.[3] It is indicated to assess postvoid residual (PRV) urine volume, detect urinary retention, determine bladder volume and thickness, and assist in bladder training.[4] Bladder ultrasonography is contraindicated in patients with open wounds in the suprapubic region that prevent scanning, women who are pregnant, and patients with ascites. Amniotic fluid and ascites interfere with visibility and interpretation of results.[5]

HOSPITAL-ACQUIRED CONDITION ALERT Keep in mind that the Centers for Medicare and Medicaid Services considers catheter-associated urinary tract infection (CAUTI) a hospital-acquired condition because it can be reasonably prevented using a variety of best practices. To reduce the risk of CAUTI when caring for a patient with an indwelling urinary catheter, be sure to follow evidence-based CAUTI prevention practices, such as performing hand hygiene before and after any catheter manipulation; maintaining a sterile, continuously closed drainage system; maintaining unobstructed urine flow; regularly emptying the collection bag; replacing the catheter and drainage system using sterile technique when breaks in sterile technique, disconnection, or leakage occurs; and discontinuing the catheter as soon as it's no longer clinically indicated.[6,7,8,9,10]

Equipment

Bladder ultrasonography unit with probe ▪ ultrasonic transmission gel ▪ gauze pads ▪ disinfectant pad ▪ Optional: washcloth, gloves.

Preparation of equipment

Inspect all equipment and supplies. If a product is expired, is defective, or has compromised integrity, remove it from patient use, label it as expired or defective, and report the expiration or defect as directed by your facility.

Calibrate the bladder ultrasonography unit, as directed, following the manufacturer's calibration instructions. Check battery functioning before performing the procedure.

Implementation

▪ Verify the practitioner's order, if required.
▪ Review the patient's history for any conditions that may affect results or contraindicate the procedure.[5]
▪ Gather and prepare the equipment.
▪ Perform hand hygiene.[11,12,13,14,15,16]
▪ Confirm the patient's identity using at least two patient identifiers.[17]
▪ Provide privacy.[18,19,20]
▪ Explain the procedure to the patient and family (if appropriate) according to their communication and learning needs *to increase understanding, allay their fears, and enhance cooperation.*[21]
▪ If this is a postvoiding scan, ask the patient to void; assist as necessary.
▪ Raise the bed to waist level before providing care *to prevent caregiver back strain.*[22]
▪ Perform hand hygiene.[11,12,13,14,15,16]
▪ Position the patient in the supine position with the head resting on a pillow *to prevent tightening of abdominal muscles, which can affect scanning.*[5]
▪ Perform hand hygiene.[11,12,13,14,15,16]
▪ Put on gloves as needed *to comply with standard precautions.*[23,24]
▪ Clean the rounded end of the ultrasonography probe with a disinfectant pad following the manufacturer's instructions.
▪ Expose the patient's suprapubic area.
▪ Turn on the bladder ultrasonography unit. If instructed by the device manufacturer's instructions for use, select the proper examination mode *to ensure the accuracy of your scan.*
▪ Place ultrasonic transmission gel on the end of the probe *to promote an airtight seal for optimal sound wave transmission.* Warn the patient that the gel will feel cold when placed on the abdomen.
▪ Locate the symphysis pubis and place the probe about 1″ (2.5 cm) superior to the symphysis pubis. If your device contains an icon (a rough figure of a patient) on the probe, make sure the head of the icon points toward the head of the patient.[5]
▪ Activate the scan following the device manufacturer's instructions for use. Hold the probe steady until the device completes the scan.[5]
▪ If present on your device, look at the aiming icon and the screen, which displays the bladder position and volume. Reposition the probe and scan until the bladder is centered in the aiming screen; then press DONE when finished. The device will save the largest measurement.
▪ Wait for the bladder ultrasonography unit to display the measured urine volume.
▪ Press PRINT to obtain a hard copy of your results, if available and required.[5]
▪ Turn off the unit. Use a gauze pad to clean the gel off the probe.
▪ Using a gauze pad or washcloth, remove the gel from the patient's skin.
▪ Remove and discard your gloves, if worn.[23,24]
▪ Perform hand hygiene.[11,12,13,14,15,16]
▪ Return the bed to the lowest position *to prevent falls and maintain patient safety.*[25]
▪ Use a disinfectant pad to clean and disinfect the unit, including the probe, according to the manufacturer's instructions.[26,27]
▪ Perform hand hygiene.[11,12,13,14,15,16]
▪ Notify the practitioner of the scan results, as indicated.[24]
▪ Document the procedure.[28,29,30,31]

Special considerations

▪ Some bladder ultrasound scanners require you to indicate the patient's gender. If the patient has had a hysterectomy, choose "male," *which allows the machine to exclude the uterus.*[5]
▪ If the PRV is more than 200 mL, assess the patient, repeat the bladder ultrasound, and encourage the patient to double void; acceptable PRV varies depending on the patient.[5]
▪ Be aware that high PRV recorded by a bladder ultrasound unit should correlate closely with the volume measurement by catheterization. Any discrepancy in PRV between these two methods may indicate cystic or pelvic issues, which can cause falsely elevated PRV readings.[32]
▪ Results may be inaccurate in patients with obesity or in a patient who has a lower abdominal scar.[5]

Documentation

If you obtained a printout, attach it to the patient's medical record. Make sure the printout contains the patient's name, the date, and the time you performed the scan.[5] In the patient's medical record, also document the date and time of the procedure, the procedure, the type of scan (prevoid or postvoid scan), voided volume (if applicable), bladder scan urine volume, intermittent catheterization volume (if applicable), the practitioner you notified of the results, and the time of notification. Also document any treatments you provided and the patient's response to those treatments. Document teaching that you provided to the patient and family (if applicable), their understanding of that teaching, and any need for follow-up teaching.

REFERENCES

1 Golubovsky, J. L., et al. (2018). Risk factors and associated complications for postoperative urinary retention after lumbar surgery for lumbar spinal stenosis. *Spine Journal, 18,* 1533–1539. (Level IV)

2 Fernandez, M. A., et al. (2014). The incidence of postoperative urinary retention in patients undergoing elective hip and knee arthroplasty. *Annals of the Royal College of Surgeons of England, 96,* 462–465. https://www.ncbi. nlm.nih.gov/pmc/articles/PMC4474200/ (Level IV)

3 Johansson, R. M., et al. (2013). Guidelines for preventing urinary retention and bladder damage during hospital care. *Journal of Clinical Nursing, 22,* 347–355. (Level VII)

4 Rachaneni, S., et al. (2016). Bladder ultrasonography for diagnosing detrusor overactivity: Test accuracy study and economic evaluation. *Health Technology Assessment, 20,* 1–150. https://www.ncbi.nlm.nih.gov/books/ NBK338657/ (Level IV)

5 Agency for Clinical Innovation. (2014). Bladder scanning (non-real time): Adult clinical guideline. https://www.aci.health.nsw.gov.au/__data/assets/ pdf_file/0019/191062/ACI_Bladder_Scanning.pdf (Level VII)

6 Agency for Healthcare Research and Quality & U.S. Department of Health and Human Services. (2015). Toolkit for reducing catheter-associated urinary tract infections in hospital units: Implementation guide. http://www.ahrq.gov/professionals/quality-patient-safety/hais/cauti-tools/ impl-guide/index.html

7 Lo, E., et al. (2014). SHEA/IDSA practice recommendation: Strategies to prevent catheter-associated urinary tract infections in acute care hospitals, 2014 update. *Infection Control and Hospital Epidemiology, 35*(5), 464–479. http://www.jstor.org/stable/10.1086/675718 (Level I)

8 Association of Professionals in Infection Control and Epidemiology. (2014). APIC implementation guide: Guide to preventing catheter-associated urinary tract infections. https://apic.org/wp-content/up-loads/2019/02/APIC_CAUTI_IG_FIN_REVD0815.pdf (Level IV)

9 Healthcare Infection Control Practices Advisory Committee. (2010, revised 2019). Guideline for prevention of catheter-associated urinary tract infections 2009. https://www.cdc.gov/infectioncontrol/pdf/guidelines/ cauti-guidelines-H.pdf (Level I)

10 The Joint Commission. (2021). Standard NPSG.07.06.01. *Comprehensive accreditation manual for hospitals.* Oakbrook Terrace, IL: The Joint Commission. (Level VII)

11 The Joint Commission. (2021). Standard NPSG.07.01.01. *Comprehensive accreditation manual for hospitals.* Oakbrook Terrace, IL: The Joint Commission. (Level VII)

12 World Health Organization (2009). WHO guidelines on hand hygiene in health care: First global patient safety challenge,

clean care is safer care. https://apps.who.int/iris/bitstream/handle/10665/44102/9789241597906_eng.pdf?sequence=1 (Level IV)

13 Centers for Disease Control and Prevention. (2002). Guideline for hand hygiene in health-care settings: Recommendations of the Healthcare Infection Control Practices Advisory Committee and the HICPAC/SHEA/APIC/IDSA Hand Hygiene Task Force. *MMWR Recommendations and Reports, 51*(RR-16), 1–45. https://www.cdc.gov/mmwr/pdf/rr/rr5116.pdf (Level II)

14 Accreditation Association for Hospitals and Health Systems. (2020). Standard 07.01.21. *Healthcare Facilities Accreditation Program: Accreditation requirements for acute care hospitals.* Chicago, IL: Accreditation Association for Hospitals and Health Systems. (Level VII)

15 Centers for Medicare and Medicaid Services, Department of Health and Human Services. (2020). Condition of participation: Infection control. 42 C.F.R. § 482.42.

16 DNV GL-Healthcare USA, Inc. (2020). IC.1.SR.1. *NIAHO® accreditation requirements, interpretive guidelines and surveyor guidance—revision 20.0.* Milford, OH: DNV GL-Healthcare USA, Inc. (Level VII)

17 The Joint Commission. (2021). Standard NPSG.01.01.01. *Comprehensive accreditation manual for hospitals.* Oakbrook Terrace, IL: The Joint Commission. (Level VII)

18 Accreditation Association for Hospitals and Health Systems. (2020). Standard 15.01.16. *Healthcare Facilities Accreditation Program: Accreditation requirements for acute care hospitals.* Chicago, IL: Accreditation Association for Hospitals and Health Systems. (Level VII)

19 The Joint Commission. (2021). Standard RI.01.01.01. *Comprehensive accreditation manual for hospitals.* Oakbrook Terrace, IL: The Joint Commission. (Level VII)

20 Centers for Medicare and Medicaid Services, Department of Health and Human Services. (2020). Condition of participation: Patient's rights. 42 C.F.R. § 482.13(c)(1).

21 The Joint Commission. (2021). Standard PC.02.01.21. *Comprehensive accreditation manual for hospitals.* Oakbrook Terrace, IL: The Joint Commission (Level VII)

22 Waters, T. R., et al. (2009). Safe patient handling training for schools of nursing. https://www.cdc.gov/niosh/docs/2009-127/pdfs/2009-127.pdf (Level VII)

23 Siegel, J. D., et al. (2007, revised 2019). 2007 guideline for isolation precautions: Preventing transmission of infectious agents in healthcare settings. https://www.cdc.gov/infectioncontrol/pdf/guidelines/isolation-guidelines-H.pdf (Level II)

24 Accreditation Association for Hospitals and Health Systems. (2020). Standard 07.01.10. *Healthcare Facilities Accreditation Program: Accreditation requirements for acute care hospitals.* Chicago, IL: Accreditation Association for Hospitals and Health Systems. (Level VII)

25 Ganz, D. A., et al. (2013, reviewed 2021). Preventing falls in hospitals: A toolkit for improving quality of care (AHRQ publication no. 13-0015-EF). https://www.ahrq.gov/professionals/systems/hospital/fallpxtoolkit/index.html (Level VII)

26 Rutala, W. A., et al. (2008, revised 2019). Guideline for disinfection and sterilization in healthcare facilities, 2008. https://www.cdc.gov/infectioncontrol/pdf/guidelines/disinfection-guidelines-H.pdf (Level I)

27 Accreditation Association for Hospitals and Health Systems. (2020). Standard 07.02.03. *Healthcare Facilities Accreditation Program: Accreditation requirements for acute care hospitals.* Chicago, IL: Accreditation Association for Hospitals and Health Systems. (Level VII)

28 The Joint Commission. (2020). Standard RC.01.03.01. *Comprehensive accreditation manual for hospitals.* Oakbrook Terrace, IL: The Joint Commission. (Level VII)

29 Accreditation Association for Hospitals and Health Systems. (2020). Standard 10.00.03. *Healthcare Facilities Accreditation Program: Accreditation requirements for acute care hospitals.* Chicago, IL: Accreditation Association for Hospitals and Health Systems. (Level VII)

30 Centers for Medicare and Medicaid Services, Department of Health and Human Services. (2020). Condition of participation: Medical record services. 42 C.F.R. § 482.24(b).

31 DNV GL-Healthcare USA, Inc. (2021). MR.2.SR.1. *NIAHO® accreditation requirements, interpretive guidelines and surveyor guidance—revision 20.0.* Milford, OH: DNV GL-Healthcare USA, Inc. (Level VII)

32 Kim, T. H., et al. (2017). Falsely elevated postvoid residual urine volume in uterine myoma. *Annals of Rehabilitation Medicine, 41,* 332–336. https://www.ncbi.nlm.nih.gov/pmc/articles/PMC5426254/ (Level IV)

BLOOD CULTURE SAMPLE COLLECTION

Blood cultures detect the presence of bacteria in the blood (bacteremia) and the systemic spread of such an infection (septicemia) through the bloodstream. Blood culture sample collection involves collecting a venous blood sample by venipuncture at the patient's bedside and transferring the sample into two bottles, one containing an anaerobic medium and the other, an aerobic medium. The bottles undergo incubation, which encourages organisms present in the sample to grow in the media. Blood cultures allow identification of about 67% of pathogens within 24 hours and up to 90% within 72 hours. If possible, blood cultures should be collected before starting antimicrobial therapy, which may interfere with bacterial growth.[1,2,3,4,5] A dedicated phlebotomy team is recommended for obtaining blood cultures by venipuncture to reduce the risk of blood culture contamination.[2,6]

Ideally, you should obtain blood specimens for culture from two or three blood draws from separate venipuncture sites, not through a vascular catheter.[1,2] Perform these blood sample collections simultaneously or within a few hours.[7] Keep in mind that blood culture specimens collected from central venous catheters are associated with higher false-positive rates,[7,8] but they may be used if you suspect a catheter-related bloodstream infection. If you suspect such an infection, withdraw one set of blood cultures through the device and one set from a separate venipuncture. Blood cultures from both the catheter and venipuncture should be positive for the same organism, with associated clinical signs and symptoms and no other recognized source. A positive culture from only the device most likely stems from a contaminant and the patient shouldn't receive treatment.[1]

Equipment

Gloves ■ antiseptic pad (alcohol, chlorhexidine-based, or tincture of iodine) ■ alcohol pads ■ winged (butterfly) or straight needle[6] ■ appropriately sized syringe(s) ■ blood culture bottles (aerobic and anaerobic) ■ laboratory biohazard transport bag ■ 2″ × 2″ (5-cm × 5-cm) gauze pads ■ small adhesive bandages ■ labels ■ needleless transfer devices ■ Optional: sterile blood culture collection kit, sterile gloves, laboratory request form, single-patient tourniquet.[6]

Note: Consider the use of a standardized sterile blood culture collection kit *to reduce the risk of sample contamination.*[6]

Preparation of equipment

Inspect all equipment and supplies. If a product is expired, is defective, or has compromised integrity, remove it from patient use, label it as expired or defective, and report the expiration or defect as directed by your facility.[9]

Implementation

- Verify the practitioner's order.
- Gather and prepare the necessary equipment and supplies.
- Perform hand hygiene.[10,11,12,13,14,15]
- Confirm the patient's identity using at least two patient identifiers.[16]
- Provide privacy.[17,18,19,20]
- Tell the patient that you need to collect a series of blood samples *to check for infection.* Explain the procedure to the patient and family (if appropriate) according to their individual communication and learning needs *to increase their understanding, allay their fears, and enhance cooperation.*[21] Explain that the procedure usually requires two blood samples collected from two different sites.
- Raise the bed to waist level before providing patient care *to prevent caregiver back strain.*[22]
- Perform hand hygiene.[10,11,12,13,14,15]
- Put on gloves *to comply with standard precautions.*[23,24,25]
- Choose a venipuncture site on the opposite extremity of an infusion. If venipuncture must be performed on the extremity with an infusion, use a vein below or distal to the site of infusion. Avoid venipuncture on the side of an axillary node dissection and in upper extremities with lymphedema,

with compromised circulation, or affected by radiation therapy or paralysis or hemiparesis from a stroke. When possible, restrict venipuncture to the dorsum of the hand in a patient with an actual or planned dialysis fistula or graft.[6]

■ Avoid use of a tourniquet, if possible.[6] If a tourniquet is necessary, apply it 2″ (5 cm) proximal to the area chosen for the venipuncture; limit tourniquet time to less than 1 minute.[6] (See the "Venipuncture" procedure.)

■ Clean the venipuncture site with an antiseptic pad following the manufacturer's instructions (if using chlorhexidine, apply using a back-and-forth scrubbing motion for at least 30 seconds), and allow it to dry completely.[1,2,26,27,28,29] Don't palpate the site again, *to avoid transfer of microorganism to the venipuncture site*. If palpation is necessary, put on a sterile glove.[29]

■ If you're also drawing blood for other laboratory tests, draw blood for culture before drawing the sample for other tests.[6] Perform a venipuncture using a straight or winged needle and discard the initial volume (1 to 5 mL) of the blood sample, if directed by your facility, *to prevent induction of contaminant organisms contained on the skin*.[6,27,29] Then draw a quantity of blood that is sufficient for isolating organisms (20 to 30 mL); follow the manufacturer's recommendations for the blood sample volume required per collection bottle.[6,27,29] Immediately release the tourniquet, if used, when blood begins to flow into the collection container.[6]

■ After you've drawn the blood sample, place a 2″ × 2″ (5-cm × 5-cm) gauze pad over the puncture site (taking care not to contaminate the needle), and slowly and gently remove the needle from the vein. Apply gentle pressure to the site for 2 to 3 minutes or until bleeding stops *to prevent extravasation into the surrounding tissue, which can cause a hematoma*. Then cover the site with a small adhesive bandage.

■ Disinfect the diaphragm tops of the culture bottles with alcohol pads and allow them to dry; avoid use of iodine-containing products *because they can degrade the diaphragm tops*.[1,6,29]

■ Divide the blood by injecting the appropriate amount into each culture bottle using a needleless transfer device *to ensure the most accurate culture results*.[1]

■ Label the culture bottles with the patient's name and identification number, the date and time of the specimen collection, and the contents of the culture bottles in the presence of the patient *to prevent mislabeling*.[16,26,28]

■ Invert the bottles 8 to 10 times gently *to mix the blood adequately with the medium inside the bottles*.[30]

■ Discard syringes and needles in a puncture-resistant sharps container.[23]

■ Return the bed to the lowest position *to prevent falls and maintain patient safety*.[31]

■ Remove and discard your gloves[23] and perform hand hygiene.[10,11,12,13,14,15]

■ Place the samples in a laboratory biohazard transport bag and, along with the laboratory request form if used by your facility, send them to the laboratory within 2 hours of collection.[2,29] Specimens should be held at room temperature. They should never be refrigerated or frozen; *doing so may kill some of the microorganisms*.[29]

■ Perform hand hygiene.[10,11,12,13,14,15]

■ Document the procedure.[32,33,34,35]

Collecting blood culture samples from a central venous access catheter

If you need to obtain two sets of blood samples from the central venous access catheter, withdraw two blood samples through different lumens, if available.[7] If only one lumen is available, withdraw two separate samples through the same lumen on separate occasions.[7]

Implementation

■ Verify the practitioner's orders.

■ Gather and prepare the necessary equipment and supplies.

■ Check the expiration dates on the culture bottles and replace outdated bottles.

■ Perform hand hygiene.[10,11,12,13,14,15,23]

■ Confirm the patient's identity using at least two patient identifiers.[16]

■ Provide privacy.[17,18,19]

■ Explain the procedure to the patient and family (if appropriate) according to their individual communication and learning needs *to increase understanding, allay their fears, and enhance communication*.[21]

■ Stop all infusions for a designated period of time, depending on the patient's condition. (Research hasn't established the length of time for stopping fluid flow; one study suggests a wait time of 10 minutes after stopping the infusion before obtaining the sample.)[6]

■ Perform hand hygiene.[10,11,12,13,14,15]

■ Put on gloves *to comply with standard precautions*.[23,24,25]

■ Clamp the catheter *to prevent accidental exposure to blood and to reduce the risk of air embolism*.[26,28]

■ Change the needleless connector of the lumen that you'll be using to obtain the blood culture sample *to reduce the risk of contamination and false-positive results*.[3,6,26,28]

■ Perform a vigorous mechanical scrub of the needleless connector for at least 5 seconds using an antiseptic pad.[36,37,38] Allow it to dry.[36,37]

■ If you're also drawing blood for other laboratory tests, draw blood for culture before drawing the sample for other tests.[6,29] Maintaining sterility of the syringe tip, connect the empty syringe to the catheter, release the clamp, and withdraw a quantity of blood that is sufficient for isolating organisms; follow the manufacturer's recommendations for the blood sample volume required per collection bottle.[1,6] Don't discard this first-drawn blood; this is the blood sample that you'll be injecting into the culture bottle.[3,6,28,29]

■ Clamp the catheter and remove the syringe.

■ Perform a vigorous mechanical scrub of the needleless connector for at least 5 seconds using an antiseptic pad.[36,37,38] Allow it to dry.[36,37]

■ Maintaining sterility of the syringe tip, connect the syringe with preservative-free normal saline solution, open the clamp, and flush and lock the device or resume the infusion, as ordered.[26,28,39] Consider using a pulsatile flushing technique *because short boluses of flush solution interrupted by short pauses may be more effective at removing deposits (for example, fibrin, drug precipitate, intraluminal bacteria) than a continuous low-flow technique*.[39]

■ If available at your facility, place a disinfectant-containing end cap on the needleless connector *to reduce the risk of vascular catheter–associated infection*.[38]

HOSPITAL-ACQUIRED CONDITION ALERT Keep in mind that the Centers for Medicare and Medicaid Services considers a vascular catheter–associated infection to be a hospital-acquired condition *because a variety of best practices can reasonably prevent it*. Use infection prevention techniques (such as performing hand hygiene, thoroughly disinfecting the needleless connector with an antiseptic pad using friction for at least 5 seconds, and using disinfectant-containing end caps, if available) *to reduce the risk of vascular catheter–associated infections*.[40,41,42,43]

■ Disinfect the diaphragm tops of the culture bottles with alcohol pads; avoid iodine-containing products *because they can degrade the diaphragm tops*.[1,6]

■ Inject the blood into each bottle using a needleless transfer device, dividing it between the two bottles.[1]

■ Label the culture bottles, including the patient's name and identification number, the date and time of sample collection, and the contents of the culture bottles, in the presence of the patient *to prevent mislabeling*.[16,26,28]

■ Invert the bottles 8 to 10 times gently to mix the blood adequately with the medium inside the bottles.[30]

■ Discard used supplies in the appropriate containers.[23]

■ Remove and discard your gloves.[23]

■ Perform hand hygiene.[10,11,12,13,14,15]

■ Place the samples in a laboratory biohazard transport bag and, along with the laboratory request form (if used by your facility), send them to the laboratory within 2 hours of collection.[2,29] Samples should be held at room temperature. They should never be refrigerated or frozen; *doing so may kill some of the microorganisms*.[29]

■ Perform hand hygiene.[10,11,12,13,14,15]

■ Document the procedure.[32,33,34,35]

Special considerations

■ Use blood conservation strategies when drawing blood *to reduce phlebotomy-related loss, which is a major cause of hospital-acquired anemia.* Collaborate with the laboratory staff about the minimum volume of blood required for each test.[6]

■ If a patient has suspected sepsis, obtain blood cultures before administering antimicrobial therapy *to optimize identification of pathogens and improve outcome.* Administration of antibiotic therapy should not be delayed in order to obtain blood cultures.[4]

■ If the patient has no obvious source of infection and you suspect catheter-related bloodstream infection, withdraw one set of samples from the distal lumen of the catheter and one set of samples peripherally.[1] (See *Collecting blood culture samples from a central venous access catheter.*)

Complications

The most common complication of venipuncture is the formation of a hematoma. Improper technique may cause false-positive results, leading to inappropriate antimicrobial use.

Documentation

Document the date and time of the venipuncture, the venipuncture site, the volume of blood collected, and the specific laboratory test. Note the patient's tolerance of the procedure. Document teaching provided to the patient and family (if applicable), their understanding of that teaching, and any need for follow-up teaching.

REFERENCES

1 Septimus, E. (2019). Collecting cultures: A clinician guide. https://www.cdc.gov/antibiotic-use/core-elements/collecting-cultures.html?CDC_AA_refVal=https%3A%2F%2Fwww.cdc.gov%2Fantibiotic-use%2Fhealthcare%2Fimplementation%2Fclinicianguide.html

2 Sivapuram, M. S. (2019). Blood culture collection: Adults. South Australia: Joanna Briggs Institute. (Level VII)

3 Standard 50. Infection. Infusion therapy standards of practice. (8th ed.). (2021). *Journal of Infusion Nursing, 44,* S153–S157. (Level VII)

4 Levy, M. M., et al. (2018). The surviving sepsis campaign bundle: 2018 update. *Critical Care Medicine, 46,* 997–1000. (Level I)

5 Cheng, M. P., et al. (2019). Blood culture results before and after antimicrobial administration in patients with severe manifestations of sepsis: A diagnostic study. *Annals of Internal Medicine, 171,* 547–554. (Level IV)

6 Standard 44. Blood sampling. Infusion therapy standards of practice. (8th ed.). (2021). *Journal of Infusion Nursing, 44,* S125–S132. (Level VII)

7 Centers for Disease Control and Prevention. (2021). Device-associated module: Bloodstream infection event (central line–associated bloodstream infection and non-central line associated bloodstream infection). https://www.cdc.gov/nhsn/pdfs/pscmanual/4psc_clabscurrent.pdf

8 Boyce, J. M., et al. (2013). Obtaining blood cultures by venipuncture versus from central lines: Impact on blood culture contamination rates and potential effect on central line-associated bloodstream infection reporting. *Infection Control and Hospital Epidemiology, 34,* 1042–1046. https://www.jstor.org/stable/10.1086/673142#metadata_info_tab_contents (Level VI)

9 Standard 12. Product evaluation, integrity, and defect reporting. Infusion therapy standards of practice (8th ed.). (2021). *Journal of Infusion Nursing, 44,* S45–S46. (Level VII)

10 The Joint Commission. (2021). Standard NPSG.07.01.01. *Comprehensive accreditation manual for hospitals.* Oakbrook Terrace, IL: The Joint Commission. (Level VII)

11 Centers for Disease Control and Prevention. (2002). Guideline for hand hygiene in health-care settings: Recommendations of the Healthcare Infection Control Practices Advisory Committee and the HICPAC/SHEA/APIC/IDSA Hand Hygiene Task Force. *MMWR Recommendations and Reports, 51*(RR-16), 1–45. https://www.cdc.gov/mmwr/pdf/rr/rr5116.pdf (Level II)

12 World Health Organization. (2009). WHO guidelines on hand hygiene in health care: First global patient safety challenge, clean care is safer care. https://apps.who.int/iris/bitstream/handle/10665/44102/9789241597906_eng.pdf (Level IV)

13 Centers for Medicare and Medicaid Services, Department of Health and Human Services. (2020). Condition of participation: Infection control. 42 C.F.R. § 482.42.

14 Accreditation Association for Hospitals and Health Systems. (2020). Standard 07.01.21. *Healthcare Facilities Accreditation Program: Accreditation requirements for acute care hospitals.* Chicago, IL: Accreditation Association for Hospitals and Health Systems. (Level VII)

15 DNV GL-Healthcare USA, Inc. (2020). IC.1.SR.1. *NIAHO® accreditation requirements, interpretive guidelines and surveyor guidance—revision 20.0.* Milford, OH: DNV GL-Healthcare USA, Inc. (Level VII)

16 The Joint Commission. (2021). Standard NPSG.01.01.01. *Comprehensive accreditation manual for hospitals.* Oakbrook Terrace, IL: The Joint Commission. (Level VII)

17 The Joint Commission. (2021). Standard RI.01.01.01. *Comprehensive accreditation manual for hospitals.* Oakbrook Terrace, IL: The Joint Commission. (Level VII)

18 Centers for Medicare and Medicaid Services, Department of Health and Human Services. (2020). Condition of participation: Patient's rights. 42 C.F.R. § 482.13(c)(1).

19 Accreditation Association for Hospitals and Health Systems. (2020). Standard 15.01.16. *Healthcare Facilities Accreditation Program: Accreditation requirements for acute care hospitals.* Chicago, IL: Accreditation Association for Hospitals and Health Systems. (Level VII)

20 DNV GL-Healthcare USA, Inc. (2020). PR.2.SR.5. *NIAHO® accreditation requirements, interpretive guidelines and surveyor guidance—revision 20.0.* Milford, OH: DNV GL-Healthcare USA, Inc. (Level VII)

21 The Joint Commission. (2021). Standard PC.02.01.21. *Comprehensive accreditation manual for hospitals.* Oakbrook Terrace, IL: The Joint Commission. (Level VII)

22 Waters, T. R., et al. (2009). Safe patient handling training for schools of nursing. https://www.cdc.gov/niosh/docs/2009-127/pdfs/2009-127.pdf (Level VII)

23 Occupational Safety and Health Administration. (2012). Bloodborne pathogens, standard number 1910.1030. https://www.osha.gov/pls/oshaweb/owadisp.show_document?p_id=10051&p_table=STANDARDS (Level VII)

24 Siegel, J. D., et al. (2007, revised 2019). 2007 guideline for isolation precautions: Preventing transmission of infectious agents in healthcare settings. https://www.cdc.gov/infectioncontrol/pdf/guidelines/isolation-guidelines-H.pdf (Level II)

25 Accreditation Association for Hospitals and Health Systems. (2020). Standard 07.01.10. *Healthcare Facilities Accreditation Program: Accreditation requirements for acute care hospitals.* Chicago, IL: Accreditation Association for Hospitals and Health Systems. (Level VII)

26 Infusion Nurses Society. (2016). *Policies and procedures for infusion therapy* (5th ed.). Boston, MA: Infusion Nurses Society.

27 Emergency Nurses Association. (2018). Clinical practice guideline: Prevention of blood culture contamination. *Journal of Emergency Nursing, 44,* 285.e1–285.e24. (Level VII)

28 Infusion Nurses Society. (2017). *Policies and procedures for infusion therapy of the older adult* (3rd ed.). Boston, MA: Infusion Nurses Society.

29 Garcia, R. A., et al. (2015). Multidisciplinary team review of best practices for collection and handling of blood cultures to determine effective interventions for increasing the yield of true-positive bacteremias, reducing contamination, and eliminating false-positive central line-associated bloodstream infections. *American Journal of Infection Control, 43,* 1222–1237. (Level VII)

30 Becton, Dickinson and Company. (2010). BD Vacutainer® order of draw for multiple tube collections. https://www.bd.com/documents/in-service-materials/specimen-collection/PAS_BC_Vacutainer-order-of-draw-for-multiple-tubes-poster_IM_EN.pdf

31 Ganz, D. A., et al. (2013-reviewed 2021). *Preventing falls in hospitals: A toolkit for improving quality of care* (AHRQ Publication No. 13-0015-EF). Rockville, MD: Agency for Healthcare Research and Quality. https://www.ahrq.gov/professionals/systems/hospital/fallpxtoolkit/index.html (Level VII)

32 The Joint Commission. (2021). Standard RC.01.03.01. *Comprehensive accreditation manual for hospitals.* Oakbrook Terrace, IL: The Joint Commission. (Level VII)

33 Centers for Medicare and Medicaid Services, Department of Health and Human Services. (2020). Condition of participation: Medical record services. 42 C.F.R. § 482.24(b).

34 Accreditation Association for Hospitals and Health Systems. (2020). Standard 10.00.03. *Healthcare Facilities Accreditation Program: Accreditation requirements for acute care hospitals.* Chicago, IL: Accreditation Association for Hospitals and Health Systems. (Level VII)

35 DNV GL-Healthcare USA, Inc. (2020). MR.2.SR.1. *NIAHO® accreditation requirements, interpretive guidelines and surveyor guidance—revision 20.0.* Milford, OH: DNV GL-Healthcare USA, Inc. (Level VII)

36 Standard 36. Needleless connectors. Infusion therapy standards of practice. (8th ed.) (2021). *Journal of Infusion Nursing, 44*, S104–S107. (Level VII)

37 Centers for Disease Control and Prevention. (2011, revised 2017). Guidelines for the prevention of intravascular catheter–related infections. https://www.cdc.gov/infectioncontrol/guidelines/bsi/index.html (Level I)

38 Marschall, J., et al. (2014). SHEA/IDSA practice recommendation: Strategies to prevent central line-associated bloodstream infections in acute care hospitals. *Infection Control and Hospital Epidemiology, 35*(7), 753–771. https://www.jstor.org/stable/10.1086/676533#metadata_info_tab_contents (Level I)

39 Standard 41. Flushing and locking. Infusion therapy standards of practice. (8th ed.). (2021). *Journal of Infusion Nursing, 44*, S113–S118. (Level VII)

40 Accreditation Association for Hospitals and Health Systems. (2020). Standard 07.01.19. *Healthcare Facilities Accreditation Program: Accreditation requirements for acute care hospitals.* Chicago, IL: Accreditation Association for Hospitals and Health Systems. (Level VII)

41 Accreditation Association for Hospitals and Health Systems. (2020). Standard 07.01.02. *Healthcare Facilities Accreditation Program: Accreditation requirements for acute care hospitals.* Chicago, IL: Accreditation Association for Hospitals and Health Systems. (Level VII)

42 The Joint Commission. (2021). Standard NPSG.07.04.01. *Comprehensive accreditation manual for hospitals.* Oakbrook Terrace, IL: The Joint Commission. (Level VII)

43 Jarrett, N., & Callaham, M. (2016). Evidence-based guidelines for selected hospital-acquired conditions: Final report. https://www.cms.gov/Medicare/Medicare-Fee-for-Service-Payment/HospitalAcqCond/Downloads/2016-HAC-Report.pdf

BLOOD GLUCOSE MONITORING

Blood glucose meters measure blood glucose concentrations. The use of a blood glucose monitor involves placing a drop of blood on a blood glucose test strip before or after inserting the strip into the meter, depending on the type of blood glucose meter used. A portable blood glucose meter provides quantitative measurements similar in accuracy to other laboratory tests. Most meters store successive test results electronically to help determine glucose patterns. If a glucose result doesn't correlate with the patient's clinical condition, the result should be confirmed through conventional laboratory sampling of blood glucose.[1]

NURSING ALERT Avoid using capillary whole blood specimens (such as those obtained by fingerstick) for glucose monitoring in patients receiving intensive medical intervention therapy *because of the risk of collection error. Specimens from patients with decreased peripheral blood flow (severe hypotension, shock, hyperosmolar-hyperglycemia, and severe dehydration) may not reflect the patient's true physiologic state.* If you obtain an arterial or venous sample for testing, use only fresh whole blood or blood collected in lithium heparin collection devices if directed by the glucose meter manufacturer.[2]

For a patient with diabetes who's receiving nutrition, perform glucose monitoring before meals. For a patient with diabetes who isn't receiving nutrition, perform blood glucose monitoring every 4 to 6 hours.[1] More frequent monitoring, ranging from every 30 minutes to every 2 hours, is required for a patient receiving an IV insulin infusion.[1]

In a hospitalized patient, hyperglycemia is defined as a blood glucose level greater than 140 mg/dL (7.8 mmol/L). Levels significantly and persistently higher than this may require treatment. The American Diabetes Association defines Level 1 hypoglycemia as a glucose value less than 70 mg/dL (3.9 mmol/L) but greater than or equal to 54 mg/dL (3 mmol/L). Level 2 hypoglycemia, defined as glucose value less than 54 mg/mL (3 mmol/L), is the level at which neuroglycopenic symptoms begin to occur and requires immediate action to resolve the hypoglycemic event. Level 3 hypoglycemia is a severe event characterized by altered mental status, physical status, or both, and requires assistance.[1] Establish a plan for preventing and treating hypoglycemia for each patient. Track hypoglycemic episodes in the hospital and document them in the medical record.[1]

For patients whom hypoglycemia or hyperglycemia is a concern, perform blood glucose monitoring based on clinical signs and symptoms.

The Centers for Disease Control and Prevention recommends that, whenever possible, blood glucose meters shouldn't be shared among patients. If a device must be shared, it should be cleaned and disinfected after every use, following the manufacturer's instructions, *to prevent carryover of blood and infectious agents.* If the manufacturer doesn't specify how the device should be cleaned and disinfected, then it shouldn't be shared.[3] Single-use, auto-disabling fingerstick devices should also be used *to prevent the spread of bloodborne pathogens.*[1,3,4,5]

Equipment

Gloves ▪ portable blood glucose meter ▪ alcohol pads ▪ facility-approved disinfectant ▪ gauze pads ▪ single-use, auto-disabling lancet[5] ▪ blood glucose test strips ▪ Optional: small adhesive bandage, warm moist compresses, soap, water, towel.

Preparation of equipment

Inspect all equipment and supplies. If a product is expired, is defective, or has compromised integrity, remove it from patient use, label it as expired or defective, and report the expiration or defect, as directed by your facility.

Make sure that the cap on the vial of strips is secured properly, and observe the strip for discoloration. *Strips are sensitive to light and humidity, and may become inactivated when exposed to these factors.* When using a blood glucose meter, calibrate it and run it with a quality-control test following the manufacturer's instructions *to ensure accurate test results.*[6] Most facility-based glucose meters must undergo quality-control tests every 24 hours. Follow the manufacturer's instructions for calibration.

Before testing, turn on the meter. If appropriate, ensure that the code strip number on the test strip matches the code number on the meter. Enter your operator identification and password, if required. Enter and then confirm the patient's identification information, either manually or by using a barcode scanner, if available; if the patient information has already been entered by another user, confirm it.

Implementation

- Verify the practitioner's order.
- Gather and prepare the necessary equipment and supplies.
- Perform hand hygiene.[7,8,9,10,11,12]
- Confirm the patient's identity using at least two patient identifiers.[13]
- Provide privacy.[14,15,16,17]
- Explain the procedure to the patient and family (if appropriate) according to their communication and learning needs, *to increase their understanding, allay their fears, and enhance cooperation.*[18]
- Perform hand hygiene.[7,8,9,10,11,12]
- Put on gloves.[19,20,21]
- Select the puncture site—usually the fingertip.[22] Some devices allow for collection from alternative sites; consult the manufacturer's instructions.
- If necessary, dilate the capillaries by applying warm, moist compresses to the area for about 10 minutes.
- If able, have the patient wash the hands with soap and water and then dry them *to remove any sugar that may remain on the patient's skin after exposure to sugar-containing products.*[23] If the patient can't wash the hands, clean the intended puncture site with an alcohol pad (as shown below) and allow it to dry completely, *because alcohol may interfere with test results if not permitted to dry completely.*[22]

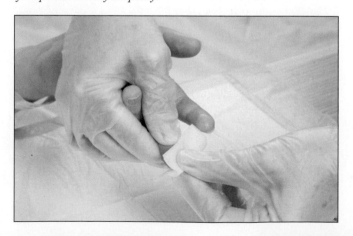

■ Insert the test strip into the blood glucose meter, according to the manufacturer's instructions. Note that some meters require that you insert the test strip after applying the blood sample (as shown below).

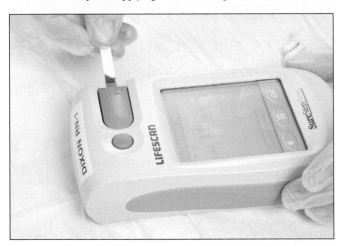

■ To collect a sample from the fingertip, use a single-use, auto-disabling lancet.[3] Position the lancet on the side of the patient's fingertip perpendicular to the lines of the fingerprints.[22] Puncture the skin with a quick, continuous, and deliberate stroke (as shown below) *to achieve a good flow of blood and to prevent the need to repeat the puncture.*[22]

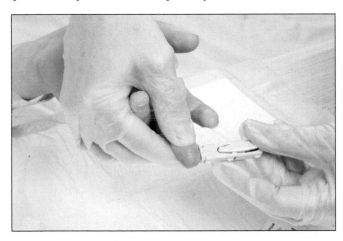

■ If required by your facility, wipe away the first drop of blood using a gauze pad, *because it may be contaminated with tissue, fluid, or debris.*[22]
■ Touch a drop of blood to the test area of the test strip; make sure the entire test area is covered. Some meters require a hanging drop of blood; refer to the manufacturer's instructions for use. Don't squeeze the patient's finger too tightly, *because doing so may dilute the specimen with plasma.*[22]
■ After collecting the blood sample, apply firm pressure to the puncture site *to stop the bleeding.*[22]
■ Read the digital display on the blood glucose meter when the alarm sounds.
■ Discard the lancet in a puncture-resistant sharps container.[3,19]
■ Remove the test strip and dispose of it properly.[19]
■ After bleeding has stopped, you may apply a small adhesive bandage to the puncture site, if necessary.
■ Remove and discard your gloves,[19] and perform hand hygiene.[7,8,9,10,11,12]
NURSING ALERT If you obtain an extremely low or high blood glucose meter result, obtain a serum blood glucose level immediately *to confirm the result.*[1,2]
■ Clean and disinfect the blood glucose meter with a disinfectant pad, following the manufacturer's instructions.[1,3,24] *Contaminated blood glucose monitoring equipment increases the risk of infection by such bloodborne pathogens as hepatitis B, hepatitis C, and human immunodeficiency viruses.*[3,25]

■ Perform hand hygiene.[7,8,9,10,11,12]
■ Notify the practitioner of critical test results within your facility's time frame *to ensure prompt treatment.*[12]
■ Document the procedure.[20,26,27,28]

Special considerations

■ Bedside blood glucose testing is considered a waived test, meaning that the U.S. Food and Drug Administration approved the test system for waiver under the Clinical Laboratory Improvement Amendments of 1988. To qualify for waived test status, the test must be simple to perform and have low risk for erroneous test results. Even so, keep in mind that errors can occur anywhere in the testing process. Be sure to follow the manufacturer's instructions for use to prevent testing errors that could result in treatment errors.[29]
■ Avoid selecting cold, cyanotic, or swollen puncture sites *to ensure an adequate blood sample.* If you can't obtain a capillary sample, perform a venipuncture and place a large drop of venous blood on the test strip. If you want to test blood from a refrigerated sample, allow the blood to return to room temperature before testing it.
■ A patient admitted with diabetes or hyperglycemia may have a hemoglobin A1c test ordered if one hasn't been performed within the past 3 months.[1]
■ *To help detect abnormal glucose metabolism and diagnose diabetes mellitus,* the practitioner may order other blood glucose tests. (See *Oral and IV glucose tolerance tests,* page 80)
■ Store the test strips away from heat and humidity, *because these conditions can affect the accuracy of the results.*

Patient teaching

If the patient will perform blood glucose monitoring at home, teach the proper use of the lancet and portable blood glucose meter, as necessary. Also teach the patient the importance of washing hands with soap and water, drying them, and then using the first drop of blood for self-monitoring of the blood glucose level. If hand washing isn't possible and the hands aren't visibly soiled or exposed to sugar-containing products, advise the patient to use the second drop of blood after wiping away the first drop.[23] Provide the patient with written instructions as well.

Complications

Complications of blood sampling include infection and injury from venipuncture or fingerstick.[3] False results from improper collection may lead to inappropriate treatment or lack of treatment.[30]

Documentation

Record the date and time of testing and the results in the patient's medical record. Document the date, time, and name of the practitioner you notified of test results, if necessary. Record any prescribed interventions and the patient's response to them. Document teaching you provided to the patient and family (if applicable), their understanding of that teaching, and any need for follow-up teaching.

REFERENCES
1 American Diabetes Association. (2021). Standards of medical care in diabetes—2021. *Diabetes Care, 44,* S1–S222. https://care.diabetesjournals. org/content/44/Supplement_1 (Level VII)
2 Nova Biomedical. (2014). *55890 StatStrip glucose hospital meter test strips package insert.* Waltham, MA: Nova Biomedical.
3 Centers for Disease Control and Prevention. (2011). Infection prevention during blood glucose monitoring and insulin administration. https://www. cdc.gov/injectionsafety/blood-glucose-monitoring.html
4 Klonoff, D. C., & Perz, J. F. (2010). Assisted monitoring of blood glucose: Special safety needs for a new paradigm in testing glucose. *Journal of Diabetes Science and Technology, 4,* 1027–1031.
5 Centers for Disease Control and Prevention. (2010). CDC clinical reminder: Use of fingerstick devices on more than one person poses risk for transmitting bloodborne pathogens. https://www.cdc.gov/injectionsafety/ Fingerstick-DevicesBGM.html

Oral and IV glucose tolerance tests

For monitoring trends in glucose metabolism, two tests—an oral glucose tolerance test and an IV glucose tolerance test—may offer benefits over test strips. For example, they may help diagnose diabetes in patients whose fasting blood glucose levels are normal, or diagnose or exclude abnormal glucose tolerance in patient without symptoms.[30,31]

Oral glucose tolerance test

The oral glucose tolerance test (OGTT) measures carbohydrate metabolism after ingestion of a challenge dose of glucose. The body absorbs this dose rapidly, causing plasma glucose levels to rise and peak within 30 minutes to 1 hour. The pancreas responds by secreting insulin, causing glucose levels to return to normal within 2 to 3 hours.[31] During this period, plasma and urine glucose levels are monitored *to assess insulin secretion and the body's ability to metabolize glucose.*

Although you may not collect the blood specimens required for this test, you will be responsible for preparing the patient for the test and monitoring the patient's physical condition during the test.

Begin by explaining the OGTT to the patient. Tell the patient to maintain a high-carbohydrate diet for 3 days; to fast for 12 to 16 hours before the test, as ordered; and to withhold drugs that may affect test results, as ordered. In addition, instruct the patient to avoid smoking, drinking coffee or alcohol, and exercising strenuously for 8 hours before or during the test. Explain that you'll obtain a fasting sample, and that the patient will then receive a challenge dose of the equivalent of 75 to 100 g of anhydrase glucose (usually a specially formulated glucose solution) to drink.[30,32]

Inform the patient who will perform the venipunctures and when, and explain that the needle punctures and the pressure of the tourniquet may cause slight discomfort. Reassure the patient that collecting each blood sample usually takes less than 3 minutes.

During the test period, watch for signs and symptoms of hypoglycemia, such as weakness, restlessness, nervousness, hunger, and sweating, and report these to the practitioner immediately.[30]

IV glucose tolerance test

■ The practitioner may choose to administer an IV glucose tolerance test for patients who can't absorb an oral dose of glucose. This procedure is rare in clinical practice and primarily in use for research.[31,32]

6 The Joint Commission. (2021). Standard WT.04.01.01. *Comprehensive accreditation manual for hospitals.* Oakbrook Terrace, IL: The Joint Commission. (Level VII)

7 The Joint Commission. (2021). Standard NPSG.07.01.01. *Comprehensive accreditation manual for hospitals.* Oakbrook Terrace, IL: The Joint Commission. (Level VII)

8 Centers for Disease Control and Prevention. (2002). Guideline for hand hygiene in health-care settings: Recommendations of the Healthcare Infection Control Practices Advisory Committee and the HICPAC/SHEA/APIC/IDSA Hand Hygiene Task Force. *MMWR Recommendations and Reports, 51*(RR-16), 1–45. https://www.cdc.gov/mmwr/pdf/rr/rr5116.pdf (Level II)

9 World Health Organization. (2009). WHO guidelines on hand hygiene in health care: First global patient safety challenge, clean care is safer care. https://apps.who.int/iris/bitstream/handle/10665/44102/9789241597906_eng.pdf?sequence=1 (Level IV)

10 Accreditation Association for Hospitals and Health Systems. (2020). Standard 07.01.21. *Healthcare Facilities Accreditation Program: Accreditation requirements for acute care hospitals.* Chicago, IL: Accreditation Association for Hospitals and Health Systems. (Level VII)

11 Centers for Medicare and Medicaid Services, Department of Health and Human Services. (2020). Condition of participation: Infection control. 42 C.F.R. § 482.42.

12 DNV GL-Healthcare USA, Inc. (2020). IC.1.SR.1. *NIAHO® accreditation requirements, interpretive guidelines and surveyor guidance—revision 20.0.* Milford, OH: DNV GL-Healthcare USA, Inc. (Level VII)

13 The Joint Commission. (2021). Standard NPSG.01.01.01. *Comprehensive accreditation manual for hospitals.* Oakbrook Terrace, IL: The Joint Commission. (Level VII)

14 Centers for Medicare and Medicaid Services, Department of Health and Human Services. (2020). Condition of participation: Patient's rights. 42 C.F.R. § 482.13(c)(1).

15 The Joint Commission. (2021). Standard RI.01.01.01. *Comprehensive accreditation manual for hospitals.* Oakbrook Terrace, IL: The Joint Commission. (Level VII)

16 Accreditation Association for Hospitals and Health Systems. (2020). Standard 15.01.16. *Healthcare Facilities Accreditation Program: Accreditation requirements for acute care hospitals.* Chicago, IL: Accreditation Association for Hospitals and Health Systems. (Level VII)

17 DNV GL-Healthcare USA, Inc. (2020). PR.2.SR.5. *NIAHO® accreditation requirements, interpretive guidelines and surveyor guidance—revision 20.0.* Milford, OH: DNV GL-Healthcare USA, Inc. (Level VII)

18 The Joint Commission. (2021). Standard PC.02.01.21. *Comprehensive accreditation manual for hospitals.* Oakbrook Terrace, IL: The Joint Commission. (Level VII)

19 Occupational Safety and Health Administration. (2012). Bloodborne pathogens, standard number 1910.1030. https://www.osha.gov/pls/oshaweb/owadisp.show_document?p_id=10051&p_table=STANDARDS (Level VII)

20 Siegel, J. D., et al. (2007, revised 2019). 2007 guideline for isolation precautions: Preventing transmission of infectious agents in healthcare settings. https://www.cdc.gov/infectioncontrol/pdf/guidelines/isolation-guidelines-H.pdf (Level II)

21 Accreditation Association for Hospitals and Health Systems. (2020). Standard 07.01.10. *Healthcare Facilities Accreditation Program: Accreditation requirements for acute care hospitals.* Chicago, IL: Accreditation Association for Hospitals and Health Systems. (Level VII)

22 World Health Organization. (2010). WHO guidelines on drawing blood: Best practices in phlebotomy. https://www.ncbi.nlm.nih.gov/books/NBK138650/ (Level VII)

23 Hortnesius, J., et al. (2011). Self-monitoring of blood glucose: The use of the first or the second drop of blood. *Diabetes Care, 34,* 556–560. https://care.diabetesjournals.org/content/34/3/556.full (Level II)

24 Rutala, W. A., et al. (2008, revised 2019). *Guideline for disinfection and sterilization in healthcare facilities, 2008.* https://www.cdc.gov/infectioncontrol/pdf/guidelines/disinfection-guidelines-H.pdf (Level I)

25 Accreditation Association for Hospitals and Health Systems. (2020). Standard 07.02.03. *Healthcare Facilities Accreditation Program: Accreditation requirements for acute care hospitals.* Chicago, IL: Accreditation Association for Hospitals and Health Systems. (Level VII)

26 The Joint Commission. (2021). Standard NPSG.02.03.01. *Comprehensive accreditation manual for hospitals.* Oakbrook Terrace, IL: The Joint Commission. (Level VII)

27 Centers for Medicare and Medicaid Services, Department of Health and Human Services. (2020). Condition of participation: Medical record services. 42 C.F.R. § 482.24(b).

28 DNV GL-Healthcare USA, Inc. (2020). MR.2.SR.1. *NIAHO® accreditation requirements, interpretive guidelines and surveyor guidance—revision 20.0.* Milford, OH: DNV GL-Healthcare USA, Inc. (Level VII)

29 Centers for Disease Control and Prevention. (2021). Clinical laboratory improvement amendments: Waived tests. https://www.cdc.gov/clia/waived-tests.html

30 Fischbach, F., & Fischbach, M. A. (2018). *A manual of laboratory and diagnostic tests* (10th ed.). Philadelphia, PA: Wolters Kluwer.

31 World Health Organization. (2006). Definition and diagnosis of diabetes mellitus and intermediate hyperglycemia. https://www.who.int/diabetes/publications/Definition%20and%20diagnosis%20of%20diabetes_new.pdf (Level VII)

32 Durnwald, C. (2021). Diabetes mellitus in pregnancy: Screening and diagnosis. In: *UpToDate,* Nathan, D. M., & Werner, E. F. (Eds.).

33 U.S. National Library of Medicine. (2020). Glucose tolerance test-non-pregnant. https://medlineplus.gov/ency/article/003466.htm

BLOOD PRESSURE MEASUREMENT

Defined as the lateral force exerted by blood on the arterial walls, blood pressure depends on the force of ventricular contractions, arterial wall elasticity, peripheral vascular resistance, and blood volume and viscosity. Systolic, or maximum, pressure occurs during left ventricular contraction and reflects the integrity of the heart, arteries, and arterioles. Diastolic, or minimum, pressure occurs during left ventricular relaxation and directly indicates blood vessel resistance.

Pulse pressure, the difference between systolic and diastolic pressures, varies inversely with arterial elasticity. Rigid vessels, incapable of distention and recoil, produce high systolic pressure and low diastolic pressure. Normally, systolic pressure exceeds diastolic pressure by about 40 mm Hg. Narrowed pulse pressure—a difference of less than 30 mm Hg—occurs when systolic pressure falls and diastolic pressure rises. These changes reflect reduced stroke volume, increased peripheral resistance, or both. Widened pulse pressure—a difference of more than 50 mm Hg between systolic and diastolic pressures—occurs when systolic pressure rises and diastolic pressure remains constant, or when systolic pressure rises and diastolic pressure falls. These changes reflect increased stroke volume, decreased peripheral resistance, or both.

Frequent blood pressure measurement is critical after serious injury, surgery, or anesthesia and during any illness or condition that threatens cardiovascular stability. (Measurement can occur manually or via an automated blood pressure device.) Frequent blood pressure measurement may also be necessary for unstable patients and for those receiving blood transfusions or oral or IV medications that stabilize blood pressure. Guidelines recommend regular measurement for patients with a history of hypertension or hypotension, and annual screening for all adults.

Measure blood pressure in the upper arm using the auscultatory or oscillatory method. When obtaining a baseline measurement, measure blood pressure in both arms. If significant differences in blood pressure exist from one arm to the other, use the arm with the higher pressure,[1,2] For subsequent measurement, monitor blood pressure in the same arm using the same device *to ensure accurate measurement.*

Equipment

Aneroid sphygmomanometer with appropriately sized cuff ▪ stethoscope ▪ disinfectant pads ▪ Optional: automated vital signs monitor.

A sphygmomanometer consists of an inflatable compression cuff linked to a manual air pump and an aneroid gauge. Use a recently calibrated aneroid gauge. Wall mounted devices require calibration at least every 6 months, while hand-held devices require calibration every 2 to 4 weeks. To obtain an accurate reading, rest the gauge in any position, but view it directly from the front.[2]

Cuffs come in sizes ranging from newborn to extra-large adult. Disposable cuffs and thigh cuffs are available. Use an appropriate-sized cuff and follow the manufacturer's instructions for proper fit and placement.[1]

An automated blood pressure device is a noninvasive device that measures pulse rate, systolic and diastolic pressures, and mean arterial pressure at preset intervals. (See *Using an automated blood pressure device.*)

Preparation of equipment

Carefully choose a cuff of appropriate size for the patient; the cuff bladder should be 75% to 100% of the measured upper arm circumference, and the bladder width should be 37% to 50% of the arm circumference (a length to width ratio of 2:1). *A cuff that is too small may cause a false-high pressure reading; a cuff that is too large may cause a false-low reading.*[2] (For information on other situations that can cause false-high or false-low readings, see *Factors affecting blood pressure measurement*, page 82.)

To use an automated vital signs monitor, collect the monitor, dual air hose, and pressure cuff. Then make sure the monitor unit is firmly positioned near the patient's bed.

Implementation

▪ Gather and prepare the necessary equipment and supplies.
▪ Perform hand hygiene.[8,9,10,11,12,13]
▪ Confirm the patient's identity using at least two patient identifiers.[14]
▪ Have the patient rest for 3 to 5 minutes before measuring the blood pressure.[2,15] Make sure the patient hasn't smoked or used other tobacco products, exercised, or had caffeine for at least 30 minutes.[2,15,16]
▪ Provide privacy.[17,18,19,20]

Using an automated blood pressure device

An automated blood pressure device enables you to track a patient's blood pressure continually without having to reapply a blood pressure cuff each time. In addition, it eliminates the need for an invasive arterial line to gather similar data.

Some automated blood pressure devices are lightweight and battery-operated, and can be attached to an IV pole for continuous monitoring even during patient transfers. Make sure you know battery capacity of the monitor you're using, and plug the machine in whenever possible *to keep it charged.* Regularly calibrate the monitor *to ensure accurate readings.*

Oscillatory devices aren't as accurate as auscultatory blood pressure measurement; they can overestimate or underestimate blood pressure measurements.[3] Before using any monitor, check its accuracy. Oscillatory devices should meet the Association for the Advancement of Medical Instrumentation standards when compared with the auscultatory method.[1]

Determine the patient's pulse rate and blood pressure manually, using the same arm you'll use for the monitor cuff. Compare your results when you get initial readings from the monitor. If the results differ, call your supply department or the manufacturer's representative.

Check the manufacturer's guidelines, *because most automated monitoring devices are intended for serial monitoring only and may be inaccurate for a one-time measurement.*

Preparing the device
▪ Explain the procedure to the patient and family (if appropriate) according to their communication and learning needs *to increase their understanding, allay their fears, and enhance cooperation.*[4] Describe the alarm system *so the patient won't be frightened if it's triggered.*
▪ Make sure the power switch is off. Then plug the monitor into a properly grounded wall outlet.
▪ Secure the dual air hose to the front of the monitor.
▪ Connect the pressure cuff's tubing into the other ends of the dual air hose, and tighten connections *to prevent air leaks.* Keep the air hose away from the patient *to avoid accidental dislodgment.*
▪ Squeeze all air from the cuff and wrap it loosely around the patient's arm about ¾" to 1" (1.9 to 2.5 cm) above the antecubital fossa. Never apply the cuff to a limb that has an IV catheter in place. Position the cuff's "artery" arrow over the palpated brachial artery. Then secure the cuff for a snug fit.[1]

Selecting parameters
▪ When you turn on the monitor, it will default to a manual mode. (In this mode, you can obtain vital signs yourself before switching to the automatic mode.) Press the AUTO/MANUAL button to select the automatic mode. The monitor will give you baseline data for the pulse rate, systolic and diastolic pressures, and mean arterial pressure.
▪ Compare your previous manual results with these baseline data. If they match, you're ready to set the alarm parameters. Press the SELECT button to blank out all displays except systolic pressure.
▪ Use the HIGH and LOW limit buttons to set the specific parameters for systolic pressure. (These limits range from a high of 240 mm Hg to a low of 0 mm Hg.) Do the same for mean arterial pressure, pulse rate, and diastolic pressure. After you've set all of the parameters, press the SELECT button again to display all current data. Note that even if you forget to do this last step, the monitor will automatically display current data 10 seconds after you set the last parameters.
▪ Make sure the alarm limits are set appropriately for the patient's condition and that the alarms are turned on, functioning properly, and audible to staff.[5,6,7]

Collecting data
▪ You also need to program the monitor to the desired frequency, according to the manufacturer's instructions. Press the SET button until you reach the desired time interval in minutes. To minimize complications, use the maximum (least frequent) cycle time for the shortest time period.[1]
▪ You can obtain a set of vital signs at any time by pressing the START button.
▪ Pressing the CANCEL button will stop the interval and deflate the cuff.
▪ You can retrieve stored data by pressing the PRIOR DATA button. The monitor will display the last data obtained, along with the time elapsed since then. Scrolling backward, you can retrieve data from the previous 99 minutes.
▪ Ensure frequent documentation of the patient's vital signs in a vital signs assessment record.

Factors affecting blood pressure measurement

Accurate blood pressure measurement relies on standardizing techniques and proper equipment.[2] When measuring blood pressure, keep the following factors in mind:

- Read the dial at eye level.
- Provide to the patient a 3- to 5-minute rest period without talking or moving before measurement.
- Place the cuff on bare skin.
- Avoid rolling shirtsleeves, *because this can cause a tourniquet effect.*
- Avoid rapid deflation, *because this can cause inaccuracies;* deflation shouldn't exceed 2 to 3 mm Hg/second.
- Ensure that the patient avoids caffeine intake, smoking, and exercise for at least 30 minutes before measurement.
- The patient's bladder should be empty.
- The patient shouldn't talk during measurement.
- The environment should be quiet.
- The patient's legs should be uncrossed.[2]

- Explain the procedure to the patient and family (if appropriate) according to their communication and learning needs *to increase their understanding, allay their fears, and enhance cooperation.*[4]
- Position the patient supine or with the head of the bed at a comfortable level, or have the patient sit erect during blood pressure measurement in the upper arms. If the patient is sitting erect, ensure the patient's back and arms are supported, legs are uncrossed, and both feet are on the floor, *because crossing the legs can increase blood pressure.*[1,2] Extend the patient's arm at heart level (the phlebostatic axis, fourth intercostal space, halfway between the anterior and posterior diameter of the chest) and provide supported.[1]

NURSING ALERT Please note that measuring blood pressure with a patient seated on an examination table or side of the bed with the back unsupported may cause false elevations in blood pressure.[2]

- Make sure the patient is relaxed and comfortable when you measure the blood pressure *so it stays at its normal level.*[2]
- Remain quiet during blood pressure measurement and instruct the patient to do the same, *because systolic and diastolic blood pressure increase with talking.*[1,2]
- Wrap the deflated cuff snugly around the patient's upper arm so that the end of the cuff is ¾" to 1¼" (2 to 3 cm) above the antecubital fossa *to enable placement of your stethoscope,* as shown below. Align the cuff to make sure that the mark on the cuff for "artery" is positioned over the artery. The cuff should fit snugly but should still allow for two fingers to slide beneath it.[2]

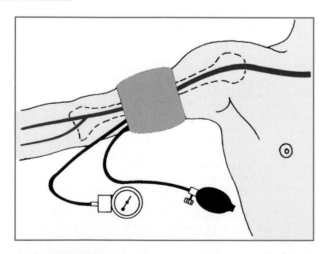

NURSING ALERT Don't measure blood pressure in an extremity with deep vein thrombosis, grafts, or ischemic changes. Don't apply a blood pressure cuff over a peripherally inserted central catheter or midline

catheter; you may apply the cuff distal to the insertion site. Avoid blood pressure measurement in extremities with a peripheral IV catheter while fluid is infusing, and in patients who have an incision or have undergone trauma. Don't measure blood pressure in an extremity that's affected by lymphedema after mastectomy or lumpectomy, *because doing so can further compromise lymphatic circulation and worsen edema.* Likewise, don't take a blood pressure measurement on the same arm as an arteriovenous fistula or hemodialysis shunt, *because blood flow through the vascular device might become compromised.*[1]

- If necessary, connect the appropriate tube to the rubber bulb of the air pump and the other tube to the gauge.
- Determine how high to pump the blood pressure cuff by estimating the systolic blood pressure by palpation. As you feel the radial artery with the fingers of one hand, inflate the cuff until the radial pulse disappears. Read this pressure on the gauge and add 30 mm Hg to it.[2] Use this sum as the target inflation *to prevent discomfort from overinflation.* Deflate the cuff.
- Locate the brachial artery by palpation. Center the diaphragm or bell of the stethoscope over the part of the artery where you detect the strongest beat and hold it in place with one hand. Place the stethoscope earpieces in your ears.[2]
- Close the valve of the sphygmomanometer. Using the thumb and index finger of your other hand, turn the thumbscrew on the rubber bulb of the air pump clockwise to close the valve.
- Pump up the cuff to the predetermined level.
- Open the valve of the air pump carefully, and then slowly deflate the cuff—between 2 and 3 mm Hg/second.[2] While releasing air, watch the mercury column or aneroid gauge and auscultate for the sound over the artery.
- When you hear the first beat or clear tapping sound, note the pressure on the column or gauge; this is the systolic pressure. The beat or tapping sound is the first of five Korotkoff sounds. The second sound resembles a murmur or swish; the third sound, crisp tapping; the fourth sound, a soft, muffled tone; and the fifth sound is when the sound disappears.[2,15]
- Continue to release air gradually while auscultating for the sound over the artery.
- Note the pressure when the sound disappears; this is the diastolic pressure: the fifth Korotkoff sound.[2,15]
- After you hear the last Korotkoff sound, deflate the cuff slowly for at least another 10 mm Hg *to ensure that no further sounds are audible.*
- Deflate the cuff rapidly and record the pressure.
- Remove the cuff.
- Check the patient's skin integrity under the blood pressure cuff.[1]
- Perform hand hygiene.[8,9,10,11,12,13]
- If the cuff isn't designated for single-patient use, clean and disinfect it with a disinfectant pad.[21,22]
- Clean and disinfect your stethoscope using an disinfectant pad.[26,27]
- Discard used supplies in appropriate receptacles.
- Perform hand hygiene.[8,9,10,11,12,13]
- Document the procedure.[24,25,26,27]

Special considerations

- If the upper arm can't be used for blood pressure measurement, or if the maximum-size cuff won't fit the patient's arm properly, measure blood pressure using the forearm. However, keep in mind that blood pressure measurements in the forearm and upper arm aren't interchangeable.[1] Studies have shown that upper arm systolic and diastolic blood pressure measurements with an appropriate-size cuff were significantly lower than forearm blood pressure measurements with a standard cuff.[28,29,30,31] When measuring blood pressure in the forearm, choose the cuff of an adequate size. (Guidelines recommend a cuff with a bladder large enough to go around 80% of the forearm.) Position the cuff midway between the elbow and the wrist, and position the forearm at heart level.[1,16]
- If you can't use the patient's upper arms and forearms, measure blood pressure using the thigh or calf.[1] Keep in mind that blood pressure measurements in the thigh or calf aren't interchangeable with upper arm measurements.[32] Use the same attention to selecting a proper cuff size as you would for blood pressure measurement at other sites. For calf blood pressure measurement, position the patient supine, and place the cuff about 1" (2.5 cm) above the malleoli. Auscultate Korotkoff sounds over the

dorsalis pedis or posterior tibial artery.[1] For thigh measurement, position the patient prone and position the cuff over the lower third of the thigh so that the lower edge of the cuff is about ¾″ to 1¼″ (2 cm to 3 cm) above the popliteal fossa. Auscultate Korotkoff sounds over the popliteal artery.[1] If the patient can't tolerate prone positioning, place the patient supine with the knee slightly bent.[1]

■ If you can't auscultate blood pressure, you may estimate systolic pressure. To do this, first palpate the brachial or radial pulse. Then inflate the cuff until you no longer detect the pulse. Slowly deflate the cuff and, when you detect the pulse again, record the pressure as the palpated systolic pressure.

■ Be aware that patients with aortic dissection, congenital heart disease, coarctation of the aorta, peripheral vascular disease, or unilateral neurologic or musculoskeletal abnormalities may demonstrate a difference in blood pressure between the two arms. If you detect such a difference, use the arm with the higher pressure.[1]

■ If the patient is crying or anxious, delay blood pressure measurement, if possible, until the patient becomes calm *to avoid falsely elevated readings.*

■ Occasionally, blood pressure must be measured in both arms or with the patient in two different positions (such as lying and standing or sitting and standing). In such cases, observe and record any significant difference between the two readings and record the blood pressure as well as the extremity and position used.[1]

■ Measure the blood pressure of patients taking antihypertensive medications while they're in a sitting position *to ensure accurate measurements.*

■ The Joint Commission issued a sentinel event alert concerning medical device alarm safety, *because alarm-related events have been associated with permanent loss of function or death.* Among the major contributing factors were improper alarm settings, alarm settings turned off inappropriately, and alarm signals that were inaudible to staff. Make sure alarm limits are set appropriately, and that alarms are turned on, functioning properly, and audible to staff. Follow facility guidelines for preventing alarm fatigue.[33]

Complications

The most common complications include bruising and skin irritation.[1] Improper technique can cause inaccurate readings, which can lead to unnecessary or inadequate treatment. Measuring blood pressure on the same arm as an arteriovenous fistula or hemodialysis shunt can compromise blood flow through the vascular device. Prolonged use of automated electronic blood pressure devices and frequent blood pressure measurement can cause pain, limb edema, phlebitis, compartment syndrome, peripheral neuropathy, thrombophlebitis, venous stasis, ecchymosis, and petechiae.[1]

Documentation

In the patient's medical record, record blood pressure as systolic over diastolic pressure, such as 120/78 mm Hg. Document an auscultatory gap, if present. If required by your facility, document blood pressures on a graph, using dots or checkmarks. Include the extremity used and the patient's position. Record the measurements to the nearest even number, and note the time of the patient's most recent blood pressure medications if any.[2] Record whom you notified about blood pressure results, the date and time of notification, prescribed interventions, and the patient's response to those interventions, if applicable. Document teaching provided to the patient and family (if applicable), their understanding of that teaching, and any need for follow-up teaching.

REFERENCES

1 American Association of Critical-Care Nurses. (2016). AACN practice alert: Obtaining accurate noninvasive blood pressure measurements in adults. https://www.aacn.org/clinical-resources/practice-alerts/obtaining-accurate-noninvasive-blood-pressure-measurements-in-adults (Level VII)

2 Munter, P., et al. (2019). Measurement of blood pressure in humans: A scientific statement from the American Heart Association. *Hypertension, 75,* e35–e66. https://www.ahajournals.org/doi/pdf/10.1161/HYP.0000000000000087 (Level I)

3 Emergency Nurses Association. (2019). Clinical practice guideline: Noninvasive blood pressure measurement with automated devices. https://www.ena.org/docs/default-source/resource-library/practice-resources/cpg/non-mbr-synopsis/nibpmsynopsis.pdf?sfvrsn=99d6971d_2 (Level VII)

4 The Joint Commission. (2021). Standard PC.02.01.21. *Comprehensive accreditation manual for hospitals.* Oakbrook Terrace, IL: The Joint Commission. (Level VII)

5 The Joint Commission. (2021). Standard NPSG.06.01.01. *Comprehensive accreditation manual for hospitals.* Oakbrook Terrace, IL: The Joint Commission. (Level VII)

6 Graham, K. C., & Cvach, M. (2010). Monitor alarm fatigue: Standardizing use of physiological monitors and decreasing nuisance alarms. *American Journal of Critical Care, 19,* 28–37. http://ajcc.aacnjournals.org/content/19/1/28.full.pdf

7 American Association of Critical-Care Nurses. (2018). AACN practice alert: Managing alarms in acute care across the life span—electrocardiography and pulse oximetry. https://www.aacn.org/clinical-resources/practice-alerts/managing-alarms-in-acute-care-across-the-life-span (Level VII)

8 The Joint Commission. (2021). Standard NPSG.07.01.01. *Comprehensive accreditation manual for hospitals.* Oakbrook Terrace, IL: The Joint Commission. (Level VII)

9 Centers for Disease Control and Prevention. (2002). Guideline for hand hygiene in health-care settings: Recommendations of the Healthcare Infection Control Practices Advisory Committee and the HICPAC/SHEA/APIC/IDSA Hand Hygiene Task Force. *MMWR Recommendations and Reports, 51*(RR-16), 1–45. https://www.cdc.gov/mmwr/pdf/rr/rr5116.pdf (Level II)

10 World Health Organization. (2009). WHO guidelines on hand hygiene in health care: First global patient safety challenge, clean care is safer care. https://apps.who.int/iris/bitstream/handle/10665/44102/9789241597906_eng.pdf?sequence=1 (Level IV)

11 Centers for Medicare and Medicaid Services, Department of Health and Human Services. (2020). Condition of participation: Infection control. 42 C.F.R. § 482.42.

12 Accreditation Association for Hospitals and Health Systems. (2020). Standard 07.01.21. *Healthcare Facilities Accreditation Program: Accreditation requirements for acute care hospitals.* Chicago, IL: Accreditation Association for Hospitals and Health Systems. (Level VII)

13 DNV GL-Healthcare USA, Inc. (2020). IC.1.SR.1. *NIAHO® accreditation requirements, interpretive guidelines and surveyor guidance—revision 20.0.* Milford, OH: DNV GL-Healthcare USA, Inc. (Level VII)

14 The Joint Commission. (2021). Standard NPSG.01.01.01. *Comprehensive accreditation manual for hospitals.* Oakbrook Terrace, IL: The Joint Commission. (Level VII)

15 Ramnarine, M. (2018). Blood pressure assessment. https://emedicine.medscape.com/article/1948157-overview

16 Kallioinen, N., et al. (2017). Sources of inaccuracy in the measurement of adult patients' resting blood pressure in clinical settings: A systematic review. *Journal of Hypertension, 35,* 421–441. https://www.ncbi.nlm.nih.gov/pmc/articles/PMC5278896/ (Level I)

17 The Joint Commission. (2021 Standard RI.01.01.01. *Comprehensive accreditation manual for hospitals.* Oakbrook Terrace, IL: The Joint Commission. (Level VII)

18 Centers for Medicare and Medicaid Services, Department of Health and Human Services. (2020). Condition of participation: Patient's rights. 42 C.F.R. § 482.13(c)(1).

19 Accreditation Association for Hospitals and Health Systems. (2020). Standard 15.01.16. *Healthcare Facilities Accreditation Program: Accreditation requirements for acute care hospitals.* Chicago, IL: Accreditation Association for Hospitals and Health Systems. (Level VII)

20 DNV GL-Healthcare USA, Inc. (2020). PR.2.SR.5. *NIAHO® accreditation requirements, interpretive guidelines and surveyor guidance—revision 20.0.* Milford, OH: DNV GL-Healthcare USA, Inc. (Level VII)

21 Rutala, W. A., et al. (2008, revised 2019). Guideline for disinfection and sterilization in healthcare facilities, 2008. https://www.cdc.gov/infection-control/pdf/guidelines/disinfection-guidelines-H.pdf (Level I)

22 Accreditation Association for Hospitals and Health Systems. (2020). Standard 07.02.03. *Healthcare Facilities Accreditation Program: Accreditation requirements for acute care hospitals.* Chicago, IL: Accreditation Association for Hospitals and Health Systems. (Level VII)

23 Occupational Safety and Health Administration. (2012). Bloodborne pathogens, standard number 1910.1030. https://www.osha.gov/pls/oshaweb/owadisp.show_document?p_id=10051&p_table=STANDARDS (Level VII)

24 The Joint Commission. (2021). Standard RC.01.03.01. *Comprehensive accreditation manual for hospitals.* Oakbrook Terrace, IL: The Joint Commission. (Level VII)

25 Centers for Medicare and Medicaid Services, Department of Health and Human Services. (2020). Condition of participation: Medical record services. 42 C.F.R. § 482.24.

26 Accreditation Association for Hospitals and Health Systems. (2020). Standard 10.00.03. *Healthcare Facilities Accreditation Program: Accreditation requirements for acute care hospitals.* Chicago, IL: Accreditation Association for Hospitals and Health Systems. (Level VII)

27 DNV GL-Healthcare USA, Inc. (2020). MR.2.SR.1. *NIAHO® accreditation requirements, interpretive guidelines and surveyor guidance—revision 20.0.* Milford, OH: DNV GL-Healthcare USA, Inc. (Level VII)

28 Pierin, A. M., et al. (2004). Blood pressure measurement in obese patients: Comparison between upper arm and forearm measurements. *Blood Pressure Monitoring, 9,* 101–105.

29 Palatini, P., et al. (2004). Wrist blood pressure over estimated blood pressure measured at the upper arm. *Blood Pressure Monitoring, 9,* 77–81.

30 Wen-Yuan, L., et al. (2013). Discrepancy of blood pressure between the brachial artery and radial artery. *World Journal of Emergency Medicine, 4,* 294–297.

31 Domiano, K., et al (2008). Comparison of upper arm and forearm blood pressure. *Clinical Nursing Research, 17,* 241–250.

32 Wilkes, J. M., & DiPalma, J. A. (2004). Brachial blood pressure monitoring versus ankle monitoring during colonoscopy. *Southern Medical Journal, 97,* 939–941.

33 The Joint Commission. (2013). Sentinel event alert 50: Medical device alarm safety in hospitals. http://www.jointcommission.org/assets/1/6/SEA_50_alarms_4_26_16.PDF (Level VII)

Body jewelry removal

Piercings and body jewelry may be present on virtually any body part. The most common sites are the ears, nose, tongue, eyebrows, lips, and umbilicus. Less common sites include the nipples and genitals.[1]

Depending on the risk to the patient and the medical interventions, the practitioner may order body jewelry removed *to reduce the risk of such complications as electrical burns, aspiration, pressure injures, surgical site infection, and tissue injuries.*[2,3,4,5,6,7] However, urgent medical care should never be delayed for the purpose of attempting to remove body jewelry.

During the process of helping a patient remove body jewelry or removing it from an unconscious patient, it's important to ensure that the patient isn't harmed and the patient's dignity is preserved. Also, you must take steps to avoid damaging the body jewelry during the removal process and to retain the jewelry for reinsertion later.

Equipment

Gloves ▪ antiseptic solution ▪ personal belongings envelope ▪ Optional: ring-opening or ring-spreading pliers, ring forceps, ball-grabber, bead tweezer, lubricating gel, inert plastic retainer, sterile dressing.

Implementation

▪ Verify the practitioner's order for body jewelry removal, if needed, and review the patient's medical record for scheduled diagnostic tests and surgical procedures.
▪ If required by your facility, ensure that informed consent has been obtained and that the signed consent form is in the patient's medical record.[8,9,10,11]
▪ Perform hand hygiene.[12,13,14,15,16,17]
▪ Confirm the patient's identity using at least two patient identifiers.[18]
▪ Provide privacy.[19,20,21,22]
▪ Ask the patient about any body jewelry, especially jewelry that isn't readily visible. If the patient is unconscious, ask the patient's family members about known body jewelry, and note the presence of body jewelry during the physical examination.
▪ Explain the procedure to the patient and family (if appropriate) according to their individual communication and learning needs *to increase their understanding, allay their fears, and enhance cooperation.*[23] Explain the reason for removing the body jewelry, and encourage the them to ask questions as needed.
▪ Determine the type of body jewelry to be removed.
▪ Ask the patient how long each piercing has been present, and if it requires a retainer to maintain its patency.
▪ Gather and prepare the necessary equipment and supplies.
▪ Perform hand hygiene[12,13,14,15,16,17] and put on gloves *to comply with standard precautions.*[24,25]
▪ Ask the patient to remove the jewelry if the patient is able; offer to assist as needed.
▪ If the patient is unconscious, remove the body jewelry following the proper technique for the type of jewelry or body piercing present. (See *Removing body jewelry.*)

NURSING ALERT When removing jewelry from the nostril, nasal septum, cheek, tongue, or lip, use special care to prevent the jewelry from slipping into the airway, *which could result in aspiration.*[26]

▪ Assess the patient's skin at the body-piercing site for signs of infection (redness, swelling, purulent drainage), *because body jewelry harbors microorganisms that can become trapped in the skin, and removal provides an opportunity for effective removal of microorganisms from the piercing site.*[26]
▪ Clean all open wounds and apply a sterile dressing, if needed.
▪ Since removing jewelry from a piercing may initiate closure of the piercing or make reinsertion difficult, help the patient insert a plastic retainer (or insert one on an unconscious patient), if necessary, *to maintain patency of the piercing.*[27]
▪ Clean soiled body jewelry with antiseptic solution, *because you should consider all piercings to be contaminated with body fluids.*
▪ Place the body jewelry in a personal belongings envelope labeled with the patient's name and identification number; give the envelope to a family member or secure it, as directed by your facility.
▪ Remove and discard your gloves[28] and perform hand hygiene.[12,13,14,15,16,17]
▪ Document the procedure.[29,30,31,32]

Special considerations

▪ If the patient refuses to remove body jewelry, notify the practitioner *for reevaluation of the risks of proceeding with any scheduled procedures.*[33]
▪ During intubation, body jewelry can prevent visualization of the airway, or aspiration can occur if body jewelry located in and around the mouth loosens and dislodges.[34]
▪ Burns can result if metal body jewelry heats up as a result of exposure to electrical currents during electrosurgery or contact with active electrodes in the operating room.[2,33]
▪ Pressure injuries can result if an unconscious patient is positioned on a body part with body jewelry in place.[4]
▪ Traumatic injury can occur if body jewelry accidentally becomes entangled in bedding or caught on equipment.[4,33]
▪ The increased risk of bacteremia during invasive surgical procedures can seed body piercings and can cause local or systemic infection.[3,34]
▪ Urethral tears may occur during urinary catheterization in patients with genital piercings.
▪ Body jewelry located on the patient's face, eyebrows, nose, or mouth should be removed while the patient is sitting upright *to minimize the risk of aspiration.*
▪ For procedures requiring electrocauterization, metal body jewelry located between the active and dispersive electrodes should be removed *to minimize the risk of burns in the operating room.*[2]
▪ Body jewelry located near the surgical site should be removed preoperatively and before the skin is prepped, *because jewelry harbors microorganisms.*[3]
▪ Notify the practitioner if your patient has a surface anchor, a type of jewelry placed under the skin. It's usually made from implant-grade materials that may not need to be removed for medical tests and procedures such as X-rays, magnetic resonance imaging, computed tomography scans, and surgical procedures.[27]

Removing body jewelry

Jewelry Type	Jewelry Description	Removal Tools	Removal Technique
Barbell (straight, curved, or circular)	Straight, curved, or circular post with balls on the ends; one or both of the balls unscrew from the rod	■ Gloves ■ Ball grabber ■ Bead tweezer ■ Ring forceps	■ Grasp the removable ball with the ball grabber, bead tweezer, or ring forceps while holding the opposite end still, and turn the ball counterclockwise to loosen it. ■ After loosening the ball, fully unscrew it by hand and pull the open end of the post toward the side of the stationary ball to remove it. ■ Use caution when pulling the post through the body part *to prevent injury from any screw threads on the end of the post.*
Captive bead ring (also called ball closure ring)	Sphere (or other shape) held in place by the tension of the ring	■ Gloves ■ Ring-opening or ring-spreading pliers	■ Insert ring-opening or ring-spreading pliers into the middle of the ring, and slowly pry the ring open. ■ Remove the ball; then remove the ring. ■ Use care when removing the ball, *which can fall when separated from the ring.*
Labret or Monroe	Straight barbell with one flat end resembling the head of a nail; the ball may be attached to the post with either internal or external threading	■ Gloves ■ Bead tweezers	■ Stabilize the stud with the bead tweezers or your gloved fingers, and rotate the ball counterclockwise. ■ Use caution when pulling the post through the body part *to prevent injury from any screw threads on the end of the post.*
Tunnel	Large, round tube usually held in place with an O-ring; the tunnel may be flared on one end	■ Gloves ■ Lubricating gel	■ If the tunnel has an O-ring, slide it off and remove the tube. ■ If the tunnel has a flared outer edge held in place by the surface tension of the skin, use gentle traction and lubricating gel during removal. ■ If the tunnel consists of two separate pieces screwed together, grasp each half (front and back) and rotate counterclockwise to separate.

Complications

Body jewelry may have rough, burred edges that may damage tissue during removal, creating a possible source of infection. Infection may also result from an incompletely healed piercing. Removing tongue jewelry can result in tissue trauma and create airway management problems.[26]

Documentation

Record any questions that the patient asked and your responses to those questions. Document whether you or the patient removed the body jewelry, the type of body jewelry removed and its location on the body, the condition of the skin at the piercing site, any drainage that you noted at the piercing site, the disposition of the body jewelry, and measures that you took to prevent closure and infection at the site. Document teaching provided to the patient and family (if applicable), their understanding of that teaching, and any need for follow-up teaching.

References

1 Desai, N. (2020). Body piercing in adolescents and young adults. In: *UpToDate*, Blake, D. (Ed.).
2 Guideline for safe use of energy-generating devices. (2021). In Wood, A. (Ed.), *Guidelines for perioperative practice, 2021 edition.* Denver, CO: AORN, Inc. (Level VII)
3 Guideline for preoperative patient skin antisepsis. (2021). In Wood, A. (Ed.), *Guidelines for perioperative practice, 2021 edition.* Denver, CO: AORN, Inc. (Level VII)
4 Guideline for positioning the patient. (2021). In Wood, A. (Ed.), *Guidelines for perioperative practice, 2021 edition.* Denver, CO: AORN, Inc. (Level VII)

5 DeBoer, S., et al. (2008). Body piercing and airway management: Photo guide to tongue jewelry removal techniques. *AANA Journal, 76,* 19–23.

6 DeBoer, S., et al. (2006). Managing body jewelry in emergency situations: Misconceptions, patient care, and removal techniques. *Journal of Emergency Nursing, 32,* 159–164.

7 DeBoer, S., et al. (2008). Puncturing myths about body piercing and tattooing. *Nursing2008, 38*(11), 50–54.

8 The Joint Commission. (2021). Standard RI.01.03.01. *Comprehensive accreditation manual for hospitals.* Oakbrook Terrace, IL: The Joint Commission. (Level VII)

9 Centers for Medicare and Medicaid Services, Department of Health and Human Services. (2020). Condition of participation: Patient's rights. 42 C.F.R. § 482.13(b).

10 DNV GL-Healthcare USA, Inc. (2020). PR.2.SR.3. *NIAHO® accreditation requirements, interpretive guidelines and surveyor guidance—revision 20.0.* Milford, OH: DNV GL-Healthcare USA, Inc. (Level VII)

11 Accreditation Association for Hospitals and Health Systems. (2020). Standard 15.01.11. *Healthcare Facilities Accreditation Program: Accreditation requirements for acute care hospitals.* Chicago, IL: Accreditation Association for Hospitals and Health Systems. (Level VII)

12 Centers for Disease Control and Prevention. (2002). Guideline for hand hygiene in health-care settings: Recommendations of the Healthcare Infection Control Practices Advisory Committee and the HICPAC/SHEA/APIC/IDSA Hand Hygiene Task Force. *MMWR Recommendations and Reports, 51*(RR-16), 1–45. https://www.cdc.gov/mmwr/pdf/rr/rr5116.pdf (Level II)

13 The Joint Commission. (2021). Standard NPSG.07.01.01. *Comprehensive accreditation manual for hospitals.* Oakbrook Terrace, IL: The Joint Commission. (Level VII)

14 World Health Organization. (2009). WHO guidelines on hand hygiene in health care: First global patient safety challenge, clean care is safer care. https://apps.who.int/iris/bitstream/handle/10665/44102/9789241597906_eng.pdf?sequence=1 (Level IV)

15 Centers for Medicare and Medicaid Services, Department of Health and Human Services. (2020). Condition of participation: Infection control. 42 C.F.R. § 482.42.

16 Accreditation Association for Hospitals and Health Systems. (2020). Standard 07.01.21. *Healthcare Facilities Accreditation Program: Accreditation requirements for acute care hospitals.* Chicago, IL: Accreditation Association for Hospitals and Health Systems. (Level VII)

17 DNV GL-Healthcare USA, Inc. (2020). IC.1.SR.1. *NIAHO® accreditation requirements, interpretive guidelines and surveyor guidance—revision 20.0.* Milford, OH: DNV GL-Healthcare USA, Inc. (Level VII)

18 The Joint Commission. (2021). Standard NPSG.01.01.01. *Comprehensive accreditation manual for hospitals.* Oakbrook Terrace, IL: The Joint Commission. (Level VII)

19 The Joint Commission. (2021). Standard RI.01.01.01. *Comprehensive accreditation manual for hospitals.* Oakbrook Terrace, IL: The Joint Commission. (Level VII)

20 Centers for Medicare and Medicaid Services, Department of Health and Human Services. (2020). Condition of participation: Patient's rights. 42 C.F.R. § 482.13(c)(1).

21 Accreditation Association for Hospitals and Health Systems. (2020). Standard 15.01.16. *Healthcare Facilities Accreditation Program: Accreditation requirements for acute care hospitals.* Chicago, IL: Accreditation Association for Hospitals and Health Systems. (Level VII)

22 DNV GL-Healthcare USA, Inc. (2020). PR.2.SR.5. *NIAHO® accreditation requirements, interpretive guidelines and surveyor guidance—revision 20.0.* Milford, OH: DNV GL-Healthcare USA, Inc. (Level VII)

23 The Joint Commission. (2021). Standard PC.02.01.21. *Comprehensive accreditation manual for hospitals.* Oakbrook Terrace, IL: The Joint Commission. (Level VII)

24 Siegel, J. D., et al. (2007, revised 2019). 2007 guideline for isolation precautions: Preventing transmission of infectious agents in healthcare settings. https://www.cdc.gov/infectioncontrol/pdf/guidelines/isolation-guidelines-H.pdf (Level II)

25 Accreditation Association for Hospitals and Health Systems. (2020). Standard 07.01.10. *Healthcare Facilities Accreditation Program: Accreditation requirements for acute care hospitals.* Chicago, IL: Accreditation Association for Hospitals and Health Systems. (Level VII)

26 De Cuyper, C., et al. (2018). *Dermatologic complications with body art.* Cham, Switzerland: Springer.

27 Association of Professional Piercers. (2013). Procedure manual 2013 Edition. https://safepiercing.org/wp-content/uploads/2020/10/APP_Procedures_2013_A_Web.pdf

28 Occupational Safety and Health Administration. (2012). Bloodborne pathogens, standard number 1910.1030 https://www.osha.gov/pls/oshaweb/owadisp.show_document?p_id=10051&p_table=STANDARDS (Level VII)

29 The Joint Commission. (2021). Standard RC.01.03.01. *Comprehensive accreditation manual for hospitals.* Oakbrook Terrace, IL: The Joint Commission. (Level VII)

30 Centers for Medicare and Medicaid Services, Department of Health and Human Services. (2020). Condition of participation: Medical record services. 42 C.F.R. § 482.24.

31 Accreditation Association for Hospitals and Health Systems. (2020). Standard 10.00.03. *Healthcare Facilities Accreditation Program: Accreditation requirements for acute care hospitals.* Chicago, IL: Accreditation Association for Hospitals and Health Systems. (Level VII)

32 DNV GL-Healthcare USA, Inc. (2020). MR.2.SR.1. *NIAHO® accreditation requirements, interpretive guidelines and surveyor guidance—revision 20.0.* Milford, OH: DNV GL-Healthcare USA, Inc. (Level VII)

33 Rothrock, J. C. (2019). *Alexander's care of the patient in surgery* (16th ed.). St. Louis, MO: Elsevier.

34 Delaisse, J., et al. (2014). Peri-operative management of the patient with body piercings. *Journal of Dermatology and Clinical Research, 2*(1), 1009.

BONE MARROW ASPIRATION AND BIOPSY, ASSISTING

Bone marrow is the major site of blood cell formation. Obtaining a specimen enables evaluation of overall blood composition, blood elements, precursor cells, and abnormal or malignant cells. A practitioner may obtain a bone marrow specimen by aspiration or needle biopsy. (See *Obtaining a bone marrow specimen.*)

Aspiration and biopsy help diagnose leukemia, multiple myeloma, anemias, and other blood disorders. They can also help assess bone marrow cellularity, cellular morphology, and maturation.[1] During aspiration, the practitioner removes cells through a needle inserted into the marrow cavity of the bone. During a biopsy, the practitioner removes a small, solid core of marrow tissue through the needle. A physician, an advanced practice nurse, or another specially trained practitioner performs both procedures, usually at the same time, to stage the disease and monitor the patient's response to treatment. Note that bone marrow biopsy is contraindicated in patients with severe bleeding disorders.[1]

Bone marrow aspiration and biopsy require a sedative, pain medication, or moderate sedation, depending on the patient's condition.[2,3,4]

Equipment

Bone marrow tray (which generally includes sterile gauze or cotton balls; sterile forceps; sterile scalpel; sterile bowl; sterile marker; antiseptic solution [chlorhexidine-based preparation][2]; two sterile fenestrated drapes; 4″ × 4″ [10-cm × 10-cm] gauze pads; 2″ × 2″ [5-cm × 5-cm] gauze pads; 10-mL or 20-mL syringes; 21G or 22G 1″ [2.5-cm] or 2″ [5-cm] needle; specimen container with appropriate fixative; bone marrow needle; biopsy needle; specimen tubes; glass slides and cover glass; sterile labels; adhesive tape; and sterile gloves) ▪ gloves ▪ sterile gown ▪ mask with face shield or masks and goggles ▪ vital signs monitoring equipment ▪ pulse oximeter and probe ▪ alcohol pads ▪ 1% or 2% lidocaine with syringe and needle ▪ labels ▪ laboratory biohazard transport bag ▪ Optional: prescribed antibiotic ointment, prescribed sedative, prescribed pain medication, emergency equipment (code cart with emergency medications, defibrillator, handheld resuscitation bag with mask, intubation equipment), moderate sedation medication, IV catheter insertion equipment, cardiac monitoring equipment.

Most of the equipment above is available in a sterile, prepackaged tray. Familiarize yourself with your facility's tray and obtain any additional equipment needed.

Preparation of equipment

Inspect all equipment and supplies. If a product is expired, is defective, or has compromised integrity, remove it from patient use, label it as expired or defective, and report the expiration or defect as directed by your facility. If the patient is receiving moderate sedation, make sure that emergency equipment is functioning properly and readily available.

Obtaining a bone marrow specimen

Aspiration removes cells through a needle inserted into the marrow cavity of the bone; a biopsy removes a small, solid core of marrow tissue through the needle. The illustration below shows the removal of bone marrow from the posterior iliac crest.

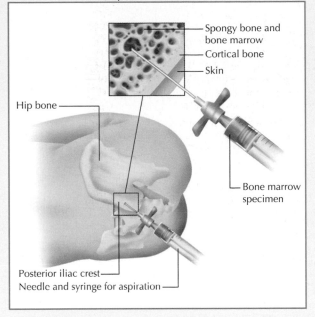

Spongy bone and bone marrow
Cortical bone
Skin
Hip bone
Bone marrow specimen
Posterior iliac crest
Needle and syringe for aspiration

Implementation

- Verify the practitioner's order.
- Gather and prepare the necessary equipment and supplies.
- Confirm that informed consent has been obtained and that the signed consent form is in the patient's medical record.[5,6,7,8]
- Check the patient's medical record for a history of allergies to the local anesthetic and pain and sedation medications.
- Assess the patient for an increased risk of bleeding, and assess coagulation studies and complete blood count, as ordered.[2]
- Conduct a preprocedure verification *to make sure that all relevant documentation, information, and equipment are available and correctly identified to the patient's identifiers.*[9,10]
- Perform hand hygiene.[11,12,13,14,15,16]
- Confirm the patient's identity by using at least two patient identifiers.[17]
- Provide privacy.[18,19,20,21]
- Reinforce the practitioner's explanation of the procedure to the patient and family (if appropriate) according to their individual communication and learning needs *to increase their understanding, allay their fears, and enhance cooperation.* Answer any questions they may have.[5,6,7,8]
- Tell the patient which bone the practitioner will aspirate. Inform patient that the practitioner will administer a local anesthetic and that the patient will feel a heavy pressure during insertion of the biopsy or aspiration needle, as well as a brief pulling sensation. Tell the patient that the practitioner may make a small incision *to avoid tearing the skin.*
- Encourage the patient to verbalize any discomfort or anxiety during the procedure.
- Explain to the patient with osteoporosis that the needle pressure may be minimal and that a drill may be necessary.
- Inform the patient that the procedure normally takes about 20 minutes, and that the practitioner may need more than one marrow specimen.
- If appropriate, make sure that the aspiration site has been marked as directed by your facility.[22]
- If the patient will be receiving moderate sedation, ensure patent IV access. (See the "IV catheter insertion and removal" procedure.)

- Attach the patient to a cardiac monitor if moderate sedation will be used and the monitor isn't already attached.[2] Make sure that alarm limits are set appropriately for the patient's current condition, and that alarms are turned on, functioning properly, and audible to staff.[23,24,25]
- Assess the patient's vital signs and oxygen saturation level by pulse oximetry *to provide baselines to monitor for changes during and after the procedure.*[2,26]
- Screen for and assess the patient's pain using facility-defined criteria that are consistent with the patient's age, condition, and ability to understand.[27]
- Perform hand hygiene.[11,12,13,14,15,16]
- The practitioner puts on a cap and mask, performs hand hygiene, and puts on a sterile gown and sterile gloves.[11,12,13,14,15,16]
- Prepare the sterile field, open the prepackaged tray, and prepare the supplies.
- Assist with labeling all medications, medication containers, and other solutions on and off the sterile field.[28,29]
- As ordered, administer a sedative, pain medication, or moderate sedation following safe medication administration practices.[2,30,31,32,33,34]
- Raise the bed to waist level before providing care, to prevent caregiver back strain.[35]
- Perform hand hygiene.[11,12,13,14,15,16]
- Put on gloves.[36,37,38]
- Position the patient according to the selected puncture site and instruct the patient to remain as still as possible. (See *Preferred site for bone marrow aspiration and biopsy,* page 88.)
- Conduct a time-out immediately before starting the procedure *to ensure identification of the correct patient, site, positioning, and procedure and that, as applicable, all relevant information and necessary equipment are available during and after the procedure.*[39]
- Using sterile forceps and sterile gauze or cotton balls, the practitioner cleans the puncture site with antiseptic solution and lets it dry. Then, the practitioner covers the area with sterile drapes.
- Assist the practitioner, as needed, during the procedure.
- To anesthetize the site, the practitioner infiltrates it with 1% or 2% lidocaine, using an appropriately sized needle to inject a small amount intradermally and then a larger 21G or 22G 1″ to 2″ (2.5-cm to 5-cm) needle *to anesthetize the tissue down to the bone.*[1,2]
- When the needle tip reaches the bone, the practitioner anesthetizes the periosteum by injecting a small amount of lidocaine in a circular area about ¾″ (2 cm) in diameter.[1] The practitioner should withdraw the needle from the periosteum after each injection.
- After allowing about 1 minute for the lidocaine to take effect, the practitioner may use a scalpel to make a small stab incision in the patient's skin to accommodate the bone marrow needle. *This technique facilitates entry and also helps avoid unnecessary skin tearing to help reduce the risk of infection and promote healing.*[1]
- Monitor vital signs, oxygen saturation, and pain levels throughout the procedure. For the patient receiving moderate sedation, see the "Moderate sedation" procedure.[2,26]

Bone marrow aspiration

- The practitioner inserts the bone marrow needle and lodges it firmly in the bone cortex. If the patient feels sharp pain instead of pressure when the needle first touches bone, the practitioner most likely inserted the needle outside the anesthetized area. If this is the case, the practitioner should withdraw the needle slightly and moved to the anesthetized area.[2]
- The practitioner advances the needle by applying an even, downward force with the heel of the hand or the palm, while twisting the needle back and forth slightly. A "giving" sensation means that the needle has entered the marrow cavity.[1,2]
- The practitioner removes the inner cannula, attaches a syringe to the needle, aspirates the required specimen (usually 3 to 5 mL), and removes the syringe.[2]
- The practitioner or assistant places a small portion of the specimen on a glass slide *to verify the presence of spicules.* The remainder of the specimen is placed in the appropriate tubes for clot sections or molecular studies.[2]

Preferred site for bone marrow aspiration and biopsy

The iliac crest is the only site at which aspiration and biopsy may be safely performed in an adult.[1] The posterior superior iliac crest (as shown below) is the preferred site for aspiration, *because this site decreases the risk of pain, increases accessibility, and isn't near any vital organs or vessels.*[1] The patient should be placed in the lateral position with one leg flexed, or in the prone position.[1,2] The practitioner may use the anterior iliac crest with a patient who can't lie prone, or when the posterior iliac crest is unapproachable or not available because of infection, injury, or morbid obesity.[1] This location is generally not preferred *because its dense cortical layer, which makes obtaining specimens more difficult, necessitates smaller specimens, and increases the risk of pain.*

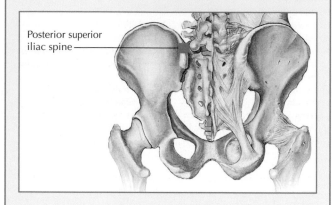

Posterior superior iliac spine

■ The practitioner attaches a second syringe and aspirates additional samples, which are placed in the appropriate tubes.[2]
■ Assist by inverting all the tubes several times *to thoroughly mix and prevent clotting.*[2]
■ Label the specimen in the presence of the patient to prevent mislabeling.[17]
■ After needle removal, if a bone marrow biopsy isn't being performed, the practitioner applies pressure to the aspiration site with a gauze pad for 5 minutes *to control bleeding.*[2]
■ Clean the area with an antiseptic solution and apply an antibiotic ointment, if prescribed.[2]
■ Apply a sterile pressure dressing.
■ Have the patient remain in a supine position for 10 to 15 minutes *to maintain pressure at the aspiration site.*[2]

Bone marrow biopsy

■ The practitioner inserts a biopsy needle into the periosteum through the same incision but at a slightly different site, and advances it steadily until the outer needle passes into the marrow cavity. The practitioner directs the biopsy needle into the marrow cavity by alternately rotating the inner needle clockwise and counterclockwise.[1]
■ The practitioner removes a plug of tissue, withdraws the needle assembly, and expels the bone core specimen on a glass slide or nonadherent dressing.[2]
■ After needle removal, the practitioner firmly presses a sterile 2″ × 2″ (5 cm × 5 cm) gauze pad against the incision for 5 minutes or until bleeding ceases.[1]
■ Clean the area around the biopsy with an antiseptic solution and apply an antibiotic ointment, if prescribed.[2]
■ Apply a sterile pressure dressing.
■ Assist the practitioner with touching the glass slides gently against the bone core biopsy sample to make imprints. Then help place the bone core sample in a specimen container with the appropriate solution (10% formalin fixative or sterile saline solution–soaked gauze) for processing.
■ Label the specimen in the presence of the patient to prevent mislabeling.[17]
■ Have the patient lie in the supine position for 10 to 15 minutes *to maintain pressure at the biopsy site.*[2]

Completing the procedure

■ Discard used supplies in appropriate receptacles.[36]
■ Assist the patient into a comfortable position.
■ Return the bed to the lowest position *to prevent falls and maintain the patient's safety.*[40]
■ Place the specimen in a biohazard transport bag and send it to the laboratory immediately.[36]
■ Remove and discard your gloves[36] and perform hand hygiene.[11,12,13,14,15,16]
■ Continue to assess the patient until fully awake.[2] Note that the duration of medications administered for sedation may extend the length of time needed to complete the procedure.
■ Reassess and respond to pain by evaluating the patient's response to treatment and progress toward pain management goals. Assess for adverse reactions and risk factors for adverse events that may result from treatment.[27]
■ Perform hand hygiene.[11,12,13,14,15,16]
■ Document the procedure.[43,44,45,46]

Special considerations

■ Faulty needle placement may yield too little aspirate. If aspiration doesn't produce a specimen, the practitioner must withdraw the needle from the bone (but not from the overlying soft tissue), replace the stylet, and insert the needle into a second site within the anesthetized field.[2]
■ The Joint Commission has issued a sentinel event alert concerning medical device alarm safety *because alarm-related events have been associated with permanent loss of function and death.* Among the major contributing factors were improper alarm settings, alarms turned off inappropriately, and alarm signals that are inaudible to staff members. Make sure that alarm limits are set appropriately, and that alarms are turned on, functioning properly, and audible to staff. Follow facility guidelines for preventing alarm fatigue.[47]
■ If the patient has received sedation, provide instruction about safety concerns and driving restrictions. Monitor the patient closely.
■ Bone marrow specimen collection shouldn't occur from irradiated areas, *because radiation may have altered or destroyed the marrow.*[1]
■ Apply ice to the site, as needed and ordered, *to reduce discomfort and the risk of bleeding.*[2]

Patient teaching

Instruct the patient and family (if applicable) to leave the sterile pressure dressing in place for 24 hours, according to the practitioner's orders.[2] Advise the patient to avoid strenuous activity, tub baths, hot tubs, swimming pools, and whirlpool baths for 48 hours after the procedure *to allow the biopsy site adequate time to heal.* Tell the patient to expect mild to moderate discomfort at the site for 24 to 48 hours. Instruct the patient to take analgesics as needed, but to avoid aspirin and nonsteroidal anti-inflammatory drugs for 24 hours *to minimize the risk of bleeding from the site.*[2] Tell the patient to call the practitioner for bleeding or fever after discharge.

Complications

Bleeding and infection are potentially life-threatening complications of aspiration and biopsy at any site. Rarely, tumor seeding or needle breakage may occur. Complications of sternal needle puncture are uncommon but include puncture of the heart and major vessels, causing severe hemorrhage; puncture of the mediastinum, causing mediastinitis or pneumomediastinum; and pulmonary emboli, sternal fracture, and puncture of the lung, causing pneumothorax.[1]

Documentation

Document the time and date of the procedure, the location of the aspiration and biopsy site, and the patient's tolerance of the procedure. Note the amount and color of aspirated marrow, ordered laboratory tests, and the time you sent the specimen to the laboratory. Record the patient's vital signs, oxygen saturation level, pain level, level of consciousness, and cardiac arrhythmias or other complications that occurred during the procedure, any prescribed interventions, and the patient's response to those interventions. Document the type of dressing applied. Document teaching provided to the patient and family (if applicable), their understanding of that teaching, and any need for follow-up teaching.

REFERENCES

1 Zehnder, J. L. (2020). Bone marrow aspiration and biopsy: Indications and technique. In: *UpToDate*, Larson, R. A. (Ed.).

2 Wiegand, D. L. (Ed.). (2017). *AACN procedure manual for high acuity, progressive, and critical care* (7th ed.). St. Louis, MO: Elsevier.

3 McGrath, P., et al. (2013). Procedural care for adult bone marrow aspiration and biopsy: Qualitative research findings from Australia. *Cancer Nursing, 36*, 309–316. (Level VI)

4 Tanasale, B., et al. (2013). Pain and anxiety during bone marrow biopsy. *Pain Management Nursing, 14*, 310–317. (Level VI)

5 The Joint Commission. (2021). Standard RI.01.03.01. *Comprehensive accreditation manual for hospitals*. Oakbrook Terrace, IL: The Joint Commission. (Level VII)

6 Accreditation Association for Hospitals and Health Systems. (2020). Standard 15.01.11. *Healthcare Facilities Accreditation Program: Accreditation requirements for acute care hospitals*. Chicago, IL: Accreditation Association for Hospitals and Health Systems. (Level VII)

7 Centers for Medicare and Medicaid Services, Department of Health and Human Services. (2020). Condition of participation: Patient's rights. 42 C.F.R. § 482.13(b)(2).

8 DNV GL-Healthcare USA, Inc. (2020). PR.2.SR.3. *NIAHO® accreditation requirements, interpretive guidelines and surveyor guidance—revision 20.0.* Milford, OH: DNV GL-Healthcare USA, Inc. (Level VII)

9 The Joint Commission. (2021). Standard UP.01.01.01. *Comprehensive accreditation manual for hospitals*. Oakbrook Terrace, IL: The Joint Commission. (Level VII)

10 Accreditation Association for Hospitals and Health Systems. (2020). Standard 30.00.14. *Healthcare Facilities Accreditation Program: Accreditation requirements for acute care hospitals*. Chicago, IL: Accreditation Association for Hospitals and Health Systems. (Level VII)

11 Centers for Disease Control and Prevention. (2002). Guideline for hand hygiene in health-care settings: Recommendations of the Healthcare Infection Control Practices Advisory Committee and the HICPAC/SHEA/APIC/IDSA Hand Hygiene Task Force. *MMWR Recommendations and Reports, 51*(RR-16), 1–45, http://www.cdc.gov/mmwr/pdf/rr/rr5116.pdf (Level II)

12 The Joint Commission. (2021). Standard NPSG.07.01.01. *Comprehensive accreditation manual for hospitals*. Oakbrook Terrace, IL: The Joint Commission. (Level VII)

13 World Health Organization. (2009). WHO guidelines on hand hygiene in health care: First global patient safety challenge, clean care is safer care. https://apps.who.int/iris/bitstream/handle/10665/44102/9789241597906_eng.pdf?sequence=1 (Level IV)

14 Centers for Medicare and Medicaid Services, Department of Health and Human Services. (2020). Condition of participation: Infection control. 42 C.F.R. § 482.42.

15 Accreditation Association for Hospitals and Health Systems. (2020). Standard 07.01.21. *Healthcare Facilities Accreditation Program: Accreditation requirements for acute care hospitals*. Chicago, IL: Accreditation Association for Hospitals and Health Systems. (Level VII)

16 DNV GL-Healthcare USA, Inc. (2020). IC.1.SR.1. *NIAHO® accreditation requirements, interpretive guidelines and surveyor guidance—revision 20.0.* Milford, OH: DNV GL-Healthcare USA, Inc. (Level VII)

17 The Joint Commission. (2021). Standard NPSG.01.01.01. *Comprehensive accreditation manual for hospitals*. Oakbrook Terrace, IL: The Joint Commission. (Level VII)

18 The Joint Commission. (2021). Standard RI.01.01.01. *Comprehensive accreditation manual for hospitals*. Oakbrook Terrace, IL: The Joint Commission. (Level VII)

19 Centers for Medicare and Medicaid Services, Department of Health and Human Services. (2020). Condition of participation: Patient's rights. 42 C.F.R. § 482.13(c)(1).

20 Accreditation Association for Hospitals and Health Systems. (2020). Standard 15.01.16. *Healthcare Facilities Accreditation Program: Accreditation requirements for acute care hospitals*. Chicago, IL: Accreditation Association for Hospitals and Health Systems. (Level VII)

21 DNV GL-Healthcare USA, Inc. (2020). PR.2.SR.5. *NIAHO® accreditation requirements, interpretive guidelines and surveyor guidance—revision 20.0.* Milford, OH: DNV GL-Healthcare USA, Inc. (Level VII)

22 The Joint Commission. (2021). Standard UP.01.02.01. *Comprehensive accreditation manual for hospitals*. Oakbrook Terrace, IL: The Joint Commission. (Level VII)

23 Graham, K. C., & Cvach, M. (2010). Monitor alarm fatigue: Standardizing use of physiological monitors and decreasing nuisance alarms. *American Journal of Critical Care, 19*, 28–37.

24 American Association of Critical-Care Nurses. (2018). AACN practice alert: Managing alarms in acute care across the life span—Electrocardiography and pulse oximetry. https://www.aacn.org/clinical-resources/practice-alerts/managing-alarms-in-acute-care-across-the-life-span (Level VII)

25 The Joint Commission. (2021). Standard NPSG.06.01.01. *Comprehensive accreditation manual for hospitals*. Oakbrook Terrace, IL: The Joint Commission. (Level VII)

26 The Joint Commission. (2021). Standard PC.01.02.03. *Comprehensive accreditation manual for hospitals*. Oakbrook Terrace, IL: The Joint Commission. (Level VII)

27 The Joint Commission. (2021). Standard PC.01.02.07. *Comprehensive accreditation manual for hospitals*. Oakbrook Terrace, IL: The Joint Commission. (Level VII)

28 The Joint Commission. (2021). Standard NPSG.03.04.01. *Comprehensive accreditation manual for hospitals*. Oakbrook Terrace, IL: The Joint Commission. (Level VII)

29 Accreditation Association for Hospitals and Health Systems. (2020). Standard 25.01.27. *Healthcare Facilities Accreditation Program: Accreditation requirements for acute care hospitals*. Chicago, IL: Accreditation Association for Hospitals and Health Systems. (Level VII)

30 Talamo, G., et al. (2010). Oral administration of analgesia and anxiolysis for pain associated with bone marrow biopsy. *Supportive Care in Cancer, 18*, 301–305.

31 The Joint Commission. (2021). Standard MM.06.01.01. *Comprehensive accreditation manual for hospitals*. Oakbrook Terrace, IL: The Joint Commission. (Level VII)

32 Centers for Medicare and Medicaid Services, Department of Health and Human Services. (2020). Condition of participation: Nursing services. 42 C.F.R. § 482.23(c).

33 Accreditation Association for Hospitals and Health Systems. (2020). Standard 16.01.03. *Healthcare Facilities Accreditation Program: Accreditation requirements for acute care hospitals*. Chicago, IL: Accreditation Association for Hospitals and Health Systems. (Level VII)

34 DNV GL-Healthcare USA, Inc. (2020). MM.1.SR.3. *NIAHO® accreditation requirements, interpretive guidelines and surveyor guidance—revision 20.0.* Milford, OH: DNV GL-Healthcare USA, Inc. (Level VII)

35 Waters, T. R., et al. (2009). Safe patient handling training for schools of nursing. https://www.cdc.gov/niosh/docs/2009-127/pdfs/2009-127.pdf (Level VII)

36 Occupational Safety and Health Administration. (2012). Bloodborne pathogens, standard number 1910.1030. https://www.osha.gov/pls/oshaweb/owadisp.show_document?p_id=10051&p_table=STANDARDS (Level VII)

37 Siegel, J. D., et al. (2007, revised 2019). 2007 guideline for isolation precautions: Preventing transmission of infectious agents in healthcare settings. https://www.cdc.gov/infectioncontrol/pdf/guidelines/isolation-guidelines-H.pdf (Level II)

38 Accreditation Association for Hospitals and Health Systems. (202-). Standard 07.01.10. *Healthcare Facilities Accreditation Program: Accreditation requirements for acute care hospitals*. Chicago, IL: Accreditation Association for Hospitals and Health Systems. (Level VII)

39 The Joint Commission. (2021). Standard UP.01.03.01. *Comprehensive accreditation manual for hospitals*. Oakbrook Terrace, IL: The Joint Commission. (Level VII)

40 Ganz, D. A., et al. (2013-reviewed 2021). *Preventing falls in hospitals: A toolkit for improving quality of care* (AHRQ Publication No. 13-0015-EF). Rockville, MD: Agency for Healthcare Research and Quality. https://www.ahrq.gov/professionals/systems/hospital/fallpxtoolkit/index.html (Level VII)

41 Accreditation Association for Hospitals and Health Systems. (2020). Standard 07.02.03. *Healthcare Facilities Accreditation Program: Accreditation requirements for acute care hospitals*. Chicago, IL: Accreditation Association for Hospitals and Health Systems. (Level VII)

42 Rutala, W. A., et al. (2008, revised 2019). Guideline for disinfection and sterilization in healthcare facilities, 2008. https://www.cdc.gov/infectioncontrol/pdf/guidelines/disinfection-guidelines-H.pdf (Level I)

43 The Joint Commission. (2021). Standard RC.01.03.01. *Comprehensive accreditation manual for hospitals*. Oakbrook Terrace, IL: The Joint Commission. (Level VII)

44 Centers for Medicare and Medicaid Services, Department of Health and Human Services. (2020). Condition of participation: Medical record services. 42 C.F.R. § 482.24(b).

45 Accreditation Association for Hospitals and Health Systems. (2020). Standard 10.00.03. *Healthcare Facilities Accreditation Program: Accreditation requirements for acute care hospitals.* Chicago, IL: Accreditation Association for Hospitals and Health Systems. (Level VII)

46 DNV GL-Healthcare USA, Inc. (2020). MR.2.SR.1. *NIAHO® accreditation requirements, interpretive guidelines and surveyor guidance—revision 20.0.* Milford, OH: DNV GL-Healthcare USA, Inc. (Level VII)

47 The Joint Commission. (2013). Sentinel event alert 50: Medical device alarm safety in hospitals. https://www.jointcommission.org/assets/1/6/SEA_50_alarms_4_26_16.pdf (Level VII)

BRAIN TISSUE OXYGEN MONITORING AND CARE

Brain tissue oxygen ($PbtO_2$) monitoring measures oxygen delivery to the cerebral tissue. It can help identify cerebral ischemia and hypoxia in patients with a brain tumor, traumatic brain injury, stroke, or aneurysmal or traumatic subarachnoid hemorrhage, as well as in those at risk for secondary brain injury.[1] Complications that result in cerebral hypoxia, including elevated intracranial pressure (ICP), shivering, agitation, seizures, fever, hypotension, hypovolemia, anemia, and hypoxia, are common causes of secondary brain injuries. Cerebral hypoxia, in turn, can lead to cerebral ischemia.

$PbtO_2$ monitoring involves the use of a $PbtO_2$ probe that the practitioner inserts through an intracranial bolt or tunnels under the scalp using a probe guide and trocar. When tunneled under the scalp, the system can measure brain tissue temperature and $PbtO_2$ saturation. When used with an intracranial bolt, the system measures ICP, brain tissue temperature, and $PbtO_2$ saturation. By detecting early changes in ICP and $PbtO_2$, this system allows treatment interventions to be performed before secondary brain injury occurs. Contraindications to $PbtO_2$ monitoring include anticoagulation therapy, insertion site infection, and coagulopathy.[1]

The normal value for $PbtO_2$ ranges between 20 and 35 mm Hg.[1] Decreased $PbtO_2$ values occur when an increase in oxygen demand or a decrease in oxygen delivery occurs.[1] Increased $PbtO_2$ values occur when oxygen delivery increases or oxygen demand decreases.[1]

Equipment

$PbtO_2$ monitor ▪ monitor-to-patient connecting cables ▪ $PbtO_2$ probe ▪ cardiopulmonary monitor ▪ vital signs monitoring equipment ▪ Optional: sedative, neuromuscular blocking agent, other prescribed medications, cooling device, cap, gown, goggles or mask with face shield, gloves.

Preparation of equipment

Inspect all equipment and supplies. If a product is expired, is defective, or has compromised integrity, remove it from patient use, label it as expired or defective, and report the expiration or defect as directed by your facility. If the $PbtO_2$ monitor that you're using isn't self-calibrating, calibrate the unit according to the manufacturer's instructions, *because failure to calibrate the device can lead to false readings.*

Implementation

▪ Verify the practitioner's order.
▪ Gather and prepare the necessary equipment and supplies.
▪ Perform hand hygiene.[2,3,4,5,6,7]
▪ Confirm the patient's identity using at least two patient identifiers.[8]
▪ Provide privacy.[9,10,11,12]
▪ Explain the procedure to the patient and family (if appropriate) according to their individual communication and learning needs *to increase their understanding, allay their fears, and enhance cooperation.*[13] Answer any questions *to promote their understanding of the information you provided.*
▪ Raise the bed to waist level *to prevent caregiver back strain.*[14]
▪ Perform hand hygiene.[2,3,4,5,6,7]
▪ Put on personal protective equipment, as needed, *to comply with standard precautions.*[15,16]

▪ Assess the patient's ICP (see the "Intracranial pressure monitoring" procedure), neurologic status, vital signs, and $PbtO_2$ *to obtain baseline measurements.* Continue to monitor these parameters every 15 minutes until the patient's condition stabilizes, then hourly or as ordered, *to provide ongoing assessment.*[1,17] Ensure that all monitor alarm limits are set appropriately for the patient's current condition, and that the alarms are turned on, functioning properly, and audible to staff.[18,19,20,21]
▪ Perform an oxygen challenge test, as ordered, if the patient's $PbtO_2$ value is unexpectedly low or if you question the $PbtO_2$ probe's accuracy. *This helps to confirm correct placement of the probe as well as probe functioning.* To perform the oxygen challenge test, set the fraction of inspired oxygen on the ventilator at 100% for 2 to 5 minutes; if the probe is accurate, the $PbtO_2$ value will increase.[1,22]
▪ Maintain the $PbtO_2$ value between 20 and 35 mm Hg, or as ordered by the practitioner.[1]
▪ Frequently assess the insertion site for signs of infection and other complications.[1]
▪ Obtain the patient's temperature every 1 to 2 hours and compare it with the cerebral temperature.[1] Institute cooling measures, according to the patient's condition and as ordered by the practitioner, *to reduce metabolic demand resulting from hyperthermia.*

NURSING ALERT The use of noninvasive and invasive cooling measures may result in patient shivering, consequently increasing skeletal muscle oxygen consumption and reducing valuable cerebral oxygen reserves. Use of a sedative and a neuromuscular blocking agent may be necessary *to maintain hypothermia and minimize systemic oxygen consumption.*

▪ Administer and titrate a sedative and neuromuscular blocking agent as ordered, following safe medication administration practices.[23,24,25,26] Maintain target sedation levels *to avoid oversedation and undersedation.* Remember that a patient receiving a neuromuscular blocking agent requires close observation *because of the inability to breathe and communicate.*
▪ Administer other medications as prescribed, such as an antipyretic or anti-inflammatory agent *to reduce hyperthermia,* following safe medication administration practices.[23,24,25,26]
▪ Remove and discard any personal protective equipment, if worn.[15,16]
▪ Return the bed to the lowest *position to prevent falls and maintain patient safety.*[27]
▪ Perform hand hygiene.[2,3,4,5,6,7]
▪ Document the procedure.[28,29,30,31]

Special considerations

▪ The Joint Commission has issued a sentinel event alert concerning medical device alarm safety, *because alarm-related events have been associated with permanent loss of function and death.* Among the major contributing factors were improper alarm settings, alarm settings turned off inappropriately, and alarm signals that are inaudible to staff. Make sure that alarm limits are set appropriately and that alarms are turned on, functioning properly, and audible to staff. Follow facility guidelines for preventing alarm fatigue.[18]
▪ $PbtO_2$ probes are compatible with magnetic resonance imaging (MRI) scanners not equipped with fiberoptic ICP devices. Follow the manufacturer's guidelines regarding MRI compatibility with the $PbtO_2$ probe. As directed, disconnect all cables and patient monitoring devices from the probe before entering the MRI environment *to avoid serious patient injury.*[32]
▪ $PbtO_2$ probes may remain in place for 5 to 7 days; check the manufacturer's guidelines.[1]

Complications

Possible complications of $PbtO_2$ monitoring include infection, cerebrospinal fluid leak, and bleeding.

Documentation

Document neurologic assessment findings, vital signs, ICP, temperature, and insertion site assessment findings. Record $PbtO_2$ values at least every hour. Document any medications that you administered, including the medication strength, dose, route of administration, and date and time of administration.[33] Also document the patient's tolerance of the procedure, any unexpected outcomes or complications, the name of the practitioner you notified, the date and time of notification, prescribed interventions, and the patient's response to those interventions. Document teaching that you provided to the patient and family (if applicable), their understanding of that teaching, and any need for follow-up teaching.

REFERENCES

1 Wiegand, D. L. (2017). *AACN procedure manual for high acuity, progressive, and critical care* (7th ed.). St. Louis, MO: Elsevier.

2 Centers for Disease Control and Prevention. (2002). Guideline for hand hygiene in health-care settings: Recommendations of the Healthcare Infection Control Practices Advisory Committee and the HICPAC/SHEA/APIC/IDSA Hand Hygiene Task Force. *MMWR Recommendations and Reports, 51*(RR-16), 1–45. https://www.cdc.gov/mmwr/pdf/rr/rr5116.pdf (Level II)

3 The Joint Commission. (2021). Standard NPSG.07.01.01. *Comprehensive accreditation manual for hospitals*. Oakbrook Terrace, IL: The Joint Commission. (Level VII)

4 World Health Organization. (2009). WHO guidelines on hand hygiene in health care: First global patient safety challenge, clean care is safer care. https://apps.who.int/iris/bitstream/handle/10665/44102/9789241597906_eng.pdf?sequence=1 (Level IV)

5 Accreditation Association for Hospitals and Health Systems. (2020). Standard 07.01.21. *Healthcare Facilities Accreditation Program: Accreditation requirements for acute care hospitals*. Chicago, IL: Accreditation Association for Hospitals and Health Systems. (Level VII)

6 Centers for Medicare and Medicaid Services, Department of Health and Human Services. (2020). Condition of participation: Infection control. 42 C.F.R. § 482.42.

7 DNV GL-Healthcare USA, Inc. (2020). IC.1.SR.1. *NIAHO® accreditation requirements, interpretive guidelines and surveyor guidance—revision 20.0*. Milford, OH: DNV GL-Healthcare USA, Inc. (Level VII)

8 The Joint Commission. (2021). Standard NPSG.01.01.01. *Comprehensive accreditation manual for hospitals*. Oakbrook Terrace, IL: The Joint Commission. (Level VII)

9 Accreditation Association for Hospitals and Health Systems. (2020). Standard 15.01.16. *Healthcare Facilities Accreditation Program: Accreditation requirements for acute care hospitals*. Chicago, IL: Accreditation Association for Hospitals and Health Systems. (Level VII)

10 Centers for Medicare and Medicaid Services, Department of Health and Human Services. (2020). Condition of participation: Patient's rights. 42 C.F.R. § 482.13(c)(1).

11 DNV GL-Healthcare USA, Inc. (2020). PR.2.SR.5. *NIAHO® accreditation requirements, interpretive guidelines and surveyor guidance—revision 20.0*. Milford, OH: DNV GL-Healthcare USA, Inc. (Level VII)

12 The Joint Commission. (2021). Standard RI.01.01.01. *Comprehensive accreditation manual for hospitals*. Oakbrook Terrace, IL: The Joint Commission. (Level VII)

13 The Joint Commission. (2021). Standard PC.02.01.21. *Comprehensive accreditation manual for hospitals*. Oakbrook Terrace, IL: The Joint Commission. (Level VII)

14 Waters, T. R., et al. (2009). Safe patient handling training for schools of nursing. https://www.cdc.gov/niosh/docs/2009-127/pdfs/2009-127.pdf (Level VII)

15 Siegel, J. D., et al. (2007, revised 2019). 2007 guideline for isolation precautions: Preventing transmission of infectious agents in healthcare settings. https://www.cdc.gov/infectioncontrol/pdf/guidelines/isolation-guidelines-H.pdf (Level II)

16 Accreditation Association for Hospitals and Health Systems. (2020). Standard 07.01.10. *Healthcare Facilities Accreditation Program: Accreditation requirements for acute care hospitals*. Chicago, IL: Accreditation Association for Hospitals and Health Systems. (Level VII)

17 American Association of Neuroscience Nurses (AANN). (2014). *Care of the patient undergoing intracranial pressure monitoring/external ventricular drainage or lumbar drainage: AANN clinical practice guideline series*. Glenview, IL: AANN. (Level VII)

18 The Joint Commission. (2013). Sentinel event alert 50: Medical device alarm safety in hospitals. https://www.jointcommission.org/assets/1/6/SEA_50_alarms_4_26_16.pdf (Level VII)

19 The Joint Commission. (2021). Standard NPSG.06.01.01. *Comprehensive accreditation manual for hospitals*. Oakbrook Terrace, IL: The Joint Commission. (Level VII)

20 American Association of Critical-Care Nurses. (2018). AACN practice alert: Managing alarms in acute care across the life span—Electrocardiography and pulse oximetry. https://www.aacn.org/clinical-resources/practice-alerts/managing-alarms-in-acute-care-across-the-life-span (Level VII)

21 Graham, K. C., & Cvach, M. (2010). Monitor alarm fatigue: Standardizing use of physiological monitors and decreasing nuisance alarms. *American Journal of Critical Care, 19*, 28–37.

22 Martini, R. P., et al. (2013). Targeting brain tissue oxygenation in traumatic brain injury. *Respiratory Care, 58*, 162–172. http://rc.rcjournal.com/content/58/1/162 (Level V)

23 Accreditation Association for Hospitals and Health Systems. (2020). Standard 16.01.03. *Healthcare Facilities Accreditation Program: Accreditation requirements for acute care hospitals*. Chicago, IL: Accreditation Association for Hospitals and Health Systems. (Level VII)

24 Centers for Medicare and Medicaid Services, Department of Health and Human Services. (2020). Condition of participation: Nursing services. 42 C.F.R. § 482.23(c).

25 The Joint Commission. (2021). Standard MM.06.01.01. *Comprehensive accreditation manual for hospitals*. Oakbrook Terrace, IL: The Joint Commission. (Level VII)

26 DNV GL-Healthcare USA, Inc. (2020). MM.1.SR.3. *NIAHO® accreditation requirements, interpretive guidelines and surveyor guidance—revision 20.0*. Milford, OH: DNV GL-Healthcare USA, Inc. (Level VII)

27 Ganz, D. A., et al. (2013-reviewed 2021). Preventing falls in hospitals: A toolkit for improving quality of care (AHRQ publication no. 13-0015-EF). https://www.ahrq.gov/professionals/systems/hospital/fallpxtoolkit/index.html (Level VII)

28 The Joint Commission. (2021). Standard RC.01.03.01. *Comprehensive accreditation manual for hospitals*. Oakbrook Terrace, IL: The Joint Commission. (Level VII)

29 Accreditation Association for Hospitals and Health Systems. (2020). Standard 10.00.03. *Healthcare Facilities Accreditation Program: Accreditation requirements for acute care hospitals*. Chicago, IL: Accreditation Association for Hospitals and Health Systems. (Level VII)

30 Centers for Medicare and Medicaid Services, Department of Health and Human Services. (2020). Condition of participation: Medical record services. 42 C.F.R. § 482.24(b).

31 DNV GL-Healthcare USA, Inc. (2020). MR.2.SR.1. *NIAHO® accreditation requirements, interpretive guidelines and surveyor guidance—revision 20.0*. Milford, OH: DNV GL-Healthcare USA, Inc. (Level VII)

32 Integra LifeSciences Corporation. (2013). Integra Licox brain tissue oxygen monitoring. https://www.integralife.com/file/general/1465323839.pdf (Level VII)

33 The Joint Commission. (2021). Standard RC.02.01.01. *Comprehensive accreditation manual for hospitals*. Oakbrook Terrace, IL: The Joint Commission. (Level VII)

BRAIN TISSUE OXYGEN MONITORING DEVICE, INSERTION, ASSISTING

Brain tissue oxygen ($PbtO_2$) monitoring measures oxygen delivery to the cerebral tissue. It can help identify cerebral ischemia and hypoxia in patients with a brain tumor, traumatic brain injury, stroke, or aneurysmal or traumatic subarachnoid hemorrhage, as well as those at risk for secondary brain injury.[1] Complications that result in cerebral hypoxia, including elevated intracranial pressure (ICP), shivering, agitation, seizures, fever, hypotension, hypovolemia, anemia, and hypoxia, are common causes of secondary brain injuries. Cerebral hypoxia, in turn, can lead to cerebral ischemia.

Use of $PbtO_2$ monitoring with ICP monitoring detects early changes in ICP and $PbtO_2$ so that treatment interventions can occur before secondary brain injury occurs. Normal values for $PbtO_2$ range from 20 to 35 mm Hg.[1] Contraindications to $PbtO_2$ monitoring include anticoagulation therapy, insertion site infection, and coagulopathy.[1]

A practitioner inserts a $PbtO_2$ probe through an intracranial bolt in a burr hole. Alternatively, the practitioner may tunnel the probe under the scalp using a probe guide and trocar. When used with an intracranial bolt, the system measures ICP, $PbtO_2$, and brain tissue temperature. The practitioner determines the insertion method and placement location after studying a computed tomography (CT) scan of the patient's brain and considering the patient's diagnosis.[2] (See *Brain tissue oxygen monitoring systems.*)

Equipment

Sterile gloves ▪ sterile gowns ▪ sterile drapes ▪ goggles and mask or mask with face shield ▪ surgical head covers ▪ antiseptic solution ▪ 4″ × 4″ (10-cm × 10-cm) gauze ▪ PbtO$_2$ monitor ▪ connecting cables from the monitor to the patient ▪ cranial access tray ▪ PbtO$_2$ probe (with smart card if using a Licox monitoring system) ▪ sterile occlusive dressing ▪ transparent adhesive dressing ▪ cardiopulmonary monitor ▪ pulse oximeter and probe ▪ blood pressure monitoring equipment ▪ prescribed sedative ▪ prescribed analgesia ▪ Optional: electric or battery-operated hair clippers with a single-use head or a reusable head that can be disinfected, tape, arm board, towels, washcloths, intracranial bolt system.

Preparation of equipment

Inspect all equipment and supplies. If a product is expired, is defective, or has compromised integrity, remove it from patient use, label it as expired or defective, and report the expiration or defect as directed by your facility. Gather a PbtO$_2$ monitor and plug it into an AC wall outlet, and then attach the cables to the PbtO$_2$ monitor. Some monitors and cables are color-coded.

Implementation

▪ Verify the practitioner's orders.
▪ Review the patient's medical record for allergies to prescribed medications or antiseptic solution and any contraindications to the procedure.[1]

Brain tissue oxygen monitoring systems

Two systems for monitoring brain tissue oxygen (PbtO$_2$) are a tunneled system and a bolt system.

Tunneled system

With the *tunneled system,* shown below, a practitioner tunnels an oxygen catheter probe under the scalp using a probe guide and trocar. Insertion of the device may occur during a cranial procedure at the margins of an existing bone flap or through a burr hole.

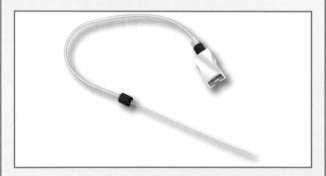

Bolt system

A practitioner inserts a *bolt system* for PbtO$_2$ monitoring, shown below, through a burr hole. This type of system has the capability of monitoring PbtO$_2$, brain tissue temperature, and intracranial pressure.

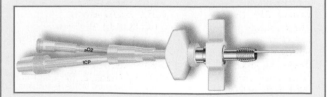

▪ Gather the necessary equipment and supplies.
▪ Confirm that informed consent has been obtained and that the signed consent form is in the patient's medical record.[1,2,3,4,5]
▪ Conduct a preprocedure verification *to make sure that all relevant documentation, related information, and equipment are available and matched correctly to the patient's identifiers.*[1,6,7]
▪ Verify that ordered laboratory and imaging studies have been completed and that the results are in the patient's medical record. Notify the practitioner of any unexpected results.
▪ Perform hand hygiene.[8,9,10,11,12,13]
▪ Confirm the patient's identity using at least two patient identifiers.[14]
▪ Provide privacy.[15,16,17,18]
▪ Explain the procedure to the patient and family (if appropriate) according to their communication and learning needs *to increase their understanding, allay their fears, and enhance cooperation.*[19]. Answer any questions *to increase their understanding of the information you provided.*
▪ Verify that the practitioner has marked the insertion site using an unambiguous mark according to the method determined by your facility.[20]
▪ Assess the patient's neurologic status before insertion *so that you can recognize any changes during and after insertion of the PbtO$_2$ probe.*[1]
▪ Attach the patient to a cardiac monitor, a pulse oximeter, and blood pressure monitoring equipment, and obtain measurements *to serve as a baseline for comparison during and after the procedure.* Make sure that alarm limits are set appropriately and that alarms are turned on, functioning properly, and audible to staff.[21,22,23,24]
▪ Before beginning the insertion procedure, administer analgesia, sedation, or both, as ordered, following safe medication administration practices, *to facilitate the insertion process.*[25,26,27,28]
▪ Keep the door to the room closed *to restrict traffic into the room and the subsequent risk of site contamination during insertion.*[29]
▪ Prepare the equipment, being careful not to contaminate the sterile field. Label all medications, medication containers, and other solutions on and off the sterile field while maintaining sterility of the sterile field.[30]
▪ Raise the patient's bed to waist level before providing patient care *to prevent caregiver back strain.*[31]
▪ Elevate the head of the bed to 30 degrees and place the patient's head in a neutral position. *This position helps decrease ICP by promoting jugular venous outflow, which provides for optimal insertion accessibility.*[1,29]
▪ Perform hand hygiene.[8,9,10,11,12,13]
▪ Immobilize the patient's head *to prevent movement and facilitate device insertion.*[29]
▪ Braid or clip the patient's hair. If you're clipping hair, use tape to remove residual hair clippings.[29]
▪ Perform hand hygiene.[8,9,10,11,12,13]
▪ Assist the practitioner with putting on a surgical head cover, a mask, protective eyewear, a sterile gown, and sterile gloves, as necessary. Put on the same personal protective equipment.[29,32,33]
▪ Assist the practitioner with site preparation using antiseptic solution *to prepare the patient for a sterile procedure.* Use antiseptic solution to clean the intended insertion site using a circular motion.[29] Make sure that the antiseptic is dry before the practitioner starts the incision.[1]
NURSING ALERT Use of chlorhexidine is controversial *because some studies suggest it's neurotoxic.*[1]
▪ Assist the practitioner with draping the patient's head, neck, and chest *to maintain a sterile field.*[1,29]
▪ Conduct a time-out immediately before starting the procedure *to perform a final assessment that the correct patient, site, positioning, and procedure are identified and that all relevant information and necessary equipment are available.*[29,34]
▪ Assist the practitioner with opening sterile trays, packaged probes (with a smart card if using a Licox monitor), and other equipment *to help maintain a sterile environment and provide efficiency.*[1]
▪ Turn on the PbtO$_2$ monitor and follow the manufacturer's guidelines *to prepare the monitor.*[1]
▪ If you are using a Licox monitor, place the smart card into the card slot located on the front of the monitor. *This monitor requires the smart*

card numbers to match those on the oxygen probe that the practitioner will insert.[1]

■ During insertion, continually monitor the patient's heart rate and rhythm, respiratory rate, and pulse oximetry; frequently monitor blood pressure; and perform neurologic assessments every 15 minutes *to ensure prompt recognition and treatment of neurologic changes.*[1,29]

■ If applicable, assist the practitioner with intracranial bolt insertion, which may occur before or after $PbtO_2$ probe insertion. (See the "Intracranial pressure monitoring" procedure.)

■ Assist the practitioner with insertion of the temperature and oxygen probes.

■ After the practitioner inserts the temperature and oxygen probes, connect them to the monitor cables.

■ Look at the monitor for temperature and $PbtO_2$ values. Note that temperature values should be accurate immediately, but $PbtO_2$ values can take as long as 2 hours to be accurate, *because brain tissue settles after the trauma of probe placement.*[1]

■ If the bedside monitor allows, use a cable to capture the values from the $PbtO_2$ monitor to the bedside monitor *to allow integration between monitoring systems.*

■ Make sure that all monitor alarm limits are set appropriately for the patient's current condition, and that the alarms are turned on, functioning properly, and audible to staff.[21,22,23,24]

■ Apply a sterile occlusive dressing at the insertion site *to reduce the risk of infection.*[1,29]

■ Secure the $PbtO_2$ monitor cables *to prevent tension at the insertion site.*[1] Anchor cables from the patient's head and shoulder with a transparent adhesive dressing. *Make sure that the entire setup is supported but that enough slack is provided for you to turn and move the patient.* Consider using an arm board *to support and secure the cables*[1] and placing towels or washcloths under the setup *for support.* Make sure that the cables aren't dragging on the ground.

■ After the patient's brain tissue has adjusted to device insertion, maintain the patient's $PbtO_2$ value between 20 and 35 mm Hg, or as ordered by the practitioner.[1] (See the "Brain tissue oxygen monitoring and care" procedure.)

■ Reassess and respond to the patient's pain by evaluating the response to treatment and progress toward pain management goals. Assess for adverse reactions and risk factors for adverse events that may result from treatment.[35]

■ Return the bed to the lowest possible position *to prevent falls and maintain patient safety.*[36]

■ Discard used supplies in the appropriate receptacles.[32,33]

■ Remove and discard your personal protective equipment.[32,33]

■ Perform hand hygiene.[8,9,10,11,12,13]

■ Document the procedure.[37,38,39,40]

Special considerations

■ The Joint Commission has issued a sentinel event alert concerning medical device alarm safety, *because alarm-related events have been associated with permanent loss of function or death.* Among the major contributing factors were improper alarm settings, alarm settings turned off inappropriately, and alarm signals that are inaudible to staff. Make sure that alarm limits are set appropriately, and that alarms are turned on, functioning properly, and audible to staff. Follow facility guidelines for preventing alarm fatigue.[23]

■ $PbtO_2$ probes are compatible with magnetic resonance imaging (MRI) machines unless they have a fiberoptic ICP device. As directed, disconnect all cables and patient monitoring devices from the probe before entering the MRI environment *to avoid serious patient injury.*[41]

■ A CT scan may be performed to confirm catheter placement.[29]

■ Probes may remain in place for 5 to 7 days. Check the manufacturer's guidelines.[1]

Complications

Possible complications include infection, cerebrospinal fluid leak, and cerebral bleeding.

Documentation

Document neurologic assessments; ICP; vital signs, including temperature; pulse oximetry; insertion site assessment findings; and medications administered. Also document the patient's tolerance of the procedure, any unexpected complications or outcomes, your interventions, and the patient's response to those interventions. Record $PbtO_2$ readings at least every hour. Document teaching provided to the patient and family (if applicable), their understanding of that teaching, and any need for follow-up teaching.

REFERENCES

1 Wiegand, D. L. (2017). *AACN procedure manual for high acuity, progressive, and critical care* (7th ed.). St. Louis, MO: Elsevier.

2 The Joint Commission. (2021). Standard RI.01.03.01. *Comprehensive accreditation manual for hospitals.* Oakbrook Terrace, IL: The Joint Commission. (Level VII)

3 Centers for Medicare and Medicaid Services, Department of Health and Human Services. (2020). Condition of participation: Patient's rights. 42 C.F.R. § 482.13.

4 Accreditation Association for Hospitals and Health Systems. (2020). Standard 15.01.11. *Healthcare Facilities Accreditation Program: Accreditation requirements for acute care hospitals.* Chicago, IL: Accreditation Association for Hospitals and Health Systems. (Level VII)

5 DNV GL-Healthcare USA, Inc. (2020). PR.2.SR.3. *NIAHO® accreditation requirements, interpretive guidelines and surveyor guidance—revision 20.0.* Milford, OH: DNV GL-Healthcare USA, Inc. (Level VII)

6 The Joint Commission. (2021). Standard UP.01.01.01. *Comprehensive accreditation manual for hospitals.* Oakbrook Terrace, IL: The Joint Commission. (Level VII)

7 Accreditation Association for Hospitals and Health Systems. (2020). Standard 30.00.14. *Healthcare Facilities Accreditation Program: Accreditation requirements for acute care hospitals.* Chicago, IL: Accreditation Association for Hospitals and Health Systems. (Level VII)

8 Centers for Disease Control and Prevention. (2002). Guideline for hand hygiene in health-care settings: Recommendations of the Healthcare Infection Control Practices Advisory Committee and the HICPAC/SHEA/APIC/ https://www.cdc.gov/mmwr/pdf/rr/rr5116.pdf (Level II)

9 The Joint Commission. (2021). Standard NPSG.07.01.01. *Comprehensive accreditation manual for hospitals.* Oakbrook Terrace, IL: The Joint Commission. (Level VII)

10 World Health Organization. (2009). WHO guidelines on hand hygiene in health care: First global patient safety challenge, clean care is safer care. https://apps.who.int/iris/bitstream/handle/10665/44102/9789241597906_eng.pdf?sequence=1 (Level IV)

11 Centers for Medicare and Medicaid Services, Department of Health and Human Services. (2020). Condition of participation: Infection control. 42 C.F.R. § 482.42.

12 Accreditation Association for Hospitals and Health Systems. (2020). Standard 07.01.21. *Healthcare Facilities Accreditation Program: Accreditation requirements for acute care hospitals.* Chicago, IL: Accreditation Association for Hospitals and Health Systems. (Level VII)

13 DNV GL-Healthcare USA, Inc. (2020). IC.1.SR.1. *NIAHO® accreditation requirements, interpretive guidelines and surveyor guidance—revision 20.0.* Milford, OH: DNV GL-Healthcare USA, Inc. (Level VII)

14 The Joint Commission. (2021). Standard NPSG.01.01.01. *Comprehensive accreditation manual for hospitals.* Oakbrook Terrace, IL: The Joint Commission. (Level VII)

15 Accreditation Association for Hospitals and Health Systems. (2020). Standard 15.01.16. *Healthcare Facilities Accreditation Program: Accreditation requirements for acute care hospitals.* Chicago, IL: Accreditation Association for Hospitals and Health Systems. (Level VII)

16 Centers for Medicare and Medicaid Services, Department of Health and Human Services. (2020). Condition of participation: Patient's rights. 42 C.F.R. § 482.13(c)(1).

17 DNV GL-Healthcare USA, Inc. (2020). PR.2.SR.5. *NIAHO® accreditation requirements, interpretive guidelines and surveyor guidance—revision 20.0.* Milford, OH: DNV GL-Healthcare USA, Inc. (Level VII)

18 The Joint Commission. (2021). Standard RI.01.01.01. *Comprehensive accreditation manual for hospitals.* Oakbrook Terrace, IL: The Joint Commission. (Level VII)

19 The Joint Commission. (2021). Standard PC.02.01.21. *Comprehensive accreditation manual for hospitals.* Oakbrook Terrace, IL: The Joint Commission. (Level VII)

20 The Joint Commission. (2021). Standard UP.01.02.01. *Comprehensive accreditation manual for hospitals.* Oakbrook Terrace, IL: The Joint Commission. (Level VII)

21 American Association of Critical-Care Nurses. (2018). AACN practice alert: Managing alarms in acute care across the life span—Electrocardiography and pulse oximetry. https://www.aacn.org/clinical-resources/practice-alerts/managing-alarms-in-acute-care-across-the-life-span (Level VII)

22 The Joint Commission. (2021). Standard NPSG.06.01.01. *Comprehensive accreditation manual for hospitals.* Oakbrook Terrace, IL: The Joint Commission. (Level VII)

23 The Joint Commission. (2013). Sentinel event alert 50: Medical device alarm safety in hospitals. https://www.jointcommission.org/assets/1/6/SEA_50_alarms_4_26_16.pdf (Level VII)

24 Graham, K. C., & Cvach, M. (2010). Monitor alarm fatigue: Standardizing use of physiological monitors and decreasing nuisance alarms. *American Journal of Critical Care, 19,* 28–37.

25 Centers for Medicare and Medicaid Services, Department of Health and Human Services. (2020). Condition of participation: Nursing services. 42 C.F.R. § 482.23(c).

26 The Joint Commission. (2021). Standard MM.06.01.01. *Comprehensive accreditation manual for hospitals.* Oakbrook Terrace, IL: The Joint Commission. (Level VII)

27 Accreditation Association for Hospitals and Health Systems. (2020). Standard 16.01.03. *Healthcare Facilities Accreditation Program: Accreditation requirements for acute care hospitals.* Chicago, IL: Accreditation Association for Hospitals and Health Systems. (Level VII)

28 DNV GL-Healthcare USA, Inc. (2020). MM.1.SR.3. *NIAHO® accreditation requirements, interpretive guidelines and surveyor guidance—revision 20.0.* Milford, OH: DNV GL Healthcare USA, Inc. (Level VII)

29 American Association of Neuroscience Nurses (AANN). (2014). *Care of the patient undergoing intracranial pressure monitoring/external ventricular drainage or lumbar drainage: AANN clinical practice guideline series.* Glenview, IL: AANN. (Level VII)

30 Accreditation Association for Hospitals and Health Systems. (2020). Standard 25.01.27. *Healthcare Facilities Accreditation Program: Accreditation requirements for acute care hospitals.* Chicago, IL: Accreditation Association for Hospitals and Health Systems. (Level VII)

31 Waters, T. R., et al. (2009). Safe patient handling training for schools of nursing. https://www.cdc.gov/niosh/docs/2009-127/pdfs/2009-127.pdf (Level VII)

32 Siegel, J. D., et al. (2007, revised 2019). 2007 guideline for isolation precautions: Preventing transmission of infectious agents in healthcare settings. https://www.cdc.gov/infectioncontrol/pdf/guidelines/isolation-guidelines-H.pdf (Level II)

33 Accreditation Association for Hospitals and Health Systems. (2020). Standard 07.01.10. *Healthcare Facilities Accreditation Program: Accreditation requirements for acute care hospitals.* Chicago, IL: Accreditation Association for Hospitals and Health Systems. (Level VII)

34 The Joint Commission. (2021). Standard UP.01.03.01. *Comprehensive accreditation manual for hospitals.* Oakbrook Terrace, IL: The Joint Commission. (Level VII)

35 The Joint Commission. (2021). Standard PC.01.02.07. *Comprehensive accreditation manual for hospitals.* Oakbrook Terrace, IL: The Joint Commission. (Level VII)

36 Ganz, D. A., et al. (2013-reviewed 2021). *Preventing falls in hospitals: A toolkit for improving quality of care* (AHRQ Publication No. 13-0015-EF). Rockville, MD: Agency for Healthcare Research and Quality. https://www.ahrq.gov/professionals/systems/hospital/fallpxtoolkit/index.html (Level VII)

37 The Joint Commission. (2021). Standard RC.01.03.01. *Comprehensive accreditation manual for hospitals.* Oakbrook Terrace, IL: The Joint Commission. (Level VII)

38 Centers for Medicare and Medicaid Services, Department of Health and Human Services. (2020). Condition of participation: Medical record services. 42 C.F.R. § 482.24(b).

39 Accreditation Association for Hospitals and Health Systems. (2020). Standard 10.00.03. *Healthcare Facilities Accreditation Program: Accreditation requirements for acute care hospitals.* Chicago, IL: Accreditation Association for Hospitals and Health Systems. (Level VII)

40 DNV GL-Healthcare USA, Inc. (2020). MR.2.SR.1. *NIAHO® accreditation requirements, interpretive guidelines and surveyor guidance—revision 20.0.* Milford, OH: DNV GL-Healthcare USA, Inc. (Level VII)

41 Integra LifeSciences Corporation. (2016). Integra Licox brain tissue oxygen monitoring. https://www.integralife.eu/products/neuro/neurocritical-care/pbto2-licox/ (Level VII)

BRONCHOSCOPY, ASSISTING

Bronchoscopy is an invasive procedure that's used to diagnose and manage various inflammatory, infectious, and malignant diseases of the airways and lungs.[1] The procedure involves using a flexible fiberoptic scope connected to a light source to visualize the upper and lower airways. (See *A look at the bronchoscope.*) Bronchoscopy may also help retrieve a foreign body or substance, obtain tissue specimens and cell washings, or perform bronchoalveolar lavage, coagulation, or laser removal of abnormal tissue.[1,2]

Bronchoscopy is indicated for various diagnostic and therapeutic purposes.[1] However, it should be performed only when the relative benefits outweigh the risks. (See *Indications for bronchoscopy.*)[1]

Bronchoscopy is contraindicated in patients with severe refractory hypoxemia, hemodynamic instability, and coagulopathy or bleeding diathesis that can't be corrected.[1]

To assist the practitioner during a bronchoscopy, you must have knowledge of the technique, the purpose of the procedure, and associated complications. Your responsibilities may include patient preparation and monitoring, handling specimens, and postprocedure care and monitoring.[1]

Equipment

Bronchoscope ▪ suction equipment ▪ specimen containers ▪ labels ▪ cytology brush ▪ biopsy forceps ▪ water-soluble lubricant ▪ sterile gauze sponges ▪ topical anesthetic (viscous lidocaine, 1% lidocaine, and 1% lidocaine with EPINEPHrine) ▪ local anesthetic spray ▪ syringes (5 mL, 10 mL, and 30 mL) ▪ pulse oximeter and probe ▪ cardiac monitor ▪ blood pressure monitor ▪ oxygen delivery equipment ▪ emergency equipment (code cart with cardiac medications, defibrillator, handheld resuscitation bag with mask, intubation equipment) ▪ personal protective equipment (gown, gloves, mask and goggles or mask with face shield) ▪ 150-mL bottle of normal saline solution ▪ prescribed

EQUIPMENT

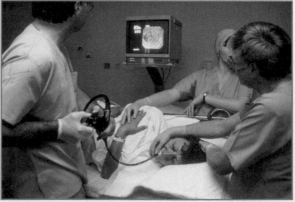

 A look at the bronchoscope

The practitioner uses the bronchoscope to view the upper and lower airways. The fiberoptic bronchoscope, equipped with a light source, transmits images to a screen to facilitate visualization, as shown below. The device also contains an irrigation channel, instrument channel, and suction apparatus to aid the examination. The practitioner can record still images, video sequences, and audio during the examination.

(© Antonia Reeve/Photo Researchers, Inc.)

Indications for bronchoscopy

Bronchoscopy helps diagnose and treat conditions that may affect the patient's airway. Bronchoscopy may be used to:
- evaluate persistent atelectasis or pulmonary infiltrates
- evaluate recurrent pneumonia
- assess upper airway patency
- assess upper airway function
- investigate the cause of hemoptysis, unexplained cough, dyspnea, localized wheezing, or stridor
- obtain lower respiratory tract secretions, cell washings, and biopsies for histologic and microbiologic evaluation
- determine the extent and location of injury from toxic inhalation or aspiration
- evaluate problems associated with endotracheal or tracheostomy tubes
- assist with difficult intubation or percutaneous tracheotomy
- determine whether mucus plugs are responsible for lobar or segmental atelectasis and removal of plugs, if necessary
- perform balloon dilatation to treat tracheobronchial stenosis
- remove abnormal endobronchial tissue or foreign material
- perform electrocoagulation, laser or argon plasma coagulation, or cryotherapy
- assess a lung transplant for infection or rejection[2]
- place a brachytherapy catheter, tracheobronchial stents, or one-way valves and coils.[1,2]

sedative and its reversal agent ■ laboratory biohazard transport bag ■ open container; fully enclosed, labeled container or watertight polyethylene bag ■ oral care supplies ■ soft, lint-free, disposable cloth or sponge ■ enzymatic detergent solution ■ stethoscope ■ disinfectant pad ■ capnography monitoring equipment ■ facility-approved disinfectant ■ Optional: bite block, ventilator, IV catheter insertion equipment, endotracheal (ET) tube adapter, prescribed medications, N-95 particulate respirator or powered air purifying respirator, lavage equipment, standardized sedation scale.

Preparation of equipment

Inspect all equipment and supplies. If a product is expired, is defective, or has compromised integrity, remove it from patient use, label it as expired or defective, and report the expiration or defect as directed by your facility.

Prepare intubation equipment if endotracheal intubation is necessary. Set up oxygen delivery equipment in case you need it. Apply water-soluble lubricant to the gauze sponges for lubricating the bronchoscope. Fill syringes with normal saline solution according to the practitioner's preference. Label all medications appropriately *to prevent medication errors.*[3] Set up and test suction apparatus and make sure it's functioning properly. Fill specimen containers with normal saline solution. Make sure other emergency equipment is functioning properly and readily available.[1,4] Make sure the sedative reversal agent is readily available.[5]

Implementation

- Verify the practitioner's orders.
- Review the patient's medical record for allergies or contraindications to the procedure.
- Gather and prepare the necessary equipment and supplies.
- If required by your facility, confirm that informed consent has been obtained and that the signed consent form is in the patient's medical record.[6,7,8,9]
- Conduct a preprocedure verification *to make sure that all relevant documentation, related information, and equipment are available and correctly matched with the patient's identifiers.*[10,11]
- Perform hand hygiene.[12,13,14,15,16,17]

- Confirm the patient's identity using at least two patient identifiers.[18]
- Provide privacy.[19,20,21,22]
- Confirm the patient's nothing-by-mouth status before the procedure. If the procedure is nonemergent, minimal fasting recommendations include 2 hours for clear liquids, 6 or more hours for a light meal or nonhuman milk, and 8 hours or more for fried or fatty foods or meat. If the need for bronchoscopy is an emergency, collaborate with the practitioner to compare the risks and benefits of the procedure, considering the amount and type of fluids or solids ingested.[23]
- Reinforce the practitioner's explanation of the procedure, and answer the patient's and family's questions *to make sure that they understand the information provided.*[6]
- Make sure that the patient has patent IV access. Insert an IV catheter if the patient doesn't already have one in place. (See the "IV catheter insertion and removal" procedure.)
- If ordered, administer preprocedure medications following safe medication administration practices.[1,24,25,26,27] Note that guidelines no longer recommend routine premedication with anticholinergics or other medications *because of insufficient evidence for their use.*[4]
- Perform hand hygiene.[12,13,14,15,16]
- Put on gloves and other personal protective equipment, including a gown, a mask (a fit-tested N-95 particulate respirator or powered air purifying respirator if the practitioner suspects or has confirmed *Mycobacterium tuberculosis*, severe acute respiratory syndrome [SARS], or avian or pandemic influenza viruses), and goggles or mask with face shield, as needed.[28,29,30]

NURSING ALERT When caring for a patient with known or suspected coronavirus disease 2019 (COVID-19), refer to the latest recommendations from the Centers for Disease Control and Prevention, available at https://www.cdc.gov/coronavirus/2019-ncov/index.html

- Make sure the patient is attached to a cardiac monitor, pulse oximeter, blood pressure monitor, and capnography monitor.[1,31] Make sure that alarm limits are set appropriately for the patient's current condition, and that the alarms are turned on, functioning properly, and audible to staff.[32,33,34]
- Remove the patient's eyeglasses and any removable devices from the mouth, such as dentures, partial plates, or retainers, if applicable.
- Provide oral care *to avoid introducing microorganisms from the patient's mouth into the airway during the procedure.*[35]
- Obtain the patient's vital signs and assess level of consciousness (LOC), breath sounds, cardiac rhythm, oxygen saturation level, and end-tidal carbon dioxide ($ETco_2$) *to serve as baselines for comparison during and after the procedure.* If the patient is receiving mechanical ventilation, also assess ventilation parameters, such as tidal volume, peak inspiratory pressure, and inspiratory flow, *to evaluate the response to the procedure.*[1]
- Position the patient in the supine position.[36]
- Conduct a time-out immediately before the procedure *to perform a final assessment that the correct patient, site, positioning, and procedure are identified and, as needed, all relevant information and necessary equipment are available.*[37]
- Administer oxygen therapy, as ordered, *to prevent hypoxia.*[31]
- Administer moderate sedation, as ordered, following safe medication administration practices, *to relieve the patient's anxiety and promote cooperation.*[24,25,26,27,31] (See the "Moderate sedation" procedure.)
- If you're using the oral route or if the patient is intubated, insert a bite block *to prevent the patient from biting down during the procedure.*[5]
- Hand the bronchoscope to the practitioner and turn on its light source. Assist with lubricating the bronchoscope, as needed.[1]
- The practitioner sprays a local anesthetic into the patient's mouth and throat.
- The practitioner introduces the bronchoscope through the patient's mouth, nose, tracheostomy, or ET tube adapter. When the bronchoscope is just above the vocal cords, the practitioner flushes lidocaine through the inner channel of the scope to the vocal cords *to anesthetize deeper areas.*
- The practitioner inspects the trachea and bronchi, observes the color of the mucosal lining, and notes masses or inflamed areas. The practitioner may use biopsy forceps *to remove a tissue specimen from a suspect area,* a

cytology brush *to obtain cells from the surface of a lesion*, or a suction apparatus *to remove foreign bodies or mucus plugs*.

■ Assist the practitioner with therapeutic treatment, if necessary. Record the lavage volumes delivered and retrieved, if appropriate.[1]

■ Assist with specimen collection. Place specimens in appropriate containers and then label in the presence of the patient *to prevent mislabeling*.[18] Send the specimens to the laboratory in a laboratory biohazard transport bag.[28]

■ Assess the patient's vital signs, LOC, subjective response to the procedure (pain, discomfort, dyspnea), breath sounds, cardiac rhythm, oxygen saturation level, and $ETco_2$ level. If the patient is intubated, monitor tidal volume, peak inspiratory pressure, and inspiratory flow. Monitor the patient continuously until the patient returns to a pre-sedation LOC. Immediately inform the practitioner of any abnormalities.[1,31,38]

■ Continuously monitor the patient's oxygen saturation. Provide supplemental oxygen when desaturation is significant, as ordered.[4,31]

■ Discard used supplies in the appropriate receptacles.[28]

■ Clean the bronchoscope and send it for formal reprocessing *to prevent transmission of microorganisms*.[39,40] Start mechanical cleaning by wiping the external surface of the bronchoscope with a soft, lint-free, disposable cloth or sponge soaked in freshly prepared enzymatic detergent solution.[41,42,43] Insert the distal portion of the bronchoscope into the solution container and use the suction device to suction the solution through the air, water, and biopsy channels. Alternate suctioning the solution and suctioning air until the return solution is visibly clean. Then flush or blow air through the channels, according to the bronchoscope manufacturer's instructions.[41,42,43]

■ Detach the bronchoscope from the light source and suction setup. If it's a video bronchoscope, attach the protective video cap to the device.[41]

■ Place the bronchoscope in a container for transportation to the reprocessing area. If the reprocessing area is adjacent to the area where the bronchoscope was used, an open container is sufficient; if the reprocessing area is distant, use a fully enclosed, labeled container or watertight polyethylene bag for transportation.[41,42,43]

■ Clean and disinfect all furniture and reusable equipment used during the procedure *to prevent transmission of microorganisms*.[41,43]

■ Remove and discard your personal protective equipment[28] and perform hand hygiene.[12,13,14,15,16,17]

■ Clean and disinfect your stethoscope using a disinfectant pad.[38,40]

■ Perform hand hygiene.[12,13,14,15,16,17]

■ Document the procedure.[44,45,46,47]

Special considerations

■ The Joint Commission issued a sentinel event alert concerning medical device alarm safety, *because alarm-related events have been associated with permanent loss of function or death*. Among the major contributing factors were improper alarm settings, alarm settings turned off inappropriately, and alarm signals that are inaudible to staff. Make sure alarm limits are set appropriately, and that alarms are turned on, functioning properly, and audible to staff. Follow facility guidelines for preventing alarm fatigue.[48]

■ In addition to standard precautions, institute airborne precautions if the practitioner suspects or has confirmation of a mycobacterial infection. (See the "Airborne precautions" procedure.) If the practitioner suspects or has confirmation of SARS or avian or pandemic influenza, institute both airborne and contact precautions.[29]

■ After the procedure, position the patient in the semi-Fowler position *to prevent aspiration*.[31] Position an unconscious patient on one side with the head of the bed elevated.

■ After the procedure, encourage the patient to expectorate saliva instead of swallowing it.

■ Notify the practitioner if the patient develops fever, chest pain or discomfort, shortness of breath, abnormal breath sounds, or hemoptysis.[1]

■ If a transbronchial biopsy was performed, arrange for a chest X-ray 1 hour after the procedure, as ordered, *to determine whether a pneumothorax is present*.[1]

■ A patient with respiratory failure who can't breathe adequately alone may require intubation and mechanical ventilation during the procedure.

■ Prior to a bronchoscopy, a nebulized bronchodilator should be considered for a patient with asthma.

Patient teaching

Provide a patient who's undergoing bronchoscopy on an outpatient basis with written instructions regarding postbronchoscopy fever, which is usually a noninfective acute inflammatory response.[4] Tell the patient that a fever that continues for longer than 24 hours or is higher than 101° F (38.3° C), requires notifying the practitioner.[49] Inform the patient about common expected short-term effects, such as a sore throat and nasal discomfort, hoarseness, cough, muscle aches, and mild hemoptysis (if the practitioner performed a biopsy).[5,49] Caution the patient to contact the health care provider with symptoms of chest pain, new or increased shortness of breath, or more than a few episodes of hemoptysis.[49] Instruct the patient not to drive or operate heavy machinery for 24 hours.[49]

Complications

Complications include bleeding, respiratory depression, airway obstruction, cardiopulmonary arrest, arrhythmias, esophagotracheal fistula, and pneumothorax. Other adverse events may include hypoxemia, hypercapnia, bronchospasm, hypotension, laryngospasm, bradycardia, epistaxis, and hemoptysis.[1,5] Transbronchial biopsies are associated with hemorrhage and pneumothorax.[49] There is an increased risk of infection for patients and health care workers from improperly processed bronchoscopes.[1,40,41]

NURSING ALERT The risk of complications from bronchoscopy is higher in patients with coagulopathy, refractory hypoxemia, and unstable hemodynamic status; however, the practitioner may still perform the procedure if the benefits outweigh the risks.[1]

Documentation

Record the date, time, and duration of the procedure. Also document vital signs before, during, and after the procedure. Document all assessment findings before and during the procedure, any medications you administered, and the patient's response to them. Document the patient's response to the procedure. After the procedure, document the patient's LOC, airway patency, respiratory rate and depth, and pulse oximetry levels; note whether the patient received supplemental oxygen. Document teaching provided to the patient and family (if applicable), their understanding of that teaching, and any need for follow-up teaching.

REFERENCES

1 American Association for Respiratory Care. (2007). AARC clinical practice guideline: Bronchoscopy assisting—2007 revision and update. *Respiratory Care, 52*, 74–80. (Level VII)

2 Islam, S. (2021). Flexible bronchoscopy in adults: Indications and contraindications. In: *UpToDate*, Colt, H. G. (Ed.)

3 Accreditation Association for Hospitals and Health Systems. (2020). Standard 25.01.18. *Healthcare Facilities Accreditation Program: Accreditation requirements for acute care hospitals*. Chicago, IL: Accreditation Association for Hospitals and Health Systems. (Level VII)

4 Du Rand, I. A., et al. (2013). British Thoracic Society guideline for diagnostic flexible bronchoscopy in adults. *Thorax, 68*(Suppl. 1), i1–i44. https://thorax.bmj.com/content/thoraxjnl/68/Suppl_1/i1.full.pdf (Level I)

5 Islam, S. (2020). Flexible bronchoscopy in adults: Preparation, procedural technique, and complications. In: *UpToDate*, Colt, H. G. (Ed.).

6 Accreditation Association for Hospitals and Health Systems. (2020). Standard 15.01.11. *Healthcare Facilities Accreditation Program: Accreditation requirements for acute care hospitals*. Chicago, IL: Accreditation Association for Hospitals and Health Systems. (Level VII)

7 The Joint Commission. (2021). Standard RI.01.03.01. *Comprehensive accreditation manual for hospitals*. Oakbrook Terrace, IL: The Joint Commission. (Level VII)

8 Centers for Medicare and Medicaid Services, Department of Health and Human Services. (2020). Condition of participation: Patient's rights. 42 C.F.R. § 482.13(b)(2).

9 DNV GL-Healthcare USA, Inc. (2020). PR.21.SR.3. *NIAHO® accreditation requirements, interpretive guidelines and surveyor guidance—revision 20.0*. Milford, OH: DNV GL-Healthcare USA, Inc. (Level VII)

10 The Joint Commission. (2021). Standard UP.01.01.01. *Comprehensive accreditation manual for hospitals*. Oakbrook Terrace, IL: The Joint Commission. (Level VII)

11 Accreditation Association for Hospitals and Health Systems. (2020). Standard 30.00.14. *Healthcare Facilities Accreditation Program: Accreditation requirements for acute care hospitals*. Chicago, IL: Accreditation Association for Hospitals and Health Systems. (Level VII)

12 Centers for Disease Control and Prevention. (2002). Guideline for hand hygiene in health-care settings: Recommendations of the Healthcare Infection Control Practices Advisory Committee and the HICPAC/SHEA/APIC/IDSA Hand Hygiene Task Force. *MMWR Recommendations and Reports, 51*(RR-16), 1–45. https://www.cdc.gov/mmwr/pdf/rr/rr5116.pdf (Level II)

13 The Joint Commission. (2021). Standard NPSG.07.01.01. *Comprehensive accreditation manual for hospitals.* Oakbrook Terrace, IL: The Joint Commission. (Level VII)

14 World Health Organization. (2009). WHO guidelines on hand hygiene in health care: First global patient safety challenge, clean care is safer care. https://apps.who.int/iris/bitstream/handle/10665/44102/9789241597906_eng.pdf?sequence=1 (Level IV)

15 Centers for Medicare and Medicaid Services, Department of Health and Human Services. (2020). Condition of participation: Infection control. 42 C.F.R. § 482.42.

16 Accreditation Association for Hospitals and Health Systems. (2020). Standard 07.01.21. *Healthcare Facilities Accreditation Program: Accreditation requirements for acute care hospitals.* Chicago, IL: Accreditation Association for Hospitals and Health Systems. (Level VII)

17 DNV GL-Healthcare USA, Inc. (2020). IC.1.SR.1. *NIAHO® accreditation requirements, interpretive guidelines and surveyor guidance—revision 20.0.* Milford, OH: DNV GL-Healthcare USA, Inc. (Level VII)

18 The Joint Commission. (2021). Standard NPSG.01.01.01. *Comprehensive accreditation manual for hospitals.* Oakbrook Terrace, IL: The Joint Commission. (Level VII)

19 The Joint Commission. (2020). Standard RI.01.01.01. *Comprehensive accreditation manual for hospitals.* Oakbrook Terrace, IL: The Joint Commission. (Level VII)

20 Centers for Medicare and Medicaid Services, Department of Health and Human Services. (2020). Condition of participation: Patient's rights. 42 C.F.R. § 482.13(c)(1).

21 Accreditation Association for Hospitals and Health Systems. (2020). Standard 15.01.16. *Healthcare Facilities Accreditation Program: Accreditation requirements for acute care hospitals.* Chicago, IL: Accreditation Association for Hospitals and Health Systems. (Level VII)

22 DNV GL-Healthcare USA, Inc. (2020). PR.21.SR.5. *NIAHO® accreditation requirements, interpretive guidelines and surveyor guidance—revision 20.0.* Milford, OH: DNV GL-Healthcare USA, Inc. (Level VII)

23 American Society of Anesthesiologists. (2017). Practice guidelines for preoperative fasting and the use of pharmacologic agents to reduce the risk of pulmonary aspiration: Application to healthy patients undergoing elective procedures. *Anesthesiology, 126,* 376–393. http://anesthesiology.pubs.asahq.org/article.aspx?articleid=2596245 (Level VII)

24 Centers for Medicare and Medicaid Services, Department of Health and Human Services. (2019). Condition of participation: Nursing services. 42 C.F.R. § 482.23(c)

25 The Joint Commission. (2021). Standard MM.06.01.01. *Comprehensive accreditation manual for hospitals.* Oakbrook Terrace, IL: The Joint Commission. (Level VII)

26 Accreditation Association for Hospitals and Health Systems. (2020). Standard 16.01.03. *Healthcare Facilities Accreditation Program: Accreditation requirements for acute care hospitals.* Chicago, IL: Accreditation Association for Hospitals and Health Systems. (Level VII)

27 DNV GL-Healthcare USA, Inc. (2020). MM.1.SR.2. *NIAHO® accreditation requirements, interpretive guidelines and surveyor guidance—revision 20.0.* Milford, OH: DNV GL-Healthcare USA, Inc. (Level VII)

28 Occupational Safety and Health Administration. (2012). Bloodborne pathogens, standard number 1910.1030. https://www.osha.gov/pls/oshaweb/owadisp.show_document?p_id=10051&p_table=STANDARDS (Level VII)

29 Siegel, J. D., et al. (2007, revised 2019). 2007 guideline for isolation precautions: Preventing transmission of infectious agents in healthcare settings. https://www.cdc.gov/infectioncontrol/pdf/guidelines/isolation-guidelines-H.pdf (Level II)

30 Accreditation Association for Hospitals and Health Systems. (2020). Standard 07.01.10. *Healthcare Facilities Accreditation Program: Accreditation requirements for acute care hospitals.* Chicago, IL: Accreditation Association for Hospitals and Health Systems. (Level VII)

31 Kacmarek, R. M., et al. (2017). *Egan's fundamentals of respiratory care* (11th ed.). St. Louis, MO: Mosby.

32 The Joint Commission. (2021). Standard NPSG.06.01.01. *Comprehensive accreditation manual for hospitals.* Oakbrook Terrace, IL: The Joint Commission. (Level VII)

33 American Association of Critical-Care Nurses. (2018). AACN practice alert: Managing alarms in acute care across the life span—Electrocardiography and pulse oximetry. https://www.aacn.org/clinical-resources/practice-alerts/managing-alarms-in-acute-care-across-the-life-span (Level VII)

34 Graham, K. C., & Cvach, M. (2010). Monitor alarm fatigue: Standardizing use of physiological monitors and decreasing nuisance alarms. *American Journal of Critical Care, 19,* 28–37.

35 Jelic, S., et al. (2008). Clinical review: Airway hygiene in the intensive care unit. *Critical Care, 12,* 209.

36 van Zwam, J. P., et al. (2010). Flexible bronchoscopy in supine or sitting position: A randomized prospective analysis of safety and patient comfort. *Journal of Bronchology and Interventional Pulmonology, 17,* 29–32. (Level II)

37 The Joint Commission. (2021). Standard UP.01.03.01. *Comprehensive accreditation manual for hospitals.* Oakbrook Terrace, IL: The Joint Commission. (Level VII)

38 Centers for Medicare and Medicaid Services. (2014). Requirements for hospital medication administration, particularly intravenous (IV) medications and post-operative care of patients receiving IV opioids. http://www.cms.gov/Medicare/Provider-Enrollment-and-Certification/SurveyCertificationGenInfo/Downloads/Survey-and-Cert-Letter-14-15.pdf

39 U.S. Food & Drug Administration. (2015). Infections associated with reprocessed flexible bronchoscope: FDA safety communication. https://www.fdanews.com/ext/resources/files/09-15/092115-safety-notice.pdf?1442508647

40 Guideline for flexible endoscopes. (2019). In Conner, R. (Ed.), *Guidelines for perioperative practice, 2019 edition.* Denver, CO: AORN, Inc. (Level VII)

41 Rutala, W. A., et al. (2008, revised 2019). Guideline for disinfection and sterilization in healthcare facilities, 2008. https://www.cdc.gov/infection-control/pdf/guidelines/disinfection-guidelines-H.pdf (Level I)

42 Mehta, A. C., et al. (2005). American College of Chest Physicians and American Association for Bronchoscopy [corrected] consensus statement: Prevention of flexible bronchoscopy-associated infection. *Chest, 128*(3), 1742–1755. https://journal.chestnet.org/article/S0012-3692(15)52213-7/fulltext

43 Accreditation Association for Hospitals and Health Systems. (2020). Standard 07.02.03. *Healthcare Facilities Accreditation Program: Accreditation requirements for acute care hospitals.* Chicago, IL: Accreditation Association for Hospitals and Health Systems. (Level VII)

44 The Joint Commission. (2021). Standard RC.01.03.01. *Comprehensive accreditation manual for hospitals.* Oakbrook Terrace, IL: The Joint Commission. (Level VII)

45 Centers for Medicare and Medicaid Services, Department of Health and Human Services. (2019). Condition of participation: Medical record services. 42 C.F.R. § 482.24(b).

46 Accreditation Association for Hospitals and Health Systems. (2020). Standard 10.00.03. *Healthcare Facilities Accreditation Program: Accreditation requirements for acute care hospitals.* Chicago, IL: Accreditation Association for Hospitals and Health Systems. (Level VII)

47 DNV GL-Healthcare USA, Inc. (2020). MR.2.SR.1. *NIAHO® accreditation requirements, interpretive guidelines and surveyor guidance—revision 20.0.* Milford, OH: DNV GL-Healthcare USA, Inc. (Level VII)

48 The Joint Commission. (2013). Sentinel event alert 50: Medical device alarm safety in hospitals. https://www.jointcommission.org/assets/1/6/SEA_50_alarms_4_26_16.pdf (Level VII)

49 Sheski, F. D. (2020). Patient information: Flexible bronchoscopy (beyond the basics). In: *UpToDate,* Colt, H. G., (Ed.).

BUCCAL AND SUBLINGUAL DRUG ADMINISTRATION

Certain drugs are given buccally or sublingually to prevent their destruction or transformation in the stomach or small intestine. These drugs act quickly, *because the oral mucosa's thin epithelium and abundant vasculature allow direct absorption into the bloodstream.*[1] Drugs reach peak blood levels within 15 minutes of their buccal or sublingual administration—typically much faster than with oral administration of the same drugs.[2]

Other benefits of buccal and sublingual administration include ease of administration in patients who refuse to swallow a tablet, such as pediatric, geriatric, and psychiatric patients; convenience of drug administration; and accurate dosing compared with liquid formulations. Because buccal and sublingual administration interferes with the patient's eating, drinking, and talking, long-term administration by these routes may be undesirable. Buccal and sublingual drugs shouldn't be administered to uncooperative or unconscious patients because this route requires the patient to be alert enough to hold the drug in the sublingual or buccal area for absorption without swallowing the drug.[1] They may be inappropriate for use in patients with dry mouth, oral cavity injuries, or cognitive impairment.[3]

Drugs given buccally include nitroglycerin and methylTES-TOSTERone; drugs given sublingually include ergotamine tartrate, isosorbide dinitrate, fentanNYL,[4] nitroglycerin, and some benzodiazepines.

Equipment

Prescribed medication ▪ gloves.

Preparation of equipment

Inspect all equipment and supplies. If a product is expired, is defective, or has compromised integrity, remove it from patient use, label it as expired or defective, and report the expiration or defect as directed by your facility.

Implementation

▪ Avoid distractions and interruptions when preparing and administering medications *to prevent medication administration errors*.[5,6]
▪ Verify the practitioner's order.[7,8,9,10]
▪ Reconcile the patient's medications when the practitioner orders a new medication *to reduce the risk of medication errors, including omissions, duplications, dosing errors, and drug interactions.*
▪ Obtain the prescribed medication.
▪ Compare the medication label with the order in the patient's medication record.[7,8,9,10]
▪ Check the patient's medical record for an allergy or contraindication to the prescribed medication. If an allergy or contraindication exists, don't administer the medication; instead, notify the practitioner.[7,8,9,10]
▪ Check the expiration date on the medication. If the medication is expired, return it to the pharmacy and obtain a new supply of the medication.[7,8,9,10]
▪ Visually inspect the medication for discoloration or other loss of integrity; don't administer the medication if integrity has been compromised.[7,8,9,10]
▪ Discuss any unresolved concerns about the medication with the patient's practitioner.[7,8,9,10]
▪ Perform hand hygiene.[11,12,13,14,15,16]
▪ Confirm the patient's identity using at least two patient identifiers.[17]
▪ Provide privacy.[18,19,20,21]
▪ Explain the procedure to the patient and family (if appropriate) according to their individual communication and learning needs *to increase their understanding, allay their fears, and enhance cooperation.*[22]
▪ If the patient is receiving the medication for the first time, teach the patient and family (if appropriate) about potential adverse reactions or any other concerns related to the medication.[7,8,9,10]
▪ Verify that the medication is being administered at the proper time, in the prescribed dose, and by the correct route *to reduce the risk of medication errors.*[7,8,9,10]
▪ If your facility uses a bar code technology, use it as directed by your facility.
▪ Raise the bed to waist level before providing care *to prevent caregiver back strain.*[23]
▪ Assist the patient to a sitting position *to avoid aspiration of the medication.*[1]
▪ Perform hand hygiene.[11,12,13,14,15,16]
▪ Put on gloves *to comply with standard precautions.*[24,25,26]
▪ Assess the patient's buccal or sublingual mucosa for redness or altered integrity. If the integrity of the mucosa is compromised, don't proceed with the medication administration. Instead, notify the practitioner.
▪ For buccal administration, place the tablet in the patient's buccal pouch, between the cheek and gum. For sublingual administration, place the tablet under the patient's tongue. (See *Placing drugs in the oral mucosa.*)
▪ Instruct the patient to keep the medication in place until it dissolves completely *to ensure absorption.*
▪ Caution the patient against chewing the tablet or touching it with the tongue *to prevent accidental swallowing.*

Placing drugs in the oral mucosa

Buccal and sublingual administration routes allow some drugs, such as nitroglycerin and methylTESTOSTERone, to enter the bloodstream rapidly without being degraded in the GI tract. To administer a drug buccally, insert it between the patient's cheek and gum (as shown below). Instruct the patient to close the mouth and hold the tablet against the cheek until absorption is complete.

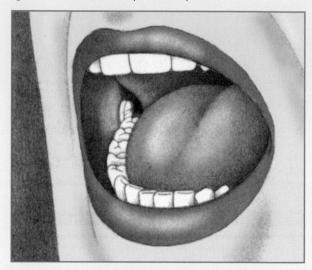

To administer a drug sublingually, place it under the patient's tongue (as shown below), and ask the patient to leave it there until it dissolves.

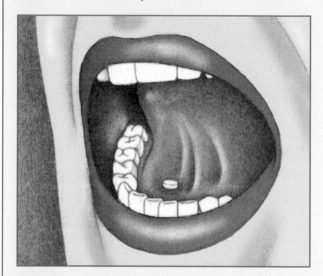

▪ If a sublingual spray is ordered, have the patient open the mouth for administration. Remind the patient not to breathe while the medication is being sprayed.
▪ Return the bed to then lowest position *to prevent falls and maintain patient safety.*[27]
▪ Remove and discard your gloves.[24]
▪ Perform hands hygiene.[11,12,13,14,15,16]
▪ Document the procedure.[28,29,30,31]

Special considerations

▪ Don't give liquids to a patient who's receiving buccal medication, *because some buccal tablets can take up to 1 hour to be absorbed.* Tell the patient not to rinse the mouth until the tablet has been absorbed.[1]
▪ Tell the patient who smokes not to do so before the drug has dissolved, *because nicotine's vasoconstrictive effects slow drug absorption.*[1]

Patient teaching

Teach the patient about the medication, dosing, correct administration technique, and any potential adverse reactions, and when to report them to the practitioner.

Complications

Some medications administered buccally may irritate the patient's oral mucosa.[1] Alternate sides of the mouth for repeat doses *to prevent continual irritation of the same site.* Some medications administered sublingually, such as nitroglycerin, may cause a tingling sensation under the tongue. If the patient finds this sensation bothersome, try placing the drug in the patient's buccal pouch instead.

Documentation

Document the name of the medication, the dose and route of administration, the date and time you administered the medication, and the patient's reaction, if any.[32] Document the appearance and integrity of the patient's oral mucosa before medication administration. Note any adverse reactions to the prescribed medication, the name of the practitioner notified, the date and time of notification, any interventions prescribed and implemented, and the patient's response to your interventions.[32] Document teaching provided to the patient and family (if applicable), their understanding of that teaching, and any need for follow-up teaching.

REFERENCES

1 Hua, S. (2019). Advances in nanoparticulate drug delivery approaches for sublingual and buccal administration. https://www.frontiersin.org/articles/10.3389/fphar.2019.01328/full

2 Narang, N., & Sharma, J. (2011). Sublingual mucosa as a route for systemic drug delivery. *International Journal of Pharmacy and Pharmaceutical Sciences, 3*(Suppl. 2), 18–22. https://innovareacademics.in/journal/ijpps/Vol3Suppl2/1092.pdf (Level V)

3 Nibha, K. P., & Pancholi, S. S. (2012). An overview on: Sublingual route for systemic drug delivery. *International Journal of Research in Pharmaceutical and Biomedical Sciences, 3*, 913–923.

4 Institute for Safe Medication Practices (2016). Look-alike drug names with recommended tall man letters. https://www.ismp.org/recommendations/tall-man-letters-list (Level VII)

5 Westbrook, J., et al. (2010). Association of interruptions with an increased risk and severity of medication administration errors. *Archives of Internal Medicine, 170*, 683–690. (Level IV)

6 Institute for Safe Medication Practices. (2012). Side tracks on the safety express: Interruptions lead to errors and unfinished...Wait, what was I doing? *Nurse Advise-ERR, 11*(2), 1–4. http://www.ismp.org/Newsletters/acutecare/showarticle.aspx?id=37

7 The Joint Commission. (2021). Standard MM.06.01.01. *Comprehensive accreditation manual for hospitals.* Oakbrook Terrace, IL: The Joint Commission. (Level VII)

8 Centers for Medicare and Medicaid Services, Department of Health and Human Services. (2020). Condition of participation: Nursing services. 42 C.F.R. § 482.23(c).

9 Accreditation Association for Hospitals and Health Systems. (2020). Standard 16.01.03. *Healthcare Facilities Accreditation Program: Accreditation requirements for acute care hospitals.* Chicago, IL: Accreditation Association for Hospitals and Health Systems. (Level VII)

10 DNV GL-Healthcare USA, Inc. (2020). MM.1.SR.3. *NIAHO® accreditation requirements, interpretive guidelines and surveyor guidance—revision 20.0.* Milford, OH: DNV GL-Healthcare USA, Inc. (Level VII)

11 The Joint Commission. (2021). Standard NPSG.07.01.01. *Comprehensive accreditation manual for hospitals.* Oakbrook Terrace, IL: The Joint Commission. (Level VII)

12 Centers for Disease Control and Prevention. (2002). Guideline for hand hygiene in health-care settings: Recommendations of the Healthcare Infection Control Practices Advisory Committee and the HICPAC/SHEA/APIC/IDSA Hand Hygiene Task Force. *MMWR Recommendations and Reports, 51*(RR-16), 1–45. https://www.cdc.gov/mmwr/pdf/rr/rr5116.pdf (Level II)

13 World Health Organization. (2009). WHO guidelines on hand hygiene in health care: First global patient safety challenge, clean care is safer care. https://apps.who.int/iris/bitstream/handle/10665/44102/9789241597906_eng.pdf?sequence=1 (Level IV)

14 Centers for Medicare and Medicaid Services, Department of Health and Human Services. (2020). Condition of participation: Infection control. 42 C.F.R. § 482.42.

15 Accreditation Association for Hospitals and Health Systems. (2020). Standard 07.01.21. *Healthcare Facilities Accreditation Program: Accreditation requirements for acute care hospitals.* Chicago, IL: Accreditation Association for Hospitals and Health Systems. (Level VII)

16 DNV GL-Healthcare USA, Inc. (2020). IC.1.SR.1. *NIAHO® accreditation requirements, interpretive guidelines and surveyor guidance—revision 20.0.* Milford, OH: DNV GL-Healthcare USA, Inc. (Level VII)

17 The Joint Commission. (2021). Standard NPSG.01.01.01. *Comprehensive accreditation manual for hospitals.* Oakbrook Terrace, IL: The Joint Commission. (Level VII)

18 The Joint Commission. (2021). Standard RI.01.01.01. *Comprehensive accreditation manual for hospitals.* Oakbrook Terrace, IL: The Joint Commission. (Level VII)

19 Centers for Medicare and Medicaid Services, Department of Health and Human Services. (2020). Condition of participation: Patient's rights. 42 C.F.R. § 482.13(c)(1).

20 Accreditation Association for Hospitals and Health Systems. (2020). Standard 15.01.16. *Healthcare Facilities Accreditation Program: Accreditation requirements for acute care hospitals.* Chicago, IL: Accreditation Association for Hospitals and Health Systems. (Level VII)

21 DNV GL-Healthcare USA, Inc. (2020). PR.2.SR.5. *NIAHO® accreditation requirements, interpretive guidelines and surveyor guidance—revision 20.0.* Milford, OH: DNV GL-Healthcare USA, Inc. (Level VII)

22 The Joint Commission. (2021). Standard PC.02.01.21. *Comprehensive accreditation manual for hospitals.* Oakbrook Terrace, IL: The Joint Commission. (Level VII)

23 Waters, T. R., et al. (2009). Safe patient handling training for schools of nursing. https://www.cdc.gov/niosh/docs/2009-127/pdfs/2009-127.pdf (Level VII)

24 Siegel, J. D., et al. (2007, revised 2019). 2007 guideline for isolation precautions: Preventing transmission of infectious agents in healthcare settings. https://www.cdc.gov/infectioncontrol/pdf/guidelines/isolation-guidelines-H.pdf (Level II)

25 Accreditation Association for Hospitals and Health Systems. (2020). Standard 07.01.10. *Healthcare Facilities Accreditation Program: Accreditation requirements for acute care hospitals.* Chicago, IL: Accreditation Association for Hospitals and Health Systems. (Level VII)

26 DNV GL-Healthcare USA, Inc. (2020). IC.1.SR.2. *NIAHO® accreditation requirements, interpretive guidelines and surveyor guidance—revision 20.0.* Milford, OH: DNV GL-Healthcare USA, Inc. (Level VII)

27 Ganz, D. A., et al. (2013, reviewed 2021). *Preventing falls in hospitals: A toolkit for improving quality of care* (AHRQ Publication No. 13-0015-EF). Rockville, MD: Agency for Healthcare Research and Quality. https://www.ahrq.gov/professionals/systems/hospital/fallpxtoolkit/index.html (Level VII)

28 The Joint Commission. (2021). Standard RC.01.03.01. *Comprehensive accreditation manual for hospitals.* Oakbrook Terrace, IL: The Joint Commission. (Level VII)

29 Centers for Medicare and Medicaid Services, Department of Health and Human Services. (2020). Condition of participation: Medical record services. 42 C.F.R. § 482.24(b).

30 Accreditation Association for Hospitals and Health Systems. (2020). Standard 10.00.03. *Healthcare Facilities Accreditation Program: Accreditation requirements for acute care hospitals.* Chicago, IL: Accreditation Association for Hospitals and Health Systems. (Level VII)

31 DNV GL-Healthcare USA, Inc. (2020). MR.2.SR.1. *NIAHO® accreditation requirements, interpretive guidelines and surveyor guidance—revision 20.0.* Milford, OH: DNV GL-Healthcare USA, Inc. (Level VII)

32 The Joint Commission. (2021). Standard RC.02.01.01. *Comprehensive accreditation manual for hospitals.* Oakbrook Terrace, IL: The Joint Commission. (Level VII)

BURN CARE

The goals of burn care are to maintain the patient's physiologic stability, repair skin integrity, prevent infection, and promote maximal functioning and psychosocial health. Competent care immediately after a burn occurs can dramatically improve the success of overall treatment. (See *Burn care at the scene*.)

During the initial evaluation, treat the burn victim as a trauma patient. Focus the evaluation on the primary trauma survey while maintaining the patient's CAB. After the primary trauma survey, perform a head-to-toe assessment, followed by efforts to stop the burn and contain the injury. The head-to-toe assessment includes an evaluation of burn severity, which is determined by the depth and extend of the burn

---

Burn care at the scene

Acting promptly when a burn injury occurs can improve a patient's chance of uncomplicated recovery. Emergency care at the scene should include steps to stop the burn from worsening; assessment of the patient's circulation, airway, and breathing (CAB); a call for help to emergency medical services (EMS); and emotional and physiologic support for the patient.

Stop the burning process

■ If the victim is on fire, tell the person to fall to the ground, cover the face, and roll *to put out the flames. (If the person panics and runs, air will fuel the flames, worsening the burn and increasing the risk of inhalation injury.)*[1] Alternatively, if you can, wrap the victim in a blanket or other large covering *to smother the flames and protect the burned area from dirt.* Keep the victim's head outside the blanket *so that the person doesn't breathe toxic fumes.* As soon as the flames are out, unwrap the person *so that the heat can dissipate.*

■ Cool the burned area with cool running water *to decrease pain and stop the burn from growing deeper and larger.*[1,2,3] Ideal water temperature for cooling is 59° F (15° C) with an acceptable range of 46.4° F to 77° F (8° C to 25° C) for 20 minutes.[1] Do not use ice to cool the burned area *because it causes vasoconstriction and hypothermia.*[1,2]

■ If possible, remove any potential sources of heat, such as jewelry, belt buckles, and some types of clothing.[1] *In addition to adding to the burning process, these items can cause constriction as edema develops.* If the person's clothing adheres to the skin, don't try to remove it. Rather, cut around it.

■ When the burn is caused by a chemical agent, remove the offending agent and irrigate the affected areas with copious amounts of cool running water for 1 to 2 hours.[1]

■ Cover the wound with a clean, dry, sheet or other smooth, nonfuzzy material. If available, cover the wound with plastic cling wrap *to protect it from bacterial colonization and excessive fluid and heat loss.*[1]

Assess the damage

■ Assess the patient's CAB and perform cardiopulmonary resuscitation, if necessary.

■ Check for other serious injuries, such as fractures, spinal cord injury, lacerations, blunt trauma, and head contusions. Estimate the extent and depth of the burns.

■ If flames caused the burns, and the injury occurred in a closed space, assess for signs of inhalation injury, such as singed nasal hairs, burns on the face or mouth, soot-stained sputum, coughing or hoarseness, wheezing, and respiratory distress. Assess for signs of carbon monoxide poisoning, such as dizziness, nausea, headache, and seizures.

Call for help

■ Call for help as quickly as possible. Send someone to contact EMS.

■ If the victim is conscious and alert, try to get a brief medical history as soon as possible.

Provide support

■ Provide a warm environment for the patient while waiting for the EMS *to prevent hypothermia, which can have a negative effect on wound healing and infection rates and can lead to complications that increase the risk of morbidity and mortality.*[2,3]

■ Reassure the patient that help is on the way. Provide emotional support by staying with the patient, answering questions, and explaining what you're doing.

■ When help arrives, give the EMS a report on the patient's status.

---

and the presence of other factors, such as age, complications, coexisting conditions, the type of first aid performed, and the source and mechanism of injury.[1]

(See *Estimating burn surfaces in adults and children* and *Evaluating burn severity,* pages 101 and 102.)

When providing ongoing care for a patient with burns, blood pressure and heart rate must be monitored to promote stability.[5] Careful monitoring of the patient's respiratory status is also necessary, especially if the patient has suffered smoke inhalation. An adult with partial- to full-thickness burns involving more than 20% of the total body surface area or a child with burns involving more than 10% of the total body surface area usually needs fluid resuscitation, which aims to support the body's compensatory mechanisms without overwhelming them.[2,5] Administration of fluids, such as a crystalloid solution like lactated Ringer solution,[6] is commonly needed to keep the patient's urine output at 1 mL/kg/hour for children and 0.3 to 0.5 mL/kg/hour for adults.[2] Interventions to control body temperature to prevent hypothermia are also necessary, *because skin loss interferes with temperature regulation.*[1] Warm fluids, heat lamps, and hyperthermia blankets might be indicated to keep the patient's temperature above 97° F (36.1° C), when possible. Another important intervention is frequent review of laboratory values, such as serum electrolyte levels, to detect early changes in the patient's condition.

Infection can increase wound depth, cause rejection of skin grafts, slow healing, worsen pain, prolong hospitalization, and even lead to death. Measures to help prevent infection include dressing the burn site as ordered; monitoring IV catheters regularly, and assessing burn extent, body system function, and the patient's emotional status carefully.

Early positioning after a burn is extremely important to prevent contractures. Careful positioning and regular exercise for burned extremities help maintain joint function and minimize deformity. When the extremities aren't being exercised, they should be maintained in maximal extension, using splints if necessary. Particular attention to the patient's hands and neck are necessary because these body areas are most prone to rapid contracture. (See *Positioning a patient with burns to prevent deformity,* page 102.)

An *escharotomy* is usually performed by the practitioner within the first 24 hours of the burn injury.[7] This procedure releases the constricting necrotic skin (eschar) and allows the body tissue and organs to maintain normal perfusion and function. *Debridement* of the wound, a procedure that removes loose necrotic tissue, is commonly performed by the practitioner 2 to 7 days after the burn injury.[7] Debridement cleans the surfaces of the wound, allowing the wound to heal more quickly. *Burn wound excision* is a procedure that removes all necrotic tissue and prepares the wound surface for closure using wound care (such as topical antimicrobials or biological or synthetic wound covers), grafting, or flap closure. These procedures are usually used by the practitioner only on deep partial-thickness or full-thickness burns.[7] In recent years, hydrosurgery has become a more precise and controlled method of burn debridement before skin grafting and may be an option for specific patients.[8,9]

Burn care requires adherence to clean technique and use of a clean gown, a cap, and a mask whenever the burn wound is exposed.[4,10] Removal of a soiled dressing and wound cleaning require the use of clean gloves; application of topical agents or inner dressings requires the use of sterile gloves and sterile instruments and dressings.[4,10] Sterile gloves are also necessary to perform sharp bedside debridement.[11] Further research is needed to determine which wound cleaning and dressing products optimize healing.[12] Most wounds require dressing changes one to three times per day.[7]

A patient may have multiple burn wounds at different stages of healing. Appropriate care requires multiple treatment modalities and daily evaluation.[7]

Equipment

Wound cleansing solution, such as normal saline solution,[13] mild pH-balanced soap solution, or wound cleanser [4,14] ■ warm water ■ sterile drape ■ sterile bowls ■ sterile tissue forceps ■ sterile scissors ■ prescribed topical medication ■ prescribed pain medication ■ prescribed eye ointment or drops ■ sterile tongue depressor ■ sterile cotton-tipped applicator

Estimating burn surfaces in adults and children

You need to use different formulas to compute burned body surface area (BSA) in adults and children, *because the proportions of BSA vary with growth*. Smaller burn areas may be estimated using the patient's palmar surface (fingers and palm), which is about 1% of the BSA.[1]

Rule of Nines

The "Rule of Nines" is a quick way to estimate the extent of an adult patient's burns. This method quantifies BSA in percentages, in fractions of nine or in multiples of nine. To use this method, mentally assess the patient's burns using the body chart shown below. Add the corresponding percentages for each body section burned. Use the total—a rough estimate of burn extent—to calculate initial fluid replacement needs.

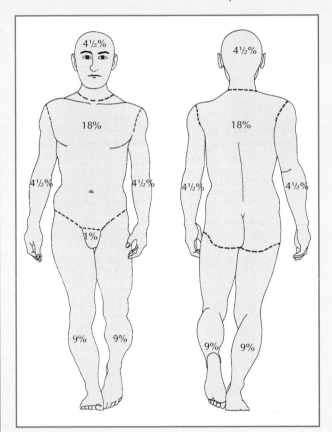

Lund and Browder chart

The Rule of Nines isn't accurate for infants and children *because their body shapes differ from those of adults*. An infant's head, for example, accounts for about 17% of total BSA, compared with 7% for an adult. The Lund and Browder chart, shown below, lists BSA percentages on the head, thigh, and leg for patients from birth to adulthood. See the figure below for these areas as well as other percentages and areas of the body for pediatric patients.

Percentage of burned body surface by age

Area	At birth	0 to 1 yr	1 to 4 yr	5 to 9 yr	10 to 15 yr	Adult
A: Half of head	9½%	8½%	6½%	5½%	4½%	3½%
B: Half of thigh	2¾%	3¼%	4%	4¼%	4½%	4¾%
C: Half of leg	2½%	2½%	2¾%	3%	3¼%	3½%

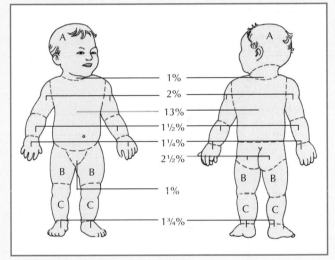

■ sterile burn dressing (for a wet dressing, use fine-mesh gauze) ■ sterile roller gauze ■ elastic netting or tape ■ sterile 4″ × 4″ (10-cm × 10-cm) gauze pads ■ gloves ■ sterile gloves ■ gowns ■ cap ■ mask and goggles or mask with face shield ■ cotton bath blanket ■ Optional: disposable hair clippers, specialty vest dressing, splint, tracheostomy ties, moisture chambers for eyes, eye dropper, pillows, elastic net slings, prescribed antimicrobial ointment.

A sterile field is required, and all equipment and supplies used when dressing the wound should be sterile.

Preparation of equipment

Inspect all equipment and supplies. If a product is expired, is defective, or has compromised integrity, remove it from patient use, label it as expired or defective, and report the expiration or defect as directed by your facility. Warm the treatment area to decrease the risk of hypothermia.[4] Make sure the treatment area has adequate light *to allow accurate wound assessment*.

Implementation

■ Verify the practitioner's orders.
■ Gather and prepare the necessary equipment and supplies.
■ Perform hand hygiene.[15,16,17,18,19,20]
■ Confirm the patient's identity using at least two patient identifiers.[21]
■ Provide privacy.[22,23,24,25]
■ Explain the procedure to the patient and family (if appropriate) according to their communication and learning needs *to increase understanding, allay their fears, and enhance cooperation*.[26]
■ Screen for and assess the patient's pain using facility-defined criteria that are consistent with the patient's age, condition, and ability to understand.[27]
■ Treat the patient's pain, as needed and ordered, using nonpharmacologic, pharmacologic, or a combination of approaches. Base treatment plan on evidence-based practices and the patient's clinical condition, past medical history, and pain management goals.[27]
■ Administer an analgesic, as prescribed, following safe medication administration practices *to increase the patient's comfort and tolerance levels*.[28,29,30,31]

Evaluating burn severity[1]

To judge a burn's severity, assess its depth and extent as well as other factors.

Superficial or epidermal (first-degree) burn

Does the burned area appear pink or red with minimal edema? Is the area sensitive to touch and temperature changes? If so, the patient most likely has a superficial or epidermal (first-degree) burn, affecting only the epidermal skin layer (shown below). Superficial burns are not included in the calculations for burn sizing.[4]

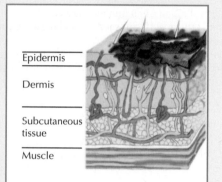

Epidermis

Dermis

Subcutaneous tissue

Muscle

Partial-thickness (second-degree) burn

Does the burned area appear pink or red, with a mottled appearance? Does the skin have large, thick-walled blisters with subcutaneous edema? Does touching the burn cause severe pain? Is the hair still present? If so, the patient most likely has a partial-thickness (second-degree) burn (shown below), affecting the epidermal and dermal layers. Superficial partial-thickness burns extend into the upper dermis and appear blistered and moist, whereas deep partial-thickness burns extend to the lower dermis, appear mottled, are drier, and do not blanch.[4]

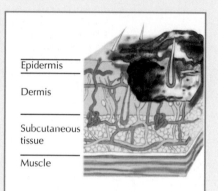

Epidermis

Dermis

Subcutaneous tissue

Muscle

Full-thickness (third-degree) burn

Does the burned area appear red, waxy white, brown, or black? Does red skin remain red with no blanching when you touch it? Is the skin leathery with extensive subcutaneous edema? Is the skin insensitive to touch? Does the hair fall out easily? If so, the patient most likely has a full-thickness (third-degree) burn that affects all skin layers (shown below). In full-thickness burns, the burn has destroyed the epidermis and all of the dermis.[4]

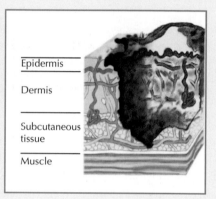

Epidermis

Dermis

Subcutaneous tissue

Muscle

Positioning a patient with burns to prevent deformity

Proper positioning of a patient with burns is necessary to help prevent deformity. This list reviews potential deformities as well as corresponding positioning and interventions that can help prevent them.

Neck flexion contracture
Preventive positioning: Extension
Nursing intervention: Remove pillow from bed.

Neck extensor contracture
Preventive positioning: Prone with head slightly raised
Nursing intervention: Place pillow or rolled towel under upper chest to flex cervical spine, or apply cervical collar, as ordered.

Axilla adduction and internal rotation
Preventive positioning: Shoulder joint in external rotation and 100- to 130-degree abduction
Nursing intervention: Use an IV pole, bedside table, or sling to suspend arm.

Axilla adduction and external rotation
Preventive positioning: Shoulder joint in forward flexion and 100- to 130-degree abduction
Nursing intervention: Use an IV pole, bedside table, or sling to suspend arm.

Shoulder protraction
Preventive positioning: Shoulders abducted and externally rotated
Nursing intervention: Remove pillow from bed.

Kyphosis
Preventive positioning: Shoulders abducted and externally rotated with hips neutral, not flexed
Nursing interventions: Avoid placing a pillow under head or legs.

Scoliosis
Preventive positioning: Supine; affected arm abducted
Nursing interventions: Place pillows, blanket rolls, or other positioning devices at sides.

Elbow flexion and pronation
Preventive positioning: Arm extended and supinated
Nursing intervention: Use an elbow splint or arm board.

Wrist flexion
Preventive positioning: Splint in 15-degree extension
Nursing interventions: Apply a wrist and hand splint.

Wrist extension
Preventive positioning: Splint in 15-degree flexion
Nursing intervention: Apply a wrist and hand splint.

Extensor tendons adhesions and loss of palmar grasp
Preventive positioning: Metacarpophalangeal joints in maximum flexion; interphalangeal joints in slight flexion; thumb in maximum abduction
Nursing intervention: Apply a hand splint; wrap fingers separately.

Hip internal rotation, flexion, and adduction
Preventive positioning: Neutral rotation and abduction; maintain extension by prone position
Nursing intervention: Place a pillow under buttocks when supine or use trochanter rolls or knee or long-leg splints.

Knee flexion
Preventive positioning: Knee extended
Nursing intervention: Apply a knee splint and avoid pillows under legs.

Plantar flexion
Preventive positioning: Ankle 90-degree dorsiflexion
Nursing intervention: Apply an ankle splint.

Administer an oral analgesic at an appropriate time before the procedure, depending on the medication's onset and peak of action. Administer an IV analgesic immediately before the procedure.

■ Raise the bed to waist level before providing patient care *to prevent caregiver back strain.*[32]
■ Perform hand hygiene.[15,16,17,18,19,20]
■ Cover the patient with a blanket *to prevent chilling.*
■ Put on a cap and mask and goggles or mask with a face shield.[33,34]
■ Perform hand hygiene.[15,16,17,18,19,20]
■ Put on a gown and gloves.[10,33,35]
■ Prepare the sterile field and supplies. Open equipment packages using sterile no-touch technique. Arrange the supplies on the sterile field in order of use. Pour the wound cleansing solution into a sterile bowl on the sterile field. If you're applying wet dressing, pour the prescribed antimicrobial agent solution into a sterile bowl.
■ Remove any old dressings and discard them in an appropriate receptacle.[34] Only remove dressings from areas that can be redressed within 30 minutes *to decrease heat loss and pain related to exposure of nerve endings to air.*[14] Complete wound care on these areas before moving to other areas of the body.
■ Remove and discard your gloves.
■ Perform hand hygiene.[15,16,17,18,19,20]
■ Put on a clean pair of gloves.[4,33,35]
■ Clean the wound with 4″ × 4″ (10-cm × 10-cm) gauze pads and wound cleansing solution, removing exudate and crusts as necessary using sterile forceps and sterile scissors.[4] If the patient has a scalp burn, clip the hair around the burn, as ordered. Clip other hair until it's about 2″ (5 cm) long *to ensure full visualization, to prevent hair from impeding the skin regeneration process of burned scalp areas.*[1] Clip the hair around an affected ear as needed. If cleaning the eyes, remove crusts and drainage.
■ Rinse the wound with warm water and pat it dry with 4″ × 4″ (10-cm × 10-cm) gauze pads.[4,14]
■ Assess the wound carefully. Focus on the wound's size, color, borders, exudate, bleeding, and odor; the type of tissue in the base; and the condition of the surrounding tissue. If the wound affects an extremity, monitor peripheral pulses, movement, and sensation, and observe for signs of pressure from splints (if used).[4]
■ Remove and discard your gloves.[34]
■ Perform hand hygiene[15,16,17,18,19,20] and put on sterile gloves.[4,10,33,35]

Providing arm and leg burn care
■ Apply prescribed topical medication to the wound using a sterile tongue depressor following safe medication administration practices.[4,28,29,30,31]
■ Wrap sterile burn dressing once around the patient's arm or leg, overlapping the edges slightly, until the wound is covered.
■ Alternatively, apply a wet dressing. If applying a wet dressing, soak fine-mesh gauze in a topical antimicrobial agent solution (such as silver nitrate), squeeze out the gauze until it is moist but not dripping, and then apply it to the wound.[4]
■ Apply a dry roller gauze dressing, wrapping from the distal area to the proximal area *to stimulate circulation.*
■ Secure the dressing with elastic netting or tape.
■ Elevate burned extremities on pillows or elastic net slings *to reduce edema.*[1,4]

Providing hand and foot burn care
■ Apply prescribed topical medication to the wound using a sterile tongue depressor[4] following safe medication administration practices.[28,29,30,31]
■ Wrap each finger or toe individually with a single layer of a sterile burn dressing[4] and then 4″ × 4″ (10-cm × 10-cm) gauze pads, or place gauze between the toes, as appropriate, to facilitate range of motion.[1,36]
■ If providing burn care for a hand, place the patient's hand in a functional position and secure this position with a dressing.
■ Apply splints as ordered.
■ Elevate burned extremities on pillows or elastic net slings *to reduce edema.*[14]

Providing chest, abdomen, and back burn care
■ Apply prescribed topical medication to the wound using a sterile tongue depressor[4] follow safe medication administration practices.[28,29,30,31]
■ Cover the entire burn area with sterile burn dressing. Alternatively, apply a wet dressing. If applying a wet dressing, soak fine-mesh gauze in a topical antimicrobial agent solution (such as silver nitrate), squeeze out the gauze until it's moist but not dripping, and then apply it to the wound.[4]
■ Wrap the area with roller gauze or apply a specialty vest dressing.
■ Secure the dressing with elastic netting or tape.
■ Make sure that the dressing doesn't restrict the patient's respiratory function.

Providing facial burn care
■ Apply prescribed topical medication to facial burns using a sterile tongue depressor following safe medication administration practices.[4,28,29,30,31]
■ Leave facial burns open to air, if possible.[1] If they require dressings, make sure that the dressings don't cover the patient's eyes, nostrils, or mouth.
■ Remove facial hair daily if it comes in contact with burned areas.

Providing ear burn care
■ Apply prescribed topical medication to ear burns using a sterile tongue depressor[4] following safe medication administration practices.[4,28,29,30,31]
■ Place a layer of 4″ × 4″ (10-cm × 10-cm) gauze behind the auricle *to prevent webbing.*[1]
■ Leave ear burns open to air, as ordered, or apply a sterile gauze burn dressing and then roller gauze. Position the patient's ears normally *to avoid damaging the auricular cartilage.*
■ Assess the patient's hearing ability.

Providing eye burn care
■ Apply prescribed eye ointment or drops using a sterile cotton-tipped applicator or eyedropper and following safe medication administration practices.[28,29,30,31] Use moisture chambers as needed, especially if the patient can't close the eyes completely.
■ Be sure to close the patient's eyes before applying eye pads *to prevent corneal abrasion.*

Providing nasal burn care
■ Check the patient's nostrils for inhalation injury, including an inflamed mucosa, singed vibrissae, and soot.[1]
■ Apply prescribed topical medication to the wound using a sterile tongue depressor[4] following safe medication administration practices.[28,29,30,31]
■ If the patient has a nasogastric tube, use tracheostomy ties *to secure the tube.* Check the ties frequently for excessive tightness resulting from swelling of facial tissue. Clean the area around the tube, as needed.

Completing burn care
■ Elevate the head of the bed *to reduce edema.*[4]
■ Reassess and respond to the patient's pain by evaluating the response to treatment and progress toward pain management goals. Assess for adverse reactions and risk factors for adverse events that may result from treatment.[27]
■ Return the bed to the lowest position *to prevent falls and maintain patient safety.*[37]
■ Discard used supplies in appropriate receptacles.[34]
■ Remove and discard your gloves and other personal protective equipment.[33,35]
■ Perform hand hygiene.[15,16,17,18,19,20]
■ Document the procedure.[38,39,40,41]

Special considerations
■ *To prevent cross-contamination,* clean and dress the cleanest areas first and the dirtiest or most contaminated areas last.[1] Make sure that you remove and discard your gloves, perform hand hygiene, and put on new gloves each time you move from one area to another. *To help prevent excessive pain and cross-contamination,* consider performing wound care in stages *to avoid exposing all wounds at the same time.*
■ Thorough assessment and documentation of the wound's appearance are essential *to detect infection and other complications.*[1] A purulent wound or green-gray exudate indicates infection, an overly dry wound suggests

dehydration, and a wound with a swollen, red edge suggests cellulitis. Suspect a fungal infection if the wound is white and powdery. Healthy granulation tissue appears clean, pinkish, and faintly shiny, and has no exudate.

■ Leave blisters intact or debride them, if ordered; studies support both interventions.[36] *Intact blisters protect underlying tissue and create a clean, moist wound environment. Debridement of blisters prevents bacterial growth and possible infection.* If ordered, debride blisters with sterile forceps or in the shower.

■ Keep in mind that the patient with healing burns has increased nutritional needs, including greater requirements for protein and carbohydrates *to accommodate an almost doubled basal metabolism.*

■ If you must manage a burn with topical medications, exposure to air, and no dressing, be sure to watch for such problems as wound adherence to bed linens, poor drainage control, and partial loss of topical medications.

■ Consider digital photography, if available at your facility, *to assist with monitoring of burn wound progress, promote ease of communication between burn units or health care facilities, and minimize prolonged exposure of the patient.*[1]

Patient teaching

Begin discharge planning as soon as the patient enters the facility *to help the patient and family (if present) make a smooth transition from facility to home. To encourage therapeutic adherence,* prepare the patient to expect scarring, teach wound management and pain control, and urge the patient to follow the prescribed exercise regimen. Provide encouragement and emotional support, and encourage the patient to join a burn survivor support group.

Successful burn self-care after discharge

You can help the patient make a successful transition from facility to home by encouraging the patient to follow the wound care and self-care guidelines below.

■ *To enhance healing,* instruct the patient to eat well-balanced meals with adequate carbohydrates and protein, to eat between-meal snacks, and to include at least one protein source in each meal and snack. Tell the patient to avoid tobacco, alcohol, and caffeine, *because these products constrict peripheral blood flow.*

■ Advise the patient to wash new skin with mild soap and water. *To prevent excessive skin dryness,* instruct the patient to use a water-based lubricating lotion and to avoid lotions containing alcohol or perfume.[10,36] Caution the patient to avoid bumping or scratching regenerated skin tissue.

■ Recommend that the patient wear nonrestrictive, nonabrasive clothing and launder it in a mild detergent. Advise the patient to wear protective clothing during cold weather *to prevent frostbite.*

■ Warn the patient not to expose new skin to strong sunlight, and to always use a sunblock with a high sun protection factor.[10,36] Also, tell the patient not to expose new skin to irritants, such as paint, solvents, strong detergents, and antiperspirants. Recommend cool baths or ice packs *to relieve itching.*

■ *To minimize scar formation,* explain to the patient the use of a pressure garment, which is usually worn for 23 hours per day for 6 months to 1 year. Instruct the patient to remove the garment only when performing daily hygiene. Tell the patient to suspect that the garment is too tight if it causes cold, numbness, or discoloration in the fingers or toes, or if its seams and zippers leave deep, red impressions for more than 10 minutes after garment removal.

■ Explain that restoring function to the burned area is a major goal for a patient with a burn. Tell the patient to follow the exercise regimens prescribed by the physical and occupational therapists and to adhere to the schedule of follow-up visits with the practitioner.[7]

■ Tell the patient to consult with the practitioner if itching occurs; explain that itching can be relieved with antihistamines, massage, cold application,[7] and other topical treatments, such as application of aloe vera, petrolatum-based creams, cocoa butter, mineral oil, hydrogel sheets, topical glucocorticoids, colloidal oatmeal in liquid paraffin, an Unna boot, local anesthetic cream, topical doxepin, silicone gel sheeting, and compression garments.[14] Tell the patient to avoid topical agents with lanolin *because they can worsen itching.*[14]

Also, teach the family and caregivers how to encourage, support, and provide care for the patient. (See *Successful burn self-care after discharge.*)

Complications

Complications include wound infection, systemic sepsis, deeper wound injury, and wound healing with unnecessary loss of function.[4] Prolonged burn care (more than 30 minutes) can cause heat loss, pain, stress, and sodium loss.[1]

Documentation

Record the date and time of all care provided. Document wound assessment findings, special dressing change techniques, preprocedure pain medication administered and its effectiveness, topical medications administered, positioning of the burned area, and the patient's tolerance of the procedure. Document teaching provided to the patient and family (if applicable), their understanding of that teaching, and any need for follow-up teaching.

REFERENCES

1 Agency for Clinical Innovation. (2019). *Clinical guidelines: Burn patient management.* (4th ed.). Chatswood, Australia: Agency for Clinical Innovation. https://www.aci.health.nsw.gov.au/__data/assets/pdf_file/0009/250020/Burn-patient-management-guidelines.pdf

2 ISBI Practice Guideline Committee, et al. (2016). ISBI practice guidelines for burn care. *Burns, 42*(5), 953–1021. https://www.sciencedirect.com/science/article/pii/S0305417916301449 (Level VII)

3 Stiles, K. (2015). Burn wound progression and the importance of first aid. *Wounds UK, 11*(2), 58–63.

4 Wiegand, D. L. (2017). *AACN procedure manual for high acuity, progressive, and critical care* (7th ed.). St. Louis, MO: Elsevier.

5 Pham, T. N., et al. (2008). American Burn Association practice guidelines: Burn shock resuscitation. *Journal of Burn Care & Research, 29,* 257–266. https://doi.org/10.1097/BCR.0b013e31815f3876 (Level VII)

6 Lewis, S. R., et al. (2018). Colloids versus crystalloids for fluid resuscitation in critically ill patients. *Cochrane Database of Systematic Reviews, 2018,* CD000567. https://www.ncbi.nlm.nih.gov/pmc/articles/PMC6513027/ (Level I)

7 Kagan, R. J., et al. (2013). Surgical management of the burn wound and use of skin substitutes: An expert panel white paper. *Journal of Burn Care & Research, 34,* e60–e79. (Level VII)

8 Legemate, C. M., et al. (2019). Application of hydrosurgery for burn wound debridement: An 8-year cohort analysis. *Burns, 45,* 88–96. (Level IV)

9 Kwa, K. A. A., et al. (2019). A systematic review on surgical and nonsurgical debridement techniques of burn wounds. *Journal of Plastic, Reconstructive & Aesthetic Surgery, 72,* 1752–1762. (Level V)

10 Knighton, J. (n.d.). Wound management: Wound care for the adult burn patient. http://burnresource.com/pdfs/wound_management.pdf

11 Wound, Ostomy and Continence Nurses Society Wound Committee & Association for Professionals in Infection Control and Epidemiology Guidelines Committee. (2011). Clean vs. sterile dressing techniques for management of chronic wounds: A fact sheet. *Journal of Wound, Ostomy and Continence Nursing, 39*(Suppl. 2), S30–S34. (Level VII)

12 Hayek, S., et al. (2010). Burn wound cleansing—a myth or a scientific practice. *Annals of Burns and Fire Disasters, 23*(1), 19–24. https://www.ncbi.nlm.nih.gov/pmc/articles/PMC3188235/

13 Wounds International. (2014). *Best practice guidelines: Effective skin and wound management of non-complex burns.* London, UK: Wounds International. https://www.woundsinternational.com/uploads/resources/5ebac-e6c70d4ea53a5d3e28ca65f1b74.pdf (Level VII)

14 Tenenhaus, M., & Rennekampff, H. O. (2020). Topical agents and dressings for local burn wound care. In: *UpToDate,* Jeschke, M. G., (Ed.).

15 The Joint Commission. (2021). Standard NPSG.07.01.01. *Comprehensive accreditation manual for hospitals.* Oakbrook Terrace, IL: The Joint Commission. (Level VII)

16 World Health Organization. (2009). WHO guidelines on hand hygiene in health care: First global patient safety challenge, clean care is safer care. https://apps.who.int/iris/bitstream/handle/10665/44102/9789241597906_eng.pdf (Level IV)

17 Centers for Disease Control and Prevention. (2002). Guideline for hand hygiene in health-care settings: Recommendations of the Healthcare

Infection Control Practices Advisory Committee and the HICPAC/SHEA/APIC/IDSA Hand Hygiene Task Force. *MMWR Recommendations and Reports, 51*(RR-16), 1–45. https://www.cdc.gov/mmwr/pdf/rr/rr5116.pdf (Level II)

18 Accreditation Association for Hospitals and Health Systems. (2020). Standard 07.01.21. *Healthcare Facilities Accreditation Program: Accreditation requirements for acute care hospitals.* Chicago, IL: Accreditation Association for Hospitals and Health Systems. (Level VII)

19 Centers for Medicare and Medicaid Services, Department of Health and Human Services. (2020). Condition of participation: Infection control. 42 C.F.R. § 482.42.

20 DNV GL-Healthcare USA, Inc. (2020). IC.1.SR.1. *NIAHO® accreditation requirements, interpretive guidelines and surveyor guidance—revision 20.0.* Milford, OH: DNV GL-Healthcare USA, Inc. (Level VII)

21 The Joint Commission. (2021). Standard NPSG.01.01.01. *Comprehensive accreditation manual for hospitals.* Oakbrook Terrace, IL: The Joint Commission. (Level VII)

22 Accreditation Association for Hospitals and Health Systems. (2020). Standard 15.01.16. *Healthcare Facilities Accreditation Program: Accreditation requirements for acute care hospitals.* Chicago, IL: Accreditation Association for Hospitals and Health Systems. (Level VII)

23 Centers for Medicare and Medicaid Services, Department of Health and Human Services. (2020). Condition of participation: Patient's rights. 42 C.F.R. § 482.13(c)(1).

24 The Joint Commission. (2021). Standard RI.01.01.01. *Comprehensive accreditation manual for hospitals.* Oakbrook Terrace, IL: The Joint Commission. (Level VII)

25 DNV GL-Healthcare USA, Inc. (2020). PR.2.SR.5. *NIAHO® accreditation requirements, interpretive guidelines and surveyor guidance—revision 20.0.* Milford, OH: DNV GL-Healthcare USA, Inc. (Level VII)

26 The Joint Commission. (2021). Standard PC.02.01.21. *Comprehensive accreditation manual for hospitals.* Oakbrook Terrace, IL: The Joint Commission.

27 The Joint Commission. (2021). Standard PC.01.02.07. *Comprehensive accreditation manual for hospitals.* Oakbrook Terrace, IL: The Joint Commission. (Level VII)

28 The Joint Commission. (2021). Standard MM.06.01.01. *Comprehensive accreditation manual for hospitals.* Oakbrook Terrace, IL: The Joint Commission. (Level VII)

29 Accreditation Association for Hospitals and Health Systems. (2020). Standard 16.01.03. *Healthcare Facilities Accreditation Program: Accreditation requirements for acute care hospitals.* Chicago, IL: Accreditation Association for Hospitals and Health Systems. (Level VII)

30 Centers for Medicare and Medicaid Services, Department of Health and Human Services. (2020). Condition of participation: Nursing services. 42 C.F.R. § 482.23(c).

31 DNV GL-Healthcare USA, Inc. (2020). MM.1.SR.3. *NIAHO® accreditation requirements, interpretive guidelines and surveyor guidance—revision 20.0.* Milford, OH: DNV GL-Healthcare USA, Inc. (Level VII)

32 Waters, T. R., et al. (2009). Safe patient handling training for schools of nursing. https://www.cdc.gov/niosh/docs/2009-127/pdfs/2009-127.pdf (Level VII)

33 Siegel, J. D., et al. (2007, revised 2019). 2007 guideline for isolation precautions: Preventing transmission of infectious agents in healthcare settings. https://www.cdc.gov/infectioncontrol/pdf/guidelines/isolation-guidelines-H.pdf (Level II)

34 Occupational Safety and Health Administration. (2012). Bloodborne pathogens, standard number 1910.1030. https://www.osha.gov/pls/oshaweb/owadisp.show_document?p_id=10051&p_table=STANDARDS (Level VII)

35 Accreditation Association for Hospitals and Health Systems. (2020). Standard 07.01.10. *Healthcare Facilities Accreditation Program: Accreditation requirements for acute care hospitals.* Chicago, IL: Accreditation Association for Hospitals and Health Systems. (Level VII)

36 Moss, L. S. (2010). Treatment of the burn patient in primary care. *Advances in Skin & Wound Care, 23*(11), 517–524. https://journals.lww.com/aswcjournal/Fulltext/2010/11000/Treatment_of_the_Burn_Patient_in_Primary_Care.8.aspx

37 Ganz, D. A., et al. (2013, reviewed 2021). *Preventing falls in hospitals: A toolkit for improving quality of care* (AHRQ Publication No. 13-0015-EF). Rockville, MD: Agency for Healthcare Research and Quality. https://www.ahrq.gov/professionals/systems/hospital/fallpxtoolkit/index.html (Level VII)

38 The Joint Commission. (2021). Standard RC.01.03.01. *Comprehensive accreditation manual for hospitals.* Oakbrook Terrace, IL: The Joint Commission. (Level VII)

39 Centers for Medicare and Medicaid Services, Department of Health and Human Services. (2020). Condition of participation: Medical record services. 42 C.F.R. § 482.24(b).

40 Accreditation Association for Hospitals and Health Systems. (2020). Standard 10.00.03. *Healthcare Facilities Accreditation Program: Accreditation requirements for acute care hospitals.* Chicago, IL: Accreditation Association for Hospitals and Health Systems. (Level VII)

41 DNV GL-Healthcare USA, Inc. (2020). MR.2.SR.1. *NIAHO® accreditation requirements, interpretive guidelines and surveyor guidance—revision 20.0.* Milford, OH: DNV GL-Healthcare USA, Inc. (Level VII)

BURN DRESSING APPLICATION, BIOLOGICAL AND SYNTHETIC

Biological dressings provide a temporary protective covering for burn wounds and for clean granulation tissue. They also secure fresh skin grafts temporarily and protect graft donor sites. In common use are three organic materials (pigskin, cadaver skin, and amniotic membrane) and one synthetic material (Biobrane). (See *Comparing biological and synthetic dressings*, page 106.) However, amniotic membrane is rarely used because of decreased availability, high cost, and risk of disease transmission.[1] In addition to stimulating rapid wound closure, biological dressings control pain, improve wound healing, and improve function and cosmetic outcomes.

Amniotic membrane or fresh cadaver skin are usually applied to the patient in the operating room (OR), although it may be applied in a treatment room. Pigskin and Biobrane may be applied in an OR or a treatment room. Before applying a biological or synthetic dressing, the caregiver must clean and debride the wound. The frequency of dressing changes depends on the type of wound and the dressing's specific function.

The use of sterile or clean technique for wound care depends on the patient's immune status; the wound status (chronic or acute), type, location, and depth; and the wound-healing environment.[4,5] For acute burn wounds, the caregiver should use sterile technique and wear a gown, a cap, and a mask whenever the burn wound is exposed.[5] The caregiver should wear a clean gown when applying dressings,[5] clean gloves to remove a soiled dressing and to clean the wound, and sterile gloves to apply topical agents and inner dressings,[2,5] and when performing sharp bedside debridement.[4]

Equipment

Two pairs of sterile gloves ▪ cap ▪ mask ▪ gown ▪ biological or synthetic dressing ▪ sterile normal saline solution ▪ sterile basin ▪ Xeroflo gauze (or similar nonadherent dressing with 3% bismuth tribromophenate in a water-in-oil emulsion), or Exu-Dry (or similar nonadherent dressing) ▪ roller gauze dressing ▪ sterile scissors ▪ tape or elastic netting ▪ Optional: prescribed analgesic, sterile forceps, sterile hemostat, gauze dressing.

Preparation of equipment

Inspect all equipment and supplies. If a product is expired, is defective, or has compromised integrity, remove it from patient use, label it as expired or defective, and report the expiration or defect as directed by your facility.

If you are using a biological dressing, pour sterile normal saline solution into a sterile basin and then place the biological dressing in the sterile basin. If you're using a synthetic dressing, open the dressing package and remove the sterile dressing packages within; then, using sterile no-touch technique, open the sterile dressing packages.[4] Make sure the treatment area has adequate light *to allow accurate wound assessment and dressing placement.*

Implementation

▪ Verify the practitioner's order.
▪ Gather and prepare the necessary equipment and supplies.
▪ Perform hand hygiene.[6,7,8,9,10,11]
▪ Confirm the patient's identity using at least two patient identifiers.[12]

Comparing biological and synthetic dressings

Type	Description and uses	Nursing considerations
Cadaver skin (allograft)	■ Obtained at autopsy up to 24 hours after death ■ Applied in the operating room or at the bedside to debrided, clean wounds ■ Available as fresh cryopreserved allografts in tissue banks nationwide ■ Provides protection, especially to granulation tissue after escharotomy ■ May be used in some patients as a test graft for autografting ■ Covers excised wounds immediately ■ Used most frequently for burns when autograft skin isn't available[2]	■ Observe for exudate. ■ Watch for signs of rejection. ■ Keep in mind that the gauze dressing may be removed every 8 hours to observe the graft.
Pigskin (heterograft or xenograft)	■ Applied in the operating room or at the bedside ■ Comes fresh or frozen in rolls or sheets ■ Can cover and protect debrided, clean wounds; mesh autografts; clean (eschar-free) partial-thickness burns; and exposed tendons	■ Reconstitute frozen form with normal saline solution 30 minutes before use. ■ Watch for signs of rejection. ■ Cover with gauze dressing or leave exposed to air, as ordered.
Amniotic membrane (homograft)	■ Must be sterile and come from an uncomplicated birth; must undergo serologic tests ■ Bacteriostatic condition doesn't require antimicrobials ■ May be used to protect partial-thickness burns or (temporarily) granulation tissue before autografting ■ Applied by the practitioner to clean wounds only	■ Change the membrane every 48 hours. ■ Cover the membrane with a gauze dressing or leave it exposed, as ordered. ■ If you apply a gauze dressing, change it every 48 hours.
Biobrane® (biosynthetic membrane)	■ Comes in sterile, prepackaged sheets in various sizes and in glove form for hand burns ■ Used to cover donor graft sites, superficial partial-thickness burns, debrided wounds awaiting autograft, and meshed autografts ■ Reduces pain ■ Applied by the nurse	■ Apply taut against the skin. ■ Leave the membrane in place until the tissue underneath is healed, typically 7 to 14 days.[3] As the burn heals, Biobrane turns white and dry and lifts away. ■ Don't use this dressing for preparing a granulation bed for subsequent autografting.

■ Provide privacy.[13,14,15,16]

■ Explain the procedure to the patient and family (if appropriate) according to their communication and learning needs *to increase their understanding, allay their fears, and enhance cooperation.*[17]

■ Screen for and assess the patient's pain using facility-defined criteria that are consistent with the patient's age, condition, and ability to understand.[18]

■ Treat the patient's pain as needed and ordered using nonpharmacologic, pharmacologic, or a combination of approaches. Base the treatment plan on evidence-based practices and the patient's clinical conditions, past medical history, and pain management goals.[18]

■ If ordered, administer an analgesic following safe medication administration practices *to increase the patient's comfort and tolerance levels.*[19,20,21,22] Administer an oral analgesic long enough before the procedure to account for the medication's onset and peak effect; administer an IV analgesic immediately before the procedure.

■ Provide a warm environment.[23]

■ Raise the patient's bed to waist level before providing patient care *to prevent caregiver back strain.*[24]

■ Perform hand hygiene.[6,7,8,9,10,11]

■ Put on a cap and a mask.[4,5,25,26]

■ Perform hand hygiene.[6,7,8,9,10,11]

■ Put on a gown and sterile gloves.[4,5,25,26]

■ Assess the burn wound, noting the color, size, odor, and depth of the wound as well as the presence of drainage, bleeding, edema, and eschar. Monitor for cellulitis in the surrounding tissue.[23]

■ Clean and debride the wound *to reduce bacteria.*[23] (See the "Sharp debridement" procedure.)

NURSING ALERT Debridement must be thorough to remove all coagulum or eschar, especially when using Biobrane, *because the dressing will not adhere to dead tissue and the presence of dead tissue may result in infection.*[3]

■ Remove and discard your gloves.[27]

■ Perform hand hygiene[6,7,8,9,10,11] and put on a new pair of sterile gloves.[4,5,25,26]

■ Place the dressing directly on the wound surface. Apply a pigskin dressing dermal (shiny) side down; apply a Biobrane dressing nylon-backed (dull) side down.[3] Roll the dressing directly onto the skin, if applicable. Place the dressing strips so that the edges touch but don't overlap. Use sterile forceps, if needed.

■ Smooth the dressing. Eliminate folds and wrinkles by rolling out the dressing with a hemostat handle, a forceps handle, or your dominant hand *to cover the wound completely and ensure adherence.*

■ Use sterile scissors to trim the dressing around the wound *so that the dressing fits the wound without overlapping adjacent areas.*

■ Place Xeroflo™ gauze directly over an allograft, pigskin graft, or amniotic membrane. Place a few layers of gauze on top *to absorb exudate*, and wrap with a roller gauze dressing. Secure the dressing with tape or elastic netting.

■ Place a nonadhesive dressing (such as Exu-Dry)[28] over a Biobrane dressing *to absorb drainage and provide stability.* Wrap the dressing with a roller gauze dressing, and secure it with tape or elastic netting.

■ Position the patient comfortably. Elevate the area if possible *to reduce edema, which can prevent the dressing from adhering.*

■ Return the bed to the lowest position *to prevent falls and maintain patient safety.*[29]

■ Reassess and respond to the patient's pain by evaluating the response to treatment and progress toward pain management goals. Assess for adverse reactions and risk factors for adverse events that may result from treatment.[18]

■ Discard used supplies in appropriate receptacles.[27]

■ Remove and discard your gloves and personal protective equipment.[25,26]

■ Perform hand hygiene.[6,7,8,9,10,11]

■ Document the procedure.[30,31,32,33]

Special considerations

■ Handle a biological or synthetic dressing as little as possible.

- During daily dressing changes, remove the dressing down to the Xeroflo gauze and replace the gauze after inspecting the Xeroflo for drainage, adherence, and signs of infection.
- For the first 24 hours after applying a Biobrane dressing, keep the outer dressing in place and don't let it get wet. After 24 hours, remove the dressing down to the Biobrane during daily dressing changes and inspect the site for signs of infection. After the Biobrane adheres (usually in 2 to 3 days), you don't need to keep it covered with an outer dressing.[3]

Patient teaching

Instruct the patient or caregiver to assess the site daily for signs of complications, such as infection, swelling, blisters, drainage, and separation. Make sure the patient knows whom to contact if any of these complications develop.

Complications

Infection can develop under a biological or synthetic dressing. Observe the wound carefully during dressing changes for signs of infection. If wound drainage appears purulent, remove the dressing; clean the area with normal saline solution or another prescribed cleaning solution, as ordered; and apply a fresh biological or synthetic dressing.

Documentation

Record the time and date of dressing changes. Note areas of application, the quality of adherence, and purulent drainage or other signs of infection. Document preprocedure pain assessment, pain medication administered, and the effectiveness of your pain management interventions. Also describe the patient's tolerance of the procedure. Document teaching provided to the patient and family (if applicable), their understanding of that teaching, and any need for follow-up teaching.

REFERENCES

1 Bezuhly, M., & Fish, J. S. (2012). Acute burn care. *Plastic and Reconstructive Surgery, 130,* 349e–358e.
2 Kagan, R. J., et al. (2013). Surgical management of the burn wound and use of skin substitutes: An expert panel white paper. *Journal of Burn Care & Research, 34,* e60–e79. (Level VII)
3 Smith & Nephew. (n.d.). Biobrane: Instructions for use. https://www.smith-nephew.com/belgique/produits-old/biobrane-/biobrane--instructions-for-use/
4 Wound, Ostomy and Continence Nurses Society Wound Committee & the Association for Professionals in Infection Control and Epidemiology 2000 Guidelines Committee. (2012). Clean vs. sterile dressing techniques for management of chronic wounds: A fact sheet. *Journal of Wound, Ostomy and Continence Nursing, 39*(Suppl. 2), S30–S34. https://www.nursingcenter.com/journalarticle?Article_ID=1320693&Journal_ID=448075&Issue_ID=1320684 (Level VII)
5 Knighton, J. (n.d.). Wound management: Wound care for the adult burn patient. http://burnresource.com/pdfs/wound_management.pdf
6 The Joint Commission. (2021). Standard NPSG.07.01.01. *Comprehensive accreditation manual for hospitals.* Oakbrook Terrace, IL: The Joint Commission. (Level VII)
7 Centers for Disease Control and Prevention. (2002). Guideline for hand hygiene in health-care settings: Recommendations of the Healthcare Infection Control Practices Advisory Committee and the HICPAC/SHEA/APIC/IDSA Hand Hygiene Task Force. *MMWR Recommendations and Reports, 51*(RR-16), 1–45. https://www.cdc.gov/mmwr/pdf/rr/rr5116.pdf (Level II)
8 World Health Organization. (2009). WHO guidelines on hand hygiene in health care: First global patient safety challenge, clean care is safer care. t https://apps.who.int/iris/bitstream/handle/10665/44102/9789241597906_eng.pdf?sequence=1 (Level IV)
9 Centers for Medicare and Medicaid Services, Department of Health and Human Services. (2020). Condition of participation: Infection control. 42 C.F.R. § 482.42.
10 Accreditation Association for Hospitals and Health Systems. (2020). Standard 07.01.21. *Healthcare Facilities Accreditation Program: Accreditation requirements for acute care hospitals.* Chicago, IL: Accreditation Association for Hospitals and Health Systems. (Level VII)
11 DNV GL-Healthcare USA, Inc. (2020). IC.1.SR.1. *NIAHO® accreditation requirements, interpretive guidelines and surveyor guidance—revision 20.0.* Milford, OH: DNV GL-Healthcare USA, Inc. (Level VII)
12 The Joint Commission. (2021). Standard NPSG.01.01.01. *Comprehensive accreditation manual for hospitals.* Oakbrook Terrace, IL: The Joint Commission. (Level VII)
13 The Joint Commission. (2021). Standard RI.01.01.01. *Comprehensive accreditation manual for hospitals.* Oakbrook Terrace, IL: The Joint Commission. (Level VII)
14 DNV GL-Healthcare USA, Inc. (2020). PR.2.SR.5. *NIAHO® accreditation requirements, interpretive guidelines and surveyor guidance—revision 20.0.* Milford, OH: DNV GL-Healthcare USA, Inc. (Level VII)
15 Centers for Medicare and Medicaid Services, Department of Health and Human Services. (2020). Condition of participation: Patient's rights. 42 C.F.R. § 482.13(c)(1).
16 Accreditation Association for Hospitals and Health Systems. (2020). Standard 15.01.16. *Healthcare Facilities Accreditation Program: Accreditation requirements for acute care hospitals.* Chicago, IL: Accreditation Association for Hospitals and Health Systems. (Level VII)
17 The Joint Commission. (2021). Standard PC.02.01.21. *Comprehensive accreditation manual for hospitals.* Oakbrook Terrace, IL: The Joint Commission. (Level VII)
18 The Joint Commission. (2021). Standard PC.01.02.07. *Comprehensive accreditation manual for hospitals.* Oakbrook Terrace, IL: The Joint Commission. (Level VII)
19 The Joint Commission. (2021). Standard MM.06.01.01. *Comprehensive accreditation manual for hospitals.* Oakbrook Terrace, IL: The Joint Commission. (Level VII)
20 Centers for Medicare and Medicaid Services, Department of Health and Human Services. (2020). Condition of participation: Nursing services. 42 C.F.R. § 482.23(c).
21 Accreditation Association for Hospitals and Health Systems. (2020). Standard 16.01.03. *Healthcare Facilities Accreditation Program: Accreditation requirements for acute care hospitals.* Chicago, IL: Accreditation Association for Hospitals and Health Systems. (Level VII)
22 DNV GL-Healthcare USA, Inc. (2020). MM.1.SR.3. *NIAHO® accreditation requirements, interpretive guidelines and surveyor guidance—revision 20.0.* Milford, OH: DNV GL-Healthcare USA, Inc. (Level VII)
23 Wiegand, D. L. (2017). *AACN procedure manual for high acuity, progressive, and critical care* (7th ed.). St. Louis, MO: Elsevier.
24 Waters, T. R., et al. (2009). Safe patient handling training for schools of nursing. https://www.cdc.gov/niosh/docs/2009-127/pdfs/2009-127.pdf (Level VII)
25 Accreditation Association for Hospitals and Health Systems. (2020). Standard 07.01.10. *Healthcare Facilities Accreditation Program: Accreditation requirements for acute care hospitals.* Chicago, IL: Accreditation Association for Hospitals and Health Systems. (Level VII)
26 Siegel, J. D., et al. (2007, revised 2019). 2007 guideline for isolation precautions: Preventing transmission of infectious agents in healthcare settings. https://www.cdc.gov/infectioncontrol/pdf/guidelines/isolation-guidelines-H.pdf (Level II)
27 Occupational Safety and Health Administration. (2012). Bloodborne pathogens, standard number 1910.1030. https://www.osha.gov/pls/oshaweb/owadisp.show_document?p_id=10051&p_table=STANDARDS (Level VII)
28 Smith & Nephew. (n.d.). EXU-DRY™. https://www.smith-nephew.com/professional/products/advanced-wound-management/exu-dry-wound-dressing/#
29 Ganz, D. A., et al. (2013, reviewed 2021). *Preventing falls in hospitals: A toolkit for improving quality of care* (AHRQ Publication No. 13-0015-EF). Rockville, MD: Agency for Healthcare Research and Quality. https://www.ahrq.gov/professionals/systems/hospital/fallpxtoolkit/index.html (Level VII)
30 The Joint Commission. (2021). Standard RC.01.03.01. *Comprehensive accreditation manual for hospitals.* Oakbrook Terrace, IL: The Joint Commission. (Level VII)
31 Centers for Medicare and Medicaid Services, Department of Health and Human Services. (2020). Condition of participation: Medical record services. 42 C.F.R. § 482.24(b).
32 Accreditation Association for Hospitals and Health Systems. (2020). Standard 10.00.03. *Healthcare Facilities Accreditation Program: Accreditation requirements for acute care hospitals.* Chicago, IL: Accreditation Association for Hospitals and Health Systems. (Level VII)
33 DNV GL-Healthcare USA, Inc. (2020). MR.2.SR.1. *NIAHO® accreditation requirements, interpretive guidelines and surveyor guidance—revision 20.0.* Milford, OH: DNV GL-Healthcare USA, Inc. (Level VII)

CANE USE TRAINING

Indicated for the patient with one-sided weakness or injury, occasional loss of balance, pain, fatigue, or joint instability, a cane provides improved balance and postural stability by widening the base of support and reduces fatigue and strain on weight-bearing joints.[1] Available in various sizes, a cane should extend from the greater trochanter to the floor and have a rubber tip to prevent slipping.[2] Canes are contraindicated for a patient with bilateral weakness; such a patient should use crutches or a walker.

Equipment

Rubber-tipped cane ▪ nonskid slippers or shoes with rubber soles ▪ Optional: gait belt, standardized fall risk assessment tool.

Although wooden canes are available, patients most commonly use one of three types of aluminum canes. A standard aluminum cane (for a patient who needs only slight assistance with walking) provides the least support. A T-handle cane (for a patient with hand weakness) has a straight-shaped handle with grips and a bent shaft. It provides greater stability than a standard cane. A three- or four-pronged (quad) cane (for a patient with poor balance or one-sided weakness and an inability to hold onto a walker with both hands) splits at the base into three or four short, splayed legs and provides greater stability than a standard cane but considerably less than a walker.

Preparation of equipment

Inspect all equipment and supplies. If a product is defective or has compromised integrity, remove it from patient use, label it as defective, and report the defect as directed by your facility. Ask the patient to hold the cane on the uninvolved side 6" (15.2 cm) from the base of the little toe. If the cane is made of aluminum, adjust its height by pushing in the metal button on the shaft and raising or lowering the shaft; if the cane is made of wood, you can remove the rubber tip and saw off the excess length. At the correct height, the handle of the cane should be level with the greater trochanter and allow approximately 30-degree flexion at the elbow.[3] If the cane is too short, the patient will have to drop the shoulder to lean on it; if it's too long, the patient will have to raise the shoulder and will have difficulty supporting weight.

Implementation

▪ Verify the practitioner's order for mobility training.
▪ Gather and prepare the necessary equipment and supplies.
▪ Perform hand hygiene.[4,5,6,7,8,9]
▪ Confirm the patient's identity using at least two patient identifiers.[10]
▪ Provide privacy.[11,12,13,14]
▪ Explain the procedure to the patient and family (if appropriate) according to their communication and learning needs *to increase their understanding, allay their fears, and enhance cooperation.*[15]
▪ Perform a fall risk assessment using a standardized fall risk assessment tool, as needed.[16,17] A fall risk assessment is generally performed on admission, on transfer within the hospital, after a significant change in the patient's condition, and after a fall.[17]
▪ Institute fall precautions: make sure that the patient is wearing nonskid slippers or shoes with rubber soles; keep the walking area uncluttered and well lit; make sure the floor is clean and dry; and keep the hospital bed and wheelchair locked.[17]

HOSPITAL-ACQUIRED CONDITION ALERT Keep in mind that the Centers for Medicare and Medicaid Services considers an injury from a fall a hospital-acquired condition *because it can be reasonably prevented using a variety of best practices.* Follow fall prevention practices (such as performing a fall risk assessment and instituting fall precautions) *to reduce the risk of injury from patient falls.*[17,18,19]

▪ Tell the patient to hold the cane close to the body and not to place the cane ahead of the toe of the affected lower extremity *to prevent leaning.* Also tell the patient to hold the cane on the uninvolved side *to promote a reciprocal gait pattern and to distribute weight away from the involved side.*[1,20]
▪ Instruct the patient to move the cane forward and the uninvolved leg forward 4" to 8" (10 to 20 cm) simultaneously, followed by the uninvolved leg.[20]
▪ Encourage the patient to keep the stride length of each leg and the timing of each step (cadence) equal.
▪ Demonstrate the technique for the patient.
▪ Have the patient return the demonstration, and provide additional teaching as needed.

Negotiating stairs

▪ Instruct the patient to always use a railing, if present, when going up or down stairs. Tell the patient to hold the cane with the other hand,[1] as shown below. To ascend stairs, tell the patient to lead with the uninvolved leg and follow with the involved leg; to descend, tell the patient to lead with the involved leg and follow with the uninvolved one. Help the patient remember by using this mnemonic device: "Up with the good; down with the bad."[1]

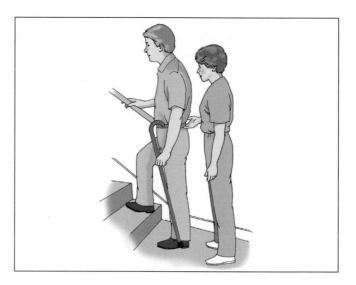

▪ To negotiate stairs without a railing, tell the patient to use the walking technique to ascend and descend the stairs. Thus, to ascend stairs, tell the patient to hold the cane on the uninvolved side, step with the uninvolved leg, advance the cane, and then move the involved leg. To descend, have the patient hold the cane on the uninvolved side, lead with the cane, advance the involved leg, and then, finally, advance the uninvolved leg.[1]
▪ Remind the patient always to move the cane just before moving the involved leg in all stair use regardless of direction.

Using a chair

▪ To teach the patient to sit down, stand by the affected side and tell the patient to place the backs of the legs against the edge of the chair seat. Then tell the patient to move the cane out from the side and to reach back with both hands to grasp the chair's armrests. Supporting the weight on the armrests, the patient can then lower down onto the seat. Have the seated patient keep the cane hooked on the armrest or the chair back.
▪ To teach the patient to get up, stand by the affected side and tell the patient to unhook the cane from the chair and hold it in the stronger hand as the patient grasps the armrests. Then tell the patient to move the uninvolved foot slightly forward, to lean slightly forward, and to push against the armrests to raise upright (as shown).

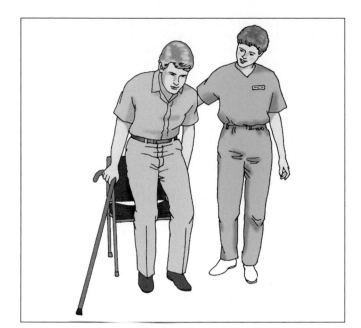

- Instruct the patient not to lean on the cane when sitting or rising from the chair, *to prevent falls.*
- Supervise the patient each time the patient gets into or out of a chair until you're both certain the patient can do so independently.
- Perform hand hygiene.[4,5,6,7,8,9]
- Document the procedure.[21,22,23,24]

Special considerations

- If the patient needs extra support during the learning period, guard the patient carefully by standing behind the patient slightly to the weaker side and putting one foot between the patient's feet and your other foot to the outside of the uninvolved leg *to prevent falls.* If necessary, use a gait belt.[1]
- Coordinate practice sessions in the physical therapy department, if necessary.[25]

Patient teaching

Instruct the patient and family to assess the patient's home environment for safety concerns. Tell them to secure or remove loose rugs, electrical cords, and clutter from the floor. Instruct the patient to use safety bars and a raised toilet seat in the bathroom, and a nonskid mat in the bathtub. Recommend that the patient use a fanny pack or backpack to carry items around the house, and to keep personal items close by.[20] Also recommend that the patient wear nonskid slippers or shoes with rubber soles and replace the tip of the cane when it's worn out.

Complications

A poorly fitted cane can cause the patient to lose balance and fall.

Documentation

Record the type of cane used, the amount of guarding required, the distance the patient walked, and the patient's understanding and tolerance of cane walking. Document teaching provided to the patient and family (if applicable), their understanding of that teaching, and any need for follow-up teaching.

REFERENCES

1 Lynn, P. (2018). *Taylor's clinical nursing skills: A nursing process approach* (5th ed.). Philadelphia, PA: Wolters Kluwer.
2 Hinkle, J. L., & Cheever, K. H. (2018). *Brunner & Suddarth's textbook of medical-surgical nursing* (14th ed.). Philadelphia, PA: Wolters Kluwer.
3 Webster, J., & Murphy, D. (2019). *Atlas of orthoses and assistive devices* (5th ed.). Philadelphia, PA: Elsevier.
4 The Joint Commission. (2021). Standard NPSG.07.01.01. *Comprehensive accreditation manual for hospitals.* Oakbrook Terrace, IL: The Joint Commission. (Level VII)
5 Centers for Disease Control and Prevention. (2002). Guideline for hand hygiene in health-care settings: Recommendations of the Healthcare Infection Control Practices Advisory Committee and the HICPAC/SHEA/APIC/IDSA Hand Hygiene Task Force. *MMWR Recommendations and Reports, 51*(RR-16), 1–45. at https://www.cdc.gov/mmwr/pdf/rr/rr5116.pdf (Level II)
6 World Health Organization. (2009). WHO guidelines on hand hygiene in health care: First global patient safety challenge, clean care is safer care. https://apps.who.int/iris/bitstream/handle/10665/44102/9789241597906_eng.pdf?sequence=1 (Level IV)
7 Centers for Medicare and Medicaid Services, Department of Health and Human Services. (2020). Condition of participation: Infection control. 42 C.F.R. § 482.42.
8 Accreditation Association for Hospitals and Health Systems. (2020). Standard 07.01.21. *Healthcare Facilities Accreditation Program: Accreditation requirements for acute care hospitals.* Chicago, IL: Accreditation Association for Hospitals and Health Systems. (Level VII)
9 DNV GL-Healthcare USA, Inc. (2020). IC.1.SR.1. *NIAHO® accreditation requirements, interpretive guidelines and surveyor guidance—revision 20.0.* Milford, OH: DNV GL-Healthcare USA, Inc. (Level VII)
10 The Joint Commission. (2021). Standard NPSG.01.01.01. *Comprehensive accreditation manual for hospitals.* Oakbrook Terrace, IL: The Joint Commission. (Level VII)
11 DNV GL-Healthcare USA, Inc. (2020). PR.2.SR.5. *NIAHO® accreditation requirements, interpretive guidelines and surveyor guidance—revision 20.0.* Milford, OH: DNV GL-Healthcare USA, Inc. (Level VII)
12 The Joint Commission. (2021). Standard RI.01.01.01. *Comprehensive accreditation manual for hospitals.* Oakbrook Terrace, IL: The Joint Commission. (Level VII)
13 Centers for Medicare and Medicaid Services, Department of Health and Human Services. (2020). Condition of participation: Patient's rights. 42 C.F.R. § 482.13(c)(1).
14 Accreditation Association for Hospitals and Health Systems. (2020). Standard 15.01.16. *Healthcare Facilities Accreditation Program: Accreditation requirements for acute care hospitals.* Chicago, IL: Accreditation Association for Hospitals and Health Systems. (Level VII)
15 The Joint Commission. (2021). Standard PC.02.01.21. *Comprehensive accreditation manual for hospitals.* Oakbrook Terrace, IL: The Joint Commission. (Level VII)
16 The Joint Commission. (2015). Sentinel event alert: Preventing falls and fall-related injuries in health-care facilities. http://www.jointcommission.org/assets/1/18/SEA_55.pdf (Level VII)
17 Ganz, D. A., et al. (2013, reviewed 2021). *Preventing falls in hospitals: A toolkit for improving quality of care* (AHRQ Publication No. 13-0015-EF). Rockville, MD: Agency for Healthcare Research and Quality. https://www.ahrq.gov/professionals/systems/hospital/fallpxtoolkit/index.html (Level VII)
18 Jarrett, N., & Callaham, M. (2016). Evidence-based guidelines for selected hospital-acquired conditions: Final report. https://www.cms.gov/Medicare/Medicare-Fee-for-Service-Payment/HospitalAcqCond/Downloads/2016-HAC-Report.pdf
19 The Joint Commission. (2021). Standard PC.01.02.08. *Comprehensive accreditation manual for hospitals.* Oakbrook Terrace, IL: The Joint Commission. (Level VII)
20 American Academy of Orthopaedic Surgeons. (2015). How to use crutches, canes, and walkers. https://orthoinfo.aaos.org/en/recovery/how-to-use-crutches-canes-and-walkers
21 The Joint Commission. (2021). Standard RC.01.03.01. *Comprehensive accreditation manual for hospitals.* Oakbrook Terrace, IL: The Joint Commission. (Level VII)
22 Accreditation Association for Hospitals and Health Systems. (2020). Standard 10.00.03. *Healthcare Facilities Accreditation Program: Accreditation requirements for acute care hospitals.* Chicago, IL: Accreditation Association for Hospitals and Health Systems. (Level VII)
23 Centers for Medicare and Medicaid Services, Department of Health and Human Services. (2020). Condition of participation: Medical record services. 42 C.F.R. § 482.24.
24 DNV GL-Healthcare USA, Inc. (2020). MR.2.SR.1. *NIAHO® accreditation requirements, interpretive guidelines and surveyor guidance—revision 20.0.* Milford, OH: DNV GL-Healthcare USA, Inc. (Level VII)
25 Craven, R. F., et al. (2021). *Fundamentals of nursing: Concepts and competencies for practice* (9th ed.). Philadelphia, PA: Wolters Kluwer.

CAPILLARY BLOOD GAS SAMPLING

An alternative to arterial blood gas (ABG) sampling, capillary blood gas sampling helps monitor a patient's respiratory status. Blood gas analysis evaluates oxygenation and ventilation by measuring blood pH and the partial pressures of arterial oxygen (Pao_2) and carbon dioxide ($Paco_2$). Blood pH measurement reveals the blood's acid–base balance. Pao_2 indicates the amount of oxygen that the lungs deliver to the blood, and $Paco_2$ indicates the lungs' capacity to eliminate carbon dioxide. Capillary blood gas sampling is used to measure acid-base balance and $Paco_2$; however, it isn't useful for measuring Pao_2. Pulse oximetry should be used to measure and evaluate oxygen saturation levels along with capillary blood gas sampling.[1]

Capillary blood gas sampling involves a simple fingerstick, and is less painful and easier to perform than an arterial puncture. The values obtained from capillary blood gas sampling are clinically significant only if the sampling site is warmed properly and if the puncture site isn't squeezed. The adequate collected sample should be free from air and clotting.[1]

Capillary blood must be collected in special balanced-heparin capillary blood gas collection tubes.[1] The laboratory should analyze samples within 15 minutes of collection.[2]

Equipment

Single use, auto-disabling sterile lancet (1.5 mm in depth) ▪ alcohol pad ▪ 2″ × 2″ (5-cm × 5-cm) sterile gauze pad ▪ gloves ▪ preheparinized capillary tube ▪ warming supplies (such as a chemical warmer or a warm cloth that's less than 109° F [42.8° C]) ▪ sealing clay, wax sealer, or cap ▪ sample collection label ▪ laboratory biohazard transport bag ▪ Optional: topical anesthetic, small adhesive bandage, crushed ice, plastic bag, laboratory request form.

Preparation of equipment

Inspect all equipment and supplies. If a product is expired, is defective, or has compromised integrity, remove it from patient use, label it as expired or defective, and report the expiration or defect as directed by your facility.

Fill a plastic bag with enough crushed ice to contain the sample if you expect a delay in analysis.[3]

Implementation

▪ Verify the practitioner's order.
▪ Gather and prepare the necessary equipment and supplies.
▪ Perform hand hygiene.[4,5,6,7,8,9]
▪ Confirm the patient's identity using at least two patient identifiers.[10]
▪ Provide privacy.[11,12,13,14]
▪ Explain the procedure to the patient and family (if appropriate), according to their individual communication and learning needs *to increase their understanding, allay their fears, and enhance cooperation.*[15]
▪ Select the capillary puncture site; avoid the earlobe, *which isn't an appropriate site for this procedure.* The finger is the preferred site in adults.[16] Select a site on the second or third finger, using the side of the finger, parallel to the side edges of the nail.[16] Avoid the finger's tip or pad *to prevent additional discomfort.*

NURSING ALERT Avoid punctures at the site of a previous puncture; through inflamed, swollen, edematous or poorly perfused tissues; at a localized area of infection; or at peripheral arteries.

▪ Apply a topical anesthetic, if indicated and if time allows, following safe medication administration practices.[17,18,19,20]

NURSING ALERT Don't use lidocaine or prilocaine if a patient is receiving methemoglobin-inducing agents, such as sulfonamides and acetaminophen, *because of the risk of methemoglobinemia.*[21]

▪ Apply a warming device to the puncture site for 5 to 10 minutes *to increase blood flow and reduce hemolysis and bruising.*[1] Don't use products warmed in a microwave oven, *because uneven heating by the microwave presents a burn risk.*
▪ Perform hand hygiene[4,5,6,7,8,9] and put on gloves *to comply with standard precautions.*[22,23,24]

▪ Remove the warming device from the puncture site.
▪ If topical anesthetic cream was used, remove it before cleaning the puncture site.
▪ Clean the puncture site with an alcohol pad and allow it to air-dry completely, *because alcohol can interfere with test results if it doesn't dry completely.*[16]
▪ Place the extremity in a dependent position and grasp it firmly.
▪ To perform the puncture, use a single-use, auto-disabling lancet *to prevent transmission of bloodborne pathogens.*[25] Puncture the skin with a quick, continuous, and deliberate stroke *to achieve good flow of blood and to prevent the need to repeat the puncture.*[16]
▪ If required by your facility, wipe off the first drop of blood with sterile gauze, *because residual alcohol and tissue fluid or debris may contaminate the blood gas sample.*[3,16]
▪ Hold the capillary tube horizontally *to fill it by capillary action and to prevent air entrapment.* Avoid squeezing the finger too tightly, *because doing so may dilute the specimen with plasma and increases the possibility of hemolysis.*[16]
▪ Fill the entire tube with blood and seal it.
▪ Apply firm pressure to the puncture site with sterile gauze *to stop the bleeding.*[16]

NURSING ALERT Patients with hematologic disorders and those receiving certain medications, such as warfarin, heparin, or aspirin, may have a prolonged clotting time.

▪ Label the sample in the presence of the patient *to prevent mislabeling.*[10] If the patient is on oxygen therapy, note the mode of oxygen therapy and flow rate on the sample label.[3]
▪ Properly dispose of contaminated equipment. Place the lancet in a sharps container and place blood soaked gauze in a biohazard bag.[3,24]
▪ Remove and discard your gloves,[24] and perform hand hygiene.[4,5,6,7,8,9]
▪ If you expect a delay in analysis, place the sample on ice *to prevent gas tension alterations due to cellular metabolism that continues after drawing the sample.*[3]
▪ Place the sample in a laboratory biohazard transport bag and send it to the laboratory immediately.[24]
▪ Evaluate the puncture site for evidence of continued bleeding. Apply a small adhesive bandage, if necessary.
▪ Keep the wound clean and dry.
▪ Perform hand hygiene.[4,5,6,7,8,9]
▪ Document the procedure.[26,27,28,29]

Special considerations

▪ For best results, the procedure should be performed when the patient is in a steady state or 20 to 30 minutes after any changes.[1]
▪ Never scoop up blood from the patient's skin, *because it may be partially coagulated, which can cause hemolysis.*
▪ Make sure there are no air bubbles in the collected sample, *because they may alter the test results.*[1]

Complications

Infection, scarring, calcified nodules, burns, hematoma, nerve damage, pain, bleeding, and bruising can occur at the puncture site.[2]

Documentation

Note the date and time of the procedure, the site of the puncture, the number of samples obtained, the amount of blood loss, and the patient's response to the procedure. Document the use of topical anesthetic, if appropriate. Document teaching provided to the patient and family (if applicable), their understanding of that teaching, and any need for follow-up teaching.

REFERENCES

1 Kacmarek, R. M., et al. (2021). *Egan's fundamentals of respiratory care* (12th ed.). St Louis, MO: Mosby.
2 American Association for Respiratory Care. (2001). AARC clinical practice guideline: Capillary blood gas sampling for neonatal and pediatric patients. *Respiratory Care, 46*, 506–513. (Level VII)
3 Fischbach, F., & Fischbach, M. A. (2018). *A manual of laboratory and diagnostic tests* (10th ed.). Philadelphia, PA: Wolters Kluwer.

4   Centers for Disease Control and Prevention. (2002). Guideline for hand hygiene in health-care settings: Recommendations of the Healthcare Infection Control Practices Advisory Committee and the HICPAC/SHEA/APIC/IDSA Hand Hygiene Task Force. *MMWR Recommendations and Reports, 51*(RR-16), 1–45. https://www.cdc.gov/mmwr/pdf/rr/rr5116.pdf (Level II)

5   The Joint Commission. (2021). Standard NPSG.07.01.01. *Comprehensive accreditation manual for hospitals.* Oakbrook Terrace, IL: The Joint Commission. (Level VII)

6   World Health Organization. (2009). WHO guidelines on hand hygiene in health care: First global patient safety challenge, clean care is safer care. https://apps.who.int/iris/bitstream/handle/10665/44102/9789241597906_eng.pdf?sequence=1 (Level IV)

7   Centers for Medicare and Medicaid Services, Department of Health and Human Services. (2020). Condition of participation: Infection control. 42 C.F.R. § 482.42.

8   American Accreditation Association for Hospitals and Health Systems. (2020). Standard 07.01.21. *Healthcare Facilities Accreditation Program: Accreditation requirements for acute care hospitals.* Chicago, IL: American Accreditation Association for Hospitals and Health Systems. (Level VII)

9   DNV GL-Healthcare USA, Inc. (2020). IC.1.SR.1. *NIAHO® accreditation requirements, interpretive guidelines and surveyor guidance—revision 20.0.* Milford, OH: DNV GL-Healthcare USA, Inc. (Level VII)

10 The Joint Commission. (2021). Standard NPSG.01.01.01. *Comprehensive accreditation manual for hospitals.* Oakbrook Terrace, IL: The Joint Commission. (Level VII)

11 American Accreditation Association for Hospitals and Health Systems. (2020). Standard 15.01.16. *Healthcare Facilities Accreditation Program: Accreditation requirements for acute care hospitals.* Chicago, IL: American Accreditation Association for Hospitals and Health Systems. (Level VII)

12 Centers for Medicare and Medicaid Services, Department of Health and Human Services. (2020). Condition of participation: Patient's rights. 42 C.F.R. § 482.13(c)(1).

13 The Joint Commission. (2021). Standard RI.01.01.01. *Comprehensive accreditation manual for hospitals.* Oakbrook Terrace, IL: The Joint Commission. (Level VII)

14 DNV GL-Healthcare USA, Inc. (2020). PR.2.SR.5. *NIAHO® accreditation requirements, interpretive guidelines and surveyor guidance—revision 20.0.* Milford, OH: DNV GL-Healthcare USA, Inc. (Level VII)

15 The Joint Commission. (2021). Standard PC.02.01.21. *Comprehensive accreditation manual for hospitals.* Oakbrook Terrace, IL: The Joint Commission. (Level VII)

16 World Health Organization (WHO). (2010). WHO guidelines on drawing blood: Best practices in phlebotomy. http://apps.who.int/iris/bitstream/handle/10665/44294/9789241599221_eng.pdf;jsessionid=D4A4E19F72CAE61361C47D5BEE8261D2?sequence=1

17 The Joint Commission. (2021). Standard MM.06.01.01. *Comprehensive accreditation manual for hospitals.* Oakbrook Terrace, IL: The Joint Commission. (Level VII)

18 Centers for Medicare and Medicaid Services, Department of Health and Human Services. (2020). Condition of participation: Nursing services. 42 C.F.R. § 482.23(c).

19 Accreditation Association for Hospitals and Health Systems. (2020). Standard 16.01.03. *Healthcare Facilities Accreditation Program: Accreditation requirements for acute care hospitals.* Chicago, IL: Accreditation Association for Hospitals and Health Systems. (Level VII)

20 DNV GL-Healthcare USA, Inc. (2020). MM.1.SR.3. *NIAHO® accreditation requirements, interpretive guidelines and surveyor guidance—revision 20.0.* Milford, OH: DNV GL-Healthcare USA, Inc. (Level VII)

21 Alanazi, M. Q. (2017). Drugs may be induced methemoglobinemia. *Journal of Hematology and Thromboembolic Diseases, 5*(3), 1000270. https://www.longdom.org/open-access/drugs-may-be-induced-methemoglobinemia-2329-8790-1000270.pdf

22 Siegel, J. D., et al. (2007, revised 2019). 2007 guideline for isolation precautions: Preventing transmission of infectious agents in healthcare settings. https://www.cdc.gov/infectioncontrol/pdf/guidelines/isolation-guidelines-H.pdf (Level II)

23 American Accreditation Association for Hospitals and Health Systems. (2020). Standard 07.01.10. *Healthcare Facilities Accreditation Program: Accreditation requirements for acute care hospitals.* Chicago, IL: American Accreditation Association for Hospitals and Health Systems. (Level VII)

24 Occupational Safety and Health Administration. (2012). Bloodborne pathogens, standard number1910.1030. https://www.osha.gov/pls/oshaweb/owadisp.show_document?p_id=10051&p_table=STANDARDS (Level VII)

25 Centers for Disease Control and Prevention. (2011). CDC clinical reminder: Use of fingerstick devices on more than one person poses risk for transmitting bloodborne pathogens. https://www.cdc.gov/injectionsafety/Fingerstick-DevicesBGM.html

26 The Joint Commission. (2021). Standard RC.01.03.01. *Comprehensive accreditation manual for hospitals.* Oakbrook Terrace, IL: The Joint Commission. (Level VII)

27 Centers for Medicare and Medicaid Services, Department of Health and Human Services. (2020). Condition of participation: Medical record services. 42 C.F.R. § 482.24(b).

28 American Accreditation Association for Hospitals and Health Systems. (2020). Standard 10.00.03. *Healthcare Facilities Accreditation Program: Accreditation requirements for acute care hospitals.* Chicago, IL: American Accreditation Association for Hospitals and Health Systems. (Level VII)

29 DNV GL-Healthcare USA, Inc. (2020). MR.2.SR.1. *NIAHO® accreditation requirements, interpretive guidelines and surveyor guidance—revision 20.0.* Milford, OH: DNV GL-Healthcare USA, Inc. (Level VII)

CARBON MONOXIDE OXIMETRY

Intermittent or continuous carbon monoxide (CO) oximetry can be performed noninvasively with a lightweight, portable display unit that's connected to a sensor probe placed on an adult's or a child's fingertip or an infant's foot. The sensor collects data about the patient's carboxyhemoglobin saturation and sends the information to the oximeter, which then displays the calculated data in the form of a percentage. A carboxyhemoglobin saturation level greater than 3% for nonsmokers and greater than 15% for smokers indicates exposure to exogenous CO.[1]

CO levels can increase as a result of chronic exposure to cigarette smoke or from acute episodes, such as from exposure to a combustion heater; inhaling spray paint or methylene chloride vapors found in paint removers, degreasers, and solvents; and inadequate ventilation of natural gas, fire, or vehicle exhaust. It may also increase with exposure to the pesticide aluminum phosphide (ALP).[2] Early clinical signs of CO poisoning include anxiety, tachypnea, dyspnea, tachycardia, arrhythmias, hypotension, hypertension followed by headache and confusion, and bradycardia followed by seizures, reduced level of consciousness, respiratory failure with pulmonary edema, coma, and death.[3]

CO poisoning is typically diagnosed using the patient's health history, physical examination findings, and laboratory test results that reveal an elevated CO level. Recent studies show that CO oximetry can also help with first-line screening and monitoring CO trends; however, further study is necessary to confirm the accuracy of these findings.[1,4,5]

Equipment

Noninvasive pulse CO oximeter ▪ appropriate sensor (according to the patient's age, weight, and digit size, and the anticipated duration of monitoring)[6] ▪ disinfectant pads ▪ Optional: nail clippers, nail polish remover, batteries, connecting cable, gloves, facility-approved disinfectant.

Preparation of equipment

Inspect all equipment and supplies. If a product is expired, is defective, or has compromised integrity, remove it from patient use, label it as expired or defective, and report the expiration or defect as directed by your facility.

Plug the CO oximeter into an electrical source, and then turn on the unit. Sensors connect directly to the device or to the connecting cable, depending on the type of sensor used. Connect a direct connect sensor directly to the oximeter unit. If using a patient cable, select a sensor that's compatible with the particular device and appropriate for the patient, and connect it to the cable.[6]

If using a portable, handheld CO oximeter, ensure that the unit is charged; replace the batteries, as needed, according to the manufacturer's instructions. Attach an appropriate patient sensor to the CO oximeter.[6] Calibrate the CO oximeter, if required, following the manufacturer's instructions.

Implementation

▪ Verify the practitioner's order for pulse CO oximetry.
▪ Gather and prepare the necessary equipment and supplies.

- Review the patient's medical record for past medical history and history of present illness.
- Perform hand hygiene.[7,8,9,10,11,12]
- Confirm the patient's identity using at least two patient identifiers.[13]
- Provide privacy.[14,15,16,17]
- Explain the procedure to the patient and family (if appropriate) according to their individual communication and learning needs *to increase their understanding, allay their fears, and enhance cooperation.*[18] Answer any questions.
- Select a finger for the test. Although the index finger is commonly used, you may use a smaller finger if the patient's index finger is too large for the equipment. Select a finger that appears to be adequately perfused. If possible, avoid choosing a finger on the hand of an arm being used for blood pressure monitoring.[19]
- **PEDIATRIC ALERT** If you're testing a neonate or small infant, wrap the probe around the foot so that the light beams and detectors align opposite each other. For a large infant, use a probe that fits on the great toe and secure it to the foot.
- *To enhance the accuracy of the measurement,* make sure the patient isn't wearing false fingernails or nail polish. If present, remove nail polish and other substances that might interfere with the transmission of light between the sensor's light source and the detector.[6]
- Clean the patient's finger and fingernail with a disinfectant pad, and allow it to dry.[19]
- Place the sensor probe on the patient's finger, making sure the light source and the detector align opposite each other.[6] If the patient has long fingernails, position the probe perpendicular to the finger, if possible, or clip the fingernail.
- Position the patient's hand at heart level *to eliminate venous pulsations and to promote accurate readings.*
- Look at the display panel on the CO oximeter; the perfusion indicator should begin registering a pulse. Adjust the sensor and sensitivity, as needed, to achieve an adequate pulse display, *because without a pulse, signal readings are erroneous.*[19]
- During oximetry, determine whether blood flow to the site is adequate by assessing the patient's pulse rate and capillary refill time. If it isn't, loosen restraints, remove tight-fitting clothes, take off the blood pressure cuff, or check arterial and IV lines, as appropriate. If none of these interventions works, consider using an alternate site.[6]
- Wait the amount of time recommended by the manufacturer before obtaining the reading.
- Monitor the patient's CO level and pulse rate on the display screen, and then obtain readings for both.
- Press the SPCO key *to obtain a CO reading.* Confirm the value as needed by placing the sensor on another finger and obtain a reading.
- For continuous monitoring, set the alarm limits appropriately for the patient's current condition, and make sure the alarms are turned on, functioning properly, and audible to staff.[20,21,22] Reposition reusable sensors at least every 4 hours; if using adhesive sensors, inspect the application site at least every 8 hours unless otherwise directed, and reapply sensors to different sites as needed.[6] Keep the monitoring site clean and dry, and make sure that the skin doesn't become irritated from the sensor.
- Report critical test results to the practitioner within the time frame established by your facility *to prevent life-threatening treatment delays.*[23]
- Record all measurements in the patient's medical record.
- Perform hand hygiene.[7,8,9,10,11,12]
- Put on gloves.[24,25]
- Clean and disinfect the oximeter, cable (as applicable), and sensor (if not disposable) with a facility-approved disinfectant, according to the manufacturer's instructions.[26,27]
- Remove and discard your gloves.[28]
- Perform hand hygiene.[7,8,9,10,11,12]
- Document the procedure.[29,30,31,32]

Special considerations

- Low CO levels don't rule out exposure, especially if the patient has already received 100% oxygen or if significant time has elapsed since exposure. In addition to CO oximetry, monitor the patient's clinical status and other laboratory parameters, such as arterial or venous blood gas values.

- Individuals who chronically smoke may have mildly elevated CO levels as high as 10%. Persistence of fetal hemoglobin may also falsely elevate levels.[1]
- The Joint Commission has issued a sentinel event alert concerning medical device alarm safety, *because alarm-related events have been associated with permanent loss of function and death.* Among the major contributing factors were improper alarm settings, inappropriately turned-off alarms, and alarm signals that weren't audible to staff. Make sure that alarm limits are appropriately set and that alarms are turned on, functioning properly, and audible to staff. Follow facility guidelines for preventing alarm fatigue.[22]

Documentation

Document the date and time that you attached the oximeter unit to the patient. Record the initial percentage of carboxyhemoglobin registered as well as pulse rate and oxygen saturation level. Record the date, time, and name of the practitioner notified of abnormal results, if applicable; the prescribed interventions; and the patient's response to those interventions. Document teaching provided to the patient and family (if applicable), their understanding of that teaching, and any need for follow-up teaching.

REFERENCES

1 Clardy, P. F., et al. (2019). Carbon monoxide poisoning. In: *UpToDate*, Traub, S. J., & Burns, M. M,. (Eds.).

2 Mashayekhian, M., et al. (2016). Elevated carboxyhaemoglobin concentrations by pulse CO-oximetry is associated with severe aluminum phosphide poisoning. *Basic and Clinical Pharmacology and Toxicology, 119*(3), 322–329. https://onlinelibrary.wiley.com/doi/full/10.1111/bcpt.12571 (Level IV)

3 Kacmarek, R. M., et al. (2021). *Egan's fundamentals of respiratory care* (12th ed.). St Louis, MO: Mosby.

4 Sebbane, M., et al. (2013). Emergency department management of suspected carbon monoxide poisoning: Role of pulse co-oximetry. *Respiratory Care, 58*(10), 1614–1620. http://rc.rcjournal.com/content/58/10/1614 (Level IV)

5 American College of Emergency Physicians, et al. (2017). Clinical policy: Critical issues in the evaluation and management of adult patients presenting to the emergency department with acute carbon monoxide poisoning. *Annals of Emergency Medicine, 69*, 98–107. https://emcrit.org/wp-content/uploads/2017/01/PIIS0196064416313452.pdf (Level I)

6 Masimo Corporation. (2011). Rad-57 operator's manual. http://vasinc.net/pdf/LAB5813D.pdf

7 The Joint Commission. (2021). Standard NPSG.07.01.01. *Comprehensive accreditation manual for hospitals.* Oakbrook Terrace, IL: The Joint Commission. (Level VII)

8 Centers for Disease Control and Prevention. (2002). Guideline for hand hygiene in health-care settings: Recommendations of the Healthcare Infection Control Practices Advisory Committee and the HICPAC/SHEA/APIC/IDSA Hand Hygiene Task Force. *MMWR Recommendations and Reports, 51*(RR-16), 1–45. https://www.cdc.gov/mmwr/pdf/rr/rr5116.pdf (Level II)

9 World Health Organization. (2009). WHO guidelines on hand hygiene in health care: First global patient safety challenge, clean care is safer care. https://apps.who.int/iris/bitstream/handle/10665/44102/9789241597906_eng.pdf?sequence=1 (Level IV)

10 Accreditation Association for Hospitals and Health Systems. (2020). Standard 07.01.21. *Healthcare Facilities Accreditation Program: Accreditation requirements for acute care hospitals.* Chicago, IL: Accreditation Association for Hospitals and Health Systems. (Level VII)

11 Centers for Medicare and Medicaid Services, Department of Health and Human Services. (2020). Condition of participation: Infection control. 42 C.F.R. § 482.42.

12 DNV GL-Healthcare USA, Inc. (2020). IC.1.SR.1. *NIAHO® accreditation requirements, interpretive guidelines and surveyor guidance—revision 20.0.* Milford, OH: DNV GL-Healthcare USA, Inc. (Level VII)

13 The Joint Commission. (2021). Standard NPSG.01.01.01. *Comprehensive accreditation manual for hospitals.* Oakbrook Terrace, IL: The Joint Commission. (Level VII)

14 Accreditation Association for Hospitals and Health Systems. (2020). Standard 15.01.16. *Healthcare Facilities Accreditation Program: Accreditation requirements for acute care hospitals.* Chicago, IL: Accreditation Association for Hospitals and Health Systems. (Level VII)

15 Centers for Medicare and Medicaid Services, Department of Health and Human Services. (2020). Condition of participation: Patient's rights. 42 C.F.R. § 482.13(c)(1).

16 DNV GL-Healthcare USA, Inc. (2020). PR.2.SR.5. *NIAHO® accreditation requirements, interpretive guidelines and surveyor guidance—revision 20.0.* Milford, OH: DNV GL-Healthcare USA, Inc. (Level VII)

17 The Joint Commission. (2021). Standard RI.01.01.01. *Comprehensive accreditation manual for hospitals.* Oakbrook Terrace, IL: The Joint Commission. (Level VII)

18 The Joint Commission. (2021). Standard PC.02.01.21. *Comprehensive accreditation manual for hospitals.* Oakbrook Terrace, IL: The Joint Commission. (Level VII)

19 World Health Organization. (2011). Pulse oximetry training manual. https://www.who.int/patientsafety/safesurgery/pulse_oximetry/who_ps_pulse_oximetry_training_manual_en.pdf?ua=1

20 The Joint Commission. (2021). Standard NPSG.06.01.01. *Comprehensive accreditation manual for hospitals.* Oakbrook Terrace, IL: The Joint Commission. (Level VII)

21 Graham, K. C., & Cvach, M. (2010). Monitor alarm fatigue: Standardizing use of physiological monitors and decreasing nuisance alarms. *American Journal of Critical Care, 19,* 28–37.

22 The Joint Commission. (2013). Sentinel event alert 50: Medical device alarm safety in hospitals. https://www.jointcommission.org/assets/1/6/SEA_50_alarms_4_26_16.pdf (Level VII)

23 The Joint Commission. (2021). Standard NPSG.02.03.01. *Comprehensive accreditation manual for hospitals.* Oakbrook Terrace, IL: The Joint Commission. (Level VII)

24 Accreditation Association for Hospitals and Health Systems. (2020). Standard 07.01.10. *Healthcare Facilities Accreditation Program: Accreditation requirements for acute care hospitals.* Chicago, IL: Accreditation Association for Hospitals and Health Systems. (Level VII)

25 Siegel, J. D., et al. (2007, revised 2019). 2007 guideline for isolation precautions: Preventing transmission of infectious agents in healthcare settings. https://www.cdc.gov/infectioncontrol/pdf/guidelines/isolation-guidelines-H.pdf (Level II)

26 Accreditation Association for Hospitals and Health Systems. (2020). Standard 07.02.03. *Healthcare Facilities Accreditation Program: Accreditation requirements for acute care hospitals.* Chicago, IL: Accreditation Association for Hospitals and Health Systems. (Level VII)

27 Rutala, W. A., et al. (2008, revised 2019). Guideline for disinfection and sterilization in healthcare facilities, 2008. https://www.cdc.gov/infectioncontrol/pdf/guidelines/disinfection-guidelines-H.pdf (Level I)

28 Occupational Safety and Health Administration. (2012). Bloodborne pathogens, standard number1910.1030. https://www.osha.gov/pls/oshaweb/owadisp.show_document?p_id=10051&p_table=STANDARDS (Level VII)

29 The Joint Commission. (2021). Standard RC.01.03.01. *Comprehensive accreditation manual for hospitals.* Oakbrook Terrace, IL: The Joint Commission. (Level VII)

30 Accreditation Association for Hospitals and Health Systems. (2020). Standard 10.00.03. *Healthcare Facilities Accreditation Program: Accreditation requirements for acute care hospitals.* Chicago, IL: Accreditation Association for Hospitals and Health Systems. (Level VII)

31 Centers for Medicare and Medicaid Services, Department of Health and Human Services. (2020). Condition of participation: Medical record services. 42 C.F.R. § 482.24(b).

32 DNV GL-Healthcare USA, Inc. (2020). MR.2.SR.1. *NIAHO® accreditation requirements, interpretive guidelines and surveyor guidance—revision 20.0.* Milford, OH: DNV GL-Healthcare USA, Inc. (Level VII)

CARDIAC MONITORING

Cardiac monitoring enables continuous observation of the heart's electrical activity in patients with conduction disturbances and in those at risk for life-threatening arrhythmias. Correct use of cardiac monitoring technology, in accordance with the manufacturer's recommendations, is necessary to reduce the number of false alarms, which can contribute to alarm fatigue during monitoring.[1]

Like other forms of electrocardiography, cardiac monitoring uses electrodes placed on the patient's chest to transmit electrical signals that are converted into a cardiac rhythm tracing on an oscilloscope. Cardiac monitoring may entail one of two types of monitoring: hardwire or telemetry. In *hardwire monitoring*, the patient is connected to a monitor

Lead selection

Select the best monitoring leads for arrhythmia identification; display two leads when possible.[3]

CLINICAL CONCERN	LEAD
Bundle branch block	V_1 or V_6
Ischemia based on the area of infarction or site of percutaneous coronary intervention: Anterior Septal Lateral Inferior Right ventricle	Varies by specific location: V_3, V_4 V_1, V_2 I, aV_L, V_5, V_6 II, III, aV_F V_{4R}
Junctional rhythm with retrograde P waves	II
Atrial activity	I, II, or Lewis leads (positive and negative electrodes at the second and fourth intercostal spaces at the right sternal border)
Ventricular ectopy, wide complex tachycardia	V_1 (may use V_6 along with V_1)
Ventricular pacing	V_1 or II

at the bedside. The rhythm display appears at the bedside, but it may also be transmitted to a console at a remote location. *Telemetry* uses a small transmitter connected to the patient to send electrical signals to another location, where they're displayed on a monitor. Battery powered and portable, telemetry frees the patient from cumbersome wires and cables, allowing the patient comfortable mobility. Telemetry is especially useful for monitoring arrhythmias that occur during sleep, rest, exercise, and stressful situations.

Regardless of the type, cardiac monitors can display the patient's heart rate and rhythm, produce a printed record of cardiac rhythm, and sound an alarm if the patient's heart rate rises above or falls below specified limits. Monitors also recognize and count abnormal heartbeats, and recognize changes in cardiac activity. For example, the ST segment represents early ventricular repolarization, and any changes in this waveform component reflect alterations in myocardial oxygenation.[2] Therefore, ST-segment monitoring can help detect myocardial ischemia, electrolyte imbalances, coronary artery spasm, and hypoxic events. Any monitoring lead that views an ischemic heart region can reveal ST-segment changes. The monitor's software establishes a template of the patient's normal PQRST pattern from the selected leads. Then the monitor displays ST-segment changes. Some monitors display such changes continuously; others, only on command. (See *Lead selection*.)

One application of bedside cardiac monitoring is the EASI system, a reduced-lead continuous, 12-lead electrocardiogram (ECG) that uses an advanced algorithm and only five electrodes placed on the torso to derive a 12-lead ECG. The system allows all 12 leads to be simultaneously displayed and recorded. (See *Understanding the EASI system*, page 114.)

Equipment

Cardiac monitor ■ lead wires ■ patient cable ■ recording paper ■ disposable pre-gelled electrodes (the number varies from three to six, depending on the monitoring system) ■ washcloth ■ soap and water ■ Optional: clippers, gloves, indelible marking pen, 4″ × 4″ (10-cm × 10-cm) gauze pads.

For telemetry monitoring

Transmitter ■ transmitter pouch ■ telemetry battery pack, leads, and electrodes.

EQUIPMENT

Understanding the EASI system

The five-lead EASI, which uses a reduced-lead, continuous, 12-lead electrocardiogram (ECG) configuration, gives a three-dimensional view of the electrical activity of the heart from the frontal, horizontal, and sagittal planes to provide 12 leads of information. The monitoring system applies a mathematical calculation to the information, creating a derived 12-lead ECG. Electrode placement for the EASI system is as follows:

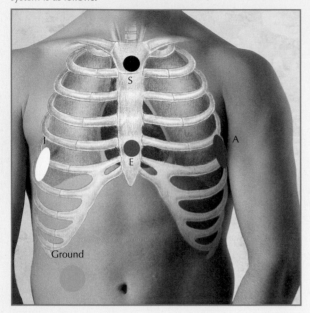

E lead	lower part of the sternum at the fifth intercostal space
A lead	left midaxillary line at the fifth intercostal space
S lead	upper part of the sternum
I lead	right midaxillary line at the fifth intercostal space
Ground	anywhere on the torso[4]

Preparation of equipment

Inspect all equipment and supplies. If a product is expired, is defective, or has compromised integrity, remove it from patient use, label it as expired or defective, and report the expiration or defect as directed by your facility.

Plug the cardiac monitor into an electrical outlet and turn it on, and insert the cable into the appropriate socket in the monitor. Connect the lead wires to the cable, if needed. In most systems, the lead wires are permanently secured to the cable. Each lead wire should indicate the location for attachment to the patient: right arm (RA), left arm (LA), right leg (RL), left leg (LL), and chest (C). This designation should appear on the lead wire, if it's permanently connected, or at the connection of the lead wires and cable to the patient. If the lead wires have a "snap" connection, connect an electrode to each of the lead wires *to prevent patient discomfort later from pushing a snap-type lead wire onto a skin electrode while the electrode is in place on the chest.*[5]

For telemetry monitoring, insert a new battery into the transmitter.[5] Match the poles on the battery with the polar markings on the transmitter case, and test the battery's charge by pressing the button at the top of the unit *to ensure that the battery and the unit are operational.* If the lead wires aren't permanently affixed to the telemetry unit, attach them securely. If they must be attached individually, connect each one to the correct outlet.

Implementation

■ Assess whether the patient has a medical history of or is at risk for a cardiac arrhythmia *to help select the best monitoring leads for arrhythmia detection.*[3,5]

■ Gather and prepare the necessary equipment and supplies.
■ Perform hand hygiene.[6,7,8,9,10,11]
■ Confirm the patient's identity using at least two patient identifiers.[12]
■ Provide privacy.[13,14,15,16]
■ Explain the procedure to the patient and family (if appropriate) according to their communication and learning needs *to increase their understanding, allay their fears, and enhance cooperation.*[17]
■ Raise the patient's bed to waist level before providing care *to prevent caregiver back strain.*[18]
■ Perform hand hygiene.[6,7,8,9,10,11]
■ Put on gloves, if needed, *to comply with standard precautions.*[19,20,21]
■ Assist the patient to the supine position and expose the patient's chest.[5]
■ Determine the electrode positions on the patient's chest based on the system and the leads you're monitoring. (See *Positioning monitoring leads.*)
■ If needed, clip the patient's hair at each electrode site *to ensure good skin contact with the electrodes.*[1,5]
■ Clean the intended electrode areas with soap and water and a washcloth. Then dry them completely with a dry washcloth or gauze pad *to enable adequate transmission of electrical impulses.* Don't use alcohol for skin preparation, *because it dries the skin.*[1]
■ Roughen the skin at the intended electrode sites by using a washcloth, a gauze pad, or the sandpaper on the electrode *to remove part of the stratum corneum or outer layer of the epidermis to facilitate electrical signal transmission.*[1]
■ If possible, use an indelible marker to mark the electrode locations *to make sure the electrode sites remain consistent if replacement becomes necessary.*[5]
■ Remove the backing from one of the pre-gelled electrodes. Check the gel for moistness. If the gel is dry, discard it and replace it with a fresh electrode.[5]
■ Apply the electrode to the appropriate site by pressing your fingers in a circular motion around the electrode *to fix the gel and stabilize the electrode.* Avoid pressing directly on the gel pad *to prevent spreading of the gel and loss of adhesion and transmission.*[5] Repeat this procedure for each electrode.

For hardwire monitoring

■ After applying all the electrodes, attach the lead wires (if not already attached). Check for a tracing on the cardiac monitor. Assess the quality of the tracing. (See *Identifying cardiac monitor problems*, page 116.)
■ *To verify that each beat is being detected by the monitor*, compare the digital heart rate display with your count of the patient's heart rate.
■ If needed, adjust the size and position of the rhythm tracing on the recording paper according to the manufacturer's instructions.
■ Select the best monitoring lead(s) for arrhythmia identification. Display two leads when possible. Use lead II to evaluate atrial activity and measure heart rate. Use V_1, if available, to assess for a wide QRS complex. A five-lead monitoring system is necessary for monitoring V leads; use modified chest lead I if a five-lead monitoring system isn't available.[3]

For telemetry monitoring

■ After applying all the electrodes, attach the lead wires (if not already attached).
■ Place the telemetry transmitter in its pouch. Tie the pouch strings around the patient's neck and waist, making sure that the pouch fits snugly without causing discomfort. If no pouch is available, place the transmitter in the patient's bathrobe pocket. Some patient gowns have a built-in pocket to hold the transmitter.[5]
■ Check the patient's waveform for clarity, position, and size. Adjust the gain and baseline, as needed. (If necessary, ask the patient to remain resting or sitting in the room while you locate the patient's ECG pattern at the central station.)
■ Select the best monitoring lead(s) for arrhythmia identification. Display two leads when possible.

Completing the procedure

■ Set the upper and lower limits of the heart rate alarm, taking into consideration the patient's current heart rate and clinical condition.[1]

Positioning monitoring leads

Proper electrode placement is necessary to ensure correct identification of arrhythmias. The illustrations below show the electrode placement for five-, six-, and three-lead systems. Before placing chest electrodes, palpate the patient's chest *to locate the intercostal spaces*.[3] Use the angle of Louis (sternal angle), formed by the junction of the manubrium and the sternum, as a clinical landmark.

Five-lead system

In the five-lead system, the electrode positions typically remain constant. *To select the leads you want to monitor*, simply use the lead selection button at the central station or on the bedside monitor. Position the electrodes as follows (shown at right):

- Place the right arm (RA) electrode near the right shoulder, close to the junction of the right arm and torso.
- Place the left arm (LA) electrode near the left shoulder, close to the junction of the left arm and torso.
- Place the right leg (RL) electrode below the level of the lowest rib on the right abdominal area.
- Place the left leg (LL) electrode below the level of the lowest rib on the left abdominal area.
- Place the chest (C) electrode in the fourth intercostal space to the right of the sternum for V_1 **or** in the fifth intercostal space in the left midaxillary line for V_6.[5]

Note: The chest electrode can be placed in any of the standard V_1 to V_6 locations, but V_1 and then V_6 are commonly used *because of their value in arrhythmia monitoring*.

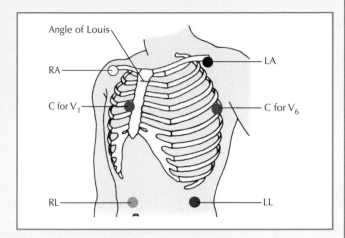

Six-lead system

The electrode positions typically remain constant in the six-lead system as well. Two chest leads monitor for arrhythmias as well as the ST segment in the anterior heart wall.[22] *To select the leads you want to monitor*, use the lead-selection button at the central station or on the bedside monitor. Position the electrodes as follows (shown above on right):

- Place the RA electrode near the right shoulder, close to the junction of the right arm and torso.
- Place the LA electrode near the left shoulder, close to the junction of the left arm and torso.
- Place the RL electrode below the level of the lowest rib on the right abdominal area.
- Place the LL electrode below the level of the lowest rib on the left abdominal area.
- Place one C electrode in the fourth intercostal space to the right of the sternum for V_1 to monitor arrhythmias; place another C electrode in the fifth intercostal space halfway between the substernal notch and the left midclavicular line for V_3 *to enhance monitoring of the anterior heart wall*.

Three-lead system

In the three-lead system, you may need to change the position of the electrodes. The first choice of leads to be monitored is modified chest lead 1 (MCL_1), followed by modified chest lead VI (MCL_6), and then lead II. For MCL_1 or MCL_6, in the three-lead system (shown below on left):

- Place the RA electrode near the left shoulder, close to the junction of the left arm and torso.[5]
- Place the LA electrode in the fourth intercostal space to the right of the sternum.[5]
- Place the LL electrode in the fifth intercostal space in the left midaxillary line.[5]
- Select lead I on the monitor to obtain MCL_1 and lead II to obtain MCL_6.[5]

For lead II in the three-lead system, position the electrodes as follows (shown below on right):

- Place the RA electrode near the right shoulder, close to the junction of the right arm and torso.
- Place the LA electrode near the left shoulder, close to the junction of the left arm and torso.
- Place the LL electrode below the level of the lowest rib on the left abdominal area.
- Select lead II on the monitor.

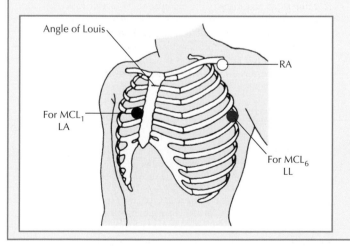

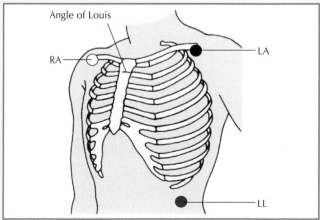

Turn on alarms and make sure they're functioning properly and audible to staff members.[23,24,25] If your system has an arrhythmia and pacemaker recognition system, follow the manufacturer's directions to set individual parameters and to activate the alarm.

- Verify that the patient's identifiers and location are correctly displayed at the central monitoring station, if appropriate.[12]

- *To obtain a rhythm strip*, press the RECORD key at the central station. Label the strip or make sure that it's labeled with the patient's name, identification number, date, time, and lead(s) recorded. Also measure and record the PR interval, QRS duration, and QT interval.

- Identify and document the rhythm. Place the rhythm strip in the appropriate location in the patient's medical record.[26]

TROUBLESHOOTING

IDENTIFYING CARDIAC MONITOR PROBLEMS

This table identifies cardiac monitor problems, their possible causes, and solutions for correcting each problem.

PROBLEM	POSSIBLE CAUSES	SOLUTIONS
False high-rate alarm	■ Monitor interpreting large T waves as QRS complexes, which doubles the rate	■ Reposition electrodes to lead where QRS complexes are taller than T waves. Decrease gain, if necessary.
	■ Skeletal muscle activity	■ Place electrodes away from major muscle masses.
False low-rate alarm	■ Shift in electrical axis from patient movement, making QRS complexes too small to register	■ Reapply electrodes. Set gain so height of complex is greater than 1 millivolt.
	■ Low amplitude of QRS	■ Increase gain.
	■ Poor contact between electrodes and skin	■ Reapply electrodes.
Low amplitude	■ Gain dial set too low	■ Increase gain.
	■ Poor contact between skin and electrodes; dried gel; broken or loose lead wires; poor connection between patient and monitor; malfunctioning monitor; physiologic loss of QRS amplitude	■ Check connections on all lead wires and monitoring cable. Replace electrodes as necessary.
Wandering baseline	■ Poor position or contact between electrodes and skin	■ Reposition or replace electrodes.
	■ Thoracic movement with respirations	■ Reposition electrodes.
Artifact (waveform interference)	■ Patient having seizures, chills, or anxiety	■ Notify practitioner and treat patient as ordered. Keep patient warm and offer reassurance.
	■ Patient movement	■ Help patient relax.
	■ Electrodes applied improperly	■ Check electrodes and reapply, if needed.
	■ Static electricity	■ Make sure cables don't have exposed connectors. Change patient's static-causing gown or pajamas.
	■ Electrical short circuit in lead wires or cable	■ Replace broken equipment. Use stress loops when applying lead wires.
	■ Interference from decreased room humidity	■ Regulate humidity to 40%.
Broken lead wires or cable	■ Stress on lead wires	■ Replace lead wires and fasten the lead wire and cable to the patient's gown, making a loop.[5]
	■ Cables and lead wires cleaned with alcohol or acetone, causing brittleness	■ Clean cable and lead wires with soapy water. Don't allow cable ends to become wet. Replace cables as needed.
60-cycle interference (fuzzy baseline)	■ Electrical interference from other equipment in room	■ Attach all electrical equipment to common ground. ■ Check plugs *to make sure prongs aren't loose.*
	■ Patient's bed improperly grounded	■ Attach bed ground to the room's common ground.
Skin excoriation under electrode	■ Patient allergic to electrode adhesive	■ Remove electrodes and apply nonallergenic electrodes and nonallergenic tape.
	■ Electrode on skin too long	■ Remove electrode, clean site, and reapply electrode at new site.

■ Return the bed to the lowest position *to prevent falls and maintain patient safety.*[27]
■ Discard the used supplies in the appropriate receptacles.[21]
■ Remove and discard your gloves, if worn.
■ Perform hand hygiene.[6,7,8,9,10,11]
■ Document the procedure.[26,28,29,30]

Special considerations

■ The Joint Commission has issued a sentinel event alert about medical device alarm safety, *because alarm-related events have been associated with permanent loss of function and death.* Among the major contributing factors were improper alarm settings, inappropriately turned-off alarms, and alarm signals not audible to staff. Make sure that alarm limits are appropriately set, and that alarms are turned on, functioning properly, and audible to staff. Follow facility guidelines for preventing alarm fatigue.[23]

■ Assess alarm settings and individualize them based on the patient's condition and age *to reduce clinically insignificant alarms.* Also, customize settings as directed by your facility.[1]
■ Check alarm settings at the start of every shift, with any change in the patient's condition, and with any change in caregiver.[1]
■ Monitor the ECG pattern continually for arrhythmias, along with the patient's response to any rhythm or heart rate change, and intervene appropriately. Obtain a rhythm strip when any rhythm change occurs.[5]
■ In patients at high risk for torsades de points, measure the QT interval and calculate the QT interval corrected for heart rate (QT_C) using a consistent lead. A QT_C greater than 0.5 second is dangerously prolonged and associated with torsades de points. Patients at risk include those who are taking antiarrhythmics, antibiotics, antipsychotics, and other medications that prolong QT_C, and those with severe bradycardia, hypokalemia, hypomagnesemia, or drug overdose.[3]

■ Ensure proper electrode placement every shift *to ensure accurate interpretation of cardiac rhythm.*[31]

■ Make sure that all electrical equipment and outlets are grounded *to avoid electric shock and interference (artifacts).* Also ensure that the patient is clean and dry *to prevent electric shock.*[31]

■ Don't open the electrode packages until just before using *to prevent the gel from drying out.*

■ Don't place the electrodes on bony prominences, hairy areas, areas where defibrillator pads will be placed, or areas for chest compression.[31]

■ Assess the electrode sites for signs of irritation or sensitivity reaction. Change electrodes daily or more often if needed.[1,3,32] Soaking the electrodes with water for at least 1 minute during the patient's bath may reduce pain during electrode removal.[33] For patients with fragile skin, such as older adults and preterm infants, daily electrode changes may not be appropriate.[1]

Complications

Complications include skin irritation or sensitivity to the electrode adhesive or gel.

Documentation

In your notes, record the date and time that monitoring began and the monitoring leads used. Document patient and family teaching provided, their understanding of that teaching, and any need for follow-up teaching. Document a rhythm strip at least every shift and with any change in the patient's condition (or as directed by your facility). Label the strip or make sure that it's labeled with the patient's name and identification number as well as the date, time, lead(s) recorded, appropriate measurements, and rhythm interpretation.

REFERENCES

1 American Association of Critical-Care Nurses. (2018). AACN practice alert: Managing alarms in acute care across the life span: Electrocardiography and pulse oximetry. https://www.aacn.org/clinical-resources/practice-alerts/managing-alarms-in-acute-care-across-the-life-span (Level VII)

2 Sandau, K. E., et al. (2017). Update to practice standards for electrocardiographic monitoring in hospital settings: A scientific statement from the American Heart Association. *Circulation, 136*, e273–e344. https://www.ahajournals.org/doi/pdf/10.1161/CIR.0000000000000527 (Level VII)

3 American Association of Critical-Care Nurses. (2016, revised 2018). AACN practice alert: Accurate dysrhythmia monitoring in adults. https://www.aacn.org/clinical-resources/practice-alerts/dysrhythmia-monitoring (Level VII)

4 Phillips Medical Systems. (2007). 12-lead ECG monitoring with EASI™ lead system. https://www.theonlinelearningcenter.com/Assets/PMDCBT/PIIC_Fundamentals_1.0/shell/viewer/swfs/assets/downloads/easi.pdf

5 Wiegand, D. L. (2017). *AACN procedure manual for high acuity, progressive, and critical care* (7th ed.). St. Louis, MO: Elsevier.

6 Centers for Disease Control and Prevention. (2002). Guideline for hand hygiene in health-care settings: Recommendations of the Healthcare Infection Control Practices Advisory Committee and the HICPAC/SHEA/APIC/IDSA Hand Hygiene Task Force. *MMWR Recommendations and Reports, 51*(RR-16), 1–45. https://www.cdc.gov/mmwr/pdf/rr/rr5116.pdf (Level II)

7 The Joint Commission. (2021). Standard NPSG.07.01.01. *Comprehensive accreditation manual for hospitals.* Oakbrook Terrace, IL: The Joint Commission. (Level VII)

8 World Health Organization. (2009). WHO guidelines on hand hygiene in health care: First global patient safety challenge, clean care is safer care. https://apps.who.int/iris/bitstream/handle/10665/44102/9789241597906_eng.pdf?sequence=1 (Level IV)

9 Centers for Medicare and Medicaid Services, Department of Health and Human Services. (2020). Condition of participation: Infection control. 42 C.F.R. § 482.42.

10 Accreditation Association for Hospitals and Health Systems. (2020). Standard 07.01.21. *Healthcare Facilities Accreditation Program: Accreditation requirements for acute care hospitals.* Chicago, IL: Accreditation Association for Hospitals and Health Systems. (Level VII)

11 DNV GL-Healthcare USA, Inc. (2020). IC.1.SR.1. *NIAHO® accreditation requirements, interpretive guidelines and surveyor guidance—revision 20.0.* Milford, OH: DNV GL-Healthcare USA, Inc. (Level VII)

12 The Joint Commission. (2021). Standard NPSG.01.01.01. *Comprehensive accreditation manual for hospitals.* Oakbrook Terrace, IL: The Joint Commission. (Level VII)

13 Centers for Medicare and Medicaid Services, Department of Health and Human Services. (2020). Condition of participation: Patient's rights. 42 C.F.R. § 482.13(c)(1).

14 Accreditation Association for Hospitals and Health Systems. (2020). Standard 15.01.16. *Healthcare Facilities Accreditation Program: Accreditation requirements for acute care hospitals.* Chicago, IL: Accreditation Association for Hospitals and Health Systems. (Level VII)

15 The Joint Commission. (2021). Standard RI.01.01.01. *Comprehensive accreditation manual for hospitals.* Oakbrook Terrace, IL: The Joint Commission. (Level VII)

16 DNV GL-Healthcare USA, Inc. (2020). PR.2.SR.5. *NIAHO® accreditation requirements, interpretive guidelines and surveyor guidance—revision 20.0.* Milford, OH: DNV GL-Healthcare USA, Inc. (Level VII)

17 The Joint Commission. (2021). Standard PC.02.01.21. *Comprehensive accreditation manual for hospitals.* Oakbrook Terrace, IL: The Joint Commission. (Level VII)

18 Waters, T. R., et al. (2009). Safe patient handling training for schools of nursing. https://www.cdc.gov/niosh/docs/2009-127/pdfs/2009-127.pdf (Level VII)

19 Siegel, J. D., et al. (2007, revised 2019). 2007 guideline for isolation precautions: Preventing transmission of infectious agents in healthcare settings. https://www.cdc.gov/infectioncontrol/pdf/guidelines/isolation-guidelines-H.pdf (Level II)

20 Accreditation Association for Hospitals and Health Systems. (2020). Standard 07.01.10. *Healthcare Facilities Accreditation Program: Accreditation requirements for acute care hospitals.* Chicago, IL: Accreditation Association for Hospitals and Health Systems. (Level VII)

21 Occupational Safety and Health Administration. (2012). Bloodborne pathogens, standard number 1910.1030. https://www.osha.gov/pls/oshaweb/owadisp.show_document?p_id=10051&p_table=STANDARDS (Level VII)

22 Nihon Kohden America. (2010). Bedside ECG monitoring for nurses: BSM 6000 series. http://edutracker.com/trktrnr/presentation/jh_newcastle_pa/n9ecgmonltor.pdf (Level VII)

23 The Joint Commission. (2013). Sentinel event alert 50: Medical device alarm safety in hospitals. https://www.jointcommission.org/assets/1/6/SEA_50_alarms_4_26_16.pdf (Level VII)

24 The Joint Commission. (2021). Standard NPSG.06.01.01. *Comprehensive accreditation manual for hospitals.* Oakbrook Terrace, IL: The Joint Commission. (Level VII)

25 Graham, K. C., & Cvach, M. (2010). Monitor alarm fatigue: Standardizing use of physiological monitors and decreasing nuisance alarms. *American Journal of Critical Care, 19*, 28–37.

26 The Joint Commission. (2021). Standard RC.01.03.01. *Comprehensive accreditation manual for hospitals.* Oakbrook Terrace, IL: The Joint Commission. (Level VII)

27 Ganz, D. A., et al. (2013, reviewed 2021). *Preventing falls in hospitals: A toolkit for improving quality of care* (AHRQ Publication No. 13-0015-EF). Rockville, MD: Agency for Healthcare Research and Quality. https://www.ahrq.gov/professionals/systems/hospital/fallpxtoolkit/index.html (Level VII)

28 Centers for Medicare and Medicaid Services, Department of Health and Human Services. (2020). Condition of participation: Medical record services. 42 C.F.R. § 482.24(b).

29 Accreditation Association for Hospitals and Health Systems. (2020). Standard 10.00.03. *Healthcare Facilities Accreditation Program: Accreditation requirements for acute care hospitals.* Chicago, IL: Accreditation Association for Hospitals and Health Systems. (Level VII)

30 DNV GL-Healthcare USA, Inc. (2020). MR.2.SR.1. *NIAHO® accreditation requirements, interpretive guidelines and surveyor guidance—revision 20.0.* Milford, OH: DNV GL-Healthcare USA, Inc. (Level VII)

31 Melendez, L. A., & Pino, R. M. (2012). Electrocardiogram interference: A thing of the past? *Biomedical Instrumentation and Technology, 46*, 470–477. (Level VI)

32 Cvach, M. M., et al. (2013). Daily electrode change and effect on cardiac monitor alarms: An evidence-based practice approach. *Journal of Nursing Care Quality, 28*, 265–271. (Level VI)

33 Dandoy, C. E., et al. (2014). A team-based approach to reducing cardiac monitor alarms. *Pediatrics, 134*, e1686–e1694. https://doi.org/10.1542/peds.2014-1162

Cardiac output measurement

Measuring cardiac output (CO)—the amount of blood ejected by the heart in 1 minute—helps evaluate cardiac function.[1] The most widely used invasive method of calculating this measurement is the bolus thermodilution technique.[2] This bedside technique evaluates the cardiac status of a critically ill patient or one suspected of having cardiac disease.

To measure CO using the bolus thermodilution technique, a quantity of solution colder than the patient's blood is injected into the right atrium through the proximal lumen on a pulmonary artery (PA) catheter. This indicator solution mixes with the blood as it travels through the right ventricle into the PA (as shown below). A thermistor near the tip of the catheter registers the change in temperature of the flowing blood. A computer then plots the temperature change over time as a curve, and calculates flow based on the area under the curve.[1,2]

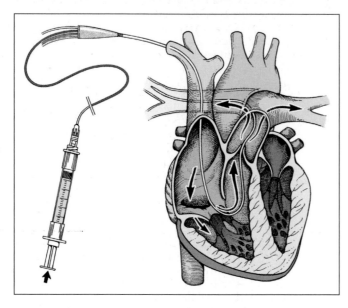

Depending on the patient's status and your facility's preference, iced or room-temperature injectate may be used. Although room-temperature injectate is more convenient and provides equally accurate measurements, iced injectate provides a stronger signal, because it's colder and may be more accurate in hypothermic patients, or when smaller volumes of injectate (3 to 5 mL) must be used, as in patients with volume restrictions.[1]

The normal CO for an adult ranges from 4 to 8 L/minute.[1] However, the adequacy of a patient's CO is better assessed by calculating cardiac index (CI), which is adjusted for the patient's body size. To calculate the CI, divide the patient's CO by body surface area (BSA), which is a function of height and weight. For example, a CO of 4 L/minute might be adequate for a 65″, 120-lb (165-cm, 54-kg) patient (normally a BSA of 1.59 and a CI of 2.5), but would be inadequate for a 74″, 230-lb (188-cm, 104-kg) patient (normally a BSA of 2.26 and a CI of 1.8). The normal CI for adults ranges from 2.5 to 4.2 L/minute/m²; for pregnant women, 3.5 to 6.5 L/minute/m²; and for older adults, 2 to 2.5 L/minute/m².[2]

Equipment

Cardiac monitoring equipment ▪ thermodilution PA catheter in position ▪ CO computer, temperature probe, and cables (or a module for the bedside cardiac monitor) ▪ closed injectate delivery system ▪ 10-mL syringe ▪ 500-mL bag of dextrose 5% in water or normal saline solution ▪ container of crushed ice and water (for iced-injectate measurement) ▪ vital signs monitoring equipment ▪ stethoscope ▪ disinfectant pad ▪ Optional: normal saline solution for flush.

Some bedside cardiac monitors measure CO continuously, using an invasive or a noninvasive method. If your bedside monitor doesn't have this capability, you'll need a free-standing CO computer.

Preparation of equipment

Inspect all equipment and supplies. If a product is expired or defective, or has compromised integrity, remove it from patient use, label it as expired or defective, and report the expiration or defect as directed by your facility.[3]

Perform hand hygiene.[4,5,6,7,8,9] Assemble the equipment at the patient's bedside. Maintain sterile no-touch technique throughout equipment preparation.[1] Insert the closed injectate system tubing into the 500-mL bag of IV solution. Connect the 10-mL syringe to the system tubing and prime the tubing with IV solution until it's free from air. Then clamp the tubing.

After clamping the system tubing, connect the primed closed injectate delivery system to the stopcock of the proximal lumen of the PA catheter. Trace the tubing from the patient to its point of origin *to make sure that you're connecting the tubing to the correct port.*[10,11] If using iced injectate, place the coiled segment into a clean container and add crushed ice and water *to cover the entire coil.* Let the solution cool for 15 to 20 minutes. If using room-temperature injectate, connect the primed closed injectate system to the stopcock of the proximal lumen of the PA catheter. Next, connect the temperature probe from the CO computer to the closed injectate system's flow-through housing device. Connect the CO computer cable to the thermistor connector on the PA catheter and verify the blood temperature reading. Lastly, turn on the CO computer and enter the correct computation constant, as recommended by the catheter's manufacturer; the computation constant varies by the type and the size of the catheter, injectate volume, and injectate temperature.[1,2]

Implementation

▪ Verify the practitioner's order or follow your facility's protocol for CO measurement.
▪ Gather and prepare the necessary equipment and supplies.
▪ Perform hand hygiene.[4,5,6,7,8,9]
▪ Confirm the patient's identity using at least two patient identifiers.[12]
▪ Provide privacy.[13,14,15,16]
▪ Explain the procedure to the patient and family (if appropriate) according to their individual communication and learning needs *to increase understanding, allay their fears, and enhance cooperation.*[17]
▪ Raise the patient's bed to waist level before providing care *to prevent caregiver back strain.*[18]
▪ Perform hand hygiene.[4,5,6,7,8,9]
▪ Obtain baseline vital signs and hemodynamic readings, and assess the patient's respiratory and cardiovascular status, including cardiac rhythm. Monitor for signs and symptoms of inadequate perfusion, including restlessness, fatigue, changes in level of consciousness, decreased capillary refill time, diminished peripheral pulses, oliguria, and pale, cool skin.[1]
▪ Make sure the patient is in a comfortable, supine position with the head of the bed elevated no more than 20 degrees. If the patient's condition prevents this position, use consistent positioning *to avoid inconsistent CO measurement.*[1] Tell the patient not to move during the procedure, *because movement can cause an error in measurement.*
▪ If you're using the proximal lumen for an infusion, flush the lumen with normal saline solution at an appropriate rate *to clear the port of infusing medication without administering a bolus of medication to the patient.* If possible, restrict infusions delivered through the introducer or other central lines, *because measurements obtained during administration of other infusions may be elevated by as much as 40%.*[1]
▪ Note the temperature of the injectant on the computer or monitor screen. The acceptable temperature range for iced injectate is 32° to 53.6° F (0° to 12° C).[1]
▪ Verify the presence of a PA waveform on the cardiac monitor *to ensure that the distal thermistor is located in the pulmonary* artery. Also observe the patient's heart rate and cardiac rhythm; *a rapid heart rate or an arrhythmia may decrease CO and lead to varying CO measurements.*[1]
▪ Turn the stopcock, unclamp the injectate system IV tubing (as shown) if required by the manufacturer, and withdraw exactly 10 mL of injectate solution into the syringe. Then, reclamp the tubing if required by the manufacturer.[1]

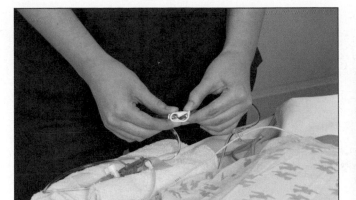

■ Inject the solution smoothly within 4 seconds at end expiration *to decrease variations in CO measurements caused by the respiratory cycle* (as shown below).[1] Make sure fluid doesn't leak at the connectors.[1]

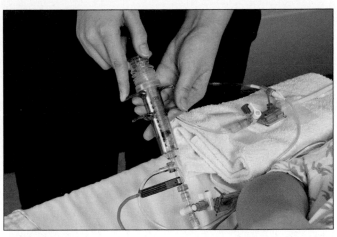

■ Turn the stopcock at the catheter proximal lumen *to open a fluid path between the proximal lumen of the PA catheter and syringe.*

■ Press the START button on the CO computer, or wait for the INJECT message to flash.

■ Observe for a steady baseline temperature before injecting the solution, *because an abnormal baseline may increase variability in CO measurement.*[1]

■ Observe and, if available, analyze the contour of the thermodilution curve on a strip chart recorder. Look for a rapid upstroke and a gradual, smooth return to baseline. (See *Analyzing thermodilution curves.*)

Analyzing thermodilution curves

A thermodilution curve provides valuable information about cardiac output (CO), injection technique, and equipment problems. When studying the curve, keep in mind that the area under the curve is inversely proportionate to the CO: The smaller the area under the curve, the higher the CO; the larger the area under the curve, the lower the CO.

In addition to providing a record of CO, the curve may indicate problems related to technique, such as erratic or slow injectate instillations, or other problems, such as respiratory variations or electrical interference. The curves below correspond to those typically seen in clinical practice.

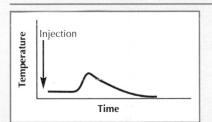

Normal thermodilution curve
With an accurate monitoring system and a patient who has adequate CO, the thermodilution curve begins with a smooth, rapid upstroke and is followed by a smooth, gradual downslope.[2] The curve shown at left indicates that the injectate instillation time was within the recommended 4 seconds, and that the temperature curve returned to baseline.

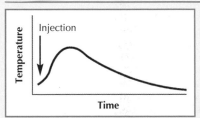

Low CO curve
A thermodilution curve representing low CO shows a rapid, smooth upstroke (from proper injection technique). However, *because the heart is ejecting blood less efficiently from the ventricles,* the injectate warms slowly and takes longer to be ejected. Consequently, the curve takes longer to return to baseline. This slow return produces a larger area under the curve, corresponding to low CO.[2]

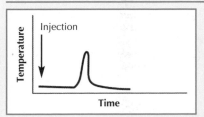

High CO curve
As with a low CO curve, the thermodilution curve representing high CO has a rapid, smooth upstroke from proper injection technique. However, because the ventricles are ejecting blood too forcefully, the injectate moves through the heart quickly and the curve returns to baseline more rapidly. The smaller area under the curve suggests higher CO.[2]

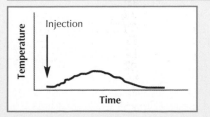

Curve reflecting poor technique
A curve reflecting poor technique results from an uneven and too-slow (taking more than 4 seconds) administration of injectate. The uneven and slower-than-normal upstroke and the larger area under the curve erroneously indicate low CO. A kinked catheter, unsteady hands during the injection, or improper placement of the proximal lumen in the introducer sheath may also cause this type of curve.

- Repeat these steps up to five times, waiting 1 minute between injections *to ensure consistency and accuracy*. Compute the average of three measurements that are within 10% of the median value, and record the patient's CO.[1,19]
- Return the stopcock to its original position, and make sure the injectate delivery system tubing is clamped *to prevent inadvertent injectate delivery to the patient* (as shown below).[1]

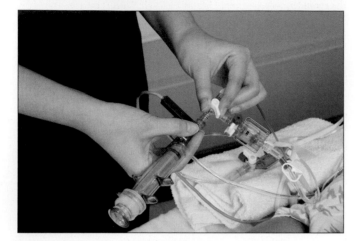

- Restart medication infusions, as ordered.[1]
- Verify the presence of a PA waveform on the cardiac monitor.[1]
- Assess the patient's vital signs and respiratory and cardiovascular status, including cardiac rhythm after the procedure, and compare your findings with baseline findings *to evaluate the patient's hemodynamic status.*[1]
- Position the patient for comfort.
- Return the bed to the lowest position *to prevent falls and maintain patient safety.*[20]
- Discard used supplies in the appropriate receptacle.[21]
- Perform hand hygiene.[4,5,6,7,8,9]
- Clean and disinfect your stethoscope with a disinfectant pad.[22,23]
- Perform hand hygiene.[4,5,6,7,8,9]
- Record the fluid volume injected for CO measurements in the patient's intake and output record.
- Document the procedure.[24,25,26,27]

Special considerations

- Certain factors can affect the accuracy and reproducibility of bolus thermodilution CO values, including variations in injectate temperatures or volumes, rapid volume infusions during bolus injections, respiratory cycle influences, an inaccurate computation constant, and thermal instability after cardiopulmonary bypass.[2]
- The Joint Commission has issued a sentinel event alert about managing risk during the transition to the new International Organization for Standardization tubing standards designed to prevent dangerous tubing misconnections, which can lead to serious patient injury and death. During the transition, be sure to trace the tubing and catheter from the patient to the point of origin before connecting or reconnecting any device or infusion, at any care transition (such as a new setting or service), and as part of the hand-off process; route tubes and catheters having different purposes in different standardized directions; when there are different access sites or several bags hanging, label the tubing at the distal and proximal ends; use tubing and equipment only as intended; and store medications for different delivery routes in separate locations.[11]
- Handle the injectate solution as little as possible *to avoid thermal indicator variations, which may alter CO values.*[1]
- Change disposable or reusable transducer systems, including continuous flush devices and flush solution used for invasive hemodynamic monitoring, every 96 hours, immediately upon suspected contamination, or when integrity of the system has been compromised. Limit the number of manipulations or entries to the system.[28]

Complications

Complications from CO measurement may include arrhythmias, inability to accurately measure CO, infection of the PA catheter site, fluid overload, and hemodynamic instability.[1]

Documentation

Document the patient's CO, CI, and other hemodynamic values as well as vital signs, cardiac rhythm, and respiratory and cardiovascular status before and after the procedure. Note the patient's position during measurement and any other complications, such as bradycardia or hemodynamic instability. Record the name of the practitioner notified of any abnormal results, the date and time of notification, prescribed interventions, and the patient's response to interventions. Document teaching provided to the patient and family (if applicable), their understanding of that teaching, and any need for follow-up teaching.

REFERENCES

1 Wiegand, D. L. (2017). *AACN procedure manual for high acuity, progressive, and critical care* (7th ed.). St. Louis, MO: Elsevier.

2 McGee, W. T., et al. (Eds.) (2018). *Edward's clinical education: Quick guide to cardiopulmonary care* (4th ed.). Irvine, CA: Edwards Lifesciences. https://education.edwards.com/quick-guide-to-cardiopulmonary-care-4th-edition/220356# (Level VII)

3 Standard 12. Product evaluation, integrity, and defect reporting. Infusion therapy standards of practice. (8th ed.). (2021). *Journal of Infusion Nursing, 44*, S45–S46. (Level VII)

4 World Health Organization. (2009). WHO guidelines on hand hygiene in health care: First global patient safety challenge, clean care is safer care. https://apps.who.int/iris/bitstream/handle/10665/44102/9789241597906_eng.pdf?sequence=1 (Level IV)

5 The Joint Commission. (2021). Standard NPSG.07.01.01. *Comprehensive accreditation manual for hospitals.* Oakbrook Terrace, IL: The Joint Commission. (Level VII)

6 Centers for Disease Control and Prevention. (2002). Guideline for hand hygiene in health-care settings: Recommendations of the Healthcare Infection Control Practices Advisory Committee and the HICPAC/SHEA/APIC/IDSA Hand Hygiene Task Force. *MMWR Recommendations and Reports, 51*(RR-16), 1–45. https://www.cdc.gov/mmwr/pdf/rr/rr5116.pdf (Level II)

7 Centers for Medicare and Medicaid Services, Department of Health and Human Services. (2020). Condition of participation: Infection control. 42 C.F.R. § 482.42.

8 Accreditation Association for Hospitals and Health Systems. (2020). Standard 07.01.21. *Healthcare Facilities Accreditation Program: Accreditation requirements for acute care hospitals.* Chicago, IL: Accreditation Association for Hospitals and Health Systems. (Level VII)

9 DNV GL-Healthcare USA, Inc. (2020). IC.1.SR.1. *NIAHO® accreditation requirements, interpretive guidelines and surveyor guidance—revision 20.0.* Milford, OH: DNV GL-Healthcare USA, Inc. (Level VII)

10 U.S. Food and Drug Administration. (2017). Examples of medical device misconnections. https://www.fda.gov/medical-devices/medical-device-connectors/examples-medical-device-misconnections

11 The Joint Commission. (2014). Sentinel event alert 53: Managing risk during transition to new ISO tubing connector standards. http://www.jointcommission.org/assets/1/6/SEA_53_Connectors_8_19_14_final.pdf (Level VII)

12 The Joint Commission. (2021). Standard NPSG.01.01.01. *Comprehensive accreditation manual for hospitals.* Oakbrook Terrace, IL: The Joint Commission. (Level VII)

13 Accreditation Association for Hospitals and Health Systems. (2020). Standard 15.01.16. *Healthcare Facilities Accreditation Program: Accreditation requirements for acute care hospitals.* Chicago, IL: Accreditation Association for Hospitals and Health Systems. (Level VII)

14 Centers for Medicare and Medicaid Services, Department of Health and Human Services. (2020). Condition of participation: Patient's rights. 42 C.F.R. § 482.13(c)(1).

15 DNV GL-Healthcare USA, Inc. (2020). PR.2.SR.5. *NIAHO® accreditation requirements, interpretive guidelines and surveyor guidance—revision 20.0.* Milford, OH: DNV GL-Healthcare USA, Inc. (Level VII)

16 The Joint Commission. (2021). Standard RI.01.01.01. *Comprehensive accreditation manual for hospitals.* Oakbrook Terrace, IL: The Joint Commission. (Level VII)

17 The Joint Commission. (2021). Standard PC.02.01.21. *Comprehensive accreditation manual for hospitals.* Oakbrook Terrace, IL: The Joint Commission. (Level VII)

18 Waters, T. R., et al. (2009). Safe patient handling training for schools of nursing. https://www.cdc.gov/niosh/docs/2009-127/pdfs/2009-127.pdf (Level VII)

19 Giraud, R., et al. (2017). Reproducibility of transpulmonary thermodilution cardiac output measurements in clinical practice: A systematic review. *Journal of Clinical Monitoring and Computing, 31,* 43–51. (Level I)

20 Ganz, D. A., et al. (2013, reviewed 2021). *Preventing falls in hospitals: A toolkit for improving quality of care* (AHRQ Publication No. 13-0015-EF). Rockville, MD: Agency for Healthcare Research and Quality. https://www.ahrq.gov/professionals/systems/hospital/fallpxtoolkit/index.html (Level VII)

21 Occupational Safety and Health Administration. (2012). Bloodborne pathogens, standard number1910.1030. https://www.osha.gov/pls/oshaweb/owadisp.show_document?p_id=10051&p_table=STANDARDS (Level VII)

22 Accreditation Association for Hospitals and Health Systems. (2020). Standard 07.02.03. *Healthcare Facilities Accreditation Program: Accreditation requirements for acute care hospitals.* Chicago, IL: Accreditation Association for Hospitals and Health Systems. (Level VII)

23 Rutala, W. A., et al. (2008, revised 2019). Guideline for disinfection and sterilization in healthcare facilities, 2008. https://www.cdc.gov/infection-control/pdf/guidelines/disinfection-guidelines-H.pdf (Level I)

24 The Joint Commission. (2021). Standard RC.01.03.01. *Comprehensive accreditation manual for hospitals.* Oakbrook Terrace, IL: The Joint Commission. (Level VII)

25 Centers for Medicare and Medicaid Services, Department of Health and Human Services. (2020). Condition of participation: Medical record services. 42 C.F.R. § 482.24(b).

26 Accreditation Association for Hospitals and Health Systems. (2020). Standard 10.00.03. *Healthcare Facilities Accreditation Program: Accreditation requirements for acute care hospitals.* Chicago, IL: Accreditation Association for Hospitals and Health Systems. (Level VII)

27 DNV GL-Healthcare USA, Inc. (2020). MR.2.SR.1. *NIAHO® accreditation requirements, interpretive guidelines and surveyor guidance—revision 20.0* Milford, OH: DNV GL-Healthcare USA, Inc. (Level VII)

28 Standard 43. Administration set management. Infusion therapy standards of practice. (8th ed.). (2021). *Journal of Infusion Nursing, 44,* S123–S125. (Level VII)

CARDIOPULMONARY RESUSCITATION, ADULT

Cardiopulmonary resuscitation (CPR) seeks to restore and maintain the patient's respirations and circulation after the heartbeat and breathing have stopped. The ultimate goal of the resuscitation process is to return a patient to prior quality of life and functional state. CPR is a basic life support (BLS) procedure for victims of cardiac arrest. The American Heart Association (AHA) Web-based integrated guidelines explain how to perform the procedure.[1]

Studies show that early CPR can improve a patient's likelihood of survival. Chest compressions are particularly important, because perfusion during CPR depends on them. To prevent a delay in chest compressions, the sequence of CPR is "C-A-B" (compressions, airway, and breathing), which gives the highest priority to chest compressions when resuscitating a patient in cardiac arrest.[1]

High-quality CPR is important not only at the onset of resuscitation but throughout the resuscitation process. Key components of high-quality CPR are minimizing chest compression interruptions, providing compressions of adequate rate and depth, allowing complete chest recoil after each compression, avoiding leaning between compressions, and avoiding excessive ventilation.[1] Integrating defibrillation and other advanced cardiac life support (ACLS) measures into the resuscitation process minimizes interruptions in CPR.[1]

Equipment

Backboard or other firm surface ■ automated external defibrillator (AED) or other defibrillator ■ Optional: barrier mask with one-way valve, gloves, other personal protective equipment, naloxone.

Implementation

The AHA created a visual algorithm that provides a step-by-step guide for CPR.

One-person CPR

The following illustrated instructions provide a step-by-step guide for CPR as currently recommended by the AHA. (See *The AHA BLS algorithm,* page 122.)

■ Put on gloves and other personal protective equipment, as needed and available, *to comply with standard precautions.*[2,3]

■ Verify the safety of the environment by quickly scanning the patient's location and surroundings for imminent physical threats, such as toxic and electrical hazards.[1]

■ Assess whether the patient is unresponsive by tapping the patient on the shoulder and shouting, "Are you all right?" (as shown below). *This helps ensure that you don't begin CPR on a conscious person.* If the patient is unresponsive, shout for help and activate the emergency response system via mobile device (if appropriate).[1]

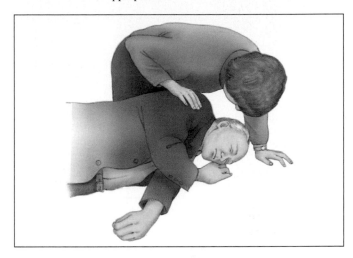

■ Check to see whether the patient is apneic or only gasping (as opposed to breathing regularly) and, if you're able, simultaneously check for a pulse *to minimize delay in detecting cardiac arrest and initiating CPR.*[1] To check for a pulse, palpate the carotid artery that's closest to you by placing your index and middle fingers in the groove between the trachea and the sternocleidomastoid muscle, as shown below. Palpate for no longer than 10 seconds.[1]

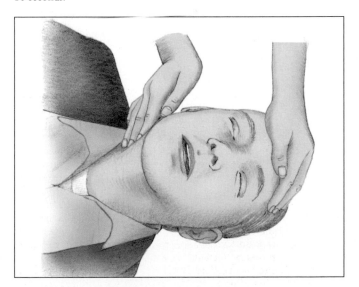

■ If the patient is breathing normally and has a pulse, monitor the patient closely until the emergency response team arrives.[1]

■ If breathing is absent or the patient is only gasping and you feel a pulse within 10 seconds, open the patient's airway using the head tilt–chin lift technique, unless you suspect a cervical spine injury, in which case use the jaw-thrust maneuver without head extension. Then provide rescue breathing by giving the patient 10 breaths/minute (1 breath every 6 seconds). Use a barrier mask with a one-way valve, if available. Give each breath over 1 second regardless of whether an advanced airway is in place; each breath should cause a minimal chest rise. Avoid excessive ventilation; *doing so minimizes the impact of positive-pressure ventilation on blood flow.* If you know of or suspect opioid overdose, administer intramuscular or intranasal naloxone, if available, according to protocol.[1]

The AHA BLS algorithm

The algorithm below illustrates the steps for basic life support (BLS) recommended by the American Heart Association (AHA).

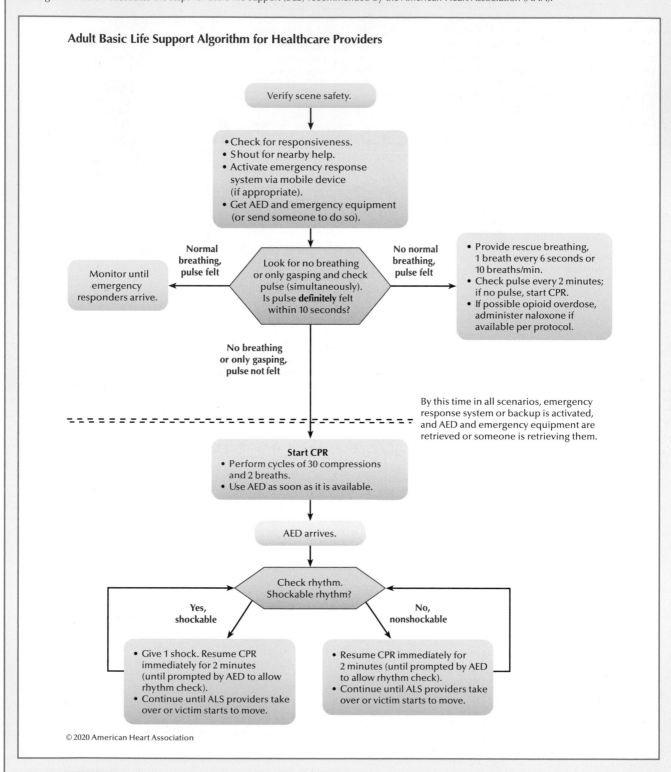

Adult Basic Life Support Algorithm for Healthcare Providers

Verify scene safety.

- Check for responsiveness.
- Shout for nearby help.
- Activate emergency response system via mobile device (if appropriate).
- Get AED and emergency equipment (or send someone to do so).

Look for no breathing or only gasping and check pulse (simultaneously). Is pulse **definitely** felt within 10 seconds?

Normal breathing, pulse felt → Monitor until emergency responders arrive.

No normal breathing, pulse felt →
- Provide rescue breathing, 1 breath every 6 seconds or 10 breaths/min.
- Check pulse every 2 minutes; if no pulse, start CPR.
- If possible opioid overdose, administer naloxone if available per protocol.

No breathing or only gasping, pulse not felt

By this time in all scenarios, emergency response system or backup is activated, and AED and emergency equipment are retrieved or someone is retrieving them.

Start CPR
- Perform cycles of 30 compressions and 2 breaths.
- Use AED as soon as it is available.

AED arrives.

Check rhythm. Shockable rhythm?

Yes, shockable
- Give 1 shock. Resume CPR immediately for 2 minutes (until prompted by AED to allow rhythm check).
- Continue until ALS providers take over or victim starts to move.

No, nonshockable
- Resume CPR immediately for 2 minutes (until prompted by AED to allow rhythm check).
- Continue until ALS providers take over or victim starts to move.

© 2020 American Heart Association

Reprinted with permission
*Circulation.*2020;142:S366-S468
©2020 American Heart Association, Inc

NURSING ALERT For patients in cardiac arrest, naloxone administration is ineffective without concomitant chest compressions to deliver the drug to the tissues. If opiate overdose is highly suspected, consider naloxone administration after initiation of CPR.[1]

■ If breathing is absent or the patient is only gasping and you don't feel a pulse within 10 seconds, have a coworker retrieve an AED or other defibrillator. If you're alone, retrieve an AED or other defibrillator and the emergency equipment. Place the patient supine on a firm surface, such as on a backboard or on the floor; if the patient is on an air-filled mattress, deflate the mattress *to maximize the effectiveness of chest compressions*. When turning the patient, roll the head and torso as a unit (as shown below); avoid twisting or pulling the patient's neck, shoulders, or hips. Don't delay the initiation of CPR by waiting to obtain and position a backboard.[1]

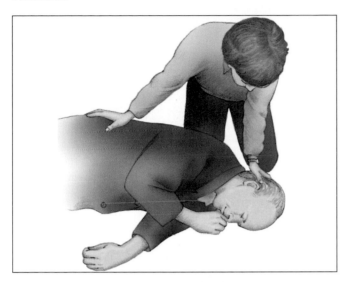

■ Place the heel of one hand on the center of the patient's chest (over the lower half of the sternum) and the heel of the second hand on top of the first so that your hands are overlapped and parallel (as shown below).[1]

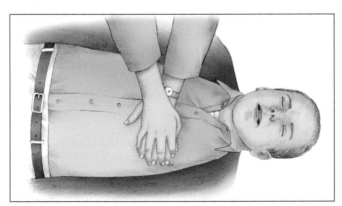

■ With your elbows locked, arms straight, and shoulders directly over your hands (shown top right), administer chest compressions. Using the weight of your upper body, compress the patient's chest at least 2″ (5 cm) but no more than 2.4″ (6 cm),[1] keeping chest compression and chest recoil duration equal. Allow the patient's chest to completely recoil after each chest compression *to create a relative negative intrathoracic pressure that promotes venous return and cardiopulmonary blood flow*.[1] Avoid leaning over the patient's chest, *which could prevent it from recoiling completely*.[1]

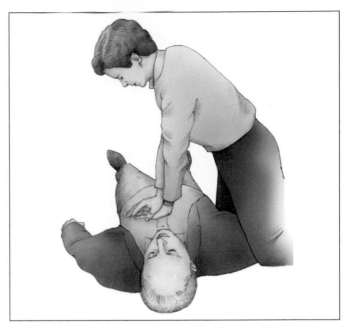

■ Administer 30 compressions at a rate of 100 to 120 compressions per minute, pushing hard and fast.[1]
■ After administering 30 compressions, open the patient's airway and give 2 ventilations. If the patient doesn't appear to have a cervical spine injury, use the head tilt–chin lift maneuver *to open the patient's airway*.[1] To perform this maneuver, first place your hand that's closer to the patient's head on the patient's forehead. Then apply enough pressure to tilt the patient's head back. Next, place the fingertips of your other hand under the bony part of the lower jaw near the chin; avoid placing your fingertips on the soft tissue under the patient's chin, *because you may inadvertently obstruct the airway you're trying to open*. At the same time, keep the patient's mouth partially open (as shown below).

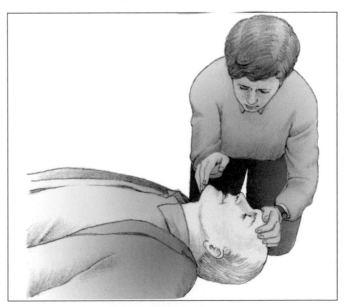

■ If you suspect a cervical spine injury, use the jaw-thrust maneuver.[1] To perform this maneuver, kneel at the patient's head with your elbows on the ground. Rest your thumbs on the patient's lower jaw near the corners of the mouth, pointing your thumbs toward the feet. Then place your fingertips around the lower jaw. To open the airway, lift the lower jaw with your fingertips (as shown on the next page).

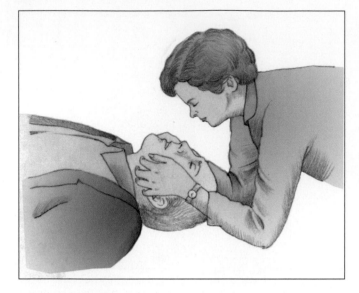

- To begin ventilations using a barrier mask with a one-way valve, position the narrow portion of the mask over the patient's nose and the wide portion above the patient's chin. Covering the nose and mouth with the mask, create a tight seal. Take a regular breath and place your mouth on the mouthpiece (as shown below). Alternatively, to begin ventilations using mouth-to-mouth rescue breathing, position yourself beside the patient's head and pinch the nostrils shut with the thumb and index finger of the hand you've had on the patient's forehead. Take a regular breath and place your mouth over the patient's mouth, creating a tight seal. Guidelines recommend a handheld resuscitation bag and mask only when a second rescuer arrives; they don't recommend use by a lone rescuer.[1]

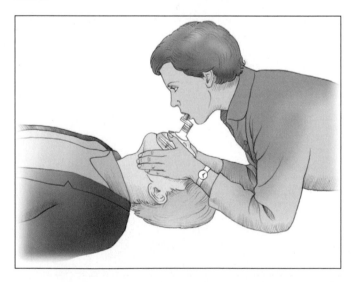

- Give two regular breaths, each over 1 second, *to promote oxygenation and to prevent overinflation of the patient's lungs.* Each ventilation should have enough volume to produce visible chest rise *to ensure adequate ventilation.*[1]
- If the first ventilation isn't successful, reposition the patient's head and try again, *because the most common cause of ventilation difficulty is an improperly opened airway.*[1] If you're still unsuccessful, the patient may have a foreign body airway obstruction.
- Administer 30 chest compressions at a rate of approximately 100 to 120 per minute.[1] Push hard and fast.
- Open the airway and give two ventilations, then find the proper hand position again and deliver 30 more compressions. Continue chest compressions until the emergency response team arrives or another rescuer arrives with a defibrillator or an AED. Interruption chest compressions as infrequently as possible. Don't interrupt chest compressions for more

than 10 seconds unless a specific intervention, such as defibrillation or advanced airway placement, is necessary *to maximize compression time and improve tissue oxygenation.*[1]
- When a second rescuer arrives, continue with two-person CPR.
- Consider switching compressors during any intervention associated with appropriate interruptions in chest compressions. Switch compressors every 2 minutes (or after about five cycles of compressions and ventilations at a ratio of 30:2) *to prevent decreases in the quality of compressions and rescuer fatigue.* Try to accomplish the switch in fewer than 5 seconds.

NURSING ALERT Avoid interruptions in chest compressions for interventions such as pulse checks *to maximize chest compression time and improve tissue oxygenation.*[1]
- Remove and discard your gloves and any other personal protective equipment, if worn,[2] and perform hand hygiene.[4,5,6,7,8,9]
- Document the procedure.[10,11,12,13]

Two-person CPR

Review the following illustrated instructions, which provide a step-by-step guide for CPR as recommended by the AHA.
- Put on gloves and other personal protective equipment as needed and available *to comply with standard precautions.*[2,14]
- Verify that the environment is safe by quickly scanning the patient's location and surroundings quickly for imminent physical threats, such as toxic and electrical hazards.[1]
- Assess the patient to determine unresponsiveness. Tap the patient on the shoulder and shout, "Are you all right?" This step ensures that you don't begin CPR on a conscious person. If the patient is unresponsive, shout for nearby help and activate the emergency response system via a mobile device (if appropriate).[1]
- Check to see whether the patient is apneic or only gasping (as opposed to breathing regularly) and, if able, simultaneously check for a pulse *to minimize delay in detecting cardiac arrest and initiating CPR.*[1] To check for a pulse, palpate the carotid artery that's closest to you by placing your index and middle fingers in the groove between the trachea and the sternocleidomastoid muscle. Palpate for no longer than 10 seconds.[1]
- If the patient is breathing normally and has a pulse, monitor the patient closely until the emergency response team arrives.[1]
- If breathing is absent or the patient is only gasping and you feel a pulse within 10 seconds, open the patient's airway; use the head tilt–chin lift technique unless you suspect a cervical spine injury, in which case you would use the jaw-thrust maneuver without head extension. Provide rescue breathing by giving the patient 10 breaths per minute (1 breath every 6 seconds). Use a barrier mask with a one-way valve, if available. Give each breath over 1 second regardless of whether there's an advanced airway in place; each breath should cause a minimal chest rise.[1] Avoid excessive ventilation *to minimize the impact of positive-pressure ventilation on blood flow.* If you know of or suspect opioid overdose, administer intramuscular or intranasal naloxone, if available, according to protocol.

NURSING ALERT For a patient in cardiac arrest, naloxone administration is ineffective without concomitant chest compressions to deliver the medication to the patient's tissues. If opioid overdose is highly suspected, consider naloxone administration after performing CPR.[1]
- If breathing is absent or the patient is only gasping and you don't feel a pulse within 10 seconds, have a coworker retrieve an AED or other defibrillator and other emergency equipment, and alert the emergency response team (if not already done).[1] Place the patient supine on a firm surface, such as on a backboard or on the floor; if the patient is on an air-filled mattress, deflate the mattress *to maximize the effectiveness of chest compressions.* When turning the patient, roll the head and torso as a unit; avoid twisting or pulling the patient's neck, shoulders, or hips. Don't delay the initiation of CPR by waiting to obtain and position a backboard.[1] Performing CPR on a patient in the prone position requires different positioning for the rescuers providing CPR.
- Make sure that your knees or feet are apart *to provide a wide base of support.*
- Place the heel of one hand on the center of the patient's chest (over the lower half of the sternum) and the heel of the second hand on top of the first so that your hands are overlapped and parallel.[1]

CPR in the prone position

Although the effectiveness of CPR in the prone position isn't completely known, the AHA recommends against turning a patient who is in the prone position with an advanced airway unless it is possible to turn without risking disconnection of equipment or aerosolization. The AHA recommends that CPR with a patient in the prone position be performed with the hands over the T7 through T10 vertebral bodies.[15,16,17] The same rate and force of compressions are recommended in the prone position as in the supine position. It is important that there is a hard surface under the patient to provide uniform force and counter-sternal pressure.[17]

Attempt to place a patient who is in the prone position without an advanced airway in the supine position for continued resuscitation.[16]

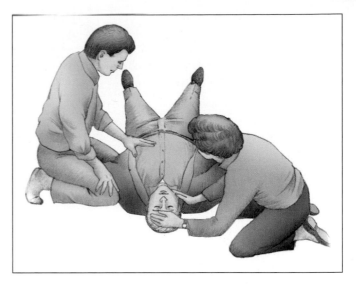

■ Immediately begin chest compressions until an AED or other defibrillator is ready for use.[1]

■ With your elbows locked, arms straight, and shoulders directly over your hands, administer chest compressions. Using the weight of your upper body, compress the patient's chest at least 2″ (5 cm) but no more than 2.4″ (6 cm),[1] keeping chest compression and chest recoil duration equal. Allow the patient's chest to completely recoil after each chest compression *to create a relative negative intrathoracic pressure that promotes venous return and cardiopulmonary blood flow.*[1] Avoid leaning over the patient's chest, *which could prevent it from recoiling completely.*[1]

■ Administer 30 compressions at a rate of 100 to 120 compressions per minute, pushing hard and fast.[1] After administering 30 compressions, open the patient's airway and give two ventilations. If the patient doesn't appear to have a cervical spine injury, use the head tilt–chin lift maneuver *to open the airway.*[1] To accomplish this, first place your hand that's closer to the patient's head on the patient's forehead. Then apply enough pressure to tilt the patient's head back. Next, place the fingertips of your other hand under the bony part of the lower jaw near the chin; avoid placing your fingertips on the soft tissue under the patient's chin, *because you may inadvertently obstruct the airway you're trying to open.* At the same time, keep the mouth partially open.

■ If you suspect a cervical spine injury, use the jaw-thrust maneuver without head extension.[1] To perform this maneuver, kneel at the patient's head with your elbows on the ground. Rest your thumbs on the lower jaw near the corners of the mouth, pointing your thumbs toward the patient's feet. Then place your fingertips under the lower jaw. To open the airway, lift the lower jaw with your fingertips.

■ To begin ventilations using a barrier mask with a one-way valve, position the narrow portion of the mask over the patient's nose and the wide portion above the patient's chin. Covering the nose and mouth with the mask, create a tight seal. Take a regular breath and then place your mouth on the mouthpiece and perform two ventilations. Alternatively, to begin ventilations using mouth-to-mouth rescue breathing, pinch the patient's nostrils shut with the thumb and index finger of the hand you've had on the patient's forehead. Take a regular breath and place your mouth over the patient's mouth, creating a tight seal.[1] Give two regular breaths, each over 1 second, *to promote oxygenation and to prevent over inflation of the patient's lungs.* Each ventilation should have enough volume to produce a minimal chest rise *to ensure adequate ventilation.*

■ Continue chest compressions until the emergency response team arrives or another rescuer arrives with an AED or another defibrillator. Use the AED or other defibrillator to evaluate the patient's rhythm as soon as it's ready. If the patient has a shockable rhythm, give one shock and then resume CPR.[1]

■ If the second rescuer is another health care professional, the two of you can perform two-person CPR. The second rescuer should start assisting after you've finished a cycle of 30 compressions and two ventilations.[1] The switch should occur in less than 5 seconds, during which the second rescuer moves into place opposite you and gets ready to begin compressions (as shown in the upper right column).[1]

■ The second rescuer should begin delivering compressions (as shown below). The compressor (at this point, the second rescuer) should count out loud so the ventilator can anticipate when to give ventilations. The rescuers should deliver 30 cycles of compressions (100 to 120 compressions per minute)[1] and two ventilations; the first rescuer should deliver ventilations during pauses in compressions and deliver each breath over 1 second.[1] Alternatively, rescue breaths can be performed during continuous chest compressions (either at a set ratio of 2 breaths : 30 compressions or asynchronously at 1 breath every 6 seconds) *to minimize interruptions in chest compressions.* Avoid excessive ventilation by performing 10 breaths/minute *to minimize the impact of positive-pressure ventilation on blood flow.*

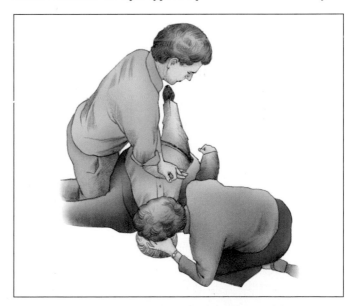

■ Switch the compressor role after five cycles of compressions and ventilations to *prevent rescuer fatigue and a subsequent decrease in compression quality*; the switch should occur in less than 5 seconds.[1] Chest compressions shouldn't be interrupted for longer than 10 seconds unless a specific intervention such as defibrillation or advanced airway placement is necessary, *to maximize compression time and improve tissue oxygenation.*[1]

■ Both rescuers should continue administering CPR until the ACLS providers take over or until normal breathing and effective circulation return.[1]

Completing the procedure

■ Remove and discard your gloves and any other personal protective equipment worn[2] and perform hand hygiene.[4,5,6,7,8,9]

■ Document the procedure.[10,11,12,13]

Potential hazards of CPR

Cardiopulmonary resuscitation (CPR) can cause various complications, including injury to bones and vital organs. This chart describes the causes of CPR hazards and lists preventive steps.

HAZARD	CAUSES	ASSESSMENT FINDINGS	PREVENTIVE MEASURES
Sternum and rib fractures	■ Osteoporosis ■ Malnutrition ■ Improper hand placement	■ Paradoxical chest movement ■ Chest pain or tenderness that increases with inspiration ■ Crepitus ■ Palpation of movable bony fragments over the sternum ■ On palpation, sternum feels unattached to surrounding ribs	■ Don't rest your hands or fingers on the patient's ribs. ■ Interlock your fingers. ■ Keep your bottom hand in contact with the chest, but release pressure after each compression. ■ Compress the sternum at the recommended depth for the patient's age.
Pneumothorax, hemothorax, or both	■ Lung puncture from fractured rib	■ Chest pain and dyspnea ■ Decreased or absent breath sounds over the affected lung ■ Tracheal deviation from midline ■ Hypotension ■ Hyperresonance to percussion over the affected area, along with shoulder pain	■ Don't rest your hands or fingers on the patient's ribs. ■ Interlock your fingers. ■ Keep your bottom hand in contact with the chest, but release pressure after each compression. ■ Compress the sternum at the recommended depth for the patient's age.
Injury to the heart and great vessels (pericardial tamponade, atrial or ventricular rupture, vessel laceration, cardiac contusion, punctures of the heart chambers)	■ Improperly performed chest compressions ■ Transvenous or transthoracic pacing attempts ■ Central line placement during resuscitation ■ Intracardiac drug administration	■ Jugular vein distention ■ Muffled heart sounds ■ Pulsus paradoxus ■ Narrowed pulse pressure ■ Electrical alternans (decreased electrical amplitude of every other QRS complex) ■ Adventitious heart sounds ■ Hypotension ■ Electrocardiogram changes (arrhythmias, ST-segment elevation, T-wave inversion, and marked decrease in QRS voltage)	■ Perform chest compressions properly.
Organ laceration (primarily liver and spleen)	■ Forceful compression ■ Sharp edge of a fractured rib or xiphoid process	■ Persistent right upper quadrant tenderness (liver injury) ■ Persistent left upper quadrant tenderness (splenic injury) ■ Increasing abdominal girth	■ Don't rest your hands or fingers on the patient's ribs. ■ Interlock your fingers. ■ Keep your bottom hand in contact with the chest, but release pressure after each compression. ■ Compress the sternum at the recommended depth for the patient's age.
Aspiration of stomach contents	■ Gastric distention and an elevated diaphragm from high ventilatory pressures	■ Fever, hypoxia, and dyspnea ■ Auscultation of wheezes and crackles ■ Increased white blood cell count ■ Changes in color and odor of lung secretions	■ Intubate early. ■ Insert a nasogastric tube and apply suction, if gastric distention is marked.

Special considerations

■ Evidence suggests that an optimal compression rate ranges between 100 and 120 compressions/minute; rates above or below this target range appear to reduce survival.[1]

■ If an arterial catheter or central venous access catheter is in place for hemodynamic monitoring, or if capnography is in use, use these devices to monitor the patient's response to CPR and the effectiveness of resuscitation efforts.[18]

■ Some health care professionals are hesitant to give mouth-to-mouth rescue breaths, however, the risk of disease transmission through mouth-to-mouth ventilation is very low, and initiation of rescue breathing is reasonable with or without a barrier device. *Because the AHA recognizes that rescuers may hesitate to give mouth-to-mouth rescue breathing,* they recommend that all health care professionals learn how to use disposable airway equipment. When using a barrier device, don't delay chest compressions while setting up the device.[1]

■ You can give bag-mask ventilation with room air or oxygen, but you should use supplemental oxygen (in a concentration greater than 40% and at a minimum flow rate of 10 L/minute) when available. Bag-mask ventilation is most effective when provided by two trained and experienced rescuers. One rescuer should open the patient's airway and seal the mask to the patient's face while the other rescuer squeezes the bag and gives the ventilations.[1]

■ After an advanced airway is in place, the compressing rescuer should perform continuous chest compressions at a rate of 100 to 120 compressions/minute without pauses for ventilation.[1] The rescuer giving ventilation can provide a breath every 6 seconds (which yields 10 breaths/minute) .[1]

■ Lay rescuers who can perform compressions and ventilations should use the head tilt–chin lift maneuver to open the airway.[1]

■ If no complications exist, give the patient's family the option of remaining at the bedside during resuscitation, *because doing so is beneficial in meeting the psychosocial needs of the patient and family in a time of crisis.*[19] Contraindications to family presence include family members who are suspected of abuse or those who demonstrate combative or violent behaviors, uncontrolled emotional outbursts, or behaviors consistent with an altered mental state associated with drug or alcohol misuse.[19]

Complications

CPR can cause certain complications—especially if the person performing the compressions doesn't place the hands properly on the sternum. These complications include fractured ribs, a lacerated liver, and punctured lungs.[20,21] Gastric distention, a common complication, results from giving too much air during ventilation.[22] (See *Potential hazards of CPR*.)

Documentation

Document all the events of resuscitation and the names of the individuals present. Record the reason CPR was initiated, whether the victim suffered from cardiac or respiratory arrest, where the arrest occurred, whether any witnesses were present, the time CPR began, and the duration of CPR. Note the patient's response, any complications, and interventions to correct complications.

If the patient also received ACLS measures, document the interventions performed, who performed them and when, the equipment used, and the results.

REFERENCES

1 American Heart Association. (2020). 2020 American Heart Association Guidelines for CPR and ECC– Part 3: Adult Basic and Advanced Life Support. https://cpr.heart.org/en/resuscitation-science/cpr-and-ecc-guidelines

2 Siegel, J. D., et al. (2007, revised 2019). 2007 guideline for isolation precautions: Preventing transmission of infectious agents in healthcare settings. https://www.cdc.gov/infectioncontrol/pdf/guidelines/isolation-guidelines-H.pdf (Level II)

3 Accreditation Association for Hospitals and Health Systems. (2020). Standard 07.01.10. *Healthcare Facilities Accreditation Program: Accreditation requirements for acute care hospitals.* Chicago, IL: Accreditation Association for Hospitals and Health Systems. (Level VII)

4 World Health Organization. (2009). WHO guidelines on hand hygiene in health care: First global patient safety challenge, clean care is safer care. https://apps.who.int/iris/bitstream/handle/10665/44102/9789241597906_eng.pdf?sequence=1 (Level IV)

5 The Joint Commission. (2021). Standard NPSG.07.01.01. *Comprehensive accreditation manual for hospitals.* Oakbrook Terrace, IL: The Joint Commission. (Level VII)

6 Centers for Disease Control and Prevention. (2002). Guideline for hand hygiene in health-care settings: Recommendations of the Healthcare Infection Control Practices Advisory Committee and the HICPAC/SHEA/APIC/IDSA Hand Hygiene Task Force. *MMWR Recommendations and Reports, 51*(RR-16), 1–45. https://www.cdc.gov/mmwr/pdf/rr/rr5116.pdf (Level II)

7 Centers for Medicare and Medicaid Services, Department of Health and Human Services. (2020). Condition of participation: Infection control. 42 C.F.R. § 482.42.

8 Accreditation Association for Hospitals and Health Systems. (2020). Standard 07.01.21. *Healthcare Facilities Accreditation Program: Accreditation requirements for acute care hospitals.* Chicago, IL: Accreditation Association for Hospitals and Health Systems. (Level VII)

9 DNV GL-Healthcare USA, Inc. (2020). IC.1.SR.1. *NIAHO® accreditation requirements, interpretive guidelines and surveyor guidance—revision 20.0.* Milford, OH: DNV GL-Healthcare USA, Inc. (Level VII)

10 The Joint Commission. (2021). Standard RC.01.03.01. *Comprehensive accreditation manual for hospitals.* Oakbrook Terrace, IL: The Joint Commission. (Level VII)

11 Centers for Medicare and Medicaid Services, Department of Health and Human Services. (2020). Condition of participation: Medical record services. 42 C.F.R. § 482.24(b).

12 Accreditation Association for Hospitals and Health Systems. (2020). Standard 10.00.03. *Healthcare Facilities Accreditation Program: Accreditation requirements for acute care hospitals.* Chicago, IL: Accreditation Association for Hospitals and Health Systems. (Level VII)

13 DNV GL-Healthcare USA, Inc. (2020). MR.2.SR.1. *NIAHO® accreditation requirements, interpretive guidelines and surveyor guidance—revision 20.0.* Milford, OH: DNV GL-Healthcare USA, Inc. (Level VII)

14 DNV GL-Healthcare USA, Inc. (2020). IC.1.SR.2. *NIAHO® accreditation requirements, interpretive guidelines and surveyor guidance—revision 20.0.* Milford, OH: DNV GL-Healthcare USA, Inc. (Level VII)

15 Cave, D. M., et al. (2010). Part 7: CPR techniques and devices: 2010 American Heart Association guidelines for cardiopulmonary resuscitation and emergency cardiovascular care. *Circulation, 122*(Suppl. 3), S720–S728. (Level II)

16 Edelson, D. P., et al. (2020). Interim Guidance for Basic and Advanced Life Support in Adults, Children, and Neonates with Suspected or Confirmed COVID-19. *Circulation, 141*(25), e933–e943. https://www.ahajournals.org/doi/10.1161/CIRCULATIONAHA.120.047463?utm_campaign=ahajournals&utm_source=phd&utm_medium=link&utm_content=phd04-09-20_circ-cpr (Level II)

17 Bhatnagar, V., et al. (2018). Cardiopulmonary resuscitation: unusual techniques for unusual situations. *Journal of Emergencies, Trauma and Shock.* 11(1), 31–37. (Level VII)

18 American Heart Association. (2020). Web-based integrated guidelines for cardiopulmonary resuscitation and emergency cardiovascular care—Part 7: Adult advanced cardiovascular life support. https://eccguidelines.heart.org/circulation/cpr-ecc-guidelines/ (Level VII)

19 American Association of Critical-Care Nurses. (2016). AACN practice alert: Family presence during resuscitation and invasive procedures. https://www.aacn.org/clinical-resources/practice-alerts/family-presence-during-resuscitation-and-invasive-procedures (Level VII)

20 Deliliga, A., et al. (2019). Cardiopulmonary resuscitation (CPR) complications encountered in forensic autopsy cases. *BMC Emergency Medicine, 19,* 23. (Level IV)

21 Kaldirim, U., et al. (2016). Complications of cardiopulmonary resuscitation in non-traumatic cases and factors affecting complications. *Egyptian Journal of Forensic Sciences, 6,* 270–274. https://www.sciencedirect.com/science/article/pii/S2090536X15000702 (Level IV)

22 Bon, C. A. (2020). Cardiopulmonary resuscitation (CPR). https://emedicine.medscape.com/article/1344081-overview#a4

CARDIOPULMONARY RESUSCITATION, CHILD

An adult who needs cardiopulmonary resuscitation (CPR) typically suffers from a primary cardiac disorder or an arrhythmia that has stopped the heart. A child who needs CPR typically suffers from hypoxia and acidosis caused by respiratory difficulty or arrest and shock.[1]

Most pediatric crises requiring CPR are preventable. They include motor vehicle collisions, drowning, burns, smoke inhalation, falls, poisoning, suffocation, and choking (typically from inhaling balloons, small objects, and certain foods, such as hot dogs, rounded candies, nuts, and grapes).[2,3,4]

The goal of CPR is the return of spontaneous circulation; however, CPR techniques differ depending on whether the patient is an adult, a child, or an infant. For CPR purposes, the American Heart Association (AHA) defines a patient by age. An infant is younger than age 1 year; a child is considered age 1 year to puberty.[4]

Survival chances improve the sooner CPR begins and the faster advanced life-support systems are implemented. However, before beginning CPR on a child, you must first determine whether the child's respiratory distress results from a mechanical obstruction or an infection, such as epiglottitis or croup. These latter conditions require immediate medical attention, not CPR. CPR is appropriate only when a child isn't breathing or is only gasping (as opposed to breathing regularly).[4]

Chest compressions are particularly important because they ensure the perfusion of vital organs during CPR. To prevent a delay in chest compressions, the sequence of CPR is "C-A-B" (compressions, airway, and breathing), which gives the highest priority to chest compressions when resuscitating a child in cardiopulmonary arrest.[4]

High-quality CPR is important not only at the outset of resuscitation, but throughout the entire resuscitation process. Key components of high-quality CPR are minimizing chest compression interruptions, administering compressions of adequate rate and depth, allowing complete recoil of the child's chest after each compression, and avoiding excessive ventilation.[4]

Equipment

Backboard or other hard surface ▪ automated external defibrillator (AED) (preferably with pediatric attenuator for children younger than age 8) or defibrillator ▪ Optional: barrier mask with one-way valve, gloves, other personal protective equipment, appropriate size bag-mask device.

Implementation

Review the following illustrated instructions, which provide a step-by-step guide for CPR as recommended by the AHA. (See *AHA BLS pediatric cardiac arrest algorithm for the single rescuer*, page 128.)

AHA BLS pediatric cardiac arrest algorithm for the single rescuer

The algorithm below illustrates the steps for basic life support for a child, as recommended by the American Heart Association.

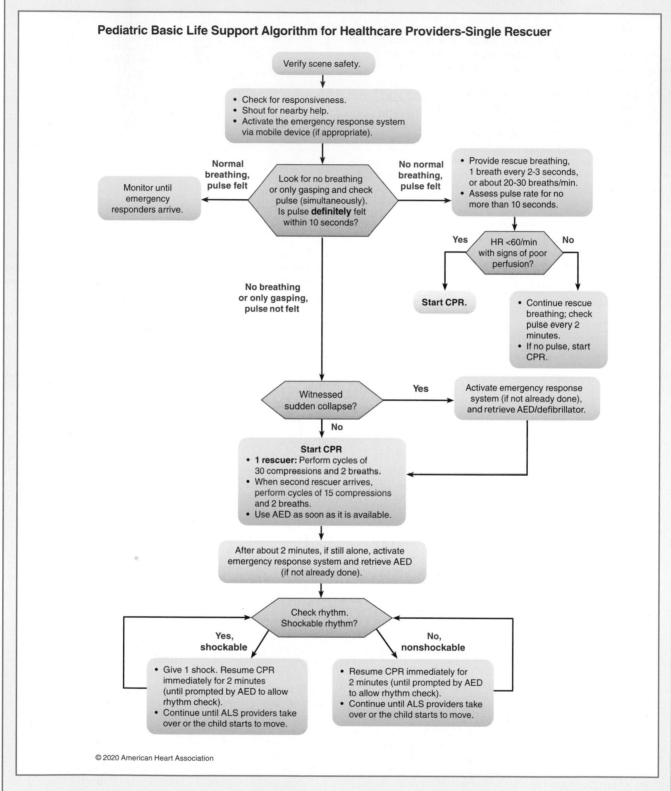

Pediatric Basic Life Support Algorithm for Healthcare Providers-Single Rescuer

Verify scene safety.

- Check for responsiveness.
- Shout for nearby help.
- Activate the emergency response system via mobile device (if appropriate).

Look for no breathing or only gasping and check pulse (simultaneously). Is pulse **definitely** felt within 10 seconds?

Normal breathing, pulse felt → Monitor until emergency responders arrive.

No normal breathing, pulse felt →
- Provide rescue breathing, 1 breath every 2-3 seconds, or about 20-30 breaths/min.
- Assess pulse rate for no more than 10 seconds.

HR <60/min with signs of poor perfusion?

Yes → **Start CPR.**

No →
- Continue rescue breathing; check pulse every 2 minutes.
- If no pulse, start CPR.

No breathing or only gasping, pulse not felt

Witnessed sudden collapse?

Yes → Activate emergency response system (if not already done), and retrieve AED/defibrillator.

No

Start CPR
- **1 rescuer:** Perform cycles of 30 compressions and 2 breaths.
- When second rescuer arrives, perform cycles of 15 compressions and 2 breaths.
- Use AED as soon as it is available.

After about 2 minutes, if still alone, activate emergency response system and retrieve AED (if not already done).

Check rhythm. Shockable rhythm?

Yes, shockable
- Give 1 shock. Resume CPR immediately for 2 minutes (until prompted by AED to allow rhythm check).
- Continue until ALS providers take over or the child starts to move.

No, nonshockable
- Resume CPR immediately for 2 minutes (until prompted by AED to allow rhythm check).
- Continue until ALS providers take over or the child starts to move.

© 2020 American Heart Association

■ Put on gloves and other personal protective equipment, as needed and available, *to comply with standard precautions and to prevent exposure to potentially infectious blood and body fluids.*[5,6,7]

■ Verify that the environment is safe by quickly scanning the location and surroundings for imminent physical threats, such as toxic and electrical hazards.[4]

■ To assess responsiveness, tap the child on the shoulder and shout, "Are you all right?" Call the child's name if you know it *to elicit a response.* If the child is unresponsive, shout for nearby help and activate the emergency response system via mobile device (if appropriate).[4]

■ Check to see whether the child is apneic or only gasping (as opposed to breathing regularly) and, if able, simultaneously check for a pulse *to minimize any delay in detecting cardiac arrest and initiating CPR. To check for a pulse,* palpate the carotid artery that's closest to you by placing your index and middle fingers in the groove formed by the trachea and the sternocleidomastoid muscle (as shown below). Alternatively, check for a femoral pulse by placing your fingers in the center of the child's groin, just below the inguinal ligament. Palpate for no longer than 10 seconds.[4]

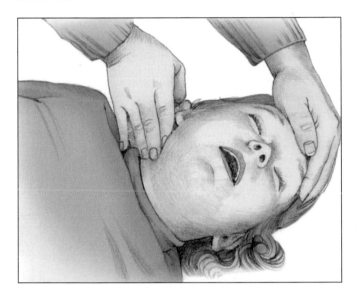

■ If the child is breathing normally and has a pulse, monitor the child closely until the emergency response team arrives.[4]

■ If breathing is absent or the child is only gasping and you feel a pulse within 10 seconds, open the child's airway. Use the head tilt–chin lift maneuver, unless you suspect a cervical spine injury, in which case you should use the jaw-thrust maneuver without head extension.[4] Provide rescue breathing by giving the child 20 to 30 breaths/minute (1 breath every 2 to 3 seconds).[4] Use a barrier mask with a one-way valve, if available. Give each breath over 1 second regardless of whether the child has an advanced airway in place; ensure that each breath causes minimal chest rise. If using bag-mask ventilation, use only the force and tidal volume necessary to just make the chest rise.[4]

■ If breathing is absent or the child is only gasping and you don't feel a pulse within 10 seconds, or the pulse is less than 60 beats/minute and the child has signs of poor perfusion (such as pallor, cyanosis, and mottling), activate the emergency response system (if not already done).[4] Have a coworker retrieve the defibrillator or AED. Alternatively, if you're alone and you witnessed the child suddenly collapse, retrieve the defibrillator or AED.[4] Place the child in the supine position on a firm, flat surface (backboard or other hard surface, such as the ground).[4] When turning the child, roll the child's head and torso as a unit (as shown above on right); avoid twisting or pulling the child's neck, shoulders, or hips. Don't delay the initiation of CPR to obtain and position a backboard.

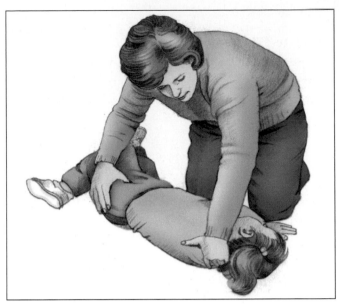

■ Kneel next to the child's chest or stand beside the bed at the child's chest, ensuring that your knees or feet are apart *to provide a wide base of support.* Place the heel of one or two hands in the center of the child's chest, directly between the child's nipples (as shown below).[4] The decision to use one or two hands depends on the size of the child and the compressor's effectiveness.

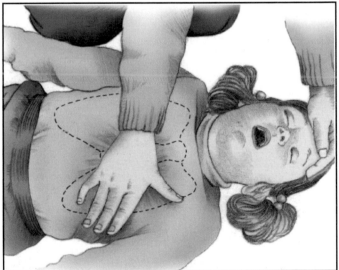

■ Immediately begin chest compressions and continue until the defibrillator or AED is ready for use.

■ With your elbows locked, arms straight, and shoulders directly over your hand(s), administer compressions. Using the weight of your upper body, compress the child's chest downward at least one-third the anterior-posterior dimensions of the chest, which is about 2″ (5 cm) in most children. Allow the child's chest to completely recoil after each compression; *incomplete chest wall recoil during CPR is associated with higher intrathoracic pressures and significantly decreased venous return, blood flow, and cerebral perfusion.*[4]

■ Administer 30 compressions at a rate of 100 to 120 compressions per minute. After administering 30 compressions, open the child's airway and prepare to give two ventilations. If the child doesn't appear to have a cervical spine injury, use the head tilt–chin lift maneuver to open the child's airway. To perform this maneuver, place your hand that's closer to the child's head on the child's forehead. Then apply enough pressure to tilt the child's head back. Next, place the fingertips of your other hand under the bony part of the child's lower jaw near the chin; avoid placing your fingertips on the soft tissue under the child's chin, *because you may inadvertently obstruct the airway you're trying to open.* At the same time, keep the child's mouth partially open (as shown below).

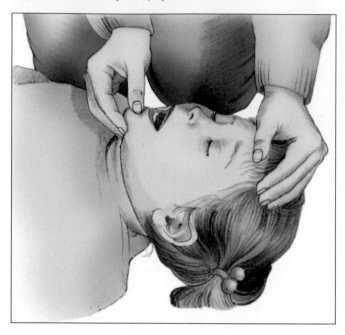

■ If you suspect a cervical spine injury, use the jaw-thrust maneuver.[4] To perform this maneuver, rest your thumbs on the child's lower jaw near the corners of the mouth, pointing your thumbs toward the child's feet. Then place your fingertips around the lower jaw. To open the airway, lift the lower jaw with your fingertips.

■ While maintaining an open airway, evaluate breathing status by placing your ear near the child's mouth and nose.[4] Look for chest movement and scan the child for breathing.

■ To begin ventilations using a barrier mask with a one-way valve, position the narrow portion of the mask over the child's nose and the wide portion above the child's chin. Covering the nose and mouth with the mask, create a tight seal. Take a regular breath and place your mouth on the mouthpiece (as shown below). Alternatively, to begin ventilations using mouth-to-mouth rescue breathing, pinch the child's nostrils shut with the thumb and index finger of the hand you've had on the child's forehead. Take a regular breath and place your mouth over the child's mouth, creating a tight seal. Keep in mind that a handheld resuscitation bag and mask is recommended only when a second rescuer arrives; *it isn't recommended for use by a lone rescuer.*[4]

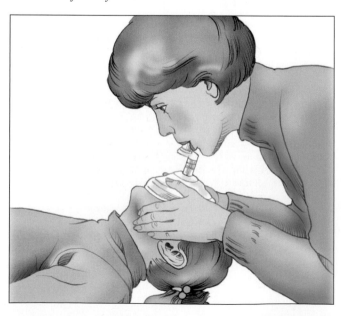

Two-person CPR

During two-person cardiopulmonary resuscitation (CPR), one rescuer administers chest compressions while the other maintains a patent airway and administers ventilations.[4] The ratio of compressions to ventilations for two-person CPR is 15:2. If available, a child-size, self-inflating bag-mask device with a volume of at least 450 mL can be used to deliver ventilations for infants and young children. For older children and adolescents, an adult-size self-inflating bag with a volume of 1,000 mL may be needed to produce adequate chest rise.

After insertion of an advanced airway, the compressor should continuously deliver 100 to 120 compressions/minute without pausing for ventilations. The rescuer delivering ventilations should deliver a breath every 2 to 3 seconds (or 20 to 30 per minute).[4]

■ Give two slow breaths, each over 1 second, *to promote oxygenation and to prevent overinflation of the child's lungs.* Use only the force and tidal volume necessary to just make the child's chest rise.[4]

■ If your first ventilation isn't successful, reposition the child's head to open the airway and try again, *because the most common cause of ventilation difficulty is an improperly opened airway.* If you're still unsuccessful, consider that the child may have a foreign body obstruction.

■ If you detect a pulse, and the pulse is greater than 60 beats/minute, continue rescue breathing with one breath every 2 to 3 seconds (20 to 30 breaths/minute). If you don't detect a pulse, continue cycles of 30 compressions to 2 ventilations until the emergency response team or another rescuer arrives with a defibrillator or AED. Use the defibrillator or AED as soon as it is available. If after about 2 minutes you're still alone, activate the emergency response system and retrieve the defibrillator or AED, if not already done.

■ When a second rescuer arrives, continue with two-person CPR. (See *Two-person CPR.*)

■ Remove and discard your gloves and other personal protective equipment, if worn.[5]

■ Perform hand hygiene.[8,9,10,11,12,13]

■ Document the procedure.[14,15,16,17]

Special considerations

■ Some health care professionals hesitate to give mouth-to-mouth rescue breaths. For this reason, the AHA recommends that all health care professionals learn how to use disposable airway equipment.[4] When using a barrier device, the rescuer shouldn't delay administering chest compressions while setting up the device.[4]

■ Compression-only CPR can be effective in children with a primary cardiac arrest. The AHA recommends compression-only CPR for children in cardiac arrest when rescuers are unwilling or unable to deliver breaths.[4]

■ *Because effective bag-and-mask ventilation requires complex steps,* it isn't recommended for use by a lone rescuer during CPR. Instead, mouth-to-barrier device techniques can be used. Bag-and-mask ventilation can be provided effectively during two-person CPR.[4]

■ A child's tongue can easily block the small airway. If this occurs, simply opening the airway may eliminate the obstruction.

■ Give the child's parents or guardians the option of remaining at the bedside during resuscitation, *because doing so helps meet the psychosocial needs of the child and family members.*[18]

Complications

CPR may cause complications, including fractured ribs, sternal fractures, liver lacerations, and pneumothorax, if the compressor doesn't place the hands on the child's sternum properly.[19,20] Gastric distention, a common complication, results from giving too much air during ventilation.[21]

Documentation

Document all of the events of resuscitation and the names of the individuals present. Record whether the child suffered cardiac or respiratory arrest and if the event was witnessed. Note the location where the arrest occurred, the time CPR began, the duration of the procedure, and the outcome. Document any complications—for example, a fractured rib, pneumothorax, or gastric distention—as well as nursing actions taken to correct them.

If the child received pediatric advanced life support, document which interventions were performed, who performed them, when they were performed, what equipment was used, and the child's response.

REFERENCES

1 Ralston, M. E. (2021). Pediatric basic life support (BLS) for health care providers. In: *UpToDate*, Torrey, S. B,. (Ed.).

2 Centers for Disease Control and Prevention. (2019). National action plan for child injury prevention. https://www.cdc.gov/safechild/nap/index.html

3 World Health Organization & UNICEF. (2008). World report on child injury prevention. https://apps.who.int/iris/bitstream/handle/10665/43851/9789241563574_eng.pdf?sequence=1

4 American Heart Association. (2020). 2020 American Heart Association Guidelines for CPR and ECC—Part 4: Pediatric Basic and Advanced Life Support. https://cpr.heart.org/en/resuscitation-science/cpr-and-ecc-guidelines

5 Siegel, J. D., et al. (2007, revised 2019). 2007 guideline for isolation precautions: Preventing transmission of infectious agents in healthcare settings. https://www.cdc.gov/infectioncontrol/pdf/guidelines/isolation-guidelines-H.pdf (Level II)

6 Accreditation Association for Hospitals and Health Systems. (2020). Standard 07.01.10. *Healthcare Facilities Accreditation Program: Accreditation requirements for acute care hospitals.* Chicago, IL: Accreditation Association for Hospitals and Health Systems. (Level VII)

7 DNV GL-Healthcare USA, Inc. (2020). IC.1.SR.2. *NIAHO® accreditation requirements, interpretive guidelines and surveyor guidance—revision 20.0.* Milford, OH: DNV GL-Healthcare USA, Inc. (Level VII)

8 World Health Organization. (2009). WHO guidelines on hand hygiene in health care: First global patient safety challenge, clean care is safer care. https://apps.who.int/iris/bitstream/handle/10665/44102/9789241597906_eng.pdf?sequence=1 (Level IV)

9 The Joint Commission. (2021). Standard NPSG.07.01.01. *Comprehensive accreditation manual for hospitals.* Oakbrook Terrace, IL: The Joint Commission. (Level VII)

10 Centers for Disease Control and Prevention. (2002). Guideline for hand hygiene in health-care settings: Recommendations of the Healthcare Infection Control Practices Advisory Committee and the HICPAC/SHEA/APIC/IDSA Hand Hygiene Task Force. *MMWR Recommendations and Reports, 51*(RR-16), 1–45. https://www.cdc.gov/mmwr/pdf/rr/rr5116.pdf (Level II)

11 Centers for Medicare and Medicaid Services, Department of Health and Human Services. (2020). Condition of participation: Infection control. 42 C.F.R. § 482.42.

12 Accreditation Association for Hospitals and Health Systems. (2020). Standard 07.01.21. *Healthcare Facilities Accreditation Program: Accreditation requirements for acute care hospitals.* Chicago, IL: Accreditation Association for Hospitals and Health Systems. (Level VII)

13 DNV GL-Healthcare USA, Inc. (2020). IC.1.SR.1. *NIAHO® accreditation requirements, interpretive guidelines and surveyor guidance—revision 20.0.* Milford, OH: DNV GL-Healthcare USA, Inc. (Level VII)

14 The Joint Commission. (2021). Standard RC.02.01.01. *Comprehensive accreditation manual for hospitals.* Oakbrook Terrace, IL: The Joint Commission. (Level VII)

15 Centers for Medicare and Medicaid Services, Department of Health and Human Services. (2020). Condition of participation: Medical record services. 42 C.F.R. § 482.24(b).

16 Accreditation Association for Hospitals and Health Systems. (2020). Standard 10.00.03. *Healthcare Facilities Accreditation Program: Accreditation requirements for acute care hospitals.* Chicago, IL: Accreditation Association for Hospitals and Health Systems. (Level VII)

17 DNV GL-Healthcare USA, Inc. (2020). MR.2.SR.1. *NIAHO® accreditation requirements, interpretive guidelines and surveyor guidance—revision 20.0.* Milford, OH: DNV GL-Healthcare USA, Inc. (Level VII)

18 American Association of Critical-Care Nurses. (2016). AACN practice alert: Family presence during resuscitation and invasive procedures. https://www.aacn.org/clinical-resources/practice-alerts/family-presence-during-resuscitation-and-invasive-procedures (Level VII)

19 Deliliga, A., et al. (2019). Cardiopulmonary resuscitation (CPR) complications encountered in forensic autopsy cases. *BMC Emergency Medicine, 19,* 23. (Level IV)

20 Kaldirim, U., et al. (2016). Complications of cardiopulmonary resuscitation in non-traumatic cases and factors affecting complications. *Egyptian Journal of Forensic Sciences, 6*(3), 270–274. https://www.sciencedirect.com/science/article/pii/S2090536X15000702 (Level IV)

21 Bon, C. A. (2020). Cardiopulmonary resuscitation (CPR). https://emedicine.medscape.com/article/1344081-overview#a4

CARDIOPULMONARY RESUSCITATION, INFANT

An adult who needs cardiopulmonary resuscitation (CPR) typically suffers from a primary cardiac disorder or an arrhythmia that has stopped the heart. An infant who needs CPR typically suffers from hypoxia and acidosis caused by respiratory difficulty or respiratory arrest and shock.[1]

In infants, the leading causes of cardiopulmonary arrest are congenital malformations, complications of prematurity, and sudden infant death syndrome. Other causes of cardiopulmonary arrest in infants include laryngospasm and edema from upper respiratory infections and choking. Liquids are the most common cause of choking in infants.[1,2]

The goal of CPR is the return of spontaneous circulation. However, CPR techniques differ depending on whether the patient is an adult, a child, or an infant. For CPR purposes, the American Heart Association (AHA) defines a patient by age. An infant is younger than age 1; a child is considered age 1 to puberty.[3]

Survival chances improve the sooner CPR begins and the faster advanced life-support systems are implemented. CPR is appropriate only when the infant isn't breathing or is only gasping (as opposed to breathing regularly).[3] Chest compressions are particularly important because perfusion to vital organs during CPR depends on them. To prevent a delay in chest compressions, the sequence of CPR is "C-A-B" (compressions, airway, and breathing), which gives the highest priority to chest compressions when resuscitating an infant in cardiac arrest.[3]

High-quality CPR is important not only at the onset of resuscitation, but throughout the entire resuscitation process. Key components of high-quality CPR are minimizing chest compression interruptions, providing compressions of adequate rate and depth, allowing complete recoil of the chest after each compression, and avoiding excessive ventilation.[3]

Equipment

Backboard or other hard surface ■ automated external defibrillator (AED) or defibrillator (a manual device is preferred for infants with a shockable rhythm; if a manual device isn't available, a device with a pediatric attenuator is preferred; if neither is available, an AED without a dose attenuator may be used) ■ Optional: gloves, other personal protective equipment, barrier mask with one-way valve.

Implementation

Review the following illustrated instructions, which provide a step-by-step guide for CPR as recommended by the AHA. (See *AHA BLS pediatric cardiac arrest algorithm for the single rescuer*, page 128.)

■ Put on gloves and other personal protective equipment, as needed and available, *to comply with standard precautions.*[4,5,6]

■ Verify that the environment is safe by quickly scanning the infant's location and surroundings for imminent physical threats, such as toxic and electrical hazards.[3]

■ Assess the infant to determine whether he or she is responsive. Gently tap the infant's foot and ask loudly, "Are you okay?" Call out the infant's name if you know it. If the infant is unresponsive, shout for nearby help and activate the emergency response system via mobile device (if appropriate).[3]

■ Check to see whether the infant is apneic or only gasping (as opposed to breathing regularly) and, if able, simultaneously check for a pulse *to minimize delay in detecting cardiac arrest and initiating CPR.* To check for a pulse, palpate the brachial artery, located inside the infant's upper arm between the elbow and the shoulder (as shown on the next page). Palpate for no longer than 10 seconds.[3]

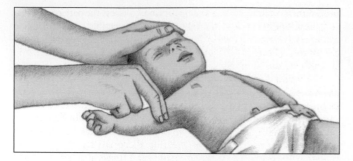

■ If the infant is breathing normally and has a pulse, monitor the infant closely until the emergency response team arrives.[3]

■ If breathing is absent or the infant is only gasping, and you feel a pulse within 10 seconds and it's 60 beats/minute or higher, open the airway using the head tilt–chin lift maneuver, unless contraindicated by trauma. If spinal injury is suspected, use the jaw-thrust maneuver. Don't hyperextend the infant's neck.[3] Provide rescue breathing by giving the infant 20 to 30 breaths/minute (1 breath every 2 to 3 seconds). To begin ventilations using a barrier mask with a one-way valve, position the narrow portion of the mask over the infant's nose and the wide portion above the infant's chin. Covering the nose and mouth with the mask, create a tight seal. Take a regular breath and place your mouth on the mouthpiece. Alternatively, take a breath and tightly seal your mouth over the infant's nose and mouth.[3]

■ If breathing is absent or the infant is only gasping and you don't feel a pulse within 10 seconds or the pulse rate is less than 60 beats/minute and the infant has signs of poor perfusion, such as pallor, cyanosis, or mottling, follow these steps: Activate the emergency response system (if not already done). Retrieve the defibrillator or AED, if you witnessed the arrest. If you didn't witness the arrest, place the infant supine on a hard surface to begin chest compressions.[7] Place two fingers on the neonate's sternum just below the nipple line (as shown below).[3] Use these two fingers to depress the sternum at least one-third the anterior-posterior chest. dimension, usually 1½″ (4 cm), at a rate of 100 to 120 compressions/minute.[3]

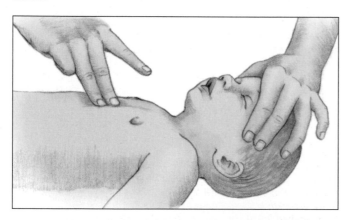

■ When performing chest compressions, take care to ensure smooth motions, and allow the chest to recoil after each compression; *incomplete chest wall recoil during CPR is associated with higher intrathoracic pressures and significantly decreased venous return, coronary perfusion, blood flow, and cerebral perfusion.*[3] Keep your fingers on the infant's chest at all times. Time your motions so that the compression and relaxation phases are equal to promote effective compressions.

■ After 30 compressions, open the airway and deliver two breaths. If the infant's chest rises and falls, then the amount of air is probably adequate. If the chest doesn't rise, reposition the infant's head, make a better seal, and try again. Avoid excessive ventilation.[3,7]

■ If you're still alone after about 2 minutes of CPR, activate the emergency response system and retrieve the defibrillator or AED (if not already done).[3]

■ Check the infant's cardiac rhythm with the defibrillator or AED. If a shockable rhythm is present, deliver a shock, as indicated.[3]

■ Resume CPR with cycles of 30 compressions to 2 ventilations. Alternatively, if a second rescuer arrives, continue with two-person CPR until the emergency response team arrives and takes over, or the infant begins breathing spontaneously.[3] (See *Two-person CPR*, page 130.)

NURSING ALERT *To maximize chest compression time and improve tissue oxygenation,* avoid interruptions to chest compressions, such as pulse checks.[3,7]

■ Continue to monitor the infant if pulse and respirations return.

■ Remove and discard your gloves and any other personal protective equipment worn.[4]

■ Perform hand hygiene.[8,9,10,11,12,13]

■ Document the procedure.[14,15,16,17]

Special considerations

■ The AHA recommends that all health care professionals learn how to use disposable airway equipment.[3] When using a barrier device, the rescuer shouldn't delay chest compressions while setting up the device.[3]

■ Compression-only CPR can be effective in infants with primary cardiac arrest. If rescuers are unwilling or unable to deliver breaths, the AHA recommends that rescuers perform compression-only CPR for infants in cardiac arrest.[3]

■ *Because effective bag-and-mask ventilation use requires complex steps*, it isn't recommended for a lone rescuer performing CPR. During CPR, the lone rescuer should use mouth-to-barrier device techniques for ventilation. Effective bag-and-mask ventilation is possible during two-person CPR.

■ An infant's tongue can easily block the small airway. If this occurs, simply opening the airway may eliminate the obstruction.

■ Give the infant's parents or guardians the option of remaining at the bedside during resuscitation, *because doing so is beneficial in meeting psychosocial needs of the infant and family in a time of crisis.*[18]

Complications

CPR can cause complications, including fractured ribs, sternal fractures, a lacerated liver, and punctured lungs if the compressor doesn't place the fingers on the sternum properly.[19,20] Gastric distention, a common complication of CPR, results from giving too much air during ventilation.[21]

Documentation

Document all of the events of resuscitation and the names of the individuals who were present. Record whether the infant suffered cardiac or respiratory arrest. Note the location where the arrest occurred and if the event was witnessed, the time CPR began, the duration of the procedure, and the outcome. Document any complications—for example, a fractured rib, a bruised mouth, or gastric distention—as well as actions taken to correct them.

If the infant received pediatric advanced life support, document which interventions the infant received, who performed those interventions, when they were performed, what equipment was used, and what the result was.

REFERENCES

1 Ralston, M. E. (2021). Pediatric basic life support (BLS) for health care providers. In: *UpToDate*, Torrey, S. B,. (Ed.).

2 American Heart Association. (2010). 2010 American Heart Association guidelines for cardiopulmonary resuscitation and emergency cardiovascular care. *Circulation, 122*(Suppl. 3), S862–S875. (Level II)

3 American Heart Association. (2020). 2020 American Heart Association Guidelines for CPR and ECC—Part 4: Pediatric Basic and Advanced Life Support. https://cpr.heart.org/en/resuscitation-science/cpr-and-ecc-guidelines

4 Siegel, J. D., et al. (2007, revised 2019). 2007 guideline for isolation precautions: Preventing transmission of infectious agents in healthcare settings. https://www.cdc.gov/infectioncontrol/pdf/guidelines/isolation-guidelines-H.pdf (Level II)

5 Accreditation Association for Hospitals and Health Systems. (2020). Standard 07.01.10. *Healthcare Facilities Accreditation Program: Accreditation requirements for acute care hospitals.* Chicago, IL: Accreditation Association for Hospitals and Health Systems. (Level VII)

6 DNV GL-Healthcare USA, Inc. (2020). IC.1.SR.2. *NIAHO® accreditation requirements, interpretive guidelines and surveyor guidance—revision 20.0.* Milford, OH: DNV GL-Healthcare USA, Inc. (Level VII)

7 American Heart Association. (2013). AHA consensus statement: Cardiopulmonary resuscitation quality—improving cardiac resuscitation outcomes both inside and outside the hospital. *Circulation, 128,* 417–435. https://www.ahajournals.org/doi/pdf/10.1161/CIR.0b013e31829d8654 (Level VII)

8 The Joint Commission. (2021). Standard NPSG.07.01.01. *Comprehensive accreditation manual for hospitals.* Oakbrook Terrace, IL: The Joint Commission. (Level VII)

9 World Health Organization. (2009). WHO guidelines on hand hygiene in health care: First global patient safety challenge, clean care is safer care. https://apps.who.int/iris/bitstream/handle/10665/44102/9789241597906_eng.pdf?sequence=1 (Level IV)

10 Centers for Disease Control and Prevention. (2002). Guideline for hand hygiene in health-care settings: Recommendations of the Healthcare Infection Control Practices Advisory Committee and the HICPAC/SHEA/APIC/IDSA Hand Hygiene Task Force. *MMWR Recommendations and Reports, 51*(RR-16), 1–45. https://www.cdc.gov/mmwr/pdf/rr/rr5116.pdf (Level II)

11 Centers for Medicare and Medicaid Services, Department of Health and Human Services. (2020). Condition of participation: Infection control. 42 C.F.R. § 482.42.

12 Accreditation Association for Hospitals and Health Systems. (2020). Standard 07.01.21. *Healthcare Facilities Accreditation Program: Accreditation requirements for acute care hospitals.* Chicago, IL: Accreditation Association for Hospitals and Health Systems. (Level VII)

13 DNV GL-Healthcare USA, Inc. (2020). IC.1.SR.1. *NIAHO® accreditation requirements, interpretive guidelines and surveyor guidance—revision 20.0.* Milford, OH: DNV GL-Healthcare USA, Inc. (Level VII)

14 The Joint Commission. (2021). Standard RC.02.01.01. *Comprehensive accreditation manual for hospitals.* Oakbrook Terrace, IL: The Joint Commission. (Level VII)

15 Centers for Medicare and Medicaid Services, Department of Health and Human Services. (2020). Condition of participation: Medical record services. 42 C.F.R. § 482.24(b).

16 Accreditation Association for Hospitals and Health Systems. (2020). Standard 10.00.03. *Healthcare Facilities Accreditation Program: Accreditation requirements for acute care hospitals.* Chicago, IL: Accreditation Association for Hospitals and Health Systems. (Level VII)

17 DNV GL-Healthcare USA, Inc. (2020). MR.2.SR.1. *NIAHO® accreditation requirements, interpretive guidelines and surveyor guidance—revision 20.0.* Milford, OH: DNV GL-Healthcare USA, Inc. (Level VII)

18 American Association of Critical-Care Nurses. (2016). AACN practice alert: Family presence during resuscitation and invasive procedures. https://www.aacn.org/clinical-resources/practice-alerts/family-presence-during-resuscitation-and-invasive-procedures (Level VII)

19 Deliliga, A., et al. (2019). Cardiopulmonary resuscitation (CPR) complications encountered in forensic autopsy cases. *BMC Emergency Medicine, 19,* 23. (Level IV)

20 Kaldirim, U., et al. (2016). Complications of cardiopulmonary resuscitation in non-traumatic cases and factors affecting complications. *Egyptian Journal of Forensic Sciences, 6,* 270–274. https://www.sciencedirect.com/science/article/pii/S2090536X15000702 (Level IV)

21 Bon, C. A. (2020). Cardiopulmonary resuscitation (CPR). https://emedicine.medscape.com/article/1344081-overview#a4

CARDIOVERSION, SYNCHRONIZED

Synchronized cardioversion delivers an electrical charge to the myocardium that's timed with the QRS complex. This charge causes immediate depolarization, interrupting reentry circuits and allowing the sinoatrial node to resume control.[1] Synchronizing the electrical charge with the QRS complex prevents delivery during the relative refractory period of the cardiac cycle, when a shock could lead to ventricular fibrillation.[2]

Synchronized cardioversion is the treatment of choice for such arrhythmias as unstable supraventricular tachycardia, unstable atrial flutter, unstable atrial fibrillation, or unstable monomorphic ventricular tachycardia with a pulse that doesn't respond to vagal maneuvers (Valsalva maneuver or carotid sinus massage) or drug therapy. The procedure can be elective or urgent depending on the patient's tolerance of the arrhythmia.[1] For example, if the patient is hemodynamically stable, the procedure is often elective, allowing for time to assess the patient's cardiac and metabolic status to determine whether a reversible cause exists that would resolve with treatment. If the patient is unstable (for example, has altered mental status, hypotension, or chest pain or is in shock), immediate cardioversion is necessary.[1]

Contraindications to synchronized cardioversion include tachycardia related to digoxin toxicity, sinus tachycardia, and multifocal atrial tachycardia. Atrial fibrillation increases the risk of stroke; therefore, cardioversion is contraindicated in patients with atrial fibrillation who aren't receiving anticoagulation, unless transesophageal imaging rules out thrombus formation.[2,3] Anticoagulant therapy is recommended for at least 3 weeks before cardioversion and for 4 weeks after cardioversion to normal sinus rhythm in patients with atrial fibrillation for 48 hours or longer or when the duration of atrial fibrillation is unknown.[4]

Practitioners using synchronized cardioversion should adhere to the American Heart Association guidelines.[1]

Equipment

Cardioverter-defibrillator ▪ self-adhesive cardioversion-defibrillation pads or anterior, posterior, or transverse paddles and conductive gel pads ▪ cardiac monitor with recording system ▪ disposable pregelled electrodes ▪ 12-lead electrocardiogram (ECG) machine ▪ oxygen administration equipment ▪ suction equipment ▪ emergency equipment (code cart with artificial airway and intubation supplies, handheld resuscitation bag and mask, emergency cardiac medications, and emergency pacing equipment) ▪ automatic blood pressure device ▪ pulse oximeter and probe ▪ stethoscope ▪ disinfectant pad ▪ facility-approved disinfectant ▪ Optional: prescribed sedation or analgesia, IV catheter insertion equipment, disposable-head clippers, prescribed cardiac medications, gloves, gown, mask with face shield, mask, goggles.

Preparation of equipment

Make sure that the cardioverter-defibrillator pads or paddles are connected to the cardioverter-defibrillator, and that the cardioverter-defibrillator battery is adequately charged or plugged into a wall outlet. Have emergency equipment and suction and intubation equipment readily available at the patient's bedside and make sure that it's functioning properly.

Inspect all equipment and supplies. If a product is expired, is defective, or has compromised integrity, remove it from patient use, label it as expired or defective, and report the expiration or defect as directed by your facility.

Implementation

▪ Verify the practitioner's orders. Check to see whether cardiac medications have been prescribed for administration before the procedure.
▪ Check the patient's medical record for recent serum potassium and magnesium levels and arterial blood gas results. Also check the patient's most recent digoxin level, as ordered. *Electrolyte imbalances, acid-base disturbances, and digoxin toxicity increase the risk of arrhythmias.*[5] Notify the practitioner of critical test results within your facility's established time frame *so that the patient can be treated promptly.*[6]
▪ If required by your facility, confirm that informed consent has been obtained and that the signed consent form is in the patient's medical record.[5,7,8,9,10]
▪ Gather and prepare the necessary equipment and supplies.
▪ Conduct a preprocedural verification *to make sure that all relevant documentation, related information, and equipment are available and correctly identified to the patient's identifiers.*[11]
▪ Perform hand hygiene.[12,13,14,15,16,17]
▪ Confirm the patient's identity using at least two patient identifiers.[18]
▪ Provide privacy.[19,20,21,22]
▪ Explain the procedure to the patient and family (if appropriate) according to their communication and learning needs *to increase their understanding, allay their fears, and enhance cooperation.*[23]
▪ If the patient's condition allows, have the patient maintain nothing-by-mouth status before the procedure; if nonemergent, minimum fasting recommendations include 2 hours for clear liquids, 6 hours or more for a light meal, and 8 hours or more for fried or fatty foods or meat.[24]

■ Raise the patient's bed to waist level before providing care *to prevent caregiver back strain.*[25]

■ Perform hand hygiene.[12,13,14,15,16,17]

■ Ensure that the patient is attached to a cardiac monitor, pulse oximeter, and automatic blood pressure device. Make sure that the alarm limits on each medical device are set appropriately for the patient's current condition, and that the alarms are turned on, functioning properly, and audible to staff.[26,27,28,29]

■ Obtain the patient's vital signs and oxygen saturation level using pulse oximetry, and assess neurologic, cardiovascular, and respiratory status *to determine whether immediate cardioversion is necessary.*[5]

■ If the patient has inadequate oxygenation or shows signs of labored breathing, notify the practitioner and administer supplemental oxygen, as prescribed.[1]

■ Perform hand hygiene.[12,13,14,15,16,17]

■ Put on gloves and other personal protective equipment, as needed, *to comply with standard precautions.*[30,31,32]

■ Make sure that the patient has patent IV access. Insert an IV catheter as needed. (See the "IV catheter insertion and removal" procedure.)

■ Obtain a 12-lead ECG *to better define the patient's heart rhythm and to serve as a baseline for comparison.* Don't delay immediate cardioversion to obtain the ECG if the patient is unstable.[1,5]

■ Administer cardiac medications, if prescribed, following safe medication administration practices.[33,34,35,36]

■ Remove all metal objects from the patient, *because metal conducts electricity and could cause burns during cardioversion.*[5]

■ If the patient has dentures, a partial plate, or another oral prosthesis, determine whether the device supports airway patency or has the potential to obstruct it. Remove the device if it increases the risk of airway obstruction.[5]

■ Make sure that the patient is in a dry environment and that the patient's chest is dry, *because if the rescuer or patient comes in contact with water, a conductor of electricity, the rescuer can receive a shock and the patient can receive a skin burn.*[5]

■ Position the patient supine *to provide access to the patient's chest during the procedure.*[5]

■ If necessary, clip hair from the patient's chest *to make sure that the electrodes adhere properly.*[5]

■ Remove transdermal medication patches from the patient's chest, if present, or make sure that the cardioversion-defibrillation pads or paddles don't touch the patches during the procedure *to prevent a chest burn during cardioversion.*[5]

■ If the patient isn't already receiving supplemental oxygen, consider preoxygenation before cardioversion *to promote myocardial oxygenation and to reduce the risk of cerebral and cardiac complications.*[5]

■ A specially trained health care provider will administer moderate sedation or anesthesia if time allows and the patient's condition permits.[1]

■ Monitor the patient's heart rate, blood pressure, and respiratory rate *to promptly detect changes in the patient's condition and, subsequently, prevent treatment delays.*

■ Conduct a time-out before starting the procedure, if the patient's condition allows, *to perform a final assessment ensuring that the correct patient, site, positioning, and procedure are identified and, as applicable, that all relevant information and necessary equipment are available.*[37]

■ Turn on the cardioverter-defibrillator.[5]

■ Apply the electrodes to the appropriate locations on the patient's chest (if not already present) and attach the monitoring lead wires on the cardioverter-defibrillator, *because the device must be able to sense the R wave to provide synchronized cardioversion.*[5] Ensure that there is an adequate cardiac rhythm tracing.[5]

■ Apply the self-adhesive cardioversion-defibrillation pads according to the manufacturer's directions. If you're using anterolateral placement, place one pad at the heart's apex just left of the nipple at the midaxillary line and the other pad just below the right clavicle to the right of the sternum. Alternatively, remove the paddles from the machine. Place the paddles and the conductive gel pads using anterolateral placement.[5] Alternative pad positions, including anteroposterior, anterior–left infrascapular, and anterior–right infrascapular, can also be used depending on the patient's individual characteristics.

■ *To decrease transthoracic resistance,* avoid placing the self-adhesive cardioversion-defibrillation pads or paddles over a female patient's breast.[5]

■ Turn on the ECG recording device to obtain a continuous printout *to document the patient's response to cardioversion.*[5]

■ Push the SYNC button *to synchronize the machine with the patient's QRS complex.* Assess the cardioverter-defibrillator waveform and make sure that a synchronized marker appears with the QRS complex and that its location is consistent from beat to beat. Also, make sure that the SYNC button flashes with each of the patient's QRS complexes; listen for audible beeps. If necessary, adjust the R wave gain until synchronization occurs. *Synchronization with the patient's QRS complex prevents the random discharge of electrical charges, which may cause ventricular fibrillation.*[5]

■ Set the energy level to the prescribed dose. Advanced cardiac life support protocols call for an initial shock of 50 to 100 joules for a patient with unstable supraventricular tachycardia, 120 to 200 joules for a patient with atrial fibrillation, 50 to 100 joules for a patient with atrial flutter, and 100 joules for a patient with monomorphic ventricular tachycardia with a pulse.[1]

■ Make sure that everyone stands clear from contact with the patient and the bed *to prevent conduction of electrical current to health care workers.*[5]

■ Charge the cardioverter-defibrillator.

■ Disconnect the oxygen source before cardioversion *to decrease the risk of combustion in the presence of electrical current.*[5]

■ Confirm that all personnel are clear of the patient and the bed.

■ If you're using cardioversion-defibrillation pads, push and hold the discharge button until the energy is delivered. Alternatively, if you're using paddles, apply firm pressure (approximately 25 to 30 lb [11.3 to 13.6 kg])[38] to each paddle against the patient's chest wall, and push and hold the discharge button until the energy is discharged. Keep in mind that the machine has to synchronize the discharge with the QRS complex.

NURSING ALERT Don't touch the bed, the patient, or any equipment attached to the patient while cardioversion is being administered *to prevent transfer of the electrical current to caregivers.*

■ Assess the patient's cardiac rhythm on the monitor.

■ If the arrhythmia fails to convert after the initial shock, repeat the procedure. Increase the energy dose in a stepwise fashion or as instructed by the practitioner.[1] Check that the synchronization mode is active after each cardioversion attempt, *because many defibrillators automatically default to the unsynchronized mode.*

■ When the patient's rhythm converts, monitor vital signs, oxygen saturation level, and cardiovascular, neurologic, and respiratory status *to evaluate patient response to the procedure.*[5] Reconnect the patient to the oxygen source, if appropriate.

■ Turn off the continuous ECG recording device.

■ Obtain a follow-up 12-lead ECG, as ordered.

■ Inspect the patient's chest for electrical burns. Treat burns as needed and prescribed.[5]

■ Screen and assess for the patient's pain using facility-defined criteria that are consistent with the patient's age, condition, and ability to understand.[39]

■ Treat the patient's pain, as needed and ordered, using nonpharmacologic, pharmacologic, or a combination of approaches. Base the treatment plan on evidence-based practices and the patient's clinical condition, past medical history, and pain management goals.[39]

■ Return the bed to the lowest position *to prevent falls and maintain patient safety.*[40]

■ Discard used supplies in the appropriate receptacles.[30]

■ Remove and discard your gloves or other personal protective equipment, if worn.[30]

■ Perform hand hygiene.[12,13,14,15,16,17]

■ Reassess and respond to the patient's pain by evaluating the response to treatment and progress toward pain management goals. Assess for adverse reactions and risk factors for adverse events that may result from treatment.[39]

■ Clean and disinfect your stethoscope using a disinfectant pad.[41,42]

■ Perform hand hygiene.[12,13,14,15,16,17]

■ Put on gloves, if needed.

■ Clean and disinfect the cardioverter-defibrillator according to the manufacturer's instructions *to prevent the spread of infection and to make sure that it's ready for its next use.*[5,41,42]

- Perform hand hygiene.[12,13,14,15,16,17]
- Document the procedure.[43,44,45,46]

Special considerations

- Synchronization to the R wave prevents the discharge of electrical energy randomly on the T wave, which can lead to ventricular tachycardia or ventricular fibrillation. If ventricular fibrillation does occur, turn off the synchronization and defibrillate according to the defibrillation procedure.[5]
- If the patient has a permanent pacemaker or an implantable cardioverter-defibrillator, don't place the pads or paddles over the device, *because doing so can impair current flow to the patient's heart and damage the device or cause it to malfunction.*[5]
- The Joint Commission issued a sentinel event alert concerning medical device alarm safety, *because alarm-related events are associated with permanent loss of function or death.* Among the contributing factors are improper alarm settings, alarm settings turned off inappropriately, and alarm signals not audible to staff. Make sure that alarm limits are set appropriately and that alarms are turned on, functioning properly, and audible to staff. Follow facility guidelines for preventing alarm fatigue.[26]

Complications

Common complications following synchronized cardioversion are altered level of consciousness, cerebral emboli, skin burns, respiratory depression, and arrhythmias.[5]

Documentation

Document the date and time that the procedure was performed, including the voltage delivered with each attempt, the patient's heart rhythm (preprocedure and postprocedure ECG rhythm strips), medications you administered, and the patient's tolerance of the procedure. Note any emergency interventions that the patient required and the patient's response to those interventions. Record the patient's vital signs and your other assessment findings. Document teaching provided to the patient and family (if applicable), their understanding of that teaching, and any need for follow-up teaching.

REFERENCES

1 American Heart Association. (2020). Web-based Integrated Guidelines for Cardiopulmonary Resuscitation and Emergency Cardiovascular Care—Part 7: Adult Advanced Cardiovascular Life Support. https://eccguidelines.heart.org/circulation/cpr-ecc-guidelines/ (Level II)

2 Beinart, S. C. (2018). Synchronized electrical cardioversion. http://emedicine.medscape.com/article/1834044-overview

3 Marchiondo, K. (2007). Transesophageal imaging and interventions: Nursing implications. *Critical Care Nurse, 27*(2), 25–36. (Level V)

4 January, C. T., et al. (2019). 2019 AHA/ACC/HRS focused update of the 2014 AHA/ACC/HRS guideline for the management of patients with atrial fibrillation: A report of the American College of Cardiology/American Heart Association Task Force on Clinical Practice Guidelines and the Heart Rhythm Society in collaboration with the Society of Thoracic Surgeons. *Circulation, 140*, e125–e151. https://www.ahajournals.org/doi/full/10.1161/CIR.0000000000000665 (Level VII)

5 Wiegand, D. L. (2017). *AACN procedure manual for high acuity, progressive, and critical care* (7th ed.). St. Louis, MO: Elsevier.

6 The Joint Commission. (2021). Standard NPSG.02.03.01. *Comprehensive accreditation manual for hospitals.* Oakbrook Terrace, IL: The Joint Commission. (Level VII)

7 The Joint Commission. (2021). Standard RI.01.03.01. *Comprehensive accreditation manual for hospitals.* Oakbrook Terrace, IL: The Joint Commission. (Level VII)

8 Centers for Medicare and Medicaid Services, Department of Health and Human Services. (2020). Condition of participation: Patient's rights. 42 C.F.R. § 482.13(b)(2).

9 Accreditation Association for Hospitals and Health Systems. (2020). Standard 30.01.11. *Healthcare Facilities Accreditation Program: Accreditation requirements for acute care hospitals.* Chicago, IL: Accreditation Association for Hospitals and Health Systems. (Level VII)

10 DNV GL-Healthcare USA, Inc. (2020). PR.2.SR.3. *NIAHO® accreditation requirements, interpretive guidelines and surveyor guidance—revision 20.0.* Milford, OH: DNV GL-Healthcare USA, Inc. (Level VII)

11 The Joint Commission. (2021). Standard UP.01.01.01. *Comprehensive accreditation manual for hospitals.* Oakbrook Terrace, IL: The Joint Commission. (Level VII)

12 The Joint Commission. (2021). Standard NPSG.07.01.01. *Comprehensive accreditation manual for hospitals.* Oakbrook Terrace, IL: The Joint Commission. (Level VII)

13 Centers for Disease Control and Prevention. (2002). Guideline for hand hygiene in health-care settings: Recommendations of the Healthcare Infection Control Practices Advisory Committee and the HICPAC/SHEA/APIC/IDSA Hand Hygiene Task Force. *MMWR Recommendations and Reports, 51*(RR-16), 1–45. https://www.cdc.gov/mmwr/pdf/rr/rr5116.pdf (Level II)

14 World Health Organization. (2009). WHO guidelines on hand hygiene in health care: First global patient safety challenge, clean care is safer care. https://apps.who.int/iris/bitstream/handle/10665/44102/9789241597906_eng.pdf?sequence=1 (Level IV)

15 Centers for Medicare and Medicaid Services, Department of Health and Human Services. (2020). Condition of participation: Infection control. 42 C.F.R. § 482.42.

16 Accreditation Association for Hospitals and Health Systems. (2020). Standard 07.01.21. *Healthcare Facilities Accreditation Program: Accreditation requirements for acute care hospitals.* Chicago, IL: Accreditation Association for Hospitals and Health Systems. (Level VII)

17 DNV GL-Healthcare USA, Inc. (2020). IC.1.SR.1. *NIAHO® accreditation requirements, interpretive guidelines and surveyor guidance—revision 20.0.* Milford, OH: DNV GL-Healthcare USA, Inc. (Level VII)

18 The Joint Commission. (2021). Standard NPSG.01.01.01. *Comprehensive accreditation manual for hospitals.* Oakbrook Terrace, IL: The Joint Commission. (Level VII)

19 Centers for Medicare and Medicaid Services, Department of Health and Human Services. (2020). Condition of participation: Patient's rights. 42 C.F.R. § 482.13(c)(1).

20 Accreditation Association for Hospitals and Health Systems. (2020). Standard 15.01.16. *Healthcare Facilities Accreditation program: Accreditation requirements for acute care hospitals.* Chicago, IL: Accreditation Association for Hospitals and Health Systems. (Level VII)

21 The Joint Commission. (2021). Standard RI.01.01.01. *Comprehensive accreditation manual for hospitals.* Oakbrook Terrace, IL: The Joint Commission. (Level VII)

22 DNV GL-Healthcare USA, Inc. (2020). PR.2.SR.5. *NIAHO® accreditation requirements, interpretive guidelines and surveyor guidance—revision 20.0.* Milford, OH: DNV GL-Healthcare USA, Inc. (Level VII)

23 The Joint Commission. (2021). Standard PC.02.01.21. *Comprehensive accreditation manual for hospitals.* Oakbrook Terrace, IL: The Joint Commission. (Level VII)

24 American Society of Anesthesiologists. (2017). Practice guidelines for preoperative fasting and the use of pharmacologic agents to reduce the risk of pulmonary aspiration: Application to healthy patients undergoing elective procedures. *Anesthesiology, 126*, 376–393. http://anesthesiology.pubs.asahq.org/article.aspx?articleid=2596245 (Level V)

25 Waters, T. R., et al. (2009). Safe patient handling training for schools of nursing. https://www.cdc.gov/niosh/docs/2009-127/pdfs/2009-127.pdf (Level VII)

26 The Joint Commission. (2013). Sentinel event alert 50: Medical device alarm safety in hospitals. https://www.jointcommission.org/assets/1/6/SEA_50_alarms_4_26_16.pdf (Level VII)

27 The Joint Commission. (2021). Standard NPSG.06.01.01. *Comprehensive accreditation manual for hospitals.* Oakbrook Terrace, IL: The Joint Commission. (Level VII)

28 Graham, K. C., & Cvach, M. (2010). Monitor alarm fatigue: Standardizing use of physiological monitors and decreasing nuisance alarms. *American Journal of Critical Care, 19*, 28–37.

29 American Association of Critical-Care Nurses. (2018). AACN practice alert: Managing alarms in acute care across the life span: Electrocardiography and pulse oximetry. https://www.aacn.org/clinical-resources/practice-alerts/managing-alarms-in-acute-care-across-the-life-span (Level VII)

30 Siegel, J. D., et al. (2007, revised 2019). 2007 guideline for isolation precautions: Preventing transmission of infectious agents in healthcare settings. https://www.cdc.gov/infectioncontrol/pdf/guidelines/isolation-guidelines-H.pdf (Level II)

31 Accreditation Association for Hospitals and Health Systems. (2020). Standard 07.01.10. *Healthcare Facilities Accreditation Program: Accreditation requirements for acute care hospitals.* Chicago, IL: Accreditation Association for Hospitals and Health Systems. (Level VII)

32 DNV GL-Healthcare USA, Inc. (2020). IC.1.SR.2. *NIAHO® accreditation requirements, interpretive guidelines and surveyor guidance—revision 20.0.* Milford, OH: DNV GL-Healthcare USA, Inc. (Level VII)

33 Centers for Medicare and Medicaid Services, Department of Health and Human Services. (2020). Condition of participation: Nursing services. 42 C.F.R. § 482.23(c).

34 Accreditation Association for Hospitals and Health Systems. (2020). Standard 16.01.03. *Healthcare Facilities Accreditation Program: Accreditation requirements for acute care hospitals*. Chicago, IL: Accreditation Association for Hospitals and Health Systems. (Level VII)

35 The Joint Commission. (2021). Standard MM.06.01.01. *Comprehensive accreditation manual for hospitals*. Oakbrook Terrace, IL: The Joint Commission. (Level VII)

36 DNV GL-Healthcare USA, Inc. (2020). MM.1.SR.3. *NIAHO® accreditation requirements, interpretive guidelines and surveyor guidance—revision 20.0*. Milford, OH: DNV GL-Healthcare USA, Inc. (Level VII)

37 The Joint Commission. (2021). Standard UP.01.03.01. *Comprehensive accreditation manual for hospitals*. Oakbrook Terrace, IL: The Joint Commission. (Level VII)

38 McKean, S. C., et al. (2016). *Principles and practice of hospital medicine* (2nd ed.). New York, NY: McGraw Hill.

39 The Joint Commission. (2021). Standard PC.01.02.07. *Comprehensive accreditation manual for hospitals*. Oakbrook Terrace, IL: The Joint Commission. (Level VII)

40 Ganz, D. A., et al. (2013, reviewed 2021). *Preventing falls in hospitals: A toolkit for improving quality of care* (AHRQ Publication No. 13-0015-EF). Rockville, MD: Agency for Healthcare Research and Quality. https://www.ahrq.gov/professionals/systems/hospital/fallpxtoolkit/index.html (Level VII)

41 Rutala, W. A., et al. (2008, revised 2019). Guideline for disinfection and sterilization in healthcare facilities, 2008. https://www.cdc.gov/infectioncontrol/pdf/guidelines/disinfection-guidelines-H.pdf (Level I)

42 Accreditation Association for Hospitals and Health Systems. (2020). Standard 07.02.03. *Healthcare Facilities Accreditation Program: Accreditation requirements for acute care hospitals*. Chicago, IL: Accreditation Association for Hospitals and Health Systems. (Level VII)

43 The Joint Commission. (2021). Standard RC.01.03.01. *Comprehensive accreditation manual for hospitals*. Oakbrook Terrace, IL: The Joint Commission. (Level VII)

44 Centers for Medicare and Medicaid Services, Department of Health and Human Services. (2020). Condition of participation: Medical record services. 42 C.F.R. § 482.24(b).

45 Accreditation Association for Hospitals and Health Systems. (2020). Standard 10.00.03. *Healthcare Facilities Accreditation Program: Accreditation requirements for acute care hospitals*. Chicago, IL: Accreditation Association for Hospitals and Health Systems. (Level VII)

46 DNV GL-Healthcare USA, Inc. (2020). MR.2.SR.1. *NIAHO® accreditation requirements, interpretive guidelines and surveyor guidance—revision 20.0*. Milford, OH: DNV GL-Healthcare USA, Inc. (Level VII)

CARE PLAN PREPARATION

A care plan directs the patient's nursing care from admission to discharge. This written action plan is based on nursing diagnoses that have been formulated after reviewing assessment findings, and it embodies the components of the nursing process: assessment, diagnosis, planning, implementation, and evaluation. (See *Elements of a nursing diagnosis*.) The care plan consists of three parts: *goals* or *expected outcomes*, which describe behaviors or results to be achieved within a specified time; appropriate *nursing actions* or *interventions* needed to achieve these goals; and *evaluations of the established goals*.[1]

A nursing care plan should be written for each patient, preferably within 24 hours of admission.[4] It's usually started by the patient's primary nurse or the nurse who admits the patient. If the care plan contains more than one nursing diagnosis, the nurse must assign priority to each one and implement those with the highest priority first. The nurse must update and revise the plan throughout the patient's stay, based on the patient's response.[5,6,7,8] The document becomes part of the permanent patient record.[9]

Some health care facilities use standardized care plans that can be modified to serve many patients. Others use computer programs to facilitate development of nursing care plans.[1]

A nursing care plan serves as a database for planning assignments, giving change-of-shift reports, conferring with the practitioner or other members of the health care team, planning patient discharge, and documenting patient care. In addition, the care plan can be a management tool to determine staffing needs and assignments.

Equipment

Nursing care plan form or care plan in electronic format ▪ patient's medical record.

Elements of a nursing diagnosis

You may identify a nursing diagnosis from an actual problem that the patient experiences, an identified risk, or a desire by the patient to improve current health status.[2]

Problem-focused diagnosis

A problem-focused nursing diagnosis contains three components: a problem, related factors, and the defining characteristics.

▪ *Human response or problem*—After analyzing the patient's condition, choose a diagnostic label from a facility-sanctioned list or create a label specific to the patient. For consistency, most facilities use NANDA-I's list of nursing diagnosis. An example of a diagnostic label is *Excess fluid volume*.

▪ *Related factors*—The second part of the nursing diagnosis lists etiologic factors that seem to influence the patient in a way that pertains to the diagnostic label. Connect these factors to the diagnostic label with the phrase "related to." For example, you might add the "related to" phrase to the previous example to read: *Excess fluid volume related to excess sodium intake*.[2,3]

▪ *Defining characteristics*—To complete the nursing diagnosis, list defining characteristics, which are signs and symptoms uncovered during assessment that help define the diagnostic label. You may list them beneath the diagnosis and related factors, or add them to the diagnostic statement and connect them with the phrase "as evidenced by." For example, you might add related factors to the previous example to read: *Excess fluid volume related to excess sodium intake as evidenced by edema, weight gain over a short time, dyspnea on exertion, and S3 heart sounds*.[2,3]

Risk diagnosis

A risk-related nursing diagnosis contains two components: the identified risk and the risk factors.

▪ *Identified risk*—After assessing the patient's condition, choose a diagnostic label from a facility-approved list, or create a specific label for the patient that describes the condition for which the patient is at risk. For example, your assessment may have identified that a patient with arthritis experiences joint stiffness, so an appropriate nursing diagnosis is *Risk for physical mobility*.[2]

▪ *Risk factors*—For a risk-related nursing diagnosis there are no related or etiological factors. You're identifying a patient's vulnerability for a potential problem, so the problem isn't yet present. Instead, list the risk factors that predispose the patient to the identified risk. For example, using the previous identified risk, you would add risk factors to identify *Risk for physical mobility related to arthritic joint pain and stiffness*.[2]

Health promotion diagnosis

A health promotion diagnosis contains two components: the health promotion diagnosis, which addresses the area of health the patient desires to improve, and the defining characteristics.

▪ *Health promotion diagnosis*—The health promotion diagnosis is the area of health that the patient desires to improve. An example of a diagnostic label is *Readiness for self-care*.

▪ *Defining characteristic(s)*—The defining characteristics in a health promotion diagnosis are evidence of the desire on the patient's part to improve current health state. For example, a health promotion diagnosis may include *Readiness for self-care as evidenced by an expressed desire to enhance self-care*.[2]

Tips for writing an effective patient care plan

How do you write a care plan that's realistic, accurate, and helpful? Here are some guidelines.

Be systematic
Avoid setting an initial outcome that's impossible to achieve. For example, suppose the outcome for a newly admitted patient with a stroke were "Patient will ambulate without assistance." Although this outcome is certainly appropriate in the long term, several short-term outcomes, such as "Patient maintains joint range-of-motion," need to be achieved first.

Be realistic
The nursing intervention should match staff resources and capabilities. For example, "Passive range-of-motion exercises to all extremities every 2 hours" may not be reasonable given the unit's staffing pattern and care requirements. The goals you set to correct a patient's problem should reflect what is reasonably possible in your setting—for example, "Passive range-of-motion exercises with a.m. care, p.m. care, and once at night."

Be clear
Remember to express goals clearly, *because you'll use these goals to evaluate the effectiveness of the care plan.*

Be specific
Include specific details in the patient's goals. For example, "Give plenty of fluids" is nonspecific because it doesn't indicate a specific amount. In contrast, an intervention that reads "Encourage fluid intake—1,000 mL/day shift, 1,000 mL/evening shift, 500 mL/night shift" allows another nurse to carry out the intervention with some assurance of correctly meeting the intended goal.

Be brief
Provide necessary details without extraneous information. An intervention that says "Follow turning schedule posted at bedside" is more readable and useful than having the entire schedule written on the nursing plan.

Implementation

- Gather the necessary equipment and supplies.
- Review the patient's medical record, especially the nursing assessment completed on admission. Review diagnostic test results, the medical plan, and other information that may affect patient care. If the patient has just been admitted, complete a nursing history and physical assessment, and add it to the patient's record.
- Perform hand hygiene.[10,11,12,13,14,15]
- Confirm the patient's identity by using at least two patient identifiers.[16]
- Provide privacy.[17,18,19,20]
- Obtain from the patient any additional subjective or objective information needed to complete your assessment.
- Based on an analysis of the data, determine which nursing diagnoses will guide your patient care.[5] Address all of the patient's significant needs when determining nursing diagnoses.
- Work with the patient to identify individualized short-term and long-term goals (expected outcomes) for each nursing diagnosis. Short-term goals can be achieved quickly; long-term goals take more time to achieve and usually involve prevention, patient teaching, and rehabilitation. A correctly written outcome expresses the desired patient behavior, the criteria for measurement, and the appropriate time and conditions under which the behavior will occur. For example, an outcome containing all these elements might read: "By Monday, using crutches, Mary Ballin will be able to walk to the end of the hall and back." *Expected outcomes serve as the basis for evaluating the effectiveness of nursing interventions.*
- Select interventions that will help the patient achieve the stated outcome for each nursing diagnosis. Include specific information, such as the frequency or particular intervention technique. *Outcomes establish criteria against which you'll judge whether further nursing actions are necessary.* (See *Tips for writing an effective patient care plan.*)
- Evaluate the patient's progress and revise the care plan as appropriate.[5,6,7,8]
- Perform hand hygiene.[10,11,12,13,14,15]
- Complete documentation of the care plan.[9,21,22,23,24]

Special considerations

- If your facility doesn't use electronic medical records, fill out the nursing care plan in ink, *because the document is part of the patient's permanent medical record.* If you must revise your plan as the patient's condition changes, fill out a new care plan and add it to the medical record.[5,9]
- Sign and date the care plan whenever you make new entries *to keep the plan current and to maintain accountability for planning the patient's care.*
- Customize a standardized care plan *to avoid "standardizing" the patient's care and to allow you to address the patient's individual concerns.*[1]
- Be aware that the patient might not meet long-term goals during hospitalization, so your planning should address postdischarge and home care needs. Interventions may include coordinating home care services.[1]
- Note that the nursing care plan may be a part of a multidisciplinary plan of care, such as a critical pathway.[1] Critical pathways address

standardized desired outcomes of care for a specific treatment or diagnosis.

Documentation

Documentation of the patient's progress (or lack of it) is required by The Joint Commission and other regulatory agencies that monitor health care quality.[5,6,7,8] Document all pertinent nursing diagnoses, expected outcomes, nursing interventions, and evaluations of expected outcomes. Write the care plan clearly and concisely so that other members of the health care team can understand it.

REFERENCES

1 Craven, R. F., et al. (2021). *Fundamentals of nursing: Concepts and competencies for practice* (9th ed.). Philadelphia, PA: Wolters Kluwer.

2 NANDA International. (n.d.). How do I write a diagnostic statement for risk, problem-focused and health promotion diagnoses? http://nanda.host4kb.com/article/AA-00492/36/English-/Frequently-Asked-Questions/Nursing-Diagnosis/Nursing-Diagnosis%3A-Learning-Using/How-do-I-write-a-diagnostic-statement-for-risk-problem-focused-and-health-promotion-diagnoses.html

3 Herdman, T. H.,, & Kamitsuru, S., (Eds.). (2018). *Nursing diagnoses: Definitions and classification 2018-2020* (11th ed.). New York, NY: Thieme Publishers.

4 DNV GL-Healthcare USA, Inc. (2020). NS.3.SR.2. *NIAHO® accreditation requirements, interpretive guidelines and surveyor guidance—revision 20.0.* Milford, OH: DNV GL-Healthcare USA, Inc. (Level VII)

5 The Joint Commission. (2021). Standard PC.01.03.01. *Comprehensive accreditation manual for hospitals.* Oakbrook Terrace, IL: The Joint Commission. (Level VII)

6 Centers for Medicare and Medicaid Services, Department of Health and Human Services. (2020). Condition of participation: Nursing services. 42 C.F.R. § 482.23(b)(4).

7 DNV GL-Healthcare USA, Inc. (2020). NS.3.SR.3. *NIAHO® accreditation requirements, interpretive guidelines and surveyor guidance—revision 20.0.* Milford, OH: DNV GL-Healthcare USA, Inc. (Level VII)

8 Accreditation Association for Hospitals and Health Systems. (2020). Standard 16.00.10. *Healthcare Facilities Accreditation Program: Accreditation requirements for acute care hospitals.* Chicago, IL: Accreditation Association for Hospitals and Health Systems. (Level VII)

9 The Joint Commission. (2021). Standard RC.02.01.01. *Comprehensive accreditation manual for hospitals.* Oakbrook Terrace, IL: The Joint Commission. (Level VII)

10 The Joint Commission. (2021). Standard NPSG.07.01.01. *Comprehensive accreditation manual for hospitals.* Oakbrook Terrace, IL: The Joint Commission. (Level VII)

11 World Health Organization. (2009). WHO guidelines on hand hygiene in health care: First global patient safety challenge, clean care is safer care. https://apps.who.int/iris/bitstream/handle/10665/44102/9789241597906_eng.pdf?sequence=1 (Level IV)

12 Centers for Disease Control and Prevention. (2002). Guideline for hand hygiene in health-care settings: Recommendations of the Healthcare Infection Control Practices Advisory Committee and the HICPAC/

SHEA/APIC/IDSA Hand Hygiene Task Force. *MMWR Recommendations and Reports, 51*(RR-16), 1–45. https://www.cdc.gov/mmwr/pdf/rr/rr5116.pdf (Level II)

13 Centers for Medicare and Medicaid Services, Department of Health and Human Services. (2020). Condition of participation: Infection control. 42 C.F.R. § 482.42.

14 Accreditation Association for Hospitals and Health Systems. (2020). Standard 07.01.21. *Healthcare Facilities Accreditation Program: Accreditation requirements for acute care hospitals.* Chicago, IL: Accreditation Association for Hospitals and Health Systems. (Level VII)

15 DNV GL-Healthcare USA, Inc. (2020). IC.1.SR.1. *NIAHO® accreditation requirements, interpretive guidelines and surveyor guidance—revision 20.0.* Milford, OH: DNV GL-Healthcare USA, Inc. (Level VII)

16 The Joint Commission. (2021). Standard NPSG.01.01.01. *Comprehensive accreditation manual for hospitals.* Oakbrook Terrace, IL: The Joint Commission. (Level VII)

17 The Joint Commission. (2021). Standard RI.01.01.01. *Comprehensive accreditation manual for hospitals.* Oakbrook Terrace, IL: The Joint Commission. (Level VII)

18 Centers for Medicare and Medicaid Services, Department of Health and Human Services. (2020). Condition of participation: Patient's rights. 42 C.F.R. § 482.13(c)(1).

19 Accreditation Association for Hospitals and Health Systems. (2020). Standard 15.01.16. *Healthcare Facilities Accreditation Program: Accreditation requirements for acute care hospitals.* Chicago, IL: Accreditation Association for Hospitals and Health Systems. (Level VII)

20 DNV GL-Healthcare USA, Inc. (2020). PR.2.SR.5. *NIAHO® accreditation requirements, interpretive guidelines and surveyor guidance—revision 20.0.* Milford, OH: DNV GL-Healthcare USA, Inc. (Level VII)

21 The Joint Commission. (2021). Standard RC.01.03.01. *Comprehensive accreditation manual for hospitals.* Oakbrook Terrace, IL: The Joint Commission. (Level VII)

22 Centers for Medicare and Medicaid Services, Department of Health and Human Services. (2020). Condition of participation: Medical record services. 42 C.F.R. § 482.24.

23 Accreditation Association for Hospitals and Health Systems. (2020). Standard 10.00.03. *Healthcare Facilities Accreditation Program: Accreditation requirements for acute care hospitals.* Chicago, IL: Accreditation Association for Hospitals and Health Systems. (Level VII)

24 DNV GL-Healthcare USA, Inc. (2020). MR.2.SR.1. *NIAHO® accreditation requirements, interpretive guidelines and surveyor guidance—revision 20.0.* Milford, OH: DNV GL-Healthcare USA, Inc. (Level VII)

Cast application

A cast is a hard mold that encases a body part, usually an extremity, to provide immobilization of bones and surrounding tissue. It can be used to treat injuries (including fractures), correct orthopedic conditions (such as deformities), or promote healing after surgery, amputation, or nerve or vascular repair. It usually remains in place until bone healing occurs, typically about 4 to 8 weeks.[1] (See *Types of cylindrical casts.*)

Casts may be constructed of cotton-polyester, plaster, fiberglass, or other synthetic materials. Plaster material used for casting is inexpensive, nontoxic, nonflammable, and easy to mold, and rarely causes allergic reactions or skin irritation. However, fiberglass, the most commonly used material, is lighter, stronger, and more resilient than plaster.[4] Fiberglass dries rapidly and is more difficult to mold, but it can bear body weight immediately if necessary and is water-resistant.[2] Typically, an orthopedist applies a cast, and a nurse prepares the patient and the equipment and assists during the procedure. With special preparation, a nurse practitioner or physician assistant may apply or change a cast and set a fracture under the direction of an orthopedist.

Equipment

Tubular stockinette ▪ cotton polyester casting material ▪ bucket of water ▪ sink equipped with a plaster trap ▪ fluid-impermeable pads ▪ cotton undercast padding ▪ gloves ▪ pillows or blankets ▪ vital signs monitoring equipment ▪ Optional: prescribed pain medication, supplies for cleaning the extremity (soap, water towels), local anesthetic, suture material, wound dressings, cast stand, fan, adhesive tape, moleskin, plaster splints.

Preparation of equipment

Inspect all equipment and supplies. If a product is expired, is defective, or has compromised integrity, remove it from patient use, label it as expired or defective, and report the expiration or defect as directed by your facility.

Gather the tubular stockinette, casting material, and plaster splints in appropriate sizes. Tubular stockinettes range from 2″ to 12″ (5 cm × 30.5 cm) wide; plaster rolls range from 2″ to 6″ (5-cm to 15.2-cm) wide; and plaster splints range from 3″ to 6″ (7.6-cm to 15.2-cm) wide.

For a cotton-polyester or fiberglass cast

Gently squeeze the packaged casting material *to make sure the envelopes don't have any air leaks. Humid air penetrating the packaging can cause the casting material to fail.* Prepare clean, fresh dipping water. Follow the manufacturer's directions for the appropriate dipping water temperature to use. For fiberglass, the temperature of the water should be cool or room temperature according to the manufacturer's instructions.[1] Place the equipment so that it's easily accessible during the procedure.

For a plaster cast

Prepare clean, fresh dipping water. The temperature of the water should be tepid or slightly warm according to the manufacturer's instructions.[1,5,6] Using water that's room temperature or slightly warmer allows the cast to set in about 7 minutes without excessive exothermia. (Cold water slows the setting rate, and may be used to facilitate molding of difficult casts; warm water speeds the setting rate, but it raises the temperature of the skin under the cast.) Place equipment so that it's easily accessible.

ELDER ALERT The chemical reaction that occurs between water and plaster casting materials produces heat, which may cause thermal injury. Be mindful of this risk when applying plaster casts to older adults, *because their skin is more temperature-sensitive than the skin of adults who are younger.*[2,7]

Implementation

▪ Verify the practitioner's order.
▪ Gather and prepare the necessary equipment and supplies.
▪ If required by your facility, confirm that informed consent has been obtained and that the signed consent form is in the patient's medical record.[8,9,10,11]
▪ Conduct a preprocedural verification *to make sure that all relevant documentation, related information, and equipment are available and correctly identified to the patient identifiers.*[12,13]
▪ Verify that the laboratory and imaging studies have been completed as ordered, and that the results are in the patient's medical record. Notify the practitioner of any unexpected results.[12]
▪ Perform hand hygiene.[14,15,16,17,18,19]
▪ Confirm the patient's identity using at least two patient identifiers.[20]
▪ Provide privacy.[21,22,23,24]
▪ Explain the procedure to the patient and family (if appropriate) according to their individual communication needs *to increase their understanding, allay their fears, and enhance cooperation.*[25]
▪ Raise the bed to waist level before providing care *to prevent caregiver back strain.*[26]
▪ Perform hand hygiene.[14,15,16,17,18,19]
▪ Put on gloves as needed *to comply with standard precautions.*[27,28]
▪ Make sure that the extremity is clean and dry. If it isn't, clean and dry it.[4]
▪ Remove jewelry from the limb to be casted. *Jewelry can interfere with circulation to the limb.*
▪ Make sure the procedure site is appropriately marked by the person performing the procedure, if indicated, *to ensure that the right site is being casted.*[12,13]
▪ Cover the appropriate parts of the patient's bedding with fluid-impermeable pads.
▪ Assess the condition of the skin of the affected limb and note any areas of abnormal color, ecchymosis, open wounds, rashes, or irritation. *This will make it easier to evaluate any patient complaints after the cast is applied.*
▪ Assess the patient's baseline neurovascular status. Palpate the pulses and assess temperature, color, capillary refill, motion, sensation, and pain in the affected and unaffected limbs.[2,4]

EQUIPMENT

Types of cylindrical casts

Made of cotton-polyester, fiberglass, plaster, or other synthetic material, casts may be applied almost anywhere on the body—to support a single finger or the entire body. Common casts are shown below.[2,3]

Long arm cast
A long arm cast is applied from the upper arm to the hand. It's used for upper, elbow, and forearm[1] fractures and to hold the arm or elbow muscles and tendons in place after surgery.

Shoulder spica cast
A shoulder spica cast is applied around the trunk of the body to the shoulder, arm, and hand. It's used for shoulder dislocations or soft tissue injury and to hold the shoulder muscles and tendons in place after surgery.

Short arm cast
A short arm cast is applied below the elbow to the hand. It's used for forearm or wrist fractures and to hold the forearm or wrist muscles and tendons in place after surgery.

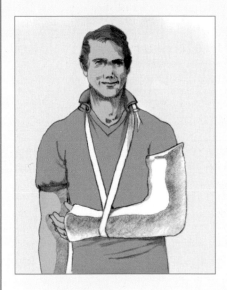

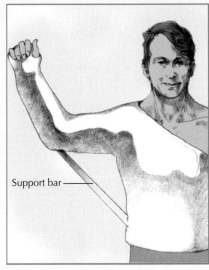

Support bar

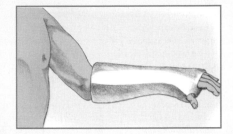

One-and-one-half hip spica cast
A one-and-one-half hip spica cast is applied from the waist or the nipple line of the chest to the foot on one leg and to the knee on the other leg. A bar is placed between the legs to keep the hips and legs immobilized. It's used for femur fractures and to hold the hip or thigh muscles and tendons in place after surgery.

Long leg cast
A long leg cast is applied to the area from the thigh to the foot. It's used for knee or lower leg fractures, knee dislocations, or ankle fractures and to hold the knee area or leg or foot muscles and tendons in place after surgery.

Short leg cast
A short leg cast is applied to the area below the knee to the foot. It's used for lower leg fractures, severe ankle sprains or strains, or ankle fractures, and to hold the leg or foot muscles or tendons in place after surgery.

Unilateral hip spica cast
A unilateral hip spica cast is applied from the waist or the nipple line on the chest to the foot on one leg. It's used for femur fractures and to hold the hip or thigh muscles in place after surgery.

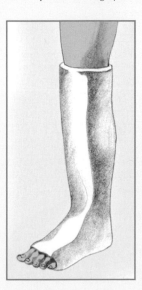

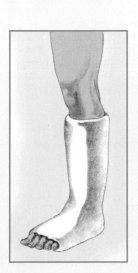

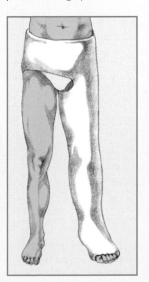

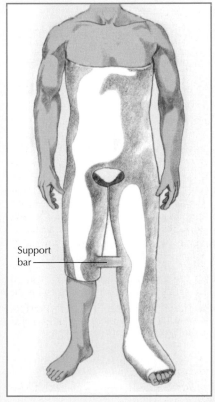

Support bar

- Assess the patient's vital signs *for baseline comparison.*
- Screen for and assess the patient's pain using facility-defined criteria that are consistent with the patient's age, condition, and ability to understand.[29]
- Treat the patient's pain as needed and ordered, using nonpharmacologic, pharmacologic, or a combination of approaches. Base the treatment on evidence-based practices and the patent's clinical condition, past medical history, and pain management goals.[29] (See the "Pain management" procedure.)
- Monitor closely if the patient is at increased risk for adverse outcomes related to opioid treatment, if prescribed.[29]
- If the patient has an open wound, assist the practitioner with administering a local anesthetic, closing the wound, and applying dressings, as needed.
- Remove and discard your gloves, if worn.[16,30]
- Perform hand hygiene [14,15,16,17,18,19] and put on gloves.
- Help the practitioner position the limb, as ordered. (The limb may be cast in a position of comfort, flexion, or extension.)[4]
- Conduct a time-out *to perform a final assessment that the correct patient, site, positioning, and procedure are identified and, as applicable, that all relevant information and necessary equipment are available.*[13,31]
- Support the limb in the prescribed position while the practitioner applies the tubular stockinette and cotton under-cast padding. The stockinette should extend beyond the ends of the cast *to pad the edges.*[4] (If the patient has an open wound or a severe contusion, the practitioner may not use a stockinette.)[1] The practitioner applies multiple layers (two to four) of cotton under-cast padding to the limb *to reduce the risk of cast saw burns during cast removal.* The padding should be an appropriate width for the size of the patient, and the practitioner should wrap it from distal to proximal. The practitioner should avoid wrinkles and overpadding *to prevent pressure points.*[1,4,6]

Applying a cotton-polyester cast
- Open the casting materials one roll at a time. Cotton and polyester casting must be applied within 3 minutes of opening, *because humidity in the air hardens the tape.*
- Immerse the roll in the bucket of cold water, and squeeze it four times *to ensure uniform saturation.*
- Remove the material from the bucket dripping wet and hand it to the practitioner.
- Tell the patient that it will be applied immediately and will feel warm, giving off heat as it sets.
- Prepare the necessary number of rolls in similar fashion.

Applying a fiberglass cast
- Open one roll at a time *to prevent opened rolls from being activated before use.* If water-activated fiberglass cast material is being used, add a minimal amount of water *to initiate the chemical reaction that causes the cast to harden. Using too much water makes the cast difficult to apply.*
- If light-cured fiberglass cast material is being used, you can unroll the material more slowly. *This material remains soft and malleable until it's exposed to ultraviolet light, which sets it.*

Applying a plaster cast
- Place a roll of plaster casting on its end in the bucket of water. Immerse it completely. When air bubbles stop rising from the roll, remove it, gently squeeze out the excess water, and hand it to the practitioner, who begins applying it to the extremity.
- As the first roll is applied, prepare a second roll in the same manner. Try to stay one roll ahead during the procedure.
- While applying each roll, the practitioner smooths it to remove wrinkles and to spread the plaster into the cloth webbing, emptying air pockets.[1] If plaster splints are used, the practitioner applies them to the middle layers of the cast. Before wrapping the last roll, the practitioner pulls the ends of the tubular stockinette over the cast edges to create a padded end, *which prevents cast crumbling and reduces skin irritation.* The final roll is wrapped *to keep the ends of the stockinette in place.*[1]

Completing the cast
- Remove and discard your gloves.
- Perform hand hygiene.[14,15,16,17,18,19]
- "Petal" the edges of the cast *to reduce roughness and cushion pressure points, as needed.* (See *How to petal a cast.*)
- Use a cast stand or your palm to support the cast in the therapeutic position until it becomes firm to touch (usually within minutes) *to prevent indentation in the cast.*
- Place the cast on a firm, smooth surface to continue drying.[4] Promote drying by leaving the cast uncovered and exposed to air; if permitted by your facility, fans can be used *to increase airflow and facilitate the drying process.*[4]

How to petal a cast

Rough cast edges can be cushioned by petaling them with adhesive tape or moleskin. To do so, first cut several 4″ × 2″ (10-cm × 5-cm) strips. Round off one end of each strip *to keep it from curling.* Then, making sure the rounded end of the strip is on the outside of the cast, tuck the straight end just inside the cast edge.

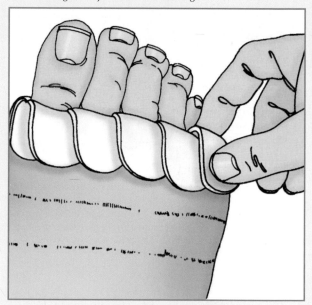

Smooth the adhesive tape or moleskin with your finger until you're sure it's secured inside and out. Repeat the procedure, overlapping the adhesive tape or moleskin pieces until you've gone all the way around the cast edge.

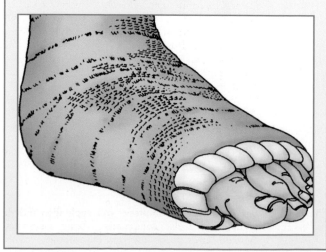

- Explain to the patient the need to limit activity while the cast dries, *because the angles of the cast must be maintained during the drying process to prevent pressure on bony processes.*
- Assess the neurovascular status of the casted limb and compare the findings bilaterally. Palpate the patient's pulses and assess the color, temperature, capillary refill, motion, and sensation of the limbs bilaterally.[2,4]
- *To facilitate venous return and reduce edema,* elevate the limb above the level of the heart using pillows or bath blankets. Make sure that the cast has matured and hardened before placing the limb on a pillow or blanket. *When a cast is allowed to mature on a pillow or blanket, temperatures beneath the cast can rise to dangerous levels, placing the patient at risk for thermal injury.*[5]
- Arrange for an X-ray of the limb *to ensure proper positioning,* if ordered.
- Reassess and respond to the patient's pain by evaluating the response to treatment and progress toward pain management goals *to ensure that the patient's pain is adequately controlled.* Assess for adverse reactions and risk factors for adverse events that may result from treatment.[29]
- Return the bed to the lowest position *to prevent falls and maintain patient safety.*[32]
- Institute fall precautions as needed, *because a cast impairs mobility, increasing the risk of falls.*[32,33,34] (See the "Fall prevention and management" procedure.)
- **HOSPITAL-ACQUIRED CONDITION ALERT** Keep in mind that the Centers for Medicare and Medicaid Services considers an injury from a fall a hospital-acquired condition *because it can be reasonably prevented using a variety of best practices.* Make sure to follow evidence-based fall prevention practices, such as performing a fall risk assessment and instituting fall precautions, *to reduce the risk of injury from falls.*[32,35]
- Discard used supplies in appropriate receptacles.[30]
- Remove and discard your gloves and perform hand hygiene.[14,15,16,17,18,19]
- Clean and disinfect your stethoscope with a disinfectant pad.[32,33]
- Perform hand hygiene.[14,15,16,17,18,19]
- Document the procedure.[36,37,38,39]

Special considerations

- Casts may need to be opened *to assess underlying skin or pulses or to relieve pressure in a specific area.* In a windowed cast, a specific area is cut out *to allow inspection of the underlying skin or to relieve pressure.* A bivalved cast is split medially and laterally, creating anterior and posterior sections. One of the sections may be removed *to prevent pressure* while the remaining section maintains the immobilization.

Patient teaching

Before discharge, teach the patient how to care for the cast. Review skin care, positioning, and activity recommendations, including the appropriate use of assistive devices. Teach the patient the signs and symptoms to report to the practitioner.

Teach the patient and family (if appropriate) about pain management strategies during discharge planning. Include information about the patient's pain management plan and adverse effects of pain management treatment. Discuss activities of daily living and items in the home environment that might exacerbate pain or reduce the effectiveness of the pain management plan, and include strategies to address these issues. Teach the patient and family (if appropriate) about safe use, storage, and disposal of opioids, if prescribed.[29]

Tell the patient that when the cast is removed, the casted limb will appear thinner with less muscle tone than the contralateral limb. The underlying skin will also appear yellow or gray from the accumulated dead skin and oils from glands near the skin's surface. If appropriate, reassure the patient that the limb will return to normal with good care and exercise.[2]

Complications

The complications associated with improper cast application include compartment syndrome, vascular compromise, disuse syndromes, thrombosis, compression neuropathy, infection, joint stiffness, muscle atrophy, and skin breakdown or thermal injury. (See *Recognizing compartment syndrome.*)[1,6]

Recognizing compartment syndrome

Compartment syndrome is a rare but serious complication that can occur if a cast is too tight. As the affected limb swells, the cast acts as a closed compartment, tightly compressing the nerves and blood vessels. The resulting decreased circulation and decreased tissue oxygenation can lead to permanent nerve damage and loss of the affected limb. Compartment syndrome is most common in the lower leg and forearm, but it can also occur in the hand, foot, thigh, and upper arm. *Because necrosis and nerve injury can occur after 6 hours of ischemia,*[40] perform frequent neurovascular assessments and be alert for complaints of increased pain or decreased effectiveness of analgesics.

Neurologic assessment of the hand is used to evaluate upper extremity injury. Assess the ulnar nerve by flexing the patient's ring and little finger and by having the patient cross the index and middle finger and abduct the fingers. Assess the median nerve by having the patient oppose the thumb to the ring finger or little finger. The radial nerve can be assessed by wrist extension, simultaneous extension of all four metacarpophalangeal joints, and thumb abduction and extension.

Assess the lower extremity by observing for loss of dorsiflexion (footdrop), loss of plantar flexion, and loss of toe dorsiflexion, and by testing for diminished sensitivity to stimulation in the space between the first and second toes.

Documentation

Record the date and time of the cast application, medications administered, and assessment of the limb, both before and after the cast was applied. Note any open wounds or abnormal skin. Note the patient's neurovascular status in the affected limb before and after cast application, and compare these findings with those of the unaffected limb. Note the location of any special devices, such as felt pads or plaster splints. Document teaching provided to the patient and family (if applicable), their understanding of that teaching, and any need for follow-up teaching.

REFERENCES

1 Boyd, A. S., et al. (2009). Splints and casts: Indications and methods. *American Family Physician, 80*(5), 491–499. https://www.aafp.org/afp/2009/0901/p491.html

2 Hinkle, J. L., & Cheever, K. H. (2017). *Brunner & Suddarth's textbook of medical-surgical nursing* (14th ed.). Philadelphia, PA: Wolters Kluwer.

3 The Children's Hospital of Philadelphia. (n.d.). Cast types and care instructions. https://www.chop.edu/conditions-diseases/cast-types-and-care-instructions

4 Satryb, S. A., et al. (2011). Casting: All wrapped up. *Orthopaedic Nursing, 30,* 37–41.

5 Shuler, F. D., & Bates, C. M. (2013). Skin temperatures generated following plaster splint application. *Orthopedics, 36*(5), 364–367. http://m4.wyanokecdn.com/f699990bf0724376a5200d9bbfbcdff1.pdf (Level VI)

6 Beutler, A. and Titus, S. (2019). General principles of acute fracture management. In: *UpToDate,* Eiff, P.,, & Asplund, C. A,. (Eds.).

7 Balentine, J. R. (2020). How to take care of a cast: Keeping it dry and clean. https://www.emedicinehealth.com/cast_care/article_em.htm

8 The Joint Commission. (2021). Standard RI.01.03.01. *Comprehensive accreditation manual for hospitals.* Oakbrook Terrace, IL: The Joint Commission. (Level VII)

9 Centers for Medicare and Medicaid Services, Department of Health and Human Services. (2020). Condition of participation: Patient's rights. 42 C.F.R. § 482.13(b)(2).

10 Accreditation Association for Hospitals and Health Systems. (2020). Standard 15.01.11. *Healthcare Facilities Accreditation Program: Accreditation requirements for acute care hospitals.* Chicago, IL: Accreditation Association for Hospitals and Health Systems. (Level VII)

11 DNV GL-Healthcare USA, Inc. (2020). PR.2.SR.3. *NIAHO® accreditation requirements, interpretive guidelines and surveyor guidance—revision 20.0.* Milford, OH: DNV GL-Healthcare USA, Inc. (Level VII)

12 The Joint Commission. (2021). Standard UP.01.01.01. *Comprehensive accreditation manual for hospitals.* Oakbrook Terrace, IL: The Joint Commission. (Level VII)

13 Accreditation Association for Hospitals and Health Systems. (2020). Standard 30.00.14. *Healthcare Facilities Accreditation Program: Accreditation requirements for acute care hospitals.* Chicago, IL: Accreditation Association for Hospitals and Health Systems. (Level VII)

14 The Joint Commission. (2021). Standard NPSG.07.01.01. *Comprehensive accreditation manual for hospitals.* Oakbrook Terrace, IL: The Joint Commission. (Level VII)

15 Centers for Disease Control and Prevention. (2002). Guideline for hand hygiene in health-care settings: Recommendations of the Healthcare Infection Control Practices Advisory Committee and the HICPAC/SHEA/APIC/IDSA Hand Hygiene Task Force. *MMWR Recommendations and Reports, 51*(RR-16), 1–45. https://www.cdc.gov/mmwr/pdf/rr/rr5116.pdf (Level II)

16 World Health Organization. (2009). WHO guidelines on hand hygiene in health care: First global patient safety challenge, clean care is safer care. https://apps.who.int/iris/bitstream/handle/10665/44102/9789241597906_eng.pdf?sequence=1 (Level IV)

17 Accreditation Association for Hospitals and Health Systems. (2020). Standard 07.01.21. *Healthcare Facilities Accreditation Program: Accreditation requirements for acute care hospitals.* Chicago, IL: Accreditation Association for Hospitals and Health Systems. (Level VII)

18 Centers for Medicare and Medicaid Services, Department of Health and Human Services. (2020). Condition of participation: Infection control. 42 C.F.R. § 482.42.

19 DNV GL-Healthcare USA, Inc. (2020). IC.1.SR.1. *NIAHO® accreditation requirements, interpretive guidelines and surveyor guidance—revision 20.0.* Milford, OH: DNV GL-Healthcare USA, Inc. (Level VII)

20 The Joint Commission. (2021). Standard NPSG.01.01.01. *Comprehensive accreditation manual for hospitals.* Oakbrook Terrace, IL: The Joint Commission. (Level VII)

21 The Joint Commission. (2021). Standard RI.01.01.01. *Comprehensive accreditation manual for hospitals.* Oakbrook Terrace, IL: The Joint Commission. (Level VII)

22 DNV GL-Healthcare USA, Inc. (2020). PR.2.SR.5. *NIAHO® accreditation requirements, interpretive guidelines and surveyor guidance—revision 20.0.* Milford, OH: DNV GL-Healthcare USA, Inc. (Level VII)

23 Accreditation Association for Hospitals and Health Systems. (2020). Standard 15.01.16. *Healthcare Facilities Accreditation Program: Accreditation requirements for acute care hospitals.* Chicago, IL: Accreditation Association for Hospitals and Health Systems. (Level VII)

24 Centers for Medicare and Medicaid Services, Department of Health and Human Services. (2020). Condition of participation: Patient's rights. 42 C.F.R. § 482.13(c)(1).

25 The Joint Commission. (2021). Standard PC.02.01.21. *Comprehensive accreditation manual for hospitals.* Oakbrook Terrace, IL: The Joint Commission. (Level VII)

26 Waters, T. R., et al. (2009). Safe patient handling training for schools of nursing. https://www.cdc.gov/niosh/docs/2009-127/pdfs/2009-127.pdf (Level VII)

27 Siegel, J. D., et al. (2007, revised 2019). 2007 guideline for isolation precautions: Preventing transmission of infectious agents in healthcare settings. https://www.cdc.gov/infectioncontrol/pdf/guidelines/isolation-guidelines-H.pdf (Level II)

28 Accreditation Association for Hospitals and Health Systems. (2020). Standard 07.01.10. *Healthcare Facilities Accreditation Program: Accreditation requirements for acute care hospitals.* Chicago, IL: Accreditation Association for Hospitals and Health Systems. (Level VII)

29 The Joint Commission. (2021). Standard PC.01.02.07. *Comprehensive accreditation manual for hospitals.* Oakbrook Terrace, IL: The Joint Commission. (Level VII)

30 Occupational Safety and Health Administration. (2012). Bloodborne pathogens, standard number1910.1030. https://www.osha.gov/pls/oshaweb/owadisp.show_document?p_id=10051&p_table=STANDARDS (Level VII)

31 The Joint Commission. (2021). Standard UP.01.03.01. *Comprehensive accreditation manual for hospitals.* Oakbrook Terrace, IL: The Joint Commission. (Level VII)

32 Ganz, D. A., et al. (2013, reviewer 2021). *Preventing falls in hospitals: A toolkit for improving quality of care* (AHRQ Publication No. 13-0015-EF). Rockville, MD: Agency for Healthcare Research and Quality. https://www.ahrq.gov/sites/default/files/publications/files/fallpxtoolkit_0.pdf (Level VII)

33 Accreditation Association for Hospitals and Health Systems. (2020). Standard 16.02.02. *Healthcare Facilities Accreditation Program: Accreditation requirements for acute care hospitals.* Chicago, IL: Accreditation Association for Hospitals and Health Systems. (Level VII)

34 The Joint Commission. (2021). Standard PC.01.02.08. *Comprehensive accreditation manual for hospitals.* Oakbrook Terrace, IL: The Joint Commission. (Level VII)

35 Jarrett, N., & Callaham, M. (2016). Evidence-based guidelines for selected hospital-acquired conditions: Final report. https://www.cms.gov/Medicare/Medicare-Fee-for-Service-Payment/HospitalAcqCond/Downloads/2016-HAC-Report.pdf

36 The Joint Commission. (2021). Standard RC.01.03.01. *Comprehensive accreditation manual for hospitals.* Oakbrook Terrace, IL: The Joint Commission. (Level VII)

37 Centers for Medicare and Medicaid Services, Department of Health and Human Services. (2020). Condition of participation: Medical record services. 42 C.F.R. § 482.24(b).

38 Accreditation Association for Hospitals and Health Systems. (2020). Standard 10.00.03. *Healthcare Facilities Accreditation Program: Accreditation requirements for acute care hospitals.* Chicago, IL: Accreditation Association for Hospitals and Health Systems. (Level VII)

39 DNV GL-Healthcare USA, Inc. (2020). MR.2.SR.1. *NIAHO® accreditation requirements, interpretive guidelines and surveyor guidance—revision 20.0.* Milford, OH: DNV GL-Healthcare USA, Inc. (Level VII)

40 Rasul, A. T., Jr. (2020). Acute compartment syndrome. https://emedicine.medscape.com/article/307668-overview

CAST REMOVAL, ASSISTING

A practitioner will typically remove a cast when a fracture heals or requires further manipulation. Less common indications include cast damage, a pressure injury under the cast, excessive drainage or bleeding, and a constrictive cast. X-rays are commonly obtained before or after cast removal to ensure that the fracture has healed properly.[1]

Cast removal requires making two parallel longitudinal cuts through several layers of casting material. The practitioner uses a cast saw to perforate the plaster or fiberglass casting material and then separates the material with a cast spreader. Then, the practitioner cuts the padding and stockinette layers with cast scissors.[2]

Equipment

Fluid-impermeable pads ▪ cast spreader ▪ cast saw (preferably with vacuum attachment) ▪ cast scissors ▪ washcloth ▪ towel ▪ soap and water ▪ facility-approved disinfectant ▪ Optional: masks and goggles, skin care supplies, ear protection.

Preparation of equipment

Inspect all equipment and supplies. If a product is expired, is defective, or has compromised integrity, remove it from patient use, label it as expired or defective, and report the expiration or defect as directed by your facility.

Ensure that the cast saw operates properly before use and that the blade is sufficiently sharp to cut through the cast. Follow the manufacturer's recommendations for use and care of the cast saw.

Implementation

- Verify the practitioner's order.
- Gather and prepare the necessary equipment and supplies.
- Perform hand hygiene.[3,4,5,6,7,8]
- Confirm the patient's identity using at least two patient identifiers.[9]
- Provide privacy.[10,11,12,13]
- Explain the procedure to the patient and family (if appropriate) according to their communication and learning needs *to increase understanding, allay their fears, and enhance cooperation.*[14] Tell the patient that the cast saw uses an oscillating blade that is designed to avoid cutting the skin, and that the patient should expect to feel some vibration and warmth when the saw cuts the cast, but must report discomfort or excessive warmth immediately during the procedure.[15] Explain that the patient must remain still during the procedure *to prevent injury.*[15] Tell the patient that after cast removal, the skin may be flaky and discolored, and the muscle may be diminished, stiff, and weak.[15]

- Raise the bed to waist level before providing care *to prevent caregiver back strain.*[16]
- Perform hand hygiene.[3,4,5,6,7,8]
- Assist the patient into a comfortable position that will allow access to the cast. For a lower limb cast, the patient should be lying down. For an upper extremity cast, the patient may be seated or lying down.[17]
- Cover the appropriate parts of the patient's bedding with fluid-impermeable pads.
- If the cast saw doesn't have a vacuum attachment to dispose of the cast dust during removal, put on a mask and goggles during the procedure and assist the patient and anyone else present with putting on a mask and goggles *to prevent inhalation and irritation from particulate cast material.*
- If needed, put on ear protection and assist the patient and anyone else present with putting on ear protection *to protect against hearing loss and reduce anxiety.*[18,19,20]
- Assist the practitioner as needed with removing the cast. The practitioner will cut one side of the cast (as shown below) and then the other.[2] The practitioner will open the cast with a cast spreader and then use cast scissors to cut through the cast padding on each side and then proceed with cutting the stockinette.[2]

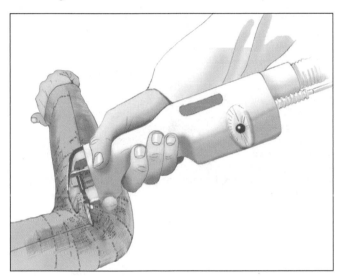

- Monitor that patient's anxiety level as the practitioner removes the cast. Provide emotional support, as needed.
- Support the extremity and inspect the patient's skin for burns, abrasions, lacerations, and pressure injuries. Provide skin care as appropriate.
- Wash the affected limb with soap and water and dry it thoroughly with a towel *to remove the accumulated dead skin.*[17]
- Remove your ear protection and mask and goggles, if worn, and assist the patient and others in doing the same, as needed.[21]
- Discard used supplies in appropriate receptacles.[21]
- Return the bed to the lowest position *to prevent falls and maintain the patient's safety.*[22]
- Perform hand hygiene.[3,4,5,6,7,8]
- Put on gloves and other personal protective equipment, as needed.[21]
- Clean and disinfect reusable equipment according to the manufacturer's instructions *to prevent the spread of infection.*[23,24]
- Remove and discard your gloves and other personal protective equipment, if worn.[21]
- Perform hand hygiene.[3,4,5,6,7,8]
- Document the procedure.[25,26,27,28]

Special considerations

- If the patient reports pain or heat during cast removal, the practitioner must discontinue saw use and cool the blade before resuming *to reduce the risk of thermal injury.* Poor cutting technique (such as the cast saw blade never leaving the cast material during cutting), fiberglass casting material, and thinner cast padding can result in significantly higher skin temperatures. Techniques for reducing the temperature of the oscillating saw blades during cast removal include cooling the blade in the ambient

air, using a vacuum attachment, and applying 70% isopropyl alcohol or water to the blade with a gauze pad. These techniques decrease the risk of skin burns.[29]

Patient teaching

Tell the patient to avoid rubbing or scratching the skin, *because doing so can damage the newly exposed skin.* Teach the patient how to perform skin care after the cast is removed. Advise the patient to follow the practitioner's instructions regarding how much and what type of activity to engage in after cast removal.[15]

Complications

The practitioner may accidentally injure the patient's skin with the cast saw, scissors, or spreader. Thermal injury may also occur due to the heat generated by the cast saw.[29]

Documentation

Record the date and time of cast removal and the patient's tolerance of the procedure. Document your neurovascular and skin assessment findings after cast removal; include any care provided. Note any complications from the procedure, your interventions, and the patient's response to those interventions. Document teaching provided to the patient and family (if applicable), their understanding of that teaching, and any need for follow-up teaching.

REFERENCES

1 Beutler, A., & Titus, S. (2019). General principles of definitive fracture management. In: *UpToDate*, Eiff, P.,, & Aplund, C. A,. (Eds.).

2 Hinkle, J. L., & Cheever, K. H. (2017). *Brunner & Suddarth's textbook of medical-surgical nursing* (14th ed.). Philadelphia, PA: Wolters Kluwer.

3 The Joint Commission. (2021). Standard NPSG.07.01.01. *Comprehensive accreditation manual for hospitals.* Oakbrook Terrace, IL: The Joint Commission. (Level VII)

4 Centers for Disease Control and Prevention. (2002). Guideline for hand hygiene in health care settings: Recommendations of the Healthcare Infection Control Practices Advisory Committee and the HICPAC/ SHEA/APIC/IDSA Hand Hygiene Task Force. *MMWR Recommendations and Reports, 51*(RR-16), 1–45. https://www.cdc.gov/mmwr/pdf/rr/rr5116. pdf (Level II)

5 World Health Organization. (2009). WHO guidelines on hand hygiene in health care: First global patient safety challenge, clean care is safer care. https://apps.who.int/iris/bitstream/handle/10665/44102/9789241597906_eng.pdf (Level IV)

6 Centers for Medicare and Medicaid Services, Department of Health and Human Services. (2020). Condition of participation: Infection control. 42 C.F.R. § 482.42.

7 Accreditation Association for Hospitals and Health Systems. (2020). Standard 07.01.21. *Healthcare Facilities Accreditation Program: Accreditation requirements for acute care hospitals.* Chicago, IL: Accreditation Association for Hospitals and Health Systems. (Level VII)

8 DNV GL-Healthcare USA, Inc. (2020). IC.1.SR.1. *NIAHO® accreditation requirements, interpretive guidelines and surveyor guidance—revision 20.0.* Milford, OH: DNV GL-Healthcare USA, Inc. (Level VII)

9 The Joint Commission. (2021). Standard NPSG.01.01.01. *Comprehensive accreditation manual for hospitals.* Oakbrook Terrace, IL: The Joint Commission. (Level VII)

10 The Joint Commission. (2021). Standard RI.01.01.01. *Comprehensive accreditation manual for hospitals.* Oakbrook Terrace, IL: The Joint Commission. (Level VII)

11 DNV GL-Healthcare USA, Inc. (2020). PR.1.SR.5. *NIAHO® accreditation requirements, interpretive guidelines and surveyor guidance—revision 20.0.* Milford, OH: DNV GL-Healthcare USA, Inc. (Level VII)

12 Accreditation Association for Hospitals and Health Systems. (2020). Standard 15.01.16. *Healthcare Facilities Accreditation Program: Accreditation requirements for acute care hospitals.* Chicago, IL: Accreditation Association for Hospitals and Health Systems. (Level VII)

13 Centers for Medicare and Medicaid Services, Department of Health and Human Services. (2020). Condition of participation: Patient's rights. 42 C.F.R. § 482.13(c)(1).

14 The Joint Commission. (2021). Standard PC.02.01.21. *Comprehensive accreditation manual for hospitals.* Oakbrook Terrace, IL: The Joint Commission. (Level VII)

15 Satryb, S. A., et al. (2011). Casting: All wrapped up. *Orthopaedic Nursing, 30*(1), 37–41.

16 Waters, T. R., et al. (2009). Safe patient handling training for schools of nursing. https://www.cdc.gov/niosh/docs/2009-127/pdfs/2009-127.pdf (Level VII)

17 Singh, A. P. (n.d.). Removal of plaster casts. https://boneandspine.com/removal-of-plaster-casts/

18 Occupational Safety and Health Administration. (n.d.). Occupational noise exposure, standard number 1910.95. https://www.osha.gov/laws-regs/regulations/standardnumber/1910/1910.95 (Level VII)

19 Marsh, J. P., et al. (2011). Noise levels in adult and pediatric orthopedic cast clinics. *American Journal of Orthopedics, 40*(7), e122–e124. https://www.researchgate.net/publication/51732261_Noise_levels_in_adult_and_pediatric_orthopedic_cast_clinics (Level VI)

20 Mahan, S. T., et al. (2017). Noise reduction to reduce anxiety during cast removal: Can we decrease patient anxiety with cast removal by wearing noise reduction headphones during cast saw use? *Orthopedic Nursing, 36*(4), 271–278. (Level VI)

21 Occupational Safety and Health Administration. (2012). Bloodborne pathogens, standard number1910.1030. https://www.osha.gov/pls/oshaweb/owadisp.show_document?p_id=10051&p_table=STANDARDS (Level VII)

22 Ganz, D. A., et al. (2013, reviewed 2021). *Preventing falls in hospitals: A toolkit for improving quality of care* (AHRQ Publication No. 13-0015-EF). Rockville, MD: Agency for Healthcare Research and Quality. https://www.ahrq.gov/professionals/systems/hospital/fallpxtoolkit/index.html (Level VII)

23 Accreditation Association for Hospitals and Health Systems. (2020). Standard 07.02.03. *Healthcare Facilities Accreditation Program: Accreditation requirements for acute care hospitals.* Chicago, IL: Accreditation Association for Hospitals and Health Systems. (Level VII)

24 Rutala, W. A., et al. (2008, revised 2019). Guideline for disinfection and sterilization in healthcare facilities, 2008. https://www.cdc.gov/infection-control/pdf/guidelines/disinfection-guidelines-H.pdf (Level I)

25 The Joint Commission. (2021). Standard RC.01.03.01. *Comprehensive accreditation manual for hospitals.* Oakbrook Terrace, IL: The Joint Commission. (Level VII)

26 Centers for Medicare and Medicaid Services, Department of Health and Human Services. (2020). Condition of participation: Medical record services. 42 C.F.R. § 482.24(b).

27 Accreditation Association for Hospitals and Health Systems. (2020). Standard 10.00.03. *Healthcare Facilities Accreditation Program: Accreditation requirements for acute care hospitals.* Chicago, IL: Accreditation Association for Hospitals and Health Systems. (Level VII)

28 DNV GL-Healthcare USA, Inc. (2020). MR.2.SR.1. *NIAHO® accreditation requirements, interpretive guidelines and surveyor guidance—revision 20.0.* Milford, OH: DNV GL-Healthcare USA, Inc. (Level VII)

29 Puddy, A. C., et al. (2014). Cast saw burns: Evaluation of simple techniques for reducing the risk of thermal injury. *Journal of Pediatric Orthopaedics, 34*(8), e63–e66. (Level VI)

CENTRAL VENOUS ACCESS CATHETER CARE

A central venous access catheter, or central venous catheter (CVC), is a sterile catheter that's inserted through a large vein to provide access to the central veins. The catheter is made of polyurethane or silicone rubber. Catheters impregnated with antiseptics (such as chlorhexidine) or antimicrobials (such as silver, carbon, platinum, minocycline, or rifampin)[1] are recommended for patients in health care facilities or in patient populations with vascular catheter–associated infection rates that are higher than facility goals, even after other vascular catheter–associated infection practices have been implemented. They may also be used in patients with limited venous access or a history of vascular catheter–associated infection, and in those at increased risk for complications from a vascular catheter–associated infection, such as patients with implanted IV devices.[2] The health care team may consider the use of an anti-infective catheter, but such devices shouldn't be used in patients with allergies to the anti-infective substances.[3] Power injectable catheters allow power injection of contrast media in patients who require computed tomography and other testing.[4]

A practitioner inserts a central venous catheter through a large vein, such as the subclavian or jugular vein, and places the tip of the catheter in the superior vena cava, ideally at or near the cavoatrial junction.[5,6] (See *Central venous access catheter pathways.*) Alternatively, the femoral vein can be used, with the tip of the catheter in the inferior vena cava above the diaphragm.[5]

By providing access to the central veins, a CVC offers several benefits. It allows monitoring of central venous pressure,[6] which indicates blood volume or pump efficiency, and permits aspiration of blood samples for diagnostic tests. It also allows for the administration of IV fluids (in large amounts if necessary) in emergencies; when decreased peripheral circulation makes peripheral vein access difficult; when prolonged IV therapy reduces the number of accessible peripheral veins; when solutions must be diluted (for large fluid volumes or irritating or hypertonic fluids such as total parenteral nutrition solutions); and when a patient requires long-term venous access.[3] Because multiple blood samples can be drawn through it without repeated venipuncture, a central venous access catheter decreases the patient's anxiety and preserves peripheral veins.

Contraindications to central venous access catheter insertion include anatomic conditions, coagulopathies, and venous obstruction.[6] Central venous access therapy increases the risk of such complications as pneumothorax, vascular catheter–associated infection, sepsis, thrombus formation, and vessel and adjacent organ perforation—all life-threatening conditions. Because of age-related changes in the immune system, older adults are more susceptible to infection than are younger adults. Remote infections may also increase the risk of vascular catheter–associated bloodstream infection in older adults.[7]

HOSPITAL-ACQUIRED CONDITION ALERT Keep in mind that the Centers for Medicare and Medicaid Services considers vascular catheter–associated infection a hospital-acquired condition, *because it can be reasonably prevented using a variety of best practices.* Make sure to follow evidence-based infection prevention practices, such as properly preparing the intended insertion site, using an all-inclusive insertion kit, using an insertion checklist, stopping the procedure for any breach in sterile technique that occurs, and instituting maximal barrier precautions, during insertion to reduce the risk of vascular catheter–associated infections.[2,8,9,10,11,12]

Blood sampling

The use of strict sterile no-touch technique is necessary to reduce the risk of vascular catheter–associated bloodstream infection. In addition, CVC blood sampling should not be performed using the same catheter lumen that is used for drug infusions.[14] Only the minimal amount of discard blood should be obtained to help prevent hospital-acquired anemia.[14] Whenever possible, multiple blood draws should be grouped together to reduce the number of times the system is accessed and thereby minimize the risk of infection.[14] Failure to adequately flush a CVC after blood withdrawal can lead to thrombotic catheter occlusion.

Flushing and locking

Aspirating for a blood return and flushing a CVC is a routine step to assess catheter patency before each infusion, to prevent mixing incompatible medications and solutions after infusion, and to prevent catheter occlusion after blood sampling.[15] Locking may be performed after the final flush to maintain patency and prevent occlusion in a device that's used intermittently. If the system is used intermittently, the flushing and locking procedure will vary by facility preference, the medication administration schedule, and the type and size of the catheter.

The flushing volume should be at least twice the internal volume of the central venous access catheter and any add-on device; a larger volume may be necessary if the catheter was used for blood sampling or transfusion, parenteral nutrition, contrast media, or other viscous solutions. All lumens of a multilumen catheter must be regularly flushed. Factors to consider when choosing the flush volume include the type and size of the catheter, age of the patient, and type of infusion therapy being given.[16] A 10-mL syringe (or a syringe specifically designed to generate lower injection pressure) is recommended to aspirate for a blood return and assess catheter patency *to reduce the risk of catheter damage.*[16,17,18,19]

Central venous access catheter pathways

The illustrations below show two common pathways for central venous access catheter insertion. Typically, a central venous access catheter is inserted in the subclavian vein or the internal jugular vein and terminates in the superior vena cava. The subclavian site is preferred over the internal jugular site in adults *to reduce the risk of infection*;[1,10,12] Patients who have a pacemaker in place should be assessed carefully *to determine the most appropriate catheter and insertion site.* Pacemakers commonly are inserted on the left side of the chest or abdomen, so the contralateral side is preferred for central venous access catheter placement. If the ipsilateral side is preferred, a peripherally inserted central catheter may be the safest option.[13]

Insertion: Subclavian vein
Termination: Superior vena cava

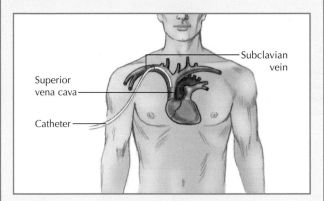

Insertion: Internal jugular vein
Termination: Superior vena cava

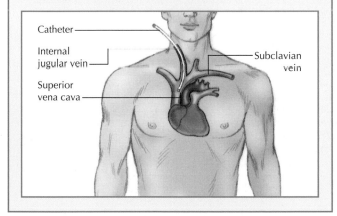

To maintain patency in catheters used intermittently, facilities may use pre-filled syringes containing heparin or preservative-free normal saline to lock the catheter, according to the directions for use for the central venous access catheter and needleless connector.[16,17] The locking solution volume should equal the internal volume of the central venous access catheter and add-on devices plus 20%.[16,17,18]

Infection prevention practices should be followed when flushing and locking a catheter *to reduce the risk of vascular catheter-associated infection.*[2,8,9,20]

Needleless connector change

Needleless connectors should be changed no more frequently than every 96 hours.[3,10] Changing connectors more frequently adds no benefit and has been shown to increase the risk of vascular access catheter-associated infection.[21] If used with a continuous infusion system, a needleless connector should be changed when the primary administration set is changed.[10,21,22,23] A needleless connector should also be changed when the connector is removed for any reason, when it has blood or debris in it, before drawing a blood sample for culturing through the device, when

the needleless connector becomes contaminated, routinely as directed by the facility, and per manufacturer's guidelines.[17,21,23]

Needleless connectors are recognized sources of bacterial contamination. Infection prevention best practices must be followed *to prevent infection.*[21]

Changing the dressing

Despite the various designs and applications of central venous access devices, certain aspects of dressing changes apply to all device types. The sterility and integrity of the device must be maintained at all times to reduce the risk of vascular catheter–associated infection.

Transparent semipermeable dressings should be changed every 5 to 7 days, and gauze dressings should be changed every 2 days.[2,10,16] If signs and symptoms of infection are present, or if the dressing becomes visibly soiled, loosened, or dislodged, change the dressing immediately and closely assess, clean, and disinfect the site.[2,10,16]

Removing a central venous access catheter

A central venous access catheter that was inserted in an emergency should be removed as soon as possible, but not later than 48 hours after insertion.[24] Catheter necessity should be routinely assessed during multidisciplinary rounds; to reduce the risk of vascular catheter–associated infection, the catheter should be removed as soon as it is no longer needed.[2,9,10,11,24] Factors to consider when deciding on removal include the patient's condition and therapy, catheter position, and catheter function. When a vascular catheter–associated infection is suspected or confirmed, the decision to remove or salvage the catheter should be based on blood culture results, the patient's condition, available vascular access sites, the effectiveness of antimicrobial therapy, and the practitioner's directive.[20,24]

The nurse removing the catheter should ensure that assistance is available *in case a complication, such as uncontrolled bleeding, occurs during catheter removal. Some vessels, such as the subclavian vein, can be difficult to compress.*

Equipment

For insertion of a central venous access catheter

Facility-approved disinfectant ▪ insertion checklist ▪ sterile gloves ▪ sterile gowns ▪ caps ▪ masks ▪ fluid-impermeable pad ▪ large sterile drape ▪ antiseptic solution or swabs (chlorhexidine-based preferred; tincture of iodine, povidone-iodine, or alcohol if chlorhexidine is contraindicated) ▪ alcohol pads ▪ 10-mL prefilled syringes containing preservative-free normal saline solution ▪ 3-mL syringe with 25G 1″ (2.5-cm) needle ▪ 1% or 2% injectable lidocaine ▪ central venous access catheter (antimicrobial impregnated, if indicated) with guide wire ▪ IV solution with administration set ▪ electronic infusion device (preferably a smart pump with dose-error reduction software and interoperability with electronic health records) ▪ sterile needleless connectors (for each catheter lumen) ▪ sterile marker ▪ sterile labels ▪ transparent semipermeable dressing ▪ sign ▪ pulse oximeter and probe ▪ cardiac monitoring equipment ▪ vital signs monitoring equipment ▪ emergency equipment (code cart with emergency medications, defibrillator, handheld resuscitation bag with mask, intubation equipment) ▪ Optional: disposable-head surgical clippers or single-patient-use scissors, sterile towel, antiseptic soap, water, prescribed sedative or analgesic, suture material, suture kit (sterile scissors, hemostat, and needle holder), disinfectant-containing end caps, chlorhexidine-impregnated sponge dressing, ultrasound device with sterile probe cover and sterile ultrasound gel, engineered stabilization device, blanket, dressings and tape specially formulated for fragile skin.

The type of catheter selected depends on the type of therapy to be used.[3] (See *Guide to central venous access catheters*, page 146.)

Use an all-inclusive insertion kit or cart that contains all of the necessary components for maintaining sterile technique during catheter insertion *to reduce the risk of catheter-related bloodstream infection.*[2,3]

For blood sampling from a central venous access catheter

Gloves ▪ 10-mL prefilled syringes of preservative-free normal saline solution (or a syringe specifically designed to generate lower injection pressure[16] ▪ antiseptic pads (chlorhexidine-based, povidone iodine, or

EQUIPMENT

Guide to central venous access catheters

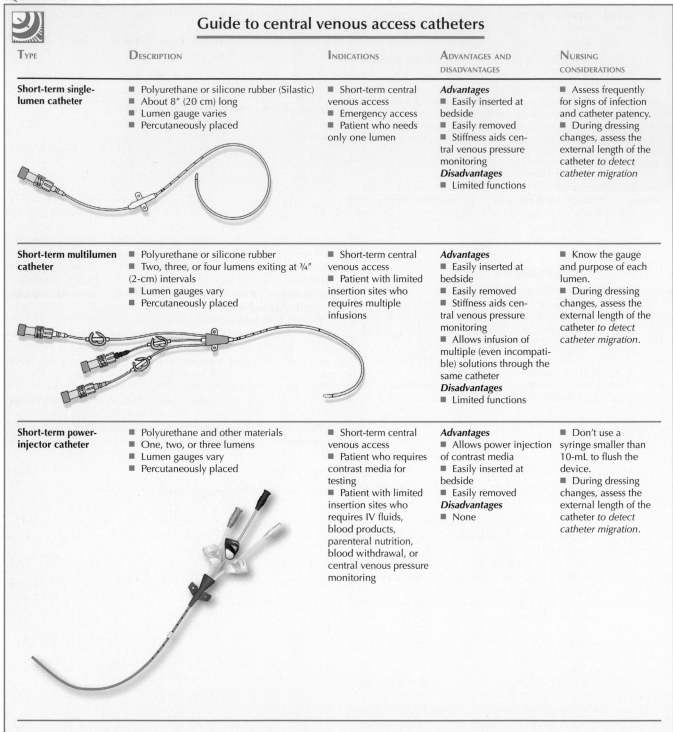

TYPE	DESCRIPTION	INDICATIONS	ADVANTAGES AND DISADVANTAGES	NURSING CONSIDERATIONS
Short-term single-lumen catheter	■ Polyurethane or silicone rubber (Silastic) ■ About 8″ (20 cm) long ■ Lumen gauge varies ■ Percutaneously placed	■ Short-term central venous access ■ Emergency access ■ Patient who needs only one lumen	*Advantages* ■ Easily inserted at bedside ■ Easily removed ■ Stiffness aids central venous pressure monitoring *Disadvantages* ■ Limited functions	■ Assess frequently for signs of infection and catheter patency. ■ During dressing changes, assess the external length of the catheter *to detect catheter migration*
Short-term multilumen catheter	■ Polyurethane or silicone rubber ■ Two, three, or four lumens exiting at ¾″ (2-cm) intervals ■ Lumen gauges vary ■ Percutaneously placed	■ Short-term central venous access ■ Patient with limited insertion sites who requires multiple infusions	*Advantages* ■ Easily inserted at bedside ■ Easily removed ■ Stiffness aids central venous pressure monitoring ■ Allows infusion of multiple (even incompatible) solutions through the same catheter *Disadvantages* ■ Limited functions	■ Know the gauge and purpose of each lumen. ■ During dressing changes, assess the external length of the catheter *to detect catheter migration*.
Short-term power-injector catheter	■ Polyurethane and other materials ■ One, two, or three lumens ■ Lumen gauges vary ■ Percutaneously placed	■ Short-term central venous access ■ Patient who requires contrast media for testing ■ Patient with limited insertion sites who requires IV fluids, blood products, parenteral nutrition, blood withdrawal, or central venous pressure monitoring	*Advantages* ■ Allows power injection of contrast media ■ Easily inserted at bedside ■ Easily removed *Disadvantages* ■ None	■ Don't use a syringe smaller than 10-mL to flush the device. ■ During dressing changes, assess the external length of the catheter *to detect catheter migration*.

alcohol) ■ appropriate-size syringes or needleless blood collection tube holder ■ blood collection tubes ■ labels ■ laboratory biohazard transport bag ■ Optional: prefilled syringe containing locking solution, gown, mask with face shield or mask and goggles, blood transfer unit, needleless connector, disinfectant-containing end cap, sterile cap, laboratory request form.

For flushing and locking a central venous access catheter

Gloves ■ 10-mL prefilled syringe(s) containing preservative-free normal saline solution (or syringe[s] specifically designed to generate lower injection pressure) ■ antiseptic pads (chlorhexidine-based, povidone iodine, or alcohol) ■ Optional: prefilled syringe with heparin lock solution (10 units/mL),[18] disinfectant-containing cap, dextrose 5% in water (D$_5$W),

IV administration set with prescribed IV fluid, prescribed IV bolus medication and administration supplies.

For changing the dressing on a central venous access catheter

Antiseptic solution (chlorhexidine preferred;[19] tincture of iodine, povidone-iodine, or alcohol if the patient is sensitive to chlorhexidine) ■ sterile transparent semipermeable dressing or sterile 4″ × 4″ (10-cm × 10-cm) gauze pad ■ sterile tape ■ sterile drape ■ skin barrier solution ■ sterile gloves ■ gloves ■ mask ■ label ■ Optional: chlorhexidine-impregnated sponge dressing, acetone-free adhesive remover, sterile disposable tape measure, facility-approved disinfectant, appropriate solution to loosen stabilization device, engineered stabilization device.

Commercially prepared central venous access device dressing change kits that include most of the equipment needed are available and recommended.[7,17]

For changing a needleless connector on a central venous access catheter

Antiseptic pad (alcohol, povidone iodine, chlorhexidine-based) ▪ sterile needleless connector ▪ gloves ▪ prefilled syringe containing preservative-free normal saline solution (10-mL syringe or a syringe specifically designed to generate lower injection pressure) ▪ Optional: disinfectant-containing end cap, prefilled syringe containing lock solution.

For removing a central venous access catheter

Gloves ▪ fluid-impermeable pads ▪ sterile 2″ × 2″ (5-cm × 5-cm) gauze pads ▪ sterile occlusive gauze dressing or sterile transparent semipermeable dressing ▪ petroleum-based ointment ▪ tape measure ▪ Optional: protective eyewear, adhesive remover, sterile suture removal set, sterile scissors and forceps, handheld resuscitation bag.

Preparation of equipment

Before insertion of a central venous access catheter, confirm catheter type and size with the practitioner; a 14G or 16G catheter is typical. Also confirm whether the practitioner intends to use ultrasound to guide insertion; if so, obtain the equipment and make sure it's functioning properly.

Perform hand hygiene.[7,17,25] Inspect all IV equipment and supplies. If a product is expired, is defective, or has compromised integrity, remove it from patient use, label it as expired or defective, and report the expiration or defect as directed by your facility.[26] Make sure emergency equipment is functioning and readily available.

Implementation

For all procedures

▪ Gather and prepare the necessary equipment and supplies.
▪ Explain the procedure to the patient and family (if appropriate) according to their individual communication and learning needs *to increase their understanding, allay their fears, and enhance cooperation.*[27,28]

Assisting with inserting a central venous access catheter

▪ Verify the practitioner's order.[17]
▪ Review the patient's medical record for a history of allergies to latex, antiseptic solution, or the local anesthetic, and for any contraindication to central venous access catheter insertion.
▪ If required by your facility, confirm that informed consent has been obtained and that the signed consent form is in the patient's medical record.[29,30,31,32,33]
▪ Reinforce the practitioner's explanation of the procedure, and answer the patient's questions.[29,30,31,32,33]
▪ Perform hand hygiene.[10,17,18,19,20,21,22,23]
▪ Confirm the patient's identity using at least two patient identifiers.[34]
▪ Provide privacy.[35,36,37,38]
▪ Provide the patient with information that addresses the rationale for device insertion, the insertion process, expected dwell time, care and maintenance of the device, and signs and symptoms of complications that should be reported.[27,28]
▪ Confirm that written informed consent has been obtained, if necessary, and that the consent form is in the patient's medical record.[39,40]
▪ Close the door to the room and place a sign on the door that reads, "Sterile Procedure in Progress—Do Not Enter."[7,17]
▪ Raise the patient's bed to waist level before providing care *to prevent caregiver back strain.*[41]
▪ Perform hand hygiene.[10,17,18,19,20,21,22,23]
▪ Attach the patient to a cardiac monitor and pulse oximeter.[6] Make sure that the alarm limits are set appropriately for the patient's current condition, and that the alarms are turned on, functioning properly, and audible to staff.[42,43,44,45]
▪ Obtain the patient's vital signs and oxygen saturation level using pulse oximetry *to serve as a baseline for comparison during and after the procedure.*[6]

▪ If ultrasound is available, assist the practitioner with the ultrasound device to evaluate the patient's vasculature *to determine the insertion site.*[7,17,46]
▪ Administer a sedative or an analgesic, if ordered, following safe medication administration practices.[6,47,48]
▪ Put on a cap and mask.[7,17]
▪ Perform hand hygiene.[10,17,18,19,20,21,22,23]
▪ Disinfect the work area (such as an overbed table) with a facility-approved disinfectant and allow it to dry completely.[7,17]
▪ Place the patient in the Trendelenburg position *to dilate the veins and to reduce the risk of air embolism.*[6]
▪ For subclavian vein insertion, place a rolled blanket lengthwise between the patient's shoulders *to increase venous distention.*[6]
▪ Place a fluid-impermeable pad under the patient *to prevent the bed from being soiled.*[6]
▪ Use an insertion checklist *to help comply with infection prevention and safety practices during insertion.*[2,9,10] Stop the procedure immediately if you observe any break in sterile technique.
▪ Turn the patient's head away from the site *to prevent possible contamination from airborne pathogens and to make the site more accessible.*[6]
▪ To prepare the insertion site, remove excess hair by using single-patient-use scissors or disposable-head surgical clippers *to facilitate dressing application.*[49] If the intended site is visibly soiled, clean the area with antiseptic soap and water.[7,14,49]
▪ Perform hand hygiene.[10,17,18,19,20,21,22,23]
▪ Establish a sterile field on a table using a sterile towel or the wrapping from the instrument tray, and assemble supplies on the sterile field.[7,17]
▪ Label all medications, medication containers, and other solutions on and off the sterile field.[50,51,52]
▪ Perform hand hygiene.[10,17,18,19,20,21,22,23]
▪ Put on a sterile gown and sterile gloves *to comply with maximal barrier precautions.*[2,10,13,53,54,55,56]
▪ Before beginning the procedure, the practitioner will put on a mask, a cap, and a sterile gown and gloves *to comply with maximal barrier precautions.*[2,10,13,53,54,55,56]
▪ Assist the practitioner as needed to prepare the insertion site. The practitioner will clean the site with a chlorhexidine sponge[7,17,49] using a vigorous side-to-side motion for 30 seconds; allow the area to air-dry.[7,17,49] If povidone-iodine solution is used, the practitioner will apply it using swabs, beginning at the intended insertion site and moving outward in concentric circles. Allow the solution to remain on the skin for at least 2 minutes until it dries completely.[7,17,49]
▪ The practitioner removes and discards gloves[54,57], performs hand hygiene[10,17,18,19,20,21,22,23], and puts on a new pair of sterile gloves.[53,54,55,56]
▪ Remove and discard your gloves[54,57], perform hand hygiene,[10,17,18,19,20,21,22,23] and put on new sterile gloves.[53,54,55,56]
▪ The practitioner drapes the patient with a large, full-body sterile drape *to create a sterile field and to comply with maximal barrier precautions.*[2,10,13]
▪ Conduct a time-out before beginning the procedure *to perform a final assessment that the correct patient, site, positioning, and procedure are identified and, as applicable, all relevant information and necessary equipment are available.*[58]
▪ Open the packaging of the 3-mL syringe and 25G 1" (2.5-cm) needle, and hand it to the practitioner using sterile technique.
▪ Disinfect the top of the local anesthetic with an alcohol pad and allow it to dry. Invert the vial and turn the vial toward the practitioner *so the fluid is visible.* The practitioner then fills the 3-mL syringe and injects the anesthetic into the site.
▪ If using ultrasound, use sterile technique to hand the practitioner the ultrasound device with the sterile probe cover. Apply sterile ultrasound gel. The practitioner locates the vessel using the device *to reduce the risk of insertion-related complications, improve success rates, and reduce the number of needle stick.*[10,13,17,46,59]
▪ Open the catheter package and inspect the device *to make sure that its integrity is intact.* Follow the manufacturer's instructions for preparing the catheter for insertion. Flush the catheter with preservative-free normal saline solution.[7,17]
▪ Hand the catheter to the practitioner using sterile technique. The practitioner then inserts the catheter.[7,17] The practitioner may use electrocardiographic (ECG) guided technology to detect the desired tip location.[5]

■ Monitor the patient's respiratory rate, heart rate, and oxygen saturation level during the procedure. Observe the cardiac monitor for arrhythmias while the guidewire and catheter are advanced.[6]

■ After the catheter is inserted and advanced to the desired tip location, the practitioner aspirates each lumen for blood return.[7,17]

■ Flush the catheter with preservative-free normal saline solution, observing for complications.[7,17] Clamp the catheter.

■ Using sterile technique, flush the needleless connector with preservative-free normal saline solution. Attach the primed needleless connectors to the catheter lumens.[7,17,21]

■ The practitioner secures the catheter with an integrated securement device, subcutaneous anchor securement system, tissue adhesive, or adhesive securement device, if available. Guidelines recommend an additional securement method beyond the primary dressing, *because these devices reduce vascular access device motion, which increases the risk of unintentional catheter dislodgment and complications requiring premature catheter removal.* Sutures should be avoided, *because they're associated with an increased risk of needle-stick injury and support the growth of biofilm, which increases the risk of catheter-related bloodstream infection.*[60]

ELDER ALERT Keep in mind that adhesive-backed tape and securement devices can cause tearing of an older adult's skin if removed improperly. An older adult can also develop sensitivities to adhesives, resulting in redness, itching, and rash, which can cause catheter dislodgment if the patient rubs, scratches, or pulls at the adhesive device.[7] If the patient has fragile skin, use dressings and tape specifically formulated for fragile skin *to prevent skin stripping and tearing during removal.*[61]

■ Use antiseptic solution to remove dried blood, *because it could harbor microorganisms.*

■ Apply a chlorhexidine-impregnated sponge dressing if required by your facility *to reduce the risk of central line–related bloodstream infection.*[2,10,59]

■ Apply a sterile transparent semipermeable dressing (as shown below).[1,10] Expect some serosanguineous drainage during the first 24 hours.[19]

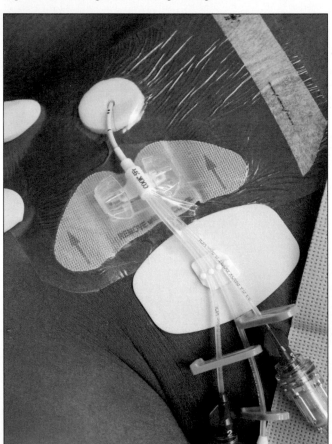

■ Label the dressing with the date of the procedure or the date when dressing change is required, as directed by your facility.[19]

■ Place the patient in a comfortable position and reassess the patient's status.

■ If insertion wasn't guided by ECG, make sure correct catheter tip location was confirmed by chest X-ray before administering medications or IV therapy, if ordered. The catheter tip should be located in the lower segment of the superior vena cava or near the cavoatrial junction. If placed in the femoral vein, the tip should be in the inferior vena cava above the diaphragm.[5,13]

■ Trace the tubing from the patient to its point of origin *to make sure that it's connected to the proper port.*[62,63,64]

■ Attach the primed IV administration set. Alternately, lock the device if ordered.

■ Route the tubing in a standardized direction if the patient has other tubing and catheters that have different purposes.[63] Label the tubing at the distal end (near the patient connection) and the proximal end (near the source container) *to reduce the risk of misconnection if multiple IV lines will be used.*[63,64]

■ Verify the electronic infusion device settings. Unclamp the catheter and administer the IV solution as ordered. Make sure that the electronic infusion device alarm limits are set according to the patient's current condition, and that the alarms are turned on, functioning properly, and audible to staff.[42,43,44]

■ Place disinfectant-containing end caps, if available at your facility, on the remaining needleless connectors *to reduce the risk of vascular catheter–associated infection.*[21,65]

Blood sampling using a central venous access catheter

■ Verify the practitioner's order.

■ Perform hand hygiene.[10,17,18,19,20,21,22,23]

■ Confirm the patient's identity using at least two patient identifiers.[34]

■ Provide privacy.[35,36,37,38]

■ Explain the procedure to the patient and family (if appropriate) according to their individual communication and learning needs *to increase their understanding, allay their fears, and enhance cooperation.*[27,28]

■ Raise the bed to waist level before providing care to prevent caregiver back strain.[41]

■ Perform hand hygiene.[10,17,18,19,20,21,22,23]

■ Put on gloves and, if splashing is likely, put on a gown and a mask with face shield or a mask and goggles.[54,55,56]

■ Trace the tubing from the patient to its point of origin *to make sure you're accessing the proper port.*[62,64]

■ Stop any infusing IV fluids, including those running through another lumen of the catheter. Follow your facility's guidance for time of cessation of fluid flow. (Research hasn't established the length of time for stopping fluid flow before obtaining the sample; one study suggests a 10-minute wait time.[66,67] The required length of time remains unknown, but may be associated with the internal volume of the catheter.[66]) Clamp the lumen, if appropriate. If necessary, detach the administration set from the needleless connector and place a sterile cap over the end of the administration set *to prevent contamination.*

■ If the patient has a multilumen catheter, select the largest lumen for blood sampling. For catheters with staggered lumen exit sites, draw the sample from the lumen exiting at the point farthest away from the heart (proximal port), or use the lumen recommended by the manufacturer.[66]

■ If no IV fluids are infusing and a disinfectant-containing end cap is covering the end of the needleless connector, remove and discard the end cap.[21]

■ Perform a vigorous mechanical scrub of the needleless connector for at least 5 seconds using an antiseptic pad; then allow it to dry completely.[2,21]

■ While maintaining the sterility of the syringe tip, attach the prefilled syringe containing preservative-free normal saline solution to the needleless connector. Use a 10-mL syringe or a syringe specifically designed to generate low injection pressure. Unclamp the catheter and slowly aspirate for blood return that's the color and consistency of whole blood. If no blood return occurs, take steps to locate an external cause of obstruction.[16] Notify the practitioner if troubleshooting is ineffective.

■ If blood return occurs, slowly inject preservative-free normal saline solution into the catheter.[66] Use a minimum volume of twice the internal volume of the catheter system.[16] Don't forcibly flush the device; further evaluate the device if you meet resistance.

■ Use the discard or push–pull method to obtain the blood sample.[66] If you're obtaining a blood sample for blood cultures, see the "Blood culture sample collection" procedure.

Discard method

Obtain a discard sample *to clear the catheter's dead space volume and to remove any blood diluted with flush solution.*

■ If you're using a needleless blood collection tube holder, clamp the catheter lumen, and then remove and discard the syringe in a puncture-resistant sharps disposal container.[7,54,57] Perform a vigorous mechanical scrub of the needleless connector for at least 5 seconds using an antiseptic pad; then allow it to dry completely.[2,21] Attach the needleless blood collection tube holder to the needleless connector, release the clamp, engage the labeled discard blood collection tube, and aspirate 4 to 5 mL of blood.[7,17]

■ If you're using a syringe, use the attached syringe you used for flushing to aspirate 4 to 5 mL of blood.[7,17]

■ Clamp the catheter, and then remove the labeled discard blood collection tube from the needleless blood collection tube holder, or remove the labeled discard syringe and discard it in a puncture-resistant sharps disposal container.[54,57] Alternatively, remove the labeled discard syringe and discard it in a puncture-resistant sharps disposal container.

■ Obtain blood samples as ordered; repeat the steps as necessary until all blood samples are obtained. If you're using a needleless blood collection tube holder, insert another blood collection tube into the needleless blood collection tube holder using the correct order of draw.[68] Unclamp the catheter and obtain the sample.

■ If you're using a syringe, perform a vigorous mechanical scrub of the needleless connector for at least 5 seconds using an antiseptic pad and allow it to dry completely.[2,21] Connect an empty syringe to the needleless connector, release the clamp, and withdraw the blood sample.[7,17,21]

■ Clamp the catheter and remove the needleless blood collection tube holder or syringe.

Push–pull method

■ Using the same syringe, aspirate 4 to 6 mL of blood.[7,17] Keeping the syringe attached to the catheter, push to reinfuse the blood into the catheter. Repeat the aspiration and reinfusion sequence three to five times (five cycles is most common).[7,17,66]

■ Clamp the catheter lumen, and then remove and discard the syringe in a puncture-resistant sharps disposal container.[54,57]

■ Perform a vigorous mechanical scrub of the needleless connector for at least 5 seconds using an antiseptic pad; then allow it to dry completely.[2,21]

■ Obtain blood samples as ordered; repeat the steps as necessary until all blood samples are obtained. If you're using a needleless blood collection tube holder, attach the needleless blood collection tube holder to the needleless connector, release the clamp, and engage the blood collection tube into the needleless blood collection tube holder using the correct order of draw.[68] Clamp the catheter and remove the needleless blood collection tube holder. If you're using a syringe, connect an empty syringe to the needleless connector, release the clamp, and withdraw the blood sample. Clamp the catheter and remove the syringe.

Completing a blood specimen collection by either method

■ Change the needleless connector according to the manufacturer's instructions. Also change the connector when the device's integrity is known or suspected to be compromised and when the connector contains blood or debris.[7,17,21]

■ Perform a vigorous mechanical scrub of the needleless connector for at least 5 seconds using an antiseptic pad. Then allow it to dry completely.[2,7,17,21]

■ While maintaining the sterility of the syringe tip, attach a prefilled syringe containing preservative-free normal saline solution to the needleless connector.[7,17,21]

■ Unclamp the catheter, slowly inject the preservative-free normal saline solution, and then reclamp the catheter.[65,7,17]

■ Remove and discard the syringe.[54,57]

■ If the patient has a continuous IV infusion prescribed, unclamp the catheter and continue the prescribed continuous IV infusion. If the administration set was detached, first perform a vigorous mechanical scrub of the needleless connector for at least 5 seconds using an antiseptic pad and allow it to dry completely.[2,21] Then remove the cap from the end of the administration set, reconnect to the catheter, and start the infusion.

■ If the patient doesn't have a continuous infusion prescribed, proceed with locking the device if required by your facility.[7,17] Perform a vigorous mechanical scrub of the needleless connector for at least 5 seconds using an antiseptic pad. Then allow it to dry completely.[2,7,17,21] While maintaining sterility of the syringe tip, attach the syringe of locking solution to the needleless connector and then unclamp the device.[7,17] Slowly inject the locking solution into the catheter.[7,17]

■ Clamp the device following the sequence required for the specific type of needleless connector used. For a positive-pressure needleless connector, clamp the catheter after disconnecting the syringe.[7,17] For a negative-pressure needleless connector, clamp the catheter while maintaining pressure on the syringe plunger, and then disconnect the syringe.[7,17] For a neutral needleless connector, clamp the catheter before or after disconnecting the syringe.[7,17] For an antireflux needleless connector, clamp the catheter and then disconnect the syringe; a specific clamping sequence isn't required.[69]

■ Discard the syringe in a puncture-resistant sharps disposal container.[54,57]

■ Place a new disinfectant-containing end cap, if available at your facility, on the needleless connector *to reduce the risk of vascular catheter–associated infection.*[2,65]

■ If you obtained blood using a syringe, use the blood transfer unit to transfer the blood into appropriate blood collection tubes.

■ Label the sample collection tubes in the presence of the patient *to prevent mislabeling.*[34,66]

■ Place the samples in a laboratory biohazard transport bag and send them immediately to the laboratory with a completed laboratory request form (if necessary).[54,66].

Flushing a central venous access catheter

■ Perform a vigorous mechanical scrub of the needleless connector for at least 5 seconds using an antiseptic pad; then allow it to dry completely.[2,21]

■ While maintaining sterility of the syringe tip, attach a prefilled syringe containing preservative-free normal saline solution to the needleless connector (use a 10-mL syringe or a syringe specifically designed to generate lower injection pressure). Unclamp the catheter, and slowly aspirate for a blood return that's the color and consistency of whole blood *to confirm the patency of the access device.*[16] If you don't obtain a blood return, take steps to locate an external cause of the obstruction.[16,70] Notify the practitioner if troubleshooting is ineffective.[7]

■ If you obtain a blood return, slowly inject preservative-free normal saline solution into the central venous access catheter. Use a minimum volume of twice the internal volume of the catheter system. Don't forcible flush the device; further evaluate the device if you meet resistance.[7,16,17]

■ Remove and discard the syringe in a puncture-resistance sharps disposable container.[54,57]

■ If indicated, proceed with locking the device.[7,17]

Locking a central venous access catheter

■ Perform a vigorous mechanical scrub of the needleless connector for at least 5 seconds using an antiseptic pad; then allow it to dry completely.[2,21]

■ While maintaining the sterility of the syringe tip, attach the syringe containing the locking solution to the needleless connector.[7,16,17]

■ Slowly inject the locking solution into the central venous access catheter.[7,17]

■ After locking the catheter, follow a clamping sequence *to reduce blood reflux* based on the type of needleless connector. Follow the manufacturer's instructions for use.[7,21,23] For a positive-pressure needleless connector, clamp the catheter after disconnecting the syringe.[7,17] For a negative-pressure needleless connector, maintain pressure on the syringe while clamping the catheter.[7,17] For a neutral needleless connector, clamp the catheter before or after disconnecting the syringe.[7,17] For an antireflux needleless connector, clamp the catheter and then disconnect the syringe; a specific clamping sequence isn't required.[69,71]

Changing a needleless connector on a central venous access catheter
- Verify the practitioner's order.
- Perform hand hygiene.[10,17,18,19,20,21,22,23]
- Put on gloves *to comply with standard precautions*.[54,55,56]
- Open the needleless connector package using sterile technique, and inspect the integrity of the device.[72] If the integrity is compromised, obtain a new device.
- While maintaining the sterility of the syringe tip, attach the prefilled syringe containing preservative-free normal saline solution to the new needleless connector. Prime the needleless connector with preservative-free normal saline solution *to purge the injection cap of air*.[7,17,73] Tap the needleless connector while priming *to purge all of the air*.[73] Leave the syringe in place.
- Trace the tubing from the patient to its point of origin *to make sure you're assessing the proper port*.[62,64]
- Close the clamp between the connector and the catheter *to prevent air from entering the catheter, which could cause air embolism*.[2]
- Remove the existing needleless connector.[7,17]
- Perform a vigorous mechanical scrub of the needleless connector for at least 5 seconds using an antiseptic pad; then allow it to dry completely.[2,21]
- Remove the protective cover from the primed needleless connector.[73]
- Attach the primed needleless connector to the catheter hub. Rotate the device to tighten it, taking care not to overtighten.[73]
- Unclamp the catheter, and slowly aspirate for a blood return that's the color and consistency whole blood. If you don't obtain a blood return, take steps to locate an external cause of the obstruction.[16] Notify the patient's practitioner if troubleshooting is ineffective.
- If you obtain a blood return, slowly inject preservative-free normal saline solution into the catheter. Use a minimum volume of twice the internal volume of the catheter system. Don't forcibly flush the device; further evaluate the device if you met resistance.[7,16,17]
- Lock the catheter, if appropriate.[7,16,17]
- Clamp the catheter and remove the syringe in the sequence appropriate for the device according to the manufacturer's instructions.[23] For a positive-pressure needleless connector, clamp the catheter after disconnecting the syringe.[7,17] For a negative-pressure needleless connector, maintain pressure on the syringe while closing the clamp.[7,17] For a neutral needleless connector, clamp before or after disconnecting the syringe.[7,17] For an antireflux needleless connector, clamp the catheter and then disconnect the syringe; a specific clamping sequence isn't required.[69,71]
- Place a new disinfectant-containing end cap (if available at your facility) on the needleless connector *to reduce the risk of vascular catheter–associated infection*.[21,65]

Changing the dressing on a central venous access catheter
- Perform hand hygiene.[10,17,18,19,20,21,22,23]
- Confirm the patient's identity using at least two patient identifiers.[34]
- Provide privacy.[35,36,37,38]
- Explain the procedure to the patient and family (if appropriate) according to their individual communication and learning needs *to increase their understanding, allay their fears, and enhance cooperation*.[27,28]
- Raise the bed to waist level before providing care *to prevent caregiver back strain*.[41]
- Perform hand hygiene.[10,17,18,19,20,21,22,23]
- Determine the date of the last dressing change.
- Put on a mask.[3,35]
- Perform hand hygiene.[8,13,14,15,16,17,18,19,20]
- Assemble the supplies on a sterile field.[3,35]
- Put on gloves *to comply with standard precautions*.[1,8,11,50,51]
- Remove the existing dressing by lifting the edge of the dressing at the catheter hub and gently pulling the dressing perpendicular to the skin toward the insertion site *to prevent catheter dislodgment and tearing or stripping of fragile skin*.[7,17] If necessary, use an acetone-free adhesive remover to remove adhesive from the patient's skin, *because acetone can harm the catheter*.[7] Discard the dressing in an appropriate receptacle.[54,57]
- If a chlorhexidine-impregnated sponge dressing was used to provide sustained antimicrobial action at the insertion site, remove and discard it in an appropriate receptacle.[54,57]

- Remove the engineered stabilization device, according to the manufacturer's instructions, and discard it in an appropriate receptacle.[7,17,22,54,57] Note that you should not remove a subcutaneous engineered stabilization device with every dressing change.[7,17] Prior to removal, use an appropriate solution to loosen the stabilization device, according to the manufacturer's instructions.[7,17]

NURSING ALERT Don't use scissors to remove vascular access device dressings, tape, or stabilization devices, *because scissors can sever the catheter or administration set and cause patient injury*.[74]

- Assess the catheter–skin junction and surrounding skin for bleeding, redness, swelling, tenderness, induration, and drainage.[10,16]
- Inspect the catheter for cracks, leakage, kinking or pinching, and mechanical problems.
- Remove and discard your gloves.[54,57]
- Perform hand hygiene.[10,17,18,19,20,21,22,23]
- Put on sterile gloves.[17,54,57]
- If you suspect catheter dislodgement, measure the external catheter length using a sterile tape measure or the incremental markings on the catheter and then compare it to the external catheter length documented at insertion.[7,16,17]
- Clean the skin with chlorhexidine swabs using a back-and-forth motion for at least 30 seconds *to provide skin antisepsis*; if the patient is sensitive to chlorhexidine, use tincture of iodine, povidone-iodine, or alcohol swabs. Allow the area to air-dry completely.[1,2,10,11,13,16,17] If povidone-iodine solution is used, apply it using swabs; begin at the catheter insertion site and move outward in concentric circles, and then allow the solution to remain on the skin until it dries completely (for at least 1½ minutes). Alternatively, use a back-and-forth motion. *No studies comparing the effectiveness of the use of concentric circles versus back-and-forth motion have been completed*.[17]
- If used in your facility, place a chlorhexidine-impregnated sponge dressing at the catheter base.[2,10,11,16] *To facilitate future removal,* position the chlorhexidine-impregnated sponge dressing with the catheter resting on or near the radial slit of the dressing. Ensure that the edges of the slit touch *to maximize antimicrobial action*.

NURSING ALERT Use chlorhexidine-impregnated dressings with caution in preterm neonates and in patients with fragile skin or complicated skin pathologies, *because contact dermatitis and pressure necrosis can occur*.[16]

- Apply a skin barrier solution according to the manufacturer's instructions *to reduce the risk of medical adhesive–related skin injury*. Don't use compound tincture of benzoin, *because it may increase the bonding of adhesives to the skin, causing skin injury when the adhesive-based engineered stabilization device is removed*.[16]
- Stabilize and secure the catheter using an engineered stabilization device, if available and as needed. An engineered stabilization device is recommended *because it reduces the risk of unintentional catheter dislodgment and complications that necessitate premature catheter removal*.[7,16,17]
- Apply a sterile transparent semipermeable dressing over the insertion site. Alternatively, apply a sterile 4″ × 4″ (10-cm × 10-cm) gauze dressing in place of the semipermeable dressing.[2,10,11,16] If the patient has fragile skin, use dressings and tape specially formulated for fragile skin *to prevent skin stripping and tearing during removal*.[61]
- Discard used supplies in appropriate receptacles.[54,57]
- Remove and discard your mask and gloves.[54,57]
- Perform hand hygiene.[10,17,18,19,20,21,22,23]
- Label the dressing with the date the dressing was changed or the date it's next due to be changed, as directed by your facility.[7,16,17]

Removing a central venous access catheter
- Verify the practitioner's order.
- Perform hand hygiene.[10,17,18,19,20,21,22,23]
- Put on gloves and, if needed, protective eyewear *to comply with standard precautions*.[10,55,56,53,54]
- Place a fluid-impermeable pad under the patient's shoulder and another close to the catheter exit site.
- Trace the tubing from the patients to its point of origin *to make sure that you're removing the proper catheter*.[62,64]
- Discontinue IV fluid administration and clamp the IV tubing.[17]

■ Position the patient in a supine flat or Trendelenburg position, unless contraindicated, so that the catheter exit site is at or below heart level *to prevent an air embolism.*[17,20,24]

■ Carefully remove the old dressing *to prevent skin stripping and tearing.*[7,17,61]

■ Discard the dressing in the appropriate receptacle.[54,57]

ELDER ALERT Remove tape and other adhesive materials carefully *to avoid skin injury, including tearing and bruising in the older adult.*[61] Use an adhesive remover if necessary *to help the removal process.*[7]

■ Remove any stabilization device or sutures present.[7,17] Prior to removal of a stabilization device, use an appropriate adhesive remover to loosen the stabilization device, according to the manufacturer's instructions.[7,17]

■ Inspect the catheter–skin junction and surrounding skin for signs of infection, such as redness, swelling, and drainage.[17]

■ Apply a sterile gauze pad to the catheter exit site.

■ With your dominant hand, slowly remove the catheter using gentle, even pressure.[7,17] If you meet resistance, don't forcibly remove the catheter, *because forcible removal can result in catheter fracture and embolization.* Consult with the practitioner *to discuss interventions for successful removal.*[24]

■ Have the patient perform the Valsalva maneuver (unless contraindicated) as you withdraw the final catheter segment *to prevent an air embolism.* If the Valsalva maneuver is contraindicated, place the patient in a Trendelenburg or left lateral decubitus position, or have the patient hold the breath, as applicable.[17,20] If the patient is receiving positive-pressure ventilation, remove the catheter during the inspiratory phase or when the patient is receiving a breath from a handheld resuscitation bag.[6]

■ Apply immediate pressure to the exit site with the sterile gauze pad until hemostasis is achieved. (Guidelines suggest applying pressure for a minimum of 30 seconds, or longer if needed to achieve homeostasis.)[6,17]

■ Apply petroleum-based ointment to the exit site; then cover it with a sterile occlusive dressing or sterile transparent semipermeable dressing for at least 24 hours *to seal the skin-to-vein tract and to decrease the risk of air embolism.*[7,17,20,75]

■ Label the dressing with the date of application or the date when change is required, as directed by your facility.[19]

■ Place the catheter on the fluid-impermeable pad. Inspect the catheter's condition and measure its length *to ensure that the entire catheter has been removed.* If you suspect that the entire catheter hasn't been completely removed, notify the practitioner immediately and closely monitor the patient for signs of distress.[76]

■ Properly discard the IV tubing and used supplies in appropriate receptacles.[54,57]

■ Encourage the patient to remain in a flat or reclining position, if able, for 30 minutes after device removal *to reduce the risk of air embolism.*[6,17,20]

After the procedure

■ After all procedures, dispose of all used supplies in the appropriate receptacles.[54,57]

■ Return the bed to the lowest position *to prevent falls and maintain patient safety.*[77]

■ Remove and discard your gloves, goggles, and mask or face shield, if worn.[54,57]

■ Perform hand hygiene.[10,17,18,19,20,21,22,23]

■ Document the procedure.[78,79,80,81,82]

Special considerations

■ If available, ultrasound technology should be used *to increase success rate and decrease complications.*[6,13,59]

■ Bathe the patient daily using a chlorhexidine wash or cloth if directed by your facility *to reduce the risk of vascular catheter–associated infection.*[2,10]

■ The Joint Commission issued a sentinel event alert concerning medical device alarm safety, *because alarm-related events have been associated with permanent loss of function or death.* Among the major contributing factors were improper alarm settings, alarm settings turned off inappropriately, and alarm signals that are inaudible to staff. Make sure that alarm limits are set appropriately and that alarms are turned on, functioning properly, and audible to staff. Follow facility guidelines for preventing alarm fatigue.[45]

■ After insertion, watch for signs and symptoms of pneumothorax, such as shortness of breath, uneven chest movement, tachycardia, and chest pain. Notify the practitioner immediately if such signs and symptoms appear.[6]

■ Teach the patient and family (if appropriate) about measures to prevent vascular catheter-associated infection, including the importance of hand hygiene. Encourage them to remind staff members who fail to comply.[28]

■ Routinely evaluate catheter necessity, and discontinue its use as soon as it's no longer needed *to reduce the risk of vascular catheter-associated infection.*[9]

■ The Joint Commission issued a sentinel event alert related to managing risk during transition to new International Organization for Standardization tubing standards that were designed to prevent dangerous tubing misconnections, which can lead to serious patient injury and death. During the transition, make sure to trace the tubing and catheter from the patient to the point of origin before connecting or reconnecting any device or infusion, at any care transition (such as a new setting or service), and as part of the hand-off process; route tubes and catheters having different purposes in different standardized directions; when there are different access sites or several bags hanging, label the tubing at both the distal and proximal ends; use tubing and equipment only as intended; and store medications for different delivery routes in separate locations.[64]

■ *Because different types of injection caps, access caps, and needleless connectors exist,* always follow the manufacturer's guidelines for flush technique and timing of clamping.[21]

■ Note that the push-pull method may be used as a blood conservation strategy *to reduce phlebotomy-associated blood loss, a significant cause of hospital-acquired anemia in patients of all ages.*[66]

■ Monitor hemoglobin and hematocrit, as appropriate, *to provide early detection of hospital-acquired anemia.*[6]

■ If you're using a heparin flush, be aware of any effects it might have on specimens, and flush the catheter before drawing a discard sample, if necessary.[16]

■ Antimicrobial locking solutions for therapeutic prophylactic purposes may be used in patients with long-term central venous access catheters, patients with a history of multiple catheter-related bloodstream infections, and high-risk patient populations, as well as at facilities that have exceptionally high rates of central line-associated bloodstream infections (CLABSI) despite using other methods to reduce CLABSI. The dwell time for antimicrobial lock solutions is unclear; up to 12 hours per day may be required. The antimicrobial locking solution should be aspirated from the catheter lumen at the end of the locking period and shouldn't be flushed into the patient's bloodstream, *because this action could increase the risk of antibiotic resistance and other adverse effects.*[16,17,18]

■ If the patient develops signs or symptoms of air embolism, immediately take steps to prevent more air from entering the bloodstream by closing, folding, or clamping the catheter. Place the patient on the left side in the Trendelenburg position or in a left decubitus position (if not contraindicated by another condition, such as increased intracranial pressure or respiratory disease). Notify the practitioner.[2]

■ Note that a gauze dressing placed underneath a transparent dressing is considered a gauze dressing and should be changed at least every 2 days.[16]

■ Visually inspect or palpate the catheter–skin junction site through the intact dressing daily *to assess for signs of infection.*[1,16]

■ Change the dressing every 24 hours until healing has occurred.[17]

■ If a catheter tip culture is required, clip 1" (2.5 cm) off the catheter tip using sterile scissors and place it in a sterile specimen container using sterile forceps. Label the container in the presence of the patient *to prevent mislabeling.*[34] Place the container in a laboratory transport bag and immediately send it to the laboratory. Keep in mind that catheter tip cultures are no longer used to determine whether a patient has a primary catheter-related bloodstream infection.[6]

Complications

Complications can occur at any time during infusion therapy. Traumatic complications, such as pneumothorax and adjacent organ perforation, typically occur on catheter insertion.[6] Systemic complications, such as sepsis, typically occur later during infusion therapy. Other complications include phlebitis (especially in peripheral central venous therapy), thrombus formation, and air embolism.[6] (See *Risks of central venous therapy*, page 152.) Complications associated with central venous catheter removal include bleeding, retained catheter fragments, air embolism, and pain.[6]

Risks of central venous therapy

SIGNS AND SYMPTOMS	POSSIBLE CAUSES	NURSING INTERVENTIONS	PREVENTION
INFECTION			
■ Redness, warmth, tenderness, or swelling at the exit site ■ Possible exudate of purulent material ■ Local rash or pustules ■ Fever, chills, and malaise ■ Leukocytosis ■ Nausea and vomiting	■ Failure to maintain sterile technique during catheter insertion or care ■ Failure to comply with dressing change protocol ■ Wet or soiled dressing remaining on the site ■ Immunosuppression ■ Irritated suture line ■ Contaminated catheter or solution ■ Frequent opening of the catheter or long-term use of a single IV access site	■ Monitor temperature frequently. ■ Monitor vital signs closely. ■ Culture the site, if indicated. ■ Re-dress using sterile technique. ■ Treat systemically with antibiotics or antifungals, depending on culture results and the practitioner's order. ■ Assist with catheter removal, if ordered ■ Collect paired cultures from a peripheral vein and the catheter, as ordered, before initiating antimicrobial therapy.[20] ■ Document interventions.[78,79,80,81,82]	■ Maintain sterile technique. Use sterile gloves, masks, and gowns when appropriate.[19] ■ Observe dressing-change protocols. ■ Change a wet, soiled, or loosened dressing immediately.[19] ■ Examine solutions for cloudiness and turbidity before infusing; check fluid containers for leaks. ■ Use a 0.2-micron filter (or a 1.2-micron filter for total parenteral nutrition solutions containing lipid injectable emulsions).[83] ■ Keep the system closed as much as possible.[20]
PNEUMOTHORAX, HEMOTHORAX, CHYLOTHORAX, OR HYDROTHORAX			
■ Decreased breath sounds on affected side ■ With hemothorax, decreased hemoglobin level because of blood pooling ■ Abnormal chest X-ray	■ Repeated or long-term use of the same vein ■ Preexisting cardiovascular disease ■ Lung puncture by the catheter during insertion or exchange over guide wire ■ Large blood vessel puncture with bleeding inside or outside lung ■ Lymph node puncture with leakage of lymph fluid ■ Infusion of solution into the chest area through an infiltrated catheter	■ Notify the practitioner. ■ Remove the catheter, or assist with removal if necessary. ■ Administer oxygen as ordered. ■ Set up and assist with chest tube insertion. ■ Document the intervention.[78,79,80,81,82]	■ Position the patient head down with a rolled blanket between the scapulae *to dilate and expose the internal jugular or subclavian vein as much as possible during insertion.* ■ Assess for early signs of fluid infiltration (swelling in the shoulder, neck, chest, and arm). ■ Ensure that the patient is immobilized and prepared for insertion. Active patients may need to be sedated or taken to the operating room.
AIR EMBOLISM			
■ Sudden onset of dyspnea ■ Gasping ■ Breathlessness ■ Tachyarrhythmias ■ Hypotension ■ Chest pain ■ Wheezing ■ Tachypnea ■ Altered mental status ■ Altered speech ■ Changes in facial appearance ■ Numbness ■ Paralysis[76]	■ Intake of air into the central venous system during catheter insertion or tubing changes ■ Inadvertent opening, cutting, or breaking of the catheter	■ Clamp, fold, or close the existing catheter or occlude the insertion site immediately.[74] ■ Place the patient on the left side in the Trendelenburg position or in a left lateral decubitus position, if not contraindicated by other conditions.[74] ■ Administer oxygen as ordered. ■ Notify the practitioner. ■ Document the patient's condition and your interventions.[78,79,80,81,82]	■ Purge all air from the administration sets and add-on devices before starting an infusion. ■ Teach the patient to perform the Valsalva maneuver during catheter insertion and tubing changes, if not contraindicated by the patient's condition.[74] ■ Use air-eliminating filters. ■ Use an infusion device with air detection capability. ■ Use Luer-lock tubing and secure all connections.[14,22]
THROMBOSIS			
■ Edema at puncture site ■ Erythema ■ Ipsilateral swelling of arm, neck, and face ■ Pain along vein ■ Fever, malaise ■ Chest pain ■ Dyspnea ■ Cyanosis	■ Sluggish flow rate ■ Composition of catheter material (polyvinyl chloride catheters are more thrombogenic) ■ Hematopoietic status of patient ■ Preexisting limb edema ■ Infusion of irritating solutions	■ Notify the practitioner. ■ Remove the catheter, if ordered. ■ Administer anticoagulant therapy as prescribed following safe medication administration practices.[47,48,49,84,85,86] ■ Verify thrombosis with diagnostic studies. ■ Apply warm, wet compresses locally. ■ Don't use the limb on the affected side for subsequent venipuncture. ■ Document interventions.[78,79,80,81,82]	■ Encourage early mobilization of the affected extremity.[86] ■ Ensure that the catheter tip is located in the lower segment of the superior vena cava or near the cavoatrial junction.[5,86] ■ Maintain a steady flow rate with an infusion pump, or flush the catheter at regular intervals. ■ Use catheters made of less thrombogenic materials *to prevent thrombosis.* ■ Dilute irritating solutions. ■ Use a 0.2-micron filter for infusions.[83]

Documentation

Record the indication for use; insertion site location; specific site preparation; local anesthetic, if used; infection prevention and safety precautions taken; type, length, size, and lot number of the catheter inserted; date and time of insertion; number of insertion attempts; device functionality; insertion method, including visualization and guidance technology; dressing; and the patient's tolerance of the procedure.

Document the date and the time the blood sample was drawn and the volume of blood withdrawn. If the patient has a multilumen catheter, document which lumen was used. Include the tests for which the sample was drawn and the time the sample was sent to the laboratory. Document the patency of the catheter, absence of signs and symptoms of complications, presence of blood return upon aspiration, lack of resistance when flushing, and the amount and types of flushes used.

Record the date and time of each dressing change, and record dressing assessment findings each shift. Document the condition of the catheter–skin junction and surrounding skin, dressing type, type of stabilization device, site care, external catheter length, and any catheter-related mechanical problems. Record any complications that occurred, the name of the practitioner notified of complications and the date and time of notification, any prescribed interventions, and the patient's response to those interventions.

Record the date and time of catheter removal and the type of ointment applied. Note the condition of the catheter exit site, the condition of the catheter and its length, the reason for catheter removal, nursing interventions during removal, the patient's response, and collection of a culture specimen, if applicable. Document teaching provided to the patient and family (if applicable), their understanding of that teaching, and any need for follow-up teaching.[79]

REFERENCES

1 American Society of Anesthesiologists. (2021). Practice guidelines for central venous access 2021: An updated report by the American Society of Anesthesiologists Task Force on Central Venous Access. *Anesthesiology, 132*(1), 8–43. https://pubs.asahq.org/anesthesiology/article/132/1/8/108838/Practice-Guidelines-for-Central-Venous-Access (Level VII)

2 Marschall, J., et al. (2014). SHEA/IDSA practice recommendations. Strategies to prevent central line–associated bloodstream infections in acute care hospitals. *Infection Control and Hospital Epidemiology, 35,* 753–771. https://www.jstor.org/stable/10.1086/676533#metadata_info_tab_ (Level I)

3 Standard 26. Vascular access device planning. Infusion therapy standards of practice (8th ed.). (2021). *Journal of Infusion Nursing, 44,* S74–S81. (Level VII)

4 Chopra, V. Central venous access devices and approach to device and site selection in adults. (2019). In: *UpToDate,* Davidson, I,. (Ed.).

5 Standard 23. Central vascular access tip location. Infusion therapy standards of practice (8th ed.). (2021). *Journal of Infusion Nursing, 44,* S65–S69. (Level VII)

6 Wiegand, D. L. (2017). *AACN procedure manual for high acuity, progressive, and critical care* (7th ed.). St. Louis, MO: Elsevier.

7 Infusion Nurses Society. (2017). *Policies and procedures for infusion therapy of the older adult* (3rd ed.). Boston, MA: Infusion Nurses Society.

8 Jarrett, N. M., & Callaham, M. (2016). Evidence-based guidelines for selected hospital-acquired conditions: Final report. https://www.cms.gov/Medicare/Medicare-Fee-for-Service-Payment/HospitalAcqCond/Downloads/2016-HAC-Report.pdf

9 The Joint Commission. (2021). Standard NPSG.07.04.01. *Comprehensive accreditation manual for hospitals.* Oakbrook Terrace, IL: The Joint Commission. (Level VII)

10 Centers for Disease Control and Prevention. (2011, revised 2017). Guidelines for the prevention of intravascular catheter-related infections. https://www.cdc.gov/infectioncontrol/guidelines/bsi/recommendations.html (Level I)

11 Association of Professionals in Infection Control and Epidemiology (APIC). (2015). Guide to preventing central line-associated bloodstream infections. https://apic.org/Resource_/TinyMceFileManager/2015/APIC_CLABSI_WEB.pdf (Level IV)

12 Standard 27. Site selection. Infusion therapy standards of practice (8th ed.). (2021). *Journal of Infusion Nursing, 44,* S81–S86. (Level VII)

13 Standard 34. Vascular access and device placement. Infusion therapy standards of practice (8th ed.). (2021). *Journal of Infusion Nursing, 44,* S97–S101. (Level VII)

14 Standard 43. Blood sampling. Infusion therapy standards of practice (8th ed.). (2021). *Journal of Infusion Nursing, 44,* S125–S133. (Level VII)

15 Goossens, G.A. (2015). Flushing and locking of venous catheters. Available evidence and evidence deficit. *Nursing Research and Practice, 2015,* 985686. https://www.ncbi.nlm.nih.gov/pmc/articles/PMC4446496/

16 Standard 41. Flushing and locking. Infusion therapy standards of practice (8th ed.). (2021). *Journal of Infusion Nursing, 44,* S113–S118. (Level VII)

17 Infusion Nurses Society. (2016). *Policies and procedures for infusion therapy* (5th ed.). Boston, MA: Infusion Nurses Society.

18 Infusion Nurses Society. (2008, revised 2016). *Infusion Nurses Society: Flushing and locking guidelines for vascular access devices.* Boston, MA: Infusion Nurses Society.

19 Standard 42. Vascular access device assessment, care, and dressing changes. Infusion therapy standards of practice (8th ed.). (2021). *Journal of Infusion Nursing, 44,* S119–S123. (Level VII)

20 Standard 50. Infection. Infusion therapy standards of practice (8th ed.). (2021). *Journal of Infusion Nursing, 44,* S153–S157. (Level VII)

21 Standard 36. Needleless connectors Infusion therapy standards of practice (8th ed.). (2021). *Journal of Infusion Nursing, 44,* S104–S107. (Level VII)

22 Standard 37. Other add-on devices. Infusion therapy standards of practice (8th ed.). (2021). *Journal of Infusion Nursing, 44,* S107–S108. (Level VII)

23 Hadaway, L. (2012). Needleless connectors for IV catheters. *American Journal of Nursing, 112*(11), 32–44.

24 Standard 45. Vascular access device removal. Infusion therapy standards of practice (8th ed.). (2021). *Journal of Infusion Nursing, 44,* S133–S137. (Level VII)

25 Association of Professionals in Infection Control and Epidemiology (APIC). (2016). APIC position paper: Safe injection, infusion, and medication vial practices in health care (2016). https://apic.org/Resource_/TinyMceFileManager/Position_Statements/2016APICSIPPositionPaper.pdf (Level IV)

26 Standard 11. Product evaluation, integrity, and defect reporting. Infusion therapy standards of practice (8th ed.). (2021). *Journal of Infusion Nursing, 44,* S45–S46. (Level VII)

27 The Joint Commission. (2021). Standard PC.02.01.21. *Comprehensive accreditation manual for hospitals.* Oakbrook Terrace, IL: The Joint Commission. (Level VII)

28 Standard 8. Patient education. Infusion therapy standards of practice (8th ed.). (2021). *Journal of Infusion Nursing, 44,* S35–S37. (Level VII)

29 The Joint Commission. (2021). Standard RI.01.03.01. *Comprehensive accreditation manual for hospitals.* Oakbrook Terrace, IL: The Joint Commission. (Level VII)

30 Centers for Medicare and Medicaid Services, Department of Health and Human Services. (2019). Condition of participation: Patient's rights. 42 C.F.R. § 482.13(b).

31 Accreditation Association for Hospitals and Health Systems. (2020). Standard 15.01.11. *Healthcare Facilities Accreditation Program: Accreditation requirements for acute care hospitals.* Chicago, IL: Accreditation Association for Hospitals and Health Systems. (Level VII)

32 Standard 9. Informed consent. Infusion therapy standards of practice (8th ed.). (2021). *Journal of Infusion Nursing, 44,* S37–S39. (Level VII)

33 DNV GL-Healthcare USA, Inc. (2020). PR.2.SR.3. *NIAHO® accreditation requirements, interpretive guidelines and surveyor guidance—revision 20.0* Milford, OH: DNV GL-Healthcare USA, Inc. (Level VII)

34 The Joint Commission. (2021). Standard NPSG.01.01.01. *Comprehensive accreditation manual for hospitals.* Oakbrook Terrace, IL: The Joint Commission. (Level VII)

35 The Joint Commission. (2021). Standard RI.01.01.01. *Comprehensive accreditation manual for hospitals.* Oakbrook Terrace, IL: The Joint Commission. (Level VII)

36 Centers for Medicare and Medicaid Services, Department of Health and Human Services. (2019). Condition of participation: Patient's rights. 42 C.F.R. § 482.13(c)(1).

37 Accreditation Association for Hospitals and Health Systems. (2020). Standard 15.01.16. *Healthcare Facilities Accreditation Program: Accreditation requirements for acute care hospitals.* Chicago, IL: Accreditation Association for Hospitals and Health Systems. (Level VII)

38 DNV GL-Healthcare USA, Inc. (2020). PR.2.SR.5. *NIAHO® accreditation requirements, interpretive guidelines and surveyor guidance—revision 20.0.* Milford, OH: DNV GL-Healthcare USA, Inc. (Level VII)

39 The Joint Commission. (2021). Standard UP.01.01.01. *Comprehensive accreditation manual for hospitals.* Oakbrook Terrace, IL: The Joint Commission. (Level VII)

40 Accreditation Association for Hospitals and Health Systems. (2018). Standard 30.00.14. *Healthcare Facilities Accreditation Program: Accreditation requirements for acute care hospitals*. Chicago, IL: Accreditation Association for Hospitals and Health Systems. (Level VII)

41 Waters, T. R., et al. (2009). Safe patient handling training for schools of nursing. https://www.cdc.gov/niosh/docs/2009-127/pdfs/2009-127.pdf (Level VII)

42 Graham, K. C., & Cvach, M. (2010). Monitor alarm fatigue: Standardizing use of physiological monitors and decreasing nuisance alarms. *American Journal of Critical Care, 19*, 28–37. http://ajcc.aacnjournals.org/content/19/1/28.full.pdf

43 American Association of Critical-Care Nurses. (2018). AACN practice alert: Managing alarms in acute care across the life span: Electrocardiography and pulse oximetry. https://www.aacn.org/clinical-resources/practice-alerts/managing-alarms-in-acute-care-across-the-life-span (Level VII)

44 The Joint Commission. (2021). Standard NPSG.06.01.01. *Comprehensive accreditation manual for hospitals*. Oakbrook Terrace, IL: The Joint Commission. (Level VII)

45 The Joint Commission. (2013). Sentinel event alert 50: Medical device alarm safety in hospitals. http://www.jointcommission.org/assets/1/6/SEA_50_alarms_4_26_16.PDF (Level VII)

46 Standard 22. Vascular visualization. Infusion therapy standards of practice (8th ed.). (2021). *Journal of Infusion Nursing, 44*, S63–S65. (Level VII)

47 Accreditation Association for Hospitals and Health Systems. (2020). Standard 16.01.03. *Healthcare Facilities Accreditation Program: Accreditation requirements for acute care hospitals*. Chicago, IL: Accreditation Association for Hospitals and Health Systems. (Level VII)

48 Centers for Medicare and Medicaid Services, Department of Health and Human Services. (2020). Condition of participation: Nursing services. 42 C.F.R. § 482.23(c).

49 Standard 33. Vascular access site preparation and skin asepsis. Infusion therapy standards of practice (8th ed.). (2021). *Journal of Infusion Nursing, 44*, S96. (Level VII)

50 The Joint Commission. (2021). Standard NPSG.03.04.01. *Comprehensive accreditation manual for hospitals*. Oakbrook Terrace, IL: The Joint Commission. (Level VII)

51 Accreditation Association for Hospitals and Health Systems. (2020). Standard 25.01.27. *Healthcare Facilities Accreditation Program: Accreditation requirements for acute care hospitals*. Chicago, IL: Accreditation Association for Hospitals and Health Systems. (Level VII)

52 Standard 13. Medication verification. Infusion therapy standards of practice (8th ed.). (2021). *Journal of Infusion Nursing, 44*, S46–S49. (Level VII)

53 Standard 17. Standard precautions. Infusion therapy standards of practice (8th ed.). (2021). *Journal of Infusion Nursing, 44*, S54–S55. (Level VII)

54 Occupational Safety and Health Administration. (2012). Bloodborne pathogens, standard number1910.1030. https://www.osha.gov/pls/oshaweb/owadisp.show_document?p_id=10051&p_table=STANDARDS (Level VII)

55 Siegel, J. D., et al. (2007, revised 2019). 2007 guideline for isolation precautions: Preventing transmission of infectious agents in healthcare settings. https://www.cdc.gov/infectioncontrol/pdf/guidelines/isolation-guidelines-H.pdf (Level II)

56 Accreditation Association for Hospitals and Health Systems. (2020). Standard 07.01.10. *Healthcare Facilities Accreditation Program: Accreditation requirements for acute care hospitals*. Chicago, IL: Accreditation Association for Hospitals and Health Systems. (Level VII)

57 Standard 21. Medical waste and sharps safety. Infusion therapy standards of practice (8th ed.). (2021). *Journal of Infusion Nursing, 44*, S60–S62. (Level VII)

58 The Joint Commission. (2021). Standard UP.01.03.01. *Comprehensive accreditation manual for hospitals*. Oakbrook Terrace, IL: The Joint Commission. (Level VII)

59 Heffner, A. C., & Androes, A. P. (2020). Overview of central venous access in adults. In: *UpToDate*, Davidson, I.,, et al. (Eds.).

60 Standard 38. Vascular access device securement. Infusion therapy standards of practice (8th ed.). (2021). *Journal of Infusion Nursing, 44*, S119–S123. (Level VII)

61 LeBlanc, K., et al. (2013). International skin tear advisory panel: A tool kit to aid in the prevention, assessment, and treatment of skin tears using a simplified classification system. *Advances in Skin & Wound Care, 26*, 459–476. (Level IV)

62 U.S. Food and Drug Administration. (2017). Examples of medical device misconnections. https://www.fda.gov/medical-devices/medical-device-connectors/examples-medical-device-misconnections

63 Standard 59. Vascular access device assessment, care, and dressing changes. Infusion therapy standards of practice (8th ed.). (2021). *Journal of Infusion Nursing, 44*, S180–S183. (Level VII)

64 The Joint Commission. (2014). Sentinel event alert 53: Managing risk during transition to new ISO tubing connector standards. http://www.jointcommission.org/assets/1/6/SEA_53_Connectors_8_19_14_final.pdf (Level VII)

65 Moreau, N. L., & Flynn, J. (2015). Disinfection of needleless connector hubs: Clinical evidence systematic review. *Nursing Research and Practice, 2015*, 1–20. https://www.ncbi.nlm.nih.gov/pmc/articles/PMC4446481/

66 Standard 44. Blood sampling. Infusion therapy standards of practice (8th ed.). (2021). *Journal of Infusion Nursing, 44*, S125–S133. (Level VII)

67 Fairholm, L., et al. (2011). Monitoring parenteral nutrition in hospitalized patients: Issues related to spurious bloodwork. *Nutrition in Clinical Practice, 26*, 700–707. (Level IV)

68 Becton, Dickinson and Company. (2010). BD Vacutainer® order of draw for multiple tube collections. https://www.bd.com/documents/in-service-materials/specimen-collection/PAS_BC_Vacutainer-order-of-draw-for-multiple-tubes-poster_IM_EN.pdf

69 Hull, G., et al. (2018). Quantitative assessment of reflux in commercially available needleless IV connectors. *Journal of Vascular Access, 19*, 12–22. (Level VI)

70 Standard 49. Central venous access device occlusion. Infusion therapy standards of practice (8th ed.). (2021). *Journal of Infusion Nursing, 44*, S149–S153. (Level VII)

71 Jasinsky, L., & Wurster, J. (2009). Occlusion reduction and heparin elimination trial using an antireflux device on peripheral and central venous catheters. *Journal of Infusion Nursing, 32*, 33–39. (Level VI)

72 Standard 12. Product evaluation, integrity, and defect reporting. Infusion therapy standards of practice (8th ed.). (2021). *Journal of Infusion Nursing, 44*, S45–S46. (Level VII)

73 CareFusion. (2012). MaxPlus® clear needleless connector: Quick reference guide. https://www.bd.com/a/35704

74 Standard 52. Air embolism. Infusion therapy standards of practice (8th ed.). (2021). *Journal of Infusion Nursing, 44*, S160–S161. (Level VII)

75 Feil, M. (2012). Reducing risk of air embolism associated with central venous access devices. *Pennsylvania Patient Safety Advisory, 9*(2), 58–65. http://patientsafety.pa.gov/ADVISORIES/Pages/201206_58.aspx

76 Standard 51. Catheter damage (embolism, repair, exchange). Infusion therapy standards of practice (8th ed.). (2021). *Journal of Infusion Nursing, 44*, S119–S123. (Level VII)

77 Ganz, D. A., et al. (2013, reviewed 2021). *Preventing falls in hospitals: A toolkit for improving quality of care* (AHRQ Publication No. 13-0015-EF). Rockville, MD: Agency for Healthcare Research and Quality. https://www.ahrq.gov/professionals/systems/hospital/fallpxtoolkit/index.html

78 The Joint Commission. (2021). Standard RC.01.03.01. *Comprehensive accreditation manual for hospitals*. Oakbrook Terrace, IL: The Joint Commission. (Level VII)

79 Standard 10. Documentation in the health record. Infusion therapy standards of practice (8th ed.). (2021). *Journal of Infusion Nursing, 44*, S39–S42. (Level VII)

80 Centers for Medicare and Medicaid Services, Department of Health and Human Services. (2020). Condition of participation: Medical service records. 42 C.F.R. § 482.24(b).

81 Accreditation Association for Hospitals and Health Systems. (2020). Standard 10.00.03. *Healthcare Facilities Accreditation Program: Accreditation requirements for acute care hospitals*. Chicago, IL: Accreditation Association for Hospitals and Health Systems. (Level VII)

82 DNV GL-Healthcare USA, Inc. (2020). MR.2.SR.1. *NIAHO® accreditation requirements, interpretive guidelines and surveyor guidance—revision 20.0*. Milford, OH: DNV GL-Healthcare USA, Inc. (Level VII)

83 Standard 35. Filtration. Infusion therapy standards of practice (8th ed.). (2021). *Journal of Infusion Nursing, 44*, S102–S104. (Level VII)

84 The Joint Commission. (2021). Standard MM.06.01.01. *Comprehensive accreditation manual for hospitals*. Oakbrook Terrace, IL: The Joint Commission. (Level VII)

85 DNV GL-Healthcare USA, Inc. (2020). MM.1.SR.3. *NIAHO® accreditation requirements, interpretive guidelines and surveyor guidance—revision 20.0*. Milford, OH: DNV GL-Healthcare USA, Inc. (Level VII)

86 Standard 53. Catheter-associated deep vein thrombosis. Infusion therapy standards of practice (8th ed.). (2021). *Journal of Infusion Nursing, 44*, S161–S164. (Level VI)

CENTRAL VENOUS PRESSURE MONITORING

In central venous pressure (CVP) monitoring, a practitioner inserts a catheter through a vein and advances it until its tip lies in the lower segment of the superior vena cava at or near the cavoatrial junction, which is the catheter tip location deemed safest.[1] The practitioner inserts the catheter percutaneously or using a cutdown method. Ultrasound-guided catheter insertion is recommended.[2,3,4] Pressure at end-diastole reflects back to the catheter, because no major valve lies at the junction of the vena cava and right atrium. When connected to a monitoring system, the catheter measures CVP, which directly reflects right atrial pressure and indirectly reflects right ventricular end-diastolic pressure.[5] A transducer system detects intravascular and intracardiac pressures and converts them to an electrical signal that transmits to a monitor.

CVP monitoring helps to assess cardiac function, evaluate venous return to the heart, and indirectly gauge the heart's pumping efficiency. The central venous (CV) catheter also provides access to a large vessel for rapid, high-volume fluid and medication administration, and allows frequent blood withdrawal for laboratory samples. (See the section entitled "Blood sampling using a central venous access catheter" in the "Central venous access catheter" procedure.)

CVP monitoring can be done intermittently or continuously. Typically, a single-lumen CVP line is used for intermittent pressure readings. A pulmonary artery (PA) catheter has a proximal lumen appropriate for continuous CVP monitoring.

Normal CVP ranges from 2 to 6 mm Hg.[5] CVP readings reflect changes in intravascular volume status and right ventricular preload status.[5] Any condition that alters venous return, circulating blood volume, or cardiac performance can affect CVP. Increased CVP may indicate vasoconstriction, increased blood volume, right ventricular failure, tricuspid insufficiency, pericardial tamponade, pulmonary embolism, obstructive pulmonary disease, or positive-pressure ventilation. Decreased CVP may indicate hypovolemia, vasodilation (as with sepsis or vasodilating medication), or increased myocardial contractility.

HOSPITAL-ACQUIRED CONDITION ALERT Keep in mind that the Centers for Medicare and Medicaid Services considers vascular catheter–associated infection a hospital-acquired condition *because it can be reasonably prevented using a variety of practices.* Be sure to follow evidence-based infection prevention practices, such as using sterile no-touch technique when accessing the device, minimizing catheter manipulations, and removing the catheter as soon as it's no longer necessary, *to reduce the risk of vascular catheter–associated* infections.[6,7,8,9,10,11]

Equipment

Cardiac monitor ▪ disposable pressure tubing with flush device and disposable pressure transducer ▪ leveling device ▪ pressure monitoring module and cable ▪ IV bag or normal saline solution ▪ pressure bag ▪ IV pole with transducer mount holder ▪ marker ▪ sterile nonvented caps ▪ gloves ▪ pulse oximeter and probe ▪ blood pressure monitoring equipment ▪ stethoscope ▪ disinfectant pad ▪ Optional: labels.

Preparation of equipment

For initial setup, turn on the monitor before gathering the equipment *to allow time for it to warm up.* Make sure that the monitor has the correct pressure module in place. Plug the pressure cable into the appropriate pressure module. Turn on the correct parameter *to visualize the correct waveform.* Set the appropriate scale for the monitored pressure *to obtain accurate pressure readings.* Note that the right atrial pressure scale is commonly set at 20 mm Hg.[5]

Perform hand hygiene.[12,13,14] Inspect all IV equipment and supplies. If a product is expired, is defective, or has compromised integrity, remove it from patient use, label it as expired or defective, and report the expiration or defect as directed by your facility.[15]

Set up the transducer system; use an IV bag of normal saline solution as the flush solution.[5] (See the "Transducer system setup"

procedure.) Place the IV bag into the pressure bag and attach the system to an IV pole.

Implementation

▪ Gather and prepare the necessary equipment and supplies.
▪ Perform hand hygiene.[8,16,17,18,19,20,21,22]
▪ Confirm the patient's identity using at least two patient identifiers.[23]
▪ Provide privacy.[24,25,26,27]
▪ Explain the procedure to the patient and family (if appropriate) according to their individual communication and learning needs *to increase their understanding, allay their fears, and enhance cooperation.*[28]
▪ Raise the bed to waist level before providing care *to prevent caregiver back strain.*[29]
▪ Perform hand hygiene.[8,16,17,18,19,20,21,22]
▪ Put on gloves *to comply with standard precautions.*[30,31,32]
▪ Ensure that the patient is attached to a cardiac monitor with pressure monitoring capability, a pulse oximeter, and blood pressure monitoring equipment, if necessary. Make sure that the alarm limits are appropriately set for the patient's current condition, and that the alarms are turned on, functioning properly, and audible to staff.[33,34,35,36]
▪ Assess the patient's cardiovascular, peripheral vascular, respiratory, and fluid status *to use as baselines for comparison.*[5]
▪ If not already in place, assist the practitioner with CV access catheter PA catheter insertion. (See the section entitled "Assisting with inserting a central venous access catheter" in the "Central venous access catheter care" procedure.)
▪ Make sure that the CV catheter or the proximal lumen of the PA catheter is attached to the transducer system. If the patient has a CV catheter with multiple lumens, the distal port may be dedicated to continuous CVP monitoring and the other lumens may be used for fluid administration and medication administration.
▪ Trace the tubing from the patient to the point of origin *to make sure that it's connected to the correct port.*[37,38,39] Route the tubing in a standardized direction if the patient has other tubing and catheters having different purposes.[38,39] If the patient has multiple IV lines in use, label the tubing at both the distal end (near the patient connection) and the proximal end (near the source container) *to reduce the risk of misconnection.*[39]
▪ Position the patient supine with the head of the bed elevated up to 60 degrees.[40,41] If the patient can't tolerate such positioning, use a prone or a 20-, 30-, or 90-degree lateral position, as appropriate.[40] Allow the patient 5 to 15 minutes to stabilize following a position change.[40]
▪ Using a leveling device, position the air-reference stopcock or the air–fluid interface of the transducer level with the phlebostatic axis (midway between the posterior chest and the sternum at the fourth intercostal space at the midaxillary line) if the patient is supine or prone.[5,40] If the patient is in a lateral position, reference the stopcock or the air–fluid interface of the transducer at the lateral angle-specific reference.[40] Mark the appropriate place on the patient's chest *so that all subsequent measurements use the same location.*[5]
▪ Turn the stopcock next to the transducer off to the patient and open to air. Remove the cap to the stopcock port.[5,40]
▪ Zero the transducer following the manufacturer's instructions.[5]
▪ Turn the stopcock so that it's in a monitoring position, with the stopcock closed to air and open to the side of the tubing that goes to the patient. Place a new sterile, nonvented cap on the stopcock *to maintain sterility.*[5]
▪ Perform a square wave test (dynamic response test) *to verify the accuracy of the pressure monitoring system.*[5,40] (See *Square-wave test*, page 156)
▪ Read the CVP value by measuring the mean of the *a* wave at end-expiration.[5] (See *Interpreting CVP measurements*, page 157.) The monitor will also provide a value on the digital display. Make sure the patient remains still when the reading is taken *to prevent artifact.* (See *Identifying hemodynamic pressure-monitoring problems*, page 158.)
▪ Monitor the CVP waveform continuously, and obtain hemodynamic values hourly and as needed, according to the patient's condition and as ordered, or according to unit protocol.[5]

Square-wave test

When using a pressure transducer system, you must ensure and document the system's accuracy. Along with leveling and zeroing the system to atmospheric pressure at the phlebostatic axis and interpreting waveforms, you can ensure accuracy by performing the square wave test, also called *a dynamic response test*. Perform a square wave test with the initial system setup and then at least once each shift, after opening the catheter system (such as for rezeroing or tubing changes), and when the waveform appears to be damped or distorted.[40]

To perform a square wave test, follow these steps:

- Activate the fast-flush device for 1 second and then release it.
- Obtain a graphic printout.
- Observe for the desired response: The pressure wave rises rapidly, squares off, and is followed by one or two oscillations (as shown below).
- Know that these oscillations should have an initial downstroke that extends below the baseline and just one to two oscillations after the initial downstroke. Usually, but not always, the first upstroke is about one-third the height of the initial downstroke.
- Be aware that the intervals between oscillations should be within 0.12 second (three small boxes).[5]

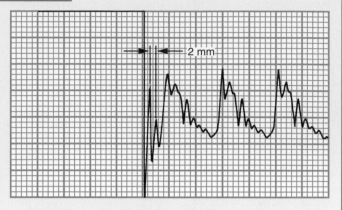

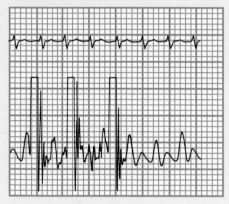

Underdamped square wave

If you observe extra oscillations after the initial downstroke or more than 0.12 second between oscillations, the waveform is underdamped (as shown above on right). This condition can cause false-high pressure readings and artifact in the waveforms. It can be corrected by:

- using large-bore, shorter tubing
- inserting a damping device (available from pressure tubing companies)
- removing air bubbles from the system.[5]

After addressing the issue, repeat the square wave test and read the pressure waveform.

Overdamped square wave

If you observe a slurred upstroke at the beginning of the square wave and a loss of oscillations after the initial downstroke, the waveform is overdamped (as shown below). This condition can cause false-low pressure readings and loss of the sharpness of waveform peaks and the dicrotic notch, which indicates pulmonic valve closure. It can be corrected by:

- clearing the system of any blood or air
- checking to make sure that the catheter has no kinks or obstructions
- using low-compliance, short monitoring equipment
- checking the bag of flush solution to make sure that the fluid remains in the bag and that the pressure is maintained at 300 mm Hg
- tightening any loose connections.[5]

After addressing the issue, repeat the square wave test and read the pressure waveform.

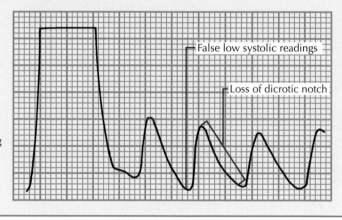

- Monitor the transducer system for the presence of air. If air is present, remove it from the system *to prevent air embolism*.[5]
- Return the bed to the lowest position *to prevent falls and maintain patient safety*.[42]
- Remove and discard your gloves.[32]
- Perform hand hygiene.[8,16,17,18,19,20,21,22]
- Clean and disinfect your stethoscope.[43,44]
- Perform hand hygiene.[8,16,17,18,19,20,21,22]
- Document the procedure.[45,46,47,48,49]

Special considerations

- To care for the insertion site, change transparent semipermeable dressings every 5 to 7 days, or change gauze dressings at least every 2 days. Change the dressing immediately to assess, clean, and disinfect the site

if signs and symptoms of infection are present or if the dressing becomes visibly soiled, loose, or dislodges. (See the section entitled "Changing the dressing on a central venous access catheter" in the "Central venous access device catheter care" procedure.)[8,52]

- Replace the IV flush solution and the pressure tubing, transducer, dome, and other components of the system, including the administration set and flush solution, every 96 hours or immediately if you suspect contamination or compromise of the product or system integrity. Label the IV solution, tubing, and dressing with the date of initiation or the date of change, as directed by your facility.[5,8,53]
- Perform a square wave test (dynamic response test) at the beginning of each shift, with a waveform change, and after the system is opened to air.[5,40]
- Zero the transducer during initial setup and before catheter insertion, when a disconnection occurs between the monitor and the monitoring

Interpreting CVP measurements

A pressure transducer set produces an intermittent or continuous CVP waveform and readout that's displayed on the patient's bedside monitor, along with the patient's electrocardiogram (shown below) and other tracings. This method allows you to continually monitor for acute and gradual changes.

When using a pressure transducer set, make sure the central venous catheter or the proximal lumen of a pulmonary artery catheter is attached to the system, and that the patient is still when the reading is taken, *to prevent artifact.*

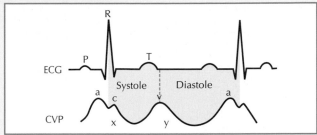

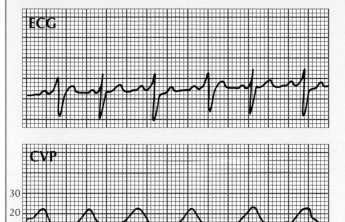

Interpretation of a CVP waveform requires awareness of three waves: *a, c,* and *v* waves (as shown above on right). Understanding the ways in which these waves relate to cardiac function is necessary to accurately interpret a CVP waveform.

■ *A* **wave (atrial contraction)**—The most prominent wave is the *a* wave, which results from atrial contraction at end-diastole. As the right atrium contracts, it forces blood into the right ventricle, causing a rise in pressure. This rise in pressure travels through the central line to the transducer, and is represented by a positive inflection on the CVP waveform. When compared with the ECG waveform produced at the same time, the *a* wave on the CVP occurs after the P wave. To measure CVP, or right atrial pressure, measure the mean of the *a* wave at end-expiration.[5]

■ *C* **wave (closure of the tricuspid valve)**—Isovolumic right ventricular contraction, which closes the tricuspid valve and causes it to bow back toward the right atrium in early systole, produces a transient increase in atrial pressure. This increase in pressure is represented by the *c* wave on the waveform.[5] The *c* wave, also a positive inflection on the CVP waveform, follows the onset of the QRS complex on the ECG.

■ *V* **wave (ventricular contraction)**—The last atrial pressure peak is the *v* wave, which is produced by a combination of atrial filling and ventricular contraction during late systole while the tricuspid valve remains closed.[5] The *v* wave peaks just after the T wave on the ECG.

In addition to the three waves, a CVP waveform has two descents that make up the rest of the CVP waveform: the *x* descent, which represents atrial diastole, and the *v* descent, which represents atrial emptying.[41]

---

cable or between the transducer and the monitoring cable, and when the values obtained don't coincide with the patient's clinical condition.[5]

■ Assess catheter necessity daily during multidisciplinary rounds. Remove the catheter as soon as it's no longer needed *to reduce the risk of central line–related bloodstream infection.*[7,8,9,10]

■ The Joint Commission issued a sentinel event alert concerning medical device alarm safety, *because alarm-related events have been associated with permanent loss of function or death.* Among the major contributing factors were improper alarm settings, alarm settings turned off inappropriately, and alarm signals that were inaudible to staff. Make sure that alarm limits are set appropriately and that alarms are turned on, functioning properly, and audible to staff. Follow facility guidelines for preventing alarm fatigue.[35]

■ The Joint Commission issued a sentinel event alert related to managing risk during transition to new International Organization for Standardization tubing standards that were designed to prevent dangerous tubing misconnections, which can lead to serious patient injury and death. During the transition, make sure to trace each tubing and catheter from the patient to its point of origin before connecting or reconnecting any device or infusion, at any care transition (such as to a new setting or service), and as part of the hand-off process; route tubes and catheters having different purposes in different standardized directions; when the patient has different access sites or several bags hanging, label tubing at both the distal

and proximal ends; use tubing and equipment only as intended; and store medications for different delivery routes in separate locations.[39]

Complications

Potential complications of CVP monitoring include pneumothorax (which may occur on catheter insertion), sepsis, thrombus, vessel or adjacent organ puncture, infection, catheter occlusion, and air embolism.

Documentation

Document the date and time of CV or PA catheter insertion, if appropriate, and the patient's tolerance of the procedure. Report all dressing, pressure tubing, and IV solution changes; the condition of the catheter exit site; and exit site care given. Document the results of the square wave test, the patient's CVP readings, the patient's position for leveling and zeroing, the practitioner notified of the CVP readings, prescribed interventions, and the patient's response to those interventions. Record any complications that occur, the name of the practitioner notified, the date and time of notification, prescribed interventions, and the patient's response to those interventions. Also document teaching provided to the patient and family (if applicable), their understanding of that teaching, and any need for follow-up teaching.

TROUBLESHOOTING

IDENTIFYING HEMODYNAMIC PRESSURE-MONITORING PROBLEMS

The table below lists various possible problems you might encounter when monitoring hemodynamic pressure, along with possible causes and nursing interventions to help solve the problem.

PROBLEM	POSSIBLE CAUSES	NURSING INTERVENTIONS
No waveform	Power supply turned off	■ Check the power supply.
	Monitor screen pressure range set too low	■ Raise the monitor screen pressure range, if necessary. ■ Rebalance and recalibrate the equipment.
	■ Loose connection in line	■ Tighten loose connections.
	■ Transducer disconnected from monitoring system	■ Check and tighten the connection
	■ Stopcock turned off to patient	■ Position the stopcock correctly.
	■ Catheter occluded or displaced from the blood vessel	■ Use the fast-flush valve to flush the line, or try to aspirate blood from the catheter. If the line remains occluded, notify the practitioner and prepare to administer thrombolytics or replace the catheter.[5,50]
Drifting waveforms	■ Electrical cable kinked or compressed	■ Place the monitor's cable where it can't be stepped on or compressed.
Line fails to flush	■ Stopcocks positioned incorrectly	■ Make sure stopcocks are positioned correctly.
	■ Inadequate pressure from pressure bag	■ Make sure the pressure bag gauge reads 300 mm Hg.[5]
	■ Kink in pressure tubing	■ Check the pressure tubing for kinks.
	■ Blood clot in catheter	■ Try to aspirate the clot with a syringe. If the line still won't flush, notify the practitioner and prepare to replace the catheter, if necessary. *Important*: Never use a syringe to flush a hemodynamic catheter.
Artifact (waveform interference)	■ Patient movement	■ Wait until the patient is quiet before taking a reading.
	■ Electrical interference	■ Make sure electrical equipment is connected and grounded correctly.
	■ Catheter fling (tip of PA catheter moving rapidly in large blood vessel in heart chamber)	■ Notify the practitioner, who may try to reposition the catheter.
False-high readings	■ Transducer balancing port positioned below patient's right atrium (phlebostatic axis)	■ Position the balancing port level with the patient's right atrium (phlebostatic axis).
	■ Flush solution flow rate too fast	■ Check the flush solution flow rate. Maintain it at 3 to 4 mL/hour.
	■ Air in system	■ Remove air from the lines and the transducer.[5]
	■ Catheter fling (tip of PA catheter moving rapidly in large blood vessel or heart chamber)	■ Notify the practitioner, who may try to reposition the catheter.
False-low readings	■ Transducer balancing port positioned above patient's right atrium	■ Position the balancing port level with the patient's right atrium.
	■ Transducer imbalance	■ Make sure the transducer's flow system isn't kinked or occluded, and rebalance and recalibrate the equipment.
	■ Loose connection	■ Tighten loose connections.
Damped waveform	■ Air bubbles	■ Secure all connections. ■ Remove air from the lines and the transducer.[5] ■ Check for and replace cracked equipment.
	■ Blood clot in catheter	■ Try to aspirate the clot with a syringe. If the line still won't flush, notify the practitioner and prepare to replace the catheter, if necessary. *Important*: Never use a syringe to flush a hemodynamic catheter.
	■ Blood flashback in line	■ Make sure stopcock positions are correct; tighten loose connections and replace cracked equipment; flush the line with the fast-flush valve; replace the transducer if blood backs up into it.
	■ Incorrect transducer position	■ Be sure to keep the transducer at the level of the right atrium at all times. *Improper levels give false-high or false-low pressure readings.*
	■ Catheter displaced from a blood vessel or pressed against a vessel wall	■ Try to aspirate blood *to confirm proper placement in the vessel.* If you can't aspirate blood, notify the practitioner, who may try to reposition the catheter if it's against the vessel wall, or prepare to replace the line.[51] ■ Notify the practitioner immediately if you note bloody drainage at the insertion site; *the catheter may be displaced.*

REFERENCES

1 Standard 23. Central vascular access device (CVAD) tip location. Infusion therapy standards of practice. (8th ed.). (2021). *Journal of Infusion Nursing, 44*, S65–S69. (Level VI)

2 American Society of Anesthesiologists. (2012). Practice guidelines for central venous access: A report by the American Society of Anesthesiologists Task Force on Central Venous Access. *Anesthesiology, 116*, 539–573. https://pubs.asahq.org/anesthesiology/article/116/3/539/12984/Practice-Guidelines-for-Central-Venous-AccessA (Level VII)

3 Standard 33. Vascular access device placement. Infusion therapy standards of practice (8th ed.) (2021). *Journal of Infusion Nursing, 44*, S97–S101. (Level VII)

4 Standard 22. Vascular visualization. Infusion therapy standards of practice. (8th ed.) (2021). *Journal of Infusion Nursing, 44*, S63–S65. (Level VII)

5 Wiegand, D. L. (2017). *AACN procedure manual for high acuity, progressive, and critical care* (7th ed.). St. Louis, MO: Elsevier.

6 Jarrett, N., & Callaham, M. (2016). Evidence-based guidelines for selected hospital-acquired conditions: Final report. https://www.cms.gov/Medicare/Medicare-Fee-for-Service-Payment/HospitalAcqCond/Downloads/2016-HAC-Report.pdf

7 Association for Professionals in Infection Control and Epidemiology. (2015). Guide to preventing central line-associated bloodstream infections. https://apic.org/Resource_/TinyMceFileManager/2015/APIC_CLABSI_WEB.pdf (Level IV)

8 Centers for Disease Control and Prevention. (2011, revised 2017). Guidelines for the prevention of intravascular catheter-related infections. https://www.cdc.gov/infectioncontrol/guidelines/bsi/recommendations.html (Level I)

9 Marschall, J., et al. (2014). SHEA/IDSA practice recommendation: Strategies to prevent central line–associated bloodstream infections in acute care hospitals. *Infection Control and Hospital Epidemiology, 35*, 753–771. https://www.jstor.org/stable/10.1086/676533#metadata_info_tab_contents (Level I)

10 The Joint Commission. (2021). Standard NPSG.07.04.01. *Comprehensive accreditation manual for hospitals*. Oakbrook Terrace, IL: The Joint Commission. (Level VII)

11 Standard 50. Infection. Infusion therapy standards of practice. (8th ed.). (2021). *Journal of Infusion Nursing, 44*, S153–S157. (Level VII)

12 Infusion Nurses Society. (2016). *Policies and procedures for infusion therapy* (5th ed.). Boston, MA: Infusion Nurses Society.

13 Infusion Nurses Society. (2016). *Policies and procedures for infusion therapy of the older adult* (3rd ed.). Boston, MA: Infusion Nurses Society.

14 Association of Professionals in Infection Control and Epidemiology (APIC). (2016). APIC position paper: Safe injection, infusion, and medication vial practices in health care (2016). https://www.apic.org/Resource_/TinyMceFileManager/Position_Statements/2016APICSIPPositionPaper.pdf (Level VII)

15 Standard 12. Product evaluation, integrity, and defect reporting. Infusion therapy standards of practice. (8th ed.) (2021). *Journal of Infusion Nursing, 44*, S45–S46. (Level VII)

16 The Joint Commission. (2021). Standard NPSG.07.01.01. *Comprehensive accreditation manual for hospitals*. Oakbrook Terrace, IL: The Joint Commission. (Level VII)

17 Centers for Disease Control and Prevention. (2002). Guideline for hand hygiene in health-care settings: Recommendations of the Healthcare Infection Control Practices Advisory Committee and the HICPAC/SHEA/APIC/IDSA Hand Hygiene Task Force. *MMWR Recommendations and Reports, 51*(RR-16), 1–45. https://www.cdc.gov/mmwr/pdf/rr/rr5116.pdf (Level II)

18 World Health Organization. (2009). WHO guidelines on hand hygiene in health care: First global patient safety challenge, clean care is safer care. https://apps.who.int/iris/bitstream/handle/10665/44102/9789241597906_eng.pdf?sequence=1 (Level IV)

19 Centers for Medicare and Medicaid Services, Department of Health and Human Services. (2020). Condition of participation: Infection control. 42 C.F.R. § 482.42.

20 Accreditation Association for Hospitals and Health Systems. (2020). Standard 07.01.21. *Healthcare Facilities Accreditation Program: Accreditation requirements for acute care hospitals*. Chicago, IL: Accreditation Association for Hospitals and Health Systems. (Level VII)

21 DNV GL-Healthcare USA, Inc. (2020). IC.1.SR.1. *NIAHO® accreditation requirements, interpretive guidelines and surveyor guidance– revision 20.0*. Milford, OH: DNV GL-Healthcare USA, Inc. (Level VII)

22 Standard 16. Hand hygiene. Infusion therapy standards of practice (8th ed.). (2021). *Journal of Infusion Nursing, 44*, S53–S54. (Level VI)

23 The Joint Commission. (2021). Standard NPSG.01.01.01. *Comprehensive accreditation manual for hospitals*. Oakbrook Terrace, IL: The Joint Commission. (Level VII)

24 DNV GL-Healthcare USA, Inc. (2020). PR.2.SR.5. *NIAHO® accreditation requirements, interpretive guidelines and surveyor guidance—revision 20.0*. Milford, OH: DNV GL-Healthcare USA, Inc. (Level VII)

25 Centers for Medicare and Medicaid Services, Department of Health and Human Services. (2020). Condition of participation: Patient's rights. 42 C.F.R. § 482.13(c)(1).

26 Accreditation Association for Hospitals and Health Systems. (2020). Standard 15.01.16. *Healthcare Facilities Accreditation Program: Accreditation requirements for acute care hospitals*. Chicago, IL: Accreditation Association for Hospitals and Health Systems. (Level VII)

27 The Joint Commission. (2021). Standard RI.01.01.01. *Comprehensive accreditation manual for hospitals*. Oakbrook Terrace, IL: The Joint Commission. (Level VII)

28 The Joint Commission. (2021). Standard PC.02.01.21. *Comprehensive accreditation manual for hospitals*. Oakbrook Terrace, IL: The Joint Commission. (Level VII)

29 Waters, T. R., et al. (2009). Safe patient handling training for schools of nursing. https://www.cdc.gov/niosh/docs/2009-127/pdfs/2009-127.pdf (Level VII)

30 Siegel, J. D., et al. (2007, revised 2019). 2007 guideline for isolation precautions: Preventing transmission of infectious agents in healthcare settings. https://www.cdc.gov/infectioncontrol/pdf/guidelines/isolation-guidelines-H.pdf (Level II)

31 Accreditation Association for Hospitals and Health Systems. (2020). Standard 07.01.10. *Healthcare Facilities Accreditation Program: Accreditation requirements for acute care hospitals*. Chicago, IL: Accreditation Association for Hospitals and Health Systems. (Level VII)

32 Occupational Safety and Health Administration. (2012). Bloodborne pathogens, standard number1910.1030. https://www.osha.gov/pls/oshaweb/owadisp.show_document?p_id=10051&p_table=STANDARDS (Level VII)

33 Graham, K. C., & Cvach, M. (2010). Monitor alarm fatigue: Standardizing use of physiological monitors and decreasing nuisance alarms. *American Journal of Critical Care, 19*, 28–37.

34 The Joint Commission. (2020). Standard NPSG.06.01.01. *Comprehensive accreditation manual for hospitals*. Oakbrook Terrace, IL: The Joint Commission. (Level VII)

35 The Joint Commission. (2013). Sentinel event alert 50: Medical device alarm safety in hospitals. https://www.jointcommission.org/assets/1/6/SEA_50_alarms_4_26_16.pdf (Level VII)

36 American Association of Critical-Care Nurses. (2018). AACN practice alert: Managing alarms in acute care across the life span: Electrocardiography and pulse oximetry. https://www.aacn.org/clinical-resources/practice-alerts/managing-alarms-in-acute-care-across-the-life-span (Level VII)

37 U.S. Food and Drug Administration. (2017). Examples of medical device misconnections. https://www.fda.gov/medical-devices/medical-device-connectors/examples-medical-device-misconnections

38 Standard 59. Infusion medication and solution administration. Infusion therapy standards of practice. (8th ed.) (2021). *Journal of Infusion Nursing, 44*, S180–S182. (Level VII)

39 The Joint Commission. (2014). Sentinel event alert 53: Managing risk during transition to new ISO tubing connector standards. http://www.jointcommission.org/assets/1/6/SEA_53_Connectors_8_19_14_final.pdf (Level VII)

40 American Association of Critical-Care Nurses. (2016). AACN practice alert: PA/CVP monitoring in adults. https://www.aacn.org/clinical-resources/practice-alerts/pulmonary-artery-pressure-measurement (Level VII)

41 McGee, W. T.,, et al. (Eds.) (2018). *Edwards clinical education: Quick guide to cardiopulmonary care* (4th ed.). Irvine, CA: Edwards Lifesciences. https://edwardsprod.blob.core.windows.net/media/Gb/devices/monitoring/hemodynamic%20monitoring/quick-guide-to-pulmonary-care-4th-edition.pdf

42 Ganz, D. A., et al. (2013, reviewed 2021). *Preventing falls in hospitals: A toolkit for improving quality of care* (AHRQ Publication No. 13-0015-EF). Rockville, MD: Agency for Healthcare Research and Quality. https://www.ahrq.gov/professionals/systems/hospital/fallpxtoolkit/index.html (Level VII)

43 Rutala, W. A., et al. (2008, revised 2019). Guideline for disinfection and sterilization in healthcare facilities, 2008. https://www.cdc.gov/infectioncontrol/pdf/guidelines/disinfection-guidelines-H.pdf

44 Accreditation association for Hospitals and Health Systems. (2020). Standard 07.02.03. *Healthcare Facilities Accreditation Programs: Accreditation requirements for acute care hospitals*. Chicago, IL: Accreditation Association for Hospitals and Health Systems. (Level VII)

45 The Joint Commission. (2021). Standard RC.01.03.01. *Comprehensive accreditation manual for hospitals.* Oakbrook Terrace, IL: The Joint Commission. (Level VII)

46 Centers for Medicare and Medicaid Services, Department of Health and Human Services. (2020). Condition of participation: Medical record services. 42 C.F.R. § 482.24(b).

47 Accreditation Association for Hospitals and Health Systems. (2020). Standard 10.00.03. *Healthcare Facilities Accreditation Program: Accreditation requirements for acute care hospitals.* Chicago, IL: Accreditation Association for Hospitals and Health Systems. (Level VII)

48 DNV GL-Healthcare USA, Inc. (2020). MR.2.SR.1. *NIAHO® accreditation requirements, interpretive guidelines and surveyor guidance—revision 20.0.* Milford, OH: DNV GL-Healthcare USA, Inc. (Level VII)

49 Standard 10. Documentation in the health record. Infusion therapy standards of practice. (8th ed.) (2021). *Journal of Infusion Nursing, 44,* S39–S42. (Level VII)

50 Standard 49. Central vascular access device occlusion. Infusion therapy standards of practice. (8th ed.) (2021). *Journal of Infusion Nursing, 44,* S149–S153. (Level VII)

51 Standard 41. Flushing and locking. Infusion therapy standards of practice (8th ed.). (2021). *Journal of Infusion Nursing, 44,* S113–S118. (Level VII)

52 Standard 42. Vascular access device assessment, care, and dressing changes. Infusion therapy standards of practice (8th ed.). (2021). *Journal of Infusion Nursing, 44,* S119–S123. (Level VII)

53 Standard 43. Administration set change. Infusion therapy standards of practice (8th ed.) (2021). *Journal of Infusion Nursing, 44,* S123–S125. (Level VII)

CEREBROSPINAL FLUID DRAINAGE MANAGEMENT

Cerebrospinal fluid (CSF) drainage aims to reduce CSF pressure to the desired level and then to maintain it at that level.[1] CSF drainage techniques fall into two categories: internal and external.

Internal drainage devices, or shunts, are surgically implanted devices that divert CSF to the abdomen or heart when proper CSF absorption is impaired or obstructed, such as with hydrocephalus.

External drainage is indicated for obstructive hydrocephalus, subarachnoid hemorrhaging resulting in acute hydrocephalus due to obstruction of the arachnoid villi, Hunt and Hess grade 3 or higher subarachnoid hemorrhage, cerebral edema, surgical mass lesions, infections (such as meningitis), Chiara malformations, shunt failure caused by mechanical disruption or infection, and brain relaxation in an operation room (OR).[1] Therapeutic uses for external CSF drainage include intracranial pressure (ICP) monitoring via the ventriculostomy; direct instillation of medications, contrast media, or air for diagnostic radiology; and aspiration of CSF for laboratory analysis.[1]

This procedure focuses on managing external ventricular CSF drainage. (See *CSF drainage.*)

Equipment

External ventricular drainage set (includes drainage tubing and sterile drainage bag) ▪ paper tape or sterile connector device ▪ IV pole ▪ leveling device ▪ label ▪ vital signs monitoring equipment ▪ gloves ▪ Optional: other personal protective equipment.

Preparation of equipment

Inspect all equipment and supplies. If a product is expired, is defective, or has compromised integrity, remove it from patient use, label it as expired or defective, and report the expiration or defect as directed by your facility. After the practitioner inserts the catheter, connect the ICP monitoring system and external ventricular drainage system to the distal tip of the catheter. (See the "External ventricular drain insertion, assisting" procedure.) Trace the tubing from the patient to its point of origin *to ensure that the tubing is connected to the correct port.* Secure the connection points with paper tape or a sterile connector device. Ensure that the drainage tubing is clearly labeled *so that it isn't mistaken for IV tubing.*[1,2,3] Place the collection system, including the drip chamber and drainage bag, on an IV pole. Level the system at the level ordered by the practitioner.[4] Note that the practitioner may order a computed tomography scan *to confirm catheter placement.*[1]

Implementation

▪ Verify the practitioner's orders.
▪ Gather and prepare the necessary equipment and supplies.

EQUIPMENT

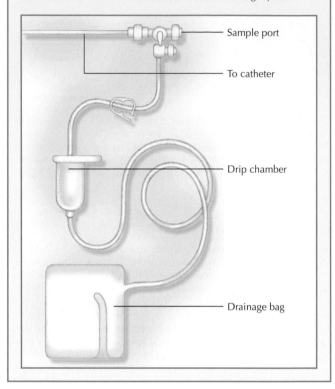

CSF drainage

Cerebrospinal fluid (CSF) drainage aims to control intracranial pressure (ICP) during treatment for traumatic injury or other conditions that cause a rise in ICP. To insert a ventricular CSF drain, a practitioner makes a burr hole in the patient's skull and inserts a catheter into the ventricle. The distal end of the catheter is connected to a closed drainage system.

▪ Perform hand hygiene.[5,6,7,8,9,10]
▪ Confirm the patient's identity using at least two patient identifiers.[11]
▪ Provide privacy.[12,13,14,15]
▪ Explain the procedure to the patient and family (if appropriate) according to their individual communication and learning needs *to increase their understanding, allay their fears, and enhance cooperation.*[16]
▪ Check the patient's positioning *to ensure that the drip chamber of the ICP monitoring system is located at the ordered reference level.*[1,4]
▪ Perform hand hygiene.[6,7,8,9,10]
▪ Put on gloves and other personal protective equipment as needed *to comply with standard precautions.*[17,18,19]
▪ Trace the drainage tubing from the patient to its point of origin *to make sure you're accessing the correct tubing.* Ensure that the drainage tubing is labeled clearly *so that it isn't mistaken for IV tubing.*[1,2,3]
▪ If the patient is active or moving around in bed, frequently assess that the ventricular drain is leveled appropriately *to prevent overdrainage and underdrainage.* The flow rate of CSF drainage is regulated by raising the pressure level on the drip chamber above the foramen of Monro, which is the zero reference level.[1,4]
▪ Ensure that the CSF drainage system is clamped or open appropriately, according to the practitioner's order. Depending on the patient's condition, the practitioner may keep the ventricular drain stopcock set to "off" to the drain and "open" to the transducer for continuous ICP monitoring. When ICP reaches a predetermined pressure, the practitioner may order the stopcock open *to drain CSF for a short period.* Alternately, the practitioner may order continuous drainage with intermittent stopcock closings for ICP readings.[1]
▪ Check the CSF drainage system for patency, as needed, by lowering the entire system briefly to assess the drip rate into the drip chamber.[1]
▪ Perform a neurologic assessment and obtain the patient's vital signs hourly, or more frequently if the patient's condition warrants. Assess for signs and symptoms of increased ICP, including decreased level of consciousness, nausea, vomiting, headache, lethargy, and agitation.[1,4]

■ Obtain mean hourly ICP, and notify the practitioner immediately if ICP exceeds the established parameter; if no parameter has been established, notify the practitioner if ICP rises above 20 mm Hg. Assess ICP in relation to the patient's mean arterial pressure *to provide an indicator of the patient's cerebral perfusion pressure.*[1] Obtain ICP more frequently if ICP is increased.[1]

NURSING ALERT To obtain accurate ICP and waveform readings, set the stopcock "off" to the drain and "open" to the transducer. Note that the ventricular drainage system can drain CSF or monitor ICP; it can't perform both functions at the same time.[1]

■ Assess the CSF drainage volume, color, and clarity, and notify the practitioner if the appearance or volume changes. If the catheter remains open to drainage, maintain a continual hourly output record of CSF *to prevent overdrainage and underdrainage.* Overdrainage can occur if the drip chamber is placed too far below the catheter insertion site. Underdrainage can result from kinked tubing, catheter displacement, clot formation, or a drip chamber placed higher than the catheter insertion site.[1,4]

■ Assess the CSF drainage system at least every 4 hours, and more frequently if the patient's condition warrants; begin the inspection at the insertion site and continue along the entire drainage system. Check for cracks in the system or fluid leaking from the insertion site, and assess the condition of the dressing *to prevent the risk of infection and overdrainage.*[20]

■ Remove and discard any other personal protective equipment worn.[17,18,19]

■ Perform hand hygiene.[5,6,7,8,9,10]

■ Document the procedure.[21,22,23,24]

Special considerations

■ Follow strict sterile technique, and wear sterile gloves and a mask with a face shield when connecting tubing, flushing the system, changing the drainage bag, obtaining specimens from the drainage system, and changing dressings *to reduce the risk of infection.*[1,4,17,18,19]

■ If a CSF specimen is needed for laboratory analysis, use strict sterile technique when accessing the external drainage system.[17,18,19] After performing hand hygiene, put on a mask and sterile gloves, and set up a sterile field. Clean the access port with a facility-approved antiseptic and allow it to dry completely.[4] Obtain the CSF specimen, label the specimen container in the presence of the patient, place it in a laboratory transport bag, and send it to the laboratory.[11,25]

■ Monitor ICP waveforms *to detect changes* and troubleshoot when necessary. (See the "Intracranial pressure monitoring" procedure.)[1]

■ Be aware that a patient may experience a chronic headache during continuous CSF drainage. Reassure the patient that this effect isn't unusual; administer analgesics, as ordered and needed, following safe medication administration practices.[26,27,28,29]

■ Avoid transferring a patient away from the patient floor to perform tests and procedures, when possible, *to prevent catheter dislodgment.* Check for the option of performing such tests and procedures at the patient's bedside. If a patient must be transported, keep the drainage system upright and aligned with the patient, and clarify with the practitioner if the drainage system needs to be turned off during transport and reopened at the destination.

■ The Joint Commission issued a sentinel event alert related to managing risk during transition to new International Organization for Standardization tubing standards that were designed to prevent dangerous tubing misconnections, which can lead to serious patient injury and death. During the transition, make sure to trace the tubing and catheter from the patient to the point of origin before connecting or reconnecting any device or infusion, at any care transition (such as a new setting or service), and as part of the hand-off process. In addition, route tubes and catheters with different purposes in different, standardized directions; label tubing at both the distal and proximal ends when the patient has different access sites or several bags hanging; use tubing and equipment only as intended; and store medications for different delivery routes in separate locations.[3]

Patient teaching

Teach the patient and family (if appropriate) about the reason for the drain. Explain that the patient's activity level must be restricted during CSF drainage. The patient may not sit up, stand, or walk when the drain is open, and the patient must ask for assistance with any movement. Instruct the patient to avoid straining, coughing, and sneezing during CSF drainage.

Complications

Signs of overdrainage of CSF include headache, tachycardia, diaphoresis, and nausea. Acute CSF overdrainage may result in collapsed ventricles, tentorial herniation, and medullary compression.

NURSING ALERT If CSF drains too rapidly, clamp the system, notify the practitioner immediately, and perform a complete neurologic assessment, *because this complication constitutes a potential neurosurgical emergency.*

Cessation of CSF drainage may indicate clot formation. If you can't quickly identify the cause of the obstruction, notify the practitioner. If CSF drainage is blocked, the patient may develop signs and symptoms of increased ICP. Failure to follow strict sterile technique can lead to infection, including meningitis.

Documentation

Record vital signs, ICP, and neurologic assessment findings at a frequency determined by your facility or the patient's condition. Document whether the drainage system remains opened or clamped, and verify the patency of the drainage system. Also document the level of the drip chamber and the anatomic landmarks used for zeroing.

Document the condition of the dressing and insertion site. Also document the color, clarity, and amount of CSF drained at a frequency determined by your facility or the patient's condition. Document any unexpected outcomes or complications, the name of the practitioner notified, the date and time of notification, any prescribed interventions, and the patient's response to those interventions. Document teaching provided to the patient and family (if applicable), their understanding of that teaching, and any need for follow-up teaching.

REFERENCES

1 American Association of Neuroscience Nurses (AANN). (2014). *Care of the patient undergoing intracranial pressure monitoring/external ventricular drainage or lumbar drainage: AANN clinical practice guideline series.* Glenview, IL: AANN. (Level VII)

2 U.S. Food and Drug Administration. (2017). Examples of medical device misconnections. https://www.fda.gov/medical-devices/medical-device-connectors/examples-medical-device-misconnections

3 The Joint Commission. (2014). Sentinel event alert: Managing risk during transition to new ISO tubing connector standards. http://www.jointcommission.org/assets/1/6/SEA_53_Connectors_8_19_14_final.pdf (Level VII)

4 Wiegand, D. L. (2017). *AACN procedure manual for high acuity, progressive, and critical care* (7th ed.). St. Louis, MO: Elsevier.

5 The Joint Commission. (2021). Standard NPSG.07.01.01. *Comprehensive accreditation manual for hospitals.* Oakbrook Terrace, IL: The Joint Commission. (Level VII)

6 Centers for Disease Control and Prevention. (2002). Guideline for hand hygiene in health-care settings: Recommendations of the Healthcare Infection Control Practices Advisory Committee and the HICPAC/SHEA/APIC/IDSA Hand Hygiene Task Force. *MMWR Recommendations and Reports, 51*(RR-16), 1–45. https://www.cdc.gov/mmwr/pdf/rr/rr5116.pdf (Level II)

7 World Health Organization. (2009). WHO guidelines on hand hygiene in health care: First global patient safety challenge, clean care is safer care. https://apps.who.int/iris/bitstream/handle/10665/44102/9789241597906_eng.pdf?sequence=1 (Level IV)

8 Accreditation Association of Hospitals and Health Systems. (2020). Standard 07.01.21. *Healthcare Facilities Accreditation Program: Accreditation requirements for acute care hospitals.* Chicago, IL: Accreditation Association of Hospitals and Health Systems. (Level VII)

9 Centers for Medicare and Medicaid Services, Department of Health and Human Services. (2020). Condition of participation: Infection control. 42 C.F.R. § 482.42.

10 DNV GL-Healthcare USA, Inc. (2020). IC.1.SR.1. *NIAHO® accreditation requirements, interpretive guidelines and surveyor guidance—revision 20.0.* Milford, OH: DNV GL-Healthcare USA, Inc. (Level VII)

11 The Joint Commission. (2021). Standard NPSG.01.01.01. *Comprehensive accreditation manual for hospitals.* Oakbrook Terrace, IL: The Joint Commission. (Level VII)

12 Accreditation Association for Hospitals and Health Systems. (2020). Standard 15.01.16. *Healthcare Facilities Accreditation Program: Accreditation requirements for acute care hospitals.* Chicago, IL: Accreditation Association for Hospitals and Health Systems. (Level VII)

162 CERVICAL COLLAR APPLICATION

13 Centers for Medicare and Medicaid Services, Department of Health and Human Services. (2020). Condition of participation: Patient's rights. 42 C.F.R. § 482.13(c)(1).

14 DNV GL-Healthcare USA, Inc. (2020). PR.2.SR.5. *NIAHO® accreditation requirements, interpretive guidelines and surveyor guidance—revision 20.0.* Milford, OH: DNV GL-Healthcare USA, Inc. (Level VII)

15 The Joint Commission. (2021). Standard RI.01.01.01. *Comprehensive accreditation manual for hospitals.* Oakbrook Terrace, IL: The Joint Commission. (Level VII)

16 The Joint Commission. (2021). Standard PC.02.01.21. *Comprehensive accreditation manual for hospitals.* Oakbrook Terrace, IL: The Joint Commission. (Level VII)

17 Siegel, J. D., et al. (2007, revised 2019). 2007 guideline for isolation precautions: Preventing transmission of infectious agents in healthcare settings. https://www.cdc.gov/infectioncontrol/pdf/guidelines/isolation-guidelines-H.pdf (Level II)

18 Accreditation Association of Hospitals and Health Systems. (2020). Standard 07.01.10. *Healthcare Facilities Accreditation Program: Accreditation requirements for acute care hospitals.* Chicago, IL: Accreditation Association of Hospitals and Health Systems. (Level VII)

19 The Joint Commission. (2021). Standard IC.02.01.01. *Comprehensive accreditation manual for hospitals.* Oakbrook Terrace, IL: The Joint Commission. (Level VII)

20 Bader, M. K., & Littlejohns, L. R., (Eds.). (2016). *AANN core curriculum for neuroscience nursing* (6th ed.). Glenview, IL: American Association of Neuroscience Nurses (AANN).

21 The Joint Commission. (2021). Standard RC.01.03.01. *Comprehensive accreditation manual for hospitals.* Oakbrook Terrace, IL: The Joint Commission. (Level VII)

22 Accreditation Association of Hospitals and Health Systems. (2020). Standard 10.00.03. *Healthcare Facilities Accreditation Program: Accreditation requirements for acute care hospitals.* Chicago, IL: Accreditation Association of Hospitals and Health Systems. (Level VII)

23 Centers for Medicare and Medicaid Services, Department of Health and Human Services. (2020). Condition of participation: Medical record services. 42 C.F.R. § 482.24(b).

24 DNV GL-Healthcare USA, Inc. (2020). MR.2.SR.1. *NIAHO® accreditation requirements, interpretive guidelines and surveyor guidance—revision 20.0.* Milford, OH: DNV GL-Healthcare USA, Inc. (Level VII)

25 Occupational Safety and Health Administration. (2012). Bloodborne pathogens, standard number1910.1030. https://www.osha.gov/pls/oshaweb/owadisp.show_document?p_id=10051&p_table=STANDARDS (Level VII)

26 Accreditation Association for Hospitals and Health Systems. (2020). Standard 16.01.03. *Healthcare Facilities Accreditation Program: Accreditation requirements for acute care hospitals.* Chicago, IL: Accreditation Association for Hospitals and Health Systems. (Level VII)

27 Centers for Medicare and Medicaid Services, Department of Health and Human Services. (2020). Condition of participation: Nursing services. 42 C.F.R. § 482.23(c).

28 DNV GL-Healthcare USA, Inc. (2020). MM.1.SR.3. *NIAHO® accreditation requirements, interpretive guidelines and surveyor guidance—revision 20.0.* Milford, OH: DNV GL-Healthcare USA, Inc. (Level VII)

29 The Joint Commission. (2021). Standard MM.06.01.01. *Comprehensive accreditation manual for hospitals.* Oakbrook Terrace, IL: The Joint Commission. (Level VII)

CERVICAL COLLAR APPLICATION

A cervical collar may be used for an nonacute injury (such as strained cervical muscles) or a chronic condition (such as arthritis or cervical metastasis). A cervical collar may also be used to prevent cervical spine fracture or spinal cord damage after an acute injury. The routine use of a cervical collar for spinal immobilization in the prehospital trauma patient is controversial because the risks may outweigh the benefits.[1,2,3]

Designed to keep the neck centrally aligned with the chin slightly elevated, the collar immobilizes the cervical spine, decreases muscle spasms, and reduces pain, prevents further injury, and promotes healing. Cervical collar size is usually based on the patient's height, weight, and physical stature. Only specially trained health care practitioners should apply and remove a cervical collar used for an acute injury. Great care is necessary when applying and removing a cervical collar in a patient with an acute injury to limit motion and protect the spinal cord

from mechanical damage.[4] At least two qualified members of the health care team must apply the initial cervical collar: One member should institute and maintain cervical spine precautions by maintaining the patient's head, neck, and airway in proper alignment, and the second should apply the collar.[5]

Equipment

Cervical collar in the appropriate size ▪ stethoscope ▪ vital signs monitoring equipment ▪ disinfectant pad ▪ Optional: gloves, gown, face shield, goggles, mask, prescribed pain medication.

Preparation of equipment

Inspect all equipment and supplies. If a product is expired, is defective, or has compromised integrity, remove it from patient use, label it as expired or defective, and report the expiration or defect as directed by your facility. Follow the manufacturer's instructions for proper sizing and cervical collar preparation.

Implementation

▪ Verify the practitioner's order.
▪ Gather and prepare the necessary equipment and supplies.
▪ Elicit the assistance of a coworker to help immobilize the patient's cervical spine. Use cervical spine precautions (such as maintaining the patient's head, neck, and airway in proper alignment).[5]
▪ Perform hand hygiene.[6,7,8,9,10,11]
▪ Confirm the patient's identity using at least two patient identifiers.[12]
▪ Provide privacy.[13,14,15,16]
▪ Explain the application procedure to the patient and the patient's family (if appropriate) according to their communication and learning needs *to increase their understanding, allay their fears, and enhance cooperation.*[17] Explain to the patient the importance of remaining still during the procedure *to prevent neurologic injury.*
▪ Obtain the patient's vital signs and assess skin integrity and neurologic and respiratory status *to serve as baselines for comparison after the procedure.*[18]
▪ Remove an appropriate-sized collar from its packaging. Identify the anterior and posterior positions of the collar. If required, assemble the collar and make sure that the padding is secure.
▪ Perform hand hygiene.[6,7,8,9,10,11]
▪ Put on gloves and other personal protective equipment *to comply with standard precautions.*[19,20,21]
▪ Position the patient with the arms at the sides, shoulders down, and head aligned centrally. Don't place a pillow under the patient's head.[5]
▪ With the help of a coworker, use cervical spine precautions and gently slide the posterior portion of the collar behind the patient's neck (as shown below), and center it.[5,22] If the patient has long hair, place it outside of the collar.[5]

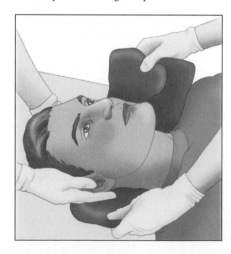

▪ Flare the sides of the anterior portion of the collar outward (as shown). Apply the anterior portion of the collar by sliding it up the patient's chest and scooping it under the chin.[5,22] Make sure that the sides of the anterior portion of the collar are oriented upward, off the trapezius muscle and toward the patient's ears.

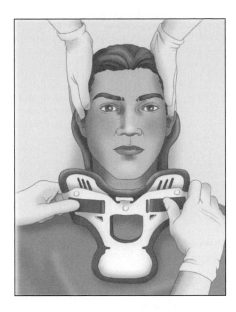

■ While holding the anterior portion of the collar securely, curl the ends snugly against the patient's neck.[5]

■ Apply the Velcro straps one side at a time (as shown below). Place the front of the collar inside the back (as directed by the manufacturer) and alternately tighten the straps, one at a time, until they're an equal length on both sides.[5] Always follow the manufacturer's instructions; some collars must be applied so that the anterior portion overlaps the posterior portion of the collar.[23]

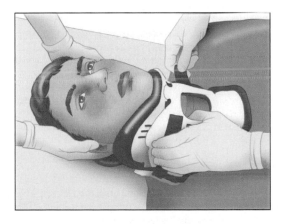

■ Assess the patient to make sure the collar fits properly; *it must fit snugly and be secure to maintain alignment and immobilization.* If the patient can slip the chin inside the collar, the collar isn't sufficiently snug.[5] Replace the collar with a better-fitting collar if you can't get the existing collar to fit snugly.

■ Obtain the patient's vital signs and reassess neurologic and respiratory status. Compare your results to baseline data *to detect complications associated with collar application. A semi-rigid cervical collar can compress the jugular veins and thus increase intracranial pressure, and possibly restrict the airway.*[24]

■ Make a final assessment *to ensure that you've properly applied the collar.* Make sure that the collar extends from the patient's jaw to just below the sternal notch; the patient's chin is centered comfortably in the chin piece; the straps are both the same length; the sides of the posterior portion of the collar overlap the sides of the anterior portion (if appropriate); the front of the collar is angled upward toward the patient's ears; the lower edges of the collar aren't resting on the patient's clavicles or digging into the shoulders; and the pads extend beyond the plastic edges.[5]

■ Screen for and assess the patient's pain using facility-defined criteria that are consistent with the patient's age, condition, and ability to understand.[25]

■ Treat the patient's pain, as needed and ordered, using nonpharmacologic, pharmacologic, or a combination of approaches. Base the treatment plan on evidence-based practices and the patient's clinical condition, past medical history, and pain management goals.[25]

■ Remove and discard your gloves and other personal protective equipment, if worn.[19]

■ Perform hand hygiene.[6,7,8,9,10,11]

■ Clean and disinfect your stethoscope with a disinfectant pad.[26,27]

■ Perform hand hygiene.[6,7,8,9,10,11]

■ Arrange for a cervical spine X-ray, if ordered, *to assess and document cervical spine alignment after the procedure.*

■ Document the procedure.[28,29,30,31]

Special considerations

■ Inspect the patient's skin under and around the cervical collar at least twice daily for signs of pressure-related injury. Conduct more frequent assessments in patients vulnerable to fluid shifts or in those who are exhibiting signs of localized or generalized edema.[32]

Patient teaching

If the patient will be going home with a cervical collar, teach the patient and family (if appropriate) how to remove the collar, provide skin care, replace moist or soiled padding, and reapply the collar. Make sure that they can perform a successful return demonstration of the procedure before discharge.

During discharge planning, teach the patient and family about pain management strategies. Include information about the patient's pain management plan and adverse effects of pain management treatment. Discuss activities of daily living and items in the home environment that may exacerbate pain or reduce the effectiveness of the pain management plan, and include strategies to address these issues. Teach the patient and family about the safe use, storage, and disposal of opioids, if prescribed.[25]

Complications

Complications associated with cervical collar application include airway compromise, skin breakdown, increased risk for aspiration, increased intracranial pressure, increased agitation, and neurologic injury.[33]

Documentation

Note the type and size of the cervical collar and the date and time of application. Record the results of neurovascular checks. Document patient comfort, the collar's snugness, and all patient instructions provided. Document any medications administered, any adverse reactions to the prescribed medications, the date and time the practitioner was notified, prescribed interventions, and the patient's response to those interventions. Document teaching provided to the patient and family (if appropriate), their understanding of that teaching, and any need for follow-up teaching.

REFERENCES

1 Sundstrøm, T., et al. (2014). Prehospital use of cervical collars in trauma patients: A critical review. *Journal of Neurotrauma, 31*(6), 531–540. https://www.ncbi.nlm.nih.gov/pmc/articles/PMC3949434/ (Level V)

2 Montrief, T. (2018). Cervical collar: Friend or foe? https://www.emra.org/emresident/article/cervical-collar/

3 American College of Emergency Physicians. (2015). EMS management of patients with potential spinal injury. *Annals of Emergency Medicine, 66*(4), 445. https://www.annemergmed.com/article/S0196-0644(15)01100-2/fulltext (Level VII)

4 Prasarn, M. L., et al. (2012). Motion generated in the unstable cervical spine during the application and removal of cervical immobilization collars. *Journal of Trauma and Acute Care Surgery, 72,* 1609–1613.

5 Össur. (2019). Miami J®: Sizing and application instructions. https://assets.ossur.com/library/41069/Miami%20J%20Instructions%20for%20use.pdf

6 The Joint Commission. (2021). Standard NPSG.07.01.01. *Comprehensive accreditation manual for hospitals.* Oakbrook Terrace, IL: The Joint Commission. (Level VII)

7 Centers for Disease Control and Prevention. (2002). Guideline for hand hygiene in health-care settings: Recommendations of the Healthcare Infection Control Practices Advisory Committee and the HICPAC/SHEA/APIC/IDSA

Hand Hygiene Task Force. *MMWR Recommendations and Reports, 51*(RR-16), 1–45. https://www.cdc.gov/mmwr/pdf/rr/rr5116.pdf (Level II)

8 World Health Organization. (2009). WHO guidelines on hand hygiene in health care: First global patient safety challenge, clean care is safer care. https://apps.who.int/iris/bitstream/handle/10665/44102/9789241597906_eng.pdf (Level IV)

9 Centers for Medicare and Medicaid Services, Department of Health and Human Services. (2020). Condition of participation: Infection control. 42 C.F.R. § 482.42.

10 Accreditation Association for Hospitals and Health Systems. (2020). Standard 07.01.21. *Healthcare Facilities Accreditation Program: Accreditation requirements for acute care hospitals.* Chicago, IL: Accreditation Association for Hospitals and Health Systems. (Level VII)

11 DNV GL-Healthcare USA, Inc. (2020). IC.1.SR.1. *NIAHO® accreditation requirements, interpretive guidelines and surveyor guidance—revision 20.0.* Milford, OH: DNV GL-Healthcare USA, Inc. (Level VII)

12 The Joint Commission. (2021). Standard NPSG.01.01.01. *Comprehensive accreditation manual for hospitals.* Oakbrook Terrace, IL: The Joint Commission. (Level VII)

13 Accreditation Association for Hospitals and Health Systems. (2020). Standard 15.01.16. *Healthcare Facilities Accreditation Program: Accreditation requirements for acute care hospitals.* Chicago, IL: Accreditation Association for Hospitals and Health Systems. (Level VII)

14 Centers for Medicare and Medicaid Services, Department of Health and Human Services. (2020). Condition of participation: Patient's rights. 42 C.F.R. § 482.13(c)(1).

15 The Joint Commission. (2021). Standard RI.01.01.01. *Comprehensive accreditation manual for hospitals.* Oakbrook Terrace, IL: The Joint Commission. (Level VII)

16 DNV GL-Healthcare USA, Inc. (2020). PR.2.SR.5. *NIAHO® accreditation requirements, interpretive guidelines and surveyor guidance—revision 20.0.* Milford, OH: DNV GL-Healthcare USA, Inc. (Level VII)

17 The Joint Commission. (2021). Standard PC.02.01.21. *Comprehensive accreditation manual for hospitals.* Oakbrook Terrace, IL: The Joint Commission. (Level VII)

18 The Joint Commission. (2021). Standard PC.01.02.01. *Comprehensive accreditation manual for hospitals.* Oakbrook Terrace, IL: The Joint Commission. (Level VII)

19 Occupational Safety and Health Administration. (2012). Bloodborne pathogens, standard number1910.1030. https://www.osha.gov/pls/oshaweb/owadisp.show_document?p_id=10051&p_table=STANDARDS (Level VII)

20 Siegel, J. D., et al. (2007, revised 2019). 2007 guideline for isolation precautions: Preventing transmission of infectious agents in healthcare settings. https://www.cdc.gov/infectioncontrol/pdf/guidelines/isolation-guidelines-H.pdf (Level II)

21 Accreditation Association for Hospitals and Health Systems. (2020). Standard 07.01.10. *Healthcare Facilities Accreditation Program: Accreditation requirements for acute care hospitals.* Chicago, IL: Accreditation Association for Hospitals and Health Systems. (Level VII)

22 Össur. (2016). NecLoc® and NecLoc® Kids: Instructions for use. https://assets.ossur.com/library/7073/NecLoc%20Extrication%20Collar%20Instructions%20for%20use.pdf

23 Össur. (2019). Adjustable Philadelphia tracheotomy collar: Instructions for use. https://assets.ossur.com/library/41183/Philadelphia%20Adjustable%20Instructions%20for%20use%20-%20Adjustable%20Philadelphia%20Tracheotomy%20Collar.pdf

24 Sparke, A., et al. (2013). The measurement of tissue interface pressures and changes in jugular venous parameters associated with cervical immobilisation devices: A systematic review. *Scandinavian Journal of Trauma, Resuscitation, and Emergency Medicine, 21*, 81. https://www.ncbi.nlm.nih.gov/pmc/articles/PMC4222127/ (Level I)

25 The Joint Commission. (2021). Standard PC.01.02.07. *Comprehensive accreditation manual for hospitals.* Oakbrook Terrace, IL: The Joint Commission. (Level VII)

26 Accreditation Association for Hospitals and Health Systems. (2020). Standard 07.02.03. *Healthcare Facilities Accreditation Program: Accreditation requirements for acute care hospitals.* Chicago, IL: Accreditation Association for Hospitals and Health Systems. (Level VII)

27 Rutala, W. A., et al. (2008, revised 2019). Guideline for disinfection and sterilization in healthcare facilities, 2008. https://www.cdc.gov/infectioncontrol/pdf/guidelines/disinfection-guidelines-H.pdf (Level I)

28 The Joint Commission. (2021). Standard RC.01.03.01. *Comprehensive accreditation manual for hospitals.* Oakbrook Terrace, IL: The Joint Commission. (Level VII)

29 Centers for Medicare and Medicaid Services, Department of Health and Human Services. (2020). Condition of participation: Medical record services. 42 C.F.R. § 482.24(b).

30 Accreditation Association for Hospitals and Health Systems. (2020). Standard 10.00.03. *Healthcare Facilities Accreditation Program: Accreditation requirements for acute care hospitals.* Chicago, IL: Accreditation Association for Hospitals and Health Systems. (Level VII)

31 DNV GL-Healthcare USA, Inc. (2020). MR.2.SR.1. *NIAHO® accreditation requirements, interpretive guidelines and surveyor guidance—revision 20.0.* Milford, OH: DNV GL-Healthcare USA, Inc. (Level VII)

32 European Pressure Ulcer Advisory Panel, et al. (2019). Prevention and treatment of pressure ulcers/injuries: Quick reference guide. http://www.internationalguideline.com/static/pdfs/Quick_Reference_Guide-10Mar2019.pdf (Level VII)

33 Ham, H. W., et al. (2014). Cervical collar-related pressure ulcers in trauma patients in intensive care unit. *Journal of Trauma Nursing, 21*, 94–102. (Level IV)

CHEST PHYSIOTHERAPY

Chest physiotherapy is a type of bronchial hygiene that helps mobilize secretions through gravity and external manipulation of a patient's chest using such techniques as effective coughing, postural drainage, and chest percussion and vibration.[1] Postural drainage uses various body positions to drain secretions from each of the patient's lung segments into the central airways, where they can be removed by coughing or suctioning.[1,2] Gravity assists drainage when patient positioning places the segmental bronchus to be drained in a more vertical position.[1] The patient is typically maintained in each position for 3 to 15 minutes (or longer for such conditions as cystic fibrosis); however, positioning should be modified according to the patient's condition and tolerance.[1] (See *Positioning patients for postural drainage.*)

Patients with copious secretions, inability to mobilize and expectorate secretions, or pulmonary conditions associated with retained secretions (such as cystic fibrosis, bronchiectasis, and ciliary dyskinetic syndromes) may benefit from chest physiotherapy.[1,2,3]

For absolute and relative contraindications to check physiotherapy, see *Contraindications to chest physiotherapy.* In patients with relative contraindications, the potential risks should be weighed against the potential benefits of therapy.[1,3,4,5]

Equipment

Vital signs monitoring equipment ▪ stethoscope ▪ pillows or towels ▪ facial tissues ▪ oral care supplies ▪ disinfectant pad ▪ suction equipment ▪ no-touch receptacle[6] ▪ Optional: pulse oximeter and probe, resuscitation bag and mask, sterile specimen collection container, labels, laboratory transport bag, gloves, gown, mask with face shield, mask, goggles, supplemental oxygen, prescribed pain medication.

Preparation of equipment

Inspect all equipment and supplies. If a product is expired, is defective, or has compromised integrity, remove it from patient use, label it as expired or defective, and report the expiration or defect as directed by your facility. Set up the suction equipment as well as the resuscitation bag and mask; make sure that they're functioning properly.

Implementation

▪ Verify the practitioner's order.
▪ Review the medical record for contraindications to the procedure and for the patient's latest chest X-ray report (if applicable) *to identify the appropriate lung lobes and segments for drainage.*[1]
▪ *To reduce the risk of gastroesophageal reflux and possible aspiration,* schedule therapy before or at least 1½ hours after meals or tube feedings, if possible.[1]
▪ Gather and prepare the necessary equipment and supplies.
▪ Perform hand hygiene.[7,8,9,10,11,12]
▪ Confirm the patient's identity using at least two patient identifiers.[13]
▪ Provide privacy.[14,15,16,17]

Positioning patients for postural drainage

The following illustrations show the various postural drainage positions and the areas of the lungs affected by each position. Before beginning, assess whether the patient can tolerate the recommended positioning; once the patient is positioned, perform ongoing assessments *to determine continued tolerance.*

Lower lobes: Posterior basal segments

Elevate the foot of the bed 30 degrees. Have the patient lie prone with head lowered. Position pillows under the chest and abdomen. Percuss the lower ribs on both sides of the spine.

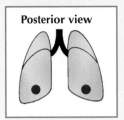

Posterior view

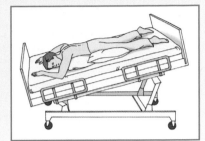

Lower lobes: Lateral basal segments

Elevate the foot of the bed 30 degrees. Instruct the patient to lie on the abdomen with head lowered and upper leg flexed over a pillow *for support.* To percuss the right lateral segment, position the patient on the left side; if percussion is to be performed on the left lateral segment, position the patient on the right side.[1] Then instruct the patient to rotate a quarter turn upward. Percuss the lower ribs on the uppermost portion of the lateral chest wall.

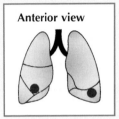

Anterior view

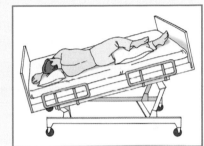

Lower lobes: Anterior basal segments

Elevate the foot of the bed 30 degrees. Instruct the patient to lie on the side with head lowered. Then place pillows under the patient's head and between the knees. Percuss with a slightly cupped hand over the lower ribs just beneath the axilla. If an acutely ill patient has trouble breathing in this position, adjust the bed to an angle the patient can tolerate. Then begin percussion.

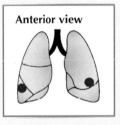

Anterior view

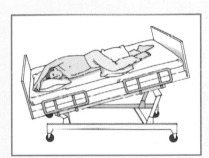

Lower lobes: Superior segments

With the bed flat, have the patient to lie prone. Place two pillows under the hips. Percuss on both sides of the spine at the lower tip of the scapulae.

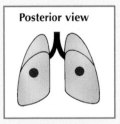

Posterior view

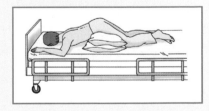

Right middle lobe: Medial and lateral segments

Elevate the foot of the bed 15 degrees. Have the patient lie on the left side with head down and knees flexed. Then have the patient rotate a quarter turn backward. Place a pillow beneath the patient to support the back and buttock area. Percuss with a moderately cupped hand under the right nipple. For a female patient, cup your hand so that its heel is under the armpit and your fingers extend forward beneath the breast.

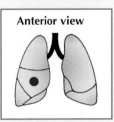

Anterior view

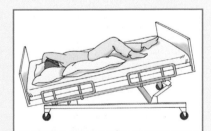

(Continued)

Positioning patients for postural drainage *(continued)*

Left upper lobe: Superior and inferior segments, lingular portion

Elevate the foot of the bed 15 degrees. Have the patient lie on the right side with head down and knees flexed. Then have the patient rotate a quarter turn backward. Place a pillow behind the patient, from shoulders to hips. Percuss with your hand moderately cupped over the left nipple. For a female patient, cup your hand so that its heel is beneath the armpit and your fingers extend forward beneath the breast.

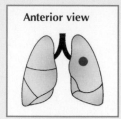

Anterior view

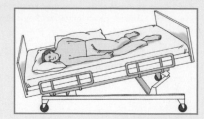

Upper lobes: Anterior segments

Ensure the bed is flat. Have the patient lie supine with a pillow folded under the knees. Then have the patient rotate slightly away from the side being drained. Percuss between clavicle and nipple.

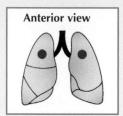

Anterior view

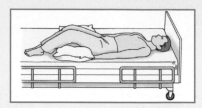

Upper lobes: Apical segments

Keep the bed flat. Assist the patient to a sitting position at the side of the bed. Instruct the patient lean back at a 30-degree angle against you and a pillow. Percuss with a cupped hand between the clavicles and the top of each scapula.

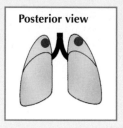

Posterior view

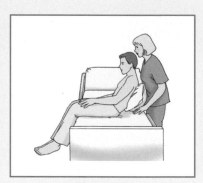

Upper lobes: Posterior segments

Keep the bed flat. Have the patient lean over a pillow at a 30-degree angle. Percuss and clap the upper back on each side.

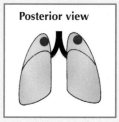

Posterior view

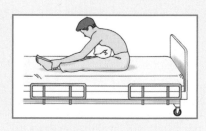

■ Explain the procedure to the patient and family (if appropriate) according to their individual communication and learning needs *to increase their understanding, allay their fears, and enhance cooperation.*[18]

■ Raise the patient's bed to waist level before providing care *to prevent caregiver back strain.*[19]

■ Perform hand hygiene.[7,8,9,10,11,12]

■ Put on gloves, a gown, and a mask with face shield or a mask and goggles, as needed, *to comply with standard precautions.*[20,21]

■ Obtain the patient's vital signs, auscultate breath sounds, and obtain oxygen saturation level by pulse oximetry (if necessary) *to determine the baseline status for monitoring the patient's response to therapy.*[1]

■ Screen for and assess the patient's pain using facility-defined criteria that are consistent with the patient's age, condition, and ability to understand.[22]

■ Treat the patient's pain, as needed and ordered, using nonpharmacologic, pharmacologic, or a combination of approaches. Base the treatment plan on evidence-based practices and the patient's clinical condition, past medical history, and pain management goals.[23,24,25,26]

■ Inspect the patient's monitoring equipment, IV catheters and tubing, oxygen therapy equipment, and other equipment *to ensure that patient repositioning doesn't cause pain or accidental disconnections.* If needed, make adjustments to the equipment or therapy.[1]

■ Position the patient for postural drainage, as indicated, *to use gravity to promote drainage from dependent lung areas to larger, more central airways.*[3] Drainage typically begins with the lower lobes, continues with the middle lobes, and ends with the upper lobes. Use pillows or towels *to ensure patient comfort and to support joints and bony prominences.*[1]

NURSING ALERT Take the necessary precautions to prevent patient falls throughout positioning.[27,28,29]

■ Ensure that the patient uses proper coughing technique during and after positioning.[30] If the patient's cough appears weak or ineffective because of pain, have the patient splint the painful area with a pillow and ensure that the patient has been medicated adequately. If pain isn't the cause, instruct the patient in coughing and diaphragmatic breathing exercises.

■ Instruct the patient to cough directly into a tissue (or, if ordered, into a sterile specimen collection container) *to promote respiratory hygiene and*

Contraindications to chest physiotherapy

The following are absolute and relative contraindications to chest physiotherapy.[1]

Absolute contraindications
Active hemorrhage with hemodynamic instability
Unstable head or neck injury

Relative contraindications

Abdominal distention	Pulmonary edema associated
Active hemoptysis	with heart failure
Bronchopleural fistula	Pulmonary embolism
Bronchospasm	Recent epidural spinal infusion
Burns of the thorax	Recent gross hemoptysis
Chest wall pain	related to recent surgery or
Coagulopathy	radiation for lung cancer
Conditions in which increased	treatment
intracranial pressure (ICP)	Recent spinal anesthesia
must be avoided (for exam-	Recent thoracic skin grafts or
ple, cerebral aneurysm,	flaps
recent eye surgery, and	Recent transvenous or subcuta-
recent neurosurgery)	neous pacemaker placement
Confusion or anxiety that pre-	Rib fracture with or without flail
vents position changes	chest
Empyema	Subcutaneous emphysema
Esophageal surgery	Suspected pulmonary
ICP greater than 20 mm Hg	tuberculosis
Lung contusion	Thoracic skin infections
Open thoracic wounds	Uncontrolled airway in a patient
Osteomyelitis of the ribs	at risk for aspiration
Osteoporosis	Uncontrolled hypertension
Pleural effusion (large volume)	

cough etiquette, and subsequently to prevent pathogen transmission.[6] (See the "Sputum collection" procedure.)

■ Instruct the patient to remain in each position, as tolerated, preferably for at least 3 minutes or longer if good sputum production results.[1,3]

■ After each position, allow pauses for relaxation and breathing control *to prevent hypoxemia.*[1]

■ Monitor the patient for pain, discomfort, dyspnea, arrhythmias, and changes in breathing pattern, skin color, sputum production, and ICP (if monitored).[1] If the patient experiences any adverse events, stop therapy, return the patient to the original position, administer supplemental oxygen (as ordered), and notify the practitioner.[1]

■ Reposition the patient to allow for coughing and expectoration. When the patient is in the head-down position, advise avoidance of strenuous coughing *because it markedly increases ICP.*[1]

■ If postural drainage alone fails to mobilize secretions, perform percussion and vibration (if needed and ordered) over the draining area, unless contraindicated.[1] Place a thin layer of cloth, such as a hospital gown or bed sheet, over the site being percussed *to promote comfort.*[1] Remove any jewelry that may cause scratching or bruising. (See *Performing percussion and vibration.*)

■ After postural drainage, percussion, or vibration, instruct the patient to deep-breathe and cough *to remove loosened secretions.* Give the patient a facial tissue. Instruct the patient to inhale deeply through the nose and then to exhale in three short huffs. Instruct the patient to inhale deeply again, cover the mouth and nose with a facial tissue, and cough and expectorate through a slightly opened mouth into the tissue.[6,20,21] Three consecutive coughs are highly effective. Alternatively, if collection of a sputum specimen is necessary, instruct the patient to expectorate into a sterile specimen container. Label the container in the presence of the patient *to prevent mislabeling.*[13] Send the specimen container to the laboratory in a laboratory transport bag. (See the "Sputum collection" procedure.) Provide a no-touch receptacle for the patient to dispose of the used facial tissue.[6]

■ If the patient's cough is ineffective, suction the patient. (See the "Oronasopharyngeal suctioning" procedure.)

Performing percussion and vibration

To perform percussion, instruct the patient to breathe slowly and deeply, using the diaphragm, *to promote relaxation.* Hold your hands in a cupped shape, with fingers flexed and thumbs pressed tightly against your index fingers (as shown below). Percuss each lung segment with your cupped hands by rhythmically alternating your hands against the patient chest over the targeted area; ideally, percuss for 3 to 5 minutes in a circular pattern over the area.[1] Listen for a hollow sound on percussion *to verify correct performance of the technique.* Refrain from percussing over tender areas and sites of trauma or surgery, and avoid percussing directly over bony prominences.[1]

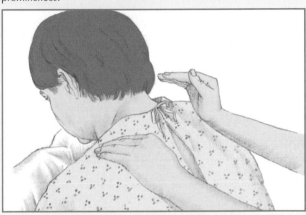

To perform vibration, ask the patient to inhale deeply and then exhale slowly through pursed lips. During exhalation, firmly press your fingers and the palms of your hands against the chest wall (as shown below). Tense the muscles of your arms and shoulders in an isometric contraction *to send fine vibrations through the chest wall.* Vibrate during five exhalations over each lung segment.

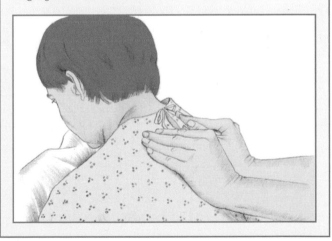

■ Monitor the patient's response to the treatment. Auscultate breath sounds and compare them to baseline findings *to evaluate the effectiveness of the therapy.* Be alert for significant skin color changes, particularly if the patient's skin becomes dusky, *which may indicate poor oxygenation.* Monitor oxygen saturation level by pulse oximetry, as needed.

■ Assist the patient with hand hygiene.[6,20]

■ Reassess and respond to the patient's pain by evaluating the patient's response to treatment and progress toward pain management goals. Assess for adverse reactions and risk factors for adverse events that may result from treatment.[31]

■ Assist the patient with or perform oral care, as needed. (See the "Oral care" procedure.)

- Return the patient's bed to the lowest position *to prevent falls and maintain safety.*[27]
- Remove and discard gloves and any other personal protective equipment, if worn.[21]
- Perform hand hygiene.[7,8,9,10,11,12]
- Clean and disinfect your stethoscope using a disinfectant pad.[32,33]
- Perform hand hygiene.[7,8,9,10,11,12]
- Document the procedure.[34,35,36,37]

Special considerations

- *For optimal effectiveness and safety,* modify chest physiotherapy according to the patient's condition. For example, initiate or increase the flow of supplemental oxygen, if indicated. If the patient tires quickly during therapy, shorten the sessions, *because fatigue leads to shallow respirations and increased hypoxia.*
- Maintain adequate hydration in the patient receiving chest physiotherapy *to prevent mucus dehydration and promote easier mobilization of secretions.* Avoid performing postural drainage immediately before or within 1½ hours after meals *to avoid nausea, vomiting, and aspiration of food or vomitus.*
- *Because chest percussion may induce bronchospasm,* ensure that any adjunct treatment (for example, intermittent positive-pressure breathing or aerosol or nebulizer therapy) precedes chest physiotherapy.

Complications

During postural drainage in head-down positions, pressure on the diaphragm by abdominal contents may increase intrathoracic pressure and lead to hypoxia. The head-down position can also lead to increased ICP, precluding the use of chest physiotherapy in a patient with head injury, elevated ICP, or acute neurologic impairment. Vigorous percussion or vibration can cause rib fracture, especially in a patient with osteoporosis. In a patient with emphysema with blebs, coughing can lead to pneumothorax. Pulmonary hemorrhage, vomiting, aspiration, bronchospasm, and arrhythmias also can occur.

Documentation

Record the date and time chest physiotherapy was performed. Document the baseline respiratory assessment and reassessment findings, evaluating the effectiveness of therapy. Note the patient positions you used for secretion drainage and the length of time each position was maintained. Note which lung segments you percussed or vibrated. Record the color, amount, odor, and viscosity of any secretions the patient produced, and note whether blood was present. Record any complications, the name of the practitioner notified, the date and time the practitioner was notified, prescribed interventions, and the patient's response to those interventions. Also document whether the patient received pain medication (and if so, its effectiveness) and the patient's tolerance of the overall procedure. Document teaching provided to the patient and family (if applicable), their understanding of that teaching, and any need for follow-up teaching.

REFERENCES

1 Kacmarek, R. M., et al. (2021). *Egan's fundamentals of respiratory care* (12th ed.). St. Louis, MO: Mosby.

2 Volsko, T. A. (2013). Airway clearance therapy: Finding the evidence. *Respiratory Care, 58*(10), 1669–1677. http://rc.rcjournal.com/content/respcare/58/10/1669.full.pdf (Level V)

3 Strickland, S. L., et al. (2013). AARC clinical practice guideline: Effectiveness of nonpharmacologic airway clearance therapies in hospitalized patients. *Respiratory Care, 58*(12), 2187–2193. http://rc.rcjournal.com/content/58/12/2187.full (Level VII)

4 Yang, M., et al. (2013). Chest physiotherapy for pneumonia in adults. *Cochrane Database of Systematic Reviews, 2013*(2), CD006338. (Level I)

5 Sethi, S., & Murphy, T. F. (2020). Management of infection in exacerbations of chronic obstructive pulmonary disease. In: *UpToDate*, Sexton, D. J,. (Ed.).

6 Centers for Disease Control and Prevention. (2009). Respiratory hygiene/cough etiquette in healthcare settings. https://www.cdc.gov/flu/professionals/infectioncontrol/resphygiene.htm (Level VII)

7 The Joint Commission. (2021). Standard NPSG.07.01.01. *Comprehensive accreditation manual for hospitals.* Oakbrook Terrace, IL: The Joint Commission. (Level VII)

8 Centers for Disease Control and Prevention. (2002). Guideline for hand hygiene in health-care settings: Recommendations of the Healthcare Infection Control Practices Advisory Committee and the HICPAC/SHEA/APIC/IDSA Hand Hygiene Task Force. *MMWR Recommendations and Reports, 51*(RR-16), 1–45. https://www.cdc.gov/mmwr/pdf/rr/rr5116.pdf (Level II)

9 World Health Organization. (2009). WHO guidelines on hand hygiene in health care: First global patient safety challenge, clean care is safer care. https://apps.who.int/iris/bitstream/handle/10665/44102/9789241597906_eng.pdf?sequence=1 (Level IV)

10 Centers for Medicare and Medicaid Services, Department of Health and Human Services. (2020). Condition of participation: Infection control. 42 C.F.R. § 482.42.

11 Accreditation Association for Hospitals and Health Systems. (2020). Standard 07.01.21. *Healthcare Facilities Accreditation Program: Accreditation requirements for acute care hospitals.* Chicago, IL: Accreditation Association for Hospitals and Health Systems. (Level VII)

12 DNV GL-Healthcare USA, Inc. (2020). IC.1.SR.1. *NIAHO® accreditation requirements, interpretive guidelines and surveyor guidance—revision 20.0.* Milford, OH: DNV GL-Healthcare USA, Inc. (Level VII)

13 The Joint Commission. (2021). Standard NPSG.01.01.01. *Comprehensive accreditation manual for hospitals.* Oakbrook Terrace, IL: The Joint Commission. (Level VII)

14 Accreditation Association for Hospitals and Health Systems. (2020). Standard 15.01.16. *Healthcare Facilities Accreditation Program: Accreditation requirements for acute care hospitals.* Chicago, IL: Accreditation Association for Hospitals and Health Systems. (Level VII)

15 The Joint Commission. (2021). Standard RI.01.01.01. *Comprehensive accreditation manual for hospitals.* Oakbrook Terrace, IL: The Joint Commission. (Level VII)

16 Centers for Medicare and Medicaid Services, Department of Health and Human Services. (2020). Condition of participation: Patient's rights. 42 C.F.R. § 482.13(c)(1).

17 DNV GL-Healthcare USA, Inc. (2020). PR.2.SR.5. *NIAHO® accreditation requirements, interpretive guidelines and surveyor guidance—revision 20.0.* Milford, OH: DNV GL-Healthcare USA, Inc. (Level VII)

18 The Joint Commission. (2021). Standard PC.02.01.21. *Comprehensive accreditation manual for hospitals.* Oakbrook Terrace, IL: The Joint Commission. (Level VII)

19 Waters, T. R., et al. (2009). Safe patient handling training for schools of nursing. http://www.cdc.gov/niosh/docs/2009-127/pdfs/2009-127.pdf (Level VII)

20 Accreditation Association for Hospitals and Health Systems. (2020). Standard 07.01.10. *Healthcare Facilities Accreditation Program: Accreditation requirements for acute care hospitals.* Chicago, IL: Accreditation Association for Hospitals and Health Systems. (Level VII)

21 Siegel, J. D., et al. (2007, revised 2019). 2007 guideline for isolation precautions: Preventing transmission of infectious agents in healthcare settings. https://www.cdc.gov/infectioncontrol/pdf/guidelines/isolation-guidelines-H.pdf (Level II)

22 The Joint Commission. (2021). Standard PC.01.02.07. *Comprehensive accreditation manual for hospitals.* Oakbrook Terrace, IL: The Joint Commission. (Level VII)

23 The Joint Commission. (2021). Standard MM.06.01.01. *Comprehensive accreditation manual for hospitals.* Oakbrook Terrace, IL: The Joint Commission. (Level VII)

24 Centers for Medicare and Medicaid Services, Department of Health and Human Services. (2020). Condition of participation: Nursing services. 42 C.F.R. § 482.23(c).

25 Accreditation Association for Hospitals and Health Systems. (2020). Standard 16.01.03. *Healthcare Facilities Accreditation Program: Accreditation requirements for acute care hospitals.* Chicago, IL: Accreditation Association for Hospitals and Health Systems. (Level VII)

26 DNV GL-Healthcare USA, Inc. (2020). MM.1.SR.3. *NIAHO® accreditation requirements, interpretive guidelines and surveyor guidance—revision 20.0.* Milford, OH: DNV GL-Healthcare USA, Inc. (Level VII)

27 Ganz, D. A., et al. (2013, reviewed 2021). *Preventing falls in hospitals: A toolkit for improving quality of care* (AHRQ Publication No. 13-0015-EF). Rockville, MD: Agency for Healthcare Research and Quality. https://www.ahrq.gov/professionals/systems/hospital/fallpxtoolkit/index.html (Level VII)

28 The Joint Commission. (2021). Standard PC.01.02.08. *Comprehensive accreditation manual for hospitals.* Oakbrook Terrace, IL: The Joint Commission. (Level VII)

29 Institute for Healthcare Improvement. (2012). How-to guide: *Reducing patient injuries from falls.* Cambridge, MA: Institute for Healthcare Improvement. (Level VII)

30 Ren, S., et al. (2020). Numerical analysis of airway mucus clearance effectiveness using assisted coughing techniques. *Scientific Reports, 10,* 2030. https://www.ncbi.nlm.nih.gov/pmc/articles/PMC7005022/ (Level IV)

31 Accreditation Association for Hospitals and Health Systems. (2020). Standard 16.02.05. *Healthcare Facilities Accreditation Program: Accreditation requirements for acute care hospitals.* Chicago, IL: Accreditation Association for Hospitals and Health Systems. (Level VII)

32 Rutala, W. A., et al. (2008, revised 2019). Guideline for disinfection and sterilization in healthcare facilities, 2008. https://www.cdc.gov/infection-control/pdf/guidelines/disinfection-guidelines-H.pdf (Level I)

33 Accreditation Association for Hospitals and Health Systems. (2020). Standard 07.02.03. *Healthcare Facilities Accreditation Program: Accreditation requirements for acute care hospitals.* Chicago, IL: Accreditation Association for Hospitals and Health Systems. (Level VII)

34 The Joint Commission. (2021). Standard RC.01.03.01. *Comprehensive accreditation manual for hospitals.* Oakbrook Terrace, IL: The Joint Commission. (Level VII)

35 Centers for Medicare and Medicaid Services, Department of Health and Human Services. (2020). Condition of participation: Medical record services. 42 C.F.R. § 482.24(b).

36 Accreditation Association for Hospitals and Health Systems. (2020). Standard 10.00.03. *Healthcare Facilities Accreditation Program: Accreditation requirements for acute care hospitals.* Chicago, IL: Accreditation Association for Hospitals and Health Systems. (Level VII)

37 DNV GL-Healthcare USA, Inc. (2020). MR.2.SR.1. *NIAHO® accreditation requirements, interpretive guidelines and surveyor guidance—revision 20.0.* Milford, OH: DNV GL-Healthcare USA, Inc. (Level VII)

CHEST TUBE DRAINAGE SYSTEM MONITORING AND CARE

Chest tube drainage systems use gravity and sometimes suction to restore negative pressure and remove air or fluid (blood, pus, or serous fluid) that collects in the pleural cavity, allowing a patient's collapsed lung to reexpand and reducing respiratory distress. A disposable drainage system combines one or more drainage collection chambers, a seal, and suction control into a single unit.

When a patient requires a chest tube to remove or drain air, blood, or fluid from the pleural cavity, nursing care focuses on maintaining and troubleshooting the chest tube drainage system to ensure that the chest tube functions properly and that the patient is protected from infection. It also includes assessing the patient's respiratory status, obtaining vital signs, monitoring for complications, and intervening appropriately when complications arise or the patient's condition changes.

Equipment

Vital signs monitoring equipment ▪ stethoscope ▪ pulse oximeter and probe ▪ disinfectant pad ▪ facility-approved disinfectant ▪ marker ▪ Optional: sterile transparent dressing; gown; mask and goggles or mask with face shield; gloves; sterile gloves; single-use, disposable, sterile chest tube drainage collection unit; sterile water; two sterile 4″ × 4″ (10-cm × 10-cm) drain dressings; sterile 4″ × 4″ (10-cm × 10-cm) gauze pads; wide paper tape; 1″ (2.5-cm) adhesive tape for connections; engineered stabilization device; prescribed pain medication; clamp.

Preparation of equipment

Inspect all equipment and supplies. If a product is expired, is defective, or has compromised integrity, remove it from patient use, label it as expired or defective, and report the expiration or defect as directed by your facility.

Implementation

▪ Verify the practitioner's orders regarding chest tube care. Note the level of suction prescribed, if ordered.

▪ Gather and prepare the necessary equipment and supplies.
▪ Perform hand hygiene.[1,2,3,4,5,6]
▪ Confirm the patient's identity using at least two patient identifiers.[7]
▪ Provide privacy.[8,9,10,11]
▪ Explain the procedure to the patient and family (if appropriate) according to their individual communication and learning needs *to enhance their understanding, allay their fears, and enhance cooperation.*[12]
▪ Screen for and assess the patient's pain using facility-defined criteria that are consistent with the patient's age, condition, and ability to understand. In collaboration with the multidisciplinary team, involve the patient in the pain management planning process.[13]
▪ Treat the patient's pain as needed and ordered using nonpharmacologic, pharmacologic, or a combination of approaches. Base the treatment plan on evidence-based practices and the patient's clinical condition, medical history, and pain management goals.[13] Administer prescribed pain medication following safe medication practices, as needed and ordered.[14,15,16,17] *Relieving the patient's pain promotes comfort, which helps facilitate deep-breathing, coughing, and range-of-motion (ROM) exercises.*
▪ Maintain sterile no-touch technique whenever you make changes in the system or alter any of the connections, *to help avoid introducing pathogens into the patient's pleural space.*[18,19,20,21,22]

For all chest tube drainage systems

▪ Monitor the color, character, consistency, and amount of drainage in the drainage collection unit chamber.[23] Notify the practitioner immediately of a sudden increase in drainage or the presence of frank bloody drainage.
▪ Mark the drainage level by writing the time and date at the drainage level on the drainage collection chamber at an interval determined by your facility or the patient's condition.[18]
▪ Observe the integrity of the drainage tubing and chest tube every 2 to 4 hours and with a change in the patient's condition *to help ensure that the drainage system is intact, with no air leaks or kinks, and to help prevent clot formation.*[18]
▪ Periodically check that the air vent in the system is working properly (if applicable).[23] *Occlusion of the air vent results in a buildup of pressure in the system that can cause the patient to develop a tension pneumothorax.*
▪ Coil the drainage system tubing and secure it to the edge of the patient's bed. Ensure that the tubing remains at the level of the patient. Avoid creating dependent loops, kinks, or pressure in the tubing, *because fluid-filled dependent loops can rapidly change pleural pressures, resulting in dramatically decreased drainage.*[18,23] Avoid lifting the drainage system above the patient's chest, *because fluid may flow back into the patient's pleural space.*[18]

NURSING ALERT Never clamp a tube to get the patient out of bed or during transportation of the patient. *Whenever the chest tube is clamped, air or fluid can't escape from the patient's pleural space, which puts the patient at risk for a tension pneumothorax.*[18]

▪ Encourage the patient to ambulate frequently and change position to perform coughing and deep breathing exercises, as ordered, *to help drain the pleural space and expand the lungs.*[18,23]
▪ Instruct the patient to sit upright *to facilitate gravity drainage of pleural fluid or optimal lung expansion;*[23] tell the patient to splint the insertion site while coughing *to minimize pain.*
▪ Monitor the patient's vital signs and oxygen saturation, and assess the rate and quality of the patient's respirations. Periodically auscultate the patient's lung fields *to assess air exchange in the affected lung;*[18] *diminished or absent breath sounds may indicate that the patient's lung hasn't reexpanded.*
▪ Instruct the patient to immediately report any breathing difficulty. Notify the practitioner immediately if the patient develops cyanosis, a decreased oxygen saturation level, rapid or shallow breathing, subcutaneous emphysema, chest pain, or excessive bleeding.
▪ Assess the chest tube dressing. Palpate the area surrounding the dressing for crepitus (a crackling feeling under the skin); *crepitus indicates the presence of subcutaneous emphysema, the leaking of air into the subcutaneous tissue surrounding the insertion site.* Change the dressing when it is soiled or as ordered by the practitioner, or at an interval determined by your facility.[18] (See *Changing a chest tube dressing,* page 170.)

Changing a chest tube dressing

Use sterile, no-touch technique when changing the chest tube dressing unless the patient's condition warrants otherwise. Follow these steps when changing a chest tube dressing:

■ Gather and prepare the necessary equipment and supplies.
■ Perform hand hygiene.[1,2,3,4,5,6]
■ Confirm the patient's identity using at least two patient identifiers.[7]
■ Provide privacy.[8,9,10,11]
■ Explain the procedure to the patient and family (if appropriate) according to their individual communication and learning needs *to enhance their understanding, allay their fears, and enhance cooperation.*[12]
■ Raise the bed to waist height before providing patient care *to prevent caregiver back strain.*[24]
■ Perform hand hygiene.[1,2,3,4,5,6]
■ Put on gloves and other personal protective equipment, if needed.[19,22]
■ Remove the existing dressing around the chest tube insertion site and discard it in an appropriate receptacle.[25] Examine the site for signs of infection or subcutaneous emphysema.[18]
■ Remove and discard your gloves[19,22] and perform hand hygiene.[1,2,3,4,5,6]
■ Open the packages containing the sterile 4″ × 4″ (10-cm × 10-cm) drain dressings and gauze pads, the sterile transparent dressing, or the dressing approved by your facility. (Note that no published research exists on chest tube insertion site dressings to directly support the use of one type of dressing over another for application over a chest tube insertion site.)
■ Perform hand hygiene.[1,2,3,4,5,6]
■ Put on sterile gloves.[19,22]
■ Clean the insertion site with sterile water or sterile normal saline solution on a sterile gauze pad or an antiseptic swab, as ordered.[26]
■ Place the two drain dressings around the insertion site, one from the top and the other from the bottom (as shown above on right), *to help seal the insertion site from any air entry and escape.*[18] Then place a gauze pad on top of the drain dressings and cover the dressing with wide paper tape *to form an occlusive dressing.*
■ Alternatively, apply a sterile transparent dressing over the chest tube insertion site *to help allow inspection of the wound.*[18]
■ Write the date, the time, and your initials on the dressing, if required by your facility.
■ Return the bed to the lowest position *to prevent falls and maintain patient safety.*[27]

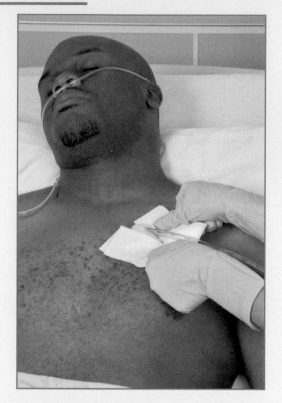

■ Discard used supplies in the appropriate receptacle.
■ Remove and discard your gloves and, if worn, other personal protective equipment.[19,22]
■ Perform hand hygiene.[1,2,3,4,5,6]
■ Document the procedure.[28,29,30,31]

■ Replace the chest tube drainage system as ordered or as needed. (See *Replacing the chest tube drainage system.*) Notify the practitioner if you must change the device because of a leak.

■ Encourage active ROM exercises or assist the patient with passive ROM exercises for the arm on the affected side. A patient with a thoracotomy usually splints the arm *to decrease discomfort.*[18]

■ Remind an ambulatory patient to keep the drainage system below the level of the chest tube *to facilitate gravity drainage,*[23] and to be careful not to disconnect the tubing *to maintain the water seal.*

■ Troubleshoot the system as needed when problems arise. (See *Troubleshooting chest tubes,* page 172.) *Early and prompt attention to system difficulties will minimize complications.*

Additional steps for a water-seal, wet-suction system
■ Check the water-seal level every shift and maintain the proper level *to ensure proper use of the chest tube drainage system, and the patient's safety.*
■ Check for fluctuation in the water-seal chamber as the patient breathes. Normal fluctuations of 2″ to 4″ (5 to 10 cm) reflect pressure changes in the pleural space during respiration. *To check for fluctuations when a suction system is being used,* momentarily disconnect the suction system so that the air vent is opened and observe for fluctuations.
■ Check for intermittent bubbling in the water-seal chamber.[23] *This bubbling occurs normally when the chest tube drainage system is removing air from the patient's pleural cavity.* If bubbling isn't readily apparent during quiet breathing, have the patient take a deep breath or cough. *Absence of bubbling indicates that the pleural space has sealed.*
■ Check the water level in the suction control chamber. Detach the chamber from the suction source; when bubbling ceases, observe the

water level. If necessary, add sterile water to bring the level to the prescribed level (typically 20 cm H_2O).
■ Check for gentle bubbling in the suction control chamber, *which indicates the proper suction level.*[23]

Additional steps for a water-seal–dry suction system
■ Check the water-seal level every shift and maintain the proper level *to help ensure that the chest tube drainage system is being used properly and to maintain the patient's safety.*[23]
■ Check for fluctuation in the water-seal chamber as the patient breathes.[23] *Normal fluctuations of 2″ to 4″ (5 to 10 cm) reflect pressure changes in the patient's pleural space during respiration. To check for fluctuations when a suction system is being used,* momentarily disconnect the suction system *so that the air vent is opened* and observe for fluctuations.
■ Check for intermittent bubbling in the water-seal chamber.[23] *This bubbling occurs normally when the system is removing air from the patient's pleural cavity.* If bubbling isn't readily apparent during quiet breathing, have the patient take a deep breath or cough. *Absence of bubbling indicates that the pleural space has sealed.*
■ Check that the rotary dry suction control dial is turned to the ordered suction mark (typically –20 cm H_2O), and verify that the appropriate indicator is present, *indicating that the chest tube drainage system has applied the desired amount of suction.* In some models, a ball or float appears in an indicator window. Other models indicate delivery of the correct amount of suction when the bellows reach the calibrated triangular mark in the suction monitor bellows window. Always refer to the manufacturer's instructions.

Replacing the chest tube drainage system

In certain circumstances, you may need to replace the chest tube drainage system. Follow these steps for replacement:
■ Gather and prepare the necessary equipment and supplies.
■ Perform hand hygiene.[1,2,3,4,5,6]
■ Confirm the patient's identity using at least two patient identifiers.[7]
■ Provide privacy.[8,9,10,11]
■ Explain the procedure to the patient and family (if appropriate) according to their individual communication and learning needs *to enhance their understanding, allay their fears, and enhance cooperation.*[12]
■ Open a new, single-use, sterile chest tube drainage collection unit.
■ If you're using a chest drainage system that has a water seal, fill the water-seal chamber with sterile water to the specified level, according to the manufacturer's instructions.
■ If you're using a dry-seal chest drainage system, fill the air-leak monitor with sterile water to the specified level, according to the manufacturer's instructions.
■ If you're using a wet suction chest drainage system, fill the suction control chamber with sterile water to the prescribed level (typically 20 cm H_2O). *The addition of suction (usually –20 cm H_2O) increases the negative intrapleural pressure and helps overcome air leakage by improving the rate of airflow out of the patient and improving fluid removal.* If you're using a dry suction chest drainage system, turn the rotary dry suction control dial to the ordered suction mark, usually –20 cm H_2O.
■ Maintain a sterile patient connection tube with the cap in place *to enable later connection of the chest tube catheter to the chest tube drainage system collection device after removal of the existing device.*
■ Place the chest tube drainage system at the bedside in the upright position, at least 1' (30 cm) below the patient's chest. *To avoid accidentally knocking over the device, hang it on the bed frame with the hangers provided, or secure it according to the manufacturer's instructions.* Ensure that the device is ready when you remove the existing device.
■ Raise the bed to waist level before providing care *to help prevent caregiver back strain.*[24]
■ Perform hand hygiene.[1,2,3,4,5,6]
■ Put on gloves and, as needed, other personal protective equipment.[19,22]
■ If using suction, turn off the suction to the current drainage system.
■ Trace the tubing from the patient to its point of origin *to ensure you're assessing the correct tube.*[32,33]
■ If the chest tube drainage system isn't equipped with an in-line connector, undo the tape or zip-tie on the connections from the existing chest tube drainage system to the chest tube catheter *to allow access to the chest tube catheter for drainage device replacement.*[23,24] Undoing the tape or ties won't be necessary if the chest tube drainage system has an in-line connector.
■ Instruct the patient to perform the Valsalva maneuver *to force air out of the pleural space and keep air from entering while you switch the tubing.* If the patient can't perform the maneuver, make the drainage system switch at the end of exhalation if the patient is breathing spontaneously or the end of inspiration of a machine-generated breath.[23]
■ Briefly clamp the chest tube close to the insertion site *to help minimize dead space and to stop air from entering and exiting the chest tube.*[18,23,34] If the chest tube drainage system has an in-line connector, also clamp the patient tube clamp.[34]
■ Using sterile no-touch technique, disconnect the old drainage system and connect the new one.
■ Unclamp the tube and instruct the patient to breathe normally *to allow fluid and air removal to begin again.*
■ Trace the tubing from the patient to its point of origin to ensure that you've attached it to the proper port.[32,33]
■ Secure the chest tube and drainage tube so that no tension is pulling on the insertion site, *to help prevent accidental tube dislodgment.* Use an engineered stabilization device, if available, *to help reduce the risk of unintentional chest tube dislodgement.*[18]
■ Tape or zip-tie the junction of the chest tube and the drainage tube as needed (as shown above on right) *to help prevent dangerous disconnections.*[18,35]

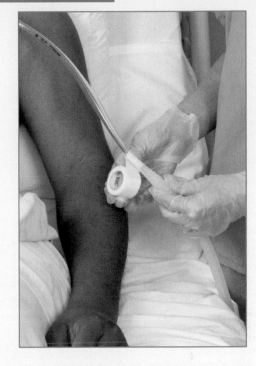

■ Discard used supplies in appropriate receptacles.[25]
■ Remove and discard your gloves and any other personal protective equipment, if worn.[19,22]
■ Perform hand hygiene.[1,2,3,4,5,6]
■ Ensure that all clamps are open and that the drainage tubing has a straight flow to the chest tube drainage collection device, and has no dependent loops or kinks.[23]
■ Ensure that the chest tube drainage system is correctly connected to the patient's chest tube; then, if appropriate, connect the suction tubing to the drainage system and the suction regulator.
■ If you're using a wet-suction chest drainage system, adjust the suction until gentle bubbling appears in the suction-control chamber. If you're using a dry-suction chest drainage system, adjust the suction regulator and verify that the appropriate indicator is present, showing that the system has applied the desired amount of suction. Verify suction operation according to the manufacturer's instructions.
■ Check the status of the drainage tubing.[23]
■ Reassess the patient after the procedure. Obtain the patient's vital signs as well as oxygen saturation; assess skin color, perfusion, level of consciousness, oxygen requirements, hemodynamic stability, and comfort and pain levels; and assess respiratory rate, pattern, and effort, *to help identify the patient's response to and tolerance of the procedure.*
■ Return the patient's bed to the lowest position *to prevent falls and maintain patient safety.*[27]
■ Perform hand hygiene.[1,2,3,4,5,6]
■ Clean and disinfect your stethoscope using a disinfectant pad.[36,37]
■ Perform hand hygiene.[1,2,3,4,5,6]
■ Put on gloves, as needed.[19,20]
■ Clean and disinfect other reusable equipment with a facility-approved disinfectant according to the manufacturer's instructions, *to prevent the spread of infection.*[36,37]
■ Remove and discard your gloves, if worn.[25]
■ Perform hand hygiene.[1,2,3,4,5,6]
■ Document the procedure.[28,29,30,31]

Additional steps for a dry-seal, dry-suction system
■ Check the air-leak monitor for right-to-left bubbling and fluctuation every shift (or more often as signs and symptoms warrant). *Fluctuation of water in the air-leak monitor chamber is a normal reflection of pressure changes in the pleural cavity during respirations. Bubbling indicates that air is leaving the system.* Keep in mind that bubbling is normal for a patient with a pneumothorax, but it could indicate an air leak.

■ Check that the rotary dry-suction control dial is turned to the ordered suction mark (typically –20 cm H_2O,) and verify that the appropriate indicator is present, *indicating the chest tube drainage system has applied the desired amount of suction.* In some models, an orange float appears in an indicator window. Other models indicate delivery of the correct amount of suction when the bellows reach the calibrated triangular mark in the suction monitor bellows window. Always refer to the manufacturer's instructions.

TROUBLESHOOTING

TROUBLESHOOTING CHEST TUBES

Use this table to determine possible causes of and interventions for common chest tube problems.

PROBLEM	POSSIBLE CAUSES	INTERVENTION
Water level in the water-seal chamber not rising and falling with breathing	Clot in chest tubing or the patient's chest	If available, incorporate an active chest tube clearance device into the drainage system *to prevent clot formation*.[38] Avoid fluid-filled dependent loops in the drainage tubing. Stripping and milking the tubing aren't recommended, *because detrimental changes in intrathoracic pressure can result*.[23]
	Dependent loop or kink in patient's tube with fluid occlusion	Straighten the catheter and tubing along its length to its connection with the collection device.[23]
	Dislodgment of the chest tube from the patient	If the chest tube accidentally dislodges and the patient has an air leak from the chest tube, immediately cover the site with a sterile dressing and tape it on three sides, allowing air to escape on the fourth side *to reduce the risk of tension pneumothorax*.[23,39] Alternatively, cover the insertion site with a sterile dressing with a one-way valve, if available. If your previous assessment revealed no leak, place a sterile occlusive dressing over the insertion site and monitor the patient closely for signs and symptoms of respiratory distress.[23] Stay with the patient and have a colleague call the practitioner immediately. Assess for signs and symptoms of tension pneumothorax (hypotension, distended jugular veins, absent or decreased breath sounds, tracheal shift, hypoxemia, weak rapid pulse, dyspnea, tachypnea, diaphoresis, and chest pain). Then ask your colleague to gather the equipment needed to reinsert the chest tube.
	Disconnection of patient's chest tube from chest tube connector	If the chest tube drainage system cracks or a tube disconnects, clamp the tube as close to the insertion site as possible. *Because no air or liquid can escape from the pleural space while the tube is clamped*, observe the patient closely for signs and symptoms of tension pneumothorax while the clamp is in place. As an alternative to clamping the tube, you can submerge the distal end of the tube in a container of normal saline solution *to create a temporary water seal* while you replace the drainage system. Notify the practitioner immediately.
	Closed clamp to the patient's chest tube	Clamp the chest tube only when indicated; otherwise, leave the tube open.
	Chest drainage tubing not positioned sufficiently below the patient's chest	Lower the chest tube *to enable gravity drainage*.[23]
	In-line connectors not properly secured, allowing for an air leak	Ensure that inline connectors are properly secured and sealed at all times; check for loose connections periodically.
Constant bubbling in the water-seal chamber	Air leak	*To determine the source of an air leak (patient or catheter connection tubing)*, momentarily clamp the chest tube close to the chest tube drain and observe the water seal chamber. If the bubbling stops, the air leak may be from the catheter connection tubing or the patient's chest. Check the catheter connection tubing and the patient's dressing for a partially withdrawn catheter. If the catheter is dislodged, follow the procedure for a dislodged chest tube, described above. If bubbling continues after temporarily clamping the patient's tube, there's a drainage system leak, which requires system replacement.
Overfilled water-seal level (water above ¾" [2-cm] limit line) or overfilled suction control chamber	Too much water in the chamber	Press and hold the negative-pressure relief valve at the top of the chest drainage system *to help vent excess negative pressure in the water-seal chamber*. Don't lower the water level in the water-seal chamber if the patient's chest tube is draining by gravity draining (not suction). Release the valve when the level of the water returns to the ¾" (2-cm) mark. *To remove water from the suction control chamber*, insert a syringe and withdraw excess.
Not enough water in the water-seal or suction control chamber	Evaporation, underfilling, or spillage	Add additional sterile water to the suction control chamber by temporarily turning off the suction source, removing the rubber stopper, and adding sterile water to the desired level. Add additional sterile water to the water-seal chamber with a 20G or smaller needle and syringe by injecting water into the grommet on the back of the water-seal chamber.
Suction control chamber not bubbling or bubbling too vigorously	Possible disconnection of suction source or too much suction-source pressure in the drainage system	Ensure that the suction tubing is connected and the suction source is turned on. A constant, gentle bubbling is normal. Vigorous bubbling causes quicker evaporation. Adjust the suction control source for gentle bubbling.
Chest tube drainage system accidentally knocked over	Human error	Set the drainage system upright and check the fluid levels in the water-seal and suction control chambers for proper volumes; adjust them accordingly. Most units have a baffle system that prevents fluids from mixing between chambers, enabling proper function after setting the system upright again.

Completing the procedure

- Reassess and respond to the patient's pain by evaluating the response to treatment and progress toward pain management goals. Assess the patient for adverse reactions and risk factors for adverse events that may result from treatment.[13]
- Perform hand hygiene.[1,2,3,4,5,6]
- Clean and disinfect your stethoscope using a disinfectant pad.[36,37]
- Perform hand hygiene.[1,2,3,4,5,6]
- Put on gloves, as needed.[19,20]
- Clean and disinfect other reusable equipment using a facility-approved disinfectant according to the manufacturer's instructions, *to prevent the spread of infection.*[36,37]
- Remove and discard your gloves, if worn.[25]
- Perform hand hygiene.[1,2,3,4,5,6]
- Document the procedure.[28,29,30,31]

Special considerations

- Instruct staff members and visitors to avoid touching the chest tube drainage system equipment *to prevent complications from separated connections.*
- The Joint Commission has issued a sentinel event alert related to managing risk during transition to new International Organization for Standardization tubing standards that were designed to prevent dangerous tubing misconnections, which can lead to serious patient injury and death. During the transition, make sure to trace each tubing and catheter from the patient to its point of origin before connecting or reconnecting any device or infusion, at any care transition (such as to a new setting or service), and as part of the hand-off process. In addition, route tubes and catheters with different purposes in different, standardized directions; label tubing at both the distal and proximal ends when the patient has different access sites or several bags hanging; use tubing and equipment only as intended; and store medications for different delivery routes in separate locations.[32]
- If the chest tube drainage system cracks, clamp the chest tube momentarily. Observe the patient for altered respirations while the tube is clamped. Then replace the damaged equipment.[23] (Prepare the new unit before clamping the tube.)
- For a patient on a ventilator with positive end-expiratory pressure (PEEP), continuous bubbling typically occurs, *because PEEP maintains positive pressure in the alveoli, resulting in air continually flowing through the lungs.* However, lack of continuous bubbling for patients on PEEP isn't abnormal.

NURSING ALERT Don't strip a chest tube drain (that is, don't occlude the chest tube with one hand while quickly squeezing and moving the other hand down the tube to move fluid down the tube into the drainage chamber), *because stripping can cause intraluminal pressures to rise to a dangerously high level, which can convert a simple pneumothorax into life-threatening pneumothorax and cause tissue trauma and unnecessary discomfort. Also, avoid other tubing manipulations, including milking, fanfolding, and tapping, which haven't been demonstrated to improve fluid drainage from the chest.*[23]

- Remember that routine clamping of the chest tube isn't recommended *because of the risk of tension pneumothorax.*[23]
- During patient transport, don't clamp the catheter tubing; instead, disconnect the suction connector tubing from the suction source. The system continues to collect fluid (by gravity) or air (by water seal). Keep the chest tube drainage collection system below the level of the chest tube at all times *to facilitate drainage.*[23]
- If you hear air leaking from the site, tape the dressing on three sides *to allow air to escape and to prevent a tension pneumothorax.* Closely monitor the patient and prepare for insertion of a new chest tube.
- If specimen collection is ordered, remove fluid using the needle and syringe from the self-sealing portion of the chest tube drainage tubing, or use a needleless syringe from the needleless site of the drainage tubing after disconnecting the tubing fluid collection site.

Complications

Complications of chest tube drainage system monitoring and care include accidental tube dislodgment, infection, pain, air leak from the insertion site, tubing disconnection, and chest tube occlusion with subsequent tension pneumothorax.

Documentation

Routine care

Record the date and time thoracic drainage began, the type of chest tube drainage system used, the amount of suction applied to the patient's pleural cavity, the presence or absence of bubbling or fluctuation in the water-seal or air-leak monitor chamber (if applicable), the initial amount and type of drainage, and the patient's respiratory status.

At the end of each shift, record the frequency of drainage system inspection; the amount, color, and consistency of drainage; the presence or absence of bubbling or fluctuation in the water-seal or air-leak monitor chamber (if applicable); the patient's respiratory status; the condition of the chest dressings; the administration of prescribed pain medication; and any complications that occurred, the practitioner notified, the date and time of notification, any interventions performed, and the patient's response to those interventions. Document teaching provided to the patient and family (if applicable), their understanding of that teaching, and any need for follow-up teaching.

Dressing change

Record the date and time and the reason for changing the insertion site dressing. Document your assessment findings before and after the procedure and the patient's response to the procedure. Record the condition of the insertion site and the patient's respiratory status and vital signs. Document teaching provided to the patient and family (if applicable), their understanding of that teaching, and any need for follow-up teaching.

Drainage system collection device change

Record the date and time and the reason for changing the chest tube drainage system. Document your assessment findings before and after the procedure and the patient's response to the procedure. Note the type of drainage system used; the amount of suction applied to the patient's pleural cavity (if applicable); the presence or absence of bubbling or fluctuation in the water-seal or air-leak monitor chamber (if applicable); the patient's respiratory status; and the amount, color, and consistency of drainage. Record the patient's respiratory status and vital signs, and the amount of drainage and its color and consistency. Document teaching provided to the patient and family (if applicable), their understanding of that teaching, and any need for follow-up teaching.

REFERENCES

1 Centers for Disease Control and Prevention. (2002). Guideline for hand hygiene in health-care settings: Recommendations of the Healthcare Infection Control Practices Advisory Committee and the HICPAC/SHEA/APIC/IDSA Hand Hygiene Task Force. *MMWR Recommendations and Reports, 51*(RR-16), 1–45. https://www.cdc.gov/mmwr/pdf/rr/rr5116.pdf (Level II)

2 The Joint Commission. (2021). Standard NPSG.07.01.01. *Comprehensive accreditation manual for hospitals.* Oakbrook Terrace, IL: The Joint Commission. (Level VII)

3 World Health Organization. (2009). WHO guidelines on hand hygiene in health care: First global patient safety challenge, clean care is safer care. https://apps.who.int/iris/bitstream/handle/10665/44102/9789241597906_eng.pdf?sequence=1 (Level IV)

4 Accreditation Association for Hospitals and Health Systems. (2020). Standard 07.01.21. *Healthcare Facilities Accreditation Program: Accreditation requirements for acute care hospitals.* Chicago, IL: Accreditation Association for Hospitals and Health Systems. (Level VII)

5 Centers for Medicare and Medicaid Services, Department of Health and Human Services. (2020). Condition of participation: Infection control. 42 C.F.R. § 482.42.

6 DNV GL-Healthcare USA, Inc. (2020). IC.1.SR.1. *NIAHO® accreditation requirements, interpretive guidelines and surveyor guidance—revision 20.0.* Milford, OH: DNV GL-Healthcare USA, Inc. (Level VII)

7 The Joint Commission. (2021). Standard NPSG.01.01.01. *Comprehensive accreditation manual for hospitals.* Oakbrook Terrace, IL: The Joint Commission. (Level VII)

8 The Joint Commission. (2021). Standard RI.01.01.01. *Comprehensive accreditation manual for hospitals.* Oakbrook Terrace, IL: The Joint Commission. (Level VII)

9 Centers for Medicare and Medicaid Services, Department of Health and Human Services. (2020). Condition of participation: Patient's rights. 42 C.F.R. § 482.13(c)(1).

10 Accreditation Association for Hospitals and Health Systems. (2020). Standard 15.01.16. *Healthcare Facilities Accreditation Program: Accreditation requirements for acute care hospitals*. Chicago, IL: Accreditation Association for Hospitals and Health Systems. (Level VII)

11 DNV GL-Healthcare USA, Inc. (2020). PR.2.SR.5. *NIAHO® accreditation requirements, interpretive guidelines and surveyor guidance—revision 20.0*. Milford, OH: DNV GL-Healthcare USA, Inc. (Level VII)

12 The Joint Commission. (2021). Standard PC.02.01.21. *Comprehensive accreditation manual for hospitals*. Oakbrook Terrace, IL: The Joint Commission. (Level VII)

13 The Joint Commission. (2021). Standard PC.01.02.07. *Comprehensive accreditation manual for hospitals*. Oakbrook Terrace, IL: The Joint Commission. (Level VII)

14 The Joint Commission. (2021). Standard MM.06.01.01. *Comprehensive accreditation manual for hospitals*. Oakbrook Terrace, IL: The Joint Commission. (Level VII)

15 DNV GL-Healthcare USA, Inc. (2020). MM.1.SR.3. *NIAHO® accreditation requirements, interpretive guidelines and surveyor guidance—revision 20.0*. Milford, OH: DNV GL-Healthcare USA, Inc. (Level VII)

16 Centers for Medicare and Medicaid Services, Department of Health and Human Services. (2020). Condition of participation: Nursing services. 42 C.F.R. § 482.23(c).

17 Accreditation Association for Hospitals and Health Systems. (2020). Standard 25.02.13. *Healthcare Facilities Accreditation Program: Accreditation requirements for acute care hospitals*. Chicago, IL: Accreditation Association for Hospitals and Health Systems. (Level VII)

18 Wiegand, D. L. (2017). *AACN procedure manual for high acuity, progressive, and critical care* (7th ed.). St. Louis, MO: Elsevier.

19 Siegel, J. D., et al. (2007, revised 2019). 2007 guideline for isolation precautions: Preventing transmission of infectious agents in healthcare settings. https://www.cdc.gov/infectioncontrol/pdf/guidelines/isolation-guidelines-H.pdf (Level II)

20 Centers for Disease Control and Prevention. (2004). Guidelines for preventing health-care-associated pneumonia, 2003: Recommendations of CDC and the Healthcare Infection Control Practices Advisory Committee. *MMWR Recommendations and Reports, 53*(RR-3), 1–36. https://www.cdc.gov/mmwr/pdf/rr/rr5303.pdf (Level II)

21 Centers for Medicare and Medicaid Services & The Joint Commission. (2020). The specifications manual for national hospital inpatient quality measures (version 5.10). https://www.qualitynet.org/inpatient/specifications-manuals#tab1

22 Accreditation Association for Hospitals and Health Systems. (2020). Standard 07.01.10. *Healthcare Facilities Accreditation Program: Accreditation requirements for acute care hospitals*. Chicago, IL: Accreditation Association for Hospitals and Health Systems. (Level VII)

23 Carroll, P. (2019). Chest tube and drainage management. https://www.rn.org/courses/coursematerial-98.pdf (Level VII)

24 Waters, T. R., et al. (2009). Safe patient handling training for schools of nursing. https://www.cdc.gov/niosh/docs/2009-127/pdfs/2009-127.pdf (Level VII)

25 Occupational Safety and Health Administration. (2012). Bloodborne pathogens, standard number1910.1030. https://www.osha.gov/pls/oshaweb/owadisp.show_document?p_id=10051&p_table=STANDARDS (Level VII)

26 Chest drains: Dressing. (2021). *The JBI EBP Database*. AN: JBI1874

27 Ganz, D. A., et al. (2013, reviewed 2021). *Preventing falls in hospitals: A toolkit for improving quality of care* (AHRQ Publication No. 13-0015-EF). Rockville, MD: Agency for Healthcare Research and Quality. https://www.ahrq.gov/professionals/systems/hospital/fallpxtoolkit/index.html (Level VII)

28 The Joint Commission. (2021). Standard RC.01.03.01. *Comprehensive accreditation manual for hospitals*. Oakbrook Terrace, IL: The Joint Commission. (Level VII)

29 Accreditation Association for Hospitals and Health Systems. (2020). Standard 10.00.03. *Healthcare Facilities Accreditation Program: Accreditation requirements for acute care hospitals*. Chicago, IL: Accreditation Association for Hospitals and Health Systems. (Level VII)

30 Centers for Medicare and Medicaid Services, Department of Health and Human Services. (2020). Condition of participation: Medical record services. 42 C.F.R. § 482.24(b).

31 DNV GL-Healthcare USA, Inc. (2020). MR.2.SR.1. *NIAHO® accreditation requirements, interpretive guidelines and surveyor guidance—revision 20.0*. Milford, OH: DNV GL-Healthcare USA, Inc. (Level VII)

32 The Joint Commission. (2014). Sentinel event alert 53: Managing risk during transition to new ISO tubing connector standards. http://www.jointcommission.org/assets/1/6/SEA_53_Connectors_8_19_14_final.pdf (Level VII)

33 U.S. Food and Drug Administration. (2017). Examples of medical device misconnections. https://www.fda.gov/medical-devices/medical-device-connectors/examples-medical-device-misconnections

34 Atrium Medical Corporation. (2015). Atrium OCEAN water seal chest drain. https://www.getinge.com/siteassets/education/chest-drains/ocean/oceanwallchart-010394-letter-size.pdf

35 Chotai, P., et al. (2020). Tube thoracostomy management. https://emedicine.medscape.com/article/1503275-overview (Level VII)

36 Rutala, W. A., et al. (2008, revised 2019). Guideline for disinfection and sterilization in healthcare facilities, 2008. https://www.cdc.gov/infection-control/pdf/guidelines/disinfection-guidelines-H.pdf (Level I)

37 Accreditation Association for Hospitals and Health Systems. (2020). Standard 07.02.03. *Healthcare Facilities Accreditation Program: Accreditation requirements for acute care hospitals*. Chicago, IL: Accreditation Association for Hospitals and Health Systems. (Level VII)

38 Perrault, L. P., et al. (2012). The PleuraFlow Active Chest Tube Clearance System: Initial clinical experience in adult cardiac surgery. *Innovations, 7*(5), 354–358. https://www.clearflow.com/wp-content/uploads/3-Perrault.The-PleuraFlow-Active-Chest-Tube-Clearance-System.2012.pdf (Level VI)

39 Mbinji, M. (2021). Evidence summary: Chest drains: Maintenance. *The JBI EBP Database*. AN: JBI1634

CHEST TUBE DRAINAGE SYSTEM SETUP

Chest tube drainage systems use gravity and sometimes suction to restore negative pressure and remove material that collects in the pleural cavity. A disposable drainage system combines drainage collection, a wet or dry seal, and suction control. The seal in the drainage system allows air and fluid to escape from the pleural cavity but doesn't allow air to reenter. Patient safety features on the device include a pressure relief valve and an air leak indicator. There are three types of chest tube drainage systems: a water seal–wet suction system, a water seal–dry suction system, and a dry seal–dry suction system.

A practitioner may order chest tube drainage to remove accumulated air, fluids (blood, pus, chyle, and serous fluids), or solids (blood clots) from the pleural cavity; to restore negative pressure in the pleural cavity; or to reexpand a partially or totally collapsed lung.

Equipment

Single-use, disposable, sterile chest drainage collection unit (water seal–wet suction system, water seal–dry-suction system, or dry seal–dry suction system) ■ sterile water ■ gloves ■ suction source ■ suction regulator ■ suction connection tubing ■ tape or zip tie ■ sterile dressing ■ Optional: commercial securement device.

Preparation of equipment

Inspect all equipment and supplies. If a product is expired, is defective, or has compromised integrity, remove it from patient use, label it as expired or defective, and report the expiration or defect as directed by your facility.

Implementation

■ Verify the practitioner's order *to determine the type of drainage system to be used and other procedural details.*
■ Gather and prepare the necessary equipment and supplies.
■ Perform hand hygiene.[1,2,3,4,5,6]
■ Confirm the patient's identity using at least two patient identifiers.[7]
■ Provide privacy.[8,9,10,11]
■ Explain the procedure to the patient and family (if appropriate) according to their individual communication and learning needs *to increase their understanding, allay their fears, and enhance cooperation.*[12]
■ Perform hand hygiene.[1,2,3,4,5,6]
■ Put on gloves *to comply with standard precautions.*[13,14]
■ Maintain sterile no-touch technique throughout the entire procedure and whenever you make changes in the system or alter connections *to avoid introducing pathogens into the pleural space.*[13,14,15,16,17]

- Open the single-use, disposable, sterile chest drainage collection unit.[15] Use the floor stand to set the unit on the floor, or use the hangers to hang it level on the bed below the level of the patient's chest tube.[18]

Water seal–wet suction system

- Use sterile water to fill the water seal chamber to the specified level according to the manufacturer's instructions.[15] The water seal chamber acts as a one-way valve to allow air to pass out of the lung, move down through a narrow channel, and bubble out through the bottom of the water seal (as shown below).

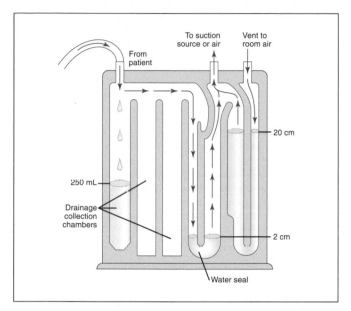

- Fill the suction control chamber with sterile water to the prescribed level (usually –10 to –20 cm H_2O).[15]
- After the practitioner inserts the chest tube, trace the chest tube from the point of origin[19] and connect it to the patient's chest tube drainage system. (See the "Chest tube insertion, assisting" procedure.)
- Secure the connection with tape or a zip tie *to ensure that the system remains airtight.*[15]
- Connect the suction tubing to the drainage system and the suction regulator if there is an order for suction.[15]
- Adjust the suction (if the chest tube is attached to suction) until gentle bubbling appears in the suction control chamber.[15] *The addition of suction increases the negative intrapleural pressure and helps overcome air leakage by improving the rate of airflow out of the patient and fluid removal.*

Water seal–dry suction system

- Use sterile water to fill the water seal chamber to the specified level according to the manufacturer's instructions.[15] The water seal chamber acts as a one-way valve to allow air to pass out of the lung, move down through a narrow channel, and bubble out through the bottom of the water seal.
- If the practitioner orders suction, turn the rotary dry suction control dial to the ordered suction mark (usually –1 to –20 cm H_2O.)[15]
- After the practitioner inserts the chest tube, trace the chest tube from the point of origin[19] and connect it to the chest tube drainage system, then secure the connection with tape or a zip tie *to ensure the system remains airtight.*[15]

- Connect the suction tubing to the drainage system if there is an order for suction.[15] Adjust the suction regulator (if the chest tube is attached to suction).[15]
- Verify suction operation according to the manufacturer's instructions. An indicator appears when the desired negative pressure is achieved by the system. In some models, an orange float appears in an indicator window. Other models indicate delivery of the correct amount of suction when the bellows reach the calibrated triangular mark in the suction monitor bellows window (as shown below). *The addition of suction increases the negative intrapleural pressure, and helps overcome air leakage by improving the rate of airflow out of the patient and fluid removal.*

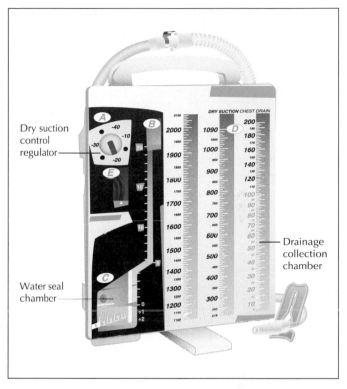

Dry seal–dry suction system

- Use sterile water to fill the air leak monitor chamber to the specified level according to the manufacturer's instructions.[15]
- If the practitioner orders suction, turn the rotary dry suction control dial to the ordered suction mark (usually –10 to –20 cm H_2O.)[15]
- After the practitioner inserts the chest tube, trace the chest tube from the point of origin[19] and connect it to the chest tube drainage system, then secure the connection with tape *to ensure the system remains airtight.* (See the "Chest tube insertion, assisting" procedure.)[15]
- Connect the suction tubing to the drainage system if there is an order for suction.[15] Adjust the suction regulator (if the chest tube is attached to suction.[15]
- Verify suction operation according to the manufacturer's instructions.[15] An indicator appears when the desired negative pressure is achieved by the system. In some models, an orange float appears in an indicator window. Other models indicate delivery of the correct amount of suction when the bellows reach the calibrated triangular mark in the suction monitor bellows window (as shown on the next page). *The addition of suction increases the negative intrapleural pressure, and helps overcome air leakage by improving the rate of airflow out of the patient and fluid removal.*

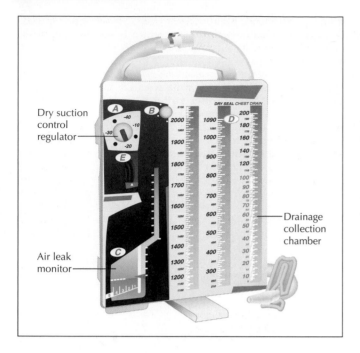

Dry suction control regulator

Air leak monitor

Drainage collection chamber

For all drainage systems

■ Place the drainage system at the bedside below the patient's chest tube in the upright position. *Placement of the device below the chest promotes optimal drainage of the tube by combining the effects of gravity with the system's negative pressure.*[15,18] *To avoid accidentally knocking over the device,* hang it on the bed frame with the hangers provided or secure it according to the manufacturer's instructions.

■ Secure the tubing to the patient's skin below the level of the dressing using a commercial securement device or tape.[15] Make sure that the tubing remains at the level of the patient. Avoid creating dependent loops, kinks, and pressure in the tubing, *because fluid-filled dependent loops can change pleural pressures rapidly, resulting in dramatically decreased drainage.*[15,18]

■ Remove and discard your gloves.[13,14]

■ Perform hand hygiene.[1,2,3,4,5,6]

■ Document the procedure.[20,21,22,23]

Special considerations

■ Don't overfill the water seal chamber. *A fluid level greater than 2 cm makes breathing more difficult.*[18] If you accidentally overfill the chamber, aspirate the excess water with a needle and syringe. Many models have a grommet to access the water seal chamber.

■ Some systems have a stopcock that can be gradually closed *to limit the suction flow into the drainage system.* If the patient's chest tube is to allow for gravity drainage, leave the stopcock in the ON or OPEN position.

■ Never block the pressure relief valve, which is usually located on the top of the unit.

■ Keep a sterile dressing and tape at the bedside in case of accidental dislodgement.

■ If excessive continuous bubbling is present in the water seal chamber, especially if you're using suction, rule out a leak in the drainage system. Try to locate the leak by momentarily clamping the tube at various points along its length. (The bubbling will stop when you clamp between the air leak and the water seal.) Begin clamping at the tube's proximal end and work down toward the drainage system, paying special attention to the seal around the connections. If a connection is loose, push it back together and tape it securely. If you clamp along the tube's entire length and the bubbling doesn't stop, the drainage system may be cracked and need replacement.[18]

■ If the chest tube and drainage system become disconnected, create a temporary water seal by immersing the end of the chest tube into a bottle of sterile water *to prevent pneumothorax.*

■ If the chest tube accidentally pulls out and the patient had an air leak from the chest tube, immediately cover the site with a sterile dressing and tape it on three sides, allowing air to escape on the fourth side *to reduce the risk of tension pneumothorax.* Alternately, cover the site with a sterile occlusive dressing with a one-way valve, if available. If your previous assessment didn't detect an air leak, place a sterile occlusive dressing over the site and monitor the patient closely for signs of respiratory distress. Stay with the patient and have a colleague call the practitioner immediately. Assess the patient for signs and symptoms of tension pneumothorax, including hypotension; distended jugular veins; absent or decreased breath sounds; tracheal shift; hypoxemia; weak, rapid pulse; dyspnea; tachypnea; diaphoresis; and chest pain. Then have your colleague gather the equipment needed to reinsert the chest tube.

■ Instruct staff members and visitors to avoid touching the equipment *to prevent complications from separated connections.*

■ *To attach a new drainage system when the existing one is full,* briefly clamp the chest tube close to the insertion site and, using sterile technique, disconnect the old drainage system, connect the new drainage system, and then unclamp the chest tube.[18]

■ The Joint Commission issued a sentinel event alert related to managing risk during transition to new International Organization for Standardization tubing standards that were designed to prevent dangerous tubing misconnections, which can lead to serious patient injury and death. During the transition, make sure to trace each tubing and catheter from the patient to its point of origin before connecting or reconnecting any device or infusion, at any care transition (such as to a new setting or service), and as part of the hand-off process; route tubes and catheters having different purposes in different standardized directions; when the patient has different access sites or several bags hanging, label tubing at both the distal and proximal ends; use tubing and equipment only as intended; and store medications for different delivery routes in separate locations.[24]

Complications

Complications associated with chest tube drainage system setup include infection, accidental chest tube dislodgement, pain, air leak from the insertion site, and tubing disconnection.

Documentation

Record the date and time that chest tube drainage began, the type of chest tube drainage system used, the amount of suction applied to the pleural cavity (if applicable), and the presence or absence of bubbling or fluctuation in the water seal chamber (if applicable). Document teaching provided to the patient and family (if applicable), their understanding of that teaching, and any need for follow-up teaching.

REFERENCES

1 Centers for Disease Control and Prevention. (2002). Guideline for hand hygiene in health-care settings: Recommendations of the Healthcare Infection Control Practices Advisory Committee and the HICPAC/SHEA/APIC/IDSA Hand Hygiene Task Force. *MMWR Recommendations and Reports, 51*(RR-16), 1–45. https://www.cdc.gov/mmwr/pdf/rr/rr5116.pdf (Level II)

2 The Joint Commission. (2021). Standard NPSG.07.01.01. *Comprehensive accreditation manual for hospitals.* Oakbrook Terrace, IL: The Joint Commission. (Level VII)

3 World Health Organization. (2009). WHO guidelines on hand hygiene in health care: First global patient safety challenge, clean care is safer care. https://apps.who.int/iris/bitstream/handle/10665/44102/9789241597906_eng.pdf?sequence=1 (Level IV)

4 Accreditation Association for Hospitals and Health Systems. (2020). Standard 07.01.21. *Healthcare Facilities Accreditation Program: Accreditation requirements for acute care hospitals.* Chicago, IL: Accreditation Association for Hospitals and Health Systems. (Level VII)

5 Centers for Medicare and Medicaid Services, Department of Health and Human Services. (2020). Condition of participation: Infection control. 42 C.F.R. § 482.42.

6 DNV GL-Healthcare USA, Inc. (2020). IC.1.SR.1. *NIAHO® accreditation requirements, interpretive guidelines and surveyor guidance—revision 20.0.* Milford, OH: DNV GL-Healthcare USA, Inc. (Level VII)

7 The Joint Commission. (2021). Standard NPSG.01.01.01. *Comprehensive accreditation manual for hospitals*. Oakbrook Terrace, IL: The Joint Commission. (Level VI)

8 The Joint Commission. (2021). Standard RI.01.01.01. *Comprehensive accreditation manual for hospitals*. Oakbrook Terrace, IL: The Joint Commission. (Level VII)

9 DNV GL-Healthcare USA, Inc. (2020). PR.2.SR.5. *NIAHO® accreditation requirements, interpretive guidelines and surveyor guidance—revision 20.0*. Milford, OH: DNV GL-Healthcare USA, Inc. (Level VII)

10 Centers for Medicare and Medicaid Services, Department of Health and Human Services. (2020). Condition of participation: Patient's rights. 42 C.F.R. § 482.13(c)(1).

11 Accreditation Association for Hospitals and Health Systems. (2020). Standard 15.01.16. *Healthcare Facilities Accreditation Program: Accreditation requirements for acute care hospitals*. Chicago, IL: Accreditation Association for Hospitals and Health Systems. (Level VII)

12 The Joint Commission. (2021). Standard PC.02.01.21. *Comprehensive accreditation manual for hospitals*. Oakbrook Terrace, IL: The Joint Commission. (Level VII)

13 Siegel, J. D., et al. (2007, revised 2019). 2007 guideline for isolation precautions: Preventing transmission of infectious agents in healthcare settings. https://www.cdc.gov/infectioncontrol/pdf/guidelines/isolation-guidelines-H.pdf (Level II)

14 Accreditation Association for Hospitals and Health Systems. (2020). Standard 07.01.10. *Healthcare Facilities Accreditation Program: Accreditation requirements for acute care hospitals*. Chicago, IL: Accreditation Association for Hospitals and Health Systems. (Level VII)

15 Wiegand, D. L. (2017). *AACN procedure manual for high acuity, progressive, and critical care* (7th ed.). Philadelphia, PA: Saunders.

16 Centers for Disease Control and Prevention. (2004). Guidelines for preventing health-care-associated pneumonia, 2003: Recommendations of CDC and the Healthcare Infection Control Practices Advisory Committee. *MMWR Recommendations and Reports, 53*(RR-3), 1–32. https://www.cdc.gov/mmwr/pdf/rr/rr5303.pdf (Level II)

17 Centers for Medicare and Medicaid Services, & The Joint Commission. (2021). The specifications manual for national hospital inpatient quality measures (version 5.10.). https://www.qualitynet.org/inpatient/specifications-manuals#tab1

18 Carroll, P. (2019). Chest tube and drainage management. https://www.rn.org/courses/coursematerial-98.pdf (Level VII)

19 U.S. Food and Drug Administration. (2017). Examples of medical device misconnections. https://www.fda.gov/medical-devices/medical-device-connectors/examples-medical-device-misconnections

20 The Joint Commission. (2021). Standard RC.01.03.01. *Comprehensive accreditation manual for hospitals*. Oakbrook Terrace, IL: The Joint Commission. (Level VII)

21 Accreditation Association for Hospitals and Health Systems. (2020). Standard 10.00.03. *Healthcare Facilities Accreditation Program: Accreditation requirements for acute care hospitals*. Chicago, IL: Accreditation Association for Hospitals and Health Systems. (Level VII)

22 Centers for Medicare and Medicaid Services, Department of Health and Human Services. (2020). Condition of participation: Medical record services. 42 C.F.R. § 482.24(b).

23 DNV GL-Healthcare USA, Inc. (2020). MR.2.SR.1. *NIAHO® accreditation requirements, interpretive guidelines and surveyor guidance—revision 20.0*. Milford, OH: DNV GL-Healthcare USA, Inc. (Level VII)

24 The Joint Commission. (2014). Sentinel event alert 53: Managing risk during transition to new ISO tubing connector standards http://www.jointcommission.org/assets/1/6/SEA_53_Connectors_8_19_14_final.pdf (Level VII)

CHEST TUBE INSERTION, ASSISTING

The pleural space in the chest cavity normally contains a thin layer of lubricating fluid that allows the visceral and parietal pleurae to move without friction during respiration. An excess of fluid (pleural effusion), air (pneumothorax), blood (hemothorax), or a combination of these elements in this space alters intrapleural pressure and causes partial or complete lung collapse. Conditions that cause an excess of fluid or air include trauma, surgery, cancer, and infection. Chest tube insertion (thoracostomy) allows drainage of air and fluid from the pleural space, which normalizes intrapleural pressure and allows the lung to reexpand. A chest tube can also be used to instill sclerosing agents to eliminate the pleural space (pleurodesis) for recurrent pleural effusion or pneumothorax.[1] Contraindications to chest tube insertion include coagulopathies, anticoagulation, bleeding diathesis, and a skin infection over the chest tube insertion site.[1]

A practitioner performs this procedure using sterile technique. During chest tube insertion, two people should be present: the practitioner performing the thoracostomy and an assistant competent in thoracostomy care. The size of the chest tube and the insertion site vary depending on the patient's size and condition. A smaller-bore tube is used to remove air, whereas a larger-bore tube is used to remove fluid.[2] In general, the smallest tube that will be effective should be used, because larger tubes cause more patient discomfort. To remove air, chest tube insertion occurs near the apex of the lung, through the second intercostal space at the midclavicular line, because air rises to the top of the intrapleural space.[2] To remove fluid, chest tube insertion occurs near the base of the lung, through the fourth or fifth intercostal space, between the anterior axillary and midaxillary lines (as shown below), because fluid settles to the lower levels of the intrapleural space.[2]

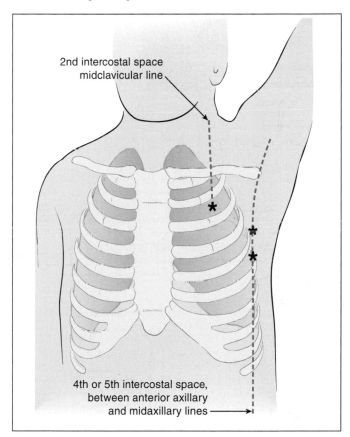

After insertion, the practitioner connects one or more chest tubes to a thoracic drainage system that removes air, fluid, or both from the pleural space and prevents backflow into that space, promoting lung reexpansion. (See the "Chest tube drainage system setup" procedure, and the "Chest tube drainage system monitoring and care" procedure.)

Equipment

Vital signs monitoring equipment ▪ lidocaine local anesthetic (0.5% or 1%) ▪ sterile gowns ▪ sterile gloves ▪ caps ▪ masks and goggles or face masks with face shields ▪ antiseptic wipes ▪ rolled towels or blanket ▪ sterile drapes and sterile towels ▪ chlorhexidine-based antiseptic swabs ▪ sterile syringes (assortment of sizes: 3 mL, 5 mL, and tuberculin) ▪ 22G and 25G needles ▪ sterile chest tube tray, which includes hemostats, forceps, trocar, scalpel, Kelly clamps, scissors, skin expanders, and sponges ▪ sterile chest tubes (#16 to #20 French catheter for air or serous fluid; #28 to #40 French catheter for blood, pus, or thick fluid) ▪ suture material (usually #2-0 to #3-0 silk with cutting needle) ▪ two sterile 4″ × 4″ (10 cm × 10 cm) drain dressings ■ sterile 4″ × 4″ (10 cm × 10 cm) or 2″ × 2″ (5 cm × 5 cm) gauze pads ■ 3″ to 4″ (7.6 to 10 cm) adhesive tape ■ 1″ (2.5 cm) adhesive tape for connections ■ sterile chest tube drainage system with tubing and connector ■ sterile marker ■ sterile labels ■ prescribed sedation ■ prescribed pain medication ■ stethoscope ■ disinfectant pad ■ sterile water ■ Optional: suction source, suction control device, suction connection tubing, sterile transparent dressing, Y connector, commercial securement device, IV catheter insertion equipment.

Prepackaged sterile chest tube trays are commercially available and contain most of the necessary equipment.

Preparation of equipment

Inspect all equipment and supplies. If a product is expired, is defective, or has compromised integrity, remove it from patient use, label it as expired or defective, and report the expiration or defect as directed by your facility. Set up the drainage system according to the manufacturer's instructions. (See the "Chest tube drainage system setup" procedure.) Place the system next to the patient's bed below the patient's chest level to facilitate drainage. Label all medications, medication containers, and other solutions on and off the sterile field.[3,4]

Implementation

■ Verify the order for chest tube insertion and the number and sizes of chest tubes needed.[5]
■ Review the patient's medical record for allergies to medications, antiseptic solution, or the local anesthetic.
■ Unless the procedure is an emergency, confirm that informed consent has been obtained and that the signed consent form is in the patient's medical record.[6,7,8,9]
■ Review the patient's medical record for abnormal chest X-ray and blood gas results. Notify the practitioner of any unexpected results.[2]
■ Review the patient's medical record for a history of chronic lung disease, spontaneous pneumothorax, and pulmonary disease, or procedures that may indicate the need for chest tube placement.[2]
■ Gather and prepare the necessary equipment and supplies.
■ Conduct a preprocedure verification *to make sure that all relevant documentation, related information, and equipment are available and correctly identified to the patient's identifiers.*[2,5,10]
■ Perform hand hygiene.[11,12,13,14,15,16]
■ Confirm the patient's identity using at least two patient identifiers.[7,17]
■ Provide privacy.[18,19,20,21]
■ Explain the procedure to the patient and family (if appropriate) according to their individual communication and learning needs *to increase their understanding, allay fears, and enhance cooperation.*[22]
■ Verify that the practitioner has marked the insertion site with initials or with another unambiguous mark designated by your facility.[23]
■ Raise the bed to waist level before providing care *to prevent caregiver back strain.*[24]
■ Perform hand hygiene.[11,12,13,14,15,16]
■ Assess the patient for signs and symptoms of respiratory distress, including tachypnea, decreased or absent breath sounds, dyspnea, cyanosis, asymmetrical chest expansion, anxiety, restlessness, shortness of breath, tachycardia, hypotension, arrhythmias, and sudden sharp chest pain.[2]
■ Obtain the patient's baseline data, including vital signs, skin color, perfusion, level of consciousness, oxygen requirements, hemodynamic stability, and respiratory rate, pattern, and effort *to identify and document acute changes that may occur during and after the procedure.*[2]
■ Ensure that the patient has adequate IV access. Insert an IV catheter, as needed, *to provide a route for medication administration.*[2]
■ Administer sedation and pain medication as ordered, following safe medication practices.[25,26,27,28] The practitioner may request sedation (benzodiazepines) and opioid analgesia *to reduce pain and to help the patient remain calm.*

Inserting a chest tube

Chest tube insertion involves these steps:
■ The practitioner puts on a cap, a mask, eye protection, a sterile gown, and sterile gloves and prepares a sterile field using sterile drapes.[2,29,30]
■ The practitioner prepares the insertion site using chlorhexidine-based antiseptic swabs.[2]
■ After the antiseptic dries completely, the practitioner drapes the patient, leaving the insertion site exposed.[2]
■ The nurse disinfects the rubber stopper of the lidocaine vial with an antiseptic pad and then inverts the bottle and holds it for the practitioner to withdraw the anesthetic.
■ The practitioner injects a local anesthetic at the site *to reduce the pain of the procedure* and waits for the anesthetic to take effect.[2]
■ The practitioner makes a skin incision about 1″ (2.5 cm) long and then inserts a hemostat through the opening *to enter the pleural space.* Typically, when the pleural space is entered, you'll see a return of pleural contents, confirming penetration.[2]
■ The practitioner spreads the hemostat open slightly *to enlarge the opening enough to accommodate the chest tube.*[2]
■ Using a finger, the practitioner creates a track for the chest tube and then clamps the chest tube with the hemostat and inserts them through the incision, guiding the hemostat and tube along the inserted finger.[2]
■ The practitioner removes the hemostat and immediately connects the chest tube to the drainage system.[2]

■ Place the patient in the lateral position (for air drainage) or supine position with the head of the bed elevated 30 degrees (for fluid drainage).[2] (Typically, the practitioner places the chest tube in the midaxillary to anterior axillary line.) It's easiest to lay the patient in the supine position, using rolled towels or a blanket to slightly rotate the upper body in a side-lying position, with the arm of the affected side raised above the head.
■ Put on a cap and mask and goggles or a mask with a face shield.[29,30]
■ Perform hand hygiene.[11,12,13,14,15,16]
■ If you're assisting in the sterile field, put on sterile gloves and a sterile gown *to maintain standard precautions and infection-prevention practices for a sterile surgical procedure.*[29,30]
■ Conduct a time-out immediately before starting the procedure *to ensure that the correct patient, site, positioning, and procedure are identified and that, as applicable, all relevant information and necessary equipment are available during and after the procedure.*[2,31]
■ If the patient can cooperate, ask the patient to take a deep breath just before tube insertion. *A deep breath displaces the diaphragm downward, minimizing the risk of injury.*
■ Assist the practitioner with the procedure, as needed, while continually assessing the patient for vital sign changes. (See *Inserting a chest tube.*)
■ Assist the practitioner in attaching the disposable sterile chest tube drainage system to the chest tube. If the practitioner inserted more than one chest tube, assist in attaching the disposable chest tube drainage system to the chest tube using a Y-connector.[2] Trace each tubing from the patient to its point of origin *to make sure it's connected to the proper port.*[32,33]
■ Assist the practitioner with suturing the chest tube securely into place.[2]
■ Remove and discard your gloves.[29,30]
■ Perform hand hygiene.[11,12,13,14,15,16]
■ Open the packages of 4″ × 4″ (10 cm × 10 cm) drain dressings and gauze pads.[2]
■ Put on new sterile gloves.[29,30]
■ Place the two 4″ × 4″ (10 cm × 10 cm) drain dressings around the insertion site, one from the top and the other from the bottom (as shown), *to seal the insertion site from any air entry or escape;*[2] place a 4″ × 4″ (10 cm × 10 cm) gauze pad on top of the drain dressings; and cover the dressing with wide adhesive tape.

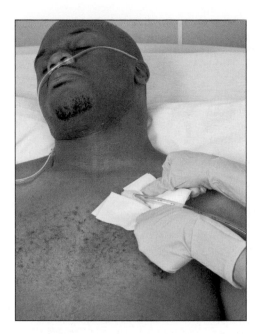

■ Alternatively, apply a sterile transparent dressing over the chest tube insertion site *to enable direct inspection of the wound.*

■ Write the date, the time, and your initials on the dressing if required by your facility.

■ Secure the chest tube and drainage tube with a commercial securement device or tape and ensure that there's no tension pulling on the insertion site *to help prevent accidental tube dislodgment.*[2]

■ Tape or zip-tie the junction of the chest tube and the drainage tube securely (as shown below) *to prevent their separation.*[2]

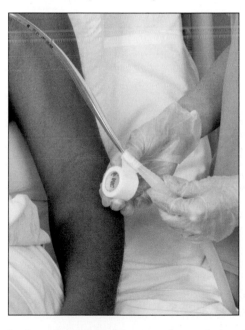

■ Secure the chest tube drainage system according to the manufacturer's instructions *to keep the drainage system from tipping over.*

■ Return the bed to the lowest position *to prevent falls and maintain patient safety.*[34]

■ Discard used supplies in the appropriate receptacles.[35]

■ Remove and discard your gloves and other personal protective equipment[29,30] and perform hand hygiene.[11,12,13,14,15,16]

■ Ensure that all clamps are open, and that the drainage tubing has a straight flow to the chest tube drainage collection system and has no dependent loops or kinks, *because fluid-filled dependent loops can rapidly change pleural pressure, resulting in dramatically decreased drainage.*[2,36]

■ Ensure that the chest tube drainage system is correctly connected to the patient's chest tube; then, if ordered, connect the suction tubing to the drainage system and the suction regulator.

■ Adjust the suction until gentle bubbling appears in the suction control chamber of a wet suction system, or ensure that the appropriate indicator appears when the dry suction system achieves the desired negative pressure.

■ Check the status of the drainage tubing.[36]

NURSING ALERT Drain large effusions slowly, *because rapid removal (removal of more than 1 L of pleural fluid during the first 30 minutes after chest tube insertion) can cause pulmonary edema.*

■ Reassess the patient after the procedure.[37] Obtain vital signs and assess skin color, perfusion, level of consciousness, oxygen requirements, hemodynamic stability, comfort level, pain level, and respiratory rate, pattern, and effort *to identify the patient's tolerance of the procedure and response to chest tube placement.*

■ Screen for and assess the patient's pain using facility-defined criteria that are consistent with the patient's age, condition, and ability to understand.[38]

■ Treat the patient's pain, as needed and ordered, using nonpharmacologic, pharmacologic, or a combination of approaches. Base the treatment plan on evidence-based practices and the patient's clinical condition, past medical history, and pain management goals.[38]

■ Arrange for a portable chest X-ray, as ordered, *to check tube position, air or fluid evacuation, and lung reexpansion.*[2]

■ Monitor the patient's vital signs at an interval determined by your facility or as indicated by the patient's condition. Auscultate breath sounds at least every 4 hours *to assess air exchange in the affected lung*. Note that diminished or absent breath sounds indicate that the lung hasn't reexpanded.

■ Record the color, character, consistency, and amount of drainage in the drainage collection chamber.[36] Notify the practitioner immediately of a sudden decrease in drainage or the presence of frank bloody drainage.

■ Mark the drainage level on the disposable chest drainage collection device at an interval determined by your facility or as indicated by the patient's condition.[7]

■ Perform hand hygiene.[11,12,13,14,15,16]

■ Clean and disinfect your stethoscope using a disinfectant pad.[39,40]

■ Perform hand hygiene.[11,12,13,14,15,16]

■ Document the procedure.[41,42,43,44]

Special considerations

NURSING ALERT Don't "strip" a chest drainage tube (occlude the chest tube with one hand while quickly squeezing and moving the other hand down the tube to move fluid down the tube into the drainage chamber) *because intraluminal pressures can rise dangerously high, which may convert a simple pneumothorax to life-threatening pneumothorax and cause tissue trauma and unnecessary discomfort. Also avoid other tubing manipulations, such as milking, fanfolding, or tapping, because these actions don't improve fluid drainage from the chest.*

■ If specimen collection is ordered, remove fluid with a needle and syringe from the self-sealing portion of the drainage tubing or with a needleless syringe from the needleless site of the drainage tubing after disinfecting the tubing collection site.

■ Avoid routine clamping of the chest tube *because of the risk of tension pneumothorax.*

■ Be aware that guidelines recommend using gravity drainage or application of minimal suction over attaching the patient's chest tube to continuous suction, *because doing so enables easier ambulation, reduces chest tube dwell time, and reduces length of stay.*

■ During patient transport, keep the chest tube drainage system below chest level. Don't clamp the chest tube during transport; instead, disconnect the suction tubing from the suction source. The system continues to collect fluid (by gravity) or air (by water seal).

■ The Joint Commission issued a sentinel event alert related to managing risk during transition to new International Organization for Standardization tubing standards that were designed to prevent dangerous tubing misconnections, which can lead to serious patient injury and death. During the transition, make sure to trace each tubing and catheter from the patient to its point of origin before connecting or reconnecting any device or infusion, at any care transition (such as to a new setting or service), and as part of the hand-off process; route tubes and catheters with different purposes in different, standardized directions; when the patient has different access sites or several bags hanging, label tubing at both the distal and proximal ends; use tubing and equipment only as intended; and store medications for different delivery routes in separate locations.[32]

■ Keep a sterile dressing and tape at the patient's bedside *in case of accidental dislodgement.*

■ If you hear air leaking from the site, tape the dressing on three sides *to allow air to escape and to prevent a tension pneumothorax.* Immediately notify the practitioner. Closely monitor the patient and prepare for insertion of a new chest tube.

Complications

Complications of chest tube insertion include bleeding (if a vessel is inadvertently nicked during the insertion process), subcutaneous emphysema from air leaking into the pleural space, and infection.

Documentation

Record the date and time of chest tube insertion, the name of the practitioner who inserted the tube, the insertion site, the size of the chest tube used, medications administered, the type of chest tube drainage system used, the suction setting, and the presence of drainage and bubbling. Document any complications that occurred, interventions performed, and the patient's response to those interventions. Record your assessment findings before and after the procedure as well as the patient's response to the procedure. Record the patient's respiratory status and vital signs and the amount of drainage and its color and consistency every 2 to 4 hours. Document teaching provided to the patient and family (if applicable), their understanding of that teaching, and any need for follow-up teaching.

REFERENCES

1 Huggins, J. T., et al. (2021). Thoracostomy tubes and catheters: Placement techniques and complications. In: *UpToDate*, Wolfson, A. B.,, et al. (Eds.)

2 Wiegand, D. L. (2017). *AACN procedure manual for high acuity, progressive, and critical care* (7th ed.). St. Louis, MO: Elsevier.

3 The Joint Commission. (2021). Standard NPSG.03.04.01. *Comprehensive accreditation manual for hospitals.* Oakbrook Terrace, IL: The Joint Commission. (Level VII)

4 Accreditation Association for Hospitals and Health Systems. (2020). Standard 25.01.27. *Healthcare Facilities Accreditation Program: Accreditation requirements for acute care hospitals.* Chicago, IL: Accreditation Association for Hospitals and Health Systems. (Level VII)

5 The Joint Commission. (2021). Standard UP.01.01.01. *Comprehensive accreditation manual for hospitals.* Oakbrook Terrace, IL: The Joint Commission. (Level VII)

6 The Joint Commission. (2021). Standard RI.01.03.01. *Comprehensive accreditation manual for hospitals.* Oakbrook Terrace, IL: The Joint Commission. (Level VII)

7 Accreditation Association for Hospitals and Health Systems. (2020). Standard 15.01.11. *Healthcare Facilities Accreditation Program: Accreditation requirements for acute care hospitals.* Chicago, IL: Accreditation Association for Hospitals and Health Systems. (Level VII)

8 Centers for Medicare and Medicaid Services, Department of Health and Human Services. (2020). Condition of participation: Patient's rights. 42 C.F.R. § 482.13.

9 DNV GL-Healthcare USA, Inc. (2020). PR.2.SR.3. *NIAHO® accreditation requirements, interpretive guidelines and surveyor guidance—revision 20.0.* Milford, OH: DNV GL-Healthcare USA, Inc. (Level VII)

10 Accreditation Association for Hospitals and Health Systems. (2020). Standard 30.00.14. *Healthcare Facilities Accreditation Program: Accreditation requirements for acute care hospitals.* Chicago, IL: Accreditation Association for Hospitals and Health Systems. (Level VII)

11 Centers for Disease Control and Prevention. (2002). Guideline for hand hygiene in health-care settings: Recommendations of the Healthcare Infection Control Practices Advisory Committee and the HICPAC/SHEA/APIC/IDSA Hand Hygiene Task Force. *MMWR Recommendations and Reports, 51*(RR-16), 1–45. https://www.cdc.gov/mmwr/pdf/rr/rr5116.pdf (Level II)

12 The Joint Commission. (2021). Standard NPSG.07.01.01. *Comprehensive accreditation manual for hospitals.* Oakbrook Terrace, IL: The Joint Commission. (Level VII)

13 World Health Organization. (2009). WHO guidelines on hand hygiene in health care: First global patient safety challenge, clean care is safer care. https://apps.who.int/iris/bitstream/handle/10665/44102/9789241597906_eng.pdf?sequence=1 (Level IV)

14 Accreditation Association for Hospitals and Health Systems. (2020). Standard 07.01.21. *Healthcare Facilities Accreditation Program: Accreditation requirements for acute care hospitals.* Chicago, IL: Accreditation Association for Hospitals and Health Systems. (Level VII)

15 Centers for Medicare and Medicaid Services, Department of Health and Human Services. (2020). Condition of participation: Infection control. 42 C.F.R. § 482.42.

16 DNV GL-Healthcare USA, Inc. (2020). IC.1.SR.1. *NIAHO® accreditation requirements: Interpretive guidelines & surveyor guidance—revision 20.0.* Milford, OH: DNV GL-Healthcare USA, Inc. (Level VII)

17 The Joint Commission. (2021). Standard NPSG.01.01.01. *Comprehensive accreditation manual for hospitals.* Oakbrook Terrace, IL: The Joint Commission. (Level VII)

18 Accreditation Association for Hospitals and Health Systems. (2020). Standard 15.01.16. *Healthcare Facilities Accreditation Program: Accreditation requirements for acute care hospitals.* Chicago, IL: Accreditation Association for Hospitals and Health Systems. (Level VII)

19 Centers for Medicare and Medicaid Services, Department of Health and Human Services. (2020). Condition of participation: Patient's rights. 42 C.F.R. § 482.13(c)(1).

20 The Joint Commission. (2021). Standard RI.01.01.01. *Comprehensive accreditation manual for hospitals.* Oakbrook Terrace, IL: The Joint Commission. (Level VII)

21 DNV GL-Healthcare USA, Inc. (2020). PR.2.SR.5. *NIAHO® accreditation requirements, interpretive guidelines and surveyor guidance—revision 20.0.* Milford, OH: DNV GL-Healthcare USA, Inc. (Level VII)

22 The Joint Commission. (2021). Standard PC.02.01.21. *Comprehensive accreditation manual for hospitals.* Oakbrook Terrace, IL: The Joint Commission. (Level VII)

23 The Joint Commission. (2021). Standard UP.01.02.01. *Comprehensive accreditation manual for hospitals.* Oakbrook Terrace, IL: The Joint Commission. (Level VII)

24 Waters, T. R., et al. (2009). Safe patient handling training for schools of nursing. https://www.cdc.gov/niosh/docs/2009-127/pdfs/2009-127.pdf (Level VII)

25 Accreditation Association for Hospitals and Health Systems. (2020). Standard 16.01.03. *Healthcare Facilities Accreditation Program: Accreditation requirements for acute care hospitals.* Chicago, IL: Accreditation Association for Hospitals and Health Systems. (Level VII)

26 Centers for Medicare and Medicaid Services, Department of Health and Human Services. (2020). Condition of participation: Nursing services. 42 C.F.R. § 482.23(c).

27 The Joint Commission. (2021). Standard MM.06.01.01. *Comprehensive accreditation manual for hospitals.* Oakbrook Terrace, IL: The Joint Commission. (Level VII)

28 DNV GL-Healthcare USA, Inc. (2020). MM.1.SR.3. *NIAHO® accreditation requirements, interpretive guidelines and surveyor guidance—revision 20.0.* Milford, OH: DNV GL-Healthcare USA, Inc. (Level VII)

29 Siegel, J. D., et al. (2007, revised 2019). 2007 guideline for isolation precautions: Preventing transmission of infectious agents in healthcare settings. https://www.cdc.gov/infectioncontrol/pdf/guidelines/isolation-guidelines-H.pdf (Level II)

30 Accreditation Association for Hospitals and Health Systems. (2020). Standard 07.01.10. *Healthcare Facilities Accreditation Program: Accreditation requirements for acute care hospitals.* Chicago, IL: Accreditation Association for Hospitals and Health Systems. (Level VII)

31 The Joint Commission. (2021). Standard UP.01.03.01. *Comprehensive accreditation manual for hospitals.* Oakbrook Terrace, IL: The Joint Commission. (Level VII)

32 The Joint Commission. (2014). Sentinel event alert 53: Managing risk during transition to new ISO tubing connector standards. http://www.jointcommission.org/assets/1/6/SEA_53_Connectors_8_19_14_final.pdf (Level VII)

33 U.S. Food and Drug Administration. (2017). Examples of medical device misconnections. https://www.fda.gov/medical-devices/medical-device-connectors/examples-medical-device-misconnections

34 Ganz, D. A., et al. (2013, reviewed 2021). *Preventing falls in hospitals: A toolkit for improving quality of care* (AHRQ Publication No. 13-0015-EF). Rockville, MD: Agency for Healthcare Research and Quality. https://www.ahrq.gov/professionals/systems/hospital/fallpxtoolkit/index.html (Level VII)

35 Occupational Safety and Health Administration. (2012). Bloodborne pathogens, standard number1910.1030. https://www.osha.gov/pls/oshaweb/owadisp.show_document?p_id=10051&p_table=STANDARDS (Level VII)

36 Carroll, P. (2019). Chest tube and drainage management. https://www.rn.org/courses/coursematerial-98.pdf (Level VII)

37 The Joint Commission. (2021). Standard PC.01.02.05. *Comprehensive accreditation manual for hospitals.* Oakbrook Terrace, IL: The Joint Commission. (Level VII)

38 The Joint Commission. (2021). Standard PC.01.02.07. *Comprehensive accreditation manual for hospitals.* Oakbrook Terrace, IL: The Joint Commission. (Level VII)

39 Rutala, W. A., et al. (2008, revised 2019). Guideline for disinfection and sterilization in healthcare facilities, 2008. https://www.cdc.gov/infection-control/pdf/guidelines/disinfection-guidelines-H.pdf (Level I)

40 Accreditation Association for Hospitals and Health Systems. (2020). Standard 07.02.03. *Healthcare Facilities Accreditation Program: Accreditation requirements for acute care hospitals.* Chicago, IL: Accreditation Association for Hospitals and Health Systems. (Level VII)

41 The Joint Commission. (2021). Standard RC.01.03.01. *Comprehensive accreditation manual for hospitals.* Oakbrook Terrace, IL: The Joint Commission. (Level VII)

42 Accreditation Association for Hospitals and Health Systems. (2020). Standard 10.00.03. *Healthcare Facilities Accreditation Program: Accreditation requirements for acute care hospitals.* Chicago, IL: Accreditation Association for Hospitals and Health Systems. (Level VII)

43 Centers for Medicare and Medicaid Services, Department of Health and Human Services. (2020). Condition of participation: Medical record services. 42 C.F.R. § 482.24(b).

44 DNV GL-Healthcare USA, Inc. (2020). MR.2.SR.1. *NIAHO® accreditation requirements, interpretive guidelines and surveyor guidance—revision 20.0.* Milford, OH: DNV GL-Healthcare USA, Inc. (Level VII)

CHEST TUBE REMOVAL, ASSISTING

Chest tube removal should occur as soon as the chest tube is no longer clinically indicated, *to prevent infection along the tube tract, reduce hospital length of stay, and prevent complications related to hospitalization.*[1] The timing of chest tube removal is based on individualized assessment of the patient. Chest tube removal occurs when drainage has diminished, an air leak no longer exists, fluctuations in the water seal chamber are minimal or absent, the patient's respiratory status has improved, breath sounds are equal and at baseline for the patient, or a chest X-ray shows the lung is reexpanded.[1,2] After lung reexpansion and drainage control have occurred, the practitioner may order tube clamping for several hours to simulate chest tube removal and assess the patient's response.[1] This approach allows time to observe the patient for signs and symptoms of respiratory distress, an indication that air or fluid remains trapped in the pleural space.

Chest tube removal is the responsibility of a physician, a nurse practitioner, an advanced practice nurse, or a physician's assistant, according to the scope of practice. A nurse assists with removal, as needed.

Equipment

Gloves ■ sterile gloves ■ goggles and masks or masks with face shield ■ gowns ■ prescribed premedication ■ suture removal kit ■ fluid-impermeable pad ■ 4″ × 4″ (10 cm × 10 cm) sterile gauze dressing ■ tape ■ antiseptic swabs ■ disinfectant pad ■ vital signs monitoring equipment ■ stethoscope ■ pulse oximeter ■ Optional: sterile petroleum gauze, prescribed pain medication, chest tube clamps.

Preparation of equipment

Inspect all equipment and supplies. If a product is expired, is defective, or has compromised integrity, remove it from patient use, label it as expired or defective, and report the expiration or defect as directed by your facility.

Implementation

■ Verify the practitioner's order for chest tube removal.
■ Gather and prepare the necessary equipment and supplies.
■ Perform hand hygiene.[3,4,5,6,7,8]
■ Confirm the patient's identity using at least two patient identifiers.[9]
■ Provide privacy.[10,11,12,13]
■ Explain the procedure to the patient and family (if appropriate) according to their individual communication and learning needs *to increase their understanding, allay their fears, and enhance cooperation.*[14]
■ Premedicate the patient, as ordered, following safe medication administration practices *to reduce the patient's discomfort.*[15,16,17,18]
■ Obtain vital signs and perform a respiratory assessment *to determine readiness for chest tube removal.*[1]
■ Raise the bed to waist level before performing patient care *to prevent caregiver back strain.*[19]
■ Perform hand hygiene[3,4,5,6,7,8] and put on a mask and goggles or mask with face shield, a gown, and gloves.[20]
■ Place the patient in the semi-Fowler position or on the unaffected side *to enhance access to the insertion site.*[1]
■ Place a fluid-impermeable pad under the affected side *to protect the linens from drainage and to provide a place to put the chest tube after removal.*
■ Prepare the suture removal kit and a sterile occlusive dressing with a 4″ × 4″ (10 cm × 10 cm) sterile gauze dressings and tape *so that the practitioner can cover the insertion site with it immediately after removing the chest tube.*[1] Note that some practitioners use petroleum gauze in addition to the sterile gauze, based on patient assessment.[1,2]
■ The practitioner performs hand hygiene and puts on goggles and a mask or a mask with a face shield, a gown, and sterile gloves.[21]
■ If instructed by the practitioner, remove the existing chest tube dressing and discard it appropriately.[22] Be careful not to dislodge the chest tube prematurely.
■ Assist the practitioner, as needed, with cleaning the area around the tubes with an antiseptic swab and removing the sutures.[1]
■ Trace the chest tube from the point of origin to the patient *to ensure removal of the proper tube.*[23] Clamp the chest tube catheter (if not already clamped) following the manufacturer's instructions *to minimize dead space and stop air from entering or exiting the catheter.*[1]
■ Assist the practitioner as necessary. The practitioner will instruct the patient to perform the Valsalva maneuver by exhaling and bearing down *to increase intrathoracic pressure and prevent air from entering the pleural space* while the practitioner removes the chest tube and covers the insertion site with the airtight dressing. If the patient can't follow instructions, the practitioner will remove the tube during peak inspiration.[1]
■ Help secure the dressing with tape. Make it as airtight as possible *to seal the insertion site from air entry.*[1]
■ Instruct the patient to breathe normally.
■ Return the bed to the lowest position *to prevent falls and maintain patient safety.*[24]
■ Discard equipment and waste in appropriate receptacles.[22]
■ Remove and discard your gloves and other personal protective equipment[20,21] and perform hand hygiene.[3,4,5,6,7,8]
■ Closely monitor the patient after the procedure *to determine the patient's response to and tolerance of the procedure.*[1] Monitor vital signs; oxygen saturation; respiratory rate, pattern, and effort; breath sounds; and symptoms of chest discomfort.[1]
■ Obtain a chest X-ray, if ordered, *to verify lung expansion.*[1] Keep in mind that a chest X-ray might not be indicated after chest tube removal unless the patient's condition changes.[1]

NURSING ALERT Notify the practitioner immediately if the patient develops acute respiratory distress, *which may indicate the need for a new chest tube.*

■ Position the patient for comfort.
■ Encourage coughing and performance of deep breathing exercises *to help prevent pneumonia and promote lung expansion.* (See *Instructions for coughing and deep breathing,* page 182.)
■ Regularly assess the chest tube site for bleeding, skin necrosis, infection, and subcutaneous emphysema (air leakage into surrounding tissue).[1] Screen for and assess the patient's pain using facility-defined criteria that are consistent with the patient's age, condition, and ability to understand.[25]

INSTRUCTIONS FOR COUGHING AND DEEP BREATHING

Coughing and "huffing" (or huff-coughing) helps break up secretions in the lungs facilitating expectorating or suctioning of mucus. Deep-breathing exercises help to expand the lungs and force better distribution of the air into all areas. The patient may initially need to lie down to do these exercises, but eventually the patient can do them while sitting upright, and then while walking.

Coughing and huffing

Help the patient to a sitting position. For a controlled cough, the patient purses the lips and takes a deep breath and hold the breath for several seconds and then briefly and gently cough twice. For huffing, the patient purses the lips and takes a deep breath. After holding the breath for several seconds, the patient exhales, using the stomach muscles to push out the air. The vocal chords remain open so that the cough has almost a whispery sound. Coughing and huffing are repeated several times per day, as needed.

Deep-breathing exercises

The patient starts by taking a deep breath through the nose, purses the lips as if to whistle, and then exhales the air slowly through pursed lips. The exhalation should take twice as long as the inhalation. For example, the patient may start by inhaling for 2 seconds and then exhaling for 4 seconds. After taking several deep breaths, the patient should breathe at a normal rhythm and then begin another cycle of deep breathing.

Combination exercises

Usually, the patient will perform coughing and deep-breathing exercises together. Instruct the patient to breathe in deeply through the nose and then exhale in three short huffs. Then have the patient inhale deeply again and cough through a slightly open mouth. Three consecutive coughs are highly effective. An effective cough sounds deep, low, and hollow; an ineffective cough is high-pitched. If possible, have the patient perform this exercise for about 1 minute and then rest for 2 minutes.

■ Treat the patient's pain, as needed and ordered, using nonpharmacologic, pharmacologic, or a combination of approaches. Base the treatment plan on evidence-based practices and on the patient's clinical condition, past medical history, and pain management goals.[25]

■ Perform hand hygiene.[3,4,5,6,7,8]

■ Clean and disinfect your stethoscope using a disinfectant pad.[26,27]

■ Perform hand hygiene.[3,4,5,6,7,8]

■ Document the procedure.[28,29,30,31]

Special considerations

■ If the patient is receiving mechanical ventilation therapy, the practitioner should remove the chest tube at peak inspiration.[1]

Complications

Potential complications of chest tube removal include infection at the site, tension pneumothorax, bleeding, skin necrosis, retained chest tube, pericardial effusion, and cardiac tamponade.[1]

Documentation

Record the date and time of chest tube removal; nursing preparation procedures; the patient's vital signs and respiratory status; and the patient's tolerance of the procedure. Also document the medications you administered, including the medication strength, dose, route of administration, date and time of administration, and effectiveness.[32] Document the condition of the insertion site and any complications that occurred, including the name of the practitioner notified, the date and time of notification, interventions performed, and the patient's response to those interventions. Document teaching provided to the patient and family (if applicable), their understanding of that teaching, and any need for follow-up teaching.

REFERENCES

1 Wiegand, D. L. (2017). *AACN procedure manual for high acuity, progressive, and critical care* (6th ed.). St: Louis, MO: Elsevier.

2 Carroll, P. (2019) Chest tube drainage and management. https://www.rn.org/courses/coursematerial-98.pdf

3 Centers for Disease Control and Prevention. (2002). Guideline for hand hygiene in health-care settings: Recommendations of the Healthcare Infection Control Practices Advisory Committee and the HICPAC/SHEA/APIC/IDSA Hand Hygiene Task Force. *MMWR Recommendations and Reports, 51*(RR-16), 1–45. https://www.cdc.gov/mmwr/pdf/rr/rr5116.pdf (Level II)

4 The Joint Commission. (2021). Standard NPSG.07.01.01. *Comprehensive accreditation manual for hospitals.* Oakbrook Terrace, IL: The Joint Commission. (Level VII)

5 World Health Organization. (2009). WHO guidelines on hand hygiene in health care: First global patient safety challenge, clean care is safer care. https://apps.who.int/iris/bitstream/handle/10665/44102/9789241597906_eng.pdf?sequence=1 (Level IV)

6 Centers for Medicare and Medicaid Services, Department of Health and Human Services. (2020). Condition of participation: Infection control. 42 C.F.R. § 482.42.

7 Accreditation Association for Hospitals and Health Systems. (2020). Standard 07.01.21. *Healthcare Facilities Accreditation Program: Accreditation requirements for acute care hospitals.* Chicago, IL: Accreditation Association for Hospitals and Health Systems. (Level VII)

8 DNV GL-Healthcare USA, Inc. (2020). IC.1.SR.1. *NIAHO® accreditation requirements, interpretive guidelines and surveyor guidance—revision 20.0.* Milford, OH: DNV GL-Healthcare USA, Inc. (Level VII)

9 The Joint Commission. (2021). Standard NPSG.01.01.01. *Comprehensive accreditation manual for hospitals.* Oakbrook Terrace, IL: The Joint Commission. (Level VII)

10 Centers for Medicare and Medicaid Services, Department of Health and Human Services. (2020). Condition of participation: Patient's rights. 42 C.F.R. § 482.13(c)(1).

11 The Joint Commission. (2021). Standard RI.01.01.01. *Comprehensive accreditation manual for hospitals.* Oakbrook Terrace, IL: The Joint Commission. (Level VII)

12 Accreditation Association for Hospitals and Health Systems. (2020). Standard 15.01.16. *Healthcare Facilities Accreditation Program: Accreditation requirements for acute care hospitals.* Chicago, IL: Accreditation Association for Hospitals and Health Systems. (Level VII)

13 DNV GL-Healthcare USA, Inc. (2020). PR.2.SR.5. *NIAHO® accreditation requirements, interpretive guidelines and surveyor guidance—revision 20.0.* Milford, OH: DNV GL-Healthcare USA, Inc. (Level VII)

14 The Joint Commission. (2021). Standard PC.02.01.21. *Comprehensive accreditation manual for hospitals.* Oakbrook Terrace, IL: The Joint Commission. (Level VII)

15 Centers for Medicare and Medicaid Services, Department of Health and Human Services. (2020). Condition of participation: Nursing services. 42 C.F.R. § 482.23(c).

16 The Joint Commission. (2021). Standard MM.06.01.01. *Comprehensive accreditation manual for hospitals.* Oakbrook Terrace, IL: The Joint Commission. (Level VII)

17 Accreditation Association for Hospitals and Health Systems. (2020). Standard 16.01.03. *Healthcare Facilities Accreditation Program: Accreditation requirements for acute care hospitals.* Chicago, IL: Accreditation Association for Hospitals and Health Systems. (Level VII)

18 DNV GL-Healthcare USA, Inc. (2020). MM.1.SR.2. *NIAHO® accreditation requirements, interpretive guidelines and surveyor guidance—revision 20.0.* Milford, OH: DNV GL-Healthcare USA, Inc. (Level VII)

19 Waters, T. R., et al. (2009). Safe patient handling training for schools of nursing. https://www.cdc.gov/niosh/docs/2009-127/pdfs/2009-127.pdf (Level VII)

20 Accreditation Association for Hospitals and Health Systems. (2020). Standard 07.01.10. *Healthcare Facilities Accreditation Program: Accreditation requirements for acute care hospitals.* Chicago, IL: Accreditation Association for Hospitals and Health Systems. (Level VII)

21 Siegel, J. D., et al. (2007, revised 2019). 2007 guideline for isolation precautions: Preventing transmission of infectious agents in healthcare settings. https://www.cdc.gov/infectioncontrol/pdf/guidelines/isolation-guidelines-H.pdf (Level II)

22 Occupational Safety and Health Administration. (2012). Bloodborne pathogens, standard number1910.1030. https://www.osha.gov/pls/oshaweb/owadisp.show_document?p_id=10051&p_table=STANDARDS (Level VII)

23 U.S. Food and Drug Administration. (2017). Examples of medical device misconnections. https://www.fda.gov/medical-devices/medical-device-connectors/examples-medical-device-misconnections

24 Ganz, D. A., et al. (2013, reviewed 2021). *Preventing falls in hospitals: A toolkit for improving quality of care* (AHRQ Publication No. 13-0015-EF). Rockville, MD: Agency for Healthcare Research and Quality. https://www.ahrq.gov/professionals/systems/hospital/fallpxtoolkit/index.html (Level VII)

25 The Joint Commission. (2021). Standard PC.01.02.07. *Comprehensive accreditation manual for hospitals.* Oakbrook Terrace, IL: The Joint Commission. (Level VII)

26 Rutala, W. A., et al. (2008, revised 2019). Guideline for disinfection and sterilization in healthcare facilities, 2008. https://www.cdc.gov/infection-control/pdf/guidelines/disinfection-guidelines-H.pdf (Level I)

27 Accreditation Association for Hospitals and Health Systems. (2020). Standard 07.02.03. *Healthcare Facilities Accreditation Program: Accreditation requirements for acute care hospitals.* Chicago, IL: Accreditation Association for Hospitals and Health Systems. (Level VII)

28 The Joint Commission. (2021). Standard RC.01.03.01. *Comprehensive accreditation manual for hospitals.* Oakbrook Terrace, IL: The Joint Commission. (Level VII)

29 Centers for Medicare and Medicaid Services, Department of Health and Human Services. (2020). Condition of participation: Medical record services. 42 C.F.R. § 482.24(b).

30 Accreditation Association for Hospitals and Health Systems. (2020). Standard 10.00.03. *Healthcare Facilities Accreditation Program: Accreditation requirements for acute care hospitals.* Chicago, IL: Accreditation Association for Hospitals and Health Systems. (Level VII)

31 DNV GL-Healthcare USA, Inc. (2020). MR.2.SR.1. *NIAHO® accreditation requirements, interpretive guidelines and surveyor guidance—revision 20.0.* Milford, OH: DNV GL-Healthcare USA, Inc. (Level VII)

32 The Joint Commission. (2021). Standard RC.02.01.01. *Comprehensive accreditation manual for hospitals.* Oakbrook Terrace, IL: The Joint Commission. (Level VII)

CLOSED-WOUND DRAIN MANAGEMENT

Closed-wound drains are typically inserted during surgery in anticipation of substantial postoperative drainage. Studies fail to show improved patient outcomes when they're inserted during clean surgical cases.[1] A closed-wound drain, commonly used after joint replacements and thyroid, breast, axillary, and abdominal procedures, prevents exudate from accumulating at the wound site.[2]

Jackson-Pratt and Hemovac closed drainage systems are used most commonly. (See *Types of closed drainage systems.*) These drains, which are considered vacuum drains, use low negative pressure. The collection chamber expands as it collects the draining fluid by exchanging negative pressure for fluid.[2,3,4]

A closed-wound drain consists of perforated tubing connected to a portable vacuum unit. The distal end of the tubing lies within the wound and usually leaves the body from a site other than the primary suture line to preserve the integrity of the surgical wound. The drain exit site is treated as an additional surgical wound; the drain is usually sutured to the skin.

The drain is emptied and its contents are measured every 4 to 8 hours or more often according to the patient's condition, the amount of drainage, and the practitioner's orders. *Removing excess drainage maintains maximum suction and avoids straining the drain's suture line.*

Equipment

Graduated cylinder ▪ antiseptic pad ▪ gloves ▪ fluid-impermeable pad ▪ Optional: gown, mask with face shield, mask, goggles, sterile specimen collection container, specimen container label, antiseptic cleaning agent or antimicrobial swabs, sterile gauze pads, tubing labels, laboratory biohazard transport bag.

Preparation of equipment

Inspect all equipment and supplies. If a product is expired, is defective, or has compromised integrity, remove it from patient use, label it as expired or defective, and report the expiration or defect as directed by your facility.

Types of closed drainage systems

There are two common types of closed drainage systems. The **Jackson-Pratt drain**, which is typically used with breast and abdominal surgery, collects exudate in a bulblike device.

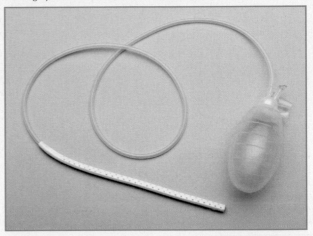

The **Hemovac drain** is used when blood drainage is expected after surgery, such as in abdominal and orthopedic surgeries.

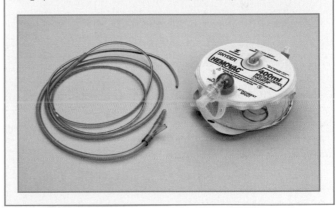

Implementation

▪ Verify the practitioner's order.
▪ Gather and prepare the necessary equipment and supplies.
▪ Perform hand hygiene.[5,6,7,8,9,10]
▪ Confirm the patient's identity using at least two patient identifiers.[11]
▪ Provide privacy.[12,13,14,15]
▪ Explain the procedure to the patient and family (if appropriate) according to their individual communication and learning needs *to increase their understanding, allay their fears, and enhance cooperation.*[16]
▪ Raise the bed to waist level before providing patient care *to prevent caregiver back strain.*[17]
▪ Put on gloves and other personal protective equipment, as needed, *to comply with standard precautions.*[18,19,20]
▪ Assess the patient's condition.
▪ If the patient has more than one closed-wound drain, number the drains *so that you can record drainage from each site.* Label each drain at the distal end (near the patient connection) and the proximal end (near the course container) *to distinguish the different drains and prevent misconnections.*[21]
▪ *Protect the patient's linens* by placing a fluid-impermeable pad under the drain.
▪ Unclip the vacuum unit from the patient's gown.
▪ Trace the tubing from the patient to its point of origin *to make sure you're emptying the correct drain.*[21,22]
▪ Release the vacuum by removing the spout plug on the collection chamber. The container expands completely as it draws in air.

■ Empty the unit's contents into a graduated cylinder and note the amount and appearance of the drainage.

■ If diagnostic tests will be performed on the fluid specimen, pour the drainage directly into a sterile laboratory container, note the amount and appearance, and label the specimen in the presence of the patient *to avoid mislabeling*.[11] Place the specimen into a laboratory biohazard transport bag[20] and send it to the laboratory.

■ Use an antiseptic pad to clean the unit's spout and plug.

■ *To reestablish the vacuum that creates the drain's suction power,* fully compress the vacuum unit with one hand and replace the spout plug with your other hand (as shown below).

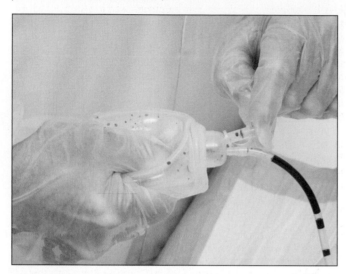

■ Check the patency of the equipment. Make sure the tubing is free of twists, kinks, and leaks, *because the drainage system must be airtight to work properly.* The vacuum unit should remain compressed when you release manual pressure; *rapid reinflation indicates an air leak.* If reinflation occurs, recompress the unit and make sure the spout plug is secure.

■ Secure the vacuum unit to the patient's gown. Fasten it below wound level *to promote drainage.* Don't apply tension on drainage tubing when fastening the unit *to prevent possible dislodgment.*

■ Remove and discard your gloves.[18,19,20]

■ Perform hand hygiene.[5,6,7,8,9,10]

■ Put on a new pair of gloves.[18,19,20]

■ Observe the sutures that secure the drain to the patient's skin; look for signs of pulling or tearing, drainage, swelling, or infection of surrounding skin. Gently clean the sutures with sterile gauze pads soaked in an antiseptic cleaning agent or with an antimicrobial swab, if ordered.

■ Properly dispose of drainage and solutions, and clean or dispose of soiled equipment and supplies.[20]

■ Return the bed to the lowest position *to prevent falls and maintain patient safety.*[23]

■ Remove and discard your gloves and any other personal protective equipment, if worn.[18,19,20]

■ Perform hand hygiene.[5,6,7,8,9,10]

■ Document the procedure.[24,25,26,27]

Special considerations

■ Check the drain frequently *to make sure suction is maintained.*[3,4]

■ Empty the drain and measure its contents before the patient ambulates *to prevent the weight of drainage from pulling on the drain as the patient ambulates.*

■ The Joint Commission issued a sentinel event alert related to managing risk during the transition to new International Organization for Standardization tubing standards that were designed to prevent dangerous tubing misconnections, which can lead to serious patient injury and death. During the transition, make sure to trace the tubing and catheter from the patient to the point of origin before connecting or reconnecting any device or infusion, at any care transition (such as a new setting or service), and as part of the hand-off process; route tubes and catheters having different purposes in different standardized directions; when there are different access sites or several bags hanging, label the tubing at both the distal and proximal ends; use tubing and equipment only as intended; and store medications for different delivery routes in separate locations.[21]

Patient teaching

If the patient will be discharged to home with a closed wound drain, teach the patient and family, if appropriate, how to empty the collection chamber, reestablish the vacuum, clean the drain exit site, and record the amount of the drainage. In addition, teach the patient about signs and symptoms to report to the practitioner, such as drain site redness, pain, swelling, drainage, or obstruction in the tubing.[28,29]

Complications

Occlusion of the tubing by fibrin, clots, or other particles can reduce or obstruct drainage. Infection may develop at the drain exit site. Other potential complications include breakage of the drain, difficulty in removal, inadvertent removal, pain, a puckering scar, and visceral perforation.[2]

Documentation

Record the date and time each time you empty the drain; the appearance of the drain exit site, including swelling or other signs of infection; equipment malfunction and subsequent nursing interventions; and the patient's tolerance of the treatment. On the intake and output sheet, record drainage color, consistency, type, and amount. If the patient has more than one closed-wound drain, number the drains and record the necessary information separately for each drainage site. Document teaching provided to the patient and family (if applicable), their understanding of that teaching, and any need for follow-up teaching.

REFERENCES

1 Reiffel, A. J., et al. (2013). A multi-disciplinary review of the potential association between closed-suction drains and surgical site infection. *Surgical Infections, 14*(3), 244–269. https://www.ncbi.nlm.nih.gov/pmc/articles/PMC3689179/ (Level V)

2 Durai, R., & Ng, P. C. H. (2010). Surgical vacuum drains: Types, uses, and complications. *AORN Journal, 91,* 266–271.

3 Khansa, I., et al. (2018). Optimal use of surgical drains: Evidence-based strategies. *Plastic and Reconstructive Surgery, 141,* 1542–1549. (Level IV)

4 Mamuyac, E. M., et al. (2019). How much blood could a JP suck if a JP could suck blood? *Laryngoscope, 129,* 1806–1809. (Level IV)

5 The Joint Commission. (2021). Standard NPSG.07.01.01. *Comprehensive accreditation manual for hospitals.* Oakbrook Terrace, IL: The Joint Commission. (Level VII)

6 World Health Organization. (2009). WHO guidelines on hand hygiene in health care: First global patient safety challenge, clean care is safer care. https://apps.who.int/iris/bitstream/handle/10665/44102/9789241597906_eng.pdf?sequence=1 (Level IV)

7 Centers for Disease Control and Prevention. (2002). Guideline for hand hygiene in health-care settings: Recommendations of the Healthcare Infection Control Practices Advisory Committee and the HICPAC/SHEA/APIC/IDSA Hand Hygiene Task Force. *MMWR Recommendations and Reports, 51*(RR-16), 1–45. https://www.cdc.gov/mmwr/pdf/rr/rr5116.pdf (Level II)

8 Centers for Medicare and Medicaid Services, Department of Health and Human Services. (2020). Condition of participation: Infection control. 42 C.F.R. § 482.42.

9 Accreditation Association for Hospitals and Health Systems. (2020). Standard 07.01.21. *Healthcare Facilities Accreditation Program: Accreditation requirements for acute care hospitals.* Chicago, IL: Accreditation Association for Hospitals and Health Systems. (Level VII)

10 DNV GL-Healthcare USA, Inc. (2020). IC.1.SR.1. *NIAHO® accreditation requirements, interpretive guidelines and surveyor guidance—revision 20.0.* Milford, OH: DNV GL-Healthcare USA, Inc. (Level VII)

11 The Joint Commission. (2021). Standard NPSG.01.01.01. *Comprehensive accreditation manual for hospitals.* Oakbrook Terrace, IL: The Joint Commission. (Level VII)

12 Centers for Medicare and Medicaid Services, Department of Health and Human Services. (2020). Condition of participation: Patient's rights. 42 C.F.R. § 482.13(c)(1).

13 Accreditation Association for Hospitals and Health Systems. (2020). Standard 15.01.16. *Healthcare Facilities Accreditation Program: Accreditation requirements for acute care hospitals.* Chicago, IL: Accreditation Association for Hospitals and Health Systems. (Level VII)

14 The Joint Commission. (2021). Standard RI.01.01.01. *Comprehensive accreditation manual for hospitals.* Oakbrook Terrace, IL: The Joint Commission. (Level VII)

15 DNV GL-Healthcare USA, Inc. (2020). PR.2.SR.5. *NIAHO® accreditation requirements, interpretive guidelines and surveyor guidance—revision 20.0.* Milford, OH: DNV GL-Healthcare USA, Inc. (Level VII)

16 The Joint Commission. (2021). Standard PC.02.01.21. *Comprehensive accreditation manual for hospitals.* Oakbrook Terrace, IL: The Joint Commission. (Level VII)

17 Waters, T. R., et al. (2009). Safe patient handling training for schools of nursing. https://www.cdc.gov/niosh/docs/2009-127/pdfs/2009-127.pdf (Level VII)

18 Siegel, J. D., et al. (2007, revised 2019). 2007 guideline for isolation precautions: Preventing transmission of infectious agents in healthcare settings. https://www.cdc.gov/infectioncontrol/pdf/guidelines/isola-tion-guidelines-H.pdf (Level II)

19 Accreditation Association for Hospitals and Health Systems. (2020). Standard 07.01.10. *Healthcare Facilities Accreditation Program: Accreditation requirements for acute care hospitals.* Chicago, IL: Accreditation Association for Hospitals and Health Systems. (Level VII)

20 Occupational Safety and Health Administration. (2012). Bloodborne pathogens, standard number1910.1030. https://www.osha.gov/pls/oshaweb/owadisp.show_document?p_id=10051&p_table=STANDARDS (Level VII)

21 The Joint Commission. (2014). Sentinel event alert 53: Managing risk during transition to new ISO tubing connector standards. https://www.jointcommission.org/assets/1/6/SEA_53_Connectors_8_19_14_final.pdf (Level VII)

22 U.S. Food and Drug Administration. (2017). Examples of medical device misconnections. https://www.fda.gov/medical-devices/medical-device-connectors/examples-medical-device-misconnections

23 Ganz, D. A., et al. (2013, reviewed 2021). *Preventing falls in hospitals: A toolkit for improving quality of care* (AHRQ Publication No. 13-0015-EF). Rockville, MD: Agency for Healthcare Research and Quality. https://www.ahrq.gov/professionals/systems/hospital/fallpxtoolkit/index.html (Level VII)

24 The Joint Commission. (2021). Standard RC.01.03.01. *Comprehensive accreditation manual for hospitals.* Oakbrook Terrace, IL: The Joint Commission. (Level VII)

25 Centers for Medicare and Medicaid Services, Department of Health and Human Services. (2020). Condition of participation: Medical record services. 42 C.F.R. § 482.24(b).

26 Accreditation Association for Hospitals and Health Systems. (2020). Standard 10.00.03. *Healthcare Facilities Accreditation Program: Accreditation requirements for acute care hospitals.* Chicago, IL: Accreditation Association for Hospitals and Health Systems. (Level VII)

27 DNV GL-Healthcare USA, Inc. (2020). MR.2.SR.1. *NIAHO® accreditation requirements, interpretive guidelines and surveyor guidance—revision 20.0.* Milford, OH: DNV GL-Healthcare USA, Inc. (Level VII)

28 National Institutes of Health Clinical Center. (2015). Patient education: How to care for the Jackson-Pratt drain. http://fliphtml5.com/lbku/rfhg/basic

29 Memorial Sloan Kettering Cancer Center. (2019). Caring for your Jackson-Pratt drain. https://www.mskcc.org/cancer-care/patient-education/caring-your-jackson-pratt-drain

CODE MANAGEMENT

A code may be called for patients with an absent pulse, apnea or inadequate breathing, ventricular fibrillation (VF), pulseless ventricular tachycardia (VT), pulseless electrical activity, or asystole. The goals of any code are to restore the patient's spontaneous heartbeat and respirations and to prevent hypoxic damage to the brain and other vital organs. Fulfilling these goals requires quick identification of a problem and rapid emergency response, optimally using a team approach to providing treatment. Ideally, the code team should consist of health care workers trained in advanced cardiac life support (ACLS), although health care workers trained in basic life support (BLS), as well as ancillary health care workers, such as laboratory and electrocardiogram technicians, may also be a part of the team. Actions during a code should be guided by the latest American Heart Association (AHA) recommendations for treatment.

According to the AHA Web-based Integrated Guidelines for Cardiopulmonary Resuscitation and Emergency Cardiovascular Care, ACLS interventions build on the foundation of BLS.[1] This foundation includes immediate recognition and activation of the emergency response system, early high-quality cardiopulmonary resuscitation (CPR), and rapid defibrillation to increase the patient's chance of survival. The recommended priority of the AHA guidelines is performing high-quality CPR chest compressions of adequate rate and depth that allow complete chest recoil after each compression with minimal interruptions as well as avoiding excessive ventilation.[1]

To prevent a delay in chest compressions, the sequence of CPR is C-A-B (compressions, airway, and breathing), which gives the highest priority to chest compressions when resuscitating a patient in cardiac arrest. In addition to high-quality CPR, the only rhythm-specific therapy known to increase survival is defibrillation. As such, defibrillation remains of primary importance in the CPR cycle when a rhythm check reveals a shockable rhythm (VF or pulseless VT). Establishing vascular access, administering medications, and inserting an advanced airway are important, but these measures shouldn't cause significant interruptions in CPR or delay defibrillation.[1]

Always be aware of a patient's code status as defined by the practitioner's orders, the patient's advance directives, and the family's wishes. Ensure that the practitioner who has ordered a "no code" or "do not resuscitate" status for the patient has written and signed the order. If these orders are established on a specific order form, have the patient or responsible family member cosign it, of possible.[2]

Equipment

Oral, nasal, and endotracheal (ET) airways ■ oxygen source ■ oxygen flowmeter ■ stethoscope ■ intubation supplies ■ tape or commercial tube holder ■ handheld resuscitation bag with mask ■ suction supplies ■ gloves ■ cardiac arrest board ■ peripheral IV supplies (14G, 18G, and 20G peripheral IV catheters) ■ IV administration sets (macrodrip and microdrip) ■ IV fluids (dextrose 5% in water [D_5W], normal saline solution, and lactated Ringer solution) ■ appropriate size syringes and needles for medication administration ■ 10-mL prefilled syringes that contain preservative free normal saline solution (or other compatible flush solution, if the medication is incompatible with normal saline solution) ■ electrocardiogram (ECG) monitor, electrodes, and leads ■ cardioverter-defibrillator ■ self-adhesive defibrillator pads and connector cable or pre-packaged gelled conduction pads ■ emergency medications (adenosine, amiodarone, atropine, diltiazem, dobutamine, dopamine, epinephrine, lidocaine, magnesium sulfate, naloxone, norepinephrine, procainamide, sodium bicarbonate, sotalol, and verapamil) ■ disinfectant pad ■ facility-approved disinfectant ■ Optional: mask and goggles or mask with face shield, gown, end-tidal carbon dioxide detector, continuous quantitative waveform capnography equipment, esophageal detector, intraosseous (IO) infusion supplies.

Preparation of equipment

Inspect all equipment and supplies. If a product is expired, is defective, or has compromised integrity, remove it from patient use, label it as expired or defective, and report the expiration or defect as directed by your facility.

Ensure that the defibrillator is charged and functioning. If the battery isn't charged, ensure that an outlet is available to plug it in. Because effective emergency care depends on reliable and accessible equipment, the equipment as well as the personnel must be ready for a code at any time. You also should be familiar with the emergency drugs you may need to administer during a code. (See *Common emergency cardiac drugs*, page 186.)

Implementation

■ Perform hand hygiene.[6,7,8,9,10,11]

■ Put on gloves and, as needed, other personal protective equipment *to follow standard precautions.*[12,13,14,15]

■ If you're the first to arrive at the scene of a code, verify that the environment is safe by quickly scanning the patient's location and surroundings for imminent physical threats, such as toxic and electrical hazards.[1]

Common emergency cardiac drugs

You may be called on to administer several drugs during a code. This chart lists the most common emergency drugs, along with their actions, indications, and dosages.

DRUG	ACTIONS	INDICATIONS	TYPICAL ADULT DOSAGE AND CONSIDERATIONS
adenosine	■ Slows conduction through atrioventricular (AV) node; may interrupt reentry through AV node ■ Shortens duration of atrial action potential during supraventricular tachycardia	■ Stable narrow complex regular tachycardia ■ Unstable narrow complex regular tachycardia ■ Stable regular monomorphic wide complex tachycardia	■ Initially, 6 mg rapid IV push over 1 to 3 seconds; if conversion hasn't occurred within 2 minutes, administer 12 mg by rapid IV push.[1] ■ Reduce initial dose to 3 mg when administered through a central venous catheter in patients receiving dipyridamole or carbamazepine and in a heart transplant recipient. ■ Immediately follow each dose with a 20-mL saline flush.[1] ■ *Caution:* Slower-than-recommended administration decreases the drug's effectiveness.[1] ■ Avoid use in patients with asthma.[1]
amiodarone	■ Thought to prolong refractory period and action potential duration	■ Cardiac arrest caused by pulseless ventricular tachycardia (VT) or ventricular fibrillation (VF) that is unresponsive to defibrillation[3] ■ Stable irregular narrow complex tachycardia (atrial fibrillation) ■ Stable regular narrow complex tachycardia ■ Stable wide complex tachycardia	■ For cardiac arrest, administer 300 mg IV push or intraosseously (IO); repeat 150 mg IV push in 3 to 5 minutes. Dilute in 20 to 30 mL of dextrose 5% in water (D_5W). Maximum dose: 2.2 g IV/24 hr.[1] ■ For narrow complex tachycardia and stable wide complex tachycardia, administer 150 mg over 10 min, followed by 1 mg/min infusion for 6 hr, and then 0.5 mg/min.[1]
atropine	■ Accelerates AV conduction and heart rate by blocking the vagus nerve	■ Symptomatic bradycardia	■ Administer 0.5 mg IV push repeated every 3 to 5 min until the patient is no longer symptomatic, up to 3 mg total.[1] ■ *Note:* Atropine is no longer recommended for use during pulseless electrical activity (PEA) or asystole,[1] and it's ineffective for type 2 AV block and new third-degree wide-complex AV block, and may cause paradoxical bradycardia in patients with these conditions.[4]
dilTIAZem	■ Slows AV node conduction and increases AV node refractoriness	■ Stable narrow complex tachycardia ■ Atrial fibrillation or atrial flutter with rapid ventricular response	■ Initially, administer 15 to 20 mg (0.25 mg/kg) IV over 2 min, followed by 20 to 25 mg (0.35 mg/kg) IV in 15 min, if needed.[1] ■ Maintenance is 5 to 15 mg/hr titrated to ventricular response.[1] ■ *Caution:* Don't use this drug to treat pre-excited atrial fibrillation or flutter.[1]
DOBUTamine	■ Increases myocardial contractility without raising oxygen demand	■ Heart failure ■ Cardiogenic shock after cardiac arrest ■ Blood pressure support after return of spontaneous circulation, if systolic blood pressure is less than 90 mm Hg after fluid bolus	■ Administer 5 to 10 mcg/kg/min by continuous IV infusion. ■ Titrate as needed to optimize blood pressure, cardiac output, and systemic perfusion.[1]
DOPamine	■ Produces inotropic effect, increasing cardiac output, blood pressure, and renal perfusion	■ Symptomatic bradycardia associated with hypotension (except when caused by hypovolemia)	■ Administer a continuous IV infusion at 2 to 20 mcg/kg/min. (*Note:* Always dilute and give IV drip, never IV push. Titrate to patient response.) ■ *Caution:* Don't administer in the same IV line with alkaline solutions.[1]
EPINEPHrine	■ Increases heart rate, peripheral resistance, and blood flow to heart (enhancing myocardial and cerebral oxygenation) ■ Strengthens myocardial contractility ■ Increases coronary perfusion pressure during cardiopulmonary resuscitation	■ VF ■ Pulseless VT ■ PEA ■ Asystole ■ Severe hypotension (secondary agent) ■ Symptomatic bradycardia	■ Initially, administer 10 mL of 1:10,000 solution (1 mg) IV push or IO; may repeat every 3 to 5 min, as needed. After each dose, flush 20 mL of IV fluid if administered peripherally.[1] ■ Administer 2 to 2½ times the IV dose given endotracheally if no IV line is available.[1] (*Note:* 1:1,000 solution contains 1 mg/mL, so it must be diluted in 9 mL of normal saline solution to provide 1 mg/10 mL.)[1] ■ For hypotension, administer 1 mg/500 mL of D_5W by continuous infusion; titrate to the desired effect (0.1 to 0.5 mcg/min). ■ For symptomatic bradycardia, administer 1 mg/500 mL of D_5W by continuous infusion; titrate to the desired effect (2 to 10 mcg/min).[1] ■ *Caution:* Don't administer in the same IV line with an alkaline solution.

Common emergency cardiac drugs *(continued)*

DRUG	ACTIONS	INDICATIONS	TYPICAL ADULT DOSAGE AND CONSIDERATIONS
lidocaine	■ Depresses automaticity and conduction of ectopic impulses in ventricles, especially in ischemic tissue ■ Raises fibrillation threshold, especially in an ischemic heart	■ Cardiac arrest from pulseless VF or VT when amiodarone isn't available[3]	■ Initially, administer 1 to 1.5 mg/kg IV push or IO; may follow with a 0.5 to 0.75 mg/kg bolus dose every 5 to 10 min, up to a total of 3 mg/kg.[1] ■ Maintenance is a continuous IV infusion of 2 g/500 mL of D_5W at 1 to 4 mg/min *to prevent recurrence of lethal arrhythmias.*[1]
magnesium sulfate	■ Decreases the influx of calcium to suppress early depolarizations to terminate the arrhythmia[5]	■ Torsades de pointe[3] ■ Treatment of hypomagnesemia	■ *Note:* Routine use of magnesium sulfate for cardiac arrest isn't recommended.[3] ■ For torsades de pointe with a pulse, initially administer 1 to 2 g in 50 to 100 mL of D_5W IV over 5 to 60 min, followed by 0.5 to 1g/hr.[5]
naloxone	■ Opioid receptor antagonist that reverses or blocks the effects of opioid drugs	■ Known or suspected opioid overdose	■ Initially administer 0.04 to 2 mg IV or IM and repeat every 3 to 5 min. ■ Administer 2 mg nebulized and give intranasal or via endotracheal tube.[1]
norepinephrine	■ Stimulates the sympathetic nervous system, resulting in vasoconstriction and cardiac stimulation	■ Systolic blood pressure less than 90 mm Hg or mean arterial pressure less than 65 mm Hg, despite fluid resuscitation after return of spontaneous circulation	■ Administer a continuous infusion at 0.1 to 0.5 mcg/kg/min titrated to desired effects up to 2 mcg/kg/min.[1]
procainamide	■ Depresses automaticity and conduction ■ Prolongs refraction in atria and ventricles	■ Premature ventricular contractions ■ Stable monomorphic VT ■ Supraventricular arrhythmias	■ Administer 20 to 50 mg/min IV infusion up to a total of 17 mg/kg, followed by a maintenance dose of 1 to 4 mg/min by IV infusion. ■ *Note:* Administration is limited by the need for slow infusion. ■ *Caution:* Avoid use in prolonged QT syndrome or heart failure.[1]
sodium bicarbonate	■ Alkalizing agent that neutralizes excess acid	■ Hyperkalemia ■ Known pre-existing bicarbonate responsive acidosis ■ Drug overdose that results in acidotic state, as with aspirin[1]	■ Administer 1 mg/kg IV push. ■ Caution: Sodium bicarbonate is not recommended for routine use in patients in cardiac arrest.[1]
sotalol	■ Depresses sinus heart rate ■ Slows conduction through the AV node ■ Prolongs the monophasic action potential	■ Spontaneously hemodynamically stable sustained monomorphic VT	■ Administer 1.5 mg/kg IV over 5 min or less.[1] ■ *Caution*: Avoid use in patients with prolonged QT interval.[1]
verapamil	■ Slows conduction through AV node ■ Causes vasodilation ■ Produces negative inotropic effect on heart, depressing myocardial contractility	■ Stable narrow complex tachycardia ■ Atrial fibrillation or atrial flutter with rapid ventricular response[1]	■ Initially, administer 2.5 to 5 mg IV push over 2 min (over 3 min in an older adult). Repeat dose of 5 to 10 mg every 15 to 30 min, if needed, to a total dose of 20 to 30 mg.[1] ■ Monitor electrocardiogram and blood pressure. ■ *Caution:* Don't use drug to treat pre-excited atrial fibrillation or flutter.[1]

Cardiopulmonary resuscitation in the prone position

Although the effectiveness of cardiopulmonary resuscitation (CPR) for a patient in the prone position is not completely known, the American Heart Association (AHA) recommends not turning a prone patient with an advanced airway, unless it is possible to turn the patient without risking disconnection of equipment or aerosolization. The AHA recommends leaving the patient in the prone position and performing CPR with the hands over the T7 through T10 vertebral bodies.[17,18,19] The AHA recommends using the same rate and force of compressions with the patient in the prone position as in the supine position. It is important to have a hard surface under the patient to provide uniform force and counter-sternal pressure.[19]

For a prone patient without an advanced airway, attempt to turn the patient to the supine position for continued resuscitation.[18]

■ Assess responsiveness by tapping the patient on the shoulder and shouting, "Are you all right?" If the patient is unresponsive, shout for nearby help and immediately activate the emergency response system via mobile device (if appropriate).[1]
■ Check to see if the patient is apneic or is only gasping (as opposed to breathing regularly), and, if able, simultaneously check for a pulse *to minimize delay in detecting cardiac arrest and initiating CPR.*[1]
■ If you don't feel a pulse within 10 seconds, begin chest compressions. (For a patient in the prone position, see *Cardiopulmonary resuscitation in the prone position.*) Depress an adult's sternum at least 2" (5 cm) but no more than 2.4" (6 cm), letting the chest completely recoil after each compression so that the heart can adequately refill with blood. Avoid leaning on the patient's chest, which could prevent it from recoiling completely.[16] Perform 30 compressions at a rate of 100 to 120 compressions/minute, followed by 2 breaths.[16] Each breath should have enough volume to produce a minimal chest rise to ensure adequate ventilation.[16]

■ After a second person arrives with a defibrillator and other emergency equipment, have that person place the cardiac arrest board under the patient (or, if the patient is on an air-filled mattress, make sure that it's deflated) and then assist with CPR.

■ Apply the self-adhesive defibrillation pads, following manufacturer's instructions, and attach their connector to the defibrillator monitor to obtain a quick look at the patient's cardiac rhythm. Alternatively, apply prepackaged gelled conduction pads and then apply the paddles to the patient's chest to quickly look at the patient's cardiac rhythm. Avoid placing pads over an implanted device, such as a pacemaker, or over medicated patches.

■ For VF or pulseless VT, follow the ACLS protocol for defibrillation as soon as possible with 360 joules (monophasic defibrillator) or 120 to 200 joules (biphasic defibrillator) according to the manufacturer's recommendations.[20] (See the "Defibrillation" procedure.)

■ After defibrillation, resume CPR immediately. Don't check the patient's rhythm at this time. Instead, check the rhythm after five cycles of CPR; perform a pulse check if you observe an organized rhythm on the monitor.

■ The second person should get into position on the other side of the patient and be ready to begin chest compressions after you complete five cycles of compressions and ventilations at a ratio of 30:2. The switch should take less than 5 seconds, *because interruptions in chest compressions can compromise vital organ perfusion.* The compressor should be relieved every 2 minutes *to prevent rescuer fatigue that could lead to inadequate compression rate or depth.*

■ Have the nurse assigned to the patient relate the patient's medical history and describe the events leading to cardiac arrest.

■ A third person—either a nurse certified in BLS or a respiratory therapist—will then attach the handheld resuscitation bag to the oxygen source.

■ Ideally, a fourth person will be available to open the patient's airway and seal the mask to the patient's face. After the mask is in place, the other person will squeeze the resuscitation bag to deliver two ventilations (each over 1 second) during a brief pause after 30 compressions. Both people will watch for the chest to rise. If a fourth person isn't available, the third person will open the patient's airway, seal the mask to the patient's face using one hand, and then, with the other hand, squeeze the resuscitation bag to deliver two ventilations during a brief pause after 30 compressions.

■ An ACLS-trained nurse will act as code leader until the practitioner arrives.

■ If not already in place, apply ECG electrodes and attach the patient to the defibrillator's cardiac monitor. Avoid placing electrodes on bony prominences and hairy areas. Also avoid the areas where the defibrillator pads will be placed and where chest compressions will be given. If you're using hands-free defibrillator pads, you'll need to apply ECG electrodes or attach them to the defibrillator (unless the patient requires synchronized cardioversion or transcutaneous pacing).

■ After five cycles of CPR, check the patient's rhythm and, if necessary, give another shock at the same energy dose (if using a monophasic defibrillator) or at the same or higher energy dose (if using a biphasic defibrillator).[1]

■ As CPR and defibrillation continue, if IV access isn't already present, insert two peripheral venous access devices using large-bore IV catheters; alternatively, IO access may be established if peripheral access isn't readily available.[1] Avoid interrupting chest compressions for IV or IO insertion. When inserting a peripheral IV catheter, use only a large vein, such as the antecubital vein, *to allow for rapid fluid administration and to prevent drug extravasation.*

■ As soon as the IV catheter is in place, begin an infusion of normal saline solution or lactated Ringer solution *to help prevent circulatory collapse.* D_5W is still acceptable, but the latest ACLS guidelines encourage the use of normal saline solution or lactated Ringer solution, *because D_5W can produce hyperglycemic effects during cardiac arrest.*

■ While one nurse obtains access for parenteral medications, another team member will set up portable or wall-suction equipment and suction the patient's oral secretions, as necessary, *to maintain an open airway.*

■ The ACLS-trained nurse will then prepare and administer emergency cardiac drugs as needed, following safe medication administration practices.[21,22,23,24] (See *AHA adult cardiac arrest algorithm,* page 189.)

Administer medications according to the AHA algorithm immediately after a rhythm check. *The AHA algorithm shows the timing of drug administration and shock administration.*[1] Keep in mind that all drugs administered IV should be followed by a 20-mL bolus of IV fluid *to facilitate the flow of the drug to central circulation.*[1]

■ If IV or IO access can't be established, you may administer medications such as epinephrine, lidocaine, and naloxone through an ET tube during cardiac arrest once the patient is intubated. (The optimal dose of most drugs given by this route is unknown, but typically the ET dose is 2 to 2½ times the recommended IV dose.) To do so, dilute the drugs in 5 to 10 mL of normal saline solution or sterile water and then instill them into the patient's ET tube. *Studies have shown that dilution with sterile water, in place of normal saline solution, may improve absorption of epinephrine and lidocaine.* Afterward, ventilate the patient manually *to improve absorption by distributing the drug throughout the bronchial tree.*[1]

■ The ACLS-trained nurse will also prepare for and assist with ET intubation or other advanced airway placement. Compression interruption should be minimized during advanced airway placement.[1]

■ Suction the patient, as needed. After the patient has been intubated, the health care provider should use clinical assessment and a confirmation device such as an end-tidal carbon dioxide ($ETco_2$) detector, continuous quantitative waveform capnography, or an esophageal detector to confirm ET tube placement. Continuous quantitative waveform capnography is recommended.[1] Assessment includes visualization of chest expansion, auscultation for equal breath sounds, and auscultation for absent breath sounds over the epigastrium. When the tube is correctly positioned, secure it with tape or a commercial tube holder. *To serve as a reference,* mark the point on the tube that's level with the patient's lips. Document the tube location on the code record.[1]

■ After the ET tube is inserted, the provider performing chest compressions should deliver 100 to 120 compressions/minute continuously without pauses for ventilations;[1,16] the provider delivering ventilations should administer 1 breath every 6 seconds (10 breaths/minute) *to avoid excessive ventilations and subsequently minimize the impact of positive-pressure ventilation on blood flow.*[1,16]

■ Meanwhile, another team member of the code team should document events and treatment. Other duties of the code team include prompting participants about when to perform certain activities (such as when to check a pulse or take vital signs), overseeing the effectiveness of CPR, keeping track of the time between therapies, and supporting the family. Each team member should know what the other participant's role is *to prevent duplicating efforts.* Lastly, someone from the team should make sure that the primary nurse's other patients are reassigned to another nurse.

■ Remove and discard your gloves and any other personal protective equipment worn.[12,13]

■ Perform hand hygiene.[6,7,8,9,10,11]

■ Clean and disinfect your stethoscope with a disinfectant pad.[25,26]

■ Perform hand hygiene.[6,7,8,9,10,11]

■ Put on gloves and, as needed, other personal protective equipment.[13]

■ Clean and disinfect other reusable equipment according to the manufacturer's instructions *to prevent the spread of infection.*[25,26]

■ Remove and discard your gloves and, if worn, other personal protective equipment.[13]

■ Perform hand hygiene.[6,7,8,9,10,11]

■ Document the procedure.[27,28,29,30]

Special considerations

■ Evidence for an optimum compression rate suggests a target of 100 to 120 compressions/minute. Rates above or below this target range appear to reduce survival to discharge.[1,16]

■ If hemodynamic monitoring, such as arterial or central venous catheters or capnography, are in place, they should be used to monitor the patient's response to CPR and the effectiveness of resuscitation efforts.[16]

■ If defibrillator gel pads aren't available, a conductive gel must be placed on defibrillator paddles before use. Place the gel on one paddle and rub the two paddles together *to spread the gel evenly between them.* Ensure that the surface of the paddle is completely covered.

■ The routine use of magnesium sulfate for cardiac arrest isn't recommended unless torsades de pointe is present.[1]

AHA adult cardiac arrest algorithm

Adult Cardiac Arrest Algorithm

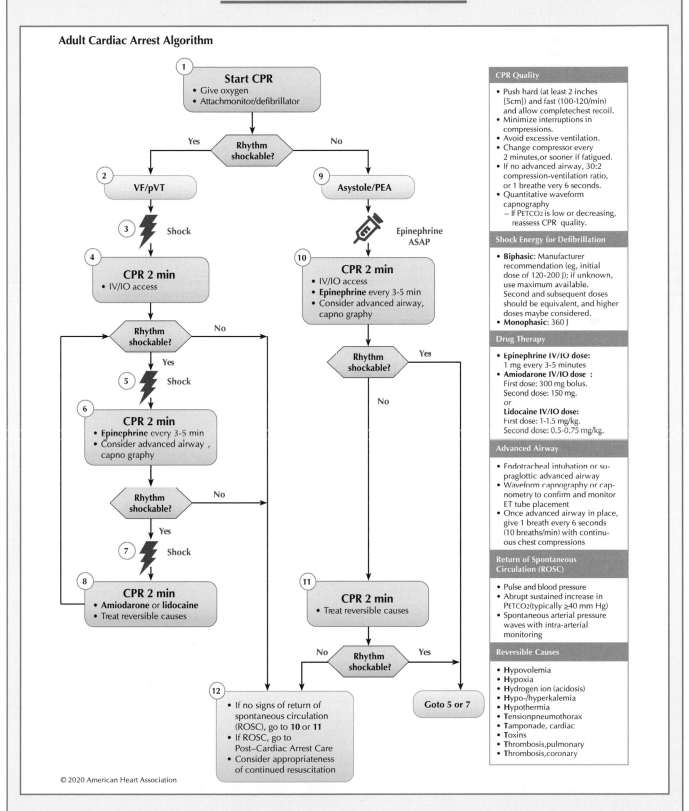

1 Start CPR
- Give oxygen
- Attach monitor/defibrillator

Rhythm shockable?

Yes → **2 VF/pVT**

No → **9 Asystole/PEA**

3 Shock

Epinephrine ASAP

4 CPR 2 min
- IV/IO access

10 CPR 2 min
- IV/IO access
- Epinephrine every 3-5 min
- Consider advanced airway, capno graphy

Rhythm shockable?

No →

Yes ↓

5 Shock

Rhythm shockable? Yes →

No ↓

6 CPR 2 min
- Epinephrine every 3-5 min
- Consider advanced airway, capno graphy

Rhythm shockable?

No →

Yes ↓

7 Shock

8 CPR 2 min
- Amiodarone or lidocaine
- Treat reversible causes

11 CPR 2 min
- Treat reversible causes

Rhythm shockable?

No ← → Yes → **Goto 5 or 7**

12
- If no signs of return of spontaneous circulation (ROSC), go to **10** or **11**
- If ROSC, go to Post–Cardiac Arrest Care
- Consider appropriateness of continued resuscitation

© 2020 American Heart Association

CPR Quality
- Push hard (at least 2 inches [5cm]) and fast (100-120/min) and allow complete chest recoil.
- Minimize interruptions in compressions.
- Avoid excessive ventilation.
- Change compressor every 2 minutes, or sooner if fatigued.
- If no advanced airway, 30:2 compression-ventilation ratio, or 1 breathe very 6 seconds.
- Quantitative waveform capnography
  – If PETCO2 is low or decreasing, reassess CPR quality.

Shock Energy for Defibrillation
- **Biphasic**: Manufacturer recommendation (eg, initial dose of 120-200 J); if unknown, use maximum available. Second and subsequent doses should be equivalent, and higher doses maybe considered.
- **Monophasic**: 360 J

Drug Therapy
- **Epinephrine IV/IO dose:** 1 mg every 3-5 minutes
- **Amiodarone IV/IO dose :** First dose: 300 mg bolus. Second dose: 150 mg. or
- **Lidocaine IV/IO dose:** First dose: 1-1.5 mg/kg. Second dose: 0.5-0.75 mg/kg.

Advanced Airway
- Endotracheal intubation or su-praglottic advanced airway
- Waveform capnography or cap-nometry to confirm and monitor ET tube placement
- Once advanced airway in place, give 1 breath every 6 seconds (10 breaths/min) with continu-ous chest compressions

Return of Spontaneous Circulation (ROSC)
- Pulse and blood pressure
- Abrupt sustained increase in PETCO2 (typically ≥40 mm Hg)
- Spontaneous arterial pressure waves with intra-arterial monitoring

Reversible Causes
- **H**ypovolemia
- **H**ypoxia
- **H**ydrogen ion (acidosis)
- **H**ypo-/hyperkalemia
- **H**ypothermia
- **T**ension pneumothorax
- **T**amponade, cardiac
- **T**oxins
- **T**hrombosis, pulmonary
- **T**hrombosis, coronary

(Continued)

- High-dose EPINEPHrine isn't recommended for routine use in patients in cardiac arrest.[1]
- Vasopressin is no longer recommended as a substitute for EPINEPHrine, but may be used with EPINEPHrine.[1,31]
- In in-hospital cardiac arrest, the combination of intra-arrest EPINEPHrine and methylPREDNISolone and post-arrest hydrocortisone may be considered.[1]
- Extracorporeal CPR may be considered among selected cardiac arrest patients who have not responded to initial conventional CPR in settings in which it can be rapidly implemented.[1]
- If family members are at the facility during the code, have someone, such as a clergy member or social worker, remain with them. Keep family members informed of the patient's status.
- Family members may be present during a code if your facility supports it. The Emergency Nurses Association and the American Association of Critical-Care Nurses support the option of family presence during invasive procedures and CPR.[32,33,34]
- If the family isn't at the facility, contact them as soon as possible. Encourage them not to drive to the facility, but offer to call someone who can give them a ride.
- When the patient's condition has stabilized, assess level of consciousness, breath sounds, heart sounds, peripheral perfusion, bowel sounds, and urine output. Also take vital signs every 15 minutes and monitor cardiac rhythm continuously.[1]
- *Because targeted temperature management (TTM) has demonstrated improved neurologic recovery*, it should be considered for any patient who is comatose (lacking meaningful response to verbal commands) after return of spontaneous circulation following a cardiac arrest. Use a target temperature for TTM that's between 89.6° and 96.8° F (32° to 36° C) and then maintain temperature constantly for at least 24 hours. Take measures to actively prevent fever in comatose patients who have received TTM.
- Make sure that the patient receives an adequate supply of oxygen, whether through a mask or a ventilator.[1] Titrate inspired oxygen to the lowest level required to achieve an arterial oxygen saturation of 94% or higher *to avoid potential oxygen toxicity*.[1]
- Check the infusion rates of all IV fluids, and use electronic infusion devices (preferably smart pumps with dose-error reduction software) to deliver vasoactive drugs. Make sure that infusion pump alarm limits are set appropriately for the patient's current condition, and that alarms are turned on, functioning properly, and audible to staff.[35,36,37]
- *To evaluate the effectiveness of fluid therapy*, insert an indwelling urinary catheter (if ordered) if the patient doesn't already have one, or use a bladder scanner to measure the volume of urine in the bladder. Also insert a nasogastric tube *to relieve or prevent gastric distention*.
- If appropriate, reassure the patient and explain what's happening. Allow the patient's family to visit as soon as possible.
- In intubated patients, failure to achieve $ETco_2$ of greater than 10 mm Hg by waveform capnography after 20 minutes of CPR may be considered in combination with other factors to help determine when to terminate resuscitation.[1] In nonintubated patients, a specific $ETco_2$ cutoff valve shouldn't be used as an indication to end resuscitation efforts at any time during CPR.[1]
- If resuscitation is unsuccessful, notify family and allow them to see the patient as soon as possible.
- *To make sure that the code team performs optimally*, schedule a time to review the code.

Complications

Even when performed correctly, CPR can cause fractured ribs, a fractured sternum, liver laceration, lung puncture, and gastric distention.[38,39,40] Defibrillation can cause burns and electric shock.[20] Emergency intubation can result in esophageal or tracheal laceration, subcutaneous emphysema, or accidental right mainstem bronchus intubation (characterized by decreased or absent breath sounds on the left side of the chest and normal breath sounds on the right), cardiac arrhythmias, broken or dislodged teeth, oral or nasal trauma, laryngeal edema, vocal cord trauma, and aspiration.[20]

Documentation

During the code, the recorder documents on the code form the events and interventions in as much detail as possible. Documentation includes whether the arrest was witnessed or unwitnessed, the time of the arrest, the time CPR began, the time the code team arrived and their names, and the total resuscitation time. Also documented are the number of defibrillations, the times they were performed, the energy dose, the patient's cardiac rhythm before and after defibrillation, and the presence or absence of a pulse.

Documentation on the code form includes all drug therapy, including dosages, administration routes, and patient response. Also included are all procedures, such as peripheral and central line insertion, pacemaker use or insertion, and ET tube insertion, with the time performed and the patient's tolerance of the procedure as well as all arterial blood gas and laboratory test results.

The recorder documents whether the patient was transferred to another unit or facility, including what the condition was at the time of transfer and whether the family was notified. Any complications and the measures taken to correct them are recorded. If the patient dies, the time of the death pronouncement is documented. When documentation on the code form is complete, the practitioner and recorder sign the form. The recorder documents teaching provided to the patient and family (if applicable), their understanding of that teaching, and any need for follow-up teaching.

REFERENCES

1 American Heart Association. (2020). 2020 American Heart Association Guidelines for CPR and ECC– Part 3: Adult Basic and Advanced Life Support. https://cpr.heart.org/en/resuscitation-science/cpr-and-ecc-guidelines

2 The Joint Commission. (2021). Standard RI.01.02.01. *Comprehensive accreditation manual for hospitals.* Oakbrook Terrace, IL: The Joint Commission. (Level VII)

3 Panchal, A. R., et al. (2018). 2018 American Heart Association focused update on advanced cardiovascular life support use of antiarrhythmic drugs during and immediately after cardiac arrest: An update to the American Heart Association guidelines for cardiopulmonary resuscitation and emergency cardiovascular care. *Circulation, 138*(23), e740–e749. https://www.ahajournals.org/doi/10.1161/CIR.0000000000000613 (Level II)

4 Field, J. M., et al. (Eds.). (2009). *The textbook of emergency cardiovascular care and CPR.* Philadelphia, PA: Lippincott Williams & Wilkins.

5 Dave, J., et al. (2017). Torsade de pointes. http://emedicine.medscape.com/article/1950863-overview#a9

6 The Joint Commission. (2021). Standard NPSG.07.01.01. *Comprehensive accreditation manual for hospitals.* Oakbrook Terrace, IL: The Joint Commission. (Level VII)

7 Centers for Disease Control and Prevention. (2002). Guideline for hand hygiene in health-care settings: Recommendations of the Healthcare Infection Control Practices Advisory Committee and the HICPAC/SHEA/APIC/IDSA Hand Hygiene Task Force. *MMWR Recommendations and Reports, 51*(RR-16), 1–45. https://www.cdc.gov/mmwr/pdf/rr/rr5116.pdf (Level II)

8 World Health Organization. (2009). WHO guidelines on hand hygiene in health care: First global patient safety challenge, clean care is safer care. https://apps.who.int/iris/bitstream/handle/10665/44102/9789241597906_eng.pdf?sequence=1 (Level IV)

9 Centers for Medicare and Medicaid Services, Department of Health and Human Services. (2020). Condition of participation: Infection control. 42 C.F.R. § 482.42.

10 Accreditation Association for Hospitals and Health Systems. (2020). Standard 07.01.21. *Healthcare Facilities Accreditation Program: Accreditation requirements for acute care hospitals.* Chicago, IL: Accreditation Association for Hospitals and Health Systems. (Level VII)

11 DNV GL-Healthcare USA, Inc. (2020). IC.1.SR.1. *NIAHO® accreditation requirements, interpretive guidelines and surveyor guidance—revision 20.0.* Milford, OH: DNV GL-Healthcare USA, Inc. (Level VII)

12 Siegel, J. D., et al. (2007, revised 2019). 2007 guideline for isolation precautions: Preventing transmission of infectious agents in healthcare settings. https://www.cdc.gov/infectioncontrol/pdf/guidelines/isolation-guidelines-H.pdf (Level II)

13 Occupational Safety and Health Administration. (2012). Bloodborne pathogens, standard number1910.1030. https://www.osha.gov/pls/oshaweb/owadisp.show_document?p_id=10051&p_table=STANDARDS (Level VII)

14 Accreditation Association for Hospitals and Health Systems. (2020). Standard 07.01.10. *Healthcare Facilities Accreditation Program: Accreditation requirements for acute care hospitals.* Chicago, IL: Accreditation Association for Hospitals and Health Systems. (Level VII)

15 DNV GL-Healthcare USA, Inc. (2020). IC.1.SR.2. *NIAHO® accreditation requirements, interpretive guidelines and surveyor guidance—revision 20.0.* Milford, OH: DNV GL-Healthcare USA, Inc. (Level VII)

16 Meaney, P. A., et al. (2013). Cardiopulmonary resuscitation quality: Improving cardiac resuscitation outcomes both inside and outside the hospital: A consensus statement from the American Heart Association. *Circulation, 128*(4), 417–435. https://www.ahajournals.org/doi/10.1161/cir.0b013e31829d8654 (Level VII)

17 American Heart Association. (2010). 2010 American Heart Association guidelines for cardiopulmonary resuscitation and emergency cardiovascular care science. *Circulation, 122,* S720–S728. (Level II)

18 American Heart Association. (2020). Interim guidance for basic and advanced life support in adults, children, and neonates with suspected or confirmed COVID-19. *Circulation, 141*(25), e933–e943. https://www.ahajournals.org/doi/10.1161/CIRCULATIONAHA.120.047463?utm_campaign=ahajournals&utm_source=phd&utm_medium=link&utm_content=phd04-09-20_circ-cpr

19 Bhatnagar, V., et al. (2018). Cardiopulmonary resuscitation: Unusual techniques for unusual situations. *Journal of Emergencies, Trauma, and Shock, 11*(1), 31–37. (Level VII)

20 Wiegand, D. L. (2017). *AACN procedure manual for high acuity, progressive, and critical care* (7th ed.). St. Louis, MO: Elsevier.

21 Centers for Medicare and Medicaid Services, Department of Health and Human Services. (2020). Condition of participation: Nursing services. 42 C.F.R. § 482.23(c).

22 Accreditation Association for Hospitals and Health Systems. (2020). Standard 16.01.03. *Healthcare Facilities Accreditation Program: Accreditation requirements for acute care hospitals.* Chicago, IL: Accreditation Association for Hospitals and Health Systems. (Level VII)

23 The Joint Commission. (2021). Standard MM.06.01.01. *Comprehensive accreditation manual for hospitals.* Oakbrook Terrace, IL: The Joint Commission. (Level VII)

24 DNV GL Healthcare USA, Inc. (2020). MM.1.SR.3. *NIAHO® accreditation requirements, interpretive guidelines and surveyor guidance—revision 20.0.* Milford, OH: DNV GL-Healthcare USA, Inc. (Level VII)

25 Accreditation Association for Hospitals and Health Systems. (2020). Standard 07.02.03. *Healthcare Facilities Accreditation Program: Accreditation requirements for acute care hospitals.* Chicago, IL: Accreditation Association for Hospitals and Health Systems. (Level VII)

26 Rutala, W. A., et al. (2008, revised 2019). Guideline for disinfection and sterilization in healthcare facilities, 2008. https://www.cdc.gov/infection-control/pdf/guidelines/disinfection-guidelines-H.pdf (Level I)

27 The Joint Commission. (2021). Standard RC.01.03.01. *Comprehensive accreditation manual for hospitals.* Oakbrook Terrace, IL: The Joint Commission. (Level VII)

28 Centers for Medicare and Medicaid Services, Department of Health and Human Services. (2020). Condition of participation: Medical record services. 42 C.F.R. § 482.24(b).

29 Accreditation Association for Hospitals and Health Systems. (2020). Standard 10.00.03. *Healthcare Facilities Accreditation Program: Accreditation requirements for acute care hospitals.* Chicago, IL: Accreditation Association for Hospitals and Health Systems. (Level VII)

30 DNV GL-Healthcare USA, Inc. (2020). MR.2.SR.1. *NIAHO® accreditation requirements, interpretive guidelines and surveyor guidance—revision 20.0.* Milford, OH: DNV GL-Healthcare USA, Inc. (Level VII)

31 Panchal, A. R., et al. (2019). 2019 American Heart Association focused update on advanced cardiovascular life support: Use of advanced airways, vasopressors, and extracorporeal cardiopulmonary resuscitation during cardiac arrest: An update to the American Heart Association guidelines for cardiopulmonary resuscitation and emergency cardiovascular care. *Circulation, 140*(24), e881–e894. https://www.ahajournals.org/doi/10.1161/CIR.0000000000000732 (Level II)

32 Emergency Nurses Association. (2012, revised 2017). Clinical practice guideline: Family presence during invasive procedures and resuscitation. https://www.ena.org/docs/default-source/resource-library/practice-resources/cpg/non-mbr-synopsis/familypresencesynopsis.pdf?sfvrsn=a95585b4_2 (Level VII)

33 American Association of Critical-Care Nurses. (2016). AACN practice alert: Family presence during resuscitation and invasive procedures. https://www.aacn.org/clinical-resources/practice-alerts/family-presence-during-resuscitation-and-invasive-procedures (Level VII)

34 Jabre, P., et al. (2014). Offering the opportunity for family to be present during cardiopulmonary resuscitation: 1-year assessment. *Intensive Care Medicine, 40*(7), 981–987. (Level II)

35 The Joint Commission. (2021). Standard NPSG.06.01.01. *Comprehensive accreditation manual for hospitals.* Oakbrook Terrace, IL: The Joint Commission. (Level VII)

36 Graham, K. C., & Cvach, M. (2010). Monitor alarm fatigue: Standardizing use of physiological monitors and decreasing nuisance alarms. *American Journal of Critical Care, 19*(1), 28–37.

37 American Association of Critical-Care Nurses. (2018). AACN practice alert: Managing alarms in acute care across the life span: Electrocardiography and pulse oximetry. https://www.aacn.org/clinical-resources/practice-alerts/managing-alarms-in-acute-care-across-the-life-span (Level VII)

38 Deliliga, A., et al. (2019). Cardiopulmonary resuscitation (CPR) complications encountered in forensic autopsy cases. *BMC Emergency Medicine, 19*(1), 2019. https://bmcemergmed.biomedcentral.com/articles/10.1186/s12873-019-0234-5#citeas

39 Kaldirim, U., et al. (2016). Complications of cardiopulmonary resuscitation in non-traumatic cases and factors affecting complications. *Egyptian Journal of Forensic Sciences, 6*(3), 270–274. https://www.sciencedirect.com/science/article/pii/S2090536X15000702

40 Bon, C. A. (2020). Cardiopulmonary resuscitation (CPR): Post procedure complications. https://emedicine.medscape.com/article/1344081-overview#a4

COLD APPLICATION

The application of cold constricts blood vessels; inhibits local circulation, suppuration, and tissue metabolism; relieves vascular congestion; slows bacterial activity in infections; affects or reduces core body temperature; and may act as a temporary anesthetic during brief, painful procedures. (See *Reducing pain with ice massage,* page 192.) Cold helps decrease edema by decreasing capillary permeability and causing vasoconstriction.[1] Because treatment with cold also relieves inflammation, reduces edema, and slows bleeding, it may provide effective initial treatment after eye injuries, strains, sprains, bruises, muscle spasms, and burns. Studies show that local application of cold may significantly reduce labor pain during the first and second phases.[2,3] Also referred to as *cryotherapy,* cold therapy is typically used to relieve pain following certain surgical procedures, including arthroscopy and total joint replacement.[4]

Cold can be applied in dry or moist forms, but cold therapy devices shouldn't be placed directly on a patient's skin because they may further damage tissue.[5] Moist application is more penetrating than dry application, *because moisture facilitates conduction.* Devices for applying dry cold include an ice bag or collar, a cold therapy system, chemical cold packs, and ice packs. Devices for applying moist cold include cold compresses for small body areas and cold packs for large areas.

Because cold treatments cause vasoconstriction, they should be used cautiously in patients with impaired circulation or high blood pressure and in patients with an area of diminished sensation, such as a patient who has been treated with local anesthesia. In addition, a cold therapy device should not be applied on an open wound.[6]

Equipment

Vital signs monitoring equipment ■ towel ■ Optional: gloves, dressings.

For an ice bag or collar

Ice bag or collar ■ cold tap water ■ crushed ice ■ insulation barrier or cloth covering and tape or roller gauze.

For a cold therapy system

Cooler control unit with tubing (differs by manufacturer) ■ water ■ cubed or chopped ice ■ appropriate cooling pad ■ power supply cord ■ insulation barrier or cloth.

For a chemical cold pack

Single-use pack for applying dry cold ■ insulation barrier or cloth covering and tape or roller gauze.

Reducing pain with ice massage

Direct application of ice to a patient's skin is normally contraindicated *because it can damage the skin surface and underlying tissues.* However, when carefully performed, this technique—called ice massage—can help patients tolerate brief, painful procedures such as bone marrow aspiration, catheterization, chest tube removal, injection into a joint, lumbar puncture, and suture removal. It can also be used to treat sore muscles, such as neck and lower back pain. Ice massage is most effective if applied within 48 hours of an injury. It reduces inflammation from the injury and slows nerve impulses, reducing pain. The goal of ice massage is to achieve numbness to the area without injuring the skin.[7]

Prepare for ice massage by gathering the ice, a porous covering to hold it in (if desired), and a cloth for wiping water from the patient as the ice melts. One option is to freeze water in a paper cup ahead of time and then remove the paper from half the cup, exposing the ice you'll use for the procedure.

Just before the procedure begins, rub the ice over the appropriate area *to numb it.*[7] Assess the site frequently; stop rubbing immediately if you detect signs of tissue intolerance. As you begin the procedure, rub the ice over a point near but not at the site. *This action distracts the patient from the procedure itself and gives the patient another stimulus to concentrate on.* Limit ice application in one area to about 5 minutes, and assess the skin frequently for damage.[7] If the procedure lasts longer than 5 minutes or if you think that tissue damage may occur, move the ice to a different site and continue massaging.[7]

If you know in advance that the procedure probably will last longer than 5 minutes, massage the site intermittently—2 minutes of massage alternating with a rest period until the skin regains its normal color. Alternatively, you can divide the area into several sites and apply ice to each one for several minutes at a time.

For a cold compress or pack
Basin of ice chips ■ container of tap water ■ bath thermometer ■ compress material (4″ × 4″ [10 cm × 10 cm] gauze pads or washcloths) or pack material (towels or flannel) ■ fluid-impermeable pad ■ waterproof covering ■ tape or roller gauze.

Preparation of equipment
Inspect all equipment and supplies. If a product is expired, is defective, or has compromised integrity, remove it from patient use, label it as expired or defective, and report the expiration or defect as directed by your facility.

Ice bag or collar
Select a device of the correct size, fill it with cold tap water, and check for leaks. Then empty the device and fill it about halfway with crushed ice, *because using small pieces of ice helps the device mold to the patient's body.* Squeeze the device *to expel air that might reduce conduction.* Fasten the cap and wipe any moisture from the outside of the device. Wrap the bag or collar in a cloth covering, and secure the cover with tape or roller gauze. *The protective cover prevents tissue trauma and absorbs condensation.*

Cold therapy system
Remove the cooler control unit lid and fill with water to the indicated fill line. Then add cubed or chopped ice to the indicated line. Replace and lock the lid. Connect the power supply cord to the device and then to the electrical outlet. Attach the cooling pad to the cooler control unit.

Chemical cold pack
Select a pack of the appropriate size and follow the manufacturer's directions (striking, squeezing, or kneading) *to activate the cold-producing chemicals.* Make certain that the container hasn't been broken during activation. Wrap the pack in a cloth cover and secure the cover with tape or roller gauze if not using an insulation barrier. Store these packs frozen until use; after exterior disinfection, you can refreeze them and use them again.

Cold compress or pack
Cool a container of tap water by placing it in a basin of ice or by adding ice to the water. Using a bath thermometer for guidance, adjust the water temperature to 59° F (15° C) or as ordered. Immerse the compress material or pack material in the water.

Implementation
- Verify the practitioner's order, as needed, based on the reason and type of cold therapy.
- Gather and prepare the necessary equipment and supplies.
- Perform hand hygiene.[8,9,10,11,12,13]
- Confirm the patient's identity using at least two patient identifiers.[14]
- Provide privacy.[15,16,17,18]
- Explain the procedure to the patient and family (if appropriate) according to their individual communication and learning needs *to increase their understanding, allay their fears, and enhance cooperation.*[19]
- Make sure the room is warm and free from drafts.
- Raise the patient's bed to waist level before providing care *to prevent caregiver back strain.*[20]
- Perform hand hygiene.[8,9,10,11,12,13]
- Record the patient's vital signs, including temperature, pulse, and respirations, *to serve as a baseline for comparison.*
- Perform hand hygiene.[8,9,10,11,12,13]
- Put on gloves, as needed, *to comply with standard precautions.*[21,22,23]
- Expose only the treatment site *to avoid chilling the patient.*
- Assess the condition of the injured or affected area and surrounding skin, including neurovascular status and skin integrity.[24]

Applying an ice bag or collar, cold therapy system, or a chemical cold pack
- Place an insulation barrier over the treatment site or a cloth cover over the cold therapy device, as appropriate.
- Place the cold device on the treatment site and begin timing the application.
- Inspect the site frequently for signs of tissue intolerance, such as blanching, mottling, cyanosis, maceration, and blisters. Also, be alert for shivering and complaints of burning or numbness. If these signs or symptoms develop, discontinue treatment and notify the practitioner.
- Refill or replace the cold device as necessary *to maintain the correct temperature.* Change the protective cover if it becomes wet.
- Remove the device after the prescribed treatment period; usually 10 minutes relieves pain and swelling in patients with soft tissue injuries.[25,26]

Applying a cold compress or pack
- Place a fluid-impermeable pad under the site.
- Remove the compress or pack from the water and wring it out *to prevent dripping.*
- Apply the compress or pack to the treatment site and begin timing the application.
- Cover the compress or pack with a waterproof covering *to provide insulation and to keep the surrounding area dry.* Secure the covering with tape or roller gauze *to prevent it from slipping.*
- Inspect the treatment site frequently for signs of tissue intolerance, such as blanching, mottling, cyanosis, maceration, and blisters. Note complaints of burning or numbness. If these issues develop, discontinue treatment and notify the practitioner.
- Change the compress or pack as needed *to maintain the correct temperature.*
- Remove the device after the prescribed treatment period; usually 10 minutes relieves pain and swelling in patients with soft tissue injuries.[25,26]

Completing the procedures
- Dry the patient's skin with a towel and re-dress the treatment site according to the practitioner's orders.
- Position the patient comfortably
- Assess the patient's vital signs, including temperature, pulse, and respirations, and compare them with baselines *to determine the patient's tolerance of the procedure.*

PATIENT TEACHING

USING COLD FOR A MUSCLE SPRAIN

For each cold application, instruct the patient to obtain enough crushed ice to cover the painful area, place it in a plastic bag, and place the bag inside a pillowcase or large piece of cloth, as shown below.

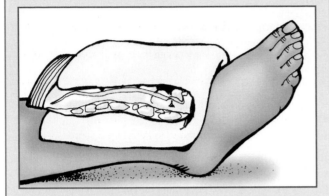

For later applications, the patient may want to fill a paper cup with water, stand a tongue blade in the cup, and place it in the freezer. After the water freezes, the patient can peel the paper off the ice and hold it with the protruding handle. If using this method, tell the patient to first cover the area with a cloth, *because applying ice directly to the skin can cause frostbite or cold shock.*

Instruct the patient to rub the ice over the painful area for the specified treatment time or not more than 20 minutes. Although ice eases pain in a joint that has begun to stiffen, the patient shouldn't let the analgesic effect encourage overuse of the joint.

After 24 to 72 hours, when pain and swelling have subsided or when cold no longer helps, the patient should switch to heat application, as directed.[6] (See the "Heat application" procedure.)

- Return the bed to the lowest position *to prevent falls and maintain patient safety.*[27]
- Discard liquids and soiled materials in appropriate receptacles.
- If treatment will be repeated, clean and store the equipment in the patient's room.
- Discard used supplies in appropriate receptacles.[28]
- Remove and discard your gloves, if worn.
- Put on gloves and, as needed, other personal protective equipment.[28]
- Clean and disinfect other reusable equipment according to the manufacturer's instructions *to prevent the spread of infection.*[29,30]
- Remove and discard your gloves and, if worn, other personal protective equipment.[28]
- Perform hand hygiene.[8,9,10,11,12,13]
- Document the procedure.[31,32,33,34]

Special considerations

- Avoid securing cooling devices with pins, *because an accidental puncture could allow extremely cold fluids to leak out and burn the patient's skin.*
- If the patient is unconscious, anesthetized, neurologically or cognitively impaired, or otherwise insensitive to cold, stay in the room throughout the treatment and check the treatment site frequently for complications.

Patient teaching

- Teach the patient how to apply cold for a muscle sprain at home, if appropriate. (See *Using cold for a muscle sprain.*) Instruct the patient and family on the use of the cold therapy system, if ordered, after an orthopedic procedure.

Complications

Intense cold can cause frostbite and tissue damage.[6]

Documentation

Record the time, date, and duration of cold application; type of device used (ice bag or collar, cold therapy system, or chemical cold pack); application site; temperature or temperature setting (if available); the patient's temperature, pulse, and respirations before and after application; treatment site skin appearance before, during, and after application; signs of complications; and the patient's tolerance of the treatment. Document teaching provided to the patient and family (if appropriate), their understanding of that teaching, and any need for follow-up teaching.

REFERENCES

1 Hsu, J. R., et al. (2019). Clinical practice guidelines for pain management in acute musculoskeletal injury. *Journal of Orthopaedic Trauma, 33*(5), e158–e182. https://www.ncbi.nlm.nih.gov/pmc/articles/PMC6485308 (Level VII)

2 Shirvani, M. A., & Ganji, Z. (2014). The influence of cold pack on labour pain relief and birth outcomes: A randomized controlled trial. *Journal of Clinical Nursing, 23*, 2473–2479. (Level II)

3 Asgar, H. P., & Yavuz, M. (2014). Effects of peripheral cold application on core body temperature and haemodynamic parameters in febrile patients. *International Journal of Nursing Practice, 20*, 156–163. (Level VI)

4 Fang, L., et al. (2012). The effects of cryotherapy in relieving postarthroscopy pain. *Journal of Clinical Nursing, 21*, 636–643. (Level VI)

5 American Academy of Orthopaedic Surgeons. (2020). Sprains, strains and other soft-tissue injuries. https://orthoinfo.aaos.org/en/diseases–conditions/sprains-strains-and-other-soft-tissue-injuries/

6 Groom, D. (n.d.). Common injury question—should I use ice or heat? https://www.issaonline.com/blog/index.cfm/2017/common-injury-question-should-i-use-ice-or-heat

7 Hochschuler, S. (2012). Ice massage for back pain relief. https://www.spine-health.com/treatment/heat-therapy-cold-therapy/ice-massage-back-pain-relief

8 The Joint Commission. (2021). Standard NPSG.07.01.01. *Comprehensive accreditation manual for hospitals.* Oakbrook Terrace, IL: The Joint Commission. (Level VII)

9 Centers for Disease Control and Prevention. (2002). Guideline for hand hygiene in health-care settings: Recommendations of the Healthcare Infection Control Practices Advisory Committee and the HICPAC/SHEA/APIC/IDSA Hand Hygiene Task Force. *MMWR Recommendations and Reports, 51*(RR-16), 1–45. https://www.cdc.gov/mmwr/pdf/rr/rr5116.pdf (Level II)

10 World Health Organization. (2009). WHO guidelines on hand hygiene in health care: First global patient safety challenge, clean care is safer care. https://apps.who.int/iris/bitstream/handle/10665/44102/9789241597906_eng.pdf?sequence=1 (Level IV)

11 Accreditation Association for Hospitals and Health Systems. (2020). Standard 07.01.21. *Healthcare Facilities Accreditation Program: Accreditation requirements for acute care hospitals.* Chicago, IL: Accreditation Association for Hospitals and Health Systems. (Level VII)

12 Centers for Medicare and Medicaid Services, Department of Health and Human Services. (2020). Condition of participation: Infection control. 42 C.F.R. § 482.42.

13 DNV GL-Healthcare USA, Inc. (2020). IC.1.SR.1. *NIAHO® accreditation requirements, interpretive guidelines and surveyor guidance—revision 20.0.* Milford, OH: DNV GL-Healthcare USA, Inc. (Level VII)

14 The Joint Commission. (2021). Standard NPSG.01.01.01. *Comprehensive accreditation manual for hospitals.* Oakbrook Terrace, IL: The Joint Commission. (Level VII)

15 Centers for Medicare and Medicaid Services, Department of Health and Human Services. (2020). Condition of participation: Patient's rights. 42 C.F.R. § 482.13(c)(1).

16 Accreditation Association for Hospitals and Health Systems. (2020). Standard 15.01.16. *Healthcare Facilities Accreditation Program: Accreditation requirements for acute care hospitals.* Chicago, IL: Accreditation Association for Hospitals and Health Systems. (Level VII)

17 DNV GL-Healthcare USA, Inc. (2020). PR.2.SR.5. *NIAHO® accreditation requirements, interpretive guidelines and surveyor guidance—revision 20.0.* Milford, OH: DNV GL-Healthcare USA, Inc. (Level VII)

18 The Joint Commission. (2021). Standard RI.01.01.01. *Comprehensive accreditation manual for hospitals.* Oakbrook Terrace, IL: The Joint Commission. (Level VII)

19 The Joint Commission. (2021). Standard PC.02.01.21. *Comprehensive accreditation manual for hospitals.* Oakbrook Terrace, IL: The Joint Commission. (Level VII)

20 Waters, T. R., et al. (2009). Safe patient handling training for schools of nursing. http://www.cdc.gov/niosh/docs/2009-127/pdfs/2009-127.pdf (Level VII)

21 Accreditation Association for Hospitals and Health Systems. (2020). Standard 07.01.10. *Healthcare Facilities Accreditation Program: Accreditation requirements for acute care hospitals.* Chicago, IL: Accreditation Association for Hospitals and Health Systems. (Level VII)

22 Siegel, J. D., et al. (2007, revised 2019). 2007 guideline for isolation precautions: Preventing transmission of infectious agents in healthcare settings. https://www.cdc.gov/infectioncontrol/pdf/guidelines/isolation-guidelines-H.pdf (Level II)

23 DNV GL-Healthcare USA, Inc. (2020). IC.1.SR.2. *NIAHO® accreditation requirements, interpretive guidelines and surveyor guidance—revision 20.0.* Milford, OH: DNV GL-Healthcare USA, Inc. (Level VII)

24 Perry, A. G., et al. (2016). *Nursing interventions and clinical skills* (6th ed.). St. Louis, MO: Elsevier.

25 Eustice, C. (2020). R.I.C.E. treatment for acute musculoskeletal injury. https://www.verywellhealth.com/what-is-rice-190446

26 Kuo, C. C., et al. (2013). Comparing the antiswelling and analgesic effects of three different ice pack therapy durations: A randomized controlled trial on cases with soft tissue injuries. *Journal of Nursing Research, 21,* 186–194. (Level II)

27 Ganz, D. A., et al. (2013, reviewed 2021). *Preventing falls in hospitals: A toolkit for improving quality of care* (AHRQ Publication No. 13-0015-EF). Rockville, MD: Agency for Healthcare Research and Quality. https://www.ahrq.gov/professionals/systems/hospital/fallpxtoolkit/index.html (Level VII)

28 Occupational Safety and Health Administration. (2012). Bloodborne pathogens, standard number 1910.1030. https://www.osha.gov/pls/oshaweb/owadisp.show_document?p_id=10051&p table=STANDARDS (Level VII)

29 Accreditation Association for Hospitals and Health Systems. (2020). Standard 07.02.03. *Healthcare Facilities Accreditation Program: Accreditation requirements for acute care hospitals.* Chicago, IL: Accreditation Association for Hospitals and Health Systems. (Level VII)

30 Rutala, W. A., et al. (2008, revised 2019). Guideline for disinfection and sterilization in healthcare facilities, 2008. https://www.cdc.gov/infection-control/pdf/guidelines/disinfection-guidelines-H.pdf (Level I)

31 The Joint Commission. (2021). Standard RC.01.03.01. *Comprehensive accreditation manual for hospitals.* Oakbrook Terrace, IL: The Joint Commission. (Level VII)

32 Accreditation Association for Hospitals and Health Systems. (2020). Standard 10.00.03. *Healthcare Facilities Accreditation Program: Accreditation requirements for acute care hospitals.* Chicago, IL: Accreditation Association for Hospitals and Health Systems. (Level VII)

33 Centers for Medicare and Medicaid Services, Department of Health and Human Services. (2020). Condition of participation: Medical record services. 42 C.F.R. § 482.24(b).

34 DNV GL-Healthcare USA, Inc. (2020). MR.2.SR.1. *NIAHO® accreditation requirements, interpretive guidelines and surveyor guidance—revision 20.0.* Milford, OH: DNV GL-Healthcare USA, Inc. (Level VII)

COLOSTOMY AND ILEOSTOMY CARE

A patient with an ascending, transverse, or descending colostomy or an ileostomy must wear an external pouch to collect emerging fecal matter, which may be watery, pasty, or formed, depending on location of the stoma. Besides collecting waste matter, the pouch helps to control odor and protect the stoma and peristomal skin.

Any pouching system should be changed immediately if a leak develops, and every pouch needs emptying when it's one-third full. The patient with an ileostomy may need to empty the pouch four or five times daily. The best time to change a pouching system is when the bowel is least active, usually in the morning before breakfast. After a few months, most patients can predict the best changing time.

The selection of a pouching system should take into consideration which system provides the best adhesive seal and skin protection for the individual patient. The type of pouch selected also depends on the stoma's location and structure, abdominal contours, availability of supplies, wear time, frequency and consistency of output, personal preference, patient or caregiver ability to manage the stoma, and cost.[1,2]

Equipment

Pouching system ■ water ■ soft cloths or gauze pads ■ gloves ■ facility-approved ostomy skin assessment tool[2,3,4] ■ stoma measuring guide ■ Optional: pen, scissors, stoma paste or moldable barrier ring, closure clamp, clippers.

Pouching systems may be disposable or reusable, drainable or closed-ended, and one-piece or two-piece. (See *Comparing ostomy pouching systems.*)

Preparation of equipment

Inspect all equipment and supplies. If a product is expired, is defective, or has compromised integrity, remove it from patient use, label it as expired or defective, and report the expiration or defect as directed by your facility.

Implementation

■ Gather and prepare the necessary equipment and supplies.
■ Perform hand hygiene.[5,6,7,8,9,10]
■ Confirm the patient's identity using at least two patient identifiers.[11]
■ Provide privacy.[12,13,14,15]
■ Explain the procedure to the patient and family (if appropriate) according to their individual communication and learning needs *to increase their understanding, allay their fears, and enhance cooperation.*[16] As you perform each step, explain what you are doing and why, *because the patient will eventually need to perform the procedure independently.* Provide emotional support, as needed.
■ Raise the bed to waist level before providing patient care *to prevent caregiver back strain.*[17]
■ Perform hand hygiene.[6,7,8,9,10]
■ Put on gloves *to comply with standard precautions.*[18,19]

Fitting the skin barrier and pouch

■ For a pouch with an attached skin barrier (one-piece pouch), measure the stoma using the measuring guide. Select the opening size that matches the stoma.
■ For an adhesive-backed pouch with a separate skin barrier (two-piece pouch), measure the stoma using the measuring guide and select the opening that matches the stoma. Trace the selected size opening onto the paper back of the skin barrier's adhesive side. Cut out the opening. If the pouch has precut openings, which can be handy for a round stoma, select an opening that's no more than ⅛" (0.32 cm) larger than the stoma. If the pouch comes without an opening, cut the hole ⅛" (0.32 cm) wider than the measured tracing (although many pouching systems can now be fit up to the stoma edge without risk of trauma to the stoma). The cut-to-fit system works best for an irregularly shaped stoma. (See *Applying a skin barrier and pouch,* page 196.)

Applying or changing the pouch

■ Empty, remove, and discard the old pouch, if applicable (as shown below).

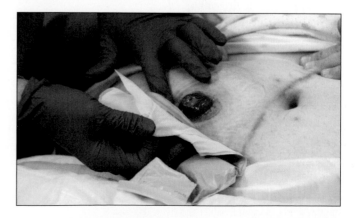

Comparing ostomy pouching systems

Manufactured in many shapes and sizes, ostomy pouches are fashioned for comfort, safety, and easy application. For example, a disposable, closed-end pouch may meet the needs of a patient who irrigates the ostomy, who wants added security, or who wants to discard the pouch after each bowel movement. Another patient may prefer a reusable, drainable pouch. Some commonly available pouches are described below.

Disposable pouches

A patient who must empty the pouch often (because of diarrhea or a new colostomy or ileostomy) may prefer a one-piece, drainable, disposable pouch with a closure clamp attached to a skin barrier (as shown below). These transparent or opaque, odor-proof plastic pouches come with attached adhesive backing. Some pouches have microporous tape edges, integrated gas filters, and belt tabs. The bottom opening allows for easy draining. This style of pouch may be used permanently or temporarily, until stoma size stabilizes.

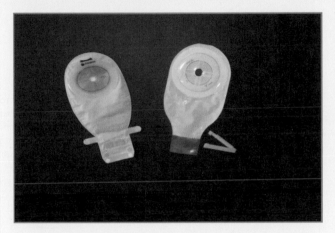

Also disposable and also made of transparent or opaque odor-proof plastic, a one-piece, disposable, closed-end pouch may come with a filter. A patient with a regular bowel elimination pattern may choose this style for additional security and confidence.

A two-piece, drainable, disposable pouch with separate skin barrier (as shown below) permits more frequent pouch changes. Also made of transparent or opaque odor-proof plastic, this style pouch comes with belt tabs and usually snaps to the skin barrier with a flange mechanism. Newer, two-piece pouches have an adhesive coupling. The pouch sticks to the wafer, allowing greater flexibility and comfort.

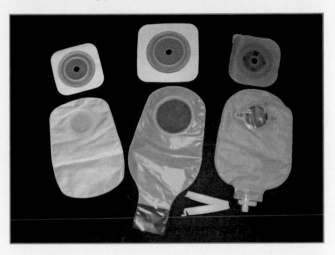

Reusable pouches

Typically manufactured from sturdy, opaque, hypoallergenic plastic, the reusable pouch comes with a separate custom-made faceplate and O-ring. The device has a 1- to 3-month life span, depending on how frequently the patient empties the pouch. Reusable equipment may benefit a patient who needs a firm faceplate or who wishes to minimize cost.

■ Wipe the stoma and peristomal skin gently with a soft cloth or gauze (as shown below).

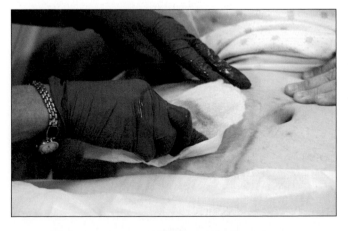

■ Carefully wash the peristomal skin with water and dry by patting gently. Allow the skin to dry thoroughly[20] (as shown to the right). If necessary, clip surrounding hair (in a direction away from the stoma) *to promote a better seal and avoid skin irritation from hair pulling against the adhesive.*

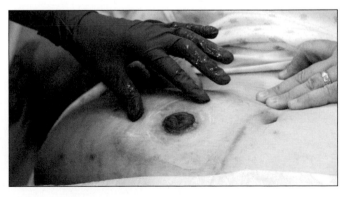

■ Inspect the peristomal skin and stoma. Use a facility-approved assessment tool *to objectively identify and track changes in peristomal skin.* Use the tool to assess for discoloration, erosion, and tissue overgrowth.[2,3,4] Observe for signs of mechanical, chemical, allergic, and infectious or disease-related complications (which may be linked to preexisting skin conditions, such as psoriasis, eczema, and seborrheic dermatitis).[3] Notify the practitioner or a wound, ostomy, and continence nurse (WOCN) of changes, as needed.
■ Consider applying a ring of stoma paste or a molded barrier ring around the opening on the back of the skin barrier (depending on the

EQUIPMENT

Applying a skin barrier and pouch

Fitting a skin barrier and ostomy pouch properly can be done in a few steps. Shown below is a one-piece pouching system with flanges.

1. Measure the stoma using a measuring guide.

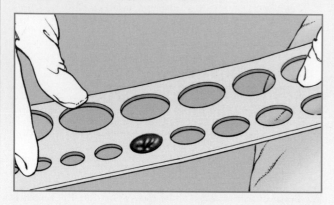

2. Trace the appropriate circle carefully on the back of the skin barrier.

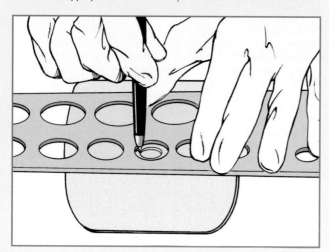

3. Cut the circular opening in the skin barrier (or cut the opening to reflect the configuration of the stoma if it's not circular). Smooth any rough edges with your finger.

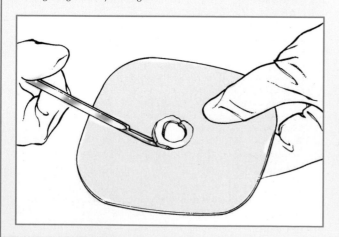

4. Remove the backing from the skin barrier and apply barrier paste or a moldable barrier ring, as needed, along the edge of the circular opening.

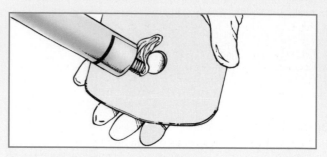

5. Center a one-piece system over the stoma, adhesive side down, and gently press it to the skin. When using a two-piece system, apply the wafer and then gently press the pouch opening onto the ring until it snaps into place. When using a two-piece adhesive coupling device, line up the adhesive portion of the pouch to the "landing zone" of the wafer. Press together *for adhesion*. The pouches used in a two-piece system can be attached to the wafer before application and applied like a one-piece system if the patient is still experiencing incisional discomfort. Other two-piece systems have a floating flange that allows the user to insert the fingers underneath *so that snapping the flange to the pouch doesn't exert pressure*.

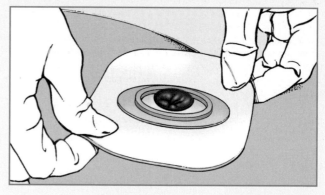

6. Close the bottom of the pouch by folding the end upward and using the clip that comes with the product, or close the integrated closure system.

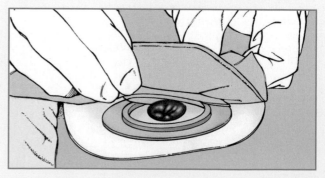

type of stoma, abdominal contours, and effluent) *to provide extra skin protection and a better seal to prevent leakage*.[21,22]

■ If applying a two-piece appliance with a separate skin barrier, peel off the paper backing of the prepared skin barrier, center the barrier over the stoma, and press gently *to ensure adhesion*.

■ For a pouching system with flanges, align the lip of the pouch flange with the bottom edge of the skin barrier flange. Gently press around the circumference of the pouch flange, beginning at the bottom, until the pouch securely adheres to the barrier flange. (The pouch will click into its secured position.) Holding the barrier against the skin, gently pull on the pouch *to confirm the seal between flanges*. When using a two-piece adhesive coupling device, line up the adhesive portion of the pouch to the "landing zone" of the wafer. Press together for adhesion. You can attach the pouches used in a two-piece system to the wafer before application if the patient is still experiencing incisional discomfort.

■ Encourage the patient to place a hand over the appliance and hold it in place for about 5 minutes after application. *The patient's body warmth helps to improve adherence and soften a rigid skin barrier.*[23]
■ Leave a bit of air in the pouch *to allow drainage to fall to the bottom*.
■ Apply the closure clamp, if necessary.
■ Return the bed to the lowest positon *to prevent falls and maintain patient safety.*[24]
■ Discard all used supplies in appropriate receptacles.[25]
■ Remove and discard your gloves.[18,19]
■ Perform hand hygiene.[5,6,7,8,9,10]
■ Document the procedure.[26,27,28,29]

Special considerations

■ When caring for a stoma during the immediate postoperative period, select an appliance with a larger opening and adjust the size of the appliance skin barrier by cutting a larger opening, or cut radial slits in the skin barrier *to allow for flexibility, because a newly created stoma may become edematous over the first 24 to 48 hours*. Use a sealant *to protect skin integrity around the opening*.[20] Adjust the size of the opening as stomal swelling subsides. Avoid cutting the opening too big after the initial postoperative period *to prevent peristomal skin complications.*[2]
■ Between 6 and 8 weeks after surgery, the stoma will shrink to its permanent size. At that point, pattern-making preparations will be unnecessary unless the patient gains weight, has additional surgery, or injures the stoma.
■ Use commercial pouch deodorants, if desired, although, most pouches are odor-free; odor should only be evident when you empty the pouch or if it leaks. Before discharge, suggest that, if desired, the patient avoid odor-causing foods, such as fish, eggs, onions, beans, cabbage, and broccoli.[30]
■ For a reusable pouching system, instruct the patient to clean the system with soap and water or a commercially prepared cleaning solution. Suggest obtaining two or more systems *so the patient can wear one while the other dries after cleaning it.*
■ Most ostomy product manufacturers will provide a patch test, if requested, *to determine whether the patient has an allergy to a specific ostomy appliance care product.*[3]

Patient teaching

After performing and explaining the procedure to the patient and caregiver, encourage the patient's increasing involvement in self-care. Before discharge, make sure that the patient and family can care for the ostomy. Provide written instructions and information about obtaining replacement equipment. Offer the patient and caregiver a pamphlet or video instructions related to ostomy care. Make sure that the patient or caregiver feels comfortable calling the practitioner, nurse, or WOCN to ask questions or discuss problems. Refer the patient to a local ostomy group. Provide counseling on nutrition, clothing, medications, body image, psychosocial issues, interpersonal relationships, and possible complications.[1,3]

Complications

Failure to fit the pouch properly over the stoma can injure the stoma and may cause leakage, which can induce peristomal skin irritation. Be alert for a possible allergic reaction to adhesives and other ostomy products.

Documentation

Record the date and time of the pouching system change; note the character of drainage, including color, amount, type, and consistency. Also describe the appearance of the stoma and the peristomal skin, using a facility-approved assessment tool if possible.[2,3,4] Document teaching provided to the patient and family (if applicable), their understanding of that teaching, and any need for follow-up teaching. Record the patient's response to self-care.

REFERENCES

1 Wound, Ostomy, and Continence Nurses (WOCN) Society, Guideline Development Task Force. (2018). WOCN Society clinical guideline: Management of the adult patient with a fecal or urinary ostomy—An executive summary. *Journal of Wound, Ostomy, and Continence Nursing, 45,* 50–58. (Level VII)
2 Australian Association of Stomal Therapy Nurses, Inc. (2013). Clinical guidelines for stomal therapy nursing practice. http://www. stomaltherapy.com/documents/AASTN_Guidelines_book_2013.pdf (Level VII)
3 Jordan, R., & Christian, M. (2013). Understanding peristomal skin complications. *Wound Care Advisor, 2*(3), 36–41. http://woundcareadvisor. com/wp-content/uploads/2013/05/Understanding_M-J13.pdf
4 Haugen, V., & Ratliff, C. R. (2013). Tools for assessing peristomal skin complications. *Journal of Wound, Ostomy, and Continence Nursing, 40*(2), 131–134. (Level VII)
5 Centers for Disease Control and Prevention. (2002). Guideline for hand hygiene in health-care settings: Recommendations of the Healthcare Infection Control Practices Advisory Committee and the HICPAC/ SHEA/APIC/IDSA Hand Hygiene Task Force. *MMWR Recommendations and Reports, 51*(RR-16), 1–45. https://www.cdc.gov/mmwr/pdf/rr/rr5116. pdf (Level II)
6 The Joint Commission. (2021) Standard NPSG.07.01.01. *Comprehensive accreditation manual for hospitals.* Oakbrook Terrace, IL: The Joint Commission. (Level VII)
7 World Health Organization. (2009). WHO guidelines on hand hygiene in health care: First global patient safety challenge, clean care is safer care. https://apps.who.int/iris/bitstream/handle/10665/44102/9789241597906_eng.pdf (Level IV)
8 Accreditation Association for Hospitals and Health Systems. (2020). Standard 07.01.21. *Healthcare Facilities Accreditation Program: Accreditation requirements for acute care hospitals.* Chicago, IL: Accreditation Association for Hospitals and Health Systems. (Level VII)
9 Centers for Medicare and Medicaid Services, Department of Health and Human Services. (2020). Condition of participation: Infection control. 42 C.F.R. § 482.42.
10 DNV GL-Healthcare USA, Inc. (2020). IC.1.SR.1. *NIAHO® accreditation requirements, interpretive guidelines and surveyor guidance—revision 20.0.* Milford, OH: DNV GL-Healthcare USA, Inc. (Level VII)
11 The Joint Commission. (2021). Standard NPSG.01.01.01. *Comprehensive accreditation manual for hospitals.* Oakbrook Terrace, IL: The Joint Commission. (Level VII)
12 Accreditation Association for Hospitals and Health Systems. (2020). Standard 15.01.16. *Healthcare Facilities Accreditation Program: Accreditation requirements for acute care hospitals.* Chicago, IL: Accreditation Association for Hospitals and Health Systems. (Level VII)
13 Centers for Medicare and Medicaid Services, Department of Health and Human Services. (2020). Condition of participation: Patient's rights. 42 C.F.R. § 482.13(c)(1).
14 The Joint Commission. (2021). Standard RI.01.01.01. *Comprehensive accreditation manual for hospitals.* Oakbrook Terrace, IL: The Joint Commission. (Level VII)
15 DNV GL-Healthcare USA, Inc. (2020). PR.2.SR.5. *NIAHO® accreditation requirements, interpretive guidelines and surveyor guidance—revision 20.0.* Milford, OH: DNV GL-Healthcare USA, Inc. (Level VII)
16 The Joint Commission. (2021). Standard PC.02.01.21. *Comprehensive accreditation manual for hospitals.* Oakbrook Terrace, IL: The Joint Commission. (Level VII)
17 Waters, T. R., et al. (2009). Safe patient handling training for schools of nursing. https://www.cdc.gov/niosh/docs/2009-127/pdfs/2009-127.pdf (Level VII)
18 Siegel, J. D., et al. (2007, revised 2019). 2007 guideline for isolation precautions: Preventing transmission of infectious agents in healthcare settings. https://www.cdc.gov/infectioncontrol/pdf/guidelines/isolation-guidelines-H.pdf (Level II)
19 Accreditation Association for Hospitals and Health Systems. (2020). Standard 07.01.10. *Healthcare Facilities Accreditation Program: Accreditation requirements for acute care hospitals.* Chicago, IL: Accreditation Association for Hospitals and Health Systems. (Level VII)
20 Wound, Ostomy and Continence Nurses Society. (2018). *Basic ostomy skin care: A guide for patients and health care providers.* Mt. Laurel, NJ: Wound, Ostomy and Continence Nurses Society. https://www.ostomy.org/ wp-content/uploads/2018/11/wocn_basic_ostomy_skin_care_2018.pdf (Level VII)

21 Hollister, Inc. (2021). Adapt skin barrier paste. https://www.hollister.com/en/products/ostomy-care-products/ostomy-accessories/stoma-pastes/adapt-skin-barrier-paste

22 Hollister, Inc. (2021). Adapt barrier rings. https://www.hollister.com/en/products/Ostomy-Care-Products/Ostomy-Accessories/Barrier-Rings-and-Strips/Adapt-Barrier-Rings

23 Lueder, W. (2018). How to change your ostomy pouch: Basic tips for changing your ostomy appliance. https://www.ostomy.org/change-ostomy-pouch/

24 Ganz, D. A., et al. (2013, reviewed 2021). *Preventing falls in hospitals: A toolkit for improving quality of care* (AHRQ Publication No. 13-0015-EF). Rockville, MD: Agency for Healthcare Research and Quality. https://www.ahrq.gov/professionals/systems/hospital/fallpxtoolkit/index.html (Level VII)

25 Occupational Safety and Health Administration. (2012). Bloodborne pathogens, standard number1910.1030. https://www.osha.gov/pls/oshaweb/owadisp.show_document?p_id=10051&p_table=STANDARDS (Level VII)

26 The Joint Commission. (2021). Standard RC.01.03.01. *Comprehensive accreditation manual for hospitals*. Oakbrook Terrace, IL: The Joint Commission. (Level VII)

27 Accreditation Association for Hospitals and Health Systems. (2020). Standard 10.00.03. *Healthcare Facilities Accreditation Program: Accreditation requirements for acute care hospitals*. Chicago, IL: Accreditation Association for Hospitals and Health Systems. (Level VII)

28 Centers for Medicare and Medicaid Services, Department of Health and Human Services. (2020). Condition of participation: Medical record services. 42 C.F.R. § 482.24(b).

29 DNV GL-Healthcare USA, Inc. (2020). MR.2.SR.1. *NIAHO® accreditation requirements, interpretive guidelines and surveyor guidance—revision 20.0*. Milford, OH: DNV GL-Healthcare USA, Inc. (Level VII)

30 United Ostomy Associations of America, Inc. (2017). Colostomy guide. https://www.ostomy.org/wp-content/uploads/2018/03/ColostomyGuide.pdf

COLOSTOMY IRRIGATION

Colostomy irrigation involves instilling warm water (irrigant) into the colon via a descending or sigmoid colostomy stoma. The warm water helps to stimulate bowel peristalsis and trains the bowel to empty at this specific time. The goal of irrigation is to prevent the passage of feces or flatus between irrigations, which may allow the patient to use only a cap, mini-pouch, or patch to protect the stoma, making the colostomy less visible through clothing. This goal can be achieved when irrigation is performed daily, or every 2 to 3 days in select patients. Colostomy irrigation may also be used to empty the large bowel before diagnostic testing (such as colonoscopy) or colon surgery.[1] The surgeon typically determines whether a patient is a candidate for colostomy irrigation.[1]

Although colostomy irrigation may begin as soon as bowel function resumes, most practitioners recommend waiting until bowel movements are more predictable. After colostomy irrigation is initiated, it may take 4 to 6 weeks before bowel emptying becomes regulated. Colostomy irrigation is most effective when performed 1 hour after a meal and at the same time each day.[1]

Colostomy irrigation is contraindicated in patients with bowel disease, irritable bowel syndrome, hernia, severe heart or kidney disease, an ascending or transverse colostomy, or an ileostomy.[1]

Equipment

Colostomy irrigation set (irrigation drain or sleeve, ostomy belt, water-soluble lubricant, drainage pouch clamp, irrigation bag with clamp with tubing and cone tip, clip) ▪ 1 L (1 qt) warm tap water ▪ IV pole or wall hook ▪ washcloth ▪ towel ▪ water ▪ gloves ▪ facility-approved ostomy skin assessment tool[2,3,4] ▪ Optional: fluid-impermeable pad, bedpan, chair, graduated measuring container, mild soap, stoma cap, ostomy appliance.

Preparation of equipment

Inspect all equipment and supplies. If a product is expired, is defective, or has compromised integrity, remove it from patient use, label it as expired or defective, and report the expiration or defect as directed by your facility.

Depending on the patient's condition, colostomy irrigation may be performed using a bedpan or in the bathroom using a chair and the toilet. Set up the irrigation bag, tubing, and cone tip. If irrigation will take place with the patient in bed, place the bedpan beside the bed and elevate the head of the bed between 45 and 90 degrees, if allowed. If irrigation will take place in the bathroom, have the patient sit on the toilet or on a chair facing the toilet, whichever the patient finds more comfortable.

Fill the irrigation bag with warm tap water. Hang the bag on the IV pole or wall hook. The bottom of the bag should be at the patient's shoulder level *to prevent the fluid from entering the bowel too quickly*. Most irrigation sets also have a clamp that regulates the flow rate. Prime the tubing with irrigant *to prevent air from entering the colon and possibly causing cramps and gas pains*.

Implementation

▪ Verify the practitioner's order, if required by your facility.
▪ Gather and prepare the necessary equipment and supplies.
▪ Perform hand hygiene.[5,6,7,8,9,10]
▪ Confirm the patient's identity using at least two patient identifiers.[11]
▪ Provide privacy.[12,13,14,15]
▪ Explain the procedure to the patient and family (if appropriate) according to their individual communication and learning needs *to increase their understanding, allay their fears, and enhance cooperation*.[16] Explain every step of the procedure to the patient, *because eventually the patient will be irrigating the colostomy independently*.
▪ If the patient is in bed, raise the bed to waist level before providing care *to prevent caregiver back strain*.[17]
▪ Perform hand hygiene.[5,6,7,8,19,10]
▪ Put on gloves *to comply with standard precautions*.[18,19]
▪ If the patient is in bed or in a chair, place a fluid-impermeable pad under the patient *to protect the sheets or chair surface from soiling*.
▪ Remove the ostomy appliance if the patient uses one.
▪ Place the irrigation sleeve over the stoma. If the sleeve doesn't have an adhesive backing, secure the sleeve with an ostomy belt. If the patient has a two-piece pouching system with flanges, snap off the pouch and save it. Snap on the irrigation sleeve.
▪ Place the open-ended bottom of the irrigation sleeve in the bedpan, toilet, or appropriate measuring container *to promote drainage by gravity*.
▪ Lubricate your gloved small finger with water-soluble lubricant and insert the finger into the stoma. If you're teaching the patient, have the patient do this step *to determine the bowel angle at which to insert the cone safely*. Expect the stoma to tighten when the finger enters the bowel and then to relax in a few seconds.
▪ Lubricate the cone with water-soluble lubricant *to prevent it from irritating the mucosa*.
▪ Insert the cone into the top opening of the irrigation sleeve and then into the stoma. Angle the cone to match the bowel angle. Insert it gently but snugly; never force it into place.
▪ Instruct the patient to take slow, deep breaths *to relax the abdominal muscles*.[20]
▪ Unclamp the irrigation tubing and allow the water to flow slowly. If you don't have a clamp to control the irrigant's flow rate, pinch the tubing *to control the flow*.[21] The water should enter the colon over 5 to 10 minutes.
▪ Explain that the patient may experience a sensation of fullness or bloating during the instillation.[20] If the patient reports cramping, slow or stop the flow, keep the cone in place, and have the patient take a few deep breaths until the cramping stops. *Cramping during irrigation may result from a bowel that's ready to empty, water that's too cold, a rapid flow rate, or air in the tubing.*
▪ When the irrigation bag is empty, close the clamp on the irrigation tubing and remove the irrigation bag, tubing, and cone and set them aside.[20]
▪ After 15 minutes, close the bottom of the irrigation sleeve with the clip provided in the irrigation kit. *The initial return of water and stool occurs within 15 minutes after irrigation*.[20] Have the patient remain stationary for 15 or 20 minutes *to allow the initial effluent to drain*.
▪ Encourage an ambulatory patient to perform activities of daily living during the next 30 to 45 minutes *to stimulate peristalsis and evacuation of*

stool.[1] Instruct a nonambulatory patient to massage the abdomen or lean forward *to stimulate peristalsis and evacuation of stool.*[1,20]

■ After 45 minutes, empty the contents of the irrigation sleeve into the bedpan, toilet, or appropriate measuring container.

■ Measure output, as ordered; subtract the amount of irrigant used from the total amount of effluent *to determine the actual output.*

■ Remove the irrigation sleeve.

■ Using a washcloth and water, gently clean the area around the stoma. Rinse it, and then dry the area thoroughly with a clean towel.

■ Inspect the peristomal skin and stoma. Use a facility-approved assessment tool if available *to objectively identify and track changes in peristomal skin.* Use the tool to assess for discoloration, erosion, and tissue overgrowth.[2,3,4] Observe for signs of mechanical, chemical, allergic, infectious, or disease-related complications (which may be linked to preexisting skin conditions, such as psoriasis, eczema, or seborrheic dermatitis). Notify the practitioner or a wound, ostomy, and continence nurse (WOCN) of changes, as needed.

■ Apply a clean ostomy appliance. (See the "Colostomy and ileostomy care" procedure.) The patient who has a regular bowel elimination pattern may prefer a small dressing, bandage, or commercial stoma cap.

■ Discard disposable equipment in an appropriate receptacle.[18,19] Rinse a reusable irrigation sleeve and irrigation bag, tubing, and cone tip with mild soap and water and hang them to dry.[20,22]

■ If the patient's bed was raised for patient care, return it to the lowest position *to prevent falls and maintain patient safety.*[23]

■ Remove and discard your gloves.[18,19]

■ Perform hand hygiene.[5,6,7,8,9,10]

■ Document the procedure.[24,25,26,27]

Special considerations

■ Irrigating a colostomy to establish a regular bowel elimination pattern doesn't work for all patients. If the bowel continues to move between irrigations, try decreasing the volume of irrigant. *Increasing the irrigant won't help because it serves only to stimulate peristalsis.* Keep a record of results. Also consider irrigating every other day.

■ Irrigation may help to regulate bowel function in patients with a descending or sigmoid colostomy, *because this is the bowel's stool storage area.* However, a patient with an ascending or transverse colostomy won't benefit from irrigation. Also, a patient with a descending or sigmoid colostomy who's missing part of the ascending or transverse colon may not be able to irrigate successfully *because the ostomy may function like an ascending or transverse colostomy.*

■ If diarrhea develops, discontinue irrigations until stools form again. Keep in mind that irrigation alone won't achieve regularity; the patient must also observe a complementary diet and exercise regimen.

■ If the patient has a strictured stoma that prohibits cone insertion, remove the cone from the irrigation tubing and replace it with a soft silicone catheter. Angle the catheter gently 2″ to 4″ (5 to 10 cm) into the bowel *to instill the irrigant.* Don't force the catheter into the stoma, and don't insert it further than the recommended length *because you may perforate the bowel.*

Patient teaching

After explaining the procedure to, and performing the procedure on, the patient, encourage the patient's increasing involvement in self-care. Discuss the patient's bathroom setup, how to hang the irrigation bag, and how to manage all of the equipment to avoid spills. Also discuss how to avoid excessive tiredness during the procedure. Teach the patient who will use reusable irrigation bags to discard the bags after 1 month (or sooner if an odor is detected). Teach the patient to monitor food intake *to determine whether certain foods are interfering with the irrigation outcomes.* Offer written instructions and information on obtaining replacement equipment.

Complications

Bowel perforation may result if a catheter is incorrectly inserted into the stoma. Fluid and electrolyte imbalances may result from using too much irrigant.

Documentation

Record the date and time of irrigation and the type and amount of irrigant. Note the stoma's color and the character of drainage, including the color, consistency, and amount. Record any patient teaching. Document teaching provided to the patient and family (if applicable), their understanding of that teaching, and any need for follow-up teaching.

REFERENCES

1 Wound, Ostomy, and Continence Nurses Society, Guideline Development Task Force. (2018). WOCN Society clinical guideline: Management of the adult patient with a fecal or urinary ostomy—An executive summary. *Journal of Wound, Ostomy, and Continence Nursing, 45,* 50–58. (Level VII)

2 Haugen, H., & Ratliff, C. R. (2013). Tools for assessing peristomal skin complications. *Journal of Wound, Ostomy, and Continence Nursing, 40*(2), 131–134. (Level VII)

3 Jordan, R., & Christian, M. (2013). Understanding peristomal skin complications. *Wound Care Advisor, 2*(3), 36–41. http://woundcareadvisor.com/wp-content/uploads/2013/05/Understanding_M-J13.pdf

4 Australian Association of Stomal Therapy Nurses, Inc. (2013). Clinical guidelines for stomal therapy nursing practice. http://www.stomaltherapy.com/documents/AASTN_Guidelines_book_2013.pdf (Level VII)

5 The Joint Commission. (2021). Standard NPSG.07.01.01. *Comprehensive accreditation manual for hospitals.* Oakbrook Terrace, IL: The Joint Commission. (Level VII)

6 Centers for Disease Control and Prevention. (2002). Guideline for hand hygiene in health-care settings: Recommendations of the Healthcare Infection Control Practices Advisory Committee and the HICPAC/SHEA/APIC/IDSA Hand Hygiene Task Force. *MMWR Recommendations and Reports, 51*(RR-16), 1–45. https://www.cdc.gov/mmwr/pdf/rr/rr5116.pdf (Level II)

7 World Health Organization. (2009). WHO guidelines on hand hygiene in health care: First global patient safety challenge, clean care is safer care. https://apps.who.int/iris/bitstream/handle/10665/44102/9789241597906_eng.pdf?sequence=1 (Level IV)

8 Accreditation Association for Hospitals and Health Systems. (2020). Standard 07.01.21. *Healthcare Facilities Accreditation Program: Accreditation requirements for acute care hospitals.* Chicago, IL: Accreditation Association for Hospitals and Health Systems. (Level VII)

9 Centers for Medicare and Medicaid Services, Department of Health and Human Services. (2020). Condition of participation: Infection control. 42 C.F.R. § 482.42.

10 DNV GL-Healthcare USA, Inc. (2020). IC.1.SR.1. *NIAHO® accreditation requirements, interpretive guidelines and surveyor guidance—revision 20.0.* Milford, OH: DNV GL-Healthcare USA, Inc. (Level VII)

11 The Joint Commission. (2021). Standard NPSG.01.01.01. *Comprehensive accreditation manual for hospitals.* Oakbrook Terrace, IL: The Joint Commission. (Level VII)

12 Accreditation Association for Hospitals and Health Systems. (2020). Standard 15.01.16. *Healthcare Facilities Accreditation Program: Accreditation requirements for acute care hospitals.* Chicago, IL: Accreditation Association for Hospitals and Health Systems. (Level VII)

13 The Joint Commission. (2021). Standard RI.01.01.01. *Comprehensive accreditation manual for hospitals.* Oakbrook Terrace, IL: The Joint Commission. (Level VII)

14 Centers for Medicare and Medicaid Services, Department of Health and Human Services. (2020). Condition of participation: Patient's rights. 42 C.F.R. § 482.13(c)(1).

15 DNV GL-Healthcare USA, Inc. (2020). PR.2.SR.5. *NIAHO® accreditation requirements, interpretive guidelines and surveyor guidance—revision 20.0.* Milford, OH: DNV GL-Healthcare USA, Inc. (Level VII)

16 The Joint Commission. (2021). Standard PC.02.01.21. *Comprehensive accreditation manual for hospitals.* Oakbrook Terrace, IL: The Joint Commission. (Level VII)

17 Waters, T. R., et al. (2009). Safe patient handling training for schools of nursing. https://www.cdc.gov/niosh/docs/2009-127/pdfs/2009-127.pdf (Level VII)

18 Siegel, J. D., et al. (2007, revised 2019). 2007 guideline for isolation precautions: Preventing transmission of infectious agents in healthcare settings. https://www.cdc.gov/infectioncontrol/pdf/guidelines/isolation-guidelines-H.pdf (Level II)

19 Accreditation Association for Hospitals and Health Systems. (2020). Standard 07.01.10. *Healthcare Facilities Accreditation Program: Accreditation requirements for acute care hospitals.* Chicago, IL: Accreditation Association for Hospitals and Health Systems. (Level VII)

20 Memorial Sloan Kettering Cancer Center. (2021). Patient and caregiver education: Irrigating your sigmoid or descending colostomy. https://www.mskcc.org/cancer-care/patient-education/colostomy-irrigation-instructions-sigmoid-descending-colostomy

21 United Ostomy Associations of America, Inc. (2017). Colostomy guide. https://www.ostomy.org/wp-content/uploads/2018/03/ColostomyGuide.pdf

22 Accreditation Association for Hospitals and Health Systems. (2020). Standard 07.02.03. *Healthcare Facilities Accreditation Program: Accreditation requirements for acute care hospitals.* Chicago, IL: Accreditation Association for Hospitals and Health Systems. (Level VII)

23 Ganz, D. A., et al. (2013, reviewed 2021). *Preventing falls in hospitals: A toolkit for improving quality of care* (AHRQ Publication No. 13-0015-EF). Rockville, MD: Agency for Healthcare Research and Quality. https://www.ahrq.gov/professionals/systems/hospital/fallpxtoolkit/index.html (Level VII)

24 The Joint Commission. (2021). Standard RC.01.03.01. *Comprehensive accreditation manual for hospitals.* Oakbrook Terrace, IL: The Joint Commission. (Level VII)

25 Accreditation Association for Hospitals and Health Systems. (2020). Standard 10.00.03. *Healthcare Facilities Accreditation Program: Accreditation requirements for acute care hospitals.* Chicago, IL: Accreditation Association for Hospitals and Health Systems. (Level VII)

26 Centers for Medicare and Medicaid Services, Department of Health and Human Services. (2020). Condition of participation: Medical record services. 42 C.F.R. § 482.24(b).

27 DNV GL-Healthcare USA, Inc. (2020). MR.2.SR.1. *NIAHO® accreditation requirements, interpretive guidelines and surveyor guidance—revision 20.0.* Milford, OH: DNV GL-Healthcare USA, Inc. (Level VII)

Contact lens care

Although most patients can remove their own contact lenses, you should be able to remove the lenses if the patient can't. Patients may present to the emergency department because of difficulty removing their own lenses or with acute ophthalmologic complications associated with contact lens use. In addition, illness or emergency treatment may require that you insert or remove and store a patient's contact lenses.[1] When a patient with an altered mental status arrives in an emergency department, a nurse must determine whether the patient wears contact lenses and remove them if they're present.

Proper handling and lens care techniques help prevent eye injury and infection as well as lens loss or damage. Appropriate lens-handling techniques depend in large part on what type of lenses the patient wears. All contact lenses float on the corneal tear layer. Soft lenses typically have diameters larger than the cornea; rigid (hard) lenses typically have diameters smaller than the cornea.[2] Because they're larger and more pliable, soft lenses tend to mold themselves more closely to the eye for a more stable fit.

Modes of lens wear vary widely. Although most patients remove and clean their lenses daily, some wear lenses overnight or for several days (sometimes up to a month) without removing them for cleaning. However, the risk of infection increases when contact lenses are worn during sleep.[3] Other patients wear disposable lenses, which means that they replace old lenses with new ones at regular intervals (a few days to a few months), possibly without removing them for cleaning between replacements.

Certain procedures are necessary when handling contact lenses, *because improper handling can lead to contamination of the eye.*

Equipment

Powder-free gloves ▪ towel ▪ lens storage case or two small specimen containers with lids (labeled LEFT and RIGHT) ▪ patient identification labels ▪ towel ▪ patient's equipment for contact lens care (a multipurpose solution or separate solutions for cleaning and disinfecting and storage)[4] ▪ Optional: flashlight, rigid contact lens remover, marker, sterile normal saline solution, hydrogen peroxide lens storage basket and case.

Preparation of equipment

Inspect all equipment and supplies. If a product is expired, is defective, or has compromised integrity, remove it from patient use, label it as expired or defective, and report the expiration or defect as directed by your facility. Inspect the patient's contact lens care equipment, and identify the

type of solution the patient uses for contact lens care. A multipurpose solution may be used for cleaning and disinfecting as well as storing lenses, or the patient may use a separate solution for each step.[4] Obtain a bottle of sterile normal saline solution if the patient doesn't have contact lens solution.[2] If a commercial lens storage case isn't available, place enough sterile normal saline solution into two small specimen containers with lids to submerge a lens in each one. To avoid confusing the left and right lenses, which may have different prescriptions, mark one cup "L" and the other cup "R." Label the patient's contact lens case or the specimen containers with a patient identification label.

Implementation

▪ Gather and prepare the necessary equipment and supplies.
▪ Perform hand hygiene.[5,6,7,8,9,10]
▪ Confirm the patient's identity using at least two patient identifiers.[11]
▪ Provide privacy.[12,13,14,15]
▪ Determine whether the patient wears soft or rigid contact lenses. *Rigid lenses are smaller in diameter than the cornea, and smaller than soft contact lenses.*[2]
▪ Explain the procedure to the patient and family (if appropriate) according to their communication and learning needs *to increase their understanding, allay their fears, and enhance cooperation.*[16]
▪ Raise the patient's bed to waist level before providing care *to prevent caregiver back strain.*[17]
▪ Put on gloves *to comply with standard precautions and help prevent ocular infection.*[18,19,20]

Inserting soft lenses
▪ Remove one of the lenses from the storage case, noting whether the lens is for the right eye or the left eye.
▪ Rinse the lens with multipurpose solution or sterile normal saline solution, as needed.
▪ Inspect the lens by placing it on the tip of your finger. Check for torn edges and damage, and make sure that the lens is right-side out by confirming that the lens forms a bowl with the edges turned up. If the lens edge points slightly inward, it's oriented correctly. If the edge points outward or the lens tends to collapse over your fingertip, it's inside out and you should reverse it.
▪ Place the lens convex side down on the tip of the index finger of your dominant hand.
▪ Instruct the patient to gaze upward slightly.
▪ Confirm that you're placing the correct lens in the correct eye.
▪ Separate the eyelids with your other thumb and index finger, and gently place the lens on the sclera just below the cornea; then gently slide the lens upward with your finger until it centers on the cornea.
▪ Using the same procedure, insert the opposite lens.

Inserting rigid lenses
▪ Remove one of the lenses from the case, noting whether the lens is for the right eye or the left eye.
▪ Wet the lens with sterile normal saline or soaking solution and then gently rub it between your thumb and index finger, or place it on your palm and rub it with your opposite index finger.[21]
▪ Rinse the lens well with the multipurpose solution, disinfecting and storage solution, or sterile normal saline solution, leaving a small amount in the lens.[21]
▪ Place the lens convex side down on the tip of the index finger of your dominant hand.
▪ Instruct the patient to gaze upward slightly.
▪ Confirm that you're placing the correct lens in the correct eye.
▪ Separate the eyelids with your other thumb and index finger, and gently place the lens directly and gently on the cornea. Don't press it to the eye; *the tear film will attract it naturally at the first touch.*
▪ Using the same procedure, insert the opposite lens.

Removing, cleaning, and disinfecting soft lenses
▪ Place the patient in a seated or supine position and place a towel under the eye *to catch the lens if it drops.*[2]
▪ Examine the eye and cornea with a flashlight, if needed, and ensure that the contact lens is present and centered on the cornea before attempting

to remove it. *Attempting to remove a contact lens that isn't there may result in a corneal abrasion.*[2]
- If the eyes appear dry, instill a few drops of sterile normal saline solution to each eye 5 to 10 minutes before removal, as needed, *to hydrate the soft lenses, making removal easier.*[2]
- Using your nondominant hand, raise the patient's upper eyelid and hold it against the orbital rim.
- Lightly place the forefinger of your other hand on the lens and move it down onto the sclera, below the cornea.
- Pinch the lens between your forefinger and thumb; the lens should pop off.
- After removal, examine the lens for tears and scratches.
- If the patient is using a multipurpose solution, clean the lens by rubbing it with the multipurpose solution and then place the lens in the proper well of the storage case (marked "L" or "R") with enough of the multipurpose solution to cover it, *to store and disinfect the lenses.* Alternatively, place the lens in a labeled specimen container with sterile normal saline solution and then secure the lid *to prevent loss of the lens.*
- If the patient is using a hydrogen peroxide solution, clean and disinfect the lens by placing it in the hydrogen peroxide storage basket, filling the case with hydrogen peroxide solution, and putting the basket in the case. Follow the manufacturer's instructions for storing the lens. Note that hydrogen peroxide solutions need a neutralizer to change the hydrogen peroxide to plain saline solution. Some cases have a built-in neutralizer, whereas others require the addition of a neutralizing tablet to the solution. Store the lens in the solution for 6 to 8 hours according to the manufacturer's instructions.
- If you don't have access to the patient's contact lens solutions, store the lens in sterile normal saline solution.[7] Note, however, that sterile saline solution will not disinfect the lens; the patient should not reuse the lens until the lens undergoes proper cleaning and disinfection.
NURSING ALERT Never store or rinse contact lenses in any type of water, including tap, bottled, distilled, or fresh water, *to reduce the risk of eye infection.*[20,21]
- Remove and care for the other lens using the same technique.

Removing, cleaning, and disinfecting rigid lenses
- Place the patient in a seated or supine position and place a towel under the eye *to catch the lens.*[2]
- Examine the patient's eye and cornea with a flashlight, if needed, and ensure that the contact lens is present and centered on the cornea before attempting to remove it. *Attempting to remove a contact lens that isn't there may result in a corneal abrasion.*[2]
- If the patient can follow directions, stretch the corner of the eyelids toward the temporal bone, *which tightens the lid edges against the glove of the eye,* and ask the patient to blink while you catch the lens in the towel.[2]
- If the patient is unable to follow directions, place one thumb against the patient's upper eyelid and the other thumb against the lower eyelid. Move the eyelids toward each other while gently pressing inward against the eye *to trap the lens edge and break the suction.* Extract the lens from the patient's eyelashes.[2]
- Alternatively, use a rigid contact lens remover *to carefully remove the lens.* Moisten the remover's suction cup with sterile normal saline solution and then gently touch it square to the center of the contact lens. Make sure to apply it directly to the lens, not the eye. After the suction cup attaches to the lens, gently twist the lens off the eye. Then carefully slide the lens off of the suction cup, *because pulling the lens directly off of the suction cup may cause the lens to warp.*[2]
- After removal, examine the lens for scratches, chips, and tears.
- Clean the lens by rubbing it with a multipurpose solution or cleaning solution designed to remove most surface deposits.[21]
- Store and disinfect the lens by placing it in the proper well of the storage case (marked "L" or "R") with enough of the multipurpose solution or disinfecting and storage solution to cover it.[21] *This step rids the lens of infectious organisms.*[22] Alternatively, place the lens in a labeled specimen container with multipurpose solution or disinfecting and storage solution and then secure the lid *to prevent loss of the lens.* Store the lens in sterile

normal saline solution if you don't have access to the patient's contact lens solutions.[2] Note, however, that sterile saline solution will not disinfect the lens; the patient should not reuse the lens until the lens undergoes proper cleaning and disinfection.[23]
- Remove and care for the opposite lens using the same technique.

Completing the procedure
- Return the bed to the lowest position *to prevent falls and maintain patient safety.*[24]
- Remove and discard your gloves.[19]
- Perform hand hygiene.[5,6,7,8,9,10]
- Document the procedure.[25,26,27,28]

Special considerations
- If you must clean a patient's lenses, use only the patient's own brand of solutions *to minimize the risk of allergic reactions to substances included in other solution brands.* Never touch the nozzle of a solution bottle to the eye lens, your fingers, or anything else *to avoid contaminating the solution in the bottle.*[21]
- If the patient's eyes appear dry or you have trouble moving the lens on the eye, instill several drops of sterile normal saline solution and wait a few minutes before trying again to remove the lens *to prevent corneal damage.* If you still can't remove the lens easily, notify the practitioner.
- Don't instill eye medication while the patient is wearing lenses, *because the lenses could trap the medication, possibly causing eye irritation or lens damage.*
- If an unconscious patient is admitted to the emergency department, check for contact lenses by opening each eyelid and searching with a small flashlight. If you detect lenses, remove them immediately, *because the patient's tears can't circulate freely beneath the lenses when the eyelids are closed, increasing the risk of corneal oxygen depletion and infection.*[1]
- If the patient has had a serious eye injury while wearing a contact lens and globe perforation is suspected, don't attempt to remove the lens; instead, the practitioner should refer the patient to an ophthalmologist. Place an eye shield (not a pad) over the eye *to minimize or prevent pressure on the globe.*[2]
- If the patient can't provide adequate care for the lenses during hospitalization, encourage the patient to send them home with a family member. If you aren't sure how to care for the lenses in the interim, store them in sterile normal saline solution until a family member can take them home.

Patient teaching
Advise contact lens wearers to carry appropriate identification *to speed lens removal and ensure proper care in an emergency.*

Complications
The main risk of contact lens removal is corneal abrasion. More significant complications are likely to result from contact lenses left in the eyes for prolonged periods and can be especially serious in patients with a reduced level of consciousness. Complications of contact lens wear include lens deposits, allergic conjunctivitis, giant papillary conjunctivitis, peripheral corneal infiltrates, microbial keratitis, and corneal neovascularization. All types of contact lenses reduce the amount of oxygen that reaches the cornea. Oxygenation is reduced further if the patient wears contact lenses when the eyes are closed.[2]

Documentation
Document the date and time of the procedure. Record the condition of the eyes before and after removal of the lenses; the time of lens insertion, removal, and cleaning; the location of stored lenses; the condition of the lenses; and, if applicable, the removal of lenses from the facility by a family member. Note the patient's tolerance of the procedure. Document teaching provided to the patient and family (if applicable), their understanding of that teaching, and any need for follow-up teaching.

REFERENCES

1 Craven, R. F., et al. (2021). *Fundamentals of nursing: Concepts and competencies for practice* (9th ed.). Philadelphia, PA: Wolters Kluwer.

2 Tatham, A. J., & Redmill, B. (2016). Contact lens removal. https://emedicine.medscape.com/article/1413506-overview

3 Cope, J. R., et al. (2017). Risk behaviors for contact lens-related eye infections among adults and adolescents—United States, 2016. *Morbidity and Mortality Weekly Report, 66*(32), 841–845. https://www.cdc.gov/mmwr/volumes/66/wr/mm6632a2.htm

4 The Joint Commission. (2021). Standard NPSG.07.01.01. *Comprehensive accreditation manual for hospitals.* Oakbrook Terrace, IL: The Joint Commission. (Level VII)

5 Centers for Disease Control and Prevention. (2002). Guideline for hand hygiene in health-care settings: Recommendations of the Healthcare Infection Control Practices Advisory Committee and the HICPAC/SHEA/APIC/IDSA Hand Hygiene Task Force. *MMWR Recommendations and Reports, 51*(RR-16), 1–45. https://www.cdc.gov/mmwr/pdf/rr/rr5116.pdf (Level II)

6 World Health Organization. (2009). WHO guidelines on hand hygiene in health care: First global patient safety challenge, clean care is safer care. http://apps.who.int/iris/bitstream/10665/44102/1/9789241597906_eng.pdf (Level IV)

7 Centers for Medicare and Medicaid Services, Department of Health and Human Services. (2020). Condition of participation: Infection control. 42 C.F.R. § 482.42.

8 Accreditation Association for Hospitals and Health Systems. (2020). Standard 07.01.21. *Healthcare Facilities Accreditation Program: Accreditation requirements for acute care hospitals.* Chicago, IL: Accreditation Association for Hospitals and Health Systems. (Level VII)

9 DNV GL-Healthcare USA, Inc. (2020). IC.1.SR.1. *NIAHO® accreditation requirements, interpretive guidelines and surveyor guidance—revision 20.0.* Milford, OH: DNV GL-Healthcare USA, Inc. (Level VII)

10 The Joint Commission. (2021). Standard NPSG.01.01.01. *Comprehensive accreditation manual for hospitals.* Oakbrook Terrace, IL: The Joint Commission. (Level VII)

11 The Joint Commission. (2021). Standard RI.01.01.01. *Comprehensive accreditation manual for hospitals.* Oakbrook Terrace, IL: The Joint Commission. (Level VII)

12 Centers for Medicare and Medicaid Services, Department of Health and Human Services. (2020). Condition of participation: Patient's rights. 42 C.F.R. § 482.13(c)(1).

13 Accreditation Association for Hospitals and Health Systems. (2020). Standard 15.01.16. *Healthcare Facilities Accreditation Program: Accreditation requirements for acute care hospitals.* Chicago, IL: Accreditation Association for Hospitals and Health Systems. (Level VII)

14 DNV GL-Healthcare USA, Inc. (2020). PR.2.SR.5. *NIAHO® accreditation requirements, interpretive guidelines and surveyor guidance—revision 20.0.* Milford, OH: DNV GL-Healthcare USA, Inc. (Level VII)

15 The Joint Commission. (2021). Standard PC.02.01.21. *Comprehensive accreditation manual for hospitals.* Oakbrook Terrace, IL: The Joint Commission. (Level VII)

16 Waters, T. R., et al. (2009). Safe patient handling training for schools of nursing. https://www.cdc.gov/niosh/docs/2009-127/pdfs/2009-127.pdf (Level VII)

17 Siegel, J. D., et al. (2007, revised 2019). 2007 guideline for isolation precautions: Preventing transmission of infectious agents in healthcare settings. https://www.cdc.gov/infectioncontrol/pdf/guidelines/isolation-guidelines-H.pdf (Level II)

18 Accreditation Association for Hospitals and Health Systems. (2020). Standard 07.01.10. *Healthcare Facilities Accreditation Program: Accreditation requirements for acute care hospitals.* Chicago, IL: Accreditation Association for Hospitals and Health Systems. (Level VII)

19 Occupational Safety and Health Administration. (2012). Bloodborne pathogens, standard number1910.1030. https://www.osha.gov/pls/oshaweb/owadisp.show_document?p_id=10051&p_table=STANDARDS (Level VII)

20 U.S. Food and Drug Administration. (2019). Contact lenses. https://www.fda.gov/medical-devices/consumer-products/contact-lenses

21 Boyd, K. (2021). How to take care of contact lenses. https://www.aao.org/eye-health/glasses-contacts/contact-lens-care

22 National Keratoconus Foundation. (n.d.). Contact lens care. https://www.nkcf.org/keratoconus-contact-lenses/contact-lens-care/

23 Centers for Disease Control and Prevention. (2020). Healthy contact lens wear and care: Contact lens care systems & solutions. https://www.cdc.gov/contactlenses/care-systems.html

24 Ganz, D. A., et al. (2013, reviewed 2021). *Preventing falls in hospitals: A toolkit for improving quality of care* (AHRQ Publication No. 13-0015-EF). Rockville, MD: Agency for Healthcare Research and Quality. https://www.ahrq.gov/professionals/systems/hospital/fallpxtoolkit/index.html (Level VII)

25 The Joint Commission. (2021). Standard RC.01.03.01. *Comprehensive accreditation manual for hospitals.* Oakbrook Terrace, IL: The Joint Commission. (Level VII)

26 Centers for Medicare and Medicaid Services, Department of Health and Human Services. (2020). Condition of participation: Medical record services. 42 C.F.R. § 482.24(b).

27 Accreditation Association for Hospitals and Health Systems. (2020). Standard 10.00.03. *Healthcare Facilities Accreditation Program: Accreditation requirements for acute care hospitals.* Chicago, IL: Accreditation Association for Hospitals and Health Systems. (Level VII)

28 DNV GL-Healthcare USA, Inc. (2020). MR.2.SR.1. *NIAHO® accreditation requirements, interpretive guidelines and surveyor guidance—revision 20.0.* Milford, OH: DNV GL-Healthcare USA, Inc. (Level VII)

CONTACT PRECAUTIONS

Contact precautions help prevent the spread of microorganisms that spread through direct or indirect contact with the patient or the patient's environment. (See *Conditions requiring contact precautions.*) Effective contact precautions require a single room, if possible, and the use of gloves and gowns by anyone having contact with the patient, the patient's support equipment, or items that have come in contact with the patient or the patient's environment. Proper hand hygiene and handling and disposal of articles that have come in contact with the patient and the patient's environment are essential.[1]

NURSING ALERT When caring for a patient with known or suspected coronavirus disease (COVID-19), please refer to the latest recommendations from the Centers for Disease Control and Prevention (CDC), located at https://www.cdc.gov/coronavirus/2019-ncov/hcp/infection-control-recommendations.html

NURSING ALERT Please refer to the latest recommendations from the Centers for Disease Control and Prevention (CDC), located at https://www.cdc.gov/vhf/ebola/healthcare-us/index.html, when caring for a patient with known or suspected Ebola virus infection.

Equipment

Gowns ▪ gloves ▪ plastic bags ▪ contact precautions sign ▪ Optional: clean dressings.

Preparation of equipment

Keep all contact precaution supplies outside the patient's room in a wall- or door-mounted cabinet, a cart, or an anteroom.

Implementation

▪ Gather and prepare the necessary equipment and supplies.

▪ Place a CONTACT PRECAUTIONS sign outside the patient's door *to notify anyone entering the room of the situation.*[1,13,14,15,16]

▪ Perform hand hygiene.[14,16,17,18,19,20]

▪ Put on a gown and gloves before entering the patient's room *to comply with contact precautions.* Instruct any visitors to do the same, as required by your facility. (See the "Personal protective equipment use" procedure.)[1,15,21]

▪ Confirm the patient's identity using at least two patient identifiers.[22]

▪ Situate the patient in a single room with private toilet facilities and an anteroom, if possible. If necessary, two patients with the same infection may share a room; however, consult with your facility's infection preventionist before placing two patients together.[1]

▪ Explain contact precautions to the patient and family (if appropriate) according to their communication and learning needs *to increase their understanding, allay their fears, and enhance cooperation.*[23]

▪ Always change gloves after contact with a contaminated body site or contact with body fluids, excretions, mucous membranes, nonintact skin, and wound dressings.[1] Perform hand hygiene after removing used gloves and before putting on new gloves.[14,15,16,17,18,20]

Conditions requiring contact precautions

The CDC recommends contact precautions for patients who are infected or colonized (positive for the microorganism without clinical signs or symptoms of infection) with epidemiologically important organisms that can be transmitted by direct or indirect contact. The table below lists common conditions that require contact precautions, along with details regarding the precautionary period and applicable special considerations.[1]

CONDITION	PRECAUTIONARY PERIOD	SPECIAL CONSIDERATIONS (IF APPLICABLE)
Abscess, major draining	■ Duration of illness, or until drainage stops or can be contained by a dressing	■ Droplet precautions should be added for the first 24 hr of appropriate antibiotic therapy if invasive group A streptococcal disease is suspected.
Acute viral (acute hemorrhagic) conjunctivitis	■ Duration of illness	■ Note that this condition is highly contagious; outbreaks can occur in pediatric and neonatal settings.
Adenovirus gastroenteritis, diapered or incontinent patient	■ Duration of illness, or a duration that's appropriate to control a facility outbreak	
Adenovirus pneumonia	■ Duration of illness	■ Droplet precautions should also be instituted. ■ Precautions should be extended in immunocompromised patients, *because viral shedding is prolonged.*
Avian influenza	■ For 14 days after onset of signs and symptoms, or until an alternate diagnosis is confirmed	■ Airborne precautions should also be implemented; use a respirator for all patient care activities.[2] ■ Eye protection should be worn.[2]
Bronchiolitis	■ Duration of illness	■ Wear a mask according to standard precautions.
Burkholderia cepacia pneumonia in a patient with cystic fibrosis	■ Unknown	■ Contact precautions should also be instituted for patients with cystic fibrosis whose respiratory tracts are colonized with bacteria. ■ Exposure to other patients with cystic fibrosis should be avoided.
Campylobacter species gastroenteritis, diapered or incontinent patient	■ Duration of illness, or a duration that's appropriate to control a facility outbreak	
Cholera gastroenteritis, diapered or incontinent patient	■ Duration of illness, or a duration that's appropriate to control a facility outbreak	
Clostridioides difficile gastroenteritis[3]	■ 48 hours after symptoms resolve, or longer; some facilities continue isolation until discharge, *because* C. difficile-*infected patients continue to shed the organism for a number of days after diarrhea ceases.*[3,4,5]	■ Avoid administering an antibiotic that was previously prescribed for the patient.[4,5] ■ Environmental cleaning and disinfection should be done consistently; consider using an Environmental Protection Agency (EPA)–registered disinfectant that has a sporicidal claim or a sodium hypochlorite solution.[4,5] ■ Note that glove use is important for preventing the spread of C. *difficile* spores via the hands of health care workers. Perform hand hygiene after removing gloves. *Alcohol doesn't kill* C. difficile *spores;* the use of soap and water or antimicrobial soap and water for hand hygiene is more effective at removing spores than the use of alcohol-based hand rubs. However, *to ensure compliance with hand hygiene,* you can use alcohol-based hand rubs instead. Consider using only soap and water in the event of an outbreak.[4,5,6,7]
Cryptosporidium species gastroenteritis, diapered or incontinent patient	■ Duration of illness, or a duration that's appropriate to control a facility outbreak	
Diphtheria, cutaneous	■ Until two cultures (obtained 24 hours apart) are negative and the patient is off antibiotics	
Escherichia coli gastroenteritis (0157:H7 and other shiga toxin–producing strains, other species), diapered or incontinent patient	■ Duration of illness, or a duration that's appropriate to control a facility outbreak	
Enteroviral infection, diapered or incontinent patient	■ Duration of illness, or a duration that's appropriate to control a facility outbreak.	
Furunculosis, staphylococcal (infants and young children)	■ Duration of illness, or when wound lesions stop draining	
Giardia lamblia gastroenteritis, diapered or incontinent patient	■ Duration of illness, or a duration that's appropriate to control a facility outbreak	

(Continued)

Conditions requiring contact precautions *(continued)*

CONDITION	PRECAUTIONARY PERIOD	SPECIAL CONSIDERATIONS (IF APPLICABLE)
Hepatitis type A	■ Duration of hospitalization in infants and children younger than age 3 years ■ For 2 weeks after the onset of signs and symptoms in children ages 3 to 14 years ■ For 1 week after the onset of signs and symptoms in children older than age 14 years	
Hepatitis type E, diapered or incontinent patient	■ Duration of illness	
Herpes simplex, mucocutaneous, disseminated or primary, severe; neonatal	■ Until lesions are dry and crusted ■ For asymptomatic, exposed neonates, until cultures obtained at 24 and 36 hours of age are negative; incubation required for 48 hours	
Herpes zoster (shingles), disseminated disease (rash affects three or more dermatomes) or localized disease in an immunocompetent or immunocompromised patient[8,9]	■ Duration of illness, or until disseminated disease is ruled out in an immunocompromised patient	■ For an immunocompetent patient with localized disease, follow standard precautions and completely cover lesions until they are dry and crusted.[9] ■ For an immunocompetent patient with disseminated disease, follow standard precautions; also implement contact and airborne precautions until lesions are dry and crusted.[9] ■ For an immunocompromised patient with localized disease, follow standard precautions; also implement contact and airborne precautions until disseminated infection is ruled out, and then follow standard precautions. Completely cover lesions until they are dry and crusted.[9] ■ For an immunocompromised patient with disseminated disease, follow standard precautions; also implement contact and airborne precautions until lesions are dry and crusted.[9] ■ Susceptible health care workers shouldn't enter the room if immune staff members are available.
Human metapneumovirus	■ Duration of illness or when wound lesions stop draining	■ Wear masks according to standard precautions.
Impetigo	■ For 24 hours after initiation of effective therapy	
Monkeypox	■ Until lesions are crusted	■ Airborne precautions should also be implemented until monkeypox is confirmed and smallpox is ruled out.
Multidrug-resistant organism (MDRO) infection or colonization (such as with methicillin-resistant *Staphylococcus aureus*, vancomycin-resistant enterococcus, vancomycin intermediate-resistant *S. aureus*, vancomycin-resistant *S. aureus*, extended beta-lactamase producers, resistant *Streptococcus pneumonia*, and carbapenem-resistant *Enterobacteriaceae*)[10]	■ Duration specified by your facility's infection control program, which is based on local, state, regional, and national recommendations	■ Note that adherence to standard precautions only may be permitted in some areas.[6] ■ For guidance concerning new or emerging MDROs, consult your state or local health department.
Mycobacterium tuberculosis, draining extrapulmonary lesion	■ Until patient improves clinically and drainage has stopped, or until three consecutive drainage cultures test negative	■ Airborne precautions should also be implemented.[11] ■ Active pulmonary tuberculosis should be ruled out.
Norovirus gastroenteritis, diapered or incontinent patient	■ Duration of illness, or a period following recovery while patient is still shedding the virus at high levels (usually 24 to 72 hours)[12]	■ Those who clean areas that are heavily contaminated with feces or vomitus should wear a mask.[12] ■ In some situations in health care facilities, isolation of exposed and potentially incubating patients may also be necessary.[12] ■ Conduct environmental cleaning and disinfecting consistently; consider using an EPA-registered disinfectant that has a sporicidal claim or sodium hypochlorite solution.
Parainfluenza virus infection, infant or young child	■ Duration of illness	■ Note that viral shedding may be prolonged in immunocompromised patients. ■ Antigen testing to determine when contact precautions can be discontinued may be unreliable.

Conditions requiring contact precautions *(continued)*

CONDITION	PRECAUTIONARY PERIOD	SPECIAL CONSIDERATIONS (IF APPLICABLE)
Pediculosis (head lice infestation)	■ For 24 hours after the initiation of effective therapy	
Poliomyelitis	■ Duration of illness or when wound lesions stop draining	
Pressure injury, infected major, draining	■ Duration of illness ■ Until wound drainage stops or can be contained	
Respiratory syncytial virus infection: infant, young child, or immunocompromised adult	■ Duration of illness, or when wound lesions stop draining	■ Note that viral shedding may be prolonged in immunocompromised patients. ■ Antigen testing to determine when contact precautions can be discontinued may be unreliable. ■ Wear a mask according to standard precautions.
Ritter disease (staphylococcal scaled skin syndrome)	■ Duration of illness, or when wound lesions stop draining	■ Note that health care workers may be a source of nursery or neonatal intensive care unit outbreaks.
Rotavirus gastroenteritis	■ Duration of illness	■ Environmental cleaning and disinfection should be done consistently. ■ Soiled diapers should be changed and disposed of frequently. ■ Note that viral shedding may be prolonged in immunocompromised pediatric and older adult patient.
Rubella, congenital syndrome	■ Until the child is 1 year old, or until nasopharyngeal and urine cultures are repeatedly negative after age 3 months	
Salmonella species gastroenteritis, diapered or incontinent patient	■ Duration of illness, or a duration that's appropriate to control a facility outbreak	
Scabies	■ For 24 hours following initiation of effective therapy	
Severe acute respiratory syndrome	■ Duration of illness plus 10 days after fever resolves (provided respiratory signs and symptoms have improved or resolved) ■ Until wound drainage stops	■ Airborne precautions should also be implemented. ■ Add droplet precautions if an airborne isolation infection room is unavailable.
Shigella species gastroenteritis, diapered or incontinent patient	■ Duration of illness, or a duration that's appropriate to control a facility outbreak	
Staphylococcus aureus enterocolitis, diapered or incontinent children	■ Duration of illness	
Staphylococcus aureus–infected draining major skin wound or burn	■ Duration of illness ■ Until wound drainage stops	
Streptococcus group A–infected draining major skin wound or burn	■ For 24 hours following initiation of effective therapy	■ Droplet precautions should also be initiated.
Vaccinia, eczema: fetal, generalized, or progressive	■ Until lesions are dry and crusted and scabs are separated	
Vaccinia blepharitis or conjunctivitis with copious drainage	■ Until drainage ceases	
Vibrio parahaemolyticus gastroenteritis, diapered or incontinent patient	■ Duration of illness, or a duration that's appropriate to control a facility outbreak	
Viral hemorrhagic fevers (Ebola, Lassa, Marburg, Crimean-Congo fever viruses)	■ Duration of illness ■ Until wound drainage stops	■ Droplet precautions should also be initiated. ■ Handle waste appropriately.
Yersinia enterocolitica gastroenteritis, diapered or incontinent patient	■ Duration of illness, or a duration that's appropriate to control a facility outbreak	

- Handle all items that have come in contact with the patient as you would for a patient on standard precautions.[1]
- Limit the patient's movement from the room. If the patient must be moved, cover any infected areas with clean dressings.[1] Notify the receiving department or area of the patient's contact precautions (and any other transmission-based precautions, if applicable) *so that the precautions will be maintained by the staff and the patient can be returned to the room promptly.*
- Teach the patient and family about the importance of hand hygiene in preventing the spread of infection, and about other measures to prevent the spread of multidrug-resistant organisms.[6,24]
- Remove and discard your gown and gloves before leaving the room.[1]
- Perform hand hygiene before leaving the patient's room.[14,15,16,17,18,20]
- Document the procedure.[25,26,27,28]

Special considerations

- Clean and disinfect equipment that must be used for different patients in between each patient use according to the manufacturer's instructions, as required by your facility, *to prevent cross-contamination.*[29,30] If *Clostridioides difficile* is confirmed or suspected, after cleaning, consider using an EPA–registered disinfectant that has a sporicidal claim or a sodium hypochlorite solution for disinfection. Notify environmental services after the patient is discharged and have them clean and disinfect the room.[1,3,4,14,29,30,31]
- Try to dedicate certain reusable equipment (thermometer, stethoscope, and blood pressure cuff) for use only with the patient on contact precautions *to reduce the risk of transmitting the infection to other patients.*[1]
- To prevent the transmission of *C. difficile*, place the patient in a private room with a toilet or in a room with other *C. difficile*-infected patients if a private room is unavailable.[3,4]

Complications

Social isolation is a complication of contact precautions.

Documentation

Record the need for contact precautions on the nursing care plan and as otherwise indicated by your facility. Document initiation and maintenance of the precautions, and the patient's tolerance of the procedure. Document teaching provided to the patient and family (if applicable), their understanding of that teaching, and any need for follow-up teaching. Note the date that you discontinued contact precautions.

REFERENCES

1 Siegel, J. D., et al. (2007, revised 2019). 2007 guideline for isolation precautions: Preventing transmission of infectious agents in healthcare settings. https://www.cdc.gov/infectioncontrol/pdf/guidelines/isolation-guidelines-H.pdf (Level II)

2 Centers for Disease Control and Prevention. (2014). Interim guidance for infection control within healthcare settings when caring for confirmed cases, probable cases, and cases under investigation for infection with novel influenza A viruses associated with severe disease. https://www.cdc.gov/flu/avianflu/novel-flu-infection-control.htm (Level VII)

3 Centers for Disease Control and Prevention. (2020). *C. diff (Clostridioides difficile).* https://www.cdc.gov/cdiff/index.html

4 Centers for Disease Control and Prevention. (2020). FAQs for clinicians about *C. diff.* https://www.cdc.gov/cdiff/clinicians/faq.html?CDC_AA_refVal=https%3A%2F%2Fwww.cdc.gov%2Fhai%2Forganisms%2Fcdiff%2Fcdiff_faqs_hcp.html

5 Dubberke, E. R., et al. (2014). SHEA/IDSA practice recommendation: Strategies to prevent Clostridium difficile infections in acute care hospitals: 2014 update. *Infection Control and Hospital Epidemiology, 35,* 628–645. (Level VII)

6 The Joint Commission. (2021). Standard NPSG.07.03.01. *Comprehensive accreditation manual for hospitals.* Oakbrook Terrace, IL: The Joint Commission. (Level VII)

7 Dubberke, E. R., & Gerding, D. N. (2011). Rationale for hand hygiene recommendations after caring for a patient with *Clostridium difficile* infection. https://www.shea-online.org/images/patients/CDI-hand-hygiene-Update.pdf (Level VII)

8 Centers for Disease Control and Prevention. (2020). Shingles (herpes zoster): Clinical overview. https://www.cdc.gov/shingles/hcp/clinical-overview.html

9 Centers for Disease Control and Prevention. (2019). Shingles (herpes zoster): Preventing varicella-zoster virus (VZV) transmission from zoster in healthcare settings—management of patients with herpes zoster. https://www.cdc.gov/shingles/hcp/hc-settings.html (Level VII)

10 Centers for Disease Control and Prevention. (2015). Facility guidance for control of carbapenem-resistant *Enterobacteriaceae* (CRE): November 2015 update—CRE toolkit. https://www.cdc.gov/hai/pdfs/cre/CRE-guidance-508.pdf (Level VII)

11 Centers for Disease Control and Prevention. (2005). Guidelines for preventing the transmission of *Mycobacterium tuberculosis* in health-care settings, 2005. *MMWR Recommendations and Reports, 54*(RR-17), 1–140. https://www.cdc.gov/mmwr/PDF/rr/rr5417.pdf (Level VII)

12 Hall, A. J., et al. (2011). Updated norovirus outbreak management and disease prevention guidelines. *MMWR Recommendations and Reports, 60*(RR-03), 1–15. https://www.cdc.gov/mmwr/preview/mmwrhtml/rr6003a1.htm?s_cid=rr6003a1_w (Level VII)

13 The Joint Commission. (2021). Standard IC.02.01.01. *Comprehensive accreditation manual for hospitals.* Oakbrook Terrace, IL: The Joint Commission. (Level VII)

14 Centers for Medicare and Medicaid Services, Department of Health and Human Services. (2020). Condition of participation: Infection control. 42 C.F.R. § 482.42.

15 Accreditation Association for Hospitals and Health Systems. (2020). Standard 07.01.10. *Healthcare Facilities Accreditation Program: Accreditation requirements for acute care hospitals.* Chicago, IL: Accreditation Association for Hospitals and Health Systems. (Level VII)

16 DNV GL-Healthcare USA, Inc. (2020). IC.1.SR.1. *NIAHO® accreditation requirements, interpretive guidelines and surveyor guidance—revision 20.0.* Milford, OH: DNV GL-Healthcare USA, Inc. (Level VII)

17 The Joint Commission. (2021). Standard NPSG.07.01.01. *Comprehensive accreditation manual for hospitals.* Oakbrook Terrace, IL: The Joint Commission. (Level VII)

18 World Health Organization. (2009). WHO guidelines on hand hygiene in health care: First global patient safety challenge, clean care is safer care. https://apps.who.int/iris/bitstream/handle/10665/44102/9789241597906_eng.pdf?sequence=1 (Level IV)

19 Centers for Disease Control and Prevention. (2002). Guideline for hand hygiene in health-care settings: Recommendations of the Healthcare Infection Control Practices Advisory Committee and the HICPAC/SHEA/APIC/IDSA Hand Hygiene Task Force. *MMWR Recommendations and Reports, 51*(RR-16), 1–45. https://www.cdc.gov/mmwr/pdf/rr/rr5116.pdf (Level II)

20 Accreditation Association for Hospitals and Health Systems. (2020). Standard 07.01.21. *Healthcare Facilities Accreditation Program: Accreditation requirements for acute care hospitals.* Chicago, IL: Accreditation Association for Hospitals and Health Systems. (Level VII)

21 Siegel, J. D., et al. (2006, revised 2017). Management of multidrug-resistant organisms in healthcare settings, 2006. https://www.cdc.gov/infectioncontrol/pdf/guidelines/mdro-guidelines.pdf (Level VII)

22 The Joint Commission. (2021). Standard NPSG.01.01.01. *Comprehensive accreditation manual for hospitals.* Oakbrook Terrace, IL: The Joint Commission. (Level VII)

23 The Joint Commission. (2021). Standard PC.02.01.21. *Comprehensive accreditation manual for hospitals.* Oakbrook Terrace, IL: The Joint Commission. (Level VII)

24 Accreditation Association for Hospitals and Health Systems. (2020). Standard 07.01.02. *Healthcare Facilities Accreditation Program: Accreditation requirements for acute care hospitals.* Chicago, IL: Accreditation Association for Hospitals and Health Systems. (Level VII)

25 The Joint Commission. (2021). Standard RC.01.03.01. *Comprehensive accreditation manual for hospitals.* Oakbrook Terrace, IL: The Joint Commission. (Level VII)

26 Centers for Medicare and Medicaid Services, Department of Health and Human Services. (2020). Condition of participation: Medical record services. 42 C.F.R. § 482.24(b).

27 Accreditation Association for Hospitals and Health Systems. (2020). Standard 10.00.03. *Healthcare Facilities Accreditation Program: Accreditation requirements for acute care hospitals.* Chicago, IL: Accreditation Association for Hospitals and Health Systems. (Level VII)

28 DNV GL-Healthcare USA, Inc. (2020). MR.2.SR.1. *NIAHO® accreditation requirements, interpretive guidelines and surveyor guidance—revision 20.0.* Milford, OH: DNV GL-Healthcare USA, Inc. (Level VII)

29 Rutala, W. A., et al. (2008, revised 2019). Guideline for disinfection and sterilization in healthcare facilities, 2008. https://www.cdc.gov/infection-control/pdf/guidelines/disinfection-guidelines-H.pdf (Level I)

30 Accreditation Association for Hospitals and Health Systems. (2020). Standard 07.02.03. *Healthcare Facilities Accreditation Program: Accreditation requirements for acute care hospitals.* Chicago, IL: Accreditation Association for Hospitals and Health Systems. (Level VII)

31 The Joint Commission. (2021). Standard IC.02.02.02. *Comprehensive accreditation manual for hospitals.* Oakbrook Terrace, IL: The Joint Commission. (Level VII)

CONTINENT ILEOSTOMY CARE

An alternative to conventional ileostomy, a continent, or pouch, ileostomy (also called a *Koch ileostomy* or an *ileal pouch*) features an internal reservoir fashioned from the terminal ileum. A continent ileostomy may be appropriate for patients who requires proctocolectomy for chronic ulcerative colitis or multiple polyposis.[1] Other patients may undergo conversion of a traditional ileostomy to a continent ileostomy. This procedure is controversial in patients with short bowel syndrome or acute severe colitis, as well as in those patients who can't handle the complex surgery and intubation.[2] Patients who need emergency surgery and those who can't care for the pouch are also unlikely to have this procedure.

The length of preoperative hospitalization varies with the patient's condition. Nursing responsibilities include providing bowel preparation, antibiotic therapy, and emotional support. After surgery, nursing responsibilities include ensuring patency of the drainage catheter, assessing GI function, caring for the stoma and peristomal skin, managing pain resulting from surgery, and, if necessary, providing perineal skin care.

Daily patient teaching on pouch intubation and drainage usually begins soon after surgery. Continuous drainage is maintained for about 2 to 6 weeks to allow the suture lines to heal.[3] A drainage catheter that uses gravity or low intermittent suction should be attached during this period. After the suture line heals, the patient learns how to drain the pouch independently.

Equipment

Bedside drainage bag ■ normal saline solution or water ■ 50-mL catheter-tip syringe ■ continent ileostomy catheter ■ 4″ × 4″ × 1″ (10 cm × 10 cm × 2.5 cm) foam dressing and Montgomery straps ■ precut drain dressing ■ scissors ■ gloves ■ water-soluble lubricant ■ graduated container ■ water ■ gauze pads, a towel, or a washcloth ■ skin sealant ■ surgical safety checklist ■ vital signs monitoring equipment ■ stethoscope ■ disinfectant pad ■ blood glucose monitoring equipment ■ pulse oximeter and probe ■ venous thromboembolism prophylaxis (unfractionated heparin, low molecular weight heparin, intermittent pneumatic compression, elastic stockings) ■ prescribed antibiotics ■ prescribed bowel preparation ■ other prescribed medications ■ facility-approved sedation scale ■ facility-approved disinfectant ■ Optional: IV catheter insertion equipment, leg drainage bag, end-tidal carbon dioxide monitor, supplemental oxygen administration supplies, facility-approved ostomy skin assessment tool, disposable head clippers, chlorhexidine solution.

Preparation of equipment

Inspect all equipment and supplies. If a product is expired, is defective, or has compromised integrity, remove it from patient use, label it as expired or defective, and report the expiration or defect as directed by your facility.

Implementation

Preoperative care

■ Verify the practitioner's orders regarding preoperative care.
■ Review the patient's medical record for the medical and surgical history, a reconciled list of current medications, any allergies, and risk factors that increase the patient's risk of adverse reactions to medications, including age, altered liver and kidney function, a history of sleep apnea, weight (obese patients may be at increased risk of apnea; underweight patients may have an increased sensitivity to dose levels of medication), asthma,

a history of smoking, drug–drug interactions, and first-time medication use.[4]
■ Gather and prepare the necessary equipment and supplies.
■ If required by your facility, confirm that informed consent has been obtained and that the signed consent form is in the patient's medical record.[5,6,7,8]
■ Conduct a preprocedural verification *to make sure that all relevant documentation, related information, and equipment are available and correctly identified to the patient's identifiers.*[9,10]
■ Verify that all laboratory and imaging studies are complete, as ordered, and that the results are in the patient's medical record. Notify the practitioner of any unexpected results.[9,10]
■ Perform hand hygiene.[11,12,13,14,15,16]
■ Confirm the patient's identity using at least two patient identifiers.[17]
■ Provide privacy.[18,19,20,21]
■ Explain the procedure to the patient and family (if appropriate) according to their communication and learning needs *to increase their understanding, allay their fears, and enhance cooperation.*[22]
■ Obtain a health history, including previous surgeries, skin condition, history of multiple drug–resistant organisms, external or implanted medical devices, sensory limitations, allergies and sensitivities (including to latex and metal), and home use of noninvasive positive-pressure ventilation or apnea monitors.[23]
■ Obtain a pain and analgesic history. Ask about measures that have been effective in relieving or controlling pain in the past. Also ask about expectations for controlling pain after surgery. *By obtaining a thorough pain history preoperatively, the health care team may be better able to control pain postoperatively.*[23]
■ Perform educational, socioeconomic, cultural, and spiritual assessments *to determine the patient's level of understanding about the surgical procedure and any special needs while in the facility.*[23,24]
■ Assess for mobility limitations and disabilities, including mental and physical impairments, *which may require the use of additional equipment or supplies.*[23,24,25] Assess and address the patient's safety needs, including the risk of falling, and implement fall-prevention interventions as needed.[23,24,25]
■ Assess the patient's risk of postoperative nausea and vomiting (PONV) *so that the practitioner can consider PONV prophylaxis to decrease postoperative discomfort.* Consider the patient's history of PONV, the duration of surgery, and the type of surgery being performed.[23]
■ Assess the patient's cognitive, mental, and cardiopulmonary status; skin condition; functional and sensory limitations; and use of any hearing or visual aids and assistive or prosthetic devices.[24]
■ Obtain other assessment data pertinent to the surgical procedure. (See the "Preoperative care" procedure.)[23]
■ Reinforce and, if necessary, supplement the practitioner's explanation of a continent ileostomy and its implications for the patient.
■ If a wound, ostomy, and continence nurse (WOCN) is available at your facility, reinforce the WOCN's preoperative teaching, which should include anatomy and physiology of the GI tract, the details of the procedure, demonstration of ostomy appliances, expected lifestyle changes, and measures to prepare psychologically for the procedure.[26] (See *Understanding pouch construction*, page 208.)
■ Assess patient and family attitudes related to the operation and to the forthcoming changes in the patient's body image.[24]
■ Provide encouragement and support.
■ Make sure the stoma site is marked preoperatively *to reduce the incidence of complications and improve self-care.*[26,27]
■ Teach the patient how to rate pain according to your facility-defined criteria. Advise the patient to report pain, and discuss such analgesic tools and methods as patient-controlled analgesia.
■ Administer bowel preparation, as ordered.
■ Monitor and control the patient's blood glucose level, as ordered, *to reduce the risk of surgical site infection.*[28]
■ Don't remove hair unless it will interfere with the surgical procedure. If hair removal is necessary, remove it by using a disposable-head hair clippers before the patient enters the operating room; don't use a razor.[28]
■ Ensure that the patient has taken a preoperative bath or shower at least the night before or the day of surgery with chlorhexidine, as ordered, to reduce the number of microorganisms on the skin, thereby reducing

Understanding pouch construction

Depending on the patient and related factors during intestinal surgery, the surgeon may construct a pouch to collect fecal matter internally. To make such a pouch, the surgeon loops about 12″ (30.5 cm) of ileum and sutures the inner sides together.[2]

The surgeon opens the loop with a U-shaped cut and seams the inside *to create a smooth lining.* Then the surgeon fashions a nipple or valve between what is becoming the pouch and what will be the stoma. The surgeon folds the open ileum over, sews the pouch closed, and fixes the pouch to the abdominal wall.

Because the pouch holds fecal matter in reserve, the patient benefits from not having to change and empty ostomy equipment. Instead, the patient empties and irrigates the pouch as needed by inserting a catheter though the stoma and into the pouch (as shown below).

Initially after surgery, the nurse performs this procedure until the patient is able to do it independently.

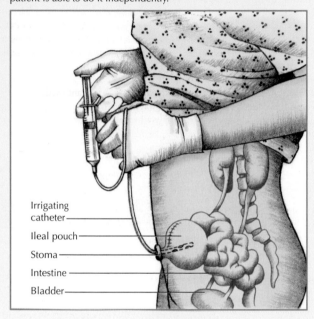

Irrigating catheter
Ileal pouch
Stoma
Intestine
Bladder

the risk of subsequent contamination of the surgical wound. Make sure that the patient has not applied any alcohol-based hair or skin products, lotions, emollients, or cosmetics.[29] Assist as needed.

■ If the patient was receiving a beta-adrenergic blocker before surgery, collaborate with the patient's practitioner *to ensure administration of the drug during the perioperative period, as appropriate.*[30]

■ Administer venous thromboembolism (VTE) prophylaxis, as ordered.[25,31] Intermittent pneumatic compression is recommended for patients at low risk for VTE; for patients at moderate risk for VTE who aren't at risk for major bleeding complications, unfractionated heparin, low-molecular-weight heparin, or intermittent pneumatic compression is recommended; for patients at high risk for VTE who aren't at high risk for major bleeding complications, unfractionated heparin, low-molecular-weight heparin, and mechanical prophylaxis with elastic stockings or intermittent pneumatic compression are recommended.[31,32]

■ Complete a surgical safety checklist *to ensure compliance with best practices to improve surgical patient safety.*[28]

■ Make sure the patient has patent IV access; insert a new IV catheter, as ordered, if necessary. (See the "IV catheter insertion and removal" procedure.)

■ Administer antibiotics, as ordered, following safe medication administration practices.[4,33,34,35] The patient should receive prophylactic antibiotics 1 hour before surgical incision (2 hours before incision is acceptable for the administration of vancomycin and fluoroquinolones) *to reduce the risk of surgical site infection.*[4,34]

■ Maintain nothing-by-mouth status, as ordered. Minimum fasting recommendations include 2 hours for clear liquids, 6 or more hours for a

light meal or nonhuman milk, and 8 hours or more for fried or fatty foods or meat.[36]

■ Maintain normothermia (95.9° F [35.5° C] or higher) during the perioperative period, *because preoperative and intraoperative warming reduces the risk of surgical site infection and intraoperative blood loss.*[28]

■ Provide hand-off communication to the person who'll be assuming responsibility for the patient's care. Ask questions as necessary *to avoid miscommunications that may cause patient care errors during transitions of care.* As part of the hand-off process, trace each tubing and catheter from the patient to its point of origin; a standardized line reconciliation process should be used.[37,38,39,40]

■ Perform hand hygiene.[11,12,13,14,15,16]

■ Document the procedure.[41,42,43,44]

Postoperative care

■ Receive hand-off communication from the person who was responsible for the patient's care; ask questions as necessary *to avoid miscommunications that may cause patient care errors during transitions of care.*[37,38] As part of the hand-off process, trace each tubing and catheter from the patient to its point of origin; a standardized line reconciliation process should be used.[40]

■ Verify the practitioner's orders regarding postoperative care.

■ Gather and prepare the necessary equipment and supplies.

■ Perform hand hygiene.[11,12,13,14,15,16]

■ Put on gloves.[45,46]

■ Confirm the patient's identity using at least two patient identifiers.[17]

■ Provide privacy.[18,19,20,21]

■ Explain the procedure to the patient and family (if applicable) according to their individual communication and learning needs *to increase their understanding, allay their fears, and enhance cooperation.*[22]

■ Perform a comprehensive postoperative assessment. (See the "Postoperative care" procedure.)

■ Administer supplemental oxygen, as needed and prescribed. *Supplemental oxygen administration is recommended during and following surgical procedures involving mechanical ventilation to optimize tissue oxygenation and subsequently reduce the risk of surgical site infection.*[28]

■ Screen for and assess the patient's pain using facility-defined criteria that are consistent with the patient's age, condition, and ability to understand.[47]

■ Treat the patient's pain, as needed and ordered, using nonpharmacologic, pharmacologic, or a combination of approaches. Base the treatment plan on evidence-based practices and the patient's clinical condition, past medical history, and pain management goals.[47] If you're administering pain medication, follow safe medication administration practices.[4,33,34,35] If you're administering the medication using an infusion device, verify proper programming of the device before administration. Advise the patient and family to notify a staff member promptly of any changes that might be a reaction to the medication.[4]

■ Monitor closely if the patient is at high risk for adverse outcomes related to opioid treatment, if prescribed.[47]

NURSING ALERT If the patient is receiving opioids to treat pain, keep in mind that these medications can cause oversedation and respiratory compromise. Failure to recognize and respond to progressive signs of respiratory compromise (somnolence, a decreased respiratory rate and oxygen saturation level) can lead to respiratory depression and death.[4] If the practitioner prescribed opioids, closely monitor the patient at high risk for adverse outcomes related to treatment.[47]

■ Monitor the patient's vital signs, oxygen saturation level by pulse oximetry, end-tidal carbon dioxide (if needed and available), respiratory status, and sedation level (using a facility-approved sedation scale) at a frequency determined by your facility and the patient's condition.[6]

■ Attach the drainage catheter emerging from the ileostomy to continuous drainage.[48,49]

■ Trace each tubing from the patient to the point of origin *to make sure that it's attached to the proper port.*[4,50] Route the tubing in a standardized direction if the patient has other tubing and catheters that have different purposes. Label the tubing at both the distal end (near the patient connection) and the proximal end (near the source container) *to reduce the risk of misconnection* if multiple IV lines will be used.[40]

■ Reassess and respond to the patient's pain by evaluating the response to treatment and progress toward pain management goals. Assess for adverse reactions and risk factors for adverse events that may result from treatment.[47]

■ Encourage early ambulation *to prevent VTE.*[32] A leg drainage bag may be attached to the patient's thigh during ambulation. Continue other prescribed methods of VTE prophylaxis.[32]

■ Ensure discontinuation of prophylactic antibiotics within 24 hours of the surgery end time.[28]

■ Irrigate the ileostomy catheter with 30 mL of normal saline solution, as ordered and needed *to prevent catheter obstruction,* and allow fluid return by gravity. During the early postoperative period, keep the pouch empty; drainage will be serosanguineous.

■ Monitor the patient's intake and output and electrolyte levels (as ordered) *to assess for fluid and electrolyte imbalances.*

■ If the patient required an indwelling urinary catheter for surgery and it wasn't removed in the postanesthesia care unit, remove it as soon as it's no longer needed *to reduce the risk of catheter-associated urinary tract infection.*[51,52,53,54]

■ Check the ileostomy catheter frequently after the patient begins eating solid food *to ensure that neither mucus nor undigested food particles block the catheter.*

■ If the patient complains of abdominal cramps, distention, and nausea—signs and symptoms of bowel obstruction—the ileostomy catheter may be clogged. Gently irrigate with 20 to 30 mL of water or normal saline solution until the ileostomy catheter drains freely. Then move the ileostomy catheter slightly or rotate it gently *to help clear the obstruction.* Finally, try milking the catheter. If these measures fail, notify the practitioner.

■ Provide stoma and peristomal skin care:

■ Remove the dressing, gently clean the peristomal area with water, and pat dry with gauze pads, a towel, or a wash cloth.

■ Inspect the peristomal skin and stoma. Use a facility-approved assessment tool, if available. *Normally pink to red, a stoma that turns dark red or blue-red may have a compromised blood supply.* Observe for signs of mechanical, chemical, allergic, infectious, or disease-related complications *to objectively identify and track changes in peristomal skin.* Notify the practitioner or your facility's WOCN about problems, as needed.[55,56,57]

■ Use a skin sealant around the stoma *to prevent skin irritation.* Apply a new stoma dressing. One technique involves slipping a precut drain dressing around the catheter *to cover the stoma.* Cut a hole slightly larger than the lumen of the catheter in the center of a 4″ × 4″ × 1″ (10 cm × 10 cm × 2.5 cm) piece of foam. Disconnect the catheter from the drainage bag and insert the distal end of the catheter through the hole in the foam. Slide the foam pad onto the dressing. Secure the foam in place with Montgomery straps. Secure the catheter by wrapping the strap ties around it or by using a commercial catheter securement device. Then reconnect the catheter to the drainage bag. (The drainage catheter will be removed by the surgeon when the surgeon determines that the suture line has healed.)

■ *To reduce discomfort from gas pain,* encourage ambulation. Also, *to minimize gas pains,* recommend that the patient avoid swallowing air by chewing food well, limiting conversation while eating, and not drinking from a straw.

■ Remove and discard your gloves.[45,46]

■ Perform hand hygiene.[11,12,13,14,15,16]

■ Clean and disinfect your stethoscope using a disinfectant pad.[58,59]

■ Perform hand hygiene.[11,12,13,14,15,16]

■ If available, consult with a WOCN *to provide ongoing postoperative education.*[26]

■ Document the procedure.[41,42,43,44]

Draining the pouch

■ Verify the practitioner's order.

■ Gather and prepare the necessary equipment and supplies.

■ Perform hand hygiene[11,12,13,14,15,16] and put on gloves.[45]

■ Confirm the patient's identity using at least two patient identifiers.[17]

■ Provide privacy.[18,19,20,21]

■ Explain the procedure to the patient and family (if applicable) according to individual communication and learning needs *to increase their understanding, allay their fears, and enhance cooperation.*[22]

■ The patient who has had a pouch conversion should sit on the toilet *to help the patient feel more at ease during the procedure.*

■ Remove the stoma dressing.

■ Encourage the patient to relax the abdominal muscles *to allow the catheter to slide easily into the pouch.*[60]

■ Lubricate the drainage catheter tip with the water-soluble lubricant and insert it with a steady, gentle pressure and a slight twisting motion into the stoma. Gently push the catheter downward. (The direction of insertion may vary depending on the patient.)[48]

■ When the catheter reaches the nipple valve of the internal pouch or reservoir (after about 2″ to 2½″ [5 cm to 6.5 cm]), you'll feel resistance. Instruct the patient to take a deep breath as you exert gentle pressure on the catheter to insert it through the valve. If this fails, have the patient lie in the supine position and rest for a few minutes. Then, with the patient still supine, try to insert the catheter again. You can also try using a smaller catheter.

■ Gently advance the catheter to the suture marking made by the surgeon.

■ Let the pouch drain completely, which usually takes 5 to 10 minutes. With thick drainage or a clogged catheter, the process may take 30 minutes.

■ If the tube clogs, irrigate with 30 mL of water or normal saline using a 50-mL catheter-tip syringe.[3] Also rotate and milk the tube. If these steps fail, remove, rinse, and reinsert the catheter.

■ Remove the catheter after completing drainage.

■ Measure the output, subtracting the amount of irrigant used.

■ Rinse the catheter thoroughly with warm water.

■ Clean the peristomal area and apply a fresh stoma dressing.

■ Remove and discard your gloves.[45]

■ Perform hand hygiene.[11,12,13,14,15,16]

■ Document the procedure.[41,42,43,44]

Special considerations

■ Encourage the patient to refrain from smoking for 30 days before the procedure *to reduce the risk of surgical site infection and reduced blood supply, which can result in necrosis.*[38]

■ Never aspirate fluid from the catheter, *because the resulting negative pressure may damage inflamed tissue.*

■ The Joint Commission issued a sentinel event alert related to managing risk during transition to new International Organization for Standardization tubing standards that were designed to prevent dangerous tubing misconnections, which can lead to serious patient injury and death. During the transition, make sure to trace the tubing and catheter from the patient to the point of origin before connecting or reconnecting any device or infusion, at any care transition (such as a new setting or service), and as part of the hand-off process; route tubes and catheters having different purposes in different standardized directions; when there are different access sites or several bags hanging, label the tubing at the distal and proximal ends; use tubing and equipment only as intended; and store medications for different delivery routes in separate locations.[40]

■ The Joint Commission issued a sentinel event alert concerning inadequate hand-off communication *because of the potential for patient harm that can result when a receiver receives inaccurate, incomplete, untimely, misinterpreted, or otherwise inadequate information. To improve hand-off communication,* standardize the critical information communicated by the sender. At a minimum, include the sender contact information; illness assessment; patient summary, including events leading up to the illness or admission, hospital course, ongoing assessment, and care plan; to-do action list; contingency plans; allergy list; code status; medication list; and dated laboratory test results and vital signs. Provide face-to-face communication whenever possible in an interruption-free location, using facility-approved, standardized tools and methods (for example, forms, templates, checklists, protocols, and mnemonics). Provide ample time and opportunity for questions, and include the multidisciplinary team members and the patient and family when appropriate.[37]

Patient teaching

Make sure the patient can properly intubate and drain the pouch. Provide the patient with the appropriate equipment. If the postoperative drainage catheter is still in place, teach the patient how to care for it properly. Make sure the patient has a pouch-draining schedule, and provide supply-appropriate pamphlets or video instructions on pouch care. Make sure that the patient feels comfortable calling the practitioner, nurse, or WOCN to ask questions or discuss problems. Tell the patient where to obtain supplies. Refer the patient to a local ostomy group. Provide counseling on nutrition, clothing, medications, body image, psychological and social issues, interpersonal relationships, and possible complications.[26]

During discharge planning, teach the patient and family (if appropriate) about pain management strategies. Include information about the patient's pain management plan and adverse effects of pain management treatment. Discuss activities of daily living and items in the home environment that might exacerbate pain or reduce the effectiveness of the pain management plan, and include strategies to address these issues. Teach about safe use, storage, and disposal of opioids, if prescribed.[47]

Complications

Common postoperative complications include hemorrhage, anastomotic leak, obstruction, fistula, pouch perforation, valve stenosis, nipple valve slippage, abdominal wall abscess, peritonitis, valve necrosis, valve prolapse, stenosis of the stoma, pouchitis, and short bowel syndrome.[2] The patient may also experience moisture-associated skin damage or infection[26] and bacterial overgrowth in the pouch.

Documentation

Record the date and time and all aspects of preoperative and postoperative care. Document the medication strength, dose, route of administration, and date and time of administration. Record any adverse reactions to the prescribed medication, the date and time the practitioner was notified, prescribed interventions, and the patient's response to those interventions. Document drainage of the pouch, noting irrigant, intubations, drainage amount and appearance, and patient tolerance. Include the condition of the stoma and peristomal skin, diet, and discharge planning. Document any complications, the name of the practitioner notified and the date and time of notification, interventions you performed, and the patient's response to those interventions. Document teaching provided to the patient and family (if applicable), their understanding of that teaching, and any need for follow-up teaching.

References

1 Jani, K., & Shah, A. (2015). Laparoscopic total proctocolectomy with ileal pouch-anal anastomosis for ulcerative colitis. *Journal of Minimal Access Surgery, 11*(3), 177–183. https://www.ncbi.nlm.nih.gov/pmc/articles/PMC4499922/ (Level VI)

2 Wu, X., et al. (2020). Continent ileostomy as an alternative to end ileostomy. *Gastroenterology Research and Practice, 2020*, 9740980. https://www.hindawi.com/journals/grp/2020/9740980/ (Level VII)

3 United Ostomy Associations of America, Inc. (2017). New ostomy patient guide. https://www.ostomy.org/wp-content/uploads/2018/05/All-In-One-New-Patient-Guide_2018.pdf

4 Centers for Medicare and Medicaid Services, Department of Health and Human Services. (2020). Condition of participation: Nursing services. 42 C.F.R. § 482.23(c).

5 The Joint Commission. (2021). Standard RI.01.03.01. *Comprehensive accreditation manual for hospitals.* Oakbrook Terrace, IL: The Joint Commission. (Level VII)

6 Centers for Medicare and Medicaid Services, Department of Health and Human Services. (2020). Condition of participation: Patient's rights. 42 C.F.R. § 482.13.

7 Accreditation Association for Hospitals and Health Systems. (2020). Standard 30.01.11. *Healthcare Facilities Accreditation Program: Accreditation requirements for acute care hospitals.* Chicago, IL: Accreditation Association for Hospitals and Health Systems. (Level VII)

8 DNV GL-Healthcare USA, Inc. (2020). PR.2.SR.3. *NIAHO® accreditation requirements, interpretive guidelines and surveyor guidance—revision 20.0.* Milford, OH: DNV GL-Healthcare USA, Inc. (Level VII)

9 The Joint Commission. (2021). Standard UP.01.01.01. *Comprehensive accreditation manual for hospitals.* Oakbrook Terrace, IL: The Joint Commission. (Level VII)

10 Accreditation Association for Hospitals and Health Systems. (2020). Standard 30.00.14. *Healthcare Facilities Accreditation Program: Accreditation requirements for acute care hospitals.* Chicago, IL: Accreditation Association for Hospitals and Health Systems. (Level VII)

11 The Joint Commission. (2021). Standard NPSG.07.01.01. *Comprehensive accreditation manual for hospitals.* Oakbrook Terrace, IL: The Joint Commission. (Level VII)

12 Centers for Disease Control and Prevention. (2002). Guideline for hand hygiene in health-care settings: Recommendations of the Healthcare Infection Control Practices Advisory Committee and the HICPAC/SHEA/APIC/IDSA Hand Hygiene Task Force. *MMWR Recommendations and Reports, 51*(RR-16), 1–45. https://www.cdc.gov/mmwr/pdf/rr/rr5116.pdf (Level II)

13 World Health Organization. (2009). WHO guidelines on hand hygiene in health care: First global patient safety challenge, clean care is safer care. https://apps.who.int/iris/bitstream/handle/10665/44102/9789241597906_eng.pdf?sequence=1 (Level IV)

14 Centers for Medicare and Medicaid Services, Department of Health and Human Services. (2020). Condition of participation: Infection control. 42 C.F.R. § 482.42.

15 Accreditation Association for Hospitals and Health Systems. (2020). Standard 07.01.21. *Healthcare Facilities Accreditation Program: Accreditation requirements for acute care hospitals.* Chicago, IL: Accreditation Association for Hospitals and Health Systems. (Level VII)

16 DNV GL-Healthcare USA, Inc. (2020). IC.1.SR.1. *NIAHO® accreditation requirements, interpretive guidelines and surveyor guidance—revision 20.0.* Milford, OH: DNV GL-Healthcare USA, Inc. (Level VII)

17 The Joint Commission. (2021). Standard NPSG.01.01.01. *Comprehensive accreditation manual for hospitals.* Oakbrook Terrace, IL: The Joint Commission. (Level VII)

18 Centers for Medicare and Medicaid Services, Department of Health and Human Services. (2020). Condition of participation: Patient's rights. 42 C.F.R. § 482.13(c)(1).

19 The Joint Commission. (2021). Standard RI.01.01.01. *Comprehensive accreditation manual for hospitals.* Oakbrook Terrace, IL: The Joint Commission. (Level VII)

20 Accreditation Association for Hospitals and Health Systems. (2020). Standard 15.01.16. *Healthcare Facilities Accreditation Program: Accreditation requirements for acute care hospitals.* Chicago, IL: Accreditation Association for Hospitals and Health Systems. (Level VII)

21 DNV GL-Healthcare USA, Inc. (2020). PR.2.SR.5. *NIAHO® accreditation requirements, interpretive guidelines and surveyor guidance—revision 20.0.* Milford, OH: DNV GL-Healthcare USA, Inc. (Level VII)

22 The Joint Commission. (2021). Standard PC.02.01.21. *Comprehensive accreditation manual for hospitals.* Oakbrook Terrace, IL: The Joint Commission. (Level VII)

23 American Society of PeriAnesthesia Nurses. (2019). *2019-2020 Perianesthesia nursing standards, practice recommendations and interpretive statements.* Cherry Hill, NJ: American Society of PeriAnesthesia Nurses. (Level VII)

24 The Joint Commission. (2010). *Advancing effective communication, cultural competence and patient- and family-centered care: A roadmap for hospitals.* Oakbrook Terrace, IL: The Joint Commission. http://www.jointcommission.org/assets/1/6/ARoadmapforHospitalsfinalversion727.pdf (Level VII)

25 Accreditation Association for Hospitals and Health Systems. (2020). Standard 16.02.02. *Healthcare Facilities Accreditation Program: Accreditation requirements for acute care hospitals.* Chicago, IL: Accreditation Association for Hospitals and Health Systems. (Level VII)

26 Wound, Ostomy and Continence Nurses Society Guideline Development Task Force. (2018). WOCN Society clinical guideline: Management of the adult patient with a fecal or urinary ostomy—An executive summary. *Journal of Wound, Ostomy and Continence Nursing, 45*, 50–58. (Level VII)

27 The Joint Commission. (2021). Standard UP.01.02.01. *Comprehensive accreditation manual for hospitals.* Oakbrook Terrace, IL: The Joint Commission. (Level VII)

28 Anderson, D. J., et al. (2014). SHEA/IDSA practice recommendation: Strategies to prevent surgical site infections in acute care hospitals: 2014 update. *Infection Control and Hospital Epidemiology, 35*(6), 605–627. https://www.jstor.org/stable/10.1086/676022#metadata_info_tab_contents (Level I)

29 Guideline for preoperative patient skin antisepsis. In A. Wood (Ed.), *Guidelines for perioperative practice, 2020 edition.* Denver, CO: AORN, Inc. (Level VII)

30 Devereaux, P. J., et al. (2020). Management of cardiac risk for noncardiac surgery. In: *UpToDate*, Pellikka, P. A.,, & Jaffe, A. S,. (Eds.).

31 Balk, E. M., et al. (2017), *Venous thromboembolism prophylaxis in major orthopedic surgery: Systematic review update.* (AHRQ Publication No. 17-EHC021-EF). Rockville, MD: Agency for Healthcare Research and Quality. https://effectivehealthcare.ahrq.gov/sites/default/files/pdf/thromboembolism-update_research-2017.pdf

32 Pai, M., & Douketis, J. D. (2021). Prevention of venous thromboembolic disease in adult nonorthopedic surgical patients. In: *UpToDate*, Leung, L. L. K.,, & Mandel, J., (Eds.)

33 DNV GL-Healthcare USA, Inc. (2020). MM.1.SR.3. *NIAHO® accreditation requirements, interpretive guidelines and surveyor guidance—revision 20.0.* Milford, OH: DNV GL-Healthcare USA, Inc. (Level VII)

34 Accreditation Association for Hospitals and Health Systems. (2020). Standard 16.01.03. *Healthcare Facilities Accreditation Program: Accreditation requirements for acute care hospitals.* Chicago, IL: Accreditation Association for Hospitals and Health Systems. (Level VII)

35 The Joint Commission. (2021). Standard MM.06.01.01. *Comprehensive accreditation manual for hospitals.* Oakbrook Terrace, IL: The Joint Commission. (Level VII)

36 American Society of Anesthesiologists. (2017). Practice guidelines for preoperative fasting and the use of pharmacologic agents to reduce the risk of pulmonary aspiration: Application to healthy patients undergoing elective procedures" *Anesthesiology, 126*, 376–393. http://anesthesiology.pubs.asahq.org/article.aspx?articleid=2596245 (Level V)

37 The Joint Commission. (2017). Sentinel event alert 58: Inadequate hand-off communication. https://www.jointcommission.org/assets/1/18/SEA_58_Hand_off_Comms_9_6_17_FINAL_(1).pdf (Level VII)

38 The Joint Commission. (2021). Standard PC.02.02.01. *Comprehensive accreditation manual for hospitals.* Oakbrook Terrace, IL: The Joint Commission. (Level VII)

39 Joint Commission Center for Transforming Healthcare. (n.d.). Hand-off communications. https://www.centerfortransforminghealthcare.org/en/improvement-topics/hand-off-communications (Level VII)

40 The Joint Commission. (2014). Sentinel event alert 53: Managing risk during transition to new ISO tubing connector standards. http://www.jointcommission.org/assets/1/6/SEA_53_Connectors_8_19_14_final.pdf (Level VII)

41 The Joint Commission. (2021). Standard RC.01.03.01. *Comprehensive accreditation manual for hospitals.* Oakbrook Terrace, IL: The Joint Commission. (Level VII)

42 Centers for Medicare and Medicaid Services, Department of Health and Human Services. (2020). Condition of participation: Medical record services. 42 C.F.R. § 482.24(b).

43 Accreditation Association for Hospitals and Health Systems. (2020). Standard 10.00.03. *Healthcare Facilities Accreditation Program: Accreditation requirements for acute care hospitals.* Chicago, IL: Accreditation Association for Hospitals and Health Systems. (Level VII)

44 DNV GL-Healthcare USA, Inc. (2020). MR.2.SR.1. *NIAHO® accreditation requirements, interpretive guidelines and surveyor guidance—revision 20.0.* Milford, OH: DNV GL-Healthcare USA, Inc. (Level VII)

45 Siegel, J. D., et al. (2007, revised 2019). 2007 guideline for isolation precautions: Preventing transmission of infectious agents in healthcare settings. https://www.cdc.gov/infectioncontrol/pdf/guidelines/isolation-guidelines-H.pdf (Level II)

46 Accreditation Association for Hospitals and Health Systems. (2020). Standard 07.01.10. *Healthcare Facilities Accreditation Program: Accreditation requirements for acute care hospitals.* Chicago, IL: Accreditation Association for Hospitals and Health Systems. (Level VII)

47 The Joint Commission. (2021). Standard PC.01.02.07. *Comprehensive accreditation manual for hospitals.* Oakbrook Terrace, IL: The Joint Commission. (Level VII)

48 Woodhouse, F. (2010, reviewed 2013). Colorectal surgery: Kock pouch operation: Information for patients. https://www.ouh.nhs.uk/patient-guide/leaflets/files/101101kochpouch.pdf

49 Beck, D. E. (2008). Continent ileostomy: Current status. *Clinics in Colon and Rectal Surgery, 21*(1), 62–70. https://www.ncbi.nlm.nih.gov/pmc/articles/PMC2780187/

50 U.S. Food and Drug Administration. (2017). Examples of medical device misconnections. https://www.fda.gov/medical-devices/medical-device-connectors/examples-medical-device-misconnections

51 Agency for Healthcare Research and Quality, & U.S. Department of Health and Human Services. (2015). Toolkit for reducing catheter-associated urinary tract infections in hospital units: Implementation guide. https://www.ahrq.gov/hai/cauti-tools/impl-guide/index.html

52 Association of Professionals in Infection Control and Epidemiology (APIC). (2014). APIC implementation guide: Guide to preventing catheter-associated urinary tract infections. https://apic.org/wp-content/uploads/2019/02/APIC_CAUTI_IG_FIN_REVD0815.pdf (Level IV)

53 Healthcare Infection Control Practices Advisory Committee. (2010, revised 2019). Guideline for prevention of catheter-associated urinary tract infections 2009. https://www.cdc.gov/infectioncontrol/pdf/guidelines/cauti-guidelines-H.pdf (Level I)

54 The Joint Commission. (2021). Standard NPSG.07.06.01. *Comprehensive accreditation manual for hospitals.* Oakbrook Terrace, IL: The Joint Commission. (Level VII)

55 Haugen, H., & Ratliff, C. R. (2013). Tools for assessing peristomal skin complications. *Journal of Wound, Ostomy and Continence Nursing, 40*, 131–134. (Level VII)

56 Jordan, R., & Christian, M. (2013). Understanding peristomal skin complications. *Wound Care Advisory, 2*(2), 36–41. http://woundcareadvisor.com/wp-content/uploads/2013/05/Understanding_M-J13.pdf (Level VII)

57 Australian Association of Stomal Therapy Nurses, Inc. (2013). Clinical guidelines for stomal therapy nursing practice. http://www.stomaltherapy.com/documents/AASTN_Guidelines_book_2013.pdf (Level VII)

58 Accreditation Association for Hospitals and Health Systems. (2020). Standard 07.02.03. *Healthcare Facilities Accreditation Program: Accreditation requirements for acute care hospitals.* Chicago, IL: Accreditation Association for Hospitals and Health Systems. (Level VII)

59 Rutala, W. A., et al. (2008, revised 2019). Guideline for disinfection and sterilization in healthcare facilities, 2008. https://www.cdc.gov/infectioncontrol/pdf/guidelines/disinfection-guidelines-H.pdf (Level I)

60 WebMD. (2020). Tips to care for your K-pouch (continent ileostomy). https://www.webmd.com/colorectal-cancer/caring-continent-ileostomy#1

Continuous bladder irrigation

Continuous bladder irrigation can help prevent urinary tract obstruction after prostate or bladder surgery by flushing out small blood clots.[1] It may also be used to treat an irritated, inflamed, or infected bladder lining.

Continuous bladder irrigation requires the placement of a triple-lumen indwelling urinary catheter. One lumen controls balloon inflation, a second lumen enables irrigant inflow, and a third enables irrigant outflow. The continuous flow of irrigation solution through the bladder creates a mild tamponade effect that may help prevent venous hemorrhage. (See *Setup for continuous bladder irrigation*, page 212.) The urinary catheter is inserted while the patient is in the operating room after prostate or bladder surgery; it may be inserted at the bedside if the patient's isn't undergoing surgery.

Unless specified otherwise by the practitioner, the patient should remain on bed rest throughout continuous bladder irrigation *to avoid kinking, dislodging, or pulling on the catheter*, which increase the risk of catheter-associated urinary tract infection (CAUTI). The urinary catheter should be removed as soon as it's no longer needed *to reduce the risk of CAUTI.*[1,2,3]

HOSPITAL-ACQUIRED CONDITION ALERT Keep in mind that the Centers for Medicare and Medicaid Services has identified CAUTI as a hospital-acquired condition *because best practices can reasonably prevent it. To reduce the risk of CAUTI,* follow CAUTI prevention practices when caring for a patient with an indwelling urinary catheter, including performing hand hygiene before and after urinary catheter manipulation; maintaining a sterile, continuously closed drainage system; maintaining unobstructed urine flow; regularly emptying the collection bag; replacing the urinary catheter and collection system using sterile technique when disconnection, leakage, or breaks in sterile technique occur; and discontinuing the urinary catheter as soon as it's no longer clinically indicated.[2,4,5,6,7]

Preparation of equipment

Inspect all equipment and supplies. If a product is expired, is defective, or has compromised integrity, remove it from patient use, label it as expired or defective, and report the expiration or defect as directed by your facility. Ensure that the irrigating solution is at room temperature to prevent bladder spasm.

Setup for continuous bladder irrigation

In continuous bladder irrigation, a triple-lumen indwelling urinary catheter is inserted through the patient's urethra and advanced to the bladder by the practitioner (as shown below). The urinary catheter enables irrigation solution to flow into the bladder through one lumen and flow out through a second lumen, as shown in the inset. The third lumen is used to inflate the balloon that holds the urinary catheter in place in the patient's bladder.

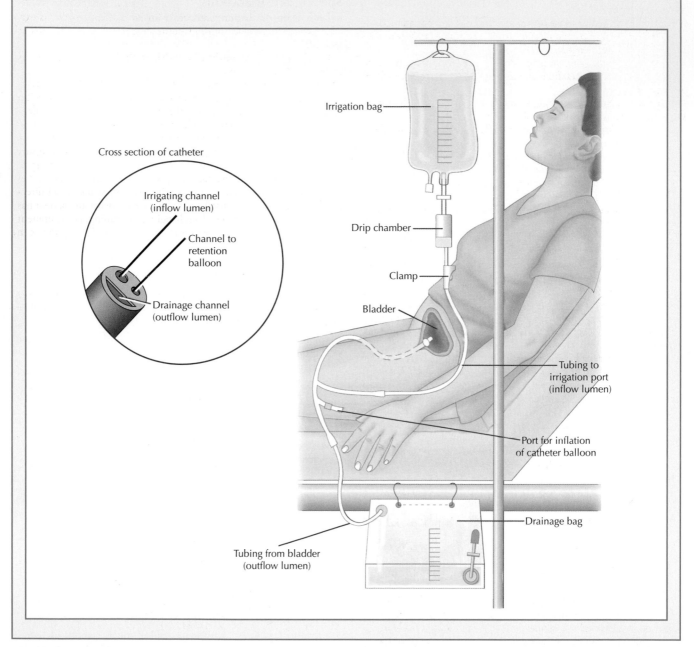

Cross section of catheter

Irrigating channel (inflow lumen)

Channel to retention balloon

Drainage channel (outflow lumen)

Irrigation bag

Drip chamber

Clamp

Bladder

Tubing to irrigation port (inflow lumen)

Port for inflation of catheter balloon

Drainage bag

Tubing from bladder (outflow lumen)

Equipment

Prescribed sterile irrigation solution ■ sterile irrigation solution administration set tubing ■ drainage bag and tubing ■ antiseptic pad ■ IV pole ■ gloves ■ vital signs monitoring equipment ■ graduated collection container ■ catheter securement device ■ Optional: gown, goggles,[8] labels.

Normal saline solution is usually prescribed for continuous bladder irrigation after prostate or bladder surgery. Large volumes of irrigating solution are usually required during the first 24 to 48 hours after prostate or bladder surgery *to prevent hemorrhage and blockage.* The irrigation solution may also contain an antibiotic.

Implementation

■ Avoid distractions and interruptions when preparing and administering the irrigation solution *to prevent administration errors.*[9,10]
■ Verify the practitioner's order in the patient's medical record.[11,12,13,14]
■ Check the patient's medical record for allergies or contraindications to the prescribed irrigation solution. If an allergy or a contraindication exists, don't administer the solution; instead, notify the practitioner.[11,12,13,14]
■ Gather and prepare the prescribed irrigation solution and supplies.
■ Compare the label on the irrigation solution with the order in the patient's medical record.[11,12,13,14]

- Check the expiration date on the irrigation solution. If the solution has expired, obtain a new supply of the irrigation solution.[11,12,13,14]
- Visually inspect the irrigation solution for particles, discoloration, or other signs of loss of integrity; don't administer the solution if its integrity has been compromised.[11,12,13,14]
- Perform hand hygiene.[15,16,17,18,19,20]
- Confirm the patient's identity using at least two patient identifiers.[21]
- Assemble all equipment at the patient's bedside.
- Provide privacy.[22,23,24,25]
- Explain the procedure to the patient and family (if appropriate) according to their individual communication and learning needs *to increase their understanding, allay their fears, and enhance cooperation.*[26]
- If the patient is receiving the irrigation solution for the first time, teach about potential adverse reactions and address any other concerns related to the solution.[11,12,13,14]
- Using sterile, no-touch technique, insert the spike of the administration set tubing into the irrigating solution bag.
- Squeeze the drip chamber on the spike of the tubing until it's about half full of irrigation solution.
- Open the flow clamp and prime the tubing *to remove air, which could cause bladder distention.* Then close the clamp.
- Hang the bag of irrigation solution on the IV pole.
- Perform hand hygiene.[15,16,17,18,10,20]
- Put on gloves and, if needed, a gown and goggles *to comply with standard precautions.*[1,8,27,28]
- Thoroughly disinfect the opening to the inflow lumen of the urinary catheter with the antiseptic pad and allow it to dry.[2,4,8]
- Using sterile, no-touch technique, insert the distal end of the administration set tubing securely into the inflow lumen of the urinary catheter. Trace the tubing from the patient to its point of origin *to make sure you've attached it to the proper port.*[29,30] If there is more than one access site, label the tubing at the distal end (near the patient connection) and proximal end (near the source container) *to distinguish the different tubing and prevent misconnections.*[30]
- Secure the urinary catheter with a catheter securement device *to prevent movement and urethral traction, which increase the risk of CAUTI.*[1,2,3,4]
- Ensure that the urinary catheter's outflow lumen is attached securely to the drainage bag tubing *to maintain a closed system, preventing disconnections that increase the risk of CAUTI.*
- Open the flow clamp under the bag of irrigation solution and set the drip rate as ordered.
- *To prevent air from entering the system,* don't allow the irrigation solution bag to empty completely before replacing it.
- Keep the drainage bag below the level of the bladder at all times *to prevent backflow of urine into the bladder, which increases the risk of CAUTI.*[1,2,4,31] Don't place the drainage bag on the floor.[1,2,3,31]
- Maintain the urinary catheter and drainage bag tubing free from kinking.[2,3]
- Empty the drainage bag regularly, using a separate collection container for each patient.[1,2,3,31] Use sterile, no-touch technique, avoid splashing, and prevent contact of the drainage spigot with the nonsterile collecting container *to decrease the risk of contamination.*[1,2,3,4,31]
- Measure the outflow volume accurately. It should equal or, allowing for urine production, exceed the inflow volume slightly. If the inflow volume exceeds the outflow volume postoperatively, suspect bladder rupture at the suture lines or kidney damage, and notify the practitioner immediately.
- Assess the outflow drainage for changes in appearance and for blood clots, especially if continuous bladder irrigation is being performed postoperatively to control bleeding. If the drainage is bright red, the irrigation solution usually should be infused rapidly (with the flow clamp wide open) until the drainage clears. Notify the practitioner immediately if you suspect hemorrhage. If the drainage appears clear, the solution is usually given at a rate of 40 to 60 drops/minute. The practitioner typically specifies the rate for irrigation solutions containing an antibiotic.
- Monitor vital signs as often as required by the patient's condition, increasing the frequency if the patient becomes unstable.
- Monitor urine output, assess for abdominal pain, and palpate for bladder distention as indicated. Notify the practitioner of abnormal findings.

- Check the inflow and outflow tubing periodically for kinks *to make sure the solution is running freely, without obstruction, which reduces the risk of CAUTI.*[1,2,4]
- Remove and discard your gloves and, if worn, gown and goggles.[27,28]
- Perform hand hygiene.[15,16,17,18,19,20]
- Document the procedure.[32,33,34,35]

Special considerations

- Don't clean the periurethral area with an antiseptic pad; instead, clean the meatal surface during routine hygiene *to reduce the risk of CAUTI.*[1,2,3]
- Encourage oral fluid intake of 2 to 3 L/day unless contraindicated by another medical condition.
- The Joint Commission issued a sentinel event alert related to managing risk during transition to new International Organization for Standardization tubing standards that were designed to prevent dangerous tubing misconnections, which can lead to serious patient injury and death. During the transition, trace each tubing and catheter from the patient to its point of origin before connecting or reconnecting any device or infusion, at any care transition (such as to a new setting or service), and as part of the hand-off process. In addition, route tubes and catheters with different purposes in different, standardized directions; label tubing at the distal and proximal ends (when the patient has different access sites or several bags hanging); use tubing and equipment only as intended; and store medications for different delivery routes in separate locations.[30]

Complications

Interruptions in a continuous bladder irrigation system can predispose the patient to infection. Obstruction in the urinary catheter's outflow lumen can cause bladder distention, spasm, or pain.

Documentation

Each time a container of irrigation solution empties, record the date, time, and amount of fluid you administered on the intake and output record. Record the time and amount of fluid each time you empty the drainage bag. Note the appearance of the outflow drainage and any complaints expressed by the patient. Note the patient's tolerance of the procedure. Document any complications that occurred, the name of the practitioner you notified, the date and time of notification, prescribed interventions, and the patient's response to those interventions. Also document teaching provided to the patient and family (if applicable), their understanding of that teaching, and any need for follow-up teaching.

REFERENCES

1 Healthcare Infection Control Practices Advisory Committee. (2010, revised 2019). Guideline for prevention of catheter-associated urinary tract infections 2009. https://www.cdc.gov/infectioncontrol/pdf/guidelines/cauti-guidelines-H.pdf (Level I)
2 Lo, E., et al. (2014). SHEA/IDSA practice recommendation: Strategies to prevent catheter-associated urinary tract infections in acute care hospitals, 2014 update. *Infection Control and Hospital Epidemiology, 35*(5), 464–479. http://www.jstor.org/stable/10.1086/675718 (Level I)
3 Association of Professionals in Infection Control and Epidemiology. (2014). APIC implementation guide: Guide to preventing catheter-associated urinary tract infections. https://apic.org/wp-content/uploads/2019/02/APIC_CAUTI_IG_FIN_REVD0815.pdf (Level IV)
4 The Joint Commission. (2021). Standard NPSG.07.06.01. *Comprehensive accreditation manual for hospitals.* Oakbrook Terrace, IL: The Joint Commission. (Level VII)
5 Centers for Medicare and Medicaid Services, Department of Health and Human Services. (2017). Appendix I: Hospital-acquired conditions (HACS) list. https://www.cms.gov/ICD10Manual/version33-full-code-cms/fullcode_cms/P0386.html
6 Jarrett, N., & Callaham, M. (2016). Evidence-based guidelines for selected hospital-acquired conditions: Final report. https://www.cms.gov/Medicare/Medicare-Fee-for-Service-Payment/HospitalAcqCond/Downloads/2016-HAC-Report.pdf

7   Accreditation Association for Hospitals and Health Systems. (2020). Standard 07.01.17. *Healthcare Facilities Accreditation Program: Accreditation requirements for acute care hospitals.* Chicago, IL: Accreditation Association for Hospital and Health Systems. (Level VII)

8   Agency for Clinical Innovation (ACI). (2019). *Bladder irrigation: Management of haematuria* (version 2). Chatswood, NSW: ACI. https://www.aci.health.nsw.gov.au/__data/assets/pdf_file/0009/497088/ACI_0195-Urology-Haem-toolkit_F.pdf (Level VII)

9   Westbrook, J., et al. (2010). Association of interruptions with an increased risk and severity of medication administration errors. *Archives of Internal Medicine, 170*, 683–690. (Level IV)

10 Institute for Safe Medication Practices. (2012). Side tracks on the safety express: Interruptions lead to errors and unfinished…Wait, what was I doing? *Nurse Advise-ERR, 11*(2), 1–4. https://www.ismp.org/resources/side-tracks-safety-express-interruptions-lead-errors-and-unfinished-wait-what-was-i-doing?id=37

11 The Joint Commission. (2021). Standard MM.06.01.01. *Comprehensive accreditation manual for hospitals.* Oakbrook Terrace, IL: The Joint Commission. (Level VII)

12 Centers for Medicare and Medicaid Services, Department of Health and Human Services. (2020). Condition of participation: Nursing services. 42 C.F.R. § 482.23(c).

13 Accreditation Association for Hospitals and Health Systems. (2020). Standard 16.01.03. *Healthcare Facilities Accreditation Program: Accreditation requirements for acute care hospitals.* Chicago, IL: Accreditation Association for Hospitals and Health Systems. (Level VII)

14 DNV GL-Healthcare USA, Inc. (2020). MM.1.SR.3. *NIAHO® accreditation requirements, interpretive guidelines and surveyor guidance—revision 20.0.* Milford, OH: DNV GL-Healthcare USA, Inc. (Level VII)

15 The Joint Commission. (2021). Standard NPSG.07.01.01. *Comprehensive accreditation manual for hospitals.* Oakbrook Terrace, IL: The Joint Commission. (Level VII)

16 Centers for Disease Control and Prevention. (2002). Guidelines for hand hygiene in health-care settings: Recommendations of the Healthcare Infection Control Practices Advisory Committee and the HICPAC/SHEA/APIC/IDSA Hand Hygiene Task Force. *MMWR Recommendations and Reports, 51*(RR-16), 1–45. https://www.cdc.gov/mmwr/pdf/rr/rr5116.pdf (Level II)

17 World Health Organization. (2009). WHO guidelines on hand hygiene in health care: First global patient safety challenge, clean care is safer care. https://apps.who.int/iris/bitstream/handle/10665/44102/9789241597906_eng.pdf?sequence=1 (Level IV)

18 Centers for Medicare and Medicaid Services, Department of Health and Human Services. (2020). Condition of participation: Infection control. 42 C.F.R. § 482.42.

19 Accreditation Association for Hospitals and Health Systems. (2020). Standard 07.01.21. *Healthcare Facilities Accreditation Program: Accreditation requirements for acute care hospitals.* Chicago, IL: Accreditation Association for Hospitals and Health Systems. (Level VII)

20 DNV GL-Healthcare USA, Inc. (2020). IC.1.SR.1. *NIAHO® accreditation requirements, interpretive guidelines and surveyor guidance—revision 20.0.* Milford, OH: DNV GL-Healthcare USA, Inc. (Level VII)

21 The Joint Commission. (2021). Standard NPSG.01.01.01. *Comprehensive accreditation manual for hospitals.* Oakbrook Terrace, IL: The Joint Commission. (Level VII)

22 Centers for Medicare and Medicaid Services, Department of Health and Human Services. (2020). Condition of participation: Patient's rights. 42 C.F.R. § 482.13(c)(1).

23 The Joint Commission. (2021). Standard RI.01.01.01. *Comprehensive accreditation manual for hospitals.* Oakbrook Terrace, IL: The Joint Commission. (Level VII)

24 Accreditation Association for Hospitals and Health Systems. (2020). Standard 15.01.16. *Healthcare Facilities Accreditation Program: Accreditation requirements for acute care hospitals.* Chicago, IL: Accreditation Association for Hospitals and Health Systems. (Level VII)

25 DNV GL-Healthcare USA, Inc. (2020). PR.2.SR.5. *NIAHO® accreditation requirements, interpretive guidelines and surveyor guidance—revision 20.0.* Milford, OH: DNV GL-Healthcare USA, Inc. (Level VII)

26 The Joint Commission. (2021). Standard PC.02.01.21. *Comprehensive accreditation manual for hospitals.* Oakbrook Terrace, IL: The Joint Commission. (Level VII)

27 Siegel, J. D., et al. (2007, revised 2019). 2007 guideline for isolation precautions: Preventing transmission of infectious agents in healthcare settings. https://www.cdc.gov/infectioncontrol/pdf/guidelines/isolation-guidelines-H.pdf (Level II)

28 Accreditation Association for Hospitals and Health Systems. (2020). Standard 07.01.10. *Healthcare Facilities Accreditation Program: Accreditation requirements for acute care hospitals.* Chicago, IL: Accreditation Association for Hospitals and Health Systems. (Level VII)

29 U.S. Food and Drug Administration. (2017). Examples of medical device misconnections. https://www.fda.gov/medical-devices/medical-device-connectors/examples-medical-device-misconnections

30 The Joint Commission. (2014). Sentinel event alert 53: Managing risk during transition to new ISO tubing connector standards. http://www.jointcommission.org/assets/1/6/SEA_53_Connectors_8_19_14_final.pdf (Level VII)

31 Moola, S. (2021). Urinary drainage bags: Emptying, changing and securing. *The JBI EBP Database.* AN: JBI1334 (Level I)

32 The Joint Commission. (2021). Standard RC.01.03.01. *Comprehensive accreditation manual for hospitals.* Oakbrook Terrace, IL: The Joint Commission. (Level VII)

33 Centers for Medicare and Medicaid Services, Department of Health and Human Services. (2020). Condition of participation: Medical record services. 42 C.F.R. § 482.24(b).

34 Accreditation Association for Hospitals and Health Systems. (2020). Standard 10.00.03. *Healthcare Facilities Accreditation Program: Accreditation requirements for acute care hospitals.* Chicago, IL: Accreditation Association for Hospitals and Health Systems. (Level VII)

35 DNV GL-Healthcare USA, Inc. (2020). MR.2.SR.1. *NIAHO® accreditation requirements, interpretive guidelines and surveyor guidance—revision 20.0.* Milford, OH: DNV GL-Healthcare USA, Inc. (Level VII)

CONTINUOUS POSITIVE AIRWAY PRESSURE USE

Continuous positive airway pressure (CPAP) provides constant pressure into the patient's airways to help hold the airway open, mobilize secretions, treat atelectasis, and generally ease the work of breathing. It's also used to treat chronic obstructive sleep apnea.[1] CPAP keeps the entire airway open, from the nares to the alveoli, thereby increasing functional residual capacity and improving gas exchange.

Although intubated patients may also receive CPAP through a ventilator, this procedure focuses on nonintubated patients who receive CPAP through a high-flow generating system, which can be used in the hospital setting or in the home and can reduce or eliminate the need for intubation. Many patients are started on CPAP in the health care facility and then continue therapy at home.

Although CPAP has traditionally been administered through a face mask, other, more comfortable methods include nasal pillows and the nasal mask.[2]

Because of increased thoracic pressure, CPAP is contraindicated in patients with increased intracranial pressure, hemodynamic instability, or recent facial, oral, or skull trauma. CPAP is also contraindicated in patients with untreated pneumothorax.[2]

Equipment

Appropriately sized nasal mask, nasal pillows, or face mask ▪ permanent marker ▪ CPAP machine ▪ washcloth ▪ water ▪ facility-approved disinfectant ▪ oral care supplies ▪ stethoscope ▪ disinfectant pad ▪ Optional: oxygen delivery tubing, oxygen source, pulse oximeter and probe, gloves, gown, mask, mask and goggles or mask with face shield, skin barrier.

Preparation of equipment

In most facilities, a respiratory therapist assumes the responsibility for setting up and administering CPAP. If a respiratory therapist isn't available and you must set up a CPAP machine, follow the manufacturer's instructions. Position the CPAP machine so that the tubing easily reaches the patient, and plug in the machine. Don't plug the CPAP machine into an outlet with another plug in it, and don't use an extension cord to reach the outlet. Connect the oxygen delivery tubing to the air outlet valve on the CPAP unit, if ordered.

Inspect all equipment and supplies. If a product is expired, is defective, or has compromised integrity, remove it from patient use, label it as expired or defective, and report the expiration or defect as directed by your facility. Check the nasal mask, nasal pillows, or face mask to ensure that the cushion isn't hard or broken. If it is, replace it.

Implementation
- Verify the practitioner's order.
- Notify the respiratory therapist (if available in your facility) of the CPAP order.
- Gather and prepare the necessary equipment and supplies.
- Perform hand hygiene.[3,4,5,6,7,8]
- Confirm the patient's identity using at least two patient identifiers.[9]
- Provide privacy.[10,11,12,13]
- Explain the procedure to the patient and family (if appropriate) according to their individual communication and learning needs *to increase their understanding, allay their fears, and enhance cooperation.*[14]
- Instruct the patient to wash the face with a washcloth and water *to remove facial oils and help achieve a better fit.*
- Perform hand hygiene.[3,4,5,6,7,8]
- Put on personal protective equipment if needed *to comply with standard precautions.*[15,16,17]
- Assess the patient's respiratory status *to establish a baseline for comparison.*

Applying a nasal mask
- Place the nasal mask so that the longer straps are located at the top of the mask (as shown below).

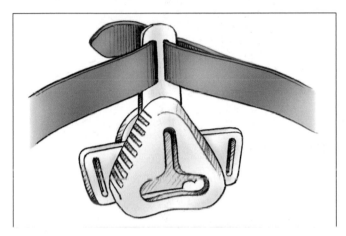

- Make sure that the Velcro is facing away from you, and thread the four tabs through the slots on the sides and top of the mask (as shown below).

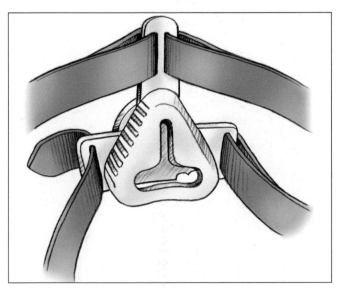

- Pull the straps through the slots and fasten them using the Velcro section.
- Place the mask over the patient's nose and position the headgear over the patient's head.
- Gradually tighten all the straps on the mask until a seal is obtained (as shown below). The mask doesn't have to be very tight to fit correctly; it just has to have a seal.

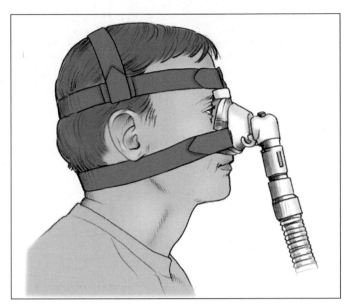

- Use the permanent marker to mark the straps with the final position *to eliminate having to fit the mask each time the patient wears it.*

Applying nasal pillows
- Insert the nasal pillows into the shell (as shown below), making sure they fit correctly and that there's no air leaking around them.

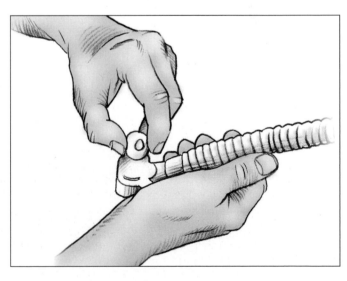

- Place the headgear around the patient's head and use the Velcro straps *to achieve the proper fit.* After the straps are in the correct place, remove the headgear without undoing the straps.

■ Attach the nasal pillows to the headgear by wrapping the Velcro strap around the tubing, leaving room for rotation (as shown below).

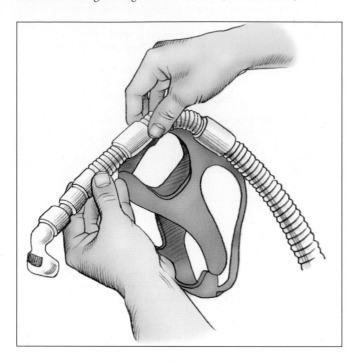

■ Place the completely assembled headgear back on the patient and position the nasal pillows comfortably.
■ Attach the shell strap across the shell and adjust the tension of the strap (as shown below) until there's a seal in both nostrils.

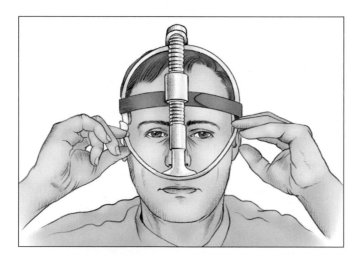

■ Be careful not to block the exhalation port on the back side of the shell.

Applying a face mask
■ Hold the mask against the patient's face and position the headgear over the head.
■ Adjust the Velcro straps as with the nasal mask (as shown above on right) until there are no leaks present.

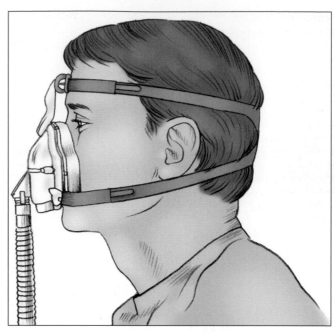

■ Connect the flexible tubing to the mask.

Administering CPAP
■ After the administration device is correctly fitted on the patient, turn on the machine's pressure generator.
■ Turn on the CPAP machine before turning on the oxygen flow (if ordered). Make sure that alarm limits are set appropriately for the patient's current condition and that the alarms are turned on, functioning properly, and audible to staff.[18,19]
■ Monitor the patient's oxygen saturation level using pulse oximetry during CPAP therapy, if ordered.
■ As ordered and tolerated, provide a CPAP mask break every 4 hours. Check strap tension and skin integrity beneath and around the mask regularly, and apply a skin barrier to pressure points as needed *to prevent device-related skin breakdown.*[20]
■ Provide frequent oral care. (See the "Oral care" procedure.) *CPAP may cause dry mouth; the oropharynx may become colonized with organisms that can be aspirated into the lungs, causing hospital-associated pneumonia.*
■ Reassess the patient's respiratory status *to ensure that the patient is tolerating CPAP therapy.*
■ Remove and discard your personal protective equipment, if worn.[15,16]
■ Perform hand hygiene.[3,4,5,6,7,8]
■ Clean and disinfect your stethoscope with a disinfectant pad.[21,22]
■ When the CPAP therapy has been completed, follow these steps. Perform hand hygiene,[3,4,5,6,7,8] put on gloves,[15,16] turn off the pressure generator, and remove the headgear and appliance from the patient. Clean and disinfect the equipment using a facility-approved disinfectant according to the manufacturer's instructions, and store it properly.[21,22] Remove and discard your gloves.[17]
■ Perform hand hygiene.[3,4,5,6,7,8]
■ Document the procedure.[23,24,25,26]

Special considerations
■ The Joint Commission issued a sentinel event alert concerning medical device alarm safety, *because alarm-related events have been associated with permanent loss of function or death.* Among the major contributing factors noted were improper alarm settings, alarm settings turned off

inappropriately, and alarm signals not audible to staff. Make sure that alarm limits are set appropriately and that alarms are turned on, functioning properly, and audible to staff. Follow facility guidelines for preventing alarm fatigue.[18]

■ When applying the mask for the first time, allow the patient to hold the mask in place *so that the patient can remove the mask quickly if the patient needs to communicate or feels claustrophobic.*[2]

■ If the patient isn't familiar with CPAP, start with the lowest pressure settings and adjust them in small increments over 1 to 2 minutes *to help the patient adjust to CPAP.*[2]

■ The patient who complains of a runny nose or dryness or burning in the nose and throat may need to use a humidifier with the CPAP unit. Discuss this option with the practitioner and obtain an order for humidification.

■ Always make sure there's air coming out of the unit when the power is turned on.

■ *Because CPAP via a mask can cause nausea and vomiting*, it shouldn't be used in a patient who's unresponsive or at risk for aspiration.

■ Such adverse effects of CPAP as dryness of the eyes, nasal stuffiness, and a leaking mask, as well as the inconvenience and noise associated with CPAP use, can lead to nonadherence.[1] For patients with obstructive sleep apnea, adherence is important for the CPAP therapy to be successful. Discuss these issues with the patient, intervene as appropriate, and encourage the patient to report persistent adverse effects.

■ If the mask isn't properly fitted, the patient may complain of dry or sore eyes. If this is the case, remove the mask and headgear and readjust them *to minimize leaks.*

■ Use a nasal pillow for a patient with a beard or mustache; leaks may occur with a nasal mask or face mask.[27]

Patient teaching

Teach the patient how to use the machine at home, including fitting the mask or nasal pillows and care of the equipment. Make sure the patient has the name and phone number of the company that will be supplying the machine for home use. Provide a contact number for the respiratory therapist, and encourage the patient to call the therapist with questions.

Complications

Most CPAP complications, including dry eyes, runny or dry nose, dry mouth, or burning in the throat or nose, result from ill-fitting masks or nasal pillows. Some patients may be allergic to the mask or nasal pillows; others may develop skin irritation from the mask or nasal pillows. Should irritation occur, apply a barrier between the mask and the nasal pillows and the patient's skin. Other complications include nosebleeds, abdominal bloating, and claustrophobia.[1]

CPAP also potentially causes decreased cardiac output due to increased intrathoracic pressure.[2]

Documentation

Document the CPAP settings, the length of time the patient was on CPAP, how the patient tolerated CPAP, and whether there were any complications. Document teaching provided to the patient and family (if applicable), their understanding of that teaching, and the need for follow-up teaching.

REFERENCES

1 Pinto, V. L., & Sharma, S. (2021). Continuous positive airway pressure (CPAP). *STATPearls*, NBK482178 https://www.ncbi.nlm.nih.gov/books/NBK482178/.

2 Kacmarek, R. M., et al. (2020). *Egan's fundamentals of respiratory care* (12th ed.). St. Louis, MO: Mosby.

3 The Joint Commission. (2021). Standard NPSG.07.01.01. *Comprehensive accreditation manual for hospitals*. Oakbrook Terrace, IL: The Joint Commission. (Level VII)

4 Centers for Disease Control and Prevention. (2002). Guideline for hand hygiene in health-care settings: Recommendations of the Healthcare Infection Control Practices Advisory Committee and the HICPAC/SHEA/APIC/IDSA Hand Hygiene Task Force. *MMWR Recommendations and Reports, 51*(RR-16), 1–45. https://www.cdc.gov/mmwr/pdf/rr/rr5116.pdf (Level II)

5 World Health Organization. (2009). WHO guidelines on hand hygiene in health care: First global patient safety challenge, clean care is safer care. https://apps.who.int/iris/bitstream/handle/10665/44102/9789241597906_eng.pdf?sequence=1 (Level IV)

6 Centers for Medicare and Medicaid Services, Department of Health and Human Services. (2020). Condition of participation: Infection control. 42 C.F.R. § 482.42.

7 Accreditation Association for Hospitals and Health Systems. (2020). Standard 07.01.21. *Healthcare Facilities Accreditation Program: Accreditation requirements for acute care hospitals*. Chicago, IL: Accreditation Association for Hospitals and Health Systems. (Level VII)

8 DNV GL-Healthcare USA, Inc. (2020). IC.1.SR.1. *NIAHO® accreditation requirements, interpretive guidelines and surveyor guidance—revision 20.0.* Milford, OH: DNV GL-Healthcare USA, Inc. (Level VII)

9 The Joint Commission. (2021). Standard NPSG.01.01.01. *Comprehensive accreditation manual for hospitals*. Oakbrook Terrace, IL: The Joint Commission. (Level VII)

10 Centers for Medicare and Medicaid Services, Department of Health and Human Services. (2020). Condition of participation: Patient's rights. 42 C.F.R. § 482.13(c)(1).

11 The Joint Commission. (2021). Standard RI.01.01.01. *Comprehensive accreditation manual for hospitals*. Oakbrook Terrace, IL: The Joint Commission. (Level VII)

12 Accreditation Association for Hospitals and Health Systems. (2020). Standard 15.01.16. *Healthcare Facilities Accreditation Program: Accreditation requirements for acute care hospitals*. Chicago, IL: Accreditation Association for Hospitals and Health Systems. (Level VII)

13 DNV GL-Healthcare USA, Inc. (2020). PR.2.SR.5. *NIAHO® accreditation requirements, interpretive guidelines and surveyor guidance—revision 20.0.* Milford, OH: DNV GL-Healthcare USA, Inc. (Level VII)

14 The Joint Commission. (2021). Standard PC.02.01.21. *Comprehensive accreditation manual for hospitals*. Oakbrook Terrace, IL: The Joint Commission. (Level VII)

15 Siegel, J. D., et al. (2007, revised 2019). 2007 guideline for isolation precautions: Preventing transmission of infectious agents in healthcare settings. https://www.cdc.gov/infectioncontrol/pdf/guidelines/isolation-guidelines-H.pdf (Level II)

16 Accreditation Association for Hospitals and Health Systems. (2020). Standard 07.01.10. *Healthcare Facilities Accreditation Program: Accreditation requirements for acute care hospitals*. Chicago, IL: Accreditation Association for Hospitals and Health Systems. (Level VII)

17 Occupational Safety and Health Administration. (2012). Bloodborne pathogens, standard number 1910.1030. https://www.osha.gov/pls/oshaweb/owadisp.show_document?p_id=10051&p_table=STANDARDS (Level VII)

18 The Joint Commission. (2013). Sentinel event alert 50: Medical device alarm safety in hospitals. https://www.jointcommission.org/assets/1/6/SEA_50_alarms_4_26_16.pdf (Level VII)

19 The Joint Commission. (2021). Standard NPSG.06.01.01. *Comprehensive accreditation manual for hospitals*. Oakbrook Terrace, IL: The Joint Commission. (Level VII)

20 Wound Ostomy and Continence Nurses Society (WOCN). (2016). *Guideline for prevention and management of pressure ulcers (injuries): WOCN clinical practice guideline series 2*. Mount Laurel, NJ: WOCN.

21 Rutala, W. A., et al. (2008, revised 2019). Guideline for disinfection and sterilization in healthcare facilities, 2008. https://www.cdc.gov/infectioncontrol/pdf/guidelines/disinfection-guidelines-H.pdf (Level I)

22 Accreditation Association for Hospitals and Health Systems. (2020). Standard 07.02.03. *Healthcare Facilities Accreditation Program: Accreditation requirements for acute care hospitals*. Chicago, IL: Accreditation Association for Hospitals and Health Systems. (Level VII)

23 The Joint Commission. (2021). Standard RC.01.03.01. *Comprehensive accreditation manual for hospitals*. Oakbrook Terrace, IL: The Joint Commission. (Level VII)

24 Centers for Medicare and Medicaid Services, Department of Health and Human Services. (2020). Condition of participation: Medical record services. 42 C.F.R. § 482.24(b).

25 Accreditation Association for Hospitals and Health Systems. (2020). Standard 10.00.03. *Healthcare Facilities Accreditation Program: Accreditation requirements for acute care hospitals*. Chicago, IL: Accreditation Association for Hospitals and Health Systems. (Level VII)

26 DNV GL-Healthcare USA, Inc. (2020). MR.2.SR.1. *NIAHO® accreditation requirements, interpretive guidelines and surveyor guidance – revision 20.0.* Milford, OH: DNV GL-Healthcare USA, Inc. (Level VII)

27 Brown, L. K., & Lee, W. (2021). Titration of positive airway pressure therapy for adults with obstructive sleep apnea In: *UpToDate*, Collop, N,. (Ed.).

CONTINUOUS RENAL REPLACEMENT THERAPY

Continuous renal replacement therapy (CRRT) is an extracorporeal purification therapy used to treat patients with acute kidney injury. Unlike the more traditional hemodialysis, CRRT is administered around the clock, providing patients with continuous therapy and sparing them the destabilizing hemodynamic and electrolytic changes characteristic of traditional hemodialysis. CCRT is a treatment for patients who can't tolerate traditional dialysis, such as those with hemodynamic instability. For such patients, CRRT is commonly the only choice of treatment.

The techniques used vary in complexity.[1] Slow continuous ultrafiltration (SCUF) uses arteriovenous or venovenous access and the patient's blood pressure to circulate blood through a hemofilter. Because the goal of this therapy is the removal of fluids, the patient doesn't receive replacement fluids to help prevent or treat fluid overload.[1] Continuous venovenous hemofiltration (CVVH) uses a double-lumen catheter to provide access to a vein, and a pump moves blood through the hemofilter. This process removes solutes and fluids primarily by convection. Replacement fluids help maintain electrolyte and acid–base balance.[2] Continuous venovenous hemodialysis (CVVHD) uses a double-lumen catheter to provide access to a vein while a pump moves dialysate solution concurrently with blood flow. This process continuously removes fluid and solutes primarily by diffusion.[2] Continuous venovenous hemodiafiltration (CVVHDF) combines the equipment and the fluid and solute removal processes of CVVH and CVVHD to continuously remove fluids and solutes by both convection and diffusion.[2] Sustained low-efficiency daily diafiltration (SLEDD) is a modification of traditional intermittent hemodialysis. SLEDD usually occurs in 4- to 12-hourtreatments,[1] administered 5 to 7 days each week. The blood flow rates range from 100 to 250 mL/minute, resulting in an extended dialysis time, decreased solute rate, and ultrafiltration.

CVVH, CVVHD, CVVHDF, or SLEDD replaces continuous arteriovenous hemofiltration (CAVH) to treat critically ill patients. CVVH in particular has several advantages over CAVH: it doesn't require arterial access, it's appropriate for patients with low mean arterial pressures, and it has a better solute clearance.

Before the procedure, the practitioner inserts a double-lumen vascular access catheter; the internal jugular vein is the preferred insertion site.[1] The practitioner should avoid the subclavian site in patients with advanced kidney disease to prevent subclavian stenosis,[3] and the femoral insertion site in patients with obesity because of its association with an increased risk of infection.[3,4]

HOSPITAL-ACQUIRED CONDITION ALERT Keep in mind that the Centers for Medicare and Medicaid Services considers vascular catheter–associated infection a hospital-acquired condition *because it can be reasonably prevented using a variety of best practices.* Make sure to follow evidence-based prevention practices, such as performing hand hygiene, properly preparing the access site, and maintaining sterile technique, when accessing the patient's double-lumen catheter *to reduce the risk of vascular catheter–associated infections.*[3,4,5,6,7,8]

Equipment

CRRT equipment (pump or other CRRT device, tubing with hemofilter) ▪ prescribed volume of normal saline flush solution ▪ prescribed dialysate solution ▪ sterile and clean gloves ▪ mask with face shield or mask and goggles ▪ gown ▪ mask for patient ▪ antiseptic pads (chlorhexidine or povidone -iodine) ▪ sterile syringes (10 mL) ▪ prefilled preservative-free normal saline flush syringes (10 mL) ▪ sterile drape ▪ cardiac monitor with leads and electrodes ▪ stethoscope ▪ vital signs monitoring equipment ▪ disinfectant pad ▪ facility-approved disinfectant ▪ pulse oximeter and probe ▪ scale ▪ securement devices ▪ prescribed anticoagulant flush ▪ Optional: prescribed replacement solution, occlusive dressing for catheter insertion sites, supplies for blood sampling, prescribed insulin, prescribed IV fluids, infusion pump (preferably a smart pump with dose-range alerts), hemodynamic monitoring equipment, extra blankets or warming blanket, prescribed thrombolytic therapy, labels.

Preparation of equipment

Inspect all equipment and supplies. If a product is expired, is defective, or has compromised integrity, remove it from patient use, label it as expired or defective, and report the expiration or defect as directed by your facility. Check the sterility of the hemofilter and blood tubing. Prime the CRRT circuit and set up the CRRT device or pump according to the manufacturer's instructions. Make sure that the CRRT device is plugged into an outlet that has an emergency power source. Ensure proper functioning of the equipment, including the blood pumps, pressure monitors, blood leak detector, air detector, and pressure safety alarms.[9] Some CRRT equipment has a screen that displays the steps for setting up the equipment. This screen may also display alarms and actions to take to correct alarms. (See *Setup for CVVH.*)

Implementation

▪ Review and verify the practitioner's CRRT treatment orders, including modality, vascular access site and type, type of CRRT device or pump, type of hemofilter, blood pump speed, anticoagulant therapy (drug, dose, infusion rate, associated laboratory tests, and anticoagulant monitoring parameters), replacement fluid (if necessary), hourly ultrafiltration rate, hourly net fluid goals, dialysate solution rate (if necessary), vital signs and hemodynamic parameter frequency, and laboratory results (including parameters for electrolyte repletion and critical values that require nephrologist notification).[8]

▪ Review the patient's medical records for a completed medical history of the patient's health, current diseases, current therapy and medications, diagnostic tests, family and social history, and allergies.[8]

▪ If required by your facility, confirm that written informed consent has been obtained and that the signed consent form is in the patient's medical record.[9,10,11,12]

▪ Verify that laboratory studies (electrolyte levels, coagulation studies, complete blood count, blood urea nitrogen, and creatinine studies) are complete as ordered, and that the results are in the patient's medical record. Notify the practitioner of any unexpected results.[8]

▪ Confirm that the practitioner verified vascular access catheter tip placement before use, if not inserted using fluoroscopy.[8]

▪ Gather and prepare the necessary equipment and supplies.

▪ If prescribed, compare the replacement fluid with the practitioner's order and make sure that the solution is sterile.[8]

▪ Verify the dialysate solution with the practitioner's order. Make sure that the solutions are clearly labeled with the date and time of expiration.[8] If any solution is expired, return it to the pharmacy and obtain new solution.[13,14,15,16]

▪ Visually inspect the solutions for particles, discoloration, or other loss of integrity; don't administer the solutions if their integrity is compromised.[13,14,15,16]

▪ Perform hand hygiene.[17,18,19,20,21,22]

▪ Confirm the patient's identity using at least two patient identifiers.[23]

▪ Provide privacy.[24,25,26,27]

▪ Explain the procedure to the patient and family (if appropriate) according to their individual communication and learning needs *to increase their understanding, allay their fears, and enhance cooperation.*[28]

▪ Make sure that the patient is attached to a cardiac monitor, blood pressure monitoring device, and pulse oximeter *to closely monitor for changes in condition.* Make sure that the alarm limits are set appropriately for the patient's current condition, and that the alarms are turned on, functioning properly, and audible to staff.[29,30,31]

▪ Obtain vital signs, including hemodynamic parameters, *to serve as a baseline for comparison.*[1,8]

▪ Assess the patient's cardiac, pulmonary, neurologic, GI, renal, hematologic, integumentary, immunologic, and psychosocial status.[8]

▪ Assess the integrity of the vascular access catheter. Assess the insertion site for redness, swelling, discoloration, bruising, drainage, bleeding, and evidence of catheter migration.[1,8]

▪ Obtain the patient's weight in kilograms *to prevent dose-related medication errors and to serve as a baseline for evaluating the effectiveness of therapy.*[1,8,32]

▪ Notify the practitioner of any assessment findings that require an alteration in the patient's treatment plan.[8]

Setup for CVVH

You'll typically perform continuous renal replacement therapy using continuous venovenous hemofiltration (CVVH). For this technique, the practitioner inserts a special catheter into a large vein, such as the internal jugular vein.[1] The practitioner then attaches tubing with a hemofilter to the catheter and uses an external pump *to move blood through the system. Because the catheter is in a vein,* the external pump moves blood through the system. The patient's venous blood moves through the arterial lumen to the pump, which then pushes the blood through the catheter to the hemofilter. The hemofilter removes fluid and toxic solutes (ultrafiltrate) from the patient's blood and drains them into a collection device. It doesn't remove blood cells *because they are too large to pass across the filter.* As the blood exits the hemofilter, the pump then pushes it through the venous lumen back to the patient.

Several components of the pump provide safety mechanisms. Pressure monitors on the pump maintain the blood flow through the circuit at a constant rate. An air detector traps air bubbles before the blood returns to the patient. A venous filter collects any blood clots that may be in the blood. A blood leak detector signals when blood is present in the dialysate. A venous clamp operates if it detects air in the circuit or if there is any disconnection in the blood line.

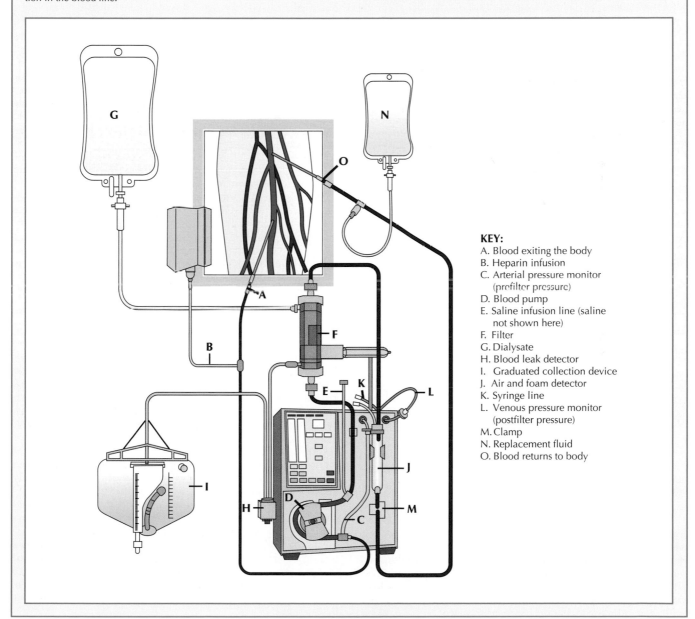

KEY:
A. Blood exiting the body
B. Heparin infusion
C. Arterial pressure monitor (profilter pressure)
D. Blood pump
E. Saline infusion line (saline not shown here)
F. Filter
G. Dialysate
H. Blood leak detector
I. Graduated collection device
J. Air and foam detector
K. Syringe line
L. Venous pressure monitor (postfilter pressure)
M. Clamp
N. Replacement fluid
O. Blood returns to body

- Position the patient for comfort.[8]
- Perform hand hygiene.[17,18,19,20,21,22]
- Put on gloves, a gown, and a mask and goggles or a mask with face shield.[33,34] Have the patient put on a mask, if possible.[8]
- Make sure that the CRRT device is set up and functioning properly. Make sure that the pressure monitors, blood leak detector, and air detector are functioning properly and that the pressure safety alarms are set, turned on, functioning properly, and audible to staff.[8,29,31]

- Prepare a sterile field. Place a sterile drape under the venous access catheter.
- Perform a vigorous mechanical scrub of the catheter hub for at least 5 seconds using a facility-approved antiseptic pad (chlorhexidine or povidone-iodine) and allow it to dry completely. (Povidone-iodine must be dry for 2 minutes.)[3,4,8,33]
- Remove your gloves and discard them in an appropriate receptacle.[34,35]
- Perform hand hygiene.[1,17,18,19,20,21,22]

Reacting in an emergency

Follow these steps if a situation arises that requires emergency intervention, such as a circuit leak, hemofilter rupture, clotting, circuit disconnection, or dialyzer or hemofilter reaction, or if the patient's condition suddenly deteriorates:[8]

- Stop the continuous renal replacement therapy (CRRT) machine's blood pump as well as the other pumps and CRRT infusions.
- Clamp and disconnect the blood lines; avoid returning the blood to the patient.
- Perform a vigorous mechanical scrub of the catheter hub using a disinfectant (2% chlorhexidine or povidone-iodine) for at least 5 seconds and allow it to dry.
- Flush each lumen of the vascular access catheter with 10 mL of preservative-free normal saline solution *to clear the lumens of blood.*
- Lock each lumen with a facility-approved flush solution and then cap them using sterile caps.
- Continue to monitor the patient's status and laboratory test results.
- Discard the CRRT system in the appropriate contaminated-waste container.
- If directed by your facility, complete an adverse occurrence report, documenting the hemofilter and blood tubing circuit lot numbers.

- Apply sterile gloves.[1,34,35]
- Attach a sterile 10-mL syringe to the arterial port and open the clamp. Withdraw the locking solution while minimizing the amount of blood withdrawn.[8] Close the clamp. Discard the waste syringe in the appropriate receptacle. Repeat this process for the venous port.[36]
- Attach a 10-mL syringe containing preservative-free normal saline flush solution to the arterial port. Open the clamp and flush with 10 mL of normal saline flush solution *to assess catheter patency and integrity.*[8] Close the clamp and repeat this process for the venous port of the access catheter.
- If catheter patency is compromised, assess for mechanical or thrombotic obstruction. If you suspect thrombotic obstruction, institute thrombolytic therapy as ordered or according to your facility's protocol.[8]
- Using sterile technique, disconnect the cap from the arterial side of the primed tubing. Trace the tubing from the patient to the point of origin and then, using sterile technique, connect the arterial line to the hemofilter circuit.[37] Repeat this process for the venous side and secure both connections.[8] Route the tubing in a standardized direction if the patient has other tubing and catheters that have different purposes. Label the tubing at the distal (near the patient connection) and proximal (near the source container) ends *to reduce the risk of misconnection* if multiple IV lines will be used.[38]
- Keep the vascular access device and connections visible at all times *to promptly detect misconnections.*[8]
- If your facility uses a bar code technology, use it as directed by your facility.

NURSING ALERT Dialysate is considered a high-alert medication *because it can cause significant harm when used in error.*[39]

- If required by your facility, have another nurse perform an independent double-check of the dialysate *to verify the patient's identity and to make sure that the correct dialysate is hanging in the prescribed concentration, the medication's indication corresponds with the patient's diagnosis, the dosage calculations are correct, the dosing formula used to derive the final dose is correct, the route of administration is safe and proper for the patient, the pump settings are correct, and the infusion lines are attached to the correct ports.*[40] Rectify any inconsistencies before beginning treatment.
- Open the clamps on the arterial and venous tubing. Turn on the blood pump and monitor the blood flow rate through the circuit.[1] Start the flow rate at half the prescribed rate (or as directed by your facility), assess the patient's response, and then increase it to the prescribed rate.[8]
- Remove the patient's mask, if worn.
- Administer an anticoagulant, as indicated and prescribed, following safe medication administration practices. Have another nurse perform an independent double-check if required by your facility. Tailor administration to the patient's response and the practitioner-ordered parameters.[1,8,13,14,15,16,41]

- Begin administering the dialysate at the prescribed rate, and start the ultrafiltration process, as indicated by the type of machine used.[8]
- Secure the hemofilter and all line connections using appropriate securement devices; keep the connections visible *to detect dangerous disconnections promptly.*[8]
- Closely monitor the patient's response to the initiation of therapy; changes in heart rate and rhythm, blood pressure, and physical condition, such as dizziness or increased anxiety, may occur.[8] Watch for signs and symptoms of dialyzer or hemofilter reaction (hypotension, pruritus, back pain, angioedema, arrhythmia, and anaphylaxis).[8]
- Monitor and record the blood flow rate and ultrafiltration flow rate at least hourly. Record changes that occur as a result of the practitioner's order or the patient's response to treatment.[8]
- Monitor the patient's temperature, blood pressure, heart rate, cardiac rhythm, respiratory status, oxygen saturation level, intravascular and extravascular fluid status, and level of consciousness. Assess central venous pressure and other hemodynamic parameters (pulmonary artery pressure, pulmonary artery wedge pressure, and cardiac output and index) if available.[8]
- If the patient exhibits signs and symptoms of decreased body temperature, such as hemodynamic instability, shivering, piloerection, skin pallor, coolness, or cyanosis, assess for factors that might be contributing to a decrease in core temperature. Adjust the CRRT machine's operational temperature as ordered and according to the manufacturer's instructions. Provide the patient with extra blankets or use a warming blanket if indicated.[8]
- Obtain blood samples for laboratory testing, as ordered or according to protocol, *to monitor blood glucose, blood urea nitrogen, and creatinine levels; coagulation and hematologic status; and acid–base and electrolyte balance.* Report critical test results to the practitioner within the time frame established by your facility *to prevent treatment delays.*[41,42]
- Adjust prescribed IV fluids, if used, *to correct electrolyte imbalances.* Administer intermittent electrolyte infusions, as ordered, *for repletion.*[8]
- If the patient's blood glucose levels are elevated, collaborate with the patient's practitioner to adjust the glucose concentration in the dialysate solution; modify the replacement fluid composition if possible and appropriate; or administer insulin as prescribed following safe medication administration practices.[8,13,14,15,16]
- Monitor the patient for signs and symptoms of dialysis disequilibrium syndrome (although rare with CRRT), such as headache, nausea or vomiting, hypertension, decreased sensorium, seizures, and coma.[8]
- Inspect the ultrafiltrate during the procedure; it should remain clear yellow with no gross blood. Pink-tinged or bloody ultrafiltrate may signal a membrane leak in the hemofilter, which permits bacterial contamination and possible exsanguination; if you observe this sign, stop the treatment. (See *Reacting in an emergency.*)[8] Prepare a new system to restart therapy, as indicated.
- Calculate the volume of required replacement fluid every hour, as ordered. Infuse the prescribed amount and type of replacement fluid through the infusion pump into the arterial side of the circuit *to achieve the planned fluid balance.*

NURSING ALERT The practitioner prescribes the targeted net fluid loss. *To calculate the volume of replacement fluid to administer,* first determine the patient's total fluid loss in the previous hour by inspecting the collection device. Then add that amount to any other fluid losses (such as blood loss, emesis, or nasogastric drainage); the sum is the total fluid loss. From the total fluid loss, subtract the patient's fluid intake from the past hour, then subtract the net fluid loss prescribed by the practitioner. This calculation will give you the volume of replacement fluid to infuse.

- Flush the CRRT circuit with the prescribed volume of normal saline solution at the prescribed interval and as needed *to maintain patency.* Be sure to include the flush solution in the patient's hourly fluid intake.[8]
- Assess the CRRT circuit and hemofilter for signs of altered patency, such as arterial and venous pressure changes, dark fibers in the hemofilter, changes in transmembrane pressure, separation of formed cells and serum in the tubing, or a decrease in hemofilter temperature. If you note such signs, prepare for a system change, as necessary.[8]
- If the hemofilter or blood tubing clots, clamp the blood lines, disconnect the CRRT system from the vascular access device, and discard the

circuit. Maintain the vascular access device *to maintain patency until you can reinitiate therapy.*

- Monitor vascular access device function at least every 30 minutes during treatment.[8]
- Perform site care and dressing changes using sterile technique if the dressing is soiled or no longer intact,[3] and at intervals determined by your facility.[3,4,5,6,7]
- Remove and discard your personal protective equipment.[34,35]
- Perform hand hygiene.[17,18,19,20,21,22]
- Clean and disinfect your stethoscope using a disinfectant pad *to prevent the spread of infection.*[43,44]
- Perform hand hygiene.[17,18,19,20,21,22]
- Put on gloves, if needed.[34,35]
- Clean and disinfect other reusable equipment according to the manufacturer's instructions *to prevent the spread of infection.*[43,44]
- Remove and discard your gloves, if worn.[36]
- Perform hand hygiene.[17,18,19,20,21,22]
- Document the procedure.[45,46,47,48]

Special considerations

- The Joint Commission issued a sentinel event alert concerning medical device alarm safety, *because alarm-related events have been associated with permanent loss of function or death.* Among the major contributing factors were improper alarm settings, alarm settings turned off inappropriately, and alarm signals not audible to staff. Make sure that alarm limits are set appropriately and that alarms are turned on, functioning properly, and audible to staff. Follow facility guidelines for preventing alarm fatigue.[29]
- The Joint Commission issued a sentinel event alert related to managing risk during transition to new International Organization for Standardization tubing standards that were designed to prevent dangerous tubing misconnections, which can lead to serious patient injury and death. During the transition, trace the tubing and catheter from the patient to the point of origin before connecting or reconnecting any device or infusion, at any care transition (such as a new setting or service), and as part of the hand-off process; route tubes and catheters having different purposes in different standardized directions; when there are different access sites or several bags hanging, label the tubing at the distal and proximal ends; use tubing and equipment only as intended; and store medications for different delivery routes in separate locations.[38]

Complications

Possible complications of CRRT include bleeding from catheter sites, hemorrhage, hemofilter occlusion, infection, hypothermia, unstable hemodynamics, vascular access limb ischemia, thrombosis, dialysis disequilibrium syndrome (decreased neurologic status, seizure activity, hypertension, nausea or vomiting, and coma), dialyzer reaction (hypotension, anaphylaxis, pruritus, angioedema, and back pain), hypoxemia, and air embolism.[1]

Documentation

Document the date and time the treatment began, the mode of therapy, and filter changes. Note the appearance of the vascular access site, patency, quality of blood flow, and ease of access. Document the type of dressing change, the condition of the insertion site, and the date and time. Record patient assessments, including vital signs, hemodynamic findings, and neurologic and respiratory assessments. Document the blood flow rate and arterial and venous monitoring pressures. Record the type of dialysate used, replacement fluids, and hourly fluid balance information. Note the anticoagulant type and dose, if used. Record the quality of pulses distal to the vascular access site. Document the patient's tolerance of the procedure, any complications that occurred, the practitioner who was notified, the date and time of notification, interventions performed, and the patient's response to those interventions. Document the patient's weight in kilograms and pertinent laboratory assessment information. Document teaching provided to the patient and family (if applicable), their understanding of that teaching, and any need for follow-up teaching.

REFERENCES

1 Wiegand, D. L. (2017). *AACN procedure manual for high acuity, progressive, and critical care* (7th ed.). St. Louis, MO: Elsevier.

2 American Nephrology Nurses Association. (2020). *Core curriculum for nephrology nursing* (7th ed.). Pitman, NJ: American Nephrology Nurses Association.

3 Centers for Disease Control and Prevention. (2011, revised 2017). Guidelines for the prevention of intravascular catheter-related infections. https://www.cdc.gov/infectioncontrol/guidelines/bsi/recommendations.html

4 Marschall, J., et al. (2014). SHEA/IDSA practice recommendation: Strategies to prevent central line–associated bloodstream infections in acute care hospitals. *Infection Control and Hospital Epidemiology, 35*(7), 753–771. https://www.jstor.org/stable/10.1086/676533#metadata_info_tab_contents (Level I)

5 Accreditation Association for Hospitals and Health Systems. (2020). Standard 07.01.19. *Healthcare Facilities Accreditation Program: Accreditation requirements for acute care hospitals.* Chicago, IL: Accreditation Association for Hospitals and Health Systems. (Level VII)

6 Accreditation Association for Hospitals and Health Systems. (2020). Standard 07.01.02. *Healthcare Facilities Accreditation Program: Accreditation requirements for acute care hospitals.* Chicago, IL: Accreditation Association for Hospitals and Health Systems. (Level VII)

7 Jarrett, N., & Callahan, M. (2016). Evidence-based guidelines for selected hospital-acquired conditions: Final report. https://www.cms.gov/Medicare/Medicare-Fee-for-Service-Payment/HospitalAcqCond/Downloads/2016-HAC-Report.pdf

8 Gomez, N., (Ed.). (2017). *Nephrology nursing scope and standards of practice* (8th ed.). Pitman, NJ: American Nephrology Nurses Association.

9 The Joint Commission. (2021). Standard RI.01.03.01. *Comprehensive accreditation manual for hospitals.* Oakbrook Terrace, IL: The Joint Commission. (Level VII)

10 Centers for Medicare and Medicaid Services, Department of Health and Human Services. (2020). Condition of participation: Patient's rights. 42 C.F.R. § 482.13.

11 Accreditation Association for Hospitals and Health Systems. (2020). Standard 15.01.11. *Healthcare Facilities Accreditation Program: Accreditation requirements for acute care hospitals.* Chicago, IL: Accreditation Association for Hospitals and Health Systems. (Level VII)

12 DNV GL-Healthcare USA, Inc. (2020). PR.2.SR.3. *NIAHO® accreditation requirements, interpretive guidelines and surveyor guidance—revision 20.0.* Milford, OH: DNV GL-Healthcare USA, Inc. (Level VII)

13 The Joint Commission. (2021). Standard MM.06.01.01. *Comprehensive accreditation manual for hospitals.* Oakbrook Terrace, IL: The Joint Commission. (Level VII)

14 Accreditation Association for Hospitals and Health Systems. (2020). Standard 16.01.03. *Healthcare Facilities Accreditation Program: Accreditation requirements for acute care hospitals.* Chicago, IL: Accreditation Association for Hospitals and Health Systems. (Level VII)

15 Centers for Medicare and Medicaid Services, Department of Health and Human Services. (2020). Condition of participation: Nursing services. 42 C.F.R. § 482.23(c).

16 DNV GL-Healthcare USA, Inc. (2020). MM.1.SR.3. *NIAHO® accreditation requirements, interpretive guidelines and surveyor guidance—revision 20.0.* Milford, OH: DNV GL-Healthcare USA, Inc. (Level VII)

17 The Joint Commission. (2021). Standard NPSG.07.01.01. *Comprehensive accreditation manual for hospitals.* Oakbrook Terrace, IL: The Joint Commission. (Level VII)

18 Centers for Disease Control and Prevention. (2002). Guideline for hand hygiene in health-care settings: Recommendations of the Healthcare Infection Control Practices Advisory Committee and the HICPAC/SHEA/APIC/IDSA Hand Hygiene Task Force. *MMWR Recommendations and Reports, 51*(RR-16), 1–45. https://www.cdc.gov/mmwr/pdf/rr/rr5116.pdf (Level II)

19 World Health Organization. (2009). WHO guidelines on hand hygiene in health care: First global patient safety challenge, clean care is safer care. https://apps.who.int/iris/bitstream/handle/10665/44102/9789241597906_eng.pdf;jsessionid=E7AA57FD101C-9C03C4E44D884F6FF02D?sequence=1 (Level IV)

20 Centers for Medicare and Medicaid Services, Department of Health and Human Services. (2020). Condition of participation: Infection control. 42 C.F.R. § 482.42.

21 Accreditation Association for Hospitals and Health Systems. (2020). Standard 07.01.21. *Healthcare Facilities Accreditation Program: Accreditation requirements for acute care hospitals.* Chicago, IL: Accreditation Association for Hospitals and Health Systems. (Level VII)

22 DNV GL-Healthcare USA, Inc. (2020). IC.1.SR.1. *NIAHO® accreditation requirements, interpretive guidelines and surveyor guidance—revision 20.0* Milford, OH: DNV GL-Healthcare USA, Inc. (Level VII)

23 The Joint Commission. (2021). Standard NPSG.01.01.01. *Comprehensive accreditation manual for hospitals.* Oakbrook Terrace, IL: The Joint Commission. (Level VII)

24 Centers for Medicare and Medicaid Services, Department of Health and Human Services. (2020). Condition of participation: Patient's rights. 42 C.F.R. § 482.13(c)(1).

25 Accreditation Association for Hospitals and Health Systems. (2020). Standard 15.01.16. *Healthcare Facilities Accreditation Program: Accreditation requirements for acute care hospitals.* Chicago, IL: Accreditation Association for Hospitals and Health Systems. (Level VII)

26 DNV GL-Healthcare USA, Inc. (2020). PR.2.SR.5. *NIAHO® accreditation requirements, interpretive guidelines and surveyor guidance—revision 20.0.* Milford, OH: DNV GL-Healthcare USA, Inc. (Level VII)

27 The Joint Commission. (2021). Standard RI.01.01.01. *Comprehensive accreditation manual for hospitals.* Oakbrook Terrace, IL: The Joint Commission. (Level VII)

28 The Joint Commission. (2021). Standard PC.02.01.21. *Comprehensive accreditation manual for hospitals.* Oakbrook Terrace, IL: The Joint Commission. (Level VII)

29 The Joint Commission. (2013). Sentinel event alert 50: Medical device alarm safety in hospitals. https://www.jointcommission.org/assets/1/6/SEA_50_alarms_4_26_16.pdf (Level VII)

30 American Association of Critical-Care Nurses. (2018). AACN practice alert: Managing alarms in acute care across the life span: Electrocardiography and pulse oximetry. https://www.aacn.org/clinical-resources/practice-alerts/managing-alarms-in-acute-care-across-the-life-span (Level VII)

31 Graham, K. C., & Cvach, M. (2010). Monitor alarm fatigue: Standardizing use of physiological monitors and decreasing nuisance alarms. *American Journal of Critical Care, 19,* 28–37.

32 Institute for Safe Medication Practices. (2020). 2020–2021 targeted medication safety best practices for hospitals. https://www.ismp.org/sites/default/files/attachments/2020-02/2020-2021%20TMSBP-%20FINAL_1.pdf

33 Standard 36. Needleless connectors. Infusion therapy standards of practice (8th ed.). (2021). *Journal of Infusion Nursing, 44,* S104–S107. (Level VII)

34 Siegel, J. D., et al. (2007, revised 2019). 2007 guideline for isolation precautions: Preventing transmission of infectious agents in healthcare settings. https://www.cdc.gov/infectioncontrol/pdf/guidelines/isolation-guidelines-H.pdf (Level II)

35 Accreditation Association for Hospitals and Health Systems. (2020). Standard 07.01.10. *Healthcare Facilities Accreditation Program: Accreditation requirements for acute care hospitals.* Chicago, IL: Accreditation Association for Hospitals and Health Systems. (Level VII)

36 Occupational Safety and Health Administration. (2012). Bloodborne pathogens, standard number1910.1030. https://www.osha.gov/pls/oshaweb/owadisp.show_document?p_id=10051&p_table=STANDARDS (Level VII)

37 U.S. Food and Drug Administration. (2017). Examples of medical device misconnections. https://www.fda.gov/medical-devices/medical-device-connectors/examples-medical-device-misconnections

38 The Joint Commission. (2014). Sentinel event alert 53: Managing risk during transition to new ISO tubing connector standards. http://www.jointcommission.org/assets/1/6/SEA_53_Connectors_8_19_14_final.pdf (Level VII)

39 Institute for Safe Medication Practices. (2018). ISMP list of high-alert medications in acute care settings. https://www.ismp.org/sites/default/files/attachments/2018-08/highAlert2018-Acute-Final.pdf (Level VII)

40 Institute for Safe Medication Practice. (2019). Independent double checks: Worth the effort if used judiciously and properly. https://www.ismp.org/resources/independent-double-checks-worth-effort-if-used-judiciously-and-properly (Level VII)

41 The Joint Commission. (2021). Standard NPSG.03.05.01. *Comprehensive accreditation manual for hospitals.* Oakbrook Terrace, IL: The Joint Commission. (Level VII)

42 The Joint Commission. (2021). Standard NPSG.02.03.01. *Comprehensive accreditation manual for hospitals.* Oakbrook Terrace, IL: The Joint Commission. (Level VII)

43 Rutala, W. A., et al. (2008, revised 2019). Guideline for disinfection and sterilization in healthcare facilities, 2008. https://www.cdc.gov/infection-control/pdf/guidelines/disinfection-guidelines-H.pdf (Level I)

44 Accreditation Association for Hospitals and Health Systems. (2020). Standard 07.02.03. *Healthcare Facilities Accreditation Program: Accreditation requirements for acute care hospitals.* Chicago, IL: Accreditation Association for Hospitals and Health Systems. (Level VII)

45 The Joint Commission. (2021). Standard RC.01.03.01. *Comprehensive accreditation manual for hospitals.* Oakbrook Terrace, IL: The Joint Commission. (Level VII)

46 Accreditation Association for Hospitals and Health Systems. (2020). Standard 10.00.03. *Healthcare Facilities Accreditation Program: Accreditation requirements for acute care hospitals.* Chicago, IL: Accreditation Association for Hospitals and Health Systems. (Level VII)

47 Centers for Medicare and Medicaid Services, Department of Health and Human Services. (2020). Condition of participation: Medical record services. 42 C.F.R. § 482.24(b).

48 DNV GL-Healthcare USA, Inc. (2020). MR.2.SR.1. *NIAHO® accreditation requirements, interpretive guidelines and surveyor guidance—revision 20.0* Milford, OH: DNV GL-Healthcare USA, Inc. (Level VII)

CRICOTHYROTOMY, ASSISTING

When endotracheal intubation or a tracheotomy can't be performed quickly and other nonsurgical methods have failed to establish an airway, an emergency cricothyrotomy may be necessary.[1] This procedure involves puncturing the trachea through the cricothyroid membrane.

Usually, your role will be to assist the physician or other specially trained practitioner responsible for airway management.[2] Ideally, cricothyrotomy is performed using sterile technique; however, sterile technique may not be possible in an emergency.

Equipment

For all types of cricothyrotomy

Gloves ▪ personal protective equipment (face mask, eye protection, gown) ▪ antiseptic solution ▪ sterile 4″ × 4″ (10 cm × 10 cm) gauze pads ▪ sterile drape ▪ sterile towels ▪ tape ▪ oxygen source ▪ oxygen delivery equipment[3] ▪ vital signs monitoring equipment ▪ pulse oximeter and probe ▪ end-tidal carbon dioxide ($ETCO_2$) detector ▪ stethoscope ▪ disinfectant pad ▪ Optional: sterile gloves, 1% lidocaine, syringe, needle.[1]

For scalpel cricothyrotomy

Scalpel ▪ #6 or smaller tracheostomy tube (if available) ▪ Trousseau dilator[1] ▪ tracheal hook[1] ▪ handheld resuscitation bag or T tube and wide-bore oxygen tubing.

For needle cricothyrotomy

14G (or larger) through-the-needle or over-the-needle catheter ▪ 10-mL syringe ▪ IV extension tubing ▪ hand-operated release valve or pressure-regulating adjustment valve.

Commercially prepared cricothyrotomy kits may be used if available at your facility.[4]

Preparation of equipment

Inspect all equipment and supplies. If a product is expired, is defective, or has compromised integrity, remove it from patient use, label it as expired or defective, and report the expiration or defect as directed by your facility.

Prepare a sterile field with the sterile drape. Pour antiseptic solution onto gauze pads. Open sterile packages and prepare the practitioner's supplies, as needed.

Implementation

▪ Have a coworker stay with the patient.
▪ Gather and prepare the necessary equipment and supplies.
▪ If possible, confirm that informed consent has been obtained and that the signed consent form is in the patient's medical record.[5,6,7,8]
▪ Perform hand hygiene.[9,10,11,12,13,14]
▪ Confirm the patient's identity using at least two patient identifiers.[15]
▪ As time permits,[4] explain the procedure to the patient and family (if appropriate) according to their individual communication and learning needs *to increase their understanding, allay their fears, and enhance cooperation.*[16]
▪ Raise the patient's bed to waist level before providing care *to prevent caregiver back strain.*[17]

■ Put on gloves and, as needed, other personal protective equipment *to comply with standard precautions.*[2,18,19]

■ Assess the patient's rate and depth of respirations, accessory muscle use, chest wall motion, and breath sounds *to identify inadequate respiratory effort.*[4]

■ Apply a pulse oximeter and ETCO₂ detector. Monitor oxygen saturation and ETCO₂ level *to identify respiratory effort.*[4]

■ Place the patient supine with the neck in a neutral position *to keep the cervical spine stabilized.*[1,2,4]

■ Administer supplemental oxygen before and throughout the procedure using the most effective delivery route (blow-by oxygen device, nasal cannula, facemask, hand-held resuscitation bag, or T-tube).[3]

■ The practitioner puts on personal protective equipment and, if available and time permits, sterile gloves. The practitioner cleans the patient's neck with antiseptic cleaning solution according to the manufacturer's instructions and allows it to dry.[2] Assist as needed.

■ Assist with draping the patient's neck with sterile towels.

■ The practitioner locates the precise insertion site by sliding the thumb and fingers down to the thyroid gland. The practitioner locates the outer borders by noting the location where the space between the fingers and thumb widens.

■ The practitioner assesses for hematomas, which may displace the trachea to the unaffected side.

■ The practitioner then moves the fingers across the center of the gland, over the anterior edge of the cricoid ring (as shown below).

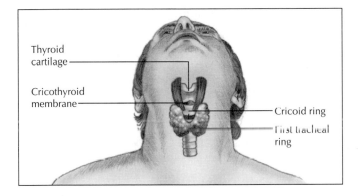

■ Assist the practitioner in anesthetizing the area with 1% lidocaine, as directed and as time allows.[1,2]

Using a scalpel

■ Hand the practitioner a scalpel. The practitioner uses the scalpel to make a horizontal incision, less than ½" (1.3 cm) long, in the cricothyroid membrane just above the cricoid ring.[1]

■ The practitioner inserts a dilator *to prevent tissue from closing around the incision.* If a dilator isn't available, the practitioner inserts the handle of the scalpel and rotates it 90 degrees[1] (as shown below).

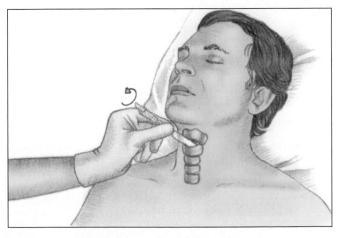

■ The practitioner inserts a tracheal hook into the opening, allowing for passage of an appropriately sized cuffed tracheostomy tube.[1] If a small tracheostomy tube (#6 or smaller) is available, the practitioner inserts it into the opening and secures it *to help maintain a patent airway*. If a tracheostomy tube isn't available, the practitioner may tape the dilator or scalpel handle in place until a tracheostomy tube is available.

■ If the patient can breathe spontaneously, attach a humidified oxygen source to the tracheostomy tube with a T tube; if the patient can't breathe, attach a handheld resuscitation bag. Trace the tubing from the patient to its point of origin *to make sure you're attaching it to the proper port.*[20,21] You'll need to inflate the cuff of the tracheostomy tube with a syringe *to provide positive-pressure ventilation.*

■ Auscultate bilaterally for breath sounds and check the patient's ETCO₂ level *to confirm tube placement.*[4]

■ Obtain the patient's vital signs.

■ Anticipate a chest X-ray *to evaluate tube placement.*

■ Discard used supplies in appropriate receptacles.[18,19]

■ Remove and discard your gloves and other personal protective equipment, in appropriate receptacles.[18,19]

■ Perform hand hygiene.[9,10,11,12,13,14]

Using a needle

■ Attach a 10-mL syringe to a 14G (or larger) through-the-needle or over-the-needle catheter.

■ Hand the catheter to the practitioner, who inserts it into the cricothyroid membrane just above the cricoid ring.

■ The practitioner directs the catheter downward at a 45-degree angle to the trachea (as shown below) *to avoid damaging the vocal cords.* The practitioner maintains negative pressure by pulling back the syringe plunger while advancing the catheter.[1]

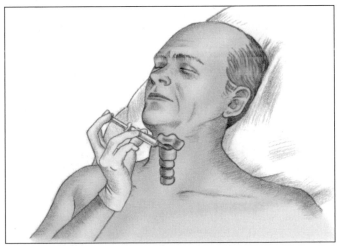

■ When the catheter reaches the trachea (when air enters the syringe), the practitioner advances it and removes the needle and syringe.[1]

■ Tape the catheter in place. Attach the catheter hub to one end of the IV extension tubing. At the other end, attach a hand-operated release valve or a pressure-regulating adjustment valve. Connect the entire assembly to an oxygen source.

■ Trace the tubing from the patient to its point of origin *to make sure that you're connecting it to the proper port.*[20,21]

■ Press the release valve to introduce oxygen into the trachea and inflate the lungs. When you can see that they're inflated, release the valve *to allow passive exhalation.* Adjust the pressure-regulating valve to the minimum pressure needed for adequate lung inflation.

■ Auscultate bilaterally for breath sounds and check the patient's ETCO₂ level *to confirm tube placement.*[4]

■ Obtain the patient's vital signs.

■ Anticipate a chest X-ray *to evaluate tube placement.*

■ Discard used supplies in appropriate receptacles.[18,19]

■ Discard your gloves and other personal protective equipment in appropriate receptacles.[18,19]

■ Perform hand hygiene.[9,10,11,12,13,14]

Completing the procedure

- Monitor the patient's heart rate, blood pressure, respiratory rate, and oxygen saturation throughout the procedure.[2]
- Check for bleeding at the insertion site; subcutaneous emphysema or inadequate ventilation, which might indicate tube displacement or an air leak; and tracheal or vocal cord damage.
- Return the patient's bed to the lowest position *to prevent falls and maintain patient safety.*[22]
- Perform hand hygiene.[9,10,11,12,13,14]
- Clean and disinfect your stethoscope using a disinfectant pad.[23,24]
- Perform hand hygiene.[9,10,11,12,13,14]
- Document the procedure.[25,26,27,28]

Special considerations

PEDIATRIC ALERT Scalpel cricothyrotomy isn't recommended for children younger than age 12 *because it could damage the cricoid cartilage*—the only circumferential support to the upper trachea.

- Whenever possible, use an ultrasound machine *to visualize the patient's anatomy* before starting the procedure.[2]
- If time allows, and if your facility indicates that cricothyrotomy falls within universal protocol guidelines, follow the necessary steps, including conducting a time-out immediately before starting the procedure, *to ensure that you have identified the correct patient, site, positioning, and procedure, and that (as applicable) all relevant information and necessary equipment are available.*[29,30,31]
- The Joint Commission issued a sentinel event alert related to managing risk during transition to new International Organization for Standardization tubing standards that were designed to prevent dangerous tubing misconnections, which can lead to serious patient injury and death. During the transition, be sure to trace each tubing and catheter from the patient to its point of origin before connecting or reconnecting any device or infusion, at any care transition (such as to a new setting or service), and as part of the hand-off process; route tubes and catheters having different purposes in different standardized directions; when the patient has different access sites or several bags hanging, label tubing at the distal and proximal ends; use tubing and equipment only as intended; and store medications for different delivery routes in separate locations.[21]

Complications

Complications include failure to obtain the airway and damage to the structures, including laceration of the thyroid cartilage, cricoid cartilage, or tracheal rings. Other complications include false passage of the tube into an extratracheal location, tracheostomy, infection, and subglottic stenosis.[2]

Documentation

Document the date and time of the procedure, circumstances necessitating the procedure, assessment findings, and the patient's vital signs before, during, and after the procedure. Document the size and type of tube the practitioner inserted and the centimeter mark at the skin opening. Document confirmation of proper tube placement (X-ray findings), $ETco_2$ level, and auscultation findings. Note whether spontaneous respirations occurred after the procedure. Record how much oxygen was administered and by what method. Note any procedures the practitioner performed (such as endotracheal intubation) after establishing the airway. Document any difficulties that occurred during the procedure, prescribed treatment, and the patient's response to the treatment. Also document any medications you administered and the patient's response.[4] Document teaching provided to the patient and family (if applicable), their understanding of that teaching, and any need for follow-up teaching.

REFERENCES

1 Markowitz, J. E. (2020). Surgical airway techniques. https://emedicine.medscape.com/article/80241-overview#a1

2 Sakles, J. C. (2021). Emergency cricothyrotomy (cricothyroidotomy). In: *UpToDate*, Wolfson, A. B,. (Ed.).

3 Apfelbaum, J. L., et al. (2013). Practice guidelines for management of the difficult airway: An updated report by the American Society of Anesthesiologists Task Force on Management of the Difficult Airway. *Anesthesiology, 118*, 251–270. (Level VII)

4 Wiegand, D. L. (2017). *AACN procedure manual for high acuity, progressive, and critical care* (7th ed.). St. Louis, MO: Elsevier.

5 The Joint Commission. (2021). Standard RI.01.03.01. *Comprehensive accreditation manual for hospitals.* Oakbrook Terrace, IL: The Joint Commission. (Level VII)

6 Centers for Medicare and Medicaid Services, Department of Health and Human Services. (2020). Condition of participation: Patient's rights. 42 C.F.R. § 482.13.

7 Accreditation Association for Hospitals and Health Systems. (2020). Standard 15.01.11. *Healthcare Facilities Accreditation Program: Accreditation requirements for acute care hospitals.* Chicago, IL: Accreditation Association for Hospitals and Health Systems. (Level VII)

8 DNV GL-Healthcare USA, Inc. (2020). PR.2.SR.3. *NIAHO® accreditation requirements, interpretive guidelines and surveyor guidance—revision 20.0.* Milford, OH: DNV GL-Healthcare USA, Inc. (Level VII)

9 The Joint Commission. (2021). Standard NPSG.07.01.01. *Comprehensive accreditation manual for hospitals.* Oakbrook Terrace, IL: The Joint Commission. (Level VII)

10 Centers for Disease Control and Prevention. (2002). Guideline for hand hygiene in health-care settings: Recommendations of the Healthcare Infection Control Practices Advisory Committee and the HICPAC/SHEA/APIC/IDSA Hand Hygiene Task Force. *MMWR Recommendations and Reports, 51*(RR-16), 1–45. https://www.cdc.gov/mmwr/pdf/rr/rr5116.pdf (Level II)

11 World Health Organization. (2009). WHO guidelines on hand hygiene in health care: First global patient safety challenge, clean care is safer care. https://apps.who.int/iris/bitstream/handle/10665/44102/9789241597906_eng.pdf?sequence=1 (Level IV)

12 Centers for Medicare and Medicaid Services, Department of Health and Human Services. (2020). Condition of participation: Infection control. 42 C.F.R. § 482.42.

13 Accreditation Association for Hospitals and Health Systems. (2020). Standard 07.01.21. *Healthcare Facilities Accreditation Program: Accreditation requirements for acute care hospitals.* Chicago, IL: Accreditation Association for Hospitals and Health Systems. (Level VII)

14 DNV GL-Healthcare USA, Inc. (2020). IC.1.SR.1. *NIAHO® accreditation requirements, interpretive guidelines and surveyor guidance—revision 20.0.* Milford, OH: DNV GL-Healthcare USA, Inc. (Level VII)

15 The Joint Commission. (2021). Standard NPSG.01.01.01. *Comprehensive accreditation manual for hospitals.* Oakbrook Terrace, IL: The Joint Commission. (Level VII)

16 The Joint Commission. (2021). Standard PC.02.01.21. *Comprehensive accreditation manual for hospitals.* Oakbrook Terrace, IL: The Joint Commission. (Level VII)

17 Waters, T. R., et al. (2009). Safe patient handling training for schools of nursing. https://www.cdc.gov/niosh/docs/2009-127/pdfs/2009-127.pdf (Level VII)

18 Siegel, J. D., et al. (2007, revised 2019). 2007 guideline for isolation precautions: Preventing transmission of infectious agents in healthcare settings. https://www.cdc.gov/infectioncontrol/pdf/guidelines/isolation-guidelines-H.pdf (Level II)

19 Accreditation Association for Hospitals and Health Systems. (2020). Standard 07.01.10. *Healthcare Facilities Accreditation Program: Accreditation requirements for acute care hospitals.* Chicago, IL: Accreditation Association for Hospitals and Health Systems. (Level VII)

20 U.S. Food and Drug Administration. (2017). Examples of medical device misconnections. https://www.fda.gov/medical-devices/medical-device-connectors/examples-medical-device-misconnections

21 The Joint Commission. (2014). Sentinel event alert 53: Managing risk during transition to new ISO tubing connector standards. http://www.jointcommission.org/assets/1/6/SEA_53_Connectors_8_19_14_final.pdf (Level VII)

22 Ganz, D. A., et al. (2013, reviewed 2021). *Preventing falls in hospitals: A toolkit for improving quality of care* (AHRQ Publication No. 13-0015-EF). Rockville, MD: Agency for Healthcare Research and Quality. https://www.ahrq.gov/professionals/systems/hospital/fallpxtoolkit/index.html (Level VII)

23 Rutala, W. A., et al. (2008, revised 2019). Guideline for disinfection and sterilization in healthcare facilities, 2008. https://www.cdc.gov/infection-control/pdf/guidelines/disinfection-guidelines-H.pdf (Level I)

24 Accreditation Association for Hospitals and Health Systems. (2020). Standard 07.02.03. *Healthcare Facilities Accreditation Program: Accreditation requirements for acute care hospitals.* Chicago, IL: Accreditation Association for Hospitals and Health Systems. (Level VII)

25 The Joint Commission. (2021). Standard RC.01.03.01. *Comprehensive accreditation manual for hospitals.* Oakbrook Terrace, IL: The Joint Commission. (Level VII)

26 Centers for Medicare and Medicaid Services, Department of Health and Human Services. (2020). Condition of participation: Medical record services. 42 C.F.R. § 482.24(b).

27 Accreditation Association for Hospitals and Health Systems. (2020). Standard 10.00.03. *Healthcare Facilities Accreditation Program: Accreditation requirements for acute care hospitals.* Chicago, IL: Accreditation Association for Hospitals and Health Systems. (Level VII)

28 DNV GL-Healthcare USA, Inc. (2020). MR.2.SR.1. *NIAHO® accreditation requirements, interpretive guidelines and surveyor guidance—revision 20.0.* Milford, OH: DNV GL-Healthcare USA, Inc. (Level VII)

29 The Joint Commission. (2021). Standard UP.01.01.01. *Comprehensive accreditation manual for hospitals.* Oakbrook Terrace, IL: The Joint Commission. (Level VII)

30 The Joint Commission. (2020). Standard UP.01.03.01. *Comprehensive accreditation manual for hospitals.* Oakbrook Terrace, IL: The Joint Commission. (Level VII)

31 Accreditation Association for Hospitals and Health Systems. (2020). Standard 30.00.14. *Healthcare Facilities Accreditation Program: Accreditation requirements for acute care hospitals.* Chicago, IL: Accreditation Association for Hospitals and Health Systems. (Level VII)

CRUTCHES USE TRAINING

Crutches improve balance, assist propulsion, and remove weight from one or both legs, enabling patients to support themselves with their hands and arms. Typically prescribed for the patient with lower extremity injury or weakness, or one who has undergone a surgical procedure on a lower limb, crutches require balance, stamina, and upper-body strength for successful use.[1] Crutch selection and walking gait depend on the patient's condition. The patient who can't use crutches may be able to use a walker.

Two types of crutches are currently prescribed by practitioners: axillary and nonaxillary. Patients with a sprain, strain, or cast should use axillary crutches, which are made of standard aluminum or wood. The primary advantage of axillary crutches is that they allow transfer of most of the patient's body weight.[2] Axillary crutches provide better trunk support than nonaxillary crutches.

Nonaxillary crutches include forearm crutches and platform crutches. These crutches are intended for long-term use.[2] Forearm crutches transfer the weight of the patient to the upper arms and are indicated for patients with good upper-body strength who have generalized weakness in the lower extremities, such as patients with paraplegia or cerebral palsy.[2] An aluminum forearm crutch has a collar that fits around the forearm and a horizontal handgrip that provides support. A wooden forearm crutch resembles wooden axillary crutches that end proximally with a closed leather band that can be situated around the proximal portion of the forearm. A platform crutch transfers the weight of the patient to the forearms.[2] It includes a platform placed on the top level of the crutch, a vertical handgrip placed at the distal end of the platform, and Velcro straps applied around the patient's forearm. This type of crutch is indicated for a patient with a painful wrist or hand condition (such as arthritis), a weak handgrip because of pain or deformity of the hand or wrist, or elbow contractures.

Equipment

Crutches with axillary or forearm pads, handgrips, and rubber suction tips ■ Optional: gait belt, full-length mirror.

Preparation of equipment

After choosing the appropriate crutches, adjust their height with the patient standing or, if necessary, recumbent. (See *Fitting a patient for crutches,* page 226.)

Implementation

■ Consult with the patient's practitioner and physical therapist *to coordinate rehabilitation orders and teaching.*
■ Determine the patient's weight-bearing status *to help determine which gait to teach the patient.*

■ Perform hand hygiene.[4,5,6,7,8,9]
■ Confirm the patient's identity using at least two patient identifiers.[10]
■ Provide privacy.[11,12,13,14]
■ Explain the procedure to the patient and family (if appropriate) according to their individual communication and learning needs *to increase their understanding, allay their fears, and enhance cooperation.*[15]
■ Place a gait belt around the patient's waist, if necessary, *to help prevent falls.* Tell the patient to position the crutches and to shift his or her weight from side to side.
■ Place the patient in front of a full-length mirror, if available, *to facilitate learning and coordination.*
■ Teach the four-point gait to the patient who can bear weight on both legs. Although this is the safest gait, *because three points are always in contact with the floor,* it requires greater coordination than other gaits *because it requires constant shifting of weight.* Use this sequence: right crutch, left foot, left crutch, right foot.[2] Suggest counting *to help develop rhythm,* and make sure each short step is of equal length. If the patient gains proficiency at this gait, teach the faster two-point gait. (See *Crutch gaits,* page 227.)
■ Teach the three-point gait to the patient who can bear only partial or no weight on one leg. Instruct the patient to advance both crutches 6″ to 8″ (15.2 to 20.3 cm) along with the affected leg. Then tell the patient to bring the unaffected leg forward and to bear the bulk of the weight on the crutches, but to put some on the affected leg, if possible and ordered.[2] Stress the importance of taking steps of equal length and duration, with no pauses.
■ Teach the two-point gait to the patient with weak legs but good coordination and arm strength. This is the most natural crutch-walking gait *because it mimics walking,* with alternating swings of the arms and legs. Instruct the patient to advance the left foot and right crutch simultaneously, followed by the right foot and left crutch.[2]
■ Teach the swing-to or swing-through gaits—the fastest ones—to the patient with complete paralysis of the hips and legs. Instruct the patient to advance both crutches simultaneously and to swing the legs parallel to (swing-to) or beyond (swing-through) the crutches.[2]
■ To teach the patient to get up from a chair, tell the patient to hold both crutches in one hand, with the tips resting firmly on the floor. The patient should then push up from the chair with the free hand while supporting the body with the crutches.
■ To teach the patient to sit down in a chair, instruct the patient to reverse the process of getting up. Tell the patient to support the body with the crutches in one hand, place the other hand on the chair, and then slowly lower the body into the chair.
■ To teach the patient to ascend stairs using the three-point gait, tell the patient to lead with the unaffected ("good") leg and to follow with both the crutches and the affected ("bad") leg. To descend stairs, the patient should lead with the crutches and the affected ("bad") leg and follow with the unaffected ("good") leg. The patient may find it helpful to remember the phrase, "up with the good; down with the bad."
■ Have the patient provide return demonstrations using the appropriate gait, using a chair, and negotiating stairs.
■ Remove the gait belt, if used
■ Perform hand hygiene.[4,5,6,7,8,9]
■ Document the procedure.[16,17,18,19]

Special considerations

■ Consult with the physical therapy department during crutch use training[20] *because, at a minimum, training should include aerobic conditioning exercises, coordination and balancing exercises, and range-of-motion and muscle strengthening of the upper and lower limbs.* Also, teach the patient two gaits if possible—one fast and one slow—*because the patient can alternate between them to prevent excessive muscle fatigue and to adjust more easily to various walking conditions.*
■ Encourage the patient to remove rugs and clutter from the floor *to decrease the risk of falls.*[20]
■ Have the patient wear shoes with nonskid soles, such as tennis shoes or other flat rubber-soled shoe, *to avoid slipping.*[20]
■ Instruct the patient not to move too fast or to swing the leg too far forward while using crutches, *because this could cause a loss of balance.*
■ Check the wing nuts or locking mechanisms on the crutches daily *to make sure they're tightened securely.*

EQUIPMENT

Fitting a patient for crutches

The procedure for fitting a patient for crutches depends on the type of crutches the patient will use.

Fitting axillary crutches

To measure for axillary crutches, position each crutch so that it extends from a point 4″ to 6″ (10.2 to 15.2 cm) to the side of the foot and 1″ to 1½″ (2.5 to 3.8 cm, or about the width of two fingers) below the axillary fold.[3]

Adjust the handgrip so that the patient's elbow is flexed at a 30-degree angle and the wrist is flexed at a 15-degree angle when the patient is standing with the crutches in the resting position.[2] The handgrip should be even with the top of the hip line. Check that the vinyl padding on the arm cuff, the rubber handgrip, and the rubber tip at the end of the crutches are secure.

Fitting forearm crutches

To fit forearm crutches, have the patient flex the elbow about 30 degrees so that the crease in the wrist is at the hip.[2] Then measure the patient's forearm from 3″ (7.6 cm) below the elbow (A) and add the distance between the wrist and the floor (B). This is the total length (C).

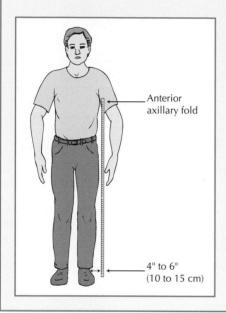
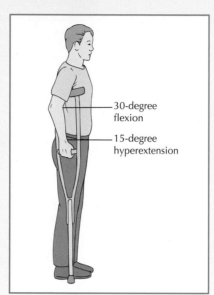
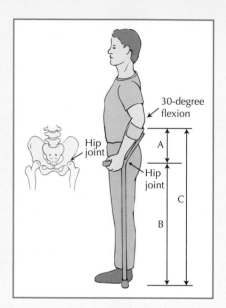

Patient teaching

Instruct the patient and family (if applicable) to contact the practitioner about any questions regarding the use of crutches or if the crutches don't fit, break, or are lost. Also instruct the patient to notify the practitioner if blisters, rashes, painful calluses, or skin breakdown of the hand, forearm, or underarm develops. Advise the patient to avoid habitually leaning on the crutches. Explain that the patient's weight should rest on the hands, not the underarm supports.[21] Instruct the patient to seek immediate care if sudden numbness of the hand or arm develops.

Complications

When used by a patient with a chronic condition, the swing-to and swing-through gaits can lead to atrophy of the hips and legs if appropriate therapeutic exercises aren't performed routinely. Prolonged pressure on the axillae can damage the brachial nerves, causing brachial nerve palsy. Crutch use can also lead to blisters, rashes, painful calluses, and skin breakdown of the hand, forearm, and underarm.

Documentation

Record the date and time of training, the type of gait, the amount of assistance required, the distance walked, and the patient's tolerance of the crutches and gait. Document teaching provided to the patient and family (if applicable), their understanding of that teaching, and any need for follow-up teaching.

REFERENCES

1 Edelstein, J. (2019). Canes, crutches, and walkers. In Webster, J. & Murphy, D. (Eds.), *Atlas of orthoses and assistive devices* (5th ed.). Philadelphia, PA: Elsevier.

2 Warees, W. M., et al. (2021). Crutches. *StatPearls*. https://www.ncbi.nlm.nih.gov/books/NBK539724/

3 American College of Foot and Ankle Surgeons. (n.d.). Instructions for using crutches. https://www.acfas.org/footankleinfo/crutches.htm

4 The Joint Commission. (2021). Standard NPSG.07.01.01. *Comprehensive accreditation manual for hospitals*. Oakbrook Terrace, IL: The Joint Commission. (Level VII)

5 Centers for Disease Control and Prevention. (2002). Guideline for hand hygiene in health-care settings: Recommendations of the Healthcare Infection Control Practices Advisory Committee and the HICPAC/SHEA/APIC/IDSA Hand Hygiene Task Force. *MMWR Recommendations and Reports, 51*(RR-16), 1–45. https://www.cdc.gov/mmwr/pdf/rr/rr5116.pdf (Level II)

6 World Health Organization. (2009). WHO guidelines on hand hygiene in health care: First global patient safety challenge, clean care is safer care. https://apps.who.int/iris/bitstream/handle/10665/44102/9789241597906_eng.pdf?sequence=1 (Level IV)

7 Centers for Medicare and Medicaid Services, Department of Health and Human Services. (2020). Condition of participation: Infection control. 42 C.F.R. § 482.42.

8 Accreditation Association for Hospitals and Health Systems. (2020). Standard 07.01.21. *Healthcare Facilities Accreditation Program: Accreditation requirements for acute care hospitals*. Chicago, IL: Accreditation Association for Hospitals and Health Systems. (Level VII)

9 DNV GL-Healthcare USA, Inc. (2020). IC.1.SR.1. *NIAHO® accreditation requirements, interpretive guidelines and surveyor guidance—revision 20.0*. Milford, OH: DNV GL-Healthcare USA, Inc. (Level VII)

10 The Joint Commission. (2021). Standard NPSG.01.01.01. *Comprehensive accreditation manual for hospitals*. Oakbrook Terrace, IL: The Joint Commission. (Level VII)

11 The Joint Commission. (2021). Standard RI.01.01.01. *Comprehensive accreditation manual for hospitals*. Oakbrook Terrace, IL: The Joint Commission. (Level VII)

12 Centers for Medicare and Medicaid Services, Department of Health and Human Services. (2020). Condition of participation: Patient's rights. 42 C.F.R. § 482.13(c)(1).

Crutch gaits

This is a guide for using the four-point, three-point, and two-point swing-to or swing-through gaits. Start at the bottom of the chart and move upward. *Note:* Shaded areas indicate weight bearing.

FOUR-POINT GAIT	TWO-POINT GAIT	THREE-POINT GAIT	THREE-POINT-PLUS-ONE GAIT
• Partial weight bearing both feet • Maximal support provided • Requires constant shift of weight	• Partial weight bearing both feet • Provides less support • Faster than a four-point gait	• Non-weight bearing on one foot • Requires good balance • Requires arm strength • Faster gait • Non-weight bearing foot moves with crutches • Can use this gait with a walker	• Partial weight bearing on one foot and full weight bearing on the second • Crutches and affected leg move together • Requires good balance • Faster than three-point gait • Dashed line indicates partial weight bearing
4. Advance right foot	4. Advance right foot and left crutch	4. Advance unaffected foot, weight on crutches only.	4. Advance unaffected leg beyond crutches again
3. Advance left crutch	3. Advance left foot and right crutch	3. Advance both crutches, weight on unaffected foot.	3. Move crutches and affected leg forward
2. Advance left foot	2. Advance right foot and left crutch	2. Advance unaffected foot, weight on crutches only.	2. Move unaffected leg forward beyond crutches
1. Advance right crutch	1. Advance left foot and right crutch	1. Advance both crutches, weight on unaffected foot.	1. Full weight on crutches and partial weight on affected leg; move crutches and affected leg forward
Beginning stance	Beginning stance	Beginning stance	Beginning stance

13 Accreditation Association for Hospitals and Health Systems. (2020). Standard 15.01.16. *Healthcare Facilities Accreditation Program: Accreditation requirements for acute care hospitals.* Chicago, IL: Accreditation Association for Hospitals and Health Systems. (Level VII)

14 DNV GL-Healthcare USA, Inc. (2020). PR.2.SR.5. *NIAHO® accreditation requirements, interpretive guidelines and surveyor guidance—revision 20.0.* Milford, OH: DNV GL-Healthcare USA, Inc. (Level VII)

15 The Joint Commission. (2021). Standard PC.02.01.21. *Comprehensive accreditation manual for hospitals.* Oakbrook Terrace, IL: The Joint Commission. (Level VII)

16 The Joint Commission. (2021). Standard RC.01.03.01. *Comprehensive accreditation manual for hospitals.* Oakbrook Terrace, IL: The Joint Commission. (Level VII)

17 Centers for Medicare and Medicaid Services, Department of Health and Human Services. (2020). Condition of participation: Medical record services. 42 C.F.R. § 482.24(b).

18 Accreditation Association for Hospitals and Health Systems. (2020). Standard 10.00.03. *Healthcare Facilities Accreditation Program: Accreditation requirements for acute care hospitals.* Chicago, IL: Accreditation Association for Hospitals and Health Systems. (Level VII)

19 DNV GL-Healthcare USA, Inc. (2020). MR.2.SR.1. *NIAHO® accreditation requirements, interpretive guidelines and surveyor guidance—revision 20.0.* Milford, OH: DNV GL-Healthcare USA, Inc. (Level VII)

20 Craven, R. F., et al. (2021). *Fundamentals of nursing: Concepts and competencies for practice.* (9th ed.). Philadelphia, PA: Wolters Kluwer.

21 American Academy of Orthopaedic Surgeons. (2015). How to use crutches, canes, and walkers. https://orthoinfo.aaos.org/en/recovery/how-to-use-crutches-canes-and-walkers

CULTURAL ASSESSMENT

Health care workers commonly care for a diverse patient population. Becoming familiar with the cultural values, beliefs, and practices of the patient population served by the facility in which they work can help health care workers ensure that each patient receives optimal care.[1]

Each patient should be treated as an individual. Beliefs and attitudes differ among patients, and affect the ways in which they perceive and respond to illness and choose a treatment plan. The patient's attitudes and beliefs may be affected by race, gender, ethnicity, language, education level, physical, cognitive, or emotional disabilities, occupation, religion, age, sexual orientation, marital and parental status, family structure, or geographic location.

A cultural assessment helps identify a patient's individual preferences so that the multidisciplinary team can collaborate with the patient to develop a culturally sensitive care plan. Health care workers should keep in mind that, regardless of membership in a particular cultural group, the patient may have individual cultural preferences and beliefs that differ from the group's.

In addition to understanding the patient's cultural influences, health care workers should understand their own cultural values and beliefs and the ways in which those values and beliefs affect their attitudes and behaviors.[1]

Equipment

Optional: glasses, hearing aid.

Implementation

■ Perform hand hygiene.[2,3,4,5,6,7]
■ Introduce yourself to the patient and ask how to address the patient.
■ Confirm the patient's identity using at least two patient identifiers.[8]
■ Provide privacy.[9,10,11,12]
■ If the patient uses a hearing aid or glasses, make sure that they're worn when needed.
■ Ask the patient about language preference. Arrange for a medical interpreter, if needed, *because the interpreter is specially trained to facilitate communication between the patient and care provider.*[13] Speak directly to the patient even if a medical interpreter is present. If a medical interpreter isn't available, use a telephonic interpreter or a video remote interpretation service, as appropriate.[14] Avoid using family members, friends, or

staff members as medical interpreters, *because errors in understanding, communication, or both may occur.*

■ Explain the procedure to the patient and family (if appropriate) according to their individual communication and learning needs *to increase their understanding, allay their fears, and enhance cooperation.*[15] Reinforce that the information gathered during the assessment is needed to develop a care plan that meets the patient's individual needs.
■ If possible, allow the patient to choose positioning during the assessment *to ensure comfort with the amount of personal space and level of eye contact.*
■ Use open-ended questions that encourage the flow of information. Give the patient time to respond to each question.
■ Perform a quick assessment of the patient *to gain insight into physical attributes, overall appearance, hygiene, and psychological status.*
■ Ask the patient to describe the illness. Encourage the patient to include information on beliefs about the cause of the illness, time when the illness started, severity of the illness, beliefs about who or what has control over the illness, preferred treatments, expected treatment results, problems caused by the illness, and biggest illness-related fear.[16,17]
■ Listen attentively to the patient's description of the illness. Use a nonjudgmental approach that encourages dialogue.
■ Inquire about the patient's common practices when ill, including whom the patient speaks to and where health information is obtained.
■ Assess the patient's verbal and nonverbal communication.
■ Ask the patient to tell you about his or her family and their traditions, rituals, and beliefs.
■ Inquire about the family's involvement in the patient's care and care-related decisions. Ask who the major decision makers are in the family.
■ Determine whether the patient would like a visit from a religious leader or clergy member.
■ Assess the degree to which the patient's beliefs and practices align with those of the patient's traditional culture. Inquire about whether the patient uses folk medicine or a native healer's services. Ask about the patient's current neighborhood and whether the patient ever leaves it to participate in a larger cultural group. Determine whether the patient wears native dress. Question the patient about religious affiliations. Ask the patient about cultural, religious, and ethnic food and nutrition preferences.
■ Question the patient about attitudes regarding personal space and touch.
■ Assess the patient's orientation to time. For example, a future-oriented patient is commonly concerned with long-term goals and interventions that will prevent illness; a present-oriented patient is more concerned with what's happening now.
■ Ask what it means to be healthy and what the patient does to stay healthy.
■ Inquire about coping strategies that the patient uses during difficult times. For example, does the patient derive support from family members, friends, prayer, meditation, music, poetry, a higher being, or a pet?
■ Collect information about the patient's socioeconomic status *to determine whether it may affect the patient's health.*
■ Perform hand hygiene.[2,3,4,5,6,7]
■ Document the procedure.[18,19,20,21]

Special considerations

■ Keep in mind that a patient may misinterpret colloquialisms, so avoid them when possible *to prevent misunderstandings.*
■ Be sensitive to the patient's response to your questions, such as hesitating to answer or averting the eyes, *because some cultures may avoid discussing certain topics or avoid discussing certain topics with the opposite sex.*[1]

Documentation

Document your assessment findings and the patient's preferences. Record the patient's preferred language and note whether a medical interpreter was needed. Document teaching provided to the patient and family (if appropriate), their understanding of that teaching, and any need for follow-up teaching.

REFERENCES

1 Hinkle, J. L., & Cheever, K. H. (2017). *Brunner & Suddarth's textbook of medical-surgical nursing* (14th ed.). Philadelphia, PA: Wolters Kluwer.

2 Centers for Disease Control and Prevention. (2002). Guideline for hand hygiene in health-care settings: Recommendations of the Healthcare Infection Control Practices Advisory Committee and the HICPAC/SHEA/APIC/IDSA Hand Hygiene Task Force. *MMWR Recommendations and Reports, 51*(RR-16), 1–45. https://www.cdc.gov/mmwr/pdf/rr/rr5116.pdf (Level II)

3 World Health Organization. (2009). WHO guidelines on hand hygiene in health care: First global patient safety challenge, clean care is safer care. https://apps.who.int/iris/bitstream/handle/10665/44102/9789241597906_eng.pdf?sequence=1 (Level IV)

4 The Joint Commission. (2021). Standard NPSG.07.01.01. *Comprehensive accreditation manual for hospitals*. Oakbrook Terrace, IL: The Joint Commission. (Level VII)

5 DNV GL-Healthcare USA, Inc. (2020). IC.1.SR.1. *NIAHO® accreditation requirements, interpretive guidelines and surveyor guidance—revision 20.0.* Milford, OH: DNV GL-Healthcare USA, Inc. (Level VII)

6 Accreditation Association for Hospitals and Health Systems. (2020). Standard 07.01.21. *Healthcare Facilities Accreditation Program: Accreditation requirements for acute care hospitals*. Chicago, IL: Accreditation Association for Hospitals and Health Systems. (Level VII)

7 Centers for Medicare and Medicaid Services, Department of Health and Human Services. (2020). Condition of participation: Infection control. 42 C.F.R. § 482.42.

8 The Joint Commission. (2021). Standard NPSG.01.01.01. *Comprehensive accreditation manual for hospitals*. Oakbrook Terrace, IL: The Joint Commission. (Level VII)

9 The Joint Commission. (2021). Standard RI.01.01.01. *Comprehensive accreditation manual for hospitals*. Oakbrook Terrace, IL: The Joint Commission. (Level VII)

10 DNV GL-Healthcare USA, Inc. (2020). PR.2.SR.5. *NIAHO® accreditation requirements, interpretive guidelines and surveyor guidance– revision 20.0.* Milford, OH: DNV GL-Healthcare USA, Inc. (Level VII)

11 Centers for Medicare and Medicaid Services, Department of Health and Human Services. (2020). Condition of participation: Patient's rights. 42 C.F.R. § 482.13(c)(1).

12 Accreditation Association for Hospitals and Health Systems. (2020). Standard 15.01.16. *Healthcare Facilities Accreditation Program: Accreditation requirements for acute care hospitals*. Chicago, IL: Accreditation Association for Hospitals and Health Systems. (Level VII)

13 The Joint Commission. (2021). Standard RI.01.01.03. *Comprehensive accreditation manual for hospitals*. Oakbrook Terrace, IL: The Joint Commission. (Level VII)

14 National Association of the Deaf. (2016). Minimum standards for video remote interpreting services in medical settings. https://www.nad.org/about-us/position-statements/minimum-standards-for-video-remote-interpreting-services-in-medical-settings/ (Level VII)

15 The Joint Commission. (2021). Standard PC.02.01.21. *Comprehensive accreditation manual for hospitals*. Oakbrook Terrace, IL: The Joint Commission. (Level VII)

16 Campinha-Bacote, J. (2011). Delivering patient-centered care in the midst of a cultural conflict: The role of cultural competence. *Online Journal of Issues in Nursing, 16*(2), 5. http://www.nursingworld.org/MainMenuCategories/ANAMarketplace/ANAPeriodicals/OJIN/TableofContents/Vol-16-2011/No2-May-2011/Delivering-Patient-Centered-Care-in-the-Midst-of-a-Cultural-Conflict.html

17 Campinha-Bacote, J. (2002). The process of cultural competence in the delivery of healthcare services: A model of care. *Journal of Transcultural Nursing, 13*, 181–184.

18 The Joint Commission. (2021). Standard RC.01.03.01. *Comprehensive accreditation manual for hospitals*. Oakbrook Terrace, IL: The Joint Commission. (Level VII)

19 DNV GL-Healthcare USA, Inc. (2020). MR.2.SR.1. *NIAHO® accreditation requirements, interpretive guidelines and surveyor guidance—revision 20.0.* Milford, OH: DNV GL-Healthcare USA, Inc. (Level VII)

20 Centers for Medicare and Medicaid Services, Department of Health and Human Services. (2020). Condition of participation: Medical record services. 42 C.F.R. § 482.24(b).

21 Accreditation Association for Hospitals and Health Systems. (2020). Standard 10.00.03. *Healthcare Facilities Accreditation Program: Accreditation requirements for acute care hospitals*. Chicago, IL: Accreditation Association for Hospitals and Health Systems. (Level VII)

DEFIBRILLATION

Defibrillation—delivery of an electrical current to the heart using paddles or pads—is indicated to treat ventricular fibrillation (VF) or pulseless ventricular tachycardia (VT). The current causes the myocardium to depolarize, which, in turn, encourages the sinoatrial node to resume control of the heart's electrical activity.[1]

A defibrillator may be monophasic or biphasic. Defibrillators with monophasic waveforms deliver current in one direction.[1] Few monophasic defibrillators are being manufactured, but some are still in use. For monophasic defibrillation to be effective, a high amount of electrical current is required.

Based on their success in arrhythmia termination, defibrillators using biphasic waveforms are preferred to monophasic defibrillators for treatment of atrial and ventricular arrhythmias.[1,2] With biphasic defibrillation, the electrical current discharged from the pads or paddles travels in a positive direction for a specified duration and then reverses and flows in a negative direction for the remaining time of the electrical discharge (as shown below). It delivers two currents of electricity and lowers the defibrillation threshold of the heart muscle, making it possible to successfully defibrillate VF with smaller amounts of energy. The biphasic defibrillator can adjust for differences in impedance or the resistance of the current through the chest. This helps reduce the number of shocks needed to terminate VF or pulseless VT. Biphasic technology uses lower energy levels and fewer shocks, which reduces the damage to the myocardial muscle.

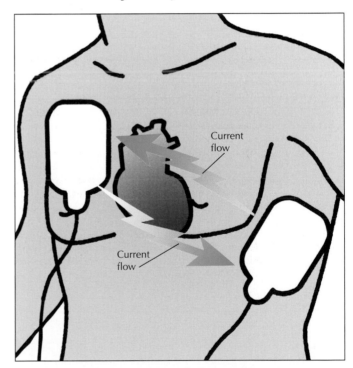

The external pads or paddles delivering the current may be placed on the patient's chest or, during cardiac surgery when the patient's chest is open, directly on the myocardium. (See *Using a defibrillator*, page 230.)

Self-adhesive defibrillation pads have been shown to be as effective as paddles, and have the advantage of delivering energy faster and safer than paddles, because energy is delivered hands-free. The pads can also be used for monitoring, and are recommended for routine use, if available.[1]

Defibrillation also can be performed using an automated external defibrillator, which commonly is used in noncritical care units and in other areas of a health care facility in which staff members have no rhythm recognition skills. (See the "Automated external defibrillation" procedure.)

EQUIPMENT

Using a defibrillator

Because ventricular fibrillation (VF) leads to death if not corrected, the success of defibrillation depends on early recognition and quick treatment of this arrhythmia. In addition to treating ventricular fibrillation (VF), defibrillation may also be used to treat ventricular tachycardia that doesn't produce a pulse.[2] *To help treat the patient as quickly as possible,* familiarize yourself with the defibrillator available at your facility. Also review the defibrillators in the photographs below to familiarize yourself with the parts of a defibrillator.

Defibrillator with self-adhesive defibrillation pads

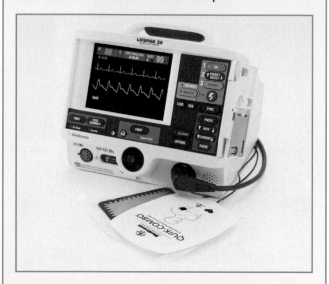

Defibrillator with paddles

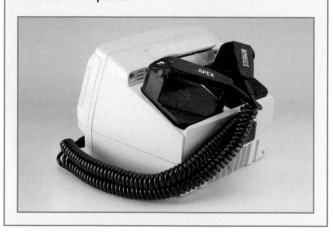

Patients with a history of VF or VT may be candidates for an implantable cardioverter-defibrillator (ICD), a sophisticated device that automatically discharges an electrical current when it senses a ventricular tachyarrhythmia. (See *Understanding the ICD.*) Defibrillation may be performed by individuals properly trained in use of the device.

Equipment

Gloves ▪ defibrillator with electrocardiogram (ECG) monitor and recorder ▪ self-adhesive defibrillation pads and connector cable, or defibrillation paddles and prepackaged gelled conduction pads ▪ emergency equipment (code cart with cardiac medications, handheld resuscitation bag with mask, suction and intubation equipment) ▪ oxygen delivery equipment ▪ facility-approved disinfectant ▪ Optional: blood pressure monitoring equipment, pulse oximeter

EQUIPMENT

Understanding the ICD

The implantable cardioverter-defibrillator (ICD) has a programmable pulse generator and lead system that monitors the heart's activity, detects ventricular bradyarrhythmias and tachyarrhythmias, and responds to each with different interventions, including antitachycardia pacing, cardioversion, defibrillation, and bradycardia pacing. Some ICDs can be programmed to pace both the atrium and ventricle or both ventricles (cardiac resynchronization therapy). Some models can also detect and correct atrial arrhythmias.

Implantation is similar to implantation of a permanent pacemaker. The cardiologist positions the lead or leads in the endocardium of the right ventricle (and the right atrium if both chambers require pacing) and then connects the other end to the generator (about the size of a wallet), which is implanted in the right or left upper chest near the collarbone. New, smaller devices can be installed through the blood vessels. These newer devices can also store information related to the arrhythmic event and perform electrophysiology testing.

and probe, stethoscope, disinfectant pads, additional prescribed medications, IV infusion equipment, supplies for obtaining a sample for arterial blood gas (ABG) analysis, supplemental oxygen supplies, 12-lead ECG machine, IV catheter insertion supplies, gown, mask with face shield or mask and goggles.

Preparation of equipment

Make sure that the defibrillation pads or paddles are connected to the defibrillator and that the defibrillator battery is adequately charged or the defibrillator electrical cord is plugged into the wall. Keep the defibrillation pads in their packages before use *to prevent the conductive gel from drying out.* Ensure that resuscitation equipment and medications are immediately available. Inspect all equipment and supplies. If a product is expired, is defective, or has compromised integrity, remove it from patient use, label it as expired or defective, and report the expiration or defect as directed by your facility.

Implementation

▪ Gather and prepare the necessary equipment and supplies.
▪ Perform hand hygiene.[3,4,5,6,7,8]
▪ Confirm the patient's identity using at least two patient identifiers.[9]
▪ Provide privacy.[10,11,12,13]
▪ If time allows, explain the procedure to the patient and family (if appropriate) according to their individual communication and learning needs *to increase their understanding, allay their fears, and enhance cooperation.*[14]
▪ Perform hand hygiene.[3,4,5,6,7,8]
▪ Put on gloves and, as needed, other personal protective equipment *to comply with standard precautions.*[15,16,17]
▪ Quickly scan the patient's location and surroundings for imminent physical threats, such as toxic or electrical hazards.[2]
▪ Assess the patient for response by tapping a shoulder and shouting, "Are you alright?" If the patient is unresponsive, shout for nearby help and immediately activate the emergency response system via mobile device (if appropriate).[2]
▪ Check for a pulse while simultaneously looking to see whether the patient is apneic or is only gasping (as opposed to breathing regularly) *to minimize delay in detecting cardiac arrest and initiating cardiopulmonary resuscitation (CPR).*[2,18]
▪ If you don't feel a pulse within 10 seconds, begin chest compressions. After 30 compressions at a rate of 100 to 120 compressions per minute,[18] open the patient's airway using a head-tilt chin-lift maneuver and give two breaths. If evidence of trauma suggests spinal injury, use a jaw-thrust maneuver to open the airway. Continue CPR until the defibrillator and emergency equipment arrive.[2,18]

■ Place the patient on a firm, flat surface as soon as possible *to make compressions more effective.*[18]

■ Make sure the environment and the patient's chest are dry, *because contact with water may cause personnel to receive a shock and the patient to receive skin burns.*[1]

■ Remove metallic objects that the patient may be wearing, *because metal conducts electricity and could cause burns during defibrillation.*[1]

■ Remove transdermal medication patches from the patient's chest (and back if using anterior–posterior placement), *because the medication may interfere with current medications and produce burns.*[1,2]

NURSING ALERT When performing defibrillation, don't place the self-adhesive pads or paddles directly over an ICD or implanted pacemaker, *because doing so may damage the device.*[1]

Defibrillation using self-adhesive defibrillation pads

■ Expose the patient's chest and apply the self-adhesive defibrillation pads. For anterolateral placement, position one pad to the right of the upper sternum, just below the right clavicle, and the other over the fifth or sixth intercostal space at the left anterior axillary line (as shown below).

Anterolateral placement

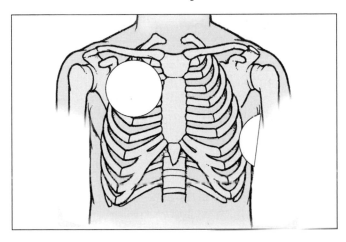

■ For anteroposterior placement, position the anterior pad directly over the heart at the precordium, to the left of the lower sternal border (as shown below).

Anterior placement

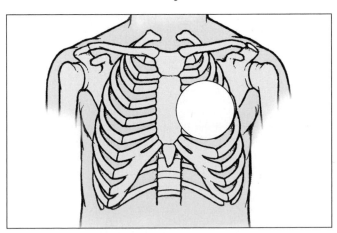

■ Place the posterior pad under the patient's body beneath the heart and immediately below the scapula but not on the vertebral column (as shown below). *Defibrillation occurs when an electrical current passes through the cardiac muscle to restore a single source of impulse production. Appropriate pad positioning maximizes the flow of electrical current through the heart.*[1]

Posterior placement

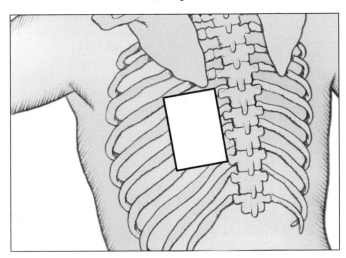

■ Turn on the defibrillator, connect the monitoring leads of the defibrillator to the patient (if needed), and assess the cardiac rhythm. If a shockable rhythm is present and you're using a biphasic defibrillator, set the clinically appropriate energy level (usually 120 to 200 joules) following the manufacturer's recommended dose.[7] If you're using a monophasic defibrillator, set the energy level for 360 joules for an adult patient.

■ Turn on the ECG recorder to document the patient's ECG and response to interventions.[1]

■ Charge the self-adhesive defibrillator pads by pressing the appropriate button on the defibrillator.

■ Reassess the patient's cardiac rhythm.

■ Disconnect the oxygen source during actual defibrillation to decrease the risk of combustion caused by arcing of the electrical current in the presence of oxygen.[1]

■ If the patient's cardiac rhythm remains in VF or pulseless VT, loudly state "all clear" or similar wording and visually verify that all personnel are clear of the patient and the bed before discharging the electrical current. *Electrical current can be conducted from the patient to anyone in contact with the patient or immediate surroundings, such as the stretcher or bed.*

■ Discharge the current by pressing the appropriate button on the defibrillator.

Defibrillation using defibrillator paddles

■ Turn on the defibrillator, expose the patient's chest, and apply the defibrillation gelled pads. For anterolateral placement, position one gelled defibrillation pad to the right of the upper sternum, just below the right clavicle, and the other over the fifth or sixth intercostal space at the left anterior axillary line. *This is the optimal pad placement when using paddles.* Alternatively, use anteroposterior pad placement, if needed. For anteroposterior placement, position the anterior gelled defibrillation pad directly over the heart at the precordium to the left of the lower sternal border. Place the posterior gelled defibrillation pad under the patient's body beneath the heart and immediately below the scapula (but not on the vertebral column). *Defibrillation occurs when an electrical current passes through the cardiac muscle to restore a single source of impulse production. Appropriate positioning of the pads maximizes the flow of electrical current through the heart.*[1]

■ Press the paddles firmly against the patient's chest on top of the gelled defibrillation pads, if available (as shown below), *to quickly view and assess the patient's cardiac rhythm on the defibrillator monitor.*[10]

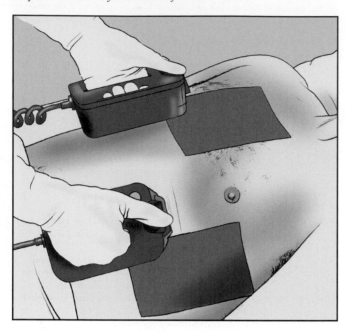

■ Connect the ECG monitoring leads of the defibrillator to the patient *to also display the cardiac rhythm.*
■ Turn on the ECG recorder to document the patient's ECG and response to interventions.
■ For a shockable rhythm, set the appropriate energy level and charge the paddles by pressing the charge buttons, located on the defibrillator or on the paddles themselves.
■ Reassess the patient's cardiac rhythm.
■ Disconnect the oxygen source before performing defibrillation *to decreases the risk of combustion caused by arcing of the electrical current in the presence of oxygen.*[1]
■ If the patient's cardiac rhythm remains in VF or pulseless VT, loudly instruct all personnel to "stand clear" of the patient and the bed. Visually verify all personnel are clear of the patient and the bed before discharging the current. *Electrical current can be conducted from the patient to anyone in contact with the patient or immediate surroundings, such as the bed.*
■ Discharge the current by pressing both paddles' charge buttons simultaneously while applying 25 lb/in² of pressure on both paddles.[19] *Using this pressure decreases transthoracic resistance.* Hold until the defibrillator delivers the electrical current.[1]

Completing the procedure
■ Resume CPR immediately after defibrillation, beginning with chest compressions. *Defibrillation is more likely to be effective if followed immediately with a cycle of chest compressions and with minimal interruption in chest compressions.*[2,18]
■ Reassess the patient's cardiac rhythm after 2 minutes (or five cycles) of CPR.
■ If the patient's cardiac rhythm remains in VF or pulseless VT, prepare to defibrillate a second time. Charge the defibrillator (monophasic at 360 joules or biphasic at 200 joules) and continue CPR while the defibrillator is charging. Announce that you're preparing to defibrillate, and follow the procedure described above.[2]
■ Resume CPR immediately after defibrillation, starting with chest compressions. Administer five cycles of CPR.[2]
■ Reassess the patient. If the patient's cardiac rhythm remains in VF or pulseless VT, defibrillate again, as needed, follow the same procedure as before.[2]
■ If defibrillation restores a normal cardiac rhythm, check the patient's central and peripheral pulses, and assess the patient's blood pressure and

heart rate. Assess the patient's respiratory status, level of consciousness, cardiac rhythm, breath sounds, skin color, and urine output. Obtain samples for baseline ABG levels and a 12-lead ECG, as ordered. Administer supplemental oxygen and ventilation, insert an IV catheter (if not already in place), and administer medications, as needed and ordered, following safe medication administration practices.[20,21,22,23] Check the patient's chest for electrical burns and treat them, as ordered. Also prepare the defibrillator for immediate reuse. (See the "IV catheter insertion and removal" procedure; the "Electrocardiogram, 12-lead" procedure; and the "Arterial puncture for blood gas analysis" procedure.)
■ Provide support and information to the patient's family, as needed. After resuscitation, inform the patient about what happened, if appropriate.
■ Discard used supplies in appropriate receptacles.[17]
■ Remove and discard your gloves and, if worn, other personal protective equipment.[17]
■ Perform hand hygiene.[3,4,5,6,7,8]
■ Clean and disinfect your stethoscope, if used, using a disinfectant wipe.[16,24]
■ Perform hand hygiene.[3,4,5,6,7,8]
■ Put on gloves and, as needed, other personal protective equipment.
■ Clean and disinfect other reusable equipment according to the manufacturer's instructions *to prevent the spread of infection.*[24,25]
■ Remove and discard your gloves and, if worn, other personal protective equipment.[17]
■ Perform hand hygiene.[3,4,5,6,7,8]
■ Document the procedure.[26,27,28,29]

Special considerations
■ The optimal sequence of advanced cardiac life support interventions isn't known, including antiarrhythmic drug administration during resuscitation and the preferred manner and timing of drug administration in relation to shock delivery.[2]
■ If defibrillation gel pads aren't available, place a conductive gel on the defibrillator paddles before use. Follow the manufacturer's instructions for use.[1]
■ Keep in mind that several factors can affect defibrillation, including the paddle size and placement, condition of the patient's myocardium, duration of the arrhythmia, chest resistance, and number of shocks delivered.[30]
■ Avoid placing a pad or paddle over a female patient's breast. Instead, place the apex of the pad or paddle at the fifth or sixth intercostal space, with the middle of the pad or paddle at the midaxillary line.[1]
■ Allow family members to remain at the bedside during resuscitation, if possible, *because it helps meet the psychosocial needs of the family and the patient in a time of crisis.*[31]
■ If the patient has a hairy chest, ensure that the self-adhesive defibrillator pads adhere to the skin by applying pressure. If the pads do not stick to the skin, quickly pull them off to remove the hair and then place new defibrillator pads on the chest.[1]

Complications
Defibrillation can cause accidental electrical shock to those providing care. Skin burns can result from using dry self-adhesive pads or applying an insufficient amount conductive medium.

Documentation
Document the procedure, including the patient's ECG rhythm before and after defibrillation; the number of times defibrillation was performed; the energy used with each attempt; whether the patient's pulse returned; the dosage, route, and time of drug administration; whether CPR was performed; how the airway was maintained; any other procedures performed; and the patient's outcome. Record the patient's vital signs and your assessment findings. Document teaching provided to the patient and family (if appropriate), their understanding of that teaching, and any need for follow-up teaching.

REFERENCES

1 Wiegand, D. (2017). *AACN procedure manual for high acuity, progressive, and critical care* (7th ed.). St. Louis, MO: Elsevier.

Dealing with a discharge against medical advice

A patient or family may demand discharge against medical advice (AMA). If this situation occurs, notify the practitioner immediately. If the practitioner fails to convince the patient to remain in the facility, the practitioner will ask the patient to sign an AMA form releasing the facility from legal responsibility for any medical problems the patient may experience after discharge.[31]

If the practitioner isn't available, discuss the discharge form with the patient and obtain the patient's signature. If the patient refuses to sign the AMA form, don't detain the patient. *Detaining the patient violates the patient's legal rights.* After the patient leaves, document the incident thoroughly in your notes and notify the practitioner.

Implementation

- Gather and prepare the necessary equipment and supplies.
- Perform hand hygiene.[20,21,22,23,24,25]
- Confirm the patient's identity using at least two patient identifiers.[26]
- Provide privacy.[27,28,29,30]
- Inform the patient and family or caregiver of the time and date of discharge as soon as it's known. Notify the social services department if the patient's family can't arrange transportation, and always confirm arranged transportation on the day of discharge.[13,14,15,16]
- Obtain a written discharge order from the practitioner. If the patient demands discharge against medical advice, obtain the appropriate form. (See *Dealing with a discharge against medical advice.*)
- If the patient requires home medical care, confirm arrangements with the appropriate facility department or community agency.[13,14,15,16]
- Review the patient's discharge care plan with the patient and family or caregiver.[13,14,15,16] List any prescribed drugs the patient is taking at the time of discharge on the discharge instruction sheet, including the dosage, prescribed time schedule, and adverse reactions to report to the practitioner. Ensure that the drug schedule is consistent with the patient's lifestyle *to promote proper administration and patient compliance.* If the patient has received a new prescription, provide an explanation of the indication, dosage, schedule, and adverse effects. Provide the patient and family or caregiver (if appropriate) with written instructions on the medications the patient should take after discharge.[32,33,34]
- Instruct the patient to provide a list of medications to the practitioner who will be caring for the patient after discharge; to update the information when the practitioner discontinues medications, changes doses, or adds new medications (including over-the-counter products); and to carry a medication list that contains all of this information at all times in the event of an emergency. Remind the patient to discard old medication lists upon returning home.[32,33]
- Review procedures the patient, family, or caregiver will need to perform at home. If necessary, demonstrate these procedures, provide written instructions, and check performance with a return demonstration.[13,14,15,16,34]
- List dietary and activity instructions, if applicable, on the discharge instruction sheet, and review the reasons for them. If the practitioner orders bed rest, make sure the patient's family or caregiver can provide daily care and obtain the necessary equipment.[13,14,15,16]
- Check with the practitioner about the patient's next office appointment; if the practitioner hasn't yet done so, inform the patient of the date, time, and location. If scheduling is your responsibility, make an appointment with the practitioner, outpatient clinic, physical therapy services, X-ray department, or other health services (as needed). Confirm the patient's ability to arrange transportation to this appointment. If the patient can't arrange transportation to these appointments, notify the social services department.[13,14,15,16]
- Retrieve the patient's valuables from the facility's safe and review each item with the patient. Then obtain the patient's signature *to document the patient's receipt of the valuables.*
- Obtain from the pharmacy any drugs the patient brought to the facility. Return these to the patient if drug therapy is unchanged.[32,33]

- If the patient is being discharged to another facility, such as an assisted-living or long-term care facility, or will receive care at home from a home health care agency, provide hand-off communication to the person who will assume responsibility for the patient's care. Allow time for questions, as necessary, *to avoid miscommunication that can cause patient care errors during transitions of care.*[35] Ensure communication of a reconciled list of the patient's medications to the next practitioner who will be caring for the patient, and that the communication is documented in the patient's medical record, *to reduce the risk of transition-related adverse medication events.* If the next practitioner is unknown, make sure that the list is given to the patient or, if appropriate, the patient's family.[32,33,36,37,38,39]
- Ask the patient, responsible family member, or caregiver to verbalize understanding of the discharge instructions.
- Ask the patient, responsible family member, or caregiver to sign the discharge instruction sheet attesting to receipt of the information.
- If required by your facility, sign and date the discharge instruction sheet and give the original copy to the patient, responsible family member, or caregiver.
- Perform hand hygiene.[20,21,22,23,24,25]
- Put on gloves, a gown, and mask with face shield or mask and goggles, as needed, *to comply with standard precautions.*[40,41,42]
- Perform a physical assessment and obtain vital signs. Notify the practitioner of any abnormal findings or the development of new symptoms, *which may warrant a change in the discharge plan.*
- Ensure proper removal of all devices discontinued by the ordering practitioner, such as IV catheters, indwelling urinary catheters, and drains, before discharge *to avoid potential complications.*
- Help the patient get dressed as needed.
- Collect the patient's personal belongings from the room, compare them with the admission inventory of belongings, and help place them in the patient's suitcase or a plastic bag.
- After checking the room for misplaced belongings, help the patient into a wheelchair and escort the patient to the exit. If the patient is leaving by ambulance, help transfer the patient onto a stretcher.
- Complete a discharge summary sheet.[19,43,44,45]
- Discard used supplies in appropriate receptacles.[42]
- Remove and discard your gloves and other personal protective equipment, if worn.[42]
- Perform hand hygiene.[20,21,22,23,24,25]
- Clean and disinfect your stethoscope with a disinfectant pad.[46,47]
- After the patient leaves the area, notify the housekeeping staff and arrange for terminal cleaning of the room.[42,46,47]
- Perform hand hygiene.[20,21,22,23,24,25]
- Document the procedure.[43,44,45,48]

Special considerations

- Involve the patient's family or caregivers in discharge planning whenever possible *so that they can better understand and perform patient care procedures.*[13,14,15,16]
- The Joint Commission issued a sentinel event alert concerning inadequate hand-off communication because of the potential for patient harm that can result when a receiver receives inaccurate, incomplete, untimely, misinterpreted, or otherwise inadequate information. To improve hand-off communication, standardize the critical information that the sender communicates. At a minimum, include the sender contact information; illness assessment; patient summary, including events leading up to the illness or admission, hospital course, ongoing assessment, and plan of care; to-do action list; contingency plans; allergy list; code status; medication list; and dated laboratory test results and vital signs. Provide face-to-face communication whenever possible in an interruption-free location, using facility-approved, standardized tools and methods (for example, forms, templates, checklists, protocols, and mnemonics). Provide ample time and opportunity for questions, and include the multidisciplinary team members and the patient and family when appropriate.[49]

Patient teaching

Patient teaching provides patients and the family or caregiver with the knowledge and skills that they need to manage the patient's health care needs after discharge. (See *Discharge teaching goals.*)

PATIENT TEACHING

DISCHARGE TEACHING GOALS

Your discharge teaching should aim to ensure that the patient:
- understands the illness
- understands and can manage medication modifications, schedules, and information
- carefully follows the ordered diet
- manages the activity level
- understands ordered treatments
- recognizes the need for rest
- knows about possible complications
- knows when and where to seek follow-up care
- is aware of available community resources (as needed).

Remember that your discharge teaching must include the patient's family members and other caregivers *to ensure that the patient receives proper home care.*[8,9,10,11,13,14,15,16]

Documentation

Your facility determines the extent and form of discharge documentation. This documentation typically includes the time and date of discharge; the patient's vital signs and physical assessment results (if applicable); devices that remain in the patient; devices removed from the patient and the patient's tolerance of the removal; family members and caregivers present for teaching; details of instructions the health care team gave to the patient, including those regarding medications, activity, diet, treatments, and the use of medical equipment; signs and symptoms to report to the practitioner; and the date, time, and location of follow-up appointments. Document teaching provided to the patient and family (if applicable), their understanding of that teaching, and any need for follow-up teaching.[19,43]

REFERENCES

1 Rochester-Eyeguokan, C. D., et al. (2016). The current landscape of transitions of care practice models: A scoping review. *Pharmacotherapy: Journal of Human Pharmacology and Drug Therapy, 36*, 117–133. (Level II)

2 Brown, M. M. (2018). Transitions of care. In Daaleman, T. P. & Helton, M. R. (Eds.), *Chronic illness care: Principles and practice* (pp. 369–373). Cham, Switzerland: Springer.

3 Sponsler, K. C., et al. (2015). Improving medication safety during hospital-based transitions of care. *Cleveland Clinic Journal of Medicine, 82*, 351–360.

4 The Joint Commission. (2021). Standard PC.04.01.01. *Comprehensive accreditation manual for hospitals.* Oakbrook Terrace, IL: The Joint Commission. (Level VII)

5 Centers for Medicare and Medicaid Services, Department of Health and Human Services. (2020). Condition of participation: Discharge planning. 42 C.F.R. § 482.43.

6 Accreditation Association for Hospitals and Health Systems. (2020). Standard 15.06.00. *Healthcare Facilities Accreditation Program: Accreditation requirements for acute care hospitals.* Chicago, IL: Accreditation Association for Hospitals and Health Systems. (Level VII)

7 DNV GL-Healthcare USA, Inc. (2020). DC.2.SR.1. *NIAHO® accreditation requirements, interpretive guidelines and surveyor guidance—revision 20.0.* Milford, OH: DNV GL-Healthcare USA, Inc. (Level VII)

8 The Joint Commission. (2021). Standard PC.04.01.03. *Comprehensive accreditation manual for hospitals.* Oakbrook Terrace, IL: The Joint Commission. (Level VII)

9 Centers for Medicare and Medicaid Services, Department of Health and Human Services. (2020). Condition of participation: Discharge planning. 42 C.F.R. § 482.43(b)(5).

10 Accreditation Association for Hospitals and Health Systems. (2020). Standard 15.06.06. *Healthcare Facilities Accreditation Program: Accreditation requirements for acute care hospitals.* Chicago, IL: Accreditation Association for Hospitals and Health Systems. (Level VII)

11 DNV GL-Healthcare USA, Inc. (2020). DC.3.SR.3. *NIAHO® accreditation requirements, interpretive guidelines and surveyor guidance—revision 20.0.* Milford, OH: DNV GL-Healthcare USA, Inc. (Level VII)

12 Cesta, T. (2014). Case management insider: Home health care—A key component of discharge planning. *Hospital Case Management, 22*, 151–154.

13 The Joint Commission. (2021). Standard PC.04.01.05. *Comprehensive accreditation manual for hospitals.* Oakbrook Terrace, IL: The Joint Commission. (Level VII)

14 Centers for Medicare and Medicaid Services, Department of Health and Human Services. (2020). Condition of participation: Discharge planning. 42 C.F.R. § 482.43(c).

15 Accreditation Association for Hospitals and Health Systems. (2020). Standard 15.06.13. *Healthcare Facilities Accreditation Program: Accreditation requirements for acute care hospitals.* Chicago, IL: Accreditation Association for Hospitals and Health Systems. (Level VII)

16 DNV GL-Healthcare USA, Inc. (2020). DC.4.SR.2. *NIAHO® accreditation requirements, interpretive guidelines and surveyor guidance—revision 20.0.* Milford, OH: DNV GL-Healthcare USA, Inc. (Level VII)

17 The Joint Commission. (2010). *Advancing effective communication, cultural competence, and patient- and family-centered care: A roadmap for hospitals.* Oakbrook Terrace, IL: The Joint Commission. https://www.jointcommission.org/assets/1/6/ARoadmapforHospitalsfinalversion727.pdf (Level VII)

18 The Joint Commission. (2021). Standard PC.02.01.21. *Comprehensive accreditation manual for hospitals.* Oakbrook Terrace, IL: The Joint Commission. (Level VII)

19 The Joint Commission. (2021). Standard RC.02.04.01. *Comprehensive accreditation manual for hospitals.* Oakbrook Terrace, IL: The Joint Commission. (Level VII)

20 The Joint Commission. (2021). Standard NPSG.07.01.01. *Comprehensive accreditation manual for hospitals.* Oakbrook Terrace, IL: The Joint Commission. (Level VII)

21 Centers for Disease Control and Prevention. (2002). Guideline for hand hygiene in health-care settings: Recommendations of the Healthcare Infection Control Practices Advisory Committee and the HICPAC/SHEA/APIC/IDSA Hand Hygiene Task Force. *MMWR Recommendations and Reports, 51*(RR-16), 1–45. https://www.cdc.gov/mmwr/pdf/rr/rr5116.pdf (Level II)

22 World Health Organization. (2009). WHO guidelines on hand hygiene in health care: First global patient safety challenge, clean care is safer care. https://apps.who.int/iris/bitstream/handle/10665/44102/9789241597906_eng.pdf?sequence=1 (Level IV)

23 Centers for Medicare and Medicaid Services, Department of Health and Human Services. (2020). Condition of participation: Infection control. 42 C.F.R. § 482.42.

24 Accreditation Association for Hospitals and Health Systems. (2020). Standard 07.01.21. *Healthcare Facilities Accreditation Program: Accreditation requirements for acute care hospitals.* Chicago, IL: Accreditation Association for Hospitals and Health Systems. (Level VII)

25 DNV GL-Healthcare USA, Inc. (2020). IC.1.SR.1. *NIAHO® accreditation requirements, interpretive guidelines and surveyor guidance—revision 20.0.* Milford, OH: DNV GL-Healthcare USA, Inc. (Level VII)

26 The Joint Commission. (2021). Standard NPSG.01.01.01. *Comprehensive accreditation manual for hospitals.* Oakbrook Terrace, IL: The Joint Commission. (Level VII)

27 Accreditation Association for Hospitals and Health Systems. (2020). Standard 15.01.16. *Healthcare Facilities Accreditation Program: Accreditation requirements for acute care hospitals.* Chicago, IL: Accreditation Association for Hospitals and Health Systems. (Level VII)

28 Centers for Medicare and Medicaid Services, Department of Health and Human Services. (2020). Condition of participation: Patient's rights. 42 C.F.R. § 482.13(c)(1).

29 DNV GL-Healthcare USA, Inc. (2020). PR.2.SR.5. *NIAHO® accreditation requirements, interpretive guidelines and surveyor guidance—revision 20.0.* Milford, OH: DNV GL-Healthcare USA, Inc. (Level VII)

30 The Joint Commission. (2021). Standard RI.01.01.01. *Comprehensive accreditation manual for hospitals.* Oakbrook Terrace, IL: The Joint Commission. (Level VII)

31 Levy, F., et al. (2012). The importance of a proper against-medical-advice (AMA) discharge. *Journal of Emergency Medicine, 43*, 516–520.

32 The Joint Commission. (2021). Standard NPSG.03.06.01. *Comprehensive accreditation manual for hospitals.* Oakbrook Terrace, IL: The Joint Commission. (Level VII)

33 Accreditation Association for Hospitals and Health Systems. (2020). Standard 25.02.13. *Healthcare Facilities Accreditation Program: Accreditation requirements for acute care hospitals.* Chicago, IL: Accreditation Association for Hospitals and Health Systems. (Level VII)

34 Accreditation Association for Hospitals and Health Systems. (2020). Standard 15.06.26. *Healthcare Facilities Accreditation Program: Accreditation requirements for acute care hospitals.* Chicago, IL: Accreditation Association for Hospitals and Health Systems. (Level VII)

35 The Joint Commission. (2021). Standard PC.02.02.01. *Comprehensive accreditation manual for hospitals.* Oakbrook Terrace, IL: The Joint Commission. (Level VII)

36 The Joint Commission. (2021). Standard PC.04.02.01. *Comprehensive accreditation manual for hospitals.* Oakbrook Terrace, IL: The Joint Commission. (Level VII)

37 Centers for Medicare and Medicaid Services, Department of Health and Human Services. (2020). Condition of participation: Discharge planning. 42 C.F.R. § 482.43(d).

38 Accreditation Association for Hospitals and Health Systems. (2020). Standard 15.06.23. *Healthcare Facilities Accreditation Program: Accreditation requirements for acute care hospitals.* Chicago, IL: Accreditation Association for Hospitals and Health Systems. (Level VII)

39 DNV GL-Healthcare USA, Inc. (2020). DC.3.SR.4. *NIAHO® accreditation requirements, interpretive guidelines and surveyor guidance—revision 20.0.* Milford, OH: DNV GL-Healthcare USA, Inc. (Level VII)

40 Siegel, J. D., et al. (2007, revised 2019). 2007 guideline for isolation precautions: Preventing transmission of infectious agents in healthcare settings. https://www.cdc.gov/infectioncontrol/pdf/guidelines/isolation-guidelines-H.pdf (Level II)

41 Accreditation Association for Hospitals and Health Systems. (2020). Standard 07.01.10. *Healthcare Facilities Accreditation Program: Accreditation requirements for acute care hospitals.* Chicago, IL: Accreditation Association for Hospitals and Health Systems. (Level VII)

42 Occupational Safety and Health Administration. (2019). Bloodborne pathogens, standard number 1910.1030. https://www.osha.gov/pls/oshaweb/owadisp.show_document?p_id=10051&p_table=STANDARDS (Level VII)

43 Centers for Medicare and Medicaid Services, Department of Health and Human Services. (2020). Condition of participation: Medical record services. 42 C.F.R. § 482.24(b).

44 Accreditation Association for Hospitals and Health Systems. (2020). Standard 10.00.03. *Healthcare Facilities Accreditation Program: Accreditation requirements for acute care hospitals.* Chicago, IL: Accreditation Association for Hospitals and Health Systems. (Level VII)

45 DNV GL-Healthcare USA, Inc. (2020). MR.2.SR.1. *NIAHO® accreditation requirements, interpretive guidelines and surveyor guidance—revision 20.0.* Milford, OH: DNV GL-Healthcare USA, Inc. (Level VII)

46 Rutala, W. A., et al. (2008, revised 2019). Guideline for disinfection and sterilization in healthcare facilities, 2008. https://www.cdc.gov/infectioncontrol/pdf/guidelines/disinfection-guidelines-H.pdf (Level I)

47 Accreditation Association for Hospitals and Health Systems. (2020). Standard 07.02.03. *Healthcare Facilities Accreditation Program: Accreditation requirements for acute care hospitals.* Chicago, IL: Accreditation Association for Hospitals and Health Systems. (Level VII)

48 The Joint Commission. (2021). Standard RC.01.03.01. *Comprehensive accreditation manual for hospitals.* Oakbrook Terrace, IL: The Joint Commission. (Level VII)

49 The Joint Commission. (2017). Sentinel event alert 58: Inadequate hand-off communication. https://www.jointcommission.org/assets/1/18/SEA_58_Hand_off_Comms_9_6_17_FINAL_(1).pdf (Level VII)

DOCUMENTATION

Documentation is the process of preparing a complete record of a patient's care, and is a vital tool for communication among health care team members.[1] Accurate, detailed documentation shows the extent and quality of the care that nurses provide, the outcomes of that care, and treatment and education that the patient still needs. Thorough, accurate documentation decreases the potential for miscommunication and errors.

Documentation is a valuable method for demonstrating that a nurse has applied nursing knowledge, skills, and judgment according to professional nursing standards.[2] In a court of law, the patient's health record serves as the legal record of the care provided to that patient. Accrediting agencies and risk managers use the medical record to evaluate the quality of care a patient receives. Insurance companies use documentation systems to verify the care received. Nursing documentation in the medical record may also aid research and education as well as quality improvement programs.[2]

Equipment

Medical record (electronic or written) ▪ Optional: pen with black or blue ink.

Preparation of equipment

Various systems are available for documentation. Because each documentation system follows specific guidelines, you should familiarize yourself with the requirements of each system. (See *Comparing documentation systems.*)

Implementation

▪ Understand your state's nurse practice act and make sure your documentation reflects the state's laws governing the scope of nursing practice.[3]

Paper-based documentation

▪ Write legibly, *because illegible entries can result in misinterpretation of information and possible patient harm.*

▪ Use blue or black ink, *because the medical record is a permanent document and ink can't be erased.*[4]

▪ Sign all entries using your first and last name and title *to clearly identify who wrote the entry.*[5,6,7,8]

▪ When signing your initials on a form, use your full signature in the appropriate place on the form *to identify yourself as the care provider.*[5,6,7,8]

▪ Make sure each sheet of the medical record is correctly labeled with the patient's identifying information *to avoid documenting on the wrong patient or mistaking the patient for another.*

▪ If you make an error, draw a single line through the mistake and make a notation, such as "documentation error." Initial the error and note the date and time, as required by your facility. Then, record the correct entry. Don't use correction fluid, erasures, or entries between lines.[4]

▪ Don't leave blank lines within and between entries. Draw a line through the blank line *to ensure that no further entries may be made.*[4]

▪ Document chronologically, using the correct time and date. Avoid block documentation, *which is vague, implies inattention to the patient, and makes it hard to determine when specific events occurred.*[6,7,8,9]

▪ When documentation continues from one page to the next, sign the bottom of the first page. At the top of the next page, write the date, the time, and "continued from previous page."[4]

▪ Document the time as required by your facility using either 24-hour military time or "a.m." or "p.m."

▪ If you need to add a late entry, such as an event that you forgot to document earlier or when the medical record wasn't available, add the entry on the next available line and label it as a "late entry" *to show it's out of sequence.* Then record the date and time of the entry as well as the date and time when the entry should have been made.

Computer-based documentation

▪ Specifically state in the body of your note the time that events occurred and the actions taken, *because most computer systems record the date and time that you make an entry.*[6,7,8,9]

▪ Document time as required by your facility, using either 24-hour military time or "a.m." or "p.m."

▪ Make sure that no one else can read the screen while you're documenting, and log off when you're finished documenting. Never share your password with anyone else.[6,7,8,10]

▪ Know that most software programs establish an electronic signature based on your personal user password.[5,6,7,8]

▪ Follow your facility's guidelines for correcting errors, such as documenting on the wrong chart.

Completing the procedure

▪ Document information as soon as possible *to ensure the accuracy of the information and to reflect ongoing care. Delayed documentation increases the potential for omissions, error, and inaccuracy due to memory lapse.*[6,7,8,10]

▪ Document only care, treatments, and medications that you've actually provided or administered; never chart in advance.[6,7,8,10]

▪ Describe observations and behaviors of the patient rather than labeling the patient. Don't offer opinions or use subjective statements or judgments.[4]

▪ Use correct spelling and grammar in your entries, *because misspelled words and poor grammar look unprofessional and can lead to errors.*[4]

▪ Use only approved abbreviations.[11] (See *Abbreviations to avoid,* page 238.)

Comparing documentation systems

Various documentation systems are available for documenting patient care, including narrative; problem-oriented medical record (POMR); problem-intervention-evaluation (PIE); focus; charting by exception (CBE); and flow sheet, assessment, concise, timely (FACT) documentation systems. Documentation systems may be paper-based or computerized.

Narrative
- Most useful in acute care, long-term care, home care, and ambulatory care settings
- Contains progress notes and flow sheets that supplement the care plan
- History and admission form used to document initial assessment; ongoing assessments documented in progress notes
- Care plan based on narrative history and progress notes
- Outcomes and evaluations documented in progress notes and discharge summaries
- Progress notes in narration form at the time of entry

POMR
- Most useful in acute care, long-term care, home care, rehabilitation, and mental health settings
- Record contains database, care plan, problem list, progress notes, and discharge summary
- Database and care plan capture details of initial assessment; ongoing assessments documented in progress notes
- Nursing care plan developed using database and primarily based on problem list
- Outcomes and evaluations documented in section E of progress note format
- Progress notes in SOAP, SOAPIE, or SOAPIER (**S**ubjective, **O**bjective, **A**ssessment, **P**lan, **I**ntervention, **E**valuation, **R**evision) format

PIE
- Most useful in acute care setting
- Record contains assessment flow sheets, progress notes, and problem list
- Initial assessment form used to document initial assessment; ongoing assessments captured on new assessment forms generated for each shift
- No care plan; problems included in section P of progress note format
- Outcomes and evaluations documented in section P of progress note format
- Progress notes in PIE (**P**roblem-**I**ntervention-**E**valuation) format

Focus
- Most useful in acute care and long-term care settings
- Record contains progress notes, flow sheets, and checklists
- Initial assessment documented in patient history and admission assessment form; ongoing assessments documented on other assessment forms
- Nursing care plan based on problems, patient concerns, or nursing diagnosis
- Outcomes and evaluations documented in section R of progress note format
- Progress notes in DAR (**D**ata-**A**ction-**R**esponse) format

CBE
- Most useful in acute care and long-term care settings
- Record contains care plan; flow sheets, including patient teaching records and discharge notes; graphic record; and progress notes
- Initial assessment entered into database assessment form; ongoing assessments documented in nursing and medical flow sheets
- Nursing care plan based on nursing diagnoses
- Outcomes and evaluations documented in section E of progress note format
- Progress notes in SOAPIE or SOAPIER (**S**ubjective, **O**bjective, **A**ssessment, **P**lan, **I**ntervention, **E**valuation, **R**evision) format

FACT
- Most useful in acute care and long-term care settings
- Record contains assessment sheet, flow sheets, and progress notes
- Initial assessment documented on baseline assessment form; ongoing assessments document on flow sheets and progress notes
- Nursing care plan based on nursing diagnoses
- Outcomes and evaluations documented in flow sheets that appear in section R of progress note format
- Progress notes in DAR (**D**ata-**A**ction-**R**esponse) format

Special considerations

- Maintain the confidentiality of the medical record at all times.[13,14,15,16] Keep the medical record closed when not in use and store it in a secure place.
- Never tamper with documentation or any part of the clinical record; tampering includes adding to a clinical note at a later date without indicating that it's a late entry, inserting inaccurate information in the record, purposely omitting information, rewriting or altering the documentation, destroying clinical record notes or other documentation, and adding to someone else's notes without indicating your identity and the date.
- If information listed on a form doesn't apply to your patient, write "N/A" (not applicable) rather than leaving the space blank. *This notation shows that you read the question and that it doesn't apply, rather than that you forgot to gather the data. It also prevents someone else from adding the information later.*

Documentation

Document the patient's vital signs, your assessment findings, the patient's care plan, your interventions, patient and family teaching, and the patient's response to your interventions according to your facility's documentation system.

REFERENCES
1 Wang, N., et al. (2011). Quality of nursing documentation and approaches to its evaluation: A mixed-method systematic review. *Journal of Advanced Nursing, 67,* 1858–1875. (Level V)
2 Craven, R. F., et al. (2021). *Fundamentals of nursing: Human health and function.* (9th ed.). Philadelphia, PA: Wolters Kluwer.
3 National Council of State Boards of Nursing. (n.d.). Nurse practice act toolkit. https://www.ncsbn.org/npa-toolkit.htm
4 Lockwood, W. (2019). Documentation: Accurate and legal. https://www.rn.org/courses/coursematerial-66.pdf
5 The Joint Commission. (2021). Standard RC.01.02.01. *Comprehensive accreditation manual for hospitals.* Oakbrook Terrace, IL: The Joint Commission. (Level VII)
6 Centers for Medicare and Medicaid Services, Department of Health and Human Services. (2020). Condition of participation: Medical record services. 42 C.F.R. § 482.24(b).
7 Accreditation Association for Hospitals and Health Systems. (2020). Standard 10.00.03. *Healthcare Facilities Accreditation Program: Accreditation requirements for acute care hospitals.* Chicago, IL: Accreditation Association for Hospitals and Health Systems. (Level VII)

Abbreviations to avoid

To reduce the risk of medical errors, The Joint Commission has created a "Do Not Use" list of abbreviations. The list applies to all orders and medication-related documentation that's handwritten, part of a free-text computer entry, or on preprinted forms.[11,12]

Abbreviation	Potential problem	Preferred term
U, u (for "unit")	Mistaken for 0 (zero), 4 (four), or cc.	Write "unit."
IU (for "International Unit")	Mistaken as IV (intravenous) or 10 (ten).	Write "International Unit."
Q.D., QD, q.d., qd (Latin abbreviation for "once daily") Q.O.D, QOD, q.o.d., qod (Latin abbreviation for "every other day")	Mistaken for each other. Period after the "Q" mistaken for "I" and "O" mistaken for "I."	Write "daily" Write "every other day."
Trailing zero (X.0 mg) (Note: Prohibited only for medication-related notations); lack of leading zero (.X mg)	Decimal point is missed.	Write X mg. Write 0.X mg.
MS MSO4 and MgSO4	Can mean "morphine sulfate" or "magnesium sulfate." Confused for one another.	Write "morphine sulfate" Write "magnesium sulfate."

© The Joint Commission, 2020. Reprinted with permission.

8 DNV GL-Healthcare USA, Inc. (2020). MR.2.SR.1. *NIAHO® accreditation requirements, interpretive guidelines and surveyor guidance—revision 20.0*. Milford, OH: DNV GL-Healthcare USA, Inc. (Level VII)

9 The Joint Commission. (2021). Standard RC.01.01.01. *Comprehensive accreditation manual for hospitals*. Oakbrook Terrace, IL: The Joint Commission. (Level VII)

10 The Joint Commission. (2021). Standard RC.01.03.01. *Comprehensive accreditation manual for hospitals*. Oakbrook Terrace, IL: The Joint Commission. (Level VII)

11 The Joint Commission. (2020). Official 'Do not use' list: The Joint Commission fact sheet. https://www.jointcommission.org/-/media/tjc/documents/fact-sheets/do-not-use-list-8-3-20.pdf?db=web&hash=2489CB1616A30CFFBDAAD1FB3F8021A5

12 The Joint Commission. (2021). Standard IM.02.02.01. *Comprehensive accreditation manual for hospitals*. Oakbrook Terrace, IL: The Joint Commission. (Level VII)

13 The Joint Commission. (2021). Standard RI.01.01.01. *Comprehensive accreditation manual for hospitals*. Oakbrook Terrace, IL: The Joint Commission. (Level VII)

14 Centers for Medicare and Medicaid Services, Department of Health and Human Services. (2020). Condition of participation: Patient's rights. 42 C.F.R. § 482.13(c)(1).

15 Accreditation Association for Hospitals and Health Systems. (2020). Standard 15.01.16. *Healthcare Facilities Accreditation Program: Accreditation requirements for acute care hospitals*. Chicago, IL: Accreditation Association for Hospitals and Health Systems. (Level VII)

16 DNV GL-Healthcare USA, Inc. (2020). PR.2.SR.5. *NIAHO® accreditation requirements, interpretive guidelines and surveyor guidance—revision 20.0*. Milford, OH: DNV GL-Healthcare USA, Inc. (Level VII)

Doppler ultrasound device use

A Doppler ultrasound device uses high-frequency sound waves to detect and measure blood flow through vessels. A thin layer of coupling (or transmission) gel placed on the patient's skin or the top of the probe (or transducer) helps transmit ultrasound waves from the device's transducer into the patient's body. The probe then collects sound waves that are reflected back from the red blood cells as they flow through the blood vessel.[1] A Doppler ultrasound device possesses greater sensitivity than palpation for detecting a weak or faint pulse, and helps determine the patient's heart rate. It may also be used to evaluate lower extremity peripheral perfusion, and to assess fetal heart sounds after the first trimester of pregnancy.[2,3,4,5]

Equipment

Doppler ultrasound device with probe (transducer) ▪ coupling or transmission gel ▪ soft cloth ▪ disinfectant spray or wipe ▪ Optional: earphones.

Preparation of equipment

Inspect the ultrasound device and probe for signs of cracks or breaks in the mechanical housing. Inspect cables and connectors for signs of wear or failure. Discontinue use of the device with any sign of loss of integrity.[6]

Implementation

▪ Gather and prepare the necessary equipment and supplies
▪ Perform hand hygiene.[7,8,9,10,11,12]
▪ Confirm the patient's identity using at least two patient identifiers.[13]
▪ Provide privacy.[14,15,16,17]
▪ Explain the procedure to the patient and family (if appropriate) according to their individual communication and learning needs *to increase their understanding, allay their fears, and enhance cooperation.*[18]
▪ Raise the patient's bed to waist level before providing patient care *to prevent caregiver back strain.*[19]
▪ Perform hand hygiene.[7,8,9,10,11,12]
▪ Expose the area intended for pulse assessment. Avoid rolling up sleeves or pant cuffs in a manner that obstructs blood flow.[6]
▪ Apply a small amount of coupling or transmission gel (not water-soluble lubricant) to the top of the probe or the patient's skin directly over the selected artery.[6]
▪ Position the probe on the skin directly over the selected artery.
▪ Turn on the Doppler ultrasound device following the manufacturer's instructions for use.[6]
▪ If the device has a speaker, adjust the audio level as needed. If your model doesn't have a speaker, plug in the earphones.
▪ *To obtain the best signal,* tilt the probe 45 degrees from the skin surface over the general location of the vessel, making sure to put gel between the skin and the probe.[6] Slowly move the probe side to side, and vary the angle of the probe until you hear vascular sounds—a pulsatile hissing noise heard with each heartbeat as blood flows through the artery.[6] Reapply more gel if it begins to dry out or is spread too thinly, creating an air gap between the probe and the skin. However, avoid applying too much gel, *because doing so makes the probe difficult to clean and doesn't improve probe performance.*[6]
▪ Count the number of pulsations produced in 60 seconds *to determine the pulse rate.*
▪ Turn off the device following the manufacturer's instructions.
▪ Wipe the gel from the patient.
▪ Return the bed to the lowest position *to prevent falls and maintain patient safety.*[20]
▪ Clean the probe and main unit of the ultrasound device following the manufacturer's instructions.[6,21,22] A cloth dampened with warm water or pre-saturated disinfectant wipes may be used to clean certain devices.[6]

■ Disinfect the probe and main ultrasound deice with a disinfectant spray, or wipe following manufacturer's instructions.[6,21,22] Don't immerse the probe or main ultrasound device.[6] Don't drop or mishandle the probe or main ultrasound device, *because damage to sensitive components is likely to occur.*[6]

■ Perform hand hygiene.[7,8,9,10,11,12]

■ Store the ultrasound device and probe in a clean area free from dust and debris.[6]

■ Perform hand hygiene.[7,8,9,10,11,12]

■ Document the procedure.[23,24,25,26]

Special considerations

■ A complete Doppler ultrasound assessment requires the clinician to listen to and interpret various signals transmitted from the Doppler probe. An experienced Doppler user can recognize the characteristic sounds of open and obstructed arteries. Doppler sounds vary in pitch (frequency) with the velocity of blood flow.[27]

Documentation

Document the location and quality of the pulse as well as the pulse rate and time of measurement. Document teaching provided to the patient and family (if appropriate), their understanding of that teaching, and any need for follow-up teaching.

REFERENCES

1 Craven, R. F., et al. (2017). *Fundamentals of nursing: Human health and function.* (8th ed.). Philadelphia, PA: Wolters Kluwer.

2 Elgendy, A., et al. (2017). Comparison of continuous-wave Doppler ultrasound monitor and echocardiography to assess cardiac output in intensive care patients. *Critical Care and Resuscitation, 19,* 222. (Level IV)

3 Zengin, S., et al. (2018). Comparison of manual pulse palpation, cardiac ultrasonography and Doppler ultrasonography to check the pulse in cardiopulmonary arrest patients. *Resuscitation, 133,* 59–64.

4 Milan, A., et al. (2019). Current assessment of pulse wave velocity: Comprehensive review of validation studies. *Journal of hypertension, 37,* 1547–1557.

5 Abdulhay, E. W., et al. (2014). Review article: Non-invasive fetal heart rate monitoring techniques. *Biomedical Science and Engineering, 2*(3), 53–67.

6 Wallach Surgical Devices. (2013). User manual for the LifeDop ABI handheld vascular system. https://www.vitalitymedical.com/pdf/lifedop-abi-user-manual.pdf

7 The Joint Commission. (2021). Standard NPSG.07.01.01. *Comprehensive accreditation manual for hospitals.* Oakbrook Terrace, IL: The Joint Commission. (Level VII)

8 Centers for Disease Control and Prevention. (2002). Guideline for hand hygiene in health-care settings: Recommendations of the Healthcare Infection Control Practices Advisory Committee and the HICPAC/SHEA/APIC/IDSA Hand Hygiene Task Force. *MMWR Recommendations and Reports, 51*(RR-16), 1–45. https://www.cdc.gov/mmwr/pdf/rr/rr5116.pdf (Level II)

9 World Health Organization. (2009). WHO guidelines on hand hygiene in health care: First global patient safety challenge, clean care is safer care. https://apps.who.int/iris/bitstream/handle/10665/44102/9789241597906_eng.pdf?sequence=1 (Level IV)

10 Accreditation Association for Hospitals and Health Systems. (2020). Standard 07.01.21. *Healthcare Facilities Accreditation Program: Accreditation requirements for acute care hospitals.* Chicago, IL: Accreditation Association for Hospitals and Health Systems. (Level VII)

11 Centers for Medicare and Medicaid Services, Department of Health and Human Services. (2020). Condition of participation: Infection control. 42 C.F.R. § 482.42.

12 DNV GL-Healthcare USA, Inc. (2020). IC.1.SR.1. *NIAHO® accreditation requirements, interpretive guidelines and surveyor guidance—revision 20.0.* Milford, OH: DNV GL-Healthcare USA, Inc. (Level VII)

13 The Joint Commission. (2021). Standard NPSG.01.01.01. *Comprehensive accreditation manual for hospitals.* Oakbrook Terrace, IL: The Joint Commission. (Level VII)

14 The Joint Commission. (2021). Standard RI.01.01.01. *Comprehensive accreditation manual for hospitals.* Oakbrook Terrace, IL: The Joint Commission. (Level VII)

15 Centers for Medicare and Medicaid Services, Department of Health and Human Services. (2020). Condition of participation: Patient's rights. 42 C.F.R. § 482.13(c)(1).

16 Accreditation Association for Hospitals and Health Systems. (2020). Standard 15.01.16. *Healthcare Facilities Accreditation Program: Accreditation requirements for acute care hospitals.* Chicago, IL: Accreditation Association for Hospitals and Health Systems. (Level VII)

17 DNV GL-Healthcare USA, Inc. (2020). PR.2.SR.5. *NIAHO® accreditation requirements, interpretive guidelines and surveyor guidance—revision 20.0.* Milford, OH: DNV GL-Healthcare USA, Inc. (Level VII)

18 The Joint Commission. (2021). Standard PC.02.01.21. *Comprehensive accreditation manual for hospitals.* Oakbrook Terrace, IL: The Joint Commission. (Level VII)

19 Waters, T. R., et al. (2009). Safe patient handling training for schools of nursing. https://www.cdc.gov/niosh/docs/2009-127/pdfs/2009-127.pdf (Level VII)

20 Ganz, D. A., et al. (2013, reviewed 2021). *Preventing falls in hospitals: A toolkit for improving quality of care (AHRQ Publication No. 13-0015-EF).* Rockville, MD: Agency for Healthcare Research and Quality. https://www.ahrq.gov/professionals/systems/hospital/fallpxtoolkit/index.html (Level VII)

21 Rutala, W. A., et al. (2008, revised 2019). Guideline for disinfection and sterilization in healthcare facilities, 2008. https://www.cdc.gov/infection-control/pdf/guidelines/disinfection-guidelines-H.pdf (Level I)

22 Accreditation Association for Hospitals and Health Systems. (2020). Standard 07.02.03. *Healthcare Facilities Accreditation Program: Accreditation requirements for acute care hospitals.* Chicago, IL: Accreditation Association for Hospitals and Health Systems. (Level VII)

23 The Joint Commission. (2021). Standard RC.0L: 1.03.01. *Comprehensive accreditation manual for hospitals.* Oakbrook Terrace, IL: The Joint Commission. (Level VII)

24 Accreditation Association for Hospitals and Health Systems. (2020). Standard 10.00.03. *Healthcare Facilities Accreditation Program: Accreditation requirements for acute care hospitals.* Chicago, IL: Accreditation Association for Hospitals and Health Systems. (Level VII)

25 Centers for Medicare and Medicaid Services, Department of Health and Human Services. (2020). Condition of participation: Medical record services. 42 C.F.R. § 482.24(b).

26 DNV GL-Healthcare USA, Inc. (2020). MR.2.SR.1. *NIAHO® accreditation requirements, interpretive guidelines and surveyor guidance—revision 20.0.* Milford, OH: DNV GL-Healthcare USA, Inc. (Level VII)

27 Beldon, P. (2010). Performing a Doppler assessment: The procedure. *Wound Essentials, 5,* 87–90. https://www.woundsinternational.com/uploads/resources/content_9496.pdf

DROPLET PRECAUTIONS

Droplet precautions prevent infectious pathogens from traveling from the respiratory tract of an infectious person to the mucous membranes of a susceptible host.[1] These pathogens, which are carried by respiratory droplets, spread when an infected person coughs, sneezes, or talks during such procedures as suctioning or endotracheal intubation. (See *Conditions requiring droplet precautions*, page 240.)

Ideally, a patient requiring droplet precautions should be placed in a single-patient room.[1] Anyone having direct contact with the patient or who will be within 3′ (1 M) of the patient should wear a surgical mask covering the nose and mouth. When exposure to a highly virulent pathogen is likely, wearing a mask when within 6′ to 10′ (2 to 3 M) of the patient or upon entering the patient's room offers further protection.[1]

NURSING ALERT Please refer to the latest recommendations from the Centers for Disease Control and Prevention (CDC), located at https://www.cdc.gov/coronavirus/2019-nCoV/hcp/index.html when caring for a patient with known or suspected Coronavirus disease (COVID-19).

NURSING ALERT Refer to the latest recommendations from the Centers for Disease Control and Prevention, located at https://www.cdc.gov/vhf/ebola/healthcare-us/index.html, when caring for the patient with known or suspected Ebola virus disease.

As a general precaution, instruct anyone who enters a health care facility with signs of a respiratory infection (such as a cough, congestion, rhinorrhea, or increased respiratory secretions) to cover both mouth and nose with a tissue when coughing and dispose of soiled tissues promptly.[2] The person should wear a surgical mask, if tolerated, and perform hand hygiene after contact with respiratory secretions.[1] If possible, separate the person by at least 3′ (1 M) from other people in common waiting areas

Conditions requiring droplet precautions

An infected patient may transmit certain conditions via respiratory droplets. Such conditions require droplet precautions.[1] The table below lists conditions that require droplet precautions, along with the precautionary period and any special considerations.

CONDITION	PRECAUTIONARY PERIOD	SPECIAL CONSIDERATIONS (AS APPLICABLE)
Adenovirus infection in infants and young children	■ Duration of illness	■ Institute contact precautions in addition to droplet precautions. ■ Prolonged viral shedding occurs in immunocompromised patients.
Diphtheria (pharyngeal)	■ Until off antibiotics and two cultures taken at least 24 hours apart are negative	
Haemophilus influenzae type b disease, including epiglottis, meningitis, pneumonia, and sepsis	■ Until 24 hours after initiation of effective therapy	
Influenza (seasonal)	■ For 7 days after onset of signs and symptoms or until 24 hours after fever and respiratory symptoms have resolved, whichever is longer.[3] ■ For duration of illness in immunocompromised patients	■ Viral shedding is prolonged in immunocompromised patients.
Mumps	■ For 5 days after onset of swelling[4]	■ Susceptible health care workers shouldn't provide care if immune caregivers are available.
Mycoplasma pneumoniae infection	■ For duration of illness	
Neisseria meningitidis disease, including meningitis, pneumonia, and sepsis	■ Until 24 hours after initiation of effective therapy	■ Household contacts should receive postexposure prophylactic antibiotic therapy. ■ Health care workers exposed to respiratory secretions should receive postexposure prophylactic antibiotic therapy. ■ A postexposure vaccine may help control outbreaks.
Parvovirus B19 (erythema infectiosum)	■ Duration of hospitalization when chronic disease occurs in immunocompromised patients ■ For 7 days in patients with transient aplastic crisis or red-cell crisis	■ Duration of precautions for immunosuppressed patients with persistently positive polymerase chain reaction is unknown, but transmission has occurred.
Pertussis (whooping cough)	■ Until 5 days after initiation of effective therapy	■ Household contacts should receive postexposure prophylaxis. ■ Health care workers with prolonged exposure to respiratory secretions should receive postexposure prophylaxis.
Pneumonic plague	■ Until 48 hours after initiation of effective therapy	■ Exposed health care workers should receive postexposure prophylactic antibiotics.
Rhinovirus	■ Duration of illness	■ Institute contact precautions if contact with copious moist secretions is likely.
Rubella (German measles)	■ Until 7 days after onset of rash	■ Susceptible health care workers shouldn't enter the room if immune caregivers are available. ■ Administer vaccine to nonpregnant susceptible individuals within 3 days of exposure. ■ Place exposed susceptible patients on droplet precautions.
Severe acute respiratory distress syndrome	■ For duration of illness plus 10 days after resolution of fever	■ Airborne precautions are preferred. ■ Institute contact precautions in addition to airborne or droplet precautions. ■ Wear eye protection. ■ Vigilant environmental disinfection is necessary.
Streptococcal group A disease, including pharyngitis (in infants and young children), pneumonia, serious invasive disease, and scarlet fever (in infants and young children)	■ Until 24 hours after initiation of effective therapy	■ If the patient has skin lesions, institute contact precautions
Viral hemorrhagic infection (Ebola, Lassa, Marburg, and Crimean-Congo fever viruses)	■ Duration of illness	■ Institute contact precautions. ■ Wear eye protection. ■ Handle wastes appropriately. ■ Use an N-95 (or higher) respirator mask when performing aerosol-generating procedures. ■ If you suspect Ebola, notify public health officials, as required by your facility

to prevent the spread of infection.[1] These actions can help prevent the spread of infectious pathogens until appropriate isolation precautions are established.

PEDIATRIC ALERT When handling infants or young children who require droplet precautions, you may also need to institute contact precautions and wear gloves and a gown *to prevent soiling of clothing from nasal and oral secretions.*

Equipment

Mask ■ tissues ■ droplet precautions sign ■ Optional: gowns, gloves, no-touch tissue disposal receptacle.

Preparation of equipment

Keep all droplet precaution supplies outside the patient's room in a cart or an anteroom.

Implementation

■ Gather and prepare the necessary equipment and supplies.
■ Put a droplet precautions sign at the patient's door *to notify anyone entering the room of the situation.*[1,5,6,7]
■ Perform hand hygiene.[6,8,9,10,11,12]
■ Put on a gown, if necessary, *to comply with standard precautions.*[1,7,13]
■ Just before entering the patient's room, put on a mask and secure the ties or elastic band at the middle of the back of your head and neck. Adjust the flexible metal nose strip to your nose bridge so it fits firmly but comfortably. Make sure the mask fits snugly to your face and below your chin.[1]
■ Put on gloves, if necessary, *to comply with standard precautions.*[1,7,13]
■ Confirm the patient's identity using at least two patient identifiers.[14]
■ Situate the patient in a single room with private toilet facilities and an anteroom, if possible. If necessary, and if approved by your facility's infection preventionist, two patients with the same infection may share a room.[1]
■ Explain droplet precautions to the patient and family (if appropriate) according to their individual communication and learning needs *to increase their understanding, allay their fears, and enhance cooperation.*[15]
■ If the patient is wearing a mask during transport to the room, remove the mask and discard it in the appropriate receptacle.[1]
■ Instruct the patient to cover both nose and mouth with a facial tissue while coughing or sneezing, dispose of the tissue immediately, and then perform hand hygiene *to prevent the spread of infectious droplets.*[2,6,8,9,10,11,12]
■ Provide the patient with a no-touch receptacle for tissue disposal, if available.[1,2]
■ Remove and discard your gloves, gown (if worn), and mask in the anteroom or, if an anteroom isn't available, at the patient's doorway just before leaving the room.[1] To remove your mask, untie the strings or remove the elastic bands and dispose of the mask while handling it by the strings or elastic bands only, *because the front of the mask is considered contaminated.*[1]
■ Perform hand hygiene.[6,8,9,10,11,12]
■ Document the procedure.[16,17,18,19]

Special considerations

■ Provide the patient with dedicated noncritical equipment (such as a stethoscope, blood pressure cuff, and thermometer) *to prevent the spread of infection.*[1] If the use of reusable equipment is necessary, clean and disinfect the equipment according to the manufacturer's instructions *to prevent the spread of infection.*[20,21]
■ Make sure all visitors wear masks when in close proximity to the patient (within 3′ [1 M]) and, if necessary, gowns and gloves.[1]
■ If the patient must leave the room for essential procedures, make sure the patient wears a surgical mask over the nose and mouth, and instruct the patient to use respiratory hygiene and proper cough etiquette.[1] Notify the receiving department or area of the patient's isolation precautions *so that the precautions will be maintained and the patient can be returned to the room promptly.*

■ It isn't necessary for health care workers to wear masks when transporting a patient on droplet precautions *because the patient is wearing a mask.*[1]
■ Because pathogens in respiratory droplets don't remain infectious over long distances (they generally drop to the ground within 3′[1 M]), special air handling and ventilation systems and an airborne-infection isolation room with negative airflow aren't necessary.[1]
■ Single-patient rooms are preferred for patients who require droplet precautions. However, when transmission continues after implementing routine infection control measures, creating patient cohorts and cohorting health care personnel may be beneficial. Consult with your infection preventionist before cohorting patients or staff members.[1]

Complications

Social isolation is a complication of droplet precautions.

Documentation

Record the need for droplet precautions on the nursing care plan and as otherwise indicated by your facility. Document initiation and maintenance of the precautions and the patient's compliance with droplet precautions. Document teaching provided to the patient and family (if applicable), their understanding of that teaching, and any need for follow-up teaching. Also document the date droplet precautions were discontinued.

REFERENCES

1 Siegel, J. D., et al. (2007, revised 2019). 2007 guideline for isolation precautions: Preventing transmission of infectious agents in healthcare settings. https://www.cdc.gov/infectioncontrol/pdf/guidelines/isolation-guidelines-H.pdf (Level II)
2 Centers for Disease Control and Prevention. (2009). Respiratory hygiene/cough etiquette in healthcare settings. https://www.cdc.gov/flu/professionals/infectioncontrol/resphygiene.htm (Level VII)
3 Centers for Disease Control and Prevention. (2021). Prevention strategies for seasonal influenza in healthcare settings. https://www.cdc.gov/flu/professionals/infectioncontrol/healthcaresettings.htm (Level VII)
4 Centers for Disease Control and Prevention. (2008). Updated recommendations for isolation of persons with mumps. https://www.cdc.gov/mmwr/preview/mmwrhtml/mm5740a3.htm (Level VII)
5 The Joint Commission. (2021). Standard IC.02.01.01. *Comprehensive accreditation manual for hospitals.* Oakbrook Terrace, IL: The Joint Commission. (Level VII)
6 Centers for Medicare and Medicaid Services, Department of Health and Human Services. (2020). Condition of participation: Infection control. 42 C.F.R. § 482.42.
7 Accreditation Association for Hospitals and Health Systems. (2020). Standard 07.01.10. *Healthcare Facilities Accreditation Program: Accreditation requirements for acute care hospitals.* Chicago, IL: Accreditation Association for Hospitals and Health Systems. (Level VII)
8 The Joint Commission. (2021). Standard NPSG.07.01.01. *Comprehensive accreditation manual for hospitals.* Oakbrook Terrace, IL: The Joint Commission. (Level VII)
9 Centers for Disease Control and Prevention. (2002). Guideline for hand hygiene in health-care settings: Recommendations of the Healthcare Infection Control Practices Advisory Committee and the HICPAC/SHEA/APIC/IDSA Hand Hygiene Task Force. *MMWR Recommendations and Reports, 51*(RR-16), 1–45. https://www.cdc.gov/mmwr/pdf/rr/rr5116.pdf (Level II)
10 World Health Organization. (2009). WHO guidelines on hand hygiene in health care: First global patient safety challenge, clean care is safer care. https://apps.who.int/iris/bitstream/handle/10665/44102/9789241597906_eng.pdf?sequence=1 (Level IV)
11 Accreditation Association for Hospitals and Health Systems. (2020). Standard 07.01.21. *Healthcare Facilities Accreditation Program: Accreditation requirements for acute care hospitals.* Chicago, IL: Accreditation Association for Hospitals and Health Systems. (Level VII)
12 DNV GL-Healthcare USA, Inc. (2020). IC.1.SR.1. *NIAHO® accreditation requirements, interpretive guidelines and surveyor guidance—revision 20.0.* Milford, OH: DNV GL-Healthcare USA, Inc. (Level VII)

13 Occupational Safety and Health Administration. (2019). Bloodborne pathogens, standard number 1910.1030. https://www.osha.gov/pls/oshaweb/owadisp.show_document?p_id=10051&p_table=STANDARDS (Level VII)

14 The Joint Commission. (2021). Standard NPSG.01.01.01. *Comprehensive accreditation manual for hospitals*. Oakbrook Terrace, IL: The Joint Commission. (Level VII)

15 The Joint Commission. (2021). Standard PC.02.01.21. *Comprehensive accreditation manual for hospitals*. Oakbrook Terrace, IL: The Joint Commission. (Level VII)

16 The Joint Commission. (2021). Standard RC.01.03.01. *Comprehensive accreditation manual for hospitals*. Oakbrook Terrace, IL: The Joint Commission. (Level VII)

17 Centers for Medicare and Medicaid Services, Department of Health and Human Services. (2020). Condition of participation: Medical record services. 42 C.F.R. § 482.24(b).

18 Accreditation Association for Hospitals and Health Systems. (2020). Standard 10.00.03. *Healthcare Facilities Accreditation Program: Accreditation requirements for acute care hospitals*. Chicago, IL: Accreditation Association for Hospitals and Health Systems. (Level VII)

19 DNV GL-Healthcare USA, Inc. (2020). MR.2.SR.1. *NIAHO® accreditation requirements, interpretive guidelines and surveyor guidance—revision 20.0*. Milford, OH: DNV GL-Healthcare USA, Inc. (Level VII)

20 Rutala, W. A., et al. (2008, revised 2019). Guideline for disinfection and sterilization in healthcare facilities, 2008. https://www.cdc.gov/infection-control/pdf/guidelines/disinfection-guidelines-H.pdf (Level I)

21 Accreditation Association for Hospitals and Health Systems. (2020). Standard 07.02.03. *Healthcare Facilities Accreditation Program: Accreditation requirements for acute care hospitals*. Chicago, IL: Accreditation Association for Hospitals and Health Systems. (Level VII)

DRUG AND ALCOHOL SPECIMEN COLLECTION

Drug and alcohol specimens are collected to help identify a patient's drug or alcohol use.[1] This information may be needed to obtain evidence for a possible criminal charges (such as after an accident), to help determine a cause of death, and to screen for employment suitability or adherence to an ongoing drug addiction rehabilitation program. It's also used to establish a differential diagnosis for a patient experiencing an altered mental state or who has signs and symptoms as slurred speech, dizziness, confusion, blurred vision, anxiety, hallucinations, memory impairment, lack of muscle coordination, or hyperthermia. The collection method and source of the specimens vary, based on the reason for testing. Because of the variability in local and state laws, each facility's guidelines must be strictly followed.

Drug testing that's performed to determine employment suitability and rehabilitation program adherence usually involves a urine sample collected under highly controlled conditions.[1] Although collection requirements may vary slightly, depending on the employer and type of employment or rehabilitation program, most include a designated collection site, security for the collection site, use of authorized personnel, privacy during collection, integrity and identity of the specimen, and chain-of-custody documentation. Some rehabilitation programs and employment circumstances may require the specimen collection to be observed. Testing is usually limited to five drug types: marijuana, cocaine, opiates, amphetamines, and phencyclidine (PCP). In the case of employment screening, if the results of the initial test are positive, a test using gas chromatography–mass spectrometry follows to confirm the results.

Depending on the reason for collection and state laws, the patient or a family member may need to provide informed consent before you obtain the sample. Consent may not be required if it's an emergency, if results will be used only for a differential diagnosis in an acute crisis, or if the patient is not in a condition to grant permission.[2] In a criminal case, a law enforcement officer can't order blood to be drawn and doesn't have the legal right to grant permission if the patient refuses consent.

Blood specimens are collected in 10-mL gray-top blood collection tubes that contain a preservative (100 mg of sodium fluoride) *to help prevent deterioration of the specimen*, including changes in alcohol concentration and the breakdown of cocaine. The tubes also contain an anticoagulant (20 mg of potassium oxalate) *to prevent the sample from clotting*.[3] The integrity and identity of the specimen must be maintained and, if indicated, chain-of-custody documentation preserved.

In general, prescription and over-the-counter drugs can be detected in blood within 4 to 24 hours and in urine for 2 to 4 days. Detection times for alcohol and other drugs vary. (See *Drug detection times*.)

This procedure focuses on drug and alcohol specimen collection for medicolegal reasons. When specimens are collected for a patient who's experiencing an altered mental state or other signs and symptoms, be sure to use the appropriate collection tubes. (See the "Venipuncture" procedure.)

Equipment

Gloves ■ chain of custody labels ■ chain of custody form with multiple copies ■ labels ■ pen ■ "limited access" signs ■ Optional: vital signs monitoring equipment, pulse oximeter and probe, secure refrigerator.

Urine specimen collection

Urine collection container with temperature measurement device attached in sealed covering ■ 90-mL plastic, screw-top specimen container in sealed covering ■ adhesive label ■ plastic sealable shipping bag ■ absorbent material ■ bluing agent for toilet water ■ lockable cabinet or box

Blood sample collection

Two 10-mL gray-top Vacutainer blood tubes containing sodium fluoride and potassium oxalate with adhesive labels ■ venipuncture supplies ■ alcohol-free swab (povidone-iodine) ■ evidence seals ■ padded transport box ■ laboratory biohazard transport bag ■ Optional: 2″ × 2″ (5 cm × 5 cm) gauze pads, soap (non-alcohol containing) and water solution.

Note: Prepackaged blood and urine collection kits are commercially available and contain everything necessary to collect and preserve the chain of custody for the specimens.

Preparation of equipment

Inspect all equipment and supplies. If a product is expired, is defective, or has compromised integrity, remove it from patient use, label it as expired or defective, and report the expiration or defect as directed by your facility. Make sure that access to collection materials and specimens is adequately restricted. Make sure that LIMITED ACCESS signs are posted in the specimen collection area *to ensure patient privacy during the specimen collection process*.

Implementation

■ Verify the practitioner's order.
■ If required by your facility, confirm that informed consent has been obtained and that the signed consent form is in the patient's medical record.[5,6,7,8]
■ Perform hand hygiene.[9,10,11,12,13,14]
■ Confirm the patient's identity using at least two patient identifiers.[15]
■ Provide privacy.[16,17,18,19]
■ Explain the procedure to the patient and family (if appropriate) according to their individual communication and learning needs *to increase their understanding, allay their fears, and enhance cooperation*.[20]
■ Perform hand hygiene.[9,10,11,12,13,14]
■ Assess the patient's level of consciousness and behavior. If applicable, obtain the patient's vital signs, including heart rate, respiratory rate, blood pressure, temperature, and oxygen saturation using pulse oximetry.
■ Obtain a thorough current and past medication history that includes prescription and nonprescription drugs as well as herbal supplements.

Urine sample collection

■ Prepare the collection site by turning off the water supply or securing water sources.[21]
■ Add bluing agent to the toilet and water tank *to prevent undetected specimen dilution by the donor*.[21]
■ Remove the waste container, soap dispenser, and any unnecessary items from the bathroom.[21]

Drug detection times

This table indicates the time it takes for specific drugs to be detectable in blood and urine. The time values in this table are only a general guideline because many variables affect the duration of drug detection, including drug metabolism and half-life, the patient's physical condition, hydration status, and frequency of ingestion.[4] Make sure to check with your facility's laboratory for specific drug detection times.

DRUG	BLOOD	URINE
Amphetamines	1 to 3 days	1 to 2 days[4]
Cocaine	5 to 6 hours (will break down in unrefrigerated blood)	2 to 4 days[4]
Ethanol	1 to 12 hours[4]	1 to 12 hours[4]
Marijuana	*Infrequent user*: 1 to 4 hours *Frequent user*: 3 to 6 hours	*Infrequent user*: 2 to 7 days[4] *Frequent user*: 1 to 2 months[4]
Opiates	1 to 4 hours	2 days[4]
Phencyclidine (PCP)	1 to 3 days	14 days; up to 30 days in chronic users[4]

■ Perform hand hygiene.[9,10,11,12,13,14]
■ Put on gloves *to comply with standard precautions.*[22,23,24]
■ Gather and prepare the necessary equipment and supplies.
■ Instruct the patient to remove any unnecessary outer clothing, such as a coat, hat, or extra shirt. If the patient refuses to remove a head covering based on religious practices, the patient may be exempt unless the collector has a visual indicator that the patient may be concealing something under the covering. Keep personal items such as a briefcase or purse with the patient's outer clothing.[21]
■ Instruct the patient to empty pockets into a lockable cabinet or box, and have the patient turn pockets inside out *to ensure that they're emptied and that the patient doesn't have anything that could be used to adulterate the specimen.* If the patient brought medications, lock them in the cabinet or box.[21]
■ Have the patient wash and dry hands.[21]
■ Provide the patient with the sealed collection kit or urine specimen container, and have the patient unwrap or break the seal on the kit or container.[21]
■ If direct observation isn't mandated for specimen collection, have the patient enter the bathroom and instruct the patient to provide a urine specimen of at least 45 mL into the collection container,[21] to not flush the toilet,[21] and to immediately leave the bathroom with the specimen and hand it to you when the patient's finished urinating.[21]
■ If direct observation is mandated, observe the patient during the collection procedure. (See *Direct observation specimen collection.*)
■ If the patient has a medical condition that requires an indwelling urinary catheter or an external urine collection bag, collect a fresh specimen. Instruct the patient to empty the urine collection bag in the bathroom and then show you the empty bag, drink sufficient fluid to provide a specimen, and pour the urine from the bag into the collection container in the privacy of the bathroom when the bag has collected at least 45 mL of urine.[21]
■ Check the specimen's temperature by reading the temperature strip, and note it on the chain-of-custody form.[21]
■ Check the specimen volume to ensure that the specimen contains the required amount of urine.[21]
■ Open the sealed screw-top specimen container and transfer the urine into the container.
■ Label the specimen container with the patient's name and identification number and the date and time in the presence of the patient *to prevent mislabeling.*[15]
■ Complete the required information on the chain-of-custody seal, initial the seal, have the patient initial the seal, and place it over the top of the specimen container.[21]
■ Turn the water on and allow the patient to wash hands.
■ Complete the chain-of-custody form and have the patient sign the form.[21]
■ Give the patient a copy of the chain-of-custody form.

■ Place the specimen, absorbent material, and completed chain-of-custody form in the plastic sealable shipping bag.
■ Seal the bag in the presence of the patient.
■ Remove and discard your gloves.[24]
■ Perform hand hygiene.[9,10,11,12,13,14]
■ Place the specimen in a secure refrigerator if it won't be immediately transported to the laboratory.
■ Make sure the person who removes the specimen for transport signs the chain-of-custody form. Retain a copy and place it in the patient's medical record.
■ Document the procedure.[25,26,27,28]

Blood sample collection
■ Perform hand hygiene.[9,10,11,12,13,14]
■ Put on gloves *to comply with standard precautions.*[22,23,24]
■ Gather and prepare the necessary equipment and supplies.
■ If applicable, ensure that the collection is observed by the law enforcement officer as required by your facility and state law.
■ Choose a venipuncture site. The most common sites are the veins in the antecubital space of the arms; however, if the patient has scarring in this area from self-injected drugs, you may need to find an alternate venipuncture site.
■ Clean the skin at the venipuncture site with an alcohol-free swab such as a povidone-iodine swab. If an alcohol-free antiseptic isn't available, use

Direct observation specimen collection

You may occasionally collect a specimen using direct observation. When an order for specimen collection mandates direct observation, the observer must be the same sex as the person producing the specimen.[21] Common reasons for mandating direct observation include the following:
■ The laboratory reports that a previously collected specimen produced invalid test results for which the medical review officer had no medical explanation.
■ The laboratory reports that the technician couldn't perform a split specimen test on a previously collected specimen.
■ The medical review officer reports a diluted test result from a previously collected specimen and the creatinine concentration of the specimen is greater than or equal to 2 mg/dL but less than or equal to 5 mg/dL.
■ Follow-up testing is required.
■ The collector observed patient conduct that indicated that the patient tampered with the previously collected specimen.
■ The temperature of a previously collected specimen was outside of the normal temperature range.

a gauze pad with a solution of soap and water, making sure that the soap doesn't contain any alcohol.

■ Use proper venipuncture technique to collect the blood sample. (See the "Venipuncture" procedure.)

■ Fill the collection tubes completely to minimize the air space above the specimen, which can change the testing results.

■ Slowly invert the tubes completely at least five times *to ensure proper mixing of the additives.* Don't shake them vigorously.

■ Label the specimen tubes with the patient's name and identification number and the date and time in the presence of the patient *to prevent mislabeling.*[15] Obtain the law enforcement officer's initials on the tubes, if applicable.

■ Complete the required information on the evidence seals, initial the seals, and have the patient initial the seals.

■ Place a completed evidence seal across the top of each tube.

■ Complete the chain-of-custody labels and form, and have the patient sign the form.

■ Place the tubes into a padded transport box and then into a biohazard laboratory transport bag.[24]

■ Seal the bag with the chain-of-custody and evidence labels.

■ Remove and discard your gloves.[24]

■ Perform hand hygiene.[9,10,11,12,13,14]

■ Attach the chain-of-custody form.

NURSING ALERT Complete all of the above steps in full view of the patient and, if applicable, the appropriate law enforcement officer.

■ Place the specimen in a secure refrigerator if it won't be immediately transported to the laboratory.

■ Perform hand hygiene.[9,10,11,12,13,14]

■ Make sure the person who removes the specimen for transport signs the chain-of-custody form. Retain a copy and place it in the patient's medical record.

■ Document the procedure.[25,26,27,28]

Special considerations

■ Consent must be obtained if your state law doesn't cover the specimen collection.

■ If the specimen is being collected for a law enforcement agency, make sure that an officer has notified the patient of the patient's rights and explained the procedure before you obtain the sample.

■ Temperature strips attached to urine collection containers allow temperature certification between 90° F and 100° F (32.2° C and 37.8° C), which are acceptable under most standards.[21] However, some testing standards require that the urine's temperature be taken with a digital thermometer and be between 96° F and 99° F (35.6° C and 37.2° C).

■ If the urine specimen volume is inadequate, discard any specimen collected and the specimen collection container used for that attempt, have the patient sit in a waiting area where you can continuously observe the patient, and provide the patient with up to 40 ounces of water to drink (which should be evenly spread out over a 3-hour period or until the patient can provide an adequate specimen). Instruct the patient to tell you when the patient feels able to provide the specimen. If, after 3 hours, the patient can't provide a specimen, the collection should be terminated and you should notify the person who requested the test.[21]

Complications

If specimen collection is performed with no subsequent medical follow-up, serious medical conditions may go unidentified, causing the patient to experience adverse effects. Mishandling of the specimen or improper documentation of the chain of custody may lead to the evidence being inaccurate or inadmissible in court.

There are many ways for patients to circumvent testing: adding adulterants to urine at the time of testing, diluting urine through excessive water ingestion, consuming substances that interfere with testing, and substituting a clean urine sample. Appropriate collection techniques and tests of specimen integrity can reduce the risk of tampering.[1]

Documentation

Record the date and time, what test was performed, the reason for the test, and the type of specimen that was obtained. Note whether a law enforcement officer was present for the specimen collection, including the

agency the officer represented and the officer's badge number. Document that the chain of custody was preserved. Document teaching provided to the patient and family (if applicable), their understanding of that teaching, and any need for follow-up teaching.

REFERENCES

1 Kale, N. (2019). Urine drug tests: Ordering and interpretation. *American Family Physician, 99*(1), 33–39. https://www.aafp.org/afp/2019/0101/p33.html (Level VII)

2 Hoffman, R. J. (2021). Testing for drugs of abuse (DOA). In: *UpToDate,* Traub, S. J., (Ed.).

3 LabCorp. (n.d.). Blood drug testing. https://www.labcorp.com/drug-testing/types-of-drug-tests/blood-drug-testing

4 LabCorp. (2016). Drugs of abuse reference guide. https://files.labcorp.com/labcorp/L1123-0216-5.pdf

5 The Joint Commission. (2021). Standard RI.01.03.01. *Comprehensive accreditation manual for hospitals.* Oakbrook Terrace, IL: The Joint Commission. (Level VII)

6 Centers for Medicare and Medicaid Services, Department of Health and Human Services. (2020). Condition of participation: Patient's rights. 42 C.F.R. § 482.13(b)(2).

7 Accreditation Association for Hospitals and Health Systems. (2020). Standard 15.01.11. *Healthcare Facilities Accreditation Program: Accreditation requirements for acute care hospitals.* Chicago, IL: Accreditation Association for Hospitals and Health Systems. (Level VII)

8 DNV GL-Healthcare USA, Inc. (2020). PR.2.SR.3. *NIAHO® accreditation requirements, interpretive guidelines and surveyor guidance—revision 20.0.* Milford, OH: DNV GL-Healthcare USA, Inc. (Level VII)

9 Centers for Disease Control and Prevention. (2002). Guideline for hand hygiene in health-care settings: Recommendations of the Healthcare Infection Control Practices Advisory Committee and the HICPAC/SHEA/APIC/IDSA Hand Hygiene Task Force. *MMWR Recommendations and Reports, 51*(RR-16), 1–45. https://www.cdc.gov/mmwr/pdf/rr/rr5116.pdf (Level II)

10 The Joint Commission. (2021). Standard NPSG.07.01.01. *Comprehensive accreditation manual for hospitals.* Oakbrook Terrace, IL: The Joint Commission. (Level VII)

11 World Health Organization. (2009). WHO guidelines on hand hygiene in health care: First global patient safety challenge, clean care is safer care. https://apps.who.int/iris/bitstream/handle/10665/44102/9789241597906_eng.pdf?sequence=1 (Level IV)

12 Centers for Medicare and Medicaid Services, Department of Health and Human Services. (2020). Condition of participation: Infection control. 42 C.F.R. § 482.42.

13 Accreditation Association for Hospitals and Health Systems. (2020). Standard 07.01.21. *Healthcare Facilities Accreditation Program: Accreditation requirements for acute care hospitals.* Chicago, IL: Accreditation Association for Hospitals and Health Systems. (Level VII)

14 DNV GL-Healthcare USA, Inc. (2020). IC.1.SR.1. *NIAHO® accreditation requirements, interpretive guidelines and surveyor guidance—revision 20.0.* Milford, OH: DNV GL-Healthcare USA, Inc. (Level VII)

15 The Joint Commission. (2021). Standard NPSG.01.01.01. *Comprehensive accreditation manual for hospitals.* Oakbrook Terrace, IL: The Joint Commission. (Level VII)

16 Centers for Medicare and Medicaid Services, Department of Health and Human Services. (2020). Condition of participation: Patient's rights. 42 C.F.R. § 482.13(c)(1).

17 Accreditation Association for Hospitals and Health Systems. (2020). Standard 15.01.16. *Healthcare Facilities Accreditation Program: Accreditation requirements for acute care hospitals.* Chicago, IL: Accreditation Association for Hospitals and Health Systems. (Level VII)

18 The Joint Commission. (2021). Standard RI.01.01.01. *Comprehensive accreditation manual for hospitals.* Oakbrook Terrace, IL: The Joint Commission. (Level VII)

19 DNV GL-Healthcare USA, Inc. (2020). PR.2.SR.5. *NIAHO® accreditation requirements, interpretive guidelines and surveyor guidance—revision 20.0.* Milford, OH: DNV GL-Healthcare USA, Inc. (Level VII)

20 The Joint Commission. (2021). Standard PC.02.01.21. *Comprehensive accreditation manual for hospitals.* Oakbrook Terrace, IL: The Joint Commission. (Level VII)

21 U.S. Department of Transportation, Office of Drug and Alcohol Policy and Compliance. (2018). Urine specimen collection guidelines. https://www.transportation.gov/sites/dot.gov/files/docs/resources/partners/drug-and-alcohol-testing/2567/urine-specimen-collection-guidelines-january-2018.pdf (Level VII)

22 Siegel, J. D., et al. (2007, revised 2019). 2007 guideline for isolation precautions: Preventing transmission of infectious agents in healthcare settings. https://www.cdc.gov/infectioncontrol/pdf/guidelines/isolation-guidelines-H.pdf (Level II)

23 Accreditation Association for Hospitals and Health Systems. (2020). Standard 07.01.10. *Healthcare Facilities Accreditation Program: Accreditation requirements for acute care hospitals.* Chicago, IL: Accreditation Association for Hospitals and Health Systems. (Level VII)

24 Occupational Safety and Health Administration. (2019). Bloodborne pathogens, standard number 1910.1030. https://www.osha.gov/pls/oshaweb/owadisp.show_document?p_id=10051&p_table=STANDARDS (Level VII)

25 The Joint Commission. (2021). Standard RC.01.03.01. *Comprehensive accreditation manual for hospitals.* Oakbrook Terrace, IL: The Joint Commission. (Level VII)

26 Centers for Medicare and Medicaid Services, Department of Health and Human Services. (2020). Condition of participation: Medical record services. 42 C.F.R. § 482.24(b).

27 Accreditation Association for Hospitals and Health Systems. (2020). Standard 10.00.03. *Healthcare Facilities Accreditation Program: Accreditation requirements for acute care hospitals.* Chicago, IL: Accreditation Association for Hospitals and Health Systems. (Level VII)

28 DNV GL-Healthcare USA, Inc. (2020). MR.2.SR.1. *NIAHO® accreditation requirements, interpretive guidelines and surveyor guidance—revision 20.0.* Milford, OH: DNV GL-Healthcare USA, Inc. (Level VII)

DYING PATIENT CARE

Death is defined as either irreversible cessation of circulatory and respiratory functions or irreversible cessation of all functions of the entire brain, including the brain stem.[1] Signs and symptoms of impending death vary and may include confusion; delirium with decreased level of consciousness; disorientation, or fluctuating symptoms of cognitive impairment,[2] agitation, hallucinations, and restlessness;[3,4] irregular or decreased respirations that may be accompanied by rattling and gurgling sounds;[3] difficulty swallowing;[3] fatigue;[3] weak or erratic pulse; decreased blood pressure; decreased socialization or social withdrawal; pale, mottled, cyanotic, diaphoretic, or cool skin; constipation; bowel and bladder incontinence; involuntary movements; and loss of reflexes in the extremities.

A patient needs intensive physical support and emotional comfort as death approaches.[5] Emotional support for the dying patient and family most commonly entails reassurance; your physical presence helps ease fear and loneliness. More intense emotional support is important at much earlier stages, especially for patients with long-term progressive illnesses who can work through the stages of dying. (See *Five stages of dying.*)

Respect the patient's wishes about extraordinary means of supporting life. The patient may have a current, signed advance directive. This document, legally binding in most states, declares the patient's wishes for end-of-life care should the patient be unable to make decisions. (See the "Advance directives" procedure.)

Equipment

Gloves ▪ warm water ▪ soap ▪ washcloth ▪ towels ▪ lotion ▪ lift sheets ▪ oral care supplies ▪ artificial tears or ophthalmic saline solution ▪ sponge-tipped oral swab ▪ vital signs monitoring equipment ▪ stethoscope ▪ disinfectant pad ▪ Optional: bed linens, patient gown, fluid-impermeable pads, indwelling urinary catheter insertion kit; suction equipment; prescribed medications; oral fluids; pressure redistribution, padding, and repositioning devices; protective barrier cream, gown, mask and goggles or mask and face shield.

Preparation of equipment

Inspect all equipment and supplies. If a product is expired, is defective, or has compromised integrity, remove it from patient use, label it as expired or defective, and report the expiration or defect as directed by your facility.

Implementation

▪ Verify the presence of a current, signed advance directive in the patient's medical record. Obtain one from the patient's family members, if indicated; offer information on advance directives as requested and required by your facility.[6,7,8,9]

Five stages of dying

According to Elisabeth Kübler-Ross, author of *On Death and Dying*, the dying patient may progress through five psychological stages in preparation for death. Although each patient experiences these stages differently, and not necessarily in this order, understanding them will help you meet your patient's needs.

Denial
When the patient first learns of the terminal illness, the patient may refuse to accept the diagnosis. The patient may experience physical signs and symptoms similar to a stress reaction—shock, fainting, pallor, sweating, tachycardia, nausea, and GI disorders. During this stage, be honest with the patient but not blunt or callous. Maintain communication so the patient can discuss feelings when the patient accepts the reality of death. Don't force the patient to confront this reality.

Anger
After the patient stops denying the impending death, the patient may show deep resentment toward those who will live on after the patient dies—to you, to the facility staff, and to family. Although you may instinctively draw back from the patient or even resent this behavior, remember that the patient is dying and has a right to be angry. After you accept the anger, you can help the patient find different ways to express it, and you can help the patient's family to understand it.

Bargaining
Although the patient acknowledges the impending death, the patient may attempt to bargain, with God or fate, for more time. The patient will probably strike this bargain secretly. If the patient does confide in you, listen.

Depression
In this stage, the patient may first experience regrets about the past and then grieve about the current condition. The patient may withdraw from friends, family, the practitioner, and you. The patient may suffer from anorexia, increased fatigue, or self-neglect. You may find the patient sitting alone, in tears. Accept the patient's sorrow, and listen. Provide comfort by touch, as appropriate. Resist the temptation to make optimistic remarks or cheerful small talk

Acceptance
The patient who reaches this last stage accepts the inevitability and imminence of death—without emotion. The patient may simply desire the quiet company of a family member or friend. If, for some reason, a family member or friend can't be present, stay with the patient to satisfy this final need. Remember, however, that many patients die before reaching this stage.

▪ Clarify and communicate goals of treatment and the patient's values with the patient's family and multidisciplinary team.
▪ Gather and prepare the necessary equipment and supplies.

Meeting physical needs
▪ Perform hand hygiene.[10,11,12,13,14,15]
▪ Confirm the patient's identity using at least two patient identifiers.[16]
▪ Provide privacy.[17,18,19,20]
▪ Explain the procedure to the patient and family (if appropriate) according to their individual communication and learning needs *to increase their understanding, allay their fears, and enhance cooperation.*
▪ Raise the patient's bed to waist level before providing care *to prevent caregiver back strain.*[21]
▪ Perform hand hygiene.[10,11,12,13,14,15]
▪ Put on gloves and, as needed, other personal protective equipment *to comply with standard precautions.*[22,23,24]
▪ Whenever moving from a contaminated to a clean area during patient care, remove and discard your gloves,[24] perform hand hygiene,[10,11,12,13,14,15] and put on new gloves.[22,24]
▪ Obtain the patient's vital signs and perform assessments, including end-of-life signs and symptoms, as indicated.
▪ Screen for and assess the patient's pain using facility-defined criteria that are consistent with the patient's age, condition, and ability to understand.[25,26]

■ Treat the patient's pain, as needed and ordered, using nonpharmacologic, pharmacologic, or a combination of approaches. Base the treatment plan on evidence-based practices and the patient's clinical condition, past medical history, and pain management goals.[25] (See the "Pain management" procedure.) Administer pain and other medications for end-of-life signs and symptoms (such as dyspnea, cough, anxiety, and delirium), as needed and prescribed, following safe medication administration practices.[27,28,29,30]

■ When the patient's vision and hearing start to fail, turn the patient's head toward the light and speak to the patient from near the head of the bed. *Because hearing may be acute despite loss of consciousness,* avoid whispering or speaking inappropriately about the patient in the patient's presence.

■ Monitor skin integrity carefully and reposition the patient as needed. Individualize turning and repositioning according to the patient's preference. Use pressure redistribution, padding, and positioning devices, as needed, *to promote comfort.*

■ Change the bed linens and the patient's gown as needed. Provide skin care during gown changes.

■ Adjust the room temperature for patient comfort, if necessary.

■ Observe for incontinence or anuria (the result of diminished neuromuscular control), decreased renal function, constipation, or diarrhea. If necessary, obtain an order to catheterize the patient, or place fluid-impermeable pads beneath the patient's buttocks. Provide perineal care using soap and warm water, a washcloth, and towels *to prevent irritation.* Apply a protective barrier cream as indicated.

■ Elevate the head of the bed *to decrease respiratory resistance.* Provide gentle suction of the patient's oropharynx, as indicated, *to remove thick, copious secretions.* As the patient's condition deteriorates, the patient may breathe mostly through the mouth.

■ Offer fluids frequently and respectfully; don't force the patient to take fluids.

■ Provide oral care frequently, taking care to moisturize the oral mucosa and lips as needed *to provide comfort.* (See the "Oral care" procedure.)

■ Provide eye care using artificial tears or ophthalmic saline solution, as ordered, to prevent corneal ulceration, which can cause blindness and prevent the use of these tissues for transplantation after the patient dies. (See the "Eye care" procedure.)

■ Reassess and respond to the patient's pain by evaluating the response to treatment and progress toward pain management goals. Assess for adverse reactions and risk factors for adverse events that may result from treatment.[75]

■ Return the bed to the lowest position to prevent falls and maintain patient safety.[31]

■ Discard used supplies in appropriate receptacles.[24]

■ Remove and discard your gloves and, if worn, other personal protective equipment.[24]

■ Perform hand hygiene.[10,11,12,13,14,15]

■ Clean and disinfect your stethoscope with a disinfectant pad.[32,33]

■ Perform hand hygiene.[10,11,12,13,14,15]

Meeting emotional needs

■ Fully explain all care and treatments to the family and patient even if the patient is unconscious, *because hearing may be intact.*[34] Answer any questions as candidly as possible while remaining sensitive and respectful.

■ Allow the patient and family to express their feelings, which may range from anger to loneliness. Take time to talk with the patient and the family. Sit near the head of the bed and avoid looking rushed or unconcerned.

■ Assure the family that care will continue before, during, and after the withdrawal of life-sustaining measures as indicated, regardless of the outcome.

■ Encourage appropriate affection among the patient and family, and provide for privacy and confidentiality.

■ Appreciate cultural, spiritual, and religious traditions related to the dying process.

■ If the family is absent, notify them when the patient wishes to see them. Let the patient and family discuss death at their own pace.

■ Offer to contact a member of the clergy, palliative care team, hospice, or social services department, if appropriate.

■ Document the procedure.[35,36,37,38]

Special considerations

■ If family remain with the patient, show them the location of bathrooms, lounges, and cafeterias. Explain the patient's needs, treatments, and care plan to them. If appropriate, offer to teach them specific skills *so that they can take part in nursing care.* Emphasize that their efforts are important and effective. As the patient's death approaches, give them emotional support.

■ Teach the family about signs and symptoms of impending death.

■ Collaborate with the multidisciplinary team *to determine whether procedures and unnecessary medications can be discontinued.* Administer necessary medications by an alternative route when the oral route becomes difficult.[39]

■ Family dynamics and cultural, religious, and spiritual beliefs may all affect the grieving experience.[5] Matters commonly expressed and discussed include questions about an afterlife, unresolved social or emotional issues, and financial concerns.

■ Respect the patient's and family's wishes regarding complementary and alternative medicine; refer to the National Institutes of Health's National Center for Complementary and Alternative Medicine, as requested.[40]

■ In caring for dying patients, nurses can experience such negative physical and psychological outcomes as moral distress, compassion fatigue, and burnout. Nurses should promote physical, emotional, and spiritual self-care techniques when caring for dying patients *to prevent negative outcomes.*[41]

■ When appropriate, contact the Organ Procurement Organization (OPO) if the patient is being evaluated for brain death or if support is being withdrawn in anticipation of imminent death *so that an OPO coordinator can discuss possible organ donation with patient's family.* Such discussions require special knowledge, training, and experience to deliver the appropriate message to family members.[42] Check the patient's records *to determine whether the patient has completed an organ donor card.* (See *Understanding organ and tissue donation.*)

Documentation

Record changes in the patient's vital signs and general status. Note the patient's pain and sign and symptom assessment, pharmacologic and nonpharmacologic pain and symptom management, and the patient's response to pain management strategies. Document end-of-life care discussions, choices, and advance directives. Obtain all necessary signatures, consents, and required copies. Note the times of cardiac arrest and the end of respiration, and document the name of the practitioner and date and time of notification when these occur. Document teaching provided to the patient and family (if applicable), their understanding of that teaching, and any need for follow-up teaching.

Understanding organ and tissue donation

A federal regulation enacted in 1998 and revised in 2004 requires health care facilities to report patients whose death is imminent or who haves died at the facility. The report must be timely and must be directed to a regional organ procurement organization.[43,44,45] This regulation attempts to ensure that no potential donor goes undetected. The regulation ensures that the family of every potential donor will understand the option to donate. According to the American Medical Association, about 25 kinds of organs and tissues are transplanted. Although donor organ requirements vary, the typical donor must be between the ages of neonate and 60 years and free from transmissible disease. Tissue donations are less restrictive, and some tissue banks will accept skin from donors up to age 75.

Collection of most organs, such as the heart, liver, kidney, or pancreas, requires that the patient be pronounced brain dead and kept physically alive until the organs are harvested. Tissue, such as eyes, skin, bone, and heart valves, may be harvested after death. Contact your regional organ procurement organization for specific organ donation criteria or to identify a potential donor. If you don't know the regional organ procurement organization in your area, call the United Network for Organ Sharing at 804-782-4800.

For more on how to register for organ donation, go to http://donatelife.net/.

REFERENCES

1 The President's Commission for the Study of Ethical Problems in Medicine and Biomedical and Behavioral Research. (1981). Defining death: Medical, legal, and ethical issues in the determination of death. https://repository.library.georgetown.edu/bitstream/handle/10822/559345/defining_death.pdf?sequence=1&isAllowed=y (Level VII)

2 Grassi, L., et al. (2015). Management of delirium in palliative care: A review. *Current Psychiatry Reports, 17*(3), 13. (Level V)

3 National Cancer Institute. (2021). Last days of life (PDQ®)-Health professional version. https://www.cancer.gov/about-cancer/advanced-cancer/caregivers/planning/last-days-hp-pdq#_7

4 Sutherland, M., & Stilos, K. K. (2019). Evaluating the pharmacological management of terminal delirium in imminently dying patients with and without the Comfort Measure Order Set. *Journal of Hospice & Palliative Nursing, 21*, 430–437. (Level IV)

5 Craven, R. F., et al. (2021). *Fundamentals of nursing: Human health and function.* (9th ed.). Philadelphia, PA: Wolters Kluwer.

6 The Joint Commission. (2021). Standard RI.01.05.01. *Comprehensive accreditation manual for hospitals.* Oakbrook Terrace, IL: The Joint Commission. (Level VII)

7 Centers for Medicare and Medicaid Services, Department of Health and Human Services. (2020). Condition of participation: Patient's rights. 42 C.F.R. § 482.13(b)(3).

8 Accreditation Association for Hospitals and Health Systems. (2020). Standard 15.01.12. *Healthcare Facilities Accreditation Program: Accreditation requirements for acute care hospitals.* Chicago, IL: Accreditation Association for Hospitals and Health Systems. (Level VII)

9 DNV GL-Healthcare USA, Inc. (2020). PR.3.SR.1a. *NIAHO® accreditation requirements, interpretive guidelines and surveyor guidance—revision 20.0.* Milford, OH: DNV GL-Healthcare USA, Inc. (Level VII)

10 The Joint Commission. (2021). Standard NPSG.07.01.01. *Comprehensive accreditation manual for hospitals.* Oakbrook Terrace, IL: The Joint Commission. (Level VII)

11 Centers for Disease Control and Prevention. (2002). Guideline for hand hygiene in health-care settings: Recommendations of the Healthcare Infection Control Practices Advisory Committee and the HICPAC/SHEA/APIC/IDSA Hand Hygiene Task Force. *MMWR Recommendations and Reports, 51*(RR-16), 1–45. https://www.cdc.gov/mmwr/pdf/rr/rr5116.pdf (Level II)

12 World Health Organization. (2009). WHO guidelines on hand hygiene in health care. First global patient safety challenge, clean care is safer care. https://apps.who.int/iris/bitstream/handle/10665/44102/9789241597906_eng.pdf?sequence=1 (Level IV)

13 Centers for Medicare and Medicaid Services, Department of Health and Human Services. (2020). Condition of participation: Infection control. 42 C.F.R. § 482.42.

14 Accreditation Association for Hospitals and Health Systems. (2020). Standard 07.01.21. *Healthcare Facilities Accreditation Program: Accreditation requirements for acute care hospitals.* Chicago, IL: Accreditation Association for Hospitals and Health Systems. (Level VII)

15 DNV GL-Healthcare USA, Inc. (2020). IC.1.SR.1. *NIAHO® accreditation requirements, interpretive guidelines and surveyor guidance—revision 20.0.* Milford, OH: DNV GL-Healthcare USA, Inc. (Level VII)

16 The Joint Commission. (2021). Standard NPSG.01.01.01. *Comprehensive accreditation manual for hospitals.* Oakbrook Terrace, IL: The Joint Commission. (Level VII)

17 The Joint Commission. (2021). Standard RI.01.01.01. *Comprehensive accreditation manual for hospitals.* Oakbrook Terrace, IL: The Joint Commission. (Level VII)

18 Centers for Medicare and Medicaid Services, Department of Health and Human Services. (2020). Condition of participation: Patient's rights. 42 C.F.R. § 482.13(c)(1).

19 Accreditation Association for Hospitals and Health Systems. (2020). Standard 15.01.16. *Healthcare Facilities Accreditation Program: Accreditation requirements for acute care hospitals.* Chicago, IL: Accreditation Association for Hospitals and Health Systems. (Level VII)

20 DNV GL-Healthcare USA, Inc. (2020). PR.2.SR.5. *NIAHO® accreditation requirements, interpretive guidelines and surveyor guidance—revision 20.0.* Milford, OH: DNV GL-Healthcare USA, Inc. (Level VII)

21 Waters, T. R., et al. (2009). Safe patient handling training for schools of nursing. https://www.cdc.gov/niosh/docs/2009-127/pdfs/2009-127.pdf (Level VII)

22 Siegel, J. D., et al. (2007, revised 2019). 2007 guideline for isolation precautions: Preventing transmission of infectious agents in healthcare settings. https://www.cdc.gov/infectioncontrol/pdf/guidelines/isolation-guidelines-H.pdf (Level II)

23 Accreditation Association for Hospitals and Health Systems. (2020). Standard 07.01.10. *Healthcare Facilities Accreditation Program: Accreditation requirements for acute care hospitals.* Chicago, IL: Accreditation Association for Hospitals and Health Systems. (Level VII)

24 Occupational Safety and Health Administration. (2019). Bloodborne pathogens, standard number 1910.1030. https://www.osha.gov/pls/oshaweb/owadisp.show_document?p_id=10051&p_table=STANDARDS (Level VII)

25 The Joint Commission. (2021). Standard PC.01.02.07. *Comprehensive accreditation manual for hospitals.* Oakbrook Terrace, IL: The Joint Commission. (Level VII)

26 Blinderman, C. D., & Billings, J. A. (2015). Comfort care for patients dying in the hospital. *New England Journal of Medicine, 373*, 2549–2561. https://www.nejm.org/doi/full/10.1056/NEJMra1411746

27 The Joint Commission. (2021). Standard MM.06.01.01. *Comprehensive accreditation manual for hospitals.* Oakbrook Terrace, IL: The Joint Commission. (Level VII)

28 Centers for Medicare and Medicaid Services, Department of Health and Human Services. (2020). Condition of participation: Nursing services. 42 C.F.R. § 482.23(c).

29 Accreditation Association for Hospitals and Health Systems. (2020). Standard 16.01.03. *Healthcare Facilities Accreditation Program: Accreditation requirements for acute care hospitals.* Chicago, IL: Accreditation Association for Hospitals and Health Systems. (Level VII)

30 DNV GL-Healthcare USA, Inc. (2020). MM.1.SR.3. *NIAHO® accreditation requirements, interpretive guidelines and surveyor guidance—revision 20.0.* Milford, OH: DNV GL-Healthcare USA, Inc. (Level VII)

31 Ganz, D. A., et al. (2013, reviewed 2021). *Preventing falls in hospitals: A toolkit for improving quality of care* (AHRQ Publication No. 13-0015-EF). Rockville, MD: Agency for Healthcare Research and Quality. https://www.ahrq.gov/professionals/systems/hospital/fallpxtoolkit/index.html (Level VII)

32 Accreditation Association for Hospitals and Health Systems. (2020). Standard 07.02.03. *Healthcare Facilities Accreditation Program: Accreditation requirements for acute care hospitals.* Chicago, IL: Accreditation Association for Hospitals and Health Systems. (Level VII)

33 Rutala, W. A., et al. (2008, revised 2019). Guideline for disinfection and sterilization in healthcare facilities, 2008. https://www.cdc.gov/infection-control/pdf/guidelines/disinfection-guidelines-H.pdf (Level I)

34 The Joint Commission. (2021). Standard PC.02.01.21. *Comprehensive accreditation manual for hospitals.* Oakbrook Terrace, IL: The Joint Commission. (Level VII)

35 The Joint Commission. (2021). Standard RC.01.03.01. *Comprehensive accreditation manual for hospitals.* Oakbrook Terrace, IL: The Joint Commission. (Level VII)

36 Centers for Medicare and Medicaid Services, Department of Health and Human Services. (2020). Condition of participation: Medical record services. 42 C.F.R. § 482.24(b).

37 Accreditation Association for Hospitals and Health Systems. (2020). Standard 10.00.03. *Healthcare Facilities Accreditation Program: Accreditation requirements for acute care hospitals.* Chicago, IL: Accreditation Association for Hospitals and Health Systems. (Level VII)

38 DNV GL-Healthcare USA, Inc. (2020). MR.2.SR.1. *NIAHO® accreditation requirements, interpretive guidelines and surveyor guidance—revision 20.0.* Milford, OH: DNV GL-Healthcare USA, Inc. (Level VII)

39 Leung, J. G., et al. (2014). Pharmacotherapy during the end of life: Caring for the actively dying patient. *AACN Advanced Critical Care, 25*, 79–88.

40 National Center for Complimentary and Integrative Health. (2021). What does NCCIH do? https://www.nccih.nih.gov

41 McAdams, J. L., & Erikson, A. (2020). Self-care in the bereavement process. *Critical Care Nursing Clinics of North America, 32*, 421–437. (Level V)

42 National Institute for Health and Care Excellence. (2011, updated 2016). Organ donation for transplantation: Improving donor identification and consent rates for deceased organ donation: Approach to the those close to the patient. https://www.nice.org.uk/guidance/cg135/chapter/1-recommendations (Level I)

43 Centers for Medicare and Medicaid Services, Department of Health and Human Services. (2020). Condition of participation: Organ, tissue, and eye procurement. 42 C.F.R. § 482.45.

44 Accreditation Association for Hospitals and Health Systems. (2020). Standard 14.00.01. *Healthcare Facilities Accreditation Program: Accreditation requirements for acute care hospitals.* Chicago, IL: Accreditation Association for Hospitals and Health Systems. (Level VII)

45 DNV GL-Healthcare USA, Inc. (2020). TO.2.SR.2. *NIAHO® accreditation requirements, interpretive guidelines and surveyor guidance—revision 20.0.* Milford, OH: DNV GL-Healthcare USA, Inc. (Level VII)

Eardrop instillation

Eardrops may be prescribed for various conditions, including infection and inflammation. They may also be used to soften cerumen for removal, produce local anesthesia, and facilitate removal of an insect or other foreign body trapped in the ear.

Instillation of eardrops is usually contraindicated if the patient has a perforated eardrum, but it may be permitted with certain medications and adherence to sterile no-touch technique. Other conditions may also prohibit instillation of certain medications into the ear. For example, instillation of drops containing hydrocortisone is contraindicated if the patient has herpes, another viral infection, or a fungal infection.[1]

Equipment

Prescribed eardrops ■ light source ■ facial tissues ■ Optional: gloves, cotton balls, cotton-tipped applicator, personal protective equipment.

Preparation of equipment

Inspect all equipment and supplies. If a product is expired, is defective, or has compromised integrity, remove it from patient use, label it as expired or defective, and report the expiration or defect as directed by your facility. Before administration, allow the medication to reach room temperature, or warm the solution by gently rotating the container in your hands. *Instilling cold eardrops can cause dizziness and nausea.*

Implementation

■ Avoid distractions and interruptions when preparing and administering the medication *to prevent medication errors.*[2,3]
■ Verify the practitioner's order.[4,5,6,7]
■ Reconcile the patient's medications when the practitioner prescribes a new medication *to reduce the risk of medication errors, including omissions, duplications, dosing errors, and drug interactions.*[8,9]
■ Gather and prepare the medication and the necessary equipment and supplies.
■ Compare the medication label with the order in the patient's medical record.[4,5,6,7]
■ Check the patient's medical record for an allergy or a contraindication to the prescribed medication. If an allergy or other contraindication exists, don't administer the medication; instead, notify the practitioner.[4,5,6,7]
■ Check the expiration date on the medication. If the medication is expired, return it to the pharmacy and obtain new medication.[4,5,6,7]
■ Visually inspect the medication for particles, discoloration, or other signs of loss of integrity; don't administer the medication if its integrity is compromised.[4,5,6,7]
■ Discuss any unresolved concerns about the medication with the patient's practitioner.[4,5,6,7]
■ Perform hand hygiene.[10,11,12,13,14,15]
■ Confirm the patient's identity using at least two patient identifiers.[16]
■ Provide privacy.[17,18,19,20]
■ Explain the procedure to the patient and family (if appropriate) according to their individual communication and learning needs *to increase their understanding, allay their fears, and enhance cooperation.*[21]
■ If the patient is receiving the medication for the first time, teach the patient and family (if appropriate) about potential adverse effects, and discuss other concerns related to the medication.[4,5,6,7]
■ Verify the medication is being administered at the proper time, in the prescribed dose, and by the correct route *to reduce the risk of medication errors.*[4,5,6,7]
■ Confirm in which ear you must administer the medication.[4,5,6,7]
■ If your facility uses bar-code technology, use it as directed by your facility.
■ Raise the bed to waist level before providing patient care *to prevent caregiver back strain.*[22]
■ Perform hand hygiene.[10,11,12,13,14,15]

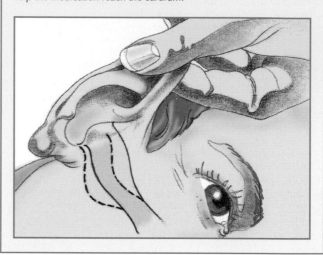

Positioning the patient for eardrop instillation

Before instilling eardrops, have the patient sit or lie with the head turned to the unaffected side. Then straighten the patient's ear canal by gently pulling the auricle (pinna) up and back (as shown below) *to help the medication reach the eardrum.*

NURSING ALERT If your facility's hazardous drug list contains the drug you're about to administer, put on personal protective equipment as directed.[23]
■ Put on gloves as needed *to comply with standard precautions.*[24,25,26]
■ Have the patient sit or lie with the head turned to the unaffected side.
■ Pull the patient's hair back, if needed, *to expose the ear.*
■ Straighten the patient's ear canal. Pull the auricle (pinna) of the ear up and back. (See *Positioning the patient for eardrop instillation.*)
■ Using a light source, examine the ear canal for drainage. If you find any, clean the outer ear with a tissue or cotton-tipped applicator.
■ *To avoid damaging the ear canal with the dropper,* gently support the hand holding the dropper against the patient's cheek or head, keeping the dropper above the ear canal and being careful not to contaminate it.
■ Squeeze the dropper slowly and firmly to instill the ordered number of drops on the side of the ear canal.
■ Massage the tragus (the fleshy part in front of the ear canal) gently with your finger, unless contraindicated because of pain. *Doing so facilitates entry of the medication into the ear canal.*
■ Have the patient remain supine with the head turned for the time specified by the medication's prescribing information (usually 1 to 5 minutes) *to allow absorption of the medication.*[27]
■ Place a cotton ball in the ear, if needed, *to prevent medication leakage.*[28]
■ Clean and dry the outer ear with a tissue.
■ If ordered, repeat the procedure on the other ear.
■ Assist the patient into a comfortable position.
■ Return the bed to the lowest position *to prevent falls and maintain patient safety.*[29]
■ Remove and discard your gloves, if worn.[26]
■ Perform hand hygiene.[10,11,12,13,14,15]
■ Document the procedure.[30,31,32,33]

Special considerations

■ Remember that some conditions make a normally tender ear canal even more sensitive, so be especially gentle when performing this procedure.
■ *To prevent injury to the eardrum,* never insert a cotton-tipped applicator or other sharp object into the ear canal.[34]

■ When the ear canal is obstructed, the practitioner may opt to enhance delivery of topical preparations by the use of aural toilet, placement of an ear wick, or both.[27]

Patient teaching

If the practitioner prescribes continued eardrop use at home, review the medication, dosage, scheduled times, expected results, and possible adverse effects with the patient and family (if appropriate). Teach the patient and family how to properly administer the medication, and observe a return demonstration of eardrop instillation (if possible).

Complications

Complications of eardrop instillation may include local reactions, such as redness and swelling of the ear canal, as well as systemic reactions. The patient may report dizziness, nausea, or discomfort if the medication is given while it's cold.

Documentation

Document the color and amount of ear drainage, if present. Document the medication strength, dose (number of eardrops instilled), administration route, ear(s) treated, and date and time of administration. Record any adverse reactions to the prescribed medication, the date and time the practitioner was notified, prescribed interventions, and the patient's response to those interventions.[35] Document teaching provided to the patient and family (if appropriate), their understanding of that teaching, and any need for follow-up teaching.

REFERENCES

1 Casper Pharma LLC. (2017). CASPORYN HC otic suspension sterile. https://www.accessdata.fda.gov/drugsatfda_docs/label/2017/060613s013lbl.pdf

2 Westbrook, J., et al. (2010). Association of interruptions with an increased risk and severity of medication administration errors. *Archives of Internal Medicine, 170*, 683–690. (Level IV)

3 Institute for Safe Medication Practices. (2012). Side tracks on the safety express: Interruptions lead to errors and unfinished…Wait, what was I doing? https://www.ismp.org/resources/side-tracks-safety-express-interruptions-lead-errors-and-unfinished-wait-what-was-i-doing?id=37

4 The Joint Commission. (2021). Standard MM.06.01.01. *Comprehensive accreditation manual for hospitals.* Oakbrook Terrace, IL: The Joint Commission. (Level VII)

5 Centers for Medicare and Medicaid Services, Department of Health and Human Services. (2020). Condition of participation: Nursing services. 42 C.F.R. § 482.23(c).

6 Accreditation Association for Hospitals and Health Systems. (2020). Standard 16.01.03. *Healthcare Facilities Accreditation Program: Accreditation requirements for acute care hospitals.* Chicago, IL: Accreditation Association for Hospitals and Health Systems. (Level VII)

7 DNV GL-Healthcare USA, Inc. (2020). MM.1.SR.3. *NIAHO® accreditation requirements, interpretive guidelines and surveyor guidance—revision 20.0.* Milford, OH: DNV GL-Healthcare USA, Inc. (Level VII)

8 The Joint Commission. (2021). Standard NPSG.03.06.01. *Comprehensive accreditation manual for hospitals.* Oakbrook Terrace, IL: The Joint Commission. (Level VII)

9 Accreditation Association for Hospitals and Health Systems. (2020). Standard 25.02.03. *Healthcare Facilities Accreditation Program: Accreditation requirements for acute care hospitals.* Chicago, IL: Accreditation Association for Hospitals and Health Systems. (Level VII)

10 The Joint Commission. (2021). Standard NPSG.07.01.01. *Comprehensive accreditation manual for hospitals.* Oakbrook Terrace, IL: The Joint Commission. (Level VII)

11 Centers for Disease Control and Prevention. (2002). Guideline for hand hygiene in health-care settings: Recommendations of the Healthcare Infection Control Practices Advisory Committee and the HICPAC/SHEA/APIC/IDSA Hand Hygiene Task Force. *MMWR Recommendations and Reports, 51*(RR-16), 1–45. https://www.cdc.gov/mmwr/pdf/rr/rr5116.pdf (Level II)

12 World Health Organization. (2009). WHO guidelines on hand hygiene in health care: First global patient safety challenge, clean care is safer care. https://apps.who.int/iris/bitstream/handle/10665/44102/9789241597906_eng.pdf?sequence=1 (Level IV)

13 Centers for Medicare and Medicaid Services, Department of Health and Human Services. (2020). Condition of participation: Infection control. 42 C.F.R. § 482.42.

14 Accreditation Association for Hospitals and Health Systems. (2020). Standard 07.01.21. *Healthcare Facilities Accreditation Program: Accreditation requirements for acute care hospitals.* Chicago, IL: Accreditation Association for Hospitals and Health Systems. (Level VII)

15 DNV GL-Healthcare USA, Inc. (2020). IC.1.SR.1. *NIAHO® accreditation requirements, interpretive guidelines and surveyor guidance—revision 20.0.* Milford, OH: DNV GL-Healthcare USA, Inc. (Level VII)

16 The Joint Commission. (2021). Standard NPSG.01.01.01. *Comprehensive accreditation manual for hospitals.* Oakbrook Terrace, IL: The Joint Commission. (Level VII)

17 Accreditation Association for Hospitals and Health Systems. (2020). Standard 15.01.16. *Healthcare Facilities Accreditation Program: Accreditation requirements for acute care hospitals.* Chicago, IL: Accreditation Association for Hospitals and Health Systems. (Level VII)

18 Centers for Medicare and Medicaid Services, Department of Health and Human Services. (2020). Condition of participation: Patient's rights. 42 C.F.R. § 482.13(c)(1).

19 DNV GL-Healthcare USA, Inc. (2020). PR.2.SR.5. *NIAHO® accreditation requirements, interpretive guidelines and surveyor guidance—revision 20.0.* Milford, OH: DNV GL-Healthcare USA, Inc. (Level VII)

20 The Joint Commission. (2021). Standard RI.01.01.01. *Comprehensive accreditation manual for hospitals.* Oakbrook Terrace, IL: The Joint Commission. (Level VII)

21 The Joint Commission. (2021). Standard PC.02.01.21. *Comprehensive accreditation manual for hospitals.* Oakbrook Terrace, IL: The Joint Commission. (Level VII)

22 Waters, T. R., et al. (2009). Safe patient handling training for schools of nursing. https://www.cdc.gov/niosh/docs/2009-127/pdfs/2009-127.pdf (Level VII)

23 United States Pharmacopeial Convention. (2019). USP general chapter <800> hazardous drugs: Handling in healthcare settings. https://www.usp.org/compounding/general-chapter-hazardous-drugs-handling-healthcare (Level VII)

24 Siegel, J. D., et al. (2007, revised 2019). 2007 guideline for isolation precautions: Preventing transmission of infectious agents in healthcare settings. https://www.cdc.gov/infectioncontrol/pdf/guidelines/isolation-guidelines-H.pdf (Level II)

25 Accreditation Association for Hospitals and Health Systems. (2020). Standard 07.01.10. *Healthcare Facilities Accreditation Program: Accreditation requirements for acute care hospitals.* Chicago, IL: Accreditation Association for Hospitals and Health Systems. (Level VII)

26 Occupational Safety and Health Administration. (2012). Bloodborne pathogens, standard number 1910.1030. https://www.osha.gov/pls/oshaweb/owadisp.show_document?p_id=10051&p_table=STANDARDS (Level VII)

27 Rosenfeld, R. M., et al. (2014). Clinical practice guideline: Acute otitis externa. *Otolaryngology—Head and Neck Surgery, 150*(1S), S1–S24. https://journals.sagepub.com/doi/pdf/10.1177/0194599813517083 (Level VII)

28 American Society of Health-System Pharmacists (ASHP). (2021). How to use ear drops. https://www.safemedication.com/-/media/SafeMed/Flyers/Ear-Drops-Flyer.pdf

29 Ganz, D. A., et al. (2013, reviewed 2021). *Preventing falls in hospitals: A toolkit for improving quality of care* (AHRQ Publication No. 13-0015-EF). Rockville, MD: Agency for Healthcare Research and Quality. https://www.ahrq.gov/professionals/systems/hospital/fallpxtoolkit/index.html (Level VII)

30 The Joint Commission. (2021). Standard RC.01.03.01. *Comprehensive accreditation manual for hospitals.* Oakbrook Terrace, IL: The Joint Commission. (Level VII)

31 Accreditation Association for Hospitals and Health Systems. (2020). Standard 10.00.03. *Healthcare Facilities Accreditation Program: Accreditation requirements for acute care hospitals.* Chicago, IL: Accreditation Association for Hospitals and Health Systems. (Level VII)

32 Centers for Medicare and Medicaid Services, Department of Health and Human Services. (2020). Condition of participation: Medical record services. 42 C.F.R. § 482.24(b).

33 DNV GL-Healthcare USA, Inc. (2020). MR.2.SR.1. *NIAHO® accreditation requirements, interpretive guidelines and surveyor guidance—revision 20.0.* Milford, OH: DNV GL-Healthcare USA, Inc. (Level VII)

34 Craven, R. F., et al. (2020). *Fundamentals of nursing: Concepts and competencies for practice* (9th ed.). Philadelphia, PA: Wolters Kluwer.

35 The Joint Commission. (2021). Standard RC.02.01.01. *Comprehensive accreditation manual for hospitals.* Oakbrook Terrace, IL: The Joint Commission. (Level VII)

EAR IRRIGATION

Ear irrigation involves washing the external auditory canal with a stream of solution to clean the canal of discharge, soften and remove impacted cerumen, or dislodge a foreign body. Sometimes, irrigation aims to relieve localized inflammation and discomfort. The procedure must be performed carefully so that it doesn't cause the patient discomfort or vertigo, and to avoid increasing the risk of otitis externa. Because irrigation may contaminate the middle ear if the tympanic membrane is ruptured, an otoscopic examination always precedes ear irrigation.[1]

NURSING ALERT This procedure is contraindicated when a vegetable (such as a pea) obstructs the auditory canal. This type of foreign body attracts and absorbs moisture. In contact with an irrigant or other solution, it swells, causing intense pain and complicating removal of the object.[2,3] Ear irrigation is also contraindicated if the patient has a cold, a fever, an ear infection, an injured or ruptured tympanic membrane, a history of ear surgery, or a cleft palate with or without surgical repair.[3] Procedural modifications may be indicated for patients with structural abnormalities, diabetes, or an immunocompromised state, or those receiving anticoagulant therapy.[3]

Equipment

Irrigation device (bulb syringe, syringe with irrigating tip, or commercial ear irrigation device) ■ otoscope with ear speculum ■ prescribed irrigating solution (water, normal saline, or other irrigating solution) ■ basin filled with hot water ■ light source ■ emesis basin ■ gloves ■ fluid-impermeable pad ■ bath towel ■ washcloth ■ 4″ × 4″ (10 cm × 10 cm) gauze pad ■ Optional: goggles or face shield.

Preparation of equipment

Inspect all equipment and supplies. If a product is expired, is defective, or has compromised integrity, remove it from patient use, label it as expired or defective, and report the expiration or defect as directed by your facility. Select an appropriate syringe and obtain the prescribed irrigating solution. Put the container of irrigating solution into the large basin filled with hot water *to warm the solution to body temperature: 98.6° F (37° C).*[1] Avoid extreme temperature changes, *because they can cause a caloric response, which can cause dizziness, nausea, vomiting, or falling.*[1,3] Test the temperature of the solution by sprinkling a few drops on your inner wrist.

Implementation

■ Verify the practitioner's order.
■ Review the patient's medical record for history of the condition, including symptoms, diseases involving the ear, and the condition of the tympanic membrane.[1]
■ Gather and prepare the necessary equipment and supplies.
■ Perform hand hygiene.[4,5,6,7,8,9]
■ Confirm the patient's identity using at least two patient identifiers.[10]
■ Provide privacy.[11,12,13,14]
■ Explain the procedure to the patient and family (if appropriate) according to their individual communication and learning needs *to increase their understanding, allay their fears, and enhance cooperation.*[15]
■ Make sure you have adequate lighting.
■ Raise the patient's bed to waist level before providing patient care *to prevent caregiver back strain.*[16]
■ Perform hand hygiene.[4,5,6,7,8,9]
■ Put on gloves *to comply with standard precautions.*[17,18,19]
■ *To avoid introducing foreign matter into the ear canal,* clean the auricle and the meatus of the auditory canal with a washcloth moistened with normal saline solution or other prescribed irrigating solution.

■ If you haven't already done so, use the otoscope with ear speculum to inspect the auditory canal to be irrigated.[1]

NURSING ALERT The ear canal is very sensitive, and instrumentation can cause pain. Use caution when examining the ear. The patient must remain still while you examine the ear and insert any instruments into the ear *to avoid ear canal damage.*

■ Help the patient to a sitting position. *To prevent the solution from running down the neck,* tilt the head slightly forward and toward the affected side. If the patient can't sit, have the patient lie on the back and tilt the head slightly forward and toward the affected ear.
■ If the patient is sitting, place the fluid-impermeable pad covered with the bath towel on the shoulder and upper arm, under the affected ear. If the patient is lying down, cover the pillow and the area under the affected ear.
■ Put on goggles or a face shield before irrigation, if necessary.[17,19]
■ Draw the irrigant into the irrigation device and expel any air.
■ Gently pull the pinna up and back *to straighten the ear canal.*[3] Have the patient hold an emesis basin beneath the ear *to catch returning irritant.*
■ Position the tip of the irrigating syringe at the meatus of the auditory canal (as shown below). Don't block the meatus, *because you'll impede backflow and raise pressure in the canal.* If using a commercial irrigation device, follow the manufacturer's instructions.

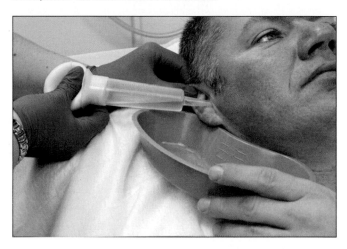

■ With the patient's head tilted toward the affected ear, point the syringe tip upward and toward the posterior ear canal. *This angle prevents damage to the tympanic membrane and guards against pushing debris farther into the ear canal.* Direct a steady stream of irrigating solution against the upper wall of the ear canal *to help clear the widening area of the ear canal next to the tympanic membrane*[20,21] (as shown below).

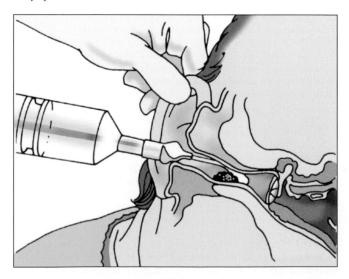

■ Check the return flow and monitor the patient's tolerance of the procedure throughout the irrigation.

NURSING ALERT During irrigation, observe the patient for signs of pain or dizziness. If the patient reports either complication, stop the procedure and recheck the temperature of the irrigating solution. Inspect the patient's ear with the otoscope, and resume irrigation, as indicated.

■ Remove the syringe when it's empty and inspect the return flow for cloudiness, cerumen, blood, or foreign matter. If necessary, refill the syringe with irrigating solution and continue the irrigation until the return flow is clear. Don't use more than 500 mL of irrigant during this procedure.[3]

■ Remove the syringe, and inspect the ear canal for cleanliness with the otoscope.

■ Dry the patient's auricle and neck.

■ Remove the bath towel and fluid-impermeable pad. Have the patient lie on the affected side with the 4" × 4" (10 cm × 10 cm) gauze pad under the ear *to promote drainage of residual debris and solution.*

■ Return the bed to the lowest position *to prevent falls and maintain patient safety.*[22]

■ Discard used supplies in the appropriate receptacles.[19]

■ Remove and discard your gloves and goggles or face shield, if worn.[19]

■ Perform hand hygiene.[4,5,6,7,8,9]

■ Document the procedure.[23,24,25,26]

Special considerations

■ Avoid dropping or squirting irrigating solution on the tympanic membrane, *which can startle the patient and cause discomfort.*

■ If the practitioner directs you to place a cotton pledget in the ear canal *to retain some of the solution*, pack the cotton loosely. Instruct the patient not to remove it.

■ If irrigation doesn't dislodge impacted cerumen, the practitioner may order you to instill several drops of glycerin, docusate, 2% acetic acid, 10% sodium bicarbonate, carbamide peroxide, or a similar preparation two to three times daily for 2 to 3 days, and then to irrigate the ear again.[1]

■ If you're performing the procedure on a patient with a hearing aid, remove the hearing aid and then inspect the ear canal with a handheld otoscope. If the patient has bilateral hearing aids, replace the first hearing aid before you examine the second ear *to facilitate communication.* Note that cerumen impaction may change hearing aid performance.[1]

Patient teaching

Discourage patients from using manual methods for cerumen removal, such as cotton-tipped applicators or an irrigator designed for teeth cleaning.[27] Measures that may be beneficial in reducing cerumen impaction include installation of prophylactic topical preparations, irrigation of the ear canal, and routine cleaning of the ear canal by a practitioner every 6 to 12 months, as indicated. Individuals who wear hearing aids are at increased risk for developing cerumen impactions; therefore, provide instructions to the patient and caregiver on proper care and cleaning of these aids. Discuss proper ear hygiene *to prevent recurrence of cerumen impaction.*[1] Advise the patient to avoid using ear candles or cones, *because evidence doesn't support their use, and they can cause serious damage to the ear canal and eardrum.*[1]

Complications

Possible complications include pain, tinnitus, vertigo, nausea, otitis externa, bleeding or injury to the canal, and otitis media (if the patient has a perforated or ruptured tympanic membrane). Forceful instillation of irrigating solution can rupture the tympanic membrane. Instilling cerumenolytic agents can also result in transient hearing loss and local irritation.[1]

Documentation

Record the date and time of irrigation, and note which ear you irrigated. Document the volume and type of irrigating solution you used, the appearance of the canal before and after irrigation, the appearance of the return flow, the patient's tolerance of the procedure, and any comments that the patient made about the condition, especially those related to the patient's hearing acuity. Document teaching provided to the patient and family (if applicable), their understanding of that teaching, and any need for follow-up teaching.

REFERENCES

1 Schwartz, S. R., et al. (2017). Clinical practice guideline (update): Earwax (cerumen impaction). *Otolaryngology—Head and Neck Surgery, 156*, S1–S29. https://journals.sagepub.com/doi/pdf/10.1177/0194599816671491 (Level VII)

2 Kwong, A. O. (2018). Ear foreign body removal procedures. https://emedicine.medscape.com/article/80507-overview

3 Hayter, K. L. (2016). Listen up for safe ear irrigation. *Nursing, 46*(6), 62–65. https://journals.lww.com/nursing/fulltext/2016/06000/Listen_up_for_safe_ear_irrigation.16.aspx

4 The Joint Commission. (2021). Standard NPSG.07.01.01. *Comprehensive accreditation manual for hospitals.* Oakbrook Terrace, IL: The Joint Commission. (Level VII)

5 Centers for Disease Control and Prevention. (2002). Guideline for hand hygiene in health-care settings: Recommendations of the Healthcare Infection Control Practices Advisory Committee and the HICPAC/SHEA/APIC/IDSA Hand Hygiene Task Force. *MMWR Recommendations and Reports, 51*(RR-16), 1–45. https://www.cdc.gov/mmwr/pdf/rr/rr5116.pdf (Level II)

6 World Health Organization. (2009). WHO guidelines on hand hygiene in health care: First global patient safety challenge, clean care is safer care. https://apps.who.int/iris/bitstream/handle/10665/44102/9789241597906_eng.pdf?sequence=1 (Level IV)

7 Centers for Medicare and Medicaid Services, Department of Health and Human Services. (2020). Condition of participation: Infection control. 42 C.F.R. § 482.42.

8 Accreditation Association for Hospitals and Health Systems. (2020). Standard 07.01.21. *Healthcare Facilities Accreditation Program: Accreditation requirements for acute care hospitals.* Chicago, IL: Accreditation Association for Hospitals and Health Systems. (Level VII)

9 DNV GL-Healthcare USA, Inc. (2020). IC.1.SR.1. *NIAHO® accreditation requirements, interpretive guidelines and surveyor guidance - revision 20.0.* Milford, OH: DNV GL-Healthcare USA, Inc. (Level VII)

10 The Joint Commission. (2021). Standard NPSG.01.01.01. *Comprehensive accreditation manual for hospitals.* Oakbrook Terrace, IL: The Joint Commission. (Level VII)

11 Centers for Medicare and Medicaid Services, Department of Health and Human Services. (2020). Condition of participation: Patient's rights. 42 C.F.R. § 482.13(c)(1).

12 Accreditation Association for Hospitals and Health Systems. (2020). Standard 15.01.16. *Healthcare Facilities Accreditation Program: Accreditation requirements for acute care hospitals.* Chicago, IL: Accreditation Association for Hospitals and Health Systems. (Level VII)

13 The Joint Commission. (2021). Standard RI.01.01.01. *Comprehensive accreditation manual for hospitals.* Oakbrook Terrace, IL: The Joint Commission. (Level VII)

14 DNV GL-Healthcare USA, Inc. (2020). PR.2.SR.5. *NIAHO® accreditation requirements, interpretive guidelines and surveyor guidance - revision 20.* Milford, OH: DNV GL-Healthcare USA, Inc. (Level VII)

15 The Joint Commission. (2021). Standard PC.02.01.21. *Comprehensive accreditation manual for hospitals.* Oakbrook Terrace, IL: The Joint Commission. (Level VII)

16 Waters, T. R., et al. (2009). Safe patient handling training for schools of nursing. https://www.cdc.gov/niosh/docs/2009-127/pdfs/2009-127.pdf (Level VII)

17 Siegel, J. D., et al. (2007, revised 2019). 2007 guideline for isolation precautions: Preventing transmission of infectious agents in healthcare settings. https://www.cdc.gov/infectioncontrol/pdf/guidelines/isolation-guidelines-H.pdf (Level II)

18 Accreditation Association for Hospitals and Health Systems. (2020). Standard 07.01.10. *Healthcare Facilities Accreditation Program: Accreditation requirements for acute care hospitals.* Chicago, IL: Accreditation Association for Hospitals and Health Systems. (Level VII)

19 Occupational Safety and Health Administration. (2012). Bloodborne pathogens, standard number 1910.1030. https://www.osha.gov/pls/oshaweb/owadisp.show_document?p_id=10051&p_table=STANDARDS (Level VII)

20 Dinces, E. A. (2021). Cerumen. In: *UpToDate*, Deschler, D. G. (Ed.).

21 Isaacson, G. C., & Ojo, A. (2020). Diagnosis and management of foreign bodies of the outer ear. In: *UpToDate*, Stack, A. M. (Ed.).

22 Ganz, D. A., et al. (2013, reviewed 2021). *Preventing falls in hospitals: A toolkit for improving quality of care* (AHRQ Publication No. 13-0015-EF). Rockville, MD: Agency for Health Research and Quality. https://www.ahrq.gov/professionals/systems/hospital/fallpxtoolkit/index.html (Level VII)

23 The Joint Commission. (2021). Standard RC.01.03.01. *Comprehensive accreditation manual for hospitals.* Oakbrook Terrace, IL: The Joint Commission. (Level VII)

24 Centers for Medicare and Medicaid Services, Department of Health and Human Services. (2020). Condition of participation: Medical record services. 42 C.F.R. § 482.24(b).

25 Accreditation Association for Hospitals and Health Systems. (2020). Standard 10.00.03. *Healthcare Facilities Accreditation Program: Accreditation requirements for acute care hospitals.* Chicago, IL: Accreditation Association for Hospitals and Health Systems. (Level VII)

26 DNV GL-Healthcare USA, Inc. (2020). MR.2.SR.1. *NIAHO® accreditation requirements, interpretive guidelines and surveyor guidance - revision 20.0.* Milford, OH: DNV GL-Healthcare USA, Inc. (Level VII)

27 Shargorodsky, J., & Zieve, D. (2020). Ear wax. https://medlineplus.gov/ency/article/000979.htm

ELASTIC COMPRESSION BANDAGE APPLICATION

Elastic compression bandages exert gentle, even pressure on a body part. They can be used to minimize joint swelling [1] and provide support after musculoskeletal trauma. When used with a splint, they can immobilize a fracture during healing. They also provide hemostatic pressure, and anchor dressings over a fresh wound or after surgical procedures, such as vein stripping.

Less commonly, elastic compression bandages are used to help promote venous return. They can prevent pooling of blood in the legs, and are sometimes used in place of antiembolism stockings to prevent venous thromboembolism, such as deep vein thrombosis and pulmonary embolism, in postoperative or bedridden patients who can't stimulate venous return through muscle activity. Elastic compression bandages may also be used to manage lower extremity edema and venous insufficiency, and to promote healing in patients with venous ulcers.[2,3]

Equipment

Elastic compression bandage of appropriate width and length ▪ tape or self-closures ▪ cleaning solution (skin cleaner, mild soap and water, or saline solution)[4] ▪ towel ▪ Optional: gloves, skin barrier cream,[4] gauze pads or absorbent cotton.

Elastic compression bandages usually come in 2″ to 6″ (5 cm to 15.2 cm) widths and 4′ and 6′ (1.2 and 1.8 M) lengths. The 3″ (7.6 cm) width is adaptable to most applications. An elastic bandage with self-closures is also available.

Preparation of equipment

Inspect all equipment and supplies. If a product is expired, is defective, or has compromised integrity, remove it from patient use, label it as expired or defective, and report the expiration or defect as directed by your facility.

Select an elastic compression bandage that wraps completely around the affected body part but isn't excessively long. Generally, use a narrower bandage for wrapping the foot, lower leg, hand, or arm and a wider bandage for the thigh or trunk. The bandage should be clean and rolled before application.

Implementation

▪ Verify the practitioner's order.
▪ Review the patient's medical record for contraindications to elastic compression bandage application.
▪ Gather and prepare the necessary equipment and supplies.
▪ Perform hand hygiene.[5,6,7,8,9,10]
▪ Confirm the patient's identity using at least two patient identifiers.[11]
▪ Provide privacy.[12,13,14,15]
▪ Explain the procedure to the patient and family (if appropriate) according to their individual communication and learning needs *to increase their understanding, allay their fears, and enhance cooperation.*[16]

▪ Raise the patient's bed to waist level before providing patient care *to prevent caregiver back strain.*[17]
▪ Position the patient comfortably, with the body part to be bandaged in normal functioning position *to promote circulation and prevent deformity and discomfort.*
▪ Perform hand hygiene.[5,6,7,8,9,10]
▪ Put on gloves as needed *to comply with standard precautions.*[18,19,20]
▪ Inspect the area to be wrapped for lesions and skin breakdown.[4] If either condition is present, consult the practitioner before applying the elastic compression bandage.
▪ Clean and dry the skin surface of the area to be wrapped; apply a skin barrier cream, as indicated.[4]
▪ If the patient requires an elastic compression wrap because of significant lower extremity edema, consult with a wound care nurse or another practitioner competent in the application of compression wraps (as needed) *to ensure proper application and reduce the risk of impaired circulation.*[4]
▪ Before applying a bandage to an extremity with significant dependent edema, elevate the extremity for 15 to 30 minutes *to facilitate venous return.*[4]
▪ Avoid allowing two adjacent skin surfaces to touch when applying an elastic compression bandage. Place gauze pads or absorbent cotton as needed between skin surfaces, such as between toes and fingers and under breasts and arms, *to prevent skin irritation.*
▪ Hold the elastic compression bandage with the roll facing up in one hand and the free end of the bandage in the other hand. Hold the bandage roll close to the part being bandaged *to ensure even tension and pressure.*
▪ When wrapping an extremity, begin wrapping at the most distal part and work proximally *to promote venous return.*
▪ Anchor the elastic compression bandage initially by circling the body part twice. *To prevent the bandage from slipping out of place on a foot,* wrap it in a figure eight around the foot, the ankle, and then the foot again before continuing. The same technique works on any joint, such as the knee. Include the heel when wrapping the foot, but don't wrap the toes unless absolutely necessary, *because the distal extremities are assessed to detect impaired circulation.*
▪ Unroll the elastic compression bandage as you wrap the body part. Never unroll the entire bandage before wrapping, *because doing so could produce uneven pressure, which may interfere with blood circulation and cell nourishment.*
▪ Overlap each layer of the elastic bandage by one-half to two-thirds the width of the strip. (See *Bandaging techniques.*)
▪ Wrap the elastic compression bandage firmly, but not too tightly. As you wrap, ask the patient to tell you if the bandage feels comfortable. If the patient reports tingling, itching, numbness, or pain, loosen the bandage.
▪ When you're finished wrapping the elastic compression bandage, secure the end of the bandage with tape or self-closures. Be careful not to scratch or pinch the patient. Avoid using metal clips, *because they typically come loose when the patient moves, and can get lost in the bed linens and injure the patient.*
▪ Assess the patient's distal circulation immediately after the bandage has been secured *because the elastic may tighten as you wrap.* Repeat this assessment every 4 hours thereafter, *because an elastic compression bandage that's too tight can cause neurovascular damage.* Lift the distal end of the bandage and assess the color, temperature, and integrity of skin underneath.
▪ If the wrapped body part is an extremity, elevate it for 15 to 30 minutes after wrapping *to facilitate venous return.*
▪ Return the bed to the lowest position *to prevent falls and maintain patient safety.*[21]
▪ Remove the elastic compression bandage every 8 hours or whenever it's loose, soiled, or wrinkled. Roll the bandage up as you unwrap it *to ready it for reuse, if appropriate.* Observe the area's skin integrity, and provide skin care before rewrapping the bandage.
▪ Replace the elastic compression bandage at least once daily. Bathe the skin with cleaning solution, dry it thoroughly, and observe for irritation or breakdown before applying a fresh bandage.
▪ Remove and discard gloves, if worn.[18]
▪ Perform hand hygiene.[5,6,7,8,9,10]
▪ Document the procedure.[22,23,24,25]

Bandaging techniques

Circular
With each turn, encircle the previous layer and cover it completely. Use this technique to anchor a bandage.

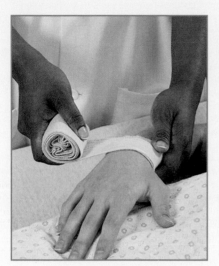

Spiral
With each turn, partially overlap the previous layer. Use this technique to wrap a long, straight body part or one of increasing circumference.

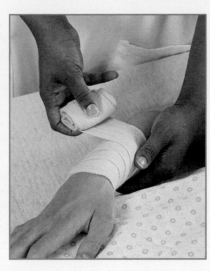

Spiral-reverse
Anchor the bandage and then reverse direction halfway through each spiral turn. Use this technique to accommodate the increasing circumference of a body part.

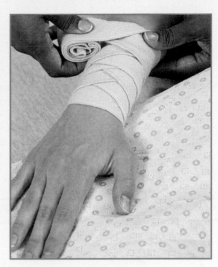

Figure eight
Anchor below the joint, and then use alternating ascending and descending turns to form a figure eight. Use this technique around joints.

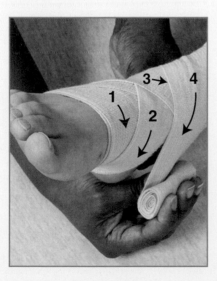

Recurrent
This technique includes a combination of recurrent and circular turns. Hold the bandage as you make each recurrent turn and then use the circular turns as a final anchor. Use this technique for a residual limb, a hand, or the scalp.

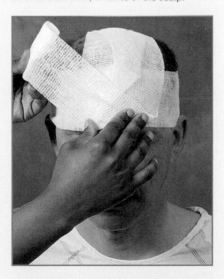

Special considerations

■ If a patient has weeping lower-extremity edema, change the elastic compression bandage frequently. Ensure that the bandage doesn't shift or crease, *which could cause constriction, particularly around the heel and ankle.*[4]

■ Avoid leaving gaps in elastic compression bandage layers, resulting in exposed skin surfaces between layers, *because doing so can result in uneven pressure on the body part.*

■ Observe the patient for an allergic reaction, *because some patients can't tolerate the sizing material in a new elastic compression bandage.* Laundering a new bandage before use reduces this risk. Use latex-free elastic bandages for patients with latex allergy.

■ Launder the elastic compression bandage daily or whenever it becomes limp *to restore the bandage's elasticity.* Always keep two bandages handy *so one can be applied while the other bandage is being laundered.*

■ When using an elastic compression bandage after a surgical procedure on an extremity (such as vein stripping) or with a splint to immobilize a fracture, remove it only as ordered rather than every 8 hours.[26]

Patient teaching

If an elastic compression bandage will be used at home, teach the patient or a family member how to apply it correctly and how to assess for impaired circulation. Demonstrate the procedure and observe a return demonstration before the patient's discharge. Tell the patient to keep two bandages available so that one is available for use while the other is being laundered. Ensure that the patient has the information needed to obtain additional supplies.

Complications

Arterial obstruction—characterized by a decreased or absent distal pulse, skin blanching or bluish discoloration, dusky nail beds, numbness and tingling or pain and cramping, and cold skin—can result from elastic compression bandage application. Edema can result from obstruction of venous return. Less serious complications include allergic reaction and skin irritation.

Documentation

Record the date and time of elastic compression bandage application and removal as well as the application site, the bandage size, skin condition before application, skin care provided after removal, and the patient's tolerance of the treatment. Note any complications, interventions performed, and the patient's response to them. Document teaching provided to the patient and family (if appropriate), their understanding of that teaching, and any need for follow-up teaching.

REFERENCES

1 Matthews, C. N., et al. (2019). Does an elastic compression bandage provide any benefit after primary TKA? *Clinical Orthopaedics and Related Research, 477*(1), 134–144. https://journals.lww.com/clinorthop/Fulltext/2019/01000/Does_an_Elastic_Compression_Bandage_Provide_Any.26.aspx (Level IV)

2 O'Meara, S., et al. (2012). Compression for venous leg ulcers. *Cochrane Database of Systematic Reviews*, 2012(11), CD000265. (Level I)

3 Mauck, K. F., et al. (2014). Comparative systematic review and meta-analysis of compression modalities for the promotion of venous ulcer healing and reducing ulcer recurrence. *Journal of Vascular Surgery, 60*(Suppl. 2), 71S–90S. https://www.jvascsurg.org/article/S0741-5214(14)00890-8/pdf (Level I)

4 Cooper, K. L. (2011). Care of the lower extremities in patients with acute decompensated heart failure. *Critical Care Nurse, 31*(4), 21–29.

5 The Joint Commission. (2021). Standard NPSG.07.01.01. *Comprehensive accreditation manual for hospitals*. Oakbrook Terrace, IL: The Joint Commission. (Level VII)

6 Centers for Disease Control and Prevention. (2002). Guideline for hand hygiene in health-care settings: Recommendations of the Healthcare Infection Control Practices Advisory Committee and the HICPAC/SHEA/APIC/IDSA Hand Hygiene Task Force. *MMWR Recommendations and Reports, 51*(RR-16), 1–45. https://www.cdc.gov/mmwr/pdf/rr/rr5116.pdf (Level II)

7 World Health Organization. (2009). WHO guidelines on hand hygiene in health care: First global patient safety challenge, clean care is safer care. https://apps.who.int/iris/bitstream/handle/10665/44102/9789241597906_eng.pdf?sequence=1 (Level IV)

8 Centers for Medicare and Medicaid Services, Department of Health and Human Services. (2020). Condition of participation: Infection control. 42 C.F.R. § 482.42.

9 Accreditation Association for Hospitals and Health Systems. (2020). Standard 07.01.21. *Healthcare Facilities Accreditation Program: Accreditation requirements for acute care hospitals*. Chicago, IL: Accreditation Association for Hospitals and Health Systems. (Level VII)

10 DNV GL-Healthcare USA, Inc. (2020). IC.1.SR.1. *NIAHO® accreditation requirements, interpretive guidelines and surveyor guidance—revision 20.0*. Milford, OH: DNV GL-Healthcare USA, Inc. (Level VII)

11 The Joint Commission. (2021). Standard NPSG.01.01.01. *Comprehensive accreditation manual for hospitals*. Oakbrook Terrace, IL: The Joint Commission. (Level VII)

12 Accreditation Association for Hospitals and Health Systems. (2020). Standard 15.01.16. *Healthcare Facilities Accreditation Program: Accreditation requirements for acute care hospitals*. Chicago, IL: Accreditation Association for Hospitals and Health Systems. (Level VII)

13 The Joint Commission. (2021). Standard RI.01.01.01. *Comprehensive accreditation manual for hospitals*. Oakbrook Terrace, IL: The Joint Commission. (Level VII)

14 DNV GL-Healthcare USA, Inc. (2020). PR.2.SR.5. *NIAHO® accreditation requirements, interpretive guidelines and surveyor guidance—revision 20.0*. Milford, OH: DNV GL-Healthcare USA, Inc. (Level VII)

15 Centers for Medicare and Medicaid Services, Department of Health and Human Services. (2020). Condition of participation: Patient's rights. 42 C.F.R. § 482.13(c)(1).

16 The Joint Commission. (2021). Standard PC.02.01.21. *Comprehensive accreditation manual for hospitals*. Oakbrook Terrace, IL: The Joint Commission. (Level VII)

17 Waters, T. R., et al. (2009). Safe patient handling training for schools of nursing. https://www.cdc.gov/niosh/docs/2009-127/pdfs/2009-127.pdf (Level VII)

18 Occupational Safety and Health Administration. (2012). Bloodborne pathogens, standard number 1910.1030. https://www.osha.gov/pls/oshaweb/owadisp.show_document?p_id=10051&p_table=STANDARDS (Level VII)

19 Siegel, J. D., et al. (2007, revised 2019). 2007 guideline for isolation precautions: Preventing transmission of infectious agents in healthcare settings. https://www.cdc.gov/infectioncontrol/pdf/guidelines/isolation-guidelines-H.pdf (Level II)

20 Accreditation Association for Hospitals and Health Systems. (2020). Standard 07.01.10. *Healthcare Facilities Accreditation Program: Accreditation requirements for acute care hospitals*. Chicago, IL: Accreditation Association for Hospitals and Health Systems. (Level VII)

21 Ganz, D. A., et al. (2013, reviewed 2021). *Preventing falls in hospitals: A toolkit for improving quality of care* (AHRQ Publication No. 13-0015-EF). Rockville, MD: Agency for Healthcare Research and Quality. https://www.ahrq.gov/professionals/systems/hospital/fallpxtoolkit/index.html (Level VII)

22 The Joint Commission. (2021). Standard RC.01.03.01. *Comprehensive accreditation manual for hospitals*. Oakbrook Terrace, IL: The Joint Commission. (Level VII)

23 Centers for Medicare and Medicaid Services, Department of Health and Human Services. (2020). Condition of participation: Medical record services. 42 C.F.R. § 482.24(b).

24 Accreditation Association for Hospitals and Health Systems. (2020). Standard 10.00.03. *Healthcare Facilities Accreditation Program: Accreditation requirements for acute care hospitals*. Chicago, IL: Accreditation Association for Hospitals and Health Systems. (Level VII)

25 DNV GL-Healthcare USA, Inc. (2020). MR.2.SR.1. *NIAHO® accreditation requirements, interpretive guidelines and surveyor guidance—revision 20.0*. Milford, OH: DNV GL-Healthcare USA, Inc. (Level VII)

26 Hinkle, J. L., & Cheever, K. H. (2017). *Brunner & Suddarth's textbook of medical-surgical nursing* (14th ed.). Philadelphia, PA: Wolters Kluwer.

ELASTOMERIC PUMP USE

An elastomeric pump (such as the ON-Q® pump), a bulblike pump attached to a wound catheter, is designed to administer a continuous infusion of medication, such as a local anesthetic, by gravity into an operative site.[1] The catheter is inserted percutaneously—directly adjacent to the peripheral nerves supplying the surgical site—so that when the infusion of the medication occurs, the patient receives site-specific analgesia. (See *A look at an elastomeric pump*.) Depending on the device, the pump can function using a manufacturer-preset rate of infusion, or it can be set to allow the patient to adjust the rate. Alternatively, it can be set to deliver a continuous (basal) infusion rate, with the option for bolus doses on demand by the patient.[2] The practitioner determines the most appropriate type of device for the patient.

Treatment delivered by an elastomeric pump is appropriate for patients who are candidates for regional anesthesia blockade, for which this type of device has been shown to improve the patient's ability to function and reduces the need for opioid pain medications. In addition, such patients can be discharged more quickly and participate in rehabilitation sooner than those who receive conventional pain management.[2,5] Elastomeric pump use in cardiovascular, thoracic, obstetric-gynecologic, orthopedic, and general surgeries has also been studied, and a limited number of studies have evaluated the use of this type of system for pain management associated with rib fractures. Elastomeric pumps can also be used for ambulatory chemotherapy.[6,7,8] Elastomeric pump use is contraindicated in patients with a preexisting neuropathy, a history of a coagulation disorder, systemic infection, or an anatomic deviation at the potential wound catheter insertion site.[9]

This procedure focuses on the use of an elastomeric pump for the infusion of a local anesthetic.

EQUIPMENT

A look at an elastomeric pump

An elastomeric pump (shown below) is a disposable pump that controls the continuous infusion of a local anesthetic directly into surgical wound tissue or along the sheath of a nerve, such as the femoral nerve. To provide a broad area of analgesia around a surgical incision, the practitioner threads a *soaker catheter,* one with multiple perforations, into the incision tissue and secures it with a sterile transparent dressing. Another option for a patient who has had knee or shoulder surgery is to place a *standard catheter* along the femoral or interscalene nerve sheath.

A needle attached to a low-voltage nerve stimulator can be used to determine the proper location for catheter insertion. Using this method, the practitioner watches for muscle twitches to determine the area of neural stimulation to the surgical site. Alternatively, the practitioner can use ultrasound to guide catheter insertion. After the practitioner identifies the correct area, the practitioner inserts the continuous infusion catheter around the target nerve bundle and secures it with a sterile transparent dressing.[3]

After catheter insertion, the disposable pump's reservoir is filled with a local anesthetic (typically bupivacaine or ropivacaine) and the pump is connected to the catheter. The pump flow rate depends on the pump manufacturer, pump size, and amount of medication placed in the pump reservoir. Overfilling or underfilling the reservoir changes the delivery rate.[3]

After the disposable pump is filled and attached to the catheter, the pump is placed in a small carrier pack so that the patient can move with it.[3] A flow restrictor located in the delivery tubing is taped to the patient's body and controls the rate of local anesthetic delivered to the patient.[4] Because the medication flow rate depends on body heat, the flow restrictor must stay in contact with the patient's skin or the medication will infuse too slowly.[3,5]

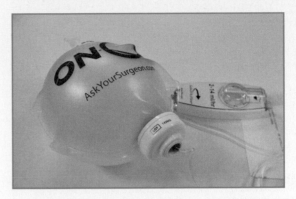

Equipment

Vital signs monitoring equipment ■ cardiac monitor ■ pulse oximeter and probe ■ elastomeric pump (including tubing, clamp, flow restrictor, and tubing cap) ■ prescribed medication ■ carrier pack ■ wound catheter (single or dual) ■ nerve stimulator or ultrasound device ■ sterile transparent dressing ■ surgical cap ■ mask ■ gloves ■ sterile drape ■ antiseptic solution ■ local anesthetic ■ 25G needle ■ syringe ■ tape ■ disinfectant pad ■ emergency equipment (code cart with emergency medications, defibrillator, handheld resuscitation bag with mask, and intubation equipment) ■ Optional: gown, sterile probe cover, prescribed preoperative medications, oxygen administration equipment, IV catheter insertion supplies, marker for skin, lipid emulsion, prescribed antiseizure medication.

Preparation of equipment

Inspect all equipment and supplies. If a product is expired, is defective, or has compromised integrity, remove it from patient use, label it as expired or defective, and report the expiration or defect as directed by your facility. Ensure that emergency equipment is functioning properly and readily available.

Fill the elastomeric pump's reservoir with the prescribed medication as directed by your facility, if necessary; note that pharmacy preparation is preferred. Ensure that the pump is labeled with the medication name and concentration, infusion rate (in milliliters per hour and dose per hour), and start date.[2] Compare the medication label with the practitioner's order in the patient's medical record.[10,11,12,13] Perform hand hygiene.[14,15,16,17,18,19] Prime the elastomeric pump tubing. Open the clamp on the tubing. Maintaining the sterility of the distal end of the elastomeric pump tubing, remove the tubing cap to begin priming. After purging all the air from the tubing and observing fluid flow at the distal end of the tubing, close the clamp, and replace the tubing cap until the set is ready for use. If the elastomeric pump tubing doesn't prime, refer to the manufacturer's instructions.[1]

Implementation

Assisting with wound catheter insertion

■ Verify the practitioner's order.
■ Review the patient's medical record for any allergies (including to latex and local anesthetics), medical and surgical history, present illness, past or present substance abuse, preoperative diagnosis, weight, current medications, use of alternative therapies, laboratory and diagnostic test results, and past problems with anesthesia.
■ If required by your facility, confirm that informed consent has been obtained and that the signed consent form is in the patient's medical record.[20,21,22,23]
■ Conduct a preprocedure verification to ensure that all relevant documentation, related information, and equipment are available and identified correctly to the patient's identifiers.[24,25]
■ Verify that ordered laboratory and imaging studies have been completed and that the results are in the patient's medical record. Notify the practitioner of any unexpected results.[24]
■ Gather and prepare the necessary equipment and supplies.
■ Perform hand hygiene.[14,15,16,17,18,19]
■ Confirm the patient's identity using at least two patient identifiers.[26]
■ Provide privacy.[27,28,29,30]
■ Reinforce the practitioner's explanation of the procedure to the patient and family (if appropriate) according to their individual communication and learning needs *to increase their understanding, allay their fears, and enhance cooperation.* Answer the patient's and family's questions.[31]
■ Assess the patient's understanding of the procedure and expectations for participation, ability to cooperate and tolerate the required positioning for the duration of the procedure, and emotional state, *because understanding what's expected will make the patient more cooperative.*[5]
■ Attach the patient to a cardiac and vital signs monitor and a pulse oximeter *to monitor the patient's condition before, during, and after the procedure.* Ensure that the alarm limits are set appropriately for the patient's current condition and that they're turned on, functioning properly, and audible to staff.[4,32,33,34,35]
■ Perform a preoperative nursing assessment, if not already done, including vital signs, oxygen saturation level, skin integrity, level of consciousness, anxiety level, sensory impairments, and pain (location, level, and description) *to serve as baselines for comparison.*[5,35]
■ Verify that a responsible person is available to drive the patient home if the patient will be discharged after the procedure.[5]
■ If not already in place, insert an IV catheter, but don't insert it into the extremity or area where the wound catheter will be inserted. (See the "IV catheter insertion and removal" procedure.)
■ Administer preoperative medications, as prescribed, following safe medication administration practices.[5,10,11,12,13]
■ Put on a surgical cap and a mask.
■ Perform hand hygiene.[14,15,16,17,18,19]

■ Put on gloves and, as needed, a gown *to comply with standard precautions.*[36,37,38]

■ Assist the practitioner with positioning the patient to gain access to the intended wound catheter insertion site.

■ If appropriate, ensure that the wound catheter insertion site is marked according to your facility's guidelines.[25,39]

■ Assist the practitioner with cleaning the intended wound catheter insertion site using antiseptic following the manufacturer's instructions. Let the antiseptic dry completely.[40,41]

■ Assist the practitioner with draping the intended wound catheter insertion site using sterile technique.[5,42]

■ Conduct a time-out immediately before starting the procedure *to perform a final assessment that the correct patient, site, positioning, and procedure are identified and, as applicable, all relevant information and necessary equipment are available.*[43]

■ Prepare the nerve stimulator or ultrasound device, according to practitioner preference, following the manufacturer's instructions. Cover the ultrasound probe with a sterile probe cover. Hand the device to the practitioner using sterile technique.[2]

■ Assist the practitioner with administering a local anesthetic and inserting the wound catheter.

■ Monitor the patient's cardiac rate and rhythm, vital signs, oxygen saturation level, pain level, anxiety level, and level of consciousness throughout the procedure *to evaluate tolerance of the procedure.*[35]

■ After wound catheter insertion, assist the practitioner with attaching the elastomeric pump tubing to the catheter and then initiating the anesthetic infusion. Verify that the elastomeric pump tubing clamp is open and the tubing isn't kinked.[1] Trace the tubing from the patient to its point of origin *to ensure that it's connected to the proper port before beginning medication administration.*[44,45]

■ Cover the wound catheter insertion site with a sterile transparent dressing.[1,46]

■ Tape the flow restrictor to the patient's skin. Don't tape over the in-line filter, *which may block the air vent and impede the infusion.*[1]

■ Ensure that the adjustable rate controller, if present, is clicked into place under the specified infusion rate.[2]

■ Assist the patient into a position that protects the wound catheter insertion site *to prevent patient injury, because sensation at the insertion site will be altered.*[46]

■ Monitor the patient for signs and symptoms of local anesthetic systemic toxicity (LAST) (such as tinnitus, metallic taste, and circumoral tingling), which may progress to motor twitching, seizure activity, coma, and respiratory arrest as blood levels of the medication rise.[35] Also monitor the patient for other adverse reactions to the medication, including dizziness, drowsiness, nausea, and vomiting.

■ Provide hand-off communication to the staff member who will assume responsibility for the patient's care. Allow time for questions as needed *to avoid miscommunication that may cause patient care errors during transitions of care.* As part of the hand-off process, allow time for the receiving staff member to trace each tubing and catheter from the patient to its point of origin using a standardized line reconciliation process.[47]

■ Remove and discard your personal protective equipment.[36]

■ Perform hand hygiene.[14,15,16,17,18,19]

■ Document the procedure.[48,49,50,51]

Providing care after wound catheter insertion

■ Perform hand hygiene.[14,15,16,17,18,19]

■ Receive hand-off communication from the person who was responsible for the patient's care. Ask questions as needed *to avoid miscommunication that may cause patient care errors during transitions of care.* As part of the hand-off process, trace each tubing and catheter from the patient to its point of origin using a standardized line reconciliation process.[47]

■ Verify the practitioner's order.

■ Review the patient's medical record for an allergy or contraindication to the prescribed medication. If an allergy or contraindication exists, don't administer the medication, and notify the practitioner.[10,11,12,13]

■ Perform hand hygiene.[14,15,16,17,18,19]

■ Put on gloves *to comply with standard precautions.*[36,37,38]

■ Confirm the patient's identity using at least two patient identifiers.[26]

Treating LAST

If the patient develops LAST, refer to the American Society of Regional Anesthesia and Pain Medicine's checklist, available at https://www.asra.com/advisory-guidelines/article/3/local-anesthetic-systemic-toxicity. Treatment commonly includes the following:

■ maintaining a patent airway
■ ventilating the patient with 100% oxygen
■ administering basic or advanced cardiac life support, as needed
■ establishing IV access, if needed
■ administering a 20% lipid emulsion based on lean body mass
■ suppressing seizures with medication, such as a benzodiazepine (if only propofol is available, use low dose [20 mg] boluses)
■ avoiding the use of vasopressin, calcium channel blockers, beta-blockers, and local anesthetics
■ reducing EPINEPHrine doses, if necessary, to less than 1 mcg/kg
■ alerting the nearest facility that has cardiopulmonary bypass capability, if not provided in your facility
■ monitoring the patient for at least 2 hours after seizure, 4 to 6 hours after cardiovascular instability, and as clinically indicated after cardiac arrest.[35,53]

■ Compare the prescribed medication label to the order in the patient's medical record.[10,11,12,13]

■ Check the expiration date on the prescribed medication. If the medication is expired, return it to the pharmacy and obtain a new supply of the medication.[10,11,12,13]

■ Obtain the patient's vital signs and oxygen saturation level, and assess the patient's cardiac rhythm and level of consciousness. Compare them with baseline findings.[35]

■ Screen for and assess the patient's pain using facility-defined criteria consistent with the patient's age, condition, and ability to understand.[52]

■ Monitor the patient for adverse reactions to the prescribed medication. Monitor a patient receiving a local anesthetic for signs and symptoms of LAST, including dizziness, tinnitus, metallic taste, circumoral numbness, confusion, slurred speech, seizures, and hypertension and tachycardia initially, followed by progressive hypotension and bradycardia. If signs and symptoms of LAST occur, call for help immediately.[35,53] Intervene as needed and ordered. (See *Treating LAST.*)

■ Ensure that the elastomeric pump tubing clamp is open and that the tubing has no kinks.[1]

■ Ensure that the transparent dressing over the wound catheter insertion site is intact.[2]

■ Maintain the elastomeric pump at room temperature, and keep it in the carrier pack outside of the patient's gown or clothing.[2]

■ Ensure that the flow restrictor is taped to the patient's skin.[1]

Removing an elastomeric pump's wound catheter

If the practitioner has ordered the removal of an elastomeric pump and its associated peripheral wound catheter, perform these steps:

✔ Verify the practitioner's order.
✔ Perform hand hygiene.[14,15,16,17,18,19]
✔ Put on gloves *to comply with standard precautions.*[36,37,38]
✔ Remove the transparent dressing and any adhesive strips carefully.[54]
✔ Hold the wound catheter near the insertion site and pull the catheter slowly without tugging. Stop the procedure and notify the practitioner if you meet resistance or the catheter stretches.[54]
✔ After removal, inspect the wound catheter tip for any signs of breakage *to ensure that the catheter was removed completely.* Notify the practitioner if you suspect catheter breakage.[54]
✔ Apply a dressing to the site as ordered.[54]

Note that you should never cut any part of the wound catheter or use force to remove it. Catheter removal should be easy and painless for the patient.[54]

■ Keep the flow restrictor away from heat and cold, *because changes in temperature affect the infusion solution's viscosity, which may result in faster or slower flow rates.*[13]

■ If a change in flow rate is prescribed during an infusion and you're permitted to do so by your facility, remove the plastic cover over the flow rate dial, insert the rate-changing key into the dial, and turn the dial until you have selected the new flow rate. Ensure that the selected flow rate setting is aligned with the milliliters per hour mark (mL/hour). Remove the key from the dial, secure the cover over the dial, and put the key in a safe place.[1]

■ Ensure that the elastomeric pump is positioned about 16" (41 cm) below the wound catheter insertion site as directed by the manufacturer. *Positioning the pump above this level increases the flow rate; positioning it below this level decreases the flow rate.*[1]

■ Monitor the appearance and size of the elastomeric pump. *As medication is delivered, the pump gradually becomes smaller; however, changes in the pump's appearance and size might not be apparent during the first 24 hours after the infusion begins.* The infusion is complete when the pump is no longer inflated.[1]

■ If the infusion is complete and the practitioner has ordered wound catheter removal, remove the catheter and discard the elastomeric pump according to your facility's instructions.[1] (See *Removing an elastomeric pump's wound catheter.*)

■ Reassess and respond to the patient's pain by evaluating the response to treatment and progress toward pain management goals. Assess the patient for adverse reactions and risk factors for adverse events that may result from treatment.[52]

■ Remove and discard your gloves.[36]

■ Perform hand hygiene.[14,15,16,17,18,19]

■ Document the procedure.[48,49,50,51]

Special considerations

■ Remove the rate-changing key from the flow rate dial if the patient is discharged to home with the elastomeric pump. The key should remain in a location designated by your facility so that the practitioner can access it if needed. Secure the plastic cover over the dial.[2]

■ The medication-containing elastomeric pump is designed for one-time use and shouldn't be refilled.[1,2]

■ The Joint Commission issued a sentinel event alert related to inadequate hand-off communication *because of the potential for patient harm that may result when a receiver receives inaccurate, incomplete, untimely, misinterpreted, or otherwise inadequate information.* To improve hand-off communication, standardize the critical information communicated by the sender. At a minimum, include the sender's contact information; illness assessment; patient summary, including events leading up to the illness or admission, hospital course, ongoing assessment, and plan of care; to-do action list; contingency plans; allergy list; code status; medication list; and dated laboratory test results and vital signs. Provide face-to-face communication whenever possible in an interruption-free location, using facility-approved, standardized tools and methods (for example, forms, templates, checklists, protocols, and mnemonics). Provide ample time and opportunity for questions, and include the multidisciplinary team members and the patient and family members when appropriate.[55]

■ The Joint Commission issued a sentinel event alert concerning medical device alarm safety, *because alarm-related events have been associated with permanent loss of function or death.* Among the major contributing factors noted were improper alarm settings, alarm settings turned off inappropriately, and alarm signals that were inaudible to staff. Ensure that alarm limits are set appropriately, and that the alarms are turned on, functioning properly, and audible to staff. Follow facility guidelines for preventing alarm fatigue.[4]

■ The Joint Commission issued a sentinel event alert related to managing risk during transition to new International Organization for Standardization tubing connector standards that were designed to prevent dangerous tubing misconnections, which may lead to serious patient injury and death. During the transition, make sure to trace each tubing and catheter from the patient to its point of origin before connecting or reconnecting any device or infusion, at any care transition (such as to a new setting or service), and as part of the hand-off process; route tubes and catheters with

different purposes in different standardized directions; when the patient has different access sites or several bags hanging, label tubing at both the distal and proximal ends; use tubing and equipment only as intended; and store medications for different delivery routes in separate locations.[45]

Patient teaching

If the patient is being discharged to home with the elastomeric pump, teach the patient and family about the pump's functioning and the items to check periodically, including the following:
■ The flow restrictor is taped to the patient's skin.
■ The pump appears to be getting smaller each day.
■ The patient's pain is under control.[2]

During discharge planning, teach the patient and family about pain management strategies. Include information about the patient's pain management plan and adverse effects of pain management treatment. Discuss activities of daily living, and items in the home environment that may exacerbate pain or reduce the effectiveness of the pain management plan; include strategies to address these issues. Also teach the patient and family about the signs of toxicity, reasons to call the practitioner, and the procedure for clamping the elastomeric pump tubing to prevent further medication administration, if necessary. Advise the patient to keep the pump away from heat and cold and to avoid squeezing the pump. Provide patient care guidelines provided by the manufacturer.[2]

Complications

Complications associated with elastomeric pump use include infection, LAST, and adverse effects of the prescribed medication.

Documentation
For wound catheter insertion
Document the preprocedure verification process; any abnormal findings; prescribed interventions, if necessary; and the patient's response to those interventions. Record the patient's vital signs, pain, and other assessment findings before, during, and immediately after the procedure. Record the time-out process, date and time of wound catheter insertion, name of the practitioner who inserted the catheter, catheter location, and the patient's tolerance of the procedure. Document the medication strength, dose, administration route, and date and time of administration. Record any adverse reactions to the prescribed medication, the name of the practitioner notified, the date and time that the practitioner was notified, any prescribed interventions, and the patient's response to those interventions.[56] Document teaching provided to the patient and family (if applicable), their understanding of that teaching, and any need for follow-up teaching.

For care after wound catheter insertion
Record your assessment findings, including the patient's vital signs and pain (location, level, and description). Document the name of the practitioner notified of the patient's condition and the date and time of notification. Record your interventions and the patient's response to those interventions. Document teaching provided to the patient and family (if applicable), their understanding of that teaching, and any need for follow-up teaching.

REFERENCES

1　Halyard Health, Inc. (2017). ON-Q pump with fixed flow rate: Instructions for use. https://avanospainmanagement.com/wp-content/uploads/AP-IFUs/IFU-ON-Q-Pump-Fixed-Flow-Rate-Insert-English-Only.pdf

2　Institute for Safe Medication Practices. (2009). Process for handling elastomeric pain relief balls (ON-Q PainBuster and others) requires safety improvements. https://www.ismp.org/resources/process-handling-elastomeric-pain-relief-balls-q-painbuster-and-others-requires-safety

3　D'Arcy, Y. (2007). New pain management options: Delivery systems and techniques. *Nursing2020, 37*(2), 26–27.

4　The Joint Commission. (2013). Sentinel event alert 50: Medical device alarm safety in hospitals. http://www.jointcommission.org/assets/1/6/SEA_50_alarms_4_26_16.pdf (Level VII)

5　Rothrock, J. C. (2019). *Alexander's care of the patient in surgery* (16th ed.). St. Louis, MO: Elsevier.

6   Salman, D., et al. (2017). Evaluation of the performance of elastomeric pumps in practice: Are we under-delivering on chemotherapy treatments? *Current Medical Research and Opinion, 33*, 2153–2159. (Level VI)

7   Shereen, N. G., & Salman, D. (2019). Delivering chemotherapy at home: How much do we know? *British Journal of Community Nursing, 24*, 482–484.

8   Baxter Corporation. (2010). Baxter elastomeric pumps: Clinician guide. https://palli-science.com/sites/default/files/PDF/baxter-elastomeric-pumps-clinician-guide11.pdf

9   Ilfeld, B. M., & Enneking, F. K. (2005). Continuous peripheral nerve blocks at home: A review. *Anesthesia & Analgesia, 100*(6), 1822–1833. http://journals.lww.com/anesthesia-analgesia/Fulltext/2005/06000/Continuous_Peripheral_Nerve-Blocks_at_Home_A.49.aspx (Level VI)

10 The Joint Commission. (2021). Standard MM.06.01.01. *Comprehensive accreditation manual for hospitals.* Oakbrook Terrace, IL: The Joint Commission. (Level VII)

11 Centers for Medicare and Medicaid Services, Department of Health and Human Services. (2020). Condition of participation: Nursing services. 42 C.F.R. § 482.23(c).

12 Accreditation Association for Hospitals and Health Systems. (2020). Standard 16.01.03. *Healthcare Facilities Accreditation Program: Accreditation requirements for acute care hospitals.* Chicago, IL: Accreditation Association for Hospitals and Health Systems. (Level VII)

13 DNV GL-Healthcare USA, Inc. (2020). MM.1.SR.3. *NIAHO® accreditation requirements, interpretive guidelines and surveyor guidance—revision 20.0.* Milford, OH: DNV GL-Healthcare USA, Inc. (Level VII)

14 Centers for Disease Control and Prevention. (2002). Guideline for hand hygiene in health-care settings: Recommendations of the Healthcare Infection Control Practices Advisory Committee and the HICPAC/SHEA/APIC/IDSA Hand Hygiene Task Force. *MMWR Recommendations and Reports, 51*(RR-16), 1–45. https://www.cdc.gov/mmwr/pdf/rr/rr5116.pdf (Level II)

15 World Health Organization. (2009). WHO guidelines on hand hygiene in health care: First global patient safety challenge, clean care is safer care. http://apps.who.int/iris/bitstream/handle/10665/44102/9789241597906_eng.pdf;jsessionid=8C7D5E862E21F485EE46762F1DC878AE?sequence=1 (Level IV)

16 The Joint Commission. (2021). Standard NPSG.07.01.01. *Comprehensive accreditation manual for hospitals.* Oakbrook Terrace, IL: The Joint Commission. (Level VII)

17 Accreditation Association for Hospitals and Health Systems. (2020). Standard 07.01.21. *Healthcare Facilities Accreditation Program: Accreditation requirements for acute care hospitals.* Chicago, IL: Accreditation Association for Hospitals and Health Systems. (Level VII)

18 Centers for Medicare and Medicaid Services, Department of Health and Human Services. (2020). Condition of participation: Infection control. 42 C.F.R. § 482.42.

19 DNV GL-Healthcare USA, Inc. (2020). IC.1.SR.1. *NIAHO® accreditation requirements, interpretive guidelines and surveyor guidance—revision 20.0.* Milford, OH: DNV GL-Healthcare USA, Inc. (Level VII)

20 Accreditation Association for Hospitals and Health Systems. (2020). Standard 30.01.11. *Healthcare Facilities Accreditation Program: Accreditation requirements for acute care hospitals.* Chicago, IL: Accreditation Association for Hospitals and Health Systems. (Level VII)

21 Centers for Medicare and Medicaid Services, Department of Health and Human Services. (2020). Condition of participation: Patient's rights. 42 C.F.R. § 482.13(b)(2).

22 DNV GL-Healthcare USA, Inc. (2020). PR.2.SR.3. *NIAHO® accreditation requirements, interpretive guidelines and surveyor guidance—revision 20.0.* Milford, OH: DNV GL-Healthcare USA, Inc. (Level VII)

23 The Joint Commission. (2021). Standard RI.01.03.01. *Comprehensive accreditation manual for hospitals.* Oakbrook Terrace, IL: The Joint Commission. (Level VII)

24 The Joint Commission. (2021). Standard UP.01.01.01. *Comprehensive accreditation manual for hospitals.* Oakbrook Terrace, IL: The Joint Commission. (Level VII)

25 Accreditation Association for Hospitals and Health Systems. (2020). Standard 30.00.14. *Healthcare Facilities Accreditation Program: Accreditation requirements for acute care hospitals.* Chicago, IL: Accreditation Association for Hospitals and Health Systems. (Level VII)

26 The Joint Commission. (2021). Standard NPSG.01.01.01. *Comprehensive accreditation manual for hospitals.* Oakbrook Terrace, IL: The Joint Commission. (Level VII)

27 Accreditation Association for Hospitals and Health Systems. (2020). Standard 15.01.16. *Healthcare Facilities Accreditation Program: Accreditation requirements for acute care hospitals.* Chicago, IL: Accreditation Association for Hospitals and Health Systems. (Level VII)

28 Centers for Medicare and Medicaid Services, Department of Health and Human Services. (2020). Condition of participation: Patient's rights. 42 C.F.R. § 482.13(c)(1).

29 DNV GL-Healthcare USA, Inc. (2020). PR.2.SR.5. *NIAHO® accreditation requirements, interpretive guidelines and surveyor guidance—revision 20.0.* Milford, OH: DNV GL-Healthcare USA, Inc. (Level VII)

30 The Joint Commission. (2021). Standard RI.01.01.01. *Comprehensive accreditation manual for hospitals.* Oakbrook Terrace, IL: The Joint Commission. (Level VII)

31 The Joint Commission. (2021). Standard PC.02.01.21. *Comprehensive accreditation manual for hospitals.* Oakbrook Terrace, IL: The Joint Commission. (Level VII)

32 The Joint Commission. (2021). Standard NPSG.06.01.01. *Comprehensive accreditation manual for hospitals.* Oakbrook Terrace, IL: The Joint Commission. (Level VII)

33 Graham, K. C., & Cvach, M. (2010). Monitor alarm fatigue: Standardizing use of physiological monitors and decreasing nuisance alarms. *American Journal of Critical Care, 19*, 28–37.

34 American Association of Critical-Care Nurses. (2018). AACN practice alert: Managing alarms in acute care across the life span: Electrocardiography and pulse oximetry. https://www.aacn.org/clinical-resources/practice-alerts/managing-alarms-in-acute-care-across-the-life-span (Level VII)

35 Guidelines for perioperative care: Local anesthesia. (2021). In Wood, A. (Ed.), *Guidelines for perioperative practice*, 2021 edition. Denver, CO: AORN, Inc. (Level VII)

36 Siegel, J. D., et al. (2007, revised 2019). 2007 guideline for isolation precautions: Preventing transmission of infectious agents in healthcare settings. https://www.cdc.gov/infectioncontrol/pdf/guidelines/isolation-guidelines-H.pdf (Level II)

37 Accreditation Association for Hospitals and Health Systems. (2020). Standard 07.01.10. *Healthcare Facilities Accreditation Program: Accreditation requirements for acute care hospitals.* Chicago, IL: Accreditation Association for Hospitals and Health Systems. (Level VII)

38 Occupational Safety and Health Administration. (2012). Bloodborne pathogens, standard number 1910.1030. https://www.osha.gov/pls/oshaweb/owadisp.show_document?p_id=10051&p_table=STANDARDS (Level VII)

39 The Joint Commission. (2021). Standard UP.01.02.01. *Comprehensive accreditation manual for hospitals.* Oakbrook Terrace, IL: The Joint Commission. (Level VII)

40 Guidelines for perioperative care: Patient skin antisepsis. (2021). In Wood, A. (Ed.), *Guidelines for perioperative practice*, 2021 edition. Denver, CO: AORN, Inc. (Level VII)

41 Anderson, D. J., et al. (2014). SHEA/IDSA practice recommendation: Strategies to prevent surgical site infections in acute care hospitals: 2014 update. *Infection Control and Hospital Epidemiology, 35*, 605–627. http://www.jstor.org/stable/10.1086/676022 (Level I)

42 Guidelines for perioperative care: Sterile technique. (2021). In Wood, A. (Ed.), *Guidelines for perioperative practice*, 2021 edition. Denver, CO: AORN, Inc. (Level VII)

43 The Joint Commission. (2021). Standard UP.01.03.01. *Comprehensive accreditation manual for hospitals.* Oakbrook Terrace, IL: The Joint Commission. (Level VII)

44 U.S. Food and Drug Administration. (2017). *Examples of medical device misconnections.* https://www.fda.gov/medical-devices/medical-device-connectors/examples-medical-device-misconnections

45 The Joint Commission. (2014). *Sentinel event alert 53: Managing risk during transition to new ISO tubing connector standards.* http://www.jointcommission.org/assets/1/6/SEA_53_Connectors_8_19_14_final.pdf (Level VII)

46 D'Arcy, Y. (2004). Using regional blockade for adjunct pain relief. *Nursing2020, 34*(11), 74–75.

47 The Joint Commission. (2021). Standard PC.02.02.01. *Comprehensive accreditation manual for hospitals.* Oakbrook Terrace, IL: The Joint Commission. (Level VII)

48 The Joint Commission. (2021). Standard RC.01.03.01. *Comprehensive accreditation manual for hospitals.* Oakbrook Terrace, IL: The Joint Commission. (Level VII)

49 Accreditation Association for Hospitals and Health Systems. (2020). Standard 10.00.03. *Healthcare Facilities Accreditation Program:*

Accreditation requirements for acute care hospitals. Chicago, IL: Accreditation Association for Hospitals and Health Systems. (Level VII)

50 Centers for Medicare and Medicaid Services, Department of Health and Human Services. (2020). Condition of participation: Medical record services. 42 C.F.R. § 482.24(b).

51 DNV GL-Healthcare USA, Inc. (2020). MR.2.SR.1. *NIAHO® accreditation requirements, interpretive guidelines and surveyor guidance revision—20.0.* Milford, OH: DNV GL-Healthcare USA, Inc. (Level VII)

52 The Joint Commission. (2021). Standard PC.01.02.07. *Comprehensive accreditation manual for hospitals.* Oakbrook Terrace, IL: The Joint Commission. (Level VII)

53 American Society of Regional Anesthesia and Pain Medicine. (2020). Local anesthetic systemic toxicity checklist. https://www.asra.com/docs/default-source/guidelines-articles/local-anesthetic-systemic-toxicity-rgb.pdf?sfvrsn=33b348e_2

54 Avanos Medical, Inc. (2018). ON-Q catheter removal. https://www.myon-q.com/wp-content/uploads/2019/09/ap_patient-brochure_catheterremoval-mk-00456-rev1_90d.pdf

55 The Joint Commission. (2017). Sentinel event alert 58: Inadequate hand-off communication. https://www.jointcommission.org/-/media/tjc/documents/resources/patient-safety-topics/sentinel-event/sea_58_hand_off_comms_9_6_17_final_(1).pdf?db=web&hash=5642D-63C1A5017BD214701514DA00139 (Level VII)

56 The Joint Commission. (2021). Standard RC.02.01.01. *Comprehensive accreditation manual for hospitals.* Oakbrook Terrace, IL: The Joint Commission. (Level VII)

ELECTRICAL BONE GROWTH STIMULATION

Electrical bone growth stimulation can accelerate healing in a fractured bone by imitating the body's natural electrical forces.[1] Electrical bone growth stimulation can also help bones grow together after fractures of the spine, femur, and tibia and in the treatment of nonunions of the foot and ankle.[2]

Direct current electrical bone growth stimulation is contraindicated in patients who are pregnant, have a demand-type pacemaker, have a cardioverter defibrillator, or have an open wound in the treatment areas. In addition, it should not be used near other equipment when potential electromagnetic or other interference may occur, such as with cell phones, magnetic resonance imaging (MRI) scanners, and electrosurgery equipment.[3,4]

Fully implantable (invasive) direct current stimulation devices and noninvasive electromagnetic coil or ultrasound stimulation devices are available. (See *Electrical bone growth stimulation devices.*) The choice of device depends on the fracture type and location, the practitioner's preference, and the patient's ability and willingness to comply with instructions. With an invasive direct-current stimulation device, implantation is performed under general anesthesia by the surgeon.[5] After the bone fragments join together, the generator and lead wire are removed under local anesthesia. The device requires no patient involvement. With noninvasive devices, the patient must manage the treatment schedule and maintain the equipment. This procedure discusses the use of noninvasive devices.

Equipment

Ordered stimulation set ▪ Optional: clippers, mineral oil, glycerin, soft cloth.

For ultrasound stimulation

The stimulation set consists of an ultrasound device with a rechargeable battery that's attached to a transducer by a cord, a strap that holds the transducer in place, a device charger, and ultrasound gel.[6]

EQUIPMENT

Electrical bone growth stimulation devices

Electrical bone growth stimulation may be invasive or noninvasive.

Invasive system
An invasive system involves placing a spiral cathode inside the bone at the fracture site. A wire leads from the cathode to a battery-powered generator, also implanted in local tissues. The patient's body completes the circuit.

Noninvasive system
A noninvasive system may include a cuff-like transducer, an ultrasound probe, or a fitted ring that wraps around the patient's limb. Electrical current or ultrasound waves penetrate the limb.

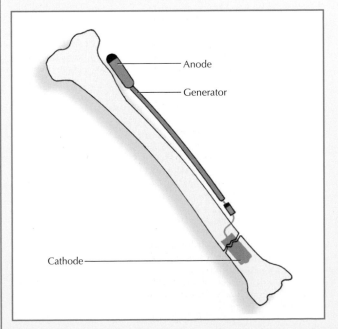

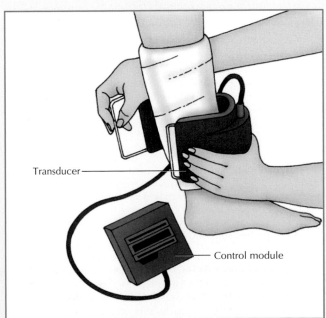

For electromagnetic stimulation

The stimulation set consists of a generator that plugs into a standard 110-volt outlet and two strong electromagnetic coils placed on either side of the injured area. The coils can be incorporated into a cast, a cuff, or an orthotic device.

Preparation of equipment

All equipment comes in sets with instructions provided by the manufacturer. Follow the instructions carefully and make sure that the equipment is operational before use.

Inspect all equipment and supplies. If a product is expired, is defective, or has compromised integrity, remove it from patient use, label it as expired or defective, and report the expiration or defect as directed by your facility.

Implementation

- Verify the practitioner's order.
- Review the patient's medical record for a history of allergies to nickel or chromium and for contraindications to the procedure. *Nickel and chromium are present in the electrical bone stimulation system.* Notify the practitioner if the patient has a known allergy to either substance or a contradiction.
- Gather and prepare the necessary equipment and supplies.
- Perform hand hygiene.[7,8,9,10,11,12]
- Confirm the patient's identity using at least two patient identifiers.[13]
- Provide privacy.[14,15,16,17]
- Explain the procedure to the patient and family (if appropriate) according to their individual communication and learning needs *to increase their understanding, allay their fears, and enhance cooperation.*[18]

Performing ultrasound stimulation

- Remove excessive body hair from the injured site using clippers, if needed.
- Apply gel to the transducer.[6]
- Apply the strap and transducer according to the manufacturer's instructions.
- Follow the manufacturer's instructions to program the device for the ordered length of time for treatment.
- Tell the patient to report local skin irritation; if it occurs, consider using mineral oil or glycerin.[6]
- After each treatment is complete, remove the strap and transducer and wipe the patient's skin, the transducer, and the strap with a soft cloth.[6]
- Teach the patient how to care for the ultrasound device according to the manufacturer's instructions.

Performing electromagnetic stimulation

- Show the patient where to place the coils.
- Tell the patient to apply the coils for 30 minutes daily, as ordered by the practitioner.[3,4] Explain that many patients find it most convenient to perform the procedure at night.
- Teach the patient how to use and care for the generator according to the manufacturer's instructions.[3,4]

Completing the procedure

- Relay the practitioner's instructions for weight bearing. Usually, the practitioner will advise against bearing weight until evidence of bone healing appears on X-rays.
- Perform hand hygiene.[7,8,9,10,11,12]
- Document the procedure.[19,20,21,22]

Special considerations

- Check the manufacturer's instructions for contraindications and precautions while using an ultrasound device. Note that pacemakers and other implantable devices may be affected while using the device. Also note that cell phones, televisions, and other devices that use radiofrequency energy can interfere with the device operation or cause the device to stop working completely.[6]

Patient teaching

Teach the patient how to care for the cast or external fixation devices as well as the electrical generator or ultrasound device. Urge the patient to follow treatment instructions faithfully.

If applicable, encourage the patient to stop smoking, provide smoking-cessation materials, and refer the patient to outpatient smoking-cessation counseling, *because smoking delays bone healing.*[23,24]

Complications

Complications associated with any surgical procedure, including infection, can occur during insertion of direct current electrical bone growth stimulation equipment. Skin irritation may occur from the gel used for ultrasound stimulation.[6] No complications are associated with use of electromagnetic stimulation.[3,4]

Documentation

Record the type of electrical bone stimulation equipment provided, including the date, time, and location, as appropriate. Note the patient's skin condition and tolerance of the procedure.[25] Document teaching provided to the patient and family (if applicable), their understanding of that teaching, and any need for follow-up teaching.

REFERENCES

1 Hannemann, P. F. W., et al. (2014). The effects of low-intensity pulsed ultrasound and pulsed electromagnetic fields bone growth stimulation in acute fractures: A systematic review and meta-analysis of randomized controlled trials. *Archives of Orthopaedic and Trauma Surgery, 134,* 1093–1106. (Level I)

2 Cook, J. J., et al. (2015). Healing in the new millennium: Bone stimulators: An overview of where we've been and where we may be heading. *Clinics in Podiatric Medicine and Surgery, 32*(1), 45–59.

3 DJO, LLC. (2015). SpinaLogic® bone growth stimulator: Physician manual and package insert. https://www.djoglobal.com/sites/default/files/13-6284_SpinaLogic%20Physician%20Manual_RevH.pdf

4 DJO, LLC. (2015). OL1000 & OL1000 SC bone growth stimulators: Physician manual and package insert. https://www.djoglobal.com/sites/default/files/13-2109_OL1000_family_RevA.pdf

5 Haglin, J. M., et al. (2017). Bone growth stimulation: A critical analysis review. *Journal of Bone and Joint Surgery, 5*(8), 1–11. https://www.researchgate.net/publication/319104836_Bone_Growth_Stimulation_A_Critical_Analysis_Review (Level V)

6 Bioventus, LLC. (2014). Exogen® user guide. https://www.exogen.com/us/exogen-user-guide-2/

7 Centers for Disease Control and Prevention. (2002). Guideline for hand hygiene in health-care settings: Recommendations of the Healthcare Infection Control Practices Advisory Committee and the HICPAC/SHEA/APIC/IDSA Hand Hygiene Task Force. *MMWR Recommendations and Reports, 51*(RR-16), 1–45. https://www.cdc.gov/mmwr/pdf/rr/rr5116.pdf (Level II)

8 World Health Organization. (2009). WHO guidelines on hand hygiene in health care: First global patient safety challenge, clean care is safer care. https://apps.who.int/iris/bitstream/handle/10665/44102/9789241597906_eng.pdf?sequence=1 (Level IV)

9 The Joint Commission. (2021). Standard NPSG.07.01.01. *Comprehensive accreditation manual for hospitals.* Oakbrook Terrace, IL: The Joint Commission. (Level VII)

10 Centers for Medicare and Medicaid Services, Department of Health and Human Services. (2020). Condition of participation: Infection control. 42 C.F.R. § 482.42.

11 Accreditation Association for Hospitals and Health Systems. (2020). Standard 07.01.21. *Healthcare Facilities Accreditation Program: Accreditation requirements for acute care hospitals.* Chicago, IL: Accreditation Association for Hospitals and Health Systems. (Level VII)

12 DNV GL-Healthcare USA, Inc. (2020). IC.1.SR.1. *NIAHO® accreditation requirements, interpretive guidelines and surveyor guidance—revision 20.0.* Milford, OH: DNV GL-Healthcare USA, Inc. (Level VII)

13 The Joint Commission. (2021). Standard NPSG.01.01.01. *Comprehensive accreditation manual for hospitals.* Oakbrook Terrace, IL: The Joint Commission. (Level VII)

14 The Joint Commission. (2021). Standard RI.01.01.01. *Comprehensive accreditation manual for hospitals.* Oakbrook Terrace, IL: The Joint Commission. (Level VII)

15 DNV GL-Healthcare USA, Inc. (2020). PR.2.SR.5. *NIAHO® accreditation requirements, interpretive guidelines and surveyor guidance—revision 20.0.* Milford, OH: DNV GL-Healthcare USA, Inc. (Level VII)

16 Centers for Medicare and Medicaid Services, Department of Health and Human Services. (2020). Condition of participation: Patient's rights. 42 C.F.R. § 482.13(c)(1).

17 Accreditation Association for Hospitals and Health Systems. (2020). Standard 15.01.16. *Healthcare Facilities Accreditation Program: Accreditation requirements for acute care hospitals.* Chicago, IL: Accreditation Association for Hospitals and Health Systems. (Level VII)

18 The Joint Commission. (2021). Standard PC.02.01.21. *Comprehensive accreditation manual for hospitals.* Oakbrook Terrace, IL: The Joint Commission.

19 The Joint Commission. (2021). Standard RC.01.03.01. *Comprehensive accreditation manual for hospitals.* Oakbrook Terrace, IL: The Joint Commission. (Level VII)

20 Centers for Medicare and Medicaid Services, Department of Health and Human Services. (2020). Condition of participation: Medical record services. 42 C.F.R. § 482.24(b).

21 Accreditation Association for Hospitals and Health Systems. (2020). Standard 10.00.03. *Healthcare Facilities Accreditation Program: Accreditation requirements for acute care hospitals.* Chicago, IL: Accreditation Association for Hospitals and Health Systems. (Level VII)

22 DNV GL-Healthcare USA, Inc. (2020). MR.2.SR.1. *NIAHO® accreditation requirements, interpretive guidelines and surveyor guidance—revision 20.0.* Milford, OH: DNV GL-Healthcare USA, Inc. (Level VII)

23 National Association of Orthopaedic Nurses (NAON). (2013). *NAON core curriculum for orthopaedic nursing* (7th ed.). Boston, MA: Pearson Custom Publishing.

24 The Joint Commission. (2020). Specifications manual for Joint Commission national quality measures (version 2020B1). https://manual.jointcommission.org/releases/TJC2020B1/

25 The Joint Commission. (2021). Standard RC.02.01.01. *Comprehensive accreditation manual for hospitals.* Oakbrook Terrace, IL: The Joint Commission. (Level VII)

ELECTROCARDIOGRAM, 12-LEAD

Coronary heart disease remains a leading cause of mortality worldwide. Promptly recognizing and treating acute coronary syndromes, such as ST-segment elevation myocardial infarction (STEMI) and non-STEMI acute coronary syndrome, can reduce and prevent cardiac arrest.[1]

One of the most valuable and frequently used diagnostic tools, an electrocardiogram (ECG) can display the heart's electrical activity as waveforms. Impulses moving through the heart's conduction system create electrical currents that can be monitored on the body's surface. Electrodes attached to the patient's skin can detect these electrical currents and transmit them to an instrument that produces a record of cardiac activity, known as the electrocardiogram. An ECG can be used to identify myocardial ischemia and infarction, rhythm and conduction disturbances, chamber enlargement, electrolyte imbalances, and drug toxicity.[2,3]

A standard 12-lead ECG uses a series of electrodes placed on the extremities and the chest wall to assess the heart from 12 different views (leads).[4] The 12 leads consist of 3 standard bipolar limb leads (designated I, II, III), 3 unipolar augmented leads (aV_R, aV_L, aV_F), and 6 unipolar precordial leads (V_1 to V_6). The limb leads and augmented leads show the heart from the frontal plane. The precordial leads show the heart from the horizontal plane.

The ECG machine measures and averages the differences between the electrical potential of the electrode sites for each lead and graphs them over time. This process creates the standard ECG complex, made up of *P-QRS-T.* The P wave represents atrial depolarization; the QRS complex, ventricular depolarization; and the T wave, ventricular repolarization. (See *Reviewing ECG waveforms and components.*)

Variations of the standard ECG include the exercise ECG (stress ECG) and ambulatory ECG (Holter monitoring). The exercise ECG monitors heart rate, blood pressure, and ECG waveforms as the patient walks on a treadmill or pedals a stationary bicycle. For the ambulatory ECG, the patient wears a portable Holter monitor to record heart activity continually over 24 hours.

Reviewing ECG waveforms and components

An electrocardiogram (ECG) waveform has three basic components: P wave, QRS complex, and T wave. These elements can be further divided into the PR interval, J point, ST segment, U wave, and QT interval.

P wave and PR interval
The P wave represents atrial depolarization. The PR interval represents the time it takes an impulse to travel from the atria through the AV nodes and bundle of His. The PR interval measures from the beginning of the P wave to the beginning of the QRS complex.

QRS complex
The QRS complex represents ventricular depolarization (the time it takes for the impulse to travel through the bundle branches to the Purkinje fibers).

The Q wave, when present, appears as the first negative deflection in the QRS complex; the R wave, as the first positive deflection. The S wave appears as the second negative deflection or the first negative deflection after the R wave.

J point and ST segment
Marking the end of the QRS complex, the J point also indicates the beginning of the ST segment. The ST segment represents part of ventricular repolarization.

T wave and U wave
Usually following the same deflection pattern as the P wave, the T wave represents ventricular repolarization. The U wave follows the T wave, but isn't always seen; its seen most frequently during bradycardia in leads V_2 and V_3.[5]

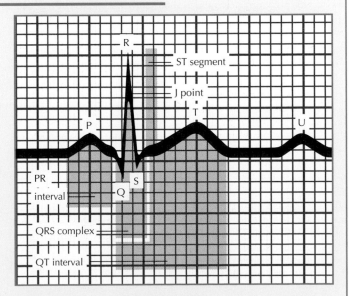

QT interval
The QT interval represents ventricular depolarization and repolarization. It extends from the beginning of the QRS complex to the end of the T wave.

The ECG is accomplished using a multichannel method. All electrodes are attached to the patient at once, and the machine prints a simultaneous view of all leads.

Equipment

ECG machine with recording paper ■ disposable pregelled electrodes ■ soap and water ■ washcloths ■ bath blanket or sheet ■ facility-approved disinfectant ■ Optional: disposable head clippers, single-patient-use scissors, indelible marking pen, gloves, alcohol pad, 4″ × 4″ (10 cm × 10 cm) gauze pads.

Preparation of equipment

Inspect all equipment and supplies. If a product is expired, is defective, or has compromised integrity, remove it from patient use, label it as expired or defective, and report the expiration or defect as directed by your facility. Place the ECG machine close to the patient's bed; check the cable and wires for fraying or breakage, and replace them or obtain another machine if necessary. Plug the cord into the wall outlet, or ensure proper functioning if the machine is battery operated. Turn on the machine, program or perform a self-test according to the manufacturer's instructions, and input the required patient information.[6] Most ECG machines have automatic settings; ensure that the paper speed selector is set to the standard 25 mm/sec, calibration set to 10 mm/mV, and filter settings set to 0.05 to 100 Hz.[6]

If the patient is already connected to a cardiac monitor, move the electrodes *to accommodate the precordial leads and to minimize electrical interference on the ECG tracing.* Keep the patient away from electrical fixtures and power cords. Depending on the type of pre-gelled electrodes used, ensure that they are moist or sticky *to promote impulse transmission.*[6]

Implementation

- Verify the practitioner's order.
- Gather and prepare the necessary equipment and supplies.
- Perform hand hygiene.[7,8,9,10,11,12]
- Put on gloves, as needed *to comply with standard precautions.*[13,14,15]
- Confirm the patient's identity using at least two patient identifiers.[16]
- Provide privacy.[17,18,19,20]
- Explain the procedure to the patient and family (if appropriate) according to their communication and learning needs *to increase their understanding, allay their fears, and enhance cooperation.*[21] Tell them the test records the heart's electrical activity, and that it may be repeated at certain intervals. Emphasize that no electrical current will enter the patient's body. Also explain that the test typically takes just a few minutes.
- Raise the bed to waist level before providing patient care *to prevent caregiver back strain.*[22]
- Place the patient in the supine position in the center of the bed with the arms at the patient's sides.[6,23] Raise the head of the patient's bed, if the patient desires, *to promote comfort.* Ensure the patient's arms and legs remain relaxed *to minimize muscle trembling, which can cause electrical interference.*[3]
- Expose the patient's arms, legs, and chest, and then cover the patient appropriately with a bath blanket or sheet.
- Select the electrode sites on the patient. Select flat, fleshy areas to place the limb lead electrodes. Avoid muscular and bony areas. If the patient has an amputated limb, choose a site on the residual limb.[4]

NURSING ALERT If the electrodes are placed incorrectly, the ECG tracing can be distorted sufficiently to cause a misdiagnosis. This can result in inappropriate treatment.[6]

- If the electrode site is excessively hairy, clip the hair using disposable head hair clippers *to promote electrode adherence to the patient's skin.*[4,6,24,25,26]
- Wash the electrode sites with soap and water and a washcloth and wipe them with a dry washcloth or gauze pad *to roughen the patient's skin, which helps remove the outer layer to facilitate electrical signal transmission.*[4,6,24,25,26] If necessary, clean any oily skin with an alcohol pad and allow it to dry.[4,26,27]
- Mark the sites with an indelible marker if serial ECGs are likely.[6]
- Apply disposable pregelled electrodes to the patient's inside forearms and to the medial aspects of the ankles or calves; *limb leads should be an*

Applying chest electrodes

To ensure proper placement of chest electrodes, use palpation to locate the correct intercostal space.[26] Palpate the point at which the sternum attaches to the clavicle (the suprasternal notch); then palpate down to identify the sternal angle, which is the bony prominence at which the second rib attaches to the sternum. The space below the second rib is the second intercostal space. Continue to palpate down the patient's sternum, counting the ribs and intercostal spaces to find the appropriate location for the chest electrodes.

To ensure accurate test results, position chest electrodes as follows:

V_1: Fourth intercostal space at right border of sternum
V_2: Fourth intercostal space at left border of sternum
V_3: Halfway between V_2 and V_4
V_4: Fifth intercostal space at midclavicular line
V_5: In the horizontal plane of V_4 at the anterior axillary line (or halfway between V_4 and V_6, if the anterior axillary line is ambiguous)
V_6: In the horizontal plane of V_4 at the midaxillary line

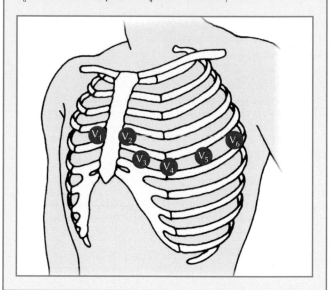

equal distance from the heart and in about the same place on each limb.[6]. Apply the pregelled electrodes directly to the prepared sites, as recommended by the manufacturer's instructions. Apply disposable electrodes on the patient's legs, with the lead connections pointing superiorly *to guarantee the best connection to the lead wire.*

- Apply a pregelled electrode at each electrode position on the patient's chest. If the patient is female, be sure to place the chest electrodes below the breast tissue.[26] (See *Applying chest electrodes.*)
- Connect the lead wires to the electrodes. Note that the tip of each lead wire is lettered and color-coded *for easy identification.* The white or RA lead wire goes to the right arm; the green or RL lead wire, to the right leg; the red or LL lead wire, to the left leg; the black or LA lead wire, to the left arm; and the brown or V_1 to V_6 lead wires, to the chest electrodes.[4]
- Instruct the patient to relax and breathe normally. Instruct the patient to lie still and to avoid talking when you record the ECG, *to minimize artifact.*[28]
- Press the AUTO or START button. The ECG machine will record all 12 leads automatically, recording 3 consecutive leads simultaneously. Some machines have a display screen so you can preview waveforms before the machine records them on paper. Observe the tracing quality.
- Repeat the ECG recording, as needed.[6]
- When the machine finishes recording the 12-lead ECG, turn off the machine, remove the electrodes, and clean the patient's skin. Disconnect the lead wires from the electrodes and dispose of the electrodes, as indicated.
- Return the bed to the lowest position *to prevent falls and maintain patient safety.*[29]
- Remove and discard your gloves, if worn.[13]

- Perform hand hygiene.[7,8,9,10,11,12]
- Put on gloves, as needed.[13]
- Clean and disinfect reusable equipment according to the manufacturer's instructions *to prevent the spread of infection.*[6,30,31]
- Remove and discard your gloves.[13]
- Perform hand hygiene.[7,8,9,10,11,12]
- Document the procedure.[32,33,34,35]

Special considerations

- During the procedure, ask the patient to breathe normally. If respirations distort the recording, ask the patient to hold the breath briefly *to reduce baseline wander in the tracing.*
- If the patient has a pacemaker, you can perform an ECG with or without a magnet, according to the practitioner's orders. Be sure to note the presence of a pacemaker and the use of the magnet on both the ECG strip and the patient's medical record.
- Record the ECG with the patient in the same position each time, *because different positions may cause differences in the tracings.* If another position is required because of the patient's condition, document the position used on the tracing and in the patient's medical record.[6,23]

Documentation

Document in the patient's medical record the date and time that the ECG was performed and any significant responses by the patient. Verify the date, time, patient's name, and assigned identification number on the ECG itself. Note any appropriate clinical information, positioning changes, and calibration variations on the ECG tracing, and place it in the patient's medical record.[6] Document teaching provided to the patient and family (if applicable), their understanding of that teaching, and any need for follow-up teaching.[32]

REFERENCES

1 American Heart Association. (2015). Part 5: Acute coronary syndromes. 2015 International consensus on cardiopulmonary resuscitation and emergency cardiovascular care science with treatment recommendations. *Circulation, 132*(16 Suppl 1), S146–S176. (Level II)

2 Kligfield, P., et al. (2007). Recommendations for the standardization and interpretation of the electrocardiogram: Part I: The electrocardiogram and its technology: A scientific statement from the American Heart Association Electrocardiography and Arrhythmias Committee, Council on Clinical Cardiology; the American College of Cardiology Foundation; and the Heart Rhythm Society endorsed by the International Society for Computerized Electrocardiology. *Circulation, 115*, 1306–1324. https://www.ahajournals.org/doi/pdf/10.1161/circulationaha.106.180200 (Level I)

3 Kadish, A. H., et al. (2001). "ACC/AHA clinical competence statement on electrocardiography and ambulatory electrocardiography: A report of the ACC/AHA/ACP-ASIM Task Force on Clinical Competence (ACC/AHA Committee to Develop a Clinical Competence Statement on Electrocardiography and Ambulatory Electrocardiography)" endorsed by the International Society for Holter and Noninvasive Electrocardiology. *Circulation, 104*, 3169–3178. https://www.ahajournals.org/doi/pdf/10.1161/circ.104.25.3169 (Level I)

4 Eggett, C., et al. (2017). Clinical guidelines by consensus: Recording a standard 12-lead electrocardiogram: An approved methodology by the Society for Cardiological Science & Technology. https://www.bmj.com/sites/default/files/response_attachments/2016/09/CAC_SCST_Recording_a_12-lead_ECG_final_version_2014_CS2v2.0.pdf (Level VII)

5 Rautaharju, P. M., et al. (2009). AHA/ACCF/HRS recommendations for the standardization and interpretation of the electrocardiogram. Part IV: The ST segment, T and U waves, and the QT interval. *Journal of the American College of Cardiology, 53*(11), 982–991. http://www.onlinejacc.org/content/53/11/982 (Level VII)

6 Wiegand, D. L. (2017). *AACN procedure manual for high acuity, progressive, and critical care* (7th ed.). St. Louis, MO: Elsevier.

7 The Joint Commission. (2021). Standard NPSG.07.01.01. *Comprehensive accreditation manual for hospitals.* Oakbrook Terrace, IL: The Joint Commission. (Level VII)

8 Centers for Disease Control and Prevention. (2002). Guideline for hand hygiene in health-care settings: Recommendations of the Healthcare Infection Control Practices Advisory Committee and the HICPAC/

SHEA/APIC/IDSA Hand Hygiene Task Force. *MMWR Recommendations and Reports, 51*(RR-16), 1–45. https://www.cdc.gov/mmwr/pdf/rr/rr5116.pdf (Level II)

9 World Health Organization. (2009). WHO guidelines on hand hygiene in health care: First global patient safety challenge, clean care is safer care. https://apps.who.int/iris/bitstream/handle/10665/44102/9789241597906_eng.pdf?sequence=1 (Level IV)

10 Centers for Medicare and Medicaid Services, Department of Health and Human Services. (2020). Condition of participation: Infection control. 42 C.F.R. § 482.42.

11 Accreditation Association for Hospitals and Health Systems. (2020). Standard 07.01.21. *Healthcare Facilities Accreditation Program: Accreditation requirements for acute care hospitals.* Chicago, IL: Accreditation Association for Hospitals and Health Systems. (Level VII)

12 DNV GL-Healthcare USA, Inc. (2020). IC.1.SR.1. *NIAHO® accreditation requirements, interpretive guidelines and surveyor guidance—revision 20.0.* Milford, OH: DNV GL-Healthcare USA, Inc. (Level VII)

13 Occupational Safety and Health Administration. (2012). Bloodborne pathogens, standard number 1910.1030. https://www.osha.gov/pls/oshaweb/owadisp.show_document?p_id=10051&p_table=STANDARDS (Level VII)

14 Siegel, J. D., et al. (2007, revised 2019). 2007 guideline for isolation precautions: Preventing transmission of infectious agents in healthcare settings. https://www.cdc.gov/infectioncontrol/pdf/guidelines/isolation-guidelines-H.pdf (Level II)

15 Accreditation Association for Hospitals and Health Systems. (2020). Standard 07.01.10. *Healthcare Facilities Accreditation Program: Accreditation requirements for acute care hospitals.* Chicago, IL: Accreditation Association for Hospitals and Health Systems. (Level VII)

16 The Joint Commission. (2021). Standard NPSG.01.01.01. *Comprehensive accreditation manual for hospitals.* Oakbrook Terrace, IL: The Joint Commission. (Level VII)

17 Accreditation Association for Hospitals and Health Systems. (2020). Standard 15.01.16. *Healthcare Facilities Accreditation Program: Accreditation requirements for acute care hospitals.* Chicago, IL: Accreditation Association for Hospitals and Health Systems. (Level VII)

18 Centers for Medicare and Medicaid Services, Department of Health and Human Services. (2020). Condition of participation: Patient's rights. 42 C.F.R. § 482.13(c)(1).

19 The Joint Commission. (2021). Standard RI.01.01.01. *Comprehensive accreditation manual for hospitals.* Oakbrook Terrace, IL: The Joint Commission. (Level VII)

20 DNV GL-Healthcare USA, Inc. (2020). PR.2.SR.5. *NIAHO® accreditation requirements, interpretive guidelines and surveyor guidance—revision 20.0.* Milford, OH: DNV GL-Healthcare USA, Inc. (Level VII)

21 The Joint Commission. (2021). Standard PC.02.01.21. *Comprehensive accreditation manual for hospitals.* Oakbrook Terrace, IL: The Joint Commission. (Level VII)

22 Waters, T. R., et al. (2009). Safe patient handling training for schools of nursing. https://www.cdc.gov/niosh/docs/2009-127/pdfs/2009-127.pdf (Level VII)

23 Garcia, T. (2015). Acquiring the 12-lead electrocardiogram: Doing it right every time. *Journal of Emergency Nursing, 41*(6), 474–478.

24 Walsh-Irwin, C., & Jurgens, C. Y. (2015). Proper skin preparation and electrode placement decreases alarms on a telemetry unit. *Dimensions of Critical Care Nursing, 34*, 134–139. (Level IV)

25 American Association of Critical-Care Nurses. (2018). AACN practice alert: Managing alarms in acute care across the life span: Electrocardiography and pulse oximetry. https://www.aacn.org/clinical-resources/practice-alerts/managing-alarms-in-acute-care-across-the-life-span (Level VII)

26 American Association of Critical-Care Nurses. (2016, updated 2018). AACN practice alert: Accurate dysrhythmia monitoring in adults. https://www.aacn.org//clinical-resources/practice-alerts/dysrhythmia-monitoring (Level VII)

27 American Association of Critical-Care Nurses. (2016, updated 2018). AACN practice alert: Ensuring accurate ST-segment monitoring. https://www.aacn.org/clinical-resources/practice-alerts/st-segment-monitoring (Level VII)

28 Physio-Control, Inc. (2015). Minimizing ECG artifact. https://www.physio-control.com/WorkArea/DownloadAsset.aspx?id=2147489452

29 Ganz, D. A., et al. (2013, reviewed 2021). *Preventing falls in hospitals: A toolkit for improving quality of care* (AHRQ Publication No. 13-0015-EF). Rockville, MD: Agency for Healthcare Research and Quality. https://www.ahrq.gov/professionals/systems/hospital/fallpxtoolkit/index.html (Level VII)

30 Rutala, W. A., et al. (2008, revised 2019). Guideline for disinfection and sterilization in healthcare facilities, 2008. https://www.cdc.gov/infection-control/pdf/guidelines/disinfection-guidelines-H.pdf (Level I)

31 Accreditation Association for Hospitals and Health Systems. (2020). Standard 07.02.03. *Healthcare Facilities Accreditation Program: Accreditation requirements for acute care hospitals.* Chicago, IL: Accreditation Association for Hospitals and Health Systems. (Level VII)

32 The Joint Commission. (2021). Standard RC.01.03.01. *Comprehensive accreditation manual for hospitals.* Oakbrook Terrace, IL: The Joint Commission. (Level VII)

33 Centers for Medicare and Medicaid Services, Department of Health and Human Services. (2020). Condition of participation: Medical record services. 42 C.F.R. § 482.24(b).

34 Accreditation Association for Hospitals and Health Systems. (2020). Standard 10.00.03. *Healthcare Facilities Accreditation Program: Accreditation requirements for acute care hospitals.* Chicago, IL: Accreditation Association for Hospitals and Health Systems. (Level VII)

35 DNV GL-Healthcare USA, Inc. (2020). MR.2.SR.1. *NIAHO® accreditation requirements, interpretive guidelines and surveyor guidance—revision 20.0.* Milford, OH: DNV GL-Healthcare USA, Inc. (Level VII)

Electrocardiogram, posterior chest lead

An electrocardiogram (ECG) is a recording of the electrical activity of the heart. The 12-lead ECG is an essential diagnostic tool in the management and treatment of ischemic heart disease, but because of the location of the heart's posterior surface, changes associated with myocardial damage may not be apparent on a standard 12-lead ECG. To help identify posterior involvement, some practitioners recommend using posterior chest leads in addition to the limb leads of the 12-lead ECG. Despite lung and muscle barriers, posterior leads may provide clues to posterior ST-elevation myocardial infarction.[1,2]

Rapid recognition of posterior infarct is important. Patients with inferior or lateral infarcts and a coexisting posterior infarction are at greater risk for complications; there should be no delay in acute therapy, including thrombolysis and percutaneous coronary intervention.[3]

Equipment

Multichannel ECG machine with attached patient cables, lead wires, and recording paper ▪ soap and water ▪ washcloths ▪ towel ▪ disposable pre-gelled electrodes ▪ 4″ × 4″ (10 cm × 10 cm) gauze pads or moist cloth ▪ bath blanket or sheet ▪ Optional: disposable-head clippers or single-patient-use scissors, indelible marker, gloves, alcohol pads.

Preparation of equipment

Inspect all equipment and supplies. If a product is expired, is defective, or has compromised integrity, remove it from patient use, label it as expired or defective, and report the expiration or defect as directed by your facility. Place the ECG machine close to the patient's bed. Verify that the cables and lead wires aren't frayed or broken; replace them if necessary. Plug the machine's cord into the wall outlet, or ensure that the machine functions if it's battery operated. Turn on the machine and input the required patient information. Keep the patient away from electrical fixtures and power cords. Depending on the type of pre-gelled electrodes you use, make sure that they're moist or sticky *to promote impulse transmission.*

Most ECG machines have automatic settings; ensure that the paper speed selector is set to the standard 25 mm/sec, calibration is set to 10 mm/mV, and the filter setting is 0.05 to 100 Hz.[4]

Implementation

▪ Verify the practitioner's order.
▪ Gather and prepare the necessary equipment and supplies.
▪ Perform hand hygiene.[5,6,7,8,9,10]
▪ Confirm the patient's identity using at least two patient identifiers.[11]
▪ Provide privacy.[12,13,14,15]
▪ Explain the procedure to the patient and family (if appropriate) according to their individual communication and learning needs *to increase their understanding, allay their fears, and enhance cooperation.*[16] Tell the patient that the test records the heart's electrical activity, and that it may

repeat at certain intervals. Emphasize that no electrical current will enter the patient's body, and tell the patient that the test typically takes about 5 minutes.

▪ Raise the bed to waist level before providing patient care *to prevent caregiver back* strain.[17]
▪ Have the patient lie supine in the center of the bed with the arms at the patient's sides.[4] Raise the head of the bed, as needed, *to promote patient comfort.* If a position other than supine is necessary, document the position on the ECG tracing.[4]
▪ Perform hand hygiene.[5,6,7,8,9,10]
▪ Put on gloves, as needed, *to comply with standard precautions.*[18,19,20]
▪ Expose the patient's arms and legs, and drape the patient appropriately with a bath blanket or sheet. The patient's arms and legs should be relaxed *to minimize muscle trembling, which can cause electrical interference.*[21]
▪ Identify the limb lead locations. Select flat, fleshy areas to place the limb lead electrodes. Avoid muscular and bony areas. If the patient has an amputated limb, choose a site on the residual limb. If an area is extremely hairy, clip the hair with a disposable-head clippers or single-use-patient scissors *to ensure that the electrode makes adequate skin contact.*[4,22,23]
▪ *To enhance limb lead electrode contact and trace quality,* prepare all the electrode sites by washing them with soap and water and drying them thoroughly, *because moist skin may prevent the electrodes from adhering.*[4] Rub the electrode sites briskly with a dry washcloth or gauze pad *to remove dead skin cells and promote impulse transmission.*[4,22,23,24] If necessary, clean oily skin with an alcohol pad and allow it to dry.[25,26]
▪ For the limb leads, apply disposable pre-gelled electrodes to the prepared sites on the patient's arms and legs, distal to the shoulders and hips, according to the manufacturer's instructions. Position them in approximately the same location on each limb.[4] *To guarantee the best connection to the lead wire,* position disposable pre-gelled electrodes on the legs with the lead connection pointing superiorly.

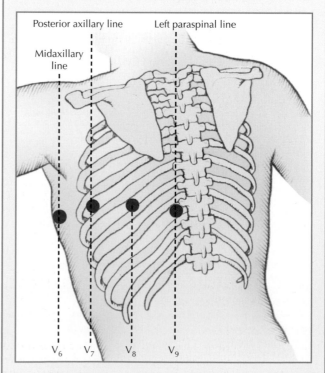

Placing electrodes for posterior ECG

To ensure an accurate electrocardiogram (ECG) reading, make sure that the posterior leads V_7, V_8, and V_9 are placed at the same level horizontally as the V_6 lead at the fifth intercostal space.[2] Place V_6 at the midaxillary line. Place lead V_7 at the posterior axillary line, lead V_9 at the left paraspinal line, and lead V_8 halfway between leads V_7 and V_9 as shown below.[4]

Midaxillary line   Posterior axillary line   Left paraspinal line

V_6 V_7 V_8 V_9

- Help the patient turn onto the right side, and expose the left side of the patient's back. Identify the electrode locations. Use disposable-head clippers or single-patient-scissors to clip hair in excessively hairy areas.[4,22,23]
- Prepare the posterior electrode application sites by washing them with soap and water and drying them thoroughly; *moist skin may prevent the electrodes from adhering.*[4] Rub the electrode sites briskly with a dry washcloth or gauze pad *to remove dead skin cells and promote impulse transmission.*[4,22,23,24] as described for the limb leads.
- If necessary, clean oily skin with an alcohol pad and allow it to dry.[25,26] Mark all the electrode sites with an indelible marker if serial ECGs are likely, *to permit accurate comparison with future tracings.*[4]
- Attach a disposable pre-gelled electrode to the V_7 position on the left posterior axillary line, fifth intercostal space, at the same level as V_6. Then attach the V_4 lead wire to the V_7 electrode.[4]
- Attach a disposable pre-gelled electrode to the patient's back at the V_9 position, just to the left of the spinal column at the left paraspinal line, at the same level as V_6 and V_7. Then, attach the V_6 lead wire to the V_9 electrode.[4]
- Attach a disposable pre-gelled electrode to the patient's back at the V_8 position, halfway between leads V_7 and V_9, at the same level as V_6 and V_7, and attach the V_5 lead wire to this electrode.[4] (See *Placing electrodes for posterior ECG.*)
- Ask the patient to breathe normally and to refrain from talking during the recording *so that muscle movement won't distort the tracing.*
- Press AUTO or START to start recording.
- Observe the tracing quality. If any part of the waveform height extends beyond the paper when you record the ECG, adjust the normal standardization to half-standardization. Note this adjustment on the ECG strip, *because the adjustment will need to be considered in interpreting the results.*
- Relabel the leads labeled V_4, V_5, and V_6 to leads V_7, V_8, and V_9, respectively.
- When the ECG is complete, turn off the machine.
- If the machine hasn't already done so, label the tracing with the date and time as well as the patient's name and identification number. Note whether the tracing is a posterior chest lead ECG. Make sure the leads are correctly labeled V_7 through V_9.[2]
- Remove the electrodes and discard them in the appropriate receptacle.
- Clean the patient's skin with a gauze pad or a moist cloth.
- Return the bed to the lowest position *to prevent falls and maintain patient safety.*[27]
- Remove and discard your gloves, if worn.[18,19]
- Perform hand hygiene.[5,6,7,8,9,10]
- Put on gloves as needed.[20]
- Clean and disinfect the ECG equipment according to the manufacturer's instructions *to prevent the spread of infection.*[28,29] Prepare the ECG equipment for future use.[4]
- Remove and discard your gloves, if worn.[20]
- Perform hand hygiene.[5,6,7,8,9,10]
- Place the ECG in the patient's medical record.
- Document the procedure.[30,31,32,33]

Special considerations

If your facility has the capability of transmitting the patient's ECG from the ECG machine to the patient's electronic medical record, verify that the ECG transmission was successful and complete. If an additional ECG is necessary, place the patient in the same position as previous ECG tracings *to ensure that any ECG changes aren't the result of body position change.*[4]

Complications

Prolonged application of the adhesive on the electrodes may cause skin irritation or tissue breakdown. Failure to correctly label the ECG leads could lead to misdiagnosis.[4]

Documentation

Document the test's date and time, the reason for the test, and the patient's tolerance of the procedure. Note any appropriate clinical information on the ECG and place it in the patient's medical record. Document teaching provided to the patient and family (if applicable), their understanding of that teaching, and any need for follow-up teaching.

REFERENCES

1 Aqel, R. A., et al. (2009). Usefulness of three posterior chest leads for the detection of posterior wall acute myocardial infarction. *American Journal of Cardiology, 103*, 159–164. (Level VI)

2 Provinse, J. F., et al. (2013). ENA's translation into practice: Right-sided and posterior electrocardiograms (ECGs). https://www.loyolamedicine.org/sites/default/files/gme/internal-medicine/rightsideecg_0.pdf (Level VII)

3 Van Gorselen, E. O. F., et al. (2007). Posterior myocardial infarction: The dark side of the moon. *Netherlands Heart Journal, 15*(1), 16–21. https://www.ncbi.nlm.nih.gov/pmc/articles/PMC1847720/ (Level V)

4 Wiegand, D. L. (2017). *AACN procedure manual for high acuity, progressive, and critical care* (7th ed.). St. Louis, MO: Elsevier.

5 The Joint Commission. (2021). Standard NPSG.07.01.01. *Comprehensive accreditation manual for hospitals.* Oakbrook Terrace, IL: The Joint Commission. (Level VII)

6 Centers for Disease Control and Prevention. (2002). Guideline for hand hygiene in health-care settings: Recommendations of the Healthcare Infection Control Practices Advisory Committee and the HICPAC/SHEA/APIC/IDSA Hand Hygiene Task Force. *MMWR Recommendations and Reports, 51*(RR-16), 1–45. https://www.cdc.gov/mmwr/pdf/rr/rr5116.pdf (Level II)

7 World Health Organization. (2009). WHO guidelines on hand hygiene in health care: First global patient safety challenge, clean care is safer care. https://apps.who.int/iris/bitstream/handle/10665/44102/9789241597906_eng.pdf?sequence=1 (Level IV)

8 Centers for Medicare and Medicaid Services, Department of Health and Human Services. (2020). Condition of participation: Infection control. 42 C.F.R. § 482.42.

9 Accreditation Association for Hospitals and Health Systems. (2020). Standard 07.01.21. *Healthcare Facilities Accreditation Program: Accreditation requirements for acute care hospitals.* Chicago, IL: Accreditation Association for Hospitals and Health Systems. (Level VII)

10 DNV GL-Healthcare USA, Inc. (2020). IC.1.SR.1. *NIAHO® accreditation requirements, interpretive guidelines and surveyor guidance—revision 20.0.* Milford, OH: DNV GL-Healthcare USA, Inc. (Level VII)

11 The Joint Commission. (2021). Standard NPSG.01.01.01. *Comprehensive accreditation manual for hospitals.* Oakbrook Terrace, IL: The Joint Commission. (Level VII)

12 Centers for Medicare and Medicaid Services, Department of Health and Human Services. (2019). Condition of participation: Patient's rights. 42 C.F.R. § 482.13(c)(1).

13 Accreditation Association for Hospitals and Health Systems. (2020). Standard 15.01.16. *Healthcare Facilities Accreditation Program: Accreditation requirements for acute care hospitals.* Chicago, IL: Accreditation Association for Hospitals and Health Systems. (Level VII)

14 The Joint Commission. (2021). Standard RI.01.01.01. *Comprehensive accreditation manual for hospitals.* Oakbrook Terrace, IL: The Joint Commission. (Level VII)

15 DNV GL-Healthcare USA, Inc. (2020). PR.2.SR.5. *NIAHO® accreditation requirements, interpretive guidelines and surveyor guidance—revision 20.0.* Milford, OH: DNV GL-Healthcare USA, Inc. (Level VII)

16 The Joint Commission. (2021). Standard PC.02.01.21. *Comprehensive accreditation manual for hospitals.* Oakbrook Terrace, IL: The Joint Commission. (Level VII)

17 Waters, T. R., et al. (2009). Safe patient handling training for schools of nursing. https://www.cdc.gov/niosh/docs/2009-127/pdfs/2009-127.pdf (Level VII)

18 Siegel, J. D., et al. (2007, revised 2019). 2007 guideline for isolation precautions: Preventing transmission of infectious agents in healthcare settings. https://www.cdc.gov/infectioncontrol/pdf/guidelines/isolation-guidelines-H.pdf (Level II)

19 Accreditation Association for Hospitals and Health Systems. (2020). Standard 07.01.10. *Healthcare Facilities Accreditation Program: Accreditation requirements for acute care hospitals.* Chicago, IL: Accreditation Association for Hospitals and Health Systems. (Level VII)

20 Occupational Safety and Health Administration. (2012). Bloodborne pathogens, standard number 1910.1030. https://www.osha.gov/pls/oshaweb/owadisp.show_document?p_id=10051&p_table=STANDARDS (Level VII)

21 American College of Cardiology/American Heart Association. (2001). ACC/AHA clinical competence statement on electrocardiography and

ambulatory electrocardiography. *Circulation, 104*, 3169–3178. https://www.ahajournals.org/doi/full/10.1161/circ.104.25.3169 (Level VII)

22 Kligfield, P., et al. (2007). Recommendations for the standardization and interpretation of the electrocardiogram: Part I: The electrocardiogram and its technology. *Circulation, 115*, 1306–1324. https://www.ahajournals.org/doi/full/10.1161/circulationaha.106.180200 (Level VII)

23 Oster, C. D. (2005). Proper skin prep helps ensure ECG trace quality. http://multimedia.3m.com/mws/media/358372O/proper-skin-prep-ecg-trace-quality-white-paper.pdf

24 American Association of Critical-Care Nurses. (2018). AACN practice alert: Managing alarms in acute care across the life span: Electrocardiography and pulse oximetry https://www.aacn.org/clinical-resources/practice-alerts/managing-alarms-in-acute-care-across-the-life-span (Level VII)

25 American Association of Critical-Care Nurses. (2018). AACN practice alert: Accurate dysrhythmia monitoring in adults. https://www.aacn.org/clinical-resources/practice-alerts/dysrhythmia-monitoring (Level VII)

26 American Association of Critical-Care Nurses. (2018). AACN practice alert: Ensuring accurate ST-segment monitoring. https://www.aacn.org/clinical-resources/practice-alerts/st-segment-monitoring (Level VII)

27 Ganz, D. A., et al. (2013, reviewed 2021). *Preventing falls in hospitals: A toolkit for improving quality of care* (AHRQ Publication No. 13-0015-EF). Rockville, MD: Agency for Healthcare Research and Quality. https://www.ahrq.gov/professionals/systems/hospital/fallpxtoolkit/index.html (Level VII)

28 Rutala, W. A., et al. (2008, revised 2019). Guideline for disinfection and sterilization in healthcare facilities, 2008. https://www.cdc.gov/infection-control/pdf/guidelines/disinfection-guidelines-H.pdf (Level I)

29 Accreditation Association for Hospitals and Health Systems. (2020). Standard 07.02.03. *Healthcare Facilities Accreditation Program: Accreditation requirements for acute care hospitals.* Chicago, IL: Accreditation Association for Hospitals and Health Systems. (Level VII)

30 The Joint Commission. (2021). Standard RC.01.03.01. *Comprehensive accreditation manual for hospitals.* Oakbrook Terrace, IL: The Joint Commission. (Level VII)

31 Centers for Medicare and Medicaid Services, Department of Health and Human Services. (2020). Condition of participation: Medical record services. 42 C.F.R. § 482.24(b).

32 Accreditation Association for Hospitals and Health Systems. (2020). Standard 10.00.03. *Healthcare Facilities Accreditation Program: Accreditation requirements for acute care hospitals.* Chicago, IL: Accreditation Association for Hospitals and Health Systems. (Level VII)

33 DNV GL-Healthcare USA, Inc. (2020). MR.2.SR.1. *NIAHO® accreditation requirements, interpretive guidelines and surveyor guidance—revision 20.0.* Milford, OH: DNV GL-Healthcare USA, Inc. (Level VII)

ELECTROCARDIOGRAM, RIGHT CHEST LEAD

An electrocardiogram (ECG) measures the electrical activity of the heart. Unlike a standard 12-lead ECG, used primarily to evaluate left ventricular function, a right chest lead ECG reflects right ventricular function and provides clues to damage or dysfunction in this chamber. You might need to perform a right chest lead ECG for a patient with an inferior wall myocardial infarction (MI) and suspected right ventricular involvement.[1] Between 10% and 50% of patients with this type of MI have right ventricular involvement.[1]

Early identification of a right ventricular MI is essential because its treatment differs from treatment for other MIs. Treatment usually requires administration of IV fluids to maintain adequate filling pressures on the right side of the heart, which helps the right ventricle eject an adequate volume of blood at an adequate pressure.[2] Diuretics, beta-adrenergic blockers, morphine, and nitrates should be avoided *to prevent a drop in blood pressure.*[3]

Equipment

Multichannel ECG machine with attached patient cable, lead wires, and recording paper ▪ soap and water ▪ washcloths ▪ towel ▪ disposable pre-gelled electrodes ▪ 4″ × 4″ (10 cm × 10 cm) gauze pads or moist cloth ▪ facility-approved disinfectant ▪ bath blanket or sheet ▪ Optional: disposable head clippers, single-patient-use scissors, indelible marking pen, gloves, alcohol pads.

Preparation of equipment

Inspect all equipment and supplies. If a product is expired, is defective, or has compromised integrity, remove it from patient use, label it as expired or defective, and report the expiration or defect as directed by your facility. Place the ECG machine close to the patient's bed. Ensure that the cable and lead wires aren't broken or frayed; replace them if necessary. Plug the machine's cord into the wall outlet, or ensure that the machine functions if it's battery operated. Turn on the machine and input the required patient information. Keep the patient away from electrical fixtures and power cords. Depending on the type of pre-gelled electrodes that you're using, make sure that they're moist or sticky *to promote impulse transmission.*

Most ECG machines have automatic settings. Ensure that the paper speed selector is set to the standard 25 mm/sec, calibration is set to 10 mm/mV, and the filter setting is 0.05 to 100 Hz.[2]

Implementation

▪ Verify the practitioner's order.
▪ Gather and prepare the necessary equipment and supplies.
▪ Perform hand hygiene.[4,5,6,7,8,9]
▪ Confirm the patient's identity using at least two patient identifiers.[10]
▪ Provide privacy.[11,12,13,14]
▪ Explain the procedure to the patient and family (if appropriate) according to their communication and learning needs *to increase their understanding, allay their fears, and enhance cooperation.*[15] Inform the patient that the practitioner has ordered a right chest lead ECG, a procedure that involves placing electrodes on the arms, legs, and chest. Reassure the patient that the test is painless and takes only a few minutes, during which the patient will need to lie quietly on the back.
▪ Raise the patient's bed to waist level before providing care *to prevent caregiver back strain.*[16]
▪ Have the patient lie supine in the center of the bed with the arms at the patient's sides.[1]
▪ Raise the head of the bed as needed *to promote patient comfort.*[17]
▪ If the patient requires a position other than supine, document the position on the ECG tracing.[2]
▪ Perform hand hygiene.[4,5,6,7,8,9]
▪ Put on gloves, if needed, *to comply with standard precautions.*[16,18,19]
▪ Expose the patient's arms, chest, and legs. Drape the patient appropriately with a bath blanket or sheet; drape a female patient's chest until you apply the chest electrodes. Ensure that the patient's arms and legs are relaxed *to minimize muscle trembling, which can cause electrical interference.*[20]
▪ Select electrode sites. Select flat, fleshy areas to place the limb lead electrodes. Avoid muscular and bony areas.[2] If the patient has an amputated limb, choose a site on the residual limb.
▪ Examine the patient's chest to locate the correct sites for chest lead placement (as shown below). If the patient is female, you'll place the electrodes under the breast tissue.[2]

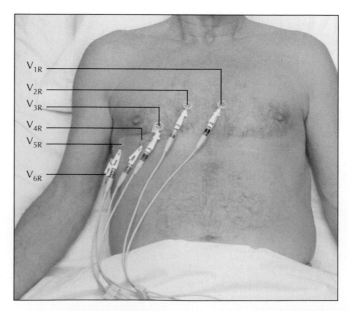

■ If an area is excessively hairy, clip the hair using a disposable-head clippers or single-patient-use scissors.[2,20,21]

■ *To enhance lead electrode contact and trace quality,* prepare all the electrode sites by washing them with soap and water and drying them thoroughly; *moist skin may prevent the electrodes from adhering.*[2] Rub the electrode sites briskly with a dry washcloth or gauze pad *to remove dead skin cells and promote impulse transmission.*[2,20,21,22] If necessary, clean oily skin with an alcohol pad and allow it to dry.[23,24]

■ Mark all the electrode sites with an indelible marker if serial ECGs are likely, *to permit accurate comparison with future tracings.*[2]

■ Apply disposable pre-gelled electrodes to the prepared sites on the patient's arms and legs, distal to the shoulders and hips, according to the manufacturer's instructions.[20] Position them in approximately the same location on each limb.[2] *To guarantee the best connection to the lead wire,* position disposable pre-gelled electrodes on the legs with the lead connection pointing superiorly.

■ Connect the lead wires to the electrodes. The lead wires are color-coded and lettered. Place the white, or right arm (RA), wire on the right arm; the black, or left arm (LA), wire on the left arm; the green, or right leg (RL), wire on the right leg; and the red, or left leg (LL), wire on the left leg.

■ Apply a pre-gelled electrode at each electrode position on the patient's chest.

■ Use your fingers to feel between the patient's ribs (the intercostal spaces). Start at the second intercostal space on the left (the notch felt at the top of the sternum, where the manubrium joins the body of the sternum). Count down two spaces to the fourth intercostal space at the left sternal border. Apply a disposable pre-gelled electrode to the site, and attach lead wire V_{1R} to that electrode.[2]

■ Move your fingers across the sternum to the fourth intercostal space at the right sternal border. Apply a disposable pre-gelled electrode to that site and attach lead V_{2R}.[2]

■ Move your finger down to the fifth intercostal space and over to the midclavicular line. Place a disposable pre-gelled electrode here and attach lead V_{4R}. Apply a disposable pre-gelled electrode midway on this line from V_{2R} and attach lead V_{3R}.[2]

■ Move your finger horizontally from V_{4R} to the right midaxillary line. Apply an electrode to this site and attach lead V_{6R}.[2]

■ Move your fingers along the same horizontal line to the midpoint between V_{4R} and V_{6R}. This is the right anterior midaxillary line. Apply a disposable pre-gelled electrode to this site and attach lead V_{5R}.[2]

■ Ask the patient to breathe normally and to refrain from talking during the recording *so that muscle movement won't distort the tracing.*

■ Make sure that the paper speed is set at 25 mm/second and the amplitude at 1 mV/10 mm.[10,11]

■ Press the AUTO or START key. The ECG machine will record all 12 leads automatically. Check your facility's policy for the number of readings to obtain. (Some facilities require at least two ECGs so that one copy can be sent out for interpretation while the other remains at the bedside.)

■ Observe the tracing quality. If any part of the waveform height extends beyond the paper when you record the ECG, adjust the normal standardization to half-standardization. Note this adjustment on the ECG strip, *because this will need to be considered in interpreting the results.*[25]

■ When you're finished recording the ECG, turn off the machine. If the ECG machine hasn't already done so, label the ECG with the date and time as well as the patient's name and identification number. Also label the tracing as RIGHT CHEST ECG *to distinguish it from a standard 12-lead ECG.*[1] Make sure that the tracings are correctly labeled V_{1R} through V_{6R}.

■ Remove the electrodes and discard them in the appropriate receptacle.

■ Clean the patient's skin with a gauze pad or moist cloth.

■ Return the bed to the lowest position *to prevent falls and maintain patients safety.*[26]

■ Remove and discard your gloves, if worn.[16,19]

■ Perform hand hygiene.[4,5,6,7,8,9]

■ Put on gloves, as needed.[19]

■ Clean and disinfect the ECG equipment according to the manufacturer's instructions *to prevent the spread of infection.*[27,28] Prepare the equipment for future use.[2]

■ Remove and discard your gloves, as needed.[19]

■ Perform hand hygiene.[4,5,6,7,8,9]

■ Place the ECG tracing in the patient's medical record.

■ Document the procedure.[29,30,31,32]

Special considerations

■ If your facility has the capability of transmitting the patient's ECG from the ECG machine to the patient's medical record, verify that the ECG transmission was successful and complete.

■ If an additional ECG is necessary, place the patient in the same position as previous ECG tracings *to ensure that any ECG changes aren't the result of body position change.*[2]

Complications

Prolonged application of the adhesive on the electrodes may cause skin irritation or tissue breakdown. Failure to identify the tracing as a right chest ECG could lead to misdiagnosis.[2]

Documentation

Document the date and time of the procedure, the reason for the test, and the patient's tolerance of it. Document teaching provided to the patient and family (if applicable), their understanding of that teaching, and any need for follow-up teaching.

REFERENCES

1 Provinse, J. F., et al. (2013). ENA's translation into practice: Right-sided and posterior electrocardiograms (ECGs). https://www.loyolamedicine.org/sites/default/files/gme/internal-medicine/rightsideecg_0.pdf (Level VII)

2 Wiegand, D. L. (2017). *AACN procedure manual for high acuity, progressive, and critical care* (7th ed.). St. Louis, MO: Elsevier.

3 Nagam, M. R., et al. (2017). ECG diagnosis: Right ventricular myocardial infarction. *The Permanente Journal, 21*, 16–105. https://www.ncbi.nlm.nih.gov/pmc/articles/PMC5267627/

4 The Joint Commission. (2021). Standard NPSG.07.01.01. *Comprehensive accreditation manual for hospitals.* Oakbrook Terrace, IL: The Joint Commission. (Level VII)

5 Centers for Disease Control and Prevention. (2002). Guideline for hand hygiene in health-care settings: Recommendations of the Healthcare Infection Control Practices Advisory Committee and the HICPAC/SHEA/APIC/IDSA Hand Hygiene Task Force. *MMWR Recommendations and Reports, 51*(RR-16), 1–45. https://www.cdc.gov/mmwr/pdf/rr/rr5116.pdf (Level II)

6 World Health Organization. (2009). WHO guidelines on hand hygiene in health care: First global patient safety challenge, clean care is safer care. https://apps.who.int/iris/bitstream/handle/10665/44102/9/89241597906_eng.pdf?sequence=1 (Level IV)

7 Centers for Medicare and Medicaid Services, Department of Health and Human Services. (2019). Condition of participation: Infection control. 42 C.F.R. § 482.42.

8 Accreditation Association for Hospitals and Health Systems. (2020). Standard 07.01.21. *Healthcare Facilities Accreditation Program: Accreditation requirements for acute care hospitals.* Chicago, IL: Accreditation Association for Hospitals and Health Systems. (Level VII)

9 DNV GL-Healthcare USA, Inc. (2020). IC.1.SR.1. *NIAHO® accreditation requirements, interpretive guidelines and surveyor guidance—revision 20.0.* Milford, OH: DNV GL-Healthcare USA, Inc. (Level VII)

10 The Joint Commission. (2021). Standard NPSG.01.01.01. *Comprehensive accreditation manual for hospitals.* Oakbrook Terrace, IL: The Joint Commission. (Level VII)

11 Centers for Medicare and Medicaid Services, Department of Health and Human Services. (2020). Condition of participation: Patient's rights. 42 C.F.R. § 482.13(c)(1).

12 Accreditation Association for Hospitals and Health Systems. (2020). Standard 15.01.16. *Healthcare Facilities Accreditation Program: Accreditation requirements for acute care hospitals.* Chicago, IL: Accreditation Association for Hospitals and Health Systems. (Level VII)

13 The Joint Commission. (2021). Standard RI.01.01.01. *Comprehensive accreditation manual for hospitals.* Oakbrook Terrace, IL: The Joint Commission. (Level VII)

14 DNV GL-Healthcare USA, Inc. (2020). PR.2.SR.5. *NIAHO® accreditation requirements, interpretive guidelines and surveyor guidance—revision 20.0.* Milford, OH: DNV GL-Healthcare USA, Inc. (Level VII)

15 The Joint Commission. (2021). Standard PC.02.01.21. *Comprehensive accreditation manual for hospitals.* Oakbrook Terrace, IL: The Joint Commission. (Level VII)

16 Siegel, J. D., et al. (2007, revised 2019). 2007 guideline for isolation precautions: Preventing transmission of infectious agents in healthcare settings. https://www.cdc.gov/infectioncontrol/pdf/guidelines/isolation-guidelines-H.pdf (Level II)

17 Waters, T. R., et al. (2009). Safe patient handling training for schools of nursing. https://www.cdc.gov/niosh/docs/2009-127/pdfs/2009-127.pdf (Level VII)

18 Accreditation Association for Hospitals and Health Systems. (2020). Standard 07.01.10. *Healthcare Facilities Accreditation Program: Accreditation requirements for acute care hospitals.* Chicago, IL: Accreditation Association for Hospitals and Health Systems. (Level VII)

19 Occupational Safety and Health Administration. (2012). Bloodborne pathogens, standard number 1910.1030. https://www.osha.gov/pls/oshaweb/owadisp.show_document?p_id=10051&p_table=STANDARDS (Level VII)

20 Kligfield, P., et al. (2007). Recommendations for the standardization and interpretation of the electrocardiogram: Part I: The electrocardiogram and its technology. *Circulation, 115*(10), 1306–1324. https://www.ahajournals.org/doi/full/10.1161/circulationaha.106.180200 (Level VII)

21 Oster, C. D. (2005). Proper skin prep helps ensure ECG trace quality. http://multimedia.3m.com/mws/media/358372O/proper-skin-prep-ecg-trace-quality-white-paper.pdf

22 American Association of Critical-Care Nurses. (2018). AACN practice alert: Managing alarms in acute care across the life span: Electrocardiography and pulse oximetry. https://www.aacn.org/clinical-resources/practice-alerts/managing-alarms-in-acute-care-across-the-life-span (Level VII)

23 American Association of Critical-Care Nurses. (2018). AACN practice alert: Accurate dysrhythmia monitoring in adults. https://www.aacn.org//clinical-resources/practice-alerts/dysrhythmia-monitoring (Level VII)

24 American Association of Critical-Care Nurses. (2018). AACN practice alert: Ensuring accurate ST-segment monitoring. https://www.aacn.org/clinical-resources/practice-alerts/st-segment-monitoring (Level VII)

25 Kadish, A. H., et al. (2001). ACC/AHA clinical competence statement on electrocardiography and ambulatory electrocardiography. *Circulation, 10*(25), 3169–3178. https://www.ahajournals.org/doi/full/10.1161/circ.104.25.3169 (Level VII)

26 Ganz, D. A., et al. (2013, reviewed 2021). *Preventing falls in hospitals: A toolkit for improving quality of care* (AHRQ Publication No. 13-0015-EF). https://www.ahrq.gov/professionals/systems/hospital/fallpxtoolkit/index.html (Level VII)

27 Rutala, W. A., et al. (2008, revised 2019). Guideline for disinfection and sterilization in healthcare facilities, 2008. https://www.cdc.gov/infection-control/pdf/guidelines/disinfection-guidelines-H.pdf (Level I)

28 Accreditation Association for Hospitals and Health Systems. (2020). Standard 07.02.03. *Healthcare Facilities Accreditation Program: Accreditation requirements for acute care hospitals.* Chicago, IL: Accreditation Association for Hospitals and Health Systems. (Level VII)

29 The Joint Commission. (2021). Standard RC.01.03.01. *Comprehensive accreditation manual for hospitals.* Oakbrook Terrace, IL: The Joint Commission. (Level VII)

30 Centers for Medicare and Medicaid Services, Department of Health and Human Services. (2020). Condition of participation: Medical record services. 42 C.F.R. § 482.24(b).

31 Accreditation Association for Hospitals and Health Systems. (2020). Standard 10.00.03. *Healthcare Facilities Accreditation Program: Accreditation requirements for acute care hospitals.* Chicago, IL: Accreditation Association for Hospitals and Health Systems. (Level VII)

32 DNV GL-Healthcare USA, Inc. (2020). MR.2.SR.1. *NIAHO® accreditation requirements, interpretive guidelines and surveyor guidance—revision 20.0.* Milford, OH: DNV GL-Healthcare USA, Inc. (Level VII)

Electrocardiogram, signal-averaged

An electrocardiogram (ECG) measures the electrical activity of the heart. A signal-averaged ECG is a more detailed type of ECG that helps identify patients at risk for re-entrant arrhythmias, such as sustained ventricular tachycardia. Because this cardiac arrhythmia can be a precursor to sudden death after a myocardial infarction (MI), the results of a signal-averaged ECG can enable appropriate preventive measures.[1,2]

Using a computer-based ECG, signal averaging detects low-amplitude signals and late electrical potentials, which reflect slow conduction or disorganized ventricular activity through abnormal or infarcted regions of the ventricles.[2] The signal-averaged ECG is developed by recording the noise-free surface ECG in three specialized leads for several hundred beats. The ECG machine gathers input from these leads and amplifies, filters, and samples the signals. The computer collects and stores data for analysis. The crucial values are those showing QRS complex duration, duration of the portion of the QRS complex with an amplitude under 40 mV, and the root mean square voltage of the last 40 msec.[3] (See *Placing electrodes for signal-averaged ECG.*)

Signal averaging enhances signals that would otherwise be missed because of increased amplitude and sensitivity to ventricular activity. For instance, on a standard 12-lead ECG, the "noise" created by muscle tissue, electronic artifacts, and electrodes masks late potentials, which have a low amplitude. This procedure identifies the risk of sustained ventricular tachycardia in patients with malignant ventricular tachycardia, a history of MI, unexplained syncope, nonischemic congestive cardiomyopathy, or nonsustained ventricular tachycardia.

Placing electrodes for signal-averaged ECG

To prepare your patient for a signal-averaged electrocardiogram (ECG), place the electrodes in the X, Y, and Z orthogonal positions, as shown below. These positions bisect one another to provide a three-dimensional, composite view of ventricular activation.

Anterior chest

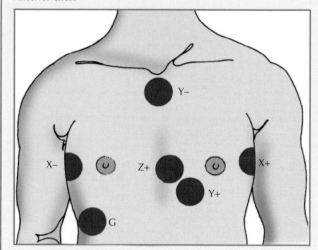

Posterior chest

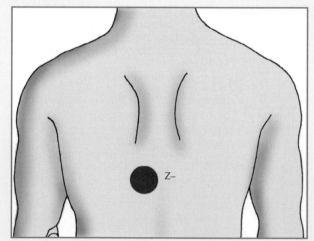

KEY

X+	Fourth intercostal space, midaxillary line, left side
X–	Fourth intercostal space, midaxillary line, right side
Y+	Standard V_3 position (or proximal left leg)
Y–	Superior aspect of manubrium
Z+	Standard V_2 position
Z–	V_2 position, posterior
G	Ground; eighth rib on right side

A signal-averaged ECG can also be used to evaluate the risk for atrial arrhythmias such as atrial fibrillation.[2,4]

Equipment

Signal-averaged ECG machine with attached patient cable, lead wires, and recording paper ■ signal-averaged computer ■ record of patient's surface ECG for 200 to 300 QRS complexes ■ soap and water ■ washcloths ■ towel ■ three bipolar disposable pre-gelled electrodes ■ 4″ × 4″ (10 cm × 10 cm) gauze pads or moist cloth ■ facility-approved disinfectant ■ bath blanket or sheet ■ Optional: disposable-head clippers or single-patient-use scissors, gloves, alcohol pads.

Preparation of equipment

Inspect all equipment and supplies. If a product is expired, is defective, or has compromised integrity, remove it from patient use, label it as expired or defective, and report the expiration or defect as directed by your facility. Place the ECG machine close to the patient's bed. Ensure that the cable and lead wires aren't broken or frayed; replace them, if necessary. Plug the machine's cord into the wall outlet, or ensure that the machine functions if it's battery operated. Turn on the machine and input the required patient information. Keep the patient away from electrical fixtures and power cords. Depending on the type of pre-gelled electrode you use, make sure that they're moist or sticky to promote impulse transmission.

Implementation

■ Verify the practitioner's order.
■ Gather and prepare the necessary equipment and supplies.
■ Perform hand hygiene.[5,6,7,8,9,10]
■ Confirm the patient's identity using at least two patient identifiers.[11]
■ Provide privacy.[12,13,14,15]
■ Explain the procedure to the patient and family (if appropriate) according to their individual communication and learning needs *to increase their understanding, allay their fears, and enhance cooperation.*[16] Inform the patient that this procedure will take 10 to 30 minutes and will help the practitioner determine the risk of a certain type of arrhythmia. If appropriate, mention that it may be done along with other tests, such as echocardiography, Holter monitoring, and a stress test.
■ Raise the patient's bed to waist level before providing patient care *to prevent caregiver back strain.*[17]
■ Perform hand hygiene.[5,6,7,8,9,10]
■ Put on gloves, as needed, *to comply with standard precautions.*[18,19,20]
■ Place the patient in the supine position, and tell the patient to remain as still as possible.[21] If a position other than supine is necessary, document the position on the ECG tracing.[22]
■ Expose the patient's chest. Drape the patient appropriately with a bath blanket or sheet. Ensure that the patient's arms and legs are relaxed *to minimize muscle trembling, which can cause electrical interference.*[23]
■ Select the electrode sites. If an area is excessively hairy, clip the hair using a disposable-head clippers or single-patient-use scissors.[1,24]
■ *To enhance electrode contact and trace quality*, prepare the electrode sites by washing them with soap and water and drying them thoroughly; *moist skin may prevent the electrodes from adhering.*[22,25] Rub the electrode sites briskly with a dry washcloth or gauze pad *to remove dead skin cells and promote impulse transmission.*[1,22,24] If necessary, clean oily skin with an alcohol pad and allow it to dry.[26,27]
■ Apply disposable pre-gelled electrodes (following the manufacturer's instructions) to the prepared electrode sites.
■ Connect the lead wires to the electrodes.
■ Place the leads in the X, Y, and Z positions.
■ Ask the patient to breathe normally and refrain from talking during the recording *so that muscle movement won't distort the tracing.*
■ Press the AUTO or START key.
■ After the ECG machine is finished recording the information, turn it off.
■ Remove and discard the electrodes in an appropriate receptacle.[20]
■ Clean the patient's skin with a gauze pad or a moist cloth.
■ Return the bed to the lowest positions *to prevent falls and maintain patient safety.*[28]

■ Remove and discard your gloves, if worn.[20]
■ Perform hand hygiene.[5,6,7,8,9,10]
■ Put on gloves, as needed.[18,20]
■ Clean, disinfect, and prepare the ECG equipment according to the manufacturer's instructions *to prevent the spread of infection.*[29,30] Prepare the ECG equipment for future use.[22]
■ Remove and discard your gloves, if worn.[20]
■ Perform hand hygiene.[5,6,7,8,9,10]
■ Place the ECG tracing in the patient's medical record for the practitioner to interpret.
■ Document the procedure.[31,32,33,34]

Special considerations

■ Results indicating low-amplitude signals include a QRS complex duration greater than 114 msec, a duration of more than 38 msec for the amplitude portion under 40 microvolts, and a root mean square voltage of less than 20 microvolts during the last 40 msec of the QRS complex.[2] However, all three factors don't need to be present to consider the result positive or negative. The final interpretation hinges on individualized patient factors.
■ Results of signal-averaged ECG help the practitioner determine whether the patient is a candidate for invasive procedures, such as electrophysiologic testing or angiography.
■ The significance of signal-averaged ECG results in patients with bundle-branch heart block is unknown, *because myocardial activation doesn't follow the usual sequence in these patients.*[2]
■ If your facility has the capability of transmitting the patient's ECG from the ECG machine to the patient's medical record, verify that the ECG transmission was successful and complete.

Complications

Prolonged application of adhesive on the electrode may cause skin irritation or tissue breakdown at the application site.[22]

Documentation

Document the date and time of the procedure, the reason for the test, and the patient's tolerance of it. Document teaching provided to the patient and family (if applicable), their understanding of that teaching, and any need for follow-up teaching.

REFERENCES

1 Kadish, A. H., et al. (2001). ACC/AHA clinical competence statement on electrocardiography and ambulatory electrocardiography: A report of the ACC/AHA/ACP-ASIM Task Force on Clinical Competence. *Circulation, 104,* 3169–3178. https://www.ahajournals.org/doi/full/10.1161/circ.104.25.3169 (Level VII)

2 Narayan, S. M., & Cain, M. E. (2019). Signal-averaged electrocardiogram: Overview of technical aspects and clinical applications. In: *UpToDate,* Goldberger, A. L. (Ed.).

3 Gatzoulis, K. A., et al. (2018). Signal-averaged electrocardiography: Past, present, and future. *Journal of Arrhythmia, 34*(3), 222–229. https://www.ncbi.nlm.nih.gov/pmc/articles/PMC6010001/

4 Tumampos, J., & Heinke, M. (2019). Spectral analysis of signal averaging electrocardiography in atrial and ventricular tachycardia arrhythmias. In Lhotska, L., et al (Eds.), *World Congress on Medical Physics and Biomedical Engineering 2018, IFMBE Proceedings, Vol 68/2,* pp. 143–147. Singapore: Springer.

5 The Joint Commission. (2021). Standard NPSG.07.01.01. *Comprehensive accreditation manual for hospitals.* Oakbrook Terrace, IL: The Joint Commission. (Level VII)

6 Centers for Disease Control and Prevention. (2002). Guidelines for hand hygiene in health-care settings: Recommendations of the Healthcare Infection Control Practices Advisory Committee and the HICPAC/SHEA/APIC/IDSA Hand Hygiene Task Force. *MMWR Recommendations and Reports, 51*(RR-16), 1–45. https://www.cdc.gov/mmwr/pdf/rr/rr5116.pdf (Level II)

7 World Health Organization. (2009). WHO guidelines on hand hygiene in health care: First global patient safety challenge, clean care is safer care. https://apps.who.int/iris/bitstream/handle/10665/44102/9789241597906_eng.pdf?sequence=1 (Level IV)

8 Centers for Medicare and Medicaid Services, Department of Health and Human Services. (2020). Condition of participation: Infection control. 42 C.F.R. § 482.42.

9 Accreditation Association for Hospitals and Health Systems. (2020). Standard 07.01.21. *Healthcare Facilities Accreditation Program: Accreditation requirements for acute care hospitals.* Chicago, IL: Accreditation Association for Hospitals and Health Systems. (Level VII)

10 DNV GL-Healthcare USA, Inc. (2020). IC.1.SR.1. *NIAHO® accreditation requirements, interpretive guidelines and surveyor guidance—revision 20.0.* Milford, OH: DNV GL-Healthcare USA, Inc. (Level VII)

11 The Joint Commission. (2021). Standard NPSG.01.01.01. *Comprehensive accreditation manual for hospitals.* Oakbrook Terrace, IL: The Joint Commission. (Level VII)

12 Accreditation Association for Hospitals and Health Systems. (2020). Standard 15.01.16. *Healthcare Facilities Accreditation Program: Accreditation requirements for acute care hospitals.* Chicago, IL: Accreditation Association for Hospitals and Health Systems. (Level VII)

13 Centers for Medicare and Medicaid Services, Department of Health and Human Services. (2020). Condition of participation: Patient's rights. 42 C.F.R. § 482.13(c)(1).

14 The Joint Commission. (2021). Standard RI.01.01.01. *Comprehensive accreditation manual for hospitals.* Oakbrook Terrace, IL: The Joint Commission. (Level VII)

15 DNV GL-Healthcare USA, Inc. (2020). PR.2.SR.5. *NIAHO® accreditation requirements, interpretive guidelines and surveyor guidance—revision 20.0.* Milford, OH: DNV GL-Healthcare USA, Inc. (Level VII)

16 The Joint Commission. (2021). Standard PC.02.01.21. *Comprehensive accreditation manual for hospitals.* Oakbrook Terrace, IL: The Joint Commission. (Level VII)

17 Waters, T. R., et al. (2009). Safe patient handling training for schools of nursing. https://www.cdc.gov/niosh/docs/2009-127/pdfs/2009-127.pdf (Level VII)

18 Siegel, J. D., et al. (2007, revised 2019). 2007 guideline for isolation precautions: Preventing transmission of infectious agents in healthcare settings. https://www.cdc.gov/infectioncontrol/pdf/guidelines/isolation-guidelines-H.pdf (Level II)

19 Accreditation Association for Hospitals and Health Systems. (2020). Standard 07.01.10. *Healthcare Facilities Accreditation Program: Accreditation requirements for acute care hospitals.* Chicago, IL: Accreditation Association for Hospitals and Health Systems. (Level VII)

20 Occupational Safety and Health Administration. (2012). Bloodborne pathogens, standard number 1910.1030. https://www.osha.gov/pls/oshaweb/owadisp.show_document?p_id=10051&p_table=STANDARDS (Level VII)

21 Feldman, T., et al. (1985). Relation of electrocardiographic R-wave amplitude to changes in left ventricular chamber size and position in normal subjects. *American Journal of Cardiology, 55,* 1168–1174. (Level VI)

22 Wiegand, D. L. (2017). *AACN procedure manual for high acuity, progressive, and critical care* (7th ed.). St. Louis, MO: Elsevier.

23 Kligfield, P., et al. (2007). Recommendations for the standardization and interpretation of the electrocardiogram: Part I: The electrocardiogram and its technology. *Circulation, 115,* 1306–1324. https://www.ahajournals.org/doi/full/10.1161/circulationaha.106.180200

24 Oster, C. D. (2005). Proper skin prep helps ensure ECG trace quality. http://multimedia.3m.com/mws/media/358372O/proper-skin-prep-ecg-trace-quality-white-paper.pdf (Level VI)

25 American Association of Critical-Care Nurses. (2018). AACN practice alert: Managing alarms in acute care across the life span: Electrocardiography and pulse oximetry. https://www.aacn.org/clinical-resources/practice-alerts/managing-alarms-in-acute-care-across-the-life-span (Level VII)

26 American Association of Critical-Care Nurses. (2018). AACN practice alert: Accurate dysrhythmia monitoring in adults. https://www.aacn.org//clinical-resources/practice-alerts/dysrhythmia-monitoring (Level VII)

27 American Association of Critical-Care Nurses. (2018). AACN practice alert: Ensuring accurate ST-segment monitoring https://www.aacn.org/clinical-resources/practice-alerts/st-segment-monitoring (Level VII)

28 Ganz, D. A., et al. (2013, reviewed 2021). *Preventing falls in hospitals: A toolkit for improving quality of care* (AHRQ Publication No. 13-0015-EF). Rockville, MD: Agency for Healthcare Research and Quality. https://www.ahrq.gov/professionals/systems/hospital/fallpxtoolkit/index.html (Level VII)

29 Rutala, W. A., et al. (2008, revised 2019). Guideline for disinfection and sterilization in healthcare facilities, 2008. https://www.cdc.gov/infection-control/pdf/guidelines/disinfection-guidelines-H.pdf (Level I)

30 Accreditation Association for Hospitals and Health Systems. (2020). Standard 07.02.03. *Healthcare Facilities Accreditation Program: Accreditation requirements for acute care hospitals.* Chicago, IL: Accreditation Association for Hospitals and Health Systems. (Level VII)

31 The Joint Commission. (2021). Standard RC.01.03.01. *Comprehensive accreditation manual for hospitals.* Oakbrook Terrace, IL: The Joint Commission. (Level VII)

32 Centers for Medicare and Medicaid Services, Department of Health and Human Services. (2020). Condition of participation: Medical record services. 42 C.F.R. § 482.24(b).

33 Accreditation Association for Hospitals and Health Systems. (2020). Standard 10.00.03. *Healthcare Facilities Accreditation Program: Accreditation requirements for acute care hospitals.* Chicago, IL: Accreditation Association for Hospitals and Health Systems. (Level VII)

34 DNV GL-Healthcare USA, Inc. (2020). MR.2.SR.1. *NIAHO® accreditation requirements, interpretive guidelines and surveyor guidance—revision 20.0.* Milford, OH: DNV GL-Healthcare USA, Inc. (Level VII)

ENDOSCOPIC THERAPY, ASSISTING

Endoscopy of the upper gastrointestinal (GI) tract, also called *esophago-gastroduodenoscopy* or *EGD*, is indicated for a range of diagnostic and therapeutic procedures.[1] This procedure focuses on endoscopic therapy to visualize the upper GI tract to help diagnose, control, or prevent bleeding and evacuate blood and clots.

During this procedure, the practitioner advances a fiberoptic endoscope through the patient's esophagus and into the stomach and duodenum to help look for a bleeding site.[2] The practitioner may also obtain tissue for biopsy. After locating the bleeding site, the practitioner may inject a sclerosing agent through an injector needle, which is inserted through a port in the endoscope. The practitioner injects the sclerosing agent into the bleeding vessel or tissue surrounding the vessel. The practitioner may also use laser or thermal therapy, or apply an esophageal band to stop bleeding.[2] A nurse assists with the procedure.

Equipment

Prescribed medications (such as anesthetic, sedative, analgesic, and sclerosing agents) ■ oral airway or bite block ■ water-soluble lubricant ■ oxygen administration equipment ■ suction apparatus ■ sterile normal saline solution or sterile water for irrigation ■ endoscope (rigid or flexible) ■ tonsil-tip suction device ■ gowns, gloves, and masks and goggles or masks with face shields ■ two 30- to 60-mL syringes ■ cardiac monitor ■ pulse oximeter and probe ■ capnography device ■ automatic blood pressure cuff ■ prescribed IV fluid ■ enzymatic detergent ■ sponge or lint-free cloth ■ facility-approved sedation scoring system ■ emergency equipment (code cart with emergency medications, defibrillator, handheld resuscitation bag with mask, intubation equipment, prescribed reversal agent) ■ labels ■ facility-approved disinfectant ■ patient goggles or waterproof covering ■ Optional: endoscopic laser or thermal equipment, endoscopic injector needle (23G to 26G, 2- to 5-mm needle), endoscopic clips, esophageal bands, specimen containers, laboratory biohazard transport bag, laboratory request form, nasogastric tube, nasogastric tube insertion supplies, IV catheter insertion equipment.

Preparation of equipment

Inspect all equipment and supplies. If a product is expired, is defective, or has compromised integrity, remove it from patient use, label it as expired or defective, and report the expiration or defect, as directed by your facility. Set up the suction apparatus and make sure that it's functioning properly.[2] Make sure that emergency equipment and oxygen administration equipment is functioning properly and readily available.[3]

Label all medications, medication containers, and other solutions on and off the sterile field. On the label, include the medication name, dosage, strength, quantity, diluent and volume (if appropriate), and expiration date and time.[4,5]

Implementation

■ Verify the practitioner's orders.
■ If your facility requires it, confirm that informed consent was obtained and that the signed consent form is in the patient's medical record.[6,7,8,9]

- Review the patient's medical record for allergies, including latex, and other contraindications to the prescribed medications. If any exist, don't administer the medications, and notify the practitioner.[10,11,12,13]
- Conduct a preprocedure verification *to make sure that all relevant documentation, related information, and equipment are available and correctly identified to the patient's identifiers.*[14,15]
- Verify that the ordered laboratory and imaging studies have been completed as ordered and that the results are in the patient's medical record. Notify the practitioner of any unexpected results. If applicable, check the patient's medical record for pregnancy test results.[16]
- Verify all medication or solution labels verbally and visually. Two individuals qualified to participate in the procedure should conduct the verification whenever the person preparing the medication or solution isn't the person who'll be administering it.[4,5]
- Review baseline coagulation studies, *because abnormal results increase the risk of bleeding.*[2] Review baseline hematocrit and hemoglobin levels.
- Perform hand hygiene.[17,18,19,20,21,22]
- Confirm the patient's identity using at least two patient identifiers.[23]
- Provide privacy.[24,25,26,27]
- Reinforce the practitioner's explanation of the procedure to the patient and family (if appropriate) according to their individual communication and learning needs *to increase their understanding, allay their fears, and enhance cooperation.*[28] Answer any questions.
- Confirm the patient's nothing-by-mouth status before the procedure. For an nonemergency procedure, minimum fasting recommendations include 2 hours for clear liquids, 6 or more hours for a light meal or non-human milk, and 8 hours or more for fried or fatty foods and meat.[2,29]
- Assess the patient for conditions that may make ventilation difficult, such as significant obesity, a history of snoring or sleep apnea, facial hair, missing teeth, or the presence of stridor.[16]
- Raise the bed to waist level before providing care *to prevent caregiver back strain.*[30]
- Perform hand hygiene.[17,18,19,20,21,22]
- Put on gloves, a gown, and a mask and goggles or a mask with a face shield, as necessary, *to comply with standard precautions.*[2,31,32,33]
- Remove the patient's dentures, if applicable, *because they can interfere with safe passage of the endoscope.* Remove and discard your gloves.[33] Perform hand hygiene and put on new gloves, as necessary.[17,18,19,20,21,22,31,33]
- Verify that the patient has an adequate-sized, patent IV catheter (an 18G catheter is preferred) *to administer sedation and any emergency medications or IV fluid, if necessary.* If an adequate catheter isn't in place, insert one. (See the "IV catheter insertion and removal" procedure.) Begin an IV infusion, as prescribed.
- Provide goggles or a waterproof covering for the patient's eyes *to protect the patient against accidental exposure to blood and sclerosing agents.*[2,31,32,33]
- Perform hand hygiene (if not wearing gloves).[17,18,19,20,21,22]
- Attach the patient to a cardiac monitor, a pulse oximeter, and an automatic blood pressure cuff *for continuous monitoring during the procedure.*[2,34] Make sure that alarm limits are set appropriately for the patient's current condition, and that the alarms are turned on, functioning properly, and audible to staff.[35,36,37,38]
- Attach the patient to a capnography (if available) *to continuously monitor exhaled carbon dioxide during the procedure.*[34] Make sure that alarm limits are set appropriately for the patient's current condition, and that the alarms are turned on, functioning properly, and audible to staff.[35,36,37,38,39]
- Obtain the patient's baseline vital signs and assess neurologic, cardiac, and respiratory status *to serve as baselines for comparison during and after the procedure.*[2,3,40]
- Determine the patient's sedation score based on vital signs, level of consciousness (LOC), and respiratory status using a facility-approved scoring system.[40,41]
- Position the patient in the left lateral position. *This position is the position of choice to prevent aspiration, enables predictable views of the stomach as the scope is advanced, and allows secretions to collect in the dependent areas of the mouth for ease of suctioning.*[2]
- Conduct a time-out immediately before starting the procedure *to perform a final assessment that the correct patient, site, positioning, and procedure are identified and, as applicable, that all relevant information and necessary equipment are available.*[15,42]

- Before endoscope insertion, administer an analgesic, a sedative, or both, as ordered, following safe medication administration practices, *to facilitate the insertion process.*[2,10,11,12,13]

NURSING ALERT Moderate sedation agents are considered high-alert medications *because they can cause significant patient harm when used in error.*[43]

- If your facility requires it, before administering moderate sedation, have another nurse perform an independent double-check *to verify the patient's identity and to make sure that you're administering the correct medication in the prescribed concentration, the medication's indication corresponds with the patient's diagnosis, the dosage calculations are correct, the dosing formula used to derive the final dose is correct, the administration route is safe and proper for the patient, and, if applicable, the pump settings are correct and the infusion line is attached to the correct port.*
- If your facility requires it, compare the results of the independent double-check. If no discrepancies exist, begin administering the medication. If discrepancies exist, rectify them before administering the medication.[44]
- Administer each medication separately in incremental doses, and titrate each it to its desired effect *to decrease the risk of overdose and respiratory and circulatory depression.*[16]
- Continuously monitor the patient's heart rate and function (using a cardiac monitor), oxygen saturation level (using pulse oximetry), and respiratory rate and adequacy of ventilation (using continual observation of clinical status and capnography, if available).[3,34,39,45]
- Obtain and evaluate the patient's blood pressure and heart rate at least every 5 minutes.[34,39,45]
- Monitor LOC by checking the patient's response to verbal commands when practical. Also monitor the patient's comfort level and skin condition at regular intervals.[16]
- If hypoxia occurs, administer supplemental oxygen, as ordered.[34] Determine the method and flow rate by the patient's optimal oxygen saturation level based on pulse oximetry.[16]
- Assist the practitioner as indicated during the procedure. If you're monitoring the patient, you can assist with minor, interruptible tasks when the patient's condition is stable. However, another trained staff member should assist with more complicated procedures.[3,46]
- The practitioner will anesthetize the posterior pharynx with a topical anesthetic agent and insert an oral airway or bite block *to prevent the patient from biting down on the endoscope.*[2]
- The practitioner will lubricate the distal end of the endoscope with a water-soluble lubricant *to facilitate passage of the endoscope.*[2] Instruct the patient to swallow while the endoscope is being advanced *to help facilitate passage into the esophagus.*[2]
- Suction the oropharynx, as needed, using a tonsil-tip suction catheter *to prevent aspiration of secretions.*[2]
- Prepare the equipment for thermal or laser coagulation therapy, as necessary, *to control bleeding.*[2]
- Assist with irrigation using sterile normal saline solution or sterile water through the endoscope *to improve visualization.*[2]
- If the site requires sclerosing, assist with the endoscopic injector needle and injecting the sclerosing agent, as requested.[2]
- Provide the practitioner with endoscopic bands or clips, as requested, if endoscopic variceal ligation (the treatment of choice for controlling variceal hemorrhage) is necessary.[47]
- If the practitioner obtains a specimen for testing, place it in the proper specimen container, label the container in the presence of the patient *to prevent mislabeling,*[23] and place the container in a laboratory transport bag.[23,33]
- The practitioner will then carefully remove the endoscope.
- Insert a nasogastric tube, if ordered, *to assess for recurrent bleeding.* (See the "Nasogastric tube insertion and removal" procedure.)[2]
- Assess the patient for gag, swallow, and cough reflexes. Maintain the patient in the left lateral position until the gag, swallow, and cough reflexes return. After these reflexes return, reposition the patient *to promote comfort.*[2]
- Return the bed to the lowest position *to prevent falls and maintain patient safety.*[48]
- Remove and discard your gloves and other personal protective equipment, if worn.[33]

- Perform hand hygiene.[17,18,19,20,21,22]
- After the procedure, continue to monitor the patient using the same monitoring parameters used during the procedure; monitor until discharge criteria are met. The patient should remain awake for at least 20 minutes without stimulation before being considered ready for discharge. The duration and frequency of monitoring should be individualized depending on the level of sedation achieved, the patient's overall condition, and the nature of the procedure. If a reversal agent was given, monitor the patient for a sufficient time (for example, 2 hours) after the last administration of an antagonist *to make sure that the patient doesn't become re-sedated after the reversal effects have worn off.*[16,34,49]
- Immediately after use, preclean the endoscope before sending it for reprocessing. Put on gloves and, as necessary, other personal protective equipment.[31,32,33] Wipe the insertion end of the endoscope with a wet sponge or lint-free cloth soaked in freshly prepared enzymatic detergent solution. Insert the distal portion of the endoscope into the solution container and use the suction device to suction the solution through the air, water, and biopsy channels. Alternate between suctioning the solution and air until the return solution is visibly clean. Flush or blow air through the channels according to the endoscope manufacturer's instructions. Detach the endoscope from the light source and suction setup. If you're using a video endoscope, attach the protective video cap to the device. Place the endoscope in a container for transport to the reprocessing area.[50,51,52,53] Remove and discard your gloves and other personal protective equipment, if worn.[33]
- Perform hand hygiene.[17,18,19,20,21,22]
- Send specimens to the laboratory in the laboratory transport bag,[33] along with a completed laboratory request form if your facility requires it.[33]
- Perform hand hygiene.[17,18,19,20,21,22]
- Put on gloves and, as necessary, other personal protective equipment *to comply with standard precautions.*[31,32]
- Clean and disinfect other reusable equipment according to the manufacturer's instructions *to prevent the spread of infection.*[50,53]
- Remove and discard your gloves and other personal protective equipment, if worn.[33]
- Perform hand hygiene.[17,18,19,20,21,22]
- Document the procedure.[54,55,56,57]

Special considerations

- Endoscope insertion and advancement may stimulate a vagal response, causing bradycardia. Closely monitor the patient.[2]
- Keep in mind that sedatives and topical anesthetics interfere with the gag reflex, placing the patient at risk for aspiration. Moderate sedation may also put the patient at risk for respiratory depression.[2]
- The Joint Commission issued a sentinel event alert concerning medical device alarm safety, *because alarm-related events have been associated with permanent loss of function or death.* Among the major contributing factors were improper alarm settings, alarm settings turned off inappropriately, and alarm signals that are inaudible to staff. Make sure that alarm limits are set appropriately, and that alarms are turned on, functioning properly, and audible to staff. Follow facility guidelines for preventing alarm fatigue.[36]
- Inspect the integrity and cleanliness of all endoscopic equipment (including accessories and valves) before, during, and after use. Remove damaged items, and reprocess soiled items.[51,52]

Complications

Complications of endoscopic therapy include respiratory depression; hypotension; bradycardia; anaphylactic reaction to medications; aspiration; bleeding; temporary dysphagia; esophageal, gastric, or duodenal perforation; and decreased LOC.[2]

Documentation

Record the patient's vital signs, oxygen saturation levels, and other assessment findings before, during, and after the procedure. Document the date and time of the procedure, analgesic or sedation you administered,

sclerosing agents you administered (if applicable), any other therapies used during the procedure, and the patient's tolerance of the procedure. If any complications occurred, record the prescribed interventions and the patient's response to them. Document teaching you provided to the patient and family (if applicable), their understanding of that teaching, and any need for follow-up teaching.

REFERENCES

1 Cohen, J., & Greenwald, D. A. (2020). Overview of upper gastrointestinal endoscopy (esophagogastroduodenoscopy). In: *UpToDate*, Howell, D. A. (Ed.).

2 Wiegand, D. L. (2017). *AACN procedure manual for high acuity, progressive, and critical care* (7th ed.). St. Louis, MO: Elsevier.

3 Society of Gastroenterology Nurses and Associates, Inc. (1991, revised 2017). *Position statement: Statement on the use of sedation and analgesia in the gastrointestinal endoscopy setting.* https://www.sgna.org/Portals/0/Practice/Sedation/Sedation_FINAL.pdf?ver=2017-10-09-110940-983 (Level VII)

4 The Joint Commission. (2021). Standard NPSG.03.04.01. *Comprehensive accreditation manual for hospitals.* Oakbrook Terrace, IL: The Joint Commission. (Level VII)

5 Accreditation Association for Hospitals and Health Systems. (2020). Standard 25.01.27. *Healthcare Facilities Accreditation Program: Accreditation requirements for acute care hospitals.* Chicago, IL: Accreditation Association for Hospitals and Health Systems. (Level VII)

6 The Joint Commission. (2021). Standard RI.01.03.01. *Comprehensive accreditation manual for hospitals.* Oakbrook Terrace, IL: The Joint Commission. (Level VII)

7 Centers for Medicare and Medicaid Services, Department of Health and Human Services. (2020). Condition of participation: Patient's rights. 42 C.F.R. § 482.13(b)(2).

8 Accreditation Association for Hospitals and Health Systems. (2020). Standard 30.01.11. *Healthcare Facilities Accreditation Program: Accreditation requirements for acute care hospitals.* Chicago, IL: Accreditation Association for Hospitals and Health Systems. (Level VII)

9 DNV GL-Healthcare USA, Inc. (2020). PR.2.SR.3. *NIAHO® accreditation requirements, interpretive guidelines and surveyor guidance—revision 20.0.* Milford, OH: DNV GL-Healthcare USA, Inc. (Level VII)

10 The Joint Commission. (2021). Standard MM.06.01.01. *Comprehensive accreditation manual for hospitals.* Oakbrook Terrace, IL: The Joint Commission. (Level VII)

11 Centers for Medicare and Medicaid Services, Department of Health and Human Services. (2020). Condition of participation: Nursing services. 42 C.F.R. § 482.23(c).

12 Accreditation Association for Hospitals and Health Systems. (2020). Standard 16.01.03. *Healthcare Facilities Accreditation Program: Accreditation requirements for acute care hospitals.* Chicago, IL: Accreditation Association for Hospitals and Health Systems. (Level VII)

13 DNV GL-Healthcare USA, Inc. (2020). MM.1.SR.3. *NIAHO® accreditation requirements, interpretive guidelines and surveyor guidance—revision 20.0.* Milford, OH: DNV GL-Healthcare USA, Inc. (Level VII)

14 The Joint Commission. (2021). Standard UP.01.01.01. *Comprehensive accreditation manual for hospitals.* Oakbrook Terrace, IL: The Joint Commission. (Level VII)

15 Accreditation Association for Hospitals and Health Systems. (2020). Standard 30.00.14. *Healthcare Facilities Accreditation Program: Accreditation requirements for acute care hospitals.* Chicago, IL: Accreditation Association for Hospitals and Health Systems. (Level VII)

16 Guideline for perioperative practice: Moderate sedation/analgesia. (2021). In Wood, A. (Ed.), *Guidelines for perioperative practice*, 2021 edition. Denver, CO: AORN, Inc. (Level VII)

17 Centers for Disease Control and Prevention. (2002). Guideline for hand hygiene in health care settings: Recommendations of the Healthcare Infection Control Practices Advisory Committee and the HICPAC/SHEA/APIC/IDSA Hand Hygiene Task Force. *MMWR Recommendations and Reports, 51*(RR-16), 1–45. https://www.cdc.gov/mmwr/pdf/rr/rr5116.pdf (Level II)

18 The Joint Commission. (2021). Standard NPSG.07.01.01. *Comprehensive accreditation manual for hospitals.* Oakbrook Terrace, IL: The Joint Commission. (Level VII)

19 World Health Organization. (2009). WHO guidelines on hand hygiene in health care: First global patient safety challenge, clean care is safer care. https://apps.who.int/iris/bitstream/handle/10665/44102/9789241597906_eng.pdf?sequence=1 (Level IV)

20 Accreditation Association for Hospitals and Health Systems. (2020). Standard 07.01.21. *Healthcare Facilities Accreditation Program: Accreditation requirements for acute care hospitals*. Chicago, IL: Accreditation Association for Hospitals and Health Systems. (Level VII)

21 Centers for Medicare and Medicaid Services, Department of Health and Human Services. (2020). Condition of participation: Infection control. 42 C.F.R. § 482.42.

22 DNV GL-Healthcare USA, Inc. (2020). IC.1.SR.1. *NIAHO® accreditation requirements, interpretive guidelines and surveyor guidance—revision 20.0*. Milford, OH: DNV GL-Healthcare USA, Inc. (Level VII)

23 The Joint Commission. (2021). Standard NPSG.01.01.01. *Comprehensive accreditation manual for hospitals*. Oakbrook Terrace, IL: The Joint Commission. (Level VII)

24 The Joint Commission. (2021). Standard RI.01.01.01. *Comprehensive accreditation manual for hospitals*. Oakbrook Terrace, IL: The Joint Commission. (Level VII)

25 Centers for Medicare and Medicaid Services, Department of Health and Human Services. (2020). Condition of participation: Patient's rights. 42 C.F.R. § 482.13(c)(1).

26 Accreditation Association for Hospitals and Health Systems. (2020). Standard 15.01.16. *Healthcare Facilities Accreditation Program: Accreditation requirements for acute care hospitals*. Chicago, IL: Accreditation Association for Hospitals and Health Systems. (Level VII)

27 DNV GL-Healthcare USA, Inc. (2020). PR.2.SR.5. *NIAHO® accreditation requirements, interpretive guidelines and surveyor guidance—revision 20.0*. Milford, OH: DNV GL-Healthcare USA, Inc. (Level VII)

28 The Joint Commission. (2021). Standard PC.02.01.21. *Comprehensive accreditation manual for hospitals*. Oakbrook Terrace, IL: The Joint Commission. (Level VII)

29 American Society of Anesthesiologists. (2017). Practice guidelines for pre-operative fasting and the use of pharmacologic agents to reduce the risk of pulmonary aspiration: Application to healthy patients undergoing elective procedures. *Anesthesiology, 126*, 376–393. https://pubs.asahq.org/anesthesiology/article/126/3/376/19733/Practice-Guidelines-for-Preoperative-Fasting-and (Level V)

30 Waters, T. R., et al. (2009). Safe patient handling training for schools of nursing. https://www.cdc.gov/niosh/docs/2009-127/pdfs/2009-127.pdf (Level VII)

31 Siegel, J. D., et al. (2007, revised 2019). 2007 guideline for isolation precautions: Preventing transmission of infectious agents in healthcare settings. https://www.cdc.gov/infectioncontrol/pdf/guidelines/isolation-guidelines-H.pdf (Level II)

32 Accreditation Association for Hospitals and Health Systems. (2020). Standard 07.01.10. *Healthcare Facilities Accreditation Program: Accreditation requirements for acute care hospitals*. Chicago, IL: Accreditation Association for Hospitals and Health Systems. (Level VII)

33 Occupational Safety and Health Administration. (2012). Bloodborne pathogens, standard number 1910.1030. https://www.osha.gov/pls/oshaweb/owadisp.show_document?p_id=10051&p_table=STANDARDS (Level VII)

34 American Society of Anesthesiologists. (2018). Practice guidelines for moderate procedural sedation and analgesia 2018. *Anesthesiology, 128*, 437–479. https://pubs.asahq.org/anesthesiology/article/128/3/437/18818/Practice-Guidelines-for-Moderate-Procedural (Level VII)

35 The Joint Commission. (2021). Standard NPSG.06.01.01. *Comprehensive accreditation manual for hospitals*. Oakbrook Terrace, IL: The Joint Commission. (Level VII)

36 The Joint Commission. (2013). Sentinel event alert 50: Medical device alarm safety in hospitals. https://www.jointcommission.org/assets/1/6/SEA_50_alarms_4_26_16.pdf (Level VII)

37 Graham, K . C., & Cvach, M. (2010). Monitor alarm fatigue: Standardizing use of physiological monitors and decreasing nuisance alarms. *American Journal of Critical Care, 19*, 28–37.

38 American Association of Critical-Care Nurses. (2018). AACN practice alert: Managing alarms in acute care across the life span: Electrocardiography and pulse oximetry. https://www.aacn.org/clinical-resources/practice-alerts/managing-alarms-in-acute-care-across-the-life-span (Level VII)

39 American Society of Anesthesiologists. (1986, last affirmed 2020). Standards for basic anesthetic monitoring. https://www.asahq.org/standards-and-guidelines/standards-for-basic-anesthetic-monitoring (Level VII)

40 The Joint Commission. (2021). Standard PC.03.01.03. *Comprehensive accreditation manual for hospitals*. Oakbrook Terrace, IL: The Joint Commission. (Level VII)

41 Centers for Medicare and Medicaid Services, Department of Health and Human Services. (2020). Condition of participation: Surgical services. 42 C.F.R. § 482.51.

42 The Joint Commission. (2021). Standard UP.01.03.01. *Comprehensive accreditation manual for hospitals*. Oakbrook Terrace, IL: The Joint Commission. (Level VII)

43 Institute for Safe Medication Practices. (2018). ISMP list of high-alert medications in acute care settings. https://www.ismp.org/sites/default/files/attachments/2018-08/highAlert2018-Acute-Final.pdf

44 Institute for Safe Medication Practice. (2019). Independent double checks: Worth the effort if used judiciously and properly. https://www.ismp.org/resources/independent-double-checks-worth-effort-if-used-judiciously-and-properly (Level VII)

45 The Joint Commission. (2021). Standard PC.03.01.05. *Comprehensive accreditation manual for hospitals*. Oakbrook Terrace, IL: The Joint Commission. (Level VII)

46 Society of Gastroenterological Nurses and Associates, Inc. (1991, revised 2017). Position statement: Manipulation of gastrointestinal endoscopes during endoscopic procedures. https://www.sgna.org/Portals/0/Manipulation%20of%20Endoscopes_FINAL.pdf?ver=2017-07-31-155327-430 (Level VII)

47 American Society for Gastrointestinal Endoscopy Standards of Practice Committee; Hwang, J. H., et al. (2014). Guideline: The role of endoscopy in the management of variceal hemorrhage. *Gastrointestinal Endoscopy, 80(2)*, 221–227. https://www.giejournal.org/article/S0016-5107(13)02139-1/fulltext (Level VII)

48 Ganz, D. A., et al. (2013, reviewed 2021). *Preventing falls in hospitals: A toolkit for improving quality of care* (AHRQ Publication No. 13-0015-EF). Rockville, MD: Agency for Healthcare Research and Quality. https://www.ahrq.gov/professionals/systems/hospital/fallpxtoolkit/index.html (Level VII)

49 The Joint Commission. (2021). Standard PC.03.01.07. *Comprehensive accreditation manual for hospitals*. Oakbrook Terrace, IL: The Joint Commission. (Level VII)

50 Rutala, W. A., et al. (2008, revised 2019). Guideline for disinfection and sterilization in healthcare facilities, 2008. https://www.cdc.gov/infection-control/pdf/guidelines/disinfection-guidelines-H.pdf (Level I)

51 Society of Gastroenterology Nurses and Associates, Inc. (2002, revised 2018). Position statement: Management of endoscopic accessories, valves, and water and irrigation bottles in the gastroenterology setting. https://www.sgna.org/Portals/0/Management%20Endoscopic%20Accessories%20Valves%20Water%20Irrigation%20bottles.pdf?ver=2018-08-20-141307-367 (Level VII)

52 American Society for Gastrointestinal Endoscopy, , Reprocessing Guideline Task Force, ; Petersen, B. T., et al. (2017). Multisociety guideline on reprocessing flexible GI endoscopes: 2016 update. *Gastrointestinal Endoscopy, 85(2)*, 282–294. https://www.giejournal.org/article/S0016-5107(16)30647-2/fulltext (Level VII)

53 Accreditation Association for Hospitals and Health Systems. (2020). Standard 07.02.03. *Healthcare Facilities Accreditation Program: Accreditation requirements for acute care hospitals*. Chicago, IL: Accreditation Association for Hospitals and Health Systems. (Level VII)

54 The Joint Commission. (2021). Standard RC.01.03.01. *Comprehensive accreditation manual for hospitals*. Oakbrook Terrace, IL: The Joint Commission. (Level VII)

55 Centers for Medicare and Medicaid Services, Department of Health and Human Services. (2020). Condition of participation: Medical record services. 42 C.F.R. § 482.24(b).

56 Accreditation Association for Hospitals and Health Systems. (2020). Standard 10.00.03. *Healthcare Facilities Accreditation Program: Accreditation requirements for acute care hospitals*. Chicago, IL: Accreditation Association for Hospitals and Health Systems. (Level VII)

57 DNV GL-Healthcare USA, Inc. (2020). MR.2.SR.1. *NIAHO® accreditation requirements, interpretive guidelines and surveyor guidance—revision 20.0*. Milford, OH: DNV GL-Healthcare USA, Inc. (Level VII)

ENDOTRACHEAL DRUG ADMINISTRATION

When IV or intraosseous (IO) access isn't readily available in an emergency, certain drugs can be administered into the respiratory system through an endotracheal (ET) tube. This route allows uninterrupted resuscitation efforts and avoids such complications as coronary artery laceration, cardiac tamponade, and pneumothorax, which can occur when emergency drugs are administered through an intrathoracic route. The five medications that can be administered in this way are lidocaine, EPINEPHrine, vasopressin, atropine, and naloxone.[1,2]

Drugs Suitable for Administration through an ET Tube

This table reviews drugs that undergo absorption by the alveoli and are suitable for administration through an endotracheal (ET) tube.[1,2]

DRUG	INDICATION	SPECIAL CONSIDERATIONS
EPINEPHrine (alpha-adrenergic stimulator)	■ Cardiac arrest ■ Beta-adrenergic blocker or calcium channel blocker overdose ■ Symptomatic bradycardia unresponsive to atropine	■ Dose of 2 to 2.5 mg via ET tube ■ Contraindicated in patients with known hypersensitivity to sympathomimetic amines or angle-closure glaucoma
Lidocaine (antiarrhythmic agent)	■ Ventricular fibrillation ■ Ventricular tachycardia	■ Contraindicated in patients with known hypersensitivity to amide anesthetics ■ Cautious use in patients with liver or kidney disease
Naloxone (opioid antagonist)	■ Opioid-induced respiratory depression ■ Known or suspected acute opioid overdose	■ Possible precipitation of acute withdrawal syndrome (body aches, fever, sweating, restlessness, tachycardia, increased blood pressure, seizures, nausea, vomiting, and diarrhea) in patients who are physically dependent on opioids ■ May cause such adverse effects as flushing, dizziness, and weakness
Atropine (anticholinergic agent)	■ Acute symptomatic bradycardia	■ Cautious use in patients with acute coronary ischemia or myocardial infarction ■ For use as a temporary measure while awaiting transcutaneous or transvenous pacing in patients with symptomatic sinus bradycardia, conduction block at the atrioventricular node, or sinus arrest ■ Implementation of pacing without delay in patients with poor perfusion ■ Usually ineffective in patients who have undergone cardiac transplantation, *because the transplanted heart lacks vagal innervation*
Vasopressin (nonadrenergic peripheral vasoconstrictor)[1,2]	■ Cardiac arrest[1,2]	■ Offers no advantage as a substitute for EPINEPHrine[3]

Drug administration via an ET tube usually produces lower or unpredictable blood levels of the drug than when the same dose is given intravenously.[2] According to the American Heart Association Guidelines for Cardiopulmonary Resuscitation (CPR) and Emergency Cardiovascular Care, studies show that these lower blood levels may be detrimental to the patient. For example, administration of EPINEPHrine via an ET tube can produce transient beta-adrenergic effects, causing vasodilation and subsequent hypotension, thus, reducing the chance of patient survival. Therefore, although administering some resuscitation drugs via ET tube is possible, IV or IO administration is preferable, because these routes provide more predictable drug delivery and pharmacologic effects.[1]

When IV or IO access can't be established, EPINEPHrine and lidocaine may be administered through an ET tube during cardiac arrest. The dose given by the ET route typically is 2 to 2½ times the recommended IV dose. The drug should be diluted in 5 to 10 mL of sterile water or normal saline solution before it is injected directly into the ET tube.[1,2] Better absorption may occur when EPINEPHrine and lidocaine are diluted in sterile water instead of normal saline solution. According to the American Heart Association Guidelines for Cardiopulmonary Resuscitation (CPR) and Emergency Cardiovascular Care, vasopressin may be administered during a cardiac arrest; however, it offers no advantage over using EPINEPHrine. In addition, EPINEPHrine and vasopressin may be given together during cardiac arrest; however, this approach offers no advantage over using EPINEPHrine alone.[1] You can also administer naloxone and atropine through an ET tube.[2] (See *Drugs suitable for administration through an ET tube.*)

A practitioner, an emergency medical technician, or a critical care nurse will usually administer endotracheal drugs. Although guidelines may vary depending on state regulations, the basic administration method is the same. Administration of ET drugs can be done using the syringe method or the adapter method. You can place a swivel adapter on the end of the ET tube and, while ventilation continues through a bag-valve device, the drug can be delivered through the closed stopcock. (See *Administering endotracheal drugs.*)

Equipment

Gloves ■ handheld resuscitation bag connected to an oxygen source ■ continuous waveform capnography device, end-tidal carbon dioxide ($ETCO_2$) detector, esophageal detection device, or tracheal ultrasound device ■ ET suctioning equipment ■ prescribed medications ■ syringe ■ needle or needleless transfer device ■ sterile water or normal saline solution ■ medication label ■ stethoscope ■ disinfectant pad ■ emergency equipment (code cart with emergency medications, defibrillator, mask for handheld resuscitation bag, intubation equipment) ■ Optional: swivel adapter, other personal protective equipment (gown, mask and goggles or mask with face shield).

Preparation of equipment

Inspect all equipment and supplies. If a product is expired, is defective, or has compromised integrity, remove it from patient use, label it as expired or defective, and report the expiration or defect as directed by your facility. Make sure emergency equipment is readily available and functioning properly.

Implementation

■ Avoid distractions and interruptions when preparing and administering the medication *to prevent medication errors.*[4,5]
■ Verify the order in the patient's medical record by checking it against the practitioner's order, if able. Use closed-loop communication in a code situation *to reduce the risk of miscommunication and errors.* In closed-loop communication, the sender of an order transmits the order verbally, the receiver of the order accepts and acknowledges the order, then the sender of the order verifies that the receiver has interpreted the order correctly.[1,2,6,7,8,9,10,11]
■ Perform hand hygiene.[12,13,14,15,16,17]
■ Gather and prepare the necessary equipment and supplies.
■ Compare the medication label to the order in the patient's medical record, if appropriate.[7,8,9,10]

Administering endotracheal drugs

In an emergency, administration of some drugs can occur through an endotracheal (ET) tube if IV or intraosseous (IO) access isn't available. You may administer the drugs using the syringe method or the adapter method. Before injecting any drug, check for proper placement of the ET tube using an end-tidal carbon dioxide detector, an esophageal detection device, or continuous waveform capnography. Auscultate breath sounds and check for equal chest expansion during manual ventilation. Make sure the patient is in the supine position with the head level with or slightly higher than the body.

Syringe method

Insert the tip of the needleless syringe into the ET tube and inject the drug deep into the tube (as shown below).

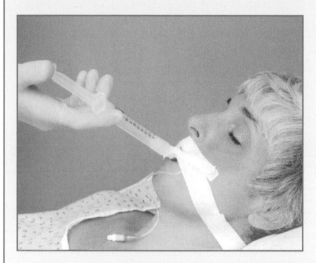

Adapter method

An adapter device for ET drug administration provides a more closed system of drug delivery than the syringe method. A special adapter placed on the end of the ET tube (as shown below) allows drug delivery through the closed stopcock.

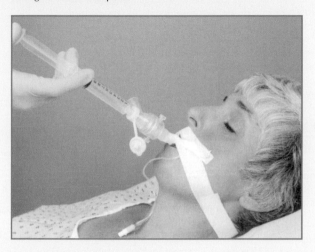

- Check the patient's medical record for an allergy or other contraindication to the prescribed medication. If an allergy or a contraindication exists, don't administer the medication, and notify the practitioner.[7,8,9,10]
- Check the expiration date on the medication. If the medication is expired, return it to the pharmacy and obtain new medication.[7,8,9,10]
- Visually inspect the medication for particles or discoloration and for other signs of loss of integrity; don't administer the medication if its integrity is compromised.[7,8,9,10]
- Discuss any unresolved concerns about the medication with the patient's practitioner.[7,8,9,10]
- If administering lidocaine, confirm the patient's weight in kilograms *to ensure accurate dosing of medication.*[18,19]
- Calculate the drug dose. Keep in mind that adult advanced cardiac life support guidelines recommend that medications given endotracheally be administered at 2 to 2½ times the recommended IV dose.[1]
- Draw up the correct amount of medication into the syringe using a needle or needleless transfer adapter. Dilute it with 5 to 10 mL of sterile water or normal saline solution. *Dilution increases drug volume and contact with the lung tissue.*
- Label the syringe with the name and the dose of the medication.[20]
- Perform hand hygiene.[12,13,14,15,16,17]
- Confirm the patient's identity using at least two patient identifiers.[21]
- Provide privacy.[22,23,24,25]
- Explain the procedure to the patient and family (if appropriate) according to their individual communication and learning needs *to increase their understanding, allay their fears, and enhance cooperation.*[26] Allow family members to remain with the patient if desired.[27,28]
- Raise the bed to waist level before providing care *to prevent caregiver back strain.*[29]
- Perform hand hygiene.[12,13,14,15,16,17]
- Put on gloves and, as needed, other personal protective equipment *to comply with standard precautions.*[30,31,32]
- Check ET tube placement by assessing chest expansion bilaterally and listening over the epigastrium (you shouldn't hear breath sounds) and by assessing the lung fields bilaterally (breath sounds should be equal and adequate). Also check placement by using a continuous waveform

capnography device, if available. If continuous waveform capnography isn't available, use an ETco₂ detector, an esophageal detector device, or a tracheal ultrasound device if an experienced ultrasound operator is available.[1]

NURSING ALERT Be aware that continuous waveform capnography combined with clinical assessment is recommended *because it's considered the most reliable method of confirming correct ET tube placement.*[1]

- Direct another health care provider to ensure that the ET tube is free from secretions. Suction, as needed. *Excessive amounts of secretions can block the airway passage and decrease the amount of medication that can be absorbed into the tracheobronchial tree.*
- If CPR is in progress, interrupt chest compressions briefly (less than 10 seconds) to administer the medication.[1,33]
- Discontinue manual ventilation with a handheld resuscitation bag momentarily.
- To administer the drug, remove the needle or needleless transfer device from the syringe, insert the tip of the syringe directly into the ET tube or swivel adapter, and inject the drug into the tube.
- After injecting the drug, reattach the resuscitation bag (if necessary) and deliver ventilations *to clear the ET tube of the drug and to disperse the drug into the airways.*
- In a code situation, communicate the type and dose of medication administered *clearly so that the recorder can document it accurately in the code and record the time, amount, and route of medication administration.*
- Discard the syringe and needle or needleless transfer device in a puncture-resistant sharps container.[32]
- Remove and discard your gloves and any other personal protective equipment worn.[32]
- Return the bed to the lowest position *to prevent falls and maintain patient safety.*[34]
- Perform hand hygiene.[12,13,14,15,16,17]
- Clean and disinfect your stethoscope with a disinfectant pad.[35,36]
- Perform hand hygiene.[12,13,14,15,16,17]
- Document the procedure.[37,38,39,40]

Special considerations

■ Don't administer nonlipid soluble medications (such as sodium bicarbonate and calcium) via the ET route *because they may injure the airway.*[1]

Complications

Potential complications of ET drug administration are related to the metabolism of the drug in the respiratory tract, which results in slow, erratic absorption and an unpredictable, reduced systemic effect.

Documentation

Document verification and methods of verification for ET tube placement. Record the date, time, and route of medication administration; the medication and dose you administered; the type and volume of diluent you used; and the patient's response to the medication.[41] Document any adverse effects, the name of the practitioner notified and the date and time of notification, any prescribed interventions, and the patient's response to those interventions. Document teaching provided to the patient and family (if applicable), their understanding of that teaching, and any need for follow-up teaching.

REFERENCES

1 American Heart Association. (2020). 2020 American Heart Association Guidelines for CPR and ECC—Part 3: Adult basic and advanced life support. https://cpr.heart.org/en/resuscitation-science/cpr-and-ecc-guidelines (Level II)

2 Pozner, C. N. (2021). Advanced cardiac life support (ACLS) in adults. In: *UpToDate*, Walls, R. M., & Page, R. L. (Eds.).

3 Panchal, A. R., et al. (2019). 2019 American Heart Association focused update on advanced cardiovascular life support: Use of advanced airways, vasopressor, and extracorporeal cardiopulmonary resuscitation during cardiac arrest: An update to the American Heart Association guidelines for cardiopulmonary resuscitation and emergency cardiovascular care. *Circulation, 140*, e881–e894. https://www.ahajournals.org/doi/10.1161/CIR.0000000000000732 (Level VII)

4 Institute for Safe Medication Practices. (2012). Side tracks on the safety express: Interruptions lead to errors and unfinished…Wait, what was I doing? *Nurse Advise-ERR, 11*(2), 1–4. https://www.ismp.org/resources/side-tracks-safety-express-interruptions-lead-errors-and-unfinished-wait-what-was-i-doing?id=37

5 Westbrook, J., et al. (2010). Association of interruptions with an increased risk and severity of medication administration errors. *Archives of Internal Medicine, 170*, 683–690. (Level IV)

6 The Joint Commission. (2021). Standard MM.04.01.01. *Comprehensive accreditation manual for hospitals.* Oakbrook Terrace, IL: The Joint Commission. (Level VII)

7 The Joint Commission. (2021). Standard MM.06.01.01. *Comprehensive accreditation manual for hospitals.* Oakbrook Terrace, IL: The Joint Commission. (Level VII)

8 Accreditation Association for Hospitals and Health Systems. (2020). Standard 16.01.03. *Healthcare Facilities Accreditation Program: Accreditation requirements for acute care hospitals.* Chicago, IL: Accreditation Association for Hospitals and Health Systems. (Level VII)

9 Centers for Medicare and Medicaid Services, Department of Health and Human Services. (2020). Condition of participation: Nursing services. 42 C.F.R. § 482.23(c).

10 DNV GL-Healthcare USA, Inc. (2020). MM.1.SR.3. *NIAHO® accreditation requirements, interpretive guidelines and surveyor guidance - revision 20.0.* Milford, OH: DNV GL-Healthcare USA, Inc. (Level VII)

11 Härgestam, M., et al. (2013). Communication interdisciplinary teams: Exploring closed-loop communication during in situ trauma team training. *BMJ Open, 3*, e003525. https://bmjopen.bmj.com/content/bmjopen/3/10/e003525.full.pdf (Level VI)

12 The Joint Commission. (2021). Standard NPSG.07.01.01. *Comprehensive accreditation manual for hospitals.* Oakbrook Terrace, IL: The Joint Commission. (Level VII)

13 World Health Organization. (2009). WHO guidelines on hand hygiene in health care: First global patient safety challenge, clean care is safer care. https://apps.who.int/iris/bitstream/handle/10665/44102/9789241597906_eng.pdf?sequence=1 (Level IV)

14 Centers for Disease Control and Prevention. (2002). Guideline for hand hygiene in health-care settings: Recommendations of the Healthcare Infection Control Practices Advisory Committee and the HICPAC/SHEA/APIC/IDSA Hand Hygiene Task Force. *MMWR Recommendations and Reports, 51*(RR-16), 1–45. https://www.cdc.gov/mmwr/pdf/rr/rr5116.pdf (Level II)

15 Accreditation Association for Hospitals and Health Systems. (2020). Standard 07.01.21. *Healthcare Facilities Accreditation Program: Accreditation requirements for acute care hospitals.* Chicago, IL: Accreditation Association for Hospitals and Health Systems. (Level VII)

16 Centers for Medicare and Medicaid Services, Department of Health and Human Services. (2020). Condition of participation: Infection control. 42 C.F.R. § 482.42.

17 DNV GL-Healthcare USA, Inc. (2020). IC.1.SR.1. *NIAHO® accreditation requirements, interpretive guidelines and surveyor guidance—revision 20.0.* Milford, OH: DNV GL-Healthcare USA, Inc. (Level VII)

18 Stone, E. (2020). Position statement: Weighing all patients in kilograms. https://www.ena.org/docs/default-source/resource-library/practice-resources/position-statements/weighingallpatientsinkilograms.pdf?sfvrsn=9c0709e_6 (Level VII)

19 Institute for Safe Medication Practices. (2020). 2020–2021 targeted medication safety best practices for hospitals. https://www.ismp.org/sites/default/files/attachments/2020-02/2020-2021%20TMSBP-%20FINAL_1.pdf

20 Accreditation Association for Hospitals and Health Systems. (2020). Standard 25.01.18. *Healthcare Facilities Accreditation Program: Accreditation requirements for acute care hospitals.* Chicago, IL: Accreditation Association for Hospitals and Health Systems. (Level VII)

21 The Joint Commission. (2021). Standard NPSG.01.01.01. *Comprehensive accreditation manual for hospitals.* Oakbrook Terrace, IL: The Joint Commission. (Level VII)

22 Accreditation Association for Hospitals and Health Systems. (2020). Standard 15.01.16. *Healthcare Facilities Accreditation Program: Accreditation requirements for acute care hospitals.* Chicago, IL: Accreditation Association for Hospitals and Health Systems. (Level VII)

23 Centers for Medicare and Medicaid Services, Department of Health and Human Services. (2020). Condition of participation: Patient's rights. 42 C.F.R. § 482.13(c)(1).

24 The Joint Commission. (2021). Standard RI.01.01.01. *Comprehensive accreditation manual for hospitals.* Oakbrook Terrace, IL: The Joint Commission. (Level VII)

25 DNV GL-Healthcare USA, Inc. (2020). PR.2.SR.5. *NIAHO® accreditation requirements, interpretive guidelines and surveyor guidance—revision 20.0.* Milford, OH: DNV GL-Healthcare USA, Inc. (Level VII)

26 The Joint Commission. (2021). Standard PC.02.01.21. *Comprehensive accreditation manual for hospitals.* Oakbrook Terrace, IL: The Joint Commission. (Level VII)

27 Emergency Nurses Association. (n.d.). Clinical practice guideline synopsis: Family presence during invasive procedures and resuscitation. https://www.ena.org/docs/default-source/resource-library/practice-resources/cpg/non-mbr-synopsis/familypresencesynopsis.pdf?sfvrsn=a95585b4_2 (Level VII)

28 American Association of Critical-Care Nurses. (2016). AACN practice alert: Family presence during resuscitation and invasive procedures. https://www.aacn.org/clinical-resources/practice-alerts/family-presence-during-resuscitation-and-invasive-procedures (Level VII)

29 Waters, T. R., et al. (2009). Safe patient handling training for schools of nursing. https://www.cdc.gov/niosh/docs/2009-127/pdfs/2009-127.pdf (Level VII)

30 Siegel, J. D., et al. (2007, revised 2019). 2007 guideline for isolation precautions: Preventing transmission of infectious agents in healthcare settings. https://www.cdc.gov/infectioncontrol/pdf/guidelines/isolation-guidelines-H.pdf (Level II)

31 Accreditation Association for Hospitals and Health Systems. (2020). Standard 07.01.10. *Healthcare Facilities Accreditation Program: Accreditation requirements for acute care hospitals.* Chicago, IL: Accreditation Association for Hospitals and Health Systems. (Level VII)

32 Occupational Safety and Health Administration. (2012). Bloodborne pathogens, standard number 1910.1030. https://www.osha.gov/pls/oshaweb/owadisp.show_document?p_id=10051&p_table=STANDARDS (Level VII)

33 Meaney, P. A., et al. (2013). Cardiopulmonary resuscitation quality: Improving cardiac resuscitation outcomes both inside and outside the hospital: A consensus statement from the American Heart Association. *Circulation, 128*(4), 417–435. https://www.ahajournals.org/doi/10.1161/CIR.0b013e31829d8654 (Level VII)

34 Ganz, D. A., et al. (2013, reviewed 2021). *Preventing falls in hospitals: A toolkit for improving quality of care* (AHRQ Publication No. 13-0015-EF). Rockville, MD: Agency for Healthcare Research and Quality. https://www.ahrq.gov/professionals/systems/hospital/fallpxtoolkit/index.html (Level VII)

35 Accreditation Association for Hospitals and Health Systems. (2020). Standard 07.02.03. *Healthcare Facilities Accreditation Program: Accreditation requirements for acute care hospitals.* Chicago, IL: Accreditation Association for Hospitals and Health Systems. (Level VII)

36 Rutala, W. A., et al. (2008, revised 2019). Guideline for disinfection and sterilization in healthcare facilities, 2008. https://www.cdc.gov/infection-control/pdf/guidelines/disinfection-guidelines-H.pdf (Level I)

37 The Joint Commission. (2021). Standard RC.01.03.01. *Comprehensive accreditation manual for hospitals.* Oakbrook Terrace, IL: The Joint Commission. (Level VII)

38 Centers for Medicare and Medicaid Services, Department of Health and Human Services. (2020). Condition of participation: Medical record services. 42 C.F.R. § 482.24(b).

39 Accreditation Association for Hospitals and Health Systems. (2020). Standard 10.00.03. *Healthcare Facilities Accreditation Program: Accreditation requirements for acute care hospitals.* Chicago, IL: Accreditation Association for Hospitals and Health Systems. (Level VII)

40 DNV GL-Healthcare USA, Inc. (2020). MR.2.SR.1. *NIAHO® accreditation requirements, interpretive guidelines and surveyor guidance—revision 20.0.* Milford, OH: DNV GL-Healthcare USA, Inc. (Level VII)

41 The Joint Commission. (2021). Standard RC.02.01.01. *Comprehensive accreditation manual for hospitals.* Oakbrook Terrace, IL: The Joint Commission. (Level VII)

ENDOTRACHEAL INTUBATION

Endotracheal (ET) intubation involves the oral or nasal insertion of a flexible tube through the larynx into the trachea for the purposes of controlling the airway and mechanically ventilating the patient. Indications include acute respiratory failure, airway protection, and inadequate oxygenation or ventilation. Additional indications include the need for general anesthesia or surgery near the airway or involving unusual positioning.[1] In most circumstances, clinicians use rapid sequence intubation to secure the patient's airway; it's the standard of care in emergency airway management when difficult intubation isn't anticipated. With rapid sequence intubation, the patient receives a rapidly acting sedative and a neuromuscular blocking agent, which cause the patient to become immediately unconscious and flaccid to facilitate emergent endotracheal intubation and minimize the risk of aspiration of stomach contents.[2,3,4,5] When not performed in an emergency, endotracheal intubation requires patient teaching and preparation.

Advantages of the procedure are that it establishes and maintains a patent airway, protects against aspiration by sealing off the trachea from the digestive tract, permits removal of tracheobronchial secretions in patients who can't cough effectively, and provides a route for mechanical ventilation. Disadvantages are that it bypasses normal respiratory defenses against infection, reduces cough effectiveness, and prevents verbal communication.[6]

Oral endotracheal intubation is preferred over nasotracheal intubation because the latter increases the risk of sinusitis, which may increase the risk of ventilator-associated pneumonia (VAP).[6] Contraindications to endotracheal intubation include trauma to the larynx and penetrating trauma of the upper airway.[1]

This procedure is performed by a practitioner or a specially trained health care professional.[7]

Equipment

Two ET tubes (one spare) of the appropriate size (normal female size is 7 to 8 mm; normal male size is 8 to 9 mm) with in-line or subglottic suctioning if available ▪ 10-mL syringe ▪ stethoscope ▪ lighted laryngoscope with a handle and blades of various sizes, curved and straight ▪ prescribed sedative ▪ local anesthetic spray ▪ overbed or other table ▪ water-soluble lubricant ▪ adhesive or other strong tape or commercial ET tube holder ▪ skin preparation product ▪ gloves ▪ mask and goggles or mask with face shield ▪ gown ▪ oral airway or bite block ▪ suction equipment ▪ cardiac monitoring equipment ▪ blood pressure monitoring equipment ▪ pulse oximeter and probe ▪ handheld resuscitation bag with sterile swivel adapter ▪ humidified oxygen source ▪ carbon dioxide detector or quantitative waveform capnography equipment ▪ oral care equipment ▪ cuff pressure manometer ▪ disinfectant pad ▪ batteries ▪ emergency equipment (code cart with emergency medications, defibrillator, handheld resuscitation bag with mask, intubation equipment) ▪ Optional: prescribed paralytic agent, prepackaged intubation tray, stylet, IV catheter insertion equipment, ventilator, disposable measuring tape, arterial blood sampling equipment.

Note: Prepackaged intubation trays that contain most of the necessary supplies may be available.

Preparation of equipment

Inspect all equipment and supplies. If a product is expired, is defective, or has compromised integrity, remove it from patient use, label it as expired or defective, and report the expiration or defect as directed by your facility. Make sure that emergency equipment is functioning properly and readily available. Check the light in the laryngoscope by snapping an appropriate-sized blade into place; if the bulb doesn't light, replace the batteries or the laryngoscope (whichever will be quicker).

Prepare the humidified oxygen source, handheld resuscitation bag with sterile swivel adapter, and suction equipment for immediate use.

Implementation

▪ Verify the practitioner's order for intubation, if not an emergency situation.
▪ Review the patient's medical record for a history of medical, surgical, and anesthetic factors that may increase the risk of difficult intubation.[8]
▪ Conduct a preprocedure verification *to make sure all relevant documentation, related information, and equipment are available and correctly identified to the patient's identifiers.*[9,10]
▪ Assess the patient's immediate history for suspected spinal cord injury or information indicating that the patient has undergone cranial surgery *to ensure that the proper intubation method is chosen.*[7]
▪ Gather and prepare the necessary equipment and supplies.
▪ Perform hand hygiene.[11,12,13,14,15,16]
▪ Confirm the patient's identity using at least two patient identifiers, if possible.[17]
▪ Provide privacy.[18,19,20,21]
▪ If the patient is in bed, remove the headboard *to provide easier access.*
▪ Raise the patient's bed to waist level before providing care *to prevent caregiver back strain.*[22]
▪ Perform hand hygiene[11,12,13,14,15,16]
▪ Put on gloves *to comply with standard precautions.*[23,24,25]
▪ Using sterile technique, open the package containing the ET tube and, if desired, open the other supplies on an overbed table.
▪ Attach the syringe to the port on the tube's exterior pilot cuff. Slowly inflate the cuff, observing for uniform inflation. Then use the syringe to deflate the cuff.
▪ If a stylet is needed to stiffen the tube, lubricate the stylet and insert it into the tube so that its distal tip lies about ½″ (1.3 cm) inside the distal end of the tube. *Lubrication eases the removal of the stylet from the tube after intubation, decreasing the risk of inadvertent extubation and trauma.*[26] Make sure that the stylet doesn't protrude from the tube *to avoid vocal cord and tracheal trauma.*[7]
▪ Lubricate the first 1″ (2.5 cm) of the distal end of the ET tube with water-soluble lubricant using sterile technique. Use only water-soluble lubricant *because it can be absorbed by the mucous membranes.*
▪ If possible, assign a staff person to provide information to the patient and family and support them throughout the procedure, according to their individual communication and learning needs;[27] offer family members the option of staying at the bedside *to allay the patient's and family's fears and to decrease anxiety.*[28]
▪ Assess the patient's oral cavity for dentures or loose teeth; remove them if possible, *because they might obstruct the airway.*[7] Inspect the patient's oral cavity, airway, head, and neck for factors that might increase the risk of difficult intubation.[8]
▪ Determine when the patient last had something to eat, *because recent food consumption increases the risk of aspiration; handheld resuscitation bag use may also increase abdominal distention, further increasing the risk of aspiration.*[7,29]

■ Assess the patient's level of consciousness, level of anxiety, and respiratory status *to determine whether the patient needs sedation, a paralytic agent, or both.*[7]

■ Attach the patient to cardiac monitoring equipment, blood pressure monitoring equipment, and a pulse oximeter *to monitor the patient's heart rhythm, blood pressure, and oxygen saturation for changes before, during, and after the procedure.*[7] Make sure alarm limits are set appropriately for the patient's current condition, and that alarms are turned on, properly functioning, and audible to staff.[30,31,32,33]

■ Insert an IV catheter if the patient doesn't already have a functioning catheter in place *to administer sedation and other emergency medications, if needed.*[7] (See the "IV catheter insertion and removal" procedure.)

■ Administer a sedative, or a sedative and paralytic agent, as ordered, following safe medication administration practices *to decrease respiratory secretions, induce amnesia or analgesia, and help calm and relax a conscious patient.*[34,35,36,37]

NURSING ALERT Sedatives and paralytic medications are considered high-alert medications *because they can cause significant harm when used in error.* If required in your facility, before administering these medications, have another nurse perform an independent double-check *to verify the patient's identity and to ensure that the correct medication is being administered in the prescribed concentration; the medication's indication corresponds with the patient's diagnosis; the dosage calculations are correct and the dosing formula used to derive the final dose is correct; the route of administration is safe and proper for the patient; and, if the medication is administered through an infusion pump, the pump settings are correct and the infusion line is attached to the correct port.*[38,39]

■ After comparing the results of the independent double-check (if required), and if no discrepancies exist, administer the medication. If discrepancies exist, rectify them before administering the medication.[38]

■ Conduct a time-out immediately before starting the procedure *to perform a final assessment that the correct patient, site, position, and procedure are identified and, as applicable, that all relevant information and necessary equipment are available.*[10,40]

■ Remove and discard your gloves.[23,25]

■ Perform hand hygiene.[11,12,13,14,15,16]

■ Put on goggles and a mask (or a mask with face shield), a gown, and gloves, *because secretions may splash during intubation.*[23,24,25]

■ Preoxygenate the patient with 100% oxygen using a handheld resuscitation bag for at least 3 minutes; continue until the tube is inserted *to prevent desaturation.*[7]

For direct visualization intubation

■ Place the patient in the supine, "sniffing" position so that the mouth, pharynx, and trachea are extended. If cervical spine injury is suspected, have an assistant maintain the patient's head in a neutral position with the spine immobilized.[7]

■ Spray a local anesthetic (such as lidocaine) deep into the posterior pharynx, if indicated, *to diminish the gag reflex and reduce patient discomfort.*

■ If necessary, suction the patient's pharynx just before tube insertion *to improve visualization of the patient's pharynx and vocal cords and to prevent aspiration of secretions.*

■ Be prepared to time each intubation attempt, limiting each attempt to less than 30 seconds *to prevent hypoxia.*[6] During cardiopulmonary resuscitation (CPR), each attempt should ideally be limited to 10 seconds.[29] Hyperoxygenate the patient between attempts, if necessary.[6,7]

■ Stand at the head of the patient's bed. Use the fingers of your right hand to open the patient's mouth *to provide access to the oral cavity.*[7]

■ Grasp the laryngoscope handle in your left hand, and gently slide the blade into the right side of the patient's mouth using the blade to push the tongue to the left *to visualize the glottis opening.*[7]

■ Advance the blade *to expose the epiglottis.* When using a straight blade, insert the tip under the epiglottis; when using a curved blade, insert the tip between the base of the tongue and the epiglottis.

■ Lift the laryngoscope handle upward and away from your body at a 45-degree angle *to reveal the vocal cords.* Avoid pivoting the laryngoscope against the patient's teeth *to avoid damaging them.*

■ Insert the ET tube into the right side of the patient's mouth.

■ Guide the tube into the vertical openings of the larynx between the vocal cords, being careful not to mistake the horizontal opening of the esophagus for the larynx. If the vocal cords are closed because of a spasm,

wait a few seconds for them to relax; then gently guide the tube past them *to avoid traumatic injury.*

■ Advance the tube until the cuff disappears beyond the vocal cords. Avoid advancing the tube farther *to avoid occluding a major bronchus and precipitating lung collapse.*[7]

■ When the ET tube is placed properly, continue to hold it securely in place at the patient's lips while withdrawing the laryngoscope blade and then the stylet, if present.[7]

For blind nasotracheal intubation

■ Position the patient with the head and neck in a neutral position.

■ Spray a local anesthetic and a mucosal vasoconstrictor into the nasal passages *to anesthetize the nasal turbinates and reduce the chance of bleeding.*[7]

■ Be prepared to time each intubation attempt, limiting each attempt to less than 30 seconds to prevent hypoxia. During CPR, each attempt should ideally be limited to 10 seconds. Hyperoxygenate the patient between attempts if necessary.[29]

■ Insert the lubricated ET tube along the floor of the nasal cavity, listening and feeling for air movement through the tube as it's advanced *to ensure that the tube is properly placed in the airway.*[6]

■ Advance the tube between the vocal cords when the patient inhales, *because the vocal cords separate on inhalation.*

■ Listen for the breath sounds to become louder when the tube is past the vocal cords. If breath sounds disappear at any time during tube advancement, withdraw the tube until they reappear.

■ When you place the ET properly, continue to hold it securely in place and withdraw the stylet, if present.[7]

After intubation

■ Inflate the tube's cuff with 5 to 10 mL of air according to the manufacturer's instructions. When the patient is mechanically ventilated, you'll use the minimal-leak technique or the minimal occlusive volume technique *to establish correct inflation of the cuff.* (For instructions, see the "Tracheal cuff-pressure measurement" procedure.) Guidelines recommend a cuff pressure between 20 and 30 cm H_2O *to ensure ventilation, prevent aspiration, and maintain tracheal perfusion.*[41,42,43,44,45]

■ Confirm ET tube placement using physical and nonphysical examination techniques. Physical examination techniques include auscultating for bilateral breath sounds, observing for bilateral chest expansion, and listening over the epigastrium (where breath sounds shouldn't be heard). The preferred nonphysical examination technique to confirm and monitor placement is continuous quantitative waveform capnography.[29]

NURSING ALERT If ET tube insertion is occurring during emergency care, avoid interrupting chest compressions when confirming tube placement.

■ If any signs of esophageal intubation are present (stomach distention, belching, or a gurgling sound), immediately deflate the cuff and remove the tube. After reoxygenating the patient *to prevent hypoxia,* repeat insertion using a sterile tube *to avoid contamination of the trachea.*

■ Auscultate bilaterally *to exclude the possibility of endobronchial intubation.* If you fail to hear breath sounds on both sides of the chest, you may have inserted the tube into one of the mainstem bronchi (usually the right one because of its wider angle at the bifurcation); such insertion occludes the other bronchus and lung and results in atelectasis on the obstructed side. It's also possible that the tube is resting on the carina, resulting in dry secretions that obstruct both bronchi. (The patient's coughing and fighting the ventilator will alert you to the problem.) To correct these situations, deflate the cuff, withdraw the tube 1 to 2 cm, auscultate for bilateral breath sounds, and then reinflate the cuff.

■ When you have confirmed correct ET tube placement, administer oxygen or initiate mechanical ventilation and suction, if indicated. During CPR, deliver ventilations using a handheld resuscitation bag at a rate of one breath every 6 seconds.[29] Insert a bite block or other oropharyngeal airway along the ET tube, if needed, *to prevent the patient from biting down on the tube.* Secure the bite block separately from the ET tube *to prevent tube dislodgement.*[7]

■ Measure the distance from the edge of the lips to the end of the tube and document the distance on the flow sheet or emergency sheet. If the tube has measurement markings on it, record the measurement where the tube exits at the lips. *By periodically monitoring this mark, you can detect tube displacement.*[11]

■ Secure the ET tube using a commercial ET tube holder or tape *to prevent inadvertent extubation.*[6] (See *Methods to secure an ET tube.*)

Methods to secure an ET tube

An endotracheal (ET) tube should be secured with tape or a tracheal tube holder as recommended by The American Heart Association. Devices and tape should be applied without compressing the neck *to prevent impaired venous return*.

To secure the tube, use one of the following methods.

Method 1
ET tube holders are available that help secure the tube in place. Made of hard plastic or of softer materials, they're available in adult and pediatric sizes, and some models come with bite blocks attached. The strap is placed around the patient's neck and secured around the tube with Velcro fasteners. *Because each model is different*, check with the manufacturer's guidelines for correct placement and care.

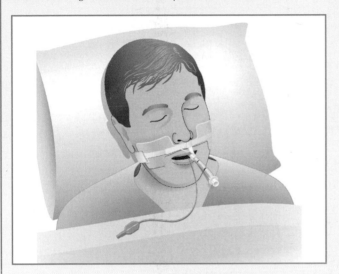

Method 2
Cut two 2" (5 cm) strips and two 15" (38.1 cm) strips of 1" (2.5 cm) cloth adhesive tape. Then cut a 13" (33 cm) slit in one end of each 15" (38.1 cm) strip (as shown below). (Some facilities require the tape to encircle the patient's head.)

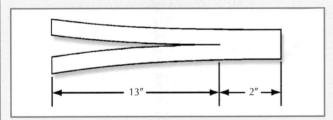

Apply compound benzoin tincture or other skin preparation product to the patient's cheeks. Place the 2" (5 cm) strips on the cheeks, creating a new surface on which to anchor the tape securing the tube. *When frequent retaping is necessary, this step helps preserve the patient's skin integrity.* If the patient's skin is excoriated or at risk, you can use a transparent semipermeable dressing to protect the skin.

Apply a skin preparation product to the part of the tube where you'll be applying the tape. On the side of the mouth where the tube will be anchored, place the unslit end of the long tape on top of the tape on the patient's cheek.

Wrap the top half of the tape around the tube twice, pulling the tape tightly around the tube. Then, directing the tape over the patient's upper lip, place the end of the tape on the patient's other cheek. Cut off any excess tape. Use the lower half of the tape to secure an oral airway, if necessary (as shown below).

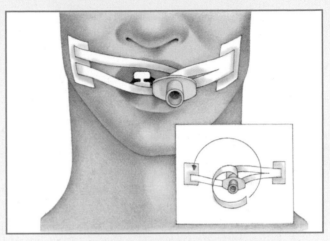

Alternatively, twist the lower half of the tape around the tube twice and attach it to the original cheek. *Taping in opposite directions places equal traction on the tube.*

If an oral airway is taped in the mouth or you're concerned about the tube's stability, apply the other 15" (38.1 cm) strip of tape in the same manner, starting on the other side of the patient's face (as shown below). If the tape around the tube is too bulky, use only the upper part of the tape and cut off the lower part. If the patient has copious oral secretions, seal the tape by cutting a 1" (2.5 cm) piece of paper tape, coating it with a skin preparation product, and placing the paper tape over the adhesive tape.

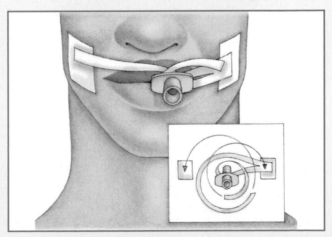

(Continued)

- Ensure that a chest X-ray is obtained *to verify tube position*.[29]
- If ordered, obtain an arterial blood sample for arterial blood gas analysis *to evaluate gas exchange*. Notify the practitioner of critical test results within your facility's established time-frame *so the patient can receive prompt treatment*.[46]
- Monitor oxygen saturation by pulse oximetry, as ordered.[7]
- Place a swivel adapter between the tube and the humidified oxygen source *to enable intermittent suctioning and to reduce tube tension*.
- Position the patient with the head elevated 30 to 45 degrees *to reduce the risk of aspiration and VAP*.[47,48]

- Provide frequent nasal and oral care *to prevent formation of pressure injuries, drying of oral mucous membranes, and VAP*. Perform oral care daily with a chlorhexidine-based mouth care solution daily, as prescribed.[47,48]
- Suction secretions through the ET tube, as the patient's condition indicates, *to clear secretions and prevent mucus plugs from obstructing the tube*.[7]
- Return the bed to the lowest position *to prevent falls and maintain patient safety*.[49]
- Remove and discard your gloves and other personal protective equipment.[23,25]

Methods to secure an ET tube *(continued)*

Method 3

Cut one piece of 1″ (2.5 cm) cloth adhesive tape long enough to wrap around the patient's head and overlap in front. Then cut an 8″ (20.3 cm) piece of tape and center it on the longer piece, sticky sides together. Next, cut a 5″ (12.7 cm) slit in each end of the longer tape (as shown below).

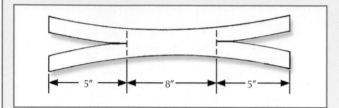

Apply a skin preparation product to the patient's cheeks, under the nose, and under the lower lip. If you're using benzoin, don't spray it directly on the patient's face, *because vapors can be irritating if inhaled and can also harm the eyes.*

Place the top half of one end of the tape under the patient's nose and wrap the lower half around the ET tube. Place the lower half of the other end of the tape along the patient's lower lip and wrap the top half around the tube (as shown below).

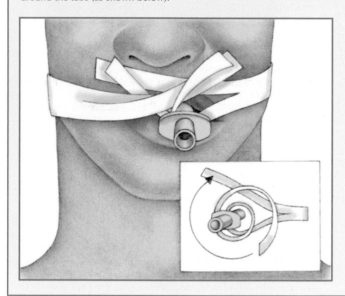

Method 4

Cut a tracheostomy tie in two pieces, one a few inches longer than the other, and cut two 6″ (15.2 cm) pieces of 1″ (2.5 cm) cloth adhesive tape. Then cut a 2″ (5 cm) slit in one end of both pieces of tape. Fold back the other end of the tape ½″ (1.3 cm) so that the sticky sides are together, and cut a small hole in it (as shown below).

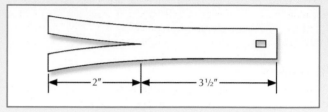

Apply a skin preparation product to the part of the ET tube that will be taped. Wrap the split ends of each piece of tape around the tube, one piece on each side. Overlap the tape *to secure it.*

Apply the free ends of the tape to both sides of the patient's face. Then insert tracheostomy ties through the holes in the tape and knot the ties (as shown below).

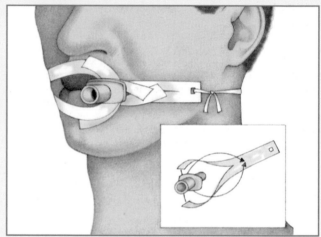

Bring the longer tie behind the patient's neck. *Knotting the ties on the side prevents the patient from lying on the knot and developing a pressure injury.*

- Perform hand hygiene.[11,12,13,14,15,16]
- Clean and disinfect your stethoscope using a disinfectant pad.[50,51]
- Perform hand hygiene.[11,12,13,14,15,16]
- Document the procedure.[52,53,54,55]

Special considerations

- The Joint Commission has issued a sentinel event alert concerning medical device alarm safety, *because alarm-related events have been associated with permanent loss of function and death.* Among the major contributing factors were improper alarm settings, inappropriately turned-off alarms, and alarm signals not audible to staff. Make sure that alarm limits are appropriately set, and that alarms are turned on, functioning properly, and audible to staff. Follow facility guidelines for preventing alarm fatigue.[33]
- Intubation performed during cardiac arrest shouldn't delay initial CPR and defibrillation for ventricular fibrillation.
- Orotracheal intubation is preferred in emergencies, *because insertion is easier and faster than it is with nasotracheal intubation, and has less risk of sinusitis and VAP.* However, maintaining exact tube placement is more difficult, and the tube must be well secured *to avoid kinking and to prevent bronchial obstruction or accidental extubation.*[6]
- The American Heart Association does not recommend the routine use of cricoid pressure in tracheal intubation.[29]
- Although low-pressure cuffs have significantly reduced the incidence of tracheal erosion and necrosis caused by cuff pressure on the tracheal wall, overinflation of a low-pressure cuff can negate the benefit. Use the minimal-leak technique *to avoid these complications.* Inflating the cuff a bit more to make a complete seal with the least amount of air is the next most desirable method. A gradual increase in cuff volume indicates tracheal dilatation or erosion. A sudden increase in volume indicates rupture of the cuff, and requires immediate reintubation if the patient is being ventilated or if the patient requires continuous cuff inflation to maintain a high concentration of delivered oxygen. A minimal pressure of 20 cm H_2O is recommended *to prevent aspiration and VAP.*[41]
- Always record the volume of air needed to inflate the cuff. Cuff pressure should be monitored at least every 8 hours *to avoid overinflation and underinflation.*[41]
- If the patient requires mechanical ventilation, interrupt the patient's sedation daily, using a multidisciplinary approach, and assess the patient's

readiness to wean. *Doing so reduces the amount of time the patient spends on a ventilator and reduces the risk of VAP.*[47,56] Make sure that the patient received deep vein thrombosis prophylaxis (unless contraindicated), as prescribed, as well as peptic ulcer disease prophylaxis. *When combined with head-of-bed elevation, oral care, daily sedation interruption, and assessment of the readiness to wean, this measure reduces the incidence of VAP.*[47,56]

■ Teach the patient and family about measures to prevent VAP, including performing hand hygiene and keeping the head of the bed elevated 30 to 45 degrees.[47]

■ Other techniques for managing a difficult airway include fiberoptic intubation, use of an intubating stylet or a tube changer, insertion of a supraglottic airway as an intubating conduit, use of laryngoscope blades of varying design and size, and use of a light wand or videolaryngoscope.[8]

Complications

ET intubation can result in apnea caused by reflex breath holding or interruption of oxygen delivery; bronchospasm; aspiration of blood, secretions, or gastric contents; tooth damage or loss; and injury to the lips, mouth, pharynx, or vocal cords. It can also result in laryngeal edema and, with long-term intubation, tracheal stenosis, erosion, and necrosis. Nasotracheal intubation can result in nasal bleeding, laceration, sinusitis, otitis media, and VAP. Incorrect placement of an ET tube can result in hypoxia, pneumothorax, vocal cord paralysis, and even death.[1,2,7]

Documentation

Record the date and time of the procedure; its indication; success or failure of the intubation, including management of a difficult airway, as indicated;[8] tube type and size; cuff size; nostril used; location in centimeters at the exit of the nostril; amount of inflation and inflation technique; administration of medication; initiation of supplemental oxygen or ventilation therapy; results of physical and nonphysical examination techniques used to confirm tube placement; complications that occurred and nursing actions taken; and the patient's tolerance of the procedure. Document teaching provided to the patient and family (if applicable), their understanding of that teaching, and any need for follow-up teaching.

REFERENCES

1 Orebaugh, S., & Snyder, J. V. (2020). Direct laryngoscopy and endotracheal intubation in adults. In: *UpToDate*, Wolfson, A. B., & Hagberg, C. A. (Eds.).

2 Brown, C. A., & Sakles, J. C. (2020). Rapid sequence intubation for adults outside the operating room. In: *UpToDate*, Walls, R. M. (Ed.).

3 Sagarin, M. J., et al. (2005). Airway management by US and Canadian emergency medicine residents: A multicenter analysis of more than 6,000 endotracheal intubation attempts. *Annals of Emergency Medicine, 46,* 328–336. (Level VI)

4 Brown, C. A., et al. (2015). Techniques, success, and adverse events in the emergency department adult intubations. *Annals of Emergency Medicine, 65,* 363–370. (Level VI)

5 Goto, T., et al. (2015). Multiple failed intubation attempts are associated with decreased success rates on the first rescue intubation in the emergency department: A retrospective analysis of multicentre observational data. *Scandinavian Journal of Trauma, Resuscitation and Emergency Medicine, 23,* 5. https://link.springer.com/article/10.1186/s13049-014-0085-8 (Level IV)

6 Kacmarek, R. M., et al. (2021). *Egan's fundamentals of respiratory care* (12th ed.). St. Louis, MO: Mosby.

7 Wiegand, D. L. (2017). *AACN procedure manual for high acuity, progressive and critical care* (7th ed.). St. Louis, MO: Elsevier.

8 American Society of Anesthesiologists. (2013). Practice guidelines for management of the difficult airway: An updated report by the American Society of Anesthesiologists Task Force on Management of the Difficult Airway. *Anesthesiology, 118,* 251–270. https://anesthesiology.pubs.asahq.org/Article.aspx?articleid=1918684 (Level VII)

9 The Joint Commission. (2021). Standard UP.01.01.01. *Comprehensive accreditation manual for hospitals.* Oakbrook Terrace, IL: The Joint Commission. (Level VII)

10 Accreditation Association for Hospitals and Health Systems. (2020). Standard 30.00.14. *Healthcare Facilities Accreditation Program: Accreditation requirements for acute care hospitals.* Chicago, IL: Accreditation Association for Hospitals and Health Systems. (Level VII)

11 The Joint Commission. (2021). Standard NPSG.07.01.01. *Comprehensive accreditation manual for hospitals.* Oakbrook Terrace, IL: The Joint Commission. (Level VII)

12 Centers for Disease Control and Prevention. (2002). Guideline for hand hygiene in health-care settings: Recommendations of the Healthcare Infection Control Practices Advisory Committee and the HICPAC/SHEA/APIC/IDSA Hand Hygiene Task Force. *MMWR Recommendations and Reports, 51*(RR-16), 1–45. https://www.cdc.gov/mmwr/pdf/rr/rr5116.pdf (Level II)

13 Centers for Medicare and Medicaid Services, Department of Health and Human Services. (2020). Condition of participation: Infection control. 42 C.F.R. § 482.42.

14 DNV GL-Healthcare USA, Inc. (2020). IC.1.SR.1. *NIAHO® accreditation requirements, interpretive guidelines and surveyor guidance—revision 20.0.* Milford, OH: DNV GL-Healthcare USA, Inc. (Level VII)

15 World Health Organization. (2009). WHO guidelines on hand hygiene in health care: First global patient safety challenge, clean care is safer care. https://apps.who.int/iris/bitstream/handle/10665/44102/9789241597906_eng.pdf?sequence=1 (Level IV)

16 Accreditation Association for Hospitals and Health Systems. (2020). Standard 07.01.21. *Healthcare Facilities Accreditation Program: Accreditation requirements for acute care hospitals.* Chicago, IL: Accreditation Association for Hospitals and Health Systems. (Level VII)

17 The Joint Commission. (2021). Standard NPSG.01.01.01. *Comprehensive accreditation manual for hospitals.* Oakbrook Terrace, IL: The Joint Commission. (Level VII)

18 The Joint Commission. (2021). Standard RI.01.01.01. *Comprehensive accreditation manual for hospitals.* Oakbrook Terrace, IL: The Joint Commission. (Level VII)

19 DNV GL-Healthcare USA, Inc. (2020). PR.2.SR.5. *NIAHO® accreditation requirements, interpretive guidelines and surveyor guidance—revision 20.0.* Milford, OH: DNV GL-Healthcare USA, Inc. (Level VII)

20 Centers for Medicare and Medicaid Services, Department of Health and Human Services. (2020). Condition of participation: Patient's rights. 42 C.F.R. § 482.13(c)(1).

21 Accreditation Association for Hospitals and Health Systems. (2020). Standard 15.01.16. *Healthcare Facilities Accreditation Program: Accreditation requirements for acute care hospitals.* Chicago, IL: Accreditation Association for Hospitals and Health Systems. (Level VII)

22 Waters, T. R., et al. (2009). Safe patient handling training for schools of nursing. https://www.cdc.gov/niosh/docs/2009-127/pdfs/2009-127.pdf (Level VII)

23 Siegel, J. D., et al. (2007, revised 2019). 2007 guideline for isolation precautions: Preventing transmission of infectious agents in healthcare settings. https://www.cdc.gov/infectioncontrol/pdf/guidelines/isolation-guidelines-H.pdf (Level II)

24 Accreditation Association for Hospitals and Health Systems. (2020). Standard 07.01.10. *Healthcare Facilities Accreditation Program: Accreditation requirements for acute care hospitals.* Chicago, IL: Accreditation Association for Hospitals and Health Systems. (Level VII)

25 Occupational Safety and Health Administration. (2012). Bloodborne pathogens, standard number 1910.1030. https://www.osha.gov/pls/oshaweb/owadisp.show_document?p_id=10051&p_table=STANDARDS (Level VII)

26 Taylor, A. M., et al. (2012). Removal of the stylet from the tracheal tube: Effect of lubrication. *Anaesthesia, 67*(8), 885–888. https://onlinelibrary.wiley.com/doi/full/10.1111/j.1365-2044.2012.07192.x (Level IV)

27 The Joint Commission. (2021). Standard PC.02.01.21. *Comprehensive accreditation manual for hospitals.* Oakbrook Terrace, IL: The Joint Commission. (Level VII)

28 American Association of Critical-Care Nurses. (2016). AACN practice alert: Family presence during resuscitation and invasive procedures. https://www.aacn.org/clinical-resources/practice-alerts/family-presence-during-resuscitation-and-invasive-procedures (Level VII)

29 American Heart Association. (2015). Web-based Integrated Guidelines for Cardiopulmonary Resuscitation and Emergency Cardiovascular Care—Part 7: Adults advanced cardiovascular life support. https://ECCguidelines.heart.org (Level II)

30 Graham, K. C., & Cvach, M. (2010). Monitor alarm fatigue: Standardizing use of physiological monitors and decreasing nuisance alarms. *American Journal of Critical Care, 19,* 28–37.

31 American Association of Critical-Care Nurses. (2018). AACN practice alert: Managing alarms in acute care across the life span: Electrocardiography and pulse oximetry. https://www.aacn.org/

clinical-resources/practice-alerts/managing-alarms-in-acute-care-across-the-life-span (Level VII)

32 The Joint Commission. (2021). Standard NPSG.06.01.01. *Comprehensive accreditation manual for hospitals.* Oakbrook Terrace, IL: The Joint Commission. (Level VII)

33 The Joint Commission. (2013). Sentinel event alert 50: Medical device alarm safety in hospitals. https://www.jointcommission.org/assets/1/6/SEA_50_alarms_4_26_16.pdf (Level VII)

34 Accreditation Association for Hospitals and Health Systems. (2020). Standard 16.01.03. *Healthcare Facilities Accreditation Program: Accreditation requirements for acute care hospitals.* Chicago, IL: Accreditation Association for Hospitals and Health Systems. (Level VII)

35 Centers for Medicare and Medicaid Services, Department of Health and Human Services. (2020). Condition of participation: Nursing services. 42 C.F.R. § 482.23(c).

36 The Joint Commission. (2021). Standard MM.06.01.01. *Comprehensive accreditation manual for hospitals.* Oakbrook Terrace, IL: The Joint Commission. (Level VII)

37 DNV GL-Healthcare USA, Inc. (2020). MM.1.SR.3. *NIAHO® accreditation requirements, interpretive guidelines and surveyor guidance—revision 20.0.* Milford, OH: DNV GL-Healthcare USA, Inc. (Level VII)

38 Institute for Safe Medication Practices. (2013). Independent double checks: Undervalued and misused: Selective use of this strategy can play an important role in medication safety. https://www.ismp.org/resources/independent-double-checks-undervalued-and-misused-selective-use-strategy-can-play (Level VII)

39 Institute for Safe Medication Practices. (2018). ISMP list of high-alert medications in acute care settings. https://www.ismp.org/sites/default/files/attachments/2018-08/highAlert2018-Acute-Final.pdf (Level VII)

40 The Joint Commission. (2021). Standard UP.01.03.01. *Comprehensive accreditation manual for hospitals.* Oakbrook Terrace, IL: The Joint Commission. (Level VII)

41 Sole, M. L., et al. (2011). Evaluation of an intervention to maintain endotracheal tube cuff pressure within therapeutic range. *American Journal of Critical Care, 20*(2), 109–117. https://www.ncbi.nlm.nih.gov/pmc/articles/PMC3506174/ (Level II)

42 Asai, S., et al. (2014). Decrease in cuff pressure during the measurement procedure: A experimental study. *Journal of Intensive Care, 2,* 34. https://jintensivecare.biomedcentral.com/articles/10.1186/2052-0492-2-34 (Level VI)

43 Sengupta, P., et al. (2004). Endotracheal tube cuff pressure in three hospitals, and the volume required to produce an appropriate cuff pressure. *BMC Anesthesiology, 4,* 8. https://bmcanesthesiol.biomedcentral.com/articles/10.1186/1471-2253-4-8 (Level VI)

44 Howard, W. R. (2011). Bench study of a new device to display and maintain stable artificial airway cuff pressure. *Respiratory Care, 56*(10), 1506–1513. http://rc.rcjournal.com/content/56/10/1506 (Level VI)

45 Nseir, S., et al. (2009). Variations in endotracheal cuff pressure in intubated critically ill patients: Prevalence and risk factors. *European Journal of Anaesthesiology, 26,* 229–1513. (Level IV)

46 The Joint Commission. (2021). Standard NPSG.02.03.01. *Comprehensive accreditation manual for hospitals.* Oakbrook Terrace, IL: The Joint Commission. (Level VII)

47 Klompas, M., et al. (2014). Strategies to prevent ventilator-associated pneumonia in acute care hospitals: 2014 update. *Infection Control and Hospital Epidemiology, 35*(8), 915–936. https://www.jstor.org/stable/10.1086/677144#metadata_info_tab_contents (Level I)

48 American Association of Critical-Care Nurses. (2017). AACN practice alert: Oral care for acutely and critically ill patients. https://www.aacn.org/clinical-resources/practice-alerts/oral-care-for-acutely-and-critically-ill-patients (Level VII)

49 Ganz, D. A., et al. (2013, reviewed 2021). *Preventing falls in hospitals: A toolkit for improving quality of care* (AHRQ Publication No. 13-0015-EF). Rockville, MD: Agency for Healthcare Research and Quality. https://www.ahrq.gov/professionals/systems/hospital/fallpxtoolkit/index.html (Level VII)

50 Rutala, W. A., et al. (2008, revised 2019). Guideline for disinfection and sterilization in healthcare facilities, 2008. https://www.cdc.gov/infection-control/pdf/guidelines/disinfection-guidelines-H.pdf (Level I)

51 Accreditation Association for Hospitals and Health Systems. (2020). Standard 07.02.03. *Healthcare Facilities Accreditation Program: Accreditation requirements for acute care hospitals.* Chicago, IL: Accreditation Association for Hospitals and Health Systems. (Level VII)

52 The Joint Commission. (2021). Standard RC.01.03.01. *Comprehensive accreditation manual for hospitals.* Oakbrook Terrace, IL: The Joint Commission. (Level VII)

53 Accreditation Association for Hospitals and Health Systems. (2020). Standard 10.00.03. *Healthcare Facilities Accreditation Program: Accreditation requirements for acute care hospitals.* Chicago, IL: Accreditation Association for Hospitals and Health Systems. (Level VII)

54 Centers for Medicare and Medicaid Services, Department of Health and Human Services. (2020). Condition of participation: Medical record services. 42 C.F.R. § 482.24(b).

55 DNV GL-Healthcare USA, Inc. (2020). MR.2.SR.1. *NIAHO® accreditation requirements, interpretive guidelines and surveyor guidance—revision 20.0.* Milford, OH: DNV GL-Healthcare USA, Inc. (Level VII)

56 Accreditation Association for Hospitals and Health Systems. (2020). Standard 07.01.02. *Healthcare Facilities Accreditation Program: Accreditation requirements for acute care hospitals.* Chicago, IL: Accreditation Association for Hospitals and Health Systems. (Level VII)

ENDOTRACHEAL TUBE CARE

An intubated patient requires meticulous care to ensure airway patency and prevent complications until the patient can maintain spontaneous ventilation. Care sometimes includes repositioning the endotracheal (ET) tube if it becomes partially dislodged or a chest X-ray shows improper placement. The tip of the ET tube should lie in the trachea about 1.2" to 2" (3 to 5 cm) above the carina.

Repositioning is indicated when the ET tube is displaced. Displacement can result from coughing, suctioning, patient movement, or patient transport by facility staff. The patient requires regular clinical assessment of the ET tube position daily and as needed with any procedure that places the patient at risk for displacement.[1] Also, the ET tube should be repositioned by moving it from one side of the patient's mouth to the other to avoid a pressure injury of the lip, face, or cheek.[1,2,3] Some commercial securement devices have a mechanism to facilitate side-to-side movement without altering the tube depth.[1]

ET tube repositioning is performed by deflating the cuff, moving the ET tube, reinflating the cuff, resecuring the tube, and confirming proper tube placement with a chest X-ray.[1] Performing this procedure with two caregivers can help prevent accidental extubation.[2,3]

ET tube repositioning has no contraindications; however, it requires the use of precautions to prevent unplanned extubation and aspiration. For example, before deflating the cuff, the patient should be suctioned to prevent aspiration.[4] A patient may have a difficult airway. Your facility may have special requirements related to performing this procedure on a patient with a difficult airway, including the use of specialized equipment and anesthesia staff.[5] Some facilities require a practitioner or a respiratory therapist to reposition the ET tube.

An ET tube should be removed as soon as it's no longer needed to reduce the risk of ventilator-associated events, such as ventilator-associated pneumonia (VAP), sepsis, acute respiratory distress syndrome, pulmonary embolism, barotrauma, and pulmonary edema.[6,7] Removal should occur when the patient is hemodynamically stable, can cough and clear secretions, can complete spontaneous breathing trials successfully, can maintain adequate oxygenation, and when the condition that required mechanical ventilation is reversed or improved to the point that mechanical ventilation is no longer needed.[2,8]

No absolute contraindications to ET tube removal exist; however, some patients may require additional support after the procedure to maintain adequate gas exchange, including noninvasive ventilation, continuous positive airway pressure, the use of a high inspired oxygen fraction, or reintubation.[8] (See the "Continuous positive airway pressure use" procedure; the "Oxygen administration" procedure; and the "Endotracheal intubation" procedure.) Your facility may have special requirements related to performing this procedure on a patient with a difficult airway, including the use of specialized equipment and anesthesia staff.[5]

ET tube removal should occur where the patient can be monitored safely, and where emergency equipment and appropriately trained staff are immediately available to manage the patient's airway in case complications occur.[8] Consult the practitioner to identify what type of supplemental oxygen therapy is planned after ET tube removal. Have the supplies needed for oxygen therapy and reintubation readily available.

Equipment

10-mL syringe ▪ suction equipment ▪ gloves ▪ handheld resuscitation bag with mask ▪ oxygen equipment ▪ disinfectant pad ▪ facility-approved disinfectant ▪ pulse oximeter and probe ▪ Optional: gown, mask, goggles, mask with face shield.

For repositioning an ET tube

Stethoscope ▪ skin adhesive preparation product ▪ adhesive or hypoallergenic tape or commercial tube holder ▪ gloves ▪ handheld resuscitation bag with mask ▪ oxygen equipment ▪ ET tube cuff pressure manometer ▪ continuous waveform capnography equipment or end-tidal carbon dioxide monitoring equipment ▪ oral care supplies.

For removing an ET tube

Suction equipment ▪ supplemental oxygen equipment with humidifier[2] ▪ emergency equipment (code cart with emergency medications, defibrillator, handheld resuscitation bag with mask, intubation equipment) ▪ vital signs monitoring equipment ▪ Optional: arterial blood gas (ABG) sample supplies, racemic EPINEPHrine or other prescribed aerosols and nebulizer or other appropriate administration equipment.

Preparation of equipment

Inspect all equipment and supplies. If a product is expired, is defective, or has compromised integrity, remove it from patient use, label it as expired or defective, and report the expiration or defect as directed by your facility.

Set up the suction and oxygen delivery equipment and make sure it's functioning properly. Have a handheld resuscitation bag with a mask available in case the ET tube becomes dislodged from the patient's airway.

For removal, set up the suction and supplemental oxygen equipment and make sure that they're functioning properly. Make sure that emergency equipment is functioning properly and readily available.

Have a racemic EPINEPHrine nebulizer and aerosol equipment available, if ordered, *in case laryngeal edema and stridor occur.*[3] The handheld resuscitation bag should be attached to the oxygen source and readily available.

Implementation

▪ Verify the practitioner's order, if required, and confirm the desired position of the ET tube in centimeters at the teeth or gumline.[3]
▪ Review the patient's medical record for the reason for intubation or extubation, the patient's current condition, a history of a difficult airway, any skin breakdown or irritation, and any allergies to adhesive products or tape (if planning to secure the tube with tape).
▪ Gather and prepare the necessary equipment and supplies.
▪ Perform hand hygiene.[9,10,11,12,13,14]
▪ Confirm the patient's identify using at least two patient identifiers.[15]
▪ Provide privacy.[16,17,18,19]
▪ Explain the procedure to the patient and family (if appropriate) according to their individual communication and learning needs *to increase their understanding, allay their fears, and enhance cooperation.*[20]
▪ Raise the bed to waist level when providing care *to prevent caregiver back strain.*[21]
▪ Perform hand hygiene.[9,10,11,12,13,14]
▪ Put on gloves and other personal protective equipment as needed *to comply with standard precautions.*[22,23]

Repositioning an ET tube

▪ Obtain assistance from a respiratory therapist or another nurse *to prevent accidental extubation during the procedure if the patient coughs or becomes agitated.*[2]
▪ Elevate the head of the bed 30 to 45 degrees (unless contraindicated), if it's not already elevated, *to reduce the risk of aspiration and subsequent ventilator-associated pneumonia (VAP).*[24]
▪ Assess the patient's respiratory status, including oxygen saturation level and end-tidal carbon dioxide level (if used in your facility), *to serve as a baseline for comparison.*[25]

▪ Hyperoxygenate the patient for 30 to 60 seconds *to prevent suction-related hypoxemia.*[25]
▪ Suction the patient's trachea through the ET tube *to remove any secretions, which can cause the patient to cough during the procedure. Coughing increases the risk of trauma and tube dislodgment.* Then suction the patient's oropharynx *to remove any secretions that may have accumulated above the ET tube cuff, which helps to prevent aspiration of secretions during cuff deflation.*[2,8,4,24,26] *Aspiration increases the risk of VAP.*[27]
▪ Hyperoxygenate the patient for at least 1 minute after suctioning *to allow the oxygen saturation level to recover.*[25]
▪ *To prevent traumatic manipulation of the ET tube,* instruct the assisting nurse or respiratory therapist to hold the tube as you carefully untape the tube or unfasten the commercial tube holder (as shown below). When freeing the tube, locate the centimeter marking on the tube at the teeth or gumline *so that you have a reference point when moving the tube.*[2]

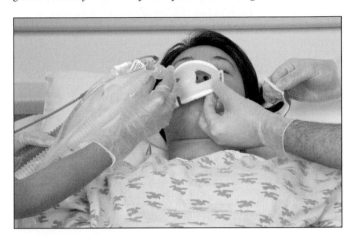

▪ Deflate the cuff by attaching a 10-mL syringe to the tube's pilot balloon port (as shown below) and aspirate air until you meet resistance and the pilot balloon deflates. *The cuff forms a seal within the trachea, and movement of an inflated cuff can damage the tracheal wall and vocal cords.*

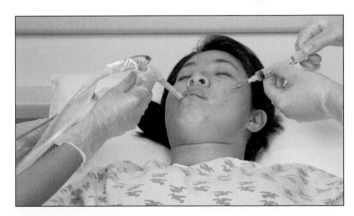

▪ Reposition the tube, as necessary, noting the centimeter marking at the teeth or gumline.[2] If performing care, shift the ET tube to the opposite side of the mouth *to prevent pressure injury.*[1]
▪ Reinflate the cuff immediately. To do this, inflate the cuff slowly using the 10-mL syringe attached to the tube's pilot balloon port. As you do this, use your stethoscope to auscultate the patient's neck *to detect an air leak.* When air leakage ceases, stop cuff inflation and, while still auscultating the patient's neck, aspirate a small amount of air until you detect a slight leak (as shown). *This maneuver creates a minimal air leak, which indicates that the cuff is inflated at the lowest pressure possible to create an adequate seal.* If the patient is mechanically ventilated, aspirate to create a minimal air leak during the inspiratory phase of respiration, *because the positive pressure of the ventilator during inspiration will create a larger leak around the cuff.*[8] Note the number of cubic centimeters of air required to achieve a minimal air leak.

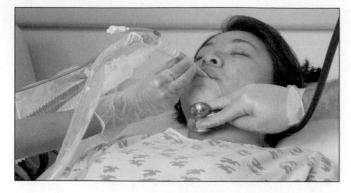

■ Attach a cuff manometer to the pilot balloon to measure the ET cuff pressure and compare the reading with previous pressure readings *to prevent over-inflation.* Cuff pressure should be maintained between 20 and 30 cm H₂O *to ensure ventilation, prevent aspiration, and maintain tracheal perfusion.*[26,28,29,30,31]

■ Confirm proper ET tube position by auscultating for bilateral breath sounds, looking for symmetrical chest wall movement, and using continuous waveform capnography. If continuous waveform capnography equipment isn't available, use clinical assessment and end-tidal carbon dioxide monitoring equipment.[32,33]

NURSING ALERT After ET tube repositioning, decreased breath sounds on the left side typically indicate that the tube has advanced into the right mainstream bronchus.[2]

■ Assess the lips, gums, and oral cavity for evidence of pressure injury or other abnormalities. Perform oral care *to prevent bacterial colonization of the oral cavity.*[2]

■ Secure the ET tube in place by applying a skin adhesive preparation product and adhesive or hypoallergenic tape, or by refastening the commercial tube holder *to prevent inadvertent dislodgement.*[2] Make sure that the tape or commercial tube holder does not compress the patient's neck, *which could impair venous return to the brain.*[2]

Removing an ET tube

■ Verify the practitioner's order or follow your facility's protocol for weaning and extubation.

■ Ensure that the patient is attached to a cardiac monitor and pulse oximeter *for continuous monitoring throughout the procedure.*[1,8] Confirm that alarm limits are set appropriately for the patient's current condition, and that alarms are turned on, functioning properly, and audible to staff.[34,35,36]

■ Obtain baseline vital signs and assess the patient's neurologic status and respiratory status, including oxygen saturation level by pulse oximeter, *to confirm that intubation is no longer necessary.*[2]

■ When you're authorized to remove the ET tube, obtain assistance from a respiratory therapist or another nurse *to prevent traumatic manipulation of the tube when it's untaped or unfastened.*

■ Position the patient in the semi-Fowler position (if it isn't contraindicated and doesn't restrict breathing) (as shown below), *because respiratory muscles are more effective in an upright position than in a supine or prone position. This position also facilitates coughing and prevents aspiration.*[2]

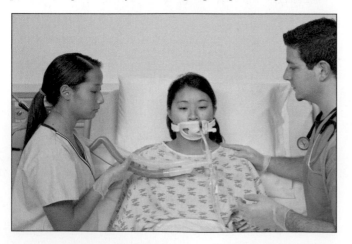

■ Hyperoxygenate the patient for 30 to 60 seconds *to prevent suctioning-related hypoxemia.*[2,25]

■ Suction the ET tube and the patient's oropharynx *to remove any accumulated secretions and to help prevent aspiration of secretions when the cuff is deflated, and subsequent VAP.*[2,6,8,24]

■ Hyperoxygenate the patient for at least 1 minute after suctioning and before ET removal *to allow the oxygen saturation levels to recover after suctioning.*[2,25]

■ Untape the ET tube or unfasten the commercial tube holder while the assistant stabilizes the tube.

■ Attach a 10-mL syringe to the pilot balloon port and aspirate air until you meet resistance and the pilot balloon deflates. If you fail to detect an air leak around the deflated cuff, notify the practitioner immediately and don't proceed with extubation. *Absence of an air leak may indicate marked tracheal edema, which can result in total airway obstruction if the ET tube is removed.*[1,8]

■ Instruct the patient to be calm and give the patient a large breath with the handheld resuscitation bag. At the peak of inspiration, *when vocal cords are maximally abducted,* remove the ET tube following the natural curve of the patient's mouth. Alternatively, remove the tube as the patient coughs.[1,2,3]

■ Administer supplemental humidified oxygen, as ordered, *to promote oxygenation and help decrease airway irritation, patient discomfort, and laryngeal edema.*[2]

■ Suction the oropharynx, if needed, and encourage the patient to cough and deep-breathe.[2] Remind the patient that a sore throat and hoarseness are to be expected, and will gradually subside.

■ Closely monitor the patient's vital signs, oxygen saturation level, neurologic status, and respiratory status, including airway patency,[2,8] *to evaluate the patient's tolerance of extubation and to watch for signs of respiratory distress.* Be alert for stridor or other evidence of upper airway obstruction. Obtain an arterial sample for blood gas analysis, if ordered.[8]

■ Administer any prescribed aerosol medications, as needed.[3]

■ Assess the patient's ability to swallow by performing a swallowing study, as indicated, *to reduce the risk of aspiration.*[2]

Completing the procedure

■ Return the bed to the lowest position *to prevent falls and maintain patient safety.*[37]

■ Discard used supplies in the appropriate receptacles.[38]

■ Remove and discard your gloves and any other personal protective equipment worn.[22]

■ Perform hand hygiene.[9,10,11,12,13,14]

■ Clean and disinfect your stethoscope with a disinfectant pad.[39,40]

■ Perform hand hygiene.[9,10,11,12,13,14]

■ Put on gloves, as needed.[22,23]

■ Clean and disinfect other reusable equipment according to the manufacturer's instructions *to prevent the spread of infection.*[39,40]

■ Remove and discard your gloves, if worn.[22]

■ Perform hand hygiene.[9,10,11,12,13,14]

■ Document the procedure.[41,42,43,44]

Special considerations

■ When repositioning an ET tube, be especially careful in patients with highly sensitive airways. Sedation may be indicated in such patients.

■ If you inadvertently cut the pilot balloon on the ET tube cuff, immediately call the person in your facility who's responsible for intubation *so that the damaged tube can be replaced with one that's intact.* Don't remove the tube, *because a tube with an air leak is better than no airway.* Provide manual ventilation, if needed, using a handheld resuscitation bag until a new ET tube is in place.

■ After repositioning an ET tube to correct dislodgement or adjust its placement, check with the practitioner to see whether a chest X-ray needs to be obtained to confirm the ET tube's new position.

■ Never remove an ET tube from a patient without the ready availability of someone skilled and authorized in insertion of advanced airway devices.[8]

■ If the patient has an oral or nasogastric tube in place, check with the practitioner to determine whether this tube should be removed when the ET tube is removed or should remain in place.[1]

Complications

Traumatic injury to the larynx or trachea may result from tube manipulation, accidental extubation, or tube slippage into the right bronchus. Tube displacement can result in respiratory distress, hypoxemia, agitation, or pneumothorax.[1,3] The patient may also aspirate secretions when the cuff is deflated, which can cause bronchospasm or VAP.[4]

Many patients experience sore throat, cough, and hoarseness after ET tube removal.[3] Patients have an increased risk of aspiration and often have difficulty clearing secretions. Edema of the glottis can cause mild to severe stridor.[8]

Documentation

After ET tube repositioning, record the date and time of the procedure, the reason for repositioning (such as malpositioning shown by chest X-ray), the centimeter marking at the teeth or gumline, cuff pressure and the total amount of air in the cuff after the procedure, and whether a chest X-ray was obtained. Document complications, including the date and time the practitioner was notified, prescribed interventions, and the patient's response to those interventions. Record oral care provided and any pressure injury identified.

Record the date and time of ET tube removal and the patient's vital signs, oxygen saturation level, and assessment findings, including the presence or absence of stridor and other signs of upper airway edema. Document the type and amount of supplemental oxygen administered, any complications that occurred, the date and time the practitioner was notified, prescribed interventions, and the patient's response to those interventions. Document teaching provided to the patient and family (if applicable), their understanding of that teaching, and any need for follow-up teaching.

REFERENCES

1 Hyzy, R. C. (2021). Complications of the endotracheal tube following initial placement: Prevention and management in adult intensive care unit patients. In: *UpToDate*, Manaker, S.(Ed.).

2 Wiegand, D. L. (2017). *AACN procedure manual for high acuity, progressive, and critical care* (7th ed.). St. Louis, MO: Elsevier.

3 Kacmarek, R. M., et al. (2021). *Egan's fundamentals of respiratory care* (12th ed.). St. Louis, MO: Mosby.

4 Centers for Disease Control and Prevention. (2004). Guidelines for preventing health-care-associated pneumonia, 2003: Recommendations of CDC and the Healthcare Infection Control Practices Advisory Committee. *MMWR Recommendations and Reports, 53*(RR-3), https://www.cdc.gov/mmwr/pdf/rr/rr5303.pdf (Level II)

5 Apfelbaum, J. L., et al. (2013). Practice guidelines for management of the difficult airway: An updated report by the American Society of Anesthesiologists Task Force on Management of the Difficult Airway. *Anesthesiology, 118*, 251–270. https://anesthesiology.pubs.asahq.org/article.aspx?articleid=1918684 (Level VII)

6 Magill, S. S., et al. (2013). Developing a new, national approach to surveillance for ventilator-associated events. *American Journal of Critical Care, 22*, 469–473. (Level VII)

7 Centers for Disease Control and Prevention. (2020). "Ventilator-associated event (VAE)" https://www.cdc.gov/nhsn/PDFs/pscManual/10-VAE_FINAL.pdf

8 American Association for Respiratory Care (AARC). (2007). AARC clinical practice guideline: Removal of the endotracheal tube—2007 revision and update. *Respiratory Care, 52*, 81–93. http://www.rcjournal.com/cpgs/pdf/removal_of_endotracheal_tube.pdf (Level I)

9 The Joint Commission. (2021). Standard NPSG.07.01.01. *Comprehensive accreditation manual for hospitals.* Oakbrook, IL: The Joint Commission. (Level VII)

10 Centers for Disease Control and Prevention. (2002). Guideline for hand hygiene in health-care settings: Recommendations of the Healthcare Infection Control Practices Advisory Committee and the HICPAC/SHEA/APIC/IDSA Hygiene Task Force. *MMWR Recommendations and Reports, 51*(RR-16), 1–45. https://www.cdc.gov/mmwr/pdf/rr/rr5116.pdf (Level II)

11 World Health Organization. (2009). WHO guidelines on hand hygiene in health care: First global patient safety challenge, clean care is safer care. https://apps.who.int/iris/bitstream/handle/10665/44102/9789241597906_eng.pdf?sequence=1 (Level IV)

12 Accreditation Association for Hospitals and Health Systems. (2020). Standard 07.01.21. *Healthcare Facilities Accreditation Program: Accreditation requirements for acute care hospitals.* Chicago, IL: Accreditation Association for Hospitals and Health Systems. (Level VII)

13 Centers for Medicare and Medicaid Services, Department of Health and Human Services. (2020). Condition of participation: Infection control. 42 C.F.R. § 482.42.

14 DNV GL-Healthcare USA, Inc. (2020). IC.1.SR.1. *NIAHO® accreditation requirements, interpretive guidelines and surveyor guidance—revision 20.0.* Milford, OH: DNV GL-Healthcare USA, Inc. (Level VII)

15 The Joint Commission. (2021). Standard NPSG.01.01.01. *Comprehensive accreditation manual for hospitals.* Oakbrook Terrace, IL: The Joint Commission. (Level VII)

16 Accreditation Association for Hospitals and Health Systems. (2020). Standard 15.01.16. *Healthcare Facilities Accreditation Program: Accreditation requirements for acute care hospitals.* Chicago, IL: Accreditation Association for Hospitals and Health Systems. (Level VII)

17 Centers for Medicare and Medicaid Services, Department of Health and Human Services. (2020). Condition of participation: Patient's rights. 42 C.F.R. § 482.13(c)(1).

18 The Joint Commission. (2021). Standard RI.01.01.01. *Comprehensive accreditation manual for hospitals.* Oakbrook, IL: The Joint Commission. (Level VII)

19 DNV GL-Healthcare USA, Inc. (2020). PR.2.SR.5. *NIAHO® accreditation requirements, interpretive guidelines and surveyor guidance—revision 20.0.* Milford, OH: DNV GL-Healthcare USA, Inc. (Level VII)

20 The Joint Commission. (2021). Standard PC.02.01.21. *Comprehensive accreditation manual for hospitals.* Oakbrook Terrace, IL: The Joint Commission. (Level VII)

21 Waters, T. R., et al. (2009). Safe patient handling training for schools of nursing. https://www.cdc.gov/niosh/docs/2009-127/pdfs/2009-127.pdf (Level VII)

22 Siegel, J. D., et al. (2007, revised 2019). 2007 guideline for isolation precautions: Preventing transmission of infectious agents in healthcare settings. https://www.cdc.gov/infectioncontrol/pdf/guidelines/isolation-guidelines-H.pdf (Level II)

23 Accreditation Association for Hospitals and Health Systems. (2020). Standard 07.01.10. *Healthcare Facilities Accreditation Program: Accreditation requirements for acute care hospitals.* Chicago, IL: Accreditation Association for Hospitals and Health Systems. (Level VII)

24 American Association of Critical-Care Nurses. (2017). AACN practice alert: Ventilator-associated pneumonia" https://www.aacn.org/clinical-resources/practice-alerts/ventilator-associated-pneumonia-vap (Level VII)

25 American Association for Respiratory Care (AARC). (2010). AARC clinical practice guidelines: Endotracheal suctioning of mechanically ventilated patients with artificial airways 2010. *Respiratory Care, 55*, 758–764. http://rc.rcjournal.com/content/55/6/758.short (Level I)

26 Sole, M. L., et al. (2011). Evaluation of an intervention to maintain endotracheal tube cuff pressure within therapeutic range. *American Journal of Critical Care, 20*, 109–118. (Level IV)

27 Klompas, M., et al. (2014). Strategies to prevent ventilator-associated pneumonia in acute care hospitals: 2014 update. *Infection Control and Hospital Epidemiology, 35*, 915–936. https://www.jstor.org/stable/10.1086/677144#metadata_info_tab_contents (Level I)

28 Asai, S., et al. (2014). Decrease in cuff pressure during the measurement procedure: An experimental study. *Journal of Intensive Care, 2*, 34. https://jintensivecare.biomedcentral.com/articles/10.1186/2052-0492-2-34 (Level VI)

29 Sengupta, P., et al. (2004). Endotracheal tube cuff pressure in three hospitals, and the volume required to produce an appropriate cuff pressure. *BMC Anesthesiology, 4*, 8. https://bmcanesthesiol.biomedcentral.com/articles/10.1186/1471-2253-4-8 (Level VI)

30 Nseir, S., et al. (2009). Variations in endotracheal cuff pressure in intubated critically ill patients: Prevalence and risk factors. *European Journal of Anaesthesiology, 26*, 229–234. (Level IV)

31 Howard, W. R. (2011). Bench study of a new device to display and maintain stable artificial airway cuff pressure. *Respiratory Care, 56*, 1506–1513. http://rc.rcjournal.com/content/respcare/56/10/1506.full.pdf (Level VI)

32 Walsh, B. K., et al. (2011). AARC clinical practice guideline: Capnography/capnometry during mechanical ventilation: 2011. *Respiratory Care, 56*, 503–509. https://www.aarc.org/wp-content/uploads/2014/08/04.11.0503.pdf (Level VII)

33 American Heart Association. Web-based integrated guidelines for cardiopulmonary resuscitation and emergency cardiovascular care—part 7:

Adult advanced cardiovascular life support. https://ECCguidelines.heart. org (Level II)

34 American Association of Critical-Care Nurses. (2018). AACN practice alert: Managing alarms in acute care across the life span: Electrocardiography and pulse oximetry. https://www.aacn.org/clinical-resources/practice-alerts/ managing-alarms-in-acute-care-across-the-life-span (Level VII)

35 The Joint Commission. (2021). Standard NPSG.06.01.01. *Comprehensive accreditation manual for hospitals.* Oakbrook Terrace, IL: The Joint Commission. (Level VII)

36 Graham, K. C., & Cvach, M. (2010). Monitor alarm fatigue: Standardizing use of physiological monitors and decreasing nuisance alarms. *American Journal of Critical Care, 19*, 28–37.

37 Ganz, D. A., et al. (2013, reviewed 2021). *Preventing falls in hospitals: A toolkit for improving quality of care* (AHRQ Publication No. 13-0015-EF). Rockville, MD: Agency for Healthcare Research and Quality. https://www. ahrq.gov/professionals/systems/hospital/fallpxtoolkit/index.html (Level VII)

38 Occupational Safety and Health Administration. (2012). Bloodborne pathogens, standard number 1910.1030. https://www.osha.gov/pls/ oshaweb/owadisp.show_document?p_id=10051&p_table=STANDARDS (Level VII)

39 Rutala, W. A., et al. (2008, revised 2019). Guideline for disinfection and sterilization in healthcare facilities, 2008. https://www.cdc.gov/infection-control/pdf/guidelines/disinfection-guidelines-H.pdf (Level I)

40 Accreditation Association for Hospitals and Health Systems. (2020). Standard 07.02.03. *Healthcare Facilities Accreditation Program: Accreditation requirements for acute care hospitals.* Chicago, IL: Accreditation Association for Hospitals and Health Systems. (Level VII)

41 The Joint Commission. (2021). Standard RC.01.03.01. *Comprehensive accreditation manual for hospitals.* Oakbrook Terrace, IL: The Joint Commission. (Level VII)

42 Accreditation Association for Hospitals and Health Systems. (2020). Standard 10.00.03. *Healthcare Facilities Accreditation Program: Accreditation requirements for acute care hospitals.* Chicago, IL: Accreditation Association for Hospitals and Health Systems. (Level VII)

43 Centers for Medicare and Medicaid Services, Department of Health and Human Services. (2020). Condition of participation: Medical record services. 42 C.F.R. § 482.24(b).

44 DNV GL-Healthcare USA, Inc. (2020). MR.2.SR.1. *NIAHO® accreditation requirements, interpretive guidelines and surveyor guidance—revision 20.0.* Milford, OH: DNV GL-Healthcare USA, Inc. (Level VII)

END-TIDAL CARBON DIOXIDE MONITORING

End-tidal carbon dioxide ($ETco_2$) monitoring determines the carbon dioxide (CO_2) concentration in exhaled gas to provide information about a patient's ventilation, perfusion, and metabolism. A sudden or gradual change in $ETco_2$ can provide valuable information about the patient's condition. An increase in $ETco_2$ can signal fever associated with sepsis, malignant hyperthermia, decreased ventilation, venous pulmonary embolism, increased carbon monoxide, return of circulation after cardiopulmonary resuscitation, chronic obstructive pulmonary disease, partial airway obstruction, neuromuscular blockade, use of respiratory depressants, or conditions causing metabolic acidosis.[1] A decrease in $ETco_2$ can indicate respiratory depression, pulmonary embolism, excess ventilation, hypometabolic state, hypotension, low cardiac output, esophageal intubation, complete airway obstruction, metabolic acidosis, or a disconnected ventilator.[1,2,3]

$ETco_2$ can be measured noninvasively using a quick, disposable method, or continuously with capnography. The disposable method uses a colorimetric CO_2 detector that relies on a color change to indicate CO_2 levels during exhalation; this method provides only a snapshot of the patient's $ETco_2$. (See *Detecting end-tidal CO_2 using a colorimetric CO_2 detector.*) The disposable method can be useful, but the litmus paper that's responsible for the color change might not function if it becomes moistened by the patient's secretions.

Capnography is the graphic display of the measurement of CO_2 in the respiratory gases.[2] Capnography uses various technologies to detect CO_2, including infrared spectroscopy, molecular correlation spectroscopy, Raman spectroscopy, mass spectroscopy, and photoacoustic spectroscopy. Each type detects CO_2 and then provides a continuous waveform and a digital readout of $ETco_2$. Infrared spectroscopy is the most commonly

EQUIPMENT

Detecting end-tidal CO_2 using a colorimetric CO_2 detector

A colorimetric carbon dioxide (CO_2) detector, such as the Easy Cap shown below, can be used during intubation *to verify proper endotracheal tube (ET) placement*, and for up to 2 hours after intubation if needed for patient transport.[4] The device attaches directly to the ET tube and responds quickly to exhaled CO_2 with a color change from purple to yellow.[4] Depending on the device you use, the meaning of color changes in the detector dome may differ from the Easy Cap detector described below. Follow the manufacturer's instructions for the specific detector you're using.

■ The rim of the Easy Cap is divided into four segments (clockwise from the top): CHECK, A, B, and C. The CHECK segment is solid purple, signifying the absence of carbon dioxide (CO_2).

■ The numbers in the other sections range from 0.03 to 5.0 and indicate the percentage of exhaled CO_2. The color should fluctuate during ventilation from purple (in section A) during inspiration to yellow (in section C) at the end of expiration. This result indicates that the $ETco_2$ levels are adequate, above 2%.

■ An end-expiratory color change from the C range to the B range may be the first sign of hemodynamic instability.

■ During cardiopulmonary resuscitation (CPR), an end-expiratory color change from the A or B range to the C range may mean the return of spontaneous ventilation.

■ During prolonged cardiac arrest, inadequate pulmonary perfusion leads to inadequate gas exchange. The patient exhales little or no CO_2, so the color stays in the purple range even with proper intubation. Ineffective CPR also leads to inadequate pulmonary perfusion.

■ Devices are available in adult and pediatric sizes.

Color indications on end-expiration

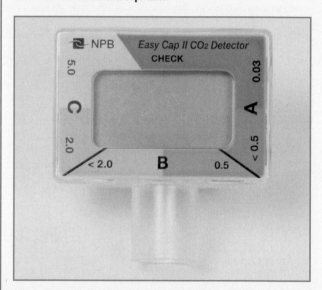

used method because it's cost effective and is found in most portable $ETco_2$ monitoring devices. (See *How continuous $ETco_2$ monitoring using infrared spectroscopy works.*)[2]

There are two methods for measuring continuous $ETco_2$: using a mainstream detector or a sidestream detector.[1] A mainstream detector is placed at the airway; it almost immediately generates a capnogram that reflects in real time the partial pressure of CO_2 within the airway. A sidestream detector attaches near the patient's mouth or nares. The device aspirates a sample of gas for analysis from the breathing circuit through a long, small-bore tube at a flow rate ranging from 50 to 250 mL/minute. Delays in sidestream analysis vary with long sampling tubes, the rate of air aspiration into the capnometer, and the efficiency of the device itself.[2]

The *American Heart Association Guidelines for Cardiopulmonary Resuscitation and Emergency Cardiovascular Care* recommend $ETco_2$ monitoring and clinical assessment to confirm initial ET tube placement in a patient in cardiac arrest when continuous quantitative waveform

How continuous ETco$_2$ monitoring using infrared spectroscopy works

With infrared spectroscopy, the optical portion of an end-tidal carbon dioxide (ETco$_2$) monitor contains an infrared light source, a sample chamber, a special carbon dioxide (CO$_2$) filter, and a photodetector. The infrared light passes through the sample chamber and is absorbed in varying amounts, depending on the amount of CO$_2$ the patient has just exhaled.[2] The photodetector measures CO$_2$ content and relays this information to the microprocessor in the monitor, which displays the continuous waveform and a digital readout of the CO$_2$ value.

Normal capnogram

Time-based capnography, the most commonly used display of ETco$_2$, depicts the respiratory phases. A normal time-based capnogram (shown below) consists of several segments, which reflect the various stages of exhalation and inhalation. Normally, any gas eliminated from the airway during early exhalation is dead-space gas, which hasn't undergone exchange at the alveolocapillary membrane. Measurements taken during this period contain no CO$_2$. As exhalation continues, CO$_2$ concentration rises sharply and rapidly. The sensor now detects gas that has undergone exchange, producing measurable quantities of CO$_2$. The final stages of alveolar emptying occur during late exhalation. During the alveolar plateau phase, CO$_2$ concentration rises more gradually, *because alveolar emptying is more constant*. The point at which the ETco$_2$ value is derived is the end of exhalation, when CO$_2$ concentration peaks. Unless an alveolar plateau is present, this value doesn't accurately estimate alveolar CO$_2$. During inhalation, the CO$_2$ concentration declines sharply to zero.[2]

Volumetric capnography, which is used less commonly than time-based capnography, measures and displays the volume of expired CO$_2$ over time. Volumetric capnography provides information about physiologic dead space and the effects of positive end-expiratory pressure on the expiratory phase.[2]

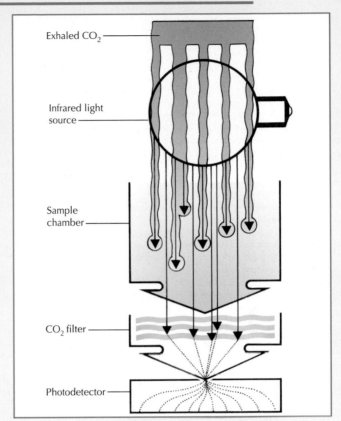

Exhaled CO$_2$

Infrared light source

Sample chamber

CO$_2$ filter

Photodetector

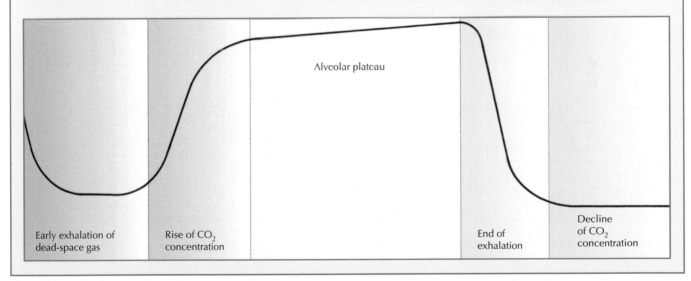

Alveolar plateau

Early exhalation of dead-space gas

Rise of CO$_2$ concentration

End of exhalation

Decline of CO$_2$ concentration

capnography isn't available.[3,5] Continuous quantitative waveform capnography can help monitor cardiopulmonary resuscitation (CPR) quality in an intubated patient during cardiac arrest, help detect the return of spontaneous circulation, and identify fatigue in a rescuer performing chest compressions.

ETco$_2$ monitoring is recommended to guide ventilator management.[3] In addition, its use can aid in the weaning of a patient without serious lung pathology off a ventilator; can help assess ventilator function; can detect ET tube displacement; has become standard during administration of anesthesia, such as moderate or deep sedation; and it is recommended during administration of epidural or patient-controlled analgesia for pain control, *because ETco$_2$ measurements can provide an indication that a patient is experiencing hypoventilation from oversedation.*[2,6,7,8]

Equipment

Gloves ▪ mainstream or sidestream CO$_2$ detector ▪ airway adapter or ETco$_2$ nasal cannula ▪ ETco$_2$ monitoring system ▪ stethoscope ▪ disinfectant pad ▪ Optional: gown, mask and goggles or mask with face shield.

Preparation of equipment

Inspect all equipment and supplies. If a product is expired, is defective, or has compromised integrity, remove it from patient use, label it as expired or defective, and report the expiration or defect as directed by your facility.

If the monitor you're using isn't self-calibrating, calibrate it as the manufacturer directs, *because failure to calibrate the device can lead to false readings.*[1] If you're using a sidestream CO$_2$ monitor, be sure to replace the water trap between patients, if directed. The trap allows humidity from exhaled gases to be condensed into an attached container. Newer sidestream models don't require water traps.

Implementation

- Verify the practitioner's order or perform the procedure as directed by your facility.
- Gather and prepare the necessary equipment and supplies.
- Perform hand hygiene.[9,10,11,12,13,14]
- Confirm the patient's identity using at least two patient identifiers.[15]
- Provide privacy.[16,17,18,19]
- Explain the procedure to the patient and family (if appropriate) according to their individual communication and learning needs *to increase their understanding, allay their fear, and enhance cooperation.*[20] Include information about the monitor, its use, and attachments.
- Raise the patient's bed to waist level before providing care *to prevent caregiver back strain.*[21]
- Perform hand hygiene.[9,10,11,12,13,14]
- Put on gloves and, as needed, other personal protective equipment *to comply with standard precautions.*[22,23,24]
- Assess the patient's cardiac and respiratory status *to serve as a baselines for comparison.*
- Plug the $ETCO_2$ monitor into a grounded outlet and then attach the cable to the display monitor. *Using a grounded outlet reduces the rate of electrical interference.*
- Assemble the airway adapter and sensor and attach them to the patient's ET tube or tracheostomy tube. If the patient isn't intubated, apply an $ETCO_2$ nasal cannula following the manufacturer's instructions.[1] Attach the airway adapter and sensor as close to the patient's ventilation connection or airway as possible *to decrease improper gas sampling.*[1]
- Observe the capnogram waveforms for quality *to make sure the readings are accurate.*[1]
- Make sure alarm limits are set properly for the patient's current condition and that alarms are turned on, functioning properly, and audible to staff.[25,26,27,28]
- Closely monitor the patient's cardiac and respiratory status, capnogram waveforms, and digital display for changes; promptly report changes in the patient's condition to the practitioner *to prevent treatment delays.*
- Return the bed to the lowest position *to prevent falls and maintain patient safety.*[29]
- Remove and discard your gloves and, if worn, any other personal protective equipment.[23,24]
- Perform hand hygiene.[9,10,11,12,13,14]
- Clean and disinfect your stethoscope with a disinfectant pad.[30,31]
- Perform hand hygiene.[9,10,11,12,13,14]
- Document the procedure.[32,33,34,35]

Special considerations

- The Joint Commission issued a sentinel event alert concerning medical device alarm safety *because alarm-related events have been associated with permanent loss of function or death.* Among the major contributing factors were improper alarm settings, alarm settings turned off inappropriately, and alarm signals not audible to staff. Make sure that alarm limits are set appropriately, and that alarms are turned on, functioning properly, and audible to staff. Follow facility guidelines for preventing alarm fatigue.[27]
- Assess for ET tube kinking, mucus plugging, and bronchospasm in a patient receiving mechanical ventilation who develops sustained decreases in $ETCO_2$.[1]
- Remember that $ETCO_2$ monitoring doesn't replace arterial blood gas (ABG) measurements. Although end-tidal measurement provides valuable information about ventilation, differences between CO_2 values obtained via capnography and those measured through ABG analysis can vary over time and may depend on patient-specific factors.[3]
- In a nonintubated patient, breath samples are obtained through both nostrils, and oxygen is delivered through nasal prongs (design depends on the manufacturer). For a patient who breathes through the mouth, use of a specially designed nasal cannula can allow the capture of exhaled gas for analysis.[1]

Complications

Inaccurate $ETCO_2$ monitoring can result from poor sampling technique, calibration drift, contamination of optics with moisture or secretions, and equipment malfunction, which can lead to misdiagnosis and improper treatment. In addition, manual resuscitation and ingestion of alcohol or carbonated beverages can alter the accuracy of a detector's findings.[5]

Documentation

Document the initial $ETCO_2$ value and all ventilator settings. Describe the waveform on the monitor and, if available, place a printout of the waveform in the patient's medical record. Document $ETCO_2$ values at least as often as vital signs, whenever significant changes in the waveform or the patient's status occur, and before and after weaning, respiratory procedures, and other interventions. Note the findings from the patient's cardiac and respiratory assessments. Record ABG levels, as ordered, and document the corresponding $ETCO_2$ values. Document abnormal readings, the name of the practitioner notified, the date and time of notification, prescribed interventions, and the patient's response to those interventions. Document teaching provided to the patient and family (if applicable), their understanding of that teaching, and any need for follow-up teaching.

References

1 Wiegand, D. L. (2017). *AACN procedure manual for high acuity, progressive, and critical care* (7th ed.). St. Louis, MO: Elsevier.

2 Spiegel, J. (2013). End-tidal carbon dioxide: The most vital of vital signs. *Anesthesiology News*, 2013, 21–27. https://www.anesthesiologynews.com/download/Capnography_ANSE13_WM.pdf

3 Walsh, B. K., et al. (2011). AARC clinical practice guideline: Capnography/capnometry during mechanical ventilation: 2011. *Respiratory Care, 56*(4), 503–509. http://rc.rcjournal.com/content/56/4/503.full.pdf (Level VII)

4 Medtronic. (2018). Nellcor™ adult/pediatric colorimetric CO_2 detector. https://www.medtronic.com/content/dam/covidien/library/us/en/product/intubation-products/nellcor-adult-pediatric-colorimetric-co2-detector-information-sheet.pdf

5 American Heart Association. (2019). Web-based integrated guidelines for cardiopulmonary resuscitation and emergency cardiovascular care—part 7: Advanced cardiac life support. https://ECCguidelines.heart.org (Level II)

6 Krauss, B., et al. (2020). Carbon dioxide monitoring (capnography). In: *UpToDate*, Walls, R. M., & Torrey, S. B. (Eds.).

7 Arrigo, R. T., et al. (2020). End-tidal capnography. http://emedicine.medscape.com/article/2116444-overview

8 Deitch, K., et al. (2010). Does end tidal CO_2 monitoring during emergency department procedural sedation and analgesia with propofol decrease the incidence of hypoxic events? A randomized, controlled trial. *Annals of Emergency Medicine, 55*, 258–264. (Level II)

9 The Joint Commission. (2021). Standard NPSG.07.01.01. *Comprehensive accreditation manual for hospitals.* Oakbrook Terrace, IL: The Joint Commission. (Level VII)

10 Centers for Disease Control and Prevention. (2002). Guideline for hand hygiene in health-care settings: Recommendations of the Healthcare Infection Control Practices Advisory Committee and the HICPAC/SHEA/APIC/IDSA Hand Hygiene Task Force. *MMWR Recommendations and Reports, 51*(RR-16), 1–45. https://www.cdc.gov/mmwr/pdf/rr/rr5116.pdf (Level II)

11 World Health Organization. (2009). WHO guidelines on hand hygiene in health care: First global patient safety challenge, clean care is safer care. https://apps.who.int/iris/bitstream/handle/10665/44102/9789241597906_eng.pdf?sequence=1 (Level IV)

12 Accreditation Association for Hospitals and Health Systems. (2020). Standard 07.01.21. *Healthcare Facilities Accreditation Program: Accreditation requirements for acute care hospitals.* Chicago, IL: Accreditation Association for Hospitals and Health Systems. (Level VII)

13 Centers for Medicare and Medicaid Services, Department of Health and Human Services. (2020). Condition of participation: Infection control. 42 C.F.R. § 482.42.

14 DNV GL-Healthcare USA, Inc. (2020). IC.1.SR.1. *NIAHO® accreditation requirements, interpretive guidelines and surveyor guidance—revision 20.0.* Milford, OH: DNV GL-Healthcare USA, Inc. (Level VII)

15 The Joint Commission. (2021). Standard NPSG.01.01.01. *Comprehensive accreditation manual for hospitals.* Oakbrook Terrace, IL: The Joint Commission. (Level VII)

16 The Joint Commission. (2021). Standard RI.01.01.01. *Comprehensive accreditation manual for hospitals.* Oakbrook Terrace, IL: The Joint Commission. (Level VII)

17 Centers for Medicare and Medicaid Services, Department of Health and Human Services. (2020). Condition of participation: Patient's rights. 42 C.F.R. § 482.13(c)(1).

18 Accreditation Association for Hospitals and Health Systems. (2020). Standard 15.01.16. *Healthcare Facilities Accreditation Program: Accreditation requirements for acute care hospitals.* Chicago, IL: Accreditation Association for Hospitals and Health Systems. (Level VII)

19 DNV GL-Healthcare USA, Inc. (2020). PR.2.SR.5. *NIAHO® accreditation requirements, interpretive guidelines and surveyor guidance—revision 20.0.* Milford, OH: DNV GL-Healthcare USA, Inc. (Level VII)

20 The Joint Commission. (2021). Standard PC.02.01.21. *Comprehensive accreditation manual for hospitals.* Oakbrook Terrace, IL: The Joint Commission. (Level VII)

21 Waters, T. R., et al. (2009). Safe patient handling training for schools of nursing. https://www.cdc.gov/niosh/docs/2009-127/pdfs/2009-127.pdf (Level VII)

22 Occupational Safety and Health Administration. (2012). Bloodborne pathogens, standard number 1910.1030. https://www.osha.gov/pls/oshaweb/owadisp.show_document?p_id=10051&p_table=STANDARDS (Level VII)

23 Siegel, J. D., et al. (2007, revised 2019). 2007 guideline for isolation precautions: Preventing transmission of infectious agents in healthcare settings. https://www.cdc.gov/infectioncontrol/pdf/guidelines/isolation-guidelines-H.pdf (Level II)

24 Accreditation Association for Hospitals and Health Systems. (2020). Standard 07.01.10. *Healthcare Facilities Accreditation Program: Accreditation requirements for acute care hospitals.* Chicago, IL: Accreditation Association for Hospitals and Health Systems. (Level VII)

25 American Association of Critical-Care Nurses. (2018). AACN practice alert: Managing alarms in acute care across the life span: Electrocardiography and pulse oximetry. https://www.aacn.org/clinical-resources/practice-alerts/managing-alarms-in-acute-care-across-the-life-span (Level VII)

26 Graham, K. C., & Cvach, M. (2010). Monitor alarm fatigue: Standardizing use of physiological monitors and decreasing nuisance alarms. *American Journal of Critical Care, 19,* 28–37.

27 The Joint Commission. (2013). Sentinel event alert 50: Medical device alarm safety in hospitals. https://www.jointcommission.org/assets/1/18/SEA_50_alarms_4_5_13_FINAL1.PDF (Level VII)

28 The Joint Commission. (2021). Standard NPSG.06.01.01. *Comprehensive accreditation manual for hospitals.* Oakbrook Terrace, IL: The Joint Commission. (Level VII)

29 Ganz, D. A., et al. (2013, reviewed 2021). *Preventing falls in hospitals: A toolkit for improving quality of care* (AHRQ Publication No. 13-0015-EF). Rockville, MD: Agency for Healthcare Quality and Research. https://www.ahrq.gov/professionals/systems/hospital/fallpxtoolkit/index.html (Level VII)

30 Accreditation Association for Hospitals and Health Systems. (2020). Standard 07.02.03. *Healthcare Facilities Accreditation Program: Accreditation requirements for acute care hospitals.* Chicago, IL: Accreditation Association for Hospitals and Health Systems. (Level VII)

31 Rutala, W. A., et al. (2008, revised 2019). Guideline for disinfection and sterilization in healthcare facilities, 2008. https://www.cdc.gov/infection-control/pdf/guidelines/disinfection-guidelines-H.pdf (Level I)

32 The Joint Commission. (2021). Standard RC.01.03.01. *Comprehensive accreditation manual for hospitals.* Oakbrook Terrace, IL: The Joint Commission. (Level VII)

33 Accreditation Association for Hospitals and Health Systems. (2020). Standard 10.00.03. *Healthcare Facilities Accreditation Program: Accreditation requirements for acute care hospitals.* Chicago, IL: Accreditation Association for Hospitals and Health Systems. (Level VII)

34 Centers for Medicare and Medicaid Services, Department of Health and Human Services. (2020). Condition of participation: Medical record services. 42 C.F.R. § 482.24(b).

35 DNV GL-Healthcare USA, Inc. (2020). MR.2.SR.1. *NIAHO® accreditation requirements, interpretive guidelines and surveyor guidance—revision 20.0.* Milford, OH: DNV GL-Healthcare USA, Inc. (Level VII)

ENEMA ADMINISTRATION

Enema administration involves instilling a solution into the rectum and colon to stimulate peristalsis by mechanical distention of the colon and stimulation of the rectal wall nerves. In a retention enema, the patient holds the solution within the rectum or colon for 30 minutes to 1 hour. With a cleansing enema, the patient expels the solution almost completely within 10 minutes.[1]

Enemas may help to clean the lower bowel in preparation for diagnostic or surgical procedures, relieve distention and promote expulsion of flatus, lubricate the rectum and colon, and soften hardened stool for removal. In addition, a retention enema may be used to administer medications such as sodium polystyrene sulfonate for treatment of hyperkalemia, lactulose for treatment of hepatic encephalopathy, and vancomycin for the treatment of severe, complicated *Clostridioides difficile* infection.[2,3,4]

Enema administration is contraindicated in patients with a recent history of bowel, rectal, or prostate gland surgery or myocardial infarction and in patients with acute abdominal conditions of unknown origin, such as suspected appendicitis. They should be administered cautiously to patients with arrhythmia or in an older adult.[1]

ELDER ALERT Enemas should be administered with caution to older adults *because people in this age-group are at greater risk for hyperphosphatemia, perforation, and sepsis.*[1]

Equipment

Prescribed solution and enema administration set or prescribed enema solution in a squeeze bottle ▪ gloves ▪ fluid-impermeable pads ▪ bath blanket ▪ bedpan or bedside commode ▪ toilet paper or moist wipes ▪ stethoscope ▪ disinfectant pad ▪ Optional: IV pole, personal protective equipment (gown, mask with goggles or mask with face shield), water-soluble lubricant, rectal balloon catheter or large urinary catheter with 30-mL balloon, prefilled syringe with 30 mL of Saline solution, clamp or catheter plug, pillows.

Prepackaged disposable enema kits are available, as are small-volume enema solutions in irrigating and retention types.

Preparation of equipment

Inspect all equipment and supplies. If a product is expired, is defective, or has compromised integrity, remove it from patient use, label it as expired or defective, and report the expiration or defect as directed by your facility. If you're using a concentrated enema solution, dilute it according to the manufacturer's instructions.[5] *Because some ingredients may be mucosal irritants,* make sure that the proportions are correct, and that you thoroughly mix the agents *to avoid local irritation.* Warm the solution until it's lukewarm to reduce patient discomfort. Clamp the tubing and fill the enema bag with the prescribed solution. Unclamp the tubing, flush the solution through the tubing, and then reclamp it. *Flushing detects leaks and removes air that could cause discomfort if introduced into the colon.* Hang the solution container on an IV pole and take all supplies to the patient's room.

No preparation is necessary if you're using an enema solution contained in a disposable squeeze bottle.

Implementation

▪ Avoid distractions and interruptions when preparing and administering an enema with or without medication, *to prevent medication errors.*[6,7]
▪ Verify the practitioner's order.[8,9,10,11]
▪ Perform hand hygiene.[12,13,14,15,16,17]
▪ Gather and prepare the necessary equipment and supplies.
▪ Compare the solution or medication label to the order in the patient's medical record.[8,9,10,11]
▪ Check the patient's medical record for allergies or other contraindications to the prescribed enema. If an allergy or another contraindication exists, don't administer the solution and notify the practitioner.[8,9,10,11]
▪ Check the expiration date on the prescribed enema. If an enema with medication is expired, return it to the pharmacy and obtain new one.[8,9,10,11]
▪ Visually inspect the solution for particles, discoloration, or other loss of integrity; don't administer the solution if its integrity is compromised.[8,9,10,11]
▪ Discuss any unresolved concerns about the enema with the patient's practitioner.[8,9,10,11]
▪ Perform hand hygiene.[12,13,14,15,16,17]
▪ Confirm the patient's identity using at least two patient identifiers.[18]
▪ Provide privacy.[19,20,21,22]

■ Explain the procedure to the patient and family (if appropriate) according to their individual communication and learning needs *to increase their understanding, allay their fears, and enhance cooperation.*[23]

■ If you're administering an enema with medication, explain that the patient must retain the medication in the colon for a prescribed amount of time (this varies by medication) and that the rectal balloon catheter or urinary catheter with balloon will remain in place for that prescribed amount of time *to assist with retention.*

■ Ask the patient about previous enemas and the patient's difficulty retaining them *to determine your equipment needs.*

■ If the patient is receiving the medication for the first time, discuss potential adverse reactions and any other patient concerns related to the medication.[8,9,10,11]

■ Verify that the medication is being administered at the proper time, in the prescribed dose, and by the correct route *to reduce the risk of medication errors.*[8,9,10,11]

■ Encourage the patient to empty the bladder, *because fluid entering the rectum may cause discomfort if the patient has a full bladder.*[24]

■ Place a bedpan or commode nearby for the patient to use. If the patient can use the bathroom, make sure that it will be available when the patient needs it. Have toilet paper or moist wipes within the patient's reach.

■ If your facility uses a bar-code technology, use it as directed by your facility.

■ Raise the bed to waist level when performing patient care *to prevent caregiver back strain.*[25]

■ Perform hand hygiene.[12,13,14,15,16,17]

NURSING ALERT If your facility's hazardous drug list contains the drug you're about to administer, put on personal protective equipment, as directed.[26]

■ Put on gloves, and as necessary, other personal protective equipment *to comply with standard precautions.*[27,28,29]

■ Remove any clothing below the patient's waist and cover the patient with a bath blanket.[24]

■ Assess the patient's GI status, noting bowel sounds and abdominal distention, *to serve as a baseline for comparison.*

■ Position the patient on the left side with the knees bent or in the knee-to-chest position *to expose the anus and ease insertion of the enema.*[5,24]

■ Place fluid-impermeable pads under the patient's buttocks *to prevent soiling the linens.*

For administration using an enema administration set

■ Remove the cap from the enema administration set and lubricate the distal tip of the administration tubing with water-soluble lubricant *to facilitate rectal insertion and reduce irritation.*[5] Alternatively, if you're using an administration set with a prelubricated tip, remove the protective covering *to expose the prelubricated tip.*

■ Gently insert the lubricated tip into the rectum, advancing it 2″ to 3″ (5 to 7.6 cm) with the tip pointing toward the umbilicus (as shown below). Don't force the tip into the rectum, *because doing so can cause injury.* During insertion, instruct the patient to bear down as if having a bowel movement, if able; *this helps relax the muscles around the anus, easing insertion.*[30]

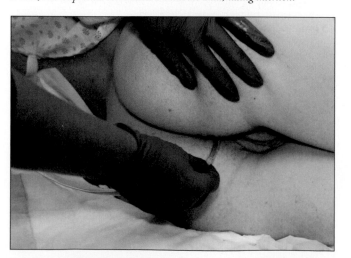

■ Unclamp the enema administration set and let the solution flow into the rectum slowly. Advise the patient to verbalize any discomfort, in which case you should slow the flow rate, *because the flow is probably too fast.*[5]

■ After infusing all the liquid, clamp the enema administration set, and slowly withdraw the tip of the enema administration set tubing *to prevent a reflex emptying of the bowel.*

■ Instruct the patient to retain the enema, as prescribed. Explain that retaining the enema may be easier while lying down.[24]

■ Return the bed to the lowest position *to prevent falls and maintain patient safety.*[31]

■ Make sure the patient has access to a call light and a bedpan, commode, or bathroom.[24]

■ If additional enemas are scheduled, clean and disinfect the reusable equipment according to the manufacturer's instructions *to prevent the spread of infection,* and store it appropriately.[32,33] If no additional enemas are scheduled, properly dispose of the enema equipment.

For administration using a squeeze bottle

■ Remove the protective covering from the disposable squeeze bottle *to expose the prelubricated tip.*

■ Expel excess air from the squeeze bottle, *because air in the colon can cause discomfort.*[30]

■ Gently insert the lubricated tip into the rectum, advancing it 2″ to 3″ (5 cm to 7.6 cm) with the tip pointing toward the umbilicus. Don't force the tip into the rectum, *because doing so can cause injury.* During insertion, instruct the patient to bear down as if having a bowel movement, if able, *to help relax the muscles around the anus, easing insertion.*[30]

■ Squeeze the bottle (as shown below) until nearly all of the solution is gone.

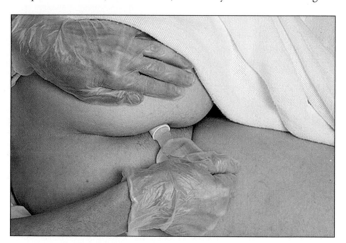

For administration using a rectal balloon catheter (retention enema)

■ Lubricate the distal tip of a rectal balloon catheter using water-soluble lubricant. Alternatively, lubricate the tip of a large urinary catheter with a 30-mL balloon.

■ Gently insert the lubricated tip into the rectum, advancing it 6″ to 8″ (15 cm to 20 cm) into the sigmoid colon. Don't force the tip into the rectum, *because doing so can cause injury.* During insertion, instruct the patient to bear down as if having a bowel movement, if able, *to help relax the muscles around the anus, easing insertion.*[30]

■ Connect the enema administration set to the rectal balloon catheter or large urinary catheter with balloon.

■ Inflate the balloon with 20 to 30 mL of saline solution, following the manufacturer's instructions, until it's snug.

■ Unclamp the enema administration set and allow the solution to flow into the rectum at the prescribed rate.

■ Advise the patient to verbalize discomfort, in which case you should slow the flow rate *because it's probably too fast.*[5]

■ After infusing all the liquid, clamp the enema administration set and slowly withdraw the tip of the enema administration set tubing. Disconnect the enema administration set from the catheter.

- Clamp or plug the rectal catheter for the ordered amount of time (dwell time varies by medication).
- If leakage occurs, elevate the patient's hips on pillows or place the patient in a temporary knee-chest position.[34]
- Dispose of the administration set appropriately.[29]
- Return the bed to the lowest position *to prevent falls and maintain patient safety.*[31]
- After the designated dwell time, deflate the balloon and remove and properly discard the rectal balloon catheter or large urinary catheter with 30-mL balloon.[29]
- Make sure the patient has access to a call light and a bedpan, commode, or bathroom.[35]

Completing the procedure
- Measure the volume of the returned solution, if possible, and assess the color and consistency of the fecal matter.
- Remove and discard your gloves and, if worn, any other personal protective equipment.[29]
- Perform hand hygiene.[11,12,13,14,15,16]
- Clean and disinfect your stethoscope with a disinfectant pad.[32,33]
- Perform hand hygiene.[12,13,14,15,16,17]
- Document the procedure.[36,37,38,39]

Special considerations
- *Because patients with a salt-retention disorder, such as heart failure or kidney failure, can absorb sodium from the saline enema solution,* administer the solution to such a patient cautiously, and monitor the patient's condition and electrolyte status. A change in electrolyte status can also cause cardiac arrhythmias.[40]

Patient teaching
Describe the procedure to the patient and family (if appropriate). Emphasize that administering an enema to a person in a sitting position or on a toilet could injure the rectal wall. Tell the patient how to prepare and care for the equipment. Discuss relaxation techniques and review measures for preventing constipation, including regular exercise, dietary modifications, and adequate fluid intake.

Complications
Enema administration can produce dizziness, faintness, excessive irritation of the colonic mucosa due to repeated administration or sensitivity to the enema ingredients, hyponatremia or hypokalemia due to repeated administration of hypotonic solutions, and cardiac arrhythmias due to vasovagal reflex stimulation after rectal tube insertion. Colonic water absorption can result from prolonged retention of hypotonic solutions, which may, in turn, cause hypervolemia or water intoxication.

Documentation
Document GI assessment findings. Record the date and time of enema administration; any special equipment you used; the type and amount of solution; the retention time; the approximate amount returned; the color, consistency, and amount of the return; any abnormalities within the return; and the patient's tolerance of the procedure. Document any complications that occurred, the name of the practitioner you notified of those complications, the date and time of notification, prescribed interventions, and the patient's response to those interventions. Document teaching provided to the patient and family (if applicable), their understanding of that teaching, and any need for follow-up teaching.

REFERENCES
1 Porritt, K. (2021). Enema administration (older person). *The JBI EBP Database.* AN: JBI1109. (Level V)
2 Feneci, P. (2021). Hepatic encephalopathy in adults: Treatment. In: *UpToDate*, Runyon, B. A. (Ed.).
3 McDonald, L. C., et al. (2018). Clinical practice guidelines for Clostridium difficile infection in adults and children: 2017 update by the Infectious Diseases Society of America and the Society for Healthcare Epidemiology of America. *Clinical Infectious Diseases, 66*(7), e1–e48. https://academic.oup.com/cid/advance-article/doi/10.1093/cid/cix1085/4855916 (Level VII)
4 Centers for Disease Control and Prevention. (2020). *Clostridioides difficile* (C. diff)https://www.cdc.gov/cdiff/index.html.
5 Institute for Safe Medication Practices. (n.d.). *Administration of rectal suppositories or enemas.* https://www.consumermedsafety.org/component/k2/item/462-administration-of-rectal-suppositories-or-enemas
6 Westbrook, J., et al. (2010). Association of interruptions with an increased risk and severity of medication administration errors. *Archives of Internal Medicine, 170*, 683–690. (Level IV)
7 Institute for Safe Medication Practices. (2012). Side tracks on the safety express: Interruptions lead to errors and unfinished...Wait, what was I doing? *Nurse Advise-ERR, 11*(2), 1–4. https://www.ismp.org/Newsletters/acutecare/showarticle.aspx?id=37
8 DNV GL-Healthcare USA, Inc. (2020). MM.1.SR.3. *NIAHO® accreditation requirements, interpretive guidelines and surveyor guidance—revision 20.0.* Milford, OH: DNV GL-Healthcare USA, Inc. (Level VII)
9 The Joint Commission. (2021). Standard MM.06.01.01. *Comprehensive accreditation manual for hospitals.* Oakbrook Terrace, IL: The Joint Commission. (Level VII)
10 Accreditation Association for Hospitals and Health Systems. (2020). Standard 16.01.03. *Healthcare Facilities Accreditation Program: Accreditation requirements for acute care hospitals.* Chicago, IL: Accreditation Association for Hospitals and Health Systems. (Level VII)
11 Centers for Medicare and Medicaid Services, Department of Health and Human Services. (2020). Condition of participation: Nursing services. 42 C.F.R. § 482.23(c).
12 DNV GL-Healthcare USA, Inc. (2020). IC.1.SR.1. *NIAHO® accreditation requirements, interpretive guidelines and surveyor guidance—revision 20.0.* Milford, OH. DNV GL-Healthcare USA, Inc. (Level VII)
13 Centers for Medicare and Medicaid Services, Department of Health and Human Services. (2020). Condition of participation: Infection control. 42 C.F.R. § 482.42.
14 Accreditation Association for Hospitals and Health Systems. (2020). Standard 07.01.21. *Healthcare Facilities Accreditation Program: Accreditation requirements for acute care hospitals.* Chicago, IL: Accreditation Association for Hospitals and Health Systems. (Level VII)
15 The Joint Commission. (2021). Standard NPSG.07.01.01. *Comprehensive accreditation manual for hospitals.* Oakbrook Terrace, IL: The Joint Commission. (Level VII)
16 World Health Organization. (2009). WHO guidelines on hand hygiene in health care: First global patient safety challenge, clean care is safer care. https://apps.who.int/iris/bitstream/handle/10665/44102/9789241597906_eng.pdf?sequence=1 (Level IV)
17 Centers for Disease Control and Prevention. (2002). Guideline for hand hygiene in health-care settings: Recommendations of the Healthcare Infection Control Practices Advisory Committee and the HICPAC/SHEA/APIC/IDSA Hand Hygiene Task Force. *MMWR Recommendations and Reports, 51*(RR-16), 1–45. https://www.cdc.gov/mmwr/pdf/rr/rr5116.pdf (Level II)
18 The Joint Commission. (2021). Standard NPSG.01.01.01. *Comprehensive accreditation manual for hospitals.* Oakbrook Terrace, IL: The Joint Commission. (Level VII)
19 The Joint Commission. (2021). Standard RI.01.01.01. *Comprehensive accreditation manual for hospitals.* Oakbrook Terrace, IL: The Joint Commission. (Level VII)
20 DNV GL-Healthcare USA, Inc. (2020). PR.2.SR.5. *NIAHO® accreditation requirements, interpretive guidelines and surveyor guidance—revision 20.0.* Milford, OH: DNV GL-Healthcare USA, Inc. (Level VII)
21 Centers for Medicare and Medicaid Services, Department of Health and Human Services. (2020). Condition of participation: Patient's rights. 42 C.F.R. § 482.13(c)(1).
22 Accreditation Association for Hospitals and Health Systems. (2020). Standard 15.01.16. *Healthcare Facilities Accreditation Program: Accreditation requirements for acute care hospitals.* Chicago, IL: Accreditation Association for Hospitals and Health Systems. (Level VII)
23 The Joint Commission. (2021). Standard PC.02.01.21. *Comprehensive accreditation manual for hospitals.* Oakbrook Terrace, IL: The Joint Commission. (Level VII)
24 Kyle, G. (2007). Bowel care, part 4: Administering an enema. *Nursing Times, 103*(45), 26–27.
25 Waters, T. R., et al. (2009). Safe patient handling training for schools of nursing. https://www.cdc.gov/niosh/docs/2009-127/pdfs/2009-127.pdf (Level VII)

26 The United States Pharmacopeial Convention. (2019). USP general chapter <800>: Hazardous drugs—handling in healthcare settings. http://www.usp.org/compounding/general-chapter-hazardous-drugs-handling-healthcare (Level VII)

27 Accreditation Association for Hospitals and Health Systems. (2020). Standard 07.01.10. *Healthcare Facilities Accreditation Program: Accreditation requirements for acute care hospitals.* Chicago, IL: Accreditation Association for Hospitals and Health Systems. (Level VII)

28 Siegel, J. D., et al. (2007, revised 2019). 2007 guideline for isolation precautions: Preventing transmission of infectious agents in healthcare settings. https://www.cdc.gov/infectioncontrol/pdf/guidelines/isolation-guidelines-H.pdf (Level II)

29 Occupational Safety and Health Administration. (2012). Bloodborne pathogens, standard number 1910.1030. https://www.osha.gov/pls/oshaweb/owadisp.show_document?p_id=10051&p_table=STANDARDS (Level VII)

30 Fleet Company, Inc. (n.d.). How to use this enema. http://fleet.stage.pml10.com/sites/fleet/files/2020-02/saline-enema-extra-uses_0.pdf

31 Ganz, D. A., et al. (2013, reviewed 2021). *Preventing falls in hospitals: A toolkit for improving quality of care* (AHRQ Publication No. 13-0015-EF). Rockville, MD: Agency for Healthcare Research and Quality. https://www.ahrq.gov/professionals/systems/hospital/fallpxtoolkit/index.html (Level VII)

32 Accreditation Association for Hospitals and Health Systems. (2020). Standard 07.02.03. *Healthcare Facilities Accreditation Program: Accreditation requirements for acute care hospitals.* Chicago, IL: Accreditation Association for Hospitals and Health Systems. (Level VII)

33 Rutala, W. A., et al. (2008, revised 2019). Guideline for disinfection and sterilization in healthcare facilities, 2008. https://www.cdc.gov/infection-control/pdf/guidelines/disinfection-guidelines-H.pdf (Level I)

34 Sanofi-Aventis Canada, Inc. (2018). Prescribing information: Kayexalate (sodium polystyrene sulfonate). http://products.sanofi.ca/en/kayexalate.pdf

35 Craven, R. F., et al. (2017). *Fundamentals of nursing: Human health and function* (8th ed.). Philadelphia, PA: Wolters Kluwer.

36 DNV GL-Healthcare USA, Inc. (2020). MR.2.SR.1. *NIAHO® accreditation requirements, interpretive guidelines and surveyor guidance—revision 20.0.* Milford, OH: DNV GL-Healthcare USA, Inc. (Level VII)

37 Accreditation Association for Hospitals and Health Systems. (2020). Standard 10.00.03. *Healthcare Facilities Accreditation Program: Accreditation requirements for acute care hospitals.* Chicago, IL: Accreditation Association for Hospitals and Health Systems. (Level VII)

38 Centers for Medicare and Medicaid Services, Department of Health and Human Services. (2020). Condition of participation: Medical record services. 42 C.F.R. § 482.24(b).

39 The Joint Commission. (2021). Standard RC.01.03.01. *Comprehensive accreditation manual for hospitals.* Oakbrook Terrace, IL: The Joint Commission. (Level VII)

40 U.S. Food and Drug Administration. (2016). FDA drug safety communication: FDA warns of possible harm from exceeding recommended dose of over-the-counter sodium phospate products to treat constipation. https://www.fda.gov/drugs/drug-safety-and-availability/fda-drug-safety-communication-fda-warns-possible-harm-exceeding-recommended-dose-over-counter-sodium

ENTERAL GASTRIC AND DUODENAL FEEDING TUBE INSERTION AND REMOVAL

Inserting an enteral feeding tube nasally or orally into the stomach or duodenum allows a patient to receive nourishment if the patient is unable to do so orally. The enteral feeding tube also permits supplemental feedings in a patient who has high nutritional requirements, such as a patient with extensive burns. The preferred feeding tube insertion route is nasal, but the oral route may be used for patients with such conditions as a head injury, a deviated septum, or another nasal injury. These feeding tubes are intended for short-term use in patients who are expected to require enteral nutrition for up to 6 weeks.[1]

A practitioner, in collaboration with other members of the health care team, decides whether the distal tip of an enteral feeding tube should be inserted into a patient's stomach (gastric feeding tube) or duodenum. Gastric feeding tubes are typically appropriate for patients with a functional stomach that's free of delayed gastric emptying, obstruction, and fistula.[1] Duodenal feeding tubes are most appropriate for patients with gastric outlet obstruction, severe gastroparesis, or a known history of reflux and aspiration of stomach contents.[1,2] Contraindications to enteral feeding tube insertion include mechanical obstruction of the GI tract,

uncorrectable coagulopathy, and bowel ischemia.[1] Traumatic injuries to the head, neck, and face and recent transsphenoidal surgery may prevent nasal insertion.[1] Relative contraindications to enteral feeding tube insertion include recent GI bleeding, hemodynamic instability, ascites, respiratory compromise, and certain anatomic anomalies.[1]

Enteral feeding tubes differ somewhat from standard nasogastric tubes. Made of silicone or polyurethane, feeding tubes have small diameters and great flexibility, and usually a water-activated coating that provides a lubricated surface. These features reduce oropharyngeal irritation, necrosis from pressure on the tracheoesophageal wall, distal esophageal irritation, and discomfort when swallowing. To facilitate passage, some feeding tubes are weighted with tungsten, and some need a guide wire to keep them from curling in the back of the throat. These small-bore tubes usually have radiopaque markings so that their position can be verified by X-ray.

Equipment
For feeding tube insertion
Enteral feeding tube (with or without a guide wire) ▪ fluid-impermeable pad or towel ▪ gloves ▪ securement device, tape, or semipermeable transparent dressing ▪ enteral syringe ▪ indelible marker ▪ stethoscope ▪ disinfectant pad ▪ water-soluble lubricant or water for lubrication ▪ Optional: penlight, cup of water, straw, pH testing equipment, alcohol pad, tape, gown, mask with face shield or mask and goggles, capnography equipment, enteral feeding pump, skin preparation product, measuring tape, protective padding, prokinetic agent.

For feeding tube removal
Gloves ▪ fluid-impermeable pad or towel ▪ enteral syringe ▪ stethoscope ▪ disinfectant pad ▪ oral care supplies ▪ Optional: adhesive remover, gown, mask with face shield or mask and goggles.

Preparation of equipment
For feeding tube insertion
Inspect all equipment and supplies. If a product is expired, is defective, or has compromised integrity, remove it from patient use, label it as expired or defective, and report the expiration or defect as directed by your facility.

Typically, the practitioner orders the smallest-bore tube that will allow free passage of the liquid feeding formula. Read the instructions on the tubing package carefully, *because tube characteristics vary according to the manufacturer.* (For example, some tubes have marks at the appropriate lengths for gastric, duodenal, and jejunal insertion.) Examine the enteral feeding tube *to ensure it's free from defects, such as cracks or rough or sharp edges.* Run water through the enteral feeding tube *to check for patency, activate the coating, and facilitate removal of the guide wire.*

Implementation
▪ Verify the practitioner's order.
▪ Review the patient's medical record for history of recent facial injury or surgery, basilar skull fracture, or transsphenoidal pituitary resection; prior nasal or upper GI surgery; esophageal stent placement; and anatomic conditions (such as deviated nasal septum or hiatal hernia) that may contraindicate nasal insertion.[3]
▪ If required in your facility, confirm that informed consent has been obtained and that the signed consent form is in the patient's medical record.[2,4,5,6]
▪ Gather and prepare the necessary equipment and supplies.
▪ Perform hand hygiene.[7,8,9,10,11,12]
▪ Confirm the patient's identity using at least two patient identifiers.[13]
▪ Provide privacy.[14,15,16,17]
▪ Explain the procedure to the patient and family (if appropriate) according to their individual communication and learning needs *to increase their understanding, allay their fears, and enhance cooperation.*[18] Ask whether the patient has a history of epistaxis or sinusitis. If so, ask whether one naris is more susceptible.[3]
▪ Agree on a signal that can be used if the patient wants you to stop briefly during the procedure.

■ Raise the patient's bed to waist level before providing care *to prevent caregiver back strain.*[19]

■ Perform hand hygiene.[7,8,9,10,11,12]

■ Assess the patient's GI status *for baseline comparison.* Assess the patient's risk of aspiration.[1,3,20]

■ Position the patient with the head of the bed elevated at least 30 degrees *to facilitate enteral feeding tube advancement into the esophagus;* if contraindicated, consider the reverse Trendelenburg position.[1]

■ *To enhance gastric motility and subsequently facilitate passage of the tube distal to the pylorus,* administer a prokinetic agent, if prescribed, following safe medication administration practices.[3]

■ Perform hand hygiene[7,8,9,10,11,12] and put on gloves and, as needed, other personal protective equipment *to comply with standard precautions.*[21,22]

■ Assess the patient's nares, if applicable, *to determine the best choice for insertion.* Use a penlight to ease visualization, as needed.

■ Determine the proper insertion length of the tube *to help ensure gastric placement.* Place the tube's distal end at the tip of the patient's nose (or mouth for oral insertion) and then extend the tube to the earlobe, down to the xiphoid process, and then midway to the umbilicus.[1] Note the corresponding incremental marking on the tube or, if the tube doesn't contain incremental markings, mark the tube or note an identifier at the intended exit point.[3]

■ Drape a fluid-impermeable pad across the patient's chest *to protect the gown and bed linens from soiling.*[3]

Inserting the enteral feeding tube nasally

■ Lubricate the curved tip of the enteral feeding tube and the tube guide wire, if appropriate, with a small amount of water-soluble lubricant *to help ease insertion and prevent tissue injury.*[3,23] Alternatively, lubricate the curved distal tip of the enteral feeding tube and the tube guidewire by immersing them in water, if appropriate.[24] Follow the manufacturer's instructions for use.

■ *To advance the enteral feeding tube,* insert the lubricated curved distal tip into the patient's more patent nostril and direct it along the nasal passage.

■ Guide the enteral feeding tube at an angle parallel to the floor of the patient's nasal canal, advancing it gently downward through the nasal passage toward the distal pharynx.[3] Instruct the patient to assume a chin-tuck position (unless contraindicated) *to help close the patient's trachea and open the esophagus.*[3] When the enteral feeding tube reaches the patient's oropharynx you'll feel some resistance.

■ Unless contraindicated, after the enteral feeding tube reaches the patient's oropharynx, allow the patient to sip water through a straw as you slowly advance the tube *to help facilitate passage of the tube into the patient's esophagus.* (If the patient in unable to swallow water safely, ask the patient to dry swallow.)[3,24]

Inserting the enteral feeding tube orally

■ Lubricate the curved distal tip of the enteral feeding tube and the tube guidewire by immersing them in water or, if appropriate, by using a small amount of water-soluble lubricant (per the manufacturer's directions) *to ease insertion and prevent tissue injury.*[3,23,24]

■ Grasp the enteral feeding tube with the distal end pointing downward, and carefully insert it into the patient's oral cavity.

■ Guide the enteral feeding tube downward toward the patient's esophagus. Instruct the patient to assume a chin-tuck position (unless contraindicated) *to close the patient's trachea and open the esophagus.*[3]

Positioning the enteral feeding tube

■ If you meet resistance, rotate the enteral feeding tube to guide it toward the patient's esophagus. If you continue to meet resistance, don't force the tube. Instead, stop the procedure and assess for barriers to tube advancement.

■ As you advance the enteral feeding tube, monitor the patient for cues (such as coughing and discomfort) that might indicate that the tube has entered the respiratory tract or has kinked or coiled in the oral cavity.[3] Immediately stop the procedure and remove the tube if you suspect

respiratory intubation. Allow the patient time to rest, and then resume the insertion procedure, as indicated.

■ Continue advancing the enteral feeding tube until you reach the predetermined insertion length at the patient's nostril or lips.[3]

■ Use at least two bedside methods to determine enteral feeding tube location during insertion.[1,25] Watch for signs of respiratory distress (such as coughing and dyspnea).[1,25] Use capnography equipment, if available, *to detect carbon dioxide in the enteral feeding tube,* which indicates inadvertent tracheal insertion.[1,25] Measure the pH of enteral feeding tube aspirate, if this procedure is performed in your facility. Fasting gastric pH is usually 5 or less, even in patients receiving gastric acid inhibitors; however, note that this method may not be reliable, *because gastric pH has a high pH occasionally.*[25] Fluid aspirated from an enteral feeding tube that has perforated the pleural space typically has a pH of 7 or higher.[1] Inspect the enteral feeding tube aspirate; fasting gastric secretions often appear grassy green or brown, or clear and colorless.[1,25] Aspirate from the pleural space typically has a pale yellow, serous appearance.[1]

■ To advance the enteral feeding tube—especially a tungsten-weighted tube—to the duodenum, position the patient on the right side *to use gravity to assist tube passage through the patient's pylorus.* Move the tube forward 2″ to 3″ (5 cm to 7.6 cm) hourly. Observe for a change in aspirate appearance as the tube progresses from the patient's stomach to the duodenum; use these findings to determine the appropriate time to obtain an order for an X-ray *to confirm duodenal placement.* Tube placement must be confirmed by X-ray before feeding begins, *because duodenal feeding can cause nausea and vomiting if enteral formula is accidentally delivered to the patient's stomach.*[1,25]

■ Ensure that enteral feeding tube placement is confirmed by X-ray and documented before initial use. *A properly obtained and interpreted X-ray is recommended to confirm correct placement of any blindly inserted enteral tube before its initial use for the administration of feedings or medication.*[1,25,26]

■ After X-ray confirmation of enteral feeding tube placement, flush the tube with up to 10 mL of water, if appropriate, *to activate the internal lubricant.*[23,24] Then, remove the guidewire (if present) with one hand while holding the tube in place at the patient's nostrils or mouth.[3]

■ Secure the enteral feeding tube with a securement device, tape, or semipermeable transparent dressing *to prevent dislodgment.* Clean the patient's skin where you intend to secure the tube.[3] For excessively oily skin, wipe the patient's skin with an alcohol pad and allow it to dry before applying the securement device.[27] Apply a skin preparation product to the skin, if needed.[3,27] Apply the securement device and secure the enteral feeding tube according to the manufacturer's instructions. Alternatively, apply the tape and secure the tube;, for a small, soft tube, use a semipermeable transparent dressing, if desired.[3] Use protective padding under enteral feeding the tube, if necessary, *to protect the patient's skin from friction and pressure.*[28] Keep the skin under the enteral feeding tube clean and dry *to prevent skin breakdown.*

■ Mark the enteral feeding tube at the patient's nostril or lips with indelible marker. Measure the external tube length or note the incremental marking on the tube where it exits the patient's nose or mouth. Document the external length in the patient's medical record *to obtain a baseline for comparison to assess for tube migration.*[1]

■ Route the tubing toward the patient's feet and place the enteral feeding pump, if used, toward the foot of the bed, *because a standardized approach of keeping IV lines routed toward the head and enteric lines routed toward the feet prevents dangerous misconnections.*[29]

■ Remove and discard the fluid-impermeable pad or towel.

■ Maintain the head of the patient's bed elevated to at least 30 degrees (unless contraindicated) *to prevent aspiration.* If elevation contraindicated, consider the reverse Trendelenburg position.[1]

■ Return the bed to the lowest position *to prevent falls and maintain the patient's safety.*[30]

Removing an enteral feeding tube

■ Trace the enteral feeding tube from the patient to its point of origin *to make sure that you're accessing the proper port.*[29,31]

■ Verify tube placement, and then use an enteral syringe to flush the enteral feeding tube with air; then clamp or pinch the tube *to prevent fluid aspiration during tube withdrawal.*[3]

■ Gently remove the securement device, tape, or semipermeable transparent dressing securing the enteral feeding tube *to prevent skin stripping or tearing.* Use adhesive remover, if needed.

■ Remove the tube with a slow, smooth, steady movement, *to prevent potential aspiration of residual formula and GI secretions during removal.*[3] If you encounter resistance while removing the enteral tube, rotate the tube and try to remove it again. If resistance continues, stop the procedure and notify the practitioner; *the location of the tube may need to be verified by X-ray.*

■ Inspect the tube *to make sure that it's intact.*[3] Notify the practitioner if the tube isn't intact.

■ Discard the tube in the appropriate receptacle.[32]

■ Assist the patient with performing oral care (or perform oral care) *to promote comfort and prevent oral colonization of microorganisms.* (See the "Oral care" procedure.)

■ Perform nasal care if the enteral feeding tube was inserted through the naris.

Completing the procedure

■ Remove and discard your gloves and (if worn) other personal protective equipment.[21,22]

■ Clean and disinfect your stethoscope using a disinfectant pad.[33,34]

■ Perform hand hygiene.[7,8,9,10,11,12]

■ Document the procedure.[35,36,37,38]

Special considerations

■ Monitor the external tube length of the enteral feeding tube before use and at least every 4 hours[1,39] *to determine whether the length of the external portion of the tube has changed, indicating that the tube has moved.* If you observe a significant increase in the external tube length, use other bedside tests *to determine whether the tube has become dislodged;* if in doubt, obtain an X-ray, as ordered, *to determine tube location.*[1]

■ The Joint Commission issued a sentinel event alert related to managing risk during transition to new International Organization for Standardization tubing standards that were designed to prevent dangerous tubing misconnections, which can lead to serious patient injury and death. During the transition, make sure to trace each tube and catheter from the patient to its point of origin before connecting or reconnecting any device or infusion, at any care transition (such as to a new setting or service), and as part of the hand-off process; route tubes and catheters having different purposes in different standardized directions; when the patient has different access sites or several bags hanging, label tubing at both the distal and proximal ends; use tubing and equipment only as intended; and store medications for different delivery routes in separate locations.[31]

Patient teaching

If the patient will use an enteral feeding tube at home, make appropriate home health care nursing referrals, and teach the patient and caregivers how to use and care for an enteral feeding tube. Teach them how to obtain equipment, insert and remove the tube, prepare and store enteral formula, and solve problems related to tube position and patency. Instruct the patient and family to contact the practitioner if the patient develops signs and symptoms of respiratory distress, nausea, vomiting, abdominal distention, food intolerance, or other signs of GI dysfunction.

Complications

Complications of insertion of an enteral feeding tube may include misplacement into the patient's bronchial tree, which can result in pneumonia, pneumonitis, and pneumothorax if not recognized.[40] Also, during insertion, the tube may coil in the esophagus or posterior pharynx, or an esophageal tear may occur.[3] Prolonged enteral feeding tube intubation may lead to sinusitis, esophagitis, esophagotracheal fistula, gastric ulceration, skin erosion at the nostril, and pulmonary and oral infection.

Complications may also include aspiration and tissue damage.[3] Forced removal of an enteral tube can cause damage to the stomach and esophagus. Respiratory distress, epistaxis, and laryngeal injury are also possible complications.[41] Stridor and vocal cord paralysis can appear up to 2 weeks after removal.[42]

Documentation

For enteral feeding tube insertion, record your assessment findings, the date and time of insertion, the enteral feeding tube type and size, the insertion site, the area of tip placement, the external tube length, and confirmation of proper placement. Document the patient's tolerance of the procedure.

For enteral feeding tube removal, record your GI assessment findings, the date and time of enteral feeding tube removal, and the patient's tolerance of the procedure. Document any adverse events related to tube removal.[3]

For insertion or removal, document teaching provided to the patient and family (if applicable), their understanding of that teaching, and any need for follow-up teaching.

REFERENCES

1 Boullata, J. I., et al. (2017). ASPEN safe practices for enteral nutrition therapy. *Journal of Parenteral & Enteral Nutrition, 41,* 15–103. https://onlinelibrary.wiley.com/doi/full/10.1177/0148607116673053 (Level VII)

2 Centers for Medicare and Medicaid Services, Department of Health and Human Services. (2020). Condition of participation: Patient's rights. 42 C.F.R. § 482.13(b)(2).

3 Wiegand, D. L. (2017). *AACN procedure manual for high acuity, progressive, and critical care* (7th ed.). St. Louis, MO: Saunders.

4 Accreditation Association for Hospitals and Health Systems. (2020). Standard 15.01.11. *Healthcare Facilities Accreditation Program: Accreditation requirements for acute care hospitals.* Chicago, IL: Accreditation Association for Hospitals and Health Systems. (Level VII)

5 DNV GL-Healthcare USA, Inc. (2020). PR.2.SR.3. *NIAHO® accreditation requirements, interpretive guidelines and surveyor guidance—revision 20.0.* Milford, OH: DNV GL-Healthcare USA, Inc. (Level VII)

6 The Joint Commission. (2021). Standard RI.01.03.01. *Comprehensive accreditation manual for hospitals.* Oakbrook Terrace, IL: The Joint Commission. (Level VII)

7 The Joint Commission. (2021). Standard NPSG.07.01.01. *Comprehensive accreditation manual for hospitals.* Oakbrook Terrace, IL: The Joint Commission. (Level VII)

8 Centers for Disease Control and Prevention. (2002). Guideline for hand hygiene in health-care settings: Recommendations of the Healthcare Infection Control Practices Advisory Committee and the HICPAC/SHEA/APIC/IDSA Hand Hygiene Task Force. *MMWR Recommendations and Reports, 51*(RR-16), 1–45. http://www.cdc.gov/mmwr/pdf/rr/rr5116.pdf (Level II)

9 World Health Organization. (2009). WHO guidelines on hand hygiene in health care: First global patient safety challenge, clean care is safer care. https://apps.who.int/iris/bitstream/handle/10665/44102/9789241597906_eng.pdf?sequence=1 (Level IV)

10 Accreditation Association for Hospitals and Health Systems. (2020). Standard 07.01.21. *Healthcare Facilities Accreditation Program: Accreditation requirements for acute care hospitals.* Chicago, IL: Accreditation Association for Hospitals and Health Systems. (Level VII)

11 Centers for Medicare and Medicaid Services, Department of Health and Human Services. (2020). Condition of participation: Infection control. 42 C.F.R. § 482.42.

12 DNV GL-Healthcare USA, Inc. (2020). IC.1.SR.1. *NIAHO® accreditation requirements, interpretive guidelines and surveyor guidance—revision 20.0.* Milford, OH: DNV GL-Healthcare USA, Inc. (Level VII)

13 The Joint Commission. (2021). Standard NPSG.01.01.01. *Comprehensive accreditation manual for hospitals.* Oakbrook Terrace, IL: The Joint Commission. (Level VII)

14 Centers for Medicare and Medicaid Services, Department of Health and Human Services. (2020). Condition of participation: Patient's rights. 42 C.F.R. § 482.13(c)(1).

15 Accreditation Association for Hospitals and Health Systems. (2020). Standard 15.01.16. *Healthcare Facilities Accreditation Program: Accreditation requirements for acute care hospitals.* Chicago, IL: Accreditation Association for Hospitals and Health Systems. (Level VII)

16 DNV GL-Healthcare USA, Inc. (2020). PR.2.SR.5. *NIAHO® accreditation requirements, interpretive guidelines and surveyor guidance—revision 20.0.* Milford, OH: DNV GL-Healthcare USA, Inc. (Level VII)

17 The Joint Commission. (2021). Standard RI.01.01.01. *Comprehensive accreditation manual for hospitals*. Oakbrook Terrace, IL: The Joint Commission. (Level VII)

18 The Joint Commission. (2021). Standard PC.02.01.21. *Comprehensive accreditation manual for hospitals*. Oakbrook Terrace, IL: The Joint Commission. (Level VII)

19 Waters, T. R., et al. (2009). Safe patient handling training for schools of nursing. https://www.cdc.gov/niosh/docs/2009-127/pdfs/2009-127.pdf (Level VII)

20 McClave, S. A., et al. (2016). Guidelines for the provision and assessment of nutrition support therapy in the adult critically ill patient: Society of Critical Care Medicine (SCCM) and American Society for Parenteral and Enteral Nutrition (A.S.P.E.N.). *Journal of Parenteral & Enteral Nutrition, 40*, 159–211. (Level VII)

21 Siegel, J. D., et al. (2007, revised 2019). 2007 guideline for isolation precautions: Preventing transmission of infectious agents in healthcare settings. https://www.cdc.gov/infectioncontrol/pdf/guidelines/isolation-guidelines-H.pdf (Level II)

22 Accreditation Association for Hospitals and Health Systems. (2020). Standard 07.01.10. *Healthcare Facilities Accreditation Program: Accreditation requirements for acute care hospitals*. Chicago, IL: Accreditation Association for Hospitals and Health Systems. (Level VII)

23 Puiggros, C., et al. (2015). Experience in bedside placement, clinical validity, and cost-efficacy of a self-propelled nasojejunal feeding tube. *Nutrition in Clinical Practice, 30*(6), 815823. https://www.ncbi.nlm.nih.gov/pmc/articles/PMC4708005/pdf/10.1177_0884533615592954.pdf

24 Corpak® Medsystems. (n.d.). Procedure for insertion of the Corflo®-ultra and controller enteral NG feeding tubes. https://iu.instructure.com/courses/1538752/files/59548650/download?wrap=1

25 American Association of Critical-Care Nurses. (2016, updated 2020). AACN practice alert: Initial and ongoing verification of feeding tube placement in adults. https://www.aacn.org/clinical-resources/practice-alerts/initial-and-ongoing-verification-of-feeding-tube-placement-in-adults (Level VII)

26 Ukleja, A., et al. (2010). Standards for nutrition support: Adult hospitalized patients. *Nutrition in Clinical Practice, 25*(4), 403–414. https://onlinelibrary.wiley.com/doi/pdf/10.1177/0884533610374200 (Level VII)

27 C. R. Bard, Inc. (2010). StatLock® nasogastric stabilization device. https://www.mnhospitals.org/Portals/0/Documents/patientsafety/Pressure%20Ulcers/NG_Stablization_Device_Procedure_Statlock.pdf

28 Camacho-Del Rio, G. (2018). Evidence-based practice: Medical device–related pressure ulcers. *American Nurse Today, 13*(10), 50–52. https://www.myamericannurse.com/medical-device-pressure-injury-prevent/

29 U.S. Food and Drug Administration. (2017). Examples of medical device misconnections. https://www.fda.gov/MedicalDevices/ProductsandMedicalProcedures/GeneralHospitalDevicesandSupplies/TubingandLuerMisconnections/ucm313275.htm

30 Ganz, D. A., et al. (2013, reviewed 2021). *Preventing falls in hospitals: A toolkit for improving quality of care* (AHRQ Publication No. 13-0015-EF). Rockville, MD: Agency for Healthcare Research and Quality. https://www.ahrq.gov/professionals/systems/hospital/fallpxtoolkit/index.html (Level VII)

31 The Joint Commission. (2014). Sentinel event alert 53: Managing risk during transition to new ISO tubing connector standards. https://www.jointcommission.org/assets/1/6/SEA_53_Connectors_8_19_14_final.pdf (Level VII)

32 Occupational Safety and Health Administration. (2019). Bloodborne pathogens, standard number 1910.1030. https://www.osha.gov/pls/oshaweb/owadisp.show_document?p_id=10051&p_table=STANDARDS (Level VII)

33 Accreditation Association for Hospitals and Health Systems. (2020). Standard 07.02.03. *Healthcare Facilities Accreditation Program: Accreditation requirements for acute care hospitals*. Chicago, IL: Accreditation Association for Hospitals and Health Systems. (Level VII)

34 Rutala, W. A., et al. (2008, revised 2019). Guideline for disinfection and sterilization in healthcare facilities, 2008. https://www.cdc.gov/infectioncontrol/pdf/guidelines/disinfection-guidelines-H.pdf (Level I)

35 The Joint Commission. (2021). Standard RC.01.03.01. *Comprehensive accreditation manual for hospitals*. Oakbrook Terrace, IL: The Joint Commission. (Level VII)

36 DNV GL-Healthcare USA, Inc. (2020). MR.2.SR.1. *NIAHO® accreditation requirements, interpretive guidelines and surveyor guidance—revision 20.0*. Milford, OH: DNV GL-Healthcare USA, Inc. (Level VII)

37 Accreditation Association for Hospitals and Health Systems. (2020). Standard 10.00.03. *Healthcare Facilities Accreditation Program: Accreditation requirements for acute care hospitals*. Chicago, IL: Accreditation Association for Hospitals and Health Systems. (Level VII)

38 Centers for Medicare and Medicaid Services, Department of Health and Human Services. (2020). Condition of participation: Medical record services. 42 C.F.R. § 482.24(b).

39 Urden, L. D., et al. (2018). *Critical care nursing: Diagnosis and management* (8th ed.). Maryland Heights, MO: Elsevier.

40 Stayner, J. L., et al. (2012). Feeding tube placement: Errors and complications. *Nutrition in Clinical Practice, 27*, 738–748. (Level V)

41 Wright, S., et al. (2014). Safe removal of knotted nasogastric tubes. *Nursing Times, 110*, 16–17. https://www.nursingtimes.net/clinical-archive/patient-safety/safe-removal-of-knotted-nasogastric-tubes-17-10-2014/

42 Prabhakaran, S., et al. (2012). Nasoenteric tube complications. *Scandinavian Journal of Surgery, 101*, 147–155. A (Level V)

ENTERAL GASTRIC, DUODENAL, AND JEJUNAL TUBE FEEDINGS

Gastric enteral tube feeding involves delivery of a liquid feeding formula directly to the stomach via an enteral tube. It's typically indicated for patients who can't eat normally because of dysphagia or oral or esophageal obstruction or injury.[1] Gastric feedings also may be given to unconscious or intubated patients or to those recovering from GI tract surgery who can't ingest food orally.[2]

Duodenal or jejunal enteral tube feeding involves delivery of a liquid feeding formula directly to the small intestine, specifically the duodenum or jejunum. Nasoduodenal or nasojejunal enteral tube feeding is indicated when the esophagus and stomach need to be bypassed, such as in cases of severe gastroesophageal reflux, recurrent emesis, or gastric dysmotility; after surgery or major trauma; and in patients who have decreased bowel sounds, are taking a paralytic agent, or are at risk for aspiration.[3] Duodenal and jejunal enteral tube feeding decreases the risk of aspiration because the formula bypasses the pylorus.

Enteral feedings should be started postoperatively in surgical patients without waiting for flatus or a bowel movement. Current literature indicates the optimal time to be within 48 hours.[4] Patients usually receive gastric feedings on an intermittent schedule; however, for duodenal or jejunal enteral feedings, rapid delivery of the formula into the intestine can cause intolerance and associated dumping syndrome.[3]

Contraindications to gastric enteral feeding include suspected bowel obstruction, upper GI bleeding, intractable vomiting or diarrhea, severe hemodynamic instability, gastrointestinal ischemia, and a high output fistula.[2,5] Liquid nutrient solutions come in various formulas for administration through a nasogastric tube, small-bore feeding tube, or gastrostomy feeding button.[4]

Duodenal and jejunal feedings are contraindicated in patients with bowel obstruction or perforation. Jejunostomy, but not insertion of a nasojejunal tube, is contraindicated in patients with pronounced ascites, coagulopathy, peritoneal dialysis, or peritoneal metastasis.[6] Insertion of a nasojejunal or duodenal tube is contraindicated in patients in whom nasal passage of a tube poses a high risk of misplacement, such as in patients with a basilar skull fracture and those who recently underwent transsphenoidal surgery.[4]

Equipment

Prescribed enteral formula ▪ enteral administration set ▪ gloves ▪ fluid-impermeable pad or towel ▪ graduated container ▪ tap or purified (sterile, distilled, ultrafiltrated, or ultraviolet-light treated) water[1] ▪ enteral syringe (20 mL or larger)[4] ▪ oral care supplies ▪ labels that state ENTERAL USE ONLY—NOT FOR IV USE ▪ tape ▪ supplies for cleaning syringe ▪ stethoscope ▪ disinfectant pad ▪ Optional: IV pole, enteral feeding pump, pH testing supplies, enteral feeding bag, facility-approved disinfectant, scale, tape measure.

An enteral infusion pump is generally required for small-bowel feedings *to ensure accurate delivery of the prescribed formula.*[4]

Preparation of equipment

Allow the formula to warm to room temperature before administration, *because feeding the patient room-temperature formula may reduce the risk of diarrhea.*[1,7]

Inspect all equipment and supplies. If a product is expired, is defective, or has compromised integrity, remove it from patient use, label it as expired or defective, and report the expiration or defect as directed by your facility.

Implementation

- Verify the practitioner's order, including the patient's identifiers, prescribed route based on the enteral tube's tip location, enteral feeding device, prescribed enteral formula, administration method, volume and rate of administration, and type, volume, and frequency of water flushes.[4]
- Review the patient's medical record for X-ray confirmation of tube placement, if needed.[4]
- Gather and prepare the necessary equipment and supplies.
- Visually inspect the enteral feeding formula for damage to the container, altered formula characteristics, and expiration date. Don't use the formula if its integrity is compromised or if it's expired. Instead, obtain a new container of the formula.[4]
- Compare the label on the enteral feeding container with the order in the patient's medical record.[4]
- Perform hand hygiene.[8,9,10,11,12,13]
- Confirm the patient's identity using at least two patient identifiers.[14]
- Provide privacy.[15,16,17,18]
- Explain the procedure to the patient and family (if appropriate) according to their individual communication and learning needs *to increase their understanding, allay their fears, and enhance cooperation.*[19]
- Raise the patient's bed to waist level before providing care *to prevent caregiver back strain.*[20]
- Assess the patient's GI status and risk for aspiration.[4,21,22]
- Position the patient with the head of the bed elevated to at least 30 degrees, or upright in a chair, *to prevent aspiration;* if this position is contraindicated, then consider a reverse Trendelenburg position.[4,21]
- If using an enteral feeding pump, attach the pump to an IV pole and plug the pump into a bedside electrical outlet.
- Perform hand hygiene.[8,9,10,11,12,13]
- Put on gloves *to comply with standard precautions.*[23,24,25]
- Open an enteral feeding bag with administration set tubing if using an open administration system. If using a closed system, open the enteral administration set tubing.
- Pour only a premeasured 4-hour volume of enteral formula into the feeding bag and hang the bag on the IV pole.[4] Set the infusion time for an open enteral nutrition feeding system to 4 to 8 hours.[4] *Limiting the volume decreases the risk of bacterial overgrowth in the formula.* Alternatively, open the sterile enteral formula container and attach it to the enteral administration set.
- If using an enteral feeding pump, attach the enteral administration set tubing to the enteral feeding pump following the manufacturer's instructions.
- Prime the enteral administration set according to the manufacturer's recommendations *to minimize the delivery of air into the GI tract.*
- Make sure that the enteral formula container is labeled with the patient's identifiers; formula name (and strength if diluted); date and time of formula preparation; date and time the formula was hung; administration route, rate, and duration (if cycled or intermittent); initials of who prepared, hung, and checked the enteral formula against the order; expiration date and time; dosing weight (if appropriate); and notation ENTERAL USE ONLY—NOT FOR IV USE.[4]
- Label the enteral administration set with the date and time that it was first hung. Change the administration set according to the manufacturer's instructions *to prevent bacterial growth.*[4]
- Place a fluid-impermeable pad or towel under the patient's feeding tube *to prevent soiling of linens.*[4]
- Verify tube placement before administration using at least two of the following methods:[4,21,26] Observe for a change in external tube length or the incremental marking where the tube exits the patient's nose or mouth *to detect tube migration.*[4,26] Observe for a change in volume of aspirate from the feeding tube, *because a persistent inability to withdraw fluid (or only a few drops of fluid) from the tube may signal the upward displacement of a gastric tube into the esophagus.*[26] Review routine chest and abdominal X-ray reports.[4,26] Aspirate contents from the tube with an enteral

syringe (as shown below) and evaluate the color of the aspirate. *Fasting gastric secretions often appear grassy-green or brown, or clear and colorless.*[4,26] If performed in your facility, measure the pH of aspirate from the tube. *Fasting gastric pH is usually 5 or less, even in patients receiving gastric acid inhibitors.*[4,26] If placement is in doubt, notify the practitioner and arrange for an X-ray, if ordered, to confirm tube location.[26]

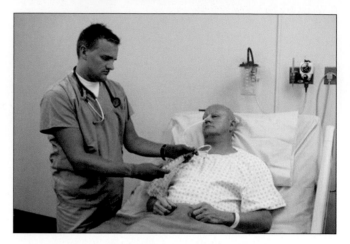

- Flush the enteral tube with at least 30 mL of water (purified water for immunocompromised or critically ill patients), as ordered.[4]
- Connect the end of the enteral administration set tubing to the end of the feeding tube (as shown below).

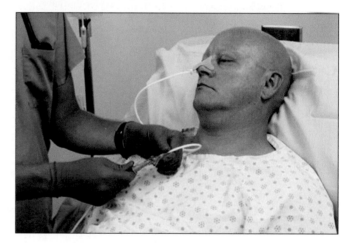

- Trace the tubing from the patient to its point of origin *to make sure you've connected it to the proper port before beginning the tube feeding.*[4,27,28] Tape the connection *to prevent accidental disconnection of the tubing.* Route the tubing toward the patient's feet and place the enteral feeding pump, if used, toward the foot of the bed, *because a standardized approach to keeping IV lines routed toward the head and enteric lines routed toward the feet prevents dangerous misconnections.* If different access sites are used, label each tubing at both the distal (near the patient connection) and proximal (near the source container) ends *to distinguish the different tubings and prevent misconnections.*[28]
- Open the enteral administration set clamp. Regulate the flow to the desired rate. If using an enteral pump, follow the manufacturer's instructions for setting the flow rate.[4] Make sure that the enteral feeding pump alarm limits are set according to the patient's current condition, and that the alarms are turned on, functioning properly, and audible to staff.[29,30,31]
- Monitor the gravity drip rate or pump infusion rate frequently *to ensure accurate delivery of the enteral formula.*
- If you're administering a continuous feeding, flush the enteral feeding tube every 4 hours with at least 30 mL of water (purified water for immunocompromised or critically ill patients), if ordered and tolerated, *to maintain patency and provide hydration.*[4]
- Monitor the patient at least every 4 hours for appropriate positioning *to prevent aspiration.*

■ Assess every 4 hours for GI intolerance to enteral tube feedings by assessing for abdominal distention, monitoring for complaints of abdominal pain, and observing for passage of flatus and stool.[4,21] Don't monitor gastric residual volume (GRV) routinely.[4,22] If GRV is used in critically ill patients, avoid holding the enteral feeding for a GRV of less than 500 mL if the patient has no other signs of feeding intolerance *to prevent inappropriate stoppage of enteral feedings.*[4]

■ To discontinue gastric feeding (depending on the equipment you're using), close the clamp on the enteral administration set tubing or turn off the enteral feeding pump. Disconnect the administration set tubing from the feeding tube. Flush the enteral feeding tube with at least 30 mL of water (purified water in immunocompromised or critically ill patients), if ordered and tolerated.[4] *Flushing maintains the tube's patency by removing excess formula, which could occlude the tubing.* Cover the end of the enteral feeding tube with its plug or cap *to prevent leakage and contamination of the tube.*

■ Perform oral care routinely *to decrease oral bacterial colonization and the risk of aspiration pneumonia.*[22]

■ Remove and discard the fluid-impermeable pad or towel.[25]

■ Monitor the patient's weight and nutritional, fluid, electrolyte, and metabolic status, as ordered, *to evaluate the effectiveness of enteral feedings.*[4]

■ Return the bed to the lowest position *to prevent falls and maintain patient safety.*[32]

■ Clean and dry the syringe and container used for flush administration.[4]
■ Remove and discard your gloves.[23,25]
■ Perform hand hygiene.[8,9,10,11,12,13]
■ Store clean equipment away from potential sources of contamination.[4]
■ Perform hand hygiene.[8,9,10,11,12,13]
■ Clean and disinfect your stethoscope with a disinfectant pad.[33,34]
■ Perform hand hygiene.[8,9,10,11,12,13]
■ If other reusable equipment is used, put on gloves, as needed.[23,24] Then, clean and disinfect other reusable equipment according to the manufacturer's instructions *to prevent the spread of infection.*[33,34] Remove and discard your gloves, if worn,[25] and perform hand hygiene.[8,9,10,11,12,13]
■ Document the procedure.[35,36,37,38]

Special considerations

■ The Joint Commission issued a sentinel event alert concerning medical device alarm safety, *because alarm-related events have been associated with permanent loss of function or death.* Among the major contributing factors were improper alarm settings, alarm settings turned off inappropriately, and alarm signals not audible to staff. Make sure that alarm limits are set appropriately, and that alarms are turned on, functioning properly, and audible to staff. Follow facility guidelines for preventing alarm fatigue.[31]

TROUBLESHOOTING

MANAGING ENTERAL TUBE FEEDING PROBLEMS

This table summarizes complications that can result from enteral tube feedings and related interventions.

COMPLICATIONS	NURSING INTERVENTIONS
Aspiration of gastric secretions	■ Elevate the head of the bed a minimum of 30 degrees, unless contraindicated.[4,21,26] ■ Avoid bolus tube feedings if the patient is at high risk for aspiration.[21] ■ Discontinue feeding immediately. ■ Perform tracheal suction of aspirated contents, if possible. ■ Notify the practitioner. ■ Verify tube placement before feeding *to prevent this complication.*[4,21,26]
Tube obstruction	■ Instill warm water into the tube using a 30- or 60-mL syringe, and apply a gentle back-and-forth motion with the plunger of the syringe. If water flushing doesn't resolve the occlusion, notify the practitioner; an enzyme declogging kit or mechanical declogging device may be ordered to resolve the occlusion. If declogging is unsuccessful, the tube may need to be replaced.[4] ■ Flush the tube with at least 30 mL of water, as ordered, to clear the tube after each feeding to remove excess sticky formula, which could occlude the tube.[4] ■ If you suspect that a small-bore feeding tube may be kinked, try changing the patient's position, or withdraw the tube a few inches and restart. Never use a guidewire to reposition the tube.[4] ■ Whenever possible, use enterally appropriate liquid forms of medications.[4] ■ Flush the tube with purified water before and after each medication administration, especially when multiple medications are administered.[4] ■ Flush the tube before and after intermittent feedings, and at standardized intervals with continuous feedings.[4]
Oral, nasal, pharyngeal, or gastrostomy site irritation or necrosis	■ Provide frequent oral care. ■ Change the tube's position. If necessary, replace the tube. ■ Provide proper skin care at the tube insertion site and use tube-anchoring devices.[4]
Vomiting, bloating, diarrhea, or cramps	■ Reduce the flow rate, if ordered. ■ Allow formula to come to room temperature before administering.[1,7] ■ Notify the practitioner, who may want to change the formula to one that's less osmotic, contains more fiber, or is lactose free; change the medication that may be causing the GI distress; or prescribe an antimotility medication, such as loperamide.[1]
Constipation	■ Provide additional fluids if the patient can tolerate them. ■ Have the patient participate in an exercise program, if possible. ■ Administer a bulk-forming laxative, as ordered, following safe medication administration practices.[40,41,42,43] ■ Review with the practitioner medications that may be causing constipation and discontinue them, as ordered. ■ Increase the fruit, vegetable, or sugar content of the feeding.
Electrolyte imbalance	■ Monitor electrolyte levels, as ordered. ■ Notify the practitioner, who may want to adjust the formula content to correct the deficiency.
Hyperglycemia	■ Monitor blood glucose levels, as ordered. ■ Notify the practitioner, who may want to adjust the sugar content of the formula. ■ Administer insulin, if ordered, following safe medication administration practices.[40,41,42,43]

■ The Joint Commission issued a sentinel event alert related to managing risk during transition to new International Organization for Standardization tubing standards that were designed to prevent dangerous tubing misconnections, which can lead to serious patient injury and death. During the transition, make sure to trace the tubing and catheters from the patient to the point of origin before connecting or reconnecting any device or infusion, at any care transition (such as a new setting or service), and as part of the hand-off process; route tubes and catheters having different purposes in different standardized directions; when there are different access sites or several bags hanging, label the tubing at the distal and proximal ends; use tubing and equipment only as intended; and store medications for different delivery routes in separate locations.[28]

■ In some cases an enteral syringe may be used to administer an enteral feeding after the patient demonstrates tolerance of gravity feeding.

■ If the patient experiences diarrhea, use risk-management algorithm, as recommended, to evaluate the patient's risk and determine the treatment plan.[7,39]

Patient teaching

If the patient will have home enteral tube feeding, provide instructions for the use of an enteral feeding pump to maintain accuracy; use of the enteral syringe or bag and enteral administration set tubing; care of the tube and exit site; and enteral formula mixing, which can be done in an electric blender according to package directions.

Teach the patient and family to discard enteral formula that's not used within 24 hours. If the enteral formula must hang for more than 4 hours, advise the patient to use an enteral feeding bag or enteral administration set with an ice pouch *to decrease the incidence of bacterial growth.* Tell the patient and family to use a new enteral feeding bag daily.

Teach the patient and family signs and symptoms to report to the practitioner or home health care nurse, as well as measures to take in an emergency.

Complications

Erosion of esophageal, tracheal, nasal, and oropharyngeal mucosa can occur if tubes are left in place for a long time. (See *Managing enteral tube feeding problems,* page 297.)

When using the gastric route, frequent or large-volume feedings can cause abdominal bloating and distention. Dehydration, diarrhea, and vomiting can cause metabolic disturbances. Glycosuria, cramping, and abdominal distention usually indicate intolerance. Other complications include aspiration; fluid and electrolyte imbalances, including hyperglycemia, glycosuria, hyperosmolar dehydration, coma, edema, hypernatremia, and essential fatty acid deficiency; constipation; and mechanical problems, such as dislodgement, occlusion, or impairment of the tube.[4,5]

Tube obstruction because of a clog is common when using the duodenal or jejunal route.

The patient may also experience dumping syndrome, in which a large amount of hyperosmotic solution in the duodenum causes excessive diffusion of fluid through the semipermeable membrane and results in nausea, vomiting, cramps, pallor, and diarrhea. In a patient with low serum albumin levels, these symptoms may result from low oncotic pressure in the duodenal mucosa.[1,4]

Documentation

Document the date, volume of formula, and volume of water. In your notes, document GI assessment findings (including the tube exit site, if appropriate), amount of residual gastric contents, if used, tube patency, and verification of tube placement. Also note the amount, type, and time of feeding. Discuss the patient's tolerance of the feeding, including whether the patient experienced nausea, vomiting, cramping, diarrhea, or distention. Note the result of blood and urine tests, hydration status, and any drugs given through the tube. Include the date and time of enteral administration set changes and oral hygiene you performed. Document any tube feeding problems, the date and time you notified the practitioner, interventions you performed, and the patient's response to those interventions. Document teaching provided to the patient and family (if applicable), their understanding of that teaching, and any need for follow-up teaching.

REFERENCES

1 Blumenstein, I., et al. (2014). Gastroenteric tube feeding: Techniques, problems and solutions. *World Journal of Gastroenterology, 20*(26), 8505–8524. https://www.ncbi.nlm.nih.gov/pmc/articles/PMC4093701/

2 Seron-Arbeola, C., et al. (2013). Enteral nutrition in critical care. *Journal of Clinical Medicine Research, 5*(1), 1–11. https://www.ncbi.nlm.nih.gov/pmc/articles/PMC3564561/

3 Heuschkel, R., & Duggan, C. (2019). Enteral feeding: Gastric versus post-pyloric. In *UpToDate,* Seres, D. (Ed.).

4 Boullata, J. I., et al. (2017). ASPEN safe practices for enteral nutrition therapy. *Journal of Parenteral and Enteral Nutrition, 41*(1), 15–103. https://onlinelibrary.wiley.com/doi/10.1177/0148607116673053 (Level VII)

5 Seres, D. (2020). Nutrition support in critically ill patients: An overview. In: *UpToDate,* Parsons, P. E.(Ed.).

6 Niv, E., et al. (2009). Post-pyloric feeding. *World Journal of Gastroenterology, 15,* 1281–1288. (Level V)

7 Nasoenteric tube: Administration of enteral feed. (2021). *The JBI EBP Database.* AN: JBI1811. (Level VII)

8 Centers for Disease Control and Prevention. (2002). Guideline for hand hygiene in health-care settings: Recommendations of the Healthcare Infection Control Practices Advisory Committee and the HICPAC/SHEA/APIC/IDSA Hand Hygiene Task Force. *MMWR Recommendations and Reports, 51*(RR-16), 1–45. https://www.cdc.gov/mmwr/pdf/rr/rr5116.pdf (Level II)

9 The Joint Commission. (2021). Standard NPSG.07.01.01. *Comprehensive accreditation manual for hospitals.* Oakbrook Terrace, IL: The Joint Commission. (Level VII)

10 World Health Organization. (2009). WHO guidelines on hand hygiene in health care: First global patient safety challenge, clean care is safer care. https://apps.who.int/iris/bitstream/handle/10665/44102/9789241597906_eng.pdf?sequence=1 (Level IV)

11 Accreditation Association for Hospitals and Health Systems. (2020). Standard 07.01.21. *Healthcare Facilities Accreditation Program: Accreditation requirements for acute care hospitals.* Chicago, IL: Accreditation Association for Hospitals and Health Systems. (Level VII)

12 Centers for Medicare and Medicaid Services, Department of Health and Human Services. (2020). Condition of participation: Infection control. 42 C.F.R. § 482.42.

13 DNV GL-Healthcare USA, Inc. (2020). IC.1.SR.1. *NIAHO® accreditation requirements, interpretive guidelines and surveyor guidance—revision 20.0.* Milford, OH: DNV GL-Healthcare USA, Inc. (Level VII)

14 The Joint Commission. (2021). Standard NPSG.01.01.01. *Comprehensive accreditation manual for hospitals.* Oakbrook Terrace, IL: The Joint Commission. (Level VII)

15 Centers for Medicare and Medicaid Services, Department of Health and Human Services. (2020). Condition of participation: Patient's rights. 42 C.F.R. § 482.13(c)(1).

16 Accreditation Association for Hospitals and Health Systems. (2020). Standard 15.01.16. *Healthcare Facilities Accreditation Program: Accreditation requirements for acute care hospitals.* Chicago, IL: Accreditation Association for Hospitals and Health Systems. (Level VII)

17 The Joint Commission. (2021). Standard RI.01.01.01. *Comprehensive accreditation manual for hospitals.* Oakbrook Terrace, IL: The Joint Commission. (Level VII)

18 DNV GL-Healthcare USA, Inc. (2020). PR.2.SR.5. *NIAHO® accreditation requirements, interpretive guidelines and surveyor guidance—revision 20.0.* Milford, OH: DNV GL-Healthcare USA, Inc. (Level VII)

19 The Joint Commission. (2021). Standard PC.02.01.21. *Comprehensive accreditation manual for hospitals.* Oakbrook Terrace, IL: The Joint Commission. (Level VII)

20 Waters, T. R., et al. (2009). Safe patient handling training for schools of nursing. https://www.cdc.gov/niosh/docs/2009-127/pdfs/2009-127.pdf (Level VII)

21 American Association of Critical-Care Nurses. (2018). AACN practice alert: Prevention of aspiration in adults. https://www.aacn.org/clinical-resources/practice-alerts/prevention-of-aspiration (Level VII)

22 McClave, S. A., et al. (2016). ACG clinical guideline: Nutrition therapy in the adult hospitalized patient. *The American Journal of Gastroenterology, 111*(3), 315–334. https://journals.lww.com/ajg/pages/articleviewer.aspx?year=2016&issue=03000&article=00014&type=Fulltext (Level VII)

23 Siegel, J. D., et al. (2007, revised 2019). 2007 guideline for isolation precautions: Preventing transmission of infectious agents in healthcare settings. https://www.cdc.gov/infectioncontrol/pdf/guidelines/isolation-guidelines-H.pdf (Level II)

24 Accreditation Association for Hospitals and Health Systems. (2020). Standard 07.01.10. *Healthcare Facilities Accreditation Program: Accreditation requirements for acute care hospitals.* Chicago, IL: Accreditation Association for Hospitals and Health Systems. (Level VII)

25 Occupational Safety and Health Administration. (2019). Bloodborne pathogens, standard number 1910.1030. https://www.osha.gov/pls/oshaweb/owadisp.show_document?p_id=10051&p_table=STANDARDS (Level VII)

26 American Association of Critical-Care Nurses. (2020). AACN practice alert: Initial and ongoing verification of feeding tube placement in adults. https://www.aacn.org/clinical-resources/practice-alerts/initial-and-ongoing-verification-of-feeding-tube-placement-in-adults (Level VII)

27 U.S. Food and Drug Administration. (2017). Examples of medical device misconnections. https://www.fda.gov/medical-devices/medical-device-connectors/examples-medical-device-misconnections

28 The Joint Commission. (2014). Sentinel event alert: Managing risk during transition to new ISO tubing connector standards. https://www.jointcommission.org/-/media/deprecated-unorganized/imported-assets/tjc/system-folders/assetmanager/sea_53_connectors_8_19_14_finalpdf.pdf?db=web&hash=5259E85202D5CE621294E9C46E8ED86C (Level VII)

29 The Joint Commission. (2021). Standard NPSG.06.01.01. *Comprehensive accreditation manual for hospitals.* Oakbrook Terrace, IL: The Joint Commission. (Level VII)

30 Graham, K. C., & Cvach, M. (2010). Monitor alarm fatigue: Standardizing use of physiological monitors and decreasing nuisance alarms. *American Journal of Critical Care, 19,* 28–37.

31 The Joint Commission. (2013). Sentinel event alert: Medical device alarm safety in hospitals. https://www.jointcommission.org/-/media/deprecated-unorganized/imported-assets/tjc/system-folders/topics-library/sea_50_alarms_4_26_16pdf.pdf?db=web&hash=D2E40EF3AE-647F592A52B98DE039F9DD (Level VII)

32 Ganz, D. A., et al. (2013). *Preventing falls in hospitals: A toolkit for improving quality of care* (AHRQ Publication No. 13-0015-EF). Rockville, MD: Agency for Healthcare Research and Quality. https://www.ahrq.gov/professionals/systems/hospital/fallpxtoolkit/index.html (Level VII)

33 Rutala, W. A., et al. (2008, revised 2019). Guideline for disinfection and sterilization in healthcare facilities, 2008. https://www.cdc.gov/infection-control/pdf/guidelines/disinfection-guidelines-H.pdf (Level I)

34 Accreditation Association for Hospitals and Health Systems. (2020). Standard 07.02.03. *Healthcare Facilities Accreditation Program: Accreditation requirements for acute care hospitals.* Chicago, IL: Accreditation Association for Hospitals and Health Systems. (Level VII)

35 The Joint Commission. (2021). Standard RC.01.03.01. *Comprehensive accreditation manual for hospitals.* Oakbrook Terrace, IL: The Joint Commission. (Level VII)

36 Centers for Medicare and Medicaid Services, Department of Health and Human Services. (2020). Condition of participation: Medical record services. 42 C.F.R. § 482.24(b).

37 Accreditation Association for Hospitals and Health Systems. (2020). Standard 10.00.03. *Healthcare Facilities Accreditation Program: Accreditation requirements for acute care hospitals.* Chicago, IL: Accreditation Association for Hospitals and Health Systems. (Level VII)

38 DNV GL-Healthcare USA, Inc. (2020). MR.2.SR.1. *NIAHO® accreditation requirements, interpretive guidelines and surveyor guidance—revision 20.0.* Milford, OH: DNV GL-Healthcare USA, Inc. (Level VII)

39 Barrett, J. S., et al. (2009). Strategies to manage gastrointestinal symptoms complicating enteral feeding. *Journal of Parenteral and Enteral Nutrition, 33,* 21–26.

40 The Joint Commission. (2021). Standard MM.06.01.01. *Comprehensive accreditation manual for hospitals.* Oakbrook Terrace, IL: The Joint Commission. (Level VII)

41 Centers for Medicare and Medicaid Services, Department of Health and Human Services. (2020). Condition of participation: Nursing services. 42 C.F.R. § 482.23(c).

42 Accreditation Association for Hospitals and Health Systems. (2020). Standard 16.01.03. *Healthcare Facilities Accreditation Program: Accreditation requirements for acute care hospitals.* Chicago, IL: Accreditation Association for Hospitals and Health Systems. (Level VII)

43 DNV GL-Healthcare USA, Inc. (2020). MM.1.SR.3. *NIAHO® accreditation requirements, interpretive guidelines and surveyor guidance—revision 20.0.* Milford, OH: DNV GL-Healthcare USA, Inc. (Level VII)

ENTERAL GASTROSTOMY AND JEJUNOSTOMY TUBE FEEDING AND CARE

To access the stomach, duodenum, or jejunum, a practitioner may place a tube through a patient's abdominal wall when enteral feedings are needed.[1] This procedure may be done surgically or percutaneously.

A gastrostomy or jejunostomy tube is usually inserted during intra-abdominal surgery. The tube may be used for feeding during the immediate postoperative period, or it may provide long-term enteral access, depending on the type of surgery. Typically, the practitioner sutures the tube in place to prevent gastric contents from leaking.

In contrast, a percutaneous endoscopic gastrostomy (PEG) or percutaneous endoscopic jejunostomy (PEJ) tube can be inserted endoscopically without the need for laparotomy or general anesthesia. Typically, the insertion is done in the endoscopy suite or in an interventional radiology department.[2] Ultrasound can be used to confirm placement. A PEG or PEJ tube may be used for nutrition, drainage, and decompression. Relative contraindications to endoscopic placement include obstruction (such as an esophageal stricture or duodenal blockage), previous gastric surgery, esophageal or gastric varices, morbid obesity, and ascites.[3] These conditions necessitate surgical placement. Long-term feeding devices should be considered when the need for enteral feeding is at least 4 weeks in adults, children, or full-term infants.[4]

With PEJ tube placement, feedings may begin after 24 hours (or when peristalsis resumes). A PEG tube can be used for feedings within several hours of placement. Current research supports PEG tube usage beginning 4 hours or less after placement in both children and adults.[4] Commercially prepared enteral administration sets and pumps allow for continuous formula administration.[4]

Contraindications to enteral feeding include bowel obstruction, severe ileus, severe upper gastrointestinal bleeding, intractable vomiting or diarrhea, severe hemodynamic instability, gastrointestinal ischemia, and a high output fistula.[5] Nursing care for patients receiving intermittent or continuous enteral tube feedings includes providing skin care at the tube site, maintaining the feeding tube, administering the enteral formula, monitoring the patient's response to feedings, adjusting the feeding schedule, and preparing the patient for self-care after discharge.

Equipment

For intermittent or continuous feeding

Fluid-impermeable pad or towel ▪ enteral syringe (20-mL or larger)[4] ▪ prescribed enteral formula ▪ tap or purified (sterile, distilled, ultrafiltrated, or ultraviolet-light treated) water[4] ▪ enteral administration set ▪ IV pole ▪ gloves ▪ labels that state ENTERAL USE ONLY—NOT FOR IV USE ▪ oral care supplies ▪ tape ▪ stethoscope ▪ disinfectant pad ▪ cleaning supplies for syringe ▪ Optional: pH testing equipment, enteral feeding pump, enteral feeding bag, scale, facility-approved disinfectant, tape measure, graduated container.

For site care

4″ × 4″ (10 cm × 10 cm) gauze pads ▪ soap and water or normal saline solution ▪ water ▪ cotton-tipped applicators ▪ hypoallergenic tape ▪ gloves ▪ label ▪ Optional: external stabilization device, sterile gauze or foam dressing, skin protectant, tape measure.

Preparation of equipment

Allow the enteral formula to warm to room temperature before administration, *because feeding the patient room-temperature formula may reduce the risk of diarrhea.*[6,7]

Inspect all equipment and supplies. If a product is expired, is defective, or has compromised integrity, remove it from patient use, label it as expired or defective, and report the expiration or defect as directed by your facility.

Implementation

▪ Verify the practitioner's order, including the patient's identifiers, the prescribed route based on the enteral tube's tip location, enteral feeding device, prescribed enteral formula, administration method, volume and rate of administration, and type, volume, and frequency of water flushes.[4]

■ Review the patient's medical record *to make sure that catheter placement was confirmed before beginning the feeding.*[4]

■ Gather and prepare the necessary equipment and supplies.

■ Visually inspect the enteral formula for damage to the container, altered formula characteristics, and expiration date. Don't use the formula if its integrity is compromised or if it's expired; instead, obtain a new container of the formula.[4]

■ Compare the label on the enteral formula container to the order in the patient's medical record.[4]

■ Perform hand hygiene.[8,9,10,11,12,13]

■ Confirm the patient's identity using at least two patient identifiers.[14]

■ Provide privacy.[15,16,17,18]

■ Explain the procedure to the patient and family (if appropriate) according to their individual communication and learning needs *to increase their understanding, allay their fears, and enhance cooperation.*[19]

■ Raise the patient's bed to waist level before providing care *to prevent caregiver back strain.*[20]

■ Assess the patient *to determine the risk for aspiration.*[4,21]

■ Position the patient with the head of the bed elevated to at least 30 degrees or upright in a chair *to prevent aspiration.* If this position is contraindicated, consider a reverse Trendelenburg position.[4,22]

■ Perform hand hygiene.[8,9,10,11,12,13]

■ Put on gloves *to comply with standard precautions.*[23,24,25]

For an intermittent or a continuous feeding

■ Open an enteral feeding bag with enteral administration set tubing if using an open administration system. If using a closed system, open the enteral administration set tubing.

■ Pour only a premeasured 4-hour volume of enteral formula into the enteral feeding bag and hang the bag on the IV pole.[4] Set infusion time for open enteral nutrition feeding systems to 4 to 8 hours.[4] *Limiting the volume decreases the risk of bacterial overgrowth in the formula.* Alternatively, open the sterile enteral formula container and attach it to the enteral administration set.

■ If using an enteral feeding pump, attach the enteral administration set tubing to the enteral feeding pump following the manufacturer's instructions.

■ Prime the enteral administration set according to the manufacturer's recommendations *to minimize air delivery into the GI tract.*

■ Make sure that the enteral formula container is labeled with the patient's identifiers; formula name (and strength if diluted); date and time of formula preparation; date and time that the formula was hung; administration route, rate, and duration (if cycled or intermittent); initials of who prepared, hung, and checked the enteral formula against the order; expiration date and time; dosing weight (if appropriate); and notation ENTERAL USE ONLY—NOT FOR IV USE.[4]

■ Label the enteral administration set with the date and time that it was first hung. Change the open-system administration set according to the manufacturer's instructions *to prevent bacterial growth.* If you're using a closed system, change the administration set according to the manufacturer's instructions.[4]

■ Place a fluid-impermeable pad or towel under the patient's feeding tube *to prevent soiling of linens.*

■ Verify tube placement by using at least two of the following methods.[4,22,26] Observe for a change in the external length or incremental marking on the tube at the exit site *to determine whether the tube has migrated.*[4,22,26] Observe for a change in volume of aspirate from the feeding tube, *because a large increase in volume may signal the upward dislocation of a small-bowel feeding tube into the stomach; persistent inability to withdrawal fluid (or only a few drops of fluid) from the tube may signal upward displacement of a gastric tube into the esophagus.*[22,26] Review routine chest and abdominal X-ray reports.[4,22,26] Aspirate tube contents and inspect the visual characteristics of the tube aspirate, *because fasting gastric secretions often appear grassy-green or brown or clear and colorless.*[4,26] If performed at your facility, measure the pH of aspirate from the tube; *fasting gastric pH is usually 5 or less, even in patients receiving gastric acid inhibitors.*[4,22,26]

■ If you suspect tube migration, don't administer the enteral feeding. Instead, notify the practitioner.

■ Flush the enteral feeding tube with at least 30 mL of water, as ordered. Use purified water for immunocompromised or critically ill patients.[4]

■ Connect the end of the enteral administration set tubing to the distal end of the enteral tube. Trace the tubing from the patient to its point of origin *to ensure that it's connected to the proper port before beginning the tube feeding.*[4,27,28]

■ Tape the connection *to prevent accidental disconnection of the tubing.* Route the enteral administration set tubing toward the patient's feet and place the enteral feeding pump toward the foot of the bed, *because a standardized approach to keeping IV lines routed toward the head and enteric lines routed toward the feet prevents dangerous misconnections.*[27,28] If the patient has different access sites or several bags hanging, label each tubing at the distal end (near the patient connection) and proximal end (near the source container) *to distinguish different tubing and prevent dangerous misconnections.*[28]

■ Open the administration set clamp. Regulate the flow to the desired rate. If using an enteral feeding pump, follow the manufacturer's instructions for setting the flow rate and starting the infusion.[4] Make sure that the enteral feeding pump alarm limits are set according to the patient's current condition, and that alarms are turned on, functioning properly, and audible to staff.[29,30,31]

■ Monitor the gravity drip rate or enteral feeding pump infusion rate frequently *to ensure accurate delivery of the enteral formula.*

■ Flush the enteral feeding tube every 4 hours with at least 30 mL of water (purified water for immunocompromised or critically ill patients), as ordered and tolerated, *to maintain patency and provide hydration.*[4]

■ Monitor the patient at least every 4 hours for appropriate positioning.[4]

■ Assess for GI intolerance of enteral tube feedings every 4 hours by assessing for abdominal distention, monitoring for reports of abdominal pain, and observing for passage of flatus and stool.[4,22] Gastric residual volume (GRV) may not need to be used routinely to monitor critically ill patients receiving enteral nutrition.[4,21] For patient care areas that still monitor GRV, avoid holding the enteral feeding for a GRV of less than 500 mL if the patient has no other signs of feeding intolerance *to prevent inappropriate stoppage of enteral feedings.*[4,32]

■ Perform oral care routinely *to decrease oral bacterial colonization and, subsequently, reduce the risk of health care–acquired pneumonia.*[33] (See the "Oral care" procedure.)

■ Remove and discard the fluid-impermeable pad or towel.[25]

■ Monitor the patient's weight and nutritional, fluid, electrolyte, and metabolic statuses, as ordered, *to evaluate the effectiveness of enteral feedings.*

For site care

■ Perform hand hygiene.[8,9,10,11,12,13]

■ Put on gloves *to comply with standard precautions.*[23,24,25]

■ Gently remove the dressing *to prevent skin stripping or tearing* and discard it in an appropriate receptacle.[19,34] Don't cut away the dressing over the catheter, *because you might cut the tube or the sutures holding the tube in place.*

■ Remove and discard your gloves.[23,24]

■ Perform hand hygiene.[8,9,10,11,12,13]

■ Put on a new pair of gloves.[23,24]

Gastrostomy or jejunostomy tube site

■ Assess the tube exit site for new or increasing pain and signs of skin breakdown, redness, edema, induration, and bleeding.[4]

■ Inspect the tube for wear and tear. *A tube that has worn out needs to be replaced.*[3,4]

■ Observe for a change in external tube length or the incremental marking at the exit site *to assess for tube migration.*[3,4]

■ Until healing occurs, clean the skin immediately around the gastrostomy or jejunostomy tube's exit site daily (and as needed) using a cotton-tipped applicator moistened with normal saline solution. Next, using a 4″ × 4″ (10 cm × 10 cm) gauze pad soaked in normal saline solution, clean the adjacent skin and pat it dry using another gauze pad. When the exit site has healed, wash the skin around it with soap and water daily. Rinse the area with water and pat it dry.[3]

■ Apply skin protectant, if necessary, *to prevent skin maceration.*[3]

■ Secure the gastrostomy or jejunostomy tube to the skin with and external stabilization device or hypoallergenic tape *to prevent peristaltic*

migration of the tube and tension on the suture that anchors the tube in place.[35]
- Coil the tube, if necessary, and tape it to the abdomen *to prevent pulling and contamination of the tube.* Rotate the taping site *to prevent skin damage.*

PEG or PEJ site care
- Slide the tube's outer bumper carefully away from the skin about ½" (1.3 cm). Depress the skin surrounding the tube gently and inspect for leakage. *Minimal wound drainage, which appears initially after implantation, should subside in about 1 week.*
- Assess the skin at the exit site for increasing pain and signs of infection, such as redness, edema, and purulent drainage.[3]
- Inspect the tube for wear and tear. *A tube that is worn out needs to be replaced.*[3,4]
- Observe for a change in external tube length or the incremental marking on the tube at the exit site *to assess for tube migration.*[3,4]
- Clean the exit site with soap and water-moistened gauze pads (as shown below), and allow it to dry.[3,36,37]

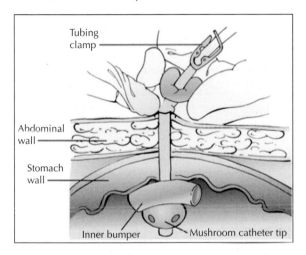

- Rotate the outer bumper 90 degrees *to avoid applying the same tension to the same skin area and to prevent pressure injury formation at the exit site,*[38] and slide the bumper back over the exit site. Ensure that the outer bumper isn't resting too tightly against the skin; one finger's breadth should fit between the skin and the outer bumper.[3]
- If leakage appears at the PEG tube exit site, or if the patient risks dislodging the tube, apply a sterile gauze or foam dressing and an external stabilization device around the site, as needed.[35] Apply the dressing over the outer bumper, *because applying it underneath the outer bumper creates pressure on the gastrostomy tube tract, which could lead to wound abscess.*[37,39]
- Label the dressing with the date, the time, and your initials.

Completing the procedure
- Discard used supplies in the appropriate receptacles.[25]
- Return the bed to the lowest position *to prevent falls and maintain the patient's safety.*[40]
- Remove and discard your gloves.[23,24]
- Perform hand hygiene.[8,9,10,11,12,13]
- Document the procedure.[41,42,43,44]

Special considerations
- The Joint Commission issued a sentinel event alert concerning medical device alarm safety, *because alarm-related events have been associated with permanent loss of function or death.* Among the major contributing factors were improper alarm settings, alarm settings turned off inappropriately, and alarm signals not audible to staff. Make sure that alarm limits are set appropriately, and that alarms are turned on, functioning properly, and audible to staff. Follow facility guidelines for preventing alarm fatigue.[31]
- The Joint Commission issued a sentinel event alert related to managing risk during transition to new International Organization for

Standardization tubing standards that were designed to prevent dangerous tubing misconnections, which can lead to serious patient injury and death. During the transition, make sure to trace the tubing and catheter from the patient to the point of origin before connecting or reconnecting any device or infusion, at any care transition (such as a new setting or service), and as part of the hand-off process; route tubes and catheters with different purposes in different standardized directions; when there are different access sites or several bags hanging, label the tubing at the distal and proximal ends; use tubing and equipment only as intended; and store medications for different delivery routes in separate locations.[28]
- If the patient has poor gastric motility and experiences early satiety, gastric pain, and gastric bloating, venting the gastrostomy tube may provide relief and increase feeding tolerance.[4]
- If the patient experiences diarrhea, a risk management algorithm is recommended *to evaluate the patient's risk and determine the treatment plan.*[6,45]
- Be aware that an enteral feeding pump is generally required for small-bowel feedings, and is preferred for gastric feedings in critically ill patients.[4]
- If skin problems develop, consult a wound, ostomy, and continence nurse (WOCN), if available.
- Ensure that the patient doesn't remove the enteral feeding tube. Consider placing an abdominal binder loosely around a confused patient's abdomen *to prevent the patient from pulling at the tube.*[3,4]
- If the patient has fragile skin, use dressings and tape specially formulated for fragile skin *to prevent skin stripping and tearing during removal.*[34]
- Don't use occlusive dressings over the tube exit site, *because they can lead to skin maceration and breakdown at the exit site.*[37]

Patient teaching
Instruct the patient and family members or other caregivers in all aspects of enteral feedings, including tube maintenance and site care. Specify signs and symptoms to report to the practitioner, define emergency situations, and review actions to take. Use the demonstration and teach-back method to assess patient and caregiver comprehension of the teaching.

When the enteral tube must be replaced, advise the patient that the practitioner may insert a replacement gastrostomy button after removing the initial feeding tube. The procedure may be done in the practitioner's office or an endoscopy or interventional radiology suite of the facility.

As the patient's tolerance of tube feeding improves, the patient may wish to try syringe feedings rather than intermittent feedings. If appropriate, teach the patient how to administer the feeding using the syringe method. (See *Teaching the patient about syringe feeding,* page 302.)

Complications
Common complications related to enteral feeding tubes include GI and other systemic problems, mechanical malfunction, and metabolic disturbances. Abdominal cramping, nausea, vomiting, bloating, and diarrhea may be related to medication, rapid infusion rate (dumping syndrome), fat malabsorption, intestinal atrophy from malnutrition, or formula contamination, osmolarity, or temperature (too cold or too warm). Constipation can result from inadequate hydration, low fiber intake, fecal impaction, or electrolyte and hormonal imbalance.[6]

Systemic problems may be caused by pulmonary aspiration, infection at the tube exit site, or contaminated formula.

Typical mechanical problems include tube dislodgment, obstruction, and impairment. For example, a PEG or PEJ tube may migrate if the external bumper loosens. Occlusion may result from incompletely crushed and liquefied medication particles or inadequate tube flushing. The tube may also rupture or crack from age, drying, or frequent manipulation.

Other complications include vitamin and mineral deficiencies, impaired glucose tolerance, and fluid and electrolyte imbalances.[5]

Documentation
Document the date, time, and amount of each enteral feeding and the water volume instilled. Maintain total volumes for enteral formula and water separately to allow calculation of nutrient intake. Document the

PATIENT TEACHING

TEACHING THE PATIENT ABOUT SYRINGE FEEDING

Teach the patient to administer tube feeding by syringe at home, as appropriate, before being discharged. Here are some points to emphasize.

Initial instructions
First, show the patient how to clamp the feeding tube, remove the syringe's bulb or plunger, and place the tip of the syringe into the feeding tube (as shown below). Then tell the patient to instill between 30 and 60 mL of water into the feeding tube *to make sure it stays open and patent.*

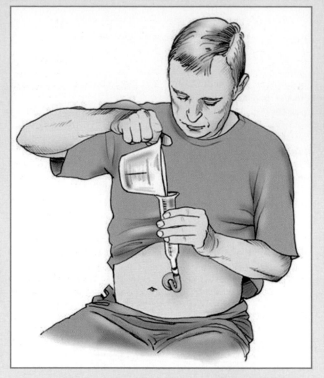

Show the patient how to increase and decrease the solution's flow rate by raising or lowering the syringe. Explain that the patient may need to dilute a thick solution *to promote free flow.*

Finishing up
Inform the patient that the feeding infusion process should take at least 15 minutes. If the process takes less than 15 minutes, dumping syndrome may result.

Show the patient the steps needed to finish the feeding, including how to flush the tube with water, clamp the tube, and clean the equipment for later use. If the patient is using disposable gear, urge the patient to discard it properly. Review instructions for storing unused feeding solution, as appropriate.

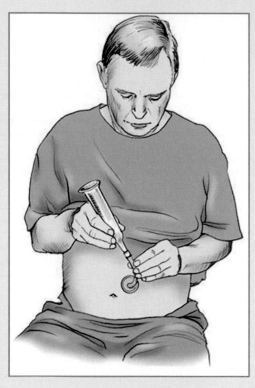

Next, tell the patient to pour the feeding solution into the syringe and begin the feeding (as shown). As the solution flows into the stomach, show the patient how to tilt the syringe *to allow air bubbles to escape.* Describe the discomfort that air bubbles may cause.

Tips for free flow
When about one-fourth of the feeding solution remains, direct the patient to refill the syringe. Caution the patient to avoid letting the syringe empty completely, *because doing so may result in abdominal cramping and gas.*

---

type of enteral formula, infusion method and rate, the patient's tolerance of the procedure and formula, and GRV (if used). Also record GI assessment findings. Document any tube feeding problems or complications, the date and time that you notified the practitioner, prescribed interventions, and the patient's response to those interventions. Note the date and time that you performed exit site care. Document the exit site care interventions. Record the appearance of the exit site and whether you noted any signs of infection, such as redness, swelling, and drainage. If you observed signs of infection, document the name of the practitioner notified, the date and time of notification, prescribed interventions, and the patient's response to those interventions. Document teaching provided to the patient and family (if applicable), their understanding of that teaching, and any need for follow-up teaching.

REFERENCES

1 Craven, R. F., et al. (2017). *Fundamentals of nursing: Human health and function* (8th ed.). Philadelphia, PA: Wolters Kluwer.

2 DeLegge, M. H. (2020). Gastrostomy tubes: Placement and routine care. In: *UpToDate*, Saltzman, J. R., & Seres, D. (Eds.).

3 Wiegand, D. L. (2017). *AACN procedure manual for high acuity, progressive, and critical care* (7th ed.). St. Louis, MO: Saunders.

4 Boullata, J. I., et al. (2017). ASPEN safe practices for enteral nutrition therapy. *Journal of Parenteral and Enteral Nutrition, 41*(1), 15–103. https://onlinelibrary.wiley.com/doi/full/10.1177/0148607116673053 (Level VII)

5 Seres, D. (2021). Nutrition support in critically ill patients: An overview. In: *UpToDate*, Parsons, P. E. (Ed.).

6 Blumenstein, I., et al. (2014). Gastroenteric tube feeding: Techniques, problems and solutions. *World Journal of Gastroenterology, 20*(26), 8505–8524. https://www.ncbi.nlm.nih.gov/pmc/articles/PMC4093701/

7 Nasoenteric tube: Administration of enteral feed. (2021). *The JBI EBP Database.* AN: JBI1811.

8 Centers for Disease Control and Prevention. (2002). Guideline for hand hygiene in health-care settings: Recommendations of the Healthcare Infection Control Practices Advisory Committee and the HICPAC/SHEA/APIC/IDSA Hand Hygiene Task Force. *MMWR Recommendations*

and Reports, 51(RR-16), 1–45. https://www.cdc.gov/mmwr/pdf/rr/rr5116. pdf (Level II)

9 The Joint Commission. (2021). Standard NPSG.07.01.01. *Comprehensive accreditation manual for hospitals.* Oakbrook Terrace, IL: The Joint Commission. (Level VII)

10 World Health Organization. (2009). WHO guidelines on hand hygiene in health care: First global patient safety challenge, clean care is safer care. https://apps.who.int/iris/bitstream/handle/10665/44102/9789241597906_eng.pdf?sequence=1 (Level IV)

11 Centers for Medicare and Medicaid Services, Department of Health and Human Services. (2020). Condition of participation: Infection control. 42 C.F.R. § 482.42.

12 Accreditation Association for Hospitals and Health Systems. (2020). Standard 07.01.21. *Healthcare Facilities Accreditation Program: Accreditation requirements for acute care hospitals.* Chicago, IL: Accreditation Association for Hospitals and Health Systems. (Level VII)

13 DNV GL-Healthcare USA, Inc. (2020). IC.1.SR.1. *NIAHO® accreditation requirements, interpretive guidelines and surveyor guidance—revision 20.0* Milford, OH: DNV GL-Healthcare USA, Inc. (Level VII)

14 The Joint Commission. (2021). Standard NPSG.01.01.01. *Comprehensive accreditation manual for hospitals.* Oakbrook Terrace, IL: The Joint Commission. (Level VII)

15 Accreditation Association for Hospitals and Health Systems. (2020). Standard 15.01.16. *Healthcare Facilities Accreditation Program: Accreditation requirements for acute care hospitals.* Chicago, IL: Accreditation Association for Hospitals and Health Systems. (Level VII)

16 Centers for Medicare and Medicaid Services, Department of Health and Human Services. (2020). Condition of participation: Patient's rights. 42 C.F.R. § 482.13(c)(1).

17 DNV GL-Healthcare USA, Inc. (2020). PR.2.SR.5. *NIAHO® accreditation requirements, interpretive guidelines and surveyor guidance—revision 20.0* Milford, OH: DNV GL-Healthcare USA, Inc. (Level VII)

18 The Joint Commission. (2021). Standard RI.01.01.01. *Comprehensive accreditation manual for hospitals.* Oakbrook Terrace, IL: The Joint Commission. (Level VII)

19 The Joint Commission. (2021). Standard PC.02.01.21. *Comprehensive accreditation manual for hospitals.* Oakbrook Terrace, IL: The Joint Commission. (Level VII)

20 Waters, T. R., et al. (2009). Safe patient handling training for schools of nursing. https://www.cdc.gov/niosh/docs/2009-127/pdfs/2009-127.pdf (Level VII)

21 McClave, S. A., et al. (2016). ACG clinical guideline: Nutrition therapy in the adult hospitalized patient. *The American Journal of Gastroenterology, 111*(3), 315–344. https://journals.lww.com/ajg/pages/articleviewer.aspx?-year=2016&issue=03000&article=00014&type=Fulltext (Level VII)

22 American Association of Critical-Care Nurses. (2018). AACN practice alert: Prevention of aspiration in adults. https://www.aacn.org/clinical-resources/practice-alerts/prevention-of-aspiration (Level VII)

23 Siegel, J. D., et al. (2007, revised 2019). 2007 guideline for isolation precautions: Preventing transmission of infectious agents in healthcare settings. https://www.cdc.gov/infectioncontrol/pdf/guidelines/isolation-guidelines-H.pdf (Level II)

24 Accreditation Association for Hospitals and Health Systems. (2020). Standard 07.01.10. *Healthcare Facilities Accreditation Program: Accreditation requirements for acute care hospitals.* Chicago, IL: Accreditation Association for Hospitals and Health Systems. (Level VII)

25 Occupational Safety and Health Administration. (2019). Bloodborne pathogens, standard number 1910.1030. https://www.osha.gov/pls/oshaweb/owadisp.show_document?p_id=10051&p_table=STANDARDS (Level VII)

26 American Association of Critical-Care Nurses (AACN). (2020). AACN practice alert: Initial and ongoing verification of feeding tube placement in adults. https://www.aacn.org/clinical-resources/practice-alerts/initial-and-ongoing-verification-of-feeding-tube-placement-in-adults (Level VII)

27 U.S. Food and Drug Administration. (2017). Examples of medical device misconnections. https://www.fda.gov/medical-devices/medical-device-connectors/examples-medical-device-misconnections

28 The Joint Commission. (2014). Sentinel event alert 53: Managing risk during transition to new ISO tubing connector standards. https://www.jointcommission.org/-/media/deprecated-unorganized/imported-assets/tjc/system-folders/assetmanager/sea_53_connectors_8_19_14_finalpdf.pdf?db=web&hash=5259E85202D5CE621294E9C46E8ED86C (Level VII)

29 The Joint Commission. (2021). Standard NPSG.06.01.01. *Comprehensive accreditation manual for hospitals.* Oakbrook Terrace, IL: (Level VII)

30 Graham, K. C., & Cvach, M. (2010). Monitor alarm fatigue: Standardizing use of physiological monitors and decreasing nuisance alarms. *American Journal of Critical Care, 19*, 28–37.

31 The Joint Commission. (2013). Sentinel event alert 50: Medical device alarm safety in hospitals. https://www.jointcommission.org/-/media/deprecated-unorganized/imported-assets/tjc/system-folders/topics-library/sea_50_alarms_4_26_16pdf.pdf?db=web&hash=D2E40EF3AE-647F592A52B98DE039F9DD (Level VII)

32 McClave, S. A., et al. (2016). Guidelines for the provision and assessment of nutrition support therapy in the adult critically ill patient: Society of Critical Care Medicine and American Society for Parenteral and Enteral Nutrition. *Journal of Parenteral and Enteral Nutrition, 40*(2), 159–211. https://onlinelibrary.wiley.com/doi/epdf/10.1177/0148607115621863 (Level VII)

33 American Association of Critical-Care Nurses. (2017). AACN practice alert: Oral care for acutely and critically ill patients. https://www.aacn.org/clinical-resources/practice-alerts/oral-care-for-acutely-and-critically-ill-patients (Level VII)

34 LeBlanc, K., et al. (2013). International skin tear advisory panel: A tool kit to aid in the prevention, assessment, and treatment of skin tears using a simplified classification system. *Advances in Skin & Wound Care, 26*, 459–476. (Level IV)

35 Fleischer, I., & Bryant, D. (2010). Techniques for preventing and managing tube-related complications. *Journal of Wound, Ostomy, and Continence Nursing, 37*, 686–690. (Level VII)

36 Heuschkel, R. B., et al. (2015). ESPGHAN position paper on management of percutaneous gastrostomy in children and adolescents. *Journal of Pediatric Gastroenterology and Nutrition, 60*, 131–141. (Level VII)

37 Itkin, M., et al. (2011). Multidisciplinary practical guidelines for gastrointestinal access for enteral nutrition and decompression from the Society of Interventional Radiology and American Gastroenterological Association (AGA) Institute, with endorsement by Canadian Interventional Radiological Association (CIRA) and Cardiovascular and Interventional Radiological Society of Europe (CIRSE). *Journal of Vascular and Interventional Radiology, 22*, 1089–1106. https://www.jvir.org/article/S1051-0443(11)00850-5/pdf (Level VII)

38 Soscia, J., & Friedman, J. N. (2011). A guide to the management of common gastrostomy and gastrojejunostomy tube problems. *Paediatrics & Child Health, 16*(5), 281–287. http://europepmc.org/articles/PMC3114992

39 DeLegge, M. H. (2019). Gastrostomy tubes: Complications and their management. In: *UpToDate*, Saltzman, J. R., & Seres, D. (Eds.).

40 Ganz, D. A., et al. (2013, reviewed 2021). *Preventing falls in hospitals: A toolkit for improving quality of care* (AHRQ Publication No. 13-0015-EF). Rockville, MD: Agency for Healthcare Research and Quality. https://www.ahrq.gov/professionals/systems/hospital/fallpxtoolkit/index.html (Level VII)

41 The Joint Commission. (2021). Standard RC.01.03.01. *Comprehensive accreditation manual for hospitals.* Oakbrook Terrace, IL: The Joint Commission. (Level VII)

42 Accreditation Association for Hospitals and Health Systems. (2020). Standard 10.00.03. *Healthcare Facilities Accreditation Program: Accreditation requirements for acute care hospitals.* Chicago, IL: Accreditation Association for Hospitals and Health Systems. (Level VII)

43 Centers for Medicare and Medicaid Services, Department of Health and Human Services. (2020). Condition of participation: Medical record services. 42 C.F.R. § 482.24(b).

44 DNV GL-Healthcare USA, Inc. (2020). MR.2.SR.1. *NIAHO® accreditation requirements, interpretive guidelines and surveyor guidance—revision 20.0.* Milford, OH: DNV GL-Healthcare USA, Inc. (Level VII)

45 Barrett, J. S., et al. (2009). Strategies to manage gastrointestinal symptoms complicating enteral feeding. *Journal of Parenteral and Enteral Nutrition, 33*, 21–26.

ENTERAL TUBE DRUG INSTILLATION

An enteral tube allows direct administration of medication into the GI system of patients who can't ingest the drug orally. Before administration, check the patency and positioning of the tube and assess the patient's GI status, *because the procedure is contraindicated if the tube is obstructed or positioned improperly, the patient is vomiting around the tube, or the patient's bowel sounds are absent because of such conditions as mesenteric ischemia, small-bowel obstruction, and paralytic ileus.*[1,2]

Administering medications via the enteral route poses risks, *because most medications given via this route weren't originally formulated for direct GI tract administration.*[3] Medications administered enterally must be given in liquid form to avoid enteral tube obstruction. They must be administered separately through an enteral tube *because of the risk of physical and chemical incompatibilities, tube obstruction, and altered therapeutic response.* They shouldn't be added directly to an enteral feeding formula.[2,4,5]

Equipment

Prescribed medication ▪ fluid-impermeable pad or towel ▪ clean enteral syringe (20 mL or larger)[2] ▪ purified water (distilled, ultrafiltrated, ultraviolet-light treated, or sterile)[2] ▪ medicine cup(s) ▪ gloves ▪ cleaning supplies for syringe and container for flushing ▪ Optional: mortar and pestle or other pill-crushing device, pH testing supplies, measuring tape, gown, mask with face shield or mask and goggles, labels.

Preparation of Equipment

Inspect all equipment and supplies. If a product is expired, is defective, or has compromised integrity, remove it from patient use, label it as expired or defective, and report the expiration or defect as directed by your facility. Consult the pharmacist if the patient receives a continuous tube feeding. You may need to withhold the feeding for at least 30 minutes before administering the medication if separation is required *to avoid altered drug bioavailability.*[2,5]

Implementation

▪ Avoid distractions and interruptions when preparing and administering the medication *to prevent medication errors.*[6,7]
▪ Verify the practitioner's order, including the drug, dose, dosage form, route, and access device.[2,8,9,10,11]
▪ Reconcile the patient's medications when the practitioner prescribes a new medication *to reduce the risk of medication errors, including omissions, duplications, dosing errors, and drug interactions.*[12]
▪ Review the patient's medical record to verify the location of the distal tube tip before administering the medication, *to ensure adequate administration and absorption of the drug.*[2,13,14]
▪ Gather and prepare the necessary equipment, supplies, and prescribed medication.
▪ Compare the medication label to the order in the patient's medical record.[8,9,10,11]
▪ Check the patient's medical record for an allergy or contraindication to the prescribed medication. If an allergy or contraindications exist, don't administer the medication, and notify the practitioner.[8,9,10,11]
▪ Check the expiration date on the medication. If the medication is expired, return it to the pharmacy and obtain new medication.[8,9,10,11]
▪ Visually inspect the solution for particles or discoloration, or other loss of integrity; don't administer the medication if integrity is compromised.[8,9,10,11]
▪ Discuss any unresolved concerns about the medication with the patient's practitioner.[8,9,10,11]
▪ Consult the pharmacist to determine the safest dosage form of the drug before administration, if needed. Use medications prepared by the pharmacy under controlled conditions whenever possible.[2] If needed and permitted by your facility, you may prepare nonhazardous and nonallergenic medications in a clean area of a medication room.[2]
▪ Use the available liquid dosage form if it's appropriate for enteral administration. Further dilute the drug before administration, as directed by the pharmacist; the volume of diluent required to further dilute liquid medication depends on the desired viscosity, osmolality, or both.[2]
▪ If the liquid form of a medication isn't appropriate or available, substitute only immediate-release dosage forms, and prepare them according to the pharmacist's instructions. This may include crushing simple compressed tablets to a fine powder using a mortar and pestle or other pill-crushing device and mixing the powder with purified water,[2] or opening hard gelatin capsules and mixing the powder containing the immediate-release medication with purified water in a medicine cup.[2]
▪ Perform hand hygiene.[15,16,17,18,19,20]

▪ Confirm the patient's identity using at least two patient identifiers.[21]
▪ Provide privacy.[22,23,24,25]
▪ If the patient is receiving the medication for the first time, teach the patient and family (if appropriate) about potential adverse reactions or other concerns related to the medication.[8,9,10,11]
▪ Explain the procedure to the patient and family (if appropriate) according to their individual communication and learning needs *to increase their understanding, allay their fears, and enhance cooperation.*[26]
▪ Verify that the medication is being administered at the proper time, in the prescribed dose, and by the correct route to reduce the risk of medication errors.[8,9,10,11]
▪ If your facility uses bar-code technology, use it as directed by your facility.
▪ Raise the bed to waist level before providing care *to prevent caregiver back strain.*[27]
▪ Place a fluid-impermeable pad or towel across the patient's chest *to avoid soiling the linens during the procedure.*
▪ Elevate the head of the bed to at least 30 degrees. If contraindications exist, consider the reverse Trendelenburg position *to reduce the risk for aspiration.*[2]
▪ Perform hand hygiene.[15,16,17,18,19,20]
▪ Put on gloves and other personal protective equipment, as needed, *to comply with standard precautions.*[28,29,30]
▪ Trace the tubing from the patient to its point of origin *to make sure that you're accessing the correct tube before beginning medication administration.*[2,31,32]
▪ Unclamp the enteral tube if not in continuous use, or (if not already done) stop the continuous enteral feeding, clamp the enteral administration set, and cap the distal end of the tubing.
▪ Verify enteral tube placement using at least two of the following.[2] Observe for a change in the external tube length or the incremental marking at the exit site.[2,14] Review chest and abdominal X-ray reports.[2,14] Aspirate tube contents and inspect the visual characteristics of the tube aspirate; fasting gastric secretions often appear grassy-green, brown, or clear and colorless. Aspirate from a tube that has perforated the pleural space typically has a pale yellow serous appearance.[2,14] Measure the pH of aspirate from the tube if your facility uses pH measurement. Fasting gastric pH is usually 5 or less, even in patients receiving gastric acid inhibitors. Fluid aspirated from a tube in the pleural space typically has a pH of 7 or higher.[2]
▪ Notify the practitioner if tube placement is in doubt. Arrange for an X-ray, if ordered.[2,14]
▪ After verifying proper tube placement, flush the tube with at least 15 mL of purified water.[2]
▪ Monitor the patient closely throughout instillation. Stop the procedure immediately and notify the practitioner if the patient shows signs of distress.

NURSING ALERT Don't mix different medications intended for administration through the enteral tube together because of the risks of physical and chemical incompatibilities, tube obstruction, and altered therapeutic drug responses.[2]

▪ Administer the medication using a clean enteral syringe (as shown below).[2]

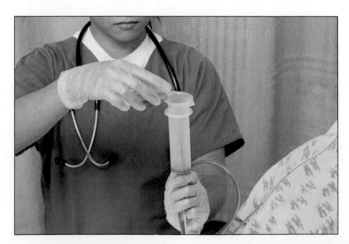

■ Flush the enteral tube again with at least 15 mL of purified water, taking into consideration the patient's fluid volume status.[2]

■ Repeat the procedure with the next medication, if prescribed.[2]

■ Flush the enteral tube one final time with at least 15 mL of purified water.[2]

■ Clamp the enteral tube and detach the syringe.

■ Replace the cap at the tip of the enteral tube. Alternatively, attach the enteral administration set tubing to the end of the enteral tube, unclamp the tube, and restart the enteral feeding, if ordered, *to avoid compromising the patient's nutrition status.* Withhold the enteral feeding for 30 minutes or more after medication administration only if separation is indicated to avoid altered drug bioavailability. Consult a pharmacist, as needed.

■ Route the tubing toward the patient's feet and place the enteral feeding pump (if used) toward the foot of the bed, *because a standardized approach of keeping IV lines routed toward the head and enteric lines routed toward the feet prevents dangerous misconnections.*[31] If different access sites are used, label each tubing at the distal end (near the patient connection) and proximal end (near the source container) *to distinguish different tubing and prevent misconnections.*[32]

■ Remove and discard the fluid-impermeable pad or towel.[30]

■ Keep the head of the bed elevated to at least 30 degrees, or have the patient sit upright in a chair. If these positions are contraindicated, consider the reverse Trendelenburg position, as ordered, *to reduce the risk of aspiration.*[2]

■ Return the bed to the lowest position *to prevent falls and maintain patient safety.*[33]

■ Clean and dry reusable equipment, including enteral syringes and containers for flushing and medication administration.[2]

■ Discard used supplies in appropriate receptacles.[30]

■ Remove and discard your gloves and, if worn, other personal protective equipment.[28,30]

■ Perform hand hygiene.[15,16,17,18,19,20]

■ Store the equipment away from potential sources of contamination.[2]

■ Perform hand hygiene.[15,16,17,18,19,20]

■ Document the procedure.[34,35,36,37]

Special considerations

■ If the patient's gastrostomy tube becomes clogged, flush the tube with water. Notify the practitioner if flushing with water is unsuccessful. A pancreatic enzyme solution, an enzymatic declogging kit, or a mechanical declogging device may be considered before exchanging the tube for a new one.[2]

■ The Joint Commission issued a sentinel event alert related to managing risk during the transition to the new International Organization for Standardization tubing standards that were designed to prevent dangerous tubing misconnections, which can lead to serious patient injury and death. During the transition, make sure to trace the tubing and catheter from the patient to the point of origin before connecting or reconnecting any device or infusion, at any care transition (such as a new setting or service), and as part of the hand-off process; route tubes and catheters with different purposes in different standardized directions; when there are different access sites or several bags hanging, label the tubing at the distal and proximal ends; use tubing and equipment only as intended; and store medications for different delivery routes in separate locations.[32]

Patient teaching

If the patient will require an enteral tube after discharge, give the patient and family (as appropriate) oral and written instructions for instilling medication through the tube. Remain with the patient when the patient or family performs the procedure the first few times *so that you can provide assistance and answer any questions.* Encourage the patient and correct errors in technique, as needed.

Complications

Potential complications of enteral drug administration include aspiration, drug–drug or drug–nutrient interactions, a clogged feeding tube, reduced drug effect, and increased drug toxicity. The risk of complications increases with inappropriate preparation or administration technique.[2]

Some medications in liquid form contain a large amount of sorbitol, which may cause abdominal cramps and diarrhea.[4]

Documentation

Document the medication strength, dose, administration route, and date and time of administration. Record any adverse reactions to the prescribed medication, the date and time that you notified the practitioner, prescribed interventions, and the patient's response to those interventions.[38] On the intake and output record, note the amount of fluid instilled. Document teaching provided to the patient and family (if applicable), their understanding of that teaching, and any need for follow-up teaching. Document whether the patient or family gave a return demonstration.

REFERENCES

1 Makic, M. B. F., et al. (2011). Evidence-based practice habits: Putting more sacred cows out to pasture. *Critical Care Nurse, 31*(2), 38–62. (Level V)

2 Boullata, J. I., et al. (2017). ASPEN safe practices for enteral nutrition therapy. *Journal of Parenteral and Enteral Nutrition, 41*(1), 15–103. https://onlinelibrary.wiley.com/doi/full/10.1177/0148607116673053 (Level VII)

3 White, R., & Bradnam, V. (2015). *Handbook of drug administration via enteral feeding tubes* (3rd ed.). London, UK: Pharmaceutical Press. https://rudiapt.files.wordpress.com/2017/11/handbook-of-drug-administration-via-enteral-feeding-tubes-2015.pdf

4 Moola, S. (2021). Enteral tubes: Administration of medication. *The JBI EBP Database.* AN: JBI19646. (Level VII)

5 Institute for Safe Medication Practices. (2010). Preventing errors when administering drugs via an enteral feeding tube. *Nurse Advise-ERR, 8*(9), 1–4. https://www.ismp.org/resources/preventing-errors-when-administering-drugs-enteral-feeding-tube

6 Westbrook, J., et al. (2010). Association of interruptions with an increased risk and severity of medication administration errors. *Archives of Internal Medicine, 170*, 683–690. (Level IV)

7 Institute for Safe Medication Practices. (2012). Side tracks on the safety express: Interruptions lead to errors and unfinished...Wait, what was I doing? *Nurse Advise-ERR, 11*(2), 1–4. https://www.ismp.org/resources/side-tracks-safety-express-interruptions-lead-errors-and-unfinished-wait-what-was-i-doing?id=3/

8 The Joint Commission. (2021). Standard MM.06.01.01. *Comprehensive accreditation manual for hospitals.* Oakbrook Terrace, IL: The Joint Commission. (Level VII)

9 Centers for Medicare and Medicaid Services, Department of Health and Human Services. (2020). Condition of participation: Nursing services. 42 C.F.R. § 482.23(c).

10 Accreditation Association for Hospitals and Health Systems. (2020). Standard 16.01.03. *Healthcare Facilities Accreditation Program: Accreditation requirements for acute care hospitals.* Chicago, IL: Accreditation Association for Hospitals and Health Systems. (Level VII)

11 DNV GL-Healthcare USA, Inc. (2020). MM.1.SR.3. *NIAHO® accreditation requirements, interpretive guidelines and surveyor guidance—revision 20.0.* Milford, OH: DNV GL-Healthcare USA, Inc. (Level VII)

12 The Joint Commission. (2021). Standard NPSG.03.06.01. *Comprehensive accreditation manual for hospitals.* Oakbrook Terrace, IL: The Joint Commission. (Level VII)

13 Wilson, N., & Best, C. (2011). Administration of medicines via an enteral feeding tube. *Nursing Times, 107*(41), 18–20.

14 American Association of Critical-Care Nurses. (2016, updated 2020). AACN practice alert: Initial and ongoing verification of feeding tube placement in adults. https://www.aacn.org/clinical-resources/practice-alerts/initial-and-ongoing-verification-of-feeding-tube-placement-in-adults (Level VII)

15 The Joint Commission. (2021). Standard NPSG.07.01.01. *Comprehensive accreditation manual for hospitals.* Oakbrook Terrace, IL: The Joint Commission. (Level VII)

16 Centers for Disease Control and Prevention. (2002). Guideline for hand hygiene in health-care settings: Recommendations of the Healthcare Infection Control Practices Advisory Committee and the HICPAC/SHEA/APIC/IDSA Hand Hygiene Task Force. *MMWR Recommendations and Reports, 51*(RR-16), 1–45. https://www.cdc.gov/mmwr/pdf/rr/rr5116.pdf (Level II)

17 World Health Organization. (2009). WHO guidelines on hand hygiene in health care: First global patient safety challenge,

clean care is safer care. https://apps.who.int/iris/bitstream/handle/10665/44102/9789241597906_eng.pdf?sequence=1 (Level IV)

18 Centers for Medicare and Medicaid Services, Department of Health and Human Services. (2020). Condition of participation: Infection control. 42 C.F.R.§ 482.42.

19 Accreditation Association for Hospitals and Health Systems. (2020). Standard 07.01.21. *Healthcare Facilities Accreditation Program: Accreditation requirements for acute care hospitals.* Chicago, IL: Accreditation Association for Hospitals and Health Systems. (Level VII)

20 DNV GL-Healthcare USA, Inc. (2020). IC.1.SR.1. *NIAHO® accreditation requirements, interpretive guidelines and surveyor guidance—revision 20.0.* Milford, OH: DNV GL-Healthcare USA, Inc. (Level VII)

21 The Joint Commission. (2021). Standard NPSG.01.01.01. *Comprehensive accreditation manual for hospitals.* Oakbrook Terrace, IL: The Joint Commission. (Level VII)

22 Centers for Medicare and Medicaid Services, Department of Health and Human Services. (2020). Condition of participation: Patient's rights. 42 C.F.R. § 482.13(c)(1).

23 Accreditation Association for Hospitals and Health Systems. (2020). Standard 15.01.16. *Healthcare Facilities Accreditation Program: Accreditation requirements for acute care hospitals.* Chicago, IL: Accreditation Association for Hospitals and Health Systems. (Level VII)

24 The Joint Commission. (2021). Standard RI.01.01.01. *Comprehensive accreditation manual for hospitals.* Oakbrook Terrace, IL: The Joint Commission. (Level VII)

25 DNV GL-Healthcare USA, Inc. (2020). PR.2.SR.5. *NIAHO® accreditation requirements, interpretive guidelines and surveyor guidance—revision 20.0.* Milford, OH: DNV GL-Healthcare USA, Inc. (Level VII)

26 The Joint Commission. (2021). Standard PC.02.01.21. *Comprehensive accreditation manual for hospitals.* Oakbrook Terrace, IL: The Joint Commission. (Level VII)

27 Waters, T. R., et al. (2009). Safe patient handling training for schools of nursing. https://www.cdc.gov/niosh/docs/2009-127/pdfs/2009-127.pdf (Level VII)

28 Siegel, J. D., et al. (2007, revised 2019). 2007 guideline for isolation precautions: Preventing transmission of infectious agents in healthcare settings. https://www.cdc.gov/infectioncontrol/pdf/guidelines/disinfection-guidelines-H.pdf (Level II)

29 Accreditation Association for Hospitals and Health Systems. (2020). Standard 07.01.10. *Healthcare Facilities Accreditation Program: Accreditation requirements for acute care hospitals.* Chicago, IL: Accreditation Association for Hospitals and Health Systems. (Level VII)

30 Occupational Safety and Health Administration. (2019). Bloodborne pathogens, standard number 1910.1030. https://www.osha.gov/pls/oshaweb/owadisp.show_document?p_id=10051&p_table=STANDARDS (Level VII)

31 U.S. Food and Drug Administration. (2017). Examples of medical device misconnections. https://www.fda.gov/medical-devices/medical-device-connectors/examples-medical-device-misconnections

32 The Joint Commission. (2014). Sentinel event alert 53: Managing risk during transition to new ISO tubing connector standards. https://www.jointcommission.org/assets/1/6/SEA_53_Connectors_8_19_14_final.pdf (Level VII)

33 Ganz, D. A., et al. (2013, reviewed 2021). *Preventing falls in hospitals: A toolkit for improving quality of care* (AHRQ Publication No. 13-0015-EF). Rockville, MD: Agency for Healthcare Research and Quality. https://www.ahrq.gov/professionals/systems/hospital/fallpxtoolkit/index.html (Level VII)

34 The Joint Commission. (2021). Standard RC.01.03.01. *Comprehensive accreditation manual for hospitals.* Oakbrook Terrace, IL: The Joint Commission. (Level VII)

35 Centers for Medicare and Medicaid Services, Department of Health and Human Services. (2020). Condition of participation: Medical record services. 42 C.F.R. § 482.24(b).

36 Accreditation Association for Hospitals and Health Systems. (2020). Standard 10.00.03. *Healthcare Facilities Accreditation Program: Accreditation requirements for acute care hospitals.* Chicago, IL: Accreditation Association for Hospitals and Health Systems. (Level VII)

37 DNV GL-Healthcare USA, Inc. (2020). MR.2.SR.1. *NIAHO® accreditation requirements, interpretive guidelines and surveyor guidance—revision 20.0.* Milford, OH: DNV GL-Healthcare USA, Inc. (Level VII)

38 The Joint Commission. (2021). Standard RC.02.01.01. *Comprehensive accreditation manual for hospitals.* Oakbrook Terrace, IL: The Joint Commission. (Level VII)

Epicardial pacing and care

Epicardial pacing wires are commonly positioned on the epicardial (outer) surface of the heart after cardiac surgery[1,2] to manage surgery-related arrhythmias. Depending on the patient's need, the surgeon may place unipolar or bipolar electrodes on the right atrium, right ventricle, or both,[3] loosely suturing the electrodes to the epicardial surface and bringing them out through the chest wall through small incisions.[3]

If the patient requires pacing, you or the practitioner will connect epicardial pacing wires to the pulse generator of a temporary pacemaker.[3] When the patient becomes hemodynamically stable and no longer requires pacing, the surgeon or a specially trained nurse removes the wires.

Equipment

For insertion and care

Pulse generator with new battery ▪ extra batteries ▪ connecting cable ▪ atrial epicardial wires ▪ ventricular epicardial wires ▪ sterile rubber finger cot, glove, or plastic cap ▪ sterile occlusive dressing ▪ label ▪ gloves ▪ cardiac monitoring equipment ▪ vital signs monitoring equipment ▪ stethoscope ▪ disinfectant pad ▪ 12-lead electrocardiogram (ECG) machine and supplies ▪ Emergency equipment (code cart with emergency medications, defibrillator, handheld resuscitation bag with mask, intubation equipment) ▪ Optional: protective plastic cover, gown, mask, goggles, mask with face shield.

For removal

Gloves ▪ prescribed analgesic ▪ sterile gauze ▪ antiseptic solution (chlorhexidine-based) ▪ tape ▪ suture removal kit ▪ cardiac monitoring equipment ▪ vital signs monitoring equipment ▪ stethoscope ▪ disinfectant pad ▪ sterile occlusive dressing ▪ emergency equipment (code cart with cardiac medications, defibrillator, handheld resuscitation bag with mask, intubation equipment) ▪ temporary transcutaneous or transvenous pacing equipment ▪ Optional: IV catheter insertion equipment, gown, mask, goggles, mask with face shield.

Preparation of equipment

Inspect all equipment and supplies. If a product is expired, is defective, or has compromised integrity, remove it from patient use, label it as expired or defective, and report the expiration or defect as directed by your facility. Make sure emergency equipment is functioning properly and readily available.

For insertion

Insert a new battery into the pulse generator and make sure it's functioning properly. Make sure extra batteries are available.[4]

For removal

Check that temporary transcutaneous or transvenous pacing equipment are readily available.

Implementation

For insertion and care

- Verify the practitioner's order.
- Gather and prepare the necessary equipment and supplies.
- If required by your facility, confirm that informed consent has been obtained and that the signed consent form is in the patient's medical record.[5,6,7,8]
- Conduct a preprocedure verification *to make sure that all relevant documentation, related information, and equipment are available and correctly identified to the patient's identifiers.*[9,10]
- Verify that the laboratory and imaging studies have been completed as ordered, and that the results are in the patient's medical record. Notify the practitioner of any unexpected results.
- Perform hand hygiene.[11,12,13,14,15,16]
- Confirm the patient's identity using at least two patient identifiers.[17]
- Provide privacy.[18,19,20,21]

- Raise the patient's bed to waist level before providing care *to prevent caregiver back strain.*[22]
- Explain the procedure to the patient and family (if appropriate) according to their individual communication and learning needs *to increase their understanding, allay their fears, and enhance cooperation.*[23] Reinforce the practitioner's explanation of the procedure and answer any questions.[5,6,7,8]
- The surgical team will conduct a time-out immediately before starting the procedure *to perform a final assessment that the correct patient, site, positioning, and procedure are identified and all relevant information and necessary equipment are available.*[24]
- The surgeon will attach epicardial wires to the epicardium just before the end of surgery. Depending on the patient's condition, the surgeon may insert atrial wires, ventricular wires, or both.[3]
- Perform hand hygiene.[11,12,13,14,15,16]
- Put on gloves and, as needed, other personal protective equipment *to comply with standard procedures and to prevent microshock.*[2,3,25,26,27]
- After wire insertion, attach the patient to the bedside cardiac monitor *to monitor the patient's heart rhythm and evaluate pacemaker function.*[3] (See the "Cardiac monitoring" procedure.) Make sure that the alarm limits are set appropriately for the patient's current condition, and that the alarms are turned on, functioning properly, and audible to staff.[28,29,30,31]
- Ensure that the pulse generator is turned off.[3,32]
- Attach the connecting cable to the pulse generator by connecting the positive pole on the cable to the positive pole on the pulse generator and the negative pole on the cable to the negative pole on the pulse generator.[3]
- Expose the epicardial pacing wires and identify the atrial and ventricular wires if both are present. Epicardial wires that exit the chest to the right of the sternum originate in the atrium; wires that exit to the left of the sternum originate in the ventricle.[3]
- Using the connecting cable, connect the epicardial wires to the pulse generator. Connect the positive electrode to the positive terminal on the pulse generator through the connecting cable; connect the negative electrode to the negative terminal.[3] Make sure that the connecting cable is tightly secured to the generator, *to ensure proper pacing and sensing to prevent accidental disconnection.*[3]
- Set the pacing mode, rate, and energy level (output or milliamperes [mA]) according to the practitioner's order, or as determined by sensitivity (the level at which intrinsic cardiac activity is sensed by electrodes) and stimulation threshold testing (the minimum amount of voltage necessary to initiate depolarization).[3] (See *Sensitivity and stimulation threshold testing.*)
- After adjusting the pacemaker settings, place the protective plastic cover over the pacemaker controls, or lock the controls.[3]
- Apply a sterile occlusive dressing over the insertion site *to prevent infection at the insertion site* and label it with the date, the time, and your initials, or as directed by your facility.[3]
- Secure the pulse generator *to prevent it from falling or becoming inadvertently detached.*[3]
- Insulate exposed wires using a sterile finger cot, glove, or plastic cap *to prevent microshock.*[3]
- Assess the patient's vital signs, skin color, level of consciousness, and peripheral pulses *to determine the effectiveness of the paced rhythm.* Perform a 12-lead electrocardiogram (ECG) *to serve as a baseline,* and then perform additional ECGs daily or with clinical changes. Also, if possible, obtain a rhythm strip before, during, and after pacemaker placement; after any adjustment in pacemaker settings; and whenever the patient receives treatment because of a pacemaker complication.[3] (See the "Electrocardiogram, 12-lead" procedure.)
- Screen for and assess the patient's pain using facility-defined criteria that are consistent with the patient's age, condition, and ability to understand.[33]
- Treat the patient's pain, as needed and ordered, using nonpharmacologic, pharmacologic, or a combination of approaches. Base the treatment plan on evidence-based practices and the patient's clinical condition, past medical history, and pain management goals.[33]
- Monitor closely if the patient at high risk for adverse outcomes related to opioid treatment, if prescribed.[33]

For removal

- Verify the practitioner's order for epicardial wire removal.
- Review laboratory data including coagulation and electrolyte results to make sure they're within normal limits, *to reduce the risk of bleeding and cardiac arrhythmias.* Notify the practitioner of abnormal values.[34,35]

Sensitivity and stimulation threshold testing

Sensitivity and stimulation threshold testing help determine the appropriate pacemaker rate and the amount of electrical current needed to initiate depolarization of the myocardium. Testing should occur on both chambers, as appropriate. Sensitivity threshold testing isn't necessary if the patient has no intrinsic rhythm. In some facilities, critical care nurses are permitted to perform sensitivity and stimulation threshold testing; in other facilities, the practitioner must perform the testing. Frequency of testing also varies by facility. Commonly, testing occurs at least every 24 hours *to make sure that the pacemaker is functioning properly and that it isn't delivering high levels of energy to the myocardium.*

Performing sensitivity threshold testing[3]
- The sensitivity threshold is the setting at which the sensing electrodes can recognize the patient's intrinsic myocardial activity. The patient must have an intrinsic rhythm.
- Turn the output dial (mA) to the lowest level *to avoid inducing a potentially lethal arrhythmia.*
- Slowly turn the sensitivity dial counterclockwise to a higher setting until the sensing indicator light stops flashing, which will occur when the device no longer senses the patient's intrinsic rhythm.
- Gradually turn the sensitivity dial clockwise to a lower setting until the sensing light begins flashing with each complex and the pacing light stops flashing; this setting is the *sensing threshold.*
- Set the sensitivity dial to the setting that's one-half the value of the sensing threshold *to provide a 2:1 safety margin.*

Performing stimulation threshold testing[3]
- The stimulation threshold is the minimum output (mA) necessary to initiate depolarization.
- Don't perform stimulation threshold testing if the sensitivity is poor or if the patient's intrinsic rate is greater than 90 beats/minute.
- In the case of dual-chambered pacing, assessment of the threshold for each chamber occurs separately.
- Set the pacing rate about 10 beats/minute above the patient's intrinsic rate.
- Beginning at 20 milliamperes (mA), slowly decrease the output until capture is lost.
- Gradually increase the mA until you see a 1:1 capture and the pacing light flashes; this is the *stimulation threshold.*
- Set the mA at least two times higher than the stimulation threshold.[1]

- Check the medication record to ensure that the patient isn't receiving anticoagulants.[3] If the patient is receiving anticoagulants, notify the practitioner to confirm wire removal, *because epicardial pacing wires aren't typically removed while the patient is receiving anticoagulant therapy owing to the risk for bleeding.*[3]
- Review the patient's medical record to confirm the number of epicardial pacing wires that you should remove, the location of the wires, and whether they're unipolar or bipolar, *to guide removal and ensure that the epicardial pacing wires are intact upon removal.*[3]
- Gather and prepare the necessary equipment and supplies.
- Perform hand hygiene.[11,12,13,14,15,16]
- Confirm the patient's identity using two patient identifiers.[17]
- Explain the procedure to the patient and family (if appropriate) according to their individual communication and learning needs *to increase their understanding, allay their fears, and enhance cooperation.*[23] Reinforce the practitioner's explanation of the procedure and answer any questions.[5,6,7,8] Tell the patient that a mild to moderate pulling sensation may be felt during wire removal.[1,36]
- Ensure that the patient is attached to a cardiac monitor. Make sure the alarm limits are set appropriately for the patient's current condition, and that the alarms are turned on, functioning properly, and audible to staff.[28,29,30,31]
- Raise the patient's bed to waist level before providing patient care *to prevent caregiver back strain.*[22]
- Obtain vital signs and an ECG rhythm strip, and assess cardiovascular status *to ensure that the patient is stable before removal of pacing wires and to provide a baseline for comparison.*[3]

■ Screen for and assess the patient's pain using facility-defined criteria that are consistent with the patient's age, condition, and ability to understand.[33]

■ Treat the patient's pain, as needed and ordered, using nonpharmacologic, pharmacologic, or a combination of approaches. Base the treatment plan on evidence-based practices and the patient's clinical condition, past medical history, and pain management goals.[33]

■ Monitor closely if the patient is at high risk for adverse outcomes related to opioid treatment, if prescribed.[33]

■ Confirm that the patient has patent IV access *in case emergency fluids or medications are required*.[3] Insert an IV catheter if patent access isn't available. (See the "IV catheter insertion and removal" procedure.)

■ Perform hand hygiene[11,12,13,14,15,16] and put on gloves and, as needed, other personal protective equipment *to comply with standard procedures and to prevent microshock.*[2,3,25,26,27]

■ Place the patient in the supine position *so that the epicardial pacing wires are readily accessible and the patient is properly positioned if emergency measures become necessary.*[23]

■ Using sterile no-touch technique, open the suture removal kit and gauze packages and place them within reach.

■ Carefully remove and discard the dressing covering the epicardial pacing wires exit site. Discard the dressing in the appropriate receptacle.[27]

■ Disconnect the epicardial pacing wires from the temporary pacemaker.

■ Remove and discard your gloves,[27] perform hand hygiene,[11,12,13,14,15,16] and put on a new pair of gloves.[25,27]

■ Clean the epicardial pacing wires exit site with antiseptic solution; clean at least a 3″ (7.6 cm) area around the exit site. Allow it to dry.[3]

■ Cut the sutures at the appropriate place and remove them. (See the "Suture removal" procedure.)[3]

■ Grasp an epicardial pacing wire and slowly and gently pull *to uncoil it from the epicardium*; repeat with each wire.[3] If you meet resistance, stop and notify the practitioner. When atrial and ventricular wires are present, remove the atrial wires first and then remove the ventricular wires. *If arrhythmias or instability occurs following atrial wire removal, you may perform ventricular pacing.*[3,35]

■ While pulling each epicardial pacing wire, observe the cardiac monitor for arrhythmias, *because arrhythmias are common during epicardial pacing wire removal.*[3]

■ Inspect the epicardial pacing wire to ensure that the entire wire is intact. Notify the practitioner and monitor the patient for complications if you see tissue in the wire.[3]

■ If you note bleeding at the epicardial pacing wire exit site, apply pressure until hemostasis is achieved.[3]

■ Observe the epicardial pacing exit site, noting drainage, redness, or skin breakdown.

■ Apply a sterile occlusive dressing over the exit sites.[3]

■ Discard used supplies in appropriate receptacles.[27]

■ Return the bed to the lowest position *to prevent falls and maintain patient safety.*[37]

■ Monitor vital signs every 15 minutes for the first hour, every 30 minutes for the next 2 hours, and then hourly for 2 hours at an interval determined by your facility and the patient's condition *to assess hemodynamic stability.* Continue arrhythmia monitoring for at least 24 hours after the wires are removed.[3]

■ Closely monitor the patient for cardiac arrhythmias and signs and symptoms of cardiac tamponade, such as the Beck triad (hypotension, muffled heart tones, and jugular vein distention), tachycardia, decreased peripheral pulses, and dyspnea.[3,35] Cardiac tamponade may not be immediately evident if bleeding is slow; therefore, you may need to monitor the patient closely for up to 2 hours.

■ Reassess and respond to the patient's pain by evaluating the response to treatment and progress toward pain management goals. Assess for adverse reactions and risk factors for adverse events that may result from treatment.[33]

■ Limit the patient's activity, as ordered.[3,38]

Completing the procedure

■ Remove and discard your gloves and, if worn, other personal protective equipment.[27]

■ Perform hand hygiene.[11,12,13,14,15,16]

■ Clean and disinfect your stethoscope using a disinfectant pad.[39,40]

■ Perform hand hygiene.[11,12,13,14,15,16]

■ Document the procedure.[41,42,43,44]

Special considerations

■ The Joint Commission issued a sentinel event alert concerning medical device alarm safety, *because alarm-related events are associated with permanent loss of function or death.* Among the major contributing factors were improper alarm settings, alarm settings turned off inappropriately, and alarm signals that were inaudible to staff. Make sure that alarm limits are set appropriately, and that alarms are turned on, functioning properly, and audible to staff. Follow facility guidelines for preventing alarm fatigue.[30]

■ Institute measures to prevent microshock, including advising the patient to avoid any electrical equipment that isn't grounded, such as electric shavers, televisions, and lamps.[32]

■ If the patient is disoriented or uncooperative, use restraints if less restrictive measures aren't effective *to prevent accidental removal of the pacemaker wires.*[45]

■ If the patient needs emergency defibrillation, make sure the pacemaker can withstand the procedure. If you're unsure, disconnect the pulse generator *to avoid damage.*[32]

■ Continuously monitor the ECG reading, noting capture, sensing, rate, intrinsic beats, and competition of paced and intrinsic rhythms. If the pacemaker is sensing correctly, the sense indicator on the pulse generator should flash with each beat. (See *Handling pacemaker malfunction.*) Continue cardiac pacing while the epicardial pacing wires are in place.[1]

■ Change the dressing at a frequency determined by your facility and the type of dressing used.[3] Clean the insertion site with an antiseptic solution, change the dressing, and label it with the date, the time, and your initials, or as directed by your facility.[3] Inspect the site for signs of infection and notify the practitioner of erythema or drainage at the site, which may necessitate pacing wire removal.[1]

■ Assess and document sensitivity and stimulation thresholds (commonly every 24 hours), as required by your facility, *to make sure that the pacemaker is functioning properly.*[3]

■ Monitor the pulse generator's battery light indicator and change the battery when necessary; *battery life varies according to the pacing energy needed.*[3]

■ If the pulse generator is no longer needed, disconnect it from the pacing wires and insulate the wires using a rubber finger cot, glove, or plastic cap *to prevent microshocks.*[3]

■ Remove pacing wires at least 24 hours before discharge *so that you can monitor the patient for complications.*[3] Continue cardiac monitoring for at least 24 hours after epicardial wire removal *to assess for possible arrhythmias.*[3,38]

■ *Because pacing wires provide a direct electrical route to the heart,* wear gloves when handling the wires *to prevent microshocks.*[3]

Complications

Complications associated with pacemaker therapy include microshock, equipment failure, competitive or fatal arrhythmias, lead dislodgement, myocardial perforation, and pulmonary embolism.[1] Epicardial pacemakers carry a risk of infection, cardiac arrest, and diaphragmatic stimulation.

Complications following epicardial pacing wire removal occur more commonly in patients with a history of heart failure, repeat heart surgery, or anticoagulant therapy. Complications include cardiac tamponade (the most serious complication), infection, hemorrhage, hematoma, arrhythmias, hemodynamic instability, myocardial ischemia, and graft site trauma.

Documentation

Record the reason for epicardial pacing, the date and time it started, locations of the electrodes, and pacemaker settings. Note the patient's response to the procedure. Record adverse events, the date and time you notified the practitioner, prescribed interventions, and the patient's response to those interventions. If possible, obtain rhythm strips before,

TROUBLESHOOTING

Handling pacemaker malfunction

Occasionally, a temporary pacemaker may fail to function appropriately. When this occurs, you need to take immediate action to correct the problem. Follow these steps when your patient's pacemaker fails to pace, capture, or sense intrinsic beats.

Failure to pace
Failure to pace occurs when the pacemaker either doesn't fire or fires too often. The pulse generator may not be working properly, or it may not be conducting the impulse to the patient.

Nursing interventions
■ If the pacing or sensing indicator flashes, check the patient, all connections, and the battery. Check the position of the pacing electrode in the patient by X-ray, if ordered.
■ If the pulse generator is turned on but the indicators still aren't flashing, change the battery. If that doesn't help, use a different pulse generator.
■ Check the settings if the pacemaker is firing too rapidly. If the rate is correct, or if increasing the sensitivity (according to the practitioner's order) doesn't help, change the pulse generator.
■ Have a transcutaneous pacemaker on standby in case the pacemaker continues to malfunction and the patient becomes symptomatic. Notify the practitioner.

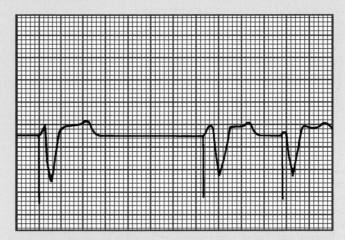

Failure to capture
In failure to capture, you can see the pacemaker spikes but the heart isn't responding. This malfunction may be caused by changes in the pacing threshold from ischemia, swelling at the insertion site, an electrolyte imbalance (high or low potassium or magnesium levels), acidosis, an adverse reaction to a medication, a perforated ventricle, fibrosis, or the electrode position.

Nursing interventions
■ Verify that the settings are correct, according to the practitioner's order.
■ If the heart isn't responding, carefully check all connections, increase the milliamperes slowly as determined by your facility, and then notify the practitioner of the failure to capture.
■ Have a transcutaneous pacemaker on standby in case the pacemaker continues to malfunction and the patient becomes symptomatic. Notify the practitioner.

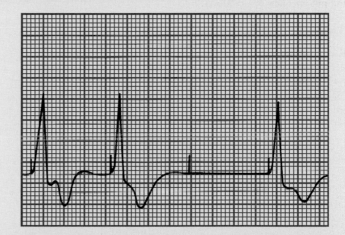

Failure to sense intrinsic beats
Failure to sense intrinsic beats could cause ventricular tachycardia or ventricular fibrillation if the pacemaker fires on the vulnerable T wave. Possible causes include the pacemaker sensing an external stimulus as a QRS complex, which could lead to asystole, or the pacemaker not being sensitive enough, which means it could fire anywhere within the cardiac cycle.

Nursing interventions
■ If the pacing is undersensing, increase the sensitivity by turning down the voltage, usually to 2 to 5 millivolts (mV). If it's oversensing, decrease the sensitivity by turning up the voltage to 5 mV or higher.
■ Change the battery and then the pulse generator if the problem persists.
■ Remove items in the room that could be causing electromechanical interference (such as razors, radios, and cautery devices). Check the ground wires on the bed and other equipment for obvious damage. Unplug each piece and see if the interference stops. When you locate the cause, notify the staff engineer to check it.
■ If the pacemaker is still firing on the T wave and all else has failed to correct it, attach the patient to a transcutaneous pacemaker, turn off the epicardial pacemaker, and notify the practitioner.

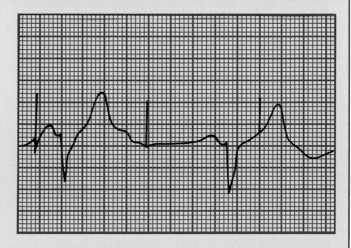

during, and after pacemaker placement; whenever pacemaker settings change; and when the patient receives treatment for a complication caused by the pacemaker. As you're monitoring the patient, record the patient's response to temporary pacing and note any changes in the patient's condition. Document your assessment findings, including the condition of pacing wire insertion sites and the patient's pain level.

Record the date and time you removed the wires. Document the patient's pain level. If you administered an analgesic, record the name of the drug; the dose, route, and time of administration; the patient's response; and any additional interventions required. Describe the condition of the exit site, the level of difficulty of wire removal, the condition of the wires (intact or not), and any tissue you noted at the end of the wires.

Include the patient's vital signs, the ECG strip, and your patient assessments before, during, and after the procedure. Record how you dressed the site. Note the patient's tolerance of the procedure. If an adverse event occurred, note the time, the name of the practitioner you notified, prescribed interventions, and the patient's response to those interventions. Document frequent assessments, as directed by your facility.

Document teaching provided to the patient and family (if appropriate), their understanding of that teaching, and any need for follow-up teaching.

REFERENCES

1 Ganz, L. I. (2019). Temporary cardiac pacing. In: *UpToDate*, Estes, N. A. M. (Ed.).

2 Sivapuram, M. A. (2019). Temporary epicardial pacing: Post-surgery. *The JBI EBP Database*. AN: JBI6671

3 Wiegand, D. L. (2017). *AACN procedure manual for high acuity, progressive, and critical care* (7th ed.). Elsevier.

4 American Heart Association. (2020). 2020 American Heart Association Guidelines for CPR and ECC—Part 3: Adult basic and advanced life support. https://cpr.heart.org/en/resuscitation-science/cpr-and-ecc-guidelines (Level II)

5 Accreditation Association for Hospitals and Health Systems. (2020). Standard 30.01.11. *Healthcare Facilities Accreditation Program: Accreditation requirements for acute care hospitals.* (Level VII)

6 Centers for Medicare and Medicaid Services, Department of Health and Human Services. (2020). Condition of participation: Patient's rights. 42 C.F.R. § 482.13(b)(2).

7 DNV GL-Healthcare USA, Inc. (2020). PR.2.SR.3. *NIAHO® accreditation requirements, interpretive guidelines and surveyor guidance—revision 20.0.* (Level VII)

8 The Joint Commission. (2021). Standard RI.01.03.01. *Comprehensive accreditation manual for hospitals.* (Level VII)

9 The Joint Commission. (2021). Standard UP.01.01.01. *Comprehensive accreditation manual for hospitals.* (Level VII)

10 Accreditation Association for Hospitals and Health Systems. (2020). Standard 30.00.14. *Healthcare Facilities Accreditation Program: Accreditation requirements for acute care hospitals.* (Level VII)

11 The Joint Commission. (2021). Standard NPSG.07.01.01. *Comprehensive accreditation manual for hospitals.* (Level VII)

12 World Health Organization. (2009). WHO guidelines on hand hygiene in health care: First global patient safety challenge, clean care is safer care. https://apps.who.int/iris/bitstream/handle/10665/44102/9789241597906_eng.pdf?sequence=1 (Level IV)

13 Centers for Disease Control and Prevention. (2002). Guideline for hand hygiene in health-care settings: Recommendations of the Healthcare Infection Control Practices Advisory Committee and the HICPAC/SHEA/APIC/IDSA Hand Hygiene Task Force. *MMWR Recommendations and Reports, 51*(RR-16), 1–45. https://www.cdc.gov/mmwr/pdf/rr/rr5116.pdf (Level II)

14 Centers for Medicare and Medicaid Services, Department of Health and Human Services. (2020). Condition of participation: Infection control. 42 C.F.R. § 482.42.

15 Accreditation Association for Hospitals and Health Systems. (2020). Standard 07.01.21. *Healthcare Facilities Accreditation Program: Accreditation requirements for acute care hospitals.* (Level VII)

16 DNV GL-Healthcare USA, Inc. (2020). IC.1.SR.1. *NIAHO® accreditation requirements, interpretive guidelines and surveyor guidance—revision 20.0.* Milford, OH: (Level VII)

17 The Joint Commission. (2021). Standard NPSG.01.01.01. *Comprehensive accreditation manual for hospitals.* (Level VII)

18 The Joint Commission. (2021). Standard RI.01.01.01. *Comprehensive accreditation manual for hospitals.* (Level VII)

19 DNV GL-Healthcare USA, Inc. (2020). PR.2.SR.5. *NIAHO® accreditation requirements, interpretive guidelines and surveyor guidance—revision 20.0.* (Level VII)

20 Centers for Medicare and Medicaid Services, Department of Health and Human Services. (2020). Condition of participation: Patient's rights. 42 C.F.R. § 482.13(c)(1).

21 Accreditation Association for Hospitals and Health Systems. (2020). Standard 15.01.16. *Healthcare Facilities Accreditation Program: Accreditation requirements for acute care hospitals.* (Level VII)

22 Waters, T. R., et al. (2009). Safe patient handling training for schools of nursing. https://www.cdc.gov/niosh/docs/2009-127/pdfs/2009-127.pdf (Level VII)

23 The Joint Commission. (2021). Standard PC.02.01.21. *Comprehensive accreditation manual for hospitals.* (Level VII)

24 The Joint Commission. (2021). Standard UP.01.03.01. *Comprehensive accreditation manual for hospitals.* (Level VII)

25 Siegel, J. D., et al. (2007, revised 2019). 2007 guideline for isolation precautions: Preventing transmission of infectious agents in healthcare settings. https://www.cdc.gov/infectioncontrol/pdf/guidelines/isolation-guidelines-H.pdf (Level II)

26 Accreditation Association for Hospitals and Health Systems. (2020). Standard 07.01.10. *Healthcare Facilities Accreditation Program: Accreditation requirements for acute care hospitals.* (Level VII)

27 Occupational Safety and Health Administration. (2019). Bloodborne pathogens, standard number 1910.1030. https://www.osha.gov/pls/oshaweb/owadisp.show_document?p_id=10051&p_table=STANDARDS (Level VII)

28 The Joint Commission. (2021). Standard NPSG.06.01.01. *Comprehensive accreditation manual for hospitals.* (Level VII)

29 Graham, K. C., & Cvach, M. (2010). Monitor alarm fatigue: Standardizing use of physiological monitors and decreasing nuisance alarms. *American Journal of Critical Care, 19*(1), 28–37. https://doi.org/10.4037/ajcc2010651

30 The Joint Commission. (2013). Sentinel event alert 50: Medical device alarm safety in hospitals. https://www.jointcommission.org/assets/1/6/SEA_50_alarms_4_26_16.pdf (Level VII)

31 American Association of Critical-Care Nurses. (2018). AACN practice alert: Managing alarms in acute care across the life span: Electrocardiography and pulse oximetry. https://www.aacn.org/clinical-resources/practice-alerts/managing-alarms-in-acute-care-across-the-life-span (Level VII)

32 Medtronic, Inc. (2016). Medtronic 5392 dual chamber temporary external pacemaker: Technical manual. https://www.manualslib.com/manual/1266418/Medtronic-5392.html

33 The Joint Commission. (2021). Standard PC.01.02.07. *Comprehensive accreditation manual for hospitals.* (Level VII)

34 The Joint Commission. (2021). Standard NPSG.02.03.01. *Comprehensive accreditation manual for hospitals.* (Level VII)

35 Temporary epicardial pacing wires: Removal. (2019). *The JBI EBP Database*. AN: JBI6672

36 Mullin, M. H., et al. (2009). Sensations during removal of epicardial pacing wires after coronary artery bypass graft surgery. *Heart and Lung, 38*(5), 377–381. https://doi.org/10.1016/j.hrtlng.2008.10.003 (Level VI)

37 Ganz, D. A., et al. (2013, reviewed 2021). *Preventing falls in hospitals: A toolkit for improving quality of care* (AHRQ publication no. 13-0015-EF). Agency for Healthcare Research and Quality. https://www.ahrq.gov/professionals/systems/hospital/fallpxtoolkit/index.html (Level VII)

38 McClurken, J. B. (2006). Minimizing complications from epicardial pacing wires after cardiac surgery. *PA-PSRS Patient Safety Advisory, 3*, 1–7. http://patientsafety.pa.gov/ADVISORIES/documents/200603_08.pdf

39 Rutala, W. A., et al. (2008, revised 2019). Guideline for disinfection and sterilization in healthcare facilities, 2008. https://www.cdc.gov/infection-control/pdf/guidelines/disinfection-guidelines-H.pdf (Level I)

40 Accreditation Association for Hospitals and Health Systems. (2020). Standard 07.02.03. *Healthcare Facilities Accreditation Program: Accreditation requirements for acute care hospitals.* (Level VII)

41 The Joint Commission. (2021). Standard RC.01.03.01. *Comprehensive accreditation manual for hospitals.* (Level VII)

42 Centers for Medicare and Medicaid Services, Department of Health and Human Services. (2020). Condition of participation: Medical record services. 42 C.F.R. § 482.24(b).

43 Accreditation Association for Hospitals and Health Systems. (2020). Standard 10.00.03. *Healthcare Facilities Accreditation Program: Accreditation requirements for acute care hospitals.* (Level VII)

44 DNV GL-Healthcare USA, Inc. (2020). MR.2.SR.1. *NIAHO® accreditation requirements, interpretive guidelines and surveyor guidance—revision 20.0.* (Level VII)

45 The Joint Commission. (2021). Standard PC.03.05.01. *Comprehensive accreditation manual for hospitals.* (Level VII)

EPIDURAL ANALGESIC ADMINISTRATION

An anesthesia practitioner, such as an anesthesiologist or a nurse anesthetist, may place an epidural catheter into the epidural space around the spinal cord to provide a route for administration of pain medication. This access can help in the short term to treat acute pain associated with surgery, procedures, trauma, or labor, or in the long term for chronic

Location of an epidural catheter

A practitioner introduces the epidural catheter via a needle through the skin, subcutaneous tissue, and ligaments between two vertebrae into the epidural space. The practitioner's choice of insertion point depends on the level where the patient requires the medication's effect. Common insertion points include thoracic and lumbar regions of the spine.

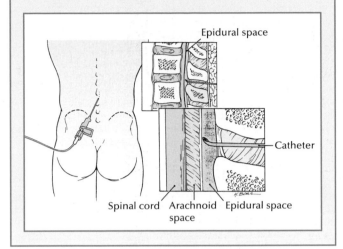

toxicity [LAST] rescue kit including 20% lipid emulsion and antiseizure medication) ▪ Optional: capnography monitoring equipment, IV catheter insertion supplies, tape measure, oxygen, standardized sedation scale.

Preparation of equipment

Ensure that the emergency equipment is functioning properly and readily available. Ensure that the pharmacy has received advance notification regarding the medication order, *because epidural solutions require special preparation.* Inspect all IV equipment and supplies. If a product is expired, is defective, or has compromised integrity, remove it from patient use, label it as expired or defective, and report the expiration or defect as directed by your facility.[9]

Implementation

▪ Avoid distractions and interruptions when preparing and administering the medication *to prevent medication errors.*[10,11]

▪ Review the practitioner's order *to make sure that the prescribed infusion solution or medication, dose, rate, and route of administration are appropriate for the patient's age, condition, and access device,* and that the infusion or medication is compatible with other solutions or medication. Make sure that the order includes any test results that require monitoring. Address concerns about the order with the practitioner, pharmacist, your supervisor, or the risk management department, or as directed by your facility.[12]

▪ Reconcile the patient's medications when the practitioner orders a new medication *to help reduce the risk of medication errors, including omissions, duplications, dosing errors, and drug interactions.*[12]

▪ Gather and prepare the necessary equipment and supplies.

▪ Obtain the prescribed medication from the pharmacy.[1]

▪ Compare the medication label with the order in the patient's medical record.[13,14,15,16]

▪ Check the patient's medical record for any allergies or contraindications to the prescribed medication. If an allergy or a contraindication exists, don't administer the medication; instead, notify the practitioner.[13,14,15,16]

▪ Check the expiration date on the medication. If the medication has expired, return it to the pharmacy and obtain a new supply of medication.[13,14,15,16]

▪ Visually inspect the solution for particulates, discoloration, and other signs of loss of integrity; don't administer the medication if its integrity is compromised.[13,14,15,16]

▪ Discuss any unresolved concerns about the medication with the patient's practitioner.[13,14,15,16]

▪ Perform hand hygiene.[17,18,19,20,21,22,23]

▪ Confirm the patient's identity using at least two patient identifiers.[24]

▪ Provide privacy.[25,26,27,28]

▪ Explain the procedure to the patient and family (if appropriate) according to their individual communication and learning needs *to increase their understanding, allay their fears, and enhance cooperation.*[29]

▪ If the patient is receiving the medication for the first time, provide teaching about the expected effects as well as potential adverse reactions and other concerns related to the medication.[13,14,15,16]

▪ Raise the patient's bed to waist level before providing patient care *to prevent caregiver back strain.*[30]

▪ Perform hand hygiene.[17,18,19,20,21,22,23]

▪ Obtain the patient's vital signs and oxygen saturation level using pulse oximetry, and assess the patient's neurologic status and sedation level *to serve as a baseline for comparison.*[1,31]

▪ Screen for and assess the patient's pain using facility-defined criteria that are consistent with the patient's age, condition, and ability to understand.[32]

▪ In collaboration with the multidisciplinary team, involve the patient in the pain management planning process. Provide education on pain management, treatment options, and the safe use of opioid and nonopioid medications, when prescribed. Develop realistic expectations and measurable goals that the patient understands regarding the degree, duration, and reduction of pain. Discuss objectives to use to evaluate treatment progress (for example, relief of pain and improved physical and psychosocial function).[32]

pain, including cancer-related pain. The primary advantage of administering pain medication through an epidural catheter is that pain can be managed with smaller doses of analgesia, thereby reducing the risks associated with larger doses of systemic analgesia.[1,2,3] Pain medication may be administered through an epidural catheter intermittently, continuously, or with a patient-controlled epidural analgesia pump. Epidural analgesic administration for chronic pain can also incorporate an implanted pump.[1] The epidural catheter is typically located in the thoracic or lumbar region of the spine. (See *Location of an epidural catheter.*)

Medications typically administered via an epidural catheter include dilute local anesthetics (such as bupivacaine or ropivacaine) and opioid analgesics (such as fentaNYL, SUFentanil, morphine, and HYDROmorphone), alone or in combination. Adjuncts, such as cloNIDine, may possibly be added to the solution. All medications administered by the epidural route must be preservative free, *because preservatives are toxic to the central nervous system.*[1,4,5]

After the anesthesia practitioner inserts the epidural catheter, administers the initial test dose, and sets the dosage parameters, a specially trained nurse may initiate the infusion, administer bolus doses, adjust infusion rates, replace empty drug containers, troubleshoot the infusion device, change the epidural infusion tubing and dressing, discontinue therapy, and, in some cases, remove the catheter. The nurse is also responsible for assessing the patient, monitoring for adverse effects, and providing teaching to the patient and family members. The nurse should check the facility's guidelines as well as with the state's nurse practice act to determine which interventions are within the nurse's scope of care.[6,7]

Equipment

Programmable electronic epidural infusion device with anti–free-flow protection[4] ▪ epidural administration set (yellow-lined epidural administration set with injection ports)[1] containing a 0.2-micron, surfactant-free, particulate-retentive filter[4] ▪ prescribed preservative-free epidural medications[4] ▪ EPIDURAL ONLY labels ▪ vital signs monitoring equipment ▪ facility-approved pain assessment scale ▪ stethoscope ▪ pulse oximeter and probe ▪ gloves ▪ mask ▪ antiseptic pads (povidone-iodine or chlorhexidine) ▪ empty 10-mL syringe ▪ 10-mL syringe containing preservative-free normal saline solution ▪ disinfectant pad ▪ facility-approved disinfectant ▪ emergency equipment (code cart with emergency medications, handheld resuscitation bag and mask, defibrillator, intubation and suction equipment, naloxone[4,8] and local anesthetic systemic

■ Treat the patient's pain, as needed and ordered, using nonpharmacologic, pharmacologic, or a combination of approaches. Base the treatment plan on evidence-based practices and the patient's clinical condition, medical history, and pain management goals.[32]

■ Closely monitor a patient who is prescribed opioid treatment and is identified as being at high risk for adverse outcomes.[32]

■ Ensure that the patient has adequate, patent IV access *to provide a route for IV fluids or emergency medications if needed*; insert a new IV catheter, if necessary. (See the "IV catheter insertion and removal" procedure.)[1,4]

■ Put on a mask.[1,4,31,33,34,35]

■ Perform hand hygiene.[17,18,19,20,21,22,23]

■ Put on gloves *to comply with standard precautions*.[1,4,31,33,34,35]

■ Assess the epidural catheter insertion site for signs of infection (tenderness, erythema, swelling, and drainage) and the insertion site dressing for moisture, leakage, and lack of intactness. Notify the practitioner of any unexpected findings.

■ Assess the epidural catheter for intactness. Routinely assess the catheter for changes in external catheter length *to help identify catheter tip dislodgement*.[4,31] Notify the practitioner of catheter damage or migration.

■ Verify that the prescribed medication is being administered at the proper time, in the prescribed dose, and by the correct route *to reduce the risk of medication errors*.[13,14,15,16]

■ If your facility uses bar-code technology, use it as directed by your facility.[12]

■ For a continuous infusion or patient-controlled epidural anesthesia:[1,2,4,31] Connect the prescribed, preservative-free medication to the epidural administration set and prime the tubing. Label the epidural administration set tubing at the distal end (near the patient connection) and proximal end (near the source container) with a label that reads EPIDURAL ONLY *to reduce the risk of misconnection*.[36] Insert the epidural administration set into the programmable electronic epidural infusion device according to the manufacturer's instructions. Program the dosage parameters according the practitioner's orders. Label the electronic epidural infusion device with a label that reads EPIDURAL ONLY.

■ Perform a vigorous mechanical scrub of the epidural catheter hub with an antiseptic pad for at least 5 seconds, and then allow it to dry completely.[1,31]

NURSING ALERT Don't use an antiseptic pad containing alcohol or acetone to disinfect the catheter hub, *because these agents can cause neurotoxic effects.* Instead, use povidone-iodine or chlorhexidine.[1,4,31]

■ Attach an empty 10-mL syringe to the epidural catheter hub and gently aspirate for blood or cerebrospinal fluid *to confirm proper epidural catheter placement.* If you aspirate more than 0.5 mL of blood or serous fluid, don't reinject the aspirate or administer the medication. Instead, notify the practitioner, *because the catheter has most likely migrated into a vein or the intrathecal space.*[1,4,31]

■ For a continuous infusion or patient-controlled epidural anesthesia: Connect the epidural administration set to the epidural catheter. Trace the epidural administration set tubing from the patient to its point of origin *to ensure that it's connected to the proper port.*[36,37] Route the epidural administration set tubing in a standardized direction if the patient has other tubing and catheters with different purposes.[36,37]

NURSING ALERT Epidural medications are considered "high-alert" medications *because they can cause significant patient harm when used in error.*[38] If required by your facility, before administering epidural analgesia, arrange for another nurse to perform an independent double-check *to verify the patient's identity and to ensure that you have the correct medication in the prescribed strength or concentration, the medication's indication corresponds with the patient's diagnosis, the dosage calculations and the dosing formula used to derive the final dose is correct, the prescribed route of administration is safe and proper for the patient, the prescribed time and frequency of administration are safe and proper for the patient, and, if an infusion, the pump settings are correct and the epidural infusion tubing is attached to the correct port.*[39]

■ If required by your facility, before administering epidural analgesia, arrange for another nurse to perform an independent double-check *to help reduce the risk of medication errors.*[39] Compare the results of the other nurse's independent double-check (if required) and, if no discrepancies exist, begin administering the medication. If discrepancies exist, rectify them before administering the medication.[39]

■ If you're administering a bolus dose of epidural analgesia:[1,31] While maintaining the sterility of the syringe tip, attach the syringe containing the prescribed, preservative-free medication to the epidural catheter hub and slowly administer the medication. If you meet excessive resistance, assess the catheter for kinks or reposition the patient. If resistance continues to impede administration, notify the practitioner.[1] After administering the bolus dose, remove the syringe from the epidural catheter hub. While maintaining sterility of the syringe tip, attach the syringe containing preservative-free normal saline solution to the epidural catheter hub. Flush the epidural catheter with 1 to 2 mL of preservative-free normal saline solution *to ensure that the medication reaches the epidural space.*

■ For a continuous infusion or patient-controlled epidural anesthesia: Ensure that the infusion device alarm limits are appropriately set for the patient's current condition, and that the alarms are turned on, functioning properly, and audible to staff.[40,41,42] Begin the infusion or set the epidural infusion device to allow the patient to self-administer doses, as appropriate. Lock the keypad on the epidural infusion device *to prevent inadvertent infusion rate changes.*[1]

■ At established intervals determined by your facility, the practitioner's orders, and the patient's condition, monitor the patient's vital signs, oxygen saturation level, end-tidal carbon dioxide level (if the practitioner orders capnography monitoring), level of sedation, and sensory and motor function.[1,2,4]

NURSING ALERT Patients at higher risk for adverse effects of epidural analgesia administration include older adults, patients with comorbidities (such as sleep apnea or psychiatric conditions), and those taking concurrent medications (such as other analgesics or sedatives). Increased vigilance while monitoring these patients is essential for promptly recognizing and treating adverse events.[4,43]

■ If the patient is receiving epidural opioid medication, frequently monitor vital signs, respiratory status, and sedation level using a standardized scale *to promptly recognize and treat oversedation and respiratory depression related to epidural opioid use.*[44]

■ If applicable, explain the sedation monitoring process to the patient and family (including the potential need to awaken the patient to assess the effects of the medication). Advise the patient and family to immediately alert staff if breathing problems or other changes that might be a reaction to the medication occur.[44]

■ Reassess and respond to the patient's pain by evaluating the response to treatment and progress toward pain management goals. Assess for adverse reactions and risk factors for adverse events that may result from treatment.[32] Reassess the patient's pain at established intervals determined by your facility, the practitioner's orders, and the patient's condition. If the patient reports moderate to severe pain, the infusion rate may require an increase. Notify the practitioner of an unacceptable pain level despite intervention.[1,4,32]

■ At established intervals determined by your facility, the practitioner's orders, and the patient's condition, monitor the patient for adverse effects of the medication, such as pruritus, nausea, vomiting, urinary retention, orthostatic hypotension, respiratory depression, oversedation, and motor block; signs and symptoms of local anesthetic systemic toxicity (LAST), including visual disturbances, ringing in the ears, tingling or numbness around the mouth, metallic taste in the mouth, and anxiety (see *Local anesthesia systemic toxicity*); signs and symptoms of catheter insertion site infection or epidural abscess, such as back pain, tenderness, erythema, swelling, drainage, fever, malaise, neck stiffness, progressive numbness, and motor block; dressing moisture, leakage, or intactness; and catheter length and intactness.[1,2,4]

■ Notify the practitioner of any adverse events or unexpected outcomes, and intervene as appropriate and as ordered.

■ For a continuous infusion or patient-controlled epidural anesthesia, monitor the programmable electronic epidural infusion device for history of analgesic use and correct administration parameters at established intervals determined by your facility, the practitioner's orders, and the patient's condition.[1,4]

■ Return the bed to the lowest position *to prevent falls and maintain patient safety.*[47]

■ Discard used supplies in appropriate receptacles.[35]

■ Remove and discard your mask and gloves.[35]

■ Perform hand hygiene.[17,18,19,20,21,22,23]

Local anesthesia systemic toxicity

Unintentional intravascular injection or systemic absorption of local anesthetics can lead to central nervous system and cardiac toxicity, resulting in disability or death. Effects of local anesthetic systemic toxicity (LAST) include syncope, seizures, coma, tachycardia, and hypertension (early), followed by bradycardia and hypotension (with increased toxicity), ventricular arrhythmias, asystole, and respiratory arrest. Prompt recognition and treatment of LAST helps increase a patient's chance of survival. Initial treatment should focus on managing the patient's airway, *because hypoxemia and acidosis intensify the effects of LAST.*[45,46]

If LAST occurs, refer to the American Society of Regional Anesthesia and Pain Medicine's checklist (shown below):

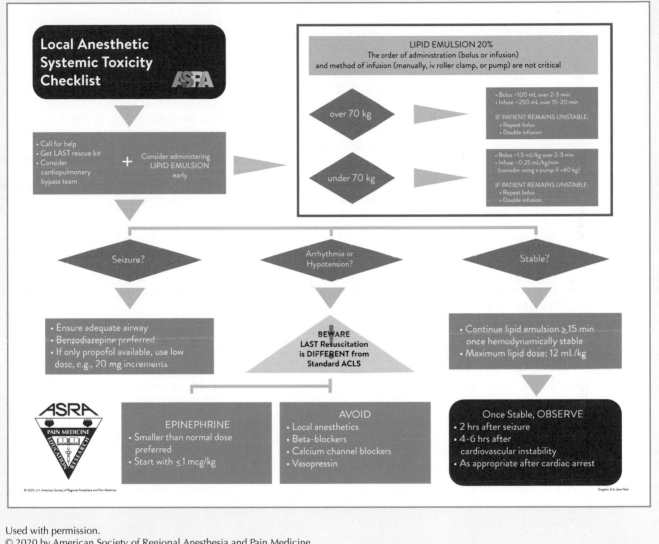

Used with permission.
© 2020 by American Society of Regional Anesthesia and Pain Medicine.

- Clean and disinfect your stethoscope with a disinfectant pad.
- Perform hand hygiene.[17,18,19,20,21,22,23]
- Put on gloves.[1,4,31,33,35]
- Clean and disinfect other reusable equipment according to the manufacturer's instructions *to prevent the spread of infection.*[48,49]
- Remove and discard your gloves.[35]
- Perform hand hygiene.[17,18,19,20,21,22,23]
- Document the procedure.[50,51,52,53]

Special considerations

- Maintain the patient's IV access for at least 24 hours after epidural catheter insertion *to facilitate the administration of IV fluids and vasopressors for hypotension, naloxone for respiratory depression or pruritus, and antiemetics for nausea and vomiting.*[1,4]
- Change the dressing on a short-term epidural catheter only if it becomes loose, wet, or soiled *due to the risk of infection and dislodgment.*

Change the dressing on a long-term epidural catheter every 7 days during the performance of catheter insertion site antisepsis.[2,31]

- Ensure that naloxone, a reversal agent for use in emergencies to treat respiratory depression associated with opioid administration, is available for administration if needed.[54,55]
- The Joint Commission has issued a sentinel event alert concerning medical device alarm safety, *because alarm-related events have been associated with permanent loss of function and death.* Among the major contributing factors were improper alarm settings, inappropriately turned-off alarms, and alarm signals not audible to staff. Make sure that alarm limits are appropriately set, and that alarms are turned on, functioning properly, and audible to staff. Follow facility guidelines for preventing alarm fatigue.[42]
- The Joint Commission has issued a sentinel event alert related to managing risk during transition to new International Organization for Standardization tubing standards that were designed to prevent dangerous tubing misconnections, which can lead to serious patient injury and

death. During the transition, make sure to trace each tubing and catheter from the patient to its point of origin before connecting or reconnecting any device or infusion, at any care transition (such as to a new setting or service), and as part of the hand-off process. In addition, route tubes and catheters with different purposes in different, standardized directions; label tubing at both the distal and proximal ends when the patient has different access sites or several bags hanging; use tubing and equipment only as intended; and store medications for different delivery routes in separate locations.[36]

Patient teaching

Teach the patient and family members about pain management strategies during discharge planning. Include information about the patient's pain management plan and adverse effects of pain management treatment. Discuss activities of daily living and items in the home environment that might exacerbate pain or reduce the effectiveness of the pain management plan, and include strategies to address these issues. Teach the patient and family members about the safe use, storage, and disposal of opioids, if prescribed.[32]

Review with the patient and family (if appropriate) signs and symptoms to report, including worsening pain or an unacceptable pain level; adverse effects of opioids, including itching, nausea, vomiting, oversedation, and respiratory depression;[1,2,4] symptoms of LAST, including visual disturbances, ringing in the ears, tingling or numbness around the mouth, metallic taste in the mouth, and anxiety;[1,45]and signs and symptoms of catheter migration or epidural hematoma or abscess, including changes in pain perception, new or worsening back pain, numbness of the extremities, loss of motor control of the lower extremities, and loss of bowel or bladder function.[1,2,4]

If the patient has a patient-controlled epidural analgesia pump, emphasize the importance of preventing overdose by allowing only the patient to administer the medication. Explain that this approach is a safeguard against oversedation, because the patient must be alert to be able to administer a dose.[1]

If the patient will be discharged with the epidural infusion device, review device care and arrange for follow-up. Emphasize the importance of reporting the use of alcohol and all medications to the practitioner *to help prevent adverse drug interactions.*[4]

Complications

Potential complications of epidural analgesic administration include adverse reactions to opioids and local anesthetics, such as pruritus, nausea, vomiting, urinary retention, decreased level of consciousness, and respiratory depression, as well as catheter-related problems, such as infection, epidural hematoma, epidural abscess, postdural puncture headache syndrome, and catheter migration.[2]

Documentation

Document your assessments before, during, and after epidural analgesic administration, including vital signs, oxygen saturation level, pain level, and sedation level. Record the epidural infusion device type and gauge, external catheter length, and insertion site and dressing condition. Record the medications you administered, including the medication strength, dose, and route of administration, and the date and time of administration.[56] Document any adverse events to the prescribed medications, the date and time that you notified the practitioner, any prescribed interventions, and the patient's response to those interventions. Also document teaching provided to the patient and family (if appropriate), their understanding of that teaching, and any need for follow-up teaching.

REFERENCES

1 Wiegand, D. L. (2017). *AACN procedure manual for high acuity, progressive and critical care* (7th ed.). St. Louis, MO: Elsevier.

2 Sawhney, M. (2012). Epidural analgesia: What nurses need to know. *Nursing, 42*(8), 36–41. https://journals.lww.com/nursing/Fulltext/2012/08000/Epidural_analgesia_What_nurses_need_to_know.15.aspx

3 Chou, R., et al. (2016). Management of postoperative pain: A clinical practice guideline from the American Pain Society, the American Society of Regional Anesthesia and Pain Medicine, and the American Society of Anesthesiologists' Committee on Regional Anesthesia, Executive Committee, and Administrative Council. *Journal of Pain, 17,* 131–157. (Level VII)

4 Standard 56. Intraspinal access devices. Infusion therapy standards of practice (8th ed.). (2021). *Journal of Infusion Nursing, 44,* S171–S174. (Level VII)

5 Ituk, U., & Wong, C. A. (2020). Epidural and combined spinal-epidural analgesia: Techniques. In: *UpToDate,* Maniker, R. (Ed.).

6 Pasero, C., et al. (2007). Registered nurse management and monitoring of analgesia by catheter techniques: Position statement. *Pain Management Nursing, 8*(2), 48–54. http://www.aspmn.org/documents/RegisteredNurseManagementandMonitoringofAnalgesiaByCatheterTechniquesPMNversion.pdf (Level VII)

7 American Association of Nurse Anesthetists (AANA). (2017). *Care of patients receiving analgesia by catheter techniques: Position statement and policy considerations.* Park Ridge, IL: AANA. https://www.aana.com/docs/default-source/practice-aana-com-web-documents-(all)/care-of-patients-receiving-analgesia-by-catheter-techniques.pdf?sfvrsn=d30049b1_2 (Level VII)

8 Institute for Safe Medication Practices. (2020). Guidelines: Targeted medication safety best practices for hospitals. https://www.ismp.org/guidelines/best-practices-hospitals

9 Standard 12. Product evaluation, integrity, and defect reporting. Infusion therapy standards of practice (8th ed.). (2021). *Journal of Infusion Nursing, 44,* S45–S46. (Level VII)

10 Westbrook, J., et al. (2010). Association of interruptions with an increased risk and severity of medication administration errors. *Archives of Internal Medicine, 170,* 683–690. (Level IV)

11 Institute for Safe Medication Practices. (2012). Side tracks on the safety express: Interruptions lead to errors and unfinished…Wait, what was I doing? https://www.ismp.org/Newsletters/acutecare/showarticle.aspx?id=37

12 Standard 13. Medication verification. Infusion therapy standards of practice (8th ed.). (2021). *Journal of Infusion Nursing, 44,* S46–S49. (Level VII)

13 The Joint Commission. (2021). Standard MM.06.01.01. *Comprehensive accreditation manual for hospitals.* Oakbrook Terrace, IL: The Joint Commission. (Level VII)

14 Centers for Medicare and Medicaid Services, Department of Health and Human Services. (2020). Condition of participation: Nursing services. 42 C.F.R. § 482.23(c).

15 Accreditation Association for Hospitals and Health Systems. (2020). Standard 16.01.03. *Healthcare Facilities Accreditation Program: Accreditation requirements for acute care hospitals.* Chicago, IL: Accreditation Association for Hospitals and Health Systems. (Level VII)

16 DNV GL-Healthcare USA, Inc. (2020). MM.1.SR.3. *NIAHO® accreditation requirements, interpretive guidelines and surveyor guidance—revision 20.0.* Milford, OH: DNV GL-Healthcare USA, Inc. (Level VII)

17 The Joint Commission. (2021). Standard NPSG.07.01.01. *Comprehensive accreditation manual for hospitals.* Oakbrook Terrace, IL: The Joint Commission. (Level VII)

18 Centers for Disease Control and Prevention. (2002). Guideline for hand hygiene in health-care settings: Recommendations of the Healthcare Infection Control Practices Advisory Committee and the HICPAC/SHEA/APIC/IDSA Hand Hygiene Task Force. *MMWR Recommendations and Reports, 51*(RR-16), 1–45. https://www.cdc.gov/mmwr/pdf/rr/rr5116.pdf (Level II)

19 World Health Organization. (2009). WHO guidelines on hand hygiene in health care: First global patient safety challenge, clean care is safer care. https://apps.who.int/iris/bitstream/handle/10665/44102/9789241597906_eng.pdf?sequence=1 (Level IV)

20 Accreditation Association for Hospitals and Health Systems. (2020). Standard 07.01.21. *Healthcare Facilities Accreditation Program: Accreditation requirements for acute care hospitals.* Chicago, IL: Accreditation Association for Hospitals and Health Systems. (Level VII)

21 Centers for Medicare and Medicaid Services, Department of Health and Human Services. (2020). Condition of participation: Infection control. 42 C.F.R. § 482.42.

22 DNV GL-Healthcare USA, Inc. (2019). IC.1.SR.1. *NIAHO® accreditation requirements, interpretive guidelines and surveyor guidance—revision 18.2.* Milford, OH: DNV GL-Healthcare USA, Inc. (Level VII)

23 Standard 16. Hand hygiene. Infusion therapy standards of practice (8th ed.). (2021). *Journal of Infusion Nursing, 44,* S53–S54. (Level VII)

24 The Joint Commission. (2021). Standard NPSG.01.01.01. *Comprehensive accreditation manual for hospitals.* Oakbrook Terrace, IL: The Joint Commission. (Level VII)

25 The Joint Commission. (2021). Standard RI.01.01.01. *Comprehensive accreditation manual for hospitals.* Oakbrook Terrace, IL: The Joint Commission. (Level VII)

26 DNV GL-Healthcare USA, Inc. (2020). PR.2.SR.5. *NIAHO® accreditation requirements, interpretive guidelines and surveyor guidance—revision 20.0.* Milford, OH: DNV GL-Healthcare USA, Inc. (Level VII)

27 Centers for Medicare and Medicaid Services, Department of Health and Human Services. (2020). Condition of participation: Patient's rights. 42 C.F.R. § 482.13(c)(1).

28 Accreditation Association for Hospitals and Health Systems. (2020). Standard 15.01.16. *Healthcare Facilities Accreditation Program: Accreditation requirements for acute care hospitals.* Chicago, IL: Accreditation Association for Hospitals and Health Systems. (Level VII)

29 The Joint Commission. (2021). Standard PC.02.01.21. *Comprehensive accreditation manual for hospitals.* Oakbrook Terrace, IL: The Joint Commission. (Level VII)

30 Waters, T. R., et al. (2009). Safe patient handling training for schools of nursing. https://www.cdc.gov/niosh/docs/2009-127/pdfs/2009-127.pdf (Level VII)

31 Infusion Nurses Society. (2016). *Policies and procedures for infusion therapy* (5th ed.). Boston, MA: Infusion Nurses Society.

32 The Joint Commission. (2021). Standard PC.01.02.07. *Comprehensive accreditation manual for hospitals.* Oakbrook Terrace, IL: The Joint Commission. (Level VII)

33 Siegel, J. D., et al. (2007, revised 2019). 2007 guideline for isolation precautions: Preventing transmission of infectious agents in healthcare settings. https://www.cdc.gov/infectioncontrol/pdf/guidelines/isolation-guidelines-H.pdf (Level II)

34 Accreditation Association for Hospitals and Health Systems. (2020). Standard 07.01.10. *Healthcare Facilities Accreditation Program: Accreditation requirements for acute care hospitals.* Chicago, IL: Accreditation Association for Hospitals and Health Systems. (Level VII)

35 Occupational Safety and Health Administration. (2019). Bloodborne pathogens, standard number 1910.1030. https://www.osha.gov/pls/oshaweb/owadisp.show_document?p_id=10051&p_table=STANDARDS (Level VII)

36 The Joint Commission. (2014). Sentinel event alert 53: Managing risk during transition to new ISO tubing connector standards. https://www.jointcommission.org/assets/1/6/SEA_53_Connectors_8_19_14_final.pdf (Level VII)

37 U.S. Food and Drug Administration. (2017). Examples of medical device misconnections. https://www.fda.gov/medical-devices/medical-device-connectors/examples-medical-device-misconnections

38 Institute for Safe Medication Practices. (2018). ISMP list of high-alert medications in acute care settings. https://www.ismp.org/sites/default/files/attachments/2018-08/highAlert2018-Acute-Final.pdf (Level VII)

39 Institute for Safe Medication Practices. (2019). Independent double checks: Worth the effort if used judiciously and properly. https://www.ismp.org/resources/independent-double-checks-undervalued-and-misused-selective-use-strategy-can-play (Level VII)

40 Graham, K. C., & Cvach, M. (2010). Monitor alarm fatigue: Standardizing use of physiological monitors and decreasing nuisance alarms. *American Journal of Critical Care, 19,* 28–37.

41 The Joint Commission. (2021). Standard NPSG.06.01.01. *Comprehensive accreditation manual for hospitals.* Oakbrook Terrace, IL: The Joint Commission. (Level VII)

42 The Joint Commission. (2013). Sentinel event alert 50: Medical device alarm safety in hospitals. https://www.jointcommission.org/assets/1/6/SEA_50_alarms_4_26_16.pdf (Level VII)

43 Standard 2. Special patient populations: neonatal, pediatric, pregnant, and older adults. Infusion therapy standards of practice (8th ed.). (2021). *Journal of Infusion Nursing, 44,* S13–S15. (Level VII)

44 Centers for Medicare and Medicaid Services. (2014). Requirements for hospital medication administration, particularly intravenous (IV) medications and post-operative care of patients receiving IV opioids. http://www.cms.gov/Medicare/Provider-Enrollment-and-Certification/SurveyCertificationGenInfo/Downloads/Survey-and-Cert-Letter-14-15.pdf

45 Neal, J. M., et al. (2021). American society of regional anesthesia and pain medicine local anesthetic systemic toxicity checklist: 2020 version. *Regional Anesthesia & Pain Medicine, 46,* 81–82. https://rapm.bmj.com/content/rapm/46/1/81.full.pdf (Level VII)

46 Guideline for perioperative practice: Local anesthesia. (2021). In Wood, A. (Ed.), *Guidelines for perioperative practice,* 2021 edition. Denver, CO: AORN, Inc. (Level VII)

47 Ganz, D. A., et al. (2013, reviewed 2021). *Preventing falls in hospitals: A toolkit for improving quality of care* (AHRQ Publication No. 13-0015-EF). Rockville, MD: Agency for Healthcare Research and Quality. https://www.ahrq.gov/professionals/systems/hospital/fallpxtoolkit/index.html (Level VII)

48 Accreditation Association for Hospitals and Health Systems. (2020). Standard 07.02.03. *Healthcare Facilities Accreditation Program: Accreditation requirements for acute care hospitals.* Chicago, IL: Accreditation Association for Hospitals and Health Systems. (Level VII)

49 Rutala, W. A., et al. (2008, revised 2019). Guideline for disinfection and sterilization in healthcare facilities, 2008. https://www.cdc.gov/infection-control/pdf/guidelines/disinfection-guidelines-H.pdf (Level I)

50 The Joint Commission. (2021). Standard RC.01.03.01. *Comprehensive accreditation manual for hospitals.* Oakbrook Terrace, IL: The Joint Commission. (Level VII)

51 Centers for Medicare and Medicaid Services, Department of Health and Human Services. (2020). Condition of participation: Medical record services. 42 C.F.R. § 482.24(b).

52 Accreditation Association for Hospitals and Health Systems. (2020). Standard 10.00.03. *Healthcare Facilities Accreditation Program: Accreditation requirements for acute care hospitals.* Chicago, IL: Accreditation Association for Hospitals and Health Systems. (Level VII)

53 DNV GL Healthcare USA, Inc. (2020). MR.2.SR.1. *NIAHO® accreditation requirements, interpretive guidelines and surveyor guidance—revision 20.0.* Milford, OH: DNV GL-Healthcare USA, Inc. (Level VII)

54 National Institute on Drug Abuse. (2021). Opioid overdose reversal with naloxone (Narcan, Evzio). https://www.drugabuse.gov/related-topics/opioid-overdose-reversal-naloxone-narcan-evzio

55 Lynn, R. R., & Galinkin, J. L. (2018). Naloxone dosage for opioid reversal: Current evidence and clinical implications. *Therapeutic Advances in Drug Safety, 9,* 63–88.

56 The Joint Commission. (2021). Standard RC.02.01.01. *Comprehensive accreditation manual for hospitals.* Oakbrook Terrace, IL: The Joint Commission. (Level VII)

ESOPHAGOGASTRIC TAMPONADE TUBE CARE

Used for the temporary control hemorrhage from esophageal or gastric varices, an esophagogastric tamponade tube is inserted nasally or orally and advanced into the esophagus or stomach. (See *Types of esophagogastric tamponade tubes,* page 316.)

Ordinarily, a practitioner inserts and removes an esophagogastric tamponade tube. However, in an emergency, a nurse may remove the tube.

After the tube is in place, a practitioner can inflate a gastric balloon located at the end of the tube, and the balloon can be drawn tightly against the cardia of the stomach. The inflated gastric balloon secures the tube and exerts pressure on the gastric cardia. The pressure, in turn, controls variceal bleeding. Most tubes also contain an esophageal balloon to control esophageal bleeding (if gastric tamponade alone is insufficient).

A basic traction frame or an esophagogastric tamponade tube is secured to a football helmet or catcher's mask to help reduce the risk of the gastric balloon slipping down or away from the patient's gastric cardia.

Esophagogastric balloon tamponade should be used as a temporary measure (for no more than 24 hours) in patients with uncontrollable bleeding who have a more definitive treatment plan.[1] If the balloon remains inflated longer than 24 hours, pressure necrosis may develop, causing further hemorrhage or perforation.

With the increasing use of endoscopic interventions, the use of esophagogastric tamponade tubes is decreasing. In fact, endoscopic variceal ligation is currently the treatment of choice for acute variceal hemorrhage. Other treatments include gastric lavage, drug therapy with octreotide or vasopressin, sclerotherapy, variceal banding, and

EQUIPMENT

Types of esophagogastric tamponade tubes

When working with a patient who has an esophagogastric tamponade tube, remember the advantages of the most common types, including the Sengstaken-Blakemore tube, Linton tube, and the Minnesota tube.

Sengstaken-Blakemore tube

A Sengstaken-Blakemore tube is a triple-lumen, double-balloon tube that has a gastric aspiration lumen, which allows you to obtain drainage from below the gastric balloon and also to instill medication.

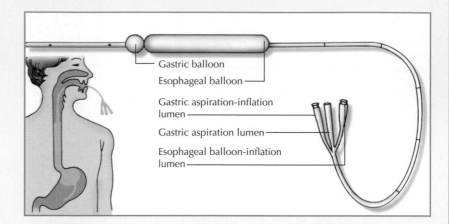

Gastric balloon
Esophageal balloon
Gastric aspiration-inflation lumen
Gastric aspiration lumen
Esophageal balloon-inflation lumen

Linton tube

A Linton tube is a triple-lumen, single-balloon tube that has one lumen for gastric aspiration and another for esophageal aspiration. The Linton tube reduces the risk of esophageal necrosis *because it doesn't have an esophageal balloon.*

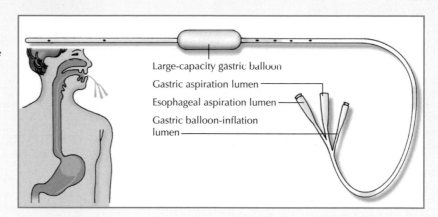

Large-capacity gastric balloon
Gastric aspiration lumen
Esophageal aspiration lumen
Gastric balloon-inflation lumen

Minnesota tube

A Minnesota esophagogastric tamponade tube is an esophageal tube that has four lumens and two balloons. The device provides pressure-monitoring ports for both balloons without the need for Y-connectors. One lumen of the four lumens is used for gastric aspiration; another is used for esophageal aspiration.

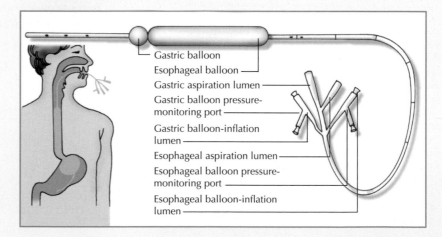

Gastric balloon
Esophageal balloon
Gastric aspiration lumen
Gastric balloon pressure-monitoring port
Gastric balloon-inflation lumen
Esophageal aspiration lumen
Esophageal balloon pressure-monitoring port
Esophageal balloon-inflation lumen

transjugular intrahepatic portosystemic shunting. Esophagogastric balloon tamponade can be used in conjunction with these therapies, but it generally isn't used unless initial endoscopic and pharmacologic treatments fail.[2]

A patient with an esophagogastric tamponade tube requires nursing care during and after insertion. Such patients typically are in the intensive care unit for close observation and constant care. Sedation can be administered, but the dose should be individualized for the patient with probable liver injury.[2]

Equipment

Vital signs monitoring equipment ▪ manometer ▪ normal saline solution ▪ irrigation set ▪ large-volume syringe ▪ washcloth ▪ warm water ▪ water-soluble lubricant ▪ cotton-tipped applicators ▪ sponge swabs or toothbrush and toothpaste ▪ oral moisturizer ▪ suction equipment ▪ gloves ▪ traction equipment (football helmet with face mask, catcher's mask, or gentle traction using a rope, 1-lb [453.6g] traction weight, or tape) ▪ scissors ▪ Optional: prescribed sedative agent, prescribed pain medication, personal protective equipment (gown and mask with goggles or mask with face shield).

Preparation of equipment

Ensure that scissors and suction equipment are present at the patient's bedside; ensure that the suction equipment is functioning properly.

Inspect all equipment and supplies. If a product is expired, is defective, or has compromised integrity, remove it from patient use, label it as expired or defective, and report the defect or expiration as directed by your facility.

Implementation

- Verify the practitioner's order.
- Gather and prepare the necessary equipment and supplies.
- Perform hand hygiene.[3,4,5,6,7,8]
- Confirm the patient's identity using at least two patient identifiers.[9]
- Provide privacy[10,11,12,13]
- Explain the procedure to the patient and family (if appropriate) according to their communication and learning needs *to increase understanding, allay their fears, and enhance cooperation.*[14]
- Raise the patient's bed to waist level before performing patient care *to prevent caregiver back strain.*[15]
- Perform hand hygiene.[3,4,5,6,7,8] Put on gloves and, as needed, other personal protective equipment *to comply with standard precautions.*[16,17,18]
- Monitor the patient's vital signs at an interval determined by the patient's condition and as ordered. *A change in vital signs may signal complications or recurrent bleeding.*
- If the patient has a Sengstaken-Blakemore or Minnesota tube, check the pressure gauge on the manometer every hour. Maintain esophageal balloon pressures at 25 to 45 mm Hg (3.3 to 6 kPa).[2]
- Assist the practitioner with reducing esophageal balloon pressure by 5 mm Hg (0.7 kPa) every 3 hours or, if permitted, perform this step as ordered until pressure is 25 mm Hg (3.3 kPa) and the patient shows no signs of bleeding. *Using the lowest possible pressure helps prevent esophageal necrosis.*[2]
- Assist the practitioner with completely deflating the esophageal balloon using a large-volume syringe for 30 minutes every 8 hours or, if permitted, perform deflation as ordered *to help prevent esophageal necrosis.*[2]
- Maintain drainage and suction on gastric and esophageal aspiration lumens, as ordered. *Fluid accumulating in the patient's stomach may cause the patient to regurgitate the tube, and fluid accumulating in the patient's esophagus may lead to vomiting and aspiration.*
- Trace the esophagogastric tamponade tube from the patient to its point of origin *to ensure that you're assessing the correct port,* and then irrigate the gastric aspiration lumen as ordered using the irrigation set and normal saline solution. *Frequent irrigation keeps the tube from clogging. Obstruction in the tube can lead to regurgitation of the tube and vomiting.*[19,20]
- *To prevent pressure injury,* clean the patient's nostrils and apply water-soluble lubricant frequently. Use a washcloth and warm water *to loosen crusted nasal secretions* before applying the lubricant with cotton-tipped applicators.
- Provide oral care frequently using sponge swabs to clean the patient's teeth, gums, and tongue, or assist the patient with brushing them with a toothbrush or toothpaste at least twice daily *to help increase patient comfort and promote a healthy oral cavity.* Encourage the patient to participate in oral care if possible.[21] (See the "Oral care" procedure.)
- Using a sponge swab, apply oral moisturizer to the patient's oral mucosa and lips every 2 to 4 hours *to help reduce oral inflammation and improve oral health.*[21,22]
- If necessary, suction the patient's oral cavity frequently, *because an esophageal balloon may prevent swallowing of secretions and saliva.*[2]
- Offer emotional support. Keep the patient as quiet as possible.
- Screen for and assess the patient's pain using facility-defined criteria that are consistent with the patient's age, condition, and ability to understand.[23]
- Treat the patient's pain as needed and ordered using nonpharmacologic, pharmacologic, or a combination of approaches. Base the treatment plan on evidence-based practices and the patient's clinical condition, medical history, and pain management goals.[23]
- Monitor the patient closely if the patient is at high risk for adverse outcomes related to opioid treatment, if ordered.[23]
- Administer a sedative agent as needed and prescribed following safe medications administration practices.[24,25,26,27]

- Ensure that the esophagogastric tamponade tube is secured. A football helmet with a face mask, a catcher's mask, or gentle traction using a traction rope, a 1-lb (0.5-kg) traction weight, or tape may be used.[2] If a traction weight is used, ensure that it hangs from the foot of the patient's bed at all times; never rest it on the bed. Instruct housekeeping staff members and other coworkers not to move the weight, *because reduced traction may change the position of the esophagogastric tamponade tube.* If using tape, tape the tube to the patient's face, *which helps provides traction.*
- Monitor the esophagogastric tamponade's external tube length *to help assess for tube migration.*
- Keep the patient on complete bed rest, *because exertion increases intra-abdominal pressure, which may trigger further bleeding.*
- Keep the head of the patient's bed elevated 30 to 45 degrees *to help minimize aspiration and to help prevent ventilator-associated pneumonia if the patient is intubated and mechanically ventilated.*[2,28]
- Observe the patient carefully for esophageal rupture, indicated by signs and symptoms of shock, increased respiratory difficulties, and increased bleeding.
- Monitor the patient's intake and output, as ordered.
- Assess the patient's sedation level, and intervene as appropriate.[23]
- Reassess and respond to the patient's pain by evaluating the response to treatment and progress toward pain management goals. Assess the patient for adverse reactions and risk factors for adverse events that may result from treatment.[23]
- Return the bed to the lowest position *to prevent falls and maintain patient safety.*[29]
- Remove and discard your gloves and any other personal protective equipment worn.[16,18]
- Perform hand hygiene.[3,4,5,6,7,8]
- Document the procedure.[30,31,32,33]

Special considerations

- Keep scissors at the bedside *so you can cut the esophagogastric tamponade tube quickly to deflate the balloons if asphyxia develops.* When performing this emergency intervention, hold the tube firmly close to the nostril before cutting.[12]
- If you're using traction, release the tension before deflating any balloons. If a traction weight is being used, remove the weight. If a football helmet with a mask, catcher's mask, or tape supplies traction, untape the esophagogastric tamponade tube from the face guard or the patient's face before deflating any balloons. *Deflating the balloon under tension triggers a rapid release of the entire tube from the nose, which may injure mucous membranes, initiate recurrent bleeding, and obstruct the airway.*
- If the practitioner orders an X-ray study to check the esophagogastric tamponade tube's position or to view the chest, lift the patient in the direction of the pulley, and then place the X-ray film behind the patient's back. Never roll the patient from side to side, *because pressure exerted on the tube in this way may shift the tube's position.* Similarly, lift the patient to make the bed or to assist with the placing the patient on a bedpan.
- *To reduce the risk of necrosis and ulceration,* the maximum recommended duration for esophagogastric balloon tamponade therapy is 24 hours.[1]
- The Joint Commission has issued a sentinel event alert related to managing risk during the transition to new International Organization for Standardization tubing connector standards that were designed to help prevent dangerous tubing misconnections, *which may lead to serious patient injury and death.* During the transition, be sure to trace the tubing and catheter from the patient to their point of origin before connecting or reconnecting any device or infusion, at any care transition (such as a new setting or service), and as part of the hand-off process; route tubes and catheters having different purposes in different standardized directions; label the tubing at the distal and proximal ends when there are different access sites presents or several bags hanging; use tubing and equipment only as intended; and store medications for different delivery routes in separate locations.[20]

Complications

Esophageal rupture, the most life-threatening complication associated with esophagogastric tamponade tube use, can occur at any time, but it's most likely to occur during intubation or inflation of the esophageal balloon. Esophageal tissue necrosis may occur if the esophageal balloon is inflated for more than 24 hours or if the balloon is overinflated.[34] Asphyxia may result if the balloon moves up the esophagus and blocks the airway. Aspiration of pooled oral secretions, other erosions, nasal tissue necrosis, and cardiac arrhythmias may also complicate the patient's condition.

Documentation

Document the patient's vital signs and esophageal pressures, any GI assessment findings, the condition of the patient's nostrils, oral care performed, and any medications administered, including the medication strength, dose, date and time, and route of administration. Note when the balloons were deflated, who deflated them, and how long they were deflated. Record the patient's tolerance of the procedure. Also, note the color, consistency, and amount of gastric return. Record any signs or symptoms of complications, the practitioner notified and the date and time of notification, any interventions prescribed, and the patient's response to those interventions. Document gastric aspiration lumen irrigations. Document any teaching provided to the patient and family members (if applicable), their understanding of that teaching, and any need for follow-up teaching.

REFERENCES

1 Garcia-Tsao, G., et al. (2017). Portal hypertensive bleeding in cirrhosis: Risk stratification, diagnosis, and management: 2016 practice guidance by the American Association for the Study of Liver Diseases. *Hepatology*, *65*(1), 310–335. https://aasldpubs.onlinelibrary.wiley.com/doi/epdf/10.1002/hep.28906 (Level VII)

2 Wiegand, D. L. (2017). *AACN procedure manual for high acuity, progressive, and critical care* (7th ed.). St. Louis, MO: Elsevier.

3 The Joint Commission. (2021). Standard NPSG.07.01.01. *Comprehensive accreditation manual for hospitals*. Oakbrook Terrace, IL: The Joint Commission. (Level VII)

4 Centers for Disease Control and Prevention. (2002). Guideline for hand hygiene in health-care settings: Recommendations of the Healthcare Infection Control Practices Advisory Committee and the HICPAC/SHEA/APIC/IDSA Hand Hygiene Task Force. *MMWR Recommendations and Reports, 51*(RR-16), 1–45. https://www.cdc.gov/mmwr/pdf/rr/rr5116.pdf (Level II)

5 World Health Organization. (2009). WHO guidelines on hand hygiene in health care: First global patient safety challenge, clean care is safer care. https://apps.who.int/iris/bitstream/handle/10665/44102/9789241597906_eng.pdf?sequence=1 (Level IV)

6 Accreditation Association for Hospitals and Health Systems. (2020). Standard 07.01.21. *Healthcare Facilities Accreditation Program: Accreditation requirements for acute care hospitals*. Chicago, IL: Accreditation Association for Hospitals and Health Systems. (Level VII)

7 Centers for Medicare and Medicaid Services, Department of Health and Human Services. (2020). Condition of participation: Infection control. 42 C.F.R. § 482.42.

8 DNV GL-Healthcare USA, Inc. (2020). IC.1.SR.1. *NIAHO® accreditation requirements, interpretive guidelines and surveyor guidance—revision 20.0*. Milford, OH: DNV GL-Healthcare USA, Inc. (Level VII)

9 The Joint Commission. (2021). Standard NPSG.01.01.01. *Comprehensive accreditation manual for hospitals*. Oakbrook Terrace, IL: The Joint Commission. (Level VII)

10 Accreditation Association for Hospitals and Health Systems. (2020). Standard 15.01.16. *Healthcare Facilities Accreditation Program: Accreditation requirements for acute care hospitals*. Chicago, IL: Accreditation Association for Hospitals and Health Systems. (Level VII)

11 Centers for Medicare and Medicaid Services, Department of Health and Human Services. (2020). Condition of participation: Patient's rights. 42 C.F.R. § 482.13(c)(1).

12 The Joint Commission. (2021). Standard RI.01.01.01. *Comprehensive accreditation manual for hospitals*. Oakbrook Terrace, IL: The Joint Commission. (Level VII)

13 DNV GL-Healthcare USA, Inc. (2020). PR.2.SR.5. *NIAHO® accreditation requirements, interpretive guidelines and surveyor guidance—revision 20.0*. Milford, OH: DNV GL-Healthcare USA, Inc. (Level VII)

14 The Joint Commission. (2021). Standard PC.02.01.21. *Comprehensive accreditation manual for hospitals*. Oakbrook Terrace, IL: The Joint Commission. (Level VII)

15 Waters, T. R., et al. (2009). Safe patient handling training for schools of nursing. https://www.cdc.gov/niosh/docs/2009-127/pdfs/2009-127.pdf (Level VII)

16 Siegel, J. D., et al. (2007, revised 2019). 2007 guideline for isolation precautions: Preventing transmission of infectious agents in healthcare settings. https://www.cdc.gov/infectioncontrol/pdf/guidelines/isolation-guidelines-H.pdf (Level II)

17 Accreditation Association for Hospitals and Health Systems. (2020). Standard 07.01.10. *Healthcare Facilities Accreditation Program: Accreditation requirements for acute care hospitals*. Chicago, IL: Accreditation Association for Hospitals and Health Systems. (Level VII)

18 Occupational Safety and Health Administration. (2019). Bloodborne pathogens, standard number 1910.1030. https://www.osha.gov/pls/oshaweb/owadisp.show_document?p_id=10051&p_table=STANDARDS (Level VII)

19 U.S. Food and Drug Administration. (2017). Examples of medical device misconnections. https://www.fda.gov/medical-devices/medical-device-connectors/examples-medical-device-misconnections

20 The Joint Commission. (2014). Sentinel event alert 53: Managing risk during transition to new ISO tubing connector standards. https://www.jointcommission.org/-/media/deprecated-unorganized/imported-assets/tjc/system-folders/assetmanager/sea_53_connectors_8_19_14_finalpdf.pdf?db=web&hash=5259E85202D5CE621294E9C46E8ED86C (Level VII)

21 American Association of Critical-Care Nurses. (2017). AACN practice alert: Oral care for acutely and critically ill patients. https://www.aacn.org/clinical-resources/practice-alerts/oral-care-for-acutely-and-critically-ill-patients (Level VII)

22 Quinn, B., & Baker, D. L. (2015). Comprehensive oral care helps prevent hospital-acquired nonventilator pneumonia. *American Nurse Today, 10*(3), 18–22. https://www.myamericannurse.com/wp-content/uploads/2015/03/ant3-CE-Oral-Care-225.pdf

23 The Joint Commission. (2021). Standard PC.01.02.07. *Comprehensive accreditation manual for hospitals*. Oakbrook Terrace, IL: The Joint Commission. (Level VII)

24 The Joint Commission. (2021). Standard MM.06.01.01. *Comprehensive accreditation manual for hospitals*. Oakbrook Terrace, IL: The Joint Commission. (Level VII)

25 Centers for Medicare and Medicaid Services, Department of Health and Human Services. (2020). Condition of participation: Nursing services. 42 C.F.R. § 482.23(c).

26 Accreditation Association for Hospitals and Health Systems. (2020). Standard 16.01.03. *Healthcare Facilities Accreditation Program: Accreditation requirements for acute care hospitals*. Chicago, IL: Accreditation Association for Hospitals and Health Systems. (Level VII)

27 DNV GL-Healthcare USA, Inc. (2020). MM.1.SR.3. *NIAHO® accreditation requirements, interpretive guidelines and surveyor guidance—revision 20.0*. Milford, OH: DNV GL-Healthcare USA, Inc. (Level VII)

28 American Association of Critical-Care Nurses. (2017). AACN practice alert: Ventilator associated pneumonia VAP. https://www.aacn.org/clinical-resources/practice-alerts/ventilator-associated-pneumonia-vap (Level VII)

29 Ganz, D. A., et al. (2013, reviewed 2021). *Preventing falls in hospitals: A toolkit for improving quality of care* (AHRQ Publication No. 13-0015-EF). Rockville, MD: Agency for Healthcare Research and Quality. https://www.ahrq.gov/professionals/systems/hospital/fallpxtoolkit/index.html (Level VII)

30 The Joint Commission. (2021). Standard RC.01.03.01. *Comprehensive accreditation manual for hospitals*. Oakbrook Terrace, IL: The Joint Commission. (Level VII)

31 Accreditation Association for Hospitals and Health Systems. (2020). Standard 10.00.03. *Healthcare Facilities Accreditation Program: Accreditation requirements for acute care hospitals*. Chicago, IL: Accreditation Association for Hospitals and Health Systems. (Level VII)

32 Centers for Medicare and Medicaid Services, Department of Health and Human Services. (2020). Condition of participation: Medical record services. 42 C.F.R. § 482.24(b).

33 DNV GL-Healthcare USA, Inc. (2019). MR.2.SR.1. *NIAHO® accreditation requirements, interpretive guidelines and surveyor guidance—revision 18.2*. Milford, OH: DNV GL-Healthcare USA, Inc. (Level VII)

34 Bajaj, J. S., & Sanyal, A. J. (2020). Methods to achieve hemostasis in patients with acute variceal hemorrhage. In: *UpToDate*, Saltzman, J. R. (Ed.).

ESOPHAGOGASTRIC TAMPONADE TUBE INSERTION AND REMOVAL

Used for the temporary control of hemorrhage from esophageal or gastric varices, an esophagogastric tamponade tube is inserted nasally or orally and advanced into the esophagus and stomach. Ordinarily, a practitioner inserts and removes the tube. However, in an emergency situation, a nurse may remove it.

After the tube is in place, a gastric balloon secured at the end of the tube can be inflated and drawn tightly against the cardia of the stomach. The inflated balloon secures the tube and exerts pressure on the cardia. The pressure, in turn, controls variceal bleeding. Most tubes also contain an esophageal balloon to control esophageal bleeding. Balloon tamponade is recommended for no longer than 24 hours in a patient with uncontrolled bleeding who has a more definitive treatment plan, *because pressure necrosis may develop and cause further hemorrhage or perforation.*[1]

With the increase in endoscopy, the use of esophagogastric tamponade tubes is decreasing. In fact, endoscopic variceal ligation is currently the treatment of choice for acute variceal hemorrhage. Other treatments include gastric lavage, drug therapy with octreotide or vasopressin, sclerotherapy, variceal banding, and transjugular intrahepatic portosystemic shunting. Balloon tamponade may be used in conjunction with these therapies but generally isn't used unless initial endoscopic and pharmacologic treatments fail.[1]

Contraindications to this procedure include a history of latex allergy, esophageal stricture, and recent esophageal or gastric surgery. Relative contraindications include heart failure, respiratory failure, hiatal hernia, severe pulmonary hypertension, and cardiac arrhythmias. However, because a patient requiring this procedure is critically ill, the practitioner must weigh the risks and benefits before inserting an esophagogastric tamponade tube in a patient with relative contraindications. Placement of an endotracheal tube before insertion of the esophagogastric tamponade tube is recommended to protect the patient's airway. Sedation may be considered for patient comfort.[2,3]

Esophagogastric tamponade tube therapy should be discontinued gradually to assess for bleeding cessation. The esophageal balloon should be deflated before the gastric balloon, *because a deflated gastric balloon may allow migration of an inflated esophageal balloon into the patient's airway, causing obstruction.*[2]

Equipment
For insertion
Esophagogastric tamponade tube ■ suction equipment (two suction sources and canisters, connecting tubing, rigid suction catheter) ■ irrigation set ■ normal saline solution ■ two 60-mL oral or enteral syringes ■ water-soluble lubricant ■ ½" or 1" (1.3- or 2.5-cm) adhesive tape ■ stethoscope ■ foam nose guard ■ traction equipment (football helmet, catcher's mask, or gentle using traction rope, a 1-lb [453.6 g] traction weight, or tape) ■ manometer ■ sphygmomanometer inflation bulb ■ basin of water ■ scissors ■ gloves ■ gown ■ goggles ■ waterproof marking pen ■ anesthetic spray ■ cardiac monitoring equipment ■ disinfectant pad ■ emergency equipment (code cart with emergency medications, defibrillator, handheld resuscitation bag with mask, and intubation equipment) ■ Optional: Y-connector tube, nasogastric (NG) tube, labels.

For removal
60-mL oral or enteral syringe ■ gloves ■ gown ■ goggles ■ manometer ■ oral care supplies.

Preparation of equipment
For insertion
Keep the traction (helmet or mask) at the bedside or attach traction equipment to the bed *so that traction is readily available after tube insertion.* Ensure that the suction source and equipment and emergency equipment are readily available and functioning properly.[2] Open the irrigation set and fill the container with normal saline solution. Place all equipment within reach. Place scissors at the bedside.

Test the balloons on the esophagogastric tamponade tube for air leaks by inflating them and submerging them in the basin of water. If no bubbles appear in the water, the balloons are intact. Remove them from the water and deflate them. Clamp the tube lumens *so that the balloons stay deflated during insertion.*

To prepare the Minnesota tube, connect the manometer to the gastric pressure monitoring port. Note the pressure when the balloon fills with 100, 200, 300, 400, and 500 mL of air.

Check the aspiration lumens for patency, and make sure they're labeled according to their purpose. If they aren't identified, label them carefully with the waterproof marking pen.

Inspect all equipment and supplies. If a product is expired, is defective, or has compromised integrity, remove it from patient use, label it as expired or defective, and report the expiration or defect as directed by your facility.

Implementation
- Verify the practitioner's order.
- Gather and prepare the necessary equipment and supplies.
- Perform hand hygiene.[4,5,6,7,8,9]
- Confirm the patient's identity using at least two patient identifiers.[10]
- Provide privacy.[11,12,13,14]
- Explain the procedure to the patient and family (if appropriate) according to their individual communication and learning needs *to increase their understanding, allay their fears, and enhance cooperation.*[15]
- Raise the bed to waist level before performing patient care *to prevent caregiver back strain.*[16]
- Attach the patient to a cardiac monitor (if not already attached) and assess the patient's cardiac rhythm.[2] (See the "Cardiac monitoring" procedure.) Ensure that the alarm limits are set appropriately for the patient's current condition, and that alarms are turned on, functioning properly, and audible to staff.[17,18,19,20] *Esophageal tube insertion can cause vagal stimulation, bradycardia, and ST-segment elevation.*[2]
- Assess the patient's baseline respiratory status *for baseline comparison.*[2]
- Perform hand hygiene.[4,5,6,7,8,9]
- Put on gloves, a gown, and goggles *to comply with standard precautions.*[21,22,23]
- Assist the patient into the semi-Fowler position. Place the patient who isn't alert in the left lateral position. *These positions facilitate esophagogastric tamponade tube passage into the stomach and help prevent aspiration.*[2]

For Insertion
- Explain that the practitioner will inspect the patient's nostrils *for patency.*
- *To determine the length of tubing needed,* hold the balloon at the patient's xiphoid process and then extend the tube to the patient's ear and forward to the nose. Using a waterproof pen, mark this point on the tubing.[2]
- Inform the patient that the practitioner will spray the throat (posterior pharynx) and nostril (if used) with an anesthetic *to minimize discomfort and gagging during intubation.*
- After lubricating the tip of the tube with water-soluble lubricant *to help reduce friction and facilitate insertion,* the practitioner will pass the tube through the more patent nostril. As the practitioner does this, the practitioner will direct the patient to tilt the chin toward the chest and to swallow when the patient senses the tip of the tube in the back of the throat. *Swallowing helps to advance the tube into the esophagus and prevents intubation of the trachea.* (If the practitioner introduces the tube orally, the practitioner will direct the patient to swallow immediately.) As the patient swallows, the practitioner quickly advances the tube at least ½" (1.3 cm) beyond the previously marked point on the tube.
- *To confirm tube placement,* the practitioner will aspirate stomach contents through the gastric port. After partially inflating the gastric balloon with 50 to 100 mL of air, the practitioner will order an X-ray of the abdomen *to confirm correct placement of the balloon.*[2] Before fully inflating the balloon, the practitioner will use the 60-mL syringe to irrigate the stomach with normal saline solution and empty the stomach as completely as possible. *This irrigation helps the patient avoid regurgitating gastric contents when the balloon inflates.*

NURSING ALERT An abdominal or chest X-ray should be performed *to ensure proper placement of an esophagogastric tamponade tube.*[2]
- After confirming tube placement, the practitioner will fully inflate the gastric balloon (250 to 500 mL of air for a Sengstaken-Blakemore tube,[24] and 700 to 800 mL of air for a Linton tube[25]) and clamp the tube. If using a Minnesota tube, the practitioner will connect the gastric pressure-monitoring port for the gastric balloon-inflation lumen to the manometer and then inflate the balloon in 100-mL increments until it fills with up to 500 mL of air.[2] While introducing the air, the

Securing an esophagogastric tamponade tube with a football helmet

If a basic traction frame isn't available, you can secure an esophagogastric tamponade tube to a football helmet or a catcher's mask *to reduce the risk of the gastric balloon's slipping down or away from the cardia of the stomach.* Tape the tube to the face guard using adhesive tape, as shown below, and fasten the chin strap.

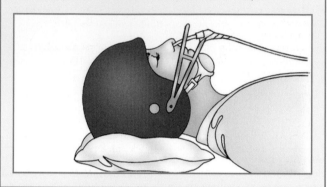

practitioner will monitor the intragastric balloon pressure *to make sure the balloon stays inflated.* Then the practitioner will clamp the inflation ports. For the Sengstaken-Blakemore or Minnesota tube, the practitioner will gently pull on the tube until feeling resistance, *which indicates that the gastric balloon is inflated and exerting pressure on the cardia of the stomach.* When sensing that the balloon is engaged, the practitioner will place the foam nose guard around the area where the tube emerges from the nostril.

■ Be ready to tape the nose guard in place around the esophagogastric tamponade tube *to help minimize pressure on the nostril from the traction and decrease the risk of necrosis.*[2]

■ With the foam nose guard secured, apply traction to the tube using the method preferred by the practitioner. Use a basic traction frame with a traction rope and a 1-lb (453.6 g) weight, or pull the tube gently and tape it tightly to the face mask of a football helmet or catcher's mask using adhesive tape. (See *Securing an esophagogastric tamponade tube with a football helmet.*) Alternatively, some facilities tape the tube to the side of the patient's face as a method of providing traction, *which helps eliminate any issues that may occur with weights or a helmet.*

■ Lavage the stomach through the gastric aspiration lumen with normal saline solution (tepid or room-temperature) until the return fluid is clear.[2] *The lavage empties the stomach of particulate matter, clots, and fresh blood. Any blood detected later in the gastric aspirate indicates that bleeding remains uncontrolled.*[26]

■ Trace the tubing from the patient to its point of origin *to ensure that you're connecting the tubing to the correct port* and attach one of the suction sources to the gastric aspiration lumen *to help empty the stomach, prevent nausea and possible vomiting, and allow continuous observation of the gastric contents for blood.*[27,28]

■ If using a Sengstaken-Blakemore or a Minnesota tube, the practitioner will inflate the esophageal and gastric balloons at the same time *to help compress the esophageal varices and control bleeding.* With a Sengstaken-Blakemore tube, the Y-connector tube is attached to the esophageal balloon-inflation lumen. Then a sphygmomanometer inflation bulb is attached to one end of the Y-connector and the manometer to the other. The esophageal balloon is inflated until the pressure gauge ranges from 25 and 45 mm Hg (3.3 and 6 kPa) and the tube is clamped.[2] With a Minnesota tube, the manometer is attached directly to the esophageal pressure-monitoring outlet. Then, using the 60-mL oral or enteral syringe and pushing the air slowly into the esophageal balloon port, the balloon is inflated until the bleeding stops, usually when the pressure gauge ranges from 35 to 45 mm Hg (4.6 to 6 kPa).

■ Set up esophageal suction *to help prevent accumulation of secretions that may cause vomiting and pulmonary aspiration. This is important, because swallowed secretions can't pass into the stomach if the patient has an inflated*

esophageal balloon in place. If the patient has a Linton or a Minnesota tube, attach the suction source to the esophageal aspiration port. If the patient has a Sengstaken-Blakemore tube, advance an NG tube through the other nostril into the esophagus to the point where the esophageal balloon begins, and attach the suction source, as ordered. Trace each tubing from the patient to its point of origin *to ensure that you're connecting the tubing to the proper port.* Route the tubing in a standardized direction if the patient has other tubing and catheters with different purposes. Label the tubing at both the distal end (near the patient connection) and proximal end (near the source container) *to help reduce the risk of misconnection* if multiple lines will be used.[27,28]

■ Assess the patient's respiratory status; observe for signs of airway obstruction.

■ Assess the patient's cardiac status.

For removal

■ The practitioner will deflate the esophageal balloon by aspirating the air using a 60-mL oral or enteral syringe. (The practitioner may order the esophageal balloon to be deflated at 5-mm Hg [0.67-kPa] increments every 3 hours.) Then, if bleeding doesn't recur, the practitioner will remove the traction from the esophagogastric tamponade tube and deflate the gastric balloon (also by aspiration). The gastric balloon is always deflated just before removing the tube *to help prevent the balloon from riding up into the esophagus or pharynx and obstructing the airway or possibly causing asphyxia or rupture.*[2]

■ After disconnecting all suction tubes, the practitioner will gently remove the esophagogastric tamponade tube. If there is resistance, the practitioner will aspirate the balloons again. (To remove a Minnesota tube, the practitioner will grasp it near the patient's nostril and cut across all four lumens approximately 3″ [7.6 cm] below that point *to ensure deflation of all balloons.*)

■ After the esophagogastric tamponade tube has been removed, assist the patient with oral care *to promote comfort and reduce bacterial colonization in the oropharynx.*

■ Discard equipment in the appropriate receptacles.[23]

Completing the procedure

■ Return the bed to the lowest position *to prevent falls and maintain patient safety.*[29]

■ Remove and discard your gloves and personal protective equipment.[21,23]

■ Perform hand hygiene.[4,5,6,7,8,9]

■ Clean and disinfect your stethoscope using a disinfectant pad.[30,31]

■ Perform hand hygiene.[4,5,6,7,8,9]

■ Document the procedure.[32,33,34,35]

Special considerations

■ The Joint Commission has issued a sentinel event alert concerning medical device alarm safety, *because alarm-related events have been associated with permanent loss of function or death.* Among the major contributing factors noted were improper alarm settings, alarm settings being turned off inappropriately, and alarm signals not being audible to staff. Ensure that alarm limits are set appropriately, and that the alarms are turned on and audible. Follow facility guidelines for preventing alarm fatigue.[17]

■ If the patient appears cyanotic, or if other signs of airway obstruction develop during tube placement, remove the tube immediately, *because it may have entered the trachea instead of the esophagus.*

■ Many practitioners will insert an endotracheal tube before inserting an esophagogastric tube *to help eliminate the possibility of aspiration during tube insertion and while the tube is in place.*

■ After insertion of an esophagogastric tamponade tube, keep scissors at the bedside. If respiratory distress or signs of airway obstruction occur, cut across all lumens while holding the tube at the patient's nostrils, and remove the tube quickly.[2]

■ Unless contraindicated, the patient can sip water through a straw during esophagogastric tamponade tube insertion *to help facilitate tube advancement.*

■ Keep in mind that the intraesophageal balloon pressure varies with respirations and esophageal contractions. Baseline pressure is the important pressure to use when monitoring for complications.

■ The esophageal balloon should stay inflated no longer than 24 hours, *because pressure necrosis of the cardia may occur.*[2] Usually, the practitioner removes the esophagogastric tamponade tube only after a trial period (lasting at least 12 hours) with the esophageal balloon deflated or with the gastric balloon tension released from the cardia *to help check for rebleeding.* In some facilities, the practitioner can deflate the esophageal balloon for 30 minutes every 8 hours *to relieve pressure on the esophageal mucosa temporarily* or decrease the pressure by 5 mm Hg every 3 hours until the pressure is 25 mm Hg.[2] Follow the manufacturer's instructions for balloon deflation.

■ The Joint Commission has issued a sentinel event alert related to managing risk during the transition to new International Organization for Standardization tubing connector standards that were designed *to prevent dangerous tubing misconnections, which may lead to serious patient injury and death.* During the transition, be sure to trace the tubing and catheter from the patient to their point of origin before connecting or reconnecting any device or infusion, at any care transition (such as a new setting or service), and as part of the hand-off process; route tubes and catheters with different purposes in different standardized directions; label the tubing at the distal and proximal ends when there are different access sites present or several bags hanging; use tubing and equipment only as intended; and store medications for different delivery routes in separate locations.[28]

■ After removal of the esophagogastric tamponade tube continue to monitor the patient for recurrence of bleeding.[2]

Complications

Aspiration is the most common complication of esophagogastric tamponade tube insertion. Erosion and perforation of the esophagus and gastric mucosa may result from the tension placed on these areas by the balloons during traction. Esophageal rupture may result if the gastric balloon accidentally inflates in the esophagus. Acute airway occlusion may result if the balloon dislodges and moves upward into the trachea. Other erosions, nasal tissue necrosis, and aspiration of oral secretions may complicate the patient's condition.[2]

Documentation

Record the date and time of esophagogastric tamponade tube insertion and removal, the type of tube used, and the name of the practitioner who performed the procedure. Record the patient's tolerance of the procedure. Document the intraesophageal balloon pressure (for a Sengstaken-Blakemore tube and a Minnesota tube), intragastric balloon pressure (for a Minnesota tube), or amount of air injected (for a Sengstaken-Blakemore tube and a Linton tube). Also, record the amount of normal saline used for gastric irrigation and the color, consistency, and amount of gastric aspirate before and after lavage. Document teaching provided to the patient and family (if appropriate), their understanding of that teaching, and any need for follow-up teaching.

REFERENCES

1 American Society for Gastrointestinal Endoscopy. (2014). Guideline: The role of endoscopy in the management of variceal hemorrhage. *Gastrointestinal Endoscopy, 80*(2), 221–227. https://www.giejournal.org/article/S0016-5107(13)02139-1/pdf (Level VII)

2 Wiegand, D. (2017). *AACN procedure manual for high acuity, progressive, and critical care* (7th ed.). St. Louis, MO: Elsevier.

3 Bajaj, J. S., & Sanyal, A. J. (2020). Methods to achieve hemostasis in patients with acute variceal hemorrhage. In: *UpToDate*, Saltzman, J. R. (Ed.).

4 The Joint Commission. (2021). Standard NPSG.07.01.01. *Comprehensive accreditation manual for hospitals.* Oakbrook Terrace, IL: The Joint Commission. (Level VII)

5 Centers for Disease Control and Prevention. (2002). Guideline for hand hygiene in health-care settings: Recommendations of the Healthcare Infection Control Practices Advisory Committee and the HICPAC/SHEA/APIC/IDSA Hand Hygiene Task Force. *MMWR Recommendations and Reports, 51*(RR-16), 1–45. at https://www.cdc.gov/mmwr/pdf/rr/rr5116.pdf (Level II)

6 World Health Organization. (2009). WHO guidelines on hand hygiene in health care: First global patient safety challenge, clean care is safer care. https://apps.who.int/iris/bitstream/handle/10665/44102/9789241597906_eng.pdf?sequence=1 (Level IV)

7 Accreditation Association for Hospitals and Health Systems. (2020). Standard 07.01.21. *Healthcare Facilities Accreditation Program: Accreditation requirements for acute care hospitals.* Chicago, IL: Accreditation Association for Hospitals and Health Systems. (Level VII)

8 Centers for Medicare and Medicaid Services, Department of Health and Human Services. (2020). Condition of participation: Infection control. 42 C.F.R. § 482.42.

9 DNV GL-Healthcare USA, Inc. (2020). IC.1.SR.1. *NIAHO® accreditation requirements, interpretive guidelines and surveyor guidance revision 20.0.* Milford, OH: DNV GL-Healthcare USA, Inc. (Level VII)

10 The Joint Commission. (2021). Standard NPSG.01.01.01. *Comprehensive accreditation manual for hospitals.* Oakbrook Terrace, IL: The Joint Commission. (Level VII)

11 Accreditation Association for Hospitals and Health Systems. (2020). Standard 15.01.16. *Healthcare Facilities Accreditation Program: Accreditation requirements for acute care hospitals.* Chicago, IL: Accreditation Association for Hospitals and Health Systems. (Level VII)

12 Centers for Medicare and Medicaid Services, Department of Health and Human Services. (2020). Condition of participation: Patient's rights. 42 C.F.R. § 482.13(c)(1).

13 The Joint Commission. (2021). Standard RI.01.01.01. *Comprehensive accreditation manual for hospitals.* Oakbrook Terrace, IL: The Joint Commission. (Level VII)

14 DNV GL-Healthcare USA, Inc. (2020). PR.2.SR.5. *NIAHO® accreditation requirements, interpretive guidelines and surveyor guidance – version 20.0.* Milford, OH: DNV GL-Healthcare USA, Inc. (Level VII)

15 The Joint Commission. (2021). Standard PC.02.01.21. *Comprehensive accreditation manual for hospitals.* Oakbrook Terrace, IL: The Joint Commission. (Level VII)

16 Waters, T. R., et al. (2009). Safe patient handling training for schools of nursing. [Online]https://www.cdc.gov/niosh/docs/2009-127/pdfs/2009-127.pdf. (Level VII)

17 The Joint Commission (2013). Sentinel event alert 50: Medical device alarm safety in hospitals. https://www.jointcommission.org/-/media/deprecated-unorganized/imported-assets/tjc/system-folders/topics-library/sea_50_alarms_4_26_16pdf.pdf?db=web&hash=D2E40EF3AE-647F592A52B98DE039F9DD (Level VII)

18 American Association of Critical-Care Nurses (AACN). (2018). AACN practice alert: Managing alarms in acute care across the life span: Electrocardiography and pulse oximetry. https://www.aacn.org/clinical-resources/practice-alerts/managing-alarms-in-acute-care-across-the life span (Level VII)

19 Graham, K. C., & Cvach, M. (2010). Monitor alarm fatigue: Standardizing use of physiological monitors and decreasing nuisance alarms. *American Journal of Critical Care, 19*, 28–37.

20 The Joint Commission. (2021). Standard NPSG.06.01.01. *Comprehensive accreditation manual for hospitals.* Oakbrook Terrace, IL: The Joint Commission. (Level VII)

21 Siegel, J. D., et al. (2007, revised 2019). 2007 guideline for isolation precautions: Preventing transmission of infectious agents in healthcare settings. https://www.cdc.gov/infectioncontrol/pdf/guidelines/isolation-guidelines-H.pdf (Level II)

22 Accreditation Association for Hospitals and Health Systems. (2020). Standard 07.01.10. *Healthcare Facilities Accreditation Program: Accreditation requirements for acute care hospitals.* Chicago, IL: Accreditation Association for Hospitals and Health Systems. (Level VII)

23 Occupational Safety and Health Administration. (2019). Bloodborne pathogens, standard number 1910.1030. https://www.osha.gov/pls/oshaweb/owadisp.show_document?p_id=10051&p_table=STANDARDS (Level VII)

24 Treger, R. (2020). Sengstaken-Blakemore tube placement technique. https://emedicine.medscape.com/article/81020-technique

25 C.R. Bard, Inc. (n.d.). Specialty tubes. https://www.crbard.com/medical/en-US/Products/Specialty-Tubes

26 Saltzman, J. R. (2021). Approach to acute upper gastrointestinal bleeding in adults. In: *UpToDate*, Feldman, M., (Eds.).

27 U.S. Food and Drug Administration. (2017). Examples of medical device misconnections. https://www.fda.gov/medical-devices/medical-device-connectors/examples-medical-device-misconnections

28 The Joint Commission. (2014). Sentinel event alert 53: Managing risk during transition to new ISO tubing connector standards. https://www.jointcommission.org/-/media/deprecated-unorganized/imported-assets/tjc/system-folders/assetmanager/sea_53_connectors_8_19_14_finalpdf.pdf?d-b=web&hash=5259E85202D5CE621294E9C46E8ED86C (Level VII)

29 Ganz, D. A., et al. (2013, reviewed 2021). *Preventing falls in hospitals: A toolkit for improving quality of care* (AHRQ Publication No. 13-0015-EF). Rockville, MD: Agency for Healthcare Research and Quality. https://www.ahrq.gov/professionals/systems/hospital/fallpxtoolkit/index.html (Level VII)

30 Rutala, W. A., et al. (2008, revised 2019). Guideline for disinfection and sterilization in healthcare facilities, 2008. https://www.cdc.gov/infection-control/pdf/guidelines/disinfection-guidelines-H.pdf (Level I)

31 Accreditation Association for Hospitals and Health Systems. (2020). Standard 07.02.03. *Healthcare Facilities Accreditation Program: Accreditation requirements for acute care hospitals.* Chicago, IL: Accreditation Association for Hospitals and Health Systems. (Level VII)

32 The Joint Commission. (2021). Standard RC.01.03.01. *Comprehensive accreditation manual for hospitals.* Oakbrook Terrace, IL: The Joint Commission. (Level VII)

33 Accreditation Association for Hospitals and Health Systems. (2020). Standard 10.00.03. *Healthcare Facilities Accreditation Program: Accreditation requirements for acute care hospitals.* Chicago, IL: Accreditation Association for Hospitals and Health Systems. (Level VII)

34 Centers for Medicare and Medicaid Services, Department of Health and Human Services. (2020). Condition of participation: Medical record services. 42 C.F.R. § 482.24(b).

35 DNV GL-Healthcare USA, Inc. (2020). MR.2.SR.1. *NIAHO® accreditation requirements, interpretive guidelines and surveyor guidance – version 20.0.* Milford, OH: DNV GL-Healthcare USA, Inc. (Level VII)

EXTERNAL FIXATION MANAGEMENT

In external fixation, a practitioner inserts metal pins and wires through skin and muscle layers into the broken bones and affixes them to an adjustable external frame that maintains their proper alignment during healing. (See *Types of external fixation devices.*) This procedure is used most commonly to treat open, unstable fractures with extensive soft-tissue damage, comminuted closed fractures, and septic, nonunion fractures. It also facilitates surgical immobilization of a joint. Specialized types of external fixators may be used to lengthen leg bones or immobilize the cervical spine.[1]

One advantage of external fixation over other immobilization techniques is that it stabilizes the fracture while allowing full visualization and access to open wounds. It also facilitates early ambulation, which reduces the risk of complications from immobilization.

Equipment

External fixation set ▪ gloves ▪ sterile container ▪ sterile cotton-tipped applicators ▪ chlorhexidine or other facility-approved solution ▪ ice pack ▪ prescribed pain medication ▪ Optional: pillow.

Equipment varies with the type of fixator and the type and location of the fracture. Typically, sets of pins, stabilizing rods, and clips are available from manufacturers.

Preparation of equipment

Inspect all equipment and supplies. If a product is expired, is defective, or has compromised integrity, remove it from patient use, label it as expired or defective, and report the expiration or defect as directed by your facility. Make sure that the external fixation set includes all the equipment it's supposed to include and that the equipment has been sterilized.

Implementation

- Verify the practitioner's order.
- Gather and prepare the necessary equipment and supplies.
- Perform hand hygiene.[5,6,7,8,9,10]
- Confirm the patient's identity using at least two patient identifiers.[11]
- Provide privacy.[12,13,14,15]

EQUIPMENT

Types of external fixation devices

The practitioner's selection of an external fixation device depends on the severity of the patient's fracture and on the type of bone alignment needed. Types include uniplanar, multiplanar, unilateral, bilateral, circular, and hybrid fixators.[2] Here are some examples of external fixation devices.

A **bilateral frame** (shown below) supports both sides of the bone, promoting stability.[2]

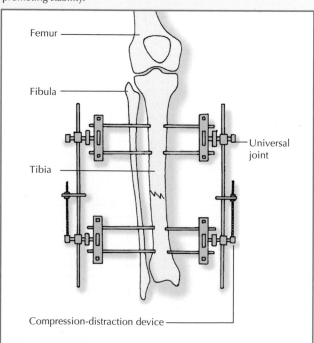

A **unilateral fixator** (shown below) supports the bone on one side.[2]

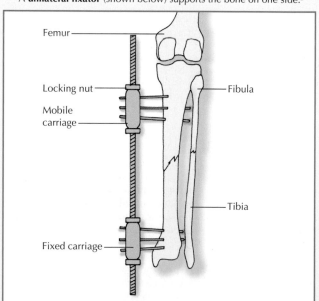

The **Ilizarov fixator** is a special type of external fixation device. This device is a combination of rings and tensioned transosseous wires used primarily in limb lengthening, bone transport, and limb salvage. Highly complex, it provides gradual distraction that results in good-quality bone formation with a minimum of complications.[3] It also provides enough stability to allow early unrestricted weight bearing.[4]

Before placement of the device

■ Explain the procedure to the patient and family (if appropriate) according to their individual communication and learning needed *to increase their understanding, allay their fears, and enhance cooperation.*[16] Emphasize that the patient will feel little pain after the fixation device is in place. Assure the patient that feelings of anxiety are normal, and that the patient will be able to adjust to the apparatus. Explain that moving about is permitted with the apparatus in place, and that it may help the patient resume normal activities more quickly.

■ Raise the patient's bed to waist level before performing patient care *to prevent caregiver back strain.*[17]

■ Screen for and assess the patient's pain using facility-defined criteria that are consistent with the patient's age, condition, and ability to understand.[18]

■ Treat the patient's pain, as needed and ordered, using nonpharmacologic, pharmacologic, or a combination of approaches. Base the treatment plan on evidence-based practices and the patient's clinical condition, past medical history, and pain management goals.[18] Administer pain medication, as ordered and indicated, following safe medication administration practices.[19,20,21,22]

■ Closely monitor any patient who is at high risk for adverse outcomes related to opioid treatment, if opioids are prescribed.[18]

After the fixation device is in place

■ Assess the patient's neurovascular status at an interval determined by your facility and the patient's condition *to assess for possible neurologic damage.* Assess color, warmth, motion, sensation, digital movement, edema, capillary refill, and pulses of the affected extremity. Compare with the unaffected side.

■ Apply an ice pack to the surgical site, as ordered, *to reduce swelling, relieve pain, and lessen bleeding.*

■ Screen for and assess the patient's pain 30 minutes to 1 hour before exercising or mobilizing the affected extremity using facility-defined criteria and techniques that are appropriate for the patient's age, condition, and ability to understand.[18] Administer pain medication, as ordered and indicated, following safe medication administration practices, *to promote comfort.*[19,20,21,22]

■ Monitor the patient for pain not relieved by analgesics and for burning, tingling, or numbness, *which may indicate nerve damage or circulatory impairment.*

■ Elevate the affected extremity on a pillow, if appropriate, *to minimize edema.*

■ Perform pin site care, as ordered. Open sterile packages and the sterile container. Pour the prescribed antiseptic solution into the sterile container. Chlorhexidine may be superior to normal saline solution as a pin site cleaning solution.[23] Povidone-iodine shouldn't be used *because it interferes with tissue healing.*[24] Perform hand hygiene.[5,6,7,8,9,10] Put on gloves *to comply with standard precautions.*[25,26,27] Using cotton-tipped applicators, clean the pin sites gently with chlorhexidine or another facility-approved solution. After the first 48 to 72 hours, pin site care may be performed daily or weekly.[23,24,28] Weekly pin-site care is supported for uninfected pin sites.[23,24] Evidence is insufficient to recommend one pin site technique over another for reducing infection and other complications.[29,30,31] Use a clean, cotton-tipped applicator for each site. Remove crusting above the level of the wound carefully during cleaning. Unless infection is suspected or confirmed, leave dried exudate sealing the pin site in place.[32] If infection is suspected or confirmed, remove crusts at the site gently during cleaning *to allow for drainage.*[33] Allow the site to dry completely.

■ Inspect the pin sites for loose pins and signs and symptoms of infection, including swelling, redness, purulent drainage, tracking (an open area where skin has pulled away from the pin), and pain at the site. Notify the practitioner if any signs or symptoms of infection develop.[33]

■ Reassess and respond to the patient's pain by evaluating the response to treatment and progress toward pain management goals. Assess for adverse reactions and risk factors for adverse events that may result from treatment.[18]

■ Return the bed to the lowest position *to prevent falls and maintain patient safety.*[34]

■ Perform hand hygiene.[5,6,7,8,9,10]

■ Document the procedure.[35,36,37,38]

Special considerations

■ The National Association of Orthopaedic Nurses recommends using 2% chlorhexidine solution for pin site care.[23]

■ As appropriate, encourage the patient to stop smoking and provide smoking-cessation materials, *because smoking delays bone healing.*[39]

Patient teaching

Before discharge, teach the patient and family members how to provide pin site care using clean technique.[23] Give them written instructions, and have them demonstrate the procedure before leaving the hospital.[23] Teach the patient to recognize and report signs of pin site infection.[23] Tell the patient to keep the affected limb elevated when sitting or lying down.

During discharge planning, teach the patient and family about pain management strategies. Include information about the patient's pain management plan and potential adverse effects of pain management treatment. Discuss activities of daily living and items in the home environment that may exacerbate pain or reduce the effectiveness of the pain management plan. Include strategies to address these issues. Teach the patient and family about the safe use, storage, and disposal of opioids, if prescribed.[18]

Complications

Complications of external fixation include loosening of pins and loss of fracture stabilization, infection of the pin tract or wound, osteomyelitis, malunion, non-union, skin breakdown, nerve damage, compartment syndrome, and refracture around the pin.[2]

Documentation

Record the patient's reaction to the apparatus. Document neurovascular status, the condition of the pin sites and surrounding skin, pin site care, and pain assessment findings. Also document pain medication administered, including the name, strength, dose, administration route, and date and time of administration. Note the patient's response to the pain medication, as appropriate. Record any adverse reactions to the prescribed medication, the name of the practitioner notified, the date and time of notification, prescribed interventions, and the patient's response to those interventions.[40] Document teaching provided to the patient and family (if applicable), their understanding of that teaching, and any need for follow-up teaching.

REFERENCES

1 Washington University Orthopedics. (n.d.). Limb lengthening using external fixation. https://www.ortho.wustl.edu/content/Patient-Care/3208/Services/Pediatric-and-Adolescent-Orthopedic-Surgery/Overview/Limb-Length-Discrepancy.aspx

2 Hadeed, A., et al. (2020). External fixation principles and overview. https://www.ncbi.nlm.nih.gov/books/NBK547694/

3 Spiegelberg, B., et al. (2010). Ilizarov principles of deformity correction. *Annals of the Royal College of Surgeons of England, 92*(2), 101–105. https://www.ncbi.nlm.nih.gov/pmc/articles/PMC3025247/

4 Ramos, T., et al. (2013). Treatment of distal tibial fractures with the Ilizarov external fixator: A prospective observational study in 39 consecutive patients. *BMC Musculoskeletal Disorders, 14*, 30. https://www.ncbi.nlm.nih.gov/pmc/articles/PMC3626620/ (Level VI)

5 The Joint Commission. (2021). Standard NPSG.07.01.01. *Comprehensive accreditation manual for hospitals.* Oakbrook Terrace, IL: The Joint Commission. (Level VII)

6 Centers for Disease Control and Prevention. (2002). Guideline for hand hygiene in health-care settings: Recommendations of the Healthcare Infection Control Practices Advisory Committee and the HICPAC/SHEA/APIC/IDSA Hand Hygiene Task Force. *MMWR Recommendations and Reports, 51*(RR-16), 1–45. https://www.cdc.gov/mmwr/pdf/rr/rr5116.pdf (Level II)

7 World Health Organization. (2009). WHO guidelines on hand hygiene in health care: First global patient safety challenge, clean care is safer care. https://apps.who.int/iris/bitstream/handle/10665/44102/9789241597906_eng.pdf (Level IV)

8 Accreditation Association for Hospitals and Health Systems. (2020). Standard 07.01.21. *Healthcare Facilities Accreditation Program: Accreditation requirements for acute care hospitals.* Chicago, IL: Accreditation Association for Hospitals and Health Systems. (Level VII)

9 Centers for Medicare and Medicaid Services, Department of Health and Human Services. (2020). Condition of participation: Infection control. 42 C.F.R. § 482.42.

10 DNV GL-Healthcare USA, Inc. (2020). IC.1.SR.1. *NIAHO® accreditation requirements, interpretive guidelines and surveyor guidance—revision 20.0.* Milford, OH: DNV GL-Healthcare USA, Inc. (Level VII)

11 The Joint Commission. (2021). Standard NPSG.01.01.01. *Comprehensive accreditation manual for hospitals.* Oakbrook Terrace, IL: The Joint Commission. (Level VII)

12 Centers for Medicare and Medicaid Services, Department of Health and Human Services. (2020). Condition of participation: Patient's rights. 42 C.F.R. § 482.13(c)(1).

13 Accreditation Association for Hospitals and Health Systems. (2020). Standard 15.01.16. *Healthcare Facilities Accreditation Program: Accreditation requirements for acute care hospitals.* Chicago, IL: Accreditation Association for Hospitals and Health Systems. (Level VII)

14 The Joint Commission. (2021). Standard RI.01.01.01. *Comprehensive accreditation manual for hospitals.* Oakbrook Terrace, IL: The Joint Commission. (Level VII)

15 DNV GL-Healthcare USA, Inc. (2020). PR.2.SR.5. *NIAHO® accreditation requirements, interpretive guidelines and surveyor guidance—revision 20.0.* Milford, OH: DNV GL-Healthcare USA, Inc. (Level VII)

16 The Joint Commission. (2021). Standard PC.02.01.21. *Comprehensive accreditation manual for hospitals.* Oakbrook Terrace, IL: The Joint Commission. (Level VII)

17 Waters, T. R., et al. (2009). Safe patient handling training for schools of nursing. https://www.cdc.gov/niosh/docs/2009-127/pdfs/2009-127.pdf (Level VII)

18 The Joint Commission. (2021). Standard PC.01.02.07. *Comprehensive accreditation manual for hospitals.* Oakbrook Terrace, IL: The Joint Commission. (Level VII)

19 The Joint Commission. (2021). Standard MM.06.01.01. *Comprehensive accreditation manual for hospitals.* Oakbrook Terrace, IL: The Joint Commission. (Level VII)

20 Centers for Medicare and Medicaid Services, Department of Health and Human Services. (2020). Condition of participation: Nursing services. 42 C.F.R. § 482.23(c).

21 Accreditation Association for Hospitals and Health Systems. (2020). Standard 16.01.03. *Healthcare Facilities Accreditation Program: Accreditation requirements for acute care hospitals.* Chicago, IL: Accreditation Association for Hospitals and Health Systems. (Level VII)

22 DNV GL-Healthcare USA, Inc. (2020). MM.1.SR.3. *NIAHO® accreditation requirements, interpretive guidelines and surveyor guidance—revision 20.0.* Milford, OH: DNV GL-Healthcare USA, Inc. (Level VII)

23 Holmes, S. B., et al. (2005). Skeletal pin site care: National Association of Orthopaedic Nurses guidelines for orthopaedic nursing. *Orthopedic Nursing, 24*(2), 99–107. (Level VII)

24 Lagerquist, D., et al. (2012). Care of external fixator pin sites. *American Journal of Critical Care, 21*(4), 288–292. (Level I)

25 Accreditation Association for Hospitals and Health Systems. (2020). Standard 07.01.10. *Healthcare Facilities Accreditation Program: Accreditation requirements for acute care hospitals.* Chicago, IL: Accreditation Association for Hospitals and Health Systems. (Level VII)

26 Occupational Safety and Health Administration. (2019). Bloodborne pathogens, standard number 1910.1030. https://www.osha.gov/pls/oshaweb/owadisp.show_document?p_id=10051&p_table=STANDARDS (Level VII)

27 Siegel, J. D., et al. (2007, revised 2019). 2007 guideline for isolation precautions: Preventing transmission of infectious agents in healthcare settings. https://www.cdc.gov/infectioncontrol/pdf/guidelines/isolation-guidelines-H.pdf (Level II)

28 Kazmers, N. H., et al. (2016). Prevention of pin site infection in external fixation: A review of the literature. *Strategies in Trauma and Limb Reconstruction, 11*(2), 75–85. https://www.ncbi.nlm.nih.gov/pmc/articles/PMC4960058/

29 Lethaby, A., et al. (2013). Pin site care for preventing infections associated with external bone fixators and pins. *Cochrane Database of Systematic Reviews*, 2013(12), CD004551. (Level I)

30 Bible, J. E., & Mir, H. R. (2015). External fixation: Principles and applications. *Journal of American Academy of Orthopaedic Surgeons, 23*, 683–690.

31 Ktistakis, I., et al. (2015). Pin-site care: Can we reduce the incidence of infections? *Injury, 46*(Suppl. 3), S35–S39. (Level VI)

32 Georgiades, D. S. (2018). A systematic integrative review of pin site crusts. *Orthopaedic Nursing, 37*(1), 36–42. (Level I)

33 Sarro, A., et al. (2010). Developing a standard of care for halo vest and pin site care including patient and family education: A collaborative approach among three greater Toronto area teaching hospitals. *Journal of Neuroscience Nursing, 42*, 169–173. (Level V)

34 Ganz, D. A., et al. (2013, reviewed 2021). *Preventing falls in hospitals: A toolkit for improving quality of care* (AHRQ Publication No. 13-0015-EF). Rockville, MD: Agency for Healthcare Research and Quality. https://www.ahrq.gov/professionals/systems/hospital/fallpxtoolkit/index.html (Level VII)

35 The Joint Commission. (2021). Standard RC.01.03.01. *Comprehensive accreditation manual for hospitals.* Oakbrook Terrace, IL: The Joint Commission. (Level VII)

36 Centers for Medicare and Medicaid Services, Department of Health and Human Services. (2020). Condition of participation: Medical record services. 42 C.F.R. § 482.24(b).

37 Accreditation Association for Hospitals and Health Systems. (2020). Standard 10.00.03. *Healthcare Facilities Accreditation Program: Accreditation requirements for acute care hospitals.* Chicago, IL: Accreditation Association for Hospitals and Health Systems. (Level VII)

38 DNV GL-Healthcare USA, Inc. (2020). MR.2.SR.1. *NIAHO® accreditation requirements, interpretive guidelines and surveyor guidance—revision 20.0.* Milford, OH: DNV GL-Healthcare USA, Inc. (Level VII)

39 Patel, R. A., et al. (2013). The effect of smoking on bone healing. *Bone & Joint Research, 2*(6), 102–111. https://www.ncbi.nlm.nih.gov/pmc/articles/PMC3686151/ (Level I)

40 The Joint Commission. (2021). Standard RC.02.01.01. *Comprehensive accreditation manual for hospitals.* Oakbrook Terrace, IL: The Joint Commission. (Level VII)

EXTERNAL URINE COLLECTION DEVICE USE

Many patients don't require an indwelling urinary catheter to manage their incontinence. External urine collection devices serve as an alternative to indwelling urinary catheters in cooperative patients who don't have signs of urinary retention or bladder outlet obstruction. An external urine collection device can prevent unnecessary indwelling catheterization, which increases the risk of catheter-associated urinary tract infection (CAUTI).[1,2,3,4] This type of device reduces the risk of CAUTI from catheterization, promotes bladder retraining when possible, prevents skin breakdown, and improves the patient's self-image.

An external urine collection device designed for male patients consists of a condom catheter or other device secured to the shaft of the penis and connected to a leg bag or drainage bag.[5] An external urine collection device designed for female patients contains an absorptive component that's placed against the urethral meatus between the patient's labia, which attaches to tubing that connects to a collection canister. The collection catheter attaches to continuous low suction to facilitate urine collection. The device may also come with an adhesive pad to keep it in place.

HOSPITAL-ACQUIRED CONDITION ALERT Keep in mind that the Centers for Medicare and Medicaid Services considers catheter-associated urinary tract infection (CAUTI) to be a hospital-acquired condition *because it can be reasonably prevented using a variety of best practices.* Use an external urine collection device instead of an indwelling urinary catheter when possible to avoid the risk of CAUTI.[1,2,3,6,7,8]

Contraindications to placement include latex allergy (unless the device is latex-free) or adhesive allergy; perineal skin irritation or breakdown, or open lesions on the glans penis or penile shaft; phimosis or paraphimosis; catheter-induced hypospadias; recent surgery of the external urogenital tract; heavy vaginal bleeding; fecal incontinence; and, if the patient is highly agitated or confused, a high risk of trauma related to improper catheter removal.[9,10] The PrimoFit device shouldn't be used for patients in a prone position or patients with female anatomy, or for stool collection.[11] Use the device with caution for patients with altered mental status.[11]

Equipment

External urine collection device of appropriate size and type[9] ■ drainage bag ■ extension tubing ■ gloves ■ nonmoisturizing soap basin ■ water ■ washcloth ■ towel ■ urine collection device (urinal or graduated cylinder) ■ fluid-impermeable pad ■ Optional: disposable-head clippers, commercial adhesive strip, skin protectant, penile clamp, FreeDerm adhesive remover, tape measure, scissors, suction source, suction control device, suction tubing disposable mesh underwear.

Preparation of equipment

Inspect all equipment and supplies. If a product is expired, is defective, or has compromised integrity, remove it from patient use, label it as expired or defective, and report the expiration or defect as directed by your facility.

Follow the manufacturer's guidelines for device sizing. Use a tape measure to determine the diameter of the penis if no one previously determined what size device is most appropriate.[9]

If the device requires suction, assemble the urine collection canister and suction tubing, and test the suction source and suction control device *to make sure that they're functioning properly.*

Implementation

- Review the patient's medical record for an allergy to latex or adhesive.[9]
- Gather and prepare the necessary equipment and supplies.
- Perform hand hygiene.[1,12,13,14,15,16,17]
- Confirm the patient's identity using at least two patient identifiers.[18]
- Provide privacy.[19,20,21,22]
- Explain the procedure to the patient and family (if appropriate) according to their individual communication and learning needs *to increase their understanding, allay their fears, and to enhance cooperation.*[23]
- Raise the bed to waist level before providing care *to prevent caregiver back strain.*[24]
- Put on gloves *to comply with standard precautions.*[25,26,27]
- Place the patient in a supine position with the legs separated. Remove the device from the packaging.

For applying and removal of external urine collection device on a male

- If necessary, apply a penile clamp (if available) *to prevent urine leakage while washing the penis.*[28]
- If the patient is circumcised, wash the penis with nonmoisturizing soap and water, rinse well, and pat dry with a towel.
- If the patient is uncircumcised, gently retract the foreskin and clean beneath it. Rinse well but don't dry, *because moisture provides lubrication and prevents friction during foreskin replacement.* Replace the foreskin *to avoid penile constriction.*
- If necessary, clip hair from the base and shaft of the penis *to prevent the adhesive strip or skin-bond cement from pulling pubic hair.*[9]
- *If applying a condom device*: Apply a skin protectant, as indicated, and allow it to dry completely.[9] If you're using a precut commercial adhesive strip for a nonadhesive-coated condom catheter, insert the glans penis through its opening and position the strip 1″ (2.5 cm) from the scrotal area. If you're using uncut adhesive for a nonadhesive-coated condom catheter, cut a strip to fit around the shaft of the penis. Remove the protective covering from one side of the adhesive strip and press this side firmly to the penis *to enhance adhesion.* Then remove the covering from the other side of the strip. If you're using an adhesive-coated condom catheter, there's no need for additional adhesive strips or securing devices. Position the rolled condom catheter at the tip of the penis, leaving ½″ (1.3 cm) between the condom end and the tip of the penis, with the drainage opening at the urinary meatus. If using a nonadhesive-coated condom catheter, unroll it upward past the adhesive strip on the shaft of the penis. Then press the sheath gently against the strip until it adheres. Using extension tubing, connect the device to the drainage. Regularly inspect the catheter and extension tubing for kinks or twists, which could obstruct urine flow and cause the catheter to balloon, eventually dislodging it.
- *For application of the Men's Liberty device*: Apply a skin protectant, as indicated, and allow it to dry completely.[9] Position the device with the vent facing upward. Align the center opening of the circular tube and petals with the urinary meatus. Remove the release papers around the petals, and attach the faceplate to the tip of the penis with the center opening directly in line with the urinary meatus. Smooth down the

petals. Position the faceplate strip under the tip of the penis and center it in the middle. Remove the adhesive backing of the faceplate strip. Make sure to position the edge of the faceplate strip over the end of the clear circular tube and the tip of the penis, and wrap the strip around each side, keeping the strip flat and wrinkle free. Using your fingers, push any ridges and grooves *to remove air pockets.* Press and hold the strip for 10 to 15 seconds *to secure the seal.*[27]

- *For application of the PrimoFit device*: Remove the liner of the base adhesive. Align the base adhesive with the patient's penis, and position the device with the adhesive toward the patient and tabs facing upward. Position the base adhesive around the penis against the skin while holding the tabs. Apply pressure all the way around to ensure adequate adhesion. Place the patient's penis into the wicking chamber. Remove the liner of the adhesive pad. Pull the device up over the patient's penis and suprapubic region, and adhere the device to the patient's abdomen. Attach suction tubing to the device at the suction tubing adapter. Secure the tubing according to facility guidelines. Set suction to low continuous suction at a minimum of 40 mmHg. Always use the minimum amount of suction needed.
- Return the patient's legs to a closed position. Assess the device periodically, especially after turning or repositioning. Perform a skin assessment every 2 hours, and document according to facility guidelines.[11]
- Regularly assess the penile skin for signs of irritation or breakdown.[9]
- *For removal of the condom device*: Soak the penis with a warm, wet washcloth for 30 seconds *to facilitate removal of the device.*[9] Simultaneously roll the device and adhesive strip off the penis and discard them. Place the patient in a supine position with the legs separated.
- *For removal of the Men's Liberty device*: Soak the seal with warm water or a warm, wet washcloth until it turns milky white and rolls gently from the skin. Alternatively, spray the edge of the adhesive with FreeDerm adhesive remover, lifting gently from the skin as you go, and continue to spray under the adhesive until you can remove it completely.[28]
- *For removal of the PrimoFit device*: Remove the adhesive pad from the abdomen, remove the penis from the wicking chamber, and remove the base adhesive gently by pulling the tabs down and away.[11]
- Clean the penis with lukewarm water, rinse thoroughly, and dry. Check for swelling or signs of skin breakdown.
- Empty the urine drainage bag into a urinal or graduated cylinder. Record the volume if you're monitoring intake and output. Close the drain clamp on the drainage bag, unlatch the leg straps (if present), and disconnect the extension tubing at the top of the bag. Disconnect the device from suction tubing, if used.[11]

For applying and removing an external urine collection device on a female

- Assist the patient to a supine or lithotomy position with the knees bent and legs abducted. Alternatively, position the patient in a knee-chest position on the side if the patient can't tolerate the supine or lithotomy position.[10,29]
- Place a fluid-impermeable pad under the patient's pelvis *to protect the bed from soiling and moisture.*
- Drape the patient with a bath blanket or sheet, exposing only the perineal area, *to maintain warmth and privacy.*
- Assess the patient's perineal area for skin irritation or breakdown, signs of fecal incontinence, and heavy vaginal bleeding. Notify the practitioner if any are present.[10,29]
- Clean and dry the perineal area as directed by your facility.[10,29] (See the "Perineal care" procedure.)
- Remove the device from its packaging and attach the proximal end to the suction tubing.[10,29]
- Separate the patient's labia and identify the urethral meatus.[10,29]
- Align the female external urine collection device vertically, with the distal end pointing toward the patient's buttocks and the proximal end with the suction tubing pointing toward the patient's pubic bone, according to the manufacturer's instructions.[10,29]
- Place the device between the patient's labia and buttocks, with the absorbent fabric against the urethral meatus.[10,29]
- If an adhesive securement pad is present on the device, remove the protective liner and apply the adhesive securement pad to the skin of the suprapubic area while holding the device in place.[10] If an adhesive

securement pad isn't present on the device, put disposable mesh underwear on the patient (as appropriate) *to secure the device in place.*[10]

- After you position and secure the device properly, position the patient's legs together.[10,29]
- Turn on continuous suction to at least 40 mm Hg, using the minimum amount of suction needed to collect the patient's urine.[10,29]
- Assess the patient's skin regularly for irritation or injury, the position of the device for proper placement (especially after turning or repositioning the patient), and the tubing for obstruction.
- Replace the device every 8 to 12 hours or whenever it becomes soiled with feces, blood, or other non-urine body fluid.[10,29] Discontinue use when the patient is able to use the toilet with assistance or independently.[10]
- Empty the urine collection canister, and measure urine output as needed or as directed by your facility. Replace the suction tubing and the urine collection canister as directed by your facility.[10,29]
- Cover the patient, as appropriate.
- Replace the device every 8 to 12 hours or whenever it becomes soiled with feces, blood, or other non-urine body fluid.
- To remove the device, assist the patient to a supine or lithotomy position with the knees bent and legs abducted.[10]
- If present, remove the adhesive securement pad gently from the skin of the patient's suprapubic area.[10]
- Separate the patient's labia and remove the device carefully by pulling it straight out (rather than pulling it against the perineal skin).[10,29]
- Clean and dry the perineal area as directed by your facility.[10,29]
- Cover the patient, as appropriate.
- Disconnect the device from the suction tubing.[10]
- Discard the device in an appropriate receptacle.[25]

Completing the procedure

- Return the bed to the lowest position *to prevent falls and maintain the patient's safety.*[30]
- Discard used supplies in appropriate receptacles.[25]
- Remove and discard your gloves.[30]
- Perform hand hygiene.[1,12,13,14,15,16,17]
- Document the procedure.[31,32,33,34]

Special considerations

- When fitting an uncircumcised male, allow adequate space within the catheter to prevent the foreskin from being drawn into the outlet during voiding.[9]
- If the penis retracts with position changes, a shorter device or different type of product may be necessary.[9]
- When using an external urine collection device to collect a clean-catch urinary specimen, collect the urine in an unused and newly applied catheter and drainage bag.[9]
- Unless the manufacturer recommends a longer wear time, remove the external collection device daily to clean and inspect the skin.[9,28]
- External urine collection devices may not function well for obese men or those with shorter penile shafts. You should consider using a penis pouch for these patients.[35]
- The PrimoFit device can be left in place for up to 24 hours. Replace the device when it's soiled with stool or body fluids other than urine.[11]
- Discontinue use of the PrimoFit device when the patient is able to toilet independently or with assistance, and when the patient is ambulating.[11]
- Don't insert the female external urine collection device into the vagina, rectum, or other body orifice; it's intended for external use only.[10,29]
- Remove the female external urine collection device and use an alternative incontinence product during ambulation.[10,29]
- Maintain suction at all time when using the female external urine collection device until the device is fully removed, *to prevent urine backflow.*[10]

Patient teaching

If the patient is being discharged with an external urine collection device, teach the patient and family (if applicable) how to perform routine device care. Also review signs and symptoms of occlusion, skin irritation, pain or discomfort, urine retention, and infection, and when to report problems to the practitioner.[9]

Complications

Complications are commonly due to equipment malfunction or trauma from improper application and removal, and can include penile irritation, skin breakdown, and edema; ischemic tissue injury; infection; and, rarely, urethral diverticulum.[9,36] A sensitivity reaction to the device materials may also occur. Improper use of a female external urine collection device can cause skin irritation, tissue injury, and urine backflow.[10]

Documentation

Record the date and time of external female external urine collection device application, replacement, and removal. Document your assessment findings before, during, and after device use. Record urine output as directed by your facility. Also document the patient's tolerance of the procedure, any interventions implemented, and the patient's response to those interventions. If you contacted the practitioner, record the date, time, and information conveyed as well as any information received. Document teaching provided to the patient and family (if applicable), their understanding of that teaching, and any need for follow-up teaching.

REFERENCES

1 Healthcare Infection Control Practices Advisory Committee. (2010, revised 2019). Guideline for prevention of catheter-associated urinary tract infections 2009. https://www.cdc.gov/infectioncontrol/pdf/guidelines/cauti-guidelines-H.pdf (Level I)

2 Meddings, J., et al. (2014). Reducing unnecessary urinary catheter use and other strategies to prevent catheter-associated urinary tract infection: An integrative review. *BMJ Quality and Safety, 23*, 277–289. https://qualitysafety.bmj.com/content/qhc/23/4/277.full.pdf (Level I)

3 Association of Professionals in Infection Control and Epidemiology (APIC). (2014). APIC implementation guide: Guide to preventing catheter-associated urinary tract infections. https://apic.org/wp-content/uploads/2019/02/APIC_CAUTI_IG_FIN_REVD0815.pdf (Level IV)

4 Kidd, M., & Makic, M. B. F. (2021). Prevention of catheter-associated urinary tract infection. In Boltz, M., et al. (Eds.), *Evidence-based geriatric nursing protocols for best practice* (6th ed.). New York, NY: Springer Publishing. (Level I)

5 Craven, R. F., et al. (2021). *Fundamentals of nursing: Concepts and competencies for practice* (9th ed.). Philadelphia, PA: Wolters Kluwer.

6 The Joint Commission. (2021). Standard NPSG.07.06.01. *Comprehensive accreditation manual for hospitals.* Oakbrook Terrace, IL: The Joint Commission. (Level VII)

7 Accreditation Association for Hospitals and Health Systems. (2020). Standard 07.01.17. *Healthcare Facilities Accreditation Program: Accreditation requirements for acute care hospitals.* Chicago, IL: Accreditation Association for Hospitals and Health Systems. (Level VII)

8 Lo, E., et al. (2014). SHEA/IDSA practice recommendation: Strategies to prevent catheter-associated urinary tract infections in acute care hospitals: 2014 update. *Infection Control and Hospital Epidemiology, 35*(5), 464–479. https://www.jstor.org/stable/10.1086/675718#metadata_info_tab_contents (Level I)

9 Wound, Ostomy and Continence Nurses Society. (2008). External catheter fact sheet. http://citeseerx.ist.psu.edu/viewdoc/download;jsessionid=BEAB30C3202F9757AB6769E047A899A4?doi=10.1.1.173.3785&rep=rep1&type=pdf (Level VII)

10 C. R. Bard, Inc. (2018). PureWick™ female external catheter: Instructions for use. https://www.crbard.com/CRBard/media/ProductAssets/BardMedicalDivision/PF10741/en-US/PF10741_BAW0319838.pdf

11 Stryker. (2020). Sage PrimoFit External urine management for the male anatomy. https://www.stryker.com/us/en/sage/products/sage-primofit.html

12 The Joint Commission. (2021). Standard NPSG.07.01.01. *Comprehensive accreditation manual for hospitals.* Oakbrook Terrace, IL: The Joint Commission. (Level VII)

13 Centers for Disease Control and Prevention. (2002). Guideline for hand hygiene in health-care settings: Recommendations of the Healthcare Infection Control Practices Advisory Committee and the HICPAC/SHEA/APIC/IDSA Hand Hygiene Task Force. *MMWR Recommendations and Reports, 51*(RR-16), 1–45. https://www.cdc.gov/mmwr/pdf/rr/rr5116.pdf (Level II)

14 World Health Organization. (2009). WHO guidelines on hand hygiene in health care: First global patient safety challenge, clean care is safer care. https://apps.who.int/iris/bitstream/handle/10665/44102/9789241597906_eng.pdf?sequence=1 (Level IV)

15 Centers for Medicare and Medicaid Services, Department of Health and Human Services. (2020). Condition of participation: Infection control. 42 C.F.R. § 482.42.

16 Accreditation Association for Hospitals and Health Systems. (2020). Standard 07.01.21. *Healthcare Facilities Accreditation Program: Accreditation requirements for acute care hospitals.* Chicago, IL: Accreditation Association for Hospitals and Health Systems. (Level VII)

17 DNV GL-Healthcare USA, Inc. (2020). IC.1.SR.1. *NIAHO® accreditation requirements, interpretive guidelines and surveyor guidance—revision 20.0.* Milford, OH: DNV GL-Healthcare USA, Inc. (Level VII)

18 The Joint Commission. (2021). Standard NPSG.01.01.01. *Comprehensive accreditation manual for hospitals.* Oakbrook Terrace, IL: The Joint Commission. (Level VII)

19 Accreditation Association for Hospitals and Health Systems. (2020). Standard 15.01.16. *Healthcare Facilities Accreditation Program: Accreditation requirements for acute care hospitals.* Chicago, IL: Accreditation Association for Hospitals and Health Systems. (Level VII)

20 Centers for Medicare and Medicaid Services, Department of Health and Human Services. (2020). Condition of participation: Patient's rights. 42 C.F.R. § 482.13(c)(1).

21 The Joint Commission. (2021). Standard RI.01.01.01. *Comprehensive accreditation manual for hospitals.* Oakbrook Terrace, IL: The Joint Commission. (Level VII)

22 DNV GL-Healthcare USA, Inc. (2020). PR.2.SR.5. *NIAHO® accreditation requirements, interpretive guidelines and surveyor guidance—revision 20.0.* Milford, OH: DNV GL-Healthcare USA, Inc. (Level VII)

23 The Joint Commission. (2021). Standard PC.02.01.21. *Comprehensive accreditation manual for hospitals.* Oakbrook Terrace, IL: The Joint Commission. (Level VII)

24 Waters, T. R., et al. (2009). Safe patient handling training for schools of nursing. https://www.cdc.gov/niosh/docs/2009-127/pdfs/2009-127.pdf (Level VII)

25 Occupational Safety and Health Administration. (2019). Bloodborne pathogens, standard number 1910.1030. https://www.osha.gov/pls/oshaweb/owadisp.show_document?p_id=10051&p_table=STANDARDS (Level VII)

26 Accreditation Association for Hospitals and Health Systems. (2020). Standard 07.01.10. *Healthcare Facilities Accreditation Program: Accreditation requirements for acute care hospitals.* Chicago, IL: Accreditation Association for Hospitals and Health Systems. (Level VII)

27 Siegel, J. D., et al. (2007, revised 2019). 2007 guideline for isolation precautions: Preventing transmission of infectious agents in healthcare settings. https://www.cdc.gov/infectioncontrol/pdf/guidelines/isolation-guidelines-H.pdf (Level II)

28 BioDerm, INC. (2018). Men's Liberty™ instructions for use. https://www.mensliberty.com/wp-content/uploads/2018/05/LT-95207-A-Mens-Liberty-IFU-New-Housing.pdf

29 Stryker. (2019). PrimaFit™ external urine management system for females: Instructions for use. https://sageproducts.com/wp-content/uploads/PrimaFit-Instructions-for-Use.pdf

30 Ganz, D. A., et al. (2013). *Preventing falls in hospitals: A toolkit for improving quality of care* (AHRQ publication no. 13-0015-EF). Rockville, MD: Agency for Healthcare Research and Quality. at https://www.ahrq.gov/professionals/systems/hospital/fallpxtoolkit/index.html (Level VII)

31 The Joint Commission. (2021). Standard RC.01.03.01. *Comprehensive accreditation manual for hospitals.* Oakbrook Terrace, IL: The Joint Commission. (Level VII)

32 Centers for Medicare and Medicaid Services, Department of Health and Human Services. (2020). Condition of participation: Medical record services. 42 C.F.R. § 482.24(b).

33 Accreditation Association for Hospitals and Health Systems. (2020). Standard 10.00.03. *Healthcare Facilities Accreditation Program: Accreditation requirements for acute care hospitals.* Chicago, IL: Accreditation Association for Hospitals and Health Systems. (Level VII)

34 DNV GL-Healthcare USA, Inc. (2020). MR.2.SR.1. *NIAHO® accreditation requirements, interpretive guidelines and surveyor guidance—revision 20.0.* Milford, OH: DNV GL-Healthcare USA, Inc. (Level VII)

35 Gray, M., et al. (2016). External collection devices as an alternative to the indwelling urinary catheter: Evidence-based review and expert clinical panel deliberations. *Journal of Wound, Ostomy, and Continence Nursing, 43*(3), 301–307. https://www.ncbi.nlm.nih.gov/pmc/articles/PMC4870965/ (Level VII)

36 Dwivedi, A. K., et al. (2014). Massive urethral diverticulum: A complication of condom catheter use. *British Journal of Nursing, 21*(9), S20–S22.

EXTERNAL VENTRICULAR DRAIN INSERTION, ASSISTING

Cerebrospinal fluid (CSF) drainage aims to reduce CSF pressure to the desired level and then to maintain it at that level. Fluid can be withdrawn from the lateral ventricle or the lumbar subarachnoid space, depending on the indication and the desired outcome, via a catheter or an external ventricular drain (EVD) attached to a sterile, closed-drainage collection system. Ventricular drainage helps to reduce intracranial pressure (ICP). In addition, ICP monitoring is possible by connecting an external transducer to the external ventricular drainage system.[1]

Indications for ventricular drain insertion include obstructive hydrocephalus, subarachnoid hemorrhage resulting in acute hydrocephalus due to obstruction of arachnoid villi, Hunt and Hess grade 3 or higher subarachnoid hemorrhage, cerebral edema, surgical mass lesions, infections (such as meningitis), Chiari malformations, shunt failure caused by mechanical disruption or infection, and brain relaxation in an operating room (OR).[2]

To insert a ventricular drain, the practitioner inserts a ventricular catheter through a burr hole in the patient's skull using sterile technique. This procedure is usually performed in the operating room with the patient receiving general anesthesia, but it can also be done in the emergency department or on the intensive care unit.

Strict sterile technique must be maintained throughout equipment setup, catheter insertion, and care of the ventricular drain, *because the catheter's location in the brain poses an increased risk of infection.*[1,2] The use of prophylactic antibiotics remains controversial because of the risk of the development of resistant microorganisms.[2]

Equipment

Overbed table ▪ gloves ▪ caps[2] ▪ sterile gloves ▪ sterile gowns ▪ masks ▪ labels ▪ cardiac monitor ▪ pulse oximeter and probe ▪ antiseptic solution or sterile preparation kit[2] ▪ sterile drapes ▪ 3-mL syringe ▪ 25G ¾" (1.9-cm) needle ▪ local anesthetic (usually 1% lidocaine) ▪ ventricular catheter[2] ▪ EVD set, including drainage tubing, drip chamber, and drainage bag[2] ▪ suture material ▪ suture scissors ▪ 18G spinal needle ▪ scalpel ▪ tape ▪ light source ▪ IV pole ▪ sterile occlusive dressing ▪ intracranial access kit[2] ▪ level or laser leveling device ▪ ICP monitoring equipment with flushless transducer setup[2] ▪ pressure cable and module ▪ sterile preservative-free normal saline solution in a 30-mL or 40-mL syringe[2] ▪ sterile nonvented dead-end caps[2] ▪ emergency equipment (code cart with emergency medications, handheld resuscitation bag and mask, defibrillator, intubation equipment) ▪ vital signs monitoring equipment ▪ facility-approved disinfectant ▪ sign ▪ Optional: prescribed sedation or analgesic, IV catheter insertion supplies, clippers, arterial catheter insertion equipment, sterile towel.

Some of the equipment may be available in a prepackaged ventriculostomy tray.

Preparation of equipment

Inspect all equipment and supplies. If a product is expired, is defective, or has compromised integrity, remove it from patient use, label it as expired or defective, and report the expiration or defect as directed by your facility. Make sure that emergency equipment is readily available and properly functioning.

If the practitioner elects to perform the procedure in an OR, prepare the equipment in that location using sterile technique. If the practitioner chooses to perform the procedure at the bedside, disinfect a work surface using a facility-approved disinfectant, as needed, to prepare for setting up a sterile field.[3,4]

Implementation

▪ Verify the practitioner's order.
▪ If required by your facility, confirm that informed consent has been obtained and that the signed consent form is in the patient's medical record.[5,6,7,8]
▪ Conduct a preprocedure verification *to make sure that all relevant documentation, related information, and equipment are available and correctly identified to the patient's identifiers.*[9,10]

- Verify that ordered laboratory and imaging studies have been completed, and that the results are in the patient's medical record. The International Normalized Ratio should range between 1.2 and 1.6 in a patient with traumatic brain injury who requires emergency ventriculostomy *to reduce the risk of hemorrhage*.[11,12] Notify the practitioner of any unexpected results.
- Check the patient's history for hypersensitivity to latex, antiseptic solution, the local anesthetic, and other medications.
- Gather and prepare the necessary equipment and supplies.
- Perform hand hygiene.[13,14,15,16,17,18]
- Confirm the patient's identity using at least two patient identifiers.[19]
- Provide privacy.[20,21,22,23]
- Reinforce the practitioner's explanation of the procedure to the patient and family (if appropriate) according to their individual communication and learning needs *to increase their understanding, allay their fears, and enhance cooperation.*[24] Answer any questions.
- Explain to the patient and family (if applicable) that the patient must restrict activity while the drain is in place.[2] The patient may not sit up, stand, or walk when the drain is open, and must ask for assistance with movement. Explain that a nurse must turn off the system when the patient is repositioning or transferring.[1] Instruct the patient to avoid straining, coughing, and sneezing.
- Make sure that the procedure room door remains closed, and limit traffic in the room *to reduce the risk of contamination.*[2]
- Raise the patient's bed to waist level before providing care *to prevent caregiver back strain.*[25]
- Perform hand hygiene.[13,14,15,16,17,18]
- Attach the patient to a cardiac monitor and pulse oximeter *to monitor heart rate and rhythm and oxygen saturation level during the procedure.*[2] Make sure alarm limits are set appropriately for the patient's current condition, and that alarms are turned on, functioning properly, and audible to staff.[26,27,28,29]
- Obtain vital signs and oxygen saturation level and perform a baseline neurologic assessment *to help detect alterations or signs of deterioration during and after the procedure.*[2]
- Make sure that the practitioner marks the catheter insertion site using the process determined by your facility. Involve the patient or family in the process, if possible, *to avoid wrong-site insertion.*[10,30]
- Assess the patency of IV access or initiate IV access, as needed and ordered. (See the "IV catheter insertion and removal" procedure.)
- Assess the patient's sedation and pain management needs in collaboration with the practitioner.[2,31] Administer sedation or analgesia, as indicated and prescribed, following safe medication administration practices, *to ensure the patient's comfort during the procedure.*[2,32,33,34,35]
- Position the patient supine with the head of the bed elevated 30 degrees. Obtain assistance, if needed, to immobilize the patient's head *to prevent movement during catheter insertion.*[2]
- Illuminate the catheter insertion area with a light source.
- Braid or clip the patient's hair, if needed, *to expose the insertion site.* If you clip the hair, use tape or another similarly sticky product to remove residual hair clippings.[2]
- Put on a cap and mask.[2] Make sure everyone in the room is wearing a cap and mask.[2]
- Perform hand hygiene.[13,14,15,16,17,18]
- Put on a gown and gloves.[36,37]
- Establish a sterile field on an overbed table using a sterile towel or the wrapping from the EVD tray, and then unwrap the EVD tray or open all supplies, using sterile technique.
- Label all medications, medication containers, and other solutions on and off the sterile field.[38,39]
- Using sterile technique, prepare the ICP monitoring equipment with flushless transducer setup by priming the pressure tubing and the EVD system with sterile preservative-free saline solution in a 30- mL or 40- mL syringe and turning the stopcocks, as needed, to prime the system. Then remove the syringe and replace it with a sterile nonvented dead-end cap.[1] (See the "Intracranial pressure monitoring" procedure.)
- If assisting with sterile supplies, remove and discard your gloves.[36,37]
- Perform hand hygiene.[13,14,15,16,17,18]
- Put on sterile gloves.[36,37]

- Assist as needed as the practitioner cleans the insertion site with antiseptic solution and allows it to dry, drapes the site with a sterile drape, and administers a local anesthetic into the scalp using a 3-mL syringe and a 25G, ¾" (1.9 cm) needle.[2]
- Conduct a time-out immediately before the start of the procedure *to perform a final assessment that the correct patient, site, positioning, and procedure are identified and that, as applicable, all relevant information and necessary equipment are available.*[2,10,40]
- During drain insertion, continuously monitor the patient's heart rate and rhythm, respiratory rate, oxygen saturation level, and blood pressure.[2] Guidelines recommend use of an arterial catheter for blood pressure monitoring *to ensure vigilant monitoring of mean arterial pressure to avoid decreased cerebral perfusion pressure.*[2]
- Assess the patient's neurologic status every 15 minutes during drain insertion. *Serial assessments are necessary for immediate identification and treatment of neurologic changes.*[2]
- Using sterile technique, assist the practitioner as needed throughout the insertion procedure.
- To insert the drain, the practitioner makes an incision in the scalp and subcutaneous tissue, drills a burr hole through the cranium, and rinses the area with sterile preservative-free normal saline solution. Next, the practitioner uses an 18G spinal needle to puncture the dura and inserts the catheter through the burr hole to the desired depth, secures it using a tunneling method through a separate incision, and sutures it. After completing EVD insertion, the practitioner covers the insertion site with a sterile occlusive dressing and secures the catheter *to prevent accidental removal.*[2]
- After the practitioner inserts the catheter, connect the prepared ICP monitoring system and the prepared EVD system to the distal tip of the catheter. Attach the pressure cables and the module, following the manufacturer's instructions for use. Trace each tube from the patient to its point of origin *to make sure that it's connected to the correct port.*[41,42] Label each tube at the distal end (near the patient) and proximal end (near the drainage bag) *to distinguish the tubing and reduce the risk of misconnections.* Secure connection points with tape or a connector *to prevent accidental disconnections.*[42]
- Return the bed to the lowest position *to prevent falls and maintain patient safety.*[43]
- Place the EVD system, including the drip chamber and collection bag, on an IV pole. Set the drip chamber manometer at the pressure level ordered by the practitioner.[1,2] Using the level or laser leveling device, level the ICP transducer at the foramen of Monro. Anatomically, the external reference point to approximate the foramen of Monro is the level of the external auditory meatus (tragus of the ear) or the outer canthus of the eye. *Maintaining the proper position of the ICP transducer ensures accurate waveform and pressure data.* Use the same landmark every time you check the zero reference level.[2]
- Ensure that the monitoring system is free from air, *which could alter the pressure reading.*
- Calibrate the pressure monitor following the manufacturer's instructions.
- After EVD insertion, monitor the patient's vital signs, oxygen saturation level, neurologic status, and ICP waveform at least every hour, according to the patient's condition, or as directed by your facility. Ensure that the drainage system is appropriately clamped or open depending on the patient's situation and the practitioner's order. Assess and record the volume, clarity, and color of CSF drainage hourly or as ordered.[2] Check the patient's position to ensure that the transducer is at the ordered reference level. If the patient is very active and moving around in the bed, frequently assess that the drainage system is leveled appropriately *to prevent overdrainage or underdrainage.* Check drain patency, as needed, by lowering the entire system briefly to assess drip rate into the graduated burette. Notify the practitioner immediately if drainage ceases and you find no external cause (for example, kinking or disconnection).[2]
- Place a sign at the head of the patient's bed that clearly identifies prescribed device height and head-of-bed elevation, as directed by your facility.
- Instruct the patient and family, if applicable, not to change the patient's position without the assistance of a nurse.[2]
- Discard used supplies in the appropriate receptacles.

- Remove and discard your gloves and other personal protective equipment.[36,37]
- Perform hand hygiene.[13,14,15,16,17,18]
- Screen and assess the patient's pain using facility-defined criteria consistent with the patient's age, condition, and ability to understand.[31] Respond appropriately.
- Perform hand hygiene.[13,14,15,16,17,18]
- Document the procedure.[44,45,46,47]

Special considerations

- Vigilant assessment of CSF drainage volume throughout each hour is essential *to prevent overdrainage and underdrainage.*[1] Overdrainage can occur if the drip chamber is placed too far below the catheter insertion site. Underdrainage may reflect kinked tubing, catheter displacement, or a drip chamber placed higher than the catheter insertion site.
- Maintain the collection system in the upright position; if you need to lay the system down, drain the CSF into the lower collection bag *to reduce the incidence of infection and backflow.*[1]
- Raising or lowering the head of the bed can affect the CSF flow rate. When changing the patient's position, level the transducer to the tragus of the ear or the outer canthus of the eye.[2]
- Patients may experience a chronic headache during continuous CSF drainage. Reassure the patient that this symptom isn't unusual; however, monitor for headache and administer analgesics, as appropriate, following safe medication administration practices.[32,33,34,35]
- Assess for signs of increased ICP, which include headache, a decrease in level of consciousness, nausea, vomiting, and lethargy or agitation.[2]
- Guidelines discourage taking the patient off the patient floor to perform tests and procedures *to avoid catheter dislodgment.* Check your facility's requirements for scheduling tests and procedures at the patient's bedside.
- Follow strict sterile technique when connecting and flushing the tubing, when taking samples from the drainage system, and during dressing changes.[1,2]
- Don't routinely change the drainage tubing; allow it to remain for the duration *to maintain sterility and reduce the risk of infection.*[2] When changing the drainage bag, wear sterile gloves and a mask *to reduce the incidence of infection.* Only change the drainage bag when it's nearly full.[2]
- Change the EVD insertion site dressing daily, as ordered, or as directed by your facility, using sterile technique *to maintain sterility and observe the insertion site.*[1]
- The Joint Commission issued a sentinel event alert concerning medical device alarm safety, *because alarm-related events have been associated with permanent loss of function or death.* Among the major contributing factors were improper alarm settings, alarm settings turned off inappropriately, and alarm signals that were inaudible to staff. Make sure that the alarm limits are set appropriately, and that the alarms are turned on, functioning properly, and audible to staff. Follow facility guidelines for preventing alarm fatigue.[29]
- The Joint Commission issued a sentinel event alert related to managing risk during transition to new International Organization for Standardization tubing standards that were designed to prevent dangerous tubing misconnections, *which can lead to serious patient injury and death.* During the transition, make sure to trace each tubing and catheter from the patient to its point of origin before connecting or reconnecting any device or infusion, at any care transition (such as to a new setting or service), and as part of the hand-off process; route tubes and catheters having different purposes in different, standardized directions; label tubing at both the distal and proximal ends when the patient has different access sites or several bags hanging; use tubing and equipment only as intended; and store medications for different delivery routes in separate locations.[42]

Complications

Complications may include infection, CSF overdrainage, aneurysmal rebleeding and hemispheric shifts from reduction in ICP, and intracranial hemorrhage or misplacement.[2]. Signs and symptoms of CSF overdrainage include postural headache that's relieved in the supine position, mental status decline, hearing changes, vertigo, facial weakness, horizontal diplopia, facial numbness, and small pupil size.[2]

NURSING ALERT If drainage accumulates too rapidly, clamp the system, notify the practitioner immediately, and perform a complete neurologic assessment. *This complication constitutes a potential neurosurgical emergency.*

Documentation

Document the preprocedure verification process and the time-out performed immediately before the procedure. Record the date and time the practitioner inserted the drain, the patient's position, and the transducer's position at the ordered reference level. Document the patient's tolerance of the insertion process, including neurologic assessments, vital signs, and oxygen saturation levels; medication administration; and ICP. Obtain an ICP pressure tracing and place it in the patient's medical record.[2] Document hourly CSF output and neurologic and hemodynamic status. Also document teaching provided to the patient and family (if applicable), their understanding of that teaching, and any need for follow-up teaching.

REFERENCES

1 Wiegand, D. L. (2017). *AACN procedure manual for high acuity, progressive, and critical care* (7th ed.). St. Louis, MO: Elsevier.

2 American Association of Neuroscience Nurses (AANN). (2014). *Care of the patient undergoing intracranial pressure monitoring/external ventricular drainage or lumbar drainage: AANN clinical practice guideline series.* Glenview, IL: AANN. (Level VII)

3 Accreditation Association for Hospitals and Health Systems. (2020). Standard 07.02.03. *Healthcare Facilities Accreditation Program: Accreditation requirements for acute care hospitals.* Chicago, IL: Accreditation Association for Hospitals and Health Systems. (Level VII)

4 Rutala, W. A., et al. (2008, revised 2019). Guideline for disinfection and sterilization in healthcare facilities, 2008. https://www.cdc.gov/infection-control/pdf/guidelines/disinfection-guidelines-H.pdf (Level I)

5 The Joint Commission. (2021). Standard RI.01.03.01. *Comprehensive accreditation manual for hospitals.* Oakbrook Terrace, IL: The Joint Commission. (Level VII)

6 Accreditation Association for Hospitals and Health Systems. (2020). Standard 30.01.11. *Healthcare Facilities Accreditation Program: Accreditation requirements for acute care hospitals.* Chicago, IL: Accreditation Association for Hospitals and Health Systems. (Level VII)

7 Centers for Medicare and Medicaid Services, Department of Health and Human Services. (2020). Condition of participation: Patient's rights. 42 C.F.R. § 482.13(b)(2).

8 DNV GL-Healthcare USA, Inc. (2020). PR.2.SR.3. *NIAHO® accreditation requirements, interpretive guidelines and surveyor guidance—revision 20.0.* Milford, OH: DNV GL-Healthcare USA, Inc. (Level VII)

9 The Joint Commission. (2021). Standard UP.01.01.01. *Comprehensive accreditation manual for hospitals.* Oakbrook Terrace, IL: The Joint Commission. (Level VII)

10 Accreditation Association for Hospitals and Health Systems. (2020). Standard 30.00.14. *Healthcare Facilities Accreditation Program: Accreditation requirements for acute care hospitals.* Chicago, IL: Accreditation Association for Hospitals and Health Systems. (Level VII)

11 Bauer, D. F., et al. (2011). The relationship between INR and development of hemorrhage with placement of ventriculostomy. *Journal of Trauma, 70*(5), 1112–1117. (Level IV)

12 Chau, C. Y. C., et al. (2019). The evolution of the role of external ventricular drainage in traumatic brain injury. *Journal of Clinical Medicine, 8*(9), 1422. https://www.ncbi.nlm.nih.gov/pmc/articles/PMC6780113/

13 The Joint Commission. (2021). Standard NPSG.07.01.01. *Comprehensive accreditation manual for hospitals.* Oakbrook Terrace, IL: The Joint Commission. (Level VII)

14 Centers for Disease Control and Prevention. (2002). Guideline for hand hygiene in health-care settings: Recommendations of the Healthcare Infection Control Practices Advisory Committee and the HICPAC/SHEA/APIC/IDSA Hand Hygiene Task Force. *MMWR Recommendations and Reports, 51*(RR-16), 1–45. https://www.cdc.gov/mmwr/pdf/rr/rr5116.pdf (Level II)

15 World Health Organization. (2009). WHO guidelines on hand hygiene in health care: First global patient safety challenge, clean care is safer care. https://apps.who.int/iris/bitstream/handle/10665/44102/9789241597906_eng.pdf (Level IV)

16 Accreditation Association for Hospitals and Health Systems. (2020). Standard 07.01.21. *Healthcare Facilities Accreditation Program: Accreditation requirements for acute care hospitals.* Chicago, IL: Accreditation Association for Hospitals and Health Systems. (Level VII)

17 Centers for Medicare and Medicaid Services, Department of Health and Human Services. (2020). Condition of participation: Infection control. 42 C.F.R. § 482.42.

18 DNV GL-Healthcare USA, Inc. (2020). IC.1.SR.1. *NIAHO® accreditation requirements, interpretive guidelines and surveyor guidance—revision 20.0.* Milford, OH: DNV GL-Healthcare USA, Inc. (Level VII)

19 The Joint Commission. (2021). Standard NPSG.01.01.01. *Comprehensive accreditation manual for hospitals.* Oakbrook Terrace, IL: The Joint Commission. (Level VII)

20 Accreditation Association for Hospitals and Health Systems. (2020). Standard 15.01.16. *Healthcare Facilities Accreditation Program: Accreditation requirements for acute care hospitals.* Chicago, IL: Accreditation Association for Hospitals and Health Systems. (Level VII)

21 Centers for Medicare and Medicaid Services, Department of Health and Human Services. (2020). Condition of participation: Patient's rights. 42 C.F.R. § 482.13(c)(1).

22 The Joint Commission. (2021). Standard RI.01.01.01. *Comprehensive accreditation manual for hospitals.* Oakbrook Terrace, IL: The Joint Commission. (Level VII)

23 DNV GL-Healthcare USA, Inc. (2020). PR.2.SR.5. *NIAHO® accreditation requirements, interpretive guidelines and surveyor guidance—revision 20.0.* Milford, OH: DNV GL-Healthcare USA, Inc. (Level VII)

24 The Joint Commission. (2021). Standard PC.02.01.21. *Comprehensive accreditation manual for hospitals.* Oakbrook Terrace, IL: The Joint Commission. (Level VII)

25 Waters, T. R., et al. (2009). Safe patient handling training for schools of nursing. https://www.cdc.gov/niosh/docs/2009-127/pdfs/2009-127.pdf (Level VII)

26 Graham, K. C., & Cvach, M. (2010). Monitor alarm fatigue: Standardizing use of physiological monitors and decreasing nuisance alarms. *American Journal of Critical Care, 19,* 28–37.

27 The Joint Commission. (2021). Standard NPSG.06.01.01. *Comprehensive accreditation manual for hospitals.* Oakbrook Terrace, IL: The Joint Commission. (Level VII)

28 American Association of Critical-Care Nurses. (2018). AACN practice alert: Managing alarms in acute care across the life span: Electrocardiography and pulse oximetry. https://www.aacn.org/clinical-resources/practice-alerts/managing-alarms-in-acute-care-across-the-life-span (Level VII)

29 The Joint Commission. (2013). Sentinel event alert 50: Medical device alarm safety in hospitals. https://www.jointcommission.org/assets/1/6/SEA_50_alarms_4_26_16.pdf (Level VII)

30 The Joint Commission. (2021). Standard UP.01.02.01. *Comprehensive accreditation manual for hospitals.* Oakbrook Terrace, IL: The Joint Commission. (Level VII)

31 The Joint Commission. (2021). Standard PC.01.02.07. *Comprehensive accreditation manual for hospitals.* Oakbrook Terrace, IL: The Joint Commission. (Level VII)

32 Accreditation Association for Hospitals and Health Systems. (2020). Standard 16.01.03. *Healthcare Facilities Accreditation Program: Accreditation requirements for acute care hospitals.* Chicago, IL: Accreditation Association for Hospitals and Health Systems. (Level VII)

33 Centers for Medicare and Medicaid Services, Department of Health and Human Services. (2020). Condition of participation: Nursing services. 42 C.F.R. § 482.23(c).

34 DNV GL-Healthcare USA, Inc. (2020). MM.1.SR.3. *NIAHO® accreditation requirements, interpretive guidelines and surveyor guidance—revision 20.0.* Milford, OH: DNV GL-Healthcare USA, Inc. (Level VII)

35 The Joint Commission. (2021). Standard MM.06.01.01. *Comprehensive accreditation manual for hospitals.* Oakbrook Terrace, IL: The Joint Commission. (Level VII)

36 Siegel, J. D., et al. (2007, revised 2019). 2007 guideline for isolation precautions: Preventing transmission of infectious agents in healthcare settings. https://www.cdc.gov/infectioncontrol/pdf/guidelines/isolation-guidelines-H.pdf (Level II)

37 Accreditation Association for Hospitals and Health Systems. (2020). Standard 07.01.10. *Healthcare Facilities Accreditation Program: Accreditation requirements for acute care hospitals.* Chicago, IL: Accreditation Association for Hospitals and Health Systems. (Level VII)

38 The Joint Commission. (2021). Standard NPSG.03.04.01. *Comprehensive accreditation manual for hospitals.* Oakbrook Terrace, IL: The Joint Commission. (Level VII)

39 Accreditation Association for Hospitals and Health Systems. (2020). Standard 25.01.27. *Healthcare Facilities Accreditation Program: Accreditation requirements for acute care hospitals.* Chicago, IL: Accreditation Association for Hospitals and Health Systems. (Level VII)

40 The Joint Commission. (2021). Standard UP.01.03.01. *Comprehensive accreditation manual for hospitals.* Oakbrook Terrace, IL: The Joint Commission. (Level VII)

41 U.S. Food and Drug Administration. (2017). Examples of medical device misconnections. https://www.fda.gov/medical-devices/medical-device-connectors/examples-medical-device-misconnections

42 The Joint Commission. (2014). Sentinel event alert 53: Managing risk during transition to new ISO tubing connector standards. http://www.jointcommission.org/assets/1/6/SEA_53_Connectors_8_19_14_final.pdf (Level VII)

43 Ganz, D. A., et al. (2013, reviewed 2021). *Preventing falls in hospitals: A toolkit for improving quality of care* (AHRQ Publication No. 13-0015-EF). Rockville, MD: Agency for Healthcare Research and Quality. https://www.ahrq.gov/professionals/systems/hospital/fallpxtoolkit/index.html (Level VII)

44 The Joint Commission. (2021). Standard RC.01.03.01. *Comprehensive accreditation manual for hospitals.* Oakbrook Terrace, IL: The Joint Commission. (Level VII)

45 Centers for Medicare and Medicaid Services, Department of Health and Human Services. (2020). Condition of participation: Medical record services. 42 C.F.R. § 482.24(b).

46 Accreditation Association for Hospitals and Health Systems. (2020). Standard 10.00.03. *Healthcare Facilities Accreditation Program: Accreditation requirements for acute care hospitals.* Chicago, IL: Accreditation Association for Hospitals and Health Systems. (Level VII)

47 DNV GL-Healthcare USA, Inc. (2020). MR.2.SR.1. *NIAHO® accreditation requirements, interpretive guidelines and surveyor guidance—revision 20.0.* Milford, OH: DNV GL-Healthcare USA, Inc. (Level VII)

Eye care

Eye care includes the practice of assessing and cleaning the eye and instilling prescribed ocular preparations. Eye care may be necessary to relieve pain and discomfort, prevent or treat infection or injury to the eye, detect disease at an early stage, detect drug-induced toxicity, prevent damage to the cornea in sedated or unconscious patients, maintain contact lenses, and care for false eye prostheses.

Eye care may be necessary to prevent ocular surface disease in patients who are unconscious, critically ill, or under sedation, or patients with paralysis with impaired ocular protective mechanisms.[1]

Prevention of ocular surface disease and its potential complications includes interventions that keep the eyelids closed to prevent dryness and concentrate the patient's tears (*tears provide antimicrobial components that prevent infection*).[1] Other interventions include providing eye lubrication and eye hygiene.[1,2] *If left untreated, ocular surface disease can lead to eye infection, corneal abrasion, corneal ulceration, and vision loss.*[1,2]

Equipment

Towel ▪ sterile drape ▪ sterile basin ▪ powder-free gloves ▪ sterile gauze pads ▪ sterile water ▪ pen light ▪ light source ▪ Optional: prescribed artificial tears or eye ointment, paper tape, polyethylene eye covers.

Preparation of equipment

Inspect all equipment and supplies. If a product is expired, is defective, or has compromised integrity, remove it from patient use, label it as expired or defective, and report the expiration or defect as directed by your facility.

Implementation

▪ Gather the necessary equipment and supplies.
▪ Ensure the lighting is adequate.
▪ Perform hand hygiene.[3,4,5,6,7,8]
▪ Confirm the patient's identity using at least two patient identifiers.[9]

Eyelid Grading System

Eyelid position assessment should be done at your initial patient assessment and then at regular intervals *to determine the type of care necessary to prevent ocular surface disease.*[1,2] Using a penlight will help reveal poor lid closure that may be masked by the eyelashes.[1]

Grade 0: Lids are completely closed.
Grade 1: The white of the eye (conjunctiva) is visible.
Grade 2: Part of the cornea is visible.

- Provide privacy.[10,11,12,13]
- Explain the procedure to the patient and family (if appropriate) according to their individual communication and learning needs *to increase their understanding, allay their fears, and enhance cooperation.*[14]
- Raise the patient's bed to waist level before providing care *to prevent caregiver back strain.*[15]
- Place the head of the patient's bed at 30 degrees, unless contraindicated by the patient's condition.
- Perform hand hygiene.[3,4,5,6,7,8]
- Ensure the patient is in a comfortable position.
- Place a towel around the patient's neck.
- Create a sterile field using a sterile drape.
- Place the sterile basin and sterile gauze pads on the sterile field.
- Pour sterile water into the sterile basin using sterile technique.[1]
- Perform hand hygiene.[3,4,5,6,7,8]
- Put on powder-free gloves *to comply with standard precautions.*[16,17,18]
- Assess the patient's eyes and periorbital area for redness, drainage, or bruising; the presence of a foreign object; pupil size and reactivity; and subjective reports of pain, vision loss, itching, sensitivity to light, or sensation of something in the eye.

NURSING ALERT Observe for corneal dullness, opacity, and chemosis (edema in the conjunctiva).[2] Notify the practitioner if you observe any of these conditions, and increase lubrication in the eye.

- *To remove secretions or crusts adhering to the eyelids and eyelashes,* first soak a sterile gauze pad in sterile water.[1,2] Instruct the patient to close the eyes; then, without applying pressure, gently wipe the patient's eye with the water-soaked gauze pad, working from the inner canthus to the outer canthus *to prevent debris and fluid from entering the nasolacrimal duct.* Use a new sterile gauze pad for each wipe until the eye is clean and you have removed all the discharge, *to prevent cross-contamination.*

NURSING ALERT Don't use swabs, tweezers, or any other materials on the eye itself, and don't use a cotton ball to clean the eyes, *because these tools can scratch the cornea.*[1]

- Repeat the procedure for the other eye.
- Perform an eyelid position assessment using a penlight and an eyelid grading system. (See *Eyelid Grading System*)
- Consult with the practitioner to determine the type of interventions needed based on the patient's eyelid assessment, or follow your facility's protocol.[1,2]
- Instill artificial tears or apply eye ointment, as ordered, following safe medication administration practices. (See the "Eye medication administration" procedure.)[19,20,21,22]
- Close the patient's eyelids gently using the back of your fingertip. Apply an eye cover, such as a polyethylene cover, as indicated, *to promote eye closure in a patient with partial or incomplete eyelid closure.*[1] Use paper tape only if necessary, and with caution, *because it can be upsetting to family members, is insufficient for eye closure, and may lead to skin irritation when removed.* If tape is used, be sure to check the position of the eyelashes so that they are clear of the cornea *to prevent abrasion.*[1,2,23]
- Return the bed to the lowest position *to prevent falls and maintain patient safety.*[24]
- Discard used supplies in appropriate receptacles.[18]
- Remove and discard your gloves.[16,18]
- Perform hand hygiene.[3,4,5,6,7,8]
- Document the procedure.[25,26,27,28]

Special considerations

- Unconscious patients lose the protective corneal reflex of blinking, increasing the risk of corneal drying, abrasions, and eye injury. In this patient population, it is important to keep the patient's eyes closed *to help maintain eye moisture and prevent injury.* Make sure to recheck the patient's eyes and apply lubricant every 4 hours, as ordered, following safe medication administration practices.[2]
- *To prevent irritation,* avoid using soap for cleaning the eyes.
- Do not use gauze pads to cover the eyes, *because this may predispose the patient to corneal abrasion.*[1]
- Avoid irrigating the patient's eyes with normal saline to wash out eye discharge, *because it can cause ocular surface disease and cross-contamination.*[1]
- Do not use Geliperm (a hydrogel wound dressing) as an eye covering, *because studies show it can worsen the severity of ocular surface disease.*[1]
- Make sure the eyes are covered when suctioning a patient at risk for ocular surface disease. Use a closed suction system, if possible, and do not withdraw the suction catheter across the face *to minimize the risk of eye infection.*[1]
- Do not cover the eye if the patient has signs of eye infection, copious secretions in the eye, or is able to blink occasionally.[1]

Documentation

Record in your notes the date, time, and type of eye care provided. Document your assessment of the eyes and periorbital areas, noting redness, drainage, and bruising; the presence of a foreign object; pupil size and reactivity; and subjective reports of pain, vision loss, itching, sensitivity to light, and the sensation of something in the eye. If applicable, record any irrigation procedure performed and the patient's tolerance of the procedure. Document the eyelid position assessment using an eyelid grading system. Document administration of eyedrops or ointment in the patient's medication record, if applicable. Document teaching provided to the patient and family (if applicable), their understanding of that teaching, and any need for follow-up teaching.

REFERENCES

1 Alansari, M. A., et al. (2015). Making a difference in eye care of the critically ill patients. *Journal of Intensive Care Medicine, 30,* 311–317. http://citeseerx.ist.psu.edu/viewdoc/download?doi=10.1.1.839.7172&rep=rep1&type=pdf

2 Hearne, B. J., et al. (2018). Eye care in the intensive care unit. *Journal of the Intensive Care Society, 19*(4), 345–350. https://www.ncbi.nlm.nih.gov/pmc/articles/PMC6259085/pdf/10.1177_1751143718764529.pdf

3 The Joint Commission. (2021). Standard NPSG.07.01.01. *Comprehensive accreditation manual for hospitals.* Oakbrook Terrace, IL: The Joint Commission. (Level VII)

4 Centers for Disease Control and Prevention. (2002). Guideline for hand hygiene in health-care settings: Recommendations of the Healthcare Infection Control Practices Advisory Committee and the HICPAC/SHEA/APIC/IDSA Hand Hygiene Task Force. *MMWR Recommendations and Reports, 51*(RR-16), 1–45. https://www.cdc.gov/mmwr/pdf/rr/rr5116.pdf (Level II)

5 World Health Organization. (2009). WHO guidelines on hand hygiene in health care: First global patient safety challenge, clean care is safer care. https://apps.who.int/iris/bitstream/handle/10665/44102/9789241597906_eng.pdf?sequence=1 (Level IV)

6 Centers for Medicare and Medicaid Services, Department of Health and Human Services. (2020). Condition of participation: Infection control. 42 C.F.R. § 482.42.

7 Accreditation Association for Hospitals and Health Systems. (2020). Standard 07.01.21. *Healthcare Facilities Accreditation Program: Accreditation requirements for acute care hospitals.* Chicago, IL: Accreditation Association for Hospitals and Health Systems. (Level VII)

8 DNV GL-Healthcare USA, Inc. (2020). IC.1.SR.1. *NIAHO® accreditation requirements, interpretive guidelines and surveyor guidance—revision 20.0.* Milford, OH: DNV GL-Healthcare USA, Inc. (Level VII)

9 The Joint Commission. (2021). Standard NPSG.01.01.01. *Comprehensive accreditation manual for hospitals.* Oakbrook Terrace, IL: The Joint Commission. (Level VII)

10 Centers for Medicare and Medicaid Services, Department of Health and Human Services. (2020). Condition of participation: Patient's rights. 42 C.F.R. § 482.13(c)(1).

11 Accreditation Association for Hospitals and Health Systems. (2020). Standard 15.01.16. *Healthcare Facilities Accreditation Program: Accreditation requirements for acute care hospitals.* Chicago, IL: Accreditation Association for Hospitals and Health Systems. (Level VII)

12 The Joint Commission. (2021). Standard RI.01.01.01. *Comprehensive accreditation manual for hospitals.* Oakbrook Terrace, IL: The Joint Commission. (Level VII)

13 DNV GL-Healthcare USA, Inc. (2020). PR.2.SR.5. *NIAHO® accreditation requirements, interpretive guidelines and surveyor guidance—revision 20.0.* Milford, OH: DNV GL-Healthcare USA, Inc. (Level VII)

14 The Joint Commission. (2021). Standard PC.02.01.21. *Comprehensive accreditation manual for hospitals.* Oakbrook Terrace, IL: The Joint Commission. (Level VII)

15 Waters, T. R., et al. (2009). Safe patient handling training for schools of nursing. https://www.cdc.gov/niosh/docs/2009-127/pdfs/2009-127.pdf (Level VII)

16 Siegel, J. D., et al. (2007, revised 2019). 2007 guideline for isolation precautions: Preventing transmission of infectious agents in healthcare settings. https://www.cdc.gov/infectioncontrol/pdf/guidelines/isolation-guidelines-H.pdf (Level II)

17 Accreditation Association for Hospitals and Health Systems. (2020). Standard 07.01.10. *Healthcare Facilities Accreditation Program: Accreditation requirements for acute care hospitals.* Chicago, IL: Accreditation Association for Hospitals and Health Systems. (Level VII)

18 Occupational Safety and Health Administration. (2019). Bloodborne pathogens, standard number 1910.1030. https://www.osha.gov/pls/oshaweb/owadisp.show_document?p_id=10051&p_table=STANDARDS (Level VII)

19 Centers for Medicare and Medicaid Services, Department of Health and Human Services. (2020). Condition of participation: Nursing services. 42 C.F.R. § 482.23(c).

20 Accreditation Association for Hospitals and Health Systems. (2020). Standard 16.01.03. *Healthcare Facilities Accreditation Program: Accreditation requirements for acute care hospitals.* Chicago, IL: Accreditation Association for Hospitals and Health Systems. (Level VII)

21 The Joint Commission. (2021). Standard MM.06.01.01. *Comprehensive accreditation manual for hospitals.* Oakbrook Terrace, IL: The Joint Commission. (Level VII)

22 DNV GL-Healthcare USA, Inc. (2020). MM.1.SR.3. *NIAHO® accreditation requirements, interpretive guidelines and surveyor guidance—revision 20.0.* Milford, OH: DNV GL-Healthcare USA, Inc. (Level VII)

23 Perry, A., et al. (2017). *Clinical nursing skills and techniques* (9th ed.). St. Louis, MO: Elsevier.

24 Ganz, D. A., et al. (2013, reviewed 2021). *Preventing falls in hospitals: A toolkit for improving quality of care* (AHRQ Publication No. 13-0015-EF). Rockville, MD: Agency for Healthcare Research and Quality. https://www.ahrq.gov/professionals/systems/hospital/fallpxtoolkit/index.html (Level VII)

25 The Joint Commission. (2021). Standard RC.01.03.01. *Comprehensive accreditation manual for hospitals.* Oakbrook Terrace, IL: The Joint Commission. (Level VII)

26 Centers for Medicare and Medicaid Services, Department of Health and Human Services. (2020). Condition of participation: Medical record services. 42 C.F.R. § 482.24(b).

27 Accreditation Association for Hospitals and Health Systems. (2020). Standard 10.00.03. *Healthcare Facilities Accreditation Program: Accreditation requirements for acute care hospitals.* Chicago, IL: Accreditation Association for Hospitals and Health Systems. (Level VII)

28 DNV GL-Healthcare USA, Inc. (2020). MR.2.SR.1. *NIAHO® accreditation requirements, interpretive guidelines and surveyor guidance—revision 20.0.* Milford, OH: DNV GL-Healthcare USA, Inc. (Level VII)

EYE COMPRESS APPLICATION

Whether applied cold or warm, eye compresses are soothing and therapeutic. Because cold numbs sensory fibers, cold compresses can reduce swelling and bleeding and relieve itching, such as with allergic conjunctivitis.[1] Cold compresses may also be ordered to ease periorbital discomfort between prescribed doses of pain medication. Because heat increases circulation, which enhances absorption and decreases inflammation, warm compresses help relieve discomfort and promote drainage of superficial infections. Warm eye compresses may be ordered for patients diagnosed with viral or bacterial conjunctivitis or blepharitis.[1,2] Warm compresses,

either dry or moist, also help patients with dry eye syndrome related to Sjögren syndrome or meibomian gland dysfunction.[3,4]

The presence of ocular infection requires the use of sterile technique for this procedure.

Equipment

Small plastic bag, ice pack, or latex-free glove ■ ice chips (for a cold compress) ■ ½″ (1.3-cm) hypoallergenic tape ■ pillow ■ towel ■ sterile 4″ × 4″ (10 cm × 10 cm) gauze pads ■ sterile water, normal saline solution, or prescribed ophthalmic irrigant ■ basin of hot tap water (for a warm compress) ■ Optional: prescribed ophthalmic ointment or eyedrops, eye patch, gloves, sterile gloves.

Preparation of equipment

Inspect all equipment and supplies. If a product is expired, is defective, or has compromised integrity, remove it from patient use, label it as expired or defective, and report the expiration or defect as directed by your facility.

For a cold compress

Place ice chips in a plastic bag, ice pack, or latex-free glove, if necessary. Keep the ice pack small *to avoid excessive pressure on the eye.* Remove excess air from the bag, pack, or glove and then knot or close the open end. Cut a piece of hypoallergenic tape *to secure the ice pack in place.* Place all equipment on the bedside stand near the patient.

For a warm compress

Place a capped bottle of sterile water or normal saline solution in a basin of hot water or under a stream of hot tap water. Allow the water or normal saline solution to become warm (no warmer than 113°F [45°C]).[5] Pour the sterile warm water or normal saline solution into a sterile basin, filling the basin about halfway. Place some of the sterile gauze pads in the basin.

Implementation

- Review the practitioner's order.
- Gather and prepare the necessary equipment and supplies.

Applying the compress

- Perform hand hygiene.[6,7,8,9,10,11]
- Confirm the patient's identity using at least two patient identifiers.[12]
- Provide privacy.[13,14,15,16]
- Explain the procedure to the patient and family (if appropriate) according to their individual communication and learning needs *to increase their understanding, allay their fears, and enhance cooperation.*[17]
- Raise the patient's bed to waist level when providing care *to prevent caregiver back strain.*[18]
- Perform hand hygiene.[6,7,8,9,10,11]
- Put on gloves, as needed, *to comply with standard precautions.*[19,20,21]
- Help the patient into the supine or semi-Fowler position; support the patient's head with a pillow and turn it slightly to the unaffected side. *This position will help hold the compress in place.*
- If the patient has an eye patch, remove and discard it.
- Inspect the eye and surrounding skin *to serve as a baseline for comparison.*
- Remove and discard your gloves (if worn,[20]) perform hand hygiene,[6,7,8,9,10,11] and put on new gloves, as needed.[20]
- Drape a towel around the patient's shoulders *to catch any spills.*

For a cold compress

- Moisten the middle of one of the sterile 4″ × 4″ (10 cm × 10 cm) gauze pads with prescribed sterile water, normal saline solution, or prescribed ophthalmic irrigant) *to help conduct the cold from the ice pack.* Keep the edges dry *so that they can absorb excess moisture.*
- Instruct the patient to close the eyes.
- Place the moist gauze pad over the affected eye, place the ice pack on top of the gauze pad, and tape it in place.

- If the patient complains of pain, remove the ice pack. *Some patients may have an adverse reaction to cold.*
- Return the patient's bed to the lowest position *to prevent falls and maintain the patient's safety.*[22]
- Remove and discard your gloves, if worn.[20]
- Perform hand hygiene.[6,7,8,9,10,11]

For a warm compress

- Remove two sterile gauze pads from the basin, and squeeze out the excess solution.
- Instruct the patient to close the eyes.
- Gently apply the pads—one on top of the other—to the affected eye. (If the patient complains that the compress feels too hot, remove it immediately.)
- Change the compress, as needed, during the prescribed length of time.
- Return the patient's bed to the lowest position *to prevent falls and maintain the patient's safety.*[22]
- Remove and discard your gloves, if worn.[20]
- Perform hand hygiene.[6,7,8,9,10,11]

For all compresses

- Use the remaining dry sterile gauze pads to clean and dry the patient's face.
- If ordered and , apply ophthalmic ointment or instill drops using safe medication practices,[23,24,25,26] or apply an eye patch. (See the "Eye medication administration" procedure.)
- Discard used supplies in appropriate receptacles.
- Remove and discard your gloves, if worn.[20]
- Perform hand hygiene.[6,7,8,9,10,11]
- Document the procedure.[27,28,29,30]

Special considerations

- When applying a warm compress, change the compress as frequently as needed—typically every 5 minutes—to maintain a constantly warm temperature *to increase vasodilation and promote discharge.*[2,5]
- Don't use a microwave to warm the solution *because of the risk of overheating the solution and causing a burn.*

Patient teaching

When teaching about how to apply cold eye compresses at home, explain that the patient can substitute a clean basin and clean washcloth for the sterile equipment. Explain that the patient must wash the hands thoroughly before and after treating the eye and, if both eyes require treatment, between treating each eye, *to help prevent infection.* Tell the patient to use a different clean washcloth for each eye *to prevent cross-contamination.* Also, teach the patient and family (if appropriate) how to instill eyedrops or ophthalmic ointment, and how to avoid contaminating the medication container.

Documentation

Record the time and duration of the procedure. Describe the eye's appearance before and after treatment. Note any ointment or eye patch you applied to the eye and any eyedrops you instilled. Record the patient's tolerance of the procedure. Document teaching provided to the patient and family (if applicable), their understanding of that teaching, and any need for follow-up teaching.

References

1 American Optometric Association. (n.d.). Conjunctivitis. https://www.aoa.org/patients-and-public/eye-and-vision-problems/glossary-of-eye-and-vision-conditions/conjunctivitis
2 American Optometric Association. (n.d.). Blepharitis. https://www.aoa.org/patients-and-public/eye-and-vision-problems/glossary-of-eye-and-vision-conditions/blepharitis?sso=y
3 Murakami, D. K., et al. (2015). All warm compresses are not equally efficacious. *Optometry and Vision Science, 92,* e327–e333. (Level VI)
4 Sjögren's Syndrome Foundation. (n.d.). Patient education sheet: Simple solutions for dry eye. https://www.sjogrens.org/sites/default/files/inline-files/Dry%20Eye%20Patient%20Education%20Sheet.pdf
5 Blackie, C. A., et al. (2008). Inner eyelid surface temperature as a function of warm compress methodology. *Optometry and Vision Science, 85,* 675–683. (Level II)
6 The Joint Commission. (2021). Standard NPSG.07.01.01. *Comprehensive accreditation manual for hospitals.* Oakbrook Terrace, IL: The Joint Commission. (Level VII)
7 World Health Organization. (2009). WHO guidelines on hand hygiene in health care: First global patient safety challenge, clean care is safer care. https://apps.who.int/iris/bitstream/handle/10665/44102/9789241597906_eng.pdf?sequence=1 (Level IV)
8 Centers for Disease Control and Prevention. (2002). Guideline for hand hygiene in health-care settings: Recommendations of the Healthcare Infection Control Practices Advisory Committee and the HICPAC/SHEA/APIC/IDSA Hand Hygiene Task Force. *MMWR Recommendations and Reports, 51*(RR-16), 1–45. https://www.cdc.gov/mmwr/pdf/rr/rr5116.pdf (Level II)
9 Centers for Medicare and Medicaid Services, Department of Health and Human Services. (2020). Condition of participation: Infection control. 42 C.F.R. § 482.42.
10 Accreditation Association for Hospitals and Health Systems. (2020). Standard 07.01.21. *Healthcare Facilities Accreditation Program: Accreditation requirements for acute care hospitals.* Chicago, IL: Accreditation Association for Hospitals and Health Systems. (Level VII)
11 DNV GL-Healthcare USA, Inc. (2020). IC.1.SR.1. *NIAHO® accreditation requirements, interpretive guidelines and surveyor guidance—revision 20.0.* Milford, OH: DNV GL-Healthcare USA, Inc. (Level VII)
12 The Joint Commission. (2021). Standard NPSG.01.01.01. *Comprehensive accreditation manual for hospitals.* Oakbrook Terrace, IL: The Joint Commission. (Level VII)
13 Centers for Medicare and Medicaid Services, Department of Health and Human Services. (2020). Condition of participation: Patient's rights. 42 C.F.R. § 482.13(c)(1).
14 Accreditation Association for Hospitals and Health Systems. (2020). Standard 15.01.16. *Healthcare Facilities Accreditation Program: Accreditation requirements for acute care hospitals.* Chicago, IL: Accreditation Association for Hospitals and Health Systems. (Level VII)
15 The Joint Commission. (2021). Standard RI.01.01.01. *Comprehensive accreditation manual for hospitals.* Oakbrook Terrace, IL: The Joint Commission. (Level VII)
16 DNV GL-Healthcare USA, Inc. (2020). PR.2.SR.5. *NIAHO® accreditation requirements, interpretive guidelines and surveyor guidance—revision 20.0.* Milford, OH: DNV GL-Healthcare USA, Inc. (Level VII)
17 The Joint Commission. (2021). Standard PC.02.01.21. *Comprehensive accreditation manual for hospitals.* Oakbrook Terrace, IL: The Joint Commission. (Level VII)
18 Waters, T. R., et al. (2009). Safe patient handling training for schools of nursing. https://www.cdc.gov/niosh/docs/2009-127/pdfs/2009-127.pdf (Level VII)
19 Occupational Safety and Health Administration. (2019). Bloodborne pathogens, standard number 1910.1030. https://www.osha.gov/pls/oshaweb/owadisp.show_document?p_id=10051&p_table=STANDARDS (Level VII)
20 Siegel, J. D., et al. (2007, revised 2019). 2007 guideline for isolation precautions: Preventing transmission of infectious agents in healthcare settings. https://www.cdc.gov/infectioncontrol/pdf/guidelines/isolation-guidelines-H.pdf (Level II)
21 Accreditation Association for Hospitals and Health Systems. (2020). Standard 07.01.10. *Healthcare Facilities Accreditation Program: Accreditation requirements for acute care hospitals.* Chicago, IL: Accreditation Association for Hospitals and Health Systems. (Level VII)
22 Ganz, D. A., et al. (2013). *Preventing falls in hospitals: A toolkit for improving quality of care* (AHRQ Publication No. 13-0015-EF). Rockville, MD: Agency for Healthcare Research and Quality. https://www.ahrq.gov/professionals/systems/hospital/fallpxtoolkit/index.html (Level VII)
23 The Joint Commission. (2021). Standard MM.06.01.01. *Comprehensive accreditation manual for hospitals.* Oakbrook Terrace, IL: The Joint Commission. (Level VII)
24 Centers for Medicare and Medicaid Services, Department of Health and Human Services. (2020). Condition of participation: Nursing services. 42 C.F.R. § 482.23(c).
25 Accreditation Association for Hospitals and Health Systems. (2020). Standard 16.01.03. *Healthcare Facilities Accreditation Program: Accreditation requirements for acute care hospitals.* Chicago, IL: Accreditation Association for Hospitals and Health Systems. (Level VII)

26 DNV GL-Healthcare USA, Inc. (2020). MM 1.SR.2. *NIAHO® accreditation requirements, interpretive guidelines and surveyor guidance—revision 20.0.* Milford, OH: DNV GL-Healthcare USA, Inc. (Level VII)

27 The Joint Commission. (2021). Standard RC.01.03.01. *Comprehensive accreditation manual for hospitals.* Oakbrook Terrace, IL: The Joint Commission. (Level VII)

28 Centers for Medicare and Medicaid Services, Department of Health and Human Services. (2020). Condition of participation: Medical record services. 42 C.F.R. § 482.24(b).

29 Accreditation Association for Hospitals and Health Systems. (2020). Standard 10.00.03. *Healthcare Facilities Accreditation Program: Accreditation requirements for acute care hospitals.* Chicago, IL: Accreditation Association for Hospitals and Health Systems. (Level VII)

30 DNV GL-Healthcare USA, Inc. (2020). MR.2.SR.1. *NIAHO® accreditation requirements, interpretive guidelines and surveyor guidance—revision 20.0.* Milford, OH: DNV GL-Healthcare USA, Inc. (Level VII)

EYE IRRIGATION

Used mainly to flush secretions, chemicals, and foreign bodies from the eye, eye irrigation also provides a way to administer medications for corneal and conjunctival disorders. This procedure typically involves the use of sterile water, normal saline solution, or lactated Ringer solution. However, a practitioner may order other solutions in special circumstances.[1,2,3,4] In an emergency, tap water may serve as an irrigant.[2]

The amount of solution needed to irrigate an eye depends on the contaminant. Secretions require a moderate volume; major chemical burns require a copious amount. Immediate water irrigation is contraindicated for exposure to such substances as dry lime, phenols, and elemental metals. Therefore, identification of the chemical causing the burn is necessary before irrigation.[1] (See *Three devices for eye irrigation*.)

Equipment

Gloves ■ fluid-impermeable pad ■ sterile gauze pads ■ emesis basin ■ towel ■ Optional: goggles, eyelid retractor, prescribed ophthalmic anesthetic eyedrops.

For moderate-volume irrigation

Prescribed sterile ophthalmic irrigant ■ sterile basin or irrigation bottle ■ 50- or 60-mL syringe or squeeze bottle.

For copious irrigation

One or more 1,000-mL bags of sterile water, normal saline solution, or lactated Ringer solution[1,2,3,4] ■ standard IV infusion set ■ IV pole.

Commercially prepared bottles of sterile ophthalmic irrigant are available.

Preparation of equipment

Inspect all equipment and supplies. If a product is expired, is defective, or has compromised integrity, remove it from patient use, label it as expired or defective, and report the expiration or defect as directed by your facility. Read the label on the irrigant and compare it with the practitioner's order. Double-check its sterility, strength, and expiration date. If possible, warm all solutions to between 90° F to 100° F (32.2° C to 37.8° C) *to promote patient comfort.*[5]

For moderate-volume irrigation

Pour the sterile irrigant into the irrigation bottle or sterile basin. Fill the syringe or squeeze bottle with 30 to 60 mL of irrigant. If you're using a commercially prepared bottle of sterile irrigant, remove the cap from the irrigant container and place the container within reach. Be sure to keep the tip of the container sterile.

For copious irrigation

Use sterile technique to set up the IV infusion set and the bag of sterile water, normal saline solution, or lactated Ringer solution.[1,2,3,4] Hang the container on an IV pole, fill the IV tubing with the solution, and adjust the drip regulator valve *to ensure an adequate but not forceful flow.*

Place all other equipment within easy reach.

Implementation

- Verify the practitioner's order.
- Gather and prepare the necessary equipment and supplies.
- Perform hand hygiene.[6,7,8,9,10,11]
- Confirm the patient's identity using at least two patient identifiers.[12]
- Provide privacy.[13,14,15,16]
- Explain the procedure to the patient and family (if appropriate) according to their individual communication and learning needs *to increase their understanding, allay their fears, and enhance cooperation.*[17] If the patient has a chemical burn, ease the patient's anxiety by explaining that irrigation prevents further damage.
- Raise the patient's bed to waist level before providing care *to prevent caregiver back strain.*[18]
- Perform hand hygiene.[6,7,8,9,10,11]
- Help the patient into the supine position with the head of the bed elevated.
- Perform hand hygiene.[6,7,8,9,10,11]
- Put on gloves and, if splashing is likely, goggles *to comply with standard precautions.*[19,20,21]
- If the patient is wearing contact lenses, remove and discard them immediately *to prevent further damage and to facilitate irrigation.*

NURSING ALERT If the patient has been exposed to an acid or alkali, irrigate the eye immediately and then perform a complete eye examination. *The extent of the injury depends on the amount of exposure. Irrigating immediately reduces damage.*[22]

- Gently remove visible external discharge or debris from the eye with sterile gauze pads. Wipe from the inner canthus to the outer canthus *to avoid washing debris into the eye.* Use a new sterile gauze pad with each wipe *to prevent cross-contamination.*
- Turn the patient's head slightly toward the affected side *to prevent cross-contamination from the solution flowing over the patient's nose and into the other eye.*
- Place a fluid-impermeable pad under the patient's head, and place an emesis basin against the affected side of the patient's head (as shown below) *to catch excess solution.*[23]

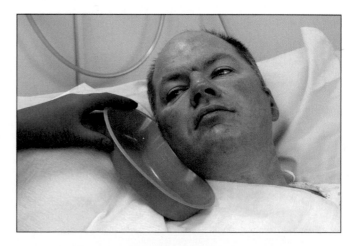

Three devices for eye irrigation

Depending on the type and extent of injury, you may need a specific device to irrigate the patient's eye, such as a syringe or squeeze bottle, IV tubing, or a Morgan lens.

Syringe or squeeze bottle

For moderate-volume irrigation—to remove eye secretions, for example—apply sterile ophthalmic irrigant to the eye directly from a 50- or 60-mL syringe or squeeze bottle (as shown) filled with ophthalmic irrigant. Direct the stream at the inner canthus, and position the patient so the stream washes across the cornea and exits at the outer canthus.

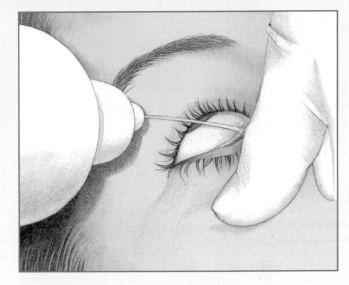

IV tubing

For copious irrigation—to treat chemical burns, for example—set up an IV bag and tubing. Direct a constant, gentle stream of irrigant at the inner canthus so that the solution flows across the cornea to the outer canthus. Flush the eye (as shown) for 30 to 60 minutes, until the pH of the eye returns to normal.[4]

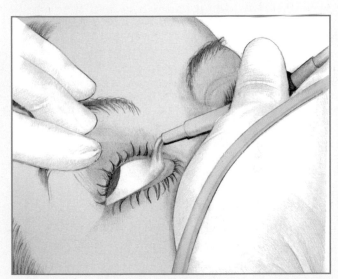

Morgan lens

Attached to IV tubing that's connected to a bag of IV fluid, a Morgan lens permits continuous lavage and also delivers medication to the eye. Begin the irrigation at the prescribed flow rate. To insert the device, ask the patient to look down as you insert the lens under the upper eyelid (as shown). Then have the patient look up as you retract and release the lower eyelid over the lens. Use of a Morgan lens is contraindicated if a penetrating injury or globe rupture is suspected.[1]

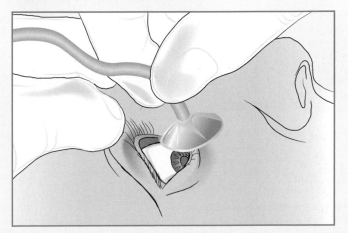

■ Using the thumb and index finger of your nondominant hand, separate the patient's eyelids (as shown below).

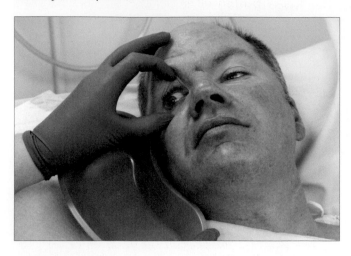

■ If ordered, instill ophthalmic anesthetic eyedrops, following safe medication practices, *as a comfort measure.*[23,24,25,26,27] Use them only once, *because repeated use slows healing.*
■ To irrigate the conjunctival cul-de-sac, continue holding the eyelids apart with your thumb and index finger.
■ To irrigate the upper eyelid (the superior fornix), use an eyelid retractor. Steady the hand holding the retractor by resting it on the patient's forehead. *The retractor prevents the eyelid from closing involuntarily when solution touches the cornea and conjunctiva.*

Administering moderate-volume irrigation

■ Holding the syringe or squeeze bottle of sterile ophthalmic irrigant about 1" (2.5 cm) from the eye, direct a constant, gentle stream at the inner canthus (as shown below) *so that the solution flows across the cornea to the outer canthus.* Use only enough force to gently remove secretions from the conjunctiva.

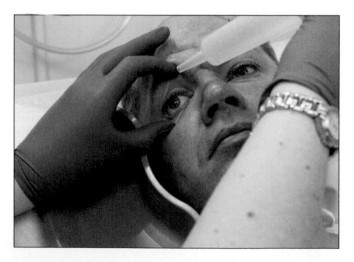

■ Avoid touching the eye with the irrigation tip or pressing on the eyeball, *to prevent unnecessary discomfort and possible further injury.*
■ Evert the lower eyelid and then the upper eyelid *to inspect for retained foreign particles.*

Administering copious irrigation

■ Hold the control valve on the IV tubing about 1" (2.5 cm) above the patient's eye, and direct a constant, gentle stream of solution at the inner canthus *so that the solution flows across the cornea to the outer canthus.*
■ Ask the patient to rotate the eye periodically while you continue the irrigation. *This action can help dislodge foreign particles and ensures irrigation of the entire eye.*

■ Evert the lower eyelid and then the upper eyelid *to inspect for retained foreign particles.* (This inspection is especially important when the patient has caustic lime in the eye.)

Completing the procedure
■ Remove any foreign particles by gently touching the conjunctiva with a sterile gauze pad moistened with irrigant. Don't touch the cornea, *to prevent unnecessary discomfort and possible further injury.*
■ Resume irrigating the eye until irrigation has removed all visible foreign particles.
■ After irrigation is complete, gently dry the patient's eyelid with a sterile gauze pad, wiping from the inner to the outer canthus. Use a new sterile gauze pad for each wipe. *This action reduces the patient's urge to rub the eye.*
■ Offer the patient a towel for drying the face and neck.
■ Return the bed to the lowest position *to prevent falls and maintain patient safety.*[28]
■ Discard used supplies in the appropriate receptacle.[19]
■ Remove and discard your gloves, and remove your goggles, if worn.[20]
■ Perform hand hygiene.[6,7,8,9,10,11]
■ Document the procedure.[29,30,31,32]

Special considerations
■ Arrange for follow-up care, when needed.
■ When irrigating both eyes, have the patient tilt the head toward the side being irrigated *to avoid cross-contamination.*
■ For chemical burns, irrigate the affected eye for 30 minutes *to dilute and wash out the harsh chemical.*[1] After irrigation, close the patient's eye for about 5 minutes and then test its pH by touching the pH test strip to the fornix (the area between the conjunctiva and the lower eyelid).[1] Continue irrigation until a neutral pH is achieved and maintained for at least 30 minutes.[1,22,33] Note that pH measurement can vary, and depends on the measurement method. When measured by litmus paper, typical eye pH can be 6.5 to 7.5.[1] After irrigating any chemical, note the time, date, and chemical for your own reference *in case you develop contact dermatitis.*[22] For further information on chemicals, contact the American Association of Poison Control Centers at 1-800-222-1222, or access their Web site at https://www.aapcc.org.
■ Studies have shown that the most comfortable method of irrigation for patients is the Morgan lens in combination with a lidocaine-saline solution.[34]
■ If you're using a Morgan lens, follow the manufacturer's guidelines. Flow of solution must start before instillation and continue while you're removing the lens.[35]

Patient teaching

If you use an ophthalmic anesthetic agent, instruct the patient to avoid touching the eye. *Touching the eye before the anesthetic wears off can result in damage to the cornea or conjunctiva.*

Complications

Corneal injuries (scratches and tears) can occur if the irrigation tip touches the eye.[33]

Documentation

Note the form of irrigation used, duration of irrigation, type and amount of solution used, and drainage characteristics. Record your assessment of the patient's eye before and after irrigation and the patient's tolerance of the procedure. Document the presence and removal of contact lenses, as appropriate. Note the chemical to which the patient was exposed, as applicable. Record the pH of the eye before irrigation and any subsequent pH values, as appropriate. Document teaching provided to the patient and family (if applicable), their understanding of that teaching, and any need for follow-up teaching.

REFERENCES

1 Kaushik, S., & Bird, S. (2020). Topical chemical burns: Initial assessment and management. In: *UpToDate*, Traub, S. J., et al. (Eds.).
2 Ventocilla, M. (2019). Ophthalmologic approach to chemical burns. https://emedicine.medscape.com/article/1215950-overview#a5
3 Ramponi, D. R. (2017). Chemical burns of the eye. *Advanced Emergency Nursing Journal, 39*, 193–198.

4 Gardiner, M. F. (2021). Overview of eye injuries in the emergency department. In: *UpToDate*, Torrey, S. B., & Jacobs, D. S. (Eds.).

5 Ernst, A. A., et al. (1998). Warmed versus room temperature saline solution for ocular irrigation: A randomized clinical trial. *Annals of Emergency Medicine, 32*, 676–679. (Level II)

6 The Joint Commission. (2021). Standard NPSG.07.01.01. *Comprehensive accreditation manual for hospitals.* Oakbrook Terrace, IL: The Joint Commission. (Level VII)

7 World Health Organization. (2009). WHO guidelines on hand hygiene in health care: First global patient safety challenge, clean care is safer care. https://apps.who.int/iris/bitstream/handle/10665/44102/9789241597906_eng.pdf?sequence=1 (Level IV)

8 Centers for Disease Control and Prevention. (2002). Guideline for hand hygiene in health-care settings: Recommendations of the Healthcare Infection Control Practices Advisory Committee and the HICPAC/SHEA/APIC/IDSA Hand Hygiene Task Force. *MMWR Recommendations and Reports, 51*(RR-16), 1–45. https://www.cdc.gov/mmwr/pdf/rr/rr5116.pdf (Level II)

9 Centers for Medicare and Medicaid Services, Department of Health and Human Services. (2020). Condition of participation: Infection control. 42 C.F.R. § 482.42.

10 Accreditation Association for Hospitals and Health Systems. (2020). Standard 07.01.21. *Healthcare Facilities Accreditation Program: Accreditation requirements for acute care hospitals.* Chicago, IL: Accreditation Association for Hospitals and Health Systems. (Level VII)

11 DNV GL-Healthcare USA, Inc. (2020). IC.1.SR.1. *NIAHO® accreditation requirements, interpretive guidelines and surveyor guidance—revision 20.0.* Milford, OH: DNV GL-Healthcare USA, Inc. (Level VII)

12 The Joint Commission. (2021). Standard NPSG.01.01.01. *Comprehensive accreditation manual for hospitals.* Oakbrook Terrace, IL: The Joint Commission. (Level VII)

13 Centers for Medicare and Medicaid Services, Department of Health and Human Services. (2020). Condition of participation: Patient's rights. 42 C.F.R. § 482.13(c)(1).

14 Accreditation Association for Hospitals and Health Systems. (2020). Standard 15.01.16. *Healthcare Facilities Accreditation Program: Accreditation requirements for acute care hospitals.* Chicago, IL: Accreditation Association for Hospitals and Health Systems. (Level VII)

15 The Joint Commission. (2021). Standard RI.01.01.01. *Comprehensive accreditation manual for hospitals.* Oakbrook Terrace, IL: The Joint Commission. (Level VII)

16 DNV GL-Healthcare USA, Inc. (2020). PR.2.SR.5. *NIAHO® accreditation requirements, interpretive guidelines and surveyor guidance—revision 20.0.* Milford, OH: DNV GL-Healthcare USA, Inc. (Level VII)

17 The Joint Commission. (2021). Standard PC.02.01.21. *Comprehensive accreditation manual for hospitals.* Oakbrook Terrace, IL: The Joint Commission. (Level VII)

18 Waters, T. R., et al. (2009). Safe patient handling training for schools of nursing. https://www.cdc.gov/niosh/docs/2009-127/pdfs/2009-127.pdf (Level VII)

19 Occupational Safety and Health Administration. (2012). Bloodborne pathogens, standard number 1910.1030. https://www.osha.gov/pls/oshaweb/owadisp.show_document?p_id=10051&p_table=STANDARDS (Level VII)

20 Siegel, J. D., et al. (2007, revised 2019). 2007 guideline for isolation precautions: Preventing transmission of infectious agents in healthcare settings. https://www.cdc.gov/infectioncontrol/pdf/guidelines/isolation-guidelines-H.pdf (Level II)

21 Accreditation Association for Hospitals and Health Systems. (2020). Standard 07.01.10. *Healthcare Facilities Accreditation Program: Accreditation requirements for acute care hospitals.* Chicago, IL: Accreditation Association for Hospitals and Health Systems. (Level VII)

22 Pokhrel, P. K., & Loftus, S. A. (2007). Ocular emergencies. *American Family Physician, 76*(6), 829–836. https://www.aafp.org/afp/2007/0915/p829.pdf

23 Stevens, S. (2016). How to irrigate the eye. *Community Eye Health Journal, 29*(95), 56. https://www.ncbi.nlm.nih.gov/pmc/articles/PMC5340106/

24 The Joint Commission. (2021). Standard MM.06.01.01. *Comprehensive accreditation manual for hospitals.* Oakbrook Terrace, IL: The Joint Commission. (Level VII)

25 Centers for Medicare and Medicaid Services, Department of Health and Human Services. (2020). Condition of participation: Nursing services. 42 C.F.R. § 482.23(c).

26 Accreditation Association for Hospitals and Health Systems. (2020). Standard 16.01.03. *Healthcare Facilities Accreditation Program: Accreditation requirements for acute care hospitals.* Chicago, IL: Accreditation Association for Hospitals and Health Systems. (Level VII)

27 DNV GL-Healthcare USA, Inc. (2020). MM.1.SR.3. *NIAHO® accreditation requirements, interpretive guidelines and surveyor guidance—revision 20.0.* Milford, OH: DNV GL-Healthcare USA, Inc. (Level VII)

28 Ganz, D. A., et al. (2013, reviewed 2021). *Preventing falls in hospitals: A toolkit for improving quality of care* (AHRQ Publication No. 13-0015-EF). Rockville, MD: Agency for Healthcare Research and Quality. https://www.ahrq.gov/professionals/systems/hospital/fallpxtoolkit/index.html (Level VII)

29 The Joint Commission. (2021). Standard RC.01.03.01. *Comprehensive accreditation manual for hospitals.* Oakbrook Terrace, IL: The Joint Commission. (Level VII)

30 Centers for Medicare and Medicaid Services, Department of Health and Human Services. (2020). Condition of participation: Medical record services. 42 C.F.R. § 482.24(b).

31 Accreditation Association for Hospitals and Health Systems. (2020). Standard 10.00.03. *Healthcare Facilities Accreditation Program: Accreditation requirements for acute care hospitals.* Chicago, IL: Accreditation Association for Hospitals and Health Systems. (Level VII)

32 DNV GL-Healthcare USA, Inc. (2020). MR.2.SR.1. *NIAHO® accreditation requirements, interpretive guidelines and surveyor guidance—revision 20.0.* Milford, OH: DNV GL-Healthcare USA, Inc. (Level VII)

33 Willmann, D., et al. (2021). Corneal injury. In *StatPearls*. Treasure Island, FL: StatPearls Publishing. https://www.ncbi.nlm.nih.gov/books/NBK459283/

34 O'Malley, G. F., et al. (2008). Eye irrigation is more comfortable with a lidocaine-containing irrigation solution compared with normal saline. *Journal of Trauma, 64*, 1360–1362. (Level II)

35 MorTan, Inc. (2017). Morgan lens instructional chart. https://www.morganlens.com/media/1067/morgan-lens-instructional-chart-2017.pdf

EYE MEDICATION ADMINISTRATION

Practitioners may prescribe eyedrops for a variety of diagnostic and therapeutic purposes, including dilating the pupil, staining the cornea to detect abrasions or scars, anesthetizing or lubricating the eye, and treating such disorders as glaucoma and infection.[1] An ointment preparation helps keep eye medication in contact with the treatment area of the eye for as long as possible. Eye ointments treat eye diseases, prevent or treat infection or inflammation, relieve discomfort, provide lubrication, and prevent damage.[2,3]

Understanding the ocular effects of medications is important, *because certain drugs can cause eye disorders or have serious ocular effects.* For example, anticholinergics, which are commonly used during eye examinations, can precipitate acute glaucoma in patients with a predisposition to the disorder.[4]

Equipment

Prescribed eye medication (drops or ointment) ■ gloves ■ warm water or normal saline solution ■ gauze pads ■ facial tissues ■ Optional: ocular dressing, personal protective equipment.

Preparation of equipment

Inspect all equipment and supplies. If a product is expired, is defective, or has compromised integrity, remove it from patient use, label it as expired or defective, and report the expiration or defect, as directed by your facility. Make sure the medication is labeled for ophthalmic use. Date the medication container the first time you open it, *because you should use the medication within the time specified by the manufacturer once you've opened the container to prevent contamination.*[5,6] Follow your facility's direction or the manufacturer's instructions on when to discard an opened eye medication. If the tip of an eye ointment tube has crusted, turn the tip on a sterile gauze pad *to remove the crust.*

Implementation

■ Avoid distractions and interruptions when preparing and administering the medication *to prevent medication administration errors.*[7,8]
■ Verify the practitioner's order.[9,10,11,12]
■ Reconcile the patient's medications when a new medication is ordered by the practitioner *to reduce the risk of medication errors, including omissions, duplications, dosing errors, and drug interactions.*[13,14]

Instilling eyedrops

To instill eyedrops, pull the lower lid down *to expose the conjunctival sac*. Have the patient look up and away, then squeeze the prescribed number of drops into the sac. Then, release the patient's eyelid.

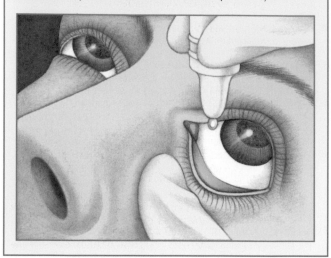

- Gather and prepare the necessary equipment and supplies.
- Compare the medication label to the order in the patient's medical record.[9,10,11,12] Confirm which eye requires treatment.

NURSING ALERT Make sure you know which eye to treat, *because the practitioner may order different medications and doses for each eye.*
- Check the patient's medical record for an allergy or other contraindication to the prescribed medication. If an allergy or contraindications exist, don't administer the medication, and notify the practitioner.[9,10,11,12]
- Check the expiration date. If the medication is expired, return it to the pharmacy and obtain new medication.[9,10,11,12]
- Visually inspect the medication for discoloration or any other loss of integrity. Don't give the medication if its integrity is compromised.[9,10,11,12]
- Discuss any unresolved concerns about the medication with the patient's practitioner.[9,10,11,12]
- Warm the medication to room temperature, as necessary.
- Perform hand hygiene.[15,16,17,18,19,20]
- Confirm the patient's identify using at least two patient identifiers.[21]
- Provide privacy.[22,23,24,25]
- Explain the procedure to the patient and family (if appropriate) according to their individual communication and learning needs *to increase their understanding, allay their fears, and enhance cooperation.*[26]
- If the patient is receiving the medication for the first time, inform the patient or family about possible significant adverse reactions, and discuss any other concerns related to the medication.[9,10,11,12]
- Verify that you're administering the medication at the proper time, in the prescribed dosage, and by the correct route *to reduce the risk of medication errors.*[9,10,11,12]
- If your facility uses a bar-code technology, use it, as directed by your facility.
- Raise the patient's bed to waist level before providing care *to prevent caregiver back strain.*[27]
- Have the patient sit or lie in the supine position.
- Perform hand hygiene.[15,16,17,18,19,20]

NURSING ALERT If your facility's hazardous drug list contains the drug you are about to administer, put on personal protective equipment, as directed.[28]
- Put on gloves *to comply with standard precautions.*[29,30,31]
- If the patient is wearing an eye dressing, remove it by gently pulling it down and away from the patient's forehead *to prevent skin shearing or tearing.*[32] Take care not to contaminate your hands.
- Perform hand hygiene[15,16,17,18,19,20] and then put on gloves.[26,27]
- Assess the patient's eye, noting any redness, edema, or discharge; note the appearance and amount of discharge.

- Remove any discharge by cleaning around the eye with gauze pads moistened with warm water or normal saline solution. With the patient's eye closed, clean from the inner to the outer canthus, using a fresh sterile gauze pad for each stroke.
- *To remove crusted secretions around the eye*, moisten a gauze pad with warm water or normal saline solution. Ask the patient to close the eye, and then place the gauze pad over it for 1 or 2 minutes. Remove the pad, and then repeat with new moist sterile gauze pads, as necessary, until the secretions are soft enough to be removed without traumatizing the mucosa.
- Remove and discard your gloves.[31]
- Perform hand hygiene.[15,16,17,18,19,20]
- Put on new gloves.[29,31]
- Instruct the patient to tilt the head back and toward the side of the affected eye *so that excess medication can flow away from the tear duct, minimizing systemic absorption through the nasal mucosa.*

For eyedrops
- Remove the bottle top from the medication container and place it on a clean, dry surface. Be careful to avoid contaminating the dropper tip or bottle top.
- Before instilling the eyedrops, instruct the patient to look up and away. *This position moves the cornea away from the lower lid and minimizes the risk of touching the cornea with the dropper if the patient blinks.*
- If necessary, steady the hand holding the dropper by resting it against the patient's forehead.[1] With your other hand, gently pull down the lower lid of the affected eye and instill the drops in the conjunctival sac. Try to avoid placing the drops directly on the eyeball *to prevent the patient from experiencing discomfort.* (See *Instilling eyedrops.*)
- After instilling the eyedrops, instruct the patient to close both eyes gently, without squeezing the lids shut.
- *To prevent systemic absorption of medication*, gently press your thumb on the inner canthus for 2 to 3 minutes while the patient closes both eyes.[32]
- Use a clean tissue to remove any excess solution leaking from the eye. Remember to use a fresh tissue for each eye *to prevent cross-contamination.*

For eye ointment
- Squeeze a small ribbon of medication on the edge of the conjunctival sac from the inner to the outer canthus.[3] If necessary, steady the hand holding the medication tube by bracing it against the patient's forehead or cheek, taking care not to touch the tip of the tube to the eye or other surface. Cut off the ribbon by turning the tube.
- Tell the patient that eye ointment may cause momentary blurring of the vision.[2]

For all eye medication
- Instruct the patient to close the eyes gently without squeezing the lids shut and to roll the eyes behind the closed lids *to help distribute the medication over the surface of the eyeball.*
- Use a clean tissue *to remove any excess solution or ointment leaking from the eye.* Remember to use a fresh tissue for each eye *to prevent cross-contamination.*
- Replace the medication cap.
- Apply a new ocular dressing, if necessary.
- Return the bed to the lowest position to prevent falls and maintain patient safety.[33]
- Return the medication to the storage area. Make sure to store it according to the label's instructions.
- Remove and discard your gloves.[31]
- Perform hand hygiene.[15,16,17,18,19,20]
- Document the procedure.[34,35,36,37]

Special considerations
- Never touch the tip of the bottle or dropper or the tip of the tube to the patient's eyeball, lids, or lashes *to maintain the drug container's sterility.*[1] If the dropper tip becomes contaminated, discard the medication and obtain another sterile medication bottle.

■ Don't use eye medication for more than one patient, if possible, *to prevent cross-contamination*; however, if permitted by your facility, you may use preserved multidose eyedrop medications in multiple patients with special infection prevention and patient safety precautions.[38]

NURSING ALERT Don't use multidose eyedrops for a patient when you've used them to treat another infectious or immunocompromised patient. [38]

NURSING ALERT Discard eyedrops immediately if contamination occurs—for example, if the dropper tip touches any part of the eye structure or surface, a staff member administering the medication touches the dropper tip, an open eyedrop container has no expiration date on it, an open eyedrop container has an expiration date that exceeds 28 days, or an eyedrop container is uncapped.[38]

NURSING ALERT *To prevent cross-contamination*, never use a container of eye medication for more than one patient.[2]

■ If you're administering eyedrops and an eye ointment, administer the drops first, *because the ointment may inhibit the action of the eyedrops*.[2] Wait times between applications vary; follow the manufacturer's prescribing information.[39]

■ Treat only the affected eye, unless otherwise ordered.[2]

Patient teaching

If the practitioner has ordered eye medication for home use, teach the patient and family (if appropriate) proper administration technique. Review the procedure, and ask for a return demonstration. Ensure that the patient has refrigeration to store the medication, if necessary . Instruct the patient to contact the practitioner if the desired medication effects don't occur within an indicated time frame, or if eye irritation or changes in vision develop. Remind the patient and family (if appropriate) not to share ophthalmic medications *to prevent cross-contamination*, and teach them about the importance of hand washing before and after administration.

Complications

Instillation of some eye medications may cause transient burning, itching, and redness. Rarely, systemic effects may occur.

Documentation

Document your assessment of the eye. Record the medication you administered, eye or eyes you treated, and date, time, and dose, according to your facility's documentation format. Note the patient's response to the procedure. Document any adverse effects that occur, the date and time you notified the practitioner, prescribed interventions, and the patient's response to those interventions. Document teaching you provided to the patient and family (if appropriate), their understanding of that teaching, and any need for follow-up teaching.

REFERENCES

1 Craven, R. F., et al. (2021). *Fundamentals of nursing: Concepts and competencies for practice* (9th ed.). Philadelphia, PA: Wolters Kluwer.

2 Shaw, M. (2014). How to administer eye drops and ointments. *Nursing Times, 110*, 16–18. https://www.nursingtimes.net/archive/how-to-administer-eye-drops-and-ointments-26-09-2014/

3 Manuel, B. (2019). Evidence summary—medication (ocular): Administration. *The JBI EBP Database*. AN: JBI22720

4 Salem, C. B., et al. (2018). Glaucoma. *The Lancet, 391*(10122), 739–740. https://www.thelancet.com/journals/lancet/article/PIIS0140-6736(18)30306-4/fulltext

5 The Joint Commission. (2021). Standard MM.05.01.09. *Comprehensive accreditation manual for hospitals*. Oakbrook Terrace, IL: The Joint Commission. (Level VII)

6 Accreditation Association for Hospitals and Health Systems. (2020). Standard 25.01.18. *Healthcare Facilities Accreditation Program: Accreditation requirements for acute care hospitals*. Chicago, IL: Accreditation Association for Hospitals and Health Systems. (Level VII)

7 Westbrook, J., et al. (2010). Association of interruptions with an increased risk and severity of medication administration errors. *Archives of Internal Medicine, 170*, 683–690. (Level IV)

8 Institute for Safe Medication Practices. (2012). Side tracks on the safety express: Interruptions lead to errors and unfinished…Wait, what was I doing? *Nurse Advise-ERR, 11*(2), 1–4. https://www.ismp.org/resources/side-tracks-safety-express-interruptions-lead-errors-and-unfinished-wait-what-was-i-doing?id=37

9 The Joint Commission. (2021). Standard MM.06.01.01. *Comprehensive accreditation manual for hospitals*. Oakbrook Terrace, IL: The Joint Commission. (Level VII)

10 Centers for Medicare and Medicaid Services, Department of Health and Human Services. (2020). Condition of participation: Nursing services. 42 C.F.R. § 482.23(c).

11 Accreditation Association for Hospitals and Health Systems. (2020). Standard 16.01.03. *Healthcare Facilities Accreditation Program: Accreditation requirements for acute care hospitals*. Chicago, IL: Accreditation Association for Hospitals and Health Systems. (Level VII)

12 DNV GL-Healthcare USA, Inc. (2020). MM.1.SR.3. *NIAHO® accreditation requirements, interpretive guidelines and surveyor guidance—revision 20.0*. Milford, OH: DNV GL-Healthcare USA, Inc. (Level VII)

13 Accreditation Association for Hospitals and Health Systems. (2020). Standard 25.02.13. *Healthcare Facilities Accreditation Program: Accreditation requirements for acute care hospitals*. Chicago, IL: Accreditation Association for Hospitals and Health Systems. (Level VII)

14 The Joint Commission. (2021). Standard NPSG.03.06.01. *Comprehensive accreditation manual for hospitals*. Oakbrook Terrace, IL: The Joint Commission. (Level VII)

15 The Joint Commission. (2021). Standard NPSG.07.01.01. *Comprehensive accreditation manual for hospitals*. Oakbrook Terrace, IL: The Joint Commission. (Level VII)

16 Centers for Disease Control and Prevention. (2002). Guideline for hand hygiene in health-care settings: Recommendations of the Healthcare Infection Control Practices Advisory Committee and the HICPAC/SHEA/APIC/IDSA Hand Hygiene Task Force. *MMWR Recommendations and Reports, 51*(RR-16), 1–45. https://www.cdc.gov/mmwr/pdf/rr/rr5116.pdf (Level II)

17 World Health Organization. (2009). WHO guidelines on hand hygiene in health care: First global patient safety challenge, clean care is safer care. https://apps.who.int/iris/bitstream/handle/10665/44102/9789241597906_eng.pdf?sequence=1 (Level IV)

18 Accreditation Association for Hospitals and Health Systems. (2020). Standard 07.01.21. *Healthcare Facilities Accreditation Program: Accreditation requirements for acute care hospitals*. Chicago, IL: Accreditation Association for Hospitals and Health Systems. (Level VII)

19 Centers for Medicare and Medicaid Services, Department of Health and Human Services. (2020). Condition of participation: Infection control. 42 C.F.R. § 482.42.

20 DNV GL-Healthcare USA, Inc. (2020). IC.1.SR.1. *NIAHO® accreditation requirements, interpretive guidelines and surveyor guidance—revision 20.0*. Milford, OH: DNV GL-Healthcare USA, Inc. (Level VII)

21 The Joint Commission. (2021). Standard NPSG.01.01.01. *Comprehensive accreditation manual for hospitals*. Oakbrook Terrace, IL: The Joint Commission. (Level VII)

22 The Joint Commission. (2021). Standard RI.01.01.01. *Comprehensive accreditation manual for hospitals*. Oakbrook Terrace, IL: The Joint Commission. (Level VII)

23 DNV GL-Healthcare USA, Inc. (2020). PR.2.SR.5. *NIAHO® accreditation requirements, interpretive guidelines and surveyor guidance—revision 20.0*. Milford, OH: DNV GL-Healthcare USA, Inc. (Level VII)

24 Centers for Medicare and Medicaid Services, Department of Health and Human Services. (2020). Condition of participation: Patient's rights. 42 C.F.R. § 482.13(c)(1).

25 Accreditation Association for Hospitals and Health Systems. (2020). Standard 15.01.16. *Healthcare Facilities Accreditation Program: Accreditation requirements for acute care hospitals*. Chicago, IL: Accreditation Association for Hospitals and Health Systems. (Level VII)

26 The Joint Commission. (2021). Standard PC.02.01.21. *Comprehensive accreditation manual for hospitals*. Oakbrook Terrace, IL: The Joint Commission. (Level VII)

27 Waters, T. R., et al. (2009). Safe patient handling training for schools of nursing. https://www.cdc.gov/niosh/docs/2009-127/pdfs/2009-127.pdf (Level VII)

28 The United States Pharmacopeial Convention. (2019). USP general chapter <800>: Hazardous drugs—handling in healthcare settings. https://www.usp.org/compounding/general-chapter-hazardous-drugs-handling-healthcare (Level VII)

29 Siegel, J. D., et al. (2007, revised 2019). 2007 guideline for isolation precautions: Preventing transmission of infectious agents in healthcare settings. https://www.cdc.gov/infectioncontrol/pdf/guidelines/isolation-guidelines-H.pdf (Level II)

30 Accreditation Association for Hospitals and Health Systems. (2020). Standard 07.01.10. *Healthcare Facilities Accreditation Program: Accreditation requirements for acute care hospitals.* Chicago, IL: Accreditation Association for Hospitals and Health Systems. (Level VII)

31 Occupational Safety and Health Administration. (2012). Bloodborne pathogens, standard number 1910.1030. https://www.osha.gov/pls/oshaweb/owadisp.show_document?p_id=10051&p_table=STANDARDS (Level VII)

32 Glaucoma Research Foundation. (2020). Eye drop tips. https://glaucoma.org/treatment/eyedrop-tips.php

33 Ganz, D. A., et al. (2013). Preventing falls in hospitals: A toolkit for improving quality of care (AHRQ publication no. 13-0015-EF). at https://www.ahrq.gov/professionals/systems/hospital/fallpxtoolkit/index.html (Level VII)

34 The Joint Commission. (2021). Standard RC.01.03.01. *Comprehensive accreditation manual for hospitals.* Oakbrook Terrace, IL: The Joint Commission. (Level VII)

35 Centers for Medicare and Medicaid Services, Department of Health and Human Services. (2020). Condition of participation: Medical record services. 42 C.F.R. § 482.24(b).

36 Accreditation Association for Hospitals and Health Systems. (2020). Standard 10.00.03. *Healthcare Facilities Accreditation Program: Accreditation requirements for acute care hospitals.* Chicago, IL: Accreditation Association for Hospitals and Health Systems. (Level VII)

37 DNV GL-Healthcare USA, Inc. (2020). MR.2.SR.1. *NIAHO® accreditation requirements, interpretive guidelines and surveyor guidance—revision 20.0.* Milford, OH: DNV GL-Healthcare USA, Inc. (Level VII)

38 Jensen, M. K., et al. (2014). Using multidose eyedrops in a health care setting: A policy and procedural approach to safe and effective treatment of patients. *JAMA Ophthalmology, 132,* 1476–1479. http://www.progressive-surgicalsolutions.com/wp-content/uploads/2016/03/3_JAMA_09042014_article.pdf

39 Hinkle, J. L., & Cheever, K. H. (2017). *Brunner and Suddarth's textbook of medical-surgical nursing* (14th ed.). Philadelphia, PA: Wolters Kluwer.

Fall prevention and management

Falls are a major cause of injury and death among older adults. Each year, one in four adults older than age 65 falls.[1] For hospitalized patients, falls are the most common safety incident, with rates of 1.7 to 25 falls per 1,000 patient stays, and 30% to 51% of falls in hospitals result in injury.[2] One-third of these falls can be prevented.[2]

Factors that contribute to falls among older adult patients include lengthy convalescent periods, incomplete recovery, medication use, increasing physical disability, and impaired vision, hearing, or mental status. For example, if an older adult's equilibrium becomes impaired, it's likely to take longer to return to normal than it would for a younger adult—and, during that extended period of disequilibrium, the older adult is at an increased risk for falling. Falls not only cause physical injuries, but also trigger such psychological issues as a loss of self-confidence, which hastens dependence and a move to a long-term care facility.

Extrinsic or environmental factors that increase the risk of falling include poor lighting, use of throw rugs, highly waxed floors, unfamiliar surroundings, and misuse of assistive devices. Intrinsic or physiologic factors include age over 80 years, lower extremity weakness, vertigo, orthostatic hypotension, depression, failing eyesight, gait or balance disorders, functional or cognitive impairment, and being female.[1,3]

You should perform a risk assessment for falls for all admitted patients[3,4,5] using a standardized, facility-approved assessment tool, such as the Hendrich II Tool, Morse Fall Scale, Johns Hopkins Tool, or STRATIFY tool.[2,4,5,6,7]

In a health care facility, an accidental fall can change a short stay for a minor problem into a prolonged stay for serious—and possibly life-threatening—problems. The risk of falling is highest during the first week of a stay in a health care or long-term care facility. (See *Who's at risk for a fall?*)

> ## Who's at risk for a fall?
>
> Fall prevention begins with identifying the patients at greatest risk. Common risk factors identified on risk assessment tools include:
> - history of falls in the past 3 months
> - mobility problems and the use of assistive devices
> - use of a large number of prescription medications or medications that cause sedation, confusion, impaired balance, or orthostatic hypotension
> - mental status disturbances, such as delirium, dementia, and psychosis
> - toileting frequency
> - environmental risks, such as being attached to medical equipment
> - impaired vision
> - orthostatic hypotension.[2]

Equipment

Vital signs monitoring equipment ▪ stethoscope ▪ standardized, validated fall risk assessment tool ▪ well-fitting nonskid footwear ▪ facility-approved disinfectant ▪ supplies for fall prevention ▪ pillows ▪ blankets ▪ Optional: gait belt, chair alarm, bed alarm, assistive device, emergency equipment (code cart with cardiac medications, defibrillator, handheld resuscitation bag with mask, and intubation equipment), other personal protective equipment, dressings, tape, prescribed analgesics, cold and warm compresses, naloxone.

Preparation of equipment

Inspect all equipment and supplies. If a product is expired, is defective, or has compromised integrity, remove it from patient use, label it as expired or defective, and report the expiration or defect as directed by your facility.

If you're helping a fallen patient, send an assistant to collect the assessment and emergency equipment you need while you stay with the patient.

Implementation

- Gather and prepare the necessary equipment and supplies.
- Perform hand hygiene.[8,9,10,11,12,13]
- Confirm the patient's identity using at least two patient identifiers.[14]

For fall prevention

- When the patient first enters the room, institute universal fall precautions *to make sure the environment is safe and the patient is comfortable.*[2] Orient the patient to the room and the call light *to help prevent falls related to an unfamiliar environment.* Have the patient perform a return demonstration on call light use.
- If the patient is age 65 or older, or demonstrates unsteadiness or difficulty walking, ask whether the patient has fallen in the past 12 months. If the patient has fallen, ask about the frequency and circumstances of the fall, and evaluate the patient for gait and balance deficits. Assess for proper use of assistive devices, if applicable.
- Assess the patient's risk of falling, using a standardized, validated fall risk assessment tool on admission and after any change in the patient's condition, transfer from another unit, or a fall, or at a frequency determined by your facility; the optimal frequency to assess fall risk hasn't been determined.[2,5,6,7] Assess such factors as the patient's history of falling, mobility, what medications the patient takes, and the patient's mental status. Note whether the patient is incontinent, has sensory deficits such as impaired vision, lives in an environment that contains fall hazards, or experiences orthostatic hypotension.[2]

HOSPITAL-ACQUIRED CONDITION ALERT Keep in mind that the Centers for Medicare and Medicaid Services considers an injury from a fall a hospital-acquired condition *because it can be reasonably prevented using a variety of best practices.* Make sure to follow evidence-based fall prevention practices, such as performing a fall risk assessment and instituting fall precautions, *to reduce the risk of injury from falls.*[2,4,6,15]

■ Be sure the patient is checked for potential dangers hourly during the daytime and evening and every 2 hours overnight *to comply with universal fall precautions.*[2] Correct potential dangers in the patient's room. Keep the call light positioned so it's within the patient's reach at all times.[2] Provide adequate nighttime lighting.[2] Place the patient's personal belongings (such as a purse or wallet, books, and tissues) and assistive devices (such as a urinal or commode, cane, or walker) within easy reach.[2]

■ Keep the bed in its lowest position *so the patient can easily reach the floor when getting out of bed. This position also reduces the distance to the floor in case the patient falls.*[2] Lock the bed's wheels.[2]

■ Keep the patient's area uncluttered.[2]

■ Keep floor surfaces clean and dry. Make sure spills are cleaned up immediately.[2]

■ Instruct the patient to rise slowly from a supine position *to avoid possible dizziness and loss of balance.*[2]

■ Advise the patient to wear well-fitting, nonskid footwear.[2]

■ Respond promptly to the patient's call light *to help limit the number of times the patient gets out of bed without help.*

■ Alert other caregivers to the patient's risk of falling and to the interventions you've implemented.[6]

■ Assess the need for one-on-one patient monitoring, and arrange for it as needed.

■ Have a gait belt readily available at the patient's bedside, if needed, *for use during ambulation or transfer.* (See the "Gait belt use" procedure.)

■ Use a chair or bed alarm, if needed, *to alert staff members that the patient is attempting to get up without assistance.*

■ Encourage the patient to perform active range-of-motion (ROM) exercises *to improve flexibility and coordination.*

■ Assist the patient with early and regular ambulation if the patient's condition allows, *because exercise reduces the risk of falling in older people.*[3] Encourage the patient to use an assistive device for ambulation, such as a walker or cane or other equipment recommended by physical or occupational therapy.

■ If needed, regularly schedule assistance with toileting.[3]

■ Review the patient's medical record for medications that may contribute to a fall.[2,3] (See *Medications associated with falls.*)

■ Perform hand hygiene.[8,9,10,11,12,13]

■ Document the procedure.[20,21,22,23]

For fall management

■ If you're with a patient as the patient falls, maintain your grip on the gait belt (if present) and place your elbow against the patient's waist or thigh *to prevent the patient from going down or to lessen the force of the fall.* If you're with a bariatric patient, move any objects out of the way that could cause injury, and try to protect the patient's head from striking any objects or the floor, *because there's very little you can do to prevent the fall.*[24] Alternatively, if you weren't with the patient when the patient fell, verify that the environment is safe by quickly scanning the patient's location and surroundings *to make sure that there are no imminent physical threats, such as toxic or electrical hazards.*[25]

■ Remain calm and stay with the patient *to prevent any further injury.*

■ Assess the patient for response. If the patient is unresponsive, shout for nearby help and activate the emergency response system via mobile device (if appropriate).[25] Check for absent breathing or only gasping and, if able, simultaneously check for a pulse *to minimize delay in detecting cardiac arrest and initiating cardiopulmonary resuscitation.*[25]

■ If the patient is breathing normally and has a pulse, monitor the patient closely until the emergency response team arrives.[25] If breathing is absent or the patient is only gasping and you feel a pulse within 10 seconds, open the patient's airway; use the head tilt-chin lift technique unless you suspect a cervical spine injury, in which case use the jaw thrust without head extension.[25] Provide rescue breathing, 1 breath every

Medications associated with falls

This table highlights some classes of drugs and the possible adverse effects of each that may increase a patient's risk of falling.[16,17,18,19]

DRUG CLASS	ADVERSE EFFECTS
Diuretics	Hypovolemia, orthostatic hypotension, electrolyte imbalance, urinary incontinence
Antihypertensives	Hypotension, syncope
Beta-adrenergic blockers	Hypotension, syncope
Nitrates	Hypotension, syncope
Vasodilators	Hypotension, syncope
Tricyclic antidepressants	Orthostatic hypotension
Antipsychotics	Orthostatic hypotension, muscle rigidity, sedation
Benzodiazepines	Excessive sedation, confusion, paradoxical agitation, loss of balance
Antihistamines	Excessive sedation, confusion, paradoxical agitation, loss of balance
Opioids	Hypotension, sedation, motor incoordination, agitation
Hypnotics	Excessive sedation, ataxia, poor balance, confusion, paradoxical agitation
Antidiabetic drugs	Acute hypoglycemia
Alcohol	Intoxication, motor incoordination, agitation, sedation, confusion

6 seconds or about 10 breaths/minute.[25] Check the patient's pulse about every 2 minutes. If you don't detect a pulse, begin chest compressions.[25] If you suspect an opioid overdose, administer naloxone intranasally or intramuscularly, if available, according to protocol.[25,26,27,28,29]

■ If breathing is absent, or the patient is only gasping and you don't feel a pulse within 10 seconds, have a coworker retrieve the defibrillator or automated external defibrillator (AED) and other emergency equipment. Alternatively, if you're alone, retrieve the defibrillator or AED and emergency equipment.[25] Immediately begin chest compressions until the defibrillator or AED is ready for use.[25] Compress an adult's chest at a rate of 100 to 120 compressions per minute, with a compression depth of at least 2″ (5 cm) for an average adult, while avoiding excessive chest compression depths (greater than 2.4″ [6 cm]). Avoid leaning on the chest between compressions *to allow full chest wall recoil.*[25] After starting compressions, open the patient's airway and deliver rescue breaths (each over about 1 second); use a ratio of 30 compressions to 2 breaths. When the defibrillator is ready for use, check the patient's rhythm and defibrillate if the patient has a shockable rhythm; otherwise, continue cardiopulmonary resuscitation.[25]

NURSING ALERT Don't move the patient until you fully evaluate the patient's status *to prevent further injury if an injury has occurred as a result of the fall.*[2]

■ To determine the extent of the patient's injuries, look for lacerations, abrasions, and obvious deformities. Note any deviations from the patient's baseline condition and notify the practitioner of them. Determine whether the patient experienced a head trauma, *because this requires further diagnostic evaluation to rule out subdural hematoma.*

NURSING ALERT Patients taking anticoagulants or on aspirin therapy who experience head trauma are at increased risk for subdural hematoma.

■ Take steps to control bleeding (if indicated), and obtain an X-ray if you suspect a fracture. Provide first aid for minor injuries, as needed.

■ If you weren't present during the fall, confirm the patient's identity using at least two patient identifiers.[14] Ask the patient or a witness what happened. Ask whether the patient experienced pain or a change in level of consciousness.

■ Provide reassurance, as needed, and observe for such signs and symptoms as confusion, tremor, weakness, pain, and dizziness.

■ Assess the patient's limb strength and motion. Don't perform ROM exercises if you suspect a fracture or if the patient complains of any odd sensations or limited movement. If you suspect an injury, don't move the patient until a practitioner examines the patient.

■ While the patient lies on the floor until the practitioner arrives, offer pillows and blankets *for comfort*. However, if you suspect a spinal cord injury, don't place a pillow under the patient's head.

■ If you don't detect any problems, return the patient to the bed with the help of another staff member. Never try to lift a patient alone, *because you may injure yourself or the patient*.

■ Even if the patient shows no signs of distress or has sustained only minor injuries, monitor vital signs and assess neurologic status frequently until the patient's condition stabilizes. Notify the practitioner if you note any change from the baseline.

■ Screen for and assess the patient's pain using facility-defined criteria that are consistent with the patient's age, condition, and ability to understand.[30]

■ Treat the patient's pain, as needed and ordered, using nonpharmacologic, pharmacologic, or a combination of approaches. Base the treatment plan on evidence-based practices and the patient's clinical condition, medical history, and pain management goals.[30] Administer analgesics, as ordered, following safe medication administration practices.[26,27,28,29] Apply cold compresses for the first 24 hours and warm compresses thereafter, as needed. (See the "Cold application" procedure, or the "Heat application" procedure.)

■ Perform a postfall assessment *to determine the root cause of the fall*.[2,6,7] Gather assessment data from the patient, staff members, and any witnesses to the fall. Review the events that preceded the fall and any contributing factors. Discuss why it occurred and how it could have been prevented. Assess the patient's environment, looking for possible causes of the fall. Review medications, such as sedatives and opioids, that may have contributed to the fall. (See *Medications associated with falls*, page 341.) Assess for gait disturbances or improper use of a cane, crutches, or a walker.

■ Monitor the patient's status for the next 48 hours or for a period determined by your facility and the patient's condition.[31]

■ Remove and discard your gloves and, if worn, other personal protective equipment.[32]

■ Perform hand hygiene.[8,9,10,11,12,13]

■ Put on gloves and, as needed, other personal protective equipment. [32]

■ Clean and disinfect other reusable equipment according to the manufacturer's instructions *to prevent the spread of infection*.[33,34]

■ Remove and discard your gloves and, if worn, other personal protective equipment.[32]

■ Perform hand hygiene.[8,9,10,11,12,13]

■ Update the patient's risk profile using a standardized, validated fall risk assessment tool. Institute fall precautions.[2,6,7,35]

■ Document the procedure.[20,21,22,23]

Special considerations

■ After a fall, review the patient's medical history *to determine the risk of other complications*. For example, if the patient hit the head, check the history to see whether the patient takes anticoagulants. If so, the patient is at greater risk for intracranial bleeding, and you'll need to monitor accordingly.

■ Consult with the practitioner and multidisciplinary team members to institute interventions to alter modifiable risk factors identified by the falls risk assessment, as ordered. Interventions may include physical therapy, nutrition therapy, medication management, psychological intervention, urinary incontinence management, environment modification, and referral to a specialist.[3]

■ If you don't already have a fall prevention program or interdisciplinary fall team in place in your facility, consider starting such a program.[2]

■ To promote patient safety, add an appropriate notation (such as "At risk for falls") in the patient's medical record, or use a special alert designated by your facility.

■ The Joint Commission issued a sentinel event alert related to preventing falls and fall-related injuries in health care facilities, *because falls are a common safety problem that can occur in patients of any age or physical ability and can result in serious injury and death*. Among the contributing factors are inadequate assessment; communication failures; failure to adhere to safety practices; inadequate staff orientation, supervision, or levels of skill mix; physical environment deficiencies; and lack of leadership. *To help prevent falls*, facilities should raise staff safety awareness; establish a falls injury prevention team; use a standardized, validated risk assessment tool; develop a plan of care for each patient based on identified fall and injury risk; engage in standardized hand-off communication; teach each patient about fall-prevention strategies; and conduct postfall management.[5]

Documentation

Record any measures you took to help prevent a fall, including teaching provided to the patient and family.

After a fall, complete a detailed incident report to help track the frequency of patient falls *so that the facility can implement prevention measures with high-risk patients*. Used primarily for your facility's insurance carrier, this report isn't considered part of the patient's record. However, a copy goes to the facility's administrator, who evaluates care given on the unit and proposes new safety policies, as appropriate. It may also go to other patient care teams, such as the fall prevention team.

Make sure that the incident report documents where and when the fall occurred, how the patient was found, and what position the patient was in. Include the events that preceded the fall, the witnesses' names, the patient's reaction to the fall, and a detailed description of the patient's condition based on assessment findings. Also include the patient's statement of the event. Note any interventions you took and the names of other staff members who helped care for the patient after the fall. Record the names of people you notified of the fall, including the practitioner and the patient's health care power of attorney, and the dates and times when you notified them. Include a copy of the practitioner's report. Also note whether the practitioner sent the patient for diagnostic tests or transferred the patient to another unit.

Include all information about the fall in the patient's record. Document vital signs and ongoing monitoring for a severe complication of the fall. Note your assessment findings, including pain, any interventions performed, and the patient's response to those interventions. Document any medications administered. Document teaching provided to the patient and family (if applicable), their understanding of that teaching, and any need for follow-up teaching.

REFERENCES

1 Centers for Disease Control and Prevention. (2017). Important facts about falls. https://www.cdc.gov/HomeandRecreationalSafety/Falls/adultfalls.html (Level VII)

2 Ganz, D. A., et al. (2013, reviewed 2021). *Preventing falls in hospitals: A toolkit for improving quality of care* (AHRQ Publication No. 13-0015-EF). Rockville, MD: Agency for Healthcare Research and Quality. https://www.ahrq.gov/professionals/systems/hospital/fallpxtoolkit/index.html (Level VII)

3 U.S. Preventive Services Task Force. (2018). Final recommendation statement: Falls prevention in community-dwelling older adults: Interventions. https://www.uspreventiveservicestaskforce.org/uspstf/recommendation/falls-prevention-in-older-adults-interventions

4 The Joint Commission. (2020). Three-step program increases patient activation and engagement in hospital fall prevention efforts. https://www.jointcommission.org/en/resources/news-and-multimedia/news/2020/02/three-step-program-increases-patient-activation-and-engagement-in-hospital-fall-prevention-efforts/

5 The Joint Commission. (2015). Sentinel event alert: Preventing falls and fall-related injuries in health care facilities. https://www.jointcommission.org/assets/1/6/SEA_55_Falls_4_26_16.pdf (Level VII)

6   The Joint Commission. (2021). Standard PC.01.02.08. *Comprehensive accreditation manual for hospitals*. Oakbrook Terrace, IL: The Joint Commission. (Level VII)

7   Accreditation Association for Hospitals and Health Systems. (2020). Standard 16.02.02. *Healthcare Facilities Accreditation Program: Accreditation requirements for acute care hospitals*. Chicago, IL: Accreditation Association for Hospitals and Health Systems. (Level VII)

8   Centers for Disease Control and Prevention. (2002). Guideline for hand hygiene in health-care settings: Recommendations of the Healthcare Infection Control Practices Advisory Committee and the HICPAC/SHEA/APIC/IDSA Hand Hygiene Task Force. *MMWR Recommendations and Reports, 51*(RR-16), 1–45. https://www.cdc.gov/mmwr/pdf/rr/rr5116.pdf (Level II)

9   World Health Organization. (2009). WHO guidelines on hand hygiene in health care: First global patient safety challenge, clean care is safer care. https://apps.who.int/iris/bitstream/handle/10665/44102/9789241597906_eng.pdf?sequence=1 (Level IV)

10 The Joint Commission. (2021). Standard NPSG.07.01.01. *Comprehensive accreditation manual for hospitals*. Oakbrook Terrace, IL: The Joint Commission. (Level VII)

11 Accreditation Association for Hospitals and Health Systems. (2020). Standard 07.01.21. *Healthcare Facilities Accreditation Program: Accreditation requirements for acute care hospitals*. Chicago, IL: American Association for Hospitals and Health Systems. (Level VII)

12 Centers for Medicare and Medicaid Services, Department of Health and Human Services. (2020). Condition of participation: Infection control. 42 C.F.R. § 482.42.

13 DNV GL-Healthcare USA, Inc. (2020). IC.1.SR.1. *NIAHO® accreditation requirements, interpretive guidelines and surveyor guidance—revision 20.0*. Milford, OH: DNV GL-Healthcare USA, Inc. (Level VII)

14 The Joint Commission. (2021). Standard NPSG.01.01.01. *Comprehensive accreditation manual for hospitals*. Oakbrook Terrace, IL: The Joint Commission. (Level VII)

15 Jarrett, N., & Callaham, M. (2016). Evidence-based guidelines for selected hospital-acquired conditions: Final report. https://www.cms.gov/Medicare/Medicare-Fee-for-Service-Payment/HospitalAcqCond/Downloads/2016-HAC-Report.pdf

16 Coggins, M. D. (2018). Medication monitor: Medications that increase fall risk. *Today's Geriatric Medicine, 11*(4), 30. https://www.todaysgeriatricmedicine.com/archive/JA18p30.shtml

17 American Geriatrics Society 2015 Beers Criteria Update Expert Panel. (2015). American Geriatrics Society 2015 updated Beers criteria for potentially inappropriate medication use in older adults. *Journal of the American Geriatrics Society, 63*(11), 2227–2246. (Level V)

18 Centers for Disease Control and Prevention. (2021). STEADI—Older adult fall prevention: Materials for healthcare providers. https://www.cdc.gov/steadi/materials.html

19 de Jong, M. R., et al. (2013). Drug-related falls in older patients: Implicated drugs, consequences, and possible prevention strategies. *Therapeutic Advances in Drug Safety, 4*, 147–154. https://www.ncbi.nlm.nih.gov/pmc/articles/PMC4125318/

20 The Joint Commission. (2021). Standard RC.01.03.01. *Comprehensive accreditation manual for hospitals*. Oakbrook Terrace, IL: The Joint Commission. (Level VII)

21 Centers for Medicare and Medicaid Services, Department of Health and Human Services. (2020). Condition of participation: Medical record services. 42 C.F.R. § 482.24(b).

22 Accreditation Association for Hospitals and Health Systems. (2020). Standard 10.00.03. *Healthcare Facilities Accreditation Program: Accreditation requirements for acute care hospitals*. Chicago, IL: Accreditation Association for Hospitals and Health Systems. (Level VII)

23 DNV GL-Healthcare USA, Inc. (2020). MR.2.SR.1. *NIAHO® accreditation requirements, interpretive guidelines and surveyor guidance—revision 20.0*. Milford, OH: DNV GL-Healthcare USA, Inc. (Level VII)

24 Waters, T. R., et al. (2009). Safe patient handling training for schools of nursing. https://www.cdc.gov/niosh/docs/2009-127/pdfs/2009-127.pdf (Level VII)

25 American Heart Association. (2020). 2020 American Heart Association guidelines for CPR and ECC– Part 3: Adult basic and advanced life support. https://cpr.heart.org/en/resuscitation-science/cpr-and-ecc-guidelines (Level II)

26 Accreditation Association for Hospitals and Health Systems. (2020). Standard 16.01.03. *Healthcare Facilities Accreditation Program: Accreditation requirements for acute care hospitals*. Chicago, IL: Accreditation Association for Hospitals and Health Systems. (Level VII)

27 Centers for Medicare and Medicaid Services, Department of Health and Human Services. (2020). Condition of participation: Nursing services. 42 C.F.R. § 482.23(c).

28 The Joint Commission. (2021). Standard MM.06.01.01. *Comprehensive accreditation manual for hospitals*. Oakbrook Terrace, IL: The Joint Commission. (Level VII)

29 DNV GL-Healthcare USA, Inc. (2020). MM.1.SR.3. *NIAHO® accreditation requirements, interpretive guidelines and surveyor guidance—revision 20.0*. Milford, OH: DNV GL-Healthcare USA, Inc. (Level VII)

30 The Joint Commission. (2021). Standard PC.01.02.07. *Comprehensive accreditation manual for hospitals*. Oakbrook Terrace, IL: The Joint Commission. (Level VII)

31 Hartford Institute for Geriatric Nursing. (2020). ConsultGeri, geriatric nursing resources, protocols, fall prevention. https://hign.org/consultgeri/resources/protocols/fall-prevention (Level VII)

32 Occupational Safety and Health Administration. (2019). Bloodborne pathogens, standard number 1910.1030. https://www.osha.gov/pls/oshaweb/owadisp.show_document?p_id=10051&p_table=STANDARDS (Level VII)

33 Accreditation Association for Hospitals and Health Systems. (2020). Standard 07.02.03. *Healthcare Facilities Accreditation Program: Accreditation requirements for acute care hospitals*. Chicago, IL: Accreditation Association for Hospitals and Health Systems. (Level VII)

34 Rutala, W. A., et al. (2008, revised 2019). Guideline for disinfection and sterilization in healthcare facilities, 2008. https://www.cdc.gov/infection-control/pdf/guidelines/disinfection-guidelines-H.pdf (Level I)

35 Christiansen, T. L., et al. (2020). Patient activation related to fall prevention: A multisite study. *The Joint Commission Journal on Quality and Patient Safety, 46*, 129–135. (Level VII)

Fᴇᴄᴀʟ ɪᴍᴘᴀᴄᴛɪᴏɴ ʀᴇᴍᴏᴠᴀʟ, ᴅɪɢɪᴛᴀʟ

Fecal impaction—a large, hard, dry mass of stool in the folds of the rectum and, at times, in the sigmoid colon—results from prolonged retention and accumulation of stool. Common causes include poor bowel habits, inactivity, dehydration, improper diet (especially inadequate fluid intake), constipation-inducing drugs, and incomplete bowel cleaning after a barium enema or barium swallow.

With newer bowel care techniques, such as transanal irrigation and digital rectal stimulation, digital removal of a fecal impaction isn't often needed.[1] However, for a small group of patients—such as those who have sustained a spinal cord injury or have a neurological condition such as multiple sclerosis or spina bifida—it may be an essential part of their bowel-care routine. Digital fecal impaction removal may also be used as an acute intervention for patients who have impacted stool that can't be resolved with medication.[1,2] Signs and symptoms of impaction may include absent or reduced evacuation of stool, abdominal bloating or distension, nausea, and pain. It may be accompanied by overflow diarrhea, in which loose stool leaks around the fecal mass.[1] Digital removal of a fecal impaction typically requires a practitioner's order.

If the patient requires digital removal of fecal impaction as part of routine bowel care, the routine shouldn't be interrupted, regardless of the setting in which care is provided. This is especially important for patients with spinal cord injury who are at risk for autonomic dysreflexia, a medical emergency that can result if the bowel becomes distended owing to impaction or constipation. Autonomic dysreflexia can lead to cerebral hemorrhage, seizures, and cardiac arrest.[1,3]

This procedure is contraindicated during pregnancy; after rectal, genitourinary, abdominal, perineal, or gynecologic reconstructive surgery; in patients with myocardial infarction, coronary insufficiency, pulmonary embolus, heart failure, heart block, and Stokes-Adams syndrome (without pacemaker treatment); and in patients with GI or vaginal bleeding, hemorrhoids, rectal polyps, or blood dyscrasias.

Equipment

Gloves ▪ fluid-impermeable pad ▪ toilet paper ▪ pH-balanced cleaner[4] or soap and water ▪ disposable cloth[4] or washcloth ▪ water-soluble lubricant ▪ bath blanket ▪ stethoscope ▪ disinfectant pad ▪ Optional: lift sheet, lift equipment, or other patient-positioning aid;[4] gown; mask with face shield or mask, goggles; prescribed lidocaine gel; vital signs monitoring equipment; bedpan or bedside commode; facility-approved disinfectant.

Preparation of equipment

Inspect all equipment and supplies. If a product is expired, is defective, or has compromised integrity, remove it from patient use, label it as expired or defective, and report the expiration or defect as directed by your facility.

Implementation

- Verify the practitioner's order.
- Gather and prepare the necessary equipment and supplies.
- Perform hand hygiene.[5,6,7,8,9,10]
- Confirm the patient's identity using at least two patient identifiers.[11]
- Provide privacy.[12,13,14,15]
- Explain the procedure to the patient and family (if appropriate) according to their individual communication and learning needs *to increase their understanding, allay their fears, and enhance cooperation.*[16] Discuss adverse effects, expected outcomes, and complications *to allow the patient to provide valid and informed consent for the procedure.*[1,2] Take the patient's religious and cultural beliefs into consideration.[1,14]
- Inform the patient that a chaperone may be present during the procedure if the patient wishes.[17]
- Offer the patient the opportunity to empty the bladder before the procedure *to promote comfort.*[17]
- Raise the patient's bed to waist level before providing care *to prevent caregiver back strain.*[18]
- Obtain vital signs for baseline comparison, *because anal stimulation may cause a vagal response, and in patients with spinal cord injury, autonomic dysreflexia may occur.*[3] If digital fecal impaction removal is routine and well-tolerated by the patient, obtaining vital signs may not be necessary.[1]
- Perform a complete GI assessment.
- Perform hand hygiene.[5,6,7,8,9,10]
- Put on gloves and, as needed, other protective equipment *to comply with standard precautions.*[19,20,21]
- Assist the patient to a Sims position (side-lying with the upper leg flexed over the lower leg).[3,17] Position the patient using a lift sheet, lift equipment, or other patient positioning aid, as needed, *to prevent friction and shear injuries of the patient's skin and caregiver injury.*[4]
- Place a fluid-impermeable pad under the patient's buttocks *to prevent soiling of the bed linens.*[3,17]
- Cover the patient with a blanket, exposing only the rectal area, *to provide privacy and warmth, and to maintain the patient's dignity.*[2]
- Inspect the perineal and perianal area for rectal prolapse, hemorrhoids, anal skin tags, wounds, discharge, anal lesions, infestations, and skin conditions. Report abnormalities to the patient's practitioner.[17]
- Moisten a gloved index finger with water-soluble lubricant *to reduce friction during insertion and avoid injury to sensitive tissue.*[17]
- Inform the patient that you are about to perform the procedure.[17] Instruct the patient to breathe deeply *to promote relaxation.*
- Gently insert your lubricated index finger beyond the anal sphincter into the rectum. Assess the fecal material by feeling for stool type (hard individual pieces, a large mass, or soft stool).[17] Rotate your finger gently around the stool and work the stool down close to the anus for removal.[3] If the patient experiences discomfort, stop the procedure, if necessary, and administer lidocaine gel, as ordered, following safe medication administration practices.[17,22,23,24,25] Wait for the lidocaine to become effective before continuing with the procedure.[17]
- Remove feces slowly with the gloved finger in a hooked or semi-hooked position *to reduce trauma to the rectal mucosa.*[17] Remove a solid mass one lump at a time. For a semi-solid mass of feces, push your gloved finger in the middle of the mass and divide it, then remove small amounts of feces in sections.[17]
- Monitor the patient closely throughout the procedure.

NURSING ALERT If the patient experiences pain, nausea, rectal bleeding, change in pulse rate or skin color, diaphoresis, or syncope, stop the procedure immediately and notify the practitioner.

- Observe the characteristics of the feces and dispose of it in the toilet. If the toilet isn't available or convenient, discard it in an appropriate receptacle.[17]

- Remove and discard your gloves.[19,20]
- Perform hand hygiene.[5,6,7,8,9,10]
- Put on gloves *to comply with standard precautions.*[19,20,21]
- Wipe residual water-soluble lubricant from the anal area with toilet paper.[17]
- Clean the perianal area with a pH-balanced cleanser and disposable cloth (if available), *because traditional soap and water and washcloths increase the risk of tissue injury.*[4] Alternatively, use soap and water and a washcloth to clean the perianal area. Gently dry the area *to prevent moisture-associated skin damage.*[4,17]
- Assist the patient with repositioning. Alternatively, reposition the patient, as needed, using an appropriate positioning aid.
- Remove and discard your gloves.[19,20]
- Perform hand hygiene.[5,6,7,8,9,10]
- Obtain the patient's vital signs, as needed, and compare them to baseline *to evaluate the patient's tolerance of the procedure.* Notify the practitioner or rapid response team if signs of autonomic dysreflexia occur.[17]
- Perform hand hygiene.[5,6,7,8,9,10]
- Put on gloves.[19,20,21]
- Offer the patient an opportunity for toileting, if necessary and appropriate, *because digital removal of a fecal impaction may stimulate peristalsis, encouraging defecation.*[17] If needed, position a bedpan under the patient and assist the patient with its use, as needed, and then return the bed to the lowest position *to prevent falls and maintain patient safety.*[26] If the patient is able to use a bedside commode, return the bed to the lowest position[26] and assist the patient to the commode, as needed. For an ambulatory patient, return the bed to the lowest position[26] and assist the patient to the toilet.
- Discard used supplies in appropriate receptacles.
- Clean and disinfect the bedpan or commode, if used, using a facility-approved disinfectant, according to manufacturer's instructions, *to prevent the spread of infection.*[27,28] Store it appropriately.
- Remove and discard your gloves and other personal protective equipment, if worn.[19,21]
- Perform hand hygiene.[5,6,7,8,9,10]
- Clean and disinfect your stethoscope with a disinfectant pad.[27,28]
- Perform hand hygiene.[5,6,7,8,9,10]
- Report any abnormalities, adverse effects, or other concerns related to the procedure to a wound, ostomy, and continence nurse or the practitioner, as appropriate.[17]
- Document the procedure.[29,30,31,32]

Special considerations

- The most important aspect of care is preventing recurrence of elimination problems by implementing a maintenance bowel regimen.[33]
- As long as there is no suspected perforation or massive bleeding, after fecal impaction removal, a warm-water enema with mineral oil may be ordered *to soften the impaction and assist with emptying the stool from the rectum.* Polyethylene glycol may also be ordered and administered orally or by nasogastric tube *to facilitate colon evacuation.*[33]

Complications

Digital removal of fecal impaction can stimulate the vagus nerve and may decrease heart rate and cause syncope. Autonomic dysreflexia may occur in the patient with spinal cord injury.[3] Potential damage to the mucous membrane lining of the bowel, which increases the risk of bleeding, inflammation, and infection, may also occur.

Documentation

Record the time and date of the procedure; the patient's response to the procedure; the color, consistency, and quantity of the stool removed; and any abnormalities. Note any complications that occurred, interventions performed, and the patient's response to them. Document teaching provided to the patient and family (if applicable), their understanding of that teaching, and any need for follow-up teaching.

REFERENCES

1 Ness, W. (2013). Digital removal of faeces. *Nursing Times, 109*(17/18), 18–20. https://www.nursingtimes.net/clinical-archive/continence/digital-removal-of-faeces-26-04-2013/

2 Sivapuram, M. (2019). Feces: Digital removal. *The JBI EBP Database.* AN: JBI23250

3 Royal College of Nursing. (2019). *Bowel care: Management of lower bowel dysfunction, including digital rectal examination and digital removal of feces: Clinical professional resource.* London, UK: Royal College of Nursing. https://www.rcn.org.uk/-/media/royal-college-of-nursing/documents/publications/2019/september/007-522.pdf?la=en (Level VII)

4 Wound, Ostomy, and Continence Nurses Society™ (WOCN®). (2016). *Guideline for prevention and management of pressure ulcers (injuries): WOCN clinical practice guideline series 2.* Mount Laurel, NJ: WOCN.

5 The Joint Commission. (2021). Standard NPSG.07.01.01. *Comprehensive accreditation manual for hospitals.* Oakbrook Terrace, IL: The Joint Commission. (Level VII)

6 Centers for Disease Control and Prevention. (2002). Guideline for hand hygiene in health-care settings: Recommendations of the Healthcare Infection Control Practices Advisory Committee and the HICPAC/SHEA/APIC/IDSA Hand Hygiene Task Force. *MMWR Recommendations and Reports, 51*(RR-16), 1–45. https://www.cdc.gov/mmwr/pdf/rr/rr5116.pdf (Level II)

7 World Health Organization. (2009). WHO guidelines on hand hygiene in health care: First global patient safety challenge, clean care is safer care. https://apps.who.int/iris/bitstream/handle/10665/44102/9789241597906_eng.pdf?sequence=1 (Level IV)

8 Centers for Medicare and Medicaid Services, Department of Health and Human Services. (2020). Condition of participation: Infection control. 42 C.F.R. § 482.42.

9 Accreditation Association for Hospitals and Health Systems. (2020). Standard 07.01.21. *Healthcare Facilities Accreditation Program: Accreditation requirements for acute care hospitals.* Chicago, IL: Accreditation Association for Hospitals and Health Systems. (Level VII)

10 DNV GL-Healthcare USA, Inc. (2020). IC.1.SR.1. *NIAHO® accreditation requirements, interpretive guidelines and surveyor guidance—revision 20.0.* Milford, OH: DNV GL-Healthcare USA, Inc. (Level VII)

11 The Joint Commission. (2021). Standard NPSG.01.01.01. *Comprehensive accreditation manual for hospitals.* Oakbrook Terrace, IL: The Joint Commission. (Level VII)

12 Accreditation Association for Hospitals and Health Systems. (2020). Standard 15.01.16. *Healthcare Facilities Accreditation Program: Accreditation requirements for acute care hospitals.* Chicago, IL: Accreditation Association for Hospitals and Health Systems. (Level VII)

13 Centers for Medicare and Medicaid Services, Department of Health and Human Services. (2020). Condition of participation: Patient's rights. 42 C.F.R. § 482.13(c)(1).

14 The Joint Commission. (2021). Standard RI.01.01.01. *Comprehensive accreditation manual for hospitals.* Oakbrook Terrace, IL: The Joint Commission. (Level VII)

15 DNV GL-Healthcare USA, Inc. (2020). PR.2.SR.5. *NIAHO® accreditation requirements, interpretive guidelines and surveyor guidance—revision 20.0.* Milford, OH: DNV GL-Healthcare USA, Inc. (Level VII)

16 The Joint Commission. (2021). Standard PC.02.01.21. *Comprehensive accreditation manual for hospitals.* Oakbrook Terrace, IL: The Joint Commission. (Level VII)

17 Trowbridge, K., & Roe, C. (2021). Digital removal of feces (neurogenic bowel or spinal cord injury): Community setting.). *The JBI EBP Database.* AN: JBI10840.

18 Waters, T. R., et al. (2009). Safe patient handling training for schools of nursing. https://www.cdc.gov/niosh/docs/2009-127/pdfs/2009-127.pdf (Level VII)

19 Siegel, J. D., et al. (2007, revised 2019). 2007 guideline for isolation precautions: Preventing transmission of infectious agents in healthcare settings. https://www.cdc.gov/infectioncontrol/pdf/guidelines/isolation-guidelines-H.pdf (Level II)

20 Accreditation Association for Hospitals and Health Systems. (2020). Standard 07.01.10. *Healthcare Facilities Accreditation Program: Accreditation requirements for acute care hospitals.* Chicago, IL: Accreditation Association for Hospitals and Health Systems. (Level VII)

21 Occupational Safety and Health Administration. (2019). Bloodborne pathogens, standard number 1910.1030. https://www.osha.gov/pls/oshaweb/owadisp.show_document?p_id=10051&p_table=STANDARDS (Level VII)

22 The Joint Commission. (2021). Standard MM.06.01.01. *Comprehensive accreditation manual for hospitals.* Oakbrook Terrace, IL: The Joint Commission. (Level VII)

23 Centers for Medicare and Medicaid Services, Department of Health and Human Services. (2020). Condition of participation: Nursing services. 42 C.F.R. § 482.23(c).

24 Accreditation Association for Hospitals and Health Systems. (2020). Standard 16.01.03. *Healthcare Facilities Accreditation Program: Accreditation requirements for acute care hospitals.* Chicago, IL: Accreditation Association for Hospitals and Health Systems. (Level VII)

25 DNV GL-Healthcare USA, Inc. (2020). MM.1.SR.3. *NIAHO® accreditation requirements, interpretive guidelines and surveyor guidance—revision 20.0.* Milford, OH: DNV GL-Healthcare USA, Inc. (Level VII)

26 Ganz, D. A., et al. (2013, reviewed 2021). *Preventing falls in hospitals: A toolkit for improving quality of care* (AHRQ Publication No. 13-0015-EF). Rockville, MD: Agency for Healthcare Research and Quality. https://www.ahrq.gov/professionals/systems/hospital/fallpxtoolkit/index.html (Level VII)

27 Rutala, W. A., et al. (2008, revised 2019). Guideline for disinfection and sterilization in healthcare facilities, 2008. https://www.cdc.gov/infection-control/pdf/guidelines/disinfection-guidelines-H.pdf (Level I)

28 Accreditation Association for Hospitals and Health Systems. (2020). Standard 07.02.03. *Healthcare Facilities Accreditation Program: Accreditation requirements for acute care hospitals.* Chicago, IL: Accreditation Association for Hospitals and Health Systems. (Level VII)

29 The Joint Commission. (2021). Standard RC.01.03.01. *Comprehensive accreditation manual for hospitals.* Oakbrook Terrace, IL: The Joint Commission. (Level VII)

30 Centers for Medicare and Medicaid Services, Department of Health and Human Services. (2020). Condition of participation: Medical record services. 42 C.F.R. § 482.24(b).

31 Accreditation Association for Hospitals and Health Systems. (2020). Standard 10.00.03. *Healthcare Facilities Accreditation Program: Accreditation requirements for acute care hospitals.* Chicago, IL: Accreditation Association for Hospitals and Health Systems. (Level VII)

32 DNV GL-Healthcare USA, Inc. (2020). MR.2.SR.1. *NIAHO® accreditation requirements, interpretive guidelines and surveyor guidance—revision 20.0.* Milford, OH: DNV GL-Healthcare USA, Inc. (Level VII)

33 Rao, S. S. C. (2020). Constipation in the older adult. In: *UpToDate,* Talley, N. J., & Schmader, K. E. (Eds.).

FECAL OCCULT BLOOD TESTS

Fecal occult blood tests (FOBTs) are helpful for detecting the presence of GI bleeding and for distinguishing between true melena and melena-like stools. (Certain medications, such as iron supplements and bismuth compounds, can darken stools so that they resemble melena.) Occult blood may be present in a patient's stool owing to colorectal cancer, gastric cancer, ulcerative colitis or other inflammatory lesions, adenoma, diaphragmatic hernia, peptic ulcer, gastritis, vasculitis, amyloidosis, or Kaposi sarcoma.[1]

A single positive test result doesn't necessarily confirm GI bleeding or indicate colorectal cancer. To confirm a positive result, the test must be repeated at least three times while the patient follows a special diet, according to the manufacturer's recommendations for the particular FOBT; however, a positive result does indicate the need for further diagnostic studies, *because blood in the stool is abnormal.*[1] FOBT can be performed easily on collected specimens or smears from digital examination.

Commonly used FOBTs include guaiac-based Hemoccult slide tests, which include Hemoccult SENSA and Hemoccult II. Hemoccult SENSA has greater sensitivity for cancer and advanced adenomas. Both tests produce a blue reaction in a fecal smear if occult blood loss exceeds 2 mL in 24 hours.

Another type of FOBT is the fecal immunochemical test (FIT), such as the InSure FIT, which detects human globin, a protein that, along with heme, constitutes human hemoglobin.[2,3] This makes the FIT more specific for human blood than guaiac-based tests. The FIT is also more specific for lower GI bleeding, which makes it more specific for detecting colorectal cancer.[1,3] FIT testing requires only one stool specimen and no dietary restrictions prior to the test.[2,3] In some facilities, the nurse collects the stool specimen, prepares the test slide, develops it with developing solution, and interprets the results. In other facilities the nurse collects the stool specimen, prepares the test slide, and sends it to the laboratory for interpretation. Follow your facility's process for fecal occult blood testing.

Equipment
Gloves.

For a guaiac-based slide test
Guaiac test slide with quality-control monitors ■ guaiac developing solution ■ specimen applicator sticks ■ Optional: label, laboratory biohazard transport bag, laboratory request form.

For a FIT
FIT kit with long-handled brushes ■ test card ■ label ■ laboratory transport bag ■ Optional: laboratory request form.

Preparation of equipment
Inspect all equipment and supplies. If a product is expired, is defective, or has compromised integrity, remove it from patient use, label it as expired or defective, and report the expiration or defect as directed by your facility. Hemoccult SENSA test slides contain guaiac paper; keep the cover flap of the slide sealed until ready to use.[1,4]

Implementation
■ Verify the practitioner's order.
■ Check the patient's history for medications and conditions that may interfere with the test results.
■ Gather and prepare the necessary equipment and supplies.
■ Perform hand hygiene.[5,6,7,8,9,10]
■ Confirm the patient's identity using at least two patient identifiers.[11]
■ Provide privacy.[12,13,14,15]
■ Explain the procedure to the patient and family (if appropriate) according to their individual communication and learning needs to increase their understanding, allay their fears, and enhance cooperation.[16]
■ Perform hand hygiene.[5,6,7,8,9,10]
■ Put on gloves *to comply with standard precautions.*[17,18,19]
■ Collect a stool specimen. (See the "Stool specimen collection" procedure.) If collecting a specimen for FIT testing from the toilet, flush the toilet before the patient defecates and instruct the patient to avoid placing used toilet paper in the toilet bowl *to ensure accurate test results.*[2]

To perform a guaiac-based slide test
■ Open the flap on the slide packet.[4]
■ Use a specimen applicator stick to apply a thin smear of the stool specimen to the guaiac-impregnated filter paper exposed in box A. Alternatively, after performing a digital rectal examination, wipe the finger you used for the examination on a square of the filter paper.[4]
■ Apply a second smear from another part of the specimen to the filter paper exposed in box B, *because some parts of the specimen may not contain blood.*[4]
■ For bedside interpretation, allow the specimen to dry for 3 to 5 minutes.[4] Open the flap on the reverse side of the slide package.[4] Place two drops of guaiac developing solution on the paper over each smear.[4] Wait for a reaction; a blue reaction will appear in 30 to 60 seconds if the test is positive. Any trace of blue on or at the edge of the smear is positive for occult blood. Absence of blue at the end of 60 seconds is negative for occult blood. Wait the full 60 seconds before recording a negative result.[4] Interpret the results.
NURSING ALERT This test is visually read and requires color differentiation. You shouldn't interpret it if you have a blue color deficiency (color blindness).[4]
■ Perform a quality-control test by applying 1 drop of developer between the positive and negative quality-control areas. Read the quality-control test results within 10 seconds. If the slide and developer are functioning properly, blue will appear in the positive area and no blue will appear

in the negative area. If the quality-control test fails to react as expected after application of the developer, the patient's test results are invalid and shouldn't be documented. Repeat the procedure using new equipment.[4]
■ Record the results.
■ Discard the slide package in an appropriate receptacle.[19] *You should handle patient specimens and all materials that come in contact with them as potentially infectious and discard them using appropriate precautions.*
■ For laboratory interpretation, close the flap on the slide packet. Label the slide in the presence of the patient *to prevent mislabeling.*[11] Place the slide in a laboratory biohazard transport bag and send it immediately to the laboratory with the appropriate laboratory request form (if necessary).[19]

To perform a FIT
■ Open the flap of the test card.[2]
■ Remove one of the long-handled brushes from the kit.
■ Gently brush the surface of the stool with the brush and then rinse the brush in the toilet water surrounding the stool.[2]
■ Dab the brush onto the test card and then close the flap.[2]
■ Discard the brush in the appropriate receptacle.[19]
■ Label the specimen in the presence of the *patient to prevent mislabeling.*[11]
■ Place the labeled test card in a laboratory biohazard transport bag and send it immediately to the laboratory with the appropriate laboratory request form (if necessary).[19]

Completing the procedure
■ Remove and discard your gloves.[17,19]
■ Perform hand hygiene.[5,6,7,8,9,10]
■ Notify the practitioner of the test results.
■ Document the procedure.[20,21,22,23]

Special considerations
■ Test stool specimens as soon as possible after collection, and make sure they aren't contaminated with urine, soap solution, iodine, or toilet tissue.
■ Test samples from several different portions of the same specimen, *because occult blood from the upper GI tract isn't always evenly dispersed throughout the formed stool; likewise, blood from colorectal bleeding may occur mostly on the outer stool surface.*
■ Don't exchange developers with different manufacturers or brands.
■ Be aware that obtaining a specimen from a patient during menstruation or for 3 days after or from a patient with active bleeding from hemorrhoids or hematuria can produce false-positive results.[1]
■ If repeated testing is necessary after a positive screening test, explain the test to the patient. Instruct the patient to maintain a high-fiber diet and to refrain from eating red meat, poultry, fish, turnips, and horseradish for 48 to 72 hours before the test as well as throughout the collection period, *because these substances can alter test results.*[4]
■ As ordered, have the patient discontinue the use of iron preparations, bromides, iodides, rauwolfia derivatives, indomethacin, colchicine, salicylates, potassium, bismuth compounds, steroids, and ascorbic acid for 48 to 72 hours before the test as well as during it *to ensure accurate test results and to avoid the possible bleeding that some of these compounds can cause.*[4]
■ Guaiac slides and developer are ready for use as packaged but must be stored and used appropriately according to the manufacturer's instructions. Store products at a controlled room temperature of 59° to 86° F (15° to 30° C).[4] Don't use them past the expiration date stamped on each slide and developer bottle. Protect them from heat, light, volatile chemicals, and refrigeration temperatures.[4] Watch for signs of deterioration, including discoloration of the normally off-white guaiac paper and failure of the control system to react as expected (subsequent test results should be regarded as invalid).
■ Note that the developer is an irritant; avoid contact with the skin and eyes. If contact should occur, rinse promptly with water and consult a practitioner.[4]

Patient teaching
If the patient will be using the Hemoccult slide packet or the FIT at home, advise the patient to complete the label on the slide packet before

PATIENT TEACHING

HOME TESTS FOR FECAL OCCULT BLOOD

Although most fecal occult blood tests require the patient to collect a specimen of stool and to smear it on a slide, the ColoCARE test doesn't, making the procedure safer and simpler.[24]

If the patient will be performing the ColoCARE test at home, tell the patient to avoid red meat and vitamin C supplements for 2 days beforehand. The patient should check with the practitioner about discontinuing any medications before the test. Drugs that may interfere with test results include aspirin, indomethacin, corticosteroids, reserpine, dietary supplements, anticancer drugs, and anticoagulants. The patient should also talk to the practitioner about medical conditions to determine the timing of the test. For example, the patient who has bleeding hemorrhoids, peptic ulcers, or gastritis shouldn't take the test. In addition, patients who are at or near the time of menstruation shouldn't take the test.

To perform the test, tell the patient to follow these steps:
- Flush the toilet twice just before performing the test *to remove any toilet-cleaning chemicals from the tank*.
- Defecate into the toilet, but don't throw toilet paper into the bowl.
- Within 5 minutes, remove the test pad from its pouch and float it printed side up on the water.
- Watch the pad for 15 to 30 seconds for any evidence of blue or green color changes
- Record the result on the reply card.
- Flush the toilet to dispose of the test pad.[24]

Emphasize that the patient should perform this test with three consecutive bowel movements and then send the completed card to the practitioner. However, inform the patient that the practitioner should be called immediately if the patient notes a positive color change in the first test.

---

specimen collection. If the patient will be using a ColoCARE test packet, inform the patient that this test is a preliminary screen for occult blood in the stool. Explain that the patient will not have to obtain a stool specimen to perform the test but that the instructions should be followed carefully. (See *Home tests for fecal occult blood.*)

Documentation

Record the time and date of the test, the name and title of the person interpreting the test, the test result, and any unusual characteristics of the stool tested. Document the name of the practitioner to whom you reported the results, including the date and time of notification. Document teaching provided to the patient and family (if applicable), their understanding of that teaching, and any need for follow-up teaching.

REFERENCES

1 Fischbach, F., & Fischbach, M. A. (2018). *A manual of laboratory and diagnostic tests* (10th ed.). Philadelphia, PA: Wolters Kluwer.

2 Enterix Inc. (2017). InSure® ONE.™ one day fecal immunochemical test: Instructions for use. https://www.clinicalgenomics.com/products/insure-one/patients

3 Doubeni, C. (2020). Tests for screening for colorectal cancer. In: *UpToDate*, Elmore, J. G., & Lamont, J. T. (Eds.).

4 Beckman Coulter, Inc. (2015). Hemoccult SENSA: Product instructions. https://image.tigermedical.com/Brochures/BEC64152–20151106122841726.pdf

5 The Joint Commission. (2021). Standard NPSG.07.01.01. *Comprehensive accreditation manual for hospitals*. Oakbrook Terrace, IL: The Joint Commission. (Level VII)

6 Centers for Disease Control and Prevention. (2002). Guideline for hand hygiene in health-care settings: Recommendations of the Healthcare Infection Control Practices Advisory Committee and the HICPAC/SHEA/APIC/IDSA Hand Hygiene Task Force. *MMWR Recommendations and Reports, 51*(RR-16), 1–45. https://www.cdc.gov/mmwr/pdf/rr/rr5116.pdf (Level II)

7 World Health Organization. (2009). WHO guidelines on hand hygiene in health care: First global patient safety challenge, clean care is safer care. https://apps.who.int/iris/bitstream/handle/10665/44102/9789241597906_eng.pdf?sequence=1 (Level IV)

8 Centers for Medicare and Medicaid Services, Department of Health and Human Services. (2020). Condition of participation: Infection control. 42 C.F.R. § 482.42.

9 Accreditation Association for Hospitals and Health Systems. (2020). Standard 07.01.21. *Healthcare Facilities Accreditation Program: Accreditation requirements for acute care hospitals*. Chicago, IL: Accreditation Association for Hospitals and Health Systems. (Level VII)

10 DNV GL-Healthcare USA, Inc. (2020). IC.1.SR.1. *NIAHO® accreditation requirements, interpretive guidelines and surveyor guidance—revision 20.0*. Milford, OH: DNV GL-Healthcare USA, Inc. (Level VII)

11 The Joint Commission. (2021). Standard NPSG.01.01.01. *Comprehensive accreditation manual for hospitals*. Oakbrook Terrace, IL: The Joint Commission. (Level VII)

12 Accreditation Association for Hospitals and Health Systems. (2020). Standard 15.01.16. *Healthcare Facilities Accreditation Program: Accreditation requirements for acute care hospitals*. Chicago, IL: Accreditation Association for Hospitals and Health Systems. (Level VII)

13 Centers for Medicare and Medicaid Services, Department of Health and Human Services. (2020). Condition of participation: Patient's rights. 42 C.F.R. § 482.13(c)(1).

14 The Joint Commission. (2021). Standard RI.01.01.01. *Comprehensive accreditation manual for hospitals*. Oakbrook Terrace, IL: The Joint Commission. (Level VII)

15 DNV GL-Healthcare USA, Inc. (2020). PR.2.SR.5. *NIAHO® accreditation requirements, interpretive guidelines and surveyor guidance—revision 20.0*. Milford, OH: DNV GL-Healthcare USA, Inc. (Level VII)

16 The Joint Commission. (2021). Standard PC.02.01.21. *Comprehensive accreditation manual for hospitals*. Oakbrook Terrace, IL: The Joint Commission. (Level VII)

17 Siegel, J. D., et al. (2007, revised 2019). 2007 guideline for isolation precautions: Preventing transmission of infectious agents in healthcare settings. https://www.cdc.gov/infectioncontrol/pdf/guidelines/isolation-guidelines-H.pdf (Level II)

18 Accreditation Association for Hospitals and Health Systems. (2020). Standard 07.01.10. *Healthcare Facilities Accreditation Program: Accreditation requirements for acute care hospitals*. Chicago, IL: Accreditation Association for Hospitals and Health Systems. (Level VII)

19 Occupational Safety and Health Administration. (2019). Bloodborne pathogens, standard number 1910.1030. https://www.osha.gov/pls/oshaweb/owadisp.show_document?p_id=10051&p_table=STANDARDS (Level VII)

20 The Joint Commission. (2021). Standard RC.01.03.01. *Comprehensive accreditation manual for hospitals*. Oakbrook Terrace, IL: The Joint Commission. (Level VII)

21 Centers for Medicare and Medicaid Services, Department of Health and Human Services. (2020). Condition of participation: Medical record services. 42 C.F.R. § 482.24(b).

22 Accreditation Association for Hospitals and Health Systems. (2020). Standard 10.00.03. *Healthcare Facilities Accreditation Program: Accreditation requirements for acute care hospitals*. Chicago, IL: Accreditation Association for Hospitals and Health Systems. (Level VII)

23 DNV GL-Healthcare USA, Inc. (2020). MR.2.SR.1. *NIAHO® accreditation requirements, interpretive guidelines and surveyor guidance—revision 20.0*. Milford, OH: DNV GL-Healthcare USA, Inc. (Level VII)

24 Helena Laboratories. (2015). Your guide to occult blood testing with ColoCARE®. https://www.lfh.org/resources/content/2/5/0/5/documents/ColoCARE_Brochure_2013(1).pdf

FEEDING

A patient who can't self-feed is susceptible to malnutrition.[1] Feeding a patient improves nutritional intake and clinical outcomes.[1,2] Various disabilities and conditions may prevent a patient from self-feeding, including cognitive deficits, neuromuscular disease, cancer, obstructive lung disease, and traumatic injury. Meeting such a patient's nutritional needs requires determining food preferences in a friendly, unhurried manner; encouraging self-feeding to promote independence and dignity; and documenting intake and output.

Equipment

Meal tray with utensils ■ overbed table ■ fluid-impermeable pad ■ hand hygiene supplies ■ facility-approved disinfectant ■ oral care supplies ■ chair ■ Optional: assistive feeding devices, prescribed pain medication, clean linens, suction catheters, suction apparatus, one-way valve, napkin, towel, intake and output monitoring equipment.

Preparation of equipment

Inspect all equipment and supplies. If a product is expired, is defective, or has compromised integrity, remove it from patient use, label it as expired or defective, and report the expiration or defect as directed by your facility.

Implementation

■ Verify the practitioner's order for diet
■ Review the patient's medical record for conditions that may affect the ability to self-feed. Review the patient's medications for adverse effects that might interfere with appetite.[3]
■ Collaborate with a speech pathologist, as indicated, *to assess the patient's swallowing ability and subsequent risk of aspiration.* Follow recommendations prescribed by the speech pathologist *to reduce the patient's risk of aspiration.*[3,4]
■ Collaborate with an occupational therapist, as indicated, *to assess the patient's need for assistive feeding devices.* Follow recommendations prescribed by the occupational therapist *to encourage self-feeding.*
■ Gather and prepare the necessary equipment and supplies.
■ Perform hand hygiene.[5,6,7,8,9,10]
■ Confirm the patient's identity using at least two patient identifiers.[11]
■ Provide privacy.[12,13,14,15]
■ Perform hand hygiene.[5,6,7,8,9,10]
■ Assess the patient's neurologic status, dentition, and functional status *to determine whether oral feeding is appropriate.*
■ Collaborate with the patient and family *to determine food preferences (including ethnic foods).* Ask about the normal consistency of preferred foods as well as the timing and frequency of the meals.[3]
■ Screen for and assess the patient's pain using facility-defined criteria that are consistent with the patient's age, condition, and ability to understand.[16]
■ Treat the patient's pain, as needed and ordered, using nonpharmacologic, pharmacologic, or a combination of approaches. Base the treatment plan on evidence-based practices and the patient's clinical condition, past medical history, and pain management goals.[16]
■ Explain the procedure to the patient and family (if appropriate) according to their individual communication and learning needs *to increase their understanding, allay their fears, and enhance cooperation.*[17]
■ *Because many adults consider being fed demeaning,* allow the patient some control over mealtime, such as letting the patient set the pace of the meal or deciding the order in which the patient eats various foods.
■ Position the patient with the head of the bed elevated 30 to 45 degrees, unless contraindicated, *to ease swallowing and reduce the risk of aspiration.*[18]
■ If the patient has a tracheostomy, follow the practitioner's order and your facility's guidelines for oral feeding, including suctioning the patient's tracheostomy tube prior to eating (if necessary), maintaining cuff pressure, applying a one-way valve, positioning the patient, and applying aspiration precautions.[19]
■ Before the meal tray arrives, give the patient the opportunity to perform hand hygiene. Alternatively, wash the patient's hands or assist with hand hygiene, as needed.
■ Clean the overbed table by wiping it with a hospital-approved disinfectant.[20,21]
■ Confirm that the correct tray has been delivered to the correct patient.
■ Check the tray *to make sure it contains foods and fluids appropriate for the patient's condition.*

■ Encourage the patient to self-feed if possible.[22] If the patient is restricted to the prone or supine position but can use arms and hands, encourage the patient to try foods that can be picked up, such as sandwiches. If the patient can assume a position with the head of the bed elevated 30 to 45 degrees but has limited use of arms or hands, teach the patient how to use assistive feeding devices. (See *Using assistive feeding devices.*)
■ If necessary, tuck a napkin or towel under the patient's chin *to protect the gown from spills.* Use a fluid-impermeable pad or towel *to protect bed linens.*
■ Position a chair next to the patient's bed *so you can sit comfortably if you need to feed the patient.*
■ Face the patient during feeding, make eye contact, and use a gentle tone of voice.
■ Set up the patient's tray, remove the plate from the tray warmer, and discard all plastic wrappings. Then cut the food into bite-sized pieces (as shown below). Season food according to the patient's request, as appropriate.

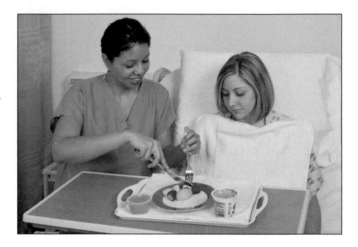

■ *To help a blind or visually impaired patient feed,* describe the placement of various foods on the plate in relation to the hours on a clock face. Maintain consistent placement for subsequent meals.
■ Ask the patient which food the patient prefers to eat first *to promote a sense of control over the meal.* Some patients prefer to eat one food at a time; others prefer to alternate foods.
■ Provide verbal encouragement to participate in eating by talking about the food's taste and smell and providing verbal prompts to chew and swallow.
■ Ask the patient to indicate when ready for each mouthful. Pause between courses and whenever the patient wants to rest. During the meal, wipe the patient's mouth and chin, as needed.
■ If the patient is at risk for aspiration, monitor closely.
■ When the patient finishes eating, remove the tray. If necessary, clean up spills and change the bed linens.
■ Provide oral care. (See the "Oral care" procedure.)
■ Perform hand hygiene.[5,6,7,8,9,10]
■ Document oral intake, as ordered. (See *Recording fluid intake and output,* page 350.)
■ Document the procedure.[23,24,25,26]

Special considerations

■ A swallow evaluation is recommended before starting oral feeding in patients who require prolonged endotracheal intubation.[18]
■ If the patient is restricted to the supine position, provide foods that can be chewed easily; feed liquids carefully, and only after the patient has swallowed any food in the mouth, *to reduce the risk of aspiration.*
■ Establish a pattern for feeding the patient, and share this information with the other staff members *so the patient doesn't need to repeatedly instruct staff members about the best way to assist with feeding.*

EQUIPMENT

Using assistive feeding devices

Various feeding devices can help the patient who has limited arm mobility, grasp, range of motion (ROM), or coordination. Before introducing the patient to an assistive feeding device, assess the patient's ability to master it. Don't introduce a device the patient can't manage. If the patient's condition is progressively disabling, encourage the use of the device only until mastery of it falters.

Introduce the assistive device before mealtime, with the patient seated in a natural position. Explain its purpose, show the patient how to use it, and encourage practice. After meals, wash the device thoroughly and store it in the patient's bedside stand. Document the patient's progress and share it with staff and family members *to help reinforce the patient's independence.*

Plate guard

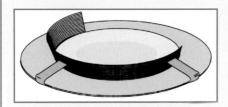

This device blocks food from spilling off the plate. Attach the guard to the side of the plate opposite the hand the patient uses to self-feed. Guiding the patient's hand, show the patient how to push food against the guard *to secure it on the utensil.* Then have the patient try again with food of a different consistency. When the patient tires, feed the patient the rest of the meal. At subsequent meals, encourage the patient to self-feed for progressively longer periods until the patient can self-feed an entire meal.

Swivel spoon

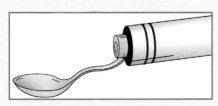

This utensil helps the patient with limited ROM in the forearm and will fit in universal cuffs.

Universal cuffs

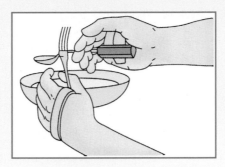

Universal cuffs are flexible bands that help the patient with flail hands or diminished grasp. Each cuff contains a slot that holds a fork or spoon. Attach the cuff to the hand the patient uses to self-feed. Then place the fork or spoon in the cuff slot. Bend the utensil *to facilitate feeding.*

Long-handled utensils

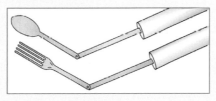

These utensils have jointed stems to help the patient with limited ROM in the elbow and shoulder.

Utensils with built-up handles

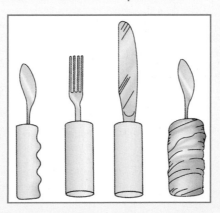

Utensils with built-up handles can help the patient with diminished grasp. They can be purchased or improvised by wrapping tape around the utensil handles.

Spouted cups

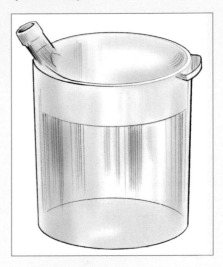

Spouted cups have a spout that can be used *to prevent spills and burns* for patients experiencing tremors or who have unsteady arms and hands.

Slotted cups

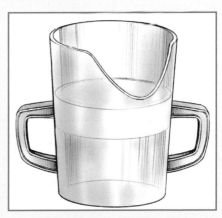

Slotted (or nosey) cups have a cutout for the nose to allow the patient to drink without bending the neck or tilting the head. Some have handles on both sides *to ensure a firm grasp.*

■ If the patient and family are willing, suggest that family members assist with feeding. *Such assistance will make the patient feel more comfortable at mealtimes and may ease discharge planning.*

Complications

Obstruction of the airway may lead to asphyxia, and aspiration of food can potentially cause hospital-acquired pneumonia.[22,27] Undernutrition may occur in the patient with feeding dependence or if the patient denies feeding difficulties.

Documentation

Describe the feeding technique used in the nursing care plan *to ensure continuity of care.* In your notes, record the amount of food and fluid consumed. Also note the amount of fluid consumed on the intake and output record, if required. Note foods that the patient consistently fails to eat and the reasons why, if known. Record the patient's level of independence. For a blind patient, record the placement of food on the plate in the nursing care plan. Document teaching provided to the patient and family (if applicable), their understanding of that teaching, and any need for follow-up teaching.

Recording fluid intake and output

Accurate intake and output records help evaluate a patient's fluid and electrolyte balance, suggest various diagnoses, and influence the choice of fluid therapy. These records are mandatory for patients with burns, renal failure, electrolyte imbalance, heart failure, or severe vomiting and diarrhea; patients who recently underwent a surgical procedure; and patients receiving diuretics or corticosteroids. Intake and output records are also significant in monitoring patients with nasogastric (NG) tubes or drainage collection devices and for those receiving IV therapy.

Fluid intake comprises all fluid entering the patient's body, including beverages, fluids contained in solid foods taken by mouth, and foods that aren't liquid at room temperature, such as flavored gelatin, custard, ice cream, and some beverages. Additional intake includes GI instillations, bladder irrigations, fluids ingested with medications, and IV fluids.

Fluid output consists of all fluid that leaves the patient's body, including urine, loose stools, vomitus, aspirated fluid loss, and drainage from surgical drains, NG tubes, and chest tubes.

When recording fluid intake and output, enlist the patient's help, if possible. Record the amount in milliliters. Measure; don't estimate. Monitor intake and output during each shift, and notify the practitioner if amounts differ significantly over a 24-hour period. Document your findings in the appropriate location; describe any fluid restrictions and the patient's compliance.

REFERENCES

1 Edwards, D., et al. (2016). Mealtime assistance for older adults in hospital settings and rehabilitation units from the perspective of patients, families and healthcare professionals: A mixed methods systematic review. *JBI Database of Systematic Reviews and Implementation Reports, 14*(9), 261–357. (Level I)

2 Tassone, E. C., et al. (2015). Should we implement mealtime assistance in the hospital setting? A systematic literature review with meta-analyses. *Journal of Clinical Nursing, 24*, 2710–2721. (Level I)

3 Vitale, C. A., et al. (2009). Strategies for improving care for patients with advanced dementia and eating problems. *Annals of Long-Term Care, 17*(5), 32–39. https://www.managedhealthcareconnect.com/content/strategies-improving-care-patients-with-advanced-dementia-and-eating-problems-full-title-bel

4 Boullata, J. I., et al. (2017). ASPEN safe practices for enteral nutrition therapy. *Journal of Parenteral and Enteral Nutrition, 41*(1), 15–103. http://journals.sagepub.com/doi/10.1177/0148607116673053 (Level VII)

5 The Joint Commission. (2021). Standard NPSG.07.01.01. *Comprehensive accreditation manual for hospitals*. Oakbrook Terrace, IL: The Joint Commission. (Level VII)

6 Centers for Disease Control and Prevention. (2002). Guideline for hand hygiene in health-care settings: Recommendations of the Healthcare Infection Control Practices Advisory Committee and the HICPAC/SHEA/APIC/IDSA Hand Hygiene Task Force. *MMWR Recommendations and Reports, 51*(RR-16), 1–45. https://www.cdc.gov/mmwr/pdf/rr/rr5116.pdf (Level II)

7 World Health Organization. (2009). WHO guidelines on hand hygiene in health care: First global patient safety challenge, clean care is safer care. https://apps.who.int/iris/bitstream/handle/10665/44102/9789241597906_eng.pdf?sequence=1 (Level IV)

8 Centers for Medicare and Medicaid Services, Department of Health and Human Services. (2020). Condition of participation: Infection control. 42 C.F.R. § 482.42.

9 Accreditation Association for Hospitals and Health Systems. (2020). Standard 07.01.21. *Healthcare Facilities Accreditation Program: Accreditation requirements for acute care hospitals*. Chicago, IL: Accreditation Association for Hospitals and Health Systems. (Level VII)

10 DNV GL-Healthcare USA, Inc. (2020). IC.1.SR.1. *NIAHO® accreditation requirements, interpretive guidelines and surveyor guidance—revision 20.0*. Milford, OH: DNV GL-Healthcare USA, Inc. (Level VII)

11 The Joint Commission. (2021). Standard NPSG.01.01.01. *Comprehensive accreditation manual for hospitals*. Oakbrook Terrace, IL: The Joint Commission. (Level VII)

12 The Joint Commission. (2021). Standard RI.01.01.01. *Comprehensive accreditation manual for hospitals*. Oakbrook Terrace, IL: The Joint Commission. (Level VII)

13 Centers for Medicare and Medicaid Services, Department of Health and Human Services. (2020). Condition of participation: Patient's rights. 42 C.F.R. § 482.13(c)(1).

14 Accreditation Association for Hospitals and Health Systems. (2020). Standard 15.01.16. *Healthcare Facilities Accreditation Program: Accreditation requirements for acute care hospitals*. Chicago, IL: Accreditation Association for Hospitals and Health Systems. (Level VII)

15 DNV GL-Healthcare USA, Inc. (2020). PR.2.SR.5. *NIAHO® accreditation requirements, interpretive guidelines and surveyor guidance—revision 20.0*. Milford, OH: DNV GL-Healthcare USA, Inc. (Level VII)

16 The Joint Commission. (2021). Standard PC.01.02.07. *Comprehensive accreditation manual for hospitals*. Oakbrook Terrace, IL: The Joint Commission. (Level VII)

17 The Joint Commission. (2021). Standard PC.02.01.21. *Comprehensive accreditation manual for hospitals*. Oakbrook Terrace, IL: The Joint Commission. (Level VII)

18 American Association of Critical-Care Nurses. (2018). AACN practice alert: Prevention of aspiration in adults. https://www.aacn.org/clinical-resources/practice-alerts/prevention-of-aspiration (Level VII)

19 John Hopkins Medicine. (n.d.). Eating with a tracheostomy. https://www.hopkinsmedicine.org/tracheostomy/living/eating.html

20 Rutala, W. A., et al. (2008, revised 2019). Guideline for disinfection and sterilization in healthcare facilities, 2008. https://www.cdc.gov/infection-control/pdf/guidelines/disinfection-guidelines-H.pdf (Level I)

21 Accreditation Association for Hospitals and Health Systems. (2020). Standard 07.02.03. *Healthcare Facilities Accreditation Program: Accreditation requirements for acute care hospitals*. Chicago, IL: Accreditation Association for Hospitals and Health Systems. (Level VII)

22 Alberta Health Services. (2017). Mealtime assistance training manual. https://nutritioncareincanada.ca/sites/default/uploads/files/TrainingManual%20Feb2017(1).pdf

23 The Joint Commission. (2021). Standard RC.01.03.01. *Comprehensive accreditation manual for hospitals*. Oakbrook Terrace, IL: The Joint Commission. (Level VII)

24 Centers for Medicare and Medicaid Services, Department of Health and Human Services. (2020). Condition of participation: Medical record services. 42 C.F.R. § 482.24(b).

25 Accreditation Association for Hospitals and Health Systems. (2020). Standard 10.00.03. *Healthcare Facilities Accreditation Program: Accreditation requirements for acute care hospitals*. Chicago, IL: Accreditation Association for Hospitals and Health Systems. (Level VII)

26 DNV GL-Healthcare USA, Inc. (2020). MR.2.SR.1. *NIAHO® accreditation requirements, interpretive guidelines and surveyor guidance—revision 20.0*. Milford, OH: DNV GL-Healthcare USA, Inc. (Level VII)

27 Klompas, M. (2021). Aspiration pneumonia in adults. In: *UpToDate*, Sexton, D. J. (Ed.).

FEMORAL COMPRESSION DEVICE USE

After a procedure involving femoral arterial access (such as cardiac catheterization or angiography), a femoral compression device is used to apply direct pressure to the arterial access site to maintains hemostasis.[1] The device, which has an inflatable dome, is attached by means of a wide strap placed under the patient's buttocks; the inflatable dome is positioned over the arterial puncture site and inflated to a set pressure.

Contraindications to femoral compression device use include severe peripheral vascular disease, limb ischemia, skin necrosis or infection, arterial injury near the inguinal ligament, an inability to compress the involved area because of hematomas or uncontrolled pain, a femoral artery or vein graft, and leg edema, femoral nerve compression, or arterial obstruction in the involved leg.[2] A practitioner or a specially trained nurse may apply and remove a femoral compression device.

Equipment

Femoral compression device strap ▪ compression arch with dome and three-way stopcock ▪ pressure inflation device ▪ sterile transparent dressing ▪ gloves ▪ mask and goggles or mask with face shield ▪ indelible marker ▪ cardiac monitoring equipment ▪ vital signs monitoring equipment ▪ emergency equipment (code cart with emergency medications, defibrillator, handheld resuscitation bag with mask, intubation equipment) ■ Optional: prescribed pain medication, Doppler ultrasound device, gown.

Preparation of equipment

Inspect all equipment and supplies. If a product is expired, is defective, or has compromised integrity, remove it from patient use, label it as expired or defective, and report the expiration or defect as directed by your facility.

Make sure the emergency equipment is readily available and functioning properly before the procedure.[1]

Implementation

■ Confirm the practitioner's order regarding the femoral compression device, including the length of time the device should remain in place.
■ Review the patient's medical record for a history of bleeding disorders. Review the patient's platelet count, prothrombin time, International Normalized Ratio, partial thromboplastin time, and complete blood count *to serve as a baseline for comparison.*[1]
■ Gather and prepare the necessary equipment and supplies.
■ Perform hand hygiene.[3,4,5,6,7,8]
■ Confirm the patient's identity using at least two patient identifiers.[9]
■ Provide privacy.[10,11,12,13]
■ Explain the procedure to the patient and family (if appropriate) according to their individual communication and learning needs *to increase their understanding, allay their fears, and enhance cooperation.*[14]
■ Raise the bed or stretcher to waist level before providing care *to prevent caregiver back strain.*[15]
■ Perform hand hygiene.[3,4,5,6,7,8]
■ Make sure the patient is positioned on the stretcher or bed with the affected leg straight and the head of the bed flat.[1]
■ Obtain the patient's vital signs and monitor cardiac rhythm *to detect bradyarrhythmias that can occur with a vasovagal reaction.*[1] Make sure that cardiac monitor alarm limits are set appropriately for the patient's current condition, and that alarms are turned on, functioning properly, and audible to staff.[16,17,18,19]
■ Screen for and assess the patient's pain using facility-defined criteria that are consistent with the patient's age, condition, and ability to understand.[20]
■ Treat the patient's pain, as needed and ordered, using nonpharmacologic, pharmacologic, or a combination of approaches. Base the treatment plan on evidence-based practices and the patient's clinical condition, past medical history, and pain management goals.[20]
■ Monitor closely if the patient is at high risk for adverse outcomes related to opioid treatment, if prescribed.[20]

Applying the femoral compression device
■ Perform hand hygiene.[3,4,5,6,7,8]
■ Put on gloves, a mask and goggles or a mask with face shield, and a gown, if needed, *to comply with standard precautions.*[1,21,22,23,24]
■ Assess the condition of the puncture site and the neurovascular status of the affected extremity. Mark the distal pulses with an indelible marker *to facilitate locating pulses during and after the procedure.*[1]
■ Place the femoral compression device strap under the patient's hips before arterial sheath removal (in cases that warrant the use of a sheath).
■ With the assistance of another nurse, position the compression arch over the arterial puncture site, not the skin puncture site. The arterial puncture site is ½″ to ¾″ (1.3 cm to 1.9 cm) above the skin puncture site, *because the practitioner inserts the arterial sheath at a 45-degree angle to the artery.*[1]
■ Apply manual pressure over the dome area while the straps are secured to the arch.
■ After the dome is properly positioned over the arterial puncture site, connect the pressure inflation device to the stopcock that's attached to the device.
■ Before inflation, verify the amplitude and location of the pedal pulse.
■ Begin to inflate the dome; the practitioner withdraws the arterial sheath when the dome is inflated between 60 and 80 mm Hg.

■ Immediately after removal of the arterial sheath, inflate the device to the ordered pressure (typically 10 to 20 mm Hg above the patient's systolic blood pressure) *to control bleeding.* (See the "Arterial and venous sheath removal" procedure.)
■ After 2 to 3 minutes, reduce the pressure following the manufacturer's recommendations and the practitioner's specific orders for pressure changes.
■ Assess the site for proper placement of the device and for signs of bleeding or hematoma.
■ Assess the distal pulses of the affected extremity and perform a neurovascular assessment. *During femoral compression device application, the distal pulses may decrease, especially during full-pressure application; however, they shouldn't be obliterated.*[1] Use a Doppler ultrasound device, if necessary.

Maintaining the device
■ Reassess the patient's vital signs, device placement, the puncture site, and peripheral vascular and neurovascular status of the affected extremity every 15 minutes for an hour, every 30 minutes over the next hour, and then hourly for the following 4 hours.[1] Afterward, continue to monitor at an interval determined by your facility and the patient's condition.
■ If the dome isn't in the proper position, perform hand hygiene and put on gloves, protective eyewear, and a gown, as needed,[3,4,5,6,7,8,21,23] and then reposition the compression arch and dome, as necessary. Using the pressure inflation device, reinflate the device to the ordered pressure.
■ Recheck the applied pressure against the pressure stated in the practitioner's order.
■ Continue to monitor the patient's cardiac rhythm *to detect bradyarrhythmias that might occur with a vasovagal reaction.*[1]
■ Confirm distal pulses after any adjustments of the device.

Removing the device
■ Perform hand hygiene.[3,4,5,6,7,8]
■ Put on gloves, a mask and goggles or a mask with face shield, and a gown, as needed.[21,22]
■ Remove the air from the dome.
■ Leave the dome in place at 0 mm Hg pressure for at least 10 minutes; then loosen the straps and remove the device by rolling it off.
■ Assess the puncture site for bleeding and hematoma after hemostasis is achieved by palpating around the site.[1]
■ Apply a sterile transparent dressing over the puncture site.
■ Frequently assess the puncture site and neurovascular status of the extremity. Watch for signs of bleeding, hematoma, and infection.
■ Discard the device in an appropriate receptacle.[23]
■ Raise the head of the bed up 30 degrees after hemostasis is achieved, as desired by the patient, *to minimize back discomfort.*[1]

Completing the procedure
■ Instruct the patient to keep the affected leg straight, to maintain the head of the bed in its prescribed position, and to splint the groin if needed to cough or sneeze. Tell the patient to call for assistance with elimination when necessary.
■ Reassess and respond to the patient's pain by evaluating the response to treatment and progress toward pain management goals. Assess for adverse reactions and risk factors for adverse events that may result from treatment.[20]
■ Return the bed or stretcher to the lowest position *to prevent falls and maintain patient safety.*[24]
■ Ensure that the patient's call light and personal belongings are within reach.
■ Remove and discard your gloves, mask and goggles or mask and face shield, and gown, if worn.[21,23]
■ Perform hand hygiene.[3,4,5,6,7,8]
■ Document the procedure.[25,26,27,28]

Special considerations
■ The Joint Commission issued a sentinel event alert concerning medical device alarm safety, *because alarm-related events have been associated with permanent loss of function or death.* Among the major contributing factors

were improper alarm settings, alarm settings turned off inappropriately, and alarm signals not audible to staff. Make sure that alarm limits are set appropriately, and that alarms are turned on, functioning properly, and audible to staff. Follow facility guidelines for preventing alarm fatigue.[19]

■ Maintain the patient on bed rest for 1 to 6 hours after arterial sheath removal.[1]

■ If you note external bleeding or signs of internal bleeding, remove the device, apply manual pressure, and notify the practitioner.[1]

■ Change the sterile transparent dressing at the puncture site every 24 to 48 hours. (The sterile transparent dressing permits inspection of the site for bleeding, drainage, or hematoma.)

■ If the patient received antiplatelet and antithrombotic regimens in conjunction with percutaneous coronary intervention, exercise caution, *because the patient is at increased risk for bleeding.*

■ The length of time it takes to achieve hemostasis varies with the patient's condition. Monitor for tissue damage, which can occur with pressure maintained for longer than 2 hours.[1]

Complications

Complications associated with femoral compression include bleeding, hematoma, retroperitoneal bleeding, and pseudoaneurysm. Other potential complications may include infection, arteriovenous fistula formation, ischemia of the extremity, thrombosis, and embolization. Tissue damage can also occur if prolonged pressure is maintained.[1,2]

Documentation

Document the date and time of the initial application of the device, sheath removal, and the patient's tolerance of the procedure. Record vital signs, cardiac rhythm, puncture site assessments, distal pulses, neurovascular assessments, periodic deflation, and any repositioning of the device. Document the date and time of the removal of the device, along with the length of time the device was in place and the appearance of the site after removal. Document any adverse events that occurred, the name of the practitioner notified, the date and time of notification, prescribed interventions, and the patient's response to those interventions. Record teaching provided to the patient and family (if appropriate), their understanding of that teaching, and any need for follow-up teaching.

REFERENCES

1 Wiegand, D. L. (2017). *AACN procedure manual for high acuity, progressive, and critical care* (7th ed.). St. Louis, MO: Elsevier.

2 Abbott. (n.d.). FemoStop™ Gold femoral compression system. https://www.cardiovascular.abbott/us/en/hcp/products/peripheral-intervention/femostop-gold.html

3 The Joint Commission. (2021). Standard NPSG.07.01.01. *Comprehensive accreditation manual for hospitals.* Oakbrook Terrace, IL: The Joint Commission. (Level VII)

4 Centers for Disease Control and Prevention. (2002). Guideline for hand hygiene in health-care settings: Recommendations of the Healthcare Infection Control Practices Advisory Committee and the HICPAC/SHEA/APIC/IDSA Hand Hygiene Task Force. *MMWR Recommendations and Reports, 51*(RR-16), 1–45. https://www.cdc.gov/mmwr/pdf/rr/rr5116.pdf (Level II)

5 World Health Organization. (2009). WHO guidelines on hand hygiene in health care: First global patient safety challenge, clean care is safer care. https://apps.who.int/iris/bitstream/handle/10665/44102/9789241597906_eng.pdf?sequence=1 (Level IV)

6 Accreditation Association for Hospitals and Health Systems. (2020). Standard 07.01.21. *Healthcare Facilities Accreditation Program: Accreditation requirements for acute care hospitals.* Chicago, IL: Accreditation Association for Hospitals and Health Systems. (Level VII)

7 Centers for Medicare and Medicaid Services, Department of Health and Human Services. (2020). Condition of participation: Infection control. 42 C.F.R. § 482.42.

8 DNV GL-Healthcare USA, Inc. (2020). IC.1.SR.1. *NIAHO® accreditation requirements, interpretive guidelines and surveyor guidance—revision 20.0.* Milford, OH: DNV GL-Healthcare USA, Inc. (Level VII)

9 The Joint Commission. (2021). Standard NPSG.01.01.01. *Comprehensive accreditation manual for hospitals.* Oakbrook Terrace, IL: The Joint Commission. (Level VII)

10 The Joint Commission. (2021). Standard RI.01.01.01. *Comprehensive accreditation manual for hospitals.* Oakbrook Terrace, IL: The Joint Commission. (Level VII)

11 DNV GL-Healthcare USA, Inc. (2020). PR.2.SR.5. *NIAHO® accreditation requirements, interpretive guidelines and surveyor guidance—revision 20.0.* Milford, OH: DNV GL-Healthcare USA, Inc. (Level VII)

12 Centers for Medicare and Medicaid Services, Department of Health and Human Services. (2020). Condition of participation: Patient's rights. 42 C.F.R. § 482.13(c)(1).

13 Accreditation Association for Hospitals and Health Systems. (2020). Standard 15.01.16. *Healthcare Facilities Accreditation Program: Accreditation requirements for acute care hospitals.* Chicago, IL: Accreditation Association for Hospitals and Health Systems. (Level VII)

14 The Joint Commission. (2021). Standard PC.02.01.21. *Comprehensive accreditation manual for hospitals.* Oakbrook Terrace, IL: The Joint Commission. (Level VII)

15 Waters, T. R., et al. (2009). Safe patient handling training for schools of nursing. https://www.cdc.gov/niosh/docs/2009-127/pdfs/2009-127.pdf (Level VII)

16 The Joint Commission. (2021). Standard NPSG.06.01.01. *Comprehensive accreditation manual for hospitals.* Oakbrook Terrace, IL: The Joint Commission. (Level VII)

17 American Association of Critical-Care Nurses. (2018). AACN practice alert: Managing alarms in acute care across the life span. Electrocardiography and pulse oximetry. https://www.aacn.org/clinical-resources/practice-alerts/managing-alarms-in-acute-care-across-the-life-span (Level VII)

18 Graham, K. C., & Cvach, M. (2010). Monitor alarm fatigue: Standardizing use of physiological monitors and decreasing nuisance alarms. *American Journal of Critical Care, 19*, 28–37.

19 The Joint Commission. (2013). Sentinel event alert 50: Medical device alarm safety in hospitals. https://www.jointcommission.org/assets/1/6/SEA_50_alarms_4_26_16.pdf (Level VII)

20 The Joint Commission. (2021). Standard PC.01.02.07. *Comprehensive accreditation manual for hospitals.* Oakbrook Terrace, IL: The Joint Commission. (Level VII)

21 Siegel, J. D., et al. (2007, revised 2019). 2007 guideline for isolation precautions: Preventing transmission of infectious agents in healthcare settings. https://www.cdc.gov/infectioncontrol/pdf/guidelines/isolation-guidelines-H.pdf (Level II)

22 Accreditation Association for Hospitals and Health Systems. (2020). Standard 07.01.10. *Healthcare Facilities Accreditation Program: Accreditation requirements for acute care hospitals.* Chicago, IL: Accreditation Association for Hospitals and Health Systems. (Level VII)

23 Occupational Safety and Health Administration. (2019). Bloodborne pathogens, standard number 1910.1030. https://www.osha.gov/pls/oshaweb/owadisp.show_document?p_id=10051&p_table=STANDARDS (Level VII)

24 Ganz, D. A., et al. (2013, reviewed 2021). *Preventing falls in hospitals: A toolkit for improving quality of care* (AHRQ Publication No. 13-0015-EF). Rockville, MD: Agency for Healthcare Research and Quality. https://www.ahrq.gov/professionals/systems/hospital/fallpxtoolkit/index.html (Level VII)

25 The Joint Commission. (2021). Standard RC.01.03.01. *Comprehensive accreditation manual for hospitals.* Oakbrook Terrace, IL: The Joint Commission. (Level VII)

26 Accreditation Association for Hospitals and Health Systems. (2020). Standard 10.00.03. *Healthcare Facilities Accreditation Program: Accreditation requirements for acute care hospitals.* Chicago, IL: Accreditation Association for Hospitals and Health Systems. (Level VII)

27 Centers for Medicare and Medicaid Services, Department of Health and Human Services. (2020). Condition of participation: Medical record services. 42 C.F.R. § 482.24(b).

28 DNV GL-Healthcare USA, Inc. (2020). MR.2.SR.1. *NIAHO® accreditation requirements, interpretive guidelines and surveyor guidance—revision 20.0.* Milford, OH: DNV GL-Healthcare USA, Inc. (Level VII)

FOOT CARE

Daily bathing of feet and regular trimming of toenails promotes cleanliness, prevents infection, stimulates peripheral circulation, and controls odor by removing debris from between toes and under toenails. It's particularly important for bedridden patients and those especially vulnerable to foot infection. Increased susceptibility may be caused by peripheral vascular disease, diabetes, poor nutritional status, arthritis, or any condition that impairs peripheral circulation. Patients with diabetes should have yearly foot examination to identify factors that increase the risk of ulcers or amputation.[1]

In at-risk patients, proper foot care should include meticulous cleanliness and regular observation for signs of skin breakdown. When you perform a foot examination, inspect the patient's foot, assess foot pulses, and test for loss of protective sensation. Ask the patient about any history of previous foot ulceration or amputation, neuropathic or peripheral vascular symptoms, impaired vision, tobacco use, and foot care practices.[1] (See *Foot care for patients with diabetes.*) Teach the at-risk patient proper foot care on at least a yearly basis.[1]

Toenail trimming is contraindicated in patients with toe infections, diabetes, neurologic disorders, kidney failure, or peripheral vascular disease, unless performed by a practitioner or a certified foot care nurse.[4] Some facilities prohibit nurses from trimming toenails. Check to see whether you're permitted by your facility before trimming the patient's toenails.

Equipment

Bath blanket ▪ large basin ▪ soap ▪ water ▪ towel ▪ fluid-impermeable pad ▪ pillow ▪ washcloth ▪ emery board ▪ cotton-tipped applicators ▪ lotion ▪ water-absorbent powder ▪ bath thermometer ▪ facility-approved disinfectant ▪ Optional: gloves, 2″ × 2″ (5 cm × 5 cm) gauze pads, heel protectors, or protective boots.

Preparation of equipment

Inspect all equipment and supplies. If a product is expired, is defective, or has compromised integrity, remove it from patient use, label it as expired or defective, and report the expiration or defect as directed by your facility.

Foot care for patients with diabetes

Because diabetes can reduce blood supply to the feet, normally minor foot injuries can lead to dangerous infection. When caring for a patient with diabetes, keep these foot care guidelines in mind:

▪ Advise the patient to exercise the feet daily *to help improve circulation.* Teach the patient to sit on the edge of the bed and point the toes upward, then downward, 10 times. The patient should then make a circle with each foot 10 times.

▪ Explain that shoes must fit properly.[1] Instruct the patient to break in new shoes gradually by increasing wearing time by 30 minutes each day. Also tell the patient to check old shoes frequently *for rough spots in the lining.*

▪ Advise high-risk patients with diabetes, including those with severe neuropathy, foot deformities, or history of amputation, that the use of specialized therapeutic footwear is recommended.[1]

▪ Tell the patient to wear clean socks daily and to avoid socks with holes, darned spots, or rough, irritating seams.[2,3]

▪ Advise the patient to avoid walking barefoot *to avoid injury.*[2]

▪ Advise the patient to see a practitioner if the patient has corns or calluses.[1] Warn the patient not to try and remove a corn or callus with over-the-counter products, *because they can burn the skin.*[3]

▪ Tell the patient to wear warm socks or slippers and to use extra blankets *to avoid cold feet.*

▪ Advise the patient to avoid heating pads or hot-water bottles, *because these items may cause burns.*

▪ Teach the patient to inspect both feet for cuts, cracks, blisters, or red, swollen areas, and to use a mirror to check the soles, as needed.[3] Inform the patient that even slight cuts on the feet should receive a practitioner's attention. As a first-aid measure, tell the patient to wash the cut thoroughly and apply a mild antiseptic. Urge the patient to avoid harsh antiseptics, such as iodine, *because they can damage tissue.*

▪ Advise the patient to avoid tight-fitting garments and activities that can decrease circulation, especially wearing elastic garters, sitting with the knees crossed, picking at sores or rough spots on the feet, walking barefoot, or applying adhesive tape to the skin on the feet.

▪ Encourage the patient to quit smoking, if applicable.[2]

Fill a large basin halfway with warm water.[2] Test water temperature with a bath thermometer, *because patients with diminished peripheral sensation could burn their feet in excessively hot water (over 105° F [40.6° C]) without feeling any warning pain.*

Implementation

▪ Gather and prepare the necessary equipment and supplies.
▪ Perform hand hygiene.[5,6,7,8,9,10]
▪ Put on gloves if needed *to comply with standard precautions.*[11,12,13]
▪ Confirm the patient's identity using at least two patient identifiers.[14]
▪ Provide privacy.[15,16,17,18]
▪ Explain the procedure to the patient and family (if appropriate) according to their individual communication and learning needs *to increase their understanding, allay their fears, and enhance cooperation.*[19]
▪ Raise the patient's bed to waist level before providing care *to prevent caregiver back strain.*[20]
▪ Cover the patient with a bath blanket. Fanfold the top linen to the foot of the bed.
▪ Place a fluid-impermeable pad and a towel under the patient's feet *to keep the bottom linen dry.* Then position the basin on the fluid-impermeable pad.
▪ Insert a pillow beneath the patient's knee *to provide support*, and cushion the rim of the basin with the edge of the towel *to prevent pressure on the patient's leg.*
▪ Immerse one foot in the basin. Allow it to soak for about 10 minutes and then wash it thoroughly with soap and water. *Soaking softens the skin and toenails, loosens debris under toenails, and comforts and refreshes the patient.*
▪ After washing the foot, rinse it, remove it from the basin, and place it on the towel.
▪ Gently and thoroughly dry the patient's foot, *especially between the toes.* Don't rub, *because doing so can cause skin breakdown.*
▪ Empty the basin and refill it with warm water at the appropriate temperature.
▪ Soak the other foot.
▪ While the second foot is soaking, give the first foot a pedicure. Using a cotton-tipped applicator, carefully clean the patient's toenails. Use an emery board to smooth the nails, as indicated, *to prevent self-inflicted skin tears.*[21]
▪ Consult a podiatrist (if required by your facility) if the patient's nails need trimming.
▪ Clean and rinse the foot that has been soaking, dry it thoroughly, and give it a pedicure.
▪ Apply lotion *to moisten dry skin.*[22] Don't apply lotion between the toes, *because lotion can cause skin maceration.*[23] Lightly dust water-absorbent powder between the toes *to absorb moisture.*[24]
▪ Remove the bath blanket and cover the patient with the top linens.
▪ Return the bed to the lowest position *to prevent falls and maintain patient safety.*[25]
▪ Empty the basin and clean and disinfect reusable equipment according to the manufacturer's instructions *to prevent the spread of infection.*[26,27]
▪ Discard used supplies in appropriate receptacles.[13]
▪ Remove and discard your gloves, if worn.[11,13]
▪ Perform hand hygiene.[5,6,7,8,9,10]
▪ Document the procedure.[28,29,30,31]

Special considerations

▪ While providing foot care, observe the color, shape, and texture of the toenails. If you see redness, drying, cracking, blisters, discoloration, or other signs of traumatic injury, especially in a patient with impaired peripheral circulation, notify the practitioner. *Because such a patient is vulnerable to infection and gangrene,* the patient needs prompt treatment.[1]
▪ If a patient's toenail grows inward at the corners, tuck a wisp of cotton under it *to relieve pressure on the toe.*
▪ When providing foot care for a bedridden patient, perform range-of-motion exercises, unless contraindicated, *to stimulate circulation and prevent foot contractures and muscle atrophy.* Tuck folded 2″ × 2″ (5 cm × 5 cm) gauze pads between overlapping toes *to protect the skin from the toenails.* Apply heel protectors or protective boots *to prevent skin breakdown.*

Patient teaching

Instruct the patient to notify the practitioner right away if the patient observes discoloration (any part of the leg or foot that turns blue or black); notes reduced sensation to pain or temperature; develops an injury that doesn't heal or becomes infected; experiences unusual numbness, tingling, cold, cramping, or pain in the feet; or develops pain while walking that's relieved by rest.

If a patient can't perform proper foot care and inspection because of visual difficulties, physical constraints that prevent movement, or cognitive problems that impair the patient's ability to assess the condition of the foot and to institute appropriate responses, educate other people (such as family members) to assist in the patient's care.[1]

Complications

Injury to the subungual skin may occur.

Documentation

Record the date and time of foot care in your notes. Record and report any abnormal findings and any nursing actions that you took in response. If toenail trimming was necessary, specify the name of the person who performed the trimming. Document teaching provided to the patient and family (if applicable), their understanding of that teaching, and any need for follow-up teaching.

REFERENCES

1 American Diabetes Association. (2020). Position statement 11. Microvascular complications and foot care: Standards of medical care in diabetes-2020. *Diabetes Care, 43*(Suppl. 1), S135–S151. https://care.diabetesjournals.org/content/43/Supplement_1/S135 (Level VII)

2 Wexler, D. J. (2020). Evaluation of the diabetic foot. In: *UpToDate*, Nathan, D. M. (Ed.).

3 American Podiatric Medical Association. (n.d.). What is diabetes? https://www.apma.org/Patients/FootHealth.cfm?ItemNumber=980

4 American Foot Care Nurses Association. (n.d.). Certification objective, rationale statement of need, foot care nurse competencies and standards. https://afcna.org/PracticeStandards

5 Centers for Disease Control and Prevention. (2002). Guideline for hand hygiene in health-care settings: Recommendations of the Healthcare Infection Control Practices Advisory Committee and the HICPAC/SHEA/APIC/IDSA Hand Hygiene Task Force. *MMWR Recommendations and Reports, 51*(RR-16), 1–45. https://www.cdc.gov/mmwr/pdf/rr/rr5116.pdf (Level II)

6 World Health Organization. (2009). WHO guidelines on hand hygiene in health care: First global patient safety challenge, clean care is safer care. https://apps.who.int/iris/bitstream/handle/10665/44102/9789241597906_eng.pdf?sequence=1 (Level IV)

7 The Joint Commission. (2021). Standard NPSG.07.01.01. *Comprehensive accreditation manual for hospitals*. Oakbrook Terrace, IL: The Joint Commission. (Level VII)

8 Centers for Medicare and Medicaid Services, Department of Health and Human Services. (2020). Condition of participation: Infection control. 42 C.F.R. § 482.42.

9 Accreditation Association for Hospitals and Health Systems. (2020). Standard 07.01.21. *Healthcare Facilities Accreditation Program: Accreditation requirements for acute care hospitals*. Chicago, IL: Accreditation Association for Hospitals and Health Systems. (Level VII)

10 DNV GL-Healthcare USA, Inc. (2020). IC.1.SR.1. *NIAHO® accreditation requirements, interpretive guidelines and surveyor guidance—revision 20.0*. Milford, OH: DNV GL-Healthcare USA, Inc. (Level VII)

11 Siegel, J. D., et al. (2007, revised 2019). 2007 guideline for isolation precautions: Preventing transmission of infectious agents in healthcare settings. https://www.cdc.gov/infectioncontrol/pdf/guidelines/isolation-guidelines-H.pdf (Level II)

12 Accreditation Association for Hospitals and Health Systems. (2020). Standard 07.01.10. *Healthcare Facilities Accreditation Program: Accreditation requirements for acute care hospitals*. Chicago, IL: Accreditation Association for Hospitals and Health Systems. (Level VII)

13 Occupational Safety and Health Administration. (2019). Bloodborne pathogens, standard number 1910.1030. https://www.osha.gov/pls/oshaweb/owadisp.show_document?p_id=10051&p_table=STANDARDS (Level VII)

14 The Joint Commission. (2021). Standard NPSG.01.01.01. *Comprehensive accreditation manual for hospitals*. Oakbrook Terrace, IL: The Joint Commission. (Level VII)

15 Centers for Medicare and Medicaid Services, Department of Health and Human Services. (2020). Condition of participation: Patient's rights. 42 C.F.R. § 482.13(c)(1).

16 Accreditation Association for Hospitals and Health Systems. (2020). Standard 15.01.16. *Healthcare Facilities Accreditation Program: Accreditation requirements for acute care hospitals*. Chicago, IL: Accreditation Association for Hospitals and Health Systems. (Level VII)

17 The Joint Commission. (2021). Standard RI.01.01.01. *Comprehensive accreditation manual for hospitals*. Oakbrook Terrace, IL: The Joint Commission. (Level VII)

18 DNV GL-Healthcare USA, Inc. (2020). PR.2.SR.5. *NIAHO® accreditation requirements, interpretive guidelines and surveyor guidance—revision 20.0*. Milford, OH: DNV GL-Healthcare USA, Inc. (Level VII)

19 The Joint Commission. (2021). Standard PC.02.01.21. *Comprehensive accreditation manual for hospitals*. Oakbrook Terrace, IL: The Joint Commission. (Level VII)

20 Waters, T. R., et al. (2009). Safe patient handling training for schools of nursing. https://www.cdc.gov/niosh/docs/2009-127/pdfs/2009-127.pdf (Level VII)

21 LeBlanc, K., et al. (2013). International skin tear advisory panel: A tool kit to aid in the prevention, assessment, and treatment of skin tears using a simplified classification system. *Advances in Skin & Wound Care, 26*, 459–476. (Level IV)

22 Wexler, D. J. (2021). Patient education: Foot care for people with diabetes mellitus (Beyond the basics). In: *UpToDate*, Nathan, D. M. (Ed.).

23 American Diabetes Association. (n.d.). Foot complications. http://www.diabetes.org/living-with-diabetes/complications/foot-complications/?loc=lwd-slabnav (Level VII)

24 National Institute of Diabetes and Digestive and Kidney Diseases. (2017). Diabetes and foot problems. https://www.niddk.nih.gov/health-information/diabetes/overview/preventing-problems/foot-problems (Level VII)

25 Ganz, D. A., et al. (2013, reviewed 2021). *Preventing falls in hospitals: A toolkit for improving quality of care* (AHRQ Publication No. 13-0015-EF). Rockville, MD: Agency for Healthcare Research and Quality. https://www.ahrq.gov/professionals/systems/hospital/fallpxtoolkit/index.html (Level VII)

26 Rutala, W. A., et al. (2008, revised 2019). Guideline for disinfection and sterilization in healthcare facilities, 2008. https://www.cdc.gov/infection-control/pdf/guidelines/disinfection-guidelines-H.pdf (Level I)

27 Accreditation Association for Hospitals and Health Systems. (2020). Standard 07.02.03. *Healthcare Facilities Accreditation Program: Accreditation requirements for acute care hospitals*. Chicago, IL: Accreditation Association for Hospitals and Health Systems. (Level VII)

28 The Joint Commission. (2021). Standard RC.01.03.01. *Comprehensive accreditation manual for hospitals*. Oakbrook Terrace, IL: The Joint Commission. (Level VII)

29 Centers for Medicare and Medicaid Services, Department of Health and Human Services. (2020). Condition of participation: Medical record services. 42 C.F.R. § 482.24(b).

30 Accreditation Association for Hospitals and Health Systems. (2020). Standard 10.00.03. *Healthcare Facilities Accreditation Program: Accreditation requirements for acute care hospitals*. Chicago, IL: Accreditation Association for Hospitals and Health Systems. (Level VII)

31 DNV GL-Healthcare USA, Inc. (2020). MR.2.SR.1. *NIAHO® accreditation requirements, interpretive guidelines and surveyor guidance—revision 20.0*. Milford, OH: DNV GL-Healthcare USA, Inc. (Level VII)

FOREIGN-BODY AIRWAY OBSTRUCTION MANAGEMENT

Most cases of foreign-body airway obstruction in adults occur while they're eating. Foreign bodies can cause mild or severe airway obstruction. In a child, foreign-body airway obstruction occurs most often when they're eating or playing and typically involves such items as balloons and small objects, or such foods as hot dogs, rounded candies, nuts, grapes, and gum. In infants, airway obstruction typically results from ingestion of a liquid.

Foreign bodies can cause mild or severe airway obstruction. If the obstruction is mild and the patient is coughing forcefully, there's no reason to intervene; spontaneous coughing and breathing typically relieve the obstruction.[1]

If severe obstruction develops, you must intervene quickly to relieve the obstruction; anoxia resulting from the obstruction may cause brain damage and death in 4 to 6 minutes.[1]

Symptoms of severe airway obstruction include a sudden inability to speak, cough, or cry; stridor; cyanosis; accessory muscle use; and agonal respirations. Intervene by administering abdominal thrusts, also called the Heimlich maneuver, which uses a subdiaphragmatic abdominal thrust to create diaphragmatic pressure in the static lung below the foreign body sufficient to expel the obstruction. Note that the performance of abdominal thrusts is indicated only for a conscious adult who can't speak, cough, or breathe and should continue until the obstruction is relieved, as long as the patient remains conscious.[1]

If abdominal thrusts are ineffective in clearing an airway, you should consider administering chest thrusts; this maneuver forces air out of the lungs, creating an artificial cough. Also use chest thrusts for an obese patient, if you're unable to encircle the patient's abdomen, and for a patient who's in the late stages of pregnancy.[1]

For infants, deliver repeated cycles of five back blows followed by five chest compressions until the foreign body is expelled or the infant becomes unresponsive. Abdominal thrusts aren't recommended for infants *because they may damage the infant's liver.*[2]

If a patient is unconscious or becomes unconscious despite your efforts, start cardiopulmonary resuscitation (CPR) immediately.[1]

Equipment

No special equipment is required.

Implementation

- Determine whether the patient is choking by asking, "Are you choking?" If the patient indicates "yes" by nodding the head without speaking, there is a severe airway obstruction.[1]
- Activate the emergency response system quickly if the patient is having difficulty breathing. If another person is present, have that person activate the system.[1]
- *To calm the patient,* talk to the patient and explain what you're doing. Tell the patient that you'll try to dislodge the foreign body.

For a conscious adult or child

- Standing behind the patient, wrap your arms around the patient's waist. Make a fist with one hand, and place the thumb side against the abdomen, slightly above the umbilicus and well below the xiphoid process. Then grasp your fist with the other hand (as shown below).

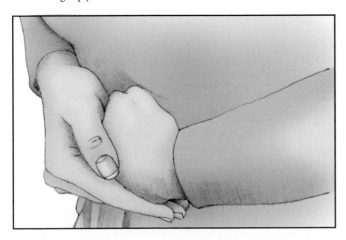

- Squeeze the patient's abdomen using quick inward and upward thrusts. Each thrust should be a separate and distinct movement; each should be forceful enough to create an artificial cough that will dislodge an obstruction. Continue the abdominal thrust in rapid sequence until the obstruction is relieved or the patient becomes unresponsive.[1]
- Make sure you have a firm grasp on the patient, *because the patient may lose consciousness and need to be lowered to the floor.*[1] Support the head and

neck *to prevent injury.* If the patient becomes unconscious, start CPR and follow the steps for an unconscious adult or child.
- Examine the patient for injuries resulting from the procedure, such as ruptured or lacerated abdominal or thoracic viscera.

For an obese or pregnant adult

- If the patient is conscious, stand behind and place your arms under the patient's armpits and around the chest.
- Place the thumb side of your clenched fist against the middle of the sternum, avoiding the margins of the ribs and the xiphoid process (as shown below).

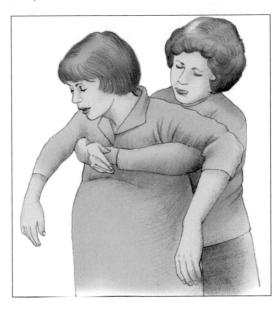

- Grasp your fist with your other hand and perform a chest thrust with enough force to expel the foreign body. Continue until the patient expels the obstruction or loses consciousness.[1] If the patient loses consciousness, carefully lower the patient to the floor, start performing CPR with chest compressions, and follow the steps outlined below for an unconscious adult or child.
- Examine the patient for injuries resulting from the procedure, such as ruptured or lacerated abdominal or thoracic viscera.
- Notify the practitioner of the patient's status, especially with loss of consciousness.

For an unconscious adult or child

- For a patient who has become unresponsive while you are trying to remove a foreign object, carefully lower the patient to the ground and call for help, or activate the emergency response system.[1]
- If you come upon an unconscious patient, establish unresponsiveness by tapping the patient and shouting, "Are you alright?" Check to see if the patient is apneic or only gasping. If the patient is unresponsive and apneic or only gasping, call for help or activate the emergency response system.[1]
- Begin CPR immediately, starting with chest compressions; use a chest compression-to-ventilation ratio of 30:2.[1] (See the "Cardiopulmonary resuscitation, adult" procedure, and the "Cardiopulmonary resuscitation, child" procedure.)
- Each time the airway is opened using a head-tilt, chin-lift maneuver, look for an object in the patient's mouth.[1] Remove the object, if seen.[1]

NURSING ALERT Never perform a blind finger-sweep to retrieve an object from a patient's airway, *because you could push the object farther into the airway instead of removing it.* Remove visible objects only.[1]

- Attempt to ventilate the patient and follow with 30 chest compressions; continue CPR until the object is expelled.[1]
- Examine the patient for injuries resulting from the procedure, such as ruptured or lacerated abdominal or thoracic viscera.

For an infant

- Determine whether the infant has a severe foreign body object obstruction. *If it's severe, the infant won't be able to cough or make a sound.*[2]
- If severe obstruction exists, place the infant face down so that the infant is straddling your arm with head lower than trunk.[2]
- Rest your forearm on your thigh and deliver five back blows with the heel of your hand between the infant's shoulder blades (as shown below).[2]

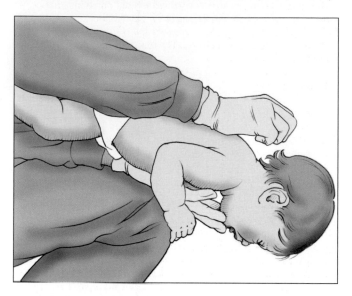

- If the back blows don't remove the obstruction, place your free hand on the infant's back.
- Supporting the neck, jaw, and chest with your other hand, turn the infant over onto your thigh, keeping the infant's head lower than the trunk.
- Imagine a line between the infant's nipples and place the index finger of your free hand on the sternum, just below this imaginary line. Then place your middle and ring fingers next to your index finger and lift the index finger off the infant's chest (as shown below).[2]

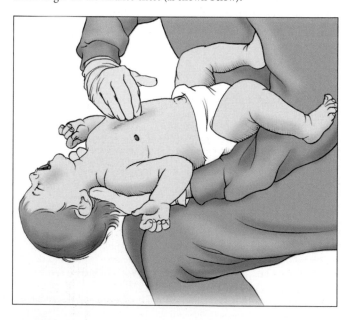

- Perform five chest thrusts as you would for chest compression, but at a slower rate.[2]
- Repeat the above steps until you've dislodged the obstruction or the infant becomes unconscious.
- If the infant becomes unconscious, call for help and start to perform CPR beginning with chest compressions.[2] (See the "Cardiopulmonary resuscitation, infant" procedure.)
- After performing 30 chest compressions, open the infant's airway.[2]

- Before performing CPR rescue breaths, look in the infant's mouth. If you see the foreign body, remove it. Never perform a blind finger-sweep on an infant, *because it may push the foreign body further back into the pharynx and damage the oropharynx.*[2]
- If you can't see the foreign object, attempt ventilations on the infant and follow with chest compressions at a rate of 30 chest compressions to two ventilations until the object is removed.[2]
- Activate the emergency response system after 2 minutes if no one else has done so.[2] Continue with CPR until the emergency response or code team arrives.

Completing the procedure
- Perform hand hygiene.[3,4,5,6,7,8]
- Document the procedure.[9,10,11,12]

Special considerations
- If the patient vomits during abdominal thrusts, quickly wipe out the patient's mouth with your fingers and resume the maneuver, as necessary.
- Even if your efforts to clear the airway don't seem to be effective, keep trying. *As oxygen deprivation increases, smooth and skeletal muscles relax, making your maneuvers more likely to succeed.*
- When performing chest compressions on most children, you should compress the chest about 2" (5 cm). On an infant, compress the chest about 1½" (4 cm). Allow complete chest recoil between compressions, and minimize interruptions. When a second rescuer arrives, perform the interventions at a rate of 15 chest compressions to 2 ventilations. Rotate who performs chest compressions every 2 minutes *to prevent fatigue.*[2]

Complications
Nausea, regurgitation, bruising, and achiness may develop after the patient can breathe independently. The patient may also be injured, possibly from incorrect placement of the rescuer's hands, or because of osteoporosis or metastatic lesions that increase the risk of fracture. Prolonged anoxia may lead to brain damage and death.

Documentation
Document all emergency response procedures in a timeline, including the names of people present, interventions you performed, and the patient's response. Record the patient's actions before the obstruction, whether anyone witnessed the event, the approximate length of time the interventions took to clear the airway, and the type and size of the object you removed. Also note your assessment findings after the procedure, any complications, the name of the practitioner you notified, the time of notification, the prescribed interventions, and the patient's response to those interventions.

REFERENCES

1 American Heart Association. Web-based integrated guidelines for cardiopulmonary resuscitation and emergency cardiovascular care—part 5: Adult basic life support and cardiopulmonary resuscitation. https://ECCguidelines.heart.org (Level II)
2 American Heart Association. Web-based integrated guidelines for cardiopulmonary resuscitation and emergency cardiovascular care—part 11: Pediatric basic life support and cardiopulmonary resuscitation quality. https://ECCguidelines.heart.org (Level II)
3 The Joint Commission. (2021). Standard NPSG.07.01.01. *Comprehensive accreditation manual for hospitals.* Oakbrook Terrace, IL: The Joint Commission. (Level VII)
4 Centers for Disease Control and Prevention. (2002). Guideline for hand hygiene in health-care settings: Recommendations of the Healthcare Infection Control Practices Advisory Committee and the HICPAC/SHEA/APIC/IDSA Hand Hygiene Task Force. *MMWR Recommendations and Reports, 51*(RR-16), 1–45. https://www.cdc.gov/mmwr/pdf/rr/rr5116.pdf (Level II)
5 World Health Organization. (2009). WHO guidelines on hand hygiene in health care: First global patient safety challenge, clean care is safer care. https://apps.who.int/iris/bitstream/handle/10665/44102/9789241597906_eng.pdf?sequence=1 (Level IV)

6 Accreditation Association for Hospitals and Health Systems. (2020). Standard 07.01.21. *Healthcare Facilities Accreditation Program: Accreditation requirements for acute care hospitals.* Chicago, IL: Accreditation Association for Hospitals and Health Systems. (Level VII)

7 Centers for Medicare and Medicaid Services, Department of Health and Human Services. (2020). Condition of participation: Infection control. 42 C.F.R. § 482.42.

8 DNV GL-Healthcare USA, Inc. (2020). IC.1.SR.1. *NIAHO® accreditation requirements, interpretive guidelines and surveyor guidance—revision 20.0.* Milford, OH: DNV GL-Healthcare USA, Inc. (Level VII)

9 The Joint Commission. (2021). Standard RC.01.03.01. *Comprehensive accreditation manual for hospitals.* Oakbrook Terrace, IL: The Joint Commission. (Level VII)

10 Accreditation Association for Hospitals and Health Systems. (2020). Standard 10.00.03. *Healthcare Facilities Accreditation Program: Accreditation requirements for acute care hospitals.* Chicago, IL: Accreditation Association for Hospitals and Health Systems. (Level VII)

11 Centers for Medicare and Medicaid Services, Department of Health and Human Services. (2020). Condition of participation: Medical record services. 42 C.F.R. § 482.24(b).

12 DNV GL-Healthcare USA, Inc. (2020). MR.2.SR.1. *NIAHO® accreditation requirements, interpretive guidelines and surveyor guidance—revision 20.0.* Milford, OH: DNV GL-Healthcare USA, Inc. (Level VII)

FUNCTIONAL ASSESSMENT

A functional assessment is used to evaluate a patient's overall well-being, mobility, and self-care abilities. It helps identify individual needs and care deficits, provides a basis for developing a care plan that enhances the abilities of an adult with coexisting disease and chronic illness, and provides feedback about treatment and rehabilitation. The goal of a functional assessment is to help a patient maintain independence by matching needs with such services as housekeeping, home health care, and day care. Several tools are available to help perform a methodical functional assessment. Become familiar with the functional assessment tool used in your facility.

The Katz Index of Independence in Activities of Daily Living is a widely used tool for evaluating a person's ability to perform six daily personal care activities: bathing, dressing, toileting, transferring, maintaining continence, and feeding. It describes functional level at a specific point in time and objectively assigns a total score based on points accrued for dependence or independence in each of the six functional areas. (See *Katz Index of Independence in Activities of Daily Living*.)

Another widely used tool, the Lawton Instrumental Activities of Daily Living Scale, evaluates a person's ability to perform more complex personal care activities. It addresses the activities needed to support independent living, such as the ability to use a telephone, cook, shop, do laundry, manage finances, take medications, and prepare meals. Each of the activities is rated on a three-point scale, ranging from independence to complete disability. When using the Lawton scale, make sure you evaluate the patient in terms of safety. For example, a person may be able to cook a small meal but may leave the stove burner on after cooking.[2,3]

The Barthel Index is commonly used in rehabilitation settings to assess the person's need for assistance with activities of daily living and to document improvement in the patient's abilities. The Barthel Index ranks functional status as either dependent or independent on the following 10 self-care functions: feeding, moving from wheelchair to bed and returning, performing personal toileting, getting on and off the toilet, bathing, walking on a level surface or propelling a wheelchair, going up and down stairs, dressing and undressing, maintaining bowel continence, and maintaining bladder control. Each item is scored according to the degree of assistance needed; over time, results reveal improvement or decline.[4] A similar scale, called the Barthel Self-Care Rating Scale, is a more detailed evaluation of function. Both tools provide information to help you determine the type of assistance needed.

Katz Index of Independence in Activities of Daily Living

Evaluation form

Name:
Date:
For each area of functioning listed below, assign a score of 1 point if the patient is independent (requires no supervision, direction, or personal assistance) and 0 points if the patient is dependent (requires supervision, direction, personal assistance, or total care).[1]

ACTIVITIES	INDEPENDENCE	DEPENDENCE
Bathing Points: _____	1 point—Bathes self completely or needs help in bathing only a single part of the body, such as the back, genital area, or disabled extremity.	0 points—Needs help with bathing more than one part of the body, with getting in or out of the tub or shower, or for total bathing.
Dressing Points: _____	1 point—Gets clothes from closets and drawers and puts on clothes and outer garments complete with fasteners; may need helping tying shoes.	0 points—Needs help with dressing self or needs to be completely dressed.
Toileting Points: _____	1 point—Goes to toilet, gets on and off, arranges clothes, and cleans genital area without help.	0 points—Needs help transferring to the toilet or cleaning self or uses a bedpan or commode.
Transferring Points: _____	1 point—Moves in and out of bed or chair unassisted; use of mechanical transferring aids is acceptable.	0 points—Needs help moving from bed to chair or requires a complete transfer.
Continence Points: _____	1 point—Exercises complete self-control over urination and defecation.	0 points—Is partially or totally incontinent of bowel or bladder.
Feeding Points: _____	1 point—Gets food from plate into mouth without help; another person may prepare the food.	0 points—Needs partial or total help with feeding or requires parenteral feeding.

Total Points: _____

6 POINTS = HIGH (PATIENT INDEPENDENT)
0 POINTS = LOW (PATIENT VERY DEPENDENT)

Adapted with permission from the Gerontological Society of America (2012).

A standardized assessment tool called the Minimum Data Set (MDS) was developed by the Centers for Medicare and Medicaid Services' (CMS's) Nursing Home Quality Initiative to make patient assessments more consistent and reliable throughout the country. The MDS includes assessment information that can be used to identify potential nutritional problems, risk factors, and potential for improved function. The use of this tool is required in all extended-care facilities that receive federal funding. MDS 3.0, the latest version of the MDS, offers better reliability and accuracy than previous versions, and includes the patient in the assessment process.[5]

The Outcome and Assessment Information Set (current version: OASIS-D1),[6] is a standardized form required by the Health Care Financing Administration for Medicare-certified agencies. The OASIS was developed to measure outcomes for adults who receive home care. It allows the collection of data to measure changes in a patient's health status over time. Providing a comprehensive assessment, this tool encompasses a patient's diagnoses, living arrangements, sensory status, skin integrity, cardiorespiratory status, bowel and bladder concerns, cognition and behavior, self-care, transferring and ambulation ability, eating and swallowing ability, communication ability, and list of medications. Typically, OASIS data are collected when a patient starts home care, at the 60-day recertification point, and when a patient is discharged or transferred to another facility, such as a hospital or subacute care facility.[7] OASIS is also used in the new Patient-Driven Grouping Model set by the CMS. It dictates the functional impairment level that, when combined with other information (such as admission source, timing of the 30-day period, clinical grouping, and comorbidity adjustment), helps determine the payment for each 30-day period.[8]

Equipment

Facility-approved functional assessment tool.

Implementation

- Perform hand hygiene.[9,10,11,12,13,14]
- Confirm the patient's identity using at least two patient identifiers.[15]
- Provide privacy.[16,17,18,19]
- Explain the procedure to the patient and family (if appropriate), including the location where it will take place (such as in a hospital room or a treatment room), according to their individual communication and learning needs *to increase their understanding, allay their fears, and enhance cooperation.*[20]
- Review the patient's health history *to obtain subjective data about the patient and insight into problem areas and subtle physical changes.*
- Obtain biographical data, including the patient's name, age, and birth date, if not already provided.
- Using a facility-approved functional assessment tool, ask the patient to answer the questions. If the patient is unable to answer, ask a caregiver to do so.
- Perform hand hygiene.[9,10,11,12,13,14]
- Document the procedure.[21,22,23,24]

Special considerations

- Physical therapists also perform functional assessments.

Documentation

Document all assessment findings according to your facility's assessment scale.

References

1 Katz, S., et al. (1970). Progress in the development of the index of ADL. *Gerontologist, 10*, 20–30.

2 Lawton, M. P., & Brody, E. M. (1969). Assessment of older people: Self-maintaining and instrumental activities of daily living. *Gerontologist, 9*, 179–186.

3 Coyne, R. (n.d.). The Lawton Instrumental Activities of Daily Living (IADL) Scale. https://hign.org/consultgeri/try-this-series/lawton-instrumental-activities-daily-living-iadl-scale

4 Mahoney, F. I., & Barthel, D. W. (1965). Functional evaluation: The Barthel Index. *Maryland State Medical Journal, 14*, 56–61. (Level VII)

5 Centers for Medicare and Medicaid Services, Department of Health and Human Services. (2020). MDS 3.0 for nursing homes and swing bed providers. https://www.cms.gov/Medicare/Quality-Initiatives-Patient-Assessment-Instruments/NursingHomeQualityInits/NHQIMDS30.html

6 Centers for Medicare and Medicaid Services, Department of Health and Human Services. (2020). OASIS-D1: OASIS update for CY 2020. https://www.cms.gov/Medicare/Quality-Initiatives-Patient-Assessment-Instruments/HomeHealthQualityInits/Downloads/OASIS-D1-Update-Memorandum_Revised_May-2019.pdf

7 Centers for Medicare and Medicaid Services, Department of Health and Human Services. (2019). OASIS user manuals. https://www.cms.gov/Medicare/Quality-Initiatives-Patient-Assessment-Instruments/HomeHealthQualityInits/HHQIOASISUserManual

8 Centers for Medicare and Medicaid Services, Department of Health and Human Services. (n.d.). Patient-driven groupings model. https://www.cms.gov/Medicare/Medicare-Fee-for-Service-Payment/HomeHealthPPS/Downloads/Overview-of-the-Patient-Driven-Groupings-Model.pdf

9 The Joint Commission. (2021). Standard NPSG.07.01.01. *Comprehensive accreditation manual for hospitals.* Oakbrook Terrace, IL: The Joint Commission. (Level VII)

10 World Health Organization. (2009). WHO guidelines on hand hygiene in health care: First global patient safety challenge, clean care is safer care. https://apps.who.int/iris/bitstream/handle/10665/44102/9789241597906_eng.pdf?sequence=1 (Level IV)

11 Centers for Disease Control and Prevention. (2002). Guideline for hand hygiene in health-care settings: Recommendations of the Healthcare Infection Control Practices Advisory Committee and the HICPAC/SHEA/APIC/IDSA Hand Hygiene Task Force. *MMWR Recommendations and Reports, 51*(RR-16), 1–45. https://www.cdc.gov/mmwr/pdf/rr/rr5116.pdf (Level II)

12 Centers for Medicare and Medicaid Services, Department of Health and Human Services. (2020). Condition of participation: Infection control. 42 C.F.R. § 482.42.

13 Accreditation Association for Hospitals and Health Systems. (2020). Standard 07.01.21. *Healthcare Facilities Accreditation Program: Accreditation requirements for acute care hospitals.* Chicago, IL: Accreditation Association for Hospitals and Health Systems. (Level VII)

14 DNV GL-Healthcare USA, Inc. (2020). IC.1.SR.1. *NIAHO® accreditation requirements, interpretive guidelines and surveyor guidance—revision 20.0.* Milford, OH: DNV GL-Healthcare USA, Inc. (Level VII)

15 The Joint Commission. (2021). Standard NPSG.01.01.01. *Comprehensive accreditation manual for hospitals.* Oakbrook Terrace, IL: The Joint Commission. (Level VII)

16 The Joint Commission. (2021). Standard RI.01.01.01. *Comprehensive accreditation manual for hospitals.* Oakbrook Terrace, IL: The Joint Commission. (Level VII)

17 Centers for Medicare and Medicaid Services, Department of Health and Human Services. (2020). Condition of participation: Patient's rights. 42 C.F.R. 482.13(c)(1).

18 Accreditation Association for Hospitals and Health Systems. (2020). Standard 15.01.16. *Healthcare Facilities Accreditation Program: Accreditation requirements for acute care hospitals.* Chicago, IL: Accreditation Association for Hospitals and Health Systems. (Level VII)

19 DNV GL-Healthcare USA, Inc. (2020). PR.2.SR.5. *NIAHO® accreditation requirements, interpretive guidelines and surveyor guidance—revision 20.0* Milford, OH: DNV GL-Healthcare USA, Inc. (Level VII)

20 The Joint Commission. (2021). Standard PC.02.01.21. *Comprehensive accreditation manual for hospitals.* Oakbrook Terrace, IL: The Joint Commission. (Level VII)

21 The Joint Commission. (2021). Standard RC.01.03.01. *Comprehensive accreditation manual for hospitals.* Oakbrook Terrace, IL: The Joint Commission. (Level VII)

22 Centers for Medicare and Medicaid Services, Department of Health and Human Services. (2020). Condition of participation: Medical record services. 42 C.F.R. § 482.24(b).

23 Accreditation Association for Hospitals and Health Systems. (2020). Standard 10.00.03. *Healthcare Facilities Accreditation Program: Accreditation requirements for acute care hospitals.* Chicago, IL: Accreditation Association for Hospitals and Health Systems. (Level VII)

24 DNV GL-Healthcare USA, Inc. (2020). MR.2.SR.1. *NIAHO® accreditation requirements, interpretive guidelines and surveyor guidance—revision 20.0.* Milford, OH: DNV GL-Healthcare USA, Inc. (Level VII)

GAIT BELT USE

A gait belt is a safety device made of cloth or plastic that buckles securely around a patient's waist. The device provides a secure grasping surface to aid with patient transfer and ambulation.[1] Commonly used for patients who are at risk for falling, a gait belt can help safely lower a patient to the ground if the patient begins to fall or loses balance during transfer or ambulation. When combined with proper body mechanics, a gait belt also improves caregiver safety by preventing back injury.

Before gait belt use, assess the patient for contraindications, including recent abdominal, back, or chest surgery or trauma; hernia; severe cardiac or respiratory conditions; abdominal aneurysm; or the presence of a gastrostomy tube or other equipment.[2]

NURSING ALERT Never use a gait belt if there is any compromise of safety to staff or the patient.[2] Such situations may include a patient demonstrating behavioral aggression (such as a patient experiencing alcohol withdrawal or possible use of the gait belt as a weapon) or patients at risk for suicide.[3]

Equipment

Shoes or slippers with nonskid soles ■ robe ■ gait belt ■ vital signs monitoring equipment ■ wheelchair, commode, or chair ■ Optional: assistive device (walker, cane, crutches), prescribed pain medication.

Preparation of equipment

Inspect all equipment and supplies. If a product is expired, is defective, or has compromised integrity, remove it from patient use, label it as expired or defective, and report the expiration or defect as directed by your facility. Check for proper buckle closure and test the buckle *to make sure that it doesn't slip when you pull on it.* Make sure that the bed and wheelchair, if used, are in a locked position.[4]

Implementation

■ Perform hand hygiene.[5,6,7,8,9,10]
■ Confirm the patient's identity using at least two patient identifiers.[11]
■ Provide privacy.[12,13,14,15]
■ Explain the procedure to the patient and family (if appropriate) according to their communication and learning needs *to increase their understanding, allay their fears, and enhance cooperation.*[16]
■ Assess the patient's risk of falling and tolerance of recent activities. Check for any conditions that would contraindicate gait belt use.[2,3,17,18]
■ Obtain the patient's vital signs *to serve as a baseline for comparison.*
■ Screen for and assess the patient's pain using facility-defined criteria that are consistent with the patient's age, condition, and ability to understand.[19]
■ Treat the patient's pain, as needed and ordered, using nonpharmacologic, pharmacologic, or a combination of approaches. Base the treatment plan on evidence-based practices and the patient's clinical condition, past medical history, and pain management goals.[19]
■ Assist the patient to a comfortable sitting position; then allow for a brief rest *to help the patient adjust to postural changes.*[20]
■ Help the patient put on a robe, *to maintain dignity,* and appropriate footwear, such as shoes or slippers with nonskid soles, *to reduce the risk of falling.*[4]
■ Wrap the gait belt around the patient's waist and over any clothing, with the buckle facing front.
■ Adjust the belt so that it fits snugly around the patient's waist (as shown above on right). Slide your open hand between the belt and the patient *to make sure that the device fits snugly but isn't too tight.*[2]

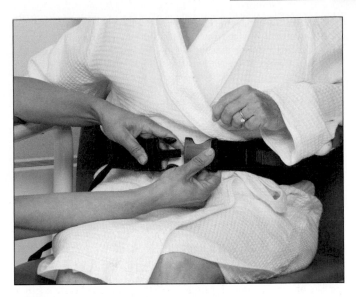

HOSPITAL-ACQUIRED CONDITION ALERT Keep in mind that the Centers for Medicare and Medicaid Services considers an injury from a fall a hospital-acquired condition, *because it can be reasonably prevented using a variety of best practices.* Make sure to follow evidence-based fall prevention practices, such as performing a fall risk assessment and instituting fall precautions, *to reduce the risk of injury from patient falls.*[4,17,21]

■ Keep clothing as wrinkle-free as possible under the gait belt *to prevent skin breakdown.*

Transferring the patient

■ If the patient has one-sided weakness, position the destination surface (wheelchair, commode, or chair) on the patient's unaffected side. If the destination surface has wheels, make sure the wheels are locked.[4]
■ Position yourself close to the patient so that you're facing each other.
■ Grasp both sides of the gait belt using an underhand grip.
■ While firmly gripping the gait belt, keep your back straight, bend your knees slightly, position your feet in a wide stance *to maintain proper body mechanics* (as shown below),[22] and begin rocking back and forth *to overcome forces resisting transfer.* Instruct the patient, on a count of three, to push off the bed or other surface *to encourage independence.*

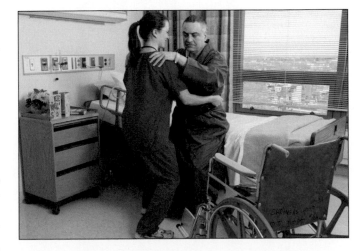

■ Allow the patient to stand for a moment *to ensure balance.*
■ Instruct the patient to pivot and to bear as much weight as possible on the unaffected side. Support the affected side, *because the patient will tend to lean to this side.*
■ Pivot on your back foot, guiding the patient to the destination surface. Make sure that the backs of the patient's legs make contact with the destination surface *to help ensure proper positioning before the patient sits.*

■ Keeping a firm grip on the gait belt, gently lower the patient onto the destination surface. Instruct the patient to reach and grasp the armrests (as shown below), using them to bear some weight, if possible. Flex your knees and hips while assisting the patient onto the destination surface. *Using good body mechanics prevents back injury by supporting weight with large muscle groups.*[22]

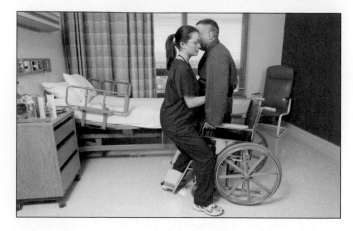

Ambulating the patient
■ Position yourself close to the patient so that you're facing each other.
■ Grasp both sides of the gait belt using an underhand grip.
■ While firmly gripping the gait belt, keep your back straight, bend your knees slightly, position your feet in a wide stance *to maintain proper body mechanics,*[22] and begin rocking back and forth *to overcome forces resisting transfer.* Instruct the patient to push off of the bed or other surface on a count of three *to encourage independence.*
■ Allow the patient to stand for a moment *to ensure balance.*
■ Place one hand under the gait belt in back of the patient. If the patient is weaker on one side, make sure to walk on that side when ambulating (as shown below), *because the patient will tend to lean to this side.* Encourage the patient to use a handrail or assistive device, if available.

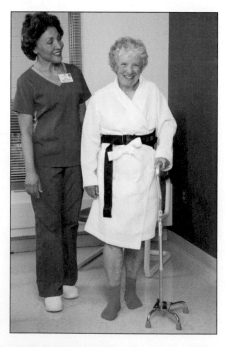

■ Walk closely behind and slightly to the side of the patient, keeping the same pattern and pace as the patient.
■ Allow for rest periods as needed.

Completing the procedure
■ Remove the gait belt after use *to prevent patient harm.*
■ Store the gait belt at the patient's bedside for immediate use.

■ Perform hand hygiene.[5,6,7,8,9,10]
■ Document the procedure.[23,24,25,26]

Special considerations
■ Don't leave a gait belt applied to a patient who's unattended in a chair or bed. *The gait belt could become displaced and result in strangulation or other patient injury.*
■ If the patient is morbidly obese or can't bear weight, consider using lift equipment to transfer the patient instead *to ensure patient safety and prevent caregiver injury.*[20]
■ If the patient loses weight-bearing ability during ambulation or transfer, maintain your grip on the gait belt,[20] pull the patient as close to your body as possible, and gently slide the patient to the floor using the large muscles in your upper leg. Call for assistance, and have the assistant help you place the patient back into the chair or bed or in another sitting position.
■ Before ambulation, decide with the patient the distance the patient can walk and your destination. *Planning helps ensure safety.*[20]

Documentation
Document the patient's tolerance of the procedure, the distance that the patient ambulated (if applicable), and any complications. If complications occurred, record the date and time you notified the practitioner, the name of the practitioner, the prescribed interventions, and the patient's response to those interventions. Document teaching provided to the patient and family (if applicable), their understanding of that teaching, and any need for follow-up teaching.

REFERENCES
1 Occupational Safety and Health Administration, Department of Labor. (2003, revised 2009). *Guidelines for nursing homes: Ergonomics for the prevention of musculoskeletal disorders* (OSHA Publication No. 3182-3R 2009). Washington, DC: Occupational Safety and Health Administration. https://www.osha.gov/sites/default/files/publications/final_nh_guidelines.pdf (Level I)
2 Posey Company. (2010). Instructions for Posey® gait and transfer belts. https://www.rehabmart.com/pdfs/m1358-posey-gait-and-transfer-belts.pdf
3 Wintersgill, W. (2019). Gait belts 101: A tool for patient and nurse safety. *American Nurse Today, 14*(5), 31–34. https://www.myamericannurse.com/wp-content/uploads/2019/05/ant5-Focus-Safety-Options-gait-belts-425.pdf
4 Ganz, D. A., et al. (2013, reviewed 2021). *Preventing falls in hospitals: A toolkit for improving quality of care* (AHRQ Publication No. 13-0015-EF). Rockville, MD: Agency for Healthcare Research and Quality. https://www.ahrq.gov/professionals/systems/hospital/fallpxtoolkit/index.html (Level VII)
5 Centers for Disease Control and Prevention. (2002). Guideline for hand hygiene in health-care settings: Recommendations of the Healthcare Infection Control Practices Advisory Committee and the HICPAC/SHEA/APIC/IDSA Hand Hygiene Task Force. *MMWR Recommendations and Reports, 51*(RR-16), 1–45. https://www.cdc.gov/mmwr/pdf/rr/rr5116.pdf (Level II)
6 World Health Organization. (2009). WHO guidelines on hand hygiene in health care: First global patient safety challenge, clean care is safer care. https://apps.who.int/iris/bitstream/handle/10665/44102/9789241597906_eng.pdf?sequence=1 (Level IV)
7 The Joint Commission. (2021). Standard NPSG.07.01.01. *Comprehensive accreditation manual for hospitals.* Oakbrook Terrace, IL: The Joint Commission. (Level VII)
8 Centers for Medicare and Medicaid Services, Department of Health and Human Services. (2020). Condition of participation: Infection control. 42 C.F.R. § 482.42.
9 Accreditation Association for Hospitals and Health Systems. (2020). Standard 07.01.21. *Healthcare Facilities Accreditation Program: Accreditation requirements for acute care hospitals.* Chicago, IL: Accreditation Association for Hospitals and Health Systems. (Level VII)
10 DNV GL-Healthcare USA, Inc. (2020). IC.1.SR.1. *NIAHO® accreditation requirements, interpretive guidelines and surveyor guidance—revision 20.0.* Milford, OH: DNV GL-Healthcare USA, Inc. (Level VII)
11 The Joint Commission. (2021). Standard NPSG.01.01.01. *Comprehensive accreditation manual for hospitals.* Oakbrook Terrace, IL: The Joint Commission. (Level VII)

12 Accreditation Association for Hospitals and Health Systems. (2020). Standard 15.01.16. *Healthcare Facilities Accreditation Program: Accreditation requirements for acute care hospitals*. Chicago, IL: Accreditation Association for Hospitals and Health Systems. (Level VII)

13 Centers for Medicare and Medicaid Services, Department of Health and Human Services. (2020). Condition of participation: Patient's rights. 42 C.F.R. § 482.13(c)(1).

14 DNV GL-Healthcare USA, Inc. (2020). PR.2.SR.5. *NIAHO® accreditation requirements, interpretive guidelines and surveyor guidance – revision 20.0*. Milford, OH: DNV GL-Healthcare USA, Inc. (Level VII)

15 The Joint Commission. (2021). Standard RI.01.01.01. *Comprehensive accreditation manual for hospitals*. Oakbrook Terrace, IL: The Joint Commission. (Level VII)

16 The Joint Commission. (2021). Standard PC.02.01.21. *Comprehensive accreditation manual for hospitals*. Oakbrook Terrace, IL: The Joint Commission. (Level VII)

17 The Joint Commission. (2021). Standard PC.01.02.08. *Comprehensive accreditation manual for hospitals*. Oakbrook Terrace, IL: The Joint Commission. (Level VII)

18 Accreditation Association for Hospitals and Health Systems. (2020). Standard 16.02.02. *Healthcare Facilities Accreditation Program: Accreditation requirements for acute care hospitals*. Chicago, IL: Accreditation Association for Hospitals and Health Systems. (Level VII)

19 The Joint Commission. (2021). Standard PC.01.02.07. *Comprehensive accreditation manual for hospitals*. Oakbrook Terrace, IL: The Joint Commission. (Level VII)

20 Craven, R. F., et al. (2020). *Fundamentals of nursing: Concepts and competencies for practice* (9th ed.). Philadelphia, PA: Wolters Kluwer.

21 Jarrett, N., & Callaham, M. (2016). Evidence-based guidelines for selected hospital-acquired conditions: Final report. https://www.cms.gov/Medicare/Medicare-Fee-for-Service-Payment/HospitalAcqCond/Downloads/2016-HAC-Report.pdf

22 Waters, T. R., et al. (2009). Safe patient handling training for schools of nursing. https://www.cdc.gov/niosh/docs/2009-127/pdfs/2009-127.pdf (Level VII)

23 The Joint Commission. (2021). Standard RC.01.03.01. *Comprehensive accreditation manual for hospitals*. Oakbrook Terrace, IL: The Joint Commission. (Level VII)

24 Accreditation Association for Hospitals and Health Systems. (2020). Standard 10.00.03. *Healthcare Facilities Accreditation Program: Accreditation requirements for acute care hospitals*. Chicago, IL: Accreditation Association for Hospitals and Health Systems. (Level VII)

25 Centers for Medicare and Medicaid Services, Department of Health and Human Services. (2020). Condition of participation: Medical record services. 42 C.F.R. § 482.24(b).

26 DNV GL-Healthcare USA, Inc. (2020). MR.2.SR.1. *NIAHO® accreditation requirements, interpretive guidelines and surveyor guidance – revision 20.0*. Milford, OH: DNV GL-Healthcare USA, Inc. (Level VII)

GASTRIC LAVAGE

Gastric lavage flushes the stomach and removes ingested substances through a tube. The procedure can help empty the stomach in preparation for endoscopic examination or after poisoning or a drug overdose, especially in patients who have an inadequate gag reflex. However, the American Academy of Clinical Toxicology and the European Association of Poison Centres and Clinical Toxicologists have concluded that routinely using gastric lavage isn't appropriate, *because the risks associated with gastric lavage outweigh the benefits in certain situations; the use of gastric lavage may delay treatment with activated charcoal and other therapies, and it may cause serious complications.*[1,2,3]

Gastric lavage should be performed in the emergency department or the intensive care unit by a practitioner, gastroenterologist, or nurse who has received proper training.[1,3,4] A large-bore lavage tube may be inserted by a gastroenterologist.

This procedure is contraindicated after ingestion of a corrosive substance (such as lye, petroleum distillates, ammonia, alkalis, or mineral acids), *because the gastric tube may perforate or cause trauma to the already compromised esophagus.*[1] It's also contraindicated for patients with an unprotected airway or craniofacial abnormalities or injuries, central nervous system depression, increased risk and severity of aspiration from lavage, and risk of hemorrhage or gastrointestinal perforation due to pathology or recent surgery, as well as when a patient resists or refuses to cooperate.[1] Gastric lavage used to manage upper GI hemorrhage is controversial.[5] Studies show that it allows endoscopy to be performed more quickly, but it doesn't affect clinical outcomes.[6]

NURSING ALERT Correct lavage tube placement is essential, *because accidental misplacement (in the lungs, for example) followed by lavage can be fatal.*

Equipment

2 to 3 L of normal saline solution, tap water, or appropriate antidote, as ordered ▪ graduated container ▪ Ewald tube or any large-lumen gastric tube, typically #34 to #40 French (See *Using wide-bore gastric tubes*, page 362.) ▪ connection tubing ▪ intermittent suction setup ▪ water-soluble lubricant or anesthetic ointment ▪ emesis basin ▪ ½″ (1.3 cm) hypoallergenic tape ▪ 60 mL enteral, oral, or prepackaged syringe irrigation kit ▪ gloves ▪ mask and goggles or mask with face shield ▪ gown ▪ fluid-impermeable pad or towel ▪ Yankauer (tonsil tip) suction device attached to suction ▪ cardiac monitor ▪ pulse oximeter and probe ▪ automated blood pressure cuff ▪ stethoscope▪ disinfectant pad ▪ emergency equipment (code cart with emergency medications, defibrillator, hand-held resuscitation bag with mask, oxygen source, intubation equipment) ▪ Optional: charcoal tablets or solution.

Preparation of equipment

Ensure emergency equipment is readily available and functioning properly. Set up the lavage and suction equipment. Lubricate the end of the gastric tube with the water-soluble lubricant or anesthetic ointment. Set up the Yankauer (tonsil tip) catheter for oropharyngeal suctioning.

Inspect all equipment and supplies. If a product has expired, is defective, or is compromised, remove it from patient use, label it as expired or defective, and report the expiration or defect as directed by your facility.

Implementation

▪ Verify the practitioner's order.
▪ Gather and prepare the appropriate equipment and supplies.
▪ Perform hand hygiene.[7,8,9,10,11,12]
▪ Confirm the patient's identity using at least two patient identifiers.[13]
▪ Provide privacy.[14,15,16,17]
▪ Explain the procedure to the patient and family members (if appropriate) according to their individual communication and learning needs *to increase their understanding, allay their fears, and enhance cooperation.*[18]
▪ Raise the patient's bed to waist level before providing patient care *to avoid caregiver back strain.*[19]
▪ Perform hand hygiene.[7,8,9,10,11,12]
▪ Attach the patient to a cardiac monitor, automated blood pressure cuff, and pulse oximeter *for monitoring during the procedure.*[20] Ensure that the alarm limits are set appropriately for the patient's current condition, and that the alarms are turned on, functioning properly, and audible to staff.[21,22,23,24]
▪ Obtain the patient's vital signs and the oxygen saturation level using pulse oximetry, and assess the patient's level of consciousness, *to serve as a baseline for comparison.*[20]
▪ Assess the patient's cardiac status (including the cardiac rhythm) and respiratory status *to serve as a baseline.*[20]
▪ Perform hand hygiene.[7,8,9,10,11,12]
▪ Put on a gown, gloves, and a mask and goggles or mask with face shield *to comply with standard precautions.*[25,26,27]
▪ Drape a fluid-impermeable pad or a towel over the patient's chest *to protect the patient's gown from soiling.*[20]
▪ Place the patient in the semi-Fowler position, ensuring the head of the bed is elevated 10 to 20 degrees, creating a slight reverse-Trendelenburg position.[20]
▪ Place the patient in the left lateral decubitus position *to increase access to the stomach, decrease pyloric emptying, and prevent aspiration should the patient vomit.*[20]
▪ Insert or wait for the practitioner to insert the gastric tube nasally or orally and then advance it slowly and gently, *because forceful insertion may injure tissues.*

EQUIPMENT

Using wide-bore gastric tubes

If you need to deliver a large volume of fluid rapidly through a gastric tube (for example, when irrigating the stomach of a patient with profuse gastric bleeding or poisoning), a wide-bore gastric tube usually serves best. Typically inserted orally, these tubes remain in place only long enough to complete the lavage and evacuate stomach contents.

Ewald tube
In an emergency, using an Ewald tube (a single-lumen tube with several openings at the distal end) allows you to aspirate large amounts of gastric contents quickly.

Levacuator tube
The Levacuator tube has two lumens. Use the larger lumen for evacuating gastric contents; use the smaller one for instilling an irrigant.

Edlich tube
The single-lumen Edlich tube has four openings near the closed distal tip. A funnel or syringe can be connected at the proximal end. Like the Ewald tube, the Edlich tube lets you withdraw large quantities of gastric contents quickly.

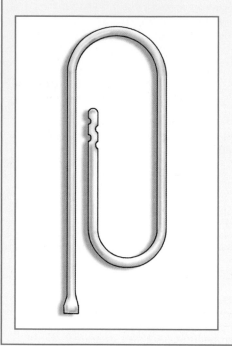 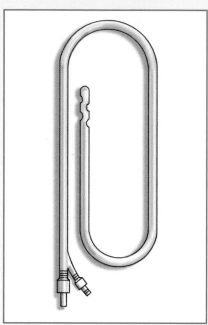 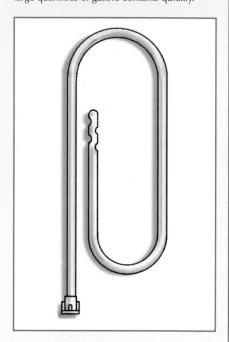

■ *Because the patient may vomit when the gastric tube reaches the posterior pharynx,* be prepared to suction the airway immediately with a Yankauer (tonsil tip) suction device.[1]

■ Confirm the gastric tube's placement by aspirating the patient's stomach contents with a 60-mL syringe and obtaining X-ray confirmation, as ordered.[20]

■ After placement is confirmed, secure the gastric tube nasally or orally with hypoallergenic tape.

■ Trace the connection tubing from the patient to its point of origin *to ensure that it's attached to the proper port to prevent dangerous misconnections.*[28,29]

■ Aspirate the patient's stomach contents using a 60-mL syringe.

■ Begin gastric lavage by slowly instilling 200 to 300 mL of fluid (for adults) using the 60-mL syringe.[20]

■ Aspirate the irrigant with the syringe and empty it into a graduated container, or connect the gastric tube to low intermittent suction.[20]

■ Measure the outflow amount to make sure it equals at least the amount of irrigant you instilled *to prevent accidental stomach distention and vomiting.* If the drainage amount falls significantly short of the instilled amount, reposition the gastric tube until sufficient solution flows out.

■ Repeat the procedure as indicated. If the procedure is being performed for hemorrhage, repeat gastric lavage intermittently until returned fluids appear clear, *signaling that bleeding has stopped.* If the procedure is being performed for a drug overdose, repeat gastric lavage intermittently until the aspirated fluid is clear of toxic substances.[20]

■ Monitor the patient's vital signs, cardiac rhythm, oxygen saturation level, and level of consciousness (LOC) during and after the procedure.[20] *Gastric lavage has been shown to cause changes in oxygen saturation and may lead to hypoxia.*[20] Notify the practitioner of any changes.

■ If ordered, remove the lavage tube by clamping the tube and then pulling it out slowly and steadily.

■ Return the patient's bed to the lowest position *to prevent falls and maintain patient safety.*[30]

■ Dispose of used supplies in the appropriate receptacles.[27]

■ Remove and discard your gloves and other personal protective equipment.[25,27]

■ Perform hand hygiene.[7,8,9,10,11,12]

■ Clean and disinfect your stethoscope using a disinfectant pad.[31,32]

■ Perform hand hygiene.[7,8,9,10,11,12]

■ Document the procedure.[33,34,35,36]

Special considerations

■ Watch closely for airway obstruction caused by vomiting or excess oral secretions. Frequently suction the oral cavity throughout gastric lavage, as necessary, *to ensure an open airway and prevent aspiration.* Be aware that the patient may require an endotracheal tube before the procedure *to ensure an open airway and prevent aspiration, or if the patient doesn't exhibit an adequate gag reflex or is comatose.*[1]

■ If ordered, after lavage to remove poisons or drugs, mix charcoal tablets or solution with the irrigant (water or normal saline solution) and administer the mixture through the gastric tube. *The charcoal will absorb any remaining toxic substances.*[20] Depending on the practitioner's orders, the tube may be clamped temporarily, allowed to drain via gravity, attached to intermittent suction, or removed.

■ When performing gastric lavage to stop bleeding, keep precise intake and output records *to determine the amount of bleeding.*

- Be aware that, as ordered, you may need to measure serum electrolyte and arterial blood gas levels during or after gastric lavage when large volumes of fluid are instilled and withdrawn.
- The Joint Commission issued a sentinel event alert concerning medical device alarm safety, *because alarm-related events have been associated with permanent loss of function and death.* Among the major contributing factors were improper alarm settings, inappropriately turned-off alarms, and alarm signals not audible to staff. Make sure that alarm limits are set appropriately, and that alarms are turned on, functioning properly, and audible to staff. Follow facility guidelines for preventing alarm fatigue.[37]
- The Joint Commission issued a sentinel event alert related to managing risk during transition to new International Organization for Standardization tubing standards designed to prevent dangerous tubing misconnections, which can lead to serious patient injury and death. During the transition, be sure to trace each tube and catheter from the patient to its point of origin before connecting or reconnecting any device or infusion, at any care transition (such as to a new setting or service), and as part of the hand-off process. In addition, route tubes and catheters with different purposes in different, standardized directions; label tubing at the distal and proximal ends when the patient has different access sites or several bags hanging; use tubing and equipment only as intended; and store medications for different delivery routes in separate locations.[29]

Complications

Complications of gastric lavage may include aspiration pneumonia, laryngospasm, arrhythmias, esophageal and stomach perforation, fluid and electrolyte imbalances, respiratory distress, and small conjunctival hemorrhages.[1,38]

Documentation

Record the date and time of gastric lavage, the size and type of gastric tube you used, and confirmation of tube placement. Document the volume and type of irrigant you used, the amount of drained gastric contents, and your observations, including the color and consistency of the drainage. Note the patient's vital signs, cardiac rhythm, oxygen saturation level, level of consciousness, and cardiac and respiratory status before, during, and after the procedure. Document any drugs you instilled through the gastric tube, the time you removed the tube, and the patient's tolerance of the procedure. Document any adverse events, the date and time you notified the practitioner, prescribed interventions, and the patient's response to those interventions. Also document teaching you provided to the patient and family (if appropriate), their understanding of that teaching, and any need for follow-up teaching.

References

1 Benson, B. E., et al. (2013). Position paper update: Gastric lavage for gastrointestinal decontamination. *Clinical Toxicology, 51,* 140–146. (Level VII)

2 Miyauchi, M., et al. (2013). Gastric lavage guided by ultrathin transnasal esophagogastroduodenoscopy in a life-threatening case of tobacco extract poisoning: A case report. *Journal of Nippon Medical School, 80,* 307–311. https://www.jstage.jst.go.jp/article/jnms/80/4/80_307/_pdf

3 Picot, E. (2021). Poisoning: Gastric lavage. *The JBI EBP Database.* AN: JBI184.

4 Mostafazadeh, B., & Farzaneh, E. (2012). A novel protocol for gastric lavage in patients with aluminum phosphide poisoning: A double-blind study. *Acta Medica Iranica, 50,* 530–534.

5 Saltzman, J. R. (2021). Approach to acute upper gastrointestinal bleeding in adults. In: *UpToDate,* Feldman, M. (Ed.).

6 Huang, E. S., et al. (2011). Impact of nasogastric lavage on outcomes in acute GI bleeding. *Gastrointestinal Endoscopy, 74,* 971–980. (Level VI)

7 Centers for Disease Control and Prevention. (2002). Guideline for hand hygiene in health-care settings: Recommendations of the Healthcare Infection Control Practices Advisory Committee and the HICPAC/SHEA/APIC/IDSA Hand Hygiene Task Force. *MMWR Recommendations and Reports, 51*(RR-16), 1–45. https://www.cdc.gov/mmwr/pdf/rr/rr5116.pdf (Level II)

8 World Health Organization. (2009). WHO guidelines on hand hygiene in health care: First global patient safety challenge, clean care is safer care. https://apps.who.int/iris/bitstream/handle/10665/44102/9789241597906_eng.pdf?sequence=1 (Level IV)

9 The Joint Commission. (2021). Standard NPSG.07.01.01. *Comprehensive accreditation manual for hospitals.* Oakbrook Terrace, IL: The Joint Commission. (Level VII)

10 Accreditation Association for Hospitals and Health Systems. (2020). Standard 07.01.21. *Healthcare Facilities Accreditation Program: Accreditation requirements for acute care hospitals.* Chicago, IL: Accreditation Association for Hospitals and Health Systems. (Level VII)

11 Centers for Medicare and Medicaid Services, Department of Health and Human Services. (2020). Condition of participation: Infection control. 42 C.F.R. § 482.42.

12 DNV GL-Healthcare USA, Inc. (2020). IC.1.SR.1. *NIAHO® accreditation requirements, interpretive guidelines and surveyor guidance—revision 20.0.* Milford, OH: DNV GL-Healthcare USA, Inc. (Level VII)

13 The Joint Commission. (2021). Standard NPSG.01.01.01. *Comprehensive accreditation manual for hospitals.* Oakbrook Terrace, IL: The Joint Commission. (Level VII)

14 Accreditation Association for Hospitals and Health Systems. (2020). Standard 15.01.16. *Healthcare Facilities Accreditation Program: Accreditation requirements for acute care hospitals.* Chicago, IL: Accreditation Association for Hospitals and Health Systems. (Level VII)

15 Centers for Medicare and Medicaid Services, Department of Health and Human Services. (2020). Condition of participation: Patient's rights. 42 C.F.R. § 482.13(c)(1).

16 The Joint Commission. (2021). Standard RI.01.01.01. *Comprehensive accreditation manual for hospitals.* Oakbrook Terrace, IL: The Joint Commission. (Level VII)

17 DNV GL-Healthcare USA, Inc. (2020). PR.2.SR.5. *NIAHO® accreditation requirements, interpretive guidelines and surveyor guidance—revision 20.0.* Milford, OH: DNV GL-Healthcare USA, Inc. (Level VII)

18 The Joint Commission. (2021). Standard PC.02.01.21. *Comprehensive accreditation manual for hospitals.* Oakbrook Terrace, IL: The Joint Commission. (Level VII)

19 Waters, T. R., et al. (2009). Safe patient handling training for schools of nursing. https://www.cdc.gov/niosh/docs/2009-127/pdfs/2009-127.pdf (Level VII)

20 Wiegand, D. L. (2017). *AACN procedure manual for high acuity, progressive, and critical care* (7th ed.). St. Louis, MO: Elsevier.

21 American Association of Critical-Care Nurses. (2018). AACN practice alert: Managing alarms in acute care across the life span—electrocardiography and pulse oximetry. https://www.aacn.org/clinical-resources/practice-alerts/managing-alarms-in-acute-care-across-the-life-span (Level VII)

22 Graham, K. C., & Cvach, M. (2010). Monitor alarm fatigue: Standardizing use of physiological monitors and decreasing nuisance alarms. *American Journal of Critical Care, 19,* 28–37.

23 The Joint Commission. (2013). Sentinel event alert: Medical device alarm safety in hospitals. https://www.jointcommission.org/assets/1/6/SEA_50_alarms_4_26_16.pdf (Level VII)

24 The Joint Commission. (2021). Standard NPSG.06.01.01. *Comprehensive accreditation manual for hospitals.* Oakbrook Terrace, IL: The Joint Commission. (Level VII)

25 Siegel, J. D., et al. (2007, revised 2019). 2007 guideline for isolation precautions: Preventing transmission of infectious agents in healthcare settings. https://www.cdc.gov/infectioncontrol/pdf/guidelines/isolation-guidelines-H.pdf (Level II)

26 Accreditation Association for Hospitals and Health Systems. (2020). Standard 07.01.10. *Healthcare Facilities Accreditation Program: Accreditation requirements for acute care hospitals.* Chicago, IL: Accreditation Association for Hospitals and Health Systems. (Level VII)

27 Occupational Safety and Health Administration. (2019). Bloodborne pathogens, standard number 1910.1030. https://www.osha.gov/pls/oshaweb/owadisp.show_document?p_id=10051&p_table=STANDARDS (Level VII)

28 U.S. Food and Drug Administration. (2017). Examples of medical device misconnections. https://www.fda.gov/medical-devices/medical-device-connectors/examples-medical-device-misconnections

29 The Joint Commission. (2014). Sentinel event alert: Managing risk during transition to new ISO tubing connector standards. https://www.jointcommission.org/assets/1/6/SEA_53_Connectors_8_19_14_final.pdf (Level VII)

30 Ganz, D. A., et al. (2013, reviewed 2021). Preventing falls in hospitals: A toolkit for improving quality of care (AHRQ publication no. 13-0015-EF). https://www.ahrq.gov/professionals/systems/hospital/fallpxtoolkit/index.html (Level VII)

31 Rutala, W. A., et al. (2008, revised 2019). Guideline for disinfection and sterilization in healthcare facilities, 2008. https://www.cdc.gov/infectioncontrol/pdf/guidelines/disinfection-guidelines-H.pdf (Level I)

32 Accreditation Association for Hospitals and Health Systems. (2020). Standard 07.02.03. *Healthcare Facilities Accreditation Program: Accreditation requirements for acute care hospitals.* Chicago, IL: Accreditation Association for Hospitals and Health Systems. (Level VII)

33 The Joint Commission. (2021). Standard RC.01.03.01. *Comprehensive accreditation manual for hospitals.* Oakbrook Terrace, IL: The Joint Commission. (Level VII)

34 Accreditation Association for Hospitals and Health Systems. (2020). Standard 10.00.03. *Healthcare Facilities Accreditation Program: Accreditation requirements for acute care hospitals.* Chicago, IL: Accreditation Association for Hospitals and Health Systems. (Level VII)

35 Centers for Medicare and Medicaid Services, Department of Health and Human Services. (2020). Condition of participation: Medical record services. 42 C.F.R. § 482.24(b).

36 DNV GL-Healthcare USA, Inc. (2020). MR.2.SR.1. *NIAHO® accreditation requirements, interpretive guidelines and surveyor guidance – revision 20.0.* Milford, OH: DNV GL-Healthcare USA, Inc. (Level VII)

37 The Joint Commission. (2013). Sentinel event alert 50: Medical device alarm safety in hospitals. https://www.jointcommission.org/assets/1/6/SEA_50_alarms_4_26_16.pdf (Level VII)

38 Hendrickson, R. G., & Kusin, S. (2021). Gastrointestinal decontamination of the poisoned patient. In: *UpToDate*, Traub, S. J., & Burns, M. M. (Eds.).

GASTROSTOMY FEEDING BUTTON REINSERTION

A gastrostomy feeding button serves as an alternative to a standard gastrostomy tube. The low-profile feeding device is generally used for an ambulatory patient or a pediatric patient who's receiving long-term enteral feedings.[1]

Low-profile feeding devices are kept in place by either a balloon or a retention dome.[2] Here we describe reinsertion of the button that has a mushroom retention dome at one end and two wing tabs and a flexible safety plug at the other. When inserted into an established stoma, the button lies almost flush with the skin,[1] with only the tabs and the top of the safety plug visible.

The button can usually be inserted into a stoma in less than 15 minutes. Besides its cosmetic appeal, the device is easy to maintain, reduces skin irritation and breakdown, and is less likely to become dislodged or migrate than an ordinary feeding tube. A one-way antireflux valve mounted just inside the mushroom dome prevents accidental leakage of gastric contents. The manufacturer's instructions specify the frequency of button replacement.[3]

The gastrostomy feeding button is contraindicated in patients who don't have a well-established stoma tract or whose stomach has not been approximated to the stomach wall, and in patients with a stoma tract longer than 1¾″ (4.4 cm).[4,5]

Equipment

Gastrostomy feeding button of the correct size (or all three sizes, if the correct one isn't known) ▪ stoma measuring device ▪ obturator ▪ washcloth ▪ mild soap and water ▪ gauze pad ▪ water-soluble lubricant ▪ gloves.

Preparation of equipment

Inspect all equipment and supplies. If a product is expired, is defective, or has compromised integrity, remove it from patient use, label it as expired or defective, and report the expiration or defect as directed by your facility.

Implementation

▪ Verify the practitioner's order.
▪ Gather and prepare the necessary equipment and supplies.
NURSING ALERT *To reduce the risk of infection,* don't reuse a feeding button that has popped out.[4]
▪ Perform hand hygiene.[5,6,7,8,9,10]
▪ Confirm the patient's identify using at least two patient identifiers.[11]
▪ Provide privacy.[12,13,14,15]

▪ Explain the procedure to the patient and family (if appropriate) according to their individual communication and learning needs *to increase their understanding, allay their fears, and enhance cooperation.*[16]
▪ Raise the bed to waist level before providing care *to prevent caregiver back strain.*[17]
▪ Perform hand hygiene.[5,6,7,8,9,10]
▪ Position the patient to allow easy access to the stoma.
▪ Perform hand hygiene.[5,6,7,8,9,10]
▪ Put on gloves *to comply with standard precautions.*[18,19,20]
▪ Inspect the stoma site for signs of infection, such as drainage, pus, inflammation, and tenderness. If any are present, don't proceed with the procedure, and notify the practitioner.[4,21]
▪ Check the depth of the stoma using a stoma measuring device *to make sure you have a feeding button of the correct size.*[3,21] If the stoma length falls between two markings, use the one that is external to the stoma tract.[4,21]
NURSING ALERT Periodic sizing is necessary, especially in growing children, *to prevent compression injuries of the gastric mucosa or epidermis.*[3]
▪ Clean the skin around the stoma with a washcloth and mild soap and water, rinse with water, and dry completely with a gauze pad *to prevent skin breakdown.*[22]
▪ Lubricate the obturator with a water-soluble lubricant, and distend the button several times *to ensure patency and function of the antireflux valve within the button.*[4]
▪ Lubricate the feeding button mushroom dome and the stoma.[4]
▪ Gently push the feeding button through the stoma into the stomach (as shown below). Don't exert too much pressure, *because excess pressure during insertion may cause the button to be pushed into the stomach.*[4,21]

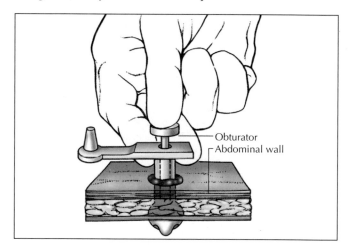

Obturator
Abdominal wall

▪ Remove the obturator by gently rotating it as you withdraw it *to keep the antireflux valve from adhering to it.*
▪ After removing the obturator, confirm placement by rotating the feeding button and gently pushing it into the stoma. If you feel no resistance, the device is properly placed.[4]
▪ Close the flexible safety plug (as shown below), which should be relatively flush with the skin surface. The feeding button is now ready for administration of enteral feedings.

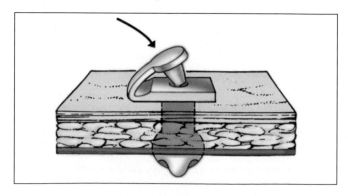

- Return the patient's bed to the lowest level *to prevent falls and maintain patient safety.*[23]
- Discard used supplies in the appropriate receptacles.[20]
- Remove and discard your gloves[20] and perform hand hygiene.[5,6,7,8,9,10]
- Document the procedure.[24,25,26,27]

Special considerations

- If the button pops out during feeding, estimate the formula already delivered, reinsert a new button, and resume feeding.
- Once daily, clean the peristomal skin with mild soap and water and then pat the skin dry with a gauze pad *to avoid skin irritation.* Also clean the site whenever spillage from the feeding bag occurs.[1,28]

Patient teaching

Before discharge, make sure the patient can insert and care for the gastrostomy feeding button. If possible, teach the patient or a family member how to reinsert the feeding button by first practicing on a model. Offer written instructions and answer questions on obtaining replacement supplies.

Complications

Complications from gastrostomy feeding button reinsertion are rare, and include irritation of the surrounding skin from leakage of gastric contents and placing or slippage of the device into the peritoneal cavity, which could cause peritonitis or sepsis.[4,21] Improper placement or excessive traction on the gastrostomy feeding button may cause misalignment of the internal dome, dislodgement, or tissue necrosis, and too much pressure on the entire device may cause it to become dislodged or be pushed into the stomach.[4,21]

Documentation

Record the date and time, reason for reinsertion, size of the feeding button you used, and patient's tolerance of the procedure. Document any complications, the name of the practitioner notified of such complications, the date and time of notification, prescribed interventions, and the patient's response to those interventions. Note the appearance of the stoma and surrounding skin. Document teaching provided to the patient and family (if appropriate), their understanding of that teaching, and any need for follow-up teaching.

REFERENCES

1 Hinkle, J. L., & Cheever, K. H. (2017). *Brunner & Suddarth's textbook of medical-surgical nursing* (14th ed.). Philadelphia, PA: Wolters Kluwer.

2 Blumenstein, I., et al. (2014). Gastroenteric tube feeding: Techniques, problems and solutions. *World Journal of Gastroenterology, 20*(26), 8505–8524. https://f6publishing.blob.core.windows.net/515a62f5-8994-4bb7-9d27-e9d7b0fa6dce/WJG-20-8505.pdf

3 Boullata, J. I., et al. (2017). ASPEN safe practices for enteral nutrition therapy. *Journal of Parenteral and Enteral Nutrition, 41*(1), 15–103. https://onlinelibrary.wiley.com/doi/full/10.1177/0148607116673053 (Level VII)

4 Bard Access Systems, Inc. (2012). BARD® button replacement gastrostomy device: Information for use. https://www.crbard.com/CRBard/media/ProductAssets/BardPeripheralVascularInc/PF10030/en-US/ua5qvrqym9p-7bqsmeue3a0wmkqc70yha.pdf

5 The Joint Commission. (2021). Standard NPSG.07.01.01. *Comprehensive accreditation manual for hospitals.* Oakbrook Terrace, IL: The Joint Commission. (Level VII)

6 Centers for Disease Control and Prevention. (2002). Guideline for hand hygiene in health-care settings: Recommendations of the Healthcare Infection Control Practices Advisory Committee and the HICPAC/SHEA/APIC/IDSA Hand Hygiene Task Force. *MMWR Recommendations and Reports, 51*(RR-16), 1–45. https://www.cdc.gov/mmwr/pdf/rr/rr5116.pdf (Level II)

7 World Health Organization. (2009). WHO guidelines on hand hygiene in health care: First global patient safety challenge, clean care is safer care. https://apps.who.int/iris/bitstream/handle/10665/44102/9789241597906_eng.pdf?sequence=1 (Level IV)

8 Accreditation Association for Hospitals and Health Systems. (2020). Standard 07.01.21. *Healthcare Facilities Accreditation Program: Accreditation requirements for acute care hospitals.* Chicago, IL: Accreditation Association for Hospitals and Health Systems. (Level VII)

9 Centers for Medicare and Medicaid Services, Department of Health and Human Services. (2020). Condition of participation: Infection control. 42 C.F.R. § 482.42.

10 DNV GL-Healthcare USA, Inc. (2020). IC.1.SR.1. *NIAHO® accreditation requirements, interpretive guidelines and surveyor guidance – revision 20.0.* Milford, OH: DNV GL-Healthcare USA, Inc. (Level VII)

11 The Joint Commission. (2021). Standard NPSG.01.01.01. *Comprehensive accreditation manual for hospitals.* Oakbrook Terrace, IL: The Joint Commission. (Level VII)

12 Accreditation Association for Hospitals and Health Systems. (2020). Standard 15.01.16. *Healthcare Facilities Accreditation Program: Accreditation requirements for acute care hospitals.* Chicago, IL: Accreditation Association for Hospitals and Health Systems. (Level VII)

13 Centers for Medicare and Medicaid Services, Department of Health and Human Services. (2020). Condition of participation: Patient's rights. 42 C.F.R. § 482.13(c)(1).

14 DNV GL-Healthcare USA, Inc. (2020). PR.2.SR.5. *NIAHO® accreditation requirements, interpretive guidelines and surveyor guidance – revision 20.0.* Milford, OH: DNV GL-Healthcare USA, Inc. (Level VII)

15 The Joint Commission. (2021). Standard RI.01.01.01. *Comprehensive accreditation manual for hospitals.* Oakbrook Terrace, IL: The Joint Commission. (Level VII)

16 The Joint Commission. (2021). Standard PC.02.01.21. *Comprehensive accreditation manual for hospitals.* Oakbrook Terrace, IL: The Joint Commission. (Level VII)

17 Waters, T. R., et al. (2009). Safe patient handling training for schools of nursing. https://www.cdc.gov/niosh/docs/2009-127/pdfs/2009-127.pdf (Level VII)

18 Siegel, J. D., et al. (2007, revised 2019). 2007 guideline for isolation precautions: Preventing transmission of infectious agents in healthcare settings. https://www.cdc.gov/infectioncontrol/pdf/guidelines/isolation-guidelines-H.pdf (Level II)

19 Accreditation Association for Hospitals and Health Systems. (2020). Standard 07.01.10. *Healthcare Facilities Accreditation Program: Accreditation requirements for acute care hospitals.* Chicago, IL: Accreditation Association for Hospitals and Health Systems. (Level VII)

20 Occupational Safety and Health Administration. (2019). Bloodborne pathogens, standard number 1910.1030. https://www.osha.gov/pls/oshaweb/owadisp.show_document?p_id=10051&p_table=STANDARDS (Level VII)

21 Bard Peripheral Vascular, Inc. (2016). Enteral feeding tube. https://www.crbard.com/CRBard/media/ProductAssets/BardPeripheralVascularInc/PF10030/en-US/vbjythyh56491gxbh-fr31iross1wrdap.pdf

22 Wound, Ostomy and Continence Nurses Society. (2016). *Peristomal skin complications: Clinical resource guide.* Mt. Laurel, NJ: WOCN.

23 Ganz, D. A., et al. (2013). *Preventing falls in hospitals: A toolkit for improving quality of care* (AHRQ publication no. 13-0015-EF). Rockville, MD: Agency for Healthcare Research and Quality. https://www.ahrq.gov/professionals/systems/hospital/fallpxtoolkit/index.html (Level VII)

24 The Joint Commission. (2021). Standard RC.01.03.01. *Comprehensive accreditation manual for hospitals.* Oakbrook Terrace, IL: The Joint Commission. (Level VII)

25 Centers for Medicare and Medicaid Services, Department of Health and Human Services. (2020). Condition of participation: Medical record services. 42 C.F.R. § 482.24(b).

26 Accreditation Association for Hospitals and Health Systems. (2020). Standard 10.00.03. *Healthcare Facilities Accreditation Program: Accreditation requirements for acute care hospitals.* Chicago, IL: Accreditation Association for Hospitals and Health Systems. (Level VII)

27 DNV GL-Healthcare USA, Inc. (2020). MR.2.SR.1. *NIAHO® accreditation requirements, interpretive guidelines and surveyor guidance – revision 20.0.* Milford, OH: DNV GL-Healthcare USA, Inc. (Level VII)

28 Wiegand, D. L. (2017). *AACN procedure manual for high acuity, progressive, and critical care* (7th ed.). St. Louis, MO: Elsevier.

Hair care

Brushing a patient's hair stimulates scalp circulation, removes dead cells and debris, and distributes hair oils along the hair shaft more effectively than combing does; however, combing the hair may be more effective for detangling and styling of short hair.[1] The frequency of hair care depends on the length and texture of the patient's hair and the patient's condition. Usually, hair should be combed and brushed daily.

Equipment

Comb ▪ brush ▪ bath towel ▪ Optional: gloves, wide-tooth comb, pick, lubricating conditioner, hair ties, hair pins, hot soapy water.

Preparation of equipment

The comb and brush should be clean. If necessary, wash them in hot, soapy water. The comb should have dull, even teeth *to prevent scratching the scalp.* The brush should have stiff bristles *to enhance vigorous brushing and stimulation of circulation.*

Implementation

▪ Gather and prepare the necessary equipment and supplies; place them on the patient's bedside stand.
▪ Perform hand hygiene.[2,3,4,5,6,7]
▪ Confirm the patient's identity using at least two patient identifiers.[8]
▪ Provide privacy.[9,10,11,12]
▪ Explain the procedure to the patient and family (if appropriate) according to their individual communication and learning needs *to increase their understanding, allay their fears, and enhance cooperation.*[13] If possible, encourage the patient to assist with brushing and combing the hair.
▪ Raise the patient's bed to waist level before providing care *to prevent caregiver back strain.*[14] If the patient's condition allows, help the patient to a sitting position by raising the head of the bed.
▪ Drape a bath towel over the patient's pillow and shoulders *to catch loose hair and dirt.*
▪ Perform hand hygiene.[2,3,4,5,6,7]
▪ Put on gloves if the patient has open scalp lesions *to comply with standard precautions.*[15,16,17]
▪ Assess the patient's hair and scalp, as needed. Notify the practitioner of any lesions, skin breakdown, or other conditions that may require special treatment or care.
▪ For short hair, comb and brush one side at a time. For long or curly hair, turn the patient's head away from you, and then part the hair down the middle from front to back. Comb and brush the hair on the side facing you. Then turn the patient's head and comb and brush the opposite side. Part hair into small sections *for easier handling.* Comb one section at a time, working from the ends toward the scalp *to remove tangles.*[1] Anchor each section of hair above the area being combed *to avoid hurting the patient.*
▪ For tightly curled hair, use a comb with wide-spaced teeth or a pick; comb through the hair working from the neckline toward the forehead.[1]
▪ If the hair is tangled, rub a small amount of lubricating conditioner on the hair strands *to loosen them.*[1] Then, comb and brush the hair, making sure to get all the tangles out.
▪ Style the hair as the patient prefers. Consider braiding long or curly hair *to help prevent it from matting in patients who must spend a lot of time in bed.*[1] To braid, part hair down the middle of the scalp and begin braiding near the face. *To avoid patient discomfort,* don't braid too tightly. Fasten the ends of the braids with hair ties. Pin the braids across the top of the patient's head or let them hang, as the patient desires, *so the finished braids don't press against the patient's scalp.*
▪ After styling the hair, carefully remove the towel by folding it inward *to prevent loose hairs and debris from falling onto the pillow or into the patient's bed.*

▪ Return the bed to the lowest position *to prevent falls and maintain patient safety.*[18]
▪ Remove and discard your gloves, if worn.[15]
▪ Perform hand hygiene.[2,3,4,5,6,7]
▪ Document the procedure.[19,20,21,22]

Special considerations

▪ Make sure each patient has a personal comb and brush *to avoid cross-contamination.*

Documentation

Describe any hair or scalp abnormalities you identified, the name of the practitioner notified, the date and time of notification, prescribed interventions, and the patient's response to those interventions. Document teaching provided to the patient and family (if applicable), their understanding of that teaching, and any need for follow-up teaching.

REFERENCES

1 Craven, R. F., et al. (2021). *Fundamentals of nursing: Concepts and competencies for practice* (9th ed.). Philadelphia, PA: Wolters Kluwer.
2 The Joint Commission. (2021). Standard NPSG.07.01.01. *Comprehensive accreditation manual for hospitals.* Oakbrook Terrace, IL: The Joint Commission. (Level VII)
3 Centers for Disease Control and Prevention. (2002). Guideline for hand hygiene in health-care settings: Recommendations of the Healthcare Infection Control Practices Advisory Committee and the HICPAC/SHEA/APIC/IDSA Hand Hygiene Task Force. *MMWR Recommendations and Reports, 51*(RR-16), 1–45. https://www.cdc.gov/mmwr/pdf/rr/rr5116.pdf (Level II)
4 World Health Organization. (2009). WHO guidelines on hand hygiene in health care: First global patient safety challenge, clean care is safer care. https://apps.who.int/iris/bitstream/handle/10665/44102/9789241597906_eng.pdf?sequence=1 (Level IV)
5 Centers for Medicare and Medicaid Services, Department of Health and Human Services. (2020). Condition of participation: Infection control. 42 C.F.R. § 482.42.
6 Accreditation Association for Hospitals and Health Systems. (2020). Standard 07.01.21. *Healthcare Facilities Accreditation Program: Accreditation requirements for acute care hospitals.* Chicago, IL: Accreditation Association for Hospitals and Health Systems. (Level VII)
7 DNV GL-Healthcare USA, Inc. (2020). IC.1.SR.1. *NIAHO® accreditation requirements, interpretive guidelines and surveyor guidance—revision 20.0.* Milford, OH: DNV GL-Healthcare USA, Inc. (Level VII)
8 The Joint Commission. (2021). Standard NPSG.01.01.01. *Comprehensive accreditation manual for hospitals.* Oakbrook Terrace, IL: The Joint Commission. (Level VII)
9 Centers for Medicare and Medicaid Services, Department of Health and Human Services. (2020). Condition of participation: Patient's rights. 42 C.F.R. § 482.13(c)(1).
10 Accreditation Association for Hospitals and Health Systems. (2020). Standard 15.01.16. *Healthcare Facilities Accreditation Program: Accreditation requirements for acute care hospitals.* Chicago, IL: Accreditation Association for Hospitals and Health Systems. (Level VII)
11 The Joint Commission. (2021). Standard RI.01.01.01. *Comprehensive accreditation manual for hospitals.* Oakbrook Terrace, IL: The Joint Commission. (Level VII)
12 DNV GL-Healthcare USA, Inc. (2020). PR.2.SR.5. *NIAHO® accreditation requirements, interpretive guidelines and surveyor guidance—revision 20.0.* Milford, OH: DNV GL-Healthcare USA, Inc. (Level VII)
13 The Joint Commission. (2021). Standard PC.02.01.21. *Comprehensive accreditation manual for hospitals.* Oakbrook Terrace, IL: The Joint Commission. (Level VII)
14 Waters, T. R., et al. (2009). Safe patient handling training for schools of nursing. https://www.cdc.gov/niosh/docs/2009-127/pdfs/2009-127.pdf (Level VII)
15 Siegel, J. D., et al. (2007, revised 2019). 2007 guideline for isolation precautions: Preventing transmission of infectious agents in healthcare settings. https://www.cdc.gov/infectioncontrol/pdf/guidelines/isolation-guidelines-H.pdf (Level II)
16 Accreditation Association for Hospitals and Health Systems. (2020). Standard 07.01.10. *Healthcare Facilities Accreditation Program: Accreditation requirements for acute care hospitals.* Chicago, IL: Accreditation Association for Hospitals and Health Systems. (Level VII)

17 Occupational Safety and Health Administration. (2019). Bloodborne pathogens, standard number 1910.1030. https://www.osha.gov/pls/oshaweb/owadisp.show_document?p_id=10051&p_table=STANDARDS (Level VII)

18 Ganz, D. A., et al. (2013, reviewed 2021). *Preventing falls in hospitals: A toolkit for improving quality of care* (AHRQ Publication No. 13-0015-EF). Rockville, MD: Agency for Healthcare Research and Quality. https://www.ahrq.gov/professionals/systems/hospital/fallpxtoolkit/index.html (Level VII)

19 The Joint Commission. (2021). Standard RC.01.03.01. *Comprehensive accreditation manual for hospitals.* Oakbrook Terrace, IL: The Joint Commission. (Level VII)

20 Centers for Medicare and Medicaid Services, Department of Health and Human Services. (2020). Condition of participation: Medical record services. 42 C.F.R. § 482.24(b).

21 Accreditation Association for Hospitals and Health Systems. (2020). Standard 10.00.03. *Healthcare Facilities Accreditation Program: Accreditation requirements for acute care hospitals.* Chicago, IL: Accreditation Association for Hospitals and Health Systems. (Level VII)

22 DNV GL-Healthcare USA, Inc. (2020). MR.2.SR.1. *NIAHO® accreditation requirements, interpretive guidelines and surveyor guidance—revision 20.0.* Milford, OH: DNV GL-Healthcare USA, Inc. (Level VII)

Halo-vest traction management

Halo-vest traction is a nonsurgical treatment used to stabilize the cervical spine after traumatic cervical vertebrae injury or destabilization.[1] It also helps treat patients who are experiencing degenerative changes from disease processes such as rheumatoid arthritis. Halo-vest traction can be a stand-alone treatment or an adjunct to a surgical procedure for spinal fracture or dislocation.[2] It can also help prevent further injury in cases of spinal cord trauma, and when surgery is involved, its preoperative use reduces spinal misalignment, and postoperatively it enables bone healing.[3]

A halo-vest traction device is a single-use item. Its components include a metal halo ring that fits over the head and a suprastructure with a rigid framework that connects the halo ring to a plastic vest that distributes the weight of the entire apparatus around the chest.[3] An orthopedic surgeon or a neurosurgeon applies the device with nursing assistance in an emergency department, a specially equipped room, an intensive care unit, or an operating room after surgical reduction of vertebral injuries. The duration of treatment varies but is usually up to 12 weeks.[3]

The advantages of this type of device are that it allows the patient to sit upright, permits the patient to mobilize out of bed (if able), and maintains the stability of the cervical spine.[2]

Halo-vest traction is contraindicated in patients with a skull fracture, infection, or severe soft-tissue injury (especially near proposed pin sites). Severe chest or multisystem trauma, barrel chest, obesity, and advanced age are relative contraindications to the procedure.[4]

Equipment
For assisting with hallo application
Vital signs monitoring equipment ▪ stethoscope ▪ halo-vest kit (vest, liner, head ring, positioning pins, skull pins, suprastructure, wrenches, and lock nuts) ▪ cap ▪ gown ▪ mask ▪ light source ▪ positioning device ▪ tape measure ▪ clippers ▪ 4″ × 4″ (10 cm × 10 cm) sterile gauze pads ▪ antiseptic solution or antiseptic swabs ▪ sterile drapes ▪ sterile gloves ▪ gloves ▪ wrench ▪ anesthetic agent ▪ alcohol pads ▪ syringe ▪ 25G needles ▪ torque screwdrivers ▪ disinfectant pad ▪ Optional: prescribed analgesic, prescribed sedative, gown, mask with face shield or mask and goggles.

For caring for the patient with a halo-vest
Chlorhexidine or another facility-approved antiseptic solution[2] ▪ basin of warm water ▪ wash cloth and towel ▪ vital signs monitoring equipment ▪ gloves ▪ cotton-tipped applicators ▪ normal saline solution ▪ torque screwdriver ▪ torque wrench ▪ crescent wrench ▪ light source ▪ shampoo ▪ stethoscope ▪ disinfectant pad ▪ Optional: prescribed pain medication, sheepskin or other vest liner, 4″ × 4″ (10 cm × 10 cm) gauze pads, plastic bag.

Preparation of equipment
The practitioner measures the patient's head at the greatest circumference of the skull (about 1 cm above the ears);[5] depending on the device type, the practitioner may also measure the mediolateral and anterior-posterior diameter of the head *to determine proper ring size. To determine the proper vest size,* the practitioner measures the patient's chest circumference at the xiphoid process.[6] Each device has specific recommendations to determine proper size.

Inspect all equipment and supplies. If a product is expired, is defective, or has compromised integrity, remove it from patient use, label it as expired or defective, and report the expiration or defect, as directed by your facility.

Implementation
▪ Verify the practitioner's order.
▪ Gather and prepare the necessary equipment and supplies.
▪ Confirm that informed consent has been obtained and that the signed consent form is in the patient's medical record.[7,8,9,10]
▪ Conduct a preprocedure verification *to make sure that all relevant documentation, related information, and equipment are available and correctly identified to the patient's identifiers.*[11,12]
▪ Verify that the laboratory and imaging studies have been completed as ordered and that the results are in the patient's medical record. Notify the practitioner of any unexpected results.
▪ Perform hand hygiene.[13,14,15,16,17,18]
▪ Confirm the patient's identity using at least two patient identifiers.[19]
▪ Provide privacy.[20,21,22,23]
▪ Reinforce the practitioner's explanation of the procedure to the patient and family (if appropriate) according to their individual communication and learning needs *to increase their understanding, allay their fears, and enhance cooperation,* and answer their questions.[24]
▪ Check the patient's history for hypersensitivity to latex or the anesthetic agent.
▪ Make sure that lighting is adequate.
▪ Raise the patient's bed to waist level before providing care *to prevent caregiver back strain.*[25]
▪ Perform hand hygiene.[13,14,15,16,17,18]
▪ Obtain baseline vital signs and assess the patient's neurologic and respiratory status *to use as baselines for comparison.* (See the "Neurologic assessment" procedure.)
▪ Screen for and assess the patient's pain using facility-defined criteria that are consistent with the patient's age, condition, and ability to understand.[26]
▪ Treat the patient's pain, as necessary and ordered, using nonpharmacologic, pharmacologic, or a combination of approaches. Base the treatment plan on evidence-based practices and the patient's clinical condition, past medical history, and pain management goals. If administering an analgesic, follow safe medication administration practices.[26]
▪ If the practitioner prescribed opioids, closely monitor the patient identified as at high risk for adverse outcomes related to opioid treatment.[26]
▪ Administer a sedative, as ordered, following safe medication administration practices *to help the patient relax during the procedure.*[27,28,29,30]

Assisting with halo application
▪ Have a coworker assist with the procedure *to maintain proper cervical spine precautions and prevent patient injury.*
▪ Remove the headboard from the bed.
▪ Maintain the patient in the supine position.
▪ Maintain cervical spine alignment by supporting the patient's head using the positioning device.
▪ The practitioner selects four pin sites: just above the lateral one-third of each eyebrow in the 1-cm (4/10″) safe zone below the equator of the skull for anterior pins and on the opposite side of the anterior pins for the posterior pins.[4] The practitioner also takes into account the degree and type of correction needed to provide proper cervical alignment.
▪ Trim the hair at the intended pin sites with clippers *to facilitate subsequent care and to help prevent infection.*[5]
▪ Perform hand hygiene.[13,14,15,16,17,18]
▪ Put on gloves and, as necessary, other personal protective equipment as needed *to comply with standard precautions.*[31,32,33]

- Establish a sterile field with sterile drapes.
- Use an antiseptic swab or 4″ × 4″ (10 cm × 10 cm) sterile gauze pads soaked in antiseptic solution to prepare the pin site areas for pin application.[6] Allow the solution to dry following the manufacturer's instructions.
- Open the halo-vest unit using sterile technique *to avoid contamination.* (See the "Sterile technique, basic" procedure.)
- The practitioner puts on a cap, a gown, a mask, and sterile gloves and then removes the halo and Allen wrench from the halo-vest kit.
- Conduct a time-out immediately before starting the procedure *to verify that the correct patient, site, positioning, and procedure are identified and, as applicable, that all relevant information and necessary equipment are available.*[12,34]
- The practitioner positions the ring on the patient's head using the positioning pins *to hold the halo ring in place temporarily,* which should accommodate access to the selected skull pin sites.
- Assist the practitioner with preparing the anesthetic agent, if necessary. Clean and disinfect the injection port of the anesthetic agent with an alcohol pad, and allow it to dry completely. Invert the vial so that the practitioner can insert a 25G needle attached to a syringe and withdraw the anesthetic.
- The practitioner injects the anesthetic at each of the four pin sites.[6] Change the needle on the syringe after each injection.
- Instruct the patient to close the eyes during skull pin application *to prevent skin bunching.*[5,6]
- Using sterile technique, the practitioner threads each skull pin through its halo ring hole until it touches the skin. The practitioner then tightens the pins by hand using one of two methods, according to the manufacturer's instructions. For an opposing pair, the pins opposite each other are tightened simultaneously;[5] for a posterior–anterior pair, the two posterior pins are tightened first and then the two anterior pins.[5]
- The practitioner visually checks the pins' positioning and then tightens them in incremental steps using the torque screwdrivers and following the manufacturer's instructions; the pins are commonly tightened 6 to 8 inch-pounds (0.49 to 1.99 newton-meters).[5]
- The practitioner removes the positioning pins and then applies and tightens the lock nuts to the pins by hand *to secure the pins in place.*[5] The practitioner applies plastic caps over the free ends of the pins *to prevent them from snagging on linens and clothing.*

Applying the vest

- Separate the anterior and posterior portions of the vest, if necessary.
- If not already in place, position the liners inside the anterior and posterior portions of the vest *to make it more comfortable to wear and to help prevent pressure injuries.*
- While the practitioner maintains the patient's head and neck position, and with assistance from a coworker, logroll the supine patient and place the posterior portion on the patient according to the manufacturer's instructions.[6] Alternatively, while the patient is supine and the practitioner maintains head and neck position, use a lifting maneuver. Lift the patient's head and upper body 6″ (15 cm) and slide the posterior portion of the vest under the patient into correct alignment, according to manufacturer's instructions.[6]
- Carefully return the patient to the supine position, and then check the position of the posterior portion of the vest for correct alignment.[6]
- The practitioner then positions the anterior portion of the vest on the patient's chest and secures it in place with the posterior portion, using the waist stabilizers and straps and the shoulder straps.[6]
- As you continue to maintain cervical spine precautions, the practitioner aligns and attaches the superstructure to the halo ring and tightens the screws or bolts.[6]
- After application is complete, help the practitioner bring the patient to a sitting position *to check that the head is in alignment with the body and that the halo superstructure is symmetrical.*
- When halo-vest traction is in place, arrange for an X-ray, as ordered, *to make sure that the desired alignment has been achieved.*[6]

NURSING ALERT If the patient complains of having difficulty swallowing or feeling pressure on top of the head, the vest may be applied too tightly, too high, or too low. Adjustments to approve patient comfort and alignment may be necessary and will be based on the results of the cervical spine X-rays.[3]

Caring for the patient

- Gather the necessary equipment at the patient's bedside.
- Perform hand hygiene.[13,14,15,16,17,18]
- Confirm the patient's identity using at least two patient identifiers.[19]
- Provide privacy.[20,21,22,23]
- Explain the procedure to the patient and family (if appropriate) according to their individual communication and learning needs *to increase their understanding, allay their fears, and enhance cooperation,* and answer their questions.[24]
- Raise the patient's bed to waist level when providing care *to prevent caregiver back strain.*[25]
- Assess the patient's vital signs and neurologic status closely for deterioration from baseline neurologic function.[2]

NURSING ALERT Notify the practitioner immediately if you observe any loss of motor function or any decreased sensation from baseline, *because these changes could indicate spinal cord trauma.*[2]

- *Because the vest limits chest expansion,* routinely assess the patient's pulmonary status, especially in a patient with pulmonary disease.

ELDER ALERT Respiratory complications from halo fixation are more common in older adult patients.[35]

- Perform hand hygiene[13,14,15,16,17,18] and put on gloves *to comply with standard precautions.*[31,32,33]
- Using cotton-tipped applicators, gently clean the pin sites with chlorhexidine or another facility-approved antiseptic solution daily or as indicated.[2,36,37] Povidone-iodine shouldn't be used *because it interferes with tissue healing.*[36]
- Use a clean cotton-tipped applicator for each site, and rinse each site afterward with normal saline solution *to remove any excess cleaning solution.*[38] *Meticulous pin site care prevents infection and removes debris that might block drainage and lead to abscess formation.*
- If crusting is present, wrap the pin site with gauze soaked in normal saline solution for 15 to 20 minutes and then remove the gauze. Using a gentle rolling motion, remove the crust with a cotton-tipped applicator that has been soaked in normal saline solution.[3]
- Observe for loose pins and signs and symptoms of infection, including swelling, redness, purulent drainage, tracking (an open area where skin has pulled away from the pin), and pain at the site. Notify the practitioner if any signs and symptoms of infection develop.[3]
- The practitioner retightens the skull pins with the torque screwdriver 24 and 48 hours after the halo is applied.[3]
- If the patient complains of a headache after the pins are tightened, administer prescribed pain medication, as ordered, following safe medication administration practices.[27,28,29,30] If pain occurs with jaw movement, or if any movement of the head or neck occurs, notify the practitioner immediately, *because this symptom may indicate that pins have slipped.*
- Examine the halo-vest unit every shift *to make sure that the unit is secure and that the patient's head is centered within the halo.*[39] If the vest fits correctly, you should be able to insert one or two fingers under the jacket at the shoulder and chest when the patient is in the supine position.
- Wash the patient's chest and back with warm water; be careful not to put any stress on the apparatus, *which could knock it out of alignment and lead to subluxation of the cervical spine.*[37] Place the patient supine. Loosen the bottom straps *so you can get to the chest and back.* Turn the patient on one side (less than 45 degrees) to wash the back. Reaching under the vest, wash and dry the skin. Check for tender, reddened areas, or pressure spots that may develop into a medical device related pressure injury.[37] If itching occurs, check to see whether the patient is allergic to sheepskin or other material that composes the vest liner, and whether any drug the patient is taking might cause a skin rash.[1] Change the vest lining, as needed. Close the vest.

NURSING ALERT Avoid the use of soap, lotion, or powder underneath the vest.[37] A cotton pillowcase or undershirt can be worn or placed under the vest for comfort and perspiration absorption; change this item regularly.[3]

- Shampoo the patient's hair regularly. Place the patient in the supine position in bed with a towel or large plastic bag along the back and shoulders of the halo vest *to protect the lining from getting wet.* The halo crown, pins, and bars can all safely get wet.[3]
- Reassess and respond to the patient's pain by evaluating the response to treatment and progress toward pain management goals. Assess for

adverse reactions and risk factors for adverse events that may result from treatment.[26]

- Verify that a torque wrench and a crescent wrench are available for use in an emergency if the patient's vest must be removed.

Completing the procedure

- Discard used supplies in the appropriate receptacles.[33]
- Remove and discard your gloves and any other personal protective equipment worn.[31,33]
- Return the bed to the lowest position *to prevent falls and maintain the patient's safety.*[40]
- Perform hand hygiene.[13,14,15,16,17,18]
- Clean and disinfect your stethoscope using a disinfectant pad.[41,42]
- Perform hand hygiene.[13,14,15,16,17,18]
- Document the procedure.[43,44,45,46]

Special considerations

NURSING ALERT Keep a torque wrench and a crescent wrench available at all times *to remove and tighten the halo vest.*[6] If the patient travels off the unit, the wrenches must accompany the patient, *because an emergency might necessitate removal of the vest.* In case of cardiac arrest, know the type of vest the patient is wearing. Some vests have a hinged front to raise the breastplate for cardiopulmonary resuscitation (CPR). If the patient doesn't have one of these vests, you'll need to use a wrench to remove the distal anterior bolts.[2] Pull the two upright bars outward, unfasten the straps, and remove the front of the vest. Use the sturdy back of the vest as a board for CPR. *To prevent subluxating a cervical injury and avoid hyperextension of the neck,* perform a jaw-thrust maneuver to open the airway. Pull the patient's mandible forward while maintaining proper head and neck alignment. *This positioning pulls the tongue forward to open the airway.*

- Be aware that there are many different types of halo and vest components. Make sure that you're familiar with the equipment used by your facility. Confirm that the device is compatible with magnetic resonance imaging, as indicated.[5,6]
- Ensure that the practitioner examines the patient about 24 hours after halo-vest application *to assess pin tightness and to check for complications.*
- The practitioner should retorque the pins 24 to 48 hours after initial application and every 2 to 3 weeks thereafter or on patient complaint of pain at the pin site.[5]

NURSING ALERT Never lift or reposition a patient by the vertical bars of a halo-vest traction device. *Doing so could strain or tear the skin at the pin sites or misalign the traction.*[2]

- If defibrillation is necessary, don't touch the bars with the defibrillator.[2]
- If you'll be applying countertraction, position the patient with the head of the bed flat and on shock blocks or in reverse Trendelenburg position.[2]
- Walk with an ambulatory patient *to prevent falls by implementing fall prevention measure.*[2,40] Remember that the patient will have trouble seeing objects at or near the feet, and that the weight of the halo-vest unit (about 10 lb [4.5 kg]) may throw the patient off balance. If the patient is in a wheelchair, lower the leg rests *to prevent the chair from tipping backward.*
- *Because the vest limits chest expansion,* routinely assess pulmonary function, especially in a patient with pulmonary disease.[2]

Patient teaching

If the patient is being discharged home with a halo-vest device, instruct the patient and family on key areas of halo-vest traction management, including vest and skin care, bathing, dressing, sleeping, ambulating, and other activities of daily living.[37] Teach the patient to turn slowly in small increments *to avoid losing balance.* Remind the patient to avoid bending forward, *because the extra weight of the halo apparatus could cause the patient to fall.* Teach the patient to bend at the knees rather than at the waist. Stress the importance of vigilant skin care; the avoidance of bending, heavy lifting, and driving; and alterations to clothing that may be necessary. Provide the patient with information regarding follow-up appointments, and instruct the patient to notify the practitioner of signs of infection, pin-site loosening or dislodgment, skin breakdown, swallowing problems, headache, malaise, visual changes, or any instances of trauma or a fall.[3] Teach the patient and family (if appropriate) about pain management strategies during discharge

planning. Include information about the patient's pain management plan and adverse effects of pain management treatment. Discuss activities of daily living and items in the home environment that might exacerbate pain or reduce the effectiveness of the pain management plan, and include strategies to address these issues. Teach the patient and family about safe use, storage, and disposal of opioids if prescribed.

Complications

The most common complication of halo-vest traction is pin loosening. Pin-site infection is also possible. Skin breakdown, irritation, and the development of pressure injuries are possible skin-related complications. Problems with balance and difficulty sleeping can also occur, particularly right after initial device application. Weakened neck muscles may become apparent after halo-vest traction removal.[1] Additional complications include respiratory distress, orthostatic hypotension, swallowing problems, and dural tears.[2,3]

Documentation

Record the date and time of halo-vest traction application and the name of the practitioner who applied it. Also note the length of the procedure and the patient's response. Record vital signs and neurologic, pain, and respiratory assessment findings. Document that you performed a pre-procedure verification and time-out. Document the appearance of the pin insertion sites. Record any medications you administered before or during the procedure, including the medication strength, dose, route of administration, and date and time of administration. Record any adverse reactions to prescribed medications, the date and time you notified the practitioner, prescribed interventions, and the patient's response to those interventions. Document pain assessment findings, any interventions you used, unexpected outcomes, related treatments, and the patient's response to those treatments. Record that the patient received a postprocedure X-ray for alignment, the X-ray results, the name of practitioner you notified of the results, and the date and time of notification. Document teaching you provided to the patient and family (if applicable), their understanding of that teaching, and any need for follow-up teaching.

REFERENCES

1 Traynelis, V., & Waziri, A. (2018). Cervical spine bracing options: Halo ring, crowns, or vest. https://www.spineuniverse.com/treatments/bracing/cervical-spine-bracing-options-halo-ring-crowns-or-vest

2 Wiegand, D. L. (2017). *AACN procedure manual for high acuity, progressive, and critical care* (7th ed.). St. Louis, MO: Elsevier.

3 Sarro, A., et al. (2010). Developing a standard of care for halo vest and pin site care including patient and family education: A collaborative approach among three greater Toronto area teaching hospitals. *Journal of Neuroscience Nursing, 42,* 169–173.

4 Abbasi, D. (2020). Orthobullets: Halo orthosis immobilization. https://www.orthobullets.com/spine/2019/halo-orthosis-immobilization

5 Anjon Holdings. (2017). Anjon Bremer crown set: Application, removal, and post-removal pin site care instructions. http://docplayer.net/90057257-Anjon-bremer-crown-set.html

6 SPS Co. (2020). Anjon Bremer classic vest: Product information, fitting halo whiteboard (video). https://www.spsco.com/anjon-bremer-classic-vest.html#description

7 The Joint Commission. (2021). Standard RI.01.03.01. *Comprehensive accreditation manual for hospitals.* Oakbrook Terrace, IL: The Joint Commission. (Level VII)

8 Centers for Medicare and Medicaid Services, Department of Health and Human Services. (2020). Condition of participation: Patient's rights. 42 C.F.R. § 482.13(b)(2).

9 Accreditation Association for Hospitals and Health Systems. (2020). Standard 30.01.11. *Healthcare Facilities Accreditation Program: Accreditation requirements for acute care hospitals.* Chicago, IL: Accreditation Association for Hospitals and Health Systems. (Level VII)

10 DNV GL-Healthcare USA, Inc. (2020). PR.2.SR.3. *NIAHO® accreditation requirements, interpretive guidelines and surveyor guidance—revision 20.0.* Milford, OH: DNV GL-Healthcare USA, Inc. (Level VII)

11 The Joint Commission. (2021). Standard UP.01.01.01. *Comprehensive accreditation manual for hospitals.* Oakbrook Terrace, IL: The Joint Commission. (Level VII)

12 Accreditation Association for Hospitals and Health Systems. (2020). Standard 30.00.14. *Healthcare Facilities Accreditation Program: Accreditation requirements for acute care hospitals.* Chicago, IL: Accreditation Association for Hospitals and Health Systems. (Level VII)

13 The Joint Commission. (2021). Standard NPSG.07.01.01. *Comprehensive accreditation manual for hospitals.* Oakbrook Terrace, IL: The Joint Commission. (Level VII)

14 Centers for Disease Control and Prevention. (2002). Guideline for hand hygiene in health-care settings: Recommendations of the Healthcare Infection Control Practices Advisory Committee and the HICPAC/SHEA/APIC/IDSA Hand Hygiene Task Force. *MMWR Recommendations and Reports, 51*(RR-16), 1–45. https://www.cdc.gov/mmwr/pdf/rr/rr5116.pdf (Level II)

15 World Health Organization. (2009). WHO guidelines on hand hygiene in health care: First global patient safety challenge, clean care is safer care. https://apps.who.int/iris/bitstream/handle/10665/44102/9789241597906_eng.pdf?sequence=1 (Level IV)

16 Accreditation Association for Hospitals and Health Systems. (2020). Standard 07.01.21. *Healthcare Facilities Accreditation Program: Accreditation requirements for acute care hospitals.* Chicago, IL: Accreditation Association for Hospitals and Health Systems. (Level VII)

17 Centers for Medicare and Medicaid Services, Department of Health and Human Services. (2020). Condition of participation: Infection control. 42 C.F.R. § 482.42.

18 DNV GL-Healthcare USA, Inc. (2020). IC.1.SR.1. *NIAHO® accreditation requirements, interpretive guidelines and surveyor guidance—revision 20.0.* Milford, OH: DNV GL-Healthcare USA, Inc. (Level VII)

19 The Joint Commission. (2021). Standard NPSG.01.01.01. *Comprehensive accreditation manual for hospitals.* Oakbrook Terrace, IL: The Joint Commission. (Level VII)

20 Accreditation Association for Hospitals and Health Systems. (2020). Standard 15.01.16. *Healthcare Facilities Accreditation Program: Accreditation requirements for acute care hospitals.* Chicago, IL: Accreditation Association for Hospitals and Health Systems. (Level VII)

21 Centers for Medicare and Medicaid Services, Department of Health and Human Services. (2020). Condition of participation: Patient's rights. 42 C.F.R. § 482.13(c)(1).

22 DNV GL-Healthcare USA, Inc. (2020). PR.2.SR.5. *NIAHO® accreditation requirements, interpretive guidelines and surveyor guidance—revision 20.0.* Milford, OH: DNV GL-Healthcare USA, Inc. (Level VII)

23 The Joint Commission. (2021). Standard RI.01.01.01. *Comprehensive accreditation manual for hospitals.* Oakbrook Terrace, IL: The Joint Commission. (Level VII)

24 The Joint Commission. (2021). Standard PC.02.01.21. *Comprehensive accreditation manual for hospitals.* Oakbrook Terrace, IL: The Joint Commission. (Level VII)

25 Waters, T. R., et al. (2009). Safe patient handling training for schools of nursing. https://www.cdc.gov/niosh/docs/2009-127/pdfs/2009-127.pdf (Level VII)

26 The Joint Commission. (2021). Standard PC.01.02.07. *Comprehensive accreditation manual for hospitals.* Oakbrook Terrace, IL: The Joint Commission. (Level VII)

27 Accreditation Association for Hospitals and Health Systems. (2020). Standard 16.01.03. *Healthcare Facilities Accreditation Program: Accreditation requirements for acute care hospitals.* Chicago, IL: Accreditation Association for Hospitals and Health Systems. (Level VII)

28 Centers for Medicare and Medicaid Services, Department of Health and Human Services. (2020). Condition of participation: Nursing services. 42 C.F.R. § 482.23(c).

29 DNV GL-Healthcare USA, Inc. (2020). MM.1.SR.3. *NIAHO® accreditation requirements, interpretive guidelines and surveyor guidance—revision 20.0.* Milford, OH: DNV GL-Healthcare USA, Inc. (Level VII)

30 The Joint Commission. (2021). Standard MM.06.01.01. *Comprehensive accreditation manual for hospitals.* Oakbrook Terrace, IL: The Joint Commission. (Level VII)

31 Accreditation Association for Hospitals and Health Systems. (2020). Standard 07.01.10. *Healthcare Facilities Accreditation Program: Accreditation requirements for acute care hospitals.* Chicago, IL: Accreditation Association for Hospitals and Health Systems. (Level VII)

32 Siegel, J. D., et al. (2007, revised 2019). 2007 guideline for isolation precautions: Preventing transmission of infectious agents in healthcare settings. https://www.cdc.gov/infectioncontrol/pdf/guidelines/isolation-guidelines-H.pdf (Level II)

33 Occupational Safety and Health Administration. (2019). Bloodborne pathogens, standard number 1910.1030. https://www.osha.gov/pls/oshaweb/owadisp.show_document?p_id=10051&p_table=STANDARDS (Level VII)

34 The Joint Commission. (2021). Standard UP.01.03.01. *Comprehensive accreditation manual for hospitals.* Oakbrook Terrace, IL: The Joint Commission. (Level VII)

35 Benzel, E. C. (2012). *The cervical spine* (5th ed.). Philadelphia, PA: Lippincott Williams & Wilkins.

36 Lagerquist, D., et al. (2012). Care of external fixator pin sites. *American Journal of Critical Care, 21,* 288–295. (Level V)

37 Reid, B. (2018). Your guide to wearing your halo vest. http://anjon-bremerhalo.com/Halo/HALOIFU/ReleasedIFU/Patient/LA0902909%20Rev%20D%20Anjon%20Bremer%20Halo%20Patient%20Guide.pdf

38 The Joint Commission. (2021). Standard NPSG.07.05.01. *Comprehensive accreditation manual for hospitals.* Oakbrook Terrace, IL: The Joint Commission. (Level VII)

39 The Joint Commission. (2021). Standard PC.01.02.01. *Comprehensive accreditation manual for hospitals.* Oakbrook Terrace, IL: The Joint Commission. (Level VII)

40 Ganz, D. A., et al. (2013, reviewed 2021). Preventing falls in hospitals: A toolkit for improving quality of care (AHRQ publication no. 13-0015-EF). https://www.ahrq.gov/professionals/systems/hospital/fallpx-toolkit/index.html (Level VII)

41 Rutala, W. A., et al. (2008, revised 2019). Guideline for disinfection and sterilization in healthcare facilities, 2008. https://www.cdc.gov/infection-control/pdf/guidelines/disinfection-guidelines-H.pdf (Level I)

42 Accreditation Association for Hospitals and Health Systems. (2020). Standard 07.02.03. *Healthcare Facilities Accreditation Program: Accreditation requirements for acute care hospitals.* Chicago, IL: Accreditation Association for Hospitals and Health Systems. (Level VII)

43 Accreditation Association for Hospitals and Health Systems. (2020). Standard 10.00.03. *Healthcare Facilities Accreditation Program: Accreditation requirements for acute care hospitals.* Chicago, IL: Accreditation Association for Hospitals and Health Systems. (Level VII)

44 Centers for Medicare and Medicaid Services, Department of Health and Human Services. (2020). Condition of participation: Medical record services. 42 C.F.R. § 482.24(b).

45 The Joint Commission. (2021). Standard RC.01.03.01. *Comprehensive accreditation manual for hospitals.* Oakbrook Terrace, IL: The Joint Commission. (Level VII)

46 DNV GL-Healthcare USA, Inc. (2020). MR.2.SR.1. *NIAHO® accreditation requirements, interpretive guidelines and surveyor guidance—revision 20.0.* Milford, OH: DNV GL-Healthcare USA, Inc. (Level VII)

HAND HYGIENE

Hand hygiene is a general term used by the Centers for Disease Control and Prevention (CDC) and the World Health Organization (WHO) to refer to hand washing, antiseptic hand washing, antiseptic hand rubbing, and surgical hand asepsis.[1,2,3,4,5,6]

The hands are the conduits for almost every transfer of potential pathogens from one patient to another, from a contaminated object to the patient, or from a staff member to the patient. Because of this, hand hygiene is the single most important procedure in preventing infection.[1] To protect patients from health care–associated infections, hand hygiene must be performed routinely and thoroughly.[4,7] In effect, clean and healthy hands with intact skin, short fingernails, and no rings minimize the risk of contamination. Artificial nails can serve as reservoirs for microorganisms, as can rough or chapped hands.[1,8]

Washing with soap and water is appropriate when hands are visibly soiled or contaminated with blood or other body fluids, when exposure to potential spore-forming pathogens (such as *Clostridioides difficile* or *Bacillus anthracis*) is strongly suspected or proven, and after using the restroom. Using an alcohol-based hand sanitizer is appropriate for decontaminating the hands before direct patient contact; before putting on gloves; before inserting an invasive device; after contact with the patient; when moving from a contaminated body site to a clean body site during patient care; after contact with body fluids, excretions, mucous membranes, nonintact skin, or wound dressings (if hands aren't visibly soiled); after removing gloves; and after contact with inanimate objects in the patient's environment.[1,2,7,9] (See *Your five moments for hand hygiene.*)

The CDC recommends performing hand hygiene with soap and water before eating,[1] and the WHO recommends using either an alcohol-based hand rub or washing with soap and water before preparing food or handling medication.[2]

Your five moments for hand hygiene

According to the World Health Organization (WHO), there are five key moments during patient care when health care workers should perform hand hygiene.

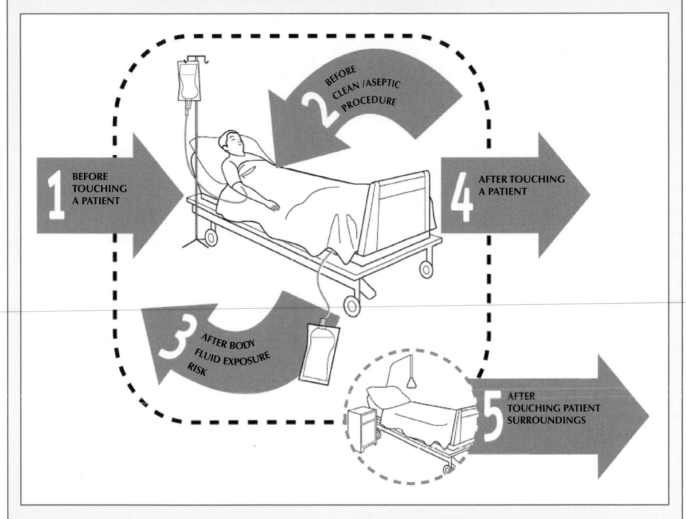

1 **BEFORE TOUCHING A PATIENT**

2 **BEFORE CLEAN / ASEPTIC PROCEDURE**

3 **AFTER BODY FLUID EXPOSURE RISK**

4 **AFTER TOUCHING A PATIENT**

5 **AFTER TOUCHING PATIENT SURROUNDINGS**

Equipment

Hand washing

Soap ■ warm running water ■ paper towels ■ Optional: emollient hand cream.

Hand sanitizing

Alcohol-based hand rub.

Preparation of equipment

Inspect all equipment and supplies. If a product is expired is defective, or has compromised integrity, remove it from patient use, label it as expired or defective, and report the expiration or defect as directed by your facility.

Implementation

Hand washing

■ Remove rings according to your facility's policy, *because they harbor dirt and microorganisms.*[1] Remove your watch and bracelets, or wear them well above the wrist. If you wear nail polish, it must be kept in good

repair *to minimize its potential to harbor microorganisms*; refer to your facility's guidelines regarding nail polish. Natural nails should be short (less than ¼" [0.6 cm]).[1]

■ With your arms angled downward toward the faucet, adjust the water temperature until it's comfortably warm (not hot).

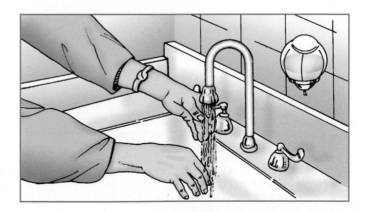

■ Wet your hands and wrists with warm water and apply soap from a dispenser.[1,2] Don't use bar soap, *because it allows cross-contamination.*[1] Hold your hands below elbow level *to prevent water from running up your arms and back down, contaminating clean areas.*
■ Work up a generous lather by rubbing your hands together vigorously for about 20 seconds.[10] *Soap and warm water reduce surface tension, which, aided by friction, loosens surface microorganisms, which wash away in the lather.*

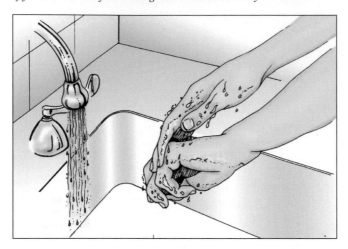

■ Pay special attention to the area under your fingernails and around your cuticles, and to your thumbs, knuckles, and the sides of your fingers and hands, *because microorganisms thrive in these protected or overlooked areas.* If you don't remove your rings, move them up and down your finger *to clean beneath them.*[1]
■ Avoid splashing water on yourself or the floor, *because microorganisms spread more easily on wet surfaces, and because slippery floors are dangerous.* Avoid touching the sink or faucets, *because they're considered contaminated.*
■ Rinse your hands and wrists well, *because running water flushes away suds, soil, and microorganisms.*
■ Pat your hands and wrists dry with a paper towel. Avoid rubbing, *which can cause abrasion and chapping.*
■ If the sink isn't equipped with knee or foot controls, turn off the faucets by gripping them with a dry paper towel *to avoid recontaminating your hands.*

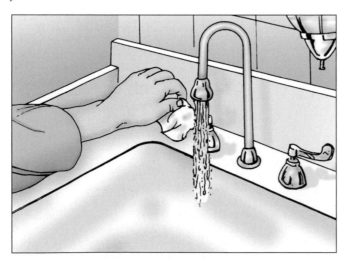

Hand sanitizing
■ Apply alcohol-based hand rub to the palm of one hand and then rub your hands together to cover all surfaces of the hands.[1,2]
■ Continue rubbing your hands together until all of the product has dried (usually about 30 seconds).[1,2]

Special considerations
■ Bundling supplies and clustering tasks reduces the number of times health care workers need to be in patients' rooms, resulting in fewer instances in which workers need to perform hand hygiene, which likely increases adherence.[11]
■ Before participating in any sterile procedure, or whenever your hands are grossly contaminated, wash your forearms as well as your hands and clean under your fingernails and in and around your cuticles. Don't use brushes, metal files, or other hard objects, *because they can injure your skin and, if reused, may be a source of contamination.*
■ The CDC hand hygiene guideline recommends that artificial nails or extenders not be worn by health care workers who have direct contact with patients at high risk for acquiring infections, such as patients on intensive care or transplant units.[1] Similarly, the WHO recommends in its publication *WHO Guidelines on Hand Hygiene in Health Care* that artificial nails or extenders not be worn by health care workers who have direct contact with patients.[2]
■ If your hands aren't visibly soiled, you can use an alcohol-based hand rub for routine decontamination.[1]
■ If you're providing care in the patient's home, bring your own supply of soap and disposable paper towels. If running water isn't available, disinfect your hands with an alcohol-based hand rub.
■ The CDC recommends that patients perform hand hygiene with soap and water or an alcohol-based hand sanitizer before or after eating food; before touching the eyes, nose, or mouth; after using the restroom; after blowing the nose, coughing, or sneezing; and after touching any surfaces in the health care facility, such as the bed rail or remote control *to decrease the spread of infection.*[12]
■ Avoid the use of triclosan-containing soaps *because of the risk of antimicrobial resistance; there's no evidence to support their superiority.*[7]
■ Keep in mind that glove use doesn't eliminate the need for hand hygiene. (See *Getting to the root of hand hygiene failure.*)
■ *To prevent your hands from becoming dry or chapped,* apply an emollient hand cream after performing hand hygiene, as needed, or switch to a different cleaning agent.[1,7] Make sure that the hand cream or lotion you use won't cause the material in your gloves to deteriorate. If you develop dermatitis, you may need to be evaluated by your employee health care provider *to determine whether you should continue to work until the condition resolves. Hands with dermatitis are more susceptible to becoming colonized with transient bacteria.*
■ Teach patients and their families about the importance of hand hygiene in preventing the spread of infection, and encourage them to remind health care workers to perform hand hygiene when necessary.[1,3]

Complications

Because frequent hand washing strips the skin of natural oils, it can result in dryness, cracking, and irritation.[1] The use of alcohol-based hand rubs can also dry the skin.[1]

REFERENCES

1 Centers for Disease Control and Prevention. (2002). Guideline for hand hygiene in health-care settings: Recommendations of the Healthcare Infection Control Practices Advisory Committee and the HICPAC/SHEA/APIC/IDSA Hand Hygiene Task Force. *MMWR Recommendations and Reports, 51*(RR-16), 1–45. https://www.cdc.gov/mmwr/pdf/rr/rr5116.pdf (Level II)

2 World Health Organization. (2009). WHO guidelines on hand hygiene in health care: First global patient safety challenge, clean care is safer care. https://apps.who.int/iris/bitstream/handle/10665/44102/9789241597906_eng.pdf?sequence=1 (Level IV)

3 The Joint Commission. (2021). Standard NPSG.07.01.01. *Comprehensive accreditation manual for hospitals.* Oakbrook Terrace, IL: The Joint Commission. (Level VII)

4 Centers for Medicare and Medicaid Services, Department of Health and Human Services. (2020). Condition of participation: Infection control. 42 C.F.R. § 482.42.

5 Accreditation Association for Hospitals and Health Systems. (2020). Standard 07.01.21. *Healthcare Facilities Accreditation Program: Accreditation requirements for acute care hospitals.* Chicago, IL: Accreditation Association for Hospitals and Health Systems. (Level VII)

6 DNV GL-Healthcare USA, Inc. (2020). IC.1.SR.1. *NIAHO® accreditation requirements, interpretive guidelines and surveyor guidance—revision 20.0.* Milford, OH: DNV GL-Healthcare USA, Inc. (Level VII)

7 Ellingson, K., et al. (2014). Strategies to prevent healthcare-associated infections through hand hygiene. *Infection Control and Hospital Epidemiology, 35*(8), 937–960. https://www.jstor.org/stable/pdf/10.1086/677145.pdf (Level VII)

8 Alberta Health Services. (2017). Artificial nails in the healthcare environment: Why we care. https://www.albertahealthservices.ca/assets/info/hp/hh/if-hp-hh-artificial-nails-in-healthcare.pdf (Level VII)

9 The Joint Commission. (2009). Measuring hand hygiene adherence: Overcoming the challenges. https://www.jointcommission.org/assets/1/18/hh_monograph.pdf (Level VII)

10 Centers for Disease Control and Prevention. (2021). When and how to wash your hands. https://www.cdc.gov/handwashing/when-how-handwashing.html (Level VII)

11 Health Research and Educational Trust. (2010). *Hand hygiene project: Best practices from hospitals participating in The Joint Commission Center for Transforming Healthcare Project.* Chicago, IL: Health Research and Educational Trust. http://www.hpoe.org/Reports-HPOE/hand_hygiene_project.pdf (Level VII)

12 Centers for Disease Control and Prevention. (2016). Clean hands count for patients. https://www.cdc.gov/handhygiene/patients/index.html

HAZARDOUS DRUG PREPARATION AND HANDLING

Nurses who handle hazardous drugs are at risk for occupational exposure, primarily through inhalation and skin contact but also through inadvertent ingestion and accidental injection.[1] Exposure can occur during drug handling activities (preparation, administration, and disposal) as well as during nondrug-related activities (handling items potentially contaminated with the drug or the patient's body fluids). Exposure to hazardous drugs places nurses at risk for acute and chronic adverse effects.

Hazardous drugs include chemotherapeutic agents, antiviral drugs, hormones, and bioengineered drugs as well as others outside these classes.[2] Hazardous drugs are categorized as antineoplastic drugs, non-antineoplastic hazardous drugs, and drugs that pose a reproductive risk.[2] This procedure focuses on non-antineoplastic hazardous drugs (see *Non-antineoplastic hazardous drugs*) and non-antineoplastic drugs that pose a reproductive risk (see *Non-antineoplastic drugs that pose a reproductive risk*, page 374).

Non-antineoplastic hazardous drugs

This table lists non-antineoplastic drug classes along with specific drugs in each class that are hazardous.[2]

Anticonvulsants
carBAMazepine
divalproex
fosphenytoin
OXcarbazepine
phenytoin

Antiparkinson agents
apomorphine
rasagiline

Antithyroid agents
methIMAzole
propylthiouracil

Antivirals
abacavir
cidofovir
entecavir
ganciclovir
nevirapine
valGANciclovir
zidovudine

Estrogen agonists-antagonists
ospemifene
raloxifene

Hormone and hormonal contraceptives
Estrogens
diethylstilbestrol
estradiol
estrogens, conjugated
estrogens, esterified
estropipate

Progesterones
medroxyPROGESTERone acetate
progesterone
Androgen
fluoxymesterone

Immunomodulatory agents
fingolimod
leflunomide
lenalidomide
teriflunomide
thalidomide
tofacitinib

Immunosuppressants
alefacept
azaTHIOprine
cycloSPORINE
mycophenolate mofetil
mycophenolic acid
sirolimus
tacrolimus

Miscellaneous agents
chloramphenicol (antibiotic)
deferiprone (chelating agent)
dexrazoxane (chemoprotective agent)
liraglutide recombinant (antidiabetic)
mipomersen (antilipid)
palifermin (human keratinocyte growth factor)
phenoxybenzamine (nonselective alpha-adrenergic blocker)
spironolactone (aldosterone antagonist diuretic)
uracil mustard

The risk of experiencing adverse effects increases with the amount and frequency of exposure and poor work practices.[1,2] The formulation of hazardous drugs also affects the risk of adverse effects. For example, powder or liquid medication poses a greater risk than coated tablets or capsules.[2] According to the Occupational Safety and Health Administration (OSHA), no acceptable levels of exposure have been determined for these drugs, and some exhibit toxicity at low doses; therefore, the goal is to prevent or minimize workplace exposure.[2,3]

OSHA, the National Institute for Occupational Safety and Health (NIOSH), the United States Pharmacopeia Convention, and the American Society of Health-System Pharmacists have established guidelines for the safe handling and administration of hazardous drugs. Adhering to these guidelines helps reduce the risk of contamination to health care workers and the environment. Using environmental and engineering controls, following good work practices, and wearing appropriate personal protective equipment properly decrease the risk of exposure. All health care workers who handle hazardous drugs must receive proper education and training in ways to reduce exposure when handling them.[1,3,4,5]

Hazardous drug preparation and handling should take place in a restricted, centralized area with negative pressure and external ventilation. A sink and eyewash station should be available in this area.[4,5] Within this area, nonsterile hazardous drugs should be prepared and handled in an enclosed class I biological safety cabinet (BSC) or a containment ventilated enclosure. Sterile hazardous drugs should be prepared and handled in an enclosed class II BSC or a compounding aseptic containment isolator.[1,3,4,5]

Use of proper personal protective equipment is essential. Personal protective equipment for preparing and handling hazardous drugs includes impermeable gowns and gloves, eye and face protection, and a NIOSH-certified fit-tested respirator. Gowns must be disposable and should be made of polyethylene-coated polypropylene, which is nonabsorbent and lint-free. Gowns should have long sleeves with elastic or knit cuffs, a full front, and a back closure.[4] Gloves should be powder-free chemotherapy gloves tested by the American Society for Testing and Materials.[4] Additional personal protective equipment, such as hair and shoe covers, may be required when compounding certain hazardous drugs, including sterile drug preparations.

Equipment

Safety data sheet (SDS) for the prescribed hazardous drug ■ prescribed drug and appropriate needles, syringes, and needleless systems required for preparation ■ polyethylene-coated polypropylene gown ■ powder-free chemotherapy gloves ■ face shield ■ goggles ■ NIOSH-certified fit-tested respirator ■ plastic-backed absorbent pad ■ facility-approved decontamination solution (such as sterile water, alcohol, peroxide, or sodium hypochlorite solution) ■ disposable towels ■ sealable plastic transport bag ■ puncture-resistant sharps container identified as hazardous waste ■ sealable hazardous waste containment bag ■ hazardous waste container with a lid ■ medication label ■ hazardous drug label (such as one with a warning stating HAZARDOUS DRUG—SPECIAL HANDLING/DISPOSAL PRECAUTIONS) ■ hazardous drug spill kit ■ ventilated cabinet ■ Optional: disposable hair and shoe covers, sterile chemotherapy gloves, 70% alcohol solution.

Preparation of equipment

Inspect all equipment and supplies. If a product is expired, is defective, or has compromised integrity, remove it from patient use, label it as

expired or defective, and report the expiration or defect as directed by your facility.

Make sure that a hazardous drug spill kit is readily available.

Implementation

■ Avoid distractions and interruptions when preparing the hazardous drug *to prevent medication errors.*[6,7]
■ Become familiar with the information in the SDS for the prescribed hazardous drug.[3]
■ Gather and prepare the necessary equipment and supplies *to avoid having to exit and re-enter the enclosed ventilated cabinet during hazardous drug preparation.* Place only the equipment and supplies essential to drug preparation in the work area.[3,5]
■ Verify the practitioner's written order and, if required by your facility, have a second practitioner independently verify the order.
■ Wash your hands with soap and water.[1,3,5]
■ Put on personal protective equipment, including two pairs of gloves, a polyethylene-coated polypropylene gown, a face shield and goggles (when splashing is possible), and a NIOSH-certified fit-tested respirator (when aerosolization is possible). Make sure that your inner glove cuff is worn under the gown cuff, and that the outer glove cuff extends over the gown cuff *to fully protect your skin.* If required by your facility, put on hair and shoe covers.[1,3,4,5]
NURSING ALERT When putting on personal protective equipment, keep in mind that eyeglasses alone don't provide adequate protection against splashes. Likewise, surgical masks don't provide adequate protection against exposure through aerosolization.[3,4,5]
■ If you're preparing a sterile drug, wear sterile chemotherapy gloves, sanitize them with a 70% alcohol solution, and allow them to dry completely.[3,8]
■ Inspect your gloves *to make sure that they're physically intact.*[1,3,5]
NURSING ALERT When working with hazardous drugs, change your gloves every 30 minutes. If you spill a drug solution on your glove or puncture or tear a glove, remove your gloves immediately. Wash your hands with soap and water before putting on new gloves and any time you remove your gloves. Likewise, change your gown immediately if it becomes damaged or contaminated.[1,3,5]
■ Wipe the internal surfaces of the enclosed ventilated cabinet with a facility-approved decontamination solution on a disposable towel. Allow the solution to dry completely. Discard the towel in a hazardous waste container. If you're preparing a sterile drug, use a 70% alcohol solution *to disinfect the cabinet surfaces.*[3,4,5]
■ Place a plastic-backed absorbent pad on the work surface of the ventilated cabinet *to absorb droplets and potential spills.* Change the pad if a spill occurs.[3,4,5]
■ Before introducing the hazardous drug into the enclosed ventilated cabinet, wipe down the outside of the drug container with a facility-approved decontamination solution on a disposable towel. Allow the solution to dry completely. Discard the towel in a hazardous waste container. If you're preparing a sterile drug, use a 70% alcohol solution *to disinfect the drug container and other supplies.*[3,4,5]
■ Prepare the hazardous drug in the enclosed ventilated cabinet according to the practitioner's order and manufacturer's instructions, paying attention to compatibility, stability, and reconstitution technique.
■ Use appropriate work practice controls to reduce exposure based on the hazardous drug's formulation *to supplement environmental design, engineering controls, and personal protective equipment.*[3,4,5] (See *Work practice controls.*)
■ After preparing the hazardous drug, wipe the outside of the drug container with a facility-approved decontamination solution on a disposable towel. Allow the solution to dry completely. Discard the towel in the hazardous waste containment bag in the enclosed ventilated cabinet.[3,5]
■ Place all contaminated supplies in a puncture-resistant sharps container or a hazardous waste containment bag (as appropriate) in the enclosed ventilated cabinet.[1]
■ Remove your outer gloves and place them in the hazardous waste containment bag in the enclosed ventilated cabinet.[3,5]

- Wipe the puncture-resistant sharps container and hazardous waste containment bag with a facility-approved decontamination solution on a disposable towel. Place the disposable towel in the hazardous waste containment bag and seal it.[1,5]
- Label the prepared drug with the patient's name and a second identifier, the drug's full generic name, drug administration route, total dose to be administered, total volume required to administer the dosage, date of administration, date and time of drug preparation, date and time of drug expiration, and special handling instructions, as appropriate. Also label the drug with a hazardous drug label.[3]
- Place the prepared hazardous drug container in a sealable plastic transport bag, taking care to avoid contaminating the outside of the transport bag. Seal the bag.[3,5]

NURSING ALERT Don't introduce the transport bag into the enclosed ventilated cabinet until after you complete the hazardous drug preparation *to prevent accidental contamination of the outside of the transport bag.*[3,5]

- Remove the transport bag containing the prepared hazardous drug from the enclosed ventilated cabinet.
- Remove the puncture-resistant sharps container (as appropriate), sealed hazardous waste containment bag, and plastic-backed absorbent pad from the enclosed ventilated cabinet. Discard them in a hazardous waste container.[1,3,5]
- Wipe the work surface of the enclosed ventilated cabinet with a facility-approved decontamination solution on a disposable towel and discard it in a hazardous waste container.[3,4,5]
- Remove your inner gloves and other personal protective equipment carefully by turning them inside out. Discard them in a hazardous waste container.[1,4]
- Wash your hands with soap and water.[1,3,5]
- Document the procedure.[4]

Special considerations

- Use resources to evaluate the hazard potential of the prescribed drug. Some resources include:[2] the drug's SDS; product labeling approved by the U.S. Food and Drug Administration (FDA); special health warnings from drug manufacturers, the FDA, and other professional organizations; reports and case studies published in medical and other health care profession journals; and evidence-based recommendations from other institutions that meet the criteria for defining hazardous drugs.
- Smoking, drinking, applying cosmetics, and eating where hazardous drugs are prepared, stored, or used is strictly prohibited. Don't place any food or drinks in the same refrigerator as hazardous drugs.[1]
- For accidental direct exposure to the skin or eyes, call for assistance, remove any contaminated clothing, and wash the affected skin with soap and water thoroughly, or rinse the affected eye with water or an isotonic eyewash solution for at least 15 minutes. Then seek medical attention.[3,5]
- For accidental ingestion, inhalation, or needlestick exposure, call for assistance and seek medical attention.[3]
- If a hazardous drug spill occurs, refer to the appropriate procedure. (See the "Hazardous drug spill management" procedure.)
- Be aware that excreta (urine, emesis, or feces) from patients who have received hazardous drugs in the last 48 hours contain varying concentrations of the drugs or their metabolic byproducts. Health care workers responsible for handling excreta must wear appropriate personal protective equipment *to prevent exposure.*[3]
- Note that any health care worker who's pregnant, trying to conceive or father a child, or breastfeeding shouldn't be exposed to hazardous drugs.[3,9]

Complications

Long-term or chronic effects of hazardous drug exposure that have been identified include damage to the liver, kidneys, bone marrow, lungs, and heart; infertility (temporary and permanent); effects on reproduction and the developing fetus; hearing impairment; and cancer.[1,3] Acute reactions to hazardous drug exposure include lightheadedness and dizziness, nausea and vomiting, skin irritation, and hair loss.[3]

Documentation

Document drug preparation and each incident of exposure as directed by your facility.

REFERENCES

1 National Institute for Occupational Safety and Health. (2004). NIOSH alert: Preventing occupational exposure to antineoplastic and other hazardous drugs in health care settings. https://www.cdc.gov/niosh/docs/2004-165/pdfs/2004-165.pdf (Level VII)

2 National Institute for Occupational Safety and Health. (2016, reviewed 2017). NIOSH list of antineoplastic and other hazardous drugs in healthcare settings, 2016 (NIOSH publication number 2014–138). https://www.cdc.gov/niosh/docs/2016-161/default.html (Level VII)

3 Occupational Safety and Health Administration. (n.d.). Controlling occupational exposure to hazardous drugs. https://www.osha.gov/hazardous-drugs/controlling-occex (Level VII)

4 United States Pharmacopeia Convention. (2019, revised 2020). USP general chapter <800> Hazardous drugs—handling in healthcare settings. https://www.usp.org/compounding/general-chapter-hazardous-drugs-handling-healthcare (Level VII)

5 American Society of Health System Pharmacists. (2018). ASHP guidelines on handling hazardous drugs. https://www.ashp.org/-/media/assets/policy-guidelines/docs/guidelines/handling-hazardous-drugs.ashx (Level VII)

6 Westbrook, J., et al. (2010). Association of interruptions with an increased risk and severity of medication administration errors. *Archives of Internal Medicine, 170,* 683–690. (Level IV)

7 Institute for Safe Medication Practices. (2012). Side tracks on the safety express: Interruptions lead to errors and unfinished...Wait, what was I doing? *Nurse Advise-ERR, 11*(2), 1–4. https://www.ismp.org/resources/side-tracks-safety-express-interruptions-lead-errors-and-unfinished-wait-what-was-i-doing?id=37

8 United States Pharmacopeia Convention. (2008). USP general chapter <797>: Pharmaceutical compounding—Sterile preparations. https://www.usp.org/compounding/general-chapter-797 (Level VII)

9 Lawson, C. C., et al. (2012). Occupational exposures among nurses and risk of spontaneous abortion. *American Journal of Obstetrics and Gynecology, 206,* 327.e1–327.e8. (Level IV)

Work practice controls

Be sure to use work practice controls during hazardous drug preparation and handling to supplement—not substitute for—environmental and engineering controls. Also ensure the proper use of personal protective equipment.[1,3,4] Work practice controls are dependent on the hazardous drug formulation and include the following:

- Always work below eye level when preparing or handling any drug formulation *to prevent accidental exposure to the eyes.*[3]
- Use closed-system transfer devices and needleless systems with locking fittings, if available, when transferring liquid hazardous drugs from their original packaging to administration equipment *to minimize aerosolization and reduce the risk of needlestick injuries.*[1,5]
- After drawing a hazardous drug into a syringe, expel any excess air or drug into a sterile vial and then pull back on the plunger *to clear the drug from the needle and hub.* Avoid filling syringes more than three-quarters full. Place a locking cap on the syringe.[3,5]
- Avoid pressurized vials and ampules whenever possible, *because the contents of these containers are difficult to control and may spill or splash.*[3]
- Prime IV sets with a non-drug-containing solution using a backflow method before introducing the hazardous drug into the solution. Don't use vented administration sets. Once the IV set is primed, don't separate the tubing from the hazardous drug container.[1,3,5]
- Avoid crushing tablets or opening capsules; use liquid formulations whenever possible.[5] If you must crush tablets, first place them in a plastic sleeve *to contain the dust particles that you generate.*[4]

Hazardous drug spill management

Nurses who prepare and administer hazardous drugs are at risk for occupational exposure, which in turn places them at risk for certain types of cancer, including leukemia; infertility and miscarriage; irritation to the skin or eyes; and allergic reactions.[1] Factors that affect the risk of exposure include preparing, administering, and disposing of hazardous drugs; the amount of drug prepared; the frequency and duration of drug handling; the potential for absorption; the use of ventilated cabinets; and work practices.[2]

The risk of experiencing adverse effects increases with the amount and frequency of exposure and poor work practices.[1] Following good work practices and using proper personal protective equipment decrease the risk of such exposure.[3]

Facilities that store, transport, prepare, and administer hazardous drugs should have emergency procedures for handling spills and exposure as part of their overall health and safety program.[3] Hazardous drug spill kits should be available wherever chemotherapeutic agents and other hazardous drugs are stored, transported, prepared, or administered.[4] All health care facility personnel who work with or handle hazardous drugs should be trained properly in spill cleanup.[2]

Equipment

Hazardous drug precaution sign ▪ disposable, low-permeability, back-closure, hemotherapy-resistant gown ▪ hazardous drug–resistant shoe covers ▪ two pairs of hazardous drug–resistant gloves ▪ face shield ▪ goggles ▪ respirator mask, appropriate for the spilled agent, approved by the National Institute for Occupational Safety and Health (NIOSH), such as fit-tested N95 or powered air-purifying respirator[4,5] ▪ disposable scoop for collecting glass fragments ▪ puncture-proof container for glass fragments ▪ heavy-duty utility gloves ▪ absorbent spill pads or absorbent plastic-backed sheets[3,4] ▪ disposable towels ▪ absorbent powder ▪ at least two large, heavy-duty, hazardous waste–labeled, sealable, disposable bags ▪ water ▪ facility-approved deactivating and decontaminating agents ▪ small, sealable plastic bag ▪ safety data sheet (SDS) ▪ cleaning agent designed to remove chemicals from stainless steel ▪ Optional: chemical cartridge-type respirator with full face piece.

Preparation of equipment

Inspect all equipment and supplies. If a product is expired, is defective, or has compromised integrity, remove it from patient use, label it as expired or defective, and report the expiration or defect as directed by your facility.

Spill kits that contain all the materials needed to clean up hazardous drug spills should be available wherever hazardous drugs are located.[4,5] Each kit should have sufficient supplies to absorb about 1,000 mL of hazardous drug. Assemble your own kit or use your facility's commercially prepared kit as appropriate.[2,3]

Access the SDS for the spilled agent *to determine if a chemical deactivator is recommended for use.*[4]

Implementation

▪ Assess the size of the hazardous drug spill and call for trained assistance, if needed.[4] If the spill is large and can't be contained with two spill kits, call for additional help.[2,3]
▪ Post a hazardous drug precaution sign immediately *to warn others of the presence of a hazardous drug spill and to limit access.*[2,3,4,5]
▪ Obtain and open a spill kit.[2,3,5]
▪ Put on gloves (inner and outer), a disposable gown, shoe covers, a face shield, goggles, and a respirator mask that's appropriate for the spilled agent.[4] The use of face shields with goggles is recommended *because they offer added skin and eye protection.* Don't use eyeglasses or safety glasses with side shields *because they don't offer adequate protection from splashes.* Put on a chemical cartridge-type respirator with a full face piece for a large spill.[2,3,5]
▪ Choose the appropriate items in the spill kit to contain the spill.[2,3]

Spills on hard surfaces

▪ Pick up any broken glass fragments with the disposable scoop or by hand wearing heavy-duty utility gloves. Place the fragments in a puncture-proof container.[2,3,4]
▪ Place an absorbent spill pad or absorbent plastic-backed sheet over the spill to wipe up a liquid. Use a damp disposable towel to wipe up powder or solids.[2,3,4]

Spills on soft surfaces

▪ Pick up any broken glass fragments with the disposable scoop or by hand wearing heavy-duty utility gloves. Place the fragments in a puncture-proof container.[2,3,4]
▪ Use an absorbent powder on the spill following the manufacturer's instructions. Don't use absorbent towels.[4]
▪ After the initial cleanup and containment, contact appropriately trained environmental services staff members to vacuum the area to remove the powder using a vacuum with a high-efficiency particulate air (HEPA) filter reserved for hazardous drug cleanup.[2,4,6]
▪ Ensure that the soft surface is cleaned as directed by your facility.[4]

Spills in a biological safety cabinet (BSC)

▪ Remove any broken glass fragments by hand wearing heavy-duty utility gloves. Place the fragments in a puncture-proof container. Be careful not to damage the fixed-glove assembly in the isolator.[2,3]
▪ Clean up a liquid spill with absorbent spill pads. For a powder or solid spill, use a damp disposable towel. Include the drain spillage trough in washing efforts.[2,3,4]
▪ Thoroughly clean and decontaminate the involved area using a cleaning agent designed to remove chemicals from stainless steel. Refer to the SDS for the cleaning agent, as needed.[2,4,7]
▪ If the HEPA filter has been contaminated by the spill, seal the BSC in a small, sealable plastic bag or plastic sheeting and label it as contaminated equipment.[4]
▪ Schedule a BSC service technician to change the HEPA filter.[4]
▪ Ensure that the BSC isn't used before the filter has been changed.[2,4]

Completing the procedure

▪ Place the puncture-proof container holding the glass fragments and all other contaminated materials into a large, heavy-duty, hazardous waste–labeled, sealable, disposable bag. Then seal the bag.[2,3,4]
▪ Place the sealed bag inside another properly labeled hazardous waste bag and leave the outer bag open.
▪ Rinse the contaminated area with water and then clean it with facility-approved deactivating and decontaminating agents following the manufacturers' instructions for use.[2,3]
▪ Rinse the contaminated area with water several more times. Place all materials used for cleanup and containment in disposable hazardous waste bags.[2,3]
▪ Seal the hazardous waste bags and put them in the appropriate container for final disposal as hazardous waste.[2,3]
▪ Remove all personal protective equipment carefully while continuing to wear your inner gloves. Consider all personal protective equipment worn during hazardous drug spill cleanup to be at least minimally contaminated with trace amounts of hazardous material.[2,3,5]
▪ Put all disposable personal protective equipment in an appropriately labeled hazardous waste disposable bag. Then seal the bag.[2,3]
▪ Remove your inner gloves.
▪ Contain your inner gloves in a small, sealable plastic bag. Then place that bag in the final container *to dispose of as hazardous waste.*[2,3]
▪ Dispose of personal protective equipment in the final hazardous waste container as trace- or bulk-contaminated waste, as determined by your facility.[4,8]
▪ Perform hand hygiene.[8,9,10,11,12,13,14]
▪ After the initial cleanup, contact your facility's environmental services department to reclean the area.[2,3]
▪ Report and document the hazardous drug spill.[4,15,16,17,18]

Special considerations

■ When cleaning hazardous drug spills, move from the area of lowest contamination to the area of highest contamination.[2,3]

■ Before use, inspect your gloves for defects, such as holes or tears. Use only gloves that are permeation-resistant to hazardous agents.[8]

■ If you have experienced direct skin or eye contact with a hazardous drug during a spill, remove any contaminated clothing immediately and wash the affected skin with soap and water, or flood the affected eye with isotonic eyewash for at least 15 minutes. Then seek medical attention.[2,3]

■ Send any nonemployee who has been exposed to the hazardous drug spill to your facility's emergency department for treatment or as directed by your facility. Then fill out your facility's incident or exposure form.[5]

Complications

Exposure to the hazardous drug is a complication of hazardous drug spill management.[2,3,4]

Documentation

Document the name of the hazardous drug and the approximate volume of drug spilled. Objectively describe how the spill occurred, the actions that were taken to manage the spill, and the procedure that was followed. Document the names of health care facility personnel and patients as well as anyone else who was exposed to the drug spill. Also document the names of facility personnel notified of the spill and the departments in which they work.

REFERENCES

1 Centers for Disease Control and Prevention, Department of Health and Human Services. (2004). NIOSH alert: Preventing occupational exposures to antineoplastic and other hazardous drugs in health care settings. https://www.cdc.gov/niosh/docs/2004-165/pdfs/2004-165.pdf (Level VII)

2 Power, L. A., & Coyne, J. W. (2018). ASHP guidelines on handling hazardous drugs. *American Journal of Health-System Pharmacy, 75,* 1996–2031. (Level VII)

3 Occupational Safety and Health Administration. (n.d.). Controlling occupational exposure to hazardous drugs. https://www.osha.gov/hazardous-drugs/controlling-occex (Level VII)

4 Olsen, M. M., et al. (Eds.). (2019). *Chemotherapy and immunotherapy guidelines and recommendations for practice.* Pittsburgh, PA: Oncology Nursing Society.

5 United States Pharmacopeial Convention (USP). (2019). USP general chapter <800> Hazardous drugs—Handling in healthcare settings. https://www.usp.org/compounding/general-chapter-hazardous-drugs-handling-healthcare

6 Esparza, D. M. (Ed.). (2014). *Oncology policies and procedures [CD-ROM].* Pittsburgh, PA: Oncology Nursing Society.

7 Lamerie, T. Q., et al. (2013). Evaluation of decontamination efficacy of cleaning solutions on stainless steel and glass surfaces contaminated by 10 antineoplastic agents. *The Annals of Occupational Hygiene, 57,* 456–469. https://academic.oup.com/annweh/article/57/4/456/158082?sid=f89 30b35-f5e0-4502-9822-b2f7290f532e (Level VI)

8 Connor, T. H., et al. (2008). Personal protective equipment for health care workers who work with hazardous drugs. https://www.cdc.gov/niosh/docs/wp-solutions/2009-106/pdfs/2009-106.pdf (Level I)

9 Centers for Disease Control and Prevention. (2002). Guideline for hand hygiene in health-care settings: Recommendations of the Healthcare Infection Control Practices Advisory Committee and the HICPAC/SHEA/APIC/IDSA Hand Hygiene Task Force. *MMWR Recommendations and Reports, 51*(RR-16), 1–45. A https://www.cdc.gov/mmwr/pdf/rr/rr5116.pdf (Level II)

10 The Joint Commission. (2021). Standard NPSG.07.01.01. *Comprehensive accreditation manual for hospitals.* Oakbrook Terrace, IL: The Joint Commission. (Level VII)

11 World Health Organization. (2009). WHO guidelines on hand hygiene in health care: First global patient safety challenge, clean care is safer care. https://apps.who.int/iris/bitstream/handle/10665/44102/9789241597906_eng.pdf?sequence=1 (Level IV)

12 Centers for Medicare and Medicaid Services, Department of Health and Human Services. (2020). Condition of participation: Infection control. 42 C.F.R. § 482.42.

13 Accreditation Association for Hospitals and Health Systems. (2020). Standard 07.01.21. *Healthcare Facilities Accreditation Program: Accreditation requirements for acute care hospitals.* Chicago, IL: Accreditation Association for Hospitals and Health Systems. (Level VII)

14 DNV GL-Healthcare USA, Inc. (2020). IC.1.SR.1. *NIAHO® accreditation requirements, interpretive guidelines and surveyor guidance—revision 20.0.* Milford, OH: DNV GL-Healthcare USA, Inc. (Level VII)

15 Centers for Medicare and Medicaid Services, Department of Health and Human Services. (2020). Condition of participation: Medical record services. 42 C.F.R. § 482.24(b).

16 Accreditation Association for Hospitals and Health Systems. (2020). Standard 10.00.03. *Healthcare Facilities Accreditation Program: Accreditation requirements for acute care hospitals.* Chicago, IL: Accreditation Association for Hospitals and Health Systems. (Level VII)

17 The Joint Commission. (2021). Standard RC.01.03.01. *Comprehensive accreditation manual for hospitals.* Oakbrook Terrace, IL: The Joint Commission. (Level VII)

18 DNV GL-Healthcare USA, Inc. (2020). MR.2.SR.1. *NIAHO® accreditation requirements, interpretive guidelines and surveyor guidance—revision 20.0.* Milford, OH: DNV GL-Healthcare USA, Inc. (Level VII)

HEARING AID CARE

Hearing loss may be congenital (developmental abnormalities of the outer, middle, or inner ear) or may be caused by disorders of the outer ear, middle ear, or inner ear. Outer ear causes of hearing loss include infection, trauma, or tumors of the external auditory canal (EAC); systemic disease such as diabetes mellitus causing occlusion of the EAC; skin diseases causing edema of the EAC; or cerumen impaction. Middle ear causes of hearing loss may include eustachian tube dysfunction, infection, tumors of the middle ear, otosclerosis, tympanic membrane perforation, or barotrauma. Inner ear causes of hearing loss include age changes (presbycusis); infection; Meniere disease; long-term exposure to loud noise; barotrauma; penetrating trauma or other injury to the inner ear; tumors; autoimmune, endocrine, systemic, neurologic, or metabolic disorders; and certain drugs (antibiotics and chemotherapeutic agents) and heavy metals.[1] Hearing aids, which are available in digital and analog form, can help some patients regain some of their lost hearing. Analog hearing aids simply amplify speech and sound; digital hearing aids provide amplification that can be individualized for the patient's type of hearing loss. All hearing aids have a microphone, a speaker, and an amplifier. There are numerous types of hearing aids:[2]

■ An *open-behind-the-ear aid* is a slim tube inserted into the external ear canal. This aid leaves the ear canal open, so it's best for mild to moderate high-frequency hearing loss in which low-frequency hearing is still normal or near normal.

■ A *behind-the-ear* aid amplifies the sound from a customized ear mold that's placed in the external ear canal. This type of aid is appropriate for almost all types of hearing loss.

■ A *full-shell aid* is custom-made and fills most of the bowl-shaped area of the outer ear. It's used for mild to severe hearing loss.

■ A *half-shell aid* is custom-made and fills the lower portion of the bowl-shaped area of the outer ear. It provides optimum performance and maximum comfort. It's used for mild to severe hearing loss.

■ A *canal aid* fits partially inside the external ear canal and is used for mild to moderately severe hearing loss.

■ A *mini-canal aid* fits almost completely inside the external ear canal and is appropriate for mild to moderately severe hearing loss.

■ A *completely-in-the-canal aid* fits deeply within the external ear canal. This type decreases wind noise, has less feedback, and provides a more natural sound. Those with mild to moderately severe hearing loss can benefit from this type of aid.

Patients generally wear hearing aids only during the day. At night and at times of rest, most patients remove their hearing aids. Because of the fragile nature of the hearing aid, the device must be cleaned properly and carefully to avoid damage.

Equipment

Hearing aid ■ facial tissue or dry cloth ■ cleaning tools based on the manufacturer's instructions ■ labeled storage container ■ towel ■ washcloth ■ warm water ■ soap ■ Optional: spare battery, hearing aid dehumidifying container, gloves.

Implementation

- Gather and prepare the necessary equipment and supplies.
- Perform hand hygiene.[3,4,5,6,7,8]
- Confirm the patient's identity using at least two patient identifiers.[9]
- Provide privacy.[10,11,12,13]
- Raise the patient's bed to waist level before providing care *to prevent caregiver back strain.*[14]
- Perform hand hygiene.[3,4,5,6,7,8]

Removing and cleaning the hearing aid

- Inspect the patient's ear. If drainage is present, put on gloves *to comply with standard precautions.*[15,16,17]
- Gently turn the hearing aid off *to prevent feedback (whistling or squealing) during removal.*
- Grasp the hearing aid and remove it, following the contour of the patient's ear.
- Wipe the outside of the hearing aid with a facial tissue or dry cloth.[18] Don't use tissues or cloths that contain lotion or aloe.[19]
- Carefully inspect the hearing aid and look for accumulated cerumen. *Cerumen can block sound and cause feedback (squealing or whistling sounds).*[18]
- Clean the hearing air following the manufacturer's instructions.
- Inspect the hearing aid for any rough areas that may irritate the ear canal.[19]
- Open the battery compartment of the hearing aid *to conserve battery life and allow internal components to air-dry.*[18,19]
- Place the hearing aid and battery in a storage container labeled with the patient's name, room number, and identification number. If possible, use a dehumidifying container to store hearing aids *to draw out moisture.*[19]
- Assess the patient's ear for drainage, redness, and irritation.
- Place a towel under the patient's ear and gently clean the ear and ear canal using a washcloth, soap, and warm water. Then dry the ear with a towel.

NURSING ALERT Don't use alcohol or other solvents on the hearing aid, *because they may cause breakdown of the material.*

Inserting the hearing aid

- Gently remove the hearing aid from the storage container.
- Close the battery compartment door.
- Cupping your hand over the hearing aid, test the battery by slowing turning the volume to high. You should hear feedback; when you do, decrease the volume. If you don't hear feedback, turn off the hearing aid and replace the battery.
- Insert the hearing aid into the appropriate ear by holding it with the thumb and index finger of your dominant hand and placing it in the ear, following the contour of the patient's ear. Note that some hearing aids are color-coded red for right and blue for left.
- Turn the volume up slowly until it reaches a comfortable level for the patient.
- If you or the patient hears feedback after insertion, decrease the volume, reposition the device, and check the ear canal for blockage from cerumen.[18]

Completing the procedure

- Return the bed to the lowest position *to prevent falls and maintain patient safety.*[20]
- Remove and discard your gloves, if worn.[15,17]
- Perform hand hygiene.[3,4,5,6,7,8]
- Document the procedure.[21,22,23,24]

Special considerations

- When communicating with a patient who has hearing loss, keep these points in mind. Many individuals with severe hearing loss have learned to read lips. Although this skill improves reception of the words, it doesn't improve the ability to hear. Face the patient when you speak, keep your hands away from your face, and speak clearly with a slightly raised voice and at a regular speed (not too slowly or too quickly).[25] Keep background noise to a minimum if possible.[25] *White noise can cause distractions, especially at higher frequencies.* Repeat and rephrase your sentences if the patient doesn't understand what you're saying. Use hand gestures and body language to assist with communication.[25]
- Avoid placing the hearing aid in direct sunlight or direct heat. Store batteries in a cool, dry place. Don't store them in the refrigerator.[18]
- Hearing aid batteries should last 1 to 2 weeks. If available, use a battery tester to check battery strength.[18]

Patient teaching

Teach the patient how to properly remove, clean, and insert the hearing aid.

ELDER ALERT Some older adult patients may have difficulty manipulating hearing aids, making it difficult to correctly insert and clean them. In such a case, refer the patient to an audiologist, who can recommend a hearing aid that will better fit the patient's abilities.

Tell the patient to keep the hearing aid in the storage case when not in use *to avoid damage.*[19] Also, tell the patient to keep the hearing aid out of reach of children and animals. Dogs are attracted to the smell of hearing aids and may damage them if they can reach them. Tell the patient to keep the hearing aid dry and to remove it before showering, swimming, or participating in an activity with water.[19] The patient should also avoid getting hairspray or cologne on the hearing aid.

Refer the patient for counseling and rehabilitative training, as needed, *to help the patient cope with hearing impairment and to learn ways to modify the environment to accommodate hearing loss.*[26]

Complications

Dropping the hearing aid may damage it; wearing a damaged device may cause ear irritation or abrasion.[19] If moisture enters the hearing aid, either during wear or during cleaning, the device might stop transmitting sound.

Documentation

Document the proper functioning, insertion, removal, and cleaning of each hearing aid. Also note skin integrity and the presence of redness, drainage, or excessive cerumen. Document the location where the hearing aid was stored. Document teaching provided to the patient and family (if applicable), their understanding of that teaching, and any need for follow-up teaching.

REFERENCES

1 Weber, P. C. (2020). Etiology of hearing loss in adults. In: *UpToDate*, Deschler, D. G. (Ed.).
2 The Mayo Clinic. (2020). Hearing aids: How to choose the right one. https://www.mayoclinic.org/diseases-conditions/hearing-loss/in-depth/hearing-aids/ART-20044116
3 The Joint Commission. (2021). Standard NPSG.07.01.01. *Comprehensive accreditation manual for hospitals.* Oakbrook Terrace, IL: The Joint Commission. (Level VII)
4 Centers for Disease Control and Prevention. (2002). Guideline for hand hygiene in health-care settings: Recommendations of the Healthcare Infection Control Practices Advisory Committee and the HICPAC/SHEA/APIC/IDSA Hand Hygiene Task Force. *MMWR Recommendations and Reports, 51*(RR-16), 1–45. https://www.cdc.gov/mmwr/pdf/rr/rr5116.pdf (Level II)
5 World Health Organization. (2009). WHO guidelines on hand hygiene in health care: First global patient safety challenge, clean care is safer care. https://apps.who.int/iris/bitstream/handle/10665/44102/9789241597906_eng.pdf?sequence=1 (Level IV)
6 Accreditation Association for Hospitals and Health Systems. (2020). Standard 07.01.21. *Healthcare Facilities Accreditation Program: Accreditation requirements for acute care hospitals.* Chicago, IL: Accreditation Association for Hospitals and Health Systems. (Level VII)
7 Centers for Medicare and Medicaid Services, Department of Health and Human Services. (2020). Condition of participation: Infection control. 42 C.F.R. § 482.42.
8 DNV GL-Healthcare USA, Inc. (2020). IC.1.SR.1. *NIAHO® accreditation requirements, interpretive guidelines and surveyor guidance—revision 20.0.* Milford, OH: DNV GL-Healthcare USA, Inc. (Level VII)

9   The Joint Commission. (2021). Standard NPSG.01.01.01. *Comprehensive accreditation manual for hospitals.* Oakbrook Terrace, IL: The Joint Commission. (Level VII)

10 The Joint Commission. (2021). Standard RI.01.01.01. *Comprehensive accreditation manual for hospitals.* Oakbrook Terrace, IL: The Joint Commission. (Level VII)

11 Centers for Medicare and Medicaid Services, Department of Health and Human Services. (2020). Condition of participation: Patient's rights. 42 C.F.R. § 482.13(c)(1).

12 Accreditation Association for Hospitals and Health Systems. (2020). Standard 15.01.16. *Healthcare Facilities Accreditation Program: Accreditation requirements for acute care hospitals.* Chicago, IL: Accreditation Association for Hospitals and Health Systems. (Level VII)

13 DNV GL-Healthcare USA, Inc. (2020). PR.2.SR.5. *NIAHO® accreditation requirements, interpretive guidelines and surveyor guidance—revision 20.0.* Milford, OH: DNV GL-Healthcare USA, Inc. (Level VII)

14 Waters, T. R., et al. (2009). Safe patient handling training for schools of nursing. https://www.cdc.gov/niosh/docs/2009-127/pdfs/2009-127.pdf (Level VII)

15 Siegel, J. D., et al. (2007, revised 2019). 2007 guideline for isolation precautions: Preventing transmission of infectious agents in healthcare settings. https://www.cdc.gov/infectioncontrol/pdf/guidelines/isolation-guidelines-H.pdf (Level II)

16 Accreditation Association for Hospitals and Health Systems. (2020). Standard 07.01.10. *Healthcare Facilities Accreditation Program: Accreditation requirements for acute care hospitals.* Chicago, IL: Accreditation Association for Hospitals and Health Systems. (Level VII)

17 Occupational Safety and Health Administration. (2019). Bloodborne pathogens, standard number 1910.1030. https://www.osha.gov/pls/oshaweb/owadisp.show_document?p_id=10051&p_table=STANDARDS (Level VII)

18 American Speech-Language-Hearing Association. (2015). Audiology information series: Daily care and troubleshooting tips for hearing aids. https://www.asha.org/uploadedFiles/AIS-Hearing-Aids-Troubleshooting.pdf#search=%22audiology%22

19 Pinkerton, C. (2016). How to properly clean and care for your hearing aids. https://www.starkey.com/blog/2016/03/hearing-aid-cleaning-tips

20 Ganz, D. A., et al. (2013, reviewed 2021). *Preventing falls in hospitals: A toolkit for improving quality of care* (AHRQ Publication No. 13-0015-EF). Rockville, MD: Agency for Healthcare Research and Quality. https://www.ahrq.gov/professionals/systems/hospital/fallpxtoolkit/index.html (Level VII)

21 The Joint Commission. (2021). Standard RC.01.03.01. *Comprehensive accreditation manual for hospitals.* Oakbrook Terrace, IL: The Joint Commission. (Level VII)

22 Accreditation Association for Hospitals and Health Systems. (2020). Standard 10.00.03. *Healthcare Facilities Accreditation Program: Accreditation requirements for acute care hospitals.* Chicago, IL: Accreditation Association for Hospitals and Health Systems. (Level VII)

23 Centers for Medicare and Medicaid Services, Department of Health and Human Services. (2020). Condition of participation: Medical record services. 42 C.F.R. § 482.24(b).

24 DNV GL-Healthcare USA, Inc. (2020). MR.2.SR.1. *NIAHO® accreditation requirements, interpretive guidelines and surveyor guidance—revision 20.0.* Milford, OH: DNV GL-Healthcare USA, Inc. (Level VII)

25 AgingCare.com. (n.d.). How to communicate with a senior who has hearing loss. https://www.agingcare.com/articles/hearing-loss-communication-techniques-144762.htm

26 Solheim, J., et al. (2016). Lack of ear care knowledge in nursing homes. *Journal of Multidisciplinary Healthcare, 9,* 481–488.

HEAT APPLICATION

Heat applied directly to the patient's body raises tissue temperature and enhances the inflammatory process by causing vasodilation and increasing local circulation, which promotes leukocytosis, suppuration, drainage, and healing. Heat also increases tissue metabolism; reduces pain caused by muscle spasm, muscle strains, or minor aches and stiffness; and decreases congestion in deep visceral organs.[1]

Direct heat may be dry or moist. Dry heat can be delivered at a higher temperature and for a longer time than moist heat. Devices for applying dry heat include the hot-water bottle, electric heating pad with or without circulating water, and chemical hot pack.[2]

Direct moist heat softens crusts and exudates, penetrates deeper than dry heat, is less drying to the skin, produces less perspiration, and is usually more comfortable for the patient.[2] Devices for applying direct moist heat include warm compresses for small body areas and warm packs for large areas.

Direct heat application can't be used on a patient at risk for hemorrhage. It also is contraindicated if the patient has a sprained limb in the acute stage (because vasodilation would increase pain and swelling) or a condition associated with acute inflammation, such as appendicitis. Direct heat should be applied cautiously to pediatric and older adult patients[2] and to patients with impaired kidney, cardiac, or respiratory function; arteriosclerosis or atherosclerosis; impaired sensation; diabetes; or a spinal cord injury. It should be applied with extreme caution to heat-sensitive areas, such as scar tissue and stomas. Don't apply heat to an open wound after trauma, to inflamed or edematous areas, to a localized malignant tumor, to the testes, to the abdomen of a pregnant woman, or over metallic implants.[2]

NURSING ALERT Don't apply direct heat over a fentanyl transdermal system or its surrounding area, *because an increase in temperature increases fentanyl release from the system, which may result in overdose and death.*[3]

Equipment

Vital signs monitoring equipment ■ watch, clock, or timer ■ Optional: gloves, towel, sterile towel, dressings, adhesive tape, or roller gauze.

For a hot-water bottle
Hot-water bottle ■ hot tap water ■ pitcher ■ bath (utility) thermometer ■ absorbent, protective cloth covering.

For an electric heating pad
Electric heating pad ■ absorbent, protective cloth covering or heating pad cover.

For a chemical hot pack (disposable)
Chemical hot pack ■ protective cloth covering.

For a warm compress or pack (sterile or nonsterile)
Warm compress or pack ■ basin or sink of hot tap water ■ container of sterile water, sterile normal saline solution, or prescribed solution ■ sterile bowl or basin ■ fluid-impermeable pad ■ sterile or nonsterile bath (utility) thermometer ■ waterproof trash bag ■ sterile or nonsterile waterproof covering ■ Optional: sterile forceps, clean container, hot-water bottle or chemical hot pack.

Preparation of equipment

Inspect all equipment and supplies. If a product is expired, is defective, or has compromised integrity, remove it from patient use, label it as expired or defective, and report the expiration or defect as directed by your facility.

Hot-water bottle
Fill the bottle with hot tap water *to detect leaks and warm the bottle;* then empty it. Run hot tap water into a pitcher and measure the water temperature with the bath (utility) thermometer. Adjust the temperature as ordered, usually to 115° to 125° F (46.1° to 51.7° C) for adults.

PEDIATRIC ALERT Adjust water temperature to between 105° and 115° F (40.6° to 46.1° C) for children younger than age 2.

ELDER ALERT Adjust water temperature to between 105° and 115° F (40.6° to 46.1° C) for older adult patients.

Next, pour hot tap water into the bottle, filling it one-half to two-thirds full. *Partially filling the bottle keeps it lightweight and flexible to mold to the treatment area.* Squeeze the bottle until the water reaches the neck *to expel any air that would make the bottle inflexible and reduce heat conduction.* Fasten the top and check the bag for leaks. Place the bag in an absorbent cloth covering, and secure the cover with tape or roller gauze.

Electric heating pad

Check the cord to ensure it is not frayed and doesn't have damaged insulation. Then plug in the pad and adjust the control switch to the desired setting. Wrap the pad in an absorbent, protective cloth covering, and secure the cover with tape or roller gauze. If the pad comes with its own cover, inspect the cover and fasteners *to ensure that all are intact.* Follow the manufacturer's instructions for use for an electric heating pad that circulates water.

Chemical hot pack

Select a disposable pack of the correct size. Then follow the manufacturer's directions (strike, squeeze, or knead) *to activate the heat-producing chemicals.* Place the pack in a protective cloth covering and secure the cover with tape or roller gauze.

Sterile warm compress or pack

Warm the container of sterile water or another solution (sterile normal saline solution or prescribed solution) by setting it in a sink or basin of hot tap water. Measure its temperature with a sterile bath (utility) thermometer. If a sterile thermometer is unavailable, pour some heated sterile solution into a clean container, check the temperature with a regular bath thermometer, and then discard the tested solution. Adjust the temperature by adding hot or cold tap water to the sink or basin until the solution reaches 120° F (48.9° C) for adults.

PEDIATRIC ALERT Adjust the water temperature to 100° F (37.8° C) for children or for an eye compress.

ELDER ALERT Adjust the water temperature to 100° F (37.8° C) for older adult patients or for an eye compress.

Pour the heated sterile solution into a sterile bowl or basin. Then, using sterile technique, soak the compress or pack in the heated solution and wring out excess solution while maintaining sterility. If necessary, prepare a hot-water bottle or chemical hot pack *to keep the compress or pack warm.*

Nonsterile warm compress or pack

Fill a bowl or basin with hot tap water, normal saline solution, or prescribed solution and measure the temperature of the solution using a nonsterile bath (utility) thermometer. Adjust the temperature as ordered, usually to 120° F (48.9° C) for adults.[3]

PEDIATRIC ALERT Adjust the water temperature to 100° F (37.8° C) for children or for an eye compress.

ELDER ALERT Adjust the water temperature to 100° F (37.8° C) for older adult or for an eye compress.

Soak the compress or pack in the hot liquid and wring out excess liquid. If necessary, prepare a hot-water bottle, K pad, or chemical hot pack *to keep the compress or pack warm.*

Implementation

- Verify the practitioner's order if needed.
- Gather and prepare the necessary equipment and supplies.
- Perform hand hygiene.[4,5,6,7,8,9]
- Confirm the patient's identity using at least two patient identifiers.[10]
- Provide privacy.[11,12,13,14]
- Explain the procedure to the patient and family (if appropriate) according to their individual communication and learning needs *to increase their understanding, allay their fears, and enhance cooperation.*[15] Tell the patient not to lean or lie directly on the heating device, *because direct contact reduces air space and increases the risk of burns.* Warn the patient against adjusting the temperature of the heating device or adding hot water to a hot-water bottle. Advise the patient to report pain immediately and to remove the device if necessary.

- Make sure the room is warm and free of drafts.
- Raise the bed to waist level before providing care *to prevent caregiver back strain.*[16]
- Perform hand hygiene.[4,5,6,7,8,9]
- Put on gloves or sterile gloves as needed *to comply with standard precautions.*[17,18,19]
- Obtain the patient's temperature, pulse, and respirations *to serve as a baseline for comparison.* If direct heat treatment is being applied to raise the patient's body temperature, monitor the patient's temperature, pulse, and respirations throughout the application.
- Expose only the treatment area, *because vasodilation will make the patient feel chilly.*
- Assess the treatment area for open lesions, edema, bleeding, and evidence of altered circulation, *because the risk of damage to tissue is increased if the area is already traumatized.*

Applying a hot-water bottle, an electric heating pad, or a chemical hot pack

- Before applying the heating device, press it against your inner forearm *to test its temperature and heat distribution.* If it heats unevenly, obtain a new device.
- Apply the device to the treatment area and, if necessary, secure it with tape or roller gauze. Begin timing the application.
- Assess the patient's skin condition frequently; remove the device if you observe increased swelling or excessive redness, blistering, maceration, or pallor, or if the patient reports discomfort. Refill the hot-water bottle as necessary *to maintain the correct temperature.*
- Remove the device after 20 to 30 minutes, or as ordered.

Applying a warm compress or pack

- Place a fluid-impermeable pad under the treatment area.
- Remove the warm compress or pack from the bowl or basin. (Use sterile forceps throughout the procedure to maintain sterility, if needed.)
- Wring excess solution from the compress or pack. *Excess moisture increases the risk of burns.*
- Apply the compress or pack gently to the treatment area. After a few seconds, lift the device and check the skin for excessive redness, maceration, or blistering. When you're sure the compress or pack isn't causing a burn, mold it firmly to the skin *to prevent air from reducing the temperature and effectiveness of the warm compress or pack.* Work quickly *so the compress or pack retains its heat.*
- Apply a waterproof covering (sterile, if necessary) to the warm compress or pack. Secure it with tape or roller gauze *to prevent it from slipping.*
- Place a hot-water bottle or chemical hot pack and waterproof covering over the compress or pack *to maintain the correct temperature.* Begin timing the application.
- Assess the patient's skin at regular intervals. Remove the heating device if you observe excessive redness, maceration, or blistering, or if the patient experiences pain or discomfort. Change the compress or pack as needed *to maintain the correct temperature.*
- After 15 or 20 minutes, or as ordered, remove the device.

Completing the procedure

- Dry the patient's skin with a towel (sterile, if necessary), as needed. Note the condition of the skin and redress the area, if necessary. Obtain the patient's temperature, pulse, and respirations *to compare with the baseline.* Then make sure the patient is comfortable.
- Return the bed to the lowest position *to prevent falls and maintain patient safety.*[20]
- Discard used supplies in appropriate receptacles.[19]
- Remove and discard your gloves, if worn,[19] and perform hand hygiene.[4,5,6,7,8,9]
- If the treatment is to be repeated, store the equipment in the patient's room, out of reach; otherwise, return it for proper cleaning and disinfection.[21,22]
- Document the procedure.[23,24,25,26]

USING MOIST HEAT TO RELIEVE MUSCLE SPASM

Tell patients to choose direct moist heat rather than dry heat when attempting to ease muscle tension or spasm. *Direct moist heat is less drying to the skin, less apt to cause burns, less likely to cause excessive fluid and salt loss through sweating, and more likely to penetrate deeper tissues.* Instruct the patient to apply heat for 20 to 30 minutes, as follows:

- Place a moist towel over the painful area.
- Cover the towel with a hot-water bottle properly filled and at the correct temperature.
- Remove the hot-water bottle and towel after 20 to 30 minutes. Don't continue the application for longer than 30 minutes, *because therapeutic value decreases after that time.*

Special considerations

- Make sure that closure devices aren't in direct contact with the skin, *because they may cause burns.*
- If the patient has decreased sensation because the patient is unconscious, anesthetized, cognitively or neurologically impaired, or insensitive to heat, stay with the patient throughout the treatment and inspect the skin frequently, *because thermal burns may occur.*[2]
- When direct heat is ordered to decrease congestion in internal organs, the application must cover a large enough area *to increase blood volume at the skin's surface.*[2] For relief of pelvic organ congestion, for example, apply direct heat over the patient's lower abdomen, hips, and thighs. *To achieve local relief,* you can concentrate heat only over the specified area. (See *Using moist heat to relieve muscle spasm.*)
- As an alternative method to apply a sterile moist compress or pack, use a bedside sterilizer *to sterilize the compress.* Saturate the compress with tap water or another solution and wring it dry. Then place the compress in the bedside sterilizer at 275°F (135°C) for 15 minutes. Remove the compress with sterile forceps or sterile gloves, and wring out the excess solution. Then place the compress in a sterile bowl, measure its temperature with a sterile thermometer, and allow it to cool to 120° F (48.9° C). Follow the manufacturer's instructions for heating compresses, and avoid overheating.

Patient teaching

If direct heat application will continue at home, teach the patient and family (if appropriate) how to use the equipment and check the equipment for safety concerns. Also, teach the patient and family to check the patient's skin at regular intervals for signs and symptoms of excessive exposure to heat.

Complications

Heat application can cause burns. Electrical shock may occur from improper use of an electric heating pad.

Documentation

Record the time and date of direct heat application; the type, temperature or heat setting, duration, and site of application; the patient's temperature, pulse, respirations, and skin condition before, during, and after treatment; and the patient's tolerance of the treatment. If complications occur, document the name of the practitioner notified, the date and time of the notification, prescribed interventions, and the patient's response to those interventions. Document teaching provided to the patient and family (if applicable), their understanding of that teaching, and any need for follow-up teaching.

REFERENCES

1 Petrofsky, J., et al. (2013). Moist heat or dry heat for delayed onset muscle soreness. *Journal of Clinical Medicine Research, 5,* 416–425. (Level VI)

2 Craven, R. F., et al. (2021). *Fundamentals of nursing: Concepts and competencies for practice* (9th ed.). Philadelphia, PA: Wolters Kluwer.

3 Janssen Pharmaceuticals, Inc. (2021). Duragesic® (fentanyl transdermal system) prescribing information. http://www.janssenlabels.com/package-insert/product-monograph/prescribing-information/DURAGESIC-pi.pdf

4 Accreditation Association for Hospitals and Health Systems. (2020). Standard 07.01.21. *Healthcare Facilities Accreditation Program: Accreditation requirements for acute care hospitals.* Chicago, IL: Accreditation Association for Hospitals and Health Systems. (Level VII)

5 Centers for Medicare and Medicaid Services, Department of Health and Human Services. (2020). Condition of participation: Infection control. 42 C.F.R. § 482.42.

6 The Joint Commission. (2021). Standard NPSG.07.01.01. *Comprehensive accreditation manual for hospitals.* Oakbrook Terrace, IL: The Joint Commission. (Level VII)

7 Centers for Disease Control and Prevention. (2002). Guideline for hand hygiene in health-care settings: Recommendations of the Healthcare Infection Control Practices Advisory Committee and the HICPAC/SHEA/APIC/IDSA Hand Hygiene Task Force. *MMWR Recommendations and Reports, 51*(RR-16), 1–45. https://www.cdc.gov/mmwr/pdf/rr/rr5116.pdf (Level II)

8 World Health Organization. (2009). WHO guidelines on hand hygiene in health care: First global patient safety challenge, clean care is safer care. https://apps.who.int/iris/bitstream/handle/10665/44102/9789241597906_eng.pdf?sequence=1 (Level IV)

9 DNV GL-Healthcare USA, Inc. (2020). IC.1.SR.1. *NIAHO® accreditation requirements, interpretive guidelines and surveyor guidance—revision 20.0.* Milford, OH: DNV GL-Healthcare USA, Inc. (Level VII)

10 The Joint Commission. (2021). Standard NPSG.01.01.01. *Comprehensive accreditation manual for hospitals.* Oakbrook Terrace, IL: The Joint Commission. (Level VII)

11 Accreditation Association for Hospitals and Health Systems. (2020). Standard 15.01.16. *Healthcare Facilities Accreditation Program: Accreditation requirements for acute care hospitals.* Chicago, IL: Accreditation Association for Hospitals and Health Systems. (Level VII)

12 Centers for Medicare and Medicaid Services, Department of Health and Human Services. (2020). Condition of participation: Patient's rights. 42 C.F.R. § 482.13(c)(1).

13 DNV GL Healthcare USA, Inc. (2020). PR.2.SR.5. *NIAHO® accreditation requirements, interpretive guidelines and surveyor guidance—revision 20.0.* Milford, OH: DNV GL-Healthcare USA, Inc. (Level VII)

14 The Joint Commission. (2021). Standard RI.01.01.01. *Comprehensive accreditation manual for hospitals.* Oakbrook Terrace, IL: The Joint Commission. (Level VII)

15 The Joint Commission. (2021). Standard PC.02.01.21. *Comprehensive accreditation manual for hospitals.* Oakbrook Terrace, IL: The Joint Commission. (Level VII)

16 Waters, T. R., et al. (2009). Safe patient handling training for schools of nursing. https://www.cdc.gov/niosh/docs/2009-127/pdfs/2009-127.pdf (Level VII)

17 Accreditation Association for Hospitals and Health Systems. (2020). Standard 07.01.10. *Healthcare Facilities Accreditation Program: Accreditation requirements for acute care hospitals.* Chicago, IL: Accreditation Association for Hospitals and Health Systems. (Level VII)

18 Siegel, J. D., et al. (2007, revised 2019). 2007 guideline for isolation precautions: Preventing transmission of infectious agents in healthcare settings. https://www.cdc.gov/infectioncontrol/pdf/guidelines/isolation-guidelines-H.pdf (Level II)

19 Occupational Safety and Health Administration. (2019). Bloodborne pathogens, standard number 1910.1030. https://www.osha.gov/pls/oshaweb/owadisp.show_document?p_id=10051&p_table=STANDARDS (Level VII)

20 Ganz, D. A., et al. (2013, reviewed 2021). *Preventing falls in hospitals: A toolkit for improving quality of care* (AHRQ Publication No. 13-0015-EF). Rockville, MD: Agency for Healthcare Research and Quality. https://www.ahrq.gov/professionals/systems/hospital/fallpxtoolkit/index.html (Level VII)

21 Accreditation Association for Hospitals and Health Systems. (2020). Standard 07.02.03. *Healthcare Facilities Accreditation Program: Accreditation requirements for acute care hospitals.* Chicago, IL: Accreditation Association for Hospitals and Health Systems. (Level VII)

22 Rutala, W. A., et al. (2008, revised 2019). Guideline for disinfection and sterilization in healthcare facilities, 2008. https://www.cdc.gov/infectioncontrol/pdf/guidelines/disinfection-guidelines-H.pdf (Level I)

23 The Joint Commission. (2021). Standard RC.01.03.01. *Comprehensive accreditation manual for hospitals.* Oakbrook Terrace, IL: The Joint Commission. (Level VII)

24 Centers for Medicare and Medicaid Services, Department of Health and Human Services. (2020). Condition of participation: Medical record services. 42 C.F.R. § 482.24(b).

25 Accreditation Association for Hospitals and Health Systems. (2020). Standard 10.00.03. *Healthcare Facilities Accreditation Program: Accreditation requirements for acute care hospitals.* Chicago, IL: Accreditation Association for Hospitals and Health Systems. (Level VII)

26 DNV GL-Healthcare USA, Inc. (2020). MR.2.SR.1. *NIAHO® accreditation requirements, interpretive guidelines and surveyor guidance—revision 20.0.* Milford, OH: DNV GL-Healthcare USA, Inc. (Level VII)

Height and weight measurement

Height and weight are routinely measured during admission to a health care facility.[1] An accurate record of the patient's height and weight is essential for calculating dosages of drugs, anesthetics, and contrast agents; assessing nutritional status and bone health;[1] and determining the height-weight ratio, body surface area, and body mass index (BMI).[2] And because body weight provides the best overall picture of fluid status, monitoring weight daily proves important for patients receiving sodium-retaining or diuretic medications.[1] Rapid weight gain may signal fluid retention; rapid weight loss, diuresis.[1] Weight should be measured rather than estimated, *because weight estimation errors can occur even when patients estimate their own weight.*

Weight can be measured with a standing scale, chair scale, portable bed scale, or built-in bed scale.[1] (See *Types of scales.*)

The Institute for Safe Medication Practices recommends that weight be measured in metric units only (kilograms for adults, adolescents, children, and infants, and grams for neonates), *because official product labeling for medications provides weight-based dosing using only the metric system.* Significant medication errors have occurred when a patient's weight was documented in nonmetric units of measure and confused with kilograms or grams. Numerous errors have been reported when health care workers convert weights from one measurement system to another, or weigh a patient in pounds but accidently record the value as kilograms in the patient's medical record, resulting in a greater than twofold dosing error.[3]

Equipment

Standing scale with measurement bar or chair scale or bed scale ▪ draw-sheet (for bed scale) ▪ facility-approved disinfectant ▪ Optional: gloves, tape measure and ruler (if scale doesn't have measuring bar), wheelchair, pillow, sheets, gown, transfer device.

Preparation of equipment

Select the appropriate scale, usually a standing scale for an ambulatory patient or a chair or bed scale for an acutely ill or debilitated patient. Then check to make sure the scale is balanced. *Standing scales and, to a lesser extent, bed scales may become unbalanced when transported.* Whichever type of scale you choose, use the same scale each time if the patient's condition allows.[2] If the department has more than one of a scale type (for example, several standing scales), make sure that each scale is marked *so that you can use of the same scale each time whenever possible.*

EQUIPMENT

Types of scales

Various scales, including standing scales, chair scales, and bed scales, are available to weigh patients.

For ambulatory patients

Standing scale

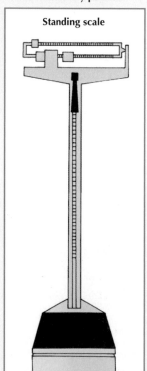

For acutely ill or debilitated patients

Chair scale   **Bed scale**

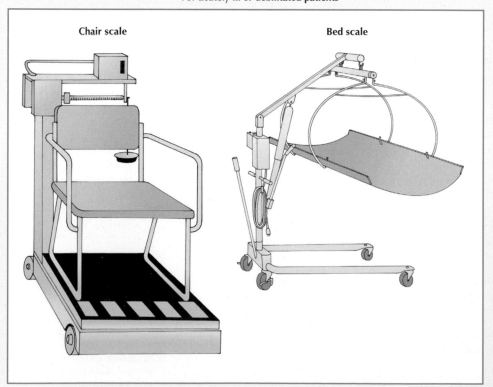

Inspect all equipment and supplies. If a product is expired, is defective, or has compromised integrity, remove it from patient use, label it as expired or defective, and report the expiration or defect as directed by your facility.

Implementation

- Gather and prepare the necessary equipment and supplies.
- Perform hand hygiene.[4,5,6,7,8,9]
- Confirm the patient's identity using at least two patient identifiers.[10]
- Explain the procedure to the patient and family (if appropriate) according to their individual communication and learning needs *to increase their understanding, allay their fears, and enhance cooperation.*[11]
- Provide privacy.[12,13,14,15]

Using a standing scale

- Check that the scale reads zero *to ensure accurate measurement.*[1,2] If you're using a digital scale, make sure it's set to display the patient's weight in kilograms. If the scale has wheels, lock them before the patient steps on *to prevent it from accidently moving.*
- Tell the patient to remove a robe or any outer clothing, if appropriate, and take off slippers or shoes.[1]
- Assist the patient onto the scale and remain close to the patient *to prevent falls.*
- If you're using an upright balance (gravity) scale, slide the lower rider to the groove representing the largest increment below the patient's estimated weight. Then slide the small upper rider until the beam balances. Add the upper and lower rider figures *to determine the patient's weight.* Return the weight holder to its proper place.
- If the scale is digital, read the display with the patient standing as still as possible.[2]
- If you're using a scale with a stadiometer (measuring bar), have the patient stand erect, with heels together and toes apart. Make sure the patient's head, shoulder blades, buttocks, and heels make contact with the bar of the stadiometer.[16] Then raise the measuring bar beyond the top of the patient's head, extend the horizontal bar, and lower the horizontal bar until it touches the top of the patient's head. Read the patient's height. Raise the horizontal bar off the patient's head and help the patient off the scale.
- Return all clothing that the patient removed for weight and height measurement.

Using a chair scale

- Transport the patient to the weighing area or the scale to the patient's bedside.
- Lock the scale in place *to prevent it from moving accidentally.*[1]
- If you're using a scale with a swing-away chair arm, unlock the arm. *When unlocked, the arm swings back 180 degrees to permit easy access.*
- Position the scale beside the patient's bed or wheelchair with the chair arm open.
- If the chair scale is digital, make sure the display reads zero before use *to ensure accurate measurement,*[1,2] and that the scale is set to display the patient's weight in kilograms.
- Transfer the patient onto the scale.
- Swing the chair arm to the front of the scale and lock the arm in place.
- Press the button and record the weight. If using a balance scale, follow the same process used with a standing scale to determine the weight.
- Transfer the patient from the chair scale to the bed or wheelchair.
- Lock the main beam *to avoid damaging the scale during transport* and unlock the wheels; remove the scale from the patient's room, if applicable.
- Perform hand hygiene.[4,5,6,7,8,9]
- Put on gloves *to comply with standard precautions.*[17,18,19]
- Clean and disinfect the scale according to the manufacturer's instructions *to prevent the spread of infection.*[20,21]
- Remove and discard your gloves.[19]

Using a portable digital bed scale

- Before using a bed scale, cover its stretcher with a drawsheet.
- Zero the scale with the drawsheet in place *to ensure accurate weighing,*[1,2] and make sure the scale is set to display the patient's weight in kilograms.

- Release the stretcher to the horizontal position; then lock it in place *to prevent it from accidently moving.*
- Remove the covered stretcher from the circular weighing arms and roll it up *to prepare for placement under the patient.*
- Raise the patient's bed to waist level when providing patient care *to prevent caregiver back strain.*[22]
- Turn the patient on the side, facing away from the scale.
- Position the stretcher under the patient.
- Roll the base of the scale under the patient's bed. Adjust the lever *to widen the base of the scale, providing stability.* Then lock the scale's wheels.
- Position the circular weighing arms of the scale over the patient and attach them securely to the stretcher bars.
- Pump the handle with long, slow strokes *to raise the patient a few inches off the bed.* Ensure that the patient doesn't lean on or touch the headboard, side rails, or other bed equipment, *because this will affect weight measurement.*
- Press the OPERATE button.
- Read the patient's weight on the digital display panel.
- Press on the scale's handle *to lower the patient.*
- Detach the circular weighing arms from the stretcher bars, roll the patient off the stretcher, and remove the stretcher.
- Position the patient comfortably in bed.
- Release the wheel lock and withdraw the scale from under the bed. Return the stretcher to its vertical position.
- Return the bed to the lowest position *to prevent falls and maintain patient safety.*[23]

Using a built-in bed scale

- Before placing the patient in a bed with a built-in scale, prepare the bed. If required by the manufacturer, place the bed in the weighing position, typically with the head of bed elevated less than 40 degrees. Make sure the bed isn't touching anything, such as the wall or medical devices, *to prevent an inaccurate reading.* Prepare the sleep surface with pillows, sheets, and any other items that don't vary in weight that the patient will be using, such as a patient gown. Place a list of these items by the patient's bedside, if needed, *to make sure the patient is weighed with these items consistently;* some facilities have a protocol that designates the specific items that should be on the bed consistently. Zero the bed scale with the items in place, making sure that no one is touching the bed during this time.
- With the assistance of coworkers and a transfer device, place the patient on the bed, making sure the patient is centered in the bed and lying still.
- If the scale doesn't function automatically, begin obtaining the patient's weight following the manufacturer's instructions.

Completing the procedure

- Perform hand hygiene.[4,5,6,7,8,9]
- Calculate the patient's BMI if necessary *to determine whether the patient is at a healthy weight.*[2] (See *Calculating and interpreting BMI,* page 384.)
- Remove and discard your gloves and perform hand hygiene.[4,5,6,7,8,9]
- Document the procedure.[25,26,27,28]

Measuring height without a scale

- Perform hand hygiene.[4,5,6,7,8,9]
- Confirm the patient's identity using at least two patient identifiers.[10]
- Provide privacy.[12,13,14,15]
- Explain the procedure to the patient and family (if appropriate) according to their individual communication and learning needs *to increase their understanding, allay their fears, and enhance cooperation.*[11]
- Have the patient stand erect against a wall with the heels together and toes apart. Make sure the patient's head, shoulder blades, buttocks, and heels touch the wall.[4] Place a ruler or other straight, level object on top of the patient's head parallel to the floor. Mark the location of the ruler on the wall. Using a tape measure, measure the distance between the mark and the floor.
- If the patient is unable to stand, place the patient supine in bed with the head of the bed flat.[29,30] Using a tape measure, measure from the top of the patient's head to the heels.[31]

Calculating and interpreting BMI

Body mass index (BMI) is a number calculated from a person's weight and height to assess the patient's status as underweight, normal, overweight, or obese. BMI allows you to compare the patient's weight status with the general population. To calculate the patient's BMI, use the following formula:

$$BMI = weight(kg) \div \left[height(m)\right]^2$$

For example, for a patient weighing 68 kg and measuring 1.65 m, the calculation is as follows:

$$68\,kg \div (1.65\,m)^2 = BMI\ of\ 25^{24}$$

For adults age 20 or older, BMI is interpreted using standard weight status categories that are the same for all ages and for both men and women. For children and adolescents, BMI interpretation is both age- and gender-specific. Use the table below to interpret BMI in adults.

BMI	Weight status
Below 18.5	Underweight
18.5 to 24.9	Normal
25 to 29.9	Overweight
30 and above	Obese

- Note the measurement in centimeters or inches, as directed by your facility.[32]
- Perform hand hygiene.[4,5,6,7,8,9]
- Document the procedure.[25,26,27,28]

Special considerations

- Reassure and steady patients who are at risk for losing their balance on a scale.[2]
- If possible, weigh the patient at the same time each day (usually before breakfast), in similar clothing, and using the same scale.[1,2] Have the patient void before being weighed, if applicable.[1,2] If the patient uses crutches, weigh the patient with the crutches, then weigh the crutches and any heavy clothing and subtract their weight from the total *to determine the patient's weight.*
- When rolling the patient onto the stretcher, be careful not to dislodge IV catheters, indwelling catheters, and other supportive equipment.[1]
- Report any change in weight of more than 1 kg (2.2 lb) per day, unless it's expected, such as after dialysis or diuretic therapy.[1]
- Measuring height can be difficult for bedbound patients, patients with structural anomalies, and patients with contractures. Alternative methods for estimating height in such patients include measuring recumbent length, knee height, forearm length, and demispan.[29,33] Use of a sliding caliper should be the method of choice, however, *because it's the closest in accuracy to standing height.*[31,34]

Complications

Inaccurate measurement can lead to errors in medication administration and other treatments.

Documentation

Record the patient's height in inches and centimeters on the nursing assessment form and in other medical records, as required by your facility.

Record the patient's weight in kilograms. Record the date and time of measurement and the type of scale used, and the scale's identification number if more than one scale of the same type is available. If the patient was weighed using a bed scale, note the items that were in place when the scale was reset to zero before use. Document teaching provided to the patient and family (if applicable), their understanding of that teaching, and any need for follow-up teaching.

References

1 Craven, R. F., et al. (2017). *Fundamentals of nursing: Human health and function* (8th ed.). Philadelphia, PA: Wolters Kluwer.

2 National Nurses Nutrition Group. (2017). Obtaining an accurate body weight measurement in adults and children in primary and secondary care settings (not babies). https://www.guidelines.co.uk/nutrition/nnng-guideline-measuring-body-weight/455172.article (Level VII)

3 Institute for Safe Medication Practices. (2018). 2018–2019 targeted medication safety best practices for hospitals. https://www.ismp.org/sites/default/files/attachments/2019-01/TMSBP-for-Hospitalsv2.pdf

4 The Joint Commission. (2021). Standard NPSG.07.01.01. *Comprehensive accreditation manual for hospitals.* Oakbrook Terrace, IL: The Joint Commission. (Level VII)

5 Centers for Disease Control and Prevention. (2002). Guideline for hand hygiene in health-care settings: Recommendations of the Healthcare Infection Control Practices Advisory Committee and the HICPAC/SHEA/APIC/IDSA Hand Hygiene Task Force. *MMWR Recommendations and Reports, 51*(RR-16), 1–45. https://www.cdc.gov/mmwr/pdf/rr/rr5116.pdf (Level II)

6 World Health Organization. (2009). WHO guidelines on hand hygiene in health care: First global patient safety challenge, clean care is safer care. https://apps.who.int/iris/bitstream/handle/10665/44102/9789241597906_eng.pdf?sequence=1 (Level IV)

7 Accreditation Association for Hospitals and Health Systems. (2020). Standard 07.01.21. *Healthcare Facilities Accreditation Program: Accreditation requirements for acute care hospitals.* Chicago, IL: Accreditation Association for Hospitals and Health Systems. (Level VII)

8 Centers for Medicare and Medicaid Services, Department of Health and Human Services. (2020). Condition of participation: Infection control. 42 C.F.R. § 482.42.

9 DNV GL-Healthcare USA, Inc. (2020). IC.1.SR.1. *NIAHO® accreditation requirements, interpretive guidelines and surveyor guidance—revision 20.0.* Milford, OH: DNV GL-Healthcare USA, Inc. (Level VII)

10 The Joint Commission. (2021). Standard NPSG.01.01.01. *Comprehensive accreditation manual for hospitals.* Oakbrook Terrace, IL: The Joint Commission. (Level VII)

11 The Joint Commission. (2021). Standard PC.02.01.21. *Comprehensive accreditation manual for hospitals.* Oakbrook Terrace, IL: The Joint Commission. (Level VII)

12 Accreditation Association for Hospitals and Health Systems. (2020). Standard 15.01.16. *Healthcare Facilities Accreditation Program: Accreditation requirements for acute care hospitals.* Chicago, IL: Accreditation Association for Hospitals and Health Systems. (Level VII)

13 Centers for Medicare and Medicaid Services, Department of Health and Human Services. (2020). Condition of participation: Patient's rights. 42 C.F.R. § 482.13(c)(1).

14 The Joint Commission. (2021). Standard RI.01.01.01. *Comprehensive accreditation manual for hospitals.* Oakbrook Terrace, IL: The Joint Commission. (Level VII)

15 DNV GL-Healthcare USA, Inc. (2020). PR.2.SR.5. *NIAHO® accreditation requirements, interpretive guidelines and surveyor guidance—revision 20.0.* Milford, OH: DNV GL-Healthcare USA, Inc. (Level VII)

16 Centers for Disease Control and Prevention. (2017). National health and nutrition examination survey (NHANES): Anthropometry procedures manual. https://www.cdc.gov/nchs/data/nhanes/2017-2018/manuals/2017_Anthropometry_Procedures_Manual.pdf (Level VII)

17 Siegel, J. D., et al. (2007, revised 2019). 2007 guideline for isolation precautions: Preventing transmission of infectious agents in healthcare settings. https://www.cdc.gov/infectioncontrol/pdf/guidelines/isolation-guidelines-H.pdf (Level II)

18 Accreditation Association for Hospitals and Health Systems. (2020). Standard 07.01.10. *Healthcare Facilities Accreditation Program: Accreditation requirements for acute care hospitals.* Chicago, IL: Accreditation Association for Hospitals and Health Systems. (Level VII)

19 Occupational Safety and Health Administration. (2019). Bloodborne pathogens, standard number 1910.1030. https://www.osha.gov/pls/oshaweb/owadisp.show_document?p_id=10051&p_table=STANDARDS (Level VII)

20 Rutala, W. A., et al. (2008, revised 2019). Guideline for disinfection and sterilization in healthcare facilities, 2008. https://www.cdc.gov/infectioncontrol/pdf/guidelines/disinfection-guidelines-H.pdf (Level I)

21 Accreditation Association for Hospitals and Health Systems. (2020). Standard 07.02.03. *Healthcare Facilities Accreditation Program: Accreditation requirements for acute care hospitals.* Chicago, IL: Accreditation Association for Hospitals and Health Systems. (Level VII)

22 Waters, T. R., et al. (2009). Safe patient handling training for schools of nursing. https://www.cdc.gov/niosh/docs/2009-127/pdfs/2009-127.pdf (Level VII)

23 Ganz, D. A., et al. (2013, reviewed 2021). *Preventing falls in hospitals: A toolkit for improving quality of care* (AHRQ Publication No. 13-0015-EF). Rockville, MD: Agency for Healthcare Research and Quality. https://www.ahrq.gov/professionals/systems/hospital/fallpxtoolkit/index.html (Level VII)

24 Centers for Disease Control and Prevention. (2020). Healthy weight: About adult BMI. http://www.cdc.gov/healthyweight/assessing/bmi/adult_bmi/index.html (Level VII)

25 The Joint Commission. (2021). Standard RC.01.03.01. *Comprehensive accreditation manual for hospitals.* Oakbrook Terrace, IL: The Joint Commission. (Level VII)

26 Accreditation Association for Hospitals and Health Systems. (2020). Standard 10.00.03. *Healthcare Facilities Accreditation Program: Accreditation requirements for acute care hospitals.* Chicago, IL: Accreditation Association for Hospitals and Health Systems. (Level VII)

27 Centers for Medicare and Medicaid Services, Department of Health and Human Services. (2020). Condition of participation: Medical record services. 42 C.F.R. § 482.24(b).

28 DNV GL-Healthcare USA, Inc. (2020). MR.2.SR.1. *NIAHO® accreditation requirements, interpretive guidelines and surveyor guidance—revision 20.0.* Milford, OH: DNV GL-Healthcare USA, Inc. (Level VII)

29 Venkataramen, R., et al. (2015). Height measurement in the critically ill patient: A tall order in the critical care unit. *Indian Journal of Critical Care Medicine, 19,* 665–668. (Level VI)

30 Freitag, E., et al. (2010). Determination of body weight and height measurement for critically ill patients admitted to the intensive care unit: A quality improvement project. *Australian Critical Care, 23,* 197–207.

31 Dennis, D. M., et al. (2015). Measuring height in recumbent critical care patients. *American Journal of Critical Care, 24,* 41–47. (Level VI)

32 Tipton, P. H., et al. (2012). Patient safety: Consider the accuracy of height and weight measurements. *Nursing, 42*(5), 50–52. https://journals.lww.com/nursing/Fulltext/2012/05000/Consider_the_accuracy_of_height_and_weight.16.aspx

33 Froehlich-Grobe, K., et al. (2011). Measuring height without a stadiometer. *American Journal of Physical Medicine & Rehabilitation, 90,* 658–666. https://www.ncbi.nlm.nih.gov/pmc/articles/PMC3148840/ (Level VI)

34 Frid, H., et al. (2013). Agreement between different methods of measuring height in elderly patients. *Journal of Human Nutrition and Dietetics, 26,* 504–511.

HEMODIALYSIS

Hemodialysis is a lifesaving procedure that removes blood from the body, circulates it through an artificial kidney known as a *dialyzer or hemodialyzer,* and then returns it to the body.[1] Various access sites can be used for this procedure. (See *Hemodialysis access,* page 386.) The access can be temporary or long-term, depending on the various patient factors. Catheters are used for short-term access; arteriovenous (AV) fistulas and AV grafts provide more long-term access for hemodialysis.[1,2]

Double-lumen catheters for hemodialysis can be nontunneled or tunneled and cuffed. Large-bore nontunneled catheters are used most often for a short-term (up to 2 weeks) immediate need for hemodialysis, such as with an acute kidney injury or poisoning.[2] If dialysis is likely to be needed for longer than a week, such as for patients who don't have functional permanent access (an AV fistula or AV graft), then a cuffed, tunneled catheter may be placed. When permanent access becomes functional, the catheter is removed.[8] The use of tunneled, cuffed catheters is associated with several complications, including vascular catheter–associated infections.[9]

HOSPITAL-ACQUIRED ALERT Keep in mind that the Centers for Medicare and Medicaid Services considers vascular catheter–associated infection a hospital-acquired condition *because it can be reasonably prevented using a variety of best practices.* Make sure to follow evidence-based infection prevention practices, such as performing hand hygiene, performing a vigorous mechanical scrub of catheter hubs, and using sterile technique, *to reduce the risk of vascular catheter–associated infections.*[5,10,11]

AV fistulas are preferred for long-term access because research shows they result in the longest survival, fewer access-related procedures, fewer hospitalizations due to infection, and lower overall costs of care. The Centers for Medicare and Medicaid Services, the National Kidney Foundation, and other kidney disease organizations have developed *Fistula First Catheter Last,* a national campaign to increase the use of AV fistulas over catheters in patients who require hemodialysis.[12,13] However, using an AV fistula requires advance planning, because the fistula must mature before a patient with stage 4 chronic kidney disease progresses to stage 5 chronic kidney disease.[14]

The underlying mechanism in hemodialysis is differential diffusion across a semipermeable membrane, which extracts the by-products of protein metabolism (urea) as well as creatinine and excess water. The semipermeable membrane doesn't permit diffusion of large molecules such as blood cells and plasma proteins. This process restores or maintains the balance of the body's buffer system and electrolytes. Hemodialysis promotes a rapid return to normal serum values and helps prevent complications associated with uremia. (See *How hemodialysis works,* page 387.)

Hemodialysis provides temporary support for patients with acute kidney injury and regular, long-term treatment of patients with stage 5 chronic kidney disease. Hemodialysis may also be necessary to remove toxic substances from the blood in patients suffering from various acute poisonings or barbiturate or analgesic overdose.[1] The patient's condition, along with such variables as the rate of creatinine accumulation and weight gain, determines the number and duration of hemodialysis treatments. To determine the patient's ultrafiltration requirements, the patient's present weight is compared with the weight after the prior dialysis treatment and the target weight. Blood pressure and hemodynamic status are also considered.

Hemodialysis is typically performed on a hemodialysis unit by specially trained personnel. However, if the patient is acutely ill and unstable, it can be performed at the bedside or in an intensive care unit.

Currently, alteplase is the only thrombolytic agent approved by the U.S. Food and Drug Administration for the restoration of central venous access device function.[15] Similar to naturally produced human tissue plasminogen activator, alteplase acts specifically on fibrin-rich clots in the occluded catheter and converts plasminogen to plasmin. Plasmin then dissolves the clot's fibrin, which promotes thrombotic breakdown. Residual debris can be aspirated from the catheter after the clot dissolves, restoring central venous access. Salvage of a central venous access device with alteplase is effective in 75% of cases, although some patients require two doses to restore line patency.[16]

Alteplase should be prescribed with caution in the presence of known or suspected vascular catheter–associated infection, *because alteplase administration can cause the release of organisms from the catheter into the systemic circulation.*[16] In addition, alteplase should be used with caution in any patient who has a known bleeding disorder, who has active internal bleeding, or who has had within the previous 48 hours surgery, an obstetric delivery, percutaneous biopsy of viscera or deep tissue, or puncture of a noncompressible vessel, *because of the risk of bleeding associated with the use of thrombolytics.*[16]

Complete occlusion requires the use of the single syringe or stopcock method of declotting, *because these methods use a negative-pressure approach.* The direct instillation method is indicated for partial thrombotic occlusions when the double-lumen catheter can still be flushed but catheter flow is sluggish or aspiration of blood isn't possible.[17]

Equipment

For initiating dialysis

Stethoscope ■ vital signs monitoring equipment ■ scale ■ gown ■ mask with face shield or mask and goggles ■ patient mask ■ pulse oximeter and probe ■ emergency equipment (code cart with emergency medications, defibrillator, handheld resuscitation bag with mask, intubation

Hemodialysis access

Hemodialysis requires vascular access.[1] The site and type of access may vary, depending on the expected duration of dialysis, the practitioner's preference, and the patient's condition.

Internal jugular vein catheterization

The internal jugular vein is the typical site for placement of a double-lumen catheter.[3] If the internal jugular vein isn't appropriate, then the external jugular, femoral, subclavian, or lumbar vein is preferable (listed in order of preference).[2] Guidelines don't recommend the use of the subclavian vein for catheter placement in a patient who requires a permanent arteriovenous (AV) fistula, because the risk of thrombosis can compromise AV fistula creation.[1,4]

A practitioner inserts an introducer needle into the internal jugular or subclavian vein using the Seldinger technique. The practitioner then inserts a guidewire through the introducer needle and removes the needle. Using the guidewire, the practitioner threads a 5″ to 12″ (13 cm to 30 cm) plastic or Teflon catheter (with a Y hub) into the patient's vein (as shown below).

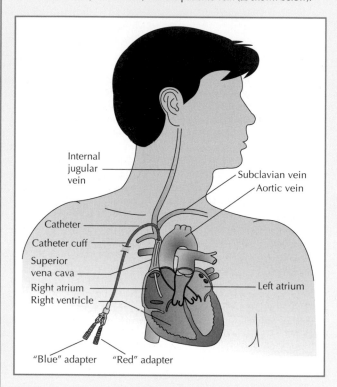

Several types of double-lumen catheters are appropriate for dialysis access, depending on the patient's condition, the practitioner's preference, and the anticipated length of time that the catheter will be necessary. The internal diameter of each lumen is about 12G to enable high flow rates. The catheters have two ports: one red and one blue. The red port is used for withdrawing the patient's blood and sending it to the dialyzer, and the blue port is used for returning dialyzed blood to the patient.

Most double-lumen catheters are appropriate for temporary dialysis accesses. However, a double-lumen tunneled catheter with a Dacron cuff is appropriate for extended use (months).[5] This type of catheter is tunneled from the skin insertion site to the selected vein, and the Dacron cuff on the catheter under the skin acts as a barrier to infection.

Femoral vein catheterization

Using the Seldinger technique, the practitioner inserts an introducer needle into the left or right femoral vein, then inserts a guidewire through the introducer needle and removes the needle.

Using the guidewire, the practitioner then threads a 5″ to 12″ (13 cm to 30 cm) plastic or Teflon catheter with a Y hub or two catheters, one for inflow and another placed about ½″ (1 cm) distal to the first for outflow, into the patient's vein. The femoral vein should be used only when no other access site is available, *because it's associated with an increased risk of infection and deep vein thrombosis.*[6]

Arteriovenous fistula

To create an AV fistula, a surgeon makes an incision into the patient's wrist or lower forearm and then makes two additional small incisions, one in the side of an artery and another in the side of a vein. The surgeon sutures the edges of the incisions together to make a common opening 0.12″ to 0.3″ (3 mm to 7 mm) long. The minimum amount of time for maturation of an AV fistula is 1 month, but guidelines generally recommend longer times (such as 6 to 12 months).[7] Therefore, creation of the fistula is preferable before hemodialysis is needed *so that the fistula is matured and ready for use when necessary.*

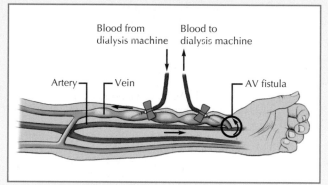

Arteriovenous graft

To create an AV graft, a surgeon makes an incision in the patient's forearm, upper arm, or thigh. The surgeon then tunnels a natural or synthetic graft under the skin and sutures the distal end to an artery and the proximal end to a vein.

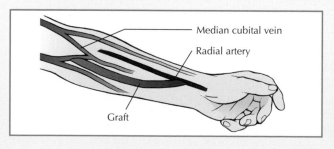

equipment) ■ hemodialysis machine with appropriate dialyzer ■ prescribed dialysate ■ fluid-impermeable pad or sterile towel ■ antiseptic pads (chlorhexidine-based solution, or povidone-iodine, preferable with alcohol, if chlorhexidine is contraindicated)[2,15,16] ■ 10-mL syringes with preservative-free normal saline solution ■ syringes ■ prescribed medications ■ supplies for blood sampling ■ Optional: prescribed anticoagulant, bioimpedance cardiography, pulmonary artery pressure or central venous pressure monitoring equipment.

For initiating hemodialysis with a double-lumen catheter

Scale ■ hemodialysis machine with appropriate dialyzer and dialysate ■ gloves ■ gown ■ mask with face shield or mask and goggles ■ antiseptic pads (chlorhexidine, povidone-iodine, or 70% alcohol)[13] ■ stethoscope ■ vital signs monitoring equipment ■ 10-mL syringes with preservative-free normal saline solution ■ syringes ■ prescribed medications ■ supplies for blood sampling ■ Optional: prescribed anticoagulant.

EQUIPMENT

How hemodialysis works

In hemodialysis, blood flows from the patient to an external dialyzer (or artificial kidney) through an access site. Inside the dialyzer, blood and dialysate flow countercurrently, divided by a semipermeable membrane. The composition of the dialysate resembles normal extracellular fluid. The blood contains an excess of specific solutes (metabolic waste products and some electrolytes), and the dialysate contains electrolytes that may be at abnormal levels in the patient's bloodstream. The dialysate's electrolyte composition can be modified to raise or lower electrolyte levels, depending on need.

Excretory function and electrolyte homeostasis are achieved by *diffusion*, the movement of a molecule across the dialyzer's semipermeable membrane from an area of higher solute concentration to an area of lower concentration.[1] Water (solvent) crosses the membrane from the blood into the dialysate by *ultrafiltration*. This process removes excess water, waste products, and other metabolites through *osmotic pressure* and *hydrostatic pressure*. Osmotic pressure is the movement of water across the semipermeable membrane from an area of lesser solute concentration to one of greater solute concentration.[1] Hydrostatic pressure forces water from the blood compartment into the dialysate compartment. Cleaned of impurities and excess water, the blood returns to the body through a venous site.

Dialyzer

The hollow-fiber dialyzer, the most common type of dialyzer, contains fine capillaries, with a semipermeable membrane enclosed in a plastic cylinder. Blood flows through these capillaries as the system pumps dialysate in the opposite direction on the outside of the capillaries.

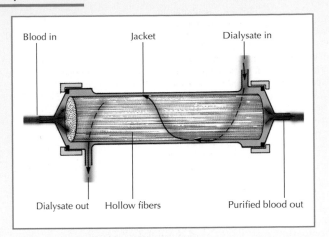

Dialysate delivery systems

Three system types can be used to deliver dialysate. The *batch system* uses a reservoir for recirculating dialysate. The *regenerative system* uses sorbents to purify and regenerate recirculating dialysate. The *proportioning system* (the most common) mixes concentrate with water to form dialysate, which then circulates through the dialyzer and goes down a drain after a single pass, followed by fresh dialysate.

For declotting a double-lumen catheter

Gloves ▪ mask ▪ 2-mg vials of alteplase ▪ 10-mL vial of sterile water for injection ▪ 3-mL syringe with needle or blunt-tip needleless device ▪ 10-mL syringe with blunt-tip or needleless device ▪ 10-mL syringes ▪ prefilled 10-mL syringes of preservative-free normal saline ▪ antiseptic pads (chlorhexidine-based solution, or povidone-iodine, preferably with alcohol, if chlorhexidine is contraindicated)[2,15,16] ▪ labels ▪ fluid-impermeable pad or sterile towel ▪ Optional: prescribed IV fluids or medications, stopcock, prefilled syringe containing locking solution, disinfectant-containing end caps, tape, needleless connectors.

For discontinuing hemodialysis

Gloves ▪ gown ▪ mask with face shield or mask and goggles ▪ mask for patient ▪ scale ▪ vital signs monitoring equipment ▪ stethoscope ▪ 10-mL syringes with preservative-free normal saline solution ▪ syringes ▪ prescribed locking solution ▪ two sterile Luer-lock caps ▪ antiseptic pads (chlorhexidine, alcohol, or povidone-iodine) ▪ disinfectant pad ▪ facility-approved disinfectant ▪ Optional: sterile specimen container; povidone-iodine ointment, polymyxin B, bacitracin zinc, or gramicidin ointment; sterile transparent semipermeable dressing or sterile 4″ × 4″ (10 cm × 10 cm) gauze pads and tape.

NURSING ALERT Use strict sterile, no-touch technique during machine and dialysis circuit preparation *to avoid a pyrogenic reaction and bacteremia with septicemia resulting from contamination.* Discard equipment that has been disconnected and exposed to the air.[18]

Preparation of equipment

Inspect all IV equipment and supplies. If a product is expired, is defective, or has compromised integrity, remove it from patient use, label it as expired or defective, and report the expiration or defect as directed by your facility.

Make sure emergency equipment is functioning properly and readily available.

Prepare and test the hemodialysis equipment following the manufacturer's instructions. *To maintain catheter patency,* carefully follow the manufacturer's instructions for specific catheter care and flushing procedures. Maintain sterile, no-touch technique *to prevent introducing pathogens into the patient's bloodstream during dialysis.* Be sure to test the dialyzer and dialysis machine for residual disinfectant after rinsing. Note that testing

for residual disinfectant may require a double-check by a second nurse or technician.[19] Make sure that the dialysis machine alarm limits are set appropriately, and that the alarms are functioning properly, turned on, and audible to staff.[20,21]

Before declotting, reconstitute the alteplase mixture immediately before use, *because it contains no antibacterial preservatives.* However, the solution may be used for up to 8 hours after reconstitution if stored between 35.6° F and 86° F (2° C and 30° C).[16]

Implementation

▪ Review the patient's medical record for advance directive and resuscitation status, isolation precautions (including the reason for isolation, date and source of culture, organisms cultured and their sensitivity, and type of isolation required), reason for admission, current problem list (including current medical diagnosis, recent surgical interventions, and recent diagnostic procedures), and medications.

▪ If required by your facility, confirm that informed consent has been obtained and that the signed consent form is in the patient's medical record.[22,23,24,25]

▪ Avoid distractions and interruptions when preparing and administering the dialysate *to prevent administration errors.*[26,27]

▪ Verify the practitioner's order. The hemodialysis order may include vascular access, treatment duration, dialyzer type, blood flow rate, dialysate flow rate, dialysate composition, dialysate temperature, frequency, target weight, anticoagulation medication (if necessary), laboratory testing, maximum ultrafiltration rate, ultrafiltration profile, sodium profile, falls risk score, allergies, and the language the patient speaks and understands.[28]

▪ Perform hand hygiene.[29,30,31,32,33,34]

▪ Confirm the patient's identity using at least two patient identifiers.[35]

▪ Provide privacy.[36,37,38,39]

▪ Explain the procedure to the patient and family (if appropriate) according to their individual communication and learning needs *to increase their understanding, allay their fears, and enhance cooperation.*[40]

▪ Raise the patient's bed to waist level (if applicable) before providing patient care *to prevent caregiver back strain.*[41]

▪ Perform hand hygiene.[29,30,31,32,33,34]

▪ Put on gloves and, as necessary, other personal protective equipment *to comply with standard precautions.* Institute transmission-based precautions, as needed.[28,42,43,44]

Performing prehemodialysis patient assessment

- Assess the patient for mobility, affect, hygiene, shortness of breath, pain, and overall well-being.[28]
- Obtain the patient's blood pressure. Obtain both sitting and standing blood pressures, as the patient's condition permits, *to detect orthostatic changes.*[28] For an immobile patient, obtain blood pressure with the head of bed down flat and then with the head of bed elevated 80 to 90 degrees, unless contraindicated. Keep the head of bed elevated at least 30 degrees for a patient with increased intracranial pressure. If the patient receives an antihypertensive medication, determine whether the pretreatment dose was held or administration times were changed.
- Obtain the patient's temperature. Keep in mind that uremic patients often have a body temperature of less than 98.6° F (37° C), and setting the dialysis solution temperature higher than the patient's temperature can cause vasodilation and subsequent hypotension.[28] Elevated temperature may indicate infection and increases insensible fluid loss.[28]
- Assess the patient's heart rate and rhythm. Auscultate heart sounds and report new findings to the practitioner.[28] Bradycardia may indicate digoxin toxicity or hyperkalemia, requiring an adjustment in dialysate *to prevent arrhythmias* and a review of medications *to check for other medications that can cause bradycardia.*
- Assess the patient's fluid balance, including intake (IV infusions, oral intake, and enteral feedings) and output (urine, removed ultrafiltrate, stool, drainage [for example, from chest tubes, a nasogastric tube, and wound drains], and insensible fluid losses caused by burns, wounds, ventilation, and temperature elevation).[28]
- Weigh the patient (in kilograms) at the same time daily. If using a bed scale, use standardized linens on the bed and bed positioning. Compare the daily weight to the prescribed "dry" weight obtained from outpatient records, if available, or to the hospital admission weight, *to additionally assess volume status.*[28]
- Assess for edema. If present, grade the severity using a scale, such as 0 = no pitting; 1+ = trace; 2+ = mild; 3+ moderate; and +4 = severe.[28] Inspect dependent areas for edema (sacral area for a patient positioned supine; legs, feet, and scrotum for a sitting or ambulatory patient; and facial and periorbital area for a patient who is reclined or positioned prone), and assess for facial and upper extremity edema, which may indicate occlusion of the subclavian and jugular veins. Assess for brawny edema (dark-colored skin that appears distended and becomes so tight with fluid that the fluid can't be displaced by applied pressure) and anasarca (generalized edema).[28]
- Assess for ascites and neck vein distention.[28]
- Assess the patient's mucous membranes and skin turgor and integrity. Dry mucous membranes and skin tenting indicate volume depletion.[28]
- Monitor hemodynamic status using bioimpedance, impedance cardiography, pulmonary artery pressure, or central venous pressure, if ordered.[28]
- Assess pulmonary status by assessing respiratory rate, rhythm, and pattern; auscultating breath sounds; assessing for cyanosis; obtaining oxygen saturation level by pulse oximetry; assessing fraction of inspired oxygen (if applicable); and reviewing current arterial blood gas values and trends and chest X-ray results.[28]
- Assess the patient's GI status, including the presence of bowel sounds and stool output. Hold anticoagulation and notify the practitioner if you suspect GI bleeding.
- Assess the patient's genitourinary status, including the primary cause of acute kidney injury or chronic kidney disease.[28]
- Assess the patient's endocrine status by reviewing blood glucose level stability and evaluating hemoglobin A1c value, if ordered. Monitor the use of systemic insulin for a patient who requires intensive care.
- Assess the patient's neurologic status, including level of consciousness; risk factors associated with hemodialysis, such as disequilibrium syndrome, use of anticoagulation, and intracranial bleed; and the presence of brain injury for which the patient requires intracranial pressure monitoring.
- Assess the patient's current laboratory test results (sodium, potassium, glucose, calcium, phosphorus, calcium phosphorus product, magnesium, carbon dioxide, blood urea nitrogen, creatinine, albumin, cholesterol, triglyceride, transaminase, ferritin, and iron levels; total iron-binding capacity; transferrin saturation; complete blood count; prothrombin time; D-dimer; heparin-induced thromboplastin antibody; and digoxin level), as needed and ordered.[28]
- If applicable, determine whether the patient had any problems with the prior dialysis treatment and inquire about posttreatment recovery time.
- Compare your assessment findings to previous treatment records (if applicable) *to detect changes in the patient's status that may require further evaluation and reporting.*[28]
- Remove and discard your gloves and other personal protective equipment, if worn.[44]
- Perform hand hygiene.[29,30,31,32,33,34]

Initiating hemodialysis with AV access

- Collaborate with the practitioner to form the patient's treatment plan based on laboratory test results and predialysis assessment findings.[25]
- Perform hand hygiene.[29,30,31,32,33,34]
- Gather and prepare the necessary equipment and supplies.
- Assist the patient into a comfortable position (supine or sitting in a recliner with the feet elevated).
- Apply a topical anesthetic to the AV puncture site, as ordered, approximately 45 to 60 minutes before cannulation, following safe medication administration practices.[45,46,47,48] If using ethyl chloride, whose anesthetic effect lasts 1 to 2 minutes, apply it immediately before cannulation.[49]
- Perform hand hygiene.[29,30,31,32,33,34]
- Wash the site with antibacterial soap or scrub and water.[2]
- Perform hand hygiene.[29,30,31,32,33,34]
- Put on gloves, a gown, and a mask with face shield or a mask and goggles *to comply with standard precautions.*[28,42,43,44]
- Place the patient's AV access limb on a fluid-impermeable pad.[1]
- Clean the skin over the AV access site with the antiseptic used in your facility, following the manufacturer's instructions.[19] Apply a chlorhexidine-based solution using a back-and-forth friction scrub for 30 seconds and allow it to dry.[1] Apply alcohol using a circular friction motion for 1 minute and allow it to dry.[1] Apply povidone-iodine solution for 2 to 3 minutes and allow it to dry.[1]
- Remove and discard your gloves.[43,44]
- Perform hand hygiene.[29,30,31,32,33,34]
- Put on new gloves.[28,42,43,44]
- Choose an appropriate-sized needle to cannulate the fistula.
- Draw up normal saline solution into each 10-mL syringe.[1,4]
- Apply a tourniquet to the upper portion of the arm containing the fistula *to increase venous pressure, enlarge and stabilize the vein, and ease cannulation.*[1]
- Lightly place the thumb and forefinger of your hand that isn't holding the needle on either side of the vessel *to prevent the vessel from moving.*
- Pull the skin taut in the direction opposite of needle insertion; stabilize the vessel but avoid placing excess pressure.[4]
- Grasp the butterfly needle by the wings, prime the needle with normal saline solution until all of the air is purged, and then clamp the needle.[1]
- Remove the protective cap and immediately cannulate the fistula. The arterial needle can be inserted in the direction of blood flow in the fistula (antegrade) or against the direction of blood flow (retrograde). Insert the needle at a 45-degree angle with the bevel up. As you advance the needle, watch for blood flashback.[1]
- Remove the tourniquet and unclamp the tubing.[1]
- Aspirate 1 mL to 5 mL of blood with a 10-mL syringe, flush the needle with normal saline solution, and then clamp it. Observe for signs and symptoms of infiltration.[1]
- Secure the needle with tape. Tape the needle at the same angle of insertion *to prevent moving the tip of the needle from the desired location within the vessel lumen.*[7]
- Cannulate the fistula with the venous needle a few inches beyond the arterial needle (farther from the AV anastomosis), inserting the needle in the same direction as the blood flow. Follow the steps used for the arterial needle.
- Remove the syringe from the end of the arterial needle tubing, uncap the arterial dialyzer tubing, and connect the two lines. Tape the connection securely *to prevent accidental separation of the tubing.*

■ Remove the syringe from the end of the venous needle tubing, uncap the venous dialyzer tubing, and connect the two lines. Tape the connection securely *to prevent accidental separation of the tubing.*

NURSING ALERT Dialysate is considered a high-alert medication *because it can cause the patient significant harm when used in error.*[50,51]

■ If required by your facility, before beginning hemodialysis, have another nurse perform an independent double-check *to verify the patient's identity and to make sure that the correct dialysate is hanging in the prescribed concentration, the dosage calculations are correct, the dialysis machine settings are correct, and the infusion line is attached to the correct port.*[51,52]

■ Compare the results of the independent double-check with the other nurse (if required) and, if no discrepancies exist, unclamp the tubing and begin the hemodialysis treatment. Keep the access and connections visible at all times. If discrepancies exist, rectify them before beginning hemodialysis.

■ Monitor the hemodialysis equipment parameters continuously.[1] Verify that all lines are open and connections are intact and secure.[7] Observe the color of blood in the dialyzer (dark color can precede filter clotting; cherry red may indicate hemolysis). Check pressure readings, including venous pressure, arterial pressure, and transmembrane pressure. Venous pressure shouldn't exceed 250 mm Hg. *High venous pressure may indicate clotting in the venous chamber, blood line, or venous needle; low venous pressure may indicate disconnection.* Arterial pressure shouldn't exceed −250 mm Hg. *Low arterial pressure indicates hypotension, excess suction on the access wall, or a clotted arterial needle or access port; a sudden drop in arterial pressure may indicate needle migration or infiltration. High arterial pressure may indicate dialyzer or system clotting.* Transmembrane pressure (venous pressure minus the dialysate pressure in millimeters of mercury) should rise slowly throughout hemodialysis in response to ultrafiltration, with subsequent increased blood viscosity. Observe the anticoagulant pump *to make sure the anticoagulant is administered as prescribed.* Monitor the system and the patient's response to the anticoagulant through direct observation and blood specimen testing, as indicated.[1,28] Check the blood and dialysate flow rates to ensure delivery of prescribed rates *to achieve the desired patient solute clearance.*[1] Monitor and adjust the ultrafiltration rate according to the patient's response to treatment.[1] Monitor dialysate conductivity to ensure delivery of dialysis solution with an electrolyte concentration that won't cause hemolysis or crenation of red blood cells.

■ Closely monitor the patient's vital signs, oxygen saturation level, pain level, intake and output, anticoagulant administration, and laboratory test results, as well as any complaints or changes in the patient's behavior throughout the treatment session *to promptly recognize changes in the patient's condition or vascular access.* Intervene quickly to resolve any treatment complications.

■ Watch for signs and symptoms of complications, including muscle cramps, air embolism, dialyzer reaction (hypotension, pruritus, back pain, angioedema, anaphylaxis), hypoxemia, and dialysis disequilibrium syndrome (such as headache, nausea, vomiting, hypertension, decreased sensorium, seizures, and coma).[1] If any of these signs or symptoms develops, notify the practitioner and intervene as ordered. The hemodialysis treatment may need to be discontinued or the efficiency of diffusion reduced.

■ Administer prescribed medications, as ordered, following safe medication administration practices.[45,46,47,48]

■ Obtain blood samples for coagulation studies, as ordered.[1]

■ Return the bed to the lowest position *to prevent falls and maintain patient safety.*[53]

■ Discard used equipment in appropriate receptacles.[44]

Initiating hemodialysis with a double-lumen catheter

■ Collaborate with the practitioner to form the patient's treatment plan, based on laboratory test results and predialysis assessment findings.[25]

■ Perform hand hygiene.[29,30,31,32,33,34]

■ Gather and prepare the necessary equipment and supplies.

■ Assist the patient into a comfortable position (supine or sitting in a recliner with the feet elevated) that also facilitates blood flow. *Different access sites may necessitate different positions.*[1] Position the patient's face away from the catheter.[2]

■ Perform hand hygiene.[29,30,31,32,33,34]

■ Remove any tape or gauze securing the catheter ports and place a clean, fluid-impermeable pad or sterile towel under the ports to prevent the catheter hubs from touching a dirty surface.[2]

■ Put on gloves, a gown, and a mask with face shield or a mask and goggles as necessary *to comply with standard precautions.*[28,42,43,44]

■ Have the patient put on a mask.[2]

■ Prepare the preservative-free normal saline flush solution in the 10-mL syringes, as indicated.

■ Assess the catheter exit site for signs and symptoms of dysfunction, infection, and other complications.[2,54]

■ Identify the red (arterial) and blue (venous) ports.

■ Clamp the catheter *to prevent air from entering either lumen of the catheter.*[2,55]

■ Remove the caps, then disinfect the catheter hubs using a new antiseptic pad for each hub. Scrub the sides (threads) and end of each hub thoroughly using friction, making sure to remove any residue. Continue disinfecting the catheter limbs using friction, moving from each hub to at least several centimeters toward the patient's body. Hold the catheter limbs while the antiseptic dries.[55] Discard the antiseptic pads.[44]

■ Don't allow the catheter hubs to touch unsterile surfaces.[2]

■ While maintaining sterility of the syringe tip, attach a syringe to the red port catheter hub, unclamp the catheter, withdraw the locking solution, clamp the catheter, and remove the syringe.[2,56]

■ Perform a vigorous mechanical scrub of the red port catheter hub for at least 5 seconds using an antiseptic pad. Then allow it to dry completely.[6,55,57]

■ While maintaining sterility of the syringe tip, attach a 10-mL prefilled syringe containing preservative-free normal saline solution to the red port, unclamp the port, gently instill the solution, and then reclamp the red port.[2,56]

■ While maintaining sterility of the syringe tip, attach another syringe to the blue port catheter hub, unclamp the catheter, withdraw the locking solution, clamp the catheter, and remove the syringe.[2,56]

■ Perform a vigorous mechanical scrub of the blue port catheter hub for at least 5 seconds using an antiseptic pad. Then allow it to dry completely.[6,55,57]

■ While maintaining sterility of the syringe tip, attach another 10-mL prefilled syringe containing preservative-free normal saline solution to the blue port, unclamp the port, gently instill the solution, and then reclamp the blue port.[55,58]

■ If catheter patency is in question, assess for mechanical or thrombotic dysfunction; institute thrombolytic therapy, as ordered, if thrombotic dysfunction is present.

■ Remove the syringe from the red port and then, maintaining sterile technique, attach the red port to the line leading to the arterial port of the dialyzer.[55]

■ Trace the tubing from the patient to its point of origin *to make sure you've connected it to the proper port.*[59,60]

■ Remove the syringe from the blue port and then, maintaining sterile technique, attach the blue port to the line leading to the venous port of the dialyzer.[55]

■ Trace the tubing from the patient to its point of origin *to make sure you've connected it to the proper port.*[59,60]

■ Secure the tubing to the patient *to reduce tension on the connections and to prevent trauma to the catheter insertion site.*

■ Open the clamps to the arterial and venous dialyzer tubing.

■ Remove the patient's mask.

■ Begin the hemodialysis treatment. Keep the access and connections visible at all times.[7]

Discontinuing hemodialysis with AV access

■ Perform hand hygiene.[29,30,31,32,33,34]

■ Put on gloves, a gown, and a mask with face shield or a mask and goggles, as necessary, *to comply with standard precautions.*[28,42,43,44]

■ Turn the blood pump on the hemodialysis machine to 50 to 100 mL/minute

■ Raise the patient's bed to waist level (if applicable) before providing patient care *to prevent caregiver back strain.*[41]

■ Remove the tape from the connection site of the arterial lines.

■ Clamp the needle tubing and then disconnect the lines. Note that the blood in the arterial line will continue to flow toward the dialyzer, followed by normal saline solution. Clamp the blood line just before the blood reaches the point where the saline solution enters the line.

■ Unclamp the saline solution and allow a small amount of saline solution to flow through the line.

■ Unclamp the dialyzer line and allow all of the blood to flow into the dialyzer, where it passes through the filter and back to the patient through the venous line.

■ After the blood is retransfused by the dialyzer, clamp the venous needle tubing and the dialyzer's venous line and turn off the blood pump.

■ Remove the tape from the connection site of the venous lines and disconnect the lines.

■ Apply a folded 4″ × 4″ (10 cm × 10 cm) sterile gauze pad over the needle site, but don't apply pressure.

■ Carefully remove the needles (one at a time *to prevent unnecessary loss of blood due to the force of pressure in the access*)[1] at approximately the same angle as needle insertion *to prevent dragging the needle across the patient's skin and to avoid puncturing the vein wall.*

■ Apply moderate pressure to the site with the folded 4″ × 4″ (10 cm × 10 cm) sterile gauze pad using two fingers until the bleeding stops.[1] Note that application of inadequate pressure can result in hematoma formation; excessive pressure can result in thrombosis. You should be able to continue to feel a thrill both above and below the compression site while holding pressure. Bleeding usually stops within 10 minutes.

■ Cover the site with a dry sterile dressing.[5,19] Avoid circumferential taping of the dressing.

■ When dialysis is complete, weigh the patient in kilograms, obtain vital signs (including blood pressure sitting and standing, if possible), and assess neurologic status.[50] Compare these findings with the predialysis assessment data.

■ Return the bed to the lowest position *to prevent falls and maintain patient safety.*[53]

Discontinuing hemodialysis with a double-lumen catheter

■ Perform hand hygiene.[29,30,31,32,33,34]

■ Put on gloves, a gown, and a mask with face shield or a mask and goggles *to comply with standard precautions.*[28,42,43,44]

■ Have the patient put on a mask.[2]

■ Turn the blood pump on the hemodialysis machine to 50 to 100 mL/minute.

■ Raise the patient's bed to waist level (if applicable) before providing patient care *to prevent caregiver back strain.*[41]

■ Clamp the catheter lumens *to prevent air from entering either lumen of the catheter.*[2,55]

■ Disinfect the connections between the catheter hubs and the lines leading to the dialyzer, using a separate antiseptic pad for each connection; then allow them to dry completely.[5,55]

■ Disconnect the dialysis line from the red port of the catheter.[2]

■ Perform a vigorous mechanical scrub of the hub for at least 5 seconds using an antiseptic pad. Scrub the sides (threads) and the end of the hub thoroughly using friction, making sure to remove any residue. Then allow it to dry completely.[2,5,44,55]

■ While maintaining sterility of the syringe tip, attach a 10-mL prefilled syringe containing preservative-free normal saline solution to the red catheter port, unclamp the catheter lumen, and then slowly flush the lumen. Then clamp the catheter lumen and remove and discard the syringe.[2,60]

■ Perform a vigorous mechanical scrub of the catheter hub for at least 5 seconds using an antiseptic pad. Then allow it to dry completely.[2,5,44,55]

■ While maintaining sterility of the syringe tip, attach a syringe containing the prescribed locking solution, unclamp the catheter lumen, and lock the port following unit protocol. Then clamp the catheter lumen and remove and discard the syringe.[2,60]

■ Perform a vigorous mechanical scrub of the red port for at least 5 seconds using an antiseptic pad and then allow it to dry completely.[2,5,44,55] Cap the port with a new sterile Luer-lock cap.[2,55]

■ Disconnect the dialysis line from the blue catheter port and perform a vigorous mechanical scrub of the hub for at least 5 seconds using an antiseptic pad. Scrub the sides (threads) and the end of the hub thoroughly

using friction, making sure to remove any residue. Allow it to dry completely.[2,5,55]

■ While maintaining sterility of the syringe tip, attach a 10-mL syringe containing preservative-free normal saline solution to the blue catheter port, unclamp the catheter lumen, and slowly flush the lumen. Then clamp the catheter lumen and remove and discard the syringe.[2,60]

■ Perform a vigorous mechanical scrub of the catheter hub for at least 5 seconds using an antiseptic pad. Then allow it to dry completely.[1,5,44,55]

■ While maintaining sterility of the syringe tip, attach a syringe containing the prescribed locking solution and lock the port following unit protocol.[2] Then clamp the catheter lumen and remove and discard the syringe.

■ Perform a vigorous mechanical scrub of the blue port for at least 5 seconds using an antiseptic pad and then allow it to dry completely.[2,5,44,55] Cap the port with a new sterile Luer-lock cap.[2,55]

■ Place the patient in the supine position, with the head facing away from the catheter.[2]

■ If necessary, perform catheter exit site care and apply a sterile transparent semipermeable (or sterile gauze and tape) dressing to the catheter exit site.[1,2] If compatible with the hemodialysis catheter material, apply povidone-iodine, polymyxin B, bacitracin zinc, or gramicidin ointment (as prescribed) to the catheter exit site *to reduce the risk of vascular catheter–associated infection.*[2,5]

■ Remove the patient's mask.

■ Assess the patient's postdialysis weight (in kilograms), vital signs, and neurologic, respiratory, and cardiac status;[50] compare your findings to predialysis baseline findings.

■ Remove and discard your gloves.[43,44]

■ Return the bed to the lowest position (if applicable) *to prevent falls and maintain patient safety.*[53]

■ Perform hand hygiene.[29,30,31,32,33,34]

■ Put on new gloves.[43,44]

■ Rinse and disinfect the dialysis delivery system.[61,62]

Declotting a double-lumen catheter

■ Perform hand hygiene.[29,30,31,32,33,34]

■ Thoroughly disinfect the top of the sterile water-for-injection vial with an antiseptic pad using friction. Allow it to dry completely.

■ Using a 3-mL syringe and needle or blunt-tip needleless device, draw up 2.2 mL of sterile water for injection.[16,17]

■ Thoroughly disinfect the top of the alteplase vial with an antiseptic pad using friction. Allow it to dry completely.[17]

■ Inject the sterile water into the alteplase vial, directing the diluent stream into the powder. Gently swirl the vial until the contents are completely dissolved (this should occur within 3 minutes). Don't shake the vial. Be aware that slight foaming may occur. Let the vial stand undisturbed to allow large bubbles to dissipate. The reconstituted preparation will be a transparent and colorless or pale yellow solution with a final concentration of 1 mg/mL. Inspect the product for foreign material and discoloration.[58]

■ Thoroughly disinfect the top of the alteplase vial with an antiseptic pad using friction. Allow it to dry completely.[17]

■ Using a 10-mL syringe, withdraw the ordered dose of reconstituted alteplase solution from the vial.

■ Trace the catheter from the patient to the point of origin *to make sure you're accessing the proper port to prevent dangerous misconnections.*[59,60,63]

For the single syringe method (use with complete occlusion)

■ Remove the cap, if present, and perform a vigorous mechanical scrub of the needleless connector or hub for at least 5 seconds using an antiseptic pad. Scrub the sides (threads) and end of the hub thoroughly using friction, being sure to remove any residue. Continue disinfecting the catheter limb using friction, moving from the hub to at least several centimeters toward the patient's body. Hold the catheter limb while the antiseptic dries.[55]

■ Don't allow the catheter hub to touch unsterile surfaces.[2]

■ Place a needleless connector on the hub, if needed, maintaining aseptic technique.

- Clamp the double-lumen catheter, if appropriate.[17]
- Remove the needle or blunt-tip needleless device from the syringe containing alteplase. While maintaining the sterility of the syringe tip, attach the alteplase-filled syringe to the needleless connector. Alternatively, remove the needleless connector, perform a vigorous mechanical scrub of the catheter hub for at least 5 seconds using an antiseptic pad, allow it to dry completely, and attach the alteplase-filled syringe to the catheter hub.[6,64]
- Unclamp the double-lumen catheter while holding the syringe vertically. Gently pull the plunger back to about the 8-mL mark.[55]
- While keeping the syringe in a vertical position, slowly release the plunger; make sure that the solution is in the end of the syringe closest to the double-lumen catheter.[17] Instill the appropriate dose of alteplase into the occluded catheter. Don't apply pressure to the plunger, *because such force could rupture the catheter or expel the clot into circulation.*[16,17]
- Clamp the device, leave the syringe in place, and secure it with tape.[17]
- Label the syringe DO NOT USE—DECLOTTING, and include the date, the time, and your initials.[17]
- After 30 minutes of drug dwell time, assess catheter function.[16] Unclamp the device and attempt to aspirate for blood return.[16,17] Brisk blood return indicates that declotting was successful; sluggish or no blood return indicates that the clot is still present.

For the stopcock method (use with complete occlusion)

- Remove the cap, if present, and perform a vigorous mechanical scrub of the needleless connector or hub for at least 5 seconds using an antiseptic pad. Scrub the sides (threads) and end of the hub thoroughly using friction, being sure to remove any residue. Continue disinfecting the catheter limb using friction, moving from the hub to at least several centimeters toward the patient's body. Hold the catheter limb while the antiseptic dries.[55]
- Don't allow the catheter hub to touch unsterile surfaces.[2]
- Clamp the catheter, remove the needleless connector, and attach a sterile stopcock to the device hub. Turn the stopcock off from the patient to the device hub.[17]
- While maintaining the sterility of the syringe tip, attach an empty 10-mL syringe to a stopcock port.[17]
- Remove the needle or blunt-tip needleless device from the syringe containing alteplase. While maintaining the sterility of the syringe tip, attach the alteplase-filled syringe to the remaining stopcock port.[17]
- Open the stopcock to the port connected to the empty syringe.[17]
- Unclamp the double-lumen catheter while holding the syringe vertically, and gently pull the plunger back to about the 8-mL mark. While maintaining the plunger position, close the stopcock to the port to create negative pressure within the central venous access device lumen.[17]
- Open the stopcock to the port to which the syringe containing alteplase is connected. Allow solution to enter the double-lumen catheter. Open the stopcock to the port where the syringe containing alteplase is connected. (You may need to repeat the process of opening the stopcock to the empty syringe, pulling back on the syringe plunger, closing the stopcock to that port, and then opening the stopcock to the port containing the alteplase until the alteplase dose is pulled into the double-lumen catheter.)[17]
- Clamp the device, leave the syringe in place, and secure it with tape, or clamp the double-lumen catheter and remove the stopcock and syringes. Thoroughly disinfect the device hub with an antiseptic pad for at least 5 seconds, allow it to dry, and attach a needleless connector to the device hub during the dwell time.[6,17]
- Label the device DO NOT USE—DECLOTTING, and include the date, the time, and your initials.[17]
- After 30 minutes of drug dwell time, assess catheter function.[16] If the syringe was left in place, unclamp the device and attempt to aspirate for blood return. Brisk blood return indicates that declotting was successful; sluggish or no blood return indicates that the clot is still present.
- If a needleless connector was attached, perform a vigorous mechanical scrub of the needleless connector for at least 5 seconds using an antiseptic pad. Allow it to dry completely.[6,55] While maintaining the sterility of the syringe tip, connect an empty 10-mL syringe to the needleless connector, unclamp the device, and attempt to aspirate for blood return. Brisk blood return indicates that declotting was successful; sluggish or no blood return indicates that the clot is still present.

For the direct instillation method (use with partial thrombotic occlusion)

- Remove the cap, if present, and perform a vigorous mechanical scrub of the needleless connector or hub for at least 5 seconds using an antiseptic pad. Scrub the sides (threads) and end of the hub thoroughly using friction, being sure to remove any residue. Continue disinfecting the catheter limb using friction, moving from the hub to at least several centimeters toward the patient's body. Hold the catheter limb while the antiseptic dries.[55]
- Don't allow the catheter hub to touch unsterile surfaces.[2]
- Place a needleless connector on the hub, if needed, maintaining aseptic technique.
- While maintaining the sterility of the syringe tip, attach the syringe containing alteplase to the needleless connector.[17]
- Unclamp the double-lumen catheter, if appropriate, and slowly inject the alteplase into the catheter; don't force the solution into the device.[17]
- Clamp the device and remove and discard the syringe.
- Label the device DO NOT USE—DECLOTTING, and include the date, the time, and your initials.[17]
- After 30 minutes of drug dwell time, assess catheter function.[16] Perform a vigorous mechanical scrub of the needleless connector for at least 5 seconds using an antiseptic pad. Allow it to dry completely.[6,17,57]
- While maintaining the sterility of the syringe tip, attach an empty 10-mL syringe to the needleless connector, unclamp the device, and attempt to aspirate for blood return. Brisk blood return indicates patency; sluggish or no blood return indicates that the occlusion is still present.

Completing the declotting procedure
If declotting was successful after 30 minutes

- Use the 10-mL syringe to withdraw 4 to 5 mL of blood (3 mL in patients who weigh less than 10 kg) to remove the alteplase.[16]
- Clamp the double-lumen catheter.[17] Remove and discard the syringe containing the blood and residual medication in a puncture-resistant sharps disposal container.[17,44,64]
- Perform a vigorous mechanical scrub of the needleless connector for at least 5 seconds using an antiseptic pad. Scrub the sides (threads) and end of the hub thoroughly using friction, being sure to remove any residue. Continue disinfecting the catheter limb using friction, moving from the hub to at least several centimeters toward the patient's body. Hold the catheter limb while the antiseptic dries.[6,55]
- While maintaining the sterility of the syringe tip, attach a 10-mL syringe filled with preservative-free normal saline solution, then gently irrigate the catheter.[16,17]
- Restart any ordered hemodialysis or lock the catheter, as indicated. To lock the device, perform a vigorous mechanical scrub of the needleless connector for at least 5 seconds using an antiseptic pad and then allow it to dry completely.[2,6,55] While maintaining the sterility of the syringe tip, attach the syringe containing the locking solution to the needleless connector and inject the locking solution into the double-lumen catheter following facility protocol.[2] After locking the catheter, clamp the catheter lumen and remove and discard the syringe.
- If you locked the catheter, place a disinfectant-containing end cap (if available at your facility) on the needleless connector to reduce the risk of vascular catheter–associated infection.[57]

If declotting was unsuccessful after 30 minutes

- Repeat the procedure and then reassess catheter function after a total of 120 minutes of alteplase dwell time by attempting to aspirate for a blood return.[16]
- If the catheter is functional, follow the steps above for withdrawing blood, irrigating the catheter, and restarting the hemodialysis or locking device.[16]
- If the catheter remains occluded 120 minutes after alteplase administration, instill a second dose of alteplase according to the initial method used, checking for patency at 30 and 120 minutes.[16]
- If the second declotting attempt was successful and the catheter is functional, follow the steps above for withdrawing blood, irrigating the catheter, and restarting the infusion or locking the device.

- If the catheter remains occluded 120 minutes after administration of the second alteplase dose, notify the practitioner.[17]

Completing the procedure

- Remove and discard your gloves and other personal protective equipment, if worn.[43,44]
- Perform hand hygiene.[29,30,31,32,33,34]
- Document the procedure.[65,66,67,68]

Special considerations

- Don't inject IV fluids or medications into either port of the double-lumen catheter. Avoid using the double-lumen catheter for routine blood sampling.[56]
- The Joint Commission issued a sentinel event alert concerning medical device alarm safety, *because alarm-related events have been associated with permanent loss of function or death.* Among the major contributing factors were improper alarm settings, alarm settings turned off inappropriately, and alarm signals not audible to staff. Make sure that alarm limits are set appropriately, and that alarms are turned on, functioning properly, and audible to staff. Follow facility guidelines for preventing alarm fatigue.[21]
- The Joint Commission issued a sentinel event alert related to managing risk during transition to new International Organization for Standardization tubing standards that were designed to prevent dangerous tubing misconnections, which can lead to serious patient injury and death. During the transition, make sure to trace each tube and catheter from the patient to its point of origin before connecting or reconnecting any device or infusion, at any care transition (such as to a new setting or service), and as part of the hand-off process; route tubes and catheters having different purposes in different, standardized directions; when the patient has different access sites or several bags hanging, label tubing at the distal and proximal ends; use tubing and equipment only as intended; and store medications for different delivery routes in separate locations.[60]

NURSING ALERT Make sure you complete each step in the hemodialysis procedure correctly. *Overlooking a single step or performing it incorrectly can cause unnecessary blood loss or inefficient treatment from poor clearances or inadequate fluid removal.* For example, when preparing the equipment, never allow a normal saline solution bag to run dry while priming *because that could cause air to enter the patient portion of the dialysate system.* Failure to perform accurate hemodialysis therapy can lead to patient injury or death.

- If catheter function isn't restored after two alteplase doses, other strategies, such as replacing the catheter, should be considered.[69]
- When administering alteplase for a double-lumen catheter declotting according to the manufacturer's instructions, circulating systemic levels are not expected to reach clinically significant concentrations.[16]

Complications

Complications that can occur as a result of hemodialysis include hypotension, cramps, nausea and vomiting, headache, angina, back pain, itching, fever, and chills. Hemolysis, usually related to problems with the dialysate solution, can occur and may present as chest or back pain. Arrhythmias, likely as a result of rapid electrolyte and fluid changes, are also possible. Disconnection can result in air embolism.[70]

Dialysis disequilibrium syndrome (DDS) is a rare syndrome presenting with neurologic symptoms thought to be caused by cerebral edema. This condition usually occurs when a patient is first started on dialysis.[71] Access site infection is also a potential complication.[72]

Tissue plasminogen activator is a naturally occurring component of the human clotting cascade, so allergic reactions are rare; however, intracatheter alteplase shouldn't be administered to patients with known hypersensitivity to alteplase or to any other component of the formulation. Serious adverse events after intracatheter use of alteplase are rare, and include sepsis, bleeding, and venous thrombosis.[16]

Documentation

Record the time that the treatment began, along with the patient's predialysis assessment data and vital signs. Record ongoing assessment data, including vital signs you obtained during treatment. Note any complications, the name of the practitioner and the date and time you notified the practitioner, your interventions, and the patient's response to those interventions. Note any blood samples you sent and the laboratory results you obtained. Record the time the treatment was completed and the patient's response to it. Record the condition of the catheter insertion site, the date and time of the dressing change, and any culture specimens you obtained.

Document the catheter's reduced or occluded blood flow. Briefly describe the declotting procedure, including drug dwell time and catheter status after alteplase instillation. Record alteplase administration and flushes in the patient's medication record. Also document flush volumes in the patient's intake and output record. Note the patient's response to the procedure, any adverse events, interventions taken, and the patient's response to those interventions

Document teaching provided to the patient and family (if applicable), their understanding of that teaching, and any need for follow-up teaching.

REFERENCES

1 Wiegand, D. L. (2017). *AACN procedure manual for high acuity, progressive, and critical care* (7th ed.). St. Louis, MO: Elsevier.

2 Lok, C. E., et al. (2020). KDOQI clinical practice guideline for vascular access: 2019 update. *American Journal of Kidney Disease, 4*(2), S1–S164. https://www.ajkd.org/action/showPdf?pii=S0272-6386%2819%2931137-0 (Level VII)

3 Aydin, Z., et al. (2012). Placement of hemodialysis catheters with a technical, functional, and anatomical viewpoint. *International Journal of Nephrology,* 2012, 302826. http://www.hindawi.com/journals/ijn/2012/302826/ (Level VI)

4 National Kidney Foundation. (2015). KDOQI clinical practice guideline for hemodialysis adequacy: 2015 update. *American Journal of Kidney Disease,* 66, 884–930. http://www.ajkd.org/article/S0272-6386(15)01019-7/pdf (Level VII)

5 Centers for Disease Control and Prevention. (2011, revised 2017). Guidelines for the prevention of intravascular catheter-related infections. https://www.cdc.gov/infectioncontrol/guidelines/bsi/recommendations.html (Level I)

6 Marschall, J., et al. (2014). SHEA/IDSA practice recommendation: Strategies to prevent central line-associated bloodstream infections in acute care hospitals. *Infection Control and Hospital Epidemiology, 35*(7), 753–771. http://www.jstor.org/stable/10.1086/676533 (Level I)

7 Woo, K. (2020). Arteriovenous fistula creation for hemodialysis and its complications. In: *UpToDate,* Dillavou, E. D., & Berns, J. S. (Eds.).

8 Bander, S. J., & You, T. H. (2020). Central catheters for acute and chronic hemodialysis access and their management. In: *UpToDate,* Davidson, I., & Berns, J. S. (Eds.).

9 Allon, M., & Sexton, D. J. (2020). Tunneled hemodialysis catheter-related bloodstream infection (CRBSI): Management and prevention. In: *UpToDate,* Berns, J. S. (Ed.).

10 Jarrett, N., & Callaham, M. (2016). Evidence based guidelines for selected hospital-acquired conditions: Final report. https://www.cms.gov/Medicare/Medicare-Fee-for-Service-Payment/HospitalAcqCond/Downloads/2016-HAC-Report.pdf

11 Standard 50. Infection. Infusion therapy standards of practice (8th ed.). (2021). *Journal of Infusion Nursing,* 44, S153–S157. (Level VII)

12 End Stage Renal Disease National Coordinating Center. (n.d.). Fistula first catheter last. https://www.esrdncc.org/en/fistula-first-catheter-last

13 National Kidney Foundation. (n.d.). NKF and the fistula first breakthrough initiative. https://www.kidney.org/patients/pfc/DialysisEducation

14 Vassalotti, J. A., et al. (2012). Fistula first breakthrough initiative: Targeting catheter last in fistula first. *Seminars in Dialysis,* 25, 303–310. (Level VII)

15 Rivera-Bou, W. L., et al. (2017). Thrombolytic therapy. https://emedicine.medscape.com/article/811234-overview#a2

16 Genentech, Inc. (2019). Cathflo® Activase® (Alteplase). https://www.gene.com/download/pdf/cathflo_prescribing.pdf

17 Infusion Nurses Society. (2016). *Policies and procedures for infusion therapy* (5th ed.). Boston, MA: Infusion Nurses Society.

18 National Kidney Foundation. (2015). KDOQI clinical practice guideline for hemodialysis adequacy: 2015 update. http://www.ajkd.org/article/S0272-6386(15)01019-7/pdf (Level VII)

19 Centers for Disease Control and Prevention. (2016). Dialysis safety: Core interventions. https://www.cdc.gov/dialysis/prevention-tools/core-interventions.html

20 The Joint Commission. (2021). Standard NPSG.06.01.01. *Comprehensive accreditation manual for hospitals.* Oakbrook Terrace, IL: The Joint Commission. (Level VII)

21 The Joint Commission. (2014). Sentinel event alert 50: Medical device alarm safety in hospitals. https://www.jointcommission.org/assets/1/6/SEA_50_alarms_4_26_16.pdf (Level VII)

22 The Joint Commission. (2021). Standard RI.01.03.01. *Comprehensive accreditation manual for hospitals.* Oakbrook Terrace, IL: The Joint Commission. (Level VII)

23 Centers for Medicare and Medicaid Services, Department of Health and Human Services. (2020). Condition of participation: Patient's rights. 42 C.F.R. § 482.13(b)(2).

24 Accreditation Association for Hospitals and Health Systems. (2020). Standard 15.01.11. *Healthcare Facilities Accreditation Program Accreditation requirements for acute care hospitals.* Chicago, IL: Accreditation Association for Hospitals and Health Systems. (Level (VII)

25 DNV GL-Healthcare USA, Inc. (2020). PR.2.SR.3. *NIAHO® accreditation requirements, interpretive guidelines and surveyor guidance—revision 20.0.* Milford, OH: DNV GL-Healthcare USA, Inc. (Level VII)

26 Westbrook, J., et al. (2010). Association of interruptions with an increased risk and severity of medication administration errors. *Archives of Internal Medicine, 170,* 683–690.

27 Institute for Safe Medication Practices. (2012). Side tracks on the safety express: Interruptions lead to errors and unfinished…Wait, what was I doing? *Nurse Advise-ERR, 11*(2), 1–4. https://www.ismp.org/Newsletters/acutecare/showarticle.aspx?id=37

28 American Nephrology Nurses' Association. (2020). *Core curriculum for nephrology nursing* (7th ed.). Pitman, NJ: ANNA.

29 The Joint Commission. (2021). Standard NPSG.07.01.01. *Comprehensive accreditation manual for hospitals.* Oakbrook Terrace, IL: The Joint Commission. (Level VII)

30 Centers for Disease Control and Prevention. (2002). Guideline for hand hygiene in health-care settings: Recommendations of the Healthcare Infection Control Practices Advisory Committee and the HICPAC/SHEA/APIC/IDSA Hand Hygiene Task Force. *MMWR Recommendations and Reports, 51*(RR-16), 1–45. http://www.cdc.gov/mmwr/pdf/rr/rr5116.pdf (Level II)

31 World Health Organization. (2009). WHO guidelines on hand hygiene in health care: First global patient safety challenge, clean care is safer care. https://apps.who.int/iris/bitstream/handle/10665/44102/9789241597906_eng.pdf?sequence=1 (Level IV)

32 Accreditation Association for Hospitals and Health Systems. (2020). Standard 07.01.21. *Healthcare Facilities Accreditation Program: Accreditation requirements for acute care hospitals.* Chicago, IL: Accreditation Association for Hospitals and Health Systems. (Level VII)

33 Centers for Medicare and Medicaid Services, Department of Health and Human Services. (2020). Condition of participation: Infection control. 42 C.F.R. § 482.42.

34 DNV GL-Healthcare USA, Inc. (2020). IC.1.SR.1. *NIAHO® accreditation requirements, interpretive guidelines and surveyor guidance—revision 20.0.* Milford, OH: DNV GL-Healthcare USA, Inc. (Level VII)

35 The Joint Commission. (2021). Standard NPSG.01.01.01. *Comprehensive accreditation manual for hospitals.* Oakbrook Terrace, IL: The Joint Commission. (Level VII)

36 The Joint Commission. (2021). Standard RI.01.01.01. *Comprehensive accreditation manual for hospitals.* Oakbrook Terrace, IL: The Joint Commission. (Level VII)

37 Centers for Medicare and Medicaid Services, Department of Health and Human Services. (2020). Condition of participation: Patient's rights. 42 C.F.R. § 482.13(c)(1).

38 DNV GL-Healthcare USA, Inc. (2019). PR.2.SR.5. *NIAHO® accreditation requirements, interpretive guidelines and surveyor guidance—revision 18.2.* Milford, OH: DNV GL-Healthcare USA, Inc. (Level VII)

39 Accreditation Association for Hospitals and Health Systems. (2020). Standard 15.01.16. *Healthcare Facilities Accreditation Program: Accreditation requirements for acute care hospitals.* Chicago, IL: Accreditation Association for Hospitals and Health Systems. (Level VII)

40 The Joint Commission. (2021). Standard PC.02.01.21. *Comprehensive accreditation manual for hospitals.* Oakbrook Terrace, IL: The Joint Commission. (Level VII)

41 Waters, T. R., et al. (2009). Safe patient handling training for schools of nursing. [Online]. https://www.cdc.gov/niosh/docs/2009-127/pdfs/2009-127.pdf (Level VII)

42 Accreditation Association for Hospitals and Health Systems. (2020). Standard 07.01.10. *Healthcare Facilities Accreditation Program: Accreditation requirements for acute care hospitals.* Chicago, IL: Accreditation Association for Hospitals and Health Systems. (Level VII)

43 Siegel, J. D., et al. (2007, revised 2019). 2007 guideline for isolation precautions: Preventing transmission of infectious agents in healthcare settings. https://www.cdc.gov/infectioncontrol/pdf/guidelines/isolation-guidelines-H.pdf (Level II)

44 Occupational Safety and Health Administration. (2019). Bloodborne pathogens, standard number 1910.1030. https://www.osha.gov/pls/oshaweb/owadisp.show_document?p_id=10051&p_table=STANDARDS (Level VII)

45 The Joint Commission. (2021). Standard MM.06.01.01. *Comprehensive accreditation manual for hospitals.* Oakbrook Terrace, IL: The Joint Commission. (Level VII)

46 Accreditation Association for Hospitals and Health Systems. (2020). Standard 16.01.03. *Healthcare Facilities Accreditation Program: Accreditation requirements for acute care hospitals.* Chicago, IL: Accreditation Association for Hospitals and Health Systems. (Level VII)

47 Centers for Medicare and Medicaid Services, Department of Health and Human Services. (2020). Condition of participation: Nursing services. 42 C.F.R. § 482.23(c).

48 DNV GL-Healthcare USA, Inc. (2020). MM.1.SR.3. *NIAHO® accreditation requirements, interpretive guidelines and surveyor guidance—revision 20.0.* Milford, OH: DNV GL-Healthcare USA, Inc. (Level VII)

49 Gebauer Company. (n.d.) Gebauer's ethyl chloride. http://cdn2.hubspot.net/hubfs/150313/docs/Ethyl_Chloride/Application/EC_English_IFU.pdf

50 Institute for Safe Medication Practices. (2020). 2020–2021 targeted medication safety best practices for hospitals. https://www.ismp.org/sites/default/files/attachments/2020-02/2020-2021%20TMSBP-%20FINAL_1.pdf

51 Institute for Safe Medication Practices. (2018). ISMP list of high-alert medications in acute care settings. https://www.ismp.org/sites/default/files/attachments/2018-08/highAlert2018-Acute-Final.pdf

52 Institute for Safe Medication Practices. (2013). Independent double-checks: Undervalued and misused: Selective use of this strategy can play an important role in medication safety. https://www.ismp.org/resources/independent-double-checks-undervalued-and-misused-selective-use-strategy-can-play (Level VII)

53 Ganz, D. A., et al. (2013). Preventing falls in hospitals: A toolkit for improving quality of care (AHRQ publication no. 13-0015-EF). https://www.ahrq.gov/professionals/systems/hospital/fallpxtoolkit/index.html (Level VII)

54 Standard 42. Vascular access device. Infusion therapy standards of practice (8th ed.). (2021). *Journal of Infusion Nursing, 44,* S119–S123. (Level VII)

55 Centers for Disease Control and Prevention. (n.d.). Hemodialysis central venous catheter scrub-the-hub protocol. https://www.cdc.gov/dialysis/PDFs/collaborative/Hemodialysis-Central-Venous-Catheter-STH-Protocol.pdf

56 Standard 29. Vascular access and hemodialysis. Infusion therapy standards of practice (8th ed.). (2021). *Journal of Infusion Nursing, 44,* S89–S90. (Level VII)

57 Standard 36. Needleless connectors. Infusion therapy standards of practice (8th ed.). (2021). *Journal of Infusion Nursing, 44,* S104–S107. (Level VII)

58 Standard 41. Flushing and locking. Infusion therapy standards of practice (8th ed.). (2021). *Journal of Infusion Nursing, 44,* S113–S118. (Level VII)

59 U.S. Food and Drug Administration. (2017). Examples of medical device misconnections. https://www.fda.gov/medical-devices/medical-device-connectors/examples-medical-device-misconnections

60 The Joint Commission. (2014). Sentinel event alert 53: Managing risk during transition to new ISO tubing connector standards. http://www.jointcommission.org/assets/1/6/SEA_53_Connectors_8_19_14_final.pdf (Level VII)

61 Accreditation Association for Hospitals and Health Systems. (2020). Standard 07.02.03. *Healthcare Facilities Accreditation Program: Accreditation requirements for acute care hospitals.* Chicago, IL: Accreditation Association for Hospitals and Health Systems. (Level VII)

62 Rutala, W. A., et al. (2008, revised 2019). Guideline for disinfection and sterilization in healthcare facilities, 2008. https://www.cdc.gov/infection-control/pdf/guidelines/disinfection-guidelines-H.pdf (Level I)

63 Standard 59. Infusion medication and solution administration. Infusion therapy standards of practice (8th ed.). (2021). *Journal of Infusion Nursing, 44,* S180–S183. (Level VII)

64 Standard 21. Medical waste and sharps safety. Infusion therapy standards of practice (8th ed.). (2021). *Journal of Infusion Nursing, 44,* S60–S162. (Level VII)

65   The Joint Commission. (2021). Standard RC.01.03.01. *Comprehensive accreditation manual for hospital*. Oakbrook Terrace, IL: The Joint Commission. (Level VII)

66   Accreditation Association for Hospitals and Health Systems. (2020). Standard 10.00.03. *Healthcare Facilities Accreditation Program: Accreditation requirements for acute care hospitals*. Chicago, IL: Accreditation Association for Hospitals and Health Systems. (Level VII)

67   Centers for Medicare and Medicaid Services, Department of Health and Human Services. (2020). Condition of participation: Medical record services. 42 C.F.R. § 482.24(b).

68   DNV GL-Healthcare USA, Inc. (2020). MR.2.SR.1. *NIAHO® accreditation requirements, interpretive guidelines and surveyor guidance—revision 20.0*. Milford, OH: DNV GL-Healthcare USA, Inc. (Level VII)

69   Standard 49. Central venous access device occlusion. Infusion therapy standards of practice (8th ed.). (2021). *Journal of Infusion Nursing, 44*, S149–S153. (Level VII)

70   Holley, J. L. (2020). Acute complications during hemodialysis. In: *UpToDate*, Berns, J. S. (Ed.).

71   Agarwal, R. (2020). Dialysis disequilibrium syndrome. In: *UpToDate*, Berns, J. S. (Ed.).

72   Berns, J. S. (2021). Patient education: Hemodialysis (beyond the basics). In: *UpToDate*, Schwab, S. J. (Ed.).

HEMOGLOBIN TESTING, BEDSIDE

Hemoglobin level can be measured at the patient's bedside using a portable photometer device.[1] This method involves obtaining a fingerstick specimen and placing it in the device, which immediately determines the hemoglobin level and allows for prompt intervention, if necessary. In contrast, the traditional method involves obtaining a blood specimen using venipuncture (or a vascular access device) and then sending the sample to the laboratory for interpretation.

Several portable testing systems are available for bedside hemoglobin monitoring. These systems are also convenient for the patient's home use. At home or at the bedside, using single-use, autodisabling fingerstick devices prevents the spread of bloodborne pathogens.[2]

Normal hemoglobin values for adults range from 12 to 16 mg/dL (120 to 160 g/L) for women and 14 to 17.4 g/dL (140 to 174 g/L) for men.[3] Normal hemoglobin ranges vary by age in children. A below-normal hemoglobin value may indicate anemia, recent hemorrhage, or fluid retention, all of which result in hemodilution. An elevated hemoglobin value suggests hemoconcentration from polycythemia or dehydration.[3]

Equipment

Portable photometer ■ single-use, auto-disabling lancet[2] ■ microcuvette ■ two pairs of gloves ■ alcohol pads ■ gauze pads ■ facility-approved disinfectant ■ Optional: warm, moist compresses.

Preparation of equipment

Inspect all equipment and supplies. If a product is expired, is defective, or has compromised integrity, remove it from patient use, label it as expired or defective, and report the expiration or defect as directed by your facility.

If you're opening the vial for the first time, label the vial with the date and time you opened it. Microcuvettes can be stored for up to 2 years; however, after the vial is opened, the shelf life of the microcuvettes is 90 days (or as specified by the manufacturer.) Turn on the photometer. If the photometer hasn't been used recently, insert the control microcuvette *to make sure that the photometer is working properly*.

Implementation

- Verify the practitioner's order.
- Gather the necessary equipment and supplies.
- Perform hand hygiene.[4,5,6,7,8,9]
- Confirm the patient's identity using at least two patient identifiers.[10]
- Provide privacy.[11,12,13,14]
- Explain the procedure to the patient and family (if appropriate) according to their individual communication and learning needs *to increase their understanding, allay their fears, and enhance cooperation*.[15] Explain that the patient will feel a pinprick in the finger during blood sampling.
- If needed, plug the photometer into the wall.
- Perform hand hygiene.[4,5,6,7,8,9]
- Put on gloves *to comply with standard precautions*.[16,17,18]
- Select an appropriate puncture site. In most cases, use the fingertip for an adult or child, and the heel or the great toe for an infant.[19] For an adult, the third and fourth fingers are the best choices, *because the second finger is usually the most sensitive, and the thumb may have thickened skin or calluses*. Blood should circulate freely in the finger from which you're drawing blood, so avoid using a ring-bearing finger. *To ensure an adequate blood sample*, don't use a cold, cyanotic, or swollen area as the puncture site.
- If necessary, dilate the capillaries by applying warm, moist compresses to the area for about 10 minutes.
- Clean the intended puncture site with an alcohol pad and allow it to air-dry completely, *because any remaining alcohol may interfere with the test results*.[19]
- To collect the sample from the fingertip, use a single-use, auto-disabling lancet.[2] Position the lancet on the side of the patient's fingertip, perpendicular to the lines of the fingerprints.[19] Puncture the skin with a quick, continuous, and deliberate stroke *to achieve a good flow of blood and to prevent the need to repeat the puncture*.[19]
- If required by your facility, wipe away the first drop of blood using a gauze pad, *because it may be contaminated with tissue, fluid, or debris*.[19]
- Apply the microcuvette, which automatically collects a precise amount of blood. Don't squeeze the patient's finger too tightly, *because doing so may dilute the specimen with plasma and increase the risk of obtaining a hemolyzed sample*.[19]
- Insert the microcuvette into the photometer and then watch for the hemoglobin results to appear on the photometer screen within the time period specified by the manufacturer.
- Place a gauze pad over the puncture site and apply firm pressure *to stop bleeding*.[19]
- Discard the lancet and microcuvette in appropriate containers.[16]
- Remove and discard your gloves[16] and perform hand hygiene.[4,5,6,7,8,9]
- Put on a pair of new gloves[16,17,18] and clean and disinfect reusable equipment according to the manufacturer's instructions *to prevent the spread of infection*.[20,21]
- Remove and discard your gloves[16] and perform hand hygiene.[4,5,6,7,8,9]
- Notify the practitioner if the test result is outside the expected parameters.[22]
- Document the procedure.[23,24,25,26]

Special considerations

- Bedside hemoglobin testing is a waived test, meaning the test system was approved for waiver under the Clinical Laboratory Improvement Amendments of 1988 by the U.S. Food and Drug Administration. To qualify for waived test status, the test must be simple to perform and have low risk for erroneous test results. However, keep in mind that errors can occur anywhere in the testing process; make sure you follow the manufacturer's instructions for use *to prevent testing errors that could result in treatment errors*.[27]
- A recent study suggested that bedside hemoglobin testing underestimated the clinical laboratory measurement of hemoglobin, and that these two methods should not be considered interchangeable. In addition, consideration for blood transfusions should also be based on the patient's clinical findings.[28]

Complications

Complications of capillary sampling include hematoma, scarring, inadvertent arterial puncture, infection, nerve damage, necrosis, and skin breakdown from repeated application of adhesive tape.[19]

Documentation

Document the values that you obtained from the photometer as well as the date and time of the test. If applicable, record the name of the practitioner and the date and time of notification of test results outside the expected parameters, any prescribed interventions, and the patient's response to those interventions. Document teaching provided to the patient and family (if applicable), their understanding of that teaching, and any need for follow-up teaching.

REFERENCES

1 Whitehead, R. D., et al. (2019). Methods and analyzers for hemoglobin measurement in clinical laboratories and field settings. *Annals of the New York Academy of Sciences, 1450*(1), 147–171. https://www.ncbi.nlm.nih.gov/pmc/articles/PMC6709845/ (Level I)

2 Centers for Disease Control and Prevention. (n.d.). CDC clinical reminder: Use of fingerstick devices on more than one person poses risk for transmitting bloodborne pathogens. https://www.cdc.gov/injectionsafety/pdf/Clinical_Reminder_Fingerstick_Devices_RiskBBP.pdf

3 Fischbach, F., & Fischbach, M. A. (2018). *A manual of laboratory and diagnostic tests* (10th ed.). Philadelphia, PA: Wolters Kluwer.

4 The Joint Commission. (2021). Standard NPSG.07.01.01. *Comprehensive accreditation manual for hospitals.* Oakbrook Terrace, IL: The Joint Commission. (Level VII)

5 Centers for Disease Control and Prevention. (2002). Guideline for hand hygiene in health-care settings: Recommendations of the Healthcare Infection Control Practices Advisory Committee and the HICPAC/SHEA/APIC/IDSA Hand Hygiene Task Force. *MMWR Recommendations and Reports, 51*(RR-16), 1–45. https://www.cdc.gov/mmwr/pdf/rr/rr5116.pdf (Level II)

6 World Health Organization. (2009). WHO guidelines on hand hygiene in health care: First global patient safety challenge, clean care is safer care. https://apps.who.int/iris/bitstream/handle/10665/44102/9789241597906_eng.pdf?sequence=1 (Level IV)

7 Centers for Medicare and Medicaid Services, Department of Health and Human Services. (2020). Condition of participation: Infection control. 42 C.F.R. § 482.42.

8 Accreditation Association for Hospitals and Health Systems. (2020). Standard 07.01.21. *Healthcare Facilities Accreditation Program: Accreditation requirements for acute care hospitals.* Chicago, IL: Accreditation Association for Hospitals and Health Systems. (Level VII)

9 DNV GL-Healthcare USA, Inc. (2020). IC.1.SR.1. *NIAHO® accreditation requirements, interpretive guidelines and surveyor guidance - revision 20.0.* Milford, OH: DNV GL-Healthcare USA, Inc. (Level VII)

10 The Joint Commission. (2021). Standard NPSG.01.01.01. *Comprehensive accreditation manual for hospitals.* Oakbrook Terrace, IL: The Joint Commission. (Level VII)

11 Accreditation Association for Hospitals and Health Systems. (2020). Standard 15.01.16. *Healthcare Facilities Accreditation Program: Accreditation requirements for acute care hospitals.* Chicago, IL: Accreditation Association for Hospitals and Health Systems. (Level VII)

12 Centers for Medicare and Medicaid Services, Department of Health and Human Services. (2020). Condition of participation: Patient's rights. 42 C.F.R. § 482.13(c)(1).

13 The Joint Commission. (2021). Standard RI.01.01.01. *Comprehensive accreditation manual for hospitals.* Oakbrook Terrace, IL: The Joint Commission. (Level VII)

14 DNV GL-Healthcare USA, Inc. (2020). PR.21.SR.5. *NIAHO® accreditation requirements, interpretive guidelines and surveyor guidance - revision 20.0.* Milford, OH: DNV GL-Healthcare USA, Inc. (Level VII)

15 The Joint Commission. (2021). Standard PC.02.01.21. *Comprehensive accreditation manual for hospitals.* Oakbrook Terrace, IL: The Joint Commission. (Level VII)

16 Occupational Safety and Health Administration. (2019). Bloodborne pathogens, standard number 1910.1030. https://www.osha.gov/pls/oshaweb/owadisp.show_document?p_id=10051&p_table=STANDARDS (Level VII)

17 Siegel, J. D., et al. (2007, revised 2019). 2007 guideline for isolation precautions: Preventing transmission of infectious agents in healthcare settings. https://www.cdc.gov/infectioncontrol/pdf/guidelines/isolation-guidelines-H.pdf (Level II)

18 Accreditation Association for Hospitals and Health Systems. (2020). Standard 07.01.10. *Healthcare Facilities Accreditation Program: Accreditation requirements for acute care hospitals.* Chicago, IL: Accreditation Association for Hospitals and Health Systems. (Level VII)

19 World Health Organization. (2010). WHO guidelines on drawing blood: Best practices in phlebotomy. https://apps.who.int/iris/bitstream/handle/10665/44294/9789241599221_eng.pdf;jsessionid=53D3FEB817C-CD5D876334C11439BE790?sequence=1 (Level IV)

20 Rutala, W. A., et al. (2008, revised 2019). Guideline for disinfection and sterilization in healthcare facilities, 2008. https://www.cdc.gov/infectioncontrol/pdf/guidelines/disinfection-guidelines-H.pdf (Level I)

21 Accreditation Association for Hospitals and Health Systems. (2020). Standard 07.02.03. *Healthcare Facilities Accreditation Program: Accreditation requirements for acute care hospitals.* Chicago, IL: Accreditation Association for Hospitals and Health Systems. (Level VII)

22 The Joint Commission. (2021). Standard NPSG.02.03.01. *Comprehensive accreditation manual for hospitals.* Oakbrook Terrace, IL: The Joint Commission. (Level VII)

23 The Joint Commission. (2021). Standard RC.01.03.01. *Comprehensive accreditation manual for hospitals.* Oakbrook Terrace, IL: The Joint Commission. (Level VII)

24 Centers for Medicare and Medicaid Services, Department of Health and Human Services. (2020). Condition of participation: Medical record services. 42 C.F.R. § 482.24.

25 Accreditation Association for Hospitals and Health Systems. (2020). Standard 10.00.03. *Healthcare Facilities Accreditation Program: Accreditation requirements for acute care hospitals.* Chicago, IL: Accreditation Association for Hospitals and Health Systems. (Level VII)

26 DNV GL-Healthcare USA, Inc. (2020). MR.2.SR.1. *NIAHO® accreditation requirements, interpretive guidelines and surveyor guidance - revision 20.0.* Milford, OH: DNV GL-Healthcare USA, Inc. (Level VII)

27 Centers for Disease Control and Prevention. (2021). Clinical laboratory improvement amendments (CLIA): Waived tests. https://www.cdc.gov/labquality/waived-tests.html

28 Johnson, M., et al. (2020). Comparison of hemoglobin measurements by 3 point-of-care devices with standard laboratory values and reliability regarding decisions for blood transfusions. *Anesthesia and Analgesia, 131,* 640–649. (Level VI)

Hip arthroplasty care

Hip arthroplasty involves surgical replacement of the hip joint. It may be total (replacing the femoral head and acetabulum) or partial (replacing only one joint component). (See *Total hip replacement,* page 396.)

Hip arthroplasty is performed to decrease or eliminate pain and improve functional status. It's most commonly used to treat osteoarthritis. Other indications include rheumatoid arthritis, avascular necrosis, traumatic arthritis, hip fractures, benign and malignant bone tumors, ankylosing spondylitis, and juvenile rheumatoid arthritis.

Arthroplasty postprocedure care includes providing routine postoperative care, implementing measures to prevent complications such as venous thromboembolism (VTE), maintaining alignment of the affected joint, and assisting with exercises. Other nursing responsibility includes teaching about safe mobility and exercises that may continue for several years at home.

HOSPITAL-ACQUIRED CONDITION ALERT Keep in mind that the Centers for Medicare and Medicaid Services considers VTE in patients who underwent hip replacement a hospital-acquired condition *because it can be reasonably prevented using a variety of best practices. To reduce the risk of VTE,* make sure to follow evidence-based VTE prevention practices, such as using mechanical compression devices (including antiembolism stockings, an intermittent pneumatic compression device, or an arterial-venous impulse foot compression device), early ambulation, and pharmacologic prophylaxis.[1,2,3]

Equipment

Antiembolism stockings, sequential compression device, or arterial-venous impulse foot compression device ▪ ice bag ▪ hypoallergenic moisturizer[4] ▪ warm water ▪ crutches or walker ▪ closed-wound drainage system ▪ marker ▪ over-the-bed trapeze bar ▪ prescribed anticoagulant ▪ prescribed pain medication ▪ vital signs monitoring equipment ▪ stethoscope ▪ disinfectant pad ▪ graduated cylinder ▪ Optional: gloves, electronic infusion device (preferably a smart pump with dose-error reduction software), sterile dressings, hypoallergenic tape, prescribed beta-adrenergic agent, pulse oximeter and probe, capnography device, sedation scale, abduction splint or pillow.

Total hip replacement

To form a totally artificial hip, the surgeon cements a femoral head prosthesis in place to articulate with a cup, which is then cemented into the deepened acetabulum. The surgeon may avoid using cement by implanting a prosthesis with a porous coating that promotes bony ingrowth.

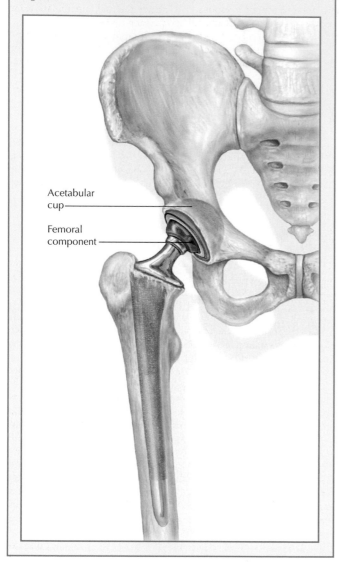

Acetabular cup

Femoral component

Implementation

- Receive hand-off communication from the person who was responsible for the patient's care. Ask questions, as necessary, *to avoid miscommunications that can cause patient care errors during transitions of care.*[5] As part of the hand-off process, trace each tubing and catheter from the patient to its point of origin using a standardized line reconciliation process.[6]
- Verify the practitioner's orders.
- Gather and prepare the necessary equipment and supplies.
- Perform hand hygiene.[7,8,9,10,11,12]
- Confirm the patient's identity using at least two patient identifiers.[13]
- Provide privacy.[14,15,16,17]
- Explain all postprocedure care to the patient and family (if appropriate) according to their individual communication and learning needs *to increase their understanding, allay their fears, and enhance cooperation.*[18]
- Raise the patient's bed to waist level before providing patient care *to prevent caregiver back strain.*[19]
- Perform hand hygiene.[7,8,9,10,11,12]
- Put on gloves, as needed, *to comply with standard precautions.*[20,21,22]

- Monitor vital signs at an interval determined by your facility and the patient's condition; *no evidence-based research is available to dictate the best practice for the frequency of vital signs monitoring.*[23] Promptly report changes in vital signs, *because these changes may indicate the presence of infection, hemorrhage, and other postoperative complications.*
- Screen for and assess the patient's pain using facility-defined criteria that are consistent for the patient's age, condition, and ability to understand.[24]
- Treat the patient's pain as needed and ordered using nonpharmacologic or pharmacologic measures, or a combination of approaches. Base the treatment plan on evidence-based practices and the patient's clinical condition, past medical history, and pain management goals.[24]
- If the patient is receiving IV opioid medication, frequently monitor vital signs, respiratory status (including oxygen saturation level using pulse oximetry, and end-tidal carbon dioxide level using a capnography device, if available), and sedation level *to enable prompt recognition and treatment of oversedation and respiratory depression related to IV opioid use.*
- Explain the monitoring process to the patient and family, and inform them that it might be necessary to awaken the patient to assess the effects of the medication. Advise the patient and family to alert staff immediately if the patient develops breathing problems or other changes that might indicate a reaction to the medication.[25,26]
- Assess the patient for postoperative nausea and vomiting, and intervene as needed.[23]
- Perform bilateral neurovascular assessments regularly, as needed,[23] *to monitor for signs and symptoms of complications.* Assess the affected leg for color, temperature, toe movement, sensation, edema, capillary filling, and pedal pulse. Investigate complaints of pain, burning, numbness and tingling.[27]
- Assess and address the patient's safety needs *to reduce the risk of patient harm.*[23]
- Assess the patient's respiratory status.[23] Direct the patient to perform deep-breathing and coughing exercises *to prevent postprocedure pneumonia.*
- Apply antiembolism stockings or a sequential compression device to the patient's lower extremities, or an arterial-venous impulse foot compression device to the patient's feet, as ordered, *to promote venous return and prevent VTE.*[28,29] (See the "Antiembolism stocking application" procedure and the "Sequential compression therapy" procedure.)
- Make sure baseline coagulation studies have been obtained and are documented in the patient's medical record.
- Administer thromboembolic pharmacoprophylaxis, as ordered, following safe medication administration practices, *to minimize the risk of VTE.*[25,28,29,30] Monitor International Normalized Ratio (INR) if the patient is receiving warfarin. If a continuous infusion of heparin is prescribed, administer it using an electronic infusion device (preferably a smart pump with dose-reduction software) *to provide consistent and accurate dosing.*[28,31] Monitor laboratory results, such as complete blood count, prothrombin time, partial thromboplastin time, and INR.[28] Notify the practitioner of critical test results within your facility's established time frame *to ensure that the patient receives prompt treatment.*[32]
- Observe the patient for bleeding and signs and symptoms of phlebitis, such as warmth, swelling, tenderness, and redness.[28]
- Inspect the dressings for excessive bleeding. Circle any drainage on the dressing and mark it with your initials, the date, and the time.
- As needed, apply more sterile dressings using hypoallergenic tape. Report excessive bleeding to the patient's practitioner.
- Observe the closed-wound drainage system for proper functioning and monitor discharge color. (See the "Closed-wound drain management" procedure.) *Proper drainage prevents hematoma. Purulent discharge and fever may indicate infection.* Empty and measure drainage, as ordered, using clean technique *to prevent infection.*
- Monitor fluid intake and output daily (including wound drainage in the output measurement) and electrolyte levels, as ordered, *to promptly detect and treat fluid and electrolyte imbalances.*[25,26] Notify the practitioner of critical test results within your facility's established time frame *to ensure that the patient receives prompt treatment.*[32]
- If an indwelling urinary catheter was inserted for surgery, remove the catheter on postoperative day 1 or 2 (with the day of surgery considered

day 0), or as soon as it's no longer needed, *to reduce the risk of catheter-associated urinary tract infection.*[28,33,34] (See the "Indwelling urinary catheter care and removal" procedure.)

HOSPITAL-ACQUIRED CONDITION ALERT Keep in mind that the Centers for Medicare and Medicaid Services considers catheter-associated urinary tract infection (CAUTI) a hospital-acquired condition *because it can be reasonably prevented using best practices.* Make sure to follow evidence-based CAUTI prevention practices—such as performing hand hygiene before and after any catheter manipulation; maintaining a sterile, continuously closed drainage system; maintaining unobstructed urine flow; regularly emptying the collection bag; replacing the catheter and drainage system using sterile technique when breaks in sterile technique, disconnection, or leakage occurs; and discontinuing the catheter as soon as it's no longer clinically indicated—when caring for a patient with an indwelling urinary catheter *to reduce the risk of CAUTI.*[33,34,35,36,37]

- Make sure prophylactic antibiotics are discontinued within 24 hours after surgery.[28,38,39]
- Apply an ice bag, as ordered, to the affected site for the first 48 hours *to reduce swelling, relieve pain, and control bleeding.*[40,41]
- Help the patient use the trapeze bar for repositioning, as ordered. *Position changes enhance comfort, prevent pressure injuries, and help prevent respiratory complications.*
- Hydrate the patient's skin, after bathing with warm water, by applying a hypoallergenic moisturizer while the skin is still damp, as indicated, *to prevent skin breakdown.*[4]
- Position the patient according to the surgical approach used and the surgeon's preference. Depending on the surgical approach and provider preference, an abduction splint or pillow may be necessary *to keep the hip in a neutral position.*[42,43] Remind the patient to avoid crossing the legs when in bed or a chair.[42]
- Encourage the patient to begin plantar flexion and dorsiflexion exercises of the ankles and feet *to prevent VTE.*[44]
- Collaborate with physical therapy professionals, as appropriate, *to formulate an individualized exercise plan for the patient.*
- Before ambulation, assess the patient's pain and administer pain medication, as ordered and indicated, following safe medication administration practices,[25,30,45,46] *because movement is very painful.* Encourage the patient during exercise.
- Help the patient with progressive ambulation, using assistive devices such as crutches or a walker when needed.[44]
- If the patient was receiving a beta-adrenergic blocker before surgery, collaborate with the patient's practitioner to make sure the patient receives it during the perioperative period, as appropriate.[47]
- Reassess and respond to the patient's pain by evaluating the response to treatment and progress toward pain management goals. Assess for adverse reactions and risk factors for adverse events that may result from treatment.[24]
- Educate the patient and family about measures to prevent surgical site infection.[39,48]
- Return the patient's bed to the lowest position *to prevent falls and maintain patient safety.*[49]
- Remove and discard your gloves, if worn.[20,22]
- Perform hand hygiene.[7,8,9,10,11,12]
- Clean and disinfect your stethoscope using a disinfectant pad.[50,51]
- Perform hand hygiene.[7,8,9,10,11,12]
- Document the procedure.[52,53,54,55]

Special considerations

- Progressive ambulation protocols vary. Most patients may to begin transfer and progressive ambulation with assistive devices on the first day. Collaborate with physical therapy professionals, as appropriate. *Early ambulation decreases the risk of postoperative, complications such as VTEs, constipation, respiratory compromise, and pressure injuries.*[56,57]
- The Joint Commission issued a sentinel event alert concerning inadequate hand-off communication *because of the potential for patient harm that can result when a receiver receives inaccurate, incomplete, untimely, misinterpreted, or otherwise inadequate information. To improve hand-off communication,* standardize the critical information communicated

by the sender. At a minimum, include the sender contact information; illness assessment; patient summary, including events leading up to the illness or admission, hospital course, ongoing assessment, and care plan; to-do action list; contingency plans; allergy list; code status; medication list; and dated laboratory test results and vital signs. Provide face-to-face communication whenever possible in an interruption-free location using facility-approved, standardized tools and methods (for example, forms, templates, checklists, protocols, and mnemonics). Provide ample time and opportunity for questions, and include the multidisciplinary team members and the patient and family when appropriate.[58]

- The Joint Commission issued a sentinel event alert related to managing risk during transition to new International Organization for Standardization tubing standards that were designed to prevent dangerous tubing misconnections, which can lead to serious patient injury and death. During the transition, make sure to trace each tubing and catheter from the patient to its point of origin before connecting or reconnecting any device or infusion, at any care transition (such as to a new setting or service), and as part of the hand-off process; route tubes and catheters having different purposes in different standardized directions; when the patient has different access sites or several bags hanging, label the tubing at both the distal and proximal ends; use tubing and equipment only as intended; and store medications for different delivery routes in separate locations.[6]

Patient teaching

During discharge teaching, instruct the patient to:
- take prescribed medications as ordered
- adhere to the ordered schedule for follow-up blood testing (usually twice weekly) until discontinued by the practitioner
- keep follow-up appointments with the surgeon
- immediately report signs or symptoms of deep vein thrombosis, such as increasing calf pain, tenderness, or swelling above or below the knee and increased swelling in the calf, ankle, or foot
- immediately report warning signs of a blood clot that has traveled to a lung, including a sudden increase in shortness of breath, sudden chest pain, and localized chest pain with coughing
- promptly report signs and symptoms of possible infection, such as fever (temperature above 101° F [38.3° C]), shaking chills, excessive incisional drainage, unusual warmth or swelling around the incision, and increasing hip pain.

Teach the patient and family about pain management strategies during discharge planning. Include information about the patient's pain management plan and adverse effects of pain management treatment. Discuss activities of daily living and items in the home environment that might exacerbate pain or reduce the effectiveness of the pain management plan, and include strategies to address these issues. Teach the patient and family about safe use, storage, and disposal of opioids if prescribed.[24]

Stress the importance of continuing with rehabilitation, not only to maintain physical function but also to prevent complications. Caution the patient about the risk of falling, and teach the patient to avoid stairs until able to keep a strong and mobile balance. Urge the patient to wear strong, sturdy shoes, and emphasize that assistive devices are an important part of rehabilitation. Explain that the patient may need periodic X-rays to evaluate for loosening or wearing out of prosthesis components, as indicated.[29]

Complications

Surgical complications of hip arthroplasty include hematoma, nerve injury, intraoperative fracture, leg length discrepancy, and (rarely) bone cement implantation syndrome.[59] Immobility after arthroplasty can result in such complications as pulmonary embolism, pneumonia, deep vein phlebitis, paralytic ileus, urine retention, constipation, and bowel impaction.[59,60] Incomplete pain control can prolong recuperation and increase the risk for chronic pain.[61] A deep wound or infection at the prosthesis site is a serious complication that can force revision or removal of the prosthesis.[59] Although these are the most common complications, the use of prophylactic antibiotics, anticoagulants, and early mobilization has significantly reduced their occurrence. Dislocation of a total hip prosthesis may occur after violent hip flexion or adduction or during internal rotation. Signs of dislocation include inability to rotate the hip or bear weight, shortening of the leg, and increased pain.

Fat embolism, a potentially fatal complication resulting from release of fat molecules in response to increased intramedullary canal pressure from the prosthesis, may develop within 72 hours after surgery. Watch for such signs and symptoms as apprehension, diaphoresis, fever, tachypnea, dyspnea, hypoxia, pulmonary effusion, tachycardia, cyanosis, seizures, decreased level of consciousness, and a petechial rash on the chest and shoulders; hypoxia is an early sign that may occur hours before the onset of respiratory complaints.[62,63]

Documentation

Record the patient's postoperative assessment findings, including vital signs, respiratory status, sedation level (if applicable), and nausea and vomiting assessment. Document signs and symptoms of infection. Record the patient's neurovascular status and the use of VTE prevention practices. Document the patient's pain assessment findings and response to pain medication. Describe the patient's position (especially the position of the affected leg), skin care and condition, and postprocedure pneumonia prevention practices. Document all exercises that the patient performed and their effect; also record the patient's ambulatory efforts and the type of support that the patient used. Document teaching provided to the patient and family (if applicable), their understanding of that teaching, and any need for follow-up teaching.

On an appropriate flowchart, record vital signs and fluid intake and output. Note the turning and skin care schedule and the current exercise and ambulation program. Record discharge instructions that you provided as well as the patient's understanding of those instructions.

REFERENCES

1 Jarrett, N., & Callaham, M. (2016). Evidence-based guidelines for selected hospital-acquired conditions: Final report. https://www.cms.gov/Medicare/Medicare-Fee-for-Service-Payment/HospitalAcqCond/Downloads/2016-HAC-Report.pdf

2 Falck-Ytter, Y., et al. (2012). Prevention of VTE in orthopedic surgery patients: antithrombotic therapy and prevention of thrombosis, 9th ed.: American College of Chest Physicians evidence-based clinical practice guidelines. *Chest, 141*(2 Suppl.), e278S–e325S. https://www.ncbi.nlm.nih.gov/pmc/articles/PMC3278063/

3 Balk, E. M., et al. (2017). *Venous thromboembolism prophylaxis in major orthopedic surgery: Systematic review update.* (AHRQ Publication No. 17-EHC021-EF). Rockville, MD: Agency for Healthcare Research and Quality. https://effectivehealthcare.ahrq.gov/products/thromboembolism-update/research-2017 (Level I)

4 LeBlanc, K., et al. (2013). International skin tear advisory panel: A tool kit to aid in the prevention, assessment, and treatment of skin tears using a simplified classification system. *Advances in Skin and Wound Care, 26,* 459–476. (Level IV)

5 The Joint Commission. (2021). Standard PC.02.02.01. *Comprehensive accreditation manual for hospitals.* Oakbrook Terrace, IL: The Joint Commission. (Level VII)

6 The Joint Commission. (2014). Sentinel event alert 53: Managing risk during transition to new ISO tubing connector standards. https://www.jointcommission.org/assets/1/6/SEA_53_Connectors_8_19_14_final.pdf (Level VII)

7 The Joint Commission. (2021). Standard NPSG.07.01.01. *Comprehensive accreditation manual for hospitals.* Oakbrook Terrace, IL: The Joint Commission. (Level VII)

8 World Health Organization. (2009). WHO guidelines on hand hygiene in health care: First global patient safety challenge, clean care is safer care. https://apps.who.int/iris/bitstream/handle/10665/44102/9789241597906_eng.pdf?sequence=1 (Level IV)

9 Centers for Disease Control and Prevention. (2002). Guideline for hand hygiene in health-care settings: Recommendations of the Healthcare Infection Control Practices Advisory Committee and the HICPAC/SHEA/APIC/IDSA Hand Hygiene Task Force. *MMWR Recommendations and Reports, 51*(RR-16), 1–45. https://www.cdc.gov/mmwr/pdf/rr/rr5116.pdf (Level II)

10 Centers for Medicare and Medicaid Services, Department of Health and Human Services. (2020). Condition of participation: Infection control. 42 C.F.R. § 482.42.

11 Accreditation Association for Hospitals and Health Systems. (2020). Standard 07.01.21. *Healthcare Facilities Accreditation Program: Accreditation requirements for acute care hospitals.* Chicago, IL: Accreditation Association for Hospitals and Health Systems. (Level VII)

12 DNV GL-Healthcare USA, Inc. (2020). IC.1.SR.1. *NIAHO® accreditation requirements, interpretive guidelines and surveyor guidance—revision 20.0.* Milford, OH: DNV GL-Healthcare USA, Inc. (Level VII)

13 The Joint Commission. (2021). Standard NPSG.01.01.01. *Comprehensive accreditation manual for hospitals.* Oakbrook Terrace, IL: The Joint Commission. (Level VII)

14 Accreditation Association for Hospitals and Health Systems. (2020). Standard 15.01.16. *Healthcare Facilities Accreditation Program: Accreditation requirements for acute care hospitals.* Chicago, IL: Accreditation Association for Hospitals and Health Systems. (Level VII)

15 Centers for Medicare and Medicaid Services, Department of Health and Human Services. (2020). Condition of participation: Patient's rights. 42 C.F.R. § 482.13(c)(1).

16 The Joint Commission. (2021). Standard RI.01.01.01. *Comprehensive accreditation manual for hospitals.* Oakbrook Terrace, IL: The Joint Commission. (Level VII)

17 DNV GL-Healthcare USA, Inc. (2020). PR.2.SR.5. *NIAHO® accreditation requirements, interpretive guidelines and surveyor guidance—revision 20.0.* Milford, OH: DNV GL-Healthcare USA, Inc. (Level VII)

18 The Joint Commission. (2021). Standard PC.02.01.21. *Comprehensive accreditation manual for hospitals.* Oakbrook Terrace, IL: The Joint Commission. (Level VII)

19 Waters, T. R., et al. (2009). Safe patient handling training for schools of nursing. https://www.cdc.gov/niosh/docs/2009-127/pdfs/2009-127.pdf (Level VII)

20 Siegel, J. D., et al. (2007, revised 2019). 2007 guideline for isolation precautions: Preventing transmission of infectious agents in healthcare settings. https://www.cdc.gov/infectioncontrol/pdf/guidelines/isolation-guidelines-H.pdf (Level II)

21 Accreditation Association for Hospitals and Health Systems. (2020). Standard 07.01.10. *Healthcare Facilities Accreditation Program: Accreditation requirements for acute care hospitals.* Chicago, IL: Accreditation Association for Hospitals and Health Systems. (Level VII)

22 Occupational Safety and Health Administration. (2019). Bloodborne pathogens, standard number 1910.1030. https://www.osha.gov/pls/oshaweb/owadisp.show_document?p_id=10051&p_table=STANDARDS (Level VII)

23 American Society of PeriAnesthesia Nurses. (2019). *2019-2020 Perianesthesia nursing standards, practice recommendations and interpretive statements.* Cherry Hill, NJ: American Society of PeriAnesthesia Nurses. (Level VII)

24 The Joint Commission. (2021). Standard PC.01.02.07. *Comprehensive accreditation manual for hospitals.* Oakbrook Terrace, IL: The Joint Commission. (Level VII)

25 Centers for Medicare and Medicaid Services, Department of Health and Human Services. (2020). Condition of participation: Nursing services. 42 C.F.R. § 482.23(c).

26 Centers for Medicare and Medicaid Services, Department of Health and Human Services. (2014). Requirements for hospital medication administration, particularly intravenous medications and post-operative care of patients receiving IV opioids. https://www.cms.gov/Medicare/Provider-Enrollment-and-Certification/SurveyCertificationGenInfo/Downloads/Survey-and-Cert-Letter-14-15.pdf

27 Slade, S. (2020). Evidence summary. Neurovascular assessment. *The JBI EBP Database.* AN: JBI188

28 Centers for Medicare and Medicaid Services & The Joint Commission. (2022). The specifications manual for national hospital inpatient quality measures (version 5.11). https://www.qualitynet.org/inpatient/specifications-manuals#tab1

29 American Academy of Orthopaedic Surgeons. (2011). Preventing venous thromboembolic disease in patients undergoing elective hip and knee arthroplasty. *American Academy of Orthopaedic Surgeon, 19*(12), 768–776. (Level VII)

30 Accreditation Association for Hospitals and Health Systems. (2020). Standard 16.01.03. *Healthcare Facilities Accreditation Program: Accreditation requirements for acute care hospitals.* Chicago, IL: Accreditation Association for Hospitals and Health Systems. (Level VII)

31 The Joint Commission. (2021). Standard NPSG.03.05.01. *Comprehensive accreditation manual for hospitals.* Oakbrook Terrace, IL: The Joint Commission. (Level VII)

32 The Joint Commission. (2021). Standard NPSG.02.03.01. *Comprehensive accreditation manual for hospitals.* Oakbrook Terrace, IL: The Joint Commission. (Level VII)

33 Healthcare Infection Control Practices Advisory Committee. (2010, revised 2019). Guideline for prevention of catheter-associated urinary tract infections 2009. https://www.cdc.gov/infectioncontrol/pdf/guidelines/cauti-guidelines-H.pdf (Level I)

34 Association of Professionals in Infection Control and Epidemiology. (2014). APIC implementation guide: Guide to preventing catheter-associated urinary tract infections. https://apic.org/wp-content/uploads/2019/02/APIC_CAUTI_IG_FIN_REVD0815.pdf (Level IV)

35 Lo, E., et al. (2014). SHEA/IDSA practice recommendation: Strategies to prevent catheter-associated urinary tract infections in acute care hospitals: 2014 update. *Infection Control and Hospital Epidemiology, 35,* 464–479. https://www.jstor.org/stable/10.1086/675718#metadata_info_tab_contents (Level I)

36 The Joint Commission. (2021). Standard NPSG.07.06.01. *Comprehensive accreditation manual for hospitals.* Oakbrook Terrace, IL: The Joint Commission.

37 Agency for Healthcare Research and Quality, & U.S. Department of Health and Human Services. (2015). Toolkit for reducing catheter-associated urinary tract infections in hospital units: Implementation guide. https://www.ahrq.gov/hai/cauti-tools/impl-guide/index.html

38 World Health Organization. (2016). Global guidelines for the prevention of surgical site infection. https://www.who.int/gpsc/global-guidelines-web.pdf (Level VII)

39 Anderson, D. J., et al. (2014). SHEA/IDSA practice recommendation: Strategies to prevent surgical site infections in acute care hospitals: 2014 update. *Infection Control and Hospital Epidemiology, 35*(6), 605–627. http://www.jstor.org/stable/10.1086/676022 (Level I)

40 Iwakiri, K., et al. (2019). Efficacy of continuous local cryotherapy following total hip arthroplasty. *SICOT-J, 5,* 13. https://www.ncbi.nlm.nih.gov/pmc/articles/PMC6498864/ (Level VI)

41 Ni, S. H., et al. (2015). Cryotherapy on postoperative rehabilitation of joint arthroplasty. *Knee Surgery, Sport Traumatology, Arthroscopy, 12,* 3354–3361. (Level VI)

42 Foran, J. R. H. (2018). Activities after hip replacement. https://orthoinfo.aaos.org/en/recovery/activities-after-hip-replacement/

43 Erens, G. A., et al. (2021). Total hip arthroplasty. In: *UpToDate,* Hunter, D., et al. (Ed.).

44 Foran, J. R. H. (2017). Total hip replacement exercise guide. https://orthoinfo.aaos.org/en/recovery/total-hip-replacement-exercise-guide/

45 The Joint Commission. (2021). Standard MM.06.01.01.01. *Comprehensive accreditation manual for hospitals.* Oakbrook Terrace, IL: The Joint Commission. (Level VII)

46 DNV GL-Healthcare USA, Inc. (2020). MM.1.SR.3. *NIAHO® accreditation requirements, interpretive guidelines and surveyor guidance—revision 20.0.* Milford, OH: DNV GL-Healthcare USA, Inc. (Level VII)

47 Devereaux, P. J., et al. (2020). Management of cardiac risk for noncardiac surgery. In: *UpToDate,* Pellikka, P. A., & Jaffe, A. S. (Eds.).

48 The Joint Commission. (2021). Standard NPSG.07.05.01. *Comprehensive accreditation manual for hospitals.* Oakbrook Terrace, IL: The Joint Commission. (Level VII)

49 Ganz, D. A., et al. (2013, reviewed 2021). Preventing falls in hospitals: A toolkit for improving quality of care (AHRQ Publication No. 13-0015-EF). https://www.ahrq.gov/professionals/systems/hospital/fallpxtoolkit/index.html (Level VII)

50 Rutala, W. A., et al. (2008, revised 2019). Guideline for disinfection and sterilization in healthcare facilities, 2008. https://www.cdc.gov/infectioncontrol/pdf/guidelines/disinfection-guidelines-H.pdf (Level I)

51 Accreditation Association for Hospitals and Health Systems. (2020). Standard 07.02.03. *Healthcare Facilities Accreditation Program: Accreditation requirements for acute care hospitals.* Chicago, IL: Accreditation Association for Hospitals and Health Systems. (Level VII)

52 The Joint Commission. (2021). Standard RC.01.03.01. *Comprehensive accreditation manual for hospitals.* Oakbrook Terrace, IL: The Joint Commission. (Level VII)

53 Centers for Medicare and Medicaid Services, Department of Health and Human Services. (2020). Condition of participation: Medical record services. 42 C.F.R. § 482.24(b).

54 Accreditation Association for Hospitals and Health Systems. (2020). Standard 10.00.03. *Healthcare Facilities Accreditation Program: Accreditation requirements for acute care hospitals.* Chicago, IL: Accreditation Association for Hospitals and Health Systems. (Level VII)

55 DNV GL-Healthcare USA, Inc. (2020). MR.2.SR.1. *NIAHO® accreditation requirements, interpretive guidelines and surveyor guidance—revision 20.0.* Milford, OH: DNV GL-Healthcare USA, Inc. (Level VII)

56 Craven, H. (Ed.). (2016). *Core curriculum for medical-surgical nursing* (5th ed.). Pitman, NJ: Academy of Medical-Surgical Nurses.

57 Wainwright, T.W., et al. (2020). Consensus statement for perioperative care in total hip replacement and total knee replacement surgery: Enhanced Recovery After Surgery (ERAS) Society recommendations. *Acta Orthopaedica, 91*(1), 3–19. https://www.ncbi.nlm.nih.gov/pmc/articles/PMC7006728/ (Level VII)

58 The Joint Commission. (2017). Sentinel event alert, Issue 58: Inadequate hand-off communication. https://www.jointcommission.org/-/media/tjc/documents/resources/patient-safety-topics/sentinel-event/sea_58_hand_off_comms_9_6_17_final_(1).pdf?db=web&hash=5642D63C1A5017BD214701514DA00139

59 Erens, G. A., & Walter, B. (2020). Complications of total hip arthroplasty. In: *UpToDate,* Hunter, D. (Ed.)

60 Rothrock, J. C. (2019). *Alexander's care of the patient in surgery* (16th ed.). St. Louis, MO: Elsevier.

61 Gan, T. G. (2017). Poorly controlled postoperative pain: Prevalence, consequences and prevention. *Journal of Pain Research, 10,* 2287–2298. https://www.ncbi.nlm.nih.gov/pmc/articles/PMC5626380/ (Level I)

62 Weinhouse, G. L. (2019). Fat embolism syndrome. In: *UpToDate,* Parsons, P. E. (Ed.).

63 Shaikh, N. (2009). Emergency management of fat embolism syndrome. *Journal of Emergencies, Trauma, and Shock, 2*(1), 29–33. http://www.onlinejets.org/article.asp?issn=0974-2700%3Byear=2009%3Bvolume=2%3Bissue=1%3Bspage=29%3Bepage=33%3Baulast=Shaikh (Level V)

HOUR-OF-SLEEP CARE

Adequate sleep is essential for overall health, and that need increases when the patient is dealing with disease or injury.[1] Hour-of-sleep care meets the patient's physical and psychological needs in preparation for sleep. It includes providing for the patient's hygiene, making the bed clean and comfortable, and ensuring safety. For example, raising the bed's side rails can prevent the drowsy or sedated patient from falling out. This type of care also provides an opportunity to answer the patient's questions about the next day's tests and procedures and to discuss worries and concerns.

Effective hour-of-sleep care prepares the patient for a good night's sleep. Ineffective care may contribute to sleeplessness, which can intensify patient anxiety and interfere with treatment and recuperation. Promoting the patient's sleep in the challenging environment of a nursing unit dictates not only that you be sensitive to the patient's needs and attuned to the environment, but also that you have the tools and resources necessary to implement effective strategies. (See *Targeted interventions for sleep promotion,* page 400.)

Equipment

Bedpan, urinal, or commode ▪ basin (single use or disposable)[11,12] ▪ skin cleaner ▪ towel ▪ washcloth or prewarmed disposable bath wipes ▪ oral hygiene supplies ▪ lotion ▪ facial tissues ▪ Optional: gloves, earplugs, eye mask, white-noise machine, prescribed medications, clean linens, extra pillow, extra blanket, patient gown, labeled denture cup, commercial denture cleaner, container for water.

Preparation of equipment

Inspect all equipment and supplies. If a product is expired, is defective, or has compromised integrity, remove it from patient use, label it as expired or defective, and report the expiration or defect as directed by your facility.

Implementation

▪ Gather and prepare the necessary equipment and supplies.
▪ Perform hand hygiene[13,14,15,16,17,18] and put on gloves, if needed, *to comply with standard precautions.*[19,20,21]
▪ Confirm the patient's identity using at least two patient identifiers.[22]
▪ Provide privacy.[23,24,25,26]
▪ Explain the procedure to the patient and family (if appropriate) according to their individual communication and learning needs *to increase their understanding, allay their fears, and enhance cooperation.*[27]

Targeted interventions for sleep promotion

Consider the following interventions to promote sleep in your patients:

- Provide large clocks and calendars.
- Plan care to provide blocks of time for uninterrupted sleep, and cluster care as much as possible. Evaluate the need for care interruptions.[2,3,4]
- Establish a unit-wide designated quiet time.
- Have earplugs and an eye mask available.[5,6]
- Review the patient's sleep history and quality of sleep, if possible.
- Provide the opportunity to listen to music.[7,8]
- Provide a 5-minute back rub before sleep.
- Consider using white noise, such as the sound of rainfall or ocean waves.[9]
- If appropriate to your role, manage the patient's pain using prescribed pharmacologic and nonpharmacologic strategies.[3,10]
- Position the patient comfortably using pillows and other positioning devices.
- Avoid bathing the patient in the middle of the night, despite its possible convenience for the nursing staff.
- Reduce environmental stimuli by turning down lights, turning down alarms, and decreasing noise from television and talking.[10]
- At bedtime, provide information to lower anxiety. Review the day, and remind the patient of progress made toward recovery; then add what to expect for the next day.[1,10]
- Assist the patient with brushing the teeth and washing the face and hands before bedtime.
- Allow the family to remain with the patient, if necessary.[3]
- Use relaxation techniques and guided imagery.[10]
- Provide privacy by closing the patient's door or curtains.[1]
- Post a sign on the patient's door at designated times to indicate that the patient is sleeping.

- Raise the patient's bed to waist level before providing care *to prevent caregiver back strain.*[28]
- Offer a bedpan or urinal to a patient on bed rest. Alternatively, assist the ambulatory patient to the bathroom or commode.
- Fill the basin with warm water or use prewarmed disposable bath wipes, if available. Bring the basin or disposable bath wipes to the patient's bedside or use prewarmed disposable bath wipes, if available. Offer the skin cleaner and encourage the patient to bathe, if possible, *to promote independence.* Otherwise, wash the patient's face and hands and dry them thoroughly.
- Provide a toothbrush and toothpaste or a properly labeled denture cup and commercial denture cleaner. Assist the patient with oral hygiene as necessary. (See the "Oral care" procedure.) If the patient prefers to wear dentures until bedtime, leave denture care items within easy reach.
- After providing oral care, turn the patient onto the side or stomach. With the washcloth or prewarmed disposable bath wipe, wash and rinse the patient's back and buttocks and dry with the towel. Massage the patient's back with lotion *to help the patient relax.*
- While providing back care, observe the skin for redness, cracking, or other signs of breakdown; notify the appropriate team member if found. If the patient's gown is soiled or damp, provide a clean one and help the patient put it on, if necessary.
- Check dressings, binders, antiembolism stockings, or other aids, changing or readjusting them as needed.
- If the patient is allowed liquids, refill the water container and place it and a box of facial tissues within the patient's easy reach *to prevent falls in case the patient needs to reach for these items.*
- Straighten or change bed linens, as necessary, and fluff the patient's pillow. Clean linens are only needed if the linen is soiled. Cover the patient with a blanket or place one within easy reach *to prevent chills during the night.* Then position the patient comfortably.
- Offer the patient ear plugs, if appropriate and available, *to help block noise from the unit,* and an eye mask *if light bothers the patient.*[5,6,9]

- If the patient appears distressed, restless, or in pain, administer medications as needed and ordered following safe medication administration practices.[29,30,31,32]
- After making the patient comfortable, evaluate the patient's mental and physical condition.
- Return the bed to the lowest position and, if appropriate, raise the side rails *to prevent falls and maintain the patient's safety.*[33]
- Place the call light within the patient's easy reach, and instruct the patient to use it whenever necessary.
- Move all breakables from the overbed table out of the patient's reach, and remove any equipment and supplies that could cause a fall if the patient gets up during the night.
- Turn off the lights.[34]
- Decrease the volume of monitor and equipment alarms as medically appropriate.

NURSING ALERT Monitor alarms should be on, set appropriately, and audible to staff; volumes should never be decreased if contraindicated by the patient's clinical status.[35,36,37]

- Remove and discard your gloves, if worn.[19,21]
- Perform hand hygiene.[13,14,15,16,17,18]
- Close the patient's door if not contraindicated.
- Document the procedure.[38,39,40,41]

Special considerations

- Ask about the patient's sleep routine at home and, whenever possible, let the patient follow it while taking into consideration the patient's social and cultural background, *because sleep, while biological, can also be shaped by societal and cultural values and beliefs.*[1,42]
- Try to observe certain rituals, such as a bedtime snack, *which can aid sleep.* A back massage, a tub bath, or a shower can also help relax the patient and promote a restful night. If the patient normally bathes or showers before bedtime, encourage this activity if the patient's condition and the practitioner's orders permit it.[43]
- *Because of the nature of the intensive care unit,* provide periods of quiet time that coincide with circadian rhythms, as possible. *Efforts to reduce controllable noise and light at particular times throughout the day have been shown to contribute to patient sleep, even during day-shift hours.*[44,45,46]
- The Joint Commission issued a sentinel event alert concerning medical device alarm safety, *because alarm-related events have been associated with permanent loss of function or death.* Among the major contributing factors were improper alarm settings, alarm settings turned off inappropriately, and alarm signals not audible to staff. Make sure alarm limits are set appropriately, and that alarms are turned on, functioning properly, and audible to staff. Follow facility guidelines for preventing alarm fatigue.[37]

Documentation

Record the time and type of hour-of-sleep care in your notes. Note your skin assessment findings. Document any medications administered. Include use of any special procedures, such as relaxation techniques.

References

1 Gellerstedt, L., et al. (2014). Patients' experiences of sleep in hospital: A qualitative interview study. *Journal of Research in Nursing, 19,* 176–188. (Level VI)

2 Salzmann-Erikson, M., et al. (2016). Keep calm and have a good night: Nurses' strategies to promote inpatients' sleep in the hospital environment. *Scandinavian Journal of Caring Sciences, 30,* 356–364. (Level VI)

3 Hopper, K., et al. (2015). Health care worker attitudes and identified barriers to patient sleep in the medical intensive care unit. *Heart & Lung, 44,* 95–99. (Level VI)

4 Lopez, M., et al. (2018). Minimizing sleep disturbances to improve patient outcomes. *Medsurg Nursing, 27,* 368–371.

5 Litton, E., et al. (2016). The efficacy of earplugs as a sleep hygiene strategy for reducing delirium in the ICU: A systematic review and meta-analysis. *Critical Care Medicine, 44,* 992–999. (Level I)

6 Demoule, A., et al. (2017). Impact of earplugs and eye mask on sleep in critically ill patients: A prospective randomized study. *Critical Care, 21,* 284. https://ccforum.biomedcentral.com/articles/10.1186/s13054-017-1865-0 (Level II)

7 Shaw, R. (2016). Using music to promote sleep for hospitalized adults. *American Journal of Critical Care, 25*(2), 181–184. http://ajcc.aacnjournals.org/content/25/2/181 (Level I)

8 Wang, C. F., et al. (2014). Music therapy improves sleep quality in acute and chronic sleep disorders: A meta-analysis of 10 randomized studies. *International Journal of Nursing Studies, 51*(1), 51–62. (Level I)

9 Afshar, P. F., et al. (2016). Effect of white noise on sleep in patients admitted to a coronary care. *Journal of Caring Sciences, 5*(2), 103–109. https://www.ncbi.nlm.nih.gov/pmc/articles/PMC4923834/ (Level VI)

10 Tan, X., et al. (2019). A narrative review of interventions for improving sleep and reducing circadian disruption in medical inpatients. *Sleep Medicine, 59*, 42–50. https://www.sciencedirect.com/science/article/pii/S1389945718303149 (Level I)

11 Johnson, D., et al. (2009). Patients' bath basins as potential sources of infection: A multicenter sampling study. *American Journal of Critical Care, 18*(1), 31–40. http://ajcc.aacnjournals.org/content/18/1/31.full.pdf+html (Level IV)

12 Powers, J., et al. (2012). Chlorhexidine bathing and microbial contamination in patients' bath basins. *American Journal of Critical Care, 21*(5), 338–342. http://ajcc.aacnjournals.org/content/21/5/338.full (Level IV)

13 The Joint Commission. (2021). Standard NPSG.07.01.01. *Comprehensive accreditation manual for hospitals*. Oakbrook Terrace, IL: The Joint Commission. (Level VII)

14 Centers for Disease Control and Prevention. (2002). Guideline for hand hygiene in health-care settings: Recommendations of the Healthcare Infection Control Practices Advisory Committee and the HICPAC/SHEA/APIC/IDSA Hand Hygiene Task Force. *MMWR Recommendations and Reports, 51*(RR-16), 1–45. https://www.cdc.gov/mmwr/pdf/rr/rr5116.pdf (Level II)

15 World Health Organization. (2009). WHO guidelines on hand hygiene in health care: First global patient safety challenge, clean care is safer care. http://apps.who.int/iris/bitstream/10665/44102/1/9789241597906_eng.pdf (Level IV)

16 Accreditation Association for Hospitals and Health Systems. (2020). Standard 07.01.21. *Healthcare Facilities Accreditation Program: Accreditation requirements for acute care hospitals*. Chicago, IL: Accreditation Association for Hospitals and Health Systems. (Level VII)

17 Centers for Medicare and Medicaid Services, Department of Health and Human Services. (2020). Condition of participation: Infection control. 42 C.F.R. § 482.42.

18 DNV GL-Healthcare USA, Inc. (2020). IC.1.SR.1. *NIAHO® accreditation requirements, interpretive guidelines and surveyor guidance—revision 20.0*. Milford, OH: DNV GL-Healthcare USA, Inc. (Level VII)

19 Siegel, J. D., et al. (2007, revised 2019). 2007 guideline for isolation precautions: Preventing transmission of infectious agents in healthcare settings. https://www.cdc.gov/infectioncontrol/pdf/guidelines/isolation-guidelines-H.pdf (Level II)

20 Accreditation Association for Hospitals and Health Systems. (2020). Standard 07.01.10. *Healthcare Facilities Accreditation Program: Accreditation requirements for acute care hospitals*. Chicago, IL: Accreditation Association for Hospitals and Health Systems. (Level VII)

21 Occupational Safety and Health Administration. (2019). Bloodborne pathogens, standard number 1910.1030. https://www.osha.gov/pls/oshaweb/owadisp.show_document?p_id=10051&p_table=STANDARDS (Level VII)

22 The Joint Commission. (2021). Standard NPSG.01.01.01. *Comprehensive accreditation manual for hospitals*. Oakbrook Terrace, IL: The Joint Commission. (Level VII)

23 Centers for Medicare and Medicaid Services, Department of Health and Human Services. (2020). Condition of participation: Patient's rights. 42 C.F.R. § 482.13(c)(1).

24 Accreditation Association for Hospitals and Health Systems. (2020). Standard 15.01.16. *Healthcare Facilities Accreditation Program: Accreditation requirements for acute care hospitals*. Chicago, IL: Accreditation Association for Hospitals and Health Systems. (Level VII)

25 The Joint Commission. (2021). Standard RI.01.01.01. *Comprehensive accreditation manual for hospitals*. Oakbrook Terrace, IL: The Joint Commission. (Level VII)

26 DNV GL-Healthcare USA, Inc. (2020). PR.2.SR.5. *NIAHO® accreditation requirements, interpretive guidelines and surveyor guidance—revision 20.0*. Milford, OH: DNV GL-Healthcare USA, Inc. (Level VII)

27 The Joint Commission. (2021). Standard PC.02.01.21. *Comprehensive accreditation manual for hospitals*. Oakbrook Terrace, IL: The Joint Commission. (Level VII)

28 Waters, T. R., et al. (2009). Safe patient handling training for schools of nursing. https://www.cdc.gov/niosh/docs/2009-127/pdfs/2009-127.pdf (Level VII)

29 Accreditation Association for Hospitals and Health Systems. (2020). Standard 16.01.03. *Healthcare Facilities Accreditation Program: Accreditation requirements for acute care hospitals*. Chicago, IL: Accreditation Association for Hospitals and Health Systems. (Level VII)

30 Centers for Medicare and Medicaid Services, Department of Health and Human Services. (2020). Condition of participation: Nursing services. 42 C.F.R. § 482.23(c).

31 The Joint Commission. (2021). Standard MM.06.01.01. *Comprehensive accreditation manual for hospitals*. Oakbrook Terrace, IL: The Joint Commission. (Level VII)

32 DNV GL-Healthcare USA, Inc. (2020). MM.1.SR.3. *NIAHO® accreditation requirements, interpretive guidelines and surveyor guidance—revision 20.0*. Milford, OH: DNV GL-Healthcare USA, Inc. (Level VII)

33 Ganz, D. A., et al. (2013, reviewed 2021). *Preventing falls in hospitals: A toolkit for improving quality of care* (AHRQ Publication No. 13-0015-EF). Rockville, MD: Agency for Healthcare Research and Quality. https://www.ahrq.gov/professionals/systems/hospital/fallpxtoolkit/index.html (Level VII)

34 Thomas, K. P., et al. (2012). Sleep rounds: A multidisciplinary approach to optimize sleep quality and satisfaction in hospitalized patients. *Journal of Hospital Medicine, 7*, 508–512. (Level IV)

35 The Joint Commission. (2021). Standard NPSG.06.01.01. *Comprehensive accreditation manual for hospitals*. Oakbrook Terrace, IL: The Joint Commission. (Level VII)

36 American Association of Critical-Care Nurses. (2018). AACN practice alert: Managing alarms in acute care across the life span: Electrocardiography and pulse oximetry. https://www.aacn.org/clinical-resources/practice-alerts/managing-alarms-in-acute-care-across-the-life-span (Level VII)

37 The Joint Commission. (2013). Sentinel event alert 50: Medical device alarm safety in hospitals. https://www.jointcommission.org/assets/1/6/SEA_50_alarms_4_26_16.pdf (Level VII)

38 The Joint Commission. (2021). Standard RC.01.03.01. *Comprehensive accreditation manual for hospitals*. Oakbrook Terrace, IL: The Joint Commission. (Level VII)

39 Accreditation Association for Hospitals and Health Systems. (2020). Standard 10.00.03. *Healthcare Facilities Accreditation Program: Accreditation requirements for acute care hospitals*. Chicago, IL: Accreditation Association for Hospitals and Health Systems. (Level VII)

40 Centers for Medicare and Medicaid Services, Department of Health and Human Services. (2020). Condition of participation: Medical record services. 42 C.F.R. § 482.24(b).

41 DNV GL-Healthcare USA, Inc. (2020). MR.2.SR.1. *NIAHO® accreditation requirements, interpretive guidelines and surveyor guidance—revision 20.0*. Milford, OH: DNV GL-Healthcare USA, Inc. (Level VII)

42 Williams, N. J., et al. (2015). Racial/ethnic disparities in sleep health and health care: Importance of the sociocultural context. *Sleep Health, 1*, 28–35.

43 American Alliance for Healthy Sleep. (2020). Healthy sleep habits. http://sleepeducation.org/essentials-in-sleep/healthy-sleep-habits

44 Hedges, C., et al. (2019). Quiet time improves the patient experience. *Journal of Nursing Care Quality, 34*(3), 197–202. https://journals.lww.com/jncqjournal/Abstract/2019/07000/Quiet_Time_Improves_the_Patient_Experience.4.aspx (Level VI)

45 Applebaum, D., et al. (2016). Implementation of quiet time for noise reduction on a medical-surgical unit. *Journal of Nursing Administration, 46*, 669–674.

46 Wilson, C., et al. (2017). Improving the patient's experience with a multimodal quiet-at-night initiative. *Journal of Nursing Care Quality, 32*(2), 134–140. https://journals.lww.com/jncqjournal/Abstract/2017/04000/Improving_the_Patient_s_Experience_With_a.8.aspx

HUMIDIFIER THERAPY

Humidifiers add molecules of water to gas. They can add moisture to room air or inhaled medical gases in an active or passive manner, sometimes using heat. Active humidifiers work by adding additional heat, water, or both. Passive humidifiers reuse the exhaled heat and water from the patient.[1]

Humidification is indicated for any patient receiving medical gases, such as oxygen, to reduce heat and water loss and help maintain the normal function of the mucociliary transport system. In addition, humidifier therapy is indicated for any patient for whom the upper airway is bypassed, such as one who is breathing with an endotracheal or tracheostomy tube. Humidification can also be used to treat bronchospasm caused by inhaling cold air or by exercising. Humidifiers help soothe irritated and inflamed airways in conditions such as croup, epiglottitis, and postextubation stridor. They can also help loosen thick, tenacious secretions. Heated humidification can also be used in treating or preventing hypothermia. No contraindications exist to humidifier therapy in patients with an artificial airway; however, the use of a heat and moisture exchanger, which is a passive humidifier, is contraindicated in certain patients.[1]

Multiple types of humidifiers are available. Unheated active bubble humidifiers are most often used with oxygen delivery devices that use diffusion; this type of humidifier works by breaking underwater gas streams into small bubbles. Active bubble humidifiers incorporate a pop-off valve that releases pressure to warn of obstruction and prevent the system from bursting. Heating the water can increase the humidity level; however, this is not recommended, *because condensation that forms as the air cools can obstruct the oxygen tubing.*[1] Active heated bubble humidifier devices are no longer used for patients with an artificial airway.[2] With a pass-over type of humidifier, air flows over water and gains humidity from the interface of the gas and water. This type of humidifier is used in-line for a patient receiving mechanical ventilation. The ventilator circuit is directly connected to the humidifier; excess water can condense in the ventilator tubing, requiring water traps or reservoirs in the circuit.[2] For invasive mechanical ventilation, the water is usually heated to add heat to the air as well. For noninvasive mechanical ventilation, heated or room-temperature water may be used.[1]

A bedside humidifier uses a spinning disk or ultrasonic vibration to produce a cool mist. A vaporizer heats the water to create steam and release mist into the air. Vaporizers can cause burns if the water is spilled. Bedside humidifiers and vaporizers can harbor bacteria and mold if not cleaned properly.[3]

Passive humidification is usually delivered to a patient with an artificial airway using a device called a heat and moisture exchanger (HME). This device is sometimes described as an "artificial nose."[1] HMEs can be used in a patient with an endotracheal or tracheostomy tube who may be receiving mechanical ventilation or breathing spontaneously.[1]

Equipment

Appropriate humidifier or HME ▪ sterile water (for bubble, active pass-over, and bedside)[3] or commercially prepared disposable unit ▪ gloves[4] ▪ thermometer with audible alarm (for active pass-over humidifier).

Preparation of equipment

Inspect all equipment and supplies. If a product is expired, is defective, or has compromised integrity, remove it from patient use, label it as expired or defective, and report the expiration or defect as directed by your facility.

For a bedside humidifier

Open the reservoir, add sterile water to the fill line, and then close the reservoir. Do not allow the humidifier to run unattended in a closed room, *because the air may become saturated and leave condensation on the walls and furniture.* Leave the door partially open or follow the manufacturer's recommendations.

For an active bubble humidifier

Unscrew the humidifier reservoir and add sterile water to the appropriate level. If you're using a disposable unit, screw the cap with the extension onto the top of the unit. Then screw the reservoir back onto the humidifier and attach the flowmeter to the oxygen source.

Screw the humidifier onto the flowmeter until the seal is tight. Then set the flowmeter at a rate of 2 L/minute and check for gentle bubbling, *which indicates that the flowmeter is working properly.* Next, check the positive-pressure release valve by occluding the end valve on the humidifier; the pressure should back up into the humidifier, signaled by a high-pitched whistle. If this whistle doesn't occur, tighten all connections and try again.[1] Make sure that the device is set up and functioning properly.

For an active pass-over humidifier

Install the humidifier in the ventilator circuit according to the manufacturer's instructions. Add sterile water to the fill line. Then screw the top back onto the reservoir. For routine use on an intubated patient, plug in the heater unit and set the gas temperature to between 93.2° F (34° C) and 105.8° F (41° C) at the circuit Y-piece.[5] Use an audible temperature alarm, as recommended and applicable. Set the high-temperature alarm no higher than 105.8° F (41° C), with a 109.4° F (43° C) over-temperature limit; set the low-temperature alarm no lower than 35.6° F (2° C) below the desired temperature at the circuit Y-piece. Test the device and alarm periodically for proper functioning.[5] Make sure that alarm limits are set appropriately for the patient's current condition, and that alarms are turned on, functioning properly, and audible to staff.[6,7,8]

Implementation

- Verify the practitioner's order.
- Gather and prepare the necessary equipment and supplies.
- Perform hand hygiene.[9,10,11,12,13,14]
- Confirm the patient's identity using at least two patient identifiers.[15]
- Provide privacy.[16,17,18,19]
- Explain the procedure to the patient and family (if appropriate) according to their individual communication and learning needs *to increase their understanding, allay their fears, and enhance cooperation.*[20]
- Put on gloves, if needed, *to comply with standard precautions.*[21,22,23]

Bedside humidifier

- Place the humidifier on a firm, flat, and waterproof surface. Place the humidifier a safe distance from the patient and away from the wall according to the manufacturer's recommendations. Plug the humidifier into an electrical outlet and then turn on the unit. Make sure the device is functioning properly.

NURSING ALERT Position the cord out of the way *to prevent it from becoming a fall hazard.*

- Check for a fine mist emission from the nozzle, *which indicates proper operation.*
- Direct the humidifier unit's nozzle toward the patient but away from the patient's face *for effective treatment.*
- Check the unit frequently for proper operation and water level.
- Clean and refill the unit daily and as needed *to reduce the risk of bacterial growth.* Unplug the unit and discard the old water. Clean and disinfect the unit using sterilization or high-level disinfection according to the manufacturer's instructions.[4,24,25]

NURSING ALERT To prevent health care–associated Legionnaires disease, room air humidifiers that use a spinning disk or ultrasonic vibration should not be used unless they can undergo sterilization or high-level disinfection at least daily.[4]

Active pass-over humidifier

- Assess the temperature of the inspired gas near the patient's airway every 2 hours or as determined by your facility. If the humidifier becomes too hot, check the heater unit and reset, or replace the unit as necessary, *because overheated water vapor can cause respiratory tract burns.*
- Check the reservoir's water level frequently and refill it as necessary.[2,5]
- Frequently check for condensation buildup in the tubing.[2]
- Empty the condensate in the tubing as necessary *so it can't drain into the patient's respiratory tract, encourage growth of microorganisms, or obstruct dependent sections of tubing.* Follow the manufacturer's recommendations for removing condensation from the patient circuit. Don't drain the condensate back into the humidifier, *because condensate is infectious waste.*[4,5]
- Assess the quantity and consistency of the patient's secretions *to evaluate the effectiveness of treatment.*[5]

Active bubble humidifier

- Attach the oxygen delivery device to the humidifier and then to the patient. Adjust the flowmeter to the appropriate oxygen flow rate and look for a gentle bubbling.
- If appropriate, add a drainage bag to the low point of the tubing *to prevent condensate from accumulating in the tubing.*

■ Check the reservoir every 4 hours or as directed by your facility. If the water level drops too low, empty the remaining water, rinse the reservoir, and refill it with sterile water. Alternately, replace a commercially prepared disposable unit at its low water mark. *As the reservoir water level decreases, the evaporation of water in the gas decreases, reducing humidification of the delivered gas.*[2]

■ Assess the patient's sputum periodically; *sputum that's too thick can hinder mobilization and expectoration.* If thick sputum occurs, the patient requires a device that can provide higher humidity.

Heat and moisture exchanger

■ Place the HME in the circuit before the "Y" *so that the device contacts inspired and expired air during each cycle.*[2] Connect the HME directly to the airway in a patient who isn't mechanically ventilated.

■ Assess the quantity and consistency of respiratory secretions. Report copious and tenacious secretions to the practitioner.[5]

Completing the procedure

■ Remove and discard your gloves, if worn.[21,23]
■ Perform hand hygiene.[9,10,11,12,13,14]
■ Document the procedure.[26,27,28,29]

Special considerations

■ Change the humidifier tubing, oxygen delivery device, or ventilator circuit when it malfunctions or becomes visibly contaminated.[4,5]

■ Follow the manufacturer's instructions for the humidifier model you are using.

■ Ensure that the tubing is draining water away from the artificial airway and that water traps are placed correctly. Never fill above the recommended level or drain water toward the humidification chamber.[2]

■ The Joint Commission issued a sentinel event alert concerning medical device alarm safety, *because alarm-related events have been associated with permanent loss of function or death.* Among the major contributing factors were improper alarm settings, alarm settings turned off inappropriately, and alarm signals not audible to staff. Make sure that alarm limits are set appropriately, and that alarms are turned on, functioning properly, and audible to staff. Follow facility guidelines for preventing alarm fatigue.[6]

■ HME performance and specifications can vary among brands. Performance standards are set by the International Organization for Standardization (ISO). HMEs should ideally operate efficiently, have standard connections, have low compliance, and add minimal weight, dead space, and flow resistance.[1]

■ Compared with active humidification systems, HMEs reduce bacterial colonization in the ventilator circuit by eliminating condensation in the circuit.[1]

■ HMEs don't require daily changing; you can use them safely for 48 hours. You may be able to use some devices for up to 1 week.[5] Follow the manufacturer's recommendations for changing intervals or change the HME when it's visibly soiled or impacted with secretions.[2]

Patient teaching

If the patient will use the humidifier at home, teach the patient and family (if appropriate) how to use the equipment and give them specific written guidelines about all aspects of home care. Have them teach back what they have learned to evaluate their comprehension.

Complications

Improper care and maintenance of humidifiers may cause infection, such as pneumonia or Legionnaires disease and mold growth, which may aggravate respiratory problems, especially in people who are allergic to molds.[4,30] Water accumulation in the ventilator tubing can lead to auto-triggering, misreading of ventilator parameters, or drainage of contaminated water into the patient's airway.[2] Pass-over humidifiers have the potential to deliver an electrical shock, cause hypothermia or hyperthermia, and cause thermal airway injury if the temperature is not set and monitored appropriately. Burns to the patient or the caregiver can occur if the equipment is not monitored correctly. Risk of increased work of breathing exists due to potential increase in dead space or from mucus plugging caused by inadequate humidification levels.[5] Vaporizers contain hot water and are a risk for burns if the water is spilled.[3]

Documentation

Record the date and time when humidification began and was discontinued, the type of humidifier used, and the patient's response to humidification. Document any complications, the name of the practitioner notified, the date and time of notification, prescribed interventions, and the patient's response to these interventions. Document teaching provided to the patient and family (if appropriate), their understanding of that teaching, and any need for follow-up teaching.

REFERENCES

1 Kacmarek, R. M., et al. (2021). *Egan's fundamentals of respiratory care* (12th ed.). St. Louis, MO: Mosby.

2 Plotnikow, G. A., et al. (2018). Humidification and heating of inhaled gas in patients with artificial airway: A narrative review. *Revista Brasileira de Terapia Intensiva, 30*(1), 86–97. https://www.ncbi.nlm.nih.gov/pmc/articles/PMC5885236/pdf/rbti-30-01-0086.pdf (Level V)

3 Mayo Clinic Staff. (2021). Humidifiers: Ease skin, breathing symptoms. https://www.mayoclinic.org/diseases-conditions/common-cold/in-depth/humidifiers/art-20048021

4 Centers for Disease Control and Prevention. (2004). Guidelines for preventing health-care-associated pneumonia, 2003: Recommendations of CDC and the Healthcare Infection Control Practices Advisory Committee. *MMWR Recommendations and Reports, 53*(RR-3), 1–32. https://www.cdc.gov/mmwr/pdf/rr/rr5303.pdf (Level II)

5 Restrepo, R. D., & Walsh, B. K. (2012). AARC clinical practice guideline: Humidification during invasive and noninvasive mechanical ventilation: 2012. *Respiratory Care, 57*(5), 782–788. https://www.aarc.org/wp-content/uploads/2014/08/12.05.0782.pdf (Level VII)

6 The Joint Commission. (2013). Sentinel event alert 50: Medical device alarm safety in hospitals. https://www.jointcommission.org/assets/1/6/SEA_50_alarms_4_26_16.pdf (Level VII)

7 The Joint Commission. (2021). Standard NPSG.06.01.01. *Comprehensive accreditation manual for hospitals.* Oakbrook Terrace, IL: The Joint Commission. (Level VII)

8 Graham, K. C., & Cvach, M. (2010). Monitor alarm fatigue. Standardizing use of physiological monitors and decreasing nuisance alarms. *American Journal of Critical Care, 19*, 28–37.

9 The Joint Commission. (2021). Standard NPSG.07.01.01. *Comprehensive accreditation manual for hospitals.* Oakbrook Terrace, IL: The Joint Commission. (Level VII)

10 Centers for Disease Control and Prevention. (2002). Guideline for hand hygiene in health-care settings: Recommendations of the Healthcare Infection Control Practices Advisory Committee and the HICPAC/SHEA/APIC/IDSA Hand Hygiene Task Force. *MMWR Recommendations and Reports, 51*(RR-16), 1–45. https://www.cdc.gov/mmwr/pdf/rr/rr5116.pdf (Level II)

11 World Health Organization. (2009). WHO guidelines on hand hygiene in health care: First global patient safety challenge, clean care is safer care. https://apps.who.int/iris/bitstream/handle/10665/44102/9789241597906_eng.pdf?sequence=1 (Level IV)

12 Accreditation Association for Hospitals and Health Systems. (2020). Standard 07.01.21. *Healthcare Facilities Accreditation Program: Accreditation requirements for acute care hospitals.* Chicago, IL: Accreditation Association for Hospitals and Health Systems. (Level VII)

13 Centers for Medicare and Medicaid Services, Department of Health and Human Services. (2020). Condition of participation: Infection control. 42 C.F.R. § 482.42.

14 DNV GL-Healthcare USA, Inc. (2020). IC.1.SR.1. *NIAHO® accreditation requirements, interpretive guidelines and surveyor guidance—revision 20.0.* Milford, OH: DNV GL-Healthcare USA, Inc. (Level VII)

15 The Joint Commission. (2021). Standard NPSG.01.01.01. *Comprehensive accreditation manual for hospitals.* Oakbrook Terrace, IL: The Joint Commission. (Level VII)

16 The Joint Commission. (2021). Standard RI.01.01.01. *Comprehensive accreditation manual for hospitals.* Oakbrook Terrace, IL: The Joint Commission. (Level VII)

17 Centers for Medicare and Medicaid Services, Department of Health and Human Services. (2020). Condition of participation: Patient's rights. 42 C.F.R. § 482.13(c)(1).

18 Accreditation Association for Hospitals and Health Systems. (2020). Standard 15.01.16. *Healthcare Facilities Accreditation Program: Accreditation requirements for acute care hospitals.* Chicago, IL: Accreditation Association for Hospitals and Health Systems. (Level VII)

19 DNV GL-Healthcare USA, Inc. (2020). PR.2.SR.5. *NIAHO® accreditation requirements, interpretive guidelines and surveyor guidance—revision 20.0.* Milford, OH: DNV GL-Healthcare USA, Inc. (Level VII)

20 The Joint Commission. (2021). Standard PC.02.01.21. *Comprehensive accreditation manual for hospitals.* Oakbrook Terrace, IL: The Joint Commission. (Level VII)

21 Siegel, J. D., et al. (2007, revised 2019). 2007 guideline for isolation precautions: Preventing transmission of infectious agents in healthcare settings. https://www.cdc.gov/infectioncontrol/pdf/guidelines/isolation-guidelines-H.pdf (Level II)

22 Accreditation Association for Hospitals and Health Systems. (2020). Standard 07.01.10. *Healthcare Facilities Accreditation Program: Accreditation requirements for acute care hospitals.* Chicago, IL: Accreditation Association for Hospitals and Health Systems. (Level VII)

23 Occupational Safety and Health Administration. (2019). Bloodborne pathogens, standard number 1910.1030. https://www.osha.gov/pls/oshaweb/owadisp.show_document?p_id=10051&p_table=STANDARDS (Level VII)

24 Accreditation Association for Hospitals and Health Systems. (2020). Standard 07.02.03. *Healthcare Facilities Accreditation Program: Accreditation requirements for acute care hospitals.* Chicago, IL: Accreditation Association for Hospitals and Health Systems. (Level VII)

25 Public Health Agency of Canada. (2019). Legionella. https://www.canada.ca/en/public-health/services/infectious-diseases/legionella.html (Level VII)

26 The Joint Commission. (2021). Standard RC.01.03.01. *Comprehensive accreditation manual for hospitals.* Oakbrook Terrace, IL: The Joint Commission. (Level VII)

27 Accreditation Association for Hospitals and Health Systems. (2020). Standard 10.00.03. *Healthcare Facilities Accreditation Program: Accreditation requirements for acute care hospitals.* Chicago, IL: Accreditation Association for Hospitals and Health Systems. (Level VII)

28 Centers for Medicare and Medicaid Services, Department of Health and Human Services. (2020). Condition of participation: Medical record services. 42 C.F.R. § 482.24(b).

29 DNV GL-Healthcare USA, Inc. (2020). MR.2.SR.1. *NIAHO® accreditation requirements, interpretive guidelines and surveyor guidance—revision 20.0* Milford, OH: DNV GL-Healthcare USA, Inc. (Level VII)

30 Miller, R. L. (2020). Patient education: Trigger avoidance in asthma (beyond the basics). In: *UpToDate,* Bochner, B. S. (Ed.).

Hyperthermia–hypothermia blanket use

A hyperthermia-hypothermia blanket raises, lowers, or maintains body temperature through conductive heat or cold transfer between the blanket and the patient.[1] It can be operated manually or automatically.

In manual operation, a nurse or the practitioner sets the temperature on the unit. The blanket reaches and maintains this temperature regardless of the patient's temperature. The temperature setting must be adjusted manually to reach a different setting. The patient's body temperature is monitored with a conventional thermometer, or with a bladder thermometer if the patient has an indwelling urinary catheter with a temperature transducer.[2]

In automatic operation, the unit directly and continually monitors the patient's temperature by means of a thermistor probe (rectal, esophageal, or nasopharyngeal), and alternates heating and cooling cycles as necessary to achieve and maintain the desired body temperature.[1] The thermistor probe also may be used in conjunction with manual operation but isn't essential. The unit is equipped with an alarm to warn of abnormal temperature fluctuations and a circuit breaker that protects against current overload.

The blanket is used most commonly to reduce high fever when more conservative measures, such as baths, ice packs, and antipyretics, have been unsuccessful. Its other uses include maintaining normothermia during surgery or shock;[2] managing targeted temperature during surgery or after cardiac arrest to decrease metabolic activity and thereby reduce oxygen requirements; reducing intracranial pressure; controlling bleeding and intractable pain in patients with amputations, burns, or cancer; and providing warmth in cases of mild to moderate hypothermia.[3]

Equipment

Hyperthermia-hypothermia control unit ▪ distilled water ▪ thermistor probe (rectal, esophageal, or nasopharyngeal) ▪ water-soluble lubricant ▪ one or two hyperthermia-hypothermia blankets ▪ one or two disposable blanket covers (or one or two sheets or bath blankets) ▪ adhesive tape ▪ vital signs monitoring equipment ▪ stethoscope ▪ disinfectant pads ▪ pillow ▪ Optional: gloves, hospital gown (with cloth ties, if possible), cardiac monitoring equipment, protective wraps for the patient's hands and feet, prescribed sedation, prescribed analgesia.

Disposable hyperthermia-hypothermia blankets are available for single-patient use.

Preparation of equipment

First, read the operation manual. Inspect all equipment and supplies. If a product is expired, is defective, or has compromised integrity, remove it from patient use, label it as expired or defective, and report the expiration or defect as directed by your facility.

Connect the blanket to the control unit, and set the controls for manual or automatic operation and for the desired blanket or body temperature. Make sure the machine is properly grounded before plugging it in. Turn on the machine and add the distilled water to the unit reservoir, if necessary, to fill the blanket.[1] Allow the blanket to preheat or precool *so that the patient receives immediate thermal benefit.*

Implementation

▪ Verify the practitioner's order.
▪ Gather and prepare the necessary equipment and supplies.
▪ If required by your facility, confirm that informed consent has been obtained and that the signed consent form is in the patient's medical record.[1,4,5,6,7]
▪ Perform hand hygiene.[8,9,10,11,12,13]
▪ Confirm the patient's identity using at least two patient identifiers.[14]
▪ Provide privacy.[15,16,17,18]
▪ Make sure the room is warm and free from drafts if using the blanket to warm the patient, *to prevent heat loss through convection.*
▪ Make sure that the patient is properly dressed for the type of system being used. If the patient will be receiving therapy with a water-based system and isn't already wearing a hospital gown, ask the patient to put one on (if able), or put one on the patient, as appropriate. Use a gown with cloth ties rather than metal snaps or pins *to prevent heat or cold injury.* If the patient is wearing a gown and receiving therapy with an air-based system, help the patient remove the gown.[1]
▪ Explain the procedure to the patient and family (if appropriate) according to their individual communication and learning needs *to increase their understanding, allay their fears, and enhance cooperation.*[19]
▪ Raise the bed to waist level before providing care *to prevent caregiver back strain.*[20]
▪ Perform hand hygiene.[8,9,10,11,12,13]
▪ Put on gloves, as needed, *to comply with standard precautions.*[21,22,23]
▪ If ordered, attach the patient to a cardiac monitor for continuous monitoring *to observe for cardiac arrhythmias.*[1] Make sure that alarm limits are set appropriately for the patient's current condition, and that alarms are turned on, functioning properly, and audible to staff.[24,25,26,27] (See the "Cardiac monitoring" procedure.)
▪ Obtain the patient's vital signs and assess cardiac rhythm, respiratory status, level of consciousness, neurologic status, and skin condition *to serve as baselines for comparison.*[1]
▪ Administer sedation, analgesia, or both, as ordered, following safe medication administration practices.[28,29,30,31]
▪ If you're using a water-based system, position the patient on the blanket. Keeping the bottom sheet in place and the patient recumbent, roll the patient to one side and slide the blanket halfway underneath so that its top edge aligns with the patient's neck. Roll the patient back and pull and flatten the blanket across the bed. Place a pillow under the patient's head. Use a disposable cover, sheet, or bath blanket as insulation between the patient and the blanket if using a water-based system *to absorb perspiration and condensation, which can cause tissue breakdown if left on the skin.* (See *Types of hyperthermia–hypothermia systems.*)

EQUIPMENT

Types of hyperthermia–hypothermia systems

There are two main types of hyperthermia-hypothermia systems: water-based and air-based.

Water-based system

A water-based hyperthermia-hypothermia system pumps warmed or cooled water through circulating coils in the blanket to modify the patient's temperature through conduction. While the blanket is in use, you must monitor the patient's temperature. The blanket's temperature can be adjusted to help keep the patient's temperature in the ordered range.

Air-based system

Like a large hair dryer, the warming unit draws air through a filter, warms or cools the air to the desired temperature, and circulates it through a hose to a blanket placed over the patient. When using an air-based system, be sure to place the blanket directly over the patient with the paper side facing down and the clear tubular side facing up. The patient shouldn't be wearing a gown. Make sure the connection hose is at the foot of the bed.

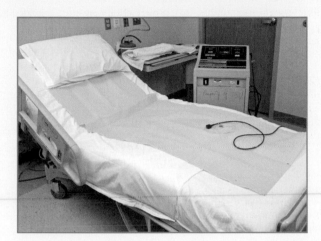

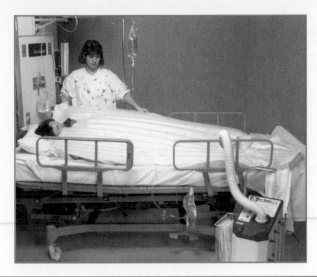

■ Alternatively, if you're using an air-based system, place the blanket directly over the patient according to the manufacturer's instructions.[1]

■ If you're using an automatic system, insert the thermistor probe in the patient's rectum using a water-soluble lubricant *to ease insertion* and tape it in place *to prevent accidental dislodgment*. If rectal insertion is contraindicated, an alternate site of temperature monitoring may be needed, such as the esophagus or nasopharynx. Verify the thermistor probe temperature measurement by comparing it to the patient's temperature obtained through another method *to ensure accuracy*.[1]

■ Remove and discard your gloves, if worn,[23] perform hand hygiene,[8,9,10,11,12,13] and plug the other end of the probe into the correct jack on the unit's control panel, if applicable.

■ Place a sheet or, if ordered, the second hyperthermia-hypothermia blanket over the patient *to increase the thermal benefit by trapping cooled or heated air or to keep the air-blanket in place*.[1]

■ If you are using the blanket to warm the patient, wrap hands and feet *to promote comfort.*

■ Monitor the patient's vital signs, cardiac rhythm, respiratory status, neurologic status, and skin integrity at regular intervals, as indicated by the patient's condition, the device manufacturer's instructions, and the practitioner's order.[1]

■ *To prevent pressure injuries*, reposition the patient at an interval determined by the patient's tissue tolerance, level of activity and mobility, skin condition, overall medical condition, treatment goals, support surface in use (if applicable), and comfort.[32] Keep the patient's skin, bedclothes, and blanket cover free of perspiration and condensation.[33]

HOSPITAL-ACQUIRED CONDITION ALERT Keep in mind that the Centers for Medicare and Medicaid Services considers a stage 3 or stage 4 pressure injury a hospital-acquired condition, *because various best practices can reasonably prevent it.* Be sure to follow evidence-based pressure injury prevention practices, such as assessing skin integrity, managing moisture, and repositioning the patient *to reduce the risk of pressure injury.*[32,33,34]

Discontinuing hyperthermia-hypothermia blanket use

■ When target temperature has been maintained for the prescribed period and the patient's condition warrants it, discontinue the hyperthermia-hypothermia blanket, as ordered. If the blanket was ordered for targeted temperature management, rewarm the patient slowly (maximum rate of 0.45° F [0.25° C] per hour).[35]

■ After turning off the machine, follow the manufacturer's directions for discontinuing use of the equipment. *Some units must remain plugged in for at least 30 minutes to allow the condenser fan to remove water vapor from the mechanism.* Continue to monitor the patient's temperature until it stabilizes, *because body temperature can drift up or down after discontinuation.*[1]

■ Remove all equipment from the bed. Discard used supplies in the appropriate receptacles.[23]

■ Dry off the patient and make the patient comfortable. Supply a fresh hospital gown, if necessary. Cover the patient as appropriate for the involved condition.

■ Return the bed to the lowest position *to prevent falls and maintain patient safety.*[36]

■ Continue to monitor the patient's vital signs and condition regularly, as indicated.

Completing the procedure

■ Perform hand hygiene.[8,9,10,11,12,13]

■ Clean and disinfect your stethoscope with a disinfectant pad.[37,38]

■ Perform hand hygiene.[8,9,10,11,12,13]

■ Put on gloves, if needed.[21,23]

■ Clean and disinfect other reusable equipment according to the manufacturer's instructions *to prevent the spread of infection.*[37,38]

■ Remove and discard your gloves, if worn.[23]

■ Perform hand hygiene.[8,9,10,11,12,13]

■ Document the procedure.[39,40,41,42]

Special considerations

■ If the patient experiences shivering during targeted temperature management, notify the practitioner immediately. *Sedation and neuromuscular blockade may be necessary to control shivering, because shivering elevates body temperature, increases metabolism, increases oxygen consumption, and negates the effects of targeted temperature management.*[43,44]

■ With hyperthermia or hypothermia therapy, the patient may experience a secondary defense reaction (vasoconstriction or vasodilation, respectively) that causes body temperature to rebound, negating the treatment's purpose.

■ Don't use pins to secure catheters, tubes, or blanket covers, *because an accidental puncture can result in fluid leakage and burns.*

■ After use, if the patient requires transmission-based isolation precautions, place the blanket, blanket cover, and probe in a plastic bag clearly marked with the type of isolation precautions *so that the central supply department can give it special handling.* If the blanket is disposable, discard it, following appropriate precautions.[21]

■ The Joint Commission has issued a sentinel event alert concerning medical device alarm safety, *because alarm-related events have been associated with permanent loss of function and death.* Among the major contributing factors are improper alarm settings, alarms turned off inappropriately, and alarm signals not audible to staff. Make sure that alarm limits are set appropriately, and that alarms are turned on, functioning properly, and audible to staff. Follow facility guidelines for preventing alarm fatigue.[27]

Complications

Use of a hyperthermia-hypothermia blanket can cause marked changes in vital signs, increased intracranial pressure, respiratory distress or arrest, and cardiac arrest. Hyperglycemia, hypokalemia, arrhythmias, hypotension, impaired coagulation, and infection have been reported as common adverse events associated with targeted temperature management after cardiac arrest.[43,45]

Documentation

Document the type of hyperthermia-hypothermia unit used, the control settings (manual or automatic mode and temperature setting), and the time, date, and duration of treatment. Record the patient's vital signs, including the temperature and the site of temperature assessment,[1,2] cardiac rhythm, respiratory status, level of consciousness, neurologic status, and skin assessment. Note the patient's tolerance of the treatment, any unexpected outcomes, any prescribed interventions, and the patient's response to those interventions. Document teaching provided to the patient and family (if applicable), their understanding of that teaching, and any need for follow-up teaching.

REFERENCES

1 Wiegand, D. L. (2017). *AACN procedure manual for high acuity, progressive, and critical care* (7th ed.). St. Louis, MO: Elsevier.

2 Guideline for the prevention of hypothermia. (2020). In Wood, A. (Ed.), *Guidelines for perioperative practice*, 2020 edition. Denver, CO: AORN, Inc. (Level VII)

3 Mathiesen, C., et al. (2015). Caring for patients treated with therapeutic hypothermia. *Critical Care Nurse, 35*(5), e1–e12. (Level VI)

4 The Joint Commission. (2021). Standard RI.01.03.01. *Comprehensive accreditation manual for hospitals.* Oakbrook Terrace, IL: The Joint Commission. (Level VII)

5 Accreditation Association for Hospitals and Health Systems. (2020). Standard 15.01.11. *Healthcare Facilities Accreditation Program: Accreditation requirements for acute care hospitals.* Chicago, IL: Accreditation Association for Hospitals and Health Systems. (Level VII)

6 DNV GL-Healthcare USA, Inc. (2020). PR.2.SR.3. *NIAHO® accreditation requirements, interpretive guidelines and surveyor guidance—revision 20.0.* Milford, OH: DNV GL-Healthcare USA, Inc. (Level VII)

7 Centers for Medicare and Medicaid Services, Department of Health and Human Services. (2020). Condition of participation: Patient's rights. 42 C.F.R. § 482.13(b)(2)

8 The Joint Commission. (2021). Standard NPSG.07.01.01. *Comprehensive accreditation manual for hospitals.* Oakbrook Terrace, IL: The Joint Commission. (Level VII)

9 Centers for Disease Control and Prevention. (2002). Guideline for hand hygiene in health-care settings: Recommendations of the Healthcare Infection Control Practices Advisory Committee and the HICPAC/SHEA/APIC/IDSA Hand Hygiene Task Force. *MMWR Recommendations and Reports, 51*(RR-16), 1–45. https://www.cdc.gov/mmwr/pdf/rr/rr5116.pdf (Level II)

10 World Health Organization. (2009). WHO guidelines on hand hygiene in health care: First global patient safety challenge, clean care is safer care. https://apps.who.int/iris/bitstream/handle/10665/44102/9789241597906_eng.pdf?sequence=1 (Level IV)

11 Accreditation Association for Hospitals and Health Systems. (2020). Standard 07.01.21. *Healthcare Facilities Accreditation Program: Accreditation requirements for acute care hospitals.* Chicago, IL: Accreditation Association for Hospitals and Health Systems. (Level VII)

12 Centers for Medicare and Medicaid Services, Department of Health and Human Services. (2020). Condition of participation: Infection control. 42 C.F.R. § 482.42.

13 DNV GL-Healthcare USA, Inc. (2020). IC.1.SR.1. *NIAHO® accreditation requirements, interpretive guidelines and surveyor guidance—revision 20.0* Milford, OH: DNV GL-Healthcare USA, Inc. (Level VII)

14 The Joint Commission. (2021). Standard NPSG.01.01.01. *Comprehensive accreditation manual for hospitals.* Oakbrook Terrace, IL: The Joint Commission. (Level VII)

15 The Joint Commission. (2021). Standard RI.01.01.01. *Comprehensive accreditation manual for hospitals.* Oakbrook Terrace, IL: The Joint Commission. (Level VII)

16 DNV GL-Healthcare USA, Inc. (2020). PR.2.SR.5. *NIAHO® accreditation requirements, interpretive guidelines and surveyor guidance—revision 20.0.* Milford, OH: DNV GL-Healthcare USA, Inc. (Level VII)

17 Centers for Medicare and Medicaid Services, Department of Health and Human Services. (2020). Condition of participation: Patient's rights. 42 C.F.R. § 482.13(c)(1).

18 Accreditation Association for Hospitals and Health Systems. (2020). Standard 15.01.16. *Healthcare Facilities Accreditation Program: Accreditation requirements for acute care hospitals.* Chicago, IL: Accreditation Association for Hospitals and Health Systems. (Level VII)

19 The Joint Commission. (2021). Standard PC.02.01.21. *Comprehensive accreditation manual for hospitals.* Oakbrook Terrace, IL: The Joint Commission. (Level VII)

20 Waters, T. R., et al. (2009). Safe patient handling training for schools of nursing. https://www.cdc.gov/niosh/docs/2009-127/pdfs/2009-127.pdf (Level VII)

21 Siegel, J. D., et al. (2007, revised 2019). 2007 guideline for isolation precautions: Preventing transmission of infectious agents in healthcare settings. https://www.cdc.gov/infectioncontrol/pdf/guidelines/isolation-guidelines-H.pdf (Level II)

22 Accreditation Association for Hospitals and Health Systems. (2020). Standard 07.01.10. *Healthcare Facilities Accreditation Program: Accreditation requirements for acute care hospitals.* Chicago, IL: Accreditation Association for Hospitals and Health Systems. (Level VII)

23 Occupational Safety and Health Administration. (2019). Bloodborne pathogens, standard number 1910.1030. https://www.osha.gov/pls/oshaweb/owadisp.show_document?p_id=10051&p_table=STANDARDS (Level VII)

24 Graham, K. C., & Cvach, M. (2010). Monitor alarm fatigue: Standardizing use of physiological monitors and decreasing nuisance alarms. *American Journal of Critical Care, 19,* 28–37.

25 The Joint Commission. (2021). Standard NPSG.06.01.01. *Comprehensive accreditation manual for hospitals.* Oakbrook Terrace, IL: The Joint Commission. (Level VII)

26 American Association of Critical-Care Nurses. (2018). AACN practice alert: Managing alarms in acute care across the life span: Electrocardiography and pulse oximetry. https://www.aacn.org/clinical-resources/practice-alerts/managing-alarms-in-acute-care-across-the-life-span (Level VII)

27 The Joint Commission. (2013). Sentinel event alert 50: Medical device alarm safety in hospitals. https://www.jointcommission.org/assets/1/6/SEA_50_alarms_4_26_16.pdf (Level VII)

28 Accreditation Association for Hospitals and Health Systems. (2020). Standard 16.01.03. *Healthcare Facilities Accreditation Program: Accreditation requirements for acute care hospitals.* Chicago, IL: Accreditation Association for Hospitals and Health Systems. (Level VII)

29 Centers for Medicare and Medicaid Services, Department of Health and Human Services. (2020). Condition of participation: Nursing services. 42 C.F.R. § 482.23.

30 DNV GL-Healthcare USA, Inc. (2020). MM.1.SR.3. *NIAHO® accreditation requirements, interpretive guidelines and surveyor guidance—revision 20.0.* Milford, OH: DNV GL-Healthcare USA, Inc. (Level VII)

31 The Joint Commission. (2021). Standard MM.06.01.01. *Comprehensive accreditation manual for hospitals.* Oakbrook Terrace, IL: The Joint Commission. (Level VII)

32 Wound Ostomy and Continence Nurses Society (WOCN). (2016). *Guideline for prevention and management of pressure ulcers (injuries): WOCN clinical practice guideline series 2.* Mount Laurel, NJ; WOCN.

33 European Pressure Ulcer Advisory Panel, et al. (2019). Prevention and treatment of pressure ulcers/injuries: Quick reference guide. http://www.internationalguideline.com/static/pdfs/Quick_Reference_Guide-10Mar2019.pdf (Level VII)

34 Jarrett, N., & Callaham, M. (2016). Evidence-based guidelines for selected hospital-acquired conditions: Final report. https://www.cms.gov/Medicare/Medicare-Fee-for-Service-Payment/HospitalAcqCond/Downloads/2016-HAC-Report.pdf

35 American Heart Association. Web-based integrated guidelines for cardiopulmonary resuscitation and emergency cardiovascular care—Part 8: Post-cardiac arrest care. https://eccguidelines.heart.org (Level II).

36 Ganz, D. A., et al. (2013, reviewed 2021). *Preventing falls in hospitals: A toolkit for improving quality of care* (AHRQ Publication No. 13-0015-EF). Rockville, MD: Agency for Healthcare Research and Quality. https://www.ahrq.gov/professionals/systems/hospital/fallpxtoolkit/index.html (Level VII)

37 Rutala, W. A., et al. (2008, revised 2019). Guideline for disinfection and sterilization in healthcare facilities, 2008. https://www.cdc.gov/infection-control/pdf/guidelines/disinfection-guidelines-H.pdf

38 Accreditation Association for Hospitals and Health Systems. (2020). Standard 07.02.03. *Healthcare Facilities Accreditation Program: Accreditation requirements for acute care hospitals.* Chicago, IL: Accreditation Association for Hospitals and Health Systems. (Level VII)

39 The Joint Commission. (2021). Standard RC 01.03.01. *Comprehensive accreditation manual for hospitals.* Oakbrook Terrace, IL: The Joint Commission. (Level VII)

40 Centers for Medicare and Medicaid Services, Department of Health and Human Services. (2020). Condition of participation: Medical record services. 42 C.F.R. § 482.24(b).

41 Accreditation Association for Hospitals and Health Systems. (2020). Standard 10.00.03. *Healthcare Facilities Accreditation Program: Accreditation requirements for acute care hospitals.* Chicago, IL: Accreditation Association for Hospitals and Health Systems. (Level VII)

42 DNV GL-Healthcare USA, Inc. (2020). MR.2.SR.1. *NIAHO® accreditation requirements, interpretive guidelines and surveyor guidance—revision 20.0.* Milford, OH: DNV GL-Healthcare USA, Inc. (Level VII)

43 Polderman, K. H., et al. (2009). Therapeutic hypothermia and controlled normothermia in the intensive care unit: Practical considerations, side effects, and cooling methods. *Critical Care Medicine, 37,* 1101–1119.

44 Elmer, J., Rittenberger, J. C. (2021). Initial assessment and management of the adult post-cardiac arrest patient. In: *UpToDate,* Walls, R. M. (Ed.).

45 Kim, Y. M., et al. (2015). Adverse events associated with poor neurological outcome during targeted temperature management and advanced critical care after out-of-hospital cardiac arrest. *Critical Care, 19,* 283. (Level VI)

IM INJECTION

Intramuscular (IM) injections deposit medication deep into muscle tissue. This route of administration provides rapid systemic action and absorption of relatively large doses (up to 5 mL in appropriate sites).[1] IM injections are recommended for patients who can't take medication orally, when IV administration is inappropriate or inaccessible, and for drugs that are altered by digestive juices. Because muscle tissue has few sensory nerves, IM injections allow less painful administration of irritating drugs.

The site for an IM injection must be chosen carefully, taking into account the patient's general physical status and the purpose of the injection.[2] IM injections shouldn't be administered at inflamed, edematous, or irritated sites or at sites that contain moles, birthmarks, scar tissue, or other lesions.[1] IM injections may also be contraindicated in patients with impaired coagulation mechanisms, occlusive peripheral vascular disease, edema, and shock, as well as after thrombolytic therapy and during an acute myocardial infarction (MI), because these conditions impair peripheral absorption. IM injections require sterile technique to maintain the integrity of muscle tissue.

The Z-track method is preferred for administering IM injections. Leaving a zigzag path that seals the needle track prevents drug leakage into the subcutaneous tissue, helps seal the drug in the muscle, and minimizes irritation.[1]

Equipment

Patient's medication administration record ■ prescribed medication ■ single-use sterile syringe and needle of appropriate size and gauge (a self-sheathing needle is recommended)[3] ■ alcohol pads ■ gauze pads ■ Optional: 1″ (2.5-cm) tape, ice or cold compress, filter needle, gloves, adhesive bandage, personal protective equipment.

The prescribed medication must be sterile. The needle may be packaged separately or already attached to the syringe. (See *Selecting the appropriate syringe and needle,* page 408.)

Preparation of equipment

Choose equipment appropriate to the prescribed medication and injection site. Inspect all equipment and supplies. If a product is expired, is defective, or has compromised integrity, remove it from patient use, label it as expired or defective, and report the expiration or defect as directed by your facility. Make sure that the needle is straight, smooth, and free from burrs.

Implementation

■ Avoid distractions and interruptions when preparing and administering medications *to prevent medication errors.*[7,8]

■ Verify the practitioner's order.[9,10,11,12]

■ Reconcile the patient's medications when a new medication is ordered *to reduce the risk of medication errors, including omissions, duplications, dosing errors, and drug interactions.*[13,14]

■ Perform hand hygiene.[15]

NURSING ALERT If your facility's hazardous drug list contains the drug that you are about to administer, put on personal protective equipment, as directed.[16]

■ Gather and prepare the necessary equipment and supplies and obtain the prescribed medication.

■ Compare the medication label with the order in the patient's medical record.[9,10,11,12]

■ Check the patient's medical record for an allergy or a contraindication to the prescribed medication. If an allergy or contraindications exist, don't administer the medication; instead, notify the practitioner.[9,10,11,12]

■ Check the expiration date on the medication. If the medication is expired, return it to the pharmacy and obtain new medication.[9,10,11,12]

■ Visually inspect the solution for particles, discoloration, or other loss of integrity; don't administer the medication if its integrity is compromised.[9,10,11,12]

■ Discuss any unresolved concerns about the medication with the patient's practitioner.[9,10,11,12]

■ Perform hand hygiene.[15,17,18,19,20,21,22,23]

■ Carefully calculate the dose. If it's a high-alert medication that can cause significant patient harm when used in error, perform an independent double-check with another nurse if required by your facility.[24,25]

■ Read the medication label again as you draw up the medication for injection, if needed. (See *Drawing up medication for injection,* page 408.)

■ Perform hand hygiene.[15,17,18,19,20,21,22,23]

■ Confirm the patient's identity using at least two patient identifiers.[29]

■ Provide privacy.[30,31,32,33]

■ Explain the procedure to the patient and family (if appropriate) according to their individual communication and learning needs *to increase their understanding, allay their fears, and enhance cooperation.*[34]

■ If the patient is receiving the medication for the first time, discuss potential adverse reactions and any other concerns related to the medication.[9,10,11,12]

■ Verify that the medication is being administered at the proper time, in the prescribed dose, and by the correct route *to reduce the risk of medication errors.*[9,10,11,12]

■ If your facility uses a bar-code technology, use it, as directed by your facility.

■ Raise the patient's bed to waist level before providing patient care *to prevent caregiver back strain.*[35]

■ Perform hand hygiene.[15,17,18,19,20,21,22,23]

■ Put on gloves if contact with blood or body fluids is likely, or if your skin or the patient's skin isn't intact.[3,36,37] *Gloves aren't required for routine IM injection because they don't protect against needle-stick injury.*[23]

■ Select an appropriate injection site. The ventrogluteal site is used most commonly for large-volume IM injection in an adult, although the deltoid muscle may be used for a small-volume injection (2 mL or less). (See *Locating IM injection sites.*) Remember to always rotate injection sites for patients who require repeated injections.

NURSING ALERT If using the ventrogluteal site, take care to correctly identify anatomic landmarks before administration. *Use of the dorsogluteal site isn't recommended because of the potential for nerve damage.*[1,38,39]

■ Position and drape the patient appropriately using the bed linens, making sure the site is well exposed and lighting is adequate (as shown below).

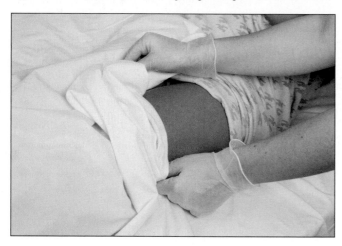

■ After selecting the injection site, clean the skin with an alcohol pad.[23] Move the pad outward in a circular motion to a circumference of about 2″ (5 cm) from the injection site and allow the skin to dry completely (as shown below).[23]

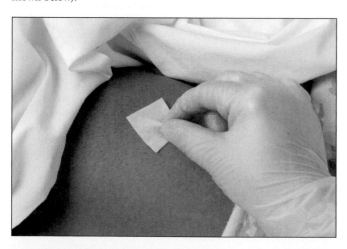

■ Remove the needle sheath. With the thumb and index finger of your nondominant hand, gently displace the skin and subcutaneous tissue of the injection site by pulling the skin laterally for the Z-track technique.[1] (See the "Z-track injection" procedure.)

■ Position the syringe at a 90-degree angle to the skin surface, with the needle a couple of inches from the skin. Tell the patient that a prick will be felt as you insert the needle. Then quickly and smoothly insert the needle through the skin and subcutaneous tissue, deep into the muscle at a 90-degree angle.

■ Support the syringe with your nondominant hand if desired. Slowly inject the medication into the muscle. *A slow, steady injection rate allows the muscle to distend gradually and accept the medication under minimal pressure. You should feel little or no resistance against the force of the injection.*

Selecting the appropriate syringe and needle

For an IM injection, the size of the syringe and the gauge and length of the needle are determined by several factors, including the amount and viscosity of the medication, the injection site chosen, and the patient's weight and amount of adipose tissue. Needles used for IM injections are longer than subcutaneous needles *because they must reach deep into the muscle.*

The volume of medication administered IM is usually 1 mL to 4 mL, so a 3-mL or 5-mL syringe is usually appropriate. The appropriate gauge of the needle is determined by the medication being administered. Biological agents and medications in aqueous solutions should be administered with a 20G to 25G needle. Medications in oil-based solutions should be administered with an 18G to 25G needle.

Needle length depends on the injection site, the patient's size, and the amount of subcutaneous fat covering the muscle. Patients who are obese may require a longer needle (1½″ [3.8 cm] or longer), and thin or emaciated patients may require a shorter needle (½″ to 1″ [1.25 cm to 2.5 cm]).[4] When choosing the needle size and injection site, take into consideration muscle size, thickness of adipose tissue at the injection site, volume of the material to be administered, injection technique, and depth below the muscle surface into which you'll inject the medication:[5,6]

■ Vastus lateralis: ½″ to 1″ (1.3 cm to 2.5 cm)

■ Deltoid: ½″ to 1½″ (1.3 cm to 3.8 cm)

■ Ventrogluteal: ½″ to 1½″ (1.3 cm to 3.8 cm)

Drawing up medication for injection

Your technique for drawing up the medication will vary according to the type of container that houses the medication. Prepare the medication in a clean, dry work space that is free of clutter and contamination.[15] Follow aseptic technique during preparation *to prevent the transfer of microorganisms to the patient.*[15]

For single-dose ampules: Disinfect the neck of the ampule with an alcohol pad before breaking it.[15] Wrap an alcohol pad around the ampule's neck and snap off the ampule's head into an ampule breaker and snap off the top, directing the force away from your body. Attach a filter needle to the syringe and withdraw the medication, keeping the needle's bevel tip below the level of the solution. Tap the syringe *to clear air from it.* Cover the needle with the needle sheath.

Before discarding the ampule, check the medication label against the patient's medication record.[9,10,11,12] Discard the filter needle and the ampule in a puncture-resistant sharps disposal container.[23] Attach the appropriate needle to the syringe.

For single-dose or multidose vials: Whenever possible, use a single-dose vial instead of a multidose vial, especially when medications will be administered to multiple patients.[26] Dedicate multidose medication vials to one patient whenever possible *to reduce the risk of bloodborne pathogen transmission and infection.* If you must use multidose vials for more than one patient, you should keep and access them in a dedicated medication preparation area that is away from immediate patient treatment areas. *Doing so prevents inadvertent contamination of the vial through direct or indirect contact with potentially contaminated surfaces or equipment that could lead to infections in subsequent patients.*[15,27,28]

Reconstitute powdered drugs according to instructions. Make sure all crystals have dissolved in the solution. Warm the vial by rolling it between your palms *to help the drug dissolve faster.*

Wipe the stopper of the medication vial with an alcohol pad and allow it to dry completely.[15] Draw up the prescribed amount of medication. Read the medication label as you select the medication, as you draw it up, and after you have drawn it up *to verify the correct dosage.*

Don't use an air bubble in the syringe. *Modern, disposable syringes are calibrated to give the correct dose without an air bubble.* Change the needle if it has become damaged or contaminated; cover the needle with the needle sheath.[3] Store all multidose vials according to the manufacturer's guidelines.

Locating IM injection sites

Deltoid

Have the patient sit or stand. Find the lower edge of the acromial process and the point on the lateral arm in line with the axilla. Insert the needle 1″ to 2″ (2.5 to 5 cm) below the acromial process, usually two or three fingerbreadths, at a 90-degree angle or angled slightly toward the process. The maximum injection volume for this site is 2 mL.[1]

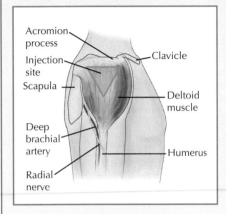

Ventrogluteal

Have the patient sit, stand, lie laterally, or lie supine. Locate the greater trochanter of the femur with the heel of your hand. Then spread your index and middle fingers from the anterior superior iliac spine to as far along the iliac crest as you can reach. Insert the needle between the two fingers at a 90-degree angle to the muscle. (Remove your fingers before inserting the needle.) The maximum injection volume for this site is 5 mL.[1]

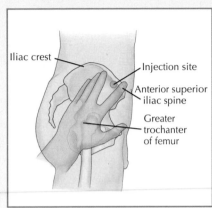

Vastus lateralis

Have the patient sit or lie supine. The patient's knee may be slightly flexed and the foot may be externally rotated *to help relax the muscle.* Use the lateral muscle of the quadriceps group, from a handbreadth below the greater trochanter to a handbreadth above the knee. Insert the needle into the middle third of the muscle parallel to the surface on which the patient is lying. The maximum injection volume for this site is 5 mL.[1]

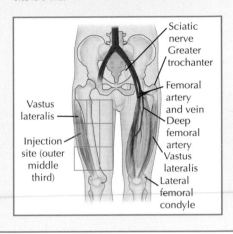

■ After the injection, wait 10 seconds *to allow the medication to begin to diffuse into the surrounding muscle tissue;* then withdraw the needle slowly at a 90-degree angle.[1,40] If present, activate the needle's safety mechanism *to prevent accidental needle-stick injury.*[3,41]

■ Release the displaced skin and subcutaneous tissue *to seal the needle track.*

■ Cover the injection site immediately with a gauze pad (as shown below), and apply gentle pressure.

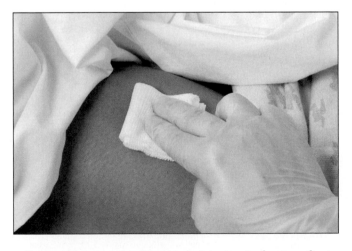

■ Remove the gauze pad and inspect the injection site for signs of active bleeding or bruising. If bleeding continues, apply pressure to the site; if bruising occurs, you may apply ice or a cold compress.

■ Return the bed to the lowest position *to prevent falls and maintain patient safety.*[42]

■ Monitor for adverse reactions at the site for 10 to 30 minutes after the injection.[43]

ELDER ALERT An older adult patient may bleed or ooze from the site after the injection *because of decreased tissue elasticity.* Applying a small pressure bandage may be helpful.

■ Discard all equipment appropriately.[3] Don't recap needles; dispose of them in an appropriate sharps container *to avoid needle-stick injuries.*[23]

■ Remove and discard your gloves, if worn,[3] and perform hand hygiene.[15,17,18,19,20,21,22,23]

■ Document the procedure.[44,45,46,47]

Special considerations

■ The Joint Commission has issued a sentinel event alert concerning the transmission of pathogens related to the misuse of vials that have caused viral and bacterial infections, including hepatitis B, hepatitis C, meningitis, and epidural abscesses. The commission has attributed these infections to the reuse of single-dose vials that typically don't contain preservatives, re-entering multidose vials with used syringes and needles, and using multidose vials for multiple patients. To prevent these infections, follow evidence-based best practices, such as disinfecting the vial's rubber stopper before piercing, using single-dose vials only once and then discarding the vial, dedicating multidose vials to a single patient, and using a new syringe and needle when re-entering a multidose vial. Assign the appropriate "beyond-use" date when first entering a multidose vial, and store multidose vials as directed by your facility and according to the manufacturer's instructions.[28]

■ *To slow their absorption,* some drugs for IM administration are dissolved in oil or other special solutions. Mix these preparations well before drawing them into the syringe.[2]

■ Although not routine, aspiration for blood may be indicated for IM injections of certain medications that, if injected systemically, would have fatal adverse effects. Consult the medication's prescribing information before administration.[48]

■ Keep a rotation record that lists all available injection sites, divided into various body areas, for patients who require repeated injections.[2] Rotate from a site in the first area to a site in each of the other areas. Then return to a site in the first area that's at least 1″ (2.5 cm) away from the previous injection site in that area.

■ Always encourage the patient to relax the muscle you'll be injecting, *because injections into tense muscles are typically more painful and may cause the site to bleed more readily.*[2]

■ IM injections can damage local muscle cells, causing elevations in serum enzyme levels (creatine kinase [CK]) that can be confused with elevations resulting from damage to cardiac muscle, as in MI. *To distinguish*

Documenting administration of controlled substances

Some facilities use a computerized system that confirms the count for each opioid drug as it's used or removed from the system via a secure identification code. This system eliminates the need for opioid counts during the day.

Before administering a controlled substance, regardless of the system being used, always verify the amount of drug in the container and sign out the medication as required by your facility. A second nurse may be required to document your activity and observe you if part of a controlled substance dose must be wasted.

What to report: If you discover a discrepancy in the controlled substance count, report it as required by your facility. You'll need to file an occurrence report as well. An investigation will follow.

between skeletal and cardiac muscle damage, diagnostic tests for suspected MI must identify the isoenzyme of CK specific to cardiac muscle (CK-MB) and include tests to determine lactate dehydrogenase and aspartate aminotransferase levels.[49] If it's important to measure these enzyme levels, suggest that the practitioner switch to IV administration and adjust dosages accordingly.

■ Prepare the injectable medication as close as possible to the time of administration—at least within 1 hour of administration.[15]

■ If the medication isn't going to be administered immediately, clearly label the medication syringe *to prevent a medication error*. An immediately administered medication is one that's prepared, taken directly to the patient, and administered without any break in the process.[50,51,52]

Complications

Accidental injection of concentrated or irritating medications into subcutaneous tissue or other areas where they can't be fully absorbed can cause sterile abscesses to develop. Failure to rotate sites in patients who require repeated injections can lead to deposits of unabsorbed medications, which can reduce the desired pharmacologic effect, and may lead to abscess formation or tissue fibrosis. Improper technique can also result in injury to bone, blood vessels, and peripheral nerves.[1]

ELDER ALERT *Because older adult patients typically have decreased muscle mass*, IM medications may be absorbed more quickly than expected.

Documentation

Document the drug you administered, its strength, the dose, the date, time, and route of administration, and the injection site, according to your facility's documentation format. Record any adverse reactions to the prescribed medication, the date and time that you notified the practitioner, prescribed interventions, and the patient's response to those interventions. If you're documenting immunization administration, include the lot number and expiration date. Document teaching you provided to the patient and family (if applicable), their understanding of that teaching, and any need for follow-up teaching. (See *Documenting administration of controlled substances*.)

REFERENCES

1 Hopkins, U., & Arias, C. Y. (2013). Large-volume IM injections: A review of best practices. *Oncology Nurse Advisor*, 2013, 32–37. http://media.oncologynurseadvisor.com/documents/44/ona_feature0213_injections_10767.pdf

2 Craven, R. F., et al. (2021). *Fundamentals of nursing: Concepts and competencies for practice* (9th ed.). Philadelphia, PA: Wolters Kluwer.

3 Occupational Safety and Health Administration. (2012). Bloodborne pathogens, standard number 1910.1030. https://www.osha.gov/pls/oshaweb/owadisp.show_document?p_id=10051&p_table=STANDARDS (Level VII)

4 Tanioka, T., et al. (2013). Optimal needle insertion length for intramuscular injection of risperidone long-acting injectable (RLAI). *Health, 5*(12), 1939–1945. https://file.scirp.org/Html/40471.html (Level VI)

5 Centers for Disease Control and Prevention. (2011). General recommendations on immunization: Recommendations of the Advisory Committee on Immunization Practices. *MMWR Recommendations and Reports, 60*(RR-02), 1–60. https://www.cdc.gov/mmwr/pdf/rr/rr6002.pdf (Level II)

6 Zaybak, A., et al. (2015). Examination of subcutaneous tissue thickness in the thigh site for intramuscular injection in obese individuals. *Journal of Ultrasound in Medicine, 34*(9), 1657–1662. https://onlinelibrary.wiley.com/doi/epdf/10.7863/ultra.15.14.09005 (Level IV)

7 Westbrook, J., et al. (2010). Association of interruptions with an increased risk and severity of medication administration errors. *Archives of Internal Medicine, 170*, 683–690. (Level IV)

8 Institute for Safe Medication Practices. (2012). Side tracks on the safety express: Interruptions lead to errors and unfinished…Wait, what was I doing? https://www.ismp.org/resources/side-tracks-safety-express-interruptions-lead-errors-and-unfinished-wait-what-was-i-doing?id=37 (Level VII)

9 The Joint Commission. (2021). Standard MM.06.01.01. *Comprehensive accreditation manual for hospitals*. Oakbrook Terrace, IL: The Joint Commission. (Level VII)

10 Accreditation Association for Hospitals and Health Systems. (2020). Standard 16.01.03. *Healthcare Facilities Accreditation Program: Accreditation requirements for acute care hospitals*. Chicago, IL: Accreditation Association for Hospitals and Health Systems. (Level VII)

11 Centers for Medicare and Medicaid Services, Department of Health and Human Services. (2020). Condition of participation: Nursing services. 42 C.F.R. § 482.23(c).

12 DNV GL-Healthcare USA, Inc. (2020). MM.1.SR.3. *NIAHO® accreditation requirements, interpretive guidelines and surveyor guidance—revision 20.0*. Milford, OH: DNV GL-Healthcare USA, Inc. (Level VII)

13 The Joint Commission. (2021). Standard NPSG.03.06.01. *Comprehensive accreditation manual for hospitals*. Oakbrook Terrace, IL: The Joint Commission. (Level VII)

14 Accreditation Association for Hospitals and Health Systems. (2020). Standard 25.02.13. *Healthcare Facilities Accreditation Program: Accreditation requirements for acute care hospitals*. Chicago, IL: Accreditation Association for Hospitals and Health Systems. (Level VII)

15 Dolan, S., et al. (2016). APIC position paper: Safe injection, infusion, and medication practices in health care. *American Journal of Infection Control, 44*(7), 750–757. (Level VII)

16 The United States Pharmacopeial Convention. (2019). USP general chapter <800>: Hazardous drugs—handling in healthcare settings. https://www.usp.org/compounding/general-chapter-hazardous-drugs-handling-healthcare (Level VII)

17 The Joint Commission. (2021). Standard NPSG.07.01.01. *Comprehensive accreditation manual for hospitals*. Oakbrook Terrace, IL: The Joint Commission. (Level VII)

18 Centers for Disease Control and Prevention. (2002). Guideline for hand hygiene in health-care settings: Recommendations of the Healthcare Infection Control Practices Advisory Committee and the HICPAC/SHEA/APIC/IDSA Hand Hygiene Task Force. *MMWR Recommendations and Reports, 51*(RR-16), 1–45. https://www.cdc.gov/mmwr/pdf/rr/rr5116.pdf (Level II)

19 World Health Organization. (2009). WHO guidelines on hand hygiene in health care: First global patient safety challenge, clean care is safer care. https://apps.who.int/iris/bitstream/handle/10665/44102/9789241597906_eng.pdf?sequence=1 (Level IV)

20 Accreditation Association for Hospitals and Health Systems. (2020). Standard 07.01.21. *Healthcare Facilities Accreditation Program: Accreditation requirements for acute care hospitals*. Chicago, IL: Accreditation Association for Hospitals and Health Systems. (Level VII)

21 Centers for Medicare and Medicaid Services, Department of Health and Human Services. (2020). Condition of participation: Infection control. 42 C.F.R. § 482.42.

22 DNV GL-Healthcare USA, Inc. (2020). IC.1.SR.1. *NIAHO® accreditation requirements, interpretive guidelines and surveyor guidance—revision 20.0*. Milford, OH: DNV GL-Healthcare USA, Inc. (Level VII)

23 World Health Organization. (2010). WHO best practices for injections and related procedures toolkit. http://apps.who.int/iris/bitstream/10665/44298/1/9789241599252_eng.pdf (Level IV)

24 Institute for Safe Medication Practices. (2018). ISMP list of high-alert medications in acute care settings. https://www.ismp.org/sites/default/files/attachments/2018-08/highAlert2018-Acute-Final.pdf (Level VII)

25 Institute for Safe Medication Practices. (2019). Independent double checks: Worth the effort if used judiciously and properly. https://www.

ismp.org/resources/independent-double-checks-worth-effort-if-used-judiciously-and-properly (Level VII)

26 Centers for Disease Control and Prevention. (2011). Safe injection practices to prevent transmission of infections to patients. https://www.cdc.gov/injectionsafety/IP07_standardPrecaution.html (Level II)

27 Centers for Disease Control and Prevention. (2019).Injection safety: Questions about multi-dose vials—frequently asked questions (FAQs) regarding safe practices for medical injections. https://www.cdc.gov/injectionsafety/providers/provider_faqs_multivials.html

28 The Joint Commission. (2014). Sentinel event alert, issue 52: Preventing infection from the misuse of vials. https://www.jointcommission.org/-/media/deprecated-unorganized/imported-assets/tjc/system-folders/assetmanager/sea_52pdf.pdf?db=web&hash=45D132407D5F06D-35C75767A9087B176 (Level VII)

29 The Joint Commission. (2021). Standard NPSG.01.01.01. *Comprehensive accreditation manual for hospitals.* Oakbrook Terrace, IL: The Joint Commission. (Level VII)

30 Accreditation Association for Hospitals and Health Systems. (2020). Standard 15.01.16. *Healthcare Facilities Accreditation Program: Accreditation requirements for acute care hospitals.* Chicago, IL: Accreditation Association for Hospitals and Health Systems. (Level VII)

31 Centers for Medicare and Medicaid Services, Department of Health and Human Services. (2020). Condition of participation: Patient's rights. 42 C.F.R. § 482.13(c)(1).

32 DNV GL-Healthcare USA, Inc. (2020). PR.2.SR.5. *NIAHO® accreditation requirements, interpretive guidelines and surveyor guidance—revision 20.0.* Milford, OH: DNV GL-Healthcare USA, Inc. (Level VII)

33 The Joint Commission. (2021). Standard RI.01.01.01. *Comprehensive accreditation manual for hospitals.* Oakbrook Terrace, IL: The Joint Commission. (Level VII)

34 The Joint Commission. (2021). Standard PC.02.01.21. *Comprehensive accreditation manual for hospitals.* Oakbrook Terrace, IL: The Joint Commission. (Level VII)

35 Waters, T. R., et al. (2009). Safe patient handling training for schools of nursing. https://www.cdc.gov/niosh/docs/2009-127/pdfs/2009-127.pdf (Level VII)

36 Siegel, J. D., et al. (2007, revised 2019). 2007 guideline for isolation precautions: Preventing transmission of infectious agents in healthcare settings. https://www.cdc.gov/Infectioncontrol/pdf/guidelines/isolation-guidelines-H.pdf (Level II)

37 Accreditation Association for Hospitals and Health Systems. (2020). Standard 07.01.10. *Healthcare Facilities Accreditation Program: Accreditation requirements for acute care hospitals.* Chicago, IL: Accreditation Association for Hospitals and Health Systems. (Level VII)

38 Mishra, P., & Stringer, M. D. (2010). Sciatic nerve injury from intramuscular injection: A persistent and global problem. *International Journal of Clinical Practice, 64,* 1573–1579. https://onlinelibrary.wiley.com/doi/full/10.1111/j.1742-1241.2009.02177.x (Level V)

39 Cocoman, A., & Murray, J. (2010). Recognizing the evidence and changing practice on injection sites. *British Journal of Nursing, 19,* 1170–1174. (Level V)

40 Nicoll, L. H., & Hesby, A. (2002). Intramuscular injection: An integrative research review and guideline for evidence-based practice. *Applied Nursing Research, 15,* 149–162. (Level V)

41 Occupational Safety and Health Administration. (n.d.). Safety and health topics: Bloodborne pathogens and needlestick prevention. https://www.osha.gov/SLTC/bloodbornepathogens (Level VII)

42 Ganz, D. A., et al. (2013, reviewed 2021). Preventing falls in hospitals: A toolkit for improving quality of care (AHRQ publication no. 13-0015-EF). https://www.ahrq.gov/professionals/systems/hospital/fallpxtoolkit/index.html (Level VII)

43 The Joint Commission. (2021). Standard MM.07.01.03. *Comprehensive accreditation manual for hospitals.* Oakbrook Terrace, IL: The Joint Commission. (Level VII)

44 The Joint Commission. (2021). Standard RC.01.03.01. *Comprehensive accreditation manual for hospitals.* Oakbrook Terrace, IL: The Joint Commission. (Level VII)

45 Accreditation Association for Hospitals and Health Systems. (2020). Standard 10.00.03. *Healthcare Facilities Accreditation Program: Accreditation requirements for acute care hospitals.* Chicago, IL: Accreditation Association for Hospitals and Health Systems. (Level VII)

46 Centers for Medicare and Medicaid Services, Department of Health and Human Services. (2020). Condition of participation: Medical record services. 42 C.F.R. § 482.24(b).

47 DNV GL-Healthcare USA, Inc. (2020). MR.2.SR.1. *NIAHO® accreditation requirements, interpretive guidelines and surveyor guidance—revision 20.0.* Milford, OH: DNV GL-Healthcare USA, Inc. (Level VII)

48 Sepah, Y., et al. (2017). Aspiration in injections: Should we continue or abandon the practice? https://www.ncbi.nlm.nih.gov/pmc/articles/PMC5333604/

49 Hinkle, J. L., & Cheever, K. H. (2018). *Brunner and Suddarth's textbook of medical-surgical nursing* (14th ed.). Philadelphia, PA: Wolters Kluwer.

50 The Joint Commission. (2021). Standard MM.05.01.09. *Comprehensive accreditation manual for hospitals.* Oakbrook Terrace, IL: The Joint Commission. (Level VII)

51 Accreditation Association for Hospitals and Health Systems. (2020). Standard 25.01.18. *Healthcare Facilities Accreditation Program: Accreditation requirements for acute care hospitals.* Chicago, IL: Accreditation Association for Hospitals and Health Systems. (Level VII)

52 The Joint Commission. (2021). Standard NPSG.03.04.01. *Comprehensive accreditation manual for hospitals.* Oakbrook Terrace, IL: The Joint Commission. (Level VII)

IMPAIRED SWALLOWING AND ASPIRATION PRECAUTIONS

Patients may experience impaired swallowing as a result of several specific problems. The first of these—oropharyngeal dysphagia—is impaired swallowing associated with deficits in oral and pharyngeal structure or function. Patients with oropharyngeal dysphagia are at especially high risk for aspiration, and many of them have silent aspiration (aspiration without visible signs of swallowing difficulty such as coughing or gagging before, during, or after swallowing).[1] Patients at risk for oropharyngeal dysphagia include those with nervous system damage, such as from stroke, head injury, or spinal cord injury; those with neuromuscular diseases, such as muscular dystrophy or cerebral palsy; those with progressive neurologic diseases, such as Parkinson disease, multiple sclerosis, amyotrophic lateral sclerosis, or dementia; those with facial, oral, or neck surgery or trauma; those with head and neck cancer; and those who have been intubated for longer than 3 days.[2,3]

The second impaired swallowing problem is associated with esophageal dysphagia and aspiration due to gastroesophageal reflux disease, esophageal dysmotility or structural abnormality, delayed gastric emptying, and radiation esophagitis or stricture.[4] Similarly, the presence of a nasogastric tube may lead to reflux, regurgitation, and subsequent aspiration.[5]

Lastly, impaired swallowing can be associated with tracheostomy or ventilation support that results in decreased sensation of the oral and pharyngeal cavities, decreased sensation of food or fluids penetrating the laryngeal vestibule (dropping below the level of the vocal cords) and being aspirated, decreased ability to cough aspirated material off the vocal cords, and decreased laryngeal elevation and airway closure. Secretions may pool above the tracheostomy or endotracheal tube cuff and be aspirated if they aren't removed by suctioning before cuff deflation.[2,6] The placement of a speaking valve can promote the return of laryngeal and pharyngeal sensation by directing airflow through the upper airway, enabling restoration of the cough reflex and safe swallowing. Speaking valves can reduce tracheal secretions and reduce the incidence of aspiration.[7]

Additionally, patients receiving sedation are at risk for aspiration, because sedation reduces cough and gag reflexes, and can interfere with the patient's ability to handle oropharyngeal secretions and refluxed gastric contents. Sedation may slow gastric emptying, increasing the risk for aspiration.[2]

Equipment

Meal and supplements ▪ wall suction or portable suction apparatus ▪ suction kit ▪ gloves ▪ oral care supplies ▪ swallowing precautions and feeding instructions information sheet ▪ stethoscope ▪ pulse oximeter and probe ▪ scale ▪ disinfectant pad ▪ facility-approved disinfectant ▪ Optional: mask with face shield or mask and goggles, adaptive feeding devices, mortar and pestle or other appropriate medication crushing supplies, appropriate vehicle for crushed pills (applesauce or pudding), thickening agent for food, irrigation tray with 50- or 60-mL piston syringe, pH strips, glucose test stripes.

Implementation

- Gather the necessary equipment and supplies.
- Perform hand hygiene.[8,9,10,11,12,13]
- Confirm the patient's identity using at least two patient identifiers.[14]
- Provide privacy.[15,16,17,18]
- Explain the procedure to the patient and family (if appropriate) according to their individual communication and learning needs *to increase their communication, allay fears, and enhance cooperation.*[19]
- Perform hand hygiene.[8,9,10,11,12,13]
- Put on gloves and, if needed, a mask with face shield or mask with goggles *to comply with standard precautions.*[20,21,22]
- Request a referral for and assist with a bedside swallow evaluation (usually conducted by a speech-language pathologist), as indicated.[2,23] *A swallowing evaluation using a facility-approved assessment tool such as the Yale Swallow Protocol, can determine if the patient is at risk for aspiration.*

Managing impaired swallowing due to oropharyngeal dysphagia

- After the swallowing evaluation is completed, develop a multidisciplinary management plan that includes common swallowing strategies and takes into consideration the patient's nutritional status and required supervision.[23,24]

Using common swallowing strategies

- Have suction equipment available at the bedside.
- Verify the patient's diet modifications, as ordered.[23,25]
- Place the patient in an upright seated position at a 90-degree angle during meals *to decrease the risk of aspiration.*[26] Otherwise, maintain the head of the patient's bed at 30 to 45 degrees unless contraindicated by the patient's condition.[2] Alternatively, consider using the reverse Trendelenburg position to elevate the head of the bed (unless contraindicated) if the patient can't tolerate backrest elevation.[2]
- Implement additional strategies of body positioning and posture, as recommended, *to alter the speed and flow direction of a food or liquid bolus, with the intent of protecting the airway to facilitate a safe swallow.*[23,24,26,27]
- Instruct the patient to sit up for 30 minutes, as recommended, after meals.[27]
- Assist with or perform oral care using appropriate oral care supplies before and after meals, and check for food residue.[26]
- If applicable, ensure that dentures are in place, free from debris, and fit well.
- Ensure the patient uses any recommended adaptive devices, and provide assistance as needed.[23] (See the "Feeding" procedure.)
- Obtain an order for the liquid form of oral medications, if needed and available. If a liquid form isn't available, open the capsule or crush the medication with a mortar and pestle or other medication-crushing equipment, if appropriate, and mix the medication in an appropriate vehicle, such as applesauce, as required. Alternatively, consult with the pharmacist, who may be able to compound medication to create a medication form, such as powder, inhaler, liquid, lozenge, or suppository, that's tailored to the patient's specialized needs.[28]
- **NURSING ALERT** While it may be necessary to open a capsule or crush oral medications for patients at risk for aspiration, it is equally necessary to ensure that only appropriate medications are opened or crushed. Consult the practitioner and your facility's pharmacist if unsure.[29]
- Avoid mixed consistencies of food.
- If applicable, ensure that the temperature, consistency, and amount of foods and liquids are appropriate. Chill water; avoid tepid liquids or food.
- Minimize distractions when the patient is eating and drinking.[26]
- Encourage small sips with liquids and slow intake with adequate chewing.
- If one side of the patient's face is paralyzed, place food on the unaffected side. Check the affected side of the mouth for food that may lodge in the cheek during and after meals. If appropriate, teach the patient to perform a finger-sweep.
- Employ swallowing maneuvers, as recommended, *to improve the safety or efficiency of swallow function.*[23,27]
- If fatigue impairs swallowing, provide rest periods before and during meals, as needed.[26]

- Assess swallowing between bites by feeling the rise and fall of the larynx (Adam's apple).
- Be alert for patient feedback during meals, and modify the presentation and pace of feeding as needed.[23,26]
- Avoid medications that dry up secretions, *which may make swallowing more difficult for the patient.*[26]
- Post swallowing precautions and feeding instructions in the patient's room.

Monitoring nutritional status

- Ask the dietitian to conduct a nutrition evaluation.
- Monitor the patient's hydration and nutrition. *Poor compliance with modified diets may lead to reduced food and fluid intake and an increased risk of malnutrition and dehydration.*[23]
- Implement calorie counts as ordered.
- Weigh the patient daily or as ordered.
- Consult with the patient and family regarding food and fluid preferences.
- Provide small, frequent meals and supplements.
- Praise the patient for achieving nutritional goals.

Using one-on-one supervision

- Ensure that someone remains with the patient throughout every meal.
- Provide feeding assistance or cueing for feeding and swallowing strategies during the entire meal, or ensure that a family member does so.[23]
- Encourage the patient to take 30 to 45 minutes to eat. *Patients with dysphagia typically need to eat slowly.*
- Monitor the patient for signs of aspiration, such as coughing and gagging.

Using close supervision

- Check on the patient frequently during the meal; spend 3 to 5 minutes each time by providing cues and reminding the patient to use swallowing strategies.
- Monitor the patient for signs of aspiration such as coughing and gagging.
- Encourage the patient to increase oral intake, if needed, and provide other options *to maximize safety and nutritional intake.*
- Keep the call light within reach.

Using distant supervision

- Provide initial cueing *to initiate swallowing strategies.*
- Check on the patient by walking past the room frequently.
- Monitor the patient for signs of aspiration such as coughing and gagging.
- Assess the patient's progress at least two to three times during meals.
- Keep the call light within reach.

Managing impaired swallowing due to esophageal dysphagia

- Monitor for reflux and aspiration risks related to esophageal dysphagia.
- Consult with a speech-language pathologist and registered dietitian *to determine the need for alternative nutrition.*
- Monitor respiratory rate and depth; monitor breath sounds for crackles or wheezes with a stethoscope, *which may indicate aspiration and airway obstruction.* Monitor for dyspnea and cyanosis.
- Monitor the patient's GI status for factors that may increase the risk of reflux and subsequent aspiration, such as abdominal distention or firmness, large gastric residual volume (GRV), feeling of fullness, or nausea. Note that GRV shouldn't be used routinely for monitoring.[30,31]
- Monitor the patient's intake and output and daily weight. *Weight loss may indicate an esophageal problem.*
- Implement strategies for oral intake.
- Position the patient sitting upright at a 90-degree angle during oral feeding and maintain the position for at least 30 minutes after the meal *to decrease the risk of reflux, regurgitation, and aspiration.*[27] Otherwise, maintain the head of the patient's bed at 30 to 45 degrees unless contraindicated by the patient's condition. Alternatively, consider using the reverse Trendelenburg position to elevate the head of the bed (unless contraindicated) if the patient can't tolerate backrest elevation.[2]
- Offer thickened liquids and pureed and moist foods that may be easier to swallow if esophageal dysmotility exists.[25]

- Feed the patient slowly; allow adequate time for esophageal emptying.
- If the patient feels full quickly, offer small, frequent meals of high-calorie foods.
- Alternate liquids and solids during feedings *to improve esophageal emptying of solids.*
- Avoid spicy and acidic foods, and decrease caffeine intake *to decrease reflux.*
- Instruct the patient to avoid eating before bed.

Managing a patient with a feeding tube
- Consult a dietician.
- Provide oral care for the patient who is on nothing-by-mouth (NPO) status *to decrease colonization of bacteria in the mouth, because the patient is at risk for secretion aspiration.*
- After feeding tube insertion, confirm tube placement by X-ray. *X-ray confirmation of placement, especially of small-bore feeding tubes, is the gold standard for safe placement.*
- Trace the tubing from the patient to its point of origin before administering the feeding through the feeding tube *to make sure the feeding is administered through the proper port.*[32,33] Route the tubing in a standardized direction if the patient has other tubing and catheters that have different purposes. If you'll be using multiple lines, label the tubing at the distal end (near the patient connection) and at the proximal end (near the source container) *to reduce the risk of misconnection.*[31,33]
- Assess placement of the feeding tube before feeding and every 4 hours for a patient with a continuous feeding using the following methods.[2,31,34,35] Observe for a change in the external feeding tube length or in the incremental markings on the feeding tube at the exit site *indicating tube migration.* Aspirate gastric contents from the feeding tube with a 50- or 60-mL piston syringe and irrigation set, and observe for changes in volume, appearance, and color of the aspirate.[2] If performed in your facility, test the pH of the aspirate with pH strips. Fasting gastric pH is usually 5 or less, even in patient's receiving gastric acid inhibitors.[2] Review routine chest and abdominal X-rays for placement. If tube placement is in doubt, obtain an X-ray *to confirm placement,* as ordered.[2,34]
- If the assessment indicates the possibility of feeding solution in mucus coughed or suctioned from the trachea, test the mucus for glucose with glucose test strips. *A positive result may indicate tube displacement and aspiration of feeding solution.*
- Assess the patient for GI intolerance of enteral tube feedings every 4 hours by assessing abdominal distention, monitoring for abdominal pain, and observing for passage of flatus and stool.[2] Don't monitor GRV routinely.[30,31] If GRV is assessed in critically ill patients, avoid holding the enteral feeding for a GRV of less than 500 mL if no other signs of feeding intolerance exist *to prevent inappropriate stoppage of enteral.*[31,36] If the patient vomits, stop the feeding and notify the practitioner.
- Unless contraindicated by the patient's condition, maintain the head of the bed elevated 30 to 45 degrees *to facilitate movement of feeding solution through the patient's stomach and into the small intestine, thus decreasing the risk of regurgitation and aspiration.* Alternatively, if the patient can't tolerate backrest elevation, consider using the reverse Trendelenburg position *to help elevate the head of the patient's bed* (unless contraindicated).[2,26]

Managing impaired swallowing due to a tracheostomy or an endotracheal tube
- Maintain the head of the bed at an angle of 30 to 45 degrees, unless contraindicated by the patient's condition.[2,26]
- Use sedatives as sparingly as feasible, *because sedation causes reduced cough and gag reflexes, may interfere with the patient's ability to handle secretions and refluxed gastric contents, and may slow gastric emptying.*[2,26]
- Maintain tracheal cuff pressures, as indicated. Suction secretions from above the cuff before deflating the cuff *to help prevent aspiration of secretions and subsequent health care–associated pneumonia.*[2]
- Suction the patient as needed *to maintain a patent airway.*
- Obtain a practitioner's order for speaking valve trials, as appropriate.

Managing impaired swallowing due to speaking valve trials
- Maintain the head of the bed at an angle of 30 to 45 degrees, unless contraindicated by the patient's condition.[2]

- Have the speech-language pathologist assess the patient's tolerance for the speaking valve. *The speaking valve permits hands-free speech and can return oropharyngeal sensation and taste.*[7]
- Deflate the tracheal cuff before placing the speaking valve. Monitor the patient's oxygen saturation level using pulse oximetry before speaking valve placement (as a baseline), with the valve in place, and after valve removal.
- Follow speaking valve recommendations for cleaning and wearing schedules.
- Ensure the speaking valve is in place during meals (according to the speech-language pathologist's recommendations), *because it's usually safer to eat with the valve in place. The patient's ability to cough material off the vocal cords is increased.*

Completing the procedure
- Remove and discard your gloves and, if worn, other personal protective equipment.[22]
- Perform hand hygiene.[8,9,10,11,12,13]
- Clean and disinfect your stethoscope with a disinfectant pad.[37,38]
- Perform hand hygiene.[8,9,10,11,12,13]
- Put on gloves and other personal protective equipment, as needed.[22]
- Clean and disinfect other reusable equipment according to the manufacturer's instructions *to prevent the spread of infection.*[37,38]
- Perform hand hygiene.[8,9,10,11,12,13]
- Document the procedure.[39,40,41,42]

Special considerations
- Patients with ischemic or hemorrhagic stroke should undergo dysphagia screening with an evidence-based, facility-approved bedside testing protocol before being given food, fluids, or medication by mouth.[43]
- Videofluoroscopic and videoendoscopic evaluations are currently the most accurate methods of diagnosing aspiration.[24,27] Monitor the patient for signs and symptoms of swallowing problems and aspiration. These include coughing before, during, or after eating; wet or "gurgling" voice; increased chest congestion after eating; multiple swallows on one mouthful or the needing to wash down food with liquids; complaints of food getting "stuck" or painful swallowing; unexplained changes in the amount of food or rate of eating; drooling or spitting food out of the mouth; difficulty breathing during meals; weight loss and poor oral intake; recurrent pneumonia; low-grade temperatures shortly after meals; increased white blood cell counts; and leakage from the tracheostomy site.
- Small-bowel feedings are recommended when patients are intolerant of gastric feedings or have documented aspiration.[2]
- Patients on modified diets may have reduced food intake, increasing the risk of malnutrition.[23,27]
- Medications in liquid form may contain large amounts of sorbitol, which may cause abdominal cramping and diarrhea.[44]

Patient teaching
If needed, a patient with dysphagia may require instructions on exercises to improve oral control or the overall strength, coordination, and initiation of oropharyngeal swallowing; how to use adaptive feeding devices; and overall strategies to reduce the risk of aspiration.

Train and supervise the family to feed the patient according to the speech therapist's and the practitioner's recommendations. Teach family members how to perform abdominal thrusts and how to use suction equipment, as needed.

Complications
Patients with impaired swallowing are more prone to airway obstruction and aspiration during meals. Aspiration may result in pneumonitis or pneumonia. Difficulty swallowing may result in decreased oral intake and eventually lead to dehydration and malnutrition.[23]

Documentation
Record the patient's amount of intake, daily weight, food preferences, progress with meals, and any techniques effective in helping the

swallowing process. Document patient tolerance of tube feedings, volume of gastric residual volume, and pH values, as indicated. Record any aspiration precautions implemented and the patient's tolerance of them. Document teaching provided to the patient and family (if applicable), their understanding of that teaching, and any need for follow-up teaching.

REFERENCES

1 Eisenstadt, E. S. (2010). Dysphagia and aspiration pneumonia in older adults. *Journal of the American Academy of Nurse Practitioners, 22*, 17–22. (Level V)

2 American Association of Critical-Care Nurses. (2018). AACN practice alert: Prevention of aspiration in adults. https://www.aacn.org/clinical-resources/practice-alerts/prevention-of-aspiration (Level VII)

3 American Speech-Language-Hearing Association. (n.d.). Dysphagia (Adult): Causes. https://www.asha.org/practice-portal/clinical-topics/adult-dysphagia/

4 Fass, R. (2020). Approach to the evaluation of dysphagia in adults. In: *UpToDate*, Feldman, M. (Ed.).

5 Sun, W., et al. (2020). Development and validation of two aspiration prediction models in patients receiving nasogastric feeding. *Journal of Nursing Management, 28*(6), 1372–1380. (Level VI)

6 Kacmarek, R. M., et al. (2021). *Egan's fundamentals of respiratory care* (12th ed.). St. Louis, MO: Elsevier.

7 Kobak, J., et al. (2016). Swallowing and patients on mechanical ventilation: Something to chew on. https://dysphagiacafe.com/2016/11/14/swallowing-patients-mechanical-ventilation-something-chew/

8 The Joint Commission. (2021). Standard NPSG.07.01.01. *Comprehensive accreditation manual for hospitals*. Oakbrook Terrace, IL: The Joint Commission. (Level VII)

9 Centers for Disease Control and Prevention. (2002). Guideline for hand hygiene in health-care settings: Recommendations of the Healthcare Infection Control Practices Advisory Committee and the HICPAC/SHEA/APIC/IDSA Hand Hygiene Task Force. *MMWR Recommendations and Reports, 51*(RR-16), 1–45. https://www.cdc.gov/mmwr/pdf/rr/rr5116.pdf (Level II)

10 World Health Organization. (2009). WHO guidelines on hand hygiene in health care: First global patient safety challenge, clean care is safer care. https://apps.who.int/iris/bitstream/handle/10665/44102/9789241597906_eng.pdf?sequence=1 (Level IV)

11 Accreditation Association for Hospitals and Health Systems. (2020). Standard 07.01.21. *Healthcare Facilities Accreditation Program: Accreditation requirements for acute care hospitals*. Chicago, IL: Accreditation Association for Hospitals and Health Systems. (Level VII)

12 Centers for Medicare and Medicaid Services, Department of Health and Human Services. (2020). Condition of participation: Infection control. 42 C.F.R. § 482.42.

13 DNV GL-Healthcare USA, Inc. (2020). IC.1.SR.1. *NIAHO® accreditation requirements, interpretive guidelines and surveyor guidance—revision 20.0*. Milford, OH: DNV GL-Healthcare USA, Inc. (Level VII)

14 The Joint Commission. (2021). Standard NPSG.01.01.01. *Comprehensive accreditation manual for hospitals*. Oakbrook Terrace, IL: The Joint Commission. (Level VII)

15 Accreditation Association for Hospitals and Health Systems. (2020). Standard 15.01.16. *Healthcare Facilities Accreditation Program: Accreditation requirements for acute care hospitals*. Chicago, IL: Accreditation Association for Hospitals and Health Systems. (Level VII)

16 Centers for Medicare and Medicaid Services, Department of Health and Human Services. (2020). Condition of participation: Patient's rights. 42 C.F.R. § 482.13(c)(1).

17 DNV GL-Healthcare USA, Inc. (2020). PR.2.SR.5. *NIAHO® accreditation requirements, interpretive guidelines and surveyor guidance—revision 20.0*. Milford, OH: DNV GL-Healthcare USA, Inc. (Level VII)

18 The Joint Commission. (2021). Standard RI.01.01.01. *Comprehensive accreditation manual for hospitals*. Oakbrook Terrace, IL: The Joint Commission. (Level VII)

19 The Joint Commission. (2021). Standard PC.02.01.21. *Comprehensive accreditation manual for hospitals*. Oakbrook Terrace, IL: The Joint Commission. (Level VII)

20 Siegel, J. D., et al. (2007, revised 2019). 2007 guideline for isolation and precautions: Preventing transmission of infectious agents in healthcare settings. https://www.cdc.gov/infectioncontrol/pdf/guidelines/isolation-guidelines-H.pdf (Level II)

21 Accreditation Association for Hospitals and Health Systems. (2020). Standard 07.01.10. *Healthcare Facilities Accreditation Program: Accreditation requirements for acute care hospitals*. Chicago, IL: Accreditation Association for Hospitals and Health Systems. (Level VII)

22 Occupational Safety and Health Administration. (2012). Bloodborne pathogens, standard number 1910.1030. https://www.osha.gov/pls/oshaweb/owadisp.show_document?p_id=10051&p_table=STANDARDS (Level VII)

23 Sura, L., et al. (2012). Dysphagia in the elderly: Management and nutritional considerations. *Clinical Interventions in Aging, 7*, 287–298. https://www.ncbi.nlm.nih.gov/pmc/articles/PMC3426263/ (Level V)

24 Accreditation Association for Hospitals and Health Systems. (2020). Standard 16.02.02. *Healthcare Facilities Accreditation Program: Accreditation requirements for acute care hospitals*. Chicago, IL: Accreditation Association for Hospitals and Health Systems. (Level VII)

25 Holdoway, A., & Smith, A. (2020). Meeting nutritional need and managing patients with dysphagia. *JCN, 34*(2), 52–59.

26 Metheny, N. A. (2018). Preventing aspiration in older adults with dysphagia. https://hign.org/consultgeri/try-this-series/preventing-aspiration-older-adults-dysphagia (Level VII)

27 Baijens, L. W. J., et al. (2016). European Society for Swallowing Disorders – European Union Geriatric Medicine Society white paper: Oropharyngeal dysphagia as a geriatric syndrome. *Clinical Interventions in Aging, 11*, 1403–1428. https://www.ncbi.nlm.nih.gov/pmc/articles/PMC5063605 (Level VII)

28 Goldsmith, T., & Cohen, A. K. (2020). Swallowing disorders and aspiration in palliative care: Assessment and strategies for management. In: *UpToDate*, Schmader, K. E., et al. (Eds.).

29 Institute for Safe Medication Practices. (2020). Oral dosage forms that should not be crushed. https://www.ismp.org/recommendations/do-not-crush

30 McClave, S. A., et al. (2016). ACG clinical guideline: Nutrition therapy in the adult hospitalized patient. *The American Journal of Gastroenterology, 111*(3), 315–334. https://journals.lww.com/ajg/fulltext/2016/03000/ACG_Clinical_Guideline__Nutrition_Therapy_in_the.14.aspx

31 Boullata, J. I., et al. (2017). ASPEN safe practices for enteral nutrition therapy. *Journal of Parenteral and Enteral Nutrition, 41*(1), 15–103. https://onlinelibrary.wiley.com/doi/full/10.1177/0148607116673053 (Level VII)

32 U.S. Food and Drug Administration. (2017). Examples of medical device misconnections. https://www.fda.gov/medical-devices/medical-device-connectors/examples-medical-device-misconnections

33 The Joint Commission. (2014). Sentinel event alert 53: Managing risk during transition to new ISO tubing connector standards. https://www.jointcommission.org/assets/1/6/SEA_53_Connectors_8_19_14_final.pdf (Level VII)

34 Simons, S. R., & Abdallah, L. M. (2012). Bedside assessment of enteral tube placement: Aligning practice with evidence. *American Journal of Nursing, 112*(2), 40–46. (Level V)

35 American Association of Critical-Care Nurses. (2016, updated 2020). AACN practice alert: Initial and ongoing verification of feeding tube placement in adults. https://www.aacn.org/clinical-resources/practice-alerts/initial-and-ongoing-verification-of-feeding-tube-placement-in-adults

36 McClave, S. A., et al. (2016). Guidelines for the provision and assessment of nutrition support therapy in the adult critically ill patient: Society of Critical Care Medicine (SCCM) and American Society for Parenteral and Enteral Nutrition (A.S.P.E.N.). *Journal of Parenteral and Enteral Nutrition, 40*, 159–211. https://onlinelibrary.wiley.com/doi/full/10.1177/0148607115621863

37 Accreditation Association for Hospitals and Health Systems. (2020). Standard 07.02.03. *Healthcare Facilities Accreditation Program: Accreditation requirements for acute care hospitals*. Chicago, IL: Accreditation Association for Hospitals and Health Systems. (Level VII)

38 Rutala, W. A., et al. (2008, updated 2019). Guideline for disinfection and sterilization in healthcare facilities, 2008. https://www.cdc.gov/infection-control/pdf/guidelines/disinfection-guidelines-H.pdf (Level I)

39 The Joint Commission. (2021). Standard RC.01.03.01. *Comprehensive accreditation manual for hospitals*. Oakbrook Terrace, IL: The Joint Commission. (Level VII)

40 Centers for Medicare and Medicaid Services, Department of Health and Human Services. (2020). Condition of participation: Medical record services. 42 C.F.R. § 482.24(b).

41 Accreditation Association for Hospitals and Health Systems. (2020). Standard 10.00.03. *Healthcare Facilities Accreditation Program: Accreditation requirements for acute care hospitals*. Chicago, IL: Accreditation Association for Hospitals and Health Systems. (Level VII)

42 DNV GL-Healthcare USA, Inc. (2020). MR.2.SR.1. *NIAHO® accredi-tation requirements, interpretive guidelines and surveyor guidance—revision 20.0*. Milford, OH: DNV GL-Healthcare USA, Inc. (Level VII)

43 The Joint Commission. (2016). Disease-specific care certification program: Comprehensive stroke performance measurement implementation guide. https://www.jointcommission.org/-/media/deprecated-unorganized/ imported-assets/tjc/system-folders/assetmanager/cstkmanual2016october-pdf.pdf?db=web&hash=8BF6C90D2E4B573DAA464FFF13F81BCD

44 Nasoenteric tube feeding (adults): Care and daily management. (2021). *The JBI EBP Database*. AN: JBI1809. (Level VII)

IMPLANTED PORT USE

Surgically implanted by a surgeon or interventional radiologist using local anesthesia, an implanted port, also known as a *vascular access device* or a *vascular access port*, is a type of central venous access device. It consists of a Silastic or polyurethane catheter attached to a reservoir, which is covered with a self-sealing silicone septum. The practitioner places the catheter in the central venous system and typically implants the reservoir in a subcutaneous pocket in the upper anterior chest wall. Alternatively, the practitioner may place the reservoir in the upper arm, abdomen, side, back, or lower extremity.[1]

Use of an implanted port is most common when some type of long-term IV therapy is required and an external central venous device isn't appropriate or desirable. Depending on patient needs, the type of port selected may have one or two lumens.[1,2] A port can be used immediately after placement is confirmed, although some edema and tenderness may persist for about 72 hours, making the device initially difficult to palpate and slightly uncomfortable for the patient.[3] (See *Understanding implanted ports*.)

For a patient who requires repeated computerized tomography scans with contrast, the practitioner may implant a port specially developed to withstand the high pressures of power injectors. Use of a power injector requires a specialized access needle and tubing approved for power injection to ensure that the tubing and connections won't rupture or separate.[4]

Central venous therapy increases the risk of complications, such as pneumothorax, vascular catheter–associated infection, sepsis, thrombus formation, and vessel and adjacent organ perforation (all life-threatening conditions). Because of age-related changes in the immune system, older adults are more susceptible to infection than younger adults. Remote infections can also increase the risk of vascular catheter–associated bloodstream infections in older adults.[5]

HOSPITAL-ACQUIRED CONDITION ALERT The Centers for Medicare and Medicaid Services considers vascular catheter–associated infection a hospital-acquired condition *because it can be reasonably prevented using a variety of best practices*. Follow evidence-based infection prevention practices, such as properly preparing the intended insertion site, instituting maximal barrier precautions, and following sterile technique, *to reduce the risk of vascular catheter–associated infections*.[6,7,8,9,10,11]

Equipment

For assisting with insertion

Insertion checklist ▪ sterile gloves ▪ sterile gown ▪ masks ▪ caps ▪ gowns ▪ sterile drapes ▪ sterile towel ▪ chlorhexidine-based antiseptic sponges ▪ noncoring needles of appropriate type and gauge ▪ extension tubing set ▪ implanted port and guidewire ▪ local anesthetic (lidocaine without epinephrine) ▪ prefilled syringes of heparin flush solution ▪ prefilled syringes of preservative-free normal saline flush solution ▪ sterile occlusive dressings (gauze or transparent semipermeable membrane) ▪ needleless connector(s) ▪ skin closure devices (suture material, surgical glue, adhesive skin closures) ▪ X-ray equipment ▪ labels ▪ fluid-impermeable pad ▪ sign stating STERILE PROCEDURE IN PROGRESS. DO NOT ENTER. ▪ Optional: prescribed prophylactic antibiotics, general anesthetic agent, other surgical equipment, ultrasound device with sterile probe cover, sterile ultrasound gel, disinfectant-containing end cap, chlorhexidine-impregnated sponge dressing, antiseptic soap and water, single-patient-use scissors, disposable-head surgical clippers.

For accessing a top-entry port

Gloves ▪ masks ▪ sterile gloves ▪ sterile drape ▪ noncoring needle with attached extension set tubing[6,12] ▪ antiseptic pad or applicator

EQUIPMENT

Understanding implanted ports

Typically, an implanted port is used to deliver intermittent infusions of medication, parenteral nutrition, chemotherapy, and blood products.[6] A port can also provide access for collection of blood samples. The patient's skin covers the device completely, reducing the risk of extrinsic contamination. Patients may prefer this type of central line *because it doesn't alter body image, requires less routine catheter care, only minimally restricts patient activity, and carries a decreased risk of infection compared with other central venous access devices.* The implanted port consists of a catheter connected to a small reservoir. A septum designed to withstand multiple punctures seals the reservoir. To access the port, a special noncoring needle is inserted perpendicular to the reservoir.

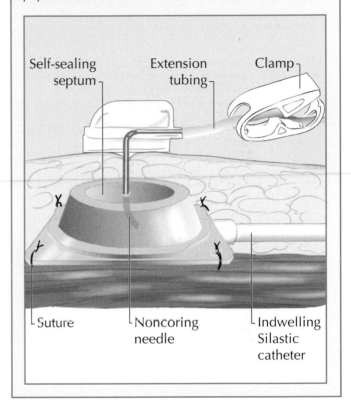

(chlorhexidine-based preferred; tincture of iodine, povidone-iodine, or alcohol if chlorhexidine is contraindicated) ▪ sterile 10-mL syringes prefilled with preservative-free normal saline solution ▪ sterile transparent semipermeable dressing ▪ sterile needleless connector ▪ engineered stabilization device ▪ labels ▪ Optional: prescribed local anesthetic, prescribed locking solution such as prefilled heparinized saline flush solution syringe (10 units/mL),[6,12] ordered IV fluid, primed IV administration set, sterile 2″ × 2″ (5 cm × 5 cm) gauze, sterile tape, chlorhexidine-impregnated sponge dressing, disinfectant-containing end cap.

Some facilities use an implantable port access kit.

For obtaining a blood sample

Gloves ▪ antiseptic pads (chlorhexidine-based, povidone iodine, or alcohol) ▪ appropriate-size syringes or needleless blood collection tube holder ▪ 10-mL syringes prefilled with preservative-free normal saline solution (use a 10-mL syringe or a syringe specifically designed to generate lower injection pressure)[13] ▪ blood collection tubes ▪ labels ▪ laboratory biohazard transport bag ▪ Optional: mask with face shield or mask and goggles, sterile IV end cap, 10-mL syringe, prefilled, containing prescribed locking solution (such as heparin lock solution), blood transfer unit, sterile needleless connector, disinfectant-containing end cap, laboratory request form.

For administering a bolus injection

Prescribed medication in a syringe ■ gloves ■ 10-mL syringes (or a syringe specifically designed to generate lower injection pressure) prefilled with preservative-free normal saline solution ■ antiseptic pads (chlorhexidine-based, povidone iodine, or alcohol) ■ Optional: 10-mL syringe prefilled with prescribed locking solution such as heparin lock solution (10 units/mL),[13] disinfectant-containing end cap, noncoring needle, diluent, dextrose 5% in water, sedation scale, pulse oximeter and probe, capnography equipment.

For administering a continuous infusion

Prescribed IV solution ■ IV administration set ■ IV pole ■ gloves ■ antiseptic pads (chlorhexidine-based, povidone iodine, or alcohol) ■ 10-mL syringe (or a syringe specifically designed to generate low injection pressure) prefilled with preservative-free normal saline solution ■ labels ■ electronic infusion device (preferably a smart pump with dose-error reduction software) ■ Optional: noncoring needle.

For a dressing change

Mask ■ antiseptic (chlorhexidine preferred; tincture of iodine, povidone-iodine, or alcohol if the patient is sensitive to chlorhexidine) ■ skin barrier solution ■ sterile transparent semipermeable dressing or sterile 4" × 4" (10-cm × 10-cm) gauze pad and tape ■ gloves ■ sterile gloves ■ label ■ Optional: sterile drape, supplies for reaccessing the implanted port, chlorhexidine-impregnated sponge dressing, engineered stabilization device, sterile gauze or foam pad for padding under the wings of the noncoring needle, dressings and tape specially formulated for fragile skin.

Commercially prepared central venous access device dressing change kits that include most of the necessary equipment are available and are recommended.[12]

For assisting with removal

Gloves ■ 10-mL prefilled syringe containing preservative-free normal saline flush solution (or a syringe specifically designed to generate lower injection pressure)[4] ■ 10-mL prefilled syringe (or a syringe specifically designed to generate lower injection pressure)[4] containing prescribed locking solution (preservative-free normal saline solution or heparinized saline flush solution [10 units/mL concentration])[13] ■ antiseptic pads (chlorhexidine and alcohol, alcohol, or tincture of iodine) ■ sterile 2" × 2" (5 cm × 5 cm) gauze pad ■ Optional: sterile cap, sterile gauze dressing, paper tape.

Preparation of equipment

Inspect all IV equipment and supplies. If a product is expired, is defective, or has compromised integrity, remove it from patient use, label it as expired or defective, and report the expiration or defect as directed by your facility.[14]

For assisting with insertion

Confirm with the practitioner the size and type of the device and the insertion site. Using a prefilled syringe with preservative-free flush solution, prime the noncoring needle with the extension set. Use strict sterile no-touch technique for all priming, and ensure all tubing is free of air.[4] After you've primed the tubing, recheck all connections for tightness. Make sure that sealed caps cover all open end.

For administering a bolus injection

If needed, access the port using the appropriate noncoring needle. Review the medication monograph so that you know the actions, adverse effects, and administration rate of the medication you'll be injecting.[5,12,15]

If needed, draw up the prescribed medication in the syringe and dilute it. Whenever possible, administer pharmacy-prepared or commercially available products.[16,17] Many medications come in unit-dose syringes.

For administering a continuous infusion

Review the patient's medical record *to determine the location of the implanted port and whether it's currently accessed with a noncoring needle.* If needed, access the port using the appropriate noncoring needle. Make sure the electronic infusion device is in good working order.[18]

For obtaining a blood sample

If necessary, contact the laboratory for questions regarding specimen tubes, order of draw, and recommended transport environment for proper collection of the ordered tests.

Implementation

Assisting with insertion

■ Conduct a preprocedure verification *to make sure that all relevant documentation, related information, and equipment are available and correctly identified to the patient's identifiers.*[19]

■ Confirm that informed consent has been obtained and that the signed consent form is in the patient's medical record.[20,21,22,23,24]

■ Gather and prepare the necessary equipment and supplies.

■ Use an insertion checklist *to adhere to infection prevention and safety practices during insertion.*[6,8,9,10,24,25] Stop the procedure immediately if you observe any breaks in sterile technique.

■ Perform hand hygiene.[6,10,26,27,28,29,30,31,32]

■ Confirm the patient's identity using at least two patient identifiers.[33]

■ Provide privacy.[34,35,36,37]

■ Reinforce to the patient the practitioner's explanation to the patient and family (if appropriate) according to their individual communication and learning needs *to increase their understanding, allay their fears, and enhance cooperation.*[21,22,23,24,38]

■ Answer questions about movement restrictions, cosmetic concerns, and management regimens *to allay the patient's fears.*

■ Administer an antibiotic, if prescribed, following safe medication administration practices.[15,17,39,40]

■ Close the door to the room, and place a sign on the door that reads STERILE PROCEDURE IN PROGRESS. DO NOT ENTER.[5,12]

■ Raise the bed to waist level before providing care *to prevent caregiver back strain.*[41]

■ Put on a cap and mask.[5,6]

■ Place a fluid-impermeable pad under the patient *to protect the bed from becoming soiled.*

■ If the intended site is visibly soiled, clean the area with antiseptic soap and water.[12,25]

■ Remove excess hair from the intended insertion site, if needed, using single-patient-use scissors or disposable-head surgical clippers *to facilitate dressing application.*[12,25]

■ Perform hand hygiene.[6,10,26,27,28,29,30,31,32]

■ Establish a sterile field on a table, and assemble supplies on the sterile field.

■ Label all medications, medication containers, and other solutions on and off the sterile field.[42,43]

■ Perform hand hygiene.[6,10,26,27,28,29,30,31,32]

■ Put on a gown and sterile gloves *to comply with maximal barrier precautions.*[5,6,8,10,44,45,46]

■ Assist the practitioner as needed with administration of a local anesthetic. Keep in mind that a general anesthetic may occasionally be administered instead.[47]

■ Prepare the insertion site using chlorhexidine-based antiseptic sponges, and allow it to dry completely.[6,9]

■ Before beginning the procedure, the practitioner will put on a mask and a cap, perform hand hygiene, put on a sterile gown and gloves, and drape the patient from head to toe *to comply with maximal barrier precautions.*[6,9] During the procedure, you may be responsible for handing equipment and supplies to the practitioner.

■ Conduct a time-out immediately before the procedure starts *to perform a final assessment that the correct patient, site, positioning, and procedure are identified and, as applicable, all relevant information and necessary equipment are available.*[19]

■ If requested by the practitioner, using sterile technique, hand the practitioner the ultrasound device with the sterile probe cover and apply sterile ultrasound gel. The practitioner locates the vessel using the device *to reduce the risk of insertion-related complications.*[48,49]

■ Assist as needed while the practitioner inserts the device. The practitioner makes a small incision and introduces the guide wire and catheter, which the practitioner typically advances into the subclavian vein, terminating in the superior vena cava. After X-ray or fluoroscopy confirms correct placement of the catheter tip, the practitioner creates a subcutaneous pocket over a bony prominence in the chest wall. The practitioner then tunnels the catheter to the pocket. Next, the practitioner connects the catheter to the reservoir, places the reservoir in the pocket, flushes it with preservative-free saline solution, and then instills heparin flush solution. Lastly, the practitioner sutures the reservoir to the underlying fasciae and closes the incision with the preferred skin closure device.

■ Access the implanted port with a noncoring needle and attach the primed extension set and needleless connector as ordered. If available at your facility, place a disinfectant-containing end cap on the needleless connector.[50,51]

■ Apply a chlorhexidine-impregnated sponge dressing, if required by your facility, *to reduce the risk of central line–related bloodstream infection.*[50]

■ Apply a sterile occlusive dressing over the site.[4]

■ Discard used supplies in appropriate receptacles.[46,52]

■ Return the bed to the lowest position *to prevent falls and maintain patient safety.*[53]

■ Remove and discard your personal protective equipment.[44,46,52]

■ Perform hand hygiene.[6,10,26,27,28,29,30,31,32]

■ Document the procedure.[54,55,56,57,58]

Accessing a top-entry port

■ Review the patient's medical record *to determine the type (such as a power-injectable device or single or double port) and location of the implanted port, whether it has been previously accessed, and the patient's response to the procedure.* If a power injection will be performed using the implanted port, the non-coring Huber needle used to access the port must be identified as power-injection compatible.[12]

■ Ensure that placement of the catheter tip has been confirmed.

■ Verify the practitioner's order, if required by your facility.

■ Determine whether the patient has a history of allergies or contraindications to the antiseptic, anesthetic, or prescribed solution.[12]

■ Gather and prepare the necessary equipment and supplies.

■ Perform hand hygiene.[6,10,26,27,28,29,30,31,32]

■ Confirm the patient's identity using at least two patient identifiers.[33]

■ Provide privacy.[34,35,36,37]

■ Explain the procedure to the patient and family (if appropriate) according to their individual communication and learning needs *to increase their understanding, allay their fears, and enhance cooperation.*[21,22,23,24,38]

■ Assess the patient's pain tolerance and discuss the patient's preferences for using a local anesthetic before accessing the port.[4,5,12]

■ Administer a topical anesthetic, as needed and prescribed, following safe medication administration practices.[5,12,39,40,59,60]

■ If appropriate, raise the bed to waist level before providing care *to prevent caregiver back strain.*[41]

■ Perform hand hygiene.[6,10,26,27,28,29,30,31,32]

■ Put on gloves *to comply with standard precautions.*[44,45,46]

■ Position the patient for comfort with head turned away from the implanted port.[5,12,61] Alternatively, put a mask on the patient.[61]

■ Assess the skin overlying the port and the tissue surrounding the port.[5] Observe for signs of infection or thrombosis. Don't insert the noncoring needle if erythema, inflammation, exudate, supraclavicular swelling, or venous distention is present. Instead, notify the practitioner.

■ Palpate and locate the septum; assess for device rotation.[5,12,61]

■ Remove and discard your gloves.[44,46,52]

■ Perform hand hygiene.[6,10,26,27,28,29,30,31,32]

■ Put on a mask.[5,12,44,61]

■ Open the supplies and prepare a sterile field using a sterile drape. Using sterile technique, place the supplies on the sterile field.[5,12]

■ Perform hand hygiene.[6,10,26,27,28,29,30,31,32]

■ Put on sterile gloves.[5,12,44,46]

■ Clean the implanted port access site with an antiseptic solution following the manufacturer's instructions. For chlorhexidine (preferred), apply with an applicator using a vigorous side-to-side motion for 30 seconds, and allow to dry completely. For povidone-iodine solution, apply using a swab. Begin at the intended insertion site, moving outward in

concentric circles. Allow the solution to dry completely, typically at least 2 minutes.[5,12,25]

■ Attach a needleless connector to the extension set, which is connected to the noncoring needle.[5,12]

■ Maintaining sterility of the syringe tip, attach a syringe containing preservative-free normal saline solution to the needleless connector and prime the extension set and noncoring needle with preservative-free normal saline solution.[5,12] Clamp the extension tubing.[61]

■ With your nondominant hand, palpate and stabilize the implanted port.[5,12]

■ Grasp the noncoring needle with your dominant hand, and insert the noncoring needle perpendicular to the skin through the septum of the port until the needle tip comes in contact with the back of the port.[5,12,61] Consider orienting the bevel of the noncoring needle in the opposite direction from the outflow channel where the catheter is attached to the port body; *this bevel orientation allows for removal of a greater amount of protein when flushing.*[4,62]

■ Unclamp the extension tubing. Aspirate for blood return that's the color and consistency of whole blood *to confirm device patency.* If you don't obtain any blood return, take steps to locate an external cause of obstruction.[13]

■ If you obtain blood return, slowly inject preservative-free normal saline solution into the port. Use a minimum volume of twice the internal volume of the catheter system. Don't forcibly flush the device; further evaluate the device if you meet resistance.[5,12,13] Troubleshoot the system and notify the patient's practitioner if you can't confirm patency.

NURSING ALERT If you can't aspirate blood return to confirm needle placement, have the patient change positions, raise the arms, cough, or perform the Valsalva maneuver *to increase thoracic pressure and increase yield for a blood return.* If you still can't obtain blood return or confirm needle placement, clamp the tubing and notify the practitioner before proceeding.[12] (See *Troubleshooting an implanted port,* page 418.)

■ Secure the noncoring needle with sterile tape with an engineered stabilization device, if available. An engineered stabilization device is recommended *to reduce vascular access device motion, which increases the risk of unintentional catheter dislodgement and complications requiring premature catheter removal.*[61,63] Support the wings of the noncoring needle (if present) with sterile gauze; make sure the gauze doesn't prevent visualization of the needle insertion site.[5,12]

■ If applicable, place a chlorhexidine-impregnated sponge dressing beneath the needle. The edges of the radial slit of the sponge dressing must touch *to maximize antimicrobial action.* Always follow the manufacturer's directions.[6,68,69,70]

■ Apply a sterile transparent semipermeable dressing over the insertion site, noncoring needle, and upper portion of the extension tubing *to maintain sterility of the system and enable visualization of the needle and insertion site.*[5,12]

■ Perform a vigorous mechanical scrub of the needleless connector device for at least 5 seconds with an antiseptic pad and allow it to dry completely.[5,8,12,50]

■ Attach the primed IV administration set to the needleless connector. Trace the tubing from the patient to its point of origin *to make sure that you are attaching the tubing to the correct port before beginning the infusion.*[15,71,72] Route the tubing in a standardized direction if the patient has other tubing and catheters that have different purposes. Label the tubing at both the distal end (near the patient connection) and proximal end (near the source container) *to reduce the risk of misconnection* if multiple IV lines will be used.[15] Begin infusion therapy, as ordered. Alternatively, lock the device with prescribed locking solution[5,13] and place a disinfectant-containing end cap on the needleless connector, if available, *to reduce the risk of vascular catheter-associated infection.*[51,52]

■ Label the dressing with the current date or the date the dressing is due to be changed, as directly by your facility.[12]

■ Discard used supplies in appropriate receptacles.[45,51]

■ Return the bed to the lowest position *to prevent falls and maintain patient safety.*[52]

■ Remove and discard your gloves and mask[43,45,51] and perform hand hygiene.[6,10,26,27,28,29,30,31,32]

■ Document the procedure.[53,54,55,56,57]

TROUBLESHOOTING

TROUBLESHOOTING AN IMPLANTED PORT

Follow these tips to troubleshoot an implanted port.

Inability to flush or draw blood
- Examine the line for external mechanical obstruction; ensure that the clamps are open and that the noncoring needle extension tubing or IV tubing isn't kinked.[64]
- If the port is located in the patient's upper anterior chest wall, move the patient's arm, shoulder, and head and attempt to aspirate for blood. Notify the practitioner if aspiration only occurs in a certain position. The patient may need to be evaluated for "pinch-off" of the catheter.[2]
- Verify the correct needle length was used and is properly placed. Replace the needle as necessary.[2]
- Occlusion can occur as a result of external or internal mechanical obstruction, including nonthrombotic occlusions (such as drug precipitates) or thrombotic occlusions caused by fibrin deposits or blood clots (thrombosis).
- If you suspect occlusion from precipitation, attempt to aspirate to clear the port or tubing. If you're successful, flush the port with sterile preservative-free normal saline solution between all medications. If you're unsuccessful, obtain a practitioner's order for an appropriate catheter clearance agent to dissolve the precipitate. Ensure that the instilled volume of the agent to clear precipitates doesn't exceed the internal volume of the port system so that the catheter clearance agent stays in the port and doesn't go into the patient's bloodstream.[64]
- If occlusion is due to thrombosis, instill low-dose alteplase as prescribed.[64,65]
- If the patient reports pain or if complete resistance is met, discontinue the flush procedure. Consult with the practitioner about performing a dye study to further define the problem. Determine which staff member is qualified to perform declotting of central venous devices in your facility.

Infiltration or extravasation
- Stop the infusion immediately.[66,67]

- Assess for a dislodged catheter, a dislodged noncoring needle, or a rupture or leak from the external catheter.[12]
- Aspirate for blood; don't attempt to flush to prevent moving additional medication into the surrounding tissue.[67]
- Assess the extent of infiltration or extravasation using a standardized scale.[67]
- Aspirate fluid from the catheter using a small syringe.[67]
- Estimate the volume of fluid that has escaped into the tissue based on the rate of injection or infusion and the time of your last assessment.[67]
- Remove the noncoring needle.[66] Don't attempt reaccess the port until you can treat the problem appropriately and swelling resolves. Consult the practitioner as indicated.
- Consult the pharmacist or practitioner to determine whether to apply cold or warm compresses.[66,67]
- If necessary, administer the appropriate antidote, as prescribed.[67]

Local infection
- Assess the skin surrounding the port and noncoring needle for erythema, inflammation, tenderness, drainage, and skin breakdown.
- Monitor the patient's temperature and vital signs.
- Notify the practitioner of signs and symptoms of localized infection.
- Obtain culture specimens as ordered.[11]

Systemic infection
- Monitor the patient's temperature and vital signs.
- Notify the practitioner of signs and symptoms of systemic infection.
- Obtain blood culture specimens as ordered.[11]
- Administer antibiotics as prescribed (after obtaining culture specimens).[65]

Extrusion
- Notify the practitioner that the port reservoir is extruding and is visible through the patient's skin *to determine whether port removal is required.*

Obtaining a blood sample
- Verify the practitioner's order for blood sampling.[73]
- Perform hand hygiene.[6,10,26,27,28,29,30,31,32]
- Confirm the patient's identity using at least two patient identifiers.[33]
- Explain the procedure to the patient and family (if appropriate) according to their individual communication and learning needs *to increase their understanding, allay their fears, and enhance cooperation.*[21,22,23,24,38]
- If fasting is required before testing, verify that the patient has fasted. If any other preparations (such as administering or holding medication) are required before testing, make sure that they were completed.[73]
- Raise the bed to waist level before providing care *to prevent caregiver back strain.*[41]
- Perform hand hygiene.[6,10,26,27,28,29,30,31,32]
- Unless contraindicated, place the patient in the supine position with head slightly elevated *to allow for optimal access.*
- If they aren't already marked clearly, label the preservative-free normal saline flush syringes.
- If you're using a needleless blood collection tube holder with the discard method, label the discard blood collection tube *to prevent confusing it with the actual specimen.* If you're using a syringe with the discard method, label one of the preservative-free normal saline flush syringes as a flush-and-discard syringe and use it to both flush the port and obtain the discard sample *to avoid re-accessing the needleless connector.*[73]
- Perform hand hygiene.[6,10,26,27,28,29,30,31,32]
- Put on gloves; also put on protective eyewear or a mask with face shield if splashing is likely.[43,45,46]
- Locate the noncoring needle extension tubing.[4]
- Stop infusions that are infusing through the port before drawing the blood sample *to prevent inaccurate blood test results.* Research hasn't established the appropriate length of time for stopping fluid flow; one study suggests a 10-minute wait time before drawing the sample.[73] Trace the

tubing from the patient to its point of origin *to make sure you've stopped the proper infusion.*[71,72] Close the clamp on the extension tubing, and clamp and disconnect the IV tubing, maintaining sterility. Cover the IV tubing end with a sterile cap.[73]
- Assess the skin overlying the port, the tissue surrounding the port, and the site of needle entry. Observe for signs of infection, thrombosis, device rotation, and skin erosion. Hold the procedure and call the practitioner if you observe any complications.[74]
- Close the clamp on the extension tubing.
- If a disinfectant-containing end cap is covering the end of the needleless connector, remove and discard it.[50,51]
- Perform a vigorous mechanical scrub of the needleless connector for at least 5 seconds using an antiseptic pad and then allow it to dry completely.[8,50,75]
- Maintaining the sterility of the syringe tip, attach a prefilled syringe containing preservative-free normal saline solution to the needleless connector. (Use a 10-mL syringe or a syringe specifically designed to generate lower injection pressure.) Unclamp the extension tubing and slowly aspirate for a blood return that is the color and consistency of whole blood. If you don't obtain a blood return, take steps to locate an external cause of the obstruction.[5,12,13]
- If you obtain a blood return, slowly inject preservative-free normal saline solution into the port. Use a minimum volume of twice the internal volume of the catheter system. Don't forcibly flush the device; further evaluate the device if you meet resistance.[5,12,13]
- Use the discard or push-pull method to obtain the blood sample.[73] If you're obtaining a sample for blood cultures, see the "Blood culture sample collection" procedure.

Discard method
- Obtain a discard sample *to clear the catheter's dead space volume and remove any blood diluted with flush solution.*

■ If you're using a needleless blood collection tube holder: Reclamp the tubing, and then remove and discard the syringe in a puncture-resistant sharps disposal container.[52] Perform a vigorous mechanical scrub of the needleless connector for at least 5 seconds using an antiseptic pad; then allow it to dry completely.[8,50,75] Attach the blood collection tube holder to the needleless connector, release the clamp, and engage the labeled discard blood collection tube. Limit the discard as directed by your facility *to ensure that a minimal amount of blood is taken from the patient as waste.*[12]

■ If you're using a syringe: Use the attached syringe you used for flushing and aspirate the discard volume. Minimum discard volumes aren't established, so limit discard volume as directed by your facility *to ensure that a minimal amount of blood is taken from the patient as waste.*[12,73]

■ Clamp the extension tubing, and then remove the labeled discard blood collection tube from the needleless blood collection tube holder, or remove the labeled discard syringe and discard it in a puncture-resistant sharps disposal container.[46,52]

■ Obtain blood samples, as ordered. If you're using a needleless blood collection tube holder, insert another blood collection tube into the needleless blood collection tube holder, unclamp the tubing, and follow the correct order of draw. If you're using a syringe, perform a vigorous mechanical scrub of the needleless connector for at least 5 seconds using an antiseptic pad and allow it to dry completely,[8,50] connect an empty syringe to the needleless connector, release the clamp, and withdraw the blood sample. Repeat the steps until you obtain all of the necessary blood samples.

■ Clamp the extension tubing and remove the needleless blood collection tube holder or the syringe.

Push-pull method

■ Using the attached syringe that you used for flushing, aspirate 4 to 6 mL of blood.[76]

■ Keeping the syringe attached to the tubing, push to reinfuse the blood into the port.

■ Repeat the aspiration and reinfusion sequence three to five times (five cycles is most common).[73,76]

■ Clamp the extension tubing, and then remove and discard the syringe in a puncture-resistant sharps disposal container.[46,52]

■ Perform a vigorous mechanical scrub of the needleless connector for at least 5 seconds using an antiseptic pad; then allow it to dry completely.[8,50]

■ Obtain blood samples, as ordered. If you're using a needleless blood collection tube holder, attach the needleless blood collection tube holder to the needleless connector, release the clamp, and engage the blood collection tube into the needleless blood collection tube holder using the correct order of draw. If you're using a syringe, connect an empty syringe to the needleless connector, release the clamp, and withdraw the blood sample. Repeat the steps until you obtain all necessary blood samples.

■ Clamp the catheter and remove the needleless blood collection tube holder or the syringe.

Completing the procedure

■ Label the samples with the patient's name, identification number, name of the test, and date and time of collection in the presence of the patient *to prevent mislabeling.*[73,77]

■ Place all blood collection tubes in a laboratory biohazard transport bag and send them to the laboratory with a completed laboratory request form.[46]

■ Discard used supplies in appropriate receptacles.[45,51]

■ Remove and discard your gloves and mask[43,45,51] and perform hand hygiene.[6,10,26,27,28,29,30,31,32]

■ Document the procedure.[53,54,55,56,57]

Administering a bolus injection

■ Review the patient's medical record *to determine the location of the implanted port, whether it's currently accessed with a noncoring needle, and the patient's response to previous procedures.*

■ Ensure that the placement of the catheter tip has been confirmed.

■ Compare the medication label with the order in the patient's medical record.[15,17,41,60,78]

■ Check the patient's medical record for an allergy or contraindication to the prescribed medication. If an allergy or contraindication exists, don't administer the medication; instead, notify the practitioner.[15,17,40,60,78]

■ Check the expiration date on the medication. If the medication is expired, return it to the pharmacy and obtain new medication.[15,17,40,60,78]

■ Visually inspect the solution for particles, discoloration, or other loss of integrity; don't administer the medication if its integrity is compromised.[15,17,40,60,78]

■ Discuss any unresolved concerns about the medication with the patient's practitioner.[15,17,40,60,78]

■ Verify that the medication is being administered at the proper time, in the prescribed dose, and by the correct route *to reduce the risk of medication errors.*[15,17,40,60,78]

NURSING ALERT Some bolus injections are considered high-alert medications *because they can cause significant patient harm when used in error.*[79] If required by your facility, before administering a bolus injection, have another nurse perform an independent double-check *to verify the patient's identity and make sure you have the correct medication in the prescribed concentration, the medication's indication corresponds with the patient's diagnosis, the dosage calculations are correct and the dosing formula used to derive the final dose is correct, and the prescribed route of administration is safe and proper for the patient.*[80,81]

■ Review the patient's baseline vital signs and observe for changes that may indicate a local or systemic infection.

■ Perform hand hygiene.[6,10,26,27,28,29,30,31,32]

■ Confirm the patient's identity using at least two patient identifiers.[33]

■ Explain the procedure to the patient and family (if appropriate) according to their individual communication and learning needs *to increase their understanding, allay their fears, and enhance cooperation.*[21,22,23,24,38]

■ If the patient is receiving the medication for the first time, teach the patient and family (if appropriate) about potential adverse reactions and any other concerns related to the medication.[8]

■ If your facility uses a bar code technology, use it as directed by your facility.[81]

■ Raise the bed to waist level before providing care *to prevent caregiver back strain.*[41]

■ Perform hand hygiene.[6,10,26,27,28,29,30,31,32]

■ Put on gloves *to comply with standard precautions.*[44,45,46]

■ If a disinfectant-containing end cap is in place at the end of the needleless connector, remove and discard it.[50,51]

■ Perform a vigorous mechanical scrub of the needleless connector for at least 5 seconds using an antiseptic pad; then allow it to dry completely.[8,50,75]

■ Maintaining the sterility of the syringe tip, attach a prefilled syringe containing preservative-free normal saline solution to the needleless connector. (Use a 10-mL syringe or a syringe specifically designed to generate lower injection pressure.) Unclamp the extension tubing and slowly aspirate for a blood return that is the color and consistency of whole blood. If you don't obtain a blood return, take steps to locate an external cause of the obstruction.[5,12,13]

■ If you obtain a blood return, slowly inject preservative-free normal saline solution into the port. Use a minimum volume of twice the internal volume of the catheter system. Don't forcibly flush the device; further evaluate the device if you meet resistance.[5,12,13]

■ Examine the skin surrounding the needle for signs of infiltration, such as swelling and tenderness. If you note these signs, stop the injection and intervene appropriately.

■ Remove and discard the saline syringe.[46,52]

■ Perform a vigorous mechanical scrub of the needleless connector for at least 5 seconds using an antiseptic pad; then allow it to dry completely.[8,50,75]

■ Maintaining the sterility of the syringe tip, connect the syringe with the medication for the IV bolus injection into the injection port of the needleless connector.[13]

NURSING ALERT After confirming patency of the vascular access device by using a 10-mL syringe (or a syringe specifically designed to generate lower injection pressure) filled with preservative-free normal saline solution, the medication can be administered by IV bolus injection in a syringe of appropriate size to measure and administer the required medication dose.[13,82] Don't transfer the medication to a larger syringe.[13]

■ Inject the medication at the rate indicated on the label; consult with the pharmacist before injection if a rate isn't present.[5,12]

■ Remove the syringe from the needleless connector.

■ Thoroughly disinfect the needleless connector of the access tubing with an antiseptic pad.

■ Perform a vigorous mechanical scrub of the needleless connector for at least 5 seconds using an antiseptic pad; then allow it to dry completely.[8,50,75]

■ While maintaining the sterility of the syringe tip, attach a prefilled syringe containing preservative-free normal saline solution to the needleless connector. (Use a 10-mL syringe or a syringe specifically designed to generate lower injection pressure). Unclamp the catheter and inject preservative-free normal saline solution into the catheter at the same rate of injection as the prescribed medication. Use the amount of flush solution needed to adequately clear the medication from the administration set lumen and the catheter. Don't forcibly flush the device; further evaluate the device if resistance is met. Consider using a pulsatile flushing technique, *because short boluses of the flush solution interrupted by short pauses may be more effective at removing deposits (such as fibrin, drug precipitate, and intraluminal bacteria) than a continuous low-flow technique.* Alternatively, if the medication is incompatible with normal saline solution, use dextrose 5% in water (D_5W), followed by preservative-free normal saline solution. Don't allow D_5W to remain in the catheter lumen, *because it provides nutrients for biofilm growth.*[13]

■ Remove and discard the syringe.[46,52]

■ Proceed with locking the device, if necessary. Perform a vigorous mechanical scrub of the needleless connector for at least 5 seconds using an antiseptic pad; then allow it to dry completely.[8,50,75] While maintaining the sterility of the syringe tip, attach a syringe containing locking solution (such as a heparin lock solution) to the needleless connector.[13] Slowly inject the locking solution.[13]

■ Close the clamp on the access tubing according to the type of needleless connector used *to reduce blood reflux.* For a positive-pressure needleless connector, clamp the catheter after disconnecting the syringe.[5,12] For a negative-pressure needleless connector, maintain pressure on the syringe while clamping the catheter.[5,12] For a neutral needleless connector, clamp the catheter before or after disconnecting the syringe.[5,12] For an antireflux needleless connector, clamp the catheter and disconnect the syringe; specific clamping sequence isn't required.[83,84]

■ Place a new disinfectant-containing end cap, if available,[50,51] or deaccess the implanted port, if indicated.

■ Discard used supplies in appropriate receptacles.[45,51]

■ Return the bed to the lowest position *to prevent falls and maintain patient safety.*[52]

■ Remove and discard your gloves.[43,45,51]

■ Perform hand hygiene.[6,10,26,27,28,29,30,31,32]

■ Monitor the patient for adverse reactions to the prescribed medication.[12,85]

■ If the patient is receiving IV opioid medication, frequently monitor the patient's respiratory rate, oxygen saturation level by pulse oximetry, end-tidal carbon dioxide level by capnography (if available), and sedation level using a standardized sedation scale *to decrease the risk of adverse events associated with IV opioid use.*[85,86] Explain the assessment and monitoring process to the patient and family. Tell them to alert a staff member if any breathing problem or sedation occurs.[85]

■ Perform hand hygiene.[6,10,26,27,28,29,30,31,32]

■ Document the procedure.[53,54,55,56,57]

Administering a continuous infusion

■ Make sure that confirmation of the placement of the catheter tip has been obtained.

■ Verify the practitioner's order for the type of infusion to be administered.

■ Review the patient's baseline vital signs and observe for changes that may indicate a local or systemic infection.

■ Gather and prepare the necessary equipment and supplies

■ Compare the IV solution label with the order in the patient's medical record.[15,17,39,40,60]

■ Check the patient's medical record for an allergy or contraindication to the prescribed solution or medication. If an allergy or contraindication exists, don't administer the medication; notify the practitioner.[15,17,39,40,60]

■ Discuss any unresolved concerns about the solution or medication with the patient's practitioner.[15,17,39,40,60]

■ Check the expiration date on the IV solution. If the solution is expired, return it to the pharmacy and obtain a new soliton.

■ Visually inspect the IV solution for particulates, discoloration, or other loss of integrity, and check the expiration date. Replace the solution if the integrity is compromised or if it's expired.[15,17,39,40,60]

■ Perform hand hygiene.[6,10,26,27,28,29,30,31,32]

■ Confirm the patient's identity using at least two patient identifiers.[33]

■ Provide privacy.[34,35,36,37]

■ Explain the procedure to the patient and family (if appropriate) according to their individual communication and learning needs *to increase their understanding, allay their fears, and enhance cooperation.*[21,22,23,24,38]

■ Raise the bed to waist level before providing care *to prevent caregiver back strain.*[41]

■ Perform hand hygiene.[6,10,26,27,28,29,30,31,32]

■ Locate the noncoring needle extension tubing under the patient's gown.

■ Assess the skin overlying the port, the tissue surrounding the port, and the site of needle entry. Observe for signs of infection, thrombosis, device rotation, and skin erosion. Hold the procedure and notify the practitioner if you observe any complications.

■ If your facility uses a bar code technology, use it as directed by your facility.

■ Perform hand hygiene.[6,10,26,27,28,29,30,31,32]

■ Put on gloves *to comply with standard precautions.*[44,45,46]

■ Close the clamp on the IV administration set tubing, remove the protective cover from the administration set's spike and the IV infusion container, insert the spike into the solution container, and hang the container on an IV pole.[5,12]

■ Prime the administration set tubing of the IV administration set *to purge the tubing of air.* (See the "IV therapy preparation" procedure.)

■ If a disinfectant-containing end cap is in place, remove it from the end of the needleless connector and discard it.[50,51]

■ Perform a vigorous mechanical scrub of the needleless connector for at least 5 seconds using an antiseptic pad; then allow it to dry completely.[8,50,75]

■ Maintaining the sterility of the syringe tip, attach a prefilled syringe containing preservative-free normal saline solution to the needleless connector. (Use a 10-mL syringe or a syringe specifically designed to generate lower injection pressure.) Unclamp the catheter and slowly aspirate for a blood return that is the color and consistency of whole blood. If you don't obtain a blood return, take steps to locate an external cause of the obstruction.[5,12,13] Have the patient change positions, raise the arms over the head, take a deep breath and hold it, or cough *to increase intrathoracic pressure and increase yield for blood return.*[12] If you still can't obtain a blood return or confirm noncoring needle placement, notify the practitioner.

■ If you obtain a blood return, slowly inject preservative-free normal saline solution into the port. Use a minimum volume of twice the internal volume of the catheter system. Don't forcibly flush the device; further evaluate the device if you meet resistance.[5,12,13]

■ Remove the syringe.

■ Perform a vigorous mechanical scrub of the needleless connector for at least 5 seconds using an antiseptic pad; then allow it to dry completely.[8,50,75]

■ Connect and secure the IV administration set tubing of the prescribed IV solution to the needleless connector of the extension tubing.

■ Trace the tubing from the patient to its point of origin *to make sure it's connected to the proper port before beginning the infusion.*[15,71,72] Route the tubing in a standardized direction if the patient has other tubing and catheters that have different purposes. Label the tubing at both the distal end (near the patient connection) and proximal end (near the source container) *to reduce the risk of misconnection* if multiple IV lines will be used.[72]

■ Following the directions for the specific infusion device, turn on the device and enter the desired infusion rate and volume according to the practitioner's order.[5,12]

- Confirm that the infusion device's display screen is displaying the correct information.
- Set the correct electronic device parameters according to the practitioner's orders and the manufacturer's instructions.[5,12] Make sure that the alarm limits are set properly, and that alarms are turned on, functioning properly, and audible to staff.[87,88,89]
- If the infusion is a high-alert medication,[79] have another nurse perform an independent double-check (if required by your facility) *to verify the patient's identity and to make sure that the correct medication is hanging in the prescribed concentration, the medication's indication corresponds with the patient's diagnosis, the dosage calculations and the dosing formula used to derive the final dose are correct, the route of administration is safe and proper for the patient, the pump settings are correct, and the infusion line is attached to the correct port.*[80]
- Compare the results of the independent double-check with the other nurse, if required, and begin the infusion if there are no discrepancies. If discrepancies exist, rectify them before beginning the infusion.[80]
- Examine the skin surrounding the implanted port for signs of extravasation or infiltration, such as swelling and tenderness. If you note these signs, or if the patient complains of stinging, burning, or pain at the site, stop the infusion and intervene appropriately.[67]
- Label the IV tubing with the date of initiation or the date it's due to be changed, as directed by your facility.[15]
- Return the bed to the lowest position *to prevent falls and maintain patient safety.*[52]
- Discard used supplies in appropriate receptacles.[45,51]
- Remove and discard your gloves and mask[43,45,51] and perform hand hygiene.[6,10,26,27,28,29,30,31,32]
- Monitor the patient's intake and output and electrolyte levels, as ordered, *to promptly recognize fluid and electrolyte imbalances.*[17,85]
- Monitor the rate of infusion, site condition, and patency at a rate indicated by the prescribed infusion or patient factors.[5,12]
- Document the procedure.[53,54,55,56,57]

Dressing change

- Review the patient's medical record for information related to the implanted port and allergies to the planned antiseptic or any adhesives.[12]
- Gather and prepare the necessary equipment and supplies.
- Perform hand hygiene.[6,10,26,27,28,29,30,31,32]
- Confirm the patient's identity using at least two patient identifiers.[33]
- Provide privacy.[34,35,36,37]
- Explain the procedure to the patient and family (if appropriate) according to their individual communication and learning needs *to increase their understanding, allay their fears, and enhance cooperation.*[21,22,23,24,38]
- Raise the bed to waist level before providing care *to prevent caregiver back strain.*[42]
- Put on a mask.[12]
- Perform hand hygiene.[6,10,26,27,28,29,30,31,32]
- Assemble the supplies on a sterile field.[12]
- Perform hand hygiene.[6,10,26,27,28,29,30,31,32]
- Put on gloves *to comply with standard precautions.*[44,45,46]
- Assess the implanted port site for bleeding, redness, swelling, tenderness, induration, and drainage. Notify the practitioner of any concerns.[12]
- Remove the existing dressing by lifting the edge of the dressing and gently pulling the dressing perpendicular to the skin toward the access site *to prevent needle dislodgment and tearing or stripping of fragile skin.*[13]
- Discard the dressing in an appropriate receptacle.[46,52]
- If a chlorhexidine-impregnated sponge dressing is in place to provide sustained antimicrobial action at the insertion site, remove it and discard it in an appropriate receptacle.[46,52]
- Remove the engineered stabilization device (if used and appropriate) according to the manufacturer's instructions, and then discard it in an appropriate receptacle.[12]
- If you are changing the noncoring needle, deaccess the implanted port and then reaccess the port.

NURSING ALERT The noncoring needle should be changed at least every 7 days when the implanted port is being used for infusion.[12]

- Remove and discard your gloves.[12,46]

- Perform hand hygiene.[6,10,26,27,28,29,30,31,32]
- Put on sterile gloves.[12]
- Clean the site with chlorhexidine using a back-and-forth motion for at least 30 seconds *to provide skin antisepsis.* Chlorhexidine is the preferred antiseptic.[12] If the patient is sensitive to chlorhexidine, use tincture of iodine, povidone-iodine, or alcohol swabs.[74] If you use povidone-iodine solution, apply it using swabs, and allow it to remain on the skin for at least 1½ minutes or, if necessary, a longer time until it dries. Take care not to dislodge the noncoring needle. Allow the area to air-dry completely.[12]
- If used in your facility, place a chlorhexidine-impregnated sponge dressing beneath the noncoring needle according to the manufacturer's instructions.[27]
- Apply a skin barrier solution according to the manufacturer's instructions *to reduce the risk of medical adhesive–related skin injury.* Don't use compound tincture of benzoin, *because it may increase the bonding of adhesives to the skin, causing skin injury when removal of the adhesive-based engineered stabilization device occurs.* Don't apply skin barrier solution beneath the chlorhexidine-impregnated sponge dressing or the gel component of the dressing (if used).[32]
- Secure the noncoring needle and tubing with an engineered stabilization device, if available and used at your facility.[12] *Guidelines recommend using an engineered stabilization device because it reduces vascular access device motion; such motion increases the risk of unintentional catheter dislodgment and complications that can lead to the need for premature catheter removal.*[63]
- Support the wings of the noncoring needle with sterile gauze or foam, if needed; make sure that the gauze doesn't prevent visualization of the needle insertion site.[26]
- Apply a sterile transparent semipermeable dressing over the insertion site, noncoring needle, and upper portion of the extension tubing *to maintain the sterility of the system while enabling visualization of the needle and insertion site.*[12] Alternatively, apply a sterile 4" × 4" (10 cm × 10 cm) gauze dressing in place of the semipermeable dressing.[12,46] If the patient has fragile skin, use dressings and tape specially formulated for fragile skin *to prevent skin stripping and tearing during removal.*[90]
- Label the dressing with the current date or the date the dressing is next due to be changed, as directed by your facility.[12]
- Return the bed to the lowest position *to prevent falls and maintain patient safety.*[52]
- Discard used supplies in appropriate receptacles.[45,46]
- Remove and discard your gloves and mask.[12,46]
- Perform hand hygiene.[6,10,26,27,28,29,30,31,32]
- Document the procedure.[53,54,55,56,57]

Assisting with removal

- Review the patient's medical record to determine the type and location of the implanted port, the patient's response to previous procedures, any history of allergies or medical conditions that would contraindicate heparin use, and the patient's baseline vital signs and any changes that may indicate a local or systemic infection.
- Gather and prepare the necessary equipment and supplies.
- Perform hand hygiene.[6,10,26,27,28,29,30,31,32]
- Confirm the patient's identity using at least two patient identifiers.[33]
- Provide privacy.[34,35,36,37]
- Assess the cognitive levels of the patient and family as well as their readiness and ability to process information. Be aware that the ability to learn may be impaired as a result of age, stress, or anxiety.
- Explain the procedure to the patient and family (if appropriate) according to their individual communication and learning needs *to increase their understanding, allay their fears, and enhance cooperation.*[21,22,23,24,38]
- Raise the bed to waist level before providing care *to prevent caregiver back strain.*[41]
- Perform hand hygiene.[6,10,26,27,28,29,30,31,32]
- Locate the noncoring needle extension tubing under the patient's gown.
- Assess the skin surrounding the implanted port and the noncoring needle for signs of infection, thrombosis, device rotation, skin erosion, and other complications. Stop the procedure, and notify the practitioner if you observe any signs of complications.[74]

- Establish a clean work area, and open the supplies using sterile technique.
- Perform hand hygiene.[6,10,26,27,28,29,30,31,32]
- Put on gloves *to comply with standard precautions*.[44,45,46] If the implanted port has an IV solution infusing, trace the tubing from the patient to the point of origin *to ensure that you're handling the correct tubing*,[71] close the clamp on the extension tubing, stop the infusion, and then disconnect the IV tubing while maintaining sterility. If you're replacing the noncoring needle, cover the IV tubing end with a sterile cap for the next IV infusion. Alternatively, if a disinfectant-containing end cap is in place, remove it from the end of the needleless connector.[50,51]
- Perform a vigorous mechanical scrub of the needleless connector for at least 5 seconds using an antiseptic pad. Allow it to dry completely.[8,50,75]
- While maintaining sterility of the syringe tip, attach a prefilled syringe containing preservative-free normal saline solution to the needleless connector. (Use a 10-mL syringe or a syringe specifically designed to generate lower injection pressure.) Unclamp the catheter and slowly aspirate for a blood return that's the color and consistency of whole blood. If you can't obtain a blood return, take steps to locate an external cause of obstruction.[5,12,13] If you can't obtain a blood return and needle placement is correct, don't proceed; instead, clamp the tubing and notify the practitioner immediately *to ensure prompt intervention. Diagnostic tests may be required to identify the cause of internal obstruction*.[13]
- If you obtain a blood return, slowly inject preservative-free normal saline solution into the catheter. Use a minimum volume of twice the internal volume of the catheter system. Don't forcibly flush the device; further evaluate the device if you meet resistance.[5,12,13]
- Inspect the skin surrounding the noncoring needle for signs of infiltration or extravasation, such as swelling and tenderness.
- Close the clamp on the extension tubing.
- Remove and discard the syringe.[46,52]
- Perform a vigorous mechanical scrub of the needleless connector for at least 5 seconds using an antiseptic pad. Allow it to dry completely.[46,52]
- While maintaining sterility of the syringe tip, attach the syringe of prescribed locking solution to the needleless connector, unclamp the extension tubing, and then slowly inject the solution.[5,12,13] Use a volume of locking solution equal to the internal volume of the catheter and add-on devices plus 20%; follow the catheter manufacturer's instructions for use.[13]
- *To reduce blood reflux*, follow the appropriate clamping sequence according to the type of needleless connector that you used. For a positive-pressure needleless connector, clamp the device after disconnecting the syringe.[5,12] For a negative-pressure needleless connector, maintain pressure on the syringe plunger while closing the clamp on the device or extension set before disconnecting the syringe.[5,12] For a neutral needleless connector, clamp the device before or after disconnecting the syringe.[5,12] For an antireflux needleless connector, clamp the catheter and then disconnect the syringe; a specific clamping sequence isn't required.[83,84]
- Remove the existing semipermeable transparent dressing carefully while stabilizing the port and noncoring needle. Remove the dressing by pulling the dressing perpendicular to the skin gently toward the insertion site *to prevent the skin from tearing or stripping*.[5,12,90]
- Visually inspect the needle insertion site and surrounding skin, and note the presence or absence of redness, swelling, drainage, or tenderness. Notify the practitioner of any signs of skin breakdown, infection, infiltration, extravasation, or occlusion.[6,12]
- With your nondominant hand, stabilize the port reservoir between your thumb and forefinger on the overlying skin.[12]
- Grasp the noncoring needle with your dominant hand, holding the hub of the needle between your thumb and forefinger, and remove the device.[12]
- Engage the safety mechanism and then discard the needle in a puncture-resistant sharps container.[12,46,52]
- Blot the needle insertion site with a sterile gauze pad, and apply a sterile gauze dressing if bleeding occurs.[12]
- Discard used supplies in appropriate receptacles.[43,45,51]
- Return the bed to the lowest position *to prevent falls and maintain patient safety*.[52]
- Remove and discard your gloves.[43,45,51]
- Perform hand hygiene.[6,10,26,27,28,29,30,31,32]
- Determine whether the patient or caregiver has any concerns.
- Document the procedure.[53,54,55,56,57]

Special considerations

- Assess the implantation site for infection by visually monitoring and palpating the site through an intact dressing. If the patient has a fever without an obvious source, tenderness at the insertion site, or other signs or symptoms suggesting local or bloodstream infection, remove the dressing and inspect the site thoroughly.
- Always use the smallest noncoring size needle necessary to accommodate the infusion *to prolong the life of the port and lessen the amount of pain experienced by the patient*.[4] Use a noncoring needle of a length that allows the needle to sit flush to the skin and securely within the port *to reduce the risk of needle dislodgment during access*.[4]
- Change the transparent semipermeable dressing and the needle every 5 to 7 days.[74] Gauze dressings should be changed every 48 hours. However, any dressing should be changed immediately if its integrity is compromised. If gauze is used to support the wings of an access needle and it doesn't obscure the insertion site under the transparent semipermeable dressing, it can be changed every 7 days.[4,6,74]
- Alternative pain management strategies, such as distraction or relaxation techniques, may be helpful.
- Assess for catheter function before each use, observing for such clinical signs and symptoms as lack of blood return, difficulty or inability to flush, edema, the patient's reports of hearing gurgling, flow stream sounds with flushing, paresthesia, and neurologic effects. Also assess the implantation site for signs of infection, device rotation, and skin erosion.[6,74,87]
- Assess the implantation site for infection by visually monitoring and palpating the site through an intact dressing. If the patient has a fever without an obvious source, tenderness at the insertion site, or other signs or symptoms suggestive of local or bloodstream infection, remove the dressing and inspect the site thoroughly.[9,69,74]
- Assess for and identify signs of central venous access device occlusion, including sluggish flow and the inability to withdraw blood, flush, or infuse through the device. If clotting threatens to occlude the implanted port, the practitioner may order a fibrinolytic agent *to clear the catheter*.[64,66] *Because such agents increase the risk of bleeding*, this intervention may be contraindicated in patients who have had surgery within the past 10 days, who have active internal bleeding such as GI bleeding, or who have experienced central nervous system damage, such as infarction, hemorrhage, traumatic injury, surgery, or primary or metastatic disease within the past 2 months.
- The Joint Commission issued a sentinel event alert related to managing risk during transition to new International Organization for Standardization tubing standards that were designed to prevent dangerous tubing misconnections, *which can lead to serious patient injury and death*. During the transition, trace the tubing and catheter from the patient to the point of origin before connecting or reconnecting any device or infusion, at any care transition (such as a new setting or service), and as part of the hand-off process; route tubes and catheters having different purposes in different standardized directions; when there are different access sites or several bags hanging, label the tubing at the distal and proximal ends; use tubing and equipment only as intended; and store medications for different delivery routes in separate locations.[72]
- Avoid obtaining blood samples from ports with parenteral nutrition infusing *to reduce the risk of central line–associated bloodstream infections*.[73]
- Blood drawn from an implanted port isn't recommended for blood cultures, unless the port is suspected to be the source of infection.[73] If blood cultures are drawn from the port, replace the needleless connector with a new one before obtaining the blood cultures, or draw the blood cultures directly from the port.[73]
- When drawing blood for therapeutic drug levels, draw blood from a lumen other than the lumen being used for the drug infusion when possible. Use caution in interpreting results when therapeutic drug levels are drawn from the same lumen being used to administer the medication.[73]
- Always follow the manufacturer's guidelines for flush technique and when to clamp.
- If you're having difficulty aspirating blood, have the patient change position, cough, move the arms above the head, or take a deep breath and hold it.[5]
- If using a heparin flush, be aware of any effects it may have on specimens, and flush the catheter before drawing a discard sample, if necessary.

■ Change primary or secondary continuous infusion administration sets no more frequently than every 96 hours, but at least every 7 days, and immediately upon suspected contamination or when the integrity of the product or system has been compromised.[91]

Patient teaching

If the patient is going home, thorough teaching about procedures, as well as follow-up visits from a home care nurse, will be needed *to ensure safety and successful treatment.* Tell the patient what type of port is in place, and explain the importance of carrying a port identification card.

If the patient will be accessing the port, explain that the most uncomfortable part of the procedure is the actual insertion of the needle into the skin. Once the needle has penetrated the skin, the patient will feel mostly pressure. Eventually, the skin over the port will become desensitized from frequent needle punctures. Until then, the patient may want to use a topical anesthetic.

Stress the importance of pushing the needle into the port until the patient feels the needle bevel touch the back of the port. *Many patients tend to stop short of the back of the port, leaving the needle bevel in the rubber septum.* Also stress the importance of monthly flushes when no more infusions are scheduled.

If possible, instruct a family member in all aspects of care. If the patient is receiving an infusion at home, teach the patient and family member about checking the dressing daily. Also instruct the patient to be careful to avoid needle dislodgement during activities of daily living, such as dressing, bathing, and using a seatbelt; to protect the site during bathing; and to immediately report pain, burning, stinging, or soreness at the site.[4]

Complications

Complications related to implantation include individual risk associated with local or general anesthesia, pneumothorax, perforation or laceration of vessel, air embolism, brachial plexus injury, infection, cardiac arrhythmia, and cardiac tamponade.[2] A patient with an implanted port faces risks similar to those associated with other central venous access devices, including infection, infiltration or extravasation, thrombus formation, catheter malposition, and occlusion.[12]

Be alert for signs and symptoms of air embolism, such as sudden onset of dyspnea, gasping, breathlessness, weak pulse, increased central venous pressure, loss of consciousness, chest pain, jugular vein distention, wheezing, altered mental status, altered speech, numbness, paralysis, coughing, and tachyarrhythmias. If any of these signs or symptoms occurs, place the patient on the left side in the Trendelenburg position or in a left lateral decubitus position and notify the practitioner.[92] Also be alert for signs and symptoms of sepsis and catheter-related infection (redness, drainage, edema, or tenderness at the exit site).[11]

Documentation

Record your assessment findings and interventions. Document the type, amount, rate, and duration of the infusion; appearance of the site; and any adverse reactions. Record the date and time you notified the practitioner of any complications, the practitioner's name, prescribed interventions, and the patient's response to those interventions. Note the type and amount of flush solution used, the presence or absence of blood return, any resistance to flushing, and the interventions implemented.[55]

Document the date and time you drew the sample and the volume of blood you withdrew. Include the tests for which you drew the sample and the time you sent the sample to the laboratory. Document the patency of the catheter, the absence of signs or symptoms of complications, the presence of a blood return upon aspiration, the lack of resistance when flushing, and the amount and types of flushes you used. Also note the patient's tolerance of the procedure.

When administering a bolus injection, document the medication's strength, dose, route and rate of administration, and date and time of administration. Record the patient's response to the medication as well as any adverse reactions, the date and time the practitioner was notified, prescribed interventions, and the patient's response to those interventions. Record the type and amount of flush solution used. Document the presence of a blood return and the condition of the site.

Record the date and time of each dressing change and your assessment findings during the dressing change, including the condition of the skin, dressing type, type of stabilization device (if any), site care provided, and any mechanical problems.

Document teaching provided to the patient and family (if applicable), their understanding of that teaching, and any need for follow-up teaching.

REFERENCES

1 Chopra, V. (2021). Central venous access devices and approach to selection in adults. In: *UpToDate*, Cochran, A., & Davidson, I. (Eds.)

2 Bard, C. R. (2010). Nursing guide: PowerPort® implantable port/PowerLoc® safety infusion set. https://www.bd.com/assets/documents/PDH/PF10414-MC-0475-01_PowerPort_Nursing_Guide.pdf

3 Camp-Sorrell, D. & Matey, L. (2017). *Access device standards of practice for oncology nursing.* Pittsburgh, PA: Oncology Nursing Society.

4 Standard 28. Implanted vascular access ports. Infusion therapy standards of practice. (8th ed.) (2021). *Journal of Infusion Nursing, 44,* S86–S89. (Level VII)

5 Infusion Nurses Society. (2017). *Policies and procedures for infusion therapy of the older adult* (3rd ed.). Boston, MA: Infusion Nurses Society.

6 Centers for Disease Control and Prevention. (2011, revised 2017). Guidelines for the prevention of intravascular catheter–related infections. https://www.cdc.gov/infectioncontrol/guidelines/bsi/recommendations.html (Level I)

7 Jarrett, N., & Callaham, M. (2016). Evidence-based guidelines for selected hospital-acquired conditions: Final report. https://www.cms.gov/Medicare/Medicare-Fee-for-Service-Payment/HospitalAcqCond/Downloads/2016-HAC-Report.pdf

8 Marschall, J., et al. (2014). SHEA/IDSA practice recommendation: Strategies to prevent central line–associated bloodstream infections in acute care hospitals. *Infection Control and Hospital Epidemiology, 35*(7), 753–771. https://www.jstor.org/stable/10.1086/676533#metadata_info_tab_contents (Level I)

9 Association of Professionals in Infection Control and Epidemiology (APIC). (2015). Guide to preventing central line–associated bloodstream infections. http://apic.org/Resource_/TinyMceFileManager/2015/APIC_CLABSI_WEB.pdf (Level IV)

10 The Joint Commission. (2021). Standard NPSG.07.04.01. *Comprehensive accreditation manual for hospitals.* Oakbrook Terrace, IL: The Joint Commission. (Level VII)

11 Standard 50. Infection. Infusion therapy standards of practice. (8th ed.) (2021). *Journal of Infusion Nursing, 44,* S153–S157. (Level VII)

12 Infusion Nurses Society. (2016). *Policies and procedures for infusion therapy* (5th ed.). Boston, MA: Infusion Nurses Society.

13 Standard 41. Flushing and locking. Infusion therapy standards of practice. (8th ed.) (2021). *Journal of Infusion Nursing, 44,* S113–S119. (Level VII)

14 Standard 12. Product evaluation, integrity, and defect reporting. Infusion therapy standards of practice. (8th ed.) (2021). *Journal of Infusion Nursing, 44,* S45–S46. (Level VII)

15 Standard 59. Infusion medication and solution administration. Infusion therapy standards of practice. (8th ed.) (2021). *Journal of Infusion Nursing, 44,* S180–S183. (Level VII)

16 Standard 20. Compounding and preparation of parenteral solutions and medications. Infusion therapy standards of practice. (8th ed.) (2021). *Journal of Infusion Nursing, 44,* S59–S60. (Level VII)

17 Centers for Medicare and Medicaid Services, Department of Health and Human Services. (2020). Condition of participation: Nursing services. 42 C.F.R. § 482.23(c).

18 Standard 24. Flow-control devices. Infusion therapy standards of practice. (2016). *Journal of Infusion Nursing, 39,* S69–S72. (Level VII)

19 The Joint Commission. (2021). Standard UP.01.01.01. *Comprehensive accreditation manual for hospitals.* Oakbrook Terrace, IL: The Joint Commission. (Level VII)

20 Standard 9. Informed consent. Infusion therapy standards of practice. (8th ed.) (2021). *Journal of Infusion Nursing, 44,* S37–S39. (Level VII)

21 The Joint Commission. (2021). Standard RI.01.03.01. *Comprehensive accreditation manual for hospitals.* Oakbrook Terrace, IL: The Joint Commission. (Level VII)

22 Centers for Medicare and Medicaid Services, Department of Health and Human Services. (2020). Condition of participation: Patient's rights. 42 C.F.R. § 482.13(b)(2).

23 Accreditation Association for Hospitals and Health Systems. (2018). Standard 15.01.11. *Healthcare Facilities Accreditation Program:*

Accreditation requirements for acute care hospitals. Chicago, IL: Accreditation Association for Hospitals and Health Systems. (Level VII)

24 DNV GL-Healthcare USA, Inc. (2020). PR.2.SR.3. *NIAHO® accreditation requirements, interpretive guidelines and surveyor guidance—revision 20.0.* Milford, OH: DNV GL-Healthcare USA, Inc. (Level VII)

25 Standard 33. Vascular access site preparation and skin antisepsis. Infusion therapy standards of practice. (8th ed.) (2021). *Journal of Infusion Nursing, 44,* S96–S97. (Level VII)

26 Centers for Disease Control and Prevention. (2002). Guideline for hand hygiene in health-care settings: Recommendations of the Healthcare Infection Control Practices Advisory Committee and the HICPAC/SHEA/APIC/IDSA Hand Hygiene Task Force. *MMWR Recommendations and Reports, 51*(RR-16), 1–45. https://www.cdc.gov/mmwr/pdf/rr/rr5116.pdf (Level II)

27 The Joint Commission. (2021). Standard NPSG.07.01.01. *Comprehensive accreditation manual for hospitals.* Oakbrook Terrace, IL: The Joint Commission. (Level VII)

28 Standard 16. Hand hygiene. Infusion therapy standards of practice. (8th ed.) (2021). *Journal of Infusion Nursing, 44,* S53–S54. (Level VII)

29 World Health Organization. (2009). WHO guidelines on hand hygiene in health care: First global patient safety challenge, clean care is safer care. https://apps.who.int/iris/bitstream/handle/10665/44102/9789241597906_eng.pdf?sequence=1 (Level IV)

30 Centers for Medicare and Medicaid Services, Department of Health and Human Services. (2020). Condition of participation: Infection control. 42 C.F.R. § 482.42.

31 Accreditation Association for Hospitals and Health Systems. (2018). Standard 07.01.21. *Healthcare Facilities Accreditation Program: Accreditation requirements for acute care hospitals.* Chicago, IL: Accreditation Association for Hospitals and Health Systems. (Level VII)

32 DNV GL-Healthcare USA, Inc. (2020). IC.1.SR.1. *NIAHO® accreditation requirements, interpretive guidelines and surveyor guidance—revision 20.0.* Milford, OH: DNV GL-Healthcare USA, Inc. (Level VII)

33 The Joint Commission. (2021). Standard NPSG.01.03.01. *Comprehensive accreditation manual for hospitals.* Oakbrook Terrace, IL: The Joint Commission. (Level VII)

34 Accreditation Association for Hospitals and Health Systems. (2020). Standard 15.01.16. *Healthcare Facilities Accreditation Program: Accreditation requirements for acute care hospitals.* Chicago, IL: Accreditation Association for Hospitals and Health Systems. (Level VII)

35 Centers for Medicare and Medicaid Services, Department of Health and Human Services. (2019). Condition of participation: Patient's rights. 42 C.F.R. § 482.13(c)(1).

36 The Joint Commission. (2021). Standard RI.01.01.01. *Comprehensive accreditation manual for hospitals.* Oakbrook Terrace, IL: The Joint Commission. (Level VII)

37 DNV GL-Healthcare USA, Inc. (2020). PR.2.SR.5. *NIAHO® accreditation requirements, interpretive guidelines and surveyor guidance—revision 20.0.* Milford, OH: DNV GL-Healthcare USA, Inc. (Level VII)

38 Standard 8. Patient education. Infusion therapy standards of practice. (8th ed.) (2021). *Journal of Infusion Nursing, 44,* S35–S37. (Level VII)

39 DNV GL-Healthcare USA, Inc. (2020). MM.1.SR.3. *NIAHO® accreditation requirements, interpretive guidelines and surveyor guidance—revision 20.0.* Milford, OH: DNV GL-Healthcare USA, Inc. (Level VII)

40 The Joint Commission. (2021). Standard MM.06.01.01. *Comprehensive accreditation manual for hospitals.* Oakbrook Terrace, IL: The Joint Commission. (Level VII)

41 Waters, T. R., et al. (2009). Safe patient handling training for schools of nursing. https://www.cdc.gov/niosh/docs/2009-127/pdfs/2009-127.pdf (Level VII)

42 Accreditation Association for Hospitals and Health Systems. (2020). Standard 25.01.27. *Healthcare Facilities Accreditation Program: Accreditation requirements for acute care hospitals.* Chicago, IL: Accreditation Association for Hospitals and Health Systems. (Level VII)

43 The Joint Commission. (2021). Standard NPSG.03.04.01. *Comprehensive accreditation manual for hospitals.* Oakbrook Terrace, IL: The Joint Commission. (Level VII)

44 Siegel, J. D., et al. (2007, revised 2019). 2007 guideline for isolation precautions: Preventing transmission of infectious agents in healthcare settings. https://www.cdc.gov/infectioncontrol/pdf/guidelines/isolation-guidelines-H.pdf (Level II)

45 Accreditation Association for Hospitals and Health Systems. (2018). Standard 07.01.10. *Healthcare Facilities Accreditation Program: Accreditation requirements for acute care hospitals.* Chicago, IL: Accreditation Association for Hospitals and Health Systems. (Level VII)

46 Occupational Safety and Health Administration. (2012). Bloodborne pathogens, standard number 1910.1030. https://www.osha.gov/pls/oshaweb/owadisp.show_document?p_id=10051&p_table=STANDARDS (Level VII)

47 Heffner, A. C., & Androes, M. P. (2021). Overview of central venous access in adults. In: *UpToDate,* Davidson, I., et al. (Eds.).

48 Granziera, E., et al. (2014). Totally implantable venous access devices: Retrospective analysis of different insertion techniques and predictors of complications in 796 devices implanted in a single institution. *BMC Surgery, 14,* 27. (Level IV)

49 Standard 22. Vascular visualization. Infusion therapy standards of practice. (8th ed.) (2021). *Journal of Infusion Nursing, 44,* S63–S65. (Level VII)

50 Standard 36. Needleless connectors. Infusion therapy standards of practice. (8th ed.) (2021). *Journal of Infusion Nursing, 44,* S104–S107. (Level VII)

51 Moureau, N. L., & Flynn, J. (2015). Disinfection of needleless connector hubs: Clinical evidence systematic review. *Nursing Research and Practice,* 2015, 1–20. https://www.hindawi.com/journals/nrp/2015/796762/

52 Standard 21. Medical waste and sharps safety. Infusion therapy standards of practice. (8th ed.) (2021). *Journal of Infusion Nursing, 44,* S60–S63. (Level VII)

53 Ganz, D. A., et al. (2013, reviewed 2021). *Preventing falls in hospitals: A toolkit for improving quality of care* (AHRQ Publication No. 13-0015-EF). Rockville, MD: Agency for Healthcare Research and Quality. https://www.ahrq.gov/professionals/systems/hospital/fallpxtoolkit/index.html (Level VII)

54 The Joint Commission. (2021). Standard RC.01.03.01. *Comprehensive accreditation manual for hospitals.* Oakbrook Terrace, IL: The Joint Commission. (Level VII)

55 Standard 10. Documentation in the health record. Infusion therapy standards of practice. (8th ed.) (2021). *Journal of Infusion Nursing, 44,* S39–S43. (Level VII)

56 Centers for Medicare and Medicaid Services, Department of Health and Human Services. (2020). Condition of participation: Medical record services. 42 C.F.R. § 482.24.

57 Accreditation Association for Hospitals and Health Systems. (2020). Standard 10.00.03. *Healthcare Facilities Accreditation Program: Accreditation requirements for acute care hospitals.* Chicago, IL: Accreditation Association for Hospitals and Health Systems. (Level VII)

58 DNV GL-Healthcare USA, Inc. (2020). MR.2.SR.1. *NIAHO® accreditation requirements, interpretive guidelines and surveyor guidance—revision 20.0.* Milford, OH: DNV GL-Healthcare USA, Inc. (Level VII)

59 Standard 32. Pain management for venipuncture and vascular access procedures. Infusion therapy standards of practice. (8th ed.) (2021). *Journal of Infusion Nursing, 44,* S94–S96. (Level VII)

60 Accreditation Association for Hospitals and Health Systems. (2020). Standard 16.01.03. *Healthcare Facilities Accreditation Program: Accreditation requirements for acute care hospitals.* Chicago, IL: Accreditation Association for Hospitals and Health Systems. (Level VII)

61 Esparza, D. M. (2014). *Oncology policies and procedures.* Pittsburgh, PA: Oncology Nursing Society.

62 Guiffant, G., et al. (2012). Flushing ports of totally implantable venous access devices, and impact of the Huber point needle bevel orientation: Experimental tests and numerical computation. *Medical Devices: Evidence and Research, 5,* 31–37. (Level VI)

63 Standard 38. Vascular access device securement. Infusion therapy standards of practice. (8th ed.) (2021). *Journal of Infusion Nursing, 44,* S108–S111. (Level VII)

64 Standard 49. Central vascular access device occlusion. Infusion therapy standards of practice. (8th ed.) (2021). *Journal of Infusion Nursing, 44,* S149–S153. (Level VII)

65 Schiffer, C. A., et al. (2013). Central venous catheter care for the patient with cancer: American Society of Clinical Oncology clinical practice guideline. *Journal of Clinical Oncology, 31*(10), 1357–1370. https://asco-pubs.org/doi/full/10.1200/jco.2012.45.5733 (Level VII)

66 Olsen, M. M., et al. (Eds.). (2019). Chemotherapy and immunotherapy guidelines and recommendations for practice. Pittsburgh, PA: Oncology Nursing Society.

67 Standard 47. Infiltration and extravasation. Infusion therapy standards of practice. (8th ed.) (2021). *Journal of Infusion Nursing, 44,* S142–S147. (Level VII)

68 The Nebraska Medical Center. (2012). *Standardizing central venous catheter care: Hospital to home* (2nd ed.). https://www.nebraskamed.com/sites/default/files/documents/scorch-guidelines.pdf

69 The Joint Commission. (2012). Preventing central line–associated blood-stream infections: A global challenge, a global perspective. https://www.jointcommission.org/assets/1/18/CLABSI_Monograph.pdf (Level VII)

70 American Society of Anesthesiologists. (2012). Practice guidelines for central venous access: A report by the American Society of Anesthesiologists Task Force on Central Venous Access. *Anesthesiology, 116*, 539–573. https://anesthesiology.pubs.asahq.org/article.aspx?articleid=2443415#106430691 (Level I)

71 U.S. Food and Drug Administration. (2017). Examples of medical device misconnections. https://www.fda.gov/medical-devices/medical-device-connectors/examples-medical-device-misconnections

72 The Joint Commission. (2014). Sentinel event alert 53: Managing risk during transition to new ISO tubing connector standards. https://www.jointcommission.org/assets/1/6/SEA_53_Connectors_8_19_14_final.pdf

73 Standard 44. Blood sampling. Infusion therapy standards of practice. (8th ed.) (2021). *Journal of Infusion Nursing, 44*, S125–S133. (Level VII)

74 Standard 42. Vascular access device assessment, care, and dressing changes. Infusion therapy standards of practice. (8th ed.) (2021). *Journal of Infusion Nursing, 44*, S119–S123. (Level VII)

75 The Joint Commission. (2013). CLABSI toolkit—Preventing central-line associated bloodstream infections: Useful tools, an international perspective. https://www.jointcommission.org/topics/clabsi_toolkit.aspx (Level VII)

76 Adlard, K. (2008). Examining the push-pull method of blood sampling from central venous access devices. *Journal of Pediatric Oncology Nursing, 25*, 200–207. https://www.choc.org/userfiles/file/jpedoncolnursing25-2.pdf (Level II)

77 The Joint Commission. (2021). Standard NPSG.01.01.01. *Comprehensive accreditation manual for hospitals.* Oakbrook Terrace, IL: The Joint Commission. (Level VII)

78 Institute for Safe Medication Practices. (2012). Side tracks on the safety express: Interruptions lead to errors and unfinished…Wait, what was I doing? *Nurse Advise-ERR, 11*(2), 1–4. https://www.ismp.org/resources/side-tracks-safety-express-interruptions-lead-errors-and-unfinished-wait-what-was-i-doing?id=37

79 Institute for Safe Medication Practices. (2018). ISMP list of high-alert medications in acute care settings. https://www.ismp.org/sites/default/files/attachments/2018-08/highAlert2018-Acute-Final.pdf (Level VII)

80 Institute for Safe Medication Practices. (2013). Independent double-checks: Undervalued and misused. Selective use of this strategy can play an important role in medication safety. https://www.ismp.org/resources/independent-double-checks-undervalued-and-misused-selective-use-strategy-can-play (Level VII)

81 Standard 13. Medication verification. Infusion therapy standards of practice. (8th ed.) (2021). *Journal of Infusion Nursing, 44*, S46–S49. (Level VII)

82 Institute for Safe Medication Practices (ISMP). (2015). Safe practice guidelines for adult IV push medications. https://www.ismp.org/guidelines/iv-push (Level VII)

83 Hull, G. J., et al. (2018). Quantitative assessment of reflux in commercially available needle-free IV connectors. *Journal of Vascular Access, 19*, 12–22. (Level VI)

84 Jasinsky, L. M., & Wurster, J. (2009). Occlusion reduction and heparin elimination trial using an antireflux device on peripheral and central venous catheters. *Journal of Infusion Nursing, 32*, 33–39. (Level VI)

85 Centers for Medicare and Medicaid Services. (2014). Requirements for hospital medication administration, particularly intravenous (IV) medications and post-operative care of patients receiving IV opioids. https://www.cms.gov/Medicare/Provider-Enrollment-and-Certification/SurveyCertificationGenInfo/Downloads/Survey-and-Cert-Letter-14-15.pdf

86 The Joint Commission. (2021). Standard PC.01.02.07. *Comprehensive accreditation manual for hospitals.* Oakbrook Terrace, IL: The Joint Commission. (Level VII)

87 Graham, K. C., & Cvach, M. (2010). Monitor alarm fatigue: Standardizing use of physiological monitors and decreasing nuisance alarms. *American Journal of Critical Care, 19*(1), 28–37. https://doi.org/10.4037/ajcc2010651

88 The Joint Commission. (2021). Standard NPSG.06.01.01. *Comprehensive accreditation manual for hospitals.* Oakbrook Terrace, IL: The Joint Commission. (Level VII)

89 The Joint Commission. (2013). Sentinel event alert 50: Medical device alarm safety in hospitals. https://www.jointcommission.org/assets/1/6/SEA_50_alarms_4_26_16.pdf (Level VII)

90 LeBlanc, K., et al. (2013). International skin tear advisory panel: A tool kit to aid in the prevention, assessment, and treatment of skin tears using a simplified classification system. *Advances in Skin & Wound Care, 26*, 459–476. (Level IV)

91 Standard 43. Administration set management. Infusion therapy standards of practice (8th ed.). (2021). *Journal of Infusion Nursing, 44*(Suppl. 1), S123–S125. (Level VII)

92 Standard 52. Air embolism. Infusion therapy standards of practice (8th ed.). (2021). *Journal of Infusion Nursing, 44*(Suppl. 1), S160–S161. (Level VII)

INCENTIVE SPIROMETRY

Incentive spirometry involves using a device to help the patient achieve maximal ventilation by providing feedback on respiratory effort. The device measures respiratory flow or respiratory volume, and induces the patient to take a deep breath and hold it for several seconds. This deep breath increases lung volume, boosts alveolar inflation, and promotes venous return. Incentive spirometry is designed to replicate the natural mechanisms of sighing or yawning, preventing and reversing the alveolar collapse that causes atelectasis and pneumonitis.

Devices used for incentive spirometry provide an immediate visual incentive to breathe deeply. Some are piston-activated when the patient inhales a certain volume of air; the device's cylinder then indicates the amount of air inhaled. Flow-oriented incentive spirometers measure and visually indicate the degree of inspiratory flow—for example, by plastic floats that rise according to the amount of air the patient pulls through the device during inhalation.[1]

Incentive spirometry is indicated for patients with atelectasis, conditions that predispose patients to atelectasis, such as upper abdominal surgery, thoracic surgery, and surgery in patients with chronic obstructive pulmonary disease (COPD). It's also indicated for patients with a restrictive lung defect associated with quadriplegia or a dysfunctional diaphragm.[2] It can be used to complement deep breathing, directed coughing, early mobilization, and postoperative analgesia to prevent and treat pulmonary complications.[1] However, current evidence has found that its use doesn't prevent postoperative pulmonary complications.[3,4] It's contraindicated in patients who are unable to cooperate, who can't receive instruction on or supervision of the proper use of the device, and who can't generate adequate inspiration because of pain, diaphragmatic dysfunction, or opiate analgesic use.[1]

Direct supervision of incentive spirometry use isn't necessary after the patient is able to demonstrate proper technique. However, periodic reassessment is necessary to make sure the patient complies with proper technique.[1,5]

Equipment

Flow or volume incentive spirometer, as indicated, with disposable tube and mouthpiece ▪ stethoscope ▪ gloves ▪ disinfectant pad ▪ plastic storage bag ▪ facility-approved disinfectant ▪ tissues ▪ Optional: pillow, prescription pain medication, gown, mask and goggles or mask with face shield.

Preparation of equipment

Inspect all equipment and supplies. If a product is expired, is defective, or has compromised integrity, remove it from patient use, label it as expired or defective, and report the expiration or defect as directed by your facility.

Read the manufacturer's instructions for spirometer setup and operation. Label the device with the patient's name. Remove the sterile flow tube and mouthpiece from the package and attach them to the device according to the manufacturer's instructions. Set the flow rate or volume goal as determined by the practitioner or respiratory therapist and based on the patient's preoperative performance; *inaccurate flow rate or volume goal may cause pulmonary hyperventilation.*

Implementation

▪ Verify the practitioner's order.
▪ Gather and prepare the necessary equipment and supplies.

- Perform hand hygiene.[6,7,8,9,10,11]
- Confirm the patient's identity using at least two patient identifiers.[12]
- Provide privacy.[13,14,15,16]
- Explain the procedure to the patient and family (if appropriate) according to their individual communication and learning needs *to increase their understanding, allay their fears, and enhance cooperation.*[17] Make sure that the patient understands the importance of performing this exercise regularly to maintain alveolar inflation. Advise the patient to avoid incentive spirometry exercises at mealtime *to prevent nausea.*
- Screen for and assess the patient's pain using facility-defined criteria that are consistent with the patient's age, condition, and ability to understand.[18]
- Treat the patient's pain, as needed and ordered, using nonpharmacologic, pharmacologic, or a combination of approaches. Base the treatment plan on evidence-based practices and the patient's clinical condition, past medical history, and pain management goals.[18]
- Raise the patient's bed to waist level before providing care *to prevent caregiver back strain.*[19]
- Perform hand hygiene.[6,7,8,9,10,11]
- Put on gloves, a gown, and a mask with face shield or a mask and goggles, if needed, *to comply with standard precautions.*[20,21,22]
- Assess the patient's condition and breath sounds *to provide a baseline for comparison with posttreatment assessment findings.*
- Help the patient sit comfortably or assume the semi-Fowler position *to promote optimal lung expansion.* If the patient can't assume or maintain this position, the patient can perform the procedure in any position as long as the device remains upright. *Tilting a flow incentive spirometer decreases the required patient effort and reduces the exercise's effectiveness.*
- Have the patient who has an incision splint the incision with a pillow.
- Instruct the patient to exhale normally, insert the mouthpiece, and close the lips tightly around the mouthpiece (as shown below), *because a weak seal can alter flow and volume readings.* Instruct the patient to then inhale as slowly and as deeply as possible. If the patient has difficulty with this step, tell the patient to suck as through a straw but more slowly. Ask the patient to retain the entire volume of air inhaled for at least 5 seconds or, if you're using a device with a light indicator, until the light turns off. This deep breath creates sustained transpulmonary pressure near the end of inspiration and is sometimes called a *sustained maximal inspiration.*[1]

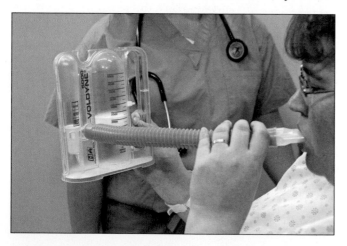

- Tell the patient to remove the mouthpiece and exhale normally. Allow the patient to relax and take several normal breaths before attempting another breath with the spirometer. Note the volumes.
- After proper instruction and return demonstration, encourage the patient to use the incentive spirometer independently.[1] The patient may take 10 breaths every 1 to 2 hours while awake, 10 breaths five times per day, or 15 breaths every 4 hours; *there is a lack of evidence for specific frequency of use.*[1]
- Evaluate the patient's ability to cough effectively, and encourage coughing during and after each incentive spirometry session, *because deep lung inflation can loosen secretions, facilitating their removal.*[23]
- Inspect any expectorated secretions.
- Auscultate the patient's breath sounds. Compare the findings with baseline auscultation findings.

- Reassess and respond to pain by evaluating the patient's response to treatment and progress toward pain management goals. Assess for adverse reactions and risk factors for adverse events that may result from treatment.[18]
- Return the bed to the lowest position *to prevent falls and maintain patient safety.*[24]
- Perform hand hygiene.[6,7,8,9,10,11]
- Put on gloves, if you haven't already done so.[20,22]
- Remove the mouthpiece from the spirometer and clean it according to manufacturer's instructions *to prevent the spread of infection.*[1] Avoid immersing the spirometer itself in water, *because water enhances bacterial growth and impairs the internal filter's effectiveness in preventing inhalation of extraneous material.*
- Let the device dry completely and then place the mouthpiece in a plastic storage bag between exercises, and label it and the spirometer, if applicable, with the patient's name *to avoid inadvertent use by another patient.*[1] Keep the incentive spirometer within the patient's reach.
- Remove and discard your gloves and, if worn, other personal protective equipment.[20,22]
- Perform hand hygiene.[6,7,8,9,10,11]
- Clean and disinfect your stethoscope using a disinfectant pad.[25,26]
- Perform hand hygiene.[6,7,8,9,10,11]
- Document the procedure.[27,28,29,30]

Special considerations

- If the patient is scheduled for surgery, make a preoperative assessment of the patient's respiratory pattern and capability *to ensure the development of appropriate postoperative goals.*[2] Teach the patient how to use the spirometer before surgery *so that the patient can concentrate on your instructions and practice the exercise.*
- Provide paper and a pencil *so the patient can note exercise times.*
- Note that some spirometers can be adapted for use by patients who have a tracheal stoma.
- If applicable, remove the patient's dentures *to create a better seal.*

Patient teaching

If the patient is learning the skill preoperatively and taking the instrument home, provide oral and written instructions for use, including cleaning and storage, frequency of sessions, and volumes desired. Demonstrate the procedure and observe return demonstrations.

Instruct the patient to contact the practitioner if shortness of breath, dizziness, extreme exacerbation of coughing, or extreme fatigue or pain associated with use of the incentive spirometer occur.

Complications

Complications of incentive spirometry include hyperventilation, which could lead to respiratory alkalosis; hypoxemia secondary to interruption of prescribed oxygen; fatigue; and pain. Incentive spirometry can be ineffective if not performed as instructed.[1]

Documentation

Document the flow or volume levels, date and time of the procedure, type of spirometer, and number of breaths taken. Also record the patient's

---

Documenting flow and volume levels

Documentation for flow and volume levels in incentive spirometry depends on the type of spirometer the patient is using.

If the patient is using a flow incentive spirometer, compute the volume by multiplying the setting by the duration that the patient kept the ball (or balls) suspended. For example, if the patient suspended the ball for 3 seconds at a setting of 500 mL during each of 10 breaths, multiply 500 mL by 3 seconds and then record this total (1,500 mL) and the number of breaths as 1,500 mL × 10 breaths.

If the patient is using a volume incentive spirometer, take the volume reading directly from the spirometer. For example, record 1,000 mL × 5 breaths.

assessment results before and after the procedure, the patient's tolerance of the procedure, and the results of preprocedure and postprocedure auscultation. Document any complications, the name of the practitioner notified, the date and time of notification, prescribed interventions, and the patient's response to those interventions. Document teaching provided to the patient and family (if applicable), their understanding of that teaching, and any need for follow-up teaching. (See *Documenting flow and volume levels*, page 426.)

REFERENCES

1 Restrepo, R. D., et al. (2011). AARC clinical practice guideline. Incentive spirometry: 2011. *Respiratory Care, 56*(10), 1600–1604. http://rc.rcjournal.com/content/respcare/56/10/1600.full.pdf (Level VII)

2 Kacmarek, R. M., et al. (2021). *Egan's fundamentals of respiratory care* (12th ed.). St. Louis, MO: Mosby.

3 Jayasekara, R. (2020). Postoperative pulmonary complications: Postoperative strategies. *JBI EBP Database.* AN: JBI15886 (Level II)

4 Pantel, H., et al. (2017). Effect of incentive spirometry on postoperative hypoxemia and pulmonary complications after bariatric surgery: A randomized clinical trial. *JAMA Surgery, 152*, 422–428. (Level I)

5 Hassanzadeh, H., et al. (2012). Postoperative incentive spirometry use. *Orthopedics, 35*, e927–e931. (Level VI)

6 Accreditation Association for Hospitals and Health Systems. (2020). Standard 07.01.21. *Healthcare Facilities Accreditation Program: Accreditation requirements for acute care hospitals.* Chicago, IL: Accreditation Association for Hospitals and Health Systems. (Level VII)

7 The Joint Commission. (2021). Standard NPSG.07.01.01. *Comprehensive accreditation manual for hospitals.* Oakbrook Terrace, IL: The Joint Commission. (Level VII)

8 Centers for Disease Control and Prevention. (2002). Guideline for hand hygiene in health-care settings: Recommendations of the Healthcare Infection Control Practices Advisory Committee and the HICPAC/SHEA/APIC/IDSA Hand Hygiene Task Force. *MMWR Recommendations and Reports, 51*(RR-16), 1–45. https://www.cdc.gov/mmwr/pdf/rr/rr5116.pdf (Level II)

9 World Health Organization. (2009). WHO guidelines on hand hygiene in health care: First global patient safety challenge, clean care is safer care. https://apps.who.int/iris/bitstream/handle/10665/44102/9789241597906_eng.pdf?sequence=1 (Level IV)

10 DNV GL Healthcare USA, Inc. (2020). IC.1.SR.1. *NIAHO® accreditation requirements, interpretive guidelines and surveyor guidance—revision 20.0.* Milford, OH: DNV GL-Healthcare USA, Inc. (Level VII)

11 Centers for Medicare and Medicaid Services, Department of Health and Human Services. (2020). Condition of participation: Infection control. 42 C.F.R. § 482.42.

12 The Joint Commission. (2021). Standard NPSG.01.01.01. *Comprehensive accreditation manual for hospitals.* Oakbrook Terrace, IL: The Joint Commission. (Level VII)

13 The Joint Commission. (2021). Standard RI.01.01.01. *Comprehensive accreditation manual for hospitals.* Oakbrook Terrace, IL: The Joint Commission. (Level VII)

14 Centers for Medicare and Medicaid Services, Department of Health and Human Services. (2020). Condition of participation: Patient's rights. 42 C.F.R. § 482.13(c)(1).

15 Accreditation Association for Hospitals and Health Systems. (2020). Standard 15.01.16. *Healthcare Facilities Accreditation Program: Accreditation requirements for acute care hospitals.* Chicago, IL: Accreditation Association for Hospitals and Health Systems. (Level VII)

16 DNV GL-Healthcare USA, Inc. (2020). PR.2.SR.5. *NIAHO® accreditation requirements, interpretive guidelines and surveyor guidance—revision 20.0* Milford, OH: DNV GL-Healthcare USA, Inc. (Level VII)

17 The Joint Commission. (2021). Standard PC.02.01.21. *Comprehensive accreditation manual for hospitals.* Oakbrook Terrace, IL: The Joint Commission. (Level VII)

18 The Joint Commission. (2021). Standard PC.01.02.07. *Comprehensive accreditation manual for hospitals.* Oakbrook Terrace, IL: The Joint Commission. (Level VII)

19 Waters, T. R., et al. (2009). Safe patient handling training for schools of nursing. https://www.cdc.gov/niosh/docs/2009-127/pdfs/2009-127.pdf (Level VII)

20 Siegel, J. D., et al. (2007, revised 2019). 2007 guideline for isolation precautions: Preventing transmission of infectious agents in healthcare settings. https://www.cdc.gov/infectioncontrol/pdf/guidelines/isolation-guidelines-H.pdf (Level II)

21 Accreditation Association for Hospitals and Health Systems. (2020). Standard 07.01.10. *Healthcare Facilities Accreditation Program: Accreditation requirements for acute care hospitals.* Chicago, IL: Accreditation Association for Hospitals and Health Systems. (Level VII)

22 Occupational Safety and Health Administration. (2012). Bloodborne pathogens, standard number 1910.1030. https://www.osha.gov/pls/oshaweb/owadisp.show_document?p_id=10051&p_table=STANDARDS (Level VII)

23 Centers for Disease Control and Prevention. (2020). Coughing and sneezing. https://www.cdc.gov/healthywater/hygiene/etiquette/coughing_sneezing.html

24 Ganz, D. A., et al. (2013, reviewed 2021). *Preventing falls in hospitals: A toolkit for improving quality of care* (AHRQ Publication No. 13-0015-EF). Rockville, MD: Agency for Healthcare Research and Quality. https://www.ahrq.gov/professionals/systems/hospital/fallpxtoolkit/index.html (Level VII)

25 Rutala, W. A., et al. (2008, revised 2019). Guideline for disinfection and sterilization in healthcare facilities, 2008. https://www.cdc.gov/infection-control/pdf/guidelines/disinfection-guidelines-H.pdf (Level I)

26 Accreditation Association for Hospitals and Health Systems. (2020). Standard 07.02.03. *Healthcare Facilities Accreditation Program: Accreditation requirements for acute care hospitals.* Chicago, IL: Accreditation Association for Hospitals and Health Systems. (Level VII)

27 The Joint Commission. (2021). Standard RC.01.03.01. *Comprehensive accreditation manual for hospitals.* Oakbrook Terrace, IL: The Joint Commission. (Level VII)

28 Accreditation Association for Hospitals and Health Systems. (2020). Standard 10.00.03. *Healthcare Facilities Accreditation Program: Accreditation requirements for acute care hospitals.* Chicago, IL: Accreditation Association for Hospitals and Health Systems. (Level VII)

29 DNV GL-Healthcare USA, Inc. (2020). MR.2.SR.1. *NIAHO® accreditation requirements, interpretive guidelines and surveyor guidance—revision 20.0.* Milford, OH: DNV GL-Healthcare USA, Inc. (Level VII)

30 Centers for Medicare and Medicaid Services, Department of Health and Human Services. (2020). Condition of participation: Medical record services. 42 C.F.R. § 482.24(b).

INCONTINENCE MANAGEMENT, FECAL

Fecal incontinence is the involuntary passage of feces, which may occur gradually (as in dementia) or suddenly (as in spinal cord injury). Urge incontinence occurs when the patient is aware of the need to defecate but is incontinent despite effort to retain the stool. Passive incontinence occurs when the patient lacks awareness of the need to defecate before being incontinent.[1] Risk factors for fecal incontinence include advanced age, diarrhea, fecal urgency, urinary incontinence, diabetes mellitus, and hormone therapy in postmenopausal women.[1]

In older adult patients, fecal incontinence may be transient or permanent, and affects up to 14% of patients in assisted living and extended care facilities.[1] Although it's not usually a sign of serious illness, fecal incontinence can seriously impair an older adult patient's physical and psychological well-being. Patients with fecal or urinary incontinence are at risk for incontinence-associated dermatitis, which can result in the development of pressure injuries and secondary skin infection.[2]

Successful management of these patients depends on identifying and treating the underlying cause or causes.[1,2,3] Most cases can be treated; some can even be cured. Treatment aims to control the condition through bowel retraining or other behavioral management techniques, diet modification, drug therapy, pessaries, and possibly surgery.[3,4] Despite appropriate management, some patients may remain incontinent because of dementia, immobility, or comorbid issues. In such cases, management aims to prevent associated complications.[5]

Equipment

Gloves ▪ stethoscope ▪ skin barrier or skin protectant ▪ appropriate skin cleaner and cloth (preferably a no-rinse cleanser) ▪ incontinence pads ▪ bedside commode or bedpan ▪ disinfectant pad ▪ Optional: skin moisturizer, fecal incontinence collector or fecal management system, superabsorbent adult disposable briefs, specimen container, label, laboratory biohazard transport bag, clean linens.

Implementation

- Gather and prepare the necessary equipment and supplies.
- Perform hand hygiene.[6,7,8,9,10,11]
- Confirm the patient's identity using at least two patient identifiers.[12]
- Provide privacy.[13,14,15,16]
- Obtain an incontinence history. Ask the patient to identify the onset, duration, and severity of the fecal incontinence as well as any identified patterns (such as whether it occurs at night or with diarrhea). Focus the history on GI, neurologic, and psychological disorders. Assess for chronic constipation or laxative abuse.[1,17]
- Assess the patient's medication regimen. Check for drugs that affect bowel activity, such as antibiotics, aspirin, some anticholinergic antiparkinsonian agents, aluminum hydroxide, calcium carbonate antacids, diuretics, iron preparations, opiates, sedatives, tricyclic antidepressants, and phenothiazines.
- Review the patient's diet.[4,18] Note whether the patient receives enteral nutrition and, if so, be sure to include the type, volume, and frequency of administration, *because osmotic diarrhea-induced incontinence should be considered.*[5]
- Note the frequency, consistency, and volume of stools passed in the past 24 hours.
- Raise the patient's bed to waist level before providing patient care *to prevent caregiver back strain.*[19]
- Perform hand hygiene.[6,7,8,9,10,11]
- Put on gloves *to comply with standard precautions.*[20,21,22]
- Protect the patient's bed with an incontinence pad. Ensure that the pads aren't layered and are without wrinkles *to reduce pressure risk and subsequent skin damage.*

NURSING ALERT Guidelines recommend use of an incontinence pad when the patient is in bed and a superabsorbent adult disposable brief when the patient's out of bed, as needed.[22] A superabsorbent adult disposable brief is designed to absorb and wick moisture from incontinence away from the skin when the patient is ambulating. However, note that this type of brief can become heavy when full; it can make ambulation difficult in a mobility-impaired patient and may increase the risk of falls. Change the superabsorbent adult disposable brief after each incontinence episode.[2]

- Inspect the abdomen for distention, and auscultate the abdomen for bowel sounds. If not contraindicated, check for fecal impaction (a factor in overflow incontinence), as ordered.
- Obtain a stool specimen, if ordered. Label the specimen in the presence of the patient *to prevent mislabeling.*[12] Send the specimen to the laboratory in a laboratory biohazard transport bag with a completed laboratory request form (if used in your facility). (See the "Stool specimen collection" procedure.)
- Provide ongoing assessment of the perineal skin, including risk factors for skin breakdown and general condition, such as visible areas of skin redness and erosion.[22,23]
- Maintain effective hygienic care *to increase the patient's comfort and prevent skin breakdown and infection.*[4,23,24] Clean the perineal area frequently with an appropriate skin cleaner; if possible, use a no-rinse skin cleaner with a pH range similar to that of normal skin, instead of soap and water, *to help prevent incontinence-associated dermatitis.*[2] If a moisturizer isn't already incorporated into the skin cleaner, apply a moisturizer daily, as needed.[18] Apply a skin barrier or skin protectant after every incontinence episode *to protect the skin from constant moisture.*[2] Use measures to control odor.

NURSING ALERT Clean the skin gently, using care to avoid rigorous scrubbing or friction *to minimize the risk of compromising the skin barrier function.* If dried or difficult-to-remove feces are present, gently apply a moistened cloth on the area and softly pat it around as needed *to remove the feces.*[22]

- Provide bowel retraining for a neurologically capable patient with chronic incontinence. Offer the patient the toilet, commode, or bedpan every 1 to 2 hours, as appropriate.
- If the patient has intact perineal skin, apply a fecal incontinence collector or fecal management system, as indicated and ordered.[18]
- Check the patient's incontinence pad (if applicable) at least every 2 hours *to ensure that it's dry. Because the skin lying on an underpad is commonly moist,* expose this area to air when turning the patient *to allow*

moisture to evaporate and the skin surface to dry.[2] Regularly and promptly remove soil and irritants from the skin *to help prevent or minimize exposure of the skin to damaging irritants.*[22]

- Replace soiled linens promptly.
- Return the patient's bed to the lowest position *to prevent falls and maintain patient safety.*[25]
- Remove and discard your gloves.[21,26]
- Perform hand hygiene.[6,7,8,9,10,11]
- Clean and disinfect your stethoscope using a disinfectant pad.[27,28]
- Perform hand hygiene.[6,7,8,9,10,11]
- Document the procedure.[29,30,31,32]

Special considerations

- Schedule extra time to provide encouragement and support for the patient, *because the patient may feel shame, embarrassment, and powerlessness from loss of control.*
- Minimize the use of incontinence pads and superabsorbent adult disposable briefs when possible, *because they can trap heat and moisture and advance skin damage.*[23]
- Antifungal products, steroid-based topical anti-inflammatory products, and topical antibiotics to treat incontinence-associated dermatitis are recommended only in specific situations.[23,24]
- Be aware that patients with fecal incontinence might be unable to reposition themselves. Reposition the patient as needed *to reduce pressure-related injury risk.*[2]

Complications

Skin breakdown and infection may result from incontinence.[18,22] Psychological problems resulting from incontinence include social isolation, shame, embarrassment, worsened sexual function, increased economic burden, lowered self-esteem, anxiety, and depression.[18,33]

Documentation

Document your assessment findings. Record all bladder and bowel retraining efforts, noting scheduled bathroom times, food and fluid intake, and elimination amounts, as appropriate. Document the duration of continent periods. Note any complications, including emotional problems and signs of skin breakdown and infection, as well as the treatments given for them and the patient's response to those treatments. Document teaching provided to the patient and family (if applicable), their understanding of that teaching, and any need for follow-up teaching.

REFERENCES

1 Robson, K. M., & Lembo, A. J. (2020). Fecal incontinence in adults: Etiology and evaluation. In: *UpToDate*, Talley, N. J. (Ed.).

2 Zulkowski, K. (2012). Diagnosing and treating moisture-associated skin damage. *Advances in Skin and Wound Care, 25*, 231–236. https://journals.lww.com/aswcjournal/Fulltext/2012/05000/Diagnosing_and_Treating_Moisture_Associated_Skin.9.aspx

3 Wald, A. (2016). Update on the management of fecal incontinence for the gastroenterologist. *Gastroenterology and Hepatology (NY), 12*(3), 155–164. https://www.ncbi.nlm.nih.gov/pmc/articles/PMC4872843/

4 Robson, K. M., & Lembo, A. J. (2020). Fecal incontinence in adults: Management. In: *UpToDate*, Talley, N. J. (Ed.).

5 Leung, F. W., & Rao, S. S. (2011). Approach to fecal incontinence and constipation in older hospitalized patients. *Hospital Practice* (1995), 39, 97–104. (Level V)

6 Centers for Disease Control and Prevention. (2002). Guideline for hand hygiene in health-care settings: Recommendations of the Healthcare Infection Control Practices Advisory Committee and the HICPAC/SHEA/APIC/IDSA Hand Hygiene Task Force. *MMWR Recommendations and Reports, 51*(RR-16), 1–45. https://www.cdc.gov/mmwr/pdf/rr/rr5116.pdf (Level II)

7 World Health Organization. (2009). WHO guidelines on hand hygiene in health care: First global patient safety challenge, clean care is safer care. https://apps.who.int/iris/bitstream/handle/10665/44102/9789241597906_eng.pdf?sequence=1 (Level IV)

8 The Joint Commission. (2021). Standard NPSG.07.01.01. *Comprehensive accreditation manual for hospitals.* Oakbrook Terrace, IL: The Joint Commission. (Level VII)

9 Centers for Medicare and Medicaid Services, Department of Health and Human Services. (2020). Condition of participation: Infection control. 42 C.F.R. § 482.42.

10 Accreditation Association for Hospitals and Health Systems. (2020). Standard 07.01.21. *Healthcare Facilities Accreditation Program: Accreditation requirements for acute care hospitals.* Chicago, IL: Accreditation Association for Hospitals and Health Systems. (Level VII)

11 DNV GL-Healthcare USA, Inc. (2020). IC.1.SR.1. *NIAHO® accreditation requirements, interpretive guidelines and surveyor guidance—revision 20.0.* Milford, OH: DNV GL-Healthcare USA, Inc. (Level VII)

12 The Joint Commission. (2021). Standard NPSG.01.01.01. *Comprehensive accreditation manual for hospitals.* Oakbrook Terrace, IL: The Joint Commission. (Level VII)

13 The Joint Commission. (2021). Standard RI.01.01.01. *Comprehensive accreditation manual for hospitals.* Oakbrook Terrace, IL: The Joint Commission. (Level VII)

14 Centers for Medicare and Medicaid Services, Department of Health and Human Services. (2020). Condition of participation: Patient's rights. 42 C.F.R. § 482.13(c)(1).

15 Accreditation Association for Hospitals and Health Systems. (2020). Standard 15.01.16. *Healthcare Facilities Accreditation Program: Accreditation requirements for acute care hospitals.* Chicago, IL: Accreditation Association for Hospitals and Health Systems. (Level VII)

16 DNV GL-Healthcare USA, Inc. (2020). PR.2.SR.5. *NIAHO® accreditation requirements, interpretive guidelines and surveyor guidance—revision 20.0.* Milford, OH: DNV GL-Healthcare USA, Inc. (Level VII)

17 Whitehead, W. E., et al. (2009). Fecal incontinence in US adults: Epidemiology and risk factors. *Gastroenterology, 137*(2), 512–517. https://www.gastrojournal.org/article/S0016-5085(09)00721-5/pdf (Level VI)

18 WOCN® Society's Continence Committee. (2013). *A quick reference guide for managing fecal incontinence.* Mount Laurel, NJ: Wound, Ostomy and Continence Nurses Society. (Level VII)

19 Waters, T. R., et al. (2009). Safe patient handling training for schools of nursing. https://www.cdc.gov/niosh/docs/2009-127/pdfs/2009-127.pdf (Level VII)

20 Accreditation Association for Hospitals and Health Systems. (2020). Standard 07.01.10. *Healthcare Facilities Accreditation Program: Accreditation requirements for acute care hospitals.* Chicago, IL: Accreditation Association for Hospitals and Health Systems. (Level VII)

21 Occupational Safety and Health Administration. (2012). Bloodborne pathogens, standard number 1910.1030. https://www.osha.gov/pls/oshaweb/owadisp.show_document?p_id=10051&p_table=STANDARDS (Level VII)

22 Beeckman, D., et al. (2015). Best practice principles: Incontinence-associated dermatitis. Moving prevention forward. https://www.woundsinternational.com/resources/details/incontinence-associated-dermatitis-moving-prevention-forward (Level VII)

23 Chatham, N., & Carls, C. (2012). How to manage incontinence-associated dermatitis. *Wound Care Advisor, 1*(1), 7–10. http://woundcareadvisor.com/wp-content/uploads/2012/05/WCA_M-J-2012_Dermatitis.pdf

24 Gray, M., et al. (2012). Incontinence-associated dermatitis: A comprehensive review and update. *Journal of Wound, Ostomy and Continence Nursing, 39*, 61–74. (Level V)

25 Ganz, D. A., et al. (2013, reviewed 2021). *Preventing falls in hospitals: A toolkit for improving quality of care* (AHRQ Publication No. 13-0015-EF). Rockville, MD: Agency for Healthcare Research and Quality. https://www.ahrq.gov/professionals/systems/hospital/fallpxtoolkit/index.html (Level VII)

26 Siegel, J. D., et al. (2007, revised 2019). 2007 guideline for isolation precautions: Preventing transmission of infectious agents in healthcare settings. https://www.cdc.gov/infectioncontrol/pdf/guidelines/isolation-guidelines-H.pdf (Level II)

27 Rutala, W. A., et al. (2008, revised 2019). Guideline for disinfection and sterilization in healthcare facilities, 2008. https://www.cdc.gov/infection-control/pdf/guidelines/disinfection-guidelines-H.pdf (Level I)

28 Accreditation Association for Hospitals and Health Systems. (2020). Standard 07.02.03. *Healthcare Facilities Accreditation Program: Accreditation requirements for acute care hospitals.* Chicago, IL: Accreditation Association for Hospitals and Health Systems. (Level VII)

29 The Joint Commission. (2021). Standard RC.01.03.01. *Comprehensive accreditation manual for hospitals.* Oakbrook Terrace, IL: The Joint Commission. (Level VII)

30 Centers for Medicare and Medicaid Services, Department of Health and Human Services. (2020). Condition of participation: Medical record services. 42 C.F.R. § 482.24(b).

31 Accreditation Association for Hospitals and Health Systems. (2020). Standard 10.00.03. *Healthcare Facilities Accreditation Program: Accreditation requirements for acute care hospitals.* Chicago, IL: Accreditation Association for Hospitals and Health Systems. (Level VII)

32 DNV GL-Healthcare USA, Inc. (2020). MR.2.SR.1. *NIAHO® accreditation requirements, interpretive guidelines and surveyor guidance—revision 20.0* Milford, OH: DNV GL-Healthcare USA, Inc. (Level VII)

33 The American College of Obstetricians and Gynecologists. (2019). ACOG practice bulletin no. 210: Fecal incontinence. *Obstetrics & Gynecology, 133*, e260–e273. (Level VII)

INCONTINENCE MANAGEMENT, URINARY

Urinary incontinence, the involuntary loss of urine, affects both male and female patients.[1] In older adult patients, urinary incontinence commonly follows any loss or impairment of urinary sphincter control. It may be transient or permanent. About 13 million adults experience some form of urinary incontinence, including half of homebound adults.[2]

Contrary to popular opinion, urinary incontinence is neither a disease nor a normal part of aging. It isn't inevitable, and can be avoided or reversed with support and interventions. Urinary incontinence may be caused by childbirth, confusion, dehydration, fecal impaction, or restricted mobility. It may also be a sign of various disorders, such as prostatic hyperplasia, bladder calculus, bladder cancer, urinary tract infection (UTI), stroke, diabetic neuropathy, Guillain-Barré syndrome, multiple sclerosis, prostatic cancer, prostatitis, spinal cord injury, and urethral stricture. It may also result from urethral sphincter damage after prostatectomy. In addition, certain drugs, including diuretics, hypnotics, sedatives, anticholinergics, antihypertensives, and alpha antagonists, may trigger urinary incontinence.

Urinary incontinence is classified as acute or chronic. Acute urinary incontinence results from disorders that are potentially reversible, such as delirium, dehydration, urinary retention, restricted mobility, fecal impaction, infection or inflammation, drug reactions, and polyuria.

Chronic urinary incontinence occurs as five distinct types: stress, overflow, urge, mixed, reflex, and functional (total) incontinence. In *stress urinary incontinence*, leakage results from a sudden physical strain, such as a sneeze, cough, or quick movement. In *overflow urinary incontinence*, urine retention causes dribbling because the distended bladder can't contract strongly enough to force a urine stream. In *urge urinary incontinence* (also called *overactive bladder with incontinence*), the patient can't control the impulse to urinate.[3] In *functional urinary incontinence*, urine leaks despite a normally functioning bladder and urethra; it is usually related to cognitive or mobility factors that prevent the patient from getting to the bathroom in a timely fashion.[3,4] In addition, the patient may have symptoms of both stress urinary incontinence and urge urinary incontinence, known as *mixed incontinence* or *overactive bladder syndrome with incontinence*.[4,5]

Patients with urinary incontinence should be carefully assessed for underlying disorders. Most can be treated; some can even be cured. Treatment aims to control the condition through bladder retraining or other behavioral management techniques, diet modification, medication therapy, pessaries, and possibly surgery. Corrective surgery for stress urinary incontinence in female patients includes various types of midurethral slings, and bladder neck slings.[6] Corrective surgery for urinary incontinence in male patients includes the injection of transurethral bulking agents, a perineal sling, and an artificial urinary sphincter implant.[4]

Equipment

Bladder management record ▪ gloves ▪ appropriate skin cleanser ▪ skin protectant or skin barrier product ▪ incontinence pads or adult briefs[7] ▪ Optional: bedside commode, skin moisturizer, clean linens, specimen collection container and label, laboratory biohazard transport bag.

Implementation

▪ Gather and prepare the necessary equipment and supplies.
▪ Perform hand hygiene.[8,9,10,11,12,13]

- Confirm the patient's identity using at least two patient identifiers.[14]
- Provide privacy.[15,16,17,18]
- Obtain an incontinence history as needed. Ask when the patient first noticed urine leakage and whether it began suddenly or gradually. Have the patient describe the typical urinary pattern: Does the patient usually experience incontinence during the day or at night? Does the patient get the urge to go again immediately after emptying the bladder? Does the patient get strong urges to go? Ask the patient to rate the degree of urinary control: Does the patient have moderate control, or is the patient completely incontinent? If the patient sometimes urinates with control, ask the patient to identify when and how much the patient usually urinates. Ask the patient to describe any previous treatment received for incontinence or measures the patient has performed independently.
- Assess for related problems, such as urinary hesitancy, frequency, or urgency; nocturia; and decreased force or interruption of the urine stream. Ask about medication regimens, including nonprescription drugs.
- Assess the patient's environment. Is a toilet or commode readily available? How long does the patient take to reach it? Assess the patient's manual dexterity in the bathroom—for example, how easily does the patient manipulate clothing?
- Evaluate the patient's mental status and cognitive function.
- Quantify the patient's normal daily fluid intake.
- Review the patient's medication and diet history for drugs and foods that affect digestion and elimination.
- Review or obtain the patient's medical history, noting especially any incidence of UTI, diabetes, spinal injury or tumor, stroke, and bladder or pelvic surgery. For a female patient, also note the number and route of births and whether she's had a hysterectomy; for a male, note any prostate disorders or prostate surgery. Assess for such disorders as delirium, dehydration, urine retention, restricted mobility, fecal impaction, infection, inflammation, and polyuria.[3,4]
- Raise the patient's bed to waist level before providing patient care *to prevent caregiver back strain.*[19]
- Perform hand hygiene[8,9,10,11,12,13] and put on gloves *to comply with standard precautions.*[20,21,22]
- Select an incontinence pad or adult brief that is absorbent enough *to wick urinary incontinence moisture away from the patient's skin and prevent maceration.*[7]
- Inspect the urethral meatus for obvious inflammation or anatomic defects. Have a female patient bear down while you note any urine leakage.
- Gently palpate the abdomen for bladder distention, which signals urine retention.
- Assess for costovertebral angle tenderness. If possible, have the patient examined by a urologist.
- Obtain specimens for appropriate laboratory tests, as ordered. (See the "Urine specimen collection" procedure.) Label the specimens in the presence of the patient *to prevent mislabeling.*[14] Place the specimens in a laboratory biohazard transport bag and send them to the laboratory immediately.
- Have the patient complete a 3-day voiding diary (bladder management record) *to help develop an individualized bladder management program for the patient.*[23]
- Begin urinary incontinence management by implementing a bladder retraining program, as appropriate.[7] (See *Correcting urinary incontinence with bladder management.*)
- *To manage stress urinary incontinence,* begin an exercise program to help strengthen the pelvic floor muscles.[23] (See *Strengthening the pelvic floor muscles.*)
- *To manage functional incontinence,* frequently assess the patient's mental and functional status. Regularly remind the patient to void. Respond to calls promptly, and help the patient get to the bathroom quickly.
- Assess the patient's perineal area for signs of breakdown, including risk factors for skin breakdown and general condition, such as visible areas of skin redness and erosion.[27,28]
- Check the patient's incontinence pad or adult brief at least every 2 hours *to ensure that it's dry.* When turning the patient, expose the area that comes in contact with the incontinence pad to air *to promote drying of the skin surface.*[27,29]
- Replace soiled linens promptly.

- Maintain effective hygienic care *to increase the patient's comfort and prevent skin breakdown and infection.*[28,30] Clean the perineal area frequently with an appropriate skin cleaner—preferably a no-rinse skin cleaner with a pH range similar to that of normal skin instead of soap and water—*to help prevent incontinence-associated dermatitis.*[29] If a moisturizer isn't already incorporated into the skin cleaner, apply a moisturizer daily, as needed. Apply a skin barrier or skin protectant product after every incontinence episode *to protect the skin from constant moisture.*[29] Use measures to control odors.

PATIENT TEACHING

STRENGTHENING THE PELVIC FLOOR MUSCLES

Stress urinary incontinence, the most common kind of urinary incontinence in women, usually results from weakening of the urethral sphincter. In men, it may sometimes occur after a radical prostatectomy. You can help male and female patients prevent or minimize stress urinary incontinence by teaching pelvic floor muscle training (PFMT) or Kegel exercises to strengthen the pubococcygeal muscles.[26]

Learning PFMT exercises

First, explain how to locate the muscles of the pelvic floor. To identify this area initially, teach the patient to tighten the muscles of the pelvic floor to stop the flow of urine while urinating and then to release the muscles to restart the flow. Then explain to the patient that PFMT exercises are a series of contractions and relaxations of the pelvic floor muscles that are essential to muscle retraining. Once learned, these exercises can be done anywhere. Although these exercises shouldn't be done while urinating, they can be done at any other time.

Establishing a regimen

Suggest that the patient start out by contracting the pelvic floor muscles for 5 seconds, relaxing for 5 seconds, and then repeating the procedure as often as needed. Typically, the patient starts with 10 contractions in the morning and 10 at night, gradually increasing the relaxation and contraction time.

Advise the patient not to use stomach, leg, or buttock muscles. Also discourage leg crossing or breath holding during these exercises.

NURSING ALERT Clean the skin gently, using care to avoid rigorous scrubbing or friction *to minimize the risk of compromising the skin barrier function.*[27]

■ Return the patient's bed to the lowest position *to prevent falls and maintain patient safety.*[31]

■ Remove and discard your gloves[20,22] and perform hand hygiene.[8,9,10,11,12,13]

■ Document the procedure.[32,33,34,35]

Special considerations

■ External male catheters or external female catheter products may be indicated to prevent wetness and incontinence-associated dermatitis that results from temporary or chronic urinary incontinence.[4,28,36] External catheters may be preferred over indwelling catheters, *because external devices are less invasive and carry less risk of urinary complications associated with instrumentation of the patient's urethra.* Male patients with bladder dysfunction who use an external catheter should undergo urodynamic testing to determine that bladder storage pressures remain low *to help avoid progressive renal damage.*[4]

■ Minimize the use of incontinence pads and adult briefs when possible, *because they can trap heat and moisture and advance skin damage.*[28]

■ Note that the use of antifungal products, steroid-based topical anti-inflammatory products, and topical antibiotics to treat incontinence-associated dermatitis is recommended only in specific situations.[28,30]

■ *To ensure healthful hydration and to prevent UTIs,* encourage the patient to maintain an adequate daily intake of fluids (six to eight 8-oz [0.24-L] glasses). Restrict oral fluid intake after 6 p.m., as appropriate.

■ Schedule extra time to provide encouragement and support for the patient, *because the patient may feel shame, embarrassment, and powerlessness from loss of control.*

Patient teaching

Teach the patient and family member or other caregiver about normal lower urinary tract function, the patient's particular type of incontinence, the benefits versus the risks of the available treatment alternatives, and the fact that symptom control may require trials of multiple therapeutic options.[37]

Complications

Skin breakdown and infection may result from incontinence.[27,28] Psychological problems resulting from urinary incontinence include social isolation, loss of independence, lowered self-esteem, incontinence-related sexual dysfunction, and depression.[3,4]

Documentation

Document your assessment findings. Record all bladder management efforts, noting scheduled bathroom times, food and fluid intake, and elimination amounts, as appropriate. Document the duration of urinary continent periods. Note any complications, including emotional problems and signs of skin breakdown and infection, as well as the treatments you provided for them. Document teaching provided to the patient and family (if applicable), their understanding of that teaching, and any need for follow-up teaching.

REFERENCES

1 Nazarko, L. (2017). Beyond the bladder: Holistic care when urinary incontinence develops. *British Journal of Community Nursing, 22,* 662–666.

2 Craven, H. (Ed.). (2016). *Core curriculum for medical-surgical nursing* (5th ed.). Pitman, NJ: Academy of Medical-Surgical Nurses.

3 Lukacz, E. S. (2021). Evaluation of females with urinary incontinence. In: *UpToDate,* Brubaker, L., & Schmader, K.E. (Eds.).

4 Clemens, J. Q. (2019). Urinary incontinence in men. In: *UpToDate,* O'Leary, M. P. (Ed.).

5 Wakamatsu, M. M., et al. (2017). *Better bladder and bowel control: Practical strategies for managing incontinence.* Boston, MA: Harvard Health Publications.

6 Jelovsek, J. E., & Reddy, J. (2020). Surgical management of stress urinary incontinence in women: Choosing a type of midurethral sling. In: *UpToDate,* Brubaker, L. (Ed.).

7 Wound Ostomy and Continence Nurses Society (WOCN). (2016). *Guideline for prevention and management of pressure ulcers (injuries): WOCN clinical practice guideline series 2.* Mount Laurel, NJ: WOCN.

8 Centers for Disease Control and Prevention. (2002). Guideline for hand hygiene in health-care settings: Recommendations of the Healthcare Infection Control Practices Advisory Committee and the HICPAC/SHEA/APIC/IDSA Hand Hygiene Task Force. *MMWR Recommendations and Reports, 51*(RR-16), 1–45. https://www.cdc.gov/mmwr/pdf/rr/rr5116.pdf (Level II)

9 World Health Organization. (2009). WHO guidelines on hand hygiene in health care: First global patient safety challenge, clean care is safer care. https://apps.who.int/iris/bitstream/handle/10665/44102/9789241597906_eng.pdf?sequence=1 (Level IV)

10 The Joint Commission. (2021). Standard NPSG.07.01.01. *Comprehensive accreditation manual for hospitals.* Oakbrook Terrace, IL: The Joint Commission. (Level VII)

11 Centers for Medicare and Medicaid Services, Department of Health and Human Services. (2020. Condition of participation: Infection control. 42 C.F.R. § 482.42.

12 Accreditation Association for Hospitals and Health Systems. (2020). Standard 07.01.21. *Healthcare Facilities Accreditation Program: Accreditation requirements for acute care hospitals.* Chicago, IL: Accreditation Association for Hospitals and Health Systems. (Level VII)

13 DNV GL-Healthcare USA, Inc. (2020). IC.1.SR.1. *NIAHO® accreditation requirements, interpretive guidelines and surveyor guidance—revision 20.0.* Milford, OH: DNV GL-Healthcare USA, Inc. (Level VII)

14 The Joint Commission. (2021). Standard NPSG.01.01.01. *Comprehensive accreditation manual for hospitals.* Oakbrook Terrace, IL: The Joint Commission. (Level VII)

15 The Joint Commission. (2021). Standard RI.01.01.01. *Comprehensive accreditation manual for hospitals.* Oakbrook Terrace, IL: The Joint Commission. (Level VII)

16 Centers for Medicare and Medicaid Services, Department of Health and Human Services. (2020). Condition of participation: Patient's rights. 42 C.F.R. § 482.13(c)(1).

17 Accreditation Association for Hospitals and Health Systems. (2020). Standard 15.01.16. *Healthcare Facilities Accreditation Program: Accreditation requirements for acute care hospitals.* Chicago, IL: Accreditation Association for Hospitals and Health Systems. (Level VII)

18 DNV GL-Healthcare USA, Inc. (2020). PR.2.SR.5. *NIAHO® accreditation requirements, interpretive guidelines and surveyor guidance—revision 20.0.* Milford, OH: DNV GL-Healthcare USA, Inc. (Level VII)

19 Waters, T. R., et al. (2009). Safe patient handling training for schools of nursing. https://www.cdc.gov/niosh/docs/2009-127/pdfs/2009-127.pdf (Level VII)

20 Siegel, J. D., et al. (2007, revised 2019). 2007 guideline for isolation precautions: Preventing transmission of infectious agents in healthcare settings. https://www.cdc.gov/infectioncontrol/pdf/guidelines/isolation-guidelines-H.pdf (Level II)

21 Accreditation Association for Hospitals and Health Systems. (2020). Standard 07.01.10. *Healthcare Facilities Accreditation Program: Accreditation requirements for acute care hospitals.* Chicago, IL: Accreditation Association for Hospitals and Health Systems. (Level VII)

22 Occupational Safety and Health Administration. (2012). Bloodborne pathogens, standard number 1910.1030. https://www.osha.gov/pls/oshaweb/owadisp.show_document?p_id=10051&p_table=STANDARDS (Level VII)

23 Elmer, C., et al. (2017). Twenty-four–hour voiding diaries versus 3-day voiding diaries: A clinical comparison. *Female Pelvic Medicine and Reconstructive Surgery, 23,* 429–432.

24 Hooton, T. M., & Gupta, K. (2021). Recurrent simple cystitis in women. In: *UpToDate*, Calderwood, S. B. (Ed.).

25 Lukacz, E. S. (2020). Treatment of urinary incontinence in females. In: *UpToDate*, Brubaker, L., & Schmader, K. E. (Eds.).

26 Qaseem, A., et al. (2014). Nonsurgical management of urinary incontinence in women: A clinical practice guideline from the American College of Physicians. *Annals of Internal Medicine, 161*(6), 429–440. https://www.acpjournals.org/doi/10.7326/M13-2410 (Level VII)

27 Langemo, D., et al. (2011). Incontinence and incontinence-associated dermatitis. *Advances in Skin and Wound Care, 24,* 126–140.

28 Chatham, N., & Carls, C. (2012). How to manage incontinence-associated dermatitis. *Wound Care Advisor, 1*(1), 7–11.

29 Zulkowski, K. (2012). Diagnosing and treating moisture-associated skin damage. *Advances in Skin and Wound Care, 25*(5), 231–236. https://journals.lww.com/aswcjournal/Fulltext/2012/05000/Diagnosing_and_Treating_Moisture_Associated_Skin.9.aspx

30 Gray, M., et al. (2012). Incontinence-associated dermatitis: A comprehensive review and update. *Journal of Wound, Ostomy and Continence Nursing, 39,* 61–74. (Level V)

31 Ganz, D. A., et al. (2013, reviewed 2021). *Preventing falls in hospitals: A toolkit for improving quality of care* (AHRQ Publication No. 13-0015-EF). Rockville, MD: Agency for Healthcare Research and Quality. https://www.ahrq.gov/professionals/systems/hospital/fallpxtoolkit/index.html (Level VII)

32 The Joint Commission. (2021). Standard RC.01.03.01. *Comprehensive accreditation manual for hospitals.* Oakbrook Terrace, IL: The Joint Commission. (Level VII)

33 Centers for Medicare and Medicaid Services, Department of Health and Human Services. (2020). Condition of participation: Medical record services. 42 C.F.R. § 482.24(b).

34 Accreditation Association for Hospitals and Health Systems. (2020). Standard 10.00.03. *Healthcare Facilities Accreditation Program: Accreditation requirements for acute care hospitals.* Chicago, IL: Accreditation Association for Hospitals and Health Systems. (Level VII)

35 DNV GL-Healthcare USA, Inc. (2020). MR.2.SR.1. *NIAHO® accreditation requirements, interpretive guidelines and surveyor guidance—revision 20.0.* Milford, OH: DNV GL-Healthcare USA, Inc. (Level VII)

36 Beeson, T. & Davis, C. (2018). Urinary management with an external female collection device. *Journal of Wound, Ostomy and Continence Nursing, 45*(2), 187–189. https://journals.lww.com/jwocnonline/fulltext/2018/03000/Urinary_Management_With_an_External_Female.15.aspx

37 Lightner, D. J., et al. (2012, amended 2019). Diagnosis and treatment of non-neurogenic overactive bladder (OAB) in adults: AUA/SUFU guideline (2019). *Journal of Urology, 202,* 588–563. https://www.auanet.org/guidelines/overactive-bladder-(oab)-guideline (Level VII)

Indwelling urinary catheter care and removal

The Centers for Disease Control and Prevention estimates that 15% to 25% of hospitalized patients have an indwelling urinary (Foley) catheter inserted at some time during their hospitalization.[1] Catheters are often inserted for inappropriate indications.[2,3] Consider alternatives to indwelling urinary catheterization when appropriate, such as external catheter application, bladder ultrasonography, intermittent catheterization, use of optimal incontinence products, prompted toileting, urinal and bedside commode use, and daily weights as alternative methods to collect and measure urine and monitor fluid balance.[4] Appropriate indications for catheter use include perioperative use for selected surgical procedures, such as urologic surgery or surgery on contiguous structures of the genitourinary tract, prolonged surgery, large-volume infusions or diuretic use during surgery, or when intraoperative urine output monitoring is needed; prolonged immobilization, such as for an unstable thoracic or lumbar spine or multiple trauma injuries, including pelvic fractures; hourly urine output measurement in critically ill patients; acute urinary retention or urinary obstruction; assistance in healing of open pressure injuries or skin grafts for selected patients with urinary incontinence; and at the patient's request to improve comfort during end-of-life care.[5]

Inappropriate or unnecessary use of an indwelling urinary catheter can result in catheter-associated urinary tract infection (CAUTI). CAUTI is the most common type of health care–associated infection in adult patients.[3,6] Researchers estimate that as much as 70% of these infections are preventable by following a variety of evidence-based practices.[3,6,7]

HOSPITAL-ACQUIRED CONDITION ALERT Keep in mind that the Centers for Medicare and Medicaid Services considers CAUTI a hospital-acquired condition *because various best practices can reasonably prevent it. To reduce the risk of CAUTI* when caring for a patient with an indwelling urinary catheter, be sure to follow evidence-based CAUTI prevention practices, such as performing hand hygiene before and after any catheter manipulation; maintaining a sterile, continuously closed drainage system; maintaining unobstructed urine flow; regularly emptying the collection bag; replacing the catheter and drainage system using sterile technique when breaks in sterile technique, disconnection, or leakage occurs; and discontinuing the catheter as soon as it's no longer clinically indicated.[5,8,9,10,11,12,13]

Equipment

Gloves ▪ washcloth and soap and water or plain disposable wipe ▪ urine collection container ▪ Optional: light source, tape, gown, goggles, mask, mask with face shield, perineal cleaner, catheter securement device.

For catheter removal

Fluid-impermeable pad ▪ gloves ▪ drape ▪ 10-mL Luer lock syringe ▪ perineal care supplies ▪ graduated container ▪ Optional: gown, mask and goggles or mask with face shield, adhesive remover, cotton-tipped applicator, gauze pads, oral fluids.

Preparation of equipment

Inspect all equipment and supplies. If a product is expired, is defective, or has compromised integrity, remove it from patient use, label it as expired or defective, and report the expiration or defect as directed by your facility.

Implementation

Catheter care

- Gather and prepare the necessary equipment and supplies.
- Perform hand hygiene.[5,13,14,15,16,17,18]
- Confirm the patient's identity using at least two patient identifiers.[19]
- Provide privacy.[20,21,22,23]
- Explain the procedure to the patient and family (if appropriate) according to their individual communication and learning needs *to increase their understanding, allay their fears, and enhance cooperation.*[24] Discuss the risks associated with indwelling urinary catheter use and the measures necessary to reduce the risk of CAUTI.[3,6,11] Advise the patient to remind staff to perform hand hygiene before and after handling the catheter if they fail to do so.[3,6,11]
- Make sure the lighting is adequate *so that you can clearly see the perineum and catheter tubing.*

- Review the necessity of continued urinary catheter use; remove the catheter (as ordered or according to facility protocol) as soon as it's no longer clinically indicated *to reduce the risk of CAUTI*.[5,8,10,11,25]
- Raise the patient's bed to waist level before performing patient care *to prevent caregiver back strain*.[26]
- Perform hand hygiene.[5,13,14,15,16,17,18]
- Put on gloves and other personal protective equipment, as needed, *to comply with standard precautions*.[27,28,29]
- Inspect the urinary catheter system for disconnections and leakage, *because a sterile, continuously closed system is required to reduce the risk of CAUTI*. Replace the catheter and drainage system using sterile no-touch technique when a break in sterile technique, disconnection, or leakage occurs.[5,8,10,11,30]
- Provide routine hygiene for meatal care; note that cleaning the meatal area with antiseptic solutions isn't necessary.[5,8,11,30] *To avoid contaminating the urinary tract*, always clean by wiping away from—never toward—the urinary meatus. Use a washcloth and soap and water (or a perineal cleaner, if used in your facility) or a plain disposable wipe to clean the periurethral area.[25,31] Clean after each bowel movement; avoid frequent and vigorous cleaning of the area.[31] Gently retract the foreskin of an uncircumcised male and clean the area, and then return the foreskin to its normal position.[31]

NURSING ALERT When cleaning the periurethral area, clean the area carefully *to prevent catheter movement and urethral traction, which increase the risk of CAUTI*.[31]

- Inspect the periurethral area for signs of inflammation and infection.
- Make sure the catheter is properly secured.[8,32] Assess the securement device daily, and change it when clinically indicated and as recommended by the manufacturer.[33] If a new securement device is needed, connect it to the catheter before applying the device to the skin.[32] If a securement device isn't available, use a piece of adhesive tape to secure the catheter.[34] If using tape, retape the catheter on the side opposite from where it was previously *to prevent skin hypersensitivity and irritation*.

NURSING ALERT Provide enough slack before securing the catheter to prevent tension on the tubing, *which could injure the urethral lumen and bladder wall*.[5]

- Monitor intake and output, as ordered. Monitor for changes in urine output, including volume and color.[35] Notify the practitioner of abnormal changes.
- Empty the drainage bag regularly when it becomes one-half to two-thirds full *to prevent undue traction on the urethra from the weight of urine in the bag*. Use a separate collecting container to empty the drainage for each patient. During emptying, avoid splashing, and don't allow the drainage spigot to come in contact with the nonsterile collecting container.[5,8,10,31,36]
- Keep the catheter and drainage tubing free from kinks and avoid dependent loops *to allow the free flow of urine*.[11,25]
- Keep the drainage bag below the level of the patient's bladder *to prevent backflow of urine into the bladder, which increases the risk of CAUTI*.[3,5,8,10,25,36] Don't place the drainage bag on the floor, *to reduce the risk of contamination and subsequent CAUTI*.[10,37]
- Return the bed to the lowest position *to prevent falls and maintain patient safety*.[38]
- Discard used supplies in appropriate receptacles.[29]
- Remove and discard your gloves and any other personal protective equipment worn.[27,29]
- Perform hand hygiene.[13,14,15,16,17,18]
- Document the procedure.[39,40,41,42]

Catheter removal

- Verify the practitioner's order, if necessary, or follow your facility's protocol for indwelling urinary catheter removal.
- Gather and prepare the necessary equipment and supplies.
- Perform hand hygiene.[5,13,14,15,16,17,18]
- Confirm the patient's identity using at least two patient identifiers.[19]
- Explain the procedure to the patient and family (if appropriate) according to their individual communication and learning needs *to increase their understanding, allay their fears, and enhance cooperation*.[24] Tell the patient to expect slight discomfort.
- Provide privacy.[20,21,22,23]

- Raise the patient's bed to waist level before performing patient care *to prevent caregiver back strain*.[26]
- Perform hand hygiene.[5,13,14,15,16,17,18]
- Put on gloves and other personal protective equipment, as necessary, *to comply with standard precautions*.[27,28,29]
- Place a fluid-impermeable pad under the patient *to protect the bed linens*.
- Position the patient for easy access to the urinary catheter, and drape the patient for privacy.
- Remove the urinary catheter securement device gently according to the manufacturer's directions, or remove the tape that secures the catheter and catheter tubing. Apply adhesive remover with a cotton-tipped applicator or gauze pad, if needed, *to assist with removal and to prevent skin tearing or shearing*.
- Assess the patient's perineum and meatus for redness, irritation, or discharge.
- Trace the tubing from the patient to the point of origin *to make sure that you're accessing the proper port*.[43] Attach a 10-mL Luer-lock syringe to the Luer-lock mechanism on the urinary catheter.
- Allow the pressure within the urinary catheter's balloon to force the plunger back and to fill the syringe with all of the sterile water in the balloon *to deflate the balloon*. The amount of sterile water injected usually is indicated on the tip of the catheter's balloon lumen and in the patient's medical record. Avoid vigorous aspiration, *because this may cause the balloon inflation lumen to collapse*; use only gentle aspiration, if needed, *to encourage deflation*. Allow adequate time (about 30 seconds) for the pressure within the balloon to fill the syringe. If the balloon doesn't deflate or if deflation is slow, remove and reapply the syringe to the Luer-lock mechanism. If the balloon still doesn't deflate, consider severing the balloon valve arm, if permitted by your facility. If necessary, contact the practitioner or other specially trained professional for assistance, as indicated by your facility.[44]
- Ask the patient to take a deep breath in and then out *to help relax the pelvic floor muscles*; as the patient exhales, gently remove the catheter by withdrawing it slowly and evenly. If you meet resistance while withdrawing the catheter, stop and notify the practitioner. Warn a male patients that he may feel discomfort as the deflated balloon passes through the prostatic urethra.[45]
- If the patient is able to perform perineal self-care, provide the necessary supplies. If not, provide perineal care.[45]
- Remove and discard the fluid-impermeable pad, and position the patient for comfort.
- Measure and record the amount of urine in the collection bag before discarding it.
- Encourage the patient whose condition allows it to maintain an oral intake of 30 mL/kg/day *to flush the bladder of microorganisms that might be associated with indwelling urinary catheter use*.[45]
- Return the bed to the lowest position *to prevent falls and maintain patient safety*.[38]
- Discard used supplies in the appropriate receptacles.[29]
- Remove and discard your gloves and any other personal protective equipment worn.[27,29]
- Perform hand hygiene.[13,14,15,16,17,18]
- Monitor the patient for first voiding after indwelling urinary catheter removal. Assess the volume and characteristics of the voided urine.
- Perform hand hygiene.[13,14,15,16,17,18]
- Document the procedure.[39,40,41,42]

Special considerations

- Unless obstruction is anticipated (for example, from bleeding after prostate or bladder surgery), bladder irrigation isn't recommended. If obstruction is anticipated, continuous irrigation is suggested *to prevent obstruction*.[31]
- If you need to collect a small urine specimen or culture, thoroughly disinfect the needleless sampling port with a disinfectant pad and then allow it to dry completely. Collect the sample by aspirating urine from the needleless sampling port with a sterile syringe or sterile urine collection tube system and a cannula adapter.[5,8,31] (See the "Urine specimen collection" procedure.)
- If a large volume of urine is needed for special analysis, obtain the sample from the drainage bag using sterile technique.[8,31]

PATIENT TEACHING

Teaching about leg bags

A urine drainage bag attached to the leg provides the catheterized patient with greater mobility. *Because the bag is hidden under clothing,* it may also help the patient feel more comfortable about catheterization. Leg bags are usually worn during the day and are replaced at night with a standard drainage bag.

If the patient will be discharged with an indwelling urinary catheter, teach the patient how to attach and remove a leg bag. To demonstrate, you'll need a bag with a short drainage tube, two straps, an alcohol pad, adhesive tape, and a screw clamp or hemostat.

Attaching the leg bag
■ Perform hand hygiene and instruct the patient to do so as well.[13,14,15,16,17,18]
■ Provide privacy.[20,21,22,23]
■ Explain the procedure according to the patient's individual communication and learning needs.[24] Describe the advantages of a leg bag, but caution the patient that a leg bag is smaller than a standard drainage bag and may have to be emptied more frequently.
■ Remove the protective covering from the tip of the drainage tube. Then show the patient how to clean the tip with an alcohol pad, wiping away from the opening *to avoid contaminating the tube.*
■ Show the patient how to attach the tube to the catheter.
■ Place the drainage bag on the patient's calf or thigh. Have the patient fasten the straps securely (as shown at right), and then show the patient how to tape the catheter to the leg. Emphasize that the patient must leave slack in the catheter *to minimize pressure on the bladder, urethra, and related structures. Excessive pressure or tension can lead to tissue breakdown.*

Avoiding complications
■ Although most leg bags have a valve in the drainage tube that prevents urine reflux into the bladder, urge the patient to keep the drainage bag lower than the bladder at all times, *because urine in the bag is a perfect growth medium for bacteria.* Caution the patient also not to go to bed or take long naps while wearing the leg bag.

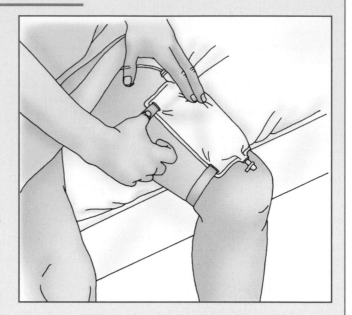

■ *To prevent a full leg bag from damaging the bladder wall and urethra,* encourage the patient to empty the bag when it's half full, or every 3 to 6 hours.[34] The patient should also inspect the catheter and drainage tube periodically for compression or kinking, *which could obstruct urine flow and result in bladder distention.*
■ Instruct the patient to avoid fastening the straps too tightly, *because doing so may impede circulation.*
■ Tell the patient to wash the leg bag with soap and water or a bacteriostatic solution before each use *to prevent infection.*

■ When possible, attach a leg bag *to allow the patient greater mobility.*
■ Encourage a patient with unrestricted fluid intake to increase intake to at least 30 mL/kg/day *to help flush the urinary system and reduce sediment formation.*[34,46]
■ Unless otherwise clinically indicated, consider using the smallest bore catheter possible, consistent with good drainage, *to minimize bladder neck and urethral trauma.*[8,25,31]
■ After catheter removal, assess the patient for incontinence, dribbling, urgency, persistent dysuria or bladder spasms, fever, chills, and palpable bladder distention. Report these conditions to the practitioner.
■ The Joint Commission issued a sentinel event alert related to managing risk during transition to new International Organization for Standardization tubing standards that were designed to prevent dangerous tubing misconnections, which can lead to serious patient injury and death. During the transition, make sure to trace the tubing and catheter from the patient to the point of origin before connecting or reconnecting any device or infusion, at any care transition (such as a new setting or service), and as part of the hand-off process; route tubes and catheters having different purposes in different standardized directions; when there are different access sites or several bags hanging, label the tubing at the distal and proximal ends; use tubing and equipment only as intended; and store medications for different delivery routes in separate locations.[43]

Patient teaching
If the patient will be discharged with an indwelling catheter, teach the patient how to use a leg bag. (See *Teaching about leg bags.*) Instruct the patient to wash the urinary meatus and perineal area with soap and water as part of routine hygiene, and to wash the anal area after each bowel movement. Provide the patient and family (if appropriate) with information regarding additional methods of infection control as well as the signs and symptoms of urinary tract infection and obstruction.[46] Also review with the patient reasons to notify the practitioner.

Inform the patient that transient incontinence, urinary urgency and frequency, dysuria, discomfort, and urine retention can occur after indwelling urinary catheter removal. Advise the patient to notify the practitioner if these signs and symptoms persist for more than 48 hours.[45]

Complications
Complications associated with indwelling urinary catheter use include CAUTI, genitourinary trauma, epididymitis (in men), retained balloon fragments, bladder fistula (with prolonged use), bladder stone formation, and incontinence.[47,48]

Indwelling urinary catheter balloon rupture can occur during indwelling urinary catheter removal. If resistance is met, failure to stop the procedure can lead to trauma, bleeding, and scar tissue formation, which can lead to urethral stricture.

Documentation
Document the indication that necessitates continued catheter use, the maintenance care you provided, and your assessment findings.[8,11,25] Document teaching you provided to the patient and family (if appropriate), their understanding of that teaching, and any need for follow-up teaching. Also record any specimens you collected and the collection method you used.

Document the date and time you removed the indwelling urinary catheter, the amount of sterile water removed from the urinary catheter balloon, perineal assessment findings, and the patient's tolerance of the procedure. Record any complications of catheter removal, your interventions, and the patient's response to those interventions. Also record the time, volume, and characteristics of the patient's first voiding after indwelling urinary catheter removal. Document teaching provided to the patient and family (if applicable), their understanding of that teaching, and any need for follow-up teaching.

REFERENCES

1 Centers for Disease Control and Prevention. (2015). Catheter-associated urinary tract infections (CAUTI). https://www.cdc.gov/hai/ca_uti/uti.html

2 Gould, C. (n.d.). Catheter-associated urinary tract infection (CAUTI) toolkit. http://www.cdc.gov/HAI/pdfs/toolkits/CAUTItoolkit_3_10.pdf

3 Carter, N. M., et al. (2014). An evidence-based approach to the prevention of catheter-associated urinary tract infections. *Urologic Nursing, 34,* 238–245.

4 American Hospital Association & Health Research and Educational Trust. (n.d.). Catheter associated urinary tract infection (CAUTI) top ten checklist. http://patientcarelink.org/wp-content/uploads/2015/11/CAUTI-Top-Ten-checklist_2014.pdf

5 Healthcare Infection Control Practices Advisory Committee. (2010, revised 2019). Guideline for prevention of catheter-associated urinary tract infections 2009. https://www.cdc.gov/infectioncontrol/pdf/guidelines/cauti-guidelines-H.pdf (Level I)

6 Halm, M. A., & O'Connor, N. (2014). Do system-based interventions affect catheter-associated urinary tract infection? *American Journal of Critical Care, 23,* 505–509. (Level V)

7 Seckel, M. A. (2013). Maintaining urinary catheters: What does the evidence say? *Nursing2013, 43*(2), 63–65. http://journals.lww.com/nursing/Pages/articleviewer.aspx?year=2013&issue=02000&article=00018&type=Fulltext

8 Lo, E., et al. (2014). SHEA/IDSA practice recommendation. Strategies to prevent catheter-associated urinary tract infections in acute care hospitals: 2014 update. *Infection Control and Hospital Epidemiology, 35*(5), 464–479. https://www.jstor.org/stable/10.1086/675718#metadata_info_tab_contents (Level I)

9 Jarrett, N., & Callaham, M. (2016). Evidence-based guidelines for selected hospital-acquired conditions: Final report. https://www.cms.gov/Medicare/Medicare-Fee-for-Service-Payment/HospitalAcqCond/Downloads/2016-HAC-Report.pdf

10 The Joint Commission. (2021). Standard NPSG.07.06.01. *Comprehensive accreditation manual for hospitals.* Oakbrook Terrace, IL: The Joint Commission. (Level VII)

11 Association of Professionals in Infection Control and Epidemiology. (2014). APIC implementation guide: Guide to preventing catheter-associated urinary tract infections. https://apic.org/wp-content/uploads/2019/02/APIC_CAUTI_IG_FIN_REVD0815.pdf (Level IV)

12 Agency for Healthcare Research and Quality & U.S. Department of Health and Human Services. (2015). Toolkit for reducing catheter-associated urinary tract infections in hospital units: Implementation guide. https://www.ahrq.gov/hai/cauti-tools/impl-guide/index.html

13 Centers for Disease Control and Prevention. (2002). Guideline for hand hygiene in health-care settings: Recommendations of the Healthcare Infection Control Practices Advisory Committee and the HICPAC/SHEA/APIC/IDSA Hand Hygiene Task Force. *MMWR Recommendations and Reports, 51*(RR-16), 1–45. https://www.cdc.gov/mmwr/pdf/rr/rr5116.pdf (Level II)

14 The Joint Commission. (2021). Standard NPSG.07.01.01. *Comprehensive accreditation manual for hospitals.* Oakbrook Terrace, IL: The Joint Commission. (Level VII)

15 World Health Organization. (2009). WHO guidelines on hand hygiene in health care: First global patient safety challenge, clean care is safer care. https://apps.who.int/iris/bitstream/handle/10665/44102/9789241597906_eng.pdf?sequence=1 (Level IV)

16 Accreditation Association for Hospitals and Health Systems. (2020). Standard 07.01.21. *Healthcare Facilities Accreditation Program: Accreditation requirements for acute care hospitals.* Chicago, IL: Accreditation Association for Hospitals and Health Systems. (Level VII)

17 Centers for Medicare and Medicaid Services, Department of Health and Human Services. (2020). Condition of participation: Infection control. 42 C.F.R. § 482.42.

18 DNV GL-Healthcare USA, Inc. (2020). IC.1.SR.1. *NIAHO® accreditation requirements, interpretive guidelines and surveyor guidance—revision 20.0.* Milford, OH: DNV GL-Healthcare USA, Inc. (Level VII)

19 The Joint Commission. (2021). Standard NPSG.01.01.01. *Comprehensive accreditation manual for hospitals.* Oakbrook Terrace, IL: The Joint Commission. (Level VII)

20 Accreditation Association for Hospitals and Health Systems. (2020). Standard 15.01.16. *Healthcare Facilities Accreditation Program: Accreditation requirements for acute care hospitals.* Chicago, IL: Accreditation Association for Hospitals and Health Systems. (Level VII)

21 Centers for Medicare and Medicaid Services, Department of Health and Human Services. (2020). Condition of participation: Patient's rights. 42 C.F.R. § 482.13(c)(1).

22 DNV GL-Healthcare USA, Inc. (2020). PR.2.SR.5. *NIAHO® accreditation requirements, interpretive guidelines and surveyor guidance—revision 20.0.* Milford, OH: DNV GL-Healthcare USA, Inc. (Level VII)

23 The Joint Commission. (2021). Standard RI.01.01.01. *Comprehensive accreditation manual for hospitals.* Oakbrook Terrace, IL: The Joint Commission. (Level VII)

24 The Joint Commission. (2021). Standard PC.02.01.21. *Comprehensive accreditation manual for hospitals.* Oakbrook Terrace, IL: The Joint Commission. (Level VII)

25 American Association of Critical-Care Nurses. (2017). AACN practice alert: Prevention of CAUTI in adults. https://www.aacn.org/~/media/aacn-website/clincial-resources/practice-alerts/adultcauti2017practicealert.pdf (Level VII)

26 Waters, T. R., et al. (2009). Safe patient handling training for schools of nursing. https://www.cdc.gov/niosh/docs/2009-127/pdfs/2009-127.pdf (Level VII)

27 Siegel, J. D., et al. (2007, revised 2019). 2007 guideline for isolation precautions: Preventing transmission of infectious agents in healthcare settings. https://www.cdc.gov/infectioncontrol/pdf/guidelines/isolation-guidelines-H.pdf (Level II)

28 Accreditation Association for Hospitals and Health Systems. (2020). Standard 07.01.10. *Healthcare Facilities Accreditation Program: Accreditation requirements for acute care hospitals.* Chicago, IL: Accreditation Association for Hospitals and Health Systems. (Level VII)

29 Occupational Safety and Health Administration. (2012). Bloodborne pathogens, standard number 1910.1030. https://www.osha.gov/pls/oshaweb/owadisp.show_document?p_id=10051&p_table=STANDARDS (Level VII)

30 Porche, D. J. (2021). Urinary tract infection (catheter related): Prevention strategies. *The JBI EBP Database.* AN: JBI14392 (Level V)

31 Quallich, S. A., et al. (2021) Insertion of an indwelling urinary catheter in the adult female. *Urologic Nursing, 41*(2), 65–69. (Level VII)

32 Payne, D. (2014). Safe and secure: Catheter fixation. *Nursing and Residential Care, 16,* 608–610.

33 Bard, C. R. (2017). StatLock® Foley stabilization devices: Instructions for use. https://www.crbard.com/CRBard/media/ProductAssets/BardMedicalDivision/PF10225/en-US/w09j05g0k3nw9x9p115ya5tnp-pvu02co.pdf

34 Quallich, S. A., et al. (2021) Insertion of an indwelling urinary catheter in the adult male. *Urologic Nursing, 41*(2), 86–109. (Level VII)

35 Craven, H. (Ed.). (2016). *Core curriculum for medical-surgical nursing* (5th ed.). Pitman, NJ: Academy of Medical-Surgical Nurses.

36 Moola, S. (2021). Urinary drainage bags: Emptying, changing, and securing. *The JBI EBP Database.* AN: JBI1334 (Level V)

37 Smith, J. M. (2003). Indwelling catheter management: From habit-based to evidence-based practice. *Ostomy/Wound Management, 49*(12), 34–45. http://www.o-wm.com/content/indwelling-catheter-management-from-habit-based-evidence-based-practice

38 Ganz, D. A., et al. (2013, reviewed 2021). *Preventing falls in hospitals: A toolkit for improving quality of care* (AHRQ Publication No. 13-0015-EF). Rockville, MD: Agency for Healthcare Research and Quality. https://www.ahrq.gov/professionals/systems/hospital/fallpxtoolkit/index.html (Level VII)

39 The Joint Commission. (2021). Standard RC.01.03.01. *Comprehensive accreditation manual for hospitals.* Oakbrook Terrace, IL: The Joint Commission. (Level VII)

40 Accreditation Association for Hospitals and Health Systems. (2020). Standard 10.00.03. *Healthcare Facilities Accreditation Program: Accreditation requirements for acute care hospitals.* Chicago, IL: Accreditation Association for Hospitals and Health Systems. (Level VII)

41 Centers for Medicare and Medicaid Services, Department of Health and Human Services. (2020). Condition of participation: Medical record services. 42 C.F.R. § 482.24(b).

42 DNV GL-Healthcare USA, Inc. (2020). MR.2.SR.1. *NIAHO® accreditation requirements, interpretive guidelines and surveyor guidance—revision 20.0.* Milford, OH: DNV GL-Healthcare USA, Inc. (Level VII)

43 The Joint Commission. (2014). Sentinel event alert 53: Managing risk during transition to new ISO tubing connector standards.

http://www.jointcommission.org/assets/1/6/SEA_53_Connectors_8_19_14_final.pdf (Level VII)

44 C. R. Bard, Inc. (n.d.). SureStep™ Foley tray system: Insertion and removal skills training checklist. http://surestep.bardmedical.com/media/675882/ud_surestep_insertionremovalchecklist.pdf

45 European Association of Urology Nurses. (2012). Evidence-based guidelines for best practice in urological health care. Catheterisation: Indwelling catheters in adults. Urethral and suprapubic. https://www.nursing.nl/PageFiles/11870/001_1391694991387.pdf (Level VII)

46 Herter, R., & Kazer, M. W. (2010). Best practices in urinary catheter care. *Home Healthcare Nurse, 28*(6), 342–349. https://journals.lww.com/homehealthcarenurseonline/Fulltext/2010/06000/Best_Practices_in_Urin

47 Leuck, A. M., et al. (2012). Complications of Foley catheters: Is infection the greatest risk? *Journal of Urology, 187*, 1662–1666. (Level VI)

48 Schaeffer, A. J. (2021). Complications of urinary bladder catheters and preventive strategies. In: *UpToDate*, Richie, J. P. (Ed.).

INDWELLING URINARY CATHETER INSERTION

An indwelling urinary (Foley) catheter remains in the bladder to provide continuous urine drainage. A balloon inflated at the catheter's distal end prevents it from slipping out of the bladder after insertion.

An indwelling urinary catheter should be inserted only when absolutely necessary, *because its use is associated with an increased risk of developing a urinary tract infection, with the risk increasing with each day of use.*[1,2] Catheter-associated urinary tract infection (CAUTI) is the most common type of health care–associated infection in the United States, accounting for 35% of all such infections.[3]

HOSPITAL-ACQUIRED CONDITION ALERT Keep in mind that the Centers for Medicare and Medicaid Services considers CAUTI a hospital-acquired condition, *because best practices can reasonably prevent it.* To reduce the risk of CAUTI when caring for a patient with an indwelling urinary catheter, be sure to follow CAUTI prevention practices, such as performing hand hygiene before and after any catheter manipulation; maintaining a sterile, continuously closed drainage system; maintaining unobstructed urine flow; emptying the collection bag regularly; replacing the catheter and collection system using sterile technique when a break in sterile technique, disconnection, or leakage occurs; and discontinuing the catheter as soon as it's no longer clinically indicated.[1,4,5,6,7,8]

To reduce the risk of CAUTI, consider alternatives to indwelling urinary catheterization when appropriate, such as external catheter application, bladder ultrasonography, intermittent catheterization, use of optimal incontinent products, prompted toileting, urinal and bedside commode use, and daily weight as alternative methods for collecting and measuring urine and monitoring fluid balance.[9] Insert an indwelling urinary catheter only for appropriate indications, such as acute urinary retention or bladder outlet obstruction; the need for accurate urine output measurements in a critically ill patient; perioperative use for a patient undergoing urologic surgery or another procedure on structures of the genitourinary tract; prolonged surgery (with removal of catheters inserted for this purpose in the postanesthesia care unit); large-volume infusions or diuretic administration anticipated during surgery; intraoperative monitoring of urinary output; assistance in the healing of open sacral or perineal wounds or skin grafts in certain incontinent patients;[5] prolonged immobilization (such as potentially unstable thoracic or lumbar spine and multiple traumatic injuries, including pelvic fractures); and improved comfort for end-of-life care, if needed.[2]

Indwelling urinary catheter insertion is contraindicated in a patient who has a urethral injury, which is typically associated with pelvic trauma. Relative contraindications include urethral stricture, recent urinary tract surgery (such as urethra or bladder surgery), and the presence of an artificial sphincter. For these issues, a practitioner should be consulted to perform the procedure.[10,11]

Use sterile technique when inserting, manipulating, and maintaining the indwelling urinary catheter. Maintain a sterile, continuously closed drainage system; don't disconnect the catheter from the drainage bag unless absolutely necessary.[12] Avoid irrigation unless necessary.[1] When the patient has an indwelling urinary catheter inserted for surgery, ensure

its discontinuation within 24 hours of surgery unless another indication exists. Review the need for the indwelling urinary catheter daily, and remove it as soon as it's no longer necessary.[1,2,3,4,5,6,8]

Equipment

Sterile indwelling urinary catheter (smallest-bore catheter possible that will support adequate urine drainage) ■ syringe filled with 10 mL of sterile water ■ fluid-impermeable pad ■ gloves ■ sterile gloves ■ sterile drape ■ sterile fenestrated drape ■ sterile, presaturated antiseptic swabs; or antiseptic solution, sterile water, or sterile saline and either sterile swabs or sterile cotton balls and plastic forceps[2,5] ■ single-use packets of soap-containing wipes, or soap and water and a washcloth ■ single-use packet of sterile water-soluble lubricant ■ sterile drainage collection device ■ catheter securement device or tape ■ Optional: insertion checklist, towel, examination light or flashlight, bladder ultrasonography device, gown, mask with face shield or mask and goggles.

Prepackaged sterile disposable kits that usually contain all the necessary equipment are available.

Preparation of equipment

Inspect all equipment and supplies. If a product is expired, is defective, or has compromised integrity, remove it from patient use, label it as expired or defective, and report the expiration or defect, as directed by your facility.

Implementation

■ Verify the practitioner's order.

■ Assess the patient to make sure that an indwelling urinary catheter is indicated; assess for alternatives to indwelling urinary catheter use.[13] If necessary, use bladder ultrasonography to measure the volume of urine in the patient's bladder *to avoid unnecessary catheterization.*[2] (See the "Bladder ultrasonography" procedure.)

■ Check the patient's medical record for allergies, including to latex and iodine.[14]

■ Gather and prepare the necessary equipment and supplies. Use the smallest bore catheter possible that will support adequate urine drainage (unless otherwise clinically indicated) *to minimize bladder neck and urethral trauma.*[5,15]

■ Obtain the assistance of a coworker, as necessary, to help with patient positioning and to ensure that sterile technique is maintained during insertion.[1,16]

■ Ensure adequate lighting.

■ Use an insertion checklist if available in your facility *to guide the insertion process.*

■ Perform hand hygiene.[2,17,18,19,20,21,22,23]

■ Confirm the patient's identity using at least two patient identifiers.[24]

■ Provide privacy.[25,26,27,28]

■ Explain the procedure to the patient and family (if appropriate) according to their individual communication and learning needs *to increase their understanding, allay their fears, and enhance cooperation.*[29] Inform them of the reason for catheterization and what to expect in the way of discomfort.[17] Discuss the risks associated with indwelling urinary catheter use and the necessary measures to reduce the risk of CAUTI.[3,8] Advise the patient and family to remind staff to perform hand hygiene before and after handling the catheter if not done.

■ Raise the patient's bed to waist level before providing care *to prevent caregiver back strain.*[30]

■ Perform hand hygiene.[2,17,18,19,20,21,22,23]

■ Put on gloves and personal protective equipment, as needed, *to comply with standard precautions.*[31,32,33]

For a female patient

■ Place the patient in the supine or lithotomy position with her knees bent and legs abducted *to allow visualization of the urinary meatus.*[17] Alternatively, position the patient on her side in a knee-chest position if she's unable to tolerate supine or lithotomy positioning.

■ Place a fluid-impermeable pad on the bed between the patient's legs and under her hips *to avoid soiling the linens.*

■ Open the outer packaging of the prepackaged insertion kit and place it between the patient's legs.

■ Wash the patient's periurethral area with soap-containing wipes. Alternatively, clean the area with warm water and soap using a washcloth. Rinse and dry thoroughly.[1,7,9]

■ Remove and discard your gloves.[31,32]

■ Perform hand hygiene.[2,17,18,19,20,21,22,23]

■ Using sterile no-touch technique, open the insertion kit wrap.[34]

■ Put on sterile gloves.[1,2,5,7,19,31,32]

■ Place a sterile underpad beneath the patient; shield your gloves by cuffing the drape material under your gloved hands *to prevent contamination.*[34]

■ Place a sterile fenestrated drape over the perineal area *to create a sterile field* (as shown below).[17] Take care not to contaminate your gloves.

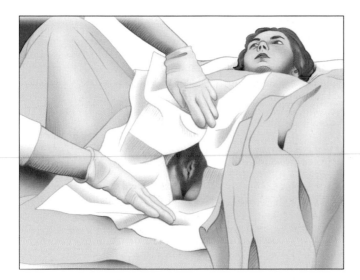

■ Tear open the packet of presaturated antiseptic swabs, or saturate sterile swabs of cotton balls with antiseptic solution, sterile water, or sterile saline as directed by your facility. Be careful not to spill the solution on the equipment.

■ Open the packet of water-soluble lubricant and deposit the lubricant into the insertion kit tray.

■ Open the catheter and place it on the tray with the lubricant.

■ If the drainage bag is not preconnected, attach it to the other end of the catheter.

■ Attach the syringe filled with sterile water to the balloon inflation port. Don't inflate the balloon before insertion unless directed by the manufacturer, *because doing so can cause microtears, which increase the risk of infection.*

■ Separate the labia majora and labia minora as widely as possible with the thumb, middle, and index fingers of your nondominant hand *so you have a full view of the urinary meatus.* Keep the labia well separated throughout the procedure *so they don't obscure the urinary meatus or contaminate the area when it's cleaned.*

■ With your dominant hand, use an antiseptic swab or, using plastic forceps, pick up a cotton ball soaked with sterile antiseptic, sterile water, or sterile saline to clean the labium minus furthest from you using a downward stroke; then discard the swab or cotton ball. Repeat for the labium closest to you. Use another antiseptic swab or solution-soaked cotton ball to clean the area between the labia minora.[17]

■ Maintaining sterile technique, pick up the catheter with your dominant hand and lubricate the catheter tip with the water-soluble lubricant.[17]

■ Hold the catheter 2″ to 3″ (5 cm to 7.6 cm) from the tip and slowly insert the lubricated catheter tip into the urinary meatus (as shown); expect to be able to advance the catheter without meeting resistance.[17]

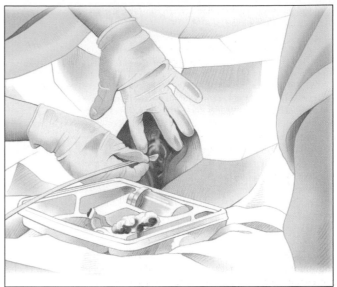

■ Continue to hold the labia apart until urine begins to flow, and advance the catheter about 2″ to 3″ (5 to 7.6 cm) further *to make sure the balloon is in the bladder and not in the urethra.*[17] If urine doesn't begin to flow, ask your coworker to apply gentle pressure to the suprapubic region, which may initiate urine flow.[11] If the catheter is inadvertently inserted into the vagina, leave it there as a landmark, then begin the procedure over again using new supplies.

■ Inflate the balloon using the water-filled syringe (as shown below), instilling the recommended amount of sterile water specified on the catheter *to secure the catheter inside the bladder.*[17] Gently pull the catheter until the inflated balloon is snug against the bladder neck.

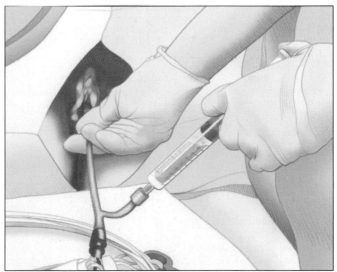

■ Secure the catheter to the patient's thigh using a securement device (or tape if a securement device isn't available) *to prevent possible tension on the urogenital trigone.*[2,17]

■ Keep the catheter and drainage tube free from kinking *to prevent obstruction of urinary flow.*[1,2,5,6]

■ Position the drainage bag below the level of the patient's bladder *to facilitate drainage and prevent stasis of urine, which increases the risk of CAUTI.*[1,2] Don't place the drainage bag on the floor, *to reduce the risk of contamination and subsequent CAUTI.*[2]

■ Return the bed to the lowest position *to prevent falls and maintain patient safety.*[35]

■ Discard used supplies in the appropriate receptacles.[33]

■ Remove and discard your gloves and any other personal protective equipment worn.[31,33]

- Perform hand hygiene.[2,17,18,19,20,21,22,23]
- Document the procedure.[36,37,38,39]

For a male patient

- Position the patient in the supine position with his legs extended and flat on the bed or his knees flexed and legs apart.[40] Ask the patient to hold the position *to give you a clear view of the urinary meatus and to prevent contamination of the sterile field.*
- Place a fluid-impermeable pad on the bed between the patient's legs and under his hips *to avoid soiling the linens.*
- Open the outer packaging of the prepackaged insertion kit and place it between the patient's legs.
- Wash the patient's periurethral area using soap-containing wipes. Alternatively, you may clean the area with warm water and soap using a washcloth. Rinse and dry the area thoroughly.[1,7,9]
- Remove and discard your gloves.[31,33]
- Perform hand hygiene.[2,17,18,19,20,21,22,23]
- Using sterile no-touch technique, open the insertion kit wrap.[34]
- Put on sterile gloves.[1,2,5,7,9,31,33]
- Place a sterile underpad beneath the patient; shield your gloves by cuffing the drape material under your gloved hands *to prevent contamination.*[34]
- Place a sterile fenestrated drape over the patient's lower abdomen and upper thighs so that only the genital area remains exposed (as shown below).[40] Take care not to contaminate your gloves.

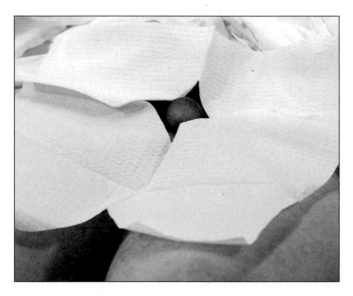

- Tear open the packet of presaturated antiseptic swabs, or saturate the sterile swabs or cotton balls with antiseptic solution, sterile water, or sterile saline solution as directed by your facility.[2,5] Be careful not to spill the solution on the equipment.
- Open the container of water-soluble lubricant and deposit the lubricant into the insertion kit tray. Open the catheter and place it in the tray with the lubricant.
- If the drainage bag is not preconnected, attach it to the other end of the catheter.
- Attach the syringe filled with sterile water to the balloon inflation port. Don't inflate the balloon before insertion unless directed by the manufacturer, *because doing so can cause microtears, which increase the risk of infection.*
- Hold the penis with your nondominant hand. If the patient is uncircumcised, retract the foreskin. Then gently lift and stretch the penis to a 60- to 90-degree angle.[40] Hold the penis this way throughout the procedure *to straighten the urethra and maintain a sterile field.*
- Use your dominant hand to clean the glans with a sterile, antiseptic swab or solution-soaked sterile cotton ball held in the forceps. Clean in a circular motion, starting at the urinary meatus and working outward (as shown above on right).[40]

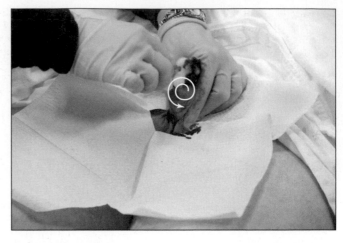

- Repeat the procedure, using another antiseptic swab or solution-soaked cotton ball, taking care not to contaminate your sterile glove.
- Maintaining sterile technique, pick up the catheter with your dominant hand and lubricate the catheter tip with the water-soluble lubricant.[40] Additionally, if ordered, instill 5 mL to 10 mL of sterile water-soluble lubricant into the urethra *to prevent trauma to the urethral lining and to facilitate insertion.*[40]
- Hold the catheter 2″ to 3″ (5 cm to 7.6 cm) from the tip and prepare to insert the lubricated tip into the urinary meatus (as shown below). *To facilitate insertion by relaxing the sphincter,* ask the patient to cough as you insert the catheter. Tell him to breathe deeply and slowly *to further relax the sphincter and help prevent spasms.*[40]

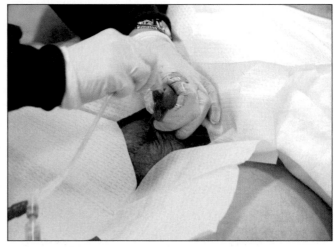

- Continue to advance the catheter to the catheter bifurcation and check for urine flow.[40] If urine fails to flow, ask a coworker to apply gently pressure to the suprapubic area. If the foreskin was retracted, replace it *to prevent compromised circulation and painful swelling.*
- Once urine starts to flow, inflate the balloon using the water-filled syringe attached to the inflation port, instilling the recommended amount of sterile water specified on the catheter. Gently pull the catheter until the inflated balloon is snug against the bladder neck.[40]

NURSING ALERT Never inflate a balloon without first establishing urine flow, *which confirms that the catheter is in the bladder.*

- Secure the catheter using a catheter securement device.[2,40,41] If a securement device isn't available, tape the catheter to the patient's abdomen or thigh *to prevent pressure on the urethra at the penoscrotal junction, which can lead to formation of urethrocutaneous fistulas. Taping this way also prevents traction on the bladder and alteration in the normal direction of urine flow in males.*
- Keep the catheter and drainage tube free from kinking and avoid dependent loops *to prevent obstruction of urine flow.*[1,2,5,6]
- Hang the collection bag below the level of the patient's bladder *to prevent urine reflux into the bladder, which can cause CAUTI, and to facilitate gravity drainage of the bladder.*[2,5,6,41] Don't place the drainage bag on the floor.[5]

- Return the bed to the lowest position *to prevent falls and maintain patient safety.*[35]
- Discard used supplies in appropriate receptacles.[33]
- Remove and discard your gloves and any other personal protective equipment worn.[31,33]
- Perform hand hygiene.[2,17,18,19,20,21,22,23]
- Document the procedure.[36,37,38,39]

Special considerations

- Patients at high risk for latex hypersensitivity include those with spina bifida, spinal cord injury, atopy, certain food allergies, and occupational exposure. Provide these patients with a latex-free environment by avoiding all products containing latex proteins, including gloves, catheters, condoms, drains, and injection ports.[14]
- In addition to hypersensitivity reactions, latex urethral catheters have been associated with an increased risk of cytotoxicity, urethritis, stricture, urinary tract infection, and encrustation. Selection of an alternative material, such as 100% silicone, reduces these risks, particularly when you anticipate long-term catheterization.[14]
- Empty the drainage bag at least once per shift using a separate, clean collecting container for each patient; avoid splashing, and prevent contact of the drainage spigot with the collecting container.[1,2,8]
- If you need a small urine sample for laboratory examination (for culture or urinalysis), thoroughly disinfect the needleless sampling port with a disinfectant pad and allow it to dry, and aspirate urine from the sampling port using a sterile adapter or syringe. If you need a large volume for special analysis (not culture), obtain the sample from the drainage bag using sterile technique.[3]
- Monitor and record the patient's intake and output.[1,3]
- Intermittent catheterization is preferable to indwelling urethral catheters in patients with bladder emptying dysfunction.[2]
- After the first unsuccessful insertion attempt, a urologist (or a nurse in some facilities) may use an #18 French Coudé catheter.[42]
- Explain the basic principles of gravity drainage *so that the patient realizes the importance of keeping the drainage tubing and collection bag lower than the bladder at all times.*[2,5]

Patient teaching

If the patient will be discharged with a long-term indwelling catheter, teach the patient and family (if appropriate) all aspects of daily catheter maintenance, including care of the skin and urinary meatus, signs and symptoms of urinary tract infection or obstruction, how to irrigate the catheter (if appropriate), and the importance of adequate fluid intake to maintain patency.[3,15]

Complications

Complications associated with indwelling urinary catheter use include CAUTI, genitourinary trauma, retained balloon fragments, bladder fistula (with prolonged use), bladder stone formation, and incontinence.[3,11,42]

Documentation

Document your assessment findings and the indication for catheter use. Record the date and time of insertion, the size and type of catheter you used, and the amount of sterile water you used to inflate the balloon. Record the patient's intake and output. Note the characteristics of the urine you obtained. Document any complications, the date and time that you notified the practitioner, the prescribed interventions, and the patient's response to those interventions. Document teaching provided to the patient and family (if applicable), their understanding of that teaching, and any need for follow-up teaching.

REFERENCES

1 Agency for Healthcare Research and Quality & U.S. Department of Health and Human Services. (2015). Toolkit for reducing catheter-associated urinary tract infections in hospital units: Implementation guide. https://www.ahrq.gov/hai/cauti-tools/impl-guide/index.html (Level VII)

2 Healthcare Infection Control Practices Advisory Committee. (2010, revised 2019). Guideline for prevention of catheter-associated urinary tract infections 2009. https://www.cdc.gov/infectioncontrol/pdf/guidelines/cauti-guidelines-H.pdf (Level I)

3 Carter, N. M., et al. (2014). An evidence-based approach to the prevention of catheter-associated urinary tract infections. *Urologic Nursing, 34*(5), 238–245.

4 Jarrett, N., & Callaham, M. (2016). Evidence-based guidelines for selected hospital-acquired conditions: Final report. https://www.cms.gov/Medicare/Medicare-Fee-for-Service-Payment/HospitalAcqCond/Downloads/2016-HAC-Report.pdf

5 Lo, E., et al. (2014). SHEA/IDSA practice recommendation: Strategies to prevent catheter-associated urinary tract infections in acute care hospitals. *Infection Control and Hospital Epidemiology, 35*(5), 464–479. https://www.jstor.org/stable/10.1086/675718#metadata_info_tab_contents (Level I)

6 The Joint Commission. (2021). Standard NPSG.07.06.01. *Comprehensive accreditation manual for hospitals.* Oakbrook Terrace, IL: The Joint Commission. (Level VII)

7 Association of Professionals in Infection Control and Epidemiology. (2014). APIC implementation guide: Guide to preventing catheter-associated urinary tract infections. https://apic.org/wp-content/uploads/2019/02/APIC_CAUTI_IG_FIN_REVD0815.pdf (Level IV)

8 Halm, M. A., & O'Connor, N. (2014). Do system-based interventions affect catheter-associated urinary tract infection? *American Journal of Critical Care, 23*(6), 505–509. (Level V)

9 American Hospital Association & Health Research and Educational Trust. (n.d.). Catheter-associated urinary tract infections (CAUTI) top ten checklist. http://patientcarelink.org/wp-content/uploads/2015/11/CAUTI-Top-Ten-checklist_2014.pdf

10 Wound, Ostomy and Continence Nurses Society. (2016). *Care and management of patients with urinary catheters: A clinical resource guide.* Mount Laurel, NJ: WOCN.

11 Schaeffer, A. J. (2021). Placement and management of urinary bladder catheters in adults. In: *UpToDate,* Richie, J. P. (Ed.).

12 Porche, D. (2021). Urinary tract infection (catheter related): Prevention strategies. *The JBI EBP Database.* AN: JBI14392 (Level V)

13 American Association of Critical-Care Nurses. (2016). AACN practice alert: Prevention of CAUTI in adults. https://www.aacn.org/clinical-resources/practice-alerts/prevention-of-cauti-in-adults (Level VII)

14 Achmetov, T., & Gray, M. (2008). Adverse reactions to latex in the clinical setting: A urologic perspective. *Infection Control Resource, 2*(2), 1, 4–6http://www.grovemedical.com/customer/grmein/pdf/latex_reactions.pdf

15 Herter, R., & Kazer, M. W. (2010). Best practices in urinary catheter care. *Home Healthcare Nurse, 28*(6), 342–349. http://journals.lww.com/homehealthcarenurseonline/pages/articleviewer.aspx?year=2010&issue=06000&article=00005&type=Fulltext

16 Fletcher-Gutowski, S., & Cecil, J. (2019). Is two-person urinary catheter insertion effective in reducing CAUTI? *American Journal of Infection Control, 47*(12), 1508–1509. (Level VI)

17 Quallich, S. A., et al. (2021) Insertion of an indwelling urinary catheter in the adult female. *Urologic Nursing, 41*(2), 65–69 (Level VII)

18 The Joint Commission. (2021). Standard NPSG.07.01.01. *Comprehensive accreditation manual for hospitals.* Oakbrook Terrace, IL: The Joint Commission. (Level VII)

19 Centers for Disease Control and Prevention. (2002). Guideline for hand hygiene in health-care settings: Recommendations of the Healthcare Infection Control Practices Advisory Committee and the HICPAC/SHEA/APIC/IDSA Hand Hygiene Task Force. *MMWR Recommendations and Reports, 51*(RR-16), 1–45. https://www.cdc.gov/mmwr/pdf/rr/rr5116.pdf (Level II)

20 World Health Organization. (2009). WHO guidelines on hand hygiene in health care: First global patient safety challenge, clean care is safer care. https://apps.who.int/iris/bitstream/handle/10665/44102/9789241597906_eng.pdf?sequence=1 (Level IV)

21 Accreditation Association for Hospitals and Health Systems. (2020). Standard 07.01.21. *Healthcare Facilities Accreditation Program: Accreditation requirements for acute care hospitals.* Chicago, IL: Accreditation Association for Hospitals and Health Systems. (Level VII)

22 Centers for Medicare and Medicaid Services, Department of Health and Human Services. (2020). Condition of participation: Infection control. 42 C.F.R. § 482.42.

23 DNV GL-Healthcare USA, Inc. (2020). IC.1.SR.1. *NIAHO® accreditation requirements, interpretive guidelines and surveyor guidance—revision 20.0.* Milford, OH: DNV GL-Healthcare USA, Inc. (Level VII)

24 The Joint Commission. (2021). Standard NPSG.01.01.01. *Comprehensive accreditation manual for hospitals.* Oakbrook Terrace, IL: The Joint Commission. (Level VII)

25 Accreditation Association for Hospitals and Health Systems. (2020). Standard 15.01.16. *Healthcare Facilities Accreditation Program: Accreditation requirements for acute care hospitals.* Chicago, IL: Accreditation Association for Hospitals and Health Systems. (Level VII)

26 Centers for Medicare and Medicaid Services, Department of Health and Human Services. (2020). Condition of participation: Patient's rights. 42 C.F.R. § 482.13(c)(1).

27 The Joint Commission. (2021). Standard RI.01.01.01. *Comprehensive accreditation manual for hospitals.* Oakbrook Terrace, IL: The Joint Commission. (Level VII)

28 DNV GL-Healthcare USA, Inc. (2020). PR.2.SR.5. *NIAHO® accreditation requirements, interpretive guidelines and surveyor guidance—revision 20.0.* Milford, OH: DNV GL-Healthcare USA, Inc. (Level VII)

29 The Joint Commission. (2021). Standard PC.02.01.21. *Comprehensive accreditation manual for hospitals.* Oakbrook Terrace, IL: The Joint Commission. (Level VII)

30 Waters, T. R., et al. (2009). Safe patient handling training for schools of nursing. https://www.cdc.gov/niosh/docs/2009-127/pdfs/2009-127.pdf (Level VII)

31 Siegel, J. D., et al. (2007, revised 2019). 2007 guideline for isolation precautions: Preventing transmission of infectious agents in healthcare settings. https://www.cdc.gov/infectioncontrol/pdf/guidelines/isolation-guidelines-H.pdf (Level II)

32 Accreditation Association for Hospitals and Health Systems. (2020). Standard 07.01.10. *Healthcare Facilities Accreditation Program: Accreditation requirements for acute care hospitals.* Chicago, IL: Accreditation Association for Hospitals and Health Systems. (Level VII)

33 Occupational Safety and Health Administration. (2012.). Bloodborne pathogens, standard number 1910.1030. [https://www.osha.gov/pls/oshaweb/owadisp.show_document?p_id=10051&p_table=STANDARDS (Level VII)

34 Guideline for perioperative practice: Sterile technique. (2020). In Wood, A. (Ed.), *Guidelines for perioperative practice*, 2020 edition. Denver, CO: AORN, Inc. (Level VII)

35 Ganz, D. A., et al. (2013). Preventing falls in hospitals: A toolkit for improving quality of care (AHRQ publication no. 13-0015-EF). https://www.ahrq.gov/professionals/systems/hospital/fallpxtoolkit/index.html (Level VII)

36 The Joint Commission. (2021). Standard RC.01.03.01. *Comprehensive accreditation manual for hospitals.* Oakbrook Terrace, IL: The Joint Commission. (Level VII)

37 Accreditation Association for Hospitals and Health Systems. (2020). Standard 10.00.03. *Healthcare Facilities Accreditation Program: Accreditation requirements for acute care hospitals.* Chicago, IL: Accreditation Association for Hospitals and Health Systems. (Level VII)

38 Centers for Medicare and Medicaid Services, Department of Health and Human Services. (2020). Condition of participation: Medical record services. 42 C.F.R. § 482.24(b).

39 DNV GL-Healthcare USA, Inc. (2020). MR.2.SR.1. *NIAHO® accreditation requirements, interpretive guidelines and surveyor guidance—revision 20.0.* Milford, OH: DNV GL-Healthcare USA, Inc. (Level VII)

40 Quallich, S. A., et al. (2021) Insertion of an indwelling urinary catheter in the adult male. *Urologic Nursing, 41*(2), 86–109 (Level VII)

41 Payne, D. (2014). Safe and secure: Catheter fixation. *Nursing and Residential Care, 16*, 608–610.

42 Leuck, A. M., et al. (2012). Complications of Foley catheters—is infection the greatest risk? *Journal of Urology, 187*(5), 1662–1666. https://www.auajournals.org/article/S0022-5347(11)06062-9/pdf (Level IV)

INDWELLING URINARY CATHETER IRRIGATION

Indwelling urinary (Foley) catheter irrigation shouldn't be performed routinely. However, obstructions sometimes occur and require irrigation. To relieve an obstruction resulting from clots, mucus, or other causes, an intermittent method of irrigation may be used.[1] Whenever possible, the catheter should be irrigated through a closed system to decrease the risk of infection.[2] If an obstruction is anticipated, closed continuous irrigation may be used to prevent it. (See the "Continuous bladder irrigation" procedure.)

Signs and symptoms that a catheter might be obstructed include absence of urine flow from the catheter, urine flow bypassing the catheter, and suprapubic pain that becomes more pronounced as the bladder fills. If the obstruction remains unrelieved, vasovagal signs such as sweating, tachycardia, and hypotension can also occur.[3]

Before initiating catheter irrigation, a bladder scanner may be used to confirm whether a decrease in urine output results from a blockage or reduced urine in the bladder, decreasing the number of unnecessary irrigations and minimizing breaks in the closed drainage system.[4]

If an obstruction occurs and it's likely that the catheter material is contributing to obstruction, change the catheter.[2] To prevent catheter-associated urinary tract infection (CAUTI), review the need for the catheter daily, and remove the catheter as soon as it's no longer needed.[1,2,4,5,6]

HOSPITAL-ACQUIRED CONDITION ALERT Keep in mind that the Centers for Medicare and Medicaid Services considers CAUTI a hospital-acquired condition *because it can be reasonably prevented using a variety of best practices.* Make sure to follow evidence-based CAUTI prevention practices—such as performing hand hygiene before and after any catheter manipulation; maintaining a sterile, continuously closed drainage system; maintaining unobstructed urine flow; emptying the collection bag regularly; replacing the catheter and drainage system using sterile technique when breaks in sterile technique, disconnection, or leakage occur; and discontinuing the catheter as soon as it's no longer clinically indicated—when caring for a patient with an indwelling urinary catheter *to reduce the risk of CAUTI.*[1,2,4,5,7]

Equipment

Prescribed irrigating solution (such as normal saline solution) ▪ sterile basin ▪ 30- to 60-mL syringes ▪ antiseptic pads ▪ gloves ▪ fluid-impermeable pad ▪ intake and output record ▪ clamp ▪ graduated receptacle ▪ sterile drape ▪ Optional: gown, mask, goggles or mask with face shield, 18G blunt-end needle, commercially packaged irrigation kit.

Commercially packaged kits containing sterile irrigating solution, a graduated receptacle, and a 50-mL catheter tip syringe may be available in some facilities.

Preparation of equipment

Inspect all equipment and supplies. If a product is expired, is defective, or has compromised integrity, remove it from patient use, label it as expired or defective, and report the expiration or defect as directed by your facility.

To prevent vesical spasms during instillation of solution, warm it to room temperature. Never heat the solution on a burner or in a microwave oven; *hot irrigating solution can injure the patient's bladder.*

Implementation

▪ Verify the practitioner's order.
▪ Gather and prepare the appropriate equipment.
▪ Perform hand hygiene.[8,9,10,11,12,13]
▪ Confirm the patient's identity using at least two patient identifiers.[14]
▪ Provide privacy.[15,16,17,18]
▪ Explain the procedure to the patient and family (if appropriate) according to their individual communication and learning needs *to increase their understanding, allay their fears, and enhance cooperation.*[19]
▪ Raise the patient's bed to waist level before providing care *to prevent caregiver back strain.*[20]
▪ Perform hand hygiene.[8,9,10,11,12,13]
▪ Put on gloves and other protective equipment as needed *to comply with standard precautions.*[21,22,23]
▪ Empty the catheter drainage bag into a graduated receptacle. During emptying, avoid splashing, and don't allow the drain spigot to come in contact with the nonsterile collecting container.[1,2,24] Measure the amount of urine, noting the color and characteristics before irrigation.
▪ Remove and discard your gloves.[22,23]
▪ Perform hand hygiene.[8,9,10,11,12,13]
▪ Put on a new set of gloves.[22,23]

■ Expose the catheter's aspiration port and place a fluid-impermeable pad under it *to protect the bed linens.*[3]
■ Clamp the catheter tubing below the aspiration port (as shown below).

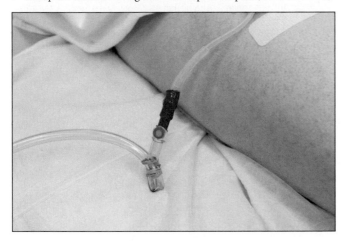

■ Create a sterile field at the patient's bedside using a sterile drape.
■ Using a sterile no-touch technique, pour the prescribed amount of sterile irrigating solution into a sterile basin.
■ Place the tip of the syringe into the solution and fill the syringe with the appropriate amount (as shown below).

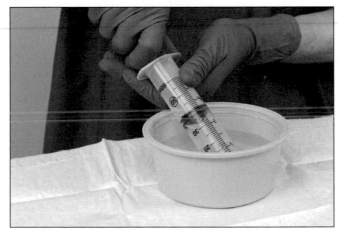

■ Trace the tubing to its point of origin *to make sure you're accessing the correct port before beginning irrigation.*[25,26]

For irrigation through the aspiration port (if permitted by the device manufacturer)
■ Thoroughly disinfect the aspiration port with an antiseptic pad (as shown below) and then allow it to dry *to remove as many bacterial contaminants as possible.*

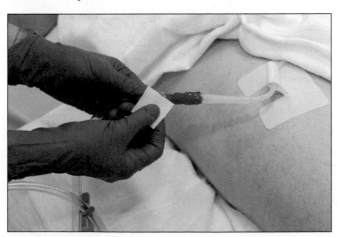

■ While maintaining the sterility of the syringe tip, attach the syringe to the aspiration port.
■ Instill the irrigating solution into the catheter. If necessary, repeat the procedure until you've instilled the prescribed amount of irrigating solution.
■ Remove the syringe and unclamp the drainage tube *to allow the irrigating solution and urine to flow into the drainage bag.* Note the color and characteristics of the drainage, and measure it *to make sure the patient isn't retaining the irrigating solution.*

For open manual irrigation through the drainage port
■ Disconnect the catheter from the drainage bag.[3]
■ Disinfect the catheter drainage port thoroughly with an antiseptic pad and allow it to dry.[3]
■ While maintaining the sterility of the syringe tip, attach the syringe to the drainage port.
■ Instill the irrigating solution into the catheter, as directed, and then draw back on the plunger to *evacuate any clot or debris.*[3]
■ Empty the syringe into the graduated container.
■ Continue to irrigate as directed until you achieve a clear or clot-free return.[3]
■ Connect a new drainage bag as directed.[3]

Completing the procedure
■ Make sure the catheter tubing is secured to the patient's leg, and that the catheter and drainage tube are free from kinking and dependent loops *to allow free flow of urine.* Keep the drainage bag below the level of the bladder *to prevent backflow of urine into the bladder, which increases the risk of CAUTI.*[2,5]
■ Return the bed to the lowest level *to prevent falls and maintain patient safety.*[27]
■ Discard used supplies in appropriate receptacles.[23]
■ Remove your gloves and any other personal protective equipment, if worn.[22,23]
■ Perform hand hygiene.[8,9,10,11,12,13]
■ Document the procedure.[28,29,30,31]

Special considerations
■ If you encounter any resistance during instillation of the irrigating solution, don't try to force the solution into the bladder. Instead, stop the procedure and notify the practitioner. If an indwelling catheter becomes totally obstructed, obtain an order to remove it and replace it with a new one *to prevent bladder distention, acute renal failure, urinary stasis, and subsequent infection.*
■ Use caution if the patient has had open bladder surgery or renal transplantation, *because increased pressure on the suture lines can result in suture line disruption and extravasation of urine.*[3]
■ Encourage a catheterized patient who isn't on restricted fluid intake to increase intake to 30 mL/kg/day *to help flush the urinary system and reduce sediment formation.*
■ The Joint Commission issued a sentinel event alert related to managing risk during transition to new International Organization for Standardization tubing standards that were designed to prevent dangerous tubing misconnections, which can lead to serious patient injury and death. During the transition, make sure to trace each tubing and catheter from the patient to the point of origin before connecting or reconnecting any device or infusion, at any care transition (such as a new setting or service), and as part of the hand-off process; route tubes and catheters having different purposes in different standardized directions; when there are different access sites or several bags hanging, label the tubing at both the distal and proximal ends; use tubing and equipment only as intended; and store medications for different delivery routes in separate locations.[26]

Complications
CAUTI is a complication associated with indwelling urinary catheter irrigation. Other complications include bladder spasm, lower abdominal pain, leakage around the catheter, and altered fluid balance.[3]

Documentation

Document the date and time of irrigation as well as the type and volume of irrigating solution instilled. Note the amount, color, and consistency of return urine flow, and document the patient's tolerance of the procedure. Also note any resistance during instillation of the solution. If the return flow volume was less than the amount of solution instilled, note this finding in the intake and output record and in your notes. Document teaching provided to the patient and family (if applicable), their understanding of that teaching, and any need for follow-up teaching.

REFERENCES

1 Lo, E., et al. (2014). SHEA/IDSA practice recommendation. Strategies to prevent catheter-associated urinary tract infections in acute care hospitals: 2014 update. *Infection Control and Hospital Epidemiology, 35*(5), 464–479. https://www.jstor.org/stable/10.1086/675718#metadata_info_tab_contents (Level I)

2 Healthcare Infection Control Practices Advisory Committee. (2010, revised 2019). Guideline for prevention of catheter-associated urinary tract infections 2009. https://www.cdc.gov/infectioncontrol/pdf/guidelines/cauti-guidelines-H.pdf (Level I)

3 Agency for Clinical Innovation. (2019). Bladder irrigation: Management of haematuria. https://www.aci.health.nsw.gov.au/__data/assets/pdf_file/0009/497088/ACI_0195-Urology-Haem-toolkit_F.pdf (Level VII)

4 Association of Professionals in Infection Control and Epidemiology (APIC). (2014). APIC implementation guide: Guide to preventing catheter-associated urinary tract infections. https://apic.org/wp-content/uploads/2019/02/APIC_CAUTI_IG_FIN_REVD0815.pdf (Level IV)

5 The Joint Commission. (2021). Standard NPSG.07.06.01. *Comprehensive accreditation manual for hospitals.* Oakbrook Terrace, IL: The Joint Commission. (Level VII)

6 Herter, R., & Kazer, M. W. (2010). Best practices in urinary catheter care. *Home Healthcare Nurse, 28,* 342–349.

7 Jarrett, N., & Callaham, M. (2016). Evidence-based guidelines for selected hospital-acquired conditions: Final report. https://www.cms.gov/Medicare/Medicare-Fee-for-Service-Payment/HospitalAcqCond/Downloads/2016-HAC-Report.pdf

8 The Joint Commission. (2021). Standard NPSG.07.01.01. *Comprehensive accreditation manual for hospitals.* Oakbrook Terrace, IL: The Joint Commission. (Level VII)

9 Centers for Disease Control and Prevention. (2002). Guideline for hand hygiene in health-care settings: Recommendations of the Healthcare Infection Control Practices Advisory Committee and the HICPAC/SHEA/APIC/IDSA Hand Hygiene Task Force. *MMWR Recommendations and Reports, 51*(RR-16), 1–45. https://www.cdc.gov/mmwr/pdf/rr/rr5116.pdf (Level II)

10 World Health Organization. (2009). WHO guidelines on hand hygiene in health care: First global patient safety challenge, clean care is safer care. https://apps.who.int/iris/bitstream/handle/10665/44102/9789241597906_eng.pdf?sequence=1 (Level IV)

11 Accreditation Association for Hospitals and Health Systems. (2020). Standard 07.01.21. *Healthcare Facilities Accreditation Program: Accreditation requirements for acute care hospitals.* Chicago, IL: Accreditation Association for Hospitals and Health Systems. (Level VII)

12 Centers for Medicare and Medicaid Services, Department of Health and Human Services. (2020). Condition of participation: Infection control. 42 C.F.R. § 482.42.

13 DNV GL-Healthcare USA, Inc. (2020). IC.1.SR.1. *NIAHO® accreditation requirements, interpretive guidelines and surveyor guidance—revision 20.0.* Milford, OH: DNV GL-Healthcare USA, Inc. (Level VII)

14 The Joint Commission. (2021). Standard NPSG.01.01.01. *Comprehensive accreditation manual for hospitals.* Oakbrook Terrace, IL: The Joint Commission. (Level VII)

15 Accreditation Association for Hospitals and Health Systems. (2020). Standard 15.01.16. *Healthcare Facilities Accreditation Program: Accreditation requirements for acute care hospitals.* Chicago, IL: Accreditation Association for Hospitals and Health Systems. (Level VII)

16 Centers for Medicare and Medicaid Services, Department of Health and Human Services. (2020). Condition of participation: Patient's rights. 42 C.F.R. § 482.13(c)(1).

17 The Joint Commission. (2021). Standard RI.01.01.01. *Comprehensive accreditation manual for hospitals.* Oakbrook Terrace, IL: The Joint Commission. (Level VII)

18 DNV GL-Healthcare USA, Inc. (2020). PR.2.SR.5. *NIAHO® accreditation requirements, interpretive guidelines and surveyor guidance—revision 20.0.* Milford, OH: DNV GL-Healthcare USA, Inc. (Level VII)

19 The Joint Commission. (2021). Standard PC.02.01.21. *Comprehensive accreditation manual for hospitals.* Oakbrook Terrace, IL: The Joint Commission. (Level VII)

20 Waters, T. R., et al. (2009). Safe patient handling training for schools of nursing. https://www.cdc.gov/niosh/docs/2009-127/pdfs/2009-127.pdf (Level VII)

21 Accreditation Association for Hospitals and Health Systems. (2020). Standard 07.01.10. *Healthcare Facilities Accreditation Program: Accreditation requirements for acute care hospitals.* Chicago, IL: Accreditation Association for Hospitals and Health Systems. (Level VII)

22 Siegel, J. D., et al. (2007, revised 2019). 2007 guideline for isolation precautions: Preventing transmission of infectious agents in healthcare settings. https://www.cdc.gov/infectioncontrol/pdf/guidelines/isolation-guidelines-H.pdf (Level II)

23 Occupational Safety and Health Administration. (2012). Bloodborne pathogens, standard number 1910.1030. https://www.osha.gov/pls/oshaweb/owadisp.show_document?p_id=10051&p_table=STANDARDS (Level VII)

24 Moola, S. (2021). Urinary drainage bags: Emptying, changing, and securing. *The JBI EBP Database.* AN: JBI1334 (Level V)

25 U.S. Food and Drug Administration. (2017). Examples of medical device misconnections. https://www.fda.gov/medical-devices/medical-device-connectors/examples-medical-device-misconnections

26 The Joint Commission. (2014). Sentinel event alert 53: Managing risk during transition to new ISO tubing connector standards. http://www.jointcommission.org/assets/1/6/SEA_53_Connectors_8_19_14_final.pdf (Level VII)

27 Ganz, D. A., et al. (2013). *Preventing falls in hospitals: A toolkit for improving quality of care* (AHRQ Publication No. 13-0015-EF). Rockville, MD: Agency for Healthcare Research and Quality. https://www.ahrq.gov/professionals/systems/hospital/fallpxtoolkit/index.html (Level VII)

28 The Joint Commission. (2021). Standard RC.01.03.01. *Comprehensive accreditation manual for hospitals.* Oakbrook Terrace, IL: The Joint Commission. (Level VII)

29 Accreditation Association for Hospitals and Health Systems. (2020). Standard 10.00.03. *Healthcare Facilities Accreditation Program: Accreditation requirements for acute care hospitals.* Chicago, IL: Accreditation Association for Hospitals and Health Systems. (Level VII)

30 Centers for Medicare and Medicaid Services, Department of Health and Human Services. (2020). Condition of participation: Medical record services. 42 C.F.R. § 482.24(b).

31 DNV GL-Healthcare USA, Inc. (2020). MR.2.SR.1. *NIAHO® accreditation requirements, interpretive guidelines and surveyor guidance—revision 20.0.* Milford, OH: DNV GL-Healthcare USA, Inc. (Level VII)

INTERMITTENT INFUSION DEVICE DRUG ADMINISTRATION

An intermittent infusion device, or *saline lock*, eliminates the need for multiple venipunctures or maintaining venous access with a continuous IV infusion. This device allows intermittent administration by infusion or by the IV bolus injection method.

When administering IV fluids to older adults, keep in mind that these patients commonly have compromised cardiac, hepatic, or renal systems, which puts them at high risk for heart failure, shock, or cardiac arrest if IV fluids are administered too rapidly or in too great a volume. Furthermore, older adult patients in particular may be unable to articulate symptoms because of such underlying conditions as stroke, intubation, tracheostomy, dementia, or delirium; monitor these patients closely during all IV infusions. Speed shock may also result from rapid administration of a bolus medication or an infusion. Symptoms of speed shock, such as dizziness and headache, occur rapidly, which may make it difficult for the older adult patient to articulate them. These early symptoms may progress to chest tightness, hypotension, irregular pulse, and anaphylactic shock. Close observation and careful control of medication or solutions administered parentally to older adults is crucial.[1]

Sterile no-touch technique should always be used when administering a drug through an intermittent infusion device *to reduce the risk of vascular catheter–associated infection.*

Equipment

Gloves ■ antiseptic pads (chlorhexidine-based, povidone iodine, or alcohol) ■ 10-mL syringe(s) prefilled with preservative-free normal saline solution ■ prescribed medication in an IV container (for IV infusion) or in a syringe (for IV bolus injection) ■ IV administration set ■ needleless connector(s) ■ sterile male Luer covering device ■ Optional: electronic infusion device, pulse oximeter and probe, capnography equipment, standardized sedation scale, disinfectant-containing end cap.

Preparation of equipment

Inspect all IV equipment and supplies. If a product is expired, is defective, or has compromised integrity, remove it from patient use, label it as expired or defective, and report the expiration or defect as directed by your facility.[5]

Implementation

■ Avoid distractions and interruptions when preparing and administering medications *to prevent medication errors.*[6,7]

■ Verify the practitioner's order.[8,9,10,11,12]

■ Gather and prepare the necessary equipment and supplies.

■ Compare the medication label with the order in the patient's medical record.[8,9,10,11,12,13]

■ Check the patient's medication record for an allergy or other contraindication to the prescribed medication. If an allergy or other contraindication exists, don't administer the medication; instead, notify the practitioner.[8,9,10,11,12]

■ Check the expiration date on the medication. If it has expired, return the medication to the pharmacy and obtain a new medication.[8,9,10,11,12]

■ Visually inspect the medication for particles, discoloration, or any other loss of integrity; don't administer the medication if its integrity is compromised.[8,9,10,11,12]

■ Discuss any unresolved concerns about the medication with the patient's practitioner.[9,10,11,12]

■ Verify that you're administering the medication at the proper time, in the prescribed dose, and by the correct route *to reduce the risk of medication errors.*[9,10,11,12]

■ Perform hand hygiene.[3,14,15,16,17,18,19,20]

■ Confirm the patient's identity using at least two patient identifiers.[21]

■ Provide privacy.[22,23,24,25]

■ Explain the procedure to the patient and family (if appropriate) according to their individual communication and learning needs *to increase their understanding, allay their fears, and enhance cooperation.*[26] If the patient is receiving the medication for the first time, teach the patient about potential adverse reactions and discuss any other concerns related to the medication.[27]

■ Raise the patient's bed to waist level before providing patient care *to prevent caregiver back strain.*[28]

■ Perform hand hygiene.[3,14,15,16,17,18,19,20]

■ Put on gloves *to comply with standard precautions.*[29,30,31]

■ Prepare the medication and administration set: For an IV infusion, remove the protective cover of the administration set's spike and the infusion container, insert the spike from the administration set into the infusion container, attach a needleless connector to the opposite end of the administration set tubing, and then prime the tubing and needleless connector.[1,32] For an IV bolus injection, attach a needleless connector to the syringe containing the prescribed medication and prime the needleless connector.[1,32]

■ Assess the intermittent infusion device site *to ensure that it's free from signs of infection (tenderness, erythema, and induration within 2 cm of the insertion site, and purulent drainage at the exit site), phlebitis (tenderness at the site, erythema, warmth, swelling, induration, purulent drainage, and palpable venous cord), and infiltration (blanching, bruising, or redness around the insertion site); edema in any direction from the insertion site; skin temperature changes; pain, burning, or stinging with injection or infusion; blisters; impaired mobility; numbness or tingling; slowed capillary refill time; and fluid leaking from the insertion site.*[1,32,33]

■ If your facility uses a bar code technology, use it as directed by your facility.

■ If required by your facility, before administering a high-alert medication,[34] have another nurse perform an independent double-check *to verify the patient's identity and make sure you have the correct medication in the prescribed strength or concentration; the medication's indication corresponds with the patient's diagnosis; the dosage calculations are correct and the dosing formula used to derive the final dose is correct; the prescribed route of administration is safe and proper for the patient; and the prescribed time and frequency of administration are safe and proper for the patient.*[35]

■ After comparing results of the independent double-check with the other nurse (if required), administer the medication if there are no discrepancies. If discrepancies exist, rectify them before administering the medication.[35]

■ If a disinfectant-containing end cap is covering the end of the needleless connector, remove and discard it.[36,37]

■ Perform a vigorous mechanical scrub of the needleless connector for at least 5 seconds using an antiseptic pad. Allow it to dry completely.[36,38]

■ While maintaining sterility of the syringe tip, attach a prefilled syringe containing preservative-free normal saline solution to the needleless connector. (Use a 10-mL syringe or a syringe specifically designed to generate lower injection pressure.) Unclamp the device clamp, if present, and slowly aspirate for blood return that is the color and consistency of whole blood. If no blood return is obtained, take steps to locate an external cause of the obstruction.[39]

■ If a blood return is obtained, slowly inject preservative-free normal saline solution into the intermittent infusion device. Use a minimum volume of twice the internal volume of the catheter system. Don't forcibly flush the device; further evaluate the device if resistance is met.[39] Insert a new intermittent infusion device at another location if needed. (See the "Intermittent infusion device insertion" procedure.)[1,32]

■ Remove and discard the syringe.[29,40]

■ Perform a vigorous scrub of the needleless connector for at least 5 seconds using an antiseptic pad. Allow it to dry completely.[36,38]

Administering an IV bolus injection

■ Attach the syringe containing the prescribed medication to the needleless connector of the intermittent infusion device.[1,32]

NURSING ALERT After confirming patency of the vascular access device by using a 10-mL syringe (or a syringe designed specifically to generate lower injection pressure) filled with preservative-free normal saline solution, administer the medication by IV bolus injection in a syringe of an appropriate size that allows you to measure and administer the required medication dose.[41] Do not transfer the medication to a larger syringe.[39]

■ Administer the medication at the rate indicated on the medication label; consult with the pharmacist if the rate isn't specified.[1,32]

■ Remove and discard the syringe.[29,40]

Administering an IV drug infusion

■ Remove the protective cover from the distal end of the administration set tubing.[1,32]

■ Connect the IV administration set tubing to the intermittent infusion device's needleless connector.[1,32]

■ Trace the tubing from the patient to its point of origin *to make sure that you're connecting it to the proper port.*[8,42] Route the tubing in a standardized direction if the patient has other tubing and catheters that have different purposes. Label the tubing at the distal end (near the patient connection) and proximal end (near the source container) *to reduce the risk of misconnection* if multiple IV lines will be used.[8,42]

■ Slowly open the clamp of the administration set tubing, and adjust the flow rate to begin the infusion. Alternatively, turn on the electronic infusion device and begin the infusion at the prescribed flow rate.[1,32] Use an electronic infusion device for infusions that require precise flow control *to maintain patient safety*. Consider the use of a smart pump with dose-error reduction software and interoperability with electronic health records *to reduce the risk for infusion-related medication errors*.[43] Make sure alarm limits are set appropriately and that alarms are turned on, functioning properly, and audible to staff.[43,44,45]

■ If using a gravity-flow administration set, monitor the drops per minute by counting the drops and using a clock with a second hand; if using an electronic infusion pump, watch the device display for 1 to 2 minutes *to ensure the proper administration rate*.[1,32]

■ When the infusion is complete, clamp the IV administration set tubing and disconnect the tubing from the intermittent infusion device. If you're reusing the IV administration set tubing, close the clamp on the tubing and aseptically attach a new, sterile, compatible covering device to the male Luer end of the administration set. Don't attach the exposed end of the administration set to a port on the same set.[44] If you won't reuse the tubing, discard it appropriately with the IV container.[29,40]

Completing the procedure

■ Perform a vigorous mechanical scrub of the needleless connector for at least 5 seconds using an antiseptic pad. Allow it to dry completely.[36,38]

■ While maintaining sterility of the syringe tip, attach a prefilled syringe containing preservative-free normal saline solution to the intermittent infusion device's needleless connector. (Use a 10-mL syringe or a syringe specifically designed to generate lower injection pressure). Unclamp the catheter and inject preservative-free normal saline solution into the catheter at the same rate of injection as the prescribed medication. Use the amount of flush solution needed to adequately clear the medication from the administration set lumen and the catheter. Don't forcibly flush the device; further evaluate the device if resistance is met.

■ Consider using a pulsatile flushing technique, *because short boluses of the flush solution interrupted by short pauses may be more effective at removing deposits (e.g., fibrin, drug precipitate, intraluminal bacteria) than a continuous low-flow technique*. Alternatively, if the medication is incompatible with normal saline solution, use dextrose 5% in water followed by preservative-free normal saline solution. Don't allow dextrose 5% in water to remain in the catheter lumen, *because it provides nutrients for biofilm growth*.[39]

■ Close the clamp and remove the syringe according to the needleless connector used, following the manufacturer's instructions. For a positive-pressure needleless connector, clamp the catheter after disconnecting the syringe.[1,32] For a negative-pressure needleless connector, maintain pressure on the syringe while clamping the catheter.[1,32] For a neutral needleless connector, clamp the catheter before or after disconnecting the syringe.[1,32] For an antireflux needleless connector, clamp the catheter and then disconnect the syringe; a specific clamping sequence isn't required.[45,46]

■ If available in your facility, place a new disinfectant-containing end cap on the end of the needleless connector *to reduce the risk of vascular catheter-associated infection*.[36,37]

■ Return the bed to the lowest position *to prevent falls and maintain patient safety*.[47]

■ Discard used supplies in appropriate receptacles.[29,40]

■ Remove and discard your gloves.[29,30,40]

■ Perform hand hygiene.[13,14,15,16,17,18,19,20]

■ Monitor the patient closely for adverse reactions to the prescribed medication.[8,48]

■ If the patient is receiving an IV opioid medication, frequently monitor the patient's respiratory rate, oxygen saturation level by pulse oximetry, end-tidal carbon dioxide level by capnography (if available), and sedation level using a standardized sedation scale *to decrease the risk of adverse events associated with IV opioid use*.[48]

■ If the patient is receiving an IV opioid medication, explain the assessment and monitoring processes to the patient and family members and tell them to alert staff if breathing problems or sedation occurs.[27,48]

■ Perform hand hygiene.[14,15,17,18,19,20]

■ Document the procedure.[49,50,51,52,53]

Special considerations

■ Before administering an injectable drug, make sure you know the prescribed infusion rate and infusion time period.[8]

■ The Joint Commission issued a sentinel event alert related to managing risk during transition to new International Organization for Standardization tubing standards that were designed to prevent dangerous tubing misconnections, which can lead to serious patient injury and death. During the transition, make sure to trace each tubing and catheter from the patient to the point of origin before connecting or reconnecting any device or infusion, at any care transition (such as to a new setting or service), and as part of the hand-off process; route tubes and catheters having different purposes in different, standardized directions; when the patient has different access sites or several bags hanging, label tubing at both the distal and proximal ends; use tubing and equipment only as intended; and store medications for different delivery routes in separate locations.[42]

■ The Joint Commission issued a sentinel event alert concerning the transmission of pathogens related to the misuse of vials that have caused viral and bacterial infections, including hepatitis B, hepatitis C, meningitis, and epidural abscesses. These infections have been attributed to the reuse of single-dose vials that typically don't contain preservatives, re-entering multidose vials with used syringes and needles, and using multidose vials for multiple patients. To prevent these infections, follow evidence-based best practices, such as disinfecting the vial's rubber stopper before piercing it, using single-dose vials only once and then discarding them, dedicating multidose vials to a single patient, and using a new syringe and needle when re-entering a multidose vial. Assign the appropriate "beyond-use" date when first entering a multidose vial, and store multidose vials as directed by your facility and according to the manufacturer's instructions.[54]

Complications

Infiltration, infection, phlebitis, and reactions specific to the infused medication are the most common complications.

Documentation

Document the type, concentration, dosage, and volume of drug administered and the time of administration. Document the date, time, amount, and type of flush solution used, patency of the catheter, presence of blood return, lack of resistance when flushing, and absence of signs and symptoms of complications. Record any adverse reactions to the prescribed medication, the name of the practitioner notified, the date and time of notification, your interventions, and the patient's response to those interventions.[55] Document teaching provided to the patient and family (if appropriate), their understanding of that teaching, and any need for follow-up teaching. On the intake record, record the type and volume of all IV solutions used to dilute the medication and to flush the line.[50]

REFERENCES

1 Infusion Nurses Society. (2017). *Policies and procedures for infusion therapy of the older adult* (3rd ed.). Boston, MA: Infusion Nurses Society.

2 Jarrett, N., & Callaham, M. (2016). Evidence-based guidelines for selected hospital-acquired conditions: Final report. https://www.cms.gov/Medicare/Medicare-Fee-for-Service-Payment/HospitalAcqCond/Downloads/2016-HAC-Report.pdf

3 Centers for Disease Control and Prevention. (2011, revised 2017). Guidelines for the prevention of intravascular catheter-related infections. https://www.cdc.gov/infectioncontrol/guidelines/bsi/recommendations.html (Level I)

4 Standard 50. Infection. Infusion therapy standards of practice. (8th ed.). (2021). *Journal of Infusion Nursing, 44*, S153–S156. (Level VII)

5 Standard 12. Product evaluation, integrity, and defect reporting. Infusion therapy standards of practice. (8th ed.). (2021). *Journal of Infusion Nursing, 44*, S45–S46. (Level VII)

6 Westbrook, J., et al. (2010). Association of interruptions with an increased risk and severity of medication administration errors. *Archives of Internal Medicine, 170*, 683–690. (Level IV)

7 Institute for Safe Medication Practices. (2012). Side tracks on the safety express: Interruptions lead to errors and unfinished…Wait, what was I

doing? *Nurse Advise-ERR, 11*(2), 1–4. https://www.ismp.org/resources/side-tracks-safety-express-interruptions-lead-errors-and-unfinished-wait-what-was-i-doing?id=37

8   Standard 20. Compounding and preparation of parenteral solutions and medications. Infusion therapy standards of practice. (8th ed.). (2021). *Journal of Infusion Nursing, 44,* S59–S60. (Level VII)

9   Accreditation Association for Hospitals and Health Systems. (2020). Standard 16.01.03. *Healthcare Facilities Accreditation Program: Accreditation requirements for acute care hospitals.* Chicago, IL: Accreditation Association for Hospitals and Health Systems. (Level VII)

10 DNV GL-Healthcare USA, Inc. (2020). MM.1.SR.3. *NIAHO® accreditation requirements, interpretive guidelines and surveyor guidance—revision 20.0.* Milford, OH: DNV GL-Healthcare USA, Inc. (Level VII)

11 Centers for Medicare and Medicaid Services, Department of Health and Human Services. (2020). Condition of participation: Nursing services. 42 C.F.R. § 482.23(c).

12 The Joint Commission. (2021). Standard MM.06.01.01. *Comprehensive accreditation manual for hospitals.* Oakbrook Terrace, IL: The Joint Commission. (Level VII)

13 Standard 13. Medication verification. Infusion therapy standards of practice. (8th ed.). (2021). *Journal of Infusion Nursing, 44,* S46–S149. (Level VII)

14 Centers for Disease Control and Prevention. (2002). Guideline for hand hygiene in health-care settings: Recommendations of the Healthcare Infection Control Practices Advisory Committee and the HICPAC/SHEA/APIC/IDSA Hand Hygiene Task Force. *MMWR Recommendations and Reports, 51*(RR-16), 1–45. https://www.cdc.gov/mmwr/pdf/rr/rr5116.pdf (Level II)

15 The Joint Commission. (2021). Standard NPSG.07.01.01. *Comprehensive accreditation manual for hospitals.* Oakbrook Terrace, IL: The Joint Commission. (Level VII)

16 Standard 16. Hand hygiene. Infusion therapy standards of practice. (8th ed.). (2021). *Journal of Infusion Nursing, 44,* S53–S54. (Level VII)

17 World Health Organization. (2009). WHO guidelines on hand hygiene in health care: First global patient safety challenge, clean care is safer care. https://apps.who.int/iris/bitstream/handle/10665/44102/9789241597906_eng.pdf?sequence=1(Level IV)

18 Accreditation Association for Hospitals and Health Systems. (2020). Standard 07.01.21. *Healthcare Facilities Accreditation Program: Accreditation requirements for acute care hospitals.* Chicago, IL: Accreditation Association for Hospitals and Health Systems. (Level VII)

19 Centers for Medicare and Medicaid Services, Department of Health and Human Services. (2020). Condition of participation: Infection control. 42 C.F.R. § 482.42.

20 DNV GL-Healthcare USA, Inc. (2020). IC.1.SR.1. *NIAHO® accreditation requirements, interpretive guidelines and surveyor guidance—revision 20.0.* Milford, OH: DNV GL-Healthcare USA, Inc. (Level VII)

21 The Joint Commission. (2021). Standard NPSG.01.01.01. *Comprehensive accreditation manual for hospitals.* Oakbrook Terrace, IL: The Joint Commission. (Level VII)

22 The Joint Commission. (2021). Standard RI.01.01.01. *Comprehensive accreditation manual for hospitals.* Oakbrook Terrace, IL: The Joint Commission. (Level VII)

23 DNV GL-Healthcare USA, Inc. (2020). PR.2.SR.5. *NIAHO® accreditation requirements, interpretive guidelines and surveyor guidance– revision 20.0.* Milford, OH: DNV GL-Healthcare USA, Inc. (Level VII)

24 Centers for Medicare and Medicaid Services, Department of Health and Human Services. (2020). Condition of participation: Patient's rights. 42 C.F.R. § 482.13(c)(1).

25 Accreditation Association for Hospitals and Health Systems. (2020). Standard 15.01.16. *Healthcare Facilities Accreditation Program: Accreditation requirements for acute care hospitals.* Chicago, IL: Accreditation Association for Hospitals and Health Systems. (Level VII)

26 The Joint Commission. (2021). Standard PC.02.01.21. *Comprehensive accreditation manual for hospitals.* Oakbrook Terrace, IL: The Joint Commission. (Level VII)

27 Standard 8. Patient education. Infusion therapy standards of practice. (8th ed.). (2021). *Journal of Infusion Nursing, 44,* S35–S37. (Level VII)

28 Waters, T. R., et al. (2009). Safe patient handling training for schools of nursing. https://www.cdc.gov/niosh/docs/2009-127/pdfs/2009-127.pdf (Level VII)

29 Occupational Safety and Health Administration. (2012). Bloodborne pathogens, standard number 1910.1030. https://www.osha.gov/pls/oshaweb/owadisp.show_document?p_id=10051&p_table=STANDARDS (Level VII)

30 Siegel, J. D., et al. (2007, revised 2019). 2007 guideline for isolation precautions: Preventing transmission of infectious agents in healthcare settings. https://www.cdc.gov/infectioncontrol/pdf/guidelines/isolation-guidelines-H.pdf (Level II)

31 Accreditation Association for Hospitals and Health Systems. (2020). Standard 07.01.10. *Healthcare Facilities Accreditation Program: Accreditation requirements for acute care hospitals.* Chicago, IL: (Level VII)

32 Infusion Nurses Society. (2016). *Policies and procedures for infusion therapy* (5th ed.). Boston, MA: Infusion Nurses Society.

33 Standard 46. Infiltration and extravasation. Infusion therapy standards of practice. (8th ed.). (2021). *Journal of Infusion Nursing, 39,* S98–S102. (Level VII)

34 Institute for Safe Medication Practices. (2018). ISMP list of high-alert medications in acute care settings. https://www.ismp.org/sites/default/files/attachments/2018-08/highAlert2018-Acute-Final.pdf (Level VII)

35 Institute for Safe Medication Practices. (2013). Independent double-checks: Undervalued and misused. Selective use of this strategy can play an important role in medication safety. https://www.ismp.org/resources/independent-double-checks-undervalued-and-misused-selective-use-strategy-can-play (Level VII)

36 Standard 36. Needleless connectors. Infusion therapy standards of practice. (8th ed.). (2021). *Journal of Infusion Nursing, 44,* S104–S107. (Level VII)

37 Moureau, N. L., & Flynn, J. (2015). Disinfection of needleless connector hubs: Clinical evidence systematic review. *Nursing Research and Practice,* 2015, 1–20. https://www.hindawi.com/journals/nrp/2015/796762/

38 Marschall, J., et al. (2014). SHEA/IDSA practice recommendation: Strategies to prevent central line-associated bloodstream infections in acute care hospitals. *Infection Control and Hospital Epidemiology, 35,* 753–771. https://www.jstor.org/stable/10.1086/676533#metadata_info_tab_contents (Level I)

39 Standard 41. Flushing and locking. Infusion therapy standards of practice. (8th ed.). (2021). *Journal of Infusion Nursing, 44,* S113–S119. (Level VII)

40 Standard 21. Medical waste and sharps safety. Infusion therapy standards of practice. (2016). *Journal of Infusion Nursing, 44,* S60–S63. (Level VII)

41 Institute for Safe Medication Practices (ISMP). (2015). ISMP safe practice guidelines for adult IV push medications. https://www.ismp.org/guidelines/iv-push (Level VII)

42 The Joint Commission. (2014). Sentinel event alert: Managing risk during transition to new ISO tubing connector standards. https://www.jointcommission.org/assets/1/6/SEA_53_Connectors_8_19_14_final.pdf (Level VII)

43 U.S. Food and Drug Administration. (2017). Examples of medical device misconnections. https://www.fda.gov/medical-devices/medical-device-connectors/examples-medical-device-misconnections

44 Standard 43. Administration set change. Infusion therapy standards of practice. (8th ed.). (2021). *Journal of Infusion Nursing, 44,* S123–S125. (Level VII)

45 Hull, G., et al. (2018). Quantitative assessment of reflux in commercially available needle-free IV connectors. *Journal of Vascular Access, 19,* 12–22. (Level VI)

46 Jasinsky, L., & Wurster, J. (2009). Occlusion reduction and heparin elimination trial using an antireflux device on peripheral and central venous catheters. *Journal of Infusion Nursing, 32*(1), 33–39. (Level VI)

47 Ganz, D. A., et al. (2013, reviewed 2021). *Preventing falls in hospitals: A toolkit for improving quality of care* (AHRQ Publication No. 13-0015-EF). Rockville, MD: Agency for Healthcare Research and Quality. https://www.ahrq.gov/professionals/systems/hospital/fallpxtoolkit/index.html (Level VII)

48 Centers for Medicare and Medicaid Services. (2014). Requirements for hospital medication administration, particularly intravenous (IV) medications and post-operative care of patients receiving IV opioids. https://www.cms.gov/Medicare/Provider-Enrollment-and-Certification/SurveyCertificationGenInfo/Downloads/Survey-and-Cert-Letter-14-15.pdf

49 The Joint Commission. (2021). Standard RC.01.03.01. *Comprehensive accreditation manual for hospitals.* Oakbrook Terrace, IL: The Joint Commission. (Level VII)

50 Standard 10. Documentation in the health record. Infusion therapy standards of practice. (8th ed.). (2021). *Journal of Infusion Nursing, 44,* S39–S43. (Level VII)

51 Centers for Medicare and Medicaid Services, Department of Health and Human Services. (2020). Condition of participation: Medical record services. 42 C.F.R. § 482.24(b).

52 Accreditation Association for Hospitals and health Systems. (2018). Standard 10.00.03. *Healthcare Facilities Accreditation Program:*

Accreditation requirements for acute care hospitals. Chicago, IL: Accreditation Association for Hospitals and Health Systems. (Level VII)

53 DNV GL-Healthcare USA, Inc. (2020). MR.2.SR.1. *NIAHO® accreditation requirements, interpretive guidelines and surveyor guidance—revision 20.0*. Milford, OH: DNV GL-Healthcare USA, Inc. (Level VII)

54 The Joint Commission. (2014). Sentinel event alert 52: Preventing infection from the misuse of vials. https://www.jointcommission.org/en/resources/patient-safety-topics/sentinel-event/sentinel-event-alert-newsletters/sentinel-event-alert-issue-52-preventing-infection-from-the-misuse-of-vials/ (Level VII)

55 The Joint Commission. (2021). Standard RC.02.01.01. *Comprehensive accreditation manual for hospitals*. Oakbrook Terrace, IL: The Joint Commission. (Level VII)

Intermittent infusion device flushing and locking

An intermittent infusion device consists of an IV catheter with a needleless connector attached. This device is used to maintain venous access in patients receiving IV medications intermittently as well as in those who might need medications if an emergency situation arises.

An intermittent infusion device should be flushed before each infusion, after each infusion (to prevent the mixing of incompatible medications and solutions), and after blood sampling.[1,2] The volume of flush solution required for flushing depends on the type and size of IV catheter and the type of infusion therapy prescribed. A volume equal to twice the internal volume of the IV catheter system is recommended, but a larger volume may be required after blood sampling or transfusion.[1,2,3] Never forcibly flush an intermittent infusion device. To prevent catheter damage, use a 10-mL syringe to assess patency, unless a smaller syringe designed to generate a lower amount of pressure is available.[1,2,3] Use sterile technique when flushing an intermittent infusion device *to reduce the risk of vascular catheter–associated infection*. Lock an intermittent infusion device immediately after each use with preservative-free normal saline solution.[3]

HOSPITAL-ACQUIRED CONDITION ALERT Keep in mind that the Centers for Medicare and Medicaid Services considers vascular catheter–associated infection a hospital-acquired condition *because it can be reasonably prevented using a variety of best practices*. Make sure to follow evidence-based infection prevention practices, such as performing hand hygiene, using sterile technique, and performing a vigorous mechanical scrub of needleless connectors, when flushing an intermittent infusion device *to reduce the risk of vascular catheter–associated infections*.[4,5,6]

Needlesticks and other sharps-related injuries that expose health care workers to bloodborne pathogens continue to be a significant hazard for hospital employees. The Occupational Safety and Health Administration recommends the use of safer medical devices, such as needleless systems, that isolate or remove the bloodborne pathogens hazard from the workplace.[7]

Equipment

Antiseptic pads (chlorhexidine-based, povidone iodine, or alcohol) ▪ prefilled 10-mL syringe with preservative-free normal saline solution, or smaller syringe designed to generate lower injection pressure ▪ gloves ▪ Optional: disinfectant-containing end cap.

Preparation of equipment

Inspect all IV equipment and supplies. If a product is expired, is defective, or has compromised integrity, remove it from patient use, label it as expired or defective, and report the expiration or defect as directed by your facility.[8]

Implementation

▪ Verify the practitioner's order and the patient's medication administration record for time intervals for flushing the IV catheter, *which helps improve the duration of IV catheter patency*.
▪ Gather and prepare the necessary equipment and supplies.
▪ Perform hand hygiene.[6,9,10,11,12,13,14,15]

▪ Confirm the patient's identity using at least two patient identifiers.[16]
▪ Provide privacy.[17,18,19,20]
▪ Explain the procedure to the patient and family (if appropriate) according to their individual communication and learning needs *to increase their understanding, allay their fears, and enhance communication*.[21]
▪ Raise the patient's bed to waist level before providing care *to prevent caregiver back strain*.[22]
▪ Perform hand hygiene.[6,9,10,11,12,13,14,15]
▪ Put on gloves *to comply with standard precautions*.[7,23,24]
▪ Assess the IV catheter insertion site *to ensure that it's free from signs of infection, infiltration, and phlebitis*.[25,26] (See *Complications of IV therapy*.)
▪ If a disinfectant-containing end cap is covering the injection cap, remove and discard it.[29,30]
▪ Perform a vigorous mechanical scrub of the needleless connector for at least 5 seconds using an antiseptic pad. Allow it to dry completely.[29,31]
▪ While maintaining the sterility of the syringe tip, attach a prefilled syringe containing preservative-free normal saline solution to the needleless connector. (Use a 10-mL syringe or a syringe specifically designed to generate lower injection pressure.) Unclamp the catheter and slowly aspirate for a blood return that is the color and consistency of whole blood. If you don't obtain a blood return, take steps to locate an external cause of the obstruction.[3]
▪ If you obtain a blood return, slowly inject the preservative-free normal saline solution into the catheter. Use a minimum volume of twice the internal volume of the IV catheter system. Don't forcibly flush the catheter; further evaluate the device if you meet resistance.[3]
▪ Close the clamp and remove the syringe according to the type of needleless injection cap used. For a positive-pressure needleless cap, clamp after the syringe is disconnected.[1,2] For a negative-pressure needleless cap, maintain pressure on the syringe plunger while closing the clamp.[1,2] For a neutral needleless cap, clamp before or after syringe disconnection.[1,2] For an antireflux needleless connector, clamp the catheter and then disconnect the syringe; a specific clamping sequence isn't required.[32,33]
▪ Attach a new disinfectant-containing end cap, if used in your facility, *to reduce the risk of vascular catheter-associated infection*.[29,30]
▪ Assess the IV catheter insertion site after any manipulation of the IV catheter *to check for infiltration at the cannula insertion site*.[26]
▪ Return the bed to the lowest position *to prevent falls and maintain patient safety*.[34]
▪ Discard the syringe in an appropriate receptacle.[7,35]
▪ Remove and discard your gloves.[7,23,24,35]
▪ Perform hand hygiene.[6,9,10,11,12,13,14,15]
▪ Document the procedure.[36,37,38,39,40]

Special considerations

▪ If the patient reports a burning sensation during injection of the flush solution, stop the injection and check cannula placement.[26] If the cannula is in the vein, inject the flush at a slower rate *to minimize irritation*.
▪ Change needleless connectors no more frequently than every 96 hours, but at least every 7 days, *because changing the device more frequently increases the risk of vascular catheter–associated infection*. If used within a continuous infusion system, change the needleless connector when changing the primary administration set. Additionally, change the needleless connector if it's removed for any reason, if there's blood or debris within the connector, before drawing a blood culture through a vascular access device, or if the needleless connector becomes contaminated. In addition, change it routinely as directed by your facility.[6]
▪ You'll typically flush an intermittent infusion device with preservative-free normal saline solution. However, when the medication to be infused is incompatible with preservative-free normal saline solution, flush the device with 5% dextrose in water (D_5W) instead; after medication administration, flush with D_5W and then follow by flushing with preservative-free normal saline solution.[3]

Patient teaching

If the patient will be discharged with an intermittent infusion device and orders for intermittent IV infusions or medications, begin discharge planning with a home health nurse as early as possible. Communicate with the home health nurse about the type of IV catheter being used,

Complications of IV therapy

This table outlines complications of IV therapy with their appropriate interventions.

COMPLICATION	NURSING INTERVENTION
Bacteremia, or bacteria in the blood, may result in the IV system being contaminated.	▪ Don't apply compresses, *because doing so may potentiate infection*. ▪ Notify the practitioner and obtain an order for antibiotics.
Bleeding, typically mild, may occur at the IV insertion site for the first 24 hours after placement.	▪ Apply a gauze dressing after initial IV placement, and change the first dressing in 24 hours. ▪ Limit movement of the extremity, using an arm board as necessary. ▪ If bleeding increases or persists after the first 24 hours, notify the practitioner.
Infiltration (the inadvertent accumulation of medication or solution in the tissue surrounding the vein) or *extravasation* (the inadvertent administration of a vesicant [an agent that may cause tissue damage when it escapes from intended vascular pathway] into surrounding tissue)[2] may be indicated by an increase in the circumference of the extremity.	▪ When assessing the IV catheter insertion site, assess along the path of the IV catheter. ▪ Measure the circumference of the extremity above the IV site, and compare serial measurements. ▪ If infiltration occurs, immediately discontinue the infusion and remove the IV catheter; institute supportive measures such as elevating the extremity, as needed.[1,2,26] ▪ If extravasation occurs, immediately discontinue the infusion. If you must remove the IV catheter, aspirate fluid using a small syringe before removing the catheter; never apply pressure to the area.[1,2,26] ▪ Estimate the volume of fluid that escaped into the tissues (based on the infusion rate and the time of your last assessment).[26] Using a skin marker, outline the area with visible signs of infiltration or extravasation to allow for assessing changes. If permitted, photograph the area *to identify progression or exacerbation of the tissue injury*.[26] ▪ Notify the practitioner of the event and obtain specific orders to treat the extravasation. Treatment depends on the type of medication and severity of the complication, and may include thermal manipulation, antidote administration, and surgical intervention.[1,2]
Hematoma formation indicates undue trauma to the vessel wall or extravasation of blood into the extravascular space.	▪ Apply a warm compress to the extremity *to help alleviate discomfort*. ▪ If symptoms increase, discontinue IV catheter use at the site.
Mechanical issues include IV catheter migration, breaks in the catheter or connective tubing, and accidental IV catheter removal.	▪ Evaluate for excessive patient movement or loose tape. ▪ Encourage the patient to limit movement of the extremity. ▪ Place the extremity with the IV catheter on an arm board, and securely fasten the IV catheter and tubing.
Nerve damage may result from trauma to an adjacent nerve during IV insertion.	▪ Evaluate for excessive patient movement. ▪ Immediately remove a peripheral IV catheter when the patient reports paresthesia-type pain during the dwell of a peripheral IV catheter.[27] ▪ Notify the practitioner.[27] ▪ Perform neurovascular assessment, observing for increased paresthesia.[27]
Phlebitis, or vein inflammation, usually results from mechanical irritation from IV catheter trauma and is an early sign of infection.	▪ Assess the severity using a standardized scale.[28] ▪ Discontinue the infusion and remove the venous access device. ▪ Determine the cause. ▪ Apply a warm compress to the extremity *to ease discomfort*.[28] ▪ Notify the practitioner. ▪ Replace the device in the opposite extremity.

including manufacturer and catheter size, if known; the date of insertion; dressing change and flush protocols taught at the facility; and any complications after placement.

Teach the patient and family (if appropriate) about hand hygiene techniques, dressing changes, device flushing, medication administration and syringe pump use (as applicable), disposal techniques for syringes, and any other relevant information about managing the intermittent infusion device.

Before discharge, demonstrate the procedure for the patient and family, and have them perform a return demonstration. In addition, *to ensure that the patient and family understand the information*, have them repeat what they have learned about the most common complications of IV therapy (for example, sepsis and accidental IV catheter removal), what signs to look for, and what to do if complications occur.[41]

Instruct the patient to contact the practitioner if the IV catheter becomes dislodged, a fever develops, or the IV insertion site becomes red or swollen or oozes fluid or blood.

Complications

Complications associated with intermittent infusion device flushing and locking include bacteremia, bleeding, hematoma, nerve damage, mechanical issues, infiltration, extravasation, and infection.

Documentation

Record the date and time of intermittent infusion device flushing, the amount and type of flush solution used, the presence or absence of a blood return and any resistance to flushing, the appearance of the insertion site (presence or absence of redness, swelling, drainage, tenderness, and streaking), and the patient's tolerance of the procedure. Record any complications that occurred, the name of the practitioner notified, the date and time of the notification, any prescribed interventions, and the patient's response to those interventions. Document teaching provided to the patient and family (if applicable), their understanding of that teaching, and any need for follow-up teaching.

REFERENCES
1 Infusion Nurses Society. (2016). *Policies and procedures for infusion therapy of the older adult* (3rd ed.). Boston, MA: Infusion Nurses Society.
2 Infusion Nurses Society. (2016). *Policies and procedures for infusion therapy* (5th ed.). Boston, MA: Infusion Nurses Society.
3 Standard 41. Flushing and locking. Infusion therapy standards of practice. (8th ed.). (2021). *Journal of Infusion Nursing, 44*, S119–S123. (Level VII)
4 Jarrett, N., & Callaham, M. (2016). Evidence-based guidelines for selected hospital-acquired conditions: Final report. https://www.cms.gov/Medicare/Medicare-Fee-for-Service-Payment/HospitalAcqCond/Downloads/2016-HAC-Report.pdf

5 Standard 50. Infection. Infusion therapy standards of practice. (8th ed.). (2021). *Journal of Infusion Nursing, 44,* S153–S157. (Level VII)

6 Centers for Disease Control and Prevention. (2011, revised 2017). Guidelines for the prevention of intravascular catheter-related infections. https://www.cdc.gov/infectioncontrol/guidelines/bsi/recommendations.html (Level I)

7 Occupational Safety and Health Administration. (2012). Bloodborne pathogens, standard number 1910.1030. https://www.osha.gov/pls/oshaweb/owadisp.show_document?p_id=10051&p_table=STANDARDS (Level VII)

8 Standard 12. Product evaluation, integrity, and defect reporting. Infusion therapy standards of practice. (8th ed.). (2021). *Journal of Infusion Nursing, 44,* S45–S46. (Level VII)

9 The Joint Commission. (2021). Standard NPSG.07.01.01. *Comprehensive accreditation manual for hospitals.* Oakbrook Terrace, IL: The Joint Commission. (Level VII)

10 Centers for Disease Control and Prevention. (2002). Guideline for hand hygiene in health-care settings: Recommendations of the Healthcare Infection Control Practices Advisory Committee and the HICPAC/SHEA/APIC/IDSA Hand Hygiene Task Force. *MMWR Recommendations and Reports, 51*(RR-16), 1–45. https://www.cdc.gov/mmwr/pdf/rr/rr5116.pdf (Level II)

11 World Health Organization. (2009). WHO guidelines on hand hygiene in health care: First global patient safety challenge, clean care is safer care. https://apps.who.int/iris/bitstream/handle/10665/44102/9789241597906_eng.pdf?sequence=1 (Level IV)

12 Standard 16. Hand hygiene. Infusion therapy standards of practice. (8th ed.). (2021). *Journal of Infusion Nursing, 44,* S53–S54. (Level VII)

13 Accreditation Association for Hospitals and Health Systems. (2020). Standard 07.01.21. *Healthcare Facilities Accreditation Program: Accreditation requirements for acute care hospitals.* Chicago, IL: Accreditation Association for Hospitals and Health Systems. (Level VII)

14 Centers for Medicare and Medicaid Services, Department of Health and Human Services. (2020). Condition of participation: Infection control. 42 C.F.R. § 482.42.

15 DNV GL-Healthcare USA, Inc. (2020). IC.1.SR.1. *NIAHO® accreditation requirements, interpretive guidelines and surveyor guidance—revision 20.0.* Milford, OH: DNV GL-Healthcare USA, Inc. (Level VII)

16 The Joint Commission. (2021). Standard NPSG.01.01.01. *Comprehensive accreditation manual for hospitals.* Oakbrook Terrace, IL: The Joint Commission. (Level VII)

17 The Joint Commission. (2021). Standard RI.01.01.01. *Comprehensive accreditation manual for hospitals.* Oakbrook Terrace, IL: The Joint Commission. (Level VII)

18 Centers for Medicare and Medicaid Services, Department of Health and Human Services. (2020). Condition of participation: Patient's rights. 42 C.F.R. § 482.13(c)(1).

19 Accreditation Association for Hospitals and Health Systems. (2020). Standard 15.01.16. *Healthcare Facilities Accreditation Program: Accreditation requirements for acute care hospitals.* Chicago, IL: Accreditation Association for Hospitals and Health Systems. (Level VII)

20 DNV GL-Healthcare USA, Inc. (2020). PR.2.SR.5. *NIAHO® accreditation requirements, interpretive guidelines and surveyor guidance—revision 20.0.* Milford, OH: DNV GL-Healthcare USA, Inc. (Level VII)

21 The Joint Commission. (2021). Standard PC.02.01.21. *Comprehensive accreditation manual for hospitals.* Oakbrook Terrace, IL: The Joint Commission. (Level VII)

22 Waters, T. R., et al. (2009). Safe patient handling training for schools of nursing. https://www.cdc.gov/niosh/docs/2009-127/pdfs/2009-127.pdf (Level VII)

23 Siegel, J. D., et al. (2007, revised 2019). 2007 guideline for isolation precautions: Preventing transmission of infectious agents in healthcare settings. https://www.cdc.gov/infectioncontrol/pdf/guidelines/isolation-guidelines-H.pdf (Level II)

24 Accreditation Association for Hospitals and Health Systems. (2020). Standard 07.01.10. *Healthcare Facilities Accreditation Program: Accreditation requirements for acute care hospitals.* Chicago, IL: Accreditation Association for Hospitals and Health Systems. (Level VII)

25 Standard 42. Vascular access device assessment, care and dressing changes. Infusion therapy standards of practice. (8th ed.). (2021). *Journal of Infusion Nursing, 44,* S119–S123. (Level VII)

26 Standard 47. Infiltration and extravasation. Infusion therapy standards of practice. (8th ed.). (2021). *Journal of Infusion Nursing, 44,* S142–S147. (Level VII)

27 Standard 48. Nerve injury. Infusion therapy standards of practice. (8th ed.). (2021). *Journal of Infusion Nursing, 44,* S147–S149. (Level VII)

28 Standard 46. Phlebitis. Infusion therapy standards of practice. (8th ed.). (2021). *Journal of Infusion Nursing, 44,* S138–S98. (Level VII)

29 Standard 36. Needleless connectors. Infusion therapy standards of practice. (8th ed.). (2021). *Journal of Infusion Nursing, 44,* S104–S107. (Level VII)

30 Moureau, N. L., & Flynn, J. (2015). Disinfection of needleless connector hubs: Clinical evidence systematic review. *Nursing Research and Practice,* 2015, 796762. https://www.hindawi.com/journals/nrp/2015/796762/

31 Marschall, J., et al. (2014). SHEA/IDSA practice recommendation: Strategies to prevent central line-associated bloodstream infections in acute care hospitals. *Infection Control and Hospital Epidemiology, 35,* 753–771. https://www.jstor.org/stable/10.1086/676533#metadata_info_tab_contents (Level I)

32 Hull, G., et al. (2018). Quantitative assessment of reflux in commercially available needleless IV connectors. *Journal of Vascular Access, 19*(1), 12–22. (Level VI)

33 Jasinsky, L., & Wurster, J. (2009). Occlusion reduction and heparin elimination trial using an antireflux device on peripheral and central venous catheters. *Journal of Infusion Nursing, 32*(1), 33–39. (Level VI)

34 Ganz, D. A., et al. (2013, reviewed 2021). *Preventing falls in hospitals: A toolkit for improving quality of care* (AHRQ Publication No. 13-0015-EF). Rockville, MD: Agency for Healthcare Research and Quality. https://www.ahrq.gov/professionals/systems/hospital/fallpxtoolkit/index.html (Level VII)

35 Standard 21. Medical waste and sharps safety. Infusion therapy standards of practice. (8th ed.). (2021). *Journal of Infusion Nursing, 44,* S60–S63. (Level VII)

36 The Joint Commission. (2021). Standard RC.01.03.01. *Comprehensive accreditation manual for hospitals.* Oakbrook Terrace, IL: The Joint Commission. (Level VII)

37 Standard 10. Documentation in the health record. Infusion therapy standards of practice. (8th ed.). (2021). *Journal of Infusion Nursing, 44,* S39–S43. (Level VII)

38 Accreditation Association for Hospitals and Health Systems. (2020). Standard 10.00.03. *Healthcare Facilities Accreditation Program: Accreditation requirements for acute care hospitals.* Chicago, IL: Accreditation Association for Hospitals and Health Systems. (Level VII)

39 Centers for Medicare and Medicaid Services, Department of Health and Human Services. (2020). Condition of participation: Medical record services. 42 C.F.R. § 482.24(b).

40 DNV GL-Healthcare USA, Inc. (2020). MR.2.SR.1. *NIAHO® accreditation requirements, interpretive guidelines and surveyor guidance—revision 20.0.* Milford, OH: DNV GL-Healthcare USA, Inc. (Level VII)

41 Standard 8. Patient education. Infusion therapy standards of practice. (8th ed.). (2021). *Journal of Infusion Nursing, 44,* S35–S37. (Level VII)

Intermittent infusion device insertion

Also called a *saline lock*, an intermittent infusion device consists of a short peripheral venous access catheter with a needleless connector attached. Filled with preservative-free normal saline solution to prevent blood clot formation, the device maintains venous access in patients who receive IV medication regularly or intermittently but who don't require continuous infusion.

An intermittent infusion device has several advantages over an IV catheter that's maintained at a moderately slow infusion rate. It minimizes the risk of fluid overload and electrolyte imbalance, cuts costs, reduces the risk of contamination by eliminating IV solution containers and administration sets, increases patient comfort and mobility, reduces patient anxiety, and, if inserted in a large vein, allows collection of multiple blood samples without repeated venipuncture.

If you anticipate long-term therapy, start with a vein at the most distal site *so that you can move proximally as needed for subsequent IV insertion sites.*[1] For infusion of an irritating medication, choose a large vein distal to any nearby joint. Cannulation of hemodialysis catheters, fistulas, and grafts for IV infusion therapy requires an order from a nephrologist or practitioner unless an emergency situation exists.[1]

Use veins on the dorsal and ventral surfaces of the upper extremities, including the metacarpal, cephalic, basilic, and median veins. If possible, choose a vein in the nondominant arm or hand.[1] Avoid using veins in an upper extremity on the side of breast surgery with axillary node dissection or with an arteriovenous fistula or graft, radiation therapy, or lymphedema, or an extremity affected by stroke.[1] If the patient has stage 4 or 5 chronic kidney disease, avoid using the upper arm or forearm veins that could be the site of dialysis access.[1] Avoid using lower extremity veins because of the increased risk of tissue damage, thrombophlebitis, and ulceration.

Avoid areas of flexion; areas where pain occurs on palpation; veins compromised by bruising, infiltration, phlebitis, sclerosis, or cord formation; and areas where procedures are planned. Avoid the lateral surface of the wrist for about 4″ to 5″ (10.2 cm to 12.7 cm) because of the risk of nerve damage; avoid the ventral surface of the wrist because of the associated pain on insertion and the risk of nerve damage. Take care to insert catheters away from open wounds. Make each successive cannulation proximal to the previous cannulation site. Collaborate with the patient and practitioner to discuss the risks and benefits of using a vein in an affected extremity if no other options exist.

For an older adult, choose an area with more subcutaneous tissue and skeletal support for better device stabilization, keeping in mind the need to conserve access for future therapy.[2] If the patient uses an ambulatory aid to maintain independence, determine on which side the patient uses the device; avoid inserting the device in the hands and in areas of flexion.[2,3] Allow an older adult to have input regarding the site of catheter insertion, because many older adults have previous experience with infusion therapy and can indicate what has been successful or unsuccessful.[2] If the patient isn't very mobile, consider using an extremity that most easily allows access to the bathroom or commode.

Follow sterile technique when inserting an IV catheter to reduce the risk of vascular catheter–associated infection.[2,4,5]

HOSPITAL-ACQUIRED CONDITION ALERT Keep in mind that the Centers for Medicare and Medicaid Services considers vascular catheter–associated infection a hospital-acquired condition *because it can be reasonably prevented using a variety of best practices.* Make sure to follow evidence-based infection prevention practices, such as performing hand hygiene, preparing the site with an antiseptic, adhering to sterile no-touch technique during insertion and maintenance, and discontinuing the device when it's no longer needed, *to reduce the risk of vascular catheter–associated infections.*[4,6,7]

Equipment

Closed IV catheter system with stabilization system and safety shield[8] ▪ needleless connector ▪ sterile 10-mL prefilled syringe of preservative-free normal saline solution ▪ single-use tourniquet (preferably latex-free) ▪ antiseptic pads (chlorhexidine-based, povidone iodine, or alcohol) ▪ chlorhexidine-based solution (tincture of iodine, povidone iodine, or alcohol if chlorhexidine is contraindicated) ▪ transparent semipermeable dressing ▪ engineered stabilization device or sterile tape ▪ dressing label or marker ▪ gloves ▪ Optional: soap and water, sterile gloves, single-patient-use scissors or disposable-head clippers, prescribed local anesthetic, warm packs, visualization technology, disinfectant-containing end cap, joint stabilization device, ultrasound device with sterile probe cover, sterile ultrasound gel, disinfectant wipes.

Preparation of equipment

Inspect all IV equipment and supplies. If a product is expired, is defective, or has compromised integrity, remove it from patient use, label it as expired or defective, and report the expiration or defect as directed by your facility.[9]

Implementation

▪ Verify the practitioner's order.
▪ Review the patient's medical record for allergies to antiseptic solutions or latex. Also review it for factors that may affect peripheral vasculature—including conditions that result in structural vessel changes (such as diabetes and hypertension), a history of frequent venipuncture or lengthy infusion therapy, skin variations, skin alterations (such as scars and tattoos), patient age, obesity, fluid volume deficit, and history of IV drug abuse—*to determine the need for vascular visualization technology.*[10]
▪ Gather and prepare the necessary equipment and supplies.

▪ Perform hand hygiene.[4,11,12,13,14,15,16,17]
▪ Confirm the patient's identity using at least two patient identifiers.[18]
▪ Provide privacy.[19,20,21,22]
▪ Explain the procedure to the patient and family (if appropriate) according to their individual communication and learning needs *to increase their understanding, allay their fears, and enhance cooperation.*[23] Describe the purpose of the intermittent infusion device. Provide the patient with information about the insertion process, expected duration of therapy, care and maintenance of the device, and signs and symptoms of complications and when to report them.[24,25,26]
▪ Raise the patient's bed to waist level before providing care *to prevent caregiver back strain.*[27]
▪ Place the patient in a comfortable reclining position, leaving the arm in a dependent position *to increase venous fill of the lower arms and hands.* If the patient's skin is cold, consider using warm packs or dry warmth *to promote vascular dilation.*[25]

Applying the tourniquet

▪ Apply a tourniquet at an appropriate location above the intended puncture site *to dilate the vein.*[2,5] Loosely apply the tourniquet or avoid its use in patients who bruise easily, are at risk for bleeding, or have compromised circulation or fragile skin.[25]
▪ Assess the patient's veins in the upper extremity and identify potential sites that are easily seen or palpated. If no access sites are visible or easily palpated, use visualization technology to help identify an appropriate insertion site. Choose an insertion site based on your assessment findings.[5]
▪ Check for a pulse distal to the tourniquet location.[2,5] If you don't detect it, release the tourniquet and reapply it with less tension *to prevent arterial occlusion.*
▪ Lightly palpate the vein with the index and middle fingers of your nondominant hand *to assess vein condition.*[2,5] Stretch the skin *to anchor the vein.* If the vein feels hard or ropelike, select another.
▪ If the vein is easily palpable but not sufficiently dilated, place the extremity in a dependent position for several seconds, or lightly stroke the vessel downward. If you have selected a vein in the arm or hand, tell the patient to open and close the fist several times.[2,5,25]
▪ Release the tourniquet for site preparation.[2,5]

Preparing the site

▪ If the intended insertion site is visibly soiled, clean it with soap and water before applying the antiseptic solution.[2,5,25]
▪ Remove excess hair from the intended insertion site, if needed, using a single-patient-use scissors or disposable-head clippers if needed *to facilitate dressing application.*[2,4,5,25]
▪ Administer a local anesthetic, as indicated and prescribed, using safe medication administration practices.[2,5,28,29,30,31,32] (See *Easing the pain of intermittent infusion device insertion,* page 450.)
▪ Perform hand hygiene[4,11,12,13,14,15,16,17] and put on gloves *to comply with standard precautions.*[33,34,35]
▪ Prepare the insertion site using a skin antiseptic agent. For chlorhexidine (preferred), apply with an applicator using a vigorous side-to-side motion for 30 seconds and allow the area to dry completely.[2,4,5,25] For povidone-iodine solution, apply using a swab. Begin at the intended insertion site, moving outward in concentric circles. Allow the solution dry completely (typically, at least 2 minutes).[2,3]
▪ If you must palpate the intended insertion site after cleaning, remove and discard your gloves, perform hand hygiene, and put on sterile gloves *to avoid contaminating the insertion site.*[5]

ELDER ALERT Keep in mind that although you should apply antiseptic agents with friction, this application can cause irritated skin to become damaged, causing discomfort in an older adult. Antiseptics can also cause stinging and irritation. Excessive amounts of alcohol may dry already-compromised skin.[2]
▪ Reapply the tourniquet.
▪ Use visualization technology such as near-infrared technology or ultrasound to locate the vein, if necessary and available.[2,5,10,25]
▪ Using the thumb of your nondominant hand, stretch the skin taut below the puncture site *to stabilize the vein.*[5]

Easing the pain of intermittent infusion device insertion

You can ease the pain of intermittent infusion device insertion by administering an anesthetic agent before insertion.[2,5] Be sure to follow these steps when administering an anesthetic agent:

- Obtain and review the practitioner's order.
- Review the patient's medical record for any history of an allergy to the prescribed anesthetic.
- Perform hand hygiene.[4,11,12,14,15,16,17]
- Confirm the patient's identity using at least two patient identifiers.[18]
- Provide the patient with information about the selected local anesthetic agent, including the benefits, potential complications, and management.[24]
- Put on gloves, as needed.[33,34,35]

For anesthetic cream

- Apply the recommended amount of anesthetic cream to the intended insertion site.[5]
- Cover the area with a transparent semipermeable dressing.[5]
- Note the time of application on the dressing with a marking pen.
- Leave the cream on the skin for the recommended application time.[5]
- After the recommended application time, remove the dressing, wipe off the cream, evaluate the effectiveness of the anesthetic, and assess for any adverse reactions to the anesthetic.[5]
- Disinfect the site with an antiseptic solution.
- Insert the device as usual.

For an anesthetic dermal patch

- Apply the dermal patch to the intended access site.[5]
- Leave the patch on the skin for the recommended application time.[5]
- Remove the patch, evaluate the effectiveness of the anesthetic, and assess the site for any adverse reactions to the anesthetic patch.[5]
- Disinfect the site with an antiseptic solution.
- Insert the device as usual

For an intradermal anesthetic

- Disinfect the skin of the intended access site with antiseptic pad and allow it to dry.[5]
- Withdraw 0.3 mL of injectable anesthetic into a 1-mL syringe.[5]
- With the needle bevel up, gently insert the needle intradermally above the intended access site.[5]
- Aspirate *to make sure that you didn't inadvertently insert the needle into a vessel.*[5]
- Inject 0.1 to 0.3 mL of the anesthetic, forming a wheal at the intended access site.[5]
- Remove the needle and discard the syringe in a puncture-resistant sharps container.[5,35]
- Evaluate the effectiveness of the anesthetic, and assess for any adverse reactions.[5]
- Disinfect the site with an antiseptic solution.
- Insert the device as usual.

For topical vapocoolant (skin refrigerant) spray

- Disinfect the skin of the intended access site with antiseptic solution and then allow it to dry.
- Spray the single-patient vapocoolant mist from the recommended distance at the intended insertion site immediately before cannulation for the recommended number of seconds or until the skin turns white, whichever occurs sooner.[36]
- Allow the liquid to evaporate from the skin.
- Insert the device as usual.

For iontophoresis

- Refer to the iontophoresis device manufacturer's instructions for use.[5]
- Evaluate the effectiveness of iontophoresis and assess for adverse reactions.[5]
- Disinfect the site with an antiseptic solution and insert the catheter as usual.

- Grasp the access cannula with your dominant hand, remove the cover, and examine the cannula tip.[25] If the edge isn't smooth, discard and replace the device.

Inserting the intermittent infusion device

- Tell the patient that you're about to insert the intermittent infusion device.
- Hold the needle bevel up and enter the skin directly over the vein at a 0- to 15-degree angle.[5]
- Puncture the skin and anterior vein wall, watching the flashback chamber or extension tubing behind the hub for blood return, *which signifies that you've properly accessed the vein.*[5] (You might not see a blood return in a small vein.)
- Level the insertion device slightly by lifting the tip of the device up *to prevent puncturing the back wall of the vein with the access device.*
- As you continue to hold the skin taut, use the device's push-off tab to separate the device from the needle stylet. Advance the catheter into the vein. *To avoid contaminating the catheter hub,* don't advance the catheter by pushing from the catheter hub.[5]
- Release the tourniquet.[5]
- Activate the device's safety mechanism following the manufacturer's instructions for use.[5]
- Clamp the extension tubing and attach a needleless connector and any other appropriate add-on devices primed with preservative-free normal saline solution.[2,5]
- Perform a vigorous mechanical scrub of the needleless connector for at least 5 seconds using an antiseptic pad. Allow it to dry completely.[37,38]
- While maintaining sterility of the syringe tip, attach a prefilled syringe containing preservative-free normal saline solution to the extension set hub. (Use a 10-mL syringe or a syringe specifically designed to generate lower injection pressure.) Slowly aspirate to remove air from the extension set and to assess for a blood return that is the color and consistency

of whole blood. If you don't obtain a blood return, take steps to locate an external cause of obstruction.[39]
- If you do obtain a blood return, slowly inject preservative-free normal saline solution into the catheter. Use a minimum volume of twice the internal volume of the catheter system. Don't forcibly flush the device; further evaluate the device if you meet resistance.[39]
- Close the clamp and remove the syringe according to the type of needleless connector used following the manufacturer's instructions.[2,5] For a positive-pressure needleless port, clamp the catheter after removing the syringe; for a negative-pressure needleless port, maintain pressure on the syringe plunger while clamping the catheter; for a neutral needleless port, clamp the device before or after disconnecting the syringe; and for an antireflux needleless connector, clamp the catheter and then disconnect the syringe (a specific clamping sequence isn't required).[40,41]
- Attach a disinfectant-containing end cap to the needless connector, if available in your facility, *to reduce the risk of vascular catheter-associated infection.*[38,42]

Dressing the site

- Secure the intermittent infusion device using an engineered stabilization device, if available. *An engineered stabilization device reduces vascular access device motion, which increases the risk for unintentional catheter dislodgement and complications requiring premature catheter removal.*[43] If an engineered stabilization device is unavailable, secure the catheter with sterile tape.[5]
- Apply a transparent semipermeable dressing.[4,44] If the patient has fragile skin, use a specially designed dressing *to prevent skin tearing or stripping.*[45]
- Secure the intermittent infusion device extension tubing using sterile tape.
- Label the dressing with the current date or the date the dressing is due to be changed, as directed by your facility.[44]

■ If the intermittent infusion device insertion site is near a movable joint, stabilize the joint using a padded joint stabilization device that supports the area of flexion and maintains the joint in a functional position. Secure the joint stabilization device following the manufacturer's instructions. Make sure that the device enables visualization and assessment of the insertion site and vascular pathway. Ensure that it doesn't exert pressure that constricts circulation or cause pressure injuries, skin impairment, or nerve damage. Periodically remove the device to assess circulation, range of motion, function, and skin integrity.[46]

■ Return the bed to the lowest position *to prevent falls and maintain patient safety.*[47]

■ Discard used supplies in the appropriate receptacle.[35,48]

■ Remove and discard your gloves.[33,35,48]

■ Perform hand hygiene[4,11,12,13,14,15,16,17]

■ Document the procedure.[49,50,51,52,53]

Special considerations

■ No more than two attempts at insertion should be made by one nurse, and total attempts should be limited to no more than four, *because multiple unsuccessful attempts cause the patient unnecessary pain, delay treatment, limit future vascular access, increase cost, and increase the risk of complications.*[25]

■ If the patient reports symptoms of paresthesia, such as radiating electrical pain, tingling, burning, a prickly feeling, or numbness, immediately stop the insertion procedure and carefully remove the catheter. Also stop the procedure upon the patient's request or when the patient's actions indicate severe pain. Notify the practitioner of the patient's report of symptoms, *because early recognition of nerve damage produces a better prognosis.* Document the details of the patient's report of symptoms in the medical record.[54]

EQUIPMENT

Converting an IV line to an intermittent infusion device

To convert an existing IV line into an intermittent infusion device, follow these steps:

■ Prime the needleless connector with preservative-free normal saline solution.[2,5]

■ Clamp the IV catheter.

■ Clamp the IV tubing, and then remove the administration set from the cannula hub.

■ Perform a vigorous mechanical scrub of the needleless connector for at least 5 seconds using an antiseptic pad. Allow it to dry completely.[37,38]

■ Remove the protective cap from the needleless connector.

■ Attach the needleless connector to the catheter hub. Rotate the device *to tighten it.*

■ Perform a vigorous mechanical scrub of the needleless connector for at least 5 seconds using an antiseptic pad. Allow it to dry completely.[37,38]

■ While maintaining the sterility of the syringe tip, attach a prefilled syringe containing preservative-free normal saline solution to the needleless connector. (Use a 10-mL syringe or a syringe specifically designed to generate lower injection pressure.) Unclamp the catheter and slowly aspirate for blood return that is the color and consistency of whole blood. If no blood return occurs, take steps to locate an external cause of obstruction.[39]

■ If blood return occurs, slowly inject preservative-free normal saline solution into the catheter. Use a minimum volume of twice the internal volume of the catheter system. Don't forcibly flush the device; further evaluate the device if you meet resistance.[39]

■ Clamp the catheter according to the type of needleless connector used.[2,5] For a positive-pressure needleless connector, clamp the catheter after removing the syringe. For a negative-pressure needleless connector, maintain pressure on the syringe plunger while clamping the catheter. For a neutral needleless connector, clamp the device before or after disconnecting the syringe.

■ For an antireflux needleless connector, clamp the catheter and disconnect the syringe; a specific clamping sequence isn't required.[40,41]

■ If the patient reports a burning sensation during the injection of the preservative-free normal saline solution, stop the injection and check catheter placement. If the catheter is in the vein, inject the preservative-free normal saline solution at a slower rate *to minimize irritation.* If the catheter isn't in the vein, remove and discard it; then select a new venipuncture site and, using fresh equipment, restart the procedure.[55]

■ If the practitioner orders discontinuing an IV infusion and orders an intermittent infusion device in its place, convert the existing line by disconnecting the IV tubing and attach a needleless connector. (See *Converting an IV line to an intermittent infusion device.*)

Complications

Complications associated with intermittent infusion device insertion include intravascular catheter–related infection, insertion site infection, phlebitis, infiltration, hematoma formation, and vasospasm.

Documentation

Record the insertion site location; specific site preparation; local anesthetic (if used); infection prevention and safety precautions taken; type, length, and gauge of the catheter you inserted; date and time of insertion; insertion method, including use of visualization and guidance technology; number of insertion attempts; type and amount of flush solution you used; device functionality; method of catheter stabilization; and the patient's tolerance of the procedure. Note any complications that occurred, subsequent interventions, and the patient's response to the interventions. Document teaching provided to the patient and family (if applicable), their understanding of that teaching, and any need for follow-up teaching.[50]

REFERENCES

1 Standard 27. Site selection. Infusion therapy standards of practice. (8th ed.). (2021). *Journal of Infusion Nursing, 44*, S81–S86. (Level VII)

2 Infusion Nurses Society. (2017). *Policies and procedures for infusion therapy of the older adult* (3rd ed.). Boston, MA: Infusion Nurses Society.

3 Vizcarra, C., et al. (2014). Recommendations for improving safety practices with short peripheral catheters. *Journal of Infusion Nursing, 37*, 121–124. (Level VII)

4 Centers for Disease Control and Prevention. (2011, revised 2017). Guidelines for the prevention of intravascular catheter-related infections. https://www.cdc.gov/infectioncontrol/guidelines/bsi/recommendations.html (Level I)

5 Infusion Nurses Society. (2016). *Policies and procedures for infusion therapy* (5th ed.). Boston, MA: Infusion Nurses Society.

6 Jarrett, N., & Callaham, M. (2016). Evidence-based guidelines for selected, candidate, and previously considered hospital-acquired conditions: Final report. https://www.cms.gov/Medicare/Medicare-Fee-for-Service-Payment/HospitalAcqCond/Downloads/2016-HAC-Report.pdf

7 Standard 50. Infection. Infusion therapy standards of practice (8th ed.). (2021). *Journal of Infusion Nursing, 44*, S153–S157. (Level VII)

8 Standard 26. Vascular access device planning. Infusion therapy standards of practice (8th ed.). (2021). *Journal of Infusion Nursing, 44*, S74–S81. (Level VII)

9 Standard 12. Product evaluation, integrity, and defect reporting (8th ed.). (2021). *Journal of Infusion Nursing, 44*, S45–S46. (Level VII)

10 Standard 22. Vascular visualization. Infusion therapy standards of practice (8th ed.). (2021). *Journal of Infusion Nursing, 44*, S63–S65. (Level VII)

11 The Joint Commission. (2021). Standard NPSG.07.01.01. *Comprehensive accreditation manual for hospitals.* Oakbrook Terrace, IL: The Joint Commission. (Level VII)

12 Standard 16. Hand hygiene. Infusion therapy standards of practice (8th ed.). (2021). *Journal of Infusion Nursing, 44*, S53–S54. (Level VII)

13 Centers for Disease Control and Prevention. (2002). Guideline for hand hygiene in health-care settings: Recommendations of the Healthcare Infection Control Practices Advisory Committee and the HICPAC/SHEA/APIC/IDSA Hand Hygiene Task Force. *MMWR Recommendations and Reports, 51*(RR-16), 1–45. https://www.cdc.gov/mmwr/pdf/rr/rr5116.pdf (Level II)

14 World Health Organization. (2009). WHO guidelines on hand hygiene in health care: First global patient safety challenge, clean care is safer care. https://apps.who.int/iris/bitstream/handle/10665/44102/9789241597906_eng.pdf?sequence=1 (Level IV)

15 Accreditation Association for Hospitals and Health Systems. (2020). Standard 07.01.21. *Healthcare Facilities Accreditation Program: Accreditation requirements for acute care hospitals.* Chicago, IL: Accreditation Association for Hospitals and Health Systems. (Level VII)

16 Centers for Medicare and Medicaid Services, Department of Health and Human Services. (2020). Condition of participation: Infection control. 42 C.F.R. § 482.42.

17 DNV GL-Healthcare USA, Inc. (2020). IC.1.SR.1. *NIAHO® accreditation requirements, interpretive guidelines and surveyor guidance—revision 20.0.* Milford, OH: DNV GL-Healthcare USA, Inc. (Level VII)

18 The Joint Commission. (2021). Standard NPSG.01.01.01. *Comprehensive accreditation manual for hospitals.* Oakbrook Terrace, IL: The Joint Commission. (Level VII)

19 Accreditation Association for Hospitals and Health Systems. (2020). Standard 15.01.16. *Healthcare Facilities Accreditation Program: Accreditation requirements for acute care hospitals.* Chicago, IL: Accreditation Association for Hospitals and Health Systems. (Level VII)

20 DNV GL-Healthcare USA, Inc. (2020). PR.1.SR.5. *NIAHO® accreditation requirements, interpretive guidelines and surveyor guidance—revision 20.0* Milford, OH: DNV GL-Healthcare USA, Inc. (Level VII)

21 Centers for Medicare and Medicaid Services, Department of Health and Human Services. (2020). Condition of participation: Patient's rights. 42 C.F.R. § 482.13(c)(1).

22 The Joint Commission. (2021). Standard RI.01.01.01. *Comprehensive accreditation manual for hospitals.* Oakbrook Terrace, IL: The Joint Commission. (Level VII)

23 The Joint Commission. (2021). Standard PC.02.01.21. *Comprehensive accreditation manual for hospitals.* Oakbrook Terrace, IL: The Joint Commission. (Level VII)

24 Standard 8. Patient education. Infusion therapy standards of practice (8th ed.). (2021). *Journal of Infusion Nursing, 44,* S35–S37. (Level VII)

25 Standard 34. Vascular access device placement (8th ed.). (2021). *Journal of Infusion Nursing, 44, Journal of Infusion Nursing, 39,* S97–S102. (Level VII)

26 The Joint Commission. (2021). Standard RI.01.01.03. *Comprehensive accreditation manual for hospitals.* Oakbrook Terrace, IL: The Joint Commission. (Level VII)

27 Waters, T. R., et al. (2009). Safe patient handling training for schools of nursing. https://www.cdc.gov/niosh/docs/2009-127/pdfs/2009-127.pdf (Level VII)

28 DNV GL-Healthcare USA, Inc. (2020). MM.1.SR.3. *NIAHO® accreditation requirements, interpretive guidelines and surveyor guidance—revision 20.0.* Milford, OH: DNV GL-Healthcare USA, Inc. (Level VII)

29 Standard 32. Pain management for venipuncture and vascular access procedures. Infusion therapy standards of practice (8th ed.). (2021). *Journal of Infusion Nursing, 44,* S94–S96. (Level VII)

30 The Joint Commission. (2021). Standard MM.06.01.01. *Comprehensive accreditation manual for hospitals.* Oakbrook Terrace, IL: The Joint Commission. (Level VII)

31 Centers for Medicare and Medicaid Services, Department of Health and Human Services. (2020). Condition of participation: Nursing services. 42 C.F.R. § 482.23(c)

32 Accreditation Association for Hospitals and Health Systems. (2020). Standard 16.01.03. *Healthcare Facilities Accreditation Program: Accreditation requirements for acute care hospitals.* Chicago, IL: Accreditation Association for Hospitals and Health Systems. (Level VII)

33 Siegel, J. D., et al. (2007, revised 2019). 2007 guideline for isolation precautions: Preventing transmission of infectious agents in healthcare settings. https://www.cdc.gov/infectioncontrol/pdf/guidelines/isolation-guidelines-H.pdf (Level II)

34 Accreditation Association for Hospitals and Health Systems. (2020). Standard 07.01.10. *Healthcare Facilities Accreditation Program: Accreditation requirements for acute care hospitals.* Chicago, IL: Accreditation Association for Hospitals and Health Systems. (Level VII)

35 Occupational Safety and Health Administration. (2012). Bloodborne pathogens, standard number 1910.1030. https://www.osha.gov/pls/oshaweb/owadisp.show_document?p_id=10051&p_table=STANDARDS (Level VII)

36 Gebauer Company (2018). Gebauer's Pain Ease® product information. https://cdn2.hubspot.net/hubfs/150313/Pain%20Ease%20Product%20Information_Application.pdf

37 Marschall, J., et al. (2014). SHEA/IDSA practice recommendation: Strategies to prevent central line-associated bloodstream infections in acute care hospitals. *Infection Control and Hospital Epidemiology, 35,* 753–771. https://www.jstor.org/stable/10.1086/676533#metadata_info_tab_contents (Level I)

38 Standard 36. Needleless connectors. Infusion therapy standards of practice (8th ed.). (2021). *Journal of Infusion Nursing, 44,* S104–S107. (Level VII)

39 Standard 41. Flushing and locking. Infusion therapy standards of practice (8th ed.). (2021). *Journal of Infusion Nursing, 44,* S113–S119. (Level VII)

40 Hull, G., et al. (2018). Quantitative assessment of reflux in commercially available needle-free IV connectors. *Journal of Vascular Access, 19,*12–22. (Level VI)

41 Jasinsky, L., & Wurster, J. (2009). Occlusion reduction and heparin elimination trial using an antireflux device on peripheral and central venous catheters. *Journal of Infusion Nursing, 32,* 33–39. (Level VI)

42 Moureau, N. L., & Flynn, J. (2015). Disinfection of needleless connector hubs: Clinical evidence systematic review. *Nursing Research and Practice, 2015,* 1–20. https://www.hindawi.com/journals/nrp/2015/796762/

43 Standard 38. Vascular access device securement. Infusion therapy standards of practice (8th ed.). (2021). *Journal of Infusion Nursing, 44,* S108–S111. (Level VII)

44 Standard 42. Vascular access device assessment, care and dressing changes. Infusion therapy standards of practice (8th ed.). (2021). *Journal of Infusion Nursing, 44,* S119–S123. (Level VII)

45 LeBlanc, K., et al. (2013). International skin tear advisory panel: A tool kit to aid in the prevention, assessment, and treatment of skin tears using a simplified classification system. *Advances in Skin & Wound Care, 26,* 459–476. (Level IV)

46 Standard 39. Joint stabilization. Infusion therapy standards of practice (8th ed.). (2021). *Journal of Infusion Nursing, 44,* S111–S112. (Level VII)

47 Ganz, D. A., et al. (2013, reviewed 2021). *Preventing falls in hospitals: A toolkit for improving quality of care* (AHRQ Publication No. 13-0015-EF). Rockville, MD: Agency for Healthcare Research and Quality. https://www.ahrq.gov/professionals/systems/hospital/fallpxtoolkit/index.html (Level VII)

48 Standard 21. Medical waste and sharps safety. Infusion therapy standards of practice (8th ed.). (2021). *Journal of Infusion Nursing, 44,* S60–S63. (Level VII)

49 The Joint Commission. (2021). Standard RC.01.03.01. *Comprehensive accreditation manual for hospitals.* Oakbrook Terrace, IL: The Joint Commission. (Level VII)

50 Standard 10. Documentation in the health record. Infusion therapy standards of practice (8th ed.). (2021). *Journal of Infusion Nursing, 44,* S39–S43. (Level VII)

51 Accreditation Association for Hospitals and Health Systems. (2020). Standard 10.00.03. *Healthcare Facilities Accreditation Program: Accreditation requirements for acute care hospitals.* Chicago, IL: Accreditation Association for Hospitals and Health Systems. (Level VII)

52 Centers for Medicare and Medicaid Services, Department of Health and Human Services. (2020). Condition of participation: Medical record services. 42 C.F.R. § 482.24(b).

53 DNV GL-Healthcare USA, Inc. (2020). MR.2.SR.1. *NIAHO® accreditation requirements, interpretive guidelines and surveyor guidance—revision 20.0.* Milford, OH: DNV GL-Healthcare USA, Inc. (Level VII)

54 Standard 48. Nerve injury. Infusion therapy standards of practice (8th ed.). (2021). *Journal of Infusion Nursing, 44,* S142–S147. (Level VII)

55 Standard 47. Infiltration and extravasation. Infusion therapy standards of practice (8th ed.). (2021). *Journal of Infusion Nursing, 44,* S142–S147. (Level VII)

INTERMITTENT URINARY CATHETERIZATION

Intermittent (straight) urinary catheter insertion involves inserting a temporary catheter into the bladder to drain urine. In contrast with an indwelling urinary catheter, an intermittent catheter is removed as soon as the urine is drained. It's a preferred alternative to indwelling urinary catheter insertion for managing patients with neurogenic bladder and urinary retention because it's associated with lower infection rates.[1,2,3,4]

Intermittent urinary catheterization has been used in patients with spinal cord injury, spinal tumors, diabetic neuropathy, multiple sclerosis, spina bifida, myelodysplasia, bladder outlet obstruction, and continent urinary diversion. It's also been used to manage incontinence and postoperative urinary retention as well as to collect urine samples for culture and sensitivity.

Intermittent urinary catheterization is used long- or short-term, depending on the patient's condition. When used routinely, it should be performed at regular intervals throughout the day according to the patient's fluid intake to prevent bladder overdistention.[2]

In the health care facility, use sterile or clean technique for insertion, as required by your facility. At home, the patient may use clean technique without increasing the risk for a urinary tract infection (UTI). This procedure focuses on using sterile technique.

Equipment

Sterile urethral catheter (#10 to #22 French) ■ single-use packets of soap-containing wipes (or soap, water, washcloth, and towel) ■ gloves ■ fluid-impermeable pads ■ sterile gloves ■ sterile drape ■ sterile fenestrated drape ■ sterile, presaturated antiseptic swabs; antiseptic solution and sterile swabs; or antiseptic solution, sterile cotton balls, and plastic forceps ■ urine drainage receptacle ■ single-use packets of sterile water-soluble lubricant ■ Optional: light source, gown, mask and goggles or mask with face shield, bladder ultrasonography unit with probe, clean and dry urinary catheter storage container, mild soap and water.

Prepackaged sterile disposable kits that usually contain all the necessary equipment are available.

Preparation of equipment

Inspect all equipment and supplies. If a product is expired, is defective, or has compromised integrity, remove it from patient use, label it as expired or defective, and report the expiration or defect as directed by your facility.

Implementation

■ Verify the practitioner's order.
■ Check the patient's medical record for a history of hypersensitivity to iodine or latex.
■ Gather and prepare the necessary equipment and supplies. Use the smallest catheter possible *to minimize urethral damage.*[3,4]
■ Obtain the assistance of a coworker if necessary *to help position the patient.*
■ Ensure adequate lighting.
■ Perform hand hygiene.[5,6,7,8,9,10]
■ Confirm the patient's identity using at least two patient identifiers.[11]
■ Provide privacy.[12,13,14,15]
■ Explain the procedure to the patient and family (if appropriate) according to their communication and learning needs *to increase understanding, allay fears, and enhance cooperation.*[16]
■ Check the patient's intake and output record *to see the time and amount of the last recent void;* confirm the time with the patient.
■ Raise the patient's bed to waist level before providing care *to prevent caregiver back strain.*[17]
■ Perform hand hygiene.[5,6,7,8,9,10]
■ Percuss and palpate the patient's bladder *to establish a baseline for comparison.* Ask if the patient feels the urge to void. If possible, measure the volume of urine in the bladder using bladder ultrasonography with a probe; *ultrasonography helps prevent unnecessary catheterization.*[2]
■ Perform hand hygiene.[5,6,7,8,9,10]
■ Put on gloves and, as needed, other personal protective equipment *to comply with standard precautions.*[18,19,20]

For a female patient

■ Place the patient in the supine position with her knees flexed and separated and her feet flat on the bed, about 2′ (60 cm) apart. If she finds this position uncomfortable, have her flex one knee and keep the other leg flat on the bed. Or have the patient lie on her side with her knees drawn up to her chest during the catheterization procedure (as shown above on right). *This position may be especially helpful for older adults and those with disabilities, such as those with severe contractures.*

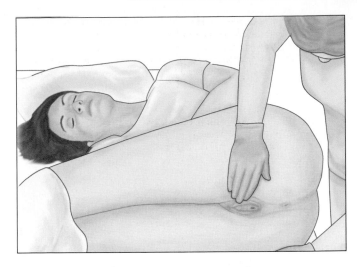

■ Ask the patient to hold her position *to give you a clear view of the urinary meatus and to prevent contamination of the sterile field.*
■ Place fluid-impermeable pads on the bed between the patient's legs and under her hips *to prevent inadvertent soiling of the patient's bed linens.*
■ Use single-use soap-containing wipes to clean the patient's periurethral area thoroughly. Alternatively, clean the area with warm, soapy water using a washcloth, rinse, and then dry the area with a towel.[2]
■ Remove and discard your gloves.[18,20]
■ Perform hand hygiene.[5,6,7,8,9,10]
■ *To create the sterile field,* open the prepackaged kit or equipment tray and place it at an area near the patient or between the patient's legs. If the sterile gloves are the first item on the top of the tray, put them on. Place the sterile drape under the patient's hips. Then drape the patient's lower abdomen with the sterile fenestrated drape so that only the genital area remains exposed (as shown below). Make sure you don't contaminate your gloves if you have them on already.[3,6,21,22]

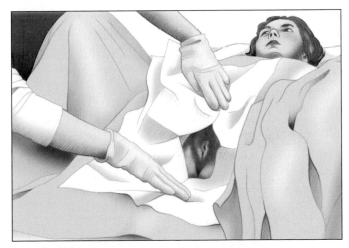

■ Open the rest of the prepackaged sterile disposable kit or equipment tray. Put on the sterile gloves if you haven't already done so.[18,20]
■ Tear open the packet of sterile, presaturated antiseptic wipes, or use antiseptic cleaning solution to saturate the sterile cotton balls or sterile swabs. Be careful not to spill the solution on the equipment.
■ Open a single-use packet of sterile, water-soluble lubricant and apply it to the catheter tip.
■ Separate the labia majora and labia minora as widely as possible with the thumb, middle, and index fingers of your nondominant hand *so you have a full view of the urinary meatus.* Keep the labia well separated throughout the procedure *so they don't obscure the urinary meatus or contaminate the area when it's cleaned.*
■ With your dominant hand, use an antiseptic swab, or pick up a sterile antiseptic-soaked cotton ball with the plastic forceps, and wipe one side

of the urinary meatus with a downward motion (as shown below), and then discard the swab or cotton ball.

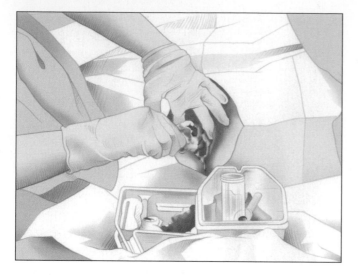

■ Wipe the other side with another sterile, presaturated antiseptic swab or antiseptic-soaked cotton ball using the same technique. Then wipe directly over the meatus with a third antiseptic swab or antiseptic-soaked cotton ball. Take care not to contaminate your sterile glove.

■ Pick up the straight catheter with your dominant hand, holding it about 2″ to 3″ (5 to 7.5 cm) from the tip, and prepare to insert the lubricated tip into the urinary meatus. *To facilitate insertion*, ask the patient to cough as you insert the catheter, *because coughing relaxes the sphincter*. If the catheter is inadvertently inserted into the vagina, leave it there as a landmark. Then begin the procedure over again using new supplies.

NURSING ALERT Never force a catheter during insertion. Maneuver it gently as the patient bears down. If you still meet resistance, stop and notify the practitioner. *Sphincter spasms, strictures, or misplacement in the vagina may cause resistance.*

■ Slowly and gently advance the catheter 2″ to 4″ (5 to 10 cm) while continuing to hold the labia apart until urine begins to flow.

■ Drain the urine into the urine receptacle.

■ Hold the catheter in place until the urine flow stops and the bladder is empty.

■ When flow has stopped, slowly remove the catheter, allowing urine to drain from the lower half of the bladder. Completely remove the catheter when there's no additional urine flow.

■ Return the bed to the lowest position *to prevent falls and maintain patient safety.*[23]

■ If the urinary catheter is disposable, discard it in the appropriate receptacle.[20] If it's reusable, clean the urinary catheter with mild soap and water and store it in a clean, dry urinary catheter storage container.[24,25]

■ Discard all the used supplies in the appropriate receptacles.[20]

■ Remove and discard your gloves and any other personal protective equipment worn.[18,20]

■ Perform hand hygiene.[5,6,7,8,9,10]

■ Document the procedure.[26,27,28,29]

For a male patient

■ Place the patient in the supine position with his legs extended and flat on the bed. Ask the patient to remain in that position *to give you a clear view of the urinary meatus and to prevent contamination of the sterile field.*

■ Place a fluid-impermeable pad on the bed between the patient's legs and under his hips *to prevent inadvertent soiling of bed linens.*

■ Use the single-use soap-containing wipes to wash the periurethral area. Alternatively, clean the area with warm, soapy water and a washcloth. Rinse the area with water and dry the area with the towel.

■ Place a new fluid-impermeable pad under the patient if the existing one is wet or soiled.

■ Remove and discard your gloves.[18,20]

■ Perform hand hygiene.[5,6,7,8,9,10]

■ *To create the sterile field*, open the prepackaged sterile disposable kit or equipment tray and place it next to the patient's hip. If the sterile gloves are the first item on the top of the tray, put them on.[18] Place the sterile drape under the patient's hips. Then drape the patient's lower abdomen with the sterile fenestrated drape so that only the genital area remains exposed. Make sure you don't contaminate your gloves if you have them on already.[3,6,21]

■ Open the rest of the prepackaged disposable kit or equipment tray. Put on the sterile gloves if you haven't already done so.[18]

■ Tear open the packet of sterile, presaturated antiseptic swabs, or use an antiseptic cleaning solution *to saturate sterile cotton balls or swabs*. Be careful not to spill the solution on the equipment.

■ Open the single-use packet of water-soluble lubricant and apply it to the urinary catheter tip.

■ Hold the penis with your nondominant hand. If the patient is uncircumcised, retract the foreskin. Then gently lift and stretch the penis to a 60- to 90-degree angle. Hold the penis this way throughout the procedure *to straighten the urethra and maintain a sterile field.*

■ Use your dominant hand to clean the glans with a sterile, presaturated antiseptic swab or an antiseptic-soaked sterile swab, or an antiseptic-soaked cotton ball you picked up with the plastic forceps. Clean in a circular motion, starting at the urinary meatus and working outward (as shown below).

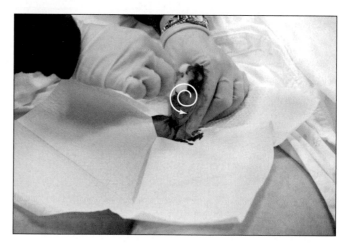

■ Repeat the procedure, using another antiseptic swab or antiseptic-soaked sterile cotton ball. Make sure that you don't contaminate your sterile glove.

■ Pick up the catheter with your dominant hand, holding it about 2″ to 3″ (5 to 7.5 cm) from the tip, and prepare to insert the lubricated tip into the urinary meatus. *To facilitate insertion*, ask the patient to cough as you insert the catheter, *because coughing will relax the sphincter*. Tell him to breathe deeply and slowly *to further relax the sphincter and reduce spasms.*[30]

■ Gently insert the catheter into the meatus, approximately 6″ to 8″ (15 to 20 cm) or until the urine begins to flow. As you reach the level of the prostate, you'll meet some resistance. Tell the patient to breathe deeply and slowly as you continue to advance the catheter.

NURSING ALERT Never force a catheter during insertion. Maneuver it gently as the patient coughs or breathes deeply and slowly. If you still meet resistance, stop and notify the practitioner. *Sphincter spasms, strictures, or an enlarged prostate may cause resistance.*[30]

■ If the foreskin was retracted, replace it *to prevent compromised circulation and painful swelling.*

■ Drain the urine into the urine receptacle.

■ Hold the catheter in place until the urine flow stops and the bladder is empty.

■ When urine flow has stopped, slowly remove the catheter, allowing urine to drain from the lower half of the bladder. Completely remove the catheter when there's no additional urine flow.

■ Return the bed to the lowest position *to prevent falls and maintain patient safety.*[23]

- If the catheter is disposable, discard it in the appropriate receptacle.[20] If it is reusable, clean the urinary catheter with mild soap and water and store it in a clean and dry urinary catheter storage container.[24,25]
- Discard used supplies in the appropriate receptacle.
- Remove and discard your gloves and any other personal protective equipment worn.[18,20]
- Perform hand hygiene.[5,6,7,8,9,10]
- Document the procedure.[26,27,28,29]

Special considerations

- Some patients may be difficult to catheterize because of difficulty viewing the patient's urinary meatus due to anatomical variations, such as presence of urethral strictures or false passages, and following surgery (in males and females),[22,30] childbirth,[22] prostatic enlargement, or postsurgical bladder neck contractures.[30] These conditions may necessitate the involvement of a urologist.
- Patients with spina bifida, spinal cord injury, atopy, certain food allergies, and occupational latex exposure are at increased risk for latex hypersensitivity. Provide these patients with a latex-free environment by avoiding all products containing latex proteins, including gloves, catheters, condoms, drains, and injection ports.
- If ordered, a topical anesthetic may be instilled directly into the urethra before catheter insertion *to prevent pain and trauma to the urethral lining.*[31]
- Some practitioners use a syringe prefilled with water-soluble lubricant and instill the lubricant directly into the male urethra instead of on the catheter tip. A topical anesthetic gel may also be instilled into the urethra before catheter insertion, if prescribed. *These methods help prevent pain and trauma to the urethral lining as well as possible urinary tract infection.*[32]
- If the practitioner orders a urine specimen for laboratory analysis, obtain it from the urine receptacle with a specimen collection container at the time of urinary catheterization, label it in the presence of the patient *to prevent mislabeling,*[11] and send it to the laboratory in a biohazard transport bag[20] with the appropriate laboratory request form (if required by your facility).

Patient teaching

Teach the patient and family (if applicable) about all aspects of urinary self-catheterization as required for discharge. Review proper handwashing technique, proper urinary catheterization technique, and daily care of the patient's urinary meatus, as well as maintenance of urinary catheter supplies. Instruct the patient to report any signs or symptoms of a UTI or an obstruction. Advise the patient to keep well hydrated so that urine is a light straw color.[33]

Complications

Complications of intermittent urinary catheter insertion include patient discomfort, urethral false passages, urethral strictures with chronic use, and bladder perforation. A UTI may result from the introduction of bacteria into the patient's bladder. Improper urinary catheter insertion may cause traumatic injury to the patient's urethral and bladder mucosa, and bleeding.[34,35]

Documentation

Record the date and time of intermittent urinary catheter insertion and the size and type of urinary catheter used. Also describe the amount, color, and other characteristics of the urine emptied from the patient's bladder. Note that your facility can require only the intake and output record for fluid balance data. Describe the patient's tolerance of the procedure. Document whether you sent a urine specimen for laboratory analysis. Document teaching provided to the patient and family (if applicable), their understanding of that teaching, and any need for follow-up teaching.

REFERENCES

1 Association of Professionals in Infection Control and Epidemiology (APIC). (2014). APIC implementation guide: Guide to preventing catheter-associated urinary tract infections. https://apic.org/wp-content/uploads/2019/02/APIC_CAUTI_IG_FIN_REVD0815.pdf (Level IV)

2 Healthcare Infection Control Practices Advisory Committee. (2010, revised 2019). Guideline for prevention of catheter-associated urinary tract infections 2009. https://www.cdc.gov/infectioncontrol/pdf/guidelines/cauti-guidelines-H.pdf (Level I)

3 Lo, E., et al. (2014). SHEA/IDSA practice recommendation. Strategies to prevent catheter-associated urinary tract infections in acute care hospitals: 2014 update. *Infection Control and Hospital Epidemiology, 35,* 464–479. https://www.jstor.org/stable/10.1086/675718#metadata_info_tab_contents (Level I)

4 Society of Urologic Nurses and Associates. (2016). Clinical practice guidelines: Prevention & control of catheter-associated urinary tract infection (CAUTI). https://www.suna.org/resource/clinical-practice?page=3 (Level VII)

5 Centers for Disease Control and Prevention. (2002). Guideline for hand hygiene in health-care settings: Recommendations of the Healthcare Infection Control Practices Advisory Committee and the HICPAC/SHEA/APIC/IDSA Hand Hygiene Task Force. *MMWR Recommendations and Reports, 51*(RR-16), 1–45. https://www.cdc.gov/mmwr/pdf/rr/rr5116.pdf (Level II)

6 The Joint Commission. (2021). Standard NPSG.07.01.01. *Comprehensive accreditation manual for hospitals.* Oakbrook Terrace, IL: The Joint Commission. (Level VII)

7 World Health Organization. (2009). WHO guidelines on hand hygiene in health care: First global patient safety challenge, clean care is safer care. https://apps.who.int/iris/bitstream/handle/10665/44102/9789241597906_eng.pdf?sequence=1 (Level IV)

8 Accreditation Association for Hospitals and Health Systems. (2020). Standard 07.01.21. *Healthcare Facilities Accreditation Program: Accreditation requirements for acute care hospitals.* Chicago, IL: Accreditation Association for Hospitals and Health Systems. (Level VII)

9 Centers for Medicare and Medicaid Services, Department of Health and Human Services. (2020). Condition of participation: Infection control. 42 C.F.R. § 482.42.

10 DNV GL-Healthcare USA, Inc. (2020). IC.1.SR.1. *NIAHO® accreditation requirements, interpretive guidelines and surveyor guidance—revision 20.0.* Milford, OH: DNV GL-Healthcare USA, Inc. (Level VII)

11 The Joint Commission. (2021). Standard NPSG.01.01.01. *Comprehensive accreditation manual for hospitals.* Oakbrook Terrace, IL: The Joint Commission. (Level VII)

12 Accreditation Association for Hospitals and Health Systems. (2020). Standard 15.01.16. *Healthcare Facilities Accreditation Program: Accreditation requirements for acute care hospitals.* Chicago, IL: Accreditation Association for Hospitals and Health Systems. (Level VII)

13 Centers for Medicare and Medicaid Services, Department of Health and Human Services. (2020). Condition of participation: Patient's rights. 42 C.F.R. § 482.13(c)(1).

14 DNV GL-Healthcare USA, Inc. (2020). PR.2.SR.5. *NIAHO® accreditation requirements, interpretive guidelines and surveyor guidance—revision 20.0.* Milford, OH: DNV GL-Healthcare USA, Inc. (Level VII)

15 The Joint Commission. (2021). Standard RI.01.01.01. *Comprehensive accreditation manual for hospitals.* Oakbrook Terrace, IL: The Joint Commission. (Level VII)

16 The Joint Commission. (2021). Standard PC.02.01.21. *Comprehensive accreditation manual for hospitals.* Oakbrook Terrace, IL: The Joint Commission. (Level VII)

17 Waters, T. R., et al. (2009). Safe patient handling training for schools of nursing. https://www.cdc.gov/niosh/docs/2009-127/pdfs/2009-127.pdf (Level VII)

18 Siegel, J. D., et al. (2007, revised 2019). 2007 guideline for isolation precautions: Preventing transmission of infectious agents in healthcare settings. https://www.cdc.gov/infectioncontrol/pdf/guidelines/isolation-guidelines-H.pdf (Level II)

19 Accreditation Association for Hospitals and Health Systems. (2020). Standard 07.01.10. *Healthcare Facilities Accreditation Program: Accreditation requirements for acute care hospitals.* Chicago, IL: Accreditation Association for Hospitals and Health Systems. (Level VII)

20 Occupational Safety and Health Administration. (2012). Bloodborne pathogens, standard number 1910.1030. https://www.osha.gov/pls/oshaweb/owadisp.show_document?p_id=10051&p_table=STANDARDS (Level VII)

21 The Joint Commission. (2021). Standard NPSG.07.06.01. *Comprehensive accreditation manual for hospitals.* Oakbrook Terrace, IL: The Joint Commission. (Level VII)

22 Quallich, S. A. et al. (2021). Urinary catheterization of the adult female. *Urologic Nursing, 41*(2), 65–69. https://www.suna.org/download/catheterizationFemaleCCP.pdf (Level VII)

23 Ganz, D. A., et al. (2013). *Preventing falls in hospitals: A toolkit for improving quality of care* (AHRQ Publication No. 13-0015-EF). Rockville, MD: Agency for Healthcare Research and Quality. https://www.ahrq.gov/professionals/systems/hospital/fallpxtoolkit/index.html (Level VII)

24 Rutala, W. A., et al. (2008, revised 2019). Guideline for disinfection and sterilization in healthcare facilities, 2008. https://www.cdc.gov/infection-control/pdf/guidelines/disinfection-guidelines-H.pdf (Level I)

25 Accreditation Association for Hospitals and Health Systems. (2020). Standard 07.02.03. *Healthcare Facilities Accreditation Program: Accreditation requirements for acute care hospitals.* Chicago, IL: Accreditation Association for Hospitals and Health Systems. (Level VII)

26 The Joint Commission. (2021). Standard RC.01.03.01. *Comprehensive accreditation manual for hospitals.* Oakbrook Terrace, IL: The Joint Commission. (Level VII)

27 Accreditation Association for Hospitals and Health Systems. (2020). Standard 10.00.03. *Healthcare Facilities Accreditation Program: Accreditation requirements for acute care hospitals.* Chicago, IL: Accreditation Association for Hospitals and Health Systems. (Level VII)

28 Centers for Medicare and Medicaid Services, Department of Health and Human Services. (2020). Condition of participation: Medical record services. 42 C.F.R. § 482.24(b).

29 DNV GL-Healthcare USA, Inc. (2020). MR.2.SR.1. *NIAHO® accreditation requirements, interpretive guidelines and surveyor guidance—revision 20.0.* Milford, OH: DNV GL-Healthcare USA, Inc. (Level VII)

30 Quallich, S. A. et al. (2021). Urinary catheterization of the adult male. *Urologic Nursing, 41*(2), 70–75. https://www.suna.org/download/catheterizationMaleCCP.pdf (Level VII)

31 Shlamovitz, G. Z. (2016). Urethral catheterization in women. https://emedicine.medscape.com/article/80735-overview

32 Villanueva, C., & Hemstreet, G. P.,III. (2008). Difficult male urethral catheterization: A review of different approaches. *International Brazilian Journal of Urology, 34*(4), 401–412. http://www.brazjurol.com.br/july_august_2008/Villanueva_ing_401_412.pdf (Level V)

33 Newman, D. K., & Wilson, M. M. (2011). Review of intermittent catheterization and current best practices. *Urologic Nursing, 31*, 12–29, 48.

34 Newman, D.K. (2021). Complications—intermittent catheters. https://www.urotoday.com/urinary-catheters-home/intermittent-catheters/complications/complications-intermittent-catheters.html

35 Schaeffer, A.J. (2021). Complications of urinary bladder catheters and preventive strategies. In: *UpToDate*, Richie, J.P. (Ed.)

INTERNAL FIXATION MANAGEMENT

In internal fixation, also known as *surgical reduction* or *open reduction–internal fixation*, the surgeon implants fixation devices to stabilize the fracture. Internal fixation devices include nails, screws, pins, wires, and rods, all of which may be used in combination with metal plates. These devices remain in the body indefinitely unless the patient experiences adverse reactions after the healing process is complete. (See *Reviewing internal fixation devices.*)

Typically, internal fixation is used to treat fractures of the face and jaw, spine, and arms and legs as well as fractures involving a joint (most commonly, the hip). Internal fixation permits earlier mobilization and can shorten hospitalization, particularly in older adult patients with hip fractures.[1]

Nursing care and management for a patient who undergoes internal fixation involves monitoring neurovascular status, administering medications, managing the patient's pain, preventing infection, and assisting with ambulation and exercises.

Equipment

Vital signs monitoring equipment ▪ ice bag ▪ compression sleeves or foot covers ▪ sequential compression device or arterial-venous impulse foot compression controller ▪ prescribed IV fluids ▪ preoperative checklist ▪ prescribed antibiotics ▪ disinfectant pad ▪ plain or antimicrobial soap, or other skin preparation product ▪ towel ▪ washcloth ▪ Optional: IV catheter insertion kit, disposable-head clippers, prescribed thrombolytic prophylactic medication, prescribed stool softener, prescribed beta-adrenergic blocker, labels, patient-controlled analgesia (PCA) pump, sedation scale, overhead frame with trapeze, pillow, crutches, walker, padded splint, capnography equipment, pressure-relief mattress, prescribed blood products.

Preparation of equipment

Inspect all equipment and supplies. If a product is expired, is defective, or has compromised integrity, remove it from patient use, label it as expired or defective, and report the expiration or defect as directed by your facility.

Implementation

Preoperative care

▪ Review the patient's medical record for relevant information, such past medical and surgical history (including postoperative nausea and vomiting), allergies (including latex), sensitivities, medication use, disabilities, substance use or abuse, physical and mental impairments, mobility limitations, external or implanted medical devices, home use of noninvasive positive-pressure ventilation, sensory limitations, and risk factors for developing postoperative delirium (for older adult patients).[2,3]

▪ Verify that laboratory and imaging studies have been completed, as ordered, and that the results are in the patient's medical record. Notify the practitioner of unexpected results.[4,5]

▪ Confirm that the practitioner has obtained written informed consent and that the signed consent form is in the patient's medical record.[6,7,8,9]

▪ Conduct a preprocedure verification *to make sure that all relevant documentation and related information or equipment are available and correctly identified to the patient's identifiers.*[4,10]

▪ Verify the practitioner's orders.

▪ Perform hand hygiene.[11,12,13,14,15,16]

▪ Confirm the patient's identity using at least two patient identifiers.[17]

▪ Provide privacy.[18,19,20,21]

▪ Obtain the patient's vital signs and oxygen saturation level *to serve as a baseline for comparison.*

▪ Assess the patient's cardiac, neurologic, and respiratory status *to serve as baselines for comparison.*

▪ Assess the neurovascular status of the affected extremity, if appropriate, and compare your results with findings in the unaffected extremity *to promptly detect signs of neurovascular compromise.*[22]

▪ Immobilize and elevate the affected extremity, if appropriate, *to reduce associated discomfort, promote venous return, and reduce swelling.* Support the extremity adequately when moving or elevating it.[22]

▪ Apply ice to the affected site, if needed and prescribed, *to promote comfort and to reduce swelling.*[22]

▪ Assess and address the patient's safety, emotional, and psychological needs.[2]

▪ Begin a preoperative checklist, such as the World Health Organization's Surgical Safety Checklist.[23]

▪ Reinforce the practitioner's explanation of the procedure and answer the patient's questions.

▪ Screen and assess the patient's pain using facility-defined criteria that are consistent with the patient's age, condition, and ability to understand.[2,24]

▪ Treat the patient's pain, as needed and ordered, using nonpharmacologic, pharmacologic, or a combination of approaches. Base the treatment plan on evidence-based practices and the patient's clinical condition, past medical history, and pain management goals.[24]

▪ Teach the patient what to expect during postoperative assessment, monitoring, and care.

▪ Teach the patient how to cough and deep breathe *to reduce the risk of postprocedure pneumonia.*[25]

▪ Prepare the patient for proposed exercise and progressive ambulation regimens if necessary.

▪ Encourage the patient to perform active range-of-motion (ROM) exercises of the uninvolved joints, unless contraindicated.[22]

▪ Confirm the patient's nothing by mouth status before the procedure. If not an emergency, minimum fasting recommendations include 2 hours for clear liquids, 6 or more hours for a light meal or nonhuman milk, and 8 hours or more for fried or fatty foods or meat.[26]

EQUIPMENT

Reviewing internal fixation devices

Hip pin
In trochanteric or subtrochanteric fractures, the surgeon may use a hip pin or nail, with or without a screw plate for internal fixation. A pin or plate with extra nails stabilizes the fracture by impacting the bone ends at the fracture site.

Intramedullary rod
In an uncomplicated fracture of the femoral shaft, the surgeon may use an intramedullary rod. The surgeon places this device through the bone lengthwise to stabilize the fractured bone ends and permits early ambulation with partial weight bearing.

Screw plate
Another choice for fixation of a long-bone fracture is a screw plate, shown here on the tibia. The surgeon will typically use a screw plate on the lower extremities to provide extra bone stability.

Humeral rod
In an arm fracture, the surgeon may fix the involved bones with a plate, rod, or nail. Most radial and ulnar fractures may be fixed with plates, whereas humeral fractures are commonly fixed with rods.

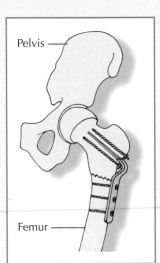

Pelvis

Femur

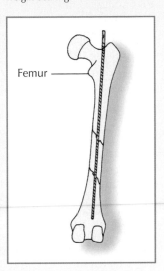

Femur

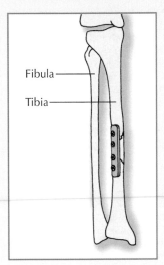

Fibula

Tibia

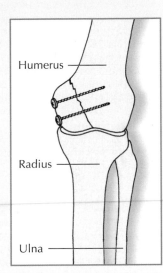

Humerus

Radius

Ulna

■ Confirm that the patient has patent IV access to administer prophylactic antibiotics (commonly administered 1 hour before the incision, or 2 hours before if vancomycin or fluoroquinolones are prescribed), IV fluids, and blood products, as prescribed.[5,27,28] Insert an IV catheter if necessary. (See the "IV catheter insertion and removal" procedure.)[29]

■ Verify the surgical procedure and site with the patient and family, if present.[10,22] If appropriate, make sure the surgical site is marked, as directed by your facility.[10,30]

■ Remove hair at the surgical site only if absolutely necessary. If hair removal is necessary, use disposable-head clippers for hair removal. Don't shave the site, *to reduce the risk of surgical site infection.*[31]

■ Assist the patient with bathing with plain or antimicrobial soap and water or another skin preparation product as ordered *to reduce the risk of surgical site* infection.[27,31]

■ Provide hand-off communication for the person who'll be assuming responsibility for the patient's care. Allow time for questions, as necessary, *to avoid miscommunications that can cause patient care errors during transitions of care.*[32] As part of the hand-off process, allow time for the receiving person to trace each tube and catheter from the patient to its point of origin. Use a standardized line reconciliation process using high-reliability practices.[33,34]

■ Perform hand hygiene.[11,12,13,14,15,16]

■ Clean and disinfect your stethoscope using a disinfectant pad.[35,36]

■ Perform hand hygiene.[11,12,13,14,15,16]

■ Document the procedure.[37,38,39,40]

Postoperative care
■ Receive hand-off communication from the person who was responsible for the patient's care. Ask questions as necessary *to avoid miscommunications that can cause patient care errors during transitions of care.*[32,41] As part of the hand-off process, trace each tube and catheter from the patient to its point of origin; use a standardized line recognition process using high-reliability practices.[33,34]

■ Verify the practitioner's orders.

■ Reconcile the patient's medications at each care transition and when the practitioner prescribes a new medication *to reduce the risk of medication errors, including omissions, duplications, dosing errors, and drug interactions.*[42,43]

■ Perform hand hygiene.[11,12,13,14,15,16]

■ Confirm the patient's identity using at least two patient identifiers.[17]

■ Provide privacy.[18,19,20,21]

■ Obtain the patient's vital signs and oxygen saturation level using pulse oximetry; assess cardiac, neurologic, and respiratory status and compare with baseline findings.

■ Monitor the patient's vital signs at an interval determined by your facility and the patient's condition, *because there's no evidence-based research to indicate the best practice for frequency of vital sign checks.*[2]

■ Assess the patency of the patient's IV catheter; insert a new one if necessary and administer IV fluids as prescribed.

■ If the patient has different IV access sites or several bags of IV fluid hanging, label the distal (near the patient connection) and proximal (near the source container) ends of the tubing.[33]

■ Monitor intake and output and electrolyte levels as ordered *to promptly detect fluid and electrolyte imbalances.* Notify the practitioner promptly if imbalances occur.[44,45]

■ Assess the patient's neurovascular status.[2] Assess color, motion, sensation, digital movement, edema, capillary refill, and pulses of the affected area. Compare your findings with the unaffected side, if appropriate. Ask about the presence of burning, tingling, and numbness in the affected area, *which may indicate impaired circulation.*

■ Apply an ice bag to the operative site, as ordered, *to reduce swelling, relieve pain, and lessen bleeding.*

■ Assess the patient's comfort level, including positioning, temperature, and postoperative nausea and vomiting.[2]

■ Screen for and assess the patient's pain using facility-defined criteria that are consistent with the patient's age, condition, and ability to understand.[2,24]

■ Treat the patient's pain as needed and ordered using nonpharmacologic, pharmacologic, or a combination of approaches. Base the treatment on evidence-based practices and the patient's clinical condition, past medical history, and pain management goals.[24] If administering pain medication, following safe administration practices *to promote comfort*.[44,46,47,48] If the patient is using PCA, instruct the patient to administer a dose before exercising or moving.

■ For a patient receiving IV opioid medication, monitor the patient closely if identified at high risk for adverse outcomes related to opioid treatment.[24] Frequently monitor the patient's respiratory rate, oxygen saturation level by pulse oximetry, end-tidal carbon dioxide level by capnography (if available), and sedation level using a standardized sedation scale *to decrease the risk of adverse events associated with IV opioid use*.[45] Explain the assessment and monitoring process to the patient and family (including that it may be necessary to awaken the patient to assess the effects of the medication). Advise the patient and family to alert a staff member immediately if breathing problems or other changes that might be a reaction to the medication occur.[44,45]

■ Assess the patient's safety needs, including the risk of falling. Implement the appropriate measures *to ensure patient safety*.[2,49,50]

HOSPITAL-ACQUIRED CONDITION ALERT Keep in mind that the Centers for Medicare and Medicaid Services considers an injury from a fall a hospital-acquired condition *because it can be reasonably prevented using best practices*. Be sure to follow evidence-based fall prevention practices, such as performing a fall risk assessment and instituting fall precautions, *to reduce the risk of injury from falls*.[49,51,52]

■ Elevate the affected limb on a pillow, if appropriate, *to minimize edema*.[22]

■ Assess the condition and color of the patient's skin.[2]

■ Monitor the patient's surgical dressings for signs of excessive drainage or bleeding.[2]

■ Assist with and encourage the patient to perform ROM and other muscle-strengthening exercises, as ordered, *to promote circulation, improve muscle tone, and maintain joint function*.

■ *To prevent postprocedure pneumonia*, have the patient cough and deep breathe.[25] Tell the patient that early ambulation and optimal pain management also reduce the risk of postoperative pulmonary complications.[31]

■ If not already in place, apply compression sleeves or a sequential compression device or foot covers and an arterial-venous impulse foot compression controller, as ordered, *to prevent venous thromboembolism (VTE)*.[53] (See the "Sequential compression therapy" procedure.)

■ If necessary, with the assistance of coworkers, position the patient on a pressure-relief mattress *to prevent skin breakdown*.

■ Teach the patient to perform early progressive ambulation and mobilization using an overhead frame with a trapeze, crutches, or a walker and splint, as appropriate.[25] (See the "Crutch use training" procedure.)

■ Continue thromboembolic pharmacologic prophylaxis as ordered by the practitioner *to prevent VTE*. Make sure baseline coagulation studies have been obtained and are documented in the patient's medical record. For the patient receiving warfarin, monitor the International Normalized Ratio.[53]

■ Ensure prophylactic antibiotics are discontinued within 24 hours after surgery.[53]

■ Encourage the patient to consume fluids, as the patient's condition allows, and administer a stool softener as ordered following safe medication administration practices, *because immobility and opioid use can slow colonic activity, causing constipation*.[44,46,47,48,54]

■ If the patient had an indwelling urinary catheter that was inserted for surgery, remove the catheter on postoperative day 1 or 2 (with the day of surgery considered day 0), according to your facility's protocol or the practitioner's order, *to reduce the risk of catheter-associated urinary tract infection*.[53,55] (See the "Indwelling urinary catheter care and removal" procedure.)

■ If the patient was receiving a beta-adrenergic blocker before surgery, collaborate with the practitioner to ensure that the patient receives it during the perioperative period, as appropriate.[3,53]

■ Reassess and respond to the patient's pain by evaluating the response to treatment and progress toward pain management goals. Assess for adverse reactions and risk factors for adverse events that may result from treatment.[2,24]

■ Perform hand hygiene.[11,12,13,14,15,16]

■ Clean and disinfect your stethoscope using a disinfectant pad.[35,36]

■ Perform hand hygiene.[11,12,13,14,15,16]

■ Document the procedure.[37,38,39,40]

Special considerations

■ Administer mupirocin nasal ointment with or without chlorhexidine body wash preoperatively, as ordered, *to prevent* Staphylococcus aureus *infection in nasal carriers*.[31]

■ After removal of the initial postoperative dressing, begin assessing the incision site for signs and symptoms of infection, such as erythema, drainage, edema, and unusual pain.

■ The Joint Commission issued a sentinel event alert related to managing risk during transition to the new International Organization for Standardization tubing standards that were designed to prevent dangerous tubing misconnections, which can lead to serious patient injury and death. During the transition, trace the tubing and catheter from the patient to the point of origin before connecting or reconnecting any device or infusion, at any care transition (such as a new setting or service), and as part of the hand-off process; route tubes and catheters with different purposes in different standardized directions; label the tubing at the distal and proximal ends (when there are different access sites or several bags hanging); use tubing and equipment only as intended; and store medications for different delivery routes in separate locations.[33]

■ The Joint Commission issued a sentinel event alert concerning inadequate hand-off communication *because of the potential for patient harm that can result when a receiver receives inaccurate, incomplete, untimely, misinterpreted, or otherwise inadequate information. To improve hand-off communication*, standardize the critical information communicated by the sender. At a minimum, include the sender contact information; illness assessment; patient summary, including events leading up to the illness or admission, hospital course, ongoing assessment, and care plan; to-do action list; contingency plans; allergy list; code status; medication list; and dated laboratory test results and vital signs. Provide face-to-face communication whenever possible in an interruption-free location using facility-approved, standardized tools and methods (for example, forms, templates, checklists, protocols, and mnemonics). Provide ample time and opportunity for questions, and include the multidisciplinary team members and the patient and family, when appropriate.[56]

Patient teaching

Before discharge, instruct the patient and family how to care for the incisional site, including the importance of proper hand hygiene and how to recognize signs and symptoms of surgical site infection. Also, instruct the patient and family about an exercise regimen (if any) and using assistive ambulation devices (such as crutches or a walker), if appropriate. Teach the patient measures to prevent postoperative pneumonia. Teach the signs and symptoms of VTE and when and how to seek treatment. Also teach the patient about the prescribed anticoagulation regimen.[28]

During discharge planning, teach the patient and family about pain management strategies; include information about the patient's pain management plan and adverse effects of pain management treatment. Discuss activities of daily living, and items in the home environment that might exacerbate pain or reduce the effectiveness of the pain management plan, and include strategies to address these issues. Teach the patient and family about safe use, storage, and disposal of opioids, if prescribed.[24]

Complications

Surgical site infection and, more critically, infection involving metal fixation devices may require reopening the incision, draining the suture line, and possibly removing the fixation device. Any such infection would require wound dressings and antibiotic therapy. Other complications may include malunion, nonunion, fat or pulmonary embolism, neurovascular impairment, compartment syndrome, and chronic pain.[54]

Documentation

Document vital signs, oxygen saturation and sedation levels, and perioperative cardiovascular, respiratory, and neurologic assessment findings. Document neurovascular assessment findings and the use of VTE prevention practices. Note all exercises that the patient performed and their effect, as well as any ambulatory effort or assistive ambulation device that you used. Document postprocedure pneumonia prevention practices that you used, and the patient's response. Record pain assessment findings, pain medications that you administered, the date and time of administration, and the patient's response. Describe wound appearance and alignment of the affected bone. Document teaching that you provided to the patient and family (if applicable), their understanding of that teaching, and any need for follow-up teaching.

REFERENCES

1 Rozell, J. C., et al. (2016). Recent advances in the treatment of hip fractures in the elderly. *F1000Research, 5*, F1000 Faculty Rev-1953. https://www.ncbi.nlm.nih.gov/pmc/articles/PMC4984486/

2 American Society of PeriAnesthesia Nurses. (2019). *2019–2020 Perianesthesia nursing standards, practice recommendations and interpretive statements.* Cherry Hill, NJ: American Society of PeriAnesthesia Nurses. (Level VII)

3 American College of Surgeons. (2012). ACS NSQIP/AGS best practice guidelines: Optimal preoperative assessment of the geriatric surgical patient. https://www.facs.org/~/media/files/quality%20programs/nsqip/acsnsqipagsgeriatric2012guidelines.ashx (Level VII)

4 The Joint Commission. (2021). Standard UP.01.01.01. *Comprehensive accreditation manual for hospitals.* Oakbrook Terrace, IL: The Joint Commission. (Level VII)

5 World Health Organization (WHO). (2009). WHO guidelines for safe surgery 2009: Safe surgery saves lives. https://apps.who.int/iris/bitstream/handle/10665/44185/9789241598552_eng.pdf;jsessionid=824E-842CA465E4F33DF4B8882901A7DC?sequence=1 (Level VII)

6 The Joint Commission. (2021). Standard RI.01.03.01. *Comprehensive accreditation manual for hospitals.* Oakbrook Terrace, IL: The Joint Commission. (Level VII)

7 Centers for Medicare and Medicaid Services, Department of Health and Human Services. (2020). Condition of participation: Patient's rights. 42 C.F.R. § 482.13(b)(2).

8 Accreditation Association for Hospitals and Health Systems. (2020). Standard 30.01.11. *Healthcare Facilities Accreditation Program: Accreditation requirements for acute care hospitals.* Chicago, IL: Accreditation Association for Hospitals and Health Systems. (Level VII)

9 DNV GL-Healthcare USA, Inc. (2020). PR.2.SR.3. *NIAHO® accreditation requirements, interpretive guidelines and surveyor guidance—revision 20.0.* Milford, OH: DNV GL-Healthcare USA, Inc. (Level VII)

10 Accreditation Association for Hospitals and Health Systems. (2020). Standard 30.00.14. *Healthcare Facilities Accreditation Program: Accreditation requirements for acute care hospitals.* Chicago, IL: Accreditation Association for Hospitals and Health Systems. (Level VII)

11 Centers for Disease Control and Prevention. (2002). Guideline for hand hygiene in health-care settings: Recommendations of the Healthcare Infection Control Practices Advisory Committee and the HICPAC/SHEA/APIC/IDSA Hand Hygiene Task Force. *MMWR Recommendations and Reports, 51*(RR-16), 1–45. https://www.cdc.gov/mmwr/pdf/rr/rr5116.pdf (Level II)

12 World Health Organization. (2009). WHO guidelines on hand hygiene in health care: First global patient safety challenge, clean care is safer care. https://apps.who.int/iris/bitstream/handle/10665/44102/9789241597906_eng.pdf?sequence=1 (Level IV)

13 The Joint Commission. (2021). Standard NPSG.07.01.01. *Comprehensive accreditation manual for hospitals.* Oakbrook Terrace, IL: The Joint Commission. (Level VII)

14 Centers for Medicare and Medicaid Services, Department of Health and Human Services. (2020). Condition of participation: Infection control. 42 C.F.R. § 482.42.

15 Accreditation Association for Hospitals and Health Systems. (2020). Standard 07.01.21. *Healthcare Facilities Accreditation Program: Accreditation requirements for acute care hospitals.* Chicago, IL: Accreditation Association for Hospitals and Health Systems. (Level VII)

16 DNV GL-Healthcare USA, Inc. (2020). IC.1.SR.1. *NIAHO® accreditation requirements, interpretive guidelines and surveyor guidance—revision 20.0.* Milford, OH: DNV GL-Healthcare USA, Inc. (Level VII)

17 The Joint Commission. (2021). Standard NPSG.01.01.01. *Comprehensive accreditation manual for hospitals.* Oakbrook Terrace, IL: The Joint Commission. (Level VII)

18 The Joint Commission. (2021). Standard RI.01.01.01. *Comprehensive accreditation manual for hospitals.* Oakbrook Terrace, IL: The Joint Commission. (Level VII)

19 Centers for Medicare and Medicaid Services, Department of Health and Human Services. (2020). Condition of participation: Patient's rights. 42.C.F.R. § 482.13(c)(1).

20 Accreditation Association for Hospitals and Health Systems. (2020). Standard 15.01.16. *Healthcare Facilities Accreditation Program: Accreditation requirements for acute care hospitals.* Chicago, IL: Accreditation Association for Hospitals and Health Systems. (Level VII)

21 DNV GL-Healthcare USA, Inc. (2020). PR.2.SR.5. *NIAHO® accreditation requirements, interpretive guidelines and surveyor guidance—revision 20.0.* Milford, OH: DNV GL-Healthcare USA, Inc. (Level VII)

22 Hinkle, J. L., & Cheever, K. H. (2018). *Brunner and Suddarth's textbook of medical-surgical nursing* (14th ed.). Philadelphia, PA: Wolters Kluwer.

23 World Health Organization. (2009). Surgical safety checklist. https://apps.who.int/iris/bitstream/handle/10665/44186/9789241598590_eng_Checklist.pdf;jsessionid=179D4C5FD5EB597F652FACB48768A462?sequence=2

24 The Joint Commission. (2021). Standard PC.01.02.07. *Comprehensive accreditation manual for hospitals.* Oakbrook Terrace, IL: The Joint Commission. (Level VII)

25 Centers for Disease Control and Prevention. (2004). Guidelines for preventing health-care-associated pneumonia, 2003: Recommendations of CDC and the Healthcare Infection Control Practices Advisory Committee. *MMWR Recommendations and Reports, 53*(RR-3), 1–32. https://www.cdc.gov/mmwr/pdf/rr/rr5303.pdf (Level II)

26 American Society of Anesthesiologists. (2017). Practice guidelines for preoperative fasting and the use of pharmacologic agents to reduce the risk of pulmonary aspiration: Application to healthy patients undergoing elective procedures. *Anesthesiology, 126*(3), 376–393. https://anesthesiology.pubs.asahq.org/article.aspx?articleid=2596245 (Level V)

27 Berríos-Torres, S. I., et al. (2017). Centers for Disease Control and Prevention guideline for the prevention of surgical site infection, 2017. *JAMA Surgery, 152*(8), 784–791. https://jamanetwork.com/journals/jamasurgery/fullarticle/2623725 (Level VII)

28 Anderson, D. J., et al. (2014). SHEA/IDSA practice recommendation. Strategies to prevent surgical site infections in acute care hospitals: 2014 update. *Infection Control and Hospital Epidemiology, 35*(6), 605–627. https://www.jstor.org/stable/10.1086/676022#metadata_info_tab_contents (Level I)

29 The Joint Commission. (2021). Standard NPSG.07.05.01. *Comprehensive accreditation manual for hospitals.* Oakbrook Terrace, IL: The Joint Commission. (Level VII)

30 The Joint Commission. (2021). Standard UP.01.02.01. *Comprehensive accreditation manual for hospitals.* Oakbrook Terrace, IL: The Joint Commission. (Level VII)

31 World Health Organization. (2016). Global guidelines for the prevention of surgical site infection. https://www.who.int/gpsc/global-guidelines-web.pdf (Level VII)

32 The Joint Commission. (2021). Standard PC.02.02.01. *Comprehensive accreditation manual for hospitals.* Oakbrook Terrace, IL: The Joint Commission. (Level VII)

33 The Joint Commission. (2014). Sentinel event alert 53: Managing risk during transition to new ISO tubing connector standards. https://www.jointcommission.org/assets/1/6/SEA_53_Connectors_8_19_14_final.pdf (Level VII)

34 U.S. Food and Drug Administration. (2017). Examples of medical device misconnections. https://www.fda.gov/medical-devices/medical-device-connectors/examples-medical-device-misconnections

35 Rutala, W. A., et al. (2008, revised 2019). Guideline for disinfection and sterilization in healthcare facilities, 2008. https://www.cdc.gov/infection-control/pdf/guidelines/disinfection-guidelines-H.pdf (Level I)

36 Accreditation Association for Hospitals and Health Systems. (2020). Standard 07.02.03. *Healthcare Facilities Accreditation Program: Accreditation requirements for acute care hospitals.* Chicago, IL: Accreditation Association for Hospitals and Health Systems. (Level VII)

37 The Joint Commission. (2021). Standard RC.01.03.01. *Comprehensive accreditation manual for hospitals.* Oakbrook Terrace, IL: The Joint Commission. (Level VII)

38 Centers for Medicare and Medicaid Services, Department of Health and Human Services. (2020). Condition of participation: Medical record services. 42 C.F.R. § 482.24(b).

39 Accreditation Association for Hospitals and Health Systems. (2020). Standard 10.00.03. *Healthcare Facilities Accreditation Program: Accreditation requirements for acute care hospitals.* Chicago, IL: Accreditation Association for Hospitals and Health Systems. (Level VII)

40 DNV GL-Healthcare USA, Inc. (2020). MR.2.SR.1. *NIAHO® accreditation requirements, interpretive guidelines and surveyor guidance—revision 20.0.* Milford, OH: DNV GL-Healthcare USA, Inc. (Level VII)

41 Guideline for perioperative practice: Team communication. (2020). In Wood, A. (Ed.), *Guidelines for perioperative practice,* 2020 edition. Denver, CO: AORN, Inc. (Level VII)

42 Accreditation Association for Hospitals and Health Systems. (2020). Standard 25.02.13. *Healthcare Facilities Accreditation Program: Accreditation requirements for acute care hospitals.* Chicago, IL: Accreditation Association for Hospitals and Health Systems. (Level VII)

43 The Joint Commission. (2021). Standard NPSG.03.06.01. *Comprehensive accreditation manual for hospitals.* Oakbrook Terrace, IL: The Joint Commission. (Level VII)

44 Centers for Medicare and Medicaid Services, Department of Health and Human Services. (2020). Condition of participation: Nursing services. 42 C.F.R. § 482.23(c).

45 Centers for Medicare and Medicaid Services. (2014). Requirements for hospital medication administration, particularly intravenous (IV) medications and post-operative care of patients receiving IV opioids. https://www.cms.gov/Medicare/Provider-Enrollment-and-Certification/SurveyCertificationGenInfo/Downloads/Survey-and-Cert-Letter-14-15.pdf

46 Accreditation Association for Hospitals and Health Systems. (2020). Standard 16.01.03. *Healthcare Facilities Accreditation Program: Accreditation requirements for acute care hospitals.* Chicago, IL: Accreditation Association for Hospitals and Health Systems. (Level VII)

47 The Joint Commission. (2021). Standard MM.06.01.01. *Comprehensive accreditation manual for hospitals.* Oakbrook Terrace, IL: The Joint Commission. (Level VII)

48 DNV GL-Healthcare USA, Inc. (2020). MM.1.SR.3. *NIAHO® accreditation requirements, interpretive guidelines and surveyor guidance—revision 20.0.* Milford, OH: DNV GL-Healthcare USA, Inc. (Level VII)

49 The Joint Commission. (2021). Standard PC.01.02.08. *Comprehensive accreditation manual for hospitals.* Oakbrook Terrace, IL: The Joint Commission. (Level VII)

50 Accreditation Association for Hospitals and Health Systems. (2020). Standard 16.02.02. *Healthcare Facilities Accreditation Program: Accreditation requirements for acute care hospitals.* Chicago, IL: Accreditation Association for Hospitals and Health Systems. (Level VII)

51 Jarrett, N., & Callaham, M. (2016). Evidence-based guidelines for selected hospital-acquired conditions: Final report. https://www.cms.gov/Medicare/Medicare-Fee-for-Service-Payment/HospitalAcqCond/Downloads/2016-HAC-Report.pdf

52 Ganz, D. A., et al. (2013, reviewed 2021). *Preventing falls in hospitals: A toolkit for improving quality of care* (AHRQ Publication No. 13-0015-EF). Rockville, MD: Agency for Healthcare Research and Quality. https://www.ahrq.gov/professionals/systems/hospital/fallpxtoolkit/index.html (Level VII)

53 Centers for Medicare and Medicaid Services & The Joint Commission. (2022). The specifications manual for national hospital inpatient quality measures (version 5.11). https://www.qualitynet.org/inpatient/specifications-manuals#tab1

54 Horn, P. L., et al. (2011). Orthopaedic trauma: Pilon fractures. *Orthopaedic Nursing, 30,* 299–300.

55 Lo, E., et al. (2014). SHEA/IDSA practice recommendation. Strategies to prevent catheter-associated urinary tract infections in acute care hospitals: 2014 update. *Infection Control and Hospital Epidemiology, 35*(5), 464–479. https://www.jstor.org/stable/10.1086/675718#metadata_info_tab_contents (Level I)

56 The Joint Commission. (2017). Sentinel event alert 58: Inadequate hand-off communication. https://www.jointcommission.org/-/media/tjc/documents/resources/patient-safety-topics/sentinel-event/sea_58_hand_off_comms_9_6_17_final_(1).pdf?db=web&hash=5642D-63C1A5017BD214701514DA00139 (Level VII)

INTRA-ABDOMINAL PRESSURE MONITORING

Intra-abdominal pressure (IAP) monitoring measures the pressure in the abdominal compartment. It can be assessed directly with an intraperitoneal catheter or indirectly with a gastric balloon or an indwelling urinary catheter. Because of such potential complications as bowel perforation and peritoneal contamination with direct methods, indirect assessment using urinary bladder pressure measurement is preferred.[1]

Pressure in the abdomen can result from many conditions, including intraperitoneal bleeding, third-spacing following fluid resuscitation, peritonitis, ascites, gaseous bowel distention, abdominal surgery, and trauma. If pressure in the abdominal cavity becomes greater than the pressure in the capillaries that perfuse the abdominal organs, ischemia and infarction may result. Increased IAP can also lead to reduced cardiac output, increased systemic vascular resistance, increased peripheral vascular resistance, reduced venous return, and increased intrathoracic pressure, which limits expansion of the diaphragm, resulting in hypoventilation and hypoxia.[2] By measuring IAP, the nurse can detect a rise in pressure and initiate lifesaving measures.[3]

The urinary catheter should be removed as soon as it's no longer needed, to reduce the risk of catheter-associated urinary tract infection (CAUTI).[4,5]

HOSPITAL-ACQUIRED CONDITION ALERT Keep in mind that the Centers for Medicare and Medicaid Services considers CAUTI a hospital-acquired condition *because it can be reasonably prevented using a variety of best practices.* Make sure to follow evidence-based CAUTI prevention practices—such as performing hand hygiene before and after catheter manipulation; maintaining a sterile, continuously closed drainage system; maintaining unobstructed urine flow; regularly emptying the collection bag; replacing the catheter and collection system using sterile technique when a break in sterile technique, disconnection, or leakage occurs; and discontinuing use of the catheter as soon as it's no longer clinically indicated—when caring for the patient with an indwelling urinary catheter *to reduce the risk of CAUTI.*[4,5,6,7,8,9]

Equipment

Indwelling urinary catheter with drainage collection bag ▪ gloves ▪ monitoring system and equipment (module, bedside monitor, and cable) ▪ IV normal saline solution (500- to 1,000-mL) ▪ commercially prepared IAP monitoring kit, with or without transducer ▪ IV pole ▪ transducer holder ▪ tape ▪ antiseptic pad ▪ leveling device ▪ Optional: preassembled disposable pressure tubing with transducer and flush device, gown, mask and goggles or mask with face shield, sterile drape.

Preparation of equipment

Inspect all equipment and supplies. If a product is expired, is defective, or has compromised integrity, remove it from patient use, label it as expired or defective, and report the expiration or defect as directed by your facility.

Implementation

- Verify the practitioner's order.
- Gather and prepare the necessary equipment and supplies.
- Perform hand hygiene.[10,11,12,13,14,15]
- Confirm the patient's identity using at least two patient identifiers.[16]
- Provide privacy.[17,18,19,20]
- Explain the procedure to the patient and family (if appropriate) according to their communication and learning needs *to increase understanding, allay fears, and enhance cooperation.*[21] Include the purpose of IAP monitoring and the anticipated duration of catheter placement.
- Raise the bed to waist level before providing care *to prevent caregiver back strain.*[22]
- Using sterile technique, insert an indwelling urinary catheter, if the patient doesn't already have one in place. (See the "Indwelling urinary catheter insertion" procedure.) If the patient has one in place, check catheter patency.
- Remove and discard your gloves.[23]
- Perform hand hygiene.[10,11,12,12,13,14]

■ Put on gloves and other personal protective equipment, as needed *to comply with standard precautions.*[23,24,25]

■ Hang the IV bag of normal saline solution on the IV pole next to the patient. Spike the IV bag with commercially prepared IAP monitoring system tubing with integrated transducer. Alternatively, attach the preassembled disposable pressure tubing with transducer and flush device to the IAP monitoring system tubing and spike the saline bag.

For a standard system

■ Mount the urinary drainage tubing on the clamp.[26]

■ Remove the cap from the distal end of the transducer and open the transducer stopcock.[26]

■ Flush the IAP monitor system tubing, transducer, and stopcock with IV normal saline solution *to prime the transducer line and remove all air bubbles.*[26]

■ Close the stopcock, and attach the transducer to the patient or the IV pole at the level of the iliac crest at the midaxillary line.[2,3,27]

■ Attach the cable from the transducer to the monitor, turn on the monitor, and select a 30-mm Hg scale for monitoring IAP.[2]

■ Remove the cap from the valve port, and flush the IAP monitoring system tubing with IV normal saline solution *to prime the valve port and remove all air bubbles.*[26]

■ Trace the tubing from the patient to its point of origin *to make sure you're accessing the correct port.*[28]

■ Thoroughly disinfect the indwelling urinary catheter sampling port with an antiseptic pad, using friction, and allow it to dry, *to reduce the risk of infection.*[5]

■ Using sterile, no-touch technique, attach the end of the valve port to the catheter sampling port.[26]

■ With the patient in the supine position and the head of the bed flat, turn the clamp handle to IAP[26] and zero the transducer to atmosphere at the level of the iliac crest at the midaxillary line *to cancel out the effect of atmospheric pressure.*[2,3,27]

■ If possible, keep the patient in the supine position with the head of the bed flat when obtaining IAP measurements *to prevent the abdominal organs from exerting pressure on the bladder.* If the patient is at risk for ventilator-associated pneumonia, you may need to elevate the head of the bed at least 30 degrees. *Because pressure measurements may differ with varying positions,* use consistent positioning for each measurement *to ensure the readings are comparable.*[2,27,29,30]

■ After zeroing the transducer, make sure that the stopcock to the transducer is open.[26]

■ Turn the clamp handle to DRAIN and allow the bladder to drain.[26]

■ Turn the clamp handle to IAP.[26]

■ Fill the IAP monitoring system syringe with 25 mL of IV normal saline solution, according to the manufacturer's instructions, and instill the normal saline solution into the bladder. *This volume won't overdistend the bladder and produce a false-high reading.*[2]

■ Allow the IAP system to equilibrate after instilling the IV normal saline solution, and then obtain the IAP reading at the end of the patient's expiration with the graphic scale on the monitor display and numeric display of the mean pressure *when the effect of respiratory pressures is minimized.*[2,26] (See *Evaluating intra-abdominal pressure.*)

■ After obtaining the IAP reading, turn the clamp to DRAIN and allow the bladder to drain.[26]

For an automated valved system

■ Prime the IAP monitoring system by flushing IV normal saline through the tubing, transducer, stopcock, and automatic valve following the manufacturer's instructions.[2]

■ Place a sterile drape under the patient's urinary drainage bag connection.[2]

■ Trace the tubing from the patient to its point of origin *to make sure you're accessing the correct port.*[28]

■ Thoroughly disinfect the indwelling urinary catheter connection with an antiseptic pad, using friction, and allow it to dry, *to reduce the risk of infection.*[5]

■ Using sterile, no-touch technique, disconnect the indwelling urinary catheter from the urinary drainage bag, holding each tube upright *to prevent urine from leaking onto the bed.*

Evaluating intra-abdominal pressure

A sustained or repeated intra-abdominal pressure (IAP) reading of 12 mm Hg or higher is considered intra-abdominal hypertension. The severity of intra-abdominal hypertension is graded according to the parameters below.[2,30]

Severity	IAP reading
Average value in critically ill patients	5 to 7 mm Hg[2]
Grade I	12 to 15 mm Hg[2]
Grade II	16 to 20 mm Hg[2]
Grade III	21 to 25 mm Hg[2]
Grade IV	Greater than 25 mm Hg[2]

■ Remove the protective covering on the valve, and attach the indwelling urinary catheter and drainage bag to appropriate locations on the automatic valve.

■ Attach the transducer to the patient or the IV pole at the level of the iliac crest at the midaxillary line.[2]

■ Attach the cable from the transducer to the monitor, turn on the monitor, and select a 30-mm Hg scale for monitoring pressure.[2]

■ Turn the stopcock off to the patient and zero the transducer at the iliac crest at the midaxillary line.[2]

■ After zeroing the transducer, turn the stopcock back to its original position facing the dead-end cap and open to the patient.[2]

■ Fill the IAP monitoring system syringe with 20 mL of IV normal saline solution, according to the manufacturer's instructions. Instill the saline solution into the bladder within 10 seconds, causing the valve to inflate, then close the connection between the indwelling urinary catheter and urinary drainage tubing.[2]

■ Allow the IAP system to equilibrate after instilling the saline solution, and then obtain the IAP reading at the end of the patient's expiration with the graphic scale on the monitor display and numeric display of the mean pressure *when the effect of respiratory pressures is minimized.*[2] Depending on the device, wait 1 to 3 minutes and the valve will automatically open, allowing the bladder to drain normally.[2]

Completing the procedure

■ Measure urine output, making sure to subtract the volume of instilled IV normal saline solution *to maintain accurate intake and output.*[2]

■ Tape the connections securely, if necessary.

■ Discard used supplies in appropriate receptacles.[23]

■ Return the bed to the lowest positions *to prevent falls and maintain patient safety.*[31]

■ Remove and discard your gloves and any other personal protective equipment worn.[23,25]

■ Perform hand hygiene.[10,11,12,12,13,14]

■ Document the procedure.[32,33,34,35]

Special considerations

■ The Joint Commission issued a sentinel event alert related to managing risk during transition to new International Organization for Standardization tubing standards that were designed to prevent dangerous tubing misconnections, which can lead to serious patient injury and death. During the transition, make sure to trace each tubing and catheter from the patient to its point of origin before connecting or reconnecting any device or infusion, at any care transition (such as to a new setting or service), and as part of the hand-off process; route tubes and catheters having different purposes in different, standardized directions; when the patient has different access sites or several bags hanging, label tubing at both the distal and proximal ends; use tubing and equipment only as intended; and store medications for different delivery routes in separate locations.[36]

■ Monitor IAP at least every 4 hours or as clinically indicated.[2] Report an increasing IAP to the practitioner. *An IAP of 12 mm Hg or greater signals intra-abdominal hypertension; an IAP above 20 mm Hg indicates abdominal compartment syndrome, which may lead to multiple organ dysfunction syndrome; decompression surgery may be needed.*[2,30]

■ IAP typically displayed on the cardiac monitor is a mean pressure that reflects the pressure during both inspiration and expiration. If noticeable differences exist in the IAP reading during inspiration and expiration, consider obtaining a more precise end-expiration IAP reading by using a printed waveform strip or the graphic scale on the cardiac monitor.[2]

■ Assess patients at risk for intra-abdominal hypertension for signs and symptoms of reduced organ perfusion, including decreased or absent urine output, increased serum creatinine levels, hypotension, reduced cardiac output, increased central venous and pulmonary artery pressures, increased intracranial pressure, increased serum lactate level, increased peak airway pressure, decreased tidal volume, hypoxemia, hypercapnia, and impaired peripheral circulation.[2,30]

■ IAP readings may not be accurate in a patient with intraperitoneal adhesions, pelvic hematomas, pelvic fractures, abdominal packs, or a neurogenic bladder, *because accurate IAP measurement requires free movement of the bladder wall.* Chronically increased IAP due to morbid obesity, pregnancy, or ascites can also complicate accurate measurement.[30]

■ Mechanical ventilation increases intrathoracic pressure, causing a direct influence on IAP as the increased pressure is transmitted across the patient's abdomen. Carefully monitor IAP in critically ill patients on mechanical ventilation, even if such patients have no other apparent risk factors for increased IAP.

■ Replace the IPA monitoring system tubing whenever you replace the urinary catheter or urinary drainage tubing.[26]

Complications

Maintaining an indwelling urinary catheter and assessing the closed system for pressure monitoring increases the risk of CAUTI.[8]

Documentation

Record the date and time and the result of the IAP reading. (Frequent IAP readings can be recorded on a frequent parameter assessment sheet.) Document whether the system was leveled and zeroed and the patient's position during the reading. Record the amount of IV normal saline solution instilled. Document the practitioner notified of an abnormal reading, any orders received, interventions performed, and the patient's response to those interventions.

Record any vital signs and other findings from assessments performed at the time of the IAP reading. Record urine output, making sure to subtract the amount of instilled normal saline solution. Document any indwelling urinary catheter care performed. If a printed waveform strip is available, label it INTRA-ABDOMINAL PRESSURE; write the date, the time, and the patient's name on the strip; and place it in the patient's medical record.

Note the patient's tolerance of the procedure. Document teaching provided to the patient and family (if applicable), their understanding of that teaching, and any need for follow-up teaching.

REFERENCES

1 Lee, R. K. (2012). Intra-abdominal hypertension and abdominal compartment syndrome: A comprehensive overview. *Critical Care Nurse, 32*(1), 19–31. https://aacnjournals.org/ccnonline/article-abstract/32/1/19/4487/Intra-abdominal-Hypertension-and-Abdominal?redirectedFrom=fulltext

2 Wiegand, D. L. (2017). *AACN procedure manual for high acuity, progressive, and critical care* (7th ed.). St. Louis, MO: Elsevier.

3 Malbrain, M. L., et al. (2006). Results from the International Conference of Experts on Intra-abdominal Hypertension and Abdominal Compartment Syndrome. I. Definitions. *Intensive Care Medicine, 32,* 1722–1732. (Level VII)

4 The Joint Commission. (2021). Standard NPSG.07.06.01. *Comprehensive accreditation manual for hospitals.* Oakbrook Terrace, IL: The Joint Commission. (Level VII)

5 Lo, E., et al. (2014). SHEA/IDSA practice recommendation. Strategies to prevent catheter-associated urinary tract infections in acute care hospitals: 2014 update. *Infection Control and Hospital Epidemiology, 35,* 464–479. https://www.jstor.org/stable/10.1086/675718#metadata_info_tab_contents (Level I)

6 Jarrett, N., & Callaham, M. (2016). Evidence-based guidelines for selected hospital-acquired conditions: Final report. https://www.cms.gov/Medicare/Medicare-Fee-for-Service-Payment/HospitalAcqCond/Downloads/2016-HAC-Report.pdf

7 Agency for Healthcare Research and Quality & U.S. Department of Health and Human Services. (2015). Toolkit for reducing catheter-associated urinary tract infections in hospital units: Implementation guide. https://www.ahrq.gov/professionals/quality-patient-safety/hais/cauti-tools/impl-guide/index.html

8 Association of Professionals in Infection Control and Epidemiology (APIC). (2014). APIC implementation guide: Guide to preventing catheter-associated urinary tract infections. https://apic.org/wp-content/uploads/2019/02/APIC_CAUTI_IG_FIN_REVD0815.pdf (Level IV)

9 Healthcare Infection Control Practices Advisory Committee. (2010, revised 2019). Guideline for prevention of catheter-associated urinary tract infections 2009. https://www.cdc.gov/infectioncontrol/pdf/guidelines/cauti-guidelines-H.pdf (Level I)

10 The Joint Commission. (2021). Standard NPSG.07.01.01. *Comprehensive accreditation manual for hospitals.* Oakbrook Terrace, IL: The Joint Commission. (Level VII)

11 World Health Organization. (2009). WHO guidelines on hand hygiene in health care: First global patient safety challenge, clean care is safer care. https://apps.who.int/iris/bitstream/handle/10665/44102/9789241597906_eng.pdf?sequence=1 (Level IV)

12 Accreditation Association for Hospitals and Health Systems. (2020). Standard 07.01.21. *Healthcare Facilities Accreditation Program: Accreditation requirements for acute care hospitals.* Chicago, IL: Accreditation Association for Hospitals and Health Systems. (Level VII)

13 Centers for Medicare and Medicaid Services, Department of Health and Human Services. (2020). Condition of participation: Infection control. 42 C.F.R. § 482.42.

14 Centers for Disease Control and Prevention. (2002). Guideline for hand hygiene in health-care settings: Recommendations of the Healthcare Infection Control Practices Advisory Committee and the HICPAC/SHEA/APIC/IDSA Hand Hygiene Task Force. *MMWR Recommendations and Reports, 51*(RR-16), 1–45. https://www.cdc.gov/mmwr/pdf/rr/rr5116.pdf (Level II)

15 DNV GL-Healthcare USA, Inc. (2020). IC.1.SR.1. *NIAHO® accreditation requirements, interpretive guidelines and surveyor guidance—revision 20.0.* Milford, OH: DNV GL-Healthcare USA, Inc. (Level VII)

16 The Joint Commission. (2021). Standard NPSG.01.01.01. *Comprehensive accreditation manual for hospitals.* Oakbrook Terrace, IL: The Joint Commission. (Level VII)

17 The Joint Commission. (2021). Standard RI.01.01.01. *Comprehensive accreditation manual for hospitals.* Oakbrook Terrace, IL: The Joint Commission. (Level VII)

18 Centers for Medicare and Medicaid Services, Department of Health and Human Services. (2020). Condition of participation: Patient's rights. 42 C.F.R. § 482.13(c)(1).

19 Accreditation Association for Hospitals and Health Systems. (2020). Standard 15.01.16. *Healthcare Facilities Accreditation Program: Accreditation requirements for acute care hospitals.* Chicago, IL: Accreditation Association for Hospitals and Health Systems. (Level VII)

20 DNV GL-Healthcare USA, Inc. (2020). PR.2.SR.5. *NIAHO® accreditation requirements, interpretive guidelines and surveyor guidance—revision 20.0.* Milford, OH: DNV GL-Healthcare USA, Inc. (Level VII)

21 The Joint Commission. (2021). Standard PC.02.01.21. *Comprehensive accreditation manual for hospitals.* Oakbrook Terrace, IL: The Joint Commission. (Level VII)

22 Waters, T. R., et al. (2009). Safe patient handling training for schools of nursing. https://www.cdc.gov/niosh/docs/2009-127/pdfs/2009-127.pdf (Level VII)

23 Occupational Safety and Health Administration. (2012). Bloodborne pathogens, standard number 1910.1030. https://www.osha.gov/pls/oshaweb/owadisp.show_document?p_id=10051&p_table=STANDARDS (Level VII)

24 Siegel, J. D., et al. (2007, revised 2019). 2007 guideline for isolation precautions: Preventing transmission of infectious agents in healthcare settings. https://www.cdc.gov/infectioncontrol/pdf/guidelines/isolation-guidelines-H.pdf (Level II)

25 Accreditation Association for Hospitals and Health Systems. (2020). Standard 07.01.10. *Healthcare Facilities Accreditation Program: Accreditation requirements for acute care hospitals.* Chicago, IL: Accreditation Association for Hospitals and Health Systems. (Level VII)

26 C. R. Bard, Inc. (2017). Intra-abdominal pressure monitoring device: Instructions for use. https://www.crbard.com/CRBard/media/ProductAssets/BardMedicalDivision/PF10351/en-US/PF10351_BAW7645966.pdf

27 Soler Morejon, C., et al. (2012). Effects of zero reference position on bladder pressure measurements: An observational study. *Annals of Intensive Care, 2*(Suppl. 1), S13. https://www.ncbi.nlm.nih.gov/pmc/articles/PMC3390299/ (Level VI)

28 U.S. Food and Drug Administration. (2017). Examples of medical device misconnections. https://www.fda.gov/medical-devices/medical-device-connectors/examples-of-medical-device-misconnections

29 Yi, M., et al. (2012). The evaluation of the effect of body positioning on intra-abdominal pressure measurement and the effect of intra-abdominal pressure at different body positioning on organ function and prognosis in critically ill patients. *Journal of Critical Care, 27*, 222.e1–222.e6. (Level IV)

30 Gestring, M. (2021). Abdominal compartment syndrome in adults. In: *UpToDate*, Cochran, A., & Bulger, E. B. (Eds.).

31 Ganz, D. A., et al. (2013, reviewed 2021). *Preventing falls in hospitals: A toolkit for improving quality of care* (AHRQ Publication No. 13-0015-EF). Rockville, MD: Agency for Healthcare Research and Quality. https://www.ahrq.gov/professionals/systems/hospital/fallpxtoolkit/index.html (Level VII)

32 The Joint Commission. (2021). Standard RC.01.03.01. *Comprehensive accreditation manual for hospitals*. Oakbrook Terrace, IL: The Joint Commission. (Level VII)

33 Accreditation Association for Hospitals and Health Systems. (2020). Standard 10.00.03. *Healthcare Facilities Accreditation Program: Accreditation requirements for acute care hospitals*. Chicago, IL: Accreditation Association for Hospitals and Health Systems. (Level VII)

34 Centers for Medicare and Medicaid Services, Department of Health and Human Services. (2020). Condition of participation: Medical record services. 42 C.F.R. § 482.24(b).

35 DNV GL-Healthcare USA, Inc. (2020). MR.2.SR.1. *NIAHO® accreditation requirements, interpretive guidelines and surveyor guidance—revision 20.0*. Milford, OH: DNV GL-Healthcare USA, Inc. (Level VII)

36 The Joint Commission. (2014). Sentinel event alert 53: Managing risk during transition to new ISO tubing connector standards. https://www.jointcommission.org/assets/1/6/SEA_53_Connectors_8_19_14_final.pdf (Level VII)

INTRA-AORTIC BALLOON COUNTERPULSATION

Providing temporary support for the heart's left ventricle, intra-aortic balloon counterpulsation (IABC) mechanically displaces blood within the aorta by means of an intra-aortic balloon (IAB) attached to an external pump console, referred to as an *intra-aortic balloon pump* (IABP). The balloon is usually inserted through the common femoral artery and positioned with its tip just distal to the left subclavian artery. It's made of polyethylene and is inflated with gas driven by the pump. Helium is commonly used because its low density facilitates rapid transfer of gas from the console to the balloon. It's also easily absorbed into the bloodstream if the balloon ruptures.[1]

When used correctly, IABC improves two key aspects of myocardial physiology: It increases the supply of oxygen-rich blood to the myocardium, and it decreases myocardial oxygen demand and consumption. Several physiologic and nonphysiologic factors can affect IABC efficacy, including the patient's cardiac function, hemodynamic conditions, the position and size of the balloon catheter used, and signal quality.[2]

IABC is indicated for patients with a wide range of low-cardiac-output disorders or cardiac instability. (See *Indications and contraindications for IABC*). Perioperatively, the technique is used to support and stabilize patients with a suspected high-grade lesion who are undergoing such procedures as angioplasty, thrombolytic therapy, cardiac surgery, and cardiac catheterization. Available evidence no longer supports routine use in patients with acute myocardial infarction complicated by cardiogenic shock who are receiving early revascularization.[3,4]

Indications and contraindications for IABC

Various indications and contraindications exist for intra-aortic balloon counterpulsation (IABC).

Indications[1]
- Acute myocardial infarction
- Refractory left ventricular failure
- Cardiogenic shock
- Refractory ventricular arrhythmias
- Acute mitral regurgitation and ventricular septal defect
- Cardiomyopathies
- Sepsis
- Refractory unstable angina
- Complex cardiac anomalies (in infants and children)
- Cardiac surgery
- Cardiac catheterization and angioplasty
- Weaning from cardiopulmonary bypass

Contraindications[5]
- Aortic regurgitation
- Aortic dissection
- Uncontrolled sepsis
- Uncontrolled bleeding disorder
- Severe peripheral artery disease
- Clinically significant abdominal aortic aneurysm

Equipment
For assisting with insertion
IAB console, cables, and appropriate-sized balloon catheters ■ IAB catheter insertion kit ■ 30-mL Luer-lock syringe ■ 10-mL sterile syringes of prefilled flush solution ■ helium gas source ■ electrocardiogram (ECG) monitor and electrodes ■ pulse oximeter and probe ■ automated blood pressure cuff ■ temperature probe ■ prescribed sedative or analgesic ■ transducer system ■ prepared bag of prescribed flush solution ■ antiseptic solution (chlorhexidine-based preferred)[6] ■ sterile drape ■ sterile gloves ■ sterile occlusive dressing ■ sterile gown ■ mask with face shield or mask and goggles ■ caps ■ sutures or other stabilization device ■ suction equipment ■ oxygen administration equipment ■ emergency equipment (code cart with emergency medications, defibrillator, handheld resuscitation bag with mask, intubation equipment) ■ temporary pacemaker equipment ■ insertion checklist[6] ■ catheter extender ■ level ■ labels ■ Optional: single-patient-use scissors or disposable-head surgical clippers, fluoroscope, backup helium supply, central venous access catheter insertion equipment, arterial catheter insertion equipment, pulmonary artery (PA) catheter insertion equipment, IV insertion and administration equipment, indwelling urinary catheter insertion equipment, arterial blood gas kit, blood sampling equipment, prescribed heparin bolus, Dacron graft (for a surgically inserted balloon), 18G angiography needle, lubrication, tubing labels.

For maintaining IABC
IABC console and balloon catheters ■ ECG monitor and electrodes ■ transducer system ■ IV flush solution ■ vital signs monitoring equipment ■ pulse oximeter and probe ■ disinfectant pad ■ oxygen administration equipment ■ emergency equipment (code cart with emergency medications, defibrillator, handheld resuscitation bag with mask, intubation equipment) ■ arterial blood gas (ABG) kits ■ equipment for obtaining laboratory samples (blood collection tubes, labels, laboratory request forms [if required], laboratory biohazard transport bag, antiseptic pads) ■ suction equipment ■ temporary pacemaker equipment ■ gloves ■ prescribed vasoactive medications ■ Optional: prescribed pain medications, mechanical ventilatory support equipment, pressure-relieving surfaces and devices.

For assisting with removal

Sterile pressure dressing materials ▪ gloves ▪ fluid-impermeable pad ▪ suture removal kit ▪ vital signs monitoring equipment ▪ Optional: protamine sulfate (as prescribed), mechanical compression device, personal protective equipment (gown, mask and goggles, or mask and face shield).

Preparation of equipment

Inspect all equipment and supplies. If a product is expired, is defective, or has compromised integrity, remove it from patient use, label it as expired or defective, and report the expiration or defect as directed by your facility.

Prepare and prime the transducer system. (See the "Transducer system setup" procedure.)

As determined by your facility, you or a perfusionist must zero and balance the pressure transducer in the IABP and calibrate the oscilloscope monitor *to ensure accuracy.* Refer to the manufacturer's instructions.

Plug the balloon pump console into a nearby power outlet and turn it on. Open the helium tank and verify that an adequate helium supply is available. Set up the IABP according to the manufacturer's instructions.

Make sure that the emergency equipment, suction setup, and temporary pacemaker setup are readily available *in case the patient develops complication (such as an arrhythmia) during insertion.*

Implementation

▪ Verify the practitioner's order.
▪ Gather and prepare the necessary equipment and supplies.
▪ Confirm that informed consent has been obtained and that the signed consent form is in the patient's medical record.[7,8,9,10]
▪ Conduct a preprocedure verification *to make sure that all relevant documentation, related information, and equipment are available and correctly identified to the patient's identifiers.*[11,12]
▪ Verify that a complete blood count, coagulation studies, and other ordered studies have been completed as ordered *to check for conditions that may increase the risk of bleeding.* Ensure that the results are in the patient's medical record.[13] Notify the practitioner of unexpected results.[14]
▪ Perform hand hygiene.[15,16,17,18,19,20]
▪ Confirm the patient's identity using at least two patient identifiers.[21]

For assisting with insertion

▪ Reinforce the practitioner's explanation of the procedure for the patient and family (if appropriate) according to their individual communication and learning needs *to increase their understanding, allay their fears, and enhance cooperation.*[7,8,9,10] Explain that the practitioner will insert a special balloon catheter into the aorta, *which increases oxygen supply to the heart, decreases the heart's workload, and increases cardiac output and perfusion of vital organs.* Briefly explain the insertion procedure, and mention that the catheter will be connected to a console next to the bed. Explain that the affected extremity will be immobilized and that the head of the bed will be no higher than 45 degrees while the catheter is in place.[13] Tell the patient that the balloon will be removed after the heart can resume an adequate workload. (See *How the intra-aortic balloon pump works.*)
▪ Provide privacy.[22,23,24,25]
▪ Raise the bed to waist level before providing patient care *to prevent caregiver back strain.*[26]
▪ Perform hand hygiene.[15,16,17,18,19,20]
▪ Make sure the patient has adequate IV access via a peripheral IV catheter or central venous access device, as prescribed, *for administering prescribed fluids and medications, as needed.*
▪ If indicated, ordered, and not already in place, assist with insertion of hemodynamic monitoring devices, such as an arterial catheter or PA catheter.
▪ Insert an indwelling urinary catheter, if ordered, *to assess fluid balance and renal function.*
▪ Connect all monitoring equipment, including the cardiac monitor, pulse oximeter, automated blood pressure cuff, temperature probe, and hemodynamic monitoring devices, as needed. Set alarm limits appropriately for the patient's current condition, and make sure alarms are turned on, functioning properly, and audible to staff.[27,28,29,30]
▪ Apply chest electrodes based on the desired trigger mode. *A trigger is the signal the IABP uses to identify the beginning of the next cardiac cycle; the R wave of the ECG is the preferred trigger source for identifying the cardiac cycle.*[13] Select the desired ECG source from the waveform selector in the IABP controls. Obtain a baseline ECG.
▪ Attach another set of ECG electrodes to the patient, unless the ECG pattern is being transmitted from the patient's bedside monitor to the IAPB through another cable, known as a slaving cable.

EQUIPMENT

How the intra-aortic balloon pump works

Made of polyurethane, the intra-aortic balloon is attached to an external pump console by means of a large-lumen catheter. These illustrations show the direction of blood flow when the pump inflates and deflates the balloon.

Balloon inflation

The balloon inflates as the aortic valve closes and diastole begins. The balloon inflation displaces blood superiorly, which in turn augments coronary artery blood flow.

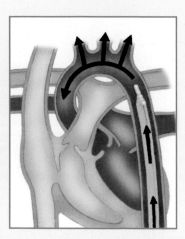

Balloon deflation

The balloon deflates before ventricular ejection, when the aortic valve opens. This deflation permits ejection of blood from the left ventricle against a lowered resistance. As a result, aortic end-diastolic pressure and afterload decrease and cardiac output rises.

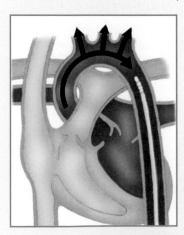

- Obtain the patient's baseline vital signs and oxygen saturation by pulse oximetry *for baseline comparison.*
- Administer supplemental oxygen as ordered and as necessary.
- Remove excess hair from the intended insertion site, if needed, using a single-patient-use scissors or disposable-head surgical clippers, *to facilitate dressing application.*[31]
- Assess and record the patient's peripheral leg pulses and document sensation, movement, color, and temperature of the legs *to help determine peripheral circulation status and the best insertion site.*
- Administer a sedative or an analgesic, as ordered, following safe medication administration practices.[32,33,34,35]
- Position the patient supine with access to the insertion site.
- Perform hand hygiene.[15,16,17,18,19,20]
- Prepare the sterile field.[6,36,37]
- Place the catheter, insertion kit, and other supplies on the sterile field as indicated.[37]
- Make sure that all medications on and off the sterile field are labeled, *to prevent medication administration errors.*[38,39]
- Put on a cap, a mask with a face shield or a mask and goggles, a sterile gown, and sterile gloves *to comply with maximal barrier precautions.*[6,13,36,37]
- The practitioner puts on a cap, a mask with a face shield or a mask and goggles, performs hand hygiene, and then puts on a sterile gown and sterile gloves. The practitioner then cleans the site with chlorhexidine-based antiseptic solution and drapes the patient using a sterile drape while observing maximal barrier precautions.[6,36,37]
- Conduct a time-out immediately before starting the procedure *to determine that the correct patient, site, positioning, and procedure are identified, and confirm, as applicable, that relevant information and necessary equipment are available.*[12,40]
- *To reduce the risk of thromboemboli related to catheter insertion,* administer a heparin bolus, if prescribed, following safe medication administration practices.[13,32,33,34]

NURSING ALERT Heparin is a high-alert medication *because it can cause significant patient harm when used in error.*[41] If required by your facility, have another nurse perform an independent double-check before administering heparin *to verify the patient's identity and to ensure that the correct medication is in the prescribed concentration or strength, the medication's indication corresponds with the patient's diagnosis, the dosage calculations are correct and the dosing formula used to derive the final dose is correct, the prescribed route of administration is safe and proper for the patient, the prescribed time and frequency of administration are safe and proper for the patient, and, if an infusion, the pump settings are correct and the infusion line is attached to the correct port.*[42]

- If required by your facility, after comparing results of the independent double-check with the other nurse, administer the medication if there are no discrepancies. If discrepancies exist, rectify them before beginning administration of the medication.[42]
- During the procedure, make sure the health care team follows infection prevention practices; use an insertion checklist to guide the insertion process *to reduce the risk of infection.*[6,37]
- Attach the 30-mL syringe with one-way valve to the distal end of the balloon lumen.
- Pull back on the syringe until all air is aspirated, and then disconnect the syringe while keeping the valve in place, *creating a vacuum.*[13]
- Lubricate the IAB catheter according to the manufacturer's instructions, as needed.[13]
- Flush the inner lumen of the IAB catheter before insertion according to the manufacturer's instructions.
- Assist the practitioner with insertion of the IAB, as appropriate.

Inserting the intra-aortic balloon percutaneously
- The practitioner may insert the balloon percutaneously into the femoral artery using Seldinger technique.[13]
- First, the practitioner accesses the vessel with an 18G angiography needle and removes the inner stylet.
- Next, the practitioner passes the guidewire through the needle and removes the needle.

- After advancing a vessel dilator over the guidewire into the vessel, the practitioner removes the vessel dilator, leaving the guidewire in place.
- Next, the practitioner passes an introducer (dilator and sheath assembly) over the guidewire into the vessel until about 1″ (2.5 cm) remains above the insertion site. The practitioner then removes the inner dilator, leaving the introducer sheath and guidewire in place.
- After passing the balloon over the guidewire into the introducer sheath, the practitioner advances the catheter into position, ⅜″ to ¾″ (1 to 2 cm) distal to the left subclavian artery, under fluoroscopic guidance.
- The practitioner secures the IAB catheter to the patient's leg using sutures or another stabilization device, as indicated.
- Apply a sterile occlusive dressing over the insertion site.

Inserting the intra-aortic balloon surgically
- If unable to insert the catheter percutaneously, the practitioner may insert it surgically using a femoral artery or subclavian artery approach. (See *Surgical insertion sites for the intra-aortic balloon.*)

Surgical insertion sites for the intra-aortic balloon

If an intra-aortic balloon can't be inserted percutaneously, the practitioner will insert it surgically, using a femoral or transthoracic approach.

Femoral artery approach
Insertion through the femoral artery requires a cutdown and an arteriotomy. The practitioner passes the balloon through a Dacron graft that has been sewn to the artery.

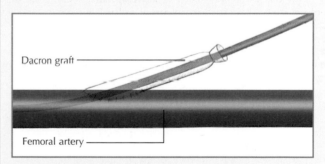

Dacron graft

Femoral artery

Subclavian artery approach
Although traditionally inserted in the femoral artery, the balloon can be inserted through the subclavian artery, which gives the patient more mobility than the femoral site.[43] For this approach, the practitioner inserts the balloon in an antegrade direction through the subclavian artery and then positions it in the descending thoracic aorta.

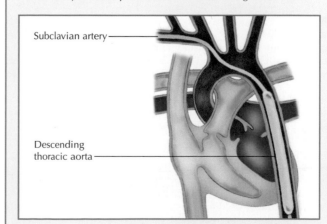

Subclavian artery

Descending thoracic aorta

Connecting the catheter to the IABP

■ The practitioner removes the one-way valve from the IAB catheter and connects the IAB catheter to a catheter extender. The practitioner or nurse then connects the catheter extender to the pneumatic module of the IABP.

■ Assist the practitioner, or connect the previously prepared and zeroed transducer system to the aortic arterial line lumen (inner lumen) of the IAB catheter. Verify blood return, gently flush the lumen using the flush device, and then level the transducer with the patient's midaxillary line and zero it *to ensure accuracy.*

■ Trace all connections from the patient to their point of origin *to make sure that they're connected to the proper ports, and to make sure that all connections are tight and secure to prevent disconnections.*[44,45]

■ Route tubing using a standardized approach if the patient has other tubing and catheters that have different purposes. Label the tubing at the distal (near the patient connection) and proximal (near the source container) ends *to reduce the risk of misconnection if you're using multiple IV lines.*[45]

■ Obtain a portable chest X-ray, as ordered, *to confirm IAB catheter placement.* Place the IABP on standby, as indicated, *for clearer visualization.*[13]

■ Initiate counterpulsation therapy, as ordered, following the manufacturer's instructions.

■ Monitor the patient's vital signs, hemodynamic parameters, and clinical status at a frequency determined by your facility and the patient's condition.[46]

Completing the procedure

■ Return the bed to the lowest position *to prevent falls and maintain patient safety.*[47]

■ Discard used supplies appropriately.[48]

■ Remove and discard your personal protective equipment.[48]

■ Perform hand hygiene.[15,16,17,18,19,20]

■ Document the procedure.[49,50,51,52]

For maintaining IABC

■ Perform hand hygiene.[15,16,17,18,19,20]

■ Put on gloves, as needed, throughout the procedure *to follow standard precautions.*[6,13,36,37]

■ Verify that the pump settings coincide with the practitioner's order.

■ Ensure that alarm limits are set appropriately for the patient's current condition, and that alarms are turned on, functioning properly, and audible to staff.[27,28,30]

■ Assess the timing of IABC with an arterial waveform *to ensure that the balloon inflation and deflation are accurately timed with the cardiac cycle.* (See *Interpreting intra-aortic balloon waveforms.*)

■ Maintain accurate IABP timing according to waveform interpretation; *proper IABP inflation and deflation balance oxygen supply and demand, reducing the risk of further ischemia and compromised contractility.*[2]

■ Monitor functioning of the IABP console, nothing mode, trigger, frequency, and alarm status with each timing assessment *to make sure that it's functioning properly.*

NURSING ALERT If the pump console malfunctions or becomes inoperable, don't allow the balloon catheter to remain dormant for more than 30 minutes, or for the length of time determined by the manufacturer.[13] Obtain another pump console and attach it to the balloon, then resume pumping. In the meantime, inflate the balloon manually, using a 60-mL syringe and room air, a minimum of once every 5 minutes *to prevent thrombus formation in the catheter.* The volume of inflation is equal to 10 mL less than the balloon size marked on the catheter. Never manually inflate the balloon if rupture is suspected.

■ Raise the bed to waist level when providing care *to prevent caregiver back strain.*[26]

■ Assess the patient's cardiovascular status and hemodynamic status every 15 to 60 minutes according to the patient's condition. Notify the practitioner immediately if you note changes.[13] Measure cardiac output (CO), cardiac index (CI), pulmonary artery pressure (PAP), and pulmonary artery occlusion pressure, as ordered, to detect changes in the patient's condition.

■ Assess the patient's peripheral vascular status every 15 to 60 minutes according to the patient's condition.[13] Note pulses, color, capillary refill, sensation, motor function, edema, and temperature in the affected limb. Notify the practitioner immediately if you detect circulatory changes, *because the balloon may need to be removed.*[46]

■ Auscultate heart and breath sounds at an interval determined by the patient's condition. If the patient's condition permits, put the IABP on standby during auscultation *so that IABP noises don't interfere with your assessment.*[13]

■ Monitor the patient's vital signs and level of consciousness at an interval determined by the patient's condition.

■ Monitor oxygen saturation level using pulse oximetry. Provide supplemental oxygen and noninvasive or invasive ventilatory support, as required and ordered.[53]

■ Assess the insertion site for hematoma, bleeding, and infection every 2 hours or at an interval determined by the patient's condition.[13,36]

■ Assess GI status regularly as warranted by the patient's condition. Check for abdominal distention and tenderness, and assess for changes in elimination patterns.

■ Monitor the patient's urine output every 15 to 60 minutes, according to the patient's condition.[13]

■ Screen for and assess the patient's pain using facility-defined criteria that are consistent with the patient's age, condition, and ability to understand.[54]

■ Treat the patient's pain, as needed and ordered, using nonpharmacologic, pharmacologic, or a combination of approaches. Base the treatment plan on evidence-based practices and the patient's clinical condition, past medical history, and pain management goals.[54]

■ Maintain the head of the bed at less than 45 degrees *to prevent kinking and migration of the catheter.*[13]

■ Avoid hip flexion; keep the affected leg still and straight.[46] *Hip flexion can put stress on the insertion site and lead to vascular complications.*

■ Assess skin integrity regularly. Reposition the patient frequently while maintaining catheter position and function. Consider the use of pressure-relief surfaces and devices.[55,56]

HOSPITAL-ACQUIRED CONDITION ALERT Keep in mind that the Centers for Medicare and Medicaid Services consider a stage 3 or 4 pressure injury a hospital-acquired condition, *because various best practices can reasonably prevent it.* Make sure to follow evidence-based pressure injury prevention practices, such as assessing skin integrity, using support surfaces, and frequently repositioning the patient, *to reduce the risk of pressure injuries.*[56,57,58]

■ Perform range-of-motion exercises as tolerated *to prevent venous stasis and muscle atrophy.*

■ As appropriate, encourage coughing and deep breathing. Provide chest physiotherapy, as tolerated and ordered.[46]

■ Monitor the patient's hematologic status. Observe for bleeding gums, blood in the urine or stools, petechiae, and bleeding or hematoma at the insertion site.[13] Monitor platelet count, hemoglobin level, and hematocrit daily. Expect to administer blood products to maintain hematocrit at 30%. If platelet count drops, expect to administer platelets.

■ If heparin is used for arterial lumen patency, monitor partial thromboplastin time (PTT) every 6 hours while the heparin dose is adjusted to maintain PTT at 1½ to 2 times the normal value, and then every 12 to 24 hours while the balloon remains in place.

NURSING ALERT Heparin is a high-alert medication *because it can cause significant patient harm when used in error.*[59] If required by your facility, before administering heparin, have another nurse perform an independent double-check *to verify the patient's identity and to ensure that you have the correct medication in the prescribed strength or concentration; the medication's indication corresponds with the patient's diagnosis; the dosage calculations are correct and the dosing formula used to derive the final dose is correct; the prescribed route of administration is safe and proper for the patient; the prescribed time and frequency of administration are safe and proper for the patient; and, if an infusion, the pump settings are correct and the infusion line is attached to the correct port.*[42]

■ After comparing the results of the independent double-check (if required) with the other nurse, administer the medication if there are no

Interpreting intra-aortic balloon waveforms

To function properly, the inflation–deflation cycle of an intra-aortic balloon pump (IABP) must be synchronized to appropriate events in the patient's cardiac cycle. During intra-aortic balloon counterpulsation (IABC), you can use electrocardiogram (ECG) and arterial pressure waveforms to determine whether the IABP is functioning properly. The central lumen of the double-lumen intra-aortic balloon catheter allows monitoring of the pressure in the descending aorta during the cardiac cycle. This arterial line provides data to the IABP console. Timing of the IABP is always performed using the arterial waveform as a guide.[13,46]

Many IABP models automatically adjust timing setting to accommodate changes in the patient's heart rate. Knowing the individuals patient's goals of therapy and the available trigger options for a particular system help optimize therapy.[2]

Normal inflation–deflation timing

Balloon inflation occurs after aortic valve closure; deflation, during isovolumetric contraction, just before the aortic valve opens. In a properly timed waveform, such as the one shown at right, the inflation point lies at or slightly above the dicrotic notch. Both inflation and deflation cause a sharp V shape. Peak diastolic pressure exceeds peak systolic pressure; peak systolic pressure exceeds assisted peak systolic pressure.

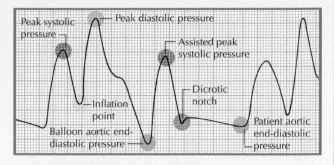

Early inflation

With early inflation, the inflation point lies before the dicrotic notch (shown at right). Early inflation dangerously increases myocardial stress and decreases cardiac output.

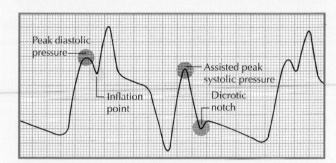

Early deflation

Early deflation results in a U shape on the arterial waveform (shown at right). Peak systolic pressure is less than or equal to assisted peak systolic pressure. Early deflation won't decrease afterload or myocardial oxygen consumption.

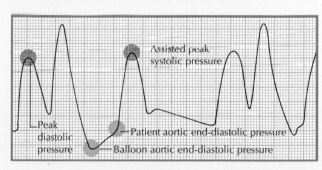

Late inflation

With late inflation, the dicrotic notch precedes the inflation point, and the notch and the inflation point create a W shape (shown at right). Late inflation can lead to a reduction in peak diastolic pressure, coronary and systemic perfusion augmentation time, and augmented coronary perfusion pressure.

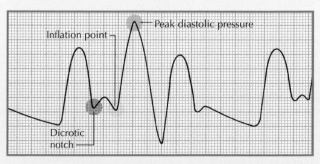

Late deflation

With late deflation, peak systolic pressure exceeds assisted peak systolic pressure (shown at right). This event threatens the patient by increasing afterload, myocardial oxygen consumption, cardiac workload, and pre-load. It occurs when the balloon has been inflated for too long or fails to receive the input signal from the ECG, indicating the start of systole (QRS complex).

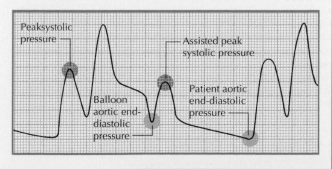

discrepancies. If discrepancies exist, rectify them before administering the medication.[42]

- Obtain samples for ABG analysis, as ordered. Notify the practitioner of critical test results within your facility's established time frame *so that the patient can be promptly treated.*[14]

- Monitor serum electrolyte levels, especially sodium and potassium, as ordered, *to assess the patient's fluid and electrolyte balance and help prevent arrhythmias.* Notify the practitioner of critical test results within your facility's established timeframe *so that the patient can be promptly treated.*[14]

NURSING ALERT Avoid sampling from the central lumen of the balloon *to avoid thrombus formation.*[46]

- Obtain an ECG, as ordered.

- Obtain a chest X-ray, if ordered, *to check catheter position to prevent complications.* Temporarily place the IABP on standby while the chest X-ray is obtained *to enhance visibility of the balloon.*[13]

- Watch for signs and symptoms of an aortic dissection,[13] including a blood pressure differential between the left and right arms, elevated blood pressure, syncope, pallor, diaphoresis, dyspnea, a throbbing abdominal mass, a reduced red blood cell count with an elevated white blood cell count, and pain in the chest, abdomen, or back. Notify the practitioner immediately if you detect any of these complications.

- Administer vasoactive medications, as prescribed, following safe medication administration practices.[32,33,34,35]

- Identify parameters that demonstrate clinical readiness to wean from IABC therapy,[13] such as resolution of signs and symptoms associated with hypoperfusion caused by low CO, including angina; CI of 2 L/minute/m² or higher that doesn't decrease by more 20%; pulmonary artery occlusion pressure that doesn't increase more than 20% above preweaning level; urine output greater than 0.5 mL/kg/hour; heart rate less than 100 beats/minute; and minimal need for positive ionotropic agents.[46]

- Reassess and respond to the patient's pain by evaluating the response to treatment and progress toward pain management goals. Assess for adverse reactions and risk factors for adverse events that may result from treatment.[54]

- Return the bed to the lowest position *to prevent falls and maintain patient safety.*[47]

- Discard used supplies in appropriate receptacles.[48]

- Remove and discard your gloves.[48]

- Perform hand hygiene.[15,16,17,18,19,20]

- Clean and disinfect your stethoscope using a disinfectant pad.[59,60]

- Perform hand hygiene.[15,16,17,18,19,20]

- Document the procedure.[49,50,51,52]

Weaning a patient from IABC

- Verify the practitioner's order.

- Perform hand hygiene.[15,16,17,18,19,20]

- Confirm the patient's identity using at least two patient identifiers.[21]

- Explain the procedure for the patient and family (if appropriate) according to their individual communication and learning needs *to increase their understanding, allay their fears, and enhance cooperation.*[7,8,9,10]

- To begin weaning, gradually decrease the frequency of balloon augmentation to 1:2, as ordered. Although each facility has its own weaning protocol, be aware that you'll usually maintain assist frequency for 1 hour or longer. If the patient's hemodynamic indices remain stable during this time, continue weaning by decreasing the frequency of balloon augmentation to 1:3, and so on.[13]

- Assess the patient's tolerance of weaning by monitoring vital signs, ECG, mental status, urine output, distal perfusion, CO, and CI.[46] Signs and symptoms of poor tolerance include hypotension, confusion, disorientation, urine output below 30 mL/hour, cold and clammy skin, chest pain, arrhythmias, ischemic ECG changes, reduced CO and CI, and elevated PAP. If the patient develops any of these problems, notify the practitioner immediately.

- Perform hand hygiene.[15,16,17,18,19,20]

- Clean and disinfect your stethoscope using a disinfectant pad.[59,60]

- Perform hand hygiene.[15,16,17,18,19,20]

- Document the procedure.[49,50,51,52]

For assisting with removal

- Verify the practitioner's order.

- Discontinue the heparin infusion 4 to 6 hours before balloon removal, or within the time frame specified by the practitioner's order. Alternatively, reverse the effects with protamine sulfate, as ordered, just before catheter removal.[13]

- Verify that coagulation study findings are within the ordered range before balloon removal *to prevent hemorrhage from the insertion site.*[46]

- Gather and prepare the necessary equipment and supplies.

- Perform hand hygiene.[15,16,17,18,19,20]

- Confirm the patient's identity using at least two patient identifiers.[21]

- Provide privacy.[22,23,24,25]

- Explain the procedure to the patient and family (if appropriate) according to their individual communication and learning needs *to increase their understanding, allay their fears, and enhance cooperation.*[7,8,9,10]

- Assess hemodynamic stability before removal.[13]

- Raise the bed to waist level *to prevent caregiver back strain.*[26]

- Perform hand hygiene.[15,16,17,18,19,20]

- Put on gloves and, as necessary, other personal protective equipment *to comply with standard precautions.*

- Place a fluid-impermeable pad under the patient's affected extremity *to help keep the bed linens clean.*

- Turn off the control system and disconnect the connection tubing from the catheter *to ensure balloon deflation.*

- Assist the practitioner with removal, as needed. The practitioner removes the sutures securing the balloon, and then withdraws the balloon until the proximal end of the catheter contacts the distal end of the introducer sheath. While applying pressure below the puncture site, the practitioner removes the balloon and introducer sheath as a unit, allowing a few seconds of free bleeding to prevent thrombus formation.

- Assess the integrity of the balloon after removal.

- Apply direct pressure to the site for 30 to 45 minutes or until bleeding stops.[13] (Note: In some facilities, applying pressure is the practitioner's responsibility.)

- Apply a mechanical compression device, as ordered.[46]

- If the balloon was inserted surgically, assist the surgeon with closure of the Dacron graft and suturing of the insertion site. A cardiologist usually removes the percutaneous catheter.

- Assess the site for bleeding or hematoma.[13] Apply a sterile pressure dressing and keep it in place for 2 to 4 hours.[13]

- Assess the patient's vital signs and hemodynamic parameters every 15 minutes for 1 hour, every 30 minutes for the next hour, and then hourly as the patient's condition warrants. Notify the practitioner of any abnormalities.[13]

- Assess the patient's pedal and posterior tibial pulses, and the color, temperature, and sensation of the affected limb immediately after removal and every 1 hour for 2 hours, then every 2 hours or according to the practitioner's orders.[13] Notify the practitioner of any abnormalities.

- Maintain the patient on bed rest, with the head of the bed elevated 30 degrees or less, as ordered. Maintain immobilization of the affected extremity as ordered or as directed by your facility.[13]

- Return the bed to the lowest position to prevent falls and maintain patient safety.[47]

- Discard used supplies in appropriate receptacles.[48]

- Remove and discard your gloves and other personal protective equipment, if worn.[48]

- Perform hand hygiene.[15,16,17,18,19,20]

- Document the procedure.[49,50,51,52]

Special considerations

- The practitioner must time inflation and deflation to the patient's cardiac cycle *to achieve optimal counterpulsation.*[13] Assess timing of the IABC with the arterial waveform. The practitioner should determine the goal of IABC therapy before choosing the best timing method, *because inappropriate timing can be detrimental to left ventricular performance.*[2]

- Some IABP manufacturers produce autotiming devices that sense the R wave on the ECG tracing and use this as the trigger source.[2,13,61]

■ The Joint Commission has issued a sentinel event alert related to managing risk during transition to new International Organization for Standardization tubing standards designed to prevent dangerous tubing misconnections, which can lead to serious patient injury and death. During the transition, be sure to trace the tubing and catheter from the patient to the point of origin before connecting or reconnecting any device or infusion, at any care transition (such as a new setting or service), and as part of the hand-off process. Route tubes and catheters with different purposes in different standardized directions. When there are different access sites or several bags hanging, label the tubing at the distal and proximal ends; use tubing and equipment only as intended; and store medications for different delivery routes in separate locations.[45]

■ The Joint Commission has issued a sentinel event alert concerning medical device alarm safety, *because alarm-related events have been associated with permanent loss of function and death.* Among the major contributing factors were improper alarm settings, inappropriately turned off alarms, and alarm signals not audible to staff. Make sure that alarm limits are set appropriately, and that alarms are turned on and audible. Follow facility guidelines for preventing alarm fatigue.[28]

■ *To prevent vascular catheter-associated infection,* perform catheter site care and dressing changes as needed according to the type of dressing used. Change a transparent semipermeable dressing at least every 7 days, and a gauze dressing every 2 days.[6,13,36,37,62] Change the dressing sooner if it's damp, loose, or visibly soiled.[6,13,36,37] Perform catheter site care with an antiseptic pad (chlorhexidine-based is preferred) and allow it to dry completely; replace the securement device (if used), and then apply a sterile occlusive dressing.[6,13,37,62]

■ Watch for pump interruptions, which may result from loose ECG electrodes or lead wires, static or 60-cycle interference, catheter kinking, or improper body alignment.

■ Keep in mind that anticoagulant use or the presence of thrombocytopenia, which can be caused by the balloon itself, increases the risk of bleeding

Complications

IABC can cause numerous complications. Potential complications include arterial embolism stemming from clot formation on the balloon surface, extension or rupture of an aortic aneurysm, femoral or iliac artery perforation, femoral artery occlusion, balloon rupture, stroke, balloon migration, sepsis, limb ischemia, cholesterol embolization, decreased platelet count, hemolysis, seromas, groin infection, and peripheral neuropathy.[5,46] Bleeding at the insertion site may become aggravated by pump-induced thrombocytopenia caused by platelet aggregation around the balloon.

Removal of and IAB can cause bleeding and hematoma formation at the insertion site. Additionally, removal may dislodge a thrombus from the catheter, leading to arterial occlusion in the extremity.[13]

Documentation

Document the date and time of insertion, the size of the catheter, balloon volume, and IABP frequency.[13] Document all aspects of patient preparation and assessment, including any teaching provide to the patient and family (if appropriate), their understanding of that teaching, and any need for follow-up teaching. Also document the procedure and the patient's response, any complications, prescribed interventions, and the patient's response to the interventions.

Document all aspects of patient assessment and management, including the patient's response to therapy and weaning. If you're responsible for the IABC device, document all routine checks, problems, and troubleshooting measures. If a technician is responsible for the IABC device, record only when and why you notified the technician as well as the results of the technician's actions on the patient, if applicable.

Document management related to removal, including the condition of the insertion site after removal, wound care performed, balloon integrity, and the patient's tolerance of the procedure.

REFERENCES

1 Krishna, M., & Zacharowski, K. (2009). Principles of intra-aortic balloon pump counterpulsation. *Continuing Education in Anaesthesia, Critical Care and Pain, 9*(1), 24–28. https://academic.oup.com/bjaed/article/9/1/24/466259

2 Hanlon-Pena, P. M., & Quaal, S. J. (2011). Intra-aortic balloon pump timing: Review of evidence supporting current practice. *American Journal of Critical Care, 20*, 323–334.

3 Thiele, H., et al. (2019). Intraaortic balloon support for myocardial infarction with cardiogenic shock: Long-term 6-year outcome of the randomized IABP-SHOCK II trial. *Circulation, 139*(3), 395–403. https://www.aha-journals.org/doi/10.1161/CIRCULATIONAHA.118.038201 (Level II)

4 Reyentovich, A. (2020). Prognosis and treatment of cardiogenic shock complicating acute myocardial infarction. In: *UpToDate,* Gersh, B. J., & Windecker, S. (Eds.).

5 Laham, R. J., & Pinto, D. S. (2020). Intraaortic balloon pump counterpulsation. In: *UpToDate*, Gersh, B. J., & Cutlip, D. (Eds.).

6 Marschall, J., et al. (2014). SHEA/IDSA practice recommendation: Strategies to prevent central line–associated bloodstream infections in acute care hospitals. *Infection Control and Hospital Epidemiology, 35*, 753–771. https://www.jstor.org/stable/10.1086/676533#metadata_info_tab_contents (Level I)

7 The Joint Commission. (2021). Standard RI.01.03.01. *Comprehensive accreditation manual for hospitals.* Oakbrook Terrace, IL: The Joint Commission. (Level VII)

8 Centers for Medicare and Medicaid Services, Department of Health and Human Services. (2020). Condition of participation: Patient's rights. 42 C.F.R. § 482.13(b)(2).

9 DNV GL-Healthcare USA, Inc. (2020). PR.2.SR.3. *NIAHO® accreditation requirements, interpretive guidelines and surveyor guidance—revision 20.0.* Milford, OH: DNV GL-Healthcare USA, Inc. (Level VII)

10 Accreditation Association for Hospitals and Health Systems. (2020). Standard 30.00.11. *Healthcare Facilities Accreditation Program: Accreditation requirements for acute care hospitals.* Chicago, IL: Accreditation Association for Hospitals and Health Systems. (Level VII)

11 The Joint Commission. (2021). Standard UP.01.01.01. *Comprehensive accreditation manual for hospitals.* Oakbrook Terrace, IL: The Joint Commission. (Level VII)

12 Accreditation Association for Hospitals and Health Systems. (2020). Standard 30.00.14. *Healthcare Facilities Accreditation Program: Accreditation requirements for acute care hospitals.* Chicago, IL: Accreditation Association for Hospitals and Health Systems. (Level VII)

13 Wiegand, D. L. (2017). *AACN procedure manual for high acuity, progressive, and critical care* (7th ed.). St. Louis, MO: Elsevier.

14 The Joint Commission. (2021). Standard NPSG.02.03.01. *Comprehensive accreditation manual for hospitals.* Oakbrook Terrace, IL: The Joint Commission. (Level VII)

15 The Joint Commission. (2021). Standard NPSG.07.01.01. *Comprehensive accreditation manual for hospitals.* Oakbrook Terrace, IL: The Joint Commission. (Level VII)

16 Centers for Disease Control and Prevention. (2002). Guideline for hand hygiene in health-care settings: Recommendations of the Healthcare Infection Control Practices Advisory Committee and the HICPAC/SHEA/APIC/IDSA Hand Hygiene Task Force. *MMWR Recommendations and Reports, 51*(RR-16), 1–45. https://www.cdc.gov/mmwr/pdf/rr/rr5116.pdf (Level II)

17 World Health Organization. (2009). WHO guidelines on hand hygiene in health care: First global patient safety challenge, clean care is safer care. https://apps.who.int/iris/bitstream/handle/10665/44102/9789241597906_eng.pdf?sequence=1 (Level IV)

18 Centers for Medicare and Medicaid Services, Department of Health and Human Services. (2020). Condition of participation: Infection control. 42 C.F.R. § 482.42.

19 Accreditation Association for Hospitals and Health Systems. (2020). Standard 07.01.21. *Healthcare Facilities Accreditation Program: Accreditation requirements for acute care hospitals.* Chicago, IL: Accreditation Association for Hospitals and Health Systems. (Level VII)

20 DNV GL-Healthcare USA, Inc. (2020). IC.1.SR.1. *NIAHO® accreditation requirements, interpretive guidelines and surveyor guidance—revision 20.0.* Milford, OH: DNV GL-Healthcare USA, Inc. (Level VII)

21 The Joint Commission. (2021). Standard NPSG.01.01.01. *Comprehensive accreditation manual for hospitals.* Oakbrook Terrace, IL: The Joint Commission. (Level VII)

22 The Joint Commission. (2021). Standard RI.01.01.01. *Comprehensive accreditation manual for hospitals.* Oakbrook Terrace, IL: The Joint Commission. (Level VII)

23 DNV GL-Healthcare USA, Inc. (2020). PR.2.SR.5. *NIAHO® accreditation requirements, interpretive guidelines and surveyor guidance—revision 20.0.* Milford, OH: DNV GL-Healthcare USA, Inc. (Level VII)

24 Centers for Medicare and Medicaid Services, Department of Health and Human Services. (2020). Condition of participation: Patient's rights. 42 C.F.R. § 482.13(c)(1).

25 Accreditation Association for Hospitals and Health Systems. (2020). Standard 15.01.16. *Healthcare Facilities Accreditation Program: Accreditation requirements for acute care hospitals.* Chicago, IL: Accreditation Association for Hospitals and Health Systems. (Level VII)

26 Waters, T. R., et al. (2009). Safe patient handling training for schools of nursing. https://www.cdc.gov/niosh/docs/2009-127/pdfs/2009-127.pdf (Level VII)

27 The Joint Commission. (2021). Standard NPSG.06.01.01. *Comprehensive accreditation manual for hospitals.* Oakbrook Terrace, IL: The Joint Commission. (Level VII)

28 The Joint Commission. (2013). Sentinel event alert 50: Medical device alarm safety in hospitals. https://www.jointcommission.org/assets/1/6/SEA_50_alarms_4_26_16.pdf (Level VII)

29 American Association of Critical-Care Nurses. (2018). AACN practice alert. Managing alarms in acute care across the life span: Electrocardiography and pulse oximetry. https://www.aacn.org/clinical-resources/practice-alerts/managing-alarms-in-acute-care-across-the-life-span (Level VII)

30 Graham, K. C., & Cvach, M. (2010). Monitor alarm fatigue: Standardizing use of physiological monitors and decreasing nuisance alarms. *American Journal of Critical Care, 19,* 28–37

31 Standard 33. Vascular access site preparation and skin asepsis. Infusion therapy standards of practice (8th ed.) (2021). *Journal of Infusion Nursing, 44,* S96–S97. (Level VII)

32 Centers for Medicare and Medicaid Services, Department of Health and Human Services. (2020). Condition of participation: Nursing services. 42 C.F.R. § 482.23(c).

33 Accreditation Association for Hospitals and Health Systems. (2020). Standard 16.01.03. *Healthcare Facilities Accreditation Program: Accreditation requirements for acute care hospitals.* Chicago, IL: Accreditation Association for Hospitals and Health Systems. (Level VII)

34 The Joint Commission. (2021). Standard MM.06.01.01. *Comprehensive accreditation manual for hospitals.* Oakbrook Terrace, IL: The Joint Commission. (Level VII)

35 DNV GL-Healthcare USA, Inc. (2020). MM.1.SR.3. *NIAHO® accreditation requirements, interpretive guidelines and surveyor guidance—revision 20.0.* Milford, OH: DNV GL-Healthcare USA, Inc. (Level VII)

36 Centers for Disease Control and Prevention. (2011, revised 2017). Guidelines for the prevention of intravascular catheter–related infections. https://www.cdc.gov/infectioncontrol/guidelines/bsi/recommendations.html (Level I)

37 The Joint Commission. (2021). Standard NPSG.07.04.01. *Comprehensive accreditation manual for hospitals.* Oakbrook Terrace, IL: The Joint Commission. (Level VII)

38 The Joint Commission. (2021). Standard NPSG.03.04.01. *Comprehensive accreditation manual for hospitals.* Oakbrook Terrace, IL: The Joint Commission. (Level VII)

39 Accreditation Association for Hospitals and Health Systems. (2020). Standard 25.01.27. *Healthcare Facilities Accreditation Program: Accreditation requirements for acute care hospitals.* Chicago, IL: Accreditation Association for Hospitals and Health Systems. (Level VII)

40 The Joint Commission. (2021). Standard UP.01.03.01. *Comprehensive accreditation manual for hospitals.* Oakbrook Terrace, IL: The Joint Commission. (Level VII)

41 Institute for Safe Medication Practices. (2018). ISMP list of high-alert medications in acute care settings. https://www.ismp.org/sites/default/files/attachments/2018-08/highAlert2018-Acute-Final.pdf

42 Institute for Safe Medication Practice. (2013). Independent double checks. Undervalued and misused: Selective use of this strategy can play an important role in medication safety. https://www.ismp.org/resources/independent-double-checks-undervalued-and-misused-selective-use-strategy-can-play (Level VII)

43 Murks, C., & Juricek, C. (2018). Balloon pumps inserted via the subclavian artery: Bridging the way to heart transplant. *AACN Advanced Critical Care, 27,* 301–315.

44 U.S. Food and Drug Administration. (2017). Examples of medical device misconnections. https://www.fda.gov/medical-devices/medical-device-connectors/examples-of-medical-device-misconnections

45 The Joint Commission. (2014). Sentinel event alert 53: Managing risk during transition to new ISO tubing connector standards. https://www.jointcommission.org/assets/1/6/SEA_53_Connectors_8_19_14_final.pdf (Level VII)

46 Goldich, G. (2011). Getting in sync with intra-aortic balloon pump therapy. *Nursing2011 Critical Care, 6*(3), 10–13. https://journals.lww.com/nursing/Fulltext/2011/10001/Getting_in_sync_with_intra_aortic_balloon_pump.3.aspx

47 Ganz, D. A., et al. (2013, reviewed 2021). *Preventing falls in hospitals: A toolkit for improving quality of care* (AHRQ Publication No. 13-0015-EF). Rockville, MD: Agency for Healthcare Research and Quality. https://www.ahrq.gov/professionals/systems/hospital/fallpxtoolkit/index.html (Level VII)

48 Occupational Safety and Health Administration. (2012). Bloodborne pathogens, standard number 1910.1030. https://www.osha.gov/pls/oshaweb/owadisp.show_document?p_id=10051&p_table=STANDARDS (Level VII)

49 The Joint Commission. (2021). Standard RC.02.01.01. *Comprehensive accreditation manual for hospitals.* Oakbrook Terrace, IL: The Joint Commission. (Level VII)

50 Centers for Medicare and Medicaid Services, Department of Health and Human Services. (2020). Condition of participation: Medical record services. 42 C.F.R. § 482.24(b).

51 Accreditation Association for Hospitals and Health Systems. (2020). Standard 10.00.03. *Healthcare Facilities Accreditation Program: Accreditation requirements for acute care hospitals.* Chicago, IL: Accreditation Association for Hospitals and Health Systems. (Level VII)

52 DNV GL-Healthcare USA, Inc. (2020). MR.2.SR.1. *NIAHO® accreditation requirements, interpretive guidelines and surveyor guidance—revision 20.0.* Milford, OH: DNV GL-Healthcare USA, Inc. (Level VII)

53 Ponikowski, P., et al. (2016). 2016 ESC guidelines for the diagnosis and treatment of acute and chronic heart failure. *European Heart Journal, 37*(27), 2129–2200. https://academic.oup.com/eurheartj/article/37/27/2129/1748921 (Level VII)

54 The Joint Commission. (2021). Standard PC.01.02.07. *Comprehensive accreditation manual for hospitals.* Oakbrook Terrace, IL: The Joint Commission. (Level VII)

55 Accreditation Association for Hospitals and Health Systems. (2020). Standard 16.02.02. *Healthcare Facilities Accreditation Program: Accreditation requirements for acute care hospitals.* Chicago, IL: Accreditation Association for Hospitals and Health Systems. (Level VII)

56 European Pressure Ulcer Advisory Panel, et al. (2019). Prevention and treatment of pressure ulcers/injuries: Quick reference guide. http://www.internationalguideline.com/static/pdfs/Quick_Reference_Guide-10Mar2019.pdf (Level VII)

57 Jarrett, N., & Callaham, M. (2016). Evidence-based guidelines for selected hospital-acquired conditions: Final report. https://www.cms.gov/Medicare/Medicare-Fee-for-Service-Payment/HospitalAcqCond/Downloads/2016-HAC-Report.pdf

58 Wound Ostomy and Continence Nurses Society (WOCN). (2016). *Guideline for prevention and management of pressure ulcers (injuries): WOCN clinical practice guideline series 2.* Mount Laurel, NJ: WOCN.

59 Rutala, W. A., et al. (2008, revised 2019). Guideline for disinfection and sterilization in healthcare facilities, 2008. https://www.cdc.gov/infection-control/pdf/guidelines/disinfection-guidelines-H.pdf (Level I)

60 Accreditation Association for Hospitals and Health Systems. (2020). Standard 07.02.03. *Healthcare Facilities Accreditation Program: Accreditation requirements for acute care hospitals.* Chicago, IL: Accreditation Association for Hospitals and Health Systems. (Level VII)

61 Yarham, G., et al. (2013). Fiber-optic intra-aortic balloon therapy and its role within cardiac surgery. *Perfusion, 28,* 97–102.

62 Standard 42. Vascular access device assessment, care, and dressing changes. Infusion therapy standards of practice (8th ed.) (2021). *Journal of Infusion Nursing, 44,* S119–S123. (Level VII)

Intracranial Pressure Monitoring

Intracranial pressure (ICP) monitoring measures pressure exerted by the brain, blood, and cerebrospinal fluid (CSF) against the inside of the skull. Indications for monitoring ICP include head trauma with bleeding or edema, overproduction or insufficient absorption of CSF, cerebral hemorrhage, and space-occupying brain lesions. ICP monitoring can detect elevated ICP early, before clinical danger signs develop.[1] Prompt intervention can then help avert or diminish neurologic damage caused by cerebral hypoxia and shifts of brain mass.

The four basic ICP monitoring methods are intraventricular catheter, subarachnoid bolt, epidural or subdural sensor, and intraparenchymal pressure monitoring. Intraventricular catheters are considered the gold standard for measuring ICP because they're inserted directly into the ventricle through a burr hole, which permits ICP monitoring and therapeutic CSF drainage to control ICP.[1] (See *Understanding ICP monitoring*, page 472.) Regardless of which system is used, the procedure is typically performed by a neurosurgeon in the operating room or emergency department, or on the intensive care unit. Insertion of an ICP monitoring device requires sterile technique to reduce the risk of central nervous system (CNS) infection. Setting up equipment for the monitoring systems also requires strict sterile technique.[1]

Equipment

Intracranial access kit ▪ catheter ▪ disposable flushless transducer ▪ pressure cable and pressure module ▪ cardiac monitor ▪ pulse oximeter and probe ▪ bedside monitor ▪ fluid-impermeable pads ▪ sterile drapes ▪ sterile towels ▪ antiseptic solution or sterile prep kit ▪ sterile gowns ▪ sterile gloves ▪ gloves ▪ gown ▪ masks ▪ caps ▪ sterile marker ▪ sterile labels ▪ preservative-free normal saline solution for injection ▪ 30-mL or 40-mL syringe[1] ▪ lidocaine local anesthetic ▪ sterile occlusive dressing supplies ▪ leveling device ▪ vital signs monitoring equipment ▪ Optional: tape, prescribed sedative agent, prescribed pain medication, prescribed osmotic diuretic, IV pole, external ventricular drainage system, arterial catheter insertion equipment, single-patient-use scissors or disposable-head clippers.

You may need to gather other equipment as instructed by the practitioner, such as the drill and bits, a scalp retractor, and a scalp staple.

Preparation of equipment

Various types of preassembled ICP monitoring units are available, each with its own setup protocols. These units are designed to reduce the risk of infection by eliminating the need for multiple stopcocks, manometers, and transducer dome assemblies.

Inspect all equipment and supplies. If a product is expired, is defective, or has compromised integrity, remove it from patient use, label it as expired or defective, and report the expiration or defect, as directed by your facility.

When preparing the equipment, label all medications, medication containers, and other solutions on and off the sterile field.[2] Prepare and set up the ICP monitoring system according to the manufacturer's instructions. (See *Setting up an ICP monitoring system*, page 473.)

Implementation

Assisting with catheter insertion

▪ Verify the practitioner's order.
▪ Gather and prepare the equipment, personnel, and supplies needed for catheter insertion.
▪ Confirm that informed consent has been obtained and that the signed consent form is in the patient's medical record.[12,13,14,15]
▪ Conduct a preprocedure verification *to make sure that all relevant documentation, related information, and equipment are available and correctly identified to the patient's identifiers.*[16,17]
▪ Verify that ordered laboratory and imaging studies have been completed and that the results are in the patient's medical record. Notify the practitioner of any unexpected results.
▪ Check the patient's history for an allergy or a hypersensitivity to iodine, latex, or the ordered local anesthetic.
▪ Perform hand hygiene.[6,7,8,9,10,11]
▪ Confirm the patient's identity using at least two patient identifiers.[18]
▪ Provide privacy.[12,13,15,19]
▪ Reinforce the practitioner's explanation of the procedure to the patient and family (if appropriate), according to their individual communication

and learning needs, *to increase their understanding, allay their fears, and enhance cooperation.*[20] Answer any questions.
▪ Raise the patient's bed to waist level before providing care *to prevent caregiver back strain.*[21]
▪ Perform hand hygiene.[6,7,8,9,10,11]
▪ Ensure the patient is attached to a cardiac monitor and pulse oximeter *to monitor heart rate and rhythm and oxygen saturation level during the procedure.*[1] Make sure the alarm limits are set appropriately for the patient's current condition, and that the alarms are turned on, functioning properly, and audible to staff.[22,23,24,25]
▪ Assist with arterial catheter insertion, if ordered, *because vigilant monitoring of mean arterial blood pressure is necessary to avoid decreased cerebral perfusion pressure (CPP).*[1] Ensure the alarm limits are set appropriately for the patient's current condition, and that the alarms are turned on, functioning properly, and audible to staff.[23,24,25]
▪ If the monitoring device is to be inserted outside the operating room (OR), ensure that conditions model the OR. Close the doors to the room where the procedure is being performed. Ensure anyone in the room wears a mask and cap.[1]
▪ Obtain baseline routine and neurologic vital signs *to aid in prompt detection of decompensation during the procedure.*[1,26]
▪ Assess the patient's sedation and pain management needs in collaboration with the practitioner.[27] Administer medications, as indicated and prescribed, following safe medication practices, *to ensure the patient's comfort during the procedure.*[1,28,29,30,31]
▪ Put on a cap and a mask.[3,4,5]
▪ Place the patient in the supine position with the head in a neutral position and the head of the bed elevated to 30 degrees (or as ordered).[1]
▪ Place fluid-impermeable pads under the patient's head.
▪ Verify that the catheter insertion site has been identified before preparing the site *to minimize the risk of preparing the wrong area.*[32]
▪ Braid or clip hair at the insertion site, as needed. If the hair is clipped, use tape or some similar sticky product *to remove residual hair clippings.*[1]
▪ Immobilize the patient's head *to prevent patient movement and facilitate catheter insertion.*[1]
▪ Perform hand hygiene.[6,7,8,9,10,11]
▪ Put on a gown and gloves.[3,4,5] The practitioner puts on a cap, a mask, a sterile gown, and sterile gloves.[1,3,26]
▪ Assist with preparing the incision site using an antiseptic solution or a sterile prep kit, following the manufacturer's instructions.[1]

NURSING ALERT Note that 2% chlorhexidine preparation isn't recommended when contact with the meninges is possible.[1,33]

▪ Assist with draping the areas surrounding the catheter insertion site with sterile drapes.[1]
▪ Conduct a time-out immediately before the practitioner begins the procedure *to perform a final assessment that the correct patient, site, positioning, and procedure have been identified and, as applicable, all relevant information and necessary equipment are available.*[17,34]
▪ The practitioner opens the interior wrap of the sterile supply tray, infiltrates the scalp with a lidocaine local anesthetic agent, and proceeds with insertion of the ICP monitoring catheter.[1] Assist with the procedure, as needed.
▪ During ICP monitoring catheter insertion, continually monitor the patient's heart rate and rhythm, respiratory rate, and oxygen saturation level. Frequently monitor the patient's blood pressure. Assess neurologic status every 15 minutes, *because serial assessments are necessary to immediately identify neurologic changes and ensure prompt treatment.*[1]
▪ After insertion, assist the practitioner with connecting the catheter to the monitoring equipment while maintaining sterility and preventing contamination of the site, catheter, and sterile field.[1] Trace the tubing from the patient to the point of origin *to make sure that it's connected to the proper port.*[35,36]
▪ Assist the practitioner with cleaning around the insertion site with antiseptic solution and then apply a sterile occlusive dressing to the site.[1]
▪ Using a sterile label and marker, clearly label the access port of an external ventricular drainage system *to indicate that it's an external ventricular drain, preventing accidental mix-up of the port with an IV line.*[1]
▪ Maintain the patient in an upright position with the head of the bed elevated 30 degrees or as ordered *to promote venous return.* Make sure that the head is at the top of the bed in a midline position to the rest of

Understanding ICP monitoring

Intracranial pressure (ICP) can be monitored using one of four types of systems.

Intraventricular catheter monitoring

For intraventricular catheter monitoring, which provides direct monitoring of ICP, the practitioner inserts a small catheter into the lateral ventricle through a burr hole. This method provides the most accurate measure of ICP, and is the only type of ICP monitoring that allows evaluation of brain compliance and drainage of significant amounts of cerebrospinal fluid (CSF); however, it carries the greatest risk of infection. Contraindications usually include stenotic cerebral ventricles, cerebral aneurysms in the path of catheter placement, and suspected vascular lesions.

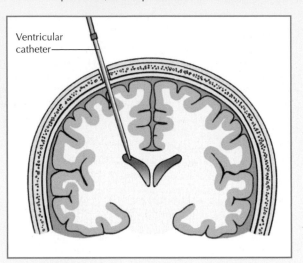

Epidural or subdural sensor monitoring

ICP can also be monitored from the epidural or subdural space. For epidural monitoring, the practitioner inserts a fiberoptic sensor into the epidural space through a burr hole. This system's main drawback is its questionable accuracy, *because it doesn't measure ICP directly from a CSF-filled space.*

For subdural monitoring, the practitioner tunnels a fiberoptic transducer-tipped catheter through a burr hole, placing its tip on brain tissue under the dura mater. The main drawback to this method is its inability to drain CSF.

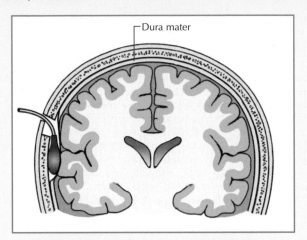

Subarachnoid bolt monitoring

Subarachnoid bolt monitoring involves insertion of a special bolt into the subarachnoid space through a twist-drill burr hole that's positioned in the front of the skull behind the hairline. Placing the bolt is easier than placing an intraventricular catheter, especially if a computed tomography scan reveals that the cerebrum has shifted or the ventricles have collapsed. This type of ICP monitoring also carries less risk of infection and parenchymal damage, *because the bolt doesn't penetrate the cerebrum.*

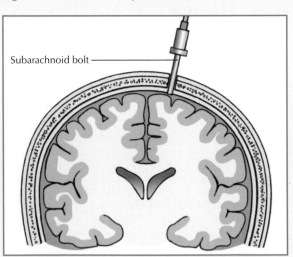

Intraparenchymal pressure monitoring

For intraparenchymal monitoring, the practitioner inserts a catheter through a small subarachnoid bolt and, after puncturing the dura mater, advances the catheter a few centimeters into the brain's white matter. One advantage of this method is that the equipment doesn't need to be balanced or calibrated after insertion. Although this method doesn't provide direct access to CSF, measurements are accurate *because brain tissue pressures correlate well with ventricular pressures.*

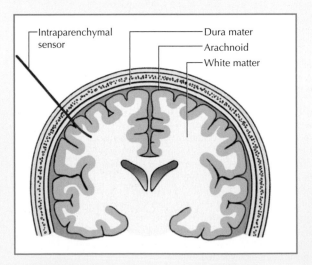

the body, *because flexion or rotation of the head or neck can obstruct venous return and thereby increase ICP.*[1]

■ Maintain the flushless transducer at the level of the patient's foramen of Monro. Anatomically, the reference point is equivalent to the level of the patient's ear or the outer canthus of the eye. *Flushless transducer*

placement at a point above or below the anatomically correct position will result in false readings.

■ Zero and calibrate the ICP monitoring catheter after insertion as required by the type of device used. If the device requires recalibration after it's in use, rezero at least every 12 hours.[1]

EQUIPMENT

Setting up an ICP monitoring system

To set up an intracranial pressure (ICP) monitoring system, use strict sterile technique. Use the two-person method when priming the tubing with normal saline solution *so that the second person can monitor the sterile technique and assist as needed*.[1] Follow these steps:

■ Put on a cap and mask.[3,4,5]

■ Perform hand hygiene.[6,7,8,9,10,11]

■ Open a sterile towel on a bedside table *to create a sterile field*.

■ On the sterile field, place a 30-mL or 40-mL syringe filled with preservative-free sterile normal saline solution and a disposable flushless transducer.[1]

■ Put on a sterile gown and sterile gloves.[3,4,5]

■ Attach the flushless transducer to the panel mount stopcock.[1]

■ Using sterile technique, attach the syringe containing sterile preservative-free normal saline solution to the stopcock at the distal end of the tubing (patient line stopcock).[1]

■ Turn the stopcock off toward the drainage device.[1]

■ Slowly inject the preservative-free sterile normal saline solution toward the distal end (patient end) of the tubing (as shown below). As the fluid reaches the distal end of the tubing, allow several drops of the solution to exit the end of the tubing *to make sure air is cleared from the tubing*.[1]

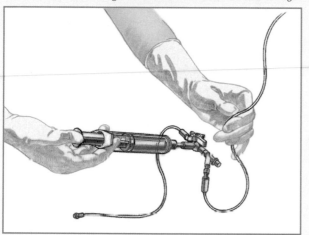

■ Turn the stopcock off to the distal end of the tubing, keeping the syringe in place. Make sure that the panel mount stopcock is open to the flushless transducer. Prime through the vented caps in the flushless transducer. Replace the vented caps with dead-end caps.[1]

■ With the syringe remaining in place, turn the stopcock off to the flushless transducer, and prime preservative-free sterile normal saline solution into the drip chamber.[1]

■ After priming the system, keep the stopcock on the distal end (patient end) of the tubing off *to make sure that no normal saline solution leaks from the system before connection*.[1]

■ Connect the flushless transducer to the bedside monitor with a pressure cable that's plugged into the designated pressure module.[1]

■ Align the zero point with the center line of the patient's head, level with the middle of the ear, using a leveling device. Keep in mind that the key to accurate ICP measurement is to use the same landmark each time you check the zero reference level.[1]

■ Lower the flow chamber to zero, and turn the stopcock off to the dead-end cap.[1]

■ Remove and discard your gloves and other personal protective equipment.[4,5]

■ Perform hand hygiene.[6,7,8,9,10,11]

■ With a clean hand, balance the ICP monitoring system according to the manufacturer's guidelines.[1]

■ Perform hand hygiene.[6,7,8,9,10,11]

■ If the patient has an external ventricular drain, maintain the drip chamber at the prescribed zero reference and pressure levels.[1]

■ Ensure that the ICP monitor's alarm limits are set appropriately for the patient's current condition, and that the alarms are turned on, functioning properly, and audible to staff.[23,24,25]

■ Begin ICP monitoring; obtain an ICP tracing and assess the ICP waveform. Use this tracing as a baseline for comparison. (See *Interpreting ICP waveforms*, page 474.) If the patient has an external ventricular drain, turn the stopcock off to the drain and open to the flushless transducer *to obtain an accurate ICP numeric value and waveform*.[1]

■ Observe ICP in relation to other hemodynamic parameters, such as mean arterial pressure.[1]

■ Dispose of insertion instruments and equipment appropriately *to prevent exposure to potentially infectious materials*.[1]

■ Remove and discard your personal protective equipment.[4,5]

■ Return the bed to the lowest position *to prevent falls and maintain patient safety*.[37]

■ Perform hand hygiene.[6,7,8,9,10,11]

■ Arrange for a computed tomography scan, if ordered, *to confirm catheter placement*.[1]

ICP monitoring and care

■ Assess the patient's neurologic status hourly, or more frequently if the patient's condition warrants. Notify the practitioner immediately if the patient's ICP exceeds established parameters. If no parameters exist, notify the practitioner if ICP exceeds 20 mm Hg. Watch for signs and symptoms of increased ICP, such as decreased level of consciousness, nausea, vomiting, headache, lethargy, and agitation.[1] (See *Managing ICP*, page 475.)

■ If the bedside monitor doesn't calculate CPP, calculate CPP hourly by subtracting the patient's ICP from the mean arterial pressure (MAP) (CPP = MAP − ICP). If CPP isn't within the specified parameters, notify the practitioner.[1]

■ Assess CSF drainage hourly for color and clarity.[1]

■ Assess external ventricular drainage system patency as needed by lowering the entire system briefly to assess drip rate into the graduated burette.[1]

■ Check the patient's position hourly to ensure that the transducer is at the ordered reference level *to prevent overdrainage or underdrainage if an external ventricular drain is in place and to ensure accurate ICP readings*.[1]

■ Assess the catheter system at least every 4 hours to ensure the system is intact and has no leaks, kinks, or clots *to decrease the risk of increased ICP related to catheter flow and drainage, and to ensure accurate pressure readings and waveforms consistent with neurologic assessment*.[1]

■ Record an ICP tracing each shift and as waveform changes occur; compare these tracings with previous tracings.[1]

■ If the patient has an external ventricular drain, inform the patient and family that the bed position should only be changed with assistance, *because raising the level of the bed with the external ventricular drain at fixed zero and reference levels can result in a large increase in CSF drainage*.[1]

■ Clamp an external ventricular drain any time there is a patient response (coughing, vomiting, or response to care) or procedure (suctioning, repositioning, and transport) that may cause CSF overdrainage.[1]

■ If an ICP waveform doesn't appear, troubleshoot the system. If the patient has an external ventricular drain, then air bubbles, clots, or debris within the drainage tubing or across the flushless transducer may be the cause. Systematically assess the system for air and debris. Make sure the drain is leveled at the appropriate landmark and the system rezeroed. If a waveform still fails to appear, replace the pressure cable, module, or transducer; change only one at a time.[1]

■ Don't routinely change the drainage tubing; leave it in place for the duration of external ventricular drainage. If the drainage tubing becomes accidently disconnected, maintain the sterility of the ventricular catheter, and obtain and connect a new sterile drainage system.[1]

■ When accessing an external ventricular drainage system, perform hand hygiene, put on a mask, set up a sterile field, and put on sterile gloves. Scrub the access port for 3 minutes using a facility-approved antiseptic solution such as povidone-iodine and follow the manufacturer's instructions for use.[1,4,5,6,7,8,9,10]

■ Maintain the external ventricular drainage system bag in an upright position. If it must be laid down, drain the CSF to the lower collection bag *to decrease the transfer of bacteria in the collection chamber to the drainage bag*. Change the drainage bag when it's nearly full, wearing sterile gloves and a mask.[1]

■ Change the catheter insertion site dressing every 48 hours, when soiled, or as directed by your facility.[1] When changing the dressing, put on a

Interpreting ICP waveforms

You must be familiar with intracranial pressure (ICP) waveforms so you can quickly identify and respond to changes that may indicate decreased intracranial compliance.

Normal waveform

A normal ICP waveform typically has three peaks: P1, P2, and P3. P1, the pressure wave, originates from choroid plexus pulsations. P2, the tidal wave, is more variable in shape and amplitude, and ends on the dicrotic notch. P3, the dicrotic wave, falls after the dicrotic notch and commonly tapers downward. P3 is caused by closure of the aortic valve. Some individuals may have additional peaks, but they aren't as clinically significant as the three main peaks. This waveform occurs continuously and indicates an ICP in the normal range, between 0 and 15 mm Hg.

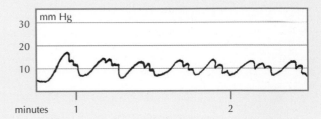

Abnormal ICP waveforms

The P2 portion of the ICP waveform most directly reflects the state of the brain's compliance. Abnormal ICP waveform trends include A, B, and C waves.

A waves

As mean ICP rises, P2 progressively elevates, causing the pulse wave to appear more rounded. The most clinically significant ICP waveforms are *A* waves, which can reach elevations of 50 to 100 mm Hg, persist for 5 to 20 minutes, and then drop sharply, signaling exhaustion of the brain's compliance mechanisms. *A* waves may come and go, spiking in response to temporary rises in thoracic pressure or to any condition that increases ICP beyond the brain's compliance limits. Certain activities, such as sustained coughing and straining during defecation, can cause temporary elevations in thoracic pressure. *Because* A *waves are an ominous sign*, they require emergency treatment.

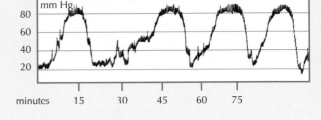

B waves

B waves, which appear sharp and rhythmic with a sawtooth pattern, occur every 1½ to 2 minutes and may reach elevations of 50 mm Hg. The clinical significance of *B* waves isn't clear, but the waves correlate with respiratory changes and may occur more frequently with decreasing compensation. *Because* B *waves sometimes precede* A *waves*, notify the practitioner if *B* waves occur frequently.

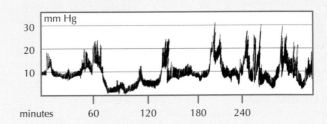

C waves

C waves are rapid and rhythmic, but not sharp, and last 1 to 2 minutes with an ICP of 20 to 50 mm Hg. Clinically insignificant, they may fluctuate with respirations or systemic blood pressure changes.

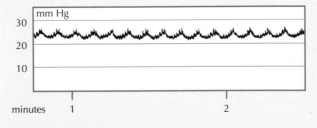

Waveform showing equipment problem

A waveform such as the one shown at right signals a problem with the flushless transducer or monitor. Check for line obstruction and determine if the transducer needs rebalancing. If the patient has a low ICP reading, this waveform may be normal.

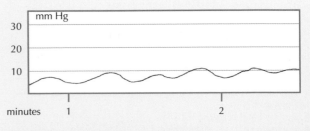

mask,[38] perform hand hygiene,[6,7,8,9,10,11] and put on sterile gloves.[4,5] Remove and discard the old dressing.[4] Then clip any hair that has grown back at the insertion site, as needed. Inspect the site for CSF leakage and signs of infection. Remove and discard your gloves,[4,5] perform hand hygiene,[6,7,8,9,10,11] put on a new pair of sterile gloves,[4,5] and place a new sterile occlusive dressing over the site.[1] Then remove and discard your gloves.[4,5]

- Perform hand hygiene.[6,7,8,9,10,11]
- Document the procedure.[39,40,41,42]

Special considerations

- The Joint Commission has issued a sentinel event alert concerning medical device alarm safety, *because alarm-related events have been associated with permanent loss of function and death*. Among the major contributing factors were improper alarm settings, inappropriately turned-off alarms, and alarm signals not audible to staff. Make sure that alarm limits are appropriately set, and that alarms are turned on, functioning properly, and audible to staff. Follow facility guidelines for preventing alarm fatigue.[25]

Managing ICP

By performing nursing care gently, slowly, and cautiously, you can best help manage—or even significantly reduce—increased intracranial pressure (ICP). If possible, urge the patient to participate in care. Here are some steps you can take to manage increased ICP.

- Plan your care to include rest periods between activities, and minimize external stimulation *to allow the patient's ICP to return to baseline, thus avoiding lengthy and cumulative pressure elevations.*
- Speak to the patient before attempting any procedures, even if the patient appears comatose. Touch the patient on an arm or leg first before touching in a more personal area, such as the face or chest. This is especially important if the patient doesn't know you, or if the patient is confused or sedated.
- Suction the patient only when it's necessary to remove secretions and maintain airway patency.
- Hyperventilate the patient with 100% oxygen as ordered. *Hyperventilation with oxygen from a handheld resuscitation bag or ventilator helps rid the patient of excess carbon dioxide, thereby constricting cerebral vessels and reducing cerebral blood volume and ICP. However, only normal brain tissues respond, because blood vessels in damaged areas have reduced vasoconstrictive ability.* Hyperventilation should only be used in an acute situation to decrease ICP until other measures can be instituted, *because it can cause ischemia.*[1]

- *To promote venous drainage,* keep the patient's head in the midline position, even when the patient is side-lying.[1] Avoid flexing the neck or hip more than 90 degrees, and keep the head of the bed elevated 30 to 45 degrees. Keep endotracheal tube ties and rigid cervical collars secure, but loose enough *to prevent compression of the jugular veins.*
- Avoid placing the patient in the prone position.
- *To avoid increasing intrathoracic pressure, which raises ICP,* discourage the Valsalva maneuver and isometric muscle contractions. *To avoid isometric contractions,* distract the patient when giving painful injections by asking the patient to wiggle the toes and by massaging the area before injection *to relax the muscle,* and have the patient concentrate on breathing through difficult procedures such as bed-to-stretcher transfers. *To keep the patient from holding the breath when moving around in bed,* tell the patient to relax as much as possible during position changes. If necessary, administer a stool softener *to help prevent constipation and unnecessary straining during defecation.*
- If the patient is heavily sedated, monitor respiratory rate and blood gas levels. *Depressed respirations will compromise ventilations and oxygen exchange. Maintaining adequate respiratory rate and volume helps reduce ICP.*

- The Joint Commission has issued a sentinel event alert related to managing risk during transition to new International Organization for Standardization tubing standards that were designed to prevent dangerous tubing misconnections, which can lead to serious patient injury and death. During the transition, make sure to trace each tubing and catheter from the patient to its point of origin before connecting or reconnecting any device or infusion, at any care transition (such as to a new setting or service), and as part of the hand-off process. In addition, route tubes and catheters with different purposes in different, standardized directions; label tubing at both the distal and proximal ends when the patient has different access sites or several bags hanging; use tubing and equipment only as intended; and store medications for different delivery routes in separate locations.[36]
- If the patient develops increased ICP, open the external ventricular drain to drain CSF, as ordered; administer hyperosmolar therapy with hypertonic saline solution or mannitol, as prescribed.[43]
- Be aware that induced hypothermia may reduce ICP initially but can cause cerebral edema during rewarming, and isn't recommended for treatment of increased ICP.[43]

Complications

CNS infection, the most common hazard of ICP monitoring, can result from contamination of the equipment setup or of the insertion site.

NURSING ALERT Excessive loss of CSF can result from faulty stopcock placement or a drip chamber that's positioned too low. Such loss can rapidly decompress the cranial contents and damage bridging cortical veins, leading to hematoma formation. Decompression can also lead to rupture of existing hematomas or aneurysms, causing hemorrhage.[1]

Watch for signs of impending or overt decompensation, such as decreasing level of consciousness; pupillary dilation (unilateral or bilateral); decreased pupillary response to light; rising systolic blood pressure and widening pulse pressure; bradycardia; slowed, irregular respirations; and, in late decompensation, decerebrate posturing.

Documentation

Record the date and time of the ICP monitoring catheter insertion procedure and the patient's response. Note the catheter insertion site and the type of ICP monitoring system used. Record the zero reference level, ICP digital values, ICP waveforms, and CPP hourly in your notes, on a flowchart, or directly on readout strips, depending on your facility's documentation format. Document any factors that might affect the patient's ICP (for example, drug therapy, stressful procedures, and sleep).

Record routine and neurologic vital signs hourly, and describe the patient's clinical status. Note the amount, character, and frequency of any CSF drainage (for example, "between 6 p.m. and 7 p.m., 15 mL

of blood-tinged CSF"). Also, record the ICP value in response to CSF drainage. Record teaching provided to the patient and family (if applicable), their understanding of that teaching, and any need for follow-up teaching.

REFERENCES

1 American Association of Neuroscience Nurses (AANN). (2014). *Care of the patient undergoing intracranial pressure monitoring/external ventricular drainage or lumbar drainage: AANN clinical practice guideline series.* Glenview, IL: AANN. (Level VII)

2 Accreditation Association for Hospitals and Health Systems. (2020). Standard 25.01.27. *Healthcare Facilities Accreditation Program: Accreditation requirements for acute care hospitals.* Chicago, IL: Accreditation Association for Hospitals and Health Systems. (Level VII)

3 Accreditation Association for Hospitals and Health Systems. (2020). Standard 07.01.10. *Healthcare Facilities Accreditation Program: Accreditation requirements for acute care hospitals.* Chicago, IL: Accreditation Association for Hospitals and Health Systems. (Level VII)

4 Occupational Safety and Health Administration. (2012). Bloodborne pathogens, standard number 1910.1030. https://www.osha.gov/pls/oshaweb/owadisp.show_document?p_id=10051&p_table=STANDARDS (Level VII)

5 Siegel, J. D., et al. (2007, revised 2019). 2007 guideline for isolation precautions: Preventing transmission of infectious agents in healthcare settings. https://www.cdc.gov/infectioncontrol/pdf/guidelines/isolation-guidelines-H.pdf (Level II)

6 The Joint Commission. (2021). Standard NPSG.07.01.01. *Comprehensive accreditation manual for hospitals.* Oakbrook Terrace, IL: The Joint Commission. (Level VII)

7 Centers for Disease Control and Prevention. (2002). Guideline for hand hygiene in health-care settings: Recommendations of the Healthcare Infection Control Practices Advisory Committee and the HICPAC/SHEA/APIC/IDSA Hand Hygiene Task Force. *MMWR Recommendations and Reports, 51*(RR-16), 1–45. https://www.cdc.gov/mmwr/pdf/rr/rr5116.pdf (Level II)

8 World Health Organization. (2009). WHO guidelines on hand hygiene in health care: First global patient safety challenge, clean care is safer care. https://apps.who.int/iris/bitstream/handle/10665/44102/9789241597906_eng.pdf?sequence=1 (Level IV)

9 Accreditation Association for Hospitals and Health Systems. (2020). Standard 07.01.21. *Healthcare Facilities Accreditation Program: Accreditation requirements for acute care hospitals.* Chicago, IL: Accreditation Association for Hospitals and Health Systems. (Level VII)

10 Centers for Medicare and Medicaid Services, Department of Health and Human Services. (2020). Condition of participation: Infection control. 42 C.F.R. § 482.42.

11 DNV GL-Healthcare USA, Inc. (2020). IC.1.SR.1. *NIAHO® accreditation requirements, interpretive guidelines and surveyor guidance—revision 20.0.* Milford, OH: DNV GL-Healthcare USA, Inc. (Level VII)

12 The Joint Commission. (2021). Standard RI.01.03.01. *Comprehensive accreditation manual for hospitals.* Oakbrook Terrace, IL: The Joint Commission. (Level VII)

13 Centers for Medicare and Medicaid Services, Department of Health and Human Services. (2020). Condition of participation: Patient's rights. 42 C.F.R. § 482.13(c)(1).

14 Accreditation Association for Hospitals and Health Systems. (2020). Standard 30.01.11. *Healthcare Facilities Accreditation Program: Accreditation requirements for acute care hospitals.* Chicago, IL: Accreditation Association for Hospitals and Health Systems. (Level VII)

15 DNV GL-Healthcare USA, Inc. (2020). PR.2.SR.3. *NIAHO® accreditation requirements, interpretive guidelines and surveyor guidance—revision 20.0.* Milford, OH: DNV GL-Healthcare USA, Inc. (Level VII)

16 The Joint Commission. (2021). Standard UP.01.01.01. *Comprehensive accreditation manual for hospitals.* Oakbrook Terrace, IL: The Joint Commission. (Level VII)

17 Accreditation Association for Hospitals and Health Systems. (2020). Standard 30.00.14. *Healthcare Facilities Accreditation Program: Accreditation requirements for acute care hospitals.* Chicago, IL: Accreditation Association for Hospitals and Health Systems. (Level VII)

18 The Joint Commission. (2021). Standard NPSG.01.01.01. *Comprehensive accreditation manual for hospitals.* Oakbrook Terrace, IL: The Joint Commission. (Level VII)

19 Accreditation Association for Hospitals and Health Systems. (2020). Standard 15.01.16. *Healthcare Facilities Accreditation Program: Accreditation requirements for acute care hospitals.* Chicago, IL: Accreditation Association for Hospitals and Health Systems. (Level VII)

20 The Joint Commission. (2021). Standard PC.02.01.21. *Comprehensive accreditation manual for hospitals.* Oakbrook Terrace, IL: The Joint Commission. (Level VII)

21 Waters, T. R., et al. (2009). Safe patient handling training for schools of nursing. https://www.cdc.gov/niosh/docs/2009-127/pdfs/2009-127.pdf (Level VII)

22 American Association of Critical-Care Nurses. (2018). AACN practice alert. Managing alarms in acute care across the life span: Electrocardiography and pulse oximetry. https://www.aacn.org/clinical-resources/practice-alerts/managing-alarms-in-acute-care-across-the-life-span (Level VII)

23 Graham, K. C., & Cvach, M. (2010). Monitor alarm fatigue: Standardizing use of physiological monitors and decreasing nuisance alarms. *American Journal of Critical Care, 19,* 28–37.

24 The Joint Commission. (2021). Standard NPSG.06.01.01. *Comprehensive accreditation manual for hospitals.* Oakbrook Terrace, IL: The Joint Commission. (Level VII)

25 The Joint Commission. (2013). Sentinel event alert 50: Medical device alarm safety in hospitals. https://www.jointcommission.org/assets/1/6/SEA_50_alarms_4_26_16.pdf (Level VII)

26 Wiegand, D. L. (2017). *AACN procedure manual for high acuity, progressive, and critical care* (7th ed.). St. Louis, MO: Elsevier.

27 The Joint Commission. (2021). Standard PC.01.02.07. *Comprehensive accreditation manual for hospitals.* Oakbrook Terrace, IL: The Joint Commission. (Level VII)

28 Accreditation Association for Hospitals and Health Systems. (2020). Standard 16.01.03. *Healthcare Facilities Accreditation Program: Accreditation requirements for acute care hospitals.* Chicago, IL: Accreditation Association for Hospitals and Health Systems. (Level VII)

29 Centers for Medicare and Medicaid Services, Department of Health and Human Services. (2020). Condition of participation: Nursing services. 42 C.F.R. § 482.23(c).

30 DNV GL-Healthcare USA, Inc. (2020). MM.1.SR.3. *NIAHO® accreditation requirements, interpretive guidelines and surveyor guidance—revision 20.0.* Milford, OH: DNV GL-Healthcare USA, Inc. (Level VII)

31 The Joint Commission. (2021). Standard MM.06.01.01. *Comprehensive accreditation manual for hospitals.* Oakbrook Terrace, IL: The Joint Commission. (Level VII)

32 The Joint Commission. (2021). Standard UP.01.02.01. *Comprehensive accreditation manual for hospitals.* Oakbrook Terrace, IL: The Joint Commission. (Level VII)

33 Becton, Dickinson and Company. (n.d.). Skin preparation. http://www.bd.com/en-us/offerings/capabilities/infection-prevention/skin-preparation

34 The Joint Commission. (2021). Standard UP.01.03.01. *Comprehensive accreditation manual for hospitals.* Oakbrook Terrace, IL: The Joint Commission. (Level VII)

35 U.S. Food and Drug Administration. (2017). Examples of medical device misconnections. https://www.fda.gov/medical-devices/medical-device-connectors/examples-medical-device-misconnections

36 The Joint Commission. (2014). Sentinel event alert 53: Managing risk during transition to new ISO tubing connector standards. http://www.jointcommission.org/assets/1/6/SEA_53_Connectors_8_19_14_final.pdf (Level VII)

37 Ganz, D. A., et al. (2013, reviewed 2021). *Preventing falls in hospitals: A toolkit for improving quality of care* (AHRQ Publication No. 13-0015-EF). Rockville, MD: Agency for Healthcare Research and Quality. https://www.ahrq.gov/professionals/systems/hospital/fallpxtoolkit/index.html (Level VII)

38 World Health Organization. (n.d.). Steps to put on personal protective equipment (PPE). https://www.who.int/csr/disease/ebola/put_on_ppequipment.pdf?ua=1

39 The Joint Commission. (2021). Standard RC.01.03.01. *Comprehensive accreditation manual for hospitals.* Oakbrook Terrace, IL: The Joint Commission. (Level VII)

40 Accreditation Association for Hospitals and Health Systems. (2020). Standard 10.00.03. *Healthcare Facilities Accreditation Program: Accreditation requirements for acute care hospitals.* Chicago, IL: Accreditation Association for Hospitals and Health Systems. (Level VII)

41 Centers for Medicare and Medicaid Services, Department of Health and Human Services. (2020). Condition of participation: Medical record services. 42 C.F.R. § 482.24(b).

42 DNV GL-Healthcare USA, Inc. (2020). MR.2.SR.1. *NIAHO® accreditation requirements, interpretive guidelines and surveyor guidance—revision 20.0.* Milford, OH: DNV GL-Healthcare USA, Inc. (Level VII)

43 Ropper, A. H. (2012). Hyperosmolar therapy for raised intracranial pressure. *New England Journal of Medicine, 367,* 746–752.

INTRADERMAL INJECTION

Because little systemic absorption of intradermally injected agents takes place, intradermal injections are used primarily to produce a local effect, as in allergy or tuberculin testing. Intradermal injections are administered in small volumes—usually 0.01 to 0.1 mL—into the outer layers of the skin.[1]

The ventral forearm is the most commonly used site for intradermal injection because of its easy accessibility and lack of hair.[1] In extensive allergy testing, the outer aspect of the upper arms may be used. (See *Intradermal injection sites.*)

Equipment

Patient's medication administration record ▪ single-use tuberculin or 1-mL syringe with a 26G or 27G, ¼″ to ½″ (0.64 cm to 1.27 cm) needle ▪ prescribed medication or antigen ▪ alcohol pads ▪ emergency equipment (code cart with emergency medications, defibrillator, handheld resuscitation bag with mask, intubation equipment) ▪ Optional: gloves, marking pen.

Preparation of equipment

Make sure that emergency equipment is functioning properly and readily available. Inspect all equipment and supplies. If a product is expired, is defective, or has compromised integrity, remove it from patient use, label it as expired or defective, and report the expiration or defect, as directed by your facility.

Implementation

▪ Avoid distractions and interruptions when preparing and administering the medication *to prevent medication errors.*[2,3]
▪ Verify the practitioner's order.[4,5,6,7]
▪ Reconcile the patient's medications when a new medication is ordered *to reduce the risk of medication errors, including omissions, duplications, dosing errors, and drug interactions.*[8,9]
▪ Perform hand hygiene.[10]
▪ Gather and prepare the necessary equipment and supplies, including the medication and an appropriate-sized syringe with needle.

Intradermal injection sites

The most common intradermal injection site is the ventral forearm. Other sites (indicated by dotted areas) include the upper chest, upper arms, and shoulder blades. Skin in these areas is usually lightly pigmented, thinly keratinized, and relatively hairless, facilitating detection of adverse reactions.

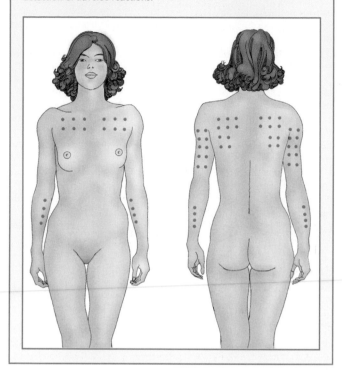

■ Compare the medication label with the order in the patient's medical record.[4,5,6,7]

■ Review the patient's medical record for drug allergies or contraindications to the prescribed medication. If an allergy or a contraindication exists, don't administer the medication; instead, notify the practitioner.[4,5,6,7])

■ Check the expiration date on the medication. If the medication is expired, return it to the pharmacy and obtain new medication.[4,5,6,7]

■ Visually inspect the prescribed medication for particles, discoloration, or other loss of integrity; don't administer the medication if its integrity is compromised.[4,5,6,7]

NURSING ALERT Never use medication that's cloudy or discolored or that contains a precipitate unless the manufacturer's instructions allow it. Remember that for some drugs (such as suspensions), the presence of drug particles is normal. When in doubt, check with the pharmacist.

■ Discuss any unresolved concerns about the medication with the patient's practitioner.[4,5,6,7]

■ Perform hand hygiene.[10,11,12,13,14,15,16,17]

■ Calculate the dose and draw up the medication in a clean, dry work space that is free of clutter and contamination.[10] Follow sterile, no-touch technique during preparation of medication *to prevent the transfer of microorganisms to the patient.*[10] Make sure to disinfect the rubber stopper of the medication vial with alcohol before inserting the needle.[10]

■ Perform hand hygiene.[10,11,12,13,14,15,16,17]

■ Confirm the patient's identity using at least two patient identifiers.[18]

■ Provide privacy.[19,20,21,22]

■ Explain the procedure to the patient and family (if appropriate) according to their individual communication and learning needs *to increase their understanding, allay their fears, and enhance cooperation.*[23] Tell the patient where you'll be giving the injection.

■ If the patient is receiving the medication for the first time, teach about potential adverse reactions and discuss any other concerns related to the medication.[4,5,6,7]

■ Verify that the medication is being administered at the proper time, in the prescribed dose, and by the correct route *to reduce the risk of medication errors.*[4,5,6,7]

■ If your facility uses a bar-code technology, use it, as directed by your facility.

■ Perform hand hygiene.[10,11,12,13,14,15,16,17]

■ Put on gloves if contact with blood or other body fluids is likely, or if your skin or the patient's skin isn't intact.[24,25,26] Gloves aren't recommended for routine intradermal injection *because they don't protect against needlestick injury.*[11]

■ Instruct the patient to sit up and to extend the arm, and support it on a flat surface with the ventral forearm exposed (as shown below).

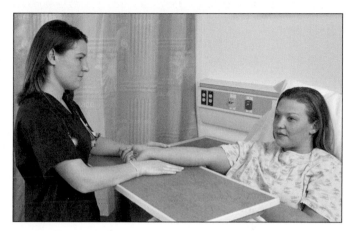

■ Select the site of injection on the ventral forearm about two or three fingerbreadths distal to the antecubital space. Be sure the test site is free of hair or blemishes.

■ With an alcohol pad, wipe the area from the center of the injection site working outward.[11] Allow the skin to dry completely before administering the injection.[11]

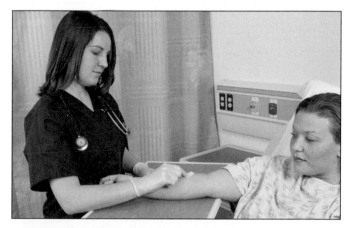

■ While holding the patient's forearm in your hand, stretch the skin taut with your thumb (as shown below).

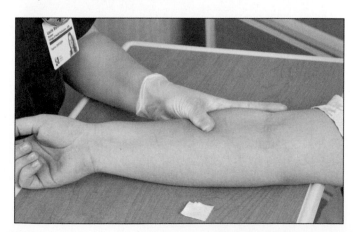

■ With your free hand, hold the needle at a 5- to 15-degree angle to the patient's arm, with its bevel up (as shown below).[27]

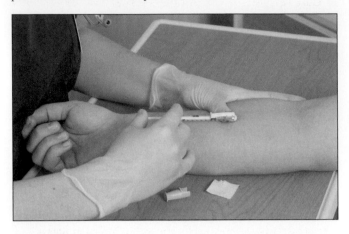

■ Insert the needle about ⅛″ (0.3 cm) below the epidermis. Stop when the needle's bevel tip is under the skin, and inject the antigen slowly. You should feel some resistance as you do this, and a wheal should form (as shown below). If no wheal forms, you have injected the antigen too deeply; withdraw the needle, and administer another test dose at least 2″ (5 cm) from the first site.

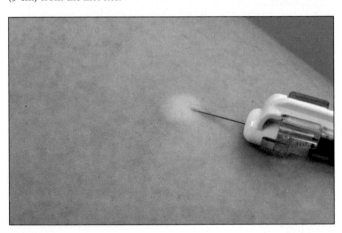

■ Withdraw the needle at the same angle you used to insert it. Don't rub the site. *Rubbing could irritate the underlying tissue, which may affect test results.*
■ Don't recap the needle. Dispose of needles and syringes in a leak-proof, puncture-resistance container.[11,24]
■ If you're administering multiple antigens, inject them at sites at least 2″ (5 cm) apart. Circle each test site with a marking pen, and label each site according to the recall antigen given. Instruct the patient to refrain from washing off the circles until the test is completed.
■ Remove and discard your gloves, if worn.[24]
■ Perform hand hygiene.[10,11,12,13,14,15,16,17]
■ Document the procedure.[28,29,30,31]

Special considerations

■ Use single-dose vials for parenteral medications whenever possible. Don't administer medications from single-dose vials or ampules to multiple patients or combine leftover contents for later use.[10,32,33]
■ Dedicate multidose medication vials to one patient whenever possible *to reduce the risk of bloodborne pathogen transmission and infection. Dedicating a multidose vial to one patient reduces infection transmission risk.* If you must use multidose vials for more than one patient, keep and access them in a dedicated medication preparation area away from immediate patient treatment areas *to prevent inadvertent contamination of the vial through direct or indirect contact with potentially contaminated surfaces or equipment that could lead to infection in subsequent patients.*[10,32,33] If you must use multidose vials, ensure that the

needle or cannula and syringe you use to access the multidose vial are sterile.[25]
■ The Joint Commission has issued a sentinel event alert concerning the transmission of pathogens related to the misuse of vials that have caused viral and bacterial infections, including hepatitis B, hepatitis C, meningitis, and epidural abscesses. These infections have been attributed to the reuse of single-dose vials that typically don't contain preservatives, reentry of multidose vials with used syringes and needles, and use of multidose vials for multiple patients. To prevent these infections, follow evidence-based best practices, such as disinfecting the vial's rubber stopper before piercing, using single-dose vials only once and then discarding the vial, dedicating multidose vials to a single patient, and using a new syringe and needle when reentering a multidose vial. Assign the appropriate "beyond-use" date when first entering a multidose vial, and store multidose vials as directed by your facility and according to the manufacturer's instructions.[32]
■ If you aren't administering the medication immediately after drawing it up, label the syringe with the patient's name, the name and amount of medication, your name or initials, the date and time of preparation, and the beyond-use date and time.[10,34]
■ Be aware that patients who are hypersensitive to test antigens can experience a severe anaphylactic response. This reaction requires immediate epinephrine injection and other emergency resuscitation procedures. Be especially alert after giving a test dose of penicillin or tetanus antitoxin.[35]
■ Assess the patient's reaction to administered antigens; for tuberculin skin testing, you should do so in 48 to 72 hours.[36]

Patient teaching

Instruct the patient to return for follow-up testing or results interpretation as indicated.

Complications

An allergic reaction or pain may occur as a result of the medication injected.

Documentation

Document the name, strength, and dose of the medication or antigen you administered; the route of administration; the lot number or expiration date, as indicated; the date and time of administration; and the injection site. Note skin reactions and other adverse reactions to the prescribed medication, the name of the practitioner you notified, the date and time of notification, prescribed interventions, and the patient's response to those interventions. Document teaching you provided to the patient and family (if appropriate), their understanding of that teaching, and any need for follow-up teaching. Document any test results according to your facility's documentation format.

References

1 Craven, R. F., et al. (2021). *Fundamentals of nursing: Concepts and competencies for practice* (9th ed.). Philadelphia, PA: Wolters Kluwer.
2 Westbrook, J., et al. (2010). Association of interruptions with an increased risk and severity of medication administration errors. *Archives of Internal Medicine, 170*, 683–690. (Level IV)
3 Institute for Safe Medication Practices. (2012). Side tracks on the safety express: Interruptions lead to errors and unfinished...Wait, what was I doing? https://www.ismp.org/resources/side-tracks-safety-express-interruptions-lead-errors-and-unfinished-wait-what-was-i-doing?id=37
4 The Joint Commission. (2021). Standard MM.06.01.01. *Comprehensive accreditation manual for hospitals.* Oakbrook Terrace, IL: The Joint Commission. (Level VII)
5 Accreditation Association for Hospitals and Health Systems. (2020). Standard 16.01.03. *Healthcare Facilities Accreditation Program: Accreditation requirements for acute care hospitals.* Chicago, IL: Accreditation Association for Hospitals and Health Systems. (Level VII)
6 Centers for Medicare and Medicaid Services, Department of Health and Human Services. (2020). Condition of participation: Nursing services. 42 C.F.R. § 482.23(c).
7 DNV GL-Healthcare USA, Inc. (2020). MM.1.SR.3. *NIAHO® accreditation requirements, interpretive guidelines and surveyor guidance—revision 20.0.* Milford, OH: DNV GL-Healthcare USA, Inc. (Level VII)

8   Accreditation Association for Hospitals and Health Systems. (2020). Standard 25.02.13. *Healthcare Facilities Accreditation Program: Accreditation requirements for acute care hospitals*. Chicago, IL: Accreditation Association for Hospitals and Health Systems. (Level VII)

9   The Joint Commission. (2021). Standard NPSG.03.06.01. *Comprehensive accreditation manual for hospitals*. Oakbrook Terrace, IL: The Joint Commission. (Level VII)

10 Dolan, S. A., et al. (2016). APIC position paper: Safe injection, infusion, and medication practices in health care. *American Journal of Infection Control, 44*(7), 750–757.

11 World Health Organization. (2010). WHO best practices for injections and related procedures toolkit. http://apps.who.int/iris/bitstream/10665/44298/1/9789241599252_eng.pdf (Level IV)

12 Accreditation Association for Hospitals and Health Systems. (2020). Standard 07.01.21. *Healthcare Facilities Accreditation Program: Accreditation requirements for acute care hospitals*. Chicago, IL: Accreditation Association for Hospitals and Health Systems. (Level VII)

13 Centers for Medicare and Medicaid Services, Department of Health and Human Services. (2020). Condition of participation: Infection control. 42 C.F.R. § 482.42.

14 The Joint Commission. (2021). Standard NPSG.07.01.01. *Comprehensive accreditation manual for hospitals*. Oakbrook Terrace, IL: The Joint Commission. (Level VII)

15 World Health Organization. (2009). WHO guidelines on hand hygiene in health care: First global patient safety challenge, clean care is safer care. https://apps.who.int/iris/bitstream/handle/10665/44102/9789241597906_eng.pdf?sequence=1 (Level IV)

16 Centers for Disease Control and Prevention. (2002). Guideline for hand hygiene in health-care settings: Recommendations of the Healthcare Infection Control Practices Advisory Committee and the HICPAC/SHEA/APIC/IDSA Hand Hygiene Task Force. *MMWR Recommendations and Reports, 51*(RR-16), 1–45. https://www.cdc.gov/mmwr/pdf/rr/rr5116.pdf (Level II)

17 DNV GL-Healthcare USA, Inc. (2020). IC.1.SR.1. *NIAHO® accreditation requirements, interpretive guidelines and surveyor guidance—revision 20.0*. Milford, OH: DNV GL-Healthcare USA, Inc. (Level VII)

18 The Joint Commission. (2021). Standard NPSG.01.01.01. *Comprehensive accreditation manual for hospitals*. Oakbrook Terrace, IL: The Joint Commission. (Level VII)

19 The Joint Commission. (2021). Standard RI.01.01.01. *Comprehensive accreditation manual for hospitals*. Oakbrook Terrace, IL: The Joint Commission. (Level VII)

20 Accreditation Association for Hospitals and Health Systems. (2020). Standard 15.01.16. *Healthcare Facilities Accreditation Program: Accreditation requirements for acute care hospitals*. Chicago, IL: Accreditation Association for Hospitals and Health Systems. (Level VII)

21 Centers for Medicare and Medicaid Services, Department of Health and Human Services. (2020). Condition of participation: Patient's rights. 42 C.F.R. § 482.13(c)(1).

22 DNV GL-Healthcare USA, Inc. (2020). PR.2.SR.5. *NIAHO® accreditation requirements, interpretive guidelines and surveyor guidance—revision 20.0*. Milford, OH: DNV GL-Healthcare USA, Inc. (Level VII)

23 The Joint Commission. (2021). Standard PC.02.01.21. *Comprehensive accreditation manual for hospitals*. Oakbrook Terrace, IL: The Joint Commission. (Level VII)

24 Occupational Safety and Health Administration. (2012). Bloodborne pathogens, standard number 1910.1030. https://www.osha.gov/pls/oshaweb/owadisp.show_document?p_id=10051&p_table=STANDARDS (Level VII)

25 Siegel, J. D., et al. (2007, revised 2019). 2007 guideline for isolation precautions: Preventing transmission of infectious agents in healthcare settings. https://www.cdc.gov/infectioncontrol/pdf/guidelines/isolation-guidelines-H.pdf (Level II)

26 Accreditation Association for Hospitals and Health Systems. (2020). Standard 07.01.10. *Healthcare Facilities Accreditation Program: Accreditation requirements for acute care hospitals*. Chicago, IL: Accreditation Association for Hospitals and Health Systems. (Level VII)

27 Tarnow, K., & King, N. (2004). Intradermal injections: Traditional bevel up versus bevel down. *Applied Nursing Research, 17*, 275–282. (Level VI)

28 The Joint Commission. (2021). Standard RC.01.03.01. *Comprehensive accreditation manual for hospitals*. Oakbrook Terrace, IL: The Joint Commission. (Level VII)

29 Accreditation Association for Hospitals and Health Systems. (2020). Standard 10.00.03. *Healthcare Facilities Accreditation Program: Accreditation requirements for acute care hospitals*. Chicago, IL: Accreditation Association for Hospitals and Health Systems. (Level VII)

30 Centers for Medicare and Medicaid Services, Department of Health and Human Services. (2020). Condition of participation: Medical record services. 42 C.F.R. § 482.24(b).

31 DNV GL-Healthcare USA, Inc. (2020). MR.2.SR.1. *NIAHO® accreditation requirements, interpretive guidelines and surveyor guidance—revision 20.0*. Milford, OH: DNV GL-Healthcare USA, Inc. (Level VII)

32 The Joint Commission. (2014). Sentinel event alert 52: Preventing infection from the misuse of vials. https://www.jointcommission.org/-/media/tjc/documents/resources/patient-safety-topics/sentinel-event/sea_52.pdf (Level VII)

33 Centers for Disease Control and Prevention. (2019). Injection safety. Questions about multi-dose vials: Frequently asked questions (FAQs) regarding safe practices for medical injections. https://www.cdc.gov/injectionsafety/providers/provider_faqs_multivials.html

34 The Joint Commission. (2021). Standard MM.05.01.09. *Comprehensive accreditation manual for hospitals*. Oakbrook Terrace, IL: The Joint Commission. (Level VII)

35 Hinkle, J. L., & Cheever, K. H. (2018). *Brunner and Suddarth's textbook of medical-surgical nursing* (14th ed.). Philadelphia, PA: Wolters Kluwer.

36 Centers for Disease Control and Prevention. (2016). Testing for tuberculosis (TB). https://www.cdc.gov/tb/publications/factsheets/testing/tb_testing.htm

INTRAOSSEOUS INFUSION

When rapid venous access is difficult or impossible, intraosseous (IO) access allows short-term delivery of fluids, medications, or blood into the bone marrow. (See *Understanding IO infusion*, page 480.) IO access may be appropriate in emergencies or urgent situations where reliable venous access can't be achieved quickly (such as in patients with shock, sepsis, status epilepticus, extensive burns, multiple trauma, or cardiopulmonary arrest) or in patients for whom IV access is medically necessary and can't be achieved by other means despite multiple attempts.[1,2,3,4,5] Insertion of an IO catheter is quicker than insertion of a central venous catheter; however, unlike with other venous access devices, an IO device should remain in place only until conventional vascular access is possible and for no longer than 24 hours, *because prolonged infusion significantly increases the risk of infection*.[2,3,4,5] All medications and fluids that can be administered through peripheral or central venous access can be administered through IO access.[6] The onset of drug action through IO administration is similar to that of IV administration, and serum drug levels are comparable for most drugs.[1,5,7,8]

There are three different types of IO devices: manually inserted needles, impact-driven devices, and battery-powered drill devices.[2,3,5,7] Whereas manually inserted needles are commonly used in pediatric patients owing to their softer bones, they are more difficult to place in adult patients. Therefore, impact-driven devices (such as the NIO, BIG, and FASTResponder) and battery-powered drills (such as the EZ-IO) are more commonly used in adults, whose bones have hardened.[2,9]

IO insertion is contraindicated at sites with previous IO access or attempted access, fractures, previous surgery, a prosthetic joint, and obscured anatomic landmarks, as well as at sites with infection, severe burns, or local vascular compromise. IO access device insertion may be contraindicated in patients with osteogenesis imperfecta, osteopetrosis, and severe osteoporosis.[2,4,5] Patients with right-to-left intracardiac shunts may be at increased risk for cerebral fat or bone-marrow emboli.[6] Only personnel trained in this procedure should perform it. With adequate training and proven competency, and in accordance with local and state regulations, a registered nurse may insert, maintain, and remove IO access devices.[2,10]

Equipment

Gloves ▪ antiseptic agent and applicator (chlorhexidine or povidone-iodine) ▪ appropriate-sized IO infusion device ▪ stabilization or protective device ▪ 5-mL syringe ▪ prefilled 10-mL syringes containing preservative-free normal saline flush solution ▪ extension set ▪ tape ▪ IV administration set and needleless connector ▪ prescribed fluids or medications ▪ sterile marker ▪ labels ▪ Optional: other personal protective

Understanding IO infusion

Intraosseous (IO) infusion devices typically are placed in the epiphysis (proximal and distal ends) of long bones *because of the thinner outer layer of compact bone and abundance of spongy cancellous bone at these sites.* Within the medullary (marrow) cavity is a vast system of blood vessels.[5,7,8]

During IO infusion, the bone marrow serves as a noncollapsible vein, allowing fluid infused into the medullary cavity of the bone to rapidly pass from this space through the vascular system and into the central circulation. The illustration shows fluid flowing through an IO infusion device positioned in the patient's proximal humerus.

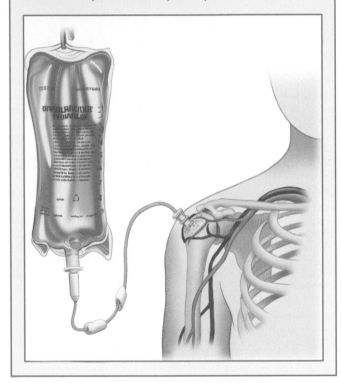

equipment (such as a gown and a mask with a face shield or a mask and goggles), soap and water, single-patient-use scissors or disposable-head clippers, local anesthetic solution (lidocaine 2% [preservative- and EPINEPHrine-free]) and administration supplies, specimen tubes, labels, laboratory biohazard transport bag, sterile occlusive dressing, electronic infusion device (preferably a smart pump with dose-error reduction software), pressure bag, stethoscope, disinfectant pad, infusion device or pressure bag, vital signs monitoring equipment, tape measure.

Some IO insertion devices come in kits with many of the necessary supplies.

Preparation of equipment

Inspect all IV equipment and supplies. If a product is expired, is defective, or has compromised integrity, remove it from patient use, label it as expired or defective, and report the expiration or defect as directed by your facility.[11] Prepare any prescribed IV fluids or medications, and prime the administration set and extension set. Using a sterile marker, label all medications, medication containers, and other solutions.[12,13] Review the IO infusion device manufacturer's instructions before insertion.

Implementation

- Verify the practitioner's order.
- If time permits, confirm that informed consent has been obtained and that the signed consent form is in the patient's medical record.[14,15,16,17]
- Review the patient's history for hypersensitivity to the local anesthetic solution, antiseptic solutions, and latex as well as contraindications to the procedure.

- If time permits, perform a preprocedure verification *to make sure that all relevant documentation, related information, and equipment are available and correctly identified to the patient's identifiers.*[18,19]
- Perform hand hygiene.[20]
- Gather and prepare the necessary equipment and supplies.
- Perform hand hygiene.[21,22,23,24,25,26]
- Confirm the patient's identity using at least two patient identifiers.[27]
- Provide privacy.[28,29,30,31]
- Explain the procedure to the patient (if conscious) and family (if appropriate) according to their individual communication and learning needs *to increase their understanding, allay fears, and enhance cooperation.*[32] Tell them which bone site will receive the IO infusion device. Inform the patient that a local anesthetic will be administered but that feeling pressure during needle insertion is to be expected.
- Raise the bed to waist level before providing patient care *to prevent caregiver back strain.*[33]
- Perform hand hygiene.[21,22,23,24,25,26]
- Identify the intended insertion site based on the patient's clinical condition and the device manufacturer's guidelines.[4,5,7]
- Common intraosseous insertion sites in adults include the proximal tibia, distal tibia, proximal humerus, and sternum.[4,5,6,7] For the proximal tibia, palpate the tibial tuberosity and move 2 cm medially and 1 cm proximally. For the distal tibia, palpate the medial malleolus and move 1 to 2 cm proximally along the medial aspect of the leg. For the proximal humerus, palpate the greater tubercle and move 2 cm distally along the lateral aspect of the arm. For the sternum, palpate the sternal notch; the site is in the manubrium (superior ⅓ of the sternum) 1.5 cm below the sternal notch.
- Position the patient in a supine position and ensure that the selected insertion site is exposed.
- If the intended insertion site is visibly soiled, put on gloves and then clean the site with soap and water.[3,34,35,36] Remove and discard your gloves and perform hand hygiene.[21,22,23,24,25,26]
- If time permits, conduct a time-out immediately before starting the procedure *to perform a final assessment that the correct patient, site, positioning, and procedure are identified and that all relevant information and necessary equipment are available.*[18,37]
- Prepare the insertion site using a skin antiseptic agent.[3,4,5] For chlorhexidine (preferred), apply with an applicator using a vigorous sided-to-side motion for 30 seconds, and then allow the area to dry completely. For povidone-iodine solution, apply using a swab, beginning at the intended insertion site and moving outward in concentric circles. Allow the solution to dry completely (typically, at least 2 minutes).
- If the patient is conscious and time permits, inject local anesthetic solution into the subcutaneous tissue at the intended site, as ordered or as directed by your facility, following safe medication administration practices.[3,4,38,39,40,41]
- If you're inserting the IO device into a limb, stabilize the limb with your nondominant hand.[3,5]
- Insert the IO device according to the manufacturer's instructions for use.

Impact-driven device

- With your nondominant hand, firmly place the device against the patient's skin at a 90-degree angle to the insertion site.
- With your dominant hand, grasp the "shoulders" of the device with your fingers and apply downward pressure with your palm until the device deploys.
- Hold the hub of the needle or catheter in place.
- Remove the insertion device and trocar (if present), leaving the needle or catheter in place.

Battery-powered drill device

- Attach an appropriate-sized needle to the drill and remove the safety cap.
- Insert the tip of the needle perpendicularly into the skin at the insertion site until you feel bone. Ensure that at least 5 mm of the catheter is visible above the skin at this point.
- Squeeze the trigger of the drill and apply slight downward pressure until the needle hub reaches the skin or you feel a decrease in resistance.

- Hold the hub of the stylet and catheter in place and detach and remove the drill by pulling it straight up from the catheter.
- Unscrew and remove the stylet from the hub, leaving the catheter in place.
- Secure the IO device to the skin with an appropriate stabilization or protective device *to prevent dislodgment.*[3,4,5]
- Attach a 5-mL syringe to the IO device and attempt to aspirate blood and bone marrow *to help confirm placement and obtain specimens for laboratory analysis.*

NURSING ALERT The presence of blood or bone marrow on aspiration confirms placement; however, the absence of blood or bone marrow on aspiration doesn't confirm improper placement, especially if the patient is severely dehydrated. Be aware that aspiration may occlude the IO catheter.[3,4,5,9]

- Replace the first syringe with a 10-mL syringe containing preservative-free normal saline flush solution, and then flush the IO device with 5 to 10 mL *to confirm placement and to clear the needle or catheter of clots and bone particles.* The flush solution should flow freely without resistance. Observe the site for swelling, leakage, and a change in skin temperature, *which indicates infiltration or extravasation.*[3,4,5]
- Cover the site with a sterile occlusive dressing, as needed, if not incorporated with the stabilization or protective device.
- Label the dressing with your name and the date and time of IO insertion.[42]
- Connect a primed extension set to the IO device, according to the manufacturer's instructions for use, and secure it to the patient's skin with tape *to avoid tension on the IO device.*[5]
- If the patient is conscious, slowly inject local anesthetic solution into the IO space after establishing access and before infusion, as ordered or as directed by your facility, following safe medication administration practices, *to prevent infusion-related pain.*[3,4,38,39,40,41]
- Attach the needleless connector from the IV administration set to the IO catheter extension set. Trace the IV administration set tubing from the patient to the point of origin *to make sure that you're connecting the tubing to the proper port.*[43] Route the tubing in a standardized direction if the patient has other tubing and catheters that have different purposes. Label the tubing at both the distal ends (near the patient connection) and proximal end (near the source container) *to reduce the risk of misconnection if multiple IV lines will be used.*[44]
- Administer fluids and medications, as ordered, following safe medication administration practices.[38,39,40,41] Use an electronic infusion device or pressure bag as needed *to regulate flow.*[8] If you're using an electronic infusion device, consider the use of a smart pump with dose-error reduction software *to reduce the risk of infusion-related medication errors.*[45]
- After administering each medication, flush the IO device with 5 to 10 mL of preservative-free normal saline flush solution *to ensure delivery of the medication into the circulation.*[5,8]
- Discourage excessive movement of the affected limb. Immobilize the affected limb as needed *to prevent accidental dislodgment.*[8]
- If you collected specimens for laboratory analysis, label them in the presence of the patient *to prevent mislabeling.*[27] Place the specimens in a laboratory biohazard transport bag and immediately send them to the laboratory.[34]
- Monitor the IO insertion site for signs of infiltration or extravasation, compartment syndrome, and infection at a frequency determined by the patient's condition, the practitioner's order, or the facility. Also monitor the limb distal to the insertion site for adequate perfusion. If complications occur, stop the infusion and notify the practitioner.[4,5,8]
- Return the patient's bed to the lowest position *to prevent falls and maintain the patient's safety.*[46]
- Discard used supplies in appropriate receptacles.[34]
- Remove and discard your gloves and, if worn, other personal protective equipment.[34,35]
- Perform hand hygiene.[21,22,23,24,25,26]
- Document the procedure.[47,48,49,50]

Maintenance

- Flush the IO catheter with 10 mL of preservative-free normal saline flush solution after administering each medication *to prevent clotting of the needle with marrow.*[8] Use dextrose 5% in water followed by

preservative-free normal saline solution when the medication is incompatible with normal saline solution.[51]

- Assess the infusion site for infiltration or extravasation. Measure the circumference of the limb distal to the infusion site and compare the result with the baseline measurement and other previous measurements, if necessary. *Swelling associated with infiltration or extravasation may be difficult to observe in obese patients or patients with chronic edema.*[8]
- Make sure the IO catheter is properly secured with an engineered stabilization device *to reduce the risk of infiltration and extravasation.*[4,52]
- Assess the infusion site for infiltration or extravasation. Measure the circumference of the limb distal to the infusion site and compare the result with the baseline measurement and other previous measurements, if necessary. *Swelling associated with infiltration or extravasation may be difficult to observe in obese patients or patients with chronic edema.*[8]
- If the IO catheter is positioned in the proximal tibia, assess for pain with movement of the toes on the same side as the infusion. *Increased pain with palpation and movement is a sign of compartment syndrome.*
- Assess the affected limb for changes in sensation, movement, color, temperature, and circulation.[4]
- Monitor for signs and symptoms of local inflammation and infection, such as erythema, edema, pain, tenderness, and drainage at the insertion site.[5]
- Monitor the patient's vital signs, *because increased temperature may indicate infection.*
- Monitor the patient's intake, output, and electrolyte levels, as ordered, *to promptly detect fluid and electrolyte imbalances.*[39]
- Remove and discard your gloves.[34,35]
- Perform hand hygiene.[21,22,23,24,25,26]
- Return the bed to the lowest position *to prevent falls and maintain the patient's safety.*[46]
- Perform hand hygiene.[21,22,23,24,25,26]
- Clean and disinfect your stethoscope with a disinfectant pad.[53,54]
- Perform hand hygiene.[21,22,23,24,25,26]
- Document the procedure.[47,48,49,50]

Special considerations

- If you need IO access during cardiac arrest, don't interrupt cardiopulmonary resuscitation for IO device insertion.[1]
- In emergency cases, the proximal tibia is the first recommended site of placement for all patients undergoing insertion of an IO device, unless contraindicated. Alternative site choices vary based on age and skeletal maturity. Placement in the sternum requires a specially designed device.[6]
- *An IO device placed in the sternum of a trauma patient may interfere with the placement of a cervical collar,* so an alternative method of cervical stabilization may be needed.[5]
- Some IO device manufacturers supply a target patch that you can affix to the patient's skin in the desired access location, such as the sternum, before IO needle insertion *to aid in placement in the appropriate location.*[7,55]
- If you're administering blood and blood products through the IO device, see the "Transfusion of blood and blood products" procedure.
- Discontinue IO infusion as soon as conventional vascular access is established (preferably within 4 hours), *because prolonged IO infusion significantly increases the risk of infection.* An IO infusion device should remain in place for no longer than 24 hours.[4]
- Note that magnetic resonance imaging is contraindicated in patients with an IO device. The IO device can cause scatter artifact on computed tomography images.[5,8]
- The Joint Commission has issued a sentinel event alert related to managing risk during transition to new International Organization for Standardization tubing standards that were designed to prevent dangerous tubing misconnections, which can lead to serious patient injury and death. During the transition, make sure to trace each tubing and catheter from the patient to its point of origin before connecting or reconnecting any device or infusion, at any care transition (such as to a new setting or service), and as part of the hand-off process. In addition, route tubes and catheters with different purposes in different, standardized directions; label tubing at both the distal and proximal ends when the patient has different access sites or several bags hanging; use tubing and equipment

only as intended; and store medications for different delivery routes in separate locations.[44]

■ The Joint Commission has issued a sentinel event alert concerning medical device alarm safety, *because alarm-related events have been associated with permanent loss of function and death.* Among the major contributing factors were improper alarm settings, inappropriately turned-off alarms, and alarm signals not audible to staff. Make sure that alarm limits are appropriately set, and that alarms are turned on, functioning properly, and audible to staff. Follow facility guidelines for preventing alarm fatigue.[56]

■ If the patient is receiving IV medication, closely monitor for adverse reactions to the medication; notify the practitioner and respond promptly if adverse reactions occur.[39]

■ If available, use an IO alert identification band *to alert staff of the IO access site.*

Complications

The most common complications of IO infusion are pain at the insertion site, and infiltration and extravasation of fluid into the subcutaneous tissue resulting from improper needle placement. Other potential complications include subperiosteal effusion resulting from failure of fluid to enter the marrow space, and clotting in the needle resulting from delayed infusion or failure to flush the needle after placement. Other complications include compartment syndrome, subcutaneous abscess, fat embolism, osteomyelitis, and fracture.[2,5,6]

Documentation

Document the indications for insertion of the IO catheter and your assessment of the insertion site. Record the date and time of insertion; specific site preparation; local anesthetic used; infection prevention and safety precautions taken; insertion method; the type, length, size, and lot number of the device inserted; and device functionality. Document verification of IO catheter placement, the presence of bone marrow aspirate, patency, and ease of flushing. Record the date, time, and type of any laboratory specimens collected. Also document the patient's tolerance of the procedure, any unexpected outcomes, interventions prescribed, and the patient's response to those interventions. Record the type and volume of fluid infused and any medications given.[4,5] Document teaching provided to the patient and family (if applicable), their understanding of that teaching, and any need for follow-up teaching.

References

1 American Heart Association. (2015). Web-based integrated guidelines for cardiopulmonary resuscitation and emergency cardiovascular care—part 7: Adult advances cardiovascular life support. https://ECCguidelines.heart.org (Level II)

2 Consortium on Intraosseous Vascular Access in Healthcare Practice. (2010). Recommendations for the use of intraosseous vascular access for emergent and nonemergent situations in various health care settings: A consensus paper. *Critical Care Nurse, 30*(6), e1–e7. (Level VII)

3 Infusion Nurses Society. (2016). *Policies and procedures for infusion therapy* (5th ed.). Boston, MA: Infusion Nurses Society.

4 Standard 57. Intraosseous access devices. Infusion therapy standards of practice (8th ed.). (2021). *Journal of Infusion Nursing, 44*, S174–S177. (Level VII)

5 Wiegand, D. L. (2017). *AACN procedure manual for high acuity, progressive, and critical care* (7th ed.). St. Louis, MO: Elsevier.

6 Perron, C. E. (2021). Intraosseous infusion. In: *UpToDate*, Stack, A. M., & Wolfson, A. B. (Eds.).

7 Day, M. W. (2011). Intraosseous devices for intravascular access in adult trauma patients. *Critical Care Nurse, 31*, 76–89.

8 Teleflex Incorporated. (2017). *The science and fundamentals of intraosseous vascular access* (3rd ed.). Wayne, PA: Teleflex Incorporated. https://www.teleflex.com/usa/en/clinical-resources/ez-io/documents/EZ-IO_Science_Fundamentals_MC-003266-Rev1-1.pdf#search='intraosseous%20vascular%20access'

9 Hunsaker, S., & Hillis, D. (2013). Intraosseous vascular access for alert patients. *American Journal of Nursing, 113*(11), 34–39.

10 Infusion Nurses Society. (2009). The role of the registered nurse in the insertion of intraosseous access devices. *Journal of Infusion Nursing, 34*, 187–188. (Level VII)

11 Standard 12. Product evaluation, integrity, and defect reporting. Infusion therapy standards of practice (8th ed.). (2021). *Journal of Infusion Nursing, 44*, S45–S46. (Level VII)

12 The Joint Commission. (2021). Standard NPSG.03.04.01. *Comprehensive accreditation manual for hospitals.* Oakbrook Terrace, IL: The Joint Commission. (Level VII)

13 Accreditation Association for Hospitals and Health Systems. (2020). Standard 25.01.27. *Healthcare Facilities Accreditation Program: Accreditation requirements for acute care hospitals.* Chicago, IL: Accreditation Association for Hospitals and Health Systems. (Level VII)

14 Accreditation Association for Hospitals and Health Systems. (2020). Standard 15.01.11. *Healthcare Facilities Accreditation Program: Accreditation requirements for acute care hospitals.* Chicago, IL: Accreditation Association for Hospitals and Health Systems. (Level VII)

15 Centers for Medicare and Medicaid Services, Department of Health and Human Services. (2020). Condition of participation: Patient's rights. 42 C.F.R. § 482.13(b)(2).

16 DNV GL-Healthcare USA, Inc. (2020). PR.2.SR.3. *NIAHO® accreditation requirements, interpretive guidelines and surveyor guidance—revision 20.0.* Milford, OH: DNV GL-Healthcare USA, Inc. (Level VII)

17 The Joint Commission. (2021). Standard RI.01.03.01. *Comprehensive accreditation manual for hospitals.* Oakbrook Terrace, IL: The Joint Commission. (Level VII)

18 Accreditation Association for Hospitals and Health Systems. (2020). Standard 30.00.14. *Healthcare Facilities Accreditation Program: Accreditation requirements for acute care hospitals.* Chicago, IL: Accreditation Association for Hospitals and Health Systems. (Level VII)

19 The Joint Commission. (2021). Standard UP.01.01.01. *Comprehensive accreditation manual for hospitals.* Oakbrook Terrace, IL: The Joint Commission. (Level VII)

20 Association of Professionals in Infection Control and Epidemiology (APIC). (2016). APIC position paper: Safe injection, infusion, and medication vial practices in health care (2016). https://apic.org/Resource_/TinyMceFileManager/Position_Statements/2016APICSIPPositionPaper.pdf (Level VII)

21 Centers for Disease Control and Prevention. (2002). Guideline for hand hygiene in health-care settings: Recommendations of the Healthcare Infection Control Practices Advisory Committee and the HICPAC/SHEA/APIC/IDSA Hand Hygiene Task Force. *MMWR Recommendations and Reports, 51*(RR-16), 1–45. https://www.cdc.gov/mmwr/pdf/rr/rr5116.pdf (Level II)

22 World Health Organization. (2009). WHO guidelines on hand hygiene in health care: First global patient safety challenge, clean care is safer care. https://apps.who.int/iris/bitstream/handle/10665/44102/9789241597906_eng.pdf?sequence=1 (Level IV)

23 The Joint Commission. (2021). Standard NPSG.07.01.01. *Comprehensive accreditation manual for hospitals.* Oakbrook Terrace, IL: The Joint Commission. (Level VII)

24 Centers for Medicare and Medicaid Services, Department of Health and Human Services. (2020). Condition of participation: Infection control. 42 C.F.R. § 482.42.

25 Accreditation Association for Hospitals and Health Systems. (2020). Standard 07.01.21. *Healthcare Facilities Accreditation Program: Accreditation requirements for acute care hospitals.* Chicago, IL: Accreditation Association for Hospitals and Health Systems. (Level VII)

26 DNV GL-Healthcare USA, Inc. (2020). IC.1.SR.1. *NIAHO® accreditation requirements, interpretive guidelines and surveyor guidance—revision 20.0.* Milford, OH: DNV GL-Healthcare USA, Inc. (Level VII)

27 The Joint Commission. (2021). Standard NPSG.01.01.01. *Comprehensive accreditation manual for hospitals.* Oakbrook Terrace, IL: The Joint Commission. (Level VII)

28 The Joint Commission. (2021). Standard RI.01.01.01. *Comprehensive accreditation manual for hospitals.* Oakbrook Terrace, IL: The Joint Commission. (Level VII)

29 Centers for Medicare and Medicaid Services, Department of Health and Human Services. (2020). Condition of participation: Patient's rights. 42 C.F.R. § 482.13(c)(1).

30 Accreditation Association for Hospitals and Health Systems. (2020). Standard 15.01.16. *Healthcare Facilities Accreditation Program: Accreditation requirements for acute care hospitals.* Chicago, IL: Accreditation Association for Hospitals and Health Systems. (Level VII)

31 DNV GL-Healthcare USA, Inc. (2020). PR.2.SR.5. *NIAHO® accreditation requirements, interpretive guidelines and surveyor guidance—revision 20.0.* Milford, OH: DNV GL-Healthcare USA, Inc. (Level VII)

32 The Joint Commission. (2021). Standard PC.02.01.21. *Comprehensive accreditation manual for hospitals.* Oakbrook Terrace, IL: The Joint Commission. (Level VII)

33 Waters, T. R., et al. (2009). Safe patient handling training for schools of nursing. https://www.cdc.gov/niosh/docs/2009-127/pdfs/2009-127.pdf (Level VII)

34 Occupational Safety and Health Administration. (2012). Bloodborne pathogens, standard number 1910.1030. https://www.osha.gov/pls/oshaweb/owadisp.show_document?p_id=10051&p_table=STANDARDS (Level VII)

35 Siegel, J. D., et al. (2007, revised 2019). 2007 guideline for isolation precautions: Preventing transmission of infectious agents in healthcare settings. https://www.cdc.gov/infectioncontrol/pdf/guidelines/isolation-guidelines-H.pdf (Level II)

36 Accreditation Association for Hospitals and Health Systems. (2020). Standard 07.01.10. *Healthcare Facilities Accreditation Program: Accreditation requirements for acute care hospitals.* Chicago, IL: Accreditation Association for Hospitals and Health Systems. (Level VII)

37 The Joint Commission. (2021). Standard UP.01.03.01. *Comprehensive accreditation manual for hospitals.* Oakbrook Terrace, IL: The Joint Commission. (Level VII)

38 Accreditation Association for Hospitals and Health Systems. (2020). Standard 16.01.03. *Healthcare Facilities Accreditation Program: Accreditation requirements for acute care hospitals.* Chicago, IL: Accreditation Association for Hospitals and Health Systems. (Level VII)

39 Centers for Medicare and Medicaid Services, Department of Health and Human Services. (2020). Condition of participation: Nursing services. 42 C.F.R. § 482.23(c).

40 DNV GL-Healthcare USA, Inc. (2020). MM.1.SR.3. *NIAHO® accreditation requirements, interpretive guidelines and surveyor guidance—revision 20.0.* Milford, OH: DNV GL-Healthcare USA, Inc. (Level VII)

41 The Joint Commission. (2021). Standard MM.06.01.01. *Comprehensive accreditation manual for hospitals.* Oakbrook Terrace, IL: The Joint Commission. (Level VII)

42 Standard 42. Vascular access device assessment, care and dressing changes. Infusion therapy standards of practice (8th ed.). (2021). *Journal of Infusion Nursing, 44,* S119–S123. (Level VII)

43 U.S. Food and Drug Administration. (2017). Examples of medical device misconnections. https://www.fda.gov/medical-devices/medical-device-connectors/examples-medical-device-misconnections

44 The Joint Commission. (2014). Sentinel event alert 53: Managing risk during transition to new ISO tubing connector standards. https://www.jointcommission.org/assets/1/6/SEA_53_Connectors_8_19_14_final.pdf (Level VII)

45 Standard 24. Flow-control devices. Infusion therapy standards of practice (8th ed.). (2021). *Journal of Infusion Nursing, 44,* S69–S72. (Level VII)

46 Ganz, D. A., et al. (2013, reviewed 2021). *Preventing falls in hospitals: A toolkit for improving quality of care* (AHRQ Publication No. 13-0015-EF). Rockville, MD: Agency for Healthcare Research and Quality. https://www.ahrq.gov/professionals/systems/hospital/fallpxtoolkit/index.html (Level VII)

47 The Joint Commission. (2021). Standard RC.01.03.01. *Comprehensive accreditation manual for hospitals.* Oakbrook Terrace, IL: The Joint Commission. (Level VII)

48 Accreditation Association for Hospitals and Health Systems. (2020). Standard 10.00.03. *Healthcare Facilities Accreditation Program: Accreditation requirements for acute care hospitals.* Chicago, IL: Accreditation Association for Hospitals and Health Systems. (Level VII)

49 Centers for Medicare and Medicaid Services, Department of Health and Human Services. (2020). Condition of participation: Medical record services. 42 C.F.R. § 482.24(b).

50 DNV GL-Healthcare USA, Inc. (2020). MR.2.SR.1. *NIAHO® accreditation requirements, interpretive guidelines and surveyor guidance—revision 20.0.* Milford, OH: DNV GL-Healthcare USA, Inc. (Level VII)

51 Standard 41. Flushing and locking. Infusion therapy standards of practice (8th ed.). (2021). *Journal of Infusion Nursing, 44,* S113–S119. (Level VII)

52 Standard 38. Vascular access device securement. Infusion therapy standards of practice (8th ed.). (2021). *Journal of Infusion Nursing, 44,* S108–S111. (Level VII)

53 Accreditation Association for Hospitals and Health Systems. (2020). Standard 07.02.03. *Healthcare Facilities Accreditation Program: Accreditation requirements for acute care hospitals.* Chicago, IL: Accreditation Association for Hospitals and Health Systems. (Level VII)

54 Rutala, W. A., et al. (2008, revised 2019). Guideline for disinfection and sterilization in healthcare facilities, 2008. https://www.cdc.gov/infection-control/pdf/guidelines/disinfection-guidelines-H.pdf (Level I)

55 Pyng Medical Corporation. (2011). FAST1 Intraosseous Infusion System: Training device instructions. http://www.pyng.com/wp/wp-content/uploads/2011/03/PM-097a%20FAST1%20Training%20Device%20Instructions.pdf

56 The Joint Commission. (2013). Sentinel event alert 50: Medical device alarm safety in hospitals. https://www.jointcommission.org/assets/1/6/SEA_50_alarms_4_26_16.pdf (Level VII)

INTRAPLEURAL DRUG ADMINISTRATION

An intrapleural drug is injected through the chest wall into the pleural space or instilled through a chest tube placed intrapleurally for drainage.[1] (For more information on chest tube insertion, see the "Chest tube insertion, assisting" procedure.) During intrapleural injection of a drug, the needle passes through the intercostal muscles and parietal pleura on its way to the pleural space. (See *Inserting an intrapleural catheter*, page 484.) Intrapleurally administered drugs diffuse across the parietal pleura and innermost intercostal muscles to affect the intercostal nerves.

Practitioners use intrapleural administration to promote analgesia, treat spontaneous pneumothorax, resolve pleural effusion, and administer chemotherapy.[1] Drugs commonly given by intrapleural injection include tetracycline, tissue plasminogen activator and deoxyribonuclease, streptokinase, anesthetics, sterile talc, biotherapy agents, and chemotherapeutic agents (to treat malignant pleural effusion or tumors).[4] Note that the use of some of these medications, such as tissue plasminogen activator, in the intrapleural space may be off-label.

Contraindications for drug administration by this route include pleural fibrosis or adhesions, which interfere with diffusion of the drug to the intended site; pleural inflammation; sepsis; and infection at the puncture site. Patients with bullous emphysema and those receiving respiratory therapy using positive end-expiratory pressure shouldn't receive intrapleural injections because they may exacerbate an already compromised pulmonary condition.

Computed tomography scans or chest X-rays of the retained pleural fluid or fluid pockets may be completed, and must be evaluated, by the practitioner before administration of certain intrapleural drugs, such as tissue plasminogen activator. Imaging may be repeated with each administration to evaluate the patient's response to therapy. Follow-up imaging and other assessment findings may be used to evaluate the effectiveness of intrapleural therapy.

Nurses should consult their state nurse practice act and facility guidelines to determine whether this procedure is within their scope of practice. Additionally, specialized training or competency measurement may also be required. Follow your facility guidelines. This procedure covers administration through an intrapleural chest tube or intrapleural catheter.

Equipment

An intrapleural drug is typically administered through a 16G to18G blunt-tipped intrapleural (epidural) needle and catheter. Accessory equipment depends on the type of access device the practitioner uses. All equipment must be sterile.

Gloves ▪ sterile gauze pads ▪ antiseptic solution ▪ prescribed medication ▪ appropriate-sized needles and syringes ▪ dressings ▪ tape ▪ chest tube clamp ▪ stethoscope ▪ marker ▪ vital sings monitoring equipment ▪ Optional: 1% lidocaine.

Preparation of equipment

Label all medications and solutions on and off the sterile field *to prevent medication administration errors.*

Inspect all equipment and supplies. If a product is expired, is defective, or has compromised integrity, remove it from patient use, label it as expired or defective, and report the expiration or defect as directed by your facility.

Follow the manufacturer's instructions for preparation of prescribed medication, if necessary.

Implementation

- Avoid distractions and interruptions when preparing and administering medications *to prevent medication administration errors.*[5,6]
- Verify the practitioner's order.[7,8,9,10]
- Review the order *to make sure that the prescribed medication dose, rate, and route of administration are appropriate for the patient's age, condition and access device.* Address concerns about the order with the practitioner, the pharmacist, or your supervisor, and, if needed, the risk management department or as directed by your facility.[7,11]
- Gather and prepare the necessary equipment and supplies.
- Compare the medication label with the order in the patient's medical record.[8,9,10,11,12]
- Check the expiration date on the medication.[11] If the medication is expired, return it to the pharmacy and obtain a new medication.[8,9,10,12]
- Check the patient's medical record for an allergy or other contraindication to the prescribed medication. If an allergy or other contraindication exists, don't administer the medication; notify the practitioner.[8,9,11,13]
- Visually inspect the medication for discoloration or other indication of loss of integrity. Don't administer the medication if its integrity is compromised.[8,9,10,11,12]

NURSING ALERT Never use a medication that's cloudy or discolored or that contains a precipitate unless the manufacturer's instructions allow it. Remember the presence of drug particles is normal for some drugs (such as suspensions). If in doubt, check with the pharmacist.

- Discuss any unresolved concerns about the medication with the patient's practitioner.[8,9,10,11]
- Coordinate with the ordering practitioner and the radiography department to ensure that a chest X-ray is obtained before medication administration, if necessary, *for use as a baseline to monitor the effect of medication.*
- Perform hand hygiene.[14,15,16,17,18,19]
- Confirm the patient's identity using at least two patient identifiers.[20]
- Provide privacy.[21,22,23,24]
- Explain the procedure to the patient and family (if appropriate) according to their individual communication and learning needs *to increase their understanding, allay their fears, and enhance cooperation.*[25]
- If the patient is receiving the medication for the first time, teach the patient and family (as appropriate) about potential adverse effects and any other concerns related to the medication.[8,9,10,12,26]
- Verify that the medication is being administered at the proper time, in the prescribed dose, and by the correct route *to reduce the risk of medication errors.*[8,9,12,13]
- If your facility uses bar-code technology, use it as directed by your facility.[11]

NURSING ALERT If required by your facility, before administering a medication by the intrapleural route, have another nurse or the practitioner perform an independent double-check to verify the patient's identity and to make sure that you have the correct medication in the prescribed strength or concentration; the medication's indication corresponds with the patient's diagnosis; the dosage calculations are correct and the dosing formula used to derive the final dose is correct; the prescribed route of administration is safe and proper for the patient; the prescribed time and frequency of administration are safe and proper for the patient; and, if an infusion, the pump settings are correct and the infusion line is attached to the correct port.[27,28]

- After comparing results of the independent double-check with the other nurse, administer the medication if there are no discrepancies. If discrepancies exist, rectify them before administering the medication.[27]
- Have the patient lie supine in the bed with the head of the bed at a comfortable level.
- Raise the bed to waist level before providing care *to prevent caregiver back strain.*[29]
- Perform hand hygiene.[14,15,16,17,18,19]
- Put on clean gloves *to comply with standard precautions.*[30,31,32]
- Obtain the patient's vital signs, including auscultation of the lungs bilaterally, *to serve as baselines for comparison.*[33]
- Screen for and assess the patient's pain using a facility-approved pain assessment tool that's consistent with the patient's age, condition, and ability to understand.[34]
- Treat the patient's pain, as needed and ordered, using nonpharmacologic, pharmacologic, or a combination of approaches. Base the treatment

---

Inserting an intrapleural catheter

In intrapleural administration, the practitioner inserts a needle into the fourth to eighth intercostal space, 3" to 4" (7.5 to 10 cm) from the posterior midline, and then advances the needle medially over the superior edge of the patient's rib through the intercostal muscles until it tangentially penetrates the parietal pleura. The practitioner advances the catheter into the pleural space through the needle, and then removes the needle. The nurse should assist the practitioner with insertion, as necessary. After inserting the catheter, the practitioner coils it to prevent kinking and then sutures it securely to the patient's skin.

The practitioner confirms placement by aspirating the catheter. Resistance indicates correct placement in the pleural space; aspirated blood means that the catheter probably is misplaced in a blood vessel, and aspirated air means that it's probably in a lung. The practitioner then orders a chest X-ray to verify placement and *to detect such complications as pneumothorax.*

After insertion, apply a sterile occlusive dressing over the insertion site *to prevent catheter dislodgment.* Monitor the patient's vital signs after the procedure at an interval determined by your facility or by the patient's condition; *no evidence-based research is available to indicate best practice for frequency of vital signs monitoring.*[2] Screen for and assess the patient's pain using facility-defined criteria that are consistent with the patient's age, condition, and ability to understand. Treat the patient's pain, as needed and ordered, using nonpharmacologic, pharmacologic, or a combination of approaches. Base the treatment plan on evidence-based practices and the patient's clinical condition, past medical history, and pain management goals.[3]

---

plan on evidence-based practices and the patient's clinical condition, past medical history, and pain management goals.[34]

- Assess the integrity of the drainage system tubing and chest tube *to ensure that the drainage system is intact, with no air leaks or kinks, and to help prevent clot formation.*[35]
- Note the character, consistency, and amount of drainage in the chest tube drainage collection unit chamber. Mark the drainage level by writing the time and date at the drainage level on the drainage collection chamber *to accurately monitor output after medication administration.*[36,37]
- Remove and discard your gloves.[30,32]
- Perform hand hygiene.[14,15,16,17,18,19]
- Put on gloves *to comply with standard precautions.*[30,31,32]
- Turn off the suction, if applicable.
- Position the patient with the affected side up to gain access to the injection port.
- Assist the practitioner with removing the dressing from the intrapleural catheter or chest tube, if indicated, and clamp the drainage tube if one is present.[36]
- Discard the dressing in the appropriate receptacle.[30]
- Remove and discard your gloves.[30]
- Perform hand hygiene.[14,15,16,17,18,19]
- Put on gloves *to comply with standard precautions.*[30,31,32]
- Trace the tubing from the patient to its point of origin *to make sure that the medication is being administered into the correct port.*[38,39]
- If a stopcock is in place, and if appropriate to the medication being administered, turn the lever to point to the chest tube drain *to stop the flow from going into the drainage collection device.*[40]
- Disinfect the access port of the catheter or chest tube with an antiseptic-soaked gauze pad and then allow it to dry.
- Connect the prepared prescribed medication to the port and administer the medication as ordered following safe medication administration practices.[36,41]
- Disinfect the access port of the catheter or chest tube with an antiseptic-soaked gauze pad and then allow it to dry.
- Flush the intrapleural chest tube or intrapleural catheter with sterile normal saline, as ordered, following safe medication administration practices.[41]
- If ordered, keep the chest tube or catheter clamped for the prescribed dwell time.[36,41,42]

■ Obtain the patient's vital signs at a frequency determined by your facility, including auscultation of lungs bilaterally, and monitor the patient for signs of discomfort.[36,42]

■ Reassess the patient's pain and assess for any adverse reactions or events from treatment. Notify the practitioner immediately if any such event occurs.[34]

■ Unclamp the chest tube after the ordered dwell time and turn the suction back on, if ordered and applicable.[41]

■ Return the stopcock lever to the open position, if applicable, *to allow drainage to collect in the drainage collection system.*[36,42]

■ Observe the type, color, and amount of drainage in the drainage collection chamber. Immediately notify the practitioner of a sudden increase in drainage or frank bloody drainage.[37]

■ Return the bed to the lowest position *to prevent falls and maintain patient safety.*[43]

■ Discard used supplies in appropriate receptacles.[30]

■ Remove and discard your gloves.[31,41]

■ Perform hand hygiene.[14,15,16,17,18,19]

■ Clean and disinfect your stethoscope using a disinfectant pad.[44,45]

■ Perform hand hygiene.[14,15,16,17,18,19]

■ Document the procedure.[46,47,48,49]

Special considerations

■ The Joint Commission issued a sentinel event alert related to managing risk during transition to new International Organization for Standardization tubing standards designed to prevent dangerous tubing misconnections, which can lead to serious patient injury and death. During the transition, trace all tubing and catheters from the patient to their points of origin before connecting or reconnecting any device or infusion, at any care transition (such as to a new setting or service), and as part of the hand-off process. Route tubes and catheters with different purposes in different, standardized directions; label the tubing at the distal and proximal ends when there are different access sites or several bags hanging; use tubing and equipment only as intended; and store medications for different delivery routes in separate locations.[39]

■ If the chest tube dislodges, cover the site at once with a sterile gauze pad and tape it in place on only three sides *to prevent the risk of pneumothorax.*[50] Stay with the patient, monitor vital signs, and observe carefully for signs and symptoms of tension pneumothorax: hypotension, distended jugular veins, absent breath sounds, tracheal shift, hypoxemia, dyspnea, tachypnea, diaphoresis, chest pain, and a weak, rapid pulse. Have another nurse call the practitioner and gather the equipment for reinsertion.

■ For a patient with a chest tube, keep clamps at the bedside. If a commercial chest tube system cracks or a tube disconnects, use the clamps to clamp the chest tube close to the insertion site.[35] As an alternative to clamping the tube, submerge the distal end of the tube in a bottle of sterile water *to create a temporary water seal while you replace the drainage system.* Notify the practitioner. Be sure to observe the patient closely for signs of tension pneumothorax, *because no air can escape from the pleural space while the tube is clamped.*[35]

Patient teaching

Advise the patient to report any difficulty with breathing, pain experienced during the procedure, or drainage from the chest tube insertion site.[42]

Complications

Pneumothorax or tension pneumothorax may occur if the practitioner accidentally injects air into the pleural cavity. These complications are more likely to occur in a patient who is on mechanical ventilation.

Accidental catheter placement in the lung can lead to respiratory distress; catheter placement within a vessel can increase the medication's effects; and laceration of intercostal vessels may cause bleeding. If the catheter fractures, lung puncture may occur.

Local anesthetic toxicity can lead to tinnitus, metallic taste, lightheadedness, somnolence, visual and auditory disturbances, restlessness, delirium, slurred speech, nystagmus, muscle tremor, seizures, arrhythmias, and cardiovascular collapse. A local anesthetic containing epinephrine can cause tachycardia and hypertension.

Failure to adhere to sterile technique may lead to infection.

Other complications specific to the medication being administered should be discussed with the patient as well.

Documentation

Document the date and time of access to the intrapleural catheter or chest tube, the practitioner's name, and the patient's tolerance of the procedure. Document any premedication that you administered before the procedure. Document all preprocedure verification, including the people involved in the verification process. For drug administration, record the date, time, drug administered, drug dosage and strength, sequence of drug administration (if appropriate), route of administration, patient's response to the treatment, and condition of the catheter or chest tube insertion site. Document the patient's vital signs before and after medication administration, as well as the volume and visual characteristics of chest tube fluid drainage before and after medication administration. Also note any adverse reactions to the medication, the date and time that you notified the practitioner, the prescribed interventions, and the patient's response to those interventions. Document teaching that you provided to the patient and family (if applicable), their understanding of that teaching, and any need for follow-up teaching.

REFERENCES

1 Olsen, M. M., et al. (Eds.). (2019). *Chemotherapy and immunotherapy guidelines and recommendations for practice.* Pittsburgh, PA: Oncology Nursing Society.

2 American Society of PeriAnesthesia Nurses. (2021). *2021–2022 perianesthesia nursing standards, practice recommendations and interpretive statements.* Cherry Hill, NJ: American Society of PeriAnesthesia Nurses. (Level VII)

3 The Joint Commission. (2021). Standard PC.01.02.07. *Comprehensive accreditation manual for hospitals.* Oakbrook Terrace, IL: The Joint Commission. (Level VII)

4 Ahmed, A. H., & Yacoub, T. E. (2010). Intrapleural therapy in management of complicated parapneumonic effusions and empyema. *Clinical Pharmacology, 2,* 213–221. https://www.ncbi.nlm.nih.gov/pmc/articles/PMC3262383/

5 Westbrook, J., et al. (2010). Association of interruptions with an increased risk and severity of medication administration errors. *Archives of Internal Medicine, 170,* 683–690. (Level IV)

6 Institute for Safe Medication Practices. (2012). Side tracks on the safety express: Interruptions lead to errors and unfinished...Wait, what was I doing? *Nurse Advise-ERR, 11*(2), 1–4. https://www.ismp.org/resources/side-tracks-safety-express-interruptions-lead-errors-and-unfinished-wait-what-was-i-doing?id=37

7 Standard 13. Medication verification. Infusion therapy standards of practice (8th ed.). (2021). *Journal of Infusion Nursing, 44,* 39, S46–S49. (Level VII)

8 Centers for Medicare and Medicaid Services, Department of Health and Human Services. (2020). Condition of participation: Nursing services. 42 C.F.R. § 482.23 (c).

9 Accreditation Association for Hospitals and Health Systems. (2020). Standard 16.01.03. *Healthcare Facilities Accreditation Program: Accreditation requirements for acute care hospitals.* Chicago, IL: Accreditation Association for Hospitals and Health Systems. (Level VII)

10 DNV GL-Healthcare USA, Inc. (2020). MM.1.SR.2. *NIAHO® accreditation requirements, interpretive guidelines and surveyor guidance—revision 20.0.* Milford, OH: DNV GL-Healthcare USA, Inc. (Level VII)

11 Standard 59. Infusion medication and solution administration. Infusion therapy standards of practice (8th ed.). (2021). *Journal of Infusion Nursing, 44,* S180–S183. (Level VII)

12 The Joint Commission. (2021). Standard MM.06.01.01. *Comprehensive accreditation manual for hospitals.* Oakbrook Terrace, IL: The Joint Commission. (Level VII)

13 DNV GL-Healthcare USA, Inc. (2020). MM.1.SR.3. *NIAHO® accreditation requirements, interpretive guidelines and surveyor guidance—revision 20.0.* Milford, OH: DNV GL-Healthcare USA, Inc. (Level VII)

14 Accreditation Association for Hospitals and Health Systems. (2020). Standard 07.01.21. *Healthcare Facilities Accreditation Program: Accreditation requirements for acute care hospitals.* Chicago, IL: Accreditation Association for Hospitals and Health Systems. (Level VII)

15 Centers for Disease Control and Prevention. (2002). Guideline for hand hygiene in health-care settings: Recommendations of the Healthcare Infection Control Practices Advisory Committee and the HICPAC/SHEA/APIC/IDSA Hand Hygiene Task Force. *MMWR Recommendations and Reports, 51*(RR-16), 1–45. https://www.cdc.gov/mmwr/pdf/rr/rr5116.pdf (Level II)

16 Centers for Medicare and Medicaid Services, Department of Health and Human Services. (2020). Condition of participation: Infection control. 42 C.F.R. § 482.42.

17 DNV GL-Healthcare USA, Inc. (2020). IC.1.SR.1. *NIAHO® accreditation requirements, interpretive guidelines, and surveyor guidance—revision 20.0.* Milford, OH: DNV GL-Healthcare USA, Inc. (Level VII)

18 The Joint Commission. (2021). Standard NPSG.07.01.01. *Comprehensive accreditation manual for hospitals.* Oakbrook Terrace, IL: The Joint Commission. (Level VII)

19 World Health Organization. (2009). WHO guidelines on hand hygiene in health care: First global patient safety challenge, clean care is safer care. https://apps.who.int/iris/bitstream/handle/10665/44102/9789241597906_eng.pdf (Level IV)

20 The Joint Commission. (2021). Standard NPSG.01.01.01. *Comprehensive accreditation manual for hospitals.* Oakbrook Terrace, IL: The Joint Commission. (Level VII)

21 Accreditation Association for Hospitals and Health Systems. (2020). Standard 15.01.16. *Healthcare Facilities Accreditation Program: Accreditation requirements for acute care hospitals.* Chicago, IL: Accreditation Association for Hospitals and Health Systems. (Level VII)

22 Centers for Medicare and Medicaid Services, Department of Health and Human Services. (2020). Condition of participation: Patient's rights. 42 C.F.R. § 482.13 (c)(1).

23 DNV GL-Healthcare USA, Inc. (2020). PR.2.SR.5. *NIAHO® accreditation requirements, interpretive guidelines and surveyor guidance—revision 20.0.* Milford, OH: DNV GL-Healthcare USA, Inc. (Level VII)

24 The Joint Commission. (2021). Standard RI.01.01.01. *Comprehensive accreditation manual for hospitals.* Oakbrook Terrace, IL: The Joint Commission. (Level VII)

25 The Joint Commission. (2021). Standard PC.02.01.21. *Comprehensive accreditation manual for hospitals.* Oakbrook Terrace, IL: The Joint Commission. (Level VII)

26 Standard 8. Patient education. Infusion standards of practice (8th ed.). (2021). *Journal of Infusion Nursing, 44*, S35–S37. (Level VII)

27 Institute for Safe Medication Practice. (2019). Independent double checks: Worth the effort if used judiciously and properly. https://www.ismp.org/resources/independent-double-checks-worth-effort-if-used-judiciously-and-properly (Level VII)

28 Institute for Safe Medication Practices. (2018). ISMP list of high-alert medications in acute care settings. https://www.ismp.org/sites/default/files/attachments/2018-08/highAlert2018-Acute-Final.pdf

29 Waters, T. R., et al. (2009). Safe patient handling training for schools of nursing. https://www.cdc.gov/niosh/docs/2009-127/pdfs/2009-127.pdf (Level VII)

30 Occupational Safety and Health Administration. (2012). Bloodborne pathogens, standard number 1910.1030. https://www.osha.gov/pls/oshaweb/owadisp.show_document?p_id=10051&p_table=STANDARDS (Level VII)

31 Siegel, J. D., et al. (2007, revised 2019). 2007 guideline for isolation precautions: Preventing transmission of infectious agents in healthcare settings. https://www.cdc.gov/infectioncontrol/pdf/guidelines/isolation-guidelines-H.pdf (Level II)

32 Accreditation Association for Hospitals and Health Systems. (2020). Standard 07.01.10. *Healthcare Facilities Accreditation Program: Accreditation requirements for acute care hospitals.* Chicago, IL: Accreditation Association for Hospitals and Health Systems. (Level VII)

33 The Joint Commission. (2021). Standard PC.01.02.03. *Comprehensive accreditation manual for hospitals.* Oakbrook Terrace, IL: The Joint Commission. (Level VII)

34 The Joint Commission. (2021). Standard PC.01.02.07. *Comprehensive accreditation manual for hospitals.* Oakbrook Terrace, IL: The Joint Commission. (Level VII)

35 Wiegand, D. L. (2017). *AACN procedure manual for high acuity, progressive, and critical care* (7th ed.). St Louis, MO: Elsevier.

36 Heimes, J., et al. (2017). The use of thrombolytics in the management of complex pleural fluid collections. *Journal of Thoracic Disease, 9*(5), 1310–1316. https://www.ncbi.nlm.nih.gov/pmc/articles/PMC5465141/

37 Chotai, P. (2020). Tube thoracostomy management. https://emedicine.medscape.com/article/1503275-overview (Level VII)

38 U.S. Food and Drug Administration. (2017). Examples of medical device misconnections. https://www.fda.gov/medical-devices/medical-device-connectors/examples-medical-device-misconnections

39 The Joint Commission. (2014). Sentinel event alert 53: Managing risk during transition to new ISO tubing connector standards. https://www.jointcommission.org/assets/1/6/SEA_53_Connectors_8_19_14_final.pdf (Level VII)

40 Noppen, M. (2021). Talc pleurodesis. In: *UpToDate.* Maldonando, F. (Ed.)

41 Kehir, F., et al. (2020). Intrapleural Fibrinolytic Therapy versus Early Medical Thoracoscopy for Treatment of Pleural Infection. *Annals of the American Thoracic Society, 17*, 958–964.

42 Piccolo, F., et al. (2015). Intrapleural tissue plasminogen activator and deoxyribonuclease therapy for pleural infection. *Journal of Thoracic Disease, 7*(6), 999–1008. https://www.ncbi.nlm.nih.gov/pmc/articles/PMC4466425/

43 Ganz, D. A., et al. (2013, reviewed 2021). *Preventing falls in hospitals: A toolkit for improving quality of care* (AHRQ Publication No. 13-0015-EF). Rockville, MD: Agency for Healthcare Research and Quality. https://www.ahrq.gov/sites/default/files/publications/files/fallpxtoolkit_0.pdf (Level VII)

44 Rutala, W. A., et al. (2008, revised 2019). Guideline for disinfection and sterilization in healthcare facilities, 2008. https://www.cdc.gov/infection-control/pdf/guidelines/disinfection-guidelines-H.pdf (Level I)

45 Accreditation Association for Hospitals and Health Systems. (2020). Standard 07.02.03. *Healthcare Facilities Accreditation Program: Accreditation requirements for acute care hospitals.* Chicago, IL: Accreditation Association for Hospitals and Health Systems. (Level VII)

46 The Joint Commission. (2021). Standard RC.01.03.01. *Comprehensive accreditation manual for hospitals.* Oakbrook Terrace, IL: The Joint Commission. (Level VII)

47 DNV GL-Healthcare USA, Inc. (2020). MR.2.SR.1. *NIAHO® accreditation requirements, interpretive guidelines and surveyor guidance—revision 20.0.* Milford, OH: DNV GL-Healthcare USA, Inc. (Level VII)

48 Centers for Medicare and Medicaid Services, Department of Health and Human Services. (2020). Condition of participation: Medical record services. 42 C.F.R. § 482.24(b).

49 Accreditation Association for Hospitals and Health Systems. (2020). Standard 10.00.03. *Healthcare Facilities Accreditation Program: Accreditation requirements for acute care hospitals.* Chicago, IL: Accreditation Association for Hospitals and Health Systems. (Level VII)

50 Mbinji, M. (2021). Chest drains: maintenance. *The JBI EBP Database.* AN: JBI-ES-1241-1

IONTOPHORESIS

Iontophoresis is a technique for delivering an ionic medication quickly with minimal discomfort. It's used as an alternative to parenteral injection for the administration of ionic medication solutions, such as local anesthetics.[1,2] An example of a device used for iontophoresis is the hand-held dual-channel Dupel device, which is powered by a 9-volt battery and capable of delivering medications with different ionic charges into the skin. A treatment electrode attached to lead wires is connected to the iontophoresis device. Current that flows through the device forces the ionic medication solution into the skin away from the like-charged electrode. If a positively charged medication solution is to be administered, the treatment electrode is attached to the positive lead wire. If a negatively charged solution is to be administered, the lead wire is attached to the negative lead wire. With the dual-channel device, one channel can deliver a negatively charge medication while the other delivers a positively charged medication simultaneously.[3] Alternatively, like-charged medications can be used in the treatment electrodes for both channels. The dose of ionic medication solution delivered depends on the current applied to the treatment electrode and the length of time that the current is applied.[3]

Local anesthetic agents, such as those administered through iontophoresis, may be considered before vascular access device insertion.[4] Lidocaine iontophoresis has been found to be 80% to 100% effective in providing anesthetic action before such procedures as injections, abrasion treatment, and laser surgery and cautery.[1] Because iontophoresis acts quickly, often within 10 minutes, it's an excellent choice for anesthetizing an IV insertion site, especially in children.[2]

Iontophoresis is contraindicated in patients who have adverse effects from applied electrical current or the prescribed medication, as well as patients who are pregnant or have electrically sensitive implanted equipment, such as a pacemaker.[3] In addition, the electrodes for iontophoresis shouldn't be placed over broken or damaged skin or newly formed scar tissue.[2,3]

Equipment

Dose-control device with battery and lead wires ▪ drug-delivery electrode kit ▪ lidocaine 2% with epinephrine 1:100,000 solution ▪ mild soap and water ▪ washcloths ▪ syringe with needle ▪ gloves ▪ tongue blade ▪ Optional: disposable-head surgical clippers, alcohol pads, single-patient-use disposable scissors, venipuncture equipment.

Preparation of equipment

Inspect all equipment and supplies. If a product is expired, is defective or has compromised integrity, remove it from patient use, label it as expired or defective, and report the expiration or defect as directed by your facility. Read the manufacturer's instructions before using the device.

Implementation

- Verify the practitioner's order.
- Perform hand hygiene.[5,6,7,8,9,10]
- Confirm the patient's identity using at least two patient identifiers.[11]
- Review the patient's medical record for a history of allergies or sensitivity to medications and contraindications to treatment.

NURSING ALERT Avoid iontophoresis in patients with cardiac pacemakers or other electrically sensitive implanted devices.[2,3]

- Explain the procedure to the patient and family (if appropriate) according to their individual communication and learning needs *to increase their understanding, allay their fears, and enhance cooperation.*[12] Tell the patient that tingling or warmth under the electrode pads might be felt while they're on the skin.
- Perform hand hygiene.[5,6,7,8,9,10]
- Put on gloves *to comply with standard precautions.*[9,13,14]
- Assess the patient's skin and select intact electrode placement sites, avoiding areas with acne, unhealed wounds, or ingrown hairs. The drug-delivery electrode should be placed over the intended procedure site; the second electrode, which drives drug ions into the skin, should be applied over a muscle 4″ to 6″ (10 to 15 cm) from the first electrode.
- Prepare the skin at the selected electrode site by cleaning with soap and water and drying thoroughly; don't use alcohol to prepare the skin unless it's excessively oily.[3]
- If necessary, trim excess body hair at the application sites using single-patient-use scissors or disposable-head surgical clippers.
- Remove the paper flap from the back of the drug-delivery electrode.
- Draw up the lidocaine with epinephrine in a syringe, as ordered, following safe medication administration practices.[15,16,17,18]
- Remove the needle from the syringe and discard it appropriately.[14]
- Saturate the drug-delivery electrode pad with the amount of lidocaine and epinephrine solution indicated on the pad (as shown below). The amount of lidocaine and epinephrine solution required to saturate the pad varies with pad size. For a standard-sized pad, use about 1 mL; for a large pad, use about 2.5 mL.

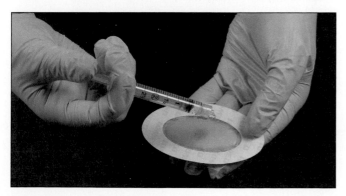

- Remove the remaining backing from the drug-delivery electrode.
- Apply the drug-delivery electrode to the selected site.
- Remove the backing from the grounding electrode, and then apply it to the second prepared site.
- Connect the lead clips to the electrodes according to the manufacturer's instructions.
- Make sure the device is turned off and then connect the lead wires to the device.
- Turn on the device.
- Set the desired treatment dosage. The device is calibrated to deliver a dose of 40 milliamps (mA). Adjust the dosage by pressing the dosage arrow keys up or down until the correct dosage is displayed.
- Set the desired level of current. Adjust the device to the desired level of current using the current knobs. If you don't know the desired level, initiate treatment at a level lower than 2 mA and adjust in 0.1-mA increments; current is commonly set between 0.5 and 4 mA.[3]
- Initiate treatment by setting the treatment mode switch. Current will ramp up to the set intensity level within 30 seconds.
- Pause the treatment as needed *to assess for patient tolerance and comfort.*
- At the end of treatment, turn off the device.
- Disconnect the lead wires and remove the electrodes.
- Assess the skin at the drug-delivery site for numbness by touching it with a blunt object, such as a tongue blade.
- Promptly prepare the site and perform the venipuncture or other procedure, *because the numbness may last only a few minutes.*
- Discard used supplies in appropriate receptacles.[14]
- Remove and discard your gloves.[14]
- Perform hand hygiene.[5,6,7,8,9,10]
- Document the procedure.[19,20,21,22]

Special considerations

- *To avoid interfering with energy emission,* don't tape or compress the electrode sites, and don't apply heat or cold to the electrode sites during treatment.
- If the device doesn't function, make sure that the battery is fresh and properly installed (check polarity markings) and that the battery contacts are clean. If a battery must be replaced during the treatment, record how much of the treatment was completed, *because this information will be lost when the battery is replaced.*[3]

Complications

Iontophoresis can cause transient erythema, inflammation, blanching, itching, burning, and a tingling sensation at the site, which usually disappears within 12 hours after treatment.[13] An allergic reaction may occur in patients sensitive to lidocaine or epinephrine.

Documentation

Document the treatment, date and time of the treatment, sites used, and effectiveness of drug delivery. Also document any adverse reactions that occur, interventions taken, and the patient's response to those interventions. Document teaching provided to the patient and family (if applicable), their understanding of that teaching, and any need for follow-up teaching.

REFERENCES

1 Tadicherla, S., & Berman, B. (2006). Percutaneous dermal drug delivery for local pain control. *Therapeutics and Clinical Risk Management, 2*(1), 99–113 https://www.ncbi.nlm.nih.gov/pmc/articles/PMC1661648

2 Bowden, V. R., & Greenberg, C. S. (2016). *Pediatric nursing procedures* (4th ed.). Philadelphia, PA: Wolters Kluwer.

3 Empi. (2010). DUPEL dual channel iontophoresis system: Instruction for use. https://manualzz.com/doc/7230048/instructions-for-use

4 Infusion Nurses Society. (2016). *Policies and procedures for infusion therapy* (5th ed.). Boston, MA: Infusion Nurses Society.

5 Centers for Disease Control and Prevention. (2002). Guideline for hand hygiene in health-care settings: Recommendations of the Healthcare Infection Control Practices Advisory Committee and the HICPAC/SHEA/APIC/IDSA Hand Hygiene Task Force. *MMWR Recommendations and Reports, 51*(RR-16), 1–45. https://www.cdc.gov/mmwr/pdf/rr/rr5116.pdf (Level II)

6   World Health Organization. (2009). WHO guidelines on hand hygiene in health care: First global patient safety challenge, clean care is safer care. https://apps.who.int/iris/bitstream/handle/10665/44102/9789241597906_eng.pdf?sequence=1 (Level IV)

7   The Joint Commission. (2021). Standard NPSG.07.01.01. *Comprehensive accreditation manual for hospitals.* Oakbrook Terrace, IL: The Joint Commission. (Level VII)

8   Centers for Medicare and Medicaid Services, Department of Health and Human Services. (2020). Condition of participation: Infection control. 42 C.F.R. § 482.42.

9   Accreditation Association for Hospitals and Health Systems. (2020). Standard 07.01.10. *Healthcare Facilities Accreditation Program: Accreditation requirements for acute care hospitals.* Chicago, IL: Accreditation Association for Hospitals and Health Systems. (Level VII)

10   DNV GL-Healthcare USA, Inc. (2020). IC.1.SR.1. *NIAHO® accreditation requirements, interpretive guidelines and surveyor guidance—revision 20.0.* Milford, OH: DNV GL-Healthcare USA, Inc. (Level VII)

11   The Joint Commission. (2021). Standard NPSG.01.01.01. *Comprehensive accreditation manual for hospitals.* Oakbrook Terrace, IL: The Joint Commission. (Level VII)

12   The Joint Commission. (2021). Standard PC.02.01.21. *Comprehensive accreditation manual for hospitals.* Oakbrook Terrace, IL: The Joint Commission. (Level VII)

13   Siegel, J. D., et al. (2007, revised 2019). 2007 guideline for isolation precautions: Preventing transmission of infectious agents in healthcare settings. https://www.cdc.gov/infectioncontrol/pdf/guidelines/isolation-guidelines-H.pdf (Level II)

14   Occupational Safety and Health Administration. (2012). Bloodborne pathogens, standard number 1910.1030. https://www.osha.gov/pls/oshaweb/owadisp.show document?p_id=10051&p_table=STANDARDS (Level VII)

15   The Joint Commission. (2021). Standard MM.06.01.01. *Comprehensive accreditation manual for hospitals.* Oakbrook Terrace, IL: The Joint Commission. (Level VII)

16   Centers for Medicare and Medicaid Services, Department of Health and Human Services. (2020). Condition of participation: Nursing services. 42 C.F.R. § 482.23(c).

17   Accreditation Association for Hospitals and Health Systems. (2020). Standard 16.01.03. *Healthcare Facilities Accreditation Program: Accreditation requirements for acute care hospitals.* Chicago, IL: Accreditation Association for Hospitals and Health Systems. (Level VII)

18   DNV GL-Healthcare USA, Inc. (2020). MM.1.SR.3. *NIAHO® accreditation requirements, interpretive guidelines and surveyor guidance—revision 20.0.* Milford, OH: DNV GL-Healthcare USA, Inc. (Level VII)

19   The Joint Commission. (2021). Standard RC.01.03.01. *Comprehensive accreditation manual for hospitals.* Oakbrook Terrace, IL: The Joint Commission. (Level VII)

20   Centers for Medicare and Medicaid Services, Department of Health and Human Services. (2020). Condition of participation: Medical record services. 42 C.F.R. § 482.24(b).

21   Accreditation Association for Hospitals and Health Systems. (2020). Standard 10.00.03. *Healthcare Facilities Accreditation Program: Accreditation requirements for acute care hospitals.* Chicago, IL: Accreditation Association for Hospitals and Health Systems. (Level VII)

22   DNV GL-Healthcare USA, Inc. (2020). MR.2.SR.1. *NIAHO® accreditation requirements, interpretive guidelines and surveyor guidance—revision 20.0.* Milford, OH: DNV GL-Healthcare USA, Inc. (Level VII)

IV BOLUS INJECTION

The IV bolus injection method allows rapid drug administration. It can be used in an emergency to provide an immediate drug effect. It can also be used to administer drugs that can't be given IM, to achieve peak drug levels in the bloodstream, and to deliver drugs that can't be diluted.

Bolus doses of medication can be injected directly through a venous access device with a continuous infusion or through a vascular access device intended for intermittent use.[1,2] Each medication has its own safe rate of injection, which is specified by the drug manufacturer.[3,4] The medication usually takes effect rapidly, so the patient must be monitored for adverse reactions, such as cardiac arrhythmias and anaphylaxis. IV bolus injections are contraindicated when rapid drug administration could cause life-threatening complications.

EQUIPMENT

Using a ready injectable

A commercially premeasured medication packaged with a syringe and needle, the ready injectable enables rapid drug administration in an emergency. Preparing a ready injectable usually takes only 15 to 20 seconds. Other advantages include the reduced risk of breaking sterile no-touch technique during administration and the easy identification of medication and dose.[4]

When using a ready injectable, be sure to give the precise dose prescribed. For example, if a 50-mg/mL cartridge is supplied but the patient's prescribed dose is 25 mg, you must administer only 0.5 mL, half of the volume contained in the cartridge. Be alert for potential medication errors whenever dispensing medications in premeasured dosage forms.

NURSING ALERT Speed shock may result from rapid bolus administration of an IV medication. Carefully administer the medication at the proper rate and closely monitor the patient during administration. Symptoms of speed shock include dizziness, headache, and other symptoms caused by the rapidity of the medication's onset. Signs and symptoms can progress to chest tightness, hypotension, irregular pulse, and anaphylactic shock. Keep in mind that an older adult patient might not be able to articulate these symptoms because of a preexisting condition, such as stroke, tracheotomy, endotracheal intubation, dementia, or delirium.[2]

Sterile no-touch technique is required during administration *to reduce the risk of vascular catheter–associated infection.*[1,2,4]

HOSPITAL-ACQUIRED CONDITION ALERT Keep in mind that the Centers for Medicare and Medicaid Services considers vascular catheter–associated infection a hospital-acquired condition *because it can be reasonably prevented using a variety of best practices.* Make sure to follow evidence-based infection prevention techniques, such as performing hand hygiene, performing a vigorous mechanical scrub of the needleless connector, following sterile no-touch technique when accessing the device, and limiting catheter manipulations, *to reduce the risk of vascular catheter–associated infections.*[5,6,7,8,9]

Equipment

Patient's medication administration record ▪ gloves ▪ syringe ▪ antiseptic pads (chlorhexidine-based, alcohol, or tincture of iodine) ▪ prescribed medication ▪ prefilled 10-mL -syringe (or a syringe designed to generate lower amounts of pressure)[10] containing preservative-free normal saline solution (or other compatible flush solution if medication is incompatible with normal saline solution)[11] ▪ vital signs monitoring equipment ▪ Optional: appropriate diluent, second prefilled syringe with preservative-free normal saline solution, prefilled syringe with locking solution, disinfectant-containing end cap, sedation scale, pulse oximeter and probe, capnography equipment, electronic infusion device, labels.

A useful dosage form is the ready injectable. (See *Using a ready injectable.*)

Preparation of equipment

Inspect all IV equipment and supplies. If a product is expired, is defective, or has compromised integrity, remove it from patient use, label it as expired or defective, and report the expiration or defect as directed by your facility.[12]

If you must dilute or reconstitute the IV bolus injection medication, do so immediately before administration in a clean, uncluttered, and functionally separate workspace (such as a medication room) using facility-approved, readily available drug information resources and sterile equipment and supplies.[4] If you transfer the medication or solution from the original packaging to another container or if you aren't going to administer it immediately, label the container with the medication name, dosage strength, quantity, diluent and volume, and expiration date as indicated.[4,13]

Implementation

- Avoid distractions and interruptions when preparing and administering medications *to prevent medication administration errors.*[14,15]
- Verify the practitioner's order.[1,2,16,17,18,19]
- Review the patient's medical record for factors that increase the patient's risk of adverse reactions and toxicity to the prescribed medication.[16,20]
- Check the patient's medical record for an allergy or other contraindication to the prescribed medication. If an allergy or contraindications exists, don't administer the medication; instead, notify the practitioner.[16,17,18,19]
- Gather and prepare the necessary equipment and supplies.
- Compare the medication label with the order in the patient's medical record.[16,17,18,19]
- Check the expiration date on the medication. If the medication is expired, return it to the pharmacy and obtain a new medication.[16,17,18,19]
- Visually inspect the medication for discoloration or any other loss of integrity; don't administer the medication if its integrity is compromised.[16,17,18,19]
- Review the drug monograph before administration (if necessary) *to ensure safe medication administration.*[1,2]
- Check the compatibility of the medication with the IV solution, other medicated infusions, and the flush solution, as appropriate.
- Discuss any unresolved concerns about the medication with the patient's practitioner.[16,17,18,19]
- Perform hand hygiene.[5,21,22,23,24,25,26,27]
- Confirm the patient's identity using at least two patient identifiers.[28]
- Provide privacy.[29,30,31,32]
- Explain the procedure to the patient and family (if appropriate) according to their individual communication and learning needs *to increase their understanding, allay their fears, and enhance cooperation.*[33]
- If the patient is receiving the medication for the first time, teach about potential adverse reactions and discuss any other concerns related to the medication.[16,17,18,19]
- Raise the bed to waist level before providing care *to prevent caregiver back strain.*[34]
- Carefully assess the patient's condition (including vital signs, body systems appropriate to the prescribed medication, and the vascular access site) *to establish baselines for comparison.*[4]
- Perform hand hygiene.[5,21,22,23,24,25,26,27]
- Put on gloves *to comply with standard precautions.*[35,36,37]
- Check the medication label three times *to prevent medication administration errors.*
- Verify that the medication is being administered at the proper time, in the prescribed dose, and by the correct route *to reduce the risk of medication errors.*[16,17,18,19]
- If your facility uses bar-code technology, use it as directed by your facility.[3,4]
- If the medication being administered is a high-alert medication,[38] have another nurse perform an independent double-check (if required by your facility) before administration *to reduce the risk of medication administration errors.* Rectify any discrepancies before administration.[39]

NURSING ALERT A high-alert medication is a medication that can cause significant patient harm when used in error.[38] If required by your facility, before administering the medication, have another nurse perform an independent double-check *to verify the patient's identity and make sure that you have the correct medication in the prescribed strength or concentration; the medication's indication corresponds with the patient's diagnosis; the dosage calculations are correct and the dosing formula used to derive the final dose is correct; the prescribed route of administration is safe and proper for the patient; and, if an infusion, the pump settings are correct and the infusion line is attached to the correct port.*[39]

For administration through a vascular access device with continuous infusion

- Trace the IV administration set tubing from the patient to its point of origin *to ensure you're accessing the proper administration set tubing and to prevent dangerous misconnections.*[3,40,41]
- Close the flow clamp of the IV administration set tubing and pause the electronic infusion device, if in use.

- Perform a vigorous mechanical scrub of the lowest needleless injection port of the administration set tubing for at least 5 seconds using an antiseptic pad; then allow it to dry completely.[6,42]
- While maintaining the sterility of the syringe tip, attach a prefilled syringe containing preservative-free normal saline or another compatible solution to the needleless connector port closest to the patient in an existing infusion *to allow the medication to reach the circulatory system as soon as possible.*[1] (Use a 10-mL syringe or a syringe specifically designed to generate lower injection pressure.) Unclamp the catheter and slowly aspirate for blood return that's the color and consistency of whole blood. If you don't obtain a blood return, take steps to locate an external cause of obstruction.[10]
- If you obtain a blood return, slowly inject preservative-free normal saline solution into the catheter. Use a minimum volume of twice the internal volume of the catheter system. Don't forcibly flush the device; further evaluate the device if you meet resistance.[10]
- Remove and discard the syringe in a puncture-resistant sharps disposal container.[37,43]
- Perform a vigorous mechanical scrub of the injection port for at least 5 seconds using an antiseptic pad; then allow it to dry completely.[6,42]
- While maintaining the sterility of the syringe tip, attach the medication syringe to the injection port.[1,2]

NURSING ALERT First, confirm the patency of the vascular access device using a 10-mL syringe filled with preservative-free normal saline solution (or a syringe designed specifically to generate lower injection pressure filled with preservative-free normal saline solution). Then, administer the medication by IV bolus injection in a syringe of the appropriate size to measure and administer the required medication dose.[4,10] Don't transfer the medication to a larger syringe.[10]

- Inject the medication as prescribed and according to the rate on the medication label; consult with the pharmacist if a rate isn't specified.[1,2]
- If the bolus medication is compatible with the patient's prescribed IV solution, open the clamp on the administration tubing, adjust the flow rate, or restart the infusion pump, as indicated.[1,2,11]
- If the bolus medication is incompatible with the patient's prescribed IV solution, perform a vigorous mechanical scrub of the lowest needleless injection port for at least 5 seconds with an antiseptic pad; then allow it to dry completely.[6,42] While maintaining the sterility of the syringe tip, attach a prefilled syringe containing preservative-free normal saline solution to the needleless injection port. Unclamp the catheter and inject preservative-free normal saline solution into the catheter at the same rate of injection as the prescribed medication. Use the amount of flush solution needed to adequately clear the medication from the administration set lumen and the catheter. Don't forcibly flush the device; further evaluate the device if you meet resistance. Consider using a pulsatile flushing technique, *because short boluses of the flush solution interrupted by short pauses may be more effective at removing deposits (such as fibrin, drug precipitate, and intraluminal bacteria) than a continuous low-flow technique.* Alternatively, if the bolus medication is incompatible with normal saline solution, use dextrose 5% in water (D_5W), followed by preservative-free normal saline solution. Don't allow D_5W to remain in the catheter lumen, *because it provides nutrients for biofilm growth.*[10] Remove and discard the syringe in a puncture-resistant sharps disposal container.[37,43] Open the clamp, adjust the flow rate, or restart the electronic infusion device, as indicated.

For administration through an intermittent vascular access device

- Trace the catheter from the patient to its point of origin *to make sure you're accessing the proper port.*[3,40,41]
- If a disinfectant-containing end cap is on the end of the needleless connector, remove and discard it.[42,44]
- Perform a vigorous mechanical scrub of the needleless connector for at least 5 seconds using an antiseptic pad; then allow it to dry completely.[1,2,6,42]
- While maintaining the sterility of the syringe tip, attach a prefilled syringe containing preservative-free normal saline or another compatible solution to the needleless connector port closest to the patient in an

existing infusion *to allow the medication to reach the circulatory system as soon as possible.* (Use a 10-mL syringe or a syringe specifically designed to generate lower injection pressure.) Unclamp the catheter and slowly aspirate for blood return that's the color and consistency of whole blood. If you don't obtain a blood return, take steps to locate an external cause of obstruction.[10]

■ If you obtain a blood return, slowly inject preservative-free normal saline solution into the catheter. Use a minimum volume of twice the internal volume of the catheter system. Don't forcibly flush the device; further evaluate the device if you meet resistance.[1,2,10]

■ Remove and discard the syringe in a puncture-resistant sharps disposal container.[37,43]

■ Perform a vigorous mechanical scrub of the needleless connector for at least 5 seconds using an antiseptic pad. Allow it to dry completely.[6,42]

■ While maintaining the sterility of the syringe tip, attach the medication syringe to the needleless connector of the venous access device.[1,2]

■ Inject the medication as prescribed and according to the rate on the medication label; consult with the pharmacist if a rate isn't specified.[1,2]

■ Remove and discard the syringe in a puncture-resistant sharps disposal container.[37,43]

■ Perform a vigorous mechanical scrub of the needleless connector for at least 5 seconds using an antiseptic pad; then allow it to dry completely.[6,42]

■ While maintaining the sterility of the syringe tip, attach a prefilled syringe containing preservative-free normal saline solution to the needleless connector. Unclamp the catheter and inject preservative-free normal saline solution into the catheter at the same rate of injection as the prescribed medication. Use the amount of flush solution needed to adequately clear the medication from the administration set lumen and the catheter. Don't forcibly flush the device; further evaluate the device if you meet resistance. Consider using a pulsatile flushing technique, *because short boluses of the flush solution interrupted by short pauses may be more effective at removing deposits (such as fibrin, drug precipitate, and intraluminal bacteria) than a continuous low-flow technique.* Alternatively, if the medication is incompatible with normal saline solution, use D_5W, followed by preservative-free normal saline solution. Don't allow D_5W to remain in the catheter lumen, *because it provides nutrients for biofilm growth.*[10]

■ If indicated, proceed with locking the catheter.[1,2] Perform a vigorous mechanical scrub of the needleless connector for at least 5 seconds using an antiseptic pad; then allow it to dry completely.[1,2,6] While maintaining the sterility of the syringe tip, attach the syringe containing the locking solution to the needleless connector.[1,2] Slowly inject the locking solution into the venous access device.[1,2] After locking the catheter, follow a clamping sequence based on the type of needleless connector. If you're using a positive-pressure needleless connector, clamp the catheter after disconnecting the syringe.[1,2] If you're using a negative-pressure needleless connector, maintain pressure on the syringe while clamping the catheter.[1,2] If you're using a neutral pressure needleless connector, clamp the catheter before or after disconnecting the syringe.[1,2] For an antireflux needleless connector, clamp the catheter and then disconnect the syringe; a specific clamping sequence isn't required.[45,46]

■ If available in your facility, apply a new disinfectant-containing end cap on the needleless connector of the venous access device *to reduce the risk of vascular catheter–associated infection.*[42,44]

Completing the procedure

■ Discard used supplies in the appropriate receptacles.[37,43]

■ Remove and discard your gloves[35,37,43] and perform hand hygiene.[5,21,22,23,24,25,26,27]

■ Return the bed to the lowest position *to prevent falls and maintain patient safety.*[47]

■ Monitor the patient closely for adverse reactions to the prescribed medication. If adverse reactions occur, notify the patient's practitioner promptly and intervene as ordered.[20]

■ If the patient is receiving IV opioid medication, frequently monitor the patient's respiratory rate, oxygen saturation level by pulse oximetry, end-tidal carbon dioxide level by capnography (if available), and sedation level using a standardized sedation scale *to decrease the risk of adverse events associated with IV opioid use.*[16,20] Explain the assessment and monitoring process to the patient and family, and instruct them to alert a staff member if the patient experiences breathing problems or sedation.[16,20]

■ Perform hand hygiene.[5,21,22,23,24,25,26,27]

■ Document the procedure.[48,49,50,51,52]

Special considerations

■ Use single-dose vials for parenteral medications whenever possible.[5,35]

■ Never administer medications from the same syringe to more than one patient.[5,35]

■ Don't enter a medication or fluid container with a used syringe.[5,35]

■ Never use medications packaged as single-dose or single-use for more than one patient. This includes ampules, bags, and bottles of IV solutions.[5,35]

■ Don't keep multidose vials in the immediate patient treatment area. Store them in accordance with the manufacturer's recommendations, and discard them if their sterility is compromised or questionable.[5,35]

■ Always use sterile no-touch technique when preparing and administering injections.[5,35]

■ Consider the use of infusion devices *to enhance the safety of IV bolus medication procedures.*

■ If you're preparing and administering more than one IV bolus injection medication to a patient, you should either completely prepare and administer one medication before preparing and administering the second, or prepare and label one medication before preparing and labeling the next one. *To decrease the risk of medication errors,* bring only one labeled syringe with a IV bolus injection medication to the bedside at a time.[4]

■ The Joint Commission issued a sentinel event alert related to managing risk during transition to new International Organization for Standardization tubing connector standards that were designed to prevent dangerous tubing misconnections, which can lead to serious patient injury and death. During the transition, make sure to trace all tubing and catheters from the patient to the points of origin before connecting or reconnecting any device or infusion, at any care transition (such as a new setting or service), and as part of the hand-off process; route tubes and catheters having different purposes in different standardized directions; when more than one access site is present or several bags are hanging, label the tubing at both the distal and proximal ends; use tubing and equipment only as intended; and store medications for different delivery routes in separate locations.[40]

Patient teaching

Teach the patient about the medication and its potential adverse effects.

Complications

Because drugs administered by IV bolus injections are delivered directly into the circulatory system and can produce an immediate effect, an acute allergic reaction or anaphylaxis can develop rapidly. If signs of anaphylaxis (dyspnea, cyanosis, seizures, and increasing respiratory distress) occur, notify the practitioner immediately and begin emergency procedures, as necessary.[1] Excessively rapid medication administration may also cause adverse effects, such as speed shock.[1] Other potential adverse effects vary depending on the medication administered. Complications such as local and systemic infection and infiltration or extravasation can occur.[53,54]

Documentation

Record the medication strength and dose administered, the date and time of administration, the route and rate of administration, the vascular access device used, the administration device used (if applicable), the condition and patency of the vascular access device before and after administration, and the patient's tolerance of the procedure.[1,2,3] Document the effects of the medication on the patient. Also note any adverse reactions to the prescribed medication, the name of the practitioner notified, the date and time of notification, any prescribed interventions, and the patient's response to those interventions. Document teaching provided to the patient and family (if applicable), their understanding of that teaching, and any need for follow-up teaching.

REFERENCES

1 Infusion Nurses Society. (2016). *Policies and procedures for infusion therapy* (5th ed.). Boston, MA: Infusion Nurses Society.

2 Infusion Nurses Society. (2017). *Policies and procedures for infusion therapy of the older adult* (3rd ed.). Boston, MA: Infusion Nurses Society.

3 Standard 59. Infusion medication and solution administration. Infusion therapy standards of practice (8th ed.). (2021). *Journal of Infusion Nursing, 44*, S180–S183. (Level VII)

4 Institute for Safe Medication Practices. (2015). Safe practice guidelines for adult IV push medications. https://www.ismp.org/guidelines/iv-push (Level VII)

5 Centers for Disease Control and Prevention. (2011, revised 2017). Guidelines for the prevention of intravascular catheter-related infections. https://www.cdc.gov/infectioncontrol/guidelines/bsi/recommendations. html (Level I)

6 Marschall, J., et al. (2014). SHEA/IDSA practice recommendation: Strategies to prevent central line–associated bloodstream infections in acute care hospitals. *Infection Control and Hospital Epidemiology, 35*, 753–771. https://www.jstor.org/stable/10.1086/676533#metadata_info_tab_contents (Level I)

7 Jarrett, N., & Callaham, M. (2016). Evidence-based guidelines for selected hospital-acquired conditions: Final report. https://www.cms.gov/Medicare/Medicare-Fee-for-Service-Payment/HospitalAcqCond/Downloads/2016-HAC-Report.pdf (Level VII)

8 The Joint Commission. (2021). Standard NPSG.07.04.01. *Comprehensive accreditation manual for hospitals.* Oakbrook Terrace, IL: The Joint Commission. (Level VII)

9 Association of Professionals in Infection Control and Epidemiology (APIC). (2015). Guide to preventing central line-associated bloodstream infections. http://apic.org/Resource_/TinyMceFileManager/2015/APIC_CLABSI_WEB.pdf (Level IV)

10 Standard 41. Flushing and locking. Infusion therapy standards of practice (8th ed.). (2021). *Journal of Infusion Nursing, 44*, S113–S119. (Level VII)

11 Loubnan, V., & Nasser, S. C. (2010). A guide on intravenous drug compatibilities based on their pH. *Pharmacie Globale, International Journal of Comprehensive Pharmacy, 5*(1), 1–9. (Level VII)

12 Standard 12. Product evaluation, integrity, and defect reporting. Infusion therapy standards of practice (8th ed.). (2021). *Journal of Infusion Nursing, 44*, S45–S46. (Level VII)

13 The Joint Commission. (2021). Standard NPSG.03.04.01. *Comprehensive accreditation manual for hospitals.* Oakbrook Terrace, IL: The Joint Commission. (Level VII)

14 Westbrook, J., et al. (2010). Association of interruptions with an increased risk and severity of medication administration errors. *Archives of Internal Medicine, 170*, 683–690. (Level IV)

15 Institute for Safe Medication Practices. (2012). Side tracks on the safety express: Interruptions lead to errors and unfinished...Wait, what was I doing? *Nurse Advise-ERR* 11(2), 1–4. https://www.ismp.org/resources/side-tracks-safety-express-interruptions-lead-errors-and-unfinished-wait-what-was-i-doing?id=37

16 Centers for Medicare and Medicaid Services, Department of Health and Human Services. (2019). Condition of participation: Nursing services. 42 C.F.R. § 482.23(c).

17 The Joint Commission. (2021). Standard MM.06.01.01. *Comprehensive accreditation manual for hospitals.* Oakbrook Terrace, IL: The Joint Commission. (Level VII)

18 Accreditation Association for Hospitals and Health Systems. (2020). Standard 16.01.03. *Healthcare Facilities Accreditation Program: Accreditation requirements for acute care hospitals.* Chicago, IL: Accreditation Association for Hospitals and Health Systems. (Level VII)

19 DNV GL-Healthcare USA, Inc. (2020). MM.1.SR.3. *NIAHO® accreditation requirements, interpretive guidelines and surveyor guidance—revision 20.0.* Milford, OH: DNV GL-Healthcare USA, Inc. (Level VII)

20 Centers for Medicare and Medicaid Services. (2014). Requirements for hospital medication administration, particularly intravenous (IV) medications and post-operative care of patients receiving IV opioids. https://www.cms.gov/Medicare/Provider-Enrollment-and-Certification/SurveyCertificationGenInfo/Downloads/Survey-and-Cert-Letter-14-15.pdf

21 Centers for Disease Control and Prevention. (2002). Guideline for hand hygiene in health-care settings: Recommendations of the Healthcare Infection Control Practices Advisory Committee and the HICPAC/SHEA/APIC/IDSA Hand Hygiene Task Force. *MMWR Recommendations and Reports, 51*(RR-16), 1–45. https://www.cdc.gov/mmwr/pdf/rr/rr5116.pdf (Level II)

22 World Health Organization. (2009). WHO guidelines on hand hygiene in health care: First global patient safety challenge, clean care is safer care. https://apps.who.int/iris/bitstream/handle/10665/44102/9789241597906_eng.pdf?sequence=1 (Level IV)

23 The Joint Commission. (2021). Standard NPSG.07.01.01. *Comprehensive accreditation manual for hospitals.* Oakbrook Terrace, IL: The Joint Commission. (Level VII)

24 Accreditation Association for Hospitals and Health Systems. (2020). Standard 07.01.21. *Healthcare Facilities Accreditation Program: Accreditation requirements for acute care hospitals.* Chicago, IL: Accreditation Association for Hospitals and Health Systems. (Level VII)

25 Centers for Medicare and Medicaid Services, Department of Health and Human Services. (2019). Condition of participation: Infection control. 42 C.F.R. § 482.42.

26 DNV GL-Healthcare USA, Inc. (2020). IC.1.SR.1. *NIAHO® accreditation requirements, interpretive guidelines and surveyor guidance—revision 20.0.* Milford, OH: DNV GL-Healthcare USA, Inc. (Level VII)

27 Standard 16. Hand hygiene. Infusion therapy standards of practice (8th ed.). (2021). *Journal of Infusion Nursing, 44*, S53–S54. (Level VII)

28 The Joint Commission. (2021). Standard NPSG.01.01.01. *Comprehensive accreditation manual for hospitals.* Oakbrook Terrace, IL: The Joint Commission. (Level VII)

29 Accreditation Association for Hospitals and Health Systems. (2020). Standard 15.01.16. *Healthcare Facilities Accreditation Program: Accreditation requirements for acute care hospitals.* Chicago, IL: Accreditation Association for Hospitals and Health Systems. (Level VII)

30 Centers for Medicare and Medicaid Services, Department of Health and Human Services. (2019). Condition of participation: Patient's rights. 42 C.F.R. § 482.13 (c)(1).

31 DNV GL-Healthcare USA, Inc. (2020). PR.2.SR.5. *NIAHO® accreditation requirements, interpretive guidelines and surveyor guidance—revision 20.0.* Milford, OH: DNV GL-Healthcare USA, Inc. (Level VII)

32 The Joint Commission. (2021). Standard RI.01.01.01. *Comprehensive accreditation manual for hospitals.* Oakbrook Terrace, IL: The Joint Commission. (Level VII)

33 The Joint Commission. (2021). Standard PC.02.01.21. *Comprehensive accreditation manual for hospitals.* Oakbrook Terrace, IL: The Joint Commission. (Level VII)

34 Waters, T. R., et al. (2009). Safe patient handling training for schools of nursing. https://www.cdc.gov/niosh/docs/2009-127/pdfs/2009-127.pdf (Level VII)

35 Siegel, J. D., et al. (2007, revised 2019). 2007 guideline for isolation precautions: Preventing transmission of infectious agents in healthcare settings. https://www.cdc.gov/infectioncontrol/pdf/guidelines/isolation-guidelines-H.pdf (Level II)

36 Accreditation Association for Hospitals and Health Systems. (2020). Standard 07.01.10. *Healthcare Facilities Accreditation Program: Accreditation requirements for acute care hospitals.* Chicago, IL: Accreditation Association for Hospitals and Health Systems. (Level VII)

37 Occupational Safety and Health Administration. (2012). Bloodborne pathogens, standard number 1910.1030. https://www.osha.gov/pls/oshaweb/owadisp.show_document?p_id=10051&p_table=STANDARDS (Level VII)

38 Institute for Safe Medication Practices. (2018). ISMP list of high-alert medications in acute care settings. https://www.ismp.org/sites/default/files/attachments/2018-08/highAlert2018-Acute-Final.pdf (Level VII)

39 Institute for Safe Medication Practices. (2013). Independent double-checks. Undervalued and misused: Selective use of this strategy can play an important role in medication safety. https://www.ismp.org/resources/independent-double-checks-undervalued-and-misused-selective-use-strategy-can-play (Level VII)

40 The Joint Commission. (2014). Sentinel event alert 53: Managing risk during transition to new ISO tubing connector standards. https://www.jointcommission.org/assets/1/6/SEA_53_Connectors_8_19_14_final.pdf (Level VII)

41 U.S. Food and Drug Administration. (2017). Examples of medical device misconnections. https://www.fda.gov/medical-devices/medical-device-connectors/examples-medical-device-misconnections

42 Standard 36. Needleless connectors. Infusion therapy standards of practice (8th ed.). (2021). *Journal of Infusion Nursing, 44*, S104–S107. (Level VII)

43 Standard 21. Medical waste and sharps safety. Infusion therapy standards of practice (8th ed.). (2021). *Journal of Infusion Nursing, 44*, S60–S63. (Level VII)

44 Moureau, N. L., & Flynn, J. (2015). Disinfection of needleless connector hubs: Clinical evidence systematic review. *Nursing Research and Practice*, 2015, 1–20. https://www.hindawi.com/journals/nrp/2015/796762/

45 Hull, G. J., et al. (2018). Quantitative assessment of reflux in commercially available needle-free IV connectors. *Journal of Vascular Access, 19*, 12–22. (Level VI)

46 Jasinsky, L., & Wurster, J. (2009). Occlusion reduction and heparin elimination trial using an anti-reflux device on peripheral and central venous catheters. *Journal of Infusion Nursing, 32*, 33–39. (Level VI)

47 Ganz, D. A., et al. (2013, reviewed 2021). *Preventing falls in hospitals: A toolkit for improving quality of care* (AHRQ Publication No. 13-0015-EF). Rockville, MD: Agency for Healthcare Research and Quality. https://www.ahrq.gov/professionals/systems/hospital/fallpxtoolkit/index.html (Level VII)

48 The Joint Commission. (2021). Standard RC.01.03.01. *Comprehensive accreditation manual for hospitals*. Oakbrook Terrace, IL: The Joint Commission. (Level VII)

49 Standard 10. Documentation in the medical record. Infusion therapy standards of practice. (2016). *Journal of Infusion Nursing, 39*, S28–S30. (Level VII)

50 Centers for Medicare and Medicaid Services, Department of Health and Human Services. (2019). Condition of participation: Medical record services. 42 C.F.R. § 482.24(b).

51 DNV GL-Healthcare USA, Inc. (2020). MR.2.SR.1. *NIAHO® accreditation requirements, interpretive guidelines and surveyor guidance—revision 20.0*. Milford, OH: DNV GL-Healthcare USA, Inc. (Level VII)

52 Accreditation Association for Hospitals and Health Systems. (2020). Standard 10.00.03. *Healthcare Facilities Accreditation Program: Accreditation requirements for acute care hospitals*. Chicago, IL: Accreditation Association for Hospitals and Health Systems. (Level VII)

53 Standard 47. Infiltration and extravasation. Infusion therapy standards of practice (8th ed.). (2021). *Journal of Infusion Nursing, 44*, S142–S147. (Level VII)

54 Standard 50. Infection. Infusion therapy standards of practice (8th ed.). (2021). *Journal of Infusion Nursing, 44*, S153–S157. (Level VII)

IV CATHETER INSERTION AND REMOVAL

Short peripheral IV catheter insertion involves selection of a venipuncture device and an insertion site, application of a tourniquet (if needed), site preparation, venipuncture, catheter securement, and dressing application. Select a venipuncture device and site according to the patient's vascular access device needs based on the prescribed therapy or treatment regimen, anticipated duration of therapy, vascular characteristics, and the patient's age, comorbidities, history of infusion therapy, preference for IV catheter location, and ability and resources available to care for the device.

A short peripheral catheter allows administration of fluids, medication, blood, and blood components, and maintains IV access to the patient. Peripheral catheters are recommended for use with infusates with an osmolality of 900 mOsm/L or less, and a therapy regimen of fewer than 6 days.[1,2] Some short peripheral catheters are available with an internal guide wire designed to minimize the need for the unnecessary needle advancement that may lead to blood vessel damage and complications. Insertion of these devices may require special training.[3]

Guidelines recommend that you select the smallest gauge short peripheral catheter that will accommodate the prescribed therapy. For example, a 20G to 24G catheter is appropriate for most infusion therapies, including blood transfusion, *because peripheral catheters larger than 20G are more likely to cause phlebitis*. For older adults, consider a 22G to 24G catheter *to minimize insertion-related trauma*. Consider a larger gauge catheter of 14G to 18G for rapid transfusion, and a 16G to 20G catheter for rapid fluid replacement, as in a trauma case or when a fenestrated catheter is needed for a contrast-based radiographic study.[1,2,4]

If you anticipate long-term therapy, start with a vein at the most distal site so that you can move proximally, as needed, for subsequent IV insertion sites. (See *Choosing an IV insertion site.*) Cannulation of dialysis fistulas and grafts for use of a hemodialysis catheter for IV infusion therapy requires an order from a nephrologist or practitioner unless an emergency situation exists.[5]

Choosing an IV insertion site

The following guidelines may be useful when choosing an appropriate peripheral IV insertion site.

■ Use veins on the dorsal and ventral surfaces of the upper extremities, including the metacarpal, cephalic, basilic, and median veins. If possible, choose a vein in the nondominant arm or hand.[5]

■ Avoid using veins in an upper extremity on the side of breast surgery with axillary node dissection or with an arteriovenous fistula or graft, radiation therapy, or lymphedema, or an extremity affected by stroke.[5]

■ If the patient has stage 4 or 5 chronic kidney disease, avoid using the upper arm or forearm veins that could be the site of dialysis access.[5]

■ Avoid using lower extremity veins *because of the increased risk of tissue damage, thrombophlebitis, and ulceration*.

■ Avoid areas of flexion; areas where pain occurs on palpation; veins compromised by bruising, infiltration, phlebitis, sclerosis, or cord formation; and areas where procedures are planned.

■ Avoid the lateral surface of the wrist for about 4″ to 5″ (10.2 cm to 12.7 cm) *because of the risk of nerve damage*; avoid the ventral surface of the wrist *because of the associated pain on insertion and the risk of nerve damage*.

■ Take care to insert catheters away from open wounds.

■ Make each successive cannulation site proximal to the previous cannulation site.

■ Collaborate with the patient and practitioner to discuss the risks and benefits of using a vein in an affected extremity if no other options exist.

■ For an older adult, choose an area with more subcutaneous tissue and skeletal support for better device stabilization, keeping in mind the need to conserve access for future therapy.[6]

■ If the patient uses an ambulatory aid to maintain independence, determine on which side the patient uses the device; avoid inserting the device in the hands and in areas of flexion.[6,7]

■ Allow an older adult to have input regarding the site of catheter insertion, *because many older adults have previous experience with infusion therapy and can indicate what has been successful or unsuccessful*.[6]

■ If the patient isn't very mobile, consider using an extremity that most easily allows access to the bathroom or commode.[6]

Sterile no-touch technique is necessary when inserting an IV catheter *to reduce the risk of vascular catheter–associated infection*.[1,4,6]

HOSPITAL-ACQUIRED CONDITION ALERT Keep in mind that the Centers for Medicare and Medicaid Services considers a vascular catheter–associated infection a hospital-acquired condition *because it can be reasonably prevented using a variety of best practices*. Make sure to follow evidence-based infection prevention practices, such as performing hand hygiene, preparing the site with an antiseptic, adhering to sterile no-touch technique during insertion and maintenance, and discontinuing the device when it's no longer needed, *to reduce the risk of vascular catheter–associated infections*.[7,8,9]

Equipment
For insertion

Chlorhexidine-based solution[10] (tincture of iodine, povidone- iodine, or alcohol may be used if chlorhexidine is contraindicated) ■ gloves ■ single-use tourniquet ■ short peripheral catheter with safety device[2] or short peripheral catheter with internal guide wire and safety device ■ antiseptic pad (chlorhexidine-based, povidone-iodine, or alcohol) ■ prescribed IV solution with attached and primed administration set ■ sterile 10-mL prefilled syringe containing preservative-free normal saline solution ■ IV pole ■ transparent semipermeable dressing ■ engineered stabilization device or sterile tape ■ Optional: soap and water, joint stabilization device, warm packs, single-use scissors, disposable-head clippers, vein stabilization device, prescribed local anesthetic, sterile gloves, short extension set (if not permanently attached to the IV catheter), electronic infusion device, manual flow-control device, ultrasound device with sterile probe cover, sterile ultrasound gel.

Commercial IV insertion kits come with or without an IV access device. In many facilities, venipuncture equipment is kept on a tray or cart, allowing more choice of access devices and easy replacement of contaminated items.[11]

For removal

Gloves ■ sterile gauze pads ■ tape ■ Optional: culture swab and tube, adhesive remover solution, nontraumatic paper or silicone tape, small adhesive dressing.

Preparation of equipment

Inspect all IV equipment and supplies. If a product is expired, is defective, or has compromised integrity, remove it from patient use, label it as expired or defective, and report the expiration or defect as directed by your facility.[12]

Prime the IV administration set with the prescribed IV solution or medication. (See the "IV therapy preparation" procedure.) Use a manual flow-control device for lower-risk infusions, an electronic infusion device for infusion therapies that require precise flow control, and a smart pump with dose-error reduction software to reduce the risk of infusion-related medication errors.[13] (See the "IV pump use" procedure.)

Implementation

■ Verify the practitioner's order for insertion of a short peripheral IV catheter. Review the order to make sure that the prescribed infusion solution or medication, dose, rate, and route of administration are appropriate for the patient's age, condition, and access device. Address concerns about the order with the practitioner, pharmacist, or your supervisor and, if needed, the risk management department, or as directed by your facility.[14]

■ Review the patient's medical record for allergies to antiseptic solutions, latex, and anesthetic agents. Also review it for factors that may affect peripheral vasculature, such as conditions that result in structural vessel changes, including diabetes or hypertension; history of frequent venipuncture or lengthy infusion therapy; skin variations; skin alterations (such as scars and tattoos); patient age; obesity; fluid volume deficit; and history of IV drug abuse, *to determine the need for vascular visualization technology*.[15]

■ Gather and prepare the necessary equipment and supplies.

■ Compare the label on the solution container to the order in the patient's medical record. Verify the name, dosage, concentration, administration route, frequency, and infusion rate.[16,17,18]

■ Check the expiration date on the solution. If the solution is expired, return it to the pharmacy and obtain new solution.

■ Visually inspect the solution for particles or discoloration or other loss of integrity; don't administer the solution if integrity is compromised.[4,6,14] Obtain a new IV solution if the integrity of the initial solution is compromised.

■ Perform hand hygiene.[1,18,19,20,21,22,23,24]

■ Confirm the patient's identity using at least two patient identifiers.[25]

■ Provide privacy.[26,27,28,29]

■ Explain the procedure to the patient and family (if appropriate) according to their individual communication and learning needs *to increase their understanding, allay their fears, and enhance cooperation*.[30] *Anxiety can cause a vasomotor response that results in venous constriction.* Provide the patient with information about the insertion process, expected duration of therapy, care and maintenance of the IV catheter, and signs and symptoms of complications as well as when to report them.[10,31]

■ If required by your facility, confirm that informed consent has been obtained and that the signed consent form is in the patient's medical record. Alternatively, obtain patient assent to perform the procedure.[4]

■ Hang the IV solution with attached primed administration set on an IV pole positioned close to the patient's bed.

■ Raise the patient's bed to waist level before providing care *to prevent caregiver back strain*.[32]

■ Place the patient in a comfortable sitting or reclining position, leaving the arm in a dependent position *to increase venous fill of the lower arms and hands*.[10]

Applying the tourniquet

■ Apply a tourniquet on an upper extremity *to dilate the veins and assess for an appropriate insertion site*. Loosely apply the tourniquet or avoid its use in patients who bruise easily, are at risk for bleeding, or have compromised circulation or fragile skin.[10]

■ Assess the patient's veins in the upper extremity and identify potential sites that are easily seen or palpated. If no access sites are visible or easily palpated, use visualization technology *to help identify an appropriate insertion site*. Choose an insertion site based on your assessment findings.[4]

■ Check for a pulse distal to the tourniquet location.[4,6] If a pulse isn't present, release the tourniquet and reapply it with less tension *to prevent arterial occlusion*.

■ Lightly palpate the vein with the index and middle fingers of your nondominant hand *to assess vein condition*.[4] Stretch the skin *to anchor the vein*. If the vein feels hard or ropelike, select another vein.

■ If the vein is easily palpable but not sufficiently dilated, place the extremity in a dependent position for several seconds or lightly stroke the vessel downward. If you have selected a vein in the arm or hand, tell the patient to open and close the fist several times, and lightly stroking the vein downward. Apply dry heat, if necessary, *to increase the likelihood of successful catheter insertion*.[4,6,10]

■ Release the tourniquet for site preparation.[4,6]

Preparing the site

■ If the intended insertion site is visibly soiled, clean it with soap and water before applying the antiseptic solution.[4,6,10]

■ Clip the hair around the insertion site, if needed, with single-patient-use scissors or disposable-head electric clippers *to facilitate dressing application after catheter insertion*.[10]

■ Administer a local anesthetic, if indicated and prescribed, following safe medication administration practices.[4,33,34] *Because there's less supportive underlying tissue in older adults*, take care not to nick or damage the vein when administering a local anesthetic; avoid inadvertently administering the anesthetic intravascularly.

■ Perform hand hygiene.[1,18,19,20,21,22,23,24]

■ Put on gloves *to comply with standard precautions*.[1,35,36,37]

■ Prepare the insertion site using an antiseptic agent *to remove flora that would otherwise be introduced into the vascular system with the venipuncture*. For chlorhexidine (preferred), apply with an applicator using a vigorous side-to-side motion for 30 seconds. Allow the area to dry completely.[4,10] For povidone-iodine solution, apply using a swab. Begin at the intended insertion site and move outward in concentric circles. Allow the solution to dry completely (typically at least 2 minutes).[4,10] If you must palpate the intended insertion site after cleaning, remove and discard your gloves, perform hand hygiene, and put on sterile gloves *to avoid contaminating the insertion site*.[4]

ELDER ALERT Be aware that, although antiseptic agents should be applied with friction, irritated skin may become more damaged, causing discomfort in older adults. Antiseptics can cause stinging and irritation. Excessive amounts of alcohol may dry already compromised skin.[6]

■ Reapply the tourniquet.[4]

■ Use visualization technology, such as near-infrared light technology (as shown below), if needed and available, *to locate a viable peripheral venous access site and decrease insertion time*, or use ultrasound technology, if available, to locate the vein in a patient with difficult venous access.[10]

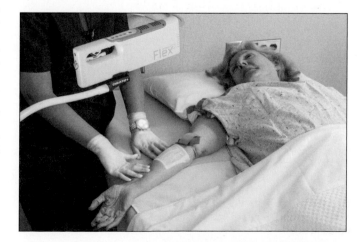

Inserting a short peripheral catheter

■ Using the thumb of your nondominant hand, stretch the skin taut below the puncture site *to stabilize the vein.*[4] If the patient is an older adult, anchor the vein distal to the intended insertion site; *the vein may be difficult to stabilize and penetrate because of the aging process.*[6]

■ Tell the patient that you are about to insert the device.

■ Place the short peripheral catheter on top of the vein at a 10- to 15-degree angle from the skin.[4]

■ Puncture the skin and anterior vein wall, watching for a blood return to appear in the catheter, flashback chamber, or both.[4]

■ As you continue to hold the skin taut, use the device's push-off tab to separate the catheter from the needle stylet. Advance the catheter into the vein. Don't advance the catheter by pushing from the catheter hub *to avoid contaminating the catheter hub.*[4]

■ Release the tourniquet.[4]

■ Activate the device's safety mechanism following the manufacturer's instructions for use.[4]

Inserting a short peripheral catheter with an internal guide wire

■ Remove the needle cover, and verify the presence of the guidewire coil. Make sure that it isn't bent, kinked, or damaged.[3]

■ To test catheter function, move the slider toward the catheter tip until it stops *to fully advance the guidewire.* Then move the slider away from the catheter tip until it stops again *to fully retract the guidewire into the needle.* Make sure that the coiled tip isn't visible.[3]

■ Stretch the skin taut below the puncture site using the thumb of your nondominant hand *to stabilize the vein.*[4] For an older adult, anchor the vein distal to the intended insertion site. *The vein may be difficult to stabilize and penetrate because of the aging process.*[6]

■ Tell the patient that you're about to insert the device.

■ Place the catheter on top of the vein at a 10- to 15-degree angle to the skin.[4]

■ Puncture the skin and anterior vein wall, watching for blood to appear in the catheter. If it's necessary to insert the needle at a steeper angle, lower the catheter and stabilize it before deploying the guidewire.[3]

■ Gently move the slider toward the catheter tip until it stops *to slowly deploy the guidewire into the vessel.* Don't force or retract the guidewire *to prevent damage to the guidewire.*[3]

■ Advance the catheter into the vessel using two fingers at the catheter hub while using the opposite hand to stabilize the device. Avoid simultaneously pulling the needle out while pushing the catheter into the vein. Once the catheter has been advanced, don't reinsert the needle back into the catheter or pull the catheter back onto the needle. If you must reposition the catheter, do so without the aid of the needle. Alternatively, remove both the catheter and the needle as a unit *to prevent the needle from damaging or shearing the catheter.*[3]

■ Depress the safety activation button while stabilizing the catheter with your opposite hand *to retract the needle and proximal portion of the guidewire into the safety chamber while leaving the coiled tip visible for inspection.* If the needle doesn't retract, depress the safety activation button again. If the needle doesn't retract on the second attempt, carefully withdraw the needle and guidewire.[3]

■ Release the tourniquet.[4]

Assessing catheter patency

■ If the catheter doesn't contain a permanently attached extension tubing and you need to attach one, compress the patient's skin well above the catheter tip to stop blood flow, attach the extension set to the catheter hub, and tighten the Luer lock, making sure the Luer lock doesn't come in contact with the patient's skin *to prevent contamination of the Luer-lock device.*[4]

■ Perform a vigorous mechanical scrub of the extension tubing hub for at least 5 seconds using an antiseptic pad. Allow it to dry completely.[38,39,40]

■ While maintaining sterility of the syringe tip, attach a prefilled syringe containing preservative-free normal saline solution to the extension hub. (Use a 10-mL syringe or a syringe specifically designed to generate lower injection pressure.) Slowly aspirate to remove air from the extension set and to assess for a blood return that is the color and consistency

of whole blood. If you don't obtain a blood return, take steps to locate an external cause of obstruction.[4,38]

■ If you do obtain a blood return, slowly inject preservative-free normal saline solution into the catheter. Use a minimum volume of twice the internal volume of the catheter system. Don't forcibly flush the device; further evaluate the device if you meet resistance.[4,38]

■ Clamp the catheter, and then remove and discard the syringe in a puncture-resistant sharps disposal container.[4]

■ Perform a vigorous mechanical scrub of the extension tubing hub for at least 5 seconds using an antiseptic pad. Allow it to dry completely.[38,39,40]

■ Attach the primed IV administration set to the hub. Trace the tubing from the patient to its point of origin *to make sure that you're connecting it to the proper port.*[14,41]

■ Unclamp the catheter and begin the infusion, as prescribed. Monitor the insertion site for swelling; remove the catheter if swelling occurs or the patient complains of discomfort or pain.[4]

Dressing the site

■ Secure the catheter with an engineered stabilization device, if available. An engineered stabilization device is recommended *because it reduces vascular access device motion, which increases the risk of unintentional catheter dislodgment and complications requiring premature catheter removal.*[31] If an engineered stabilization device is unavailable, secure the catheter with sterile tape.[4]

■ Apply a transparent semipermeable dressing over the insertion site following the manufacturer's instructions.[31] If the patient has fragile skin, use a dressing specifically formulated for fragile skin *to prevent skin stripping or tearing with removal.*[42]

■ Route the tubing in a standardized direction if the patient has other tubing and catheters that have different purposes. Label the tubing at the distal end (near the patient connection) and proximal end (near the source container) *to reduce the risk of misconnection* if you'll be using multiple IV access sites or IV bags.[43]

■ Curl the extension set to the side and tape it to the patient's arm if needed for extra securement.[3]

■ Label the dressing with the current date or the date the dressing is due to be changed, as directed by your facility.[4]

■ If the IV catheter insertion site is near a movable joint, stabilize the joint using a padded joint stabilization device that supports the area of flexion and maintains the joint in a functional position. Secure the joint stabilization device following the manufacturer's instructions. Make sure the device enables visualization and assessment of the insertion site and vascular pathway. Ensure that it doesn't exert pressure that constricts circulation or cause pressure injuries, skin impairment, or nerve damage. Periodically remove the device *to assess circulation, range of motion, function, and skin integrity.*[44]

Removing an IV catheter

■ Verify the order to remove the peripheral IV catheter.[4,45]

■ Gather and prepare the necessary equipment and supplies.

■ Perform hand hygiene.[1,18,19,20,21,22,23,24]

■ Confirm the patient's identity using at least two patient identifiers.[25]

■ Provide privacy.[26,27,28,29]

■ Explain the procedure to the patient and family (if appropriate) according to their individual communication and learning needs *to increase their understanding, allay their fears, and enhance cooperation.*[30]

■ Raise the patient's bed to waist level when providing care *to prevent caregiver back strain.*[32]

■ Place the patient in a sitting or recumbent position.[4]

■ Perform hand hygiene.[1,18,19,20,21,22,23,24]

■ Open the sterile gauze pads and place them within reach on a clean barrier.

■ Perform hand hygiene.[1,18,19,20,21,22,23,24]

■ Put on gloves *to comply with standard precautions.*[35,36,37]

■ Trace the IV administration set tubing from the patient to its point of origin *to make sure you're accessing the proper IV administration set.*[41]

■ Clamp the IV administration set tubing, the extension set, or both *to stop the flow of solution.*[4]

■ Remove the joint stabilization device, if present.

- Remove the IV insertion site protection device, if present.
- Remove the transparent dressing by gently pulling the dressing edges back toward the IV insertion site *to avoid stripping or tearing the skin.*[6,42]
- Remove the IV catheter stabilization device, if present.[4,6]
- Apply the adhesive removal solution to loosen the dressing and securement device adhesive, if necessary.[4]
- Inspect the catheter–skin junction for signs of infection or phlebitis.[4,6,9,46] If signs of vascular catheter–associated infection are present, notify the practitioner and discuss the need for obtaining specimens for culture (such as blood and drainage) before removing the IV catheter.[4] Obtain culture specimens as indicated and ordered.[4]
- Hold the gauze pad over the puncture site with one hand, and use your other hand to withdraw the cannula slowly and smoothly, keeping it parallel to the skin.[4]
- Using the gauze pad, apply pressure over the puncture site until bleeding has stopped (for a minimum of 30 seconds).[4,6]
- Tape a gauze pad to the catheter exit site, or apply a small adhesive bandage.[4] If the patient has fragile skin, use nontraumatic paper or silicone tape to secure the gauze pad *to avoid skin stripping and tearing.*[42]
- Assess the IV catheter tip after removal for damage and possible fragmentation. If damage is seen or suspected, notify the practitioner, *because a chest X-ray or further evaluation may be warranted.* Assess the patient carefully for signs and symptoms of catheter embolism (for example, palpitations, arrhythmias, dyspnea, cough, and thoracic pain that isn't associated with the patient's primary condition or comorbidities).[4]
- Return the bed to the lowest level *to prevent falls and maintain patient safety.*[47]
- Discard used supplies in an appropriate receptacle.[35,36,48,49]
- Remove and discard your gloves.[35,36,48]
- Perform hand hygiene.[1,18,19,20,21,22,23,24]
- Document the procedure.[50,51,52,53,54]

Special considerations

- One nurse should make no more than two attempts at insertion, and total attempts should be limited to no more than four, *because unsuccessful attempts limit future attempts and cause the patient unnecessary pain, delay treatment, limit future vascular access, increase cost, and increase risk of complications.*[10]
- If the patient reports symptoms of paresthesia, such as radiating electrical pain, tingling, burning, a prickly feeling, or numbness, immediately stop the insertion procedure and carefully remove the catheter. Also stop the procedure upon the patient's request or when the patient's actions indicate severe pain. Notify the practitioner of the patient's report of symptoms, *because early recognition of nerve damage produces a better prognosis.* Document the details of the patient's report of symptoms in the medical record.[55]
- If the patient reports a burning sensation during the injection of preservative-free normal saline solution, stop the injection and check catheter placement. If the catheter is in the vein, inject the preservative-free normal saline solution at a slower rate *to minimize irritation.* If the catheter isn't in the vein, remove and discard it; then select a new venipuncture site and, using fresh equipment, restart the procedure.[56]
- The Joint Commission issued a sentinel event alert related to managing risk during transition to new International Organization for Standardization tubing standards that were designed to prevent dangerous tubing misconnections, which can lead to serious patient injury and death. During the transition, make sure to trace the tubing and catheter from the patient to the point of origin before connecting or reconnecting any device or infusion, at any care transition (such as to a new setting or service), and as part of the hand-off process; route tubes and catheters having different purposes in different standardized directions; when the patient has different access sites or several bags hanging, label tubing at both the distal and proximal ends; use tubing and equipment only as intended; and store medications for different delivery routes in separate locations.[43]
- Change or remove dressing, as needed.[4]
- Monitor the site for 48 hours after removal of the IV catheter *to detect postinfusion phlebitis.*[46]

Complications

Improper insertion technique during peripheral IV catheter insertion may cause vascular catheter–associated infection, hematoma, bleeding, nerve damage, and inadvertent arterial access.[10]

Complications of IV catheter removal include hematoma, local and systemic infection, phlebitis, and catheter embolism.[4]

Documentation

Record the insertion site location; specific site preparation; local anesthetic (if used); infection prevention and safety precautions you took; type, length, and gauge of the catheter you inserted; date and time of insertion; number and location of insertion attempts; device functionality; insertion method, including the use of visualization and guidance technology; method of catheter stabilization; and patient's tolerance of the procedure. Also document the type and flow rate of the IV solution, the name and dose of medication in the solution (if any), any adverse reactions, and the patient's response to those interventions. Record teaching you provided to the patient and family (if applicable), their understanding of that teaching, and any need for follow-up teaching.[51]

Record the date and time of IV catheter removal, the site from which you removed the IV catheter, the condition of the IV insertion site and the catheter, and the patient's tolerance of the procedure.

REFERENCES

1 Centers for Disease Control and Prevention. (2011, revised 2017). Guidelines for the prevention of intravascular catheter–related infections. https://www.cdc.gov/infectioncontrol/guidelines/bsi/recommendations.html (Level I)

2 Standard 26. Vascular access device planning. Infusion therapy standards of practice (8th ed.). (2021). *Journal of Infusion Nursing, 44,* S74–S81. (Level VII)

3 C.R. Bard, Inc. (2018). AccuCath intravascular catheter. https://www.bd.com/en-us/offerings/capabilities/vascular-access/vascular-iv-catheters/peripheral-iv-catheters/accucath-ace-intravascular-catheter

4 Infusion Nurses Society. (2016). *Policies and procedures for infusion therapy* (5th ed.). Boston, MA: Infusion Nurses Society.

5 Standard 27. Site selection. Infusion therapy standards of practice (8th ed.). (2021). *Journal of Infusion Nursing, 44,* S81–S86. (Level VII)

6 Infusion Nurses Society. (2016). *Policies and procedures for infusion therapy of the older adult* (3rd ed.). Boston, MA: Infusion Nurses Society.

7 Vizcarra, C., et al. (2014). Recommendations for improving safety practices with short peripheral catheters. *Journal of Infusion Nursing, 37,* 121–124. (Level VII)

8 Jarrett, N., & Callaham, M. (2016). Evidence-based guidelines for selected hospital-acquired conditions: Final report. https://www.cms.gov/Medicare/Medicare-Fee-for-Service-Payment/HospitalAcqCond/Downloads/2016-HAC-Report.pdf

9 Standard 50. Infection. Infusion therapy standards of practice (8th ed.). (2021). *Journal of Infusion Nursing, 44,* S153–S157. (Level VII)

10 Standard 33. Vascular access site preparation and skin antisepsis. Infusion therapy standards of practice (8th ed.). (2021). *Journal of Infusion Nursing, 44,* S96–S97. (Level VII)

11 Franklin, B. D., et al. (2012). The safe insertion of peripheral intravenous catheters: A mixed methods descriptive study of the availability of the equipment needed. *Antimicrobial Resistance and Infection Control, 1,* 15. https://aricjournal.biomedcentral.com/articles/10.1186/2047-2994-1-15 (Level VII)

12 Standard 12. Product evaluation, integrity, and defect reporting. Infusion therapy standards of practice (8th ed.). (2021). *Journal of Infusion Nursing, 44,* S45–S46. (Level VII)

13 Standard 24. Flow-control devices. Infusion therapy standards of practice (8th ed.). (2021). *Journal of Infusion Nursing, 44,* S69–S72. (Level VII)

14 Standard 59. Infusion medication and solution administration. Infusion therapy standards of practice (8th ed.). (2021). *Journal of Infusion Nursing, 44,* S180–S183. (Level VII)

15 Standard 22. Vascular visualization. Infusion therapy standards of practice (8th ed.). (2021). *Journal of Infusion Nursing, 44,* S63–S65. (Level VII)

16 Centers for Medicare and Medicaid Services, Department of Health and Human Services. (2020). Condition of participation: Nursing services. 42 C.F.R. § 482.23(c).

17 Accreditation Association for Hospitals and Health Systems. (2020). Standard 16.01.03. *Healthcare Facilities Accreditation Program:*

Accreditation requirements for acute care hospitals. Chicago, IL: Accreditation Association for Hospitals and Health Systems. (Level VII)

18 The Joint Commission. (2021). Standard NPSG.07.01.01. *Comprehensive accreditation manual for hospitals.* Oakbrook Terrace, IL: The Joint Commission. (Level VII)

19 Standard 16. Hand hygiene. Infusion therapy standards of practice (8th ed.). (2021). *Journal of Infusion Nursing, 44,* S53–S54. (Level VII)

20 Centers for Disease Control and Prevention. (2002). Guideline for hand hygiene in health-care settings: Recommendations of the Healthcare Infection Control Practices Advisory Committee and the HICPAC/SHEA/APIC/IDSA Hand Hygiene Task Force. *MMWR Recommendations and Reports, 51*(RR-16), 1–45. https://www.cdc.gov/mmwr/pdf/rr/rr5116.pdf (Level II)

21 World Health Organization. (2009). WHO guidelines on hand hygiene in health care: First global patient safety challenge, clean care is safer care. https://apps.who.int/iris/bitstream/handle/10665/44102/9789241597906_eng.pdf?sequence=1 (Level IV)

22 Accreditation Association for Hospitals and Health Systems. (2020). Standard 07.01.21. *Healthcare Facilities Accreditation Program: Accreditation requirements for acute care hospitals.* Chicago, IL: Accreditation Association for Hospitals and Health Systems. (Level VII)

23 Centers for Medicare and Medicaid Services, Department of Health and Human Services. (2020). Condition of participation: Infection control. 42 C.F.R. § 482.42.

24 DNV GL-Healthcare USA, Inc. (2020). IC.1.SR.1. *NIAHO® accreditation requirements, interpretive guidelines and surveyor guidance—revision 20.0.* Milford, OH: DNV GL-Healthcare USA, Inc. (Level VII)

25 The Joint Commission. (2021). Standard NPSG.01.01.01. *Comprehensive accreditation manual for hospitals.* Oakbrook Terrace, IL: The Joint Commission. (Level VII)

26 Accreditation Association for Hospitals and Health Systems. (2020). Standard 15.01.16. *Healthcare Facilities Accreditation Program: Accreditation requirements for acute care hospitals.* Chicago, IL: Accreditation Association for Hospitals and Health Systems. (Level VII)

27 Centers for Medicare and Medicaid Services, Department of Health and Human Services. (2020). Condition of participation: Patient's rights. 42 C.F.R. § 482.13(c)(1).

28 DNV GL-Healthcare USA, Inc. (2020). PR.2.SR.5. *NIAHO® accreditation requirements, interpretive guidelines and surveyor guidance—revision 20.0.* Milford, OH: DNV GL-Healthcare USA, Inc. (Level VII)

29 The Joint Commission. (2021). Standard RI.01.01.01. *Comprehensive accreditation manual for hospitals.* Oakbrook Terrace, IL: The Joint Commission. (Level VII)

30 The Joint Commission. (2021). Standard PC.02.01.21. *Comprehensive accreditation manual for hospitals.* Oakbrook Terrace, IL: The Joint Commission. (Level VII)

31 Standard 38. Vascular access device securement. Infusion therapy standards of practice (8th ed.). (2021). *Journal of Infusion Nursing, 44,* S108–S111. (Level VII)

32 Waters, T. R., et al. (2009). Safe patient handling training for schools of nursing. https://www.cdc.gov/niosh/docs/2009-127/pdfs/2009-127.pdf (Level VII)

33 Standard 32. Pain management for venipuncture and vascular access device procedures. Infusion therapy standards of practice (8th ed.). (2021). *Journal of Infusion Nursing, 44,* S94–S96. (Level VII)

34 DNV GL-Healthcare USA, Inc. (2020). MM.1.SR.3. *NIAHO® accreditation requirements, interpretive guidelines and surveyor guidance—revision 20.0.* Milford, OH: DNV GL-Healthcare USA, Inc. (Level VII)

35 Occupational Safety and Health Administration. (2012). Bloodborne pathogens, standard number 1910.1030. https://www.osha.gov/pls/oshaweb/owadisp.show_document?p_id=10051&p_table=STANDARDS (Level VII)

36 Siegel, J. D., et al. (2007, revised 2019). 2007 guideline for isolation precautions: Preventing transmission of infectious agents in healthcare settings. https://www.cdc.gov/infectioncontrol/pdf/guidelines/isolation-guidelines-H.pdf (Level II)

37 Accreditation Association for Hospitals and Health Systems. (2020). Standard 07.01.10. *Healthcare Facilities Accreditation Program: Accreditation requirements for acute care hospitals.* Chicago, IL: Accreditation Association for Hospitals and Health Systems. (Level VII)

38 Standard 41. Flushing and locking. Infusion therapy standards of practice (8th ed.). (2021). *Journal of Infusion Nursing, 44,* S113–S119. (Level VII)

39 Marschall, J., et al. (2014). SHEA/IDSA practice recommendation: Strategies to prevent central line-associated bloodstream infections in acute care hospitals. *Infection Control and Hospital Epidemiology, 35,* 753–771. https://www.jstor.org/stable/10.1086/676533#metadata_info_tab_contents (Level I)

40 Standard 36. Needleless connectors. Infusion therapy standards of practice (8th ed.). (2021). *Journal of Infusion Nursing, 44,* S104–S107. (Level VII)

41 U.S. Food and Drug Administration. (2017). Examples of medical device misconnections. https://www.fda.gov/medical-devices/medical-device-connectors/examples-medical-device-misconnections

42 LeBlanc, K., et al. (2013). International skin tear advisory panel: A tool kit to aid in the prevention, assessment, and treatment of skin tears using a simplified classification system. *Advances in Skin & Wound Care, 26,* 459–476. (Level IV)

43 The Joint Commission. (2014). Sentinel event alert 53: Managing risk during transition to new ISO tubing connector standards. http://www.jointcommission.org/assets/1/6/SEA_53_Connectors_8_19_14_final.pdf (Level VII)

44 Standard 39. Joint stabilization. Infusion therapy standards of practice (8th ed.). (2021). *Journal of Infusion Nursing, 44,* S111–S112. (Level VII)

45 Standard 45. Vascular access device removal. Infusion therapy standards of practice (8th ed.). (2021). *Journal of Infusion Nursing, 44,* S133–S138. (Level VII)

46 Standard 46. Phlebitis. Infusion therapy standards of practice (8th ed.). (2021). *Journal of Infusion Nursing, 44,* S138–S142. (Level VII)

47 Ganz, D. A., et al. (2013, reviewed 2021). *Preventing falls in hospitals: A toolkit for improving quality of care* (AHRQ Publication No. 13-0015-EF). Rockville, MD: Agency for Healthcare Research and Quality. https://www.ahrq.gov/professionals/systems/hospital/fallpxtoolkit/index.html (Level VII)

48 Standard 21. Medical waste and sharps safety. Infusion therapy standards of practice (8th ed.). (2021). *Journal of Infusion Nursing, 44,* S60–S63. (Level VII)

49 Accreditation Association for Hospitals and Health Systems. (2020). Standard 07.03.07. *Healthcare Facilities Accreditation Program: Accreditation requirements for acute care hospitals.* Chicago, IL: Accreditation Association for Hospitals and Health Systems. (Level VII)

50 The Joint Commission. (2021). Standard RC.01.03.01. *Comprehensive accreditation manual for hospitals.* Oakbrook Terrace, IL: The Joint Commission. (Level VII)

51 Standard 10. Documentation in the health record. Infusion therapy standards of practice (8th ed.). (2021). *Journal of Infusion Nursing, 44,* S39–S43. (Level VII)

52 Centers for Medicare and Medicaid Services, Department of Health and Human Services. (2020). Condition of participation: Medical record services. 42 C.F.R. § 482.24(b).

53 Accreditation Association for Hospitals and Health Systems. (2020). Standard 10.00.03. *Healthcare Facilities Accreditation Program: Accreditation requirements for acute care hospitals.* Chicago, IL: Accreditation Association for Hospitals and Health Systems. (Level VII)

54 DNV GL-Healthcare USA, Inc. (2020). MR.2.SR.1. *NIAHO® accreditation requirements, interpretive guidelines and surveyor guidance—revision 20.0.* Milford, OH: DNV GL-Healthcare USA, Inc. (Level VII)

55 Standard 48. Nerve injury. Infusion therapy standards of practice (8th ed.). (2021). *Journal of Infusion Nursing, 44,* S147–S149. (Level VII)

56 Standard 47. Infiltration and extravasation. Infusion therapy standards of practice (8th ed.). (2021). *Journal of Infusion Nursing, 44,* S142–S147. (Level VII)

IV CATHETER MAINTENANCE

Routine maintenance of a short peripheral IV catheter insertion site includes regular assessment of the site (at least every 4 hours, or every 1 to 2 hours for a patient who's critically ill, sedated, or cognitively impaired). It also includes periodic dressing changes, which help to prevent complications, such as thrombophlebitis and infection.[1] The recommended frequency of dressing changes varies based on such factors as the type of dressing and the patient's condition.

The Infusion Nurses Society (INS) recommends that you change a gauze dressing over an IV catheter insertion site every 2 days, or immediately if the dressing becomes damp, loosened, or visibly soiled, or if you suspect infection or inflammation of the site.[1,2] The INS recommends that you change a transparent semipermeable membrane dressing every 5 to 7 days, or immediately if the dressing becomes damp, loosened, or visibly soiled, or if you suspect infection or inflammation of the site.[1,2] You should also change the dressing whenever you replace the IV device, which should occur as soon as possible (preferably in 24 to 48 hours) after insertion under suboptimal conditions (such as during an emergency),[1] as well as when clinically indicated based on the patient's condition, integrity of the vein and skin, length and type of prescribed therapy, integrity and patency of the existing catheter, and the patient's care location.[1,3]

HOSPITAL-ACQUIRED CONDITION ALERT Keep in mind that the Centers for Medicare and Medicaid Services considers vascular catheter–associated infection a hospital-acquired condition *because it can be reasonably prevented using a variety of best practices.* Make sure to use evidence-based infection prevention practices, such as performing hand hygiene, cleaning the IV insertion site properly with an antiseptic, and using sterile no-touch technique, when changing an IV dressing *to reduce the risk of vascular catheter–associated infections.*[4,5]

The need for continued use of a short peripheral IV catheter should be reassessed on a daily basis. Catheter removal should occur as soon as the catheter is no longer included in the plan of care, or when it hasn't been used for at least 24 hours.[6]

Blood sampling for laboratory testing can occur through short peripheral IV catheters, and may be an option for patients who need serial blood tests and those with poor venous access or bleeding disorders. However, you should use it only after weighing the benefits against the risks. Benefits include decreased patient anxiety and discomfort and decreased risk of local tissue injury and hematoma formation. Risks include erroneous laboratory values (when solutions are infusing), catheter occlusion, and catheter-associated bloodstream infection caused by contamination during catheter manipulation.[7]

Failure to adequately flush the IV catheter after blood withdrawal can lead to thrombotic occlusion. Group multiple blood draws whenever possible *to reduce the number of times you enter the system and minimize the risk of infection.* Don't reinfuse the discard specimen after obtaining the blood sample *because of the risk of contamination and blood clot formation in the discard syringe.*[7]

Equipment

For a dressing change

Gloves ■ antiseptic swab or pad (chlorhexidine-based solution [preferred]; tincture of iodine, povidone-iodine, or alcohol may be used if a contraindication to chlorhexidine exists)[1] ■ sterile transparent semipermeable dressing ■ engineered stabilization device ■ label ■ Optional: sterile 2″ × 2″ (5 cm × 5 cm) gauze pads, 4″ × 4″ (10 cm × 10 cm) gauze dressing, sterile tape, alcohol pad or adhesive remover solution, skin protectant solution.

Many facilities stock commercially prepared or facility-prepared sterile dressing change kits that contain the necessary supplies.

For a solution change

IV solution container ■ labels ■ Optional: time tape. antiseptic pads (chlorhexidine-based, or tincture of iodine)

For an IV administration tubing change

IV administration set ■ prescribed IV fluid ■ IV pole ■ gloves ■ antiseptic pads (chlorhexidine-based, povidone iodine, or alcohol) ■ labels ■ Optional: add-on devices, electronic infusion device, engineered stabilization device, transparent semipermeable dressing.

For using a time tape

Prescribed IV solution ■ preprinted IV time tape or approximate length of 1″ (2.5-cm) tape ■ pen ■ watch or clock.

For blood sampling

Gloves ■ 10-mL prefilled syringe of preservative-free normal saline solution ■ antiseptic pads (chlorhexidine-based, povidone-iodine, or alcohol) ■ 3-mL or 5-mL syringes, as appropriate for the volume of blood needed, or needleless blood collection tube holder ■ needleless transfer device ■ blood collection tubes ■ syringe or blood collection tube for discard

sample ■ labels ■ laboratory biohazard transport bag ■ Optional: sterile end caps, needleless connector, disinfectant-containing end cap, laboratory request forms.

Preparation of equipment

Inspect all equipment and supplies. If a product is expired, is defective, or has compromised integrity, remove it from patient use, label it as expired or defective, and report the expiration or defect as directed by your facility.[8]

Implementation

■ Review the patient's medical record for allergies, sensitivities, and contraindications to the antiseptic solution or dressing materials.[9]
■ Gather and prepare the necessary equipment and supplies.
■ Perform hand hygiene.[10,11,12,13,14,15,16]
■ Confirm the patient's identity using at least two patient identifiers.[17]
■ Provide privacy.[18,19,20,21]
■ Explain the procedure to the patient and family (if appropriate) according to their individual communication and learning needs *to increase their understanding, allay their fears, and enhance cooperation.*[22]
■ Raise the patient's bed to waist level before providing patient care *to prevent caregiver back strain.*[23]
■ Perform hand hygiene.[10,11,12,13,14,15,16]

Changing a dressing

■ Put on gloves *to comply with standard precautions.*[10,24,25,26]
■ Visually inspect the entire infusion system for clarity of the solution, integrity of the system (such as leakage and secure Luer connections), accurate flow rate, and expiration dates of the solution and administration set, as applicable.[1]
■ Assess the catheter–skin junction and surrounding area by visual inspection and palpation through an intact dressing for erythema, tenderness, swelling, and drainage. Pay attention for patient reports of pain, paresthesia, numbness, or tingling.[1,2,27]
■ Gently remove the existing dressing, beginning at the catheter hub and pulling it perpendicular to the skin toward the insertion site *to avoid catheter dislodgment and skin tearing and stripping.*[2,27,28] Use an alcohol pad or other appropriate adhesive removal solution, as needed, *to loosen the dressing.*[2]
■ Carefully remove the stabilization device, if indicated, following the manufacturer's instructions for use.[1,29]
■ Assess the skin that was underneath the dressing. If signs or symptoms of phlebitis (pain, tenderness, erythema, warmth, swelling, induration, purulence, or palpable venous cord), infiltration (pain, edema, blanching, or fluid leakage from the puncture site), or infection (erythema extending at least 1 cm from the insertion site, induration, exudate, pain or tenderness, or fever with no other obvious source of infection) are present, remove and replace the catheter (preferably in the opposite extremity).[1,30,31,32] (See the "IV catheter insertion and removal" procedure.) Notify the patient's practitioner and intervene as indicated and ordered.
■ Clean the insertion site and surrounding skin with an antiseptic solution following the manufacturer's instructions. Apply chlorhexidine using a back-and-forth motion for at least 30 seconds and allow it to dry completely.[2] Apply povidone iodine (or other iodophors) using swab sticks in a concentric circle, beginning at the catheter insertion site and moving outward. Allow the antiseptic to dry completely (typically 1½ to 2 minutes).[2]
■ Secure the catheter with an engineered stabilization device, if available. *An engineered stabilization device reduces vascular access device motion, which increases the risk of unintentional catheter dislodgement and complications that require premature catheter removal.* Apply skin protectant solution to the area before applying the engineered stabilization device according to the manufacturer's instructions *to decrease the risk of medical adhesive-related skin injury.*[2,29]
■ Place a sterile, transparent semipermeable dressing over the insertion site and catheter hub *to prevent contamination of the insertion site.* Alternately, apply a sterile 4″ × 4″ (10 cm × 10 cm) gauze dressing secured

with sterile tape.[1,2] If the patient has fragile skin, use a dressing specifically formulated for fragile skin *to prevent skin tearing and stripping.*[28]

- Label the dressing with the date you changed the dressing or the date it's next due to be changed, as directed by your facility.[1]
- Return the bed to the lowest level *to prevent falls and maintain patient safety.*[33]
- Discard used supplies in appropriate receptacles.[24,25,34,35]
- Remove and discard your gloves.[24,25,34]
- Perform hand hygiene.[10,11,12,13,14,15,16]
- Document the procedure.[36,37,38,39,40]

Changing the solution

- Gather and prepare the necessary equipment and supplies.
- Review the practitioner's order *to make sure that the prescribed infusion solution, rate, and route of administration are appropriate for the patient's age, condition, and access device.* Address concerns about the order with the practitioner, pharmacist, or your supervisor and, if needed, risk management, or as directed by your facility.[2,41,42]
- Compare the IV solution label with the order in the patient's medical record.[2,41,42]
- Perform hand hygiene.[10,11,12,13,14,15,16]
- Confirm the patient's identity using at least two patient identifiers.[17]
- Provide privacy.[18,19,20,21]
- Explain the procedure to the patient and family (if appropriate) according to their individual communication and learning needs *to increase their understanding, allay their fears, and enhance cooperation.*[22]
- If your facility uses barcode technology, use it as directed by your facility.
- Clamp the administration set tubing when inverting it *to prevent air from entering the tubing.* Keep the drip chamber filled to the level determined by the manufacturer. Place the IV infusion device in standby or pause mode.
- If you're replacing an IV solution bag, remove the seal or tab from the new bag and remove the old bag from the IV pole. Remove the spike, insert it into the new IV solution bag, trace the administration set tubing from the patient to its point of origin *to ensure that the tubing is connected to the proper port,*[41,43,44] and adjust the infusion flow rate or restart the IV infusion device.[2]
- If you're replacing an IV solution bottle, remove the cap and seal from the new bottle, disinfect the bottle's rubber port thoroughly with an antiseptic pad, and allow the port to dry. Clamp the IV line, pause the IV infusion device, remove the spike from the old bottle, and insert the spike into the new bottle. Then hang the new bottle, trace the administration set tubing from the patient to its point of origin *to ensure that the tubing is connected to the proper port,*[41,43,44] and adjust the infusion flow rate or restart the IV infusion device.

ELDER ALERT *Because older adults often have compromised cardiac, hepatic, or renal systems,* they're at risk for complications associated with IV solution administration. An older patient may not be able to articulate symptoms because of an underlying condition (such as stroke, intubation, tracheotomy, dementia, or delirium). *Infusion of a large volume of fluid or fluid delivered at a rapid rate may quickly result in heart failure, shock, or cardiac arrest,* so frequently monitor an older patient during IV infusions. An older patient is also at risk for speed shock, which results from rapid administration of a bolus medication or infusion. The patient may not be able to communicate such early symptoms as dizziness or headache, which can rapidly progress to chest tightness, hypotension, irregular pulse, and anaphylactic shock. Control IV administration rates carefully and monitor older patients closely *to reduce the risk of speed shock.*[27]

- Route the administration set tubing in a standardized direction if the patient has other tubing and IV catheters in place that have different purposes. If multiple IV lines will be used, label the tubing at the distal (near the patient connection) and proximal (near the source container) ends *to reduce the risk of misconnection.*[41,43]
- Label the new IV solution container with the date and time of change, and place a time tape on the container if required by your facility.
- Discard used supplies in the appropriate receptacles.[24,25,34,35]
- Monitor the flow-control device regularly, inspect the IV insertion site for complications, and evaluate the patient's response to therapy.[41]

- Perform hand hygiene.[10,11,12,13,14,15,16]
- Document the procedure.[36,37,38,39,40]

Changing the tubing

- Hang the solution on an IV pole.
- To prime the new administration set (including add-on devices and extension tubing, if used), squeeze the administration set's drip chamber, filling it to the level indicated by the manufacturer.[27] Then slowly open the clamp while holding the distal end of the administration set upright, allowing the filter to hang upside down.[27] Prime the entire length of the administration set and add-on devices. Alternatively, use the priming feature on the electronic infusion device.
- Clamp the administration set.[27]
- Perform hand hygiene.[10,11,12,13,14,15,16]
- Put on gloves *to comply with standard precautions.*[10,24,25,26]
- Assess the catheter–skin junction and surrounding area by visual inspection and palpation through an intact dressing for erythema, tenderness, swelling, and drainage. Pay attention for patient reports of pain, paresthesia, numbness, or tingling.[1]
- Gently remove the existing dressing, beginning at the catheter hub and pulling it perpendicular to the skin toward the insertion site as needed to access the catheter hub.[2]
- Carefully remove the stabilization device, if indicated, following the manufacturer's instructions for use.[1,29]
- Stop or pause the electronic infusion device, if indicated.
- Trace the existing tubing from the patient to its point of origin *to make sure you're accessing the proper tubing.*[41,43,44,45]
- Clamp the existing administration set.[27]
- Clamp the IV catheter *to prevent accidental exposure to blood and to reduce the risk of air embolism.*[2,27]
- Gently disconnect the existing tubing from the IV catheter hub, being careful not to dislodge the catheter.[27]
- Perform a vigorous mechanical scrub of the catheter hub for at least 5 seconds, using an antiseptic pad. Allow it to dry completely.[46]
- Remove the protective cap from the distal end of the new administration set and attach it to the catheter hub.[27] Trace the tubing from the patient to its point of origin *to make sure you've connected the new administration tubing to the proper port.*[41,43,44,45]
- Open the IV catheter clamp.[27]
- Place the administration set in the electronic infusion device and then turn on the device. Alternatively, slowly open the clamp of the administration set to begin the infusion.[27]
- Confirm that the electronic infusion device displays the correct information, unclamp the tubing, and begin the infusion. (See the "IV pump use" procedure.) If using a manual flow-control device, monitor the drops per minute manually *to ensure the proper administration rate.*
- Clean the insertion site and surrounding skin.
- Apply a new stabilization device, if needed.
- Apply a new transparent semipermeable dressing over the insertion site, if needed. (See the section above entitled "Changing a dressing.")[1,29]
- Check that all connections are secure *to prevent leakage, bleeding, contamination, and disconnections.*[43,44]
- Recheck the IV flow rate.
- Discard used supplies in an appropriate receptacle.[24,25,34,35]
- Remove and discard your gloves.[24,25,34]
- Perform hand hygiene.[10,11,12,13,14,15,16]
- Label the administration set at the proximal and distal ends *to prevent dangerous misconnections.* Route the tubing in a standardized direction if the patient has other tubing and catheters that have different purposes.[41,43]
- Label the administration set and solution container with the date of initiation or the date when change is necessary, as directed by your facility.[45]
- Monitor the patient's intake, output, and electrolyte levels, as ordered, *to promptly recognize fluid and electrolyte imbalances.* Promptly report fluid and electrolyte imbalances to the patient's practitioner *to prevent treatment delays.*[47,48]
- Perform hand hygiene.[10,11,12,13,14,15,16]
- Document the procedure.[36,37,38,39,40]

Using a time tape

- Calculate the hourly IV infusion rate.
- Place a preprinted IV time tape (or approximate length of 1″ [2.5-cm] tape) vertically on the IV solution container alongside the volume-increment markers.
- Starting at the IV solution level, identify the number of milliliters of solution to be infused, and use a pen to mark the appropriate time and a horizontal line on the IV time tape at this level. Then continue to mark the tape similarly at 1-hour intervals until you've reached the bottom of the IV solution container. Don't use a felt-tip pen to write directly on a plastic IV solution bag directly, *because the ink may penetrate the container, contaminating the IV solution.*[49]
- Monitor the flow-control device regularly, inspect the IV insertion site for complications, and evaluate the patient's response to therapy.[41]
- Compare the time with the appropriate IV infusion level on the time tape *to ensure safe and accurate delivery of the prescribed IV infusion rate and volume.*
- Perform hand hygiene.[10,11,12,13,14,15,16]
- Document the procedure.[36,37,38,39,40]

Blood sampling

- Assess the IV catheter site for signs and symptoms of complications, including edema, erythema, drainage, pain, numbness, and tingling. Don't use the site for blood sampling if complications are present.[1,2]
- If using an active IV site, trace the tubing from the patient to the point of origin *to make sure that you're accessing the proper site.*[43,44] Stop the infusion at least 2 minutes prior to collecting the sample.[7] Close the clamp on the extension set, if present.[2] Detach the IV administration tubing from the extension set and cover the end with a sterile end cap.[2]
- If using a capped IV site and a disinfectant-containing end cap is covering the end of the needleless connector, remove and discard it.[50,51]
- Perform a vigorous mechanical scrub of the needleless connector for at least 5 seconds using an antiseptic pad. Allow it to dry completely.[4,10,50,51]

If using the syringe method

- While maintaining sterility of the syringe tip, attach an empty syringe to the needleless connector or extension set hub and open the clamp, if present.[2]
- Slowly aspirate 1 to 2 mL of blood, remove the syringe, and discard it in a puncture-resistant sharps disposal container.[2,25,34]
- Perform a vigorous mechanical scrub of the needleless connector for at least 5 seconds using an antiseptic pad. Allow it to dry completely.[4,10,50,51]
- While maintaining sterility of the syringe tip, attach an empty syringe, slowly aspirate the needed blood volume, and then detach the syringe. *Using a 3- or 5-mL syringe allows better blood flow than a large, 10-mL syringe.*[2] Repeat the antiseptic scrub and blood aspiration with additional unused syringes, as necessary.
- Perform a vigorous mechanical scrub of the needleless connector for at least 5 seconds using an antiseptic pad. Allow it to dry completely.[4,10,50,51]
- While maintaining sterility of the syringe tip, attach a prefilled syringe containing preservative-free normal saline solution to the needleless connector and flush the catheter and extension set, if present.[2]
- As appropriate, reattach the administration set and trace the tubing from the patient to the point of origin *to make sure that you're accessing the proper site.* Resume the infusion, as ordered.[43,44] Alternatively, place a new disinfectant-containing end cap (if available at your facility) on the needleless connector *to reduce the risk of vascular catheter–associated infection.*[2,51]
- Fill the required blood collection tubes from the syringes using a needleless transfer device. Be careful to fill the tubes to the appropriate volume and in the correct order.
- Gently invert each tube the appropriate number of times *to mix the samples.*

If using the blood collection tube method

- While maintaining sterility of the tip, attach the blood collection tube holder to the needleless connector or extension set hub and open the clamp, if present.[2]

- Insert a blood collection tube into the holder, allow it to fill with 1 to 2 mL of blood, and discard it in a puncture-resistant sharps disposal container.[2,25,34]
- Insert the first required blood collection tube into the blood collection tube holder *to fill the tube by vacuum.*[2]
- When the first tube fills to its correct volume and blood flow ceases, remove the tube from the holder. Continue to fill the required tubes using the correct order of draw, removing one and inserting another.
- Gently invert each tube the appropriate number of times *to mix the samples.*
- Detach and discard the blood collection tube holder in a puncture-resistant sharps disposal container.[2,25,34]
- Perform a vigorous mechanical scrub of the needleless connector for at least 5 seconds using an antiseptic pad. Allow it to dry completely.[4,10,50,51]
- While maintaining sterility of the syringe tip, attach a prefilled syringe containing preservative-free normal saline solution to the needleless connector and flush the catheter and extension set if present.[2]
- As appropriate, reattach the administration set and trace the tubing from the patient to the point of origin *to make sure that you're accessing the proper site.* Resume the infusion, as ordered.[43,44] Alternatively, place a new disinfectant-containing end cap (if available at your facility) on the needleless connector *to reduce the risk of vascular catheter–associated infection.*[2,51] Label the blood collection tubes in the presence of the patient *to prevent mislabeling.*[7,17]

Completing the blood sampling procedure

- Place all blood collection tubes in a laboratory biohazard transport bag, and send them to the laboratory with a completed laboratory request form, if required in your facility.[25]
- Discard used supplies in appropriate receptacles.[24,25,34,35]
- Return the bed to the lowest position, as appropriate, *to prevent falls and maintain patient safety.*[47]
- Remove and discard your gloves.[24,25,34]
- Perform hand hygiene.[10,11,12,13,14,15,16]
- Document the procedure.[36,37,38,39,40]

Special considerations

- Change the needleless connector no more frequently than every 96 hours, *because changing the device more frequently increases the risk of intravascular catheter–associated infection.*[51] If used within a continuous infusion system, change the needleless connector when changing the primary administration set. Additionally, change the needleless connector if you remove it for any reason; if there is blood or debris within the connector; before drawing a blood culture through a vascular access device; if the needleless connector becomes contaminated; and routinely, as directed by your facility.[51]
- Change primary and secondary continuous administration sets used to administer solutions other than lipid, blood, or blood products no more frequently than every 96 hours,[45] but at least every 7 days,[52] and immediately upon suspected contamination or when the integrity of the product or system is compromised.[2,45] In addition to routine changes, change the administration set whenever you change the peripheral catheter site or when you insert a new central venous access device.[45]
- Change the transfusion administration set and filter after completion of each unit or every 4 hours; if you can infuse more than 1 unit in 4 hours, use the transfusion administration set for a 4-hour period.[45]
- *Because of the risk of contamination, accidental disconnections, and misconnections,* limit the use of add-on devices. When they must be used, change them with the catheter, with each administration set replacement, or as defined by your facility, and whenever you know or suspect that the integrity of the product is compromised.[45,53]
- When possible, change the solution and tubing at the same time *to decrease the risk of contamination.*[45]
- If the initial attempt to withdraw blood is unsuccessful, you may use a disposable tourniquet or inflated blood pressure cuff placed several inches above the catheter site *to promote venous dilation and improve blood flow. To reduce the risk of hemolysis and inaccurate test results,* you should limit venous occlusion by this method to no more than 1 minute.[2]

■ Use blood conservation techniques whenever possible, such as using small volume collection tubes, requesting the lab use previously collected samples for add-on tests, using point-of-care testing when applicable, and determining the minimum number of collections tubes necessary, *to reduce the risk of hospital-acquired anemia.*[7,54]

Complications

Potential complications include catheter dislodgment and infection.[2,52] Complications of IV solution change include air embolism, infection, and circulatory overload.[55] An excessively slow flow rate may cause insufficient intake of fluids, drugs, and nutrients; an excessively rapid rate of fluid or drug infusion may cause circulatory overload, possibly leading to heart failure and pulmonary edema as well as adverse drug effects.[2] Complications of blood sampling through an IV catheter include erroneous laboratory results due to improper collection technique, loss of catheter patency, and catheter-associated bloodstream infection caused by contamination during catheter manipulation.[7]

Documentation

For an IV dressing change, record the date and time of the dressing change, the appearance of the IV insertion site, the type of dressing you used, the type of stabilization device you used, site care you performed, and any patient reports of discomfort or pain. Document teaching provided to the patient and family (if applicable), their understanding of that teaching, and any need for follow-up teaching.

For an IV solution change, record the time and date of the solution change, the infusion rate and type of solution used, and any additives involved. Also record your assessment findings of the IV insertion site, the patient's response to therapy, and any complications, including your interventions and the patient's response to those interventions.

For a tubing change, record the date and time of the tubing change, the location and appearance of the site, the type of IV fluid you administered, the administration device used (if applicable), the rate of infusion, the type of dressing applied, and the patient's tolerance of the procedure.

When using a time tape, record the original flow rate when beginning the infusion through the peripheral IV catheter. If you adjust the rate, record the change, the date and time, and your initials.

When collecting a blood sample, document the date and time that you drew the sample and the volume of blood you withdrew. Include the tests for which you drew the sample and the time that you sent the sample to the laboratory. Document the location of the catheter, your assessment of the IV catheter site, presence of a blood return on aspiration, lack of resistance when flushing, and amount and type of flush you used. Document teaching provided to the patient and family (if applicable), their understanding of the teaching, and any need for follow-up teaching.

REFERENCES

1 Standard 42. Vascular access device assessment, care and dressing changes. Infusion therapy standards of practice (8th ed.). (2021). *Journal of Infusion Nursing, 44,* S119–S123. (Level VII)

2 Infusion Nurses Society. (2016). *Policies and procedures for infusion therapy* (5th ed.). Boston, MA: Infusion Nurses Society.

3 Rickard, C. M., et al. (2012). Routine versus clinically indicated replacement of peripheral intravenous catheters: A randomised controlled equivalence trial. *Lancet, 380,* 1066–1074. (Level I)

4 Jarrett, N., & Callaham, M. (2016). Evidence-based guidelines for selected hospital-acquired conditions: Final report. https://www.cms.gov/Medicare/Medicare-Fee-for-Service-Payment/HospitalAcqCond/Downloads/2016-HAC-Report.pdf

5 Vizcarra, C., et al. (2014). Recommendations for improving safety practices with short peripheral catheters. *Journal of Infusion Nursing, 37*(2), 121–124. (Level VII)

6 Standard 45. Vascular access device removal. Infusion therapy standards of practice (8th ed.). (2021). *Journal of Infusion Nursing, 44,* S133–S138. (Level VII)

7 Standard 44. Blood sampling. Infusion therapy standards of practice (8th ed.). (2021). *Journal of Infusion Nursing, 44,* S125–S133. (Level VII)

8 Standard 12. Product evaluation, integrity, and defect reporting. Infusion therapy standards of practice (8th ed.). (2021). *Journal of Infusion Nursing, 44,* S45–S46. (Level VII)

9 Silvestri, D. L., & McEnery-Stonelake, M. (2013). Chlorhexidine: Uses and adverse reactions. *Dermatitis, 24,* 112–118. (Level VII)

10 Centers for Disease Control and Prevention. (2011, revised 2017). Guidelines for the prevention of intravascular catheter–related infections. https://www.cdc.gov/infectioncontrol/guidelines/bsi/recommendations.html (Level I)

11 The Joint Commission. (2021). Standard NPSG.07.01.01. *Comprehensive accreditation manual for hospitals.* Oakbrook Terrace, IL: The Joint Commission. (Level VII)

12 Centers for Disease Control and Prevention. (2002). Guideline for hand hygiene in health-care settings: Recommendations of the Healthcare Infection Control Practices Advisory Committee and the HICPAC/SHEA/APIC/IDSA Hand Hygiene Task Force. *MMWR Recommendations and Reports, 51*(RR-16), 1–45. https://www.cdc.gov/mmwr/pdf/rr/rr5116.pdf (Level II)

13 World Health Organization. (2009). WHO guidelines on hand hygiene in health care: First global patient safety challenge, clean care is safer care. https://apps.who.int/iris/bitstream/handle/10665/44102/9789241597906_eng.pdf?sequence=1 (Level IV)

14 Standard 16. Hand hygiene. Infusion therapy standards of practice (8th ed.). (2021). *Journal of Infusion Nursing, 44,* S53–S5. (Level VII)

15 Accreditation Association for Hospitals and Health Systems. (2020). Standard 07.01.21. *Healthcare Facilities Accreditation Program: Accreditation requirements for acute care hospitals.* Chicago, IL: Accreditation Association for Hospitals and Health Systems. (Level VII)

16 DNV GL-Healthcare USA, Inc. (2020). IC.1.SR.1. *NIAHO® accreditation requirements, interpretive guidelines and surveyor guidance—revision 20.0.* Milford, OH: DNV GL-Healthcare USA, Inc. (Level VII)

17 The Joint Commission. (2021). Standard NPSG.01.01.01. *Comprehensive accreditation manual for hospitals.* Oakbrook Terrace, IL: The Joint Commission. (Level VII)

18 The Joint Commission. (2021). Standard RI.01.01.01. *Comprehensive accreditation manual for hospitals.* Oakbrook Terrace, IL: The Joint Commission. (Level VII)

19 DNV GL-Healthcare USA, Inc. (2020). PR.2.SR.5. *NIAHO® accreditation requirements, interpretive guidelines and surveyor guidance—revision 20.0.* Milford, OH: DNV GL-Healthcare USA, Inc. (Level VII)

20 Centers for Medicare and Medicaid Services, Department of Health and Human Services. (2020). Condition of participation: Patient's rights. 42 C.F.R. § 482.13(c)(1).

21 Accreditation Association for Hospitals and Health Systems. (2020). Standard 15.01.16. *Healthcare Facilities Accreditation Program: Accreditation requirements for acute care hospitals.* Chicago, IL: Accreditation Association for Hospitals and Health Systems. (Level VII)

22 The Joint Commission. (2021). Standard PC.02.01.21. *Comprehensive accreditation manual for hospitals.* Oakbrook Terrace, IL: The Joint Commission. (Level VII)

23 Waters, T. R., et al. (2009). Safe patient handling training for schools of nursing. https://www.cdc.gov/niosh/docs/2009-127/pdfs/2009-127.pdf (Level VII)

24 Siegel, J. D., et al. (2007, revised 2019). 2007 guideline for isolation precautions: Preventing transmission of infectious agents in healthcare settings. https://www.cdc.gov/infectioncontrol/pdf/guidelines/isolation-guidelines-H.pdf (Level II)

25 Occupational Safety and Health Administration. (2012). Bloodborne pathogens, standard number 1910.1030. https://www.osha.gov/pls/oshaweb/owadisp.show_document?p_id=10051&p_table=STANDARDS (Level VII)

26 Accreditation Association for Hospitals and Health Systems. (2020). Standard 07.01.10. *Healthcare Facilities Accreditation Program: Accreditation requirements for acute care hospitals.* Chicago, IL: Accreditation Association for Hospitals and Health Systems. (Level VII)

27 Infusion Nurses Society. (2016). *Policies and procedures for infusion therapy of the older adult* (3rd ed.). Boston, MA: Infusion Nurses Society.

28 LeBlanc, K., et al. (2013). International skin tear advisory panel: A tool kit to aid in the prevention, assessment, and treatment of skin tears using a simplified classification system. *Advances in Skin & Wound Care, 26,* 459–476. (Level IV)

29 Standard 38. Vascular access device securement. Infusion therapy standards of practice (8th ed.). (2021). *Journal of Infusion Nursing, 44,* S108–S111. (Level VII)

30 Standard 50. Infection. Infusion therapy standards of practice (8th ed.). (2021). *Journal of Infusion Nursing, 44,* S153–S157. (Level VII)

31 Standard 46. Phlebitis. Infusion therapy standards of practice (8th ed.). (2021). *Journal of Infusion Nursing, 44*, S138–S142.

32 Standard 47. Infiltration and extravasation. Infusion therapy standards of practice (8th ed.). (2021). *Journal of Infusion Nursing, 44*, S142–S147. (Level VII)

33 Ganz, D. A., et al. (2013). *Preventing falls in hospitals: A toolkit for improving quality of care* (AHRQ Publication No. 13-0015-EF). Rockville, MD: Agency for Healthcare Research and Quality. https://www.ahrq.gov/professionals/systems/hospital/fallpxtoolkit/index.html (Level VII)

34 Standard 21. Medical waste and sharps safety. Infusion therapy standards of practice (8th ed.). (2021). *Journal of Infusion Nursing, 44*, S60–S63. (Level VII)

35 Accreditation Association for Hospitals and Health systems. (2020). Standard 07.03.07. *Healthcare Facilities Accreditation Program: Accreditation requirements for acute care hospitals*. Chicago, IL: Accreditation Association for Hospitals and Health Systems. (Level VII)

36 The Joint Commission. (2021). Standard RC.01.03.01. *Comprehensive accreditation manual for hospitals*. Oakbrook Terrace, IL: The Joint Commission. (Level VII)

37 Standard 10. Documentation in the health record. Infusion therapy standards of practice (8th ed.). (2021). *Journal of Infusion Nursing, 44*, S39–S43. (Level VII)

38 Centers for Medicare and Medicaid Services, Department of Health and Human Services. (2020). Condition of participation: Medical record services. 42 C.F.R. § 482.24(b).

39 Accreditation Association for Hospitals and Health Systems. (2020). Standard 10.00.03. *Healthcare Facilities Accreditation Program: Accreditation requirements for acute care hospitals*. Chicago, IL: Accreditation Association for Hospitals and Health Systems. (Level VII)

40 DNV GL-Healthcare USA, Inc. (2020). MR.2.SR.1. *NIAHO® accreditation requirements, interpretive guidelines and surveyor guidance—revision 20.0*. Milford, OH: DNV GL-Healthcare USA, Inc. (Level VII)

41 Standard 59. Infusion medication and solution administration. Infusion therapy standards of practice (8th ed.). (2021). *Journal of Infusion Nursing, 44*, S180–S183. (Level VII)

42 The Joint Commission. (2021). Standard PC.02.01.03. *Comprehensive accreditation manual for hospitals*. Oakbrook Terrace, IL: The Joint Commission. (Level VII)

43 The Joint Commission. (2014). Sentinel event alert 53: Managing risk during transition to new ISO tubing connector standards. http://www.jointcommission.org/assets/1/6/SEA_53_Connectors_8_19_14_final.pdf (Level VII)

44 U.S. Food and Drug Administration. (2017). Examples of medical device misconnections. https://www.fda.gov/medical-devices/medical-device-connectors/examples-medical-device-misconnections

45 Standard 43. Administration set management. Infusion therapy standards of practice (8th ed.). (2021). *Journal of Infusion Nursing, 44*, S123–S125. (Level VII)

46 Marschall, J., et al. (2014). SHEA/IDSA practice recommendation: Strategies to prevent central line–associated bloodstream infections in acute care hospitals. *Infection Control and Hospital Epidemiology, 35*, 753–771. https://www.jstor.org/stable/10.1086/676533#metadata_info_tab_contents (Level I)

47 Centers for Medicare and Medicaid Services. (2014). Requirements for hospital medication administration, particularly intravenous (IV) medications and post-operative care of patients receiving IV opioids. http://www.cms.gov/Medicare/Provider-Enrollment-and-Certification/SurveyCertificationGenInfo/Downloads/Survey-and-Cert-Letter-14-15.pdf

48 Centers for Medicare and Medicaid Services, Department of Health and Human Services. (2020). Condition of participation: Nursing services. 42 C.F.R. § 482.23(c).

49 Smith, S. F., et al. (2017). *Clinical nursing skills: Basic to advanced skills* (9th ed.). Hoboken, NJ: Pearson Education.

50 Moureau, N. L., & Flynn, J. (2015). Disinfection of needleless connector hubs: Clinical evidence systematic review. *Nursing Research and Practice, 2015*, 1–20. https://www.hindawi.com/journals/nrp/2015/796762/ (Level I)

51 Standard 36. Needleless connectors. Infusion therapy standards of practice (8th ed.). (2021). *Journal of Infusion Nursing, 44*, S104–S107. (Level VII)

52 Association for Professionals in Infection Control and Epidemiology (APIC). (2015). Guide to preventing central line-associated bloodstream infections. http://apic.org/Resource_/TinyMceFileManager/2015/APIC_CLABSI_WEB.pdf (Level IV)

53 Standard 37. Other add-on devices. Infusion therapy standards of practice (8th ed.). (2021). *Journal of Infusion Nursing, 44*, S107–S108. (Level VII)

54 Noguez, J. (2016). Tackling hospital-acquired anemia: Lab based intervention to reduce diagnostic blood loss. https://www.aacc.org/publications/cln/articles/2016/april/tackling-hospital-acquired-anemia-lab-based-interventions-to-reduce-diagnostic-blood-loss

55 Standard 52. Air embolism. Infusion therapy standards of practice (8th ed.). (2021). *Journal of Infusion Nursing, 44*, S160–S161. (Level VII)

IV INFUSION RATES AND MANUAL CONTROL

Calculated from a practitioner's order, flow rate is usually expressed as the total volume of IV solution infused over a prescribed interval, or as the total volume given in milliliters per hour. Many devices can regulate the flow of IV solution, including several types of clamps, an IV flow regulator, and an electronic infusion device. (See *Using IV clamps*.)

When regulated by a clamp, flow rate is usually measured in drops per minute; by an infusion pump, in milliliters per hour. Flow regulators can be set to deliver the desired amount of solution, also in milliliters per hour. Less accurate than an electronic infusion pump, flow regulators are most reliable when used with inactive adult patients. With any flow

EQUIPMENT

Using IV clamps

With a **roller clamp**, you can increase or decrease the flow through the IV line by turning a wheel.

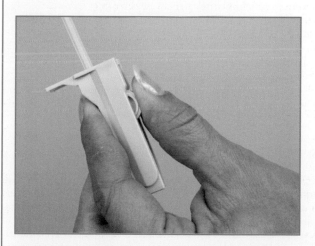

With a **slide clamp**, you can open or close the line by moving the clamp horizontally. However, you can't make fine adjustments to the flow rate.

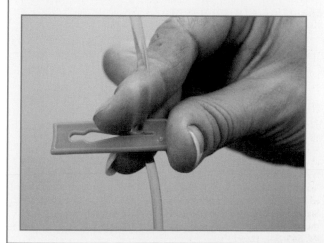

Calculating IV flow rates

When calculating the IV flow rate of infused solutions, remember that the number of drops required to deliver 1 mL varies with the type and manufacturer of the IV administration set used. To calculate the IV flow rate, you must know the calibration of the IV drip rate for each manufacturer's product. Use this formula to calculate specific drip rates:

$$\frac{\text{volume of infusion (in mL)}}{\text{time of infusion (in minutes)}} \times \text{drip factor (in drops/mL)} = \text{drops/minute}$$

Macrodrip administration set
A standard (macrodrip) administration set delivers from 10 to 20 drops/mL.

Microdrip administration set
A pediatric (microdrip) administration set delivers about 60 drops/mL

Blood transfusion set
A blood transfusion set delivers about 10 drops/mL.

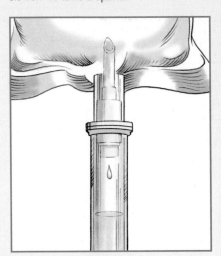

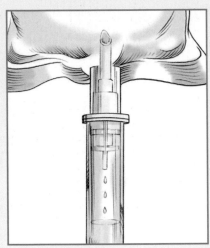

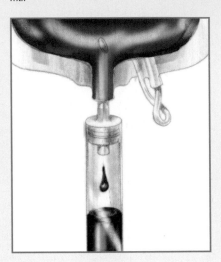

regulating device, IV flow rate can easily be monitored by using a time tape, which indicates the prescribed IV solution level at hourly intervals. (See the "IV catheter maintenance" procedure.)

Equipment

Watch with second hand ▪ labels ▪ Optional: drip rate chart.

Check the label on the IV administration set to determine how many drops per unit it delivers. A standard macrodrip IV administration set delivers from 10 to 20 drops/mL, depending on the manufacturer. A microdrip IV administration set delivers about 60 drops/mL. A blood transfusion set delivers about 10 drops/mL. A commercial adapter is available that converts a macrodrip set to a microdrip system.

Preparation of equipment

Inspect all IV equipment and supplies. If a product is expired, is defective, or has compromised integrity, remove it from patient use, label it as expired or defective, and report the expiration or defect as directed by your facility.[1]

Implementation

▪ Verify the practitioner's order for the prescribed IV flow rate.[2]
▪ Gather and prepare the necessary equipment and supplies.
▪ Perform hand hygiene.[3,4,5,6,7,8,9,10]
▪ Confirm the patient's identity using at least two patient identifiers.[11]
▪ Provide privacy.[12,13,14,15]
▪ Explain the procedure to the patient and family (if appropriate) according to their individual communication and learning needs *to increase their understanding, allay their fears, and enhance cooperation.*[16]
▪ Calculate the proper drip rate, or use a drip rate chart (if available). (See *Calculating IV flow rates.*)

▪ After calculating the desired IV drip rate, remove your watch and hold it next to the IV drip chamber *so that you can observe the watch and drops simultaneously.*
▪ Release the IV clamp and regulate the flow to the approximate drip rate. Then count drops for 1 minute *to account for flow irregularities and ensure the proper administration rate.*[17,18]
▪ Adjust the IV clamp as necessary, and count drops for 1 minute. Continue to adjust the IV clamp and count drops until the correct IV flow rate is achieved.
▪ Closely monitor the IV flow rate, inspect the IV site for complications, and assess the patient's response to therapy.
▪ Perform hand hygiene.[3,4,5,6,7,8,9,10]
▪ Document the procedure.[19,20,21,22,23]

Special considerations

▪ Use an electronic infusion device for infusions that require precise flow control *to maintain patient safety.* Consider the use of a smart pump with dose error-reduction software and interoperability with electronic health records *to reduce the risk of infusion-related medication errors.* Make sure that alarm limits are set properly and that alarms are turned on, functioning properly, and audible to staff.[2,24]
▪ The Joint Commission issued a sentinel event alert related to managing risk during transition to new International Organization for Standardization tubing standards that were designed to prevent dangerous tubing misconnections, which can lead to serious patient injury and death. During the transition, make sure to trace the tubing and catheter from the patient to the point of origin before connecting or reconnecting any device or infusion, at any care transition (such as a new setting or service), and as part of the hand-off process; route tubes and catheters having different purposes in different standardized directions; when there are different access sites or several bags hanging, label the tubing at the distal and proximal ends; use tubing and equipment only as intended; and store medications for different delivery routes in separate locations.[25]

Complications

An excessively slow IV flow rate may cause insufficient intake of fluids, drugs, and nutrients; an excessively rapid IV flow rate of fluid or drug infusion may cause circulatory overload—possibly leading to heart failure and pulmonary edema—as well as other adverse drug effects.

Documentation

Record the original IV flow rate when setting up a peripheral IV line. If you adjust the IV flow rate, record the change, the date and time, and your initials. Document the patient's response to therapy, any complications, interventions provided, and the patient's response to those interventions. Document teaching provided to the patient and family (if applicable), their understanding of that teaching, and any need for follow-up teaching.

REFERENCES

1 Standard 12. Product evaluation, integrity, and defect reporting. Infusion therapy standards of practice (8th ed.). (2021). *Journal of Infusion Nursing, 44*, S45–S46. (Level VII)

2 Standard 59. Infusion medication and solution administration. Infusion therapy standards of practice (8th ed.). (2021). *Journal of Infusion Nursing, 44*, S180–S183. (Level VII)

3 The Joint Commission. (2021). Standard NPSG.07.01.01. *Comprehensive accreditation manual for hospitals.* Oakbrook Terrace, IL: The Joint Commission. (Level VII)

4 Centers for Disease Control and Prevention. (2002). Guideline for hand hygiene in health-care settings: Recommendations of the Healthcare Infection Control Practices Advisory Committee and the HICPAC/SHEA/APIC/IDSA Hand Hygiene Task Force. *MMWR Recommendations and Reports, 51*(RR-16), 1–45. https://www.cdc.gov/mmwr/pdf/rr/rr5116.pdf (Level II)

5 World Health Organization. (2009). WHO guidelines on hand hygiene in health care: First global patient safety challenge, clean care is safer care. https://apps.who.int/iris/bitstream/handle/10665/44102/9789241597906_eng.pdf?sequence=1 (Level IV)

6 Standard 16. Hand hygiene. Infusion therapy standards of practice (8th ed.). (2021). *Journal of Infusion Nursing, 44*, S53–S54. (Level VII)

7 Centers for Disease Control and Prevention. (2011, revised 2017). Guidelines for the prevention of intravascular catheter-related infections. https://www.cdc.gov/infectioncontrol/guidelines/bsi/recommendations.html (Level I)

8 Centers for Medicare and Medicaid Services, Department of Health and Human Services. (2020). Condition of participation: Infection control. 42 C.F.R. § 482.42.

9 Accreditation Association for Hospitals and Health Systems. (2020). Standard 07.01.21. *Healthcare Facilities Accreditation Program: Accreditation requirements for acute care hospitals.* (Level VII)

10 DNV GL-Healthcare USA, Inc. (2020). IC.1.SR.1. *NIAHO® accreditation requirements, interpretive guidelines and surveyor guidance—revision 20.0.* Milford, OH: DNV GL-Healthcare USA, Inc. (Level VII)

11 The Joint Commission. (2021). Standard NPSG.01.01.01. *Comprehensive accreditation manual for hospitals.* Oakbrook Terrace, IL: The Joint Commission. (Level VII)

12 Accreditation Association for Hospitals and Health Systems. (2020). Standard 15.01.16. *Healthcare Facilities Accreditation Program: Accreditation requirements for acute care hospitals.* (Level VII)

13 Centers for Medicare and Medicaid Services, Department of Health and Human Services. (2020). Condition of participation: Patient's rights. 42 C.F.R. § 482.13(c)(1).

14 DNV GL-Healthcare USA, Inc. (2020). PR.2.SR.5. *NIAHO® accreditation requirements, interpretive guidelines and surveyor guidance—revision 20.0.* Milford, OH: DNV GL-Healthcare USA, Inc. (Level VII)

15 The Joint Commission. (2021). Standard RI.01.01.01. *Comprehensive accreditation manual for hospitals.* Oakbrook Terrace, IL: The Joint Commission. (Level VII)

16 The Joint Commission. (2021). Standard PC.02.01.21. *Comprehensive accreditation manual for hospitals.* Oakbrook Terrace, IL: The Joint Commission. (Level VII)

17 Infusion Nurses Society. (2016). *Policies and procedures for infusion therapy* (5th ed.). Boston, MA: Infusion Nurses Society.

18 Infusion Nurses Society. (2016). *Policies and procedures for infusion therapy of the older adult* (3rd ed.). Boston, MA: Infusion Nurses Society.

19 The Joint Commission. (2021). Standard RC.01.03.01. *Comprehensive accreditation manual for hospitals.* Oakbrook Terrace, IL: The Joint Commission. (Level VII)

20 Standard 10. Documentation in the health record. Infusion therapy standards of practice (8th ed.). (2021). *Journal of Infusion Nursing, 44*, S39–S42. (Level VII)

21 Centers for Medicare and Medicaid Services, Department of Health and Human Services. (2020). Condition of participation: Medical record services. 42 C.F.R. § 482.24(b).

22 Accreditation Association for Hospitals and Health Systems. (2020). Standard 10.00.03. *Healthcare Facilities Accreditation Program: Accreditation requirements for acute care hospitals.* (Level VII)

23 DNV GL-Healthcare USA, Inc. (2020). MR.2.SR.1. *NIAHO® accreditation requirements, interpretive guidelines and surveyor guidance — revision 20.0.* Milford, OH: DNV GL-Healthcare USA, Inc. (Level VII)

24 Standard 24. Flow-control devices. Infusion therapy standards of practice (8th ed.). (2021). *Journal of Infusion Nursing, 44*, S69–S73. (Level VII)

25 The Joint Commission. (2014). Sentinel event alert 53: Managing risk during transition to new ISO tubing connector standards. http://www.jointcommission.org/assets/1/6/SEA_53_Connectors_8_19_14_final.pdf (Level VII)

IV PUMP USE

Various types of pumps electronically regulate the flow of IV solutions or drugs with great accuracy. Volumetric IV pumps, used for high-pressure infusion of drugs or for highly accurate delivery of fluids or drugs, have mechanisms to propel the solution at the desired rate under pressure. (Pressure is applied only when gravity flow rates are insufficient to maintain preset infusion rates.) The peristaltic IV pump applies pressure to the IV tubing to force the solution through it. (Not all peristaltic IV pumps are volumetric; some count drops.) The piston-cylinder IV pump pushes the solution through special disposable cassettes. Most of these IV pumps operate at high pressures (up to 45 psi), delivering from 1 to 999 mL/hour with about 98% accuracy. The portable syringe pump delivers very small amounts of fluid over a long period of time. It's used for administering fluids to infants and for delivering intra-arterial drugs.

Other specialized devices include barcode-automated programming devices, smart pumps, the controlled-release infusion system, the secondary syringe converter, and patient controlled analgesia. (See *Understanding smart pumps*, page 504.)

IV pumps also have various detectors and alarms that automatically signal or respond to the completion of an infusion, air in the line, low battery power, and occlusion or inability to deliver at the set rate.

ELDER ALERT Keep in mind that older adults commonly have compromised cardiac, hepatic, or renal systems, placing them at risk for heart failure, shock, or cardiac arrest during IV fluid administration if infusions are too rapid or the volume is too great. An older adult may be unable to articulate symptoms because of underlying conditions, including stroke, intubation, tracheostomy, dementia, and delirium. Monitor older adult patients closely during all IV infusions. Rapid administration of a bolus medication or infusion can cause speed shock; symptoms associated with speed shock, such as dizziness and headache, occur rapidly, making it difficult for the patient to articulate such symptoms. Early symptoms of speed shock may progress to chest tightness, hypotension, irregular pulse, and anaphylactic shock. Carefully control any parenteral medication or solution and observe older adult patients closely.[2]

Equipment

IV pump ▪ IV pole ▪ prescribed IV solution ▪ sterile administration set ▪ antiseptic pad (alcohol, tincture of iodine, or chlorhexidine-based) ▪ prefilled syringe containing preservative-free normal saline ▪ gloves ▪ Optional: needleless connector, IV catheter insertion kit.

Preparation of equipment

Inspect all IV equipment and supplies. If a product is expired, is defective, or has compromised integrity, remove it from patient use, label it as expired or defective, and report the expiration or defect as directed by your facility.[3] Attach the IV pump to the IV pole.

EQUIPMENT

Understanding smart pumps

Conventional, general-purpose infusion pumps allow nurses to program an hourly infusion rate and volume. A smart pump has software that enables nurses to choose infusion parameters from a facility's customized drug library, which can help prevent serious infusion errors. Before smart pumps are used at the bedside, a facility programs the pumps with its own specific information. These profiles specify the infusion requirements for different types of patients, such as adults and children, and care areas, such as pediatric, maternal, oncology, intensive care, and postanesthesia care units. Each profile includes a drug library that contains facility-defined drug infusion parameters, such as acceptable concentrations, infusion rates, dosing units, and maximum and minimum loading and maintenance dose bolus limits. The maximum rate and pressure at which the infusion will run can also be programmed into the software. A team that typically consist of pharmacists, practitioners, and nurses within each facility sets up and manages these profiles based on the facility's own best-practice guidelines.

Smart pumps vary by manufacturer, with some pumps even incorporating barcode technology on each IV medication bag. The barcode automatically programs the pump according to a current drug order. When you turn on a typical smart pump, it asks you to designate the specific patient care area you're going to use it in. Then it automatically configures itself to provide you with the infusion parameters for that area. Because a pump may be used in different types of patient care units and departments throughout the facility, this feature adds an extra layer of safety.

You then program the pump by choosing the intended drug and concentration from the smart pump's list and entering the ordered dose and infusion rate. The pump checks this information against the drug library. If the parameters you've programmed match those in the pump's drug library for that patient care area, the pump allows the infusion to begin. However, if what you've programmed is outside of the specified limits, the pump alerts you with a visual and audible alarm and lets you know which parameter lies outside of the recommended range.

A smart pump also logs and tracks all alerts, recording the time, date, drug, concentration, and infusion rate, as well as your action—including whether you overrode the alert or reprogrammed the pump with different settings. This provides your facility with data it can use to shape current practice guidelines and identify process improvements.

The Institute for Safe Medication Practices recommends that, before deploying a smart pump, a facility should follow these steps:
- Standardize and limit concentrations within the facility; *asking a nurse to choose from several concentrations increases the risk of selection error.*
- Use commercially prepared, premixed drug infusion products when available and appropriate.
- Standardize dosing units for a given drug; for instance, always use either micrograms per minute or micrograms per kilogram per minute for nitroglycerin, but not both.
- Standardize definitions for terms used in IV drug administration (such as *bolus, intermittent infusion, continuous infusion*).
- Ensure that the concentrations, dose units, and nomenclature used in the smart pump are consistent with those used in the medication administration record, pharmacy computer system, and electronic medical record.
- Use an interdisciplinary team to develop and update the drug library at least quarterly, and create a process for reviewing the drug library content that includes literature review, practice changes, facility requests, formulary changes, and quality data.
- Monitor overrides of alerts to assess whether the alerts have been properly configured or whether additional quality intervention is required.
- Ensure the pump's "smart" feature is used in all parts of the facility; for instance, if the operating room sets up the IV pump volumetrically without the "smart" feature, but the intensive care unit uses the "smart" feature, an error may occur if the IV pump isn't reprogrammed properly.
- Ensure that the upper and lower dose limits are set for bolus doses, when applicable.
- Involve frontline staff in a risk assessment to identify new opportunities for failure before receiving smart pumps.
- Limit the ability to manually program continuous infusions
- Deploy the smart pump throughout all areas of the hospital so that people in all departments are trained to use it properly.[1]

Implementation

- Avoid distractions and interruptions when preparing and administering medications *to prevent medication errors.*[4,5,6]
- Review the practitioner's order to make sure that the prescribed infusion solution or medication, dose, rate, and route of administration is appropriate for the patient's age, condition, and access device, and that the infusion or medication is compatible with other solutions or medication. Make sure the order includes any test results that require monitoring. Address concerns about the order with the practitioner, pharmacist, your supervisor, the risk management department, or as directed by your facility.[4,7]
- Perform a medication reconciliation when the practitioner orders a new medication *to reduce the risk of medication errors, including omissions, duplications, dosing errors, and drug interactions.*[7]
- Check the patient's medical record for an allergy or contraindication to the prescribed medication. If an allergy or contraindication exists, don't administer the medication; instead, notify the practitioner.[8,9,10,11]
- Gather and prepare the necessary equipment and supplies
- Check the expiration date on the IV solution. If the solution is expired, return it to the pharmacy and obtain new solution.[8,9,10,11]
- Visually inspect the IV solution for particles or discoloration, or other loss of integrity; don't administer the solution if integrity is compromised.[2,8,9,10,11,12]
- Discuss any unresolved concerns about the medication with the patient's practitioner.[8,9,10,11]
- Verify that you're administering the medication at the proper time, in the prescribed dose, and by the correct route *to reduce the risk of medication errors.*[8,9,10,11]
- Perform hand hygiene.[13,14,15,16,17,18,19]
- Confirm the patient's identity using at least two patient identifiers.[20]
- Provide privacy.[21,22,23,24]

- Explain the procedure to the patient and family (if appropriate) according to their individual communication and learning needs *to increase their understanding, allay their fears, and enhance cooperation.*[25]
- If the patient is receiving the medication for the first time, teach the patient and family (if appropriate) about potential adverse reactions and other concerns related to the medication.[8,9,10,11]
- If your facility uses bar-code technology, use it as directed by your facility.[7]
- Access the port on the IV container and perform a vigorous mechanical scrub using an antiseptic pad, if appropriate, and allow it to dry completely. (See the "IV therapy preparation" procedure.)
- Insert the administration set spike, and fill the drip chamber to the manufacturer's mark *to prevent air bubbles from entering the tubing.*[2,12]
- Slowly open the clamp to prime the administration set tubing while holding the distal end of the administration set upright, permitting the filter to hang upside down. Prime the entire length of the administration set tubing, and then close the clamp.[2,12] Place the administration set tubing into the IV pump following the manufacturer's instructions.
- Alternatively, insert the administration set tubing into the IV pump and use the pump's priming function to prime the administration set tubing.
- Position the IV pump on the same side of the bed as the vascular access device or the anticipated IV insertion site *to avoid misconnections.*[26]
- Plug in the IV pump.
- Raise the patient bed to waist level before providing care *to prevent caregiver back strain.*[27]
- Perform hand hygiene.[13,14,15,16,17,18,19]
- Put on gloves *to comply with standard precautions.*[14,28,29,30]
- Assess the IV insertion site.[4]
- If a disinfectant-containing end cap is in place at the end of the needleless connector, remove and discard it.[31]

■ Perform a vigorous mechanical scrub of the needleless connector for at least 5 seconds using an antiseptic and allow it to dry completely.[2,12,32,33]

■ While maintaining sterility of the syringe tip, attach a prefilled syringe containing preservative-free normal saline solution to the needleless connector. Use a 10-mL syringe or a syringe specifically designed to generate low injection pressure. Unclamp the catheter and slowly aspirate for blood return that is the color and consistency of whole blood. If no blood return occurs, take steps to locate an external cause of obstruction.[34]

■ If blood return occurs, slowly inject preservative-free normal saline solution into the catheter. Use a minimum volume of twice the internal volume of the catheter system. Don't forcibly flush the device; further evaluate the device if you meet resistance.[34]

■ Clamp the IV catheter, and remove and discard the syringe in a puncture-resistant sharps disposal container.[29]

■ Perform a vigorous mechanical scrub of the IV catheter hub or needleless connector for at least 5 seconds using an antiseptic pad; then allow it to dry completely.[33]

■ Trace the sterile administration set tubing from the patient to its point of origin *to ensure that you're connecting the tubing to the correct port.*[4,26,35]

■ Remove the protective cap from the distal end of the sterile administration set tubing and attach the administration set tubing to the IV catheter hub using sterile technique.[2,12] If you're infusing an IV solution or medication via a secondary IV line, attach the secondary IV administration set tubing to an injection port with a needleless connector above or below the pumping mechanism as appropriate.[12] (See the "IV secondary line drug infusion" procedure.)

■ Route the tubing in a standardized direction if the patient has other tubing and catheters that have different purposes. If multiple IV access sites or IV bags will be used, label the tubing at both the distal end (near the patient connection) and proximal end (near the source container) *to reduce the risk of misconnection.*[35]

■ Turn on the IV pump and enter the desired drug infusion rate and volume settings, following specific operating instructions.

■ Confirm that the IV pump's display screen displays the right information.

■ Open the IV catheter (if appropriate) and sterile administration set tubing clamps, and then push the RUN or START button.

■ Ensure that the alarm limits are set appropriately and that the alarms are turned on, functioning properly, and audible to staff.[36,37,38] Explain the alarm system to the patient and family (if appropriate) *to prevent anxiety when the alarm is activated.* Don't rely on the IV pump to detect IV infiltration or extravasation, *because these alarms aren't intended to detect IV fluid flow disruption.*[39,40]

■ Check that all connections are secure *to prevent leakage, bleeding, contamination, and disconnections.*[26,35]

■ Recheck the patency of the IV catheter and watch the IV insertion site for infiltration.[4,37]

■ Observe the IV pump for 1 to 2 minutes *to make sure it's delivering the infusion at the proper rate.*[4,39]

■ Return the bed to the lowest position *to prevent falls and maintain patient safety.*[41]

■ Discard used supplies in the appropriate receptacles.[29]

■ Remove and discard your gloves.[28,29]

■ Perform hand hygiene.[13,14,15,16,17,18,19]

■ Frequently monitor the IV pump and the patient *to ensure the device's correct operation and flow rate and to detect complications, including infiltration, infection, and air embolism.*[39]

■ Monitor the patient's intake and output and electrolyte levels, as ordered, *to detect fluid and electrolyte imbalances.* Promptly notify the practitioner of imbalances *to prevent treatment delays.*[9,42]

■ Perform hand hygiene.[13,14,15,16,17,18,19]

■ Document the procedure.[43,44,45,46,47]

Special considerations

■ The Joint Commission issued a sentinel event alert concerning medical device alarm safety, *because alarm-related events have been associated with permanent loss of function or death.* Among the major contributing factors were improper alarm settings, alarm settings turned off inappropriately, and alarm signals not audible to staff. Make sure that alarm limits are set appropriately, and that alarms are turned on, functioning properly, and audible to staff. Follow facility guidelines for preventing alarm fatigue.[38]

■ The Joint Commission issued a sentinel event alert related to managing risk during transition to new International Organization for Standardization tubing standards that were designed to prevent dangerous tubing misconnections, which can lead to serious patient injury and death. During the transition, make sure to trace each tubing and catheter from the patient to the point of origin before connecting or reconnecting any device or infusion, at any care transition (such as to a new setting or service), and as part of the hand-off process; route tubes and catheters having different purposes in different standardized directions; when the patient has different access sites or several bags hanging, label tubing at both the distal and proximal ends; use tubing and equipment only as intended; and store medications for different delivery routes in separate locations.[35]

Complications

Complications associated with IV solution and medication infusion via an IV pump can include circulatory overload and adverse effects related to specific medications. General complications associated with IV infusion include infiltration, extravasation, phlebitis, infection, and air embolism.[40,48,49,50] Keep in mind that infiltration can develop rapidly with infusion by a volumetric pump *because the increased subcutaneous pressure won't slow the infusion rate until significant edema occurs.* Never rely on infusion pump alarms to detect the presence of infiltration.[40]

Documentation

In addition to routine documentation of the IV solution or medication infusion, record the use of an IV pump. Also record the patient's response to the infusion. Document teaching provided to the patient and family (if applicable), their understanding of that teaching, and any need for follow-up teaching.

REFERENCES

1 Institute for Safe Medication Practices. (2020). Guidelines for optimizing safe implementation and use of smart infusion pumps. https://www.ismp.org/guidelines/safe-implementation-and-use-smart-pumps (Level VII)

2 Infusion Nurses Society. (2017). *Policies and procedures for infusion therapy of the older adult* (3rd ed.). Boston, MA: Infusion Nurses Society.

3 Standard 12. Product evaluation, integrity, and defect reporting. Infusion therapy standards of practice (8th ed.). (2021). *Journal of Infusion Nursing, 44,* S45–S46. (Level VII)

4 Standard 59. Infusion medication and solution administration. Infusion therapy standards of practice (8th ed.). (2021). *Journal of Infusion Nursing, 44,* S180–S183. (Level VII)

5 Institute for Safe Medication Practices. (2012). Side tracks on the safety express: Interruptions lead to errors and unfinished…Wait, what was I doing? *Nurse Advise-ERR, 11*(2), 1–4. https://www.ismp.org/Newsletters/acutecare/showarticle.aspx?id=37

6 Westbrook, J., et al. (2010). Association of interruptions with an increased risk and severity of medication administration errors. *Archives of Internal Medicine, 170,* 683–690. (Level IV)

7 Standard 13. Medication verification. Infusion therapy standards of practice (8th ed.). (2021). *Journal of Infusion Nursing, 44*(Suppl. 1), S46–S49. https://doi.org/10.1097/NAN.0000000000000396 (Level VII)

8 The Joint Commission. (2021). Standard MM.06.01.01. *Comprehensive accreditation manual for hospitals.* Oakbrook Terrace, IL: The Joint Commission. (Level VII)

9 Centers for Medicare and Medicaid Services, Department of Health and Human Services. (2020). Condition of participation: Nursing services. 42 C.F.R. § 482.23(c).

10 Accreditation Association for Hospitals and Health Systems. (2020). Standard 16.01.03. *Healthcare Facilities Accreditation Program: Accreditation requirements for acute care hospitals.* Chicago, IL: Accreditation Association for Hospitals and Health Systems. (Level VII)

11 DNV GL-Healthcare USA, Inc. (2020). MM.1.SR.3. *NIAHO® accreditation requirements, interpretive guidelines and surveyor guidance—revision 20.0.* (Level VII)

12 Infusion Nurses Society. (2016). *Policies and procedures for infusion therapy* (5th ed.). Boston, MA: Infusion Nurses Society.

13 Centers for Disease Control and Prevention. (2002). Guideline for hand hygiene in health-care settings: Recommendations of the Healthcare Infection Control Practices Advisory Committee and the HICPAC/SHEA/APIC/IDSA Hand Hygiene Task Force. *MMWR Recommendations and Reports, 51*(RR-16), 1–45. https://www.cdc.gov/mmwr/pdf/rr/rr5116.pdf (Level II)

14 Centers for Disease Control and Prevention. (2011, revised 2017). Guidelines for the prevention of intravascular catheter–related infections. https://www.cdc.gov/infectioncontrol/guidelines/bsi/recommendations.html (Level I)

15 Standard 16. Hand hygiene. Infusion therapy standards of practice (8th ed.). (2021). *Journal of Infusion Nursing, 44,* S53–S54. (Level VII)

16 The Joint Commission. (2021). Standard NPSG.07.01.01. *Comprehensive accreditation manual for hospitals.* Oakbrook Terrace, IL: The Joint Commission. (Level VII)

17 World Health Organization. (2009). WHO guidelines on hand hygiene in health care: First global patient safety challenge, clean care is safer care. https://apps.who.int/iris/bitstream/handle/10665/44102/9789241597906_eng.pdf?sequence=1(Level IV)

18 Accreditation Association for Hospitals and Health Systems. (2020). Standard 07.01.21. *Healthcare Facilities Accreditation Program: Accreditation requirements for acute care hospitals.* Chicago, IL: Accreditation Association for Hospitals and Health Systems. (Level VII)

19 DNV GL-Healthcare USA, Inc. (2020). IC.1.SR.1. *NIAHO® accreditation requirements, interpretive guidelines and surveyor guidance—revision 20.0.* Milford, OH: DNV GL-Healthcare USA, Inc. (Level VII)

20 The Joint Commission. (2021). Standard NPSG.01.01.01. *Comprehensive accreditation manual for hospitals.* Oakbrook Terrace, IL: The Joint Commission. (Level VII)

21 The Joint Commission. (2021). Standard RI.01.01.01. *Comprehensive accreditation manual for hospitals.* Oakbrook Terrace, IL: The Joint Commission. (Level VII)

22 Centers for Medicare and Medicaid Services, Department of Health and Human Services. (2020). Condition of participation: Patient's rights. 42 C.F.R. § 482.13(c)(1).

23 DNV GL-Healthcare USA, Inc. (2020). PR.2.SR.5. *NIAHO® accreditation requirements, interpretive guidelines and surveyor guidance—revision 20.0.* Milford, OH: DNV GL-Healthcare USA, Inc. (Level VII)

24 Accreditation Association for Hospitals and Health Systems. (2020). Standard 15.01.16. *Healthcare Facilities Accreditation Program: Accreditation requirements for acute care hospitals.* Chicago, IL: Accreditation Association for Hospitals and Health Systems. (Level VII)

25 The Joint Commission. (2021). Standard PC.02.01.21. *Comprehensive accreditation manual for hospitals.* Oakbrook Terrace, IL: The Joint Commission. (Level VII)

26 U.S. Food and Drug Administration. (2017). Examples of medical device misconnections. https://www.fda.gov/medical-devices/medical-device-connectors/examples-medical-device-misconnections

27 Waters, T. R., et al. (2009). Safe patient handling training for schools of nursing. https://www.cdc.gov/niosh/docs/2009-127/pdfs/2009-127.pdf (Level VII)

28 Siegel, J. D., et al. (2007, revised 2019). 2007 guideline for isolation precautions: Preventing transmission of infectious agents in healthcare settings. https://www.cdc.gov/infectioncontrol/pdf/guidelines/isolation-guidelines-H.pdf (Level II)

29 Occupational Safety and Health Administration. (2012). Bloodborne pathogens, standard number 1910.1030. https://www.osha.gov/pls/oshaweb/owadisp.show_document?p_id=10051&p_table=STANDARDS (Level VII)

30 Accreditation Association for Hospitals and Health Systems. (2020). Standard 07.01.10. *Healthcare Facilities Accreditation Program: Accreditation requirements for acute care hospitals.* Chicago, IL: Accreditation Association for Hospitals and Health Systems. (Level VII)

31 Moureau, N. L., & Flynn, J. (2015). Disinfection of needleless connector hubs: Clinical evidence systematic review. *Nursing Research and Practice, 2015,* 796762. https://www.hindawi.com/journals/nrp/2015/796762 (Level I)

32 Marschall, J., et al. (2014). SHEA/IDSA practice recommendation: Strategies to prevent central line–associated bloodstream infections in acute care hospitals. *Infection Control and Hospital Epidemiology, 35,* 753–771. https://www.jstor.org/stable/10.1086/676533#metadata_info_tab_contents (Level I)

33 Standard 36. Needleless connectors. Infusion therapy standards of practice (8th ed.). (2021). *Journal of Infusion Nursing, 44,* S104–S107. (Level VII)

34 Standard 41. Flushing and locking. Infusion therapy standards of practice (8th ed.). (2021). *Journal of Infusion Nursing, 44,* S113–S119. (Level VII)

35 The Joint Commission. (2014). Sentinel event alert 53: Managing risk during transition to new ISO tubing connector standards. http://www.jointcommission.org/assets/1/6/SEA_53_Connectors_8_19_14_final.pdf (Level VII)

36 The Joint Commission. (2021). Standard NPSG.06.01.01. *Comprehensive accreditation manual for hospitals.* Oakbrook Terrace, IL: The Joint Commission. (Level VII)

37 Graham, K. C., & Cvach, M. (2010). Monitor alarm fatigue: Standardizing use of physiological monitors and decreasing nuisance alarms. *American Journal of Critical Care, 19,* 28–37. http://ajcc.aacnjournals.org/content/19/1/28.full.pdf

38 The Joint Commission. (2013). Sentinel event alert 50: Medical device alarm safety in hospitals. https://www.jointcommission.org/assets/1/6/SEA_50_alarms_4_26_16.pdf (Level VII)

39 Standard 24. Flow-control devices. Infusion therapy standards of practice (8th ed.). (2021). *Journal of Infusion Nursing, 44,* S69–S72. (Level VII)

40 Standard 47. Infiltration and extravasation. Infusion therapy standards of practice (8th ed.). (2021). *Journal of Infusion Nursing, 44,* S142–S147. (Level VII)

41 Ganz, D. A., et al. (2013, reviewed 2021). *Preventing falls in hospitals: A toolkit for improving quality of care* (AHRQ Publication No. 13-0015-EF). Rockville, MD: Agency for Healthcare Research and Quality. https://www.ahrq.gov/professionals/systems/hospital/fallpxtoolkit/index.html (Level VII)

42 Centers for Medicare and Medicaid Services. (2014). Requirements for hospital medication administration, particularly intravenous (IV) medications and post-operative care of patients receiving IV opioids. http://www.cms.gov/Medicare/Provider-Enrollment-and-Certification/SurveyCertificationGenInfo/Downloads/Survey-and-Cert-Letter-14-15.pdf

43 The Joint Commission. (2021). Standard RC.01.03.01. *Comprehensive accreditation manual for hospitals.* Oakbrook Terrace, IL: The Joint Commission. (Level VII)

44 Standard 10. Documentation in the health record. Infusion therapy standards of practice (8th ed.). (2021). *Journal of Infusion Nursing, 44,* S39–S43. (Level VII)

45 Centers for Medicare and Medicaid Services, Department of Health and Human Services. (2020). Condition of participation: Medical record services. 42 C.F.R. § 482.24(b).

46 Accreditation Association for Hospitals and Health Systems. (2020). Standard 10.00.03. *Healthcare Facilities Accreditation Program: Accreditation requirements for acute care hospitals.* Chicago, IL: Accreditation Association for Hospitals and Health Systems. (Level VII)

47 DNV GL-Healthcare USA, Inc. (2020). MR.2.SR.1. *NIAHO® accreditation requirements, interpretive guidelines and surveyor guidance—revision 20.0.* Milford, OH: DNV GL-Healthcare USA, Inc. (Level VII)

48 Standard 46. Phlebitis. Infusion therapy standards of practice (8th ed.). (2021). *Journal of Infusion Nursing, 44,* S138–S142. (Level VII)

49 Standard 50. Infection. Infusion therapy standards of practice (8th ed.). (2021). *Journal of Infusion Nursing, 44,* S153–S157. (Level VII)

50 Standard 52. Air embolism. Infusion therapy standards of practice (8th ed.). (2021). *Journal of Infusion Nursing, 44,* S160–S161. (Level VII)

IV SECONDARY LINE DRUG INFUSION

A secondary IV line is a complete IV set, container, tubing, and microdrip or macrodrip system connected to the lower Y port (secondary port) of a primary line instead of to the IV catheter. It can be used for continuous or intermittent drug infusion. When used continuously, a secondary IV line permits drug infusion and titration while the primary line maintains a constant total infusion rate.

A secondary IV line used for intermittent infusions is commonly called a *piggyback set*. In this case, the primary line maintains venous access between drug doses. Typically, a piggyback set includes a small IV container, short tubing, and a macrodrip system. The volume is typically 25 to 250 mL. This set connects to the primary line's upper Y port, also called a *piggyback port*. You should position the primary IV solution below the secondary solution to facilitate infusion. (The manufacturer provides an extension hook for that purpose.)

You should change a secondary administration set used to continuously administer fluids other than lipids, blood, or blood products at least every 7 days but no more frequently than every 96 hours, unless it becomes contaminated or otherwise compromised. If the secondary administration set is detached from the primary administration set, it's considered a primary intermittent administration set, and you should change it every 24 hours. The administration set must also be changed when the vascular access device is changed or when a new vascular access device is inserted.[1]

HOSPITAL-ACQUIRED CONDITION ALERT Keep in mind that the Centers for Medicare and Medicaid Services considers vascular catheter–associated infection a hospital-acquired condition *because it can be reasonably prevented using a variety of best practices.* Make sure to follow evidence-based infection prevention practices, such as performing hand hygiene, performing a vigorous mechanical scrub of the needleless connectors, limiting catheter access, and following sterile no-touch technique, during IV secondary line drug infusion *to reduce the risk of vascular catheter–associated infections.*[2,3]

Equipment

Gloves ■ prescribed IV medication ■ administration set with secondary injection port (Luer-lock design recommended) or volume-controlled administration set[1] ■ needleless adapter ■ antiseptic pads (chlorhexidine-based, alcohol, or tincture of iodine) ■ 10-mL prefilled syringe containing preservative-free normal saline solution ■ IV pole ■ labels ■ Optional: extension hook, electronic infusion device (preferably a smart pump with dose-error reduction software).

For intermittent infusion, the primary line typically has a piggyback port with a back check valve that stops the flow from the primary line during drug infusion and returns to the primary flow after infusion. You can also use a volume-control set with an intermittent infusion line.

Preparation of equipment

Inspect all IV equipment and supplies. If a product is expired, is defective, or has compromised integrity, remove it from patient use, label it as expired or defective, and report the expiration or defect as directed by your facility.[4] Confirm that the primary administration set contains a secondary port.

Check drug compatibility with the primary solution.[5] If necessary, add the drug to the secondary IV solution. (Whenever possible, administer pharmacy-prepared or commercially available products.) To do so, perform hand hygiene,[6] remove any seals from the secondary container, perform a vigorous mechanical scrub of the main port for at least 5 seconds with an antiseptic pad, and allow it to dry completely.[3] Inject the prescribed medication using safe medication administration practices, and gently agitate the solution *to mix the medication thoroughly.* Properly label the mixed IV solution as required by your facility. In a perioperative or procedural setting, the label should contain the medication name, strength, and quantity; diluent type and volume; and the expiration date.[7]

Insert the administration set spike and attach the needleless system. Open the flow clamp, prime the line, and then close the flow clamp. Initiate immediate-use medications within 1 hour of preparation or discard them.[8]

Implementation

■ Avoid distractions and interruptions when preparing and administering medications *to prevent medication errors.*[9,10]
■ Review the practitioner's order *to make sure that the prescribed infusion solution or medication, dose, rate, route of administration, and frequency and duration of administration are appropriate for the patient's age, condition, and access device, and that the infusion or medication is compatible with other solutions or medication.* Make sure that the order includes any test results that require monitoring. Address concerns about the order with the practitioner,[10,11] pharmacist, your supervisor, the risk management department, or as directed by your facility.[5,11,12,13,14,15,16]
■ Reconcile the patient's medications when a new medication is ordered *to reduce the risk of medications errors, including omissions, duplications, dosing errors, and drug interactions.*[17]

■ Check the patient's medical record for an allergy or a contraindication to the prescribed medication. If an allergy or contraindication exists, don't administer the medication; instead, notify the practitioner.[10,11,15,18]
■ Gather and prepare the prescribed medication and the necessary equipment and supplies.
■ Compare the medication label with the order in the patient's medical record.[10,11,12,14,15,17,18,19]
■ Check the expiration date on the medication. If the medication is expired, return it to the pharmacy and obtain a new medication.[10,11,12,15,18]
■ Visually inspect the solution for particles, discoloration, or other loss of integrity; don't administer the medication if its integrity is compromised.[10,11,12,15,18]
■ Verify that you're administering the medication at the proper time, in the prescribed dose, and by the correct route *to reduce the risk of medication errors.*[10,11,12,15,18]
■ Perform hand hygiene.[20,21,22,23,24,25,26]
■ Confirm the patient's identity using at least two patient identifiers.[27]
■ Provide privacy.[28,29,30,31]
■ Explain the procedure to the patient and family (if appropriate) according to their individual communication and learning needs *to increase their understanding, allay their fears, and enhance cooperation.*[32]
■ If the patient is receiving the medication for the first time, teach the patient and family (if appropriate) about the potential adverse reactions and discuss any other concerns related to the medication.[10,11,15,18,33]
■ If your facility uses a bar code technology, use it as directed by your facility.[17]
■ Perform hand hygiene.[20,21,22,23,24,25,26]
■ Put on gloves *to comply with standard precautions.*[20,34,35,36]
■ If the prescribed drug is incompatible with the primary IV solution, replace the primary solution with a fluid that's compatible with both solutions, as ordered.[37]
■ Assess the patient's IV site for pain, redness, or swelling.[5,12,16,38]
■ If a disinfectant-containing cap is in place at the end of the needleless connector, remove and discard it.[39,40]
■ Perform a vigorous mechanical scrub of the needleless connector for at least 5 seconds with an antiseptic pad[3] and allow it to dry completely.[3,5,16,40,41]
■ While maintaining sterility of the syringe tip, attach a prefilled syringe containing preservative-free normal saline solution to the needleless connector; use a 10-mL syringe or a syringe specifically designed to generate lower injection pressure. If necessary, unclamp the catheter and slowly aspirate for a blood return that's the color and consistency of whole blood. If you don't obtain a blood return, take steps to locate an external cause of obstruction.[5,12,16,42]
■ If you obtain a blood return, slowly inject preservative-free normal saline solution into the catheter *to assess catheter function.* Use a minimum volume of twice the internal volume of the catheter system. Don't forcibly flush the device; further evaluate the device if you meet resistance.[5,16,42]
■ If needed, insert a new IV catheter, or notify the practitioner if the patient has a central venous access catheter and you see signs of complications at the insertion site, or if you detect catheter function is compromise. (See the "IV catheter insertion and removal" procedure.)[12]

NURSING ALERT Don't administer continuous high-alert medications as a secondary infusion. Don't piggyback a secondary infusion into a primary infusion containing a high-alert drug, *to avoid adverse drug events caused by infusion at indeterminate rates or pump programming errors.*[10,43]

■ Hang the secondary set's container on the IV pole.
■ Perform a vigorous mechanical scrub of the needleless connector of the primary line that's closest to the vascular access catheter for at least 5 seconds with an antiseptic pad,[3] and allow it to dry completely.[3,5,16,40,41]
■ Trace the tubing from the patient to its point of origin *to make sure that you're connecting it to the proper port.* Route the tubing in a standardized direction if the patient has other tubing and catheters that have different purposes. Label the tubing at the distal (near the patient connection) and proximal ends (near the source container) *to reduce the risk of misconnection if multiple IV lines will be used.*[1,12,44]

EQUIPMENT

Assembling a piggyback set

A piggyback set is useful for intermittent drug infusion. For the set to work properly, you must position the secondary set's container higher than the primary set's container.

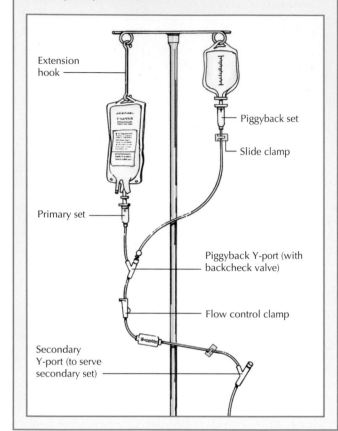

- Extension hook
- Piggyback set
- Slide clamp
- Primary set
- Piggyback Y-port (with backcheck valve)
- Flow control clamp
- Secondary Y-port (to serve secondary set)

■ Insert the needleless adapter from the secondary line into the needleless connector, verify a proper connection, and secure it to the primary line, as needed.[45]

■ To run the secondary set's container by itself, lower the primary set's container with an extension hook. To run both containers simultaneously, place them at the same height. (See *Assembling a piggyback set.*)

■ Open the clamp and adjust the drip rate.

■ For continuous infusion, set the secondary solution to the desired drip rate; then adjust the primary solution *to achieve the desired total infusion rate.*

■ For intermittent infusion, perform a visual inspection of the drip chambers *to verify that the secondary infusion is active and that the primary infusion is not active.* Adjust the primary drip rate, as required, on completion of the secondary solution. If you're reusing the secondary solution tubing, close the clamp on the tubing. Don't detach the secondary administration set from the injection port or remove the empty secondary solution container. Allow this set to remain connected, and use the back priming method to administer the next medication dose using the same administration set.[5] If you won't reuse the tubing, discard it appropriately with the IV container. When the next dose of medication is to be infused, hold the empty secondary solution container below the primary IV solution container and allow primary solution to backflow through the secondary administration set, filling it with solution and moving air into the empty secondary solution container. Remove the cover from the new mediation container. Detach the secondary solution container and insert the spike from the secondary administration set into the new container, being careful not to contaminate the spike. Hang the secondary

solution container above the primary container, open the clamp, and regulate the flow rate as appropriate.[5]

■ Use an electronic infusion device for infusions that require precise flow control *to maintain patient safety.* Consider the use of a smart pump with dose-error reduction software and interoperability with electronic health records *to reduce the risk of infusion-related medication errors.* Make sure alarm limits are set appropriately for the patient's current condition, and that alarms are turned on, properly functioning, and audible to staff members.[46]

■ Discard used supplies in appropriate receptacles.[34,35,47]

■ Remove and discard your gloves.[34,35,47]

■ Perform hand hygiene.[20,21,22,23,24,25,26]

■ Monitor the infusion regularly, inspect the IV insertion site for complications, and evaluate the patient's response to therapy.[12]

■ Document the procedure.[48,49,50,51,52]

Special considerations

■ Use an electronic infusion device for medication infusion *to maintain a constant infusion rate.* (See the "IV pump use" procedure.)

■ Inadequate height differential between the primary and secondary infusion can result in both infusions running at the same rate, unpredictable rates, or potentially the secondary infusion not infusing at all. Newer smart pumps are now available that do not depend on height differential.[53] Be aware of what technology is available at your facility.

■ The Joint Commission issued a sentinel event alert related to managing risk during transition to new International Organization for Standardization tubing standards that were designed to prevent dangerous tubing misconnections, which can lead to serious patient injury and death. During the transition, trace all tubing and catheters from the patient to the points of origin before connecting or reconnecting any device or infusion, at any care transition (such as to a new setting or service), and as part of the hand-off process; route tubes and catheters having different purposes in different standardized directions; when there are different access sites or several bags hanging, label the tubing at both the distal and proximal ends; use tubing and equipment only as intended; and store medications for different delivery routes in separate locations.[44]

Complications

The patient may experience an adverse reaction to the infused drug. In addition, repeated punctures of the secondary injection port can damage the seal, possibly allowing leakage or contamination.

General complications of infusion therapy include phlebitis, infiltration, extravasation, air embolism, infection, and circulatory overload.[54,55,56]

Documentation

Document the amount and type of medication administered and the amount of IV solution on the intake and output and medication records, noting the date, time, and the duration and rate of infusion. Record the access site used for the administration and the administration device used.[12] Record any adverse reactions to the prescribed medication, the date and time the practitioner was notified, prescribed interventions, and the patient's response to those interventions.[57] Document teaching provided to the patient and family (if applicable), their understanding of that teaching, and any need for follow-up teaching.[49]

REFERENCES

1　Standard 43. Administration set management. Infusion therapy standards of practice (8th ed.). (2021). *Journal of Infusion Nursing, 44,* S123–S125. (Level VII)

2　Jarrett, N., & Callaham, M. (2016). Evidence-based guidelines for selected hospital-acquired conditions: Final report. https://www.cms.gov/Medicare/Medicare-Fee-for-Service-Payment/HospitalAcqCond/Downloads/2016-HAC-Report.pdf

3　Marschall, J., et al. (2014). SHEA/IDSA practice recommendation: Strategies to prevent central line–associated bloodstream infections in acute care hospitals. *Infection Control and Hospital Epidemiology, 35,*

753–771. https://www.jstor.org/stable/10.1086/676533#metadata_info_tab_contents (Level I)

4 Standard 12. Product evaluation, integrity, and defect reporting. Infusion therapy standards of practice (8th ed.). (2021). *Journal of Infusion Nursing, 44,* S45–S46. (Level VII)

5 Infusion Nurses Society. (2016). *Policies and procedures for infusion therapy* (5th ed.). Boston, MA: Infusion Nurses Society.

6 Centers for Disease Control and Prevention. (2019). Medication preparation questions: FAQs regarding safe practices for medical injections. https://www.cdc.gov/injectionsafety/providers/provider_faqs_med-prep.html

7 The Joint Commission. (2021). Standard NPSG.03.04.01. *Comprehensive accreditation manual for hospitals.* Oakbrook Terrace, IL: The Joint Commission. (Level VII)

8 Standard 20. Compounding and preparation of parenteral solutions and medications. Infusion therapy standards of practice (8th ed.). (2021). *Journal of Infusion Nursing, 44,* S59–S60. (Level VII)

9 Westbrook, J., et al. (2010). Association of interruptions with an increased risk and severity of medication administration errors. *Archives of Internal Medicine, 170,* 683–690. (Level IV)

10 Centers for Medicare and Medicaid Services, Department of Health and Human Services. (2020). Condition of participation: Nursing services. 42 C.F.R. § 482.23(c).

11 The Joint Commission. (2021). Standard MM.06.01.01. *Comprehensive accreditation manual for hospitals.* Oakbrook Terrace, IL: The Joint Commission. (Level VII)

12 Standard 59. Infusion medication and solution administration. Infusion therapy standards of practice (8th ed.). (2021). *Journal of Infusion Nursing, 44,* S180–S183. (Level VII)

13 The Joint Commission. (2021). Standard MM.04.01.01. *Comprehensive accreditation manual for hospitals.* Oakbrook Terrace, IL: The Joint Commission. (Level VII)

14 Centers for Medicare and Medicaid Services, Department of Health and Human Services. (2020). Condition of participation: Pharmaceutical services. 42 C.F.R. § 482.25.

15 DNV GL-Healthcare USA, Inc. (2020). MM.1.SR.3. *NIAHO® accreditation requirements, interpretive guidelines and surveyor guidance—revision 20.0.* Milford, OH: DNV GL-Healthcare USA, Inc. (Level VII)

16 Infusion Nurses Society. (2017). *Policies and procedures for infusion therapy of the older adult* (3rd ed.). Boston, MA: Infusion Nurses Society.

17 Standard 13. Medication verification. Infusion therapy standards of practice (8th ed.). (2021). *Journal of Infusion Nursing, 44,* S46–S49. (Level VII)

18 Accreditation Association for Hospitals and Health Systems. (2020). Standard 16.01.03. *Healthcare Facilities Accreditation Program: Accreditation requirements for acute care hospitals.* Chicago, IL: Accreditation Association for Hospitals and Health Systems. (Level VII)

19 Accreditation Association for Hospitals and Health Systems. (2020). Standard 25.01.18. *Healthcare Facilities Accreditation Program: Accreditation requirements for acute care hospitals.* Chicago, IL: Accreditation Association for Hospitals and Health Systems. (Level VII)

20 Centers for Disease Control and Prevention. (2011, revised 2017). Guidelines for the prevention of intravascular catheter-related infections. https://www.cdc.gov/infectioncontrol/guidelines/bsi/recommendations.html (Level I)

21 The Joint Commission. (2021). Standard NPSG.07.01.01. *Comprehensive accreditation manual for hospitals.* Oakbrook Terrace, IL: The Joint Commission. (Level VII)

22 Standard 16. Hand hygiene. Infusion therapy standards of practice (8th ed.). (2021). *Journal of Infusion Nursing, 44,* S53–S54. (Level VII)

23 Centers for Disease Control and Prevention. (2002). Guideline for hand hygiene in health-care settings: Recommendations of the Healthcare Infection Control Practices Advisory Committee and the HICPAC/SHEA/APIC/IDSA Hand Hygiene Task Force. *MMWR Recommendations and Reports, 51*(RR-16), 1–45. https://www.cdc.gov/mmwr/pdf/rr/rr5116.pdf (Level II)

24 World Health Organization. (2009). WHO guidelines on hand hygiene in health care: First global patient safety challenge, clean care is safer care. https://apps.who.int/iris/bitstream/handle/10665/44102/9789241597906_eng.pdf?sequence=1 (Level IV)

25 Accreditation Association for Hospitals and Health Systems. (2020). Standard 07.01.21. *Healthcare Facilities Accreditation Program: Accreditation requirements for acute care hospitals.* Chicago, IL:

Accreditation Association for Hospitals and Health Systems. (Level VII)

26 DNV GL-Healthcare USA, Inc. (2020). IC.1.SR.1. *NIAHO® accreditation requirements, interpretive guidelines and surveyor guidance—revision 20.0.* Milford, OH: DNV GL-Healthcare USA, Inc. (Level VII)

27 The Joint Commission. (2021). Standard NPSG.01.01.01. *Comprehensive accreditation manual for hospitals.* Oakbrook Terrace, IL: The Joint Commission. (Level VII)

28 Accreditation Association for Hospitals and Health Systems. (2020). Standard 15.01.16. *Healthcare Facilities Accreditation Program: Accreditation requirements for acute care hospitals.* Chicago, IL: Accreditation Association for Hospitals and Health Systems. (Level VII)

29 Centers for Medicare and Medicaid Services, Department of Health and Human Services. (2020). Condition of participation: Patient's rights. 42 C.F.R. § 482.13(c)(1).

30 DNV GL-Healthcare USA, Inc. (2020). PR.2.SR.5. *NIAHO® accreditation requirements, interpretive guidelines and surveyor guidance—revision 20.0.* Milford, OH: DNV GL-Healthcare USA, Inc. (Level VII)

31 The Joint Commission. (2021). Standard RI.01.01.01. *Comprehensive accreditation manual for hospitals.* Oakbrook Terrace, IL: The Joint Commission. (Level VII)

32 The Joint Commission. (2021). Standard PC.02.01.21. *Comprehensive accreditation manual for hospitals.* Oakbrook Terrace, IL: The Joint Commission. (Level VII)

33 Standard 8. Patient education. Infusion therapy standards of practice (8th ed.). (2021). *Journal of Infusion Nursing, 44,* S35–S37. (Level VII)

34 Occupational Safety and Health Administration. (2012). Bloodborne pathogens, standard number 1910.1030. https://www.osha.gov/pls/oshaweb/owadisp.show_document?p_id=10051&p_table=STANDARDS (Level VII)

35 Siegel, J. D., et al. (2007, revised 2019). 2007 guideline for isolation precautions: Preventing transmission of infectious agents in healthcare settings. https://www.cdc.gov/infectioncontrol/pdf/guidelines/isolation-guidelines-H.pdf (Level II)

36 Accreditation Association for Hospitals and Health Systems. (2020). Standard 07.01.10. *Healthcare Facilities Accreditation Program: Accreditation requirements for acute care hospitals.* Chicago, IL: Accreditation Association for Hospitals and Health Systems. (Level VII)

37 Loubnan, V., & Nasser, S. C. (2010). A guide on intravenous drug compatibilities based on their pH. *Pharmacie Globale, 5*(1), 1–9. (Level VII)

38 Standard 42. Vascular access device assessment, care and dressing changes. Infusion therapy standards of practice (8th ed.). (2021). *Journal of Infusion Nursing, 44,* S119–S123. (Level VII)

39 Moureau, N. L., & Flynn, J. (2015). Disinfection of needleless connector hubs: Clinical evidence systematic review. *Nursing Research and Practice, 2015,* 796762. https://www.hindawi.com/journals/nrp/2015/796762/

40 Standard 36. Needleless connectors. Infusion therapy standards of practice (8th ed.). (2021). *Journal of Infusion Nursing, 44,* S104–S107. (Level VII)

41 The Joint Commission. (2013). Central line–associated bloodstream infections toolkit and monograph: Preventing central line–associated bloodstream infections. https://www.jointcommission.org/-/media/tjc/documents/resources/hai/clabsi_monographpdf.pdf (Level VII)

42 Standard 41. Flushing and locking. Infusion therapy standards of practice (8th ed.). (2021). *Journal of Infusion Nursing, 44,* S113–S119. (Level VII)

43 The Joint Commission. (2021). Standard MM.01.01.03. *Comprehensive accreditation manual for hospitals.* Oakbrook Terrace, IL: The Joint Commission. (Level VII)

44 The Joint Commission. (2014). Sentinel event alert 53: Managing risk during transition to new ISO tubing connector standards. http://www.jointcommission.org/assets/1/6/SEA_53_Connectors_8_19_14_final.pdf (Level VII)

45 U.S. Food and Drug Administration. (2017). Examples of medical device misconnections. https://www.fda.gov/medical-devices/medical-device-connectors/examples-medical-device-misconnections

46 Standard 24. Flow-control devices. Infusion therapy standards of practice (8th ed.). (2021). *Journal of Infusion Nursing, 44,* S69–S72. (Level VII)

47 Standard 21. Medical waste and sharps safety. Infusion therapy standards of practice (8th ed.). (2021). *Journal of Infusion Nursing, 44,* S60–S63. (Level VII)

48 The Joint Commission. (2021). Standard RC.01.03.01. *Comprehensive accreditation manual for hospitals.* Oakbrook Terrace, IL: The Joint Commission. (Level VII)

49 Standard 10. Documentation in the health record. Infusion therapy standards of practice (8th ed.). (2021). *Journal of Infusion Nursing, 44*, S39–S43. (Level VII)

50 Centers for Medicare and Medicaid Services, Department of Health and Human Services. (2020). Condition of participation: Medical record services. 42 C.F.R. § 482.24(b).

51 Accreditation Association for Hospitals and Health Systems. (2018). Standard 10.00.03. *Healthcare Facilities Accreditation Program: Accreditation requirements for acute care hospitals.* Chicago, IL: Accreditation Association for Hospitals and Health Systems. (Level VII)

52 DNV GL-Healthcare USA, Inc. (2020). MR.2.SR.1. *NIAHO® accreditation requirements, interpretive guidelines and surveyor guidance—revision 20.0.* Milford, OH: DNV GL-Healthcare USA, Inc. (Level VII)

53 Institute for Safe Medication Practices. (2020). Guidelines for optimizing safe implementation and use of smart infusion pumps. https://www.ismp.org/guidelines/safe-implementation-and-use-smart-pumps (Level VII)

54 Standard 57. Infiltration and extravasation. Infusion therapy standards of practice (8th ed.). (2021). *Journal of Infusion Nursing, 44*, S142–S147. (Level VII)

55 Standard 50. Infection. Infusion therapy standards of practice (8th ed.). (2021). *Journal of Infusion Nursing, 44*, S153–S157. (Level VII)

56 Standard 52. Air embolism. Infusion therapy standards of practice (8th ed.). (2021). *Journal of Infusion Nursing, 44*, S160–S161. (Level VII)

57 The Joint Commission. (2021). Standard RC.02.01.01. *Comprehensive accreditation manual for hospitals.* Oakbrook Terrace, IL: The Joint Commission. (Level VII)

IV THERAPY PREPARATION

Selection and preparation of appropriate equipment are essential for accurate delivery of an IV solution. IV bag preparation is necessary before administering parenteral medication or solutions. Solutions and medications should be prepared and dispensed from the pharmacy or as commercially prepared solutions.[1] If a solution is prepared outside of the pharmacy, initiation of administration should begin within 1 hour after the start of preparation. IV bag preparation requires sterile no-touch technique to prevent contamination and reduce the risk of vascular catheter–associated infection.[2]

NURSING ALERT Keep in mind that the Centers for Medicare and Medicaid Services considers vascular catheter–associated infection a hospital-acquired condition *because it can be reasonably prevented using a variety of best practices.* Make sure to follow evidence-based infection prevention techniques, such as performing hand hygiene and following sterile no-touch technique, *to reduce the risk of vascular catheter–associated infections.*[3,4,5,6,7,8]

Because certain IV solutions and medications are unstable in plastic fluid containers, they're prepared in bottles. Before such a solution or medication can be administered, however, the nonvented IV bottle must be prepared.[1] A vented IV administration set should be used to administer the solution or medication. The pharmacy should prepare and dispense these IV solutions and medications, or a commercially prepared solution should be used.[2] If an IV solution or medication has been prepared outside the pharmacy, administration should begin within 1 hour of the start of preparation.[1]

There's insufficient evidence to recommend the frequency of routine replacement of IV solution containers (without post-manufacturer additives), with the exception of parenteral nutrition solutions, which should be replaced every 24 hours. Replacing other IV solution containers less frequently than every 24 hours can be considered in times of product shortages, but the decision should be weighed against the risk of infection.[2]

Equipment

IV solution bag ▪ IV administration set ▪ IV pole ▪ labels ▪ Optional: prescribed medication, flow-control device.

Preparation of equipment

Inspect all IV equipment and supplies. If a product is expired, is defective, or has compromised integrity, remove it from patient use, label it as expired or defective, and report the expiration or defect as directed by your facility.[9]

Implementation

Preparing the bag

▪ Slide the flow clamp of the administration set tubing down to the drip chamber or injection port and close the clamp.
▪ Remove the protective cap or tear the tab from the tubing insertion port (as shown below).

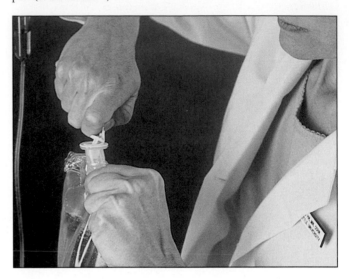

▪ Remove the protective cap from the administration set spike.
▪ Hold the port firmly with one hand and insert the spike with your other hand (as shown below). Be careful not to contaminate the IV bag insertion port or the IV tubing spike.

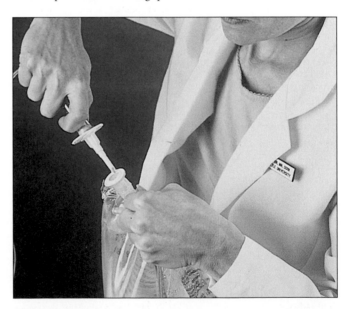

▪ Hang the bag on the IV pole and squeeze the drip chamber, filling it to the level recommended by the manufacturer (usually about one-half full).
▪ Prime the IV administration tubing. (See the section entitled "Priming the tubing.") Attach a flow-control device, if needed, following the manufacturer's instructions. (See the "IV pump use" procedure.) Choose a flow-control device that's appropriate for the severity of the illness, the type of therapy, dosing considerations, health care setting, risk of adverse effects to therapy, and the patient's age, acuity, and mobility.[9]
▪ Label the IV bag with the patient's name and identification number, date and time, the bag number (if applicable), ordered rate and duration of infusion, and your initials.

EQUIPMENT

Using in-line filters

In-line filters are used to prevent undesirable substances from entering the vascular system. The size and type of filter required is determined by the type of infusate; follow the manufacturer's instructions for use. The filter may be an add-on device or part of the IV administration set tubing. Consult the information below about filter use, or check with a pharmacist and the manufacturer's specific recommendations if you're unsure about the type of filter to use or whether a filter is required.[23,24,25]

- Apply or replace an in-line filter with each change of the IV administration set.
- When administering lipid infusions or 3-in-1 parenteral nutrition solutions, use a 1.2-micron filter, which retains particles and eliminates air.
- When administering nonlipid-containing solutions that require filtration, use a 0.2-micron filter, which retains bacteria and particulates and eliminates air.
- When using an electronic infusion device, ensure that the pounds per square inch (psi) rating of the filter exceeds the psi exerted by the electronic infusion device.
- Don't administer small-volume infusions of 5 mL or less over 24 hours through a 0.2-micron filter.
- Don't administer IV push medications through a 0.2-micron filter.

- Label the tubing as IV ROUTE at the proximal and distal ends *to avoid misconnections to a different route of entry into the body*.[10]
- Maintain the sterility of the male Luer end of the administration set before and during connection to the vascular access device.
- Perform hand hygiene.[11,12,13,14,15,16,17]
- Document the procedure.[18,19,20,21,22]

Preparing a bottle
- Close the flow or roller clamp on the IV administration set tubing.
- For a nonvented bottle, remove the IV bottle's metal cap and inner disk, if present. For a vented bottle, remove the bottle's metal cap and latex diaphragm *to release the vacuum*. If the vacuum isn't intact, discard the bottle and begin again.
- Place the IV bottle on a stable surface and disinfect the rubber stopper with an antiseptic pad using friction, and allow it to dry completely.
- Remove the protective cap from the administration set spike, and push the spike through the center of the nonvented bottle's rubber stopper. If using a vented bottle, push the spike through the insertion port next to the air vent tube opening. Avoid twisting or angling the spike *to prevent pieces of the stopper from breaking off and falling into the solution*.
- Invert the nonvented bottle. If its vacuum is intact, you'll hear a hissing sound and see air bubbles rise (this may not occur if you've already added medication). If the vacuum isn't intact, discard the bottle and begin again.
- Hang the bottle on the IV pole.
- Squeeze the drip chamber to the level recommended by the manufacturer.
- Reclamp the IV administration set.
- Perform hand hygiene.[11,12,13,14,15,16,17]
- Document the procedure.[18,19,20,21,22]

Priming the tubing
- Hang the solution container on the IV pole, if you haven't already, and squeeze the drip chamber until it's half full or according to the manufacturer's instructions.
- Leave the protective cover on the end of the tubing, hold the tubing above waist level, aim the distal end of the tubing over a wastebasket or sink, and slowly open the flow clamp.
- If an in-line filter is necessary, purge the tubing before attaching it *to avoid forcing air into the filter and possibly clogging some filter channels*. Attach an add-on filter to the end of the IV administration set tubing as close to the catheter site as possible. Then, follow the manufacturer's instructions for filling and priming it.[23] (See *Using in-line filters*.)
- Leave the clamp open until the IV solution flows through the entire length of tubing *to release trapped air bubbles and force out all the air*.
- Invert all Y-ports and backcheck valves and tap them, if necessary, *to fill them with solution*.

- Loop the IV administration set tubing over the IV pole until you're prepared to attach the tubing to the venous access device.
- Attach a flow-control device, if needed, following the manufacturer's instructions. (See the "IV pump use" procedure.) Choose a flow-control device that's appropriate for the severity of illness, type of therapy, dosing considerations, health care setting, risk of therapy adverse effects, and the patient's age, acuity, and mobility.[9]
- Label the IV administration set tubing with the date of initiation or the date when change is required, as directed by your facility.[24,25,26]
- Label the tubing with the infusing solution or medication at both the proximal and distal ends *to avoid misconnections to a different route of entry into the body*, if appropriate.[10]
- Perform hand hygiene.[11,12,13,14,15,16,17]
- Document the procedure.[18,19,20,21,22]

Special considerations
- The Joint Commission issued a sentinel event alert related to managing risk during transition to new International Organization for Standardization tubing standards that were designed to prevent dangerous tubing misconnections, which can lead to serious patient injury and death. During the transition, make sure to trace the tubing and catheter from the patient to the point of origin before connecting or reconnecting any device or infusion, at any care transition (such as a new setting or service), and as part of the hand-off process; route tubes and catheters having different purposes in different standardized directions; when there are different access sites or several bags hanging, label the tubing at the distal and proximal ends; use tubing and equipment only as intended; and store medications for different delivery routes in separate locations.[10]
- Replace a primary or secondary continuous IV administration set for administering solutions other than lipids, blood, or blood products no more frequently than every 96 hours but at least every 7 days, and immediately upon suspected contamination or when the integrity of the product or system is compromised. Also, replace an IV administration set whenever the peripheral catheter site is changed or when a new central venous access device is inserted.[3,26]
- Replace a secondary IV administration set that's detached from the primary administration set every 24 hours.[26]
- Replace an IV administration set for administering parenteral nutrition at least every 24 hours as well as when hanging a new parenteral nutrition container.[26]
- Replace an IV administration set for administering IV fat emulsions that are infused separately every 12 hours as well as when hanging a new fat emulsion container.[26]

Documentation
Document the type of therapy, medication, and dose (if applicable), administration rate, time, route, and method of administration.[2]

REFERENCES

1 Standard 20. Compounding and preparation of parenteral solutions and medications. Infusion therapy standards of practice (8th ed.). (2021). *Journal of Infusion Nursing, 44*, S59–S60. (Level VII)

2 Standard 59. Infusion medication and solution administration. Infusion therapy standards of practice (8th ed.). (2021). *Journal of Infusion Nursing, 44*, S180–S183. (Level VII)

3 Centers for Disease Control and Prevention. (2011, revised 2017). Guidelines for the prevention of intravascular catheter-related infections. https://www.cdc.gov/infectioncontrol/guidelines/bsi/recommendations.html (Level I)

4 The Joint Commission. (2021). Standard NPSG.07.04.01. *Comprehensive accreditation manual for hospitals.* Oakbrook Terrace, IL: The Joint Commission. (Level VII)

5 Marschall, J., et al. (2014). SHEA/IDSA practice recommendation: Strategies to prevent central line–associated bloodstream infections in acute care hospitals. *Infection Control and Hospital Epidemiology, 35*, 753–771. https://www.jstor.org/stable/10.1086/676533#metadata_info_tab_contents (Level I)

6 Jarrett, N., & Callaham, M. (2016). Evidence-based guidelines for selected hospital-acquired conditions: Final report. https://www.cms.gov/Medicare/Medicare-Fee-for-Service-Payment/HospitalAcqCond/Downloads/2016-HAC-Report.pdf

7 Association of Professionals in Infection Control and Epidemiology (APIC). (2015). Guide to preventing central line–associated bloodstream infections. http://apic.org/Resource_/TinyMceFileManager/2015/APIC_CLABSI_WEB.pdf (Level IV)

8 Standard 50. Infection. Infusion therapy standards of practice (8th ed.). (2021). *Journal of Infusion Nursing, 44*, S153–S157. (Level VII)

9 Standard 24. Flow-control devices. Infusion therapy standards of practice (8th ed.). (2021). *Journal of Infusion Nursing, 44*, S69–S72. (Level VII)

10 The Joint Commission. (2014). Sentinel event alert 53: Managing risk during transition to new ISO tubing connector standards. https://www.jointcommission.org/assets/1/6/SEA_53_Connectors_8_19_14_final.pdf (Level VII)

11 The Joint Commission. (2021). Standard NPSG.07.01.01. *Comprehensive accreditation manual for hospitals.* Oakbrook Terrace, IL: The Joint Commission. (Level VII)

12 Standard 16. Hand hygiene. Infusion therapy standards of practice (8th ed.). (2021). *Journal of Infusion Nursing, 44*, S53–S54. (Level VII)

13 Centers for Disease Control and Prevention. (2002). Guideline for hand hygiene in health-care settings: Recommendations of the Healthcare Infection Control Practices Advisory Committee and the HICPAC/SHEA/APIC/IDSA Hand Hygiene Task Force. *MMWR Recommendations and Reports, 51*(RR-16), 1–45. https://www.cdc.gov/mmwr/pdf/rr/rr5116.pdf (Level II)

14 World Health Organization. (2009). WHO guidelines on hand hygiene in health care: First global patient safety challenge, clean care is safer care https://apps.who.int/iris/bitstream/handle/10665/44102/9789241597906_eng.pdf?sequence=1 (Level IV)

15 Accreditation Association for Hospitals and Health Systems. (2020). Standard 07.01.21. *Healthcare Facilities Accreditation Program: Accreditation requirements for acute care hospitals.* Chicago, IL: Accreditation Association for Hospitals and Health Systems. (Level VII)

16 Centers for Medicare and Medicaid Services, Department of Health and Human Services. (2020). Condition of participation: Infection control. 42 C.F.R. § 482.42.

17 DNV GL-Healthcare USA, Inc. (2020). IC.1.SR.1. *NIAHO® accreditation requirements, interpretive guidelines and surveyor guidance—revision 20.0.* Milford, OH: DNV GL-Healthcare USA, Inc. (Level VII)

18 The Joint Commission. (2021). Standard RC.01.03.01. *Comprehensive accreditation manual for hospitals.* Oakbrook Terrace, IL: The Joint Commission. (Level VII)

19 Standard 10. Documentation in the health record. Infusion therapy standards of practice (8th ed.). (2021). *Journal of Infusion Nursing, 44*, S39–S43. (Level VII)

20 Centers for Medicare and Medicaid Services, Department of Health and Human Services. (2020). Condition of participation: Medical record services. 42 C.F.R. § 482.24(b).

21 Accreditation Association for Hospitals and Health Systems. (2020). Standard 10.00.03. *Healthcare Facilities Accreditation Program: Accreditation requirements for acute care hospitals.* Chicago, IL: Accreditation Association for Hospitals and Health Systems. (Level VII)

22 DNV GL-Healthcare USA, Inc. (2020). MR.2.SR.1. *NIAHO® accreditation requirements, interpretive guidelines and surveyor guidance—revision 20.0.* Milford, OH: DNV GL-Healthcare USA, Inc. (Level VII)

23 Standard 35. Filtration. Infusion therapy standards of practice (8th ed.). (2021). *Journal of Infusion Nursing, 44*, S102–S104. (Level VII)

24 Infusion Nurses Society. (2017). *Policies and procedures for infusion therapy of the older adult* (3rd ed.). Boston, MA: Infusion Nurses Society.

25 Infusion Nurses Society. (2016). *Policies and procedures for infusion therapy* (5th ed.). Boston, MA: Infusion Nurses Society.

26 Standard 43. Administration set management. Infusion therapy standards of practice (8th ed.). (2021). *Journal of Infusion Nursing, 44*, S123–S125. (Level VII)

JUGULAR VENOUS OXYGEN SATURATION MONITORING

Jugular venous oxygen saturation ($Sjvo_2$) monitoring measures the venous oxygenation saturation of blood as it leaves the brain using a catheter inserted into the jugular vein, which reflects the oxygen saturation of blood after cerebral perfusion has taken place.[1] Comparing $Sjvo_2$ with the arterial venous oxygenation can help to determine whether blood flow to the brain matches the brain's metabolic demand. Indications for $Sjvo_2$ monitoring include any neurologic injury in which ischemia is a threat, intraoperative monitoring, subarachnoid hemorrhage, and postacute head injury with increased intracranial pressure (ICP).

The normal range for $Sjvo_2$ is 55% to 75%. Values higher than 75% indicate hyperperfusion (as seen with cerebral vasodilation, hypercapnia, or hypertension) or decreased oxygen demand (as seen in deep sedation, coma, cerebral infarction, or hypothermia). Values below 54% indicate hypoperfusion (as seen with hypotension, cerebral vasoconstriction, or anemia) or increased oxygen demand (as seen with fever, agitation, pain, or seizures), and the brain is at risk for ischemia.[2,3] If an $Sjvo_2$ of less than 50% lasts for 10 minutes or more, it is considered cerebral desaturation and suggests a mismatch between O_2 delivery and demand, which is associated with poor outcomes.[1,2]

$Sjvo_2$ monitoring commonly is used with other types of cerebral hemodynamic monitoring—such as ICP monitoring—to provide detailed information regarding pressure and perfusion states during treatment. Treatment regimens can be titrated to enhance pressure and perfusion, allowing maximal balance between cerebral perfusion, oxygenation, and metabolism.

Data from monitoring can also be used to calculate the following:

- cerebral extraction of oxygen (CEo_2 = arterial oxygen saturation [Sao_2] – $Sjvo_2$)
- cerebral arterial oxygen content (Cao_2 = 1.34 × hemoglobin [Hgb] × Sao_2 + 0.0031 × partial pressure of arterial oxygen [Pao_2])
- global cerebral oxygen extraction ratio (O_2ER = Sao_2 – $Sjvo_2/Sao_2$) and jugular venous oxygen content saturation ($Cjvo_2$ = 1.34 × Hgb × $Sjvo_2$ + 0.0031 × jugular venous oxygen tension [$Pjvo_2$])
- arteriovenous jugular oxygen content ($AVjDo_2$ = Cao_2 – $Cjvo_2$).

These calculations help determine cerebral oxygen use, metabolic demand, and adequacy of oxygen delivery.

Insertion of the catheter for $Sjvo_2$ monitoring is contraindicated in patients with coagulopathies. Catheter insertion may be difficult in patients with cervical spine injury, local neck trauma, or a tracheostomy.[2]

HOSPITAL-ACQUIRED CONDITION ALERT Keep in mind that the Centers for Medicare and Medicaid Services considers vascular catheter–associated infection a hospital-acquired condition because it can be reasonably prevented using a variety of best practices. Make sure to follow evidence-based infection prevention practices, such as performing hand hygiene, following sterile technique when accessing the device, and removing the catheter as soon as it's no longer needed, to reduce the risk of vascular catheter–associated infections.[4,5,6,7,8,9]

Equipment

Monitoring equipment with cable for fiberoptic $Sjvo_2$ catheter ■ catheter, tubing, pressure bag system ■ gloves ■ facility-approved pain assessment tool ■ vital signs monitoring equipment ■ Optional: gown, mask with face shield, mask, goggles, supplies for venous blood sampling, prescribed pain medication.

Preparation of equipment

Inspect all equipment and supplies. If a product is expired, is defective, or has compromised integrity, remove it from patient use, label it as expired or defective, and report the expiration or defect as directed by your facility.

Implementation

- Verify the practitioner's order.
- Gather and prepare the necessary equipment and supplies.
- Perform hand hygiene.[10,11,12,13,14,15]
- Confirm the patient's identity using at least two patient identifiers.[16]
- Provide privacy.[17,18,19,20]
- Explain the procedure to the patient and family (if appropriate) according to their individual communication and learning needs *to increase their understanding, allay their fears, and enhance cooperation.*[21]
- Raise the bed to waist level before providing care *to prevent caregiver back strain.*[22]

TROUBLESHOOTING

COMMON CAUSES OF DESATURATION

During jugular venous oxygen saturation monitoring, you may encounter periods of desaturation and need to be prepared to take action. Below are common causes of desaturation and appropriate interventions.

CAUSE	NURSING INTERVENTIONS
■ Systemic hypoxemia (one of the most common causes of cerebral hypoxia)	■ If the oxygen saturation is less than 90%, increase the oxygen percentage or fraction of inspired oxygen and adjust the ventilator settings as ordered.
■ Anemia (hemoglobin less than 9 g/L)	■ Report abnormal results to the practitioner, and administer a blood transfusion if ordered.
■ Systemic hypotension (mean blood pressure less than 70 mm Hg)	■ Report abnormal results to the practitioner, and administer a fluid challenge or vasopressors following safe medication administration practices,[27,28,29,30] if ordered.
■ Increased intracranial pressure (greater than 20 mm Hg)	■ Elevate the head of the bed 30 degrees, decrease external stimuli, administer osmotic diuretics (such as mannitol) or a hypertonic saline solution bolus, as ordered, following safe medication administration practices.[27,28,29,30] Adjust the ventilator settings *to produce mild hyperventilation (partial pressure of arterial carbon dioxide of 26 to 30 mm Hg)*, as ordered.[37] Other measures may include drainage of cerebrospinal fluid and methods to reduce cerebral oxygen demand, such as sedation, neuromuscular blockade, or barbiturate coma.[37]

■ Perform hand hygiene.[10,11,12,13,14,15]
■ Put on gloves and other personal protective equipment, as needed, *to comply with standard precautions.*[23,24,25]
■ Monitor the patient's neurologic status, vital signs, and ICP *to promptly detect changes in the patient's condition.*

NURSING ALERT *Because the catheter in the jugular bulb can inhibit venous outflow,* a sustained ICP of more than 5 mm Hg over preinsertion baseline may be an indication for catheter removal.

■ Screen for and assess the patient's pain using facility-defined criteria that are consistent with the patient's age, condition, and ability to understand.[26]
■ Treat the patient's pain, as needed and ordered, using nonpharmacologic, pharmacologic, or a combination of approaches. Base the treatment plan on evidence-based practices and the patient's clinical condition, past medical history, and pain management goals.[26] If pharmacologic treatment is indicated and ordered, administer sedation or analgesia following safe medication administration practices *to maintain, monitor, and enhance cerebral perfusion pressure (CPP).*[27,28,29,30]
■ Make sure that the monitor alarm limits are set appropriately for the patient's current condition, and that the alarms are turned on, functioning properly, and audible to staff.[31,32,33,34]
■ Obtain a jugular venous blood gas sample and perform in vivo calibration according to the manufacturer's instructions and at intervals indicated by the manufacturer.[35] *In vivo calibration is necessary to ensure reliability of the data.*
■ Obtain blood samples for laboratory testing, as ordered; *hemoglobin and hematocrit values may be necessary to interpret $Sjvo_2$ and to calculate other hemodynamic parameters.*[36]
■ Monitor catheter, tubing, and pressure bag system integrity, and monitor the insertion site for signs of infection, infiltration, and bleeding *to detect possible complications and catheter dislodgment.*
■ Record baseline parameters for $Sjvo_2$,[36] and calculate and record baseline arteriovenous jugular oxygen ($AVjDo_2$), cerebral extraction of oxygen (CEo_2), and global cerebral oxygen extraction ratio (O_2ER) values.[36]
■ Continuously monitor $Sjvo_2$ and ICP values *to promptly identify changes in the patient's condition and prevent treatment delays.* Monitor for $Sjvo_2$ desaturations (see *Common causes of desaturation*) and note the correlation between the ICP and $Sjvo_2$, *because increased ICP is a frequent cause of desaturation in patients with brain injury.* Notify the practitioner if desaturations occur.
■ Recalculate and record $AVjDo_2$, CEo_2, and O_2ER, as indicated.
■ Reassess and respond to the patient's pain by evaluating the response to treatment and progress toward pain management goals. Assess for adverse reactions and risk factors for adverse events that may result from treatment.[26]
■ Return the bed to the lowest position *to prevent falls and maintain the patient's safety.*[38]
■ Discard used supplies in appropriate receptacles.[25]

■ Remove and discard your gloves and other personal protective equipment, if worn.[23,25]
■ Perform hand hygiene.[10,11,12,13,14,15]
■ Document the procedure.[39,40,41,42]

Special considerations

■ Maintain a safe environment during monitoring *to prevent accidental dislodgment of the catheter.*
■ Change the dressing using sterile technique if it becomes soiled or loosened and at the interval determined by your facility.
■ Change the disposable or reusable transducer systems, including administration set, continuous flush device, and flush solution used for invasive hemodynamic pressure monitoring every 96 hours, immediately upon suspected contamination, or when the integrity of the system has been compromised. Limit the number of manipulations and entries to the system.[5,43]
■ For an $Sjvo_2$ catheter with low light intensity, check the fiberoptics for obstruction, occlusion, and damage. Aspirate the catheter until blood can be freely sampled and normal light intensity is displayed. If you can't aspirate a blood sample, check whether the catheter needs to be replaced.
■ For an $Sjvo_2$ catheter with high light intensity, adjust the patient's head *to ensure neutral neck position. High light intensity indicates a vessel wall artifact and is usually encountered during patient repositioning.*
■ *To assess for catheter coiling,* identify rhythmic fluctuations in $Sjvo_2$ trends. Those unrelated to changes in ICP, CPP, or systemic blood pressure signify coiling of the catheter. Obtain a lateral cervical spine or lateral skull X-ray *to assess the position of the catheter in the external jugular vein (compare to X-ray done on insertion).* If coiling is confirmed, the practitioner may consider replacing the catheter.

Complications

This is an invasive procedure with potential complications related to catheter insertion, including carotid puncture and hematoma or injury to the vessel wall or jugular bulb. The catheter has potential to be malpositioned, which would result in inaccurate measurements. Intravascular catheter–related infection, thrombosis, and kinking of the catheter are also possible.[2]

Documentation

Record the baseline $SjvO_2$ reading and initial CEo_2, $AvjDo_2$, and O_2ER calculations. Record $Sjvo_2$ and ICP hourly. Record subsequent CEo_2, $AvjDo_2$, and O_2ER, when indicated. Document your assessment findings; the date, time, and name of the practitioner notified of any abnormalities; prescribed interventions; and the patient's response to those interventions. Document any medications administered, including the medication strength, dose, and route of administration and date and time of administration. Document teaching provided to the patient and family (if applicable), their understanding of that teaching, and any need for follow-up teaching.

References

1 Rajajee, V. (2021). Management of acute moderate and severe traumatic brain injury. In: *UpToDate*, Aminoff, M. J., et al. (Eds.).

2 Bhardwaj, A., et al. (2015). Jugular venous oximetry. *Journal of Neuroanaesthesiology and Critical Care, 2*(3), 225–231. https://www.thieme-connect.com/products/ejournals/html/10.4103/2348-0548.165046#N68787

3 Wiegand, D. L. (2017). *AACN procedure manual for high acuity, progressive, and critical care* (7th ed.). St. Louis, MO: Elsevier.

4 Jarrett, N., & Callaham, M. (2016). Evidence-based guidelines for selected hospital-acquired conditions: Final report. https://www.cms.gov/Medicare/Medicare-Fee-for-Service-Payment/HospitalAcqCond/Downloads/2016-HAC-Report.pdf

5 Centers for Disease Control and Prevention. (2011, revised 2017). Guidelines for the prevention of intravascular catheter-related infections. https://www.cdc.gov/infectioncontrol/guidelines/bsi/recommendations.html (Level I)

6 Standard 50. Infection. Infusion therapy standards of practice. (8th ed.). (2021). *Journal of Infusion Nursing, 44*, S153–S157. (Level VII)

7 Association of Professionals in Infection Control and Epidemiology (APIC). (2015). Guide to preventing central line-associated bloodstream infections. http://apic.org/Resource_/TinyMceFileManager/2015/APIC_CLABSI_WEB.pdf (Level IV)

8 Marschall, J., et al. (2014). SHEA/IDSA practice recommendation: Strategies to prevent central line-associated bloodstream infections in acute care hospitals. *Infection Control and Hospital Epidemiology, 35*, 753–771. https://www.jstor.org/stable/10.1086/676533#metadata_info_tab_contents (Level I)

9 The Joint Commission. (2021). Standard NPSG.07.04.01. *Comprehensive accreditation manual for hospitals.* Oakbrook Terrace, IL: The Joint Commission. (Level VII)

10 The Joint Commission. (2021). Standard NPSG.07.01.01. *Comprehensive accreditation manual for hospitals.* Oakbrook Terrace, IL: The Joint Commission. (Level VII)

11 Centers for Disease Control and Prevention. (2002). Guideline for hand hygiene in health-care settings: Recommendations of the Healthcare Infection Control Practices Advisory Committee and the HICPAC/SHEA/APIC/IDSA Hand Hygiene Task Force. *MMWR Recommendations and Reports, 51*(RR-16), 1–45. https://www.cdc.gov/mmwr/pdf/rr/rr5116.pdf (Level II)

12 World Health Organization. (2009). WHO guidelines on hand hygiene in health care: First global patient safety challenge, clean care is safer care. https://apps.who.int/iris/bitstream/handle/10665/44102/9789241597906_eng.pdf?sequence=1 (Level IV)

13 Accreditation Association for Hospitals and Health Systems. (2020). Standard 07.01.21. *Healthcare Facilities Accreditation Program: Accreditation requirements for acute care hospitals.* Chicago, IL: Accreditation Association for Hospitals and Health Systems. (Level VII)

14 Centers for Medicare and Medicaid Services, Department of Health and Human Services. (2020). Condition of participation: Infection control. 42 C.F.R. § 482.42.

15 DNV GL-Healthcare USA, Inc. (2020). IC.1.SR.1. *NIAHO® accreditation requirements, interpretive guidelines and surveyor guidance—revision 20.0.* Milford, OH: DNV GL-Healthcare USA, Inc. (Level VII)

16 The Joint Commission. (2021). Standard NPSG.01.01.01. *Comprehensive accreditation manual for hospitals.* Oakbrook Terrace, IL: The Joint Commission. (Level VII)

17 DNV GL-Healthcare USA, Inc. (2020). PR.2.SR.5. *NIAHO® accreditation requirements, interpretive guidelines and surveyor guidance—revision 20.0.* Milford, OH: DNV GL-Healthcare USA, Inc. (Level VII)

18 Centers for Medicare and Medicaid Services, Department of Health and Human Services. (2020). Condition of participation: Patient's rights. 42 C.F.R. § 482.13(c)(1).

19 The Joint Commission. (2021). Standard RI.01.01.01. *Comprehensive accreditation manual for hospitals.* Oakbrook Terrace, IL: The Joint Commission. (Level VII)

20 Accreditation Association for Hospitals and Health Systems. (2020). Standard 15.01.16. *Healthcare Facilities Accreditation Program: Accreditation requirements for acute care hospitals.* Chicago, IL: Accreditation Association for Hospitals and Health Systems. (Level VII)

21 The Joint Commission. (2021). Standard PC.02.01.21. *Comprehensive accreditation manual for hospitals.* Oakbrook Terrace, IL: The Joint Commission. (Level VII)

22 Waters, T. R., et al. (2009). Safe patient handling training for schools of nursing. https://www.cdc.gov/niosh/docs/2009-127/pdfs/2009-127.pdf (Level VII)

23 Siegel, J. D., et al. (2007, revised 2019). 2007 guideline for isolation precautions: Preventing transmission of infectious agents in healthcare settings. https://www.cdc.gov/infectioncontrol/pdf/guidelines/isolation-guidelines-H.pdf (Level II)

24 Accreditation Association for Hospitals and Health Systems. (2020). Standard 07.01.10. *Healthcare Facilities Accreditation Program: Accreditation requirements for acute care hospitals.* Chicago, IL: Accreditation Association for Hospitals and Health Systems. (Level VII)

25 Occupational Safety and Health Administration. (2012). Bloodborne pathogens, standard number 1910.1030. https://www.osha.gov/pls/oshaweb/owadisp.show_document?p_id=10051&p_table=STANDARDS (Level VII)

26 The Joint Commission. (2021). Standard PC.01.02.07. *Comprehensive accreditation manual for hospitals.* Oakbrook Terrace, IL: The Joint Commission. (Level VII)

27 The Joint Commission. (2021). Standard MM.06.01.01. *Comprehensive accreditation manual for hospitals.* Oakbrook Terrace, IL: The Joint Commission. (Level VII)

28 DNV GL-Healthcare USA, Inc. (2020). MM.1.SR.3. *NIAHO® accreditation requirements, interpretive guidelines and surveyor guidance—revision 20.0.* Milford, OH: DNV GL-Healthcare USA, Inc. (Level VII)

29 Centers for Medicare and Medicaid Services, Department of Health and Human Services. (2020). Condition of participation: Nursing services. 42 C.F.R. § 482.23(c).

30 Accreditation Association for Hospitals and Health Systems. (2020). Standard 16.01.03. *Healthcare Facilities Accreditation Program: Accreditation requirements for acute care hospitals.* Chicago, IL: Accreditation Association for Hospitals and Health Systems. (Level VII)

31 The Joint Commission. (2013). Sentinel event alert 50: Medical device alarm safety in hospitals. https://www.jointcommission.org/-/media/tjc/documents/resources/patient-safety-topics/sentinel-event/sea_50_alarms_4_26_16.pdf (Level VII)

32 Graham, K. C., & Cvach, M. (2010). Monitor alarm fatigue: Standardizing use of physiological monitors and decreasing nuisance alarms. *American Journal of Critical Care, 19*, 28–37.

33 American Association of Critical-Care Nurses. (2018). AACN practice alert: Managing alarms in acute care across the life span: Electrocardiography and pulse oximetry. https://www.aacn.org/clinical-resources/practice-alerts/managing-alarms-in-acute-care-across-the-life-span (Level VII)

34 The Joint Commission. (2021). Standard NPSG.06.01.01. *Comprehensive accreditation manual for hospitals.* Oakbrook Terrace, IL: The Joint Commission. (Level VII)

35 Manno, E. M. (Ed.). (2012). *Emergency management in neurocritical care.* Hoboken, NJ: Wiley-Blackwell.

36 Cyrous, A., et al. (2012). New approaches to bedside monitoring in stroke. *Expert Review of Neurotherapeutics, 12*, 915–928.

37 Smith, E. R., & Amin-Hanjani, S. (2019). Evaluation and management of elevated intracranial pressure in adults. In: *UpToDate*, Aminoff, M. J. (Ed.)

38 Ganz, D. A., et al. (2013, reviewed 2021). *Preventing falls in hospitals: A toolkit for improving quality of care* (AHRQ Publication No. 13-0015-EF). Rockville, MD: Agency for Healthcare Research and Quality. https://www.ahrq.gov/professionals/systems/hospital/fallpxtoolkit/index.html (Level VII)

39 The Joint Commission. (2021). Standard RC.01.03.01. *Comprehensive accreditation manual for hospitals.* Oakbrook Terrace, IL: The Joint Commission. (Level VII)

40 Accreditation Association for Hospitals and Health Systems. (2020). Standard 10.00.03. *Healthcare Facilities Accreditation Program: Accreditation requirements for acute care hospitals.* Chicago, IL: Accreditation Association for Hospitals and Health Systems. (Level VII)

41 Centers for Medicare and Medicaid Services, Department of Health and Human Services. (2020). Condition of participation: Medical record services. 42 C.F.R. § 482.24(b).

42 DNV GL-Healthcare USA, Inc. (2020). MR.2.SR.1. *NIAHO® accreditation requirements, interpretive guidelines and surveyor guidance—revision 20.0.* Milford, OH: DNV GL-Healthcare USA, Inc. (Level VII)

43 Standard 43. Administration set change. Infusion therapy standards of practice (8th ed.). (2021). *Journal of Infusion Nursing, 44*, S123–S125. (Level VII)

44 The Joint Commission. (2014). Sentinel event alert 53: Managing risk during transition to new ISO tubing connector standards. https://www.jointcommission.org/-/media/tjc/documents/resources/patient-safety-topics/sentinel-event/sea_53_connectors_8_19_14_final.pdf (Level VII)

Knee arthroplasty postprocedure care

Knee arthroplasty involves surgical replacement of all or part of the knee joint. In partial knee replacement, either the medial or lateral compartment of the knee joint is replaced. Total knee replacement is commonly used to relieve severe arthritic pain, treat joint contractures, or treat deterioration of joint surfaces, conditions that prohibit full extension or flexion.[1]

Arthroplasty postprocedure care includes maintaining alignment of the affected joint, assisting with exercises, and providing routine postoperative care. Nursing responsibilities include teaching, assisting with safe mobility, coordinating home care, and assisting with exercises that may continue for several years.

HOSPITAL-ACQUIRED CONDITION ALERT Keep in mind that the Centers for Medicare and Medicaid Services considers venous thromboembolism (VTE) in patients who underwent total knee replacement a hospital-acquired condition, *because use of best practices can reasonably prevent it.* Be sure to follow evidence-based VTE prevention practices, such as using mechanical compression devices (including antiembolism stockings or an intermittent pneumatic compression device), early ambulation, and pharmacologic prophylaxis *to reduce the risk of VTE.*[2,3,4]

Equipment

Arterial-venous foot compression controller and foot covers, or sequential compression device and sleeves ■ gloves ■ hypoallergenic moisturizer ■ warm water ■ skin cleanser ■ over-the-bed trapeze bar ■ crutches or walker ■ prescribed pain medications ■ prescribed anticoagulants ■ stethoscope ■ vital signs monitoring equipment ■ pillow ■ disinfectant pad ■ Optional: ice pack, knee immobilizer, closed wound drainage system, measuring container, electronic infusion device (preferably a smart pump with dose-error reduction software), capnography equipment, prescribed beta-adrenergic blocker, pulse oximeter and probe, standardized sedation scale.

Implementation

■ Receive hand-off communication from the person who was responsible previously for the patient's care. Ask questions as necessary *to help avoid miscommunications that can cause patient care errors during transition of care.*[5] Trace the tubing and catheter from the patient to its point of origin as part of the hand-off process; use a standardized line reconciliation process using high-reliability practices.[6,7]
■ Verify the practitioner's orders.
■ Perform hand hygiene.[8,9,10,11,12,13]
■ Confirm the patient's identity using at least two patient identifiers.[14]
■ Provide privacy.[15,16,17,18]
■ Explain all the procedures to the patient and family members (if appropriate) according to their individual communication and learning needs *to help increase their understanding, allay their fears, and enhance cooperation.*[19]
■ Perform hand hygiene.[8,9,10,11,12,13]
■ Put on gloves as necessary *to comply with standard precautions.*[20,21,22]
■ Monitor vital signs according to the patient's condition and at an interval determined by your facility and the patient's condition; *no evidence-based research exists to indicate best practices for the frequency of vital signs assessment.*[23] Report changes in vital signs, *because they may indicate infection, hemorrhage, or postoperative complications.*
■ Assess the patient's respiratory status.[23] Encourage the patient to perform deep-breathing and coughing exercises *to help prevent postprocedure pneumonia.*
■ Assess the patient's bilateral neurovascular status regularly at an interval determined by your facility and the patient's condition, *to help detect signs of complications.* Check the patient's affected leg for color, temperature, toe movement, sensation, edema, capillary filling, and pedal pulse. Investigate any complaints of pain, burning, numbness, or tingling.[23,24]

■ If not already in place, apply a sequential compression device to the patient's lower extremities or an arterial-venous impulse foot compression device to the patient's feet, as ordered, to help prevent VTE.[25,26] (See the "Sequential compression therapy" procedure.) Remove the sleeves or foot covers regularly to inspect the patient's skin for breakdown, and then reapply the sleeves or foot covers.
■ Screen and assess pain using facility-defined criteria that are consistent with the patient's age, condition, and ability to understand.[27]
■ In collaboration with the multidisciplinary team, involve the patient in the pain management planning process. Provide education on pain management, treatment options, and the safe use of opioid and nonopioid medications when prescribed. Develop realistic expectations and measurable goals that the patient understands for the degree, duration, and reduction of pain. Discuss objectives used to evaluate treatment progress (for example, relief of pain and improved physical and psychosocial function).[27]
■ Treat the patient's pain as needed and ordered using nonpharmacologic or pharmacologic methods, or a combination of approaches. Base the treatment plan on evidence-based practices and the patient's clinical condition, medical history, and pain management goals.[27]
■ If the patient is receiving IV opioid medication, take these steps: Frequently monitor the patient's respiratory status, oxygen saturation level by pulse oximetry, end-tidal carbon dioxide level by capnography (if available), and sedation level using a standardized sedation scale *to help promptly recognize and treat oversedation and respiratory depression related to IV opioid medication use.*[28] Explain the monitoring process to the patient and family members (including that it may be necessary to awaken the patient to assess the effects of the medication). Advise the patient and family members to alert staff immediately if breathing problems, sedation, or other changes occur that might be a reaction to the medication.[28,29]
■ If the patient was receiving a beta-adrenergic blocker before surgery, collaborate with the practitioner to ensure that the patient receives it during the perioperative period as appropriate.[30]
■ Ensure that prophylactic antibiotics are discontinued within 24 hours after surgery.[26,31,32]
■ Administer thromboembolic pharmacologic prophylaxis, as ordered, following safe medication administration practices, *to minimize the risk of VTE.*[25,29,33,34,35,36] If the practitioner prescribes a continuous infusion of heparin, administer it using an electronic infusion device (preferably a smart pump with dose-error-reduction software) *to help provide consistent, accurate dosing.*
■ Observe the patient for bleeding and symptoms of phlebitis, such as warmth, swelling, tenderness, and redness. Monitor laboratory results, such as complete blood count, prothrombin time, International Normalized Ratio, and partial thromboplastin time.[26] Notify the practitioner of critical test results within your facility's established time frame *so that the patient can be treated promptly.*[33]
■ Monitor the patient's dressings for excessive bleeding; notify the practitioner of excessive bleeding if present.

NURSING ALERT During inspection, pay special attention to the incisional area. Monitor for bruising, and report redness, warmth, or swelling of the surgical site. Record drainage amounts, and report excess drainage immediately, *because this could signal bleeding into the joint.* Be aware that many patients complain of slight numbness or tingling and mild swelling at the incision site.

■ Observe the closed-wound drainage system for discharge color. (See the "Closed-wound drain management" procedure.) *Proper drainage prevents hematoma. Purulent discharge and fever may indicate infection.* Empty and measure drainage, as ordered, using clean technique *to prevent infection.*
■ Monitor the patient's fluid intake and output (include wound drainage in the output measurement) and electrolyte levels as ordered *to help detect and treat fluid and electrolyte imbalances promptly.* Notify the practitioner of critical test results within your facility's established time frame *so that the patient can receive prompt treatment.*[33]
■ If the patient has an indwelling urinary catheter that was inserted for surgery, remove the catheter on postoperative day 1 or 2 (with the day of surgery considered day 0), according to your facility's protocol or the practitioner's order, *to reduce the risk of catheter-associated urinary tract infection.*[26,37] (See the "Indwelling urinary catheter care and removal" procedure.)

- If ordered, apply an ice pack to the patient's affected surgical site for the first 48 hours; however, be aware that the potential benefits of cold therapy on blood loss, postoperative pain, and range of motion may be too insignificant to justify its use.[38,39]
- Help the patient use the trapeze to reposition every 2 hours. *These position changes enhance comfort, prevent pressure injuries, and help prevent respiratory complications.*
- Provide skin care for the patient's back and buttocks, using warm water and skin cleanser for bathing. While the patient's skin is still damp, hydrate the skin with a hypoallergenic moisturizer as indicated *to help prevent skin tearing.*[40]
- Instruct the patient to perform muscle-strengthening exercises for the affected and unaffected extremities, as ordered, *to help maintain muscle strength and range of motion and to help prevent phlebitis.* Collaborate with physical therapy professionals, as appropriate.
- Instruct the patient to begin quadriceps exercises and straight-leg raises when ordered (usually as soon as the patient is able).
- Encourage the patient to begin flexion-extension exercises when ordered.[1] Collaborate with physical therapy professionals, as appropriate.
- Elevate the patient's affected leg, as ordered, *to reduce swelling.*[41]
- Before ambulation, ensure adequate pain management, *because movement is very painful after arthroplasty.*[1] Encourage the patient during exercise.
- Help the patient with progressive ambulation, using adjustable crutches or a walker when necessary, depending on the practitioner's orders. Some patients may have weight-bearing restrictions.[41]
- Reassess and respond to the patient's pain by evaluating the response to treatment and the progress toward pain management goals. Assess the patient for adverse reactions as well as for risk factors for adverse events that may result from treatment.[27]
- Teach the patient and family about measures to prevent surgical site infection.[31,42]
- Remove and discard your gloves if worn.[20,22]
- Perform hand hygiene.[8,9,10,11,12,13]
- Clean and disinfect your stethoscope using a disinfectant pad.[43,44]
- Perform hand hygiene.[8,9,10,11,12,13]
- Document the procedure.[45,46,47,48]

Special considerations

- Fever within the first 48 hours after surgery is commonly due to the normal inflammatory response.[49,50] In superficial wound infections, it commonly takes 4 to 6 days for fever to develop.
- Studies involving patients with total knee arthroplasty suggest that continuous passive motion doesn't improve active knee flexion, pain, function, or quality of life, and does not reduce VTE. Thus, guidelines don't recommend routine use for postoperative uncomplicated total knee replacement.[51,52,53,54]

Complications

Immobility after arthroplasty may result in such complications as DVT, pulmonary embolism, pneumonia, phlebitis, paralytic ileus, urine retention, and bowel impaction.[55,56] A deep wound or infection at the prosthesis site is a serious complication that may require revision or removal of the prosthesis.[55] Incomplete pain control may prolong recuperation and increase the risk of chronic pain.[57]

Fat embolism syndrome may develop within 72 hours after surgery. Watch for such signs and symptoms as apprehension, diaphoresis, fever, dyspnea, hypoxia, tachypnea, hypotension, cyanosis, seizures, decreased level of consciousness, and a petechial rash on the head, subconjunctiva, chest, and shoulders.[58]

Other complications include patellofemoral instability, patellar component loosening or failure, patella fracture, patellar clunk syndrome, and rupture of the extensor mechanism. Injury to the peroneal nerve may cause paresthesia, numbness, and extensor weakness (drop foot).

Documentation

Record the patient's neurovascular status and describe the patient's position (especially the position of the affected leg), skin care and condition,
respiratory care and condition, and the use of a sequential compression device, if ordered. Document all exercises the patient performed and their effect. Also record the patient's ambulation efforts, the type of support the patient used, and the amount of traction weight. Record assessment of the patient's pain, interventions you provided, and the patient's response to those interventions.

Record the patient's vital signs and fluid intake and output on the appropriate flowcharts. Note the patient's turning and skin care schedule and the patient's current exercise and ambulation program. Document teaching you provided to the patient and family (if applicable), their understanding of that teaching, and any need for follow-up teaching.

REFERENCES

1 Martin, G. M., & Harris, I. (2020). Total knee arthroplasty. In: *UpToDate*, Hunter, D. (Ed.).

2 Jarrett, N., & Callaham, M. (2016). Evidence-based guidelines for selected hospital-acquired conditions: Final report. https://www.cms.gov/Medicare/Medicare-Fee-for-Service-Payment/HospitalAcqCond/Downloads/2016-HAC-Report.pdf

3 Balk, E. M., et al. (2017). Venous thromboembolism prophylaxis in major orthopedic surgery: Systematic review update (AHRQ publication no. 17-EHC021-EF). https://effectivehealthcare.ahrq.gov/topics/thromboembolism-update/research-2017

4 Falck-Ytter, Y., et al. (2012). Prevention of VTE in orthopedic surgery patients: Antithrombotic therapy and prevention of thrombosis (9th ed.). *Chest, 141,* e278S–e325S. (Level VII)

5 The Joint Commission. (2021). Standard PC.02.02.01. *Comprehensive accreditation manual for hospitals.* Oakbrook Terrace, IL: The Joint Commission. (Level VII)

6 U.S. Food and Drug Administration. (2017). Examples of medical device misconnections. https://www.fda.gov/medical-devices/medical-device-connectors/examples-medical-device-misconnections

7 The Joint Commission. (2014). Sentinel event alert 53: Managing risk during transition to new ISO tubing connector standards. https://www.jointcommission.org/-/media/tjc/documents/resources/patient-safety-topics/sentinel-event/sea_53_connectors_8_19_14_final.pdf (Level VII)

8 DNV GL-Healthcare USA, Inc. (2020). IC.1.SR.1. *NIAHO® accreditation requirements, interpretive guidelines and surveyor guidance—revision 20.0.* Milford, OH: DNV GL-Healthcare USA, Inc. (Level VII)

9 The Joint Commission. (2021). Standard NPSG.07.01.01. *Comprehensive accreditation manual for hospitals.* Oakbrook Terrace, IL: The Joint Commission. (Level VII)

10 Centers for Disease Control and Prevention. (2002). Guideline for hand hygiene in health-care settings: Recommendations of the Healthcare Infection Control Practices Advisory Committee and the HICPAC/SHEA/APIC/IDSA Hand Hygiene Task Force. *MMWR Recommendations and Reports, 51*(RR-16), 1–45. https://www.cdc.gov/mmwr/pdf/rr/rr5116.pdf (Level II)

11 World Health Organization. (2009). WHO guidelines on hand hygiene in health care: First global patient safety challenge, clean care is safer care. https://apps.who.int/iris/bitstream/handle/10665/44102/9789241597906_eng.pdf?sequence=1 (Level IV)

12 Centers for Medicare and Medicaid Services, Department of Health and Human Services. (2020). Condition of participation: Infection control. 42 C.F.R. § 482.42.

13 Accreditation Association for Hospitals and Health Systems. (2020). Standard 07.01.21. *Healthcare Facilities Accreditation Program: Accreditation requirements for acute care hospitals.* Chicago, IL: Accreditation Association for Hospitals and Health Systems. (Level VII)

14 The Joint Commission. (2021). Standard NPSG.01.01.01. *Comprehensive accreditation manual for hospitals.* Oakbrook Terrace, IL: The Joint Commission. (Level VII)

15 The Joint Commission. (2021). Standard RI.01.01.01. *Comprehensive accreditation manual for hospitals.* Oakbrook Terrace, IL: The Joint Commission. (Level VII)

16 Centers for Medicare and Medicaid Services, Department of Health and Human Services. (2020). Condition of participation: Patient's rights. 42 C.F.R. § 482.13(c)(1).

17 Accreditation Association for Hospitals and Health Systems. (2020). Standard 15.01.16. *Healthcare Facilities Accreditation Program: Accreditation requirements for acute care hospitals.* Chicago, IL: Accreditation Association for Hospitals and Health Systems. (Level VII)

18 DNV GL-Healthcare USA, Inc. (2020). PR.2.SR.5. *NIAHO® accreditation requirements, interpretive guidelines and surveyor guidance—revision 20.0.* Milford, OH: DNV GL-Healthcare USA, Inc. (Level VII)

19 The Joint Commission. (2021). Standard PC.02.01.21. *Comprehensive accreditation manual for hospitals.* Oakbrook Terrace, IL: The Joint Commission. (Level VII)

20 Siegel, J. D., et al. (2007, revised 2019). 2007 guideline for isolation precautions: Preventing transmission of infectious agents in healthcare settings. https://www.cdc.gov/infectioncontrol/pdf/guidelines/isolation-guidelines-H.pdf (Level II)

21 Accreditation Association for Hospitals and Health Systems. (2020). Standard 07.01.10. *Healthcare Facilities Accreditation Program: Accreditation requirements for acute care hospitals.* Chicago, IL: Accreditation Association for Hospitals and Health Systems. (Level VII)

22 Occupational Safety and Health Administration. (2012). Bloodborne pathogens, standard number 1910.1030. https://www.osha.gov/pls/oshaweb/owadisp.show_document?p_id=10051&p_table=STANDARDS (Level VII)

23 American Society of PeriAnesthesia Nurses. (2019). *2019-2020 Perianesthesia nursing standards, practice recommendations and interpretive statements.* Cherry Hill, NJ: American Society of PeriAnesthesia Nurses. (Level VII)

24 Slade, S. (2020). Evidence summary: Neurovascular assessment. *JBI EBP Database.* AN: JBI188

25 American Academy of Orthopaedic Surgeons. (2011). Preventing venous thromboembolic disease in patients undergoing elective hip and knee arthroplasty: Evidence-based guideline and evidence report. https://www.aaos.org/globalassets/quality-and-practice-resources/vte/vte_full_guideline_10.31.16.pdf (Level VII)

26 Centers for Medicare and Medicaid Services & The Joint Commission. (2022). The specifications manual for national hospital inpatient quality measures (version 5.11). https://www.qualitynet.org/inpatient/specifications-manuals#tab1

27 The Joint Commission. (2021). Standard PC.01.02.07. *Comprehensive accreditation manual for hospitals.* Oakbrook Terrace, IL: The Joint Commission. (Level VII)

28 Centers for Medicare and Medicaid Services. (2014). Requirements for hospital medication administration, particularly intravenous (IV) medications and post-operative care of patients receiving IV opioids. https://www.cms.gov/Medicare/Provider-Enrollment-and-Certification/SurveyCertificationGenInfo/Downloads/Survey-and-Cert-Letter-14-15.pdf

29 Centers for Medicare and Medicaid Services, Department of Health and Human Services. (2020). Condition of participation: Nursing services. 42 C.F.R. § 482.23(c).

30 Devereaux, P. J., et al. (2020). Management of cardiac risk for noncardiac surgery. In: *UpToDate,* Pellikka, P. A., & Jaffe, A. S. (Eds.).

31 Anderson, D. J., et al. (2014). SHEA/IDSA practice recommendation: Strategies to prevent surgical site infections in acute care hospitals: 2014 update. *Infection Control and Hospital Epidemiology, 35,* 605–627. https://www.jstor.org/stable/10.1086/676022#metadata_info_tab_contents (Level I)

32 World Health Organization. (2016). Global guidelines for the prevention of surgical site infection. http://www.who.int/gpsc/global-guidelines-web.pdf (Level VII)

33 The Joint Commission. (2021). Standard NPSG.02.03.01. *Comprehensive accreditation manual for hospitals.* Oakbrook Terrace, IL: The Joint Commission. (Level VII)

34 DNV GL-Healthcare USA, Inc. (2020). MM.1.SR.3. *NIAHO® accreditation requirements, interpretive guidelines and surveyor guidance—revision 20.0.* Milford, OH: DNV GL-Healthcare USA, Inc. (Level VII)

35 Accreditation Association for Hospitals and Health Systems. (2020). Standard 16.01.03. *Healthcare Facilities Accreditation Program: Accreditation requirements for acute care hospitals.* Chicago, IL: Accreditation Association for Hospitals and Health Systems. (Level VII)

36 The Joint Commission. (2021). Standard MM.06.01.01. *Comprehensive accreditation manual for hospitals.* Oakbrook Terrace, IL: The Joint Commission. (Level VII)

37 Healthcare Infection Control Practices Advisory Committee. (2010, revised 2019). Guideline for prevention of catheter-associated urinary tract infections 2009. https://www.cdc.gov/infectioncontrol/pdf/guidelines/cauti-guidelines-H.pdf (Level I)

38 Adie, S., et al. (2012). Cryotherapy following total knee replacement. *Cochrane Database of Systematic Reviews, 2012*(9), CD007911. https://www.cochranelibrary.com/cdsr/doi/10.1002/14651858.CD007911.pub2/full (Level I)

39 Thacoor, A., & Sandiford, N. A. (2019). Cryotherapy following total knee arthroplasty: What is the evidence? *Journal of Orthopaedic Surgery (Hong Kong), 27*(1), 2309499019832752. https://journals.sagepub.com/doi/pdf/10.1177/2309499019832752 (Level I)

40 LeBlanc, K., et al. (2013). International skin tear advisory panel: A tool kit to aid in the prevention, assessment, and treatment of skin tears using a simplified classification system. *Advances in Skin and Wound Care, 26,* 459–476. (Level IV)

41 Foran, J. R. H. (2017). Total knee replacement exercise guide. https://orthoinfo.aaos.org/en/recovery/total-knee-replacement-exercise-guide/

42 The Joint Commission. (2021). Standard NPSG.07.05.01. *Comprehensive accreditation manual for hospitals.* Oakbrook Terrace, IL: The Joint Commission. (Level VII)

43 Rutala, W. A., et al. (2008, revised 2019). Guideline for disinfection and sterilization in healthcare facilities, 2008. https://www.cdc.gov/infection-control/pdf/guidelines/disinfection-guidelines-H.pdf (Level I)

44 Accreditation Association for Hospitals and Health Systems. (2020). Standard 07.02.03. *Healthcare Facilities Accreditation Program: Accreditation requirements for acute care hospitals.* Chicago, IL: Accreditation Association for Hospitals and Health Systems. (Level VII)

45 The Joint Commission. (2021). Standard RC.01.03.01. *Comprehensive accreditation manual for hospitals.* Oakbrook Terrace, IL: The Joint Commission. (Level VII)

46 Centers for Medicare and Medicaid Services, Department of Health and Human Services. (2020). Condition of participation: Medical record services. 42 C.F.R. § 482.24(b).

47 Accreditation Association for Hospitals and Health Systems. (2020). Standard 10.00.03. *Healthcare Facilities Accreditation Program: Accreditation requirements for acute care hospitals.* Chicago, IL: Accreditation Association for Hospitals and Health Systems. (Level VII)

48 DNV GL-Healthcare USA, Inc. (2020). MR.2.SR.1. *NIAHO® accreditation requirements, interpretive guidelines and surveyor guidance—revision 20.0.* Milford, OH: DNV GL-Healthcare USA, Inc. (Level VII)

49 Shaw, J. A., & Chung, R. (1999). Febrile response after knee and hip arthroplasty. *Clinical Orthopaedics and Related Research, 367,* 181–189. (Level VI)

50 Crompton, J. G., et al. (2019). Does atelectasis cause fever after surgery? Putting a damper on dogma. *JAMA Surgery, 154*(5), 375–376.

51 Harvey, L. A., et al. (2014). Continuous passive motion following total knee arthroplasty in people with arthritis. *Cochrane Database of Systematic Reviews, 2014*(2), CD004260. https://www.cochranelibrary.com/cdsr/doi/10.1002/14651858.CD004260.pub3/full (Level I)

52 He, M. L., et al. (2014). Continuous passive motion for preventing venous thromboembolism after total knee arthroplasty. *Cochrane Database of Systematic Reviews, 2014*(7), CD008207. https://www.cochranelibrary.com/cdsr/doi/10.1002/14651858.CD008207.pub3/full (Level I)

53 Tabor, D. (2013). An empirical study using range of motion and pain score as determinants for continuous passive motion: Outcomes following total knee replacement surgery in an adult population. *Orthopedic Nursing, 32,* 261–265. (Level VI)

54 Choosing Wisely. (2014). American Physical Therapy Association: Don't use continuous passive motion machines for the postoperative management of patients following uncomplicated total knee replacement. https://www.choosingwisely.org/clinician-lists/american-physical-therapy-association-continuous-passive-motion-machines-following-uncomplicated-total-knee-replacement/

55 Martin, G. M., & Harris, I. (2020). Complications of total knee arthroplasty. In: *UpToDate,* Hunter, D. (Ed.).

56 Wainwright, T. W., et al. (2020). Consensus statement for perioperative care in total hip replacement and total knee replacement surgery: Enhanced Recovery After Surgery (ERAS) Society recommendations. *Acta Orthopaedica, 91*(1), 3–19. https://www.ncbi.nlm.nih.gov/pmc/articles/PMC7006728/ (Level VII)

57 Gan, T. J. (2017). Poorly controlled postoperative pain: Prevalence, consequences, and prevention. *Journal of Pain Research, 10,* 2287-2298. https://www.ncbi.nlm.nih.gov/pmc/articles/PMC5626380/ (Level I)

58 Weinhouse, G. L. (2021). Fat embolism syndrome. In: *UpToDate,* Parsons, P. E. (Ed.).

Laryngeal mask airway insertion

The laryngeal mask airway (LMA) establishes and maintains a patent airway in the unconscious patient. It's appropriate for emergency airway and ventilatory support when endotracheal (ET) intubation isn't immediately possible, and to secure an airway in known or suspected difficult airway situations. Nurses and other health care practitioners with special training in the use of the LMA may also use it in place of a face mask during adult, pediatric, and neonatal resuscitation. [1,2,3,4,5]

First- and second-generation LMAs exist. Some are reusable, and must be cleaned and sterilized between uses; others are disposable, made for single-patient use. First-generation LMAs (such as the LMA Unique) consist of a semirigid tube attached to an inflatable polyvinylchloride cuff. [4] Second-generation LMAs (such as the LMA Supreme) consist of an anatomically shaped airway tube with an inflatable polyvinylchloride cuff, along with a separate drainage tube for passage of a gastric tube to the stomach and an incorporated bite block. [5] The cuff is placed into the patient's mouth and advanced blindly until it rests above the larynx. The patient may then breathe spontaneously or be assisted with moderate positive-pressure ventilation. In addition, some second-generation LMAs have noninflatable gel cuffs (such as the I-Gel LMA), and others are designed to facilitate intubation (such as the Air-Q LMA).

The LMA may not protect the patient from regurgitation and aspiration; however, when compared with the bag-valve-mask device, regurgitation is less likely and aspiration uncommon. [1] Because of the risks of regurgitation and aspiration, LMAs should be used in patients with full stomachs only in emergency situations in which intubation isn't possible, or if ventilation by face mask is ineffective. The benefits of using an LMA must be weighed against the risk of aspiration. [4,5] LMAs may be contraindicated in patients who have not fasted or in whom you can't confirm fasting, patients with severe obesity, patients greater than 14 weeks pregnant, those with sustained multiple or massive injuries or acute abdominal or thoracic injuries, those with any condition that results in delayed gastric emptying, and those who have recently received opiate medication. [6] Other possible contraindications to first-generation LMAs include fixed decreased pulmonary compliance or peak inspiratory pressure exceeding 20 cm H_2O. [4] Other potential contraindications for second-generation LMAs include radiotherapy to the neck involving the hypopharynx, head or neck surgery in which adequate access is unobtainable, and ingestion of caustic substances. [5] Always follow the manufacturer's indications and instructions for use. [4,5]

This procedure only discusses first- and second-generation disposable LMAs with inflatable cuffs that are inserted as an emergency airway device.

Equipment

Two appropriately-sized LMAs based on the patient's weight (see *LMA specifications*.) ▪ syringe of appropriate size for cuff deflation and inflation ▪ water-soluble lubricant ▪ gloves ▪ oxygen administration equipment ▪ handheld resuscitation bag with mask ▪ tape or commercial device to secure the tube ▪ stethoscope ▪ pulse oximeter and probe ▪ capnometer ▪ disinfectant pad ▪ folded towel or blanket ▪ suction equipment ▪ emergency equipment (code cart with emergency medications, defibrillator, intubation equipment) ▪ Optional: other personal protective equipment (gown, goggles and mask or mask with face shield), bite block, orogastric tube, denture cup.

Preparation of equipment

Inspect all equipment and supplies. If a product is expired, is defective, or has compromised integrity, remove it from patient use, label it as expired or defective, and report the expiration or defect, as directed by your facility. Assemble suction equipment and check that it's working properly *in case you can't adequately ventilate the patient with the LMA after successful insertion.* Make sure supplies for endotracheal intubation are readily available *in case they're needed.* [1] Also, make sure that emergency equipment is functioning properly and readily available.

LMA specifications

The following table will help you choose the right size laryngeal mask airway (LMA) for your patient. This applies to both first- and second-generation LMAs (LMA Unique and LMA Supreme).

LMA SIZE	PATIENT SIZE
1	Up to 5 kg
1.5	5 to10 kg
2	10 to 20 kg
2.5	20 to 30 kg
3	30 to 50 kg
4	50 to 70 kg
5	70 to100 kg

For a first-generation LMA

Perform hand hygiene and then put on gloves. [7,8,9,10,11,12,13,14,15] Remove the LMA from its package and visually inspect it for discoloration, cracks, kinks, and visible foreign particles; also make sure it's the right size. Inspect the airway opening and check that the aperture bars are intact. Manually tighten the connector, if needed, and gently pull the inflation line *to ensure it's securely attached.* [4]

Flex the airway tube to increase its curvature up to but not exceeding 180 degrees. If the tube kinks, discard the device and use a new one. [4] Test the integrity of the cuff. [4] (See *Performing a cuff test: First-generation LMA.*)

For a second-generation LMA

Perform hand hygiene and then put on gloves. [7,8,9,10,11,12,13,14,15] Remove the LMA from its package, and visually inspect the surface of the airway tube and the drain tube for discoloration, cracks, or kinks; also, make sure it's the right size. Inspect the interior of the airway tube and the drain tube for any loose particles or blockages. If present, remove loose particles. Completely deflate the cuff. [5] (See *Cuff deflation technique.*)

Performing a cuff test: First-generation LMA

To perform a cuff test on a first-generation laryngeal mask airway (LMA Unique), first withdraw all air and then reinflate the cuff using an appropriate-size syringe; inject air through the pilot balloon at an overinflation volume indicated by the manufacturer. While the cuff is inflated, visually inspect it for leaks, herniations, and symmetry, and then completely deflate it. Don't use the LMA if it's leaking air or if you note asymmetry when you inflate the cuff. [4]

LMA SIZE	MAXIMAL CUFF INFLATION VOLUME	OVERINFLATION VOLUME FOR CUFF TEST
1	4 mL	6 mL
1.5	7 mL	10 mL
2	10 mL	15 mL
2.5	14 mL	21 mL
3	20 mL	30 mL
4	30 mL	45 mL
5	40 mL	60 mL

EQUIPMENT

Cuff deflation technique

Follow these steps to properly deflate a laryngeal mask airway cuff:[5]
- Firmly attach a syringe that is at least 50 mL to the inflation port.
- Compress the distal end of the device in between the thumb and index finger (as shown below).

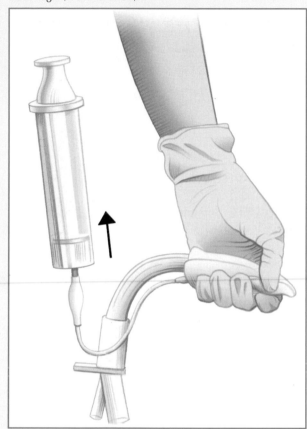

- Apply slight tension to the inflation line so that it's slightly stretched.
- Draw back on the syringe plunger, withdrawing all the air and creating a palpable vacuum.
- Disconnect the syringe.
- Check that the cuff doesn't spontaneously reinflate. If it does, discard the device and use a new one.

NURSING ALERT Don't use a device that fails any of the inspections or tests. Always have a second device available to use in case of failure.[4,5]

Implementation

- Gather and prepare the necessary equipment and supplies.
- Perform hand hygiene.[7,8,9,10,11,12]
- Confirm the patient's identity using at least two patient identifiers.[16]
- Assess the patient's level of consciousness. The patient should be unconscious and unresponsive, *because the LMA shouldn't be inserted into a patient who may resist insertion owing to stimulation of the gag reflex.*[6,17]
- If time allows, explain the procedure to the family according to their individual communication and learning needs *to increase their understanding, allay their fears, and enhance cooperation.*[18]
- Give the family the option to be present at the bedside, *because family presence during resuscitation and invasive procedures fosters medical decision making, patient care, and communication with family members.*[19]
- Perform hand hygiene.[7,8,9,10,11,12]
- Put on gloves and, as needed, other personal protective equipment *to comply with standard precautions.*[13,14,15]
- While a coworker prepares the equipment, use a handheld resuscitation bag with mask to ventilate and oxygenate the patient with 100%

oxygen for several minutes before LMA insertion, if possible, *to facilitate more time to place the airway and increase patient safety.*[6]
- Remove any removable dental work from the patient's mouth, if present.[4,5,6]
- Lubricate the posterior surface of the LMA using a water-soluble lubricant *to ease insertion.*[4,5] Avoid getting the lubricant on the anterior surface of the cuff, *because the lubricant may be aspirated.*
- Place the patient in the supine position with a folded towel or blanket under the head to flex the neck and extend the head (the "sniffing position") *to ease insertion of the LMA.*
- Stand behind the patient's head and place your nondominant hand under the patient's head, lifting the head slightly and keeping upward pressure.[6]

Inserting a first-generation device
- Hold the LMA in your dominant hand like a pencil, with your index finger placed at the junction of the mask and the tube (as shown below). The lumen of the LMA should be facing up, with the lubricated posterior surface facing the floor.[4]

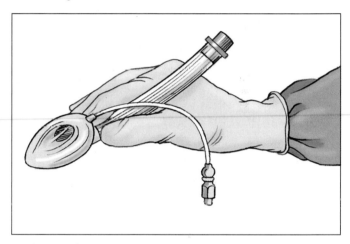

- Extend the patient's head while flexing the neck and flatten the LMA against the patient's hard palate.[4,6] Use your middle finger to gently press down on the patient's jaw.
- Flex your wrist fully so that the tip of the LMA points toward the patient's head and down, and use your index finger to insert the tip of the LMA into the patient's mouth (as shown below).[4]

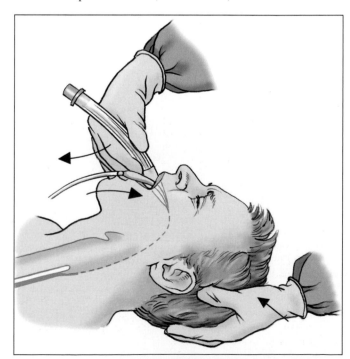

■ Press the posterior surface of the LMA against the hard palate and advance it into the oropharynx (as shown below).[4,6] *By applying pressure up against the hard palate, the LMA will advance to the proper position.*

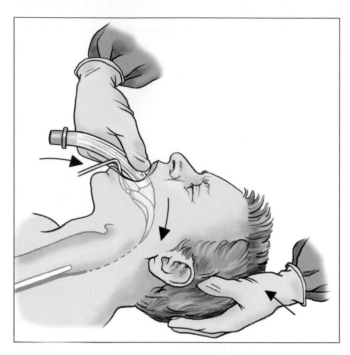

■ Use your middle finger to open the patient's jaw and check that the cuff is compressed against the hard palate. If the cuff isn't flattened against the hard palate, remove the LMA and insert it again.

■ While maintaining pressure on the LMA so that it stays pressed against the hard palate, extend your index finger fully while continuing to advance the LMA until you meet resistance at the hypopharynx (as shown below). The LMA should now be in the correct position.[4,6]

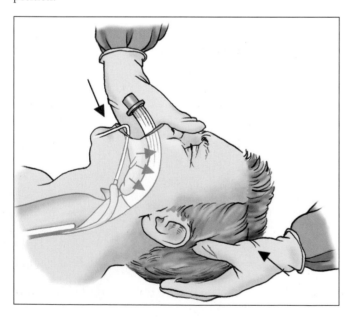

■ Remove your nondominant hand from under the patient's head, and use it to hold the LMA in place while removing your index finger (as shown above on right).[4,6]

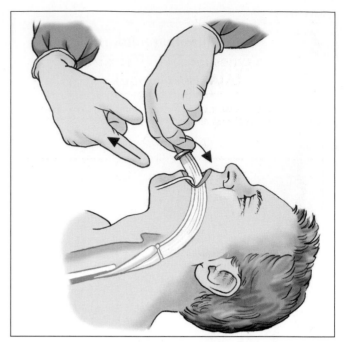

■ Without holding the LMA, use the syringe to inflate the cuff to an intracuff pressure of no more than 60 cm H_2O.[4,6,17] Note that making a seal requires only one-half the maximum inflation volume. *Inflating the cuff without holding the tube allows it to settle itself into the correct position during cuff inflation.* Don't overinflate the cuff.

■ Check the patient's mouth to make sure the cuff isn't visible, and observe for minor outward movement of the tube and minor neck bulging in the area of the cricothyroid, *indicating proper tube placement and cuff inflation.*

■ Insert a bite block *to keep the patient from biting on the tube, which may cause it to become occluded or move out of proper position.*[4,6]

■ Tape the LMA and bite block securely to the patient's face, or use a commercial device to secure the tube.

Inserting a second-generation device

■ Holding the proximal end of the device with the connector pointing downward to the chest and the distal tip pointing toward the palate (as shown below), press the distal tip against the inner aspect of the upper teeth or gums.[5]

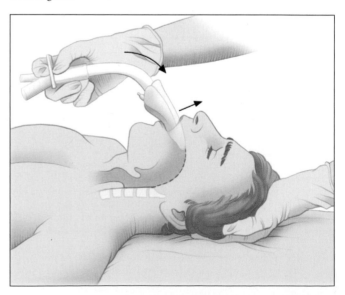

EQUIPMENT

Maximum cuff inflation volumes for first-generation LMA (LMA Unique)

This table represents the maximum cuff inflation volume for a first-generation laryngeal mask airway (LMA) by LMA size.[4]

LMA SIZE	MAXIMUM CUFF INFLATION VOLUME
1	4 mL
1.5	7 mL
2	10 mL
2.5	14 mL
3	20 mL
4	30 mL
5	40 mL

■ Begin sliding the device inward against the hard palate using a slight diagonal approach. (Direct the tip away from the midline.) While maintaining pressure against the palate, continue to slide inward, rotating the hand in a circular motion so that the device follows the curvature of the hard and soft palates behind the tongue (as shown below).[5]

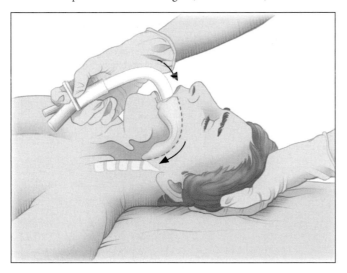

■ Continue until you feel resistance, which indicates contact with the upper esophageal sphincter (as shown below).[5]

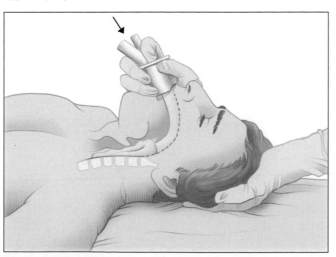

■ While maintaining inward pressure, secure the device using a 12″ to 16″ (30 to 40 cm) piece of adhesive tape. Press the tape transversely across the fixation tab, taping cheek to cheek. The tape should gently press the device downward (as shown below). Don't rotate the tape around the proximal end of the device.[5]

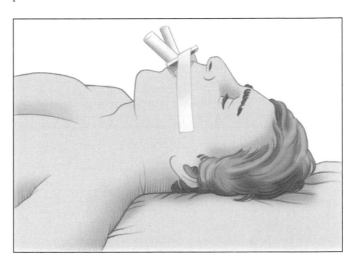

■ Inflate the cuff with the minimal amount of air to achieve an effective seal. (See *Maximum cuff inflation volumes and orogastric tube size for second-generation LMA [LMA Supreme]*, page 522.) The intracuff pressure shouldn't exceed 60 cm H_2O.[5]
■ Check the bite block position. The integrated bite block should lie between the teeth.[5]
■ Perform a suprasternal notch test *to confirm placement*. Place a small drop (1 to 2 mL) of water-soluble lubricant on the proximal end of the gastric drain tube and watch for a slight up-and-down meniscus movement of the lubricant following the application and release of gentle pressure on the suprasternal notch.[5]
■ Pass a well-lubricated orogastric tube slowly through the drain tube into the stomach, as indicated, *to facilitate gastric drainage*.[5]

Completing the procedure

■ Verify correct placement by capnography, by auscultating for bilateral breath sounds using a stethoscope, and by oxygen saturation level using pulse oximetry.[1,20]
■ Use a handheld resuscitation bag connected to an oxygen source, if indicated, to gently deliver ventilations using a peak airway pressure less than 20 cm H_2O and a tidal volume of 8 mL/kg of body weight or less. *Using low pressure ventilations avoids exceeding cuff pressure and reduces the risk of forcing air into the stomach.*
■ Remove and discard your gloves and other personal protective equipment, if worn.[15]
■ Perform hand hygiene.[7,8,9,10,11,12]
■ Clean and disinfect your stethoscope using a disinfectant pad.[21,22]
■ Perform hand hygiene.[7,8,9,10,11,12]
■ Document the procedure.[23,24,25,26]

Special considerations

■ If there's a risk that the patient may have neck trauma, insert the LMA with the patient's neck in a neutral position.[6]
■ If the patient vomits, turn the patient to the side *to allow for drainage of contents* and suction the airway.[6]

Complications

Aspiration of stomach contents is a risk, *because the LMA doesn't protect the airway*. Use of excessive force during insertion can result in trauma to the mouth, teeth, or pharynx, including lacerations, bleeding, edema, and laryngospasm. Use of excessive air to inflate the cuff can result in edema or nerve damage. Other complications include hoarseness, dysphagia, stridor, dysarthria, and dysphonia.

EQUIPMENT

Maximum cuff inflation volumes and orogastric tube size for second-generation LMA (LMA Supreme)

This table supplies the maximum cuff inflation volume and orogastric tube size for a second-generation laryngeal mask airway (LMA) by LMA size.[5]

LMA SIZE	MAXIMAL CUFF INFLATION VOLUME	MAXIMUM OROGASTRIC TUBE SIZE
1	5 mL	6 Fr
1.5	8 mL	6 Fr
2	12 mL	10 Fr
2.5	20 mL	10 Fr
3	30 mL	14 Fr
4	45 mL	14 Fr
5	45 mL	14 Fr

Documentation

Document the reason for LMA insertion. Record the method of ventilation and oxygenation you used while preparing for LMA insertion. Note that you tested the cuff for patency and visually inspected the device and found no irregularities. Record the date and time you performed the procedure. Include the size of the LMA, volume of air you used to inflate the cuff, and number of attempts necessary to achieve proper placement. Record the methods you used to determine proper device placement and secure the device. As appropriate, include placement of the bite block and the method used to secure the bite block and device. If appropriate, document the size of the orogastric tube you inserted. Document whether the patient is breathing spontaneously or receiving assisted or controlled ventilations. Include the amount of oxygen being delivered. Also document any evidence of airway trauma from LMA insertion. Record frequent assessments of tube placement and respiratory status on a patient assessment record using the appropriate documentation format. Document teaching you provided to the patient and family (if appropriate), their understanding of that teaching, and any need for follow-up teaching.

REFERENCES

1 Berg, K. M., et al. (2020). 2020 American Heart Association guidelines for cardiopulmonary resuscitation and emergency cardiovascular care, part 7: Adult advanced cardiovascular life support. *Circulation, 142*(16), S580–S604. https://www.ahajournals.org/doi/10.1161/CIR.0000000000000899 (Level II)

2 Topjian, A. A., et al (2020). Part 4: Pediatric basic and advanced life support: 2020 American Heart Association guidelines for cardiopulmonary resuscitation and emergency cardiovascular care. *Circulation, 142*(16), S469–S523. https://www.ahajournals.org/doi/10.1161/CIR.0000000000000901 (Level II)

3 Aziz, K., et al. (2020). Part 5: Neonatal resuscitation: 2020 American Heart Association guidelines for cardiopulmonary resuscitation and emergency cardiovascular care. *Circulation, 142*(16), S524–S550. https://www.ahajournals.org/doi/10.1161/CIR.0000000000000902 (Level II)

4 Teleflex Medical. (2015). Instructions for use: LMA Unique (Silicone Cuff) & LMA Unique (Silicone Cuff) Cuff Pilot. https://www.lmaco-ifu.com/sites/default/files/node/8872/ifu/revision/11723/pbq2100000auk-ifu-lma-unique-silicone-cuff.pdf

5 Teleflex Medical. (2015). Instructions for use—LMA Supreme. http://www.lmaco-ifu.com/sites/default/files/node/438/ifu/revision/3593/ifu-lma-supreme-paj2100002buk.pdf

6 Wiegand, D. L. (2017). *AACN procedure manual for high acuity, progressive, and critical care* (7th ed.). St. Louis, MO: Elsevier.

7 The Joint Commission. (2021). Standard NPSG.07.01.01. *Comprehensive accreditation manual for hospitals.* Oakbrook Terrace, IL: The Joint Commission. (Level VII)

8 Centers for Disease Control and Prevention. (2002). Guideline for hand hygiene in health-care settings: Recommendations of the Healthcare Infection Control Practices Advisory Committee and the HICPAC/SHEA/APIC/IDSA Hand Hygiene Task Force. *MMWR Recommendations and Reports, 51*(RR-16), 1–45. https://www.cdc.gov/mmwr/pdf/rr/rr5116.pdf (Level II)

9 World Health Organization. (2009). WHO guidelines on hand hygiene in health care: First global patient safety challenge, clean care is safer care. https://apps.who.int/iris/bitstream/handle/10665/44102/9789241597906_eng.pdf?sequence=1 (Level IV)

10 Accreditation Association for Hospitals and Health Systems. (2020). Standard 07.21.10. *Healthcare Facilities Accreditation Program: Accreditation requirements for acute care hospitals.* Chicago, IL: Accreditation Association for Hospitals and Health Systems. (Level VII)

11 Centers for Medicare and Medicaid Services, Department of Health and Human Services. (2020). Condition of participation: Infection control. 42 C.F.R. § 482.42.

12 DNV GL-Healthcare USA, Inc. (2020). IC.1.SR.1. *NIAHO® accreditation requirements, interpretive guidelines and surveyor guidance—revision 20.0.* Milford, OH: DNV GL-Healthcare USA, Inc. (Level VII)

13 Accreditation Association for Hospitals and Health Systems. (2020). Standard 07.01.10. *Healthcare Facilities Accreditation Program: Accreditation requirements for acute care hospitals.* Chicago, IL: Accreditation Association for Hospitals and Health Systems. (Level VII)

14 Siegel, J. D., et al. (2007, revised 2019). 2007 guideline for isolation precautions: Preventing transmission of infectious agents in healthcare settings. https://www.cdc.gov/infectioncontrol/pdf/guidelines/isolation-guidelines-H.pdf (Level II)

15 Occupational Safety and Health Administration. (2012). Bloodborne pathogens, standard number 1910.1030. https://www.osha.gov/pls/oshaweb/owadisp.show_document?p_id=10051&p_table=STANDARDS (Level VII)

16 The Joint Commission. (2021). Standard NPSG.01.01.01. *Comprehensive accreditation manual for hospitals.* Oakbrook Terrace, IL: The Joint Commission. (Level VII)

17 Kacmarek, R. M., et al. (2019). *Egan's fundamentals of respiratory care* (12th ed.). St Louis, MO: Mosby.

18 The Joint Commission. (2021). Standard PC.02.01.21. *Comprehensive accreditation manual for hospitals.* Oakbrook Terrace, IL: The Joint Commission. (Level VII)

19 American Association of Critical-Care Nurses. (2016). AACN practice alert: Family presence during resuscitation and invasive procedures. https://www.aacn.org/clinical-resources/practice-alerts/family-presence-during-resuscitation-and-invasive-procedures (Level VII)

20 American Society of Anesthesiologists. (2003, revised 2013). Practice guidelines for management of the difficult airway: An updated report by the American Society of Anesthesiologists Task Force on Management of the Difficult Airway. *Anesthesiology, 118,* 251–270. https://anesthesiology.pubs.asahq.org/article.aspx?articleid=1918684 (Level IV)

21 Rutala, W. A., et al. (2008, revised 2019). Guideline for disinfection and sterilization in healthcare facilities, 2008. https://www.cdc.gov/infection-control/pdf/guidelines/disinfection-guidelines-H.pdf (Level I)

22 Accreditation Association for Hospitals and Health Systems. (2020). Standard 07.02.03. *Healthcare Facilities Accreditation Program: Accreditation requirements for acute care hospitals.* Chicago, IL: Accreditation Association for Hospitals and Health Systems. (Level VII)

23 The Joint Commission. (2021). Standard RC.01.03.01. *Comprehensive accreditation manual for hospitals.* Oakbrook Terrace, IL: The Joint Commission. (Level VII)

24 Accreditation Association for Hospitals and Health Systems. (2020). Standard 10.00.03. *Healthcare Facilities Accreditation Program: Accreditation requirements for acute care hospitals.* Chicago, IL: Accreditation Association for Hospitals and Health Systems. (Level VII)

25 Centers for Medicare and Medicaid Services, Department of Health and Human Services. (2020). Condition of participation: Medical record services. 42 C.F.R. § 482.24(b).

26 DNV GL-Healthcare USA, Inc. (2020). MR.2.SR.1. *NIAHO® accreditation requirements, interpretive guidelines and surveyor guidance—revision 20.0.* Milford, OH: DNV GL-Healthcare USA, Inc. (Level VII)

LASER THERAPY, ASSISTING

Using the highly focused and intense energy of a laser beam, the surgeon can treat various skin lesions. Laser therapy has several advantages. As a surgical instrument, the laser offers precise control. It spares normal tissue, speeds healing, and deters infection by sterilizing the operative site. In addition, by sealing tiny blood vessels as it vaporizes tissue, the laser beam leaves a nearly bloodless operative field.

Laser therapy can be performed on an outpatient basis. The lasers used most commonly to treat skin lesions are vascular, pigment, and carbon dioxide (CO_2) lasers. (See *Understanding types of laser therapy*.)

In general, laser surgery is safe, although bleeding and scarring can occur. One pronounced hazard, to the patient and treatment staff alike, is eye damage or other injury caused by unintended laser beam reflection. For this reason, anyone in the surgical suite, including the patient, must wear special goggles to filter laser light, and the surgeon must use special nonreflective instruments. Access to the room must be strictly controlled, and all windows must be covered.

Equipment

Laser ▪ high-filtration face masks ▪ appropriate protective eyewear approved by the laser safety officer (LSO)[1] ▪ laser smoke evacuator ▪ extra vacuum filters for evacuator ▪ surgical drape ▪ skin preparation product ▪ prescribed cleaning solution ▪ sterile gauze ▪ normal saline solution ▪ nonadherent dressings ▪ surgical tape ▪ sterile scissors ▪ sterile cotton-tipped applicators ▪ nonreflective surgical instruments ▪ gowns ▪ cap ▪ sterile gloves ▪ prescribed local anesthetic ▪ sterile basin of water ▪ sterile towels ▪ fire extinguisher ▪ door warning signs ▪ covers for walls, windows, and doors.

Preparation of equipment

Inspect all equipment and supplies. If a product is expired, is defective, or has compromised integrity, remove it from patient use, label it as expired or defective, and report the expiration or defect, as directed by your facility. Carefully inspect protective eyewear for damage and scratches before use. Don't use damaged eyewear.[1]

Prepare a surgical field, which should include a local anesthetic, as ordered, as well as both dry and wet sterile gauze; normal saline solution; a basin of water; and wet towels.[2] *The gauze is used to control bleeding, protect healthy tissue, and abrade and remove any eschar that would otherwise inhibit laser absorption.* Prepare nonreflective surgical instruments as needed.

Cover all the windows in the surgical suite (including windows in doors as well as in walls) *to prevent the laser beam from escaping through the windows, creating a potential for exposure.*[1,3]

Make sure all laser equipment is tested according to the manufacturer's recommendations by trained personnel before the patient enters the procedure room. Only lasers that successfully pass the beam alignment verification should be used for procedures.[3]

Make sure that water, normal saline solution, and a fire extinguisher are readily available for use during the procedure.[1,2] Keep in mind that fire is a significant hazard during laser use. Never use a laser in an oxygen-rich environment. Exercise caution when using a laser near flammable solutions or volatile or combustible chemicals or liquids.[4] Refer to the manufacturer's instructions for use and fire safety information.[4]

Implementation

▪ If your facility requires it, make sure a written informed consent has been obtained and that the signed consent form is in the patient's medical record.[5,6,7,8]
▪ Conduct a preprocedure verification *to make sure that all relevant documentation, related information, and equipment are available and correctly identified to the patient's identifiers.*[9,10]
▪ Perform hand hygiene.[11,12,13,14,15,16]
▪ Gather and prepare the necessary equipment and supplies.
▪ Perform hand hygiene.[11,12,13,14,15,16]

Understanding types of laser therapy

Laser therapy is now an essential tool for treating many types of skin lesions. The number of lasers used in dermatology continues to grow, with different types used for specific conditions.

The term *laser* is an acronym for **L**ight **A**mplification by the **S**timulated **E**mission of **R**adiation. When directed toward the skin, most of this light energy is absorbed by *chromophores*, substances that absorb specific wavelengths of light. This is the basis of selective photothermolysis, which has revolutionized cutaneous laser surgery. Melanin is the target chromophore in pigmented lesions, and oxyhemoglobin within microvessels is the target chromophore in vascular lesions.

Make sure you're familiar with the various types of lasers and the indications for each.

Lasers for treating vascular lesions
The laser most commonly used for vascular lesions is the pulsed dye laser (PDL). Other lasers used for vascular lesions include copper vapor, argon, argon-pumped tunable dye, potassium-titanyl-phosphate (KTP), krypton, and neodymium: yttrium-aluminum-garnet (Nd:YAG). Vascular lesions appropriate for laser therapy include port-wine stains, hemangiomas, venous lakes, rosacea, telangiectasia, and Kaposi sarcoma.

Lasers for treating pigmented lesions
Lasers that are effective in treating tattoos and dermal and epidermal pigmented lesions include Q-switched ruby, Q-switched Nd:YAG, Q-switched alexandrite, and PDL. Pigmented lesions appropriate for laser treatment include tattoos, freckles, and birthmarks, including nevi of Ota, melasma, solar lentigines, café-au-lait spots, Becker nevi, and epidermal nevi.

Lasers for hair removal
Lasers used to eliminate unwanted hair include ruby, alexandrite, and Nd:YAG. Laser treatment is only effective in removing dark-colored hair; it doesn't effectively remove blonde, red, white, or gray hair.

▪ Confirm the patient's identity using at least two patient identifiers.[17]
▪ Reinforce the surgeon's explanation of the procedure according to the patient's individual communication and learning needs *to increase understanding, allay fears, and enhance cooperation.*[18] Answer the patient's questions. Discuss with the patient how the laser works and point out the equipment *to help allay the patient's concerns.*
▪ Put on a cap and gown *to comply with standard precautions*, a high-filtration face mask, and protective eyewear.[3,19,20,21]
▪ Ensure that the surgical site is marked, as directed by your facility.[22]
▪ Position the patient comfortably. Drape the patient and place sterile gauze saturated with normal saline solution over exposed tissue around the operative site, if needed. *To avoid thermal injuries and reduce the risk of fire*, ensure that all surgical drapes at the site are moist.
▪ Place protective eyewear on the patient: goggles or glasses designed for the type of laser, if the patient will remain awake during the procedure; wet eye pads, laser-specific eye shields, or as designated by the LSO if the patient will undergo general anesthesia; or metal corneal eye shields if the patient will undergo laser surgery on or around the eyelids.[1]
▪ Confirm that everyone in the room, including the patient, is wearing protective eyewear *to filter the laser light.*[1,2]
▪ Keep the door to the surgical suite closed and post warning signs regarding the type of laser used at all entrances to the surgical suite *to keep unprotected people from inadvertently entering the room.*[1]
▪ Make sure that the skin preparation product and hand antiseptic agents are completely dry before the laser is turned on *to prevent surgical fires. Use of nonflammable preparation agents minimizes the risk.*[1]
▪ Keep drapes near the surgical site moist *to reduce the risk of fire.* Ensure that wet towels and normal saline solution are available on the sterile field *to extinguish a fire if one occurs.*[1]

NURSING ALERT With high-enough energy and absorption, laser beams can ignite clothing, hair, or paper products. The risk increases in the presence of oxygen, methane, and alcohol. Take such precautions as removing or protecting hair and clothing within the treatment areas *to help reduce this risk.* The high voltage required by lasers can also result in electric shock. Proper wiring during installation is critical.[23]

■ Conduct a time-out immediately before the procedure *to perform a final assessment that the correct patient, site, positioning, and procedure are identified and, as applicable, all relevant information and necessary equipment are available.*[10,24]

■ After the surgeon administers the anesthetic and it takes effect, activate the laser smoke evacuator. The CO_2 laser has a vacuum hose attached to a separate apparatus *to clear the surgical site of laser smoke plume during laser therapy.* The vacuum has a filter that traps and collects most of the vaporized tissue. Change the filter whenever suction decreases, and follow facility guidelines for filter disposal.

■ When the surgeon completes the procedure, perform hand hygiene, put on sterile gloves, and apply direct pressure with a sterile gauze pad to any bleeding wound until hemostasis is achieved.[11,12,13,14,15,16,19,21] If a wound continues to bleed, notify the surgeon.

■ When the bleeding is controlled, use sterile technique to clean the area with a cotton-tipped applicator dipped in the prescribed cleaning solution. Then size and cut a nonadherent dressing. Secure the dressing with surgical tape.

■ Remove the patient's protective eyewear.

■ Discard used equipment and supplies in the appropriate receptacles.[21]

■ Remove and discard your gloves and other personal protective equipment.[19,21]

■ Perform hand hygiene.[11,12,13,14,15,16]

■ Document the procedure.[25,26,27,28]

Special considerations

■ Evidence shows that surgical smoke contains toxic gases and vapors as well as bacterial and viral contaminants.[29] The National Institute for Occupational Safety and Health, the Occupational Safety and Health Administration, the Laser Institute of America, the Association of periOperative Registered Nurses, and the American Society for Laser Medicine and Surgery recommend that surgical smoke be filtered and evacuated through the use of room ventilation, smoke evacuators, and room suction systems.[29,30,31,32] Staff should wear high-filtration face masks to filter particulates.[2]

Complications

Pain, bruising, erythema, and blistering can occur after laser surgery. Scarring, pigment changes, and infection are rare complications. Delayed wound healing and allergic reaction are also potential complications of certain types of laser therapies.[23]

Potential laser safety-related complications include ocular damage, burns, and electric shock. Depending on the laser and its indication, laser-tissue interaction may produce a smoke plume, tissue splatter, or both, potentially transmitting infectious microorganisms.[23]

Documentation

Note the patient's skin condition before and after the procedure. Document the safety measures taken before and during the procedure, the type of laser used, and the laser time and energy level.[3] Also document any bleeding, the type of dressing applied, and any complaints by the patient of pain and the interventions implemented. Document home care instructions provided to the patient, the patient's understanding of those instructions, and whether any follow-up teaching was needed.

REFERENCES

1 Guideline for perioperative practice: Energy-generating devices. (2020). In Wood, A. (Ed.), *Guidelines for perioperative practice, 2020 edition.* Denver, CO: AORN. (Level VII)

2 Castelluccio, D. (2012). Implementing AORN recommended practices for laser safety. *AORN Journal, 95*, 612–627. (Level VII)

3 Occupational Safety and Health Administration. (n.d.). OSHA technical manual, section III, chapter 6: Laser hazards. https://www.osha.gov/otm/section-3-health-hazards/chapter-6 (Level VII)

4 Guideline for perioperative practice: Environment of care. (2020). In Wood, A. (Ed.), *Guidelines for perioperative practice,* 2020 edition. Denver, CO: AORN, Inc. (Level VII)

5 The Joint Commission. (2021). Standard RI.01.03.01. *Comprehensive accreditation manual for hospitals.* Oakbrook Terrace, IL: The Joint Commission. (Level VII)

6 Centers for Medicare and Medicaid Services, Department of Health and Human Services. (2020). Condition of participation: Patient's rights. 42 C.F.R. § 482.13(b)(2).

7 Accreditation Association for Hospitals and Health Systems. (2020). Standard 30.01.11. *Healthcare Facilities Accreditation Program: Accreditation requirements for acute care hospitals.* Chicago, IL: Accreditation Association for Hospitals and Health Systems. (Level VII)

8 DNV GL-Healthcare USA, Inc. (2020). PR.2.SR.3. *NIAHO® accreditation requirements, interpretive guidelines and surveyor guidance—revision 20.0.* Milford, OH: DNV GL-Healthcare USA, Inc. (Level VII)

9 The Joint Commission. (2021). Standard UP.01.01.01. *Comprehensive accreditation manual for hospitals.* Oakbrook Terrace, IL: The Joint Commission. (Level VII)

10 Accreditation Association for Hospitals and Health Systems. (2020). Standard 30.00.14. *Healthcare Facilities Accreditation Program: Accreditation requirements for acute care hospitals.* Chicago, IL: Accreditation Association for Hospitals and Health Systems. (Level VII)

11 Centers for Disease Control and Prevention. (2002). Guideline for hand hygiene in health-care settings: Recommendations of the Healthcare Infection Control Practices Advisory Committee and the HICPAC/SHEA/APIC/IDSA Hand Hygiene Task Force. *MMWR Recommendations and Reports, 51*(RR-16), 1–45. https://www.cdc.gov/mmwr/pdf/rr/rr5116.pdf (Level II)

12 World Health Organization. (2009). WHO guidelines on hand hygiene in health care: First global patient safety challenge, clean care is safer care. https://apps.who.int/iris/bitstream/handle/10665/44102/9789241597906_eng.pdf?sequence=1 (Level IV)

13 The Joint Commission. (2021). Standard NPSG.07.01.01. *Comprehensive accreditation manual for hospitals.* Oakbrook Terrace, IL: The Joint Commission. (Level VII)

14 Centers for Medicare and Medicaid Services, Department of Health and Human Services. (2020). Condition of participation: Infection control. 42 C.F.R. § 482.42.

15 Accreditation Association for Hospitals and Health Systems. (2020). Standard 07.01.21. *Healthcare Facilities Accreditation Program: Accreditation requirements for acute care hospitals.* Chicago, IL: Accreditation Association for Hospitals and Health Systems. (Level VII)

16 DNV GL-Healthcare USA, Inc. (2020). IC.1.SR.1. *NIAHO® accreditation requirements, interpretive guidelines and surveyor guidance—revision 20.0.* Milford, OH: DNV GL-Healthcare USA, Inc. (Level VII)

17 The Joint Commission. (2021). Standard NPSG.01.01.01. *Comprehensive accreditation manual for hospitals.* Oakbrook Terrace, IL: The Joint Commission. (Level VII)

18 The Joint Commission. (2021). Standard PC.02.01.21. *Comprehensive accreditation manual for hospitals.* Oakbrook Terrace, IL: The Joint Commission. (Level VII)

19 Siegel, J. D., et al. (2007, revised 2019). 2007 guideline for isolation precautions: Preventing transmission of infectious agents in healthcare settings. https://www.cdc.gov/infectioncontrol/pdf/guidelines/isolation-guidelines-H.pdf (Level II)

20 Accreditation Association for Hospitals and Health Systems. (2020). Standard 07.01.10. *Healthcare Facilities Accreditation Program: Accreditation requirements for acute care hospitals.* Chicago, IL: Accreditation Association for Hospitals and Health Systems. (Level VII)

21 Occupational Safety and Health Administration. (2012). Bloodborne pathogens, standard number 1910.1030. https://www.osha.gov/pls/oshaweb/owadisp.show_document?p_id=10051&p_table=STANDARDS (Level VII)

22 The Joint Commission. (2021). Standard UP.01.02.01. *Comprehensive accreditation manual for hospitals.* Oakbrook Terrace, IL: The Joint Commission. (Level VII)

23 Brown, C. W., Jr. (2019). Complications of dermatologic laser surgery. https://emedicine.medscape.com/article/1120837-overview

24 The Joint Commission. (2021). Standard UP.01.03.01. *Comprehensive accreditation manual for hospitals.* Oakbrook Terrace, IL: The Joint Commission. (Level VII)

25 The Joint Commission. (2021). Standard RC.01.03.01. *Comprehensive accreditation manual for hospitals.* Oakbrook Terrace, IL: The Joint Commission. (Level VII)

26 Centers for Medicare and Medicaid Services, Department of Health and Human Services. (2020). Condition of participation: Medical record services. 42 C.F.R. § 482.24(b).

27 Accreditation Association for Hospitals and Health Systems. (2020). Standard 10.00.03. *Healthcare Facilities Accreditation Program: Accreditation requirements for acute care hospitals.* Chicago, IL: Accreditation Association for Hospitals and Health Systems. (Level VII)

28 DNV GL-Healthcare USA, Inc. (2020). MR.2.SR.1. *NIAHO® accreditation requirements, interpretive guidelines and surveyor guidance—revision 20.0.* Milford, OH: DNV GL-Healthcare USA, Inc. (Level VII)

29 Guideline for perioperative practice: Surgical smoke safety. (2020). In Wood, A. (Ed.), *Guidelines for perioperative practice,* 2020 edition. Denver, CO: AORN, Inc. (Level VII)

30 National Institute for Occupational Safety and Health. (2014). Control of smoke from laser/electric surgical procedures. https://www.cdc.gov/niosh/docs/hazardcontrol/hc11.html

31 Laser Institute of America. (n.d.). ANSI Z136 standards: Guidelines for implement a safe laser program. https://www.lia.org/resources/laser-safety-information/laser-safety-standards/ansi-z136-standards

32 American Society for Laser Medicine and Surgery, Inc. (2017). ASLMS laser and energy device plume position statement. https://www.aslms.org/for-professionals/professional-resources/safety-and-complications/aslms-laser-and-energy-device-plume-position-statement

LATEX ALLERGY PRECAUTIONS

Latex—a natural product of the rubber tree—is used in many products in the health care field. With the increased use of latex in barrier protection and medical equipment, more nurses and patients are becoming hypersensitive to it. Certain groups of people are at increased risk for developing latex allergy. These groups include people who have had or will undergo multiple surgical procedures (such as those with a history of spina bifida), health care workers (especially those who work in emergency departments and operating rooms), workers who manufacture latex and latex-containing products, and people with a genetic predisposition to latex allergy.[1] Some studies also suggest that pregnant patients are at a greater risk for latex allergy.[2]

People allergic to certain foods, including bananas, avocados, chestnuts, apples, carrots, celery, papaya, potatoes, kiwis, melons, and tomatoes, may also be allergic to latex.[3] Exposure to latex elicits an allergic response similar to the one that occurs with these foods; thus, these foods are termed cross-reactive. Inclusion of latex allergy–specific questions during the health history helps identify patients at risk for latex allergy. (See *Latex allergy screening*.)

For people with latex allergy, latex becomes a hazard when the protein in latex comes in direct contact with mucous membranes or is inhaled, which happens with the use of powdered latex surgical gloves. Manipulation of the powder in the latex surgical gloves can trigger rhinitis and asthma signs and symptoms.[3,4]

Latex allergy can produce a myriad of signs and symptoms, including generalized itching (such as on the hands and arms); itchy, watery, or burning eyes; sneezing and coughing (hay fever–type signs and symptoms); rash; hives; bronchial asthma, scratchy throat, or difficulty breathing; edema of the face, hands, or neck; and anaphylaxis.[1]

The diagnosis of latex allergy is based on the patient's history and physical examination findings. The patient should undergo laboratory testing to confirm or eliminate the diagnosis. Laboratory tests include skin testing, such as the skin-prick or patch test; the latex-specific immunoglobulin E testing using ImmunoCAP or Immulite analyzers, and other serum blood tests, such as Pharmacia CAP, AlaSTAT, and HYTEC.[4,5]

If you determine that the patient has a sensitivity to latex, ensure that the patient doesn't come in contact with latex, because such contact could result in a life-threatening hypersensitivity reaction. Creating a latex-safe environment is the only way to safeguard the patient. Many facilities now have nonlatex equipment and supplies on hand, which is usually kept on a cart that can be moved into the patient's room.

Equipment

Latex-free equipment, including room contents ▪ anaphylaxis kit ▪ latex allergy sign or other facility-specific alert ▪ appropriate warning labels ▪ latex-free supply kit ▪ latex-free emergency equipment (code cart with

---

Latex allergy screening

To determine if the patient has a latex sensitivity or allergy, ask the following screening questions:

▪ What is your occupation?

▪ Have you experienced an allergic reaction, local sensitivity, or itching following exposure to any latex products, such as balloons, dishwashing gloves, or condoms?

▪ Have you experienced shortness of breath or wheezing after blowing up balloons or after a dental visit?

▪ Have you experienced itching in or around your mouth after eating a banana?

   If the patient answers *yes* to any of these questions, proceed with the following questions:

▪ Do you have a history of allergies, dermatitis, or asthma? If so, what type of reaction do you have?

▪ Do you have any congenital abnormalities? If yes, explain.

▪ Do you have any food allergies? If so, what specific allergies do you have? Describe your reaction.

▪ If you experience shortness of breath or wheezing when blowing up latex balloons, describe your reaction.

▪ Have you had any previous surgical procedures? Did you experience associated complications? If so, describe them.

▪ Have you had previous dental procedures? Did you experience associated complications? If so, describe them.

▪ Are you exposed to latex in your occupation, and have you ever had a reaction to these products? If so, describe your reaction.

---

emergency medications, defibrillator, handheld resuscitation bag with mask, and intubation equipment) ▪ Optional: face mask with latex-free ties, latex-allergy patient identification wristband or bracelet, latex-free transparent dressing, latex-free gown.

Preparation of equipment

Inspect all equipment and supplies. If a product is expired, is defective, or has compromised integrity, remove it from patient use, label it as expired or defective, and report the expiration or defect as directed by your facility. Place all equipment on a supply cart, and make sure the supply cart is readily available. Make sure latex-free emergency equipment and an anaphylaxis kit are readily available *so that you can act immediately if the patient has an allergic reaction to latex.* Make sure that the emergency equipment functions properly.

Implementation

▪ Review the patient's medical record for a latex allergy, factors that increase the risk of a latex allergy, or a history of signs and symptoms of contact dermatitis (especially of the hands), contact urticaria, hay fever, rhinitis, or asthma.[6]

▪ Perform hand hygiene.[7,8,9,10,11,12]

▪ If the patient is suspected of having or confirmed to have a latex sensitivity or allergy, and you've used latex products, put on a gown before entering the patient's room *to reduce the risk of potential patient exposure to residual latex powder.*

▪ Confirm the patient's identify using at least two patient identifiers.[13]

▪ If a latex allergy hasn't been identified, assess the patient for factors that increase the risk of latex sensitivity, as well as for signs and symptoms associated with contact dermatitis, contact urticaria, hay fever, rhinitis, or asthma.[6,14]

▪ Gather and prepare the appropriate equipment.

▪ Explain latex allergy precautions to the patient and family (if appropriate) according to their communication and learning needs *to increase understanding, allay fears, and enhance cooperation.*[15]

▪ If a latex allergy has been identified, arrange for the patient to be admitted to a latex-safe room. Make sure latex products aren't used for other patients in the room if the room isn't private.

▪ Post a latex allergy sign (or other facility-specific alert) at the room entrance *to prevent personnel from entering the patient's room with supplies that contain latex.*[6]

■ If your facility requires that the patient wear a latex allergy identification wristband or bracelet, place it on the patient.[6]

■ Make sure that there's a visual alert on the front of the patient's medical record *to alert staff members immediately to the patient's latex allergy.*[6]

■ Label the patient's bed (if directed by your facility) *to alert staff members to the patient's latex allergy.*[6]

■ If the patient requires surgery, document the patient's latex sensitivity or allergy and communicate this information to the perioperative team.[6]

■ If the health care facility's electronic medical record system doesn't automatically alert other departments (such as the dietary and central supply departments and the pharmacy) to the patient's allergy to latex, notify them of the patient's allergy.

■ Ensure that dietary personnel are notified of the patient's latex allergy, and verify that dietary personnel wear latex-free gloves when preparing food. *Patients who have a latex allergy have reportedly reacted to latex-contaminated foods that were prepared using latex gloves.*

■ If you must transport the patient to another area of the facility, make sure that the latex-free supply cart accompanies the patient, and that all health care workers who come in contact with the patient wear latex-free gloves. The patient may need to wear a face mask with latex-free ties when leaving the room *for protection from inhaling airborne latex particles.*

■ Review labels on all medical devices, equipment, and supplies (such as adhesives, tape, IV equipment, electrocardiogram electrodes, and dressing supplies) for latex content.[14] Use latex-free products whenever possible. When a latex-safe alternative isn't available, cover latex-containing equipment that comes in contact with the patient.[6]

■ Puncture medication vials only once when withdrawing medication, *because multiple punctures increase the risk of introducing latex proteins into the contents.*[6] Don't remove the rubber stopper from a medication vial when withdrawing medication, *because removing the stopper doesn't reduce contamination of the contents with latex protein, and the medication may already contain latex absorbed from the stopper during transport and storage.*[6]

■ If the patient requires pulse oximetry and the oximeter probe contains latex, cover the patient's skin with a transparent dressing before applying the probe *to create a barrier and prevent latex exposure.*

■ Perform hand hygiene.[7,8,9,10,11,12]

■ Document the procedure.[16,17,18,19]

Special considerations

■ If the patient requires surgery or another invasive procedure that can't be performed in a latex-safe room, staff members performing the procedure should remove all latex-containing products from the room the evening before the procedure (if possible), except for those that are sealed or contained;[6] schedule an elective procedure as the first procedure of the day *to allow time for the room air to be completely exchanged after terminal cleaning;*[6] restrict traffic and equipment in the operating room before and during the procedure *to help reduce the release of latex particles;*[6] and cover latex-containing equipment that will come in direct contact with the patient with stockinettes *to provide a barrier between the equipment and the patient's skin.*[6]

■ Remember that signs and symptoms of latex allergy usually occur within 30 minutes of anesthesia induction. However, the time of onset can range from 10 minutes to several hours.

Documentation

Document the results of latex allergy screening, the date and time of screening, and notification of staff members of the patient's status. Document the placement of latex allergy signs and warning labels. Document teaching provided to the patient and family (if applicable), their understanding of that teaching, and any need for follow-up teaching.

REFERENCES

1 American Association of Nurse Anesthetists. (1993, reaffirmed 2018). Latex allergy management: Guidelines. https://www.aana.com/docs/default-source/practice-aana-com-web-documents-(all)/latex-allergy-management.pdf?sfvrsn=9c0049b1_2 (Level VII)

2 Draisci, G., et al. (2011). Latex sensitization: A special risk for the obstetric population? *Anesthesiology, 114*, 565–569. https://anesthesiology.pubs.asahq.org/article.aspx?articleid=1933469 (Level VI)

3 Asthma and Allergy Foundation of America. (2015). Latex allergy. https://www.aafa.org/latex-allergy/

4 Hamilton, R. G. (2019). Latex allergy: Epidemiology, clinical manifestations, and diagnosis. In: *UpToDate*, Bochner, B. S. (Ed.).

5 Stokes, J., & Casale, T. B. (2020). The biology of IgE. In: *UpToDate*, Bochner, B. S. (Ed.).

6 Guideline for perioperative practice: Environment of care. (2021). In Wood, A. (Ed.), *Guidelines for perioperative practice*, 2021 edition. Denver, CO: AORN, Inc. (Level VII)

7 The Joint Commission. (2021). Standard NPSG.07.01.01. *Comprehensive accreditation manual for hospitals.* Oakbrook Terrace, IL: The Joint Commission. (Level VII)

8 Centers for Disease Control and Prevention. (2002). Guideline for hand hygiene in health-care settings: Recommendations of the Healthcare Infection Control Practices Advisory Committee and the HICPAC/SHEA/APIC/IDSA Hand Hygiene Task Force. *MMWR Recommendations and Reports, 51*(RR-16), 1–45. https://www.cdc.gov/mmwr/pdf/rr/rr5116.pdf (Level II)

9 World Health Organization. (2009). WHO guidelines on hand hygiene in health care: First global patient safety challenge, clean care is safer care. https://apps.who.int/iris/bitstream/handle/10665/44102/9789241597906_eng.pdf?sequence=1 (Level IV)

10 Centers for Medicare and Medicaid Services, Department of Health and Human Services. (2020). Condition of participation: Infection control. 42 C.F.R. § 482.42.

11 DNV GL-Healthcare USA, Inc. (2020). IC.1.SR.1. *NIAHO® accreditation requirements, interpretive guidelines and surveyor guidance—revision 20.0.* Milford, OH: DNV GL-Healthcare USA, Inc. (Level VII)

12 Accreditation Association for Hospitals and Health Systems. (2020). Standard 07.01.21. *Healthcare Facilities Accreditation Program: Accreditation requirements for acute care hospitals.* Chicago, IL: Accreditation Association for Hospitals and Health Systems. (Level VII)

13 The Joint Commission. (2021). Standard NPSG.01.01.01. *Comprehensive accreditation manual for hospitals.* Oakbrook Terrace, IL: The Joint Commission. (Level VII)

14 Standard 14. Latex sensitivity or allergy. Infusion therapy standards of practice (8th ed.) (2021). *Journal of Infusion Nursing, 44*, 49–S50. (Level VII)

15 The Joint Commission. (2021). Standard PC.02.01.21. *Comprehensive accreditation manual for hospitals.* Oakbrook Terrace, IL: The Joint Commission. (Level VII)

16 The Joint Commission. (2021). Standard RC.01.03.01. *Comprehensive accreditation manual for hospitals.* Oakbrook Terrace, IL: The Joint Commission. (Level VII)

17 Centers for Medicare and Medicaid Services, Department of Health and Human Services. (2020). Condition of participation: Medical record services. 42 C.F.R. § 482.24(b).

18 DNV GL-Healthcare USA, Inc. (2020). MR.2.SR.1. *NIAHO® accreditation requirements, interpretive guidelines and surveyor guidance—revision 20.0.* Milford, OH: DNV GL-Healthcare USA, Inc. (Level VII)

19 Accreditation Association for Hospitals and Health Systems. (2020). Standard 10.00.03. *Healthcare Facilities Accreditation Program: Accreditation requirements for acute care hospitals.* Chicago, IL: Accreditation Association for Hospitals and Health Systems. (Level VII)

20 Pollart, S. M., et al. (2009). Latex allergy. *American Family Physician, 80*(12), 1413–1418. https://www.aafp.org/afp/2009/1215/p1413.html

LIPID EMULSION ADMINISTRATION

Given as a separate solution in conjunction with parenteral nutrition or as a component of a total nutrient admixture or three-in-one solution, lipid emulsions are a source of calories and essential fatty acids. A deficiency in essential fatty acids can hinder wound healing, adversely affect production of red blood cells, and impair prostaglandin synthesis.

Currently, all of the IV lipid emulsions available in the United States are soybean oil–based; however, other countries have used alternative oil-based lipid emulsions containing olives and fish.[1] Studies show that these alternative lipid emulsions may have fewer proinflammatory effects, less immune suppression, and more antioxidant effects than the standard soybean oil products.[2,3] Further research is needed to develop specific guidelines for their use.[3]

When given alone, lipid emulsions can be administered through a peripheral or a central venous access catheter. Central venous access is preferred when lipid emulsion administration accompanies hypertonic parenteral nutrition solution administration.[4] Follow sterile no-touch technique when administering a lipid emulsion *to reduce the risk of vascular catheter-associated infection.*

HOSPITAL-ACQUIRED CONDITION ALERT Keep in mind that the Centers for Medicare and Medicaid Services considers vascular catheter–associated infection a hospital-acquired condition *because it can be reasonably prevented using a variety of best practices.* Make sure to follow evidence-based infection prevention practices, such as performing hand hygiene, performing a vigorous mechanical scrub of the needleless connector, and following sterile no-touch technique, *to reduce the risk of vascular catheter-associated infections.*[5,6,7,8,9]

Lipid emulsions are contraindicated in patients who have a condition that disrupts normal fat metabolism, such as pathologic hyperlipidemia, lipid nephrosis, and acute pancreatitis. They also can't be given to patients with severe egg allergies.[10,11] They must be used cautiously in patients who have liver disease,[11] pulmonary anemia disease, or coagulation disorders as well as in those who are at risk for developing a fat embolism.[10]

Equipment

Medication administration record ■ prescribed lipid emulsion ■ diethylhexyl phthalate (DEHP)–free lipid administration set[12] ■ filter (1.2 micron)[13] ■ prefilled syringe containing preservative-free normal saline solution (10-mL syringe or a syringe specifically designed to generate a lower injection pressure) ■ needleless connector ■ antiseptic pads (chlorhexidine-based, povidone iodine, or alcohol) ■ electronic infusion device with anti-free-flow protection and interoperability with the electronic health record[14] ■ gloves ■ labels ■ marker ■ vital signs monitoring equipment ■ intake and output monitoring equipment ■ Optional: mask, time tape.

Preparation of equipment

To prevent aggregation of fat globules, don't shake the lipid container excessively. Protect the emulsion from freezing, and never add anything to it.

Inspect all IV equipment and supplies. If a product is expired, is defective, or has compromised integrity, remove it from patient use, label it as expired or defective, and report the expiration or defect, as directed by your facility.[15]

Implementation

■ Avoid distractions and interruptions when preparing and administering lipids *to prevent medication errors.*[16,17]

■ Verify the practitioner's order, and make sure that the prescribed therapy, dose, and rate of administration are appropriate for the patient's age, condition, and access device. Check the location of the access device catheter tip location, as appropriate. Address concerns about the order with the practitioner, pharmacist, or your supervisor and, if needed, the risk management department, or as directed by your facility.[18,19]

■ Perform hand hygiene before assessing supplies and preparing medications *to prevent infection transmission.*[20]

■ Gather and prepare the necessary equipment and supplies.

■ Compare the label on the lipid emulsion with the order in the patient's medical record. The label should contain the appropriate patient identifiers, the administration date and time, the patient's current weight, the route of administration, and the complete name and prescribed amount of lipid emulsion, including the total volume to be infused, the infusion rate in milliliters per hour, the duration of the infusion, and the expiration date.[21,22,23,24,25]

■ Check the patient's medical record for an allergy or contraindication to the lipid emulsion. If an allergy or contraindication exists, don't administer the emulsion; instead, notify the practitioner.[22,23,24,25]

■ If appropriate, remove the overwrap by tearing at the notch and pulling down along the lipid emulsion container.[10,11]

■ Visually inspect the emulsion for opacity and consistency of color and texture. If the emulsion looks frothy or oily or contains particles, or if you think its stability or sterility is questionable, return the bottle to the pharmacy.[22,23,24,25]

■ Discuss unresolved concerns about lipids with the patient's practitioner.[22,23,24,25]

■ Confirm that informed consent has been obtained (if required) and that the signed consent form is in the patient's medical record.[26,27,28,29,30]

■ Perform hand hygiene.[31,32,33,34,35,36,37]

■ Confirm the patient's identity using at least two patient identifiers.[38]

■ Provide privacy.[39,40,41,42]

■ Explain the procedure to the patient and family (if appropriate) according to their individual communication and learning needs *to increase their understanding, allay their fears, and enhance cooperation.*[43]

■ If the patient is receiving lipids for the first time, teach about potential adverse reactions or other concerns.[22,23,24,25]

■ Verify that the lipid emulsion is being administered at the proper time, in the prescribed dose, and by the correct route *to reduce the risk of medication errors.*[22,23,24,25]

■ If your facility uses a bar code technology, use it as directed by your facility.[44]

■ Raise the patient's bed to waist level before providing care *to prevent caregiver back strain.*[45]

■ Perform hand hygiene.[31,32,33,34,35,36,37]

■ Put on gloves, as well as a mask if required by your facility.[46,47,48]

■ Using sterile no-touch technique, remove the protective cap from the lipid emulsion bottle, thoroughly disinfect the rubber stopper with an antiseptic pad using friction, and allow the stopper to dry. Alternatively, using sterile no-touch technique, remove the protective cover from the outlet port at the bottom of the lipid emulsion bag.[10,11]

■ Hold the lipid emulsion bottle upright and, using strict sterile no-touch technique, insert the vented spike of the administration set through the inner circle of the rubber stopper. Alternatively, insert the spike of the administration set through the outlet port at the bottom of the lipid emulsion bag according to the manufacturer's instructions.[10,11]

■ Invert the lipid emulsion container and squeeze the drip chamber until it fills to the level indicated in the tubing package instructions.

■ Open the flow clamp and prime the administration set tubing and the 1.2 micron filter.[10,13,14,21,49] *An in-line filter should be used to reduce the potential for harm from particulates, microprecipitates, microorganisms, and air emboli.*[21] Gently tap the tubing *to dislodge air bubbles trapped in the Y-ports.* If necessary, attach a time tape to the lipid emulsion container *to monitor fluid intake.*

■ Label the administration set tubing, noting the date and time of initiation or the date when change is required, as directed by your facility.[12]

■ Perform a vigorous mechanical scrub of the needleless connector for at least 5 seconds using an antiseptic pad and allow it to dry completely.[9,50]

■ Verify patency of the access device by aspirating for a blood return and flushing the catheter *to reduce the risk of infiltration and extravasation.*[19,51] While maintaining sterility of the syringe tip, attach a prefilled syringe containing preservative-free normal saline solution to the needleless connector. (Use a 10-mL syringe or a syringe specifically designed to generate lower injection pressure.) Unclamp the catheter and slowly aspirate for a blood return that is the color and consistency of whole blood. If you don't obtain a blood return, take steps to locate an external cause of obstruction.[51]

■ If you obtain a blood return, slowly inject preservative-free normal saline solution into the catheter. Use a minimum volume of twice the internal volume of the catheter system. Don't forcibly flush the device; further evaluate the device if you meet resistance. Flush the catheter with preservative-free normal saline solution according to the catheter type.[51]

■ Clamp the access device before disconnecting the syringe *to prevent air from entering the catheter.* If the catheter is a central venous (CV) access device and a clamp isn't available, ask the patient to perform the Valsalva maneuver just as you disconnect the tubing, if possible. Or, if the patient is being mechanically ventilated, disconnect the syringe immediately after the machine delivers a breath at peak inspiration. *Both of these measures increase intrathoracic pressure and prevent air embolism.*[52]

■ Using sterile no-touch technique, attach the primed lipid emulsion tubing to the needleless connector.

■ Trace the administration set tubing from the patient to its point of origin *to make sure that you're connecting it to the proper port.*[19,53] Route the tubing in a standardized direction if the patient has other tubing and catheters that have different purposes. Label the tubing at the distal (near the patient connection) and proximal (near the source container) ends *to reduce the risk of misconnection* if you'll be using multiple IV lines.[53,54]

■ Put the administration set tubing into the electronic infusion device.[14] Program the infusion pump following the manufacturer's instructions. For the patient's first lipid infusion, set the test dose at a rate of 1 mL/minute for 30 minutes, or as ordered.

NURSING ALERT A lipid infusion is considered a high-alert medication *because it can cause significant patient harm when used in error.*[55]

■ Before beginning a lipid infusion, if required by your facility, have another nurse perform an independent double-check *to verify the patient's identity and make sure that the correct medication is hanging in the prescribed concentration; the medication's indication corresponds with the patient's diagnosis; the dosage calculations are correct and the dosing formula used to derive the final dose is correct; the route of administration is safe and proper for the patient; the pump settings are correct; and the infusion line is attached to the correct port.*[21,56]

■ After comparing results of the independent double-check with another nurse (if required), begin infusing the medication if no discrepancies exist. If discrepancies exist, rectify them before beginning the infusion.

■ Unclamp the catheter and start the electronic infusion device.

■ Make sure that the infusion device alarm limits are set appropriately and that the alarms are turned on, functioning properly, and audible to staff.[14,21,57,58,59]

■ Monitor the patient's vital signs, and watch for signs and symptoms of adverse reactions, such as fever; flushing, sweating, or chills; a pressure sensation over the eyes; nausea; vomiting; headache; chest and back pain; tachycardia; dyspnea; and cyanosis. An allergic reaction usually is due to either the source of lipids or to eggs, which occur in the emulsion as egg phospholipids, an emulsifying agent.

■ Monitor the patient's intake and output *to promptly recognize fluid imbalances.*

■ If the patient has no adverse reactions to the test dose, begin the infusion at the prescribed rate after an independent double-check with another nurse, if required.[56]

■ Return the bed to the lowest position *to prevent falls and maintain patient safety.*[60]

■ Discard used supplies in appropriate receptacles.[48,61]

■ Remove and discard your gloves and mask, if worn.[48,61]

■ Perform hand hygiene.[31,32,33,34,35,36,37]

■ Document the procedure.[62,63,64,65,66]

Special considerations

■ Exercise caution when administering IV lipid emulsions to patients with severe liver damage, pulmonary disease, anemia, or blood coagulation disorders, and when a danger of fat embolism is present.[10]

■ Be aware that IV lipid emulsions contain aluminum; levels can become toxic with prolonged use in patients with kidney impairment.[10]

■ Always maintain strict sterile no-touch technique while preparing and handling equipment.[6,12]

■ If the lipid emulsion will be piggybacked into parenteral nutrition, connect it between the filter and the patient's access device; control flow rates of each infusion with separate infusion devices.[10]

■ If a multilumen catheter will be used to administer parenteral nutrition, one port should be designated exclusively for parenteral nutrition administration *to reduce the risk of catheter-associated central line infection.*[21]

■ Change the administration set used for IV lipid emulsion that are infused separately every 12 hours; change the set with a new fat emulsion container.[12] Change the administration set immediately upon suspected contamination, or when the integrity of the system has been compromised.[6]

Complications

Immediate or early adverse reactions to lipid emulsion therapy, which occur in less than 1% of patients, include fever, dyspnea, cyanosis, nausea and vomiting, headache, flushing, diaphoresis, lethargy, syncope, chest and back pain, slight pressure over the eyes, irritation at the infusion site, hyperlipidemia, hypercoagulability, and thrombocytopenia.

PEDIATRIC ALERT Thrombocytopenia has been reported in infants receiving a 20% IV lipid emulsion.

Delayed but uncommon complications associated with prolonged administration of lipid emulsion include hepatomegaly, splenomegaly, jaundice caused by central lobular cholestasis, and blood dyscrasias (such as thrombocytopenia, leukopenia, and transient increases in liver function studies). Dry or scaly skin, thinning hair, abnormal liver function tests, and thrombocytopenia may indicate a deficiency of essential fatty acids. For unknown reasons, some patients develop brown pigmentation in the reticuloendothelial system.[10]

Documentation

Record the date and time the infusion was started, the exact solution administered, the administration rate, the volume administered, and findings from assessment of the access device and insertion site. Record the patient's vital signs, intake and output, and tolerance of the procedure. Note any complications, interventions performed, and the patient's response to those interventions. Document teaching provided to the patient and family (if applicable), their understanding of that teaching, and any need for follow-up teaching.

REFERENCES

1 Spray, J. W. (2016). Review of intravenous lipid emulsion therapy. *Journal of Infusion Nursing, 39*(6), 377–380. https://www.ncbi.nlm.nih.gov/pmc/articles/PMC5102272/

2 Barbosa, V. M., et al. (2010). Effects of a fish oil containing lipid emulsion on plasma phospholipid fatty acids, inflammatory markers, and clinical outcomes in septic patients: A randomized, controlled clinical trial. *Critical Care, 14*(1), R5. https://www.ncbi.nlm.nih.gov/pmc/articles/PMC2875515/ (Level I)

3 Vanek, V. W., et al. (2012). A.S.P.E.N. position paper: Clinical role for alternative intravenous fat emulsions. *Nutrition in Clinical Practice, 27,* 150–192.

4 Standard 26. Vascular access device planning. Infusion therapy standards of practice (8th ed.). (2021). *Journal of Infusion Nursing, 44,* S74–S81. (Level VII)

5 Jarrett, N., & Callaham, M. (2016). Evidence-based guidelines for selected hospital-acquired conditions: Final report. https://www.cms.gov/Medicare/Medicare-Fee-for-Service-Payment/HospitalAcqCond/Downloads/2016-HAC-Report.pdf

6 Centers for Disease Control and Prevention. (2011, revised 2017). Guidelines for the prevention of intravascular catheter–related infections. https://www.cdc.gov/infectioncontrol/guidelines/bsi/recommendations.html (Level I)

7 Standard 50. Infection. Infusion therapy standards of practice (8th ed.). (2021). *Journal of Infusion Nursing, 44,* S153–S157. (Level VII)

8 Association of Professionals in Infection Control and Epidemiology (APIC). (2015). Guide to preventing central line-associated bloodstream infections. http://apic.org/Resource_/TinyMceFileManager/2015/APIC_CLABSI_WEB.pdf (Level IV)

9 Marschall, J., et al. (2014). SHEA/IDSA practice recommendation: Strategies to prevent central line-associated bloodstream infections in acute care hospitals. *Infection Control and Hospital Epidemiology, 35*(7), 753–771. https://www.jstor.org/stable/10.1086/676533#metadata_info_tab_contents (Level I)

10 Baxter Healthcare Corp. (2015). Intralipid® 20% prescribing information. https://www.accessdata.fda.gov/drugsatfda_docs/label/2016/020248s020lbl.pdf

11 B. Braun Medical Inc. (2014). Nutrilipid® prescribing information. https://www.accessdata.fda.gov/drugsatfda_docs/label/2014/019531s002lbl.pdf

12 Standard 43. Administration set change. Infusion therapy standards of practice (8th ed.). (2021). *Journal of Infusion Nursing, 44,* S123–S125. (Level VII)

13 Worthington, P., et al. (2021). Update on the uses of filters for parenteral nutrition: An ASPEN position paper. *Nutrition in Clinical Practice, 36*(1), 29–39. https://aspenjournals.onlinelibrary.wiley.com/doi/epdf/10.1002/ncp.10587

14 Standard 63. Parenteral nutrition. Infusion therapy standards of practice (8th ed.). (2021). *Journal of Infusion Nursing, 44,* S133–S135. (Level VII)

15 Standard 12. Product evaluation, integrity, and defect reporting. Infusion therapy standards of practice (8th ed.) (2021). *Journal of Infusion Nursing, 44,* S45–S46. (Level VII)

16 Westbrook, J., et al. (2010). Association of interruptions with an increased risk and severity of medication administration errors. *Archives of Internal Medicine, 170,* 683–690. (Level IV)

17 Institute for Safe Medication Practices. (2012). Side tracks on the safety express: Interruptions lead to errors and unfinished...Wait, what was I doing? *Nurse Advise-ERR, 11*(2), 1–4. https://www.ismp.org/resources/side-tracks-safety-express-interruptions-lead-errors-and-unfinished-wait-what-was-i-doing?id=37

18 The Joint Commission. (2021). Standard MM.04.01.01. *Comprehensive accreditation manual for hospitals.* Oakbrook Terrace, IL: The Joint Commission. (Level VII)

19 Standard 59. Infusion medication and solution administration. Infusion therapy standards of practice (8th ed.). (2021). *Journal of Infusion Nursing, 44,* S180–S183. (Level VII)

20 Dolan, S. A., et al. (2016). APIC position paper: Safe injection, infusion and medication vial practices in health care. https://www.apic.org/Resource_/TinyMceFileManager/Position_Statements/2016APICSIPPositionPaper.pdf (Level VII)

21 Ayers, P., et al. (2014). A.S.P.E.N. parenteral nutrition safety consensus recommendations. *Journal of Parenteral and Enteral Nutrition, 38,* 296–333. https://onlinelibrary.wiley.com/doi/pdf/10.1177/0148607113511992 (Level VII)

22 The Joint Commission. (2021). Standard MM.06.01.01. *Comprehensive accreditation manual for hospitals.* Oakbrook Terrace, IL: The Joint Commission. (Level VII)

23 Accreditation Association for Hospitals and Health Systems. (2020). Standard 16.01.03. *Healthcare Facilities Accreditation Program: Accreditation requirements for acute care hospitals.* Chicago, IL: Accreditation Association for Hospitals and Health Systems. (Level VII)

24 Centers for Medicare and Medicaid Services, Department of Health and Human Services. (2020). Condition of participation: Nursing services. 42 C.F.R. § 482.23(c).

25 DNV GL-Healthcare USA, Inc. (2020). MM.1.SR.3. *NIAHO® accreditation requirements, interpretive guidelines and surveyor guidance—revision 20.0.* Milford, OH: DNV GL-Healthcare USA, Inc. (Level VII)

26 Infusion Nurses Society. (2016). *Policies and procedures for infusion therapy* (5th ed.). Boston, MA: Infusion Nurses Society.

27 Accreditation Association for Hospitals and Health Systems. (2020). Standard 15.01.11. *Healthcare Facilities Accreditation Program: Accreditation requirements for acute care hospitals.* Chicago, IL: Accreditation Association for Hospitals and Health Systems. (Level VII)

28 Centers for Medicare and Medicaid Services, Department of Health and Human Services. (2020). Condition of participation: Patient's rights. 42 C.F.R. § 482.13(b)(2).

29 DNV GL-Healthcare USA, Inc. (2020). PR.2.SR.3. *NIAHO® accreditation requirements, interpretive guidelines and surveyor guidance—revision 20.0.* Milford, OH: DNV GL-Healthcare USA, Inc. (Level VII)

30 The Joint Commission. (2021). Standard RI.01.03.01. *Comprehensive accreditation manual for hospitals.* Oakbrook Terrace, IL: The Joint Commission. (Level VII)

31 The Joint Commission. (2021). Standard NPSG.07.01.01. *Comprehensive accreditation manual for hospitals.* Oakbrook Terrace, IL: The Joint Commission. (Level VII)

32 Centers for Disease Control and Prevention. (2002). Guideline for hand hygiene in health-care settings: Recommendations of the Healthcare Infection Control Practices Advisory Committee and the HICPAC/SHEA/APIC/IDSA Hand Hygiene Task Force. *MMWR Recommendations and Reports, 51*(RR-16), 1–45. https://www.cdc.gov/mmwr/pdf/rr/rr5116.pdf (Level II)

33 World Health Organization. (2009). WHO guidelines on hand hygiene in health care: First global patient safety challenge, clean care is safer care. https://apps.who.int/iris/bitstream/handle/10665/44102/9789241597906_eng.pdf?sequence=1 (Level IV)

34 Accreditation Association for Hospitals and Health Systems. (2020). Standard 07.01.21. *Healthcare Facilities Accreditation Program: Accreditation requirements for acute care hospitals.* Chicago, IL: Accreditation Association for Hospitals and Health Systems. (Level VII)

35 Centers for Medicare and Medicaid Services, Department of Health and Human Services. (2020). Condition of participation: Infection control. 42 C.F.R. § 482.42.

36 DNV GL-Healthcare USA, Inc. (2020). IC.1.SR.1. *NIAHO® accreditation requirements, interpretive guidelines and surveyor guidance—revision 20.0.* Milford, OH: DNV GL-Healthcare USA, Inc. (Level VII)

37 Standard 16. Hand hygiene. Infusion therapy standards of practice (8th ed.). (2021). *Journal of Infusion Nursing, 44,* S53–S54. (Level VII)

38 The Joint Commission. (2021). Standard NPSG.01.01.01. *Comprehensive accreditation manual for hospitals.* Oakbrook Terrace, IL: The Joint Commission. (Level VII)

39 Accreditation Association for Hospitals and Health Systems. (2020). Standard 15.01.16. *Healthcare Facilities Accreditation Program: Accreditation requirements for acute care hospitals.* Chicago, IL: Accreditation Association for Hospitals and Health Systems. (Level VII)

40 Centers for Medicare and Medicaid Services, Department of Health and Human Services. (2020). Condition of participation: Patient's rights. 42 C.F.R. § 482.13(c)(1).

41 DNV GL-Healthcare USA, Inc. (2020). PR.2.SR.5. *NIAHO® accreditation requirements, interpretive guidelines and surveyor guidance—revision 20.0.* Milford, OH: DNV GL-Healthcare USA, Inc. (Level VII)

42 The Joint Commission. (2021). Standard RI.01.01.01. *Comprehensive accreditation manual for hospitals.* Oakbrook Terrace, IL: The Joint Commission. (Level VII)

43 The Joint Commission. (2021). Standard PC.02.01.21. *Comprehensive accreditation manual for hospitals.* Oakbrook Terrace, IL: The Joint Commission. (Level VII)

44 Standard 13. Medication verification. Infusion therapy standards of practice (8th ed.). (2021). *Journal of Infusion Nursing, 44,* S46–S49. (Level VII)

45 Waters, T. R., et al. (2009). Safe patient handling training for schools of nursing. https://www.cdc.gov/niosh/docs/2009-127/pdfs/2009-127.pdf (Level VII)

46 Siegel, J. D., et al. (2007, revised 2019). 2007 guideline for isolation precautions: Preventing transmission of infectious agents in healthcare settings. https://www.cdc.gov/infectioncontrol/pdf/guidelines/isolation-guidelines-H.pdf (Level II)

47 Accreditation Association for Hospitals and Health Systems. (2020). Standard 07.01.10. *Healthcare Facilities Accreditation Program: Accreditation requirements for acute care hospitals.* Chicago, IL: Accreditation Association for Hospitals and Health Systems. (Level VII)

48 Occupational Safety and Health Administration. (2012). Bloodborne pathogens, standard number 1910.1030. https://www.osha.gov/pls/oshaweb/owadisp.show_document?p_id=10051&p_table=STANDARDS (Level VII)

49 Institute for Safe Medication Practices. (2016). IV fat emulsion needs a filter. *ISMP Medication Safety Alert! Acute Care, 21*(1), 3.

50 Standard 36. Needleless connectors. Infusion therapy standards of practice (8th ed.). (2021). *Journal of Infusion Nursing, 44,* S104–S107. (Level VII)

51 Standard 41. Flushing and locking. Infusion therapy standards of practice (8th ed.). (2021). *Journal of Infusion Nursing, 44,* S113–S118. (Level VII)

52 Standard 52. Air embolism. Infusion therapy standards of practice (8th ed.). (2021). *Journal of Infusion Nursing, 44,* 39, S160–S161. (Level VII)

53 The Joint Commission. (2014). Sentinel event alert 53: Managing risk during transition to new ISO tubing connector standards. https://www.jointcommission.org/-/media/tjc/documents/resources/patient-safety-topics/sentinel-event/sea_53_connectors_8_19_14_final.pdf (Level VII)

54 U.S. Food and Drug Administration. (2017). Examples of medical device misconnections. https://www.fda.gov/medical-devices/medical-device-connectors/examples-medical-device-misconnections

55 Institute for Safe Medication Practices. (2018). ISMP list of high-alert medications in acute care settings. https://www.ismp.org/sites/default/files/attachments/2018-08/highAlert2018-Acute-Final.pdf (Level VII)

56 Institute for Safe Medication Practices. (2013). Independent double checks: Undervalued and misused: Selective use of this strategy can play an important role in medication safety. https://www.ismp.org/resources/independent-double-checks-undervalued-and-misused-selective-use-strategy-can-play (Level VII)

57 The Joint Commission. (2021). Standard NPSG.06.01.01. *Comprehensive accreditation manual for hospitals.* Oakbrook Terrace, IL: The Joint Commission. (Level VII)

58 The Joint Commission. (2013). Sentinel event alert 50: Medical device alarm safety in hospitals. https://www.jointcommission.org/-/media/tjc/documents/resources/patient-safety-topics/sentinel-event/sea_50_alarms_4_26_16.pdf (Level VII)

59 Graham, K. C., & Cvach, M. (2010). Monitor alarm fatigue: Standardizing use of physiological monitors and decreasing nuisance alarms. *American Journal of Critical Care, 19,* 28–37.

60 Ganz, D. A., et al. (2013, reviewed 2021). *Preventing falls in hospitals: A toolkit for improving quality of care* (AHRQ Publication No. 13-0015-EF). Rockville, MD: Agency for Healthcare Research and Quality. https://www.ahrq.gov/professionals/systems/hospital/fallpxtoolkit/index.html (Level VII)

61 Standard 21. Medical waste and sharps safety. Infusion therapy standards of practice (8th ed.) (2021). *Journal of Infusion Nursing, 44,* S60–S62. (Level VII)

62 The Joint Commission. (2021). Standard RC.01.03.01. *Comprehensive accreditation manual for hospitals*. Oakbrook Terrace, IL: The Joint Commission. (Level VII)

63 Accreditation Association for Hospitals and Health Systems. (2018). Standard 10.00.03. *Healthcare Facilities Accreditation Program: Accreditation requirements for acute care hospitals*. Chicago, IL: Accreditation Association for Hospitals and Health Systems. (Level VII)

64 Centers for Medicare and Medicaid Services, Department of Health and Human Services. (2020). Condition of participation: Medical record services. 42 C.F.R. § 482.24(b).

65 DNV GL-Healthcare USA, Inc. (2020). MR.2.SR.1. *NIAHO® accreditation requirements, interpretive guidelines and surveyor guidance—revision 20.0*. Milford, OH: DNV GL-Healthcare USA, Inc. (Level VII)

66 Standard 10. Documentation in the health record. Infusion therapy standards of practice. (8th ed.) (2021). *Journal of Infusion Nursing, 44*, S39–S42. (Level VII)

67 Ukleja, A., et al. (2018). Standards for nutrition support: Adult hospitalized patients. *Nutrition in Clinical Practice, 33*(6), 906–920. https://onlinelibrary.wiley.com/doi/full/10.1002/ncp.10204

Low-air-loss therapy bed use

Low-air-loss therapy beds consist of segmented, air-filled cushions that provide surface area for pressure relief. Studies have shown that these beds are effective in preventing pressure injuries in obese patients, although recent research hasn't demonstrated that this type of support surface is superior in preventing and treating skin breakdown and minimizing pain than other support surfaces.[1] Low-air-loss therapy beds inflate to specific pressures based on the height and weight of the patient. They're indicated for patients with skin grafts and surgical flaps, pressure injuries, edema, cancer, and malnutrition, as well as patients undergoing orthopedic or transplant procedures.

The segmented air cushions, covered by a low-friction fabric, inflate and rest on a bed frame (similar to a standard bed frame), reducing pressure on skin surfaces and diminishing shearing forces when repositioning the patient. A maximum-inflate feature allows the entire surface to become firm for patient repositioning. The system is also capable of deflating quickly in emergencies. As with a standard bed frame, you can adjust the head and foot of the bed.

These beds also assist with microclimate management by circulating air, which helps to evaporate moisture and reduce temperature, reducing excess skin moisture and preventing maceration.[2] (See *Low-air-loss therapy bed*.) Although pressure redistribution devices are helpful for preventing and managing pressure injuries, they shouldn't replace repositioning protocols; instead, they should serve as adjunct therapy.[3]

Some models are equipped with pulsation or rotational capability. Pulsation promotes circulation, which improves healing; lateral rotation capability raises one lung over the other, mobilizing secretions and preventing pulmonary complications.[4] Larger beds are available for patients with obesity, and some bed models allow pressure zone and lumbar support adjustment.

Low-air-loss therapy beds are contraindicated for patients with an unstable cervical, thoracic, or lumbar fracture.[5] Patients with uncontrolled diarrhea, hemodynamic instability, severe agitation, or uncontrolled claustrophobia may not benefit from this bed.

Equipment

Low-air-loss therapy bed ▪ manufacturer-approved turning sheet ▪ assistive transfer device ▪ Optional: gloves, other personal protective equipment, pillows, foam wedges.

Preparation of equipment

Inspect all equipment and supplies. If a product is expired, is defective, or has compromised integrity, remove it from patient use, label it as expired or defective, and report the expiration or defect as directed by your facility. Usually, the manufacturer's representative or a trained staff member prepares the bed for use. The unit is plugged in and turned on *to inflate the bed*. Make sure the bed inflates properly and the equipment is in working order. If the bed isn't self-calibrating, follow the manufacturer's

Low-air-loss therapy bed

A low-air-loss therapy bed reduces pressure on skin surfaces and may be used for patients with such conditions as immobility, malnutrition, incontinence, contractures, fractures, or amputations. Some models come with special features, such as rotational or percussion options.

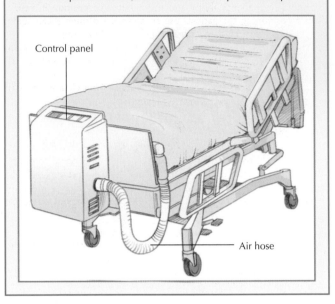

instructions for proper calibration and alarm activation for low-pressure and power-failure alarm settings.[6] Adjust additional settings, such as degree of rotation, as appropriate. Don't fully inflate the bed until the patient is moved onto it.

Implementation

- Review the patient's medical record to identify contraindications to use of the low-air-loss therapy bed.[7]
- Verify the practitioner's order.
- Gather and prepare the necessary equipment and supplies.
- Make sure that the bed is plugged in and turned on and that it inflates properly. Adjust the settings as appropriate.
- Perform hand hygiene.[8,9,10,11,12,13,14]
- Confirm the patient's identity using at least two patient identifiers.[15]
- Provide privacy.[16,17,18,19]
- Explain the use of the bed to the patient and family (if appropriate) according to their communication and learning needs *to increase their understanding, allay their fears, and enhance cooperation*.[20] If possible, demonstrate the operation of the low-air-loss therapy bed. Explain its special features, such as lumbar supports and rotation.
- Perform hand hygiene.[8,9,10,11,12,13,14]
- Put on gloves and other personal protective equipment if needed *to comply with standard precautions*.[21]
- With the help of coworkers, transfer the patient to the bed using an appropriate assistive transfer device *to prevent patient and caregiver injury*.[22]
- Start with the settings as set by the representative, monitor the patient for comfort, and ensure proper functioning of the bed.
- Adjust the inflation settings on the control panel according to the patient's comfort and therapeutic use.
- To turn and reposition the patient, use the turn-assist feature (if present), or use the maximum-inflate feature *to fully inflate the bed*. Use the turning sheet to position the patient, and place the pillows or foam wedges. Then return the bed to the correct patient settings.
- Make sure that the side rails are raised, as appropriate, and then lower the bed and lock its wheels *to ensure the patient's safety*.[23] Assess the patient's body alignment.
- Place the call light within the patient's reach.

- Remove and discard your gloves and other personal protective equipment, if worn.[13,24]
- Perform hand hygiene.[8,9,10,11,12,13,14]
- Document the procedure.[25,26,27,28]

Special considerations

- Initiate and maintain an individualized turning schedule based on risk factors and the patient's ability and willingness to reposition in bed.[29] When repositioning the patient, use an approved turning sheet; some beds come with special foam wedges to use for repositioning.
- Assess the patient's skin every 2 hours. Assess pressure injury risk on admission to the facility, at regular intervals, and with any signs of skin or wound deterioration.[3,30]
- Engage the emergency or cardiopulmonary resuscitation button during cardiac arrest *to help ensure adequate chest compressions.*[5]

Documentation

Record the duration of therapy and the patient's response to it. Document the condition of the patient's skin, including the presence of pressure injuries and other wounds. Document the patient's comfort level and tolerance of rotational angles, as applicable. Document teaching provided to the patient and family (if applicable), their understanding of that teaching, and any need for follow-up teaching.

REFERENCES

1 Saha, S., et al. (2013). Pressure ulcer treatment strategies: Comparative effectiveness. https://effectivehealthcare.ahrq.gov/sites/default/files/pdf/pressure-ulcer-treatment_research.pdf (Level V)
2 Krasner, D. L. (Ed.). (2014). *Chronic wound care: The essentials: A clinical source book for healthcare professionals.* Malvern, PA: HMP Communications.
3 Wound, Ostomy, and Continence Nurses Society (WOCN). (2016). *Guideline for prevention and management of pressure ulcers (injuries): WOCN clinical practice guideline series 2.* Mount Laurel, NJ: WOCN.
4 Bryant, R. A., & Nix, D. P. (2016). *Acute & chronic wounds: Current management concepts* (5th ed.). St. Louis, MO: Elsevier.
5 ArjoHuntleigh Getinge Group. (2013). *KinAir MedSurg: User manual.* https://www.arjo.com/DownloadFile?fileId=00000000-0000-0000-0000-000000022568
6 American National Manufacturing, Inc. (n.d.). Medical beds. http://www.americannationalmfg.com/medical-beds.html
7 McNichol, L., et al. (2015). Identifying the right surface for the right patient at the right time: Generation and content validation of an algorithm for support surface selection. *Journal of Wound, Ostomy and Continence Nursing, 42,* 19–37. (Level VII)
8 The Joint Commission. (2021). Standard NPSG.07.01.01. *Comprehensive accreditation manual for hospitals.* Oakbrook Terrace, IL: The Joint Commission. (Level VII)
9 Centers for Disease Control and Prevention. (2002). Guideline for hand hygiene in health-care settings: Recommendations of the Healthcare Infection Control Practices Advisory Committee and the HICPAC/SHEA/APIC/IDSA Hand Hygiene Task Force. *MMWR Recommendations and Reports, 51*(RR-16), 1–45. https://www.cdc.gov/mmwr/pdf/rr/rr5116.pdf (Level II)
10 World Health Organization. (2009). WHO guidelines on hand hygiene in health care: First global patient safety challenge, clean care is safer care. https://apps.who.int/iris/bitstream/handle/10665/44102/9789241597906_eng.pdf?sequence=1 (Level IV)
11 Centers for Medicare and Medicaid Services, Department of Health and Human Services. (2020). Condition of participation: Infection control. 42 C.F.R. § 482.42.
12 Accreditation Association for Hospitals and Health Systems. (2020). Standard 07.01.21. *Healthcare Facilities Accreditation Program: Accreditation requirements for acute care hospitals.* Chicago, IL: Accreditation Association for Hospitals and Health Systems. (Level VII)
13 Siegel, J. D., et al. (2007, revised 2019). 2007 guideline for isolation precautions: Preventing transmission of infectious agents in healthcare settings. https://www.cdc.gov/infectioncontrol/pdf/guidelines/isolation-guidelines-H.pdf (Level II)
14 DNV GL-Healthcare USA, Inc. (2020). IC.1.SR.1. *NIAHO® accreditation requirements, interpretive guidelines and surveyor guidance—revision 20.0.* Milford, OH: DNV GL-Healthcare USA, Inc. (Level VII)
15 The Joint Commission. (2021). Standard NPSG.01.01.01. *Comprehensive accreditation manual for hospitals.* Oakbrook Terrace, IL: The Joint Commission. (Level VII)
16 Centers for Medicare and Medicaid Services, Department of Health and Human Services. (2020). Condition of participation: Patient's rights. 42 C.F.R. § 482.13(c)(1).
17 Accreditation Association for Hospitals and Health Systems. (2020). Standard 15.01.16. *Healthcare Facilities Accreditation Program: Accreditation requirements for acute care hospitals.* Chicago, IL: Accreditation Association for Hospitals and Health Systems. (Level VII)
18 DNV GL-Healthcare USA, Inc. (2020). PR.2.SR.5. *NIAHO® accreditation requirements, interpretive guidelines and surveyor guidance—revision 20.0.* Milford, OH: DNV GL-Healthcare USA, Inc. (Level VII)
19 The Joint Commission. (2021). Standard RI.01.01.01. *Comprehensive accreditation manual for hospitals.* Oakbrook Terrace, IL: The Joint Commission. (Level VII)
20 The Joint Commission. (2021). Standard PC.02.01.21. *Comprehensive accreditation manual for hospitals.* Oakbrook Terrace, IL: The Joint Commission. (Level VII)
21 Accreditation Association for Hospitals and Health Systems. (2020). Standard 07.01.10. *Healthcare Facilities Accreditation Program: Accreditation requirements for acute care hospitals.* Chicago, IL: Accreditation Association for Hospitals and Health Systems. (Level VII)
22 Occupational Safety and Health Administration. (2009). Guidelines for nursing homes: Ergonomics for the prevention of musculoskeletal disorders. https://www.osha.gov/sites/default/files/publications/final_nh_guidelines.pdf
23 Accreditation Association for Hospitals and Health Systems. (2020). Standard 16.02.02. *Healthcare Facilities Accreditation Program: Accreditation requirements for acute care hospitals.* Chicago, IL: Accreditation Association for Hospitals and Health Systems. (Level VII)
24 Occupational Safety and Health Administration. (2012). Bloodborne pathogens, standard number 1910.1030. https://www.osha.gov/pls/oshaweb/owadisp.show_document?p_id=10051&p_table=STANDARDS (Level VII)
25 The Joint Commission. (2021). Standard RC.01.03.01. *Comprehensive accreditation manual for hospitals.* Oakbrook Terrace, IL: The Joint Commission. (Level VII)
26 Centers for Medicare and Medicaid Services, Department of Health and Human Services. (2020). Condition of participation: Patient's rights. 42 C.F.R. § 482.13(b)(2).
27 Accreditation Association for Hospitals and Health Systems. (2020). Standard 10.00.03. *Healthcare Facilities Accreditation Program: Accreditation requirements for acute care hospitals.* Chicago, IL: Accreditation Association for Hospitals and Health Systems. (Level VII)
28 DNV GL-Healthcare USA, Inc. (2020). MR.2.SR.1. *NIAHO® accreditation requirements, interpretive guidelines and surveyor guidance—revision 20.0.* Milford, OH: DNV GL-Healthcare USA, Inc. (Level VII)
29 Fletcher, J. (2017). Reposition patients effectively to prevent pressure ulcers. *Wounds International, 8*(1), 7–10. (Level VII)
30 Agency for Healthcare Research and Quality. (2014). *Preventing pressure ulcers in hospitals: A toolkit for improving quality of care.* Rockville, MD: Agency for Healthcare Research and Quality. https://www.ahrq.gov/patient-safety/settings/hospital/resource/pressureulcer/tool/index.html (Level VII)

LUMBAR PUNCTURE, ASSISTING

Lumbar puncture involves the insertion of a sterile needle into the subarachnoid space of the spinal canal, usually between the third and fourth (or fourth and fifth) lumbar vertebrae. This procedure is used to detect blood in cerebrospinal fluid (CSF), obtain CSF specimens for laboratory analysis, inject contrast media for radiologic studies, or administer drugs or anesthesia. It also involves measuring the pressure of CSF, which flows freely between the patient's brain and spinal column.

Performed by a practitioner with a nurse assisting, lumbar puncture requires sterile no-touch technique and careful patient positioning. This procedure is contraindicated in patients with increased intracranial pressure (ICP) with mass effect, a lumbar deformity, a platelet count of less than 50,000/mm³ (50 x 10⁹/L), or an International Normalized Ratio greater than 1.5, as well as in those receiving anticoagulants or who have an infection at the puncture site.[1,2]

Equipment

Overbed or procedure table ■ vital signs monitoring equipment ■ stethoscope ■ disinfectant pad ■ sterile gloves ■ caps ■ masks with face shield or mask and goggles[2,3] ■ sterile gown ■ gown ■ gloves ■ antiseptic solution ■ sterile gauze pads ■ antiseptic pads ■ sterile fenestrated drape ■ sterile 3-mL syringe ■ sterile 25G ¾″ sterile needle ■ local anesthetic (usually 1% lidocaine without EPINEPHrine) ■ sterile 22G 3½″ spinal needle with stylet[2,4] ■ three-way stopcock ■ manometer ■ sterile occlusive dressing ■ four sterile collection tubes with caps ■ labels ■ light source ■ sterile marker ■ sterile labels ■ laboratory biohazard transport bag ■ Optional: prescribed analgesia or anxiolytic, laboratory request form, antiseptic sponge, spinal anesthetic, contrast media.

Disposable lumbar puncture trays contain most of the needed sterile equipment.

Preparation of equipment

Inspect all equipment and supplies. If a product is expired, is defective, or has compromised integrity, remove it from patient use, label it as expired or defective, and report the expiration or defect as directed by your facility.

Implementation

■ Verify the practitioner's order.
■ Check the patient's medical record for any history of allergies to the local anesthetic, latex, antiseptic solution, analgesic, or anxiolytic.
■ If required by your facility, confirm that the practitioner has obtained written informed consent and that the consent is in the patient's medical record.[5,6,7]
■ Perform a preprocedure verification to make sure that all relevant documentation, related information, and equipment is available and is correctly identified to the patient's identifiers.[8,9]
■ Verify that the laboratory and imaging studies are complete, as ordered, and that the results are in the patient's medical record. Notify the practitioner of any unexpected results.
■ Perform hand hygiene.[10,11,12,13,14,15]
■ Confirm the patient's identity using at least two patient identifiers.[16]
■ Provide privacy.[17,18,19,20]
■ Reinforce the practitioner's explanation of the procedure to the patient and family (if appropriate) according to their individual communication and learning needs *to increase their understanding, allay their fears, and enhance cooperation.*[5,6,21]
■ Inform the patient that a headache may be felt after lumbar puncture, but reassure the patient that cooperation during the procedure will minimize such an effect.
■ Instruct the patient to void before the procedure.
■ Obtain the patient's vital signs and assess neurologic status *as a baseline for comparison to monitor for complications.*
■ If prescribed, administer an analgesia or anxiolytic following safe medication practices *to promote comfort and decrease anxiety so the patient can maintain the position during the procedure.*[2,22,23,24,25]
■ Perform hand hygiene.[10,11,12,13,14,15]
■ Provide adequate lighting at the puncture site.[26]
■ Raise the patient's bed to waist level before providing patient care *to prevent caregiver back strain.*[26]
■ Perform hand hygiene.[10,11,12,13,14,15]
■ Position the patient in a side-lying (lateral recumbent) or sitting position according to the practitioner's preference.
■ For a side-lying position, have the patient lie on the side at the edge of the bed, with the chin tucked to the chest and the knees drawn up to the abdomen. Make sure the head of the bed is flat and the patient has no more than a small pillow under the head.[2] Make sure the patient's spine is curved and the back is at the edge of the bed (as shown). *This position widens the spaces between the vertebrae, easing insertion of the needle. To help the patient maintain this position,* place one of your hands behind the

patient's neck and the other hand behind the knees, and pull gently. Hold the patient firmly in this position throughout the procedure *to prevent accidental needle displacement.*

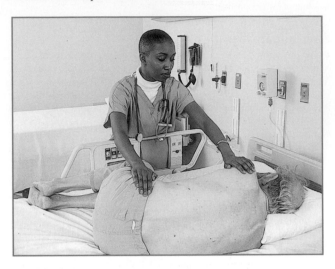

■ For a sitting position, have the patient sit on the edge of the bed, leaning over the overbed or procedure table.
■ Reemphasize the importance of remaining as still as possible *to minimize discomfort and trauma.*
■ Perform hand hygiene.[10,11,12,13,14,15]
■ Put on a cap, a mask, a gown, and gloves *to comply with standard precautions and protect equipment tray sterility.*[3,27,28,29]
■ Open the equipment tray on an overbed or procedure table, being careful not to contaminate the sterile field when you open the wrapper.
■ Label all medications, medication containers, and other solutions on and off the sterile field using a sterile marker.
■ The practitioner puts on a cap, a mask, a sterile gown, and sterile gloves. Then the practitioner cleans the puncture site with antiseptic solution and allows it to dry *to prevent contamination by the body's normal skin flora.* The practitioner then drapes the area with the sterile fenestrated drape *to provide a sterile field.* (If the practitioner uses antiseptic sponges instead of sterile gauze pads, the practitioner may remove the sterile gloves and put on another pair *to avoid introducing antiseptic solution into the subarachnoid space with the spinal needle.*)
NURSING ALERT Studies suggest that chlorhexidine is neurotoxic; its use as an antiseptic agent for skin preparation before lumbar puncture remains controversial.[2,30]
■ Conduct a time-out before starting the procedure *to perform a final assessment that the correct patient, site, positioning, and procedure are identified and all relevant information and necessary equipment are available as applicable.*[9,31]
■ If the equipment tray doesn't include an ampule of local anesthetic, disinfect the injection port of a vial of anesthetic using an antiseptic pad and allow it to dry completely. Then invert the vial 45 degrees *so that the practitioner can insert a sterile 25G needle and sterile 3-mL syringe and withdraw the anesthetic for injection.*
NURSING ALERT Dedicate multidose medication vials to one patient whenever possible *to reduce the risk of viral hepatitis transmission and other infections.*[32,33,34]
■ Before the practitioner injects the anesthetic, explain that the patient will experience a transient burning sensation and local pain. Ask the patient to report any other persistent pain or sensations, *because they may indicate irritation or puncture of a nerve root, requiring repositioning of the needle.*
■ When the practitioner inserts the sterile spinal needle into the subarachnoid space (usually between the third and fourth lumbar vertebrae, as shown, or between the fourth and fifth lumbar vertebrae), instruct the patient to remain still and breathe normally. If needed, hold the patient firmly in position *to prevent sudden movement that may displace the needle.*

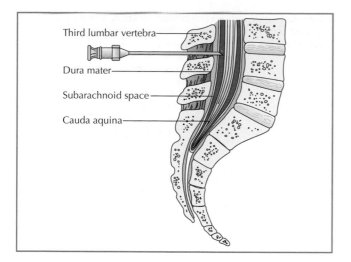

Third lumbar vertebra

Dura mater

Subarachnoid space

Cauda aquina

- Closely monitor the patient for adverse reactions, such as headache, nausea, vomiting, elevated heart rate, pallor, and clammy skin. Immediately alert the practitioner to any significant changes.
- If the lumbar puncture is being used to administer contrast media for radiologic studies or to administer a spinal anesthetic, the practitioner injects the contrast media or spinal anesthetic at this time.
- When the spinal needle is in place, the practitioner attaches a manometer with a three-way stopcock to the needle hub *to read the CSF opening pressure.* If ordered, help the patient extend the patient's legs *to provide a more accurate pressure reading.*
- The practitioner then detaches the manometer and allows CSF to drain from the needle hub into the collection tubes. When the practitioner has collected 2 to 3 mL in each tube, mark the tubes in sequence and securely cap them. Label the specimens in the presence of the patient *to prevent mislabeling.*[16]
- The practitioner removes the spinal needle and then applies a sterile occlusive dressing to the puncture site.[2]
- Assist the patient into a supine or prone position, for a length of time specified by the practitioner's order (usually 1 to 4 hours), *which acts as pressure to the site.*[2]
- Return the patient's bed to the lowest position *to prevent falls and maintain patient safety.*[35]
- Discard used supplies in the appropriate receptacles.[28]
- Remove and discard your gloves and other personal protective equipment.[3,28]
- Perform hand hygiene.[10,11,12,13,14,15]
- Place the collected CSF specimens in a laboratory biohazard transport bag and send them to the laboratory immediately, with completed laboratory request forms if used in your facility. Don't refrigerate collected CSF specimens for later transport, *because refrigeration alters results.*[36]
- Perform hand hygiene.[10,11,12,13,14,15]
- Clean and disinfect your stethoscope using a disinfectant pad.[37,38]
- Perform hand hygiene.[10,11,12,13,14,15]
- Document the procedure.[39,40,41,42]

Special considerations

- Monitor CSF test results and report critical results to the practitioner within the time frame determined by your facility *to prevent treatment delays.*[43]
- Interventions that have been shown to decrease post-lumbar puncture headache include the use of a pencil-point needle tip, use of a small-gauge needle, orientation of the needle bevel parallel to the dura during insertion, and reinsertion of the stylet before spinal needle removal.[44]
- Obtain the patient's serum glucose level as ordered, *to compare the serum and CSF glucose levels. Hyperglycemia increases CSF glucose level, and hypoglycemia decreases CSF glucose level.*[2]
- After the procedure, monitor the puncture site for redness, swelling, and drainage.
- For patients who are obese, the practitioner may use an ultrasound *to help determine accurate spinal needle placement.*[45]

Complications

Headache is the most common complication of lumbar puncture.[1] Other adverse effects may include a reaction to the anesthetic, infection (such as meningitis, epidural or subdural abscess, discitis, or vertebral osteomyelitis), bleeding into the spinal canal, CSF leakage through the dural defect remaining after spinal needle withdrawal, local pain caused by nerve root irritation, edema or hematoma at the puncture site, minor neurologic symptoms (such as radicular pain or numbness or abducens nerve palsy) and transient difficulty voiding.[1,2] The most serious complication of lumbar puncture, although rare, is cerebral herniation due to overdrainage of CSF.[1,2] A late complication is growth of epidermoid tumors of the thecal sac.[1]

Documentation

Record that you performed a time-out before the procedure to verify the correct patient, site, positioning, and procedure.[31] Document the time that the procedure started and ended; the administration of medications (including the strength, dose, route, administration rate, date and time of administration, access site used, administration devices used, and any adverse effects of the prescribed medication);[46] the number of collection tubes you filled; the color, consistency, and other characteristics of the collected specimens; and the time of specimen transport to the laboratory. Note any adverse reactions experienced by the patient during the procedure, any prescribed interventions, and the patient's response to the interventions. Also, record patient positioning after the procedure and the patient's response to the procedure. Document any teaching you provided to the patient and family members (if applicable), their understanding of that teaching, and any need for follow-up teaching.

REFERENCES

1 Johnson, K. S., & Sexton, D. J. (2018). Lumbar puncture: Technique, indications, contraindications, and complications in adults. In: *UpToDate*, Aminoff, M. J. (Ed.).

2 Wiegand, D. L. (2017). *AACN procedure manual for high acuity, progressive, and critical care* (7th ed.). St. Louis, MO: Elsevier.

3 Siegel, J. D., et al. (2007, revised 2019). 2007 guideline for isolation precautions: Preventing transmission of infectious agents in healthcare settings. https://www.cdc.gov/infectioncontrol/pdf/guidelines/isolation-guidelines-H.pdf (Level II)

4 Armon, C., & Evans, R. W. (2005). Addendum to assessment: Prevention of post–lumbar puncture headaches. *Neurology, 65*(4), 510–512. http://n.neurology.org/content/65/4/510 (Level V)

5 The Joint Commission. (2021). Standard RI.01.03.01. *Comprehensive accreditation manual for hospitals.* Oakbrook Terrace, IL: The Joint Commission. (Level VII)

6 Centers for Medicare and Medicaid Services, Department of Health and Human Services. (2020). Condition of participation: Patient's rights. 42 C.F.R. § 482.13(b)(2).

7 Accreditation Association for Hospitals and Health Systems. (2020). Standard 15.01.11. *Healthcare Facilities Accreditation Program: Accreditation requirements for acute care hospitals.* Chicago, IL: Accreditation Association for Hospitals and Health Systems. (Level VII)

8 The Joint Commission. (2021). Standard UP.01.01.01. *Comprehensive accreditation manual for hospitals.* Oakbrook Terrace, IL: The Joint Commission. (Level VII)

9 Accreditation Association for Hospitals and Health Systems. (2020). Standard 30.00.14. *Healthcare Facilities Accreditation Program: Accreditation requirements for acute care hospitals.* Chicago, IL: Accreditation Association for Hospitals and Health Systems. (Level VII)

10 The Joint Commission. (2021). Standard NPSG.07.01.01. *Comprehensive accreditation manual for hospitals.* Oakbrook Terrace, IL: The Joint Commission. (Level VII)

11 Centers for Disease Control and Prevention. (2002). Guideline for hand hygiene in health-care settings: Recommendations of the Healthcare Infection Control Practices Advisory Committee and the HICPAC/SHEA/APIC/IDSA Hand Hygiene Task Force. *MMWR Recommendations and Reports, 51*(RR-16), 1–45. https://www.cdc.gov/mmwr/pdf/rr/rr5116.pdf (Level II)

12 World Health Organization. (2009). WHO guidelines on hand hygiene in health care: First global patient safety challenge, clean care is safer care. https://apps.who.int/iris/bitstream/handle/10665/44102/9789241597906_eng.pdf?sequence=1 (Level IV)

13 Accreditation Association for Hospitals and Health Systems. (2020). Standard 07.01.21. *Healthcare Facilities Accreditation Program: Accreditation requirements for acute care hospitals.* Chicago, IL: Accreditation Association for Hospitals and Health Systems. (Level VII)

14 Centers for Medicare and Medicaid Services, Department of Health and Human Services. (2020). Condition of participation: Infection control. 42 C.F.R. § 482.42.

15 DNV GL-Healthcare USA, Inc. (2020). IC.1.SR.1. *NIAHO® accreditation requirements, interpretive guidelines and surveyor guidance—revision 20.0.* Milford, OH: DNV GL-Healthcare USA, Inc. (Level VII)

16 The Joint Commission. (2021). Standard NPSG.01.01.01. *Comprehensive accreditation manual for hospitals.* Oakbrook Terrace, IL: The Joint Commission. (Level VII)

17 Accreditation Association for Hospitals and Health Systems. (2020). Standard 15.01.16. *Healthcare Facilities Accreditation Program: Accreditation requirements for acute care hospitals.* Chicago, IL: Accreditation Association for Hospitals and Health Systems. (Level VII)

18 Centers for Medicare and Medicaid Services, Department of Health and Human Services. (2020). Condition of participation: Patient's rights. 42 C.F.R. § 482.13(c)(1).

19 DNV GL-Healthcare USA, Inc. (2020). PR.2.SR.5. *NIAHO® accreditation requirements, interpretive guidelines and surveyor guidance—revision 20.0.* Milford, OH: DNV GL-Healthcare USA, Inc. (Level VII)

20 The Joint Commission. (2021). Standard RI.01.01.01. *Comprehensive accreditation manual for hospitals.* Oakbrook Terrace, IL: The Joint Commission. (Level VII)

21 The Joint Commission. (2021). Standard PC.02.01.21. *Comprehensive accreditation manual for hospitals.* Oakbrook Terrace, IL: The Joint Commission. (Level VII)

22 The Joint Commission. (2021). Standard MM.06.01.01. *Comprehensive accreditation manual for hospitals.* Oakbrook Terrace, IL: The Joint Commission. (Level VII)

23 Accreditation Association for Hospitals and Health Systems. (2020). Standard 16.01.03. *Healthcare Facilities Accreditation Program: Accreditation requirements for acute care hospitals.* Chicago, IL: Accreditation Association for Hospitals and Health Systems. (Level VII)

24 Centers for Medicare and Medicaid Services, Department of Health and Human Services. (2020). Condition of participation: Nursing services. 42 C.F.R. § 482.23(c).

25 DNV GL-Healthcare USA, Inc. (2020). MM.1.SR.3. *NIAHO® accreditation requirements, interpretive guidelines and surveyor guidance—revision 20.0.* Milford, OH: DNV GL-Healthcare USA, Inc. (Level VII)

26 Waters, T. R., et al. (2009). Safe patient handling training for schools of nursing. https://www.cdc.gov/niosh/docs/2009-127/pdfs/2009-127.pdf (Level VII)

27 Accreditation Association for Hospitals and Health Systems. (2020). Standard 07.01.10. *Healthcare Facilities Accreditation Program: Accreditation requirements for acute care hospitals.* Chicago, IL: Accreditation Association for Hospitals and Health Systems. (Level VII)

28 Occupational Safety and Health Administration. (2012). Bloodborne pathogens, standard number 1910.1030. https://www.osha.gov/pls/oshaweb/owadisp.show_document?p_id=10051&p_table=STANDARDS (Level VII)

29 Rothrock, J. C. (2019). *Alexander's care of the patient in surgery* (16th ed.). St. Louis, MO: Elsevier.

30 Guideline for perioperative practice: Patient skin antisepsis. (2021). In Wood, A. (Ed.), *Guidelines for perioperative practice*, 2021 edition. Denver, CO: AORN, Inc. (Level VII)

31 The Joint Commission. (2021). Standard UP.01.03.01. *Comprehensive accreditation manual for hospitals.* Oakbrook Terrace, IL: The Joint Commission. (Level VII)

32 Dolan, S. A. (2016). APIC position paper: Safe injection, infusion, and medication practices in health care (2016). http://www.apic.org/Resource_/TinyMceFileManager/Position_Statements/2016APICSIPPositionPaper.pdf

33 Centers for Disease Control and Prevention. (2019). FAQs regarding safe practices for medical injections: Questions about multi-dose vials. https://www.cdc.gov/injectionsafety/providers/provider_faqs_multivials.html

34 The Joint Commission. (2014). Sentinel event alert 52: Preventing infection from the misuse of vials. https://www.jointcommission.org/-/media/tjc/documents/resources/patient-safety-topics/sentinel-event/sea_52.pdf (Level VII)

35 Ganz, D. A., et al. (2013, reviewed 2021). *Preventing falls in hospitals: A toolkit for improving quality of care* (AHRQ Publication No. 13-0015-EF). Rockville, MD: Agency for Healthcare Research and Quality. https://www.ahrq.gov/professionals/systems/hospital/fallpxtoolkit/index.html (Level VII)

36 Fischbach, F., & Fischbach, M. A. (2018). *A manual of laboratory and diagnostic tests* (10th ed.). Philadelphia, PA: Wolters Kluwer.

37 Rutala, W. A., et al. (2008, revised 2019). Guideline for disinfection and sterilization in healthcare facilities, 2008. https://www.cdc.gov/infection-control/pdf/guidelines/disinfection-guidelines-H.pdf (Level I)

38 Accreditation Association for Hospitals and Health Systems. (2020). Standard 07.02.03. *Healthcare Facilities Accreditation Program: Accreditation requirements for acute care hospitals.* Chicago, IL: Accreditation Association for Hospitals and Health Systems. (Level VII)

39 The Joint Commission. (2021). Standard RC.01.03.01. *Comprehensive accreditation manual for hospitals.* Oakbrook Terrace, IL: The Joint Commission. (Level VII)

40 Accreditation Association for Hospitals and Health Systems. (2020). Standard 10.00.03. *Healthcare Facilities Accreditation Program: Accreditation requirements for acute care hospitals.* Chicago, IL: Accreditation Association for Hospitals and Health Systems. (Level VII)

41 Centers for Medicare and Medicaid Services, Department of Health and Human Services. (2020). Condition of participation: Medical record services. 42 C.F.R. § 482.24(b).

42 DNV GL-Healthcare USA, Inc. (2020). MR.2.SR.1. *NIAHO® accreditation requirements, interpretive guidelines and surveyor guidance—revision 20.0.* Milford, OH: DNV GL-Healthcare USA, Inc. (Level VII)

43 The Joint Commission. (2021). Standard NPSG.02.03.01. *Comprehensive accreditation manual for hospitals.* Oakbrook Terrace, IL: The Joint Commission. (Level VII)

44 Bateman, B. T., et al. (2021). Post dural puncture headache. In: *UpToDate*, Hepner, D. L., & Swanson, J. W. (Eds.).

45 Strony, R. (2010). Ultrasound-assisted lumbar puncture in obese patients. *Critical Care Clinics, 26*, 661–664.

46 The Joint Commission. (2021). Standard RC.02.01.01. *Comprehensive accreditation manual for hospitals.* Oakbrook Terrace, IL: The Joint Commission. (Level VII)

MANUAL VENTILATION

A handheld resuscitation bag is a self-inflating device that can be attached to a face mask or directly to an endotracheal (ET) or tracheostomy tube[1], allowing manual delivery of oxygen or room air to the lungs of a patient with absent or inadequate respirations.

During cardiopulmonary resuscitation (CPR), using a handheld resuscitation bag to administer rescue breaths is less important than providing high-quality chest compressions. Lone rescuers should begin chest compressions first. After 30 compressions, the rescuer should then administer two breaths. When a second person arrives, that person can use a handheld resuscitation bag to administer two breaths after every 30 compressions. After an advanced airway (endotracheal tube or supraglottic device) is inserted, one breath can be delivered every 6 seconds. Whenever an advanced airway is inserted during CPR, rescuers may perform continuous compressions with positive pressure ventilation delivered through the handheld resuscitation bag without pausing chest compressions.[2]

Equipment

Handheld resuscitation bag with mask ▪ oxygen source ▪ oxygen tubing ▪ nipple adapter attached to oxygen flowmeter ▪ gloves ▪ suction equipment ▪ emergency resuscitation equipment (code cart with emergency medications, defibrillator, and intubation equipment) ▪ Optional: gown, mask and goggles or mask and face shield, oropharyngeal airway, nasopharyngeal airway, oxygen accumulator (oxygen reservoir).

Preparation of equipment

Unless the patient is intubated or has a tracheostomy, select a mask that fits snugly over the mouth and nose. Attach the mask to the resuscitation bag.

If oxygen is readily available, connect the handheld resuscitation bag to the oxygen. Attach one end of the tubing to the bottom of the bag and the other end to the nipple adapter on the flowmeter of the oxygen source.

Turn on the oxygen and adjust the flow rate to 15 L/minute.[3] The patient who has a low partial pressure of arterial oxygen will need a higher fraction of inspired oxygen (FIO_2). *To increase the concentration of inspired oxygen,* you can add an oxygen accumulator (also called an oxygen reservoir). This device, which attaches to an adapter on the bottom of the bag, permits an FIO_2 of up to 100%. If time allows, set up suction equipment. Make sure emergency resuscitation equipment is readily available.

Implementation

- Gather and prepare the necessary equipment and supplies
- Perform hand hygiene.[4,5,6,7,8,9]
- Confirm the patient's identity using at least two patient identifiers.[10]
- Provide privacy.[11,12,13,14]
- Explain the procedure to the patient and family, if they're present and time allows, according to their individual communication and learning needs, *to increase their understanding, allay their fears, and enhance cooperation.*[15]
- Raise the bed to waist level before providing care *to prevent caregiver back strain.*[16]
- Put on gloves and other personal protective equipment, as needed, *to comply with standard precautions.*[17,18,19]
- Before using the handheld resuscitation bag, inspect the patient's upper airway for foreign objects. If present, remove them, *because doing so may restore spontaneous respirations in some instances, and because foreign matter or secretions can obstruct the airway and impede resuscitation efforts.*
- Suction the patient *to remove any secretions that may obstruct the airway.* If necessary, insert an oropharyngeal or nasopharyngeal airway *to maintain airway patency.* If the patient has a tracheostomy or ET tube in place, suction the tube.
- If appropriate, remove the bed's headboard and stand at the head of the bed *to help keep the patient's neck extended and to free space at the side of the bed for other activities, such as CPR.*

- Unless the patient shows evidence of head or neck trauma, use the head-tilt, chin-lift maneuver to open the patient's airway *to move the tongue away from the base of the pharynx and prevent obstruction of the airway.*[20]
- Apply the mask to the patient's face. (See *How to apply a handheld resuscitation bag and mask.*)
- Keeping your nondominant hand on the patient's mask, exert downward pressure *to seal the mask against the face.* For the adult patient, use your dominant hand to compress the bag to deliver 600 mL of air over 1 second *to produce a rise in the patient's chest.*[20]
- Deliver breaths with the patient's own inspiratory effort, if any is present. Don't attempt to deliver a breath as the patient exhales. During CPR, deliver cycles of 30 compressions and two breaths; deliver breaths during pauses in compressions, and deliver each breath over 1 second.[20]
- Observe the patient's chest *to ensure that it rises and falls with each ventilation.*[20] If ventilation fails to occur, check the fit of the mask and the patency of the patient's airway; if necessary, reposition the patient's head and ensure patency with an oral airway.
- Assist with advanced airway insertion, if necessary. (See the "Endotracheal intubation" procedure.) After advanced airway insertion, remove the mask, connect the handheld resuscitation bag to the tube, and provide one breath every 6 seconds. During CPR, deliver ventilations through the advanced airway without having the second rescuer pause chest compressions.[2]
- Remove and discard your gloves and any other personal protective equipment worn.[19]
- Return the bed to the lowest position *to prevent falls and maintain patient safety.*[21]
- Perform hand hygiene.[4,5,6,7,8,9]
- Document the procedure.[22,23,24,25]

Special considerations

- Observe for vomiting through the clear part of the mask.[20] If vomiting occurs, stop the procedure immediately, lift the mask, wipe and suction vomitus, and resume resuscitation.
- It isn't possible to deliver an accurate or exact tidal volume while using a handheld resuscitation bag and mask.[26]

EQUIPMENT

How to apply a handheld resuscitation bag and mask

Place the mask over the patient's face so that the apex of the triangle covers the bridge of the nose and the base lies between the lower lip and chin *to create a tight seal.* Hold the mask in place (as shown below).

Using your nondominant hand, create a C shape with the thumb and index finger over the top of the mask and apply gentle downward pressure. Hook the remaining fingers around the mandible and lift it upward toward the mask, creating an E shape (as shown below). Make sure that the patient's mouth remains open underneath the mask. Attach the resuscitation bag to the mask and the tubing leading to the oxygen source. Alternatively, if the patient has a tracheostomy or endotracheal tube in place, remove the mask from the bag and attach the handheld resuscitation bag directly to the tube.

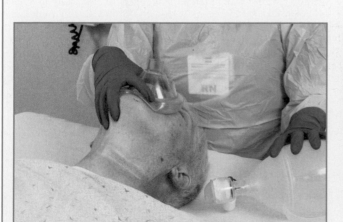

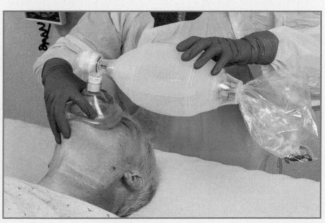

■ Give the family the option to remain at the bedside during the procedure, *because doing so helps meet the psychosocial needs of the patient and family in a time of crisis.*[27]

Complications

Complications may include aspiration of vomitus, pneumonia, gastric distention, and increased intrathoracic pressure with a subsequent decrease in coronary and cerebral perfusion pressures.

Documentation

In an emergency, record the date and time of the procedure, the reason for initiating the procedure, any complications, interventions taken, and the patient's response to treatment using your facility's documentation system or cardiopulmonary resuscitation flow sheet.

If it isn't an emergency, record the date and time of the procedure as well as the reason and length of time the patient was disconnected from mechanical ventilation and received manual ventilation. Note the patient's tolerance of the procedure, along with any complications, interventions taken, and the patient's response to those interventions. Document teaching provided to the patient and family (if appropriate), their understanding of that teaching, and any need for follow-up teaching.

REFERENCES

1 Craven, R. F., et al. (2020). *Fundamentals of nursing: Concepts and competencies for practice* (9th ed.). Philadelphia, PA: Wolters Kluwer.

2 Kleinman, M. E., et al. (2018). 2017 American Heart Association focused update on adult basic life support and cardiopulmonary resuscitation quality: An update to the American Heart Association guidelines for cardiopulmonary resuscitation and emergency cardiovascular care, *Circulation, 137*, e7–e13. https://www.ahajournals.org/doi/pdf/10.1161/CIR.0000000000000539 (Level VII)

3 Wiegand, D. L. (2017). *AACN procedure manual for high acuity, progressive, and critical care* (7th ed.). St. Louis, MO: Elsevier.

4 The Joint Commission. (2021). Standard NPSG.07.01.01. *Comprehensive accreditation manual for hospitals*. Oakbrook Terrace, IL: The Joint Commission. (Level VII)

5 Centers for Disease Control and Prevention. (2002). Guideline for hand hygiene in health-care settings: Recommendations of the Healthcare Infection Control Practices Advisory Committee and the HICPAC/SHEA/APIC/IDSA Hand Hygiene Task Force. *MMWR Recommendations and Reports, 51*(RR-16), 1–45. https://www.cdc.gov/mmwr/pdf/rr/rr5116.pdf (Level II)

6 World Health Organization. (2009). WHO guidelines on hand hygiene in health care: First global patient safety challenge, clean care is safer care. https://apps.who.int/iris/bitstream/handle/10665/44102/9789241597906_eng.pdf?sequence=1 (Level IV)

7 Accreditation Association for Hospitals and Health Systems. (2020). Standard 07.01.21. *Healthcare Facilities Accreditation Program: Accreditation requirements for acute care hospitals*. Chicago, IL: Accreditation Association for Hospitals and Health Systems. (Level VII)

8 Centers for Medicare and Medicaid Services, Department of Health and Human Services. (2020). Condition of participation: Infection control. 42 C.F.R. § 482.42.

9 DNV GL-Healthcare USA, Inc. (2020). IC.1.SR.1. *NIAHO® accreditation requirements, interpretive guidelines and surveyor guidance—revision 20.0*. Milford, OH: DNV GL-Healthcare USA, Inc. (Level VII)

10 The Joint Commission. (2021). Standard NPSG.01.01.01. *Comprehensive accreditation manual for hospitals*. Oakbrook Terrace, IL: The Joint Commission. (Level VII)

11 Accreditation Association for Hospitals and Health Systems. (2020). Standard 15.01.16. *Healthcare Facilities Accreditation Program: Accreditation requirements for acute care hospitals*. Chicago, IL: Accreditation Association for Hospitals and Health Systems. (Level VII)

12 Centers for Medicare and Medicaid Services, Department of Health and Human Services. (2020). Condition of participation: Patient's rights. 42 C.F.R. § 482.13(c)(1).

13 DNV GL-Healthcare USA, Inc. (2020). PR.2.SR.5. *NIAHO® accreditation requirements, interpretive guidelines and surveyor guidance—revision 20.0*. Milford, OH: DNV GL-Healthcare USA, Inc. (Level VII)

14 The Joint Commission. (2021). Standard RI.01.01.01. *Comprehensive accreditation manual for hospitals*. Oakbrook Terrace, IL: The Joint Commission. (Level VII)

15 The Joint Commission. (2021). Standard PC.02.01.21. *Comprehensive accreditation manual for hospitals*. Oakbrook Terrace, IL: The Joint Commission. (Level VII)

16 Waters, T. R., et al. (2009). Safe patient handling training for schools of nursing. https://www.cdc.gov/niosh/docs/2009-127/pdfs/2009-127.pdf (Level VII)

17 Siegel, J. D., et al. (2007, revised 2019). 2007 guideline for isolation precautions: Preventing transmission of infectious agents in healthcare settings. https://www.cdc.gov/infectioncontrol/pdf/guidelines/isolation-guidelines-H.pdf (Level II)

18 Accreditation Association for Hospitals and Health Systems. (2020). Standard 07.01.10. *Healthcare Facilities Accreditation Program: Accreditation requirements for acute care hospitals*. Chicago, IL: Accreditation Association for Hospitals and Health Systems. (Level VII)

19 Occupational Safety and Health Administration. (2012). Bloodborne pathogens, standard number 1910.1030. https://www.osha.gov/pls/oshaweb/owadisp.show_document?p_id=10051&p_table=STANDARDS (Level VII)

20 Panchal, A. R., et al. (2020). 2020 American Heart Association Guidelines for Cardiopulmonary Resuscitation and Emergency Cardiovascular Care, Part 3: Adult basic and advanced life support. *Circulation, 142*(6), S358–S365. https://www.ahajournals.org/doi/10.1161/CIR.0000000000000898 (Level II)

21 Ganz, D. A., et al. (2013, reviewed 2021). *Preventing falls in hospitals: A toolkit for improving quality of care* (AHRQ Publication No. 13-0015-EF). Rockville, MD: Agency for Healthcare Research and Quality. https://www.ahrq.gov/professionals/systems/hospital/fallpxtoolkit/index.html (Level VII)

22 The Joint Commission. (2021). Standard RC.02.01.01. *Comprehensive accreditation manual for hospitals*. Oakbrook Terrace, IL: The Joint Commission. (Level VII)

23 Centers for Medicare and Medicaid Services, Department of Health and Human Services. (2020). Condition of participation: Medical record services. 42 C.F.R. § 482.24(b).

24 Accreditation Association for Hospitals and Health Systems. (2020). Standard 10.00.03. *Healthcare Facilities Accreditation Program: Accreditation requirements for acute care hospitals*. Chicago, IL: Accreditation Association for Hospitals and Health Systems. (Level VII)

25 DNV GL-Healthcare USA, Inc. (2020). MR.2.SR.1. *NIAHO® accreditation requirements, interpretive guidelines and surveyor guidance—revision 20.0*. Milford, OH: DNV GL-Healthcare USA, Inc. (Level VII)

26 Lee, H. M., et al. (2008). Can you deliver accurate tidal volume by manual resuscitator? *Emergency Medicine Journal, 25*, 632–634. (Level VI)

27 American Association of Critical-Care Nurses. (2016). AACN practice alert: Family presence during resuscitation and invasive procedures. https://www.aacn.org/clinical-resources/practice-alerts/family-presence-during-resuscitation-and-invasive-procedures (Level VII)

MASSIVE INFUSION DEVICE USE

A massive infusion device is a mechanical device used in patients who need rapid fluid replacement with IV fluids or blood products. It can warm IV fluids or blood products to room temperature to prevent hypothermia and then administer the fluid rapidly at rates of up to 45,000 mL/hour.[1] The device requires specialized IV tubing that expands under pressure.[2]

Examples of a massive infusion device include the Level 1 infuser, the Belmont infuser, and the ThermaCor 1200 Rapid Infuser. The Level 1 infuser warms fluids through a sealed heat exchanger that contains recirculating solution. Pressure chambers apply pressure and deliver the prescribed fluids at a rapid rate. The administration set tubing contains a gas vent filter and the heat exchanger. An air detector clamp monitors for the presence of air; when it detects air, the clamp closes off the line and alerts the clinician of the presence of air in the system.[3] The Belmont infuser administers the prescribed fluids through the administration set tubing using a roller-type peristaltic fluid pump. Fluid passes through a heat exchanger that consists of a plastic device housing stainless steel rings, which transfer heat to the fluid. The infuser also contains a pressure sensor that monitors the line pressure of the infusate. If the sensor detects pressure that exceeds the limit set by the clinician, the pump automatically slows the infusion. If line pressure suddenly increases, the device shuts down and an alarm sounds.[1] The ThermaCor 1200 Rapid Infusor has a single-use disposable cassette that warms the fluid and provides an administration set with single and dual patient lines. The system has an air-trapping capability that triggers the air volume sensors when enough air is trapped.[4]

Patients with life-threatening conditions such as severe trauma, burns, or GI, postoperative, or postpartum hemorrhage may require the use of a rapid infusion device to receive large volumes of fluids within a short period.[2] Sterile no-touch technique is required during massive infusion administration to reduce the risk of vascular catheter-associated infection. **HOSPITAL-ACQUIRED CONDITION ALERT** Keep in mind that the Centers for Medicare and Medicaid Services considers vascular catheter–associated infection to be a hospital-acquired condition *because it can be reasonably prevented using best practices.* Follow evidence-based infection prevention practices, such as performing a vigorous mechanical scrub of the needleless connector and using sterile no-touch technique, *to reduce the risk of vascular catheter–associated infections.*[5,6,7,8]

Equipment

Massive infusion device ▪ prescribed IV fluids or blood products ▪ prefilled 10-mL syringe (or a syringe specifically designed to generate lower injection pressure) containing preservative-free normal saline solution ▪ appropriate administration set with warming device or heat exchanger[1,3] ▪ replacement filter or vent or large-capacity reservoir, as indicated[1,3] ▪ IV pole ▪ gloves ▪ antiseptic pads (chlorhexidine-based, povidone iodine, or alcohol) ▪ labels ▪ blankets ▪ stethoscope ▪ vital signs monitoring equipment ▪ disinfectant pad ▪ Optional: indwelling urinary catheter, central venous access catheter or pulmonary artery catheter insertion and monitoring equipment, arterial catheter insertion and monitoring equipment, supplies for blood gas sampling, gown, mask with face shield or mask and goggles.

Preparation of equipment

Make sure that the equipment is safe for massive, rapid, or pressurized infusion.

Inspect all IV equipment and supplies; if a product is expired, is defective, or has compromised integrity, remove it from patient use, label it as expired or defective, and report the expiration or defect as directed by your facility.[9]

Set up and use the massive infusion device, warming device, or heat exchanger following the manufacturer's instructions for use. Make sure that the system is plugged into an outlet *to ensure that the infused fluid is heated properly.*[1,3] Make sure that the device alarm limits are set appropriately, and that the alarms are turned on, functioning properly, and audible to staff.[10,11] Troubleshoot alarms according to the specific manufacturer's instructions for use.[1,3]

Implementation

▪ Verify that the practitioner's orders for the prescribed solution, rate, and route of administration are appropriate for the patient's age, condition, and access device. Address concerns about the order with the practitioner, the pharmacist, or your supervisor, and (if needed) the risk management department, or as directed by your facility.[12]
▪ Verify the baseline coagulation studies and hematocrit, electrolyte, and hemoglobin levels, and results of coagulation and other studies, as ordered, *to serve as benchmarks for comparison and help guide fluid replacement.*[2]
▪ Check the patient history for allergies, as indicated.
▪ Perform hand hygiene.[13,14,15,16,17,18]
▪ Confirm the patient's identity using at least two patient identifiers.[19]
▪ Provide privacy.[20,21,22,23]
▪ Reinforce the practitioner's explanation of the procedure according to the patient's and family's individual communication and learning needs *to increase communication, allay their fears, and enhance cooperation.*[24] Answer any questions.
▪ Raise the bed to waist level before providing care *to prevent caregiver back strain.*[25]
▪ Perform a baseline physical assessment (before obtaining blood for transfusion, if ordered), including vital signs and respiratory status. Assess

for conditions that can increase the risk of adverse effects of therapy, such as heart failure, fever, kidney disease, and risk of fluid volume excess.[26]
▪ If the patient doesn't already have one in place, insert an indwelling urinary catheter, as ordered, *to help monitor fluid resuscitation efforts.* (See the "Indwelling urinary catheter insertion" procedure.)
▪ Perform hand hygiene.[13,14,15,16,17,18]
▪ Put on gloves and other personal protective equipment as needed *to comply with standard precautions.*[27,28]
▪ Make sure the patient has two patent, large-bore (14G to 18G) IV catheters.[15] If not, insert two IV catheters *to administer IV fluid and medications, as needed, until a central venous catheter is possible.*[29] (See the "IV catheter insertion and removal" procedure.) If you're unable to establish venous access, initiate intraosseous access, if indicated.[2,30] (See the "Intraosseous infusion" procedure.)
▪ Assist the practitioner, as needed, with insertion of a central venous or pulmonary artery catheter *to facilitate administration of large fluid volumes and to help monitor the patient's hemodynamic status.*[2]
▪ Assist the practitioner, as needed, with arterial catheter insertion *for continuous blood pressure assessment.*[2]
▪ Turn on the infusion device according to the manufacturer's instructions *to allow the system to warm up.*[2]
▪ If you're infusing blood products, perform a pretransfusion blood verification with another qualified health care provider. *A pretransfusion verification by two qualified health care providers is required to prevent life-threatening blood incompatibility errors.*[19,26,31] (See the "Transfusion of blood and blood products" procedure.)
HOSPITAL-ACQUIRED CONDITION ALERT Keep in mind that the Centers for Medicare and Medicaid Services considers blood incompatibility errors to be a hospital-acquired condition *because they can be reasonably prevented using best practices.* Be sure to follow evidence-based prevention practices, such as carefully identifying the patient and the blood sample for compatibility testing and participating in a two-person verification process before blood and blood products administration, *to reduce the risk of blood incompatibility errors.*[5]
▪ Remove the appropriate administration set from its packaging. Inspect the administration sets for loose or missing Luer and spike caps *to ensure sterility.*[1,3]

Using the Level 1 infuser

▪ Install the appropriate administration set into the infusion device according to the manufacturer's instructions.[3]
▪ Secure the heat exchanger and gas vent filter in their proper positions and turn them on, following the manufacturer's instructions.[2,3]
▪ Close all of the clamps on the Y-administration set.[3]
▪ Invert and spike the fluid or blood product bag. Squeeze the bag *to remove all air* and connect the ordered fluid or blood product to the Y-set. Then hang the bag on the hooks provided within the rapid infuser pressure chambers.[2] Close the pressure chamber door and secure the latch. Repeat for each fluid line you'll use.[3]
▪ Open the clamps above the drip chamber for each IV fluid bag you'll use.[3] Fill the drip chambers on the administration set halfway by squeezing them *to prevent air from entering the tubing.*[2] Repeat with each fluid line, as indicated.
▪ Open the remaining clamps above the heat exchanger *so that fluid will flow into the gas vent filter assembly.*[3]
▪ Gently tap the gas vent filter assembly *to dislodge air bubbles from the filter screen,* according to the manufacturer's instructions. Inspect the tubing and filter when finished *to make sure there are no air bubbles.*[2]
▪ Remove the male Luer cap from the distal end of the administration set tubing.[3]
▪ Open the pinch clamp below the gas vent filter assembly. Allow fluid to flow until you no longer observe air in the tubing and the line is primed with fluid *to prevent air embolism.* Then close the roller clamp. Put a new needleless connector on the end of the tubing.[3,32]
▪ Perform a vigorous mechanical scrub of the needleless connector on the vascular access device for at least 5 seconds using an antiseptic pad, and allow it to dry completely.[6,32]
▪ While maintaining sterility of the syringe tip, attach a 10-mL syringe or a syringe specifically designed to generate low injection pressure containing preservative-free normal saline solution to the needleless connector.

Unclamp the catheter and slowly aspirate for blood return that is the color and consistency of whole blood. If no blood return occurs, take steps to locate an external cause of obstruction.[33]

■ If blood return occurs, slowly inject preservative-free normal saline solution into the catheter. Use a minimum volume of twice the internal volume of the catheter system. Don't forcibly flush the device; further evaluate the device if you meet resistance.[33]

■ Clamp the catheter and remove and discard the syringe in a puncture-resistant sharps disposal container.[34]

■ Carefully remove the needleless connector from the vascular access device. Perform a vigorous mechanical scrub of the catheter hub for at least 5 seconds using an antiseptic pad; then allow it to dry completely.[6,35,36]

■ Trace the tubing from the patient to its point of origin *to make sure that you're attaching the tubing to the proper port.*[37,38]

■ Connect the distal end of the tubing to the patient's vascular access catheter. If the patient has other tubing and catheters that have different purposes, route the tubing using a standardized approach. If you're using multiple IV lines, label each tubing at the distal end (near the patient connection) and the proximal end (near the source container) *to reduce the risk of misconnection.*[38]

■ Complete functional testing of all audible and visual alarms according to the manufacturer's instructions. If any visual indicator doesn't illuminate or the audible signal doesn't sound, remove the device from service immediately.[3,39,40]

■ After confirming proper infusion device operation, unclamp the tubing and begin the infusion, adjusting the infusion rate as needed.[2]

Using the Belmont infuser

■ Install the appropriate administration set into the infusion device according to the manufacturer's instructions.[1]

■ Confirm that the heat exchanger is secured properly.[1]

■ As needed for infusion of larger volumes of fluid, replace the reservoir chamber with the larger-capacity reservoir. Using sterile technique, remove the reservoir chamber from the administration set by disconnecting the Luer connectors.[1]

■ Attach the reservoir holder onto the IV pole and place the larger reservoir into the holder.[1]

■ Attach the three fluid supply tails onto the top of the larger reservoir to be used.[1]

■ Connect the larger reservoir to the administration set. Adjust the reservoir holder *to make sure that the connection leads underneath the reservoir aren't stretched or kinked.*[1]

■ Hang the fluid bag on the IV pole.[1]

■ Close the bag clamps and remove the bag spike cap. Perform a vigorous mechanical scrub of the port with an antiseptic pad for at least 5 seconds and allow it to dry completely. Then spike the fluid bag, piercing it fully *to ensure that fluids flow freely.*[1]

■ Repeat with additional fluid lines that you'll use.[1]

■ Open the bag clamps.[1]

■ Prime the main system by pressing the PRIME button to recirculate 100 mL of fluid at 500 mL/minute *to remove air and replace the main system with fluid.*[1]

■ Prime the remainder of the administration tubing by opening the roller clamp and removing the male Luer cap at the distal end of the tubing. Press the PT. LINE PRIME button once *to prime at 50 mL/minute* and press and hold the button *to prime at 200 mL/minute*. Press the STOP button after inspecting the tubing *to make sure there are no air bubbles*. Press the PT. LINE PRIME button again *to remove any remaining air.*[1]

■ Perform a vigorous mechanical scrub of the needleless connector of the vascular access device for at least 5 seconds with an antiseptic pad, and allow it to dry completely.[6,32,35,36]

■ While maintaining sterility of the syringe tip, attach a prefilled 10-mL syringe or a syringe specifically designed to generate low injection pressure containing preservative-free normal saline solution to the needleless connector. Unclamp the catheter and slowly aspirate for blood return that is the color and consistency of whole blood. If no blood return occurs, take steps to locate an external cause of obstruction.[33,35,36]

■ If blood return occurs, slowly inject preservative-free normal saline solution into the catheter. Use a minimum volume of twice the internal

volume of the catheter system. Don't forcibly flush the device; further evaluate the device if you meet resistance.[33]

■ Clamp the catheter and remove and discard the syringe in a puncture-resistant sharps disposal container.[34]

■ Carefully remove the needleless connector from the vascular access device. Perform a vigorous mechanical scrub of the catheter hub for at least 5 seconds using an antiseptic pad; then allow it to dry completely.[32,35,36]

■ Trace the tubing from the patient to its point of origin *to make sure that you're attaching the tubing to the proper port.*[37,38]

■ Connect the distal end of the tubing to the patient's vascular access catheter.[1] If the patient has other tubing and catheters that have different purposes, route the tubing using a standardized approach. If you're using multiple IV lines, label each tubing at the distal end (near the patient connection) and the proximal end (near the source container) *to reduce the risk of misconnection.*[38]

■ Unclamp the catheter, press INFUSE *to start infusing*, and adjust the flow rate, as needed.[1]

Using the ThermaCor 1200 Rapid Infuser

■ Unlatch and remove the component guard from the unit.[41]

■ Turn the latch into the load position. Place the cassette on the load bar (at the bottom of the unit) at a 45-degree angle and then lift and press the cassette directly into the unit. Close the latch into the lock position.[41]

■ Open the roller pump door and push the roller tubing all the way to the back *to reduce the incidence of improper loading of the tubing*. Close the pump door.[41]

■ Connect the three-spike in-flow set to the cassette by following the color-coded caps. *Connect the blue to blue and the yellow to yellow.*[41]

■ Connect the patient line by following the color-coded caps. Connect the red to red.[41]

■ Connect one or more of the spikes from the in-flow set to an IV fluid bag and hang it on the pole.[41]

■ Open the clamp closest to the fluid or blood bag and observe for fluid filling the filter. When the filter is ⅔ full, push the PRIME button for the system to autoprime. As needed for infusion of larger volumes of fluid, replace the fluid infusion bag with the larger-capacity reservoir.[41]

■ When the system beeps, push and hold the PRIME button and observe as fluid primes the tubing that connects to the patient *to ensure that all air is removed from the system.*[41]

■ Perform a vigorous mechanical scrub of the needleless connector on the vascular access device for at least 5 seconds using an antiseptic pad. Then let it dry completely.[6,32,35,36]

■ While maintaining sterility of the syringe tip, attach a prefilled 10-mL syringe or a syringe specifically designed to generate lower injection pressure containing preservative-free normal saline solution to the needleless connector. Unclamp the catheter and slowly aspirate for a blood return that's the color and consistency of whole blood. If you don't obtain a blood return, take steps to locate an external cause of obstruction.[33,35,36]

■ If you obtain a blood return, inject preservative-free normal saline solution slowly into the catheter. Use a minimum volume of twice the internal volume of the catheter system. Don't forcibly flush the device; further evaluate the device if you meet resistance.[33]

■ Clamp the catheter and remove and discard the syringe in a puncture-resistant sharps disposal container.[34]

■ Carefully remove the needleless connector from the vascular access device. Perform a vigorous mechanical scrub of the catheter hub for at least 5 seconds using an antiseptic pad. Then let it dry completely.[32,35,36]

■ Trace the tubing from the patient to its point of origin *to make sure that you're attaching the tubing to the proper port.*[37,38]

■ Connect the distal end of the tubing to the patient's vascular access catheter. If the patient has other tubing and catheters that have different purposes, route the tubing using a standardized approach. If you're using multiple IV lines, label each tubing at the distal end (near the patient connection) and the proximal end (near the source container) *to reduce the risk of misconnection.*[38]

■ Choose the mode of operation (slow, rapid, or bolus) for fluid delivery and then push the start button.[41]

Completing the procedure

■ Monitor the patient's vital signs every 5 to 15 minutes, as indicated. As the patient's condition stabilizes, monitor vital signs less frequently (every 30 minutes until the patient's blood pressure is stable for longer than 2 hours).[2]

■ Monitor core temperature every 15 to 30 minutes and maintain a core temperature no lower than 96.8° F (36° C) *to prevent hypothermia-induced coagulopathies.*[2]

■ Assess the patient's hemodynamic parameters every 15 to 30 minutes and urine output every 30 to 60 minutes, as ordered, *to evaluate the patient's fluid volume status, which indicates the effectiveness of fluid resuscitation and can be used to guide therapy.*[2]

■ Inspect IV sites every 15 minutes, *because rapid infusion increases the risk of infiltration.*[2]

■ If the patient is receiving blood products, monitor closely for signs of a transfusion reaction, such as fever, chills, flushing, nausea, chest tightness, restlessness, apprehension, and back pain.[2,26]

■ Obtain an arterial blood gas sample, as ordered, *to monitor oxygenation and acid-base balance.* (See the "Arterial puncture for blood gas analysis" procedure.)

■ When the infusion is complete, change the IV fluid or blood bag according to the specific manufacturer's instructions.

■ Discard the empty infusion bag in the proper receptacle[27,34] or, if required by your facility, return empty blood transfusion bags to the blood bank.

■ Obtain blood samples for hemoglobin level, hematocrit, lactic acid level, and electrolyte levels, and for coagulation studies and thromboelastography, as ordered. (See the "Venipuncture" procedure.)

■ Report all critical test results to the practitioner within the time frame established by your facility *to prevent life-threatening treatment delays.*[42]

■ Return the bed to the lowest position *to prevent falls and maintain patient safety.*[43]

■ Discard used supplies in appropriate receptacles.[27,34,44]

■ Provide warming measures, such as additional blankets, *to keep the patient warm and prevent hypothermia.*[2]

■ Remove and discard your gloves and other personal protective equipment, if worn.[27,34,45]

■ Perform hand hygiene.[13,14,15,16,17,18]

■ Clean and disinfect your stethoscope with a disinfectant pad.[46,47]

■ Perform hand hygiene.[13,14,15,16,17,18]

■ Document the procedure.[48,49,50,51]

Special considerations

■ Replace gas vent filters and reservoirs according to the manufacturer's instructions.[1,3] Change the tubing and filter of a Level 1 transfuser according to the manufacturer's recommendations.[52] Clean and disinfect the device according to the manufacturer's recommendations.

■ If you're administering blood products, prime the system with a compatible IV solution; don't prime with the blood product.[1,3]

Complications

Possible complications include electrolyte imbalances, fluid overload, acid-base imbalance, infiltration or extravasation, pulmonary edema, heart failure, interstitial edema, acute respiratory distress syndrome, and hypothermia.[2]

Documentation

Document the transfusion of all blood products in the patient's record, including the product type, date and time of the infusion, and unique number or lot number for blood products. Document the infusion site used, access device, and site condition. Record the patient's core temperature before the start of a massive infusion and at intervals during and after the procedure. Documentation should include a meticulous account of the amounts and types of fluids and correlating vital signs. Record the patient's response to the procedure, the practitioner notified of any complications of the procedure, and actions taken to address the complications. Incorporate documentation of massive fluid infusion into the existing required documentation protocol for resuscitation documentation.[48,49] Record teaching provided to the patient and family (if applicable), their understanding of that teaching, and any need for follow-up teaching.

REFERENCES

1 Belmont Instrument Corporation. (n.d.). The Belmont® Rapid Infuser, FMS2000: Operator's manual. http://derriforded.weebly.com/uploads/1/5/2/4/15247360/belmont.pdf

2 Wiegand, D. L. (2017). *AACN procedure manual for high acuity, progressive, and critical care* (7th ed.). Elsevier.

3 Smiths Medical. (2006). Level 1® H-1200 Fast Flow Fluid Warmer: Operator's manual. https://www.medwrench.com/documents/view/724/smiths-medical-level-1-h-1200-fast-flow-operators-manual

4 Smisson-Cartledge Biomedical. (n.d.). Why ThermaCor 1200 Rapid Infuser. https://www.thermacor1200.com/why-thermacor.cms

5 Jarrett, N., & Callaham, M. (2016). Evidence-based guidelines for selected hospital-acquired conditions: Final report. https://www.cms.gov/Medicare/Medicare-Fee-for-Service-Payment/HospitalAcqCond/Downloads/2016-HAC-Report.pdf

6 Marschall, J., et al. (2014). SHEA/IDSA practice recommendation: Strategies to prevent central line–associated bloodstream infections in acute care hospitals. *Infection Control and Hospital Epidemiology, 35*(7), 753–771. https://www.jstor.org/stable/10.1086/676533#metadata_info_tab_contents (Level I)

7 Accreditation Association for Hospitals and Health Systems. (2020). Standard 07.01.02. *Healthcare Facilities Accreditation Program: Accreditation requirements for acute care hospitals.* (Level VII)

8 Accreditation Association for Hospitals and Health Systems. (2020). Standard 07.01.19. *Healthcare Facilities Accreditation Program: Accreditation requirements for acute care hospitals.* (Level VII)

9 Standard 12. Product evaluation, integrity, and defect reporting. Infusion therapy standards of practice (8th ed.). (2021). *Journal of Infusion Nursing, 44*(Suppl. 1), S45–S46. (Level VII)

10 Zoremba, N., et al. (2011). Air elimination capability in rapid infusion systems. *Anaesthesia, 66*(11), 1031–1034. https://doi.org/10.1111/j.1365-2044.2011.06899.x (Level IV)

11 The Joint Commission. (2021). Standard NPSG.06.01.01. *Comprehensive accreditation manual for hospitals.* (Level VII)

12 Standard 59. Infusion medication and solution administration. Infusion therapy standards of practice (8th ed.). (2021). *Journal of Infusion Nursing, 44*(Suppl. 1), S180–S183. (Level VII)

13 Centers for Disease Control and Prevention. (2002). Guideline for hand hygiene in health-care settings: Recommendations of the Healthcare Infection Control Practices Advisory Committee and the HICPAC/SHEA/APIC/IDSA Hand Hygiene Task Force. *MMWR Recommendations and Reports, 51*(RR-16), 1–45. https://www.cdc.gov/mmwr/pdf/rr/rr5116.pdf (Level II)

14 The Joint Commission. (2021). Standard NPSG.07.01.01. *Comprehensive accreditation manual for hospitals.* (Level VII)

15 Standard 16. Hand hygiene. Infusion therapy standards of practice (8th ed.). (2021). *Journal of Infusion Nursing, 44*(Suppl. 1), S53–S54. (Level VII)

16 World Health Organization. (2009). WHO guidelines on hand hygiene in health care: First global patient safety challenge, clean care is safer care. https://apps.who.int/iris/bitstream/handle/10665/44102/9789241597906_eng.pdf?sequence=1 (Level IV)

17 Centers for Medicare and Medicaid Services, Department of Health and Human Services. (2020). Condition of participation: Infection control. 42 C.F.R. § 482.42.

18 DNV GL-Healthcare USA, Inc. (2020). IC.1.SR.1. *NIAHO® accreditation requirements, interpretive guidelines and surveyor guidance—revision 20.0.* (Level VII)

19 The Joint Commission. (2021). Standard NPSG.01.01.01. *Comprehensive accreditation manual for hospitals.* (Level VII)

20 Accreditation Association for Hospitals and Health Systems. (2020). Standard 15.01.16. *Healthcare Facilities Accreditation Program: Accreditation requirements for acute care hospitals.* (Level VII)

21 Centers for Medicare and Medicaid Services, Department of Health and Human Services. (2020). Condition of participation: Patient's rights. 42 C.F.R. § 482.13(c)(1).

22 DNV GL-Healthcare USA, Inc. (2020). PR.2.SR.5. *NIAHO® accreditation requirements, interpretive guidelines and surveyor guidance—revision 20.0.* (Level VII)

23 The Joint Commission. (2021). Standard RI.01.01.01. *Comprehensive accreditation manual for hospitals.* (Level VII)

24 The Joint Commission. (2021). Standard PC.02.01.21. *Comprehensive accreditation manual for hospitals.* (Level VII)

25 Waters, T. R., et al. (2009). Safe patient handling training for schools of nursing. https://www.cdc.gov/niosh/docs/2009-127/pdfs/2009-127.pdf (Level VII)

26 Standard 64. Blood administration. Infusion therapy standards of practice (8th ed.). (2021). *Journal of Infusion Nursing, 44*(Suppl. 1), S191–S194. (Level VII)

27 Occupational Safety and Health Administration. (2012). Bloodborne pathogens, standard number 1910.1030. https://www.osha.gov/pls/oshaweb/owadisp.show_document?p_id=10051&p_table=STANDARDS (Level VII)

28 Siegel, J. D., et al. (2007, revised 2019). 2007 guideline for isolation precautions: Preventing transmission of infectious agents in healthcare settings. https://www.cdc.gov/infectioncontrol/pdf/guidelines/isolation-guidelines-H.pdf (Level II)

29 American College of Surgeons Committee on Trauma. (2012). *Advanced trauma life support: Student course manual* (9th edition). American College of Surgeons.

30 Perron, C. E. (2021). Intraosseous infusion. In: *UpToDate*, Stack, A. M., & Wolfson, A. B. (Eds.).

31 The Joint Commission. (2021). Standard NPSG.01.03.01. *Comprehensive accreditation manual for hospitals.* (Level VII)

32 Standard 36. Needleless connectors. Infusion therapy standards of practice (8th ed.). (2021). *Journal of Infusion Nursing, 44*(Suppl. 1), S104–S107. (Level VII)

33 Standard 41. Flushing and locking. Infusion therapy standards of practice (8th ed.). (2021). *Journal of Infusion Nursing, 44*(Suppl. 1), S113–S118. (Level VII)

34 Standard 21. Medical waste and sharps safety. Infusion therapy standards of practice (8th ed.). (2021). *Journal of Infusion Nursing, 44*(Suppl. 1), S460–S62. (Level VII)

35 Infusion Nurses Society. (2016). *Policies and procedures for infusion therapy* (5th ed.). Infusion Nurses Society.

36 Infusion Nurses Society. (2017). *Policies and procedures for infusion therapy of the older adult* (3rd ed.). Infusion Nurses Society.

37 U.S. Food and Drug Administration. (2017). Examples of medical device misconnections. https://www.fda.gov/medical-devices/medical-device-connectors/examples-medical-device-misconnections

38 The Joint Commission. (2014). Sentinel event alert: Managing risk during transition to new ISO tubing connector standards. https://www.joint-commission.org/-/media/tjc/documents/resources/patient-safety-topics/sentinel-event/sea_53_connectors_8_19_14_final.pdf (Level VII)

39 Graham, K. C., & Cvach, M. (2010). Monitor alarm fatigue: Standardizing use of physiological monitors and decreasing nuisance alarms. *American Journal of Critical Care, 19*(1), 28–37. https://aacnjournals.org/ajcconline/article-abstract/19/1/28/5720/Monitor-Alarm-Fatigue-Standardizing-Use-of?redirectedFrom=fulltext

40 The Joint Commission. (2013). Sentinel event alert 50: Medical device alarm safety in hospitals. https://www.jointcommission.org/-/media/tjc/documents/resources/patient-safety-topics/sentinel-event/sea_50_alarms_4_26_16.pdf (Level VII)

41 Medical Solutions, Inc. (n.d.). ThermaCor® 1200 videos. https://www.msi-healthcare.com/our-products-thermacor-1200-videos/

42 The Joint Commission. (2021). Standard NPSG.02.03.01. *Comprehensive accreditation manual for hospitals.* (Level VII)

43 Ganz, D. A., et al. (2013, reviewed 2021). *Preventing falls in hospitals: A toolkit for improving quality of care* (AHRQ Publication No. 13-0015-EF). Agency for Healthcare Research and Quality. https://www.ahrq.gov/professionals/systems/hospital/fallpxtoolkit/index.html (Level VII)

44 Accreditation Association for Hospitals and Health Systems. (2020). Standard 07.03.07. *Healthcare Facilities Accreditation Program: Accreditation requirements for acute care hospitals.* (Level VII)

45 Accreditation Association for Hospitals and Health Systems. (2020). Standard 07.01.10. *Healthcare Facilities Accreditation Program: Accreditation requirements for acute care hospitals.* (Level VII)

46 Accreditation Association for Hospitals and Health Systems. (2020). Standard 07.02.03. *Healthcare Facilities Accreditation Program: Accreditation requirements for acute care hospitals.* (Level VII)

47 Rutala, W. A., et al. (2008, revised 2019). Guideline for disinfection and sterilization in healthcare facilities, 2008. https://www.cdc.gov/infection-control/pdf/guidelines/disinfection-guidelines-H.pdf (Level I)

48 The Joint Commission. (2021). Standard RC.01.03.01. *Comprehensive accreditation manual for hospitals.* (Level VII)

49 Standard 10. Documentation in the medical record. Infusion therapy standards of practice (8th ed.). (2021). *Journal of Infusion Nursing, 44*(Suppl. 1), S39–S42. (Level VII)

50 Centers for Medicare and Medicaid Services, Department of Health and Human Services. (2020). Condition of participation: Medical record services. 42 C.F.R. § 482.24(b).

51 DNV GL-Healthcare USA, Inc. (2020). MR.2.SR.1. *NIAHO® accreditation requirements, interpretive guidelines and surveyor guidance—revision 20.0.* (Level VII)

52 Smiths Medical. (2013). Level 1® H-1200 Fast Flow Fluid Warmer. https://m.smiths-medical.com/~/media/M/Smiths-medical_com/Files/Import%20Files/TM194848EN-102013_LR.pdf

MECHANICAL VENTILATION, POSITIVE PRESSURE

Positive pressure mechanical ventilation promotes gas exchange in the lungs by producing positive intrathoracic pressure and positive airway pressure. An endotracheal (ET) or tracheostomy tube delivers positive pressure mechanical ventilation to airways. The amount of gas exchange depends on the resistance and compliance of the lung itself. Mechanical ventilators deliver ventilation according to a specific mode. The mode may deliver a preset amount of tidal volume (V_T), a preset amount of peak inspiratory pressure, or rates at high frequency through oscillation. Newer, more sophisticated modes of positive pressure ventilation are currently evolving.[1]

Positive pressure ventilation is indicated for the patient with apnea, ventilatory failure or impending failure, severe hypoxemia, and respiratory muscle fatigue.[1] These signs and symptoms may result from acute or chronic lung injury; laryngeal angioedema; neurologic disorders; trauma; chemical or medical respiratory depressants, such as sedation, anesthesia, or opioids; multiple organ dysfunction syndrome; or such disease states as cardiogenic pulmonary edema, pulmonary hemorrhage, pulmonary thromboembolism, acute severe asthma, sepsis, and septic shock.[2]

The goals of positive pressure ventilation include maintaining adequate alveolar ventilation and oxygenation, correcting hypoxemia and acid-base balance, and decreasing the work of breathing while providing adequate respirations and respiratory muscle rest, and minimizing complications for the patient.[1,3] The practitioner may prescribe intermittent administration of continuous infusion of a sedative or pain medication and a paralytic agent to decrease the patient's work of breathing and enable the ventilator to work effectively.

A practitioner orders mechanical ventilation and, in collaboration with the respiratory therapist, sets ventilatory parameters to maintain pH, partial pressure of arterial carbon dioxide, partial pressure of arterial oxygen, and arterial oxygen saturation. The practitioner, respiratory therapist, and nurse must collaborate to manage the moment-to-moment ventilatory needs of the patient. The nurse must know how to assess, monitor, and care for patients on mechanical ventilation and understand basic ventilator mechanisms of action. (See *Mechanical ventilation terminology.*)

Equipment

Oxygen source ▪ compressed air source ▪ flow meters ▪ blender or Y-connector ▪ large- and small-bore oxygen tubing (sterile) ▪ mechanical ventilator unit (with heated filtered humidifier, manometer and in-line thermometer) ▪ ventilator circuit tubing, connectors, and adapters ▪ condensation collection trap ▪ gloves ▪ handheld resuscitation bag with reservoir and mask ▪ suction equipment ▪ sterile distilled water ▪ equipment for arterial blood gas (ABG) analysis ▪ vital signs monitoring equipment ▪ stethoscope ▪ disinfectant pad ▪ pulse oximeter and probe ▪ capnography device ▪ cardiac monitoring equipment ▪ oral care supplies ▪ emergency resuscitation equipment (code cart with emergency medications, defibrillator, intubation equipment) ▪ ET tube securement supplies (tape, securement device or skin-barrier product, hydrocolloid dressing, or soft silicone dressing) ▪ Optional: prescribed sedative, neuromuscular blocking agent, and other medications; gown, mask and goggles or mask with face shield; peripheral nerve stimulation equipment; communication board; eye covering; eye lubricant; exhaled carbon dioxide detector

Mechanical ventilation terminology

Make sure you're familiar with the following mechanical ventilation terminologies:

Assist-control mode: The ventilator delivers a preset tidal volume (V_T) at a preset rate; however, the patient can initiate additional breaths, which trigger the ventilator to deliver the preset V_T at positive pressure.[1]

Continuous positive airway pressure (CPAP): This setting prompts the ventilator to deliver positive pressure to the airway throughout the respiratory cycle. It works only on patients who can breathe spontaneously.[3]

Control mode: The ventilator delivers all of the patient's minute ventilation with a preset V_T at a fixed rate, regardless of whether the patient is breathing spontaneously. This mode isn't a standard mode on modern ventilators.[1]

Fraction of inspired oxygen (FIO₂): This is the percentage of oxygen delivered to the patient by the ventilator. The dial or digital display on the ventilator that sets this percentage is labeled OXYGEN CONCENTRATION or OXYGEN PERCENTAGE. You should use the lowest possible FIO_2 to meet the patient's oxygenation goal.[2]

Inspiratory-expiratory (I:E) ratio: This ratio compares the duration of inspiration to the duration of expiration. The I:E ratio of normal, spontaneous breathing is 1:2, meaning that expiration is twice as long as inspiration.[3]

Inspiratory flow rate (IFR): The IFR denotes the V_T delivered within a certain time. Its value can range from 20 to 120 L/minute. You should adjust the ventilator to meet or exceed the IFR on the patient's spontaneous breaths.[3]

Minute ventilation or minute volume (VE): This measurement results from the multiplication of respiratory rate and V_T. Minute ventilation is equivalent to the total volume per minute entering and exiting the lungs.[3]

Peak inspiratory pressure (PIP): Measured by the pressure manometer on the ventilator, PIP reflects the amount of pressure required to deliver a preset V_T. It's the highest pressure produced during inspiration.[3]

Plateau pressure: Airway pressure measured after a 0.5 second pause at the end of inspiration, plateau pressure indicates the stiffness of the lungs.[3]

Positive end-expiratory pressure (PEEP): In PEEP mode, the ventilator is set to maintain positive pressure at the end of each expiration to increase the area for oxygen exchange by helping to inflate and keep open collapsed alveoli. The practitioner typically initiates PEEP at 5 cm H_2O but possibly as high as 24 cm H_2O in acute respiratory distress syndrome (ARDS).[2,4]

Pressure support: A ventilator adjunct, pressure support delivers positive pressure, supplementing the spontaneous breath of a patient on the ventilator. It's used to reduce the work of breathing associated with the artificial airway or increase the volume of the patient's spontaneous breath.[3]

Respiratory rate: The number of breaths per minute delivered by the ventilator; also called *frequency*. The rate set is dependent on the patient's condition and the ventilator mode, but it's typically 12 to 16 breaths per minute.[2]

Sensitivity setting: A setting that determines the amount of effort the patient must exert to trigger the inspiratory cycle.[3]

Sigh volume: A ventilator-delivered breath that's 1¼ times as large as the patient's V_T.

Synchronized intermittent mandatory ventilation (SIMV): The ventilator delivers a preset number of breaths at a specific V_T. The patient's own breaths may supplement these mechanical ventilations, in which case the patient's inspiratory ability determines the V_T and rate.[1]

Tidal volume (VT): This refers to the volume of air delivered to the patient with each cycle, usually 8 to 10 mL/kg. Low V_T ventilation of 6 to 8 mL/kg predicted body weight has been associated with decreased mortality and improved outcomes in patients with acute respiratory failure and ARDS.[2]

---

or esophageal carbon dioxide detector; replacement inserts or filters for heat and moisture exchangers; positive end-expiratory pressure (PEEP) valve for resuscitation bag.

Preparation of equipment

Inspect all equipment and supplies. If a product is expired, is defective, or has compromised integrity, remove it from use, label it as expired or defective, and report the expiration or defect, as directed by your facility. In most facilities, respiratory therapists assume responsibility for setting up a ventilator. If necessary, however, check the manufacturer's instructions for setting it up. In some cases, you'll need to add sterile distilled water to the humidifier and connect the ventilator to the appropriate gas source.

Plug the ventilator into an emergency electrical outlet (with generator backup) and turn it on. Adjust the settings on the ventilator, as ordered. Make sure the ventilator's alarms are set appropriately for the ventilator settings and the patient's current condition, and that the alarms are turned on, functioning properly, and audible to staff.[5,6,7] Make sure that the humidifier is filled with sterile distilled water, and that the heated humidifier is set to deliver an inspired gas temperature of greater than or equal to 93.2° F (34° C) but less than 105.8° F (41° C) at the circuit Y-piece and provide a minimum of 33 mg/L of water vapor.[8]

Attach a capnography device to measure carbon dioxide levels *to confirm placement of the ET tube and detect any disconnection from the ventilator or other complications.*[9]

Make sure that emergency equipment is functioning properly and readily available *in case the ventilator malfunctions or the patients is extubated accidently.*

Implementation

- Verify the practitioner's order.
- If the patient isn't already intubated, prepare the patient for intubation.
- Gather and prepare the necessary equipment and supplies.
- Perform hand hygiene.[10,11,12,13,14,15]
- Confirm the patient's identity using at least two patient identifiers.[16]

- Provide privacy.[17,18,19,20]
- When possible, explain the procedure to the patient and family (if appropriate) according to their individual communication and learning needs *to increase their understanding, allay their fears, and enhance cooperation.*[21] Assure them that staff members are nearby to provide care.
- Make sure the patient is being adequately oxygenated.
- Raise the patient's bed to waist level before providing patient care *to prevent caregiver back strain.*[22]
- Perform hand hygiene.[10,11,12,13,14,15]
- Put on gloves and other personal protective equipment as needed *to comply with standard precautions.*[23,24,25,26]
- As the patient's condition allows, perform a complete physical assessment and obtain blood for ABG analysis *to establish baselines for comparison.*
- Assist with intubation (if necessary) and then connect the ET tube to the ventilator circuit. Trace the ventilator circuit from the patient to its point of origin *to make sure it's connected properly.*[27,28]
- Observe for chest expansion and auscultate for bilateral breath sounds *to verify that the patient is being ventilated.*[23]
- Apply a skin barrier product, hydrocolloid dressing, or soft silicone dressing to the skin *to prevent skin breakdown*, and then tape the tube securely *to prevent accidental dislodgement.* Alternatively, use an ET tube securement device.[1,29]
- Monitor the patient's oxygen saturation level by pulse oximetry; make sure that the alarm limits are set appropriately for the patient's current condition, and that the alarms are turned on, functioning properly, and audible to staff.[5,6,7,30]
- Use waveform capnography, an exhaled-carbon dioxide detector, or an esophageal detector device in addition to a chest X-ray *to confirm ET tube placement.*[31,32]
- Position the patient with the head of the bed elevated 30 to 45 degrees, unless contraindicated by the patient's condition, *to reduce the risk of aspiration and consequent ventilator-associated pneumonia (VAP).* If the patient can't bend at the waist, use a reverse Trendelenburg position.[33]
- Suction the patient's airway when necessary *to maintain airway patency by removing accumulated pulmonary secretions.*[32] Before performing

suctioning, hyperoxygenate the patient, as needed, with 100% oxygen for 30 to 60 seconds. Suction the patient with a closed-suction catheter, limiting suctioning to 15 seconds. After suctioning, hyperoxygenate the patient for at least 1 minute using the same technique you used before suctioning.[32]

■ Observe the amount and consistency of the patient's secretions.

■ Monitor the patient's ABG values after the initial ventilator setup, after changes in ventilator settings, and as the patient's condition indicates, if ordered, *to determine whether the patient is being adequately ventilated and to avoid oxygen toxicity*. Be prepared to adjust ventilator settings based on ABG analysis. Notify the practitioner of critical test results within your facility's established time frame *so the patient can receive prompt treatment*.[34]

■ Check the ventilator tubing frequently for condensation, *which can cause resistance to airflow and which the patient may aspirate*. As needed, drain the condensate into a collection trap. Keep the circuit closed during condensate drainage *to prevent bacterial contamination*. Don't drain the condensate into the humidifier, *because the condensate may be contaminated with the patient's secretions*. Also avoid accidental drainage of condensation into the patient's airway when moving the tubing or the patient, *because condensate is considered infectious waste*.[8,23]

■ Inspect heat and moisture exchangers, and replace inserts or filters contaminated by secretions.

■ Check the in-line thermometer *to make sure the temperature of the air delivered to the patient is close to body temperature*.

■ If you're using a heated humidifier, monitor the inspired air temperature as close to the patient's airway as possible. The heated humidifier should be set to deliver an inspired gas temperature of 93.2° F (34° C) or above, but less than 105.8° F (41° C), with a 109.4° F (43° C) over-limit temperature, and the low temperature alarm should be set no lower than 3.6° F (2° C) below the desired temperature at the circuit Y-piece.[8]

■ Change, clean, or dispose of the ventilator tubing and equipment when it's visibly soiled or malfunctioning, or at an interval determined by your facility, *to reduce the risk of bacterial contamination*.[8,23]

■ Monitor the patient's vital signs and respiratory status at an interval determined by the patient's condition and your facility. When monitoring the patient's vital signs, count spontaneous breaths as well as ventilator-delivered breaths.

■ Provide emotional support to the patient during all phases of mechanical ventilation *to reduce anxiety and promote successful treatment*. Even if the patient is unresponsive, continue to explain all procedures and treatments.

■ Confirm that the ventilator alarms are set appropriately for the patient's current condition. Make sure that the alarms are turned on, functioning, and audible to staff.[5,6,7,30]

■ Unless contraindicated, turn the patient from side to side every 1 to 2 hours *to facilitate lung expansion and removal of secretions*, and perform active or passive range-of-motion exercises for all extremities *to reduce the hazards of immobility*.

■ Assess the patient's peripheral circulation, and monitor intake and output *to assess for signs of decreased cardiac output*. Watch for signs and symptoms of fluid volume excess or dehydration.

■ Brush the patient's teeth, gums, and tongue at least twice a day using a soft toothbrush *to prevent VAP*.[35,36]

■ Use a chlorhexidine rinse twice daily, as prescribed, *to reduce colonization of the oropharynx and prevent subsequent VAP*.[35,36,37] For a patient undergoing cardiac surgery, use the rinse before intubation and postoperatively twice a day.[35]

■ Moisten the patient's lips and oral mucosa every 2 to 4 hours *to reduce oral inflammation and improve oral health*.[35,36]

■ Institute measures to prevent venous thromboembolism (VTE) and peptic ulcer disease (PUD), if prescribed.[36]

NURSING ALERT Make sure that you follow evidence-based infection-prevention techniques (such as performing hand hygiene, providing oral care, positioning the patient with the head of the bed elevated 30 to 45 degrees) when caring for the patient receiving mechanical ventilation *to reduce the risk of VAP*.[23,38]

■ Place the call light within the patient's reach, and establish a method of communication, such as a communication board, *because intubation and mechanical ventilation impair the patient's ability to speak*.[1]

■ Administer and titrate the patient's sedative or neuromuscular blocking agent as ordered following safe medication administration practices.[39,40,41,42] Maintain target sedation levels *to avoid oversedation*.[43] Remember that the patient receiving a neuromuscular blocking agent requires close observation, such as by using peripheral nerve stimulation, *because of the inability to breathe spontaneously or communicate*.[1] (See the "Peripheral nerve stimulation" procedure.)

■ Return the bed to the lowest position *to prevent falls and maintain patient safety*.[44]

■ Take steps to ensure the patient's safety, such as raising the side rails of the bed while turning the patient, and covering and lubricating the patient's eyes.

■ Discard used supplies in the appropriate receptacle.[26]

■ Remove and discard your gloves and any other personal protective equipment.[24,26]

■ Perform hand hygiene.[10,11,12,13,14,15]

■ Clean and disinfect your stethoscope using a disinfectant pad.[45,46]

■ Perform hand hygiene.[10,11,12,13,14,15]

■ Document the procedure.[47,48,49,50]

Special considerations

■ If signs of respiratory distress or hypoxemia develop, or if an alarm sounds and you can't easily identify the problem, disconnect the patient from the ventilator and use a handheld resuscitation bag to ventilate the patient. (See *Responding to ventilator alarms*.)

■ In a postoperative patient, screen for and assess for pain using facility-defined criteria that are consistent with the patient's age, condition, and ability to understand. Treat the patient's pain, as needed and ordered, using nonpharmacologic or pharmacologic approaches or a combination of approaches. Base the treatment plan on evidence-based practices and the patient's clinical condition, past medical history, and pain management goals.[51]

■ If the patient is receiving enteral feedings, position the patient with the head of the bed elevated 30 to 45 degrees, unless contraindicated by the patient's condition, *to reduce the risk of aspiration*.[52]

Complications

Mechanical ventilation can cause damage to lungs as well as hemodynamic changes within in the body. Complications include lung injuries, pneumothorax, pneumomediastinum, pneumopericardium, pneumoperitoneum, and subcutaneous emphysema. Positive pressure ventilation reduces venous return and increases pulmonary vascular resistance, which can decrease cardiac output. Ventilator-associated pneumonia may also occur.[1,33] Gastric bleeding from stress ulcers is also a potential complication.[2]

Documentation

Document the date and time of initiation of mechanical ventilation. Name the type of ventilator you used for the patient and note its settings. Record the artificial airway type and size, the method used to secure the airway, and the tube's location (such as oral, nasal, or tracheal.) Describe the patient's response to mechanical ventilation, including vital signs, breath sounds, assessment findings, and oxygen saturation levels. List any complications and nursing interventions you took and the patient's response to those interventions. Record all pertinent laboratory data, including ABG analysis results. Describe the patient's LOC, respiratory effort, and skin color. Note the patient's need for suctioning and the color and amount of secretions. Document interventions, such as head-of-bed elevation, oral care, sedation interruption, and weaning. Record the patient's response to these interventions. Document teaching you provided to the patient and family (if applicable), their understanding of that teaching, and any need for follow-up teaching.

If the patient was receiving pressure-support ventilation (PSV) or using a T-piece or tracheostomy collar, note the duration of spontaneous breathing and the patient's ability to maintain the weaning schedule. If you're using intermittent mandatory ventilation with or without PSV, record the control breath rate, time of each breath reduction, and rate of spontaneous respirations.

TROUBLESHOOTING

RESPONDING TO VENTILATOR ALARMS

Ventilator alarms alert the nursing staff to potentially hazardous conditions and changes in the patient's status. Use this table as a guide to possible causes of ventilator alarms and how to respond.

SIGNAL	POSSIBLE CAUSE	NURSING INTERVENTIONS
Low-pressure alarm	■ Endotracheal (ET) tube disconnected from ventilator	■ Reconnect the ET tube to the ventilator.
	■ ET tube displaced above vocal cords or tracheostomy tube extubated	■ Check ET tube placement and reposition if needed. If extubation or displacement has occurred, ventilate the patient manually and call the practitioner immediately.
	■ Leaking tidal volume from low cuff pressure (from an underinflated or ruptured cuff or a leak in the cuff or one-way valve)	■ Listen for a whooshing sound around the ET tube, indicating an air leak. If you hear one, check cuff pressure. If you can't maintain pressure, call the practitioner, who may need to insert a new tube.
	■ Ventilator malfunction	■ Disconnect the patient from the ventilator and ventilate manually if necessary. Obtain another ventilator.
	■ Leak in ventilator circuitry (from loose connection or hole in tubing, loss of temperature-sensitive device, or cracked humidification device)	■ Make sure all connections are intact. Check for holes or leaks in the tubing and replace if necessary. Check the humidification device and replace if cracked.
High-pressure alarm	■ Increased airway pressure or decreased lung compliance caused by worsening disease	■ Auscultate breath sounds for evidence of increasing lung consolidation, barotrauma, or wheezing. Notify the practitioner if indicated.
	■ Patient biting on oral ET tube	■ Insert a bite block if needed. ■ Consider pain medication or sedation if appropriate.
	■ Secretions in airway	■ Look for secretions in the airway; suction the patient's airway or have the patient cough to remove secretions as necessary.
	■ Condensate in large-bore tubing	■ Check tubing for condensate and drain the condensate from the tubing as necessary.
	■ Intubation of right mainstem bronchus	■ Auscultate for diminished or absent breath sounds in the left lung fields.
	■ Patient coughing, gagging, or attempting to talk	■ Check tube position. If it has become displaced, call the practitioner, who may need to reposition it.
	■ Chest wall resistance	■ If the patient's breathing is asynchronous with the ventilator, the practitioner may order a sedative or neuromuscular blocking agent and sedative.
	■ Failure of high-pressure relief valve	■ Reposition the patient to improve chest expansion. ■ Administer the prescribed analgesic if needed following safe medication administration practices.[39,40,41,42] ■ Replace faulty equipment.
	■ Bronchospasm	■ Assess the patient to try to determine the cause. Report your findings to the practitioner, and treat the patient as ordered.

REFERENCES

1 Wiegand, D. L. (2017). *AACN procedure manual for high acuity, progressive, and critical care* (7th ed.). St. Louis, MO: Elsevier.

2 Hyzy, R. C., & McSparron, J. I. (2021). Overview of initiating invasive mechanical ventilation in adults in the intensive care unit. In: *UpToDate*, Parsons, P. E. (Ed.).

3 Kacmarek, R. M., et al. (2021). *Egan's fundamentals of respiratory care* (12th ed.). St. Louis, MO: Mosby.

4 ARDSnet. (n.d.). NIH NHLBI ARDS clinical network mechanical ventilation protocol summary. http://www.ardsnet.org/files/ventilator_protocol_2008-07.pdf (Level VII)

5 The Joint Commission. (2013). Sentinel event alert 50: Medical device alarm safety in hospitals. https://www.jointcommission.org/-/media/tjc/documents/resources/patient-safety-topics/sentinel-event/sea_50_alarms_4_26_16.pdf (Level VII)

6 Graham, K. C., & Cvach, M. (2010). Monitor alarm fatigue: Standardizing use of physiological monitors and decreasing nuisance alarms. *American Journal of Critical Care, 19*, 28–37.

7 The Joint Commission. (2021). Standard NPSG.06.01.01. *Comprehensive accreditation manual for hospitals.* Oakbrook Terrace, IL: The Joint Commission. (Level VII)

8 Restrepo, R. D., & Walsh, B. K. (2012). AARC clinical practice guideline: Humidification during invasive and noninvasive mechanical ventilation, 2012. *Respiratory Care, 57*(5), 782–788. http://rc.rcjournal.com/content/respcare/57/5/782.full.pdf (Level VII)

9 American Heart Association. (2020). 2020 American Heart Association Guidelines for CPR and ECC– Part 3: Adult Basic and Advances Life Support: Advanced Techniques for Resuscitation. https://cpr.heart.org/en/resuscitation-science/cpr-and-ecc-guidelines

10 The Joint Commission. (2021). Standard NPSG.07.01.01. *Comprehensive accreditation manual for hospitals.* Oakbrook Terrace, IL: The Joint Commission. (Level VII)

11 Centers for Disease Control and Prevention. (2002). Guideline for hand hygiene in health-care settings: Recommendations of the Healthcare Infection Control Practices Advisory Committee and the HICPAC/SHEA/APIC/IDSA Hand Hygiene Task Force. *MMWR Recommendations*

and Reports, 51(RR-16), 1–45. https://www.cdc.gov/mmwr/pdf/rr/rr5116.pdf (Level II)

12 World Health Organization. (2009). WHO guidelines on hand hygiene in health care: First global patient safety challenge, clean care is safer care. https://apps.who.int/iris/bitstream/handle/10665/44102/9789241597906_eng.pdf?sequence=1 (Level IV)

13 Centers for Medicare and Medicaid Services, Department of Health and Human Services. (2020). Condition of participation: Infection control. 42 C.F.R. § 482.42.

14 Accreditation Association for Hospitals and Health Systems. (2020). Standard 07.01.21. *Healthcare Facilities Accreditation Program: Accreditation requirements for acute care hospitals.* Chicago, IL: Accreditation Association for Hospitals and Health Systems. (Level VII)

15 DNV GL-Healthcare USA, Inc. (2020). IC.1.SR.1. *NIAHO® accreditation requirements, interpretive guidelines and surveyor guidance—revision 20.0.* Milford, OH: DNV GL-Healthcare USA, Inc. (Level VII)

16 The Joint Commission. (2021). Standard NPSG.01.01.01. *Comprehensive accreditation manual for hospitals.* Oakbrook Terrace, IL: The Joint Commission. (Level VII)

17 The Joint Commission. (2021). Standard RI.01.01.01. *Comprehensive accreditation manual for hospitals.* Oakbrook Terrace, IL: The Joint Commission. (Level VII)

18 Centers for Medicare and Medicaid Services, Department of Health and Human Services. (2020). Condition of participation: Patient's rights. 42 C.F.R. § 482.13(c)(1).

19 Accreditation Association for Hospitals and Health Systems. (2020). Standard 15.01.16. *Healthcare Facilities Accreditation Program: Accreditation requirements for acute care hospitals.* Chicago, IL: Accreditation Association for Hospitals and Health Systems. (Level VII)

20 DNV GL-Healthcare USA, Inc. (2020). PR.2.SR.5. *NIAHO® accreditation requirements, interpretive guidelines and surveyor guidance—revision 20.0.* Milford, OH: DNV GL-Healthcare USA, Inc. (Level VII)

21 The Joint Commission. (2021). Standard PC.02.01.21. *Comprehensive accreditation manual for hospitals.* Oakbrook Terrace, IL: The Joint Commission. (Level VII)

22 Waters, T. R., et al. (2009). Safe patient handling training for schools of nursing. https://www.cdc.gov/niosh/docs/2009-127/pdfs/2009-127.pdf (Level VII)

23 Centers for Disease Control and Prevention. (2004). Guidelines for preventing health-care–associated pneumonia, 2003: Recommendations of CDC and the Healthcare Infection Control Practices Advisory Committee. *MMWR Recommendations and Reports, 53*(RR-3), 1–32. https://www.cdc.gov/mmwr/pdf/rr/rr5303.pdf (Level II)

24 Siegel, J. D., et al. (2007, revised 2019). 2007 guideline for isolation precautions: Preventing transmission of infectious agents in healthcare settings. https://www.cdc.gov/infectioncontrol/pdf/guidelines/isolation-guidelines-H.pdf (Level II)

25 Accreditation Association for Hospitals and Health Systems. (2020). Standard 07.01.10. *Healthcare Facilities Accreditation Program: Accreditation requirements for acute care hospitals.* Chicago, IL: Accreditation Association for Hospitals and Health Systems. (Level VII)

26 Occupational Safety and Health Administration. (2012). Bloodborne pathogens, standard number 1910.1030. https://www.osha.gov/pls/oshaweb/owadisp.show_document?p_id=10051&p_table=STANDARDS (Level VII)

27 U.S. Food and Drug Administration. (2017). Examples of medical device misconnections. https://www.fda.gov/medical-devices/medical-device-connectors/examples-medical-device-misconnections

28 The Joint Commission. (2014). Sentinel event alert 53: Managing risk during transition to new ISO tubing connector standards. https://www.jointcommission.org/-/media/tjc/documents/resources/patient-safety-topics/sentinel-event/sea_53_connectors_8_19_14_final.pdf (Level VII)

29 LeBlanc, K., et al. (2013). International skin tear advisory panel: A tool kit to aid in the prevention, assessment, and treatment of skin tears using a simplified classification system. *Advances in Skin and Wound Care, 26,* 459–476. (Level IV)

30 American Association of Critical-Care Nurses. (2018). AACN practice alert: Managing alarms in acute care across the life span—electrocardiography and pulse oximetry. https://www.aacn.org/clinical-resources/practice-alerts/managing-alarms-in-acute-care-across-the-life-span (Level VII)

31 Walsh, B. K., et al. (2011). Capnography/capnometry during mechanical ventilation, 2011. *Respiratory Care, 56*(4), 503–509. http://rc.rcjournal.com/content/respcare/56/4/503.full.pdf (Level VII)

32 American Association for Respiratory Care. (2010). AARC clinical practice guidelines: Endotracheal suctioning of mechanically ventilated patients with artificial airways 2010. *Respiratory Care, 55*(6), 758–764. http://rc.rcjournal.com/content/respcare/55/6/758.full.pdf (Level VII)

33 American Association of Critical-Care Nurses. (2017). AACN practice alert: Ventilator associated pneumonia. https://www.aacn.org/clinical-resources/practice-alerts/ventilator-associated-pneumonia-vap (Level VII)

34 The Joint Commission. (2021). Standard NPSG.02.03.01. *Comprehensive accreditation manual for hospitals.* Oakbrook Terrace, IL: The Joint Commission. (Level VII)

35 American Association of Critical-Care Nurses. (2017). AACN practice alert: Oral care for acutely and critically ill patients. https://www.aacn.org/clinical-resources/practice-alerts/oral-care-for-acutely-and-critically-ill-patients (Level VII)

36 Accreditation Association for Hospitals and Health Systems. (2020). Standard 07.01.02. *Healthcare Facilities Accreditation Program: Accreditation requirements for acute care hospitals.* Chicago, IL: Accreditation Association for Hospitals and Health Systems. (Level VII)

37 Hillier, B., et al. (2013). Preventing ventilator-associated pneumonia through oral care, product selection, and application method: A literature review. *AACN Advanced Critical Care, 24,* 38–58. (Level I)

38 Klompas, M., et al. (2014). Strategies to prevent ventilator-associated pneumonia in acute care hospitals: 2014 update. *Infection Control and Hospital Epidemiology, 35*(8), 915–936. https://www.jstor.org/stable/pdf/10.1086/677144.pdf?refreqid=excelsior%3A05d9aad-de774900c567534d3dbc7bf2e (Level I)

39 Centers for Medicare and Medicaid Services, Department of Health and Human Services. (2020). Condition of participation: Nursing services. 42 C.F.R. § 482.23(c).

40 Accreditation Association for Hospitals and Health Systems. (2020). Standard 16.01.03. *Healthcare Facilities Accreditation Program: Accreditation requirements for acute care hospitals.* Chicago, IL: Accreditation Association for Hospitals and Health Systems. (Level VII)

41 The Joint Commission. (2021). Standard MM.06.01.01. *Comprehensive accreditation manual for hospitals.* Oakbrook Terrace, IL: The Joint Commission. (Level VII)

42 DNV GL-Healthcare USA, Inc. (2020). MM.1.SR.3. *NIAHO® accreditation requirements, interpretive guidelines and surveyor guidance—revision 20.0.* Milford, OH: DNV GL-Healthcare USA, Inc. (Level VII)

43 Grap, M. J., et al. (2012). Sedation in adults receiving mechanical ventilation: Physiological and comfort outcomes. *American Journal of Critical Care, 21*(3), e53–e64. https://www.ncbi.nlm.nih.gov/pmc/articles/PMC3703630/ (Level VI)

44 Ganz, D. A., et al. (2013, reviewed 2021). Preventing falls in hospitals: A toolkit for improving quality of care (AHRQ publication no. 13-0015-EF). https://www.ahrq.gov/professionals/systems/hospital/fallpxtoolkit/index.html (Level VII)

45 Rutala, W. A., et al. (2008, revised 2019). Guideline for disinfection and sterilization in healthcare facilities, 2008. https://www.cdc.gov/infectioncontrol/pdf/guidelines/disinfection-guidelines-H.pdf (Level I)

46 Accreditation Association for Hospitals and Health Systems. (2020). Standard 07.02.03. *Healthcare Facilities Accreditation Program: Accreditation requirements for acute care hospitals.* Chicago, IL: Accreditation Association for Hospitals and Health Systems. (Level VII)

47 The Joint Commission. (2021). Standard RC.01.03.01. *Comprehensive accreditation manual for hospitals.* Oakbrook Terrace, IL: The Joint Commission. (Level VII)

48 Centers for Medicare and Medicaid Services, Department of Health and Human Services. (2020). Condition of participation: Medical record services. 42 C.F.R. § 482.24(b).

49 Accreditation Association for Hospitals and Health Systems. (2020). Standard 10.00.03. *Healthcare Facilities Accreditation Program: Accreditation requirements for acute care hospitals.* Chicago, IL: Accreditation Association for Hospitals and Health Systems. (Level VII)

50 DNV GL-Healthcare USA, Inc. (2020). MR.2.SR.1. *NIAHO® accreditation requirements, interpretive guidelines and surveyor guidance—revision 20.0.* Milford, OH: DNV GL-Healthcare USA, Inc. (Level VII)

51 The Joint Commission. (2021). Standard PC.01.02.07. *Comprehensive accreditation manual for hospitals.* Oakbrook Terrace, IL: The Joint Commission. (Level VII)

52 Boullata, J. I., et al. (2017). ASPEN safe practices for enteral nutrition therapy. *Journal of Parenteral and Enteral Nutrition, 41,* 15–103. https://onlinelibrary.wiley.com/doi/full/10.1177/0148607116673053 (Level VII)

METERED-DOSE INHALER USE

A metered-dose inhaler (MDI) delivers topical medications to the respiratory tract, producing local and systemic effects.[1,2] The mucosal lining of the respiratory tract absorbs the inhalant almost immediately. Examples of common inhalants include bronchodilators, which improve airway patency and facilitate drainage of mucus; mucolytics, which attain a high local concentration to liquefy tenacious bronchial secretions; and corticosteroids, which decrease inflammation in the respiratory tract.[3]

The use of MDIs may be contraindicated in patients who can't form an airtight seal around the device and in those who lack the coordination or clear vision to assemble the device. Some patients use an MDI spacer to assist them with the airtight seal.[3] Specific inhalants may also be contraindicated.[4] For example, bronchodilators are contraindicated in patients with tachycardia or a history of cardiac arrhythmias associated with tachycardia.

Equipment

Prescribed MDI with mouthpiece ▪ stethoscope ▪ disinfectant pad ▪ Optional: gloves, MDI spacer, water for gargling, emesis basin.

Implementation

▪ Avoid distractions and interruptions when preparing and administering medication *to prevent medication errors.*[5,6]
▪ Verify the practitioner's order.[7,8,9,10]
▪ Reconcile the patient's medications when the practitioner prescribes a new medication *to help reduce the risk of medication errors, including omissions, duplications, dosing errors, and drug interactions.*
▪ Perform hand hygiene.[11,12,13,14,15,16]
▪ Gather and prepare the necessary equipment and supplies.
▪ Compare the medication label with the order in the patient's medical record.[7,8,9,10]
▪ Check the patient's medical record for an allergy or other contraindication to the medication. If an allergy or a contraindication exists, don't administer the medication; notify the practitioner.[7,8,9,10]
▪ Check the expiration date on the medication. If the medication has expired, return it to the pharmacy and obtain new medication.[7,8,9,10]
▪ Inspect the medication container and MDI visually for loss of integrity; don't administer the medication if integrity has been compromised.[7,8,9,10]
▪ Discuss any unresolved concerns about the medication with the practitioner.[7,8,9,10]
▪ Perform hand hygiene.[11,12,13,14,15,16]
▪ Confirm the patient's identity using at least two patient identifiers.[17]
▪ Provide privacy.[18,19,20,21]
▪ Explain the procedure to the patient and family members (if appropriate) according to their individual communication and learning needs *to increase their understanding, allay their fears, and enhance cooperation.*[22]
▪ Teach the patient who is using the medication for the first time about potential adverse reactions, and discuss any other concerns related to the medication.[7,8,9,10]
▪ Verify that the medication is being administered at the proper time, in the prescribed dose, and by the correct route *to reduce the risk of medication errors.*[7,8,9,10]
▪ If your facility uses bar code technology, use it as directed by your facility.
▪ Raise the patient's bed to waist level before providing care *to help prevent caregiver back strain.*[23]
▪ Perform hand hygiene.[11,12,13,14,15,16]
▪ Put on gloves, if needed, *to comply with standard precautions.*[24,25,26]
▪ Assess the patient's respiratory status, including respiratory rate, breath sounds, and accessory muscle use, *to obtain a baseline for comparison.*[27]
▪ Insert the metal stem of the prescribed MDI into the small hole on the flattened portion of the mouthpiece.
▪ Shake the prescribed MDI *to mix the medication and aerosol propellant.* Prime the MDI, as needed, according to the manufacturer's instructions. *Requirements for priming an MDI (spraying one or more puffs into the air before use) vary among devices and ensure that the MDI is ready to use and will dispense the correct amount of medication.*[28]

▪ Remove the mouthpiece cap. Attach the prescribed MDI to the spacer as indicated, making sure not to touch the mouthpiece. Note that some MDIs have a spacer built in.
▪ Instruct the patient to exhale fully and then place the prescribed MDI or spacer into the patient's mouth, and tell the patient to close the lips around it using a closed mouth technique (as shown below).[1,29,30] Alternatively, if directed by the practitioner, use an open-mouth technique by holding the prescribed MDI 1″ to 2″ (2.5 cm to 5 cm) in front of the patient's mouth.[29,30]

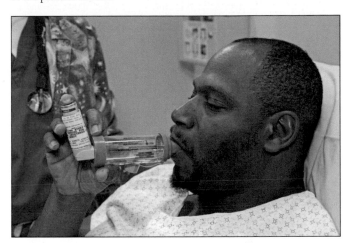

▪ Instruct the patient to press down on the prescribed MDI one time as the patient starts breathing in through the mouth slowly. (If a spacer is being used, instruct the patient to press down on the prescribed MDI first and then begin to breathe in slowly within 5 seconds.)
▪ Instruct the patient to continue breathing in slowly, as deeply as possible.[1] *This action draws the medication into the lungs.*
▪ Remove the mouthpiece from the patient's mouth, and instruct the patient to hold the breath and count to 10 slowly, if possible, *to allow the medication to reach the alveoli.*[1,28]
▪ Instruct the patient to exhale slowly through pursed lips *to keep the distal bronchioles open, allowing increased absorption and diffusion of the drug and better gas exchange.*
▪ When inhaled corticosteroids (such as beclomethasone, budesonide, ciclesonide, flunisolide, fluticasone, and triamcinolone) are administered, instruct the patient to rinse and gargle with water and then to expectorate using an emesis basin, if necessary, after each dose *to help prevent an infection in the mouth.*[2,3,28]
▪ When inhaled quick-relief medications (beta$_2$-adrenergic agonists) are administered, the patient should wait about 15 to 30 seconds between inhalations. There's no need to wait between inhalations for other medications.
▪ When all the ordered inhalations have been administered, remove the spacer (if used) from the MDI, and wash the spacer and mouthpiece according to the manufacturer's instructions.
▪ Put the cap back on the prescribed MDI after each use. Store the MDI and spacer, if used, with the patient's medication.
▪ Assess the patient's respiratory status, including respiratory rate, breath sounds, and accessory muscle use after medication administration *to determine the response to the medication.*[27]
▪ Allow the patient to gargle with water, if desired, *to remove the medication from the mouth and the back of the throat.*
▪ Return the bed to the lowest position *to prevent falls and maintain patient safety.*[31]
▪ Remove and discard your gloves, if worn.[24,26]
▪ Perform hand hygiene.[11,12,13,14,15,16]
▪ Clean and disinfect your stethoscope using a disinfectant pad.[32,33]
▪ Perform hand hygiene.[11,12,13,14,15,16]
▪ Document the procedure.[34,35,36,37]

Special considerations

▪ MDIs with spacers may be recommended *to provide greater therapeutic benefit for children and for patients who have difficulty with coordination.*

A spacer attachment is an extension to the MDIs mouthpiece that provides more dead-air space for mixing the medication. Some MDIs have built-in spacers.[4]

■ Some spacers have built-in whistles. If a whistling sound is heard, the patient is inhaling too fast or too strongly.[28]

Complications

Complications are related to the medication being administered by the MDI. Incorrect use of an MDI can cause overdosing or underdosing of the prescribed medication.[38]

Documentation

Document the medication strength, dose, and route of administration and the date and time of its administration. Document respiratory status findings before and after MDI use and the patient's response to treatment. Document any adverse reactions that occur, the date and time the practitioner was notified, any prescribed interventions, and the patient's response to those interventions.[39] Document any teaching provided to the patient and family (if applicable), their understanding of the teaching, and any need for follow-up teaching.

References

1 National Heart, Lung, and Blood Institute & National Asthma Education and Prevention Program. (2007). Expert panel report 3: Guidelines for the diagnosis and management of asthma (NIH publication no. 07-4051). https://www.ncbi.nlm.nih.gov/books/NBK7232/ (Level VII)

2 National Asthma Education and Prevention Program. (2013). How to use a metered-dose inhaler. https://www.nhlbi.nih.gov/files/docs/public/lung/asthma_tipsheets.pdf

3 American Academy of Allergy, Asthma and Immunology. (2020). Inhaled asthma medications. https://www.aaaai.org/conditions-and-treatments/library/asthma-library/inhaled-asthma-medications

4 Ari, A., & Restrepo, R. D. (2012). AARC clinical practice guideline: Aerosol delivery device selection for spontaneously breathing patients—2012. *Respiratory Care, 57*(4), 613–626. https://www.aarc.org/wp-content/uploads/2014/08/aerosol_delivery_2012.pdf (Level VII)

5 Westbrook, J., et al. (2010). Association of interruptions with an increased risk and severity of medication administration errors. *Archives of Internal Medicine, 170*, 683–690. (Level IV)

6 Institute for Safe Medication Practices. (2012). Side tracks on the safety express: Interruptions lead to errors and unfinished…Wait, what was I doing? *Nurse Advise-ERR, 11*(2), 1–4. https://www.ismp.org/resources/side-tracks-safety-express-interruptions-lead-errors-and-unfinished-wait-what-was-i-doing?id=37

7 The Joint Commission. (2021). Standard MM.06.01.01. *Comprehensive accreditation manual for hospitals.* Oakbrook Terrace, IL: The Joint Commission. (Level VII)

8 Centers for Medicare and Medicaid Services, Department of Health and Human Services. (2020). Condition of participation: Nursing services. 42 C.F.R. § 482.23(c).

9 Accreditation Association for Hospitals and Health Systems. (2020). Standard 16.01.03. *Healthcare Facilities Accreditation Program: Accreditation requirements for acute care hospitals.* Chicago, IL: Accreditation Association for Hospitals and Health Systems. (Level VII)

10 DNV GL-Healthcare USA, Inc. (2020). MM.1.SR.3. *NIAHO® accreditation requirements, interpretive guidelines and surveyor guidance—revision 20.0.* Milford, OH: DNV GL-Healthcare USA, Inc. (Level VII)

11 Centers for Disease Control and Prevention. (2002). Guideline for hand hygiene in health-care settings: Recommendations of the Healthcare Infection Control Practices Advisory Committee and the HICPAC/SHEA/APIC/IDSA Hand Hygiene Task Force. *MMWR Recommendations and Reports, 51*(RR-16), 1–45. https://www.cdc.gov/mmwr/pdf/rr/rr5116.pdf (Level II)

12 World Health Organization. (2009). WHO guidelines on hand hygiene in health care: First global patient safety challenge, clean care is safer care. https://apps.who.int/iris/bitstream/handle/10665/44102/9789241597906_eng.pdf?sequence=1 (Level IV)

13 The Joint Commission. (2021). Standard NPSG.07.01.01. *Comprehensive accreditation manual for hospitals.* Oakbrook Terrace, IL: The Joint Commission. (Level VII)

14 Centers for Medicare and Medicaid Services, Department of Health and Human Services. (2020). Condition of participation: Infection control. 42 C.F.R. § 482.42.

15 Accreditation Association for Hospitals and Health Systems. (2020). Standard 07.01.21. *Healthcare Facilities Accreditation Program: Accreditation requirements for acute care hospitals.* Chicago, IL: Accreditation Association for Hospitals and Health Systems. (Level VII)

16 DNV GL-Healthcare USA, Inc. (2020). IC.1.SR.1. *NIAHO® accreditation requirements, interpretive guidelines and surveyor guidance—revision 20.0.* Milford, OH: DNV GL-Healthcare USA, Inc. (Level VII)

17 The Joint Commission. (2021). Standard NPSG.01.01.01. *Comprehensive accreditation manual for hospitals.* Oakbrook Terrace, IL: The Joint Commission. (Level VII)

18 The Joint Commission. (2021). Standard RI.01.01.01. *Comprehensive accreditation manual for hospitals.* Oakbrook Terrace, IL: The Joint Commission. (Level VII)

19 Centers for Medicare and Medicaid Services, Department of Health and Human Services. (2020). Condition of participation: Patient's rights. 42 C.F.R. § 482.13(c)(1).

20 Accreditation Association for Hospitals and Health Systems. (2020). Standard 15.01.16. *Healthcare Facilities Accreditation Program: Accreditation requirements for acute care hospitals.* Chicago, IL: Accreditation Association for Hospitals and Health Systems. (Level VII)

21 DNV GL-Healthcare USA, Inc. (2020). PR.2.SR.5. *NIAHO accreditation requirements, interpretive guidelines and surveyor guidance—revision 20.0.* Milford, OH: DNV GL-Healthcare USA, Inc. (Level VII)

22 The Joint Commission. (2021). Standard PC.02.01.21. *Comprehensive accreditation manual for hospitals.* Oakbrook Terrace, IL: The Joint Commission. (Level VII)

23 Waters, T. R., et al. (2009). Safe patient handling training for schools of nursing. https://www.cdc.gov/niosh/docs/2009-127/pdfs/2009-127.pdf (Level VII)

24 Siegel, J. D., et al. (2007, revised 2019). 2007 guideline for isolation precautions: Preventing transmission of infectious agents in healthcare settings. https://www.cdc.gov/infectioncontrol/pdf/guidelines/isolation-guidelines-H.pdf (Level II)

25 Accreditation Association for Hospitals and Health Systems. (2020). Standard 07.01.10. *Healthcare Facilities Accreditation Program: Accreditation requirements for acute care hospitals.* Chicago, IL: Accreditation Association for Hospitals and Health Systems. (Level VII)

26 Occupational Safety and Health Administration. (2012). Bloodborne pathogens, standard number 1910.1030. https://www.osha.gov/pls/oshaweb/owadisp.show_document?p_id=10051&p_table=STANDARDS (Level VII)

27 Craven, R. F., et al. (2020). *Fundamentals of nursing: Concepts and competencies for practice.* (9th ed.). Philadelphia, PA: Wolters Kluwer.

28 American Thoracic Society. (2020). Patient information series: Using your metered dose inhaler (MDI). https://www.thoracic.org/patients/patient-resources/resources/metered-dose-inhaler-mdi.pdf

29 American College of Chest Physicians (2006). Using your MDI—Open-mouth technique. http://www.myallergyasthma.com/images/Open_Mouth_inhaler_method.pdf

30 Hess, D., & Dhand, R. (2020). The use of inhaler devices in adults. In: *UpToDate,* Bochner, B. S. (Ed).

31 Ganz, D. A., et al. (2013, reviewed 2021). *Preventing falls in hospitals: A toolkit for improving quality of care* (AHRQ publication no. 13-0015-EF). Rockville, MD: Agency for Healthcare Research and Quality. https://www.ahrq.gov/professionals/systems/hospital/fallpxtoolkit/index.html (Level VII)

32 Rutala, W. A., et al. (2008, revised 2019). Guideline for disinfection and sterilization in healthcare facilities, 2008. https://www.cdc.gov/infection-control/pdf/guidelines/disinfection-guidelines-H.pdf (Level I)

33 Accreditation Association for Hospitals and Health Systems. (2020). Standard 07.02.03. *Healthcare Facilities Accreditation Program: Accreditation requirements for acute care hospitals.* Chicago, IL: Accreditation Association for Hospitals and Health Systems. (Level VII)

34 The Joint Commission. (2021). Standard RC.01.03.01. *Comprehensive accreditation manual for hospitals.* Oakbrook Terrace, IL: The Joint Commission. (Level VII)

35 Centers for Medicare and Medicaid Services, Department of Health and Human Services. (2020). Condition of participation: Medical record services. 42 C.F.R. § 482.24(b).

36 Accreditation Association for Hospitals and Health Systems. (2020). Standard 10.00.03. *Healthcare Facilities Accreditation Program: Accreditation requirements for acute care hospitals.* Chicago, IL: Accreditation Association for Hospitals and Health Systems. (Level VII)

37 DNV GL Healthcare USA, Inc. (2020). MR.2.SR.1. *NIAHO accreditation requirements, interpretive guidelines and surveyor guidance—revision 20.0.* Milford, OH: DNV GL-Healthcare USA, Inc. (Level VII)

38 Cho-Reyes, S., et al. (2019). Inhalation technique errors with metered-dose inhalers among patients with obstructive lung diseases: A systematic review and meta-analysis of U.S. studies. *Chronic Obstructive Pulmonary Diseases, 6*(3), 267–280. https://journal.copdfoundation.org/jcopdf/id/1241/Inhalation-Technique-Errors-with-Metered-Dose-Inhalers-Among-Patients-with-Obstructive-Lung-Diseases-A-Systematic-Review-and-Meta-Analysis-of-US-Studies (Level I)

39 The Joint Commission. (2021). Standard RC.02.01.01. *Comprehensive accreditation manual for hospitals.* Oakbrook Terrace, IL: The Joint Commission. (Level VII)

MIXED VENOUS OXYGEN SATURATION MONITORING

Mixed venous oxygen saturation (SVO_2) monitoring involves the use of a fiberoptic thermodilution pulmonary artery (PA) catheter to continuously monitor oxygen delivery to tissues and oxygen consumption by tissues. Monitoring of SVO_2 allows rapid detection of impaired oxygen delivery, such as from decreased cardiac output, hemoglobin level, or arterial oxygen saturation. It also helps evaluate a patient's response to drug therapy, endotracheal tube suctioning, ventilator setting changes, positive end-expiratory pressure (PEEP), and fraction of inspired oxygen. SVO_2 usually ranges from 60% to 80%.[1]

NURSING ALERT Keep in mind that the Centers for Medicare and Medicaid Services considers vascular catheter–associated infection a hospital-acquired condition *because it can be reasonably prevented using a variety of best practices.* Make sure to follow evidence-based infection prevention techniques, such as performing hand hygiene, using sterile technique when accessing the device, and removing the catheter as soon as it's no longer necessary, *to reduce the risk of vascular catheter–associated infections.*[2,3,4,5,6,7]

Equipment

Fiberoptic PA catheter ▪ co-oximeter (monitor) ▪ optical module and cable ▪ gloves ▪ mixed venous blood sampling equipment ▪ laboratory biohazard bag ▪ label ▪ Optional: gown, protective eyewear, laboratory request form.

Preparation of equipment

Inspect all equipment and supplies. If a product is expired, is defective, or has compromised integrity, remove it from patient use, label it as expired or defective, and report the expiration or defect as directed by your facility.

Review the manufacturer's instructions for assembly and use of the fiberoptic PA catheter. Connect the optical module and cable to the monitor. Next, peel back the wrapping covering the catheter just enough to uncover the fiberoptic connector. Attach the fiberoptic connector to the optical module while allowing the rest of the catheter to remain in its sterile wrapping. Calibrate the fiberoptic catheter by following the manufacturer's instructions. Enter the patient's most recent hemoglobin level during the calibration process.[8]

To prepare for the rest of the procedure, follow the instructions for PA catheter insertion, as described in the "Pulmonary artery pressure and pulmonary artery occlusion pressure monitoring" procedure. (See *SVO_2 monitoring equipment*, page 548.)

Implementation

▪ Verify the practitioner's order.
▪ Gather and prepare the necessary equipment and supplies.
▪ Perform hand hygiene.[10,11,12,13,14,15]
▪ Confirm the patient's identity using at least two patient identifiers.[16]
▪ Provide privacy.[17,18,19,20]
▪ Explain the procedure to the patient and family (if appropriate) according to their individual communication and learning needs *to increase their understanding, allay their fears, and enhance cooperation.*[21]
▪ Raise the bed to waist level before providing care *to prevent caregiver back strain.*[22]
▪ Perform hand hygiene.[10,11,12,13,14,15]

▪ Put on gloves and other personal protective equipment, including a gown and protective eyewear, if indicated, *to comply with standard precautions.*[23,24]
▪ Assist with the insertion of the fiberoptic catheter just as you would for a PA catheter insertion.
▪ After the fiberoptic PA catheter is inserted, confirm that the light intensity tracing on the graphic printout is within normal range *to ensure correct positioning and function of the catheter.*
▪ Observe the digital readout and record the SVO_2 on the graph paper or as required by your facility. Repeat readings at least once each hour *to monitor and document trends.*
▪ Make sure the alarms limits are set appropriately for the patient's current condition, and that the alarms are turned on, functioning, and audible to staff.[25,26,27,28]

Recalibrating the monitor

▪ Trace the tubing from the patient to the point of origin *to make sure that you're accessing the correct port.*[29,30] Draw a mixed venous blood sample from the distal port of the PA catheter.
▪ Label the specimen in the presence of the patient *to prevent mislabeling.*[16] Place it in a laboratory biohazard transport bag and send it to the laboratory immediately with the appropriate laboratory request forms (if necessary).[24]
▪ Compare the laboratory's SVO_2 reading with that of the fiberoptic PA catheter. If the fiberoptic PA catheter SVO_2 values and the laboratory values differ by more than 4%, follow the manufacturer's instructions to enter the SVO_2 value obtained by the laboratory into the co-oximeter.
▪ Recalibrate the monitor every 24 hours and whenever the catheter has been disconnected from the optical module.

Completing the procedure

▪ Return the bed to the lowest position *to prevent falls and maintain patient safety.*[31]
▪ Remove and discard your gloves and other personal protective equipment, if worn.[24]
▪ Perform hand hygiene.[10,11,12,13,14,15]
▪ Document the procedure.[32,33,34,35]

Special considerations

▪ If the patient's SVO_2 drops below 60% or varies by more than 10% for 3 minutes or longer, reassess the patient. If the SVO_2 doesn't return to the baseline value after nursing interventions, notify the practitioner. *A decreasing SVO_2, or a value less than 60%, indicates impaired oxygen delivery, which can occur in hemorrhage, hypoxia, shock, sepsis, arrhythmias, and suctioning.* SVO_2 can also decrease as a result of increased oxygen demand from hyperthermia, shivering, and seizures.[1,8,36,37]
▪ If the intensity of the tracing is low, ensure that all connections between the catheter and co-oximeter are secure, and that the catheter is patent and not kinked.[1,38]
▪ If the tracing is damped or erratic, try to aspirate blood from the catheter *to check for patency.* If you can't aspirate blood, notify the practitioner *to replace the catheter.* Also check the PA waveform *to determine whether the catheter has wedged.*[1,9,38] If the catheter has wedged, ensure that the balloon is fully deflated, and turn the patient from side to side and instruct the patient to cough.[1] If the catheter remains wedged, notify the practitioner immediately.[1]

Complications

Potential complications may include catheter-related infection, catheter migration, and thromboembolism. Complications such as pneumothorax, hemothorax, or arrhythmias can occur during catheter placement.[1]

Documentation

Document the date and time of the SVO_2 value and place a waveform tracing in the documentation. Note significant changes in the patient's status, the name of the practitioner notified, the date and time of notification, prescribed interventions, and the patient's response to those interventions. For comparison, note the SVO_2 as measured by the fiberoptic PA catheter whenever a blood sample is obtained for laboratory

EQUIPMENT

SVO₂ monitoring equipment

A mixed venous oxygen saturation (SVO₂) monitoring system consists of a flow-directed pulmonary artery (PA) catheter with fiberoptic filaments, an optical module, and a co-oximeter. The co-oximeter displays a continuous digital SVO₂ value; the strip recorder prints a permanent record.

Catheter insertion follows the same technique as with any thermodilution flow-directed PA catheter. The distal lumen connects to an external PA pressure monitoring system, the proximal or central venous pressure lumen connects to another monitoring system or to a continuous flow administration unit, and the optical module connects to the co-oximeter unit.[9]

Normal SVO₂ waveform

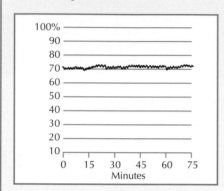

SVO₂ with patient activities

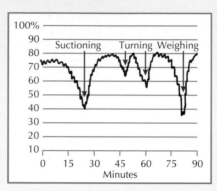

SVO₂ with positive end-expiratory pressure (PEEP) and fraction of inspired oxygen (FIO₂) changes

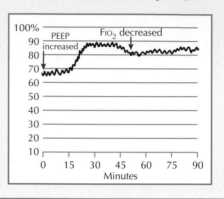

analysis of SVO₂. Document teaching provided to the patient and family (if applicable), their understanding of that teaching, and any need for follow-up teaching.

REFERENCES

1 Wiegand, D. L. (2017). *AACN procedure manual for high acuity, progressive, and critical care* (7th ed.). St. Louis, MO: Elsevier.

2 Jarrett, N., & Callaham, M. (2016). Evidence-based guidelines for selected hospital-acquired conditions: Final report. https://www.cms.gov/Medicare/Medicare-Fee-for-Service-Payment/HospitalAcqCond/Downloads/2016-HAC-Report.pdf

3 Association of Professionals in Infection Control and Epidemiology (APIC). (2015). Guide to preventing central line-associated bloodstream infections. http://apic.org/Resource_/TinyMceFileManager/2015/APIC_CLABSI_WEB.pdf (Level IV)

4 Marschall, J., et al. (2014). SHEA/IDSA practice recommendation: Strategies to prevent central line-associated bloodstream infections in acute care hospitals. *Infection Control and Hospital Epidemiology, 35,* 753–771. https://www.jstor.org/stable/10.1086/676533#metadata_info_tab_contents (Level I)

5 Centers for Disease Control and Prevention. (2011, revised 2017). Guidelines for the prevention of intravascular catheter-related infections, 2011. https://www.cdc.gov/infectioncontrol/pdf/guidelines/bsi-guidelines-H.pdf (Level I)

6 Standard 50. Infection. Infusion therapy standards of practice. (8th ed.) (2021). *Journal of Infusion Nursing, 44,* S153–S157. (Level VII)

7 The Joint Commission. (2021). Standard NPSG.07.04.01. *Comprehensive accreditation manual for hospitals.* Oakbrook Terrace, IL: The Joint Commission. (Level VII)

8 Edwards Lifesciences. (n.d.). Swan-Ganz pulmonary artery catheters. https://www.edwards.com/devices/hemodynamic-monitoring/swan-ganz-catheters

9 Edwards Lifesciences. (2018). *Edwards clinical education: Quick guide to cardiopulmonary care* (4th ed.). https://education.edwards.com/quick-guide-to-cardiopulmonary-care-4th-edition/220356#

10 The Joint Commission. (2021). Standard NPSG.07.01.01. *Comprehensive accreditation manual for hospitals.* Oakbrook Terrace, IL: The Joint Commission. (Level VII)

11 Centers for Disease Control and Prevention. (2002). Guideline for hand hygiene in health-care settings: Recommendations of the Healthcare Infection Control Practices Advisory Committee and the HICPAC/SHEA/APIC/IDSA Hand Hygiene Task Force. *MMWR Recommendations and Reports, 51*(RR-16), 1–45. https://www.cdc.gov/mmwr/pdf/rr/rr5116.pdf (Level II)

12 World Health Organization. (2009). WHO guidelines on hand hygiene in health care: First global patient safety challenge, clean care is safer care. https://apps.who.int/iris/bitstream/handle/10665/44102/9789241597906_eng.pdf?sequence=1 (Level IV)

13 Centers for Medicare and Medicaid Services, Department of Health and Human Services. (2020). Condition of participation: Infection control. 42 C.F.R. § 482.42.

14 Accreditation Association for Hospitals and Health Systems. (2020). Standard 07.01.21. *Healthcare Facilities Accreditation Program: Accreditation requirements for acute care hospitals.* Chicago, IL: Accreditation Association for Hospitals and Health Systems. (Level VII)

15 DNV GL-Healthcare USA, Inc. (2020). IC.1.SR.1. *NIAHO® accreditation requirements, interpretive guidelines and surveyor guidance—revision 20.0.* Milford, OH: DNV GL-Healthcare USA, Inc. (Level VII)

16 The Joint Commission. (2021). Standard NPSG.01.01.01. *Comprehensive accreditation manual for hospitals.* Oakbrook Terrace, IL: The Joint Commission. (Level VII)

17 The Joint Commission. (2021). Standard RI.01.01.01. *Comprehensive accreditation manual for hospitals.* Oakbrook Terrace, IL: The Joint Commission. (Level VII)

18 Centers for Medicare and Medicaid Services, Department of Health and Human Services. (2020). Condition of participation: Patient's rights. 42 C.F.R. § 482.13(c)(1).

19 Accreditation Association for Hospitals and Health Systems. (2020). Standard 15.01.16. *Healthcare Facilities Accreditation Program: Accreditation requirements for acute care hospitals.* Chicago, IL: Accreditation Association for Hospitals and Health Systems. (Level VII)

20 DNV GL-Healthcare USA, Inc. (2020). PR.2.SR.5. *NIAHO® accreditation requirements, interpretive guidelines and surveyor guidance—revision 20.0.* Milford, OH: DNV GL-Healthcare USA, Inc. (Level VII)

21 The Joint Commission. (2021). Standard PC.02.01.21. *Comprehensive accreditation manual for hospitals.* Oakbrook Terrace, IL: The Joint Commission. (Level VII)

22 Waters, T. R., et al. (2009). Safe patient handling training for schools of nursing. https://www.cdc.gov/niosh/docs/2009-127/pdfs/2009-127.pdf (Level VII)

23 Accreditation Association for Hospitals and Health Systems. (2020). Standard 07.01.10. *Healthcare Facilities Accreditation Program: Accreditation requirements for acute care hospitals.* Chicago, IL: Accreditation Association for Hospitals and Health Systems. (Level VII)

24 Occupational Safety and Health Administration. (2012). Bloodborne pathogens, standard number 1910.1030. https://www.osha.gov/pls/oshaweb/owadisp.show_document?p_id=10051&p_table=STANDARDS (Level VII)

25 American Association of Critical-Care Nurses. (2018). AACN practice alert: Managing alarms in acute care across the life span: Electrocardiography and pulse oximetry. https://www.aacn.org/clinical-resources/practice-alerts/managing-alarms-in-acute-care-across-the-life-span (Level VII)

26 The Joint Commission. (2013). Sentinel event alert: Medical device alarm safety in hospitals. https://www.jointcommission.org/-/media/tjc/documents/resources/patient-safety-topics/sentinel-event/sea_50_alarms_4_26_16.pdf (Level VII)

27 The Joint Commission. (2021). Standard NPSG.06.01.01. *Comprehensive accreditation manual for hospitals*. Oakbrook Terrace, IL: The Joint Commission. (Level VII)

28 Graham, K. C., & Cvach, M. (2010). Monitor alarm fatigue: Standardizing use of physiological monitors and decreasing nuisance alarms. *American Journal of Critical Care, 19*, 28–37.

29 U.S. Food and Drug Administration. (2017). Examples of medical device misconnections. https://www.fda.gov/medical-devices/medical-device-connectors/examples-medical-device-misconnections

30 The Joint Commission. (2014). Sentinel event alert: Managing risk during transition to new ISO tubing connector standards. https://www.jointcommission.org/-/media/tjc/documents/resources/patient-safety-topics/sentinel-event/sea_53_connectors_8_19_14_final.pdf (Level VII)

31 Ganz, D. A., et al. (2013, reviewed 2021). *Preventing falls in hospitals: A toolkit for improving quality of care* (AHRQ Publication No. 13-0015-EF). Rockville, MD: Agency for Healthcare Research and Quality. https://www.ahrq.gov/professionals/systems/hospital/fallpxtoolkit/index.html (Level VII)

32 The Joint Commission. (2021). Standard RC.01.03.01. *Comprehensive accreditation manual for hospitals*. Oakbrook Terrace, IL: The Joint Commission. (Level VII)

33 Centers for Medicare and Medicaid Services, Department of Health and Human Services. (2020). Condition of participation: Medical record services. 42 C.F.R. § 482.24(b).

34 Accreditation Association for Hospitals and Health Systems. (2020). Standard 10.00.03. *Healthcare Facilities Accreditation Program: Accreditation requirements for acute care hospitals*. Chicago, IL; Accreditation Association for Hospitals and Health Systems. (Level VII)

35 DNV GL-Healthcare USA, Inc. (2020). MR.2.SR.1. *NIAHO® accreditation requirements, interpretive guidelines and surveyor guidance—revision 20.0*. Milford, OH: DNV GL-Healthcare USA, Inc. (Level VII)

36 Rhodes, A., et al. (2017). Surviving sepsis campaign: International guidelines for management of severe sepsis and septic shock: 2016. *Critical Care Medicine, 45*, 486–552. (Level VII)

37 Lee, C., & Bora, V. (2021). Anesthesia monitoring of mixed venous saturation. https://www.ncbi.nlm.nih.gov/books/NBK539835/

38 Edwards Lifesciences. (2012). Vigilance II monitor: Quick reference guide. https://edwardsprod.blob.core.windows.net/media/De/devices/monitoring/hemodynamic%20monitoring/ar07822-vigilance_ii_monitor_sell-sheet_6x9alr.pdf

MODERATE SEDATION

Previously referred to as *conscious sedation*, moderate sedation is a drug-induced depression of consciousness in which the patient responds purposefully to verbal commands, either spontaneously or with light tactile stimulation. With moderate sedation, the patient can maintain a patent airway, protective reflexes (such as the ability to handle secretions without aspiration), adequate spontaneous ventilations, and cardiovascular function without interventions.[1,2]

Moderate sedation is commonly administered to relieve anxiety, discomfort, or pain so that patients can tolerate unpleasant procedures.[1] In children and uncooperative adults, it may be used to expedite procedures that aren't particularly uncomfortable but that require the patient to remain still.

Because predicting a patient's response to sedation isn't always possible, health care providers must have an understanding of the different levels of sedation. (See *Levels of sedation*, page 550.)

In addition to the health care practitioner administering moderate sedation, this procedure requires the presence of at least one other person capable of establishing a patent airway, administering positive pressure ventilation to the patient, and summoning additional assistance if necessary. A person with advanced life support skills should be immediately available.[1,4]

A patient receiving moderate sedation requires sedation monitoring before the procedure, throughout the procedure, and during the recovery period. Health care practitioners who are permitted by their scope of practice to administer moderate sedation should receive special training.[2,4,5,6]

Those administering the sedation and who are responsible for the patient's care should understand the pharmacology of the agents as well as the role of reversal agents. Those monitoring the patient receiving moderate sedation should be able to recognize associated complications, such as apnea and airway obstruction.[1] The health care practitioner responsible for monitoring a patient receiving moderate sedation or analgesia shouldn't have other responsibilities that would require leaving the patient unattended or that would compromise continuous monitoring during the procedure.[2,4]

Some patients who require a procedure may not be appropriate candidates for moderate sedation and may require anesthesia that's monitored by an anesthesia care provider. The American Society of Anesthesiologists (ASA) devised the ASA physical status classification system to provide a uniform guideline for evaluating the severity of systemic diseases, physiologic dysfunction, and anatomic abnormalities to determine a patient's risk of developing complications.[7] (See *ASA physical status classification system*, page 550.) Patients classified as ASA I, ASA II, and medically stable ASA III are commonly considered appropriate for registered nurse–administered moderate sedation.[4]

Moderate sedation is commonly administered for procedures that are performed in many settings outside the operating room, including GI procedure units, interventional radiology suites, bronchoscopy suites, emergency departments, interventional cardiology suites, and critical care units. Regardless of the location, adequately trained staff and appropriate monitoring equipment must be available to ensure the patient's safety.

Equipment

Facility-approved sedation scale ■ positive pressure oxygen delivery system ■ supplemental oxygen administration equipment[1] ■ suction apparatus ■ suction catheter ■ pulse oximeter and probe ■ vital signs monitoring equipment ■ capnometer ■ stethoscope ■ cardiac monitoring equipment ■ disinfectant pad ■ emergency equipment (code cart with emergency medications, defibrillator, handheld resuscitation bag with mask, and intubation equipment)[1,2] ■ prescribed medications and reversal agents ■ Optional: gloves and other personal protective equipment, IV catheter insertion equipment.

Preparation of equipment

Make sure the room where the patient will be receiving the sedation has all the necessary equipment, including emergency care supplies.[1,2,6] Make sure all emergency equipment is readily available and functioning properly.[6] Inspect all equipment and supplies *to ensure that they're in proper working order* before attaching them to the patient.[1] If a product is expired, is defective, or has compromised integrity, remove it from patient use, label it as expired or defective, and report the expiration or defect as directed by your facility.

Implementation

■ Avoid distractions and interruptions when preparing and administering medication *to prevent medication errors*.[9,10]

■ Verify the practitioner's order for the prescribed medication.[11,12,13,14]

■ Review the patient's medical record and verify documentation of pre-existing medical conditions; a history of tobacco, alcohol, or substance use or abuse; previous anesthesia and sedation experiences; history of a difficult airway; current medications; allergies; frequent or repeated exposure to sedation or analgesia agents; the last time the patient ate or had oral fluids; a recent height and weight (in metric units);[15] and physical examination findings, including evaluation of the airway, cardiac and respiratory assessments, and vital signs.[1,2,4,6,16,17]

NURSING ALERT Contact the anesthesia care provider if the patient has any of the following conditions: a history of respiratory or hemodynamic instability; one or more significant comorbidities; pregnancy; sleep apnea; inability to communicate or cooperate; multiple drug allergies; multiple medications with potential for drug interactions with sedative analgesia; or current substance abuse. Extra precautions may need to be taken with these patients, including additional monitoring and medication management.[4]

NURSING ALERT Patients with obesity have special needs during moderate sedation because they're at increased risk for complications *owing to altered physiology*. Consult with the anesthesia care provider.[1]

■ Check the patient's medical record for pregnancy test results, if applicable.[4]

■ Confirm that written informed consent has been obtained and that the signed consent form is in the patient's medical record.[2,4,6,18,19,20,21]

■ Conduct a preprocedure verification *to make sure that all relevant documentation, related information, and equipment are available and correctly identified to the patient's identifiers.*[22,23]

■ Verify that the laboratory studies have been completed as ordered and that the results are in the patient's medical record *to evaluate whether the results will affect the management of moderate sedation.* Notify the practitioner of any unexpected results.[1]

■ Compare the medication label with the order in the patient's medical record.[11,12,13,14]

■ Check the patient's medical record for allergy or a contraindication to the prescribed medication. If an allergy or a contraindication exists, don't administer the medication, and notify the practitioner.[11,12,13,14]

■ Check the expiration date on the medication. If the medication is expired, return it to the pharmacy and obtain new medication.[11,12,13,14]

■ Visually inspect the solution for particles or discoloration or other loss of integrity; don't administer the medication if its integrity is compromised.[11,12,13,14]

■ Discuss any unresolved concerns about the medication with the patient's practitioner.[11,12,13,14]

■ Perform hand hygiene.[24,25,26,27,28,29]

■ Confirm the patient's identity using at least two patient identifiers.[30]

■ Provide privacy.[31,32,33,34]

■ Verify the scheduled invasive procedure and the correct site as stated by the patient, and compare it with the medical record.[22]

■ Reinforce the practitioner's explanation of the sedation administration procedure to the patient and family (if appropriate) according to their individual communication and learning needs *to increase their understanding, allay their fears, and enhance cooperation.*[35] Answer their questions. Teach the patient and family about potential adverse reactions or other concerns related to the medication.[11,12,13,14]

■ If the patient is to be discharged after receiving sedation within a time frame determined by your facility (up to 24 hours after completion of the procedure), verify that arrangements have been made to transport the patient home, and that an adult will be available in case complications arise.[1,2]

■ Confirm the patient's nothing-by-mouth status before the procedure;[6] if the procedure is not an emergency, minimum fasting recommendations include 2 hours for clear liquids, 6 or more hours for a light meal or nonhuman milk, and 8 or more hours for fried or fatty foods or meat. If the need for the procedure is an emergency, collaborate with the practitioner to compare the risks and benefits of the procedure, considering the amount and type of liquids or solids ingested.[36]

■ Assess the patient for conditions that might make ventilation difficult, such as significant obesity, history of snoring or sleep apnea, facial hair, missing teeth, and stridor.[4]

■ When the patient is in the room where sedation will be administered, perform hand hygiene.[24,25,26,27,28,29]

■ Put on gloves and other personal protective equipment as needed *to comply with standard precautions.*[37,38]

■ Attach the patient to a pulse oximeter *to monitor the patient's oxygen saturation level.* Make sure that the alarm limits are set appropriately for the patient's current condition, and that the alarms are turned on, functioning properly, and audible to staff.[4,39,40,41,42,43]

■ Attach the patient to a cardiac monitor *to monitor heart rate and rhythm.*[4,39] Make sure that the alarm limits are set appropriately for the patient's current condition, and that the alarms are turned on, functioning properly, and audible to staff.[1,40,41,42,43]

■ Attach the patient to a capnometer *to continuously monitor exhaled carbon dioxide during the procedure.* Make sure that the alarm limits are set appropriately for the patient's current condition, and that alarms are turned on, functioning properly, and audible to staff.[1,4,6,39,40,41,42]

■ Obtain the patient's pulse, blood pressure, respiratory rate, exhaled carbon dioxide level by capnography, and oxygen saturation level, and assess level of consciousness (LOC), pain level, and anxiety level *to use as a baseline for comparison during and after the procedure.*[4,16]

■ Ensure that the patient has patent IV access. If a patent IV catheter isn't present, insert one.[1,6] (See the "IV catheter insertion and removal" procedure.)

Levels of sedation

Because a patient receiving sedation might not always respond as intended, make sure you can recognize the different levels of sedation. The American Society of Anesthesiologists describes levels of sedation as follows:[3]

■ **Minimal sedation (anxiolysis)** is a drug-induced state during which a patient responds normally to verbal commands. Cognitive function and physical coordination may be impaired, but airway reflexes and ventilatory and cardiovascular functions aren't affected.

■ **Moderate sedation/analgesia (conscious sedation)** is a drug-induced depression of consciousness during which a patient responds purposefully to verbal commands, unaided or accompanied by light tactile stimulation. (Reflex withdrawal from a painful stimulus isn't considered a purposeful response.) The patient doesn't require intervention to maintain a patent airway, has adequate spontaneous ventilation, and maintains cardiovascular function.

■ **Deep sedation/analgesia** is a drug-induced depression of consciousness during which a patient can't be easily aroused but responds purposefully to repeated or painful stimulation. The patient's ability to independently maintain ventilatory function may be impaired. The patient may require assistance to maintain a patent airway and may not have adequate spontaneous ventilation, but typically maintains cardiovascular function.

■ **General anesthesia** is a drug-induced loss of consciousness during which a patient can't be aroused, even by painful stimulation. The patient's ability to maintain ventilatory and cardiovascular function independently is typically impaired. The patient is likely to require assistance to maintain a patent airway, and may need positive pressure ventilation because of depressed spontaneous ventilation or drug-induced depression of neuromuscular function.

ASA physical status classification system

The American Society of Anesthesiologists (ASA) physical status classification system is widely used to estimate a patient's risk of developing complications.[8]

ASA I: normal, healthy patient
ASA II: patient with mild systemic disease
ASA III: patient with severe systemic disease
ASA IV: patient with severe systemic disease that's a constant threat to life
ASA V: moribund patient who isn't expected to survive without the procedure
ASA VI: patient declared brain dead whose organs are being removed for donation

■ Confirm that the procedure site has been marked appropriately by the practitioner, if indicated. Involve the patient in the process if possible.[23,44]

■ Confirm the medication dosage calculations based on the patient's weight or body surface area.

■ If your facility uses a bar-code technology, use it as directed by your facility.

■ After the patient is prepared and draped for the procedure, conduct a time-out immediately before starting the procedure *to perform a final assessment that the correct patient, site, positioning, and procedure are identified and, as applicable, all relevant information and necessary equipment are available.*[45]

NURSING ALERT Medications used for moderate sedation are considered high-alert medications *because they can cause significant patient harm when used in error.*[46,47]

■ Before administering moderate sedation, have another nurse perform an independent double-check *to verify the patient's identity and to make sure that the correct medication is being administered in the prescribed concentration, the medication's indication corresponds with the patient's diagnosis, the dosage calculations are correct and the dosing formula used to derive the final dose is correct, and the route of administration is safe and proper for the patient.*[48]

■ Compare the results of the independent double-check with the other nurse and, if no discrepancies exist, begin administering the medication. If discrepancies exist, rectify them before administering the medication.[48]

TROUBLESHOOTING

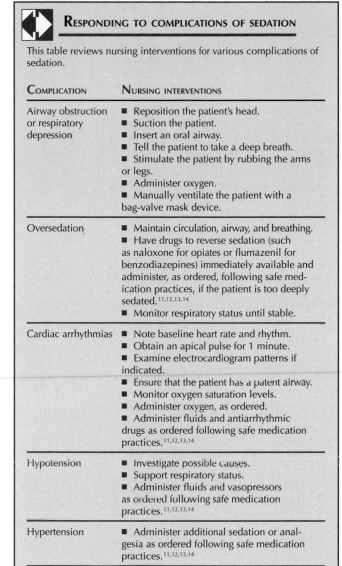

RESPONDING TO COMPLICATIONS OF SEDATION

This table reviews nursing interventions for various complications of sedation.

COMPLICATION	NURSING INTERVENTIONS
Airway obstruction or respiratory depression	■ Reposition the patient's head. ■ Suction the patient. ■ Insert an oral airway. ■ Tell the patient to take a deep breath. ■ Stimulate the patient by rubbing the arms or legs. ■ Administer oxygen. ■ Manually ventilate the patient with a bag-valve mask device.
Oversedation	■ Maintain circulation, airway, and breathing. ■ Have drugs to reverse sedation (such as naloxone for opiates or flumazenil for benzodiazepines) immediately available and administer, as ordered, following safe medication practices, if the patient is too deeply sedated.[11,12,13,14] ■ Monitor respiratory status until stable.
Cardiac arrhythmias	■ Note baseline heart rate and rhythm. ■ Obtain an apical pulse for 1 minute. ■ Examine electrocardiogram patterns if indicated. ■ Ensure that the patient has a patent airway. ■ Monitor oxygen saturation levels. ■ Administer oxygen, as ordered. ■ Administer fluids and antiarrhythmic drugs as ordered following safe medication practices.[11,12,13,14]
Hypotension	■ Investigate possible causes. ■ Support respiratory status. ■ Administer fluids and vasopressors as ordered following safe medication practices.[11,12,13,14]
Hypertension	■ Administer additional sedation or analgesia as ordered following safe medication practices.[11,12,13,14]

■ Administer each medication separately in incremental doses and titrate it to the desired effect following safe medication administration practices *to decrease the risk of overdose and respiratory and circulatory depression.*[4,11,12,13,14]

■ Continuously monitor the patient's heart rate and rhythm (using a cardiac monitor), oxygenation (using pulse oximetry), and respiratory rate and adequacy of ventilation (using continual observation of clinical status and capnography).[1,4,6,49]

■ Determine and evaluate the patient's blood pressure and heart rate at least every 5 minutes.[1,39,49]

■ Monitor the patient's LOC (by checking response to verbal commands when practical), depth of sedation (using a facility-approved sedation scale), comfort level, and skin condition at regular intervals.[1,4,49]

■ Administer supplemental oxygen, as ordered, unless specifically contraindicated for the patient's condition or the procedure.[1] Determine the method and rate of flow using the patient's optimal oxygen saturation level according to pulse oximetry.[4] *Hypoxemia may cause cardiopulmonary complications.*[4]

■ Monitor the patient's temperature when clinically significant changes in body temperature are intended, anticipated, or suspected.[39,49]

■ Monitor the patient for complications; intervene as indicated.[2,49]

■ When sedation administration is complete, use the same monitoring parameters used during the procedure and monitor the patient until discharge criteria are met. The patient should remain awake for at least 20 minutes without stimulation before being considered ready for discharge. The duration and frequency of monitoring should be individualized, depending on the level of sedation achieved, the patient's overall condition, and the nature of the procedure for which sedation was administered. If a reversal agent was given, monitor the patient for a sufficient time interval (for example, 2 hours) after the last administration of an antagonist *to make sure that the patient doesn't become resedated after the reversal effects have worn off.*[1,4]

■ Remove and discard your gloves and other personal protective equipment, if worn.[37]

■ Perform hand hygiene.[24,25,26,27,28,29]

■ Clean and disinfect your stethoscope using a disinfectant pad.[50,51]

■ Perform hand hygiene.[24,25,26,27,28,29]

■ Document the procedure.[52,53,54,55,56]

Special considerations

■ The State Board of Nursing may have guidelines about the registered nurses' role in administering moderate sedation or caring for a patient who has received moderate sedation. Check the regulations in your state.

■ Use a recovery and discharge criteria scoring system, such as the Aldrete Post-Anesthesia Recovery Score and the Post-Anesthesia Discharge Scoring System, *to monitor the patient's status and to help determine when the patient is ready for discharge*; tailor use of the scoring system to the patient's specific needs.[4]

■ Before discharge, the patient should meet certain criteria, which may include a return to preprocedural baseline LOC and stable vital signs; a sufficient time interval (for example, 2 hours) since the last administration of an antagonist; the use of an objective patient assessment scoring system; absence of protracted nausea; intact protective reflexes (for example, gag or cough reflex); adequate pain control; and return of sensory and motor control.[4]

Complications

The patient can become oversedated during moderate sedation. Other complications of moderate sedation include aspiration of gastric contents, respiratory depression or failure, and adverse reactions to the medication. Observe the patient for airway obstruction, respiratory depression, hypotension, and drug-specific complications.

Age and general health, in addition to such preexisting respiratory conditions as chronic obstructive pulmonary disease and asthma, and hepatic or renal dysfunction can increase the patient's risk of adverse reactions. In general, older adults, because of decreased renal and hepatic function and relative loss of muscle, are at greater risk. Drug interactions may occur; opioids when used in combination with sedatives may produce a synergistic effect. (See *Responding to complications of sedation.*)

Documentation

Document according to your facility's documentation system and stated parameters, including preprocedure assessment findings, procedure and site verification, and time-out procedure; the name, dose, route, time, and effects of all medications administered; the patient's LOC, ventilation, and oxygenation status; and the procedure start and end times. Documentation should also include vital signs at intervals determined by the type and quantity of medication administered and the patient's condition.[4] Record any adverse reactions, the date and time a practitioner was notified, prescribed interventions, and the patient's response to the interventions. Document teaching provided to the patient and family (if applicable), their understanding of that teaching, and any need for follow-up teaching.

REFERENCES

1 American Society of Anesthesiologists. (2018). Practice guidelines for moderate procedural sedation and analgesia 2018. *Anesthesiology, 128*, 437–479. https://anesthesiology.pubs.asahq.org/article.aspx?articleid=2670190 (Level VII)

2 American Society of PeriAnesthesia Nurses. (2020). *2021-2022 Perianesthesia nursing standards, practice recommendations and interpretive statements.* Cherry Hill, NJ: American Society of PeriAnesthesia Nurses. (Level VII)

3 American Society of Anesthesiologists. (2019). Continuum of depth of sedation: Definition of general anesthesia and levels of sedation/analgesia. https://www.asahq.org/standards-and-guidelines/continuum-of-depth-of-sedation-definition-of-general-anesthesia-and-levels-of-sedationanalgesia (Level VII)

4 Guideline for perioperative practice: Moderate sedation/analgesia. (2021). In Wood, A. (Ed.), *Guidelines for perioperative practice*, 2021 edition. Denver, CO: AORN, Inc. (Level VII)

5 Accreditation Association for Hospitals and Health Systems. (2020). Standard 30.01.04. *Healthcare Facilities Accreditation Program: Accreditation requirements for acute care hospitals.* Chicago, IL: Accreditation Association for Hospitals and Health Systems. (Level VII)

6 Standard 65. Moderate sedation/analgesia using intravenous infusion. Infusion therapy standards of practice (8th ed.). (2021). *Journal of Infusion Nursing, 44*, S194–S1195. (Level VII)

7 Rothrock, J. C. (2019). *Alexander's care of the patient in surgery* (16th ed.). St. Louis, MO: Elsevier.

8 American Society of Anesthesiologists. (2020). ASA physical status classification system. https://www.asahq.org/standards-and-guidelines/asa-physical-status-classification-system (Level VII)

9 Westbrook, J., et al. (2010). Association of interruptions with an increased risk and severity of medication administration errors. *Archives of Internal Medicine, 170*, 683–690. (Level IV)

10 Institute for Safe Medication Practices. (2012). Side tracks on the safety express: Interruptions lead to errors and unfinished...Wait, what was I doing? *Nurse Advise-ERR, 11*(2), 1–4. https://www.ismp.org/resources/side-tracks-safety-express-interruptions-lead-errors-and-unfinished-wait-what-was-i-doing?id=37

11 The Joint Commission. (2021). Standard MM.06.01.01. *Comprehensive accreditation manual for hospitals.* Oakbrook Terrace, IL: The Joint Commission. (Level VII)

12 Centers for Medicare and Medicaid Services, Department of Health and Human Services. (2020). Condition of participation: Nursing services. 42 C.F.R. § 482.23(c).

13 Accreditation Association for Hospitals and Health Systems. (2020). Standard 16.01.03. *Healthcare Facilities Accreditation Program: Accreditation requirements for acute care hospitals.* Chicago, IL: Accreditation Association for Hospitals and Health Systems. (Level VII)

14 DNV GL-Healthcare USA, Inc. (2020). MM.1.SR.3. *NIAHO® accreditation requirements, interpretive guidelines and surveyor guidance—revision 20.0.* Milford, OH: DNV GL-Healthcare USA, Inc. (Level VII)

15 Institute for Safe Medication Practices. (2020). 2020-2021 targeted medication safety best practices for hospitals. https://www.ismp.org/sites/default/files/attachments/2020-02/2020-2021%20TMSBP-%20FINAL_1.pdf

16 The Joint Commission. (2021). Standard PC.03.01.03. *Comprehensive accreditation manual for hospitals.* Oakbrook Terrace, IL: The Joint Commission. (Level VII)

17 Accreditation Association for Hospitals and Health Systems. (2020). Standard 30.01.06. *Healthcare Facilities Accreditation Program: Accreditation requirements for acute care hospitals.* Chicago, IL: Accreditation Association for Hospitals and Health Systems. (Level VII)

18 DNV GL-Healthcare USA, Inc. (2020). PR.2.SR.3. *NIAHO® accreditation requirements, interpretive guidelines and surveyor guidance—revision 20.0.* Milford, OH: DNV GL-Healthcare USA, Inc. (Level VII)

19 The Joint Commission. (2021). Standard RI.01.03.01. *Comprehensive accreditation manual for hospitals.* Oakbrook Terrace, IL: The Joint Commission. (Level VII)

20 Centers for Medicare and Medicaid Services, Department of Health and Human Services. (2020). Condition of participation: Patient's rights. 42 C.F.R. § 482.13(b)(2).

21 Accreditation Association for Hospitals and Health Systems. (2020). Standard 15.01.11. *Healthcare Facilities Accreditation Program: Accreditation requirements for acute care hospitals.* Chicago, IL: Accreditation Association for Hospitals and Health Systems. (Level VII)

22 The Joint Commission. (2021). Standard UP.01.01.01. *Comprehensive accreditation manual for hospitals.* Oakbrook Terrace, IL: The Joint Commission. (Level VII)

23 Accreditation Association for Hospitals and Health Systems. (2020). Standard 30.00.14. *Healthcare Facilities Accreditation Program: Accreditation requirements for acute care hospitals.* Chicago, IL: Accreditation Association for Hospitals and Health Systems. (Level VII)

24 The Joint Commission. (2021). Standard NPSG.07.01.01. *Comprehensive accreditation manual for hospitals.* Oakbrook Terrace, IL: The Joint Commission. (Level VII)

25 Centers for Disease Control and Prevention. (2002). Guideline for hand hygiene in health-care settings: Recommendations of the Healthcare Infection Control Practices Advisory Committee and the HICPAC/SHEA/APIC/IDSA Hand Hygiene Task Force. *MMWR Recommendations and Reports, 51*(RR-16), 1–45. https://www.cdc.gov/mmwr/pdf/rr/rr5116.pdf (Level II)

26 World Health Organization. (2009). WHO guidelines on hand hygiene in health care: First global patient safety challenge, clean care is safer care. https://apps.who.int/iris/bitstream/handle/10665/44102/9789241597906_eng.pdf?sequence=1 (Level IV)

27 Centers for Medicare and Medicaid Services, Department of Health and Human Services. (2020). Condition of participation: Infection control. 42 C.F.R. § 482.42.

28 Accreditation Association for Hospitals and Health Systems. (2020). Standard 07.01.21. *Healthcare Facilities Accreditation Program: Accreditation requirements for acute care hospitals.* Chicago, IL: Accreditation Association for Hospitals and Health Systems. (Level VII)

29 DNV GL-Healthcare USA, Inc. (2020). IC.1.SR.1. *NIAHO® accreditation requirements, interpretive guidelines and surveyor guidance—revision 20.0.* Milford, OH: DNV GL-Healthcare USA, Inc. (Level VII)

30 The Joint Commission. (2021). Standard NPSG.01.01.01. *Comprehensive accreditation manual for hospitals.* Oakbrook Terrace, IL: The Joint Commission. (Level VII)

31 Accreditation Association for Hospitals and Health Systems. (2020). Standard 15.01.16. *Healthcare Facilities Accreditation Program: Accreditation requirements for acute care hospitals.* Chicago, IL: Accreditation Association for Hospitals and Health Systems. (Level VII)

32 Centers for Medicare and Medicaid Services, Department of Health and Human Services. (2020). Condition of participation: Patient's rights. 42 C.F.R. § 482.13(c)(1).

33 DNV GL-Healthcare USA, Inc. (2020). PR.2.SR.5. *NIAHO® accreditation requirements, interpretive guidelines and surveyor guidance—revision 20.0.* Milford, OH: DNV GL-Healthcare USA, Inc. (Level VII)

34 The Joint Commission. (2021). Standard RI.01.01.01. *Comprehensive accreditation manual for hospitals.* Oakbrook Terrace, IL: The Joint Commission. (Level VII)

35 The Joint Commission. (2021). Standard PC.02.01.21. *Comprehensive accreditation manual for hospitals.* Oakbrook Terrace, IL: The Joint Commission. (Level VII)

36 American Society of Anesthesiologists. (2017). Practice guidelines for preoperative fasting and the use of pharmacologic agents to reduce the risk of pulmonary aspiration: Application to healthy patients undergoing elective procedures. *Anesthesiology, 126*, 376–393. https://anesthesiology.pubs.asahq.org/article.aspx?articleid=2596245 (Level V)

37 Siegel, J. D., et al. (2007, revised 2019). 2007 guideline for isolation precautions: Preventing transmission of infectious agents in healthcare settings. https://www.cdc.gov/infectioncontrol/pdf/guidelines/isolation-guidelines-H.pdf (Level II)

38 Accreditation Association for Hospitals and Health Systems. (2020). Standard 07.01.10. *Healthcare Facilities Accreditation Program: Accreditation requirements for acute care hospitals.* Chicago, IL: Accreditation Association for Hospitals and Health Systems. (Level VII)

39 American Society of Anesthesiologists. (2020). Standards for basic anesthetic monitoring. https://www.asahq.org/standards-and-guidelines/standards-for-basic-anesthetic-monitoring (Level VII)

40 The Joint Commission. (2013). Sentinel event alert 50: Medical device alarm safety in hospitals. https://www.jointcommission.org/-/media/tjc/documents/resources/patient-safety-topics/sentinel-event/sea_50_alarms_4_26_16.pdf (Level VII)

41 Graham, K. C., & Cvach, M. (2010). Monitor alarm fatigue: Standardizing use of physiological monitors and decreasing nuisance alarms. *American Journal of Critical Care, 19*, 28–37.

42 The Joint Commission. (2021). Standard NPSG.06.01.01. *Comprehensive accreditation manual for hospitals.* Oakbrook Terrace, IL: The Joint Commission. (Level VII)

43 American Association of Critical Care Nurses. (2018). AACN practice alert: Managing alarms in acute care across the life span: Electrocardiography and pulse oximetry. https://www.aacn.org/clinical-resources/practice-alerts/managing-alarms-in-acute-care-across-the-life-span (Level VII)

44 The Joint Commission. (2021). Standard UP.01.02.01. *Comprehensive accreditation manual for hospitals.* Oakbrook Terrace, IL: The Joint Commission. (Level VII)

45 The Joint Commission. (2021). Standard UP.01.03.01. *Comprehensive accreditation manual for hospitals.* Oakbrook Terrace, IL: The Joint Commission. (Level VII)

46 Institute for Safe Medication Practices. (2018). ISMP list of high-alert medications in acute care settings. https://www.ismp.org/sites/default/files/attachments/2018-08/highAlert2018-Acute-Final.pdf (Level VII)

47 Institute for Safe Medication Practices. (2019). Safety enhancements every hospital must consider in wake of another tragic neuromuscular

blocker event. https://www.ismp.org/resources/safety-enhancements-every-hospital-must-consider-wake-another-tragic-neuromuscular

48 Institute for Safe Medication Practices. (2019). Independent double-checks: Worth the effort if used judiciously and properly. https://www.ismp.org/resources/independent-double-checks-worth-effort-if-used-judiciously-and-properly (Level VII)

49 The Joint Commission. (2021). Standard PC.03.01.05. *Comprehensive accreditation manual for hospitals.* Oakbrook Terrace, IL: The Joint Commission. (Level VII)

50 Rutala, W. A., et al. (2008, revised 2019). Guideline for disinfection and sterilization in healthcare facilities, 2008. https://www.cdc.gov/infection-control/pdf/guidelines/disinfection-guidelines-H.pdf (Level I)

51 Accreditation Association for Hospitals and Health Systems. (2020). Standard 17.02.03. *Healthcare Facilities Accreditation Program: Accreditation requirements for acute care hospitals.* Chicago, IL: Accreditation Association for Hospitals and Health Systems. (Level VII)

52 The Joint Commission. (2021). Standard RC.01.03.01. *Comprehensive accreditation manual for hospitals.* Oakbrook Terrace, IL: The Joint Commission. (Level VII)

53 The Joint Commission. (2021). Standard RC.02.01.03. *Comprehensive accreditation manual for hospitals.* Oakbrook Terrace, IL: The Joint Commission. (Level VII)

54 Centers for Medicare and Medicaid Services, Department of Health and Human Services. (2020). Condition of participation: Medical record services. 42 C.F.R. § 482.24(b).

55 Accreditation Association for Hospitals and Health Systems. (2020). Standard 10.00.03. *Healthcare Facilities Accreditation Program: Accreditation requirements for acute care hospitals.* Chicago, IL: Accreditation Association for Hospitals and Health Systems. (Level VII)

56 DNV GL-Healthcare USA, Inc. (2020). MR.2.SR.1. *NIAHO® accreditation requirements, interpretive guidelines and surveyor guidance—revision 20.0.* Milford, OH: DNV GL-Healthcare USA, Inc. (Level VII)

MUCUS CLEARANCE DEVICE

Patients with chronic respiratory disorders, such as cystic fibrosis, bronchitis, and bronchiectasis, require therapy to mobilize and remove mucus secretions from the lungs. A handheld mucus clearance device can help such patients cough up secretions more easily. The use of a mucus clearing device in patients with chronic obstructive pulmonary disease has been shown to improve the response to bronchodilators when the device is used before bronchodilator therapy.[1,2]

Currently, multiple types of mucus clearance devices are available on the market. These devices take a variety of forms, including mouth pieces, masks, and vests, and they use various methods. They are designed to either increase the amount of air that moves behind the obstruction or to modulate expiratory airflow so that secretions propel upward.[3] For example, some devices contain a valve that vibrates as the patient exhales vigorously through it. The vibrations propagate throughout the patient's airways during expiration, which loosens the mucus. As the patient repeats this process several times, the mucus progressively moves up the airways until the patient can easily cough it out. Examples of mucus clearance devices include the Flutter, the Acapella, and the Aerobika.

A licensed practitioner should individualize mucus clearance device use, including frequency and duration, according to the patient's clinical, functional, and social factors.[3] A recent systematic review found no clear evidence that oscillation was a better intervention than other forms of chest physiotherapy for people with cystic fibrosis.[4]

Mucus clearance device use is contraindicated in patients with known pneumothorax or overt right-sided heart failure.[2] These devices should be used with caution in patients with intolerance to the increased work of breathing; hemodynamic instability; increased intracranial pressure; acute sinusitis; recent facial, oral, or skull surgery or trauma; epistaxis; esophageal surgery; active hemoptysis; nausea; or known or suspected tympanic membrane rupture or other middle ear pathology.[5]

Equipment

Mucus clearance device ■ emesis basin or tissues ■ gloves ■ stethoscope ■ disinfectant pad ■ facility-approved disinfectant ■ oral care supplies (see the "Oral care" procedure) ■ Optional: gown, mask and goggles or mask with face shield.

Preparation of equipment

Inspect all equipment and supplies. If a product is expired, is defective, or has compromised integrity, remove it from patient use, label it as expired or defective, and report the expiration or defect as directed by your facility.

Implementation

- Verify the practitioner's order.
- Gather and prepare the necessary equipment and supplies.
- Perform hand hygiene.[6,7,8,9,10,11]
- Confirm the patient's identity using at least two patient identifiers.[12]
- Provide privacy.[13,14,15,16]
- Explain the procedure to the patient and family (if appropriate) according to their individual communication and learning needs *to increase their understanding, allay their fears, and enhance cooperation.*[17] Tell the patient that using the mucus clearance device will help move the mucus through the airways so that it can eventually be expectorated.
- Perform hand hygiene.[6,7,8,9,10,11]
- Put on gloves as needed *to comply with standard precautions.*[18,19]
- Auscultate the patient's breath sounds *to obtain a baseline assessment for comparison.*
- Instruct the patient to sit with the back straight and head tilted backward slightly so that the throat and trachea are wide open. *This position allows exhaled air to flow smoothly from the lungs and out through the device.* If the patient prefers, the patient may place the elbows on a table at a height that prevents slouching, *which would interfere with smooth breathing.*
- For the Flutter mucus clearance device, tell the patient to hold the device so that the stem is parallel to the floor. *This position places the interior cone of the device at a 30-degree tilt, which allows the ball valve inside the device to bounce and roll freely in the cone.*[2] For the Acapella mucus clearance device, make sure the resistance dial is set as ordered, and tell the patient to hold the device parallel with the floor.[5] For the Aerobika mucus clearance device, make sure the resistance indicator is set as ordered; this device is not dependent on the patient maintaining it in a specific position.[20]
- Instruct the patient to draw a deep breath and hold it for 2 to 3 seconds. This inhalation step is important, *because it evenly distributes the inspired air throughout the lungs, especially in the small airways, where infection and airway damage can occur.*
- After 2 to 3 seconds, instruct the patient to place the device in the mouth and then exhale at a steady rate for as long as possible. *Breathing out too quickly and forcefully, may cause the vibrations to be ineffective.*
- Instruct the patient to keep the cheeks as flat and hard as possible while exhaling *to direct the air out through the mucus clearance device most effectively.*[20] Suggest that the patient hold the cheeks lightly with the other hand *to help learn the proper technique.*
- After the patient has completely exhaled, instruct the patient to repeat the use of the device for the number of breaths recommended by the practitioner. Generally, the recommendation is 5 to 10 breaths for the Flutter device and 10 to 20 breaths for the Acapella and Aerobika devices.[2,5,20]
- Instruct the patient to remove the mucus clearance device from the mouth and then perform two or three coughs to clear the airway.[2,5,20]
- Instruct the patient to expectorate the mucus into an emesis basin or tissue.
- Instruct the patient to repeat the entire procedure several times or as recommended by the practitioner.
- Observe the type, amount, color, viscosity, and odor of expectorated secretions.
- Dispose of expectorated mucus appropriately.[18]
- Auscultate the patient's breath sounds *to determine the effectiveness of coughing,* and compare your findings with the baseline assessment.
- Instruct the patient to perform oral care.
- Remove and discard your gloves, if worn.[18]
- Perform hand hygiene.[6,7,8,9,10,11]
- Put on gloves *to comply with standard precautions.*[18,19]
- Using a facility-approved disinfectant, clean and disinfect the device according to the manufacturer's instructions.
- Remove and discard your gloves.[18]

- Perform hand hygiene.[6,7,8,9,10,11]
- Clean and disinfect your stethoscope using a disinfectant pad.[21,22]
- Perform hand hygiene.[6,7,8,9,10,11]
- Document the procedure.[23,24,25,26]

Special considerations

- Patients routinely perform multiple sets of 10 to 15 exhalations over 12 to 20 minutes. After each series of exhalations, the patient is instructed to "huff" (perform repeated, controlled, short, rapid exhalations) and cough, *which aids expectoration.*[20,27,28]
- Observe the patient over several sets and evaluate the patient's ability to self-administer the treatment.
- For the Flutter mucus clearance device, the oscillation frequency can be regulated by moving the device slightly up or down from its horizontal position.[27]
- All models of the Acapella mucus clearance device can be used with a mask or mouthpiece or in line with a nebulizer.[27]
- The Aerobika mucus clearance device may be used with a small volume nebulizer.[29]
- Patients with severe airway obstruction may not be able to generate sufficient airflow to cause the steel ball within the Flutter® device to vibrate, limiting its effectiveness.[29]

Complications

The increased work of breathing caused by the use of a mucus clearance device may lead to hypoventilation and hypercarbia. Other potential adverse events include increased intracranial pressure, cardiovascular compromise (myocardial ischemia, decreased venous return), claustrophobia, and pulmonary barotrauma. Patients may also swallow excess air, increasing the likelihood of vomiting and aspiration.[5]

Documentation

Record the date, time, type of mucus clearance device, and patient's tolerance of the procedure. Record the amount, color, viscosity, and odor of secretions that the patient expectorates. Document the patient's breath sounds before and after using the mucus clearance device and coughing. Also record the number of times the patient repeated the procedure and the success of the coughing efforts. Document teaching provided to the patient and family (if applicable), their understanding of that teaching, and any need for follow-up teaching.

References

1 Wolkove, N., et al. (2004). A randomized trial to evaluate the sustained efficacy of a mucus clearance device in ambulatory patients with chronic obstructive pulmonary disease. *Canadian Respiratory Journal, 11*, 567–572. (Level II)

2 Aptalis Pharma US, Inc. (2013). FLUTTER® mucus clearance device: Instructions for use. https://media.allergan.com/actavis/actavis/media/allergan-pdf-documents/product-prescribing/Flutter.pdf

3 McIlwaine, M., et al. (2017). Personalising airway clearance in chronic lung disease. *European Respiratory Review, 26*(143), 160086.

4 Morrison, L., & Milroy, S. (2020). Oscillating devices for airway clearance in people with cystic fibrosis. *Cochrane Database of Systematic Reviews, 4*(4), CD006842. (Level I)

5 Smiths Medical ASD, Inc. (2014). Acapella® Vibratory PEP Therapy System: Reference guide. https://www.smiths-medical.com/-/media/M/Smiths-medical_com/Files/Import-Files/RE194317EN-102014_LR.pdf

6 The Joint Commission. (2021). Standard NPSG.07.01.01. *Comprehensive accreditation manual for hospitals.* Oakbrook Terrace, IL: The Joint Commission. (Level VII)

7 Centers for Disease Control and Prevention. (2002). Guideline for hand hygiene in health-care settings: Recommendations of the Healthcare Infection Control Practices Advisory Committee and the HICPAC/SHEA/APIC/IDSA Hand Hygiene Task Force. *MMWR Recommendations and Reports, 51*(RR-16), 1–45. https://www.cdc.gov/mmwr/pdf/rr/rr5116.pdf (Level II)

8 World Health Organization. (2009). WHO guidelines on hand hygiene in health care: First global patient safety challenge,

clean care is safer care. https://apps.who.int/iris/bitstream/handle/10665/44102/9789241597906_eng.pdf?sequence=1 (Level IV)

9 Centers for Medicare and Medicaid Services, Department of Health and Human Services. (2020). Condition of participation: Infection control. 42 C.F.R. § 482.42.

10 Accreditation Association for Hospitals and Health Systems. (2020). Standard 07.01.21. *Healthcare Facilities Accreditation Program: Accreditation requirements for acute care hospitals.* Chicago, IL: Accreditation Association for Hospitals and Health Systems. (Level VII)

11 DNV GL-Healthcare USA, Inc. (2020). IC.1.SR.1. *NIAHO® accreditation requirements, interpretive guidelines and surveyor guidance—revision 20.0.* Milford, OH: DNV GL-Healthcare USA, Inc. (Level VII)

12 The Joint Commission. (2021). Standard NPSG.01.01.01. *Comprehensive accreditation manual for hospitals.* Oakbrook Terrace, IL: The Joint Commission. (Level VII)

13 Centers for Medicare and Medicaid Services, Department of Health and Human Services. (2020). Condition of participation: Patient's rights. 42 C.F.R. § 482.13(c)(1).

14 Accreditation Association for Hospitals and Health Systems. (2020). Standard 15.01.16. *Healthcare Facilities Accreditation Program: Accreditation requirements for acute care hospitals.* Chicago, IL: Accreditation Association for Hospitals and Health Systems. (Level VII)

15 The Joint Commission. (2021). Standard RI.01.01.01. *Comprehensive accreditation manual for hospitals.* Oakbrook Terrace, IL: The Joint Commission. (Level VII)

16 DNV GL-Healthcare USA, Inc. (2020). PR.2.SR.5. *NIAHO® accreditation requirements, interpretive guidelines and surveyor guidance—revision 20.0.* Milford, OH: DNV GL-Healthcare USA, Inc. (Level VII)

17 The Joint Commission. (2021). Standard PC.02.01.21. *Comprehensive accreditation manual for hospitals.* Oakbrook Terrace, IL: The Joint Commission. (Level VII)

18 Siegel, J. D., et al. (2007, revised 2019). 2007 guideline for isolation precautions: Preventing transmission of infectious agents in healthcare settings. https://www.cdc.gov/infectioncontrol/pdf/guidelines/isolation-guidelines-H.pdf (Level II)

19 Accreditation Association for Hospitals and Health Systems. (2020). Standard 07.01.10. *Healthcare Facilities Accreditation Program: Accreditation requirements for acute care hospitals.* Chicago, IL: Accreditation Association for Hospitals and Health Systems. (Level VII)

20 Monaghan Medical Corporation. (n.d.). Aerobika OPEP. https://www.monaghanmed.com/Aerobika-OPEP#1540812069002-acaba3d3-ddd2d628-9b4b

21 Rutala, W. A., et al. (2008, revised 2019). Guideline for disinfection and sterilization in healthcare facilities, 2008. https://www.cdc.gov/infectioncontrol/pdf/guidelines/disinfection-guidelines-H.pdf (Level I)

22 Accreditation Association for Hospitals and Health Systems. (2020). Standard 07.02.03. *Healthcare Facilities Accreditation Program: Accreditation requirements for acute care hospitals.* Chicago, IL: Accreditation Association for Hospitals and Health Systems. (Level VII)

23 The Joint Commission. (2021). Standard RC.01.03.01. *Comprehensive accreditation manual for hospitals.* Oakbrook Terrace, IL: The Joint Commission. (Level VII)

24 Centers for Medicare and Medicaid Services, Department of Health and Human Services. (2020). Condition of participation: Medical record services. 42 C.F.R. § 482.24(b).

25 Accreditation Association for Hospitals and Health Systems. (2020). Standard 10.00.03. *Healthcare Facilities Accreditation Program: Accreditation requirements for acute care hospitals,* Chicago, IL: Accreditation Association for Hospitals and Health Systems. (Level VII)

26 DNV GL-Healthcare USA, Inc. (2020). MR.2.SR.1. *NIAHO® accreditation requirements, interpretive guidelines and surveyor guidance—revision 20.0.* Milford, OH: DNV GL-Healthcare USA, Inc. (Level VII)

27 Hristara-Papadopoulou, A., et al. (2008). Current devices of respiratory physiotherapy. *Hippokratia, 12*(4), 211–220. https://www.ncbi.nlm.nih.gov/pmc/articles/PMC2580042/ (Level V)

28 Lester, M. K., & Flume, P. A. (2009). Airway-clearance therapy guidelines and implementation. *Respiratory Care, 54*(6), 733–753. http://rc.rcjournal.com/content/respgcare/54/6/733.full.pdf (Level VII)

29 Jane and Leonard Korman Respiratory Institute—Jefferson Health and National Jewish Health. (2017). Medfacts: Using the Aerobika. https://hospitals.jefferson.edu/content/dam/health/PDFs/departments/korman-NJH/using-the-aerobika.pdf

NASAL BRIDLE INSERTION AND REMOVAL

A nasal bridle is used to secure a nasally inserted gastric or enteral feeding tube *to prevent the tube's inadvertent dislodgment or removal.*[1,2] It's more effective than traditional tape, thus reducing the need for repeated X-ray exposure to verify tube placement after inadvertent dislodgment or removal.[3] Additionally, the use of a nasal bridle reduces the risk of skin breakdown, *because tape isn't needed to secure the tube.*[1]

Nasal bridle use is contraindicated in patients with a nasal airway abnormality or obstruction, and in those with facial or cranial fractures, thrombocytopenia, or a graft vomer bone.[1,2] It also shouldn't be used following septoplasty or in patients who may pull on the bridle hard enough to cause injury.[1,2]

Before a nasal bridal is inserted, the practitioner should perform a nasal examination to ensure that the patient has adequate bone in the posterior septum to support the bridle system.[1,2] A nasal bridle should be inserted only by those who have been specially trained in the insertion technique and have demonstrated competency in performing insertion.

Equipment

For nasal bridle with umbilical tape and stylet
Gloves ▪ bridle catheter with attached cloth umbilical tape and stylet ▪ clip (preattached to umbilical tape) ▪ retrieval probe ▪ water-soluble lubricant ▪ scissors ▪ Optional: skin barrier, clip reopening tool, gown, mask and goggles or mask with face shield.

For nasal bridle with flexible tubing and stylet
Gloves ▪ flexible bridle tubing with stylet ▪ clip (attached to flexible tubing) ▪ retrieval probe ▪ scissors ▪ Optional: skin barrier, clip reopening tool, gown, mask and goggles or mask with face shield, water-soluble lubricant or water for lubrication.

For nasal bridle with umbilical tape
Gloves ▪ bridle catheter with attached cloth umbilical tape and stylet ▪ clip ▪ retrieval probe ▪ water-soluble lubricant ▪ scissors ▪ Optional: skin barrier, clip reopening tool, gown, mask and goggles or mask with face shield.

Preparation of equipment
Inspect all equipment and supplies. If a product is expired, is defective, or has compromised integrity, remove it from patient use, label it as expired or defective, and report the expiration or defect as directed by your facility.

Implementation
▪ Verify the practitioner's order.
▪ Review the patient's medical record for a history of contraindications to the procedure, such as facial or cranial fractures, nasal airway abnormalities or obstructions, septoplasty, thrombocytopenia, or a graft vomer bone.[1,2]
▪ If required by your facility, confirm that informed consent has been obtained from the patient and that the signed consent form is in the patient's medical record.[4,5,6,7]
▪ Gather and prepare the necessary equipment and supplies.
▪ Perform hand hygiene.[8,9,10,11,12,13]
▪ Confirm the patient's identity using at least two patient identifiers.[14]
▪ Provide privacy.[15,16,17,18]
▪ Explain the procedure to the patient and family (if appropriate) according to their individual communication and learning needs *to help increase their understanding, allay their fears, and enhance cooperation.*[19]
▪ Raise the patient's bed to waist level before providing care *to help prevent caregiver back strain.*[20]
▪ Place the patient in a supine or sitting position *to help ease insertion.*[1]
▪ Perform hand hygiene.[8,9,10,11,12,13]
▪ Put on gloves and other personal protective equipment as needed *to comply with standard precautions.*[21,22,23]

Inserting a nasal bridle with umbilical tape and stylet
▪ Lubricate the nasal bridle retrieval probe, catheter, and umbilical tape with water-soluble lubricant.[1]
▪ Insert the retrieval probe (blue) into the patient's nostril; if the nasogastric or nasoenteral feeding tube is already in place, insert the probe in the nostril opposite the existing tube (as shown below) until the second rib is at the base of the nostril; make adjustments for a smaller patient.[1]

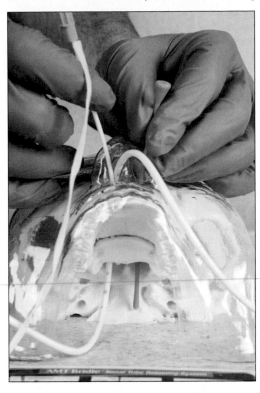

▪ Insert the nasal bridle catheter (white) into the opposite nostril to allow the magnets to meet (as shown below).[1]

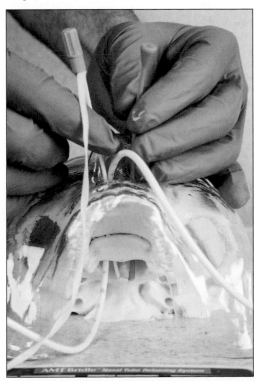

▪ Pull back on the nasal bridle stylet (orange) about ½" (1.3 cm) until the magnets connect; you should hear or feel the click of the magnets as they connect. Check that equal lengths of both probes, minus the orange stylet, are exposed.[1] If necessary, twist the retrieval probe and nasal bridle catheter gently from side to side or up and down *to encourage contact between the magnets*. If contact still doesn't occur, advance the retrieval probe (blue) and bridle catheter (white).[1]

■ Remove the stylet (orange) completely from the nasal bridle catheter (white) when the magnets connect (as shown below).[1]

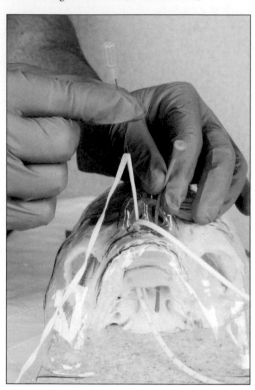

■ Slowly withdraw the retrieval probe (blue) (as shown below), and allow the nasal bridle catheter (white) to advance through the nose; continue until the cloth umbilical tape is in the nose, creating a loop or bridle around the vomer bone. If the catheter and umbilical tape don't advance out of the opposite nostril, remove the catheter, replace the stylet, and repeat the procedure.[1]

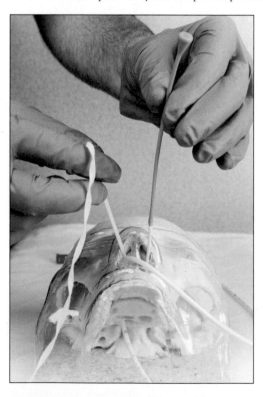

■ Using scissors, cut the nasal bridle catheter portion from the umbilical tape. Discard the catheter (white) and retrieval probe (blue).[1]

■ If the nasogastric or nasoenteral feeding tube hasn't been inserted, insert it now.[1] (See the "Enteral gastric and duodenal feeding tube insertion and removal" procedure.)

■ Place the clip about ½″ (1.3 cm) or one finger's width from the nostril (as shown below); make sure that the clip doesn't touch the nostril.[1]

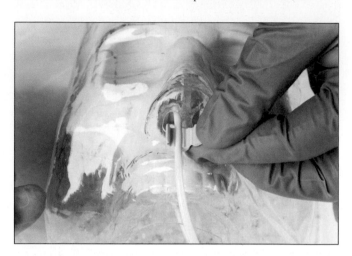

NURSING ALERT Use caution when handling the bridle clip near the patient's mouth; consider covering the patient's mouth to prevent the clip from falling into the patient's mouth should you accidentally drop it.[1]

■ For a #5 to #12 French clip, ensure that the nasogastric or nasoenteral feeding tube fits securely in the clip's channel, and then place both strands of the umbilical tape near the hinge of the clip, keeping the tape flat.[1] For a #14 to #18 French clip, ensure that the nasogastric or nasoenteral feeding tube fits securely in the clip's channel. Place both strands of umbilical tape between the soft inner portion of the clip and the outer, more rigid plastic section.[1]

■ Close the clip by folding over the plastic edge (as shown below) and firmly snapping it shut. Keep in mind that the clip is difficult to reopen, so be sure to position the nasogastric or nasoenteral feeding tube, umbilical tape, and clip properly before closing the clip. Don't use another object to open or close the clip, *because the clip may become damaged, making it less secure*. If the clip becomes damaged, use a new one.[1]

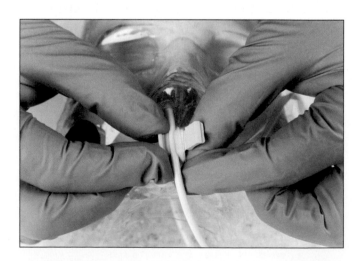

■ After closing the clip completely, tie the two umbilical tape strands together (excluding the tube) in a simple knot (as shown). Knot the tape ends two to three times, and then cut the excess umbilical tape.

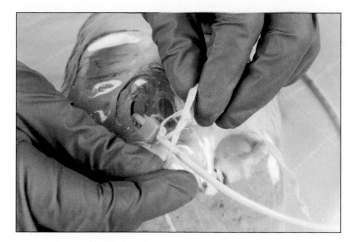

Inserting a nasal bridle with flexible tubing and stylet

■ If desired, lubricate the probe or top of the bridle tube using water or water-soluble lubricant. Although lubricant isn't necessary with this system, you can use it if desired.[1]

■ Insert the retrieval probe into the patient's nostril. If the nasogastric or nasoenteral feeding tube is already in place, insert the probe into the nostril opposite the existing tube. Insert the probe until the second rib of the probe appears level with the base of the nostril. Make adjustments for a smaller patient.[1]

■ Insert the bridle tubing into the opposite nostril to approximate the depth of the magnets.[1]

■ Pull back on the stylet ½″ (1.3 cm) until you hear or feel the magnets connect. Ensure that the exposed portions of the probes remain equal in length (minus the length of the stylet).[1]

■ Twist the probe from side to side, up and down, or in both directions as necessary to encourage magnetic contact. If contact doesn't occur, advance the retrieval probe and bridle tubing.

■ Remove the stylet completely from the bridle tubing after magnetic contact occurs.

■ Withdraw the retrieval probe slowly and allow the bridle tubing to advance through the nose. Continue withdrawing until the two black markings on the bridle tubing are completely pulled through the insertion nostril and a few inches outside the opposite nostril. This positioning creates the loop or bridle around the vomer bone. If the bridle tubing doesn't advance, remove the retrieval probe and tubing and reinsert them.[1]

■ Cut the bridle tubing to remove the magnet and black markings.[1]

■ If the nasal tube isn't in place, insert it now.[1]

■ Slide the clip until it's ½″ (1.3 cm), or one finger's width, from the patient's nostril, ensuring that the clip doesn't touch the nostril.[1]

■ Ensure that the nasal tube fits securely within the clip. For #5 to #6 French clips and #8 to #10 French clips, place the tubing between the clear flats and below the circular region of the clip. For #8, #10, or #12 French clips, place the tubing in the clip's hinge. For #14, #16, or #18 French clips, place the tubing between the soft inner portion and the outer, more rigid plastic portions of the clip.[1]

■ Close the clip. For #5 to #6 French clips and #8 to #10 French clips, grip near the base of the clip and then firmly snap the clip closed. For #8, #10, #12, #14, #16, and #18 French clips, fold over the plastic edge and firmly snap the clip closed.[1] Keep in mind that the clip is difficult to reopen; properly position the nasogastric or nasoenteral feeding tube, umbilical tape, and clip before closing it. Don't use another object to open or close the clip, *because the clip may become damaged, making it less secure.* If the clip becomes damaged, use a new one.[1]

■ While holding the nasal tube in place, pull gently on the bridle tubing ends to ensure proper clip closure. When the clip is fully closed, tie the bridle tubing ends together in a simple knot below the clip. Cut the excess tubing about ½″ (1.3 cm) from the knot.

Inserting a nasal bridle with umbilical tape

■ Remove the clear protective covering of the retrieval catheter and the nasal bridle catheter.

■ Lubricate the distal tip of both catheters thoroughly with water-soluble lubricant. Avoid lubricating the magnetic tips.[2]

■ Insert the retrieval catheter in the desired nostril to the desired depth, using the centimeter markings on the catheter as a guide. Don't exert force during catheter insertion *to avoid damaging the sinus cavity.*[2]

■ Insert the bridle catheter into the opposite nostril to the same insertion depth as the retrieval catheter.[2]

■ Manipulate the catheters gently until you feel or hear the magnets connect behind the vomer bone.[2]

■ After the magnets connect, withdraw the bridle catheter slowly until the tape becomes visible and the catheter is fully outside of the nostril.[2]

■ Remove the retrieval catheter until the tape becomes visible outside the opposite nostril and the catheter is fully outside of the nostril.[2]

■ Pull the bridle catheter until the umbilical tape comes completely out of the catheter.[2]

■ Disconnect the retrieval catheter from the magnet, and adjust the umbilical tape so that an equal length extends from each nostril.[2]

■ If the nasal tube isn't in place, insert it now.[2]

■ Insert the nasal tube into the groove of the clip, and place one or both sides of umbilical tape onto the flat area of the clamp in front of the nasal tube.[2]

■ Slide the clip up to approximately ½″ (1.3 cm) below the nostril.[2]

■ Lock the clip in place by pinching the clip closed.[2]

■ Tie the ends of umbilical tape in a double or triple knot, excluding the nasal tube.[2]

■ Trim the umbilical tape approximately ½″ (1.3 cm) below the knot, and discard the remaining tape and magnet.[2]

NURSING ALERT Don't secure the clip over the patient's mouth or allow it to touch the patient's nostril.

Completing the procedure

■ Perform a thorough nasal examination after inserting the nasal bridle *to ensure that the umbilical tape loop has passed behind the nasal septum, not through a septal perforation.*[1]

■ Regularly monitor the position of the nasogastric or nasoenteral feeding tube and clip for signs of tube migration.[1,2,24]

■ Monitor the insertion site for redness, swelling, drainage, and skin irritation. Use a skin barrier as necessary.[25]

■ Monitor the clip for signs of damage or loose attachment to the nasogastric or nasoenteral feeding tube; replace the clip if necessary.[1]

■ Return the patient's bed to the lowest position *to prevent falls and maintain patient safety.*[26]

Removing a nasal bridle

To remove a nasal bridle and nasogastric or nasoenteral tube together

■ Using scissors, cut one strand of the umbilical tape or flexible tubing.[26]

■ Pull the nasal bridle and nasogastric or nasoenteral tube gently out of the patient's nose.[26]

To remove a nasal bridle alone

■ Leaving the nasal clip in place, cut both ends of the umbilical tape near the clip.[1,2]

■ Open the clip with the clip reopening tool, and pull gently on the open end clip *to remove the flexible tubing or umbilical tape from the nose.*[1,2]

■ Take care to prevent accidental swallowing of the umbilical tape or flexible tubing, *because the tape and tubing can easily slide back into the nose.*[1,2]

Completing the procedure

■ Assess the condition of the umbilical tape or flexible tubing, *because it may degrade over time, resulting in pieces being left in the patient's nose.*[1,2]

■ Assess the patient's skin around the nares and upper lip for signs of bleeding, skin breakdown, and irritation.

- Return the bed to the lowest position *to prevent falls and maintain the patient's safety.*[26]
- Discard used supplies in the appropriate receptacle.[23]
- Remove and discard your gloves and any other personal protective equipment worn.[22,23]
- Perform hand hygiene.[8,9,10,11,12,13]
- Document the procedure.[27,28,29,30]

Special considerations

- The nasal bridle can remain in place for up to 30 days of continuous use before requiring replacement.[1,2]
- Keep magnets at least 6" (15 cm) away from pacemakers and other implanted devices, such as defibrillators, *because direct contact with some magnets can interfere with these devices.*[2]

Complications

If the nasal bridle is secured too tightly, damage may occur to the internal and external tissues. If the nasal bridle is secured too loosely, the nasogastric or nasoenteral feeding tube may become dislodged and increase the risk of aspiration, pneumothorax, and sinusitis.[1,24]

Documentation

Document that the practitioner assessed the patient's nose before the procedure. Record the type of bridle you used, size of the clip, position of the nasogastric or nasoenteral feeding tube, condition of the patient's nose, and patient's tolerance of the procedure. Document teaching provided to the patient and family (if applicable), their understanding of that teaching, and any need for follow-up teaching.

REFERENCES

1 Applied Medical Technology, Inc. (2018). AMT Bridle: Directions, indications, & contraindications for use. https://www.appliedmedical.net/resources/directions/en/Bridle-DFU_C-4615-Rev-B-01_18_Digital.pdf

2 Halyard Health, Inc. (2015, revised 2017). Corgrip NG/NI Feeding Tube Retention System: Instructions for use. http://docplayer.fr/189064887-Corgrip-ng-ni-feeding-tube-retention-system-instructions-for-use.html

3 Bechtold, M. L., et al. (2014). Nasal bridles for securing nasoenteric tubes: A meta-analysis. *Nutrition in Clinical Practice, 29*(5), 667–671. https://www.ncbi.nlm.nih.gov/pmc/articles/PMC4304091/ (Level I)

4 The Joint Commission. (2021). Standard RI.01.03.01. *Comprehensive accreditation manual for hospitals.* Oakbrook Terrace, IL: The Joint Commission. (Level VII)

5 Centers for Medicare and Medicaid Services, Department of Health and Human Services. (2020). Condition of participation: Patient's rights. 42 C.F.R. § 482.13(b)(2).

6 Accreditation Association for Hospitals and Health Systems. (2020). Standard 15.01.11. *Healthcare Facilities Accreditation Program: Accreditation requirements for acute care hospitals.* Chicago, IL: Accreditation Association for Hospitals and Health Systems. (Level VII)

7 DNV GL-Healthcare USA, Inc. (2020). PR.2.SR.3. *NIAHO® accreditation requirements, interpretive guidelines and surveyor guidance—revision 20.0.* Milford, OH: DNV GL-Healthcare USA, Inc. (Level VII)

8 The Joint Commission. (2021). Standard NPSG.07.01.01. *Comprehensive accreditation manual for hospitals.* Oakbrook Terrace, IL: The Joint Commission. (Level VII)

9 Centers for Disease Control and Prevention. (2002). Guideline for hand hygiene in health-care settings: Recommendations of the Healthcare Infection Control Practices Advisory Committee and the HICPAC/SHEA/APIC/IDSA Hand Hygiene Task Force. *MMWR Recommendations and Reports, 51*(RR-16), 1–45. https://www.cdc.gov/mmwr/pdf/rr/rr5116.pdf (Level II)

10 World Health Organization. (2009). WHO guidelines on hand hygiene in health care: First global patient safety challenge, clean care is safer care. https://apps.who.int/iris/bitstream/handle/10665/44102/9789241597906_eng.pdf?sequence=1 (Level IV)

11 Accreditation Association for Hospitals and Health Systems. (2020). Standard 07.01.21. *Healthcare Facilities Accreditation Program: Accreditation requirements for acute care hospitals.* Chicago, IL: Accreditation Association for Hospitals and Health Systems. (Level VII)

12 Centers for Medicare and Medicaid Services, Department of Health and Human Services. (2020). Condition of participation: Infection control. 42 C.F.R. § 482.42.

13 DNV GL-Healthcare USA, Inc. (2020). IC.1.SR.1. *NIAHO® accreditation requirements, interpretive guidelines and surveyor guidance—revision 20.0.* Milford, OH: DNV GL-Healthcare USA, Inc. (Level VII)

14 The Joint Commission. (2021). Standard NPSG.01.01.01. *Comprehensive accreditation manual for hospitals.* Oakbrook Terrace, IL: The Joint Commission. (Level VII)

15 The Joint Commission. (2021). Standard RI.01.01.01. *Comprehensive accreditation manual for hospitals.* Oakbrook Terrace, IL: The Joint Commission. (Level VII)

16 Centers for Medicare and Medicaid Services, Department of Health and Human Services. (2020). Condition of participation: Patient's rights. 42 C.F.R. § 482.13(c)(1).

17 Accreditation Association for Hospitals and Health Systems. (2020). Standard 15.01.16. *Healthcare Facilities Accreditation Program: Accreditation requirements for acute care hospitals.* Chicago, IL: Accreditation Association for Hospitals and Health Systems. (Level VII)

18 DNV GL-Healthcare USA, Inc. (2020). PR.2.SR.5. *NIAHO® accreditation requirements, interpretive guidelines and surveyor guidance—revision 20.0.* Milford, OH: DNV GL-Healthcare USA, Inc. (Level VII)

19 The Joint Commission. (2021). Standard PC.02.01.21. *Comprehensive accreditation manual for hospitals.* Oakbrook Terrace, IL: The Joint Commission. (Level VII)

20 Waters, T. R., et al. (2009). Safe patient handling training for schools of nursing. https://www.cdc.gov/niosh/docs/2009-127/pdfs/2009-127.pdf (Level VII)

21 Siegel, J. D., et al. (2007, revised 2019). 2007 guideline for isolation precautions: Preventing transmission of infectious agents in healthcare settings. https://www.cdc.gov/infectioncontrol/pdf/guidelines/isolation-guidelines-H.pdf (Level II)

22 Accreditation Association for Hospitals and Health Systems. (2020). Standard 07.01.10. *Healthcare Facilities Accreditation Program: Accreditation requirements for acute care hospitals.* Chicago, IL: Accreditation Association for Hospitals and Health Systems. (Level VII)

23 Occupational Safety and Health Administration. (2012). Bloodborne pathogens, standard number 1910.1030. https://www.osha.gov/pls/oshaweb/owadisp.show_document?p_id=10051&p_table=STANDARDS (Level VII)

24 McGinnis, C. (2011). The feeding tube bridle: One inexpensive, safe, and effective method to prevent inadvertent feeding tube dislodgement. *Nutrition in Clinical Practice, 26*, 70–77.

25 Wiegand, D. L. (2017). *AACN procedure manual for high acuity, progressive, and critical care* (7th ed.). St. Louis, MO: Elsevier.

26 Ganz, D. A., et al. (2013, Reviewed 2021). *Preventing falls in hospitals: A toolkit for improving quality of care* (AHRQ publication no. 13-0015-EF). https://www.ahrq.gov/professionals/systems/hospital/fallpxtoolkit/index.html (Level VII)

27 The Joint Commission. (2021). Standard RC.01.03.01. *Comprehensive accreditation manual for hospitals.* Oakbrook Terrace, IL: The Joint Commission. (Level VII)

28 Centers for Medicare and Medicaid Services, Department of Health and Human Services. (2020). Condition of participation: Medical record services. 42 C.F.R. § 482.24(b).

29 Accreditation Association for Hospitals and Health Systems. (2020). Standard 10.00.03. *Healthcare Facilities Accreditation Program: Accreditation requirements for acute care hospitals.* Chicago, IL: Accreditation Association for Hospitals and Health Systems. (Level VII)

30 DNV GL-Healthcare USA, Inc. (2020). MR.2.SR.1. *NIAHO® accreditation requirements, interpretive guidelines and surveyor guidance—revision 20.0.* Milford, OH: DNV GL-Healthcare USA, Inc. (Level VII)

NASAL DECOLONIZATION

Patients who are colonized with a pathogen carry the pathogen on a body surface, such as the skin, mouth, nose, intestines, or airway, without actually having the disease. Infection occurs when the pathogen invades the body, causing the disease. The process of decolonization can prevent the pathogen from causing infection. It's believed that patients infected or colonized with methicillin-resistant *Staphylococcus aureus* (MRSA) are a major source of MRSA being introduced into health care facilities.[1]

Research shows that nasal carriage increases the risk of bacteremia and other infections caused by the pathogen, including surgical site infections.[1] Moreover, it's the most common indication for total knee arthroplasty revision and the third most common indication in total hip arthroplasty revision.[2] Nasal decolonization strategies have proven effective in reducing not only *S. aureus* colonization but also *S. aureus* surgical site infections.[3] Guidelines recommend nasal decolonization for patients undergoing high-risk surgeries, including orthopedic surgery, cardiothoracic surgery, and neurosurgery.[4,5] Universal decolonization in intensive care units has also been effective in reducing bloodstream infections.[6]

Mupirocin, administered to the nares twice a day for 5 days preoperatively, has become the gold standard topical antibacterial agent for nasal decolonization. It's effective against staphylococci and many gram-negative bacteria.[3] Povidone-iodine and alcohol can also be used.[7] Povidone-iodine has a broad spectrum of activity against many grampositive organisms, including methicillin-susceptible *S. aureus*, MRSA, and many gram-negative organisms.[8] It has some advantages over mupirocin in that it's bactericidal within 10 to 20 seconds, and there's no evidence that bacteria can develop resistance to it; however, mupirocin has a more persistent bactericidal effect than povidone-iodine.[3] Alcohol has activity against a wide range of gram-positive and gram-negative bacteria, including such resistant organisms as MRSA. It's rapidly bactericidal but has almost no residual bactericidal effects after application.

Equipment

Prescribed decolonization agent (mupirocin 2% ointment, povidoneiodine 10% swab stick, alcohol 62%) ■ gloves ■ tissues ■ Optional: gown, cotton-tipped swab.

Implementation

■ Verify the practitioner's order.
■ Review the patient's medical record for history of colonization with a resistant organism and allergies to the prescribed decolonization agent or its ingredients.
■ Gather the necessary equipment and supplies.
■ Perform hand hygiene.[9,10,11,12,13,14]
■ Put on gloves and, as needed, other personal protective equipment *to comply with standard precautions.*[15,16,17]
■ Confirm the patient's identity using at least two patient identifiers.[18]
■ Provide privacy.[19,20,21,22]
■ Explain the procedure to the patient and family (if appropriate) according to their individual communication and learning needs *to increase their understanding, allay their fears, and enhance cooperation.*[23]
■ Ask the patient to tilt the head back *to gain access to the nares.*
■ Clean the inside of both nostrils with a tissue, including the inside tips of the nostrils. Discard the tissue in an appropriate receptacle.[24,25]

For decolonization with mupirocin

■ Apply one-half of the mupirocin nasal ointment from a single-use tube into one nostril and the other half into the other nostril.[26]

NURSING ALERT Avoid contact between mupirocin nasal ointment and the patient's eyes. If accidental contact occurs, rinse well with water *to prevent burning and tearing.*[26]

■ Close the nostrils by pressing together and releasing the sides of the nose repetitively for about 1 minute *to spread the ointment throughout the nares.*[26]
■ Discard the tube after use; don't reuse.[26]
■ Apply the ointment twice daily (morning and night) for 5 days, as ordered.[26]
■ Avoid concurrent administration of any other intranasal products during the treatment period.[26]
■ Monitor the patient for such adverse effects as headache, rhinitis, pharyngitis, respiratory disorders, taste perversion, burning, stinging, cough, and pruritus.[3,26]

For decolonization with a povidone-iodine swab stick

■ Hold the applicator tube between the thumb and forefinger with the tube in a vertical position with the tip or handle up. Tap the swab stick gently against a firm surface *to push any excess solution to the bottom of the swab stick tube.*[25]

■ Place the thumb and forefinger of the other hand at the base of the handle or tip (thumb-to-thumb).[25]
■ Bend and snap the swab stick away from yourself at the score line.[25]
■ Bend and snap the swab stick in the opposite direction *to disconnect the swab stick.*[25]
■ Remove the swab stick from the tube and discard the tube in an appropriate receptacle.[25] Don't place the swab stick back into the tube, *because the swab stick is presaturated with the correct volume of solution at the time of removal from the tube.*[25]
■ Insert the swab stick comfortably into one nostril.[25]
■ For a total of 15 seconds, rotate the swab stick around the circumference of the nostril. Then rotate the swab stick in the anterior nares for a least six complete revolutions, applying slight pressure and covering all surfaces. Repeat the procedure in the same nostril, using a new swab stick.[25]
■ Complete the swab insertion two times in the other nostril.[25]
■ If the solution drips from the nose, wipe it gently with a tissue; don't allow the patient to blow the nose.[25]
■ Discard the swab sticks in an appropriate receptacle.[25]

For decolonization with alcohol using an ampule

■ Holding the ampule by the cardboard sleeve, shake it for 4 to 5 seconds until the solution becomes emulsified.[27]
■ Remove the ampule from the cardboard sleeve to expose the swab's tip.[27]
■ Reinsert the ampule into the cardboard sleeve with the swab's tip exposed. Avoid touching the swab tip with your fingers.[27]
■ Hold the ampule by the cardboard sleeve and press firmly near the middle, at the blue dot, *to crush the ampule.*[27]
■ Pointing the swab tip downward, squeeze the ampule *to saturate the swab tip.*[27]
■ Insert the swab tip into the right nostril, to a distance no deeper than the tip of the swab.[27]
■ While applying moderate pressure, swab the right nostril six times clockwise and then six times counterclockwise. Make sure to swab the inside front pocket of the right nostril.[27]
■ Turn the swab upside down, and then squeeze the ampule gently and repeatedly *to resaturate the swab tip.*[27]
■ Repeat the application in the left nostril.[27]
■ Discard the ampule and sleeve in an appropriate receptacle.[27]
■ Repeat the application in both nostrils using all three ampules in the pack, within 1 hour before surgery.[27]

For decolonization with alcohol using a cotton-tipped swab

■ Shake the multidose bottle well and then remove the cap.[28]
■ Apply four drops of alcohol solution onto the tip of a cotton-tipped swab.[28]
■ Insert the swab tip into the patient's right nostril to a distance no deeper than the tip of the swab.[28]
■ While applying moderate pressure, swab the right nostril six times clockwise and then six times counterclockwise. Make sure to swab all surfaces of the nostril, including the inside tip of the nostril.[28]
■ Resaturate the swab tip of the cotton-tipped swab by applying two drops of alcohol solution.[28]
■ Repeat the application in the left nostril.[28]
■ Discard the cotton-tipped swab in an appropriate receptacle.

Completing the procedure

■ Remove and discard your gloves and, if worn, other personal protective equipment.
■ Perform hand hygiene.[9,10,11,12,13,14]
■ Document the procedure.[29,30,31,32]

Special considerations

■ Data are insufficient to recommend mupirocin nasal ointment for general prophylaxis of an infection in any patient population.[2]

Complications

Improper technique can result in continued colonization, increasing the risk of infection. Another potential complication is allergic reaction to the prescribed decolonization agent.

Documentation

Document the decolonization agent's name and strength and the date and time of administration. Include the route and site you used, such as the right and left nares. Record any adverse reactions to the prescribed agent, the date and time you notified the practitioner, prescribed interventions, and the patient's response to those interventions. Document teaching provided to the patient and family (if applicable), their understanding of that teaching, and any need for follow-up teaching.

REFERENCES

1 Association of Professionals in Infection Control and Epidemiology (APIC). (2014). *APIC text of infection control and epidemiology* (4th ed.). Arlington, VA: APIC.

2 Berríos-Torres, S. I., et al. (2017). Centers for Disease Control and Prevention guideline for the prevention of surgical site infection, 2017. *JAMA, 152*(8), 784–791. https://jamanetwork.com/journals/jamasurgery/fullarticle/2623725?appId=scweb

3 Brock, J. (2019). Nasal decolonization: Potential alternatives for SSI prevention. *Infectious Diseases News*, Julyhttps://www.healio.com/news/infectious-disease/20190702/nasal-decolonization-potential-mupirocin-alternatives-for-ssi-prevention.

4 World Health Organization. (2016). Global guidelines for the prevention of surgical site infection. https://apps.who.int/iris/bitstream/handle/10665/250680/9789241549882-eng.pdf?sequence=8 (Level IV)

5 Centers for Disease Control and Prevention. (2019). Strategies to prevent hospital-onset *Staphylococcus aureus* bloodstream infections in acute care facilities. https://www.cdc.gov/hai/prevent/staph-prevention-strategies.html

6 Huang, S. S., et al. (2013). Targeted versus universal decolonization to prevent ICU infection. *New England Journal of Medicine, 368*, 2255–2265. (Level I)

7 Septimus, E. J., & Schweizer, M. L. (2016). Decolonization in prevention of health care-associated infections. *Clinical Microbiology Reviews, 29*, 201–222.

8 Ghaddara, H. A., et al. (2019). Efficacy of a povidone iodine preparation in reducing nasal methicillin-resistant *Staphylococcus aureus* in colonized patients. *American Journal of Infection Control, 48*, 456–459.

9 Accreditation Association for Hospitals and Health Systems. (2020). Standard 07.01.21. *Healthcare Facilities Accreditation Program: Accreditation requirements for acute care hospitals.* Chicago, IL: Accreditation Association for Hospitals and Health Systems. (Level VII)

10 Centers for Disease Control and Prevention. (2002). Guideline for hand hygiene in health-care settings: Recommendations of the Healthcare Infection Control Practices Advisory Committee and the HICPAC/SHEA/APIC/IDSA Hand Hygiene Task Force. *MMWR Recommendations and Reports, 51*(RR-16), 1–45. https://www.cdc.gov/mmwr/pdf/rr/rr5116.pdf (Level II)

11 Centers for Medicare and Medicaid Services, Department of Health and Human Services. (2020). Condition of participation: Infection control. 42 C.F.R. § 482.42.

12 DNV GL-Healthcare USA, Inc. (2020). IC.1.SR.1. *NIAHO® accreditation requirements: Interpretive guidelines & surveyor guidance—revision 20.0.* Milford, OH: DNV GL-Healthcare USA, Inc. (Level VII)

13 The Joint Commission. (2021). Standard NPSG.07.01.01. *Comprehensive accreditation manual for hospitals.* Oakbrook Terrace, IL: The Joint Commission. (Level VII)

14 World Health Organization. (2009). WHO guidelines on hand hygiene in health care: First global patient safety challenge, clean care is safer care. https://apps.who.int/iris/bitstream/handle/10665/44102/9789241597906_eng.pdf?sequence=1 (Level IV)

15 Accreditation Association for Hospitals and Health Systems. (2020). Standard 07.01.10. *Healthcare Facilities Accreditation Program: Accreditation requirements for acute care hospitals.* Chicago, IL: Accreditation Association for Hospitals and Health Systems. (Level VII)

16 Occupational Safety and Health Administration. (2012). Bloodborne pathogens, standard number 1910.1030. https://www.osha.gov/pls/oshaweb/owadisp.show_document?p_id=10051&p_table=STANDARDS (Level VII)

17 Siegel, J. D., et al. (2007, revised 2019). 2007 guideline for isolation precautions: Preventing transmission of infectious agents in healthcare settings. https://www.cdc.gov/infectioncontrol/pdf/guidelines/isolation-guidelines-H.pdf (Level II)

18 The Joint Commission. (2021). Standard NPSG.01.01.01. *Comprehensive accreditation manual for hospitals.* Oakbrook Terrace, IL: The Joint Commission. (Level VII)

19 Accreditation Association for Hospitals and Health Systems. (2020). Standard 15.01.16. *Healthcare Facilities Accreditation Program: Accreditation requirements for acute care hospitals.* Chicago, IL: Accreditation Association for Hospitals and Health Systems. (Level VII)

20 Centers for Medicare and Medicaid Services, Department of Health and Human Services. (2020). Condition of participation: Patient's rights. 42 C.F.R. § 482.13 (c)(1).

21 DNV GL-Healthcare USA, Inc. (2020). PR.2.SR.5. *NIAHO® accreditation requirements: Interpretive guidelines & surveyor guidance—revision 20.0.* Milford, OH: DNV GL-Healthcare USA, Inc. (Level VII)

22 The Joint Commission. (2021). Standard RI.01.01.01. *Comprehensive accreditation manual for hospitals.* Oakbrook Terrace, IL: The Joint Commission. (Level VII)

23 The Joint Commission. (2021). Standard PC.02.01.21. *Comprehensive accreditation manual for hospitals.* Oakbrook Terrace, IL: The Joint Commission. (Level VII)

24 Global Life Technologies Corp. (2017). Nozin Nasal Sanitizer Popswab Ampule instructions for use. https://www.nozin.com/wp-content/uploads/Poster-Nozin-Daily-Decolonization-8x8_v66.x61666.pdf

25 PDI. (2018). Profend nasal decolonization kit: General guidelines for use for nasal application. https://pdihc.com/wp-content/uploads/2018/09/PDI-Profend-IFU_05189933.pdf

26 GlaxoSmithKline. (2017). Bactroban nasal ointment prescribing information. https://www.accessdata.fda.gov/drugsatfda_docs/label/2017/050703s017lbl.pdf

27 Global Life Technologies Corp. (2017). Pre-Op: Nozin Nasal Sanitizer preoperative pack instructions for use. https://www.nozin.com/wp-content/uploads/IFU_PreOp_Ampule_VF.x61666.pdf

28 Global Life Technologies Corp. (2017). Nozin Nasal Sanitizer multidose 12mL bottle instructions for use. https://www.nozin.com/wp-content/uploads/IFU-POSTER-Multidose-Bottle-6x6-v56.x61666.pdf

29 Accreditation Association for Hospitals and Health Systems. (2020). Standard 10.00.03. *Healthcare Facilities Accreditation Program: Accreditation requirements for acute care hospitals.* Chicago, IL: Accreditation Association for Hospitals and Health Systems. (Level VII)

30 Centers for Medicare and Medicaid Services, Department of Health and Human Services. (2020). Condition of participation: Medical record services. 42 C.F.R. § 482.24 (b).

31 DNV GL-Healthcare USA, Inc. (2020). MR.2.SR.1. *NIAHO® accreditation requirements: Interpretive guidelines & surveyor guidance—revision 20.0.* Milford, OH: DNV GL-Healthcare USA, Inc. (Level VII)

32 The Joint Commission. (2021). Standard RC.01.03.01. *Comprehensive accreditation manual for hospitals.* Oakbrook Terrace, IL: The Joint Commission. (Level VII)

NASAL IRRIGATION

Irrigation of the nasal passages soothes irritated mucous membranes and washes away crusted mucus, secretions, and foreign matter. Left unattended, these deposits may impede sinus drainage and nasal airflow and cause headaches, infections, and unpleasant odors. Irrigation may be done with a bulb syringe or an electronic irrigating device.

Nasal irrigation benefits patients with acute or chronic nasal conditions, including sinusitis, rhinitis, Wegener granulomatosis, and Sjögren syndrome.[1,2] The procedure may also help people who regularly inhale toxins or allergens—paint fumes, sawdust, pesticides, or coal dust.[3] Nasal irrigation is routinely recommended after some nasal surgeries to enhance healing by removing postoperative eschar and to aid remucosolization of the sinus cavities and ostia.[4]

Possible contraindications for nasal irrigation may include advanced destruction of the sinuses, frequent nosebleeds, and foreign bodies in the nasal passages (which could be driven farther into the passages by the irrigant). However, some patients with these conditions may benefit from irrigation. Other contraindications to the procedure include facial trauma and neurologic or musculoskeletal problems that may increase the risk of aspiration.[1]

Equipment

Bulb syringe, squeeze bottle, or electronic irrigation device ■ rigid or flexible disposable irrigation tips (for single-patient use) ■ normal saline solution ■ fluid-impermeable pad ■ towels ■ facial tissues ■ bath basin or sink ■ gloves ■ soap ■ water ■ facility-approved disinfectant.

Preparation of equipment

Inspect all equipment and supplies. If a product is expired, is defective, or has compromised integrity, remove it from patient use, label it as expired or defective, and report the expiration or defect as directed by your facility.

Attach the disposable nasal irrigation tip to the irrigation delivery device, as needed.

Warm the normal saline solution to room temperature.[5] If you'll be irrigating with a bulb syringe, draw some irrigant into the bulb and then expel it *to rinse any residual solution from the previous irrigation and to warm the bulb.*

If you're using an electronic irrigating device, plug the instrument into an electrical outlet in an area near the patient. Then run about 1 cup (240 mL) of normal saline solution through the tubing *to rinse residual solution from the lines and to warm the tubing.* Next, fill the reservoir of the device with warm saline solution.

Implementation

- Verify the practitioner's order, if required.
- Gather and prepare the necessary equipment.
- Perform hand hygiene.[6,7,8,9,10,11]
- Confirm the patient's identity using at least two patient identifiers.[12]
- Provide privacy.[13,14,15,16]
- Explain the procedure to the patient and family members (if appropriate) according to their individual communication and learning needs *to increase their understanding, allay their fears, and enhance cooperation.*[17]
- Raise the patient's bed to waist level before providing care *to help prevent caregiver back strain.*[18]
- Perform hand hygiene.[6,7,8,9,10,11]
- Put on gloves *to comply with standard precautions.*[19,20,21]
- Place a towel on the patient's upper body *to protect clothing from getting wet.* Place a fluid-impermeable pad on the bed if indicated.
- Have the patient sit comfortably near the equipment in a position that allows the bulb syringe, squeeze bottle, or irrigating tip to enter the nose and the draining irrigant to flow into the bath basin or sink. (See *Positioning the patient for nasal irrigation.*)
- Instruct the patient to keep the mouth open and to breathe rhythmically during irrigation. *This action causes the soft palate to seal the throat, allowing the irrigant to stream out the opposite nostril and carry discharge with it.*
- Instruct the patient not to speak or swallow during the irrigation *to avoid forcing infectious material into the sinuses or eustachian tubes.*
- *To avoid injuring the nasal mucosa,* remove the irrigating tip from the nostril if the patient reports the need to sneeze or cough.

Using a bulb syringe or squeeze bottle

- Fill the bulb syringe with saline solution and insert the tip about ½″ (1.3 cm) into the patient's nostril. Alternatively, fill the squeeze bottle with normal saline solution (unless using a prefilled bottle) and insert the tip according to the manufacturer's instructions.[22]
- Squeeze the bulb syringe or squeeze bottle until a gentle stream of warm irrigant washes through the nose. Avoid forceful squeezing, *which may drive debris from the nasal passages into the sinuses or eustachian tubes and introduce infection.* Alternate irrigating each nostril until the draining irrigant runs clear.

Using an electronic irrigation device

- Insert the irrigation tip into the nostril about ½″ to 1″ (1.3 to 2.5 cm) into the patient's nostril.
- Turn on the electronic irrigating device. Begin with a low pressure setting, increasing the pressure as needed *to obtain a gentle stream of irrigant.* Be careful not to drive material from the nose into the sinuses or eustachian tubes. Irrigate both nostrils until the draining irrigant runs clear.

Positioning the patient for nasal irrigation

Whether you're helping a patient to perform nasal irrigation with a bulb syringe, squeeze bottle, or an electronic irrigating device, the irrigation will progress more easily once the patient learns how to hold the head for optimal safety, comfort, and effectiveness.

Help the patient to sit upright with the head bent forward over the basin or sink and well-flexed on the chest. The patient's nose and ear should be on the same vertical plane (as shown below).

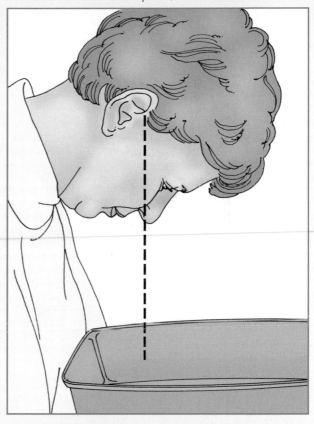

Explain that the patient is less likely to breathe in the irrigant when holding the head in this position. This position should also keep the irrigant from entering the eustachian tubes, which will now lie above the level of the irrigation stream.

Completing the procedure

- Inspect the draining irrigant for purulence (*which may indicate infection*), *bleeding, or foreign bodies.* Report unexpected findings to the practitioner.
- After irrigation, have the patient wait a few minutes before blowing excess fluid from both nostrils at once. *Gentle blowing through both nostrils prevents fluid or pressure buildup in the sinuses. This action also helps to loosen and expel crusted secretions and mucus.*
- Return the patient's bed to the lowest position *to prevent falls and maintain patient safety.*[23]
- Remove and discard the disposable irrigation tip in an appropriate receptacle.[21]
- Clean the bulb syringe, squeeze bottle, or electronic irrigation device with soap and water and then disinfect it, as recommended. Rinse and dry the device.[24,25] Clean the basin or sink with facility-approved disinfectant.[24,25]
- Remove and discard your gloves.[19,21]
- Perform hand hygiene.[6,7,8,9,10,11]
- Document the procedure.[26,27,28,29]

Special considerations

■ Nasal irrigation with normal saline solution can be used prior to administration of other intranasal medications *to improve absorption by cleansing mucosa.*[30]

■ Expect fluid to drain from the patient's nose for a brief time after irrigation and before blowing the nose.

■ Insert the irrigation tip far enough to ensure that the irrigant cleans the nasal membranes before draining out.

Patient teaching

■ To continue nasal irrigations at home, teach the patient how to prepare saline solution. Tell the patient to fill a clean 1-L plastic bottle (4 cups + 1 oz = 1L) with bottled or distilled water, add 1 tsp of salt, and shake the solution until the salt dissolves. Stress to the patient that tap water obtained from the faucet directly isn't safe for use in nasal irrigation due to the increased risk of infection and nasal mucosal irritation associated with tap water use.[31] Only distilled or sterile water or boiled and cooled tap water should be used for nasal irrigation.[31]

■ If the patient will use a commercial nasal rinsing device, teach the necessary steps,[31] beginning with washing and drying the hands; ensuring that the device is clean and completely dry before use; using the appropriate irrigant as recommended by the device manufacturer (normal saline solution, sterile or distilled water, boiled [for 1 to 3 minutes] and cooled tap water, or filtered tap water); following the manufacturer's directions for use; cleaning the device with distilled, sterile, or boiled and cooled tap water; and finally drying the inside with a paper towel or letting it air-dry between uses. Prepared solutions should be refrigerated and should not be stored for longer than 7 days.[32,33]

■ Instruct the patient to notify the practitioner if signs and symptoms worsen or if fever, headaches, or nosebleeds develop.[31]

Complications

Use of nasal irrigation devices can lead to ear fullness, stinging of the nasal mucosa, sinus discomfort, nosebleeds, and injury to the anterior nose.[1,3] Infection is possible with improper use of the device.[31,33]

Documentation

Document the date, time, and duration of the nasal irrigation procedure and the amount of irrigant used. Describe the appearance of the drained solution. Note the patient's tolerance of the procedure. Document teaching provided to the patient and family (if applicable), their understanding of that teaching, and any need for follow-up teaching.

REFERENCES

1 Rabago, D., & Zgierska, A. (2009). Saline nasal irrigation for upper respiratory conditions. *American Family Physician, 80*(10), 1117–1119. https://www.aafp.org/afp/2009/1115/p1117.html

2 Rosenfeld, R. M., et al (2015). Clinical practice guideline (update): Adult sinusitis. *Otolaryngology—Head and Neck Surgery, 152*(Suppl. 2), S1–S39. https://journals.sagepub.com/doi/pdf/10.1177/0194599815572097

3 Hermelingmeier, K. E., et al. (2012). Nasal irrigation as an adjunctive treatment in allergic rhinitis: A systematic review and meta-analysis. *American Journal of Rhinology & Allergy, 26*(5), e119–e125. https://www.ncbi.nlm.nih.gov/pmc/articles/PMC3904042/ (Level I)

4 Low, T. H., et al. (2014). A double-blind randomized controlled trial of normal saline, lactated Ringer's, and hypertonic saline nasal irrigation solution after endoscopic sinus surgery. *American Journal of Rhinology & Allergy, 28*, 225–231. (Level II)

5 Nimsakul, S., et al. (2018). Does heating up saline for nasal irrigation improve mucociliary function in chronic rhinosinusitis? *American Journal of Rhinology & Allergy, 32*, 106–111. (Level II)

6 Centers for Disease Control and Prevention. (2002). Guideline for hand hygiene in health-care settings: Recommendations of the Healthcare Infection Control Practices Advisory Committee and the HICPAC/SHEA/APIC/IDSA Hand Hygiene Task Force. *MMWR Recommendations and Reports, 51*(RR-16), 1–45. https://www.cdc.gov/mmwr/pdf/rr/rr5116.pdf (Level II)

7 World Health Organization. (2009). WHO guidelines on hand hygiene in health care: First global patient safety challenge, clean care is safer care. https://apps.who.int/iris/bitstream/handle/10665/44102/9789241597906_eng.pdf?sequence=1(Level IV)

8 The Joint Commission. (2021). Standard NPSG.07.01.01. *Comprehensive accreditation manual for hospitals.* Oakbrook Terrace, IL: The Joint Commission. (Level VII)

9 Centers for Medicare and Medicaid Services, Department of Health and Human Services. (2020). Condition of participation: Infection control. 42 C.F.R. § 482.42.

10 Accreditation Association for Hospitals and Health Systems. (2020). Standard 07.01.21. *Healthcare Facilities Accreditation Program: Accreditation requirements for acute care hospitals.* Chicago, IL: Accreditation Association for Hospitals and Health Systems. (Level VII)

11 DNV GL-Healthcare USA, Inc. (2020). IC.1.SR.1. *NIAHO® accreditation requirements, interpretive guidelines and surveyor guidance—revision 20.0.* Milford, OH: DNV GL-Healthcare USA, Inc. (Level VII)

12 The Joint Commission. (2021). Standard NPSG.01.01.01. *Comprehensive accreditation manual for hospitals.* Oakbrook Terrace, IL: The Joint Commission. (Level VII)

13 Centers for Medicare and Medicaid Services, Department of Health and Human Services. (2020). Condition of participation: Patient's rights. 42 C.F.R. § 482.13(c)(1).

14 Accreditation Association for Hospitals and Health Systems. (2020). Standard 15.01.16. *Healthcare Facilities Accreditation Program: Accreditation requirements for acute care hospitals.* Chicago, IL: Accreditation Association for Hospitals and Health Systems. (Level VII)

15 The Joint Commission. (2021). Standard RI.01.01.01. *Comprehensive accreditation manual for hospitals.* Oakbrook Terrace IL: The Joint Commission. (Level VII)

16 DNV GL-Healthcare USA, Inc. (2020). PR.2.SR.5. *NIAHO® accreditation requirements, interpretive guidelines and surveyor guidance—revision 20.0.* Milford, OH: DNV GL-Healthcare USA, Inc. (Level VII)

17 The Joint Commission. (2021). Standard PC.02.01.21. *Comprehensive accreditation manual for hospitals.* Oakbrook Terrace, IL: The Joint Commission. (Level VII)

18 Waters, T. R., et al. (2009). Safe patient handling training for schools of nursing. https://www.cdc.gov/niosh/docs/2009-127/pdfs/2009-127.pdf (Level VII)

19 Siegel, J. D., et al. (2007, revised 2019). 2007 guideline for isolation precautions: Preventing transmission of infectious agents in healthcare settings. https://www.cdc.gov/infectioncontrol/pdf/guidelines/isolation-guidelines-H.pdf (Level II)

20 Accreditation Association for Hospitals and Health Systems. (2020). Standard 07.01.10. *Healthcare Facilities Accreditation Program: Accreditation requirements for acute care hospitals.* Chicago, IL: Accreditation Association for Hospitals and Health Systems. (Level VII)

21 Occupational Safety and Health Administration. (2012). Bloodborne pathogens, standard number 1910.1030. https://www.osha.gov/pls/oshaweb/owadisp.show_document?p_id=10051&p_table=STANDARDS (Level VII)

22 NeilMed Pharmaceuticals, Inc. (n.d.). Directions for use & warnings: Sinus rinse. http://www.neilmed.com/usa/directions-for-use.php

23 Ganz, D. A., et al. (2013, Reviewed 2021). *Preventing falls in hospitals: A toolkit for improving quality of care* (AHRQ Publication No. 13-0015-EF). Rockville, MD: Agency for Healthcare Research and Quality. https://www.ahrq.gov/professionals/systems/hospital/fallpxtoolkit/index.html (Level VII)

24 Rutala, W. A., et al. (2008, revised 2019). Guideline for disinfection and sterilization in healthcare facilities, 2008. https://www.cdc.gov/infection-control/pdf/guidelines/disinfection-guidelines-H.pdf (Level I)

25 Accreditation Association for Hospitals and Health Systems. (2020). Standard 07.02.03. *Healthcare Facilities Accreditation Program: Accreditation requirements for acute care hospitals.* Chicago, IL: Accreditation Association for Hospitals and Health Systems. (Level VII)

26 The Joint Commission. (2021). Standard RC.01.03.01. *Comprehensive accreditation manual for hospitals.* Oakbrook Terrace, IL: The Joint Commission. (Level VII)

27 Centers for Medicare and Medicaid Services, Department of Health and Human Services. (2020). Condition of participation: Medical record services. 42 C.F.R. § 482.24(b).

28 Accreditation Association for Hospitals and Health Systems. (2020). Standard 10.00.03. *Healthcare Facilities Accreditation Program: Accreditation requirements for acute care hospitals.* Chicago, IL: Accreditation Association for Hospitals and Health Systems. (Level VII)

29 DNV GL-Healthcare USA, Inc. (2020). MR.2.SR.1. *NIAHO® accreditation requirements, interpretive guidelines and surveyor guidance—revision 20.0.* Milford, OH: DNV GL-Healthcare USA, Inc. (Level VII)

30 Hamilos, D. L., & Holbrook, E. H. (2021). Chronic rhinosinusitis: Management. In: *UpToDate*, Corren, J., & Deschler, D. G. (Eds.)

31 U.S. Food and Drug Administration. (2021). Is rinsing your sinuses with neti pots safe? https://www.fda.gov/consumers/consumer-updates/rinsing-your-sinuses-neti-pots-safe?source=govdelivery

32 Succar, E. F., et al. (2019). Nasal saline irrigation: A clinical update. *International Forum of Allergy& Rhinology, 9*, S4–S8. https://onlinelibrary.wiley.com/doi/epdf/10.1002/alr.22330

33 Centers for Disease Control and Prevention. (2017). Sinus rinsing for health or religious practice. https://www.cdc.gov/parasites/naegleria/sinus-rinsing.html

NASAL MEDICATION ADMINISTRATION

Medications can be instilled into the nostril as nose drops, via a nasal inhaler, or as a spray. This noninvasive, essentially painless method avoids GI breakdown and adverse effects as well as hepatic first-pass metabolism of the drug.[1,2]

Most nasal medications are vasoconstrictors, which relieve nasal congestion by coating and shrinking swollen mucous membranes; an example is phenylephrine. Because vasoconstrictors such as phenylephrine can be absorbed systemically, they are usually contraindicated in hypertensive patients. Other types of nasal medications include antiseptics, anesthetics, opioids, and corticosteroids. Local anesthetics may be administered to promote patient comfort during rhinolaryngologic examination, laryngoscopy, bronchoscopy, and endotracheal intubation. Nasal corticosteroids may be prescribed to reduce inflammation in patients with allergic or inflammatory conditions and those with nasal polyps.

Medication can also be administered using a nasal inhaler, which delivers topical medications to the respiratory tract, producing local and systemic effects.[3] The mucosal lining of the respiratory tract absorbs the inhalant almost immediately. Examples of common inhalants are bronchodilators, which improve airway patency and facilitate mucous drainage; mucolytics, which attain a high local concentration to liquefy tenacious bronchial secretions; and corticosteroids, which decrease inflammation.

Nasal spray, a third method of delivery, diffuses liquid medication throughout the nasal passages.[1,3] This method results in increased local effects with minimal systemic effects; it is noninvasive, essentially painless, and helpful in rapid absorption and effect.[1,2]

Nasal delivery of medications avoids gastrointestinal (GI) breakdown, adverse GI reactions, and first-pass metabolism of the drug by the liver.[2,3] It can be used for local therapy of nasal diseases as well as for systemic drug delivery.[1,2,3] It's especially useful in the treatment of central nervous system diseases, *because this method allows the medication to be transported to the brain through the olfactory, trigeminal, and vascular pathways.*[3]

Equipment

For nose drop instillation
Prescribed medication ▪ medication administration record ▪ dropper or appropriate-sized syringe ▪ emesis basin ▪ facial tissues ▪ label ▪ Optional: pillow, gloves, other personal protective equipment.

For nasal inhaler
Prescribed medication ▪ medication administration record ▪ facial tissues ▪ normal saline solution (or water) ▪ Optional: gloves, emesis basin.

For nasal spray
Prescribed medication ▪ medication administration record ▪ emesis basin ▪ facial tissues ▪ Optional: gloves, other personal protective equipment.

Preparation of equipment

If you are using the inhaler or nasal spray for the first time, follow the manufacturer's instructions for priming it.[4,5,6]

Implementation

▪ Avoid distractions and interruptions when preparing and administering medications *to prevent medication administration errors.*[7,8]
▪ Verify the order on the patient's medication record by checking it against the practitioner's order.[9,10,11,12]
▪ Reconcile the patient's medications when a new medication is ordered *to reduce the risk of medication errors, including omissions, duplications, dosing errors, and drug interactions.*
▪ Gather and the necessary equipment and supplies.
▪ Compare the medication label with the practitioner's order *to verify the correct medication, indication, dose, route, and time of administration.*[9,10,11,12] Verify the correct concentration of the medication. Phenylephrine, for example, is available in concentrations from 0.125% to 1%.[13]
▪ Check the expiration date on the medication. If the medication is expired, return it to the pharmacy and obtain new medication.[9,10,11,12]
▪ Check the patient's medical record for an allergy or other contraindication to the prescribed medication. If an allergy or other contraindication exists, don't administer the medication; instead, notify the practitioner.[9,10,11,12]
▪ Visually inspect the medication for discoloration or other loss of integrity. Don't give the medication if its integrity is compromised.[9,10,11,12]
▪ Discuss any unresolved concerns about the medication with the patient's practitioner.[9,10,11,12]
▪ Perform hand hygiene.[14,15,16,17,18,19]
▪ Confirm the patient's identity using at least two patient identifiers.[20]
▪ Provide privacy.[21,22,23,24]
▪ Explain the procedure to the patient and family (if appropriate) according to their individual communication and learning needs *to increase their understanding, allay their fears, and enhance cooperation.*[25]
▪ If the patient is receiving the medication for the first time, inform the patient or family about significant adverse reactions and discuss any other concerns related to the medication.[9,10,11,12]
▪ Verify that the medication is being administered at the proper time, in the prescribed dose, and by the correct route *to reduce the risk of medication errors.*[9,10,11,12]
▪ If your facility uses a bar-code technology, use it as directed by your facility.
▪ Raise the patient's bed to waist level when providing care *to prevent caregiver back strain.*[26]
▪ Perform hand hygiene.[14,15,16,17,18,19]

NURSING ALERT If your facility's hazardous drug list contains the drug you are about to administer, put on personal protective equipment as directed.[27]

▪ Put on gloves, if needed, *to comply with standard precautions.*[28,29]

For nose drop instillation
▪ Provide a facial tissue and ask the patient to blow the nose before instilling nose drops, as appropriate.[30]
▪ When possible, position the patient so that the drops flow back into the nostrils, toward the affected area. (See *Positioning the patient for nose drop instillation*, page 564.)
▪ Draw the medication into the dropper or an appropriate-sized syringe.
▪ Push up the tip of the patient's nose slightly. Position the dropper just above the nostril and direct its tip toward the midline of the nose *so that the drops flow toward the back of the nasal cavity rather than down the throat.*
▪ Insert the dropper about ⅜″ (1 cm) into the nostril. Don't let the dropper or syringe touch the sides of the nostril, *because this would contaminate the dropper or could cause the patient to sneeze.*
▪ Instill the prescribed number of drops or milliliters, observing the patient carefully for signs of discomfort.
▪ *To prevent the drops from leaking out of the nostrils*, ask the patient to keep the head tilted back for at least 5 minutes and to breathe through the mouth. *This also allows sufficient time for the medication to constrict mucous membranes.*
▪ Keep an emesis basin handy *so that the patient can expectorate any medication that flows into the oropharynx and mouth.* Use a facial tissue to wipe any excess medication from the patient's nostrils and face.

Positioning the patient for nose drop instillation

To reach the ethmoid and sphenoid sinuses, have the patient lie on the back with the neck hyperextended and the head tilted back over the edge of the bed. Support the head with one hand *to prevent neck strain*.

To reach the maxillary and frontal sinuses, have the patient lie on the back with the head toward the affected side and hanging slightly over the edge of the bed. Ask the patient to rotate the head laterally after hyperextension, and support the head with one hand *to prevent neck strain*.

To administer drops for relief of ordinary nasal congestion, help the patient to a reclining or supine position with the head tilted slightly toward the affected side. Aim the dropper upward, toward the patient's eye, rather than downward, toward the ear.

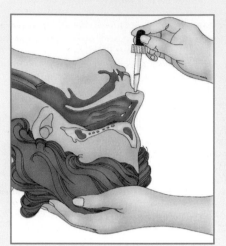
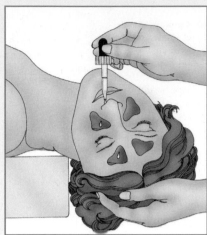
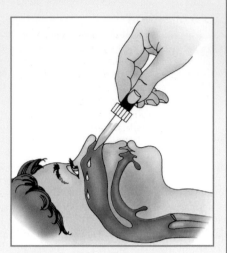

■ If used, clean the dropper by separating the plunger and pipette (or a syringe by separating it from the plunger) and flushing them with warm water. Allow them to air-dry completely, and label and store them appropriately .

For nasal inhaler
■ Agitate the contents of the medication bottle for an aqueous spray inhaler, as directed. Follow the manufacturer's instructions for loading and activating a dry-powdered inhaler.[4]
■ Remove the protective cap from the applicator tip.
■ Have the patient tilt the head slightly forward.
■ Tell the patient to keep the medication container upright and to place the applicator tip into one nostril, pointing it slightly away from the nasal septum, while occluding the other nostril with a finger.
■ For an aqueous spray inhaler, instruct the patient to place the thumb at the bottom of the container and the middle and index fingers on either side of the spray tip, and then to press down firmly and quickly on the inhaler while inhaling deeply with the mouth closed. For a dry-powder inhaler, instruct the patient to breathe in quickly and forcefully *to release a premeasured, loaded dose of medication*.[4]
■ Tell the patient to remove the inhaler from the nostril and to hold the breath for a few seconds.
■ Have the patient exhale through the mouth.
■ Have the patient repeat the procedure in the other nostril, as directed.
■ Have the patient tilt the head back for a few seconds and gargle with normal saline solution or water *to remove the medication from the mouth and throat*.[5] Offer the patient an emesis basin, as needed.
■ Instruct the patient to avoid blowing the nose for 15 minutes after medication administration.[6]

For nasal spray instillation
■ Agitate the contents of the medication container according to the manufacturer's instructions.
■ Remove the protective cap from the spray nozzle.
■ *To prevent air from entering the nasal cavity and to allow the medication to flow properly*, occlude one of the patient's nostrils with your finger.[31] Insert the atomizer tip into the open nostril.

■ Instruct the patient to inhale with the mouth closed. As the patient inhales, squeeze the atomizer once, quickly and firmly. Use just enough force to coat the inside of the patient's nose with the medication. Then tell the patient to exhale through the mouth.[31]
■ If ordered, spray the nostril again. Then repeat the procedure in the other nostril, if ordered.
■ Instruct the patient to keep the head tilted back for several minutes and to breathe slowly through the nose *so that the medication has time to work*. Tell the patient to avoid nose blowing for 15 minutes after nasal spray instillation.
■ Keep an emesis basin handy *so that the patient can expectorate any medication that flows into the oropharynx and mouth*. Use a facial tissue to wipe any excess medication from the patient's nostrils and face.

Completing the procedure
■ Return the bed to the lowest position *to prevent falls and maintain patient safety*.[32]
■ Discard used supplies in the appropriate receptacles.[33]
■ Remove and discard your gloves and other personal protective equipment, if worn.[28,33]
■ Perform hand hygiene.[14,15,16,17,18,19]
■ Document the procedure.[34,35,36,37]

Special considerations
■ To administer nasal medications more easily to a child or uncooperative patient, attach a small piece of tubing or an atomizer to a prefilled syringe of medication. *An atomizer device allows for atomization of the medication in any position*. Always follow the manufacturer's instructions for atomization device used.[38]
■ *To prevent cross-contamination*, label the medication bottle so that it will be used only for that patient.[39]
■ If using a metered-dose pump spray system, prime the delivery system with four sprays (or as directed by the manufacturer), or until a fine mist appears. Repeat the process to prime the system, as directed. Newer delivery system designs may reduce the need for priming and repriming, and may provide safety features to enhance dosing control. Always follow the manufacturer's instructions for use.[1]

Complications

Complications may include infection and local reactions, such as redness or swelling of the nares, bleeding, a burning sensation, an odd taste in the mouth after administration, drying of the nasal membranes, or epistaxis.[40] Adverse effects depend on the drug being administered. Long-term use of some glucocorticoid preparations may result in adrenal suppression, slow growth in children, decreased bone mineral density, glaucoma, or cataracts.[41]

Documentation

Document the name of the medication and its concentration, the number of drops or milliliters you administered, the time and date of each instillation, whether you instilled the medication in one or both nostrils, and the patient's tolerance of the procedure. Record any adverse reactions to the prescribed medication, the date and time that you notified the practitioner, prescribed interventions, and the patient's response to those interventions. Document teaching provided to the patient and family (if applicable), their understanding of that teaching, and any need for follow-up teaching.

REFERENCES

1 Djupesland, P. G. (2013). Nasal drug delivery devices: Characteristics and performance in a clinical perspective—a review. *Drug Delivery and Translational Research, 3*, 42–62. https://link.springer.com/article/10.1007/s13346-012-0108-9

2 Bitter, C., et al. (2011). Nasal drug delivery in humans. *Current Problems in Dermatology, 40*, 20–35.

3 Gao, M., et al. (2020). Factors influencing drug deposition in the nasal cavity upon delivery via nasal sprays. *Journal of Pharmaceutical Investigation, 50*, 251–259. https://link.springer.com/article/10.1007/s40005-020-00482-z

4 AstraZeneca. (2018). Rhinocort Turbuhaler. https://pdf.hres.ca/dpd_pm/00045951.PDF

5 Mayo Clinic. (2021). Corticosteroid (inhalation route), proper use. https://www.mayoclinic.org/drugs-supplements/corticosteroid-inhalation-route/proper-use/drg-20070533

6 Teva Respiratory, LLC. (2018). Prescribing information: Qnasl (beclomethasone dipropionate) nasal aerosol. https://www.qnasl.com/wp-content/uploads/primeless-valve-pi.pdf

7 Westbrook, J., et al. (2010). Association of interruptions with an increased risk and severity of medication administration errors. *Archives of Internal Medicine, 170*, 683–690. (Level IV)

8 Institute for Safe Medication Practices. (2012). Side tracks on the safety express: Interruptions lead to errors and unfinished…Wait, what was I doing? *Nurse Advise-ERR, 11*(2), 1–4. https://www.ismp.org/resources/side-tracks-safety-express-interruptions-lead-errors-and-unfinished-wait-what-was-i-doing?id=37

9 The Joint Commission. (2021). Standard MM.06.01.01. *Comprehensive accreditation manual for hospitals.* Oakbrook Terrace, IL: The Joint Commission. (Level VII)

10 Accreditation Association for Hospitals and Health Systems. (2020). Standard 16.01.03. *Healthcare Facilities Accreditation Program: Accreditation requirements for acute care hospitals.* Chicago, IL: Accreditation Association for Hospitals and Health Systems. (Level VII)

11 Centers for Medicare and Medicaid Services, Department of Health and Human Services. (2020). Condition of participation: Nursing services. 42 C.F.R. § 482.23(c).

12 DNV GL-Healthcare USA, Inc. (2020). MM.1.SR.3. *NIAHO® accreditation requirements, interpretive guidelines and surveyor guidance—revision 20.0.* Milford, OH: DNV GL-Healthcare USA, Inc. (Level VII)

13 U.S. National Library of Medicine. (2016). Phenylephrine nasal spray. https://medlineplus.gov/druginfo/meds/a616049.html

14 The Joint Commission. (2021). Standard NPSG.07.01.01. *Comprehensive accreditation manual for hospitals.* Oakbrook Terrace, IL: The Joint Commission. (Level VII)

15 Centers for Disease Control and Prevention. (2002). Guideline for hand hygiene in health-care settings: Recommendations of the Healthcare Infection Control Practices Advisory Committee and the HICPAC/SHEA/APIC/IDSA Hand Hygiene Task Force. *MMWR Recommendations and Reports, 51*(RR-16), 1–45. https://www.cdc.gov/mmwr/pdf/rr/rr5116.pdf (Level II)

16 World Health Organization. (2009). WHO guidelines on hand hygiene in health care: First global patient safety challenge, clean care is safer care. https://apps.who.int/iris/bitstream/handle/10665/44102/9789241597906_eng.pdf?sequence=1 (Level IV)

17 Accreditation Association for Hospitals and Health Systems. (2020). Standard 07.01.21. *Healthcare Facilities Accreditation Program: Accreditation requirements for acute care hospitals.* Chicago, IL: Accreditation Association for Hospitals and Health Systems. (Level VII)

18 Centers for Medicare and Medicaid Services, Department of Health and Human Services. (2020). Condition of participation: Infection control. 42 C.F.R. § 482.42.

19 DNV GL-Healthcare USA, Inc. (2020). IC.1.SR.1. *NIAHO® accreditation requirements, interpretive guidelines and surveyor guidance—revision 20.0.* Milford, OH: DNV GL-Healthcare USA, Inc. (Level VII)

20 The Joint Commission. (2021). Standard NPSG.01.01.01. *Comprehensive accreditation manual for hospitals.* Oakbrook Terrace, IL: The Joint Commission. (Level VII)

21 Accreditation Association for Hospitals and Health Systems. (2020). Standard 15.01.16. *Healthcare Facilities Accreditation Program: Accreditation requirements for acute care hospitals.* Chicago, IL: Accreditation Association for Hospitals and Health Systems. (Level VII)

22 Centers for Medicare and Medicaid Services, Department of Health and Human Services. (2020). Condition of participation: Patient's rights. 42 C.F.R. § 482.13(c)(1).

23 DNV GL-Healthcare USA, Inc. (2020). PR.2.SR.5. *NIAHO® accreditation requirements, interpretive guidelines and surveyor guidance—revision 20.0.* Milford, OH: DNV GL-Healthcare USA, Inc. (Level VII)

24 The Joint Commission. (2021). Standard RI.01.01.01. *Comprehensive accreditation manual for hospitals.* Oakbrook Terrace, IL: The Joint Commission. (Level VII)

25 The Joint Commission. (2021). Standard PC.02.01.21. *Comprehensive accreditation manual for hospitals.* Oakbrook Terrace, IL: The Joint Commission. (Level VII)

26 Waters, T. R., et al. (2009). Safe patient handling training for schools of nursing. https://www.cdc.gov/niosh/docs/2009-127/pdfs/2009-127.pdf (Level VII)

27 The United States Pharmacopeial Convention. (2020). USP general chapter <800> Hazardous drugs—Handling in healthcare settings. https://www.usp.org/compounding/general-chapter-hazardous-drugs-handling-healthcare (Level VII)

28 Siegel, J. D., et al. (2007, revised 2019). 2007 guideline for isolation precautions: Preventing transmission of infectious agents in healthcare settings. https://www.cdc.gov/infectioncontrol/pdf/guidelines/isolation-guidelines-H.pdf (Level II)

29 Accreditation Association for Hospitals and Health Systems. (2020). Standard 07.01.10. *Healthcare Facilities Accreditation Program: Accreditation requirements for acute care hospitals.* Chicago, IL: Accreditation Association for Hospitals and Health Systems. (Level VII)

30 American Society of Health-System Pharmacists. (2021). How to use nose drops. https://www.safemedication.com/-/media/SafeMed/Flyers/Nose-Drops-Flyer.pdf

31 GlaxoSmithKline. (2017). Highlights of prescribing information: Imitrex® (sumatriptan) nasal spray. https://www.gsksource.com/pharma/content/dam/GlaxoSmithKline/US/en/Prescribing_Information/Imitrex_Nasal_Spray/pdf/IMITREX-NASAL-SPRAY-PI-PIL.PDF

32 Ganz, D. A., et al. (2013, reviewed 2021). *Preventing falls in hospitals: A toolkit for improving quality of care* (AHRQ publication no. 13-0015-EF). Rockville, MD: Agency for Healthcare Research and Quality. https://www.ahrq.gov/professionals/systems/hospital/fallpxtoolkit/index.html (Level VII)

33 Occupational Safety and Health Administration. (2012). Bloodborne pathogens, standard number 1910.1030. https://www.osha.gov/pls/oshaweb/owadisp.show_document?p_id=10051&p_table=STANDARDS (Level VII)

34 The Joint Commission. (2021). Standard RC.01.03.01. *Comprehensive accreditation manual for hospitals.* Oakbrook Terrace, IL: The Joint Commission. (Level VII)

35 Accreditation Association for Hospitals and Health Systems. (2020). Standard 10.00.03. *Healthcare Facilities Accreditation Program: Accreditation requirements for acute care hospitals.* Chicago, IL: Accreditation Association for Hospitals and Health Systems. (Level VII)

36 Centers for Medicare and Medicaid Services, Department of Health and Human Services. (2020). Condition of participation: Medical record services. 42 C.F.R. § 482.24(b).

37 DNV GL-Healthcare USA, Inc. (2020). MR.2.SR.1. *NIAHO® accreditation requirements, interpretive guidelines and surveyor guidance—revision 20.0.* Milford, OH: DNV GL-Healthcare USA, Inc. (Level VII)

38 Teleflex Incorporated. (2017). MAD Nasal™ intranasal mucosal atomization device: User guide. https://www.teleflex.com/usa/en/product-areas/anesthesia/atomization/mad-nasal-device/AN_ATM_Anesthesia-MAD-Nasal-User-Guide_MC_MC-001925_Rev1.pdf

39 Accreditation Association for Hospitals and Health Systems. (2020). Standard 25.01.18. *Healthcare Facilities Accreditation Program: Accreditation requirements for acute care hospitals.* Chicago, IL: Accreditation Association for Hospitals and Health Systems. (Level VII)

40 Peden, D. (2020). An overview of rhinitis. In: *UpToDate*, Corren, J. (Ed.).

41 deShazo, R. D., & Kemp, S. F. (2021). Pharmacotherapy of allergic rhinitis. In: *UpToDate*, Corren, J. (Ed.).

Nasal packing, assisting

In the highly vascular nasal mucosa, even seemingly minor injuries can cause major bleeding and blood loss. Initial treatment for nasal bleeding begins with ensuring a secure airway and hemodynamic stability.

Most nasal bleeding originates at a plexus of arterioles and venules in the anteroinferior septum. About 90% of nosebleeds are anterior and can be controlled by pinching the anterior aspect of the nose.[1] Initially, direct pressure is applied for about 20 minutes. When direct pressure alone doesn't stop bleeding, topical vasoconstrictive drugs such as oxymetazoline or chemical cautery with silver nitrate sticks may be effective.[2] Silver nitrate sticks are rolled over the area for 5 to 10 seconds until a gray eschar forms; then antibiotic ointment is applied to the area.[1]

If these steps are unsuccessful, nasal packing is typically the next step for persistent bleeding.[1,2,3] The patient may have to undergo nasal packing to stop anterior bleeding (which runs out of the nose) or posterior bleeding (which runs down the throat).[2,3] If blood drains into the nasopharyngeal area or lacrimal ducts, the patient may also appear to bleed from the mouth and eyes. Only about 1 in 10 nosebleeds occurs in the posterior nose, which usually bleeds more heavily than the anterior location.[1] Posterior nasal packing is contraindicated in patients with facial trauma. If the patient can't protect the airway because of shock, altered mental status, or another condition, the airway should be secured before posterior nasal packing insertion.[3]

The nurse typically assists a practitioner with anterior or posterior nasal packing. Commercially available balloons are relatively easy to insert and quite effective for anterior bleeding. Whichever procedure is used, the patient will need ongoing encouragement and support to reduce discomfort and anxiety, as well as ongoing assessment to determine whether the procedure succeeded and to detect possible complications.

Equipment

Gowns ▪ mask and goggles or mask with face shield ▪ gloves ▪ drape ▪ emesis basin ▪ nasal speculum ▪ light source (headlamp or fiberoptic nasal endoscope) ▪ suction apparatus ▪ normal saline solution ▪ prescribed anesthetic agent ▪ cotton balls or gauze pad ▪ nasal balloon device or nasal tampon ▪ vital signs monitoring equipment ▪ disinfectant pad ▪ oral care supplies ▪ stethoscope ▪ tape ▪ pulse oximeter and probe ▪ sterile nasal aspirator tip ▪ nasal speculum and tongue blades (may be in a preassembled head and neck examination kit) ▪ vial of 2% lidocaine ▪ sterile normal saline solution (1-g container and 60-mL syringe with Luer-lock tip or 5-mL bullets for moistening nasal tampons) ▪ antibiotic ointment ▪ prescribed medications ▪ Kelly clamp or Bayonet forceps ▪ Optional: epistaxis tray, supplemental humidified oxygen and face mask, arterial blood gas kit, facial tissues, tongue blade, syringe, hemostats, nasal dressing holder, topical nasal vasoconstrictor (such as 0.5% phenylephrine), 20-mL syringe, prescribed sedative, supplies for blood sampling, sterile water, water-soluble lubricant, facial tissues.

Preparation of equipment

Inspect all equipment and supplies. If a product is expired, is defective, or has compromised integrity, remove it from patient use, label it as expired or defective, and report the expiration or defect as directed by your facility.

Make sure that the light source functions properly, *because good lighting is essential.*[3] Prepare the suction equipment and make sure that it's functioning properly. Have normal saline solution readily available *to flush the suction tubing, as needed.*

Implementation

▪ Gather and prepare the necessary equipment and supplies.
▪ Perform hand hygiene.[4,5,6,7,8,9]
▪ Confirm the patient's identity using at least two patient identifiers.[10]
▪ Provide privacy.[11,12,13,14]
▪ Explain the procedure to the patient and family (if appropriate) according to their individual communication and learning needs *to increase their understanding, allay their fears, and enhance cooperation.*[15]
▪ Raise the patient's bed to waist level before providing care *to prevent caregiver back strain.*[16]
▪ Perform hand hygiene.[4,5,6,7,8,9]
▪ Obtain the patient's vital signs and observe for hypotension with postural changes. *Hypotension and tachycardia suggest significant blood loss.*
▪ Obtain the patient's oxygen saturation level using pulse oximetry.
▪ Monitor airway patency and provide the patient with an emesis basin, *because the patient will be at risk for aspirating or vomiting swallowed blood.*
▪ Screen for and assess the patient's pain using facility-defined criteria that are consistent with the patient's age, condition, and ability to understand.[17]
▪ Treat the patient's pain, as needed and ordered, using nonpharmacologic or pharmacologic approaches, or a combination of approaches. Base the treatment plan on evidence-based practices and the patient's clinical condition, past medical history, and pain management goals.[18] Monitor the patient closely if identified as at high risk for adverse outcomes related to opioid treatment, if opioids are prescribed.[17]

Inserting posterior nasal packing

Posterior packing consists of a gauze roll shaped and secured by three sutures (one suture at each end and one in the middle), or a balloon-type catheter. To insert the packing, the practitioner advances one or two soft catheters into the patient's nostrils (as shown below). When the catheter tips appear in the nasopharynx, the practitioner grasps them with a Kelly clamp or bayonet forceps and pulls them forward through the mouth. The practitioner secures the two end sutures to the catheter tip and draws the catheter back through the nostrils. This step brings the packing into place with the end sutures hanging from the patient's nostril. (The middle suture emerges from the patient's mouth to free the packing, when needed.)

The practitioner may weigh the nose sutures with a clamp. Then the practitioner will pull the packing securely into place behind the soft palate and against the posterior end of the septum (nasal choana).

Secure the strings to the patient's face with tape *to prevent migration or aspiration of the packing.*[29]

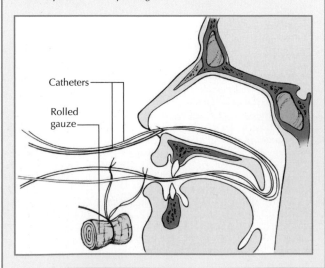

Catheters

Rolled gauze

Inserting anterior nasal packing

If bleeding persists despite chemical cautery, assist the practitioner with insertion of nasal packing to stop the bleeding. You may use a commercially available inflatable balloon or nasal tampon to pack the area.

Inflatable balloon device

An inflatable balloon device has a balloon that's coated with a carboxymethylcellulose hydrocolloid compound, which acts as a platelet aggregator. The substance also creates a lubricant when it comes in contact with water *to ease insertion*. After soaking the device in sterile water, the practitioner inserts the device along the superior aspect of the hard palate until the fabric ring is well into the naris (as shown below). Then, using a 20-mL syringe, the practitioner inflates the balloon until the pilot cuff becomes rounded and feels firm when squeezed.[27]

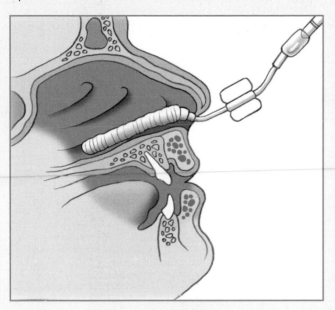

Reassess the device 15 to 20 minutes after insertion. If necessary, reinflate the cuff *to ensure proper pressure*. Tape the pilot balloon to the

patient's cheek away from the upper lip. The device can remain in place for up to 72 hours, as needed.[30]

Nasal tampon

To insert a nasal tampon, after coating the tampon with water-soluble lubricant or antibiotic ointment, as prescribed, the practitioner grabs the string end with gloved fingers or forceps. The practitioner inserts the tampon gently and quickly along the floor of the nasal cavity until the string reaches the naris (as shown below).[3]

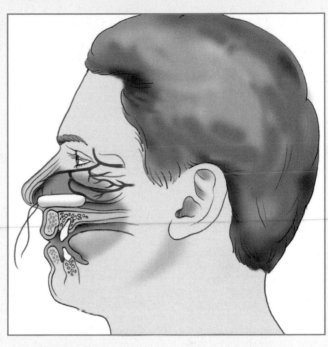

If the tampon doesn't expand within 30 seconds of insertion, the practitioner irrigates it with 10 mL of saline solution or water *so that the tampon expands*. Tape the string to the patient's nose *to secure the device in place*, and trim the ends of the string, if necessary.

■ If ordered, administer a mild sedative, following safe medication administration practices, *to reduce the patient's anxiety and decrease sympathetic stimulation, which can exacerbate a nosebleed.*[18,19,20,21]

■ Perform hand hygiene.[4,5,6,7,8,9]

■ Put on gloves, a gown, and a mask and goggles or a mask with face shield *to comply with standard precautions.*[22,23,24]

■ Help the patient sit with the head tilted forward *to minimize blood drainage into the throat and prevent aspiration.*[2,3]

■ Drape the patient as necessary.

■ At the bedside, create a sterile field using sterile no-touch technique. Open and place all sterile equipment on the sterile field, including the sterile nasal aspirating tip. Label all medications, medication containers, and solutions on and off the sterile field.[25,26] Thoroughly lubricate the posterior packing with antibiotic ointment, as ordered.[3] Alternatively, the practitioner will lubricate the catheters.

■ To inspect the nasal cavity, the practitioner will use a nasal speculum and an external light source such as a headlamp or a fiberoptic nasal endoscope. *To remove collected blood and help visualize the bleeding vessel*, the practitioner may ask the patient to blow the nose gently, or the practitioner may use suction.[27] The practitioner may treat the nose early with a vasoconstrictor, such as phenylephrine, *to slow bleeding and aid visualization.*[28]

■ Instruct the patient to open and breathe normally through the mouth during catheter insertion *to minimize gagging as the catheters pass through the nostril.*

■ Assist with administering an anesthetic agent, if needed. This step may include administration of a solution containing lidocaine, EPINEPHrine, and tetracaine applied to cotton balls or a gauze pad, which the practitioner will then place in the nostrils for 10 minutes, or the application of lidocaine spray.[3]

■ Assist the practitioner with insertion of packing, as directed. (See *Inserting posterior nasal packing* and *Inserting anterior nasal packing*.)

■ After insertion, help the patient assume a comfortable position with head elevated 45 to 90 degrees.[3]

■ Monitor the patient's vital signs *to detect changes in condition*.

■ Monitor the patient's respiratory status *to make sure the airway is patent*; monitor oxygen saturation level by pulse oximetry *to detect hypoxemia*. Make sure that the alarm limits are set appropriately for the patient's current condition, and that the alarms are turned on, functioning properly, and audible to staff.[31,32,33,34]

■ Administer supplemental humidified oxygen by face mask, as needed and ordered.

■ Provide emotional support, *because mouth breathing, which is necessary with the packing in place, may cause anxiety and hyperventilation.*

■ If severe or recurrent bleeding or an underlying medical condition is present, obtain a blood sample for complete blood count and blood compatibility testing, as ordered.[27] If the patient has renal or hepatic dysfunction, or if the patient was taking an anticoagulant, obtain a specimen for coagulation studies, as ordered.[27] Notify the practitioner of critical test results within your facility's established timeframe *so the patient can receive prompt treatment.*[35]

- Check the posterior oropharynx frequently *to see whether there's bleeding into the back of the throat or whether the packing has slipped out of position.*
- Maintain the head of the bed at 30 degrees or higher.[27]
- *Because a patient with nasal packing must breathe through the mouth,* provide frequent oral care. Artificial saliva, room humidification, and ample fluid intake also relieve dryness caused by mouth breathing.
- As ordered, administer an antiemetic, a decongestant, a sedative, and a prophylactic antibiotic following safe medication administration practices.[18,19,20,21,27,28]
- Reassess and respond to the patient's pain by evaluating the response to treatment and progress toward pain management goals. Assess for adverse reactions and risk factors for adverse events that may result from treatment.[17]
- Return the patient's bed to the lowest position *to prevent falls and maintain patient safety.*[36]
- Discard used supplies in the appropriate receptacles.[23]
- Remove and discard your gloves and other personal protective equipment.[22,23]
- Perform hand hygiene.[4,5,6,7,8,9]
- Clean and disinfect your stethoscope using a disinfectant pad.[37,38]
- Perform hand hygiene.[4,5,6,7,8,9]
- Document the procedure.[39,40,41,42]

Special considerations

- Keep emergency equipment (flashlight, tongue blade, syringe, and hemostat) at the patient's bedside *to expedite packing removal if it becomes displaced and occludes the airway.*
- Avoid administration of aspirin and nonsteroidal anti-inflammatory drugs for a few days *to reduce the risk of bleeding.*[27,28]
- After the packing is in place, compile assessment data carefully *to help detect the underlying cause of nosebleeds.* Mechanical factors include a deviated septum, injury, and a foreign body. Environmental factors include drying and erosion of the nasal mucosa, which can occur with nasal oxygen delivery or intranasal cocaine use.[2,43] Other possible causes include upper respiratory tract infection, anticoagulant or salicylate therapy, blood dyscrasias, cardiovascular or hepatic disorders, tumors of the nasal cavity or paranasal sinuses, chronic nephritis, human immunodeficiency virus infection, and familial hemorrhagic telangiectasia.
- The patient should remain on modified bed rest until removal of the pack.[3] The practitioner will usually remove nasal packing in 3 to 4 days.[2,3]

Patient teaching

Advise the patient to eat soft foods, *because nasal packing can impair the ability to eat and swallow.* Instruct the patient to drink fluids often or to use artificial saliva *to cope with dry mouth.* Teach the patient measures to prevent nosebleeds, and instruct the patient to seek medical help if these measures fail to stop bleeding.[2]

Complications

Airway obstruction can occur if an anterior or posterior pack slips backward.[1] The patient may complain of difficulty swallowing, pain, or discomfort.[28] Other possible complications include continued bleeding despite packing, aspiration of blood, hypoxia, infection, intranasal adhesions, and pressure necrosis of nasal structures, especially the septum.[1,2,3] Bradyarrhythmias can develop because of stimulation of the posterior oropharynx related to the packing.[3] Sedation can cause hypotension in a patient with significant blood loss and can also increase the patient's risk of aspiration and hypoxemia.

Documentation

Record the date and time of the procedure and the type of packing used *to ensure its removal at the appropriate time.* On the intake and output record, document the estimated blood loss and all fluids administered. Note the patient's vital signs and oxygen saturation level; the results of all laboratory tests; all drugs administered, including topical agents; and the patient's response to sedation, analgesics, and position changes. Record any complications that occur, interventions taken, and the patient's response to those interventions. Document teaching provided to the patient and family (if applicable), discharge instructions, and clinical follow-up plans; their understanding of that information; and any need for follow-up teaching.

REFERENCES

1 Alter, H. (2021). Approach to the adult with epistaxis. In: *UpToDate,* Wolfson, A. B., & Deschler, D. G. (Eds.).

2 Smith, J., et al. (2019). Community-based management of epistaxis: Who bloody knows? *Canadian Pharmacists Journal, 152*(3), 164–176. https://www.ncbi.nlm.nih.gov/pmc/articles/PMC6512189/

3 Goralnick, E. (2018). Anterior nasal packing for epistaxis. https://emedicine.medscape.com/article/80526-overview

4 Centers for Disease Control and Prevention. (2002). Guideline for hand hygiene in health-care settings: Recommendations of the Healthcare Infection Control Practices Advisory Committee and the HICPAC/SHEA/APIC/IDSA Hand Hygiene Task Force. *MMWR Recommendations and Reports, 51*(RR-16), 1–45. https://www.cdc.gov/mmwr/pdf/rr/rr5116.pdf (Level II)

5 World Health Organization. (2009). WHO guidelines on hand hygiene in health care: First global patient safety challenge, clean care is safer care. https://apps.who.int/iris/bitstream/handle/10665/44102/9789241597906_eng.pdf?sequence=1 (Level IV)

6 The Joint Commission. (2021). Standard NPSG.07.01.01. *Comprehensive accreditation manual for hospitals.* Oakbrook Terrace, IL: The Joint Commission. (Level VII)

7 Centers for Medicare and Medicaid Services, Department of Health and Human Services. (2020). Condition of participation: Infection control. 42 C.F.R. § 482.42.

8 Accreditation Association for Hospitals and Health Systems. (2020). Standard 07.01.21. *Healthcare Facilities Accreditation Program: Accreditation requirements for acute care hospitals.* Chicago, IL: Accreditation Association for Hospitals and Health Systems. (Level VII)

9 DNV GL-Healthcare USA, Inc. (2020). IC.1.SR.1. *NIAHO® accreditation requirements, interpretive guidelines and surveyor guidance—revision 20.0.* Milford, OH: DNV GL-Healthcare USA, Inc. (Level VII)

10 The Joint Commission. (2021). Standard NPSG.01.01.01. *Comprehensive accreditation manual for hospitals.* Oakbrook Terrace, IL: The Joint Commission. (Level VII)

11 The Joint Commission. (2021). Standard RI.01.01.01. *Comprehensive accreditation manual for hospitals.* Oakbrook Terrace, IL: The Joint Commission. (Level VII)

12 Centers for Medicare and Medicaid Services, Department of Health and Human Services. (2020). Condition of participation: Patient's rights. 42 C.F.R. § 482.13(c)(1).

13 Accreditation Association for Hospitals and Health Systems. (2020). Standard 15.01.16. *Healthcare Facilities Accreditation Program: Accreditation requirements for acute care hospitals.* Chicago, IL: Accreditation Association for Hospitals and Health Systems. (Level VII)

14 DNV GL-Healthcare USA, Inc. (2020). PR.2.SR.5. *NIAHO® accreditation requirements, interpretive guidelines and surveyor guidance—revision 20.0.* Milford, OH: DNV GL-Healthcare USA, Inc. (Level VII)

15 The Joint Commission. (2021). Standard PC.02.01.21. *Comprehensive accreditation manual for hospitals.* Oakbrook Terrace, IL: The Joint Commission. (Level VII)

16 Waters, T. R., et al. (2009). Safe patient handling training for schools of nursing. https://www.cdc.gov/niosh/docs/2009-127/pdfs/2009-127.pdf (Level VII)

17 The Joint Commission. (2021). Standard PC.01.02.07. *Comprehensive accreditation manual for hospitals.* Oakbrook Terrace, IL: The Joint Commission. (Level VII)

18 Centers for Medicare and Medicaid Services, Department of Health and Human Services. (2020). Condition of participation: Nursing services. 42 C.F.R. § 482.23(c).

19 Accreditation Association for Hospitals and Health Systems. (2020). Standard 16.01.03. *Healthcare Facilities Accreditation Program: Accreditation requirements for acute care hospitals.* Chicago, IL: Accreditation Association for Hospitals and Health Systems. (Level VII)

20 The Joint Commission. (2021). Standard MM.06.01.01. *Comprehensive accreditation manual for hospitals.* Oakbrook Terrace, IL: The Joint Commission. (Level VII)

21 DNV GL-Healthcare USA, Inc. (2020). MM.1.SR.3. *NIAHO® accreditation requirements, interpretive guidelines and surveyor guidance—revision 20.0*. Milford, OH: DNV GL-Healthcare USA, Inc. (Level VII)

22 Siegel, J. D., et al. (2007, revised 2019). 2007 guideline for isolation precautions: Preventing transmission of infectious agents in healthcare settings. https://www.cdc.gov/infectioncontrol/pdf/guidelines/isolation-guidelines-H.pdf (Level II)

23 Occupational Safety and Health Administration. (2012). Bloodborne pathogens, standard number 1910.1030. https://www.osha.gov/pls/oshaweb/owa-disp.show_document?p_id=10051&p_table=STANDARDS (Level VII)

24 Accreditation Association for Hospitals and Health Systems. (2020). Standard 07.01.10. *Healthcare Facilities Accreditation Program: Accreditation requirements for acute care hospitals*. Chicago, IL: Accreditation Association for Hospitals and Health Systems. (Level VII)

25 The Joint Commission. (2021). Standard NPSG.03.04.01. *Comprehensive accreditation manual for hospitals*. Oakbrook Terrace, IL: The Joint Commission. (Level VII)

26 Accreditation Association for Hospitals and Health Systems. (2020). Standard 25.01.27. *Healthcare Facilities Accreditation Program: Accreditation requirements for acute care hospitals*. Chicago, IL: Accreditation Association for Hospitals and Health Systems. (Level VII)

27 Gilman, C., & Solomon, R. C. (2009). Treatment of epistaxis. *ACEP News, 28*(6). https://www.acepnow.com/article/treatment-epistaxis/

28 Nguyen, Q. A. (2020). Epistaxis treatment and management. https://emedicine.medscape.com/article/863220-treatment

29 Killick, N., et al. (2014). Nasal packing for epistaxis: An evidence-based review. *British Journal of Hospital Medicine, 75*, 143–147. (Level V)

30 Smith & Nephew, Inc. (2015). RAPID RHINO epistaxis products. http://www.smith-nephew.com/global/ent/rr_epistaxis_solutions_brochure_rr117l.pdf

31 The Joint Commission. (2013). Sentinel event alert 50: Medical device alarm safety in hospitals. https://www.jointcommission.org/-/media/tjc/documents/resources/patient-safety-topics/sentinel-event/sea_50_alarms_4_26_16.pdf (Level VII)

32 The Joint Commission. (2021). Standard NPSG.06.01.01. *Comprehensive accreditation manual for hospitals*. Oakbrook Terrace, IL: The Joint Commission. (Level VII)

33 Graham, K. C., & Cvach, M. (2010). Monitor alarm fatigue: Standardizing use of physiological monitors and decreasing nuisance alarms. *American Journal of Critical Care, 19*, 28–37.

34 American Association of Critical-Care Nurses. (2018). AACN practice alert: Managing alarms in acute care across the life span: Electrocardiography and pulse oximetry. https://www.aacn.org/clinical-resources/practice-alerts/managing-alarms-in-acute-care-across-the-life-span (Level VII)

35 The Joint Commission. (2021). Standard NPSG.02.03.01. *Comprehensive accreditation manual for hospitals*. Oakbrook Terrace, IL: The Joint Commission. (Level VII)

36 Ganz, D. A., et al. (2013, reviewed 2021). *Preventing falls in hospitals: A toolkit for improving quality of care* (AHRQ Publication No. 13-0015-EF). Rockville, MD: Agency for Healthcare Research and Quality. https://www.ahrq.gov/professionals/systems/hospital/fallpxtoolkit/index.html (Level VII)

37 Rutala, W. A., et al. (2008, revised 2019). Guideline for disinfection and sterilization in healthcare facilities, 2008. https://www.cdc.gov/infection-control/pdf/guidelines/disinfection-guidelines-H.pdf (Level I)

38 Accreditation Association for Hospitals and Health Systems. (2020). Standard 07.02.03. *Healthcare Facilities Accreditation Program: Accreditation requirements for acute care hospitals*. Chicago, IL: Accreditation Association for Hospitals and Health Systems. (Level VII)

39 The Joint Commission. (2021). Standard RC.01.03.01. *Comprehensive accreditation manual for hospitals*. Oakbrook Terrace, IL: The Joint Commission. (Level VII)

40 Centers for Medicare and Medicaid Services, Department of Health and Human Services. (2020). Condition of participation: Medical record services. 42 C.F.R. § 482.24(b).

41 Accreditation Association for Hospitals and Health Systems. (2020). Standard 10.00.03. *Healthcare Facilities Accreditation Program: Accreditation requirements for acute care hospitals*. Chicago, IL: Accreditation Association for Hospitals and Health Systems. (Level VII)

42 DNV GL-Healthcare USA, Inc. (2020). MR.2.SR.1. *NIAHO® accreditation requirements, interpretive guidelines and surveyor guidance—revision 20.0*. Milford, OH: DNV GL-Healthcare USA, Inc. (Level VII)

43 Womack, J. P., et al. (2018). Epistaxis: Outpatient management. *American Family Physician, 98*(4), 240–245. https://www.aafp.org/afp/2018/0815/p240.html

NASOENTERIC-DECOMPRESSION TUBE CARE

A nasoenteric-decompression tube is used to aspirate intestinal contents for analysis and to treat intestinal obstruction or a GI fistula.[1] The tube may also help to prevent nausea, vomiting, and abdominal distention after GI surgery.

The patient with a nasoenteric-decompression tube needs special care, including precise intake-and-output records, as well as continuous monitoring to ensure tube patency, maintain suction and bowel decompression, and detect such complications as fluid and electrolyte imbalances related to aspiration of intestinal contents. The patient will also need frequent oral care and monitoring of the tube's exit site to provide comfort and prevent skin breakdown, and encouragement and support during tube insertion and removal and while the tube is in place.

Equipment

Suction apparatus with intermittent suction capability and appropriate connectors ▪ gloves ▪ oral care supplies ▪ stethoscope ▪ disinfectant pad ▪ securement device or tape ▪ Optional: protective padding, gown, mask and goggles or mask with face shield, irrigation set, normal saline solution, blood sampling supplies, irrigation set, tape specially formulated for fragile skin, skin preparation product, measuring tape.

Preparation of equipment

Inspect all equipment and supplies. If a product is expired, is defective, or has compromised integrity, remove it from patient use, label it as expired or defective, and report the expiration or defect as directed by your facility.

Assemble the suction apparatus and set up the suction unit. If indicated, test the unit by turning it on and placing the end of the suction tubing in a container of water. If the tubing draws in water, the unit works.

Implementation

▪ Gather and prepare the necessary equipment and supplies.
▪ Verify that tube placement has been confirmed by X-ray or electromagnetic placement device.[1,2,3,4]
▪ Perform hand hygiene.[5,6,7,8,9,10]
▪ Confirm the patient's identity using at least two patient identifiers.[11]
▪ Provide privacy.[12,13,14,15]
▪ Explain the procedure to the patient and family (if appropriate) according to their individual communication and learning needs *to increase their understanding, allay their fears, and enhance cooperation.*[16]
▪ Raise the patient's bed to waist level before performing care *to prevent caregiver back strain.*[17]
▪ Keep the head of the patient's bed elevated at least 30 degrees; if contraindicated, consider the reverse Trendelenburg position.[18]
▪ Perform hand hygiene.[5,6,7,8,9,10]
▪ Put on gloves and, as needed, other personal protective equipment *to comply with standard precautions.*[19,20,21,22]
▪ Trace the tubing from the patient to its point of origin *to make sure that you're accessing the correct tube.*[23,24]
▪ Assess for tube migration at least every 4 hours by checking the external tube length or the incremental marking at the tube's exit site and comparing it with the baseline.[18]
▪ Assess the patient's GI status at least every 4 hours and as indicated by the patient's condition *to promptly recognize changes in the patient's condition.*[18]
▪ Inspect the skin under the tube by gently lifting and repositioning it at the naris at least twice daily (but preferably more frequently) *to assess for pressure injury formation, redistribute pressure, and decrease shear force.*[18,25]
▪ Ask the patient whether the tube causes pain or discomfort at the naris or whether the securement device or tape feels too tight. For a patient who is unable to communicate, observe for agitation, pulling, itching, or grabbing, *which may be a sign that the tube causes discomfort.*
▪ Clean the skin and apply fresh tape (at least daily) or a new securement device (at least weekly according to the manufacturer's instructions), as needed. Apply a skin preparation product to the skin, if needed.[18] Enlist the help of a co-worker, if necessary, *to avoid dislodging the tube.*[26]

■ Avoid securing the tube toward the top of the patient's head *to avoid pressure on the naris from the tube.*[25]

■ Use protective padding under the device, if needed, *to protect the skin from friction and pressure.* Keep the skin under the tube clean and dry.[25]

NURSING ALERT If the patient has fragile skin and you're using tape to secure the tube, use tape specifically formulated for fragile skin *to prevent skin stripping and tearing during removal.*[27]

■ Ensure that the tube is attached to suction, as prescribed.[18] Monitor the suction device for proper functioning.

■ Monitor the patient's intake and output at an interval determined by the patient's condition and your facility. Note the characteristics of the nasoenteric decompression tube drainage.[18] If drainage isn't accumulating in the collection container, suspect an obstruction in the tube. Notify the practitioner and then irrigate the tube with normal saline solution *to clear the obstruction.* Include the instilled volume in the patient's intake. Notify the practitioner if you're unable to establish tube patency.

■ Obtain blood samples for laboratory testing, as ordered, *to monitor fluids, electrolytes, and blood loss.*[28] (See the "Venipuncture" procedure.) Notify the practitioner of critical test results within your facility's established time frame so the patient can be promptly treated.[29]

■ Correlate the patient's output with laboratory test results *to detect a trend toward dehydration, electrolyte imbalance, or both.*[18]

■ Provide oral care regularly *to promote comfort and prevent oral colonization, to decrease the risk for health care-associated pneumonia.* (See the "Oral care" procedure.)[26,30]

■ Return the bed to the lowest position *to prevent falls and to maintain patient safety.*[31]

■ Remove and discard your gloves and any other personal protective equipment, if worn.[19,20]

■ Perform hand hygiene.[5,6,7,8,9,10]

■ Clean and disinfect your stethoscope using a disinfectant pad.[32,33]

■ Perform hand hygiene.[5,6,7,8,9,10]

■ Document the procedure.[34,35,36,37]

Special considerations

■ The Joint Commission issued a sentinel event alert related to managing risk during transition to new International Organization for Standardization tubing standards that were designed to prevent dangerous tubing misconnections, which can lead to serious patient injury and death. During the transition, make sure to trace each tubing and catheter from the patient to its point of origin before connecting or reconnecting any device or infusion, at any care transition (such as to a new setting or service), and as part of the hand-off process; route tubes and catheters with different purposes in different standardized directions; when there are different access sites or several bags hanging, label tubing at both the distal and proximal ends; use tubing and equipment only as intended; and store medications for different delivery routes in separate locations.[23]

Complications

Complications may be mechanical, such as an obstructed or clogged tube or tube breakage. Other potential complications include laryngospasm, aspiration, pneumonia, pneumonitis, mucosal erosion and bleeding, aorto-esophageal fistula, stricture formation, throat pain, stridor, dysphagia, vocal cord paralysis, rhinitis, and sinusitis.[4,38] Dehydration and electrolyte imbalances can result from the removal of body fluids and electrolytes by suctioning.

Documentation

Document your assessment findings, the external tube length, the condition of the patient's naris, the volume and characteristics of drainage, suction applied, and oral care provided. Record any complications, the name of the practitioner notified, and the date and time of the notification, prescribed interventions, and the patient's response to those interventions. Document teaching provided to the patient and family (if applicable), their understanding of that teaching, and any need for follow-up teaching.

REFERENCES

1 Itkin, M., et al. (2011). Multidisciplinary practical guidelines for gastrointestinal access for enteral nutrition and decompression from the Society of Interventional Radiology and American Gastroenterological Association (AGA) Institute, with endorsement by Canadian Interventional Radiological Association (CIRA) and Cardiovascular and Interventional Radiological Society of Europe (CIRSE). *Journal of Vascular and Interventional Radiology, 22*, 1089–1106. https://www.jvir.org/article/S1051-0443(11)00850-5/pdf (Level VII)

2 American Association of Critical-Care Nurses. (2016). AACN practice alert: Initial and ongoing verification of feeding tube placement in adults. https://www.aacn.org/clinical-resources/practice-alerts/initial-and-ongoing-verification-of-feeding-tube-placement-in-adults (Level VII)

3 Boullata, J. I., et al. (2016). ASPEN safe practices for enteral nutrition therapy. *Journal of Parenteral and Enteral Nutrition, 41*(1), 15–103. https://onlinelibrary.wiley.com/doi/pdf/10.1177/0148607116673053 (Level VII)

4 Prabhakaran, S., et al. (2012). Nasoenteric tube complications. *Scandinavian Journal of Surgery, 101*, 147–155. https://journals.sagepub.com/doi/pdf/10.1177/145749691210100302

5 The Joint Commission. (2021). Standard NPSG.07.01.01. *Comprehensive accreditation manual for hospitals.* Oakbrook Terrace, IL: The Joint Commission. (Level VII)

6 Centers for Disease Control and Prevention. (2002). Guideline for hand hygiene in health-care settings: Recommendations of the Healthcare Infection Control Practices Advisory Committee and the HICPAC/SHEA/APIC/IDSA Hand Hygiene Task Force. *MMWR Recommendations and Reports, 51*(RR-16), 1–45. https://www.cdc.gov/mmwr/pdf/rr/rr5116.pdf (Level II)

7 World Health Organization. (2009). WHO guidelines on hand hygiene in health care: First global patient safety challenge, clean care is safer care. https://apps.who.int/iris/bitstream/handle/10665/44102/9789241597906_eng.pdf?sequence=1 (Level IV)

8 Centers for Medicare and Medicaid Services, Department of Health and Human Services. (2020). Condition of participation: Infection control. 42 C.F.R. § 482.42.

9 Accreditation Association for Hospitals and Health Systems. (2020). Standard 07.01.21. *Healthcare Facilities Accreditation Program: Accreditation requirements for acute care hospitals.* Chicago, IL: Accreditation Association for Hospitals and Health Systems. (Level VII)

10 DNV GL-Healthcare USA, Inc. (2020). IC.1.SR.1. *NIAHO® accreditation requirements, interpretive guidelines and surveyor guidance—revision 20.0.* Milford, OH: DNV GL-Healthcare USA, Inc. (Level VII)

11 The Joint Commission. (2021). Standard NPSG.01.01.01. *Comprehensive accreditation manual for hospitals.* Oakbrook Terrace, IL: The Joint Commission. (Level VII)

12 The Joint Commission. (2021). Standard RI.01.01.01. *Comprehensive accreditation manual for hospitals.* Oakbrook Terrace, IL: The Joint Commission. (Level VII)

13 Centers for Medicare and Medicaid Services, Department of Health and Human Services. (2020). Condition of participation: Patient's rights. 42 C.F.R. § 482.13(c)(1).

14 Accreditation Association for Hospitals and Health Systems. (2020). Standard 15.01.16. *Healthcare Facilities Accreditation Program: Accreditation requirements for acute care hospitals.* Chicago, IL: Accreditation Association for Hospitals and Health Systems. (Level VII)

15 DNV GL-Healthcare USA, Inc. (2020). PR.2.SR.5. *NIAHO® accreditation requirements, interpretive guidelines and surveyor guidance—revision 20.0.* Milford, OH: DNV GL-Healthcare USA, Inc. (Level VII)

16 The Joint Commission. (2021). Standard PC.02.01.21. *Comprehensive accreditation manual for hospitals.* Oakbrook Terrace, IL: The Joint Commission. (Level VII)

17 Waters, T. R., et al. (2009). Safe patient handling training for schools of nursing. https://www.cdc.gov/niosh/docs/2009-127/pdfs/2009-127.pdf (Level VII)

18 Wiegand, D. L. (2017). *AACN procedure manual for high acuity, progressive, and critical care* (7th ed.). St. Louis, MO: Elsevier.

19 Siegel, J. D., et al. (2007, revised 2019). 2007 guideline for isolation precautions: Preventing transmission of infectious agents in healthcare settings. https://www.cdc.gov/infectioncontrol/pdf/guidelines/isolation-guidelines-H.pdf (Level II)

20 Occupational Safety and Health Administration. (2012). Bloodborne pathogens, standard number 1910.1030. https://www.osha.gov/pls/oshaweb/owadisp.show_document?p_id=10051&p_table=STANDARDS (Level VII)

21 Accreditation Association for Hospitals and Health Systems. (2020). Standard 07.01.10. *Healthcare Facilities Accreditation Program: Accreditation requirements for acute care hospitals*. Chicago, IL: Accreditation Association for Hospitals and Health Systems. (Level VII)

22 DNV GL-Healthcare USA, Inc. (2020). IC.1.SR.2. *NIAHO® accreditation requirements, interpretive guidelines and surveyor guidance—revision 20.0*. Milford, OH: DNV GL-Healthcare USA, Inc. (Level VII)

23 The Joint Commission. (2014). Sentinel event alert 53: Managing risk during transition to new ISO tubing connector standards. https://www.jointcommission.org/-/media/tjc/documents/resources/patient-safety-topics/sentinel-event/sea_53_connectors_8_19_14_final.pdf (Level VII)

24 U.S. Food and Drug Administration. (2017). Examples of medical device misconnections. https://www.fda.gov/medical-devices/medical-device-connectors/examples-medical-device-misconnections

25 European Pressure Ulcer Advisory Panel, et al. (2019). Prevention and treatment of pressure ulcers/injuries: Quick reference guide. http://www.internationalguideline.com/static/pdfs/Quick_Reference_Guide-10Mar2019.pdf (Level VII)

26 Nasoenteric tube feeding (adults): Care and daily management. (2021). *JBI EBP Database*. AN: JBI1809 (Level VII)

27 LeBlanc, K., et al. (2013). International skin tear advisory panel: A toolkit to aid in the prevention, assessment, and treatment of skin tears using a simplified classification system. *Advances in Skin & Wound Care, 26*, 459–476. (Level IV)

28 Jackson, P., & Cruz, M. V. (2018). Intestinal obstruction: Evaluation and management. *American Family Physician, 98*(6), 362–367. https://www.aafp.org/afp/2018/0915/p362.html

29 The Joint Commission. (2021). Standard NPSG.02.03.01. *Comprehensive accreditation manual for hospitals*. Oakbrook Terrace, IL: The Joint Commission. (Level VII)

30 Maeda, K., & Akagi, J. (2014). Oral care may reduce pneumonia in the tube-fed elderly: A preliminary study. *Dysphagia, 29*, 616–621. (Level VI)

31 Ganz, D. A., et al. (2013, reviewed 2021). *Preventing falls in hospitals: A toolkit for improving quality of care* (AHRQ Publication No. 13-0015-EF). Rockville, MD: Agency for Healthcare Research and Quality. https://www.ahrq.gov/professionals/systems/hospital/fallpxtoolkit/index.html (Level VII)

32 Rutala, W. A., et al. (2008, revised 2019). Guideline for disinfection and sterilization in healthcare facilities, 2008. https://www.cdc.gov/infection-control/pdf/guidelines/disinfection-guidelines-H.pdf (Level I)

33 Accreditation Association for Hospitals and Health Systems. (2020). Standard 07.02.03. *Healthcare Facilities Accreditation Program: Accreditation requirements for acute care hospitals*. Chicago, IL: Accreditation Association for Hospitals and Health Systems. (Level VII)

34 The Joint Commission. (2021). Standard RC.01.03.01. *Comprehensive accreditation manual for hospitals*. Oakbrook Terrace, IL: The Joint Commission. (Level VII)

35 Centers for Medicare and Medicaid Services, Department of Health and Human Services. (2020). Condition of participation: Medical record services. 42 C.F.R. § 482.24(b).

36 Accreditation Association for Hospitals and Health Systems. (2020). Standard 10.00.03. *Healthcare Facilities Accreditation Program: Accreditation requirements for acute care hospitals*. Chicago, IL: Accreditation Association for Hospitals and Health Systems. (Level VII)

37 DNV GL-Healthcare USA, Inc. (2020). MR.2.SR.1. *NIAHO® accreditation requirements, interpretive guidelines and surveyor guidance—revision 20.0*. Milford, OH: DNV GL-Healthcare USA, Inc. (Level VII)

38 Hodin, R. A., & Bordeianou, L. (2020). Inpatient placement and management of nasogastric and nasoenteric tubes in adults. In: *UpToDate*, Cochran, A. (Ed.).

Nasoenteric-decompression tube insertion and removal

A nasoenteric-decompression tube, inserted nasally and advanced beyond the stomach into the intestinal tract, aspirates intestinal contents for analysis and to treat intestinal obstruction or GI fistula.[1,2] The tube can also help prevent nausea, vomiting, and abdominal distention after GI surgery. A practitioner usually inserts and removes a nasoenteric-decompression tube; however, a nurse may remove it in an emergency. An oroenteric-decompression tube is a good substitute if the patient has facial trauma, a nasal injury, or abnormal nasal anatomy.[1]

EQUIPMENT

Nasoenteric-decompression tubes

The type of nasoenteric-decompression tube chosen for the patient depends on the size of the patient and the nostrils, the estimated duration of intubation, and the reason for the procedure. For example, to remove viscous material from the patient's intestinal tract, the practitioner may select a tube with a wide bore and a single lumen. Typically, a #14 or #16 French tube is appropriate.

Such tubes as the preweighted Andersen Miller-Abbot type intestinal tube (shown below), have a tungsten-weighted inflatable latex balloon tip designed for temporary management of mechanical obstruction in the small or large intestines.

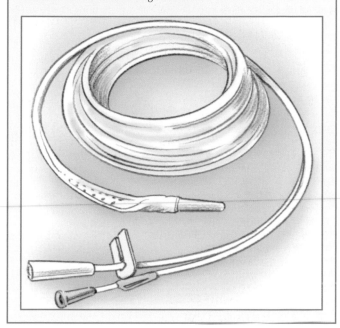

Some nasoenteric-decompression tubes have a preweighted tip and balloon at one end of the tube that holds air or water to stimulate peristalsis and facilitate the tube's passage through the pylorus and into the intestinal tract. (See *Nasoenteric-decompression tubes*.)

Equipment

For insertion
Nasoenteric-decompression tube ▪ suction apparatus with intermittent suction capability ▪ suction tubing and appropriate connectors ▪ light source ▪ gloves ▪ towel or fluid-impermeable pad ▪ water-soluble lubricant ▪ securement device ▪ tape ▪ oral care supplies ▪ washcloth and towel ▪ stethoscope ▪ disinfectant pad ▪ Optional: penlight, anesthetic agent, gown, mask and goggles or mask with face shield, tape specially formulated for fragile skin, pen with indelible ink, pH testing supplies, cup of water, straw, capnography equipment, skin preparation product, transparent semipermeable dressings, protective padding, tape measure.

For removal
Gloves ▪ fluid-impermeable pad or towel ▪ clamp ▪ oral care supplies ▪ supplies for cleaning the naris ▪ Optional: 10-mL syringe, adhesive remover.

Preparation of equipment

Inspect all equipment and supplies. If a product is expired, is defective, or has compromised integrity, remove it from patient use, label it expired or defective, and report the expiration or defect as directed by your facility.

Prepare the nasoenteric-decompression tube according to the manufacturer's instructions. Set up the suction apparatus, as ordered, and make sure that it's functioning properly.

Implementation

- Verify the practitioner's order.
- Review the patient's medical record for a history of nausea, vomiting, intestinal obstruction or fistula, allergies to adhesives or nasoenteric tube material, and contraindications to the procedure.
- Gather and prepare the necessary equipment and supplies.
- Perform hand hygiene.[3,4,5,6,7,8]
- Confirm the patient's identity using at least two patient identifiers.[9]
- Provide privacy.[10,11,12,13]
- Explain the procedure to the patient and family (if appropriate) according to their individual communication and learning needs *to increase their understanding, allay their fears, and enhance cooperation.*[14]
- Make sure that lighting is adequate.
- Raise the patient's bed to waist level when performing care *to prevent caregiver back strain.*[15]
- Perform hand hygiene.[3,4,5,6,7,8]

Inserting a nasoenteric-decompression tube

- Put on gloves and other personal protective equipment as needed *to comply with standard precautions.*[16,17,18]
- Assess the patient's GI status *to serve as a baseline for comparison.*
- Position the patient as the practitioner specifies, usually in the semi-Fowler or high Fowler position.[19]
- Place a fluid-impermeable pad or towel across the patient's chest *to protect the patient from soiling during tube insertion.*
- Agree with the patient on a signal that can be used to stop the insertion briefly if necessary.
- The practitioner assesses the patency of the patient's nostrils, using a penlight if needed.
- Administer an anesthetic agent, if prescribed, following safe medication administration practices.[19,20,21,22,23]
- *To determine the insertion depth of the tube to ensure it reaches the stomach,* the practitioner places the tube's distal end at the tip of the patient's nose and then extends the tube to the earlobe and down to the xiphoid process, and then midway to the umbilicus.[19] The practitioner marks the tube with an indelible pen or holds it at this point.[19]
- The practitioner applies water-soluble lubricant to the distal end of the tube *to facilitate insertion.*[19]
- Assist the practitioner with insertion, as needed.
- Advise the patient to breathe through the mouth as the balloon enters the nostril.
- After the balloon begins its descent, the practitioner releases the grip on it, allowing the weight of the fluid or the preweighted tip to pull the tube into the nasopharynx.
- When the tube reaches the nasopharynx, the practitioner instructs the patient to lower the chin in a chin-tuck position (unless contraindicated) and to swallow. In some cases, the practitioner instructs the patient to sip water through a straw after the tube is in the oropharynx *to facilitate tube insertion with swallowing.*[19] If it's unsafe for the patient to swallow water, the practitioner may encourage dry swallowing, if desired.[19]
- The practitioner continues to advance the tube slowly *to prevent it from curling or kinking in the stomach.*
- *To confirm the tube's passage into the stomach,* assist the practitioner with using at least two bedside methods to determine tube location during insertion,[24] including watching for signs of respiratory distress (coughing and dyspnea);[24] using capnography, if available, to detect carbon dioxide, which indicates inadvertent tracheal insertion;[24] measuring pH aspirate from the tube if pH strips are available and pH measurement is performed in your facility (fasting gastric pH is usually 5 or less, even in patients receiving gastric acid inhibitors; however, this method isn't reliable enough to exclude the need for X-ray placement verification, *because gastric content occasionally has a high pH*);[24] and inspecting the visual characteristics of the tube aspirate (fasting gastric secretions commonly appear grassy-green or clear and colorless).[24]
- Position the patient as directed *to help advance the tube.* The patient will typically lie on the right side until the tube clears the pylorus (about 2 hours).
- After the tube clears the pylorus, the practitioner may direct you to advance it 2″ to 3″ (5 cm to 7.5 cm) every hour and to reposition the patient until the premeasured mark reaches the patient's nostril. Gravity and peristalsis will help advance the tube. (Notify the practitioner if you can't advance the tube.)

NURSING ALERT Don't secure the tube while it advances to the premeasured mark unless instructed to do so by the practitioner.

- Keep the remaining premeasured length of tube well lubricated *to ease passage and prevent irritation.*
- After the tube progresses the necessary distance, the practitioner will order an X-ray; most tubes are impregnated with a radiopaque mark so that you can easily confirm placement by X-ray or other imaging technique.[24]
- Secure the tube with a securement device or tape *to prevent displacement.* Clean the patient's skin where you intend to secure the tube with soap and water, and dry with a towel. Apply a skin preparation product to the skin, if needed.[19] Avoid securing the tube toward the top of the patient's head *to avoid putting pressure on the naris.*[19] Apply the securement device and secure the tube following the manufacturer's instructions. Alternatively, apply the tape and secure the tube or, for a small soft tube, use transparent semipermeable dressings to secure the tube, if desired.[19] Use protective padding under the tube if necessary *to protect the skin from friction and pressure.*[25] Keep the skin under the tube clean and dry.[26]

NURSING ALERT If the patient has fragile skin and you're using tape to secure the tube, use tape specially formulated for fragile skin *to prevent stripping and tearing during removal.*[27]

- Measure the external tube length or note the incremental marking on the tube where it exits the patient's nose; document the external tube length in the patient's medical record *to establish a baseline for comparison to assess for tube migration.*
- Trace the tubing from the patient to its point of origin *to make sure that you're accessing the correct tube,* and then attach the tube to intermittent suction, as ordered.[28] Tape the connection *to prevent accidental disconnection of the tubing.* Route the tubing toward the foot of the bed, *because a standardized approach of keeping IV lines routed toward the head and enteric lines routed toward the feet prevents dangerous misconnections.* If you're using different access sites, label each tubing at the distal and proximal ends *to distinguish them and to prevent misconnections.*[29,30]
- Provide oral care and continue to do so regularly *to promote comfort and prevent oral colonization with microorganisms that may contribute to health care–associated pneumonia.*
- Remove and discard the towel or fluid-impermeable pad.
- Inspect the skin under the tube by gently lifting and repositioning it at the naris at least twice daily, but preferably more frequently, *to assess for pressure injury formation, redistribute pressure, and decrease shear force.*[19,31]
- Return the bed to the lowest position *to prevent falls and maintain patient safety.*[32]

Removing a nasoenteric-decompression tube

- Put on gloves *to comply with standard precautions.*[16,17,18]
- Position the patient as the practitioner specifies, typically in the semi-Fowler or high Fowler position. You may also need to help the patient hold the neck in a hyperextended position, as needed.
- Protect the patient from soiling during tube removal by placing a fluid-impermeable pad or towel on top of the patient's chest.
- Trace the tubing from the patient to its point of origin *to make sure you're accessing the correct tube.*[29] Clamp the tube and disconnect it from suction *to prevent the patient from aspirating gastric contents that leak from the tube during withdrawal.*
- Remove the securement device or tape carefully from the patient's nose *to prevent skin stripping and tearing.*[27] Use adhesive remover, if needed, *to assist with removal and prevent skin breakdown.*[31]
- If the patient has a tube with an inflated balloon tip, attach a 10-mL syringe to the balloon port and withdraw the air or water. Don't deflate the balloon until you're ready to remove the tube.
- Slowly withdraw 6″ to 8″ (15 cm to 20 cm) of the tube. Wait 10 minutes, then withdraw another 6″ to 8″ (15 cm to 20 cm). Continue this procedure until the tube reaches the patient's esophagus (with 18″ [45 cm] of the tube remaining inside the patient). At this point, gently withdraw the tube completely.

NURSING ALERT If the tube doesn't come out easily, don't force it. Notify the practitioner.[33]

■ Inspect the tube *to ensure that it's intact*. If the tube isn't intact, notify the practitioner.[19]

Completing the procedure

■ Return the bed to the lowest position *to prevent falls and maintain patient safety*.[32]
■ Discard used supplies in appropriate receptacles.[16,17]
■ Remove and discard your gloves and, if worn, other personal protective equipment.[16,17]
■ Perform hand hygiene.[3,4,5,6,7,8]
■ Clean and disinfect your stethoscope using a disinfectant pad.[34,35]
■ Perform hand hygiene.[3,4,5,6,7,8]
■ Document the procedure.[36,37,38,39]

Special considerations

■ For a double- or triple-lumen tube, label which lumen accommodates balloon inflation and which accommodates drainage.

Complications

Nasoenteric-decompression tubes may cause reflux esophagitis, nasal or oral inflammation, and nasal, laryngeal, or esophageal ulceration. Misplacement into the bronchial tree can result in pneumonitis, pneumonia, and pneumothorax if not recognized.[28,40]

Nasoenteric-decompression tube removal can cause aspiration of residual gastric fluid in the tube and skin injury from removal of the securement device or tape.[19,31]

Documentation

Document the procedure; the date and time of insertion; the name of the practitioner who inserted the tube; the length, size, and type of nasoenteric tube inserted; the nostril used to place the tube; the amount of suction applied; the type of securement device used to secure the tube; and a description of the gastric contents aspirated. Record the patient's tolerance of the procedure, method used to confirm tube placement, external tube length, and GI assessment findings.

Record the date and time of tube removal, the indication for removal, and the patient's tolerance of the procedure. Record the color, consistency, and amount of drainage. Document teaching provided to the patient and family (if applicable), their understanding of that teaching, and any need for follow-up teaching.

REFERENCES

1 Itkin, M., et al. (2011). Multidisciplinary practical guidelines for gastrointestinal access for enteral nutrition and decompression from the Society of Interventional Radiology and American Gastroenterological Association (AGA) Institute, with endorsement by Canadian Interventional Radiological Association (CIRA) and Cardiovascular and Interventional Radiological Society of Europe (CIRSE). *Journal of Vascular and Interventional Radiology, 22,* 1089–1106. https://www.jvir.org/article/S1051-0443(11)00850-5/pdf (Level VII)

2 Jackson, P., & Cruz, M. V. (2018). Intestinal obstructions: Evaluation and management. *American Family Physician, 98*(6), 362–367. https://www.aafp.org/afp/2018/0915/p362.html

3 The Joint Commission. (2021). Standard NPSG.07.01.01. *Comprehensive accreditation manual for hospitals.* Oakbrook Terrace, IL: The Joint Commission. (Level VII)

4 Centers for Disease Control and Prevention. (2002). Guideline for hand hygiene in health-care settings: Recommendations of the Healthcare Infection Control Practices Advisory Committee and the HICPAC/SHEA/APIC/IDSA Hand Hygiene Task Force. *MMWR Recommendations and Reports, 51*(RR-16), 1–45. https://www.cdc.gov/mmwr/pdf/rr/rr5116.pdf (Level II)

5 World Health Organization. (2009). WHO guidelines on hand hygiene in health care: First global patient safety challenge, clean care is safer care. https://apps.who.int/iris/bitstream/handle/10665/44102/9789241597906_eng.pdf?sequence=1 (Level IV)

6 Centers for Medicare and Medicaid Services, Department of Health and Human Services. (2020). Condition of participation: Infection control. 42 C.F.R. § 482.42.

7 Accreditation Association for Hospitals and Health Systems. (2020). Standard 07.01.21. *Healthcare Facilities Accreditation Program: Accreditation requirements for acute care hospitals.* Chicago, IL: Accreditation Association for Hospitals and Health Systems. (Level VII)

8 DNV GL-Healthcare USA, Inc. (2020). IC.1.SR.1. *NIAHO® accreditation requirements, interpretive guidelines and surveyor guidance—revision 20.0.* Milford, OH: DNV GL-Healthcare USA, Inc. (Level VII)

9 The Joint Commission. (2021). Standard NPSG.01.01.01. *Comprehensive accreditation manual for hospitals.* Oakbrook Terrace, IL: The Joint Commission. (Level VII)

10 Centers for Medicare and Medicaid Services, Department of Health and Human Services. (2020). Condition of participation: Patient's rights. 42 C.F.R. § 482.13(c)(1).

11 Accreditation Association for Hospitals and Health Systems. (2020). Standard 15.01.16. *Healthcare Facilities Accreditation Program: Accreditation requirements for acute care hospitals.* Chicago, IL: Accreditation Association for Hospitals and Health Systems. (Level VII)

12 The Joint Commission. (2021). Standard RI.01.01.01. *Comprehensive accreditation manual for hospitals.* Oakbrook Terrace, IL: The Joint Commission. (Level VII)

13 DNV GL-Healthcare USA, Inc. (2020). PR.2.SR.5. *NIAHO® accreditation requirements, interpretive guidelines and surveyor guidance—revision 20.0.* Milford, OH: DNV GL-Healthcare USA, Inc. (Level VII)

14 The Joint Commission. (2021). Standard PC.02.01.21. *Comprehensive accreditation manual for hospitals.* Oakbrook Terrace, IL: The Joint Commission. (Level VII)

15 Waters, T. R., et al. (2009). Safe patient handling training for schools of nursing. https://www.cdc.gov/niosh/docs/2009-127/pdfs/2009-127.pdf (Level VII)

16 Siegel, J. D., et al. (2007, revised 2019). 2007 guideline for isolation precautions: Preventing transmission of infectious agents in health care settings. https://www.cdc.gov/infectioncontrol/pdf/guidelines/isolation-guidelines-H.pdf (Level II)

17 Occupational Safety and Health Administration. (2012). Bloodborne pathogens, standard number 1910.1030. https://www.osha.gov/pls/oshaweb/owadisp.show_document?p_id=10051&p_table=STANDARDS (Level VII)

18 Accreditation Association for Hospitals and Health Systems. (2020). Standard 07.01.10, *Healthcare Facilities Accreditation Program: Accreditation requirements for acute care hospitals.* Chicago, IL: Accreditation Association for Hospitals and Health Systems. (Level VII)

19 Wiegand, D. L. (2017). *AACN procedure manual for high acuity, progressive, and critical care* (7th ed.). St. Louis, MO: Elsevier.

20 The Joint Commission. (2021). Standard MM.06.01.01. *Comprehensive accreditation manual for hospitals.* Oakbrook Terrace, IL: The Joint Commission. (Level VII)

21 Centers for Medicare and Medicaid Services, Department of Health and Human Services. (2020). Condition of participation: Nursing services. 42 C.F.R. § 482.23(c).

22 Accreditation Association for Hospitals and Health Systems. (2020). Standard 16.01.03. *Healthcare Facilities Accreditation Program: Accreditation requirements for acute care hospitals.* Chicago, IL: Accreditation Association for Hospitals and Health Systems. (Level VII)

23 DNV GL-Healthcare USA, Inc. (2020). MM.1.SR.3. *NIAHO® accreditation requirements, interpretive guidelines and surveyor guidance—revision 20.0.* Milford, OH: DNV GL-Healthcare USA, Inc. (Level VII)

24 American Association of Critical-Care Nurses. (2016, updated 2020). AACN practice alert: Initial and ongoing verification of feeding tube placement in adults. https://www.aacn.org/clinical-resources/practice-alerts/initial-and-ongoing-verification-of-feeding-tube-placement-in-adults (Level VII)

25 Black, J. M., & Kalowes, P. (2016). Medical device-related pressure ulcers. *Chronic Wound Care Management and Research, 3,* 91–99. https://www.dovepress.com/medical-device-related-pressure-ulcers-peer-reviewed-fulltext-article-CWCMR

26 C. R. Bard, Inc. (2009). StatLock® nasogastric stabilization devices: Catheter stabilization device. https://www.crbard.com/CRBard/media/ProductAssets/BardMedicalDivision/PF10228/en-US/e2ggy5vl57pe-jw8u6xm87dvb40cu2nde.pdf

27 LeBlanc, K., et al. (2013). International skin tear advisory panel: A tool kit to aid in the prevention, assessment, and treatment of skin tears using a simplified classification system. *Advances in Skin & Wound Care, 26,* 459–476. (Level IV)

28 Hodin, R. A., & Bordeianou, L. (2020). Inpatient placement and management of nasogastric and nasoenteric tubes in adults. In: *UpToDate*, Cochran, A. (Ed.).

29 U.S. Food and Drug Administration. (2017). Examples of medical device misconnections. https://www.fda.gov/medical-devices/medical-device-connectors/examples-medical-device-misconnections

30 The Joint Commission. (2014). Sentinel event alert 53: Managing risk during transition to new ISO tubing connector standards. http://www.jointcommission.org/assets/1/6/SEA_53_Connectors_8_19_14_final.pdf (Level VII)

31 European Pressure Ulcer Advisory Panel, et al. (2019). Prevention and treatment of pressure ulcers/injuries: Quick reference guide. http://www.internationalguideline.com/static/pdfs/Quick_Reference_Guide-10Mar2019.pdf (Level VII)

32 Ganz, D. A., et al. (2013, reviewed 2021). *Preventing falls in hospitals: A toolkit for improving quality of care* (AHRQ Publication No. 13-0015-EF). Rockville, MD: Agency for Healthcare Research and Quality. https://www.ahrq.gov/professionals/systems/hospital/fallpxtoolkit/index.html (Level VII)

33 Hinkle, J. L., & Cheever, K. H. (2018). *Brunner and Suddarth's textbook of medical-surgical nursing* (14th ed.). Philadelphia, PA: Wolters Kluwer.

34 Rutala, W. A., et al. (2008, revised 2019). Guideline for disinfection and sterilization in healthcare facilities, 2008. https://www.cdc.gov/infection-control/pdf/guidelines/disinfection-guidelines-H.pdf (Level I)

35 Accreditation Association for Hospitals and Health Systems. (2020). Standard 07.02.03. *Healthcare Facilities Accreditation Program: Accreditation requirements for acute care hospitals.* Chicago, IL: Accreditation Association for Hospitals and Health Systems. (Level VII)

36 The Joint Commission. (2021). Standard RC.01.03.01. *Comprehensive accreditation manual for hospitals.* Oakbrook Terrace, IL: The Joint Commission. (Level VII)

37 Centers for Medicare and Medicaid Services, Department of Health and Human Services. (2020). Condition of participation: Medical record services. 42 C.F.R. § 482.24(b).

38 Accreditation Association for Hospitals and Health Systems. (2020). Standard 10.00.03. *Healthcare Facilities Accreditation Program: Accreditation requirements for acute care hospitals.* Chicago, IL: Accreditation Association for Hospitals and Health Systems. (Level VII)

39 DNV GL-Healthcare USA, Inc. (2020). MR.2.SR.1. *NIAHO® accreditation requirements, interpretive guidelines and surveyor guidance—revision 20.0.* Milford, OH: DNV GL-Healthcare USA, Inc. (Level VII)

40 Stayner, J. L., et al. (2012). Feeding tube placement: Errors and complications. *Nutrition in Clinical Practice, 27,* 738–748. (Level V)

NASOGASTRIC TUBE CARE

Providing effective nasogastric (NG) tube care requires meticulous monitoring of the patient and the equipment. Monitoring the patient involves assessing GI function, including volume and appearance of the NG tube drainage. Monitoring the equipment involves verifying correct tube placement and function.

Equipment

Gloves ■ stethoscope ■ commercial securement device or tape ■ graduated container ■ disinfectant pad ■ Optional: skin preparation product, irrigation supplies, fluid-impermeable pad, towel, catheter-tip syringe, alcohol pad, protective padding, tape specially formulated for fragile skin.

Preparation of equipment

If the practitioner ordered suction, for a Salem sump tube, make sure that the larger primary lumen (for drainage and suction) is connected to the suction equipment and the ordered setting has been selected (usually low intermittent suction *to prevent tissue damage*).[1] If the practitioner didn't specify the setting, follow the manufacturer's instructions. A Levin tube usually calls for intermittent low suction.

Check the suction device *to make sure it's functioning properly.* If using a thermotic pump (such as the Gomco gastric drainage pump), make sure the device is plugged into a grounded outlet. Make sure the collection chamber is assembled properly, and that the connecting tubing to the bacteria filter is without moisture. Make sure that the suction tubing is

attached to the collection chamber and that the selector switch is set to the prescribed suction, usually 90 to 120 mm Hg.[2]

If using wall suction, make sure the suction device and collection chamber are connected to the suction source. Verify that the suction tubing is attached to the collection chamber. Ensure that the suction setting is correct (intermittent or continuous) and that it's set to the prescribed suction, usually 30 to 40 mm Hg.[3]

Implementation

■ Gather and prepare the necessary equipment and supplies.

■ Perform hand hygiene.[4,5,6,7,8,9]

■ Confirm the patient's identity using at least two patient identifiers.[10]

■ Provide privacy.[11,12,13,14]

■ Explain the procedure to the patient, and family (if appropriate) according to their individual communication and learning needs *to increase their understanding, allay their fears, and enhance cooperation.*[15]

■ Raise the patient's bed to waist level before providing patient care *to prevent caregiver back strain.*[16]

■ Maintain the patient with the head of the bed elevated at least 30 degrees; if contraindicated, consider the reverse Trendelenburg position *to prevent aspiration.*[1,17]

■ Perform hand hygiene.[4,5,6,7,8,9]

■ Put on gloves *to comply with standard precautions.*[18,19,20,21]

■ Assess the patient's GI status at an interval determined by the patient's condition and your facility.[1]

■ Ask the patient whether the NG tube causes pain or discomfort at the naris or whether the securement device or tape feels too tight. For a patient who is unable to communicate, observe for agitation, pulling, itching, or grabbing, which may be a sign that the NG tube causes discomfort.[22]

■ Inspect the skin under the NG tube by gently lifting and repositioning it at the naris at least daily *to prevent medical device-related pressure injury.*[23]

■ Clean the skin and apply fresh tape (at least daily) or a new securement device (at least weekly according to the manufacturer's instructions), as needed.[24] Wipe excessively oily skin with an alcohol pad and allow it to dry completely before applying the securement device.[24] Apply a skin barrier preparation product to the skin if necessary.[1] Avoid securing the NG tube toward the top of the patient's head *to prevent pulling of the tube upward against the nares.*[1] Use protective padding under the device, if necessary, *to prevent medical device-related pressure injury.*[25] Keep the skin under the NG tube clean and dry.[25] Enlist the assistance of a coworker, as necessary, *to prevent tube dislodgement.*[26]

NURSING ALERT If the patient has fragile skin and you're using tape to secure the tube, use tape specifically formulated for fragile skin *to prevent skin stripping and tearing during removal.*[27]

■ Trace the tubing from the patient to its point of origin *to make sure that you're accessing the correct tube.*[17,28,29]

■ Confirm accurate NG tube placement regularly and before instilling any type of solution into the tube using one of these methods.[30] Observe the incremental marking on the tube at the exit site, or measure the external tube length and compare it to the baseline documented in the medical records at the time of insertion *to assess for tube migration.*[1,17,30] Review chest and abdominal X-ray reports *for notations about the tube's location.*[17,30] Inspect the visual characteristics of the tube aspirate; fasting gastric secretions commonly appear grassy-green, brown, or clear and colorless, whereas fluid withdrawn from the tube that has perforated into the pleural space typically has a pale yellow, serous appearance.[17] Measure the pH of aspirate from the tube if pH strips are available and pH measurement is performed in your facility; fasting gastric pH is usually 5 or less, even in patients receiving gastric acid inhibitors.[17,30] Arrange for an X-ray, as ordered, if the tube's placement is uncertain.[17,30]

■ Irrigate the tube, as ordered or necessary, *to maintain tube patency.*[1]

■ Monitor the patient's intake and output at an interval determined by the patient's condition and your facility.[26] Monitor the patient's fluid and electrolyte status *to enable prompt recognition of fluid and electrolyte imbalances.* Keep in mind that patients with large-volume NG output are at risk for acid-base imbalances. Report imbalances to the patient's practitioner promptly.[1]

- Monitor the appearance of gastric drainage; report bloody or coffee-ground-color drainage, which may indicate bleeding.[31]
- Provide oral care regularly *to promote comfort and prevent oral colonization, and to decrease the risk of hospital-associated pneumonia.*[26,32] (See the "Oral care" procedure.)
- Return the bed to the lowest position *to prevent falls and maintain patient safety.*[33]
- Remove and discard your gloves.[18,19]
- Perform hand hygiene.[4,5,6,7,8,9]
- Clean and disinfect your stethoscope using a disinfectant pad.[34,35]
- Perform hand hygiene.[4,5,6,7,8,9]
- Document the procedure.[36,37,38,39]

Special considerations

- If necessary, irrigate the NG tube and instill at least 15 mL of air into the vent tube *to maintain patency.*[3] Don't attempt to stop reflux by clamping the vent tube. Unless contraindicated, elevate the patient's torso more than 30 degrees, and keep the vent tube above the patient's midline *to prevent a siphoning effect.*[3]

Complications

Epigastric or abdominal pain and vomiting can result from a clogged or improperly placed tube. Any NG tube—the Levin tube in particular—can move and aggravate esophagitis, ulcers, or esophageal varices, causing hemorrhage. Dehydration and electrolyte imbalances can result from removing body fluids and electrolytes by suctioning. NG intubation can cause oral and nasal skin breakdown, discomfort, and increased mucous secretions. Aspiration pneumonia can result from gastric reflux. Vigorous suction can damage the gastric mucosa and cause significant bleeding, possibly interfering with endoscopic assessment and diagnosis.[1,3,31]

Documentation

Document your GI assessment findings, including the volume and description of drainage. Record intake and output. Note the condition of the patient's naris and skin under and surrounding the tube and securement device, the skin care provided, and whether the securement device was changed (if applicable). Document the methods used to confirm NG tube placement. Record oral care provided. Document teaching provided to the patient and family (if applicable), their understanding of that teaching, and any need for follow-up teaching.

REFERENCES

1 Wiegand, D. L. (2017). *AACN procedure manual for high acuity, progressive, and critical care* (7th ed.). St. Louis, MO: Elsevier.
2 Allied Healthcare Products, Inc. (2018) Gomco suction equipment. https://alliedhpi.com/wp-content/uploads/2021/08/21-00-0000-Gomco-Suction-Equipment-Rev-May-2018-1.pdf
3 C. R. Bard, Inc. (2017). BARD® nasogastric sump tubes: Instructions for use. https://www.crbard.com/CRBard/media/ProductAssets/BardMedicalDivision/PF10357/en-US/UCC-BG-gastric-NGtubes_PF10357-IFU.pdf
4 Centers for Disease Control and Prevention. (2002). Guideline for hand hygiene in health-care settings: Recommendations of the Healthcare Infection Control Practices Advisory Committee and the HICPAC/SHEA/APIC/IDSA Hand Hygiene Task Force. *MMWR Recommendations and Reports, 51*(RR-16), 1–45. https://www.cdc.gov/mmwr/pdf/rr/rr5116.pdf (Level II)
5 World Health Organization. (2009). WHO guidelines on hand hygiene in health care: First global patient safety challenge, clean care is safer care. https://apps.who.int/iris/bitstream/handle/10665/44102/9789241597906_eng.pdf?sequence=1 (Level IV)
6 The Joint Commission. (2021). Standard NPSG.07.01.01. *Comprehensive accreditation manual for hospitals.* Oakbrook Terrace, IL: The Joint Commission. (Level VII)
7 Centers for Medicare and Medicaid Services, Department of Health and Human Services. (2020). Condition of participation: Infection control. 42 C.F.R. § 482.42.
8 Accreditation Association for Hospitals and Health Systems. (2020). Standard 07.01.21. *Healthcare Facilities Accreditation Program: Accreditation requirements for acute care hospitals.* Chicago, IL: Accreditation Association for Hospitals and Health Systems. (Level VII)
9 DNV GL-Healthcare USA, Inc. (2020). IC.1.SR.1. *NIAHO® accreditation requirements, interpretive guidelines and surveyor guidance—revision 20.0.* Milford, OH: DNV GL-Healthcare USA, Inc. (Level VII)
10 The Joint Commission. (2021). Standard NPSG.01.01.01. *Comprehensive accreditation manual for hospitals.* Oakbrook Terrace, IL: The Joint Commission. (Level VII)
11 Centers for Medicare and Medicaid Services, Department of Health and Human Services. (2020). Condition of participation: Patient's rights. 42 C.F.R. § 482.13(c)(1).
12 Accreditation Association for Hospitals and Health Systems. (2020). Standard 15.01.16. *Healthcare Facilities Accreditation Program: Accreditation requirements for acute care hospitals.* Chicago, IL: Accreditation Association for Hospitals and Health Systems. (Level VII)
13 The Joint Commission. (2021). Standard RI.01.01.01. *Comprehensive accreditation manual for hospitals.* Oakbrook Terrace, IL: The Joint Commission. (Level VII)
14 DNV GL-Healthcare USA, Inc. (2020). PR.2.SR.5. *NIAHO® accreditation requirements, interpretive guidelines and surveyor guidance—revision 20.0.* Milford, OH: DNV GL-Healthcare USA, Inc. (Level VII)
15 The Joint Commission. (2021). Standard PC.02.01.21. *Comprehensive accreditation manual for hospitals.* Oakbrook Terrace, IL: The Joint Commission. (Level VII)
16 Waters, T. R., et al. (2009). Safe patient handling training for schools of nursing. https://www.cdc.gov/niosh/docs/2009-127/pdfs/2009-127.pdf (Level VII)
17 Boullata, J. I., et al. (2016). ASPEN safe practices for enteral nutrition therapy. *Journal of Parenteral and Enteral Nutrition, 41*(1), 15–103. https://onlinelibrary.wiley.com/doi/pdf/10.1177/0148607116673053 (Level VII)
18 Siegel, J. D., et al. (2007, revised 2019). 2007 guideline for isolation precautions: Preventing transmission of infectious agents in healthcare settings. https://www.cdc.gov/infectioncontrol/pdf/guidelines/isolation-guidelines-H.pdf (Level II)
19 Occupational Safety and Health Administration. (2012). Bloodborne pathogens, standard number 1910.1030. https://www.osha.gov/pls/oshaweb/owadisp.show_document?p_id=10051&p_table=STANDARDS (Level VII)
20 Accreditation Association for Hospitals and Health Systems. (2020). Standard 07.01.10. *Healthcare Facilities Accreditation Program: Accreditation requirements for acute care hospitals.* Chicago, IL: Accreditation Association for Hospitals and Health Systems. (Level VII)
21 DNV GL-Healthcare USA, Inc. (2020). IC.1.SR.2. *NIAHO® accreditation requirements, interpretive guidelines and surveyor guidance—revision 20.0.* Milford, OH: DNV GL-Healthcare USA, Inc. (Level VII)
22 American Society for Pain Management Nursing. (2011). Pain assessment in the patient unable to self-report: Position statement with clinical practice recommendations. *Pain Management Nursing, 12*(4), 230–250. http://www.aspmn.org/documents/PainAssessmentinthePatientUnabletoSelfReport.pdf (Level VII)
23 Baranoski, S., & Ayello, E. A. (2020). *Wound care essentials: Practice principles* (5th ed.). Philadelphia, PA: Wolters Kluwer.
24 C. R. Bard, Inc. (2009). StatLock® nasogastric stabilization devices: Catheter stabilization device. https://www.crbard.com/CRBard/media/ProductAssets/BardMedicalDivision/PF10228/en-US/e2ggy5vl57pe-jw8u6xm87dvb40cu2nde.pdf
25 European Pressure Ulcer Advisory Panel, et al. (2021). Prevention and treatment of pressure ulcers/injuries: Quick reference guide. http://www.internationalguideline.com/static/pdfs/Quick_Reference_Guide-10Mar2019.pdf (Level VII)
26 Nasoenteric tube feeding (adults): Care and daily management. (2021). *JBI EBP Database.* AN: JBI1809 (Level VII)
27 LeBlanc, K., et al. (2013). International skin tear advisory panel: A toolkit to aid in the prevention, assessment, and treatment of skin tears using a simplified classification system. *Advances in Skin and Wound Care, 26,* 459–476. (Level IV)
28 U.S. Food and Drug Administration. (2017). Examples of medical device misconnections. https://www.fda.gov/medical-devices/medical-device-connectors/examples-medical-device-misconnections
29 The Joint Commission. (2014). Sentinel event alert 53: Managing risk during transition to new ISO tubing connector standards. https://www.jointcommission.org/-/media/tjc/documents/resources/patient-safety-topics/sentinel-event/sea_53_connectors_8_19_14_final.pdf (Level VII)

30 American Association of Critical-Care Nurses. (2016). AACN practice alert: Initial and ongoing verification of feeding tube placement in adults. https://www.aacn.org/clinical-resources/practice-alerts/initial-and-ongoing-verification-of-feeding-tube-placement-in-adults (Level VII)

31 Hodin, R. A., & Bordeianou, L. (2020). Inpatient placement and management of nasogastric and nasoenteric tubes in adults. In: *UpToDate*, Cochran, A. (Ed.)

32 Maeda, K., & Akagi, J. (2014). Oral care may reduce pneumonia in the tube-fed elderly: A preliminary study. *Dysphagia, 29*, 616–621. (Level VI)

33 Ganz, D. A., et al. (2013, reviewed 2021). Preventing falls in hospitals: A toolkit for improving quality of care (AHRQ publication no. 13-0015-EF). https://www.ahrq.gov/professionals/systems/hospital/fallpxtoolkit/index.html (Level VII)

34 Rutala, W. A., et al. (2008, revised 2019). Guideline for disinfection and sterilization in healthcare facilities, 2008. https://www.cdc.gov/infection-control/pdf/guidelines/disinfection-guidelines-H.pdf (Level I)

35 Accreditation Association for Hospitals and Health Systems. (2020). Standard 07.02.03. *Healthcare Facilities Accreditation Program: Accreditation requirements for acute care hospitals.* Chicago, IL: Accreditation Association for Hospitals and Health Systems. (Level VII)

36 The Joint Commission. (2021). Standard RC.01.03.01. *Comprehensive accreditation manual for hospitals.* Oakbrook Terrace, IL: The Joint Commission. (Level VII)

37 Centers for Medicare and Medicaid Services, Department of Health and Human Services. (2020). Condition of participation: Medical record services. 42 C.F.R. § 482.24(b).

38 Accreditation Association for Hospitals and Health Systems. (2020). Standard 10.00.03. *Healthcare Facilities Accreditation Program: Accreditation requirements for acute care hospitals.* Chicago, IL: Accreditation Association for Hospitals and Health Systems. (Level VII)

39 DNV GL-Healthcare USA, Inc. (2020). MR.2.SR.1. *NIAHO® accreditation requirements, interpretive guidelines and surveyor guidance—revision 20.0.* Milford, OH: DNV GL-Healthcare USA, Inc. (Level VII)

NASOGASTRIC TUBE INSERTION AND REMOVAL

Usually inserted to decompress the stomach, a nasogastric (NG) tube can prevent vomiting after major surgery. An NG tube is typically in place for 48 to 72 hours after surgery, by which time peristalsis usually resumes. It may remain in place for shorter or longer periods depending on its use.

An NG tube has other diagnostic and therapeutic applications, especially in assessing and treating upper GI bleeding, collecting gastric contents for analysis, performing gastric lavage, aspirating gastric secretions, and administering medications and nutrients.[1]

Inserting an NG tube requires close observation of the patient and verification of proper placement. The NG tube position and patency must be confirmed before initial use of the tube for nutrition or medication administration.[2]

Most NG tubes have a radiopaque marker or strip at the distal end so that the tube's position can be verified by X-ray. If the position can't be confirmed, the practitioner may order fluoroscopy to verify placement.

The most common NG tubes are the Levin tube, which has one lumen, and the Salem sump tube, which has two lumens—one for suction and drainage and a smaller one for ventilation. Air flows through the vent lumen continuously, which protects the delicate gastric mucosa by preventing a vacuum from forming should the tube adhere to the stomach lining.

Contraindications to NG tube placement include a basilar skull or facial fracture, a history of recent facial surgery or transsphenoidal pituitary resection, upper GI surgery, esophageal stricture or stet placement, or anatomic conditions (such as a deviated nasal septum or hiatal hernia) that may contraindicate insertion. Guidelines don't recommend use in patients with esophageal varices or a bleeding disorder.[1,3] (See *Types of NG tubes.*)

When an NG tube is no longer needed, a nurse can remove it with a practitioner's order.

Equipment

For insertion

NG tube (usually #12, #14, #16, or #18 French for an average adult) ■ fluid-impermeable pad or towel ■ securement device, tape, or transparent semipermeable dressing ■ gloves ■ water-soluble lubricant ■ enteral catheter-tip syringe or irrigation set with syringe ■ oral care supplies ■ stethoscope ■ disinfectant pad ■ Optional: penlight, prescribed anesthetic, cup of water, straw, mask and goggles or mask with face shield, basin of warm water or ice water, labels, carbon dioxide detector, pH testing equipment, suction equipment, indelible marker, alcohol pad, protective padding, skin preparation product, tape specially formulated for fragile skin.

For removal

Stethoscope ■ catheter-tip syringe ■ fluid-impermeable pad or towel ■ gloves ■ supplies for cleaning the naris ■ oral care supplies ■ disinfectant pad. Optional: gown, mask and goggles or mask with face shield, adhesive remover.

Preparation of equipment

Inspect all equipment and supplies. If a product is expired, is defective, or has compromised integrity, remove it from patient use, label it as expired or defective, and report the expiration or defect as directed by your facility.

Inspect the NG tube for defects, such as rough edges or partially closed lumens. Then check the tube's patency by flushing it with water. If you need to increase the tube's flexibility *to ease insertion*, coil it around your gloved fingers for a few seconds or dip it in warm water. If the tube is too flaccid, stiffen it by filling the tube with water and then freezing it or dipping the tube in ice water.[4]

If the practitioner orders it, set up suction equipment. If using a thermotic pump (such as the Gomco gastric drainage pump), plug the device into a grounded outlet. Make sure the collection chamber is assembled properly and the connecting tubing to the bacteria filter is without moisture. Attach the suction tubing to the collection chamber. Set the selector switch to the prescribed suction, usually 90 to 120 mm Hg.[5] Follow the manufacturer's directions for use.

If using wall suction, connect the suction device and collection chamber to the suction source. Attach the suction tubing to the collection chamber. Choose the prescribed suction setting (intermittent or continuous) and set to the prescribed suction, usually 30 to 40 mm Hg.[6]

Make sure the suction device functions properly.

Implementation

- Verify the practitioner's order.
- Review the patient's medical record for contraindications to NG tube insertion.[3]
- Gather and prepare the necessary equipment and supplies.
- Perform hand hygiene.[7,8,9,10,11,12]
- Confirm the patient's identity using at least two patient identifiers.[13]
- Provide privacy.[14,15,16,17]
- Explain the procedure to the patient and family (if appropriate) according to their individual communication and learning needs *to increase their understanding, allay their fears, and enhance cooperation.*[18]

Inserting an NG tube

- Ask the patient whether there is a history of epistaxis or sinusitis. If so, ask whether one naris is more susceptible.[3]
- Agree on a signal that the patient can use to stop the procedure briefly.
- Raise the patient's bed to waist level when providing care *to prevent caregiver back strain.*[19]
- Assess the patient's GI status *to establish a baseline for comparison.*[3]
- Position the patient with the head of the bed elevated at least 30 degrees; if contraindicated, consider the reverse Trendelenburg position.[2,3]
- Perform hand hygiene.[7,8,9,10,11,12]
- Put on gloves and, as needed, other personal protective equipment *to comply with standard precautions*).[20,21,22,23]
- Assess the patient's nares to determine the best choice for insertion. Use a penlight to ease visualization, as needed.
- Determine the insertion length of the tube *to help ensure gastric placement*. Place the tube's distal end at the tip of the patient's nose (as shown), or mouth for oral insertion, and then extend the tube to the earlobe,

EQUIPMENT

Types of NG tubes

The practitioner will choose the type and diameter of nasogastric (NG) tube that best suits the patient's needs, such as lavage, aspiration, enteral therapy, or stomach decompression. Choices may include the Levin or Salem sump tubes.

Levin tube
The Levin tube is a rubber or plastic tube that has a single lumen, a length of 42″ to 50″ (106.7 cm to 127 cm), and holes at the tip and along the side.

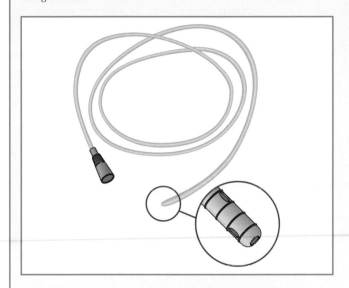

Salem sump tube
A Salem sump tube is a double-lumen NG tube that's made of clear plastic and has a blue sump port (pigtail) that allows atmospheric air to enter the patient's stomach. This air allows the tube to float freely and not adhere to or damage gastric mucosa. The larger port of this 48″ (122-cm) tube serves as the main suction conduit. The tube has openings at 45, 55, 65, and 75 cm as well as a radiopaque line *to verify placement.*

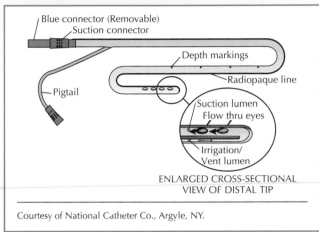

Courtesy of National Catheter Co., Argyle, NY.

down to the xiphoid process, and then midway to the umbilicus.[3] Note the corresponding incremental marking on the tube, or if the tube doesn't contain incremental markings, mark the tube or note an identifier at the intended exit point.[3]

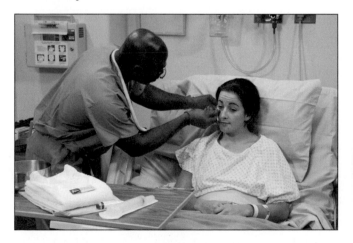

■ Place a fluid-impermeable pad or towel over the patient's chest *to protect the gown and bed linens from soiling.*[3]
■ Administer an anesthetic agent, if ordered, following safe medication administration practices.[24,25,26,27,28,29]
■ Lubricate the distal tip of the tube with water-soluble lubricant.[3] Alternatively, if the tube is impregnated with water-activated lubricant, activate the lubricant by dipping the tip in water.
■ Grasp the tube with the distal end pointing downward, curve it if necessary, and carefully insert it into the more patent nostril (as shown).

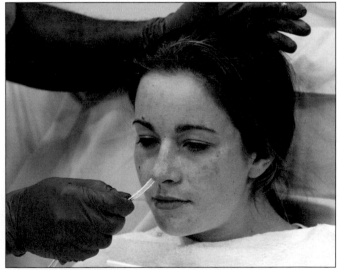

■ Instruct the patient to flex the head forward (if not contraindicated) and tuck the chin *to close the trachea and open the esophagus.*[3]
■ Guide the tube at an angle parallel to the floor of the nasal canal, and guide it gently downward as the tube advances through the nasal passage toward the distal pharynx.[3] If you meet resistance, try to gently rotate the tip of the tube until it advances past the nasal passage. If you continue to meet resistance, don't force the tube. Instead, withdraw the tube and allow the patient to rest, relubricate the tube, and retry, or insert the tube in the other naris.[3]
■ Unless contraindicated, after the tube reaches the oropharynx, allow the patient to sip water through a straw (as shown) as you slowly advance

the tube *to facilitate passage of the tube into the esophagus.* (If the patient isn't able to safely swallow water, ask the patient to dry swallow.) Although swallowing may be helpful, it isn't necessary for successful NG tube insertion. Some patients may prefer rapid insertion without swallowing.[3]

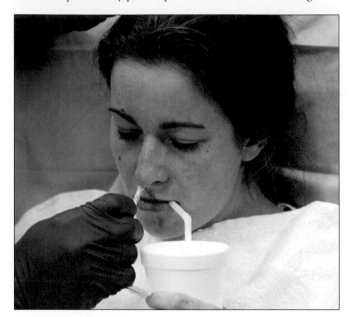

■ As you advance the tube, monitor the patient for cues (such as coughing or discomfort) that might indicate that the tube entered the respiratory tract or kinked or coiled in the oral cavity.[3]
■ Continue to advance the tube to the predetermined length.[3]
■ After you insert the tube to the predetermined length, confirm the tube's placement in the stomach, using at least two of the following bedside methods:[2,30] Watch for signs of respiratory distress (coughing and dyspnea).[2,30] Use capnography, if available, to detect carbon dioxide, *which indicates inadvertent tracheal insertion.*[2,30,31] Measure pH of aspirate from the tube if your facility uses pH measurement.[2,30,32] (Fasting gastric pH is typically 5 or less, even in patients receiving gastric acid inhibitors; however, this method isn't reliable enough to exclude the need for X-ray placement verification, *because gastric aspirate occasionally has a high pH.*[30] Fluid aspirated from a tube that has perforated the pleural space typically has a pH of 7 or higher.)[2] Aspirate secretions from the tube with an enteral syringe (as shown below), and inspect the visual characteristics of the tube aspirate; fasting gastric secretions commonly appear grassy-green, brown, or clear and colorless,[2,30] whereas aspirate from the pleural space typically has a pale yellow serous appearance.[2]

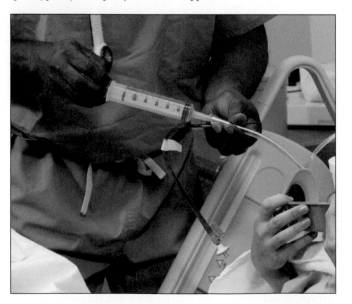

■ Arrange for an X-ray, if ordered, *to verify placement.*[2,30] Ensure that proper tube placement has been confirmed by X-ray and documented before initial use for feedings or medication administration *to prevent complications associated with blind tube insertion.*[2]
■ Secure the tube with a securement device, tape (as shown), or transparent semipermeable dressing *to prevent displacement:* Clean the patient's skin where you intend to secure the tube.[3] Wipe excessively oily skin with an alcohol pad and let it dry before applying the securement device.[33] Apply a skin preparation product to the skin if needed.[3] Avoid securing the tube toward the top of the patient's head to avoid putting pressure on the naris.[1] Apply the securement device and secure the tube following the manufacturer's instructions. Alternatively, apply the tape and secure the tube or, for a small soft tube, use a transparent semipermeable dressing to secure the tube, if desired.[3] Use protective padding under the tube, if necessary, *to protect the skin from friction and pressure.*[34]

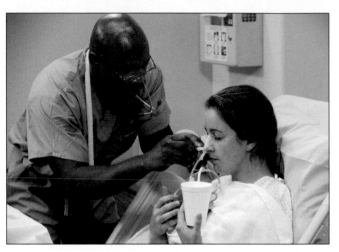

■ Keep the skin under the tube clean and dry *to prevent skin breakdown.*[35]
NURSING ALERT If the patient has fragile skin and you're using tape to secure the tube, use tape specifically formulated for fragile skin *to prevent skin stripping and tearing during removal.*[36]
■ Mark the tube at the patient's naris with an indelible marker. Measure the external tube length or note the incremental marking on the tube where it exits the patient's nose; document the external tube length in the patient's medical record *to establish a baseline for comparison to assess for tube migration.*[3]
■ Trace the tubing from the patient to its point of origin *to make sure that you're connecting the correct tubing,* and then attach it to suction equipment, if ordered, and verify the designated suction pressure.[37,38] Route the tubing toward the patient's feet, *because a standardized approach of keeping IV lines routed toward the head and enteric lines routed toward the feet prevents dangerous misconnections.* If you're using different access sites, label each tubing at the distal and proximal ends *to distinguish the different tubing and prevent misconnections.*[38]
■ Provide oral care, and continue to do so regularly *to promote comfort and prevent oral colonization with microorganisms that may contribute to health care–associated pneumonia.*
■ Remove and discard the fluid-impermeable pad or towel.[21]
■ Keep the head of the bed elevated at least 30 degrees (unless contraindicated) *to prevent aspiration.* If contraindicated, consider the reverse Trendelenburg position.[2,3]

Removing an NG tube
■ Position the patient with the head of the bed elevated at least 30 degrees *to prevent aspiration.* If contraindicated, consider the reverse Trendelenburg position.[2]
■ Assess the patient's GI function by assessing for nausea, vomiting, abdominal distention, abdominal discomfort, and ability to pass flatus or stools. Notify the practitioner of abnormal findings, which may suggest that the patient is not ready for tube removal.[2]
■ Place a fluid-impermeable pad or towel across the patient's chest, as shown, *to protect the gown and bed linens from spills.*[2,3]

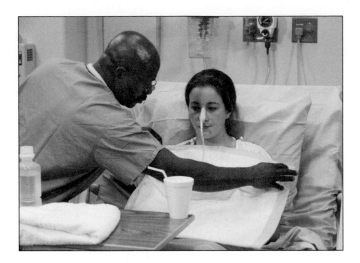

- Discontinue gastric suction, as needed, *to prepare for NG tube removal.*[3]
- Perform hand hygiene.[7,8,9,10,11,12]
- Put on gloves and, if needed, other personal protective equipment *to comply with standard precautions.*[20,21,22,23]
- Trace the tubing from the patient to its point of origin *to make sure that you're accessing the correct tube.*[2,37]
- Verify tube placement, and then use a catheter-tip syringe to flush the tube with a small bolus of air *to clear the tube of any remaining gastric contents and subsequently prevent aspiration.*[3]
- Gently remove the securement device or tape from the patient's nose *to prevent skin stripping and tearing.*[36] Use adhesive remover, if necessary, *to assist with removal and to prevent skin breakdown.*
- Fold over or clamp the proximal end of the tube *to prevent backflow of gastric contents from the tube during removal.*[3]
- Ask the patient to hold the breath *to close the epiglottis.* Then withdraw the tube gently and steadily. (When the distal end of the tube reaches the nasopharynx, you can pull the remainder quickly.) Inspect the tube *to be sure it's intact.*[3]
- Discard the tube in an appropriate receptacle.[21]

Completing the procedure
- Return the bed to the lowest position *to prevent falls and maintain patient safety.*[39]
- Discard used supplies in the appropriate receptacle.[21]
- Remove and discard your gloves and any other personal protective equipment worn.[20,21]
- Perform hand hygiene.[7,8,9,10,11,12]
- Clean and disinfect your stethoscope using a disinfectant pad.[40,41]
- Perform hand hygiene.[7,8,9,10,11,12]
- Document the procedure.[42,43,44,45]

Special considerations
- When using a Salem-sump tube with suction, connect the larger primary lumen (for drainage and suction) to the suction equipment and select the appropriate setting, as ordered (usually low suction). If the practitioner doesn't specify the setting, follow the manufacturer's instructions. A Levin tube usually calls for intermittent suction.
- The Joint Commission issued a sentinel event alert related to managing risk during transition to new International Organization for Standardization tubing standards that were designed to prevent dangerous tubing misconnections, which can lead to serious patient injury and death. During the transition, make sure to trace each tube and catheter from the patient to its point of origin before connecting or reconnecting any device or infusion, at any care transition (such as to a new setting or service), and as part of the hand-off process; route tubes and catheters having different purposes in different, standardized directions; when the patient has different access sites or several bags hanging, label tubing at the distal and proximal ends; use tubing and equipment only as intended; and store medications for different delivery routes in separate locations.[38]

- Monitor the patient for signs of GI dysfunction, including nausea, vomiting, abdominal distention or discomfort, and food intolerance. GI dysfunction may necessitate reinsertion of the NG tube.

Complications
Potential complications of prolonged intubation with an NG tube include skin erosion at the nostril, sinusitis, esophagitis, esophagotracheal fistula, gastric ulceration, and pulmonary and oral infection.[3,6,34] Complications that can result from suctioning include electrolyte imbalances and dehydration.[3]

Documentation
Record the type and size of the NG tube as well as the date and time of insertion, the insertion route, and the tube's external length measurement or centimeter mark. Include the method you used to confirm tube placement. Also note the type and amount of suction (if you used it) and describe the drainage, including the amount, color, character, consistency, and odor. Note the patient's tolerance of the procedure. Include in your notes any signs and symptoms of complications, such as nausea, vomiting, and abdominal distention; the person you notified of any complications and the date and time of notification; interventions you performed; and the patient's response to those interventions. Document subsequent irrigation procedures and continuing problems after irrigation.

Document the patient's GI status before tube removal. Record the date and time of NG tube removal. Describe the color, consistency, and amount of gastric drainage. Note unusual events after NG tube removal, such as nausea, vomiting, abdominal distention, and food intolerance. Note the patient's tolerance of the procedure. Document teaching provided to the patient and family (if applicable), their understanding of that teaching, and any need for follow-up teaching.

REFERENCES
1 Hodin, R. A., & Bordeianou, L. (2020). Inpatient placement and management of nasogastric and nasoenteric tubes in adults. In: *UpToDate*, Cochran, A. (Ed.).
2 Boullata, J. I., et al. (2016). ASPEN safe practices for enteral nutrition therapy. *Journal of Parenteral and Enteral Nutrition, 41*, 15–103. https://onlinelibrary.wiley.com/doi/pdf/10.1177/0148607116673053 (Level VII)
3 Wiegand, D. L. (2017). *AACN procedure manual for high acuity, progressive, and critical care* (7th ed.). St. Louis, MO: Elsevier.
4 Chun, D. H., et al. (2009). A randomized, clinical trial of frozen versus standard nasogastric tube placement. *World Journal of Surgery, 33*, 1789–1792. (Level II)
5 Allied Healthcare Products, Inc. (2018). Gomco suction equipment. https://alliedhpi.com/wp-content/uploads/2021/08/21-00-0000-Gomco-Suction-Equipment-Rev-May-2018-1.pdf
6 C. R. Bard, Inc. (2017). BARD® nasogastric sump tubes: Instructions for use. https://www.crbard.com/CRBard/media/ProductAssets/BardMedicalDivision/PF10357/en-US/UCC-BG-gastric-NGtubes_PF10357-IFU.pdf
7 The Joint Commission. (2021). Standard NPSG.07.01.01. *Comprehensive accreditation manual for hospitals.* Oakbrook Terrace, IL: The Joint Commission. (Level VII)
8 Centers for Disease Control and Prevention. (2002). Guideline for hand hygiene in health-care settings: Recommendations of the Healthcare Infection Control Practices Advisory Committee and the HICPAC/SHEA/APIC/IDSA Hand Hygiene Task Force. *MMWR Recommendations and Reports, 51*(RR-16), 1–45. https://www.cdc.gov/mmwr/pdf/rr/rr5116.pdf (Level II)
9 World Health Organization. (2009). WHO guidelines on hand hygiene in health care: First global patient safety challenge, clean care is safer care. https://apps.who.int/iris/bitstream/handle/10665/44102/9789241597906_eng.pdf?sequence=1 (Level IV)
10 Centers for Medicare and Medicaid Services, Department of Health and Human Services. (2020). Condition of participation: Infection control. 42 C.F.R. § 482.42.
11 Accreditation Association for Hospitals and Health Systems. (2020). Standard 07.01.21. *Healthcare Facilities Accreditation Program: Accreditation requirements for acute care hospitals.* Chicago, IL: Accreditation Association for Hospitals and Health Systems. (Level VII)

12 DNV GL-Healthcare USA, Inc. (2020). IC.1.SR.1. *NIAHO® accreditation requirements, interpretive guidelines and surveyor guidance—revision 20.0.* Milford, OH: DNV GL-Healthcare USA, Inc. (Level VII)

13 The Joint Commission. (2021). Standard NPSG.01.01.01. *Comprehensive accreditation manual for hospitals.* Oakbrook Terrace, IL: The Joint Commission. (Level VII)

14 Centers for Medicare and Medicaid Services, Department of Health and Human Services. (2020). Condition of participation: Patient's rights. 42 C.F.R. § 482.13(c)(1).

15 Accreditation Association for Hospitals and Health Systems. (2020). Standard 15.01.16. *Healthcare Facilities Accreditation Program: Accreditation requirements for acute care hospitals.* Chicago, IL: Accreditation Association for Hospitals and Health Systems. (Level VII)

16 The Joint Commission. (2021). Standard RI.01.01.01. *Comprehensive accreditation manual for hospitals.* Oakbrook Terrace, IL: The Joint Commission. (Level VII)

17 DNV GL-Healthcare USA, Inc. (2020). PR.2.SR.5. *NIAHO® accreditation requirements, interpretive guidelines and surveyor guidance—revision 20.0.* Milford, OH: DNV GL-Healthcare USA, Inc. (Level VII)

18 The Joint Commission. (2021). Standard PC.02.01.21. *Comprehensive accreditation manual for hospitals.* Oakbrook Terrace, IL: The Joint Commission. (Level VII)

19 Waters, T. R., et al. (2009). Safe patient handling training for schools of nursing. https://www.cdc.gov/niosh/docs/2009-127/pdfs/2009-127.pdf (Level VII)

20 Siegel, J. D., et al. (2007, revised 2019). 2007 guideline for isolation precautions: Preventing transmission of infectious agents in healthcare settings. https://www.cdc.gov/infectioncontrol/pdf/guidelines/isolation-guidelines-H.pdf (Level II)

21 Occupational Safety and Health Administration. (2012). Bloodborne pathogens, standard number 1910.1030. https://www.osha.gov/pls/oshaweb/owadisp.show_document?p_id=10051&p_table=STANDARDS (Level VII)

22 Accreditation Association for Hospitals and Health Systems. (2020). Standard 07.01.10. *Healthcare Facilities Accreditation Program: Accreditation requirements for acute care hospitals.* Chicago, IL: Accreditation Association for Hospitals and Health Systems. (Level VII)

23 DNV GL-Healthcare USA, Inc. (2020). IC.1.SR.2. *NIAHO® accreditation requirements, interpretive guidelines and surveyor guidance—revision 20.0.* Milford, OH: DNV GL-Healthcare USA, Inc. (Level VII)

24 Uri, O., et al. (2011). Lidocaine gel as an anesthetic protocol for nasogastric tube insertion in the ED. *American Journal of Emergency Medicine, 29,* 386–390. (Level IV)

25 Kuo, Y., et al. (2010). Reducing the pain of nasogastric tube intubation with nebulized and atomized lidocaine: A systematic review and meta-analysis. *Journal of Pain and Symptom Management, 40*(4), 613–620. https://www.jpsmjournal.com/article/S0885-3924(10)00398-2/fulltext (Level I)

26 Centers for Medicare and Medicaid Services, Department of Health and Human Services. (2020). Condition of participation: Nursing services. 42 C.F.R. § 482.23(c).

27 Accreditation Association for Hospitals and Health Systems. (2020). Standard 16.01.03. *Healthcare Facilities Accreditation Program: Accreditation requirements for acute care hospitals.* Chicago, IL: Accreditation Association for Hospitals and Health Systems. (Level VII)

28 The Joint Commission. (2021). Standard MM.06.01.01. *Comprehensive accreditation manual for hospitals.* Oakbrook Terrace, IL: The Joint Commission. (Level VII)

29 DNV GL-Healthcare USA, Inc. (2020). MM.1.SR.3. *NIAHO® accreditation requirements, interpretive guidelines and surveyor guidance—revision 20.0.* Milford, OH: DNV GL-Healthcare USA, Inc. (Level VII)

30 American Association of Critical Care Nurses. (2016). AACN practice alert: Initial and ongoing verification of feeding tube placement in adults. https://www.aacn.org/clinical-resources/practice-alerts/initial-and-ongoing-verification-of-feeding-tube-placement-in-adults (Level VII)

31 Galbois, A., et al. (2011). Colorimetric capnography, a new procedure to ensure correct feeding tube placement in the intensive care unit: An evaluation of a local protocol. *Journal of Critical Care, 26,* 411–414. (Level IV)

32 Emergency Nurses Association. (2019). Clinical practice guideline: Gastric tube placement verification. *Journal of Emergency Nursing, 45*(3), 306. (Level VII)

33 C. R. Bard, Inc. (2009). StatLock nasogastric stabilization devices: Catheter stabilization device. https://www.crbard.com/CRBard/media/ProductAssets/BardMedicalDivision/PF10228/en-US/e2ggy5vl57pe-jw8u6xm87dvb40cu2nde.pdf

34 Black, J. M., & Kalowes, P. (2016). Medical device-related pressure ulcers. *Chronic Wound Care Management and Research, 3,* 91–99. https://www.dovepress.com/medical-device-related-pressure-ulcers-peer-reviewed-fulltext-article-CWCMR

35 Baranoski, S., & Ayello, E. A. (2020). *Wound care essentials: Practice principles* (5th ed.). Philadelphia, PA: Wolters Kluwer.

36 LeBlanc, K., et al. (2013). International skin tear advisory panel: A tool kit to aid in the prevention, assessment, and treatment of skin tears using a simplified classification system. *Advances in Skin and Wound Care, 26,* 459–476. (Level IV)

37 U.S. Food and Drug Administration. (2017). Examples of medical device misconnections. https://www.fda.gov/medical-devices/medical-device-connectors/examples-medical-device-misconnections

38 The Joint Commission. (2014). Sentinel event alert 53: Managing risk during transition to new ISO tubing connector standards. https://www.jointcommission.org/-/media/tjc/documents/resources/patient-safety-topics/sentinel-event/sea_53_connectors_8_19_14_final.pdf (Level VII)

39 Ganz, D. A., et al. (2013, reviewed 2021). Preventing falls in hospitals: A toolkit for improving quality of care (AHRQ publication no. 13-0015-EF). https://www.ahrq.gov/professionals/systems/hospital/fallpx-toolkit/index.html (Level VII)

40 Rutala, W. A., et al. (2008, revised 2019). Guideline for disinfection and sterilization in healthcare facilities, 2008. https://www.cdc.gov/infection-control/pdf/guidelines/disinfection-guidelines-H.pdf (Level I)

41 Accreditation Association for Hospitals and Health Systems. (2020). Standard 07.02.03. *Healthcare Facilities Accreditation Program: Accreditation requirements for acute care hospitals.* Chicago, IL: Accreditation Association for Hospitals and Health Systems. (Level VII)

42 The Joint Commission. (2021). Standard RC.01.03.01. *Comprehensive accreditation manual for hospitals.* Oakbrook Terrace, IL: The Joint Commission. (Level VII)

43 Centers for Medicare and Medicaid Services, Department of Health and Human Services. (2020). Condition of participation: Medical record services. 42 C.F.R. § 482.24(b).

44 Accreditation Association for Hospitals and Health Systems. (2020). Standard 10.00.03. *Healthcare Facilities Accreditation Program: Accreditation requirements for acute care hospitals.* Chicago, IL: Accreditation Association for Hospitals and Health Systems. (Level VII)

45 DNV GL-Healthcare USA, Inc. (2020). MR.2.SR.1. *NIAHO® accreditation requirements, interpretive guidelines and surveyor guidance—revision 20.0.* Milford, OH: DNV GL-Healthcare USA, Inc. (Level VII)

NASOPHARYNGEAL AIRWAY INSERTION AND CARE

Insertion of a nasopharyngeal airway—a soft rubber or latex uncuffed catheter—establishes or maintains a patent airway by displacing the tongue or soft palate from the pharyngeal air passages.[1] The airway follows the curvature of the nasopharynx, passing through the nose and extending from the nostril to the posterior pharynx. The bevel-shaped pharyngeal end of the airway facilitates insertion, and its funnel-shaped nasal end helps prevent slippage.

This airway is the typical choice for patients with airway obstruction or the risk of developing airway obstruction when conditions such as a clenched jaw or oral problems prevent placement of an oral airway.[2] It's also used to protect the nasal mucosa from injury when the patient needs frequent nasotracheal suctioning. Unconscious patients as well as consciously sedated patients may tolerate a nasopharyngeal airway better than an oral airway.[1]

Insertion of a nasopharyngeal airway is preferred when an oropharyngeal airway is contraindicated or fails to maintain a patent airway. A nasopharyngeal airway is contraindicated for patients with pathologic nasopharyngeal deformities, those receiving anticoagulation therapy, and those prone to epistaxis.[1,3] An oropharyngeal airway is preferred for patients who have or are suspected of having traumatic brain injury, central facial fractures, basal skull fractures, severe coagulopathy, or anticoagulation therapy.[2,3,4]

Equipment

Nasopharyngeal airway of proper size ▪ tongue blade ▪ water-soluble lubricant ▪ gloves ▪ stethoscope ▪ disinfectant pad ▪ oral care supplies ▪ suction equipment (suction apparatus, connection tubing, suction catheter kit) ▪ Optional: resuscitation mask, handheld resuscitation bag, or oxygen-powered breathing device, flashlight, prescribed topical anesthetic with a vasoconstrictor, sterile water or normal saline solution.

Preparation of equipment

Inspect all equipment and supplies. If a product is expired, is defective, or has compromised integrity, remove it from patient use, label it as expired or defective, and report the expiration or defect as directed by your facility. Make sure suction equipment is readily available and properly functioning.

Implementation

- Verify the practitioner's order.
- Gather and prepare the necessary equipment and supplies.
- Perform hand hygiene.[5,6,7,8,9,10]
- Confirm the patient's identity using at least two patient identifiers.[11]
- Provide privacy.[12,13,14,15]
- In nonemergency situations, explain the procedure to the patient and family (if appropriate) according to their individual communication and learning needs *to increase their understanding, allay their fears, and enhance cooperation.*[16]
- Raise the patient's bed to waist level before providing patient care *to prevent caregiver back strain.*[17]
- Perform hand hygiene.[5,6,7,8,9,10]
- Put on gloves *to comply with standard precautions.*[18,19]
- Measure the diameter of the patient's nostril and the distance from the tip of the nose to the earlobe *to ensure that the airway is the correct size.*
- Select an airway diameter that is slightly smaller than that of the nostril and a length that is the patient's measurement from the nose tip to the earlobe.[3] Airway sizes are labeled according to their internal diameter. The recommended airway size for a large adult is 8 to 9 mm; for a medium-sized adult, 7 to 8 mm; for a small adult, 6 to 7 mm.[3]
- If necessary, suction the patient's mouth and nostrils.
- Apply a topical anesthetic with a vasoconstrictor to the nasal mucosa, if ordered, *to shrink the mucosa and decrease trauma.*[3]
- Lubricate the distal half of the airway's surface with a water-soluble lubricant *to prevent traumatic injury during insertion.*[3]
- Properly insert the airway. (See *Inserting a nasopharyngeal airway.*)
- Immediately after insertion, auscultate the patient's breath sounds. If they're absent or inadequate, initiate artificial positive-pressure ventilation with a mouth-to-mask technique, a handheld resuscitation bag, or an oxygen-powered breathing device.
- Suction the patient's airway as needed *to remove secretions.*
- Reassess the patient's respiratory status following suctioning and at an interval determined by the patient's condition and your facility.[3]
- Assess the patient's skin surrounding the nasopharyngeal airway regularly for redness, swelling, drainage, bleeding, and skin breakdown.[3,20]
- Check the airway regularly *to detect dislodgment or obstruction.*
- Provide oral care, moisturizing the oral mucosa and lips every 2 to 4 hours and as needed. Brush the patient's teeth, gums, and tongue at least twice a day *to reduce the risk of pneumonia.*[21]
- Return the bed to the lowest position *to prevent falls and maintain patient safety.*[22]
- Remove and discard your gloves.[18]
- Perform hand hygiene.[5,6,7,8,9,10]
- Clean and disinfect your stethoscope using a disinfectant pad.[23,24]
- Perform hand hygiene.[5,6,7,8,9,10]
- Document the procedure.[25,26,27,28]

Special considerations

- Every 8 hours, remove and clean the airway *to check for skin breakdown.* Clean the airway according to the manufacturer's instructions. Reinsert the clean airway. Consider rotating to the other nostril *to prevent skin breakdown.*[3]

Inserting a nasopharyngeal airway

First, hold the airway beside the patient's face *to make sure it's the proper size* (as shown below). It should be slightly smaller than the patient's nostril diameter and slightly longer than the distance from the tip of the nose to the earlobe.[3]

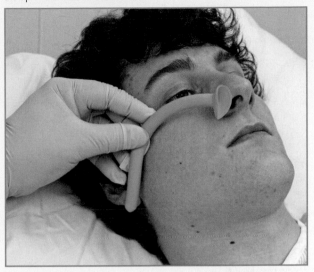

To insert the airway, hyperextend the patient's neck using a chin-lift or jaw-thrust technique *to anteriorly displace the patient's mandible* (unless contraindicated). Position the bevel of the airway toward the center of the nose and then push up the tip of the nose and pass the airway into the nostril (as shown below). Avoid pushing against any resistance *to prevent tissue trauma and airway kinking.*

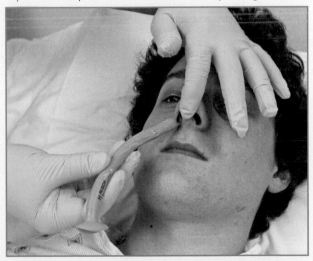

To check for correct airway placement, first close the patient's mouth. Then, place your finger over the tube's opening *to detect air exchange.* Also, open the patient's mouth, depress the patient's tongue with a tongue blade, and look for the airway tip behind the uvula. Use a flashlight to illuminate the oral cavity if necessary.[3]

Complications

Complications of nasopharyngeal airway insertion include injury of the nasal mucosa, skin breakdown of the nares, bleeding, and possibly aspiration of blood into the trachea.[3,20,29] After airway insertion, sinus infection can result from obstruction of sinus drainage.[29] If the tube is too long, it can enter the esophagus and cause gastric distention and hypoventilation during artificial ventilation.[3,29] Although semiconscious patients usually tolerate this type of airway better than conscious patients do, they may still experience laryngospasm and vomiting.

Documentation

Document the date and time of airway insertion, the size of the airway, removal and cleaning of the airway, shifts from one nostril to the other, the condition of the mucous membranes, and suctioning. Record complications that occur, nursing interventions you performed, and the patient's tolerance of the procedure. Document teaching provided to the patient and family (if appropriate), their understanding of that teaching, and any need for follow-up teaching.

References

1 Becker, D. E., et al. (2014). Essentials of airway management, oxygenation, and ventilation, part 1: Basic equipment and devices. *Anesthesia Progress, 61*(12), 78–83. https://www.ncbi.nlm.nih.gov/pmc/articles/PMC4068090/

2 American Heart Association. (2020). 2020 American Heart Association Guidelines for CPR and ECC– Part 7: Systems of Care. *Circulation, 142*(16), 78–83. https://cpr.heart.org/en/resuscitation-science/cpr-and-ecc-guidelines (Level II)

3 Wiegand, D. L. (2017). *AACN procedure manual for high acuity, progressive, and critical care* (7th ed.). St. Louis, MO: Elsevier.

4 Bullard, D., et al. (2012). Contraindications to nasopharyngeal airway insertion. *Nursing, 42*(10), 66–67. https://journals.lww.com/nursing/Fulltext/2012/10000/Contraindications_to_nasopharyngeal_airway.21.aspx (Level V)

5 The Joint Commission. (2021). Standard NPSG.07.01.01. *Comprehensive accreditation manual for hospitals.* Oakbrook Terrace, IL: The Joint Commission. (Level VII)

6 Centers for Disease Control and Prevention. (2002). Guideline for hand hygiene in health-care settings: Recommendations of the Healthcare Infection Control Practices Advisory Committee and the HICPAC/SHEA/APIC/IDSA Hand Hygiene Task Force. *MMWR Recommendations and Reports, 51*(RR-16), 1–45. https://www.cdc.gov/mmwr/pdf/rr/rr5303.pdf (Level II)

7 World Health Organization. (2009). WHO guidelines on hand hygiene in health care: First global patient safety challenge, clean care is safer care. https://apps.who.int/iris/bitstream/handle/10665/44102/9789241597906_eng.pdf?sequence=1 (Level IV)

8 Centers for Medicare and Medicaid Services, Department of Health and Human Services. (2020). Condition of participation: Infection control. 42 C.F.R. § 482.42.

9 Accreditation Association for Hospitals and Health Systems. (2020). Standard 07.01.21. *Healthcare Facilities Accreditation Program: Accreditation requirements for acute care hospitals.* Chicago, IL: Accreditation Association for Hospitals and Health Systems. (Level VII)

10 DNV GL-Healthcare USA, Inc. (2020). IC.1.SR.1. *NIAHO® accreditation requirements, interpretive guidelines and surveyor guidance—revision 20.0.* Milford, OH: DNV GL-Healthcare USA, Inc. (Level VII)

11 The Joint Commission. (2021). Standard NPSG.01.01.01. *Comprehensive accreditation manual for hospitals.* Oakbrook Terrace, IL: The Joint Commission. (Level VII)

12 The Joint Commission. (2021). Standard RI.01.01.01. *Comprehensive accreditation manual for hospitals.* Oakbrook Terrace, IL: The Joint Commission. (Level VII)

13 Centers for Medicare and Medicaid Services, Department of Health and Human Services. (2020). Condition of participation: Patient's rights. 42 C.F.R. § 482.13(c)(1).

14 Accreditation Association for Hospitals and Health Systems. (2020). Standard 15.01.16. *Healthcare Facilities Accreditation Program: Accreditation requirements for acute care hospitals.* Chicago, IL: Accreditation Association for Hospitals and Health Systems. (Level VII)

15 DNV GL-Healthcare USA, Inc. (2020). PR.2.SR.5. *NIAHO® accreditation requirements, interpretive guidelines and surveyor guidance—revision 20.0.* Milford, OH: DNV GL-Healthcare USA, Inc. (Level VII)

16 The Joint Commission. (2021). Standard PC.02.01.21. *Comprehensive accreditation manual for hospitals.* Oakbrook Terrace, IL: The Joint Commission. (Level VII)

17 Waters, T. R., et al. (2009). Safe patient handling training for schools of nursing. https://www.cdc.gov/niosh/docs/2009-127/pdfs/2009-127.pdf (Level VII)

18 Siegel, J. D., et al. (2007, revised 2019). 2007 guideline for isolation precautions: Preventing transmission of infectious agents in healthcare settings. https://www.cdc.gov/infectioncontrol/pdf/guidelines/isolation-guidelines-H.pdf (Level II)

19 Accreditation Association for Hospitals and Health Systems. (2020). Standard 07.01.10. *Healthcare Facilities Accreditation Program: Accreditation requirements for acute care hospitals.* Chicago, IL: Accreditation Association for Hospitals and Health Systems. (Level VII)

20 European Pressure Ulcer Advisory Panel, et al. (2019). Prevention and treatment of pressure ulcers/injuries: Quick reference guide. http://www.internationalguideline.com/static/pdfs/Quick_Reference_Guide-10Mar2019.pdf (Level VII)

21 American Association of Critical-Care Nurses. (2017). AACN practice alert: Oral care for acutely and critically ill patients. https://www.aacn.org/clinical-resources/practice-alerts/oral-care-for-acutely-and-critically-ill-patients (Level VII)

22 Ganz, D. A., et al. (2013, reviewed 2021). Preventing falls in hospitals: A toolkit for improving quality of care (AHRQ publication no. 13-0015-EF). https://www.ahrq.gov/professionals/systems/hospital/fallpxtoolkit/index.html (Level VII)

23 Rutala, W. A., et al. (2008, revised 2019). Guideline for disinfection and sterilization in healthcare facilities, 2008. https://www.cdc.gov/infection-control/pdf/guidelines/disinfection-guidelines-H.pdf (Level I)

24 Accreditation Association for Hospitals and Health Systems. (2020). Standard 07.02.03. *Healthcare Facilities Accreditation Program: Accreditation requirements for acute care hospitals.* Chicago, IL: Accreditation Association for Hospitals and Health Systems. (Level VII)

25 The Joint Commission. (2021). Standard RC.01.03.01. *Comprehensive accreditation manual for hospitals.* Oakbrook Terrace, IL: The Joint Commission. (Level VII)

26 Centers for Medicare and Medicaid Services, Department of Health and Human Services. (2020). Condition of participation: Medical record services. 42 C.F.R. § 482.24(b).

27 Accreditation Association for Hospitals and Health Systems. (2020). Standard 10.00.03. *Healthcare Facilities Accreditation Program: Accreditation requirements for acute care hospitals.* Chicago, IL: Accreditation Association for Hospitals and Health Systems. (Level VII)

28 DNV GL-Healthcare USA, Inc. (2020). MR.2.SR.1. *NIAHO® accreditation requirements, interpretive guidelines and surveyor guidance—revision 20.0.* Milford, OH: DNV GL-Healthcare USA, Inc. (Level VII)

29 Atanelov, Z., et al. (2020). Nasopharyngeal airway. https://www.ncbi.nlm.nih.gov/books/NBK513220/

Nebulizer therapy

An established component of respiratory care, nebulizer therapy aids bronchial hygiene by hydrating dried and retained secretions, promoting expectoration of secretions, humidifying inspired oxygen, and delivering medications to the lower respiratory tract. Medications delivered directly to lung tissue can be administered at lower doses and cause fewer adverse reactions than systemically delivered medications. Therapy may be administered through nebulizers that have a large or small volume, are connected to ventilator tubing, or are ultrasonic.[1,2]

Large-volume nebulizers, such as the Venturi jet, are used to provide long-term 100% humidity for an artificial airway such as a tracheostomy or for certain pulmonary conditions such as cystic fibrosis. (See *Large-volume nebulizer.*) Cool aerosols can be used to treat upper airway disorders, such as croup, epiglottiditis, and postextubation edema.[1] Heated aerosols are used whenever the upper airway is bypassed, such as in patients who are intubated or have a tracheostomy, *to prevent the dry gas from causing damage to the bronchial airways.*[1] The aerosol mist can be delivered via mist tent, hood, mouthpiece, mask, T-piece, face tent, or tracheostomy collar. The amount of aerosol the nebulizer delivers varies depending on the design, gas flow, air entrainment port, and temperature.[1] Small-volume nebulizers are also used to deliver medications such as bronchodilators to the upper and lower airways.[1,2]

In-line nebulizers are used to deliver medications to patients who are being mechanically ventilated. In such cases, the nebulizer is placed in the inspiratory side of the ventilatory circuit.

Ultrasonic nebulizers are electrically driven and use high-frequency vibrations to break up surface water into particles.[1] The resultant dense mist works to penetrate smaller airways and is useful for hydrating secretions, thereby inducing a cough and sputum expectoration. The aerosol mist can be delivered to the patient via mist tent, hood, mouthpiece, mask, T-piece, face tent, or tracheostomy collar.[1] Some ultrasonic

EQUIPMENT

Large-volume nebulizer

Connected to a flowmeter and pneumatically powered, an air entrainment port allows oxygen and air to mix to deliver a reliable oxygen concentration through a jet orifice. When the nebulizer is connected to a liquid chamber, liquid is siphoned into the jet flow and creates an aerosol.[1] The amount of aerosol delivered varies depending on the nebulizer design, gas flow, air entrapment port, and temperature.[1] The following are advantages and disadvantages to using a large-volume nebulizer.

Advantages
- Provides oxygen and aerosol therapy
- Can be used for long-term therapy

Disadvantages
- Increases the risk of bacterial growth (reusable units)
- Allows condensate collection in large-bore tubing
- May cause mucosal irritation from breathing hot, dry air (if the water level isn't maintained correctly in the reservoir)
- Increases the risk of overhydration by mist (in infants, children, and patients with delicate fluid balance)

nebulizers are also capable of aerosolizing medications, but this application hasn't been shown to be superior to a standard jet nebulizer.[1]

Standard precautions should be used for all patients on nebulizer therapy *to prevent exposure to body fluids.* Airborne precautions should be implemented for patients with known or suspected tuberculosis, including enclosing and containing aerosol administration and filtering aerosols that bypass or are exhaled by the patient.[3,4]

Equipment
For large-volume nebulizer therapy
Stethoscope ▪ pressurized gas source ▪ flowmeter ▪ patient interface device (such as a mask or collar) ▪ large-bore oxygen tubing ▪ nebulizer ▪ sterile distilled water[1] ▪ tissues and emesis basin or other container (for collection or disposal of expectorated sputum) ▪ suction source and supplies ▪ gloves ▪ vital signs monitoring equipment ▪ disinfectant pad ▪ oral care supplies ▪ Optional: oxygen blender (if a built-in adjustable oxygen controller isn't available), heating device, in-line thermometer (if using a heater), gown, mask and goggles or mask with face shield.

For small-volume nebulizer therapy
Stethoscope ▪ pressurized gas source ▪ flowmeter ▪ vital signs monitoring equipment ▪ nebulizer with tubing ▪ mouthpiece or mask ▪ prescribed medication ▪ syringe and needle or needleless device ▪ antiseptic pad ▪ tissues and emesis basin or other container (for collection or disposal of expectorated sputum) ▪ oral care supplies ▪ gloves ▪ disinfectant pad ▪ Optional: sterile normal saline solution,[1] spirometer or peak flow meter, suction source and supplies, sterile water, gown, mask and goggles or mask with face shield.

For in-line nebulizer therapy
Syringe and needle or needleless device ▪ disinfectant pad ▪ pressurized gas source ▪ in-line nebulizer ▪ prescribed medication and sterile diluent ▪ gloves ▪ stethoscope ▪ pulse oximeter and probe ▪ vital signs monitoring equipment ▪ sterile or distilled water ▪ Optional: gown, mask and goggles or mask with face shield, suction source and supplies, flowmeter, suction equipment.

For ultrasonic nebulizer therapy
Stethoscope ▪ ultrasonic gas-delivery device ▪ large-bore oxygen tubing ▪ patient interface device, such as a mask, mouthpiece, or collar[2] ▪ nebulizer couplet compartment ▪ tissues and emesis basin or other container (for collection or disposal of expectorated sputum) ▪ disinfectant pad ▪

prescribed medications for inhalation ▪ oral care supplies ▪ gloves ▪ vital signs monitoring equipment ▪ Optional: sterile distilled water, spirometer or peak flow meter, sterile normal saline solution, suction source and supplies, gown, mask and goggles or mask with face shield.

Preparation of equipment
Inspect all equipment and supplies; if a product is expired, is defective, or has compromised integrity, remove it from patient use, label it as expired or defective, and report the expiration or defect as directed by your facility. Assemble the nebulizer according to the manufacturer's instructions.

Assemble the ultrasonic nebulizer according to the manufacturer's instructions. *To ensure proper operation of the nebulizer,* check the connections with the AC adapter and electrical output or battery installation. Reconnect or reinstall, as needed.[2]

Depending on the manufacturer, fill the reservoir of the device with sterile distilled water until it reaches exactly the level marked. *This amount of water serves as a conductor for the ultrasonic waves and medication and will never be nebulized.*[5]

Implementation
For large-volume nebulizer therapy
- Verify the practitioner's order.
- Gather and prepare the necessary equipment and supplies.
- Perform hand hygiene.[6,7,8,9,10,11]
- Confirm the patient's identity using at least two patient identifiers.[12]
- Provide privacy.[13,14,15,16]
- Explain the procedure to the patient and family (if appropriate) according to their individual communication and learning needs *to increase their understanding, allay their fears, and enhance cooperation.*[17]
- Raise the patient's bed to waist level when providing patient care *to prevent caregiver back strain.*[18]
- Perform hand hygiene.[6,7,8,9,10,11]
- Put on gloves and, as needed, other personal protective equipment *to comply with standard precautions.*[3,19]
- Obtain the patient's vital signs and perform a respiratory assessment *to establish a baseline.*
- If possible, place the patient in a sitting or high Fowler position *to encourage full lung expansion and promote aerosol dispersion.*
- Attach the flowmeter to the pressurized gas source.
- Fill the nebulizer water chamber to the indicated level with sterile distilled water.[1] *To prevent corrosion,* avoid using saline solution.
- Attach the nebulizer tubing to the flowmeter.
- Add a heating device, if ordered, and place an in-line thermometer between the outlet port and the patient, as close to the patient as possible, *to monitor the actual temperature of the inhaled gas and to avoid burning the patient.*
- If the nebulizer will also supply oxygen to the patient, set the air entrainment port or adjust the external oxygen blender to the ordered oxygen concentration and analyze the flow at the patient's end of the tubing *to ensure delivery of the prescribed oxygen percentage.*
- Attach the delivery device to the patient.
- Encourage the patient to cough and expectorate sputum, and suction as needed.
- Check the water level in the nebulizer at frequent intervals and refill or replace, as indicated. When refilling a reusable container, discard the old water *to prevent infection from bacterial or fungal growth,* and refill the container to the indicator line with sterile distilled water.[1]
- If the aerosol is heated, use the in-line thermometer to monitor the temperature of the gas the patient is inhaling; tell the patient to report warmth, discomfort, or hot tubing, *because these may indicate a heater malfunction.* If you turn off the flow for more than 5 minutes, unplug the heater *to avoid overheating the water and burning the patient when the aerosol is resumed.*
- Obtain the patient's vital signs and assess respiratory status *to evaluate the effectiveness of therapy.*
- Change the nebulizer unit and tubing at an interval determined by your facility *to prevent bacterial contamination.*
- Assist the patient with oral care, as needed. (See the "Oral care" procedure.)

■ Return the bed to the lowest position *to prevent falls and maintain patient safety*.[20]

■ Remove and discard your gloves and any other personal protective equipment worn.[3]

■ Perform hand hygiene.[6,7,8,9,10,11]

■ Clean and disinfect your stethoscope using a disinfectant pad.[21,22]

■ Perform hand hygiene.[6,7,8,9,10,11]

■ Document the procedure.[23,24,25,26]

For small-volume, in-line, or ultrasonic nebulizer therapy

■ Avoid distractions and interruptions when preparing and administering medications *to prevent medication errors*.[27,28]

■ Verify the practitioner's order.[29,30,31,32]

■ Reconcile the patient's medications when the practitioner orders a new medication *to reduce the risk of medication errors, including omissions, dosing errors, and drug interactions*.[33]

■ Gather and prepare the necessary equipment and supplies.

■ Compare the medication label with the order in the patient's medical record.[29,30,31,32]

■ Check the patient's medical record for an allergy or a contraindication to the prescribed medication. If an allergy or a contraindications exists, don't administer the medication; notify the practitioner.[29,30,31,32]

■ Check the expiration date on the medication. If the medication is expired, return it to the pharmacy and obtain new medication.[29,30,31,32]

■ Visually inspect the medication for particles or discoloration or other signs of loss of integrity; don't administer the medication if its integrity is compromised.[29,30,31,32]

■ Label all medications, medication containers, and other solutions and handle them using sterile technique.[34,35]

■ Discuss any unresolved concerns about the medication with the patient's practitioner.[29,30,31,32]

■ Perform hand hygiene.[6,7,8,9,10,11]

■ Confirm the patient's identity using at least two patient identifiers.[12]

■ Provide privacy.[13,14,15,16]

■ Explain the procedure to the patient and family (if appropriate) according to their individual communication and learning needs *to increase their understanding, allay their fears, and enhance cooperation*.[17]

■ If the patient is receiving the medication for the first time, teach about potential adverse effects and discuss any other concerns related to the medication.[29,30,31,32]

■ Raise the patient's bed to waist level when providing patient care *to prevent back strain*.[18]

■ Perform hand hygiene.[6,7,8,9,10,11]

■ Put on gloves and, as needed, other personal protective equipment *to comply with standard precautions*.[3,19]

■ Obtain the patient's vital signs, perform a respiratory assessment, and obtain a spirometry or peak flow reading, as ordered, *to establish a baseline*.[36,37]

■ Suction the patient as needed to clear the airway.[1]

■ If possible, place the patient in a sitting or high Fowler position *to encourage full lung expansion and promote aerosol dispersion*.[2]

■ Verify that the medication is being administered at the proper time, in the prescribed dose, and by the correct route *to reduce the risk of medication errors*.[29,30,31,32]

■ If your facility uses a bar code technology, use it as directed by your facility.

For small-volume therapy

■ Draw up the prescribed medication and inject it into the nebulizer cup. *To prevent contamination, don't touch the interior of the nebulizer.*

■ Add sterile normal saline solution to the prescribed dose volume according to the drug manufacturer's prescribing information.[1,2]

■ After attaching the flowmeter to the gas source, attach the nebulizer to the flowmeter and then adjust the flow according to the manufacturer's recommendations, usually 6 to 10 L/minute (as shown above on right).[1]

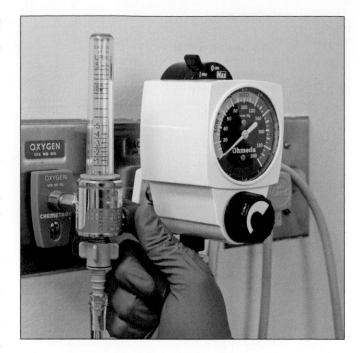

■ Check the outflow port *to ensure adequate misting.*

■ Assist the patient with the mouthpiece or mask, as needed, depending on the delivery system and patient-related factors such as age and physical and cognitive ability.[2] Instruct the patient to inhale slowly through the mouth at a normal tidal volume (as shown below).[1]

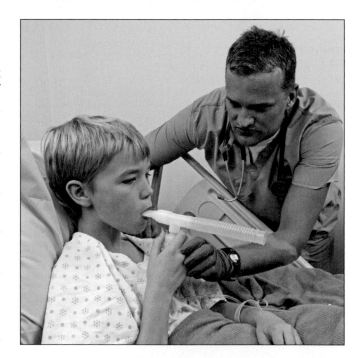

■ Remain with the patient and continue the treatment until the nebulizer begins to sputter.[1,2,38]

■ Monitor heart rate and respiratory status during the procedure *to detect any adverse reactions to the medication*.[39]

■ After treatment, obtain the patient's vital signs, assess the respiratory status, and obtain a spirometry or peak flow measurement as indicated *to detect any adverse reactions to the medication*.[36,37]

■ Encourage the patient to cough and expectorate, or suction the patient's airway as needed.[39]

■ Assist the patient with oral care.

- Return the bed to the lowest position *to prevent falls and maintain patient safety.*[20]
- Rinse the nebulizer with sterile water and allow it to air-dry, or discard it after the treatment.[1]

For in-line nebulizer therapy

- Draw up the medication and diluent, open the in-line nebulizer cup, inject the medication, and then replace the lid. Attach the cup to the gas source with the attached tubing.
- Insert the in-line nebulizer into the inspiratory limb of the ventilator circuit following the manufacturer's instructions.[1]
- Remove the heat-moisture exchanger from the ventilator if it's attached.[1]
- Initiate gas flow by using the nebulizer function on the ventilator, if available. If this function isn't available, initiate gas flow from an external source *to create a mist.*[1]

NURSING ALERT Adding an external gas flow to the ventilator can affect gas flow and volume delivery to the patient, causing alarms to trigger. Monitor the patient closely during a nebulizer treatment, and return ventilator settings to pretreatment levels as soon as possible after treatment.[1]

- If the patient is being ventilated using a spontaneous pressure mode, encourage the patient to take slow, even breaths during the treatment.
- Remain with the patient during the treatment, which typically lasts 15 to 20 minutes, and monitor vital signs, oxygen saturation level, and ventilator parameters *to detect any adverse reaction to the medication.*[1]
- Discontinue treatment when all of the medication has been aerosolized. Remove the in-line nebulizer cup from the ventilatory circuit.[1]
- Encourage the patient to cough, and suction excess secretions as needed.
- Perform a respiratory assessment *to evaluate the effectiveness of therapy.*[36,37]
- Return the bed to the lowest position *to prevent falls and maintain patient safety.*[20]
- Rinse the nebulizer cup with sterile or distilled water, shake off excess water, and allow it to air-dry. Then store it in a clean, dry place according to the manufacturer's instructions.[1]

For ultrasonic nebulizer therapy

- Fill the couplet compartment on the nebulizer with the prescribed medication or sterile normal saline solution to the level indicated.[1] If the dose to be inhaled is larger than the maximum capacity of the compartment, divide it into several separate inhalations.[5]
- Before beginning, administer an inhaled bronchodilator (via metered-dose inhaler or small-volume nebulizer) *to prevent bronchospasm,* as ordered, following safe medication administration practices.[29,30,31,32]
- Turn on the nebulizer machine and check the outflow port *to ensure proper misting.*
- As needed, assist the patient with applying a mouthpiece, mask, or collar, as necessary, depending on the delivery system and patient-related factors such as age and physical and cognitive ability.[2]
- Encourage the patient to take slow, even breaths through the mouth.[1]
- Remain with the patient during the procedure until all of the medication in the nebulizer cup has been aerosolized *to observe for adverse reactions.* Watch for labored respirations, *because ultrasonic nebulizer therapy may hydrate retained secretions and obstruct airways.* Observe for wheezing resulting from irritation of the airways.[40]
- When medication delivery is complete, turn off the nebulizer.
- Clean and store the nebulizer and tubing appropriately *to prevent bacterial contamination.*[2]
- Obtain the patient's vital signs, assess respiratory status, and obtain a spirometry or peak flow measurement, as ordered, *to determine the efficacy of treatment.*[36,37]
- Encourage the patient to cough and expectorate, or suction the airway as needed.
- Dispose of sputum properly or send an ordered specimen to the laboratory immediately. (See the "Sputum collection" procedure.)
- Assist the patient with oral care.
- Return the bed to the lowest position *to prevent falls and maintain patient safety.*[20]

Completing the procedure

- Dispose of used supplies in the appropriate receptacle.
- Remove and discard your gloves and any other personal protective equipment worn.[3]
- Perform hand hygiene.[6,7,8,9,10,11]
- Clean and disinfect your stethoscope using a disinfectant pad.[21,22]
- Perform hand hygiene.[6,7,8,9,10,11]
- Document the procedure.[23,24,25,26]

Special considerations

- If a nebulizer device is for single-patient use, use it only for a single patient, label it with the proper patient identifiers, and discard it at the end of the patient's stay *to prevent cross-contamination.*[2,41]
- A nose clip may be used if the patient has difficulty remembering to breathe through the mouth.
- Use only sterile fluids for nebulization *to reduce the risk of infection.*[1]
- Don't leave the in-line nebulizer cup in the ventilator circuit between treatments, *because doing so increases the risk of a pressure leak in the system.*
- You should typically consider the treatment over with the onset of nebulizer sputtering. Some nebulizers will sputter for extended periods after administration of the majority of the inhaled dose. Evidence suggests that after the onset of sputter, the patient inhales very little additional drug. A newer electronic nebulizer may use a microprocessor that monitors how much dose the nebulizer has administered and automatically turns off the nebulizer at the end of each dose.[2]
- Humidification in the ventilator circuit decreases aerosol delivery of medication as particles are deposited in the circuit. Medications delivered to patients during mechanical ventilation may require increased dosage to achieve a therapeutic effect.[38]
- Be aware that specialized equipment (such as filters for the expiratory port of the ventilation circuit during nebulization) may be available to minimize aerosolization into the room.[41] Follow the manufacturer's instructions for use or the directions of your facility when appropriate.

Complications

Nebulized particulates can irritate the mucosa and cause bronchospasm and dyspnea.[2] Other complications include airway burns (when a heating element is used), infection from contaminated equipment (rare), adverse reactions to the prescribed medication,[38] and drug deliver to the eyes if using a face mask.[2]

Documentation

Record the date, time, and duration of therapy; the medication, strength, and dose; FIO_2 or oxygen flow rate, if administered; baseline and subsequent vital signs, oxygen saturation levels, ventilator parameters, and respiratory assessment findings; peak flow or spirometry readings before and after treatment; and the patient's response to treatment. Record any adverse reactions to the prescribed medication, the name of the practitioner notified, the date and time of notification, prescribed interventions, and the patient's response to those interventions. Document teaching provided to the patient and the family (if appropriate), their understanding of that teaching, and any need for follow-up teaching.

REFERENCES

1 Kacmarek, R. M., et al. (2021). *Egan's fundamentals of respiratory care* (12th ed.). St. Louis, MO: Mosby.
2 Gregory, K. L., et al. (2017). *Pulmonary disease aerosol delivery devices: A guide for physicians, nurses, pharmacists, and other health care professionals* (3rd ed.). Irving, TX: American Association for Respiratory Care (AARC). https://www.aarc.org/wp-content/uploads/2018/03/aersol-guides-for-hcp.pdf (Level VII)
3 Siegel, J. D., et al. (2007, revised 2019). 2007 guideline for isolation precautions: Preventing transmission of infectious agents in healthcare settings. https://www.cdc.gov/infectioncontrol/pdf/guidelines/isolation-guidelines-H.pdf (Level II)
4 Jensen, P. A., et al. (2005). Guidelines for preventing the transmission of *Mycobacterium tuberculosis* in health-care settings, 2005. *Morbidity and Mortality Weekly Report, 54*(RR17), 1–141. https://www.cdc.gov/mmwr/preview/mmwrhtml/rr5417a1.htm?s_cid=rr5417a1_e (Level II)

5 GF Health Products, Inc. (2008). Lumiscope: Portable ultrasonic nebulizer model 6700: User manual. http://www.grahamfield.com/nosync/producti-magesV2/ProductAdditionalInfoItemOriginal2220.PDF

6 Centers for Disease Control and Prevention. (2002). Guideline for hand hygiene in health-care settings: Recommendations of the Healthcare Infection Control Practices Advisory Committee and the HICPAC/SHEA/APIC/IDSA Hand Hygiene Task Force. *MMWR Recommendations and Reports, 51*(RR-16), 1–45. https://www.cdc.gov/mmwr/pdf/rr/rr5116.pdf (Level II)

7 World Health Organization. (2009). WHO guidelines on hand hygiene in health care: First global patient safety challenge, clean care is safer care. https://apps.who.int/iris/bitstream/handle/10665/44102/9789241597906_eng.pdf?sequence=1 (Level IV)

8 The Joint Commission. (2021). Standard NPSG.07.01.01. *Comprehensive accreditation manual for hospitals.* Oakbrook Terrace, IL: The Joint Commission. (Level VII)

9 Centers for Medicare and Medicaid Services, Department of Health and Human Services. (2020). Condition of participation: Infection control. 42 C.F.R. § 482.42.

10 Accreditation Association for Hospitals and Health Systems. (2020). Standard 07.01.21. *Healthcare Facilities Accreditation Program: Accreditation requirements for acute care hospitals.* Chicago, IL: Accreditation Association for Hospitals and Health Systems. (Level VII)

11 DNV GL-Healthcare USA, Inc. (2020). IC.1.SR.1. *NIAHO® accreditation requirements, interpretive guidelines and surveyor guidance—revision 20.0.* Milford, OH: DNV GL-Healthcare USA, Inc. (Level VII)

12 The Joint Commission. (2021). Standard NPSG.01.01.01. *Comprehensive accreditation manual for hospitals.* Oakbrook Terrace, IL: The Joint Commission. (Level VII)

13 The Joint Commission. (2021). Standard RI.01.01.01. *Comprehensive accreditation manual for hospitals.* Oakbrook Terrace, IL: The Joint Commission. (Level VII)

14 Centers for Medicare and Medicaid Services, Department of Health and Human Services. (2020). Condition of participation: Patient's rights. 42 C.F.R. § 482.13(c)(1).

15 Accreditation Association for Hospitals and Health Systems. (2020). Standard 15.01.16. *Healthcare Facilities Accreditation Program: Accreditation requirements for acute care hospitals.* Chicago, IL: Accreditation Association for Hospitals and Health Systems. (Level VII)

16 DNV GL-Healthcare USA, Inc. (2020). PR.2.SR.5. *NIAHO® accreditation requirements, interpretive guidelines and surveyor guidance—revision 20.0.* Milford, OH: DNV GL-Healthcare USA, Inc. (Level VII)

17 The Joint Commission. (2021). Standard PC.02.01.21. *Comprehensive accreditation manual for hospitals.* Oakbrook Terrace, IL: The Joint Commission. (Level VII)

18 Waters, T. R., et al. (2009). Safe patient handling training for schools of nursing. https://www.cdc.gov/niosh/docs/2009-127/pdfs/2009-127.pdf

19 Accreditation Association for Hospitals and Health Systems. (2020). Standard 07.01.10. *Healthcare Facilities Accreditation Program: Accreditation requirements for acute care hospitals.* Chicago, IL: Accreditation Association for Hospitals and Health Systems. (Level VII)

20 Ganz, D. A., et al. (2013, reviewed 2021). *Preventing falls in hospitals: A toolkit for improving quality of care* (AHRQ Publication No. 13-0015-EF). Rockville, MD: Agency for Healthcare Research and Quality. https://www.ahrq.gov/professionals/systems/hospital/fallpxtoolkit/index.html (Level VII)

21 Rutala, W. A., et al. (2008, revised 2019). Guideline for disinfection and sterilization in healthcare facilities, 2008. https://www.cdc.gov/infection-control/pdf/guidelines/disinfection-guidelines-H.pdf (Level I)

22 Accreditation Association for Hospitals and Health Systems. (2020). Standard 07.02.03. *Healthcare Facilities Accreditation Program: Accreditation requirements for acute care hospitals.* Chicago, IL: Accreditation Association for Hospitals and Health Systems. (Level VII)

23 The Joint Commission. (2021). Standard RC.01.03.01. *Comprehensive accreditation manual for hospitals.* Oakbrook Terrace, IL: The Joint Commission. (Level VII)

24 Centers for Medicare and Medicaid Services, Department of Health and Human Services. (2020). Condition of participation: Medical record services. 42 C.F.R. § 482.24(b).

25 Accreditation Association for Hospitals and Health Systems. (2020). Standard 10.00.03. *Healthcare Facilities Accreditation Program: Accreditation requirements for acute care hospitals.* Chicago, IL: Accreditation Association for Hospitals and Health Systems. (Level VII)

26 DNV GL-Healthcare USA, Inc. (2020). MR.2.SR.1. *NIAHO® accreditation requirements, interpretive guidelines and surveyor guidance—revision 20.0.* Milford, OH: DNV GL-Healthcare USA, Inc. (Level VII)

27 Westbrook, J., et al. (2010). Association of interruptions with an increased risk and severity of medication administration errors. *Archives of Internal Medicine, 170,* 683–690. (Level IV)

28 Institute for Safe Medication Practices. (2012). Side tracks on the safety express: Interruptions lead to errors and unfinished…Wait, what was I doing? *Nurse Advise-ERR, 11*(2), 1–4. https://www.ismp.org/resources/side-tracks-safety-express-interruptions-lead-errors-and-unfinished-wait-what-was-i-doing?id=37

29 The Joint Commission. (2021). Standard MM.06.01.01. *Comprehensive accreditation manual for hospitals.* Oakbrook Terrace, IL: The Joint Commission. (Level VII)

30 Centers for Medicare and Medicaid Services, Department of Health and Human Services. (2020). Condition of participation: Nursing services. 42 C.F.R. § 482.23(c).

31 Accreditation Association for Hospitals and Health Systems. (2020). Standard 16.01.03. *Healthcare Facilities Accreditation Program: Accreditation requirements for acute care hospitals.* Chicago, IL: Accreditation Association for Hospitals and Health Systems. (Level VII)

32 DNV GL-Healthcare USA, Inc. (2020). MM.1.SR.3. *NIAHO® accreditation requirements, interpretive guidelines and surveyor guidance—revision 20.0.* Milford, OH: DNV GL-Healthcare USA, Inc. (Level VII)

33 Institute for Healthcare Improvement. (2011). *How-to guide: Prevent adverse drug events (medication reconciliation).* Cambridge, MA: Institute for Healthcare Improvement. http://www.ihi.org/resources/Pages/Tools/HowtoGuidePreventAdverseDrugEvents.aspx (Level VII)

34 The Joint Commission. (2021). Standard MM.05.01.09. *Comprehensive accreditation manual for hospitals.* Oakbrook Terrace, IL: The Joint Commission. (Level VII)

35 Accreditation Association for Hospitals and Health Systems. (2020). Standard 25.01.18. *Healthcare Facilities Accreditation Program: Accreditation requirements for acute care hospitals.* Chicago, IL: Accreditation Association for Hospitals and Health Systems. (Level VII)

36 Fanta, C. H. (2022). Acute exacerbations of asthma in adults: Emergency department and inpatient management. In: *UpToDate,* Bochner, B. S., & Hockberger, R. S. (Eds.).

37 Global Initiative for Chronic Obstructive Lung Disease. (2020). 2020 global strategy for the diagnosis, management, and prevention of chronic obstructive pulmonary disease. https://goldcopd.org/wp-content/uploads/2019/12/GOLD-2020-FINAL-ver1.2-03Dec19_WMV.pdf (Level VII)

38 Hess, D., & Dhand, R. (2020). Delivery of inhaled medication in adults. In: *UpToDate,* Bochner, B. S. (Ed.)

39 Ari, A., & Restrepo, R. D. (2012). AARC clinical practice guideline: Aerosol delivery device selection for spontaneously breathing patients: 2012. *Respiratory Care, 57*(4), 613–626. https://www.aarc.org/wp-content/uploads/2014/08/aerosol_delivery_2012.pdf (Level VII)

40 Hoisington, E. R., et al. (2009). A comparison of respiratory care workload with 2 different nebulizers. *Respiratory Care, 54*(4), 495–499. http://rc.rcjournal.com/content/respcare/54/4/495.full.pdf (Level VI)

41 Gardenhire, D. S., et al. (2017). *A guide to aerosol delivery devices for respiratory therapists* (4th ed.). Irving, TX: American Association for Respiratory Care (AARC). https://www.aarc.org/wp-content/uploads/2018/03/aerosol-guides-for-rts.pdf

NEGATIVE-PRESSURE WOUND THERAPY

Negative-pressure wound therapy encourages healing of acute and chronic wounds by applying continuous or intermittent subatmospheric pressure to the surface of a wound using a well-sealed dressing.[1,2] Doing so removes excess wound fluids that can cause maceration and delay healing, reduces edema and bacterial colonization, and stimulates the formation of healthy granulation tissue. It also increases local blood flow and draws wound edges together. (See *Understanding negative-pressure wound therapy.*)

Negative-pressure wound therapy is indicated for acute and traumatic wounds, pressure injuries, and chronic open wounds, such as diabetic ulcers, dehisced surgical wounds, partial-thickness burns, meshed grafts, and skin flaps.[1,3] It's contraindicated in patients with exposed vital organs, necrotic tissue wounds with eschar, untreated osteomyelitis, malignancy disease in the wound, nonenteric and unexplored fistula, wounds with

Understanding negative-pressure wound therapy

When a wound fails to heal in a timely manner, negative-pressure wound therapy is an option to help enhance delayed or impaired wound healing. It involves placing a special dressing in a wound or over a graft or flap and using a vacuum-assisted closure device to create negative pressure within the wound bed, which dilates arterioles within the wound bed, increasing circulation and improving proliferations of granulation tissue.[2]

Depending on the type of wound, the selected manufacturer's equipment, and the practitioner's preference, gauze or foam packing will be used.

Gauze packing
Gauze packing, as shown below, is typically used in circumferential and tunneling wounds and explored enteric fistulas. Gauze fits most wounds and tends to be more comfortable for the patient during application and removal.

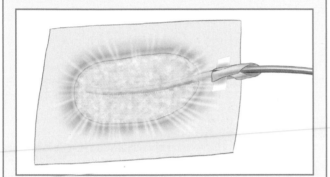

Foam packing
Foam packing, as shown below, is typically used in wounds with a lot of exudate. It's available in various sizes to fit a wide range of wound types, and can be cut to accommodate any wound size.

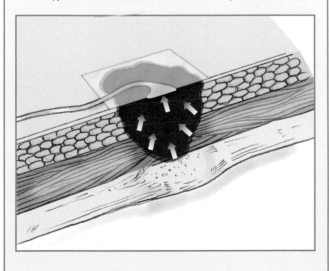

inadequate debridement, an untreated coagulopathy, or an allergy to any component of the procedure. This therapy should be used cautiously in patients with active bleeding, in those taking anticoagulants or platelet aggregate inhibitors, and when achieving wound hemostasis has been difficult.[4,5]

There are negative pressure wound therapy units that enable continuous wound irrigation to the wound bed. Also available are portable, single-patient-use, and disposable negative pressure wound therapy units. The use of such devices promotes patient mobility, increases the ease of performing activities of daily living, and facilitates early hospital discharge.[6]

No consensus of expert opinion exists regarding the use of clean or sterile technique when caring for chronic wounds.[7]

Equipment
Emesis basin ■ sterile normal saline irrigating solution ■ gloves ■ sterile gloves ■ fluid-impermeable pad ■ irrigation kit with syringe ■ suction tubing ■ evacuation canister tubing ■ skin protectant wipe ■ evacuation canister ■ negative-pressure wound therapy unit ■ wound assessment tool and guide ■ label ■ Optional: gown, goggles, prescribed pain medication, scale, prescribed cleansing agent, additional skin barrier product, prescribed wound irrigation solution, irrigation tubing set.

For foam packing
Sterile scissors ■ foam packing ■ transparent dressing therapy drape ■ transparent semipermeable dressing.

For gauze packing
Nonadherent gauze ■ antimicrobial gauze packing moistened with sterile normal saline solution ■ drain ■ ostomy strip paste ■ transparent dressings.

Preparation of equipment
Inspect all equipment and supplies. If a product is expired, is defective, or has compromised integrity, remove it from patient use, label it as expired or defective, and report the expiration or defect as directed by your facility.

Assemble the negative-pressure wound therapy unit at the bedside according to the manufacturer's instructions. Make sure the unit functions properly and the tubing and canister are appropriate for the unit and the patient's size, weight, condition, and wound characteristics. A large canister shouldn't be used for an older adult patient, a patient at high risk of bleeding, or a patient who can't tolerate large-volume fluid loss.[4] Set negative pressure according to the practitioner's order and the manufacturer's instructions (25 to 200 mm Hg). Prepare a place for the supplies that's within reach.

Warm the sterile irrigating solution to 90° F to 95° F (32.2° C to 37.8° C) *to promote comfort. Studies show that warm solutions may be more comfortable for patients than room-temperature solutions.*[8] Pour irrigating solution into the container of the irrigation kit.

Implementation
■ Verify the practitioner's order for the appropriate wound cleaning agent, frequency of dressing change, type of negative-pressure unit, type of wound packing, and settings for the negative-pressure device.[9]
■ Review the patient's medical record for allergies or contraindications to treatment. Also assess the patient's bleeding risk before initiation of therapy.[4,9,10]
■ Confirm that informed consent has been obtained and that the signed consent form is in the patient's medical record, as required.[11,12,13,14]
■ Gather and prepare necessary equipment and supplies.
■ Perform hand hygiene.[15,16,17,18,19,20]
■ Confirm the patient's identity using at least two patient identifiers.[21]
■ Provide privacy.[22,23,24,25]
■ Explain the procedure to the patient and family (if appropriate) according to their individual communication and learning needs *to increase their understanding, allay their fears, and enhance cooperation.*[26]
■ Assess the patient's condition.
■ Screen for and assess the patient's pain using facility-defined criteria that are consistent with the patient's age, condition, and ability to understand.[27]
■ Treat the patient's pain as needed and ordered using nonpharmacologic, pharmacologic, or a combination of approaches. Base the treatment plan on evidence-based practices and the patient's clinical condition, past medical history, and pain management goals.[27]
■ Closely monitor the patient at high risk for adverse outcomes related to opioid treatment (if prescribed).[27]

- Raise the patient's bed to waist level before providing patient care *to prevent caregiver back strain.*[28]
- Perform hand hygiene.[15,16,17,18,19,20]
- Put on gloves and, if necessary, a gown and goggles *to comply with standard precautions, and protect yourself from wound drainage and contamination.*[29,30]
- Place a fluid-impermeable pad under the patient *to catch any spills and avoid linen changes.*
- Position the patient *to allow maximum wound exposure and patient comfort.*
- Place the emesis basin under the wound *to collect any drainage.*
- Using sterile technique, prepare a sterile field and place all the supplies on it.
- Remove the soiled dressing and weigh it as ordered. Verify that the number of removed pieces correlates with the number documented in the patient's medical record.[4] Then discard them in an appropriate receptacle.[31]
- Thoroughly inspect the wound *to ensure that all pieces of dressing components have been removed.*
- Remove and discard your gloves[29,31] and perform hand hygiene.[15,16,17,18,19,20]
- Replace your gown as needed and put on a new pair of gloves.[29,31]
- Irrigate the wound thoroughly using normal saline solution and an irrigation syringe. (See the "Wound irrigation" procedure.)
- Clean the area around the wound with normal saline solution or ordered cleansing agent.[9]
- Wipe the intact skin with a skin protectant wipe and allow it to dry *to prevent blistering when removing the dressing.* Apply an additional skin barrier product, as indicated.[2,4]
- Remove and discard your gloves[29] and perform hand hygiene.[15,16,17,18,19,20]
- Put on sterile gloves.[29,31]
- Assess the wound. Note the wound's precise location, any tunneling, tissue type and loss, size, color, odor, and the presence of warmth, edema, or drainage. Also observe for signs and symptoms of wound infection, including increased pain, fever, and elevated white blood cell count.[2]

ELDER ALERT Closely monitor older adult patients, certain small adults, and those with large exudating wounds in relation to body size and weight for fluid loss and dehydration. When monitoring fluid output, consider the volume of fluid in both the tubing and canister and the weight of the dressing removed.[4]

- Measure the wound (length, depth, and width) using your facility's assessment tool and guide. Obtain measurements at the baseline assessment, with the first dressing change, weekly, and when negative-pressure wound therapy is discontinued.
- If your gloves are contaminated, remove and discard them, perform hand hygiene, and put on a new pair of sterile gloves.[15,16,17,18,19,20,29,31]

Using foam packing
- Using sterile scissors, cut the foam to the shape and measurement of the wound *to help maintain negative pressure to the entire wound.* More than one piece of foam may be necessary, depending on the size of the wound. Don't cut the foam directly over the wound *to prevent foam fragments from falling into the wound.* If a tunnel is present, cut the foam longer than the tunnel *to ensure the foam makes contact with the wound.*
- Carefully place the foam in the wound, ensuring that the foam is in contact with the wound bed, margins, and any tunneled area or areas of undermining. (If there's a groove in the foam, apply it with the groove side up.) The foam shouldn't overlap intact skin. Don't pack the foam tightly into any areas of the wound, *because doing so may cause pressure on granulation tissue, which may delay healing.*
- Count the number of foam pieces you use and document the number on the dressing and in the patient's medical record.[4,10] Confirm the count with another nurse if available.
- Apply the transparent therapy dressing drape over the foam, leaving a 1″ to 2″ (3 cm to 5 cm) margin of intact skin covered by the dressing around the wound *to ensure that the wound is covered completely and that the negative-pressure seal will be intact.*[4]

- If continuous wound irrigation isn't prescribed, pinch the transparent therapy dressing drape and carefully cut a hole no larger than 1″ (2.5 cm) in the center of the drape (over the groove in the foam, if present). Do not cut a slit, *because it could seal during therapy.*[4] The hole in the drape is the insertion point for the suction tubing. Depending on the equipment your facility uses, the tubing may be attached to an adhesive pad that you attach to this site. If you're not using a preattached system, place the suction tubing into the center of the foam. *The embedded tubing delivers negative pressure to the wound.* Apply a transparent semipermeable dressing over the insertion point of the suction tubing.
- If continuous wound irrigation is prescribed, connect the administration set to the prescribed irrigation solution bag and hang it on the device's hanger arm. Select the instillation pad application site, giving consideration to fluid flow and tubing positioning *to allow for optimal flow and exudate removal.*[5] Pinch the transparent therapy dressing drape and carefully cut a hole (based on manufacturer's directions) no larger than 1″ (2.5 cm) in the selected location. Do not cut a slit, *because it could seal during therapy.* The hole must be large enough to allow for the input of the irrigant.[5] Peel the backing from the instillation pad and apply it over the hole in the transparent therapy dressing drape.
- Select the vacuum pad application site, giving consideration to fluid flow and tubing positioning *to allow for optimal flow and exudate removal.* Avoid placing over bony prominences or within tissue creases.[5] Pinch the transparent therapy dressing drape and carefully cut another hole (based on manufacturer's directions) no larger than 1″ (2.5 cm) in the selected location. Do not cut a slit, *because it could seal during therapy.* The hole must be large enough to allow for the removal of fluid and exudate.[5] Peel the backing from the vacuum pad and apply it over the hole in the transparent therapy dressing drape. Connect the tubing from the irrigation bag to the instillation pad following the manufacturer's instructions. Connect the tubing from the vacuum pad to the device's collection canister following the manufacturer's instructions.

Using gauze packing
- Using sterile scissors, trim a single layer of nonadherent gauze.
- Lay the nonadherent gauze across the wound bed.
- Apply saline-moistened antimicrobial gauze loosely into the wound, ensuring that the gauze is in contact with the nonadherent gauze, margins, and any tunneled area or areas of undermining. Don't overpack the wound, *because doing so can delay healing.*
- Count the number of gauze pads or rolls used and document that number on the dressing and in the patient's medical record.[10] Confirm the count with another nurse if available.
- Position the drain tubing on top of the gauze. If a channel drain (a small, cylindrical drain) or round drain (a round, perforated drain) is used, wrap a layer of saline-moistened gauze around the drain.
- Apply ostomy strip paste to a small portion of the wound edge at the location where the drain tubing exits the wound *to secure the tubing's position.* Position the drain tubing on top of the ostomy strip paste. Apply the ostomy strip paste over the top of the tubing and pinch it in place *to secure the tubing's position.*
- Apply one or more transparent semipermeable dressing(s) over the wound. Reinforce the seal by pinching the transparent occlusive film and ostomy strip paste together.

Completing the procedure
- Connect the free end of the drain tubing to the canister tubing at the adapter.
- Position the drain tubing on flat surfaces, away from the perineal area, bony prominences, or pressure areas *to prevent additional skin breakdown.*[4]
- Anchor the drain tubing several inches away from the dressing *to prevent tension on the suction tubing.*
- Label the dressing with the date, time, and number of dressings you used.
- Discard used supplies in appropriate receptacles.[31]

- Remove and discard your gloves and any other personal protective equipment worn,[29,31] and perform hand hygiene.[15,16,17,18,19,20]
- Turn on the negative-pressure unit. Make sure the transparent dressing drape shrinks to the foam or gauze and the skin *to ensure a good seal*, as evidenced by a raisin-like appearance of the dressing. Failure of the dressing drape to shrink to the foam or gauze under negative pressure indicates a break in the seal and will trigger the device's alarm. If administering continuous irrigation, set the instillation rate per the practitioner's order.
- Make sure the device alarm limits are set appropriately, and that the alarms are turned on, functioning properly, and audible to staff.[32,33,34]
- Reassess and respond to the patient's pain by evaluating the response to treatment and progress toward pain management goals. Assess for adverse reactions and risk factors for adverse events that may result from treatment.[27]
- Make sure the patient is comfortable.
- Return the bed to the lowest position *to prevent falls and maintain patient safety.*[35]
- Monitor the patient closely; monitor and record the drainage at an interval determined by your facility and the patient's condition.
- Perform hand hygiene.[15,16,17,18,19,20]
- Document the procedure.[36,37,38,39]

Special considerations

- Many manufacturers have dressing kits that contain the necessary equipment. Make sure that you're using the correct kit for your patient's needs.
- Change the dressing according to the manufacturer's directions, usually 48 hours after the beginning of treatment and then two to three times per week.[7] More frequent dressing changes may be necessary if the wound has heavy drainage or drainage with sediment, or if the wound is infected. Try to coordinate the dressing change with the practitioner's visit *so the practitioner can inspect the wound.*
- Change the evacuation canister once per week or when it's full according to the manufacturer's instructions and as directed by your facility.[4] Never leave the dressing in place without suction. If the machine malfunctions, replace the dressing with a wet-to-damp dressing until the machine is repaired or replaced. *Leaving the dressing in place without suction puts the patient at high risk for infection.*[9]
- Evaluate the effectiveness of negative-pressure wound therapy weekly using a comprehensive wound assessment tool and wound measurements. If the wound shows no response or improvement within 2 weeks, or if the wound worsens, reevaluate the use of negative-pressure wound therapy.[4]
- If the patient experiences pain from the negative-pressure wound therapy or dressing changes, consider premedicating the patient, decreasing the pressure settings, using continuous instead of intermittent suction, changing the type of filler dressing, applying a contact layer to the wound surface before inserting the foam, and instilling normal saline solution before removing the dressing.[40]
- For best results, ensure that the patient receives uninterrupted therapy for at least 22 hours daily.[4] If therapy is interrupted for more than 2 hours, remove the old dressing and irrigate the wound. Apply a new sterile dressing and reapply the therapy. Alternatively, if ordered, apply a sterile wet-to-moist gauze dressing to the wound.[4]

Complications

Local skin irritation may occur. Serious complications include bleeding and excessive fluid loss.[10] Cleaning and care of wounds may temporarily increase the patient's pain and increases the risk of infection.[10]

Documentation

Document the date and time; wound assessment, including signs and symptoms of infection; wound measurements; pain assessment and any intervention; and the patient's response. Record the weight of soiled dressings (if appropriate). Note the type and number of dressings used and the settings for the negative pressure wound therapy unit.[4,10] Record the verification of components removed from the wound.[4] Document the patient's tolerance of the procedure. Document teaching you provided to the patient and family (if applicable), their understanding of that teaching, and any need for follow-up teaching.

REFERENCES

1 Gestring, M. (2020). Negative pressure wound therapy. In: *UpToDate*, Berman, R. S., & Cochran, A. (Eds.).
2 Baranoski, S., & Ayello, E. A. (2020). *Wound care essentials: Practice principles* (5th ed.). Philadelphia, PA: Wolters Kluwer.
3 Sandoz, H. (2015). Negative pressure wound therapy: Clinical utility. *Chronic Wound Care Management and Research, 2*, 71–79. https://www.dovepress.com/negative-pressure-wound-therapy-clinical-utility-peer-reviewed-fulltext-article-CWCMR
4 KCI® Licensing, Inc. (2015). V.A.C.™ therapy clinical guidelines: A reference source for clinicians. https://www.acelity.com/-/media/Project/Acelity/Acelity-Base-Sites/shared/PDF/2-b-128h-vac-clinical-guidelines-web.pdf/#EN (Level VII)
5 Cardinal Health. (2019). SVED clinical user manual. https://www.cardinalhealth.com/content/dam/corp/web/documents/Manual/cardinal-health-sved-clinician-user-manual.pdf
6 Brandon, T. (2015). A portable, disposable system for negative-pressure wound therapy. *British Journal of Nursing, 24*, 98–106.
7 Wound Ostomy and Continence Nurses Society. (2012). Clean vs. sterile dressing techniques for management of chronic wounds: A fact sheet. *Journal of Wound Ostomy Continence Nursing, 39*(25), S30–S34. https://journals.lww.com/jwocnonline/Fulltext/2012/03001/Clean_vs__Sterile_Dressing_Techniques_for.7.aspx (Level VII)
8 Health Service Executive. (2018). HSE National wound management guidelines 2018. https://healthservice.hse.ie/filelibrary/onmsd/hse-wound-management-guidelines-2018.pdf (Level VII)
9 Martindell, D. (2012). Safety monitor: The safe use of negative-pressure wound therapy. *American Journal of Nursing, 112*(6), 59–63.
10 U.S. Food and Drug Administration. (2009). Negative pressure wound devices draw notice, advice. https://www.medpagetoday.com/upload/2009/12/11/UCM193750.pdf
11 The Joint Commission. (2021). Standard RI.01.03.01. *Comprehensive accreditation manual for hospitals*. Oakbrook Terrace, IL: The Joint Commission. (Level VII)
12 Centers for Medicare and Medicaid Services, Department of Health and Human Services. (2020). Condition of participation: Patient's rights. 42 C.F.R. § 482.13(b)(2).
13 Accreditation Association for Hospitals and Health Systems. (2020). Standard 15.01.11. *Healthcare Facilities Accreditation Program: Accreditation requirements for acute care hospitals*. Chicago, IL: Accreditation Association for Hospitals and Health Systems. (Level VII)
14 DNV GL-Healthcare USA, Inc. (2020). PR.2.SR.3. *NIAHO® accreditation requirements, interpretive guidelines and surveyor guidance—revision 20.0*. Milford, OH: DNV GL-Healthcare USA, Inc. (Level VII)
15 The Joint Commission. (2021). Standard NPSG.07.01.01. *Comprehensive accreditation manual for hospitals*. Oakbrook Terrace, IL: The Joint Commission. (Level VII)
16 Centers for Disease Control and Prevention. (2002). Guideline for hand hygiene in health-care settings: Recommendations of the Healthcare Infection Control Practices Advisory Committee and the HICPAC/SHEA/APIC/IDSA Hand Hygiene Task Force. *MMWR Recommendations and Reports, 51*(RR-16), 1–45. https://www.cdc.gov/mmwr/pdf/rr/rr5116.pdf (Level II)
17 World Health Organization. (2009). WHO guidelines on hand hygiene in health care: First global patient safety challenge, clean care is safer care. https://apps.who.int/iris/bitstream/handle/10665/44102/9789241597906_eng.pdf?sequence=1 (Level IV)
18 Accreditation Association for Hospitals and Health Systems. (2020). Standard 07.01.21. *Healthcare Facilities Accreditation Program: Accreditation requirements for acute care hospitals*. Chicago, IL: Accreditation Association for Hospitals and Health Systems. (Level VII)
19 Centers for Medicare and Medicaid Services, Department of Health and Human Services. (2020). Condition of participation: Infection control. 42 C.F.R. § 482.42.

20 DNV GL-Healthcare USA, Inc. (2020). IC.1.SR.1. *NIAHO® accreditation requirements, interpretive guidelines and surveyor guidance—revision 20.0.* Milford, OH: DNV GL-Healthcare USA, Inc. (Level VII)

21 The Joint Commission. (2021). Standard NPSG.01.01.01. *Comprehensive accreditation manual for hospitals.* Oakbrook Terrace, IL: The Joint Commission. (Level VII)

22 Accreditation Association for Hospitals and Health Systems. (2020). Standard 15.01.16. *Healthcare Facilities Accreditation Program: Accreditation requirements for acute care hospitals.* Chicago, IL: Accreditation Association for Hospitals and Health Systems. (Level VII)

23 Centers for Medicare and Medicaid Services, Department of Health and Human Services. (2020). Condition of participation: Patient's rights. 42 C.F.R. § 482.13(c)(1).

24 DNV GL-Healthcare USA, Inc. (2020). PR.2.SR.5. *NIAHO® accreditation requirements, interpretive guidelines and surveyor guidance—revision 20.0.* Milford, OH: DNV GL-Healthcare USA, Inc. (Level VII)

25 The Joint Commission. (2021). Standard RI.01.01.01. *Comprehensive accreditation manual for hospitals.* Oakbrook Terrace, IL: The Joint Commission. (Level VII)

26 The Joint Commission. (2021). Standard PC.02.01.21. *Comprehensive accreditation manual for hospitals.* Oakbrook Terrace, IL: The Joint Commission. (Level VII)

27 The Joint Commission. (2021). Standard PC.01.02.07. *Comprehensive accreditation manual for hospitals.* Oakbrook Terrace, IL: The Joint Commission. (Level VII)

28 Waters, T. R., et al. (2009). Safe patient handling training for schools of nursing. https://www.cdc.gov/niosh/docs/2009-127/pdfs/2009-127.pdf (Level VII)

29 Siegel, J. D., et al. (2007, revision 2019). 2007 guideline for isolation precautions: Preventing transmission of infectious agents in healthcare settings. https://www.cdc.gov/infectioncontrol/pdf/guidelines/isolation-guidelines-H.pdf (Level II)

30 Accreditation Association for Hospitals and Health Systems. (2018). Standard 07.01.10. *Healthcare Facilities Accreditation Program: Accreditation requirements for acute care hospitals.* Chicago, IL: Accreditation Association for Hospitals and Health Systems. (Level VII)

31 Occupational Safety and Health Administration. (2012). Bloodborne pathogens, standard number 1910.1030. https://www.osha.gov/pls/oshaweb/owadisp.show_document?p_id=10051&p_table=STANDARDS (Level VII)

32 The Joint Commission. (2013). Sentinel event alert 50: Medical device alarm safety in hospitals. https://www.jointcommission.org/-/media/tjc/documents/resources/patient-safety-topics/sentinel-event/sea_50_alarms_4_26_16.pdf (Level VII)

33 The Joint Commission. (2021). Standard NPSG.06.01.01. *Comprehensive accreditation manual for hospitals.* Oakbrook Terrace, IL: The Joint Commission. (Level VII)

34 Graham, K. C., & Cvach, M. (2010). Monitor alarm fatigue: Standardizing use of physiological monitors and decreasing nuisance alarms. *American Journal of Critical Care, 19,* 28–37.

35 Ganz, D. A., et al. (2013, reviewed 2021). Preventing falls in hospitals: A toolkit for improving quality of care (AHRQ publication no. 13-0015-EF). https://www.ahrq.gov/professionals/systems/hospital/fallpxtoolkit/index.html (Level VII)

36 The Joint Commission. (2021). Standard RC.01.03.01. *Comprehensive accreditation manual for hospitals.* Oakbrook Terrace, IL: The Joint Commission. (Level VII)

37 Accreditation Association for Hospitals and Health Systems. (2020). Standard 10.00.03. *Healthcare Facilities Accreditation Program: Accreditation requirements for acute care hospitals.* Chicago, IL: Accreditation Association for Hospitals and Health Systems. (Level VII)

38 Centers for Medicare and Medicaid Services, Department of Health and Human Services. (2020). Condition of participation: Medical record services. 42 C.F.R. § 482.24(b).

39 DNV GL-Healthcare USA, Inc. (2020). MR.2.SR.1. *NIAHO® accreditation requirements, interpretive guidelines and surveyor guidance—revision 20.0.* Milford, OH: DNV GL-Healthcare USA, Inc. (Level VII)

40 Bryant, R. A., & Nix, D. P. (Eds.). (2015). *Acute and chronic wounds: Current management concepts* (5th ed.). St. Louis, MO: Mosby.

Nephrostomy and cystostomy tube dressing changes

Two urinary diversion techniques—nephrostomy and cystostomy—ensure temporary or permanent drainage from the kidneys or bladder and help prevent urinary tract infection or kidney injury. (See *Urinary diversion techniques*.)

A nephrostomy tube drains urine directly from a kidney when a disorder inhibits the normal flow of urine. Practitioners usually place the tube percutaneously, although they sometimes insert it surgically through the renal cortex and medulla into the renal pelvis from a lateral flank incision.[1,2] The practitioner will usually place the tube because of obstructive problems, such as ureteral or ureteropelvic junction calculi or tumors, and access to the kidney for radiologic procedures, such as ureteral stent placement or direct infusion of medications.[1,3,4] Diverting urine with a nephrostomy tube also allows kidney tissue damaged from obstructive disease to heal end ensures drainage of infected urine.[5]

A cystostomy tube drains urine from the bladder, diverting it from the urethra. The practitioner will use this type of tube after certain

Urinary diversion techniques

A cystostomy or a nephrostomy can be used to create a permanent diversion to relieve obstruction from an inoperable tumor or provide an outlet for urine after cystectomy. A temporary diversion can relieve obstruction from a calculus or ureteral edema.

Cystostomy
In a cystostomy, the practitioner inserts a catheter percutaneously through the suprapubic area into the bladder, as shown below.

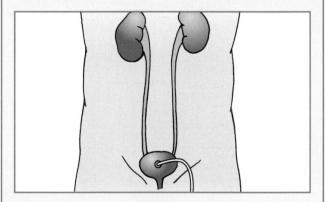

Nephrostomy
In a nephrostomy, the practitioner inserts a catheter percutaneously through the flank into the renal pelvis, as shown below.

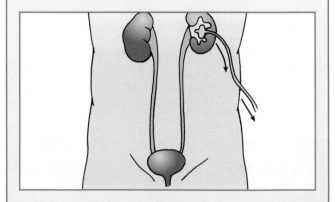

gynecologic procedures, bladder surgery, prostatectomy, severe urethral strictures, or traumatic injury. The practitioner inserts the tube into the bladder approximately 2″ (5 cm) above the pubic symphysis.[6]

Equipment

Sterile saline solution ▪ sterile gauze pads ▪ sterile bowl ▪ fluid-impermeable pad ▪ gloves ▪ sterile gloves ▪ sterile precut 4″ × 4″ (10 cm × 10-cm) drain dressings or transparent semipermeable dressing ▪ hypoallergenic adhesive tape or other securement device ▪ Optional: antiseptic swabs.

Preparation of equipment

Inspect all equipment and supplies. If a product is expired, is defective, or has compromised integrity, remove it from patient use, label it as expired or defective, and report the expiration or defect as directed by your facility.

Implementation

- Verify the practitioner's order.
- Gather and prepare the necessary equipment and supplies.
- Perform hand hygiene.[7,8,9,10,11,12]
- Confirm the patient's identity using at least two patient identifiers.[13]
- Provide privacy.[14,15,16,17]
- Explain the procedure to the patient and family (if appropriate) according to their individual communication and learning needs *to increase their understanding, allay their fears, and enhance cooperation.*[18]
- Raise the patient's bed to waist level before providing patient care *to prevent caregiver back strain.*[19]
- Perform hand hygiene.[7,8,9,10,11,12]
- Put on gloves *to comply with standard precautions.*[20,21]
- Position the patient *so you can clearly see the tube exit site.* If the patient has a nephrostomy tube, have the patient lie on the side opposite the tube. If the patient has a cystostomy tube, have the patient lie supine.
- Place the fluid-impermeable pad under the patient *to absorb excess drainage and keep the patient dry*
- Carefully remove the tape around the tube, and remove the wet or soiled dressing.
- Note the markings on the tube at the insertion site *to check for accidental dislodgment.*
- Assess the tube exit site for redness, swelling, warmth, tenderness, or drainage *to detect signs of infection and skin breakdown;*[22] if any signs are present, report them to the practitioner.
- Discard used supplies in the appropriate receptacle.[23]
- Remove and discard your gloves[23] and perform hand hygiene.[7,8,9,10,11,12]
- Open the sterile saline solution, gauze pads, sterile bowl, antiseptic swabs (as needed), the sterile precut 4″ × 4″ (10 cm × 10 cm) drain dressings or transparent semipermeable dressing, and the sterile gloves using sterile no-touch technique.
- Perform hand hygiene.[7,8,9,10,11,12]
- Put on sterile gloves.[20,21]
- Use a saline-moistened gauze pad *to clean the skin,* wiping from the tube exit site outward.[22] If drainage is present, use an antiseptic swab.
- Discard the gauze pad or swab appropriately, being careful not to contaminate your gloves.
- Repeat the skin cleaning procedure, if needed.
- Dry the site with gauze pads or let it air-dry.
- Place a sterile precut 4″ × 4″ (10 cm × 10 cm) drain dressing around the tube exit site. If necessary, overlap two drain dressings *for maximum absorption.* Alternatively, apply a transparent semipermeable dressing over the tube exit site *to enable observation of the site without removing the dressing.*
- Secure the dressing with hypoallergenic tape or other securement device. Tape the tube to the patient's lateral abdomen *to prevent tension on the tube.*

NURSING ALERT If the patient has fragile skin, use dressings and tape specifically formulated for fragile skin *to prevent skin stripping and tearing during removal.*[24]

- Remove and discard your gloves.[23]
- Perform hand hygiene.[7,8,9,10,11,12]
- Help the patient to a comfortable position.
- Return the bed to the lowest position *to prevent falls and maintain safety.*[25]
- Perform hand hygiene.[7,8,9,10,11,12]
- Document the procedure.[26,27,28,29]

Special considerations

- Change the dressings daily as needed.[22]
- Keep the drainage bag below the level of the kidney at all times *to prevent urine reflux.*[4]

Patient teaching

Teach the patient and family how to care for the tube after discharge. Instruct them how to clean the tube exit site with soap and water, check for skin breakdown, change the dressing daily, and wash hands before and after dressing and drainage bag changes.[4] Also teach them how to change the drainage bag or leg bag and perform irrigation, as indicated. Explain that the patient can use a leg bag during the day and a larger drainage bag at night.

Tell the patient that showering is permitted but that baths and swimming are not. Stress the importance of reporting to the practitioner any signs of infection (including red skin and white, yellow, or green drainage at the insertion site), an oral temperature above 100.4° F (38° C), tube displacement (drainage that smells like urine), and severe flank pain.

Encourage patients with unrestricted fluid intake to follow the practitioner's directions for fluid intake *to prevent complications.*

Complications

The patient has an increased risk of infection, *because nephrostomy and cystostomy tubes provide a direct opening to the kidneys and bladder.*[2,3] Skin irritation and breakdown may also occur.[22,24]

Documentation

Document the date and time of dressing change and the patient's tolerance of the procedure. Describe the color and amount of drainage from the nephrostomy or cystostomy tube, and record any color changes as they occur. Note the markings on the tube at the tube exit site and the presence of any signs of infection or skin breakdown. If the patient has more than one tube, describe the drainage (color, amount, and character) from each separate tube. Record any complications, interventions, and the patient's response to the interventions. Document teaching provided to the patient and family (if applicable), their understanding of that teaching, and any need for follow-up teaching.

REFERENCES

1 Siddiqi, N. H. (2017). Percutaneous nephrostomy. *Medscape.* https://emedicine.medscape.com/article/1821504-overview
2 Hautmann, S. H. (2018). Nephrostomy treatment and management. *Medscape.* https://emedicine.medscape.com/article/445893-treatment#d10
3 Nakada, S., & Patel, S. (2019). Placement and management of indwelling ureteral stents. In: *UpToDate,* Richie, J. P. (Ed.).
4 Agency for Clinical Innovation. (2012). *Nursing management of patients with nephrostomy tubes: Guidelines and patient information templates.* https://www.aci.health.nsw.gov.au/__data/assets/pdf_file/0011/165917/Nephrostomy-Tubes-Toolkit.pdf (Level VII)
5 Preminger, G. M. (2021). Kidney stones in adults: Surgical management of kidney and ureteral stones. In: *UpToDate,* Goldfarb, S., & O'Leary, M. P. (Eds.).
6 Fisher, J. S. (2021). Suprapubic cystostomy. *Medscape.* https://emedicine.medscape.com/article/1893882-overview

7 The Joint Commission. (2021). Standard NPSG.07.01.01. *Comprehensive accreditation manual for hospitals.* Oakbrook Terrace, IL: The Joint Commission. (Level VII)

8 Centers for Disease Control and Prevention. (2002). Guideline for hand hygiene in health-care settings: Recommendations of the Healthcare Infection Control Practices Advisory Committee and the HICPAC/SHEA/APIC/IDSA Hand Hygiene Task Force. *MMWR Recommendations and Reports, 51*(RR-16), 1–45. https://www.cdc.gov/mmwr/pdf/rr/rr5116.pdf (Level II)

9 World Health Organization. (2009). WHO guidelines on hand hygiene in health care: First global patient safety challenge, clean care is safer care. https://apps.who.int/iris/bitstream/handle/10665/44102/9789241597906_eng.pdf?sequence=1 (Level IV)

10 Centers for Medicare and Medicaid Services, Department of Health and Human Services. (2020). Condition of participation: Infection control. 42 C.F.R. § 482.42.

11 Accreditation Association for Hospitals and Health Systems. (2020). Standard 07.01.21. *Healthcare Facilities Accreditation Program: Accreditation requirements for acute care hospitals.* Chicago, IL: Accreditation Association for Hospitals and Health Systems. (Level VII)

12 DNV GL-Healthcare USA, Inc. (2020). IC.1.SR.1. *NIAHO® accreditation requirements, interpretive guidelines and surveyor guidance—revision 20.0.* Milford, OH: DNV GL-Healthcare USA, Inc. (Level VII)

13 The Joint Commission. (2021). Standard NPSG.01.01.01. *Comprehensive accreditation manual for hospitals.* Oakbrook Terrace, IL: The Joint Commission. (Level VII)

14 Centers for Medicare and Medicaid Services, Department of Health and Human Services. (2020). Condition of participation: Patient's rights. 42 C.F.R. § 482.13(c)(1).

15 Accreditation Association for Hospitals and Health Systems. (2020). Standard 15.01.16. *Healthcare Facilities Accreditation Program: Accreditation requirements for acute care hospitals.* Chicago, IL: Accreditation Association for Hospitals and Health Systems. (Level VII)

16 The Joint Commission. (2021). Standard RI.01.01.01. *Comprehensive accreditation manual for hospitals.* Oakbrook Terrace, IL: The Joint Commission. (Level VII)

17 DNV GL-Healthcare USA, Inc. (2020). PR.2.SR.5. *NIAHO® accreditation requirements, interpretive guidelines and surveyor guidance—revision 20.0.* Milford, OH: DNV GL-Healthcare USA, Inc. (Level VII)

18 The Joint Commission. (2021). Standard PC.02.01.21. *Comprehensive accreditation manual for hospitals.* Oakbrook Terrace, IL: The Joint Commission. (Level VII)

19 Waters, T. R., et al. (2009). Safe patient handling training for schools of nursing. https://www.cdc.gov/niosh/docs/2009-127/pdfs/2009-127.pdf (Level VII)

20 Siegel, J. D., et al. (2007, revised 2019). 2007 guideline for isolation precautions: Preventing transmission of infectious agents in healthcare settings. https://www.cdc.gov/infectioncontrol/pdf/guidelines/isolation-guidelines-H.pdf (Level II)

21 Accreditation Association for Hospitals and Health Systems. (2020). Standard 07.01.10. *Healthcare Facilities Accreditation Program: Accreditation requirements for acute care hospitals.* Chicago, IL: Accreditation Association for Hospitals and Health Systems. (Level VII)

22 Baranoski, S., & Ayello, E. A. (2020). *Wound care essentials: Practice principles* (5th ed.). Philadelphia, PA: Wolters Kluwer.

23 Occupational Safety and Health Administration. (2012). Bloodborne pathogens, standard number 1910.1030. https://www.osha.gov/pls/oshaweb/owadisp.show_document?p_id=10051&p_table=STANDARDS (Level VII)

24 LeBlanc, K., et al. (2013). International skin tear advisory panel: A tool kit to aid in the prevention, assessment, and treatment of skin tears using a simplified classification system. *Advances in Skin & Wound Care, 26,* 459–476. (Level IV)

25 Ganz, D. A., et al. (2013, reviewed 2021). *Preventing falls in hospitals: A toolkit for improving quality of care* (AHRQ Publication No. 13-0015-EF). Rockville, MD: Agency for Healthcare Research and Quality. https://www.ahrq.gov/professionals/systems/hospital/fallpxtoolkit/index.html (Level VII)

26 The Joint Commission. (2021). Standard RC.01.03.01. *Comprehensive accreditation manual for hospitals.* Oakbrook Terrace, IL: The Joint Commission. (Level VII)

27 Centers for Medicare and Medicaid Services, Department of Health and Human Services. (2020). Condition of participation: Medical record services. 42 C.F.R. § 482.24(b).

28 Accreditation Association for Hospitals and Health Systems. (2020). Standard 10.00.03. *Healthcare Facilities Accreditation Program: Accreditation requirements for acute care hospitals.* Chicago, IL: Accreditation Association for Hospitals and Health Systems. (Level VII)

29 DNV GL-Healthcare USA, Inc. (2020). MR.2.SR.1. *NIAHO® accreditation requirements, interpretive guidelines and surveyor guidance—revision 20.0.* Milford, OH: DNV GL-Healthcare USA, Inc. (Level VII)

NEUROLOGIC ASSESSMENT

Neurologic vital signs supplement the routine measurement of temperature, pulse rate, blood pressure, and respirations by evaluating the patient's level of consciousness (LOC), pupillary activity, and orientation to time, place, and person. They provide a simple, indispensable tool for checking the patient's neurologic status quickly.

A measure of environmental awareness and self-awareness, LOC reflects cortical function and usually provides the first sign of central nervous system deterioration. Changes in pupillary activity (pupil size, shape, equality, and response to light) may signal increased intracranial pressure (ICP) associated with a space-occupying lesion. Evaluating muscle strength and tone, reflexes, and posture also may help identify nervous system damage.

Equipment

Low-pitched tuning fork ■ penlight ■ vital signs monitoring equipment ■ sterile cotton ball ■ pupil size chart or pupillometer with headrest ■ pencil or pen ■ paperclip or key ■ safety pin ■ disinfectant pad ■ Optional: gloves, gown, mask, goggles, mask with face shield.

Preparation of Equipment

Inspect all equipment and supplies. If a product is expired, is defective, or has compromised integrity, remove it from patient use, label it as expired or defective, and report the expiration or defect as directed by your facility.

Implementation

■ Review the patient's medical record for the medical diagnosis, medical and surgical history, and medication history *to help determine whether neurologic changes are consistent with the current medical condition.*
■ Review the results of the patient's last neurologic assessment, if available, *to provide baseline data.*
■ Gather and prepare the necessary equipment and supplies.
■ Perform hand hygiene.[1,2,3,4,5,6]
■ Put on gloves and, as needed, other personal protective equipment *to comply with standard precautions.*[7,8,9]
■ Confirm the patient's identity using at least two patient identifiers.[10]
■ Provide privacy.[11,12,13,14]
■ Explain the procedure to the patient (even if unresponsive) and family (if appropriate) according to their individual communication and learning needs *to increase their understanding, allay their fears, and enhance cooperation.*[15]
■ Raise the patient's bed to waist level before providing care *to prevent caregiver back strain.*[16]
■ Obtain the patient's temperature, pulse rate, respiratory rate, and blood pressure. The patient's pulse pressure (the difference between the systolic and diastolic pressure) is especially important *because widening pulse pressure can indicate increased ICP.*
■ Perform hand hygiene.[1,2,3,4,5,6]

Using the Glasgow Coma Scale

In an effort to improve the accuracy, reliability, and communication of the Glasgow Coma Scale after 40 years of use, the scale has undergone revision to follow a new structured approach to assessment (check, observe, stimulate, and rate).[17] The scale provides a standard reference for level of consciousness in response to defined stimuli. It can describe an impairment of consciousness from any cause, but has been most useful in cases of suspected or confirmed brain injury.[18]

The scale measures three responses to stimuli—eye opening, verbal response, and best motor response—and assigns a letter and number to each of the possible responses within these categories. Documenting serial findings on a coma scale chart allows for clear communication of observations and rapid appreciation of trends, which makes clear any improvement or deterioration in a patient's condition.[19]

In addition to plotting trends on a coma scale chart, documenting a patient's ratings numerically in shorthand (such as E2V4M6) helps to record and communicate findings quickly. However, when describing the patient in this way, use of the full criteria alongside the numbers is always necessary to ensure that others will accurately understand the assessment findings.[19] Adding the shorthand numbers together provides a total coma score (for example, E2V4M6 = 12), which provides a summary of the severity of the patient's condition; however, this score doesn't communicate the more informative detailed description of each response, which should always be used in addition to the score. For example, a total score of 8 could be E2V2M4 or E1V1M6, which have very different implications for the severity of a patient's condition.[19] Importantly, reporting of a total score should not occur when a component rating is *Not testable*, because the total score will be low, which could be confusing to the multidisciplinary team and might imply that a patient's condition is worse than it actually is.[18]

For a patient who doesn't obey commands, a central stimulus is necessary to assess the motor component of the coma scale (best motor response). Use a trapezius pinch first; if this pinch doesn't elicit a response, apply a supraorbital notch press. To perform a trapezius pinch, place your hand over the patient's shoulder and press your fingers into the muscle above the shoulder blade; apply increasing intensity for up to 10 seconds and observe the patient's best response. To perform a supraorbital notch press, place your hand on the patient's forehead with your thumb over the upper rim of the orbit; feel for the notch in the supraorbital margin and apply increasing pressure for up to 10 seconds, again observing for the patient's best response. Don't use a supraorbital notch press if the patient has facial injuries close to the testing area.[20,21]

If the patient exhibits different responses on different sides, record the response from the better side.[21] Guidelines strongly discourage stimulation by rubbing the knuckles on the sternum, because this practice can cause bruising and responses can be difficult to interpret.[20]

CRITERION	RATING	RESPONSE
EYE OPENING		
Open before stimulus	Spontaneous	E4
After spoken or shouted request	To sound	E3
After fingertip stimulus (press on the fingertip with increasing intensity up to 10 seconds)[21]	To pressure	E2
Not opening at any time, no interfering factor	None	E1
Closed by local factor (such as swelling)	Not testable	NT
VERBAL RESPONSE		
Correctly gives name, place, and date	Oriented	V5
Not oriented but communicates coherently	Confused	V4
Intelligible single words	Words	V3
Only moans or groans	Sounds	V2
No audible response, no interfering factor	None	V1
Factors interfering with communication	Not testable	NT
BEST MOTOR RESPONSE		
Obeys 2-part request (grasps and releases your fingers with hand; opens mouth and sticks out tongue)[21]	Obeys commands	M6
Brings hand above clavicle to stimulus on head or neck	Localizing	M5
Bends arm at elbow rapidly but features not predominantly abnormal (elbow bends and arm moves rapidly away from body)[21]	Normal flexion	M4
Bends arm at elbow but features predominantly abnormal (arm slowly moves across chest, forearm rotates, thumb clenched, leg extends)[21]	Abnormal flexion	M3
Extends arm at elbow	Extension	M2
No movement in arms or legs, no interfering factor	None	M1
Paralyzed or other limiting factor	Not testable	NT

Using the Rancho Los Amigos Cognitive Scale

Widely used to classify brain-injured patients according to their behavior, the Rancho Los Amigos Cognitive Scale describes the phases of recovery—from coma to independent functioning—on a scale of I (unresponsive) to VIII (purposeful, appropriate, alert, and oriented). This table is useful when assessing patients with posttraumatic amnesia.

LEVEL	RESPONSE	CHARACTERISTICS
I	None	The patient is unresponsive to any stimulus, including pain.
II	Generalized	The patient makes limited, inconsistent, nonpurposeful responses, often to pain only.
III	Localized	The patient can localize and withdraw from painful stimuli, can make purposeful responses and focus on presented objects, and may follow simple commands, but inconsistently and in a delayed manner.
IV	Confused and agitated	The patient is alert but agitated, confused, disoriented, and aggressive. The patient can't perform self-care and has no awareness of present events. Bizarre behavior is likely; agitation appears related to internal confusion.
V	Confused and inappropriate	The patient is alert and responds to commands but is easily distracted and can't concentrate on tasks or learn new information. The patient becomes agitated in response to external stimuli, and behavior and speech are inappropriate. The patient has a severely impaired memory and can't carry over learning from one situation to another.
VI	Confused and appropriate	The patient has some awareness of self and others but is inconsistently oriented. The patient can follow simple directions consistently with cueing and can relearn some old skills, such as activities of daily living, but continues to have serious memory problems (especially short-term memory).
VII	Automatic and appropriate	The patient is consistently oriented with little or no confusion, but frequently appears robotic when performing daily routines. Although awareness of self and interaction with the environment are increased, the patient lacks insight, judgment, problem-solving skills, and the ability to plan realistically.
VIII	Purposeful and appropriate	The patient is alert and oriented, recalls and integrates past events, learns new activities, and performs activities of daily living independently; however, deficits in stress tolerance, judgment, and abstract reasoning persist. The patient may function in society at a reduced level.

Assessing LOC and orientation

■ Assess the patient's LOC by evaluating the responses. Use standard methods such as the Glasgow Coma Scale (see *Using the Glasgow Coma Scale*, page 593.) and the Rancho Los Amigos Cognitive Scale (see *Using the Rancho Los Amigos Cognitive Scale*.). Begin by measuring the patient's response to verbal, light tactile (touch), or painful (nail bed pressure) stimuli. First, ask the patient's full name. If the patient responds appropriately, assess orientation to time, place, and person. Ask the patient the place and then what day, season, and year it is. (Expect disorientation to affect the sense of date first, then time, place, caregivers, and lastly self.) Assess the quality of the patient's replies. For example, garbled words indicate difficulty with the motor nerves that govern speech muscles. Rambling responses indicate difficulty with thought processing and organization.

ELDER ALERT Because of decreased hearing, vision, and tactile sensation with aging, cues in the environment are an important feedback mechanism for older adults. When an older adult experiences a change in environment, such as admission to a hospital or other health care facility or a transfer from one unit to another, neurologic functioning may be affected negatively. Orienting the patient to the environment and planning for other needs, such as providing adequate lighting without glare, visual and auditory clues, and appropriate assistive devices, may maximize the patient's functioning within the environment.

■ Assess the patient's ability to understand and follow one-step commands that require a motor response. For example, ask the patient to open and close the eyes or stick out the tongue (as shown on right). Note whether the patient can maintain LOC. If you must gently shake the patient to keep the patient focused on your verbal commands, the patient may be neurologically compromised.

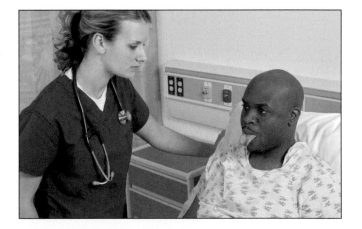

■ If the patient doesn't respond to commands or touch, apply a painful stimulus. Painful stimuli are classified as central (response via the brain) or peripheral (response via the spine). Apply a peripheral stimulus to all four extremities *to establish a baseline.* With moderate pressure, squeeze the nail beds on the patient's finger and toes and note the response. Check motor responses bilaterally *to rule out monoplegia (paralysis of a single area) and hemiplegia (paralysis of one side of the body.)* If the patient doesn't respond to peripheral stimuli, apply a central stimulus and note the patient's response. Acceptable central stimuli include squeezing the trapezius muscle or applying supraorbital pressure. Application of mandibular pressure and rubbing the sternum re not recommended by the guidelines.[20]

Assessing the pupils

Two methods can be used to assess pupil size and reactivity to light: the manual method and the automated method. The automated method uses a pupillometer, which eliminates subjectivity. Use the method chosen by your facility.

Manual assessment method

To evaluate pupil size by the manual method, use a chart showing the various pupil sizes in increments of 1 mm, with the normal diameter ranging from 3 to 5 mm, as shown below. Remember, pupil size varies considerably, and some patients have normally unequal pupils (anisocoria).[22]

To test the pupillary reaction to light, slightly darken the room, ask the patient to look into the distance, and shine a penlight obliquely into each pupil in turn (as shown).[22] Observe for direct reaction (pupillary constriction in the same eye) and consensual reaction (pupillary constriction in the opposite eye).[22] The pupil should react quickly when you shine the light into it and then dilate when you move the light away. Grade the light reactions as "brisk," "sluggish," or "nonreactive."

Next, test accommodation by placing your finger about 4″ (10 cm) from the bridge of the patient's nose. Ask the patient to look at a fixed object in the distance and then to look at your finger. The patient's eyes should converge and the pupils should constrict.[22]

To more accurately measure pupil size and reactivity to light, use a pupillometer. This noninvasive, handheld device provides an objective measurement of pupil size and reactivity to light using an LED light source and infrared camera.[23]

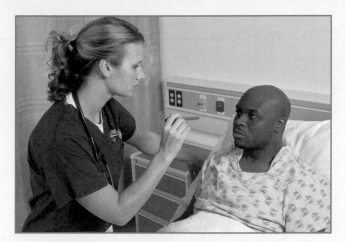

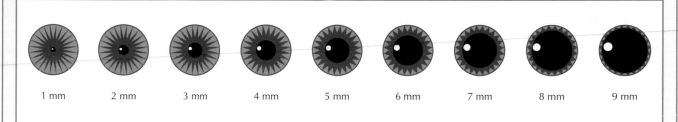

| 1 mm | 2 mm | 3 mm | 4 mm | 5 mm | 6 mm | 7 mm | 8 mm | 9 mm |

Automated method using a pupillometer

To use a pupillometer, remove the device from the docking or charging station.[23,24] If you're using it on the patient for the first time, obtain a new single-patient-use headrest, connect the headrest to the pupillometer, and then input the patient's identification either manually or using the bar-code scanner. Follow the manufacturer's instructions for use.[23,24]

Ask the patient to open the eyes and look straight ahead, if able. Alternatively, open the patient's eye by gently lifting the eyelid with your finger or thumb, making sure to open the eyelid far enough to expose the entire pupil.[23]

Position the pupillometer with the headrest against one of the patient's cheek bones at a right angle to the axis of vision.[23,24] Avoid tilting the device. If testing the left eye first, press and hold the left button until the left eye becomes centered on the pupillometer's touchscreen and a green circle appears around the pupil. Alternatively, if testing the right eye first, press and hold the right button until the right eye becomes centered on the pupillometer's touchscreen and a green circle appears around the pupil. After the green circle appears, release the button and wait for the result to appear on the display screen. Repeat the procedure for the patient's other eye to complete the bilateral pupil assessment.[24] After completing the bilateral eye assessment, obtain the pupil measurement parameters and pupillary light reflex waveform from the display screen.[23,24] Upload the measurements to the patient's electronic medical record, if directed by your facility.[23,24]

The pupillometer measures neurologic pupil index (NPi), which uses an algorithm to compare the patient's pupil measurements (such as size, latency, constriction velocity, and dilation velocity) against a normative model of pupillary reaction to light. An individual measurement is rated on a scale between 0 and 5. An NPi of 3 or above is considered normal or "brisk," less than 3 is considered abnormal or "sluggish," and 0 is considered atypical or "nonreactive."[24]

After use, remove and store the headrest. Clean and disinfect the pupillometer following the manufacturer's instructions, and then return it to the docking or charging station.[23,24]

Examining pupils and eye movement

■ Ask the patient to open the eyes. If the patient doesn't (or can't) respond, gently lift the upper eyelids.

■ Assess the pupils. Inspect each pupil for size and shape and compare the two *for equality;* then test the pupillary response to light. (See *Assessing the pupils.*) Also see if the pupils are positioned in, or deviated from, the midline.

■ Brighten the room and have the conscious patient open the eyes. Observe the eyelids for ptosis or drooping. Then check extraocular movements. Hold up one finger and ask the patient to follow it with the eyes alone. As you move the finger up, down, laterally, and obliquely, see if the patient's eyes track together to follow your finger (conjugate gaze). Watch for involuntary jerking or oscillating eye movements (nystagmus).

■ Bring a pencil or other object in from the side and have the patient state when the object enters the field of vision. *This tests the peripheral field.*

■ Test the corneal reflex by touching a wisp of cotton ball to the cornea. *This test normally causes an immediate blink reflex.* Repeat for the other eye.

NURSING ALERT Excessive testing of the corneal reflex can cause corneal damage. Perform this assessment carefully.

■ If the patient is unconscious, test the oculocephalic (doll's eye) reflex. Hold the patient's eyelids open, then quickly but gently turn the patient's head to one side and then the other. If the patient's eyes move in the opposite direction from the side to which you turn the head, the reflex is intact.

NURSING ALERT Never test the doll's eye reflex if you know or suspect that the patient has a cervical spine injury, *because permanent spinal cord damage can result.*

Evaluating motor function

■ If the patient is conscious, test grip strength in both hands at the same time. Extend your hands, ask the patient to squeeze your fingers as hard as possible, and compare the strength of each hand. Grip strength is usually slightly stronger in the dominant hand.

■ Test arm strength by having the patient close the eyes and hold the arms straight out in front with the palms up (as shown below). See if either arm drifts downward or pronates, *indicating muscle weakness.*

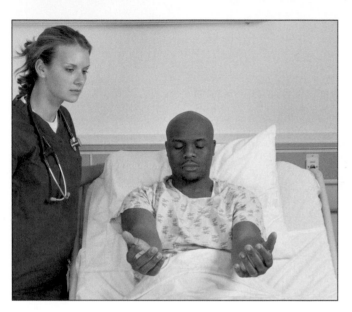

■ Test leg strength by having the patient raise the legs, one at a time (as shown below), against gentle downward pressure from your hand. Gently push down on each leg at the midpoint of the thigh *to evaluate muscle strength.*

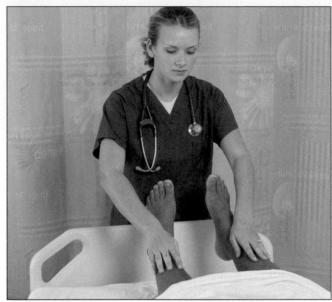

NURSING ALERT If decorticate or decerebrate posturing develops in response to stimuli, notify the practitioner immediately. (See *Identifying warning postures.*)

■ Evaluate muscle tone by having the patient flex and extend the extremities on both sides.

■ Test the plantar reflex. To do so, stroke the lateral aspect of the sole of the patient's foot with your thumbnail or another moderately sharp object. *Normally, this elicits flexion of all toes* (as shown). Watch for a positive Babinski sign—dorsiflexion of the great toe with fanning of the other toes—*which indicates an upper motor neuron lesion.*

Identifying warning postures

Decorticate and decerebrate postures are ominous signs of central nervous system deterioration.

Decorticate (abnormal flexion)
In the decorticate posture, the patient's arms are adducted and flexed, with the wrists and fingers flexed on the chest. The legs may be stiffly extended and internally rotated, with plantar flexion of the feet.

 The decorticate posture may indicate a lesion of the frontal lobe, internal capsule, or cerebral peduncles.

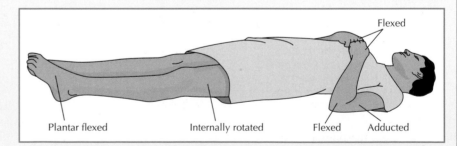

Flexed

Plantar flexed   Internally rotated   Flexed   Adducted

Decerebrate (extension)
In the decerebrate posture, the patient's arms are adducted and extended with the wrists pronated and the fingers flexed. One or both legs may be stiffly extended, with plantar flexion of the feet.

 The decerebrate posture may indicate lesions of the upper brain stem.

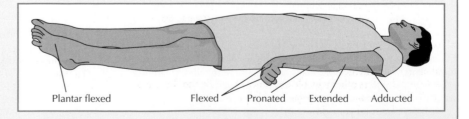

Plantar flexed   Flexed   Pronated   Extended   Adducted

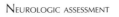

- Perform hand hygiene.[1,2,3,4,5,6]
- Notify the practitioner of abnormalities identified in your assessment or a deterioration in the findings from a previous assessment.
- Document the procedure.[29,30,31,32]

Special considerations

NURSING ALERT If a previously stable patient suddenly develops a change in neurologic or routine vital signs, further assess the patient's condition and notify the practitioner immediately. *One of the earliest changes that may occur with increased ICP is a change in LOC. Changes in pulse and blood pressure do occur, but generally late in the course of increasing ICP.*

- If you suspect the patient has had a stroke, use the National Institutes of Health Stroke Scale to evaluate the patient.[33]

Documentation

Document detailed baseline data; subsequent notes can be brief, unless the patient's condition changes. Record the patient's LOC and orientation, pupillary activity, motor function, sensory function, and routine vital signs. Note the Glasgow Coma Scale or Rancho Los Amigos Cognitive Scale score, if used. Describe the patient's behavior—for example, "difficult to arouse by gentle shaking," "sleepy," or "unresponsive to painful stimuli." Document the practitioner notified of any changes in the patient's condition, the date and time of notification, prescribed interventions, and the patient's response to those interventions. Document teaching provided to the patient and family (if applicable), their understanding of that teaching, and any need for follow-up teaching.

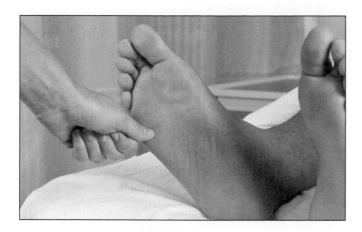

Evaluating sensory function

- To test for pain sensation, start by having the patient close the eyes. Then, using a safety pin, gently touch various areas of the patient's body, alternating between the sharp and dull end of the pin. Ask the patient "Is this sharp or dull?" as you proceed. Compare corresponding areas on the two sides of the body. Start with both shoulders and then proceed with the inner and outer aspects of the forearms, the thumbs and little fingers, the fronts of the thighs, the medial and lateral aspects of both calves, the little toes, and the medial aspect of the buttock *to test most of the dermatomes and major peripheral nerves.*[22]
- Test the patient's sense of light touch by touching the skin lightly with a wisp of cotton while the patient's eyes remain closed. Ask the patient to respond whenever a touch is felt. Compare corresponding areas on the two sides of the body.[22]
- To test vibratory sense, apply a tuning fork over different bony prominences while the patient keeps the eyes closed. Tap the tuning fork on the heel of your hand and place it firmly over a distal interphalangeal joint of the patient's finger, and then over the interphalangeal joint of the big toe. Ask the patient to tell you when the sensation stops; then touch the fork to stop it.[25]
- Assess position sense (proprioception) by grasping the patient's big toe, holding it by its sides between your thumb and index finger, and then pulling it away from the other toes. Show the patient "up" and "down" as you move the toe clearly upward and downward. Then, have the patient close the eyes and ask the patient to tell you whether you're moving the toe up or down as you move the large toe in an arc. Repeat several times on each side.[22]
- To test stereognosis, have the patient close the eyes. Place a familiar object, such as a paperclip or key, in the patient's hand and have the patient identify it. If motor impairment prevents the patient from identifying the object in this manner, use a blunt end of a pen or pencil to draw a number in the patient's palm and have the patient identify it.[22]
- Test point localization by having the patient close the eyes; then touch one of the patient's limbs and ask the patient where you touched.
- Test two-point discrimination by touching the patient simultaneously in two contralateral areas with an opened paperclip. Find the minimal distance at which the patient can discriminate one from two points.[22]

Completing the neurologic examination

- Return the bed to the lowest position *to prevent falls and maintain patient safety.*[26]
- Discard used supplies in appropriate receptacles.[8]
- Remove and discard your gloves and, if worn, other personal protective equipment.[8]
- Perform hand hygiene.[1,2,3,4,5,6]
- Clean and disinfect your stethoscope using a disinfectant pad
- Put on gloves. as needed.[8]
- Clean and disinfect other reusable equipment according to the manufacturer's instruction *to prevent the spread of infection.*[27,28]
- Remove and discard your gloves.[8]

REFERENCES

1. World Health Organization. (2009). WHO guidelines on hand hygiene in health care: First global patient safety challenge, clean care is safer care. https://apps.who.int/iris/bitstream/handle/10665/44102/9789241597906_eng.pdf?sequence=1 (Level IV)
2. The Joint Commission. (2021). Standard NPSG.07.01.01. *Comprehensive accreditation manual for hospitals.* Oakbrook Terrace, IL: The Joint Commission. (Level VII)
3. Centers for Disease Control and Prevention. (2002). Guideline for hand hygiene in health-care settings: Recommendations of the Healthcare Infection Control Practices Advisory Committee and the HICPAC/SHEA/APIC/IDSA Hand Hygiene Task Force. *MMWR Recommendations and Reports, 51*(RR-16), 1–45. https://www.cdc.gov/mmwr/pdf/rr/rr5116.pdf (Level II)
4. Centers for Medicare and Medicaid Services, Department of Health and Human Services. (2020). Condition of participation: Infection control. 42 C.F.R. § 482.42.
5. Accreditation Association for Hospitals and Health Systems. (2020). Standard 07.01.21. *Healthcare Facilities Accreditation Program: Accreditation requirements for acute care hospitals.* Chicago, IL: Accreditation Association for Hospitals and Health Systems. (Level VII)
6. DNV GL-Healthcare USA, Inc. (2020). IC.1.SR.1. *NIAHO® accreditation requirements, interpretive guidelines and surveyor guidance—revision 20.0.* Milford, OH: DNV GL-Healthcare USA, Inc. (Level VII)
7. Accreditation Association for Hospitals and Health Systems. (2020). Standard 07.01.10. *Healthcare Facilities Accreditation Program: Accreditation requirements for acute care hospitals.* Chicago, IL: Accreditation Association for Hospitals and Health Systems. (Level VII)
8. Occupational Safety and Health Administration. (2012). Bloodborne pathogens, standard number 1910.1030. https://www.osha.gov/pls/oshaweb/owadisp.show_document?p_id=10051&p_table=STANDARDS (Level VII)
9. Siegel, J. D., et al. (2007, revised 2019). 2007 guideline for isolation precautions: Preventing transmission of infectious agents in healthcare settings. https://www.cdc.gov/infectioncontrol/pdf/guidelines/isolation-guidelines-H.pdf (Level II)
10. The Joint Commission. (2021). Standard NPSG.01.01.01. *Comprehensive accreditation manual for hospitals.* Oakbrook Terrace, IL: The Joint Commission. (Level VII)

11 Centers for Medicare and Medicaid Services, Department of Health and Human Services. (2020). Condition of participation: Patient's rights. 42 C.F.R. § 482.13(c)(1).

12 Accreditation Association for Hospitals and Health Systems. (2020). Standard 15.01.16. *Healthcare Facilities Accreditation Program: Accreditation requirements for acute care hospitals*. Chicago, IL: Accreditation Association for Hospitals and Health Systems. (Level VII)

13 The Joint Commission. (2021). Standard RI.01.01.01. *Comprehensive accreditation manual for hospitals*. Oakbrook Terrace, IL: The Joint Commission. (Level VII)

14 DNV GL-Healthcare USA, Inc. (2020). PR.2. SR.5. *NIAHO® accreditation requirements, interpretive guidelines and surveyor guidance—revision 20.0*. Milford, OH: DNV GL-Healthcare USA, Inc. (Level VII)

15 The Joint Commission. (2021). Standard PC.02.01.21. *Comprehensive accreditation manual for hospitals*. Oakbrook Terrace, IL: The Joint Commission. (Level VII)

16 Waters, T. R., et al. (2009). Safe patient handling training for schools of nursing. https://www.cdc.gov/niosh/docs/2009-127/pdfs/2009-127.pdf (Level VII)

17 Teasdale, G. (2015). Glasgow Coma Scale: Do it this way. https://www.glasgowcomascale.org/downloads/GCS-Assessment-Aid-English.pdf?v=2

18 Royal College of Physicians and Surgeons of Glasgow. (n.d.). Frequently asked questions. https://www.glasgowcomascale.org/faq/

19 Royal College of Physicians and Surgeons of Glasgow. (n.d.). Recording the Glasgow Coma Scale. https://www.glasgowcomascale.org/recording-gcs/

20 Royal College of Physicians and Surgeons of Glasgow. (n.d.). GCS aid. https://www.glasgowcomascale.org/gcs-aid/

21 Royal College of Physicians and Surgeons of Glasgow. (n.d.). Glasgow Coma Scale at 40: The new approach to Glasgow Coma Scale assessment (video). https://www.glasgowcomascale.org/#video

22 Bickley, L. (2017). *Bates' guide to physical examination and history taking* (12th ed.). Philadelphia, PA: Wolters Kluwer.

23 Wiegand, D. L. (2017). *AACN procedure manual for high acuity, progressive, and critical care* (7th ed.). St. Louis, MO: Elsevier.

24 NeurOptics, Inc. (2019). NPi®-200 pupillometer system: Quick start guide. https://www.neurovisio.de/wp-content/uploads/2019/06/NPi2_QuickStart_HOMA-A9VP25-RevJ-web.pdf

25 Hickey, J. V. (2019). *The clinical practice of neurological and neurosurgical nursing* (8th ed.). Philadelphia, PA: Wolters Kluwer.

26 Ganz, D. A., et al. (2013, reviewed 2021). *Preventing falls in hospitals: A toolkit for improving quality of care* (AHRQ Publication No. 13-0015-EF). Rockville, MD: Agency for Healthcare Research and Quality. https://www.ahrq.gov/professionals/systems/hospital/fallpxtoolkit/index.html (Level VII)

27 Rutala, W. A., et al. (2008, revised 2019). Guideline for disinfection and sterilization in healthcare facilities. https://www.cdc.gov/infectioncontrol/pdf/guidelines/disinfection-guidelines-H.pdf (Level I)

28 Accreditation Association for Hospitals and Health Systems. (2020). Standard 07.02.03. *Healthcare Facilities Accreditation Program: Accreditation requirements for acute care hospitals*. Chicago, IL: Accreditation Association for Hospitals and Health Systems. (Level VII)

29 The Joint Commission. (2021). Standard RC.01.03.01. *Comprehensive accreditation manual for hospitals*. Oakbrook Terrace, IL: The Joint Commission. (Level VII)

30 Centers for Medicare and Medicaid Services, Department of Health and Human Services. (2020). Condition of participation: Medical record services. 42 C.F.R. § 482.24(b).

31 Accreditation Association for Hospitals and Health Systems. (2020). Standard 10.00.03. *Healthcare Facilities Accreditation Program: Accreditation requirements for acute care hospitals*. Chicago, IL: Accreditation Association for Hospitals and Health Systems. (Level VII)

32 DNV GL-Healthcare USA, Inc. (2020). MR.2. SR.1. *NIAHO® accreditation requirements, interpretive guidelines and surveyor guidance—revision 20.0*. Milford, OH: DNV GL-Healthcare USA, Inc. (Level VII)

33 National Institute of Neurological Disorders and Stroke. (n.d.). NIH Stroke Scale. https://www.ninds.nih.gov/sites/default/files/NIH_Stroke_Scale_Booklet.pdf

Nutritional screening

Nutritional screening may identify malnutrition or risk factors associated with malnutrition.[1,2] Malnutrition is associated with negative clinical outcomes, including increased mortality rate, longer hospital stays, increased complications, and more frequent hospital readmissions.[2] You can evaluate a patient's nutritional status by examining information from several sources, such as the patient's medical history, physical assessment findings, and laboratory results. If nutritional screening determines that the patient is at risk for a nutritional disorder, you should conduct a comprehensive nutritional assessment to set goals and determine interventions to correct actual or potential imbalances.[3,4]

Nutritional screening also provides information about the status of acute and chronic conditions.[5] It examines certain variables to determine the risk of problems in specific populations, such as pregnant women, older adults, and those with chronic diseases (for example, cardiac disorders or diabetes), to detect deficiencies or potential imbalances.

If warranted by the patient's needs or condition, complete a nutritional screening within 24 hours of the patient's admission to an acute care center.[3]

Equipment

Scale with stadiometer ▪ nutritional screening tool[6] ▪ tape measure ▪ Optional: chair or bed scale, sliding calipers.[6]

Preparation of equipment

Select the appropriate scale—usually, a standing scale for an ambulatory patient or a chair or bed scale for an acutely ill or debilitated patient. Ensure the scale is balanced according to the manufacturer's instructions. Inspect all equipment and supplies. If a product is expired, is defective, or has compromised integrity, remove it from patient use, label it as expired or defective, and report the expiration or defect as directed by your facility.

Implementation

- Perform hand hygiene.[7,8,9,10,11,12]
- Confirm the patient's identity using at least two patient identifiers.[13]
- Provide privacy.[14,15,16,17]
- Explain the procedure to the patient and family (if appropriate) according to their individual communication and learning needs *to increase their understanding, allay their fears, and enhance cooperation.*[6,18]
- Ask the patient to remove shoes (if appropriate) and obtain the patient's weight using a standing, chair, or bed scale, as appropriate. *Weight provides a rough estimate of body composition.*
- Ask about unplanned or unintentional weight change. Determine how much weight the patient lost or gained and over what period. A weight loss of more than 5% of body weight in 30 days or 10% in 180 days, or a weight gain of 10 lb (4.5 kg) or more in 180 days places the patient at nutritional risk.[19]
- Measure the patient's height while the patient is standing erect without shoes, using the measuring bar on the scale. If the patient can't stand, approximate height by measuring "wingspan." (See *Overcoming height measurement problems.*)

Overcoming height measurement problems

A patient confined to a wheelchair or one who can't stand up straight because of such orthopedic problems as kyphosis or scoliosis poses a challenge for accurate height measurement. Alternative methods include measurement of recumbent length, knee height, forearm length, and demi-span.[20] However, sliding calipers is the method of choice *because it is closest in accuracy to measuring standing height.*[21]

- Calculate or estimate body mass index (BMI) *to evaluate weight in relation to height.* (See *Calculating BMI.*)[22]

Calculating BMI

Use one of the formulas below to calculate your patient's body mass index (BMI).

$$BMI = \left(\frac{weight\ in\ pounds}{height\ in\ inches \times height\ in\ inches} \right) \times 703$$

OR

$$BMI = \left(\frac{weight\ in\ kilograms}{height\ in\ centimeters \times height\ in\ centimeters} \right) \times 10{,}000$$

- Explain BMI to the patient. (See *Determining BMI.*)

Determining BMI

Body mass index (BMI) measures weight in relation to height. The BMI ranges discussed here are for adults. Although these ranges don't provide an exact guide for healthy or unhealthy weight, studies show that health risks increase with increasing weight and obesity. A BMI of less than 18.5 kg/m² defines underweight; 18.8 to 24.9 kg/m², a healthy weight; 25 to 29.9 kg/m², overweight; and 30 kg/m² or more, obesity.[23]

- Evaluate the patient's weight distribution by measuring waist circumference around the patient's abdomen at the level of the iliac crest. Before reading the tape measure, ensure that the tape is snug but doesn't compress the skin and is parallel to the floor. If the measurement is greater than 35″ (89 cm) for a woman or 40″ (102 cm) for a man (with a normal BMI), the patient is at greater risk for health problems.[3] People with a high distribution of fat around their waists as opposed to their hips and thighs are at greater risk for such diseases as type 2 diabetes, dyslipidemia, hypertension, and cardiovascular disease.[24]
- Question the patient about eating habits, living environment, and functional status. *A problem in any of these areas places the patient at risk for nutritional problems and requires further nutritional assessment.*
- Review the medical record and interview the patient *to determine whether the present illness or medical history places the patient at nutritional risk.* Use a nutritional screening tool if available.
- Review physical assessment findings for signs of poor nutrition. (See *Evaluating nutritional disorders,* page 600.)
- Make a referral to a registered dietitian if a nutritional screening suggests the patient is at risk for nutritional problems.[3] *A registered dietitian will perform a comprehensive nutritional assessment.*
- Perform hand hygiene.[7,8,9,10,11,12]
- Document the procedure.[26,27,28,29]

Special considerations

- The nutritional screening is typically performed during the initial nursing history and physical assessment, but should be completed within 24 hours of admission.[3,30,31]
- When measuring height, note the growth of children as well as diminishing height of older adults. Growth of children may be noted on standardized charts *to assess growth patterns for possible abnormalities.* Diminishing height of older adults may be related to osteoporotic changes and should be investigated.[6]

Documentation

Record the date and time of the nutritional screening. Record the patient's height and weight on the screening form as well as the graphic sheet or patient care flow sheet. Note the type of scale used. Complete the screening tool as recommended. Calculate and record the patient's BMI. Use a progress note to record information that doesn't have a space on the screening tool. Record whether the patient has experienced any weight loss, the time over which the loss occurred, and how much weight was lost.

Make sure laboratory results are documented, including the name of anyone you notified of abnormal results, and whether orders were given. Note any nutritional problems detected during the physical examination and review of the patient's medical record. For patients at nutritional risk, record the date and time, names of the people notified and whether those who were notified came to see the patient, any orders received, and your nursing interventions and the patient's response. Document teaching you provided to the patient and family (if applicable), their understanding of that teaching, and any need for follow-up teaching.

REFERENCES

1 Omidvari, A. H., et al. (2013). Nutritional screening for improving professional practice for patient outcomes in hospital and primary care settings. *Cochrane Database of Systematic Reviews, 2013*(6), CD005539. https://www.cochranelibrary.com/cdsr/doi/10.1002/14651858.CD005539.pub2/full (Level I)

2 Mogensen, K. M., et al. (2019). Academy of Nutrition and Dietetics/American Society for Parenteral and Enteral Nutrition consensus malnutrition characteristics: Usability and association with outcomes. *Nutrition in Clinical Practice, 34*(5), 657–665. (Level VII)

3 Mueller, C., et al. (2011). A.S.P.E.N. clinical guidelines: Nutrition screening, assessment, and intervention in adults. *Journal of Parenteral and Enteral Nutrition, 35,* 16–24. https://onlinelibrary.wiley.com/doi/pdf/10.1177/0148607110389335 (Level I)

4 Kirkland, L., et al. (2013). Nutrition in the hospitalized patient. *Journal of Hospital Medicine, 8,* 52–58. (Level VII)

5 Lilamand, M., et al. (2015). The mini nutritional assessment short form and mortality in nursing home residents: Results from the INCUR study. *Journal of Nutrition, Health and Aging, 19,* 383–388. (Level IV)

6 Potter, P., et al. (2021). *Fundamentals of nursing* (10th ed.). St. Louis, MO: Elsevier.

7 The Joint Commission. (2021). Standard NPSG.07.01.01. *Comprehensive accreditation manual for hospitals.* Oakbrook Terrace, IL: The Joint Commission. (Level VII)

8 Centers for Disease Control and Prevention. (2002). Guideline for hand hygiene in health-care settings: Recommendations of the Healthcare Infection Control Practices Advisory Committee and the HICPAC/SHEA/APIC/IDSA Hand Hygiene Task Force. *MMWR Recommendations and Reports, 51*(RR-16), 1–45. https://www.cdc.gov/mmwr/pdf/rr/rr5116.pdf (Level II)

9 World Health Organization. (2009). WHO guidelines on hand hygiene in health care: First global patient safety challenge, clean care is safer care. https://apps.who.int/iris/bitstream/handle/10665/44102/9789241597906_eng.pdf?sequence=1 (Level IV)

10 Accreditation Association for Hospitals and Health Systems. (2020). Standard 07.01.21. *Healthcare Facilities Accreditation Program: Accreditation requirements for acute care hospitals.* Chicago, IL: Accreditation Association for Hospitals and Health Systems. (Level VII)

11 Centers for Medicare and Medicaid Services, Department of Health and Human Services. (2020). Condition of participation: Infection control. 42 C.F.R. § 482.42.

12 DNV GL-Healthcare USA, Inc. (2020). IC.1.SR.1. *NIAHO® accreditation requirements, interpretive guidelines and surveyor guidance—revision 20.0.* Milford, OH: DNV GL-Healthcare USA, Inc. (Level VII)

13 The Joint Commission. (2021). Standard NPSG.01.01.01. *Comprehensive accreditation manual for hospitals.* Oakbrook Terrace, IL: The Joint Commission. (Level VII)

14 Accreditation Association for Hospitals and Health Systems. (2020). Standard 15.01.16. *Healthcare Facilities Accreditation Program: Accreditation requirements for acute care hospitals.* Chicago, IL: Accreditation Association for Hospitals and Health Systems. (Level VII)

15 Centers for Medicare and Medicaid Services, Department of Health and Human Services. (2020). Condition of participation: Patient's rights. 42 C.F.R. § 482.13 (c)(1).

Evaluating nutritional disorders

Physical examination findings throughout various body systems can indicate poor nutrition. The table below lists body systems or regions, along with signs and symptoms that appear in that area when the patient has poor nutrition, and their implications.

BODY SYSTEM OR REGION	SIGN OR SYMPTOM	IMPLICATIONS
General	■ Weakness and fatigue	■ Anemia or electrolyte imbalance
	■ Weight loss	■ Decreased calorie intake, increased calorie use, or inadequate nutrient intake or absorption
Skin, hair, and nails	■ Dry, flaky skin	■ Vitamin A, vitamin B complex, or linoleic acid deficiency
	■ Dry skin with poor turgor	■ Dehydration
	■ Rough, scaly skin with bumps	■ Vitamin A deficiency
	■ Petechiae or ecchymoses	■ Vitamin C or K deficiency
	■ Sore that won't heal	■ Protein, vitamin C, or zinc deficiency
	■ Thinning, dry hair	■ Protein deficiency
	■ Spoon-shaped, brittle, or ridged nails	■ Iron deficiency
Eyes	■ Night blindness; corneal swelling, softening, or dryness; Bitot spots (gray triangular patches on the conjunctiva)	■ Vitamin A deficiency
	■ Red conjunctiva	■ Riboflavin deficiency
Throat and mouth	■ Cracks at the corner of the mouth	■ Riboflavin or niacin deficiency
	■ Magenta tongue	■ Riboflavin deficiency
	■ Beefy, red tongue	■ Vitamin B_{12} deficiency
	■ Soft, spongy, bleeding gums	■ Vitamin C deficiency
	■ Poor dentition	■ Overconsumption of refined sugars or acidic carbonated beverages; illicit drug use[25]
	■ Swollen neck (goiter)	■ Iodine deficiency
Cardiovascular	■ Edema, shortness of breath, third and fourth heart sounds, murmur	■ Protein deficiency, thiamine deficiency
	■ Tachycardia, irregular rhythm	■ Fluid volume deficit, electrolyte imbalance, anemia
GI	■ Ascites	■ Protein deficiency
Musculoskeletal	■ Bone pain and bow leg	■ Vitamin D or calcium deficiency
	■ Muscle wasting	■ Protein, carbohydrate, and fat deficiency
Neurologic	■ Altered mental status, ataxia	■ Dehydration and thiamine or vitamin B_{12} deficiency
	■ Paresthesia, neuropathies	■ Vitamin B_{12}, pyridoxine, thiamine, or niacin deficiency; electrolyte imbalance

16 DNV GL-Healthcare USA, Inc. (2020). PR.2.SR.5. *NIAHO® accreditation requirements, interpretive guidelines and surveyor guidance—revision 20.0*. Milford, OH: DNV GL-Healthcare USA, Inc. (Level VII)

17 The Joint Commission. (2021). Standard RI.01.01.01. *Comprehensive accreditation manual for hospitals*. Oakbrook Terrace, IL: The Joint Commission. (Level VII)

18 The Joint Commission. (2021). Standard PC.02.01.21. *Comprehensive accreditation manual for hospitals*. Oakbrook Terrace, IL: The Joint Commission. (Level VII)

19 White, J. V., et al. (2012). Consensus statement of the Academy of Nutrition and Dietetics and American Society for Parenteral and Enteral Nutrition: Characteristics recommended for the identification and documentation of adult malnutrition (undernutrition). *Journal of Parenteral and Enteral Nutrition, 36*, 275–283. https://dietitian-sondemand.com/wp-content/uploads/2017/09/ASPEN-AND-2012-Consensus-Statement-Regarding-Malnutrition-Diagnosis-1.pdf (Level VII)

20 Froehlich-Grobe, K., et al. (2011). Measuring height without a stadiometer. *American Journal of Physical Medicine and Rehabilitation, 90*(8), 658–666. https://www.ncbi.nlm.nih.gov/pmc/articles/PMC3148840 (Level IV)

21 Frid, H., et al. (2013). Agreement between different methods of measuring height in elderly patients. *Journal of Human Nutrition and Dietetics, 26*(5), 504–511. (Level IV)

22 Centers for Disease Control and Prevention. (2021). About adult BMI. https://www.cdc.gov/healthyweight/assessing/bmi/adult_bmi/index.html#Interpreted

23 U.S. Department of Health and Human Services & U.S. Department of Agriculture. (2015). *Dietary guidelines for Americans: 2015–2020* (8th ed.). https://health.gov/sites/default/files/2019-09/2015-2020_Dietary_Guidelines.pdf (Level VII)

24 U.S. Department of Health and Human Services, National Heart, Lung, and Blood Institute. (2012). Integrated guidelines for cardiovascular health and risk reduction in children and adolescents. https://www.nhlbi.nih.gov/health-topics/integrated-guidelines-for-cardiovascular-health-and-risk-reduction-in-children-and-adolescents (Level I)

25 Bassiouny, M. A. (2013). Dental erosion due to abuse of illicit drugs and acidic carbonated beverages. *General Dentistry, 61*, 38–44. (Level VI)

26 The Joint Commission. (2021). Standard RC.01.03.01. *Comprehensive accreditation manual for hospitals.* Oakbrook Terrace, IL: The Joint Commission. (Level VII)

27 Centers for Medicare and Medicaid Services, Department of Health and Human Services. (2020). Condition of participation: Medical record services. 42 C.F.R. § 482.24(b).

28 Accreditation Association for Hospitals and Health Systems. (2020). Standard 10.00.03. *Healthcare Facilities Accreditation Program: Accreditation requirements for acute care hospitals.* Chicago, IL: Accreditation Association for Hospitals and Health Systems. (Level VII)

29 DNV GL-Healthcare USA, Inc. (2020). MR.2.SR.1. *NIAHO® accreditation requirements, interpretive guidelines and surveyor guidance—revision 20.0.* Milford, OH: DNV GL-Healthcare USA, Inc. (Level VII)

30 The Joint Commission. (2021). Standard PC.01.02.03. *Comprehensive accreditation manual for hospitals.* Oakbrook Terrace, IL: The Joint Commission. (Level VII)

31 Accreditation Association for Hospitals and Health Systems. (2020). Standard 10.01.24. *Healthcare Facilities Accreditation Program: Accreditation requirements for acute care hospitals.* Chicago, IL: Accreditation Association for Hospitals and Health Systems. (Level VII)

OMMAYA RESERVOIR DRUG INFUSION

Also known as a *subcutaneous cerebrospinal fluid (CSF) reservoir*, the Ommaya reservoir allows delivery of long-term drug therapy to the CSF by way of the brain's ventricles. It's most commonly used for chemotherapy and pain management, specifically for treating central nervous system (CNS) lymphoma, malignant CNS disease, and meningeal carcinomatosis. The reservoir spares the patient repeated lumbar punctures to administer chemotherapeutic drugs, analgesics, antibiotics, and antifungals.[1,2]

The reservoir is a mushroom-shaped silicone apparatus with an attached catheter. It's surgically implanted beneath the patient's scalp, and the catheter is threaded into the ventricle through a burr hole in the skull. (See *How the Ommaya reservoir works.*) Besides providing convenient, comparatively painless access to CSF, the Ommaya reservoir permits consistent and predictable drug distribution throughout the subarachnoid space and CNS. It also allows for measurement of intracranial pressure (ICP).

Before reservoir insertion, the patient may receive a local or general anesthetic, depending on the patient's condition and the practitioner's preference. After an X-ray confirms placement of the reservoir, a pressure dressing is applied for 24 hours. The sutures may be removed in about 10 days. However, the reservoir can be used within 48 hours to deliver drugs, measure CSF pressure, drain CSF, and withdraw CSF specimens.

The practitioner usually injects drugs into the Ommaya reservoir, but a specially trained nurse may perform this procedure if permitted by the facility and the state's nurse practice act. This sterile procedure usually takes 15 to 30 minutes.

Equipment

Equipment varies but may include the following: Preservative-free prescribed drug ▪ personal protective equipment (sterile gloves, gown, mask and goggles or mask with face shield) ▪ antiseptic solution (avoid antiseptics containing alcohol or acetone) ▪ 10-mL syringe ▪ two 3-mL syringes ▪ 25G 5/8″ butterfly needle or Huber needle ▪ 10-mL prefilled syringe containing preservative-free normal saline solution ▪ sterile drape ▪ sterile gauze pads ▪ vital signs monitoring equipment ▪ stethoscope ▪ disinfectant pad ▪ Optional: CSF collection tubes, label, laboratory biohazard transport bag, hair clippers, additional medications as prescribed.

EQUIPMENT

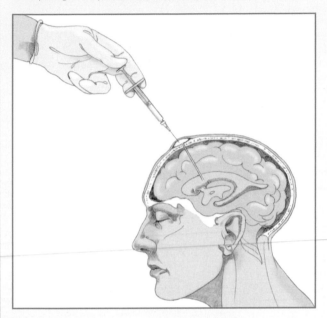

How the Ommaya reservoir works

To insert an Ommaya reservoir, the practitioner drills a burr hole and inserts the device's catheter through the patient's nondominant frontal lobe into the lateral ventricle. The reservoir, which has a self-sealing silicone injection dome, rests over the burr hole under a scalp flap. This creates a slight, soft bulge on the scalp about the size of a quarter. Usually, drugs are injected into the dome with a syringe.

For chemotherapy

Safety data sheet for prescribed chemotherapy drug ▪ prescribed chemotherapy drug ▪ powder-free chemotherapy gloves ▪ nonlinting, nonabsorbent disposable gown ▪ face shield ▪ syringes with Luer-lock connector ▪ chemotherapy sharps container ▪ hazardous-waste container approved for cytotoxic waste ▪ hazardous-drug spill kit ▪ emergency equipment (code cart with emergency drugs, defibrillator, handheld resuscitation bag with mask, intubation equipment) ▪ Optional: National Institute of Occupational Safety and Health–approved respirator mask (if aerosolization is likely)

Preparation of equipment

Inspect all equipment and supplies. If a product is expired, is defective, or has compromised integrity, remove it from patient use, label it as expired or defective, and report the expiration or defect as directed by your facility. Make sure that the emergency equipment is readily available and functioning properly.

Make sure that a hazardous drug spill kit is readily available if administering chemotherapy.

Bring the drug to be administered to room temperature as needed.

Implementation

▪ Perform hand hygiene.[3,4,5,6,7,8]
▪ Gather the prescribe medication and the appropriate equipment.
▪ Avoid distractions and interruptions when preparing and administering medications *to prevent medication administration errors.*[9,10]

Preparing for nonchemotherapy drug administration

▪ Verify the practitioner's order.[11,12,13,14]
▪ Compare the medication label to the order in the patient's medical record.[11,12,13,14]
▪ Check the patient's medical record for allergies and other contraindications to the prescribed drug. If an allergy or another contraindication exists, don't administer the drug; notify the practitioner.[11,12,13,14]

- Review an accurate list of all the patient's medications and supplements.[15,16,17,18]
- Check the expiration date on the drug. If the drug is expired, return it to the pharmacy and obtain new drug.[11,12,13,14]
- Visually inspect the solution for particles, discoloration, or other loss of integrity; don't administer the drug if its integrity is compromised.[11,12,13,14]
- Discuss any unresolved concerns about the drug with the patient's practitioner.[11,12,13,14]
- Perform hand hygiene.[3,4,5,6,7,8]
- Confirm the patient's identity using two patient identifiers.[19]
- Provide privacy.[20,21,22,23]
- If the patient is receiving the medication for the first time, teach about the potential adverse reactions and discuss any other concerns related to the drug.[11,12,13,14]
- Assess the patient's baseline vital signs and neurologic status; if any are altered, stop the procedure and notify the practitioner.
- Screen for and assess pain using facility-defined criteria that are consistent with the patient's age, condition, and ability to understand.[24]
- Treat the patient's pain, as needed and ordered, using nonpharmacologic, pharmacologic, or a combination of approaches. Base the treatment plan on evidence-based practices and the patient's clinical condition, medical history, and pain management goals.[24]
- Remove hair over the reservoir site using clippers, as necessary; don't shave the hair.[15]

Preparing for chemotherapy drug administration

- Review the patient's medical record for initial cancer diagnosis and staging or current cancer status; recent treatments, including surgery, radiation therapy, hormone therapy, cytotoxic therapy, and complementary therapy; medical, psychiatric, and surgical history; history of allergic or hypersensitivity reactions; pregnancy and reproductive status, including the last menstrual period if applicable; laboratory and radiologic test results required by the chemotherapy protocol, as ordered; and physical examination findings, including assessment of organ function as appropriate for the planned treatment regimen.[15,16,25]
- Review an accurate list of all the patient's drugs and supplements.[15,16,17,18,25]
- Confirm that informed consent has been obtained and that the signed consent form is in the patient's medical record.[15,26,27,28,29]
- Check that the order is written and contains the following information: patient's complete name and a second identifier,[15,16,25] the date,[25] the patient's diagnosis,[15] any allergies,[15,25] regimen name or protocol name and number,[15,16,25] cycle number and day (if applicable,[15,16,25] full generic name of the drug ordered,[15,25] drug dose,[15,16,25] patient's height and weight in kilograms[30] and any other variables used to calculate the dose,[15,16,25] method of calculation,[15,25] administration route,[15,16,25] frequency or dates of administration,[15,25] administration rate,[15,16,25] length of infusion (if applicable),[15] supportive care measures (premedications for hypersensitivity and nausea, if needed, and hydration, if applicable),[15,25] criteria to administer or parameters to hold or modify a dose (such as laboratory or diagnostic test results and the patient's clinical status),[15,25] sequence of medication administration (if applicable),[15,25] and planned duration of treatment, such as the number of cycles for which the order is valid.[25]
- Review the patient's height, weight (in kilograms), and double-check the body surface area (BSA). If a recent weight isn't available, weigh the patient.[15,16]
- Recalculate and verify the dose using the patient's BSA and weight, if applicable. Check your calculations against the written order.
- Have a second qualified individual verify the chemotherapy order before drug preparation, which should include confirming the two patient identifiers; drug name, dose, volume, and administration route; dose calculation; and treatment cycle and day of cycle.[15,16]
- Verify that the prescribed drug dose is appropriate for the patient, diagnosis, and treatment plan. If you have concerns, consult the prescribing practitioner or pharmacist.[11,12,13,14,15,16]
- Review the information in the safety data sheet for the prescribed drug.[31,32]
- In collaboration with the multidisciplinary team, review the patient's test results, specifically those for complete blood count, blood urea nitrogen level, platelet count, and liver function studies.[33]

- Compare the drug label to the order in the patient's medical record.[11,12,13,14]
- Verify that the drug is properly labeled when you receive it from the pharmacy, and that this information includes the patient's full name and second identifier, full generic drug name, administration route, total dose to be given, total volume required to administer the dosage, date of administration, and date and time of preparation and expiration. Make sure that it also contains any special handling instructions and a label that clearly identifies the drug as hazardous and for intrathecal use only.[15,25]
- Check the expiration date on the drug. If the drug is expired, return it to the pharmacy and obtain a replacement.[11,12,13,14]
- Visually inspect the solution for particles, discoloration, or other loss of integrity; don't administer the drug if its integrity is compromised.[11,12,13,14]
- Discuss any unresolved concerns about the drug with the patient's practitioner.[11,12,13,14]
- Perform hand hygiene.[3,4,5,6,7,8]
- Confirm the patient's identity using at least two patient identifiers.[19]
- Provide privacy.[20,21,22,23]
- Confirm that the patient has received verbal and written or electronic information about the cancer diagnosis and associated chemotherapy regimen, its short- and long-term adverse effects (including fertility risks, as appropriate), therapy goals, and the continuing care plan.[25] If the patient is receiving the drug for the first time, teach about potential adverse reactions and discuss other concerns related to the drug.[11,12,13,14]
- Verify with the patient any allergies, previous reactions, and treatment-related toxicities.[25]
- Monitor any cumulative chemotherapy dose *to ensure that the patient hasn't reached the maximum lifetime dose.*[33]
- Ask the patient about any psychosocial concerns or cultural or spiritual issues that may affect treatment, and take action as indicated.[25]
- Confirm the treatment plan, administration route, and symptom management plan with the patient.[15]
- Assess the patient's clinical and performance status.[25]
- Obtain the patient's vital signs *to use as a baseline for comparison.*[15,16,33]
- Screen for and assess pain using facility-defined criteria that are consistent with the patient's age, condition, and ability to understand.[24]
- Treat the patient's pain, as needed and ordered, using nonpharmacologic, pharmacologic, or a combination of approaches. Base the treatment plan on evidence-based practices and the patient's clinical condition, medical history, and pain management goals.[24] Administer pain medication, as needed and prescribed, following safe medication administration practices.[11,12,13,14]
- Remove hair over the reservoir site using clippers, as necessary; don't shave the hair.[15]

Administering the medication or chemotherapeutic agent

- Ensure that placement of the Ommaya reservoir has been confirmed before initial use.
- If required, conduct a preprocedure verification *to make sure that all relevant documentation, related information, and equipment are available and correctly identified to the patient's identifiers.*[34,35]
- Explain the procedure to the patient and family (if appropriate) according to their individual communication and learning needs *to increase their understanding, allay their fears, and enhance cooperation.*[36]
- Determine whether the practitioner has ordered any premedications *to combat adverse effects of the prescribed medication or chemotherapeutic agent,* and administer them as prescribed following safe medication administration practices.[11,14]
- If your facility uses a bar code technology, use it as directed by your facility.
- Raise the patient's bed to waist level before providing patient care *to prevent caregiver back strain.*[37]
- Position the patient in a sitting or reclining position.
- Perform hand hygiene.[3,4,5,6,7,8]
- Open a sterile tray and prepare a sterile field on a work surface close to the patient.
- Place the prescribed drug and necessary supplies on the sterile field. Make sure that all drugs on and off the sterile field are clearly labeled.[38,39]
- Perform hand hygiene.[3,4,5,6,7,8]

■ Put on a mask, sterile gloves, and other personal protective equipment, as necessary.[15,40] Maintain strict sterile technique throughout the procedure.[15] If you're administering a chemotherapeutic drug, wear two pairs of sterile gloves, a mask, a face shield (if splashing is likely), and a respirator (if needed).[15,32,41] Make sure that your inner glove cuff is worn under the gown cuff and that the outer glove cuff extends over the gown cuff *to fully protect your skin.* Inspect your gloves *to make sure that they're physically intact.*

■ Conduct a time-out immediately before starting the procedure *to ensure that the correct patient, site, positioning, and procedure are identified and, as applicable, that all relevant information and necessary equipment are available.*[42]

■ Examine the area over the reservoir for signs of infection or trauma. Notify the practitioner if any are present.

■ *To confirm placement and to fill the reservoir,* gently palpate the reservoir and pump it three or four times; expect free flow of CSF from the ventricle into the reservoir.

■ Drape the reservoir site with a sterile drape and prepare the patient's scalp with an antiseptic solution, as directed by your facility, working in a circular motion from the center outward. Allow the solution to dry completely *to achieve its maximum effect.*

NURSING ALERT Chemotherapeutic drugs are considered high-alert medications *because they can cause significant patient harm if used in error.* Never administer a chemotherapeutic drug without performing an independent double-check with another practitioner who is qualified to prepare or administer chemotherapy.[15,25,43]

NURSING ALERT Vinca alkaloids such as vinCRIStine are never given in an Ommaya reservoir *because of potentially lethal neurotoxicity, including coma and death.*[15]

■ Verify that the prescribed medication is being administered at the proper time, in the prescribed dose, and by the correct route *to reduce the risk of medication errors.*[11,12,13,14]

■ If administering a chemotherapeutic agent, have another practitioner who is qualified to prepare or administer chemotherapy perform an independent double-check *to verify the patient's identity and to make sure that the correct drug is prepared in the prescribed concentration and volume, the drug hasn't expired, the drug's indication corresponds with the patient's diagnosis, the dosage calculations are correct and the dosing formula used to derive the final dose is correct, the route of administration is safe and proper for the patient, and the drug's integrity is intact.*[44] Both of you should sign the patient's medical record indicating that the verification took place.[15,25]

■ Compare the results of the independent double-check with the other practitioner (if necessary) and, if no discrepancies exist, begin administering the drug. If discrepancies exist, rectify them before administering the drug.[44]

■ Using sterile technique, attach a 10-mL syringe to the butterfly needle. Consider using a stopcock between the butterfly needle and syringe to avoid changing multiple syringes.[1]

■ Place the butterfly needle at a 45-degree angle and insert it into the reservoir. Alternatively, puncture the reservoir with the Huber needle.

■ Slowly and gently aspirate 3 mL of CSF into the attached syringe *to make sure that it's clear and doesn't contain blood.*[45] If the aspirate isn't clear, or if you can't aspirate fluid and you suspect reservoir catheter malfunction, notify the practitioner before continuing.

■ If a CSF sample is needed for laboratory testing, clamp the tubing, discard the CSF, and, using a new syringe, withdraw the appropriate amount of CSF.

NURSING ALERT Don't use a Vacutainer to aspirate CSF, *because rapidly withdrawing CSF with this device could damage the ventricle's choroid plexus.*

■ Continue to aspirate as many milliliters of CSF as the volume of drug to be instilled. (Some facilities use the CSF instead of a preservative-free diluent to deliver the drug.)

■ Detach the syringe from the needle hub.

■ Attach the drug syringe.

■ Instill the prescribed drug slowly, monitoring the patient for headache, nausea, dizziness, and other change in neurologic status.

■ Clamp the tubing and then detach the syringe.

■ Attach the prefilled syringe containing preservative-free normal saline solution and slowly flush the reservoir.

■ Withdraw the needle.

■ Cover the site with a sterile gauze pad and apply gentle pressure for 1 to 2 minutes until superficial bleeding stops.

■ Gently pump the reservoir *to distribute the drug.*

■ Discard the needle and syringe in an appropriate sharps disposal container;[46] use a chemotherapy sharps container if the drug was a chemotherapeutic drug.[16,47]

■ If laboratory testing is ordered, place the CSF reserved for laboratory testing in the collection tubes and label the tubes in the presence of the patient *to prevent mislabeling.*[19] Then discard the syringe in an appropriate sharps container.[46]

■ Return the bed to the lowest position *to prevent falls and maintain patient safety.*[48]

■ If a hazardous drug was administered, clean and decontaminate all work surfaces that may have come into contact with the hazardous drug.[15,32,49]

Completing the procedure

■ Remove and discard used supplies in appropriate waste receptacles.[32,46,47,50]

■ Remove your personal protective equipment and discard it in an appropriate receptacle.[40] If you administered chemotherapy, discard your equipment in the hazardous waste container for cytotoxic waste.[32,47]

■ Wash your hands with soap and water if you administered a chemotherapy drug.[5,15,25,32,49] Perform hand hygiene if you didn't.[3,4,5,6,7,8]

■ Instruct the patient to lie quietly for about 15 to 30 minutes after the procedure *to prevent meningeal irritation, which can lead to nausea and vomiting.*

■ Monitor the patient for adverse drug reactions and signs and symptoms of increased ICP (such as vital sign changes, nausea, vomiting, pain, and dizziness) every 30 minutes for 2 hours, every hour for 2 hours, every 4 hours for 24 hours, and then every 8 hours for the duration of care, or as directed by your facility.[51]

■ Reassess and respond to the patient's pain by evaluating the response to treatment and progress toward pain management goals. Assess for adverse reactions and risk factors for adverse events that may result from treatment.[24]

■ If a laboratory specimen was obtained, place it in a laboratory biohazard transport bag[50] and immediately send it to the laboratory.

■ Perform hand hygiene.[3,4,5,6,7,8]

■ With a disinfectant pad, disinfect equipment that isn't for single-patient use.[52,53]

■ Perform hand hygiene.[3,4,5,6,7,8]

■ Document the procedure.[54,55,56,57]

Special considerations

■ Be aware that the practitioner may prescribe an antiemetic to be administered 30 minutes before the procedure *to control nausea and vomiting.*

■ For patients receiving chemotherapy in a health care setting, measure weight (in kilograms) at least weekly[25] or as directed by your facility.[15] Measure height at least weekly and when appropriate for the treatment[25] or as directed by your facility.[15]

■ If some of the chemotherapy drug comes in contact with your skin, wash your skin thoroughly with soap (not a germicidal agent) and water. If eye contact occurs, flood your eye with water or saline solution for at least 15 minutes while holding your eyelid open. Obtain a medical evaluation as soon as possible after accidental exposure.[15,31,32]

■ If a spill occurs, manage it properly. (See the "Hazardous drug spill management" procedure).

■ Note that any health care worker who is pregnant, trying to conceive, or breast-feeding shouldn't be exposed to chemotherapeutic drugs.[15,31]

Complications

Ommaya reservoir device complications include infection, which usually can be treated with antibiotics injected directly into the reservoir; however, persistent infection may require reservoir removal.[60] Noninfectious complications, such as catheter migration and blockage, neurologic complications (including seizures, focal neurologic deficit, and cranial nerve palsies), cerebrospinal fluid leakage, and hemorrhage can also occur.[2,61,62] Adverse reactions specific to the drug infused can also occur.

Documentation

Document your assessment findings; the type and size of needle used; patient tolerance of the procedure; CSF characteristics; drug, dose, and volume administered; amount of CSF withdrawn; specimens collected and results; and any complications, interventions performed, and the patient's response to those interventions. Also record the appearance of the reservoir insertion site before and after access. Record pain assessment findings, any prescribed pain medication administered, and the patient's response. Note any adverse effects of the drug, the name of the practitioner who was notified, the date and time of notification, prescribed interventions, and the patient's response to those interventions. Document patient and family teaching provided, their understanding of the teaching, and any need for follow-up teaching.

Rᴇꜰᴇʀᴇɴᴄᴇꜱ

1 Anwar, A., et al. (2021). Carcinomatous meningitis. https://www.ncbi. nlm.nih.gov/books/NBK560816/

2 Cohen-Pfeffer, J. L., et al. (2017). Intracerebroventricular delivery as a safe, long-term route of drug administration. *Pediatric Neurology, 67*, 23–35. https://www.pedneur.com/article/S0887-8994(16)30280-6/pdf (Level I)

3 Centers for Disease Control and Prevention. (2002). Guideline for hand hygiene in health-care settings: Recommendations of the Healthcare Infection Control Practices Advisory Committee and the HICPAC/SHEA/APIC/IDSA Hand Hygiene Task Force. *MMWR Recommendations and Reports, 51*(RR-16), 1–45. https://www.cdc.gov/mmwr/pdf/rr/rr5116. pdf (Level II)

4 World Health Organization. (2009). WHO guidelines on hand hygiene in health care: First global patient safety challenge, clean care is safer care. https://apps.who.int/iris/bitstream/handle/10665/44102/9789241597906_eng.pdf?sequence=1 (Level IV)

5 The Joint Commission. (2021). Standard NPSG.07.01.01. *Comprehensive accreditation manual for hospitals*. Oakbrook Terrace, IL: The Joint Commission. (Level VII)

6 Accreditation Association for Hospitals and Health Systems. (2020). Standard 07.01.21. *Healthcare Facilities Accreditation Program: Accreditation requirements for acute care hospitals*. Chicago, IL: Accreditation Association for Hospitals and Health Systems. (Level VII)

7 Centers for Medicare and Medicaid Services, Department of Health and Human Services. (2020). Condition of participation: Infection control. 42 C.F.R. § 482.42.

8 DNV GL-Healthcare USA, Inc. (2020). IC.1.SR.1. *NIAHO® accreditation requirements, interpretive guidelines and surveyor guidance—revision 20.0.* Milford, OH: DNV GL-Healthcare USA, Inc. (Level VII)

9 Westbrook, J., et al. (2010). Association of interruptions with an increased risk and severity of medication administration errors. *Archives of Internal Medicine, 170*, 683–690. (Level IV)

10 Institute for Safe Medication Practices. (2012). Side tracks on the safety express: Interruptions lead to errors and unfinished…Wait, what was I doing? *Nurse Advise-ERR, 11*(2), 1–4. https://www.ismp.org/resources/side-tracks-safety-express-interruptions-lead-errors-and-unfinished-wait-what-was-i-doing?id=37

11 The Joint Commission. (2021). Standard MM.06.01.01. *Comprehensive accreditation manual for hospitals*. Oakbrook Terrace, IL: The Joint Commission. (Level VII)

12 Accreditation Association for Hospitals and Health Systems. (2020). Standard 16.01.03. *Healthcare Facilities Accreditation Program: Accreditation requirements for acute care hospitals*. Chicago, IL: Accreditation Association for Hospitals and Health Systems. (Level VII)

13 Centers for Medicare and Medicaid Services, Department of Health and Human Services. (2020). Condition of participation: Nursing services. 42 C.F.R. § 482.23(c).

14 DNV GL-Healthcare USA, Inc. (2020). MM.1.SR.3. *NIAHO® accreditation requirements, interpretive guidelines and surveyor guidance—revision 20.0.* Milford, OH: DNV GL-Healthcare USA, Inc. (Level VII)

15 Olsen, M. M., et al. (Eds.). (2019). *Chemotherapy and immunotherapy guidelines and recommendations for practice.* Pittsburgh, PA: Oncology Nursing Society.

16 Esparza, D. M. (Ed.). (2019). *Oncology policies and procedures* (2nd ed.). Pittsburgh, PA: Oncology Nursing Society.

17 The Joint Commission. (2021). Standard NPSG.03.06.01. *Comprehensive accreditation manual for hospitals*. Oakbrook Terrace, IL: The Joint Commission. (Level VII)

18 Accreditation Association for Hospitals and Health Systems. (2020). Standard 25.02.03. *Healthcare Facilities Accreditation Program: Accreditation requirements for acute care hospitals*. Chicago, IL: Accreditation Association for Hospitals and Health Systems. (Level VII)

19 The Joint Commission. (2021). Standard NPSG.01.01.01. *Comprehensive accreditation manual for hospitals*. Oakbrook Terrace, IL: The Joint Commission. (Level VII)

20 The Joint Commission. (2021). Standard RI.01.01.01. *Comprehensive accreditation manual for hospitals*. Oakbrook Terrace, IL: The Joint Commission. (Level VII)

21 Accreditation Association for Hospitals and Health Systems. (2020). Standard 15.01.16. *Healthcare Facilities Accreditation Program: Accreditation requirements for acute care hospitals*. Chicago, IL: Accreditation Association for Hospitals and Health Systems. (Level VII)

22 Centers for Medicare and Medicaid Services, Department of Health and Human Services. (2020). Condition of participation: Patient's rights. 42 C.F.R. § 482.13(c)(1).

23 DNV GL-Healthcare USA, Inc. (2020). PR.2.SR.5. *NIAHO® accreditation requirements, interpretive guidelines and surveyor guidance—revision 20.0.* Milford, OH: DNV GL-Healthcare USA, Inc. (Level VII)

24 The Joint Commission. (2021). Standard PC.01.02.07. *Comprehensive accreditation manual for hospitals*. Oakbrook Terrace, IL: The Joint Commission. (Level VII)

25 Neuss, M. N., et al. (2017). 2016 Updated American Society of Clinical Oncology/Oncology Nursing Society chemotherapy administration safety standards, including standards for pediatric oncology. *Oncology Nursing Forum, 44*(1), A1–A13. https://www.ons.org/sites/default/files/2016%20 ASCO_ONS%20Chemo%20Standards.pdf (Level VII)

26 Centers for Medicare and Medicaid Services, Department of Health and Human Services. (2020). Condition of participation: Patient's rights. 42 C.F.R. § 482.13(b)(2).

27 DNV GL-Healthcare USA, Inc. (2020). PR.2.SR.3. *NIAHO® accreditation requirements, interpretive guidelines and surveyor guidance—revision 20.0.* Milford, OH: DNV GL-Healthcare USA, Inc. (Level VII)

28 The Joint Commission. (2021). Standard RI.01.03.01. *Comprehensive accreditation manual for hospitals*. Oakbrook Terrace, IL: The Joint Commission. (Level VII)

29 Accreditation Association for Hospitals and Health Systems. (2020). Standard 15.01.11. *Healthcare Facilities Accreditation Program: Accreditation requirements for acute care hospitals*. Chicago, IL: Accreditation Association for Hospitals and Health Systems. (Level VII)

30 Institute for Safe Medication Practices. (2020). 2020-2021 targeted medication safety best practices for hospitals. https://www.ismp.org/sites/default/files/attachments/2020-02/2020-2021%20TMSBP-%20 FINAL_1.pdf

31 Occupational Safety and Health Administration. (n.d.). Controlling occupational exposure to hazardous drugs. https://www.osha.gov/hazardous-drugs/controlling-occex (Level VII)

32 National Institute for Occupational Safety and Health (NIOSH). (2004). NIOSH alert: Preventing occupational exposures to antineoplastic and other hazardous drugs in health care settings. https://www.cdc.gov/niosh/docs/2004-165/pdfs/2004-165.pdf (Level VII)

33 Standard 60. Antineoplastic therapy. Infusion therapy standards of practice (8th ed.). (2021). *Journal of Infusion Nursing, 44*, S183–S185. (Level VII)

34 The Joint Commission. (2021). Standard UP.01.01.01. *Comprehensive accreditation manual for hospitals*. Oakbrook Terrace, IL: The Joint Commission. (Level VII)

35 Accreditation Association for Hospitals and Health Systems. (2020). Standard 30.00.14. *Healthcare Facilities Accreditation Program: Accreditation requirements for acute care hospitals*. Chicago, IL: Accreditation Association for Hospitals and Health Systems. (Level VII)

36 The Joint Commission. (2021). Standard PC.02.01.21. *Comprehensive accreditation manual for hospitals*. Oakbrook Terrace, IL: The Joint Commission. (Level VII)

37 Waters, T. R., et al. (2009). Safe patient handling training for schools of nursing. https://www.cdc.gov/niosh/docs/2009-127/pdfs/2009-127.pdf (Level VII)

38 The Joint Commission. (2021). Standard NPSG.03.04.01. *Comprehensive accreditation manual for hospitals*. Oakbrook Terrace, IL: The Joint Commission. (Level VII)

39 Accreditation Association for Hospitals and Health Systems. (2020). Standard 25.01.27. *Healthcare Facilities Accreditation Program: Accreditation requirements for acute care hospitals*. Chicago, IL: Accreditation Association for Hospitals and Health Systems. (Level VII)

40 Siegel, J. D., et al. (2007, revised 2019). 2007 guideline for isolation precautions: Preventing transmission of infectious agents in healthcare settings. https://www.cdc.gov/infectioncontrol/pdf/guidelines/isolation-guidelines-H.pdf (Level II)

41 National Institute for Occupational Safety and Health. (2008). Personal protective equipment for health care workers who work with hazardous drugs. Centers for Disease Control and Prevention. https://www.cdc.gov/niosh/docs/wp-solutions/2009-106/pdfs/2009-106.pdf. (Level VII)

42 The Joint Commission. (2021). Standard UP.01.03.01. *Comprehensive accreditation manual for hospitals*. Oakbrook Terrace, IL: The Joint Commission. (Level VII)

43 Institute for Safe Medication Practices. (2018). ISMP list of high-alert medications in acute care settings. https://www.ismp.org/sites/default/files/attachments/2018-08/highAlert2018-Acute-Final.pdf (Level VII)

44 Institute for Safe Medication Practice. (2019). Independent double checks: Worth the effort if used judiciously and properly. https://www.ismp.org/resources/independent-double-checks-worth-effort-if-used-judiciously-and-properly (Level VII)

45 Standard 56. Intraspinal access devices. Infusion therapy standards of practice (8th ed.). (2021). *Journal of Infusion Nursing, 44*, S171–S174. (Level VII)

46 Standard 21. Medical waste and sharps safety. Infusion therapy standards of practice (8th ed.). (2021). *Journal of Infusion Nursing, 44*, S460–S62. (Level VII)

47 Standard 15. Hazardous drugs and waste. Infusion therapy standards of practice (8th ed.). (2021). *Journal of Infusion Nursing, 44*, S50–S52. (Level VII)

48 Ganz, D. A., et al. (2013, reviewed 2021). *Preventing falls in hospitals: A toolkit for improving quality of care* (AHRQ Publication No. 13-0015-EF). Rockville, MD: Agency for Healthcare Research and Quality. https://www.ahrq.gov/patient-safety/settings/hospital/fall-prevention/toolkit/index.html (Level VII)

49 United States Pharmacopeial (USP) Convention. (2019). USP general chapter <800> Hazardous drugs—Handling in healthcare settings. http://www.usp.org/compounding/general-chapter-hazardous-drugs-handling-healthcare (Level VII)

50 Occupational Safety and Health Administration. (2019). Bloodborne pathogens, standard number 1910 1030. https://www.osha.gov/pls/oshaweb/owadisp.show_document?p_id=10051&p_table=STANDARDS (Level VII)

51 Aiello-Laws, L., & Rutledge, D. N. (2008). Management of adult patients receiving intraventricular chemotherapy for the treatment of leptomeningeal metastasis. *Clinical Journal of Oncology Nursing, 12*, 429–435.

52 Rutala, W. A., et al. (2008, revised 2019). Guideline for disinfection and sterilization in healthcare facilities, 2008. https://www.cdc.gov/infection-control/pdf/guidelines/disinfection-guidelines-H.pdf (Level I)

53 Accreditation Association for Hospitals and Health Systems. (2020). Standard 07.02.03. *Healthcare Facilities Accreditation Program: Accreditation requirements for acute care hospitals*. Chicago, IL: Accreditation Association for Hospitals and Health Systems. (Level VII)

54 The Joint Commission. (2021). Standard RC.01.03.01. *Comprehensive accreditation manual for hospitals*. Oakbrook Terrace, IL: The Joint Commission. (Level VII)

55 Accreditation Association for Hospitals and Health Systems. (2020). Standard 10.00.03. *Healthcare Facilities Accreditation Program: Accreditation requirements for acute care hospitals*. Chicago, IL: Accreditation Association for Hospitals and Health Systems. (Level VII)

56 Centers for Medicare and Medicaid Services, Department of Health and Human Services. (2020). Condition of participation: Medical record services. 42 C.F.R. § 482.24(b).

57 DNV GL-Healthcare USA, Inc. (2020). MR.2.SR.1. *NIAHO® accreditation requirements, interpretive guidelines and surveyor guidance—revision 20.0*. Milford, OH: DNV GL-Healthcare USA, Inc. (Level VII)

58 Moraff, A. M., et al. (2017). Real-time fluoroscopic and C-arm computed tomography evaluation of Ommaya reservoir integrity. *Cureus, 9*(3), e1097. https://www.ncbi.nlm.nih.gov/pmc/articles/PMC5392038/

59 Ozerov, S., et al. (2018). The use of a smartphone-assisted ventricle catheter guide for Ommaya reservoir placement: Experience of a retrospective bi-center study. *Child's Nervous System, 34*, 853–859. https://link.springer.com/article/10.1007/s00381-017-3713-6

60 Baddour, L. M., et al. (2020). Infections of cerebrospinal fluid shunts and other devices. In: *UpToDate*, Edwards, M. S., & Tunkel, A. R. (Eds.).

61 Azka, A., et al. (2019). Ommaya reservoir related complications: A single center experience and review of current literature. *International Journal of Clinical Oncology and Cancer Research, 4*(2), 10–24. (Level I)

62 Bosse, R., et al. (2018). A retrospective review of complication rates of Ommaya reservoir placement for intrathecal medication administration. *Journal of Clinical Oncology, 36*(Suppl. 15), e18532. (Level VI)

OPIOID WITHDRAWAL MANAGEMENT

Opioid withdrawal syndrome occurs after the abrupt reduction or discontinuation of opioids after heavy, prolonged use (also known as *spontaneous withdrawal*) or the administration of an opioid antagonist (such as naloxone) to a patient who's physically dependent on opioids (also known as *precipitated withdrawal*).[1] The onset of opioid withdrawal varies, depending on the opioid and whether the withdrawal is spontaneous or precipitated. Opioid withdrawal commonly occurs within 6 to 12 hours after the last dose of short-acting opioids (such as heroin or oxyCODONE) and within 30 hours after the last dose of long-acting opioids (such as methadone).[1,2] After administration of naloxone to an opioid-dependent patient, opioid withdrawal can occur within minutes.[1]

Although rarely life-threatening, opioid withdrawal causes uncomfortable symptoms for the patient and results in opioid cravings that may lead to relapse.[1,2] (See *Signs and symptoms of opioid withdrawal*.)

Pharmacologic management of opioid withdrawal typically consists of a tapering dose of a long-acting opioid substitute or a nonopioid adjunct in combination with nonopioid medications to treat the patient's symptoms. Although pharmacologic management of opioid withdrawal can ease the patient's symptoms, it isn't a cure for opioid use disorder, which requires psychosocial treatment with long-term, medication-assisted therapy using methadone, buprenorphine, or naltrexone.[1,2,3]

Equipment

Vital signs monitoring equipment ■ stethoscope ■ facility-approved opioid withdrawal assessment tool ■ prescribed medications and administration supplies ■ disinfectant pad ■ emergency equipment (code cart with emergency medications, defibrillator, handheld resuscitation bag with mask, intubation equipment) ■ Optional: gloves, gown, mask and goggles or mask with face shield, cardiac monitor, pulse oximeter and probe, laboratory specimen collection supplies, laboratory biohazard transport bag, prescribed IV fluid and administration supplies.

Signs and symptoms of opioid withdrawal

Signs and symptoms of opioid withdrawal include sympathetic nervous system effects, central nervous system effects, flulike symptoms, and gastrointestinal upset.[1,2]

Sympathetic nervous system effects
- Hypertension (mild)
- Tachycardia (mild)
- Mydriasis (dilated pupils)
- Excessive yawning
- Tremor

Central nervous system effects
- Anxiety
- Agitation
- Restlessness
- Irritability
- Insomnia

Flulike symptoms
- Lacrimation (tearing)
- Rhinorrhea (runny nose)
- Sneezing
- Myalgia (muscle aches)
- Arthralgia (joint pain)
- Diaphoresis (sweating)
- Chills
- Piloerection (gooseflesh)

Gastrointestinal upset
- Abdominal cramps
- Diarrhea
- Nausea
- Vomiting

Preparation of equipment

Inspect all equipment and supplies. If a product is expired, is defective, or has compromised integrity, remove it from patient use, label it as expired or defective, and report the expiration or defect, as directed by your facility.

Make sure emergency equipment is readily available and functioning properly.

Implementation

- Review the patient's medical record for a history of opioid use, previous withdrawal episodes, common comorbidities (such as substance abuse of alcohol or other drugs and psychiatric disorders), and conditions that may increase the risk of complications and death during opioid withdrawal (such as coronary artery disease, heart failure, insulin-dependent diabetes mellitus, epilepsy, and liver failure).[1,2]
- Perform hand hygiene.[4,5,6,7,8,9]
- Confirm the patient's identity using at least two patient identifiers.[10]
- Provide privacy.[11,12,13,14]
- Provide nonjudgmental, supportive, empathetic, comprehensive emotional care.

NURSING ALERT *Because opioid withdrawal can cause the patient to experience anxiety, agitation, restlessness, and irritability, the patient may become aggressive to health care workers. Provide emotional support and display empathy, which may diffuse aggression and help promote a therapeutic relationship.*[2]

- Explain the procedure to the patient and family (if appropriate) according to their individual communication and learning needs *to increase their understanding, allay their fears, and enhance cooperation.*[15]
- Ask the patient about opioid use. Determine the opioid amount, frequency, length of use, and date and time of last use. Note that patients experiencing opioid withdrawal commonly describe themselves as "sick" from not using opioids.[16]
- Raise the bed to waist level before providing care *to prevent caregiver back strain.*[17]

- Perform hand hygiene.[4,5,6,7,8,9]
- Put on gloves and other personal protective equipment, as necessary, *to comply with standard precautions.*[18,19,20]
- Obtain the patient's vital signs *to identify hypertension and tachycardia associated with opioid withdrawal.*[2] Monitor the patient's vital signs at a frequency determined by your facility or the practitioner's order, and according to the patient's condition.
- If the patient is at high risk for complications during opioid withdrawal, attach a continuous cardiac monitor and pulse oximeter *to monitor closely for changes in condition.*[1,2] Make sure that alarm limits are set appropriately for the patient's current condition, and that alarms are turned on, functioning properly, and audible to staff.[21,22,23]
- Assess the patient for signs and symptoms of opioid withdrawal using a facility-approved opioid withdrawal tool, such as the commonly used Clinical Opioid Withdrawal Scale (COWS).[24,25] Other validated tools include the Clinical Institute Narcotic Assessment (CINA) Scale, the Objective Opioid Withdrawal Scale (OOWS), and the Subjective Opioid Withdrawal Scale (SOWS). Perform serial assessments using the same tool at a frequency determined by your facility or the practitioner's order, and according to the patient's condition, *to identify trends and gauge treatment efficacy.*[1,2,3]
- Obtain laboratory specimens, if ordered, *to identify fluid and electrolyte imbalances resulting from vomiting and diarrhea.*[2,16] Label all specimens in the presence of the patient *to prevent mislabeling.*[10] Place the specimens in a laboratory biohazard transport bag and send them to the laboratory immediately. Notify the practitioner of critical test results within your facility's established time frame *so that the patient can receive prompt treatment.*[26]
- Monitor the patient's intake and output. Administer IV fluids, if prescribed, *to replace fluids lost through vomiting and diarrhea and help correct electrolyte imbalances.*[2,16]
- Administer prescribed medications following safe medication administration practices *to control the patient's symptoms of opioid withdrawal.*[27,28,29,30] (See *Common medications for treating opioid withdrawal.*)

Common medications for treating opioid withdrawal

Typical management of opioid withdrawal includes administration of a tapering dose of a long-acting opioid agonist, such as methadone, buprenorphine, or an alpha-2 adrenergic agonist, such as cloNIDine, with medications targeted to the patient's specific symptoms. The table below lists common medications for treating opioid withdrawal, along with their class, action or use, and special considerations. Note that the use of some of these medications for opioid withdrawal may be off-label.[1,2,3,31]

Medication	Action or use	Special considerations
Opioid agonists		
Methadone	Competes with opioids for mu receptors	- Possible precipitated withdrawal with concurrent administration of opioid antagonists, agonists, or partial agonists - Many drug interactions - Possible respiratory depression, hypotension, profound sedation, coma, or death with concurrent use with central nervous system (CNS) depressants, including alcohol - Possible withdrawal syndrome with abrupt discontinuation - Possible QT-interval prolongation[32]
Buprenorphine	Partially competes with opioids for mu receptors	- Not for use in precipitated withdrawal - Fewer drug interactions than methadone - Possible precipitation of opioid withdrawal symptoms with administration before onset of moderate opioid withdrawal symptoms - Possible respiratory depression, hypotension, profound sedation, coma, or death with concurrent use with CNS depressants, including alcohol[33]
Opioid antagonists		
Naloxone	Competes with opioids at the mu-receptors	- Combination medication product with oral buprenorphine naloxone; deterrent to IV buprenorphine abuse (precipitating withdrawal symptoms)[34,35]
Naltrexone	Competes with opioids at the mu receptors	- Acceleration of withdrawal in some treatment protocols, reducing treatment time - Close monitoring of the patient and careful management of resulting withdrawal symptoms necessary with accelerated treatment[34]

Common medications for treating opioid withdrawal *(continued)*

MEDICATION	ACTION OR USE	SPECIAL CONSIDERATIONS
ALPHA-2 ADRENERGIC AGONIST		
CloNIDine	Suppresses overactivity of the brain's noradrenergic system	■ Less effective than opioid agonists ■ Possible cause of hypotension and bradycardia
Lofexidine	Suppresses overactivity of the brain's noradrenergic system	■ Possible cause of hypotension, bradycardia, and syncope ■ Possible QT-interval prolongation ■ Possible potentiation of the effects of other CNS depressants ■ Essential to taper administration gradually, avoiding abrupt discontinuation ■ Common adjunctive therapy for symptom control rather than primary therapy[34,36]
SYMPTOM MANAGEMENT		
DiazePAM (and other benzodiazepines)	Anxiety, restlessness, irritability, insomnia	■ Possible oversedation with opioid agonists
HydrOXYzine	Anxiety, restlessness, insomnia, nausea, vomiting	■ Possible oversedation with opioid agonists
DiphenhydrAMINE	Anxiety, restlessness, insomnia, nausea, vomiting	■ Possible oversedation with opioid agonists
TiZANidine	Muscle spasms	■ Possible respiratory depression with other CNS depressants, including alcohol ■ Possible hypotension and sedation ■ Contraindicated for use with other alpha-2 adrenergic agonists[34,37]
Ondansetron	Nausea, vomiting	■ Possible QT-interval prolongation[38]
Loperamide	Diarrhea	■ Possible cardiac arrhythmias at high doses
Bismuth-salicylate	Diarrhea, GI upset	■ Not for use in patients allergic to salicylates (including aspirin)
Ibuprofen (and other nonsteroidal anti-inflammatory drugs)	Muscle and joint pain	■ Not for use in patients with known allergy to ibuprofen or aspirin[39] ■ Possible severe gastric bleeding, especially in patients age 60 or older and in those with a history of stomach ulcers or bleeding disorders[39] ■ Possible severe gastric bleeding when used with anticoagulants, corticosteroids, or other nonsteroidal anti-inflammatory drugs[39]
Acetaminophen	Muscle and joint pain	■ Possible severe liver damage in patients who consume alcohol and take acetaminophen in excess of 4,000 mg in 24 hours[40] ■ Not for use with other medications containing acetaminophen[40]

■ Provide one-on-one supervision, if necessary, *to ensure the safety of the patient, staff, and visitors.*
■ Return the bed to the lowest position *to prevent falls and maintain patient safety.*[41]
■ Discard used supplies in appropriate receptacles.[19]
■ Remove and discard your gloves and other personal protective equipment you wore.[19]
■ Perform hand hygiene.[4,5,6,7,8,9]
■ Clean and disinfect your stethoscope with a disinfectant pad.[42,43]
■ Perform hand hygiene.[4,5,6,7,8,9]
■ Coordinate care with other services, such as social work, case management, and community resources, as appropriate, to plan for comprehensive outpatient care with medication-assisted therapy and psychosocial support after withdrawal symptoms have subsided.[1,2]
■ Document the procedure.[44,45,46,47]

Special considerations

■ Pregnant women with opioid use disorder experiencing withdrawal should receive long-term treatment throughout the pregnancy with an opioid agonist, rather than a tapered dose or abstinence, *because opioid withdrawal poses a risk to the fetus.*[1]
■ If the patient exhibits signs of violent or aggressive behavior, use de-escalation strategies or provide crisis intervention. Report violence or a credible threat to leadership and facility security staff (and, as necessary, to law enforcement), following the channels designated by your facility.[48,49] (See *De-escalation strategies.*)

Consider referring the patient to mutual-help programs, such as Narcotics Anonymous (NA), Methadone Anonymous (MA), Self-Management and Recovery Therapy (SMART), and Moderation

De-escalation strategies

Patients who are experiencing opioid withdrawal may display violent or aggressive behavior. Early recognition and use of de-escalation strategies aimed at defusing a volatile situation is the preferred approach to protecting the safety of the patient, staff, and visitors. In such a situation, institute these de-escalation strategies:[49,50,51]

■ Be empathetic and nonjudgmental when the patient says or does something that you perceive as irrational.
■ Respect the patient's personal space by standing 1½' to 3' (46 to 91.5 cm) away from the escalating patient. If you must enter the patient's personal space to provide care, explain your actions *so the patient feels less confused or frightened.*
■ Use nonthreatening nonverbal communication. Be aware of your facial expressions, gestures, movements, and tone of voice.
■ Don't overreact; instead, remain calm, rational, and professional.
■ Pay attention to the patient's feelings. Be aware that some patients have trouble identifying how they feel about what's happening to them.
■ Ignore challenging questions by the patient that could result in a power struggle. If the patient challenges your authority, redirect the patient's attention to the real issue *so you can work together to solve the problem.*
■ Set limits with the patient that are clear, simple, and enforceable, *because the patient may not be able to focus on everything you say.* Offer the patient respectful and concise choices and consequences.
■ Choose wisely which rules are negotiable and which aren't. *You may be able to avoid unnecessary altercations by offering the patient options and flexibility.*
■ Allow periods of silence *to give the patient a chance to reflect on what's happening and what the patient needs to proceed.*
■ Permit time for decisions. *The patient's stress level may rise if the patient feels rushed.*

Management.[1] Also consider referring family members to a program specifically for friends and family of patients with opioid use disorder, such as Nar-Anon.

Complications

Medications for opioid withdrawal management can cause various adverse effects, depending on the agent. Without adequate treatment, excessive vomiting and diarrhea can lead to volume depletion and electrolyte imbalances, possibly resulting in hypotension, cardiac arrhythmias, and death, especially in a patient with comorbidities.[2,52]

Documentation

Document the patient's history of opioid use, including the name of the opioid, amount, frequency, length of use, and date and time of last use. Record the patient's vital signs, your assessment findings (including the scores of your facility's opioid withdrawal assessment tool), the patient's intake and output, and any laboratory test results. Document medications you administered, the patient's response to those medications, and any adverse effects. Record your interventions and the patient's response to those interventions. Document any teaching you provided to the patient and family, their understanding of the teaching, and any need for follow-up teaching.

REFERENCES

1 American Society of Addiction Medicine (ASAM). (2015). *The national practice guideline for the use of medications in the treatment of addiction involving opioid use.* Chevy Chase, MD: ASAM. https://www.asam.org/docs/default-source/practice-support/guidelines-and-consensus-docs/asam-national-practice-guideline-supplement.pdf (Level VII)

2 Duber, H. C., et al. (2018). Identification, management, and transition of care for patients with opioid use disorder in the emergency department. *Annals of Emergency Medicine, 72,* 420–431.

3 Schuckit, M. A. (2016). Treatment of opioid-use disorders. *New England Journal of Medicine, 374,* 357–368.

4 Accreditation Association for Hospitals and Health Systems. (2020). Standard 07.01.21. *Healthcare Facilities Accreditation Program: Accreditation requirements for acute care hospitals.* Chicago, IL: Accreditation Association for Hospitals and Health Systems. (Level VII)

5 Centers for Disease Control and Prevention. (2002). Guideline for hand hygiene in health-care settings: Recommendations of the Healthcare Infection Control Practices Advisory Committee and the HICPAC/SHEA/APIC/IDSA Hand Hygiene Task Force. *MMWR Recommendations and Reports, 51*(RR-16), 1–45. https://www.cdc.gov/mmwr/pdf/rr/rr5116.pdf (Level II)

6 Centers for Medicare and Medicaid Services, Department of Health and Human Services. (2020). Condition of participation: Infection control. 42 C.F.R. § 482.42.

7 DNV GL-Healthcare USA, Inc. (2020). IC.1.SR.1. *NIAHO® accreditation requirements, interpretive guidelines and surveyor guidance—revision 20.0.* Milford, OH: DNV GL-Healthcare USA, Inc. (Level VII)

8 The Joint Commission. (2021). Standard NPSG.07.01.01. *Comprehensive accreditation manual for hospitals.* Oakbrook Terrace, IL: The Joint Commission. (Level VII)

9 World Health Organization. (2009). WHO guidelines on hand hygiene in health care: First global patient safety challenge, clean care is safer care. https://apps.who.int/iris/bitstream/handle/10665/44102/9789241597906_eng.pdf?sequence=1 (Level IV)

10 The Joint Commission. (2021). Standard NPSG.01.01.01. *Comprehensive accreditation manual for hospitals.* Oakbrook Terrace, IL: The Joint Commission. (Level VII)

11 Accreditation Association for Hospitals and Health Systems. (2020). Standard 15.01.16. *Healthcare Facilities Accreditation Program: Accreditation requirements for acute care hospitals.* Chicago, IL: Accreditation Association for Hospitals and Health Systems. (Level VII)

12 Centers for Medicare and Medicaid Services, Department of Health and Human Services. (2020). Condition of participation: Patient's rights. 42 C.F.R. § 482.13 (c)(1).

13 DNV GL-Healthcare USA, Inc. (2020). PR.2.SR.5. *NIAHO® accreditation requirements, interpretive guidelines and surveyor guidance—revision 20.0.* Milford, OH: DNV GL-Healthcare USA, Inc. (Level VII)

14 The Joint Commission. (2021). Standard RI.01.01.01. *Comprehensive accreditation manual for hospitals.* Oakbrook Terrace, IL: The Joint Commission. (Level VII)

15 The Joint Commission. (2021). Standard PC.02.01.21. *Comprehensive accreditation manual for hospitals.* Oakbrook Terrace, IL: The Joint Commission. (Level VII)

16 Stolbach, A., & Hoffman, R. S. (2020). Opioid withdrawal in the emergency setting. In: *UpToDate,* Traub, S. J. (Ed.).

17 Waters, T. R., et al. (2009). Safe patient handling training for schools of nursing. https://www.cdc.gov/niosh/docs/2009-127/pdfs/2009-127.pdf (Level VII)

18 Accreditation Association for Hospitals and Health Systems. (2020). Standard 07.01.10. *Healthcare Facilities Accreditation Program: Accreditation requirements for acute care hospitals.* Chicago, IL: Accreditation Association for Hospitals and Health Systems. (Level VII)

19 Occupational Safety and Health Administration. (2012). Bloodborne pathogens, standard number 1910.1030. https://www.osha.gov/pls/oshaweb/owadisp.show_document?p_id=10051&p_table=STANDARDS (Level VII)

20 Siegel, J. D., et al. (2007, revised 2019). 2007 guideline for isolation precautions: Preventing transmission of infectious agents in healthcare settings. https://www.cdc.gov/infectioncontrol/pdf/guidelines/isolation-guidelines-H.pdf (Level II)

21 American Association of Critical-Care Nurses. (2018). AACN practice alert: Managing alarms in acute care across the life span—electrocardiography and pulse oximetry. https://www.aacn.org/clinical-resources/practice-alerts/managing-alarms-in-acute-care-across-the-life-span (Level VII)

22 The Joint Commission. (2021). Standard NPSG.06.01.01. *Comprehensive accreditation manual for hospitals.* Oakbrook Terrace, IL: The Joint Commission. (Level VII)

23 Graham, K. C., & Cvach, M. (2010). Monitor alarm fatigue: Standardizing use of physiological monitors and decreasing nuisance alarms. *American Journal of Critical Care, 19,* 28–37. https://aacnjournals.org/ajcconline/article-abstract/19/1/28/5720/Monitor-Alarm-Fatigue-Standardizing-Use-of?redirectedFrom=fulltext

24 Wesson, D. R., & Ling, W. (2003). The Clinical Opiate Withdrawal Scale (COWS). *Journal of Psychoactive Drugs, 35*(2), 253–259.

25 Tompkins, D. A., et al. (2009). Concurrent validation of the Clinical Opiate Withdrawal Scale (COWS) and single-item indices against the Clinical Institute Narcotic Assessment (CINA) opioid withdrawal instrument. *Drug and Alcohol Dependence, 105*(1–2), 154–159. (Level II)

26 The Joint Commission. (2021). Standard NPSG.02.03.01. *Comprehensive accreditation manual for hospitals.* Oakbrook Terrace, IL: The Joint Commission. (Level VII)

27 Accreditation Association for Hospitals and Health Systems. (2020). Standard 16.01.03. *Healthcare Facilities Accreditation Program: Accreditation requirements for acute care hospitals.* Chicago, IL: Accreditation Association for Hospitals and Health Systems. (Level VII)

28 Centers for Medicare and Medicaid Services, Department of Health and Human Services. (2020). Condition of participation: Nursing services. 42 C.F.R. § 482.23 (c).

29 DNV GL-Healthcare USA, Inc. (2020). MM.1.SR.3. *NIAHO® accreditation requirements, interpretive guidelines and surveyor guidance– revision 20.0.* Milford, OH: DNV GL-Healthcare USA, Inc. (Level VII)

30 The Joint Commission. (2021). Standard MM.06.01.01. *Comprehensive accreditation manual for hospitals.* Oakbrook Terrace, IL: The Joint Commission. (Level VII)

31 Broglio, K., & Matzo, M. (2018). Acute pain management for people with opioid use disorder. *American Journal of Nursing, 118*(10), 30–38.

32 Lexicomp. (2020). Methadone (Lexi-Drugs). Wolters Kluwer Clinical Drug Information, Inc.

33 Lexicomp. (2020). Buprenorphine (Lexi-Drugs). Wolters Kluwer Clinical Drug Information, Inc.

34 Sevarino, K. A. (2020). Medically supervised opioid withdrawal during treatment for addiction. In: *UpToDate.* Saxon, A. J. (Ed.)

35 BioDelivery Sciences International. (2019). Bunavail® (buprenorphine and naloxone buccal film) prescribing information. https://www.accessdata.fda.gov/drugsatfda_docs/label/2019/205637s020lbl.pdf

36 US WorldMeds. (2018). Lucemyra™ (lofexidine) prescribing information. https://www.accessdata.fda.gov/drugsatfda_docs/label/2018/209229s000lbl.pdf

37 Acorda Therapeutics. (2013). Zanaflex Capsules® (tizanidine hydrochloride) prescribing information. https://www.accessdata.fda.gov/drugsatfda_docs/label/2013/021447s011_020397s026lbl.pdf

38 Novartis Pharmaceuticals Corporation. (2017). Zofran® (ondansetron hydrochloride) prescribing information. https://www.accessdata.fda.gov/drugsatfda_docs/label/2017/020103s036,020605s020,020781s020lbl.pdf

39 Pfizer. (2018). Advil tablets label. https://www.accessdata.fda.gov/drugsatfda_docs/label/2018/018989Orig1s090lbl.pdf

40 Johnson and Johnson Consumer, Inc. (n.d.). Tylenol safety profile. https://www.tylenolprofessional.com/safety-and-efficacy/safety

41 Ganz, D. A., et al. (2013). Preventing falls in hospitals: A toolkit for improving quality of care (AHRQ publication no. 13-0015-EF). https://www.ahrq.gov/professionals/systems/hospital/fallpxtoolkit/index.html (Level VII)

42 Accreditation Association for Hospitals and Health Systems. (2020). Standard 07.02.03. *Healthcare Facilities Accreditation Program: Accreditation requirements for acute care hospitals.* Chicago, IL: Accreditation Association for Hospitals and Health Systems. (Level VII)

43 Rutala, W. A., et al. (2008, revised 2019). Guideline for disinfection and sterilization in healthcare facilities, 2008. https://www.cdc.gov/infection-control/pdf/guidelines/disinfection-guidelines-H.pdf (Level I)

44 Accreditation Association for Hospitals and Health Systems. (2020). Standard 10.00.03. *Healthcare Facilities Accreditation Program: Accreditation requirements for acute care hospitals.* Chicago, IL: Accreditation Association for Hospitals and Health Systems. (Level VII)

45 Centers for Medicare and Medicaid Services, Department of Health and Human Services. (2020). Condition of participation: Medical record services. 42 C.F.R. § 482.24 (b).

46 DNV GL-Healthcare USA, Inc. (2020). MR.2.SR.1. *NIAHO® accreditation requirements, interpretive guidelines and surveyor guidance—revision 20.0.* Milford, OH: DNV GL-Healthcare USA, Inc. (Level VII)

47 The Joint Commission. (2021). Standard RC.01.03.01. *Comprehensive accreditation manual for hospitals.* Oakbrook Terrace, IL: The Joint Commission. (Level VII)

48 The Joint Commission. (2018). Sentinel event alert 59: Physical and verbal violence against health care workers. https://www.jointcommission.org/-/media/tjc/documents/resources/patient-safety-topics/sentinel-event/sea-59-workplace-violence-final2.pdf (Level VII)

49 Crisis Prevention Institute, Inc. (2020). CPI's top 10 de-escalation tips. https://www.crisisprevention.com/Blog/CPI-s-Top-10-De-Escalation-Tips-Revisited (Level VII)

50 Boyd, M. A. (2018). *Psychiatric nursing: Contemporary practice* (6th ed.). Philadelphia, PA: Wolters Kluwer.

51 The Joint Commission. (2019). De-escalation in health care. *Quick Safety, 47*, 1–5. https://www.jointcommission.org/-/media/tjc/documents/resources/workplace-violence/qs_deescalation_1_28_18_final.pdf?

52 Darke, S., et al. (2017). Yes, people can die from opiate withdrawal. *Addiction, 112*, 199–200.

ORAL CARE

Oral care promotes patient comfort, nutritional intake, and oral health, and reduces dental plaque, oral colonization, and mucosal inflammation.[1,2] Research shows that changes in oral bacterial colonization can occur within 48 hours of hospitalization.[3,4] Aspiration of small droplets of secretions while sleeping can occur even in healthy adults from such causes as supine positioning and medications that suppress the central nervous system. Aspiration of small droplets doesn't usually cause pneumonia; however, in combination with decreased mobility and changes in oral colonization, patients are at an increased risk for infection due to organism growth in the respiratory tract.[5] Without effective oral care, a patient can develop hospital-acquired pneumonia and other infections as well as reduced nutritional intake, which can increase mortality and hospital length of stay.[5,6]

Without effective oral care, a patient who is intubated can develop ventilator-associated pneumonia (VAP) and other infections, which can increase mortality and the length of hospital stay.[5,6] To reduce the risk of VAP, expect to perform oral care and other interventions, such as elevating the patient's head 30 to 45 degrees, assessing readiness to extubate through daily spontaneous awakening and breathing trials, implementing subglottic suctioning in patients who are expected to be intubated for more than 48 hours, engaging in early mobilization and exercise, and changing ventilator circuits only if visibly soiled.[7]

Providing oral care—including brushing the teeth, gums, and tongue with a soft, compact-head toothbrush; using an oral rinse; and moisturizing the oral mucosa—is essential for maintaining the patient's general health.[7]

Equipment

Gloves ▪ oral moisturizer ▪ swabs ▪ soft, compact-head toothbrush ▪ toothpaste (preferably plaque-removing)[8] ▪ oral rinse (preferably alcohol-free)[9] ▪ Optional: mask, goggles, mask with face shield, gown, facility-approved oral assessment tool, flossing device, emesis basin.

For a patient who can't expectorate or is dependent for oral care

Suction equipment ▪ suction toothbrush or tonsil-tip catheter ▪ Optional: bite block or mouth prop.[9]

For a patient with dentures or no teeth

Denture cup ▪ paper towel ▪ Optional: commercial denture cleanser, denture adhesive.

For an intubated patient

Gloves ▪ oral moisturizer ▪ swabs ▪ soft, compact-head toothbrush ▪ toothpaste (preferably plaque-removing)[8] ▪ suction equipment ▪ Optional: chlorhexidine oral rinse, bite block, oropharyngeal airway, facility-approved oral assessment tool, gown, mask, goggles, mask with face shield.

Preparation of equipment

Inspect all equipment and supplies. If a product is expired, is defective, or has compromised integrity, remove it from patient use, label it as expired or defective, and report the expiration or defect as directed by your facility. Set up suction equipment (if necessary) and ensure its proper functioning *to prevent aspiration during oral care.*

Implementation

▪ Gather and prepare the necessary equipment and supplies.
▪ Perform hand hygiene.[10,11,12,13,14,15]
▪ Confirm the patient's identity using at least two patient identifiers.[16]
▪ Explain the procedure to the patient and family (if appropriate) according to their individual communication and learning needs *to increase their understanding, allay their fears, and enhance cooperation.*[17]
▪ Provide privacy.[18,19,20]
▪ Raise the patient's bed to waist level before providing patient care *to prevent caregiver back strain.*[21]
▪ Perform hand hygiene.[10,11,12,13,14,15]
▪ Put on gloves and other personal protective equipment, as needed, *to comply with standard precautions.*[22,23,24]
▪ Assess the patient's current oral hygiene regimen and self-care ability *to help determine the level of oral care necessary.*[9]
▪ Assess the patient's oral health using a facility-approved assessment tool (if used in your facility) *to assess the condition of the teeth gums, tongue, lips, mucosa, and saliva.*[8,25]

For a patient who can expectorate and perform self-care

▪ Set up oral care supplies for the patient at a sink or on an overbed table.
▪ Instruct the patient to brush the teeth, gums, and tongue with a soft, compact-head toothbrush and toothpaste at least twice per day, but ideally four times per day (after each meal and at bedtime; or morning, midday, evening, and bedtime for the patient unable to receive oral intake). Brush the teeth for at least 2 minutes at each session.[1,4,26,27] Place the toothbrush at a 45-degree angle to the gums.[27] Move the brush back and forth gently using short strokes.[27] Brush the outer, inner, and then chewing surfaces of all teeth.[27] Tilt the brush vertically and make several up-and-down strokes to clean the inside surface of the front teeth.[27] Brush the gums and tongue *to remove bacteria.*[27]
▪ Instruct the patient to clean between the teeth daily using string floss (as shown on next page), a water flosser, or other flossing device. Advise the patient to clean before or after brushing at a time of day preferred

by the patient, *because there is no optimal time for cleaning between the teeth.*[28] Use about 18" (45 cm) of floss wound around one of the middle fingers with the rest wound around the opposite middle finger.[29] Hold the floss tightly between the thumbs and forefingers and gently insert it between the teeth.[29] Curve the floss into a "C" shape against the side of the tooth.[29] Rub the floss gently up and down, keeping it pressed against the tooth; don't jerk or snap the floss.[29] Floss all of the teeth, including behind the back teeth.[29]

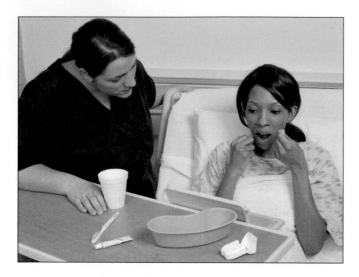

■ Instruct the patient to swish oral rinse in the mouth and then spit it into the sink or emesis basin.[8]
■ Tell the patient to moisturize the oral mucosa and lips every 2 to 4 hours, if desired, *to reduce oral inflammation and improve oral health.*[1,8]

For a patient who can't expectorate or is dependent for oral care
■ If necessary, insert a bite block or mouth prop *to hold the patient's mouth open during oral care.*[9]
■ Brush the patient's teeth, gums, and tongue with a soft, compact-head toothbrush and toothpaste at least twice per day but ideally four times per day. Brush the teeth for at least 2 minutes at each session using the brushing method described above.[1,4,8,27] Suction the patient's oral cavity using a tonsil-tip suction device *to prevent aspiration of secretions and debris.* Alternatively, moisten a suction toothbrush in oral rinse and then brush the patient's teeth, gums, and tongue with the toothbrush attached to continuous suction *to prevent aspiration.*[8]
■ If performed as part of oral care in your facility, clean between the patient's teeth daily using string floss, a water flosser, or other flossing device. Use the method described above for cleaning between the teeth. Clean before or after brushing at a time of day preferred by the patient, *because there is no optimal time for cleaning between the teeth.*[28]
■ Using a moistened swab, apply oral rinse *to reduce microbial colonization.*[4]
■ Using a swab, apply moisturizer to the oral mucosa and lips every 2 to 4 hours *to reduce oral inflammation and improve oral health.*[8]

For a patient with dentures or no teeth
■ Instruct the patient to remove the dentures, if present, and place them in a labeled denture cup. Alternatively, if the patient is unable, remove the dentures (if present) and place them in a labeled denture cup.[8]
■ Brush the patient's palate, buccal surfaces, gums, and tongue with a soft toothbrush or swab at least twice per day but ideally four times per day.[8]
■ Instruct the patient to swish oral rinse around in the mouth and then to spit it into the sink or emesis basin.[8]
■ Before adding water to the sink, line the sink with a paper towel *to cushion the dentures in case someone drops them.*[8]

■ Carefully brush the dentures using a soft toothbrush and warm water; don't use toothpaste, *because it may scratch the dentures.*[8]
■ If the patient requires denture adhesive to hold the dentures firmly in place, apply it according to the manufacturer's instructions.[8] Assist the patient with putting the dentures into the mouth. Alternatively, soak the dentures in commercial cleanser in the labeled denture cup if the patient desires.[8]
■ Using a swab, apply moisturizer to the oral mucosa and lips every 2 to 4 hours *to reduce oral inflammation and improve oral health.*[8]

For a patient who is intubated
■ Position the patient with the head of the bed elevated 30 to 45 degrees, unless contraindicated by the patient's condition, *to reduce the risk of aspiration and consequent VAP.* If the patient can't bend at the waist, use a reverse Trendelenburg position.[7,30]
■ Assess the patient's level of consciousness. If the patient is unconscious or disoriented, the patient may reflexively bite down when you introduce something into the mouth. Use a bite block or oropharyngeal airway, as necessary, *to keep the mouth open.*[25]
■ Assess the patient's oral health using a facility-approved oral assessment tool (if used in your facility) *to assess the condition of the teeth, gums, lips, mucosa, and saliva.*[25] For a patient with oral intubation, assess the skin under the endotracheal (ET) tube at least once per shift *to reduce the risk of device-associated pressure injury.*
■ Suction the patient as necessary before and during the procedure *to remove debris and oropharyngeal secretions.*[8]
■ Brush the patient's teeth, gums, and tongue with a soft, compact-head toothbrush and toothpaste at least twice per day. Brush the teeth for at least 2 minutes at each session (if tolerated).[1,26,27] Place the toothbrush at a 45-degree angle to the gums.[27] Move the brush back and forth gently using short strokes.[27] Brush the outer, inner, and then chewing surfaces of all teeth.[27] Tilt the brush vertically and make several up-and-down strokes to clean the inside surface of the front teeth.[27] Brush the gums and tongue to remove bacteria.
■ For a patient with no teeth, brush the palate, buccal surfaces, gums, and tongue with a soft toothbrush or swab at least twice per day.[8]
■ For a patient with oral intubation, carefully clean the portion of the ET tube in the oral cavity as part of oral care, *because plaque and bacterial biofilm can form on the tube's surface.*[25]
■ Moisturize the oral mucosa and lips every 2 to 4 hours *to reduce oral inflammation and improve oral health.*[1,31]
■ Use chlorhexidine oral rinse twice per day, if ordered or as directed by your facility, *to reduce microbial colonization.*[1] Apply it with a moistened swab.

After oral care
■ Reassess the patient's mouth for cleanliness and tooth and tissue condition.
■ Return the patient's bed to the low position *to maintain patient safety.*[32]
■ Discard used supplies in appropriate receptacles.[22]
■ Remove and discard your gloves and any other personal protective equipment worn.[22]
■ Perform hand hygiene.[10,11,12,13,14,15]
■ Put on gloves, as necessary.[22]
■ Clean and disinfect other reusable equipment according to the manufacturer's instructions *to prevent the spread of infection.*[33,34]
■ Remove and discard your gloves.[22]
■ Perform hand hygiene.[10,11,12,13,14,15]
■ Refer the patient to a dental professional, as indicated.[9]
■ Document the procedure.[35,36,37,38]

Special considerations
■ Move the ET tube to the other side of the mouth at least daily *to reduce pressure on the lips and oral cavity and subsequently reduce the risk of medical device–associated pressure injury.* Suction the patient's oropharynx before deflating the ET tube cuff and moving the tube. Replace the bite block or oropharyngeal airway along the ET tube, if necessary, *to prevent biting.*[4]

Patient teaching

Instruct the patient as needed in proper oral hygiene and the need for regular follow-up with a dental professional.[9]

Complications

Oral care may cause bleeding or pain in patients with gum disease, loose teeth, or ulcerations in the mouth. If the patient has loose teeth, oral care may cause further dislodgement.

Documentation

Record the date and time of oral care, whether the patient assisted in performing oral care, the type of oral care you administered, and the patient's response to the procedure. Record successful strategies in the patient's oral hygiene care plan.[9] Also document unusual conditions, such as bleeding, edema, mouth odor, excessive secretions, loose teeth, and plaque on the tongue. Document teaching you provided to the patient and family (if applicable), their understanding of that teaching, and any need for follow-up teaching.

REFERENCES

1 American Association of Critical-Care Nurses. (2017). AACN practice alert: Oral care for acutely and critically ill patients. *Critical Care Nurse, 37*(3), e19–e21. https://www.aacn.org/clinical-resources/practice-alerts/oral-care-for-acutely-and-critically-ill-patients

2 Salamone, K., et al. (2013). Oral care of hospitalised older patients in the acute medical setting. *Nursing Research and Practice, 2013*, 827670. https://www.ncbi.nlm.nih.gov/pmc/articles/PMC3683489

3 Heo, S. M., et al. (2008). A genetic relationship between respiratory pathogens isolated from dental plaque and bronchoalveolar lavage fluid from patients in the intensive care unit undergoing mechanical ventilation. *Clinical Infectious Diseases, 47*(12), 1562–1570. https://www.ncbi.nlm.nih.gov/pmc/articles/PMC3582026/ (Level IV)

4 Wiegand, D. L. (2017). *AACN procedure manual for high acuity, progressive, and critical care* (7th ed.). St. Louis, MO: Elsevier.

5 Quinn, B., & Baker, D. (2015). Using oral care to prevent nonventilator hospital-acquired pneumonia. https://www.myamericannurse.com/using-oral-care-prevent-nonventilator-hospital-acquired-pneumonia/

6 Murray, J., & Scholten, I. (2018). An oral hygiene protocol improves oral health for patients in inpatient stroke rehabilitation. *Gerodontology, 35*, 18–24.

7 American Association of Critical-Care Nurses. (2017). AACN practice alert: Ventilator-associated pneumonia. https://www.aacn.org/clinical-resources/practice-alerts/ventilator-associated-pneumonia-vap (Level VII)

8 Quinn, B., & Baker, D. L. (2015). Comprehensive oral care helps prevent hospital-acquired nonventilator pneumonia. *American Nurse Today, 10*(3), 18–22. https://www.myamericannurse.com/wp-content/uploads/2015/03/ant3-CE-Oral-Care-225.pdf

9 Johnson, V. B. (2012). Evidence-based practice guideline: Oral hygiene care for functionally dependent and cognitively impaired older adults. *Journal of Gerontological Nursing, 38*(11), 11–19. (Level I)

10 The Joint Commission. (2021). Standard NPSG.07.01.01. *Comprehensive accreditation manual for hospitals.* Oakbrook Terrace, IL: The Joint Commission. (Level VII)

11 World Health Organization. (2009). WHO guidelines on hand hygiene in health care: First global patient safety challenge, clean care is safer care. https://apps.who.int/iris/bitstream/handle/10665/44102/9789241597906_eng.pdf?sequence=1 (Level IV)

12 Centers for Disease Control and Prevention. (2002). Guideline for hand hygiene in health-care settings: Recommendations of the Healthcare Infection Control Practices Advisory Committee and the HICPAC/SHEA/APIC/IDSA Hand Hygiene Task Force. *MMWR Recommendations and Reports, 51*(RR-16), 1–45. https://www.cdc.gov/mmwr/pdf/rr/rr5116.pdf (Level II)

13 Centers for Medicare and Medicaid Services, Department of Health and Human Services. (2020). Condition of participation: Infection control. 42 C.F.R. § 482.42.

14 Accreditation Association for Hospitals and Health Systems. (2020). Standard 07.01.21. *Healthcare Facilities Accreditation Program: Accreditation requirements for acute care hospitals.* Chicago, IL: Accreditation Association for Hospitals and Health Systems. (Level VII)

15 DNV GL-Healthcare USA, Inc. (2020). IC.1.SR.1. *NIAHO® accreditation requirements, interpretive guidelines and surveyor guidance—revision 20.0.* Milford, OH: DNV GL-Healthcare USA, Inc. (Level VII)

16 The Joint Commission. (2021). Standard NPSG.01.01.01. *Comprehensive accreditation manual for hospitals.* Oakbrook Terrace, IL: The Joint Commission. (Level VII)

17 The Joint Commission. (2021). Standard PC.02.01.21. *Comprehensive accreditation manual for hospitals.* Oakbrook Terrace, IL: The Joint Commission. (Level VII)

18 Accreditation Association for Hospitals and Health Systems. (2020). Standard 15.01.16. *Healthcare Facilities Accreditation Program: Accreditation requirements for acute care hospitals.* Chicago, IL: Accreditation Association for Hospitals and Health Systems. (Level VII)

19 Centers for Medicare and Medicaid Services, Department of Health and Human Services. (2020). Condition of participation: Patient's rights. 42 C.F.R. § 482.13(c)(1).

20 The Joint Commission. (2021). Standard RI.01.01.01. *Comprehensive accreditation manual for hospitals.* Oakbrook Terrace, IL: The Joint Commission. (Level VII)

21 Waters, T. R., et al. (2009). Safe patient handling training for schools of nursing. https://www.cdc.gov/niosh/docs/2009-127/pdfs/2009-127.pdf

22 Occupational Safety and Health Administration. (2019). Bloodborne pathogens, standard number 1910.1030. https://www.osha.gov/pls/oshaweb/owadisp.show_document?p_id=10051&p_table=STANDARDS (Level VII)

23 Siegel, J. D., et al. (2007, revised 2019). 2007 guideline for isolation precautions: Preventing transmission of infectious agents in healthcare settings. https://www.cdc.gov/infectioncontrol/pdf/guidelines/isolation-guidelines-H.pdf (Level II)

24 Accreditation Association for Hospitals and Health Systems. (2020). Standard 07.01.10. *Healthcare Facilities Accreditation Program: Accreditation requirements for acute care hospitals.* Chicago, IL: Accreditation Association for Hospitals and Health Systems. (Level VII)

25 Ames, N. J., et al. (2011). Effects of systematic oral care in critically ill patients: A multicenter study. *American Journal of Critical Care, 20*, e103–e114.

26 American Dental Association. (n.d.). Brushing your teeth. https://www.mouthhealthy.org/en/az-topics/b/brushing-your-teeth

27 American Dental Association. (2012). How to brush. https://www.mouthhealthy.org/-/media/MouthHealthy/Files/Kids_Section/ADAHowToBrush_Eng.pdf?la=en

28 American Dental Association. (n.d.). Flossing. https://www.mouthhealthy.org/en/az-topics/f/flossing

29 American Dental Association. (n.d.). 5 steps to a flawless floss. https://www.mouthhealthy.org/en/az-topics/f/flossing-steps

30 Klompas, M., et al. (2014). Strategies to prevent ventilator-associated pneumonia in acute care hospitals: 2014 update. *Infection Control and Hospital Epidemiology, 35*(8), 915–936. https://www.jstor.org/stable/10.1086/677144?seq=1#page_scan_tab_contents (Level I)

31 Kiyoshi-Teo, H., & Blegen, M. (2015). Influences of institutional guidelines on oral hygiene practices in intensive care units. *American Journal of Critical Care, 24*, 309–318. (Level IV)

32 Ganz, D. A., et al. (2013, reviewed 2021). Preventing falls in hospitals: A toolkit for improving quality of care (AHRQ publication no. 13-0015-EF). https://www.ahrq.gov/professionals/systems/hospital/fallpxtoolkit/index.html (Level VII)

33 Accreditation Association for Hospitals and Health Systems. (2020). Standard 07.02.03. *Healthcare Facilities Accreditation Program: Accreditation requirements for acute care hospitals.* Chicago, IL: Accreditation Association for Hospitals and Health Systems. (Level VII)

34 Rutala, W. A., et al. (2008, revised 2019). Guideline for disinfection and sterilization in healthcare facilities, 2008. https://www.cdc.gov/infectioncontrol/pdf/guidelines/disinfection-guidelines-H.pdf (Level I)

35 The Joint Commission. (2021). Standard RC.01.03.01. *Comprehensive accreditation manual for hospitals.* Oakbrook Terrace, IL: The Joint Commission. (Level VII)

36 Centers for Medicare and Medicaid Services, Department of Health and Human Services. (2020). Condition of participation: Medical record services. 42 C.F.R. § 482.24(b).

37 Accreditation Association for Hospitals and Health Systems. (2020). Standard 10.00.03. *Healthcare Facilities Accreditation Program: Accreditation requirements for acute care hospitals.* Chicago, IL: Accreditation Association for Hospitals and Health Systems. (Level VII)

38 DNV GL-Healthcare USA, Inc. (2020). MR.2.SR.1. *NIAHO® accreditation requirements, interpretive guidelines and surveyor guidance—revision 20.0.* Milford, OH: DNV GL-Healthcare USA, Inc. (Level VII)

ORAL DRUG ADMINISTRATION

Because oral administration is usually the safest, most convenient, and least expensive method, most drugs are administered by this route. Drugs for oral administration are available in many forms: tablets, enteric-coated tablets, capsules, syrups, elixirs, oils, liquids, suspensions, powders, and granules. Some require special preparation before administration, such as mixing with juice to make them more palatable; oils, powders, and granules most often require such preparation.[1]

Sometimes oral drugs are prescribed in higher dosages than their parenteral equivalents, because after absorption through the GI system, they are immediately broken down by the liver before they reach the systemic circulation.

ELDER ALERT Oral dosages normally prescribed for adults may be dangerous for older adult patients because of decreased hepatic and renal clearance.[2]

Oral administration is contraindicated for unconscious patients; it may also be contraindicated in patients with nausea and vomiting and in those who can't swallow.

Make sure you understand the pharmacology behind the medications administered *to prevent potential error and patient harm.*[3]

Equipment

Patient's medication record ▪ prescribed drug ▪ medication cup ▪ water ▪ Optional: personal protective equipment, appropriate vehicle (such as pudding or applesauce) for crushed pills (commonly used with older adult patients), preferred beverage, pill-crushing device.

Implementation

▪ Avoid distractions and interruptions when preparing and administering medication *to prevent medication administration errors.*[4,5]

▪ Verify the order on the patient's medication record by checking it against the practitioner's order.[6,7,8,9]

▪ Reconcile the patient's medications when a new medication is ordered *to reduce the risk of medication errors, including omissions, duplications, dosing errors, and drug interactions.*

▪ Perform hand hygiene.[10,11,12,13,14,15]

NURSING ALERT If your facility's hazardous drug list contains the drug you're about to administer, put on personal protective equipment, as directed.[16]

▪ Gather and prepare the necessary equipment and supplies.

▪ Compare the medication label against the order in the patient's medical record.[6,7,8,9]

▪ Check the patient's medical record for an allergy or a contraindication to the prescribed medication. If an allergy or a contraindication exists, don't administer the medication; notify the practitioner.[6,7,8,9]

NURSING ALERT Cardiovascular agents, antibiotics, antifungals, antiretrovirals, diuretics, anticoagulants, antidiabetics, steroids, opioids, anticholinergics, benzodiazepines, and nonsteroidal anti-inflammatory drugs most commonly cause drug interactions. *To avoid drug interactions,* review with the patient all current prescribed and over-the-counter medications, dietary supplements, and herbal preparations. Notify the patient's practitioner and your facility's pharmacy of any potential interactions.[2,3,17,18,19]

▪ Check the expiration date on the medication (as shown below). If the medication is expired, return it to the pharmacy and obtain new medication.[6,7,8,9]

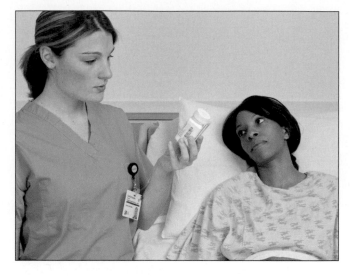

▪ Visually inspect the medication for any loss of integrity; don't administer the medication if its integrity is compromised.[6,7,8,9]

▪ Discuss any unresolved concerns about the medication with the patient's practitioner.[6,7,8,9]

▪ Perform hand hygiene.[10,11,12,13,14,15]

▪ Confirm the patient's identity using at least two patient identifiers.[20]

▪ Provide privacy.[21,22,23,24]

▪ Explain the procedure to the patient and family (if appropriate) according to their individual communication and learning needs *to increase their understanding, allay their fears, and enhance cooperation.*[25]

▪ If the patient is receiving the medication for the first time, teach about significant adverse reactions and discuss any other concerns related to the medication.[6,7,8,9]

▪ Assess the patient's condition *to determine the need for the medication and the effectiveness of previous therapy.*

▪ Carefully observe the patient for a rash, pruritus, cough, or other signs of an adverse reaction to a previously administered drug.

▪ Verify that the medication is being administered at the proper time, in the prescribed dose, and by the correct route *to reduce the risk of medication errors.*[6,7,8,9,26]

▪ If your facility uses a bar-code technology, use it as directed by your facility.

▪ Administer the medication to the patient (as shown below) along with an appropriate vehicle or liquid, as needed, *to aid swallowing, minimize adverse effects, or promote absorption.* For example, give cyclophosphamide with adequate amounts of fluids *to force diuresis and subsequently reduce the risk of urinary tract toxicity;*[27] give antitussive cough syrup without a fluid *to avoid diluting its soothing effect on the throat.*

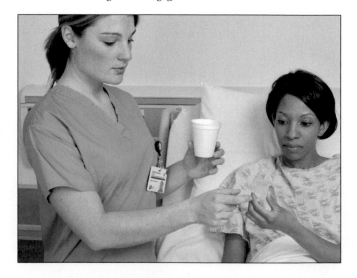

■ If the patient can't swallow a whole tablet or capsule, ask the pharmacist whether the drug is available in liquid form or can be administered by another route. If not, request a crushed tablet (if appropriate) or discuss whether you can crush the tablet yourself or open the capsule and mix it with food. Keep in mind that many enteric-coated timed-release medications and gelatin capsules shouldn't be crushed *to prevent possible adverse effects*. Contact the practitioner for an order to change the route of administration when necessary.

■ Stay with the patient until the drug has been swallowed. If the patient seems confused or disoriented, check the mouth *to make sure that the drug has been swallowed*.

■ Monitor the patient for adverse reactions and respond appropriately.[28]

■ Discard used supplies in appropriate receptacles.[29]

■ Perform hand hygiene.[10,11,12,13,14,15]

■ Document the procedure.[30,31,32,33]

Special considerations

■ Notify the practitioner about any medication that the patient refuses or that you withheld.

■ Assess parameters such as blood pressure and pulse as needed before administering a medication with dose-holding parameters.

■ Evaluate appropriate current laboratory test results (including potassium and digoxin levels), as needed and ordered, before administering medication affected by these values.

■ Have the pharmacy prepare and dispense an oral solution in a single-dose oral syringe whenever possible.[34] If not available, use care when measuring the prescribed dose of liquid oral medication. (See *Measuring liquid medications*.)

■ Don't administer medication from a poorly labeled or unlabeled container. Don't attempt to label or reinforce drug labels yourself; *this must be done by a pharmacist*.[35,36]

■ Never administer a medication prepared by someone else.

■ Never return unwrapped or prepared medications to stock containers; instead, dispose of them or return them to the pharmacy. Keep in mind that the disposal of any controlled substance must be cosigned by another nurse, as mandated by law.

■ If the patient questions you about the medication or dosage, check the medication record again. If the medication is correct, reassure the patient. Explain any changes in the medication or dosage. Teach the patient and family (if appropriate) about possible adverse effects. Ask the patient to report anything perceived as a possible adverse effect.

■ *To avoid damaging or staining the patient's teeth*, administer iron preparations through a straw.

■ An unpleasant-tasting liquid can usually be made more palatable if taken through a straw, *because the liquid contacts fewer taste buds, making it more palatable*.

■ When tablets must be split, request the pharmacy to split and repackage them before dispensing the medication *to prevent medication errors*.

Patient teaching

Teach the patient about the prescribed oral medications, including the indication; dosage; potential interactions with other drugs, foods, and herbal and dietary supplements; adverse effects; and special administration guidelines. Provide a completely reconciled list of medications and written information about those medications at discharge.[37,38]

Make sure you meet the communication and health literacy needs of the patient and caregiver (if appropriate) when providing discharge instructions.[39] To assist those with functional, cognitive, or memory deficits, provide detailed medication templates or pictorial aids; assist the patient and caregiver with memory aids and dispensing devices, as needed.[40]

Take special care when teaching older adult patients, who are at risk for polypharmacy. (See *Reducing medication risks in older adult patients*.)

Complications

Complications of oral medication administration include aspiration, adverse effects of the prescribed drug, and medication administration errors.

Measuring liquid medications

To pour liquids, hold the medication cup at eye level. Use your thumb to mark off the correct level on the cup (as shown below).

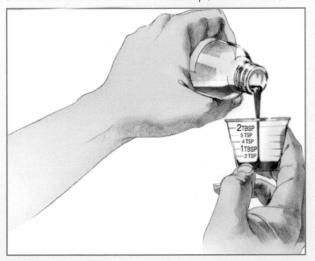

Then put the cup down and read the bottom of the meniscus (the curved surface of the liquid) at eye level *to ensure accuracy*. If you've poured too much medication into the cup, discard the excess; don't return it to the bottle. Here are a few additional tips:

■ Hold the container so that the medication flows from the side opposite the label *so it won't run down the container and stain or obscure the label*. Remove drips from the lip of the bottle first and then from the sides, using a clean, damp paper towel.

■ For a liquid measured in drops, use only the dropper supplied with the medication.

Reducing medication risks in older adult patients

To help prevent polypharmacy, you can help older adult patients manage and adhere to their medication regimens by instructing them (and caregivers, as appropriate) to take the following actions:[18]

■ Maintain an accurate list of all medications, including over-the-counter and prescribed drugs (generic and brand-names), dietary supplements, and herbal remedies; note dosages, dosing frequency, and the reason for use.

■ Maintain a complete list of practitioners and their contact information.

■ Bring all current medications to each practitioner's appointment.

■ Post the name and telephone number of the local pharmacy where it can be easily seen.

■ Adhere to dietary restrictions.

■ Understand potential medication-related problems that warrant emergency care.

■ Take medications exactly as directed.

■ Link dosing schedules to routine activities of daily living.

■ Use only one pharmacy to obtain medications.

■ Don't share medications with others.

■ Store medications in a secure, dry location away from sunlight.

■ Refrigerate medications, if necessary.

■ Properly dispose of old medications.

Documentation

Document the medication strength, dose, administration route, and date and time of administration.[41] Record pertinent assessment data you obtained before administration, such as the heart rate or symptoms that warranted the use of an as-needed medication. Record any adverse reactions to the prescribed medication, the date and time you notified the practitioner, prescribed interventions, and the patient's response to those interventions.[41] If the patient refuses a medication, document the refusal and the name of the practitioner you notified. Also note whether you omitted or withheld a medication for other reasons, such as for radiology or laboratory tests or if, in your judgment, the drug was contraindicated at the ordered time. Verify and sign out all controlled substances according to your facility's controlled substance documentation system. Document teaching you provided to the patient and family (if applicable), their understanding of that teaching, and any need for follow-up teaching.

REFERENCES

1 Emblin, K. (2013). Drug formulations and delivery systems. *Nurse Prescribing, 11*(2), 83–88.

2 Davies, E. A., & O'Mahony, M. S. (2015). Adverse drug reactions in special populations—The elderly. *British Journal of Clinical Pharmacology, 80*(4), 796–807. https://bpspubs.onlinelibrary.wiley.com/doi/epdf/10.1111/bcp.12596 (Level V)

3 Ndosi, M. E., & Newell, R. (2009). Nurses' knowledge of pharmacology behind drugs they commonly administer. *Journal of Clinical Nursing, 18,* 570–580. (Level VI)

4 Westbrook, J., et al. (2010). Association of interruptions with an increased risk and severity of medication administration errors. *Archives of Internal Medicine, 170,* 683–690. (Level IV)

5 Institute for Safe Medication Practices. (2012). Side tracks on the safety express: Interruptions lead to errors and unfinished…Wait, what was I doing? *Nurse Advise-ERR, 11*(2), 1–4. https://www.ismp.org/resources/side-tracks-safety-express-interruptions-lead-errors-and-unfinished-wait-what-was-i-doing?id=37

6 The Joint Commission. (2021). Standard MM.06.01.01. *Comprehensive accreditation manual for hospitals.* Oakbrook Terrace, IL: The Joint Commission. (Level VII)

7 Accreditation Association for Hospitals and Health Systems. (2020). Standard 16.01.03. *Healthcare Facilities Accreditation Program: Accreditation requirements for acute care hospitals.* Chicago, IL: Accreditation Association for Hospitals and Health Systems. (Level VII)

8 Centers for Medicare and Medicaid Services, Department of Health and Human Services. (2020). Condition of participation: Nursing services. 42 C.F.R. § 482.23(c).

9 DNV GL-Healthcare USA, Inc. (2020). MM.1.SR.3. *NIAHO® accreditation requirements, interpretive guidelines and surveyor guidance—revision 20.0.* Milford, OH: DNV GL-Healthcare USA, Inc. (Level VII)

10 The Joint Commission. (2021). Standard NPSG.07.01.01. *Comprehensive accreditation manual for hospitals.* Oakbrook Terrace, IL: The Joint Commission. (Level VII)

11 Centers for Disease Control and Prevention. (2002). Guideline for hand hygiene in health-care settings: Recommendations of the Healthcare Infection Control Practices Advisory Committee and the HICPAC/SHEA/APIC/IDSA Hand Hygiene Task Force. *MMWR Recommendations and Reports, 51*(RR-16), 1–45. https://www.cdc.gov/mmwr/pdf/rr/rr5116.pdf (Level II)

12 World Health Organization. (2009). WHO guidelines on hand hygiene in health care: First global patient safety challenge, clean care is safer care. https://apps.who.int/iris/bitstream/handle/10665/44102/9789241597906_eng.pdf?sequence=1 (Level IV)

13 Accreditation Association for Hospitals and Health Systems. (2020). Standard 07.01.21. *Healthcare Facilities Accreditation Program: Accreditation requirements for acute care hospitals.* Chicago, IL: Accreditation Association for Hospitals and Health Systems. (Level VII)

14 Centers for Medicare and Medicaid Services, Department of Health and Human Services. (2020). Condition of participation: Infection control. 42 C.F.R. § 482.42.

15 DNV GL-Healthcare USA, Inc. (2020). IC.1.SR.1. *NIAHO® accreditation requirements, interpretive guidelines and surveyor guidance—revision 20.0.* Milford, OH: DNV GL-Healthcare USA, Inc. (Level VII)

16 United States Pharmacopeial Convention. (2019). USP general chapter <800> Hazardous drugs—Handling in healthcare settings. https://www.usp.org/compounding/general-chapter-hazardous-drugs-handling-healthcare (Level VII)

17 Gabe, M. E., et al. (2011). Adverse drug reactions: Treatment burdens and nurse-led medication monitoring. *Journal of Nursing Management, 19,* 377–392. (Level V)

18 Woodruff, K. (2010). Preventing polypharmacy in older adults. *American Nurse, 5*(10). https://www.myamericannurse.com/preventing-polypharmacy-in-older-adults/

19 Runganga, M., et al. (2014). Multiple medication use in older patients in post-acute transitional care: A prospective cohort study. *Clinical Interventions in Aging, 9,* 1453–1462. https://www.ncbi.nlm.nih.gov/pmc/articles/PMC4158998/ (Level IV)

20 The Joint Commission. (2021). Standard NPSG.01.01.01. *Comprehensive accreditation manual for hospitals.* Oakbrook Terrace, IL: The Joint Commission. (Level VII)

21 Centers for Medicare and Medicaid Services, Department of Health and Human Services. (2020). Condition of participation: Patient's rights. 42 C.F.R. § 482.13(c)(1).

22 Accreditation Association for Hospitals and Health Systems. (2020). Standard 15.01.16. *Healthcare Facilities Accreditation Program: Accreditation requirements for acute care hospitals.* Chicago, IL: Accreditation Association for Hospitals and Health Systems. (Level VII)

23 DNV GL-Healthcare USA, Inc. (2020). PR.2.SR.5. *NIAHO® accreditation requirements, interpretive guidelines and surveyor guidance—revision 20.0.* Milford, OH: DNV GL-Healthcare USA, Inc. (Level VII)

24 The Joint Commission. (2021). Standard RI.01.01.01. *Comprehensive accreditation manual for hospitals.* Oakbrook Terrace, IL: The Joint Commission. (Level VII)

25 The Joint Commission. (2021). Standard PC.02.01.21. *Comprehensive accreditation manual for hospitals.* Oakbrook Terrace, IL: The Joint Commission. (Level VII)

26 Edwards, S., & Axe, S. (2015). The 10 'R's of safe multidisciplinary drug administration. *Nurse Prescribing, 13,* 398–406.

27 Roxane Laboratories, Inc. (2013). Cyclophosphamide capsules, for oral use. https://www.accessdata.fda.gov/drugsatfda_docs/label/2013/203856s000lbl.pdf

28 The Joint Commission. (2021). Standard MM.07.01.03. *Comprehensive accreditation manual for hospitals.* Oakbrook Terrace, IL: The Joint Commission. (Level VII)

29 Occupational Safety and Health Administration. (2012). Bloodborne pathogens, standard number 1910.1030. https://www.osha.gov/pls/oshaweb/owadisp.show_document?p_id=10051&p_table=STANDARDS

30 The Joint Commission. (2021). Standard RC.01.03.01. *Comprehensive accreditation manual for hospitals.* Oakbrook Terrace, IL: The Joint Commission. (Level VII)

31 Accreditation Association for Hospitals and Health Systems. (2020). Standard 10.00.03. *Healthcare Facilities Accreditation Program: Accreditation requirements for acute care hospitals.* Chicago, IL: Accreditation Association for Hospitals and Health Systems. (Level VII)

32 Centers for Medicare and Medicaid Services, Department of Health and Human Services. (2020). Condition of participation: Medical record services. 42 C.F.R. § 482.24(b).

33 DNV GL-Healthcare USA, Inc. (2020). MR.2.SR.1. *NIAHO® accreditation requirements, interpretive guidelines and surveyor guidance—revision 20.0.* Milford, OH: DNV GL-Healthcare USA, Inc. (Level VII)

34 Institute for Safe Medication Practices (ISMP). (2020). 2020-2021 targeted medication safety best practices for hospitals. https://www.ismp.org/sites/default/files/attachments/2020-02/2020-2021%20TMSBP-%20FINAL_1.pdf

35 The Joint Commission. (2021). Standard MM.05.01.09. *Comprehensive accreditation manual for hospitals.* Oakbrook Terrace, IL: The Joint Commission. (Level VII)

36 Accreditation Association for Hospitals and Health Systems. (2020). Standard 25.01.18. *Healthcare Facilities Accreditation Program: Accreditation requirements for acute care hospitals.* Chicago, IL: Accreditation Association for Hospitals and Health Systems. (Level VII)

37 Accreditation Association for Hospitals and Health Systems. (2020). Standard 25.02.13. *Healthcare Facilities Accreditation Program: Accreditation requirements for acute care hospitals.* Chicago, IL: Accreditation Association for Hospitals and Health Systems. (Level VII)

38 The Joint Commission. (2021). Standard NPSG.03.06.01. *Comprehensive accreditation manual for hospitals.* Oakbrook Terrace, IL: The Joint Commission. (Level VII)

39 The Joint Commission. (2010). *Advancing effective communication, cultural competence, and patient- and family-centered care: A roadmap for hospitals.* Oakbrook Terrace, IL: The Joint Commission. https://www. jointcommission.org/-/media/tjc/documents/resources/patient-safety-topics/health-equity/aroadmapforhospitalsfinalversion727pdf.pdf?d-b=web&hash=AC3AC4BED1D973713C2CA6B2E5ACD01B (Level VII)

40 Hesselink, G., et al. (2012). Are patients discharged with care? A qualitative study of perceptions and experiences of patients, family members, and care providers. *BMJ Quality and Safety, 21*(Suppl. 1), i39–i49. https://qualitysafety.bmj.com/content/21/Suppl_1/i39 (Level VI)

41 The Joint Commission. (2021). Standard RC.02.01.01. *Comprehensive accreditation manual for hospitals.* Oakbrook Terrace, IL: The Joint Commission. (Level VII)

ORGAN DONOR, IDENTIFICATION

In 1984, the U.S. Congress passed the National Organ Transplant Act, which established the Organ Procurement and Transplant Network, a national registry for organ matching.[1] This act was created to address the critical shortage of organ donations and to improve the organ matching and placement process. With passage of this act, it's now a federal requirement for U.S. health care facilities to identify potential organ donors.

In addition to requirements of the National Organ Transplant Act, the U.S. Department of Health and Human Services requires U.S. health care facilities to report every death or imminent death to the Organ Procurement Organization (OPO) as part of the health care facility's condition of participation and eligibility to receive Medicare funds. The Joint Commission has also addressed organ donation in its accreditation requirements.[2]

As part of the process of identifying a potential organ donor, to help elicit a more positive response from the family, the practitioner should keep the family members informed about the patient's condition and provide them with information about realistic expectations for the patient's outcome.[3,4] Separating brain death notification from the discussion of organ donation results in as much as an eight-times-greater chance that the family will consent to donation than when discussed together.[4] The hospital and OPO should agree when a referral to the OPO should be made. Guidelines vary on what criteria to use, but they generally stipulate that referral to the OPO should occur when a patient scores less than a 4 or 5 on the Glasgow Coma Scale[5,6] or in the absence of a patient's brain stem reflexes.[3,6]

As the need for organ donation continues to surge, timely identification and maintenance of potential organ donors becomes even more critical to saving lives. Innovative programs are needed to provide an effective model for identifying donors, creating decision protocols, and integrating organ donation into the end-of-life continuum of care.

Equipment

Organ donation information materials ▪ appropriate consent forms ▪ monitoring equipment ▪ Optional: personal protective equipment, laboratory specimen collection supplies, labels, laboratory biohazard transport bag, laboratory request forms.

Preparation of equipment

Have information regarding organ donation and appropriate consent forms readily available. Ensure that the information is provided in a language and at a literacy level that the family members can understand.[7,8,9]

Implementation

▪ Determine whether the patient has an advance directive that addresses organ donation or is listed in a donor registry (such as on a driver's license), *because these legal documents, which are supported in most states, may influence the family's ultimate decision.*[2,7,10,11,12]
▪ Keep the family informed of the patient's medical condition *to prepare them for realistic patient outcomes.*[3,4]
▪ Arrange for an interdisciplinary meeting with the family in a quiet, nonthreatening environment, if needed, *to further help the family realize the diagnosis and prognosis.*[6]

▪ Assess the family's spiritual needs, resources, and preferences. Refer the family to spiritual care services, as needed.[13,14]
▪ Consult the OPO coordinator in your area when the patient's death is imminent and before brain death testing begins *to convey that your facility is evaluating a potential candidate for organ donation, so that the coordinator can be present to guide staff members through the preparation process when appropriate.*[6]
▪ Collaborate with the OPO staff member in the exchange of critical information *to ensure that the family's unique needs are met. Planning with the OPO helps improve donation rates.*[6,15]
▪ Perform hand hygiene.[16,17,18,19,20,21]
▪ Confirm the patient's identity using at least two patient identifiers.[22]
▪ Put on personal protective equipment, including gloves, a gown, and eye protection, if indicated, *to comply with standard precautions.*[19,23,24]
▪ Collect laboratory samples as indicated *to provide data for the assessment of organ function.* Tests may include complete blood count, liver and renal function tests, electrolyte levels, and hepatitis and human immunodeficiency virus tests.[3,25] Label the specimens in the presence of the patient *to prevent mislabeling.*[22] Place the specimens in a laboratory biohazard transport bag and send them immediately to the laboratory with the appropriate laboratory request form, if necessary.[24]
▪ Monitor the patient's vital signs and hemodynamic and fluid status, *because a patient with decreased organ perfusion may not be eligible to donate an organ.*[3,25]
▪ Assist with examining the patient for the determination of brain death.[26]
▪ As applicable, ensure appropriate declaration and documentation of the patient's brain death. Many states have certain criteria that must be followed, as well as guidelines on what type of practitioner can make the declaration, before the OPO coordinator can officially approach family members and determine their willingness to discuss organ donation.[25]
▪ Contact the OPO coordinator if the patient is being evaluated for brain death or if support is being withdrawn in anticipation of imminent death *so that the coordinator can discuss organ donation with the family. An OPO coordinator has the special knowledge, training, and experience to be able to deliver the appropriate message to family.*[6]
▪ If the family agrees to proceed with organ donation, the OPO coordinator obtains dated and timed witnessed consent and then coordinates the process with the health care team.[7,9,27]
▪ Encourage the family to be at the bedside as much as possible and keep them informed as procedures and preparations are taking place *to help promote family time and facilitate closure.* Assure the family that the primary focus is on the care and dignity of the patient, whether or not the donation occurs.[6]
▪ Make sure that the family knows what to expect regarding end-of-life care, including when drugs are discontinued and ventilator or other therapies are withdrawn, *to help prevent additional grief or anxiety.*[6]
▪ Discard used supplies in the appropriate receptacles.[24]
▪ Remove and discard your gloves and personal protective equipment, if worn.[23,24]
▪ Perform hand hygiene.[16,17,18,19,20,21]
▪ Document the procedure.[28,29,30,31]

Special considerations

▪ Be sure to provide explanations to the family according to their individual communication and learning needs *to increase their understanding, allay their fears, and enhance cooperation.*[32]
▪ Guidelines and practices for the determination of brain death and laws regarding consents and procedures for organ procurement can vary by state, international region, and patient age.[5,26,33,34]

Complications

If communication with the OPO coordinator isn't established early enough, trust may be lost between the professional caregivers and the family, and organ donation may be denied. Other negative outcomes that may result include the patient's wishes not being honored, obtaining consent for organs that aren't viable, and identifying a donor who isn't medically suitable for organ donation.[3,15]

Documentation

Document any interactions you have with the family, such as multidisciplinary conferences and contact with the OPO coordinator. After brain death has been determined, record the date and time of the determination as well as the name of the practitioner who made the declaration. Include all methods used to determine brain death. Document teaching provided to the family, their understanding of that teaching, and any need for follow-up teaching. Also document any family contact, visitation, requests, or further teaching that takes place after organ donation occurs.

REFERENCES

1 U.S. Department of Health and Human Services. (2020). Organ Procurement and Transplantation Network (OPTN) policies. https://optn.transplant.hrsa.gov/media/1200/optn_policies.pdf (Level VII)

2 The Joint Commission. (2021). Standard RI.01.05.01. *Comprehensive accreditation manual for hospitals.* Oakbrook Terrace, IL: The Joint Commission. (Level VII)

3 Wiegand, D. L. (2017). *AACN procedure manual for high acuity, progressive and critical care* (7th ed.). St. Louis, MO: Elsevier.

4 Robey, T. E., & Marcolini, E. G. (2013). Organ donation after acute brain death: Addressing limitations of time and resources in the emergency department. *Yale Journal of Biology and Medicine, 86*(3), 333–342. https://www.ncbi.nlm.nih.gov/pmc/articles/PMC3767218 (Level VII)

5 Rudge, C., et al. (2012). International practices of organ donation. *British Journal of Anaesthesia, 108*(Suppl. 1), i48–i55. https://academic.oup.com/bja/article/108/suppl_1/i48/237865 (Level V)

6 Alban, R. F., et al. (2016). Improving donor conversion rates at a level one trauma center: Impact of best practice guidelines. *Cureus, 8*(11), e891. https://www.ncbi.nlm.nih.gov/pmc/articles/PMC5178983/ (Level IV)

7 Centers for Medicare and Medicaid Services, Department of Health and Human Services. (2020). Condition of participation: Patient's rights. 42 C.F.R. § 482.13(b)(2).

8 The Joint Commission. (2010). Advancing effective communication, cultural competence, and patient- and family-centered care: A roadmap for hospitals. http://www.jointcommission.org/assets/1/6/aroadmapforhospitalsfinalversion727.pdf (Level VII)

9 Accreditation Association for Hospitals and Health Systems. (2020). Standard 30.01.11. *Healthcare Facilities Accreditation Program: Accreditation requirements for acute care hospitals.* Chicago, IL: Accreditation Association for Hospitals and Health Systems. (Level VII)

10 U.S. Department of Health and Human Services. (n.d.). How organ donation works. https://organdonor.gov/about/process.html (Level VII)

11 Accreditation Association for Hospitals and Health Systems. (2020). Standard 15.01.12. *Healthcare Facilities Accreditation Program: Accreditation requirements for acute care hospitals.* Chicago, IL: Accreditation Association for Hospitals and Health Systems. (Level VII)

12 DNV GL-Healthcare USA, Inc. (2020). PR.3.SR.1. *NIAHO® accreditation requirements, interpretive guidelines and surveyor guidance—revision 20.0.* Milford, OH: DNV GL-Healthcare USA, Inc. (Level VII)

13 Johnson, J. R., et al. (2014). The association of spiritual care providers' activities with family members' satisfaction with care after a death in the ICU. *Critical Care Medicine, 42,* 1991–2000. (Level IV)

14 Prommer, E. (2014). Organ donation and palliative care: Can palliative care make a difference? *Journal of Palliative Medicine, 17,* 368–371. (Level VII)

15 Ehrle, R. (2006). Timely referral of potential organ donors. *Critical Care Nurse, 26*(2), 88–93. (Level V)

16 Centers for Disease Control and Prevention. (2002). Guideline for hand hygiene in health-care settings: Recommendations of the Healthcare Infection Control Practices Advisory Committee and the HICPAC/SHEA/APIC/IDSA Hand Hygiene Task Force. *MMWR Recommendations and Reports, 51*(RR-16), 1–45. A https://www.cdc.gov/mmwr/pdf/rr/rr5116.pdf (Level II)

17 The Joint Commission. (2021). Standard NPSG.07.01.01. *Comprehensive accreditation manual for hospitals.* Oakbrook Terrace, IL: The Joint Commission. (Level VII)

18 World Health Organization. (2009). WHO guidelines on hand hygiene in health care: First global patient safety challenge, clean care is safer care. https://apps.who.int/iris/bitstream/handle/10665/44102/9789241597906_eng.pdf?sequence=1 (Level IV)

19 Accreditation Association for Hospitals and Health Systems. (2020). Standard 07.01.10. *Healthcare Facilities Accreditation Program: Accreditation requirements for acute care hospitals.* Chicago, IL: Accreditation Association for Hospitals and Health Systems. (Level VII)

20 Centers for Medicare and Medicaid Services, Department of Health and Human Services. (2020). Condition of participation: Infection control. 42 C.F.R. § 482.42.

21 DNV GL-Healthcare USA, Inc. (2020). IC.1.SR.1. *NIAHO® accreditation requirements, interpretive guidelines and surveyor guidance—revision 20.0.* Milford, OH: DNV GL-Healthcare USA, Inc. (Level VII)

22 The Joint Commission. (2021). Standard NPSG.01.01.01. *Comprehensive accreditation manual for hospitals.* Oakbrook Terrace, IL: The Joint Commission. (Level VII)

23 Siegel, J. D., et al. (2007, revised 2019). 2007 guideline for isolation precautions: Preventing transmission of infectious agents in healthcare settings. https://www.cdc.gov/infectioncontrol/pdf/guidelines/isolation-guidelines-H.pdf (Level II)

24 Occupational Safety and Health Administration. (2019). Bloodborne pathogens, standard number 1910.1030. https://www.osha.gov/pls/oshaweb/owadisp.show_document?p_id=10051&p_table=STANDARDS (Level VII)

25 McKeown, D. W., et al. (2012). Management of the heartbeating brain-dead organ donor. *British Journal of Anaesthesia, 108*(Suppl. 1), i96–i107. https://academic.oup.com/bja/article/108/suppl_1/i96/237125 (Level VII)

26 Wijdicks, E. F. M., et al. (2010). Evidence-based guideline update: Determining brain death in adults: Report of the Quality Standards Subcommittee of the American Academy of Neurology. *Neurology, 74*(23), 1911–1918. https://n.neurology.org/content/74/23/1911 (Level I)

27 DNV GL-Healthcare USA, Inc. (2020). PR.2.SR.3. *NIAHO® accreditation requirements, interpretive guidelines and surveyor guidance—revision 20.0.* Milford, OH: DNV GL-Healthcare USA, Inc. (Level VII)

28 The Joint Commission. (2021). Standard RC.01.03.01. *Comprehensive accreditation manual for hospitals.* Oakbrook Terrace, IL: The Joint Commission. (Level VII)

29 Accreditation Association for Hospitals and Health Systems. (2020). Standard 10.00.03. *Healthcare Facilities Accreditation Program: Accreditation requirements for acute care hospitals.* Chicago, IL: Accreditation Association for Hospitals and Health Systems. (Level VII)

30 Centers for Medicare and Medicaid Services, Department of Health and Human Services. (2020). Condition of participation: Medical record services. 42 C.F.R. § 482.24(b).

31 DNV GL-Healthcare USA, Inc. (2020). MR.2.SR.1. *NIAHO® accreditation requirements, interpretive guidelines and surveyor guidance—revision 20.0.* Milford, OH: DNV GL-Healthcare USA, Inc. (Level VII)

32 The Joint Commission. (2021). Standard PC.02.01.21. *Comprehensive accreditation manual for hospitals.* Oakbrook Terrace, IL: The Joint Commission. (Level VII)

33 Wijdicks, E. F. (2012). The transatlantic divide over brain death determination and the debate. *Brain, 135,* 1321–1331. (Level V)

34 Nakagawa, T. A., et al. (2011, reaffirmed 2019). American Academy of Pediatrics: Guidelines for the determination of brain death in infants and children: An update of the 1987 task force recommendations. *Pediatrics, 128*(3), e720–e740. http://pediatrics.aappublications.org/content/128/3/e720.full (Level I)

ORONASOPHARYNGEAL SUCTIONING

Oronasopharyngeal suctioning removes secretions from the pharynx by a suction catheter inserted through the mouth or nostril. Used to maintain a patent airway, this procedure helps the patient who can't clear the airway effectively with coughing and expectoration, such as the unconscious or severely debilitated patient. The procedure should be performed as often as necessary, depending on the patient's condition. Including oral suctioning as part of standard oral hygiene practice in patients who require intubation may reduce the risk of ventilator-associated pneumonia.[1,2]

Because the catheter may inadvertently slip into the lower airway or esophagus, oronasopharyngeal suction is a sterile procedure that requires sterile equipment. However, clean technique is sufficient for a tonsil-tip suction device. In fact, an alert patient can use a tonsil-tip suction device independently to remove secretions.

Equipment

Wall suction or portable suction unit with connecting tubing ▪ water-soluble lubricant ▪ sterile normal saline solution ▪ disposable sterile container ▪ sterile suction catheter (#10 to #16 French) ▪ sterile gloves ▪ overbed table ▪ towel ▪ stethoscope ▪ disinfectant pad ▪ Optional: tongue blade, tonsil-tip suction device, nasopharyngeal or oropharyngeal airway (optional for frequent suctioning), gown, mask and goggles or mask with face shield.

A commercially prepared kit contains a sterile catheter, a disposable container, and sterile gloves.

Preparation of equipment

Inspect all equipment and supplies. If a product is expired, is defective, or has compromised integrity, remove it from patient use, label it as expired or defective, and report the expiration or defect as directed by your facility.

Gather and place the suction equipment on the patient's overbed table or bedside stand. Position the table or stand on your preferred side of the bed *to facilitate suctioning*. Connect the tubing to the suctioning unit. Date and then open the bottle of normal saline solution.

Implementation

■ Verify the practitioner's order for oropharyngeal suctioning if your facility requires one.
■ Review the patient's arterial blood gas or oxygen saturation values and vital signs.
■ Check the patient's history for contraindications, such as a deviated septum, nasal polyps, nasal obstruction, traumatic injury, facial trauma, epistaxis, or mucosal swelling.
■ Gather and prepare the necessary equipment and supplies.
■ Perform hand hygiene.[3,4,5,6,7,8]
■ Confirm the patient's identity using at least two patient identifiers.[9]
■ Provide privacy.[10,11,12,13]
■ Explain the procedure to the patient (even if unresponsive) and family (if appropriate) according to their individual communication and learning needs *to increase their understanding, allay their fears, and enhance cooperation*.[14] Inform the patient that suctioning may stimulate transient coughing or gagging, but that coughing helps to mobilize secretions. If the patient has been suctioned before, summarize the reasons for the procedure. Provide reassurance throughout the procedure *to minimize anxiety and fear, which can increase oxygen consumption*.
■ Raise the patient's bed to waist level during patient care *to prevent caregiver back strain*.[15]
■ Perform hand hygiene.[3,4,5,6,7,8]
■ Put on personal protective equipment, as appropriate, *to comply with standard precautions*.[16,17,18] A gown and a mask and goggles or a face shield are recommended even for patients not suspected of being infectious.[16]
■ Evaluate the patient's respiratory status and ability to cough and deep-breathe *to determine the patient's ability to move secretions up the tracheobronchial tree*.
■ If you are suctioning through the nose, determine which nostril is more patent.
■ Place the patient in the semi-Fowler or high Fowler position, if tolerated, *to promote lung expansion and effective coughing*. If the patient is unconscious, use the side-lying position with the patient facing you *to help promote drainage of secretions*.
■ Place a towel across the patient's chest.
■ Turn on the suction from the wall or portable unit and set the pressure, typically to between 100 and 120 mm Hg; *higher pressures cause excessive trauma without enhancing secretion removal*.[19]
■ Occlude the end of the connecting tubing *to check suction pressure*.
■ Using sterile technique, open the suction catheter kit or the packages containing the sterile catheter, container, and gloves.
■ Perform hand hygiene.[3,4,5,6,7,8]
■ Put on sterile gloves;[16,18] consider your dominant hand sterile and your nondominant hand nonsterile.
■ Using your nondominant hand, pour the normal saline solution into the sterile container.
■ With your nondominant hand, place a small amount of water-soluble lubricant on the sterile area of the catheter. *The lubricant facilitates passage of the catheter during nasopharyngeal suctioning to minimize traumatic injury*.

■ Pick up the catheter with your dominant (sterile) hand and attach it to the connecting tubing (as shown below). Use your nondominant hand to control the suction valve while your dominant hand manipulates the catheter.

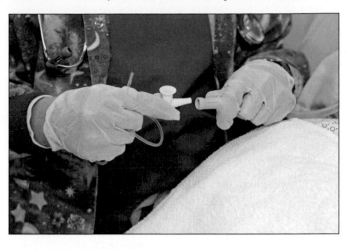

■ Dip the catheter into the sterile normal saline solution (as shown below) *to moisten the inside of the catheter*.

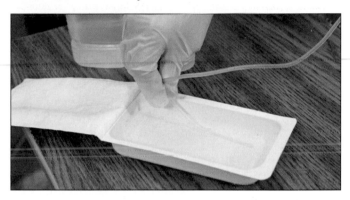

Instruct the patient to cough and to breathe slowly and deeply several times before you begin suctioning. *Coughing helps loosen secretions and may decrease the amount of suction necessary, while deep breathing helps minimize or prevent hypoxia*.

For nasal insertion

■ Raise the tip of the patient's nose with your nondominant hand *to straighten the passageway and facilitate insertion of the catheter*.
■ Without applying suction, gently insert the suction catheter into the patient's nostril (as shown below). Roll the catheter between your fingers *to help it advance through the turbinates*. Continue to advance the catheter approximately 5″ to 6″ (12.7 to 15.2 cm) until you reach the pool of secretions or the patient begins to cough.

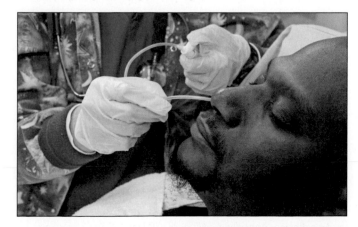

For oral insertion

■ Without applying suction, gently insert the catheter into the patient's mouth. Advance it 3″ to 4″ (7.6 to 10.2 cm) along the side of the patient's mouth until you reach the pool of secretions or the patient begins to cough. Suction both sides of the patient's mouth and pharyngeal area.

Completing the procedure

■ Using intermittent suction, withdraw the catheter from either the mouth or the nose with a continuous rotating motion *to minimize invagination of the mucosa into the catheter's tip and side ports.* Apply suction for no longer than 10 seconds at a time *to minimize tissue trauma.*

■ Assess the volume, color, consistency, and odor of the suctioned respiratory secretions.[20]

■ Between passes, wrap the catheter around your dominant hand *to prevent contamination.*

■ If secretions are thick, clear the lumen of the catheter by dipping it in normal saline solution and applying suction.

■ Repeat the procedure, up to three times, until gurgling or bubbling sounds stop and respirations are quiet. Allow 30 seconds to 1 minute *to allow reoxygenation and reventilation.*

■ After completing suctioning, pull your sterile glove off over the coiled catheter and discard it.[16,18]

■ Flush the connecting tubing with normal saline solution. Discard the container of normal saline solution and remove and discard your other glove.[16,18]

■ Return the bed to the lowest position *to prevent falls and maintain patient safety.*[21]

■ Remove and discard other personal protective equipment, if worn.[16,18]

■ Perform hand hygiene.[3,4,5,6,7,8]

■ Reassess the patient's respiratory status *to evaluate the patient's tolerance and the effectiveness of the procedure.*

■ Clean and disinfect your stethoscope using a disinfectant pad.[22,23]

■ Perform hand hygiene.[3,4,5,6,7,8]

■ Document the procedure.[24,25,26,27]

Special considerations

■ If the patient has no history of nasal problems, alternate suctioning between nostrils *to minimize traumatic injury.*

■ If the patient requires repeated oronasopharyngeal suctioning, the use of a nasopharyngeal or oropharyngeal airway will help with catheter insertion, reduce traumatic injury, and promote a patent airway. (See the "Nasopharyngeal airway insertion and care" and "Oropharyngeal airway insertion and care" procedures.)

■ If the patient has excessive oral secretions, consider using a tonsil-tip suction device, *which allows the patient to remove oral secretions independently.*

■ Let the patient rest after suctioning while you continue to observe. The frequency and duration of suctioning depend on the patient's tolerance of the procedure and any complications that occurred.

Patient teaching

Oronasopharyngeal suctioning may be performed in the home using a portable suction machine. Under these circumstances, suctioning is a clean rather than a sterile procedure. Properly cleaned catheters can be reused, putting less financial strain on the patient. Whether the patient requires disposable or reusable suction equipment, make sure that the patient and caregivers have received proper teaching and support.

Complications

Increased dyspnea caused by hypoxia and anxiety may result from this procedure. Hypoxia may occur *because suction removes oxygen from the oronasopharynx along with the secretions.* In addition, bloody aspirate can result from prolonged or traumatic suctioning. The procedure can cause pain and discomfort.[28]

Documentation

Record the date, time, reason for suctioning, and technique used; the amount, color, consistency, and odor (if any) of the secretions; the patient's respiratory status before and after the procedure; the patient's tolerance of the procedure; any complications and the interventions taken; and the patient's response to the interventions. Document teaching provided to the patient and family (if applicable), their understanding of that teaching, and any need for follow-up teaching.

REFERENCES

1 Larrow, V., & Klich-Heartt, E. (2016). Prevention of ventilator-associated pneumonia in the intensive care unit: Beyond the basics. *Journal of Neuroscience Nursing, 48,* 160–165.

2 Sole, M. L., et al. (2011). Oropharyngeal secretion volume in intubated patients: The importance of oral suctioning. *American Journal of Critical Care, 20*(6), e141–e145. https://doi.org/10.4037/ajcc2011178 (Level IV)

3 The Joint Commission. (2021). Standard NPSG.07.01.01. *Comprehensive accreditation manual for hospitals.* Oakbrook Terrace, IL: The Joint Commission. (Level VII)

4 Centers for Disease Control and Prevention. (2002). Guideline for hand hygiene in health-care settings: Recommendations of the Healthcare Infection Control Practices Advisory Committee and the HICPAC/ SHEA/APIC/IDSA Hand Hygiene Task Force. *MMWR Recommendations and Reports, 51*(RR-16), 1–45. https://www.cdc.gov/mmwr/pdf/rr/rr5116. pdf (Level II)

5 World Health Organization. (2009). WHO guidelines on hand hygiene in health care: First global patient safety challenge, clean care is safer care. https://apps.who.int/iris/bitstream/handle/10665/44102/9789241597906_eng.pdf?sequence=1 (Level IV)

6 Centers for Medicare and Medicaid Services, Department of Health and Human Services. (2020). Condition of participation: Infection control. 42 C.F.R. 482.42.

7 Accreditation Association for Hospitals and Health Systems. (2020). Standard 07.01.21. *Healthcare Facilities Accreditation Program: Accreditation requirements for acute care hospitals.* Chicago, IL: Accreditation Association for Hospitals and Health Systems. (Level VII)

8 DNV GL-Healthcare USA, Inc. (2020). IC.1.SR.1. *NIAHO® accreditation requirements, interpretive guidelines and surveyor guidance—revision 20.0.* Milford, OH: DNV GL-Healthcare USA, Inc. (Level VII)

9 The Joint Commission. (2021). Standard NPSG.01.01.01. *Comprehensive accreditation manual for hospitals.* Oakbrook Terrace, IL: The Joint Commission. (Level VII)

10 The Joint Commission. (2021). Standard RI.01.01.01. *Comprehensive accreditation manual for hospitals.* Oakbrook Terrace, IL: The Joint Commission. (Level VII)

11 Centers for Medicare and Medicaid Services, Department of Health and Human Services. (2020). Condition of participation: Patient's rights. 42 C.F.R. § 482.13(c)(1).

12 Accreditation Association for Hospitals and Health Systems. (2020). Standard 15.01.16. *Healthcare Facilities Accreditation Program: Accreditation requirements for acute care hospitals.* Chicago, IL: Accreditation Association for Hospitals and Health Systems. (Level VII)

13 DNV GL-Healthcare USA, Inc. (2020). PR.2.SR.5. *NIAHO® accreditation requirements, interpretive guidelines and surveyor guidance—revision 20.0.* Milford, OH: DNV GL-Healthcare USA, Inc. (Level VII)

14 The Joint Commission. (2021). Standard PC.02.01.21. *Comprehensive accreditation manual for hospitals.* Oakbrook Terrace, IL: The Joint Commission. (Level VII)

15 Waters, T. R., et al. (2009). Safe patient handling training for schools of nursing. https://www.cdc.gov/niosh/docs/2009-127/pdfs/2009-127.pdf (Level VII)

16 Siegel, J. D., et al. (2007, revised 2019). 2007 guideline for isolation precautions: Preventing transmission of infectious agents in healthcare settings. https://www.cdc.gov/infectioncontrol/pdf/guidelines/isolation-guidelines-H.pdf (Level II)

17 Accreditation Association for Hospitals and Health Systems. (2020). Standard 07.01.10. *Healthcare Facilities Accreditation Program: Accreditation requirements for acute care hospitals.* Chicago, IL: Accreditation Association for Hospitals and Health Systems. (Level VII)

18 Occupational Safety and Health Administration. (2012). Bloodborne pathogens, standard number 1910.1030. https://www.osha.gov/pls/oshaweb/owadisp.show_document?p_id=10051&p_table=STANDARDS (Level VII)

19 Wiegand, D. L. (2017). *AACN procedure manual for high acuity, progressive, and critical care* (7th ed.). St. Louis, MO: Elsevier.

20 Craven, H. (Ed.). (2016). *Core curriculum for medical-surgical nursing* (5th ed.). Pitman, NJ: Academy of Medical-Surgical Nurses.

21 Ganz, D. A., et al. (2013, reviewed 2021). *Preventing falls in hospitals: A toolkit for improving quality of care* (AHRQ publication no. 13-0015-EF). https://www.ahrq.gov/professionals/systems/hospital/fallpx-toolkit/index.html (Level VII)

22 Rutala, W. A., et al. (2008, revised 2019). Guideline for disinfection and sterilization in healthcare facilities, 2008. https://www.cdc.gov/infection-control/pdf/guidelines/disinfection-guidelines-H.pdf (Level I)

23 Accreditation Association for Hospitals and Health Systems. (2020). Standard 07.02.03. *Healthcare Facilities Accreditation Program: Accreditation requirements for acute care hospitals.* Chicago, IL: Accreditation Association for Hospitals and Health Systems. (Level VII)

24 The Joint Commission. (2021). Standard RC.01.03.01. *Comprehensive accreditation manual for hospitals.* Oakbrook Terrace, IL: The Joint Commission. (Level VII)

25 Centers for Medicare and Medicaid Services, Department of Health and Human Services. (2020). Condition of participation: Medical record services. 42 C.F.R. § 482.24(b).

26 Accreditation Association for Hospitals and Health Systems. (2020). Standard 10.00.03. *Healthcare Facilities Accreditation Program: Accreditation requirements for acute care hospitals.* Chicago, IL: Accreditation Association for Hospitals and Health Systems. (Level VII)

27 DNV GL-Healthcare USA, Inc. (2020). MR.2.SR.1. *NIAHO® accreditation requirements, interpretive guidelines and surveyor guidance—revision 20.0.* Milford, OH: DNV GL-Healthcare USA, Inc. (Level VII)

28 Kacmarek, R. M., et al. (2021). *Egan's fundamentals of respiratory care* (12th ed.). St Louis, MO: Mosby.

OROPHARYNGEAL AIRWAY INSERTION AND CARE

An oropharyngeal airway, a curved plastic device, is inserted into the mouth to the posterior pharynx to establish or maintain a patent airway. In an unconscious patient, the tongue usually obstructs the posterior pharynx. The oropharyngeal airway conforms to the curvature of the palate, removing the obstruction and allowing air to pass around and through the tube. It also facilitates oropharyngeal suctioning.

The oropharyngeal airway is intended for short-term use and should be used only in an unresponsive patient who can't maintain the airway. It may be left in place longer as an airway adjunct to prevent the orally intubated patient from biting the endotracheal tube. The oropharyngeal airway isn't the airway of choice for the patient with loose or avulsed teeth or who has undergone recent oral surgery. The presence of a foreign body or space-occupying lesion in the pharynx or mouth or traumatic injury to the oral cavity, mandible, or maxillary bones also precludes the use of an oropharyngeal airway.[1]

NURSING ALERT Inserting this airway in a conscious or semiconscious patient may stimulate vomiting and laryngospasm; use only in unresponsive patients who don't have a cough or gag reflex.[2]

Equipment
For inserting
Oropharyngeal airway of appropriate size ▪ tongue blade ▪ gloves ▪ tape or other securement device ▪ stethoscope ▪ disinfectant pad ▪ oral care supplies ▪ Optional: suction equipment, resuscitation mask, handheld resuscitation bag or oxygen-powered breathing device, mask and goggles or mask with face shield, gown.

For reflex testing
Cotton-tipped applicator.

Preparation of equipment
Select an appropriate-sized airway for the patient; *an oversized airway can obstruct breathing.*[3] Typically, you'll select a medium size (size 4 or 5) for an adult of average size and a large size (size 6) for a large adult. Be sure to confirm the correct size of the airway by placing the airway flange beside the patient's cheek, parallel to the maxillary incisors.[3] If the airway is the right size, the airway curve should reach to the angle of the jaw.

Inspect all equipment and supplies. If a product is expired, is defective, or has compromised integrity, remove it from patient use, label it as expired or defective, and report the expiration or defect as directed by your facility.

Implementation
- Verify the practitioner's order.
- Gather and prepare the necessary equipment and supplies.
- Perform hand hygiene.[4,5,6,7,8,9]
- Confirm the patient's identity using at least two patient identifiers.[10]
- Provide privacy.[11,12,13,14]
- Explain the procedure to the patient and family (if appropriate) according to their individual communication and learning needs *to increase their understanding, allay their fears, and enhance cooperation.*[15]
- Raise the patient's bed to waist level before performing patient care *to prevent caregiver back strain.*[16]
- Perform hand hygiene.[4,5,6,7,8,9]

EQUIPMENT

Inserting an oral airway

Unless this position is contraindicated, hyperextend the patient's head (as shown below) before using either the cross-finger or tongue-blade insertion method.

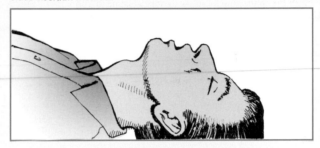

To insert an oropharyngeal airway using the cross-finger method, place your thumb on the patient's lower teeth and your index finger on the upper teeth. Gently open the mouth by pushing the teeth apart (as shown below).

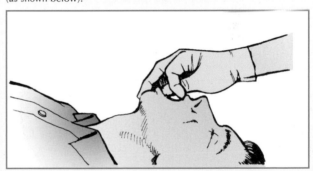

Insert the airway upside down *to avoid pushing the tongue toward the pharynx,* and slide it over the tongue toward the back of the mouth. Rotate the airway as it approaches the posterior wall of the pharynx so that it points downward (as shown below).

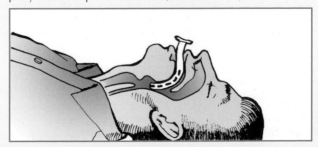

To use the tongue blade technique, open the patient's mouth and depress the tongue with the blade. Guide the airway over the back of the tongue as you did for the cross-finger technique.

- Put on gloves as necessary *to comply with standard precautions*. Also put on a gown and mask and goggles or a mask with face shield if secretions are copious.[17,18,19,20]
- If the patient wears dentures, remove them *so they don't cause further airway obstruction*.
- Suction the patient if necessary *to remove secretions*. (See the "Oronasopharyngeal suction" procedure.)
- Place the patient in the supine position with the neck hyperextended, unless contraindicated. Otherwise, use the jaw-thrust maneuver for suspected cervical spine injury or other contraindication to neck hyperextension.[2]
- Insert the oropharyngeal airway using the cross-finger or the tongue-blade technique. (See *Inserting an oral airway*, page 619.)
- Immediately after airway insertion, auscultate breath sounds and assess the patient's respirations. If respirations are absent or inadequate, initiate artificial positive-pressure ventilation with a mouth-to-mask technique, a handheld resuscitation bag, or an oxygen-powered breathing device *to ensure adequate ventilation*. Stridor, gasping respirations, or snoring may indicate inadequate airway placement.[17]
- Secure the airway with tape or other securement device, if indicated, *to prevent expulsion of the airway*; leave the airway unsecured in patients who need to be able to cough out the airway if gagging occurs.[17]
- Position the patient in a side-lying position *to decrease the risk of aspiration of vomitus*.
- Frequently check the position of the airway *to ensure correct placement*. Make sure that the patient's lips and tongue aren't between the teeth and airway *to prevent traumatic injury*.
- Suction the patient as needed *to remove secretions*.
- Reassess the patient's respiratory status following suctioning and at an interval determined by the patient's condition and your facility.[17]
- Brush the patient's teeth, gums, and tongue at least twice per day using a soft toothbrush. Moisturize the oral mucosa and lips every 2 to 4 hours.[21] Inspect the mucous membranes of the patient's mouth for tissue irritation, *which can result from prolonged airway use*. (See the "Oral care" procedure.)
- Return the bed top the lowest position *to prevent falls and maintain patient safety*.[22]
- Remove and discard your gloves and, if worn, other personal protective equipment.[18,20]
- Perform hand hygiene.[4,5,6,7,8,9]
- Clean and disinfect your stethoscope with a disinfectant pad.[23,24]
- Perform hand hygiene.[4,5,6,7,8,9]
- Document the procedure.[25,26,27,28]

Special considerations

- Evaluate the patient's behavior *to provide the cue for airway removal*. The patient is likely to gag or cough as the patient becomes more alert, indicating that the airway is no longer needed.
- When the patient regains consciousness and can swallow, remove the airway by pulling it outward and downward, following the mouth's natural curvature.
- Remove the oropharyngeal airway every 8 hours or as needed. Clean the airway according to the manufacturer's instructions and reinsert the clean airway.[17]
- After removing the airway, test the patient's cough and gag reflexes *to ensure that removal of the airway wasn't premature and that the patient can maintain the airway*. To test for the gag reflex, use a cotton-tipped applicator to touch both sides of the posterior pharynx. To test for the cough reflex, gently touch the posterior oropharynx with the cotton-tipped applicator.

Complications

Reflex gagging, vomiting, aspiration, and laryngeal spasms may occur with oropharyngeal airway insertion.[1,29] Tooth damage or loss, tissue damage, and bleeding may result from airway insertion.[29] If the airway is too long, it may cause traumatic injury to the laryngeal structures. If it is too short, the distal end may be obstructed by the tongue, worsening airway obstruction.[3] If the airway isn't inserted properly, it may push the tongue posteriorly, aggravating the problem of upper airway obstruction.[2]

Documentation

Record the date and time of the airway's insertion, size of the airway, removal and cleaning of the airway, condition of mucous membranes, any suctioning performed, respiratory assessment findings, adverse reactions, nursing interventions performed, and the patient's tolerance of the procedure. Document teaching provided to the patient and family (if applicable), their understanding of that teaching, and any need for follow-up teaching.

REFERENCES

1 Kacmarek, R. M., et al. (2021). *Egan's fundamentals of respiratory care* (12th ed.). St. Louis, MO: Mosby.
2 American Heart Association. (2020). 2020 American Heart Association Guidelines for CPR and ECC–Part 3: Adult basic and advanced life support. https://cpr.heart.org/en/resuscitation-science/cpr-and-ecc-guidelines
3 Kim, H. J., et al. (2016). Determination of the appropriate sizes of oropharyngeal airways in adults: Correlation with external facial measurements: A randomized crossover study. *European Journal of Anaesthesiology, 33*, 936–942. https://journals.lww.com/ejanaesthesiology/Fulltext/2016/12000/Determination_of_the_appropriate_sizes_of.9.aspx (Level II)
4 The Joint Commission. (2021). Standard NPSG.07.01.01. *Comprehensive accreditation manual for hospitals.* Oakbrook Terrace, IL: The Joint Commission. (Level VII)
5 Centers for Disease Control and Prevention. (2002). Guideline for hand hygiene in health-care settings: Recommendations of the Healthcare Infection Control Practices Advisory Committee and the HICPAC/SHEA/APIC/IDSA Hand Hygiene Task Force. *MMWR Recommendations and Reports, 51*(RR-16), 1–45. https://www.cdc.gov/mmwr/pdf/rr/rr5116.pdf (Level II)
6 World Health Organization. (2009). WHO guidelines on hand hygiene in health care: First global patient safety challenge, clean care is safer care. https://apps.who.int/iris/bitstream/handle/10665/44102/9789241597906_eng.pdf?sequence=1 (Level IV)
7 Centers for Medicare and Medicaid Services, Department of Health and Human Services. (2020). Condition of participation: Infection control. 42 C.F.R. § 482.42.
8 Accreditation Association for Hospitals and Health Systems. (2020). Standard 07.01.21. *Healthcare Facilities Accreditation Program: Accreditation requirements for acute care hospitals.* Chicago, IL: Accreditation Association for Hospitals and Health Systems. (Level VII)
9 DNV GL-Healthcare USA, Inc. (2020). IC.1.SR.1. *NIAHO® accreditation requirements, interpretive guidelines and surveyor guidance—revision 20.0.* Milford, OH: DNV GL-Healthcare USA, Inc. (Level VII)
10 The Joint Commission. (2021). Standard NPSG.01.01.01. *Comprehensive accreditation manual for hospitals.* Oakbrook Terrace, IL: The Joint Commission. (Level VII)
11 Centers for Medicare and Medicaid Services, Department of Health and Human Services. (2020). Condition of participation: Patient's rights. 42 C.F.R. § 482.13(c)(1).
12 Accreditation Association for Hospitals and Health Systems. (2020). Standard 15.01.16. *Healthcare Facilities Accreditation Program: Accreditation requirements for acute care hospitals.* Chicago, IL: Accreditation Association for Hospitals and Health Systems. (Level VII)
13 The Joint Commission. (2021). Standard RI.01.01.01. *Comprehensive accreditation manual for hospitals.* Oakbrook Terrace, IL: The Joint Commission. (Level VII)
14 DNV GL-Healthcare USA, Inc. (2020). PR.2.SR.5. *NIAHO® accreditation requirements, interpretive guidelines and surveyor guidance—revision 20.0.* Milford, OH: DNV GL-Healthcare USA, Inc. (Level VII)
15 The Joint Commission. (2021). Standard PC.02.01.21. *Comprehensive accreditation manual for hospitals.* Oakbrook Terrace, IL: The Joint Commission. (Level VII)
16 Waters, T. R., et al. (2009). Safe patient handling training for schools of nursing. https://www.cdc.gov/niosh/docs/2009-127/pdfs/2009-127.pdf (Level VII)
17 Wiegand, D. L. (2017). *AACN procedure manual for high acuity, progressive, and critical care* (7th ed.). St. Louis, MO: Elsevier.
18 Siegel, J. D., et al. (2007, revised 2019). 2007 guideline for isolation precautions: Preventing transmission of infectious agents in healthcare settings. https://www.cdc.gov/infectioncontrol/pdf/guidelines/isolation-guidelines-H.pdf (Level II)

19 Accreditation Association for Hospitals and Health Systems. (2020). Standard 07.01.10. *Healthcare Facilities Accreditation Program: Accreditation requirements for acute care hospitals.* Chicago, IL: Accreditation Association for Hospitals and Health Systems. (Level VII)

20 Occupational Safety and Health Administration. (2019). Bloodborne pathogens, standard number 1910.1030. https://www.osha.gov/pls/oshaweb/owadisp.show_document?p_id=10051&p_table=STANDARDS (Level VII)

21 American Association of Critical-Care Nurses. (2017). AACN practice alert: Oral care for acutely and critically ill patients. https://www.aacn.org/clinical-resources/practice-alerts/oral-care-for-acutely-and-critically-ill-patients (Level VII)

22 Ganz, D. A., et al. (2013, reviewed 2021). *Preventing falls in hospitals: A toolkit for improving quality of care* (AHRQ Publication No. 13-0015-EF). Rockville, MD: Agency for Healthcare Research and Quality. https://www.ahrq.gov/professionals/systems/hospital/fallpxtoolkit/index.html (Level VII)

23 Rutala, W. A., et al. (2008, revised 2019). Guideline for disinfection and sterilization in healthcare facilities, 2008. https://www.cdc.gov/infection-control/pdf/guidelines/disinfection-guidelines-H.pdf (Level I)

24 Accreditation Association for Hospitals and Health Systems. (2020). Standard 07.02.03. *Healthcare Facilities Accreditation Program: Accreditation requirements for acute care hospitals.* Chicago, IL: Accreditation Association for Hospitals and Health Systems. (Level VII)

25 The Joint Commission. (2021). Standard RC.01.03.01. *Comprehensive accreditation manual for hospitals.* Oakbrook Terrace, IL: The Joint Commission. (Level VII)

26 Centers for Medicare and Medicaid Services, Department of Health and Human Services. (2020). Condition of participation: Medical record services. 42 C.F.R. § 482.24(b).

27 Accreditation Association for Hospitals and Health Systems. (2020). Standard 10.00.03. *Healthcare Facilities Accreditation Program: Accreditation requirements for acute care hospitals.* Chicago, IL: Accreditation Association for Hospitals and Health Systems. (Level VII)

28 DNV GL-Healthcare USA, Inc. (2020). MR.2.SR.1. *NIAHO® accreditation requirements, interpretive guidelines and surveyor guidance—revision 20.0* Milford, OH: DNV GL-Healthcare USA, Inc. (Level VII)

29 Castro, D., & Freeman, L. A. (2021). Oropharyngeal airway https://www.ncbi.nlm.nih.gov/books/NBK470198/

OXYGEN ADMINISTRATION

Oxygen administration helps relieve hypoxemia and maintain adequate oxygenation of tissues and vital organs. In patients with hypoxemia, the cardiopulmonary system compensates by increasing ventilation and cardiac output. Oxygen administration increases blood oxygen content so that the heart doesn't have to pump as much blood per minute to meet tissue demands. Reducing cardiac workload is especially important when disease or injury, such as myocardial infarction, sepsis, or trauma, is already stressing the heart. Hypoxemia causes pulmonary vasoconstriction and subsequent pulmonary hypertension, which increases workload in the right side of the heart. Oxygen administration can reverse pulmonary vasoconstriction, thereby decreasing right ventricular workload.[1] Oxygen administration has only limited benefit for treatment of hypoxia caused by anemia because of the blood's limited oxygen-carrying capacity.

Indications for oxygen administration include:
- documented hypoxemia (partial pressure of arterial oxygen [PaO_2] less than 60 mm Hg or arterial oxygen saturation [SaO_2] less than 90% on room air, or PaO_2 or SaO_2 below desirable range for the particular clinical situation)
- acute care situations suggestive of hypoxemia
- severe trauma
- acute myocardial infarction
- short-term therapy or surgical intervention (for example, postanesthesia recovery).[1,2]

When indications are present, there are no contraindications to oxygen administration.[2]

Various methods of oxygen delivery are available. The patient's disease, physical condition, and age help determine the most appropriate method of administration. The adequacy of oxygen therapy is determined by arterial blood gas (ABG) analysis, oxygen saturation monitoring, and clinical examination.

Equipment

The equipment needed depends on the type of delivery system ordered. (See *Guide to oxygen delivery systems,* page 622.) Equipment includes selections from the following list: Oxygen source (wall unit, cylinder, liquid tank, or concentrator) ■ flowmeter ■ adapter (if using a wall unit) or a pressure-reduction gauge (if using a cylinder) ■ sterile humidity bottle and adapters ■ appropriate oxygen delivery system (nasal cannula, simple mask, high-flow nasal cannula, humidified high-flow nasal cannula, simple mask, or nonrebreather mask for low-flow and variable oxygen concentrations; Venturi mask, aerosol mask, T-tube, tracheostomy collar, tent, or oxygen hood for high-flow and specific oxygen concentrations) ■ small- or large-diameter connection tubing ■ stethoscope ■ disinfectant pad ■ vital signs monitoring equipment ■ pulse oximeter and probe ■ Optional: gloves, mask and goggles or mask with face shield, gauze pads, tape, oxygen analyzer, ABG kit, jet adapter for Venturi mask, OXYGEN PRECAUTIONS sign.[3]

Preparation of equipment

Although a respiratory therapist typically is responsible for setting up, maintaining, and managing the equipment, you'll need a working knowledge of the oxygen system being used.

Check the oxygen outlet port *to verify flow.* All oxygen delivery systems should be checked at least once each day by the respiratory therapist; some systems require more frequent checks using a calibrated analyzer.[2]

Implementation

- Verify the practitioner's order for the oxygen therapy, *because oxygen is considered a medication or therapy and should be prescribed.*[5]
- Gather and prepare the necessary equipment and supplies.
- Perform hand hygiene.[6,7,8,9,10,11]
- Confirm the patient's identity using at least two patient identifiers.[12]
- Provide privacy.[13,14,15,16]
- Explain the procedure to the patient and family (if appropriate) according to their individual communication and learning needs *to increase their understanding, allay their fears, and enhance cooperation.*[17]
- Raise the patient's bed to waist level before providing patient care *to prevent caregiver back strain.*[18]
- Elevate the head of the bed 30 to 45 degrees (unless contraindicated) *to prevent health care–associated pneumonia.*[19,20]
- Perform hand hygiene.[6,7,8,9,10,11]
- Put on gloves and, as needed, other personal protective equipment *to comply with standard precautions.*[21,22,23]
- Perform a baseline assessment, including vital signs, breath sounds, oxygen saturation level using pulse oximetry, and physical assessment. In an emergency, verify that the patient has a patent airway before administering oxygen.
- Select the most appropriate oxygen delivery device based on the practitioner's order and the patient's status.
- Check the patient's room *to make sure it's safe for oxygen administration.* Whenever possible, replace electrical devices with nonelectrical ones *to reduce the risk of fire.*
- If the patient care area isn't already clearly labeled and your facility requires it, place an OXYGEN PRECAUTIONS sign on the door to the patient's room.
- Help place the oxygen delivery device on the patient. Make sure it fits properly and is stable.
- Monitor the patient's oxygen saturation level using pulse oximetry *to assess the response to oxygen therapy.* Make sure that the alarm limits are set appropriately for the patient's current condition, and that alarms are turned on, functioning properly, and audible to staff.[24,25,26,27]
- If the practitioner has ordered an ABG analysis to evaluate ventilation, acid-base balance, oxygenation status, or oxygen-carrying capacity, obtain an arterial sample after allowing sufficient time for the patient's oxygenation to return to a steady state. (See the "Arterial puncture for blood gas analysis" procedure.) A patient with healthy lungs may achieve a steady state within 5 minutes after a change in therapy; a patient with chronic obstructive pulmonary disease (COPD) may require 20 to 30 minutes.[1] Notify the practitioner of critical test results within your facility's established time frame *so that the patient can be promptly treated.*[28]

Guide to oxygen delivery systems

Patients may receive oxygen through one of several administration systems. Each has its own benefits, drawbacks, and indications for use. The advantages and disadvantages of each system are described below.

Nasal cannula

Oxygen is delivered through plastic cannulas in the patient's nostrils.

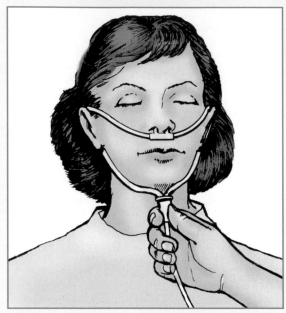

Advantages: Safe and simple, comfortable, and easily tolerated; nasal prongs can be shaped to fit any face; effective for low oxygen concentrations; allows movement, eating, and talking; inexpensive and disposable.

Disadvantages: Maximum concentration delivery of 40%; can't be used in complete nasal obstruction; may cause headaches or dry mucous membranes if flow rate exceeds 6 L/minute; can dislodge easily.[2]

Administration guidelines: Place the nasal cannula interface on the patient, fitting the prongs to the patient's nares. Hook the cannula tubing behind the patient's ears and under the chin. Slide the adjuster upward under the chin *to secure the tubing*. If using an elastic strap to secure the cannula, position it over the ears and around the back of the head. Don't apply it too tightly, *because doing so can result in excess pressure on facial structures and cannula occlusion as well*. With a nasal cannula, oral breathers achieve the same oxygen delivery as nasal breathers. Provide humidification at a flow rate greater than 4 L/minute.[2] Use care estimating the fraction of inspired oxygen (FIO$_2$) to deliver to patients, *because this low-flow system can have great fluctuations*.[2]

High-flow nasal cannula

A high-flow nasal cannula consists of a cannula that attaches to large-bore tubing (shown below) connected to a heated humidifier and an oxygen source.

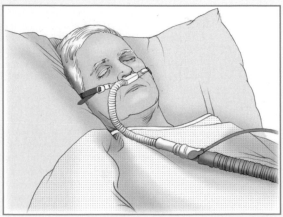

Advantages: Comfortable and easier to tolerate than a mask in patients who require higher doses of supplemental oxygen than a

conventional nasal cannula delivers; possible to deliver FIO$_2$ of 50% to 92% with relative humidity of 95% to 100% at a flow rate of 15 to 60 L/minute, depending on the system.[4]

Disadvantages: Not appropriate for patients with maxillofacial trauma, complete nasal obstruction, or a suspected skull fracture.

Administration guidelines: Turn on the humidifier; set the target temperature at 98.6° F (37° C) at the nares to optimize humidification, and allow 10 to 15 minutes for the device to warm up to the target temperature. Place the nasal cannula interface on the patient, fitting the prongs to the patient's nares and making sure that the prongs don't take up more than half of the opening of the nares to avoid inadvertently creating continuous positive airway pressure (CPAP).[1] Place the elastic strap around the back of the patient's head above the ears. Adjust the strap so that it fits snugly but not too tightly to prevent skin breakdown. Set the blender to the prescribed FIO$_2$. Gradually increase the flowmeter to the prescribed flow rate, allowing time for the patient to acclimate to the increased flow.

Simple mask

Oxygen flows through an entry port at the bottom of the mask and exits through large holes on the sides of the mask, allowing exhaled gases to escape.

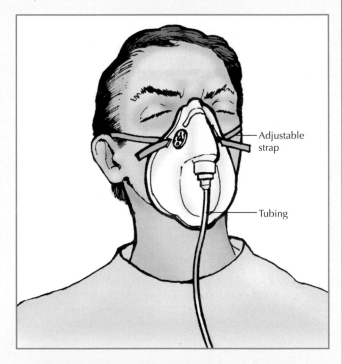

Adjustable strap

Tubing

Advantages: Can deliver concentrations of 35% to 50%.[2]

Disadvantages: Hot and confining; may irritate patient's skin; tight seal, is required for higher oxygen concentrations; interferes with talking and eating; impractical for long-term therapy because of its imprecision.

Administration guidelines: Select the mask size that offers the best fit. Place the mask over the patient's nose, mouth, and chin, and mold the flexible metal edge to the bridge of the nose. Adjust the elastic band around the head *to hold the mask firmly but comfortably over the cheeks, chin, and bridge of the nose*. For an older adult or a patient with cachexia who has sunken cheeks, tape gauze pads to the mask over the cheek area *to try to create an airtight seal*. *Without this seal, room air dilutes the oxygen, preventing delivery of the prescribed concentration.* All masks require a minimum of 5 L/minute *to flush expired carbon dioxide from the mask so that the patient doesn't rebreathe it.*[2]

Nonrebreather mask

On inhalation, the one-way valve opens, directing oxygen from a reservoir bag into the mask. On exhalation, gas exits the mask through the one-way expiratory valve and enters the atmosphere. The patient breathes gas only from the bag.

Guide to oxygen delivery systems *(continued)*

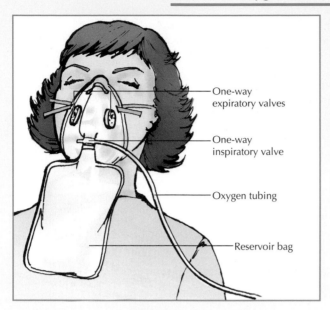

One-way expiratory valves

One-way inspiratory valve

Oxygen tubing

Reservoir bag

Advantages: Noninvasively improves arterial oxygenation by increasing functional residual capacity; possible for the patient to avoid intubation; allows the patient to talk and cough without interrupting positive pressure.

Disadvantages: Requires a tight fit, which may cause discomfort; interferes with eating and talking; increases the risk of aspiration if the patient vomits; increases the risk of pneumothorax, diminished cardiac output, and gastric distention.

Administration guidelines: Place one strap behind the patient's head and the other strap over the head *to ensure a snug fit.* Attach one latex strap to the connector prong on one side of the mask. Then, use one hand to position the mask on the patient's face while using the other hand to connect the strap to the other side of the mask. After the mask is applied, assess the patient's respiratory, circulatory, and GI function every hour. Watch for signs of pneumothorax, decreased cardiac output, a drop in blood pressure, and gastric distention. Use cautiously in patients with chronic obstructive pulmonary disease, bullous lung disease, low cardiac output, or tension pneumothorax.

Transtracheal oxygen

The patient receives oxygen through a catheter inserted into the tracheal cartilage through a small permanent opening in the base of the neck in a simple outpatient procedure.

Advantages: Delivers the highest possible oxygen concentration (60% to 80%) short of intubation and mechanical ventilation; effective for short-term therapy; can be converted to a partial rebreather mask, if necessary, by removing the one-way valve.

Disadvantages: Requires a tight seal, which may be difficult to maintain and may cause discomfort; may irritate the patient's skin; interferes with talking and eating; impractical for long-term therapy.

Administration guidelines: Follow procedures listed for the simple mask. Make sure that the mask fits very snugly and that the one-way valves are secure and functioning. Provide a minimum flow rate of 10 L/minute.? *Because the mask excludes room air,* valve malfunction can cause carbon dioxide buildup and suffocate an unconscious patient. If the reservoir bag collapses more than slightly during inspiration, raise the flow rate until you see only a slight deflation. *Marked or complete deflation indicates an insufficient flow rate.* Keep the reservoir bag from twisting or kinking. *Ensure free expansion* by making sure the bag lies outside the patient's gown and bedcovers.

CPAP mask

This system allows the spontaneously breathing patient to receive continuous positive airway pressure (CPAP), with or without an artificial airway. A positive end-expiratory pressure valve may be fitted to the mask on the lower expiratory port *to allow expired gases to be exhaled under a fixed valve pressure.*

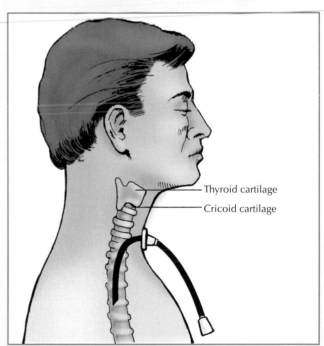

Thyroid cartilage

Cricoid cartilage

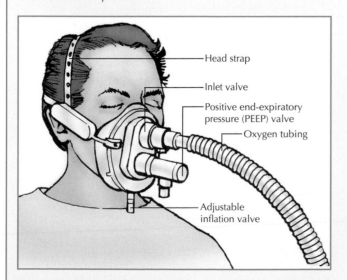

Head strap

Inlet valve

Positive end-expiratory pressure (PEEP) valve

Oxygen tubing

Adjustable inflation valve

Advantages: Supplies oxygen to the lungs throughout the respiratory cycle; provides continuous oxygen without hindering mobility; doesn't interfere with eating or talking; doesn't dry mucous membranes; catheter can easily be concealed by a shirt or scarf.

Disadvantages: Not suitable for use in patients at risk for bleeding or those with severe bronchospasm, uncompensated respiratory acidosis, pleural herniation into the base of the neck, or high corticosteroid dosages.

Administration guidelines: After insertion, obtain a chest X-ray *to confirm placement.* Monitor the patient for bleeding, respiratory distress, pneumothorax, pain, coughing, or hoarseness. Don't use the catheter for about 1 week after insertion *to decrease the risk of subcutaneous emphysema.*

(Continued)

Guide to oxygen delivery systems *(continued)*

Venturi mask

The mask is connected to a Venturi device, which mixes a specific volume of air and oxygen.

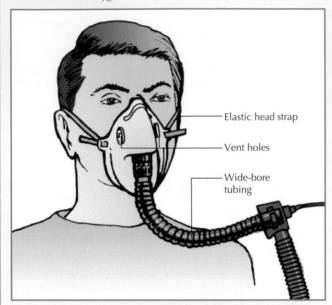

- Elastic head strap
- Vent holes
- Wide-bore tubing

Advantages: Delivers highly accurate oxygen concentration despite the patient's respiratory pattern, *because the same amount of air is always entrained*; dilute jets can be changed or the dial turned to change oxygen concentration; doesn't dry mucous membranes; humidity or aerosol can be added.

Disadvantages: Confining, and may irritate skin; oxygen concentration may be altered if mask fits loosely, tubing kinks, oxygen intake ports become blocked, flow is insufficient, or patient is hyperpneic; interferes with eating and talking; condensate may collect and drip on the patient if humidification is used.

Administration guidelines: Make sure that the oxygen flow rate is set at the amount specified on each mask and that the Venturi valve is set for the desired FIO_2.

Aerosols

An aerosol, such as a face mask, hood, tent, or tracheostomy tube or collar, is connected to wide-bore tubing that receives aerosolized oxygen from a jet nebulizer. The jet nebulizer, which is attached near the oxygen source, adjusts air entrainment in a manner similar to the Venturi device.

Advantages: Administers high humidity; gas can be heated (when delivered through an artificial airway) or cooled (when delivered through a tent).

Disadvantages: Condensate collected in the tracheostomy collar or T tube may drain into the tracheostomy; the weight of the T tube can put stress on the tracheostomy tube.

Administration guidelines: Guidelines vary with the type of nebulizer used—the ultrasonic, large-volume, small-volume, or in-line. When using a high-output nebulizer, watch for signs of overhydration, pulmonary edema, crackles, and electrolyte imbalance.

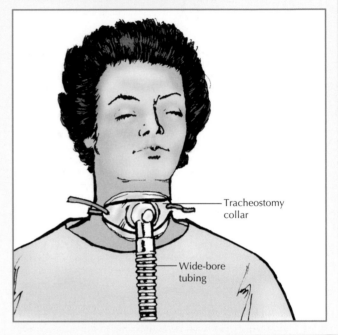

- Tracheostomy collar
- Wide-bore tubing

- Assess the patient frequently for signs of hypoxia, such as restlessness, decreased level of consciousness, increased heart rate, arrhythmias, perspiration, dyspnea, use of accessory muscles, yawning, flared nostrils, cyanosis, and cool, clammy skin. Obtain vital signs, as needed.
- Regularly monitor the patient's skin integrity around the oxygen delivery device *to prevent medical device–related skin injury.* Wipe moisture or perspiration from the patient's face and from the mask, and pad pressure areas if needed.
- Return the bed to the lowest position *to prevent falls and maintain patient safety.*[29]
- Remove and discard your personal protective equipment, if worn.[21,23]
- Perform hand hygiene.[6,7,8,9,10,11]
- Clean and disinfect your stethoscope using a disinfectant pad *to prevent transmission of microorganisms.*[30,31]
- Perform hand hygiene.[6,7,8,9,10,11]
- Document the procedure.[32,33,34,35]

Special considerations

- Maintain the patient's target oxygen saturation level within the recommended range of 94% to 98%, unless otherwise specified. If the patient has COPD or another risk factor for hypercapnic respiratory failure, a saturation of 88% to 92% may be necessary.
- Be aware that flowmeters, which connect to an oxygen or compressed air source, are color-coded so that oxygen (green) isn't confused with compressed air (yellow).

Patient teaching

Before discharging a patient who will receive oxygen therapy at home, make sure you know the types of oxygen therapy, the types of services that are available, and the service schedules offered by local home suppliers. Together with the practitioner and the patient, choose the device best suited to the patient. (See *Types of home oxygen therapy.*)

If the patient will be using transtracheal oxygen therapy, teach the patient how to properly clean and care for the catheter. Advise the patient to keep the skin surrounding the insertion site clean and dry *to prevent infection.*

No matter which device the patient uses, you'll need to evaluate the ability and motivation of the patient and family members to administer oxygen therapy at home. Make sure they understand the reason the patient is receiving oxygen and the safety issues involved in oxygen administration. Teach them how to properly use and clean the equipment and supplies.

If the patient will be discharged with oxygen for the first time, make sure the patient's health insurance covers home oxygen. If it doesn't, find out what criteria the patient must meet to obtain coverage. Without a third-party payer, the patient may not be able to afford home oxygen therapy.

Complications

Oxygen use increases the risk of fires.[2,36] Humidification systems may become contaminated, increasing the risk of infection.[2] With a

EQUIPMENT

Types of home oxygen therapy

Oxygen therapy can be administered at home using an oxygen tank, an oxygen concentrator, or liquid oxygen.

Oxygen tank
Commonly used for patients who need oxygen on a standby basis or who need a ventilator at home, the oxygen tank has several disadvantages, including its cumbersome design and the need for frequent replacement. *Because oxygen is stored under high pressure,* the oxygen tank also poses a potential hazard.

Oxygen concentrator
The oxygen concentrator extracts oxygen molecules from room air. It can be used for low oxygen flow (less than 4 L/minute) and doesn't need to be refilled with oxygen. However, *because the oxygen concentrator runs on electricity,* it won't function during a power failure.

Liquid oxygen
This option is commonly used by patients who are oxygen-dependent but still mobile. The system includes a large liquid reservoir for home use. When the patient wants to leave the house, the patient fills a portable unit worn over the shoulder; this supplies oxygen for up to several hours, depending on the liter flow.

---

fraction of inspired oxygen of greater than 50%, absorption atelectasis, oxygen toxicity, and depression of ciliary or leukocytic function can occur.[2] Hypothermia and increased oxygen consumption can result from administering cool oxygen.[37] Pressure injuries can develop on the patient's head and face and around the nose during prolonged oxygen administration.[38]

Documentation

Record the date and time of oxygen administration; the type of delivery device; the oxygen flow rate; the patient's vital signs, skin color, respiratory effort, and breath sounds; the patient's response before and after initiation of therapy; and any complications that occur, interventions you took, and the patient's response to those interventions. Document teaching that you provided to the patient and family (if applicable), their understanding of that teaching, and any need for follow-up teaching.

REFERENCES

1 Kacmarek, R. M., et al. (2021). *Egan's fundamentals of respiratory care* (12th ed.). St. Louis, MO: Mosby.

2 American Association for Respiratory Care. (2002). AARC clinical practice guideline: Oxygen therapy for adults in the acute care facility—2002 revision and update. *Respiratory Care, 47*(6), 717–720. https://www.aarc.org/wp-content/uploads/2014/08/06.02.717.pdf (Level VII)

3 World Health Organization. (2009). Glove use information leaflet. https://www.who.int/gpsc/5may/Glove_Use_Information_Leaflet.pdf (Level VII)

4 Spoletini, G., et al. (2015). Heated humidified high-flow nasal oxygen in adults: Mechanisms of action and clinical implications. *CHEST Journal, 148*(1), 253–261. https://emcrit.org/wp-content/uploads/2011/10/CHEST-2015-Spoletini.pdf

5 U. S. Food and Drug Administration. (2019). Medical gases. 21 CFR§201.161. https://www.accessdata.fda.gov/scripts/cdrh/cfdocs/cfCFR/CFRSearch.cfm?fr=201.161

6 The Joint Commission. (2021). Standard NPSG.07.01.01. *Comprehensive accreditation manual for hospitals.* Oakbrook Terrace, IL: The Joint Commission. (Level VII)

7 Centers for Disease Control and Prevention. (2002). Guideline for hand hygiene in health-care settings: Recommendations of the Healthcare Infection Control Practices Advisory Committee and the HICPAC/SHEA/APIC/IDSA Hand Hygiene Task Force. *MMWR Recommendations and Reports, 51*(RR-16), 1–45. https://www.cdc.gov/mmwr/pdf/rr/rr5116.pdf (Level II)

8 World Health Organization. (2009). WHO guidelines on hand hygiene in health care: First global patient safety challenge, clean care is safer care. https://apps.who.int/iris/bitstream/handle/10665/44102/9789241597906_eng.pdf?sequence=1 (Level IV)

9 Centers for Medicare and Medicaid Services, Department of Health and Human Services. (2020). Condition of participation: Infection control. 42 C.F.R. § 482.42.

10 Accreditation Association for Hospitals and Health Systems. (2020). Standard 07.01.21. *Healthcare Facilities Accreditation Program: Accreditation requirements for acute care hospitals.* Chicago, IL: Accreditation Association for Hospitals and Health Systems. (Level VII)

11 DNV GL-Healthcare USA, Inc. (2020). IC.1.SR.1. *NIAHO® accreditation requirements, interpretive guidelines and surveyor guidance—revision 20.0.* Milford, OH: DNV GL-Healthcare USA, Inc. (Level VII)

12 The Joint Commission. (2021). Standard NPSG.01.01.01. *Comprehensive accreditation manual for hospitals.* Oakbrook Terrace, IL: The Joint Commission. (Level VII)

13 The Joint Commission. (2021). Standard RI.01.01.01. *Comprehensive accreditation manual for hospitals.* Oakbrook Terrace, IL: The Joint Commission. (Level VII)

14 Centers for Medicare and Medicaid Services, Department of Health and Human Services. (2020). Condition of participation: Patient's rights. 42 C.F.R. § 482.13(c)(1).

15 Accreditation Association for Hospitals and Health Systems. (2020). Standard 15.01.16. *Healthcare Facilities Accreditation Program: Accreditation requirements for acute care hospitals.* Chicago, IL: Accreditation Association for Hospitals and Health Systems. (Level VII)

16 DNV GL-Healthcare USA, Inc. (2020). PR.2.SR.5. *NIAHO® accreditation requirements, interpretive guidelines and surveyor guidance—revision 20.0.* Milford, OH: DNV GL-Healthcare USA, Inc. (Level VII)

17 The Joint Commission. (2021). Standard PC.02.01.21. *Comprehensive accreditation manual for hospitals.* Oakbrook Terrace, IL: The Joint Commission. (Level VII)

18 Waters, T. R., et al. (2009). Safe patient handling training for schools of nursing. https://www.cdc.gov/niosh/docs/2009-127/pdfs/2009-127.pdf (Level VII)

19 Centers for Disease Control and Prevention. (2004). Guidelines for preventing health-care–associated pneumonia, 2003: Recommendations of CDC and the Healthcare Infection Control Practices Advisory Committee. *MMWR Recommendations and Reports, 53*(RR-3), 1–32. https://www.cdc.gov/mmwr/pdf/rr/rr5303.pdf (Level II)

20 Klompas, M., et al. (2014). Strategies to prevent ventilator-associated pneumonia in acute care hospitals: 2014 update. *Infection Control and Hospitals Epidemiology, 35*(8), 915–936. https://www.jstor.org/stable/10.1086/677144?seq=1#page_scan_tab_contents (Level I)

21 Siegel, J. D., et al. (2007, revised 2019). 2007 guideline for isolation precautions: Preventing transmission of infectious agents in healthcare settings. https://www.cdc.gov/infectioncontrol/pdf/guidelines/isolation-guidelines-H.pdf (Level II)

22 Accreditation Association for Hospitals and Health Systems. (2020). Standard 07.01.10. *Healthcare Facilities Accreditation Program: Accreditation requirements for acute care hospitals.* Chicago, IL: Accreditation Association for Hospitals and Health Systems. (Level VII)

23 Occupational Safety and Health Administration. (2019). Bloodborne pathogens, standard number 1910.1030. https://www.osha.gov/pls/oshaweb/owadisp.show_document?p_id=10051&p_table=STANDARDS (Level VII)

24 The Joint Commission. (2013). Sentinel event alert 50: Medical device alarm safety in hospitals. https://www.jointcommission.org/-/media/tjc/documents/resources/patient-safety-topics/sentinel-event/sea_50_alarms_4_26_16.pdf (Level VII)

25 The Joint Commission. (2021). Standard NPSG.06.01.01. *Comprehensive accreditation manual for hospitals.* Oakbrook Terrace, IL: The Joint Commission. (Level VII)

26 Graham, K. C., & Cvach, M. (2010). Monitor alarm fatigue: Standardizing use of physiological monitors and decreasing nuisance alarms. *American Journal of Critical Care, 19*, 28–37.

27 American Association of Critical-Care Nurses. (2018). AACN practice alert: Managing alarms in acute care across the life span: Electrocardiography and pulse oximetry. https://www.aacn.org/clinical-resources/practice-alerts/managing-alarms-in-acute-care-across-the-life-span (Level VII)

28 The Joint Commission. (2021). Standard NPSG.02.03.01. *Comprehensive accreditation manual for hospitals*. Oakbrook Terrace, IL: The Joint Commission. (Level VII)

29 Ganz, D. A., et al. (2013, reviewed 2021). Preventing falls in hospitals: A toolkit for improving quality of care (AHRQ publication no. 13-0015-EF). https://www.ahrq.gov/professionals/systems/hospital/fallpxtoolkit/index.html (Level VII)

30 Rutala, W. A., et al. (2008, revised 2019). Guideline for disinfection and sterilization in healthcare facilities, 2008. https://www.cdc.gov/infection-control/pdf/guidelines/disinfection-guidelines-H.pdf (Level I)

31 Accreditation Association for Hospitals and Health Systems. (2020). Standard 07.02.03. *Healthcare Facilities Accreditation Program: Accreditation requirements for acute care hospitals*. Chicago, IL: Accreditation Association for Hospitals and Health Systems. (Level VII)

32 The Joint Commission. (2021). Standard RC.01.03.01. *Comprehensive accreditation manual for hospitals*. Oakbrook Terrace, IL: The Joint Commission. (Level VII)

33 Centers for Medicare and Medicaid Services, Department of Health and Human Services. (2020). Condition of participation: Medical record services. 42 C.F.R. § 482.24(b).

34 Accreditation Association for Hospitals and Health Systems. (2020). Standard 10.00.03. *Healthcare Facilities Accreditation Program: Accreditation requirements for acute care hospitals*. Chicago, IL: Accreditation Association for Hospitals and Health Systems. (Level VII)

35 DNV GL-Healthcare USA, Inc. (2020). MR.2.SR.1. *NIAHO® accreditation requirements, interpretive guidelines and surveyor guidance—revision 20.0*. Milford, OH: DNV GL-Healthcare USA, Inc. (Level VII)

36 National Heart, Lung, and Blood Institute. (2016). Oxygen therapy. https://www.nhlbi.nih.gov/health-topics/oxygen-therapy

37 Weekley, M. S., & Bland, L. E. (2021). Oxygen administration. https://www.ncbi.nlm.nih.gov/books/NBK551617/

38 Black, J. M., & Kalowes, P. (2016). Medical device-related pressure ulcers. *Chronic Wound Care Management and Research, 3*, 91–99. https://www.dovepress.com/medical-device-related-pressure-ulcers-peer-reviewed-fulltext-article-CWCMR

PAIN MANAGEMENT

Defined as the sensory and emotional experience associated with actual or potential tissue damage, pain includes not only the perception of an uncomfortable stimulus, but also the response to that perception.

The patient's report of pain is the most reliable indicator of the existence of pain.[1,2] With severe pain, a patient commonly seeks medical help for pain relief and may believe that the pain signals a serious problem.. This perception produces anxiety, which, in turn, can increase the pain. To assess and manage pain properly, the nurse must both listen to the person's subjective description and make use of objective tools.

Each facility should have defined criteria to screen, assess, and reassess pain.[3] These criteria should be consistent with the patient's age, condition, and ability to understand.[3] Pain assessment should include personal, cultural, spiritual, and ethnic beliefs. Patients and families should be educated about their role in pain management. They should also be informed about potential limitations and adverse effects of pain treatment. It's important to reassess pain at designated intervals and the effectiveness of the type of pain intervention used (for example, oral, IV, or transdermal route) to evaluate progress toward pain management goals.

Several interventions can be used to manage pain, including administering analgesics, providing emotional support and comfort measures, and using complementary and alternative therapies, such as cognitive techniques to distract the patient and Reiki or aromatherapy to promote relaxation. Severe pain usually requires an opioid analgesic. Invasive measures, such as epidural analgesia or patient-controlled analgesia (PCA), may also be required.

Equipment

Facility-approved pain assessment tool or scale ▪ oral care supplies ▪ water ▪ soap ▪ washcloth and towel ▪ glass or cup of fresh water ▪ prescribed nonopioid analgesic (such as aspirin or acetaminophen) ▪ Optional: PCA device, prescribed mild opioid (such as codeine), prescribed strong opioid (such as morphine or HYDROmorphone), pulse oximeter and probe, capnography equipment, sedation scale, pillow, cold compresses, lotion, radio or other device to listen to music.

Preparation of equipment

Inspect all equipment and supplies. If a product is expired, is defective, or has compromised integrity, remove it from patient use, label it as expired or defective, and report the expiration or defect as directed by your facility.

Implementation

▪ Review the patient's medical record for information related to the patient's current clinical condition, past medical history, and pain management goals, when available.[3]
▪ Review the patient's pain history, including previous use or abuse of analgesics, possible adverse effects associated with potential opioid tolerance or intolerance, and previous pain level, when available.[4]
▪ Perform hand hygiene.[5,6,7,8,9,10]
▪ Confirm the patient's identity using at least two patient identifiers.[11]
▪ Provide privacy.[12,13,14,15]
▪ Obtain the assistance of a medical interpreter as needed.[16,17]
▪ Raise the patient's bed to waist level before providing patient care *to prevent caregiver back strain*.[18]
▪ Perform hand hygiene.[5,6,7,8,9,10]
▪ Screen and assess the patient's pain using facility-defined criteria that are consistent with the patient's age, condition, and ability to understand.[3] As directed, use a facility-approved pain assessment tool or scale.
▪ Ask key questions and note the patient's response.[3] For example, ask the patient to describe the pain's duration, severity, and location. Look for physiologic or behavioral clues to the pain's severity.[19] (See *How to assess pain*.)
▪ In collaboration with the multidisciplinary team, involve the patient in the pain management planning process. Provide education on pain management, treatment options, and the safe use of opioid and nonopioid medications when prescribed. Develop realistic expectations and measurable goals that the patient understands for the degree, duration, and reduction of pain. Discuss objectives used to evaluate treatment progress (for example, relief of pain and improved physical and psychosocial function).[3]
▪ Treat the patient's pain as needed and ordered using nonpharmacologic or pharmacologic approaches, or a combination of approaches. Base the treatment plan on evidence-based practices and the patient's clinical condition, past medical history, and pain management goals.[3]

Providing emotional support
▪ Show your concern by spending time talking with the patient. Because of the pain and the inability to manage it, the patient may be anxious and frustrated. Such feelings can worsen pain.
▪ Assess the patient's spiritual and cultural needs, and incorporate spiritual and cultural practices as desired by the patient.

Performing comfort measures
▪ Perform hand hygiene.[5,6,7,8,9,10]
▪ Reposition the patient periodically *to reduce muscle spasms and tension and to relieve pressure on bony prominences*. Increasing the angle of the bed can reduce pull on an abdominal incision, diminishing pain. If appropriate, elevate a limb *to reduce swelling, inflammation, and pain*.
▪ Encourage the patient to splint or support abdominal and chest incisions with a pillow when coughing or changing position *to help decrease pain*.
▪ Apply cold compresses as appropriate *to decrease discomfort*.[19]
▪ Give the patient a back massage *to help relax tense muscles*.[19]

How to assess pain

To assess pain properly, you need to consider the patient's description and your observations of the patient's physical and behavioral responses. A comprehensive, culturally sensitive pain assessment tool can help capture the effects of cultural norms on the patient's pain experiences, examine the meaning that the pain has to the patient, and determine the patient's treatment preferences (such as herbs, home remedies, complementary therapies, or the services of alternative or cultural healers).[16]

Start by asking the following questions, bearing in mind that the patient's responses will be shaped by previous experiences, self-image, and beliefs about the condition:
- Where is the pain located? How long does it last? How often does it occur?
- How would you describe the pain?
- What brings the pain on?
- What relieves the pain or makes it worse?
- What do you think is causing your pain?
- What do you fear most about the pain?
- What problems does the pain cause you?
- Who else have you consulted about the pain? Family members? A traditional healer?
- What treatments do you think might help you with the pain?

Ask the patient to rank the pain on a scale from 0 to 10, with 0 denoting lack of pain and 10 denoting the worst pain possible. Establish with the patient what would be considered a low pain level, usually 4 or lower on a 0-to-10 scale.

Observe the patient's behavioral and physiologic (sympathetic or parasympathetic) responses to pain:
- **Behavioral responses** include altered body position, moaning, sighing, grimacing, withdrawal, crying, restlessness, muscle twitching, and immobility.
- **Sympathetic responses** are commonly associated with mild to moderate pain, and include pallor, elevated blood pressure, dilated pupils, skeletal muscle tension, dyspnea, tachycardia, and diaphoresis.
- **Parasympathetic responses** are commonly associated with severe, deep pain, and include pallor, decreased blood pressure, bradycardia, nausea, vomiting, weakness, dizziness, and loss of consciousness.

- Perform passive range-of-motion exercises *to prevent stiffness and further loss of mobility, relax tense muscles, and provide comfort.* (See the "Passive range-of-motion exercises" procedure.)
- Provide oral care (see the "Oral care" procedure). Keep a glass or cup of fresh water at the bedside, *because many pain medications tend to dry out the mouth.*
- Wash the patient's face and hands *to soothe the patient, which may reduce the perception of pain.*

Using complementary and alternative techniques
- Help the patient enhance the effect of analgesics by using such techniques as distraction, guided imagery, deep breathing, music therapy, muscle relaxation, and visual concentration and rhythmic massage.[19] Choose the method the patient prefers. If possible, start these techniques when the patient feels little or no pain. If the patient feels persistent pain, begin with short, simple exercises. Before beginning, dim the lights, remove the patient's restrictive clothing, and eliminate noise from the environment.
- For *distraction*, have the patient recall a pleasant experience or focus attention on an enjoyable activity. Note, however, that distraction is mainly helpful in relieving pain lasting for brief episodes or for painful procedures of short duration.[4]
- For *imagery*, help the patient concentrate on a peaceful, pleasant image, such as walking on the beach. Encourage the patient to concentrate on the details of that image by asking about the associated sights, sounds, smells, tastes, and touch. *The positive emotions evoked by this exercise minimize pain.*[4]
- For *deep breathing*, have the patient focus on an object, then slowly inhale and exhale while maintaining a comfortable rate and rhythm. Have the patient concentrate on the rise and fall of the abdomen. Encourage

the patient to feel more and more weightless with each breath and to concentrate on the rhythm of breathing, or on any restful image.[4]
- For *music therapy*, play music that the patient prefers. Consult with a music therapist if available. Music therapy has been associated with statistically significant reduction in opioid and nonopioid analgesic use.[20,21]
- For *muscle relaxation*, have the patient focus on a particular muscle group. Then ask the patient to tense the muscles and note the sensation. After 5 to 7 seconds, tell the patient to relax the muscles and concentrate on the relaxed state. Have the patient note the difference between the tense and relaxed states. After the patient tenses and relaxes one muscle group, have the patient proceed to another and then another, until the patient has covered the entire body.[4]
- For *visual concentration and rhythmic massage*, have the patient stare at an object or close the eyes and think of a peaceful, calm scene. Then instruct the patient to firmly massage the area near the painful body part using a circular motion with the palm of the hand. Tell the patient to avoid red or swollen areas. A family member can perform the massage as well.[4]

Giving medications
- Perform hand hygiene.[5,6,7,8,9,10]
- If the patient's condition allows oral medications, begin with a nonopioid analgesic, such as acetaminophen or aspirin, every 4 to 6 hours as ordered, following safe medication administration practices.[22,23,24,25,26]
- If the patient needs more relief than a nonopioid analgesic provides, administer a mild opioid (such as oxyCODONE or codeine) as ordered, following safe medication administration practices.[22,23,24,25,26]
- If the patient needs still more pain relief, administer a strong opioid (such as morphine or HYDROmorphone), as ordered (administer oral medications if possible), following safe medication administration practices.[22,23,24,25,26]
- For the patient receiving IV opioid medication, monitor the patient closely if identified as high risk for adverse outcomes related to opioid treatment.[3] Frequently monitor the patient's respiratory rate, oxygen saturation level by pulse oximetry, end-tidal carbon dioxide level by capnography (if available), and sedation level using a standardized sedation scale, *to decrease the risk of adverse events associated with IV opioid use.*[23,27] Explain the assessment and monitoring process to the patient and family members according to their individual communication and learning needs *to increase their understanding, allay their fears, and enhance cooperation.*[17] Tell them to alert staff if breathing problems or other changes occur that might be a reaction to the medication.[23,27]
- If ordered, teach the patient to use a PCA device, which can help manage the pain and decrease anxiety. (See the "Patient-controlled analgesia" procedure.)

Completing the procedure
- Reassess and respond to the patient's pain by evaluating the response to treatment and progress toward pain management goals. Assess for adverse reactions and risk factors for adverse events that may result from treatment.
- Return the bed to the lowest position *to prevent falls and maintain the patient's safety.*[28]
- Perform hand hygiene.[5,6,7,8,9,10]
- Document the procedure.[29,30,31,32]

Special considerations
- Pain shouldn't be considered a normal part of the aging process. Provide pain relief for older adult patients using pharmacologic and nonpharmacologic approaches. Remember, safety is a special concern, especially the risk of falls resulting from impaired mobility due to pain and from adverse effects of pain medications.[33]
- Identify age-related factors that affect assessment and pain management in older adult patients.[33]

ELDER ALERT *Because of the potential for adverse effects,* certain medications (such as meperidine and methadone) and prolonged use of nonsteroidal-anti-inflammatory drugs should be avoided in older adult patients.[34,35]

■ Cultural remedies for pain, such as the involvement of extended family and the use of complementary therapies such as acupuncture, should be permitted and even encouraged. *Research indicates that family support improves patient outcomes, and that acupuncture can be effective in managing pain.*[16]

■ The U.S. Food and Drug Administration has required a boxed warning be added to the prescribing information for all opioid drugs advising that opioids are not be stopped abruptly. Opioids should be withdrawn slowly according to an individualized and gradual taper plan *to prevent signs and symptoms of withdrawal, worsening of pain, and psychological distress in physically dependent patients.* Refer to the manufacturer's label for specific tapering instructions.

■ When tapering opioids, monitor patients closely for signs and symptoms of opioid withdrawal, such as restlessness, lacrimation, rhinorrhea, yawning, perspiration, chills, myalgia, mydriasis, irritability, anxiety, insomnia, backache, joint pain, weakness, abdominal cramps, anorexia, nausea, vomiting, diarrhea, increased blood pressure or heart rate, and increased respiratory rate. Such symptoms may indicate a need to taper more slowly. Also monitor for suicidal thoughts, use of other substances, or changes in mood.

■ Don't assume that the patient who has dementia or another cognitive impairment can't understand the pain scale or communicate about pain. Experiment with several pain scales to find one that works. A scale featuring faces, such as the Wong-Baker FACES® Pain Rating Scale, is a good choice for many cognitively impaired patients and those with limited language skills. (See *Visual pain rating scale.*)

Complications

When left untreated, pain can have negative consequences, including multisystem complications and the development of chronic disabling pain, which may seriously affect the patient's functioning, quality of life, and well-being.[2] In fact, pain may actually accelerate death by limiting mobility, increasing physiologic stress, and increasing the risk of complications such as pneumonia and thromboembolism.[1] Adverse effects of opioids or other medications used to treat pain include respiratory depression (the most serious), drowsiness or sedation, constipation, nausea, vomiting, and addiction.[36]

Documentation

Document each step of the nursing process. Describe the subjective information you elicited from the patient, using the patient's own words. Note the location, quality, and duration of the pain as well as precipitating factors.

Record the pain-relief methods selected and the patient's rating of the pain before and after pain management interventions. Summarize your actions, including the name and dosage of any medications given and the patient's response. If the patient's pain wasn't relieved, note alternative treatments ordered and ways to revise the treatment plan. Also record any complications of drug therapy. Document teaching provided to the patient and family (if applicable), their understanding of that teaching, and any need for follow-up teaching.

REFERENCES

1 Herr, K., et al. (2011). Position statement: Pain assessment in the patient unable to self-report: Position statement with clinical practice recommendations. *Pain Management Nursing, 12*(4), 230–250. http://www.aspmn.org/documents/PainAssessmentinthePatientUnabletoSelfReport.pdf

2 American Association of Critical-Care Nurses. (2018). AACN practice alert: Assessing pain in the critically ill adult. https://www.aacn.org/clinical-resources/practice-alerts/assessing-pain-in-critically-ill-adults (Level VII)

3 The Joint Commission. (2021). Standard PC.01.02.07. *Comprehensive accreditation manual for hospitals.* Oakbrook Terrace, IL: The Joint Commission. (Level VII)

4 American Cancer Society. (2019). Non-medical treatments for pain. https://www.cancer.org/treatment/treatments-and-side-effects/physical-side-effects/pain/non-medical-treatments-for-cancer-pain.html

5 The Joint Commission. (2021). Standard NPSG.07.01.01. *Comprehensive accreditation manual for hospitals.* Oakbrook Terrace, IL: The Joint Commission. (Level VII)

6 Centers for Disease Control and Prevention. (2002). Guideline for hand hygiene in health-care settings: Recommendations of the Healthcare Infection Control Practices Advisory Committee and the HICPAC/SHEA/APIC/IDSA Hand Hygiene Task Force. *MMWR Recommendations and Reports, 51*(RR-16), 1–45. https://www.cdc.gov/mmwr/pdf/rr/rr5116.pdf (Level II)

7 World Health Organization. (2009). WHO guidelines on hand hygiene in health care: First global patient safety challenge, clean care is safer care. https://apps.who.int/iris/bitstream/handle/10665/44102/9789241597906_eng.pdf?sequence=1 (Level IV)

8 Centers for Medicare and Medicaid Services, Department of Health and Human Services. (2020). Condition of participation: Infection control. 42 C.F.R. § 482.42.

9 Accreditation Association for Hospitals and Health Systems. (2020). Standard 07.01.21. *Healthcare Facilities Accreditation Program: Accreditation requirements for acute care hospitals.* Chicago, IL: Accreditation Association for Hospitals and Health Systems. (Level VII)

10 DNV GL-Healthcare USA, Inc. (2020). IC.1.SR.1. *NIAHO® accreditation requirements, interpretive guidelines and surveyor guidance—revision 20.0.* Milford, OH: DNV GL-Healthcare USA, Inc. (Level VII)

11 The Joint Commission. (2021). Standard NPSG.01.01.01. *Comprehensive accreditation manual for hospitals.* Oakbrook Terrace, IL: The Joint Commission. (Level VII)

12 The Joint Commission. (2021). Standard RI.01.01.01. *Comprehensive accreditation manual for hospitals.* Oakbrook Terrace, IL: The Joint Commission. (Level VII)

13 Centers for Medicare and Medicaid Services, Department of Health and Human Services. (2020). Condition of participation: Patient's rights. 42. C.F.R. § 482.13(c)(1).

14 Accreditation Association for Hospitals and Health Systems. (2020). Standard 15.01.16. *Healthcare Facilities Accreditation Program: Accreditation requirements for acute care hospitals.* Chicago, IL: Accreditation Association for Hospitals and Health Systems. (Level VII)

15 DNV GL-Healthcare USA, Inc. (2020). PR.2.SR.5. *NIAHO® accreditation requirements, interpretive guidelines and surveyor guidance—revision 20.0.* Milford, OH: DNV GL-Healthcare USA, Inc. (Level VII)

16 Narayan, M. C. (2010). Culture's effects on pain assessment and management. *American Journal of Nursing, 110*(4), 38–47.

17 The Joint Commission. (2021). Standard PC.02.01.21. *Comprehensive accreditation manual for hospitals.* Oakbrook Terrace, IL: The Joint Commission. (Level VII)

Visual pain rating scale

Patients with language difficulties can indicate pain using many instruments. One such instrument is the Wong-Baker FACES® Pain Rating Scale (shown below), which uses six faces to help the patient describe the level of pain. It's used with a 0 to 10 scale. Explain to the patient what each face means before having the patient rate the pain.

To use the FACES® scale, explain to the patient that each face represents a person who feels happy because of having no pain or is sad because of having some or a lot of pain. Face 0 is very happy because nothing hurts. Face 2 hurts just a little bit. Face 4 hurts a little more. Face 6 hurts even more. Face 8 hurts a whole lot. Face 10 hurts as much as you can imagine, although you don't have to be crying to feel this bad. Ask the patient to choose the face that best describes how the patient is feeling

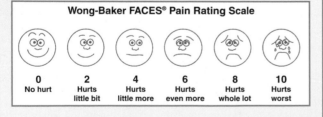

Wong-Baker FACES® Pain Rating Scale

0	2	4	6	8	10
No hurt	Hurts little bit	Hurts little more	Hurts even more	Hurts whole lot	Hurts worst

© 1983 Wong-Baker FACES Foundation. www.WongBakerFACES.org. Used with permission. Originally published in *Whaley & Wong's Nursing Care of Infants and Children.* © Elsevier Inc.

18 Waters, T. T., et al. (2009). Safe patient handling training for schools of nursing. https://www.cdc.gov/niosh/docs/2009-127/pdfs/2009-127.pdf (Level VII)

19 American Society of PeriAnesthesia Nurses. (2003). ASPAN pain and comfort clinical guideline. *Journal of PeriAnesthesia Nursing, 18*(4), 232–236. http://www.aspan.org/Portals/6/docs/ClinicalPractice/Guidelines/ASPAN_ClinicalGuideline_PainComfort.pdf (Level VII)

20 The Joint Commission. (2018). Quick safety: Non-pharmacologic and non-opioid solutions for pain management. https://www.jointcommission.org/resources/news-and-multimedia/newsletters/newsletters/quick-safety/quick-safety-44-nonpharmacologic-and-nonopioid-solutions-for-pain-management/

21 Lee, J. H. (2016). The effects of music on pain: A meta-analysis. *Journal of Music Therapy, 53*, 430–477.

22 World Health Organization (WHO). (n.d.). WHO's guidelines for the management of cancer pain. https://www.who.int/ncds/management/palliative-care/Infographic-cancer-pain-lowres.pdf

23 Centers for Medicare and Medicaid Services, Department of Health and Human Services. (2020). Condition of participation: Nursing services. 42 C.F.R. § 482.23(c).

24 Accreditation Association for Hospitals and Health Systems. (2020). Standard 16.01.03. *Healthcare Facilities Accreditation Program: Accreditation requirements for acute care hospitals.* Chicago, IL: Accreditation Association for Hospitals and Health Systems. (Level VII)

25 The Joint Commission. (2021). Standard MM.06.01.01. *Comprehensive accreditation manual for hospitals.* Oakbrook Terrace, IL: The Joint Commission. (Level VII)

26 DNV GL-Healthcare USA, Inc. (2020). MM.1.SR.3. *NIAHO® accreditation requirements, interpretive guidelines and surveyor guidance—revision 20.0.* Milford, OH: DNV GL-Healthcare USA, Inc. (Level VII)

27 Centers for Medicare and Medicaid Services. (2014). Requirements for hospital medication administration, particularly intravenous (IV) medications and post-operative care of patients receiving IV opioids. https://www.cms.gov/Medicare/Provider-Enrollment-and-Certification/SurveyCertificationGenInfo/Downloads/Survey-and-Cert-Letter-14-15.pdf

28 Ganz, D. A., et al. (2013. Reviewed 2021). *Preventing falls in hospitals: A toolkit for improving quality of care* (AHRQ Publication No. 13-0015-EF). Rockville, MD: Agency for Healthcare Research and Quality. https://www.ahrq.gov/professionals/systems/hospital/fallpxtoolkit/index.html (Level VII)

29 The Joint Commission (2021). Standard RC.01.03.01. *Comprehensive accreditation manual for hospitals.* Oakbrook Terrace, IL: The Joint Commission. (Level VII)

30 Centers for Medicare and Medicaid Services, Department of Health and Human Services. (2020). Condition of participation: Medical record services. 42 C.F.R. § 482.24(b).

31 Accreditation Association for Hospitals and Health Systems. (2020). Standard 10.00.03. *Healthcare Facilities Accreditation Program: Accreditation requirements for acute care hospitals.* Chicago, IL: Accreditation Association for Hospitals and Health Systems. (Level VII)

32 DNV GL-Healthcare USA, Inc. (2020). MR.2.SR.1. *NIAHO® accreditation requirements, interpretive guidelines and surveyor guidance—revision 20.0.* Milford, OH: DNV GL-Healthcare USA, Inc. (Level VII)

33 Harmon, J. R., et al. (2012). Efficacy of the use of evidence-based algorithmic guidelines in the acute care setting for pain assessment and management in older people: A critical review of the literature. *International Journal of Older People Nursing, 7*, 127–140. (Level V)

34 Cavalieri, T. A. (2007). Managing pain in geriatric patients. *Journal of the American Osteopathic Association, 107*(6), ES10–ES16. https://www.degruyter.com/document/doi/10.7556/jaoa.2007.20014/html

35 Galicia-Castillo, M. C., & Weiner, D. K. (2019). Treatment of chronic non-cancer pain in older adults. In: *UpToDate*, Schmader, K. E. & Fishman, S. (Eds.)

36 U.S. National Library of Medicine. (2020). Opioid misuse and addiction. https://medlineplus.gov/opioidmisuseandaddiction.html

PARENTERAL NUTRITION ADMINISTRATION

The patient who can't meet nutritional needs by oral or enteral feedings may require IV nutritional support, or parenteral nutrition (PN). The patient's diagnosis, history, and prognosis determine the need for PN. Generally, this treatment is prescribed in collaboration with the patient and the heath care team, depending upon the goals of care.[1] Specific indications include debilitating illness lasting longer than 2 weeks; loss of 10% or more of pre-illness weight; serum albumin level below 3.5 g/dL; excessive nitrogen loss from wound infection, fistulas, or abscesses; kidney or liver failure; or a nonfunctioning GI tract for more than 5 days in a patient experiencing severe catabolism.

Common illnesses that can trigger the need for PN include inflammatory bowel disease, radiation enteritis, severe diarrhea, intractable vomiting, and moderate to severe pancreatitis. A massive small-bowel resection, bone marrow transplantation, high-dose chemotherapy or radiation therapy, and major surgery can also hinder a patient's ability to absorb nutrients, requiring PN.[2]

PN shouldn't be given to patients with a normally functioning GI tract, and it has limited value for well-nourished patients whose GI tract will resume normal function within 10 days. It also may be inappropriate for patients with a poor prognosis or if the risks of PN outweigh the benefits.

PN may be administered through a peripheral or central venous (CV) access device depending on the solution's osmolarity and the expected duration of treatment.[3] The solution prescribed varies by whether it's used to boost the patient's caloric intake, supply full caloric needs, or surpass the patient's caloric requirements.

The type of PN prescribed depends on the patient's condition and metabolic needs and on the administration route. The solution usually contains protein, carbohydrates, electrolytes, vitamins, and trace minerals. A lipid emulsion provides necessary fat. Standard IV solutions, such as dextrose 5% in water, dextrose 10% in water, and normal saline solution, are nutritionally incomplete and don't provide sufficient calories to maintain a patient's nutritional status. (See *Types of parenteral nutrition*, page 630.)

Total parenteral nutrition (TPN) refers to any nutrient solution, including lipids, given through a CV access device. Peripheral parenteral nutrition (PPN), which is given through a peripheral catheter, supplies sufficient calories for weight maintenance while avoiding the risks that accompany CV access. To keep from sclerosing the vein through which it's administered, the dextrose in PPN solution must be limited to 10%, and the osmolarity must be less than 900 mOsm/L.[1] Therefore, the success of PPN depends on the patient's tolerance of the large volume of fluid necessary to supply nutritional needs.

In many cases, the patient may need an increase in the dextrose content and osmolarity beyond the level a peripheral vein can handle. For example, most TPN solutions are six times more concentrated than blood. As a result, they must be delivered into a central vein with a high blood flow rate to dilute the solution. The most common delivery route for TPN is through a CV access device into the superior vena cava. Follow sterile no-touch technique when administering PN to reduce the risk of vascular catheter–associated infection.

HOSPITAL-ACQUIRED CONDITION ALERT Keep in mind that the Centers for Medicare and Medicaid Services considers vascular catheter–associated infection a hospital-acquired condition *because it can be reasonably prevented using a variety of best practices.* Make sure to follow evidence-based infection prevention practices, such as performing hand hygiene, performing a vigorous mechanical scrub of the needleless connector, and using sterile no-touch technique *to reduce the risk of vascular catheter–associated bloodstream infections.*[5,6,7]

Equipment

Prescribed PN solution ■ sterile IV administration set for the infusion device ■ 1.2-micron filter[8] ■ 10-mL syringe with preservative-free normal saline solution (or a syringe specifically designed to generate lower injection pressure) ■ antiseptic pads (chlorhexidine-based, povidone iodine, or alcohol) ■ electronic infusion device (preferably a smart pump with dose-error reduction software and interoperability with the electronic health records) with anti-free-flow protection[1] ■ gloves ■ scale ■ intake-and-output monitoring supplies ■ labels ■ facility-approved disinfectant ■ Optional: mask, glucometer, supplies for blood specimen collection.

Preparation of equipment

Keep the PN solution refrigerated and protected from light until 1 hour before use *to prevent vitamin oxidation.* Remove the PN solution from the refrigerator 60 minutes before use *to reduce the risk of hypothermia, venospasm, and pain.*[9]

Types of parenteral nutrition

Type	Solution components/liter	Uses	Special considerations
Total parenteral nutrition (TPN) by way of central venous (CV) access	▪ Dextrose 15% in water ($D_{15}W$) to $D_{25}W$ (1 L of dextrose 25% = 850 nonprotein calories) ▪ Crystalline amino acids 2.5% to 8.5% ▪ Electrolytes, vitamins, trace elements, and insulin, as ordered ▪ Lipid emulsion 10% to 20% (usually infused as a separate solution)	▪ Two weeks or more ▪ For patients with high caloric and nutrient needs ▪ Provides calories, restores nitrogen balance, and replaces essential vitamins, electrolytes, minerals, and trace elements ▪ Promotes tissue synthesis, wound healing, and normal metabolic function ▪ Allows bowel rest and healing; reduces activity in the gallbladder, pancreas, and small intestine ▪ Improves tolerance of surgery	**Basic solution** ▪ Nutritionally complete ▪ Requires minor surgical procedure for CV access insertion and radiologic placement verification ▪ Highly hypertonic solution ▪ May cause metabolic complications (glucose intolerance, electrolyte imbalance, essential fatty acid deficiency) **IV lipid emulsion** ▪ May interfere with immune mechanisms[4] ▪ Administered via CV access device; irritates peripheral vein in long-term use
Total nutrient admixture	▪ One day's nutrients contained in a single bag (also called *3:1 solution*) ▪ Combines lipid emulsion with other parenteral solution components	▪ Two weeks or more ▪ For relatively stable patients ▪ For patients with large caloric and nutrient needs ▪ Provides calories, restores nitrogen balance, and replaces essential vitamins, electrolytes, minerals, and trace elements ▪ Promotes tissue synthesis, wound healing, and normal metabolic function ▪ Allows bowel rest and healing; reduces activity in the gallbladder, pancreas, and small intestine ▪ Improves tolerance of surgery	▪ Nutritionally complete ▪ Requires minor surgical procedure for CV access insertion and radiologic placement verification ▪ Highly hypertonic solution ▪ May cause metabolic complications (glucose intolerance, electrolyte imbalance) ▪ Reduces need to handle bag, reducing contamination risk ▪ Decreases nursing time and reduces need for infusion sets and electronic devices, lowering facility costs, increasing patient mobility, and allowing easier adjustment to home care ▪ Has limited use because not all types and amounts of components are compatible
Peripheral parenteral nutrition (PPN)	▪ D_5W to $D_{10}W$ ▪ Crystalline amino acids 2.5% to 5% ▪ Electrolytes, minerals, vitamins, and trace elements, as ordered ▪ Lipid emulsion 10% or 20% (1 L of dextrose 10% and amino acids 3.5% infused at the same time as 1 L of lipid emulsion = 1,440 nonprotein calories)	▪ Two weeks or less ▪ Provides up to 2,000 calories/day ▪ Maintains adequate nutritional status in patients who can tolerate relatively high fluid volume, in those who usually resume bowel function and oral feedings after a few days, and in those susceptible to infections associated with a CV access device	**Basic solution** ▪ Nutritionally complete for a short time ▪ Can't be used long term in nutritionally depleted patients ▪ Used for weight maintenance, not weight gain ▪ Avoids insertion and care of CV access device but requires adequate venous access ▪ Delivers less hypertonic solutions than TPN ▪ May cause phlebitis ▪ Less chance of metabolic complications than with TPN **IV lipid emulsion** ▪ As effective as dextrose for caloric source ▪ Diminishes phlebitis if infused at the same time as basic nutrient solution

Inspect all IV equipment and supplies; if a product is expired, is defective, or has compromised integrity, remove it from patient use, label it as expired or defective, and report the expiration or defect as directed by your facility.[10] Ensure that any administration set to be used for lipids is di-(2-ethylhexyl)phthalate (DEHP)-free.[1]

Implementation

▪ Avoid distractions and interruptions when preparing and administering the PN solution *to prevent administration errors*.[11,12]

▪ Verify the practitioner's order. Make sure that the prescribed therapy is appropriate for the patient's age, condition, and vascular access device, and that the infusion or medication is compatible with other solutions and medication. Make sure that the order includes any test results that require monitoring. Confirm the access device catheter tip, as appropriate. Also confirm that the dose, rate, and administration route are appropriate. Address concerns about the order with the practitioner, pharmacist, your supervisor, the risk management department, or as directed by your facility.[13,14,15,16,17,18,19]

▪ Gather and prepare the necessary equipment and supplies.

▪ Make sure that the solution container is labeled with the patient's identifiers and weight, administration date and time, expiration date, administration route (central or peripheral), dextrose concentration, and component names and dosages. (All components should be labeled as amount per day and listed in the same sequence and same unit of measure as the practitioner's order.) Make sure the total volume of solution and the infusion rate are included, as well as the duration of the infusion (continuous or cycled) and the appropriate size filter to use.

▪ Visually inspect the integrity of the container and solution, and check the expiration date. Return the solution to the pharmacy if the integrity of the container is compromised or if the solution is cloudy, separated, contains particles, or is expired.[13,14,15,16,18]

▪ If required by your facility, confirm that informed consent has been obtained, and that the signed consent form is in the patient's medical record.[9,20,21,22,23]

▪ Perform hand hygiene.[6,24,25,26,27,28,29,30]

▪ Confirm the patient's identity using at least two patient identifiers.[18,31]

▪ Provide privacy.[32,33,34,35]

▪ Explain the procedure to the patient and family (if appropriate) according to their individual communication and learning needs *to increase their understanding, allay their fears, and enhance cooperation*.[36] Answer any questions the patient has about PN.[21,22]

▪ Compare the patient's name and second patient identifier on the solution container against the name and second patient identifier on the patient's identification band.

- If your facility uses a bar-code technology, use it as directed by your facility.[19]
- Raise the bed to waist level when providing care *to prevent caregiver back strain.*[37]
- Perform hand hygiene.[6,24,25,26,27,28,29,30]
- Put on gloves and, if required by your facility, a mask *to comply with standard precautions.*[38,39]
- Connect the IV administration set and micron filter. Insert the filter as close to the catheter insertion site as possible.[8,40]

NURSING ALERT Guidelines recommend a 1.2-micron filter for all parenteral nutrition regimens, including dextrose-amino acid admixtures, total nutrient admixtures, and lipid injectable emulsions. (If the manufacturer requires a specific filter, consult with the manufacturer's instruction for use.) If administering a dextrose-amino acid admixture and lipid injectable emulsion as separate infusions, the filter should be located below the Y-site where the infusions meet.[8]

- Squeeze the IV administration set drip chamber and, holding the drip chamber upright, insert the IV administration set spike into the IV bag or bottle. Then release the drip chamber.
- Prime the IV administration set by opening the roller clamp. Let the solution fill the filter and the tubing; gently tap the tubing, filter, and Y-ports *to dislodge trapped air and prevent air embolism.*[41] Don't invert the filter during priming to allow the vented side of the housing to fill before flowing to the patient side of the device; follow the manufacturer's instructions for priming the filter.[8]
- Attach the IV administration set to the infusion pump following the manufacturer's instructions.
- Set the infusion rate, concentration, and volume to be infused. Make sure the alarms limits are set appropriately for the patient's current condition, and that the alarms are turned on, functioning, and audible to staff.[18,42,43,44]
- Label the container and IV administration set with the date of initiation or the date when change is required, as directed by your facility.[45]
- Perform a vigorous mechanical scrub of the needleless connector for at least 5 seconds using an antiseptic pad. Allow it to dry completely.[7,46]
- Verify patency of the access device by aspirating for blood return and flushing the catheter *to reduce the risk of infiltration and extravasation.*[17,47]
- While maintaining sterility of the syringe tip, attach a prefilled 10-mL syringe or a syringe specifically designed to generate lower injection pressure containing preservative-free normal saline solution to the needleless connector. Unclamp the catheter and slowly aspirate for a blood return that's the color and consistency of whole blood. If you don't obtain a blood return, take steps to locate an external cause of obstruction.[47]
- If you do obtain a blood return, inject preservative-free normal saline solution slowly into the catheter. Use a minimum volume of twice the internal volume of the catheter system. Don't forcibly flush the device; further evaluate the device if you meet resistance. Flush the catheter with preservative-free normal saline solution according to the catheter type.[47]
- Clamp the access device before disconnecting it *to prevent air from entering the catheter.* If the catheter is a CV access device and a clamp isn't available, ask the patient to perform the Valsalva maneuver just as you change the tubing, if possible. Or, if the patient is being mechanically ventilated, change the IV tubing immediately after the machine delivers a breath at peak inspiration. *Both of these measures increase intrathoracic pressure and prevent air embolism.*[41]
- Perform a vigorous mechanical scrub of the needleless connector for at least 5 seconds using an antiseptic pad. Allow it to dry completely.[7,46]
- Attach the IV administration set to the needleless connector using sterile no-touch technique.
- Trace the tubing from the patient to its point of origin *to make sure that you've connected it to the proper port.* Route the tubing in a standardized direction if the patient has other tubing and catheters that have different purposes. Label the tubing at the distal (near the patient connection) and proximal (near the source container) ends *to reduce the risk of misconnection* if you'll be using multiple IV lines.[17,45,48]
- After connecting the tubing, remove the clamp, if applicable. Secure all connections *to prevent harmful disconnections.*

NURSING ALERT Parenteral nutrition preparations are considered high-alert medications *because they can cause significant harm when used in error.*[49]

- If required by your facility, before beginning the PN infusion, have another nurse perform an independent double-check *to verify the patient's identity and to make sure that the correct solution is hanging in the prescribed concentration, the solution's indication corresponds with the patient's diagnosis, the dosage calculations are correct and the dosing formula used to derive the final dose is correct, the prescribed route of administration is safe and proper for the patient, the prescribed time and frequency of administration are safe and proper for the patient, the infusion pump settings are correct, and the infusion line is attached to the correct port.*[18,50]
- After comparing the results of the independent double-check with the other nurse, open the clamp and begin infusing the PN, as ordered, if there are no discrepancies. If discrepancies exist, rectify them before beginning the infusion.[50]

NURSING ALERT It's important to maintain PN infusions at the prescribed rate *to avoid blood glucose fluctuations.*[18] Avoid interrupting the infusion for routine care or patient transport. Don't adjust the rate for off-schedule infusion starts or alter the infusion rate in response to changes in fluid needs.[51]

- Return the bed to the lowest position *to prevent falls and maintain the patient's safety.*[52]
- Discard used supplies in the appropriate receptacles.[38,39,53]
- Remove and discard your gloves and, if worn, your mask.[38,39,53]
- Perform hand hygiene.[6,24,25,26,27,28,29,30]
- Monitor the patient's glucose level according to the ordered parameters.[1] Notify the practitioner of abnormal blood glucose results. *Insulin may be added to the PN solution; however, you may also need to administer additional subcutaneous doses if insulin is ordered.*
- Obtain blood specimens for laboratory analysis according to the ordered parameters *to monitor the patient's metabolic status.* Report abnormalities to the practitioner.
- Monitor intake and output, assess for edema, and weigh the patient daily at the same time each morning, after the patient voids if possible.[18] Suspect fluid imbalance if the patient gains more than 0.5 kg daily.
- Perform hand hygiene.[24,25,26,27,28,29,30]
- Put on gloves.[39]
- Clean and disinfect reusable equipment according to the manufacturer's instructions *to prevent the spread of infection.*[54,55]
- Remove and discard your gloves.[39]
- Perform hand hygiene.[6,24,25,26,27,28,29,30]
- Document the procedure.[56,57,58,59,60]

Special considerations

- Change administration sets, including in-line and add-on filters used for parenteral nutrition (with or without lipids), at least every 24 hours. Change the set with each new parenteral container. Change administration sets used for injectable lipid emulsions that are infused separately every 12 hours; change the set with each new lipid emulsion container. Change administration sets immediately if you suspect contamination or when the integrity of the product or system has been compromised. In addition to routine changes, change the administrations set whenever the vascular access device is changed or when a new vascular access device is inserted[45]
- Closely monitor the catheter site for signs of catheter site infection and local tissue swelling, which may indicate infiltration.[61,62] *Extravasation of PN solution can lead to tissue necrosis.* For patients at risk for refeeding syndrome, administer IV potassium, phosphate, and magnesium supplements as ordered. Monitor serum electrolyte levels daily or more frequently as ordered.[2,51]
- Seek compatibility information or consult the facility pharmacist before co-administering medications with PN.

Patient teaching

Patients who require prolonged or indefinite PN may be able to receive the therapy at home. Home PN reduces the length of hospitalization and allows the patient to resume normal activities. Make a home care referral and begin patient teaching before discharge *to make sure the patient knows how to perform the administration procedure and how to handle complications.*

Complications

Metabolic, mechanical, and other complications can occur during PN administration.[63]

Documentation

Document the type and location of the access device used, including catheter tip confirmation, as appropriate; the PN formulation and additives; the volume of solution administered; the infusion rate; the independent-double check process; the condition of the catheter insertion site; presence of blood return; your assessment findings; and the patient's response to therapy, any complications and interventions, and the patient's response to those interventions. If you discontinued the CV access device or peripheral IV catheter used for PN, document the date and time you removed the catheter, the condition of the catheter insertion site, and the type of dressing applied. Document teaching provided to the patient and family (if applicable, their understanding of that teaching, and any need for follow-up teaching.[18,57]

References

1 Standard 63. Parenteral nutrition. Infusion therapy standards of practice (8th ed.). (2021). *Journal of Infusion Nursing, 44*(Suppl.1), S190–S191. (Level VII)

2 Fletcher, J. (2013). Parenteral nutrition: Indications, risks and nursing care. *Nursing Standard, 27*(46), 50–57.

3 Ukleja, A., et al. (2018). Standards for nutrition support: Adult hospitalized patients. *Nutrition in Clinical Practice, 33*(6), 906–920. https://onlinelibrary.wiley.com/doi/full/10.1002/ncp.10204 (Level VII)

4 Spray, J. (2016). Review of intravenous lipid emulsion therapy. *Journal of Infusion Nursing, 39*(6), 377–380. https://journals.lww.com/journalofinfusionnursing/Fulltext/2016/11000/Review_of_Intravenous_Lipid_Emulsion_Therapy.6.aspx

5 Jarrett, N., & Callaham, M. (2016). Evidence-based guidelines for selected hospital-acquired conditions: Final report. https://www.cms.gov/Medicare/Medicare-Fee-for-Service-Payment/HospitalAcqCond/Downloads/2016-HAC-Report.pdf

6 Centers for Disease Control and Prevention. (2011, revised 2017). Guidelines for the prevention of intravascular catheter–related infections. https://www.cdc.gov/infectioncontrol/guidelines/bsi/recommendations.html (Level I)

7 Marschall, J., et al. (2014). SHEA/IDSA practice recommendation: Strategies to prevent central line-associated bloodstream infections in acute care hospitals. *Infection Control and Hospital Epidemiology, 35*, 753–771. https://www.jstor.org/stable/10.1086/676533#metadata_info_tab_contents (Level I)

8 Worthington, P., et al. (2020). Update on the use of filters for parenteral nutrition: An ASPEN position paper. *Nutrition in Clinical Practice, 36*(1), 29–39. https://aspenjournals.onlinelibrary.wiley.com/doi/10.1002/ncp.10587 (Level VII)

9 Infusion Nurses Society. (2016). *Policies and procedures for infusion therapy* (5th ed.). Boston, MA: Infusion Nurses Society.

10 Standard 12. Product evaluation, integrity, and defect reporting. Infusion therapy standards of practice (8th ed.). (2021). *Journal of Infusion Nursing, 44*(Suppl.1), S45–S46. (Level VII)

11 Westbrook, J., et al. (2010). Association of interruptions with an increased risk and severity of medication administration errors. *Archives of Internal Medicine, 170*, 683–690. (Level IV)

12 Institute for Safe Medication Practices. (2012). Side tracks on the safety express: Interruptions lead to errors and unfinished…Wait, what was I doing? *Nurse Advise-ERR, 11*(2), 1–4. https://www.ismp.org/resources/side-tracks-safety-express-interruptions-lead-errors-and-unfinished-wait-what-was-i-doing?id=37

13 The Joint Commission. (2021). Standard MM.06.01.01. *Comprehensive accreditation manual for hospitals.* Oakbrook Terrace, IL: The Joint Commission. (Level VII)

14 Centers for Medicare and Medicaid Services, Department of Health and Human Services. (2020). Condition of participation: Nursing services. 42 C.F.R. § 482.23(c).

15 Accreditation Association for Hospitals and Health Systems. (2020). Standard 16.01.03. *Healthcare Facilities Accreditation Program: Accreditation requirements for acute care hospitals.* Chicago, IL: Accreditation Association for Hospitals and Health Systems. (Level VII)

16 DNV GL-Healthcare USA, Inc. (2020). MM.1.SR.3. *NIAHO® accreditation requirements, interpretive guidelines and surveyor guidance—revision 20.0.* Milford, OH: DNV GL-Healthcare USA, Inc. (Level VII)

17 Standard 59. Infusion medication and solution administration. Infusion therapy standards of practice (8th ed.). (2021). *Journal of Infusion Nursing, 44*(Suppl.1), S180–S183. (Level VII)

18 Ayers, P., et al. (2014). A.S.P.E.N. parenteral nutrition safety consensus recommendations. *Journal of Parenteral and Enteral Nutrition, 38*(3), 296–333. https://onlinelibrary.wiley.com/doi/pdf/10.1177/0148607113511992 (Level VII)

19 Standard 13. Medication verification. Infusion therapy standards of practice (8th ed.). (2021). *Journal of Infusion Nursing, 44*(Suppl.1), S46–S49. (Level VII)

20 Accreditation Association for Hospitals and Health Systems. (2020). Standard 15.01.11. *Healthcare Facilities Accreditation Program: Accreditation requirements for acute care hospitals.* Chicago, IL: Accreditation Association for Hospitals and Health Systems. (Level VII)

21 Centers for Medicare and Medicaid Services, Department of Health and Human Services. (2020). Condition of participation: Patient's rights. 42 C.F.R. § 482.13(b)(2).

22 The Joint Commission. (2021). Standard RI.01.03.01. *Comprehensive accreditation manual for hospitals.* Oakbrook Terrace, IL: The Joint Commission. (Level VII)

23 DNV GL-Healthcare USA, Inc. (2020). PR.2.SR.3. *NIAHO® accreditation requirements, interpretive guidelines and surveyor guidance—revision 20.0.* Milford, OH: DNV GL-Healthcare USA, Inc. (Level VII)

24 Centers for Disease Control and Prevention. (2002). Guideline for hand hygiene in health-care settings: Recommendations of the Healthcare Infection Control Practices Advisory Committee and the HICPAC/SHEA/APIC/IDSA Hand Hygiene Task Force. *MMWR Recommendations and Reports, 51*(RR-16), 1–45. https://www.cdc.gov/mmwr/pdf/rr/rr5116.pdf (Level II)

25 World Health Organization. (2009). WHO guidelines on hand hygiene in health care: First global patient safety challenge, clean care is safer care. https://apps.who.int/iris/bitstream/handle/10665/44102/9789241597906_eng.pdf?sequence=1 (Level IV)

26 The Joint Commission. (2021). Standard NPSG.07.01.01. *Comprehensive accreditation manual for hospitals.* Oakbrook Terrace, IL: The Joint Commission. (Level VII)

27 Standard 16. Hand hygiene. Infusion therapy standards of practice (8th ed.). (2021). *Journal of Infusion Nursing, 44*(Suppl.1), S53–S54. (Level VII)

28 Accreditation Association for Hospitals and Health Systems. (2020). Standard 07.01.21. *Healthcare Facilities Accreditation Program: Accreditation requirements for acute care hospitals.* Chicago, IL: Accreditation Association for Hospitals and Health Systems. (Level VII)

29 Centers for Medicare and Medicaid Services, Department of Health and Human Services. (2020). Condition of participation: Infection control. 42 C.F.R. § 482.42.

30 DNV GL-Healthcare USA, Inc. (2020). IC.1.SR.1. *NIAHO® accreditation requirements, interpretive guidelines and surveyor guidance—revision 20.0.* Milford, OH: DNV GL-Healthcare USA, Inc. (Level VII)

31 The Joint Commission. (2021). Standard NPSG.01.01.01. *Comprehensive accreditation manual for hospitals.* Oakbrook Terrace, IL: The Joint Commission. (Level VII)

32 Accreditation Association for Hospitals and Health Systems. (2020). Standard 15.01.16. *Healthcare Facilities Accreditation Program: Accreditation requirements for acute care hospitals.* Chicago, IL: Accreditation Association for Hospitals and Health Systems. (Level VII)

33 Centers for Medicare and Medicaid Services, Department of Health and Human Services. (2020). Condition of participation: Patient's rights. 42 C.F.R. § 482.13(c)(1).

34 DNV GL-Healthcare USA, Inc. (2020). PR.2.SR.5. *NIAHO® accreditation requirements, interpretive guidelines and surveyor guidance—revision 20.0.* Milford, OH: DNV GL-Healthcare USA, Inc. (Level VII)

35 The Joint Commission. (2021). Standard RI.01.01.01. *Comprehensive accreditation manual for hospitals.* Oakbrook Terrace, IL: The Joint Commission. (Level VII)

36 The Joint Commission. (2021). Standard PC.02.01.21. *Comprehensive accreditation manual for hospitals.* Oakbrook Terrace, IL: The Joint Commission. (Level VII)

37 Waters, T. R., et al. (2009). Safe patient handling training for schools of nursing. https://www.cdc.gov/niosh/docs/2009-127/pdfs/2009-127.pdf (Level VII)

38 Siegel, J. D., et al. (2007, revised 2019). 2007 guideline for isolation precautions: Preventing transmission of infectious agents in healthcare settings. https://www.cdc.gov/infectioncontrol/pdf/guidelines/isolation-guidelines-H.pdf (Level II)

39 Occupational Safety and Health Administration. (2019). Bloodborne pathogens, standard number 1910.1030. https://www.osha.gov/pls/oshaweb/owadisp.show_document?p_id=10051&p_table=STANDARDS (Level VII)

40 Standard 35. Filtration. Infusion therapy standards of practice (8th ed.). (2021). *Journal of Infusion Nursing, 44*(Suppl.1), S102–S104. (Level VII)

41 Standard 52. Air embolism. Infusion therapy standards of practice (8th ed.). (2021). *Journal of Infusion Nursing, 44*(Suppl.1), S160–S161. (Level VII)

42 The Joint Commission. (2013). Sentinel event alert 50: Medical device alarm safety in hospitals. https://www.jointcommission.org/-/media/tjc/documents/resources/patient-safety-topics/sentinel-event/sea_50_alarms_4_26_16.pdf (Level VII)

43 The Joint Commission. (2021). Standard NPSG.06.01.01. *Comprehensive accreditation manual for hospitals.* Oakbrook Terrace, IL: The Joint Commission. (Level VII)

44 Graham, K. C., & Cvach, M. (2010). Monitor alarm fatigue: Standardizing use of physiological monitors and decreasing nuisance alarms. *American Journal of Critical Care, 19*(1), 28–37.

45 Standard 43. Administration set management. Infusion therapy standards of practice (8th ed.). (2021). *Journal of Infusion Nursing, 44*(Suppl.1), S104–S107. (Level VII)

46 Standard 36. Needleless connectors. Infusion therapy standards of practice. (2016). *Journal of Infusion Nursing, 39,* S68–S70. (Level VII)

47 Standard 41. Flushing and locking. Infusion therapy standards of practice (8th ed.). (2021). *Journal of Infusion Nursing, 44*(Suppl.1), S113–S118. (Level VII)

48 The Joint Commission. (2014). Sentinel event alert 53: Managing risk during transition to new ISO tubing connector standards" https://www.jointcommission.org/-/media/tjc/documents/resources/patient-safety-topics/sentinel-event/sea_53_connectors_8_19_14_final.pdf (Level VII)

49 Institute for Safe Medication Practices. (2018). ISMP list of high-alert medications in acute care settings. https://www.ismp.org/sites/default/files/attachments/2018-08/highAlert2018 Acute-Final.pdf

50 Institute for Safe Medication Practices. (2013). Independent double checks: Undervalued and misused: Selective use of this strategy can play an important role in medication safety. https://www.ismp.org/resources/independent-double-checks-undervalued-and-misused-selective-use-strategy-can-play (Level VII)

51 Agency for Clinical Innovation. (2011). Parenteral nutrition pocketbook: For adults. https://www.aci.health.nsw.gov.au/__data/assets/pdf_file/0010/159805/aci_parenteral_nutrition_pb.pdf

52 Ganz, D. A., et al. (2013, reviewed 2021). *Preventing falls in hospitals: A toolkit for improving quality of care* (AHRQ Publication No. 13-0015-EF). Rockville, MD: Agency for Healthcare Research and Quality. https://www.ahrq.gov/professionals/systems/hospital/fallpxtoolkit/index.html (Level VII)

53 Standard 21. Medical waste and sharps safety. Infusion therapy standards of practice (8th ed.). (2021). *Journal of Infusion Nursing, 44*(Suppl.1), S60–S62. (Level VII)

54 Accreditation Association for Hospitals and Health Systems. (2020). Standard 07.02.03. *Healthcare Facilities Accreditation Program: Accreditation requirements for acute care hospitals.* Chicago, IL: Accreditation Association for Hospitals and Health Systems. (Level VII)

55 Rutala, W. A., et al. (2008, revised 2019). Guideline for disinfection and sterilization in healthcare facilities, 2008. https://www.cdc.gov/infection-control/pdf/guidelines/disinfection-guidelines-H.pdf (Level I)

56 The Joint Commission. (2021). Standard RC.01.03.01. *Comprehensive accreditation manual for hospitals.* Oakbrook Terrace, IL: The Joint Commission. (Level VII)

57 Standard 10. Documentation in the health record. Infusion therapy standards of practice (8th ed.). (2021). *Journal of Infusion Nursing, 44*(Suppl.1), S39–S42. (Level VII)

58 Accreditation Association for Hospitals and Health Systems. (2020). Standard 10.00.03. *Healthcare Facilities Accreditation Program:*

Accreditation requirements for acute care hospitals. Chicago, IL: Accreditation Association for Hospitals and Health Systems. (Level VII)

59 Centers for Medicare and Medicaid Services, Department of Health and Human Services. (2020). Condition of participation: Medical record services. 42 C.F.R. § 482.24(b).

60 DNV GL-Healthcare USA, Inc. (2020). MR.2.SR.1. *NIAHO® accreditation requirements, interpretive guidelines and surveyor guidance—revision 20.0.* Milford, OH: DNV GL-Healthcare USA, Inc. (Level VII)

61 Standard 47. Infiltration and extravasation. Infusion therapy standards of practice (8th ed.). (2021). *Journal of Infusion Nursing, 44*(Suppl.1), S142–S147. (Level VII)

62 Centers for Medicare and Medicaid Services. (2022). *Specifications manual for national hospital inpatient quality measures* (version 5.11a). https://www.qualitynet.org/inpatient/specifications-manuals#tab1

63 Hamdan, M., & Puckett, Y. (2021). Total parenteral nutrition. https://www.ncbi.nlm.nih.gov/books/NBK559036/

PARENTERAL NUTRITION MONITORING

A patient receiving parenteral nutrition (PN) requires careful monitoring.[1,2,3] Because the typical patient is in a protein-wasting state, PN therapy causes marked changes in fluid and electrolyte status and glucose, amino acid, mineral, and vitamin levels. Administration of a lipid emulsion can also cause the patient's lipid level to rise. Careful monitoring can help detect adverse reactions and signs and symptoms of other complications, which require practitioner notification. The PN regimen can be changed as needed with a practitioner's order.

Monitoring a patient's condition during PN therapy requires recognition of the signs and symptoms of possible complications, understanding of laboratory test results, and careful record keeping. Assessing a patient's nutritional status includes a physical examination and a review of body weight, body composition, somatic and visceral protein stores, and laboratory values. Because a PN solution has a high dextrose content, the infusion must be started slowly to allow the patient's pancreatic beta cells to adapt to it by increasing insulin output. Within the first 5 days of PN therapy, an adult patient can typically tolerate 3 L of solution daily without adverse reactions.

Monitoring the venous access device during PN administration is also essential because of the risk of vascular catheter–associated infection and other access device complications.[1,2,4]

HOSPITAL-ACQUIRED CONDITION ALERT Keep in mind that the Centers for Medicare and Medicaid Services considers a vascular catheter–associated infection a hospital-acquired condition *because it can be reasonably prevented using a variety of best practices.* Make sure to follow evidence-based infection prevention practices, such as performing hand hygiene and using sterile no-touch technique, *to reduce the risk of vascular catheter–associated infections.*[5,6,7,8,9,10]

Equipment

Prescribed PN solution ▪ electronic infusion device (preferably a smart pump with dose-error reduction software and interoperability with electronic medical records) with anti-free-flow protection[11] ▪ sterile IV administration set ▪ 1.2-micron filter[12] ▪ glucometer and related supplies ▪ vital signs monitoring equipment ▪ stethoscope ▪ scale ▪ input and output record ▪ supplies for blood specimen collection ▪ disinfectant pad ▪ oral care supplies ▪ gloves ▪ facility-approved disinfectant ▪ Optional: dressing change kit, 24-hour urine collection supplies, prescribed IV dextrose solution, prescribed insulin, tape measure.

Preparation of equipment

For information on preparing the infusion pump and PN solution, see the "Parenteral nutrition administration" procedure. Inspect all equipment and supplies. If a product is expired, is defective, or has compromised integrity, remove it from patient use, label it as expired or defective, and report the expiration or defect as directed by your facility.[13]

Implementation

- Gather and prepare the necessary equipment and supplies.
- Perform hand hygiene.[7,14,15,16,17,18,19,20]
- Confirm the patient's identity using at least two patient identifiers.[3,21]
- Provide privacy.[22,23,24,25]
- Explain the procedure to the patient and family (if appropriate) according to their individual communication and learning needs *to increase their understanding, allay their fears, and enhance cooperation.*[26] Instruct the patient to report any unusual sensations during the infusion.
- Raise the bed to waist level before providing care *to prevent caregiver back strain.*[27]
- Perform hand hygiene.[7,14,15,16,17,18,19,20]
- Put on gloves as needed *to comply with standard precautions.*[28,29,30]
- Monitor the patient's vital signs at an interval determined by the patient's condition *to promptly recognize changes in the patient's condition.*
- Make sure that each PN bag or bottle has a label listing the patient's identifiers and weight, administration date and time, expiration date, administration route (central or peripheral), dextrose concentration, and component names and dosages. All components should be listed in the same sequence and same unit of measure as the practitioner's order. All components should be ordered and labeled as amounts per day for adults and amounts per kilogram per day for children. The total volume of solution and the infusion rate should be included, as well as the duration of the infusion (continuous or cycled) and the appropriate-size filter to use.[3] (If the bag or bottle is damaged and you don't have an immediate replacement, hang a bag of dextrose 10% in water, as prescribed, until the new container is ready.)
- Change administration sets, including in-line and add-on filters used for parenteral nutrition (with or without lipids), at least every 24 hours. Change the set with each new parenteral nutrition container. Change administration sets used for injectable lipid emulsions that are infused separately every 12 hours; change the set with each new fat emulsion container. Change the IV administration set with each new container and at least every 12 hours. Change the IV administration set immediately if you suspect contamination or when the integrity of the product or system has been compromised. In addition to routine changes, change the administration set whenever the vascular access device is changed or when a new vascular access device is inserted.[31]
- Using sterile no-touch technique, perform site care and dressing changes according to the type of dressing:[32] Change transparent semipermeable dressings at least every 7 days and gauze dressings at least every 2 days. Additionally, change the dressing immediately if it becomes visibly soiled, loosened, or dislodged, or if there is any moisture, drainage, blood, or compromised skin integrity beneath the dressing. (See the "IV catheter maintenance" or the "Central venous access catheter care" procedure.)[32]
- Assess the patient:[11] Monitor for signs of peripheral and pulmonary edema. Inspect the vascular catheter exit site. Palpate for tenderness through the intact dressing. Remove the dressing and examine the site thoroughly if fever, tenderness, or other findings suggest a local or bloodstream infection.[4,7,32] If ordered, measure the patient's upper-arm circumference 10 cm above the antecubital fossa. Compare the finding to the baseline measurement *to assess for edema and possible deep vein thrombosis.*[32]
- Weigh the patient (in kilograms) at the same time each morning after the patient voids, in similar-weight clothing, and on the same scale. Compare the patient's weight with the fluid intake and output record.[2,11] *Weight gain, particularly early in treatment, may indicate fluid overload rather than increasing fat and protein stores.* A patient shouldn't gain more than 1.5 kg per week; a weight gain of 0.5 kg per week is a reasonable goal for most patients; suspect fluid imbalance if the patient gains more than 0.5 kg daily.
- Monitor the patient's bowel function by auscultating bowel sounds and assessing the number, volume, and consistency of bowel movements.[4]
- Monitor the patient for signs and symptoms of glucose metabolism disturbance, fluid and electrolyte imbalances, and nutritional aberrations.[1,2,3,11] Note that some patients may require supplemental insulin for the duration of PN; the pharmacy should add insulin directly to the PN solution.[3] Monitor electrolyte levels frequently—daily at first.[2,11] Monitor serum albumin levels weekly. (See *Laboratory monitoring of*

Laboratory monitoring of parenteral nutrition

Laboratory tests are typically ordered by the practitioner as part of monitoring for a patient receiving parenteral nutrition (PN). The American Society for Parenteral and Enteral Nutrition recommends that facilities standardize PN monitoring parameters.[3] When collecting specimens for laboratory testing, be sure to label them in the presence of the patient to prevent mislabeling.[21] Notify the practitioner of critical test results within your facility's established time frame *so that the patient can receive prompt treatment.*[33]

Baseline tests

Baseline tests include complete blood count (CBC); comprehensive metabolic panel (CMP*); cholesterol and triglyceride levels; liver function tests (LFTs), including prothrombin time (PT), International Normalized Ratio (INR), lactate dehydrogenase level, and bilirubin level; and magnesium, phosphate, and transferrin levels. Possible additional tests at the initiation of PN include trace elements and vitamin levels.[2,34]

Daily tests and measurements

Daily tests include weight, intake and output, and glucose by fingerstick every 6 hours until stable and then as directed. Also expect the practitioner to order a basic metabolic panel (BMP**), magnesium and phosphate levels, and LFTs daily until the patient is stable, and then two to three times per week as directed.[2]

Weekly tests

Weekly tests include CBC, CMP, PT, and INR, and cholesterol, triglyceride, C-reactive protein, and transferrin levels.[2]

Additional tests

For a patient receiving long-term PN, the practitioner may also order additional tests as indicated, including bone mineral density assessment, liver ultrasound, and zinc, copper, selenium, manganese, folate, ferratin iron, and vitamin A, B$_{12}$, and E levels.[2,35]

---

*CMP includes blood urea nitrogen (BUN), creatinine, sodium, chloride, carbon dioxide (CO_2), glucose, potassium, calcium, albumin, total protein, alkaline phosphatase, alanine transaminase, aspartate transaminase, and bilirubin levels.
**BMP includes BUN, creatinine, sodium, chloride, CO_2, glucose, and potassium levels.

parenteral nutrition.) Later, as the patient's condition stabilizes, reduce the frequency of monitoring these values, as indicated. (Be aware that in a severely dehydrated patient, albumin levels may actually drop initially as treatment restores hydration.)

- Monitor the potassium, magnesium, phosphate, and calcium levels. If these electrolytes were added to the PN solution, the dosage may need adjusting *to maintain normal serum levels.*[2]
- Monitor serum glucose levels every 6 hours initially, and then once daily or according to the ordered parameters.[3] Watch for signs and symptoms of hyperglycemia, such as thirst, hunger, and polyuria. Confirm glucometer readings with laboratory tests periodically.
- Assess renal function by monitoring the blood urea nitrogen and creatinine levels, *because increases can indicate excess amino acid intake.* Also assess nitrogen balance with 24-hour urine collection, as ordered.[2]
- Assess liver function by periodically monitoring liver enzyme, bilirubin, triglyceride, and cholesterol levels. *Abnormal values may indicate an intolerance or excess of lipid emulsions, or problems with metabolizing the protein or glucose in the PN formula.*[2]
- Provide emotional support. *Patients tend to associate eating with positive feelings and can become disturbed when eating is prohibited.*[11]
- Provide frequent oral care. (See the "Oral care" procedure.)
- Keep the patient active *to enable the body to use nutrients more fully.*
- When discontinuing PN, taper the infusion rate, as ordered or as directed by the facility. For adults receiving insulin, closely monitor the

patient's glucose level; adjust the insulin, as needed and ordered, *to reduce the risk of hyperinsulinemia and subsequent hypoglycemia.* If you must stop PN abruptly, begin a dextrose infusion, as ordered, *to reduce the risk of hypoglycemia.*[2]

■ While weaning the patient from PN, document the dietary intake, and work with the nutritionist *to determine the total calorie and protein intake.* Also teach other health care staff caring for the patient the importance of recording food intake. Use percentages of food consumed (such as "ate 50% of a baked potato") instead of subjective descriptions (such as "had a good appetite") *to provide a more accurate account of patient intake.*

■ Return the bed to the lowest position *to prevent falls and maintain patient safety.*[36]

■ Discard used supplies in appropriate receptacles.[30]

■ Remove and discard your gloves, if worn.[30]

■ Perform hand hygiene.[14,15,16,17,18,19,20]

■ Put on gloves.[30]

■ Clean and disinfect other reusable equipment according to the manufacturer's instructions *to prevent the spread of infection.*[37,38]

■ Remove and discard your gloves.[29,30]

■ Perform hand hygiene.[14,15,16,17,18,19,20]

■ Clean and disinfect your stethoscope using a disinfectant pad.[37,38]

■ Perform hand hygiene.[14,15,16,17,18,19,20]

■ Document the procedure.[39,40,41,42,43]

Special considerations

■ During daily multidisciplinary rounds, discuss the patient's readiness for enteral feeding; switch to enteral feeding as soon as the patient's condition warrants. Make sure the CV access device is removed as soon as it's no longer needed *to reduce the risk of vascular catheter–related bloodstream infection.*[7]

■ When using a filter, position it as close to the access site as possible.[12,44] Check the filter's porosity and pounds-per-square-inch (psi) capacity *to make sure it exceeds the number of psi exerted by the infusion pump.*

■ When a patient is severely malnourished, starting PN may spark refeeding syndrome, which includes a rapid drop in potassium, magnesium, and phosphorus levels. *To avoid compromising cardiac function,* initiate feeding slowly and monitor the patient's blood test results closely until they stabilize.[2]

■ Teach the patient and family (if appropriate) about measures to prevent intravascular catheter–related infections, including the importance of hand hygiene.[8] Encourage the patient and family to remind staff members if they fail to perform hand hygiene before delivering care. Teach the patient about signs and symptoms of complications and to report them immediately.

Complications

Metabolic, mechanical, and other complications can occur during PN administration.[45] (See the "Parenteral nutrition administration" procedure.)

Documentation

Document the type and location of the access device used, the PN formulation and additives, the volume of solution administered, the infusion rate, assessment findings, and the patient's response to therapy. Note laboratory test results, the name of the practitioner notified, the date and time of notification, any prescribed interventions, and the patient's response to those interventions. Record any adverse effects that occur, the name of the practitioner notified, the date and time of notification, any prescribed interventions, and the patient's response to those interventions.[46] Document teaching provided to the patient and family (if applicable), their understanding of that teaching, and any need for follow-up teaching.

REFERENCES

1 Ukleja, A., et al. (2018). Standards for nutrition support: Adult hospitalized patients. *Nutrition in Clinical Practice, 33*(6), 906–920. https://onlinelibrary.wiley.com/doi/full/10.1002/ncp.10204 (Level VII)

2 Agency for Clinical Innovation. (2011). Parenteral nutrition pocketbook: For adults. https://www.aci.health.nsw.gov.au/__data/assets/pdf_file/0010/159805/aci_parenteral_nutrition_pb.pdf

3 Ayers, P., et al. (2014). A.S.P.E.N. parenteral nutrition safety consensus recommendations. *Journal of Parenteral and Enteral Nutrition, 38*(3), 296–333. https://onlinelibrary.wiley.com/doi/pdf/10.1177/0148607113511992 (Level VII)

4 Centers for Medicare and Medicaid Services. (2022). *Specifications manual for national hospital inpatient quality measures* (version 5.11a.). https://www.qualitynet.org/inpatient/specifications-manuals#tab1

5 Jarrett, N., & Callaham, M. (2016). Evidence-based guidelines for selected hospital-acquired conditions: Final report. https://www.cms.gov/Medicare/Medicare-Fee-for-Service-Payment/HospitalAcqCond/Downloads/2016-HAC-Report.pdf

6 Standard 50. Infection. Infusion therapy standards of practice (8th ed.). (2021). *Journal of Infusion Nursing, 44*(Suppl.1), S153–S157. (Level VII)

7 Centers for Disease Control and Prevention. (2011, revised 2017). Guidelines for the prevention of intravascular catheter–related infections. https://www.cdc.gov/infectioncontrol/guidelines/bsi/recommendations.html (Level I)

8 The Joint Commission. (2021). Standard NPSG.07.04.01. *Comprehensive accreditation manual for hospitals.* Oakbrook Terrace, IL: The Joint Commission. (Level VII)

9 Association of Professionals in Infection Control and Epidemiology (APIC). (2015). Guide to preventing central line-associated bloodstream infections. http://apic.org/Resource_/TinyMceFileManager/2015/APIC_CLABSI_WEB.pdf (Level IV)

10 Marschall, J., et al. (2014). SHEA/IDSA practice recommendation: Strategies to prevent central line-associated bloodstream infections in acute care hospitals. *Infection Control and Hospital Epidemiology, 35,* 753–771. https://www.jstor.org/stable/10.1086/676533#metadata_info_tab_contents (Level I)

11 Standard 63. Parenteral nutrition. Infusion therapy standards of practice (8th ed.). (2021). *Journal of Infusion Nursing, 44*(Suppl.1), S190–S191. (Level VII)

12 Standard 12. Product evaluation, integrity, and defect reporting. Infusion therapy standards of practice (8th ed.). (2021). *Journal of Infusion Nursing, 44*(Suppl.1), S32–S34. (Level VII)

13 Worthington, P., et al. (2020). Update on the use of filters for parenteral nutrition: An ASPEN position paper. *Nutrition in Clinical Practice, 36*(1), 29–39. https://aspenjournals.onlinelibrary.wiley.com/doi/10.1002/ncp.10587 (Level VII)

14 Centers for Disease Control and Prevention. (2002). Guideline for hand hygiene in health-care settings: Recommendations of the Healthcare Infection Control Practices Advisory Committee and the HICPAC/SHEA/APIC/IDSA Hand Hygiene Task Force. *MMWR Recommendations and Reports, 51*(RR–16), 1–45. https://www.cdc.gov/mmwr/pdf/rr/rr5116.pdf (Level II)

15 World Health Organization. (2009). WHO guidelines on hand hygiene in health care: First global patient safety challenge, clean care is safer care. https://apps.who.int/iris/bitstream/handle/10665/44102/9789241597906_eng.pdf?sequence=1 (Level IV)

16 The Joint Commission. (2021). Standard NPSG.07.01.01. *Comprehensive accreditation manual for hospitals.* Oakbrook Terrace, IL: The Joint Commission. (Level VII)

17 Standard 16. Hand hygiene. Infusion therapy standards of practice (8th ed.). (2021). *Journal of Infusion Nursing, 44*(Suppl.1), S53–S54. (Level VII)

18 Centers for Medicare and Medicaid Services, Department of Health and Human Services. (2020). Condition of participation: Infection control. 42 C.F.R. § 482.42.

19 Accreditation Association for Hospitals and Health Systems. (2020). Standard 07.01.21. *Healthcare Facilities Accreditation Program: Accreditation requirements for acute care hospitals.* Chicago, IL: Accreditation Association for Hospitals and Health Systems. (Level VII)

20 DNV GL-Healthcare USA, Inc. (2020). IC.1.SR.1. *NIAHO® accreditation requirements, interpretive guidelines and surveyor guidance—revision 20.0* Milford, OH: DNV GL-Healthcare USA, Inc. (Level VII)

21 The Joint Commission. (2021). Standard NPSG.01.01.01. *Comprehensive accreditation manual for hospitals.* Oakbrook Terrace, IL: The Joint Commission. (Level VII)

22 Accreditation Association for Hospitals and Health Systems. (2020). Standard 15.01.16. *Healthcare Facilities Accreditation Program: Accreditation requirements for acute care hospitals.* Chicago, IL: Accreditation Association for Hospitals and Health Systems. (Level VII)

23 Centers for Medicare and Medicaid Services, Department of Health and Human Services. (2020). Condition of participation: Patient's rights. 42 C.F.R. § 482.13(c)(1).

24 DNV GL-Healthcare USA, Inc. (2020). PR.2.SR.5. *NIAHO® accreditation requirements, interpretive guidelines and surveyor guidance—revision 20.0.* Milford, OH: DNV GL-Healthcare USA, Inc. (Level VII)

25 The Joint Commission. (2021). Standard RI.01.01.01. *Comprehensive accreditation manual for hospitals.* Oakbrook Terrace, IL: The Joint Commission. (Level VII)

26 The Joint Commission. (2021). Standard PC.02.01.21. *Comprehensive accreditation manual for hospitals.* Oakbrook Terrace, IL: The Joint Commission. (Level VII)

27 Waters, T. R., et al. (2009). Safe patient handling training for schools of nursing. https://www.cdc.gov/niosh/docs/2009-127/pdfs/2009-127.pdf (Level VII)

28 Accreditation Association for Hospitals and Health Systems. (2020). Standard 07.01.10. *Healthcare Facilities Accreditation Program: Accreditation requirements for acute care hospitals.* Chicago, IL: Accreditation Association for Hospitals and Health Systems. (Level VII)

29 Siegel, J. D., et al. (2007, revised 2019). 2007 guideline for isolation precautions: Preventing transmission of infectious agents in healthcare settings. https://www.cdc.gov/infectioncontrol/pdf/guidelines/isolation-guidelines-H.pdf (Level II)

30 Occupational Safety and Health Administration. (2019). Bloodborne pathogens, standard number 1910.1030. https://www.osha.gov/pls/oshaweb/owadisp.show_document?p_id=10051&p_table=STANDARDS (Level VII)

31 Standard 43. Administration set management. Infusion therapy standards of practice (8th ed.). (2021). *Journal of Infusion Nursing, 44*(Suppl.1), S123–S125. (Level VII)

32 Standard 42. Vascular access device assessment, care and dressing changes. Infusion therapy standards of practice (8th ed.). (2021). *Journal of Infusion Nursing, 44*(Suppl.1), S119–S123. (Level VII)

33 The Joint Commission. (2021). Standard NPSG.02.03.01. *Comprehensive accreditation manual for hospitals.* Oakbrook Terrace, IL: The Joint Commission. (Level VII)

34 Fessler, T. A. (2013). Trace elements in parenteral nutrition: A practical guide for dosage and monitoring for adult patients. *Nutrition in Clinical Practice, 28*, 722–729.

35 Pironi, L., et al. (2020). ESPEN guidelines on home parenteral nutrition. *Clinical Nutrition, 39*(6), 1645–1666. http://espen.info/documents/0909/Home%20Parenteral%20Nutrition%20in%20adults.pdf (Level VII)

36 Ganz, D. A., et al. (2013, reviewed 2021). *Preventing falls in hospitals: A toolkit for improving quality of care* (AHRQ Publication No. 13-0015-EF). Rockville, MD: Agency for Healthcare Research and Quality. https://www.ahrq.gov/professionals/systems/hospital/fallpxtoolkit/index.html (Level VII)

37 Accreditation Association for Hospitals and Health Systems. (2020). Standard 07.02.03. *Healthcare Facilities Accreditation Program: Accreditation requirements for acute care hospitals.* Chicago, IL: Accreditation Association for Hospitals and Health Systems. (Level VII)

38 Rutala, W. A., et al. (2008, revised 2019). Guideline for disinfection and sterilization in healthcare facilities, 2008. https://www.cdc.gov/infection-control/pdf/guidelines/disinfection-guidelines-H.pdf (Level I)

39 The Joint Commission. (2021). Standard RC.01.03.01. *Comprehensive accreditation manual for hospitals.* Oakbrook Terrace, IL: The Joint Commission. (Level VII)

40 Standard 10. Documentation in the health record. Infusion therapy standards of practice (8th ed.). (2021). *Journal of Infusion Nursing, 44*(Suppl.1), S39–S42. (Level VII)

41 Centers for Medicare and Medicaid Services, Department of Health and Human Services. (2020). Condition of participation: Medical record services. 42 C.F.R. § 482.24(b).

42 Accreditation Association for Hospitals and Health Systems. (2020). Standard 10.00.03. *Healthcare Facilities Accreditation Program: Accreditation requirements for acute care hospitals.* Chicago, IL: Accreditation Association for Hospitals and Health Systems. (Level VII)

43 DNV GL-Healthcare USA, Inc. (2020). MR.2.SR.1. *NIAHO® accreditation requirements, interpretive guidelines and surveyor guidance—revision 20.0.* Milford, OH: DNV GL-Healthcare USA, Inc. (Level VII)

44 Standard 35. Filtration. Infusion therapy standards of practice (8th ed.). (2021). *Journal of Infusion Nursing, 44*(Suppl.1), S102–S104. (Level VII)

45 Hamdan, M., & Puckett, Y. (2021). Total parenteral nutrition. https://www.ncbi.nlm.nih.gov/books/NBK559036/

46 The Joint Commission. (2021). Standard RC.02.01.01. *Comprehensive accreditation manual for hospitals.* Oakbrook Terrace, IL: The Joint Commission. (Level VII)

PASSIVE RANGE-OF-MOTION EXERCISES

Passive range-of-motion (ROM) exercises involve the movement of a joint through partial or complete range of activity with the assistance of a health care provider. Full ROM involves flexion, extension, abduction, adduction, and rotation of the affected joint. ROM exercises are indicated for a patient who has temporary or permanent loss of mobility, sensation, or consciousness. These exercises have been shown to improve or maintain joint mobility, strength, and endurance and prepare the patient for ambulation.[1]

When included as a key component of care, ROM exercises can enhance patient outcomes, improve gas exchange, reduce rates of ventilator-associated pneumonia, shorten the duration of mechanical ventilation, reduce the risk of contractures,[2,3] and enhance long-term functional ability.

The exercises described here treat all joints, but they do not have to be performed in the order given or all at once. You can schedule them over the course of a day, whenever the patient is in the most convenient position. You'll typically perform these exercises three times for each joint, at least twice a day.[1] Perform all exercises slowly, gently, and to the end of the normal ROM or to the point of pain but no further.[1] (See *Glossary of joint movements.*) Hold each position for 1 to 2 seconds. It is important to note that passive ROM exercises require recognition of the patient's limits of motion and support of all joints during movements.

Passive ROM exercises are contraindicated in patients with septic joints (until infection subsides), bone tumors or metastases, acute myocardial infarction, or recent trauma with possible hidden fractures or internal injuries.[1,4]

Equipment

Optional: gloves, other personal protective equipment (gown, mask and goggle or mask and face shield).

Implementation

- Determine the joints that need ROM exercises.
- Consult the practitioner or physical therapist about limitations or precautions for specific exercises.
- Perform hand hygiene.[5,6,7,8,9,10]
- Confirm the patient's identity using at least two patient identifiers.[11]
- Provide privacy.[12,13,14,15]
- Explain the procedure to the patient and family (if appropriate) according to their individual communication and learning needs *to increase their understanding, allay their fears, and enhance cooperation.*[16]
- Raise the patient's bed to waist level before providing patient care *to prevent caregiver back strain.*[17]
- Put on gloves and other personal protective equipment, as needed, *to comply with standard precautions.*[18,19,20]

Exercising the neck

- While supporting the patient's head with your hands, extend the neck, flex the chin to the chest, and tilt the head laterally toward each shoulder.
- Rotate the patient's head from right to left (as shown below).

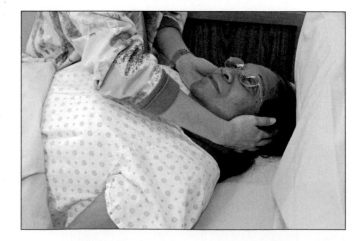

Glossary of joint movements

The different joint movements, illustrated in the images below, include abduction and adduction, dorsiflexion and plantar flexion, extension and flexion, external and internal rotation, eversion and inversion, and supination and pronation.

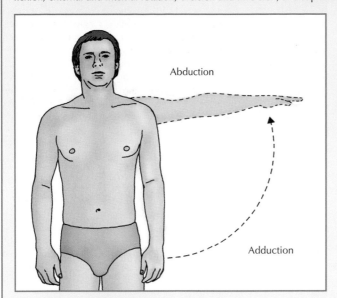

Abduction

Adduction

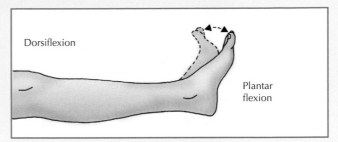

Dorsiflexion

Plantar flexion

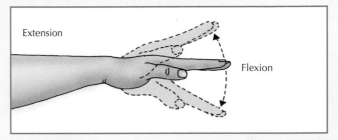

Extension

Flexion

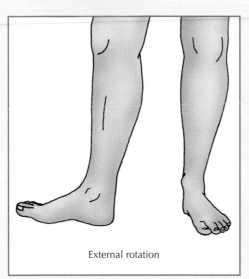

External rotation

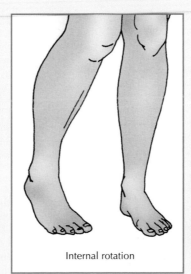

Internal rotation

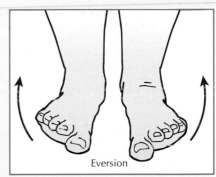

Eversion

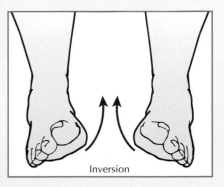

Inversion

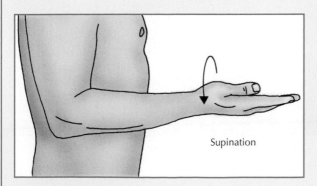

Supination

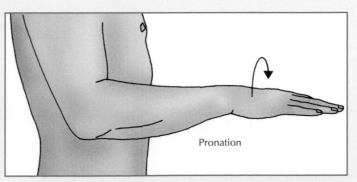

Pronation

Exercising the shoulders
■ Support the patient's arm in an extended, neutral position; then extend the forearm and flex it back.
■ Abduct the patient's arm outward from the side of the body, and then adduct it back to the side.
■ Rotate the shoulder so that the patient's arm crosses the midline, and then bend the elbow so that the hand touches the opposite shoulder and then touches the mattress for complete internal rotation.
■ Return the patient's shoulder to a neutral position and, with elbow bent, push the patient's arm backward so that the back of the hand touches the mattress for complete external rotation (as shown below).

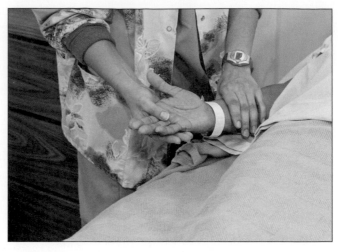

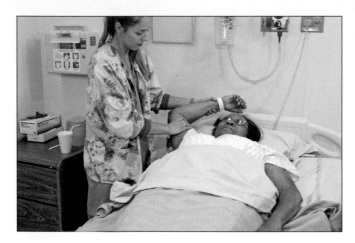

Exercising the elbow
■ Place the patient's arm at the side with palm facing up.
■ Flex and extend the patient's arm at the elbow (as shown below).

Exercising the wrist
■ Stabilize the patient's forearm, and then flex and extend the wrist.
■ Rock the patient's hand sideways for lateral flexion.
■ Rotate the patient's hand in a circular motion (as shown below).

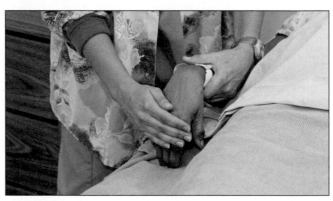

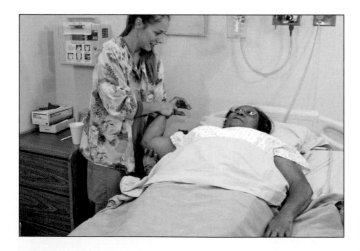

Exercising the fingers and thumb
■ Extend the patient's fingers, and then flex the hand into a fist; repeat extension and flexion of each joint of each finger and thumb separately.
■ Spread two adjoining fingers apart (abduction, as shown below), and then bring them together (adduction).
■ Oppose each fingertip to the patient's thumb.
■ Rotate the thumb and each finger in a circle.

Exercising the forearm
■ Stabilize the patient's elbow, and then twist the hand to bring the palm up (supination, as shown on top right).
■ Twist it back again to bring the palm down (pronation).

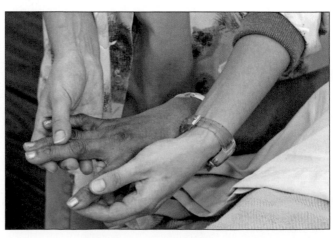

Exercising the hip and knee

■ Fully extend the patient's leg, and then bend the hip and knee toward the chest, allowing full joint flexion.
■ Move the patient's straight leg sideways, out and away from the other leg (abduction), and then back, over, and across it (adduction).
■ Rotate the patient's straight leg internally toward the midline (as shown below), and then externally away from the midline.

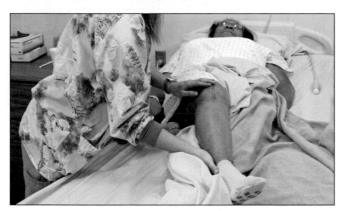

Exercising the ankle

■ Bend the patient's foot so that the toes push upward (dorsiflexion), and then bend the foot so that the toes push downward (plantar flexion).
■ Rotate the ankle in a circular motion.
■ Invert the patient's ankle so that the sole of the foot faces the midline (as shown below), and evert the ankle so that the sole faces away from the midline.

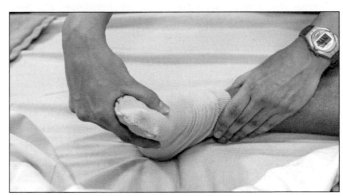

Learning about isometric exercises

Patients can strengthen and increase muscle tone by contracting muscles against resistance (from other muscles or from a stationary object, such as a bed or a wall) without joint movement. These exercises require only a comfortable position—standing, sitting, or lying down—and proper body alignment. For each exercise, instruct the patient to hold each contraction for 2 to 5 seconds and to repeat it three to four times daily, below peak contraction level for the first week and at peak level thereafter.

Neck rotators

The patient places the heel of the hand above one ear, then pushes the head toward the hand as forcefully as possible, without moving the head, neck, or arm. The patient then repeats the exercise on the other side.

Neck flexors

The patient places both palms on the forehead. Without moving the neck, the patient pushes the head forward while resisting with the palms.

Neck extensors

The patient clasps the fingers behind the head, and then pushes the head against the clasped hands without moving the neck.

Shoulder elevators

Holding the right arm straight down at the side, the patient grasps the right wrist with the left hand. The patient then tries to shrug the right shoulder, but prevents it from moving by holding the arm in place. The patient repeats this exercise, alternating arms.

Shoulder, chest, and scapular musculature

The patient places the right fist in the left palm and raises both arms to shoulder height. The patient pushes the fist into the palm as forcefully as possible without moving either arm. Then, with the arms in the same position, the patient clasps the fingers and tries to pull the hands apart. The patient repeats the pattern, beginning with the left fist in the right palm.

Elbow flexors and extensors

With the right elbow bent 90 degrees and the right palm facing upward, the patient places the left fist against the right palm. The patient tries to bend the right elbow further while resisting with the left fist. The patient repeats the pattern, bending the left elbow.

Abdomen

The patient assumes a sitting position and bends slightly forward, with the hands in front of the middle of the thighs. The patient tries to bend forward further, resisting by pressing the palms against the thighs.

Alternatively, in the supine position, the patient clasps the hands behind the head. Then the patient raises the shoulders about 1" (2.5 cm), holding this position for a few seconds.

Back extensors

In a sitting position, the patient bends forward and places the hands under the buttocks. The patient tries to stand up, resisting with both hands.

Hip abductors

While standing, the patient squeezes the inner thighs together as tightly as possible. Placing a pillow between the knees supplies resistance and increases the effectiveness of this exercise.

Hip extensors

The patient squeezes the buttocks together as tightly as possible.

Knee extensors

The patient straightens the knee fully. Then the patient vigorously tightens the muscle above the knee so that it moves the kneecap upward. The patient repeats this exercise, alternating legs.

Ankle flexors and extensors

The patient pulls the toes upward, holding briefly. Then the patient pushes them down as far as possible, again holding briefly.

Exercising the toes
■ Flex the patient's toes toward the sole, and then extend them back toward the top of the foot.
■ Spread two adjoining toes apart (abduction, as shown below), and bring them together (adduction).

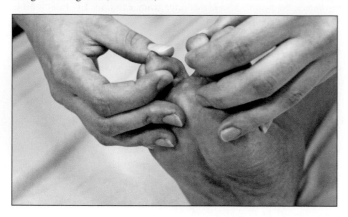

Completing the procedure
■ Return the bed to the lowest position *to prevent falls and maintain patient safety.*[21]
■ Assess the patient's comfort level and response to ROM.
■ Remove and discard your gloves and other personal protective equipment, if worn.[20]
■ Perform hand hygiene.[5,6,7,8,9,10]
■ Document the procedure.[22,23,24,25]

Special considerations
■ *Because changes in joints can begin within 3 days of immobility,* start passive ROM exercises as soon as possible.[26]
■ Patients on prolonged bed rest or limited activity without profound weakness can also be taught to perform ROM exercises on their own (called *active ROM*),[26] or they may benefit from isometric exercises. (See *Learning about isometric exercises,* page 639.)
■ If a patient who is disabled requires long-term rehabilitation after discharge, consult with a physical therapist and teach a family member or caregiver to perform passive ROM exercises.

Complications
Complications may include pain or muscle spasms.[1,26]

Documentation
Document the date and time and the joints that you exercised, the presence of edema or pressure areas, any pain resulting from the exercises, any limitation of ROM, and the patient's tolerance of the exercises. Document teaching provided to the patient and family (if applicable), their understanding of that teaching, and any need for follow-up teaching.

REFERENCES

1 Hinkle, J. L., & Cheever, K. H. (2018). *Brunner and Suddarth's textbook of medical-surgical nursing* (14th ed.). Philadelphia, PA: Wolters Kluwer.

2 Skalsky, A. J., & McDonald, C. M. (2012). Prevention and management of limb contractures in neuromuscular diseases. *Physical Medicine and Rehabilitation Clinics of North America, 23*(3), 675–687. https://www.ncbi.nlm.nih.gov/pmc/articles/PMC3482407/

3 Amidei, C., & Sole, M. L. (2013). Physiological responses to passive exercise in adults receiving mechanical ventilation. *American Journal of Critical Care, 22*, 337–348. (Level VI)

4 Kisner, C., et al. (2018). *Therapeutic exercise: Foundations and techniques* (7th ed.). Philadelphia, PA: F. A. Davis Company.

5 The Joint Commission. (2021). Standard NPSG.07.01.01. *Comprehensive accreditation manual for hospitals.* Oakbrook Terrace, IL: The Joint Commission. (Level VII)

6 Centers for Disease Control and Prevention. (2002). Guideline for hand hygiene in health-care settings: Recommendations of the Healthcare Infection Control Practices Advisory Committee and the HICPAC/SHEA/APIC/IDSA Hand Hygiene Task Force. *MMWR Recommendations and Reports, 51*(RR-16), 1–45. https://www.cdc.gov/mmwr/pdf/rr/rr5116.pdf (Level II)

7 World Health Organization. (2009). WHO guidelines on hand hygiene in health care: First global patient safety challenge, clean care is safer care. https://apps.who.int/iris/bitstream/handle/10665/44102/9789241597906_eng.pdf?sequence=1 (Level IV)

8 Accreditation Association for Hospitals and Health Systems. (2020). Standard 07.01.21. *Healthcare Facilities Accreditation Program: Accreditation requirements for acute care hospitals.* Chicago, IL: Accreditation Association for Hospitals and Health Systems. (Level VII)

9 Centers for Medicare and Medicaid Services, Department of Health and Human Services. (2020). Condition of participation: Infection control. 42 C.F.R. § 482.42.

10 DNV GL-Healthcare USA, Inc. (2020). IC.1.SR.1. *NIAHO® accreditation requirements, interpretive guidelines and surveyor guidance—revision 20.0.* Milford, OH: DNV GL-Healthcare USA, Inc. (Level VII)

11 The Joint Commission. (2021). Standard NPSG.01.01.01. *Comprehensive accreditation manual for hospitals.* Oakbrook Terrace, IL: The Joint Commission. (Level VII)

12 The Joint Commission. (2021). Standard RI.01.03.01. *Comprehensive accreditation manual for hospitals.* Oakbrook Terrace, IL: The Joint Commission. (Level VII)

13 Accreditation Association for Hospitals and Health Systems. (2020). Standard 15.01.16. *Healthcare Facilities Accreditation Program: Accreditation requirements for acute care hospitals.* Chicago, IL: Accreditation Association for Hospitals and Health Systems. (Level VII)

14 Centers for Medicare and Medicaid Services, Department of Health and Human Services. (2020). Condition of participation: Patient's rights. 42 C.F.R. § 482.13(c)(1).

15 DNV GL-Healthcare USA, Inc. (2020). PR.2.SR.5. *NIAHO® accreditation requirements, interpretive guidelines and surveyor guidance—revision 20.0.* Milford, OH: DNV GL-Healthcare USA, Inc. (Level VII)

16 The Joint Commission. (2021). Standard PC.02.01.21. *Comprehensive accreditation manual for hospitals.* Oakbrook Terrace, IL: The Joint Commission. (Level VII)

17 Waters, T. R., et al. (2009). Safe patient handling training for schools of nursing. https://www.cdc.gov/niosh/docs/2009-127/pdfs/2009-127.pdf (Level VII)

18 Accreditation Association for Hospitals and Health Systems. (2020). Standard 07.01.10. *Healthcare Facilities Accreditation Program: Accreditation requirements for acute care hospitals.* Chicago, IL: Accreditation Association for Hospitals and Health Systems. (Level VII)

19 Siegel, J. D., et al. (2007, revised 2019). 2007 guideline for isolation precautions: Preventing transmission of infectious agents in healthcare settings. https://www.cdc.gov/infectioncontrol/pdf/guidelines/isolation-guidelines-H.pdf (Level II)

20 Occupational Safety and Health Administration. (2019). Bloodborne pathogens, standard number 1910.1030. https://www.osha.gov/pls/oshaweb/owadisp.show_document?p_id=10051&p_table=STANDARDS (Level VII)

21 Ganz, D. A., et al. (2013, reviewed 2021). Preventing falls in hospitals: A toolkit for improving quality of care (AHRQ publication no. 13-0015-EF). https://www.ahrq.gov/professionals/systems/hospital/fallpxtoolkit/index.html (Level VII)

22 The Joint Commission. (2021). Standard RC.01.03.01. *Comprehensive accreditation manual for hospitals.* Oakbrook Terrace, IL: The Joint Commission. (Level VII)

23 Centers for Medicare and Medicaid Services, Department of Health and Human Services. (20209). Condition of participation: Medical record services. 42 C.F.R. § 482.24(b).

24 Accreditation Association for Hospitals and Health Systems. (2020). Standard 10.00.03. *Healthcare Facilities Accreditation Program: Accreditation requirements for acute care hospitals.* Chicago, IL: Accreditation Association for Hospitals and Health Systems. (Level VII)

25 DNV GL-Healthcare USA, Inc. (2020). MR.2.SR.1. *NIAHO® accreditation requirements, interpretive guidelines and surveyor guidance—revision 20.0.* Milford, OH: DNV GL-Healthcare USA, Inc. (Level VII)

26 Craven, R. F., et al. (2020). *Fundamentals of nursing: Concepts and competencies for practice* (9th ed.). Philadelphia, PA: Wolters Kluwer.

PATIENT-CONTROLLED ANALGESIA

Patient-controlled analgesia (PCA) is a drug delivery system providing IV analgesia, when the patient presses a button at the end of a cord. This type of delivery system allows analgesics to be provided at the level and time needed by the patient. A PCA device prevents the patient from accidentally overdosing by imposing a lockout time between doses, usually 6 to 10 minutes. During this interval, the device won't deliver a bolus of analgesic, even if the patient pushes the button. Another key safety feature of PCA is that a sedated patient can't press the PCA button to deliver additional doses of analgesia.[1]

A PCA system can also be programmed to administer a continuous analgesia infusion at a prescribed basal rate.[2,3] Morphine is the drug most commonly administered via this method, although HYDROmorphone and fentaNYL may also be prescribed for patients with renal insufficiency.[4] FentaNYL is preferred for patients with renal and hepatic insufficiency.[5]

NURSING ALERT Basal infusion of opioids isn't routinely recommended in patients who are opioid-naive *because of the increased risk of nausea, vomiting, and respiratory depression.* Evidence hasn't shown that a basal infusion improves analgesia compared with PCA without a basal infusion.[3,5]

PCA offers several advantages. It eliminates the need for IM analgesics, provides pain relief tailored to each patient's size and pain tolerance, gives the patient a sense of control over pain, and allows the patient to sleep at night with minimal daytime drowsiness. It also improves postoperative deep breathing, coughing, and ambulation and reduces opioid use.

PCA is typically given to patients postoperatively and to those with terminal cancer or other chronic diseases. To receive PCA therapy, a patient must be mentally alert and able to understand and adhere to instructions and procedures, and have no history of allergy to the analgesic.

To ensure patient safety, standardized medication concentrations and standardized or preprinted order sets for PCA are recommended.[6,7] Although PCA is intended to be patient-controlled, authorized agent–controlled analgesia for those who can't use PCA independently offers a safe alternative through an authorized, educated agent such as a nurse. Recommendations for increased safety of authorized agent–controlled analgesia include proper identification and education of authorized agents, accurate clinical documentation, careful adherence to facility guidelines, and careful selection of eligible patients and their agents.[8] To avoid analgesic administration by unauthorized individuals (PCA by proxy), nursing interventions should include placing hazard warnings on PCA equipment and teaching family members and health care practitioners about the potential dangers of administering PCA without authorization.[7] The Institute for Safe Medication Practices, The Joint Commission, and the American Society for Pain Management Nursing don't support PCA by proxy because of the risk of adverse events, such as respiratory depression, oversedation, cardiopulmonary arrest, and death.[1,8]

Equipment

Patient's medication administration record ▪ programmable PCA pump ▪ PCA administration set ▪ syringe, cassette, or bag with prescribed medication ▪ antiseptic pads (chlorhexidine-based, povidone-iodine, or alcohol) ▪ compatible IV solution ▪ gloves ▪ labels ▪ naloxone ▪ facility-approved standardized sedation scale ▪ facility-approved pain assessment scale ▪ oxygen administration setup and equipment ▪ vital signs monitoring equipment ▪ emergency equipment (code cart with emergency medications, defibrillator, handheld resuscitation bag with mask, intubation and suction equipment) ▪ Optional: pulse oximeter with probe, capnography monitoring equipment, IV catheter insertion equipment, personal protective equipment.

Preparation of equipment

Inspect all IV equipment and supplies; if a product is expired, is defective, or has compromised integrity, remove it from patient use, label it as expired or defective, and report the expiration or defect as directed by your facility.[9]

Numerous types of PCA devices are available, so follow the manufacturer's instructions for setting up the device. Plug the PCA device into an electrical outlet, if applicable. If the device is battery-operated, make sure that the battery is fully charged and working.

Have oxygen and naloxone readily available *in case the patient develops respiratory depression.*[7] Make sure emergency equipment is functioning and readily available.

Implementation

▪ Avoid distractions and interruptions when preparing and administering medication *to prevent medication administration errors.*[10,11]

▪ Review the practitioner's order to make sure that the prescribed infusion solution or medication, dose, rate, and administration route are appropriate for the patient's age, condition, and access device, and that the infusion medication is compatible with other solutions or medications. Address concerns about the order with the practitioner, the pharmacist, your supervisor, or the risk management department, as directed by your facility.[12,13,14,15,16,17]

▪ Reconcile the patient's medications when a new medication is ordered *to reduce the risk of medication errors, including omissions, duplications, dosing errors, and drug interactions.*[17]

▪ Review the patient's medical record for factors that place the patient at risk for respiratory depression and other adverse events; risk factors include advanced age, morbid obesity, obstructive sleep apnea, chronic obstructive pulmonary disease, cardiac disease, impaired liver function, and renal insufficiency.[6]

▪ Gather and prepare the necessary equipment and supplies.

▪ Compare the medication label with the order in the patient's medical record.[12,13,14,15]

▪ Check the patient's medical record for an allergy or a contraindication to the prescribed medication. If an allergy or a contraindication exists, don't administer the medication; instead, notify the practitioner.[12,13,14,15]

▪ Check the expiration date on the medication. If the medication is expired, return it to the pharmacy and obtain new medication.[12,13,14,15]

▪ Visually inspect the solution for particles, discoloration, or other loss of integrity; don't administer the medication if its integrity is compromised.[12,13,14,15]

▪ Discuss any unresolved concerns about the medication with the patient's practitioner.[12,13,14,15]

▪ Perform hand hygiene.[18,19,20,21,22,23,24,25]

▪ Confirm the patient's identity using at least two patient identifiers.[26]

▪ Provide privacy.[27,28,29,30]

▪ Explain the procedure to the patient and family (if appropriate) according to their individual communication and learning needs *to increase their understanding, allay their fears, and enhance cooperation.*[31,32]

▪ If the patient is receiving the medication for the first time, teach the patient about potential adverse reactions and discuss any other concerns related to the medication.[12,13,14,15]

▪ Teach the patient how to use the PCA device, and assess the patient's comprehension by using the teach-back method. Notify the practitioner if the patient can't participate safely in PCA therapy.[6,33]

▪ Verify that the medication is being administered at the proper time, in the prescribed dose, and by the correct route *to reduce the risk of medication errors.*[12,13,14,15]

▪ Raise the bed to waist level when providing care *to prevent caregiver back strain.*[34]

▪ Screen for and assess the patient's pain using facility-defined criteria that are consistent with the patient's age, condition, and ability to understand.[35]

▪ Obtain vital signs *to serve as a baseline for comparison.*

▪ Perform hand hygiene.[18,19,20,21,22,23,24,25]

NURSING ALERT If your facility's hazardous drug list contains the drug you are about to administer, put on personal protective equipment, as directed.[36]

▪ Put on gloves *to comply with standard precautions.*[37,38,39]

▪ Assess the patency of the patient's vascular access device; insert a new catheter, if needed.[16] (See the "IV catheter insertion and removal" procedure.)

- Prime the PCA administration set according to the manufacturer's instructions.
- Program the pump to deliver the prescribed parameters, such as loading dose, basal rate, bolus amount, bolus lockout period, and maximum limit. Have a second nurse confirm these settings *to prevent possible errors.*[6,7]
- Perform a vigorous mechanical scrub of the lowest needleless port of the patient's primary IV administration set for at least 5 seconds using an antiseptic pad. Then allow it to dry completely.[40,41]
- Attach the needleless connector from the PCA administration set to the lowest needleless port on the primary IV administration set.[7]
- Trace the tubing from the patient to its point of origin *to make sure that it's connected to the correct port.* Route the tubing in a standardized direction if the patient has other tubing and catheters that have different purposes. If multiple IV lines will be used, label the tubing at both the distal end (near the patient connection) and proximal end (near the source container) *to reduce the risk of misconnection.*[16,42,43]
- Have another nurse perform an independent double-check, if required by your facility, *to verify the patient's identity, allergies, correct medication and concentration, loading dose, basal rate (if applicable), bolus amount, bolus lockout period, and maximum limit.*[6,7]

NURSING ALERT Opioids are considered high-alert medications *because they can cause significant patient harm when used in error.*[44] Before beginning an opioid infusion, have another nurse perform an independent double-check, if required by your facility, *to verify the patient's identity and to make sure that the correct medication is in the syringe in the prescribed concentration, the medication's indication corresponds with the patient's diagnosis, the dosage calculations are correct, the route of administration is safe and proper for the patient, the pump settings are correct, and the infusion line is attached to the correct port.*[45]

- Compare the results of the independent double-check with another nurse if required. If discrepancies exist, rectify them before beginning PCA; if none exist, begin infusing the medication.[45]
- If your facility uses a bar code scanning system, use it as directed by your facility.
- Label the PCA pump, PCA administration set, and IV administration set tubing with the date of initiation or date of change, as directed by your facility.[43]
- Instruct the patient to push the button each time pain occurs and the patient needs relief.[6]
- Frequently monitor the patient's vital signs, sedation level (using a standardized sedation scale), and respiratory status (including oxygen saturation level and carbon dioxide level by capnography, if ordered) *to identify adverse effects related to IV opioid use, such as respiratory depression and oversedation.*[6,46] Be aware of the amount of analgesia the patient receives when the device is activated and the maximum amount the patient can receive within a specified time frame (if an adjustable device is used).[7]
- For a patient who is receiving an IV opioid medication, explain the assessment and monitoring process to the patient and family, and tell them to alert staff if a breathing problem or sedation occurs.[47]

NURSING ALERT *If the respiratory rate falls below 8 breaths/minute or the patient becomes overly sedated, becomes unarousable, has a change in cognition, or has an adverse reaction to the medication,* suspend the use of PCA and notify the practitioner.[2]

- Reassess and respond to the patient's pain by evaluating the response to treatment and progress toward pain management goals. Assess for adverse reactions and risk factors for adverse events that may result from treatment.[6,7,5,48] Notify the practitioner if the patient's pain isn't being adequately relieved.
- Monitor the vascular access site for signs of infection, infiltration, and catheter-associated venous thrombosis.
- Return the bed to the lowest position *to prevent falls and maintain patient safety.*[49]
- Discard used supplies in appropriate receptacles.[39,50]
- Remove and discard your gloves.[37,39,50]
- Perform hand hygiene.[18,19,20,21,22,23,24,25]
- Document the procedure.[51,52,53,54,55]

Special considerations

- Establish a bowel regimen if the patient experiences opioid-induced constipation.[3]
- Administer an antiemetic, as needed and prescribed, following safe medication administration practices if the patient develops nausea related to PCA therapy.[12,13,14,15]
- Verify PCA pump settings at the beginning of each shift and during or immediately after receiving hand-off communications.[7]

Complications

Potential complications include infection, IV infiltration, and adverse reactions to the prescribed medication, including respiratory depression, oversedation, nausea, vomiting, constipation, urine retention, and pruritus.[2,3,5]

Documentation

Record the date and time of PCA therapy initiation; the IV access device used and its location; baseline vital signs and pain assessment findings; medication (concentration, loading dose, basal rate, bolus amount, bolus lockout period, maximum limit, and total dose delivered); and ongoing assessments of vital signs, pain, sedation level, respiratory status (including oxygen saturation and carbon dioxide level, if monitored), and the IV site. Record any adverse reactions to the prescribed medication, the date and time the practitioner was notified, prescribed interventions, and the patient's response to those interventions.[56] Document the patient's tolerance of the procedure, any unexpected outcomes, nursing interventions provided, and the patient's response to them. Document teaching provided to the patient and family (if applicable), their understanding of that teaching, and any need for follow-up teaching.

References

1 Institute for Safe Medication Practices. (2016). Worth repeating… recent PCA by proxy event suggests reassessment of practices that may have fallen by the wayside. https://www.ismp.org/resources/worth-repeating-recent-pca-proxy-event-suggests-reassessment-practices-may-have-fallen?id=1149

2 Infusion Nurses Society. (2016). *Policies and procedures for infusion therapy* (5th ed.). Boston, MA: Infusion Nurses Society.

3 Chou, R., et al. (2016). Management of postoperative pain: A clinical practice guideline from the American Pain Society, the American Society of Regional Anesthesia and Pain Medicine, and the American Society of Anesthesiologists' Committee on Regional Anesthesia, Executive Committee, and Administrative Council. *Journal of Pain, 17*(2), 131–157. https://www.jpain.org/article/S1526-5900(15)00995-5/fulltext (Level VII)

4 Stewart, D. (2017). Pearls and pitfalls of patient-controlled analgesia. *US Pharmacist, 42*(3), HS24–HS27. https://www.uspharmacist.com/article/pearls-and-pitfalls-of-patientcontrolled-analgesia

5 Mariano, E. R. (2021). Management of acute perioperative pain. In: *UpToDate.* Fishman, S. (Ed.)

6 Standard 62. Patient-controlled analgesia. Infusion therapy standards of practice (8th ed.). (2021). *Journal of Infusion Nursing, 44*(Suppl. 1), S187–S190. (Level VII)

7 Institute for Safe Medication Practices. (2003). Safety issues with PCA part II—How to prevent errors. https://www.ismp.org/resources/safety-issues-pca-part-ii-how-prevent-errors (Level VII)

8 Cooney, M. F., et al. (2013). American Society for Pain Management Nursing position statement with clinical practice guidelines: Authorized agent controlled analgesia. *Pain Management Nursing, 14*(3), 176–181. http://www.aspmn.org/documents/AuthorizedAgentControlledAnalgesia_PMN_August2013.pdf (Level VII)

9 Standard 12. Product evaluation, integrity, and defect reporting. Infusion therapy standards of practice (8th ed.). (2021). *Journal of Infusion Nursing, 44*(Suppl. 1), S45–S46. (Level VII)

10 Westbrook, J., et al. (2010). Association of interruptions with an increased risk and severity of medication administration errors. *Archives of Internal Medicine, 170*(1), 683–690. https://doi.org/10.1001/archinternmed.2010.65 (Level IV)

11 Institute for Safe Medication Practices. (2012). Side tracks on the safety express: Interruptions lead to errors and unfinished…Wait, what was I doing? *Nurse Advise-ERR, 11*(2), 1–4. https://www.ismp.org/resources/side-tracks-safety-express-interruptions-lead-errors-and-unfinished-wait-what-was-i-doing?id=37

12 The Joint Commission. (2021). Standard MM.06.01.01. *Comprehensive accreditation manual for hospitals.* (Level VII)

13 Accreditation Association for Hospitals and Health Systems. (2020). Standard 16.01.03. *Healthcare Facilities Accreditation Program: Accreditation requirements for acute care hospitals.* (Level VII)

14 Centers for Medicare and Medicaid Services, Department of Health and Human Services. (2020). Condition of participation: Nursing services. 42 C.F.R. § 482.23(c).

15 DNV GL-Healthcare USA, Inc. (2020). MM.1.SR.3. *NIAHO® accreditation requirements, interpretive guidelines and surveyor guidance—revision 20.0.* (Level VII)

16 Standard 59. Infusion medication and solution administration. Infusion therapy standards of practice (8th ed.). (2021). *Journal of Infusion Nursing, 44*(Suppl. 1), S180–S183. (Level VII)

17 Standard 13. Medication verification. Infusion therapy standards of practice (8th ed.). (2021). *Journal of Infusion Nursing, 44*(Suppl. 1), S46–S49. (Level VII)

18 The Joint Commission. (2021). Standard NPSG.07.01.01. *Comprehensive accreditation manual for hospitals.* (Level VII)

19 World Health Organization. (2009). WHO guidelines on hand hygiene in health care: First global patient safety challenge, clean care is safer care. https://apps.who.int/iris/bitstream/handle/10665/44102/9789241597906_eng.pdf?sequence=1 (Level IV)

20 Centers for Disease Control and Prevention. (2002). Guideline for hand hygiene in health-care settings: Recommendations of the Healthcare Infection Control Practices Advisory Committee and the HICPAC/SHEA/APIC/IDSA Hand Hygiene Task Force. *MMWR Recommendations and Reports, 51*(RR-16), 1–45. https://www.cdc.gov/mmwr/pdf/rr/rr5116.pdf (Level II)

21 Standard 16. Hand hygiene. Infusion therapy standards of practice (8th ed.). (2021). *Journal of Infusion Nursing, 44*(Suppl. 1), S53–S54. (Level VII)

22 Centers for Disease Control and Prevention. (2011, revised 2017). Guidelines for the prevention of intravascular catheter-related infections. https://www.cdc.gov/infectioncontrol/guidelines/bsi/recommendations.html (Level I)

23 Accreditation Association for Hospitals and Health Systems. (2020). Standard 07.01.21. *Healthcare Facilities Accreditation Program: Accreditation requirements for acute care hospitals.* (Level VII)

24 Centers for Medicare and Medicaid Services, Department of Health and Human Services. (2020). Condition of participation: Infection control. 42 C.F.R. § 482.42.

25 DNV GL-Healthcare USA, Inc. (2020). IC.1.SR.1. *NIAHO® accreditation requirements, interpretive guidelines and surveyor guidance—revision 20.0.* (Level VII)

26 The Joint Commission. (2021). Standard NPSG.01.01.01. *Comprehensive accreditation manual for hospitals.* (Level VII)

27 The Joint Commission. (2021). Standard RI.01.01.01. *Comprehensive accreditation manual for hospitals.* (Level VII)

28 Centers for Medicare and Medicaid Services, Department of Health and Human Services. (2020). Condition of participation: Patient's rights. 42 C.F.R. § 482.13(c)(1).

29 DNV GL-Healthcare USA, Inc. (2020). PR.2.SR.5. *NIAHO® accreditation requirements, interpretive guidelines and surveyor guidance—revision 20.0.* (Level VII)

30 Accreditation Association for Hospitals and Health Systems. (2020). Standard 15.01.16. *Healthcare Facilities Accreditation Program: Accreditation requirements for acute care hospitals.* (Level VII)

31 The Joint Commission. (2021). Standard PC.02.01.21. *Comprehensive accreditation manual for hospitals.* (Level VII)

32 The Joint Commission. (2010). *Advancing effective communication, cultural competence, and patient- and family-centered care: A roadmap for hospitals.* Oakbrook Terrace, IL: The Joint Commission. https://www.jointcommission.org/-/media/tjc/documents/resources/patient-safety-topics/health-equity/aroadmapforhospitalsfinalversion727pdf.pdf?db=web&hash=AC3AC4BED1D973713C2CA6B2E5ACD01B (Level VII)

33 Standard 8. Patient education. Infusion therapy standards of practice (8th ed.). (2021). *Journal of Infusion Nursing, 44*(Suppl. 1), S35–S37. (Level VII)

34 Waters, T. R., et al. (2009). Safe patient handling training for schools of nursing. https://www.cdc.gov/niosh/docs/2009-127/pdfs/2009-127.pdf (Level VII)

35 The Joint Commission. (2021). Standard PC.01.02.07. *Comprehensive accreditation manual for hospitals.* (Level VII)

36 The United States Pharmacopeial Convention. (2019). USP general chapter <800> hazardous drugs: Handling in healthcare centers. https://www.usp.org/compounding/general-chapter-hazardous-drugs-handling-healthcare?gclid=EAIaIQobChMIiJisgpXu2QIVwrfACh3jBAupEAAYASAAEgJMDfD_BwE (Level VII)

37 Siegel, J. D., et al. (2007, revised 2019). 2007 guideline for isolation precautions: Preventing transmission of infectious agents in healthcare settings. https://www.cdc.gov/infectioncontrol/pdf/guidelines/isolation-guidelines-H.pdf (Level II)

38 Accreditation Association for Hospitals and Health Systems. (2020). Standard 07.01.10. *Healthcare Facilities Accreditation Program: Accreditation requirements for acute care hospitals.* (Level VII)

39 Occupational Safety and Health Administration. (2019). Bloodborne pathogens, standard number 1910.1030. https://www.osha.gov/pls/oshaweb/owadisp.show_document?p_id=10051&p_table=STANDARDS (Level VII)

40 Marschall, J., et al. (2014). SHEA/IDSA practice recommendation: Strategies to prevent central line–associated bloodstream infections in acute care hospitals. *Infection Control and Hospital Epidemiology, 35*(7), 753–771. https://www.jstor.org/stable/10.1086/676533#metadata_info_tab_contents (Level I)

41 Standard 36. Needleless connectors. Infusion therapy standards of practice (8th ed.). (2021). *Journal of Infusion Nursing, 44*(Suppl. 1), S104–S107. (Level VII)

42 The Joint Commission. (2014). Sentinel event alert: Managing risk during transition to new ISO tubing connector standards. http://www.jointcommission.org/assets/1/6/SEA_53_Connectors_8_19_14_final.pdf (Level VII)

43 Standard 43. Administration set management. Infusion therapy standards of practice (8th ed.). (2021). *Journal of Infusion Nursing, 44*(Suppl. 1), S123–S125. (Level VII)

44 Institute for Safe Medication Practices. (2018). ISMP list of high-alert medications in acute care settings. https://www.ismp.org/sites/default/files/attachments/2018-08/highAlert2018-Acute-Final.pdf (Level VII)

45 Institute for Safe Medication Practice. (2019). Independent double checks: Worth the effort if used judiciously and properly. https://www.ismp.org/resources/independent-double-checks-worth-effort-if-used-judiciously-and-properly (Level VII)

46 Jarzyna, D., et al. (2011). American Society for Pain Management Nursing guidelines on monitoring for opioid-induced sedation and respiratory depression. *Pain Management Nursing, 12*(3), 118–145. http://www.aspmn.org/documents/GuidelinesonMonitoringforOpioid-InducedSedationandRespiratoryDepression.pdf (Level VII)

47 Centers for Medicare and Medicaid Services. (2014). Requirements for hospital medication administration, particularly intravenous (IV) medications and post-operative care of patients receiving IV opioids. https://www.cms.gov/Medicare/Provider-Enrollment-and-Certification/SurveyCertificationGenInfo/Downloads/Survey-and-Cert-Letter-14-15.pdf

48 Accreditation Association for Hospitals and Health Systems. (2020). Standard 16.02.05. *Healthcare Facilities Accreditation Program: Accreditation requirements for acute care hospitals.* (Level VII)

49 Ganz, D. A., et al. (2013, reviewed 2021). *Preventing falls in hospitals: A toolkit for improving quality of care* (AHRQ Publication No. 13-0015-EF). Agency for Healthcare Research and Quality. https://www.ahrq.gov/professionals/systems/hospital/fallpxtoolkit/index.html (Level VII)

50 Standard 21. Medical waste and sharps safety. Infusion therapy standards of practice (8th ed.). (2021). *Journal of Infusion Nursing, 44*(Suppl. 1), S460–S62. (Level VII)

51 The Joint Commission. (2021). Standard RC.01.03.01. *Comprehensive accreditation manual for hospitals.* (Level VII)

52 Accreditation Association for Hospitals and Health Systems. (2020). Standard 10.00.03. *Healthcare Facilities Accreditation Program: Accreditation requirements for acute care hospitals.* (Level VII)

53 Centers for Medicare and Medicaid Services, Department of Health and Human Services. (2020). Condition of participation: Medical record services. 42 C.F.R. § 482.24(b).

54 DNV GL-Healthcare USA, Inc. (2020). MR.2.SR.1. *NIAHO® accreditation requirements, interpretive guidelines and surveyor guidance—revision 20.0.* (Level VII)

55 Standard 10. Documentation in the medical record. Infusion therapy standards of practice (8th ed.). (2021). *Journal of Infusion Nursing, 44*(Suppl. 1), S39–S42. (Level VII)

56 The Joint Commission. (2021). Standard RC.02.01.01. *Comprehensive accreditation manual for hospitals.* (Level VII)

Percutaneous coronary intervention care

Percutaneous coronary intervention (PCI), also referred to as *percutaneous transluminal coronary angioplasty,* is a procedure to open narrowed or occluded coronary arteries and restore blood flow to the heart in patients with coronary artery disease. PCI is commonly performed in a cardiac catheterization laboratory. (See *Understanding PCI.*) The American Heart Association recommends performing PCI emergently for managing ST-elevation myocardial infarction (STEMI).[1] The period of time from arrival at the emergency department until PCI is performed is commonly referred to as *door-to-balloon* time. When door-to-balloon time is 90 minutes or less, mortality rates are lower.[2]

When PCI is used to treat STEMI, it may be performed with or without stent placement. However, when a stent is placed, it decreases the risk of target vessel revascularization, and may reduce the risk of myocardial reinfarction. For these reasons, stent placement has become routine during PCI in patients with STEMI.[3] Drug-eluting stents are inserted more commonly than are bare metal stents, because drug-eluting stents are associated with low restenosis rates.[4]

PCI provides an alternative for patients who are poor surgical candidates because of chronic medical problems. It's also useful for patients who have total coronary occlusion, unstable angina, and plaque buildup in several areas, and for those with poor left ventricular function.

Equipment

Vital signs monitoring equipment ▪ antiseptic solution (preferably chlorhexidine-based) ▪ local anesthetic ▪ prescribed IV solution ▪ IV administration set ▪ cardiac monitor and electrodes ▪ oxygen and oxygen delivery system ▪ clippers ▪ prescribed antiplatelet medication ▪ prescribed sedative ▪ contrast medium ▪ emergency equipment (code cart with emergency medications, defibrillator, handheld resuscitation bag, intubation equipment) ▪ heparin (or other prescribed anticoagulant) for injection[6] ▪ introducer kit for PCI catheter ▪ sterile gloves ▪ sterile gown ▪ sterile drapes ▪ surgical cap ▪ mask with goggles or mask and face shield ▪ Optional: Doppler ultrasound device, nitroglycerin, pulmonary artery catheter, IV catheter insertion supplies, statin medication (if prescribed).

Preparation of equipment

Inspect all equipment and supplies. If a product is expired, is defective, or has compromised integrity, remove it from patient use, label it as expired or defective, and report the expiration or defect as directed by your facility.

Make sure that emergency equipment is available and functioning properly.

Implementation
Before PCI
▪ Verify the practitioner's orders.
▪ Check the patient's medical record for allergies (including any to the prescribed medications, contrast medium, latex, or the local anesthetic) and contraindications; if the patient has any allergies or contraindications, notify the practitioner.[5,7,8,9,10]
▪ If required by your facility, confirm that informed consent has been obtained and that the signed consent form is in the patient's medical record.[11,12,13,14]
▪ Conduct a preprocedure verification *to make sure that all relevant documentation, related information, and equipment are available and correctly identified with the patient's identifiers.*[15,16]
▪ Verify that laboratory and imaging studies have been completed as ordered and that the results are in the patient's medical record. Notify the practitioner of any unexpected results.[16]

Understanding PCI

Percutaneous coronary intervention (PCI) begins with cardiac catheterization, which involves inserting a sheath and a guide catheter through a vessel in the groin or arm (commonly the femoral or radial artery) and advancing the catheter into the heart. A radial artery approach is particularly useful in patients with coagulopathy, elevated International Normalized Ratio, or morbid obesity, *because this approach reduces the risk of bleeding.*[4,5]

After the catheter is advanced into the heart, an imaging technique called coronary angiography or coronary arteriography is performed. Contrast medium is injected through the catheter into the heart's vascular system *to allow visualization of the coronary arteries and identify areas of occlusion, narrowing, and other abnormalities of the coronary arteries.* If narrowing or blockage is identified during cardiac catheterization, PCI may be performed *to open up the narrowed or blocked vessel.* During this procedure, the practitioner directs a balloon through the guide catheter into the narrowed artery. When the balloon is in place (shown below), the practitioner alternately inflates and deflates it, compressing the plaque against the vessel wall and subsequently restoring blood flow through the vessel.

During PCI, the practitioner may also insert a stent (shown below) to prevent vessel reclosure and restenosis. A bare-metal or drug-eluting stent may be used. A bare-metal stent is most commonly made of stainless steel. A drug-eluting stent is coated with a medication or polymer. The medication coating is released at the implantation site *to reduce the risk of restenosis.* The polymer coating acts to decrease platelet aggregation; some polymers also contain medication. The polymer allows the medication to be released gradually *to help reduce inflammation at the site,* which reduces the risk of restenosis. However, the medication's effect is localized.

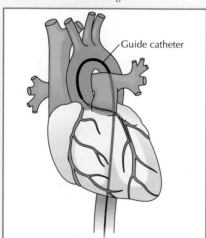

Guide catheter

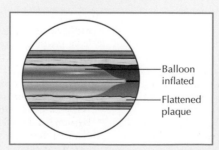

Balloon inflated
Flattened plaque

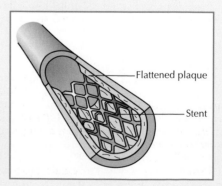

Flattened plaque
Stent

■ Ensure that the results of coagulation studies, complete blood count, serum electrolyte studies, and blood typing and cross-matching are available.[15] Notify the practitioner of any critical test results within your facility's established time frame *so that the patient can be promptly treated.*[5,17]

■ Review baseline hemodynamic parameters and patient medications for contraindications to the procedure.[18,19]

■ Perform hand hygiene.[20,21,22,23,24,25]

■ Confirm the patient's identity using at least two patient identifiers.[19,26]

■ Provide privacy.[27,28,29,30]

■ Reinforce the practitioner's explanation of the procedure according to the patient's individual communication and learning needs *to increase their understanding, allay their fears, and enhance cooperation.* Answer the patient's questions.[31]

■ Inform the patient that the procedure can last from 1 to 4 hours and that some discomfort may occur from lying on a hard table for that long.

■ Tell the patient that the practitioner will insert a catheter into an artery or a vein in the groin or wrist, and that pressure may be felt as the catheter moves along the vessel.

■ Explain that although the patient will be awake during the procedure, a sedative will be given. Explain that the practitioner or nurse may ask how the patient feels during the procedure; encourage the patient to report any experiences of angina.

■ Explain that the practitioner will inject a contrast medium through the catheter *to help visualize the heart structures.* Warn the patient that a hot, flushing sensation or transient nausea may occur during the injection.

■ Administer a statin medication, as prescribed, following safe medication administration practices *to reduce the risk of periprocedural myocardial infarction (MI).*[5,7,8,9,10]

■ If the procedure isn't an emergency, confirm the patient's nothing-by-mouth status before the procedure; minimum fasting recommendations are 2 hours for clear liquids, 6 or more hours for nonhuman milk or a light meal, and 8 hours or more for fried or fatty foods or meat.[32]

■ Perform hand hygiene.[20,21,22,23,24,25]

■ Insert an IV catheter, as needed, *in case emergency medications are required.* (See the "IV catheter insertion and removal" procedure.)

■ Following safe medication administration practices, administer antiplatelet drugs (such as aspirin and a $P2Y_{12}$ inhibitor), as ordered, *to reduce the risk of periprocedure mortality and stroke.*[3,7,8,9,10,18]

■ Clip hair from the insertion site, as needed.

■ Clean the insertion site with antiseptic solution.

■ Administer a sedative, as prescribed, following safe medication administration practices.[7,8,9,10]

■ Obtain vital signs *to serve as a baseline for comparison during and after the procedure.*

■ Assess for the presence and quality of distal pulses *to evaluate the neurovascular status of the patient's extremities.* If the pulses are weak or nonpalpable, use a portable Doppler ultrasound device *to detect and assess pulses.* (See the "Doppler ultrasound device use" procedure.)[19]

■ Perform hand hygiene.[20,21,22,23,24,25]

■ Provide hand-off communication about the patient's history, condition, and care to the person who will assume responsibility for the patient's care during the procedure. Allow time for questions, as necessary, *to avoid miscommunications that can cause patient care errors during transition of care.* As part of the hand-off process, allow time for the receiving staff member to trace each tubing and catheter from the patient to its point of origin using a standardized line reconciliation process.[33,34,35]

■ Document the procedure.[36,37,38,39]

During PCI

■ Receive hand-off communication from the person who was responsible for the patient's care before the procedure. Ask questions, as necessary, *to avoid miscommunications that can cause patient care errors during transitions of care. As part of the hand-off process,* trace each tubing and catheter from the patient to its point of origin; use a standardized line reconciliation process.[33,34,35]

■ Perform hand hygiene.[20,21,22,23,24,25]

■ When the patient arrives at the cardiac catheterization laboratory, confirm the patient's identity using at least two patient identifiers.[26]

■ Conduct a preprocedure verification *to make sure that all relevant documentation, related information, and equipment are available and correctly identified with the patient's identifiers.*[15]

■ Attach the patient to a cardiac monitor. Make sure that alarm limits are set appropriately for the patient's current condition, and that alarms are turned on, functioning properly, and audible to staff.[40,41,42,43]

■ Ensure that the IV catheter is patent.

■ Administer oxygen through an appropriate oxygen delivery device, as ordered.[5]

■ The practitioner puts on a surgical cap, a sterile gown, a mask, eye protection, and sterile gloves if needed. Put on the same personal protective equipment.[44,45,46,47]

■ Open the sterile supplies and label all medications, medication containers, and other solutions on and off the sterile field.[48,49]

■ The practitioner prepares the site, injects a local anesthetic, and then drapes the patient from head to toe, leaving the insertion site exposed. *Maximal barrier precautions prevent infection.*[44]

■ Conduct a time-out immediately before starting the procedure *to ensure that the correct patient, site, positioning, and procedure are identified, and, as applicable, that all relevant information and necessary equipment are available.*[50]

■ The practitioner inserts a sheath and a guide catheter through a vessel in the patient's groin or arm (commonly the femoral or radial artery) and advances the catheter into the heart.

■ The practitioner injects contrast medium through the catheter into the heart's vascular system *to allow visualization of the coronary arteries and help identify areas of occlusion, narrowing, and other abnormalities of the coronary arteries.* The practitioner also injects heparin or another anticoagulant[6] *to prevent the catheter from clotting,* and, if needed, intracoronary nitroglycerin *to dilate the coronary vessels and prevent spasms.*[51]

NURSING ALERT *Because coronary spasms can occur during or after PCI,* monitor the patient's electrocardiogram for ST-segment and T-wave changes, and obtain vital signs frequently.[52] Be alert for signs of ischemia, which requires emergency coronary revascularization.

■ The practitioner directs a balloon through the guide catheter into the narrowed artery. When the balloon is in place, the practitioner alternately inflates and deflates it, compressing the plaque against the vessel wall and subsequently restoring blood flow through the vessel.

■ The practitioner inserts a stent, if needed, *to prevent reclosure and restenosis of the vessel.*[4]

■ Assist with coronary angiography *to help determine the effectiveness of treatment.*

■ Monitor the insertion site for bleeding throughout the procedure.

■ Monitor the patient's International Normalized Ratio, prothrombin time, partial thromboplastin time, activated clotting time, and platelet count, as ordered.[6,19]

■ The practitioner removes the guide catheter. Note that the practitioner may leave the sheath in place *until the effects of any anticoagulant medication given during the procedure wear off.*[53] The sheath is generally removed 4 to 6 hours after the procedure;[53] assist with suturing it in place, as appropriate. (See the "Arterial and venous sheath removal" procedure.)

■ Discard used supplies in appropriate receptacles.[45,46]

■ Remove and discard your gloves and other personal protective equipment.[45,46]

■ Perform hand hygiene.[20,21,22,23,24,25]

■ Document the procedure.[36,37,38,39]

After PCI

■ Receive hand-off communication from the person who was responsible for the patient's care during the procedure. Ask questions as necessary *to avoid miscommunications that can cause patient care errors during transitions of care.* As part of the hand-off process, trace each tubing and catheter from the patient to its point of origin; use a standardized line reconciliation process.[33,34,35]

■ Verify the practitioner's orders.

■ Perform hand hygiene.[20,21,22,23,24,25]

■ Confirm the patient's identity using at least two patient identifiers.[19,26]

■ Provide privacy.[27,28,29,30]

- Explain the procedure to the patient and family (if appropriate) according to their individual communication and learning needs *to increase their understanding, allay their fears, and enhance cooperation.*[31]
- Raise the bed to waist level before providing care *to prevent caregiver back strain.*[54]
- Perform hand hygiene.[20,21,22,23,24,25]
- Put on gloves and, as needed, other personal protective *equipment to comply with standard precautions.*[45,46,47]
- Assess the catheter insertion site for bleeding. If the patient is bleeding at the catheter insertion site, confirm the presence of a compression device, *which is used to prevent hematoma formation,* or apply manual pressure approximately 1″ (2.5 cm) above the puncture site.[55]
- Attach the patient to a cardiac monitor and monitor the electrocardiogram (ECG) rhythm and arterial pressures. Make sure that alarm limits are set appropriately for the patient's current condition, and that alarms are turned on, functioning properly, and audible to staff.[40,41,42,43]
- Monitor the patient's vital signs according to the patient's condition and at an interval determined by your facility. *Practice varies, and ranges from every 5 to 15 minutes. Expert opinion recommends vital sign measurement at least every 15 minutes during phase I recovery.*[56]
- Monitor neurovascular status distal to the catheter insertion site, including peripheral pulses, color, temperature, and capillary refill time of the affected extremity. Watch for signs of neurovascular compromise; if present, notify the practitioner.[57] Immediate surgical consultation may be necessary if compartment syndrome develops after a radial approach.

NURSING ALERT *Because coronary artery spasm can occur during or after PCI,* monitor the patient's ECG for ST-segment and T-wave changes, and take vital signs frequently. Be alert for signs and symptoms of ischemia, which requires emergency coronary revascularization.[5]

- Instruct the patient to remain in bed for the amount of time specified by the practitioner, and to keep the affected extremity straight and immobilized while on bed rest. Elevate the head of the bed 15 to 30 degrees, as ordered. *Bed positioning and rest times vary depending on the arterial site selected, the technique used for closure during PCI, the size of the sheath used, and the patient's receipt of antiplatelet therapy after the procedure.*
- Assess the catheter insertion site for hematoma or hemorrhage. If a hematoma develops, apply pressure to the site, mark the area to evaluate for any change in size, and notify the patient's practitioner. If hemorrhage develops, apply pressure to the site and notify the practitioner. For hematoma or hemorrhage, interrupt anticoagulant and antiplatelet medications, as ordered; prolong bed rest, as needed; monitor serial complete blood counts, as prescribed; and administer a blood transfusion, if indicated and ordered.[6,58]
- Administer IV fluids, as ordered (usually 100 mL/hour), *to promote excretion of the contrast medium.* Monitor for signs of fluid overload (jugular vein distention, atrial and ventricular gallops, dyspnea, pulmonary congestion, tachycardia, hypertension, and hypoxemia).
- Monitor intake and output and electrolyte levels, as ordered, *to promptly recognize fluid and electrolyte imbalances.*[8,59] Notify the practitioner of critical test results within your facility's established timeframe *so the patient can be promptly treated.*[17]

When the catheter is ready for removal:
- Perform hand hygiene.[20,21,22,23,24,25]
- Put on gloves *to comply with standard precautions.*[45,46,47]
- Remove the catheter and apply direct pressure for at least 10 minutes; apply a compression or hemostatic device or a topical hemostatic agent, as ordered.[57,60,61]
- For a femoral artery approach, assess pedal pulses regularly during compression, as directed by your facility.[55]
- Monitor the site frequently and place a dressing over the site, preferably a transparent semipermeable dressing.[62]
- Discard used supplies in appropriate receptacles.[46]
- Remove and discard your gloves and other personal protective equipment, if worn.[46]
- Perform hand hygiene.[20,21,22,23,24,25]
- Clean and disinfect your stethoscope with an antiseptic pad.[63,64]
- Perform hand hygiene.[20,21,22,23,24,25]
- Document the procedure.[36,37,38,39]

Special considerations
- Devices to prevent lower extremity embolism, such as a sequential compression device or an embolic capture device, are recommended for use during PCI for a saphenous vein graft.[5,65]
- The current recommendation is to administer clopidogrel 75 mg daily, prasugrel 10 mg daily, or ticagrelor 90 mg twice daily after the procedure for a period of 1 to 12 months, depending on the exact procedure completed. If the patient isn't already receiving long-term aspirin therapy, the recommendation is for the practitioner to prescribe a maintenance dose of 81 mg of aspirin to be continued indefinitely, depending on the patient's condition and history.[3,5,64,66,67]
- If the patient exhibits signs and symptoms of an MI after the procedure, expect the practitioner to order a 12-lead ECG as well as laboratory tests to assess creatinine kinase-MB and troponin levels.[5]

Documentation
Note the patient's status before the procedure, and responses during the procedure and condition after it. Include vital signs, fluid intake and output, and neurovascular assessment findings in the extremity distal to the catheter insertion site, as well as your assessment of the insertion site. Document any complications that occurred before or during the procedure, the practitioner notified, date and time of notification, any interventions performed for those complications, and the patient's response to those interventions. Record teaching provided to the patient and family (if applicable), their understanding of that teaching, and any need for follow-up teaching.

REFERENCES

1 American Heart Association. (2020). 2020 American Heart Association Guidelines for CPR and ECC—Part 3: Adult basic and advanced life support. https://cpr.heart.org/en/resuscitation-science/cpr-and-ecc-guidelines (Level II)

2 Brodie, B. R., et al. (2010). When is door-to-balloon time critical? Analysis from the HORIZONS-AMI (Harmonizing Outcomes with Revascularization and Stents in Acute Myocardial Infarction) and CADILLAC (Controlled Abciximab and Device Investigation to Lower Late Angioplasty Complications) trials. *Journal of the American College of Cardiology, 56*(5), 407–413. https://www.sciencedirect.com/science/article/pii/S0735109710019066 (Level II)

3 O'Gara, P. T., et al. (2013). 2013 ACCF/AHA guideline for the management of ST-elevation myocardial infarction: Executive summary. A report of the American College of Cardiology Foundation/American Heart Association Task Force on Practice Guidelines. *Circulation, 127*(4), 529–555. https://www.ahajournals.org/doi/full/10.1161/CIR.0b013e3182742c84 (Level VII)

4 Gibson, C. M., et al. (2020). Primary percutaneous coronary intervention in acute ST elevation myocardial infarction: Periprocedural management. In: *UpToDate,* Cutlip, D. (Ed.).

5 Levine, G. N., et al. (2011). 2011 ACCF/AHA/SCAI guideline for percutaneous coronary intervention: A report of the American College of Cardiology Foundation/American Heart Association task force on practice guidelines and the Society for Cardiovascular Angiography and Interventions. *Circulation, 124*(23), e574–e651. https://www.ahajournals.org/doi/pdf/10.1161/CIR.0b013e31823ba622 (Level VII)

6 Merriweather, N., & Sulzbach-Hoke, L. M. (2012). Managing risk of complications at femoral vascular access sites in percutaneous coronary intervention. *Critical Care Nurse, 32*(5), 16–29.

7 The Joint Commission. (2021). Standard MM.06.01.01. *Comprehensive accreditation manual for hospitals.* (Level VII)

8 Centers for Medicare and Medicaid Services, Department of Health and Human Services. (2020). Condition of participation: Nursing services. 42 C.F.R. § 482.23(c).

9 Accreditation Association for Hospitals and Health Systems. (2020). Standard 16.01.03. *Healthcare Facilities Accreditation Program: Accreditation requirements for acute care hospitals.* (Level VII)

10 DNV GL-Healthcare USA, Inc. (2020). MM.1.SR.3. *NIAHO® accreditation requirements, interpretive guidelines and surveyor guidance—revision 20.0.* (Level VII)

11 The Joint Commission. (2021). Standard RI.01.03.01. *Comprehensive accreditation manual for hospitals.* (Level VII)

12 Centers for Medicare and Medicaid Services, Department of Health and Human Services. (2020). Condition of participation: Patient's rights. 42 C.F.R. § 482.13(b)(2).

13 Accreditation Association for Hospitals and Health Systems. (2020). Standard 30.01.11. *Healthcare Facilities Accreditation Program: Accreditation requirements for acute care hospitals.* (Level VII)

14 DNV GL-Healthcare USA, Inc. (2020). PR.2.SR.3. *NIAHO® accreditation requirements, interpretive guidelines and surveyor guidance—revision 20.0.* (Level VII)

15 The Joint Commission. (2021). Standard UP.01.01.01. *Comprehensive accreditation manual for hospitals.* (Level VII)

16 Accreditation Association for Hospitals and Health Systems. (2020). Standard 30.00.14. *Healthcare Facilities Accreditation Program: Accreditation requirements for acute care hospitals.* (Level VII)

17 The Joint Commission. (2021). Standard NPSG.02.03.01. *Comprehensive accreditation manual for hospitals.* (Level VII)

18 Levine, G. N., et al. (2015). 2015 ACC/AHA/SCAI focused update on primary percutaneous coronary intervention for patients with ST-elevation myocardial infarction: An update of the 2011 ACCF/AHA/SCAI guideline for percutaneous coronary intervention and the 2013 ACCF/AHA guideline for the management of ST-elevation myocardial infarction. *Circulation, 133*(6), 1135–1147. https://www.ahajournals.org/doi/pdf/10.1161/CIR.0000000000000336 (Level VII)

19 Gulanick, M., & Myers, J. L. (2017). *Nursing care plans: Diagnosis, interventions, and outcomes* (9th ed.). St. Louis, MO: Elsevier.

20 The Joint Commission. (2021). Standard NPSG.07.01.01. *Comprehensive accreditation manual for hospitals.* (Level VII)

21 World Health Organization. (2009). WHO guidelines on hand hygiene in health care: First global patient safety challenge, clean care is safer care. https://apps.who.int/iris/bitstream/handle/10665/44102/9/89241597906_eng.pdf?sequence=1 (Level IV)

22 Centers for Disease Control and Prevention. (2002). Guideline for hand hygiene in health-care settings: Recommendations of the Healthcare Infection Control Practices Advisory Committee and the HICPAC/SHEA/APIC/IDSA Hand Hygiene Task Force. *MMWR Recommendations and Reports, 51*(RR-16), 1–45. https://www.cdc.gov/mmwr/pdf/rr/rr5116.pdf (Level II)

23 Centers for Medicare and Medicaid Services, Department of Health and Human Services. (2020). Condition of participation: Infection control. 42 C.F.R. § 482.42.

24 Accreditation Association for Hospitals and Health Systems. (2020). Standard 07.01.21. *Healthcare Facilities Accreditation Program: Accreditation requirements for acute care hospitals.* (Level VII)

25 DNV GL-Healthcare USA, Inc. (2020). IC.1.SR.1. *NIAHO® accreditation requirements, interpretive guidelines and surveyor guidance—revision 20.0.* (Level VII)

26 The Joint Commission. (2021). Standard NPSG.01.01.01. *Comprehensive accreditation manual for hospitals.* (Level VII)

27 The Joint Commission. (2021). Standard RI.01.01.01. *Comprehensive accreditation manual for hospitals.* (Level VII)

28 Centers for Medicare and Medicaid Services, Department of Health and Human Services. (2020). Condition of participation: Patient's rights. 42 C.F.R. § 482.13(c)(1).

29 Accreditation Association for Hospitals and Health Systems. (2020). Standard 15.01.16. *Healthcare Facilities Accreditation Program: Accreditation requirements for acute care hospitals.* (Level VII)

30 DNV GL-Healthcare USA, Inc. (2020). PR.2.SR.5. *NIAHO® accreditation requirements, interpretive guidelines and surveyor guidance—revision 20.0.* (Level VII)

31 The Joint Commission. (2021). Standard PC.02.01.21. *Comprehensive accreditation manual for hospitals.* (Level VII)

32 American Society of Anesthesiologists. (2017). Practice guidelines for preoperative fasting and the use of pharmacologic agents to reduce the risk of pulmonary aspiration: Application to healthy patients undergoing elective procedures. *Anesthesiology, 126*(3), 376–393. https://anesthesiology.pubs.asahq.org/article.aspx?articleid=2596245 (Level V)

33 The Joint Commission. (2021). Standard PC.02.02.01. *Comprehensive accreditation manual for hospitals.* (Level VII)

34 The Joint Commission. (2014). Sentinel event alert: Managing risk during transition to new ISO tubing connector standards. https://www.jointcommission.org/-/media/tjc/documents/resources/patient-safety-topics/sentinel-event/sea_53_connectors_8_19_14_final.pdf (Level VII)

35 U.S. Food and Drug Administration. (2017). Examples of medical device misconnections. https://www.fda.gov/medical-devices/medical-device-connectors/examples-medical-device-misconnections

36 The Joint Commission. (2021). Standard RC.01.03.01. *Comprehensive accreditation manual for hospitals.* (Level VII)

37 Centers for Medicare and Medicaid Services, Department of Health and Human Services. (2020). Condition of participation: Medical record services. 42 C.F.R. § 482.24(b).

38 Accreditation Association for Hospitals and Health Systems. (2020). Standard 10.00.03. *Healthcare Facilities Accreditation Program: Accreditation requirements for acute care hospitals.* (Level VII)

39 DNV GL-Healthcare USA, Inc. (2020). MR.2.SR.1. *NIAHO® accreditation requirements, interpretive guidelines and surveyor guidance—revision 20.0.* (Level VII)

40 The Joint Commission. (2013). Sentinel event alert 50: Medical device alarm safety in hospitals. https://www.jointcommission.org/-/media/tjc/documents/resources/patient-safety-topics/sentinel-event/sea_50_alarms_4_26_16.pdf (Level VII)

41 The Joint Commission. (2021). Standard NPSG.06.01.01. *Comprehensive accreditation manual for hospitals.* (Level VII)

42 Graham, K. C., & Cvach, M. (2010). Monitor alarm fatigue: Standardizing use of physiological monitors and decreasing nuisance alarms. *American Journal of Critical Care, 19*(1), 28–37. https://aacnjournals.org/ajcconline/article-abstract/19/1/28/5720/Monitor-Alarm-Fatigue-Standardizing-Use-of?redirectedFrom=fulltext

43 American Association of Critical-Care Nurses. (2018). AACN practice alert: Managing alarms in acute care across the life span: Electrocardiography and pulse oximetry. https://www.aacn.org/clinical-resources/practice-alerts/managing-alarms-in-acute-care-across-the-life-span (Level VII)

44 Centers for Disease Control and Prevention. (2011, revised 2017). Guidelines for the prevention of intravascular catheter-related infections. https://www.cdc.gov/infectioncontrol/guidelines/bsi/recommendations.html (Level I)

45 Siegel, J. D., et al. (2007, revised 2019). 2007 guideline for isolation precautions: Preventing transmission of infectious agents in healthcare settings. https://www.cdc.gov/infectioncontrol/pdf/guidelines/isolation-guidelines-H.pdf (Level II)

46 Occupational Safety and Health Administration. (2019). Bloodborne pathogens, standard number 1910.1030. https://www.osha.gov/pls/oshaweb/owadisp.show_document?p_id=10051&p_table=STANDARDS (Level VII)

47 Accreditation Association for Hospitals and Health Systems. (2020). Standard 07.01.10. *Healthcare Facilities Accreditation Program: Accreditation requirements for acute care hospitals.* (Level VII)

48 The Joint Commission. (2021). Standard NPSG.03.04.01. *Comprehensive accreditation manual for hospitals.* (Level VII)

49 Accreditation Association for Hospitals and Health Systems. (2020). Standard 25.01.27. *Healthcare Facilities Accreditation Program: Accreditation requirements for acute care hospitals.* (Level VII)

50 The Joint Commission. (2021). Standard UP.01.03.01. *Comprehensive accreditation manual for hospitals.* (Level VII)

51 Vishnevsky, A., et al. (2017). Unrecognized coronary vasospasm in patients referred for percutaneous coronary intervention: Intracoronary nitroglycerin, the forgotten stepchild of cardiovascular guidelines. *Catheterization and Cardiovascular Interventions, 90*(7), 1086–1090. (Level VI)

52 Carrozza, J. P., & Levin, T. (2021). Periprocedural complications of percutaneous coronary intervention. In: *UpToDate*, Cutlip, D. (Ed.).

53 John Hopkins Medicine Health Library. (n.d.). Angioplasty and stent placement for the heart. https://www.hopkinsmedicine.org/health/treatment-tests-and-therapies/angioplasty-and-stent-placement-for-the-heart

54 Waters, T. R., et al. (2009). Safe patient handling training for schools of nursing. https://www.cdc.gov/niosh/docs/2009-127/pdfs/2009-127.pdf (Level VII)

55 Kern, M. (2013). Back to basics: Femoral artery access and hemostasis. *Cath Lab Digest, 21*(10). https://www.cathlabdigest.com/articles/Back-Basics-Femoral-Artery-Access-Hemostasis

56 American Society of PeriAnesthesia Nurses. (2020). *2021–2022 Perianesthesia nursing standards, practice recommendations and interpretive statements.* Cherry Hill, NJ: American Society of PeriAnesthesia Nurses. (Level VII)

57 Mason, P. J., et al. (2018). An update on radial artery access and best practices for transradial coronary angiography and intervention in acute coronary syndrome: A scientific statement from the American Heart Association. *Circulation: Cardiovascular Interventions, 11*, 9. https://www.ahajournals.org/doi/10.1161/HCV.0000000000000035 (Level VII)

58 Shoulders-Odom, B. (2008). Management of patients after percutaneous coronary interventions. *Critical Care Nurse, 28*(5), 26–40.

59 Centers for Medicare and Medicaid Services. (2014). Requirements for hospital medication administration, particularly intravenous (IV) medications and post-operative care of patients receiving IV opioids. http://www.cms.gov/Medicare/Provider-Enrollment-and-Certification/SurveyCertificationGenInfo/Downloads/Survey-and-Cert-Letter-14-15.pdf

60 Kordestani, S. S., et al. (2012). A randomized controlled trial on the hemostasis of femoral artery using topical hemostatic agent. *Clinical and Applied Thrombosis/Hemostasis, 18*(5), 501–505. (Level II)

61 Altin, S. E., & Singh, V. P. (2012). Managing radial access complications. *Cardiac Interventions Today, 3*, 48–52. http://bmctoday.net/citoday/pdfs/cit0512_F5_Singh.pdf (Level V)

62 Mcle, S., et al. (2009). Transparent film dressing vs pressure dressing after percutaneous transluminal coronary angiography. *American Journal of Critical Care, 18*(1), 14–20. (Level II)

63 Accreditation Association for Hospitals and Health Systems. (2020). Standard 07.02.03. *Healthcare Facilities Accreditation Program: Accreditation requirements for acute care hospitals.* (Level VII)

64 Rutala, W. A., et al. (2008, revised 2019). Guideline for disinfection and sterilization in healthcare facilities, 2008. https://www.cdc.gov/infectioncontrol/pdf/guidelines/disinfection-guidelines-H.pdf (Level I)

65 Zankar, A., et al. (2011). Embolic capture angioplasty of lower extremity lesion following distal embolization. *Cardiovascular Revascularization Medicine, 12*, 337–340.

66 Levine, G. N., et al. (2016). 2016 ACC/AHA guideline focused update on duration of dual antiplatelet therapy in patients with coronary artery disease: A report of the American College of Cardiology/ American Heart Association Task Force on Clinical Practice Guidelines. *Circulation, 134*(10), e123–e155. https://www.ahajournals.org/doi/full/10.1161/CIR.0000000000000404 (Level VII)

67 Cutlip, D., & Levin, T. (2020). Antithrombotic therapy for elective percutaneous coronary intervention: General use. In: *UpToDate*, Windecker, S. (Ed.)

Pericardiocentesis, assisting

Pericardiocentesis is needle aspiration of pericardial fluid. Echocardiogram imaging or ultrasound generally guides needle insertion.[1,2,3] This procedure can be therapeutic and diagnostic, but is most useful as an emergency measure to relieve cardiac tamponade.[2] It can also provide a fluid sample to confirm and identify the cause of pericardial effusion (excess pericardial fluid) and help determine appropriate therapy.

Normally, small amounts of plasma-derived fluid within the pericardium lubricate the heart, reducing friction for the beating heart. The pericardium normally contains up to 50 mL of sterile fluid.[2,4] Pericardial fluid is clear and straw-colored, without evidence of pathogens, blood, or malignant cells. The white blood cell count in the fluid is usually less than 1,000/mm[3]. Its glucose concentration should approximate the glucose levels in blood.[5]

Excess pericardial fluid may accumulate after inflammation, cardiac surgery, rupture, or penetrating trauma of the pericardium (such as a gunshot or stab wound). Rapidly forming effusions, such as those that develop after cardiac surgery or penetrating trauma, may induce cardiac tamponade, a potentially lethal syndrome marked by increased intrapericardial pressure that prevents complete ventricular filling and thus reduces cardiac output. Slowly forming effusions (such as those that occur in pericarditis, metastatic cancer, or tuberculosis) typically pose less immediate danger because they allow the pericardium more time to adapt to the accumulating fluid, and may be better managed medically or surgically.[1,6,7,8]

> ## Pericardial effusions: Transudates and exudates
>
> ***Transudates*** are protein-poor effusions that usually arise from mechanical factors altering fluid formation or resorption, such as increased hydrostatic pressure, decreased plasma oncotic pressure, or obstruction of the pericardial lymphatic drainage system by a tumor.
>
> Most ***exudates*** result from inflammation and contain large amounts of protein. Inflammation damages the capillary membrane, allowing protein molecules to leak into the pericardial fluid.
>
> Both effusion types occur in pericarditis, neoplasms, acute myocardial infarction, tuberculosis, rheumatoid disease, and systemic lupus erythematosus.

Pericardial effusions are typically classified as transudates or exudates. (See *Pericardial effusions: Transudates and exudates.*)

Pericardiocentesis may also be performed using fluoroscopy-guided technique in a cardiac catheterization laboratory or interventional radiology department.[2] This procedure focuses on pericardiocentesis using echocardiography.

Equipment

Prepackaged pericardiocentesis tray ▪ vital signs monitoring equipment ▪ oxygen source ▪ supplemental oxygen delivery equipment ▪ pulse oximeter and probe ▪ stethoscope ▪ Kelly clamp ▪ two-dimensional echocardiography equipment and echocontrast medium ▪ emergency equipment (code cart with cardiac medications, handheld resuscitation bag and mask, defibrillator, intubation and suction equipment, and temporary pacemaker[2] ▪ sterile gloves ▪ sterile marker ▪ sterile labels ▪ gloves ▪ masks and goggles or mask and face shields ▪ surgical caps ▪ sterile gowns ▪ electrocardiograph (ECG) or bedside monitor ▪ prescribed sedative ▪ disinfectant pad ▪ Optional: single-patient-use scissors or disposable-head surgical clippers, light source, hemodynamic monitoring equipment, nasogastric tube, ultrasound equipment.

If a prepackaged equipment tray isn't available, you'll need the following: antiseptic solution (2% chlorhexidine-based solution) ▪ 1% lidocaine for local anesthetic ▪ 3-mL and 5-mL syringes ▪ sterile needles (25G for anesthetic and 14G, 16G, and 18G 4″ or 5″ [10 to 12.7 cm] cardiac or spinal needles)[1] ▪ 50- or 60-mL syringe with Luer-lock tip ▪ sterile specimen container for culture ▪ laboratory biohazard transport bags ▪ sterile drapes and towels ▪ 4″ × 4″ (10 cm × 10 cm) sterile gauze pads ▪ sterile occlusive dressing ▪ three-way stopcock ▪ Optional: laboratory specimen tubes, laboratory request form.

Preparation of equipment

Inspect all equipment and supplies. If a product is expired, is defective, or has compromised integrity, remove it from patient use, label it as expired or defective, and report the expiration or defect as directed by your facility. Make sure emergency equipment is functioning properly and readily available. Assist the practitioner with arterial catheter insertion for hemodynamic monitoring, as required.[1]

Implementation

- Verify the practitioner's order.
- Review the patient's medical record for history of allergies to latex or the local anesthetic.
- Gather and prepare the necessary equipment and supplies.
- Conduct a preprocedure verification process *to make sure that all relevant documentation, related information, and equipment are available and correctly identified to the patient's identifiers.*[9,10]
- Verify that the laboratory and imaging studies are complete and that the results are in the patient's medical record. Notify the practitioner of any unexpected results.[9]
- Confirm that informed consent has been obtained and that the signed consent form is in the patient's medical record.[11,12,13,14]

- Perform hand hygiene.[15,16,17,18,19,20]
- Confirm the patient's identity using at least two patient identifiers.[21]
- Provide privacy.[22,23,24,25]
- Reinforce the practitioner's explanation of the procedure, and answer the patient and family's questions (if applicable) according to their individual communication and learning needs *to increase their understanding, allay their fears, and to enhance cooperation.*[11,12,13,14] Inform the patient that some pressure may be felt when the needle is inserted into the pericardial sac.
- Confirm the patient's nothing-by-mouth status before the procedure, if possible, based on the patient's condition, *to allow sufficient time for gastric emptying to prevent pulmonary aspiration*; if the situation is nonemergent, minimum fasting recommendations include 2 hours for clear liquids, 6 or more hours for a light meal or nonhuman milk, and 8 hours or more for fried or fatty foods or meat.[26]
- Raise the patient's bed to waist level before providing patient care *to prevent caregiver back strain.*[27]
- Perform hand hygiene.[15,16,17,18,19,20]
- Put on gloves and other personal protective equipment, as needed, *to comply with standard precautions.*[28,29,30]
- Verify patent IV access *in case fluids and medications are needed during the procedure.*
- If not already done, connect the patient to the bedside monitor, which is set to read lead V_1. Also connect the patient to a pulse oximeter.[7] Make sure the alarm limits are set appropriately for the patient's current condition, and that the alarms are turned on, functioning properly, and audible to staff.[31,32,33,34]
- Obtain the patient's vital signs and oxygen saturation level using pulse oximetry, and assess heart sounds, respiratory status, and neurologic status *to serve as a baseline for comparison during and after the procedure.*[2]
- Administer supplemental oxygen, as ordered.[7]
- Insert a nasogastric tube, as ordered and as time allows, *to decompress the stomach and decrease the risk of gastric perforation.* (See the "Nasogastric tube insertion and removal" procedure.)
- Remove excess hair from the intended insertions site, if needed, using single-patient-use scissors or disposable-head surgical clippers *to facilitate dressing application.*[2,35]
- Administer sedation as ordered following safe medication administration practices.[7,36,37,38,39]
- Remove and discard your gloves and other personal protective equipment, if worn.[29]
- Perform hand hygiene.[15,16,17,18,19,20]
- Prepare a sterile field by carefully opening the equipment tray on the overbed table. Be careful not to contaminate the sterile field as you open the wrapper.[2] Label all medications, medication containers, and other solutions on and off the sterile field, maintaining the sterility of the sterile field.[40,41]
- Provide adequate lighting at the puncture site.
- Place the patient in the supine position with the head of the bed elevated 30 to 45 degrees, if not contraindicated, *to facilitate breathing and bring the heart closer to the anterior chest wall, which eases fluid aspiration.*[1,2,7,8]
- Attach the cardiac monitoring leads, if not already attached. Monitor the patient's cardiac rhythm *to evaluate the patient's response to the procedure.*
- Perform hand hygiene.[15,16,17,18,19,20]
- Assist the practitioner, as necessary, with putting on a mask and goggles or a mask and face shield, a surgical cap, a sterile gown, and sterile gloves. Then put on the same personal protective equipment.[28,29,30]
- The practitioner cleans the skin with sterile gauze pads soaked in antiseptic solution from the left costal margin to the xiphoid process. Assist with fully draping the patient with only the site exposed.[2] *Using maximum barrier precautions helps prevent infection.*
- Conduct a time-out immediately before starting the procedure *to ensure that the correct patient, site, positioning, and procedure are identified, and that, as applicable, all relevant information and necessary equipment are available.*[42]
- If the anesthetic is only available in a multidose vial, clean the injection port of the vial with an alcohol pad. Then invert the vial 45 degrees *so*

that the practitioner can insert a 25G needle and syringe and withdraw the anesthetic for injection.
- Before the practitioner injects the anesthetic, tell the patient that a transient burning sensation and local pain may occur.
- The practitioner attaches a 50- or 60-mL syringe to one end of a three-way stopcock and the cardiac or spinal needle to the other end.[2]
- Assist the practitioner and the echocardiogram or ultrasound technician, as needed. The practitioner may inject echocontrast medium *to verify needle placement.*
- The practitioner inserts the needle through the chest wall into the pericardial sac, maintaining gentle aspiration until fluid appears in the syringe. The practitioner angles the needle 35 to 45 degrees toward the tip of the right scapula between the left costal margin and the xiphoid process. *This subxiphoid approach minimizes the risk of lacerating the coronary vessels and the pleura.*
- Carefully observe the ECG tracing when the practitioner inserts the needle; *ST-segment elevation indicates that the needle has reached the epicardial surface, and the practitioner should retract it slightly; an abnormally shaped QRS complex may indicate perforation of the myocardium. Premature ventricular contractions usually indicate that the needle has touched the ventricular wall.*
- After the needle is positioned properly, the practitioner attaches a Kelly clamp to the skin surface *so that the needle won't advance any further.*
- Assist the practitioner during aspiration of the pericardial fluid and labeling and numbering of the specimen containers. (See *Aspirating pericardial fluid*, page 650.)
- If required, and if bacterial culture and sensitivity tests are scheduled, record on the laboratory request any antimicrobial drugs the patient is receiving. If you suspect anaerobic organisms, consult the laboratory about proper collection technique *to avoid exposing the aspirate to air.* Label all specimens in the presence of the patient *to prevent mislabeling.*[21] Make sure that the containers are clearly labeled with the source of the specimen. Send them to the laboratory immediately in a laboratory biohazard transport bag.[29]
- When the practitioner withdraws the needle, immediately apply pressure to the site with sterile gauze pads for 3 to 5 minutes. Clean the area around the site with an antiseptic solution and then apply a sterile occlusive dressing.[2]
- Return the bed to the lowest position *to prevent falls and maintain patient safety.*[43]
- Remove and discard personal protective equipment[29] and perform hand hygiene.[15,16,17,18,19,20]
- Arrange for a portable chest X-ray immediately after the procedure *to assess for pneumothorax and hemothorax.*[2]
- Monitor blood pressure, pulse, respiratory rate, oxygen saturation level, heart sounds, and respiratory and neurologic status every 15 minutes until the patient's condition stabilizes *to assess for complications.*[2] (Your facility may require more frequent monitoring.) Reassure the patient that such monitoring is routine.
- Monitor the puncture site for bleeding every 15 minutes until the patient's condition stabilizes, and then every 4 hours for 24 hours.[2]
- Monitor continually for cardiac arrhythmias, and document rhythm strips.
- Notify the practitioner of any changes in the patient's vital signs, cardiac rhythm, or condition.
- Monitor hemoglobin level, hematocrit, and coagulation levels, as ordered and indicated, *to assess for effusion recurrence or bleeding at the pericardiocentesis site.*[2] Notify the practitioner of critical test results within your facility's established time frame *so that the patient can be treated promptly.*[44]
- Screen for and assess the patient's pain using facility-defined criteria that are consistent with the patient's age, condition, and ability to understand.[45]
- Treat the patient's pain, as needed and ordered, using nonpharmacologic, pharmacologic, or a combination of approaches. Base the treatment plan on evidence-based practices and the patient's clinical condition, past medical history, and pain management goals.[45]
- *To show the effectiveness of the procedure,* arrange for an echocardiogram within several hours of the procedure, as ordered.[2]
- Discard used supplies in appropriate receptacles.[29]
- Perform hand hygiene.[15,16,17,18,19,20]

Aspirating pericardial fluid

In pericardiocentesis, the practitioner inserts a needle and syringe assembly through the chest wall into the pericardial sac (as illustrated below). Electrocardiographic (ECG) monitoring, with a lead wire attached to the needle and electrodes placed on the limbs (right arm [RA], right leg [RL], left arm [LA], and left leg [LL]), helps ensure proper needle placement and reduces the risk of damage to the heart.

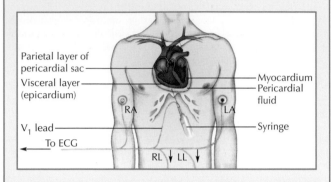

Parietal layer of pericardial sac

Visceral layer (epicardium)

RA

LA

V_1 lead

To ECG

RL ↓ LL

Myocardium

Pericardial fluid

Syringe

- Put on gloves and other personal protective equipment as needed.[28,29]
- Clean and disinfect reusable equipment according to the manufacturer's instructions *to prevent the spread of infection.*[46,47]
- Remove and discard your personal protective equipment, if worn.[29]
- Perform hand hygiene.[15,16,17,18,19,20]
- Clean and disinfect your stethoscope using a disinfectant pad.[46,47]
- Perform hand hygiene.[15,16,17,18,19,20]
- Document the procedure.[48,49,50,51]

Special considerations

- *To minimize the risk of complications,* echocardiography should precede pericardiocentesis *to determine the extent of pericardial effusion and identify the appropriate puncture site.* After the procedure, echocardiography may be performed *to evaluate the effectiveness of the procedure and to assess for complications.*[52]
- Watch for grossly bloody fluid aspirate, *which may indicate inadvertent puncture of a cardiac chamber.*
- After the procedure, be alert for respiratory and cardiac distress. Watch especially for signs of cardiac tamponade, which include muffled and distant heart sounds, distended jugular veins, paradoxical pulse, and shock. *Cardiac tamponade can result from rapid accumulation of pericardial fluid or puncture of a coronary vessel, causing bleeding into the pericardial sac.*[8]
- Depending on the patient's condition, the practitioner may place a catheter in the pericardium *to enable continuous drainage.* Monitor and record the amount and appearance of any drainage collected.[1,8]

Complications

Pericardiocentesis should be performed cautiously *because of the risk of potentially fatal complications, such as laceration of the myocardium, a coronary artery, or an intraabdominal blood vessel.* Other possible complications include ventricular fibrillation or vasovagal arrest; supraventricular arrhythmias; hemodynamic instability; air embolism; ventricular dysfunction; pleural infection; accidental puncture of the lung (pneumothorax or hemothorax), liver, or stomach; hematoma or hemorrhage at the needle insertion site; recurrent pericardial effusion; and cardiac tamponade.[2,7]

Documentation

Record the initiation and completion time of the procedure, the patient's response, vital signs, cardiac rhythm, and any medications administered. Also record and document ECG recording strips from before, during, and after the procedure. Document the amount, color, and consistency of the fluid; the number of specimen containers collected; and the time of transport to the laboratory. Document any complications that occur, prescribed interventions, and the patient's response to the interventions. Document teaching provided to the patient and family (if applicable), their understanding of that teaching, and any need for follow-up teaching.

REFERENCES

1 Fitch, M. T., et al. (2012). Emergency pericardiocentesis. *New England Journal of Medicine, 366,* e17–e21. https://doi.org/10.1056/NEJMvcm0907841

2 Wiegand, D. L. (2017). *AACN procedure manual for high acuity, progressive, and critical care* (7th ed.). St. Louis, MO: Elsevier.

3 Salazar, M., et al. (2012). Use of contrast echocardiography to detect displacement of the needle during pericardiocentesis. *Echocardiography, 29*(3), E60–E61. https://doi.org/10.1111/j.1540-8175.2011.01572.x

4 Phelan, D., et al. (2015). Disease management: Pericardial disease. http://www.clevelandclinicmeded.com/medicalpubs/diseasemanagement/cardiology/pericardial-disease/

5 American Association for Clinical Chemistry. (2020). Pericardial fluid analysis. https://labtestsonline.org/tests/pericardial-fluid-analysis

6 Lee, T. H., et al. (2013). Pericardiocentesis in trauma: A systematic review. *Journal of Trauma and Acute Care Surgery, 75*(4), 543–549. https://doi.org/10.1097/TA.0b013e3182a1fea2 (Level I)

7 Heffner, A. C. (2021). Emergency pericardiocentesis. In: *UpToDate,* Wolfson, A. B. & Stack, A. M. (Eds.).

8 Shiavone, W. A. (2013). Cardiac tamponade: 12 pearls in diagnosis and management. *Cleveland Clinic Journal of Medicine, 80*(2), 109–116. https://doi.org/10.3949/ccjm.80a.12052

9 The Joint Commission. (2021). Standard UP.01.01.01. *Comprehensive accreditation manual for hospitals.* (Level VII)

10 Accreditation Association for Hospitals and Health Systems. (2020). Standard 30.00.14. *Healthcare Facilities Accreditation Program: Accreditation requirements for acute care hospitals.* (Level VII)

11 The Joint Commission. (2021). Standard RI.01.03.01. *Comprehensive accreditation manual for hospitals.* (Level VII)

12 Centers for Medicare and Medicaid Services, Department of Health and Human Services. (2020). Condition of participation: Patient's rights. 42 C.F.R. § 482.13.

13 Accreditation Association for Hospitals and Health Systems. (2020). Standard 15.01.11. *Healthcare Facilities Accreditation Program: Accreditation requirements for acute care hospitals.* (Level VII)

14 DNV GL-Healthcare USA, Inc. (2020). PR.2.SR.3. *NIAHO® accreditation requirements, interpretive guidelines and surveyor guidance—revision 20.0.* (Level VII)

15 The Joint Commission. (2021). Standard NPSG.07.01.01. *Comprehensive accreditation manual for hospitals.* (Level VII)

16 Centers for Disease Control and Prevention. (2002). Guideline for hand hygiene in health-care settings: Recommendations of the Healthcare Infection Control Practices Advisory Committee and the HICPAC/SHEA/APIC/IDSA Hand Hygiene Task Force. *MMWR Recommendations and Reports, 51*(RR-16), 1–45. https://www.cdc.gov/mmwr/pdf/rr/rr5116.pdf (Level II)

17 World Health Organization. (2009). WHO guidelines on hand hygiene in health care: First global patient safety challenge, clean care is safer care. https://apps.who.int/iris/bitstream/handle/10665/44102/9789241597906_eng.pdf?sequence=1 (Level IV)

18 Accreditation Association for Hospitals and Health Systems. (2020). Standard 07.01.21. *Healthcare Facilities Accreditation Program: Accreditation requirements for acute care hospitals.* (Level VII)

19 Centers for Medicare and Medicaid Services, Department of Health and Human Services. (2020). Condition of participation: Infection control. 42 C.F.R. § 482.42.

20 DNV GL-Healthcare USA, Inc. (2020). IC.1.SR.1. *NIAHO® accreditation requirements, interpretive guidelines and surveyor guidance—revision 20.0.* (Level VII)

21 The Joint Commission. (2021). Standard NPSG.01.01.01. *Comprehensive accreditation manual for hospitals.* (Level VII)

22 Accreditation Association for Hospitals and Health Systems. (2020). Standard 15.01.16. *Healthcare Facilities Accreditation Program: Accreditation requirements for acute care hospitals.* (Level VII)

23 Centers for Medicare and Medicaid Services, Department of Health and Human Services. (2020). Condition of participation: Patient's rights. 42 C.F.R. § 482.13(c)(1).

24 The Joint Commission. (2021). Standard RI.01.01.01. *Comprehensive accreditation manual for hospitals.* (Level VII)

25 DNV GL-Healthcare USA, Inc. (2020). PR.2.SR.5. *NIAHO® accreditation requirements, interpretive guidelines and surveyor guidance—revision 20.0.* (Level VII)

26 American Society of Anesthesiologists. (2017). Practice guidelines for pre-operative fasting and the use of pharmacologic agents to reduce the risk of pulmonary aspiration: Application to healthy patients undergoing elective procedures. *Anesthesiology, 126*(3), 378–393. http://anesthesiology.pubs.asahq.org/article.aspx?articleid=2596245 (Level V)

27 Waters, T. R., et al. (2009). Safe patient handling training for schools of nursing. https://www.cdc.gov/niosh/docs/2009-127/pdfs/2009-127.pdf (Level VII)

28 Siegel, J. D., et al. (2007, reviewed 2019). 2007 guideline for isolation precautions: Preventing transmission of infectious agents in healthcare settings. https://www.cdc.gov/infectioncontrol/pdf/guidelines/isolation-guidelines-H.pdf (Level II)

29 Occupational Safety and Health Administration. (2019). Bloodborne pathogens, standard number 1910.1030. https://www.osha.gov/pls/oshaweb/owadisp.show_document?p_id=10051&p_table=STANDARDS (Level VII)

30 Accreditation Association for Hospitals and Health Systems. (2020). Standard 07.01.10. *Healthcare Facilities Accreditation Program: Accreditation requirements for acute care hospitals.* (Level VII)

31 American Association of Critical-Care Nurses. (2018). AACN practice alert: Managing alarms in acute care across the life span: Electrocardiography and pulse oximetry. https://www.aacn.org/clinical-resources/practice-alerts/managing-alarms-in-acute-care-across-the-life-span (Level VII)

32 The Joint Commission. (2021). Standard NPSG.06.01.01. *Comprehensive accreditation manual for hospitals.* (Level VII)

33 Graham, K. C., & Cvach, M. (2010). Monitor alarm fatigue: Standardizing use of physiological monitors and decreasing nuisance alarms. *American Journal of Critical Care, 19*(1), 28–37. https://doi.org/10.4037/ajcc2010651

34 The Joint Commission. (2013). Sentinel event alert 50: Medical device alarm safety in hospitals. https://www.jointcommission.org/-/media/tjc/documents/resources/patient-safety-topics/sentinel-event/sea_50_alarms_4_26_16.pdf (Level VII)

35 The Joint Commission. (2021). Standard NPSG.07.05.01. *Comprehensive accreditation manual for hospitals.* (Level VII)

36 Accreditation Association for Hospitals and Health Systems. (2020). Standard 16.01.03. *Healthcare Facilities Accreditation Program: Accreditation requirements for acute care hospitals.* (Level VII)

37 The Joint Commission. (2021). Standard MM.06.01.01. *Comprehensive accreditation manual for hospitals.* (Level VII)

38 Centers for Medicare and Medicaid Services, Department of Health and Human Services. (2020). Condition of participation: Nursing services. 42 C.F.R. § 482.23(c).

39 DNV GL-Healthcare USA, Inc. (2020). MM.1.SR.3. *NIAHO® accreditation requirements, interpretive guidelines and surveyor guidance—revision 20.0.* (Level VII)

40 The Joint Commission. (2021). Standard NPSG.03.04.01. *Comprehensive accreditation manual for hospitals.* (Level VII)

41 Accreditation Association for Hospitals and Health Systems. (2020). Standard 25.01.27. *Healthcare Facilities Accreditation Program: Accreditation requirements for acute care hospitals.* (Level VII)

42 The Joint Commission. (2021). Standard UP.01.03.01. *Comprehensive accreditation manual for hospitals.* (Level VII)

43 Ganz, D. A., et al. (2013, reviewed 2021). *Preventing falls in hospitals: A toolkit for improving quality of care* (AHRQ Publication No. 13-0015-EF). Agency for Healthcare Research and Quality. https://www.ahrq.gov/professionals/systems/hospital/fallpxtoolkit/index.html (Level VII)

44 The Joint Commission. (2021). Standard NPSG.02.03.01. *Comprehensive accreditation manual for hospitals.* (Level VII)

45 The Joint Commission. (2021). Standard PC.01.02.07. *Comprehensive accreditation manual for hospitals.* (Level VII)

46 Accreditation Association for Hospitals and Health Systems. (2020). Standard 07.02.03. *Healthcare Facilities Accreditation Program: Accreditation requirements for acute care hospitals.* (Level VII)

47 Rutala, W. A., et al. (2008, revised 2019). Guideline for disinfection and sterilization in healthcare facilities, 2008. https://www.cdc.gov/infection-control/pdf/guidelines/disinfection-guidelines-H.pdf (Level I)

48 The Joint Commission. (2021). Standard RC.01.03.01. *Comprehensive accreditation manual for hospitals.* (Level VII)

49 Accreditation Association for Hospitals and Health Systems. (2020). Standard 10.00.03. *Healthcare Facilities Accreditation Program: Accreditation requirements for acute care hospitals.* (Level VII)

50 Centers for Medicare and Medicaid Services, Department of Health and Human Services. (2020). Condition of participation: Medical record services. 42 C.F.R. § 482.24(b).

51 DNV GL-Healthcare USA, Inc. (2020). MR.2.SR.1. *NIAHO® accreditation requirements, interpretive guidelines and surveyor guidance—revision 20.0.* (Level VII)

52 Fuster, V., et al. (2017). *Hurst's the heart* (14th ed.). McGraw-Hill Education.

PERINEAL CARE

Perineal care, which includes care of the external genitalia and the anal area, should occur during the daily bath and if the patient is incontinent for urine or stool. The procedure promotes cleanliness and prevents infection. It also removes irritating and odorous secretions, such as smegma, a cheese-like substance that collects under the foreskin of the penis and the inner surface of the labia. For a patient with perineal skin breakdown, frequent bathing followed by application of a moisture-barrier skin protectant aids healing.

Standard precautions must be followed when providing perineal care, with great consideration for the patient's privacy.[1,2,3]

Equipment

Gloves ■ bathing supplies (disposable cleaning cloths, prepackaged bath product, or washcloths, a towel, and mild soap or pH-balanced skin cleanser) ■ bath blanket, sheet, or towel ■ fluid-impermeable pad ■ Optional: facility-approved disinfectant, bath basin, moisture-barrier skin protectant, absorbent underpad or brief, gown and mask.

After genital or rectal surgery, you may need to use sterile supplies, including sterile gloves, gauze, and cotton balls.

Preparation of equipment

Inspect all equipment and supplies. If a product is expired, is defective, or has compromised integrity, remove it from patient use, label it as expired or defective, and report the expiration or defect as directed by your facility. Obtain ointment or cream, as needed. If you're using a basin, fill it two-thirds full with warm water. If using a prepackaged bath product, warm the product, if desired, according to the manufacturer's instructions, or use at room temperature.

NURSING ALERT Studies have shown that patients' bath basins are a reservoir for bacteria, and may be a source of transmission of health care facility–acquired infections.[4] Clean and disinfect the basin after use with a facility-approved disinfectant and allow it to dry thoroughly before storing.[5,6]

Implementation

■ Gather and prepare the necessary equipment and supplies.
■ Perform hand hygiene.[7,8,9,10,11,12]
■ Confirm the patient's identity using at least two patient identifiers.[13]
■ Provide privacy.[14,15,16,17]
■ Explain the procedure to the patient and family (if appropriate) according to their individual communication and learning needs *to increase their understanding, allay their fears, and enhance cooperation.*[18]
■ Raise the patient's bed to waist level before performing patient care *to prevent back strain.*[19]
■ Perform hand hygiene.[7,8,9,10,11,12]
■ Put on gloves, gown, and mask, as needed, *to comply with standard precautions.*[1,2,3]
■ Help the patient into a supine position. Place a fluid-impermeable pad under the patient's buttocks *to protect the bed from stains and moisture.* Lower the head of the bed, if appropriate.
■ Drape the patient with a towel, bath blanket, or sheet exposing only the perineum, *to minimize exposure and embarrassment.*

■ Assess the patient's perineal area for color changes, skin breakdown, drainage, discharge, or tenderness. Notify the practitioner and the wound ostomy continence nurse, as needed.

■ Wet the washcloth with warm water from a running spigot (or from a clean and disinfected bath basin) and apply mild soap. If you're using disposable cleaning cloths or a prepackaged bath product, open the packages and obtain the wet cloths. If warmed, check the temperature before applying it to the patient's skin. If there's any indication that the cloth is excessively hot, don't use it until it cools to a comfortable temperature. Be aware that gloves affect the perception of heat.[20]

For a female patient

■ Ask the patient to bend her knees slightly and to spread her legs.

■ Separate the patient's labia with one hand. If the patient has an indwelling urinary catheter in place, use the other hand to clean the urethral meatus with the washcloth *to reduce the risk of catheter-associated urinary tract infection.* Avoid traction on the catheter. Don't aggressively clean the meatal area; *aggressive cleaning can lead to meatal irritation, increasing the risk of infection.*[21]

■ Using gentle downward strokes, clean from the front to the back of the perineum *to prevent intestinal organisms from contaminating the urethra or vagina.* Avoid the area around the anus, and use a clean section of washcloth for each stroke by folding each used section inward. *This method prevents the spread of contaminated secretions or discharge.*

■ If you're using soap and water, wet a clean washcloth and rinse the perineum thoroughly from front to back, *because soap residue can cause skin irritation.* Pat the area dry with a bath towel, *because moisture can also cause skin irritation and discomfort.*

■ Turn the patient on her side to the Sims position, if possible, *to expose the anal area.*

■ Clean, rinse, and dry the anal area, starting at the posterior vaginal opening and wiping from front to back.

■ After cleaning the perineum, apply a moisture-barrier skin protectant as needed (cream, ointment, or film-forming skin protectant) *to protect and maintain intact skin or to treat nonintact skin.*[22]

For a male patient

■ Hold the shaft of the penis with one hand. If the patient has an indwelling urinary catheter in place, use the other hand to clean the urethral meatus with the washcloth *to reduce the risk of catheter-associated urinary tract infection.*[21] Avoid tension on the catheter. Don't aggressively clean the meatal area; *aggressive cleaning can lead to meatal irritation, increasing the risk of infection.*

■ Wash the penis with the washcloth, beginning at the tip and working in a circular motion from the center to the periphery (as shown below) *to avoid introducing microorganisms into the urethra.* Use a clean section of washcloth for each stroke *to prevent the spread of contaminated secretions or discharge.* For an uncircumcised patient, gently retract the foreskin and clean beneath it.

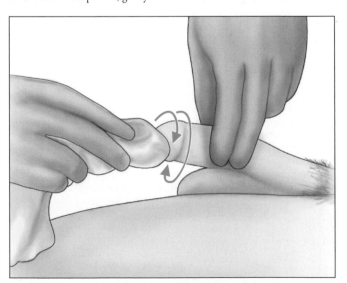

■ If you're using soap and water, wet a clean washcloth and rinse thoroughly, using the same circular motion.

■ If the patient is uncircumcised, rinse well but don't dry, *because moisture provides lubrication and prevents friction when replacing the foreskin.* Replace the foreskin *to avoid constriction of the penis, which causes edema and tissue damage.*

■ Clean the top and sides of the scrotum; rinse thoroughly and pat dry. Handle the scrotum gently *to avoid causing discomfort.*

■ Clean the bottom of the scrotum and the anal area. If appropriate, rinse well and pat dry.

■ After cleaning the perineum, apply a moisture-barrier skin protectant (cream, ointment, or film-forming skin protectant) as needed *to protect and maintain intact skin or to treat nonintact skin.*[22]

Completing the procedure

■ Reposition the patient comfortably.

■ Remove the bath blanket, sheet, or towel and fluid-impermeable pad, and then replace the bed linens if necessary.

■ Return the bed to the lowest position *to prevent falls and to maintain the patient's safety.*[23]

■ Dispose of soiled articles in the appropriate receptacle.[3] Don't flush disposable cloths down the toilet.

■ Remove and discard your gloves, gown, and mask, if worn.[1,3]

■ Perform hand hygiene.[7,8,9,10,11,12]

■ If you used a bath basin: Put on gloves.[1,3] Clean and disinfect the basin using a facility-approved disinfectant,[5,6] and allow it to dry thoroughly before storing. Remove and discard your gloves[1,3] and perform hand hygiene.[7,8,9,10,11,12]

■ Document the procedure.[24,25,26,27]

Special considerations

■ If the patient is incontinent, gently clean the skin with water or pH-balanced skin cleaner. *Note:* Soap, an alkaline, can strip the skin of natural oils and lead to secondary infection from fungi and bacteria; therefore, pH-balanced skin cleansers are recommended by the guidelines for patients at risk for incontinence-associated dermatitis.[22] Avoid excessive friction and scrubbing, *which can further traumatize the patient's skin.*[22]

Documentation

Record perineal care and any special treatment you provided. Document the need for continued treatment, if necessary. Describe perineal skin condition and odor or discharge. Document teaching you provided to the patient and family (if applicable), their understanding of that teaching, and any need for follow-up teaching.

REFERENCES

1 Siegel, J. D., et al. (2007, revised 2019). 2007 guideline for isolation precautions: Preventing transmission of infectious agents in healthcare settings. https://www.cdc.gov/infectioncontrol/pdf/guidelines/isolation-guidelines-H.pdf (Level II)

2 Accreditation Association for Hospitals and Health Systems. (2020). Standard 07.01.10. *Healthcare Facilities Accreditation Program: Accreditation requirements for acute care hospitals.* Chicago, IL: Accreditation Association for Hospitals and Health Systems. (Level VII)

3 Occupational Safety and Health Administration. (2019). Bloodborne pathogens, standard number 1910.1030. https://www.osha.gov/pls/oshaweb/owadisp.show_document?p_id=10051&p_table=STANDARDS (Level VII)

4 Johnson, D., et al. (2009). Patients' bath basins as potential sources of infection: A multicenter sampling study. *American Journal of Critical Care, 18*(1), 31–41. http://ajcc.aacnjournals.org/content/18/1/31.full (Level IV)

5 Rutala, W. A., et al. (2008, revised 2019). Guideline for disinfection and sterilization in healthcare facilities, 2008. https://www.cdc.gov/infection-control/pdf/guidelines/disinfection-guidelines-H.pdf (Level I)

6 Accreditation Association for Hospitals and Health Systems. (2020). Standard 07.02.03. *Healthcare Facilities Accreditation Program: Accreditation requirements for acute care hospitals.* Chicago, IL: Accreditation Association for Hospitals and Health Systems. (Level VII)

7 Centers for Disease Control and Prevention. (2002). Guideline for hand hygiene in health-care settings: Recommendations of the Healthcare Infection Control Practices Advisory Committee and the HICPAC/SHEA/APIC/IDSA Hand Hygiene Task Force. *MMWR Recommendations and Reports, 51*(RR–16), 1–45. https://www.cdc.gov/mmwr/pdf/rr/rr5116.pdf (Level II)

8 The Joint Commission. (2021). Standard NPSG.07.01.01. *Comprehensive accreditation manual for hospitals.* Oakbrook Terrace, IL: The Joint Commission. (Level VII)

9 World Health Organization. (2009). WHO guidelines on hand hygiene in health care: First global patient safety challenge, clean care is safer care. https://apps.who.int/iris/bitstream/handle/10665/44102/9789241597906_eng.pdf?sequence=1 (Level IV)

10 Centers for Medicare and Medicaid Services, Department of Health and Human Services. (2020). Condition of participation: Infection control. 42 C.F.R. § 482.42.

11 Accreditation Association for Hospitals and Health Systems. (2020). Standard 07.01.21. *Healthcare Facilities Accreditation Program: Accreditation requirements for acute care hospitals.* Chicago, IL: Accreditation Association for Hospitals and Health Systems. (Level VII)

12 DNV GL-Healthcare USA, Inc. (2020). IC.1.SR.1. *NIAHO® accreditation requirements, interpretive guidelines and surveyor guidance—revision 20.0.* Milford, OH: DNV GL-Healthcare USA, Inc. (Level VII)

13 The Joint Commission. (2021). Standard NPSG.01.01.01. *Comprehensive accreditation manual for hospitals.* Oakbrook Terrace, IL: The Joint Commission. (Level VII)

14 Centers for Medicare and Medicaid Services, Department of Health and Human Services. (2020). Condition of participation: Patient's rights. 42 C.F.R. § 482.13(c)(1).

15 Accreditation Association for Hospitals and Health Systems. (2020). Standard 15.01.16. *Healthcare Facilities Accreditation Program: Accreditation requirements for acute care hospitals.* Chicago, IL: Accreditation Association for Hospitals and Health Systems. (Level VII)

16 The Joint Commission. (2021). Standard RI.01.01.01. *Comprehensive accreditation manual for hospitals.* Oakbrook Terrace, IL: The Joint Commission. (Level VII)

17 DNV GL-Healthcare USA, Inc. (2020). PR.2.SR.5. *NIAHO® accreditation requirements, interpretive guidelines and surveyor guidance—revision 18.2.* Milford, OH: DNV GL-Healthcare USA, Inc. (Level VII)

18 The Joint Commission. (2021). Standard PC.02.01.21. *Comprehensive accreditation manual for hospitals.* Oakbrook Terrace, IL: The Joint Commission. (Level VII)

19 Waters, T. R., et al. (2009). Safe patient handling training for schools of nursing. https://www.cdc.gov/niosh/docs/2009-127/pdfs/2009-127.pdf (Level VII)

20 Agency for Healthcare Research and Quality. (2013). Universal ICU decolonization: An enhanced protocol: Appendix E. Training and education materials. https://www.ahrq.gov/hai/universal-icu-decolonization/universal-icu-ape4.html

21 Society of Urologic Nurses and Associates. (2015). *Clinical practice guidelines: Care of the patient with an indwelling catheter.* Pitman, NJ: Society of Urologic Nurses and Associates. https://www.suna.org/resource/clinical-practice (Level VII)

22 Beeckman, D., et al. (2016). Interventions for preventing and treating incontinence-associated dermatitis in adults. *Cochrane Database of Systematic Reviews, 2016*(11), CD011627. https://www.ncbi.nlm.nih.gov/pmc/articles/PMC6464993/ (Level I)

23 Ganz, D. A., et al. (2013, reviewed 2021). *Preventing falls in hospitals: A toolkit for improving quality of care* (AHRQ publication no. 13-0015-EF). Rockville, MD: Agency for Healthcare Research and Quality. https://www.ahrq.gov/professionals/systems/hospital/fallpxtoolkit/index.html (Level VII)

24 The Joint Commission. (2021). Standard RC.01.03.01. *Comprehensive accreditation manual for hospitals.* Oakbrook Terrace, IL: The Joint Commission. (Level VII)

25 Centers for Medicare and Medicaid Services, Department of Health and Human Services. (2020). Condition of participation: Medical record services. 42 C.F.R. § 482.24(b).

26 Accreditation Association for Hospitals and Health Systems. (2020). Standard 10.00.03. *Healthcare Facilities Accreditation Program: Accreditation requirements for acute care hospitals.* Chicago, IL: Accreditation Association for Hospitals and Health Systems. (Level VII)

27 DNV GL-Healthcare USA, Inc. (2020). MR.2.SR.1. *NIAHO® accreditation requirements, interpretive guidelines and surveyor guidance—revision 20.0.* Milford, OH: DNV GL-Healthcare USA, Inc. (Level VII)

PERIPHERALLY INSERTED CENTRAL CATHETER USE

For a patient who needs long-term central venous (CV) infusion therapy or requires repeated venous access, a peripherally inserted central catheter (PICC) may be the best option. It provides safe, reliable access for drug administration and other infusions as well as for blood sampling. Infusions commonly given by PICC include total parenteral nutrition, chemotherapy, blood and blood products, antibiotics, intermittent inotropes, fluids, and analgesics. The decision to insert a PICC is part of a collaboration with the patient and caregiver and is based on the prescribed therapy and treatment plan.[1,2]

PICCs are made of silicone or polyurethane and vary in diameter and length. They're available in single-, double-, and triple-lumen versions. You should use a PICC with the minimal number of lumens essential for managing the patient's care.[2,3] The type and size of the PICC depends on the patient's size and anatomic measurements and the required therapy. Power injection–capable PICCs are also available for patients who require injection of contrast media for computed tomography and other studies.[4]

Most PICCs are manufactured with smooth, rounded tips to reduce trauma on the vein wall during insertion. To avoid the need to trim a PICC, the best option is to select a catheter length that's as close to the desired patient length measurement as possible. Groshong PICCs shouldn't be trimmed; instead, subtract the desired patient length from the total length of the PICC, and leave any length outside the insertion site, safely secured.

Most PICCs have a preloaded stylet wire inside the catheter to add stiffness to the soft catheter, easing its advancement through the vein. The stylet terminates 1 to 2 cm away from the catheter tip. If the catheter length does require trimming, you must withdraw and reposition the stylet 1 to 2 cm from the cut end. You should never cut the stylet; rather, remove it after insertion.

PICC devices are easier to insert than other CV access devices and are considered medium-term venous access devices, which can be used for several months.[5,6] You may use a single catheter for the entire course of therapy with greater convenience and reduced cost. If the state nurse practice act permits, a nurse with proper training may insert a PICC, although the nurse may have to demonstrate competence every year, according to facility guidelines.[7]

A PICC may be inserted using a modified Seldinger technique (discussed here), or with a through-the-introducer technique. Veins you may consider for PICC insertion include the basilic (preferred), cephalic, and brachial veins. When selecting a site, avoid areas that are painful on palpation and those compromised by bruising, infiltration, phlebitis, sclerosing, or cording. Also avoid using the arm on the side of breast surgery with axillary node dissection, on the side with lymphedema, on the side where a pacemaker has been inserted, and on a side affected by stroke or radiation therapy.[2,8] Use of an ultrasound device to guide insertion increases the rate of success and reduces the risk of insertion-related complications.[2,8,9,10,11] (See *Bedside ultrasound for PICC insertion*, page 654.) After insertion, advance the catheter until it reaches the cavoatrial junction.[2,9] *To reduce the risk of vascular catheter–associated infection*, PICC insertion requires the use of maximal barrier precautions.[3]

HOSPITAL-ACQUIRED CONDITION ALERT Keep in mind that the Centers for Medicare and Medicaid Services considers vascular catheter–associated infection a hospital-acquired condition *because it can be reasonably prevented using a variety of best practices.* Make sure to follow evidence-based infection-prevention techniques, such as performing hand hygiene, using maximal barrier precautions, following sterile technique, and properly preparing the insertion site, *to reduce the risk of vascular catheter–associated infections.*[3,12,13,14,15,16]

PICC insertion is contraindicated in patients with chronic kidney disease *because of the risk of central vein stenosis, and because of the possible need for a future fistula.*

Equipment
For insertion
PICC insertion kit ▪ PICC catheter ▪ insertion checklist ▪ antiseptic swabs (alcohol-based chlorhexidine preferred; if contraindicated, an iodophor may be used [such as povidone-iodine or 70% alcohol]) ▪ two sterile

---

Bedside ultrasound for PICC insertion

Although the use of bedside ultrasound requires special training, it helps provide safer, more efficient insertion of a peripherally inserted central catheter (PICC). Since the introduction of ultrasound, the placement of PICCs using visualization and palpation alone is rare. Advantages of using ultrasound include:

- the ability to locate the exact position of veins that are neither visible nor palpable
- the ability to detect possible anatomic variations or thrombosis in the vessel
- a successful cannulation rate of more than 90% on the first attempt
- the possibility of inserting a PICC in a location away from the antecubital fossa, which can limit or eliminate such complications as mechanical phlebitis
- a reduction in complications related to traumatic placement.

---

and clean single-use disposable measuring tapes ▪ 10-mL syringes prefilled with preservative-free normal saline solution ▪ syringes and needles of appropriate size ▪ sterile gauze pads ▪ fluid-impermeable pads ▪ sterile drapes ▪ disposable skin marker ▪ single-patient-use tourniquet ▪ sterile marker ▪ sterile labels ▪ clean gloves ▪ sterile gloves ▪ sterile gown ▪ mask ▪ protective eyewear ▪ head cover ▪ 1% lidocaine without EPINEPHrine ▪ sterile transparent semipermeable dressing (may be chlorhexidine-impregnated) ▪ sterile 2″ × 2″ (5 cm × 5 cm) gauze pad ▪ door sign ▪ facility-approved disinfectant ▪ Optional: bedside ultrasound equipment, sterile and clean disposable ultrasound probe covers, ultrasound gel, tip-locator technology, chlorhexidine-impregnated sponge dressing, topical anesthetic cream, sterile needleless connectors, prefilled 10-mL syringe of heparin lock solution (10 units/mL), single-patient-use scissors or disposable-head surgical clippers, skin barrier solution, primed extension set, safety scalpel, gauze pad, soap and water, washcloth, antiseptic wipe, disinfectant-containing end cap, integrated securement device, subcutaneous anchor securement system, tissue adhesive, adhesive securement device.

Use an all-inclusive insertion kit or cart that contains all of the necessary components for maintaining sterile technique during catheter insertion *to reduce the risk of catheter-related bloodstream infection.*[9,15,17]

For flushing

Gloves ▪ syringe prefilled with preservative-free normal saline solution (10 mL syringe or syringe designed to generate lower injection pressure) ▪ antiseptic pads (chlorhexidine-based, povidone iodine, or alcohol) ▪ Optional: prescribed locking solution (such as heparin lock solution), prescribed IV fluid, disinfectant-containing end cap.

For a dressing change

Gloves ▪ sterile gloves ▪ masks ▪ sterile drape ▪ antiseptic agent (alcohol-based chlorhexidine-preferred; if contraindicated, use an iodophor [such as povidone-iodine or 70% alcohol]) ▪ transparent semipermeable dressing (may be chlorhexidine-impregnated) ▪ sterile disposable tape measure ▪ label ▪ Optional: sterile 4″ × 4″ (10 cm × 10 cm) gauze dressing, chlorhexidine-impregnated sponge dressing, alcohol-free skin barrier product, sterile measuring tape, integrated securement device, subcutaneous anchor securement system, tissue adhesive, adhesive securement device.

Many facilities stock commercially prepared or facility-prepared sterile dressing change kits that contains the necessary supplies.

For drug administration

Gloves ▪ prescribed medication in an IV container with administration set (for infusion) or in a syringe (for IV bolus) ▪ 10-mL syringes prefilled with preservative-free normal saline solution (or a syringe specifically designed to generate lower injection pressure) ▪ antiseptic pads (chlorhexidine-based, povidone iodine, or alcohol) ▪ Optional: vital signs monitoring equipment, locking solution, electronic infusion device,

pulse oximeter and probe, capnography equipment, facility-approved standardized sedation scale, disinfectant-containing end cap.

For blood sampling

Gloves ▪ 10-mL prefilled syringes of preservative-free normal saline solution (or one specifically designed to generate lower injection pressure) ▪ antiseptic pads (chlorhexidine-based, povidone iodine, or alcohol) ▪ appropriately sized syringes or needleless blood collection tube holder ▪ blood collection tubes ▪ labels ▪ laboratory biohazard transport bag ▪ Optional: prefilled syringe containing locking solution, mask with face shield or mask and goggles, blood transfer unit, needleless connector, disinfectant-containing end cap.

For removal

Gloves ▪ fluid-impermeable pad ▪ sterile transparent semipermeable dressing ▪ petroleum-based ointment ▪ tape ▪ sterile gauze pads ▪ tape measure ▪ emergency equipment (code cart with emergency medications, handheld resuscitation bag with mask, intubation equipment) ▪ Optional: gown, mask and goggles or mask with face shield, single-patient-use tourniquet, suture removal kit, warm compress.

Preparation of equipment

Inspect all IV equipment and supplies. If a product is expired, is defective, or has compromised integrity, remove it from patient use, label it as expired or defective, and report the expiration or defect as directed by your facility.[18]

Implementation
Inserting a PICC

▪ Verify the practitioner's order for PICC insertion. If necessary, before placing the PICC, collaborate with the practitioner about any relative contraindications to placement.[2]

▪ Review the patient's medical record for a history of allergies, including allergies to latex, local anesthetics, and antiseptics, *to prevent anaphylaxis.*[2]

▪ If required by your facility, confirm that informed consent has been obtained and that the signed consent form is in the patient's medical record.[17,19,20,21,22]

▪ Gather and prepare the necessary equipment and supplies.

▪ Conduct a preprocedure verification *to make sure that all relevant documentation, related information, and equipment are available and correctly identified to the patient's identifiers.*[23,24]

▪ Verify that laboratory and imaging studies have been completed, and that the results are in the patient's medical record. Notify the practitioner of any unexpected results.[23]

▪ Obtain the assistance of a second nurse or appropriate assistant who's been properly trained *to make sure that sterile technique is maintained during the procedure.*[16]

▪ Close the door to the room and put a sign on the door that states STERILE PROCEDURE IN PROGRESS. DO NOT ENTER.[2]

▪ Perform hand hygiene.[3,14,25,26,27,28,29,30,31]

▪ Confirm the patient's identity using at least two patient identifiers.[32]

▪ Provide privacy.[33,34,35,36]

▪ Explain the procedure to the patient and family (if appropriate) according to their individual communication and learning needs *to increase their understanding, allay their fears, and enhance cooperation.*[37]

▪ Provide the patient with information related to the PICC insertion procedure, including the benefits, management, and potential risks. Teach the patient and family about measures to prevent vascular catheter–associated infections, including the importance of hand hygiene.[2,38] Encourage them to remind staff members to perform hand hygiene and to follow infection prevention practices when providing care.[15]

▪ Use an insertion checklist *to help adhere to infection prevention and safety practices during insertion.*[2,15,16,25] Have your assistant stop the procedure immediately if any breaks in sterile technique occur.

▪ Raise the patient's bed to waist level before providing patient care *to prevent caregiver back strain.*[39]

- Position the patient in a supine flat position, with the arm extended at a 90-degree angle away from the body. If the patient can't tolerate a flat position, raise the head of the bed for patient comfort.[2]
- Assess the patient's upper extremities and chest for a contraindication to PICC placement.[2,40]
- If you're using ultrasound, disinfect the ultrasound probe with an antiseptic wipe and place a clean disposable cover on it.[2]
- Perform hand hygiene.[3,14,25,26,27,28,29,30,31]
- Put on clean gloves.[41,42,43]
- Apply a liberal amount of ultrasound gel to the patient's arm, and use the probe to locate the veins, arteries, and nerves surrounding the proposed insertion site.[2]
- Without a tourniquet in place, assess veins for size, path, shape, and compressibility. Healthy veins should compress easily when you apply light, downward pressure with the probe. Determine the depth of the intended vein for venipuncture and measure its diameter.[2] Use this information to select a catheter with a catheter-to-vein ratio of 45% or less *to prevent thrombosis.*[2,44]
- Mark the level of the expected insertion site with a single-use disposable skin marker on the outer aspect of the arm *to avoid leaving ink under the dressing and enable appropriate skin cleansing.*[2]
- Remove the ultrasound gel from the patient's skin using a gauze pad.
- Using a clean, single-use measuring tape, measure the upper-arm circumference of the selected extremity *to provide a baseline measurement.* Take this measurement 4" (10 cm) above the antecubital fossa.[2,40]
- Measure the distance from the intended insertion site to the clavicular head on the right side and then down to the bottom of the third intercostal space on the right (desired terminal tip location) to determine insertion depth. Add length, as needed, to accommodate use of the stabilization device.[2]
- Clean the intended insertion site with soap and water if it's visibly soiled.[2,9,16,40]
- Remove excess hair from the intended insertion site, if needed, using single-patient-use scissors or disposable-head surgical clippers *to facilitate dressing application.*[2,6,10,21]
- If you're using a topical anesthetic cream: Apply the anesthetic cream to the insertion site following safe medication administration practices.[45,46,47,48] Cover the site with a sterile transparent semipermeable dressing. Note the time of application on a label and then place the label on the dressing. Wait the recommended period of time (per the manufacturer's directions), usually 15 to 60 minutes, *to allow the cream to work.*[2] While waiting, return the bed to the lowest position *to prevent falls and maintain patient safety,*[39] and position the patient for comfort. Remove and discard your gloves.[41,49] Perform hand hygiene.[3,14,25,26,27,28,29,30,31] After the recommended application time, perform hand hygiene, put on gloves *to avoid touching the cream,* remove the dressing, wipe off the cream, evaluate the effectiveness of the anesthetic, and assess for adverse reactions to the anesthetic.[40] Remove and discard your gloves. Perform hand hygiene.[3,14,25,26,27,28,29,30,31]
- Place a fluid-impermeable pad under the arm.[2,40]
- Put on a surgical head cover, protective eyewear, and a mask. Have the second person do the same.[3,16,41,42,50]
- Perform hand hygiene.[3,14,25,26,27,28,29,30,31]
- Disinfect your work area using a hospital-grade disinfectant, and then allow it to dry.[2,40]
- Prepare a sterile field using a sterile drape.
- Set up the PICC supplies on the sterile field.[2]
- If you didn't use a topical anesthetic, prepare a lidocaine injection.
- Label all medications, medication containers, and other solutions on and off the sterile field using a sterile marker and labels.[51,52]
- Perform hand hygiene.[3,14,25,26,27,28,29,30,31]
- Put on a sterile gown and two pairs of sterile gloves.[2,40,42,43]
- Follow the manufacturer's recommendations and guidelines for using the stylet wire and altering the device length if the device requires trimming. Don't use scissors to adjust the PICC length, *because trimming with scissors causes rough, irregular surfaces.*[2]
- Prepare the catheter according to the manufacturer's recommendations; flush the device and extension set (if needed) with preservative-free normal saline solution.[2,40]
- Place the catheter on the sterile field.

- Place a sterile drape under the patient's arm. If using the external jugular insertion site, place the sterile drape under the patient's shoulder.[2]
- Prepare the insertion site by scrubbing with an antiseptic agent (alcohol-based chlorhexidine preferred; if contraindicated, use iodophor [such as povidone-iodine or 70% alcohol]). Apply the antiseptic solution using a sterile applicator. Allow the solution to dry completely without fanning, wiping, or blowing.[9] Apply alcohol-based chlorhexidine with an applicator using a vigorous side-to-side motion for 30 seconds. Allow the area to dry completely.[9,53] Apply povidone-iodine using a swab beginning at the intended insertion site and moving outward in concentric circles. Allow the solution to dry completely (typically at least 2 minutes).[9,54]
- Apply a single-patient-use tourniquet about 4" (10 cm) above the antecubital fossa. Make sure that an arterial pulse is easily palpable distal to the tourniquet.[2]
- Remove the outer set of gloves.[2]
- Place a full body drape over the patient from head to toe. Cover everything except the insertion site *to comply with maximal barrier precautions, thereby reducing the risk of vascular catheter–associated infection.*[2,40] If the patient can't tolerate having the face covered, tent the drape and have the patient wear a mask or turn the head away from the insertion site.[2]
- If using ultrasound, place and secure a sterile probe cover on the ultrasound probe *to prevent cross-contamination between patients.* If using a locator system, follow the manufacturer's directions regarding its use.[2]
- Conduct a time-out immediately before starting the procedure *to determine that the correct patient, site, positioning, and procedure are identified, and to confirm, as applicable, that relevant information and necessary equipment are available.*[23,55]
- If using ultrasound, apply sterile ultrasound gel to the probe and use it to locate the appropriate vein as well as the adjacent artery and nerve. Verify that the vein is nonpulsatile and compressible.[2]
- If you didn't use a topical anesthetic cream, anesthetize the area with lidocaine following safe medication administration practices *to provide for patient comfort during insertion.*[2,40,45,46,47,48]
- While visualizing the vessel, insert the micro-introducer needle through the skin at a 45-degree angle. The micro-introducer needle will appear as an echogenic white dot on the ultrasound screen. Move the ultrasound probe and needle in the same direction, keeping the needle tip in view on the ultrasound screen as it approaches the vein. Align the path of the needle to enter the centermost superficial area of the vein wall. Observe for blood return, and visualize the needle tip in the center of the vein on the ultrasound screen.[2]
- Put the ultrasound probe down on the sterile field.[2]
- Reduce the angle of the micro-introducer needle and stabilize it.[2]
- Insert the guidewire into the micro-introducer and carefully advance it at least 4" (10 cm) but not more than 6" (15 cm) into the vein.[2] Stop advancing the guidewire if you meet resistance, and don't advance it past the axilla.[2,40]
- Gently remove the micro-introducer needle, taking care not to dislodge or damage the guidewire.[2,40] Secure the guidewire with your nondominant hand *to prevent migration in or out of the vein.*[2]
- If necessary, using a safety scalpel, make a small skin nick at the insertion site *to facilitate the advancement of the peel-away dilator-introducer.*[2]
- Thread the peel-away dilator-introducer over the guidewire until you're sure the tip is well within the vein. After successful vein entry, you should see blood return.[2]
- Carefully remove the guidewire and place it on the sterile field.[2,10]
- Release the tourniquet, being careful not to break sterile technique.[2,40]
- Confirm the preinsertion measurement for the desired catheter insertion depth.[2,40]
- Carefully separate and remove the dilator from the peel-away introducer while holding the introducer still.[2,40] *To minimize blood loss,* try applying finger pressure on the vein just beyond the distal end of the introducer sheath, or place a finger over the opening of the introducer.
- If using a locator system, activate it now and follow the manufacturer's directions, or use electrocardiographic (ECG)-guided technology *to detect the desired tip location.*[2,56] (See *Understanding ECG-guided technology,* page 656.) Advance the catheter through the introducer sheath at a slow, steady pace until it's in position at the premeasured length.[2,40]
- If you aren't using tip-location technology, withdraw the stylet wire from the catheter lumen, using air emboli precautions.[2]

Understanding ECG-guided technology

You can use electrocardiogram (ECG) technology to guide central venous access catheter insertion. This technique requires a metal guidewire or column of normal saline solution inside the catheter lumen. During insertion, the catheter itself functions as an intracavitary traveling electrode. As the catheter advances toward the sinoatrial node, P-wave changes occur on the ECG monitor tracing. You can identify the catheter tip location by the following ECG waveform changes:

- If no P-wave changes are evident, the catheter tip isn't in an acceptable location.
- When the P waves appear at maximal height, the catheter tip is in the lower one-third of the superior vena cava, at the right atrial junction or cavoatrial junction, which is the desired catheter tip location.
- If a downward deflection appears on the leading edge of the P waves, the catheter tip is entering the right atrium.
- If biphasic P waves appear, the catheter tip is within the right atrium.
- An inverted P wave indicates that the catheter is approaching the right ventricle.
- You can adjust the catheter position in real time during insertion, allowing for accurate tip placement; a post-insertion chest X-ray isn't necessary to confirm catheter tip placement, eliminating patient exposure to radiation and reducing costs.
- ECG-guided technology is contraindicated in patients with an abnormal ECG rhythm in which P waves are absent or altered (such as those with a pacemaker, atrial fibrillation, or extreme tachycardia). Follow the manufacturers' directions for use in the appropriate patient populations.

- Attach a prefilled syringe with preservative-free normal saline solution and aspirate for blood return; if blood is present, flush the catheter *to determine patency*.[2]
- Grasp the tabs of the introducer sheath and flex them toward its distal end *to split the sheath*. Peel the introducer away from the catheter while pulling away from the insertion site. Take care to ensure that the catheter tip remains at its terminal tip location.[2,40]
- If appropriate, connect a primed extension set to the catheter hub.[2]
- Attach a needleless connector to each lumen.[2]
- If available at your facility, apply a disinfectant-containing end cap to the end of the needleless connector *to reduce the risk of vascular catheter-associated infection*.[57,58]
- Clean the site and secure the catheter with an integrated securement device, subcutaneous anchor securement system, tissue adhesive, or adhesive securement device, if available. Guidelines recommend an additional securement method beyond the primary dressing *to reduce vascular access device motion, which increases the risk of unintentional catheter dislodgment and other complications that require premature catheter removal.* Sutures should be avoided whenever possible *because they're associated with an increased risk of needlestick injury and support the growth of biofilm, which increases the risk of catheter-related bloodstream infection.*[59] If appropriate, first apply a skin barrier solution to the area to be covered and allow it to dry. If using a chlorhexidine-impregnated sponge dressing, don't apply the skin barrier solution directly under the sponge, *because the solution will block its action at the puncture site*.[2]
- If necessary, apply a sterile 2″ × 2″ (5 cm × 5 cm) gauze pad directly over the site and a sterile transparent semipermeable dressing over the gauze pad. Leave this dressing in place for 24 hours.[2]
- Lock the catheter with the prescribed locking solution or as directed by your facility.[2,40]
- Return the bed to the lowest position *to prevent falls and maintain patient safety*.[60]
- Discard used supplies in appropriate receptacles.[41,49]
- Remove and discard your gloves and other personal protective equipment.[41,49]
- Perform hand hygiene.[3,14,25,26,27,28,29,30,31]
- Label the dressing with the date you performed the procedure or the date the dressing is next due to be changed, as directed by your facility.[2,61]

- If you didn't use a tip-locating device or ECG-guided technology, obtain a chest X-ray, as ordered, *to verify proper placement* before initiating an infusion.[2,9]
- Perform hand hygiene.[3,14,25,26,27,28,29,30,31]
- Put on gloves.[41,42]
- Clean and disinfect reusable equipment according to the manufacturer's instructions *to prevent the spread of infection*.[62,63]
- Remove and discard your gloves.[41,49]
- Perform hand hygiene.[25,26,27,28,29,30,31,32,41]
- Document the procedure.[64,65,66,67,68]

Flushing a PICC

- Review the patient's medical record to confirm the type and size of the catheter and the location of the catheter tip, *because the flush protocol depends on the type and size of the catheter.*
- Gather and prepare the necessary equipment and supplies.
- Perform hand hygiene.[3,14,25,26,27,28,29,30,31]
- Confirm the patient's identity using at least two patient identifiers.[32]
- Provide privacy.[33,34,35,36]
- Explain the procedure to the patient and family (if appropriate) according to their individual communication and learning needs *to increase their understanding, allay their fears, and enhance cooperation.*[37]
- Raise the patient's bed to waist level before providing patient care *to prevent caregiver back strain*.[39]
- Perform hand hygiene.[3,14,25,26,27,28,29,30,31]
- Put on gloves *to comply with standard precautions*.[41,42]
- If a disinfectant-containing end cap is covering the needleless connector, remove and discard it.[57,58]
- Perform a vigorous mechanical scrub of the needleless connector for at least 5 seconds using an antiseptic pad; allow it to dry completely.[3,16,21,40,57]
- Trace the tubing from the patient to its point of origin *to make sure that you're accessing the correct port*.[69,70]
- While maintaining the sterility of the syringe tip, attach a prefilled 10-mL syringe containing preservative-free normal saline solution to the needleless connector. (A syringe specifically designed to generate lower injection pressure may be used instead.) Unclamp the catheter and slowly aspirate for a blood return that's the color and consistency of whole blood. If you don't obtain a blood return, take steps to locate an external cause of obstruction.[2,40,71]
- If you obtain a blood return, slowly inject preservative-free normal saline solution into the catheter. Use a minimum volume of twice the internal volume of the catheter system. Don't forcibly flush the device; further evaluate the device if you meet resistance.[2,40,71]
- Remove and discard the syringe.[2,40,41,57]
- Perform a vigorous mechanical scrub of the needleless connector for at least 5 seconds using an antiseptic pad; allow it to dry completely.[3,16,21,40,57]
- Administer IV fluid through the catheter, as prescribed, or proceed with locking the device if indicated.

Locking a PICC

- While maintaining sterility of the syringe tip, attach a syringe with facility-approved locking solution (heparin flush or preservative-free normal saline solution, as required) to the needleless connector.[2,40] Use a volume equal to the internal volume of the PICC and any add-on devices, plus 20%.[71]
- Slowly inject the solution into the catheter.[71,57,2,40]
- Clamp the device according to the type of needleless connector used.[57]
- For a positive-pressure needleless connector, disconnect the syringe and then clamp the catheter. For a negative-pressure needleless connector, clamp the catheter while maintaining pressure on the syringe plunger and then disconnect the syringe.[57] For a neutral needleless connector or an anti-reflux needleless connector, clamp the catheter before or after removing the syringe; a specific clamping sequence isn't required.[2,40,57,72]
- If available at your facility, place a disinfectant-containing end cap on the needleless connector *to reduce the risk of vascular catheter–associated infection*.[57,58]
- Double-check all connections *to prevent tubing misconnections and air embolism*.[73]
- Discard the syringe and other used supplies in appropriate receptacles.[41,49]

Completing the procedure

- Return the bed to the lowest position *to prevent falls and maintain patient safety*.[60]
- Remove and discard your gloves.[41,42,49]
- Perform hand hygiene.[25,26,27,28,29,30,31]
- Document the procedure.[64,65,66,67,68]

Performing a PICC dressing change

- Gather and prepare the necessary equipment and supplies.
- Perform hand hygiene.[3,14,25,26,27,28,29,30,31]
- Confirm the patient's identity using at least two patient identifiers.[32]
- Provide privacy.[33,34,35,36]
- Explain the procedure to the patient and family (if appropriate) according to their individual communication and learning needs *to increase their understanding, allay their fears, and enhance cooperation*.[37]
- Raise the bed to waist before providing patient care *to prevent caregiver back strain*.[39]
- Put on a mask.[3,2,40]
- Perform hand hygiene.[3,14,25,26,27,28,29,30,31]
- Assemble your supplies on a sterile field.[2,40]
- Perform hand hygiene.[3,14,25,26,27,28,29,30,31]
- Put on gloves to comply with standard precautions.[41,42,43]
- Position the patient with arm extended away from the body *to gain access to the insertion site*. Ensure that the insertion site is below heart level *to reduce the risk of air embolism*.[2,40,74]
- Visually inspect the entire infusion system for clarity of the solution, integrity of the system (such as absence of leakage and secure Luer lock connections), accurate flow rate, and expiration dates of the solution and administration set, as applicable.[61]
- Inspect the catheter–skin junction and surrounding area, and palpate through the intact dressing for redness, tenderness, swelling, and drainage. Pay attention to the patient's reports of pain, paresthesias, numbness, or tingling.[61]
- Remove the existing dressing beginning at the device hub, and gently pulling the dressing perpendicular to the skin toward the insertion site *to prevent catheter dislodgment and tearing or stripping of fragile skin*.[2,40,75]
- If you used a chlorhexidine-impregnated sponge dressing *to provide sustained antimicrobial action at the insertion site*, remove and discard it in the appropriate receptacle.[41,49]
- Remove and discard the adhesive-based securement device if present.[41,49,61]
- Inspect the integrity of the catheter and hub *to detect any defects, such as cracks or splits*.
- Remove and discard your gloves.[41,49]
- Perform hand hygiene.[3,14,25,26,27,28,29,30,31]
- Put on sterile gloves.[2,3,40,41,42,43]
- Use a sterile measuring tape or the incremental markings on the catheter to measure the external length of the catheter from hub to skin entry *to make sure that the catheter hasn't migrated*.[2,40,61]
- Clean the skin using an antiseptic agent (alcohol-based chlorhexidine preferred; if contraindicated, use an iodophor [such as povidone-iodine or 70% alcohol]). Apply the antiseptic agent using a single-use applicator. Allow the solution to dry completely without fanning, wiping, or blowing.[61]
- Apply alcohol-based chlorhexidine with an applicator using a vigorous side-to-side motion for 30 seconds. Allow the area to dry completely.
- Apply povidone-iodine solution using a swab. Begin at the insertion site and move outward in concentric circles. Allow the solution to dry completely (typically at least 2 minutes).
- If applicable, apply a chlorhexidine-impregnated sponge dressing at the catheter base.[2,40,61] Position it with the catheter resting on or near the radial slit of the disk. The edges of the slit must touch *to maximize antimicrobial action*. Always follow the manufacturer's directions.
- If applicable, apply an alcohol-free skin barrier product *to protect at-risk skin*.[61] Follow the manufacturer's directions for use.[61]
- Secure the catheter with an integrated securement device, subcutaneous anchor securement system, tissue adhesive, or adhesive securement device, if available. Guidelines recommend an additional securement method beyond the primary dressing *to reduce motion of the vascular

access device, which increases the risk of unintentional catheter dislodgment and complications requiring premature catheter removal*. Sutures should be avoided whenever possible *because they're associated with an increased risk of needlestick injury and support the growth of biofilm, which increases the risk of catheter-related bloodstream infection*.[59]
- Apply a transparent semipermeable (or gauze and tape) dressing to the insertion site.[61]
- Measure upper arm circumference when clinically indicated to assess for the presence of edema and deep vein thrombosis; take the measurement 4" (10 cm) above the antecubital fossa and compare this measurement to the baseline.[2,40]
- Label the dressing with the date of the dressing change or the date it's next due to be changes, as directed by your facility. Don't place the label over the insertion site.[61]
- Discard used supplies in appropriate receptacles.[41,49]
- Return the bed to the lowest level *to prevent falls and maintain the patient's safety*.[60]
- Remove and discard your gloves and mask.[41,49]
- Perform hand hygiene.[25,26,27,28,29,30,31,32,41]
- Document the procedure.[64,65,66,67,68]

Administering drugs using a PICC

- Avoid distractions and interruptions when preparing and administering medications *to prevent medication errors*.[76,77,78]
- Review the practitioner's order to make sure that the prescribed infusion solution or medication, dose, and route of administration are appropriate for the patient's age, condition, and access device, and that the infusion or medication is compatible with other solutions or medications. Make sure that the order includes any test results that require monitoring.[2,40,45,46,47,48,76,79] Address concerns about the order with the practitioner, pharmacist, your supervisor, the risk management department, or as directed by your facility.[65,79]
- Check the patient's medical record for an allergy or a contraindication to the prescribed medication. If one exists, don't administer the medication; notify the practitioner.[45,46,47,48]
- Review the patient's medical record for confirmation of catheter type, size, and tip location. Review laboratory test results and assess the appropriateness of therapy.[2]
- Reconcile the patient's medication when the practitioner orders a new medication *to reduce the risk of medication errors, including omissions, duplications, dosing errors, and drug interactions*.[76,79]
- Gather the necessary equipment, including a prefilled syringe or a prepared infusion container of the prescribed medication.
- Compare the medication label with the practitioner's order *to verify the correct medication, indication, dose, route, and time of administration*.[45,46,47,48,76]
- Check the expiration date on the medication. If the medication has expired, return it to the pharmacy and obtain new medication.[45,46,47,48,76]
- Visually inspect the solution for particles, discoloration, and other signs of loss of integrity; don't administer the medication if its integrity is compromised.[45,46,47,48,76]
- Discuss any unresolved concerns about the medication with the patient's practitioner.[45,46,47,48,76]
- Perform hand hygiene.[3,14,25,26,27,28,29,30,31]
- Confirm the patient's identity using at least two patient identifiers.[32]
- Provide privacy.[33,34,35,36]
- Explain the procedure to the patient and family (if appropriate) according to their individual communication and learning needs *to increase their understanding, allay their fears, and enhance cooperation*.[37]
- If the patient is receiving the medication for the first time, teach the patient or family (if appropriate) about potential adverse reactions, and discuss any other concerns related to the medication.[38,45,46,47,48]
- Raise the patient's bed to waist level before providing patient care *to prevent caregiver back strain*.[39]
- Perform hand hygiene.[3,14,25,26,27,28,29,30,31]
- Obtain the patient's vital signs and assess the patient's condition, if applicable.[2,40]
- Verify that you are administering the medication at the proper time, in the prescribed dose, and by the correct route *to reduce the risk of medication errors*.[45,46,47,48,76]

- If your facility uses bar-code technology, use it as directed by your facility.[76]
- If the medication you are administering is a high-alert medication. Have another nurse perform an independent double-check (if required by your facility) before administration *to help the risk of medication administration errors.*[79,80]

NURSING ALERT Some medications may be considered high-alert medications *because they can cause significant patient harm when used in error.*[81] If required by your facility, before beginning an infusion or administering a bolus injection, have another nurse perform an independent double-check *to verify the patient's identity and to ensure that you're administering the correct medication in the prescribed strength or concentration; the medication's indication corresponds with the patient's diagnosis; the dosage calculations are correct and the dosing formula used to derive the final dose is correct; the prescribed route of administration is safe and proper for the patient; the prescribed time and frequency of administration are safe and proper for the patient; and, if using an infusion, the pump settings are and the infusion line is attached to the correct port.*[76,79,80]

- After comparing results of the independent double-check with the other nurse, administer the medication if there are no discrepancies. If discrepancies exist, rectify them before beginning administering the medication.[80]
- Perform hand hygiene.[3,14,25,26,27,28,29,30,31]
- Put on gloves *to comply with standard precautions.*[41,42,43]
- If a disinfectant-containing cap is in place at the end of the needleless connector, remove and discard it.[57,58]
- Perform a vigorous mechanical scrub of the needleless connector for at least 5 seconds using an antiseptic pad. Allow it to dry completely.[2,40,41,57]
- While maintaining sterility of the syringe tip, attach a prefilled 10-mL syringe containing preservative-free normal saline solution to the needleless connector. (A syringe specifically designed to generate lower injection pressure may be used instead of a 10-mL syringe.) Unclamp the catheter, and slowly aspirate for a blood return that is the color and consistency of whole blood. If you don't obtain a blood return, take steps to locate an external cause of obstruction.[2,40,71]
- If you obtain a blood return, slowly inject preservative-free normal saline solution into the catheter. Use a minimum volume of twice the internal volume of the catheter system. Don't forcibly flush the device. Further evaluate the device if you meet resistance.[2,40,71]
- Remove and discard the syringe in the appropriate container.[41,49]
- Perform a vigorous mechanical scrub of the needleless connector for at least 5 seconds using an antiseptic pad. Allow it to dry completely.[2,40,41,57]

Administering an IV bolus injection

- Attach the syringe containing the prescribed medication for IV bolus injection to the needleless connector.[2,40]

NURSING ALERT After using a 10-mL syringe (or a syringe designed to generate lower injection pressure) filled with preservative-free normal saline solution to confirm patency of the vascular access device, you can administer the medication by IV bolus injection in a syringe of appropriate size to measure and administer the required medication dose.[71,81,82] Don't transfer the medication to a larger syringe.[71]

- Inject the medication into the PICC at the rate indicated on the medication label. Consult with the pharmacist if a rate isn't specified.[2,40]
- Remove and discard the syringe in the appropriate container.[2,40,41,57]

Administering an infusion

- Spike the IV infusion container and prime the IV administration set tubing, as directed. Insert the IV administration set tubing into an electronic infusion device
- Perform a vigorous mechanical scrub of the needleless connector for at least 5 seconds using an antiseptic pad. Allow it to dry completely.[3,16,21,40,57]
- Clamp the PICC.
- Connect the IV administration set tubing to the PICC.
- Trace the tubing from the patient to its point of origin *to make sure that you're connecting the tubing to the correct port.* Route the tubing in a standardized direction if the patient has other tubing and catheters that have

different purposes. If you'll be using multiple IV lines, label the tubing at the distal end (near the patient connection) and the proximal end (near the source container) *to reduce the risk of misconnection.*[69,70,76]

- Set the electronic infusion device according to the practitioner's order. Make sure that the alarm limits are set appropriately, and that the alarms are turned on, functioning properly, and audible to staff.[83,84,85]
- Unclamp the PICC and administration set tubing; begin the infusion, as ordered.
- When the infusion is complete, clamp the catheter and disconnect the administration set tubing.

Completing the procedure

- Proceed with flushing the device *to prevent mixing of incompatible medications and solutions:*
  - Perform a vigorous mechanical scrub of the needleless connector for at least 5 seconds using an antiseptic pad. Allow it to dry completely.[3,16,21,40,57]
  - While maintaining sterility of the syringe tip, attach a syringe containing preservative-free normal saline solution to the needleless connector. (Use a 10-mL syringe or a syringe specifically designed to generate lower injection pressure.) Unclamp the catheter and inject preservative-free normal saline solution into the catheter at the same rate of injection as the prescribed medication. Use the amount of flush solution needed to adequately clear the medication from the administration set lumen and catheter. Don't forcibly flush the device; further evaluate the device if you meet resistance. Consider a pulsatile flushing technique, *because short boluses of flush solution interrupted by short pauses may be more effective at removing deposits (such as fibrin, drug precipitate, and intraluminal bacteria) than a continuous low-flow technique.* Alternatively, if the medication is incompatible with normal saline solution, use dextrose 5% in water (D_5W) followed by preservative-free normal saline solution. Don't allow D_5W to remain in the catheter lumen, *because it provides nutrients for biofilm growth.*[18,71]
  - Remove and discard the syringe in the appropriate container.[2,40,41,57]
- If necessary, proceed with locking the device. Perform a vigorous mechanical scrub of the needleless connector for at least 5 seconds using an antiseptic pad. Allow it to dry completely.[16,57] Maintaining sterility of the syringe tip, attach a syringe containing locking solution to the needleless connector.[18,71] Slowly inject the locking solution into the PICC.[18,71]
- Clamp the PICC according to the type of needleless connector. Follow the manufacturer's directions for use. Use the following sequence if directions aren't available.[57] For a positive-pressure needleless connector, clamp the device after disconnecting the syringe. For a negative-pressure needleless connector, maintain pressure on the syringe plunger while closing the PICC clamp and then disconnect the syringe. For a neutral displacement needleless connector or for an anti-reflux needleless connector, clamp the PICC before or after syringe disconnection; a specific clamping sequence isn't required.[57]
- If available at your facility, place a disinfectant-containing end cap on the needleless connector *to reduce the risk of vascular catheter-associated infection.*[57,58]
- Return the bed to the lowest level *to prevent falls and maintain the patient's safety.*[60]
- Discard used supplies in appropriate receptacles.[41,49]
- Remove and discard your gloves.[41,49]
- Perform hand hygiene.[25,26,27,28,29,30,31,32,41]
- Closely monitor the patient for adverse reactions to the prescribed medication.[76,86]
- If the patient is receiving IV opioid medication, frequently monitor the patient's respiratory rate, oxygen saturation level by pulse oximetry, end-tidal carbon dioxide level by capnography (if available), and sedation level using a facility-approved standardized sedation scale *to decrease the risk of adverse events associated with IV opioid use.*[46,86]
- For a patient receiving IV opioid medication, explain to the patient and family members about the assessment and monitoring process, and tell them to alert staff if breathing problems or sedation occurs.[46,86]
- Perform hand hygiene.[25,26,27,28,29,30,31,32,41]
- Document the procedure.[64,65,66,67,68]

Obtaining a blood sample

- Verify the practitioner's order.
- Gather and prepare the necessary equipment and supplies.
- Perform hand hygiene.[25,26,27,28,29,30,31,32,41]
- Confirm the patient's identity using at least two patient identifiers.[32]
- Provide privacy.[33,34,35,36]
- Explain the procedure to the patient and family (if appropriate) according to their individual communication and learning needs *to increase their understanding, allay their fears, and enhance cooperation.*[37]
- If fasting was necessary for the ordered test, confirm that the patient has observed fasting.[87]
- Raise the bed to waist level before providing care *to prevent caregiver back strain.*[39]
- Perform hand hygiene.[25,26,27,28,29,30,31,32,41]
- Put on gloves and, if splashing is likely, a mask with a face shield or a mask and goggles *to comply with standard precautions.*[41,42,43]
- Trace the tubing from the patient to its point of origin *to make sure that you're accessing the proper port.*[69,70]
- Stop any infusing IV fluids, including those running through another lumen of the catheter. Research hasn't established the length of time for stopping fluid flow before obtaining the sample; however, that time would be associated with the internal volume of the specific catheter.[87] Clamp the lumen if appropriate.
- Select the largest lumen for blood sampling if you're using a multiple-lumen catheter.[87]
- If a disinfectant-containing end cap is covering the end of the needleless connector, remove and discard it.[57,58]
- Perform a vigorous mechanical scrub of the needleless connector for at least 5 seconds using an antiseptic pad. Allow it to dry completely.[3,16,21,40,57]
- While maintaining sterility of the syringe tip, attach a prefilled 10-mL syringe that contains preservative-free normal saline solution to the needleless connector. (You may instead use a syringe specifically designed to generate lower injection pressure.) Unclamp the catheter and slowly aspirate for a blood return that's the color and consistency of whole blood. If you don't obtain a blood return, take steps to locate an external cause of obstruction.[2,40,71] Notify the practitioner if troubleshooting is ineffective.
- If you obtain a blood return, slowly inject preservative-free normal saline solution into the catheter. Use a minimum volume of twice the internal volume of the catheter system. Don't forcibly flush the device; further evaluate the device if you meet resistance.[2,40,71]
- Use the discard or push-pull method to obtain the blood sample.[87] (If you're obtaining a blood sample for blood cultures, see the "Blood culture sample collection" procedure.)

Discard method

- Obtain a discard sample *to clear the catheter's dead space volume and remove any blood diluted with flush solution:*
- If you're using a needleless blood collection tube holder: Clamp the catheter lumen, and remove and discard the syringe in a puncture-resistant sharps disposal container.[2,41,49] Perform a vigorous mechanical scrub of the needleless connector for at least 5 seconds using an antiseptic pad. Allow it to dry completely.[3,16,21,40,57] Attach the needleless blood collection tube holder to the needleless connector, release the clamp, engage the labeled discard blood collection tube, and aspirate 2 to 25 mL of blood, depending on the internal volume of the catheter, saline flushing prior to drawing the discard volume, and specific laboratory tests ordered.[87]
- If you're using a syringe: Use the attached syringe you used for flushing to aspirate 2 to 25 mL of blood, depending on the internal volume of the catheter, saline flushing prior to drawing the discard volume, and specific laboratory tests ordered.[87]
- Clamp the catheter. If you're using a closed-loop blood collection system to allow return of discard, keep the discard syringe attached for reinfusion after obtaining blood samples.[87] Otherwise, remove the labeled discard blood collection tube from the needleless blood collection tube holder, or remove the labeled discard syringe, and discard it in a puncture-resistant sharps disposal container.[2,40,41,49]

- Obtain blood samples, as ordered. Repeat the steps, as necessary, until you obtain all blood samples. If you're using a needleless blood collection tube holder, insert another blood collection tube into the needleless blood collection tube holder using the correct order of draw.[87] Unclamp the catheter and obtain the sample. If you're using a syringe, perform a vigorous mechanical scrub of the needleless connector for at least 5 seconds using an antiseptic pad. Allow it to dry completely.[16,57] Connect an empty syringe to the needleless connector, release the clamp, and withdraw the blood sample.[2,40]
- Clamp the catheter, and remove the needleless blood collection tube holder or syringe.
- If you're using the closed-loop blood collection system, return any blood you drew *for the purpose of clearing the catheter lumen* before removing the discard syringe.[87]

NURSING ALERT Don't reinfuse any discard sample from a disconnected syringe, *because doing so can increase the risk of contamination and blood clot formation.*[87]

Push-pull method

- Using the same syringe, aspirate 4 to 6 mL of blood.[87] Keeping the syringe attached to the catheter, push to reinfuse the blood into the catheter. Repeat the aspiration and reinfusion sequence four times.[87]
- Clamp the catheter lumen, and remove and discard the syringe in a puncture-resistant sharps disposal container.[2,40,41,49]
- Perform a vigorous mechanical scrub of the needleless connector for at least 5 seconds using an antiseptic pad. Allow it to dry completely.[3,16,21,40,57]
- Obtain blood samples, as ordered. Repeat the steps, as necessary, until you obtain all blood samples. If you're using a needleless blood collection tube holder, attach it to the needleless connector, release the clamp, and engage the blood collection tube into the needleless blood collection tube holder using the correct order of draw.[87] If you're using a syringe, connect an empty syringe to the needleless connector, release the clamp, and withdraw the blood sample.[2,40]
- Clamp the catheter and remove the needleless blood collection tube holder or the syringe.

Completing the procedure

- Change the needleless connector according to the manufacturer's instructions, if you know or suspect that the device's integrity is compromised, or if there's blood or debris in the connector.[2,57,40]
- Perform a vigorous mechanical scrub of the needleless connector for at least 5 seconds using an antiseptic pad. Allow it to dry completely.[3,16,21,40,57]
- While maintaining sterility of the syringe tip, attach a prefilled syringe containing preservative-free normal saline solution to the needleless connector.[2,40,71]
- Unclamp the catheter and slowly inject the preservative-free normal saline solution into the catheter. Use a minimum volume of twice the internal volume of the catheter system.[71] Then reclamp the catheter.[2,71]
- Remove and discard the syringe.[2,40,41,49]
- If the practitioner prescribed a continuous IV infusion, unclamp the catheter and continue the prescribed continuous IV infusion. If the practitioner didn't prescribe a continuous infusion, proceed with locking the device if required by your facility.[2,40] (See "Locking a PICC," page 656.)
- If you obtained blood using a syringe, use the blood transfer unit to transfer the blood into the appropriate blood collection tubes.
- Label the samples in the presence of the patient *to prevent mislabeling.*[32,87]
- Place the samples in a laboratory biohazard transport bag and send them immediately to the laboratory with the appropriate laboratory request forms (if necessary).[41]
- Discard used supplies in appropriate receptacles.[41,49]
- Return the bed to the lowest position *to prevent falls and maintain patient safety.*[60]
- Remove and discard your gloves as well as your mask with face shield or mask and goggles if you wore them.[41,42,49]
- Perform hand hygiene.[25,26,27,28,29,30,31,32,41]
- Document the procedure.[64,65,66,67,68]

Removing a PICC

- Verify the practitioner's order to discontinue the catheter.
- Gather and prepare the necessary equipment and supplies.
- Perform hand hygiene.[25,26,27,28,29,30,31,41]
- Confirm the patient's identity using at least two patient identifiers.[32]
- Provide privacy.[33,34,35,36]
- Explain the procedure to the patient and family (if appropriate) according to their individual communication and learning needs *to increase their understanding, allay their fears, and enhance cooperation*.[37]
- Raise the bed to waist level before providing care *to prevent caregiver back strain*.[39]
- Perform hand hygiene.[25,26,27,28,29,30,31,32,41]
- Position the patient in a supine flat or Trendelenburg position, unless contraindicated, so that the insertion site is at or below heart level *to reduce the risk of air embolism*.[73,88]
- Perform hand hygiene.[25,26,27,28,29,30,31,32,41]
- Put on gloves and, as needed, other personal protective equipment *to comply with standard precautions*.[41,42,43]
- Trace the catheter from the patient to its point of origin *to make sure that you're removing the proper catheter*.[69,70]
- Discontinue all infusions, and document the volume infused in the patient's intake and output record.[2,8,40]
- Place a fluid-impermeable pad under the patient's arm.
- Teach the patient how to perform the Valsalva maneuver during removal, unless contraindicated, *to prevent air embolism*.[74]
- Stabilize the catheter at the hub with one hand.
- Carefully remove the dressing with your other hand, beginning at the device hub and gently pulling the dressing perpendicular to the skin toward the insertion site, *to prevent skin tearing or stripping*.[2,8,40]
- If a securement device holds the catheter in place, remove the device. If the catheter is secured with sutures, carefully cut and remove them.[2]
- Assess the site for signs of infection, including swelling, drainage, redness, and inflammation.[2]
- Apply gauze to the insertion site; with your dominant hand, slowly withdraw the catheter using gentle, even pressure (as shown below).[2,88]

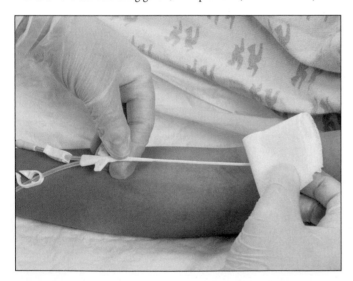

- If you meet resistance, don't remove the catheter forcibly, *because forcible removal can result in catheter fracture and embolism*.[2,88] Instead, stop the removal procedure and cover the catheter site with a sterile dressing. Perform interventions such as applying a warm compress above the exit site, having the patient perform relaxation techniques, and elevating the limb, and reattempt removal after 15 to 30 minutes. Consult with the practitioner to discuss interventions for successful removal.[2,40]
- Have the patient perform the Valsalva maneuver as you withdraw the final catheter segment, *to prevent air embolism*. If the Valsalva maneuver is contraindicated, use the Trendelenburg or left lateral decubitus position, or have the patient hold the breath, as applicable.[2,74,88]

- After successful removal of the catheter, apply manual pressure to the site and just above the site with a sterile gauze pad for a minimum of 30 seconds or until hemostasis is achieved.[2,40,73,88]
- Cover the site with a petroleum-based ointment and a sterile dressing for at least 24 hours *to seal the skin-to-vein tract and reduce the risk of air embolus*.[2,40,73,74,88]
- Assess the integrity of the removed catheter. Compare the length of the catheter with the original insertion length (as shown below) *to ensure that the entire catheter has been removed*.[2,88] If you note any damage, notify the practitioner or the rapid response team immediately, and monitor the patient for signs and symptoms of catheter embolism (palpitations, arrhythmia, dyspnea, cough, and thoracic pain). Note that a chest X-ray may be needed *for further evaluation*.[2,40,89]

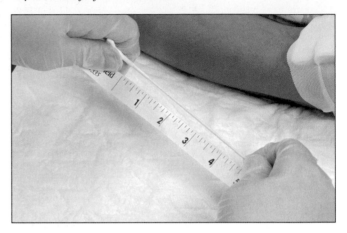

NURSING ALERT If a PICC isn't intact after removal, apply a tourniquet to the upper arm, above the insertion site, close to the axilla, *to prevent the advancement of the broken piece into the right atrium*. Maintain the patient on strict bed rest, notify the practitioner (or the rapid response team) immediately, and monitor the patient closely for signs of distress. Have emergency resuscitative equipment available. If radiographic extraction of the catheter embolus is necessary, explain the procedure to the patient.[2,10]

- Return the bed to the lowest position *to prevent falls and maintain patient safety*.[60]
- Instruct the patient to remain in a flat or reclining position for at least 30 minutes after device removal *to reduce the risk of air embolism*.[2,88]
- Discard used supplies in the appropriate receptacles.[41,49]
- Remove and discard your gloves and any other personal protective equipment worn.[41,49]
- Perform hand hygiene.[25,26,27,28,29,30,31,32,41]
- Document the procedure.[64,65,66,67,68]

Special considerations

- After insertion, you may withdraw a PICC using a sterile dressing change procedure to ensure proper tip location; however, you should never advance a PICC *because the sterility of the catheter can't be ensured*.[2,90]
- Changes in the eye, such as pupil constriction with equal light reaction and upper eyelid drooping, are signs of nerve injury. PICCs and jugular-inserted catheters have been reported to produce eye changes, which may indicate inflammation of cervical sympathetic nerves (Horner syndrome) caused by trauma from insertion technique and vein thrombosis.[91]
- PICC therapy works best when introduced early in treatment; it shouldn't be considered a last resort for patients with sclerotic or repeatedly punctured veins.
- Confirm a venous blood return and catheter patency before initiating any infusion.[71]
- Assess the catheter insertion site daily by inspection and palpation through the transparent semipermeable dressing *to discern tenderness*.[3,61] Look at the catheter and cannula pathway, and check for bleeding, redness, drainage, and swelling.[61] Although oozing is common for the first 24 hours after insertion, excessive bleeding after that period should be evaluated. Ask the patient about pain associated with therapy.

TROUBLESHOOTING

TROUBLESHOOTING A **PICC**

PROBLEM	INTERVENTION
Inability to flush or draw blood	■ Examine the catheter *to ensure that clamps (if used or as part of extension tubing) are open, and to confirm the catheter isn't kinked.*[93] ■ If sutures are present, make sure they aren't causing obstruction. ■ Assess for catheter occlusion, which may result from the patient's position; external or internal mechanical obstruction (kinked catheter under the dressing, catheter migration, precipitation, thrombosis); nonthrombotic factors, such as drug precipitates; thrombotic factors, such as fibrin deposits and blood clots; catheter pinch-off resulting from an area of compression between the first rib and clavicle; or the medication itself and its compatibilities. ■ Note when the catheter was last functioning and when the last blood return was documented. ■ Extend or raise the patient's arm overhead. *This may help move the catheter away from the vessel wall.* If the catheter remains positional, notify the practitioner. *An X-ray or other diagnostic test may be needed to determine tip placement.* ■ If you suspect occlusion from precipitation, attempt to aspirate *to clear the catheter.* If successful, flush the catheter with preservative-free normal saline solution between all medications. If unsuccessful, obtain a practitioner's order for an agent to treat the precipitates.[93] Consult with the pharmacy and determine who is permitted to perform this procedure in your facility. The instilled volume of the solution to clear precipitates shouldn't exceed the internal volume of the catheter *to avoid pushing precipitate into the bloodstream.* Instillation, aspiration, and flushing should be done using a method that doesn't exceed the catheter manufacturer's maximum pressure limits *to avoid line rupture.* ■ If occlusion is due to thrombosis, obtain a practitioner's order for a thrombolytic declotting agent; follow the manufacturer's recommendations, and determine who is permitted to administer the declotting agent in your facility.[93]
Infiltration or extravasation (suspected or actual)	■ Always assess along the path of the catheter when performing IV site checks.[94] ■ Assess the extent of infiltration or extravasation using a standardized scale.[94] ■ Discontinue the infusion and remove the administration set, but don't remove the PICC. Aspirate fluid from the catheter using a small syringe.[94] ■ Notify the practitioner of the extravasation or infiltration; report the solution or medications infusing at the time of the complication, the estimated volume of fluid that escaped into the tissue, and the site's appearance.[94] ■ Assess for changes by using measurement or photography as appropriate.[94] ■ Obtain a practitioner's order, in collaboration with the pharmacy, for an agent to treat the infiltration or extravasation, as needed. Treatment depends on the properties of the infiltrated medication or solution, the manufacturer's guidelines for that agent, and the severity of the problem.
Phlebitis	■ Use a standardized phlebitis scale *to assess phlebitis.*[95] ■ Elevate the affected limb.[95] ■ Apply warm compresses to the extremity *to ease discomfort.*[95] ■ If signs or symptoms increase, or if streak formation or a palpable cord is present, notify the practitioner. ■ If pain at the access site and erythema or edema accompany the phlebitis, the PICC may need to be removed.
Catheter migration (suspected or actual)	■ Be aware that catheter migration may be caused by excessive sneezing, coughing, or vomiting. Suspect migration of the PICC distally if the patient complains of chest pain or hears a noise during flushing of the PICC. ■ If migration is internal, or if external PICC migration is greater than ¾" (2 cm), notify the practitioner. ■ Obtain an order for an X-ray or other diagnostic test *to confirm tip placement.* ■ Be aware that external migration may necessitate replacement of a PICC or a change in therapy; internal migration requires manipulation or removal.
Leaking or damaged catheter	■ Clamp and secure the catheter *to prevent migration and possible embolization of a catheter fragment.* Catheter embolization is an emergency and may require surgical intervention. ■ Determine the extent and location of damage. ■ A registered nurse competent in this procedure using the manufacturer's repair kit and guidelines may repair the PICC line, as ordered. Note that not all PICC manufacturers provide repair kits; repair with other materials may lead to catheter separation and migration or embolization. ■ Be aware that inability to repair the PICC necessitates its removal. ■ Report a defective catheter using the proper channels established by your facility.[18]
Bleeding at insertion site	■ Apply a gauze dressing after initial placement of the PICC, and change the first dressing in 24 hours. Be aware that mild bleeding at the site may occur for the first 24 hours after PICC placement. ■ Apply a product containing hydrophilic polymer and potassium ferrate, if available at your facility.[96] ■ Limit movement of the extremity using an arm board, as necessary. ■ If bleeding increases or persists past the first 24 hours, notify the practitioner.

■ For catheters that aren't being used routinely, flush nonvalved catheters at least every 24 hours and valved catheters at least weekly.[92] Flush the catheter with preservative-free normal saline solution; lock with heparin (10 units/mL) if applicable.[71]

■ If necessary, use a declotting agent to clear a clotted PICC, but make sure you read the manufacturer's recommendations first. (See *Troubleshooting a PICC.*)

■ When a medication is incompatible with preservative-free normal saline solution, flush the device with dextrose 5% in water and then follow by flushing with preservative-free normal saline solution. Dextrose 5% in water should be flushed from the catheter, *because it provides nutrients for biofilm growth, which increases the risk of vascular catheter–associated infection.*[55]

■ Consider using a pulsatile flushing technique, which consists of short boluses of the flush solution interrupted by short pauses, *because this technique may be more effective at removing deposits (such as fibrin, drug precipitate, and intraluminal bacteria) than a continuous low-flow technique.*[71,97]

- Follow the PICC manufacturer's flushing instructions after the administration of contrast media.[98]
- *To prevent catheter damage when flushing and locking a PICC,* use the syringe size recommended by the manufacturer. Assess patency using a minimum 10-mL syringe filled with preservative-free normal saline solution, unless a flush syringe that holds a smaller volume and is specifically designed to generate lower pressure is available.[71]
- If you can't flush the PICC, follow a series of troubleshooting measures *to identify the source of the problem.* Notify the practitioner if you still can't flush the PICC.
- Encourage the patient to report changes in the catheter site or any new discomfort.[3]
- Assess catheter necessity daily during multidisciplinary rounds, and discontinue the PICC as soon as it's no longer needed *to reduce the risk of vascular catheter–associated infection.*[15,16,88]
- If you inadvertently withdraw the catheter a significant amount during a dressing change, measure from the exit site to the hub and reapply a sterile dressing. Never advance the catheter back inside the insertion site, *because contact with the skin can introduce microorganisms to the catheter.* Notify the practitioner, and prepare for a chest X-ray or other diagnostic test *to determine the position of the PICC tip.*[90]

Complications

PICCs are associated with higher rates of deep vein thrombosis (DVT) than other CV access devices *owing to insertion into veins with a smaller diameter and greater movement in the upper extremity.* Critical care patients and those with cancer are also at greater risk for DVT with PICCs when compared with other CV access devices.[44] Infection and catheter breakage on removal are other possible complications.[99] Critical care patients may also have a tendency for a higher rate of malposition on PICC insertion because of difficulty in patient positioning, use of mechanical ventilation, and different venous blood flow characteristics.[90] Power injection can result in catheter tip malposition.[2] Nerve injury can occur related to trauma from insertion or vein thrombosis.[91] Air embolism, always a potential risk of venipuncture, is less likely with PICC therapy than with traditional CV access devices, *because you insert the line below heart level.*

The patient may experience adverse reactions to the particular drug you administer.

Catheter tip migration may occur with vigorous flushing. Patients receiving chemotherapy are most vulnerable to this complication *because of frequent nausea and vomiting and subsequent changes in intrathoracic pressure.* Infection, thrombosis, and air embolism may also occur.[73,100]

Possible complications during PICC removal include air embolism, venospasm, thrombosis, and catheter breakage.

Documentation

For PICC insertion, record the indication for use; insertion site location; specific site preparation; local anesthetic, if used; infection prevention and safety precautions taken; type, length, and gauge of the catheter inserted; external catheter length and length of the catheter inserted; date and time of insertion; number of insertion attempts; device functionality; insertion method, including visualization and guidance technology; condition of the site; method of catheter stabilization; dressing; and the patient's tolerance of the procedure. Document teaching provided to the patient and family (if applicable), their understanding of that teaching, and any need for follow-up teaching.[2,65]

For flushing and locking, document the site's appearance as well as the date, time, and type and amount of flush solution used. Document patency, absence of signs and symptoms of complications, lack of resistance when flushing, and presence of a blood return on aspiration if the PICC functions correctly.[65] Document signs and symptoms of complications or if the PICC fails to function appropriately, steps taken to troubleshoot the problem, the date and time the practitioner was notified (if applicable), prescribed interventions, and the response to those interventions. Document whether the patient experienced pain or discomfort during flushing.

For dressing change, document the condition and length of the external catheter, the appearance of the site, and any reports of pain or tenderness. Record the date and the time of the dressing change, site care,

dressing type, securement device type, any unexpected outcomes, and your interventions.

For drug administrations, document the type of therapy, drug, dose, rate, time, route, and method of administration. Include the condition and patency of the site before and after administration. When multiple catheter lumens are in use, document which solutions and medications are infusing through each lumen. Note the patient's response to infusion therapy, including symptoms, adverse effects, adverse events, and laboratory tests (as appropriate). Record the date and time you notified the practitioner of any adverse reactions to the prescribed medication, prescribed interventions, and the patient's response to those interventions. If any complications occurred, note them and your interventions.[65]

For blood sampling, Document the date and time that you drew the sample and the volume of blood you drew. If fasting was necessary, document if the patient observed fasting. If you're using a multi-lumen catheter, document which lumen you used. Include the tests for which you drew the sample and the time that you sent the sample to the laboratory. Record the patency of the catheter, absence of signs and symptoms of complications, presence of a blood return on aspiration, lack of resistance when flushing, and amount and types of flushes you used.

For PICC removal, document the date and time of removal, the condition of the insertion site, the condition and length of the catheter, the reason you removed the device, and the patient's tolerance of the procedure. Record any nursing interventions that were necessary during removal, the patient's response to those interventions, and the type of petroleum-based ointment and dressing you applied to the site. Also document teaching provided to the patient and family (if appropriate), their understanding of that teaching, and any need for follow-up teaching.

REFERENCES

1 Standard 26. Vascular access device planning. Infusion therapy standards of practice (8th ed.). (2021). *Journal of Infusion Nursing, 44*, S74–S81. (Level VII)

2 Infusion Nurses Society. (2016). *Policies and procedures for infusion therapy* (5th ed.). Boston, MA: Infusion Nurses Society.

3 Centers for Disease Control and Prevention. (2011, revised 2017). Guidelines for the prevention of intravascular catheter–related infections. https://www.cdc.gov/infectioncontrol/guidelines/bsi/recommendations.html (Level I)

4 Wiegand, D. L. (2017). *AACN procedure manual for high acuity, progressive, and critical care* (7th ed.). St. Louis, MO: Elsevier.

5 Chopra, V. (2021). Central venous access devices and approach to device and site selection in adults. In: *UpToDate*, Cochran, A. & Davidson, I. (Eds.).

6 Gonzalez, R., & Cassaro, S. (2020). Percutaneous central catheter. https://www.ncbi.nlm.nih.gov/books/NBK459338/

7 Standard 5. Competency and competency assessment. Infusion therapy standards of practice (8th ed.). (2021). *Journal of Infusion Nursing, 44*, S26–S31. (Level VII)

8 Standard 27. Site selection. Infusion therapy standards of practice (8th ed.). (2021). *Journal of Infusion Nursing, 44*, S81–S86. (Level VII)

9 Standard 33. Vascular access site preparation and skin antisepsis. Infusion therapy standards of practice (8th ed.). (2021). *Journal of Infusion Nursing, 44*, S96. (Level VII)

10 Standard 22. Vascular visualization. Infusion therapy standards of practice (8th ed.). (2021). *Journal of Infusion Nursing, 44*, S63–S65. (Level VII)

11 Li, Z., & Chen, L. (2015). Comparison of ultrasound-guided modified Seldinger technique versus blind puncture for peripherally inserted central catheter: A meta-analysis of randomized controlled trials. *Critical Care, 19*(1), 64. https://www.ncbi.nlm.nih.gov/pmc/articles/PMC4328546/ (Level I)

12 Standard 50. Infection. Infusion therapy standards of practice (8th ed.). (2021). *Journal of Infusion Nursing, 44*, S153–S157. (Level VII)

13 Jarrett, N., & Callaham, M. (2016). Evidence-based guidelines for selected hospital-acquired conditions: Final report. at https://www.cms.gov/Medicare/Medicare-Fee-for-Service-Payment/HospitalAcqCond/Downloads/2016-HAC-Report.pdf

14 Association of Professionals in Infection Control and Epidemiology (APIC). (2015). Guide to preventing central line-associated bloodstream infections. http://apic.org/Resource_/TinyMceFileManager/2015/APIC_CLABSI_WEB.pdf (Level IV)

15 The Joint Commission. (2021). Standard NPSG.07.04.01. *Comprehensive accreditation manual for hospitals.* Oakbrook Terrace, IL: The Joint Commission. (Level VII)

16 Marschall, J., et al. (2014). SHEA/IDSA practice recommendation: Strategies to prevent central line–associated bloodstream infections in acute care hospitals. *Infection Control and Hospital Epidemiology, 35,* 753–771. https://www.jstor.org/stable/10.1086/676533#metadata_info_tab_contents (Level I)

17 The Joint Commission. (2021). Standard RI.01.03.01. *Comprehensive accreditation manual for hospitals.* Oakbrook Terrace, IL: The Joint Commission. (Level VII)

18 Standard 12. Product evaluation, integrity, and defect reporting. Infusion therapy standards of practice (8th ed.). (2021). *Journal of Infusion Nursing, 44,* S45–S46. (Level VII)

19 Standard 9. Informed consent. Infusion therapy standards of practice (8th ed.). (2021). *Journal of Infusion Nursing, 44,* S37–S39. (Level VII)

20 Centers for Medicare and Medicaid Services, Department of Health and Human Services. (2020). Condition of participation: Patient's rights. 42 C.F.R. § 482.13.

21 Accreditation Association for Hospitals and Health Systems. (2020). Standard 15.01.11. *Healthcare Facilities Accreditation Program: Accreditation requirements for acute care hospitals.* Chicago, IL: Accreditation Association for Hospitals and Health Systems. (Level VII)

22 DNV GL-Healthcare USA, Inc. (2020). PR.2.SR.3. *NIAHO® accreditation requirements, interpretive guidelines and surveyor guidance—revision 20.0.* Milford, OH: DNV GL-Healthcare USA, Inc. (Level VII)

23 Accreditation Association for Hospitals and Health Systems. (2020). Standard 30.00.14. *Healthcare Facilities Accreditation Program: Accreditation requirements for acute care hospitals.* Chicago, IL: Accreditation Association for Hospitals and Health Systems. (Level VII)

24 The Joint Commission. (2021). Standard UP.01.01.01. *Comprehensive accreditation manual for hospitals.* Oakbrook Terrace, IL: The Joint Commission. (Level VII)

25 The Joint Commission. (2021). Standard NPSG.07.01.01. *Comprehensive accreditation manual for hospitals.* Oakbrook Terrace, IL: The Joint Commission. (Level VII)

26 Centers for Disease Control and Prevention. (2002). Guideline for hand hygiene in health-care settings: Recommendations of the Healthcare Infection Control Practices Advisory Committee and the HICPAC/SHEA/APIC/IDSA Hand Hygiene Task Force. *MMWR Recommendations and Reports, 51*(RR-16), 1–45. https://www.cdc.gov/mmwr/pdf/rr/rr5116.pdf (Level II)

27 World Health Organization. (2009). WHO guidelines on hand hygiene in health care: First global patient safety challenge, clean care is safer care. https://apps.who.int/iris/bitstream/handle/10665/44102/9789241597906_eng.pdf?sequence=1 (Level IV)

28 Standard 16. Hand hygiene. Infusion therapy standards of practice (8th ed.). (2021). *Journal of Infusion Nursing, 44,* S53–S54. (Level VII)

29 Accreditation Association for Hospitals and Health Systems. (2020). Standard 07.01.21. *Healthcare Facilities Accreditation Program: Accreditation requirements for acute care hospitals.* Chicago, IL: Accreditation Association for Hospitals and Health Systems. (Level VII)

30 Centers for Medicare and Medicaid Services, Department of Health and Human Services. (2020). Condition of participation: Infection control. 42 C.F.R. § 482.42.

31 DNV GL-Healthcare USA, Inc. (2020). IC.1.SR.1. *NIAHO® accreditation requirements, interpretive guidelines and surveyor guidance—revision 20.0.* Milford, OH: DNV GL-Healthcare USA, Inc. (Level VII)

32 The Joint Commission. (2021). Standard NPSG.01.01.01. *Comprehensive accreditation manual for hospitals.* Oakbrook Terrace, IL: The Joint Commission. (Level VII)

33 The Joint Commission. (2021). Standard RI.01.01.01. *Comprehensive accreditation manual for hospitals.* Oakbrook Terrace, IL: The Joint Commission. (Level VII)

34 Centers for Medicare and Medicaid Services, Department of Health and Human Services. (2020). Condition of participation: Patient's rights. 42 C.F.R. § 482.13(c)(1).

35 DNV GL-Healthcare USA, Inc. (2020). PR.2.SR.5. *NIAHO® accreditation requirements, interpretive guidelines and surveyor guidance—revision 20.0.* Milford, OH: DNV GL-Healthcare USA, Inc. (Level VII)

36 Accreditation Association for Hospitals and Health Systems. (2020). Standard 15.01.16. *Healthcare Facilities Accreditation Program: Accreditation requirements for acute care hospitals.* Chicago, IL: Accreditation Association for Hospitals and Health Systems. (Level VII)

37 The Joint Commission. (2021). Standard PC.02.01.21. *Comprehensive accreditation manual for hospitals.* Oakbrook Terrace, IL: The Joint Commission. (Level VII)

38 Standard 8. Patient education. Infusion therapy standards of practice (8th ed.). (2021). *Journal of Infusion Nursing, 44,* S35–S37. (Level VII)

39 Waters, T. R., et al. (2009). Safe patient handling training for schools of nursing. https://www.cdc.gov/niosh/docs/2009-127/pdfs/2009-127.pdf (Level VII)

40 Infusion Nurses Society. (2017). *Policies and procedures for infusion therapy of the older adult* (3rd ed.). Boston, MA: Infusion Nurses Society.

41 Occupational Safety and Health Administration. (2019). Bloodborne pathogens, standard number 1910.1030. https://www.osha.gov/pls/oshaweb/owadisp.show_document?p_id=10051&p_table=STANDARDS (Level VII)

42 Siegel, J. D., et al. (2007, revised 2019). 2007 guideline for isolation precautions: Preventing transmission of infectious agents in healthcare settings. https://www.cdc.gov/infectioncontrol/pdf/guidelines/isolation-guidelines-H.pdf (Level II)

43 Accreditation Association for Hospitals and Health Systems. (2020). Standard 07.01.10. *Healthcare Facilities Accreditation Program: Accreditation requirements for acute care hospitals.* Chicago, IL: Accreditation Association for Hospitals and Health Systems. (Level VII)

44 Standard 53. Catheter-associated deep vein thrombosis. Infusion therapy standards of practice (8th ed.). (2021). *Journal of Infusion Nursing, 44,* S161–S164. (Level VII)

45 The Joint Commission. (2021). Standard MM.06.01.01. *Comprehensive accreditation manual for hospitals.* Oakbrook Terrace, IL: The Joint Commission. (Level VII)

46 Centers for Medicare and Medicaid Services, Department of Health and Human Services. (2020). Condition of participation: Nursing services. 42 C.F.R. § 482.23(c).

47 Accreditation Association for Hospitals and Health Systems. (2020). Standard 16.01.03. *Healthcare Facilities Accreditation Program: Accreditation requirements for acute care hospitals.* Chicago, IL: Accreditation Association for Hospitals and Health Systems. (Level VII)

48 DNV GL-Healthcare USA, Inc. (2020). MM.1.SR.3. *NIAHO® accreditation requirements, interpretive guidelines and surveyor guidance—revision 20.0.* Milford, OH: DNV GL-Healthcare USA, Inc. (Level VII)

49 Standard 21. Medical waste and sharps safety. Infusion therapy standards of practice (8th ed.). (2021). *Journal of Infusion Nursing, 44,* S60–S62. (Level VII)

50 Standard 17. Standard precautions. Infusion therapy standards of practice (8th ed.). (2021). *Journal of Infusion Nursing, 44,* S54–S55. (Level VII)

51 Accreditation Association for Hospitals and Health Systems. (2020). Standard 25.01.27. *Healthcare Facilities Accreditation Program: Accreditation requirements for acute care hospitals.* Chicago, IL: Accreditation Association for Hospitals and Health Systems. (Level VII)

52 The Joint Commission. (2021). Standard NPSG.03.04.01. *Comprehensive accreditation manual for hospitals.* Oakbrook Terrace, IL: The Joint Commission. (Level VII)

53 CareFusion. (2021). ChloraPrep Single Swabstick/ChloraPrep Triple Swabstick. https://go.bd.com/ChloraPrep-PurPrep-Portfolio.html?utm_source=google&utm_medium=cpc&utm_content=su-purprep-portf-google-ads-fy21&utm_campaign=7014W000001B0Ts&gclid=CjwKCAjwmqKJBhAWEiwAMvGt6MdrLdgnTTUxtub-KQNCISj5ZRxoAOWos1AfFDQY2bd5dln8EboJwhoCUA8QAvD_BwE

54 CareFusion. (n.d.). Scrub Care 10% povidone-iodine, paint. https://www.bd.com/documents/labels/IP_PVP-I-Topical-Solution-10-Percent-2-oz-29906-002_PL_EN.pdf

55 The Joint Commission. (2021). Standard UP.01.03.01. *Comprehensive accreditation manual for hospitals.* Oakbrook Terrace, IL: The Joint Commission. (Level VII)

56 Standard 23. Central vascular access device (CVAD) tip location. Infusion therapy standards of practice (8th ed.). (2021). *Journal of Infusion Nursing, 44,* S65–S69. (Level VII)

57 Standard 36. Needleless connectors. Infusion therapy standards of practice (8th ed.). (2021). *Journal of Infusion Nursing, 44,* S104–S107. (Level VII)

58 Moureau, N. L., & Flynn, J. (2015). Disinfection of needleless connector hubs: Clinical evidence systematic review. *Nursing Research and Practice, 2015,* 1–20.

59 Standard 38. Vascular access device securement. Infusion therapy standards of practice (8th ed.). (2021). *Journal of Infusion Nursing, 44,* S108–S111. (Level VII)

60 Ganz, D. A., et al. (2013, reviewed 2021). *Preventing falls in hospitals: A toolkit for improving quality of care* (AHRQ Publication No. 13-0015-EF). Rockville, MD: Agency for Healthcare Research and Quality. https://www.ahrq.gov/patient-safety/settings/hospital/fall-prevention/toolkit/index.html (Level VII)

61 Standard 42. Vascular access device assessment, care and dressing changes. Infusion therapy standards of practice (8th ed.). (2021). *Journal of Infusion Nursing, 44*, S119–S123. (Level VII)

62 Accreditation Association for Hospitals and Health Systems. (2020). Standard 07.02.03. *Healthcare Facilities Accreditation Program: Accreditation requirements for acute care hospitals.* Chicago, IL: Accreditation Association for Hospitals and Health Systems. (Level VII)

63 Rutala, W. A., et al. (2008, revised 2019). Guideline for disinfection and sterilization in healthcare facilities, 2008. https://www.cdc.gov/infection-control/pdf/guidelines/disinfection-guidelines-H.pdf (Level I)

64 The Joint Commission. (2021). Standard RC.01.03.01. *Comprehensive accreditation manual for hospitals.* Oakbrook Terrace, IL: The Joint Commission. (Level VII)

65 Standard 10. Documentation in the health record. Infusion therapy standards of practice (8th ed.). (2021). *Journal of Infusion Nursing, 44*, S39–S42. (Level VII)

66 Accreditation Association for Hospitals and Health Systems. (2020). Standard 10.00.03. *Healthcare Facilities Accreditation Program: Accreditation requirements for acute care hospitals.* Chicago, IL: Accreditation Association for Hospitals and Health Systems. (Level VII)

67 Centers for Medicare and Medicaid Services, Department of Health and Human Services. (2020). Condition of participation: Medical record services. 42 C.F.R. § 482.24(b).

68 DNV GL-Healthcare USA, Inc. (2020). MR.2.SR.1. *NIAHO® accreditation requirements, interpretive guidelines and surveyor guidance—revision 20.0.* Milford, OH: DNV GL-Healthcare USA, Inc. (Level VII)

69 The Joint Commission. (2014). Sentinel event alert: Managing risk during transition to new ISO tubing connector standards. https://www.joint-commission.org/-/media/tjc/documents/resources/patient-safety-topics/sentinel-event/sea_53_connectors_8_19_14_final.pdf (Level VII)

70 U.S. Food and Drug Administration. (2017). Examples of medical device misconnections. https://www.fda.gov/medical-devices/medical-device-connectors/examples-medical-device-misconnections

71 Standard 41. Flushing and locking. Infusion therapy standards of practice (8th ed.). (2021). *Journal of Infusion Nursing, 44*(Suppl. 1), S113–S118. (Level VII)

72 Hull, G. J., et al. (2018). Quantitative assessment of reflux in commercially available needleless IV connectors. *Journal of Vascular Access, 19*(1), 12–22. https://journals.sagepub.com/doi/pdf/10.5301/jva.5000781?casa_token=tM64lszfNzMAAAAA:K2yFquq_vLVY5q6alBhkBPL9Q5bnsio7K-zrAW3Ffi-V21QNUzoqVTXuVnw7bnP-O2OgPks4yVc6VA (Level VI)

73 Feil, M. (2012). Reducing risk of air embolism associated with central venous access devices. *Pennsylvania Patient Safety Advisory, 9*(2), 58–64. http://patientsafety.pa.gov/ADVISORIES/Pages/201206_58.aspx

74 Standard 52. Air embolism. Infusion therapy standards of practice (8th ed.). (2021). *Journal of Infusion Nursing, 44*(Suppl. 1), S160–S161. (Level VII)

75 LeBlanc, K., et al. (2013). International skin tear advisory panel: A tool kit to aid in the prevention, assessment, and treatment of skin tears using a simplified classification system. *Advances in Skin and Wound Care, 26*, 459–476. (Level IV)

76 Standard 59. Infusion medication and solution administration. Infusion therapy standards of practice (8th ed.). (2021). *Journal of Infusion Nursing, 44*(Suppl. 1), S180–S183. (Level VII)

77 Westbrook, J., et al. (2010). Association of interruptions with an increased risk and severity of medication administration errors. *Archives of Internal Medicine, 170*(8), 683–690. https://doi.org/10.1001/archinternmed.2010.65 (Level IV)

78 Institute for Safe Medication Practices. (2012). Side tracks on the safety express: Interruptions lead to errors and unfinished…Wait what was I doing? *Nurse Advise-ERR, 11*(2), 1–4. https://www.ismp.org/resources/side-tracks-safety-express-interruptions-lead-errors-and-unfinished-wait-what-was-i-doing?id=37

79 Standard 13. Medication verification. Infusion therapy standards of practice (8th ed.). (2021). *Journal of Infusion Nursing, 44*(Suppl. 1), S46–S49. (Level VII)

80 Institute for Safe Medication Practices. (2019). Independent double checks: Worth the effort if used judiciously and properly. https://www.ismp.org/resources/independent-double-checks-worth-effort-if-used-judiciously-and-properly (Level VII)

81 Institute for Safe Medication Practices. (2018). ISMP list of high-alert medications in acute care settings. https://www.ismp.org/sites/default/files/attachments/2018-08/highAlert2018-Acute-Final.pdf

82 Institute for Safe Medication Practices. (2015). ISMP safe practice guidelines for adult IV push medications. https://www.ismp.org/guidelines/iv-push (Level VII)

83 The Joint Commission. (2013). Sentinel event alert 50: Medical device alarm safety in hospitals. https://www.jointcommission.org/-/media/tjc/documents/resources/patient-safety-topics/sentinel-event/sea_50_alarms_4_26_16.pdf (Level VII)

84 The Joint Commission. (2021). Standard NPSG.06.01.01. *Comprehensive accreditation manual for hospitals.* (Level VII)

85 Graham, K. C., & Cvach, M. (2010). Monitor alarm fatigue: Standardizing use of physiological monitors and decreasing nuisance alarms. *American Journal of Critical Care, 19*(1), 28–37. https://doi.org/10.4037/ajcc2010651

86 Centers for Medicare and Medicaid Services. (2014). Requirements for hospital medication administration, particularly intravenous (IV) medications and post-operative care of patients receiving IV opioids. https://www.cms.gov/Medicare/Provider-Enrollment-and-Certification/SurveyCertificationGenInfo/Downloads/Survey-and-Cert-Letter-14-15.pdf

87 Standard 44. Blood sampling. Infusion therapy standards of practice (8th ed.). (2021). *Journal of Infusion Nursing, 44*(Suppl. 1), S125–S133. (Level VII)

88 Standard 45. Vascular access device removal. Infusion therapy standards of practice (8th ed.). (2021). *Journal of Infusion Nursing, 44*(Suppl. 1), S133–S137. (Level VII)

89 Standard 51. Catheter damage (embolism, repair, exchange). Infusion therapy standards of practice (8th ed.). (2021). *Journal of Infusion Nursing, 44*(Suppl. 1), S157–S160. (Level VII)

90 Standard 54. Central venous access device malposition. Infusion therapy standards of practice (8th ed.). (2021). *Journal of Infusion Nursing, 44*(Suppl. 1), S164–S167. (Level VII)

91 Standard 48. Nerve injury. Infusion therapy standards of practice (8th ed.). (2021). *Journal of Infusion Nursing, 44*(Suppl. 1), S147–S149. (Level VII)

92 Infusion Nurses Society. (2008, revised 2016). *Infusion Nurses Society: Flushing and locking guidelines for vascular access devices.* Boston, MA: Infusion Nurses Society.

93 Standard 49. Central vascular access device occlusion. Infusion therapy standards of practice (8th ed.). (2021). *Journal of Infusion Nursing, 44*(Suppl. 1), S149–S153. (Level VII)

94 Standard 47. Infiltration and extravasation. Infusion therapy standards of practice (8th ed.). (2021). *Journal of Infusion Nursing, 44*(Suppl. 1), S142–S147. (Level VII)

95 Standard 46. Phlebitis. Infusion therapy standards of practice (8th ed.). (2021). *Journal of Infusion Nursing, 44*(Suppl. 1), S138–S142. (Level VII)

96 Biolife, LLC. (n.d.). StatSeal. http://statseal.com/wp-content/uploads/2015/08/SPF01r1_85_11.pdf

97 Pan, M., et al. (2019). Nursing interventions to reduce peripherally inserted central catheter occlusion for cancer patients: A systematic review of literature. *Cancer Nursing, 42*(6), E49–E58. https://journals.lww.com/cancernursingonline/fulltext/2019/11000/Nursing_Interventions_to_Reduce_Peripherally.19.aspx (Level I)

98 American College of Radiology (ACR). (2020). ACR manual on contrast media. https://www.acr.org/-/media/ACR/Files/Clinical-Resources/Contrast_Media.pdf

99 Liem, T. K., et al. (2012). Peripherally inserted central catheter usage patterns and associated symptomatic upper extremity venous thrombosis. *Journal of Vascular Surgery, 55*, 761–767. (Level IV)

100 Chopra, V., et al. (2012). Bloodstream infection, venous thrombosis, and peripherally inserted central catheters: Reappraising the evidence. *American Journal of Medicine, 125*, 733–741. (Level VII)

Peripheral nerve stimulation

Peripheral nerve stimulation is used to assess the transmission of nerve impulses at the neuromuscular junction of certain skeletal muscles to monitor the depth of neuromuscular blockade in patients receiving neuromuscular-blocking drugs.[1] Neuromuscular-blocking drugs produce paralysis to help synchronize breathing and mechanical ventilation in patients with severe lung injury; assist with the treatment of severe muscle spasms in patients with seizures, tetanus, or drug overdose; and help in the management of increased intracranial pressure in patients with head injury.[1,2]

A peripheral nerve stimulator (PNS) helps to evaluate the level of neuromuscular blockade and determine the lowest therapeutic dose of the neuromuscular-blocking drug needed to produce paralysis.[3] A PNS works by stimulating a peripheral nerve with a series of brief electrical pulses to produce a muscle response or twitch.

The train of four (TOF) method is the most commonly used method for monitoring neuromuscular blockade.[2] In this method, a series of four electrical impulses are delivered to a particular peripheral nerve by the PNS and the muscle response is evaluated. The ulnar nerve site is the recommended and most commonly used location for the test, but the facial and posterior tibial nerves may also be used.[1] If four twitches occur in response to the PNS, then up to 70% of the receptors are blocked. Three twitches occur when about 75% of the receptors are blocked. One or two twitches correspond to approximately 80% to 90% neuromuscular blockade.[1] After the neuromuscular-blocking drug is administered, it's titrated so that each set of four electrical impulses produces one or two muscle twitches. The absence of twitches may indicate that 100% of the receptors are blocked, exceeding the desired level of neuromuscular blockade.[1]

Equipment

PNS ■ two electrode gel patches ■ two lead wires ■ alcohol pads ■ Optional: clippers.

Preparation of Equipment

Inspect all equipment and supplies. If a product is expired, is defective, or has compromised integrity, remove it from patient use, label it as expired or defective, and report the expiration or defect as directed by your facility.

Implementation

■ Verify the practitioner's order.
■ Perform hand hygiene.[4,5,6,7,8,9]
■ Confirm the patient's identity using at least two patient identifiers.[10]
■ Provide privacy.[11,12,13,14]
■ Explain the procedure to the patient and family (if appropriate) according to their individual communication and learning needs *to increase their understanding, allay their fears, and enhance cooperation.*[15]
■ Raise the bed to waist level before performing patient care *to prevent caregiver back strain.*[16]
■ Perform hand hygiene.[4,5,6,7,8,9]
■ Select a site for electrode placement that's accessible and without edema, wounds, catheters, or dressings *to ensure optimum placement for conduction of stimulating current.* (The preferred monitoring site is the ulnar nerve, but if it isn't accessible, other sites may be used.)
■ If the patient has excessive hair where an electrode is to be placed, remove the hair with clippers *to improve contact of the pad with the skin.*[1]

Ulnar nerve stimulation

■ Use an alcohol pad to clean the site on the patient's arm where the electrodes are to be placed, and allow the site to dry *to reduce skin resistance.*
■ Place the patient's arm in a relaxed position with the palm up *so that the ulnar nerve is easily accessible.*
■ Place one electrode over the ulnar nerve at the crease of the wrist and the other electrode 0.4″ to 0.8″ (1 to 2 cm) away, parallel to the carpi ulnaris tendon (as shown below) *to ensure stimulation of the ulnar nerve.*

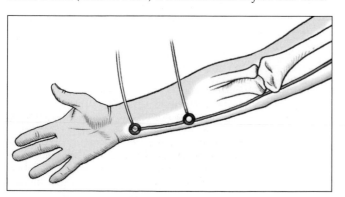

■ Attach the lead wires to the PNS.
■ Connect the black lead (negative) to the electrode nearest the wrist and the red lead (positive) to the electrode on the forearm.
■ Turn on the PNS on and choose a low amplitude—commonly 10 to 20 milliampere (mA)—*because higher current can cause overstimulation of the nerve and rhythmic nerve firing.*[1]
■ Press the TOF button to initiate the four impulses. Count the number of thumb adductions or twitches that the stimulator produces while lightly feeling for twitches. Don't count finger movement that's caused by muscle stimulation.
■ Turn off the PNS.
■ Perform hand hygiene.[4,5,6,7,8,9]

Facial nerve stimulation

■ Use an alcohol pad to clean the site on the patient's face where the electrodes are to be placed, and allow the site to dry *to improve contact of the electrode with the skin.*
■ Place one electrode near the outer canthus of the eye and a second electrode 0.8″ (2 cm) below and at the level of the tragus of the ear (as shown below) *to ensure stimulation of the facial nerve.*

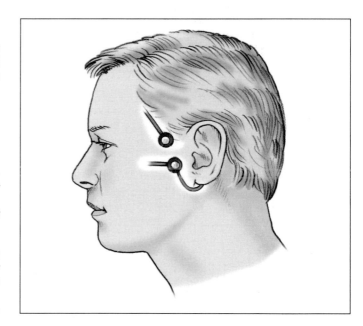

■ Attach the lead wires to the PNS
■ Connect the black lead (negative) to the electrode nearest the tragus and the red lead (positive) to the electrode near the outer canthus of the eye.
■ Turn on the PNS on and choose a low amplitude—commonly 10 to 20 mA—*because higher current can cause overstimulation of the nerve and rhythmic nerve firing.*
■ Press the TOF button to initiate the four impulses. Count the number of twitches you observe while lightly feeling for twitches.
■ Turn off the PNS.
■ Perform hand hygiene.[4,5,6,7,8,9]

Posterior tibial nerve stimulation

■ Use an alcohol pad to clean the site on the patient's foot where the electrodes are to be placed and allow it to dry *to improve contact of the electrode with the skin.*
■ Place one electrode 0.8″ (2 cm) behind the medial malleolus and a second electrode 0.8″ (2 cm) above the first electrode (as shown) *to ensure stimulation of the posterior tibial nerve.*

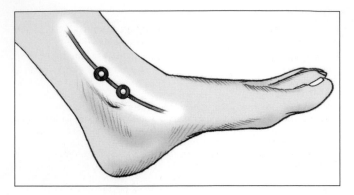

- Attach the lead wires to the PNS.
- Connect the black lead (negative) to the electrode behind the medial malleolus and the red lead (positive) to the electrode above the first.
- Turn on the PNS on and choose a low mA—commonly 10 to 20 mA—*because higher current can cause overstimulation of the nerve and rhythmic nerve firing.*
- Press the TOF button to initiate the four impulses. Note plantar flexion of the great toe and count the number of twitches that the stimulation produces.
- Turn off the PNS.
- Perform hand hygiene.[4,5,6,7,8,9]

Establishing supramaximal stimulation

- *To determine the baseline amplitude setting for a patient who hasn't received neuromuscular blockade,* set the amplitude to 5 mA and press the TOF button to initiate the stimulus.[1]
- Note the number of twitches produced.
- Increase the amplitude 5 mA at a time until four muscle twitches are produced by the TOF stimulation. *This step establishes the amount of current that should be used for peripheral nerve stimulation and enhances the reliability of testing.*[1]

Establishing TOF after neuromuscular blockade

- Determine the TOF 10 to 15 minutes following a bolus dose or any change in neuromuscular drug administration *to assess the level of neuromuscular blockade.*[1]
- If no twitches occur, troubleshoot the equipment. Next, increase the stimulating current and then retest another nerve. If there's still no response, check the neuromuscular blocker infusion rate, concentration, and dose, and then hold the bolus dose or reduce the infusion rate, as ordered. Retest the TOF in 10 to 15 minutes.[1]
- If one or two twitches occur, continue the current rate of the infusion.
- If three or four twitches occur, increase the rate of the neuromuscular blockade and then retest the TOF in 10 to 15 minutes.

Ongoing care

- Perform respiratory, cardiovascular, and neurologic assessments before any increase in the level of neuromuscular blockade.
- Perform neurovascular checks hourly.
- Change electrodes daily, or more frequently if they become loose or the gel has dried out, *to ensure optimum conduction.*[1]
- Assess the skin under the electrodes for signs of irritation or breakdown, *which could impede conduction.*
- Reevaluate the level of neuromuscular blockade every 4 to 8 hours during therapy with neuromuscular-blocking drugs after the patient is stable and an adequate level of neuromuscular blockade is reached, as ordered or as directed by your facility.[1]
- Return the bed to the lowest position *to prevent falls and maintain patient safety.*[17]
- Perform hand hygiene.[4,5,6,7,8,9]
- Document the procedure.[18,19,20,21]

Special considerations

- *Because neuromuscular-blocking drugs don't produce amnesia, sedation, or analgesia,* sedative and analgesic drugs should always be administered before giving a neuromuscular-blocking drug.[1,2,3]
- Assess the patient's baseline electrolyte, blood urea nitrogen, and creatinine levels, *because imbalances may potentiate the effects of neuromuscular-blocking drugs.*[1]
- *To avoid complications of neuromuscular blockade,* the patient will require routine frequent oral care and suctioning, deep vein thrombosis prophylaxis (as ordered), GI prophylaxis (as ordered), eye lubrication, and footdrop prevention measures.[2]
- Check the site of electrode placement carefully, *because incorrect placement can lead to muscle, rather than nerve, stimulation.*[1]
- If no twitches are elicited at a level that previously elicited a response, troubleshoot the PNS before decreasing the level of neuromuscular blockade. Check the polarity of the leads, battery charge, electrode contact with the skin, condition of electrode gel pads, and lead wire connections.[1]

Complications

Excessive neuromuscular blockade can cause protracted paralysis and muscle weakness.[3] During TOF testing, the patient may experience mild discomfort or tingling.[1] Skin irritation and breakdown can occur under the electrode pads.[1] Cardiac arrhythmias can result if the PNS lead wires come in contact with an external pacing catheter or lead wire.[1]

Documentation

Record the date and time of the assessment. Record the initial TOF assessment, amplitude used, and dose of neuromuscular-blocking drug being administered. Document each subsequent TOF assessment on the appropriate flow sheet as a ratio of twitches per four stimulations—for example, 0/4, 1/4, 2/4, 3/4, 4/4.

Note the current used, as well as any bolus doses or changes in the rate of infusion of the neuromuscular-blocking drug. Record respiratory, cardiovascular, neurologic, and neurovascular assessments on a frequent assessment form. Note any adverse effects of neuromuscular blockade, the time and name of the practitioner notified, orders given, nursing interventions performed, and the patient's response to those interventions. Document teaching you provided to the patient and family (if applicable), their understanding of that teaching, and any need for follow-up teaching.

REFERENCES

1 Wiegand, D. L. (2017). *AACN procedure manual for high acuity, progressive, and critical care* (7th ed.). St. Louis, MO: Elsevier.

2 Bittner, E. A. (2019). Neuromuscular blocking agents in critically ill patients: Use, agent selection, administration, and adverse effects. In: *UpToDate,* Parsons, P. E. (Ed.).

3 Brull, S. J., & Kopman, A. F. (2017) Current status of neuromuscular reversal and monitoring: Challenges and opportunities. *Anesthesiology, 126,* 173–190. https://anesthesiology.pubs.asahq.org/article.aspx?articleid=2583391

4 The Joint Commission. (2021). Standard NPSG.07.01.01. *Comprehensive accreditation manual for hospitals.* Oakbrook Terrace, IL: The Joint Commission. (Level VII)

5 Centers for Disease Control and Prevention. (2002). Guideline for hand hygiene in health-care settings: Recommendations of the Healthcare Infection Control Practices Advisory Committee and the HICPAC/SHEA/APIC/IDSA Hand Hygiene Task Force. *MMWR Recommendations and Reports, 51*(RR-16), 1–45. https://www.cdc.gov/mmwr/pdf/rr/rr5116.pdf (Level II)

6 World Health Organization. (2009). WHO guidelines on hand hygiene in health care: First global patient safety challenge, clean care is safer care. https://apps.who.int/iris/bitstream/handle/10665/44102/9789241597906_eng.pdf?sequence=1 (Level IV)

7 Centers for Medicare and Medicaid Services, Department of Health and Human Services. (2020). Condition of participation: Infection control. 42 C.F.R. § 482.42.

8 Accreditation Association for Hospitals and Health Systems. (2020). Standard 07.01.21. *Healthcare Facilities Accreditation Program: Accreditation requirements for acute care hospitals.* Chicago, IL: Accreditation Association for Hospitals and Health Systems. (Level VII)

9 DNV GL-Healthcare USA, Inc. (2020). IC.1.SR.1. *NIAHO® accreditation requirements, interpretive guidelines and surveyor guidance—revision 20.0.* Milford, OH: DNV GL-Healthcare USA, Inc. (Level VII)

10 The Joint Commission. (2021). Standard NPSG.01.01.01. *Comprehensive accreditation manual for hospitals.* Oakbrook Terrace, IL: The Joint Commission. (Level VII)

11 Centers for Medicare and Medicaid Services, Department of Health and Human Services. (2020). Condition of participation: Patient's rights. 42 C.F.R. § 482.13(c)(1).

12 Accreditation Association for Hospitals and Health Systems. (2020). Standard 15.01.16. *Healthcare Facilities Accreditation Program: Accreditation requirements for acute care hospitals.* Chicago, IL: Accreditation Association for Hospitals and Health Systems. (Level VII)

13 The Joint Commission. (2021). Standard RI.01.01.01. *Comprehensive accreditation manual for hospitals.* Oakbrook Terrace, IL: The Joint Commission. (Level VII)

14 DNV GL-Healthcare USA, Inc. (2020). PR.2.SR.5. *NIAHO® accreditation requirements, interpretive guidelines and surveyor guidance—revision 20.0.* Milford, OH: DNV GL-Healthcare USA, Inc. (Level VII)

15 The Joint Commission. (2021). Standard PC.02.01.21. *Comprehensive accreditation manual for hospitals.* Oakbrook Terrace, IL: The Joint Commission. (Level VII)

16 Waters, T. R., et al. (2009). Safe patient handling training for schools of nursing. https://www.cdc.gov/niosh/docs/2009-127/pdfs/2009-127.pdf (Level VII)

17 Ganz, D. A., et al. (2013, reviewed 2021). *Preventing falls in hospitals: A toolkit for improving quality of care* (AHRQ Publication No. 13-0015-EF). Rockville, MD: Agency for Healthcare Research and Quality. https://www.ahrq.gov/professionals/systems/hospital/fallpxtoolkit/index.html (Level VII)

18 The Joint Commission. (2021). Standard RC.01.03.01. *Comprehensive accreditation manual for hospitals.* Oakbrook Terrace, IL: The Joint Commission. (Level VII)

19 Centers for Medicare and Medicaid Services, Department of Health and Human Services. (2020). Condition of participation: Medical record services. 42 C.F.R. § 482.24(b).

20 Accreditation Association for Hospitals and Health Systems. (2020). Standard 10.00.03. *Healthcare Facilities Accreditation Program: Accreditation requirements for acute care hospitals.* Chicago, IL: Accreditation Association for Hospitals and Health Systems. (Level VII)

21 DNV GL-Healthcare USA, Inc. (2020). MR.2.SR.1. *NIAHO® accreditation requirements, interpretive guidelines and surveyor guidance—revision 20.0.* Milford, OH: DNV GL-Healthcare USA, Inc. (Level VII)

PERITONEAL DIALYSIS

Peritoneal dialysis requires insertion of a peritoneal catheter (such as a Tenckhoff catheter) to circulate dialysate in the peritoneal cavity.[1] The practitioner inserts a catheter under general or local anesthesia, sutures it in place, and tunnels the distal portion subcutaneously to the skin surface. There, it serves as a port for the dialysate solution (the solution instilled into the peritoneal cavity through the catheter), which draws waste products, excess fluid, and electrolytes from the blood across the semipermeable peritoneal membrane.[2] After a prescribed period, dialysate drains from the peritoneal cavity. (See *How peritoneal dialysis works*.)

Each solution change is called an *exchange* or *cycle;* each exchange or cycle involves three phases:

■ During the *instillation,* or the *fill phase,* dialysate infuses through the catheter into the abdominal cavity. It typically takes 5 to 10 minutes for the dialysate to infuse and fill the abdominal cavity.

■ During the *dwell phase,* the dialysate remains in the abdominal cavity, allowing osmosis and diffusion to occur. The dwell time varies (as prescribed and determined by the patient's condition and delivery method) but typically ranges from 30 minutes to 4 hours.

■ In the *drain phase,* dialysate and excess extracellular fluid, waste, and electrolytes drain from the abdominal cavity via the catheter, typically over 15 to 20 minutes.[2]

How peritoneal dialysis works

Peritoneal dialysis works through a combination of diffusion and osmosis.

Diffusion

In diffusion, particles move through a semipermeable membrane from an area of high-solute concentration to an area of low-solute concentration. In peritoneal dialysis, the water-based dialysate being infused contains glucose, sodium chloride, calcium, magnesium, acetate or lactate, and no waste products. Therefore, the waste products and excess electrolytes in the blood cross through the semipermeable peritoneal membrane into the dialysate. Removing the waste-filled dialysate and replacing it with fresh solution keeps the waste concentration low and encourages further diffusion.

Osmosis

In osmosis, fluids move through a semipermeable membrane from an area of low-solute concentration to an area of high-solute concentration. In peritoneal dialysis, dextrose is added to the dialysate to give it a higher solute concentration than the blood, creating a high osmotic gradient. Water migrates from the blood through the membrane at the beginning of each infusion, when the osmotic gradient is highest.

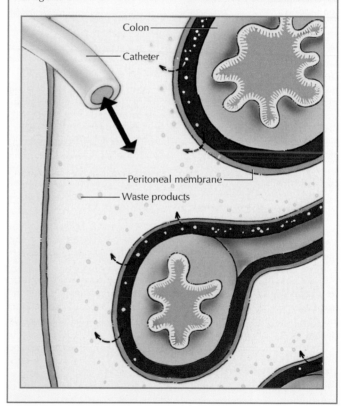

If this is the patient's first time receiving peritoneal dialysis, the instillation phase occurs first. For patients who have been receiving therapy, the drain phase must be completed first, followed by the instillation and then the dwell phase.[2]

The procedure is indicated for patients with stage 5 chronic kidney disease, or an earlier stage of kidney disease when signs and symptoms become severe.[3,4] Patients with acute kidney injury, hemodialysis vascular access issues, chronic heart failure, coagulation abnormalities, or ischemic heart disease can also benefit from peritoneal dialysis.[4,5]

Peritoneal dialysis gives the patient more independence, requires less travel for treatments, and results in more stable fluid and electrolyte levels than conventional hemodialysis. Because the patient can resume normal daily activities between dialysate solution changes, peritoneal dialysis helps the patient return to a near-normal lifestyle. It also costs less than hemodialysis. Peritoneal dialysis may be manual or automated.[2]

The manual method requires a tubing and bag setup that fills and drains by gravity. The automated method uses a machine that uses gravity or a pump to drain dialysate.

Contraindications to peritoneal dialysis include inability to self-care or lack of a capable caregiver to assist with peritoneal dialysis after discharge, recent major intra-abdominal surgery, and severe morbid obesity (body mass index greater than 40).[6] Extraperitoneal procedures, such as nephrectomy, aren't necessarily contraindications.[6] Contraindications to urgent peritoneal dialysis for acute kidney injury include ileus, appendicitis, ischemic bowel, intestinal obstruction or perforation, bacterial or fungal peritonitis, new aortic grafts, abdominal or diaphragmatic fistulae, abdominal burns, cellulitis, severe hypercatabolic states, and profound metabolic acidosis.[6]

The practitioner may insert the catheter in the operating room or in the interventional radiology department under sterile conditions. Peritoneal dialysis may be performed by a nephrology nurse, an acute care hemodialysis nurse, an acute care dialysis technician with nurse supervision, a critical care nurse, an expert medical-surgical nurse, or a contracted nurse from an agency who is trained and competent to perform peritoneal dialysis.[6] Know who may perform peritoneal dialysis in your facility. (See *Comparing peritoneal dialysis catheters.*)

Equipment

Scale ▪ vital signs monitoring equipment ▪ stethoscope ▪ disinfectant pad.

To instill and drain dialysate

Prescribed dialysate solution ▪ peritoneal dialysis administration set (usually a closed system with attached drainage bag)[2] ▪ transfer set ▪ heating pad or commercial warmer ▪ IV pole ▪ masks ▪ gloves ▪ sterile gloves ▪ sterile 4″ × 4″ (10 cm × 10 cm) gauze pads ▪ antiseptic solution (povidone-iodine, hypochlorite, or chlorhexidine)[2,7] ▪ hypoallergenic tape or catheter securement device ▪ facility-approved disinfectant ▪ sterile drape ▪ Optional: gown, mask with face shield or mask and goggles, prescribed medication, labels, peritoneal dialysis machine, sterile container, transfer set change kit with patient connector, sterile caps or disinfectant-containing disconnect cap, sterile swabs, specimen container or sterile culture tube with transport medium, specimen label, laboratory biohazard transport bag, laboratory request form.

For catheter dressing change

Sterile drape ▪ sterile 4″ × 4″ (10 cm × 10 cm) gauze pads ▪ dressing ▪ masks ▪ hypoallergenic tape or catheter securement device ▪ antiseptic solution ▪ sterile gloves ▪ sterile cap ▪ Optional: gown, mask with face shield or mask and goggles, sterile container, disinfectant-containing disconnect cap, prescribed antibiotic ointment.

Commercially prepared sterile continuous ambulatory peritoneal dialysis kits are available.

Preparation of equipment

Inspect all equipment and supplies. If a product is expired, is defective, or has compromised integrity, remove it from patient use, label it as expired or defective, and report the expiration or defect as directed by your facility.[2] If medications are prescribed for the peritoneal dialysis solution and the pharmacy can't add them into the dialysis solution bag using a laminar airflow hood, add them using sterile technique *to prevent bacterial and fungal contamination of the solution bag.*[6] Mix the solution by inverting the bag several times.[6] After adding the medication, label the solution bag with the name and dose of the medication, the time and date of the addition, your initials, and whether refrigeration is needed.[6] Warm the dialysis solution bags to body temperature using dry heat *to prevent patient discomfort and abdominal pain.*[1,8]

Implementation

▪ Avoid distractions and interruptions when preparing and administering dialysate solution *to prevent administration errors.*[9,10]
▪ Review the patient's medical record for primary kidney disease and other comorbid conditions, response to prior peritoneal dialysis

Comparing peritoneal dialysis catheters

The first step in any type of peritoneal dialysis is insertion of a catheter *to allow instillation of dialyzing solution.* The surgeon may insert one of the three catheters described here.

Tenckhoff catheter

To implant a Tenckhoff catheter, the surgeon inserts the first 6¾″ (17 cm) of the catheter into the patient's abdomen. The next 2¾″ (7-cm) segment, which may have a Dacron cuff at one or both ends, is embedded subcutaneously. Within a few days after insertion, the patient's tissues grow around the cuffs, forming a tight barrier against bacterial infiltration. The remaining 4″ (10 cm) of the catheter extends outside of the abdomen and is equipped with a metal adapter at the tip that connects to dialyzer tubing.

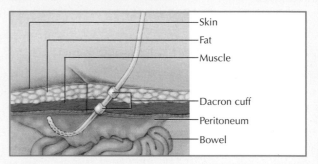

Flanged-collar catheter

To insert this kind of catheter, the surgeon positions its flanged collar just below the skin so that the device extends through the abdominal wall, keeping the distal end of the cuff from extending into the peritoneum, where it could cause adhesions.

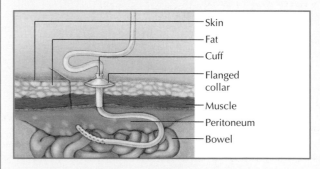

Column-disk peritoneal catheter

To insert a column-disk peritoneal catheter (CDPC), the surgeon rolls up the flexible disk section of the implant, inserts it into the peritoneal cavity, and retracts it against the abdominal wall. The implant's first cuff rests just outside the peritoneal membrane, and its second cuff rests just underneath the skin.

Because the CDPC doesn't float freely in the peritoneal cavity, it keeps inflowing dialyzing solution from being directed at the sensitive organs, which increases patient comfort during dialysis.

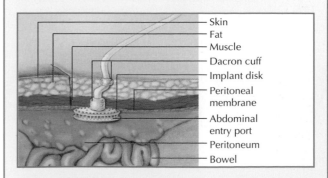

treatments (if applicable), medication history, and pertinent laboratory test results (blood urea nitrogen, serum creatinine, albumin, bicarbonate, glucose, potassium, and hemoglobin levels; hematocrit; and white blood cell and platelet counts).[2,3]

■ Verify the practitioner's order, which should include the number of daily exchanges, frequency of exchanges, fill volume, dialysis solution type, dextrose and calcium concentrations, and added medications.[2,6,11,12,13,14]

■ Compare the dialysate solution label with the order in the patient's medical record.[11,12,13,14]

■ Check the patient's medical record for an allergy or a contraindication to the prescribed dialysate solution or its additives. If an allergy or a contraindication exists, don't administer the dialysate solution, and notify the practitioner.[11,12,13,14]

■ Inspect the dialysate solution visually for particles, discoloration, or other signs of loss of integrity; don't administer the dialysate solution if its integrity has been compromised.[11,12,13,14]

■ Discuss any unresolved concerns about the dialysate solution with the patient's practitioner.[11,12,13,14]

■ Gather and prepare the necessary equipment and supplies.

■ Perform hand hygiene.[15,16,17,18,19,20]

■ Confirm the patient's identity using at least two patient identifiers.[21]

■ Close the door to the room or pull the curtain around the bedside *to minimize airborne contaminants.*

■ Provide privacy.[22,23,24,25]

■ Explain the procedure to the patient and family (if appropriate) according to their individual communication and learning needs *to increase their understanding, allay their fears, and enhance cooperation.*[26] If the patient previously received peritoneal dialysis, ask about the response to previous treatment.

■ Assess the patient's respiratory and abdominal status.[2] Assess for signs of dehydration and for unusual insensible fluid loss.[6]

■ Obtain the patient's baseline weight (in kilograms) before initiation of peritoneal dialysis therapy, and then weigh the patient daily. Obtain the patient's weight consistently with or without fluid dwelling. Use the same scale and make sure the patient wears similar clothing *to ensure consistency for accurate weight measurement.*[6]

■ Clean and disinfect your identified work surface.[2]

■ If you're using an automated peritoneal dialysis machine, program the machine as prescribed and according to the manufacturer's instructions for use.

For the instillation phase

■ Perform hand hygiene.[15,16,17,18,19,20]

■ Raise the patient's bed to waist level when providing care *to prevent caregiver back strain.*[27]

■ Position the patient with the head and upper torso elevated during infusion and drainage of dialysate, if possible, *to prevent respiratory compromise when infusing dialysate and to maximize gravity effect when draining dialysate.*[6] Position the patient supine if peritoneal dialysis becomes necessary during the first 2 weeks after catheter insertion.

■ Perform hand hygiene.[15,16,17,18,19,20]

■ Hang the dialysate solution bag on an IV pole, and connect the peritoneal dialysis administration set to the dialysate; prime the dialysis administration set tubing with the dialysate to purge the system of air, *because air in the peritoneum can cause pain and interfere with filling.* Clamp the tubing between the dialysate bag and the patient.[2]

■ Place the drainage bag on a clean surface below the mid-abdominal area *to facilitate drainage.*[2]

■ Put on a mask and assist the patient with putting on a mask.[2,6]

■ Perform hand hygiene.[15,16,17,18,19,20]

■ Prepare a sterile field using a sterile drape. Open a sterile container package or sterile 4″ × 4″ (10 cm × 10 cm) gauze pads. Pour antiseptic solution into a sterile container or onto the gauze pads.[2]

■ Put on gloves and, as needed, other personal protective equipment *to comply with standard precautions.*[28,29,30]

■ If there's a dressing covering the peritoneal catheter, carefully remove the dressing without pulling on the catheter, and then discard the dressing.[2,29]

■ Check the skin integrity at the catheter exit site and assess for signs of infection, such as purulent drainage, redness, or edema. If drainage is present, notify the practitioner. Obtain a specimen, if ordered, using a sterile swab, put it in a specimen container or a sterile culture tube with transport medium, and label the specimen in the presence of the patient *to prevent mislabeling.*[2,21]

■ Palpate the catheter exit site and subcutaneous tunnel route for tenderness or pain. If these symptoms occur, notify the practitioner.[2]

■ Remove and discard your gloves.[29]

■ Perform hand hygiene.[15,16,17,18,19,20]

■ Put on sterile gloves.[2,6,28,29]

■ Scrub the catheter–cap connection using a gauze pad soaked in antiseptic solution.[6] The antiseptic solution effectiveness depends on the length of scrub time. Povidone-iodine requires 2 to 3 minutes, hypochlorite requires 1 minute, and chlorhexidine requires 30 seconds. Follow the manufacturer's instructions for the correct disinfectant to use.[2]

■ Wrap another antiseptic-soaked gauze pad around the distal end of the transfer set–cap connection and leave it in place for 5 minutes *to reduce the transmission of microorganisms.*[6]

■ Remove and discard the used gauze pad and allow the catheter–cap connection to dry.[2,6,29]

■ Remove the cap and wrap another antiseptic-soaked gauze pad around the catheter adapter *to disinfect the open catheter adapter.*[6]

■ Using sterile technique, attach the dialysate administration set to the transfer set. Be sure to secure the Luer-lock connector tightly.[6]

■ Trace the tubing from the patient to its point of origin *to make sure that you're connecting the tubing to the correct port* (shown below).[31,32]

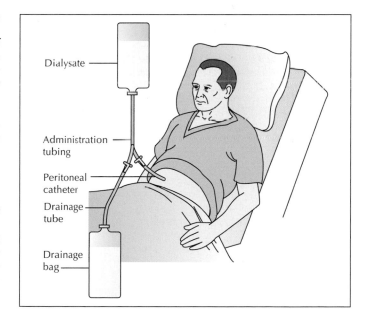

■ Unclamp the catheter and dialysate administration set tubing and instill the dialysate as ordered. Alternatively, unclamp the catheter and allow the peritoneal dialysis machine to instill the dialysate.[2]

■ Monitor the flow of the dialysate, making sure the catheter isn't kinked or occluded.

■ Remove and discard the patient's mask.[29]

■ Return the bed to the lowest position *to prevent falls and maintain the patient's safety.*[33]

■ Monitor the patient's vital signs, as ordered or according to the patient's condition, *to assess for signs of hypovolemia (hypotension and tachycardia) and sudden release of intraperitoneal pressure.* Notify the practitioner if the patient develops hypotension, tachycardia, or abdominal pain.[2]

■ Discard used supplies in the appropriate receptacles.[29]

■ Remove and discard your gloves, mask, and other personal protective equipment if worn.[29]

■ Perform hand hygiene.[15,16,17,18,19,20]

For the dwell phase

- If you're using a manual system, after the dialysate infuses, close the clamp on the transfer set and peritoneal dialysis administration set tubing *to make sure that air doesn't enter the patient's peritoneum.*
- If the patient's schedule requires disconnection from the system during the dwell phase, disconnect the patient from the system.
- Put on a mask and have the patient put on a mask.[2]
- Perform hand hygiene.[15,16,17,18,19,20]
- Put on sterile gloves and, as needed, other personal protective equipment.[28,29]
- Thoroughly disinfect the catheter connection as directed by your facility and according to the manufacturer's instructions.[2]
- Using a sterile gauze pad, disconnect the peritoneal dialysis administration set tubing from the transfer set.
- Using sterile technique, carefully connect the catheter cap to the transfer set.
- Secure the catheter to the patient's abdomen.
- Remove and discard the patient's mask.[29]
- Remove and discard your gloves, mask, and other personal protective equipment if worn.[29]
- Perform hand hygiene.[15,16,17,18,19,20]
- Allow the solution to dwell for the prescribed dwell time.
- Explain that the patient may resume normal activities during the prescribed dialysate solution dwell time.

For the drain phase

- If the patient was disconnected from the system during the prescribed dwell time, reconnect the patient to the peritoneal dialysis catheter following the attachment steps after the prescribed dwell time elapses.
- If you're using a manual system, place the drainage bag below the patient's mid-abdominal area *to enhance gravity flow;* unclamp the transfer set and drainage bag tubing and allow the drainage to flow from the patient's peritoneal cavity.[2] Alternatively, make sure that the peritoneal dialysis machine is functioning according to the drain phase.
- Assist the patient with position changes as needed *to facilitate drainage.*[2]
- Observe the appearance of the effluent; the fluid may be bloody or pink after catheter insertion but should become clear and colorless to light yellow after the first few exchanges. Suspect peritonitis if the fluid appears cloudy; notify the practitioner and obtain a specimen for laboratory testing if ordered. Label the specimen in the presence of the patient *to prevent mislabeling.*[21] Place the specimen in a laboratory biohazard transport bag and send it to the laboratory immediately with the appropriate laboratory request form (if necessary).[29]
- If you're using a manual system, clamp or close the transfer set and clamp the drainage bag tubing after the peritoneal fluid drains completely.
- Obtain the weight of the drainage bag or measure the drainage volume as ordered *to ensure adequate drainage and assess intake and output.*[2]

Completing the procedure

- Perform hand hygiene.[15,16,17,18,19,20]
- Raise the patient's bed to waist level before providing care *to prevent caregiver back strain.*[27]
- Perform hand hygiene.[15,16,17,18,19,20]
- Put on a mask and assist the patient in putting on a mask.[2,6]
- Perform hand hygiene.[15,16,17,18,19,20]
- Set up a sterile field using a sterile drape. Open a sterile container package or sterile 4″ × 4″ (10 cm × 10 cm) gauze pads. Pour antiseptic solution into a sterile container or onto the gauze pads.[6]
- Put on sterile gloves and, as needed, other personal protective equipment.[6,28,29]
- Disconnect the peritoneal dialysis administration set tubing from the transfer set.[34]
- If required by your facility, disinfect the end of the transfer set.[6] Some facilities don't require disinfection of the catheter if a new sterile cap is attached to the transfer set.[34] If using a disinfectant-containing disconnect cap, visually inspect the cap *to ensure wetness.*
- With the transfer set pointing downward, attach the cap to the transfer set using sterile no-touch technique.[2,34]

- Using the antiseptic-soaked gauze pads, clean the catheter and exit site junction (following the antiseptic manufacturer's instructions) and then allow them to air-dry.[2]
- Apply an antibiotic ointment to the catheter exit site if ordered following safe medication administration practices.[7,11,12,13,14]
- Apply a new dressing to the catheter exit site if needed.[35]
- Secure the catheter and transfer set to the patient's abdomen using hypoallergenic tape or other securement device *to prevent accidental dislodgment.*[2]
- Remove and discard the patient's mask.[29]
- Return the bed to the lowest position *to prevent falls and maintain the patient's safety.*[33]
- Discard used supplies in the appropriate receptacles.[2,29]
- Remove and discard your gloves, mask, and other personal protective equipment if worn.[29]
- Perform hand hygiene.[15,16,17,18,19,20]
- Clean and disinfect your stethoscope using a disinfectant pad.[36,37]
- Perform hand hygiene.[15,16,17,18,19,20]
- Document the procedure.[38,39,40,41]

Special considerations

- Change the catheter dressing at an interval determined by your facility or whenever it becomes wet or soiled.[2,35]

NURSING ALERT If the patient suffers severe respiratory distress during the dwell phase of dialysis, immediately drain the peritoneal cavity and notify the practitioner. Carefully monitor any patient on peritoneal dialysis who's being weaned from a ventilator.

- Dialysate is available in three concentrations: 4.25%, 2.5%, and 1.5% dextrose.[6] The 4.25% solution usually removes the largest amount of fluid from the blood *because its glucose concentration is highest.*[2] If your patient receives this concentrated solution, monitor the patient carefully *to prevent excess fluid loss.* Also, some of the glucose in the 4.25% solution may enter the patient's bloodstream, causing hyperglycemia severe enough to require an insulin injection or an insulin addition to the dialysate.
- Patients with low serum potassium levels may require the addition of potassium to the dialysate solution *to prevent further losses.*[42]
- Heparin is commonly added to the dialysate *to prevent occlusion of fibrin in the dialysis catheter.*[2,42]
- *To reduce the risk of peritonitis,* use strict sterile technique during the catheter insertion, dialysate exchanges, and dressing changes. Ensure all personnel and the patient wear masks in the room whenever the dialysis system is opened or entered.[2]
- Monitor the patient's hemodynamic status.[2] Note the patient's fluid balance at the end of each infusion–dwell–drain cycle. (The fluid balance is positive if the patient retains fluid at the end of an exchange and negative if you recover more fluid than was instilled with the exchange.) Notify the practitioner if the patient retains 500 mL or more of fluid for three consecutive cycles or loses 1 L of fluid for three consecutive cycles.
- If dialysate instillation or drainage is slow or absent, check all of the tubing for kinks. You can also try raising the IV pole or repositioning the patient *to increase the inflow rate.* Repositioning the patient or applying manual pressure to the lateral aspects of the patient's abdomen may also help increase drainage. If these maneuvers fail, notify the practitioner, *because the catheter may be improperly positioned or an accumulation of fibrin may be obstructing the catheter.*[2]
- Always examine the drained fluid from each exchange (effluent) for color and clarity. Normally, the fluid is clear or pale yellow, but pink-tinged effluent may appear during the first three or four cycles.[1] If the effluent remains pink-tinged or if it's grossly bloody, suspect bleeding into the peritoneal cavity and notify the practitioner.[2] Also notify the practitioner if the effluent contains feces, which suggests bowel perforation; if it's cloudy, which suggests peritonitis; or if fibrin is present. Obtain a specimen for culture and Gram stain, as ordered. Place the specimen in a labeled specimen container, place the container in a laboratory biohazard transport bag, and send it to the laboratory with a laboratory request form (if necessary).

- Expect patient discomfort at the start of the procedure. If the patient experiences pain during the procedure, determine when it occurs, its quality and duration, and whether it radiates to other body parts, and notify the practitioner. Pain during infusion usually results from a dialysate that's too cool or acidic.[1] Pain may also result from rapid instillation; slowing the inflow rate may reduce the pain. Severe, diffuse pain with rebound tenderness and cloudy effluent may indicate peritoneal infection.[1] Pain that radiates to the shoulder often results from air accumulation under the diaphragm. Severe, persistent perineal or rectal pain can result from improper catheter placement.
- During and after dialysis, monitor the patient; assess abdominal and respiratory status and response to treatment.[2]
- Monitor the patient's vital signs according to the patient's condition and at an interval determined by your facility; *there's no evidence-based research to indicate best practice for frequency of vital signs assessment.*[43] Notify the practitioner of any abrupt changes in the patient's condition.
- Monitor the patient's fluid and electrolyte status.[2] Report unexpected results to the practitioner and administer fluids and electrolytes, as prescribed.
- Check whether your facility has a clearly developed curriculum for peritoneal dialysis training.[35]
- Keep in mind that the patient who requires peritoneal dialysis will need your support related to a potential alteration in body image and ability to live a satisfying lifestyle. Encourage the patient and caregiver to build a support system or to use available support systems.[44,45]

Patient teaching

If the patient or a caregiver is to perform peritoneal dialysis in the home, begin teaching about its purpose and indications, as well as appropriate techniques for preparation, instillation, and drainage of dialysate, and methods to troubleshoot complications. Ensure that the patient is aware of the importance of infection control, proper diet and hydration, routine care and maintenance of the catheter and insertion site, and compliance with the prescribed regimen. Review potential complications, and instruct the patient or caregiver to immediately report cloudy effluent, abdominal pain, and fever, and to save any drained, cloudy dialysate to bring to the dialysis clinic.[46] Provide the patient with contact information to report complications, and additional educational information and resources as indicated.

Complications

Complications of peritoneal dialysis may include peritonitis, mild abdominal pain or bloating, intra-abdominal bleeding, leakage around the catheter site, inadequate drainage, and bowel perforation. Respiratory distress can occur when dialysate in the peritoneal cavity increases pressure on the diaphragm, which decreases lung expansion, leading to atelectasis and pneumonia. Pleural effusion, gastroesophageal reflux, and aspiration are also possible. Protein depletion can result from the diffusion of protein in the blood into the dialysate solution through the peritoneal membrane. Excessive fluid loss can cause hypovolemia, hypotension, and shock. Excessive fluid retention can lead to blood volume expansion, hypertension, peripheral edema, and even pulmonary edema and heart failure. Other possible complications include glucose and electrolyte imbalances as well as arrhythmias.[5]

Documentation

Record the type and amount of dialysate infused and drained, any medications added to the dialysate solution, and the color and character of the effluent. Record the patient's daily weight and fluid balance. Use a peritoneal dialysis flowchart to compute total fluid balance after each exchange. Note your assessment findings, including the patient's vital signs and tolerance of the treatment, as well as other pertinent observations. Note any complications, the name of the practitioner notified, the date and time of notification, any prescribed interventions, and the patient's response to the interventions. Document teaching provided to the patient and family (if applicable), their understanding of that teaching, and any need for follow-up teaching.

REFERENCES

1 Hinkle, J. L., & Cheever, K. H. (2018). *Brunner & Suddarth's textbook of medical-surgical nursing* (14th ed.). Philadelphia, PA: Wolters Kluwer.
2 Wiegand, D. L. (2017). *AACN procedure manual for high acuity, progressive, and critical care* (7th ed.). St. Louis, MO: Elsevier.
3 American Nephrology Nurses Association. (2017). *Nephrology nursing: Scope and standards of practice* (8th ed.). Pitman, NJ: American Nephrology Nurses Association.
4 National Kidney Foundation. (2006). Clinical practice guidelines and clinical practice recommendations: 2006 updates: Peritoneal dialysis adequacy. http://kidneyfoundation.cachefly.net/professionals/KDOQI/guideline_upHD_PD_VA/index.htm (Level VII)
5 Golper, T. A., & Ponce, D. (2020). Use of peritoneal dialysis (PD) for the treatment of acute kidney injury (AKI) in adults. In: *UpToDate*, Schwab, S. J. (Ed.).
6 American Nephrology Nurses Association. (2020). *Core curriculum for nephrology nurses* (7th ed.). Pitman, NJ: American Nephrology Nurses Association.
7 Szeto, C., et al. (2017). ISPD catheter-related infection recommendations: 2017 update. *Peritoneal Dialysis International, 37*(2), 141–154. https://journals.sagepub.com/doi/pdf/10.3747/pdi.2016.00120 (Level VII)
8 National Institute of Diabetes and Digestive and Kidney Diseases. (2018). Peritoneal dialysis. https://www.niddk.nih.gov/health-information/kidney-disease/kidney-failure/peritoneal-dialysis
9 Westbrook, J., et al. (2010). Association of interruptions with an increased risk and severity of medication administration errors. *Archives of Internal Medicine, 170*(8), 683–690. https://doi.org/10.1001/archinternmed.2010.65 (Level IV)
10 Institute for Safe Medication Practices. (2012). Side tracks on the safety express: Interruptions lead to errors and unfinished...Wait, what was I doing? *Nurse Advise-ERR, 11*(2), 1–4. https://www.ismp.org/Newsletters/acutecare/showarticle.aspx?id=37
11 Accreditation Association for Hospitals and Health Systems. (2020). Standard 16.01.03. *Healthcare Facilities Accreditation Program: Accreditation requirements for acute care hospitals.* (Level VII)
12 Centers for Medicare and Medicaid Services, Department of Health and Human Services. (2020). Condition of participation: Nursing services. 42 C.F.R. § 482.23(c).
13 The Joint Commission. (2021). Standard MM.06.01.01. *Comprehensive accreditation manual for hospitals.* (Level VII)
14 DNV GL-Healthcare USA, Inc. (2020). MM.1.SR.3. *NIAHO® accreditation requirements, interpretive guidelines and surveyor guidance—revision 20.0.* (Level VII)
15 Centers for Disease Control and Prevention. (2002). Guideline for hand hygiene in health-care settings: Recommendations of the Healthcare Infection Control Practices Advisory Committee and the HICPAC/SHEA/APIC/IDSA Hand Hygiene Task Force. *MMWR Recommendations and Reports, 51*(RR-16), 1–45. https://www.cdc.gov/mmwr/pdf/rr/rr5116.pdf (Level II)
16 World Health Organization (WHO). (2009). WHO guidelines on hand hygiene in health care: First global patient safety challenge, clean care is safer care. https://apps.who.int/iris/bitstream/handle/10665/44102/9789241597906_eng.pdf?sequence=1 (Level IV)
17 The Joint Commission. (2021). Standard NPSG.07.01.01. *Comprehensive accreditation manual for hospitals.* (Level VII)
18 Centers for Medicare and Medicaid Services, Department of Health and Human Services. (2020). Condition of participation: Infection control. 42 C.F.R. § 482.42.
19 Accreditation Association for Hospitals and Health Systems. (2020). Standard 07.01.21. *Healthcare Facilities Accreditation Program: Accreditation requirements for acute care hospitals.* (Level VII)
20 DNV GL-Healthcare USA, Inc. (2020). IC.1.SR.1. *NIAHO® accreditation requirements, interpretive guidelines and surveyor guidance—revision 20.0.* (Level VII)
21 The Joint Commission. (2021). Standard NPSG.01.01.01. *Comprehensive accreditation manual for hospitals.* (Level VII)
22 Centers for Medicare and Medicaid Services, Department of Health and Human Services. (2020). Condition of participation: Patient's rights. 42 C.F.R. § 482.13(c)(1).
23 Accreditation Association for Hospitals and Health Systems. (2020). Standard 15.01.16. *Healthcare Facilities Accreditation Program: Accreditation requirements for acute care hospitals.* (Level VII)

24 The Joint Commission. (2021). Standard RI.01.01.01. *Comprehensive accreditation manual for hospitals.* (Level VII)

25 DNV GL-Healthcare USA, Inc. (2020). PR.2.SR.5. *NIAHO® accreditation requirements, interpretive guidelines and surveyor guidance—revision 20.0.* (Level VII)

26 The Joint Commission. (2021). Standard PC.02.01.21. *Comprehensive accreditation manual for hospitals.* (Level VII)

27 Waters, T. R., et al. (2009). Safe patient handling training for schools of nursing. https://www.cdc.gov/niosh/docs/2009-127/pdfs/2009-127.pdf (Level VII)

28 Siegel, J. D., et al. (2007, revised 2019). 2007 guideline for isolation precautions: Preventing transmission of infectious agents in healthcare settings. https://www.cdc.gov/infectioncontrol/pdf/guidelines/isolation-guidelines-H.pdf (Level II)

29 Occupational Safety and Health Administration. (2019). Bloodborne pathogens, standard number 1910.1030. https://www.osha.gov/pls/oshaweb/owadisp.show_document?p_id=10051&p_table=STANDARDS (Level VII)

30 Accreditation Association for Hospitals and Health Systems. (2020). Standard 07.01.10. *Healthcare Facilities Accreditation Program: Accreditation requirements for acute care hospitals.* (Level VII)

31 U.S. Food and Drug Administration. (2017). Examples of medical device misconnections. https://www.fda.gov/medical-devices/medical-device-connectors/examples-medical-device-misconnections

32 The Joint Commission. (2014). Sentinel event alert 53: Managing risk during transition to new ISO tubing connector standards. https://www.jointcommission.org/-/media/tjc/documents/resources/patient-safety-topics/sentinel-event/sea_53_connectors_8_19_14_final.pdf (Level VII)

33 Ganz, D. A., et al. (2013, Reviewed 2021). *Preventing falls in hospitals: A toolkit for improving quality of care* (AHRQ Publication No. 13-0015-EF). Agency for Healthcare Research and Quality. https://www.ahrq.gov/professionals/systems/hospital/fallpxtoolkit/index.html (Level VII)

34 Baxter. (2007). Ultrabag aseptic exchange procedure. http://www.capd.org.tw/4_2/UltraBagusa.pdf

35 Piraino, B., et al. (2011). ISPD position statement on reducing the risks of peritoneal dialysis–related infections. *Peritoneal Dialysis International, 31*(6), 614–630. https://ispd.org/media/pdf/Perit_Dial_Int-2011-Piraino-614-30.pdf (Level VII)

36 Rutala, W. A., et al. (2008, revised 2019). Guideline for disinfection and sterilization in healthcare facilities, 2008. https://www.cdc.gov/infectioncontrol/pdf/guidelines/disinfection-guidelines-H.pdf (Level I)

37 Accreditation Association for Hospitals and Health Systems. (2020). Standard 07.02.03. *Healthcare Facilities Accreditation Program: Accreditation requirements for acute care hospitals.* (Level VII)

38 The Joint Commission. (2021). Standard RC.01.03.01. *Comprehensive accreditation manual for hospitals.* (Level VII)

39 Centers for Medicare and Medicaid Services, Department of Health and Human Services. (2020). Condition of participation: Medical record services. 42 C.F.R. § 482.24(b).

40 Accreditation Association for Hospitals and Health Systems. (2020). Standard 10.00.03. *Healthcare Facilities Accreditation Program: Accreditation requirements for acute care hospitals.* (Level VII)

41 DNV GL-Healthcare USA, Inc. (2020). MR.2.SR.1. *NIAHO® accreditation requirements, interpretive guidelines and surveyor guidance—revision 20.0.* (Level VII)

42 Alam, M., & Krause, M. W. (2021). Peritoneal dialysis solutions. In: *UpToDate*, Golper, T. A. (Ed.).

43 American Society of PeriAnesthesia Nurses (ASPAN). (2020). *2021–2022 Perianesthesia nursing standards, practice recommendations and interpretive statements.* Cherry Hill, NJ: ASPAN. (Level VII)

44 Moore, R., & Teitelbaum, I. (2009). Preventing burnout in peritoneal dialysis patients. *Advances in Peritoneal Dialysis, 25*, 92–95. http://www.advancesinpd.com/adv09/308a-Moore-Final.pdf (Level V)

45 Burkart, J. M. (2021). Patient education: Peritoneal dialysis (beyond the basics). In: *UpToDate*, Golper, T. A. (Ed.).

46 Li, P. K., et al. (2016). ISPD peritonitis recommendations: 2016 update on prevention and treatment. *Peritoneal Dialysis International, 36*(5), 481–508. https://journals.sagepub.com/doi/pdf/10.3747/pdi.2016.00078 (Level VII)

PERITONEAL LAVAGE, ASSISTING

Peritoneal lavage may be used by the practitioner for both diagnostic and therapeutic purposes.[1] It's used mainly as a diagnostic tool in patients who have blunt abdominal trauma to help detect bleeding in the peritoneal cavity, or for obtaining cytology specimens in patients with cancer. It's used therapeutically in patients with hypothermia to warm the abdominal cavity, and in those with peritonitis or intra-abdominal abscess to provide irrigation.[1]

The test may proceed through several steps. Initially, the practitioner inserts a trocar or catheter through the abdominal wall into the peritoneal cavity and aspirates the peritoneal fluid with a syringe. If blood isn't visible in the aspirated fluid, a warmed lavage solution is infused and then siphoned from the cavity. The practitioner inspects the siphoned fluid for blood and also sends fluid samples to the laboratory for microscopic examination. When possible, the patient may undergo abdominal ultrasound before peritoneal lavage for assessment of fluid in the abdominal cavity, or during the procedure for assistance with catheter placement.[1]

The health care team maintains strict sterile technique throughout this procedure to avoid introducing microorganisms into the peritoneum and causing peritonitis. (See *Tapping the peritoneal cavity.*)

Because of the widespread availability of computed tomography (CT) scanning and focused assessment with sonography for trauma patients (FAST), peritoneal lavage is no longer used as commonly as it was in

---

Tapping the peritoneal cavity

After preparing the patient's skin with an antiseptic solution and administering a local anesthetic *to numb the area near the patient's umbilicus,* the practitioner will make a small incision (about ¾" [2 cm]) through the skin and subcutaneous tissues of the abdominal wall. The practitioner will retract the tissue, ligate several blood vessels, and use sterile 4" × 4" (10 cm × 10 cm) gauze pads to absorb incisional blood and keep it from entering the wound and producing a false-positive test result. Next, the practitioner directs a trocar or catheter through the incision into the pelvic midline until the instrument enters the peritoneum. Then the practitioner advances the trocar or catheter 6" to 8" (15 to 20 cm) into the pelvis.

Using a syringe attached to the trocar or catheter, the practitioner aspirates fluid from the peritoneal cavity and looks for blood or other abnormal findings.

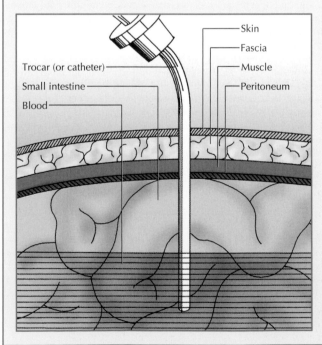

the past. In trauma patients, it remains most useful in hemodynamically unstable patients with a negative or uncertain FAST.[2,3]

Peritoneal lavage is contraindicated in a patient who requires immediate laparotomy.[1,2] Relative contraindications include multiple abdominal surgeries (owing to adhesions, especially in pelvic surgery), severe bowel distention, abdominal wall hematoma, medical instability, severe obesity, advanced cirrhosis, obvious infection at the intended site of catheter insertion, coagulopathies, or inability to perform urinary catheterization before the procedure.[1] The procedure is also contraindicated in a patient whose stomach and bladder can't be decompressed. The procedure requires great caution, and a different technique if the patient is pregnant or has a suspected pelvic fracture because of potential false-positive results.[1]

Equipment

Vital signs monitoring equipment ▪ cardiac monitoring equipment ▪ pulse oximeter and probe ▪ indwelling urinary (Foley) catheter insertion equipment ▪ nasogastric (NG) tube insertion equipment ▪ gastric suction machine ▪ IV pole ▪ macrodrip IV administration set ▪ 1 mL of warmed lavage solution (typically, sterile lactated Ringer normal saline solution) ▪ peritoneal lavage tray ▪ sterile gloves ▪ gown ▪ masks with face shields or goggles ▪ gloves ▪ caps ▪ antiseptic solution (povidone-iodine or chlorhexidine) ▪ 3-mL syringe with 25G 1″ (2.5-cm) needle ▪ sterile towels or drapes ▪ specimen collection containers, including one sterile tube for a culture and sensitivity testing ▪ labels ▪ sterile 4″ × 4″ (10 cm × 10 cm) gauze pads ▪ antiseptic pads ▪ 1″ (2.5 cm) hypoallergenic tape ▪ 2-0 and 3-0 sutures ▪ laboratory biohazard transport bag ▪ trocar or catheter ▪ emergency equipment (code cart with emergency medications, defibrillator, handheld resuscitation bag and mask, and intubation equipment) ▪ Optional: single-patient-use scissors or disposable-head surgical clippers, prescribed analgesic, prescribed sedative, laboratory request form, 1% lidocaine with EPINEPHrine, three-way stopcock, drainage collection bag, IV catheter insertion equipment, sterile marking pen, sterile ultrasound equipment and supplies.

If using a commercially prepared peritoneal lavage kit, ensure the macrodrip IV administration set doesn't have a reverse-flow (or back-check) valve that prevents infused fluid from draining out of the peritoneal cavity.

Preparation of equipment

Inspect all equipment and supplies. If a product is expired, is defective, or has compromised integrity, remove it from patient use, label it as expired or defective, and report the expiration or defect as directed by your facility. Make sure emergency equipment is functioning properly and readily available.

Implementation

▪ Gather and prepare the necessary equipment and supplies.
▪ If required by your facility, confirm that written informed consent was obtained and that the signed consent form is in the patient's medical record.[4,5,6,7]
▪ Review the patient's medical record for a history of any allergies to medications or latex and any contraindications to the procedure.
▪ Conduct a preprocedure verification *to make sure that all relevant documentation, related information, and equipment are available and correctly identified to the patient's identifiers.*[8,9]
▪ Verify that the laboratory and imaging studies have been completed as ordered, and that the results are in the patient's medical record. Notify the practitioner of any unexpected results.[9]
▪ Perform hand hygiene.[10,11,12,13,14,15]
▪ Confirm the patient's identity using at least two patient identifiers.[16]
▪ Provide privacy.[17,18,19,20]
▪ Reinforce the practitioner's explanation of the procedure to the patient and family (if appropriate) according to their individual communication and learning needs *to increase their understanding, allay their fears, and enhance cooperation.*[21] Answer any questions. Tell the patient to expect a sensation of abdominal fullness and possibly a chill if the lavage solution hasn't been warmed or doesn't reach body temperature.

▪ Confirm that the correct procedure has been identified for the correct patient at the correct site.[8]
▪ Raise the patient's bed to waist level before providing patient care *to prevent caregiver back strain.*[22]
▪ Perform hand hygiene.[10,11,12,13,14,15]
▪ Put on gloves as necessary *to comply with standard precautions.*[23,24,25]
▪ Ensure that the patient is attached to a cardiac monitor and pulse oximeter *for monitoring throughout the procedure.* Ensure that the alarm limits are set appropriately for the patient's current condition, and that the alarms are turned on, functioning properly, and audible to staff.[26,27,28]
▪ Obtain the patient's vital signs and oxygen saturation level using pulse oximetry *to serve as a baseline for comparison during and after the procedure.*
▪ If family members will remain present for the procedure, ask them to perform hand hygiene and to put on gowns, gloves, masks, a cap, and goggles.[1,29]
▪ Insert an indwelling urinary catheter and attach it to a drainage collection bag, as ordered, *to decompress the bladder and decrease the risk of the practitioner accidentally perforating the bladder during the procedure.*[1,2] (See the "Indwelling urinary catheter insertion" procedure.)
▪ Insert an NG tube, as ordered.[1,2] (See the "Nasogastric tube insertion and removal" procedure.) Trace the NG tubing from the patient to its point of origin *to make sure that you're assessing the correct tubing.*[30,31] Attach the tubing to the gastric suction machine (set for low intermittent suction) *to drain the patient's stomach contents. Decompressing the stomach prevents vomiting and subsequent aspiration, and minimizes the possibility of bowel perforation during trocar or catheter insertion.* Ensure an X-ray is obtained *to verify placement of the NG tube.*
▪ Confirm the patient has patent IV access. Insert an IV catheter as necessary.
▪ Remove hair, as necessary, from the insertion site using single-patient-use scissors or disposable-head surgical clippers.[1,32]
▪ Remove and discard your gloves, if worn.[24]
▪ Perform hand hygiene.[10,11,12,13,14,15]
▪ Set up the peritoneal lavage equipment. Attach macrodrip IV tubing to the warmed lavage solution and prime the system *to avoid introducing air into the peritoneal cavity during lavage.*[1] Place the setup on an IV pole. If you're using a drainage collection bag, attach a three-way stopcock to the end of the macrodrip IV administration set and attach the drainage collection bag to the other port of the stopcock. Alternatively, plan to use the lavage solution bag as the drainage collection bag.
▪ Place the patient in the supine position.[1]
▪ Administer analgesics or sedatives, if ordered and indicated, following safe medication administration practices.[33,34,35,36] Pain or agitation in the patient may indicate the need for analgesia or sedation *to facilitate patient comfort, safety, and cooperation.*
▪ Perform hand hygiene.[10,11,12,13,14,15]
▪ Using sterile no-touch technique, open the peritoneal lavage tray. Label all medications, medication containers, and other solutions on and off the sterile field.[37,38]
▪ Put on a gown, a mask and goggles or a mask with face shield, and gloves *to comply with standard precautions.*[1,23,24,25]
▪ Assist the practitioner with setting up the sterile field and putting on personal protective equipment. The practitioner disinfects the patient's abdomen from the costal margin to the pubic area and from flank to flank using an antiseptic solution and allows it to dry. The practitioner drapes the area with sterile towels or drapes *to create a sterile field.* The practitioner can consider using ultrasound *to aid in catheter insertion.*[1]
▪ The practitioner can mark the insertion site using a sterile marking pen.[1] The standard site for insertion is 2 cm to 3 cm below the patient's umbilicus, but alternative sites may be necessary depending on the clinical situation.[1,2]
▪ Conduct a time-out immediately before starting the procedure *to determine that the correct patient, site, positioning, and procedure are identified and, as applicable, that relevant information and necessary equipment are available.*[39]
▪ Using sterile technique, hand the practitioner the 3-mL syringe and the 25G 1″ (2.5 cm) needle. If the peritoneal lavage tray doesn't contain a sterile ampule of local anesthetic, disinfect the top of a multidose vial of 1% lidocaine with EPINEPHrine using an antiseptic pad and allow

Interpreting peritoneal lavage results

If test findings in peritoneal lavage are abnormal, the patient may need laparotomy and further treatment. The most common abnormal findings include:

■ unclotted blood, bile, or intestinal contents in aspirated peritoneal fluid (20 mL in an adult)

■ bloody or pinkish-red fluid returned from lavage—dark enough to obscure reading newsprint through it (if you can read newsprint through the fluid, test results are considered negative, although the practitioner may order more tests)

■ green, cloudy, turbid, or milky peritoneal fluid return (it normally appears clear to pale yellow)

■ red blood cell count greater than 100,000/mm³

■ white blood cell count greater than 500/mm³

■ bacteria in fluid (identified by culture and sensitivity or Gram stain testing).

If the patient's condition is stable, borderline positive results may suggest the need for additional tests, such as ultrasound or arteriogram. If test results are questionable or inconclusive, the practitioner may leave the catheter in place to repeat the procedure.

it to dry. Then, invert the vial at a 45-degree angle *to allow the practitioner to insert the needle and withdraw the anesthetic without touching the nonsterile vial.*

■ The practitioner injects the anesthetic directly below the umbilicus (or at an adjacent site if the patient has a surgical scar). After the area is anesthetized, the practitioner makes an incision, inserts the catheter or trocar, attaches a 20-mL syringe, and aspirates a lavage fluid specimen.[1]

■ If the results are positive for blood, the procedure will stop. As appropriate, prepare the patient for laparotomy and further measures. (See *Interpreting peritoneal lavage results.*)

■ If ordered, attach a peritoneal lavage catheter to the three-way stopcock, if used, or directly to the IV administration set.[1] Trace the IV administration set tubing from the patient to its point of origin *to make sure that you're connecting it to the proper port.*[30]

■ If ordered, instill 700 to 1,000 mL (10 mL/kg body weight) of the warmed lavage solution into the peritoneal cavity over 10 to 15 minutes by turning the stopcock off to the drainage collection bag, if used, and opening the clamp on the IV administration set. Then, clamp the IV tubing after instillation of the lavage solution.[1]

■ Unless contraindicated by the patient's injuries (such as a spinal cord injury, fractured ribs, or unstable pelvic fracture), gently tilt the patient from side to side *to distribute the fluid throughout the peritoneal cavity.* If the patient's condition contraindicates tilting, the practitioner may gently palpate the sides of the abdomen *to distribute the fluid.*[1]

■ After 5 to 10 minutes, drain the lavage fluid by turning the stopcock off to the IV tubing, if you're using a drainage collection bag, and allow the fluid to drain from the patient's peritoneal cavity. Alternatively, lower the lavage solution bag to the patient and unclamp the IV tubing *to facilitate drainage.*[1] Typically, the first 100 mL of lavage fluid is sent for laboratory analysis.[1]

■ Rotate the patient gently from side to side, if not contraindicated, *to drain fluid that may have settled in pockets in the patient's peritoneal cavity.*[1] Be careful not to disconnect the tubing from the catheter. The peritoneal cavity may take 20 to 30 minutes to drain completely.

■ Repeat the peritoneal lavage as needed *to cleanse the patient's peritoneal space.*[1]

■ Disconnect the peritoneal lavage catheter from the drainage tubing.[2]

■ After lavage fluid removal, the practitioner removes the peritoneal lavage catheter and closes the wound with sutures.[1]

■ Dress the insertion site with a sterile 4″ × 4″ (10 cm × 10 cm) gauze pad and secure the pad with 1″ (2.5 cm) hypoallergenic tape.

NURSING ALERT If the patient has fragile skin, use dressings and tape formulated specifically for fragile skin *to prevent skin tripping and tearing during removal.*[40]

■ Deposit the lavage fluid specimens in specimen collection containers for culture and sensitivity analysis; red and white blood cell counts;

amylase, lipase, and alkaline phosphatase level determinations; and spundown sediment evaluation, or as ordered.[1]

■ Label the collected specimens in the presence of the patient *to prevent mislabeling* and send them to the laboratory immediately in a laboratory biohazard transport bag.[16,24] If required, indicate the ordered tests on the laboratory request form.

■ Discard used supplies in the appropriate receptacles.[24]

■ Remove and discard your gloves and other personal protective equipment.[24]

■ Perform hand hygiene.[10,11,12,13,14,15]

■ Monitor vital signs according to the patient's condition and at an interval determined by your facility; *there's no evidence-based research to indicate best practice for frequency of vital signs assessment.*[41] Watch for and report signs and symptoms of shock (tachycardia, decreased blood pressure, diaphoresis, dyspnea, and vertigo) immediately.

■ Monitor the insertion site for bleeding, the oxygen saturation level using pulse oximetry, and the pulmonary status frequently.[1]

■ Screen and assess for the patient's pain using facility-defined criteria that are consistent with the patient's age, condition, and ability to understand.[42]

■ Treat the patient's pain as needed and ordered using nonpharmacologic, pharmacologic, or a combination of approaches. Base the treatment plan on evidence-based practices and the patient's clinical conditions, past medical history, and pain management goals.[42]

■ Return the patient's bed to the lowest position *to prevent falls and maintain patient safety.*[43]

■ Perform hand hygiene.[10,11,12,13,14,15]

■ Put on gloves.[23,24]

■ Clean and disinfect reusable equipment according to the manufacturer's instructions *to prevent the spread of infection.*[44,45]

■ Remove and discard your gloves.[24]

■ Perform hand hygiene.[10,11,12,13,14,15]

■ Document the procedure.[46,47,48,49]

Special considerations

■ Diagnostic peritoneal lavage may not identify a retroperitoneal bleed.[3,50]

Complications

Complications from peritoneal lavage may include bleeding from lacerated blood vessels at the incision site or intra-abdominally; bladder, stomach, or bowel perforation; local or systemic infection; hypovolemia; hypotension; bleeding from the insertion site; inadequate drainage of lavage fluid; respiratory compromise; and unrelieved pain.[1,2] False-positive results may occur due to misplacement of the trocar or catheter, injury to the diaphragm, or adhesions.[2]

Documentation

Record the date and time of the peritoneal lavage procedure, the type and size of the peritoneal lavage catheter used, the type and amount of lavage solution instilled and withdrawn from the patient's peritoneal cavity, and the amount and color of the fluid returned. Document whether the lavage fluid flowed freely into and out of the patient's abdomen. Note which specimens you obtained and sent to the laboratory. Document X-rays you obtained and results. Record all preprocedure and postprocedure assessments, including the patient's tolerance of the procedure. Also, note any complications, any interventions the practitioner ordered, and the patient's response to the interventions. Document any teaching you provided to the patient and family members (if applicable), their understanding of that teaching, and any need for follow-up teaching.

References

1 Wiegand, D. L. (2017). *AACN procedure manual for high acuity, progressive, and critical care* (7th ed.). St. Louis, MO: Elsevier.

2 Simon, R. J. (2020). Diagnostic peritoneal lavage. In: *UpToDate*, Bulger, E. M. (Ed.).

3 Jagminas, L. (2021). Diagnostic peritoneal lavage. https://emedicine.medscape.com/article/82888-overview

4 The Joint Commission. (2021). Standard RI.01.03.01. *Comprehensive accreditation manual for hospitals*. Oakbrook Terrace, IL: The Joint Commission. (Level VII)

5 DNV GL-Healthcare USA, Inc. (2020). PR.2.SR.3. *NIAHO® accreditation requirements, interpretive guidelines and surveyor guidance—revision 20.0*. Milford, OH: DNV GL-Healthcare USA, Inc. (Level VII)

6 Centers for Medicare and Medicaid Services, Department of Health and Human Services. (2020). Condition of participation: Patient's rights. 42 C.F.R. § 482.13(b)(2).

7 Accreditation Association for Hospitals and Health Systems. (2020). Standard 15.01.11. *Healthcare Facilities Accreditation Program: Accreditation requirements for acute care hospitals*. Chicago, IL: Accreditation Association for Hospitals and Health Systems. (Level VII)

8 The Joint Commission. (2021). Standard UP.01.01.01. *Comprehensive accreditation manual for hospitals*. Oakbrook Terrace, IL: The Joint Commission. (Level VII)

9 Accreditation Association for Hospitals and Health Systems. (2020). Standard 30.00.14. *Healthcare Facilities Accreditation Program: Accreditation requirements for acute care hospitals*. Chicago, IL: Accreditation Association for Hospitals and Health Systems. (Level VII)

10 Centers for Disease Control and Prevention. (2002). Guideline for hand hygiene in health-care settings: Recommendations of the Healthcare Infection Control Practices Advisory Committee and the HICPAC/SHEA/APIC/IDSA Hand Hygiene Task Force. *MMWR Recommendations and Reports, 51*(RR-16), 1–45. https://www.cdc.gov/mmwr/pdf/rr/rr5116.pdf (Level II)

11 World Health Organization. (2009). WHO guidelines on hand hygiene in health care: First global patient safety challenge, clean care is safer care. https://apps.who.int/iris/bitstream/handle/10665/44102/9789241597906_eng.pdf?sequence=1 (Level IV)

12 The Joint Commission. (2021). Standard NPSG.07.01.01. *Comprehensive accreditation manual for hospitals*. Oakbrook Terrace, IL: The Joint Commission. (Level VII)

13 Centers for Medicare and Medicaid Services, Department of Health and Human Services. (2020). Condition of participation: Infection control. 42 C.F.R. § 482.42.

14 Accreditation Association for Hospitals and Health Systems. (2020). Standard 07.01.21. *Healthcare Facilities Accreditation Program: Accreditation requirements for acute care hospitals*. Chicago, IL: Accreditation Association for Hospitals and Health Systems. (Level VII)

15 DNV GL-Healthcare USA, Inc. (2020). IC.1.SR.1. *NIAHO® accreditation requirements, interpretive guidelines and surveyor guidance—revision 20.0*. Milford, OH: DNV GL-Healthcare USA, Inc. (Level VII)

16 The Joint Commission. (2021). Standard NPSG.01.01.01. *Comprehensive accreditation manual for hospitals*. Oakbrook Terrace, IL: The Joint Commission. (Level VII)

17 Centers for Medicare and Medicaid Services, Department of Health and Human Services. (2020). Condition of participation: Patient's rights. 42 C.F.R. § 482.13(c)(1).

18 Accreditation Association for Hospitals and Health Systems. (2020). Standard 15.01.16. *Healthcare Facilities Accreditation Program: Accreditation requirements for acute care hospitals*. Chicago, IL: Accreditation Association for Hospitals and Health Systems. (Level VII)

19 The Joint Commission. (2021). Standard RI.01.01.01. *Comprehensive accreditation manual for hospitals*. Oakbrook Terrace, IL: The Joint Commission. (Level VII)

20 DNV GL-Healthcare USA, Inc. (2020). PR.2.SR.5. *NIAHO® accreditation requirements, interpretive guidelines and surveyor guidance—revision 20.0*. Milford, OH: DNV GL-Healthcare USA, Inc. (Level VII)

21 The Joint Commission. (2021). Standard PC.02.01.21. *Comprehensive accreditation manual for hospitals*. Oakbrook Terrace, IL: The Joint Commission. (Level VII)

22 Waters, T. R., et al. (2009). Safe patient handling training for schools of nursing. https://www.cdc.gov/niosh/docs/2009-127/pdfs/2009-127.pdf (Level VII)

23 Siegel, J. D., et al. (2007, revised 2019). 2007 guideline for isolation precautions: Preventing transmission of infectious agents in healthcare settings. https://www.cdc.gov/infectioncontrol/pdf/guidelines/isolation-guidelines-H.pdf (Level II)

24 Occupational Safety and Health Administration. (2019). Bloodborne pathogens, standard number 1910.1030. https://www.osha.gov/pls/oshaweb/owadisp.show_document?p_id=10051&p_table=STANDARDS (Level VII)

25 Accreditation Association for Hospitals and Health Systems. (2020). Standard 07.01.10. *Healthcare Facilities Accreditation Program: Accreditation requirements for acute care hospitals*. Chicago, IL: Accreditation Association for Hospitals and Health Systems. (Level VII)

26 American Association of Critical-Care Nurses. (2018). AACN practice alert: Managing alarms in acute care across the life span: Electrocardiography and pulse oximetry. https://www.aacn.org/clinical-resources/practice-alerts/managing-alarms-in-acute-care-across-the-life-span (Level VII)

27 The Joint Commission. (2021). Standard NPSG.06.01.01. *Comprehensive accreditation manual for hospitals*. Oakbrook Terrace, IL: The Joint Commission. (Level VII)

28 Graham, K. C., & Cvach, M. (2010). Monitor alarm fatigue: Standardizing use of physiological monitors and decreasing nuisance alarms. *American Journal of Critical Care, 19*, 28–37. https://aacnjournals.org/ajcconline/article-abstract/19/1/28/5720/Monitor-Alarm-Fatigue-Standardizing-Use-of?redirectedFrom=fulltext

29 American Association of Critical-Care Nurses. (2016). AACN practice alert: Family presence during resuscitation and invasive procedures. https://www.aacn.org/clinical-resources/practice-alerts/family-presence-during-resuscitation-and-invasive-procedures (Level VII)

30 U.S. Food and Drug Administration. (2017). Examples of medical device misconnections. https://www.fda.gov/medical-devices/medical-device-connectors/examples-medical-device-misconnections

31 The Joint Commission. (2014). Sentinel event alert 53: Managing risk during transition to new ISO tubing connector standards. https://www.jointcommission.org/-/media/tjc/documents/resources/patient-safety-topics/sentinel-event/sea_53_connectors_8_19_14_final.pdf (Level VII)

32 Guideline for perioperative practice: Preoperative patient skin antisepsis. (2020). In Wood, A. (Ed.), *Guidelines for perioperative practice*, 2020 edition. Denver, CO: AORN, Inc.

33 Centers for Medicare and Medicaid Services, Department of Health and Human Services. (2020). Condition of participation: Nursing services. 42 C.F.R. § 482.23(c).

34 Accreditation Association for Hospitals and Health Systems. (2020). Standard 16.01.03. *Healthcare Facilities Accreditation Program: Accreditation requirements for acute care hospitals*. Chicago, IL: Accreditation Association for Hospitals and Health Systems. (Level VII)

35 The Joint Commission. (2021). MM.06.01.01. *Comprehensive accreditation manual for hospitals*. Oakbrook Terrace, IL: The Joint Commission. (Level VII)

36 DNV GL-Healthcare USA, Inc. (2020). MM.1.SR.3. *NIAHO® accreditation requirements, interpretive guidelines and surveyor guidance—revision 20.0*. Milford, OH: DNV GL-Healthcare USA, Inc. (Level VII)

37 The Joint Commission. (2021). Standard NPSG.03.04.01. *Comprehensive accreditation manual for hospitals*. Oakbrook Terrace, IL: The Joint Commission. (Level VII)

38 Accreditation Association for Hospitals and Health Systems. (2020). Standard 25.01.27. *Healthcare Facilities Accreditation Program: Accreditation requirements for acute care hospitals*. Chicago, IL: Accreditation Association for Hospitals and Health Systems. (Level VII)

39 The Joint Commission. (2021). Standard UP.01.03.01. *Comprehensive accreditation manual for hospitals*. Oakbrook Terrace, IL: The Joint Commission. (Level VII)

40 LeBlanc, K., et al. (2013). International skin tear advisory panel: A tool kit to aid in the prevention, assessment, and treatment of skin tears using a simplified classification system. *Advances in Skin & Wound Care, 26*, 459–476. (Level IV)

41 American Society of PeriAnesthesia Nurses. (2019). *2019-2020 Perianesthesia nursing standards, practice recommendations and interpretive statements*. Cherry Hill, NJ: American Society of PeriAnesthesia Nurses. (Level VII)

42 The Joint Commission. (2021). Standard PC.01.02.07. *Comprehensive accreditation manual for hospitals*. Oakbrook Terrace, IL: The Joint Commission. (Level VII)

43 Ganz, D. A., et al. (2013, Reviewed 2021). *Preventing falls in hospitals: A toolkit for improving quality of care* (AHRQ publication no. 13-0015-EF). Rockville, MD: Agency for Healthcare Research and Quality. https://www.ahrq.gov/sites/default/files/publications/files/fallpxtoolkit_0.pdf (Level VII)

44 Rutala, W. A., et al. (2008, revised 2019). Guideline for disinfection and sterilization in healthcare facilities, 2008. https://www.cdc.gov/infection-control/pdf/guidelines/disinfection-guidelines-H.pdf (Level I)

45 Accreditation Association for Hospitals and Health Systems. (2020). Standard 07.02.03. *Healthcare Facilities Accreditation Program: Accreditation requirements for acute care hospitals.* Chicago, IL: Accreditation Association for Hospitals and Health Systems. (Level VII)

46 The Joint Commission. (2021). Standard RC.01.03.01. *Comprehensive accreditation manual for hospitals.* Oakbrook Terrace, IL: The Joint Commission. (Level VII)

47 Centers for Medicare and Medicaid Services, Department of Health and Human Services. (2020). Condition of participation: Medical record services. 42 C.F.R. § 482.24(b).

48 Accreditation Association for Hospitals and Health Systems. (2020). Standard 10.00.03. *Healthcare Facilities Accreditation Program: Accreditation requirements for acute care hospitals.* Chicago, IL: Accreditation Association for Hospitals and Health Systems. (Level VII)

49 DNV GL-Healthcare USA, Inc. (2020). MR.2.SR.1. *NIAHO® accreditation requirements, interpretive guidelines and surveyor guidance—revision 20.0.* Milford, OH: DNV GL-Healthcare USA, Inc. (Level VII)

50 Rothrock, J. C. (2019). *Alexander's care of the patient in surgery* (16th ed.). St. Louis, MO: Elsevier.

51 The Joint Commission. (2013). Sentinel event alert 50: Medical device alarm safety in hospitals. https://www.jointcommission.org/assets/1/6/SEA_50_alarms_4_26_16.pdf (Level VII)

Permanent pacemaker care

A permanent pacemaker is an implanted electronic device that provides electrical stimulation to the myocardium. Pacemakers are designed to last 5 to 15 years before requiring battery replacement, depending on the device and the amount of pacing it performs.[1,2] The surgeon implants the pacemaker in a pocket beneath the patient's skin. This procedure is usually done in the operating room, an electrophysiology laboratory, or a cardiac catheterization laboratory.

HOSPITAL-ACQUIRED CONDITION ALERT Keep in mind that the Centers for Medicare and Medicaid Services considers a surgical site infection after electronic cardiac device implantation a hospital-acquired infection *because it can be reasonably prevented using a variety of best practices.* Make sure to follow evidence-based infection prevention techniques, such as performing hand hygiene, advising the patient to shower or bathe with soap or an antiseptic agent the day before surgery, administering prophylactic antibiotics, maintaining glycemic control, and preparing the skin with an alcohol-based antiseptic agent (unless contraindicated) *to reduce the risk of surgical site infection.*[3,4]

Permanent pacemakers function in the demand mode, allowing the patient's heart to beat on its own but preventing it from falling below a preset rate. Pacing electrodes can be placed in the atria, the ventricles, or both chambers (atrioventricular [AV] sequential, dual chamber). (See *Understanding pacemaker codes.*) The most common pacing codes are VVI for single-chamber pacing and DDD for dual-chamber pacing.

Candidates for permanent pacemakers include patients with bradycardia due to symptomatic sinus node dysfunction, some acquired atrioventricular (AV) block disorders, conduction disorders, adult heart failure, acute myocardial infarction, epilepsy, and certain congenital heart diseases, and some patients after certain cardiac surgeries.[5]

A biventricular pacemaker is effective in patients with heart failure who have intraventricular conductor defects. This device differs from a standard pacemaker in that it has three leads instead of one or two. One lead is placed in the right atrium and the others are placed in each of the ventricles, where they simultaneously stimulate the right and left ventricle. This allows the ventricles to coordinate their pumping action, making the heart more efficient.

Equipment

Vital signs monitoring equipment ■ stethoscope ■ facility-approved pain assessment tool ■ pulse oximeter and probe ■ cardiac monitor with leads and electrodes ■ gloves ■ sterile gauze dressing ■ hypoallergenic tape ■ IV catheter insertion equipment ■ prescribed IV fluids ■ disinfectant pads ■ prescribed antibiotics ■ prescribed sedation ■ backup pacing device[6] ■ emergency equipment (code cart with emergency medications, defibrillation, handheld resuscitation bag with mask, intubation equipment)[6] ■ Optional: prescribed analgesic, prescribed antiseptic ointment, disposable-head clippers, ice pack.

Preparation of equipment

Make sure emergency equipment is functioning properly and readily available. Ensure that backup pacing device is readily available and functioning *in the event of pacemaker failure.*[6]

Inspect all equipment and supplies. If a product is expired, is defective, or has compromised integrity, remove it from patient use, label it as expired or defective, and report the expiration or defect as directed by your facility.

Implementation
Preoperative care
■ Verify the practitioner's order.

Understanding pacemaker codes

A permanent pacemaker's three-letter (or sometimes five-letter) code simply refers to how it's programmed. The first letter represents the chamber that is paced; the second letter, the chamber that is sensed; and the third letter, how the pulse generator responds. The fourth letter describes rate modulation, and the fifth letter specifies the location or absence of multisite pacing. Typically, only the first three letters are shown.

First letter	*Second letter*	*Third letter*	*Fourth letter*	*Fifth letter*
A = atrium	A = atrium	I = inhibited	R = rate modulation—a sensor adjusts the programmed heart rate in response to patient activity.	O = none
V = ventricle	V = ventricle	T = triggered		A = atrium or atria
D = dual (both chambers)	D = dual (both chambers)	D = dual (inhibited and triggered)		V = ventricle or ventricles
O = not applicable	O = not applicable	O = not applicable	O = none	D = dual site
S = single	S = single			

Examples of two common programming codes
DDD
Pace: atrium and ventricle
Sense: atrium and ventricle
Response: inhibited and triggered
This is a fully automatic, or universal, pacemaker.

VVI
Pace: ventricle
Sense: ventricle
Response: inhibited
This is a demand pacemaker, inhibited.

- Gather and prepare the necessary equipment and supplies.
- If required by your facility, confirm that written informed consent has been obtained and that the signed consent form is in the patient's medical record.[7,8,9,10]
- Review the patient's medical records for allergies to local anesthetics, iodine, or latex.
- Conduct a preprocedure verification *to make sure that all relevant documentation, related information, and equipment are available and correctly identified to the patient's identifiers.*[11,12]
- Verify that ordered laboratory and imaging studies are complete and that the results are in the patient's medical record. Notify the practitioner of any unexpected results.[11]
- Perform hand hygiene.[13,14,15,16,17,18]
- Confirm the patient's identity using at least two patient identifiers.[19]
- Provide privacy.[20,21,22,23]
- Reinforce the practitioner's explanation of the procedure to the patient and family (if appropriate) according to their individual communication and learning needs *to increase their understanding, allay their fears, and enhance cooperation.*[24] Answer any questions. Provide and review literature from the manufacturer or from the American Heart Association *so that the patient can learn about the pacemaker and how it works.* Emphasize that the pacemaker merely augments the patient's natural heart rate.
- Raise the patient's bed to waist level before providing patient care *to prevent caregiver back strain.*[25]
- Perform hand hygiene[13,14,15,16,17,18] and put on gloves *to comply with standard precautions.*[26,27,28]
- Obtain the patient's vital signs, oxygen saturation level using pulse oximetry and an electrocardiogram (ECG) tracing, and assess the level of consciousness, skin color, and cardiac and respiratory status *to serve as a baseline for comparison during and after the procedure.*
- Using disposable-head clippers, remove chest hair from the axilla to the midline and from the clavicle to the nipple line on the side selected by the surgeon, if necessary.
- Insert an IV catheter if the patient doesn't already have one, and administer IV fluids as ordered. (See the "IV catheter insertion and removal" procedure.)
- Confirm the patient's nothing-by-mouth status before the procedure; minimum fasting recommendations include 2 hours for clear liquids, 6 or more hours for a light meal or nonhuman milk, and 8 hours or more for fried or fatty foods or meat.[29]
- Administer antibiotics, as ordered, following safe medication administration practices.[30,31,32,33,34]
- Administer sedation, as ordered, following safe medication administration practices.[31,32,33,34]
- Return the bed to the lowest position *to prevent falls and maintain patient safety.*[35]
- Discard all used supplies in appropriate receptacles.[27]
- Remove and discard your gloves[27] and perform hand hygiene.[13,14,15,16,17,18]
- Disinfect your stethoscope using a disinfectant pad.[36,37]
- Perform hand hygiene.[13,14,15,16,17,18]
- Provide hand-off communication to the person who will assume responsibility for the patient's care during the procedure. Allow time for questions, as necessary, *to avoid miscommunications that may cause patient care errors during transitions of care.*[38,39,40] Use a hand-off communication technique, such as the situation-background-assessment-recommendation (SBAR) or another facility-approved communication technique, *to improve communication and reduce errors.*[39,40] As part of the hand-off process, allow time for the receiving staff member to trace each tubing and catheter from the patient to its point of origin; a standardized line reconciliation process should be used.[38,40,41,42]
- Document the procedure.[43,44,45,46]

Postoperative care

- Receive hand-off communication from the person who was responsible for the patient's care during the procedure. Ask questions, as necessary, *to avoid miscommunications that can cause patient care errors during transitions of care.* As part of the hand-off process, trace each tubing and catheter from the patient to its point of origin; a standardized line reconciliation process should be used.[38,40,41,42]

- Verify the practitioner's orders.
- Perform hand hygiene.[13,14,15,16,17,18]
- Confirm the patient's identity using at least two patient identifiers.[19]
- Raise the patient's bed to waist level before providing patient care *to prevent caregiver back strain.*[25]
- Perform hand hygiene.[13,14,15,16,17,18]
- Put on gloves *to comply with standard precautions.*[26,27,28]
- Verify and document the manufacturer as well as the device code and pacemaker settings and parameters, including pacing mode, heart rate parameters, output, pulse width, and sensitivity. For dual-chamber pacemakers, verify and document postventricular atrial refractory periods and AV intervals.[47]
- Attach the patient to a cardiac monitor. Make sure that alarm limits are set appropriately for the patient's current condition, and that alarms are turned on, functioning properly, and audible to staff.[48,49,50,51]
- Monitor the patient's ECG tracing *to check for arrhythmias and to ensure correct pacemaker functioning.* Inspect the ECG tracing for pacemaker spikes, and evaluate for evidence of failure to sense or failure to capture.[2] Monitor the patient for signs of pacemaker malfunction, such as pulse generator failure and decreased cardiac output, including decreased level of consciousness, fatigue, dizziness, shortness of breath, pallor, diaphoresis, chest pain, and decreased blood pressure.[2]
- Obtain a chest X-ray as ordered *to verify lead placement and to check for lead fragmentation, generator or lead dislodgment, and heart enlargement.*[52]
- Obtain a 12-lead ECG, as ordered.
- Monitor the IV flow rate; the IV catheter is usually kept in place for 24 to 48 hours postoperatively *to allow for possible treatment of arrhythmias.*
- Inspect the dressing bleeding, and regularly assess the incision site for signs of infection (swelling, redness, and exudate).[2]
- Change the dressing and apply antiseptic ointment to the incision line, as ordered.[47] If the dressing becomes soiled or the site is exposed to air, change the dressing immediately.
- Monitor vital signs as required by the patient's condition and your facility. *Practice varies and ranges from every 5 to every 15 minutes. Expert opinion recommends vital sign measurement at least every 15 minutes during phase I recovery.*[53]
- Monitor the patient's level of consciousness, cardiac status, and respiratory status, as required by your facility and the patient's condition.

ELDER ALERT Confused older adult patients with second-degree heart block won't show immediate improvement in level of consciousness.

- Screen for and assess the patient's pain using facility-defined criteria that are consistent with the patient's age, condition, and ability to understand.[54]
- Treat the patient's pain, as needed and ordered, using nonpharmacologic, pharmacologic, or a combination of approaches. Base the treatment plan on evidence-based practices and the patient's clinical condition, medical history, and pain management goals.[54] As indicated, provide nonpharmacologic pain relief interventions, such as repositioning the patient and applying an ice pack. Also, administer an analgesic, as indicated and ordered, following safe medication administration practices.[31,32,33,34]
- Return the bed to the lowest position *to prevent falls and maintain patient safety.*[35]
- Discard used supplies in appropriate receptacles.[27]
- Remove and discard your gloves[26,27] and perform hand hygiene.[13,14,15,16,17,18]
- Clean and disinfect your stethoscope using a disinfectant pad.[36,37]
- Perform hand hygiene.[13,14,15,16,17,18]
- Document the procedure.[43,44,45,46]

Special considerations

- Be aware that electromagnetic interference may occur with implanted electronic devices. Take the necessary precautions *to prevent interference.*[2]

NURSING ALERT Health care team members must plan carefully before scheduling magnetic resonance imaging (MRI) for a patient with a pacemaker. Be aware that, although many pacemakers and pacemaker leads placed today are MRI-conditional, this classification isn't the same as MRI-safe. No MRI-safe cardiac pacing devices exist. Patients with MRI-conditional pacemakers can undergo an MRI as long as certain conditions are met, such as proper evaluation and programming of the pacemaker just before and after the MRI; proper cardiac monitoring during the MRI; and availability of a cardiologist with expertise in cardiac device management before, during, and after the scan. Patients without an MRI-conditional pacing system should be approved to undergo an MRI only in urgent situations when the benefit of the information gained from the MRI outweighs the risk. An MRI-conditional pacing system can be identified by the patient's pacemaker identification card.[55,56,57,58]

■ If the patient returns to the facility to determine if the pacemaker battery must be replaced, a specially trained nurse can record an ECG rhythm strip with a pacemaker magnet placed over the pacemaker, if permitted in your facility. Placing a magnet over most permanent pacemakers reprograms the pacemaker temporarily into asynchronous mode; it doesn't turn the pacemaker off. Evaluating the pacing rate during a magnet test can determine whether the pacemaker's battery needs replacement. Contact the pacemaker's manufacturer to determine the appropriate magnet rate for the patient's pacemaker. Removing the magnet returns the pacemaker to its pre-magnet application state.[47]

■ Recently, leadless self-contained right ventricular single-chamber pacemakers have become available. They're implanted via a femoral percutaneous approach and eliminate lead and device pocket-related complications.[59]

■ In end-of-life circumstances, the patient can choose to have the pacemaker deactivated.[60]

Patient teaching

Teach the patient and family about pacemaker precautions and care. Instruct the patient and family (if appropriate) to report syncope or near-syncope; muscle twitching over the pacemaker site; frequent hiccups; a pulse rate lower than the pacemaker's lowest preset limit; and any redness, pain, swelling, or discharge from incision sites or over the pacemaker pocket. Tell them that if they can't palpate the pacemaker at the insertion site, then the pacemaker may have migrated and the patient will require follow-up medical care.

Instruct the patient to avoid close contact with machinery and to avoid placing cellular devices directly over the pacemaker *because of electromagnetic interference.* Teach them that pacemakers require regular follow-up care *to assess battery and pacemaker function.*[2] The practitioner can assess the pacemaker during follow-up visits or by remote monitoring via telephone, a mobile device, or a secure Web-based system.[61,62] (See *Teaching the patient who has a permanent pacemaker.*)

Make sure that the patient receives a pacemaker identification card with the pacemaker information, including the type and manufacturer, serial number, pacemaker rate setting, date implanted, and the practitioner's name. Instruct the patient to keep the card on hand at all times and to present it at all medical appointments, including emergency department visits. Suggest obtaining a medical identification bracelet or necklace that states that the patient has a pacemaker.

Complications

NURSING ALERT Watch for signs and symptoms of a perforated ventricle with resultant cardiac tamponade. These signs and symptoms include tachycardia, distant heart sounds, pulsus paradoxus, hypotension with narrow pulse pressure, increased venous pressure, cyanosis, distended jugular veins, decreased urine output, restlessness, and chest pain or a feeling of fullness in the chest. If the patient develops any of these, notify the practitioner immediately.[66]

Complications of having a permanent pacemaker include ventricle perforation from endocardial leads, infection, pneumothorax or hemorrhage from insertion, inadequate pacing or sensing, pacemaker malfunction, battery depletion, and lead fracture or displacement.[67] Rarely, an allergic reaction to the device may occur and can present as localized or generalized dermatitis or mimic signs and symptoms of infection.[68]

Documentation

Document the type of pacemaker used, the model and serial numbers, the manufacturer's name, the pacing rate, the date and site of implantation,

---

TEACHING THE PATIENT WHO HAS A PERMANENT PACEMAKER

If your patient is going home with a permanent pacemaker, teach the patient about daily care, safety and activity guidelines, and other precautions. Be sure to cover the instructions listed below.

Daily care
■ Clean your pacemaker site gently with soap and water when you take a shower or a bath. Leave the incision exposed to the air.
■ Inspect your skin around the incision. A slight bulge is normal, but call your practitioner if you feel discomfort or notice swelling, redness, a discharge, or other problems.[63,64]
■ Check your pulse for 1 minute as your nurse or practitioner showed you: on the side of your neck, inside your elbow, or on the thumb side of your wrist. Your pulse rate should be the same as your pacemaker rate or faster. Contact your practitioner if you think your heart is beating too fast or too slow.
■ Take your medications, including those for pain, as prescribed. Even with a pacemaker, you still need the medication that your practitioner ordered.

Safety and activity
■ Keep your pacemaker instruction booklet handy, and carry your pacemaker identification card at all times. This card has your pacemaker model number and other information needed by health care personnel who treat you.
■ You can resume most of your usual activities when you feel comfortable doing so, but don't drive until the practitioner gives you permission. Also avoid heavy lifting and stretching exercises for at least 6 weeks or as directed by your practitioner.
■ Use both arms equally to prevent stiffness. Check with your practitioner before you golf, swim, play tennis, or perform other strenuous activities.

Electromagnetic interference
■ Today's pacemakers are designed and insulated to eliminate most electrical interference. You can safely operate common household electrical devices, including microwave ovens, razors, and sewing machines. And you can ride in or operate a motor vehicle without it affecting your pacemaker.

■ Avoid direct contact with large running motors, high-powered CB radios and similar equipment, welding machinery, and radar devices.
■ Electromagnetic anti-theft security systems, located near workplaces, airports, and courthouses, are unlikely to cause clinical interference; however, you should be aware of their location, move through them at a normal pace, and avoid leaning or standing close to the system.[65]
■ If your pacemaker activates a metal detector in an airport, show your pacemaker identification card to the security official.[61]
■ *Because the metal in your pacemaker makes you ineligible for certain diagnostic studies,* such as magnetic resonance imaging, be sure to inform your practitioners, dentist, and other health care personnel that you have a pacemaker.

Special precautions
■ If you feel lightheaded or dizzy when you're near any electrical equipment, moving away from the device should restore normal pacemaker function.[65] Ask your practitioner about particular electrical devices.
■ Notify your practitioner if you experience any signs of pacemaker failure, such as palpitations, a fast heart rate, a slow heart rate (5 to 10 beats less than the pacemaker's setting), dizziness, fainting, shortness of breath, swollen ankles or feet, anxiety, forgetfulness, or confusion.
■ If you feel like you're going to faint, call the emergency calling number for emergency assistance immediately and lie down to prevent falling.

Checkups
■ Be sure to schedule a follow-up visit, and keep regular checkup appointments with your practitioner.
■ If your practitioner monitors your pacemaker status remotely by wireless telemetry, keep your transmission schedule and instructions handy.[5]

and the surgeon's name from the implantation record. Record your assessment findings, the condition of the pacemaker insertion site, vital signs, and completion of an X-ray for verification of lead placement. If the patient's ECG tracing is being monitored, place a rhythm strip in the patient's medical record each shift and with any change in the patient's condition, and note any loss of sensing or capture. Note communication with other health care team members, including reporting of abnormal assessment findings, the presence of the pacemaker, and upcoming procedures. Include any assessments of the pacemaker and changes in pacemaker programming performed by the cardiology team. Record the patient's pain assessment, interventions performed, and the patient's response to those interventions. Document teaching provided to the patient and family (if applicable), their understanding of that teaching, and any need for follow-up teaching.

REFERENCES

1 Mayo Clinic. (n.d.). Pacemaker. https://www.mayoclinic.org/tests-procedures/pacemaker/about/pac-20384689

2 Wiegand, D. L. (2017). *AACN procedure manual for high acuity, progressive, and critical care* (7th ed.). St. Louis, MO: Elsevier.

3 Jarrett, N., & Callaham, M. (2016). Evidence-based guidelines for selected hospital-acquired conditions: Final report. https://www.cms.gov/Medicare/Medicare-Fee-for-Service-Payment/HospitalAcqCond/Downloads/2016-HAC-Report.pdf

4 Berríos-Torres, S. I., et al. (2017). Centers for Disease Control and Prevention guideline for the prevention of surgical site infection, 2017. https://jamanetwork.com/journals/jamasurgery/fullarticle/2623725 (Level VII)

5 Kusumoto, F. M., et al. (2018). 2018 ACC/AHA/HRS guideline on the evaluation and management of patients with bradycardia and cardiac conduction delay: Executive summary: A report of the American College of Cardiology/American Heart Association Task Force on Practice Guidelines, and the Heart Rhythm Society. *HeartRhythm, 16*(9), e227–e279. https://www.heartrhythmjournal.com/article/S1547-5271(18)31126-3/fulltext (Level VII)

6 American Society of Anesthesiologists Task Force on Perioperative Management of Patients with Cardiac Implantable Electronic Devices. (2011). Practice advisory for the perioperative management of patients with cardiac implantable electronic devices: Pacemakers and implantable cardioverter-defibrillators. *Anesthesiology, 114*(2), 247–261. https://pubs.asahq.org/anesthesiology/article/114/2/247/10965/Practice-Advisory-for-the-Perioperative-Management (Level VII)

7 The Joint Commission. (2021). Standard RI.01.03.01. *Comprehensive accreditation manual for hospitals.* (Level VII)

8 Centers for Medicare and Medicaid Services, Department of Health and Human Services. (2020). Condition of participation: Patient's rights. 42 C. F. R. § 482.13(b)(2).

9 Accreditation Association for Hospitals and Health Systems. (2020). Standard 30.01.11. *Healthcare Facilities Accreditation Program: Accreditation requirements for acute care hospitals.* (Level VII)

10 DNV GL-Healthcare USA, Inc. (2020). PR.2.SR.3. *NIAHO® accreditation requirements, interpretive guidelines and surveyor guidance—revision 20.0.* (Level VII)

11 The Joint Commission. (2021). Standard UP.01.01.01. *Comprehensive accreditation manual for hospitals.* (Level VII)

12 Accreditation Association for Hospitals and Health Systems. (2020). Standard 30.00.14. *Healthcare Facilities Accreditation Program: Accreditation requirements for acute care hospitals.* (Level VII)

13 Centers for Disease Control and Prevention. (2002). Guideline for hand hygiene in health-care settings: Recommendations of the Healthcare Infection Control Practices Advisory Committee and the HICPAC/SHEA/APIC/IDSA Hand Hygiene Task Force. *MMWR Recommendations and Reports, 51*(RR-16), 1–45. https://www.cdc.gov/mmwr/pdf/rr/rr5116.pdf (Level II)

14 The Joint Commission. (2021). Standard NPSG.07.01.01. *Comprehensive accreditation manual for hospitals.* (Level VII)

15 World Health Organization. (2009). WHO guidelines on hand hygiene in health care: First global patient safety challenge, clean care is safer care. https://apps.who.int/iris/bitstream/handle/10665/44102/9789241597906_eng.pdf?sequence=1 (Level IV)

16 Accreditation Association for Hospitals and Health Systems. (2020). Standard 07.01.21. *Healthcare Facilities Accreditation Program: Accreditation requirements for acute care hospitals.* (Level VII)

17 Centers for Medicare and Medicaid Services, Department of Health and Human Services. (2020). Condition of participation: Infection control. 42 C.F.R. § 482.42.

18 DNV GL-Healthcare USA, Inc. (2020). IC.1.SR.1. *NIAHO® accreditation requirements, interpretive guidelines and surveyor guidance—revision 20.0.* (Level VII)

19 The Joint Commission. (2021). Standard NPSG.01.01.01. *Comprehensive accreditation manual for hospitals.* (Level VII)

20 The Joint Commission. (2021). Standard RI.01.01.01. *Comprehensive accreditation manual for hospitals.* (Level VII)

21 Centers for Medicare and Medicaid Services, Department of Health and Human Services. (2020). Condition of participation: Patient's rights. 42 C.F.R. § 482.13(c)(1).

22 Accreditation Association for Hospitals and Health Systems. (2020). Standard 15.01.16. *Healthcare Facilities Accreditation Program: Accreditation requirements for acute care hospitals.* (Level VII)

23 DNV GL-Healthcare USA, Inc. (2020). PR.2.SR.5. *NIAHO® accreditation requirements, interpretive guidelines and surveyor guidance—revision 20.0.* (Level VII)

24 The Joint Commission. (2021). Standard PC.02.01.21. *Comprehensive accreditation manual for hospitals.* (Level VII)

25 Waters, T. R., et al. (2009). Safe patient handling training for schools of nursing. https://www.cdc.gov/niosh/docs/2009-127/pdfs/2009-127.pdf (Level VII)

26 Siegel, J. D., et al. (2007, revised 2019). 2007 guideline for isolation precautions: Preventing transmission of infectious agents in healthcare settings. https://www.cdc.gov/infectioncontrol/pdf/guidelines/isolation-guidelines-H.pdf (Level II)

27 Occupational Safety and Health Administration. (2019). Bloodborne pathogens, standard number 1910.1030. https://www.osha.gov/pls/oshaweb/owadisp.show_document?p_id=10051&p_table=STANDARDS (Level VII)

28 Accreditation Association for Hospitals and Health Systems. (2020). Standard 07.01.10. *Healthcare Facilities Accreditation Program: Accreditation requirements for acute care hospitals.* (Level VII)

29 American Society of Anesthesiologists. (2017). Practice guidelines for preoperative fasting and the use of pharmacologic agents to reduce the risk of pulmonary aspiration: Application to healthy patients undergoing elective procedures. *Anesthesiology, 126*(3), 376–393. https://pubs.asahq.org/anesthesiology/article/126/3/376/19733/Practice-Guidelines-for-Preoperative-Fasting (Level VII)

30 Anderson, D. J., & Sexton, D. J. (2019). Antimicrobial prophylaxis for prevention of surgical site infection in adults. In: *UpToDate*, Harris, A. (Ed.).

31 Accreditation Association for Hospitals and Health Systems. (2020). Standard 16.01.03. *Healthcare Facilities Accreditation Program: Accreditation requirements for acute care hospitals.* (Level VII)

32 The Joint Commission. (2021). Standard MM.06.01.01. *Comprehensive accreditation manual for hospitals.* (Level VII)

33 Centers for Medicare and Medicaid Services, Department of Health and Human Services. (2020). Condition of participation: Nursing services. 42 C.F.R. § 482.23(c).

34 DNV GL-Healthcare USA, Inc. (2020). MM.1.SR.3. *NIAHO® accreditation requirements, interpretive guidelines and surveyor guidance—revision 20.0.* (Level VII)

35 Ganz, D. A., et al. (2013, reviewed 2021). *Preventing falls in hospitals: A toolkit for improving quality of care* (AHRQ Publication No. 13-0015-EF). Agency for Healthcare Research and Quality. https://www.ahrq.gov/professionals/systems/hospital/fallpxtoolkit/index.html (Level VII)

36 Rutala, W. A., et al. (2008, revised 2019). Guideline for disinfection and sterilization in healthcare facilities, 2008. https://www.cdc.gov/infectioncontrol/pdf/guidelines/disinfection-guidelines-H.pdf (Level I)

37 Accreditation Association for Hospitals and Health Systems. (2020). Standard 07.02.03. *Healthcare Facilities Accreditation Program: Accreditation requirements for acute care hospitals.* (Level VII)

38 The Joint Commission. (2021). Standard PC.02.02.01. *Comprehensive accreditation manual for hospitals.* (Level VII)

39 The Joint Commission. (2021). Standard PC.04.02.01. *Comprehensive accreditation manual for hospitals.* (Level VII)

40 The Joint Commission. (2017). Sentinel event alert 58: Inadequate hand-off communication. https://www.jointcommission.org/-/media/tjc/documents/resources/patient-safety-topics/sentinel-event/sea_58_hand-off_comms_9_6_17_final_(1).pdf (Level VII)

41 U.S. Food and Drug Administration. (2017). Examples of medical device misconnections. https://www.fda.gov/medical-devices/medical-device-connectors/examples-medical-device-misconnections

42 The Joint Commission. (2014). Sentinel event alert 53: Managing risk during transition to new ISO tubing connector standards. https://www.jointcommission.org/-/media/tjc/documents/resources/patient-safety-topics/sentinel-event/sea_53_connectors_8_19_14_final.pdf (Level VII)

43 The Joint Commission. (2021). Standard RC.01.03.01. *Comprehensive accreditation manual for hospitals.* (Level VII)

44 Accreditation Association for Hospitals and Health Systems. (2020). Standard 10.00.03. *Healthcare Facilities Accreditation Program: Accreditation requirements for acute care hospitals.* (Level VII)

45 Centers for Medicare and Medicaid Services, Department of Health and Human Services. (2020). Condition of participation: Medical record services. 42 C.F.R. § 482.24(b).

46 DNV GL-Healthcare USA, Inc. (2020). MR.2.SR.1. *NIAHO® accreditation requirements, interpretive guidelines and surveyor guidance—revision 20.0.* (Level VII)

47 Ellenbogen, K. A., et al. (2017). *Clinical cardiac pacing, defibrillation, and resynchronization therapy* (5th ed.). St. Louis, MO: Elsevier.

48 The Joint Commission. (2013). Sentinel event alert 50: Medical device alarm safety in https://www.jointcommission.org/-/media/tjc/documents/resources/patient-safety-topics/sentinel-event/sea_50_alarms_4_26_16.pdf (Level VII)

49 The Joint Commission. (2021). Standard NPSG.06.01.01. *Comprehensive accreditation manual for hospitals.* (Level VII)

50 American Association of Critical-Care Nurses. (2018). AACN practice alert: Managing alarms in acute care across the life span: Electrocardiography and pulse oximetry. https://www.aacn.org/clinical-resources/practice-alerts/managing-alarms-in-acute-care-across-the-life-span (Level VII)

51 Graham, K. C., & Cvach, M. (2010). Monitor alarm fatigue: Standardizing use of physiological monitors and decreasing nuisance alarms. *American Journal of Critical Care, 19*(1), 28–37. https://doi.org/10.4037/ajcc2010651

52 Dissmann, R., et al. (2013). Double left ventricular pacing following accidental malpositioning of the right ventricular electrode during implantation of a cardiac resynchronization therapy device. *Journal of Cardiothoracic Surgery, 8,* Article 162https://doi.org/10.1186/1749-8090-8-162.

53 American Society of PeriAnesthesia Nurses. (2020). *2021-2022 Perianesthesia nursing standards, practice recommendations and interpretive statements.* (Level VII)

54 The Joint Commission. (2021). Standard PC.01.02.07. *Comprehensive accreditation manual for hospitals.* (Level VII)

55 Sethi, K. K., & Chutani, S. K. (2018). Magnetic resonance imaging-conditional devices: Where have we reached today? *International Journal of Heart Rhythm, 3*(1), 16–24. http://www.ijhronline.org/article.asp?issn=2352-4197;year=2018;volume=3;issue=1;spage=16;epage=24;aulast=Sethi

56 Korutz, A. W., et al. (2017). Pacemakers in MRI for the neuroradiologist. *American Journal of Neuroradiology, 38*(12), 2222–2230. http://www.ajnr.org/content/38/12/2222

57 Medtronic. (n.d.). Getting an MRI: MRI and your cardiac device. https://www.medtronic.com/us-en/patients/treatments-therapies/living-with-heart-device/mri/getting-scan.html

58 Medtronic. (n.d.). MRI resources: For clinicians who have a Medtronic system. https://www.medtronic.com/us-en/healthcare-professionals/mri-resources.html

59 Tjong, F. V. Y., & Reddy, V. Y. (2017). Permanent leadless cardiac pacemaker therapy. *Circulation, 135*(15), 1458–1470. from https://www.ahajournals.org/doi/10.1161/CIRCULATIONAHA.116.025037

60 Lampert, R., et al. (2010). HRS expert consensus statement on the management of cardiovascular implantable electronic devices (CIEDs) in patients nearing end of life or requesting withdrawal of therapy. *Heart Rhythm, 7*(7), 1008–1026. https://www.sciencedirect.com/science/article/pii/S154752711000408X?via%3Dihub (Level VII)

61 Olshansky, B. (2021). Patient education: Pacemakers (Beyond the basics). In: *UpToDate,* Ganz, L. I. (Ed.).

62 Zeitler, E. P., & Piccini, J. P. (2016). Remote monitoring of cardiac implantable electronic devices (CIED). *Trends in Cardiovascular Medicine, 26*(6), 568–577. https://www.ncbi.nlm.nih.gov/pmc/articles/PMC4958580/

63 Karchmer, A. W., & Chu, V. H. (2021). Infections involving cardiac implantable electronic devices: Epidemiology, microbiology, clinical manifestations, and diagnosis. In: *UpToDate,* Calderwood, S. B. & Ganz, L. I. (Eds.).

64 Baddour, L. M., et al. (2010). Update on cardiovascular implantable electronic device infections and their management: A scientific statement from the American Heart Association. *Circulation, 121*(3), 458–477. https://www.ahajournals.org/doi/full/10.1161/circulationaha.109.192665 (Level VII)

65 Medtronic. (2017). Answers to questions about implantable cardiac devices: Electromagnetic compatibility guide. https://www.medtronic.com/content/dam/medtronic-com/01_crhf/cc/pdfs/emc_pt_brochure_f.pdf

66 Hoit, B. D. (2019). Cardiac tamponade. In: *UpToDate,* Gersh, B. J. & Hoekstra, J. (Eds.)

67 Gillis, A. M., et al. (2012). HRS/ACCF expert consensus statement on pacemaker device and mode selection. *Heart Rhythm, 9*(8), 1344–1365. https://doi.org/10.1016/j.hrthm.2012.06.026 (Level VII)

68 Ganz, L. I. (2021). Cardiac implantable electronic devices: Long-term complications. In: *UpToDate,* Piccini, J. (Ed.)

PERSONAL PROTECTIVE EQUIPMENT USE

Standard and transmission-based precautions help to prevent the spread of infection from patient to patient, from patient to health care worker, and from health care worker to patient.[1,2,3,4,5] They also reduce the risk of infection in immunocompromised patients. Central to the success of these procedures is the selection of the proper personal protective equipment (PPE), such as gowns, gloves, masks, and eye protection, as well as adequate training of those who use it.[6]

NURSING ALERT For information on Coronavirus disease (COVID-19), please refer to the latest recommendations from the Centers for Disease Control and Prevention (CDC), located at https://www.cdc.gov/coronavirus/2019-ncov/hcp/infection-control-recommendations.html, when caring for a patient with known or suspected Coronavirus disease.

NURSING ALERT Please refer to the latest recommendations from the Centers for Disease Control and Prevention, located at http://www.cdc.gov/vhf/ebola/hcp/index.html, when caring for a patient with known or suspected Ebola virus disease.

Equipment

Materials required for standard and transmission-based isolation typically include PPE, a cart or anteroom for storing equipment, and a door card or sign alerting staff members and others entering the room that isolation precautions are in effect.

Personal protective equipment

Fluid-resistant gown ▪ gloves ▪ goggles or face shield ▪ mask or respirator (each staff member must be trained in its proper use).

Preparation of equipment

Inspect all equipment and supplies. If a product is expired, is defective, or has compromised integrity, remove it from patient use, label it as expired or defective, and report the expiration or defect as directed by your facility. Remove the cover from the isolation cart if necessary and set up the work area. Check the cart or anteroom *to make sure an adequate amount of the proper isolation supplies are available for the designated transmission-based precautions category.*

Implementation
Donning PPE

▪ Remove your watch (or push it well up on your arm) and your rings if required by your facility. *These actions help to prevent the spread of microorganisms hidden under these adornments.*

▪ Perform hand hygiene.[2,7,8,9,10,11]

▪ Pick up the fluid-resistant gown and allow it to unfold in front of you without touching areas of your body that may be contaminated, *to minimize the transmission of microorganisms.*

▪ Put on the gown and wrap it around the back of your uniform, making sure it overlaps and completely covers your uniform, *to prevent contact*

with the patient or the patient's environment.[3,5,12] Tie the strings or fasten the snaps or pressure-sensitive tabs at the neck. Then tie the waist strings.
■ Place the mask snugly over your nose and mouth and below your chin.[5,12] Secure the ear loops around your ears or tie the strings at the middle of the back of your head and neck *so the mask won't slip off.* If the mask has a metal strip, squeeze it to fit your nose firmly but comfortably.[3,5] (See *Putting on a face mask.*) If you wear eyeglasses, tuck the upper edge of the mask under the lower edge of the glasses *to minimize the likelihood of clouding your glasses.*
■ Choose eye protection according to your risk of exposure. Although goggles provide eye protection, they don't protect the rest of the face from splashing of potentially infectious substances. Wear a face shield for any procedures that may involve spraying or splashing of respiratory secretions or other body fluids.[3,5,6]
■ Select gloves according to your hand size *to make sure they fit securely.* Put on the gloves and pull them over the cuffs of your gown *to cover the edges of the gown's sleeves.*[12]

Removing PPE
■ After completing patient care, prepare to leave the room by collecting items that need to be removed.
■ Remember that the outside surfaces of your goggles or face shield, mask or respirator, and barrier clothes (such as a gown) are contaminated.[3,5]
■ Except for a respirator mask, remove all PPE at the patient's doorway or in the anteroom. Remove a respirator mask after leaving the patient's room and closing the door.[3,5,12]
■ Remove your gloves using the appropriate technique. (See *Removing contaminated gloves.*) Don't touch any of your skin surfaces with the outside of either glove.[13]
■ Discard your gloves in the appropriate receptacle.[3,5,14]
■ Perform hand hygiene.[6,7,8,9,10,11]
■ To remove your gown, untie the neck straps and then the waist ties.[13] Pull the gown away from your neck and shoulders, touching only the inside of the gown. Turn the gown inside out as you remove it, folding it or rolling it into a bundle *to help ensure containment of pathogens.*[13] Discard the gown in the appropriate receptacle.[3,5,6,12,14] (See *Removing your gown and gloves together.*)
■ To remove your goggles or face shield, grasp the ear pieces or headband and remove the goggles or face shield carefully.[13] Place the equipment in the appropriate receptacle for reprocessing, or discard it in the appropriate receptacle.[3,5,6,12,13,14]
■ To remove your mask or respirator, grasp the bottom tie or elastic and lift it over your head.[13] Then grasp the top tie or elastic and carefully remove the mask or respirator. *To help prevent contamination,* don't touch the front of the mask.[13] Discard the mask or respirator in the appropriate receptacle.[3,5,12,14]
■ Perform hand hygiene immediately.[6,7,8,9,10,11]

EQUIPMENT

Putting on a face mask

To avoid exposure to infectious agents and potentially infections blood or body fluids, put on a face mask.[5] Position the mask to cover your nose and mouth, and secure it high enough *to ensure stability.* Tie the top strings at the back of your head above the ears. Then tie the bottom strings at the base of your neck. Alternatively, if the mask has ear loops, secure them around your ears.[3,6]

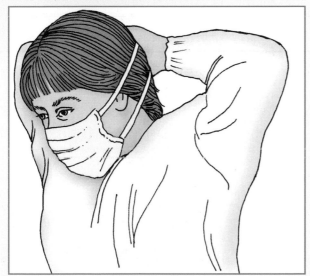

Adjust the metal nose strip if the mask has one.[3,6]

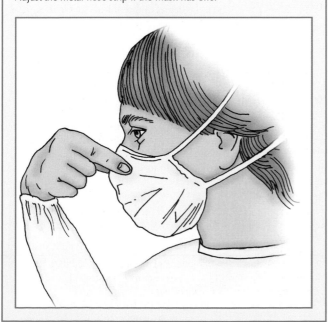

Removing contaminated gloves

Proper removal techniques are essential for helping to prevent the spread of pathogens from your gloves to your skin surfaces. Follow these steps carefully to remove your contaminated gloves properly:[5,6]
■ Grasp the outside of one glove with your opposite gloved hand and peel it off, turning the glove inside out as you pull it off. Hold the removed glove in your remaining gloved hand.[6]
■ Slide two fingers of your ungloved hand under the remaining glove at the wrist, taking care not to touch the outer surface of the glove.[6]
■ Peel off the glove over the first removed glove, containing the one glove inside the other.[6]
■ Discard your gloves in the appropriate receptacle.[3,5,6,14]
■ Perform hand hygiene.[6,7,8,9,10,11]

Removing your gown and gloves together

The CDC discusses an alternate method for removing your gown and gloves. In this method, a disposable gown is used, and the gown and gloves are removed together.[12] Follow these steps to remove your gown and gloves together:
■ With your gloved hands, grasp the gown in the front.
■ Pull the gown away from your body so that the ties break.
■ While removing the gown, fold or roll the gown inside-out into a bundle.
■ As you remove the gown, peel off your gloves at the same time; touch only the inside of your gloves and gown with your bare hands.
■ Discard the gown and gloves in the appropriate receptacle.[3,5,12,14]
■ Perform hand hygiene immediately.[6,7,8,9,10,11]

Special considerations

■ If airborne precautions are required, an N95 or higher level particulate respirator approved by the Occupational Safety and Health Administration should be worn rather than a surgical mask.[3,4,15] (See the "Airborne precautions" procedure.) Employees who wear respirators must be properly fit-tested initially, and then periodically thereafter according to federal, state, and local regulations.[16,17]

■ If your respirator device is reusable, retain it for further personal use unless it's contaminated or damaged or it fails to form a good seal.[17] Store it as directed by your facility. Reuse of respiratory protection may consist of removing and putting on the device again between patient encounters. *To avoid a transmission risk,* adhere to stringent hand hygiene before and after handling the respiratory protection device.[17]

■ Always perform hand hygiene before putting on gloves *to avoid contaminating the gloves with microorganisms from your hands.*[2,7,8,9,10]

■ Use gloves only once.[3,5] If a glove tears, remove it, perform hand hygiene, and put on a new pair of gloves.[5,6]

■ Be aware that isolation garb loses its effectiveness when wet, *because moisture permits organisms to seep through the material.* Change masks and gowns as soon as moisture is noticeable, or according to the manufacturer's recommendations or your facility's guidelines.[3,5,18]

■ Keep PPE and other isolation precaution supplies stocked *so they're readily available for those who must enter the patient's room.*[5]

Documentation

None needed.

REFERENCES

1 The Joint Commission. (2021). Standard IC.02.01.01. *Comprehensive accreditation manual for hospitals.* (Level VII)

2 Centers for Medicare and Medicaid Services, Department of Health and Human Services. (2020). Condition of participation: Infection control. 42 C.F.R. § 482.42.

3 Accreditation Association for Hospitals and Health Systems. (2020). Standard 07.01.10. *Healthcare Facilities Accreditation Program: Accreditation requirements for acute care hospitals.* (Level VII)

4 DNV GL-Healthcare USA, Inc. (2020). IC.1.SR.2. *NIAHO® accreditation requirements, interpretive guidelines and surveyor guidance—revision 20.0.* (Level VII)

5 Siegel, J. D., et al. (2007, revised 2019). 2007 guideline for isolation precautions: Preventing transmission of infectious agents in healthcare settings. https://www.cdc.gov/infectioncontrol/pdf/guidelines/isolation-guidelines-H.pdf (Level II)

6 Centers for Disease Control and Prevention. (n.d.). Guidance for the selection and use of personal protective equipment (PPE) in healthcare settings. https://www.cdc.gov/HAI/pdfs/ppe/PPEslides6-29-04.pdf (Level VII)

7 The Joint Commission. (2021). Standard NPSG.07.01.01. *Comprehensive accreditation manual for hospitals.* (Level VII)

8 Centers for Disease Control and Prevention. (2002). Guideline for hand hygiene in health-care settings: Recommendations of the Healthcare Infection Control Practices Advisory Committee and the HICPAC/SHEA/APIC/IDSA Hand Hygiene Task Force. *MMWR Recommendations and Reports, 51*(RR-16), 1–45. https://www.cdc.gov/mmwr/pdf/rr/rr5116.pdf (Level II)

9 World Health Organization. (2009). WHO guidelines on hand hygiene in health care: First global patient safety challenge, clean care is safer care. https://apps.who.int/iris/bitstream/handle/10665/44102/9789241597906_eng.pdf?sequence=1 (Level IV)

10 Accreditation Association for Hospitals and Health Systems. (2020). Standard 07.01.21. *Healthcare Facilities Accreditation Program: Accreditation requirements for acute care hospitals.* (Level VII)

11 DNV GL-Healthcare USA, Inc. (2020). IC.1.SR.1. *NIAHO® accreditation requirements, interpretive guidelines and surveyor guidance—revision 20.0.* (Level VII)

12 Centers for Disease Control and Prevention. (n.d.). Sequence for donning personal protective equipment (PPE). https://www.cdc.gov/HAI/pdfs/ppe/ppeposter1322.pdf

13 Centers for Disease Control and Prevention. (2020). Using personal protective equipment. https://www.cdc.gov/coronavirus/2019-ncov/hcp/using-ppe.html

14 Accreditation Association for Hospitals and Health Systems. (2020). Standard 07.03.07. *Healthcare Facilities Accreditation Program: Accreditation requirements for acute care hospitals.* (Level VII)

15 Occupational Safety and Health Administration. (2011). Respiratory protection, standard number 1910.134. https://www.osha.gov/laws-regs/regulations/standardnumber/1910/1910.134 (Level VII)

16 Centers for Disease Control and Prevention. (2005). Guidelines for preventing the transmission of Mycobacterium tuberculosis in health-care settings, 2005. *MMWR Recommendations and Reports, 54*(RR-17), 1–141. https://www.cdc.gov/mmwr/pdf/rr/rr5417.pdf (Level I)

17 Rebmann, T., et al. (2009). APIC position paper: Extending the use and/or reusing respiratory protection in healthcare settings during disasters. http://www.apic.org/Resource_/TinyMceFileManager/Advocacy-PDFs/APIC_Position_Ext_the_Use_and_or_Reus_Resp_Prot_in_Hlthcare_Settings1209l.pdf (Level VII)

18 Occupational Health and Safety Administration. (2019). Bloodborne pathogens, standard number 1910.1030. https://www.osha.gov/pls/oshaweb/owadisp.show_document?p_id=10051&p_table=STANDARDS (Level VII)

POSTMORTEM CARE

After a patient dies, care includes preparing the body for family viewing, arranging transportation to the morgue or funeral home, and determining the disposition of the patient's belongings.[1,2] In addition, postmortem care entails comforting and supporting the patient's family and friends and providing for their privacy.[1] Before performing postmortem care, ask the family members if they have any special cultural or spiritual requests.[1,2,3] The family members should also be asked if they want to participate in postmortem care.[1] Postmortem care usually begins after a practitioner certifies the patient's death; you must perform postmortem care as soon as possible to prevent discoloration, tissue damage, and deformity.[1] If the patient died violently or under suspicious circumstances, postmortem care may be postponed until the medical examiner completes an autopsy.[1]

Equipment

Gloves ■ bath supplies (towels, washcloths, water-filled basin, and soap) ■ cotton balls ■ shroud kit (includes three identification tags, a plastic shroud or body wrap, chin straps, and gauze or soft string ties) ■ pillow or rolled towel ■ clean sheet ■ plastic bag for belongings ■ stretcher or morgue cart ■ Optional: tape, personal protective equipment (gown, mask and goggles or mask with face shield), dressings, organ procurement consent, clean gown, absorbent pads, gauze, normal saline solution.

Implementation

■ Gather and prepare the necessary equipment and supplies.

■ Notify the appropriate facility personnel (such as the nursing supervisor) that the patient has been pronounced dead.

■ If an autopsy is necessary, speak with the medical examiner to determine whether tubes and catheters must remain intact *to avoid altering the body before the autopsy.* Ensure that the practitioner or another member of the health care team has explained the need for an autopsy to the family members and that consent has been obtained, if indicated.

■ Notify support services (such as the clergy person or social worker) as needed *to assist the family.*

■ Identify any spiritual, cultural, or other wishes of the deceased patient and family members, including immediate release of the deceased patient's body for burial or cremation.[1,2,3]

■ Notify the local organ procurement agency of the patient's death, if applicable.[4,5,6,7]

■ Provide privacy by pulling curtains and closing doors *to maintain patient dignity.*[1,8,9,10,11]

■ Explain the procedure to the family according to their individual communication and learning needs *to increase their understanding, allay their fears, and enhance cooperation.*[12]

■ Offer comfort and emotional support to the family members and intimate friends.[2]

■ Perform hand hygiene.[13,14,15,16,17,18]

■ Put on gloves and other personal protective equipment as needed *to comply with standard precautions*, or maintain isolation precautions if they were being used. Offer personal protective equipment to other staff and family members as required *to ensure the health and safety of all people coming in contact with the patient's body.*[1,19,20,21]

■ Help any family members who are present to approach and touch the patient. *They may feel that they need permission to touch the patient.*

■ Determine whether family members would like to remain and assist with caring for the body.[1] *Helping with postmortem care provides bonding time for family members and may be part of the family's cultural and spiritual beliefs.*

■ Raise the bed to waist level *to prevent caregiver back strain.*[22]

■ Place the deceased patient's body in the supine position. Straighten the limbs (if possible), with the arms at the sides and the head on a pillow, *to support alignment and help keep the jaw closed.*[1] Then elevate the head of the bed 30 degrees *to prevent discoloration from blood settling in the face.*

■ Close the eyes by pressing gently on the eyelids with your fingertips for 30 seconds.[1] If they don't stay closed, place moist cotton balls on the eyelids for a few minutes and then try again to close them. If the deceased patient is a cornea donor, cover the closed eyes with gauze soaked in normal saline solution.[23]

■ Clean the mouth *to remove secretions and debris.*[1] If the patient wore dentures, clean and replace them as soon after death as possible. If you can't replace them, send them with the deceased in a clearly identified receptacle.[1]

■ Place a pillow or rolled towel under the chin *to keep the jaw closed.*[1]

■ Turn off all equipment.

■ If an autopsy is to be performed, leave tubes and catheters intact, if instructed by the medical examiner.[1] If no autopsy is to be performed, remove all tubes and catheters.[24,25]

■ Apply gauze and tape to puncture sites. Cover any exuding wound or unhealed surgical incision with a clean, absorbent dressing and secure it with an occlusive dressing.[1] Avoid using strongly adhesive tape, *because it can be difficult to remove and can leave a permanent mark.*[1]

■ Ask family members if they would prefer to leave the patient's jewelry (if present) on the body, and collect all the patient's valuables *to prevent loss.* If you can't remove a ring, cover it with gauze, tape it in place, and tie the gauze to the wrist *to prevent slippage and subsequent loss.*

■ If family members wish to remain with and assist with caring for the body or perform after-death rituals because of ethnic, religious, or cultural requirements, allow them to do so.[1,26]

■ Bathe the deceased body thoroughly, using soap, a water-filled basin, and washcloths, or as directed by your facility.

■ Place a pad between the buttocks *to absorb any fluid that may leak from the urethra, vagina, or rectum.*[1]

■ Cover the deceased patient's body up to the chin with a clean sheet.

■ Return the deceased patient's bed to the lowest position.[27]

■ Remove and discard your gloves and other personal protective equipment, if worn.[21]

■ Perform hand hygiene.[13,14,15,16,17,18]

■ Be mindful of other patients and families on the unit when transferring the body to the morgue. Close the doors of adjacent rooms, if possible. Then take the body to the morgue, using corridors that aren't crowded and, if possible, a service elevator.

■ Perform hand hygiene.[13,14,15,16,17,18]

■ Document the procedure.[28,29,30,31]

Special considerations

■ Honor the spiritual or cultural wishes of the deceased patient and the family and caregivers while ensuring that legal obligations are met.[1,32]

■ Give the deceased patient's personal belongings to the family or bring them to the morgue. If you give the family jewelry or money, make sure a coworker is present as a witness. Obtain the signature of an adult family member *to verify receipt of valuables or to state their preference that jewelry remain on the patient.*[1]

■ When a patient's family members can't view the body within the designated time frame on the hospital unit, make arrangements for viewing the body at another appropriate location, if desired.[1]

■ If the mortuary transport team transports the body directly from the room, complete the necessary documentation and have the mortuary transport team sign the forms, as indicated.[1]

Documentation

Document in the patient's medical record the events and care provided at the time of death. Document the time of death, who was notified of the death, and any special instructions given. Record any tubes and catheters you removed from the body. If an autopsy is required, document any tubes or catheters that remain intact and any care you performed on the body. Although the extent of documentation varies among facilities, always record the disposition of the patient's possessions, especially jewelry and money. Also note the date and time that the deceased patient was transported to the morgue and the name of the person who received the body.

REFERENCES

1　Hospice UK & National Nurse Consultant Group (Palliative Care). (2015). Care after death: Guidance for staff responsible for care after death (3rd ed.). https://www.hospiceuk.org/what-we-offer/publications?cat=72e54312-4ccd-608d-ad24-ff0000fd3330 (Level V II)

2　National Consensus Project for Quality Palliative Care. (2018). *Clinical practice guidelines for quality palliative care* (4th ed.). Pittsburgh, PA: National Consensus Project for Quality Palliative Care. https://www.nationalcoalitionhpc.org/wp-content/uploads/2018/10/NCHPC-NCPGuidelines_4thED_web_FINAL.pdf (Level VII)

3　The Joint Commission. (2021). Standard PC.02.02.13. *Comprehensive accreditation manual for hospitals.* Oakbrook Terrace, IL: The Joint Commission. (Level VII)

4　Centers for Medicare and Medicaid Services, Department of Health and Human Services. (2020). Condition of participation: Organ, tissue, and eye procurement. 42 C.F.R. § 482.45(a)(1).

5　Accreditation Association for Hospitals and Health Systems. (2020). Standard 14.00.02. *Healthcare Facilities Accreditation Program: Accreditation requirements for acute care hospitals.* Chicago, IL: Accreditation Association for Hospitals and Health Systems. (Level VII)

6　DNV GL-Healthcare USA, Inc. (2020). TO.1.SR.2. *NIAHO® accreditation requirements, interpretive guidelines and surveyor guidance—revision 20.0.* Milford, OH: DNV GL Healthcare USA, Inc. (Level VII)

7　The Joint Commission. (2021). Standard TS.01.01.01. *Comprehensive accreditation manual for hospitals.* Oakbrook Terrace, IL: The Joint Commission. (Level VII)

8　Accreditation Association for Hospitals and Health Systems. (2020). Standard 15.01.16. *Healthcare Facilities Accreditation Program: Accreditation requirements for acute care hospitals.* Chicago, IL: Accreditation Association for Hospitals and Health Systems. (Level VII)

9　Centers for Medicare and Medicaid Services, Department of Health and Human Services. (2020). Condition of participation: Patient's rights. 42 C.F.R. § 482.13(c)(1).

10　The Joint Commission. (2021). Standard RI.01.01.01. *Comprehensive accreditation manual for hospitals.* Oakbrook Terrace, IL: The Joint Commission. (Level VII)

11　DNV GL-Healthcare USA, Inc. (2020). PR.2.SR.5. *NIAHO® accreditation requirements, interpretive guidelines and surveyor guidance—revision 20.0.* Milford, OH: DNV GL-Healthcare USA, Inc. (Level VII)

12　The Joint Commission. (2021). Standard PC.02.01.21. *Comprehensive accreditation manual for hospitals.* Oakbrook Terrace, IL: The Joint Commission. (Level VII)

13　Centers for Disease Control and Prevention. (2002). Guideline for hand hygiene in health-care settings: Recommendations of the Healthcare Infection Control Practices Advisory Committee and the HICPAC/SHEA/APIC/IDSA Hand Hygiene Task Force. *MMWR Recommendations and Reports, 51*(RR-16), 1–45. https://www.cdc.gov/mmwr/pdf/rr/rr5116.pdf (Level II)

14　Centers for Medicare and Medicaid Services, Department of Health and Human Services. (2020). Condition of participation: Infection control. 42 C.F.R. § 482.42.

15　Accreditation Association for Hospitals and Health Systems. (2020). Standard 07.01.21. *Healthcare Facilities Accreditation Program: Accreditation requirements for acute care hospitals.* Chicago, IL: Accreditation Association for Hospitals and Health Systems. (Level VII)

16　World Health Organization. (2009). WHO guidelines on hand hygiene in health care: First global patient safety challenge,

clean care is safer care. https://apps.who.int/iris/bitstream/handle/10665/44102/9789241597906_eng.pdf?sequence=1 (Level IV)

17 The Joint Commission. (2021). Standard NPSG.07.01.01. *Comprehensive accreditation manual for hospitals*. Oakbrook Terrace, IL: The Joint Commission. (Level VII)

18 DNV GL-Healthcare USA, Inc. (2020). IC.1.SR.1. *NIAHO® accreditation requirements, interpretive guidelines and surveyor guidance—revision 20.0*. Milford, OH: DNV GL-Healthcare USA, Inc. (Level VII)

19 Accreditation Association for Hospitals and Health Systems. (2020). Standard 07.01.10. *Healthcare Facilities Accreditation Program: Accreditation requirements for acute care hospitals*. Chicago, IL: Accreditation Association for Hospitals and Health Systems. (Level VII)

20 Siegel, J. D., et al. (2007, revised 2019). 2007 guideline for isolation precautions: Preventing transmission of infectious agents in healthcare settings. https://www.cdc.gov/infectioncontrol/pdf/guidelines/isolation-guidelines-H.pdf (Level II)

21 Occupational Safety and Health Administration. (2019). Bloodborne pathogens, standard number 1910.1030. https://www.osha.gov/pls/oshaweb/owadisp.show_document?p_id=10051&p_table=STANDARDS (Level VII)

22 Waters, T. R., et al. (2009). Safe patient handling training for schools of nursing. https://www.cdc.gov/niosh/docs/2009-127/pdfs/2009-127.pdf (Level VII)

23 Rocky Mountain Lions Eye Bank. (n.d.). Post-mortem eye care for the potential eye donor. https://corneas.org/userfiles/1389/files/postmortemeyecare.pdf

24 Schreiber, M. L. (2020). The patient at death: Nursing responsibilities and expectations during postmortem care. *MEDSURG Nursing, 29*, 419–422. (Level VII)

25 Craven, R. F., et al. (2021). *Fundamentals of nursing: Concepts and competencies for practice* (9th ed.). Philadelphia, PA: Wolters Kluwer.

26 National Institute on Aging. (2020). What to do after someone dies. https://www.nia.nih.gov/health/what-do-after-someone-dies

27 Ganz, D. A., et al. (2013, reviewed 2021). Preventing falls in hospitals: A toolkit for improving quality of care (AHRQ publication no. 13-0015-EF). https://www.ahrq.gov/professionals/systems/hospital/fallpxtoolkit/index.html (Level VII)

28 The Joint Commission. (2021). Standard RC.01.03.01. *Comprehensive accreditation manual for hospitals*. Oakbrook Terrace, IL: The Joint Commission. (Level VII)

29 Centers for Medicare and Medicaid Services, Department of Health and Human Services. (2020). Condition of participation: Medical record services. 42 C.F.R. § 482.24(b).

30 Accreditation Association for Hospitals and Health Systems. (2020). Standard 10.00.03. *Healthcare Facilities Accreditation Program: Accreditation requirements for acute care hospitals*. Chicago, IL: Accreditation Association for Hospitals and Health Systems. (Level VII)

31 DNV GL-Healthcare USA, Inc. (2020). MR.2.SR.1. *NIAHO® accreditation requirements, interpretive guidelines and surveyor guidance—revision 20.0*. Milford, OH: DNV GL-Healthcare USA, Inc. (Level VII)

32 Hand, M. W. (2014). Lasting impressions: Using the perspective of the funeral director to guide post mortem nursing care practice. *Medsurg Nursing, 23*(6), 4–6. (Level VII)

POSTOPERATIVE CARE

Postoperative care begins when the patient arrives on the postanesthesia care unit (PACU) and continues as the patient moves to the short procedure unit, medical-surgical unit, or critical care area. The purpose of postoperative care is to minimize postoperative complications, such as pain, inadequate oxygenation, or adverse physiologic effects of sudden movement, through early detection and prompt treatment.[1]

Recovery from general anesthesia takes longer than its induction because the anesthetic is retained in fat and muscle. Because fat has a meager blood supply, it releases the anesthetic slowly, providing enough anesthesia to maintain adequate blood and brain levels during surgery. The patient's recovery time varies with the amount of body fat,[2] the patient's overall condition, the premedication regimen, and the type, dosage, and duration of anesthesia.

Equipment

Gloves ▪ vital signs monitoring equipment ▪ stethoscope ▪ pulse oximeter and probe ▪ facility-approved assessment tools ▪ blood glucose monitor and supplies ▪ prescribed medications and fluids ▪ disinfectant pad ▪ emergency equipment (code care with emergency medications, defibrillator, handheld resuscitation bag with mask, intubation equipment) ▪ Optional: transfer device, oxygen, oxygen delivery equipment, suction equipment, other personal protective equipment, cardiac monitoring equipment, capnography equipment, incentive spirometer, dressings, sequential compression device, active warming devices, electronic infusion device.

Implementation

▪ Gather and prepare the necessary equipment and supplies.
▪ Perform hand hygiene.[3,4,5,6,7,8]
▪ Put on gloves and other personal protective equipment as needed *to comply with standard precautions.*[9,10,11]
▪ Confirm the patient's identity using at least two patient identifiers.[12]
▪ Receive hand-off communication from the perianesthesia nurse *to obtain information about the patient's intraoperative status, immediate postoperative condition before admission to the PACU, and condition during the patient's stay in the PACU. Ask questions as necessary to avoid miscommunication that may cause patient care errors during the transition of care.*[13,14] As part of the hand-off process, trace each tubing and catheter from the patient to its point of origin *to make sure they're attached to the proper port*; also use a standardized line reconciliation process.[14,15,16] Hand-off communication should include relevant preoperative status, operative procedure, estimated fluid and blood loss and replacement, medications administered, anesthesia or sedation technique and agents administered, length of time anesthesia or sedation was administered, complications that occurred during the course of anesthesia and treatment (including the time at which reversal agents were given), pain and comfort management interventions and plan, and emotional status.[13]
▪ Provide privacy.[17,18,19,20]
▪ Transfer the patient from the PACU stretcher to the bed and position the patient properly. Get a coworker to help, if necessary. When moving the patient, raise the patient's bed to hip level *to prevent caregiver back strain,*[21] and keep transfer movements smooth *to minimize pain and postoperative complications.* Use a transfer device as needed.[22]
▪ Raise the bed's side rails *to ensure the patient's safety.*[23]

NURSING ALERT For the patient who has had orthopedic surgery, always have coworkers help with transfers. Ask one coworker to move only the affected extremity. If the patient is in skeletal traction, you may receive special orders for transferring. If you must move the patient, have one coworker move the weights as you and another coworker move the patient.

▪ Monitor the patient's respiratory status by assessing airway patency, chest wall movement, depth of respirations, breath sounds, and oxygen saturation level using pulse oximetry. Administer supplemental oxygen, as ordered, for a patient at risk for hypoxemia.[24] Simple oxygen face masks are generally used until the patient is more awake.
▪ Monitor the patient's vital signs at a frequency determined by your facility and the patient's condition. *There's no evidence-based research to indicate best practice for frequency of vital signs checks; therefore, frequency is determined by each facility.*[25]
▪ Monitor the patient's pulse rate, which should be strong and easily palpable. The heart rate should be within 20% of the preoperative heart rate. Monitor the patient's cardiac rhythm, if indicated.[24]
▪ Compare postoperative blood pressure with preoperative blood pressure. It should be within 20% of the preoperative level unless the patient suffered a hypotensive episode during surgery.
▪ Elevate the head of the bed, if not contraindicated, *to improve ventilation and to prevent aspiration of secretions.*[22]
▪ At frequent intervals, assess the patient's level of consciousness. *A patient who's somnolent or disoriented is unable to protect the airway or interact properly with the environment, and is at risk of aspiration, hypoventilation, poor pain management, and falls.*
▪ Obtain the patient's core body temperature, *because anesthesia lowers body temperature.* If the patient has a temperature lower than 96.8° F (36° C) or is shivering or demonstrating other signs of hypothermia, use active rewarming measures, and assess the patient's temperature and thermal comfort level at a minimum of every 15 minutes until the patient

achieves normothermia.[26] *Hypothermia adversely affects many systems and inhibits the metabolism of inhaled, IV, and regional anesthetics, and increases the risk of surgical site infection.*[25,26,27,28]

■ Perform a neurologic assessment, particularly in a patient who has undergone a surgical procedure involving components of the neurologic system.

■ Monitor blood glucose levels, as ordered. *Postoperative control of blood glucose levels is linked to surgical site infection prevention, especially after cardiac surgery.*[28,29]

HOSPITAL-ACQUIRED CONDITION ALERT Keep in mind that the Centers for Medicare and Medicaid Services considers a surgical site infection after certain cardiac surgeries, bariatric surgeries, or orthopedic procedures a hospital-acquired condition, *because various best practices can reasonably prevent it.* Be sure to follow evidence-based infection prevention techniques, such as performing hand hygiene, monitoring the blood glucose level postoperatively, and maintaining normothermia, *to reduce the risk of surgical site infection.*[28,30,31]

■ Complete a GI assessment and verify the patency of any nasogastric or orogastric drainage tubes present. Also verify whether they should be connected to suction; after connecting to suction, if ordered, trace the tubing from the patient to its point of origin *to make sure that you've connected it to the proper port.*[16] Assess the patient's bowel sounds, especially if the patient underwent surgery involving the abdomen.

■ Assess for nausea as soon as the patient awakens and regularly thereafter. If nausea is present, quantify the severity using a facility-approved assessment tool. *Nausea and vomiting should be treated early and aggressively.*[24,32,33]

■ Perform a genitourinary assessment. If the patient has an indwelling urinary catheter, assess the color, quantity, and quality of urine. Ensure that the catheter is secure and that there are no dependent loops in the drainage tubing. Maintain the drainage bag below the level of the bladder and hips *to prevent backflow of urine into the bladder, which increases the risk of catheter-associated urinary tract infection (CAUTI).* Remove the catheter as ordered or according to facility protocol as soon as it's no longer needed *to reduce the risk of CAUTI.*[34,35,36,37]

NURSING ALERT Keep in mind that the Centers for Medicare and Medicaid Services considers catheter-associated urinary tract infection (CAUTI) a hospital-acquired condition *because it can be reasonably prevented using various best practices.* Be sure to follow evidence-based CAUTI prevention practices—such as performing hand hygiene before and after any catheter manipulation; maintaining a sterile, continuously closed drainage system; maintaining unobstructed urine flow; regularly emptying the collection bag; replacing the catheter and drainage system using sterile technique when a break in sterile technique, disconnection, or leakage occurs; and discontinuing the catheter as soon as it's no longer clinically indicated—when caring for a patient with an indwelling urinary catheter *to reduce the risk of CAUTI.*[31,35,36,37,38,39]

■ Some patients who undergo urinary tract surgery may require continuous bladder irrigation to control bleeding and reduce the chance of blockage or clots forming in the bladder. Maintain continuous bladder irrigation as ordered by the practitioner.[40]

■ Screen for and assess pain using facility-defined criteria that are consistent with the patient's age, condition, and ability to understand.[41] Assess pain type, location, frequency, and duration. Also assess other sources of discomfort, such as nausea, vomiting, positioning, and anxiety.

■ Treat the patient's pain, as needed and ordered, using nonpharmacologic, pharmacologic, or a combination of approaches. Base the treatment plan on evidence-based practices and the patient's clinical condition, medical history, and pain management goals.[41] Guidelines recommend a multimodal pain management approach that may include opioid and nonopioid therapy, positioning, cold or heat application, and treatment for anxiety.[42] (See the "Pain management" procedure.) Assess the patient's pain level before and after intervention.

■ For a patient receiving IV opioid medication, frequently monitor respiratory rate, oxygen saturation level by pulse oximetry, end-tidal carbon dioxide level by capnography (if available), and sedation levels using a standardized sedation scale *to decrease the risk of adverse events associated with IV opioid use.*[43,44]

■ For a patient receiving IV opioid medication, explain to the patient and family members about the assessment and monitoring process, and tell them to alert staff if breathing problems or sedation occur.[43,44]

■ Assess the patient's infusion sites for redness, pain, swelling, or drainage. *These findings indicate infiltration, and require discontinuing the IV line and restarting it at another site.*[45] Trace each tubing from the patient to its point of origin *to make sure it's attached to the proper port to prevent dangerous misconnections.*[16]

■ Assess surgical wound dressings; they should be clean and dry. If they're soiled, assess the characteristics of the drainage and outline the soiled area. Note the date and time of assessment on the dressing. Assess the soiled area frequently; if it enlarges, reinforce the dressing and alert the practitioner.[46]

■ Note the presence and condition of any drains and tubes. Note the color, type, odor, and amount of drainage. Make sure all drains are properly connected and free from kinks and obstructions.

■ If the patient has had vascular or orthopedic surgery, assess the appropriate extremity, or all extremities, depending on the surgical procedure. Perform a neurovascular assessment, including color, temperature, sensation, movement, and presence and quality of pulses, and notify the practitioner of any abnormalities.

■ Continue venous thromboembolism (VTE) prophylaxis, such as using sequential compression sleeves or boots, according to the practitioner's order or facility protocol.[34]

HOSPITAL-ACQUIRED CONDITION ALERT Keep in mind that the Centers for Medicare and Medicaid Services considers VTE in patients who underwent total knee replacement a hospital-acquired condition *because it can be prevented using various best practices.* Be sure to follow evidence-based VTE prevention practices, such as using mechanical compression devices (including antiembolism stockings or an intermittent pneumatic compression device), early ambulation, and pharmacologic prophylaxis, *to reduce the risk of VTE.*[31,46,47]

■ Encourage coughing and deep-breathing exercises (unless the patient has just had nasal, ophthalmic, or neurologic surgery) and incentive spirometry use, as indicated and prescribed.[48]

■ Administer IV fluids[5] and medications, such as antibiotics, analgesics, antiemetics, or reversal agents, as ordered and appropriate following safe medication administration practices.[43,49,50,51]

■ If the patient was receiving a beta-adrenergic blocker before surgery, collaborate with the patient's practitioner to make sure that the patient receives it during the perioperative period, as appropriate.[34]

■ If administering IV fluids or medications through an electronic infusion device, make sure that alarm limits are set according to the patient's current condition, and that the alarms are turned on, functioning properly, and audible to staff.[52,53,54]

■ Assess and address the patient's safety needs.[25]

■ Remove all oral fluids from the bedside until the patient is alert enough to eat and drink.

■ Monitor the patient's intake and output.

■ Remove and discard your gloves and other personal protective equipment, if worn.[11]

■ Perform hand hygiene.[3,4,5,6,7,8]

■ Clean and disinfect your stethoscope using a disinfectant pad.[55,56]

■ Perform hand hygiene.[3,4,5,6,7,8]

■ Document the procedure.[57,58,59,60]

Special considerations

■ Notify the anesthesia practitioner if the patient reports awareness while under general anesthesia. This rare condition, known as anesthetic awareness or intraoperative awareness, occurs when surgical patients can recall their surroundings or an event (sometimes even pressure or pain) related to their surgery while they are under general anesthesia. Severe cases of anesthetic awareness happen infrequently, but researchers are trying to determine a cause to prevent it from happening. When it does occur, patients should be encouraged to discuss the experience and personal feelings with the anesthesia practitioner. Early counseling after an episode of awareness is important to lessening feelings of stress, confusion, or trauma associated with the experience. Rarely, patients develop posttraumatic stress disorder, which is associated with repetitive nightmares, anxiety, irritability, and preoccupation with death.[61]

■ Fear, pain, anxiety, hypothermia, confusion, and immobility can upset the patient and jeopardize safety and postoperative status. Offer emotional support to the patient and family.[2] Keep in mind that the patient who has lost a body part or who has been diagnosed with an incurable disease will need ongoing emotional support. Refer the patient and family for counseling as needed.

■ As the patient recovers from general anesthesia, reflexes appear in reverse order to that in which they disappeared. Hearing recovers first, so avoid holding inappropriate conversations.

■ A patient under general anesthesia can't protect the airway *because of muscle relaxation.*[2] As the patient recovers, cough and gag reflexes reappear. The patient who can lift the head without assistance can usually breathe independently.

■ If the anesthesia provider administered spinal anesthesia, the patient may require supine positioning[2] with the bed adjusted to between 0 and 20 degrees for at least 6 hours *to reduce the risk of spinal headache from leakage of cerebrospinal fluid.* The patient won't be able to move the legs, so reassure the patient that sensation and mobility will return. (See *Assessing level of blockade from spinal anesthesia.*)

■ If the patient has had an epidural analgesia infusion for postoperative pain control, monitor respiratory status closely.[2] *Respiratory arrest may result from the respiratory depressant effects of the opioid.* Also monitor the patient's blood pressure, heart rate, and arterial oxygen saturation at an interval determined by your facility or the patient's condition. The patient may also suffer from nausea, vomiting, or itching. Epidural analgesia may also include administering a local anesthetic with the opioid. (See the "Epidural analgesic administration" procedure.) Assess the patient's lower-extremity motor strength every 2 to 4 hours. If sensorimotor loss occurs (numbness or weakness of the legs), notify the practitioner, *because the dosage may need to be decreased.*

■ If the patient will be using a patient-controlled analgesia unit, make sure the patient understands how to use it.[2] Caution the patient to activate it only when experiencing pain, not when feeling sleepy or pain-free. (See the "Patient-controlled analgesia" procedure.)

ELDER ALERT If the patient is older, be aware of age-related changes that will alter your assessment. Monitor cardiovascular status carefully, *because blood loss, pain, bed rest, and fluid and electrolyte imbalances can alter it.* Monitor fluid and electrolyte status closely. Encourage early mobilization *to reduce the risks associated with prolonged bedrest.* Also carefully monitor respiratory status, *because ventilation and oxygenation can be altered by age-related changes or years of smoking or chronic diseases.* Encourage coughing and deep breathing exercises. Closely monitor level of consciousness and pain, *because mental status changes can affect these and make pain control more difficult.* Drug metabolism slows

Assessing level of blockade from spinal anesthesia

Spinal anesthesia produces a sympathetic, sensory, and motor block. If the patient received spinal anesthesia, be ready to assess the downward progression of the level of blockade. Using a dermatome chart aids this assessment. Each dermatome represents a specific body area supplied with nerve fibers from an individual spinal root (cervical, thoracic, lumbar, or sacral). To document the patient's sensory and motor function, mentally divide the patient's body into dermatomes. Anatomic reference points include the nipple line at T4, xiphoid at T6, umbilicus at T10, and groin at L1.

Anterior view

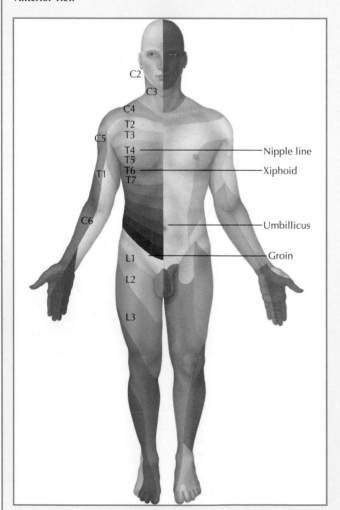

Posterior view

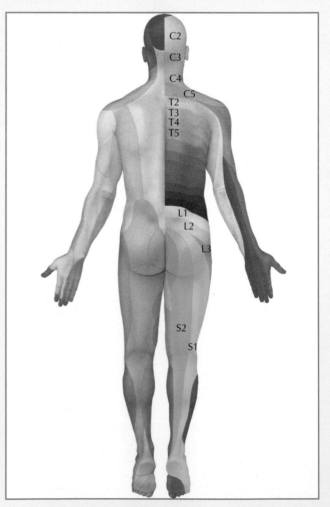

with age, so monitor the older adult's risk of drug reactions, toxicity, and interactions. Monitor intake and output carefully, and watch for urinary tract infections (UTIs), *because decreased renal functioning and decreased bladder capacity increase the risk of UTIs.* Position the older patient carefully, and prevent postoperative falls, *because the patient may have osteoporosis and may be prone to fractures.* Also monitor for signs and symptoms of infection, *because the risk of infection increases with age.*

Complications

Postoperative complications may include airway obstruction, laryngospasm, bronchospasm, obstructive sleep apnea, cardiac arrhythmias, delirium, alterations in blood pressure, alterations in temperature, hypovolemia, aspiration, nausea and vomiting, and acute pain.[62] Less immediate postoperative complications include septicemia, septic shock, atelectasis, pneumonia, thrombophlebitis, pulmonary embolism, urine retention, wound infection, wound dehiscence, evisceration, abdominal distention, paralytic ileus, constipation, and altered body image.[62]

Documentation

Document vital signs and all assessment findings according to your facility's documentation format. Record the condition of dressings and drains and characteristics of drainage. Document all pain assessment findings, interventions performed to alleviate pain and anxiety, and the patient's responses to those interventions. Record all medications that you administered. Document any complications, interventions performed, and the patient's response to those interventions. Document teaching provided to the patient and family (if applicable), their understanding of that teaching, and any need for follow-up teaching.

REFERENCES

1 The Joint Commission. (2021). Standard PC.03.01.07. *Comprehensive accreditation manual for hospitals.* Oakbrook Terrace, IL: The Joint Commission. (Level VII)

2 Hinkle, J. L., & Cheever, K. H. (2018). *Brunner & Suddarth's textbook of medical-surgical nursing* (14th ed.). Philadelphia, PA: Wolters Kluwer.

3 The Joint Commission. (2021). Standard NPSG.07.01.01. *Comprehensive accreditation manual for hospitals.* Oakbrook Terrace, IL: The Joint Commission. (Level VII)

4 Centers for Disease Control and Prevention. (2002). Guideline for hand hygiene in health-care settings: Recommendations of the Healthcare Infection Control Practices Advisory Committee and the HICPAC/SHEA/APIC/IDSA Hand Hygiene Task Force. *MMWR Recommendations and Reports, 51*(RR-16), 1–45. https://www.cdc.gov/mmwr/pdf/rr/rr5116.pdf (Level II)

5 World Health Organization. (2009). WHO guidelines on hand hygiene in health care: First global patient safety challenge, clean care is safer care. https://apps.who.int/iris/bitstream/handle/10665/44102/9789241597906_eng.pdf (Level IV)

6 Centers for Medicare and Medicaid Services, Department of Health and Human Services. (2020). Condition of participation: Infection control. 42 C.F.R. § 482.42.

7 Accreditation Association for Hospitals and Health Systems. (2020). Standard 07.01.21. *Healthcare Facilities Accreditation Program: Accreditation requirements for acute care hospitals.* Chicago, IL: Accreditation Association for Hospitals and Health Systems. (Level VII)

8 DNV GL-Healthcare USA, Inc. (2020). IC.1.SR.1. *NIAHO® accreditation requirements, interpretive guidelines and surveyor guidance—revision 20.0.* Milford, OH: DNV GL-Healthcare USA, Inc. (Level VII)

9 Siegel, J. D., et al. (2007, revised 2019). 2007 guideline for isolation precautions: Preventing transmission of infectious agents in healthcare settings. https://www.cdc.gov/infectioncontrol/pdf/guidelines/isolation-guidelines-H.pdf (Level II)

10 Accreditation Association for Hospitals and Health Systems. (2020). Standard 07.01.10. *Healthcare Facilities Accreditation Program: Accreditation requirements for acute care hospitals.* Chicago, IL: Accreditation Association for Hospitals and Health Systems. (Level VII)

11 Occupational Safety and Health Administration. (2019). Bloodborne pathogens, standard number 1910.1030. https://www.osha.gov/pls/oshaweb/owadisp.show_document?p_id=10051&p_table=STANDARDS (Level VII)

12 The Joint Commission. (2021). Standard NPSG.01.01.01. *Comprehensive accreditation manual for hospitals.* Oakbrook Terrace, IL: The Joint Commission. (Level VII)

13 Guideline for perioperative practice: Team communication. (2020). In Wood, A. (Ed.), *Guidelines for perioperative practice,* 2020 edition. Denver, CO: AORN, Inc. (Level VII)

14 The Joint Commission. (2021). Standard PC.02.02.01. *Comprehensive accreditation manual for hospitals.* Oakbrook Terrace, IL: The Joint Commission. (Level VII)

15 The Joint Commission. (2014). Sentinel event alert 53: Managing risk during transition to new ISO tubing connector standards. https://www.jointcommission.org/-/media/tjc/documents/resources/patient-safety-topics/sentinel-event/sea_53_connectors_8_19_14_final.pdf (Level VII)

16 U.S. Food and Drug Administration. (2017). Examples of medical device misconnections. https://www.fda.gov/medical-devices/medical-device-connectors/examples-medical-device-misconnections

17 Accreditation Association for Hospitals and Health Systems. (2020). Standard 15.01.16. *Healthcare Facilities Accreditation Program: Accreditation requirements for acute care hospitals.* Chicago, IL: Accreditation Association for Hospitals and Health Systems. (Level VII)

18 The Joint Commission. (2021). Standard RI.01.01.01. *Comprehensive accreditation manual for hospitals.* Oakbrook Terrace, IL: The Joint Commission. (Level VII)

19 DNV GL-Healthcare USA, Inc. (2020). PR.2.SR.5. *NIAHO® accreditation requirements, interpretive guidelines and surveyor guidance—revision 20.0.* Milford, OH: DNV GL-Healthcare USA, Inc. (Level VII)

20 Centers for Medicare and Medicaid Services, Department of Health and Human Services. (2020). Condition of participation: Patient's rights. 42 C.F.R. § 482.13(c)(1).

21 Waters, T. R., et al. (2009). Safe patient handling training for schools of nursing. https://www.cdc.gov/niosh/docs/2009-127/pdfs/2009-127.pdf (Level VII)

22 Guideline for perioperative practice: Positioning the patient. (2020). In Wood, A. (Ed.), *Guidelines for perioperative practice,* 2020 edition. Denver, CO: AORN, Inc. (Level VII)

23 Ganz, D. A., et al. (2013, reviewed 2021). *Preventing falls in hospitals: A toolkit for improving quality of care* (AHRQ Publication No. 13-0015-EF). Rockville, MD: Agency for Healthcare Research and Quality. https://www.ahrq.gov/professionals/systems/hospital/fallpxtoolkit/index.html (Level VII)

24 American Society of Anesthesiologists Task Force on Postanesthetic Care. (2013). Practice guidelines for postanesthetic care: An updated report by the American Society of Anesthesiologists Task Force on Postanesthetic Care. *Anesthesiology, 118*(2), 291–307. https://anesthesiology.pubs.asahq.org/article.aspx?articleid=1918686 (Level VII)

25 American Society of PeriAnesthesia Nurses. (2019). *2019-2020 Perianesthesia nursing standards, practice recommendations and interpretive statements.* Cherry Hill, NJ: American Society of PeriAnesthesia Nurses. (Level VII)

26 Hooper, V. D. (2010). ASPAN's evidence-based clinical practice guideline for the promotion of perioperative normothermia: Second edition. *Journal of PeriAnesthesia Nursing, 25*(6), 346–365. http://www.aspan.org/Portals/6/docs/ClinicalPractice/Guidelines/Normothermia_Guideline_12-10_JoPAN.pdf (Level VII)

27 Guideline for perioperative practice: Hypothermia. (2020). In Wood, A. (Ed.), *Guidelines for perioperative practice,* 2020 edition. Denver, CO: AORN, Inc. (Level VII)

28 Berríos-Torres, S. I., et al. (2017). Centers for Disease Control and Prevention guideline for the prevention of surgical site infection, 2017. *JAMA Surgery, 152*(8), 784–791. https://jamanetwork.com/journals/jamasurgery/fullarticle/2623725 (Level VII)

29 Accreditation Association for Hospitals and Health Systems. (2020). Standard 07.01.20. *Healthcare Facilities Accreditation Program: Accreditation requirements for acute care hospitals.* Chicago, IL: Accreditation Association for Hospitals and Health Systems. (Level VII)

30 The Joint Commission. (2021). Standard NPSG.07.05.01. *Comprehensive accreditation manual for hospitals.* Oakbrook Terrace, IL: The Joint Commission. (Level VII)

31 Jarrett, N., & Callaham, M. (2016). Evidence-based guidelines for selected hospital-acquired conditions: Final report. https://www.cms.gov/Medicare/Medicare-Fee-for-Service-Payment/HospitalAcqCond/Downloads/2016-HAC-Report.pdf

32 American Society of PeriAnesthesia Nurses. (2006). ASPAN'S evidence-based clinical practice guideline for the prevention and/or management of PONV/PDNV. *Journal of PeriAnesthesia Nursing, 21*(4), 230–250. http://www.aspan.org/Portals/6/docs/ClinicalPractice/Guidelines/PONV-PDNV_Clinical_Guideline_Aug_2006_JoPAN.pdf (Level VII)

33 Habib, A. S., et al. (2006). Postoperative nausea and vomiting following inpatient surgeries in a teaching hospital: A retrospective database analysis. *Current Medical Research and Opinion, 22*, 1093–1099. (Level IV)

34 Centers for Medicare and Medicaid Services, & The Joint Commission. (2022). The specifications manual for national hospital inpatient quality measures (version 5.11). https://www.qualitynet.org/inpatient/specifications-manuals#tab1

35 Association of Professionals in Infection Control and Epidemiology. (2014). APIC implementation guide: Guide to preventing catheter-associated urinary tract infections. https://apic.org/wp-content/uploads/2019/02/APIC_CAUTI_IG_FIN_REVD0815.pdf (Level IV)

36 Healthcare Infection Control Practices Advisory Committee. (2010, revised 2019). Guideline for prevention of catheter-associated urinary tract infections 2009. https://www.cdc.gov/infectioncontrol/pdf/guidelines/cauti-guidelines-H.pdf (Level I)

37 The Joint Commission. (2021). Standard NPSG.07.06.01. *Comprehensive accreditation manual for hospitals.* Oakbrook Terrace, IL: The Joint Commission. (Level VII)

38 Agency for Healthcare Research and Quality & U.S. Department of Health and Human Services. (2015). Toolkit for reducing catheter-associated urinary tract infections in hospital units: Implementation guide. https://www.ahrq.gov/professionals/quality-patient-safety/hais/cauti-tools/impl-guide/index.html

39 Lo, E., et al. (2014). SHEA/IDSA practice recommendation: Strategies to prevent catheter-associated urinary tract infections in acute care hospitals: 2014 update. *Infection Control and Hospital Epidemiology, 35*(5), 464–479. https://www.jstor.org/stable/10.1086/675718#metadata_info_tab_contents (Level I)

40 Feliciano, T., et al. (2008). A retrospective, descriptive, exploratory study evaluating incidence of postoperative urinary retention after spinal anesthesia and its effect on PACU discharge. *Journal of Perianesthesia Nursing, 23*, 394–400. (Level IV)

41 The Joint Commission. (2021). Standard PC.01.02.07. *Comprehensive accreditation manual for hospitals.* Oakbrook Terrace, IL: The Joint Commission. (Level VII)

42 American Society of Anesthesiologists Task Force on Acute Pain Management. (2012). Practice guidelines for acute pain management in the perioperative setting: An updated report by the American Society of Anesthesiologists Task Force on Acute Pain Management. *Anesthesiology, 116*, 248–273. https://anesthesiology.pubs.asahq.org/article.aspx?articleid=1933589 (Level VII)

43 Centers for Medicare and Medicaid Services, Department of Health and Human Services. (2020). Condition of participation: Nursing services. 42 C.F.R. § 482.23(c).

44 Centers for Medicare and Medicaid Services. (2014). Requirements for hospital medication administration, particularly intravenous (IV) medications and post-operative care of patients receiving IV opioids. http://www.cms.gov/Medicare/Provider-Enrollment-and-Certification/SurveyCertificationGenInfo/Downloads/Survey-and-Cert-Letter-14-15.pdf

45 Standard 47. Infiltration and extravasation. Infusion therapy standards of practice (8th ed.). (2021). *Journal of Infusion Nursing, 44*, S142–S147. (Level VII)

46 Falck-Ytter, Y., et al. (2012). Prevention of VTE in orthopedic surgery patients: Antithrombotic therapy and prevention of thrombosis (9th ed.): American College of Chest Physicians evidence-based clinical practice guidelines. *Chest, 141*(Suppl. 2), e278S–e325S. https://www.ncbi.nlm.nih.gov/pmc/articles/PMC3278063/

47 Balk, E. M., et al. (2017). *Venous thromboembolism prophylaxis in major orthopedic surgery: Systematic review update.* (AHRQ Publication No. 17-EHC021-EF). Rockville, MD: Agency for Healthcare Research and Quality. https://effectivehealthcare.ahrq.gov/products/thromboembolism-update/research-2017 (Level I)

48 Restrepo, R. D., et al. (2011). AARC clinical practice guideline: Incentive spirometry: 2011. *Respiratory Care, 56*(10), 1600–1604. http://rc.rcjournal.com/content/respcare/56/10/1600.full.pdf (Level VII)

49 Accreditation Association for Hospitals and Health Systems. (2020). Standard 16.01.03. *Healthcare Facilities Accreditation Program: Accreditation requirements for acute care hospitals.* Chicago, IL: Accreditation Association for Hospitals and Health Systems. (Level VII)

50 DNV GL-Healthcare USA, Inc. (2020). MM.1.SR.3. *NIAHO® accreditation requirements, interpretive guidelines and surveyor guidance—revision 20.0.* Milford, OH: DNV GL-Healthcare USA, Inc. (Level VII)

51 The Joint Commission. (2021). Standard MM.06.01.01. *Comprehensive accreditation manual for hospitals.* Oakbrook Terrace, IL: The Joint Commission. (Level VII)

52 The Joint Commission. (2021). Standard NPSG.06.01.01. *Comprehensive accreditation manual for hospitals.* Oakbrook Terrace, IL: The Joint Commission. (Level VII)

53 Graham, K. C., & Cvach, M. (2010). Monitor alarm fatigue: Standardizing use of physiological monitors and decreasing nuisance alarms. *American Journal of Critical Care, 19*, 28–37. https://aacnjournals.org/ajcconline/article-abstract/19/1/28/5720/Monitor-Alarm-Fatigue-Standardizing-Use-of?redirectedFrom=fulltext

54 The Joint Commission. (2013). Sentinel event alert 50: Medical device alarm safety in hospitals. https://www.jointcommission.org/-/media/tjc/documents/resources/patient-safety-topics/sentinel-event/sea_50_alarms_4_26_16.pdf (Level VII)

55 Rutala, W. A., et al. (2008, revised 2019). Guideline for disinfection and sterilization in healthcare facilities, 2008. https://www.cdc.gov/infection-control/pdf/guidelines/disinfection-guidelines-H.pdf (Level I)

56 Accreditation Association for Hospitals and Health Systems. (2020). Standard 07.02.03. *Healthcare Facilities Accreditation Program: Accreditation requirements for acute care hospitals.* Chicago, IL: Accreditation Association for Hospitals and Health Systems. (Level VII)

57 The Joint Commission. (2021). Standard RC.01.03.01. *Comprehensive accreditation manual for hospitals.* Oakbrook Terrace, IL: The Joint Commission. (Level VII)

58 Centers for Medicare and Medicaid Services, Department of Health and Human Services. (2020). Condition of participation: Medical record services. 42 C.F.R. § 482.24(b).

59 Accreditation Association for Hospitals and Health Systems. (2020). Standard 10.00.03. *Healthcare Facilities Accreditation Program: Accreditation requirements for acute care hospitals.* Chicago, IL: Accreditation Association for Hospitals and Health Systems. (Level VII)

60 DNV GL-Healthcare USA, Inc. (2020). MR.2.SR.1. *NIAHO® accreditation requirements, interpretive guidelines and surveyor guidance—revision 20.0.* Milford, OH: DNV GL-Healthcare USA, Inc. (Level VII)

61 American Association of Nurse Anesthetists. (n.d.). Anesthetic awareness. https://www.aana.com/patients/all-about-anesthesia/anesthetic-awareness

62 Rothrock, J. C. (2019). *Alexander's care of the surgical patient* (16th ed.). St. Louis, MO: Elsevier.

POSTTRAUMATIC STRESS DISORDER ASSESSMENT

Posttraumatic stress disorder (PTSD) occurs in some individuals after they experience a traumatic event, such as assault, combat, or disaster. Individuals cope differently with psychological stress. Although most people exposed to traumatic events don't develop PTSD, others progress to the complete syndrome. Trauma isn't an external incident open to objective interpretation. Similar to pain, the traumatic experience is filtered through cognitive and emotional processes before it becomes perceived as an extreme threat to the individual. People have different trauma thresholds; some are more vulnerable than others to developing clinical symptoms after exposure to extremely stressful situations.[1]

For patients with PTSD, the traumatic event remains a dominating psychological experience that evokes despair, dread, grief, panic, or terror. These emotions may occur during intrusive daytime images of the event, nightmares, and vivid flashbacks. Trauma-related stimuli that trigger memories of the original event can evoke emotional responses and physiologic reactions associated with the trauma.[1]

In response, patients with PTSD often use avoidance to reduce the risk of exposure to trauma-related stimuli. They avoid any thought or situation that is likely to produce distressing traumatic memories. For example, a patient may be afraid to leave the house for fear of encountering reminders of the traumatic event. Patients with PTSD often have a wide variety of negative emotional states, such as anger, guilt, and shame. Additionally, they're unable to experience positive feelings, such as love, pleasure, or enjoyment, making close interpersonal relationships difficult.[1]

Other symptoms of PTSD, such as insomnia and cognitive impairment, closely resemble those seen in panic and generalized anxiety disorders, while hypervigilance and the startle response are more characteristic symptoms of PTSD. To meet criteria for PTSD, symptoms must persist for at least a month, and the patient must experience significant social, occupational, or other distress as a result of the symptoms. Medication, substance use and abuse, or other illness should be ruled out as causes of the symptoms.[1]

Equipment

Facility-approved PTSD assessment tool ▪ Optional: facility-approved substance use screening tool, facility-approved suicide risk assessment tool.

Implementation

▪ Review the patient's medical record for a history of trauma as well as substance use disorder, dissociative symptoms, sleep disturbances, panic and generalized anxiety disorders, intrusive experiences, or other trauma-related effects.[2]
▪ Gather the assessment tools needed to perform a comprehensive PTSD assessment. *Advanced preparation allows you to be fully present and demonstrate respect for the patient during the assessment.*
▪ Allow a period of time for the assessment in order to avoid rushing through the interview.
▪ Perform hand hygiene.[3,4,5,6,7,8]
▪ Confirm the patient's identity using at least two patient identifiers.[9]
▪ Select a quiet, private setting that's free from interruptions and distractions. *A private setting promotes an environment in which you can establish rapport and a sense of trust with the patient and protect confidentiality. In a calm setting, patients are more likely to speak freely, feel heard, and sense that the nurse cares about their needs and health care.*[10,11]
▪ Ensure that the assessment location has comfortable seating. Arrange the seating so that you're at an angle to the patient in a position that promotes comfortable eye contact *to show that you're fully engaged in the interview.*
▪ Position yourself so that you have direct access to an exit in case the patient's behavior becomes inappropriate, intimidating, or threatening.
▪ Be familiar with facility safeguards that permit you to obtain assistance, if needed.
▪ Address the patient by name, and then introduce yourself to the patient.
▪ Explain the procedure to the patient and family (if appropriate) according to their individual communication and learning needs *to increase their understanding, allay their fears, and enhance cooperation.*[12,13]
▪ Ask the patient's permission to conduct the PTSD assessment.
▪ Perform the PTSD assessment using a facility-approved assessment tool, such as the PTSD Checklist–Civilian Version or the PTSD Checklist for DSM-5 (PCL-5).[13]
▪ Use therapeutic communication and motivational interviewing techniques *to engage the patient in conversation and facilitate a therapeutic process.*
▪ As the patient shares information, listen actively, maintain eye contact, verbalize concern, and respond with interest *to convey empathy and promote a sense of trust.*
▪ Observe the patient's coping strategies.
▪ Watch for the presence of—or an escalation in—the patient's anger, agitation, or unsafe behavior *to prevent a dangerous situation.* Implement de-escalation techniques, if needed, *to prevent violence.*[14,15]
▪ Obtain assistance, if needed, *to ensure personal and patient safety.*[15]
▪ Depending on your preliminary PTSD assessment findings, assess the patient for substance use and suicide risk using facility-approved assessment tools.[16,17,18,19]
▪ Report your findings to the treatment team and collaborate with the team on the patient's treatment plan, if indicated.
▪ Perform hand hygiene.[3,4,5,6,7,8]
▪ Document the procedure.[20,21,22,23]

Special considerations

▪ Early assessment and intervention can improve outcomes in patients with PTSD.

▪ Trauma-focused psychotherapies, such as prolonged exposure, cognitive processing therapy, and eye movement desensitization and reprocessing, are the most highly recommended therapies for PTSD. These therapies use different techniques to help the patient process the traumatic experience.[24]
▪ The sympathetic nervous system releases hormones in response to stress that, according to magnetic resonance imaging, alter areas of the brain and may impair functioning in patients with PTSD.[25]

Complications

Posttraumatic stress disorder assessment may trigger adverse physical and psychological events.

Documentation

Record your assessment findings, any interventions, and the patient's response to those interventions. Document teaching provided to the patient and family (if applicable), their understanding of that teaching, and any need for follow-up teaching.

References

1 U.S. Department of Veterans Affairs. (n.d.). PTSD history and overview. https://www.ptsd.va.gov/professional/treat/essentials/history_ptsd.asp
2 Substance Abuse and Mental Health Services Administration. (2014). A treatment improvement protocol: Trauma-informed care in behavioral health services: Tip 57. https://store.samhsa.gov/sites/default/files/d7/priv/sma14-4816.pdf
3 Accreditation Association for Hospitals and Health Systems. (2020). Standard 07.01.21. *Healthcare Facilities Accreditation Program: Accreditation requirements for acute care hospitals.* Chicago, IL: Accreditation Association for Hospitals and Health Systems. (Level VII)
4 Centers for Disease Control and Prevention. (2002). Guideline for hand hygiene in health-care settings: Recommendations of the Healthcare Infection Control Practices Advisory Committee and the HICPAC/SHEA/APIC/IDSA Hand Hygiene Task Force. *MMWR Recommendations and Reports, 51*(RR-16), 1–45. https://www.cdc.gov/mmwr/pdf/rr/rr5116.pdf (Level II)
5 Centers for Medicare and Medicaid Services, Department of Health and Human Services. (2020). Condition of participation: Infection control. 42 C.F.R. § 482.42.
6 DNV GL-Healthcare USA, Inc. (2020). IC.1.SR.1. *NIAHO® accreditation requirements, interpretive guidelines and surveyor guidance—revision 20.0.* Milford, OH: DNV GL-Healthcare USA, Inc. (Level VII)
7 The Joint Commission. (2021). Standard NPSG.07.01.01. *Comprehensive accreditation manual for hospitals.* Oakbrook Terrace, IL: The Joint Commission. (Level VII)
8 World Health Organization. (2009). WHO guidelines on hand hygiene in health care: First global patient safety challenge, clean care is safer care. https://apps.who.int/iris/bitstream/handle/10665/44102/9789241597906_eng.pdf?sequence=1 (Level IV)
9 The Joint Commission. (2021). Standard NPSG.01.01.01. *Comprehensive accreditation manual for hospitals.* Oakbrook Terrace, IL: The Joint Commission. (Level VII)
10 Centers for Medicare and Medicaid Services, Department of Health and Human Services. (2020). Condition of participation: Patient's rights. 42 C.F.R. § 482.13(c)(1).
11 DNV GL-Healthcare USA, Inc. (2020). PR.2.SR.5. *NIAHO® accreditation requirements, interpretive guidelines and surveyor guidance—revision 20.0.* Milford, OH: DNV GL-Healthcare USA, Inc. (Level VII)
12 The Joint Commission. (2021). Standard PC.02.01.21. *Comprehensive accreditation manual for hospitals.* Oakbrook Terrace, IL: The Joint Commission. (Level VII)
13 U.S. Department of Veterans Affairs. (2019). PTSD: National Center for PTSD: Assessment. https://www.ptsd.va.gov/professional/assessment/index.asp
14 Hallett, N., & Dickens, G. L. (2017). De-escalation of aggressive behaviour in healthcare settings: Concept analysis. *International Journal of Nursing Studies, 75,* 10–20.
15 Brous, E. (2018). Workplace violence. *American Journal of Nursing, 118*(10), 51–55.
16 National Institute of Mental Health. (n.d.). Ask suicide-screening questions (ASQ) toolkit. https://www.nimh.nih.gov/research/research-conducted-at-nimh/asq-toolkit-materials/index.shtml

17 Rahm, A. K., et al. (2015). Facilitators and barriers to implementing screening, brief intervention, and referral to treatment (SBIRT) in primary care in integrated health care settings. *Substance Abuse, 36,* 281–288.

18 Bush, K., et al. (1998). The AUDIT alcohol consumption questions (AUDIT-C): An effective brief screening test for problem drinking: Ambulatory Care Quality Improvement Project (ACQUIP): Alcohol use disorders identification test. *Archives of Internal Medicine, 158,* 1789–1795.

19 The Joint Commission. (2021). Standard NPSG.15.01.01. *Comprehensive accreditation manual for hospitals.* Oakbrook Terrace, IL: The Joint Commission.

20 Accreditation Association for Hospitals and Health Systems. (2020). Standard 10.00.03. *Healthcare Facilities Accreditation Program: Accreditation requirements for acute care hospitals.* Chicago, IL: Accreditation Association for Hospitals and Health Systems. (Level VII)

21 Centers for Medicare and Medicaid Services, Department of Health and Human Services. (2020). Condition of participation: Medical record services. 42 C.F.R. § 482.24(b).

22 DNV GL-Healthcare USA, Inc. (2020). MR.2.SR.1. *NIAHO® accreditation requirements, interpretive guidelines and surveyor guidance—revision 20.0.* Milford, OH: DNV GL-Healthcare USA, Inc. (Level VII)

23 The Joint Commission. (2021). Standard RC.01.03.01. *Comprehensive accreditation manual for hospitals.* Oakbrook Terrace, IL: The Joint Commission. (Level VII)

24 U.S. Department of Veterans Affairs. (2020). PTSD treatment basics. https://www.ptsd.va.gov/understand_tx/tx_basics.asp

25 Kunimatsu, A., et al. (2020). MRI findings in posttraumatic stress disorder. *Journal of Magnetic Resonance Imaging, 52,* 380–396.

PREOPERATIVE CARE

Preoperative care is the preparation and management of a patient before surgery. Preoperative care begins when surgery is planned and ends with the administration of anesthesia. This phase of care includes a preoperative interview and assessment to collect baseline subjective and objective data from the patient and family; diagnostic tests such as urinalysis, electrocardiography (ECG), and chest radiography; preoperative teaching; informed consent from the patient; and physical preparation.[1]

If the patient is having same-day surgery, nursing interventions include providing instructions before the day of surgery that cover the arrival time to the facility, the need to leave all jewelry and valuables at home, the need to have someone accompany and stay with the patient after surgery, fasting guidelines, medication use, and any prescribed surgical preparation, such as showering with an antimicrobial cleaner.[1]

The nurse is responsible for performing a patient assessment and ensuring collection, documentation, and communication of all data.[2]

Equipment

Vital signs monitoring equipment ▪ stethoscope ▪ pulse oximetry and probe ▪ scale ▪ tape measure ▪ patient gown ▪ facility-approved pain assessment scale ▪ preoperative checklist ▪ prescribed medications ▪ prescribed IV fluids ▪ patient education materials ▪ blood glucose monitoring supplies ▪ disinfectant pad ▪ Optional: gloves, gown , mask with face shield or mask and goggles, IV catheter insertion supplies, cardiac monitor, specimen collection supplies, disposable-head clippers, antiseptic mouthwash.

Implementation

▪ Verify the practitioner's orders.
▪ Gather and prepare the necessary equipment and supplies.
▪ Review the patient's preadmission assessment findings, including X-rays, laboratory test results, and other preoperative test findings, as indicated.[3,4]
▪ Perform hand hygiene.[5,6,7,8,9,10]
▪ Put on personal protective equipment as needed *to comply with standard precautions.*[11,12,13]
▪ Confirm the patient's identity using at least two patient identifiers.[14]
▪ If the patient is having same-day surgery, ensure that arrangements are in place for someone to accompany the patient home after surgery.[2]
▪ Provide privacy.[15,16,17,18]

▪ Explain all procedures to the patient and family (if appropriate) according to their individual communication and learning needs *to increase their understanding, allay their fears, and enhance cooperation.*[19]
▪ Obtain a health history, including previous surgery, recent myocardial infarction (within the previous 60 days),[3] skin condition, immunization status, history of multiple drug-resistant organisms, external or implanted medical devices, sensory limitations, and home use of noninvasive positive-pressure ventilation or apnea monitors.[2,20] Use your facility's preoperative surgical assessment database, if available, to gather this information.
▪ Assess the patient's knowledge, perceptions, and expectations about the planned surgery.[3]
▪ Ask whether the patient has known allergies to latex, medications, food, or other substances *to determine the risk of an allergic reaction.*[2,20]
▪ Ask whether the patient has a personal or family history of a serious reaction to anesthesia or intraoperative awareness (also known as anesthetic awareness).[2]
▪ Obtain a complete list of medications the patient uses, including prescription drugs, over-the-counter medications, herbal preparations and supplements, alcohol, tobacco, and illicit drugs.[2,3,20,21,22] *It may be necessary to adjust or continue medications whose sudden cessation may provoke a withdrawal syndrome.*[23] *In addition, certain herbs (nutraceuticals) have unknown interactions with anesthetic drugs and effects on blood coagulation.* Consult with the practitioner about discontinuation before surgery and continuation after surgery for any medications the patient takes.
▪ If the patient was receiving a beta-adrenergic blocker, collaborate with the practitioner to make sure the patient receives it during the perioperative period, as appropriate.[24]
▪ Ask whether the patient has an advance directive.[25,26] Provide information about advance directives as appropriate. (See the "Advance directives" procedure.)
▪ Obtain the patient's height, weight (in kilograms), vital signs, and oxygen saturation level using pulse oximetry.[2,20]
▪ Screen for and assess the patient's pain using facility-defined criteria that are consistent with the patient's age, condition, and ability to understand.[23,27]
▪ Obtain a pain and analgesic history; ask about measures that have helped to effectively relieve or control pain in the past. Also ask about expectations for controlling pain after surgery. *By obtaining a thorough pain history preoperatively, the health care team may be able to better control pain postoperatively.*[2,20]
▪ Perform educational, socioeconomic, cultural, and spiritual assessments *to determine the patient's level of understanding about the surgical procedure and whether the patient has special needs while in the facility.*[2,20]
▪ Assess for mobility limitations and disabilities, including mental and physical impairments, *which may require the use of additional equipment or supplies.*
▪ Assess and address the patient's safety needs, including the risk of falling, and implement fall prevention interventions as needed.[2,20,22,28]
▪ Assess the patient's risk of postoperative nausea and vomiting (PONV) *to help determine whether PONV prophylaxis should be administered to decrease postoperative discomfort.* Use a facility approved PONV assessment tool, if available. Consider such risk factors as the patient's history of PONV and motion sickness, gender, and smoking history; the duration and type of surgery and anesthesia; and the potential use of postoperative opioids.[2,20,29,30]
▪ Assess the patient's cognitive and mental status, cardiopulmonary status,[22,31] skin condition, functional and sensory limitations, and use of any hearing or visual aids and assistive or prosthetic devices. Obtain other assessment data as pertinent to the surgical procedure.[2,3,20]
▪ Perform a suicide risk assessment.[2]
▪ Identify risk factors that may interfere with a positive expected outcome. Consider age, general health, medications, mobility, nutritional status, fluid and electrolyte disturbances, and lifestyle. Also consider the location, nature, and extent of the surgical procedure.[20]

ELDER ALERT Be aware that the development of postoperative delirium is a common complication of surgery in older adult patients.[22]

▪ Provide patient education using methods appropriate to the patient's and caregiver's preference, reading level, and level of understanding, addressing any potential visual impairments.[32] Include typical events that the patient can expect. Explain the incision, dressings, and staples or sutures that the surgeon typically uses. Use the teach-back method *to assess comprehension and guide additional teaching, if needed.*[2] *Preoperative teaching can help reduce postoperative anxiety and pain, increase patient adherence, hasten recovery, and decrease length of stay.*[20]

■ Teach the patient how to use a pain assessment scale that's appropriate for the patient's age, condition, and ability to understand. Tell the patient how to rate and report pain, and discuss analgesic tools and methods such as patient-controlled analgesia.[20,23,27,33]

■ Provide patient and family education on behavioral pain control techniques, such as biofeedback and progressive relaxation, *to help the patient manage perioperative pain and anxiety.*[2,20]

■ Discuss possible postoperative equipment, such as nasogastric tubes and IV equipment.[2,20]

■ Determine whether the patient will require home health care services and, if so, help make the necessary arrangements.[2,20]

■ Teach the patient the importance of performing coughing and deep breathing exercises after surgery (while splinting the incision, if necessary) *to minimize respiratory and circulatory complications.*

■ Explain the importance of frequent repositioning, extremity exercises, and early progressive ambulation after surgery *to minimize complications associated with immobility.*[20,34]

NURSING ALERT Be aware that a patient who is undergoing ophthalmic or neurologic surgery should avoid coughing, *because coughing increases intracranial pressure.*

■ Talk the patient through the sequence of events from the operating room (OR), to the postanesthesia care unit, and back to the patient's room or to an intensive care unit or surgical care unit, as appropriate, *to allay the patient's anxiety.*[20]

■ When discussing transfer procedures and techniques, describe sensations the patient will experience. Tell the patient that the use of a stretcher is necessary for travel to the OR, and explain the procedure for transfer from the stretcher to the OR table. Explain that, for safety reasons, the patient will be held securely to the table with soft straps.

■ Tell the patient that the OR may feel cool.

■ Explain that the OR nurses will check the patient's vital signs frequently, and electrodes may be put on the chest *to monitor heart rate during surgery.*

■ Describe the drowsy, floating sensation the patient will feel as the anesthetic takes effect. Tell the patient it's important to relax at this time.

■ Tell the patient about the need to fast before the procedure, according to the practitioner's order, *to reduce vomiting and the risk of aspiration.* Minimum fasting recommendations include 2 hours for clear liquids, 6 or more hours for a light meal or nonhuman milk, and 8 hours or more for fried or fatty foods or meat.[35]

■ If the patient is undergoing colorectal surgery, administer a combination of parenteral and oral antimicrobial agents, if ordered by the practitioner, following safe medication administration practices.[36,37,38,39] If ordered, administer mechanical bowel preparation in combination with oral antimicrobial agents. *Research supports the use of oral antimicrobials in combination with mechanical bowel preparation to reduce the risk of surgical site infection.*[40] Be aware that routine use of vancomycin isn't recommended for antimicrobial prophylaxis; instead, it should be reserved for special clinical situations.[40]

■ Advise the patient not to shave or remove hair at or near the surgical site before surgery *to prevent the risk of surgical site infection.*[41] Also tell the patient to clean the skin the night before or the morning of surgery. *Some studies support the use of 2% chlorhexidine cloths wiped on the surgical site the night before and the morning of surgery for specific procedures, such as cardiothoracic and total joint procedures.*[3,40]

■ If ordered, administer an antiseptic mouthwash and have the patient gargle with it, *because research supports gargling with bactericidal mouthwash to reduce bioburden in the oropharynx.*[42]

■ Obtain IV access, as needed and ordered, and begin IV fluid administration *to provide a route for medication administration and prevent dehydration caused by the required nothing-by-mouth status.*

■ Remove and discard your personal protective equipment if worn.[13]

■ Perform hand hygiene.[5,6,7,8,9,10]

■ Clean and disinfect your stethoscope with a disinfectant pad.[43,44]

■ Perform hand hygiene.[5,6,7,8,9,10]

■ Document the procedure.[45,46,47,48]

On the day of surgery

■ Verify the practitioner's orders.

■ Confirm that informed consent was obtained and that the signed consent form is in the patient's medical record.[49,50,51,52]

■ Conduct a preprocedure verification *to make sure that all documentation, related information, and equipment are available and correctly identified to the patient's identifiers.*[4,53]

■ Verify that the laboratory and imaging studies have been completed, as ordered, and that the results are in the patient's medical record. Notify the practitioner of any unexpected results.

■ If ordered, confirm completion of blood typing and cross-matching, and verify that appropriate blood is available and ready for possible transfusion.[1]

■ Perform hand hygiene.[5,6,7,8,9,10]

■ Confirm the patient's identity using at least two patient identifiers.[14]

■ Assess vital signs *to serve as a baseline for comparison during and after the procedure.*

■ Collect additional laboratory specimens and perform other tests as indicated and ordered, such as an ECG.[2]

■ Ensure patent IV access.

■ Implement measures *to prevent surgical site infection.* Don't remove hair at the operative site unless the presence of hair will interfere with the operative procedure. If hair removal is necessary, remove the hair using disposable-head clippers; don't use a razor.[3,40,41] Administer a prophylactic antibiotic within 1 hour before incision (2 hours for fluoroquinolones and vancomycin), as prescribed, following safe medication administration practices, *to maximize tissue concentration.*[36,37,38,39,40,41] Obtain the patient's blood glucose level, as ordered, *to identify hyperglycemia*; initiate treatment as needed and ordered.[41]

HOSPITAL-ACQUIRED CONDITION ALERT Keep in mind that the Centers for Medicare and Medicaid Services considers surgical site infection following certain cardiac surgeries, bariatric surgeries, or orthopedic procedures a hospital-acquired condition, *because using best practices can prevent it.* Be sure to follow evidence-based infection-prevention techniques (such as using clippers for hair removal, administering prophylactic antibiotics before incision, maintaining normothermia, and monitoring for hyperglycemia) *to reduce the risk of surgical site infection.*[41,54,55]

■ Administer ordered preoperative medications, including analgesics as part of a multimodal analgesic pain-management program, following safe medication administration practices.[23,36,37,38,39]

■ Complete a preoperative checklist, such as the World Health Organization's Surgical Safety checklist.

■ Provide support to the patient and family.

■ Notify the surgeon and anesthesia care provider about any abnormal assessment findings, and document responding orders.[2]

■ Assess the patient's retention of preoperative teaching and reinforce education, as indicated.[2,20]

■ Make sure that the patient is accompanied by a responsible adult who can provide transportation home and assume the patient's care after discharge. Instruct the patient not to drive *to maintain patient safety.*[2]

■ Allow loved ones time to be with the patient before surgery *so that the patient feels comforted and supported from the physical and emotional presence of the family preoperatively.*[56]

Just before moving the patient to the surgical area

■ Make sure that the patient's vital signs are documented in the patient's medical record.

■ Make sure the patient is wearing a hospital gown and identification band.

■ Provide a warm blanket *to reduce the risk of hypothermia.*[57]

■ Verify that no hearing aid(s), glasses, hair accessories, nail polish, body piercing accessories, or jewelry remains on the patient.[58]

■ Note whether dentures, contact lenses, or prosthetic devices have been removed or left in place.

■ Verify with the patient that the surgeon has marked the correct surgical site, as directed by your facility.[53,59,60]

■ Provide hand-off communication to the staff member who will assume responsibility for the patient in the OR. As part of the hand-off process, allow time for the receiving staff member to trace each tubing and catheter from the patient to its point of origin using a standardized line reconciliation process.[35,61,62,63,64] Allow time for questions as necessary *to avoid miscommunication that can cause patient care errors during transition of care.*

- Perform hand hygiene.[5,6,7,8,9,10]
- Clean and disinfect your stethoscope with a disinfectant pad.[43,44]
- Perform hand hygiene.[5,6,7,8,9,10]
- Document the procedure.[45,46,47,48]

Special considerations

- The patient may benefit from receiving a tour of the areas in which perioperative events will occur. Arrange such a tour, as time allows and as permitted by the facility.
- If the patient smokes, as appropriate, emphasize the benefits of smoking cessation before surgery, including improved blood flow and oxygen delivery to the tissues. Recommend that the patient quit smoking 8 weeks prior to the surgery, if possible.[65]
- If the patient's family or friends are present, direct them to the appropriate waiting area and offer support as needed.[56]

Complications

Incomplete or inadequate preoperative patient assessment and care can result in cancellation of the surgical procedure, patient injury, and postoperative complications.[1]

Documentation

Complete the preoperative checklist used by your facility. Record all nursing care measures that you performed, preoperative medications that you administered, results of diagnostic tests, and the time that the patient was transferred to the surgical area. Record teaching provided to the patient and family (if applicable), their understanding of that teaching, and any need for follow-up teaching. Make sure that the patient's medical record and the surgical checklist accompany the patient to surgery.

REFERENCES

1 Hinkle, J. L., & Cheever, K. H. (2018). *Brunner & Suddarth's textbook of medical-surgical nursing* (14th ed.). Philadelphia, PA: Wolters Kluwer.

2 American Society of PeriAnesthesia Nurses. (2019). *2019-2020 Perianesthesia nursing standards, practice recommendations and interpretative statements.* Cherry Hill, NJ: American Society of PeriAnesthesia Nurses. (Level VII)

3 Institute for Clinical Systems Improvement (ICSI). (2019). ICSI health care guideline: Perioperative protocol (6th ed.). ICSI. https://www.icsi.org/guideline/perioperative-protocol/ (Level VII)

4 The Joint Commission. (2021). Standard UP.01.01.01. *Comprehensive accreditation manual for hospitals.* Oakbrook Terrace, IL: The Joint Commission. (Level VII)

5 Centers for Disease Control and Prevention. (2002). Guideline for hand hygiene in health-care settings: Recommendations of the Healthcare Infection Control Practices Advisory Committee and the HICPAC/SHEA/APIC/IDSA Hand Hygiene Task Force. *MMWR Recommendations and Reports, 51*(RR-16), 1–45. https://www.cdc.gov/mmwr/pdf/rr/rr5116.pdf (Level II)

6 World Health Organization. (2009). WHO guidelines on hand hygiene in health care: First global patient safety challenge, clean care is safer care. https://apps.who.int/iris/bitstream/handle/10665/44102/9789241597906_eng.pdf?sequence=1 (Level IV)

7 The Joint Commission. (2021). Standard NPSG.07.01.01. *Comprehensive accreditation manual for hospitals.* Oakbrook Terrace, IL: The Joint Commission. (Level VII)

8 Centers for Medicare and Medicaid Services, Department of Health and Human Services. (2020). Condition of participation: Infection control. 42 C.F.R. § 482.42.

9 Accreditation Association for Hospitals and Health Systems. (2020). Standard 07.01.21. *Healthcare Facilities Accreditation Program: Accreditation requirements for acute care hospitals.* Chicago, IL: Accreditation Association for Hospitals and Health Systems. (Level VII)

10 DNV GL-Healthcare USA, Inc. (2020). IC.1.SR.1. *NIAHO® accreditation requirements, interpretive guidelines and surveyor guidance—revision 20.0.* Milford, OH: DNV GL-Healthcare USA, Inc. (Level VII)

11 Siegel, J. D., et al. (2007, revised 2019). 2007 guideline for isolation precautions: Preventing transmission of infectious agents in healthcare settings. https://www.cdc.gov/infectioncontrol/pdf/guidelines/isolation-guidelines-H.pdf (Level II)

12 Accreditation Association for Hospitals and Health Systems. (2020). Standard 07.01.10. *Healthcare Facilities Accreditation Program: Accreditation requirements for acute care hospitals.* Chicago, IL: Accreditation Association for Hospitals and Health Systems. (Level VII)

13 Occupational Safety and Health Administration. (2019). Bloodborne pathogens, standard number 1910.1030. https://www.osha.gov/pls/oshaweb/owadisp.show_document?p_id=10051&p_table=STANDARDS (Level VII)

14 The Joint Commission. (2021). Standard NPSG.01.01.01. *Comprehensive accreditation manual for hospitals.* Oakbrook Terrace, IL: The Joint Commission. (Level VII)

15 Accreditation Association for Hospitals and Health Systems. (2020). Standard 15.01.16. *Healthcare Facilities Accreditation Program: Accreditation requirements for acute care hospitals.* Chicago, IL: Accreditation Association for Hospitals and Health Systems. (Level VII)

16 Centers for Medicare and Medicaid Services, Department of Health and Human Services. (2020). Condition of participation: Patient's rights. 42 C.F.R. § 482.13(c)(1).

17 DNV GL-Healthcare USA, Inc. (2020). PR.2.SR.5. *NIAHO® accreditation requirements, interpretive guidelines and surveyor guidance—revision 20.0.* Milford, OH: DNV GL-Healthcare USA, Inc. (Level VII)

18 The Joint Commission. (2021). Standard RI.01.01.01. *Comprehensive accreditation manual for hospitals.* Oakbrook Terrace, IL: The Joint Commission. (Level VII)

19 The Joint Commission. (2021). Standard PC.02.01.21. *Comprehensive accreditation manual for hospitals.* Oakbrook Terrace, IL: The Joint Commission. (Level VII)

20 The Joint Commission. (2021). Standard PC.03.01.03. *Comprehensive accreditation manual for hospitals.* Oakbrook Terrace, IL: The Joint Commission. (Level VII)

21 The Joint Commission. (2021). Standard NPSG.03.06.01. *Comprehensive accreditation manual for hospitals.* Oakbrook Terrace, IL: The Joint Commission. (Level VII)

22 American College of Surgeons (ACS) National Surgical Quality Improvement Program (NSQIP). (2012). ACS NSQIP®/AGS best practice guidelines: Optimal preoperative assessment of the geriatric surgical patient. https://www.facs.org/-/media/files/quality%20programs/nsqip/acsnsqipagsgeriatric2012guidelines.ashx (Level VII)

23 American Society of Anesthesiologists Committee on Standards and Practice Parameters. (2012). Practice guidelines for acute pain management in the perioperative setting: An updated report by the American Society of Anesthesiologists Task Force on Acute Pain Management. *Anesthesiology, 116,* 248–273. https://anesthesiology.pubs.asahq.org/article.aspx?articleid=1933589 (Level VII)

24 Centers for Medicare and Medicaid Services & The Joint Commission. (2022). The specifications manual for national hospital inpatient quality measures (version 5.11a). https://www.qualitynet.org/inpatient/specifications-manuals#tab1

25 The Joint Commission. (2021). Standard RI.01.05.01. *Comprehensive accreditation manual for hospitals.* Oakbrook Terrace, IL: The Joint Commission. (Level VII)

26 Accreditation Association for Hospitals and Health Systems. (2020). Standard 15.01.12. *Healthcare Facilities Accreditation Program: Accreditation requirements for acute care hospitals.* Chicago, IL: Accreditation Association for Hospitals and Health Systems. (Level VII)

27 The Joint Commission. (2021). Standard PC.01.02.07. *Comprehensive accreditation manual for hospitals.* Oakbrook Terrace, IL: The Joint Commission. (Level VII)

28 The Joint Commission. (2021). Standard PC.01.02.08. *Comprehensive accreditation manual for hospitals.* Oakbrook Terrace, IL: The Joint Commission. (Level VII)

29 Feinleib, J., et al. (2021). Postoperative nausea and vomiting. In: *UpToDate,* Holt, N. F. & Davidson, A. (Eds.).

30 Apfel, C. C., et al. (1999). A simplified risk score for predicting postoperative nausea and vomiting: Conclusions from cross-validations between two centers. *Anesthesiology, 91,* 693. https://anesthesiology.pubs.asahq.org/article.aspx?articleid=1946036 (Level IV)

31 Fleisher, L. A., et al. (2014). 2014 ACC/AHA guideline on perioperative cardiovascular evaluation and management of patients undergoing noncardiac surgery: A report of the American College of Cardiology/ American

Heart Association Task Force on Practice Guidelines. *Journal of the American College of Cardiology, 64*(22), e77–e137. http://www.onlinejacc.org/content/64/22/e77 (Level VII)

32 The Joint Commission. (2021). Standard PC.02.01.21. *Comprehensive accreditation manual for hospitals.* Oakbrook Terrace, IL: The Joint Commission. (Level VII)

33 American Society of PeriAnesthesia Nurses (ASPAN). (2003). ASPAN pain and comfort clinical guideline. *Journal of PeriAnesthesia Nursing, 18*(4), 232–236. http://www.aspan.org/Portals/6/docs/ClinicalPractice/Guidelines/ASPAN_ClinicalGuideline_PainComfort.pdf (Level VII)

34 Clarke, H. D., et al. (2012). Preoperative patient education reduces in-hospital falls after total knee arthroplasty. *Clinical Orthopaedics and Related Research, 470*(1), 244–249. https://www.ncbi.nlm.nih.gov/pmc/articles/PMC3237968/ (Level III)

35 American Society of Anesthesiologists. (2017). Practice guidelines for preoperative fasting and the use of pharmacologic agents to reduce the risk of pulmonary aspiration: Application to healthy patients undergoing elective procedures. *Anesthesiology, 126*, 376–393. https://anesthesiology.pubs.asahq.org/article.aspx?articleid=2596245 (Level VII)

36 The Joint Commission. (2021). Standard MM.06.01.01. *Comprehensive accreditation manual for hospitals.* Oakbrook Terrace, IL: The Joint Commission. (Level VII)

37 Centers for Medicare and Medicaid Services, Department of Health and Human Services. (2020). Condition of participation: Nursing services. 42 C.F.R. § 482.23(c).

38 Accreditation Association for Hospitals and Health Systems. (2020). Standard 16.01.03. *Healthcare Facilities Accreditation Program: Accreditation requirements for acute care hospitals.* Chicago, IL: Accreditation Association for Hospitals and Health Systems. (Level VII)

39 DNV GL-Healthcare USA, Inc. (2020). MM.1.SR.3. *NIAHO® accreditation requirements, interpretive guidelines and surveyor guidance—revision 20.0.* Milford, OH: DNV GL-Healthcare USA, Inc. (Level VII)

40 Anderson, D. J., et al. (2014). SHEA/IDSA practice recommendation: Strategies to prevent surgical site infections in acute care hospitals: 2014 update. *Infection Control and Hospital Epidemiology, 35*(6), 605–627. https://www.jstor.org/stable/10.1086/676022#metadata_info_tab_contents (Level I)

41 Berríos-Torres, S. I., et al. (2017). Centers for Disease Control and Prevention guideline for the prevention of surgical site infection, 2017. *JAMA Surgery, 152*, 784–791. https://jamanetwork.com/journals/jamasurgery/fullarticle/2623725 (Level VII)

42 Suzuki, T., et al. (2012). Bactericidal activity of topical antiseptics and their gargles against *Bordetella pertussis. Journal of Infection and Chemotherapy, 18*, 272–275. (Level VI)

43 Rutala, W. A., et al. (2008, revised 2019). Guideline for disinfection and sterilization in healthcare facilities, 2008. https://www.cdc.gov/infection-control/pdf/guidelines/disinfection-guidelines-H.pdf (Level I)

44 Accreditation Association for Hospitals and Health Systems. (2020). Standard 07.02.03. *Healthcare Facilities Accreditation Program: Accreditation requirements for acute care hospitals.* Chicago, IL: Accreditation Association for Hospitals and Health Systems. (Level VII)

45 Centers for Medicare and Medicaid Services, Department of Health and Human Services. (2020). Condition of participation: Medical record services. 42 C.F.R. § 482.24(b).

46 Accreditation Association for Hospitals and Health Systems. (2020). Standard 10.00.03. *Healthcare Facilities Accreditation Program: Accreditation requirements for acute care hospitals.* Chicago, IL: Accreditation Association for Hospitals and Health Systems. (Level VII)

47 DNV GL-Healthcare USA, Inc. (2020). MR.2.SR.1. *NIAHO® accreditation requirements, interpretive guidelines and surveyor guidance—revision 18.2.* Milford, OH: DNV GL-Healthcare USA, Inc. (Level VII)

48 The Joint Commission. (2021). Standard RC.01.03.01. *Comprehensive accreditation manual for hospitals.* Oakbrook Terrace, IL: The Joint Commission. (Level VII)

49 Accreditation Association for Hospitals and Health Systems. (2020). Standard 30.01.11. *Healthcare Facilities Accreditation Program: Accreditation requirements for acute care hospitals.* Chicago, IL: Accreditation Association for Hospitals and Health Systems. (Level VII)

50 The Joint Commission. (2021). Standard RI.01.03.01. *Comprehensive accreditation manual for hospitals.* Oakbrook Terrace, IL: The Joint Commission. (Level VII)

51 Centers for Medicare and Medicaid Services, Department of Health and Human Services. (2020). Condition of participation: Patient's rights. 42 C.F.R. § 482.13.

52 DNV GL-Healthcare USA, Inc. (2020). PR.2.SR.3. *NIAHO® accreditation requirements, interpretive guidelines and surveyor guidance—revision 20.0.* Milford, OH: DNV GL-Healthcare USA, Inc. (Level VII)

53 Accreditation Association for Hospitals and Health Systems. (2020). Standard 30.00.14. *Healthcare Facilities Accreditation Program: Accreditation requirements for acute care hospitals.* Chicago, IL: Accreditation Association for Hospitals and Health Systems. (Level VII)

54 The Joint Commission. (2021). Standard NPSG.07.05.01. *Comprehensive accreditation manual for hospitals.* Oakbrook Terrace, IL: The Joint Commission. (Level VII)

55 Jarrett, N., & Callaham, M. (2016). Evidence-based guidelines for selected hospital-acquired conditions: Final report. https://www.cms.gov/Medicare/Medicare-Fee-for-Service-Payment/HospitalAcqCond/Downloads/2016-HAC-Report.pdf (Level VII)

56 Trimm, D. R., & Sanford, J. T. (2010). The process of family waiting during surgery. *Journal of Family Nursing, 16*, 435–461. (Level VI)

57 Guideline for perioperative practice: Prevention of hypothermia. (2020). In Wood, A. (Ed.), *Guidelines for perioperative practice*, 2020 edition. Denver, CO: AORN, Inc. (Level VII)

58 Guideline for perioperative practice: Positioning the patient. (2020). In Wood, A. (Ed.), *Guidelines for perioperative practice*, 2020 edition. Denver, CO: AORN, Inc. (Level VII)

59 The Joint Commission. (2021). Standard UP.01.02.01. *Comprehensive accreditation manual for hospitals.* Oakbrook Terrace, IL: The Joint Commission. (Level VII)

60 Guideline for perioperative practice: Team communication. (2020). In Wood, A. (Ed.), *Guidelines for perioperative practice*, 2020 edition. Denver, CO: AORN, Inc. (Level VII)

61 The Joint Commission. (2021). Standard PC.02.02.01. *Comprehensive accreditation manual for hospitals.* Oakbrook Terrace, IL: The Joint Commission. (Level VII)

62 Center for Patient Safety. (2021). Hot topics in health care: Transitions of care: The need for more effective approach to continuing patient care. https://www.centerforpatientsafety.org/resource/hot-topics-in-healthcare-transitions-of-care-the-need-for-a-more-effective-approach-to-continuing-patient-care/ (Level VII)

63 The Joint Commission. (2014). Sentinel event alert 53: Managing risk during transition to new ISO tubing connector standards. https://www.jointcommission.org/-/media/tjc/documents/resources/patient-safety-topics/sentinel event/sea_53_connectors_8_19_14_final.pdf (Level VII)

64 U.S. Food and Drug Administration. (2017). Examples of medical device misconnections. https://www.fda.gov/medical-devices/medical-device-connectors/examples-medical-device-misconnections (Level VII)

65 Arnold, M. J., & Beer, J. (2016). Preoperative evaluation: A time-saving algorithm. *Journal of Family Practice, 65*(10), 702–710. https://www.mdedge.com/familymedicine/article/113361/practice-management/preoperative-evaluation-time-saving-algorithm (Level VII)

PREOPERATIVE SKIN PREPARATION

Proper preparation of the patient's skin for surgery renders it as free as possible from microorganisms, which reduces the risk of infection at the incision site.[1]

Unless contraindicated, before undergoing a surgical procedure, the patient should be instructed to take (or assisted with) a preoperative bath or shower the night before or the day of surgery with soap or prescribed skin antiseptic, such as 4% chlorhexidine gluconate, *to reduce the number of microorganisms on the skin and to decrease the risk of contaminating the surgical incision.* The patient's skin should be dried with a fresh, clean, dry towel, and the patient should put on clean clothing *to reduce the risk of reintroducing microorganisms to clean skin.* The patient shouldn't apply any body lotion, emollients, or cosmetics after the shower *because they may impede the antiseptic effectiveness of the bath or shower or affect the ability of adhesive products such as monitor leads to adhere to the patient's skin.* Patients should also avoid alcohol-based skin products, *because they may pose a fire risk in the operating room.* Patients undergoing a procedure involving the axilla shouldn't apply deodorant.[1]

Patients undergoing surgery of the head or neck should be instructed in or assisted to wash the hair with shampoo or a prescribed antiseptic shampoo product. Contact with the eyes, ears, and other mucous membranes should be avoided. Alcohol-based hair products, conditioners and other hair care products should be avoided after shampooing.[1]

If hair removal is necessary, it should occur on the day of surgery in a location outside of the operating or procedure room *to decrease the risk of surgical site infection.*[1,2]

The area of preparation always exceeds that of the expected incision *to minimize the number of microorganisms in the areas adjacent to the proposed incision, to allow surgical draping of the patient without contamination, and to allow for the potential of additional incisions and drains.*[1] The skin preparation procedure described here doesn't duplicate or replace the full sterile preparation that immediately precedes surgery. Instead, it covers preparation of the skin when preoperative baths or showers haven't been performed. Because the efficacy of antiseptic agents depends on the cleanliness of the skin, any superficial soil, debris, and transient microbes should be removed first to reduce the risk of wound contamination.[1]

Equipment

4% chlorhexidine gluconate antiseptic skin cleaner ■ gloves ■ tap water ■ bath blanket ■ fluid-impermeable pad ■ washcloth(s) ■ towel ■ basin ■ adjustable light ■ Optional: 4″ × 4″ (10 cm × 10 cm) gauze pads, cotton-tipped applicators, nail polish remover, nonirritating makeup remover, plastic or paper trash bag, electric or battery-operated hair clippers with a single head or with a reusable head that can be disinfected, other personal protective equipment.

Preparation of equipment

Ensure the patient's bath basin has been thoroughly disinfected before use; *studies indicate that bath basins may be a source of microbial contamination.*[3,4] Pour plain, warm tap water into a basin for rinsing. Use warm water, *because heat reduces the skin's surface tension and facilitates the removal of soil and hair.* Inspect all equipment and supplies. If a product is expired, is defective, or has compromised integrity, remove it from patient use, label it as expired or defective, and report the expiration or defect as directed by your facility.

Implementation

- Verify the practitioner's order.
- Review the patient's medical record for an allergy or a sensitivity to chlorhexidine. Use an alternative antiseptic agent if indicated.[1]
- Gather and prepare the necessary equipment and supplies.
- Perform hand hygiene.[5,6,7,8,9,10]
- Confirm the patient's identity using at least two patient identifiers.[11]
- Provide privacy.[12,13,14,15]
- Explain the procedure to the patient and family (if appropriate) according to their individual communication and learning needs *to increase their understanding, allay their fears, and enhance cooperation.*[16]
- Raise the patient's bed to waist level before providing patient care *to prevent caregiver back strain.*[17]
- Perform hand hygiene.[5,6,7,8,9,10]
- Put on gloves and, if needed, other personal protective equipment.[18,19,20]
- Place the patient in a comfortable position, drape the patient with the bath blanket, and expose the preparation area. *To ensure privacy and avoid chilling the patient,* expose only one small area at a time while performing skin preparation.
- Place a fluid-impermeable pad beneath the patient *to catch spills and avoid linen changes.*
- Adjust the light *to illuminate the preparation area.*
- Assess skin condition in the preparation area, and report any rash, abrasion, or laceration to the practitioner before beginning the procedure. *Any break in the skin increases the risk of infection and could cause cancellation of planned surgery.*[1]
- Instruct the patient to remove all jewelry.[1] Have the patient give the jewelry to a family member or caregiver, or secure it as directed by your facility *to prevent loss.*

- Remove cosmetics using a nonirritating agent *to facilitate securing an endotracheal tube, if needed, and to provide adequate skin assessment during surgery.*[1]
- Clean under the patient's fingernails and remove nail polish, if necessary. If the patient is having hand or wrist surgery, make sure that the nails are short and natural, with no artificial nail surfaces, such as extensions, overlays, acrylic, silk wraps, or enhancements.[1]
- When hair removal is necessary, remove it using a hair clipper. Only hair that interferes with the surgical procedure should be removed, *because hair removal may increase the risk of infection.*[1,21,22] Limit the amount of clipping *to reduce the risk of microscopic nicks, which may increase the risk of surgical site infection.*[1]
- Wash the skin around the surgical site *to remove gross contaminants and oils that might block the penetration of the antiseptic agent used during the sterile prep before surgery.*[1] Carefully clean skin folds and crevices, *because they harbor greater numbers of microorganisms.* Clean anatomic areas that contain more debris separately *to prevent the distribution of microorganisms from these areas to the surgical site.*[1]
- If the patient is undergoing abdominal surgery, clean the umbilicus.[1] If needed, instill soap and water, or antiseptic solutions such as chlorhexidine, into the umbilicus *to soften debris.* Then remove the debris using a cotton-tipped applicator, *because debris within the umbilicus is a contaminant and can't be adequately disinfected.*
- If an intestinal or urinary stoma is within the surgical field, clean the area gently and separately from the rest of the prepped area *to remove organic material that might interfere with the effectiveness of the antiseptic agent.*[1]
- For a surgical field that includes the penis, retract the foreskin, if present, and then gently clean the penis, *because organic material and microorganisms accumulate under the foreskin.*[1] After cleaning the foreskin, pull it back over the glans *to prevent circulatory compromise.*
- Dry the area with a clean towel and remove the fluid-impermeable pad.
- Return the bed to the lowest position *to prevent falls and maintain patient safety.*[23]
- Give the patient any special instructions for care of the prepared area, and remind the patient to keep the area clean for surgery. Make sure that the patient is comfortable.
- Discard used supplies in appropriate receptacles.[20]
- Remove and discard your gloves and any other personal protective equipment worn.[20]
- Perform hand hygiene.[5,6,7,8,9,10]
- Document the procedure.[24,25,26,27]

Special considerations

- In cases of head surgery, verify the surgical site before hair removal. The practitioner should identify the surgical site in advance of the surgical time-out *to ensure that the correct site is prepared, reducing the risk of wrong-site surgery.*[28]
- Scalp hair removal is usually performed in the operating room, but if you're required to prepare the patient's scalp, put all hair in a plastic or paper trash bag and store it with the patient's possessions.
- Depilatory cream can also be used to remove hair. Although this method produces clean, intact skin without risking lacerations or abrasions, it can cause skin irritation or rash, especially in the groin area.[1] Perform a skin test first in an area away from the surgical site *to determine whether the cream irritates the skin.*[1] If no irritation develops, proceed with applying the depilatory cream according to the manufacturer's instructions.

Complications

Complications include rashes, nicks, lacerations, and abrasions, which may increase the risk of postoperative infection.

Documentation

Document the date and time of skin preparation, the product used, the area prepared, and the skin condition before and after preparation. Also record hair removal if performed, including the time, method, and area of removal.[1] Record removal and disposition of jewelry.[1] Document teaching provided to the patient and family (if appropriate), their understanding of that teaching, and any need for follow-up teaching.

REFERENCES

1 Guideline for perioperative practice: Patient skin antisepsis. (2021). In Wood, A. (Ed.). *Guidelines for perioperative practice*, 2021 edition. Denver, CO: AORN, Inc. (Level VII)
2 Anderson, D. J., et al. (2014). SHEA/IDSA practice recommendation: Strategies to prevent surgical site infections in acute care hospitals: 2014 update. *Infection Control and Hospital Epidemiology, 35*(6), 605–627. http://www.jstor.org/stable/10.1086/676022 (Level I)
3 Powers, J., et al. (2012). Chlorhexidine bathing and microbial contamination in patients' bath basins. *American Journal of Critical Care, 21*, 338–342. (Level III)
4 Johnson, D., et al. (2009). Patients' bath basins as potential sources of infection: A multicenter sampling study. *American Journal of Critical Care, 18*(41), 34–38. (Level III)
5 Centers for Disease Control and Prevention. (2002). Guideline for hand hygiene in health-care settings: Recommendations of the Healthcare Infection Control Practices Advisory Committee and the HICPAC/SHEA/APIC/IDSA Hand Hygiene Task Force. *MMWR Recommendations and Reports, 51*(RR-16), 1–45. https://www.cdc.gov/mmwr/pdf/rr/rr5116.pdf (Level II)
6 The Joint Commission. (2021). Standard NPSG.07.01.01. *Comprehensive accreditation manual for hospitals.* Oakbrook Terrace, IL: The Joint Commission. (Level VII)
7 World Health Organization. (2009). WHO guidelines on hand hygiene in health care: First global patient safety challenge, clean care is safer care. https://apps.who.int/iris/bitstream/handle/10665/44102/9789241597906_eng.pdf?sequence=1 (Level IV)
8 Accreditation Association for Hospitals and Health Systems. (2020). Standard 07.01.21. *Healthcare Facilities Accreditation Program: Accreditation requirements for acute care hospitals.* Chicago, IL: Accreditation Association for Hospitals and Health Systems. (Level VII)
9 Centers for Medicare and Medicaid Services, Department of Health and Human Services. (2020). Condition of participation: Infection control. 42 C.F.R. § 482.42.
10 DNV GL-Healthcare USA, Inc. (2020). IC.1.SR.1. *NIAHO® accreditation requirements, interpretive guidelines and surveyor guidance—revision 20.0.* Milford, OH: DNV GL-Healthcare USA, Inc. (Level VII)
11 The Joint Commission. (2021). Standard NPSG.01.01.01. *Comprehensive accreditation manual for hospitals.* Oakbrook Terrace, IL: The Joint Commission. (Level VII)
12 Accreditation Association for Hospitals and Health Systems. (2020). Standard 15.01.16. *Healthcare Facilities Accreditation Program: Accreditation requirements for acute care hospitals.* Chicago, IL: Accreditation Association for Hospitals and Health Systems. (Level VII)
13 Centers for Medicare and Medicaid Services, Department of Health and Human Services. (2020). Condition of participation: Patient's rights. 42 C.F.R. § 482.13(c)(1).
14 The Joint Commission. (2021). Standard RI.01.01.01. *Comprehensive accreditation manual for hospitals.* Oakbrook Terrace, IL: The Joint Commission. (Level VII)
15 DNV GL-Healthcare USA, Inc. (2020). PR.2.SR.5. *NIAHO® accreditation requirements, interpretive guidelines and surveyor guidance—revision 20.0.* Milford, OH: DNV GL-Healthcare USA, Inc. (Level VII)
16 The Joint Commission. (2021). Standard PC.02.01.21. *Comprehensive accreditation manual for hospitals.* Oakbrook Terrace, IL: The Joint Commission. (Level VII)
17 Waters, T. R., et al. (2009). Safe patient handling training for schools of nursing. https://www.cdc.gov/niosh/docs/2009-127/pdfs/2009-127.pdf (Level VII)
18 Accreditation Association for Hospitals and Health Systems. (2020). Standard 07.01.10. *Healthcare Facilities Accreditation Program: Accreditation requirements for acute care hospitals.* Chicago, IL: Accreditation Association for Hospitals and Health Systems. (Level VII)
19 Siegel, J. D., et al. (2007, revised 2019). 2007 guideline for isolation precautions: Preventing transmission of infectious agents in healthcare settings. https://www.cdc.gov/infectioncontrol/pdf/guidelines/isolation-guidelines-H.pdf (Level II)
20 Occupational Safety and Health Administration. (2019). Bloodborne pathogens, standard number 1910.1030. https://www.osha.gov/pls/oshaweb/owadisp.show_document?p_id=10051&p_table=STANDARDS (Level VII)
21 World Health Organization. (2016). Global guidelines for the prevention of surgical site infection. https://apps.who.int/iris/bitstream/handle/10665/250680/9789241549882-eng.pdf (Level IV)
22 Tanner, J., et al. (2011). Preoperative hair removal to reduce surgical site infection. *Cochrane Database of Systematic Reviews, 2011*(11), CD004122. (Level II)
23 Ganz, D. A., et al. (2013, reviewed 2021). *Preventing falls in hospitals: A toolkit for improving quality of care* (AHRQ Publication No. 13-0015-EF). Rockville, MD: Agency for Healthcare Research and Quality. https://www.ahrq.gov/professionals/systems/hospital/fallpxtoolkit/index.html (Level VII)
24 The Joint Commission. (2021). Standard RC.01.03.01. *Comprehensive accreditation manual for hospitals.* Oakbrook Terrace, IL: The Joint Commission. (Level VII)
25 Centers for Medicare and Medicaid Services, Department of Health and Human Services. (2020). Condition of participation: Medical record services. 42 C.F.R. § 482.24(b).
26 DNV GL-Healthcare USA, Inc. (2020). MR.2.SR.1. *NIAHO® accreditation requirements, interpretive guidelines and surveyor guidance—revision 20.0.* Milford, OH: DNV GL-Healthcare USA, Inc. (Level VII)
27 Accreditation Association for Hospitals and Health Systems. (2020). Standard 10.00.03. *Healthcare Facilities Accreditation Program: Accreditation requirements for acute care hospitals.* Chicago, IL: Accreditation Association for Hospitals and Health Systems. (Level VII)
28 The Joint Commission. (2021). Standard UP.01.02.01. *Comprehensive accreditation manual for hospitals.* Oakbrook Terrace, IL: The Joint Commission. (Level VII)

PRESSURE DRESSING APPLICATION

To control capillary or small-vein bleeding, a nurse can apply pressure directly over a wound with a bulk dressing held by a glove protected hand or bound into place with a pressure bandage.[1,2] A pressure dressing requires frequent inspection for wound drainage to determine its effectiveness in controlling bleeding. The wound shouldn't be cleaned until the bleeding stops.

Equipment

Two or more sterile gauze pads ▪ roller gauze ▪ adhesive tape ▪ gloves ▪ metric ruler.

Preparation of equipment

Obtain the pressure dressing quickly *to avoid excessive blood loss.* Use clean cloth for the dressing if sterile gauze pads are unavailable.

Implementation

▪ Gather and prepare the necessary equipment and supplies
▪ Perform hand hygiene.[3,4,5,6,7,8]
▪ Put on gloves and other personal protective equipment as needed *to comply with standard precautions.*[9,10,11]
▪ Explain the procedure to the patient and family (if appropriate) according to their individual communication and learning needs *to increase their understanding, allay their fears, and enhance cooperation.*[12]
▪ Immobilize the injured body part *to help reduce bleeding.*
▪ Place enough gauze pads over the wound to cover it.
▪ For an extremity or a trunk wound, hold the gauze pad dressing firmly over the wound, and wrap the roller gauze tightly across it and around the body part *to provide pressure on the wound.* Secure the bandage with adhesive tape.
▪ To apply a dressing to the neck, the shoulder, or another location that can't be tightly wrapped, don't use roller gauze. Instead, apply tape directly over the gauze pad dressings *to provide the necessary pressure at the wound site.*
▪ Assess the patient's pulses, capillary refill, and skin temperature, sensation, and color distal to the wound site, *because excessive pressure can compromise circulation.*
▪ Inspect the dressing frequently *to monitor wound drainage.* Use the metric standard of measurement to determine the amount of drainage, and document these serial measurements for later reference. Don't circle

a potentially wet dressing with ink, *because such markings don't provide permanent documentation in the medical record and also risk contaminating the dressing.*

- If the dressing becomes saturated, don't remove it; *removal would interfere with the pressure.* Instead, apply an additional dressing over the saturated one and continue to monitor and record drainage.
- Obtain additional medical care as soon as possible.
- Remove and discard your gloves and any other personal protective equipment worn.[10]
- Perform hand hygiene.[3,4,5,6,7,8]
- Document the procedure.[13,14,15,16]

Special considerations

- Apply pressure directly to the wound with your gloved hand if sterile gauze pads and clean cloth are unavailable.
- Avoid using an elastic bandage to bind the dressing, *because it can't be wrapped tightly enough to create pressure on the wound site.*

Complications

A pressure dressing that's applied too tightly can impair circulation.

Documentation

When the bleeding is controlled, record the date and time of dressing application, site of the wound, circulation assessment findings distal to the wound, amount of wound drainage, and the patient's tolerance of the procedure. Document teaching provided to the patient and family (if applicable), their understanding of that teaching, and any need for follow-up teaching.

REFERENCES

1. Pelligrino, J. L., et al. (2020). 2020 American Heart Association and American Red Cross focused update for first aid. *Circulation, 142*(17), e287–e303. https://www.ahajournals.org/doi/full/10.1161/CIR.0000000000000900 (Level VII)

2. Singletary, E. M., et al. (2020). 2020 International Consensus on First Aid Science with treatment recommendations. *Resuscitation, 156*, A240–A282. https://www.resuscitationjournal.com/article/S0300-9572(20)30464-0/fulltext (Level VII)

3. The Joint Commission. (2021). Standard NPSG.07.01.01. *Comprehensive accreditation manual for hospitals.* (Level VII)

4. Centers for Disease Control and Prevention. (2002). Guideline for hand hygiene in health-care settings: Recommendations of the Healthcare Infection Control Practices Advisory Committee and the HICPAC/SHEA/APIC/IDSA Hand Hygiene Task Force. *MMWR Recommendations and Reports, 51*(RR-16), 1–45. https://www.cdc.gov/mmwr/pdf/rr/rr5116.pdf (Level II)

5. World Health Organization. (2009). WHO guidelines on hand hygiene in health care: First global patient safety challenge, clean care is safer care. https://apps.who.int/iris/bitstream/handle/10665/44102/9789241597906_eng.pdf?sequence=1 (Level IV)

6. Accreditation Association for Hospitals and Health Systems. (2020). Standard 07.01.21. *Healthcare Facilities Accreditation Program: Accreditation requirements for acute care hospitals.* (Level VII)

7. Centers for Medicare and Medicaid Services, Department of Health and Human Services. (2020). Condition of participation: Infection control. 42 C.F.R. § 482.42.

8. DNV GL-Healthcare USA, Inc. (2020). IC.1.SR.1. *NIAHO® accreditation requirements, interpretive guidelines and surveyor guidance—revision 20.0.* (Level VII)

9. Siegel, J. D., et al. (2007, revised 2019). 2007 guideline for isolation precautions: Preventing transmission of infectious agents in healthcare settings. https://www.cdc.gov/infectioncontrol/pdf/guidelines/isolation-guidelines-H.pdf (Level II)

10. Occupational Safety and Health Administration. (2019). Bloodborne pathogens, standard number 1910.1030. https://www.osha.gov/pls/oshaweb/owadisp.show_document?p_id=10051&p_table=STANDARDS (Level VII)

11. Accreditation Association for Hospitals and Health Systems. (2020). Standard 07.01.10. *Healthcare Facilities Accreditation Program: Accreditation requirements for acute care hospitals.* (Level VII)

12. The Joint Commission. (2021). Standard PC.02.01.21. *Comprehensive accreditation manual for hospitals.* (Level VII)

13. The Joint Commission. (2021). Standard RC.01.03.01. *Comprehensive accreditation manual for hospitals.* (Level VII)

14. Accreditation Association for Hospitals and Health Systems. (2020). Standard 10.00.03. *Healthcare Facilities Accreditation Program: Accreditation requirements for acute care hospitals.* (Level VII)

15. Centers for Medicare and Medicaid Services, Department of Health and Human Services. (2020). Condition of participation: Medical record services. 42 C.F.R. § 482.24(b).

16. DNV GL-Healthcare USA, Inc. (2020). MR.2.SR.1. *NIAHO® accreditation requirements, interpretive guidelines and surveyor guidance—revision 20.0.* (Level VII)

PRESSURE INJURY PREVENTION

As the name implies, pressure injuries result when pressure—applied with great force for a short period or with less force over a long period—impairs circulation, depriving tissues of oxygen and other life-sustaining nutrients. This process damages skin and underlying structures. Untreated, resulting ischemic lesions can lead to serious infection.

Most pressure injuries develop over bony prominences, where friction and shearing force combine with pressure to break down skin and underlying tissues.[1] Persistent pressure on bony prominences obstructs capillary blood flow, leading to tissue necrosis. Common sites include the sacrum, coccyx, ischial tuberosities, and greater trochanters. Other common sites include the skin over the vertebrae, scapulae, elbows, knees, and heels in bedridden and relatively immobile patients.

Successful pressure injury treatment involves relieving pressure, restoring circulation, promoting adequate nutrition and, if possible, resolving or managing related disorders.[2] Typically, the effectiveness and duration of treatment depend on the pressure injury's characteristics. To describe the pressure injuries, the nurse should use a staging tool, such as the classification system developed by the National Pressure Injury Advisory Panel (NPIAP), available at https://npiap.com/page/PressureInjuryStages.

Prevention is the key to avoiding extensive therapy. Preventive measures include off-loading pressure, maintaining adequate nourishment, and ensuring mobility to relieve pressure and promote circulation.[2] A risk assessment may be an important part of an overall prevention plan.[1] Several risk assessment tools are available. (See *Braden scale: Predicting pressure injury risk.*)

When a pressure injury develops despite preventive efforts, treatment includes methods to decrease pressure, such as frequent repositioning to shorten pressure duration and the use of special equipment to reduce pressure intensity. Treatment also may involve pressure-redistribution devices, such as special beds, mattresses, mattress overlays, and chair cushions.[1]

Equipment

Facility-approved skin assessment tool ■ pressure-redistribution devices ■ positioning devices (pillows, foam wedges) ■ appropriate skin cleanser and bathing supplies ■ lotion ■ Optional: gloves; trapeze bar; turning sheet; heel protection devices; padding for devices, appliances, casts, or splints; protective barrier ointment or film; underpads or briefs.

Preparation of equipment

Inspect all equipment and supplies. If a product is expired, is defective, or has compromised integrity, remove it from patient use, label it as expired or defective, and report the expiration or defect as directed by your facility.

Implementation

- Gather and prepare the necessary equipment and supplies.
- Perform hand hygiene.[4,5,6,7,8,9]
- Confirm the patient's identity using at least two patient identifiers.[10]
- Provide privacy.[11,12,13,14]
- Explain the procedure to the patient and family (if appropriate) according to their individual communication and learning needs *to increase their understanding, allay their fears, and enhance cooperation.*[15]

Braden scale: Predicting pressure injury risk

The Braden scale is the most reliable of several instruments used to assess the risk of developing pressure ulcers. The numbers to the left of each description are the points to be tallied; the lower the score, the greater the risk.[3]

Patient's name: _____

Evaluator's name: _____

Sensory perception	1. Completely limited	2. Very limited	3. Slightly limited	4. No impairment	Score
Ability to respond meaningfully to pressure-related discomfort	Patient is unresponsive to painful stimuli (doesn't moan, flinch, or grasp in response) because of diminished level of consciousness or sedation. OR Patient has a limited ability to feel pain over most of body's surface.	Patient responds only to painful stimuli; can't communicate discomfort except through moaning or restlessness. OR Patient has a sensory impairment that limits ability to feel pain or discomfort over half of body.	Patient responds to verbal commands but can't always communicate discomfort or the need to be turned. OR Patient has some sensory impairment that limits ability to feel pain or discomfort in one or two extremities.	Patient responds to verbal commands; has no sensory deficit that would limit ability to feel or voice pain or discomfort.	
Moisture Degree to which skin is exposed to moisture	**1. Constantly moist** Patient's skin is kept moist almost constantly by perspiration or urine; dampness is detected every time patient is moved or turned.	**2. Very moist** Patient's skin is usually but not always moist; linen must be changed at least once per shift.	**3. Occasionally moist** Patient's skin is occasionally moist; linen requires an extra change approximately once per day.	**4. Rarely moist** Patient's skin is usually dry; linen requires changing only at routine intervals.	Score
Activity Degree of physical activity	**1. Bedfast** Patient is confined to bed.	**2. Chairfast** Patient's ability to walk is severely limited or nonexistent; can't bear own weight and must be assisted into a chair or wheelchair.	**3. Walks occasionally** Patient walks occasionally during the day, but for very short distances, with or without assistance; spends majority of each shift in a bed or chair.	**4. Walks frequently** Patient walks outside room at least twice per day and inside room at least once every 2 hours during waking hours.	Score
Mobility Ability to change and control body position	**1. Completely immobile** Patient doesn't make even slight changes in body or extremity position without assistance.	**2. Very limited** Patient makes occasional slight changes in body or extremity position but can't make frequent or significant changes independently.	**3. Slightly limited** Patient makes frequent (although slight) changes in body or extremity position independently.	**4. No limitations** Patient makes major and frequent changes in body or extremity position without assistance.	Score
Nutrition Usual food intake pattern	**1. Very poor** Patient never eats a complete meal; rarely eats more than one-third of any food offered; eats two servings or less of protein (meat or dairy products) per day; takes fluids poorly; doesn't take a liquid dietary supplement. OR Patient is NPO or maintained on clear liquids or IV fluids for more than 5 days.	**2. Probably inadequate** Patient rarely eats a complete meal and generally eats only about one-half of any food offered; protein intake includes only three servings of meat or dairy products per day; occasionally will take a dietary supplement. OR Patient receives less than optimum amount of liquid diet or tube feeding.	**3. Adequate** Patient eats more than one-half of most meals; eats four servings of protein (meat and dairy products) per day; occasionally refuses a meal but will usually take a supplement if offered. OR Patient is on a tube feeding or total parenteral nutrition regimen that probably meets most nutritional needs.	**4. Excellent** Patient eats most of every meal and never refuses a meal; usually eats four or more servings of meat and dairy products per day; occasionally eats between meals; doesn't require supplementation.	Score
Friction and shear	**1. Problem** Patient requires moderate to maximum assistance in moving; complete lifting without sliding against sheets is impossible; frequently slides down in bed or chair, requiring frequent repositioning with maximum assistance; spasticity, contractures, or agitation leads to almost constant friction.	**2. Potential problem** Patient moves feebly or requires minimum assistance during a move; skin probably slides to some extent against sheets, chair restraints, or other devices; maintains relatively good position in chair or bed most of the time but occasionally slides down.	**3. No apparent problem** Patient moves in bed and in chair independently and has sufficient muscle strength to lift up completely during move; maintains good position in bed or chair at all times.		Score

Total Score

Distinguishing between pressure injuries and moisture-associated skin damage

Distinguishing between a stage 1 or 2 pressure injury and moisture-associated skin damage is often difficult. Both conditions can occur over the buttocks of an ill person. However, pressure injuries require pressure or shear to develop. In addition, they normally occur over bony prominences and have distinct edges. Necrosis may be present in a deep tissue pressure injury.[21]

Moisture-associated skin damage presents as an area of erythema. It can extend into skinfolds, between buttocks, and down the thighs; skin damage is shallow or superficial. Scaling of the skin may be present, with papule and vesicle formation. Maceration and whitening of the skin may also be present. The wound edges are irregular or diffuse. Patients commonly report burning, itching, and pain. Necrosis isn't present in moisture-associated skin damage.[21]

Proper identification of the cause of a patient's skin damage as pressure or moisture is the key to providing adequate treatment. Keep in mind that incontinent patients who can't reposition themselves may have a condition that results from both pressure and moisture.[21]

■ Raise the bed to waist level before providing patient care *to prevent caregiver back strain.*[16]

■ Perform hand hygiene.[4,5,6,7,8,9]

■ Put on gloves as needed *to comply with standard precautions.*[17,18,19]

■ Perform a comprehensive skin assessment using a facility-approved skin assessment tool.[1] *A comprehensive skin assessment may be the first step in pressure injury prevention.*[20,21] (See *Distinguishing between pressure injuries and moisture-associated skin damage.*)

■ Turn and reposition the patient regularly and frequently unless contraindicated.[22] Base the frequency of repositioning on the patient's tissue tolerance, skin condition, mobility, medical condition, and treatment goals. When turning or repositioning the patient, inspect the skin for signs of pressure injury or damage, and avoid positioning the patient on areas that have nonblanchable erythema.[22]

■ For patients with limited mobility, use a pressure-redistribution device, such as an air, gel, or 4″ (10.2 cm) foam mattress overlay.[23] The patient's condition may indicate the need for low- or high-air-loss bed therapy *to redistribute excessive pressure and promote evaporation of excess moisture.*

■ Implement the use of trapeze bars *to facilitate mobility in a patient who can assist.*[22]

■ When turning the patient, lift rather than slide the patient, *because sliding increases friction and shear.*[1] Use a turning sheet and get help from coworkers, if necessary.

NURSING ALERT Avoid placing the patient directly on the trochanter (hip). Instead, position the patient on the side, at about a 30-degree angle.[1]

■ Use positioning devices (for example, pillows or foam wedges) *to avoid positioning the patient on a pressure injury or other area at risk for pressure.*[22] (See the "Alignment and pressure-reducing device application" procedure.)

■ Eliminate sheet wrinkles *that could increase pressure and cause discomfort.*

■ Make sure the patient's heels don't rest on the bed.[1] Apply heel protection devices, as required, *to prevent heel pressure injuries.* The devices should completely off-load pressure from the heels. If you're placing pillows under the patient's calves to decrease pressure, place each pillow longitudinally underneath the calf with the heel suspended in the air.[22]

■ Work with the patient and multidisciplinary team to implement a regular repositioning routine, *because patients at risk for pressure injuries require teaching and encouragement to perform regular repositioning movements that redistribute pressure, preventing the buildup of pressure around areas at risk.*[24] Post a repositioning schedule at the patient's bedside. Adapt position changes to the patient's situation. Emphasize the importance of regular position changes to the patient and family, and encourage their participation in the treatment and prevention of pressure injuries by

having them perform a position change correctly, after you have demonstrated the proper technique.[24]

■ As appropriate, implement active or passive range-of-motion exercises *to redistribute pressure and promote circulation. To save time,* combine these exercises with bathing, if applicable.

■ Direct a patient confined to a chair or wheelchair to shift weight every 15 minutes *to promote blood flow to compressed tissues.*[1,22]

■ Show a patient with paraplegia how to shift weight in a wheelchair by doing push-ups in the wheelchair. If the patient needs your help, sit next to the patient and help shift the weight to one buttock for 60 seconds; then repeat the procedure on the other side. Provide pressure-redistribution cushions, as appropriate; however, avoid seating the patient on a rubber or plastic doughnut, *which can increase localized pressure at vulnerable points.*

NURSING ALERT The Wound, Ostomy and Continence Nurses Society (WOCN) recommends avoiding the use of doughnuts, foam rings, foam cut-outs, and synthetic sheepskin.[22]

■ If a patient confined to a chair or wheelchair can stand, assist the patient into a standing position every hour, if possible.[24]

■ Inspect the skin under and around medical devices for signs of pressure-related injury.[1] Adjust or pad devices, appliances, casts, or splints, as needed, *to ensure proper fit and to avoid increased pressure and impaired circulation.*

■ Tell the patient to avoid using hot water, drying bar soaps, and irritating cleaning agents, such as those with fragrance or alcohol, *because these items can dry the skin.*[22] Teach the patient how to apply lotion after bathing, or help the patient do so, *to keep the skin hydrated.* Also instruct the patient to avoid vigorous massage, *because it can damage capillaries.*

■ If diarrhea develops or if the patient is incontinent, change underpants and briefs after soiling. Clean the skin with a no-rinse cleanser that has a pH similar to normal skin.[21,25] Apply a barrier ointment or barrier film *to protect the skin from constant moisture and to prevent moisture-associated skin damage.*[21,22,25]

■ If the patient's condition permits, recommend a diet that includes adequate calories, protein, and vitamins. Dietary therapy may involve nutritional consultation, food supplements, enteral feeding, or total parenteral nutrition.[26,27]

■ Consult with your facility's wound, continence, and ostomy nurse; nutritionist or registered dietician; and physical or occupational therapist, as indicated, *because pressure injury prevention requires a multidisciplinary approach.*[20,24,28]

■ Return the bed to the lowest position *to prevent falls and maintain patient safety.*[29]

■ Discard used supplies in appropriate receptacles.[19]

■ Remove and discard your gloves, if worn.[17,19]

■ Perform hand hygiene.[4,5,6,7,8,9]

■ Document the procedure.[30,31,32,33]

Special considerations

■ Comprehensive skin assessment shouldn't be a one-time event limited to admission. Repeat it regularly *to determine any changes in skin condition.* Perform a comprehensive skin assessment when the patient is admitted to the unit, daily, and on transfer or discharge. In some settings, such an assessment may be done as frequently as every shift. It may be appropriate to conduct more frequent assessments on units in which pressure injuries may develop rapidly, such as in a critical care unit. Staff on each unit should know the frequency with which they should perform comprehensive skin assessments.[20,34] The admission assessment is particularly important on arrival at the emergency department, operating room, or postanesthesia care unit.

■ Except for brief periods, avoid raising the head of the bed more than 30 degrees, *to prevent shearing forces.*[1]

■ For an incontinent patient, use absorbent underpads or undergarments that wick moisture away from the skin. The WOCN also recommends establishing a bowel and bladder management retraining program and possibly using a pouching system or a bowel or fecal containment device *to contain excessive stool output and protect the skin.* In situations in which the severity of urinary incontinence has contributed to or may contaminate a pressure injury, the WOCN recommends considering use of an indwelling catheter.[22]

- Depending on the patient's needs, repair of stage 3 and stage 4 pressure injuries may require surgical intervention, such as direct closure, skin grafting, and flaps.[1]

Complications

If left untreated, pressure injuries can become infected or necrotic. Advancing infection or cellulitis can lead to septicemia. Other complications include sinus tracts, heterotrophic calcification, a chronic inflammatory state causing amyloidosis, and squamous cell carcinoma.[35]

Documentation

Update the care plan, as required. On the clinical record, document complete skin assessment findings. Also record interventions used to prevent pressure injuries as well as the patient's response to them. If a pressure injury develops, note changes in its condition or size and elevations of skin temperature. Document the name of the practitioner you notified, when you notified the practitioner of pertinent observations of abnormalities, prescribed interventions you performed, and the patient's response to them. Document teaching provided to the patient and family (if applicable), their understanding of that teaching, and any need for follow-up teaching.

REFERENCES

1 European Pressure Ulcer Advisory Panel, et al. (2019). Prevention and treatment of pressure ulcers: Quick reference guide. http://www.internationalguideline.com/static/pdfs/Quick_Reference_Guide-10Mar2019.pdf (Level VII)

2 National Pressure Ulcer Advisory Panel. (2016). Pressure injury prevention points. https://cdn.ymaws.com/npiap.com/resource/resmgr/1a._pressure-injury-preventi.pdf

3 Braden, B., & Bergstrom, N. (1988). Braden Scale for predicting pressure sore risk. https://www.in.gov/isdh/files/Braden_Scale.pdf

4 Centers for Disease Control and Prevention. (2002). Guideline for hand hygiene in health-care settings: Recommendations of the Healthcare Infection Control Practices Advisory Committee and the HICPAC/SHEA/APIC/IDSA Hand Hygiene Task Force. *MMWR Recommendations and Reports, 51*(RR-16), 1–45. https://www.cdc.gov/mmwr/pdf/rr/rr5116.pdf (Level II)

5 World Health Organization. (2009). WHO guidelines on hand hygiene in health care: First global patient safety challenge, clean care is safer care. https://apps.who.int/iris/bitstream/handle/10665/44102/9789241597906_eng.pdf?sequence=1 (Level IV)

6 The Joint Commission. (2021). Standard NPSG.07.01.01. *Comprehensive accreditation manual for hospitals.* Oakbrook Terrace, IL: The Joint Commission. (Level VII)

7 Accreditation Association for Hospitals and Health Systems. (2020). Standard 07.01.21. *Healthcare Facilities Accreditation Program: Accreditation standards for acute care hospitals.* Chicago, IL: Accreditation Association for Hospitals and Health Systems. (Level VII)

8 Centers for Medicare and Medicaid Services, Department of Health and Human Services. (2020). Condition of participation: Infection control. 42 C.F.R. § 482.42.

9 DNV GL-Healthcare USA, Inc. (2020). IC.1.SR.1. *NIAHO® accreditation requirements, interpretive guidelines and surveyor guidance—revision 20.0.* Milford, OH: DNV GL-Healthcare USA, Inc. (Level VII)

10 The Joint Commission. (2021). Standard NPSG.01.01.01. *Comprehensive accreditation manual for hospitals.* Oakbrook Terrace, IL: The Joint Commission. (Level VII)

11 Accreditation Association for Hospitals and Health Systems. (2020). Standard 15.01.16. *Healthcare Facilities Accreditation Program: Accreditation requirements for acute care hospitals.* Chicago, IL: Accreditation Association for Hospitals and Health Systems. (Level VII)

12 The Joint Commission. (2021). Standard RI.01.01.01. *Comprehensive accreditation manual for hospitals.* Oakbrook Terrace, IL: The Joint Commission. (Level VII)

13 Centers for Medicare and Medicaid Services, Department of Health and Human Services. (2020). Condition of participation: Patient's rights. 42 C.F.R. § 482.13(c)(1).

14 DNV GL-Healthcare USA, Inc. (2020). PR.2.SR.5. *NIAHO® accreditation requirements, interpretive guidelines and surveyor guidance—revision 20.0.* Milford, OH: DNV GL-Healthcare USA, Inc. (Level VII)

15 The Joint Commission. (2021). Standard PC.02.01.21. *Comprehensive accreditation manual for hospitals.* Oakbrook Terrace, IL: The Joint Commission. (Level VII)

16 Waters, T. R., et al. (2009). Safe patient handling training for schools of nursing. https://www.cdc.gov/niosh/docs/2009-127/pdfs/2009-127.pdf (Level VII)

17 Siegel, J. D., et al. (2007, revised 2019). 2007 guideline for isolation precautions: Preventing transmission of infectious agents in healthcare settings. https://www.cdc.gov/infectioncontrol/pdf/guidelines/isolation-guidelines-H.pdf (Level II)

18 Accreditation Association for Hospitals and Health Systems. (2020). Standard 16.02.02. *Healthcare Facilities Accreditation Program: Accreditation requirements for acute care hospitals.* Chicago, IL: Accreditation Association for Hospitals and Health Systems. (Level VII)

19 Occupational Safety and Health Administration. (2019). Bloodborne pathogens, standard number 1910.1030. https://www.osha.gov/pls/oshaweb/owadisp.show_document?p_id=10051&p_table=STANDARDS (Level VII)

20 Agency for Healthcare Research and Quality. (n.d.). Preventing pressure ulcers in hospitals: A toolkit for improving quality of care. https://www.ahrq.gov/sites/default/files/publications/files/putoolkit.pdf (Level VII)

21 Zulkowski, K. (2012). Diagnosing and treating moisture-associated skin damage. *Advances in Skin and Wound Care, 25,* 231–236. (Level VII)

22 Wound Ostomy and Continence Nurses Society. (2016). *Guideline for prevention and management of pressure ulcers (injuries): WOCN clinical practice guidelines series 2.* Mount Laurel, NJ: WOCN.

23 McInnes, E., et al. (2015). Support surfaces for pressure ulcer prevention. *Cochrane Database of Systematic Reviews, 2015*(9), CD001735. (Level I)

24 Schofield, R., et al. (2013). Reviewing the literature on the effectiveness of pressure relieving movements. *Nursing Research and Practice, 2013,* 124095. https://www.hindawi.com/journals/nrp/2013/124095/ (Level V)

25 Beeckman, D., et al. (2016). Interventions for preventing and treating incontinence-associated dermatitis in adults. *Cochrane Database of Systematic Reviews, 2016*(11), CD011627. (Level I)

26 Sernekos, L. A. (2013). Nutritional treatment of pressure ulcers: What is the evidence? *Journal of the American Association of Nurse Practitioners, 25,* 281–288. (Level V)

27 Doley, J. (2010). Nutrition management of pressure ulcers. *Nutrition in Clinical Practice, 25,* 50–60. (Level VII)

28 Posthauer, M. E., et al. (2015). The role of nutrition for pressure ulcer management: National Pressure Ulcer Advisory Panel, European Pressure Ulcer Advisory Panel, and Pan Pacific Pressure Injury Alliance white paper. *Advances in Skin and Wound Care, 28,* 175–188. (Level VII)

29 Ganz, D. A., et al. (2013, reviewed 2021). *Preventing falls in hospitals: A toolkit for improving quality of care* (AHRQ Publication No. 13-0015-EF). Rockville, MD: Agency for Healthcare Research and Quality. https://www.ahrq.gov/professionals/systems/hospital/fallpxtoolkit/index.html (Level VII)

30 The Joint Commission. (2021). Standard RC.01.03.01. *Comprehensive accreditation manual for hospitals.* Oakbrook Terrace, IL: The Joint Commission. (Level VII)

31 Centers for Medicare and Medicaid Services, Department of Health and Human Services. (2020). Condition of participation: Medical record services. 42 C.F.R. § 482.24(b).

32 Accreditation Association for Hospitals and Health Systems. (2020). Standard 10.00.03. *Healthcare Facilities Accreditation Program: Accreditation requirements for acute care hospitals.* Chicago, IL: Accreditation Association for Hospitals and Health Systems. (Level VII)

33 DNV GL-Healthcare USA, Inc. (2020). MR.2.SR.1. *NIAHO® accreditation requirements, interpretive guidelines and surveyor guidance—revision 20.0.* Milford, OH: DNV GL-Healthcare USA, Inc. (Level VII)

34 Accreditation Association for Hospitals and Health Systems. (2020). Standard 10.01.24. *Healthcare Facilities Accreditation Program: Accreditation requirements for acute care hospitals.* Chicago, IL: Accreditation Association for Hospitals and Health Systems. (Level VII)

35 Berlowitz, D. (2020). Clinical staging and management of pressure-induced skin and soft tissue injury. In: *UpToDate,* Berman, R. S. & Schmader, K. E. (Eds.).

Progressive ambulation

After surgery or a period of bed rest, patients must begin the gradual return to full ambulation. When it's begun promptly and properly, progressive ambulation thwarts many of the complications of prolonged inactivity. Immobility strongly increases the risk for venous thromboembolism (VTE) in hospitalized medical, surgical, and critically ill patients. These patients should be encouraged to ambulate as soon and as often as possible.[1]

The American Academy of Orthopaedic Surgeons recommends early progressive ambulation after hip and knee arthroplasty to prevent VTE.[2] Other complications prevented by early progressive ambulation include respiratory stasis and hypostatic pneumonia; urine retention, urinary tract infection, urinary stasis, and calculus formation; abdominal distention, constipation, and decreased appetite; and sensory deprivation. Progressive ambulation also helps restore the patient's sense of equilibrium and enhances self-confidence and self-image.[3] In patients who have undergone hip replacement, early dangling and ambulation result in excellent postoperative pain management and a shortened length of stay.[3]

HOSPITAL-ACQUIRED CONDITION ALERT Keep in mind that the Centers for Medicare and Medicaid Services considers VTE in patients who underwent total knee replacement or hip replacement a hospital-acquired condition *because it can be reasonably prevented using a variety of best practices.* Make sure to follow evidence-based VTE prevention practices, such as using mechanical compression devices (including antiembolism stockings or an intermittent pneumatic compression device), early ambulation, and pharmacologic prophylaxis, *to reduce the risk of VTE.*[1,2,4,5,6,7]

Progressive ambulation begins with dangling the patient's feet over the edge of the bed and progresses to seating the patient in an armchair or wheelchair, walking around the room with the patient, and then walking with the patient in the halls until the patient can walk independently. The rate of progress depends on the patient's physical condition and tolerance. Successful return to full ambulation requires correct body mechanics, careful patient observation, and open communication among patient, practitioner, and nurse.

Equipment

Chair or wheelchair ▪ facility-approved disinfectant ▪ nonskid slippers or socks (for standing) or hard-soled shoes (for walking) ▪ Optional: robe, assistive device (cane, crutches, or walker), prescribed analgesic, vital signs monitoring equipment, disinfectant pad, gait belt, powered stand-assist lift, pillow, supplies for securing IV tubing and catheters.

If the patient requires an assistive device, the physical therapist usually selects the appropriate one and teaches about its use.

Implementation

▪ Check the patient's medical record for history, diagnosis, and therapeutic regimen.
▪ Gather and prepare the necessary equipment and supplies.
▪ Perform hand hygiene.[8,9,10,11,12,13]
▪ Confirm the patient's identity using at least two patient identifiers.[14]
▪ Provide privacy.[15,16,17,18]
▪ Screen for and assess the patient's pain using facility-defined criteria that are consistent with the patient's age, condition, and ability to understand.[19]
▪ Treat the patient's pain as needed and ordered using nonpharmacologic, pharmacologic, or a combination of approaches. Base the treatment plan on evidence-based practices and the patient's clinical condition, past medical history, and pain management goals.[20,21,22,23] Wait 30 to 60 minutes for an analgesic to take effect before attempting ambulation.

NURSING ALERT Keep in mind that certain medications may cause hypotension, dizziness, and drowsiness, increasing the patient's risk of falling. Review the patient's medications *to determine whether the patient is at an increased risk of falling.*

▪ Explain the goal of ambulation to the patient and family (if appropriate) according to their individual communication and learning needs *to increase their understanding, allay their fears, and enhance cooperation.*[24]

Provide encouragement, *because the patient may be hesitant or fearful*; provide reassurance that the patient need not attempt more than the patient can reasonably do. If the patient fears pain in an incision, demonstrate how to support the incision by placing a hand alongside or gently over the dressing site, or splint the incision for the patient, if needed.
▪ Ask a coworker for assistance, as needed.
▪ Remove equipment or other objects from the patient's path, if appropriate, *to provide a clear path and to help prevent falls.*[25,26]
▪ If the patient has IV tubing, or other tubing or catheters, secure them *to prevent accidental dislodgement.* Don't let them discourage ambulation.
▪ Lock the wheels on the bed or chair, if appropriate.[25,26]

Dangling the patient's legs
▪ Position the bed horizontally and the patient laterally, facing you.
▪ Assist with moving the patient's legs over the side of the bed.
▪ Grasp the patient's shoulders, standing with your feet apart *so you have a wide base of support.*[25]
▪ Help the patient to rise slowly. Ask the patient to help by pushing up from the bed with the arms. Then shift your weight from the foot closest to the patient's head to the other foot as you steadily raise the patient to the sitting position. Pull with your whole body, not just your arms, *to avoid straining your back and jostling the patient.* Alternatively, you can raise the head of the bed to a 45-degree angle *to allow easier elevation of the patient.* Don't use this method if the patient has trouble balancing while sitting. Ask a coworker for assistance whenever necessary.
▪ While the patient adjusts to an upright position, continue to stand facing the patient *to keep the patient from falling*, and observe the patient closely. Be alert for signs and symptoms of orthostatic hypotension, such as fainting, dizziness, and reports of blurred vision. Be prepared to respond quickly if these signs and symptoms develop *to prevent the patient from falling.*
▪ Check the patient's pulse rate and blood pressure, as needed. If the pulse rate increases more than 20 beats/minute, allow the patient to rest before slowly progressing to a standing position.

Helping the patient stand
▪ Before attempting the standing position, help the patient put on a robe (as needed) and nonskid slippers or socks (for standing only) or hard-soled shoes (for walking).
▪ Don't allow the robe, a drainage tube, or anything else to dangle around the patient's feet.

HOSPITAL-ACQUIRED CONDITION ALERT Keep in mind that the Centers for Medicare and Medicaid Services considers an injury from a fall a hospital-acquired condition *because it can be reasonably prevented using best practices.* Make sure to follow evidence-based fall prevention practices, such as performing a fall-risk assessment and instituting fall precautions, *to reduce the risk of injury from falls.*[4,5,26,27]

▪ If the patient is cooperative and can bear weight fully, have the patient place the feet flat on the floor and allow the patient to stand. Stand by for safety.[25] Alternatively, if the patient is cooperative and can partially bear weight, apply a gait belt and use another assistive device, as ordered, *to assist with standing.* (See the "Gait belt use" procedure.) If you're required to lift more than 35 lb (15.8 kg) of the patient's weight to assist with standing, use a powered stand-assist lift *to help the patient stand.*[25]
▪ Encourage the patient to look forward and not at the floor *to help maintain balance.*

Helping the patient sit
▪ Make sure the chair is secure or the wheelchair brakes are applied *to prevent the patient from falling as the patient lowers to a sitting position.*[26,27]
▪ After the patient stands, have the patient pivot and lower the body into a chair with armrests and a straight back, or into a wheelchair.
▪ Instruct the patient to sit with the lower back against the rear of the chair, feet flat on the floor, hips and knees at right angles, and upper body straight. Tell the patient to flex the elbows and rest the forearms on the armrests of the chair (as shown).

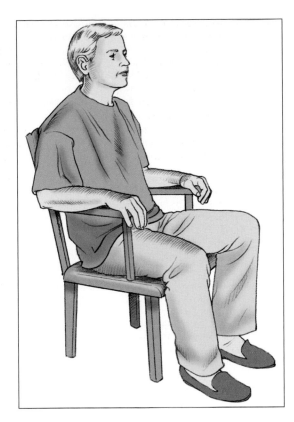

■ Make sure to provide a call light or other signal device if you leave the patient sitting in the chair *to reduce the risk of falling.*[26,27]

Helping the patient walk

■ If the patient can bear weight fully, have the patient begin walking while you stand by for safety.[25]

■ If the patient requires a gait belt, place one hand under the gait belt in back of the patient. If the patient is weaker on one side, make sure to walk on that side when ambulating (as shown below) *because the patient will tend to lean to this side.* Encourage the patient to use an assistive device if needed.[28]

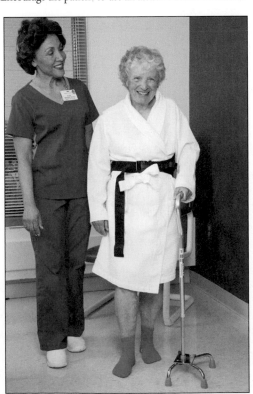

■ Walk closely behind and slightly to the side of the patient, keeping the same pattern and pace as the patient.[28]

■ Give the patient verbal and tactile cues *for encouragement.*

■ Allow for rest periods as needed.

Completing the procedure

■ Reassess and respond to the patient's pain by evaluating the response to treatment and progress toward pain management goals. Assess for adverse reactions and risk factors for adverse events that may result from treatment.[19]

■ Perform hand hygiene.[8,9,10,11,12,13]

■ Put on gloves and, as needed, other personal protective equipment *to comply with standard precautions.*[29]

■ Clean and disinfect reusable equipment according to the manufacturer's instructions *to prevent the spread of infection.*[30,31]

■ Remove and discard your gloves and, if worn, other personal protective equipment.[29]

■ Perform hand hygiene.[8,9,10,11,12,13]

■ Document the procedure.[32,33,34,35]

Special considerations

■ If the patient experiences dyspnea, diaphoresis, or orthostatic hypotension, stabilize the patient's position and obtain vital signs. Place the patient in the semi-Fowler position *to facilitate breathing.* If the patient's condition doesn't improve rapidly, notify the practitioner.

Complications

Orthostatic hypotension, dyspnea, diaphoresis, and falls are common complications of progressive ambulation.

Documentation

Record the type of transfer and assistance needed; the duration of sitting, standing, or walking; the distance walked, if applicable; the patient's response to ambulation; and any significant changes in blood pressure, pulse, and respiration. Document teaching provided to the patient and family (if applicable), their understanding of that teaching, and any need for follow-up teaching.

REFERENCES

1   American Association of Critical-Care Nurses. (2016). AACN practice alert: Preventing venous thromboembolism in adults. https://www.aacn.org/clinical-resources/practice-alerts/venous-thromboembolism-prevention (Level VII)

2   American Academy of Orthopaedic Surgeons. (2011). Preventing venous thromboembolic disease in patients undergoing elective hip and knee arthroplasty: Evidence-based clinical practice guideline. https://www.aaos.org/globalassets/quality-and-practice-resources/vte/vte_full_guideline_10.31.16.pdf (Level I)

3   Morris, B. A., et al. (2010). Clinical practice guidelines for early mobilization hours after surgery. *Orthopedic Nursing, 29*, 290–316. (Level IV)

4   Accreditation Association for Hospitals and Health Systems. (2020). Standard 16.02.02. *Healthcare Facilities Accreditation Program: Accreditation requirements for acute care hospitals.* Chicago, IL: Accreditation Association for Hospitals and Health Systems. (Level VII)

5   Jarrett, N., & Callaham, M. (2016). Evidence-based guidelines for selected hospital-acquired conditions: Final report. https://www.cms.gov/Medicare/Medicare-Fee-for-Service-Payment/HospitalAcqCond/Downloads/2016-HAC-Report.pdf

6   Falck-Ytter, Y., et al. (2012). Prevention of VTE in orthopedic surgery patients: Antithrombotic therapy and prevention of thrombosis (9th ed.): American College of Chest Physicians evidence-based clinical practice guidelines. *Chest, 141*(Suppl. 2), e278S–e325S. https://www.ncbi.nlm.nih.gov/pmc/articles/PMC3278063/ (Level VII)

7   Balk, E. M., et al. (2017). *Venous thromboembolism prophylaxis in major orthopedic surgery: Systematic review update.* (AHRQ Publication No. 17-EHC021-EF). Rockville, MD: Agency for Healthcare Research and Quality. https://effectivehealthcare.ahrq.gov/sites/default/files/pdf/thromboembolism-update_research-2017.pdf (Level V)

8 The Joint Commission. (2021). Standard NPSG.07.01.01. *Comprehensive accreditation manual for hospitals.* Oakbrook Terrace, IL: The Joint Commission. (Level VII)

9 Centers for Disease Control and Prevention. (2002). Guideline for hand hygiene in health-care settings: Recommendations of the Healthcare Infection Control Practices Advisory Committee and the HICPAC/ SHEA/APIC/IDSA Hand Hygiene Task Force. *MMWR Recommendations and Reports, 51*(RR-16), 1–45. https://www.cdc.gov/mmwr/pdf/rr/rr5116. pdf (Level II)

10 World Health Organization. (2009). WHO guidelines on hand hygiene in health care: First global patient safety challenge, clean care is safer care. https://apps.who.int/iris/bitstream/han-dle/10665/44102/9789241597906_eng.pdf?sequence=1 (Level IV)

11 Centers for Medicare and Medicaid Services, Department of Health and Human Services. (2020). Condition of participation: Infection control. 42 C.F.R. § 482.42.

12 Accreditation Association for Hospitals and Health Systems. (2020). Standard 07.01.21. *Healthcare Facilities Accreditation Program: Accreditation requirements for acute care hospitals.* Chicago, IL: Accreditation Association for Hospitals and Health Systems. (Level VII)

13 DNV GL-Healthcare USA, Inc. (2020). IC.1.SR.1. *NIAHO® accreditation requirements, interpretive guidelines and surveyor guidance—revision 20.0.* Milford, OH: DNV GL-Healthcare USA, Inc. (Level VII)

14 The Joint Commission. (2021). Standard NPSG.01.01.01. *Comprehensive accreditation manual for hospitals.* Oakbrook Terrace, IL: The Joint Commission. (Level VII)

15 The Joint Commission. (2021). Standard RI.01.01.01. *Comprehensive accreditation manual for hospitals.* Oakbrook Terrace, IL: The Joint Commission. (Level VII)

16 DNV GL-Healthcare USA, Inc. (2020). PR.2.SR.5. *NIAHO® accreditation requirements, interpretive guidelines and surveyor guidance—revision 20.0.* Milford, OH: DNV GL-Healthcare USA, Inc. (Level VII)

17 Centers for Medicare and Medicaid Services, Department of Health and Human Services. (2020). Condition of participation: Patient's rights. 42 C.F.R. § 482.13(c)(1).

18 Accreditation Association for Hospitals and Health Systems. (2020). Standard 15.01.16. *Healthcare Facilities Accreditation Program: Accreditation requirements for acute care hospitals.* Chicago, IL: Accreditation Association for Hospitals and Health Systems. (Level VII)

19 The Joint Commission. (2021). Standard PC.01.02.07. *Comprehensive accreditation manual for hospitals.* Oakbrook Terrace, IL: The Joint Commission. (Level VII)

20 Accreditation Association for Hospitals and Health Systems. (2020). Standard 16.01.03. *Healthcare Facilities Accreditation Program: Accreditation requirements for acute care hospitals.* Chicago, IL: Accreditation Association for Hospitals and Health Systems. (Level VII)

21 Centers for Medicare and Medicaid Services, Department of Health and Human Services. (2020). Condition of participation: Nursing services. 42 C.F.R. § 482.23(c).

22 The Joint Commission. (2021). Standard MM.06.01.01. *Comprehensive accreditation manual for hospitals.* Oakbrook Terrace, IL: The Joint Commission. (Level VII)

23 DNV GL-Healthcare USA, Inc. (2020). MM.1.SR.3. *NIAHO® accreditation requirements, interpretive guidelines and surveyor guidance—revision 20.0.* Milford, OH: DNV GL-Healthcare USA, Inc. (Level VII)

24 The Joint Commission. (2021). Standard PC.02.01.21. *Comprehensive accreditation manual for hospitals.* Oakbrook Terrace, IL: The Joint Commission. (Level VII)

25 Waters, T. R., et al. (2009). Safe patient handling training for schools of nursing. https://www.cdc.gov/niosh/docs/2009-127/pdfs/2009-127.pdf (Level VII)

26 Institute for Healthcare Improvement. (2012). *Transforming care at the bedside how-to guide: Reducing patient injuries from falls.* Cambridge, MA: Institute for Healthcare Improvement. (Level VII)

27 Ganz, D. A., et al. (2013, reviewed 2021). *Preventing falls in hospitals: A toolkit for improving quality of care* (AHRQ Publication No. 13-0015-EF). Rockville, MD: Agency for Healthcare Research and Quality. https://www. ahrq.gov/professionals/systems/hospital/fallpxtoolkit/index.html (Level VII)

28 O'Sullivan, S. B., et al. (2019). *Physical rehabilitation* (7th ed.). Philadelphia, PA: F.A. Davis

29 Occupational Safety and Health Administration. (2019). Bloodborne pathogens, standard number 1910.1030. https://www.osha.gov/pls/ oshaweb/owadisp.show_document?p_id=10051&p_table=STANDARDS (Level VII)

30 Accreditation Association for Hospitals and Health Systems. (2020). Standard 07.02.03. *Healthcare Facilities Accreditation Program: Accreditation requirements for acute care hospitals.* Chicago, IL: Accreditation Association for Hospitals and Health Systems. (Level VII)

31 Rutala, W. A., et al. (2008, revised 2019). Guideline for disinfection and sterilization in healthcare facilities, 2008. https://www.cdc.gov/infection-control/pdf/guidelines/disinfection-guidelines-H.pdf (Level I)

32 The Joint Commission. (2021). Standard RC.01.03.01. *Comprehensive accreditation manual for hospitals.* Oakbrook Terrace, IL: The Joint Commission. (Level VII)

33 Centers for Medicare and Medicaid Services, Department of Health and Human Services. (2020). Condition of participation: Medical record services. 42 C.F.R. § 482.24(b).

34 Accreditation Association for Hospitals and Health Systems. (2020). Standard 10.00.03. *Healthcare Facilities Accreditation Program: Accreditation requirements for acute care hospitals.* Chicago, IL: Accreditation Association for Hospitals and Health Systems. (Level VII)

35 DNV GL-Healthcare USA, Inc. (2020). MR.2.SR.1. *NIAHO® accreditation requirements, interpretive guidelines and surveyor guidance—revision 20.0.* Milford, OH: DNV GL-Healthcare USA, Inc. (Level VII)

PRONE POSITIONING

Prone positioning is a therapeutic maneuver used to improve oxygenation and pulmonary mechanics in patients with acute lung injury or mechanically ventilated patients with acute respiratory distress syndrome (ARDS)[1] who require high concentrations of inspired oxygen. Also known as *proning,* the procedure involves physically turning a patient from a supine position (on the back) to a face-down (prone) position.

The recommended criteria for using prone positioning include patients with ARDS who require high plateau pressure or a high fraction of inspired oxygen, which make mechanical ventilation potentially damaging to the lungs.[1,2]

The physical challenges of prone positioning have been a traditional barrier to its use. However, equipment innovations have helped to minimize the risks associated with moving patients and maintaining them in the prone position for several hours at a time. Several bed manufacturers have also developed automated systems designed to provide multiple intervals of prone therapy automatically over an extended time. With the appropriate equipment, prone positioning may promote better movement of the diaphragm by allowing the abdomen to expand more fully.

There isn't an established recommended timeframe for prone positioning. Most studies used repeated sessions of prone positioning that lasted either 6 to 8 hours per day or 17 to 20 hours per day, with similar results.[3] Prone positioning usually is performed until the requirement for a high concentration of inspired oxygen resolves.[4] Patients with ARDS have improved oxygenation when prone positioning is used during mechanical ventilation. Research has demonstrated increased survival rates when prone positioning is used during mechanical ventilation in patients with moderate to severe ARDS who received protective lung ventilation (tidal volume of less than 8 mL/kg).[5] In these patients, prone positioning was used for 16 or more hours per day.[5]

Prone positioning can be accomplished by manually turning the patient or by using an automated proning device, such as the RotoProne Therapy System. Prone positioning is contraindicated in patients whose heads can't be supported in a face-down position, as well as in those who can't tolerate a head-down position. Relative contraindications include increased intracranial pressure; unstable spine, chest, or pelvis; unstable bone fractures; left-sided heart failure (nonpulmonary respiratory failure); shock; bronchopleural fistula; presence of a bifurcated endotracheal tube; abdominal compartment syndrome; abdominal surgery; extreme obesity (greater than 300 lb [136 kg]); and pregnancy.[1] Thorough evaluation of hemodynamically unstable patients (systolic blood pressure less than 90 mm Hg [12 kPa] despite aggressive fluid resuscitation and vasopressors) is essential before initiating prone positioning.

Contraindications specific to RotoProne therapy include unstable cervical, thoracic, lumbar, pelvic, skull, or facial fractures; cervical or skeletal traction; uncontrolled intracranial pressure; body weight below 88 lb (40 kg) or above 350 lb (159 kg); and height less than 54″ (140.2 cm) or greater than 78″ (201.2 cm).[1,6]

Equipment

Hospital bed, specialty bed, or automated prone-positioning device ▪ small towels ▪ small pillows or rolled towels, or gel or foam positioning devices ▪ foam or other padded dressings[7] ▪ drawsheet or transfer device ▪ suction equipment ▪ oral care supplies (see the "Oral care" procedure) ▪ vital signs monitoring equipment ▪ pulse oximeter and probe ▪ stethoscope ▪ disinfectant pad ▪ cardiac monitoring equipment ▪ arterial blood gas sampling equipment ▪ emergency equipment (code cart with emergency medications, defibrillator, handheld resuscitation bag with mask, intubation equipment) ▪ facility-approved disinfectant ▪ gloves ▪ facility-approved assessment tools (such as for pain, anxiety or agitation, or delirium assessment) ▪ Optional: gown, mask and goggles or mask and face shield, wound and ostomy care supplies, skin care supplies, tape, bite block, dental mouth prop, eye lubricant, labels.

Preparation of equipment

Turn off the patient's enteral tube feeding 1 hour before prone positioning *to reduce the risk of aspiration during the turning procedure.*[1,8,9] Make sure that emergency equipment is readily available and functioning properly.[1] Using a facility-approved disinfectant, clean and disinfect the positioner between positioning turns and when discontinuing prone positioning.[10,11]

Inspect all equipment and supplies. If a product is expired, is defective, or has compromised integrity, remove it from patient use, label it as expired or defective, and report the expiration or defect as directed by your facility.

Implementation

▪ Verify the practitioner's order. If your facility requires the presence of a practitioner for initial proning, collaborate with the practitioner to set up a time for initial proning.
▪ Perform hand hygiene.[12,13,14,15,16,17]
▪ Confirm the patient's identity using at least two patient identifiers.[18]
▪ Provide privacy.[19,20,21,22]
▪ Explain the procedure the patient and family (if appropriate) according to their individual communication and learning needs *to increase their understanding, allay their fears, and enhance cooperation.*[23]

Assessing the patient

▪ Assess the patient's hemodynamic status *to determine whether the patient can tolerate the prone position.*[1]
▪ Assess the patient's neurologic status before prone positioning. Typically, the patient will be sedated heavily. Although agitation isn't a contraindication for the procedure, you must manage it effectively. Use facility-approved assessment tools to assess the patient's pain, anxiety or agitation, and delirium before, during, and after proning *to promote a safe environment for the patient.*[1,24]
▪ Determine whether the patient's size and weight will allow turning 180 degrees on a narrow critical care bed.[1] If needed, consider obtaining a wider specialty bed or the RotoProne Therapy System.

Before turning the patient

▪ Gather and prepare the necessary equipment and supplies.
▪ Perform hand hygiene.[12,13,14,15,16,17]
▪ Put on gloves or other protective equipment, as needed, *to comply with standard precautions.*[25,26,27]
▪ Provide eye care, including lubrication and horizontal taping of eyelids, if indicated.[1]
▪ Ensure that the patient's tongue is inside the mouth; if it's edematous or protruding, insert a dental mouth prop or bite block. Avoid bite blocks that fit over the tongue *because of the risk of tongue breakdown.*[1]
▪ Secure the patient's endotracheal (ET) tube or tracheotomy tube *to prevent accidental dislodgment.*[1]
▪ Perform anterior body wound care and dressing changes, as needed.[1]
▪ Use foam or other padded dressings or positioning devices to protect anterior bony prominences and other areas that are likely to have prolonged contact with bed surfaces (such as shoulders, hips, knees, anterior lower legs, great toes, outer ears and chin).[28]

▪ Empty ileostomy or colostomy drainage bags, as needed.[1]
▪ Remove anterior chest wall electrocardiogram (ECG) monitoring leads while ensuring the ability to monitor the patient's cardiac rate and rhythm. You'll position these leads on the patient's back after the patient is in the prone position.[1]
▪ Ensure that the bed's brake is engaged.[6]

Turning the patient manually

▪ Raise the bed to hip level before turning the patient *to prevent back strain.*[29]
▪ Position at least three and up to six staff members appropriately on either side of the bed and at the head of the bed, depending on the size and complexity of the patient.[1,6]
NURSING ALERT The staff member at the head of the bed is responsible for monitoring the ET tube and mechanical ventilator tubing.
▪ Adjust all patient tubing and invasive monitoring lines *to prevent dislodgment, kinking, disconnection, or contact with the patient's body during the turning procedure and while the patient remains in the prone position.*[1]
NURSING ALERT Place all lines inserted in the upper torso over the right or left shoulder, with the exception of chest tubes, which are placed at the foot of the bed. Position all lines inserted in the lower torso at the foot of the bed.[1]
▪ Turn the patient's face away from the ventilator, placing the ET tubing on the side of the patient's face that's turned away from the ventilator.[1] Loop the remaining tubing above the patient's head *to prevent disconnection of the ventilator tubing or kinking of the ET tube.*
▪ Lower the side rails of the bed and move the patient to the edge of the bed farthest away from the ventilator using a drawsheet or transfer device. The person closest to the patient maintains body contact with the bed at all times, serving as a side rail.[1]
▪ Tuck the patient's arm and hand that are resting in the center of the bed under the buttocks. Cross the leg closest to the edge of the bed over the opposite leg at the ankle, *which will help with forward motion when the turning process begins.*[1]
NURSING ALERT If you can't straighten and tuck the patient's arm under the buttocks, tuck the arm into the open space between the chest and pelvic pads.
▪ Turn the patient toward the ventilator, first turning the patient onto the side, and then roll the patient into the prone position.[1]
NURSING ALERT Always turn the patient in the direction of the mechanical ventilator.
▪ Gently move the patient's tucked arm and hand *so they're parallel to the body,* and then flex them to a comfortable position.[1] Alternatively, place one of the patient's arms up and one down, as in a swimmer's position.[1,6]
▪ Support the patient's ankles and feet with a pillow or towel roll *to provide correct flexion while prone.*[1]
▪ Pad the patient's elbows with small towels *to prevent ulnar nerve compression.*
▪ Replace ECG monitoring leads on the patient's back. Make sure that ECG alarm limits are set appropriately for the patient's current condition, and that alarms are turned on, functioning properly, and audible to staff.[30,31,32,33]
▪ Readjust all patient tubing and invasive monitoring lines. Route the tubing toward the patient's feet, and place the enteral feeding pump toward the foot of the bed, *because a standardized approach of keeping IV lines routed toward the head and enteric lines routed toward the feet helps prevent dangerous misconnections.* If multiple access sites will be used, label the tubing at both the distal end (near the patient connection) and the proximal end (near the source container) *to reduce the risk of misconnection.*[34]
▪ Readjust the bed to waist level for patient care *to prevent caregiver back strain.*[29]

Turning the patient using the RotoProne Therapy System[1,5]

▪ Ask a coworker to help you position the patient on the RotoProne device.
▪ Secure ventilator tubes and other upper body lines into the tube management system at the head of the bed.

■ Secure all lower body tubes and lines through the circular opening at the foot of the bed.

■ Make sure all tubes have enough slack and can slide freely without being pinched or compressed by the tube management system during turning.

NURSING ALERT Don't hang or attach any equipment to the side of the RotoProne Therapy System support frame.[6]

■ Secure the patient into the device following the manufacturer's instructions, as described in the following steps: Secure the patient within the side packs to prevent shear or friction injuries during turning. Secure the abdominal support mesh over the patient's abdomen. Position the lower leg packs, pelvic pack, and chest pack appropriately. Make sure the patient's head is secure within the headpiece. Place the face pack on the patient's face, making sure the top pad is above the eyebrows and the side pieces are around the mouth.

■ Remove all equipment from around the RotoProne Therapy System before turning *to prevent patient or caregiver injury.*[6]

■ Use the RotoProne touch screen *to turn the patient prone following the manufacturer's instructions.*

■ Using the touch screen, place the patient in the reverse Trendelenburg position *to elevate the head of the bed, decrease edema, and prevent aspiration.*[1]

■ Open back hatches and replace ECG monitoring leads. Make sure that alarm limits are set appropriately for the patient's current condition, and that alarms are turned on, functioning properly, and audible to staff.[30,31,32,33]

■ Readjust all patient tubing and invasive monitoring lines. Route the tubing toward the patient's feet, and place the enteral feeding pump toward the foot of the bed, *because a standardized approach of keeping IV lines routed toward the head and enteric lines routed toward the feet prevents dangerous misconnections.* If different access sites are used, label the tubing at both the distal end (near the patient connection) and the proximal end (near the source container) *to distinguish the different tubing and prevent misconnections.*[34]

Monitoring the patient

■ Monitor the patient's response to the prone position by assessing vital signs, oxygen saturation level (by pulse oximeter), and capnography. The patient's vital signs should return to normal within 10 minutes of initiating the prone position. Obtain an arterial sample for blood gas analysis, as ordered, within 30 minutes of a position change.[1]

■ Assess the patient's skin at intervals determined by the patient's condition, and provide skin care as needed. Keep the patient's skin clean and dry *to prevent pressure injuries.*[7,9,35]

■ Reposition the patient's head hourly while the patient is in the prone position *to prevent facial breakdown.* As one person lifts the patient's head, the second person moves the headpieces *to provide head support in a different position.*[1]

■ Perform range-of-motion exercises to the shoulders, arms, and legs every 2 hours.

■ If the patient was turned prone manually, adjust the patient's position frequently *to prevent skin breakdown.*[6]

HOSPITAL-ACQUIRED CONDITION ALERT Keep in mind that the Centers for Medicare and Medicaid Services considers a stage 3 or 4 pressure injury a hospital-acquired condition *because it can be reasonably prevented using best practices.* Make sure to follow evidence-based pressure injury prevention practices, such as assessing skin integrity and repositioning the patient, *to reduce the risk of pressure injuries.*[7,36,37]

■ Give frequent oral care, and suction the patient's airway as needed. *The prone position promotes postural drainage.*

■ After the patient is prone, restart the patient's tube feeding, as ordered and tolerated; *prone position involves minimal risk of aspiration because the patient is in a head-down position.*[1,9]

■ Assess the security of the ET tube or tracheostomy tube and all lines and tubes.[6]

■ Monitor the length of time the patient is prone; the duration and frequency of proning should be individualized according to the patient's tolerance or the practitioner's order, or as directed by the facility.[6]

■ Return the bed to the lowest position *to prevent falls and maintain patient safety.*[38]

■ Remove and discard your gloves and any other personal protective equipment worn,[27] and perform hand hygiene.[12,13,14,15,16,17]

Returning the patient to the supine position

■ Perform hand hygiene.[12,13,14,15,16,17]

■ Put on gloves and other personal protective equipment as needed *to comply with standard precautions.*[25,26,27]

■ Remove the posterior chest ECG leads while ensuring the ability to monitor the patient's cardiac rate and rhythm; you'll reposition the leads on the patient's chest once the patient is in the supine position.

■ *To return the patient to the supine position manually*: Raise the bed to hip level *to prevent back strain while turning the patient.*[29] Position the patient on the edge of the bed closest to the ventilator.[1] Adjust all patient tubing and monitoring lines *to prevent dislodgment.*[1] Position at least three and up to six staff members appropriately on either side of the bed and at the head of the bed, depending on the size and complexity of the patient.[1,6] Straighten the patient's arms and rest them on either side. Cross the leg closest to the edge of the bed over the opposite leg.[1] Turn the patient onto the side and then onto the back. Position the patient's arms parallel to the body.

■ *To return the patient to the supine position using the RotoProne Therapy System*: Use the touch screen and follow manufacturer's instructions to turn the patient to the supine position. Insert the locking pin.[1] Remove the face pack.[6] Using the touch screen, place the patient in the reverse Trendelenburg position *to elevate the head of the bed, decrease edema, and prevent aspiration.*[1,6]

■ Replace ECG monitoring leads on the patient's chest. Make sure that ECG alarm limits are set appropriately for the patient's current condition, and that alarms are turned on, functioning properly, and audible to staff.[30,31,32,33]

■ Readjust all patient tubing and invasive monitoring lines. Route the tubing toward the patient's feet, and place the enteral feeding pump toward the foot of the bed, *because a standardized approach of keeping IV lines routed toward the head and enteric lines routed toward the feet prevents dangerous misconnections.* If different access sites are used, label each tubing at both the distal end (near the patient connection) and the proximal end (near the source container) *to distinguish the different tubing and prevent misconnections.*[34]

■ Assess the patient's response to repositioning.[1].

■ If you raised the bed, return it to the lowest position *to prevent falls and maintain the patient's safety.*[38]

■ Remove and discard your gloves and any other personal protective equipment worn.[27]

■ Perform hand hygiene.[12,13,14,15,16,17]

■ Clean and disinfect your stethoscope.[10,11]

■ Perform hand hygiene.[12,13,14,15,16,17]

■ Document the procedure.[39,40,41,42]

Special considerations

■ You'll usually need a practitioner's order before prone positioning of a critically ill patient.

■ The procedure requires special training and established guidelines *to ensure patient safety.*[9]

■ Not all patients with ARDS respond favorably to prone positioning, and the benefit sometimes decreases over time.

■ The patient may not have an immediate positive response to the prone position. Maximum response to the position may take up to 6 hours in some patients.[1]

■ The prone-positioning schedule is generally determined by the patient's ability to maintain improvements in partial pressure of arterial oxygen while in the prone position.[1]

■ Use capnography, if possible, *to detect dislodgement of the ET tube.*[1]

■ Discontinue the procedure when the patient no longer demonstrates improved oxygenation with the position change.[1]

NURSING ALERT Lateral rotation therapy is strongly recommended with prone positioning.

Complications

Potential complications of prone positioning include inadvertent ET extubation; airway obstruction; decreased oxygen saturation; apical atelectasis; obstructed chest tube; pressure injuries on the weight-bearing parts of the body, including the knees and chest; hemodynamic instability;

dislodgment of central venous access; transient arrhythmias; reversible dependent edema of the face (forehead, eyelids, conjunctiva, lips, and tongue) and anterior chest wall; contractures; enteral feeding intolerance; aspiration of enteral feeding when repositioned; wound dehiscence; and corneal ulceration.

NURSING ALERT Critically ill patients with active intra-abdominal processes, regardless of position, are at risk for sepsis and septic shock.

Documentation

Document the patient's response to therapy, ability to tolerate the turning procedure, length of time in the position, and positioning schedule. Also document your assessments, monitoring details, any complications during or after the procedure, the name of the practitioner notified and the time and date of notification, any prescribed interventions, and the patient's response to those interventions. Record teaching provided to the patient and family (if applicable), their understanding of that teaching, and any need for follow-up teaching.

REFERENCES

1 Wiegand, D. L. (2017). *AACN procedure manual for high acuity, progressive, and critical care* (7th ed.). St. Louis, MO: Elsevier.

2 Fan, E., et al. (2017). An official American Thoracic Society/ European Society of Intensive Care Medicine/ Society of Critical Care Medicine clinical practice guideline: Mechanical ventilation in adult patients with acute respiratory distress syndrome. *American Journal of Respiratory and Critical Care Medicine, 195*(9), 1253–1263. https://www.atsjournals.org/doi/full/10.1164/rccm.201703-0548ST#readcube-epdf (Level VII)

3 Malhotra, A. (2021). Prone ventilation for adult patients with acute respiratory distress syndrome. In: *UpToDate*, Parsons, P. E. (Ed.).

4 Scholten, E. L., et al. (2017). Treatment of ARDS with prone positioning. *Chest, 151*(1), 215–224. https://journal.chestnet.org/article/S0012-3692(16)52643-9/fulltext (Level I)

5 Sud, S., et al. (2014). Effect of prone positioning during mechanical ventilation on mortality among patients with acute respiratory distress syndrome: A systematic review and meta-analysis. *Canadian Medical Association Journal, 186*(10), E381–E390. http://www.cmaj.ca/content/186/10/E381.full (Level I)

6 ArjoHuntleigh, Inc. (2016). RotoProne Therapy System user manual. https://www.arjo.com/siteassets/inriver/resources/2/208662-ah-rev-d_mnl_rotoprone_user_en

7 European Pressure Ulcer Advisory Panel, et al. (2019). Prevention and treatment of pressure ulcers/injuries: Quick reference guide. http://www.internationalguideline.com/static/pdfs/Quick_Reference_Guide-10Mar2019.pdf (Level VII)

8 Reignier, J., et al. (2010). Before-after study of a standardized ICU protocol for early enteral feeding in patients turned in the prone position. *Clinical Nutrition, 29*, 210–216. (Level VI)

9 Mitchell, D. A., & Seckel, M. A. (2018). Acute respiratory distress syndrome and prone positioning. *AACN Advanced Critical Care, 29*(4), 415–425. https://aacnjournals.org/aacnacconline/article/29/4/415/2281/Acute-Respiratory-Distress-Syndrome-and-Prone (Level VII)

10 Rutala, W. A., et al. (2008, revised 2019). Guideline for disinfection and sterilization in healthcare facilities, 2008. https://www.cdc.gov/infection-control/pdf/guidelines/disinfection-guidelines-H.pdf (Level I)

11 Accreditation Association for Hospitals and Health Systems. (2020). Standard 07.02.03. *Healthcare Facilities Accreditation Program: Accreditation requirements for acute care hospitals.* Chicago, IL: Accreditation Association for Hospitals and Health Systems. (Level VII)

12 Centers for Disease Control and Prevention. (2002). Guideline for hand hygiene in health-care settings: Recommendations of the Healthcare Infection Control Practices Advisory Committee and the HICPAC/SHEA/APIC/IDSA Hand Hygiene Task Force. *MMWR Recommendations and Reports, 51*(RR-16), 1–45. https://www.cdc.gov/mmwr/pdf/rr/rr5116.pdf (Level II)

13 World Health Organization. (2009). WHO guidelines on hand hygiene in health care: First global patient safety challenge, clean care is safer care. https://apps.who.int/iris/bitstream/handle/10665/44102/9789241597906_eng.pdf?sequence=1 (Level IV)

14 The Joint Commission. (2021). Standard NPSG.07.01.01. *Comprehensive accreditation manual for hospitals.* Oakbrook Terrace, IL: The Joint Commission. (Level VII)

15 Accreditation Association for Hospitals and Health Systems. (2020). Standard 07.01.21. *Healthcare Facilities Accreditation Program: Accreditation requirements for acute care hospitals.* Chicago, IL: Accreditation Association for Hospitals and Health Systems. (Level VII)

16 Centers for Medicare and Medicaid Services, Department of Health and Human Services. (2020). Condition of participation: Infection control. 42 C.F.R. § 482.42.

17 DNV GL-Healthcare USA, Inc. (2020). IC.1.SR.1. *NIAHO® accreditation requirements, interpretive guidelines and surveyor guidance—revision 20.0.* Milford, OH: DNV GL-Healthcare USA, Inc. (Level VII)

18 The Joint Commission. (2021). Standard NPSG.01.01.01. *Comprehensive accreditation manual for hospitals.* Oakbrook Terrace, IL: The Joint Commission. (Level VII)

19 Accreditation Association for Hospitals and Health Systems. (2020). Standard 15.01.16. *Healthcare Facilities Accreditation Program: Accreditation requirements for acute care hospitals.* Chicago, IL: Accreditation Association for Hospitals and Health Systems. (Level VII)

20 Centers for Medicare and Medicaid Services, Department of Health and Human Services. (2020). Condition of participation: Patient's rights. 42 C.F.R. § 482.13(c)(1).

21 DNV GL-Healthcare USA, Inc. (2020). PR.2.SR.5. *NIAHO® accreditation requirements, interpretive guidelines and surveyor guidance—revision 20.0.* Milford, OH: DNV GL-Healthcare USA, Inc. (Level VII)

22 The Joint Commission. (2021). Standard RI.01.01.01. *Comprehensive accreditation manual for hospitals.* Oakbrook Terrace, IL: The Joint Commission. (Level VII)

23 The Joint Commission. (2021). Standard PC.02.01.21. *Comprehensive accreditation manual for hospitals.* Oakbrook Terrace, IL: The Joint Commission. (Level VII)

24 The Joint Commission. (2021). Standard PC.01.02.07. *Comprehensive accreditation manual for hospitals.* Oakbrook Terrace, IL: The Joint Commission. (Level VII)

25 Accreditation Association for Hospitals and Health Systems. (2020). Standard 07.01.10. *Healthcare Facilities Accreditation Program: Accreditation requirements for acute care hospitals.* Chicago, IL: Accreditation Association for Hospitals and Health Systems. (Level VII)

26 Siegel, J. D., et al. (2007, revised 2019). 2007 guideline for isolation precautions: Preventing transmission of infectious agents in healthcare settings. https://www.cdc.gov/infectioncontrol/pdf/guidelines/isolation-guidelines-H.pdf (Level II)

27 Occupational Safety and Health Administration. (2019). Bloodborne pathogens, standard number 1910.1030. https://www.osha.gov/pls/oshaweb/owadisp.show_document?p_id=10051&p_table=STANDARDS (Level VII)

28 Baldi, M., et al. (2017). Prone positioning? Remember ABCDEFG. *Chest, 151*, 1184–1185. (Level VII)

29 Waters, T. R., et al. (2009). Safe patient handling training for schools of nursing. https://www.cdc.gov/niosh/docs/2009-127/pdfs/2009-127.pdf (Level VII)

30 American Association of Critical-Care Nurses. (2018). AACN practice alert: Managing alarms in acute care across the life span: Electrocardiography and pulse oximetry. https://www.aacn.org/clinical-resources/practice-alerts/managing-alarms-in-acute-care-across-the-life-span (Level VII)

31 Graham, K. C., & Cvach, M. (2010). Monitor alarm fatigue: Standardizing use of physiological monitors and decreasing nuisance alarms. *American Journal of Critical Care, 19*, 28–37.

32 The Joint Commission. (2021). Standard NPSG.06.01.01. *Comprehensive accreditation manual for hospitals.* Oakbrook Terrace, IL: The Joint Commission. (Level VII)

33 The Joint Commission. (2013). Sentinel event alert 50: Medical device alarm safety in hospitals. https://www.jointcommission.org/-/media/tjc/documents/resources/patient-safety-topics/sentinel-event/sea_50_alarms_4_26_16.pdf (Level VII)

34 The Joint Commission. (2014). Sentinel event alert 53: Managing risk during transition to new ISO tubing connector standards. https://www.jointcommission.org/-/media/tjc/documents/resources/patient-safety-topics/sentinel-event/sea_53_connectors_8_19_14_final.pdf (Level VII)

35 Accreditation Association for Hospitals and Health Systems. (2020). Standard 16.02.02. *Healthcare Facilities Accreditation Program: Accreditation requirements for acute care hospitals.* Chicago, IL: Accreditation Association for Hospitals and Health Systems. (Level VII)

36 Jarrett, N., & Callaham, M. (2016). Evidence-based guidelines for selected hospital-acquired conditions: Final report. https://www.cms.gov/Medicare/Medicare-Fee-for-Service-Payment/HospitalAcqCond/Downloads/2016-HAC-Report.pdf

37 Wound Ostomy and Continence Nurses Society (WOCN). (2016). *Guideline for prevention and management of pressure ulcers (injuries): WOCN clinical practice guideline series 2.* Mount Laurel, NJ: WOCN.

38 Ganz, D. A., et al. (2013, reviewed 2021). *Preventing falls in hospitals: A toolkit for improving quality of care* (AHRQ Publication No. 13-0015-EF). Rockville, MD: Agency for Healthcare Research and Quality. https://www.ahrq.gov/professionals/systems/hospital/fallpxtoolkit/index.html (Level VII)

39 The Joint Commission. (2021). Standard RC.01.03.01. *Comprehensive accreditation manual for hospitals.* Oakbrook Terrace, IL: The Joint Commission. (Level VII)

40 Accreditation Association for Hospitals and Health Systems. (2020). Standard 10.00.03. *Healthcare Facilities Accreditation Program: Accreditation requirements for acute care hospitals.* Chicago, IL: Accreditation Association for Hospitals and Health Systems. (Level VII)

41 Centers for Medicare and Medicaid Services, Department of Health and Human Services. (2020). Condition of participation: Medical record services. 42 C.F.R. § 482.24(b).

42 DNV GL-Healthcare USA, Inc. (2020). MR.2.SR.1. *NIAHO® accreditation requirements, interpretive guidelines and surveyor guidance—revision 20.0.* Milford, OH: DNV GL-Healthcare USA, Inc. (Level VII)

PRONE POSITIONING FOR THE AWAKE PATIENT

Prone positioning is a therapeutic maneuver used to improve oxygenation and pulmonary mechanics in patients with acute lung injury or acute respiratory distress syndrome (ARDS). Also known as *proning*, the procedure involves physically turning or assisting a patient from a supine position to a stomach-lying position with the head turned to the side. Prone positioning helps improve oxygenation by helping to recruit previously collapsed alveoli in the posterior lung fields, improving secretion management and shifting perfusion towards healthier alveoli in the anterior lung fields (which, in turn, improves ventilation-perfusion matching). When used early and in combination with noninvasive ventilation or a high-flow nasal cannula, prone positioning can help avoid the need for intubation in patients with moderate to severe ARDS.[1]

Although prone positioning may prevent the need for intubation, it can also delay intubation if a patient deteriorates further and becomes more hypoxemic, necessitating endotracheal intubation.[2] Because of this, it's important to consider the patient's trajectory before prone positioning. Prone positioning shouldn't be considered in patients with anticipated airway issues, *because such issues could further delay intubation if the patient's condition rapidly deteriorates.*

Prone positioning should be considered for patients receiving supplemental oxygen with a fraction of inspired oxygen of 28% or higher to achieve an arterial oxygen saturation of 92% to 96% (or 88% to 92% if the patient is at risk for hypercapnic respiratory failure).[3] Before implementing prone positioning, you must assess the patient *to determine the patient's ability to communicate and cooperate with the procedure, rotate to the supine position, and adjust position independently.*[3]

Absolute contraindications to prone positioning include respiratory distress, an immediate need for intubation, hemodynamic instability (a systolic blood pressure of less than 90 mm Hg), cardiac arrhythmias, agitation or altered mental status, an unstable spine, thoracic injury, and recent abdominal surgery.[3] Relative contraindications include facial injury, neurologic issues such as frequent seizures, extreme obesity, pregnancy that's in the second or third trimester, and pressure injuries.[3]

Equipment

Gloves ■ cardiac monitoring equipment ■ vital signs monitoring equipment ■ pulse oximeter and probe ■ emergency equipment (code cart with emergency medications, defibrillator, handheld resuscitation bag with mask, intubation equipment) ■ Optional: pillow, gown, mask and goggles or mask with face shield, ostomy drainage bag emptying equipment.

Preparation of equipment

Make sure that emergency equipment is functioning properly and readily available.[4]

Inspect all equipment and supplies. If a product is expired or defective or has compromised integrity, remove it from patient use, label it as expired or defective, and report the expiration or defect as directed by your facility.

Implementation

■ Verify the practitioner's order. If your facility requires the presence of a practitioner for initial prone positioning, collaborate with the practitioner to set up a time.

■ Review the patient's medical record for contraindications to prone positioning.

■ Perform hand hygiene.[5,6,7,8,9,10]

■ Confirm the patient's identity using at least two patient identifiers.[11]

■ Provide privacy.[12,13,14,15]

■ Explain the procedure to the patient and family (if appropriate) according to their individual communication and learning needs *to increase their understanding, allay their fears, and enhance and promote cooperation.*[16]

■ Raise the patient's bed to waist level before providing care *to prevent caregiver back strain.*[17]

■ Connect the patient to the cardiac monitor and pulse oximeter if not already connected.[4] Make sure that the alarm limits are set appropriately for the patient's current condition, and that the alarms are turned on, functioning properly, and audible to staff.[18,19,20,21]

■ Assess the patient's vital signs and other hemodynamic parameters *to determine whether the patient can tolerate the prone position and to serve as a baseline for comparison.*

■ Assess the patient's neurologic status before prone positioning. *Prone positioning is contraindicated in a patient with agitation or altered mental status.*[3]

■ Perform hand hygiene.[5,6,7,8,9,10]

■ Put on gloves and, as needed, other personal protective equipment *to comply with standard precautions.*[22,23,24]

■ Empty ileostomy or colostomy drainage bags as needed.[4]

■ Remove the anterior chest wall electrocardiogram (ECG) monitoring leads while ensuring the ability to monitor the patient's cardiac rate and rhythm. You'll reposition these leads on the patient's back after assisting the patient to the prone position.[4]

■ Ensure that the patient's supplemental oxygen equipment has sufficient tubing to facilitate turning.[3]

■ Adjust all patient tubing and invasive monitoring equipment *to prevent dislodgment, kinking, or disconnection during turning and while the patient remains prone.*[3]

■ Assist the patient to the prone position.[3]

NURSING ALERT Avoid sedation *to facilitate prone positioning in the awake patient.*[3]

■ Place the ECG chest leads on the patient's back.

■ Support the patient's chest with a pillow if needed *to promote comfort.*[3]

■ Place the patient's bed in the reverse Trendelenburg position, if needed, *to aid comfort.*[3]

■ Monitor the patient's oxygen saturation level for 15 minutes after each position change, *because the oxygen saturation level may decrease in response to the position change.*[3]

■ If the patient's oxygen saturation level deteriorates, make sure that the supplemental oxygen hasn't disconnected from the patient; reconnect if needed. If it hasn't disconnected, increase the inspired oxygen as needed and ordered. If there's no response, return the patient to the supine position and notify the practitioner of the change in the patient's condition.[3]

■ If the patient tolerates prone positioning, assist with position changes, with the goal of having the patient remain prone as long as possible. (See *Timing position changes.*)[3]

Timing position changes

If the patient tolerates prone positioning, consider setting up timed position changes with the patient *to maintain patient safety.* One such schedule includes:

■ lying fully prone for 30 minutes to 2 hours
■ lying on the right side with the bed flat for 30 minutes to 2 hours
■ sitting up with the head of bed elevated 30 to 60 degrees for 30 minutes to 2 hours
■ lying on the left side with the bed flat for 30 minutes to 2 hours
■ lying prone again for 30 minutes to 2 hours.[3]

Encourage the patient to repeat the cycle. Monitor the oxygen saturation level for 15 minutes after each position change. Monitor the patient closely *to promptly detect changes in the patient's condition.*[3]

- Discontinue prone positioning if the patient feels unable to tolerate the position, if the respiratory rate increases to 35 breaths/minute or higher, or if the patient appears tired or uses accessory muscles to breathe.[3]
- Remove and discard your gloves and other personal protective equipment, if worn.[23]
- Perform hand hygiene.[5,6,7,8,9,10]
- Document the procedure.[25,26]

Special considerations

- If the patient experiences cardiac arrest while in the prone position, attempt to place the patient in a supine position for continued resuscitation.[27]

Complications

Complications associated with prone positioning include pressure injuries, hemodynamic instability, transient cardiac arrhythmias, catheter dislodgment, agitation, peripheral arm nerve injury, periorbital and conjunctival edema, eye pressure or injury, vomiting, and decreased oxygen saturation level.[4,28]

Documentation

Document the patient's response to therapy, ability to tolerate the turning procedures, length of time in the prone position, and positioning schedule. Record your assessment findings, monitoring details, any complications that occurred during or after the procedure, any interventions taken, and the patient's response to those interventions. Document teaching provided to the patient and family (if applicable), their understanding of that teaching, and any need for follow-up teaching.

REFERENCES

1 Ding, L., et al. (2020). Efficacy and safety of early prone positioning combined with HFNC or NIV in moderate to severe ARDS: A multi-center prospective cohort study. *Critical Care, 24*, Article 28. https://ccforum.biomedcentral.com/articles/10.1186/s13054-020-2738-5 (Level IV)

2 Sun, Q., et al. (2020). Lower mortality of COVID-19 by early recognition and intervention: Experience from Jiangsu Province. *Annals of Intensive Care, 10*, Article 33. https://annalsofintensivecare.springeropen.com/track/pdf/10.1186/s13613-020-00650-2.pdf

3 Bamford, P., et al. (2020). ICS guidance for prone positioning of the conscious COVID patient 2020. https://emcrit.org/wp-content/uploads/2020/04/2020-04-12-Guidance-for-conscious-proning.pdf (Level VII)

4 Wiegand, D. L. (2017). *AACN procedure manual for high acuity, progressive, and critical care* (7th ed.). St. Louis, MO: Elsevier.

5 Accreditation Association for Hospitals and Health Systems. (2020). Standard 07.01.21. *Healthcare Facilities Accreditation Program: Accreditation requirements for acute care hospitals.* (Level VII)

6 Centers for Disease Control and Prevention. (2002). Guideline for hand hygiene in health-care settings: Recommendations of the Healthcare Infection Control Practices Advisory Committee and the HICPAC/SHEA/APIC/IDSA Hand Hygiene Task Force. *MMWR Recommendations and Reports, 51*(RR-16), 1–45. https://www.cdc.gov/mmwr/pdf/rr/rr5116.pdf (Level II)

7 Centers for Medicare and Medicaid Services, Department of Health and Human Services. (2020). Condition of participation: Infection control. 42 C.F.R. § 482.42.

8 DNV GL-Healthcare USA, Inc. (2020). IC.1.SR.1. *NIAHO® accreditation requirements, interpretive guidelines and surveyor guidance—revision 20.0.* (Level VII)

9 The Joint Commission. (2021). Standard NPSG.07.01.01. *Comprehensive accreditation manual for hospitals.* (Level VII)

10 World Health Organization. (2009). WHO guidelines on hand hygiene in health care: First global patient safety challenge, clean care is safer care. https://apps.who.int/iris/bitstream/handle/10665/44102/9789241597906_eng.pdf?sequence=1 (Level IV)

11 The Joint Commission. (2021). Standard NPSG.01.01.01. *Comprehensive accreditation manual for hospitals.* (Level VII)

12 The Joint Commission. (2021). Standard RI.01.01.01. *Comprehensive accreditation manual for hospitals.* (Level VII)

13 Accreditation Association for Hospitals and Health Systems. (2020). Standard 15.01.16. *Healthcare Facilities Accreditation Program: Accreditation requirements for acute care hospitals.* (Level VII)

14 Centers for Medicare and Medicaid Services, Department of Health and Human Services. (2020). Condition of participation: Patient's rights. 42 C.F.R. § 482.13(c)(1).

15 DNV GL-Healthcare USA, Inc. (2020). PR.2.SR.5. *NIAHO® accreditation requirements, interpretive guidelines and surveyor guidance—revision 20.0.* (Level VII)

16 The Joint Commission. (2021). Standard PC.02.01.21. *Comprehensive accreditation manual for hospitals.* (Level VII)

17 Waters, T. R., et al. (2009). Safe patient handling training for schools of nursing. https://www.cdc.gov/niosh/docs/2009-127/pdfs/2009-127.pdf (Level VII)

18 American Association of Critical-Care Nurses. (2018). AACN practice alert: Managing alarms in acute care across the life span: Electrocardiography and pulse oximetry. https://www.aacn.org/clinical-resources/practice-alerts/managing-alarms-in-acute-care-across-the-life-span (Level VII)

19 The Joint Commission. (2021). Standard NPSG.06.01.01. *Comprehensive accreditation manual for hospitals.* (Level VII)

20 Graham, K. C., & Cvach, M. (2010). Monitor alarm fatigue: Standardizing use of physiological monitors and decreasing nuisance alarms. *American Journal of Critical Care, 19*(1), 28–37. https://doi.org/10.4037/ajcc2010651

21 The Joint Commission. (2013). Sentinel event alert 50: Medical device alarm safety in hospitals. https://www.jointcommission.org/-/media/tjc/documents/resources/patient-safety-topics/sentinel-event/sea_50_alarms_4_26_16.pdf

22 Accreditation Association for Hospitals and Health Systems. (2020). Standard 07.01.10. *Healthcare Facilities Accreditation Program: Accreditation requirements for acute care hospitals.* (Level VII)

23 Occupational Safety and Health Administration. (2019). Bloodborne pathogens, standard number 1910.1030. https://www.osha.gov/pls/oshaweb/owadisp.show_document?p_id=10051&p_table=STANDARDS

24 Siegel, J. D., et al. (2007, revised 2019). 2007 guideline for isolation precautions: Preventing transmission of infectious agents in healthcare settings. https://www.cdc.gov/infectioncontrol/pdf/guidelines/isolation-guidelines-H.pdf (Level II)

25 The Joint Commission. (2021). Standard RC.01.03.01. *Comprehensive accreditation manual for hospitals.* (Level VII)

26 DNV GL-Healthcare USA, Inc. (2020). MR.2.SR.1. *NIAHO® accreditation requirements, interpretive guidelines and surveyor guidance—revision 20.0.* (Level VII)

27 Edelson, D. P., et al. (2020). Interim guidance for basic and advanced life support in adults, children, and neonates with suspected or confirmed COVID-19: From the Emergency Cardiovascular Care Committee and Get With the Guidelines®—Resuscitation Adult and Pediatric Task Forces of the American Heart Association. https://www.ahajournals.org/doi/10.1161/CIRCULATIONAHA.120.047463

28 Malhotra, A. (2021). Prone ventilation for adult patients with acute respiratory distress syndrome. In: *UpToDate*, Parsons, P. E. (Ed.).

PROTECTIVE ENVIRONMENT GUIDELINES

The Centers for Disease Control and Prevention (CDC) recommends that patients undergoing allogeneic hematopoietic stem cell transplantation (in which bone marrow is taken from a person other than the recipient) be placed in a protective environment (PE) to prevent the development of opportunistic infections.[1,2,3] To prevent exposure to fungal spores, an effective PE requires a positive-pressure room with the door kept closed to maintain the proper air pressure balance between the PE room and the adjoining hallway (at least 12 air changes per hour). The incoming air passes through a high-efficiency particulate air (HEPA) filtration unit before circulation.[4,5,6] Positive air pressure must be monitored daily using smoke tubes or flutter strips, with monitoring results documented.[7,8,9]

Equipment

PE precautions signs ■ gloves ■ gown ■ mask ■ disinfectant approved by the facility and the Environmental Protection Agency (EPA) ■ N95 respirator mask ■ positive-pressure room with HEPA filtration unit ■ new thermometer ■ new blood pressure cuff ■ new disposable stethoscope.

Use of the equipment should be restricted to the patient's room.

Preparation of equipment

Inspect all equipment and supplies. If a product is expired, is defective, or has compromised integrity, remove it from patient use, label it as expired or defective, and report the expiration or defect as directed by your facility. Ensure that all equipment is cleaned properly using facility- and EPA-approved disinfectant before it is taken into the room. Follow the manufacturer's guidelines for the disinfectant's use, *because products have different contact times, and are effective only if the product remains on the item to be cleaned for the appropriate amount of time*.[10] Provide the patient with a new thermometer, blood pressure cuff, and stethoscope, if available.[3]

Implementation

- Gather and prepare the necessary equipment and supplies.
- Review the patient's medical record and verify the need for a PE.
- Perform hand hygiene before putting on gloves, after removing gloves, and as indicated during patient care.[2,11,12,13,14,15,16]
- Put on gloves, a gown, and a mask according to standard and other (droplet, contact, and airborne) precautions as indicated.[3,17,18]
- Confirm the patient's identity using at least two patient identifiers.[19]
- Place the patient in the PE room, and explain the PE requirements to the patient and family (if appropriate) according to their individual communication and learning needs *to increase their understanding, allay their fears, and enhance cooperation*.[20]
- Keep the patient's door (and the anteroom door, if applicable) closed at all times *to maintain the proper air pressure balance between the PE room and the adjoining hallway*.[3]
- Place a PE precautions sign on the door of the patient's room *to notify anyone entering the room of the PE and associated requirements*.
- Screen visitors *to prevent anyone with a known or suspected infection from entering the PE room*.
- Ensure daily room cleaning with techniques that minimize dust, such as wet-dusting horizontal surfaces.[6,7,10]
- Avoid transporting the patient out of the PE room; if the patient must be moved, make sure the patient wears a regular mask until the patient returns to the PE room *to protect the patient from breathing in small particles that may cause infection*.[3] Also, notify the receiving department that the patient is on PE requirements and must be returned to the room promptly.
- Assess the patient daily for signs of anxiety or depression while in a PE.[21,22]
- Prohibit fresh flowers in water, dried flowers, and potted plants from being brought into the patient's PE room or area, *because standing water supports the growth of micro-organisms, and soil may harbor fungi*.[6,23]
- Remove and discard your gloves and other personal protective equipment.[17]
- Perform hand hygiene.[11,12,13,14,15,16]
- Document the procedure.[24,25,26,27]

Special considerations

- If the patient requires airborne precautions and the room has an anteroom, implement the precautions in the patient's room, *because air in the anteroom is filtered by a portable HEPA filtration unit*. If the patient's room does not have an anteroom, place the patient in an airborne infection isolation room with portable ventilation units and HEPA filters *to increase the filtration of fungal spores*.[3,9]
- Back-up ventilation, such as a portable unit for fans or filters, should be maintained for areas that require a PE *to provide emergency ventilation*.[6]
- HEPA filters should be replaced regularly according to the manufacturer's instructions.[9]

Complications

Failure to appropriately follow PE guidelines may cause the development of an infection in the patient. A patient may experience anxiety or depression while in a PE room.[21]

Documentation

Record the need for a PE on the patient's nursing care plan and as otherwise required by your facility. Document initiation and maintenance of the PE and the patient's tolerance of the PE. Document teaching provided to the patient and family (if applicable), their understanding of that teaching, and any need for follow-up teaching. Also document the date the protective environment was discontinued.

REFERENCES

1 Centers for Disease Control and Prevention. (2000). Guidelines for preventing opportunistic infections among hematopoietic stem cell transplant recipients. *MMWR Recommendations and Reports, 49*(RR-10), 1–125. https://www.cdc.gov/mmwr/PDF/RR/RR4910.PDF (Level I)

2 Ezzone, S. A. (Ed.) (2020). *Hematopoietic stem cell transplantation: A manual for nursing practice* (3rd ed.). Pittsburgh, PA: Oncology Nursing Society.

3 Siegel, J. D., et al. (2007, revised 2019). 2007 guideline for isolation precautions: Preventing transmission of infectious agents in healthcare settings. https://www.cdc.gov/infectioncontrol/pdf/guidelines/isolation-guidelines-H.pdf (Level II)

4 Grota, P. G., et al. (Ed.) (2014). *APIC text of infection control and epidemiology* (4th ed.). Arlington, VA: Association for Professionals in Infection Control and Epidemiology.

5 Garbin, L. M., et al. (2011). Infection prevention measures used in hematopoietic stem cell transplantation: Evidences for practice. *Revista Latino-Americana de Enfermagem, 19*(3), 640–650. https://www.scielo.br/pdf/rlae/v19n3/25.pdf (Level I)

6 Centers for Disease Control and Prevention. (2015). Components of a protective environment. Patients: Allogenic hematopoietic stem cell transplant (HSCT) only. https://www.cdc.gov/infectioncontrol/guidelines/isolation/appendix/environment.html

7 Sehulster, L., & Chinn, R. Y. W. (2003). Guidelines for environmental infection control in health-care facilities: Recommendations of CDC and the Healthcare Infection Control Practices Advisory Committee. *MMWR Recommendations and Reports, 52*(RR-10), 1–42. https://www.cdc.gov/mmwr/preview/mmwrhtml/rr5210a1.htm (Level VII)

8 Beam, E., et al. (2015). Clinical challenges in isolation care. *American Journal of Nursing, 115*(4), 44–49. (Level VI)

9 Styczynski, J., et al. (2018). Protective environment for hematopoietic cell transplant (HSCT) recipients: The Infectious Diseases Working Party EBMT analysis of global recommendations on health-care facilities. *Bone Marrow Transplantation, 53*(9), 1131–1138. https://www.nature.com/articles/s41409-018-0141-5.pdf (Level VII)

10 Rutala, W. A., et al. (2008, revised 2019). Guideline for disinfection and sterilization in healthcare facilities, 2008. https://www.cdc.gov/infection-control/pdf/guidelines/disinfection-guidelines-H.pdf (Level I)

11 Centers for Disease Control and Prevention. (2002). Guideline for hand hygiene in health-care settings: Recommendations of the Healthcare Infection Control Practices Advisory Committee and the HICPAC/SHEA/APIC/IDSA Hand Hygiene Task Force. *MMWR Recommendations and Reports, 51*(RR-16), 1–45. https://www.cdc.gov/mmwr/pdf/rr/rr5116.pdf (Level II)

12 World Health Organization. (2009). WHO guidelines on hand hygiene in health care: First global patient safety challenge, clean care is safer care. https://apps.who.int/iris/bitstream/handle/10665/44102/9789241597906_eng.pdf?sequence=1 (Level IV)

13 The Joint Commission. (2021). Standard NPSG.07.01.01. *Comprehensive accreditation manual for hospitals*. (Level VII)

14 Accreditation Association for Hospitals and Health Systems. (2020). Standard 07.01.21. *Healthcare Facilities Accreditation Program: Accreditation requirements for acute care hospitals*. (Level VII)

15 Centers for Medicare and Medicaid Services, Department of Health and Human Services. (2020). Condition of participation: Infection control. 42 C.F.R. § 482.42.

16 DNV GL-Healthcare USA, Inc. (2020). IC.1.SR.1. *NIAHO® accreditation requirements, interpretive guidelines and surveyor guidance—revision 20.0*. (Level VII)

17 Occupational Safety and Health Administration. (2019). Bloodborne pathogens, standard number 1910.1030. https://www.osha.gov/pls/oshaweb/owadisp.show_document?p_id=10051&p_table=STANDARDS (Level VII)

18 Accreditation Association for Hospitals and Health Systems. (2020). Standard 07.01.10. *Healthcare Facilities Accreditation Program: Accreditation requirements for acute care hospitals*. (Level VII)

19 The Joint Commission. (2021). Standard NPSG.01.01.01. *Comprehensive accreditation manual for hospitals*. (Level VII)

20 The Joint Commission. (2021). Standard PC.02.01.21. *Comprehensive accreditation manual for hospitals.* (Level VII)

21 Tecchio, C., et al. (2013). Predictors of anxiety and depression in hematopoietic stem cell transplant patients during protective isolation. *Psycho-Oncology, 22*(8), 1790–1797. https://doi.org/10.1002/pon.3215 (Level IV)

22 Annibali, O., et al. (2017). Protective isolation for patients with haematologic malignancies: A pilot study investigating patients' distress and use of time. *International Journal of Hematology-Oncology and Stem Cell Research, 11*, 313–318. https://www.ncbi.nlm.nih.gov/pmc/articles/PMC5767293/pdf/IJHOSCR-11-313.pdf (Level VI)

23 Craven, R. F., et al. (2021). *Fundamentals of nursing: Concepts and competencies for practice* (9th ed.). Philadelphia, PA: Wolters Kluwer.

24 The Joint Commission. (2021). Standard RC 01.03.01. *Comprehensive accreditation manual for hospitals.* The Joint Commission. (Level VII)

25 Centers for Medicare and Medicaid Services, Department of Health and Human Services. (2020). Condition of participation: Medical record services. 42 C.F.R. § 482.24(b).

26 Accreditation Association for Hospitals and Health Systems. (2020). Standard 10.00.03. *Healthcare Facilities Accreditation Program: Accreditation requirements for acute care hospitals.* (Level VII)

27 DNV GL-Healthcare USA, Inc. (2020). MR.2.SR.1. *NIAHO® accreditation requirements, interpretive guidelines and surveyor guidance—revision 20.0.* (Level VII)

PULMONARY ARTERY PRESSURE AND PULMONARY ARTERY OCCLUSION PRESSURE MONITORING

Continuous pulmonary artery pressure (PAP) and intermittent pulmonary artery occlusion pressure (PAOP) measurements provide important information about left ventricular function and preload.[1] (PAOP may also be referred to as *pulmonary artery wedge pressure.*[1]) This information is useful not only for monitoring but also for aiding diagnosis, refining assessment, guiding interventions, and projecting patient outcomes. All acutely ill patients are candidates for PAP monitoring, especially those who are hemodynamically unstable, who need fluid management or continuous cardiopulmonary assessment, or who are receiving multiple or frequently administered cardioactive drugs.

A pulmonary artery (PA) catheter is recommended for many clinical conditions, and can be used to assess intravascular volume, particularly in patients with severe pulmonary edema, heart failure, or acute kidney injury; evaluate pulmonary hypertension; guide therapy in severe refractory shock or multiple organ dysfunction syndrome; and guide therapy to maximize oxygen delivery to tissues in some selected patients.[1,2]

PA catheters can have up to six lumens, allowing more hemodynamic information to be gathered. In addition to distal and proximal lumens used to measure pressures, a PA catheter has a balloon inflation lumen that inflates the balloon for PAOP measurement, and a thermistor connector lumen that allows cardiac output measurement. Some catheters also have a pacemaker wire lumen that provides a port for pacemaker electrodes and measures continuous mixed venous oxygen saturation. (See *PA catheters: From basic to complex.*)

A practitioner inserts the PA catheter into a central vessel and directs it through the right atrium, across the tricuspid valve, and into the right ventricle until the catheter tip is positioned in the pulmonary artery, where it assesses left ventricular function indirectly.

Some facilities allow only practitioners or specially trained nurses to measure PAOP *because of the risk of pulmonary artery rupture,* a rare but life-threatening complication. If your facility permits you to perform this procedure, do so with extreme caution, and make sure that you're thoroughly familiar with intracardiac waveform interpretation beforehand.

You should remove the PA catheter, as ordered, as soon as the patient no longer needs it to reduce the risk of central line-associated bloodstream infection.[3,4]

HOSPITAL-ACQUIRED CONDITION ALERT Keep in mind that the Centers for Medicare and Medicaid Services considers a vascular catheter–associated infection a hospital–acquired condition, *because it can be reasonably prevented using a variety of best practices.* Make sure to follow evidence-based infection-prevention practices, such as performing hand hygiene, following sterile no-touch technique when accessing and changing the transducer system, and removing the PA catheter as soon as it's no longer needed *to reduce the risk of vascular catheter–associated infections.*[3,4,5,6,7,8]

EQUIPMENT

PA catheters: From basic to complex

Depending on the intended use, a pulmonary artery (PA) catheter may be basic or complex. The basic PA catheter has a distal and proximal lumen, a thermistor, and a balloon inflation valve. The distal lumen, which exits in the pulmonary artery, monitors PA pressure. Its hub usually is marked PA DISTAL. The proximal lumen exits in the right atrium or vena cava, depending on the size of the patient's heart. It monitors right atrial pressure, and can be used as the injected solution lumen for cardiac output determination and for infusing solutions. The proximal lumen hub usually is marked PROXIMAL.

The thermistor, located about 1½" (4 cm) from the distal tip, measures temperature (aiding core temperature evaluation) and allows cardiac output measurement. The thermistor connector attaches to a cardiac output connector cable and then to a cardiac output monitor. The balloon inflation lumen is used for inflating the balloon tip with air when measuring the pulmonary artery occlusion pressure. A stopcock connection may be used.

Additional lumens

Some PA catheters have additional lumens used to obtain other hemodynamic data or permit certain interventions. For instance, a proximal infusion port, which exits in the right atrium or vena cava, allows additional fluid administration. A right ventricular lumen, exiting in the right ventricle, allows fluid administration, right ventricular pressure measurement, or use of a temporary ventricular pacing lead.

Some catheters have additional right atrial and right ventricular lumens for atrioventricular pacing. A right ventricular ejection fraction test-response thermistor with PA and right ventricular sensing electrodes allows volumetric and ejection fraction measurements. Fiberoptic filaments, such as those used in pulse oximetry, exit into the pulmonary artery and permit measurement of continuous mixed venous oxygen saturation.

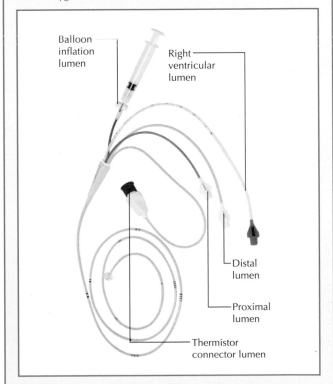

Equipment

1.5-mL syringe attached to balloon port or catheter ▪ Optional: indelible marking pen.

Preparation of equipment

Inspect all equipment and supplies. If a product is expired, is defective, or has compromised integrity, remove it from patient use, label it as expired or defective, and report the expiration or defect as directed by your facility.

Implementation

- Verify the practitioner's order for PAP and PAOP monitoring.
- Perform hand hygiene.[9,10,11,12,13,14]
- Confirm the patient's identity using at least two patient identifiers.[15]
- Provide privacy.[16,17,18,19]
- Explain the procedure to the patient and family (if appropriate) according to their individual communication and learning needs *to increase their understanding, allay their fears, and enhance cooperation.*[20]
- Raise the patient's bed to waist level before providing patient care *to prevent caregiver back strain.*[21]
- Perform hand hygiene.[9,10,11,12,13,14]
- Place the patient in the supine position with the head of the bed elevated at 0 to 60 degrees, or position the patient in a 20-, 30-, or 90-degree lateral position with the head of the bed flat. Allow the patient to stabilize for 5 to 15 minutes after the position change.[22]
- Trace the tubing from the patient to its point of origin *to make sure that you're accessing the proper port.*[23,24] Zero and calibrate the pressure monitoring system, making sure that the transducer air–fluid interface is leveled to the phlebostatic axis (located at the 4th intercostal space at one-half the anterior posterior diameter of the chest) if the patient is supine. *If the air–fluid interface is positioned below the phlebostatic axis, the readings will be erroneously high; if it's positioned above the phlebostatic axis, the readings will be erroneously low.*[22] If the patient is in a lateral position, use the following reference points: for a 30-degree lateral position, one-half the distance from the bed surface to the sternal border; for a 90-degree right lateral position, 4th intercostal space at the midsternum; and for a 90-degree left lateral position, 4th intercostal space at the left parasternal border.[25]

- Mark the phlebostatic axis or appropriate-angle specific reference point with an indelible pen, if necessary, *to ensure consistent monitoring.*[1,22]
- Make sure that the alarm limits are set appropriately for the patient's current condition, and that the alarms are turned on, functioning properly, and audible to staff.[26,27,28,29]

Obtaining a PAP measurement

- Inspect the waveform and pressure readings *to make sure that the PA catheter is in the correct location and functioning properly.*[1]
- Verify that the transducer is properly leveled and zeroed.
- Perform a square wave test (dynamic response test) at the start of each shift, with a change in the waveform configuration, or when the system is opened to air; document the results.[2,22] (See *Performing a square wave test.*)

Performing a square wave test

When using a pressure transducer system, you must ensure and document the system's accuracy. Along with leveling and zeroing the system to atmospheric pressure at the phlebostatic axis and interpreting waveforms, you can ensure accuracy by performing the square wave test (or dynamic response test).[1,2,22] To perform the test, take the following steps:

- Activate the fast-flush device for 1 second, and then release. Obtain a graphic printout.
- Observe for the desired response: The pressure wave rises rapidly, squares off, and is followed by one or two oscillations. (See illustration below.)
- Know that these oscillations should have an initial downstroke, which extends below the baseline and just 1 to 2 oscillations after the initial downstroke. Usually, but not always, the first upstroke is about one-third the height of the initial downstroke.
- Be aware that the intervals between oscillations should be within 0.12 second (3 small boxes).[1]

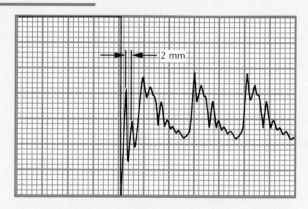

Overdamped square wave

If you observe a slurred upstroke at the beginning of the square wave and a loss of oscillations after the initial downstroke, the waveform is overdamped. (See illustration below.) This can cause falsely low pressure readings, and you can lose the sharpness of waveform peaks and the dicrotic notch. It can be corrected by:

- clearing the line of any blood or air
- checking to make sure there are no kinks or obstructions in the line
- ensuring that you're using short, low-compliance tubing
- checking to make sure that the flush bag has fluid and the pressure is maintained at 300 mm Hg
- tightening loose connections.

Repeat the square wave test and read the pressure waveform.

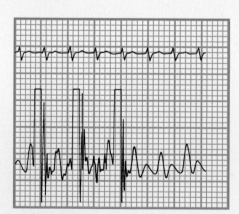

Underdamped square wave

If you observe extra oscillations after the initial downstroke or more than 0.08 second between oscillations, the waveform is underdamped. (See illustration at top right.) This can cause falsely high pressure readings and artifact in the waveforms. It can be corrected by:

- using large-bore, shorter tubing[1]
- removing air bubbles from the system[1]
- inserting a dampening device (available from pressure tubing companies).

Repeat the square wave test and read the pressure waveform.

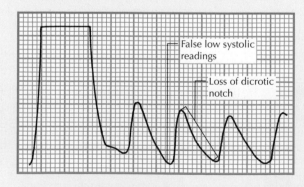

■ Monitor PA systolic and diastolic pressures continuously *to detect early changes in the patient's condition.*[1]

■ Obtain PAP values at end expiration (when the patient completely exhales).[2,22] *At end expiration, intrathoracic pressure approaches atmospheric pressure and has the least effect on PAP.*[1,2] If you obtain a reading during other phases of the respiratory cycle, respiratory interference may occur. For instance, during inspiration, when intrathoracic pressure drops, PAP may be falsely low, *because the negative pressure is transmitted to the catheter.* During expiration, when intrathoracic pressure rises, PAP may be falsely high.

■ Obtain a dual-channel electrocardiogram (ECG) strip and PA waveform trace *to identify the correct pressure readings.* If a dual-channel recording isn't available, use the cursor on the monitor to identify the pressure reading that correctly correlates with the waveform. Digital readouts may reflect pressures obtained throughout respiration and may not be accurate. Use of the monitor cursor line may be a reasonable alternative if simultaneous graphic recording of the ECG and PA waveform isn't possible.[1,22,30]

■ Make sure that the scale of the PAP tracing is set appropriately on the monitor. Most PA scales are commonly set at 40 mm Hg.[1]

■ Align the QT interval with the PA waveform. The peak of the PA waveform is the PA systolic pressure.[1]

■ Align the end of the QRS complex with the PA waveform. Measure the PA diastolic pressure at the point of the intersection of the QRS complex and the PA waveform.[1]

Obtaining a PAOP measurement

■ Verify that the transducer is properly leveled and zeroed.

■ Detach the syringe from the balloon inflation hub. Draw 1.5 mL of air into the syringe, and then reattach the syringe to the hub.

■ Begin running a dual-chamber recording of the ECG and PA waveform *to assist in the interpretation of the pressure reading.*

■ Watching the monitor, inject the air through the hub slowly and smoothly. When you see an occlusion tracing on the monitor, immediately stop inflating the balloon. (See *Observing the PAOP waveform.*)

NURSING ALERT Never inflate the balloon beyond the volume needed to obtain an occlusion pressure tracing. Never inflate the balloon for more than 15 seconds (two to four respiratory cycles) or leave the balloon inflated, *because this may cause a pulmonary infarction and rupture.*[1,2]

■ Take the pressure reading at end expiration. Note the amount of air needed to change the PA tracing to an occluded tracing (normally, 1.25 to 1.5 mL). If the occluded tracing appeared with the injection of less than 1.25 mL, *suspect that the catheter has migrated into a more distal branch and requires repositioning.* If the balloon is in a more distal branch, the tracings may move up the oscilloscope, *indicating that the catheter*

tip is recording balloon pressure rather than PAOP, which may lead to PA rupture. Notify the practitioner of this finding.[1]

■ After obtaining the PAOP measurement, detach the syringe from the balloon inflation port and allow the balloon to deflate on its own. Observe the waveform tracing and make sure the tracing returns from the wedge tracing to the normal PA tracing.

■ Expel air from the syringe and then reconnect it to the end of the balloon-inflation valve.[1]

■ Looking at the dual-channel recorded strip, identify the *a* wave of the PAOP waveform. (The *a* wave represents atrial contraction, correlates with the end of the QRS complex, and occurs approximately 20 msec after the *p* wave.) Measure the mean of the *a* wave *to obtain an accurate PAOP.*[1]

Completing the procedure

■ Return the bed to the lowest position *to prevent falls and maintain patient safety.*[31]

■ Report changes in the patient's measurements to the practitioner, and intervene as ordered.

■ Perform hand hygiene.[9,10,11,12,13,14]

■ Document the procedure.[32,33,34,35]

Special considerations

■ Advise the patient to use caution when moving about in bed *to avoid dislodging the catheter.*

■ Never inflate the balloon with more than the recommended air volume (specified on the catheter shaft), *because this action may cause loss of elasticity or balloon rupture.* With appropriate inflation volume, the balloon floats easily through the heart chambers and rests in the main branch of the pulmonary artery, producing accurate waveforms. Never inflate the balloon with fluids, *because they may not be able to be retrieved from inside the balloon, preventing deflation.*[1]

■ Be aware that the catheter may slip back into the right ventricle. *Because the tip may irritate the ventricle and cause arrhythmias,* check the monitor for a right ventricular waveform to detect this problem promptly. Immediately notify the practitioner if this waveform occurs.[1]

■ *To minimize valvular trauma,* make sure the balloon is deflated whenever the catheter is withdrawn from the pulmonary artery to the right ventricle or from the right ventricle to the right atrium.[1]

■ Never flush the PA catheter for longer than 2 seconds, *because PA rupture may occur with prolonged flushing of high-pressure fluids.*[1]

■ If you find a close correlation between the PA diastolic pressure and the PA occlusive pressure, follow the diastolic pressure *to minimize the number of times the PA catheter balloon is inflated.*

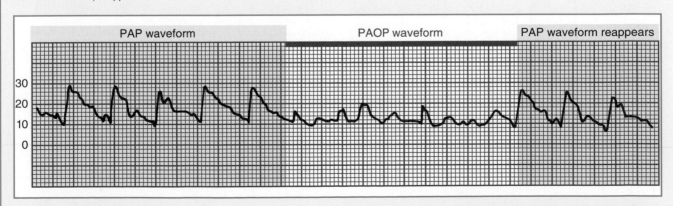

Observing the PAOP waveform

Upon balloon inflation, you should see the normal pulmonary artery pressure (PAP) waveform flatten to the characteristic pulmonary artery occlusion pressure (PAOP) waveform. Balloon inflation should be stopped upon observation of this waveform. Upon balloon deflation, the PAP waveform should immediately reappear.

■ Change transparent semipermeable dressings at least every 7 days and gauze dressings at least every 2 days. Change the dressing immediately if it becomes visibly spoiled, loosens, or dislodges, or if there is any moisture, drainage, blood, or compromised skin integrity beneath the dressing.[36]

■ Change a disposable or reusable transducer system (including the administration set, continuous flush device, and flush solution used for invasive hemodynamic pressure monitoring) every 96 hours, immediately upon suspected contamination, and when the integrity of the system has been compromised. Limit the number of manipulations and entries to the system.[3,37]

Complications

Potential complications of PA catheter monitoring include PA perforation or rupture, pulmonary infarction, catheter knotting, local and systemic infection, cardiac arrhythmias, and air embolus.[1,38]

Documentation

Document the date and time that the measurements were taken, the results of the square wave (dynamic response) test, the patient's position, the measurement results, the amount of air necessary to obtain a PAOP, and the patient's tolerance of the procedure. Record the name of the practitioner notified of the measurements, if necessary; the date and time of notification; prescribed interventions; and the patient's response to those interventions. Document teaching provided to the patient and family (if applicable), their understanding of that teaching, and any need for follow-up teaching.

References

1 Wiegand, D. L. (2017). *AACN procedure manual for high acuity, progressive, and critical care* (7th ed.). St. Louis, MO: Elsevier.

2 Edwards Lifesciences. (2018). *Edwards clinical education: Quick guide to cardiopulmonary care* (4th ed.). https://www.edwards.com/gb/pages/quick-guide-to-cardiopulmonary-care

3 Centers for Disease Control and Prevention. (2011, revised 2017). Guidelines for the prevention of intravascular catheter-related infections. https://www.cdc.gov/infectioncontrol/guidelines/bsi/recommendations.html (Level I)

4 Marschall, J., et al. (2014). SHEA/IDSA practice recommendation: Strategies to prevent central line-associated bloodstream infections in acute care hospitals. *Infection Control and Hospital Epidemiology, 35*(7), 753–771. https://www.jstor.org/stable/10.1086/676533#metadata_info_tab_contents (Level I)

5 Jarrett, N., & Callaham, M. (2016). Evidence-based guidelines for selected hospital-acquired conditions: Final report. https://www.cms.gov/Medicare/Medicare-Fee-for-Service-Payment/HospitalAcqCond/Downloads/2016-HAC-Report.pdf

6 Standard 50. Infection. Infusion therapy standards of practice (8th ed.). (2021). *Journal of Infusion Nursing, 44*(Suppl. 1), S1153–S157. (Level VII)

7 Association of Professionals in Infection Control and Epidemiology (APIC). (2015). Guide to preventing central line–associated bloodstream infections. http://apic.org/Resource_/TinyMceFileManager/2015/APIC_CLABSI_WEB.pdf (Level IV)

8 The Joint Commission. (2021). Standard NPSG.07.04.01. *Comprehensive accreditation manual for hospitals.* (Level VII)

9 The Joint Commission. (2021). Standard NPSG.07.01.01. *Comprehensive accreditation manual for hospitals.* (Level VII)

10 Centers for Disease Control and Prevention. (2002). Guideline for hand hygiene in health-care settings: Recommendations of the Healthcare Infection Control Practices Advisory Committee and the HICPAC/SHEA/APIC/IDSA Hand Hygiene Task Force. *MMWR Recommendations and Reports, 51*(RR-16), 1–45. https://www.cdc.gov/mmwr/pdf/rr/rr5116.pdf (Level II)

11 World Health Organization. (2009). WHO guidelines on hand hygiene in health care: First global patient safety challenge, clean care is safer care. https://apps.who.int/iris/bitstream/handle/10665/44102/9789241597906_eng.pdf?sequence=1 (Level IV)

12 Accreditation Association for Hospitals and Health Systems. (2020). Standard 07.01.10. *Healthcare Facilities Accreditation Program: Accreditation requirements for acute care hospitals.* (Level VII)

13 Centers for Medicare and Medicaid Services, Department of Health and Human Services. (2020). Condition of participation: Infection control. 42 C.F.R. § 482.42.

14 DNV GL-Healthcare USA, Inc. (2020). IC.1.SR.1. *NIAHO® accreditation requirements, interpretive guidelines and surveyor guidance—revision 20.0.* (Level VII)

15 The Joint Commission. (2021). Standard NPSG.01.01.01. *Comprehensive accreditation manual for hospitals.* (Level VII)

16 The Joint Commission. (2021). Standard RI.01.01.01. *Comprehensive accreditation manual for hospitals.* (Level VII)

17 Centers for Medicare and Medicaid Services, Department of Health and Human Services. (2020). Condition of participation: Patient's rights. 42 C.F.R. § 482.13(c)(1).

18 Accreditation Association for Hospitals and Health Systems. (2020). Standard 15.01.16. *Healthcare Facilities Accreditation Program: Accreditation requirements for acute care hospitals.* (Level VII)

19 DNV GL-Healthcare USA, Inc. (2020). PR.2.SR.5. *NIAHO® accreditation requirements, interpretive guidelines and surveyor guidance—revision 20.0.* (Level VII)

20 The Joint Commission. (2021). Standard PC.02.01.21. *Comprehensive accreditation manual for hospitals.* (Level VII)

21 Waters, T. R., et al. (2009). Safe patient handling training for schools of nursing. https://www.cdc.gov/niosh/docs/2009-127/pdfs/2009-127.pdf (Level VII)

22 American Association of Critical-Care Nurses (AACN). (2016). AACN practice alert: Pulmonary artery/central venous pressure monitoring in adults. https://www.aacn.org/clinical-resources/practice-alerts/pulmonary-artery-pressure-measurement (Level VII)

23 The Joint Commission. (2014). Sentinel event alert 53: Managing risk during transition to new ISO tubing connector standards. https://www.jointcommission.org/-/media/tjc/documents/resources/patient-safety-topics/sentinel-event/sea_53_connectors_8_19_14_final.pdf (Level VII)

24 U.S. Food and Drug Administration. (2017). Examples of medical device misconnections. https://www.fda.gov/medical-devices/medical-device-connectors/examples-medical-device-misconnections

25 Rauen, C. A., et al. (2009). Evidence based practice habits: Transforming research into bedside practice. *Critical Care Nurse, 29*(2), 46–59. https://doi.org/10.4037/ccn2009287

26 The Joint Commission. (2013). Sentinel event alert 50: Medical device alarm safety in hospitals. https://www.jointcommission.org/-/media/tjc/documents/resources/patient-safety-topics/sentinel-event/sea_50_alarms_4_26_16.pdf (Level VII)

27 The Joint Commission. (2021). Standard NPSG.06.01.01. *Comprehensive accreditation manual for hospitals.* Oakbrook Terrace, IL: The Joint Commission. (Level VII)

28 American Association of Critical-Care Nurses (AACN). (2018). AACN practice alert: Managing alarms in acute care across the life span: Electrocardiography and pulse oximetry. https://www.aacn.org/clinical-resources/practice-alerts/managing-alarms-in-acute-care-across-the-life-span (Level VII)

29 Graham, K. C., & Cvach, M. (2010). Monitor alarm fatigue: Standardizing use of physiological monitors and decreasing nuisance alarms. *American Journal of Critical Care, 19*(1), 28–37. https://doi.org/10.4037/ajcc2010651

30 Pasion, E., et al. (2010). Evaluation of the monitor cursor–line method for measuring pulmonary artery and central venous pressures. *American Journal of Critical Care, 19*(6), 511–521. https://doi.org/10.4037/ajcc2010502 (Level VI)

31 Ganz, D. A., et al. (2013, Reviewed 2021). *Preventing falls in hospitals: A toolkit for improving quality of care* (AHRQ Publication No. 13-0015-EF). Agency for Healthcare Research and Quality. https://www.ahrq.gov/professionals/systems/hospital/fallpxtoolkit/index.html (Level VII)

32 The Joint Commission. (2021). Standard RC.01.03.01. *Comprehensive accreditation manual for hospitals.* (Level VII)

33 Accreditation Association for Hospitals and Health Systems. (2020). Standard 10.00.03. *Healthcare Facilities Accreditation Program: Accreditation requirements for acute care hospitals.* (Level VII)

34 Centers for Medicare and Medicaid Services, Department of Health and Human Services. (2020). Condition of participation: Medical record services. 42 C.F.R. § 482.24(b).

35 DNV GL-Healthcare USA, Inc. (2020). MR.2.SR.1. *NIAHO® accreditation requirements, interpretive guidelines and surveyor guidance—revision 20.0.* (Level VII)

36 Standard 42. Vascular access device assessment, care and dressing changes. Infusion therapy standards of practice (8th ed.). (2021). *Journal of Infusion Nursing, 44*(Suppl. 1), S119–S123. (Level VII)

37 Standard 43. Administration set management. Infusion therapy standards of practice (8th ed.). (2021). *Journal of Infusion Nursing, 44*(Suppl. 1), S123–S125. (Level VII)

38 Weinhouse, G. L. (2019). Pulmonary artery catheterization: Indications, contraindications, and complications in adults. In: *UpToDate.* Parsons, P. E. (Ed.).

PULSE AMPLITUDE MONITORING

Determining the presence and strength of peripheral pulses, an essential part of cardiovascular assessment, helps you to evaluate the adequacy of peripheral perfusion. A pulse amplitude monitor simplifies this procedure. A sensor taped to the patient's skin over a pulse point sends signals to a monitor, which measures the amplitude of the pulse and displays it as a waveform on a screen. (See *Identifying a normal pulse amplitude waveform.*) The system continuously monitors the patient's peripheral pulse.

The pulse amplitude monitor can be used after peripheral vascular reconstruction on the upper or lower extremities or after percutaneous transluminal peripheral or coronary angioplasty (either with the sheaths in place or after they've been removed).

Because the sensor monitors only relatively flat pulse points, it can't be used for the posterior tibial pulse point. Also, movement distorts the waveform, so the patient must stay as still as possible during monitoring. The patient shouldn't have lesions on the skin where the pulse will be monitored, *because the sensor must be placed directly on this site; the sensor and tape could irritate the lesion, or the lesion could impair transmission of the pulse amplitude.* If the patient has a strong peripheral pulse, you'll see an adequate waveform.

Equipment

Pulse amplitude display monitor with sensor ▪ facility-approved disinfectant.

Preparation of equipment

Plug the monitor into a grounded outlet. Inspect all equipment and supplies. If a product is expired, is defective, or has compromised integrity, remove it from patient use, label it as expired or defective, and report the expiration or defect as directed by your facility.

Implementation

- Verify the practitioner's order
- Gather and prepare the necessary equipment and supplies.
- Perform hand hygiene.[1,2,3,4,5,6]
- Confirm the patient's identity using at least two patient identifiers.[7]
- Provide privacy.[8,9,10,11]
- Explain the procedure to the patient and family (if appropriate) according to their individual communication and learning needs *to increase their understanding, allay their fears, and enhance cooperation.*[12] Explain that you'll tape the sensor to a selected site, usually the foot.

Initiating monitor use

- Turn on the monitor and allow it to warm up, which may take up to 10 seconds.
- Plug the sensor cable into the monitor; then tap the sensor gently. If tapping causes interference on the display screen, you can assume the sensor–monitor connection is functioning properly.
- Raise the patient's bed to waist level before providing care *to prevent caregiver back strain.*[13]
- Perform hand hygiene.[1,2,3,4,5,6]
- Locate the peripheral pulse you want to monitor.
- Place the sensor over the strongest point of the pulse you're going to monitor. While observing the display screen, move the sensor until you see a strong upright waveform.
- Without moving the sensor from this site, peel off the adhesive strips and affix the sensor securely to the patient's foot. *The sensor must maintain proper skin contact,* so be sure to tape it firmly.
- Adjust the height of the pulse wave signal to half the height of the display screen. *This will give the waveform room to fluctuate as the pulse amplitude increases and decreases.*
- Set the low and high waveform amplitude alarms *so you'll be alerted to any waveform changes.* Make sure the alarm limits are set appropriately for the patient's current condition, and that the alarms are turned on, functioning properly, and audible to staff.[14,15,16]
- Print out a strip of the patient's waveform during every shift, and whenever you notice a change in the waveform or the patient's condition.

Discontinuing monitor use

- Print out a strip of the patient's waveform.
- Peel the sensor tape from the patient's skin and discard it.
- Turn the machine off but keep it plugged in.
- Perform hand hygiene.[1,2,3,4,5,6]
- Disinfect the monitor using a hospital-grade disinfectant.[17,18]

Completing the procedure

- Perform hand hygiene.[1,2,3,4,5,6]
- Return the bed to the lowest position *to prevent falls and maintain patient safety.*[19]

Identifying a normal pulse amplitude waveform

If the patient has adequate peripheral perfusion, the pulse amplitude monitor will usually display a normal waveform, like the one shown here. This waveform resembles the waveform seen when a patient has an arterial line.

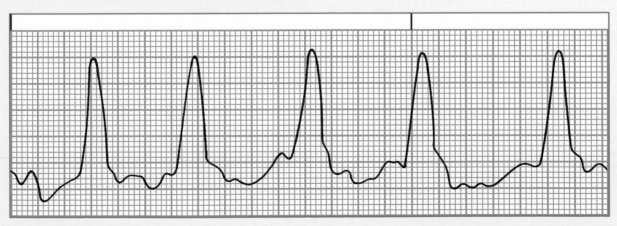

- Place the strip printout in the patient's medical record.
- Document the procedure.[20,21,22,23]

Special considerations

- Although the waveform displayed by a pulse amplitude monitor may resemble an electrocardiogram or blood pressure waveform, it's not the same, *because it is measuring a different parameter.*
- Don't apply much pressure on the pulse sensor film or press on it with a sharp object, *because such stress may warp or destroy the sensor.*
- Never place the sensor over an open wound or on ulcerated skin.
- If waveform amplitude decreases, assess the site distal to the sensor for capillary refill time, temperature, color, and sensation. The amplitude change may stem from a malfunction in the monitor itself (such as a low battery) or from a thrombus, hematoma, or significant change in the patient's hemodynamic status.
- If the display screen is blank when you turn on the machine, make sure that the monitor is plugged in. If it's plugged in but the screen remains blank, the screen may need repair.
- If the screen is functioning but no waveform appears on it, first check the sensor–monitor connection. Then check the sensor by gently tapping it to see if interference appears on the screen. If the sensor is working properly, relocate the peripheral pulse on the patient's foot, and reapply the sensor. If your interventions don't work, the screen may need servicing.

Complications

Local irritation from the sensor adhesive tape may occur. Tissue damage can occur from sensor application that is too tight or left too long in one place, or where supplemental tape is applied.[24]

Documentation

Document the date and time of the procedure, the site where the sensor was affixed, the waveform amplitude, and the patient's tolerance of the procedure. Record any waveform amplitude decreases, interventions taken, and the patient's response to those interventions. Document teaching provided to the patient and family (if applicable), their understanding of that teaching, and any need for follow-up teaching.

Include a strip of the patient's waveform in the patient's medical record. Note in your documentation the reference scale you used to measure amplitude height, usually located on the left side of the strip.

References

1 The Joint Commission. (2021). Standard NPSG.07.01.01. *Comprehensive accreditation manual for hospitals.* Oakbrook Terrace, IL: The Joint Commission. (Level VII)

2 Centers for Disease Control and Prevention. (2002). Guideline for hand hygiene in health-care settings: Recommendations of the Healthcare Infection Control Practices Advisory Committee and the HICPAC/SHEA/APIC/IDSA Hand Hygiene Task Force. *MMWR Recommendations and Reports, 51*(RR-16), 1–45. https://www.cdc.gov/mmwr/pdf/rr/rr5116.pdf (Level II)

3 World Health Organization. (2009). WHO guidelines on hand hygiene in health care: First global patient safety challenge, clean care is safer care. https://apps.who.int/iris/bitstream/handle/10665/44102/9789241597906_eng.pdf?sequence=1 (Level IV)

4 Accreditation Association for Hospitals and Health Systems. (2020). Standard 07.01.21. *Healthcare Facilities Accreditation Program: Accreditation requirements for acute care hospitals.* Chicago, IL: Accreditation Association for Hospitals and Health Systems. (Level VII)

5 Centers for Medicare and Medicaid Services, Department of Health and Human Services. (2020). Condition of participation: Infection control. 42 C.F.R. § 482.42.

6 DNV GL-Healthcare USA, Inc. (2020). IC.1.SR.1. *NIAHO® accreditation requirements, interpretive guidelines and surveyor guidance—revision 20.0.* Milford, OH: DNV GL-Healthcare USA, Inc. (Level VII)

7 The Joint Commission. (2021). Standard NPSG.01.01.01. *Comprehensive accreditation manual for hospitals.* Oakbrook Terrace, IL: The Joint Commission. (Level VII)

8 Accreditation Association for Hospitals and Health Systems. (2020). Standard 15.01.16. *Healthcare Facilities Accreditation Program: Accreditation requirements for acute care hospitals.* Chicago, IL: Accreditation Association for Hospitals and Health Systems. (Level VII)

9 DNV GL-Healthcare USA, Inc. (2020). PR.2.SR.5. *NIAHO® accreditation requirements, interpretive guidelines and surveyor guidance—revision 20.0.* Milford, OH: DNV GL-Healthcare USA, Inc. (Level VII)

10 Centers for Medicare and Medicaid Services, Department of Health and Human Services. (2020). Condition of participation: Patient's rights. 42 C.F.R. § 482.13(c)(1).

11 The Joint Commission. (2021). Standard RI.01.01.01. *Comprehensive accreditation manual for hospitals.* Oakbrook Terrace, IL: The Joint Commission. (Level VII)

12 The Joint Commission. (2021). Standard PC.02.01.21. *Comprehensive accreditation manual for hospitals.* Oakbrook Terrace, IL: The Joint Commission. (Level VII)

13 Waters, T. R., et al. (2009). Safe patient handling training for schools of nursing. https://www.cdc.gov/niosh/docs/2009-127/pdfs/2009-127.pdf (Level VII)

14 The Joint Commission. (2021). Standard NPSG.06.01.01. *Comprehensive accreditation manual for hospitals.* Oakbrook Terrace, IL: The Joint Commission. (Level VII)

15 The Joint Commission. (2013). Sentinel event alert 50: Medical device alarm safety in hospitals. https://www.jointcommission.org/-/media/tjc/documents/resources/patient-safety-topics/sentinel-event/sea_50_alarms_4_26_16.pdf (Level VII)

16 Turmell, J. W., et al. (2017). Alarm fatigue: Use of an evidence-based alarm management strategy. *Journal of Nursing Care Quality, 32*(1), 47–54.

17 Rutala, W. A., et al. (2008, revised 2019). Guideline for disinfection and sterilization in healthcare facilities, 2008. https://www.cdc.gov/infection-control/pdf/guidelines/disinfection-guidelines-H.pdf (Level I)

18 Accreditation Association for Hospitals and Health Systems. (2020). Standard 07.02.03. *Healthcare Facilities Accreditation Program: Accreditation requirements for acute care hospitals.* Chicago, IL: Accreditation Association for Hospitals and Health Systems. (Level VII)

19 Ganz, D. A., et al. (2013, reviewed 2021). *Preventing falls in hospitals: A toolkit for improving quality of care* (AHRQ Publication No. 13-0015-EF). Rockville, MD: Agency for Healthcare Research and Quality. https://www.ahrq.gov/professionals/systems/hospital/fallpxtoolkit/index.html (Level VII)

20 The Joint Commission. (2021). Standard RC.01.03.01. *Comprehensive accreditation manual for hospitals.* Oakbrook Terrace, IL: The Joint Commission. (Level VII)

21 Accreditation Association for Hospitals and Health Systems. (2020). Standard 10.00.03. *Healthcare Facilities Accreditation Program: Accreditation requirements for acute care hospitals.* Chicago, IL: Accreditation Association for Hospitals and Health Systems. (Level VII)

22 Centers for Medicare and Medicaid Services, Department of Health and Human Services. (2020). Condition of participation: Medical record services. 42 C.F.R. § 482.24(b).

23 DNV GL-Healthcare USA, Inc. (2020). MR.2.SR.1. *NIAHO® accreditation requirements, interpretive guidelines and surveyor guidance—revision 20.0.* Milford, OH: DNV GL-Healthcare USA, Inc. (Level VII)

24 Covidien. (2018). Operator's manual: Nellcor bedside SpO₂ patient monitoring system. https://www.medtronic.com/content/dam/covidien/library/us/en/product/pulse-oximetry/BedsideSpO2_OperatorsManual_en_PT00093073B00.pdf

Pulse assessment

Blood pumped into an already-full aorta during ventricular contraction creates a fluid wave that travels from the heart to the peripheral arteries. This recurring wave—called a *pulse*—is palpable at locations on the body where an artery crosses over bone or firm tissue and lies close to the skin surface.[1] The radial artery in the wrist is the most common palpation site in adults[1] and children older than age 3. (See *Pulse points.*) In infants and children younger than age 3, a stethoscope is used to listen to the heart itself rather than palpating a pulse;[2,3] because auscultation is done at the heart's apex, this is called the *apical pulse.*[1]

An apical–radial pulse is taken by simultaneously counting apical and radial beats: the first by auscultation at the apex of the heart, the second by palpation at the radial artery. Some heartbeats detected at the apex can't be detected at peripheral sites. When this occurs, the apical pulse

Pulse points

Shown below are anatomic locations where an artery crosses bone or firm tissue that can be used for pulse assessment.

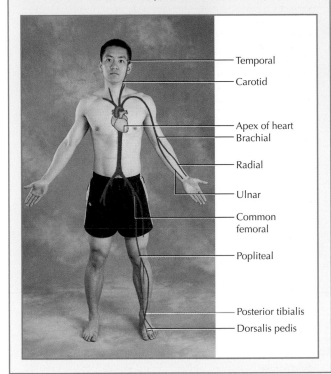

- Temporal
- Carotid
- Apex of heart
- Brachial
- Radial
- Ulnar
- Common femoral
- Popliteal
- Posterior tibialis
- Dorsalis pedis

rate is higher than the radial; the difference between the two is the *pulse deficit*.[1]

Pulse taking involves determining the rate (number of beats per minute), rhythm (pattern or regularity of the beats), and volume (amount of blood pumped with each beat).

Equipment

Clock or watch with second hand ■ Optional: blanket or sheet, stethoscope, disinfectant pads.

Preparation of equipment

Clean and disinfect the stethoscope with a disinfectant pad *to ensure it is clean and to prevent cross-contamination.*[4,5] If you aren't using your own stethoscope, also disinfect the earpieces with a disinfectant pad before and after use *to prevent cross-contamination.*[4,5]

Implementation

- Gather and prepare the necessary equipment and supplies.
- Perform hand hygiene.[6,7,8,9,10,11]
- Confirm the patient's identity using at least two patient identifiers.[12]
- Provide privacy.[13,14,15,16]
- Explain the procedure to the patient and family (if appropriate) according to their individual communication and learning needs *to increase their understanding, allay their fears, and enhance cooperation.*[17]
- Make sure the patient is comfortable and relaxed, *because an awkward, uncomfortable position may affect the heart rate.*

Taking a radial pulse

- Place the patient in a sitting or supine position, with the arm at the side or across the chest.[1]
- Gently press your index, middle, and ring fingers on the radial artery, inside the patient's wrist, using moderate pressure (as shown on top right);

excessive pressure may obstruct blood flow distal to the pulse site. Don't use your thumb to take the patient's pulse, *because your thumb's own strong pulse may be confused with the patient's pulse.*

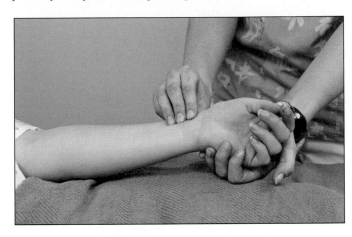

- After locating the pulse, if the rhythm is regular and the rate seems normal, count for 30 seconds and then multiply by 2. If the rate is unusually fast or slow, count for 60 seconds.
- While counting the rate, assess pulse rhythm and amplitude. If the pulse is irregular, note whether the irregularity occurs in a pattern or randomly. If you aren't sure, use your stethoscope to obtain an apical pulse.[18] (See *Identifying pulse patterns*, page 716.)
- Perform hand hygiene.[6,7,8,9,10,11]
- Document the procedure.[19,20,21,22]

Taking an apical pulse

- Help the patient to the supine position *for better accuracy in pulse counting.*[23]
- Drape the patient with a blanket or sheet, if necessary.
- Warm the diaphragm or bell of the stethoscope in your hand. *Placing a cold stethoscope against the skin may startle the patient and momentarily increase the heart rate.* Keep in mind that the bell transmits low pitched sounds more effectively than the diaphragm does.
- Place the diaphragm or bell of the stethoscope over the apex of the heart (normally located at the fifth intercostal space left of the midclavicular line). Then insert the earpieces into your ears.
- Count the beats for 60 seconds (as shown below), and note their rhythm, volume, and intensity (loudness).

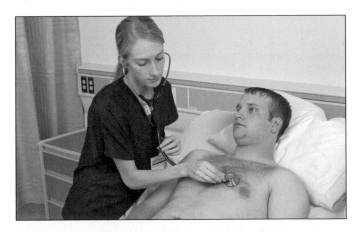

- Remove the stethoscope and make the patient comfortable.
- Perform hand hygiene.[6,7,8,9,10,11]
- Clean the stethoscope with an alcohol pad *to prevent cross-contamination.*[4,5]
- Perform hand hygiene.[6,7,8,9,10,11]
- Document the procedure.[19,20,21,22]

Identifying pulse patterns

TYPE	RATE	RHYTHM (PER 3 SECONDS)	CAUSES AND INCIDENCE
Normal	60 to 100 beats/minute	● ● ● ●	■ Varies with such factors as age, physical activity, and gender (men usually have lower pulse rates than women)
Tachycardia	More than 100 beats/minute	● ● ● ● ● ● ●	■ Accompanies stimulation of the sympathetic nervous system by emotional stress, such as anger, fear, or anxiety, or by the use of certain drugs, such as caffeine ■ May result from exercise and from certain health conditions, such as heart failure, anemia, and fever (which increases oxygen requirements and therefore pulse rate)
Bradycardia	Less than 60 beats/minute	● ● ●	■ Accompanies stimulation of the parasympathetic nervous system by drug use, especially digoxin, or such conditions as cerebral hemorrhage and heart block ■ May also be present in conditioned athletes
Irregular	Uneven time intervals between beats (for example, periods of regular rhythm interrupted by pauses or premature beats)	● ● ● ● ● ● ●	■ May indicate cardiac irritability, hypoxia, digoxin toxicity, potassium imbalance, or sometimes more serious arrhythmias if premature beats occur frequently ■ Occasional premature beats are normal

Taking an apical–radial pulse

■ Obtain the assistance of another nurse to obtain the apical–radial pulse: one person palpates the radial pulse while the other auscultates the apical pulse with a stethoscope. Both must use the same watch when counting beats.
■ Help the patient to the supine position for better accuracy.[23]
■ Drape the patient with a blanket or sheet, if necessary.
■ Locate the apical or radial pulse while the other nurse locates the other pulse.
■ Determine a time to begin counting.
■ Count beats for 60 seconds, starting at the appropriate time and using the same watch.
■ Remove the stethoscope.
■ Make the patient comfortable.
■ Perform hand hygiene.[6,7,8,9,10,11]
■ Clean and disinfect the stethoscope with a disinfectant pad *to prevent cross-contamination.*[4,5]
■ Perform hand hygiene.[6,7,8,9,10,11]
■ Document the procedure.[19,20,21,22]

Special considerations

■ If the pulse is faint or weak, use a Doppler ultrasound blood flow detector, if available.[1] (See the "Doppler ultrasound device use" procedure.) Note that a rapid, weak, or faint pulse may indicate dehydration.
■ If another nurse isn't available for an apical–radial pulse, hold the stethoscope in place with the hand that holds the watch while palpating the radial pulse with the other hand. You can then feel any discrepancies between the apical and radial pulses.

Documentation

Record the pulse rate, rhythm, and volume as well as the time of measurement. Describe the amplitude as diminished, brisk, or bounding. When recording the apical pulse, also include intensity of heart sounds. When recording the apical–radial pulse, document the rate according to the pulse site—for example, A/R 80/76. Document teaching provided to the patient and family (if applicable), their understanding of that teaching, and any need for follow-up teaching.

REFERENCES

1 Craven, R. F., et al. (2020). *Fundamentals of nursing: Concepts and competencies for practice.* (9th ed.). Philadelphia, PA: Wolters Kluwer.
2 Bowden, V. R., & Greenberg, C. S. (2016). *Pediatric nursing procedures* (4th ed.). Philadelphia, PA: Wolters Kluwer.
3 Duderstadt, K. G. (2019). *Pediatric physical examination: An illustrated handbook* (3rd ed.). St. Louis, MO: Elsevier.
4 Rutala, W. A., et al. (2008, revised 2019). Guideline for disinfection and sterilization in healthcare facilities, 2008. https://www.cdc.gov/infection-control/pdf/guidelines/disinfection-guidelines-H.pdf (Level I)
5 Accreditation Association for Hospitals and Health Systems. (2020). Standard 07.02.03. *Healthcare Facilities Accreditation Program: Accreditation requirements for acute care hospitals.* Chicago, IL: Accreditation Association for Hospitals and Health Systems. (Level VII)
6 World Health Organization. (2009). WHO guidelines on hand hygiene in health care: First global patient safety challenge, clean care is safer care. https://apps.who.int/iris/bitstream/handle/10665/44102/9789241597906_eng.pdf?sequence=1 (Level IV)
7 Centers for Disease Control and Prevention. (2002). Guideline for hand hygiene in health-care settings: Recommendations of the Healthcare Infection Control Practices Advisory Committee and the HICPAC/SHEA/APIC/IDSA Hand Hygiene Task Force. *MMWR Recommendations and Reports, 51*(RR-16), 1–45. https://www.cdc.gov/mmwr/pdf/rr/rr5116.pdf (Level II)
8 Accreditation Association for Hospitals and Health Systems. (2020). Standard 07.01.21. *Healthcare Facilities Accreditation Program: Accreditation requirements for acute care hospitals.* Chicago, IL: Accreditation Association for Hospitals and Health Systems. (Level VII)
9 Centers for Medicare and Medicaid Services, Department of Health and Human Services. (2020). Condition of participation: Infection control. 42 C.F.R. § 482.42.
10 DNV GL-Healthcare USA, Inc. (2020). IC.1.SR.1. *NIAHO® accreditation requirements, interpretive guidelines and surveyor guidance—revision 20.0.* Milford, OH: DNV GL-Healthcare USA, Inc. (Level VII)
11 The Joint Commission. (2021). Standard NPSG.07.01.01. *Comprehensive accreditation manual for hospitals.* Oakbrook Terrace, IL: The Joint Commission. (Level VII)
12 The Joint Commission. (2021). Standard NPSG.01.01.01. *Comprehensive accreditation manual for hospitals.* Oakbrook Terrace, IL: The Joint Commission. (Level VII)

13 The Joint Commission. (2021). Standard RI.01.01.01. *Comprehensive accreditation manual for hospitals.* Oakbrook Terrace, IL: The Joint Commission. (Level VII)

14 DNV GL-Healthcare USA, Inc. (2020). PR.2.SR.5. *NIAHO® accreditation requirements, interpretive guidelines and surveyor guidance—revision 20.0.* Milford, OH: DNV GL-Healthcare USA, Inc. (Level VII)

15 Centers for Medicare and Medicaid Services, Department of Health and Human Services. (2020). Condition of participation: Patient's rights. 42 C.F.R. § 482.13(c)(1).

16 Accreditation Association for Hospitals and Health Systems. (2020). Standard 15.01.16. *Healthcare Facilities Accreditation Program: Accreditation requirements for acute care hospitals.* Chicago, IL: Accreditation Association for Hospitals and Health Systems. (Level VII)

17 The Joint Commission. (2021). Standard PC.02.01.21. *Comprehensive accreditation manual for hospitals.* Oakbrook Terrace, IL: The Joint Commission. (Level VII)

18 Bickley, L. (2017). *Bates' guide to physical examination and health history taking* (12th ed.). Philadelphia, PA: Wolters Kluwer.

19 The Joint Commission. (2021). Standard RC.01.03.01. *Comprehensive accreditation manual for hospitals.* Oakbrook Terrace, IL: The Joint Commission. (Level VII)

20 Centers for Medicare and Medicaid Services, Department of Health and Human Services. (2020). Condition of participation: Medical record services. 42 C.F.R. § 482.24(b).

21 Accreditation Association for Hospitals and Health Systems. (2020). Standard 10.00.03. *Healthcare Facilities Accreditation Program: Accreditation requirements for acute care hospitals.* Chicago, IL: Accreditation Association for Hospitals and Health Systems. (Level VII)

22 DNV GL-Healthcare USA, Inc. (2020). MR.2.SR.1. *NIAHO® accreditation requirements, interpretive guidelines and surveyor guidance—revision 20.0.* Milford, OH: DNV GL-Healthcare USA, Inc. (Level VII)

23 Kobayashi, H. (2013). Effect of measurement duration on accuracy of pulse-counting. *Ergonomics, 56*(12), 1940–1944. https://www.ncbi.nlm.nih.gov/pmc/articles/PMC3877911 (Level IV)

Pulse oximetry

Performed intermittently or continuously, pulse oximetry is a relatively simple procedure used to monitor arterial oxygen saturation noninvasively. Pulse oximeters usually denote arterial oxygen saturation values with the symbol SpO_2, whereas invasively measured arterial oxygen saturation values are denoted by the symbol SaO_2.[1] Pulse oximetry can aid clinical decision-making; however, it isn't a substitute for a clinical assessment. Arterial blood gas (ABG) measurements, obtained by arterial puncture, are the gold standard for measuring oxygen saturation level.[2,3]

In pulse oximetry, two diodes send red and infrared light through a pulsating arterial vascular bed, like the one in the fingertip. A photodetector slipped over the finger measures the transmitted light as it passes through the vascular bed, detects the relative amount of color absorbed by arterial blood, and calculates the SpO_2 without interference from surrounding venous blood, skin, connective tissue, or bone. Oximetry using the ear probe works by monitoring the transmission of light waves through the vascular bed of a patient's earlobe. Results will be inaccurate if the patient's earlobe is poorly perfused, as from a low cardiac output. If a patient is hemodynamically unstable, a forehead sensor may be a better alternative for obtaining an accurate reading, *because the forehead is reasonably resistant to the vasoconstrictive effects of the sympathetic nervous system.*[4] (See *How oximetry works.*)

Equipment

Pulse oximeter ▪ finger probe, ear probe, or forehead sensor (preferably a disposable adhesive sensor)[5] ▪ facility-approved disinfectant ▪ Optional: blanket, cloth, nail polish remover, nail clipper, supplemental oxygen delivery equipment, alcohol pad, earlobe stabilizer, stethoscope.

Preparation of equipment

Inspect all equipment and supplies. If a product is expired, is defective, or has compromised integrity, remove it from patient use, label it as expired or defective, and report the expiration or defect as directed by your facility. Follow the manufacturer's guidelines for proper operation of pulse oximeters, probes, and sensors.

Implementation

- Gather and prepare the necessary equipment and supplies.
- Perform hand hygiene.[6,7,8,9,10,11]
- Confirm the patient's identity using at least two patient identifiers.[12]
- Explain the procedure to the patient and family (if appropriate) according to their individual communication and learning needs *to increase their understanding, allay their fears, and enhance cooperation.*[13]
- Select a desired sensor site that has warmth and adequate blood flow *to ensure adequate arterial pulse strength for accurate monitoring.*[4] If necessary,

EQUIPMENT

How oximetry works

The pulse oximeter allows noninvasive monitoring of the percentage of hemoglobin saturated by oxygen (SpO_2) by measuring the absorption (amplitude) of light waves as they pass through areas of the body that are highly perfused by arterial blood. Oximetry also monitors pulse rate and amplitude.

Light-emitting diodes in a transducer (photodetector) attached to the patient's body (shown below on the index finger) send red and infrared light beams through tissue. The photodetector records the relative amount of each color absorbed by arterial blood and transmits the data to a monitor, which displays the information with each heartbeat. If the SpO_2 level or pulse rate varies from preset limits, the monitor triggers visual and audible alarms.

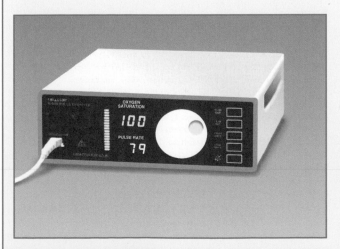

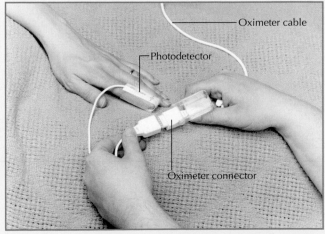

Oximeter cable

Photodetector

Oximeter connector

warm the sensor site with a cloth or blanket. Avoid placing a sensor on edematous tissue *to reduce possible loss of light transmission*. Avoid placing the sensor on the same extremity being used for automated noninvasive blood pressure monitoring *to reduce intermittent interference with pulsatility*.[14]

■ Choose a sensor according to the patient's size and level of activity, duration of use, and infection control concerns.[14]

Using a finger probe

■ Make sure the patient isn't wearing false fingernails, and remove any nail polish from the test finger.

■ Place the transducer (photodetector) probe over the patient's finger so that light beams and sensors oppose each other. If the patient has long fingernails, position the probe perpendicular to the finger, if possible, or clip the fingernail.

■ Always position the patient's hand at heart level *to eliminate venous pulsations and to promote accurate readings*.

■ Turn on the power switch (as shown below). If the device is working properly, a beep will sound, a display will light momentarily, and the pulse searchlight will flash. The SpO_2 and pulse rate displays will show stationary zeros. After four to six heartbeats, the SpO_2 and pulse rate displays will supply information with each beat, and the pulse amplitude indicator will begin tracking the pulse. Confirm that the pulse rate displayed corresponds with the patient's radial pulse *to ensure an accurate reading*.

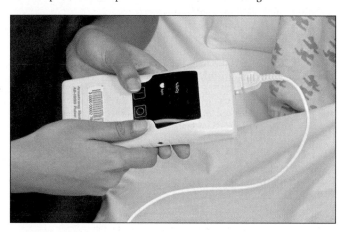

Using an ear probe

■ Clean the earlobe with an alcohol pad (as shown below), if necessary, *to remove oils from the skin,* and then allow it to dry.

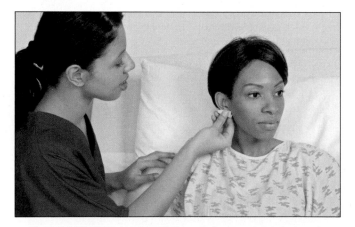

■ Following the manufacturer's instructions, attach the ear probe to the patient's earlobe or pinna. Use the ear probe stabilizer for prolonged or exercise testing. Be sure to establish good contact on the ear; *an unstable probe may set off the low-perfusion alarm*.

■ After the probe has been attached for a few seconds, watch for an SpO_2 level and pulse waveform on the oximeter's screen.

■ Leave the ear probe in place for 3 or more minutes until readings stabilize at the highest point, or take three separate readings and average them. Make sure you revascularize the patient's earlobe each time.

Using a forehead sensor

■ Clean the patient's forehead site with an alcohol pad, if necessary, *to remove oils from the skin*. Allow it to dry completely.[14]

■ Following the manufacturer's instructions, attach the forehead sensor to the patient's forehead. Don't use a disposable sensor intended for use on the fingers, *because it may produce an inaccurate reading*.[4]

■ Turn on the device.

■ After the probe has been attached for a few seconds, an SpO_2 level and pulse waveform will appear on the oximeter's screen.

Completing the procedure

■ If monitoring continuous pulse oximetry, confirm that alarm limits are set appropriately for the patient's current condition, and that the alarms are turned on, functioning properly, and audible to staff.[5,15,16,17]

■ If the pulse oximeter alarms, assess the patient's respiratory status and make sure the sensor remains attached properly.[4]

■ If you detect and confirm a low SpO_2 level, administer supplemental oxygen as needed and prescribed. Reassess the patient to evaluate the effectiveness of the supplemental oxygen therapy.

■ Regularly monitor and document the patient's SpO_2 level and the condition of the skin under the probe. Change the sensor site as needed or at an interval established by your facility *to reduce incidence of pressure injury*.[18]

■ When monitoring is completed, remove the probe, turn off and unplug the unit, and, if using a reusable probe, clean it by gently rubbing it with a disinfectant wipe or pad.[19,20]

■ Perform hand hygiene.[6,7,8,9,10,11]

■ Document the procedure.[21,22,23,24]

Special considerations

■ The pulse rate on the pulse oximeter should correspond with the patient's actual pulse. If the rates don't correspond, the SpO_2 level can't be considered accurate. Assess the patient, check the oximeter, and reposition the probe, if necessary.[25]

■ Collaborate with an interprofessional team, including biomedical engineering, *to determine the best delay and threshold settings*.[5]

■ Use disposable adhesive sensors (if available), and replace the sensors when they no longer adhere properly to the patient's skin, they become soiled or have a detectable odor, or their wires become exposed.[5,14]

■ If you've performed oximetry properly, readings are typically accurate to within plus-or-minus 2% of SaO_2 at higher levels, but may reflect SaO_2 less accurately when SpO_2 falls below 80%.[2,26]

■ Certain factors may interfere with accuracy, including[2,3,4] elevated carboxyhemoglobin or methemoglobin levels (possible in heavy smokers and urban dwellers), which can cause a falsely elevated SpO_2 reading; certain intravascular substances, such as lipid emulsions and dyes; excessive light (for example, from phototherapy, surgical lamps, direct sunlight, and excessive ambient lighting); excessive patient movement; dark skin; digital clubbing; hypothermia; hypotension; vasoconstriction; poor perfusion; and altered venous return at the sensor location.

■ Forehead sensors are a good alternative for patients with poor peripheral circulation and in patients under general anesthesia whose extremities aren't readily accessible.[2]

■ If you're using SpO_2 to guide weaning the patient from forced inspiratory oxygen, obtain samples for ABG analysis occasionally to correlate SpO_2 readings with SaO_2 levels.[4]

■ If light is a problem, cover the probes; if patient movement is a problem, move the probe or select a different probe; and if placement is a problem, reposition the probe, revascularize the site, or use a finger probe.[4] (See *Diagnosing pulse oximeter problems*.)

■ Normal SpO_2 levels aren't clearly defined *because of variations in measurement technique, sensor site, device type, patient age, altitude, and the definition of normal for each patient*.[2] However, a normal SpO_2 level for an adult generally ranges from 95% to 100%. An SpO_2 of 92% or less suggests hypoxemia,[3] in which case you should follow your facility's protocol or the practitioner's orders, which may include increasing oxygen therapy. If SpO_2 levels decrease suddenly, assess the patient immediately to determine whether you need to begin resuscitation. Notify the practitioner of any significant change in the patient's condition.

TROUBLESHOOTING

DIAGNOSING PULSE OXIMETER PROBLEMS

To maintain a continuous display of arterial oxygen saturation (SpO₂) levels, keep the monitoring site clean. Make sure the skin doesn't become irritated from adhesives used to keep disposable probes in place; you may need to change the site if this happens. Disposable probes that irritate the skin also can be replaced by nondisposable models.[4]

Another common problem with pulse oximeters is the failure of the devices to obtain a signal. If the device you're using fails to obtain a signal, first assess the patient's vital signs.[25] If they're sufficient to produce a signal, check for a poor connection, inadequate or intermittent blood flow to the site, or equipment malfunctions.

Poor connection

To check for a poor connection, make sure that the sensors are properly aligned. Make sure that wires are intact and securely fastened, and that the pulse oximeter is plugged into a power source.[14]

Inadequate or intermittent blood flow to the site

To determine inadequate or intermittent blood flow to the site, assess the patient's pulse rate and capillary refill time. If blood flow to the site is decreased, take corrective action by loosening restraints, removing tight fitting clothes, taking off a blood pressure cuff, or assessing arterial and IV catheters.[4,14] If none of these interventions works, you may need to find an alternate site. Finding a site with proper circulation may also prove challenging when a patient is receiving vasoconstrictive drugs. Refer to the manufacturer's recommendations regarding the effects of low perfusion states on pulse oximeter performance.[3]

Equipment malfunctions

If you suspect an equipment malfunction, remove the pulse oximeter from the patient, set the alarm limits, and try the instrument on yourself or another healthy person *to determine whether the equipment is working correctly.*

NURSING ALERT Be aware that anemic patients may be hypoxic but will demonstrate normal SpO₂ levels, *because total oxygen content of the arterial blood is decreased.*[4]

Complications

A potential complication of pulse oximetry is skin breakdown under the probe if the probe is left on too long or applied too tightly.[4]

Documentation

Document the date, time, patient activity level and position, probe site, amount of supplemental oxygen, method of oxygen delivery, SpO₂ level, and any interventions performed and the patient's response to those interventions. Record levels on appropriate flowcharts, if indicated. Document teaching provided to the patient and family (if applicable), their understanding of that teaching, and any need for follow-up teaching.

REFERENCES

1 Kacmarek, R. M., et al. (2021). *Egan's fundamentals of respiratory care* (12th ed.). St. Louis, MO: Elsevier.

2 Pretto, J. J., et al. (2014). Clinical use of pulse oximetry: Official guidelines from the Thoracic Society of Australia and New Zealand. *Respirology, 19*(1), 38–46. https://www.thoracic.org.au/clinical-documents/command/download_file/id/34/filename/Pretto_et_al-2014-Respirology.pdf (Level VII)

3 Mohammad, Y., et al. (2010). Clinical use of pulse oximetry: Pocket reference 2010. https://www.networks.nhs.uk/nhs-networks/south-east-coast-respiratory-programme/documents/OximetryPG.pdf

4 Wiegand, D. L. (2017). *AACN procedure manual for high acuity, progressive, and critical care* (7th ed.). St. Louis, MO: Elsevier.

5 American Association of Critical-Care Nurses. (2018). AACN practice alert: Managing alarms in acute care across the life span: Electrocardiography and pulse oximetry. https://www.aacn.org/clinical-resources/practice-alerts/managing-alarms-in-acute-care-across-the-life-span (Level VII)

6 Centers for Disease Control and Prevention. (2002). Guideline for hand hygiene in health-care settings: Recommendations of the Healthcare Infection Control Practices Advisory Committee and the HICPAC/SHEA/APIC/IDSA Hand Hygiene Task Force. *MMWR Recommendations and Reports, 51*(RR-16), 1–45. https://www.cdc.gov/mmwr/pdf/rr/rr5116.pdf (Level II)

7 World Health Organization. (2009). WHO guidelines on hand hygiene in health care: First global patient safety challenge, clean care is safer care. https://apps.who.int/iris/bitstream/handle/10665/44102/9789241597906_eng.pdf?sequence=1 (Level IV)

8 The Joint Commission. (2021). Standard NPSG.07.01.01. *Comprehensive accreditation manual for hospitals.* Oakbrook Terrace, IL: The Joint Commission. (Level VII)

9 Centers for Medicare and Medicaid Services, Department of Health and Human Services. (2020). Condition of participation: Infection control. 42 C.F.R. § 482.42.

10 Accreditation Association for Hospitals and Health Systems. (2020). Standard 07.01.21. *Healthcare Facilities Accreditation Program: Accreditation requirements for acute care hospitals.* Chicago, IL: Accreditation Association for Hospitals and Health Systems. (Level VII)

11 DNV GL-Healthcare USA, Inc. (2020). IC.1.SR.1. *NIAHO® accreditation requirements, interpretive guidelines and surveyor guidance—revision 20.0.* Milford, OH: DNV GL-Healthcare USA, Inc. (Level VII)

12 The Joint Commission. (2021). Standard NPSG.01.01.01. *Comprehensive accreditation manual for hospitals.* Oakbrook Terrace, IL: The Joint Commission. (Level VII)

13 The Joint Commission. (2021). Standard PC.02.01.21. *Comprehensive accreditation manual for hospitals.* Oakbrook Terrace, IL: The Joint Commission. (Level VII)

14 Nellcor. (n.d.). Clinician's guide to Nellcor® sensors. http://nbninfusions.com/wp-content/uploads/nbnmanuals/Ventilator%20Manuals/Nellcor%20Sensors%20Clinician's%20Manual.pdf

15 The Joint Commission. (2021). Standard NPSG.06.01.01. *Comprehensive accreditation manual for hospitals.* Oakbrook Terrace, IL: The Joint Commission. (Level VII)

16 Turmell, J. W., et al. (2017). Alarm fatigue: Use of an evidence-based alarm management strategy. *Journal of Nursing Care Quality, 32*(1), 47–54.

17 The Joint Commission. (2013). Sentinel event alert 50: Medical device alarm safety in hospitals. https://www.jointcommission.org/-/media/tjc/documents/resources/patient-safety-topics/sentinel-event/sea_50_alarms_4_26_16.pdf (Level VII)

18 European Pressure Ulcer Advisory Panel, et al. (2019). Prevention and treatment of pressure ulcers/injuries: Quick reference guide. http://www.internationalguideline.com/static/pdfs/Quick_Reference_Guide-10Mar2019.pdf (Level VII)

19 Rutala, W. A., et al. (2008, revised 2019). Guideline for disinfection and sterilization in healthcare facilities, 2008. https://www.cdc.gov/infection-control/pdf/guidelines/disinfection-guidelines-H.pdf (Level I)

20 Accreditation Association for Hospitals and Health Systems. (2020). Standard 07.02.03. *Healthcare Facilities Accreditation Program: Accreditation requirements for acute care hospitals.* Chicago, IL: Accreditation Association for Hospitals and Health Systems. (Level VII)

21 The Joint Commission. (2021). Standard RC.01.03.01. *Comprehensive accreditation manual for hospitals.* Oakbrook Terrace, IL: The Joint Commission. (Level VII)

22 Centers for Medicare and Medicaid Services, Department of Health and Human Services. (2020). Condition of participation: Medical record services. 42 C.F.R. § 482.24(b).

23 Accreditation Association for Hospitals and Health Systems. (2020). Standard 10.00.03. *Healthcare Facilities Accreditation Program: Accreditation requirements for acute care hospitals.* Chicago, IL: Accreditation Association for Hospitals and Health Systems. (Level VII)

24 DNV GL-Healthcare USA, Inc. (2020). MR.2.SR.1. *NIAHO® accreditation requirements, interpretive guidelines and surveyor guidance—revision 20.0.* Milford, OH: DNV GL-Healthcare USA, Inc. (Level VII)

25 World Health Organization. (2011). Pulse oximetry training manual. https://www.who.int/patientsafety/safesurgery/pulse_oximetry/who_ps_pulse_oxymetry_training_manual_en.pdf (Level VII)

26 Casey, G. (2011). Pulse oximetry—What are we really measuring? *Nursing New Zealand, 17*(3), 24–29. (Level VII)

RADIATION IMPLANT THERAPY

For this treatment, also called *brachytherapy*, the practitioner uses implants of radioactive isotopes (encapsulated in seeds, needles, catheters, or sutures) to deliver ionizing radiation within a body cavity or interstitially to a tumor site.[1] Common implant sites include the brain, breast, cervix, endometrium, lung, neck, oral cavity, prostate, and vagina. Implants can deliver a continuous radiation dose over several hours or days to a specific site while minimizing exposure to adjacent tissues. The implants may be permanent or temporary. Isotopes such as cesium-137 and -131, gold-198, iodine-125, iridium-192, palladium-103, and phosphorus-32 are used to treat cancers. (See *Radioisotopes and their uses*.) Radiation implant therapy is commonly combined with external radiation therapy (teletherapy) for increased effectiveness.

For treatment, the patient is usually placed in a private room (with its own bathroom) located as far away from high-traffic areas as practical. If monitoring shows an increased radiation hazard, adjacent rooms and hallways may also need to be restricted. Consult your facility's radiation safety guidelines.

Equipment

Ring or film badge ■ RADIATION PRECAUTION sign for door ■ RADIATION PRECAUTION labels ■ masking tape ■ lead-lined container ■ long-handled forceps ■ Optional: lead shield, pocket dosimeter.

For implants inserted in the oral cavity or neck

Emergency tracheotomy tray.

Preparation of equipment

Place the lead-lined container and long-handled forceps in a corner of the patient's room. Mark a "Safe line" on the floor with masking tape 6'

Radioisotopes and their uses

Unstable elements, radioisotopes emit three kinds of energy particles as they decay to a stable state. These particles are ranked by their penetrating power. *Alpha particles* possess the lowest energy level and are easily stopped by a sheet of paper. More powerful *beta particles* can be stopped by the skin's surface. *Gamma rays*, the most powerful, can be stopped only by dense shielding, such as lead. Some isotopes commonly used in cancer treatments are listed below.

RADIOISOTOPE	KEY FACTS	NURSING INTERVENTIONS
Cesium-137 (^{137}Cs) Gynecologic cancers, head and neck cancers, rectal cancers, and esophageal cancers	■ 30-year half-life ■ Emits gamma particles ■ Encased in steel capsules placed temporarily in the patient in the operating room	■ Elevate the head of the bed no more than 45 degrees. ■ Encourage fluids and implement a low-residue diet. ■ Encourage quiet activities; enforce strict bed rest, as ordered.
Iodine-125 (^{125}I) Localized or unresectable tumors, slow-growing tumors, and recurrent disease	■ 60-day half-life ■ Emits gamma particles ■ Permanently implanted as tiny seeds or sutures directly into the tumor or tumor bed	■ *Because seeds may become dislodged,* no linens, body fluids, instruments, or utensils may leave the patient's room until these items are monitored. ■ If a seed becomes dislodged and found, call the radiation oncology department; use long-handled forceps to put it in a lead-lined container in the room. ■ Monitor body fluids *to detect displaced seeds.* Give the patient a 24-hour urine container that can be closed.
Iridium-192 (^{192}Ir) Gynecologic cancers and tumors of the prostate, brain, head, neck, rectum, and breast; sarcomas	■ 74-day half-life ■ Emits gamma particles ■ Temporarily implanted as seeds strung inside special catheters implanted around the tumor	■ If a catheter becomes dislodged, call the radiation oncology department; use long-handled forceps to put the implant in a lead-lined container in the room.
Palladium-103 (^{103}Pd) Prostate cancer	■ 17-day half-life ■ Emits gamma particles ■ Permanently implanted as seeds in the tumor or tumor bed	■ *Because seeds may become dislodged,* no linens, body fluids, instruments, or utensils may leave the patient's room until these items are monitored. ■ If a seed becomes dislodged and found, call the radiation oncology department; use long-handled forceps to put it in a lead-lined container in the room. ■ Monitor body fluids *to detect displaced seeds.* Give the patient a 24-hour urine container that can be closed.
Phosphorus-32 (^{32}P) Polycythemia, leukemia, bone metastasis, and malignant ascites	■ 14-day half-life ■ Emits beta particles ■ Used as an IV solution rather than an implant *because of its low energy level*	■ No shielding is required other than an acrylic syringe shield. ■ Patients receiving ^{32}P are placed in a private room with a separate bathroom.
Gold-198 (^{198}Au) Localized male genitourinary tumors	■ 3-day half-life ■ Emits gamma particles ■ Permanently implanted as tiny seeds directly into the tumor or tumor bed	■ If a seed becomes dislodged and found, call the radiation oncology department for disposal.
Cesium-131 (^{131}Cs) Prostate, liver, head, and neck tumors	■ 10-day half-life ■ Emits gamma particles ■ Permanently implanted as tiny seeds directly into the tumor bed	■ If a seed becomes dislodged and found, call the radiation oncology department for disposal.

(1.8 M) from the patient's bed *to warn visitors to keep clear of the patient to minimize their radiation exposure.* If desired, place a portable lead shield in the back of the room *to use when providing care.* Place an emergency tracheotomy tray in the room if an implant will be inserted in the oral cavity or neck.

Inspect all equipment and supplies. If a product is expired, is defective, or has compromised integrity, remove it from patient use, label it as expired or defective, and report the expiration or defect as directed by your facility.

Implementation

- Verify the practitioner's order.
- If required by your facility, confirm that informed consent has been obtained and that the signed consent form is in the patient's medical record.[2,3,4,5,6]
- Perform hand hygiene.[7,8,9,10,11,12]
- Confirm the patient's identity using at least two patient identifiers.[13,14]
- Explain the procedure to the patient and family (if appropriate) according to their individual communication and learning needs *to increase their understanding, allay their fears, and enhance cooperation.*[15] Discuss the treatment and its goals. Before treatment begins, review your facility's radiation safety and visitation procedures, potential adverse effects, and interventions for those effects. Also review long-term concerns and home care issues.
- Verify that all laboratory tests are performed as ordered and that the results are in the patient's medical record. Notify the practitioner of any unexpected results.[14]

After radiation implantation

- Review the practitioner's orders regarding the level of shielding and patient care required for the type of radiation implant.[16]
- Place a RADIATION PRECAUTION sign on the patient's door.
- If laboratory studies are required during treatment, a technician (equipped with a ring or film badge) should obtain the specimen and label it with the patient's name, identification number, and date and time of collection in the presence of the patient *to prevent mislabeling*;[13] affix it with a RADIATION PRECAUTION label; and then alert laboratory personnel before taking the samples to the laboratory. If urine tests are needed for phosphorus-32 therapy, ask the radiation oncology department or a laboratory technician about how to safely transport these specimens.[17,18,19,20]
- Affix a RADIATION PRECAUTION label to the patient's identification wristband.
- Alert staff members that the patient is receiving radiation implant therapy by placing a RADIATION PRECAUTION warning in the patient's medical record *to prevent accidental exposure to radiation.*
- Each nurse must wear a personal, nontransferable ring or film badge placed at or above waist level for the entire shift. The badge must only be worn within the work environment.[16] *Badges document each person's cumulative lifetime radiation exposure.* Only primary caregivers are badged and allowed into the patient's room.[16] Turn in the radiation badge monthly, or as directed by your facility.
- If using a pocket dosimeter, be aware that these devices measure immediate exposures to radiation. In many facilities, these measurements aren't part of the permanent exposure record but are used to ensure that nurses receive the lowest possible exposure.
- *To minimize exposure to radiation,* use the three principles of time, distance, and shielding: Time—Limit the amount of time spent near the radiation source,[16] and plan to give care in the shortest time possible, *because less time equals less exposure.* Distance—Work as far away from the radiation source as possible; give care from the side opposite the implant or from a position allowing the greatest working distance possible, *because the intensity of radiation exposure varies inversely as the square of the distance from the source.* Shielding—Add a protective barrier between yourself and the radioactive source, if needed and desired; the type of shielding used depends on the type of radiation.[16,17,18,19,20]
- Provide essential nursing care only, limiting time in the patient's room.
- Make sure that perineal wipes, sanitary pads, and similar items are bagged correctly and monitored. (Refer to your facility's radiation guideline.)

- Keep soiled linens in the patient's room until scanned and cleared by the radiation officer.[16]
- Dressing changes over an implanted area must be supervised by the radiation technician or another designated caregiver.
- Before discharge, a patient's temporary implant must be removed and properly stored by the radiation oncology department.[17,18,19,20] A patient with a permanent implant may not be released until the radioactivity level is less than 5 millirems/hour at a distance of 3.3′ (1 M).
- Perform hand hygiene.[7,8,9,10,11,12]
- Document the procedure.[21,22,23,24]

Special considerations

- Nurses and visitors who are pregnant or trying to conceive or father a child must not care for patients receiving radiation implant therapy, *because the gonads and developing embryo and fetus are highly susceptible to the damaging effects of ionizing radiation.*
- If the patient must be moved out of the room, notify the appropriate department of the patient's status *to give receiving personnel time to make appropriate preparations to receive the patient.* When moving the patient, make sure that the route is clear of equipment and other people, and that the elevator (if there is one) is keyed and ready to receive the patient. Move the patient in a bed or wheelchair, accompanied by two caregivers equipped with badges. If the patient is delayed along the way, stand as far away from the bed as possible until you can continue.
- The radiation oncology department must monitor the patient's room, and disposables must be monitored and removed according to facility guidelines.
- If a code is called on a patient with an implant, follow your facility's code procedures as well as these steps: Notify the code team of the patient's radioactive status *to exclude any team member who is pregnant or trying to conceive or father a child.* Also notify the radiation oncology department. Cover the implant site with a strip of lead shielding, if possible. Don't allow anything to leave the patient's room until it's monitored for radiation. Limit those entering the room to personnel essential to performing code procedures. The primary care nurse must remain in the room (as far away from the patient as possible) *to act as a resource person for the patient and to provide film badges or dosimeters to code team members.*
- If the patient has radiation seeds implanted for treatment of prostate cancer, strain the urine for the seeds. Tell the patient not to allow children or young animals to sit on the patient's lap for 1 to 2 months after seed implantation. Advise a male patient to wear a condom during intercourse for 1 to 2 weeks after seed implantation, and tell him that his semen may be dark from blood.[25]
- Tell the patient who has had a cervical implant to expect slight to moderate vaginal bleeding after being discharged. This flow normally changes color from pink to brown to white. Instruct her to notify the practitioner if bleeding increases, persists for more than 48 hours, or has a foul odor. Explain to the patient that she may resume most normal activities but should avoid sexual intercourse and the use of tampons until after her follow-up visit to the practitioner (about 6 weeks after discharge). Instruct her to take showers rather than baths for 2 weeks, to avoid douching unless allowed by the practitioner, and to avoid activities that cause abdominal strain for 6 weeks.
- Refer the patient for sexual or psychological counseling if needed.
- If a patient with an implant dies on the unit, notify the radiation oncology department *so they can remove a temporary implant and store it properly.* If the implant was permanent, radiation oncology staff members will determine which precautions to follow before postmortem care can be provided and before the body can be moved to the morgue.

Complications

Depending on the implant site and total radiation dose, complications of implant therapy may include dislodgment of the radiation source or applicator, discomfort at the implant site, tissue fibrosis, xerostomia, radiation pneumonitis, muscle atrophy, sterility, vaginal dryness or stenosis, fistulas, hypothyroidism, altered bowel habits, infection, airway obstruction, diarrhea, cystitis, myelosuppression, neurotoxicity, and secondary cancers. Encourage the patient and family members to keep in contact with the radiation oncology department and to call them if concerns or physical changes occur.[26,27,28]

Documentation

Record date and time of therapy, radiation precautions taken during and after treatment, and the patient's tolerance of the procedure and radiation precautions. Document any adverse effects of therapy, any interventions taken, and the patient's response to the interventions. Document teaching provided to the patient and family (if applicable), their understanding of that teaching, and any need for follow-up teaching.

REFERENCES

1 Iwamoto, R. R., et al. (Eds.). (2012). *Manual for radiation oncology nursing practice and education* (4th ed.). Pittsburgh, PA: Oncology Nursing Society.

2 The Joint Commission. (2021). Standard RI.01.03.01. *Comprehensive accreditation manual for hospitals.* Oakbrook Terrace, IL: The Joint Commission. (Level VII)

3 Centers for Medicare and Medicaid Services, Department of Health and Human Services. (2020). Condition of participation: Patient's rights. 42 C.F.R. § 482.13(b)(2).

4 American College of Radiology (ACR). (2020). ACR-ABS-ASTRO practice parameter for the performance of radionuclide-based high-dose-rate brachytherapy. https://www.acr.org/-/media/ACR/Files/Practice-Parameters/hdr-brachyro.pdf?la=en (Level VII)

5 Accreditation Association for Hospitals and Health Systems. (2020). Standard 15.01.11. *Healthcare Facilities Accreditation Program: Accreditation requirements for acute care hospitals.* Chicago, IL: Accreditation Association for Hospitals and Health Systems. (Level VII)

6 DNV GL-Healthcare USA, Inc. (2020). PR.2.SR.3. *NIAHO® accreditation requirements, interpretive guidelines and surveyor guidance—revision 20.0.* Milford, OH: DNV GL-Healthcare USA, Inc. (Level VII)

7 Centers for Disease Control and Prevention. (2002). Guideline for hand hygiene in health-care settings: Recommendations of the Healthcare Infection Control Practices Advisory Committee and the HICPAC/SHEA/APIC/IDSA Hand Hygiene Task Force. *MMWR Recommendations and Reports, 51*(RR–16), 1–45. https://www.cdc.gov/mmwr/pdf/rr/rr5116.pdf (Level II)

8 World Health Organization (WHO). (2009). WHO guidelines on hand hygiene in health care: First global patient safety challenge, clean care is safer care. https://apps.who.int/iris/bitstream/handle/10665/44102/9789241597906_eng.pdf?sequence=1 (Level IV)

9 The Joint Commission. (2021). Standard NPSG.07.01.01. *Comprehensive accreditation manual for hospitals.* Oakbrook Terrace, IL: The Joint Commission. (Level VII)

10 Accreditation Association for Hospitals and Health Systems. (2020). Standard 07.01.21. *Healthcare Facilities Accreditation Program: Accreditation requirements for acute care hospitals.* Chicago, IL: Accreditation Association for Hospitals and Health Systems. (Level VII)

11 Centers for Medicare and Medicaid Services, Department of Health and Human Services. (2020). Condition of participation: Infection control. 42 C.F.R. § 482.42.

12 DNV GL-Healthcare USA, Inc. (2020). IC.1.SR.1. *NIAHO® accreditation requirements, interpretive guidelines and surveyor guidance—revision 20.0.* Milford, OH: DNV GL-Healthcare USA, Inc. (Level VII)

13 The Joint Commission. (2021). Standard NPSG.01.01.01. *Comprehensive accreditation manual for hospitals.* Oakbrook Terrace, IL: The Joint Commission. (Level VII)

14 Accreditation Association for Hospitals and Health Systems. (2020). Standard 30.00.14. *Healthcare Facilities Accreditation Program: Accreditation requirements for acute care hospitals.* Chicago, IL: Accreditation Association for Hospitals and Health Systems. (Level VII)

15 The Joint Commission. (2021). Standard PC.02.01.21. *Comprehensive accreditation manual for hospitals.* Oakbrook Terrace, IL: The Joint Commission. (Level VII)

16 Olsen, M. M., et al. (Eds.). (2019). *Chemotherapy and immunotherapy guidelines and recommendations for practice.* Pittsburgh, PA: Oncology Nursing Society.

17 The Joint Commission. (2021). Standard EC.02.02.01. *Comprehensive accreditation manual for hospitals.* Oakbrook Terrace, IL: The Joint Commission. (Level VII)

18 Centers for Medicare and Medicaid Services, Department of Health and Human Services. (2020). Condition of participation: Radiologic services. 42 C.F.R. § 482.26(b)(1).

19 Accreditation Association for Hospitals and Health Systems. (2020). Standard 19.00.03. *Healthcare Facilities Accreditation Program: Accreditation requirements for acute care hospitals.* Chicago, IL: Accreditation Association for Hospitals and Health Systems. (Level VII)

20 DNV GL-Healthcare USA, Inc. (2020). MI.2.SR.1. *NIAHO® accreditation requirements, interpretive guidelines and surveyor guidance—revision 20.0.* Milford, OH: DNV GL-Healthcare USA, Inc. (Level VII)

21 The Joint Commission. (2021). Standard RC.01.03.01. *Comprehensive accreditation manual for hospitals.* Oakbrook Terrace, IL: The Joint Commission. (Level VII)

22 Accreditation Association for Hospitals and Health Systems. (2020). Standard 10.00.03. *Healthcare Facilities Accreditation Program: Accreditation requirements for acute care hospitals.* Chicago, IL: Accreditation Association for Hospitals and Health Systems. (Level VII)

23 Centers for Medicare and Medicaid Services, Department of Health and Human Services. (2020). Condition of participation: Medical record services. 42 C.F.R. § 482.24(b).

24 DNV GL-Healthcare USA, Inc. (2020). MR.2.SR.1. *NIAHO® accreditation requirements, interpretive guidelines and surveyor guidance—revision 20.0.* Milford, OH: DNV GL-Healthcare USA, Inc. (Level VII)

25 Esparza, D. M. (2019). *Oncology policies & procedures* (2nd ed.). Pittsburgh, PA: Oncology Nurses Society.

26 Mitin, T. (2020). Radiation therapy techniques in cancer treatment. In: *UpToDate*, Loeffler, J. S. (Ed.).

27 American Cancer Society. (2020). Radiation therapy side effects. https://www.cancer.org/treatment/treatments-and-side-effects/treatment-types/radiation/effects-on-different-parts-of-body.html

28 American Cancer Society. (2019). Getting internal radiation therapy (brachytherapy). https://www.cancer.org/treatment/treatments-and-side-effects/treatment-types/radiation/internal-radiation-therapy-brachytherapy.html

RADIATION THERAPY, EXTERNAL

Many cancer patients are treated with some form of external radiation therapy. Also called *radiotherapy* or *external beam radiation*, this treatment delivers radiation directly to the cancer site.[1] Radiation therapy in combination with surgery and systemic therapy is gaining widespread use; when used in combination, it controls tumor growth and improves quality of life by minimizing toxicity and preserving the organs.[2]

Radiation doses are based on the type, stage, and location of the tumor as well as on the patient's size, condition, and overall treatment goals. Doses are given in increments, usually three to five times a week, until the total dose is reached, typically 5 to 8 weeks.[1] A radiation oncologist works with a radiation therapist to plan and deliver the treatment.[1]

The goals of radiation therapy include *cure*, in which the cancer is completely destroyed and not expected to recur; *control*, in which the cancer doesn't progress or regress but is expected to progress at some later time; and *palliation*, in which radiation is given to relieve symptoms (such as bone pain, seizures, bleeding, and headache) caused by the cancer.[3]

External radiation therapy is delivered by machines that aim a concentrated beam of high-energy particles (X-rays and gamma rays) at the target site. Two types of machines are commonly used: units containing cobalt or cesium as radioactive sources for gamma rays, and linear accelerators that use electricity to produce X-rays. Linear accelerators produce high energy with great penetrating ability. Radiation therapy may be augmented by chemotherapy, brachytherapy (radiation implant therapy), or surgery, as needed.[3]

Equipment

Radiation therapy machine ▪ Optional: radiation shields, individual positioning device (mold, mask, or cast).

Implementation

▪ Verify the practitioner's order.
▪ If required by your facility, confirm that informed consent has been obtained and that the signed consent form is in the patient's medical record.[4,5,6,7]
▪ Perform hand hygiene.[8,9,10,11,12,13]
▪ Confirm the patient's identity using at least two patient identifiers.[14,15]
▪ Explain the procedure to the patient and family (if appropriate) according to their individual communication and learning needs *to increase their understanding, allay their fears, and enhance cooperation.*[16] Explain that because radiation beams must be delivered to a precise location, a special

mold, mask, or cast may be needed *to help maintain positioning during therapy*.[1,3] Tell the patient that it may be necessary to mark the treatment field with semipermanent ink that will need to remain in place during therapy.[1,17] Review the treatment goals, and discuss the range of potential adverse effects as well as interventions to minimize them. Also discuss possible long-term complications and treatment issues. Educate the patient and family about local cancer services.

■ Review the patient's clinical record for recent laboratory and imaging results, and alert the radiation oncology staff to any abnormalities or pertinent results (such as myelosuppression, paraneoplastic syndromes, oncologic emergencies, and tumor progression).

■ Reassure the patient throughout the treatment planning simulation, during which the target area is mapped out on the body using a machine similar to the radiation therapy machine and is then tattooed or marked in ink on the body *to ensure accurate treatments*.

■ The radiation oncologist determines the duration and frequency of treatments, depending on the patient's body size, size of the portal, extent and location of cancer, and treatment goals.

■ The patient is positioned on the treatment table beneath the machine.[18] Radiation shields may be placed *to protect other areas of the body not receiving treatment*.[1] Treatments last from a few seconds to a few minutes. Reassure the patient that the patient won't feel anything and won't be radioactive.[1]

■ After treatment is complete, the patient may return home or be transported to the hospital room.

■ Perform hand hygiene.[8,9,10,11,12,13]

■ Document the procedure.[19,20,21,22]

Special considerations

■ Make sure that the patient is aware of how to prepare for the specified treatment, such as having a full bladder for prostate radiation, or learning to hold the breath for respiratory gating.[23]

■ Tell the patient to avoid the use of lotions, topical medications, deodorants, perfumes, and powders at the area of the body being treated, unless directed by the practitioner.[1]

■ Encourage the patient to avoid sun exposure even after treatment ends, to wear protective clothing, and to use a sunblock with a sun protection factor of 30 or higher on exposed skin.[24]

■ Refer the patient to a support group, such as a local chapter of the American Cancer Society.

Patient teaching

Emphasize the importance of keeping all scheduled radiation treatment appointments, *because missed appointments may affect treatment outcomes*.[3] Make sure that the patient is aware of how to prepare for the specified treatment, such as having a full bladder for prostate radiation, or learning to hold the breath for respiratory gating.[1,23]

Instruct the patient and family on proper skin care and management of the possible adverse effects of treatment. Instruct the patient to report any long-term adverse effects. Explain to the patient that the full benefit of radiation treatments may not occur until several weeks or months after treatments begin. Stress that the patient isn't considered radioactive at any time during or after treatment. Instruct the patient about the importance of leaving the target area markings intact *to ensure treatment accuracy*. Emphasize the importance of keeping follow-up appointments *so that the practitioner can address treatment outcomes and resolution of signs and symptoms*.

Complications

Adverse effects arise gradually and diminish gradually after treatments. They may be acute, subacute (accumulating as treatment progresses), chronic (after treatment), or long-term (arising months to years after treatment). Adverse effects are localized to the area of treatment, and their severity depends on the total radiation dosage, underlying organ sensitivity, and the patient's overall condition.

Common acute and subacute adverse effects may include altered skin integrity, alopecia, headache, altered GI function (such as xerostomia, nausea, vomiting, diarrhea, and esophagitis) and genitourinary function (such as cystitis), altered sexual function, altered bone marrow production, anxiety, fatigue, and sleep disturbances. Stomatitis and dysphagia can occur and lead to poor oral intake and dehydration.[3,25] Adverse effects during radiation therapy may be increased when the patient receives concurrent chemotherapy and biotherapy.

Long-term complications and adverse effects may include radiation pneumonitis, tissue fibrosis, neuropathy, skin and muscle atrophy, telangiectasia, fistulas, altered endocrine function, infertility, and secondary cancers.

Documentation

Document the date and time of radiation therapy, radiation precautions taken during treatment, and the patient's tolerance of the procedure. Record any adverse effects, interventions used, and the patient's response to the interventions. Document any teaching provided to the patient and family (if applicable), their understanding of that teaching, and any need for follow-up teaching. Note discharge plans and teaching and referrals to local cancer services, if applicable.

REFERENCES

1 American Cancer Society. (2019). Getting external beam radiation therapy. https://www.cancer.org/content/cancer/en/treatment/treatments-and-side-effects/treatment-types/radiation/external-beam-radiation-therapy.html

2 Loeffler, J. S., & Durante, M. (2013). Charged particle therapy—optimization, challenges and future directions. *Nature Reviews: Clinical Oncology, 10*(7), 411–424. https://doi.org/10.1038/nrclinonc.2013.79 (Level VII)

3 Mitin, T. (2020). Radiation therapy techniques in cancer treatment. In: *UpToDate*, Loeffler, J. S. (Ed.).

4 Centers for Medicare and Medicaid Services, Department of Health and Human Services. (2020). Condition of participation: Patient's rights. 42 C.F.R. § 482.13(b)(2).

5 The Joint Commission. (2021). Standard RI.01.03.01. *Comprehensive accreditation manual for hospitals*. Oakbrook Terrace, IL: The Joint Commission. (Level VII)

6 Accreditation Association for Hospitals and Health Systems. (2020). Standard 15.01.11. *Healthcare Facilities Accreditation Program: Accreditation requirements for acute care hospitals*. Chicago, IL: Accreditation Association for Hospitals and Health Systems. (Level VII)

7 DNV GL-Healthcare USA, Inc. (2020). PR.2.SR.3. *NIAHO® accreditation requirements, interpretive guidelines and surveyor guidance—revision 20.0*. Milford, OH: DNV GL-Healthcare USA, Inc. (Level VII)

8 Centers for Disease Control and Prevention. (2002). Guideline for hand hygiene in health-care settings: Recommendations of the Healthcare Infection Control Practices Advisory Committee and the HICPAC/SHEA/APIC/IDSA Hand Hygiene Task Force. *MMWR Recommendations and Reports, 51*(RR-16), 1–45. https://www.cdc.gov/mmwr/pdf/rr/rr5116.pdf (Level II)

9 World Health Organization (WHO). (2009). WHO guidelines on hand hygiene in health care: First global patient safety challenge, clean care is safer care. https://apps.who.int/iris/bitstream/handle/10665/44102/9789241597906_eng.pdf?sequence=1 (Level IV)

10 The Joint Commission. (2021). Standard NPSG.07.01.01. *Comprehensive accreditation manual for hospitals*. Oakbrook Terrace, IL: The Joint Commission. (Level VII)

11 Accreditation Association for Hospitals and Health Systems. (2020). Standard 07.01.21. *Healthcare Facilities Accreditation Program: Accreditation requirements for acute care hospitals*. Chicago, IL: Accreditation Association for Hospitals and Health Systems. (Level VII)

12 Centers for Medicare and Medicaid Services, Department of Health and Human Services. (2020). Condition of participation: Infection control. 42 C.F.R. § 482.42.

13 DNV GL-Healthcare USA, Inc. (2020). IC.1.SR.1. *NIAHO® accreditation requirements, interpretive guidelines and surveyor guidance—revision 20.0*. Milford, OH: DNV GL-Healthcare USA, Inc. (Level VII)

14 The Joint Commission. (2021). Standard NPSG.01.01.01. *Comprehensive accreditation manual for hospitals*. Oakbrook Terrace, IL: The Joint Commission. (Level VII)

15 Accreditation Association for Hospitals and Health Systems. (2020). Standard 30.00.14. *Healthcare Facilities Accreditation Program: Accreditation requirements for acute care hospitals*. Chicago, IL: Accreditation Association for Hospitals and Health Systems. (Level VII)

16 The Joint Commission. (2021). Standard PC.02.01.21. *Comprehensive accreditation manual for hospitals.* Oakbrook Terrace, IL: The Joint Commission. (Level VII)

17 National Cancer Institute. (2018). External beam radiation therapy for cancer. https://www.cancer.gov/about-cancer/treatment/types/radiation-therapy/external-beam

18 American College of Radiology (ACR). (2016). ACR practice parameter for 3D external beam radiation planning and conformal therapy. https://www.acr.org/-/media/ACR/Files/Practice-Parameters/3d-conformal.pdf?la=en (Level VII)

19 The Joint Commission. (2021). Standard RC.01.03.01. *Comprehensive accreditation manual for hospitals.* Oakbrook Terrace, IL: The Joint Commission. (Level VII)

20 Accreditation Association for Hospitals and Health Systems. (2020). Standard 10.00.03. *Healthcare Facilities Accreditation Program: Accreditation requirements for acute care hospitals.* Chicago, IL: Accreditation Association for Hospitals and Health Systems. (Level VII)

21 Centers for Medicare and Medicaid Services, Department of Health and Human Services. (2020). Condition of participation: Medical record services. 42 C.F.R. § 482.24(b).

22 DNV GL-Healthcare USA, Inc. (2020). MR.2.SR.1. *NIAHO® accreditation requirements, interpretive guidelines and surveyor guidance—revision 20.0.* Milford, OH: DNV GL-Healthcare USA, Inc. (Level VII)

23 Iwamoto, R. R., et al. (Eds.). (2012). *Manual for radiation oncology nursing practice and education* (4th ed.). Pittsburgh, PA: Oncology Nursing Society.

24 American Cancer Society. (2020). Radiation therapy: What it is, how it helps. https://www.cancer.org/content/dam/cancer-org/cancer-control/en/booklets-flyers/radiation-therapy-what-it-is-how-it-helps.pdf

25 National Cancer Institute. (2018). Radiation therapy side effects. https://www.cancer.gov/about-cancer/treatment/types/radiation-therapy/side-effects

RADIOACTIVE IODINE THERAPY

Because the thyroid gland concentrates iodine, radioactive iodine-131 (^{131}I) can be used to treat thyroid cancer. Also called *radioiodine,* this isotope is usually administered orally and used to treat postoperative residual cancer, recurrent disease, inoperable primary thyroid tumors, invasion of the thyroid capsule, and thyroid ablation, as well as cancers that have metastasized to cervical or mediastinal lymph nodes or other distant sites. Radioiodine is usually given orally as a solution or a capsule. The radioiodine is rapidly incorporated into the thyroid, and its beta-emissions result in extensive local tissue damage.[1]

Because ^{131}I is absorbed systemically, all body secretions, especially urine, must be considered radioactive. For ^{131}I treatments, the patient is usually placed in a private room (with its own bathroom) located as far away from high-traffic areas as practical. Adjacent rooms and hallways may also need to be restricted. Health care workers caring for a patient who is undergoing radioactive iodine therapy must take precautions as directed by the facility.

In lower doses, ^{131}I also may be used to treat hyperthyroidism. Most patients receive this treatment on an outpatient basis and are sent home with appropriate home care instructions.

Equipment

Patient's medical record ▪ film badges or ring badges ▪ RADIATION PRECAUTION sign for door ▪ RADIATION PRECAUTION warning labels ▪ waterproof gowns ▪ gloves ▪ hazardous-waste containers ▪ sealable leak-proof trash bags (clear and red) ▪ sealable leak-proof bags ▪ nondisposable radioresistant gloves ▪ emergency tracheotomy tray ▪ Optional: portable lead shield, pocket dosimeter.

Preparation of equipment

Gather all necessary equipment in the patient's room. Keep a hazardous-waste container lined with a clear and then a red leak-proof bag in the patient's room. Keep sealable leak-proof bags in the patient's room for containing linens. Do not remove objects from the patient's room until they've been scanned and cleared by the radiation safety officer.[2,3]

Inspect all equipment and supplies. If a product is expired, is defective, or has compromised integrity, remove it from patient use, label it as expired or defective, and report the expiration or defect as directed by your facility.

Keep an emergency tracheotomy tray just outside the room or in a handy place at the nurses' station *because of the potential for neck swelling following treatment.*

Implementation

▪ Verify the practitioner's order.
▪ Review the patient's health history for vomiting, diarrhea, productive cough, and sinus drainage, *which could increase the risk of radioactive secretions.*
▪ Check the patient's medical history for allergies to iodine-containing substances, such as contrast media and shellfish. Review the medication history for thyroid-containing or thyroid-altering drugs; for lithium carbonate, *which may increase* ^{131}I *uptake;* and for drugs with high iodine content, such as amiodarone, *which may decrease* ^{131}I *uptake.*[4]
▪ If required by your facility, confirm that informed consent has been obtained, and that the signed consent form is in the patient's medical record.[3,5,6,7,8]
▪ Perform hand hygiene.[9,10,11,12,13,14]
▪ Confirm the patient's identity using at least two patient identifiers.[15,16]
▪ Explain the procedure to the patient and family (if appropriate) according to their individual communication and learning needs *to increase their understanding, allay their fears, and enhance cooperation.*[17] Review treatment goals with the patient and family. Before treatment begins, review with the patient your facility's radiation safety and visitation procedures, potential adverse effects, interventions, and home care procedures.[3]
▪ Ensure that all ordered laboratory tests are performed before beginning treatment.[3] The American College of Radiology recommends a human chorionic gonadotropin test be performed within 24 hours of treatment of women of childbearing potential *to ensure that the patient isn't pregnant.*[18]
▪ If necessary, remove the patient's dentures *to avoid contaminating them and to reduce radioactive secretions.* Tell the patient the dentures will be returned 48 hours after treatment.

After the treatment

▪ Place the RADIATION PRECAUTION sign on the door.
▪ Place a RADIATION PRECAUTION label in the patient's medical record *to ensure staff awareness of the patient's radioactive status.*
▪ Affix a RADIATION PRECAUTION label to the patient's identification band.
▪ Notify the dietitian to supply foods and beverages only in disposable containers and with disposable utensils.[19]
▪ Encourage the patient to use the toilet rather than a bedpan or urinal, and to flush it two or three times after each use *to reduce radiation levels.*[3,18,20] *To help avoid splash and aerosol contamination,* instruct the patient to sit while urinating and close the lid or cover the toilet before flushing.[18]
▪ Tell the patient to remain in the room except for tests or procedures.[3,18] Allow the patient to ambulate.
▪ Unless contraindicated, instruct the patient to increase fluid intake to 3 qt (3 L) daily *to help flush the iodine from the body's system.*
▪ Encourage the patient to chew or suck on hard candy *to keep salivary glands stimulated and prevent them from becoming inflamed (inflammation can develop in the first 24 hours).*
▪ If laboratory testing is required, a laboratory technician equipped with a radiation badge obtains the specimen; labels it with the patient's name, identification number, and the date and time of the collection in the presence of the patient *to prevent mislabeling;*[15] affixes the specimen with a RADIATION PRECAUTION warning label; and alerts laboratory department personnel before transporting it. If urine tests are needed, ask the radiation oncology department or laboratory technician how to transport the specimens safely.
▪ Each nurse must wear a personal, nontransferable ring badge or a film badge placed at or above waist level for the entire shift.[19] The badge must only be worn within the work environment. *Badges document each person's cumulative lifetime radiation exposure.* Only primary caregivers should

have a badge and be permitted in the patient's room.[2] Turn in the radiation badge monthly or as directed by your facility, and be sure to record your exposures accurately.

■ If using a pocket dosimeter, be aware that these devices measure immediate exposures to radiation. *In many facilities, these measurements aren't part of the permanent exposure record but are used to ensure that nurses receive the lowest possible exposure.*

■ Wear gloves to touch the patient or objects in the room. Any item that the patient touches must be kept in the room.[19]

■ Wear a waterproof gown and gloves when handling the patient's body secretions (for example, when moving the emesis basin).

■ Restrict visiting time to 30 minutes every 24 hours *to limit radiation exposure.*[3,19] Stress that visitors who are pregnant or trying to conceive or father a child won't be allowed to visit the patient.

PEDIATRIC ALERT Visitors younger than age 18 shouldn't be permitted to visit a patient receiving ^{131}I therapy.[19]

■ Restrict direct contact to 30 minutes or 20 millirems per day. If the patient is receiving 200 millicuries of ^{131}I, remain with the patient only 2 to 4 minutes and stand no closer than 1' (30 cm) away. If standing 3' (1 M) away, the time limit is 20 minutes; if standing 5' (1.5 M) away, the limit is 30 minutes.

■ Perform only essential nursing care, limiting time in the room.

■ Make sure that perineal wipes, sanitary pads, and similar items are bagged correctly.

■ If the patient vomits or urinates on the floor, notify the nuclear medicine department, and use nondisposable radioresistant gloves when cleaning the floor. After cleanup, wash your gloved hands, and remove the gloves and leave them in the room. Then rewash your hands.

■ If the patient must be moved from the room, notify the appropriate department of the patient's status *so that receiving personnel can make appropriate arrangements to receive the patient.* When moving the patient, ensure that the route is clear of equipment and other people, and that the elevator (if one is present) is keyed and ready to receive the patient. Move the patient in a bed or wheelchair, accompanied by two badged caregivers. If you're delayed during transport, stand as far away from the patient as possible until you can continue.

■ Ensure the patient's room is monitored and cleaned by the radiation oncology department, not by housekeeping. The room must be monitored daily, and disposable items must be monitored and removed according to your facility's guidelines.

■ At discharge, schedule the patient for a follow-up examination. Also arrange for a whole-body scan approximately 7 to 10 days after ^{131}I treatment, as ordered.

■ Inform the patient and family of community support services for cancer patients.

■ Perform hand hygiene.[9,10,11,12,13,14]

■ Document the procedure.[21,22,23,24]

Special considerations

■ Nurses and visitors who are pregnant or trying to conceive or father a child must not attend or visit patients receiving ^{131}I therapy, *because the gonads and developing embryo and fetus are highly susceptible to the damaging effects of ionizing radiation.*

■ If a code is called on a patient undergoing ^{131}I therapy, follow your facility's guidelines.[19]

■ If the patient dies on the unit, notify the radiology safety officer, who will determine which precautions to follow before postmortem care is provided and before the body can be removed to the morgue.

Patient teaching

Teach the patient and family (if appropriate) about special precautions that will need to be followed when the patient returns home. (See *What to do after ^{131}I treatment.*)

Complications

Myelosuppression is common in patients who undergo repeated ^{131}I treatments. Radiation pulmonary fibrosis and pneumonitis may develop if extensive lung metastasis was present when ^{131}I was administered.[18]

What to do after ^{131}I treatment

■ Instruct the patient to report any long-term adverse reactions. In particular, review signs and symptoms of hypothyroidism and hyperthyroidism. Also ask the patient to report any signs and symptoms of thyroid cancer, such as enlarged lymph nodes, dyspnea, bone pain, nausea, vomiting, and abdominal discomfort.

■ Although the patient's radiation level at discharge will be safe, suggest that the patient take extra precautions during the period of time established by the practitioner, such as using separate eating utensils, sleeping in a separate bedroom, and avoiding body contact.[1,3,18]

■ Instruct the patient to follow the practitioner's directions regarding resumption of sexual intercourse after ^{131}I treatment; however, urge both male and female patients to avoid pregnancy for 6 to 12 months after treatment.[3,18] Inform a male patient that he may have decreased sperm counts and temporary infertility for 1 year or more. Provide information about the option of sperm banking before treatment begins.

■ A patient who is breastfeeding should discontinue breastfeeding at least 6 weeks before treatment because a lactating breast absorbs a large amount of radioactive iodine, which is then passed through the milk to the infant. Explain that no breastfeeding restrictions are necessary with subsequent pregnancies.[18]

Secondary malignancy and transient decreased sperm or ovarian function may also occur.[4,18]

Other potential complications include nausea, vomiting, headache, radiation thyroiditis, fever, sialadenitis, excessive tearing, loss or alteration in taste, tumor hemorrhage, and neck pain and swelling.[4,18]

Documentation

Record the date and time of therapy, radiation precautions taken during and after treatment, and the patient's tolerance of the procedure. Record any adverse effects of the therapy, any interventions taken, and the patient's response to those interventions. Document teaching provided to the patient and family (if applicable), their understanding of that teaching, and any need for follow-up teaching. Note referrals to local cancer counseling services.

REFERENCES

1 American Thyroid Association Taskforce on Radioiodine Safety, et al. (2011). Radiation safety in the treatment of patients with thyroid diseases by radioiodine 131I: Practice recommendations of the American Thyroid Association. *Thyroid, 21*(4), 335–346. http://www.thyca.org/download/document/184/ataradiation.pdf (Level VII)

2 Olsen, M. M., et al. (Eds.). (2019). *Chemotherapy and immunotherapy guidelines and recommendations for practice.* Pittsburgh, PA: Oncology Nursing Society.

3 American College of Radiology (ACR). (2015, revised 2019). ACR-ACNM-ASTRO-SNMMI practice parameter for the performance of therapy with unsealed radiopharmaceutical sources. https://www.acr.org/-/media/ACR/Files/Practice-Parameters/unsealedsources.pdf?la=en (Level VII)

4 Tuttle, R. M. (2020). Differentiated thyroid cancer: Radioiodine treatment. In: *UpToDate*, Ross, D. S. (Ed.).

5 Centers for Medicare and Medicaid Services, Department of Health and Human Services. (2020). Condition of participation: Patient's rights. 42 C.F.R. § 482.13(b)(2).

6 The Joint Commission. (2021). Standard RI.01.03.01. *Comprehensive accreditation manual for hospitals.* Oakbrook Terrace, IL: The Joint Commission. (Level VII)

7 Accreditation Association for Hospitals and Health Systems. (2020). Standard 15.01.11. *Healthcare Facilities Accreditation Program: Accreditation requirements for acute care hospitals.* Chicago, IL: Accreditation Association for Hospitals and Health Systems. (Level VII)

8 DNV GL-Healthcare USA, Inc. (2020). PR.2.SR.3. *NIAHO® accreditation requirements, interpretive guidelines and surveyor guidance—revision 20.0.* Milford, OH: DNV GL-Healthcare USA, Inc. (Level VII)

9 Centers for Disease Control and Prevention. (2002). Guideline for hand hygiene in health-care settings: Recommendations of the Healthcare Infection Control Practices Advisory Committee and the HICPAC/SHEA/APIC/IDSA Hand Hygiene Task Force. *MMWR Recommendations and Reports, 51*(RR-16), 1–45. https://www.cdc.gov/mmwr/pdf/rr/rr5116.pdf (Level II)

10 World Health Organization (WHO). (2009). WHO guidelines on hand hygiene in health care: First global patient safety challenge, clean care is safer care. https://apps.who.int/iris/bitstream/handle/10665/44102/9789241597906_eng.pdf?sequence=1 (Level IV)

11 The Joint Commission. (2021). Standard NPSG.07.01.01. *Comprehensive accreditation manual for hospitals.* Oakbrook Terrace, IL: The Joint Commission. (Level VII)

12 Accreditation Association for Hospitals and Health Systems. (2020). Standard 07.01.21. *Healthcare Facilities Accreditation Program: Accreditation requirements for acute care hospitals.* Chicago, IL: Accreditation Association for Hospitals and Health Systems. (Level VII)

13 Centers for Medicare and Medicaid Services, Department of Health and Human Services. (2020). Condition of participation: Infection control. 42 C.F.R. § 482.42.

14 DNV GL-Healthcare USA, Inc. (2020). IC.1.SR.1. *NIAHO® accreditation requirements, interpretive guidelines and surveyor guidance—revision 20.0.* Milford, OH: DNV GL-Healthcare USA, Inc. (Level VII)

15 The Joint Commission. (2021). Standard NPSG.01.01.01. *Comprehensive accreditation manual for hospitals.* Oakbrook Terrace, IL: The Joint Commission. (Level VII)

16 Accreditation Association for Hospitals and Health Systems. (2020). Standard 30.00.14. *Healthcare Facilities Accreditation Program: Accreditation requirements for acute care hospitals.* Chicago, IL: Accreditation Association for Hospitals and Health Systems. (Level VII)

17 The Joint Commission. (2021). Standard PC.02.01.21. *Comprehensive accreditation manual for hospitals.* Oakbrook Terrace, IL: The Joint Commission. (Level VII)

18 American College of Radiology (ACR). (2019). ACR-ACNM-ASTRO-SNMMI-SPR practice parameter for treatment of benign and malignant thyroid disease with I-131 sodium iodide. https://www.acr.org/-/media/ACR/Files/Practice-Parameters/I131SodiumIodide.pdf (Level VII)

19 Beck, M. (2015). Radiation safety in the management of patients undergoing radioactive iodine ablation therapy. *Clinical Journal of Oncology Nursing, 19*(1), 44. https://doi.org/10.1188/15.cjon.44-46

20 American Thyroid Association. (2014). Radioactive iodine. http://www.thyroid.org/wp-content/uploads/patients/brochures/Radioactive_iodine_brochure.pdf

21 The Joint Commission. (2021). Standard RC.01.03.01. *Comprehensive accreditation manual for hospitals.* Oakbrook Terrace, IL: The Joint Commission. (Level VII)

22 Accreditation Association for Hospitals and Health Systems. (2020). Standard 10.00.03. *Healthcare Facilities Accreditation Program: Accreditation requirements for acute care hospitals.* Chicago, IL: Accreditation Association for Hospitals and Health Systems. (Level VII)

23 Centers for Medicare and Medicaid Services, Department of Health and Human Services. (2020). Condition of participation: Medical record services. 42 C.F.R. § 482.24(b).

24 DNV GL-Healthcare USA, Inc. (2020). MR.2.SR.1. *NIAHO® accreditation requirements, interpretive guidelines and surveyor guidance—revision 20.0.* Milford, OH: DNV GL-Healthcare USA, Inc. (Level VII)

Rectal suppository and ointment administration

A rectal suppository is a small, solid, medicated mass, usually cone-shaped, with a cocoa butter or glycerin base, intended as a single-dose rectal application.[1,2] It can help stimulate peristalsis and defecation or relieve pain, vomiting, and local irritation. Rectal suppositories commonly contain drugs that reduce fever and induce relaxation but that can't be given orally *because they interact poorly with digestive enzymes or have an offensive taste.* They may also help when a patient can't take medications orally because of nausea, vomiting, or another GI condition. Rectal suppositories melt at body temperature and are absorbed slowly by the rectal mucosa. Suppositories aren't used for colon cleansing for a scheduled colonoscopy *because they only exert their effect on the distal colon.*[3]

Because insertion of a rectal suppository may stimulate the vagus nerve, this procedure is contraindicated in patients who have the potential for cardiac arrhythmias. It may also be contraindicated in patients who have active rectal bleeding or recent rectal or prostate surgery *because of the risk of local trauma or discomfort during insertion.* The rectal route for medication administration isn't recommended for use in patients with immunosuppression or thrombocytopenia *because of the risk of infection and bleeding.*[4,5]

An ointment is a semisolid medication used to produce local effects when applied externally to the anus or internally to the rectum with an applicator. Rectal ointments often contain drugs that reduce inflammation or relieve pain and itching. Rectal medications may also be used when a patient is vomiting, unable to swallow, or unconscious.[1] They should be used with caution in patients who have a history of rectal ulcers or fissures.

Equipment

Prescribed rectal suppository or ointment ▪ patient's medication administration record ▪ gloves ▪ water-soluble lubricant ▪ 4″ × 4″ (10 cm × 10 cm) gauze pads ▪ soap and water ▪ tissues ▪ Optional: bedpan, other personal protective equipment, cleansing wipes or washcloth, towel.

Implementation

▪ Avoid distractions and interruptions when preparing and administering medications *to prevent medication administration errors.*[6,7]
▪ Verify the practitioner's order.[8,9,10,11]
▪ Reconcile the patient's medications when the practitioner orders a new medication *to reduce the risk of medication errors, including omissions, duplications, dosing errors, and drug interactions.*[12,13]
▪ Gather and prepare the necessary equipment and supplies.
▪ Compare the medication label with the order in the patient's medical record.[8,9,10,11]
▪ Check the patient's medical record for an allergy or a contraindication to the prescribed medication. If an allergy or a contraindication exists, don't administer the medication and notify the practitioner.[8,9,10,11]
▪ Check the expiration date on the medication. If the medication is expired, return it to the pharmacy and obtain a new medication.[8,9,10,11]
▪ Visually inspect the medication for discoloration or any other loss of integrity; don't administer the medication if its integrity is compromised.[8,9,10,11]
▪ Discuss any unresolved concerns about the medication with the patient's practitioner.[8,9,10,11]
▪ Perform hand hygiene.[14,15,16,17,18,19]
▪ Confirm the patient's identity using at least two patient identifiers.[20]
▪ Provide privacy.[21,22,23,24]
▪ Explain the procedure to the patient and family (if appropriate) according to their individual communication and learning needs *to increase their understanding, allay their fears, and enhance cooperation.*[25]
▪ If the patient is receiving the medication for the first time, teach the patient and family (if appropriate) about potential adverse reactions and discuss any other concerns related to administering the medication.[8,9,10,11]
▪ Verify that the medication is being administered at the proper time, in the prescribed dose, and by the correct route *to reduce the risk of medication errors.*[8,9,10,11]
▪ If your facility uses a bar code technology, use it as directed by your facility.
▪ Raise the patient's bed to waist level before providing patient care *to prevent caregiver back strain.*[26]
▪ Perform hand hygiene.[14,15,16,17,18,19]

NURSING ALERT If your facility's hazardous drug list contains the medication you're about to administer, put on personal protective equipment as directed.[27]

▪ Put on gloves *to comply with standard precautions.*[28,29,30]
▪ Position the patient on the left side in the Sims position. Drape the patient with the bedcovers *to expose only the buttocks.*

Rectal suppository administration

▪ Remove the suppository from its wrapper and lubricate it with water-soluble lubricant.
▪ Lift the patient's upper buttock with your nondominant hand *to expose the anus.*

How to administer a rectal suppository

When inserting a suppository, direct its tapered end toward the side of the rectum *so that it contacts the membranes, which encourages absorption of the medication.*

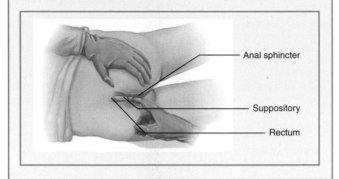

Anal sphincter

Suppository

Rectum

How to administer rectal ointment

When applying a rectal ointment internally, be sure to lubricate the applicator *to minimize pain on insertion.* Direct the applicator tip toward the patient's umbilicus.

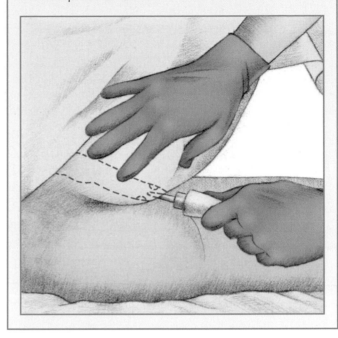

- Instruct the patient to take several deep breaths through the mouth *to help relax the anal sphincters and reduce anxiety or discomfort during insertion.*
- Using the index finger of your dominant hand, insert the suppository—tapered end first—about 1″ (2.5 cm), until you feel it pass the internal anal sphincter, *to prevent expulsion.*[31] Ensure the suppository is in direct contact with the rectal wall.[3] Direct the tapered end toward the side of the rectum *so that it contacts the membranes.* (See *How to administer a rectal suppository.*)
- Ensure the patient's comfort and make sure the patient can reach the call light. Encourage the patient to lie still and, if applicable, to squeeze or hold the buttocks together *to retain the suppository for the appropriate time.* The patient should retain a suppository administered to relieve constipation as long as possible (at least 20 minutes) to be effective. If appropriate, keep a bedpan close by to place underneath the patient in case there's difficulty retaining the suppository.

Rectal ointment administration
To apply externally
- Clean the affected area using a cleansing wipe or a washcloth, soap, and water. Gently pat or blot the area dry with a tissue or soft towel.
- Squeeze the required amount of ointment onto your gloved finger or a gauze pad. Lift the patient's upper buttock with your nondominant hand *to expose the anus.* Spread the ointment over the anal area.

To apply internally
- Expect to use about 1″ (2.5 cm) of ointment. *To gauge how much pressure to use during application,* squeeze a small amount from the tube before you attach the applicator. Then attach the applicator to the tube of ointment and coat the applicator with water-soluble lubricant.
- Lift the patient's upper buttock with your nondominant hand *to expose the anus.*
- Instruct the patient to take several deep breaths through the mouth *to relax the anal sphincters and reduce anxiety or discomfort during insertion.*
- Gently insert the applicator, directing it toward the umbilicus. (See *How to administer rectal ointment.*)
- Slowly squeeze the tube *to eject the medication.*
- Remove the applicator and place a folded 4″ × 4″ (10 cm × 10 cm) gauze pad between the patient's buttocks *to absorb excess ointment.*
- Detach the applicator from the tube and recap the tube.

Completing the procedure
- Return the bed to the lowest position *to prevent falls and maintain patient safety.*[32]
- Remove and discard your gloves and, if worn, other personal protective equipment.[28,30]

- Perform hand hygiene.[14,15,16,17,18,19]
- Document the procedure.[33,34,35,36]

Special considerations
- Store rectal suppositories in a cool, dry place *to avoid melting.* Refrigerate them if directed by the medications label.[37]
- Inform the patient that the suppository may discolor the next bowel movement. For example, hydrocortisone suppositories can give feces a silver-gray, pasty appearance.
- Advise the patient to report any increase in itching or burning in the rectal area.

Patient teaching
Some rectal suppositories and ointments are available over the counter. Teach the patient how to self-administer the suppositories or ointment if appropriate. A patient experiencing constipation may need further teaching about proper diet, hydration, daily exercise, and proper use of laxatives.[3]

Complications
Complications may be related to the action of the medication. Occasionally, vagal nerve stimulation may occur, causing a vagal reaction. Defecation can cause early expulsion of the suppository, resulting in incomplete absorption.[38] Other potential complications include local reactions, such as tissue irritation[39,40] and rectal bleeding.

Documentation
Document the medication strength, dose, administration route, and date and time of administration. Record any adverse reactions to the prescribed medication, the date and time that the practitioner was notified, prescribed interventions, and the patient's response to them.[41] Document the patient's tolerance of the procedure and response to therapy. Document teaching provided to the patient and family (if applicable), their understanding of that teaching, and any need for follow-up teaching.

References

1 Emblin, K. (2013). Drug formulations and delivery systems. *Nurse Prescribing, 11*, 83–88.

2 World Health Organization. (2020). The international pharmacopoeia (10th ed.): Rectal preparations. http://apps.who.int/phint/pdf/b/6.2.1.6.Rectal-preparations.pdf

3 Daniels, G., & Schmelzer, M. (2013). Giving laxatives safely and effectively. *MedSurg Nursing, 22*, 290–302. (Level VII)

4 Thom, K. A., et al. (2013). Infection prevention in the cancer center. *Clinical Infectious Diseases, 57*(4), 579–585. https://www.ncbi.nlm.nih.gov/pmc/articles/PMC3726067/ (Level VII)

5 OncoLink Team. (2020). Low platelet count (thrombocytopenia). https://www.oncolink.org/support/side-effects/low-blood-counts/low-platelet-count-thrombocytopenia

6 Westbrook, J., et al. (2010). Association of interruptions with an increased risk and severity of medication administration errors. *Archives of Internal Medicine, 170*, 683–690. (Level IV)

7 Institute for Safe Medication Practices. (2012). Side tracks on the safety express: Interruptions lead to errors and unfinished…Wait, what was I doing? *Nurse Advise-ERR, 11*(2), 1–4. https://www.ismp.org/resources/side-tracks-safety-express-interruptions-lead-errors-and-unfinished-wait-what-was-i-doing?id=37

8 Centers for Medicare and Medicaid Services, Department of Health and Human Services. (2020). Condition of participation: Nursing services. 42 C.F.R. § 482.23(c).

9 DNV GL-Healthcare USA, Inc. (2020). MM.1.SR.3. *NIAHO® accreditation requirements, interpretive guidelines and surveyor guidance—revision 20.0.* Milford, OH: DNV GL-Healthcare USA, Inc. (Level VII)

10 Accreditation Association for Hospitals and Health Systems. (2020). Standard 16.01.03. *Healthcare Facilities Accreditation Program: Accreditation requirements for acute care hospitals.* Chicago, IL: Accreditation Association for Hospitals and Health Systems. (Level VII)

11 The Joint Commission. (2021). Standard MM.06.01.01. *Comprehensive accreditation manual for hospitals.* Oakbrook Terrace, IL: The Joint Commission. (Level VII)

12 Accreditation Association for Hospitals and Health Systems. (2020). Standard 25.02.13. *Healthcare Facilities Accreditation Program: Accreditation requirements for acute care hospitals.* Chicago, IL: Accreditation Association for Hospitals and Health Systems. (Level VII)

13 The Joint Commission. (2021). Standard NPSG.03.06.01. *Comprehensive accreditation manual for hospitals.* Oakbrook Terrace, IL: The Joint Commission. (Level VII)

14 The Joint Commission. (2021). Standard NPSG.07.01.01. *Comprehensive accreditation manual for hospitals.* Oakbrook Terrace, IL: The Joint Commission. (Level VII)

15 Centers for Disease Control and Prevention. (2002). Guideline for hand hygiene in health-care settings: Recommendations of the Healthcare Infection Control Practices Advisory Committee and the HICPAC/SHEA/APIC/IDSA Hand Hygiene Task Force. *MMWR Recommendations and Reports, 51*(RR-16), 1–45. https://www.cdc.gov/mmwr/pdf/rr/rr5116.pdf (Level II)

16 World Health Organization. (2009). WHO guidelines on hand hygiene in health care: First global patient safety challenge, clean care is safer care. https://apps.who.int/iris/bitstream/handle/10665/44102/9789241597906_eng.pdf?sequence=1 (Level IV)

17 Accreditation Association for Hospitals and Health Systems. (2020). Standard 07.01.21. *Healthcare Facilities Accreditation Program: Accreditation requirements for acute care hospitals.* Chicago, IL: Accreditation Association for Hospitals and Health Systems. (Level VII)

18 Centers for Medicare and Medicaid Services, Department of Health and Human Services. (2020). Condition of participation: Infection control. 42 C.F.R. § 482.42.

19 DNV GL-Healthcare USA, Inc. (2020). IC.1.SR.1. *NIAHO® accreditation requirements, interpretive guidelines and surveyor guidance—revision 20.0.* Milford, OH: DNV GL-Healthcare USA, Inc. (Level VII)

20 The Joint Commission. (2021). Standard NPSG.01.01.01. *Comprehensive accreditation manual for hospitals.* Oakbrook Terrace, IL: The Joint Commission. (Level VII)

21 Centers for Medicare and Medicaid Services, Department of Health and Human Services. (2020). Condition of participation: Patient's rights. 42 C.F.R. § 482.13(c)(1).

22 DNV GL-Healthcare USA, Inc. (2020). PR.2.SR.5. *NIAHO® accreditation requirements, interpretive guidelines and surveyor guidance—revision 20.0.* Milford, OH: DNV GL-Healthcare USA, Inc. (Level VII)

23 Accreditation Association for Hospitals and Health Systems. (2020). Standard 15.01.16. *Healthcare Facilities Accreditation Program: Accreditation requirements for acute care hospitals.* Chicago, IL: Accreditation Association for Hospitals and Health Systems. (Level VII)

24 The Joint Commission. (2021). Standard RI.01.01.01. *Comprehensive accreditation manual for hospitals.* Oakbrook Terrace, IL: The Joint Commission. (Level VII)

25 The Joint Commission. (2021). Standard PC.02.01.21. *Comprehensive accreditation manual for hospitals.* Oakbrook Terrace, IL: The Joint Commission. (Level VII)

26 Waters, T. R., et al. (2009). Safe patient handling training for schools of nursing. https://www.cdc.gov/niosh/docs/2009-127/pdfs/2009-127.pdf (Level VII)

27 United States Pharmacopeial Convention. (2020). USP general chapter <800> hazardous drugs—handling in healthcare settings. https://www.usp.org/compounding/general-chapter-hazardous-drugs-handling-healthcare (Level VII)

28 Siegel, J. D., et al. (2007, revised 2019). 2007 guideline for isolation precautions: Preventing transmission of infectious agents in healthcare settings. https://www.cdc.gov/infectioncontrol/pdf/guidelines/isolation-guidelines-H.pdf (Level II)

29 Accreditation Association for Hospitals and Health Systems. (2020). Standard 07.01.10. *Healthcare Facilities Accreditation Program: Accreditation requirements for acute care hospitals.* Chicago, IL: Accreditation Association for Hospitals and Health Systems. (Level VII)

30 Occupational Safety and Health Administration. (2019). Bloodborne pathogens, standard number 1910.1030. https://www.osha.gov/pls/oshaweb/owadisp.show_document?p_id=10051&p_table=STANDARDS (Level VII)

31 Craven, R. F., et al. (2020). *Fundamentals of nursing: Concepts and competencies for practice* (9th ed.). Philadelphia, PA: Wolters Kluwer.

32 Ganz, D. A., et al. (2013, reviewed 2021). *Preventing falls in hospitals: A toolkit for improving quality of care* (AHRQ Publication No. 13-0015-EF). Rockville, MD: Agency for Healthcare Research and Quality. https://www.ahrq.gov/professionals/systems/hospital/fallpxtoolkit/index.html (Level VII)

33 Accreditation Association for Hospitals and Health Systems. (2020). Standard 10.00.03. *Healthcare Facilities Accreditation Program: Accreditation requirements for acute care hospitals.* Chicago, IL: Accreditation Association for Hospitals and Health Systems. (Level VII)

34 Centers for Medicare and Medicaid Services, Department of Health and Human Services. (2020). Condition of participation: Medical record services. 42 C.F.R. § 482.24(b).

35 DNV GL-Healthcare USA, Inc. (2020). MR.2.SR.1. *NIAHO® accreditation requirements, interpretive guidelines and surveyor guidance—revision 20.0.* Milford, OH: DNV GL-Healthcare USA, Inc. (Level VII)

36 The Joint Commission. (2021). Standard RC.01.03.01. *Comprehensive accreditation manual for hospitals.* Oakbrook Terrace, IL: The Joint Commission. (Level VII)

37 American Society of Health-System Pharmacists (ASHP). (2021). Safe medication: How to use rectal suppositories. https://www.safemedication.com/how-to-use-medication/rectal-suppositories

38 Hua, S. (2019). Physiological and pharmaceutical considerations for rectal drug formulations. *Frontiers in Pharmacology, 10*, 1196. https://www.frontiersin.org/articles/10.3389/fphar.2019.01196/full (Level V)

39 Multum, C. (2021). Hydrocortisone rectal (cream, ointment, suppository). https://www.drugs.com/mtm/hydrocortisone-rectal-cream-ointment-suppository.html

40 ProStrakan, Inc. (2011). RECTIV (nitroglycerin) ointment 0.4% for intra-anal use: Prescribing information. https://www.accessdata.fda.gov/drugsatfda_docs/label/2011/021359s000lbl.pdf

41 The Joint Commission. (2021). Standard RC.02.01.01. *Comprehensive accreditation manual for hospitals.* Oakbrook Terrace, IL: The Joint Commission. (Level VII)

Rectal tube insertion and removal

Decreased gastrointestinal (GI) motility may result from various medical or surgical conditions, certain medications (such as atropine and opioids), colonoscopy, or even swallowed air, resulting in abdominal discomfort and bloating. Inserting a rectal tube may relieve the discomfort of distention and flatus in these situations.[1]

Contraindications to rectal tube insertion include recent rectal or prostatic surgery, recent myocardial infarction, allergies to the rectal tube material, and diseases or injuries of the rectal mucosa.[2,3]

Equipment

Stethoscope ▪ fluid-impermeable pads ▪ drape ▪ water-soluble lubricant ▪ commercial kit or #22 to #34 French rectal tube of soft rubber or plastic ▪ tape ▪ gloves ▪ perineal care supplies ▪ disinfectant pad ▪ Optional: collection container, other personal protective equipment, clean linens, labels.

Implementation

- Verify the practitioner's order.
- Review the patient's medical record for a history of allergies to rectal tube materials and contraindications to rectal tube insertion.[2]
- Gather and prepare the necessary equipment and supplies.
- Perform hand hygiene.[4,5,6,7,8,9]
- Confirm the patient's identity using at least two patient identifiers.[10]
- Provide privacy.[11,12,13,14]
- Explain the procedure to the patient and family (if appropriate) according to their individual communication and learning needs *to increase their understanding, allay their fears, and enhance cooperation.*[15]
- Raise the patient's bed to waist level before providing patient care *to prevent caregiver back strain.*[16]
- Perform hand hygiene.[4,5,6,7,8,9]
- Put on gloves and, as needed, other personal protective equipment *to comply with standard precautions.*[17,18,19]
- Assess the patient for abdominal distention.
- Using the stethoscope, auscultate for bowel sounds.
- Place fluid-impermeable pads under the patient's buttocks *to absorb any drainage that may leak from the rectal tube.*[3]

Inserting the tube

- Place the patient in the left-lateral Sims position *to facilitate rectal tube insertion.*[3]
- Drape the patient's exposed buttocks *to maintain the patient's dignity and privacy.*
- Lubricate the rectal tube tip with water-soluble lubricant *to ease insertion and prevent rectal irritation.*[3,20]
- Lift the patient's right buttock *to expose the anus.*
- Insert the rectal tube tip into the patient's anus. As you insert the tube, instruct the patient to breathe slowly and deeply,[3] or suggest that the patient bear down as if having a bowel movement *to relax the anal sphincter and ease tube insertion.*
- Advance the tube 2″ to 4″ (5 to 10 cm) into the rectum (as shown below).[3,20] Direct the tube toward the umbilicus along the anatomic course of the patient's large intestine. Never force a rectal tube if you feel an obstruction.[3]

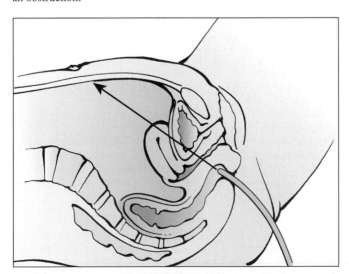

- Using tape, secure the rectal tube to the patient's buttocks.
- If necessary, attach the tube to a collection container *to collect possible leakage.*

- Route the rectal tubing in a standardized direction, if tubing and catheters for different purposes are present. Label the tubing at the distal end (near the patient connection) and proximal end (near the source container) *to reduce the risk of misconnection,* if the patient has multiple tubing and catheters.[21,22]
- Remove and discard your gloves and, if worn, other personal protective equipment.[19]
- Perform hand hygiene.[4,5,6,7,8,9]

Removing the tube

- Perform hand hygiene.[4,5,6,7,8,9]
- Put on gloves and, as needed, other personal protective equipment *to comply with standard precautions.*[17,18,19]
- Remove the tape carefully from the patient's buttocks and then remove the rectal tube after it has been in place for 20 minutes.[20] If the patient reports continued discomfort or if gas wasn't expelled, you can repeat the procedure in 2 or 3 hours if ordered.

Completing the procedure

- Perform perineal care, and replace soiled linens and fluid-impermeable pads if necessary. Ensure the patient feels as comfortable as possible.
- Assess the patient for abdominal distention and auscultate for bowel sounds.
- Return the bed to its lowest position *to prevent falls and maintain patient safety.*[23]
- Discard used supplies in appropriate receptacles.[19].
- Remove and discard your gloves and, if worn, any other personal protective equipment .[19]
- Perform hand hygiene.[4,5,6,7,8,9]
- Clean and disinfect your stethoscope using a disinfectant pad.[24,25]
- Perform hand hygiene.[4,5,6,7,8,9]
- Document the procedure.[26,27,28,29]

Special considerations

- Repeat rectal tube insertion periodically *to stimulate GI activity,* if ordered.[20] If the tube fails to relieve the patient's abdominal distention, notify the practitioner.

Complications

Leaving a rectal tube in place indefinitely may reduce sphincter responsiveness, and may lead to permanent sphincter damage or pressure necrosis of the mucosa.

Documentation

Record the date and time that you inserted the rectal tube. Record the amount, color, and consistency of any evacuated matter. Describe the patient's abdomen: hard, distended, soft, or drum-like on percussion. Note the patient's bowel sounds before and after rectal tube insertion and the patient's tolerance of the procedure. Document teaching provided to the patient and family (if applicable), their understanding of that teaching, and any need for follow-up teaching.

REFERENCES

1 Yi, C. H., et al. (2016). Influence of rectal decompression on abdominal symptoms and anorectal physiology following colonoscopy in healthy adults. *Gastroenterology Research and Practice, 2016,* 4101248. https://www.ncbi.nlm.nih.gov/pmc/articles/PMC5019887/ (Level VI)

2 Ousey, K. (2014). An easily forgotten tube. https://psnet.ahrq.gov/web-mm/easily-forgotten-tube

3 C. R. Bard, Inc. (2015). Bard® rectal tubes: Instructions for use. https://www.crbard.com/CRBard/media/ProductAssets/BardMedicalDivision/PF10210/en-US/PF10210-Rectal-tubes-plastic-IFU.pdf

4 World Health Organization. (2009). WHO guidelines on hand hygiene in health care: First global patient safety challenge, clean care is safer care. https://apps.who.int/iris/bitstream/handle/10665/44102/9789241597906_eng.pdf?sequence=1 (Level IV)

5 Centers for Disease Control and Prevention. (2002). Guideline for hand hygiene in health-care settings: Recommendations of the Healthcare Infection Control Practices Advisory Committee and the HICPAC/SHEA/APIC/IDSA Hand Hygiene Task Force. *MMWR Recommendations and Reports, 51*(RR-16), 1–45. https://www.cdc.gov/mmwr/pdf/rr/rr5116.pdf (Level II)

6 The Joint Commission. (2021). Standard NPSG.07.01.01. *Comprehensive accreditation manual for hospitals.* Oakbrook Terrace, IL: The Joint Commission. (Level VII)

7 Centers for Medicare and Medicaid Services, Department of Health and Human Services. (2020). Condition of participation: Infection control. 42 C.F.R. § 482.42.

8 Accreditation Association for Hospitals and Health Systems. (2020). Standard 07.01.21. *Healthcare Facilities Accreditation Program: Accreditation requirements for acute care hospitals.* Chicago, IL: Accreditation Association for Hospitals and Health Systems. (Level VII)

9 DNV GL-Healthcare USA, Inc. (2020). IC.1.SR.1. *NIAHO® accreditation requirements, interpretive guidelines and surveyor guidance—revision 20.0.* Milford, OH: DNV GL-Healthcare USA, Inc. (Level VII)

10 The Joint Commission. (2021). Standard NPSG.01.01.01. *Comprehensive accreditation manual for hospitals.* Oakbrook Terrace, IL: The Joint Commission. (Level VII)

11 Centers for Medicare and Medicaid Services, Department of Health and Human Services. (2020). Condition of participation: Patient's rights. 42 C.F.R. § 482.13(c)(1).

12 Accreditation Association for Hospitals and Health Systems. (2020). Standard 15.01.16. *Healthcare Facilities Accreditation Program: Accreditation requirements for acute care hospitals.* Chicago, IL: Accreditation Association for Hospitals and Health Systems. (Level VII)

13 DNV GL-Healthcare USA, Inc. (2020). PR.2.SR.5. *NIAHO® accreditation requirements, interpretive guidelines and surveyor guidance—revision 20.0.* Milford, OH: DNV GL-Healthcare USA, Inc. (Level VII)

14 The Joint Commission. (2021). Standard RI.01.01.01. *Comprehensive accreditation manual for hospitals.* Oakbrook Terrace, IL: The Joint Commission. (Level VII)

15 The Joint Commission. (2021). Standard PC.02.01.21. *Comprehensive accreditation manual for hospitals.* Oakbrook Terrace, IL: The Joint Commission. (Level VII)

16 Waters, T. R., et al. (2009). Safe patient handling training for schools of nursing. https://www.cdc.gov/niosh/docs/2009-127/pdfs/2009-127.pdf (Level VII)

17 Siegel, J. D., et al. (2007, revised 2019). 2007 guideline for isolation precautions: Preventing transmission of infectious agents in healthcare settings. https://www.cdc.gov/infectioncontrol/pdf/guidelines/isolation-guidelines-H.pdf (Level II)

18 Accreditation Association for Hospitals and Health Systems. (2020). Standard 07.01.10. *Healthcare Facilities Accreditation Program: Accreditation requirements for acute care hospitals.* Chicago, IL: Accreditation Association for Hospitals and Health Systems. (Level VII)

19 Occupational Safety and Health Administration. (2019). Bloodborne pathogens, standard number 1910.1030. https://www.osha.gov/pls/oshaweb/owadisp.show_document?p_id=10051&p_table=STANDARDS (Level VII)

20 Craven, R. F., et al. (2020). *Fundamentals of nursing: Concepts and competencies for practice.* (9th ed.). Philadelphia, PA: Wolters Kluwer.

21 The Joint Commission. (2014). Sentinel event alert: Managing risk during transition to new ISO tubing connector standards. https://www.jointcommission.org/-/media/tjc/documents/resources/patient-safety-topics/sentinel-event/sea_53_connectors_8_19_14_final.pdf (Level VII)

22 U.S. Food and Drug Administration. (2017). Examples of medical device misconnections. https://www.fda.gov/medical-devices/medical-device-connectors/examples-medical-device-misconnections (Level VII)

23 Ganz, D. A., et al. (2013, reviewed 2021). *Preventing falls in hospitals: A toolkit for improving quality of care* (AHRQ Publication No. 13-0015-EF). Rockville, MD: Agency for Healthcare Research and Quality. https://www.ahrq.gov/professionals/systems/hospital/fallpxtoolkit/index.html (Level VII)

24 Rutala, W. A., et al. (2008, revised 2019). Guideline for disinfection and sterilization in healthcare facilities, 2008. https://www.cdc.gov/infectioncontrol/pdf/guidelines/disinfection-guidelines-H.pdf (Level I)

25 Accreditation Association for Hospitals and Health Systems. (2020). Standard 07.02.03. *Healthcare Facilities Accreditation Program: Accreditation requirements for acute care hospitals.* Chicago, IL: Accreditation Association for Hospitals and Health Systems. (Level VII)

26 The Joint Commission. (2021). Standard RC.01.03.01. *Comprehensive accreditation manual for hospitals.* Oakbrook Terrace, IL: The Joint Commission. (Level VII)

27 Accreditation Association for Hospitals and Health Systems. (2020). Standard 10.00.03. *Healthcare Facilities Accreditation Program: Accreditation requirements for acute care hospitals.* Chicago, IL: Accreditation Association for Hospitals and Health Systems. (Level VII)

28 Centers for Medicare and Medicaid Services, Department of Health and Human Services. (2020). Condition of participation: Medical record services. 42 C.F.R. § 482.24(b).

29 DNV GL-Healthcare USA, Inc. (2020). MR.2.SR.1. *NIAHO® accreditation requirements, interpretive guidelines and surveyor guidance—revision 20.0.* Milford, OH: DNV GL-Healthcare USA, Inc. (Level VII)

RESIDUAL LIMB CARE

Patient care immediately after limb amputation includes monitoring drainage from the residual limb, controlling pain, reducing edema, positioning the affected limb, assisting with exercises prescribed by a physical therapist, and wrapping and conditioning the residual limb.[1] Postoperative care of the residual limb will vary slightly, depending on the amputation site (arm or leg) and the type of dressing applied to the residual limb (elastic bandage or plaster cast).

After the residual limb heals, it requires daily care, including proper hygiene and continued muscle-strengthening exercises. While recovering from the physical and psychological trauma of amputation, the patient will need to learn correct procedures for routine daily care of the residual limb.[1]

Equipment

For postoperative residual limb care

Gloves ▪ absorbent pad ▪ overhead trapeze ▪ trochanter roll (for a leg) ▪ elastic residual limb shrinker or 4″ (10 cm) elastic bandages ▪ 1″ (2.5 cm) adhesive tape or bandage clips ▪ vital signs monitoring equipment ▪ stethoscope ▪ disinfectant pad ▪ Optional: pressure dressing, tourniquet, prescribed skin and wound care products.

For ongoing residual limb care

Gentle, nondetergent soap ▪ residual limb sock ▪ washcloth ▪ towel.

Preparation of equipment

Inspect all equipment and supplies. If a product is expired, is defective, or has compromised integrity, remove it from patient use, label it as expired or defective, and report the expiration or defect as directed by your facility.

Implementation

▪ Gather and prepare the necessary equipment and supplies.
▪ Perform hand hygiene.[2,3,4,5,6,7]
▪ Confirm the patient's identity using at least two patient identifiers.[8]
▪ Provide privacy.[9,10,11,12]
▪ Explain the procedure to the patient and family (if appropriate) according to their individual communication and learning needs *to increase their understanding, allay their fears, and enhance cooperation.*[13]
▪ Raise the patient's bed to waist level before providing direct patient care *to prevent caregiver back strain.*[14]
▪ Perform hand hygiene.[2,3,4,5,6,7]
▪ Put on gloves *to comply with standard precautions.*[15,16,17]
▪ Perform routine postoperative care. Frequently assess the patient's respiratory status and level of consciousness, monitor IV infusions, assess tube patency, and provide for the patient's comfort, pain management, and safety. Monitor vital signs at an interval determined by your facility and the patient's condition; *there's no evidence-based research to indicate best practice for frequency of monitoring vital signs.* (See the "Postoperative care" procedure.)[18]

Monitoring residual limb drainage

■ *Because gravity causes fluid to accumulate at the residual limb,* frequently inspect the dressing to assess the amount of blood and drainage on the dressing. Notify the practitioner if accumulations of drainage or blood increase rapidly. If excessive bleeding occurs, notify the practitioner immediately, and apply a pressure dressing or compress the appropriate pressure points. If this doesn't control bleeding, and only as a last resort, use a tourniquet and notify the practitioner.

■ Tape an absorbent pad over the moist part of the dressing as necessary. *Doing so provides a dry area to help prevent bacterial infection.*

Positioning the extremity

■ Elevate the extremity for the first 24 to 48 hours, as ordered, *to reduce swelling and promote venous return.*[19]

■ For an arm amputation, position the patient's arm with the elbow extended and the shoulder abducted *to prevent contractures.*

■ For a leg amputation, elevate the foot of the bed slightly and place a trochanter roll against the patient's hip *to prevent external rotation.*

NURSING ALERT Don't place a pillow under the patient's thigh to flex the hip, *because this positioning can cause hip flexion contracture.* For the same reason, tell the patient to avoid prolonged sitting.[19]

■ After a below-the-knee amputation, maintain knee extension *to prevent hamstring muscle contractures.*

■ After any level of leg amputation, place the patient on a firm surface in the prone position for at least 2 hours a day, with legs close together and without pillows under the stomach, hips, knees, or residual limb, unless this position is contraindicated. *This position helps prevent hip flexion, contractures, and abduction; it also stretches the flexor muscles.*

Assisting with prescribed exercises

■ After arm amputation, encourage the patient to exercise the remaining arm *to prevent muscle contractures.* Help the patient perform isometric and range-of-motion (ROM) exercises for both shoulders, as prescribed by the physical therapist, *because use of a prosthesis requires both shoulders.*

■ After leg amputation, stand behind the patient and, if necessary, support the patient with your hands at the waist during balancing exercises.

■ Instruct the patient to exercise the affected and unaffected limbs *to maintain muscle tone and increase muscle strength.* The patient with a leg amputation may perform push-ups, as ordered (in the sitting position, arms at the sides), or pull-ups on the overhead trapeze *to strengthen the arms, shoulders, and back in preparation for using crutches.*

Wrapping and conditioning a residual limb

■ Apply an elastic residual limb shrinker *to prevent edema and shape the limb in preparation for the prosthesis.* Wrap the residual limb so that it narrows toward the distal end *to help ensure comfort when the patient wears the prosthesis.*

■ If an elastic residual limb shrinker isn't available, you can wrap the residual limb of an amputated leg in a 4″ (10 cm) elastic bandage. To do this, stretch the bandage to about two-thirds its maximum length as you wrap it diagonally around the residual limb, with the greatest pressure distally. (Depending on the size of the leg, you may need to use two 4″ [10 cm] bandages.) Secure the bandage with clips or adhesive tape. Make sure the bandage covers the residual limb smoothly, *because wrinkles or exposed areas encourage skin breakdown.* (See *Wrapping a residual limb.*)

■ To wrap an amputated arm, follow the same technique as described for the leg, using a 4″ (10 cm) elastic bandage and wrapping the patient's remaining arm using figure-eight turns until the entire residual limb is covered. Pass the bandage wrap across the patient's back and shoulders *to anchor it,* and then secure the bandage with clips or adhesive tape.

■ If the patient experiences throbbing after the residual limb is wrapped, the bandage may be too tight; remove the bandage immediately and reapply it less tightly. *Throbbing indicates impaired circulation.*

Wrapping a residual limb

Proper residual limb care helps protect the limb, reduces swelling, and prepares the limb for a prosthesis. As you perform the procedure, teach it to the patient.

Start by elevating the residual limb *to reduce edema and vascular stasis.*[19] Obtain two 4″ (10 cm) elastic bandages and center the end of the first bandage at the top of the patient's thigh. Unroll the bandage downward over the residual limb and to the back of the leg.

Make three figure-eight turns to adequately cover the ends of the residual limb. As you wrap, be sure to include the roll of flesh in the groin area. Use enough pressure to ensure that the residual limb narrows toward the end *so that it fits comfortably into the prosthesis.*

Use the second 4″ (10 cm) bandage to anchor the first bandage around the waist. For a below-the-knee amputation, use the knee to anchor the bandage in place. Secure the bandage with clips or adhesive tape. Check the residual limb bandage regularly, and rewrap it if it bunches at the end.

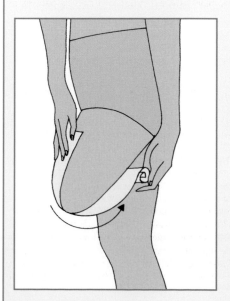
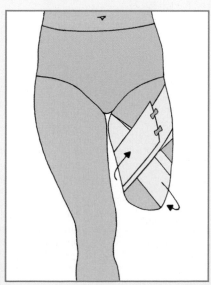
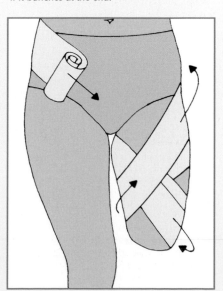

■ Unwrap the residual limb every 4 to 6 hours for the first 2 days postoperatively, as prescribed, and then at least once daily.[19] Assess for signs and symptoms of infection and skin irritation or breakdown. Assess the color, temperature, and most-proximal pulse on the residual limb, comparing findings to those on the opposite extremity.[19] Report your findings to the practitioner.

■ After removing, massage the residual limb gently, always pushing toward the suture line rather than away from it. *Massage stimulates circulation and prevents scar tissue from adhering to the bone.*[1]

■ Perform residual limb skin care and wound care as needed and prescribed.[19]

■ When healing begins, instruct the patient to push the residual limb against a pillow. Then have the patient progress gradually to pushing against harder surfaces, such as a padded chair, and then a hard chair. *These conditioning exercises will help the patient adjust to experiencing pressure and sensation in the residual limb.*[19]

Caring for the healed residual limb

■ *To shape the residual limb*, have the patient wear an elastic bandage 24 hours a day except while bathing.

■ *To prevent infection*, bathe the residual limb but never shave it. If possible, bathe the residual limb at the end of the day, *because the warm water may cause swelling, making reapplication of the prosthesis difficult.* Don't soak the residual limb for long periods.

■ Avoid applying lotions, oils, or creams to the residual limb, unless prescribed; *these may clog follicles, which increases the risk of infection.*[19]

■ Inspect the residual limb for redness, swelling, irritation, and calluses. Report any of these to the practitioner. Tell the patient to avoid putting weight on the residual limb. (The skin should be firm but not taut over the bony end of the limb.)

■ Have the patient continue muscle-strengthening exercises *to build the strength needed to control the prosthesis.*

■ Change and wash the patient's elastic bandages or sock every day *to avoid exposing the skin to excessive perspiration, which can lead to skin breakdown.*[20] Wash the elastic bandages in warm water and gentle, nondetergent soap; lay them flat on a towel to dry. *Machine washing or drying may shrink the elastic bandages.*

Completing the procedure

■ Return the bed to the lowest position *to prevent falls and maintain patient safety.*[21]

■ Discard used supplies in appropriate receptacle.[17]

■ Remove and discard your gloves.[15,17]

■ Perform hand hygiene.[2,3,4,5,6,7]

■ Clean and disinfect your stethoscope with a disinfectant pad.[22,23]

■ Perform hand hygiene.[2,3,4,5,6,7]

■ Document the procedure.[24,25,26,27]

Special considerations

■ Ensure adequate postoperative pain control. *Inadequate pain control can increase the risk of chronic amputation pain.*[28]

■ Nonpharmacological therapies, such as transcutaneous electrical nerve stimulation, acupuncture, spinal cord stimulation, virtual reality therapy, and mirror therapy, may be used to manage phantom limb pain.[28]

Complications

Postoperative complications include hemorrhage, infection, contractures, and edema in the residual limb. Skin breakdown and phantom limb pain may also occur. Altered body image and grieving can lead to withdrawal and depression.[1] Stump hematoma formation and deep vein thrombosis are also possibilities.[28]

Documentation

Record the date and time of your observations and specific procedures that you performed for all postoperative care, including the amount and type of drainage, presence and appearance of any drains, condition of the dressing, need for dressing reinforcement, appearance of the suture line and surrounding tissue, and pain assessment findings. Also note any signs of skin irritation or infection, any complications, the date and time that the practitioner was notified and the name of the practitioner notified, interventions performed, the patient's response to those interventions, the patient's tolerance of exercises, and the patient's psychological reaction to the amputation.

During routine daily care, document the date, time, type of care you gave, and condition of the skin and suture line, noting any signs of irritation, such as redness and tenderness. Also record the patient's progress in caring for the residual limb or prosthesis. Document teaching provided to the patient and family (if applicable), their understanding of that teaching, and any need for follow-up teaching.

REFERENCES

1 Hinkle, J. L., & Cheever, K. H. (2018). *Brunner & Suddarth's textbook of medical-surgical nursing* (14th ed.). Philadelphia, PA: Wolters Kluwer.

2 Centers for Disease Control and Prevention. (2002). Guideline for hand hygiene in health-care settings: Recommendations of the Healthcare Infection Control Practices Advisory Committee and the HICPAC/SHEA/APIC/IDSA Hand Hygiene Task Force. *MMWR Recommendations and Reports, 51*(RR-16), 1–45. https://www.cdc.gov/mmwr/pdf/rr/rr5116.pdf (Level II)

3 World Health Organization. (2009). WHO guidelines on hand hygiene in health care: First global patient safety challenge, clean care is safer care. https://apps.who.int/iris/bitstream/handle/10665/44102/9789241597906_eng.pdf?sequence=1 (Level IV)

4 The Joint Commission. (2021). Standard NPSG.07.01.01. *Comprehensive accreditation manual for hospitals.* Oakbrook Terrace, IL: The Joint Commission. (Level VII)

5 Centers for Medicare and Medicaid Services, Department of Health and Human Services. (2020). Condition of participation: Infection control. 42 C.F.R. § 482.42.

6 Accreditation Association for Hospitals and Health Systems. (2020). Standard 07.01.21. *Healthcare Facilities Accreditation Program: Accreditation requirements for acute care hospitals.* Chicago, IL: Accreditation Association for Hospitals and Health Systems. (Level VII)

7 DNV GL-Healthcare USA, Inc. (2020). IC.1.SR.1. *NIAHO® accreditation requirements, interpretive guidelines and surveyor guidance—revision 20.0.* Milford, OH: DNV GL-Healthcare USA, Inc. (Level VII)

8 The Joint Commission. (2021). Standard NPSG.01.01.01. *Comprehensive accreditation manual for hospitals.* Oakbrook Terrace, IL: The Joint Commission. (Level VII)

9 The Joint Commission. (2021). Standard RI.01.01.01. *Comprehensive accreditation manual for hospitals.* Oakbrook Terrace, IL: The Joint Commission. (Level VII)

10 Centers for Medicare and Medicaid Services, Department of Health and Human Services. (2020). Condition of participation: Patient's rights. 42 C.F.R. § 482.13(c)(1).

11 Accreditation Association for Hospitals and Health Systems. (2020). Standard 15.01.16. *Healthcare Facilities Accreditation Program: Accreditation requirements for acute care hospitals.* Chicago, IL: Accreditation Association for Hospitals and Health Systems. (Level VII)

12 DNV GL-Healthcare USA, Inc. (2020). PR.2.SR.5. *NIAHO® accreditation requirements, interpretive guidelines and surveyor guidance—revision 20.0.* Milford, OH: DNV GL-Healthcare USA, Inc. (Level VII)

13 The Joint Commission. (2021). Standard PC.02.01.21. *Comprehensive accreditation manual for hospitals.* Oakbrook Terrace, IL: The Joint Commission. (Level VII)

14 Waters, T. R., et al. (2009). Safe patient handling training for schools of nursing. https://www.cdc.gov/niosh/docs/2009-127/pdfs/2009-127.pdf (Level VII)

15 Siegel, J. D., et al. (2007, revised 2019). 2007 guideline for isolation precautions: Preventing transmission of infectious agents in healthcare settings. https://www.cdc.gov/infectioncontrol/pdf/guidelines/isolation-guidelines-H.pdf (Level II)

16 Accreditation Association for Hospitals and Health Systems. (2020). Standard 07.01.10. *Healthcare Facilities Accreditation Program: Accreditation requirements for acute care hospitals.* Chicago, IL: Accreditation Association for Hospitals and Health Systems. (Level VII)

17 Occupational Safety and Health Administration. (2019). Bloodborne pathogens, standard number 1910.1030. https://www.osha.gov/pls/oshaweb/owadisp.show_document?p_id=10051&p_table=STANDARDS (Level VII)

18 American Society of PeriAnesthesia Nurses. (2019). *2019-2020 Perianesthesia nursing standards, practice recommendations and interpretive statements.* Cherry Hill, NJ: American Society of PeriAnesthesia Nurses. (Level VII)

19 Pullen, R. L. (2010). Clinical queries: Caring for a patient after amputation. *Nursing, 40*(1), 15. https://journals.lww.com/nursing/Pages/articleviewer.aspx?year=2010&issue=01000&article=00008&type=Fulltext#pdf-link

20 Klute, G. K., et al. (2016). Prosthesis management of residual-limb perspiration with subatmospheric vacuum pressure. *Journal of Rehabilitation Research and Development, 53*, 721–728. (Level II)

21 Ganz, D. A., et al. (2013, reviewed 2021). *Preventing falls in hospitals: A toolkit for improving quality of care* (AHRQ Publication No. 13-0015-EF). Rockville, MD: Agency for Healthcare Research and Quality. https://www.ahrq.gov/professionals/systems/hospital/fallpxtoolkit/index.html (Level VII)

22 Accreditation Association for Hospitals and Health Systems. (2020). Standard 07.02.03. *Healthcare Facilities Accreditation Program: Accreditation requirements for acute care hospitals.* Chicago, IL: Accreditation Association for Hospitals and Health Systems. (Level VII)

23 Rutala, W. A., et al. (2008, revised 2019). Guideline for disinfection and sterilization in healthcare facilities, 2008. https://www.cdc.gov/infection-control/pdf/guidelines/disinfection-guidelines-H.pdf (Level I)

24 The Joint Commission. (2021). Standard RC.01.03.01. *Comprehensive accreditation manual for hospitals.* Oakbrook Terrace, IL: The Joint Commission. (Level VII)

25 Centers for Medicare and Medicaid Services, Department of Health and Human Services. (2020). Condition of participation: Medical record services. 42 C.F.R. § 482.24(b).

26 Accreditation Association for Hospitals and Health Systems. (2020). Standard 10.00.03. *Healthcare Facilities Accreditation Program: Accreditation requirements for acute care hospitals.* Chicago, IL: Accreditation Association for Hospitals and Health Systems. (Level VII)

27 DNV GL-Healthcare USA, Inc. (2020). MR.2.SR.1. *NIAHO® accreditation requirements, interpretive guidelines and surveyor guidance—revision 20.0.* Milford, OH: DNV GL-Healthcare USA, Inc. (Level VII)

28 Kalapatapu, V. (2021). Lower extremity amputation. In: *UpToDate,* Mills, J. L., Sr., & Eidt, J. F. (Eds.).

29 U.S. National Library of Medicine. (2020). Leg amputation: Discharge. https://medlineplus.gov/ency/patientinstructions/000014.htm

30 Urits, I., et al. (2019). Treatment strategies and effective management of phantom limb-associated pain. *Current Pain and Headache Reports, 33*(9), 64.

31 Mayo Clinic. (n.d.). Phantom pain. https://www.mayoclinic.org/diseases-conditions/phantom-pain/diagnosis-treatment/drc-20376278

RESPIRATION ASSESSMENT

Controlled by the respiratory center in the lateral medulla oblongata, respiration is the exchange of oxygen and carbon dioxide between the atmosphere and body cells. External respiration, or breathing, is accomplished by the diaphragm and chest muscles and delivers oxygen to the lower respiratory tract and alveoli.[1]

Four measures of respiration—rate, rhythm, depth, and sound—reflect the body's metabolic state, diaphragm and chest-muscle condition, and airway patency. Respiratory rate is recorded as the number of cycles (with one cycle consisting of inspiration and expiration) per minute; rhythm, as the regularity of these cycles; depth, as the volume of air inhaled and exhaled with each respiration; and sound, as the audible deviation from normal, effortless breathing. Normal respiratory rates for an adult range from 12 to 18 breaths/minute;[1] however, it's important to know the patient's normal baseline respiratory rate so that you can detect changes in the patient's condition.

The best time to assess the patient's respirations is immediately after taking the pulse rate; however you should observe the patient's breathing with each contact.[2]

Equipment

Watch or clock with second hand or digital timer ▪ stethoscope ▪ disinfectant pad ▪ Optional: gloves, personal protective equipment (gown, mask and goggles, or mask with face shield).

Implementation

▪ Gather the necessary equipment and supplies.
▪ Perform hand hygiene.[3,4,5,6,7,8] (If you performed hand hygiene before taking the patient's pulse, you don't need to repeat this step.)
▪ Confirm the patient's identity using at least two patient identifiers.[9]
▪ Provide privacy.[10,11,12,13]
▪ Explain the procedure to the patient and family (if appropriate) according to their individual communication and learning needs *to increase their understanding, allay their fears, and enhance cooperation.*[14]
▪ Perform hand hygiene.[3,4,5,6,7,8]
▪ Put on gloves and other personal protective equipment, as necessary, *to prevent contact with body fluids and comply with standard precautions.*[15,16,17]
▪ Place your fingertips over the patient's radial artery, and don't tell the patient you're counting respirations. *If you tell the patient, the patient will become conscious of respirations and the rate may change.*[1]
▪ Count respirations by observing the rise and fall of the patient's chest during breathing.[2] Alternatively, position the patient's opposite arm across the chest and count respirations by feeling its rise and fall. Consider one rise and one fall as one respiration.
▪ If the patient's respirations are regular, count the respirations for 30 seconds and multiply by two *to determine the respiratory rate.*[2] Alternatively, count the patient's respirations for 60 seconds if respirations are irregular *to account for variations in respiratory rate and pattern.*
▪ As you count respirations, be alert for stertor, stridor, wheezing, and expiratory grunting. *Stertor* is a snoring sound resulting from secretions in the trachea and large bronchi. Listen for it in patients with neurologic disorders and in those who are comatose. *Stridor* is an inspiratory crowing sound that results from upper airway obstruction. It occurs in laryngitis, croup, or the presence of a foreign body in the upper airway. *Wheezing* is a high-pitched or whistling sound that may be audible with or without a stethoscope. It occurs as a result of airway narrowing. *Expiratory grunting* is a deep, low-pitched sound heard at the end of each breath that coincides with the closure of the glottis and may indicate respiratory distress.

ELDER ALERT In older adult patients, an expiratory grunt may result from partial airway obstruction or neuromuscular reflex.

▪ Observe chest movements for depth of respirations. If the patient inhales a small volume of air, record this as shallow; record the inhalation of a large volume as deep.
▪ Listen to breathing *to determine the rhythm and sound of respirations.* (See *Identifying respiratory patterns,* page 734.)
▪ Auscultate breath sounds using a stethoscope. You'll hear four types of breath sounds over normal lungs. *Tracheal sounds* are heard over the trachea and are harsh and discontinuous. *Bronchial sounds* are usually heard over the fourth intercostal space, between the sternum and the midclavicular line; they are loud, high-pitched, and discontinuous, and loudest when the patient exhales. *Bronchovesicular sounds* are heard when the patient inhales or exhales; medium-pitched and continuous, they are best heard over the upper third of the sternum and between the scapulae. *Vesicular sounds* are heard over the rest of the lungs; soft and low-pitched, they are prolonged during inspiration and shortened during expiration.
▪ Adventitious breath sounds are abnormal no matter where you hear them over the lungs. *Crackles* are intermittent, nonmusical, brief crackling sounds caused by collapsed or fluid-filled alveoli popping open; heard primarily during inspiration, they are classified as fine or coarse, and usually don't clear with coughing unless caused by secretions. *Wheezes* are high-pitched sounds heard first during expiration due to blocked airflow; they are also heard during inspiration when airflow is severely blocked. *Rhonchi* are low-pitched, snoring, rattling sounds that occur primarily when the patient exhales, usually due to fluid or secretions in the large bronchial airways that may change or disappear with coughing. *Stridor* is a loud, high-pitched crowing sound that is heard, typically without a stethoscope, during inspiration; caused by obstruction of the upper airway, stridor requires immediate intervention. A *pleural friction rub*—a low-pitched, grating, rubbing sound heard when the patient inhales and exhales—results from pleural inflammation that causes the two layers of the pleura to rub together; it may result in pain in the areas where the sound is heard.
▪ Observe the patient for use of accessory muscles, such as the scalene, sternocleidomastoid, trapezius, and latissimus dorsi. *Use of these muscles*

Identifying respiratory patterns

Type	Characteristics	Pattern	Possible causes
Apnea	Periodic absence of breathing; may be temporary		■ Mechanical airway obstruction ■ Conditions affecting the brain's respiratory center
Bradypnea	Slow, regular respirations of equal depth		■ Normal pattern during sleep ■ Conditions affecting the respiratory center, such as tumors, metabolic disorders, and respiratory decompensation ■ Use of opiates, alcohol, or both
Cheyne-Stokes	Gradual increase in respiratory rate and tidal volume, then gradual decrease to complete apnea, which may last several seconds before gradual increase again as cycle repeats[1]		■ Brain injury or stroke ■ Heart failure ■ Kidney failure ■ Drug-induced respiratory depression ■ Cerebral anoxia ■ May occur in older adults during sleep[1,18,19]
Eupnea	Normal rate and rhythm		■ Normal respiration
Kussmaul	Rapid (over 20 breaths/minute), deep (resembling sighs), labored respirations without pause		■ Kidney failure ■ Metabolic acidosis, particularly diabetic ketoacidosis
Tachypnea	Rapid respirations; rate increase corresponds to increase in body temperature—about four breaths/minute for every 1° F (0.6° C) above normal		■ Pneumonia ■ Compensatory respiratory alkalosis ■ Respiratory insufficiency ■ Lesions in the brain's respiratory center ■ Salicylate poisoning

reflects a weakness of the diaphragm and the external intercostal muscles, the primary muscles of respiration.
- Remove and discard your gloves and other personal protective equipment, if worn.[17]
- Perform hand hygiene.[3,4,5,6,7,8]
- Clean and disinfect your stethoscope using a disinfectant pad.[20,21]
- Perform hand hygiene.[3,4,5,6,7,8]
- Document your findings.[22,23,24,25]

Special considerations

- When assessing the patient's respiratory status, consider the patient's personal and family history. Ask if the patient smokes; if the patient says yes, ask for how many years the patient smoked and how many packs per day.[1]
- A more detailed assessment (including palpating the chest for lymph node abnormalities, assessing tracheal position, and percussing for signs of fluid or trapped air in the chest) may be necessary for a patient with a respiratory disease, such as chronic obstructive pulmonary disease or asthma.[26]
- If the patient's respiratory rate suddenly increases, assess for other signs of respiratory distress, such as anxiety, nasal flaring, accessory muscle use, abnormal breath sounds, grunting, and cyanosis.[2] *To detect cyanosis,* look for characteristic bluish discoloration in the nail beds or lips, under the tongue, in the buccal mucosa, and in the conjunctiva.[27] Report your findings to the practitioner.
- If the patient's respiratory rate suddenly decreases, assess for an underlying cause.[27] Notify the practitioner, as needed.
- If you find the patient unresponsive, shout for nearby help and activate the emergency response system via mobile device (if appropriate). Check for absent breathing or only gasping while simultaneously checking for a pulse *to minimize delay in detecting cardiac arrest and initiating cardiopulmonary resuscitation (CPR).*[28] If the patient has a pulse but inadequate breathing, administer 1 rescue breath every 6 seconds; check the patient's pulse about every 2 minutes.[28] If breathing is absent, or if the patient is only gasping and you don't feel a pulse within 10 seconds, have a coworker retrieve the defibrillator (or automated external defibrillator [AED]) and other emergency equipment. If you're alone, retrieve them yourself.[28] Immediately begin chest compressions until the defibrillator or AED is ready for use. Compress an adult's chest at a rate of 100 to 120 compressions per minute, with a compression depth of at least 2″ (5 cm) for an average adult, but do not exceed a depth of 2.4″ (6 cm). Avoid leaning on the chest between compressions *to allow full chest wall recoil.*[28] After 30 compressions, open the patient's airway and deliver two breaths (with each breath over approximately 1 second); continue CPR using a ratio of 30 compressions to 2 breaths. When the defibrillator is ready for use, check the patient's rhythm, and defibrillate if the patient has a shockable rhythm; otherwise, continue CPR.[28]

Documentation

Record the date and time, and the rate, depth, rhythm, and sound of the patient's respirations. If the patient isn't breathing adequately, note the date and time, the name of the practitioner you notified, and any interventions you provided (such as oxygen therapy) and the patient's response to the interventions. Document teaching provided to the patient and family (if applicable), their understanding of that teaching, and any need for follow-up teaching.

REFERENCES

1. Kacmarek, R. M., et al. (2021). *Egan's fundamentals of respiratory care* (12th ed.). St. Louis, MO: Elsevier.
2. Craven, R. F., et al. (2020). *Fundamentals of nursing: Concepts and competencies for practice* (9th ed.). Philadelphia, PA: Wolters Kluwer.
3. The Joint Commission. (2021). Standard NPSG.07.01.01. *Comprehensive accreditation manual for hospitals.* Oakbrook Terrace, IL: The Joint Commission. (Level VII)
4. World Health Organization. (2009). WHO guidelines on hand hygiene in health care: First global patient safety challenge, clean care is safer care. https://apps.who.int/iris/bitstream/handle/10665/44102/9789241597906_eng.pdf?sequence=1 (Level IV)
5. Centers for Disease Control and Prevention. (2002). Guideline for hand hygiene in health-care settings: Recommendations of the Healthcare Infection Control Practices Advisory Committee and the HICPAC/SHEA/APIC/IDSA Hand Hygiene Task Force. *MMWR Recommendations and Reports, 51*(RR-16), 1–45. https://www.cdc.gov/mmwr/pdf/rr/rr5116.pdf (Level II)

6 Accreditation Association for Hospitals and Health Systems. (2020). Standard 07.01.21. *Healthcare Facilities Accreditation Program: Accreditation requirements for acute care hospitals.* Chicago, IL: Accreditation Association for Hospitals and Health Systems. (Level VII)

7 Centers for Medicare and Medicaid Services, Department of Health and Human Services. (2020). Condition of participation: Infection control. 42 C.F.R. § 482.42.

8 DNV GL–Healthcare USA, Inc. (2020). IC.1.SR.1. *NIAHO® accreditation requirements, interpretive guidelines and surveyor guidance—revision 20.0.* Milford, OH: DNV GL–Healthcare USA, Inc. (Level VII)

9 The Joint Commission. (2021). Standard NPSG.01.01.01. *Comprehensive accreditation manual for hospitals.* Oakbrook Terrace, IL: The Joint Commission. (Level VII)

10 The Joint Commission. (2021). Standard RI.01.01.01. *Comprehensive accreditation manual for hospitals.* Oakbrook Terrace, IL: The Joint Commission. (Level VII)

11 DNV GL–Healthcare USA, Inc. (2020). PR.2.SR.5. *NIAHO® accreditation requirements, interpretive guidelines and surveyor guidance—revision 20.0.* Milford, OH: DNV GL–Healthcare USA, Inc. (Level VII)

12 Centers for Medicare and Medicaid Services, Department of Health and Human Services. (2020). Condition of participation: Patient's rights. 42 C.F.R. § 482.13(c)(1).

13 Accreditation Association for Hospitals and Health Systems. (2020). Standard 15.01.16. *Healthcare Facilities Accreditation Program: Accreditation requirements for acute care hospitals.* Chicago, IL: Accreditation Association for Hospitals and Health Systems. (Level VII)

14 The Joint Commission. (2021). Standard PC.02.01.21. *Comprehensive accreditation manual for hospitals.* Oakbrook Terrace, IL: The Joint Commission. (Level VII)

15 Siegel, J. D., et al. (2007, revised 2019). 2007 guideline for isolation precautions: Preventing transmission of infectious agents in healthcare settings. https://www.cdc.gov/infectioncontrol/pdf/guidelines/isolation-guidelines-H.pdf (Level II)

16 Accreditation Association for Hospitals and Health Systems. (2020). Standard 07.01.10. *Healthcare Facilities Accreditation Program: Accreditation requirements for acute care hospitals.* Chicago, IL: Accreditation Association for Hospitals and Health Systems. (Level VII)

17 Occupational Safety and Health Administration. (2019). Bloodborne pathogens, standard number 1910.1030. https://www.osha.gov/pls/oshaweb/owadisp.show_document?p_id=10051&p_table=STANDARDS (Level VII)

18 Bickley, L. (2021). *Bates' guide to physical examination and health history taking* (13th ed.). Philadelphia, PA: Wolters Kluwer.

19 Rudrappa, M., et al. (2021). Cheyne-Stokes respirations. https://www.ncbi.nlm.nih.gov/books/NBK448165/#:~:text=in%20elderly%20patients.-,Pathophysiology,of%20unstable%20central%20respiratory%20control.

20 Rutala, W. A., et al. (2008, revised 2019). Guideline for disinfection and sterilization in healthcare facilities, 2008. https://www.cdc.gov/infection-control/pdf/guidelines/disinfection-guidelines-H.pdf (Level I)

21 Accreditation Association for Hospitals and Health Systems. (2020). Standard 07.02.03. *Healthcare Facilities Accreditation Program: Accreditation requirements for acute care hospitals.* Chicago, IL: Accreditation Association for Hospitals and Health Systems. (Level VII)

22 The Joint Commission. (2021). Standard RC.01.03.01. *Comprehensive accreditation manual for hospitals.* Oakbrook Terrace, IL: The Joint Commission. (Level VII)

23 Accreditation Association for Hospitals and Health Systems. (2020). Standard 10.00.03. *Healthcare Facilities Accreditation Program: Accreditation requirements for acute care hospitals.* Chicago, IL: Accreditation Association for Hospitals and Health Systems. (Level VII)

24 Centers for Medicare and Medicaid Services, Department of Health and Human Services. (2020). Condition of participation: Medical record services. 42 C.F.R. § 482.24(b).

25 DNV GL–Healthcare USA, Inc. (2020). MR.2.SR.1. *NIAHO® accreditation requirements, interpretive guidelines and surveyor guidance—revision 20.0.* Milford, OH: DNV GL–Healthcare USA, Inc. (Level VII)

26 Miller, S., et al. (2015). Physical examination of the adult patient with chronic respiratory disease. *Medsurg Nursing, 24*(3), 195–198.

27 Hinkle, J. L., & Cheever, K. H. (2018). *Brunner and Suddarth's textbook of medical-surgical nursing* (14th ed.). Philadelphia, PA: Wolters Kluwer.

28 American Heart Association. (2020). 2020 American Heart Association guidelines for CPR and ECC—Part 3: Adult basic and advanced life support. https://cpr.heart.org/en/resuscitation-science/cpr-and-ecc-guidelines

RESTRAINT APPLICATION

The Centers for Medicare and Medicaid Services (CMS) and The Joint Commission define restraints as devices that immobilize or reduce the ability of a patient to move the arms, legs, body, or head freely, except in situations involving orthopedic devices, surgical bandages, and similar devices required for the patient's care.[1,2] The Healthcare Facilities Accreditation Program (HFAP) defines physical restraint as any manual method, physical or mechanical device, material, or equipment attached or adjacent to the patient that restricts freedom of movement or normal access to one's body.[3] DNV GL–Healthcare USA defines restraint as any manual method, physical or mechanical device, material, or equipment that immobilizes or reduces the ability of the patient to move arms, legs, head, or body freely.[4]

A vest restraint can be used to prevent self-injury from falls, or to immobilize a patient to assist medical treatment. It's applied to a patient's torso over the hospital gown or clothing. The straps are then secured to the patient's bed frame (not the side rail) or chair.[5]

A limb restraint is a device consisting of a cuff, typically made of padded fabric or foam, applied to a patient's wrists or ankles with straps that are secured to the patient's bed frame. Limb restraints are used to prevent self-injury or the removal of therapeutic equipment, such as IV lines, indwelling catheters, and nasogastric tubes.

A mitt restraint is a pocket enclosure that's applied over a patient's hand to prevent self-injury or the removal of therapeutic equipment, such as IV lines, indwelling catheters, and nasogastric tubes. Mitt restraints may be padded or rigid, and may include finger separators or leave the fingers exposed. Optional straps that can be secured to the patient's bed frame or chair may be included with the device or may need to be ordered separately, if indicated. Most mitt restraints can be applied to either hand. Although some hand mitts aren't considered restraints if the hand mitts immobilizes the hands, if they're pinned or attached to the bedding, or if they're used in conjunction with the wrist restraints, they meet the definition of a restraint and the associated standards apply.[1,6]

A belt restraint consists of a strip of material—usually cotton fabric or mesh—that's applied over a patient's gown or clothing, around the waist or lap. The straps are then secured to the patient's bed frame or chair. Belt restraints can be used to prevent self-injury from falling or to immobilize a patient, if needed, during medical treatment.

A leather or leather-like restraint is made of leather or a synthetic substitute for leather, such as polyurethane or vinyl. Leather restraints are used to prevent self-injury or injury to others, and to immobilize a patient for medical treatment. The restraint is applied to a patient's wrists or ankles and then secured to a bed frame or chair.

The CMS, The Joint Commission, HFAP, and DNV GL–Healthcare USA recognize the rights of patients to be free from restraint or seclusion of any form imposed as a means of coercion, discipline, convenience, or retaliation by staff. Restraint or seclusion may only be used to ensure the immediate physical safety of the patient, a staff member, or others, and only when all other methods have failed to keep the patient from self-harm or from harming others. This standard has been established with the intent of reducing the overall use of restraint. If restraint must be used, the health care provider must choose a restraint that's the least restrictive to the patient, and discontinue restraint use at the earliest possible time.[1,2,3,4]

Only staff members trained in the use of restraints as well as less restrictive techniques aimed at avoiding restraint are permitted to evaluate the need for restraint, apply restraints, and monitor patients who are restrained.[7,8]

Interventions that can reduce the need for restraint include pain management techniques, conversation with the patient, exercise, activity involvement, meditation, prayer, contact with familiar people or places, and such therapies as massage, therapeutic touch, aromatherapy, music therapy, pet therapy, and reminiscence therapy.[9]

Equipment

Restraint device (vest, limb, mitt, belt, or leather) ▪ vital signs monitoring equipment ▪ Optional: gloves, gown, mask, eye protection, padding, straps, key, cuff liners.

Preparation of equipment

Because there are various types of body restraints, refer to the manufacturer's preparation and application instructions. Some vest restraints wrap around the patient with the straps crossing in the front, whereas other types close with a zipper at the patient's back. Check to see that you have obtained the correct size for the patient's build and weight. Some devices require that the straps be fed through the cuff before application. Check the device for damage, and obtain a new device as necessary. *Because there are various types of belt restraints,* make sure you've chosen a restraint that's appropriate for your patient. For example, a restraint may hold a patient in a stationary position or allow the patient to roll from side to side, may wrap around the pelvis in addition to the waist for additional security when sitting up, or be padded or unpadded. Some belt restraints wrap around the patient with the straps crossing in the back; others have straps that cross in the front.

If using leather or leather-like restraints, make sure the straps are unlocked and the key fits the lock. If indicated by the manufacturer, apply cuff liners to the restraint cuffs *to reduce friction between the patient's skin and the restraint, which helps prevent skin irritation and breakdown.*

Inspect the restraint for damage and obtain a new restraint if necessary. If the restraint is defective, remove it from patient use, label it as defective, and report the defect as directed by your facility.

Implementation

■ Obtain a practitioner's order for the restraint. In an emergency situation, obtain an order as soon as possible after applying the restraint.[7,10,11]
NURSING ALERT If the patient is being restrained because of violent or self-destructive behavior that jeopardizes the patient's physical safety or that of staff members or others, the doctor, clinical psychologist, or other licensed independent practitioner responsible for the patient's care must conduct an in-person evaluation within 1 hour of initiation of the restraint or seclusion. A specially trained nurse or physician's assistant may perform the face-to-face evaluation; however, the nurse or physician's assistant must consult the licensed practitioner who's responsible for the care of the patient as soon as possible after completing the face-to-face evaluation. You can't use as-needed or standing orders for restraints.[1,11,12,13,14]
■ Gather and prepare the necessary equipment and supplies.
■ Perform hand hygiene.[15,16,17,18,19]
■ Put on gloves and personal protective equipment as needed *to comply with standard precautions.*[20]
■ Confirm the patient's identity using at least two patient identifiers.[19]
■ Explain the procedure to the patient and family (if appropriate) according to their individual communication and learning needs *to increase their understanding, allay their fears, and enhance cooperation.*[21] Tell the patient that you're applying a vest restraint. Assure the patient that you're using the restraint as a protection from injury rather than a punishment. Emphasize that you'll remove the restraint as soon as it's safe to do so, and explain the criteria you'll use for discontinuing its use.
■ If necessary, obtain the assistance of additional staff members to apply the restraint.
■ If the patient's condition permits, assist the patient to a sitting position. If the patient can't sit, apply the vest restraint by rolling the patient side-to-side.
■ Smooth out the patient's gown or clothing, removing as many wrinkles as possible *to prevent skin breakdown.*
■ Slip the vest over the patient's gown or clothing.

Applying a crisscross vest restraint

■ Assist the patient in putting the arms through the armholes with the V-shape neck in front. Crisscross the straps in the front of the vest. Never crisscross the flaps in the back, *because doing so may cause the patient to choke if the patient tries to squirm out of the vest.*
■ Feed the straps through the holes in the front of the vest, as indicated by manufacturer's instructions.

Applying a zipper vest restraint

■ Place the vest over the patient with the zipper in back.

■ Assist the patient in placing the arms through the armholes.
■ Zip up the back of the restraint.
■ Adjust the vest for a comfortable fit. Make sure that the restraint doesn't compromise breathing or circulation. You should be able to slip an open, flat hand between the vest and the patient.[5]
■ If the patient is in bed, fasten the restraint straps securely to a movable part of the bed frame, out of the patient's reach. Don't fasten the straps to the bed's side rails. Alternatively, if the patient is in a chair or wheelchair, secure the restraint to a movable part of the chair frame, out of the patient's reach. Some restraints have quick-release clips or buckles, whereas others require tying a quick-release knot that you can easily release in an emergency.[5] (See *Tying a quick-release knot,* page 738) Follow the manufacturer's instructions for the type of restraint used in your facility.

Applying a limb restraint

■ Position the patient's wrist or ankle in the soft padded cuff portion of the restraint by slipping the cuff over the patient's hand or foot. If using a wrap-type device, wrap the wrist or ankle so that the fasteners are on the outside of the device.
■ If indicated, fasten the buckle or Velcro fastener.
■ Adjust the straps for a snug fit that doesn't compromise the patient's circulation. You should be able to slip two fingers (flat) between the restraint and the patient's skin. *Applying the restraint too tightly may impair circulation distal to the restraint.*[22]

Applying a mitt restraint

■ Assess for baseline hand and finger circulation *to determine the appropriateness of the device and to determine whether circulatory changes may occur after application.*
■ Insert the patient's hand into the mitt with the palm facing down according to the manufacturer's instructions. If finger separators are available in the device, separate each finger into its own slot.
■ Wrap the strap over the mitt and around the patient's wrist *to secure the mitt to the patient.*
■ Secure the strap with the device's fastener, which may be Velcro or some other type of fastener.
■ Adjust the straps for a snug fit that doesn't compromise the patient's circulation. You should be able to slip one finger between the restraint and the patient's skin. *Applying the restraint too tightly may impair circulation distal to the restraint.*[23]
■ If you must restrict arm movement, wrap a second restraint strap around the patient's wrist and fasten the restraint strap securely to a movable part of the bed frame according to the manufacturer's instructions. Don't fasten them to the side rails. Some restraints have quick-release clips or buckles; others require tying a quick-release knot that you can release easily in an emergency.[23] (See *Tying a quick-release knot,* page 738.)

Applying a belt restraint
Restraining a patient in a chair or wheelchair

■ Position the patient as far back in the seat as possible. If the patient is in a wheelchair, make sure that the wheels are locked.
NURSING ALERT Do not apply a belt restraint to a chair or wheelchair that doesn't permit proper application as directed by the manufacturer's instructions for use.
■ Wrap the belt restraint around the patient's hips and over the smoothed-out gown or clothing so that the straps end up at the back of the chair.
■ If the belt restraint is padded, place the padded side toward the patient.
■ If the belt restraint includes a pelvic holder, place the narrow side to the back of the chair, and bring the wide part of the holder up between the patient's legs and connect the straps.
■ Crisscross the straps at the back of the chair *for added security.*
■ If the chair has an adjustable seat, secure the straps to a movable part of the chair frame, out of the patient's reach.[24] Some restraints have a quick-release device, such as clips or buckles, whereas others require tying a quick-release knot that you can release easily in an emergency. (See *Tying a quick-release knot,* page 738.) Follow the manufacturer's instructions for the type of restraint used in your facility.

Restraining a patient in a bed

- Raise the patient's bed to waist level when providing patient care *to prevent caregiver back strain.*[25]
- Position the belt under the patient at waist level.
- Thread the straps through the slots at either the front or back of the patient, according to the manufacturer's directions and the desired movement limitation.
- Fasten the restraint straps securely to a movable part of the bed frame, out of the patient's reach.[24] Do not fasten the straps to the bed's side rails. Some restraints have a quick-release device, such as clips or buckles, whereas others require tying a quick-release knot that you can release easily in an emergency. (See *Tying a quick-release knot*, page 738.) Follow the manufacturer's instructions for the type of restraint used in your facility.
- Return the bed to the lowest position (if applicable) *to prevent falls and maintain patient safety.*[26]

Applying a leather or leather-like restraint

- *Ensure the safety of the patient and staff members* by having enough trained staff members available to assist in properly applying restraints. *Never attempt to apply leather restraints to a patient alone.* Give each staff member a specific task to immobilize the patient before applying the restraints.[7,27,28]
- Place the patient on the bed in the supine position, with each arm and leg securely held down *to minimize combative behavior and to prevent injury to the patient and others.* Immobilize the patient's arms and legs above and below the joints—knee, ankle, shoulder, and wrist—*to minimize movement without exerting excessive force.*
- Wrap each restraint around the extremity and adjust it to fit. Apply the restraint securely but not too tightly. You should be able to slip one finger between the restraint and the patient's skin. *A tight restraint can compromise circulation; a loose one can slip off or move up the patient's arm or leg, causing skin irritation and breakdown.*[29]
- Secure the locking mechanism and make sure that it clicks. Tug it gently *to be sure it's secure.*
- Attach the connecting strap to the restraint, and then secure the strap to the bed frame, out of the patient's reach.[30] Do not fasten the straps to the bed's side rails. Flex the patient's arm or leg slightly before locking the strap *to allow room for movement and to prevent frozen joints and dislocations.*
- Once the restraint is secure, allow the coworker to release the arm or leg. Then recheck the restraint *for proper fit.*
- Repeat the procedure for each restraint.
- Place the key in an accessible location at the nurse's station.

Completing the procedure

- Tie all the straps of the restraints securely to the frame of the bed, chair, or wheelchair and out of the patient's reach. Never secure the restraint to a bed rail. Use a knot that you can release quickly and easily in an emergency. (See *Tying a quick-release knot*, page 738.)
- Monitor the patient's physical and psychological well-being, including (but not limited to) vital signs, respiratory and circulatory status, skin integrity, and any special requirements identified during the practitioner's assessment, at a frequency determined by your facility, the patient's condition, and the type of device used.[1,30] Be alert for complications, such as impaired breathing and circulation, skin breakdown, and psychological distress. Make sure that the restraint doesn't tighten with the patient's movements. Adjust the fit if necessary. Notify the practitioner if signs and symptoms persist.
- If the patient consented to have family members (or another significant person) informed about care, notify them of the use of restraint, the patient monitoring that will be used during restraint, and the criteria for discontinuing restraint.[1,30]
- Assist the restrained patient with nutrition, hydration, hygiene, elimination, pain control, and comfort measures.
- *To prevent pressure injuries,* reposition the patient regularly based on the individual patient's risk factors and ability or willingness to self-position.[31,32] Encourage a patient who is sitting to shift weight every 15 minutes; reposition hourly if the patient can't reposition independently.[31]

- If you can do so safely and while continually monitoring the patient, release the restraint regularly as required by your facility *to allow the patient to participate in care, perform range-of-motion (ROM) exercises, turn, stretch, and breathe deeply.* Have a coworker assist as needed when releasing the restraint.
- Continue to reassess the need for restraint, and release the restraints as soon as the patient's condition permits, according to the practitioner's order.[33]
- Debrief the patient after removal of the restraint *to identify what led to use of the restraint and what could have been done differently,* and counsel the patient for physical or psychological trauma that may have resulted from the use of the restraint.[34]
- Remove and discard your gloves and personal protection equipment, if worn.[35]
- Perform hand hygiene.[15,16,17,18,19]
- Document the procedure.[36,37,38,39]

Special considerations

- Know the latest standards for restraint use from the CMS, The Joint Commission, HFAP, and DNV GL-Healthcare USA.[40,41] Make sure that you or another staff member have attempted less restrictive measures before restraint implementation, and that thorough documentation of those measures is in the patient's medical record. Aim to discontinue restraints as soon as it's safe to do so.[1,2,12]
- Use a vest restraint with caution in a patient with heart failure or a respiratory disorder.
- When the patient is at high risk for aspiration, restrain the patient on the side.
- Don't restrain a patient in the prone position. *This position limits the patient's field of vision, intensifies feelings of helplessness and vulnerability, and impairs respiration, especially if the patient has been sedated.*
- Don't apply a limb or mitt restraint above an IV site, *because the constriction may occlude the infusion or cause infiltration into surrounding tissue.*
- *To prevent skin breakdown,* ensure that you apply restraints correctly, loosen or remove the restraints regularly to assess the skin, and provide regular skin care.[42]
- If you're restraining the patient because of violent or self-destructive behavior, follow The Joint Commission, HFAP, or DNV GL-Healthcare and CMS guidelines for order limits[1,11,43,44] (unless your facility or state law has more restrictive guidelines):
  - 4 hours for adults (age 18 and older)
  - 2 hours for children and adolescents ages 9 to 17
  - 1 hour for children younger than age 9 years.[1,7,11,45]
- Note that the practitioner may renew orders for patient restraint because of violent or self-destructive behavior to the above time limits for a maximum of 24 consecutive hours. After 24 hours, the practitioner must write a new order for restraint use.[1,7,11,45]
- Follow U.S. Food and Drug Administration recommendations regarding bed safety, and be alert for a restrained patient's potential for entrapment and serious injury.[46]
- After removing restraints, disinfect them according to the manufacturer's instructions. You may wash synthetic restraints by machine or wipe them down with a disinfectant. You may clean soiled leather restraints with a disinfectant; however, you must discard leather restraints if they were exposed to blood or other body fluids.[47,48]
- Follow your facility's communication protocol for reporting to the CMS any death that occurs while a patient is in a restraint or within 24 hours of restraint removal.[49,50,51,52]

Complications

Follow the U.S. Food and Drug Administration's recommendations regarding bed safety, and be alert for a restrained patient's potential for entrapment, serious injury, and even death if the restraint is used inappropriately.[5,46] Some patients resist restraint and, in the course of resisting, may injure themselves or others.

Long periods of immobility can predispose the patient to pneumonia, urine retention and urinary tract infection, incontinence, pressure

Tying a quick-release knot

A quick-release knot allows you to quickly release the knot, using one hand, if the patient is in distress or has an emergency. Follow the steps below to tie a quick-release knot.

1. Wrap the attachment strap once around the moveable part of the bed frame (not the side rail), leaving at least an 8″ (a 20 cm) tail.
2. Fold the loose end in half *to create a loop*.

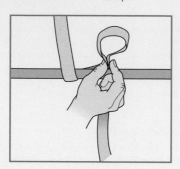

3. Cross the loop over the other end of the tie.

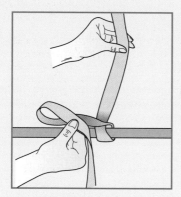

4. Insert the folded loop where the straps cross over each other. This step is similar to tying your shoes.

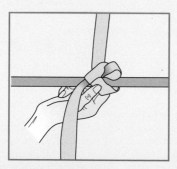

5. Pull on the loop to tighten the knot. Test to make sure that the strap is secure and won't slide in any direction.

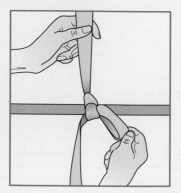

6. Create a second loop by folding the loose end in half.

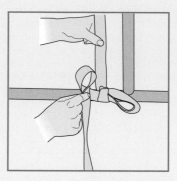

7. Insert the second loop, made of the loose end, through the first loop.

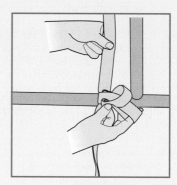

8. Pull on the remaining loop to securely tighten the knot. Test to make sure that the strap is secure and won't slide in any direction,

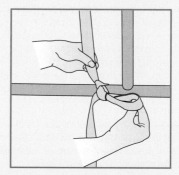

injuries, deconditioning, psychological distress,[53] constipation, and sensory deprivation. Reposition the patient and attend to elimination requirements as needed. Provide regular skin care, and make sure the patient wears garments under the vest *to protect the skin.*

Excessively tight limb restraints can reduce peripheral circulation. Apply restraints carefully and check them regularly. Skin breakdown can occur under limb restraints. *To prevent this complication,* make sure the restraint is padded around the patient's wrists and ankles, loosen or remove the restraints frequently, and provide regular skin care.

Documentation

Document each episode of the use of restraint, including the date and time that you initiated the restraint as well as the total number of minutes of physical restraint use.[54] Document the patient's symptoms, the less restrictive interventions that you tried first, your assessment of the need for restraint, and the name of the licensed independent practitioner who evaluated the patient and ordered the restraint as directed by your facility. Document the patient's response to the restraint. Include the conditions or behaviors necessary for discontinuing the restraint and whether these conditions were communicated to the patient.[55,56,57,58,59]

Document each in-person evaluation by the licensed independent practitioner.[55,60] Record regular patient assessments, including signs of injury, nutrition, hydration, circulation, ROM, vital signs, hygiene, elimination, comfort, physical and psychological status, and readiness for removing restraints. Record your interventions to help the patient meet the conditions for removing the restraint. You may use a flow sheet to record frequent assessments. Document any injuries or complications, the name of the practitioner that you notified, the time of your notification, and your actions.[55,59]

Document teaching provided to the patient and family (if applicable), their understanding of that teaching, and any need for follow-up teaching.

REFERENCES

1 Centers for Medicare and Medicaid Services. (2020). Condition of participation: Patient's rights. 42 C.F.R. § 482.13(e).

2 The Joint Commission. (2021). Standard PC.03.05.01. *Comprehensive accreditation manual for hospitals.* (Level VII)

3 Accreditation Association for Hospitals and Health Systems. (2020). Standard 32.02.01. *Healthcare Facilities Accreditation Program: Accreditation requirements for acute care hospitals.* Chicago, IL: Accreditation Association for Hospitals and Health Systems. (Level VII)

4 DNV GL-Healthcare USA, Inc. (2020). PR.7.SR.1. *NIAHO® accreditation requirements, interpretive guidelines and surveyor guidance—revision 20.0.* Milford, OH: DNV GL-Healthcare USA, Inc. (Level VII)

5 J. T. Posey Company. (2007). Application instruction sheet: Posey® jackets and vests. https://www.rehabmart.com/pdfs/jackets_and_vests.pdf

6 Accreditation Association for Hospitals and Health Systems. (2020). Standard 15.02.03. *Healthcare Facilities Accreditation Program: Accreditation requirements for acute care hospitals.* Chicago, IL: Accreditation Association for Hospitals and Health Systems. (Level VII)

7 Centers for Medicare and Medicaid Services. (2020). Condition of participation: Patient's rights. 42 C.F.R. § 482.13.

8 The Joint Commission. (2021). Standard PC.03.03.07. *Comprehensive accreditation manual for hospitals.* Oakbrook Terrace, IL: The Joint Commission. (Level VII)

9 American Nurses Association. (2012). Position statement: Reduction of patient restraint and seclusion in health care settings. https://www.nursingworld.org/~4af287/globalassets/docs/ana/ethics/ps_reduction-of-patient-restraint-and-seclusion-in-health-care-settings.pdf

10 The Joint Commission. (2021). Standard PC.03.03.13. *Comprehensive accreditation manual for hospitals.* Oakbrook Terrace, IL: The Joint Commission. (Level VII)

11 DNV GL-Healthcare USA, Inc. (2020). PR.7.SR.3. *NIAHO® accreditation requirements, interpretive guidelines and surveyor guidance—revision 20.0.* Milford, OH: DNV GL-Healthcare USA, Inc. (Level VII)

12 The Joint Commission. (2021). Standard PC.03.05.11. *Comprehensive accreditation manual for hospitals.* Oakbrook Terrace, IL: The Joint Commission. (Level VII)

13 Accreditation Association for Hospitals and Health Systems. (2020). Standard 15.02.20. *Healthcare Facilities Accreditation Program: Accreditation requirements for acute care hospitals.* Chicago, IL: Accreditation Association for Hospitals and Health Systems. (Level VII)

14 Centers for Medicare and Medicaid Services. (2020). Condition of participation: Patient's rights. 42 C.F.R. § 482.13(e)(6).

15 Centers for Disease Control and Prevention. (2002). Guideline for hand hygiene in health-care settings: Recommendations of the Healthcare Infection Control Practices Advisory Committee and the HICPAC/SHEA/APIC/IDSA Hand Hygiene Task Force. *MMWR Recommendations and Reports, 51*(RR-16), 1–45. https://www.cdc.gov/mmwr/pdf/rr/rr5116.pdf (Level II)

16 World Health Organization (WHO). (2009). WHO guidelines on hand hygiene in health care: First global patient safety challenge, clean care is safer care. https://apps.who.int/iris/bitstream/handle/10665/44102/9789241597906_eng.pdf?sequence=1 (Level IV)

17 The Joint Commission. (2021). Standard NPSG.07.01.01. *Comprehensive accreditation manual for hospitals.* Oakbrook Terrace, IL: The Joint Commission. (Level VII)

18 Accreditation Association for Hospitals and Health Systems. (2020). Standard 07.01.21. *Healthcare Facilities Accreditation Program: Accreditation requirements for acute care hospitals.* Chicago, IL: Accreditation Association for Hospitals and Health Systems. (Level VII)

19 DNV GL-Healthcare USA, Inc. (2020). IC.1.SR.1. *NIAHO® accreditation requirements, interpretive guidelines and surveyor guidance—revision 20.0.* Milford, OH: DNV GL-Healthcare USA, Inc. (Level VII)

20 The Joint Commission. (2021). Standard NPSG.01.01.01. *Comprehensive accreditation manual for hospitals.* Oakbrook Terrace, IL: The Joint Commission. (Level VII)

21 The Joint Commission. (2021). Standard PC.02.01.21. *Comprehensive accreditation manual for hospitals.* Oakbrook Terrace, IL: The Joint Commission. (Level VII)

22 Posey Company. (2012). Posey® limb holders: Application instructions. https://www.rehabmart.com/pdfs/i9209-posey-limb-holders.pdf

23 Posey Company. (2012). Posey® double-security mitts: https://www.rehabmart.com/pdfs/i9223-posey-double-security-mitts.pdf

24 Posey Company. (2016). Posey® roll belts: Application instructions. https://www.manualsdir.com/manuals/408370/posey-roll-belt.html

25 Waters, T. R., et al. (2009). Safe patient handling training for schools of nursing. https://www.cdc.gov/niosh/docs/2009-127/pdfs/2009-127.pdf (Level VII)

26 Ganz, D. A., et al. (2013, reviewed 2021). *Preventing falls in hospitals: A toolkit for improving quality of care* (AHRQ Publication No. 13-0015-EF). Agency for Healthcare Research and Quality. https://www.ahrq.gov/professionals/systems/hospital/fallpxtoolkit/index.html (Level VII)

27 DNV GL-Healthcare USA, Inc. (2020). PR.8.SR.2. *NIAHO® accreditation requirements, interpretive guidelines and surveyor guidance—revision 20.0.* Milford, OH: DNV GL-Healthcare USA, Inc. (Level VII)

28 Accreditation Association for Hospitals and Health Systems. (2020). Standard 15.02.09. *Healthcare Facilities Accreditation Program: Accreditation requirements for acute care hospitals.* Chicago, IL: Accreditation Association for Hospitals and Health Systems. (Level VII)

29 J. T. Posey Company. (2006). Application instruction sheet: Posey® limb holders. https://www.rehabmart.com/pdfs/patient_safety_restraints-3.pdf

30 The Joint Commission. (2021). Standard PC.03.05.07. *Comprehensive accreditation manual for hospitals.* Oakbrook Terrace, IL: The Joint Commission. (Level VII)

31 Wound, Ostomy, and Continence Nurses Society (WOCN). (2016). *Guideline for prevention and management of pressure ulcers (injuries): WOCN clinical practice guideline series 2.* Mt. Laurel, NJ: WOCN.

32 Fletcher, J. (2017). Reposition patients effectively to prevent pressure ulcers. *Wounds International, 8*(1), 7–10.

33 The Joint Commission. (2021). Standard PC.03.03.27. *Comprehensive accreditation manual for hospitals.* Oakbrook Terrace, IL: The Joint Commission. (Level VII)

34 The Joint Commission. (2021). Standard PC.03.03.29. *Comprehensive accreditation manual for hospitals.* Oakbrook Terrace, IL: The Joint Commission. (Level VII)

35 Occupational Safety and Health Administration. (2019). Bloodborne pathogens, standard number 1910.1030. https://www.osha.gov/pls/oshaweb/owadisp.show_document?p_id=10051&p_table=STANDARDS (Level VII)

36 The Joint Commission. (2021). Standard RC.01.03.01. *Comprehensive accreditation manual for hospitals.* Oakbrook Terrace, IL: The Joint Commission. (Level VII)

37 Accreditation Association for Hospitals and Health Systems. (2020). Standard 10.00.03. *Healthcare Facilities Accreditation Program: Accreditation requirements for acute care hospitals.* Chicago, IL: Accreditation Association for Hospitals and Health Systems. (Level VII)

38 DNV GL-Healthcare USA, Inc. (2020). MR.2.SR.1. *NIAHO® accreditation requirements, interpretive guidelines and surveyor guidance—revision 20.0.* Milford, OH: DNV GL-Healthcare USA, Inc. (Level VII)

39 Centers for Medicare and Medicaid Services. (2020). Condition of participation: Medical record services. 42 C.F.R. § 482.24(b).

40 The Joint Commission. (2021). Standard PC.03.05.09. *Comprehensive accreditation manual for hospitals.* Oakbrook Terrace, IL: The Joint Commission. (Level VII)

41 Accreditation Association for Hospitals and Health Systems. (2020). Standard 15.02.05. *Healthcare Facilities Accreditation Program: Accreditation requirements for acute care hospitals.* Chicago, IL: Accreditation Association for Hospitals and Health Systems. (Level VII)

42 American Psychiatric Nurses Association (APNA). (2018). APNA position on the use of seclusion and restraint. https://www.apna.org/resources/apna-seclusion-restraint-position-paper/ (Level VII)

43 The Joint Commission. (2021). Standard PC.03.05.05. *Comprehensive accreditation manual for hospitals.* Oakbrook Terrace, IL: The Joint Commission. (Level VII)

44 Accreditation Association for Hospitals and Health Systems. (2020). Standard 15.02.13. *Healthcare Facilities Accreditation Program: Accreditation requirements for acute care hospitals.* Chicago, IL: Accreditation Association for Hospitals and Health Systems. (Level VII)

45 Accreditation Association for Hospitals and Health Systems. (2020). Standard 15.02.14. *Healthcare Facilities Accreditation Program: Accreditation requirements for acute care hospitals.* Chicago, IL: Accreditation Association for Hospitals and Health Systems. (Level VII)

46 U.S. Food and Drug Administration. (2018). Hospital beds. https://www.fda.gov/medical-devices/general-hospital-devices-and-supplies/hospital-beds

47 Accreditation Association for Hospitals and Health Systems. (2020). Standard 07.02.03. *Healthcare Facilities Accreditation Program: Accreditation requirements for acute care hospitals.* Chicago, IL: Accreditation Association for Hospitals and Health Systems. (Level VII)

48 Rutala, W. A., et al. (2008, revised 2019). Guideline for disinfection and sterilization in healthcare facilities, 2008. https://www.cdc.gov/infection-control/pdf/guidelines/disinfection-guidelines-H.pdf (Level I)

49 Centers for Medicare and Medicaid Services, Department of Health and Human Services. (2020). Condition of participation: Patient's rights. 42 C.F.R. § 482.13(g).

50 DNV GL-Healthcare USA, Inc. (2020). PR.9.SR.1. *NIAHO® accreditation requirements, interpretive guidelines and surveyor guidance—revision 20.0.* Milford, OH: DNV GL-Healthcare USA, Inc. (Level VII)

51 The Joint Commission. (2021). Standard PC.03.05.19. *Comprehensive accreditation manual for hospitals.* Oakbrook Terrace, IL: The Joint Commission. (Level VII)

52 Accreditation Association for Hospitals and Health Systems. (2020). Standard 15.02.41. *Healthcare Facilities Accreditation Program: Accreditation requirements for acute care hospitals.* Chicago, IL: Accreditation Association for Hospitals and Health Systems. (Level VII)

53 Colling, L. G., et al. (2009). Restraining devices for patients in acute and long-term care facilities. *American Family Physician, 79*(4), 254–256. https://www.aafp.org/afp/2009/0215/p254.html

54 DNV GL-Healthcare USA, Inc. (2020). PR.7.SR.6. *NIAHO® accreditation requirements, interpretive guidelines and surveyor guidance—revision 20.0.* Milford, OH: DNV GL-Healthcare USA, Inc. (Level VII)

55 The Joint Commission. (2021). Standard PC.03.05.15. *Comprehensive accreditation manual for hospitals.* Oakbrook Terrace, IL: The Joint Commission. (Level VII)

56 Accreditation Association for Hospitals and Health Systems. (2020). Standard 15.02.25. *Healthcare Facilities Accreditation Program: Accreditation requirements for acute care hospitals.* Chicago, IL: Accreditation Association for Hospitals and Health Systems. (Level VII)

57 Accreditation Association for Hospitals and Health Systems. (2020). Standard 15.02.26. *Healthcare Facilities Accreditation Program: Accreditation requirements for acute care hospitals.* Chicago, IL: Accreditation Association for Hospitals and Health Systems. (Level VII)

58 Accreditation Association for Hospitals and Health Systems. (2020). Standard 15.02.27. *Healthcare Facilities Accreditation Program: Accreditation requirements for acute care hospitals.* Chicago, IL: Accreditation Association for Hospitals and Health Systems. (Level VII)

59 Accreditation Association for Hospitals and Health Systems. (2020). Standard 15.02.28. *Healthcare Facilities Accreditation Program: Accreditation requirements for acute care hospitals.* Chicago, IL: Accreditation Association for Hospitals and Health Systems. (Level VII)

60 Accreditation Association for Hospitals and Health Systems. (2020). Standard 15.02.24. *Healthcare Facilities Accreditation Program: Accreditation requirements for acute care hospitals.* Chicago, IL: Accreditation Association for Hospitals and Health Systems. (Level VII)

Ring removal

A ring can become excessively tight on a patient's finger or toe after an injury such as a sprain, or from some other cause of swelling such as in a localized allergic reaction, dependent extremity position, and excessive salt intake.[1] A very tight-fitting ring can obstruct lymphatic and venous drainage, causing pain and further swelling and constriction.[1] Removal may be necessary to relieve chronic or acute edema and to prevent vascular compromise, which can lead to ischemia with permanent tissue damage in a finger or toe constricted by a ring or metal or plastic band.[1]

Equipment

Ice or cold pack ▪ soap and water ▪ towel ▪ water-soluble lubricant[1] ▪ facility-approved disinfectant ▪ Optional: local anesthetic without EPINEPHrine, syringe, needles, alcohol pads, gloves, tourniquet, blood pressure cuff, Penrose drains, antibiotic ointment, adhesive bandage.[1]

Coiled-string method

String, umbilical tape, ribbon gauze, or thick suture material ▪ Optional: hemostat.

Ring-cutter method

Ring-cutter (manual, or battery- or electric-powered) ▪ pliers, hemostat, or ring spreader ▪ protective eyewear ▪ 20-mL syringe filled with water.

Preparation of equipment

Inspect all equipment and supplies. If a product is expired, is defective, or has compromised integrity, remove it from patient use, label it as expired or defective, and report the expiration or defect as directed by your facility.

Implementation

- Perform hand hygiene.[2,3,4,5,6,7]
- Confirm the patient's identity using at least two patient identifiers.[8]
- Provide privacy.[9,10,11,12]
- Explain the procedure to the patient and family (if appropriate) according to their individual communication and learning needs *to increase their understanding, allay their fears, and enhance cooperation.*[13]
- Perform hand hygiene.[2,3,4,5,6,7]
- Put on gloves as needed *to comply with standard precautions.*[14,15,16]
- Inspect the patient's digit for wounds, lacerations, fractures, and dislocations. Assess the digit's color, sensation, movement, and capillary refill. **NURSING ALERT** If you detect vascular compromise, remove the ring from the patient's digit with a ring cutter as quickly as possible.
- Screen for and assess the patient's pain using facility-defined criteria that are consistent with the patient's age, condition, and ability to understand.[17]
- Treat the patient's pain as needed and ordered using nonpharmacologic, pharmacologic, or a combination of approaches. Base the treatment plan on evidence-based practices and the patient's clinical condition, medical history, and pain management goals.[17]
- Arrange for an X-ray of the patient's digit, if ordered, and report abnormal findings to the practitioner.
- *To reduce swelling*, apply ice and elevate the affected extremity above heart level.[1] You may also use the tourniquet or Penrose drain method *to further reduce swelling.* For the tourniquet method: Apply a blood pressure cuff to the patient's affected extremity and inflate it.[1] Then wrap a tourniquet tightly from the tip of the digit proximally.[1] Elevate the extremity above the patient's heart for 10 to 15 minutes and then attempt to remove the ring manually.[1] Keep the blood pressure cuff inflated during the manual removal attempt, but remember that the total tourniquet time shouldn't exceed 60 minutes.[1,18] Deflate the cuff and remove

the tourniquet after the ring removal attempt.[1] For the Penrose drain method: Apply one Penrose drain just distal to the proximal interphalangeal (PIP) joint.[1] Wrap a second Penrose drain tightly, starting at the first drain and extending back to the ring.[1] Repeat as needed *to sufficiently reduce edema and allow for manual ring removal.* After the ring passes the PIP joint, remove the first Penrose drain.[1]

■ Lubricate the skin beneath the ring with soap and water or a water-soluble lubricant *to make it easier for the ring to be slipped off the digit.* Hold the ring with a towel, and pull with a rocking motion in an attempt to remove the ring from the patient's digit.

NURSING ALERT Even if the patient relates previous attempts to remove the object from the finger at home, it's worthwhile to attempt removal with soap and water or a water-soluble lubricant before trying other techniques. The pain from constriction often prevents the patient from applying adequate circular traction to remove the ring.

■ If the ring can't be removed using soap and water or a water-soluble lubricant, use one of the methods outlined below.

■ If required, assist the practitioner when administering digital anesthesia using a local anesthetic without EPINEPHrine.[19]

NURSING ALERT Never use products containing EPINEPHrine on a patient's finger or toe, *because EPINEPHrine exerts a vasoconstrictive effect.*[19]

Using the coiled-string method

NURSING ALERT Don't use the coiled-string method if the patient has any lacerations, fractures, or dislocations involving the affected digit; instead, use a ring cutter method.

■ While the affected digit is elevated, slip the end of a long strip of string or alternative material under the ring. Use a hemostat, if necessary, to thread the string under the ring.

■ Anchor the string with your nondominant hand, or ask the patient to anchor it.

■ Wrap the string around the patient's digit, beginning adjacent to the ring margin. Wrap the string in a snug, smooth, single layer in a clockwise fashion, slightly overlapping the previous layer, progressing in a proximal-to-distal direction until it covers the area of greatest swelling. *Because the area of the PIP joint is the most difficult area to slip the ring over,* make sure that you wrap this area firmly (as shown below).

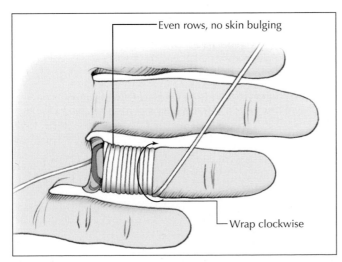

Even rows, no skin bulging

Wrap clockwise

■ When the wrapping is complete, pull the proximal end of the string against the ring and then start to unwrap the string in a clockwise direction, moving the ring toward the tip of the finger (as shown on top right). If needed, place a small amount of lubricant over the string *to facilitate sliding the ring.*

Using locking pliers

Tungsten carbide, ceramic, and natural stone rings made of onyx or jade are removed by cracking them into pieces with standard locking pliers.[30] Follow these steps:

■ Place the locking pliers over the band, and adjust the jaws to clamp lightly.

■ Release the clamp and then readjust the jaws, tightening the screw one-quarter turn to clamp it again.[30]

■ Repeat this process until you hear, see, or feel a crack. The ring or band will break into two or more pieces.[30]

■ Take care when removing the pieces. *Because the cracked edges are sharp,* don't rotate the cracked ring on the patient's digit.

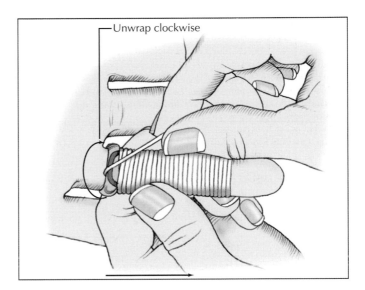

Unwrap clockwise

NURSING ALERT Moving the ring over the PIP joint will be the most difficult and may cause the most pain to the patient. It's common for this procedure to cause abrasions.

Using the manual ring-cutter method

■ Confirm that informed consent for cutting and removing the ring has been obtained and that the signed consent form is in the patient's medical record.[20,21,22,23]

■ Put on protective eyewear *to avoid possible injury caused by metal fragments.*

■ Slip the curved finger guard of the ring cutter under the ring. Use lubricant if necessary. Rotate the ring, if possible, so that the thinnest part of the band is located under the saw blade (as shown below).

■ Clamp the cutting disk down firmly on the ring, and use the turnkey to manually turn the cutting disk until the ring is severed.

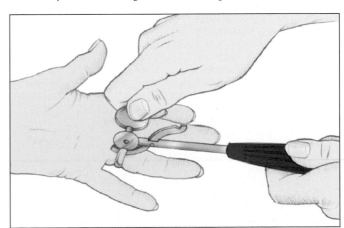

■ After the ring has been cut through, bend the ring apart with pliers, a hemostat, or a ring spreader (as shown below) *to allow ring removal.*

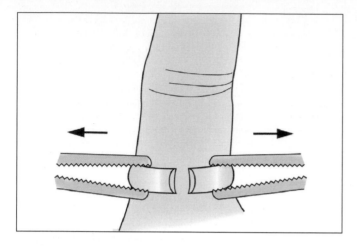

■ If the ring is a wide band, it may be necessary to make a second cut *to remove a wedge from the ring.*
■ Remove the ring.
■ Irrigate the skin with water *to remove any metal particles.*
■ Remove protective eyewear.

Using the battery- or electric-powered ring-cutter method
■ Confirm that informed consent for cutting and removing the ring has been obtained and that the signed consent form is in the patient's medical record.[20,21,22,23]
■ Put on protective eyewear *to avoid possible injury caused by metal fragments.*
■ Ensure that the correct cutting blade of the ring cutter is in place. *Some manufacturers supply different blades for different types of metals.* Always follow the manufacturer's instructions.
■ Place the finger guard of the ring cutter under the ring. Use lubricant if necessary. Rotate the ring, if possible, so that the thinnest part of the band is located under the saw blade of the ring cutter.
■ Turn on the power to the cutting blade so that it's rotating before it makes contact with the ring.
■ Apply gentle pressure to make contact between the rotating blade and the ring.

NURSING ALERT The friction caused by cutting may produce an uncomfortable amount of heat in the ring and the patient's hand. Ask if the patient is comfortable, and regularly check the temperature of the ring and cutter blade with your fingers. Stop briefly if necessary *to allow the ring and cutter to cool down.*

■ After you've cut through the ring, bend the ring apart with pliers, a hemostat, or a ring spreader *to allow removal,* or make a second cut on the opposite side of the ring and remove the wedge.
■ Remove the ring.
■ Irrigate the skin with water *to remove any metal particles.*
■ Remove your protective eyewear.

Completing the procedure
■ Reassess the neurovascular status of the patient's digit.
■ Assess for soft tissue trauma, including bruising or small cuts. Apply antibiotic ointment and an adhesive bandage, as ordered.[1]
■ Elevate the digit and apply cold packs, as ordered.
■ Return the ring or all pieces of the removed ring to the patient.
■ Discard used supplies in the appropriate receptacle.[16]
■ Remove and discard your gloves, if worn.[16]
■ Perform hand hygiene.[2,3,4,5,6,7]
■ Put on gloves, as necessary.[16]
■ Clean and disinfect reusable equipment according to the manufacturer's instructions *to prevent the spread of infection.*[24,25]
■ Remove and discard your gloves, if worn.[16]
■ Perform hand hygiene.[2,3,4,5,6,7]

■ Reassess and respond to the patient's pain by evaluating the patient's response to treatment and progress toward pain management goals. Assess for any adverse reactions and risk factors for adverse events that may result from treatment.[17]
■ Document the procedure.[26,27,28,29]

Special considerations
■ Some rings are made of tungsten carbide, ceramic, or natural stone; these rings can be removed with locking pliers (vise-grip pliers). (See *Using locking pliers,* page 741.)
■ Reassess the neurovascular status of the patient's digit frequently after ring removal. Notify the practitioner immediately of any abnormalities.
■ Clean any open wounds and cover them with a sterile dressing *to prevent infection.*
■ Administer tetanus immunization, as indicated and ordered, following safe medication administration practices.[31,32,33]
■ When removing a ring or other objects from a child's digit, use age-appropriate terms when explaining the procedure. Allow the child's parents or guardian to stay and hold the child during the procedure. Allow the child to examine the equipment, if appropriate.

Complications
Possible complications of the coiled string or ring cutter method include laceration of the skin on the patient's affected digit.

Documentation
Document your assessment findings, including the skin condition and neurovascular status of the digit before and after ring removal. Document the methods used to remove the ring, the success or failure of the methods, and the disposition of the ring. Record the patient's pain status, any interventions provided, and the patient's response to those interventions. Document teaching provided to the patient and family (if applicable), their understanding of that teaching, and any need for follow-up teaching.

REFERENCES

1 Bothner, J. (2020). Ring entrapment and removal. In: *UpToDate,* Stack, A. M., & Wolfson, A. B. (Eds.).
2 Centers for Disease Control and Prevention. (2002). Guideline for hand hygiene in health-care settings: Recommendations of the Healthcare Infection Control Practices Advisory Committee and the HICPAC/SHEA/APIC/IDSA Hand Hygiene Task Force. *MMWR Recommendations and Reports, 51*(RR-16), 1–45. https://www.cdc.gov/mmwr/pdf/rr/rr5116.pdf (Level II)
3 The Joint Commission. (2021). Standard NPSG.07.01.01. *Comprehensive accreditation manual for hospitals.* Oakbrook Terrace, IL: The Joint Commission. (Level VII)
4 World Health Organization. (2009). WHO guidelines on hand hygiene in health care: First global patient safety challenge, clean care is safer care. https://apps.who.int/iris/bitstream/handle/10665/44102/9789241597906_eng.pdf?sequence=1 (Level IV)
5 Accreditation Association for Hospitals and Health Systems. (2020). Standard 07.01.21. *Healthcare Facilities Accreditation Program: Accreditation requirements for acute care hospitals.* Chicago, IL: Accreditation Association for Hospitals and Health Systems. (Level VII)
6 Centers for Medicare and Medicaid Services, Department of Health and Human Services. (2020). Condition of participation: Infection control. 42 C.F.R. § 482.42.
7 DNV GL-Healthcare USA, Inc. (2020). IC.1.SR.1. *NIAHO® accreditation requirements, interpretive guidelines and surveyor guidance—revision 20.0.* Milford, OH: DNV GL-Healthcare USA, Inc. (Level VII)
8 The Joint Commission. (2021). Standard NPSG.01.01.01. *Comprehensive accreditation manual for hospitals.* Oakbrook Terrace, IL: The Joint Commission. (Level VII)
9 DNV GL-Healthcare USA, Inc. (2020). PR.2.SR.5. *NIAHO® accreditation requirements, interpretive guidelines and surveyor guidance—revision 20.0.* Milford, OH: DNV GL-Healthcare USA, Inc. (Level VII)
10 Centers for Medicare and Medicaid Services, Department of Health and Human Services. (2020). Condition of participation: Patient's rights. 42 C.F.R. § 482.13(c)(1).
11 Accreditation Association for Hospitals and Health Systems. (2020). Standard 15.01.16. *Healthcare Facilities Accreditation Program: Accreditation requirements for acute care hospitals.* Chicago, IL: Accreditation Association for Hospitals and Health Systems. (Level VII)

12 The Joint Commission. (2021). Standard RI.01.01.01. *Comprehensive accreditation manual for hospitals.* Oakbrook Terrace, IL: The Joint Commission. (Level VII)

13 The Joint Commission. (2021). Standard PC.02.01.21. *Comprehensive accreditation manual for hospitals.* Oakbrook Terrace, IL: The Joint Commission. (Level VII)

14 Accreditation Association for Hospitals and Health Systems. (2020). Standard 07.01.10. *Healthcare Facilities Accreditation Program: Accreditation requirements for acute care hospitals.* Chicago, IL: Accreditation Association for Hospitals and Health Systems. (Level VII)

15 Siegel, J. D., et al. (2007, revised 2019). 2007 guideline for isolation precautions: Preventing transmission of infectious agents in healthcare settings. https://www.cdc.gov/infectioncontrol/pdf/guidelines/isolation-guidelines-H.pdf (Level II)

16 Occupational Safety and Health Administration. (2019). Bloodborne pathogens, standard number 1910.1030. https://www.osha.gov/pls/oshaweb/owadisp.show_document?p_id=10051&p_table=STANDARDS (Level VII)

17 The Joint Commission. (2021). Standard PC.01.02.07. *Comprehensive accreditation manual for hospitals.* Oakbrook Terrace, IL: The Joint Commission. (Level VII)

18 Guideline for perioperative practice: Pneumatic tourniquet. (2021). In Wood, A. (Ed.), *Guidelines for perioperative practice,* 2021 edition. Denver, CO: AORN, Inc. (Level VII)

19 Baldor, R., & Mathes, B. M. (2020). Digital nerve block. In: *UpToDate,* Wolfson, A. B. (Ed.).

20 Centers for Medicare and Medicaid Services, Department of Health and Human Services. (2020). Condition of participation: Patient's rights. 42 C.F.R. § 482.13(b)(2).

21 The Joint Commission. (2021). Standard RI.01.03.01. *Comprehensive accreditation manual for hospitals.* Oakbrook Terrace, IL: The Joint Commission. (Level VII)

22 Accreditation Association for Hospitals and Health Systems. (2020). Standard 15.01.11. *Healthcare Facilities Accreditation Program: Accreditation requirements for acute care hospitals.* Chicago, IL: Accreditation Association for Hospitals and Health Systems. (Level VII)

23 DNV GL-Healthcare USA, Inc. (2020). PR.2.SR.3. *NIAHO® accreditation requirements, interpretive guidelines and surveyor guidance—revision 20.0.* Milford, OH: DNV GL-Healthcare USA, Inc. (Level VII)

24 Accreditation Association for Hospitals and Health Systems. (2020). Standard 07.02.03. *Healthcare Facilities Accreditation Program: Accreditation requirements for acute care hospitals.* Chicago, IL: Accreditation Association for Hospitals and Health Systems. (Level VII)

25 Rutala, W. A., et al. (2008, revised 2019). Guideline for disinfection and sterilization in healthcare facilities, 2008. https://www.cdc.gov/infection-control/pdf/guidelines/disinfection-guidelines-H.pdf (Level I)

26 The Joint Commission. (2021). Standard RC.01.03.01. *Comprehensive accreditation manual for hospitals.* Oakbrook Terrace, IL: The Joint Commission. (Level VII)

27 Accreditation Association for Hospitals and Health Systems. (2020). Standard 10.00.03. *Healthcare Facilities Accreditation Program: Accreditation requirements for acute care hospitals.* Chicago, IL: Accreditation Association for Hospitals and Health Systems. (Level VII)

28 Centers for Medicare and Medicaid Services, Department of Health and Human Services. (2020). Condition of participation: Medical record services. 42 C.F.R. § 482.24(b).

29 DNV GL-Healthcare USA, Inc. (2020). MR.2.SR.1. *NIAHO® accreditation requirements, interpretive guidelines and surveyor guidance—revision 20.0.* Milford, OH: DNV GL-Healthcare USA, Inc. (Level VII)

30 Moser, A., et al. (2016). Removal of a tungsten carbide ring from the finger of a pregnant patient: A case report involving 2 emergency departments and the internet. *Case Reports in Emergency Medicine, 2016,* 8164524. https://www.ncbi.nlm.nih.gov/pmc/articles/PMC4799811/

31 Accreditation Association for Hospitals and Health Systems. (2020). Standard 16.01.03. *Healthcare Facilities Accreditation Program: Accreditation requirements for acute care hospitals.* Chicago, IL: Accreditation Association for Hospitals and Health Systems. (Level VII)

32 Centers for Medicare and Medicaid Services, Department of Health and Human Services. (2020). Condition of participation: Nursing services. 42 C.F.R. § 482.23(c).

33 DNV GL-Healthcare USA, Inc. (2020). MM.1.SR.3. *NIAHO® accreditation requirements, interpretive guidelines and surveyor guidance—revision 20.0.* Milford, OH: DNV GL-Healthcare USA, Inc. (Level VII)

SAFE MEDICATION ADMINISTRATION PRACTICES,

GENERAL

An *adverse drug event* (ADE) is defined as harm to the patient, including mental harm, physical harm, or loss of function, that results from a medication error. A *medication error* is a mistake that occurs during the medication administration process. If a mistake occurs, it doesn't matter whether the patient was harmed or whether there was only a potential for injury; it's still considered a medication error.[1] An ADE is a more direct measure of harm to the patient than a medication error.

ADEs can be further defined as preventable or nonpreventable. A *preventable ADE* occurs as a result of a clinician error or a systematic error and thus could have been prevented. A *nonpreventable ADE* results from a drug's pharmacologic properties.[1] A potential ADE is also known as a *near miss* or *close call*: although the patient wasn't harmed, the potential for risk or harm was averted because of actions taken by the patient or clinician.[1]

To promote a culture of safety and to prevent medication errors, nurses must avoid distractions and interruptions when preparing and administering medications[2,3] and adhere to the "five rights" of medication administration: identify the right patient by using at least two patient-specific identifiers; select the right medication; administer the right dose; administer the medication at the right time; and administer the medication by the right route. Recent literature identifies nine rights of medication administration, which in addition to the five rights includes the right documentation, the right action (or appropriate reason for prescribing the medication), the right form, and the right response.[4,5]

Equipment

Patient's medical record ▪ patient's medication reconciliation form or list ▪ medication order sheets, preprinted or plain ▪ medication administration record (MAR) or electronic medication administration record (EMAR) ▪ Optional: conversion weight chart.

Implementation

▪ Avoid distractions and interruptions when preparing and administering medication *to prevent medication errors.*[2,3]

Verifying the medication order

▪ Follow a written or typed order or an order entered into a computer order-entry system, *because these types of orders are less likely to result in error or misunderstanding.*

▪ Make sure that the prescriber's order contains a diagnosis, a condition, or an indication for the medication.[4,6,7,8]

▪ Verify that other essential elements of the medication order are present, including the patient's name, age, and weight (in kilograms)[9]; the date and time the order was written; the name of the drug to be administered; the drug dosage; the route of administration; the frequency of administration; dose calculation requirements (when applicable); the exact strength or concentration of the drug (when applicable); the quantity of the drug or duration of administration (when applicable); specific instructions for use (when applicable); and the signature of the person writing the information.[4,6,7,8]

▪ Review the practitioner's order *to make sure that the prescribed infusion solution or medication, dose, rate, and route of administration are appropriate for the patient's age, condition, and access device (if applicable).* Address concerns about the order with the practitioner, pharmacist, or your supervisor and, if needed, the risk management department or as directed by your facility.[10]

▪ Reconcile the patient's medications when the practitioner orders a new medication *to reduce the risk of medication errors, including omissions, duplications, dosing errors, and drug interactions.*[11]

Identifying the patient

- Check the patient's medical record *to make sure that all the required documents, medication information, sensitivities, history, physical examination, diagnoses, and laboratory results are present with current information.*[12]
- Perform hand hygiene.[13,14,15,16,17,18]
- Confirm the patient's identity using at least two patient identifiers *to minimize the potential for a medication error because it is the wrong patient.*[19] Compare the information with the MAR or EMAR.
- Explain the name and purpose of each medication and when and how it the patient will take it. Discuss important and common adverse effects for each medication and what to do if the patient experiences any symptoms. Discuss any possible drug–drug, drug–food, or drug–disease interactions.[4,7,8,20,21,22]

Obtaining an accurate medication listing

- Ensure that the admitting practitioner obtained a complete list of the patient's current medications, including all prescription and over-the-counter medications and dietary supplements, as well as a history of known drug or food allergies, when the patient arrived at the facility.[12,20] If possible, involve the patient in creating this list. If the patient can't participate, obtain help from an immediate family member or another authorized person. If the list was obtained before the patient's date of admission, update it *to provide the most accurate listing of the medications that the patient is taking.*[12]
- Ensure that the medication list is readily available in the patient's medical record, and that the patient's practitioners have reviewed it. *This practice helps reduce the risk of drug interactions, allergic reactions, and dose-related errors, and helps identify contraindications.*
- Send a copy of the patient's medication list and new medication orders to the pharmacy *to enable the pharmacy to check the appropriateness of the new medication against what the patient has been taking. Doing so helps prevent drug interactions, allergic reactions, improper routes of administration, duplication of medications or types or classes of medications, and administration of a contraindicated medication.*[23,24]

Checking for medication contraindications

- Obtain and update the patient's allergy information and current medications during each admission or transfer *to ensure that all health care providers have access to the most up-to-date information.*[25]
- Communicate the patient's current allergy information to all members of the health care team.
- Send medication orders to the pharmacy before the medication is administered *so that the pharmacist can check the medication against the patient's current active medications.*[23,24]
- Have all health care providers review the list of current medications and allergies at each patient encounter *to determine the appropriateness of each medication for the intended condition.*[1,20]
- If any health care team member has questions about a medication, whether it's a new drug or part of the patient's existing regimen, that team member should contact the pharmacist before administering it.[1]

Ensuring accurate dosage calculations

- Make sure that the patient's most recent weight (in kilograms) is documented in the medical record *to enable accurate weight-related dosage calculations.*[9]
- Have a conversion chart readily available in case weight is documented in only one unit of measure.
- Calculate the correct dosage of medications that are ordered using weight-based dose schedules. Have two licensed practitioners verify these calculations.
- Use automated dosage calculations whenever possible, especially with IV infusion pumps, *to eliminate dosage calculation errors for drugs with narrow therapeutic dose ranges.*

Administering high-alert medications

- Identify high-alert medications based on your facility's approved list.[4,26] Examples of high-alert medications are adrenergic agonists, adrenergic antagonists, anesthetic agents, antiarrhythmics, antithrombic agents, cardioplegic solutions, hypertonic glucose solutions, dialysis solutions, epidural or intrathecal medications, inotropic medications, liposomal forms of drugs, moderate sedation agents, opioids, neuromuscular blocking agents, parenteral nutrition preparations, radiocontrast agents administered IV, antidiabetic agents, and chemotherapeutic drugs.[1,27]

NURSING ALERT Before administering a high-alert medication, if required by your facility, ask another nurse to perform an independent double-check *to verify the patient's identity and to make sure that the right medication is on hand, the medication's indication corresponds with the patient's diagnosis, dosage calculations are correct, the route of administration is safe and proper for the patient, and, if giving an infusion, the pump settings are correct and the infusion line is attached to the correct port.*[6]

- Monitor medication dosing carefully, especially if dosing adjustments are necessary because of narrow therapeutic windows.[1]
- Obtain and review any laboratory values required for dosing adjustments. Collaborate with the practitioner if values are out of the therapeutic range; watch for adverse effects.[1]

NURSING ALERT For patients receiving IV opioid medication, frequently monitor respiratory rate, sedation level, and oxygen saturation level by continuous pulse oximetry, or exhaled carbon dioxide by continuous capnography, *to decrease the risk of adverse events associated with IV opioid use.* If adverse reactions occur, respond promptly *to prevent treatment delays.*[5]

Handling verbal orders

- Minimize the use of verbal orders, *because verbal orders are especially susceptible to error.*[4,6]
- Have the practitioner repeat and verify the verbal order.[28,29]
- Record the verbal order in the patient's medical record, and make sure to include the date and name of the practitioner who gave the verbal order, your name as the person who received and recorded the order, and the name of the person who implemented the order.
- Read back the order to the practitioner as you have written it down *to confirm correct documentation.*[4,30]

Administering scheduled medications in a timely manner

- Maintenance doses administered according to a standard repeated cycle of frequency, such as every 4 hours or 3 times per day, are considered scheduled medications.[31]
- Identify a time-critical list of common scheduled medications specific to the patient population of the facility unit, such as the oncology unit.[31]
- Identify a time-critical list of scheduled medications that might be used on all units. Examples of time-critical scheduled medications are antibiotics, anticoagulants, insulin, anticonvulsants, immunosuppressive agents, non-IV pain medications, medications prescribed for administration within a specific time of the medication order, medications that must be administered apart from other medications for optimal therapeutic effect, and medications prescribed more frequently than every 4 hours.[4,31]
- Establish guidelines to facilitate the administration of time-critical medications to be administered 30 minutes before or after the regularly scheduled time.[8,31]
- Establish guidelines to facilitate the administration of non–time-critical daily, weekly, and monthly medications that are to be administered 2 hours before or after the scheduled time.[8,31]
- Give medications that are administered more frequently than daily but less frequently than every 4 hours (for instance, twice daily or three times per day) no more than 1 hour before or after the scheduled time.[8,31]

Completing the procedure

- Monitor and document the effectiveness of all medications administered.[32,33,34,35]
- Document any medication errors or adverse effects according to your facility's event-reporting system.[4,36]
- Dispose of all containers *to avoid cross-contamination issues.* Keep in mind that after a medication is removed from its original container, it should be used for one patient only.
- Perform hand hygiene.[13,14,15,16,17,18]

Evaluating the medication management process

■ Make sure that there's a defined method for reviewing and updating any preprinted order sheets or standing orders.[37] Routinely review this process *to look for points of failure that could contribute to a medication error.*[38]

■ Make sure that the pharmacy annually reviews the high-risk medications and look-alike and sound-alike medications it stores and uses. *The pharmacy should remove medications if they aren't being used.*[39,40,41]

■ Make sure that a list of "Do Not Use" abbreviations, symbols, and acronyms is updated regularly and posted prominently where medications are prepared.[38,42]

Special considerations

■ Maintain a nonpunitive culture for reporting medication errors *to encourage reporting compliance.*[43]

■ Adjust dosages as needed, based on the patient's age or if renal insufficiency is identified. Pediatric patients, patients with identified renal dysfunction, and patients older than age 80 are at a higher risk for ADEs.[1,20]

■ Perform a medication reconciliation at transition points, such as during admission, discharge, and transfer between units.[6,44]

■ Your facility should establish standards for a medication delivery process and ways to ensure ongoing review and evaluation.[45]

■ Use smart pump technology and standardized medication concentrations when available *to reduce the risk of IV medication infusion errors.*[9]

■ Make sure that the infusion pump alarm limits are set according to the patient's current condition, and that the alarms are turned on, functioning properly, and audible to staff.[46,47,48,49]

■ Use a bar-code technology (if available) to scan the bar codes on medications and the patient's identification bracelet (as shown below) in addition to verifying the practitioner's order entry and EMAR *to reduce medication administration errors and as a final step to intercept a medication error before drug administration.*[20]

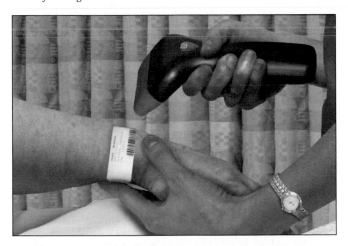

■ If indicated, include the patient's age and weight (in kilograms) in the patient's medical and medication records.[9]

■ When possible, medications should be prescribed by practitioners electronically.[1,20]

■ Handle medications brought by the patient from home as directed by your facility.[4,50]

■ If any questions arise about a prescribed medication, collaborate with the prescriber or pharmacist.[4,6,7,8,22]

■ If an automated dispensing cabinet is used to dispense medications, follow the manufacturer's instructions for use.

■ Report all medication errors and adverse effects; this includes preventable ADEs, close calls, and hazardous conditions.[4,6,43,51]

■ Investigate patient-reported medication errors and adverse events, and verify them in a timely manner *to prevent dangerous consequences.*[52]

Complications

With any medication use, there's the potential for an ADE or medication error. Familiarize yourself with all medications that you administer; be aware of potential ADEs, and know the required antidotes if indicated.

Resources should be readily available *to confirm any potential ADE if you aren't familiar with the medications being used.* Report any medication errors, adverse drug reactions, and medication incompatibilities immediately to the attending practitioner or clinical psychologist.[36]

Documentation

Document all medications administered in the patient's MAR or EMAR. Include the medication strength, dose, route of administration, and date and time of administration, as well as any access site for the medication, administration devices used, and the rate of administration.[53] If a medication wasn't administered, document the reason why, any interventions taken, practitioner notification, and the patient's response to interventions.

If the patient experiences an ADE or medication error, document the event as required by your facility. Your facility may require that you submit a medication error report to the national Medication Errors Reporting Program (MERP) operated by the Institute for Safe Medication Practices, a patient safety organization certified by the Agency for Healthcare Research and Quality. The MERP is a confidential voluntary medication error reporting program that performs expert analysis of system-based causes of medication errors.[51] Document teaching provided to the patient and family (if applicable), their understanding of that teaching, and any need for follow-up teaching.

REFERENCES

1 Zhu, J., & Weingart, S. N. (2020). Prevention of adverse drug events in hospitals. In: *UpToDate*, Auerbach, D. A. (Ed.).

2 Westbrook, J., et al. (2010). Association of interruptions with an increased risk and severity of medication administration errors. *Archives of Internal Medicine, 170*, 683–690. (Level IV)

3 Institute for Safe Medication Practices. (2012). Side tracks on the safety express: Interruptions lead to errors and unfinished...Wait what was I doing? *Nurse Advise ERR, 11*(2), 1 4. https://www.ismp.org/resources/side-tracks-safety-express-interruptions-lead-errors-and-unfinished-wait-what-was-i-doing?id=37

4 Centers for Medicare and Medicaid Services, Department of Health and Human Services. (2020). Condition of participation: Nursing services. 42 C.F.R. § 482.23(c).

5 Centers for Medicare and Medicaid Services. (2014). Requirements for hospital medication administration, particularly intravenous (IV) medications and post-operative care of patients receiving IV opioids. http://www.cms.gov/Medicare/Provider-Enrollment-and-Certification/SurveyCertificationGenInfo/Downloads/Survey-and-Cert-Letter-14-15.pdf

6 The Joint Commission. (2021). Standard MM.04.01.01. *Comprehensive accreditation manual for hospitals.* Oakbrook Terrace, IL: The Joint Commission. (Level VII)

7 Accreditation Association for Hospitals and Health Systems. (2020). Standard 16.01.03. *Healthcare Facilities Accreditation Program: Accreditation requirements for acute care hospitals.* Chicago, IL: Accreditation Association for Hospitals and Health Systems. (Level VII)

8 DNV GL-Healthcare USA, Inc. (2020). MM.1.SR.3. *NIAHO® accreditation requirements: Interpretive guidelines and surveyor guidance—revision 20.0.* Milford, OH: DNV GL-Healthcare USA, Inc. (Level VII)

9 Institute for Safe Medication Practices. (2020). 2020–2021 targeted medication safety best practices for hospitals. https://www.ismp.org/sites/default/files/attachments/2020-02/2020-2021%20TMSBP-%20FINAL_1.pdf

10 Standard 59. Infusion medication and solution administration. Infusion therapy standards of practice (8th ed.). (2021). *Journal of Infusion Nursing, 44*, S180–S183. (Level VII)

11 Standard 13. Medication verification. Infusion therapy standards of practice (8th ed.). (2021). *Journal of Infusion Nursing, 44*, S46–S49. (Level VII)

12 The Joint Commission. (2021). Standard NPSG.03.06.01. *Comprehensive accreditation manual for hospitals.* Oakbrook Terrace, IL: The Joint Commission. (Level VII)

13 The Joint Commission. (2021). Standard NPSG.07.01.01. *Comprehensive accreditation manual for hospitals.* Oakbrook Terrace, IL: The Joint Commission. (Level VII)

14 World Health Organization. (2009). WHO guidelines on hand hygiene in health care: First global patient safety challenge, clean care is safer care. https://apps.who.int/iris/bitstream/handle/10665/44102/9789241597906_eng.pdf?sequence=1 (Level IV)

15 Centers for Disease Control and Prevention. (2002). Guideline for hand hygiene in health-care settings: Recommendations of the Healthcare Infection Control Practices Advisory Committee and the HICPAC/ SHEA/APIC/IDSA Hand Hygiene Task Force. *MMWR Recommendations and Reports, 51*(RR-16), 1–45. https://www.cdc.gov/mmwr/pdf/rr/rr5116. pdf (Level II)

16 Centers for Medicare and Medicaid Services, Department of Health and Human Services. (2020). Condition of participation: Infection control. 42 C.F.R. § 482.42.

17 Accreditation Association for Hospitals and Health Systems. (2020). Standard 07.01.21. *Healthcare Facilities Accreditation Program: Accreditation requirements for acute care hospitals.* Chicago, IL: Accreditation Association for Hospitals and Health Systems. (Level VII)

18 DNV GL-Healthcare USA, Inc. (2020). IC.1.SR.1. *NIAHO® accreditation requirements: Interpretive guidelines and surveyor guidance—revision 20.0.* Milford, OH: DNV GL-Healthcare USA, Inc. (Level VII)

19 The Joint Commission. (2021). Standard NPSG.01.01.01. *Comprehensive accreditation manual for hospitals.* Oakbrook Terrace, IL: The Joint Commission. (Level VII)

20 Institute of Medicine of the National Academies Committee on Identifying and Preventing Medication Errors, Board on Health Care Services. (2007). *Preventing medication errors: Quality chasm series.* Washington, DC: National Academies Press. https://www.nap.edu/ read/11623/chapter/1#xiii

21 The Joint Commission. (2021). Standard PC.02.03.01. *Comprehensive accreditation manual for hospitals.* Oakbrook Terrace, IL: The Joint Commission. (Level VII)

22 The Joint Commission. (2021). Standard MM.06.01.01. *Comprehensive accreditation manual for hospitals.* Oakbrook Terrace, IL: The Joint Commission. (Level VII)

23 The Joint Commission. (2021). Standard MM.05.01.01. *Comprehensive accreditation manual for hospitals.* Oakbrook Terrace, IL: The Joint Commission. (Level VII)

24 Centers for Medicare and Medicaid Services, Department of Health and Human Services. (2020). Condition of participation: Pharmaceutical services. 42 C.F.R. § 482.25 (b).

25 The Joint Commission. (2021). Standard MM.01.01.01. *Comprehensive accreditation manual for hospitals.* Oakbrook Terrace, IL: The Joint Commission. (Level VII)

26 The Joint Commission. (2021). Standard MM.01.01.03. *Comprehensive accreditation manual for hospitals.* Oakbrook Terrace, IL: The Joint Commission. (Level VII)

27 Institute for Safe Medication Practices. (2018). ISMP list of high-alert medications in acute care settings. https://www.ismp.org/sites/default/files/ attachments/2018-08/highAlert2018-Acute-Final.pdf

28 Centers for Medicare and Medicaid Services, Department of Health and Human Services. (2020). Condition of participation: Nursing services. 42 C.F.R. § 482.23.

29 Institute for Safe Medication Practices. (2017). Despite technology, verbal orders persist, read back is not widespread, and errors continue. https:// www.ismp.org/resources/despite-technology-verbal-orders-persist-read- back-not-widespread-and-errors-continue?id=1167 (Level VI)

30 The Joint Commission. (2021). Standard PC.02.01.03. *Comprehensive accreditation manual for hospitals.* Oakbrook Terrace, IL: The Joint Commission. (Level VII)

31 Institute for Safe Medication Practices. (2011). Guidelines for timely administration of scheduled medications (acute). https://www.ismp.org/ guidelines/timely-administration-scheduled-medications-acute (Level VII)

32 DNV GL-Healthcare USA, Inc. (2020). MR.2.SR.1. *NIAHO® accreditation requirements: Interpretive guidelines and surveyor guidance—revision 20.0.* Milford, OH: DNV GL-Healthcare USA, Inc. (Level VII)

33 The Joint Commission. (2021). Standard RC.01.03.01. *Comprehensive accreditation manual for hospitals.* Oakbrook Terrace, IL: The Joint Commission. (Level VII)

34 Accreditation Association for Hospitals and Health Systems. (2020). Standard 10.00.03. *Healthcare Facilities Accreditation Program: Accreditation requirements for acute care hospitals.* Chicago, IL: Accreditation Association for Hospitals and Health Systems. (Level VII)

35 Centers for Medicare and Medicaid Services, Department of Health and Human Services. (2020). Condition of participation: Medical record services. 42 C.F.R. § 482.24(b).

36 The Joint Commission. (2021). Standard MM.07.01.03. *Comprehensive accreditation manual for hospitals.* Oakbrook Terrace, IL: The Joint Commission. (Level VII)

37 DNV GL-Healthcare USA, Inc. (2020). MM.1.SR.9. *NIAHO® accreditation requirements, interpretive guidelines and surveyor guidance—revision 20.0.* Milford, OH: DNV GL-Healthcare USA, Inc. (Level VII)

38 Institute for Safe Medication Practices. (2010). Guidelines for standard order sets. https://www.ismp.org/guidelines/standard-order-sets (Level VII)

39 Institute for Safe Medication Practices. (2021). List of error-prone abbreviations. https://www.ismp.org/recommendations/ error-prone-abbreviations-list

40 The Joint Commission. (2021). Standard MM.01.02.01. *Comprehensive accreditation manual for hospitals.* Oakbrook Terrace, IL: The Joint Commission. (Level VII)

41 Institute for Safe Medication Practices & Food and Drug Administration. (2016). FDA and ISMP lists of look-alike drug names with recommended tall man letters. https://www.ismp.org/sites/default/files/attach- ments/2017-11/tallmanletters.pdf (Level VII)

42 The Joint Commission. (n.d.). Do Not Use list. https://www.jointcommis- sion.org/resources/news-and-multimedia/fact-sheets/facts-about-do-not- use-list/ (Level VII)

43 Standard 11. Adverse and serious adverse events. Infusion therapy stan- dards of practice. (2016). *Journal of Infusion Nursing, 39,* S3–S32. (Level VII)

44 Accreditation Association for Hospitals and Health Systems. (2020). Standard 25.02.13. *Healthcare Facilities Accreditation Program: Accreditation requirements for acute care hospitals.* Chicago, IL: Accreditation Association for Hospitals and Health Systems. (Level VII)

45 The Joint Commission. (2021). Standard MM.08.01.01. *Comprehensive accreditation manual for hospitals.* Oakbrook Terrace, IL: The Joint Commission. (Level VII)

46 American Association of Critical-Care Nurses. (2018). AACN practice alert: Managing alarms in acute care across the life span: Electrocardiography and pulse oximetry. https://www.aacn.org/clinical- resources/practice-alerts/managing-alarms-in-acute-care-across-the-life- span (Level VII)

47 Graham, K. C., & Cvach, M. (2010). Monitor alarm fatigue: Standardizing use of physiological monitors and decreasing nuisance alarms. *American Journal of Critical Care, 19,* 28–37.

48 The Joint Commission. (2021). Standard NPSG.06.01.01. *Comprehensive accreditation manual for hospitals.* Oakbrook Terrace, IL: The Joint Commission. (Level VII)

49 The Joint Commission. (2013). Sentinel event alert: Medical device alarm safety in hospitals. https://www.jointcommission.org/assets/1/6/SEA_50_ alarms_4_26_16.pdf (Level VII)

50 The Joint Commission. (2021). Standard MM.03.01.05. *Comprehensive accreditation manual for hospitals.* Oakbrook Terrace, IL: The Joint Commission. (Level VII)

51 Institute for Safe Medication Practices. (n.d.). Report an error. https:// www.ismp.org/report-medication-error

52 Institute for Safe Medication Practices. (2015). Unverified patient-reported error: A false alarm can have real consequences. *Nurse Advise- ERR, 13*(2), 1–4.

53 The Joint Commission. (2021). Standard RC.02.01.01. *Comprehensive accreditation manual for hospitals.* Oakbrook Terrace, IL: The Joint Commission. (Level VII)

SEIZURE MANAGEMENT

Seizures are paroxysmal events associated with abnormal excessive or synchronous electrical discharges of neurons in the brain.[1] (See *Classifying seizure types.*) When a patient has a generalized motor seizure, nursing care aims to protect the patient from injury and prevent serious complications. Appropriate care also includes obser- vation of seizure characteristics to help determine the area of the brain involved.[2]

Adults who experience an initial seizure have a greater chance for a recurrent seizure within the first 2 years after the first seizure.[4] Patients considered at risk for seizures are those with a history of seizures and those with conditions that predispose them to seizures. These condi- tions include metabolic abnormalities, such as hypocalcemia, hypoglyce- mia, and pyridoxine deficiency; brain tumors or other space-occupying lesions; infections, such as meningitis, encephalitis, and brain abscess; traumatic injury, especially if the dura mater was penetrated; ingestion of toxins, such as mercury, lead, or carbon monoxide; genetic abnormalities, such as tuberous sclerosis and phenylketonuria; perinatal injuries; alcohol

Classifying seizure types

The International League Against Epilepsy (ILAE) has revised the classification system for seizure types *to provide consistent communication among health care professionals who care for patients with seizures*. The ILAE's revised classification recognizes that seizures have either a focal, generalized, or unknown onset.[1,3]

SEIZURE TYPE	MOTOR ONSET	NONMOTOR ONSET
Focal onset—the patient remains aware or has impaired awareness; seizure activity is limited to one hemisphere of the brain	■ *Automatisms*—automatic action or behavior without conscious awareness (licking lips, rubbing hands, walking, repeating meaningless phrases, undressing) ■ *Atonic*—transient loss of muscle tension or tone ■ *Clonic*—sustained rhythmic jerking of one part of the body or face; alternating muscular rigidity and relaxation ■ *Epileptic spasms*—sudden flexion or bending of the trunk with flexion or extension of the limbs that lasts less than a few seconds; often occur in clusters ■ *Hyperkinetic*—agitated thrashing or leg pedaling ■ *Myoclonic*—irregular, intermittent spasms or twitching of a muscle or muscles ■ *Tonic*—stiffening of limb or neck, causing a forced posture during the seizure	■ *Autonomic*—effects on autonomic nervous system functions (heart rate, blood pressure, sweating, skin color, GI sensations, salivation) ■ *Behavior arrest*—brief cessation of movement; applies only if arrest is the main feature throughout the entire seizure ■ *Cognitive*—impaired cognition during seizure (aphasia, apraxia, neglect, déjà vu, jamais vu, hallucinations, illusions, perceptual distortion) ■ *Emotional*—appearance of anxiety, fear, joy, or another emotion without subjective emotion (laughing, crying) ■ *Sensory*—disturbance of senses (tingling, numbness, vertigo, hot-cold feelings, sounds, smells, tastes, visual symptoms)
Generalized onset—awareness isn't used to classify this seizure type, *because most patients with generalized onset seizures present with impaired awareness or complete loss of consciousness*	■ *Tonic-clonic*—stiffening of all limbs, follow by sustained rhythmic jerking of limbs and face; patient may cry out at onset, fall, bite tongue, or experience incontinence ■ *Clonic*—rhythmic sustained jerking of the limbs and head ■ *Tonic*—stiffening of all limbs without clonic jerking ■ *Myoclonic*—bilateral, irregular, sustained jerking of the limbs, face, eyes, and eyelids ■ *Myoclonic-tonic-clonic*—initially, a few bilateral myoclonic jerks followed by tonic-clonic seizure ■ *Myoclonic-atonic*—initially, a few myoclonic jerks followed by limp drop ■ *Atonic*—sudden loss of muscle tone and strength with subsequent fall or slump ■ *Epileptic spasms*—brief seizures with flexions at the truck and flexion or extension of the limbs	■ *Typical absence*—sudden onset; activity stops with a brief pause and staring; possible eye fluttering, head nodding, or other automatic behaviors; immediate recovery ■ *Atypical absence*—slower onset and more pronounced than typical absence seizure ■ *Myoclonic absence*—initially, a few myoclonic jerks, then an absence seizure ■ *Eyelid myoclonic*—jerks of the eyelids and upward deviation of the eyes, often precipitated by closing the eyes or by light
Unknown onset—unobserved or masked by other events but with features that can still be classified	■ *Tonic-clonic*—stiffening of all limbs, follow by sustained rhythmic jerking of the limbs and face; patient may cry out at onset, fall, bite tongue, or experience incontinence ■ *Epileptic spasms*—brief seizures with flexions at the trunk and flexion or extension of the limbs	■ *Behavior arrest*—brief cessation of movement; applies only if arrest is the main feature throughout the entire seizure
Unclassified seizure—inadequate information or inability to place in other category		

use disorder; drug abuse and withdrawal; and stroke.[2] For patients at risk for seizures, precautionary measures are needed to help prevent injury if a seizure occurs.

Equipment

Stethoscope ■ vital signs monitoring equipment ■ pulse oximeter and probe ■ gloves ■ padding for side rails ■ disinfectant pad ■ clock or watch ■ emergency equipment (code cart with emergency medications, defibrillator, handheld resuscitation bag with mask, and intubation equipment) ■ Optional: oral airway, suction equipment, prescribed thiamine, seizure activity record, IV catheter insertion equipment, oxygen administration equipment, adhesive tape, perineal care supplies, prescribed medications.

Preparation of equipment

If the patient is at risk for seizures, pad the patient's side rails and have IV equipment, suction equipment, and oxygen administration equipment available at the patient's bedside. Make sure emergency equipment is functioning properly and readily available.[5]

Implementation

■ Gather and prepare the necessary equipment and supplies.
■ Perform hand hygiene.[6,7,8,9,10,11]
■ Confirm the patient's identify using at least two patient identifiers.[12]
■ Provide privacy if possible.[13,14,15,16]
■ Perform hand hygiene.[6,7,8,9,10,11]
■ Put on gloves, as needed, *to comply with standard precautions.*[17,18,19]

For focal seizures with impaired awareness

■ If you're present when the patient experiences a focal seizure with impaired awareness, guide the patient from danger.[5]
■ Time the seizure.[5] If you find the patient during a seizure, begin timing as soon as you discover the event.
■ Remain with the patient until the baseline level of consciousness returns.[5]
■ If the patient is agitated, stay a distance away but close enough to provide protection from injury until full awareness returns.[5]
■ Monitor the patient's vital signs *to promptly detect changes in condition.*[5]
■ Administer medications, as needed and prescribed, following safe medication practices.[20,21,22,23]

For a generalized seizure

■ If you're present when a generalized seizure occurs, ease the patient into bed and put up the side rails *to prevent a fall.* If you're away from the bed, ease the patient to the floor and place something soft, such as a pillow or blanket, under the patient's head *to protect it from injury.*[2,24]

HOSPITAL-ACQUIRED CONDITION ALERT Keep in mind that the Centers for Medicare and Medicaid Services considers an injury from a fall a hospital-acquired condition, *because it can be reasonably prevented using a variety of best practices.* Make sure to follow evidence-based fall prevention practices, such as performing a fall risk assessment and instituting fall precautions, *to reduce the risk of injury from patient falls.*[25,26,27]

■ Time the seizure. If you find the patient during a seizure, begin timing as soon as you observe it. If the seizure continues for more than 5 minutes, or if the patient has trouble breathing or has significant injury, call for help *to activate an emergency response.*[5]

■ Position the patient on the side as soon as possible *to maintain airway patency.*[5,24]

NURSING ALERT During a seizure, don't put anything into the patient's mouth, *to prevent patient or caregiver injury.*[5]

■ Protect the patient from injury, but don't restrain the patient, *because the force of the patient's movements against restraints could cause muscle strain or even joint dislocation.*[5]

■ Remove the patient's eyeglasses, if present.[5,24]

■ Loosen anything from around the patient's neck that might restrict breathing.[5,24]

■ Clear the area around the patient of anything hard or sharp *to prevent injury.*[24]

■ Assess the patient during the seizure. Monitor for changes in consciousness, mental status, and behaviors. *Your description may help determine the seizure's type and cause.*[5]

■ Remain with the patient until the patient's level of consciousness returns to baseline.[5]

■ If this is the patient's first seizure, notify the practitioner immediately. If the patient has had seizures before, notify the practitioner only if the seizure activity is prolonged or if the patient fails to regain consciousness. (See *Understanding status epilepticus.*)

■ If ordered, insert an IV catheter *to obtain IV access for medication administration.*[5]

NURSING ALERT Don't attempt to insert an IV catheter during an active seizure unless absolutely necessary, *because doing so can cause injuries.*

■ Administer medication, as needed and prescribed, following safe medication administration practices.[20,21,22,23]

■ If the seizure is prolonged and the patient becomes hypoxemic, administer oxygen as ordered.[5] Some patients may require endotracheal intubation. Attach the patient to a pulse oximeter as needed *to monitor oxygen saturation levels.*

■ For suspected hypoglycemia in a patient with diabetes, follow your facility's protocol for treating severe hypoglycemia.[30]

■ After the seizure, suction the patient's airway as needed *to clear secretions and maintain airway patency.*[5]

■ Assess the patient for postictal injury, specifically tongue and cheek lacerations, bruising, and fractures.[5] Notify the practitioner as needed.

■ Assess the patient for urinary incontinence that may have occurred as a result of seizure activity.[5] Provide perineal care as needed.

■ If the patient experiences postictal confusion and wandering, gently guide the patient to the bed or a chair.[5]

■ If not already done, pad the patient's side rails and place the bed in the lowest position with the wheels locked *to prevent injury should seizure activity recur.*[5]

■ For a patient known to have alcohol use disorder who may be experiencing severe withdrawal, administer thiamine, as prescribed, following safe medication administration practices.[20,21,22,23,31,32]

Completing the procedure

■ Monitor the patient's vital signs; oxygen saturation level by pulse oximetry, if needed; simple cognitive ability (orientation, response to simple motor commands, naming of objects, and recall of simple phrases); level of awareness; and responsiveness.[5]

■ Ask the patient about activities that preceded the seizure.

Understanding status epilepticus

The Commission on Classification and Terminology and the Commission on Epidemiology of the International League Against Epilepsy have proposed a new definition of status epilepticus: "Status epilepticus is a condition resulting either from the failure of the mechanisms responsible for seizure termination or from the initiation of mechanisms, which lead to abnormally prolonged seizures (after time point t_1). It is a condition, which can have long-term consequences (after time point t_2), including neuronal death, neuronal injury, and alteration of neuronal networks, depending on the type and duration of seizures." This definition is conceptual, with two operational dimensions. The first is the length of the seizure and the time point (t_1) beyond which the seizure should be regarded as "continuous seizure activity." The second time point (t_2) is the time of ongoing seizure activity after which there's a risk of long-term consequences.[28]

Always an emergency, status epilepticus is accompanied by respiratory distress. It can result from abrupt withdrawal of anticonvulsant medications, hypoxic or metabolic encephalopathy, acute head trauma, or septicemia secondary to encephalitis or meningitis.

In 2016, the American Epilepsy Society issued new guidelines for the treatment of status epilepticus using a phased treatment approach. After the initial stabilization phase, the treatment algorithm recommends a benzodiazepine as the initial therapy of choice. First-line drugs include one of the following: IM midazolam, IV LORazepam, or IV diazePAM. If none of the first-line drug options is available, then one of the following is administered: IV PHENobarbital, rectal diazePAM, or intranasal or buccal midazolam. If the seizure continues, then one of the second therapy–phase drugs should be given as a single dose. Second therapy drugs include IV fosphenytoin, IV valproic acid, and IV levETIRAcetam. If the seizure continues, then second line therapy should be repeated, or anesthetic doses of thiopental, midazolam, PENTobarbital, or propofol should be administered.[29]

■ Remove and discard your gloves.[17]
■ Perform hand hygiene.[6,7,8,9,10,11]
■ Clean and disinfect your stethoscope using a disinfectant pad.[33,34]
■ Perform hand hygiene.[6,7,8,9,10,11]
■ Document the procedure.[35,36,37,38]

Special considerations

■ *Because a seizure can indicate an underlying disorder, such as meningitis or a metabolic imbalance (especially hypoglycemia) or an electrolyte imbalance (especially hyponatremia),* the practitioner may order a complete diagnostic laboratory workup if the cause of the seizure isn't evident.[39]

■ Anticipate monitoring for therapeutic levels of any antiseizure medications that the patient is taking, if applicable.[40,41,42,43]

Complications

The patient who experiences a seizure may experience an injury, respiratory distress, and decreased mental capability. Common injuries include scrapes and bruises suffered when the patient hits objects during the seizure, and traumatic injury to the tongue and cheek caused by biting. Changes in respiratory function may include aspiration, airway obstruction, and hypoxemia.

Documentation

Document that the patient requires seizure precautions, and record all precautions taken.

If a seizure occurs, document the event on a seizure activity record (if used in your facility) or other appropriate location in the patient's medical record. Document the date and time the seizure began, as well as its duration and any precipitating factors and activities before the seizure.

Record involuntary behavior that occurred at the onset of the seizure, such as lip smacking, chewing movements, or hand and eye movements. Describe where the movement began and the parts of the body involved.

Note the progression or pattern of the activity. Document whether the patient's eyes deviated to one side and if the pupils changed in size, shape, equality, or reaction to light. Note if the patient's teeth were clenched or open. Record incontinence, vomiting, or salivation that occurred during the seizure.

Note the patient's response to the seizure. Note the patient's awareness of the event and postseizure state. Also note any medications the patient received, complications the patient experienced during the seizure, and interventions you performed. Lastly, note the patient's postseizure vital signs, oxygen saturation level, and neurologic status.

Document teaching provided to the patient and family (if appropriate), their understanding of that teaching, and any need for follow-up teaching.

REFERENCES

1 Fisher, R. S., et al. (2017). Operational classifications of seizure types by the International League Against Epilepsy: Position paper of the ILAE Commission for Classification and Terminology. *Epilepsia, 58*(4), 522–530. https://onlinelibrary.wiley.com/doi/full/10.1111/epi.13670 (Level VII)

2 Hinkle, J. L., & Cheever, K. H. (2018). *Brunner & Suddarth's textbook of medical-surgical nursing* (14th ed.). Philadelphia, PA: Wolters Kluwer.

3 Fisher, R. S., et al. (2016). Epilepsy Foundation: 2017 revised classification of seizures. https://epilepsy.com/article/2016/12/2017-revised-classification-seizures

4 Krumholz, A., et al. (2015). Evidence-based guideline: Management of an unprovoked first seizure in adults. *Neurology, 84*(16), 1705–1713. https://n.neurology.org/content/84/16/1705 (Level I)

5 American Association of Neuroscience Nurses (AANN). (2016). *AANN clinical practice guideline series: Care of adults and children with seizures and epilepsy.* Chicago, IL: AANN. (Level VII)

6 The Joint Commission. (2021). Standard NPSG.07.01.01. *Comprehensive accreditation manual for hospitals.* Oakbrook Terrace, IL: The Joint Commission. (Level VII)

7 Centers for Disease Control and Prevention. (2002). Guideline for hand hygiene in health-care settings: Recommendations of the Healthcare Infection Control Practices Advisory Committee and the HICPAC/SHEA/APIC/IDSA Hand Hygiene Task Force. *MMWR Recommendations and Reports, 51*(RR-16), 1–45. https://www.cdc.gov/mmwr/pdf/rr/rr5116.pdf (Level II)

8 World Health Organization. (2009). WHO guidelines on hand hygiene in health care: First global patient safety challenge, clean care is safer care. https://apps.who.int/iris/bitstream/handle/10665/44102/9789241597906_eng.pdf?sequence=1 (Level IV)

9 Centers for Medicare and Medicaid Services, Department of Health and Human Services. (2020). Condition of participation: Infection control. 42 C.F.R. § 482.42.

10 Accreditation Association for Hospitals and Health Systems. (2020). Standard 07.01.21. *Healthcare Facilities Accreditation Program: Accreditation requirements for acute care hospitals.* Chicago, IL: Accreditation Association for Hospitals and Health Systems. (Level VII)

11 DNV GL-Healthcare USA, Inc. (2020). IC.1.SR.1. *NIAHO® accreditation requirements, interpretive guidelines and surveyor guidance—revision 20.0.* Milford, OH: DNV GL-Healthcare USA, Inc. (Level VII)

12 The Joint Commission. (2021). Standard NPSG.01.01.01. *Comprehensive accreditation manual for hospitals.* Oakbrook Terrace, IL: The Joint Commission. (Level VII)

13 Centers for Medicare and Medicaid Services, Department of Health and Human Services. (2020). Condition of participation: Patient's rights. 42 C.F.R. § 482.13(c)(1).

14 Accreditation Association for Hospitals and Health Systems. (2020). Standard 15.01.16. *Healthcare Facilities Accreditation Program: Accreditation requirements for acute care hospitals.* Chicago, IL: Accreditation Association for Hospitals and Health Systems. (Level VII)

15 DNV GL-Healthcare USA, Inc. (2020). PR.2.SR.5. *NIAHO® accreditation requirements, interpretive guidelines and surveyor guidance—revision 20.0.* Milford, OH: DNV GL-Healthcare USA, Inc. (Level VII)

16 The Joint Commission. (2021). Standard RI.01.01.01. *Comprehensive accreditation manual for hospitals.* Oakbrook Terrace, IL: The Joint Commission. (Level VII)

17 Siegel, J. D., et al. (2007, revised 2019). 2007 guideline for isolation precautions: Preventing transmission of infectious agents in healthcare settings. https://www.cdc.gov/infectioncontrol/pdf/guidelines/isolation-guidelines-H.pdf (Level II)

18 Accreditation Association of Hospitals and Health Systems. (2020). Standard 07.01.10. *Healthcare Facilities Accreditation Program: Accreditation requirements for acute care hospitals.* Chicago, IL: Accreditation Association for Hospitals and Health Systems. (Level VII)

19 Occupational Safety and Health Administration. (2012). Bloodborne pathogens, standard number 1910.1030. https://www.osha.gov/pls/oshaweb/owadisp.show_document?p_id=10051&p_table=STANDARDS (Level VII)

20 Centers for Medicare and Medicaid Services, Department of Health and Human Services. (2020). Condition of participation: Nursing services. 42 C.F.R. § 482.23(c).

21 Accreditation Association for Hospitals and Health Systems. (2020). Standard 16.01.03. *Healthcare Facilities Accreditation Program: Accreditation requirements for acute care hospitals.* Chicago, IL: Accreditation Association for Hospitals and Health Systems. (Level VII)

22 The Joint Commission. (2021). Standard MM.06.01.01. *Comprehensive accreditation manual for hospitals.* Oakbrook Terrace, IL: The Joint Commission. (Level VII)

23 DNV GL-Healthcare USA, Inc. (2020). MM.1.SR.3. *NIAHO® accreditation requirements, interpretive guidelines and surveyor guidance—revision 20.0.* Milford, OH: DNV GL-Healthcare USA, Inc. (Level VII)

24 Centers for Disease Control and Prevention. (2020). Seizure first aid. https://www.cdc.gov/epilepsy/about/first-aid.htm

25 Jarrett, N., & Callaham, M. (2016). Evidence-based guidelines for selected hospital-acquired conditions: Final report. https://www.cms.gov/Medicare/Medicare-Fee-for-Service-Payment/HospitalAcqCond/Downloads/2016-HAC-Report.pdf

26 Ganz, D. A., et al. (2013, reviewed 2021). *Preventing falls in hospitals: A toolkit for improving quality of care* (AHRQ Publication No. 13-0015-EF). Rockville, MD: Agency for Healthcare Research and Quality. https://www.ahrq.gov/professionals/systems/hospital/fallpxtoolkit/index.html(Level VII)

27 The Joint Commission. (2021). Standard PC.01.02.08. *Comprehensive accreditation manual for hospitals.* Oakbrook Terrace, IL: The Joint Commission. (Level VII)

28 Trinka, E., et al. (2015). A definition and classification of status epilepticus—Report of the ILAE Task Force on Classification of Status Epilepticus. *Epilepsia, 56*(10), 1515–1523. https://onlinelibrary.wiley.com/doi/abs/10.1111/epi.13121 (Level VII)

29 Glauser, T., et al. (2016). Evidence-based guideline: Treatment of convulsive status epilepticus in children and adults: Report of the Guideline Committee of the American Epilepsy Society. *Epilepsy Currents, 16*(1), 48–61. https://www.ncbi.nlm.nih.gov/pmc/articles/PMC4749120/ (Level VII)

30 American Diabetes Association. (2020). American Diabetes Association standards of medical care in diabetes—2020. *Diabetes Care, 42*, S1–S193. https://care.diabetesjournals.org/content/43/Supplement_1

31 World Health Organization. (2012). Management of alcohol withdrawal. https://www.who.int/mental_health/mhgap/evidence/resource/alcohol_q2.pdf

32 Schuckit, M. A. (2014). Recognition and management of withdrawal delirium (delirium tremens). *New England Journal of Medicine, 371*, 2109–2113.

33 Rutala, W. A., et al. (2008, revised 2019). Guideline for disinfection and sterilization in healthcare facilities, 2008. https://www.cdc.gov/infection-control/pdf/guidelines/disinfection-guidelines-H.pdf (Level I)

34 Accreditation Association for Hospitals and Health Systems. (2020). Standard 07.02.03. *Healthcare Facilities Accreditation Program: Accreditation requirements for acute care hospitals.* Chicago, IL: Accreditation Association for Hospitals and Health Systems. (Level VII)

35 The Joint Commission. (2021). Standard RC.01.03.01. *Comprehensive accreditation manual for hospitals.* Oakbrook Terrace, IL: The Joint Commission. (Level VII)

36 Centers for Medicare and Medicaid Services, Department of Health and Human Services. (2020). Condition of participation: Medical record services. 42 C.F.R. § 482.24(b).

37 Accreditation Association for Hospitals and Health Systems. (2020). Standard 10.00.03. *Healthcare Facilities Accreditation Program: Accreditation requirements for acute care hospitals.* Chicago, IL: Accreditation Association for Hospitals and Health Systems. (Level VII)

38 DNV GL-Healthcare USA, Inc. (2020). MR.2.SR.1. *NIAHO® accreditation requirements, interpretive guidelines and surveyor guidance—revision 20.0.* Milford, OH: DNV GL-Healthcare USA, Inc. (Level VII)

39 Schachter, S. C. (2021). Evaluation and management of the first seizure in adults. In: *UpToDate*, Garcia, P., & Edlow, J. A. (Eds.).

40 Bonnett, L. J., et al. (2017). Breakthrough seizures—further analysis of the standard versus new antiepileptic drugs (SANAD) study. *Plos One, 12*(12), 1–16. https://journals.plos.org/plosone/article?id=10.1371/journal.pone.0190035 (Level II)

41 Ko, D. Y. (2020). Epilepsy and seizures. https://emedicine.medscape.com/article/1184846-overview

42 Epilepsy Foundation. (2019). Seizure first aid and safety. https://www.epilepsy.com/learn/seizure-first-aid-and-safety

43 Stepanova, D., & Beran, R. G. (2015). The benefits of antiepileptic drug (AED) blood level monitoring to complement clinical management of people with epilepsy. *Epilepsy and Behavior, 42*, 7–9. (Level V)

SELF-CATHETERIZATION

Self-catheterization is performed by many patients who have some form of impaired or absent bladder function. This form of intermittent catheterization involves inserting a catheter into the bladder to drain urine and then removing it after the bladder empties. This technique is preferable to an indwelling urinary catheter, because it's considered a safe and effective way of preserving renal function and poses a lower risk of infection and other complications.[1,2,3] Self-catheterization promotes independence and bladder self-management, and improves quality of life. In addition, it allows normal sexual intimacy without the fear of incontinence, decreases the chance of urinary reflux, reduces the use of aids and appliances, and in many cases allows the patient to return to work. However, patients performing self-catheterization may experience pain and bleeding on insertion, and may have difficulty inserting and removing the catheter.[4]

Intermittent self-catheterization is contraindicated in patients who have a high intravesicular pressure because of the potential for kidney reflux.[4]

Nursing responsibilities regarding self-catheterization include providing the patient with instruction and ensuring that the patient receives periodic follow-up care to maintain adherence.[1,2] Before teaching the patient, the nurse should assess for physical barriers (such as poor eyesight and reduced manual dexterity), psychological barriers (such as fear or anxiety), and cultural or religious beliefs that may interfere with teaching.[1,2,5] At home, the patient will use clean technique for self-catheterization.[2,6] In the hospital, sterile technique is recommended.[1]

Equipment

Sterile catheter (of appropriate material, diameter, and length)[1] ▪ washcloth ▪ soap and water ▪ small packet of water-soluble lubricant ▪ gloves ▪ Optional: drainage container, mirror.

Implementation

▪ Review the patient's medical record for contraindications to the procedure and any allergy or sensitivity to latex.
▪ Verify the practitioner's order.
▪ Gather and prepare the necessary equipment and supplies.
▪ Perform hand hygiene.[6,7,8,9,10,11,12]
▪ Confirm the patient's identity using at least two patient identifiers.[13]
▪ Provide privacy.[14,15,16,17]
▪ Explain the procedure to the patient and family (if appropriate) according to their individual communication and learning needs *to increase their understanding, allay their fears, and enhance cooperation.*[5] Obtain the assistance of a medical interpreter as needed.[18,19]
▪ Instruct the patient to wash the hands thoroughly with soap and water and then dry them.[4]
▪ Perform hand hygiene.[6,7,8,9,10,11,12]
▪ Put on gloves.[20,21,22]
▪ Arrange the patient's clothing so that it's out of the way.
▪ Demonstrate how the patient should perform the catheterization, explaining each step clearly and carefully.

Teaching the male patient

▪ Instruct the patient to wash and rinse the end of the penis thoroughly with soap and water. Instruct the patient to pull back the foreskin for cleaning and to keep it pulled back during the procedure, if applicable.[4]

▪ Tell the patient to lubricate the first 6" to 8" (15.3 to 20.3 cm) of the catheter, and observe this being done. Explain that dry catheters can cause excoriation in the urethra that can serve as entry points for bacterial contamination, and that copious lubricant will make the procedure more comfortable.[1]
▪ Instruct the patient to insert the catheter into the urethra and to allow all of the urine to drain. (See *Teaching the male patient self-catheterization.*)
▪ When the urine stops draining, tell the patient to remove the catheter slowly and, if necessary, pull the foreskin forward again.[4]
▪ Have the patient get dressed.

Teaching the female patient

▪ Demonstrate and explain to the patient that she should separate the vaginal folds as widely as possible with the fingers of her nondominant hand *to obtain a full view of the urinary meatus.* She may need to use a mirror *to visualize the meatus.*
▪ Instruct the patient to hold her labia open with the nondominant hand and then to use the dominant hand to wash the perineal area thoroughly with a soapy washcloth, using downward strokes. Tell her to rinse the soap from the area with another clean wet or damp washcloth using downward strokes as well.
▪ Show the patient how to squeeze some lubricant onto the first 2" to 4" (5 to 10 cm) of the catheter and then how to insert the catheter.
▪ Instruct the patient to insert the catheter into her urethra and let the urine drain. (See *Teaching the female patient self-catheterization.*)
▪ When the urine stops draining, tell the patient to remove the catheter slowly and get dressed.

PATIENT TEACHING

TEACHING THE MALE PATIENT SELF-CATHETERIZATION

Teach the male patient to find a comfortable position; some men prefer to stand for the procedure, but it can be done just as easily in the sitting position.[20] Have the patient hold his penis in his nondominant hand, at a right angle to his body. He should hold the catheter in his dominant hand as if it were a pencil or a dart and slowly insert it 6" to 8" (15.2 to 20.3 cm) into the urethra until urine begins flowing. If the patient feels resistance at the passage of the catheter at the prostatic urethra, instruct him to apply firm, gently, steady pressure to the pelvic floor muscles; the muscles should relax, allowing the catheter to pass.[20] Then the patient should gently advance the catheter about 1" (2.5 cm) further, allowing all urine to drain into the toilet or drainage container.

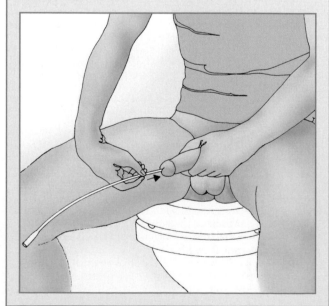

PATIENT TEACHING

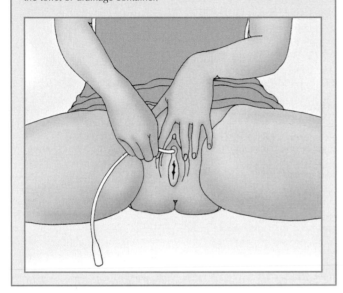

⌂ TEACHING THE FEMALE PATIENT SELF-CATHETERIZATION

Instruct the female patient to find a comfortable position and hold the catheter in her dominant hand as if it were a pencil or a dart, about ½" (1.25 cm) from its tip. Tell her to keep the vaginal folds separated and slowly insert the lubricated catheter about 2" to 4" (5 to 10 cm) into the urethra. Inform her that if she feels resistance, she should apply firm, gentle, steady pressure to the pelvic floor muscles; the muscles should then relax, allowing the catheter to pass.[20] Tell the patient to press down with her abdominal muscles *to empty the bladder*, allowing all urine to drain through the catheter and into the toilet or drainage container.

Completing the procedure

- Tell the patient to discard used equipment appropriately and to perform hand hygiene.
- Remove and discard your gloves.[22]
- Perform hand hygiene.[6,7,8,9,10,11,12]
- Document the procedure.[23,24,25,26]

Special considerations

- Avoid latex exposure in patients who require frequent catheterization.[27]
- Hydrophilic catheters might be preferable to standard catheters for patients requiring intermittent catheterization.[4,6] Catheter choice more often depends on the patient's general clinical situation—such as injury, manual dexterity, visual impairment, urethral sensibility, and age—than on the cause of the bladder dysfunction.[1,4]
- A female patient may prefer a shorter catheter of 6" to 12" (15.3 to 30.5 cm), which is easier to grasp and manipulate. *Women have shorter urethras than men, and a shorter catheter won't loop or kink, allowing urine to more easily drain through the catheter.*[1]
- Catheters with lengths of approximately 12" (about 40 cm) allow for adequate passage through a male urethra.[1]
- Curved and olive-tipped catheters are available as needed for certain clinical conditions, such as urethral strictures or enlarged prostates. Closed intermittent catheterization systems are also available and have been designed to reduce contamination of the bladder (*the catheter never comes in direct contact with the inserter's hands*).[1]
- Follow the manufacturer's instructions for catheter use. Single-use devices shouldn't be reused in any setting.[1] Instruct the patient to keep a supply of catheters at home and to use a new catheter each time.
- Explain to the patient that the timing of catheterization is critical *to prevent overdistention of the bladder, which can lead to infection*. Self-catheterization is usually performed every 4 to 6 hours around the clock (more often at first).[1]
- Stress the importance of regulating fluid intake, as ordered, *to prevent incontinence while maintaining adequate hydration*. However, explain that incontinent episodes may occur occasionally. For managing incontinence, the practitioner or a home health care nurse can help develop a plan, such as more frequent catheterizations. After an incontinence episode, tell the patient to wash with soap and water, pat the area dry with a towel, and expose the skin to the air for as long as possible. Bedding and furniture can be protected by covering them with rubber or plastic sheets and then covering the rubber or plastic with fabric.

- Explain that if the patient can't pass the catheter and can feel that the bladder is full, the patient should immediately go to the nearest urgent care center or emergency department or should contact the practitioner immediately.[20,28]

Patient teaching

At discharge, give the patient individualized written instructions regarding home care.[4,28,29] *To prevent urinary tract infections (UTIs) associated with catheterization*, emphasize the importance of hand and perineal hygiene. Also instruct the patient to perform catheterization after voiding (if the patient maintains the capacity to void spontaneously),[1] before a bowel movement *to minimize bacterial contamination of the urethra*, and right before bed *to minimize nocturia*.[4] Encourage the female patient to clean the perineal area immediately after vaginal intercourse, and to avoid the use of spermicidal lubricants, *because these products may alter vaginal and urethral flora*.[1] Also instruct the patient to use a generous amount of lubricant along the length of the catheter, *because dry catheters can cause excoriations in the urethra that provide an entry point for bacterial contamination*.[1] Advise the patient to keep a voiding diary to help evaluate bladder emptying over time.[4] If the patient has difficulty practicing self-catheterization because of limited mobility, vision, or dexterity, family members and caregivers can be taught the procedure, as appropriate. Provide the patient and family with contact information for appropriate follow-up and peer support *to enhance compliance*.[4]

Complications

Advancing the catheter too far into the bladder can cause irritation of the bladder wall, kinking of the catheter in the urethra if the catheter moves around in the bladder and then back into the urethra, and knotting of the catheter inside the bladder. Forcing the catheter can cause trauma, bleeding, and scar formation, leading to strictures, false passage, and obstruction of the urethra. Improper hand washing or equipment cleaning can cause a UTI.[1]

Documentation

Document the date and time of the procedure, amount and characteristics of urine obtained, size and description of the catheter used, and tolerance of the procedure. Document that the self-catheterization procedure was taught and the method of instruction, the names of those who received the instruction, their readiness to learn, and their understanding (knowledge and skill). Note and document whether the patient had difficulty performing a return demonstration and action taken. Record any need for follow-up teaching.

REFERENCES

1 Newman, D. K., & Wilson, M. M. (2011). Review of intermittent catheterization and current best practices. *Urology Nursing, 31*(1), 12–29. https://www.suna.org/sites/default/files/download/education/2013/article3101229.pdf (Level VII)

2 Beauchemin, L., et al. (2018). Best practices for clean intermittent catheterization. *Nursing, 48*(9), 49–54.

3 National Institute for Health and Care Excellence. (2010, revised 2015). Lower urinary tract symptoms in men: Management. https://www.nice.org.uk/Guidance/cg97 (Level VII)

4 Vahr, S., et al. (2013). *Evidence-based guidelines for best practice in urological care: Catheterisation: Urethral intermittent in adults: Dilatation, urethral intermittent in adults.* Arnhem, Netherlands: European Association of Urology Nurses. https://nurses.uroweb.org/guideline/catheterisation-urethral-intermittent-in-adults/ (Level VII)

5 The Joint Commission. (2021). Standard PC.02.01.21. *Comprehensive accreditation manual for hospitals.* Oakbrook Terrace, IL: The Joint Commission. (Level VII)

6 Healthcare Infection Control Practices Advisory Committee. (2010, revised 2019). Guideline for prevention of catheter-associated urinary tract infections 2009. https://www.cdc.gov/infectioncontrol/pdf/guidelines/cauti-guidelines-H.pdf (Level I)

7 Centers for Disease Control and Prevention. (2002). Guideline for hand hygiene in health-care settings: Recommendations of the Healthcare Infection Control Practices Advisory Committee and the HICPAC/SHEA/APIC/IDSA Hand Hygiene Task Force. *MMWR Recommendations and Reports*, 51(RR-16), 1–45. https://www.cdc.gov/mmwr/pdf/rr/rr5116.pdf (Level II)

8 World Health Organization. (2009). WHO guidelines on hand hygiene in health care: First global patient safety challenge, clean care is safer care. https://apps.who.int/iris/bitstream/handle/10665/44102/9789241597906_eng.pdf?sequence=1 (Level IV)

9 The Joint Commission. (2021). Standard NPSG.07.01.01. *Comprehensive accreditation manual for hospitals.* Oakbrook Terrace, IL: The Joint Commission. (Level VII)

10 Accreditation Association for Hospitals and Health Systems. (2020). Standard 07.01.21. *Healthcare Facilities Accreditation Program: Accreditation requirements for acute care hospitals.* Chicago, IL: Accreditation Association for Hospitals and Health Systems. (Level VII)

11 Centers for Medicare and Medicaid Services, Department of Health and Human Services. (2020). Condition of participation: Infection control. 42 C.F.R. § 482.42.

12 DNV GL-Healthcare USA, Inc. (2020). IC.1.SR.1. *NIAHO® accreditation requirements, interpretive guidelines and surveyor guidance—revision 20.0.* Milford, OH: DNV GL-Healthcare USA, Inc. (Level VII)

13 The Joint Commission. (2021). Standard NPSG.01.01.01. *Comprehensive accreditation manual for hospitals.* Oakbrook Terrace, IL: The Joint Commission. (Level VII)

14 The Joint Commission. (2021). Standard RI.01.01.01. *Comprehensive accreditation manual for hospitals.* Oakbrook Terrace, IL: The Joint Commission. (Level VII)

15 Accreditation Association for Hospitals and Health Systems. (2020). Standard 15.01.16. *Healthcare Facilities Accreditation Program: Accreditation requirements for acute care hospitals.* Chicago, IL: Accreditation Association for Hospitals and Health Systems. (Level VII)

16 Centers for Medicare and Medicaid Services, Department of Health and Human Services. (2020). Condition of participation: Patient's rights. 42 C.F.R. § 482.13(c)(1).

17 DNV GL-Healthcare USA, Inc. (2020). PR.2.SR.5. *NIAHO® accreditation requirements, interpretive guidelines and surveyor guidance—revision 20.0.* Milford, OH: DNV GL-Healthcare USA, Inc (Level VII)

18 The Joint Commission. (2021). Standard PC.02.03.01. *Comprehensive accreditation manual for hospitals.* Oakbrook Terrace, IL: The Joint Commission. (Level VII)

19 The Joint Commission. (2010). *Advancing effective communication, cultural competence, and patient- and family-centered care: A roadmap for hospitals.* Oakbrook Terrace, IL: The Joint Commission. https://www.jointcommission.org/assets/1/6/ARoadmapforHospitalsfinalversion727.pdf (Level VII)

20 Society of Urologic Nurses and Associates. (2006). Clinical practice guidelines: Adult clean intermittent catheterization. https://www.suna.org/resources/adultCICGuide.pdf (Level VII)

21 Accreditation Association for Hospitals and Health Systems. (2020). Standard 07.01.10. *Healthcare Facilities Accreditation Program: Accreditation requirements for acute care hospitals.* Chicago, IL: Accreditation Association for Hospitals and Health Systems. (Level VII)

22 Occupational Safety and Health Administration. (2012). Bloodborne pathogens, standard number 1910.1030. https://www.osha.gov/pls/oshaweb/owadisp.show_document?p_id=10051&p_table=STANDARDS (Level VII)

23 The Joint Commission. (2021). Standard RC.01.03.01. *Comprehensive accreditation manual for hospitals.* Oakbrook Terrace, IL: The Joint Commission. (Level VII)

24 Centers for Medicare and Medicaid Services, Department of Health and Human Services. (2020). Condition of participation: Medical record services. 42 C.F.R. § 482.24(b).

25 Accreditation Association for Hospitals and Health Systems. (2020). Standard 10.00.03. *Healthcare Facilities Accreditation Program: Accreditation requirements for acute care hospitals.* Chicago, IL: Accreditation Association for Hospitals and Health Systems. (Level VII)

26 DNV GL-Healthcare USA, Inc. (2020). MR.2.SR.1. *NIAHO® accreditation requirements, interpretive guidelines and surveyor guidance—revision 20.0.* Milford, OH: DNV GL-Healthcare USA, Inc. (Level VII)

27 Hamilton, R. G. (2020). Latex allergy: Management. In: *UpToDate*, Bochner, B. S. (Ed.).

28 Centers for Medicare and Medicaid Services, Department of Health and Human Services. (2020). Condition of participation: Discharge planning. 42 C.F.R. § 482.43.

29 DNV GL-Healthcare USA, Inc. (2020). DC.1.SR.1. *NIAHO® accreditation requirements, interpretive guidelines and surveyor guidance—revision 20.0.* Milford, OH: DNV GL-Healthcare USA, Inc. (Level VII)

Sepsis, emergency patient care

The latest Surviving Sepsis Campaign guidelines use the Sepsis-3 definition, which defines sepsis as a life-threatening organ dysfunction that occurs when the body has a dysregulated response to infection.[1] Organ dysfunction distinguishes uncomplicated infection from sepsis. Early identification and treatment of patients with or at risk for sepsis improves patient survival.[1,2]

A tool known as the *quick Sequential (Sepsis-Related) Organ Failure Assessment (qSOFA)* helps clinicians quickly identify patients at risk for sepsis. The tool directs clinicians to look for the following warning signs in a patient with suspected infection: altered mental status (Glasgow coma scale score less than 15), systolic blood pressure 100 mm Hg or less, and respiratory rate 22 breaths/minute or more.[2,3,4] A patient with two or more of these signs should be assessed for organ dysfunction. Conversely, a patient who presents with signs of organ dysfunction should be evaluated for infection.[2]

Septic shock is defined as "a subset of sepsis, in which underlying circulatory, cellular, and metabolic abnormalities are associated with a greater risk of mortality than sepsis alone."[3] Clinical criteria used to identify patients with septic shock include persistent hypotension that requires vasopressors to maintain a mean arterial pressure (MAP) of 65 mm Hg or higher, and blood lactate level that exceeds 18 mg/dL (2 mmol/L) despite adequate volume resuscitation.[1,2,3]

The Centers for Medicare and Medicaid Services (CMS) core measure entitled *Severe Sepsis and Septic Shock: Management Bundle* doesn't use the Sepsis-3 definitions. Instead, it defines severe sepsis as systemic inflammatory response syndrome (SIRS) due to infection. SIRS is defined as two or more of the following: temperature greater than 100.4° F (38° C) or less than 96.8° F (36° C); heart rate greater than 90 beats/minute; respiratory rate greater than 20 breaths/minute or partial pressure of carbon dioxide less than 32 mm Hg (4.3 kPa); and white blood cell count greater than 12,000/mm^3 (12 × 10^9) or less than 4,000/mm^3 (4 × 10^9/L), or greater than 10% immature bands.[1]

The CMS defines septic shock as severe sepsis with hypoperfusion despite adequate fluid resuscitation or a lactate level greater than 36 mg/dL (4 mmol/L).[1]

Sepsis is the leading cause of death from infection, and its reported incidence continues to rise. The mortality rate for patients who meet the clinical criteria for septic shock exceeds 40%, which is four times higher than the rate for patients with sepsis alone.[2] Early recognition and transfer to the intensive care unit (ICU) for immediate treatment that includes fluid resuscitation and antibiotic therapy improves a patient's chance of survival.[5] The Society of Critical Care Medicine and the European Society of Intensive Medicine recommend using an "hour-1 bundle" with the intention of beginning resuscitation and management immediately.[5] Use your facility's criteria to screen patients for sepsis.

Equipment

Gloves ▪ facility-approved sepsis screening tool ▪ vital signs monitoring equipment ▪ stethoscope ▪ oxygen administration equipment ▪ oxygen source ▪ emergency equipment (code cart with emergency medications, defibrillator, handheld resuscitation bag with mask, intubation equipment) ▪ prescribed IV fluids (crystalloids recommended)[6] ▪ IV administration set ▪ electronic infusion device (preferably a smart pump with dose-error reduction software and interoperability with the electronic health record) ▪ venipuncture supplies and collection tubes ▪ blood culture bottles ▪ labels ▪ laboratory biohazard transport bag ▪ cardiac monitoring equipment ▪ pulse oximeter and probe ▪ prescribed antibiotics ▪ facility-approved delirium assessment tool ▪ facility-approved pressure injury risk assessment tool ▪ graduated measuring container ▪

disinfectant pad ■ Optional: IV catheter insertion equipment, prescribed insulin, blood glucose testing equipment, prescribed venous thrombo-embolism (VTE) prevention medication and equipment, arterial catheter insertion and monitoring equipment, central venous pressure (CVP) monitoring equipment, urine, sputum, and wound culture specimen kits, central venous access device insertion kit, pressure tubing, norepinephrine, EPINEPHrine, vasopressin, DOBUTamine, prescribed corticosteroid, sterile gloves, gown, mask and goggles or mask with face shield, enteral feeding supplies, bedside cardiovascular ultrasound equipment, support surfaces.

Preparation of equipment

Make sure that emergency equipment is functioning properly and readily available. Inspect all equipment and supplies. If a product is expired or defective or has compromised integrity, remove it from patient use, label it as expired or defective, and report the expiration or defect as directed by your facility.

Implementation

■ Review the patient's medical record for factors that increase the risk of sepsis.
■ Verify the practitioner's orders.
■ Gather and prepare the necessary equipment and supplies.
■ Perform hand hygiene.[7,8,9,10,11,12]
■ Confirm the patient's identity using at least two patient identifiers.[13]
■ Provide privacy.[14,15,16,17]
■ Explain the procedure to the patient and family (if appropriate) according to their individual communication and learning needs *to increase their understanding, allay their fears, and enhance cooperation.*[18]
■ Raise the patient's bed to waist level before providing care *to prevent caregiver back strain.*[19]
■ Perform hand hygiene.[7,8,9,10,11,12]
■ Put on gloves and, as necessary, other personal protective equipment *to comply with standard precautions.*[20,21,22]
■ Attach the patient to the cardiac monitor, pulse oximeter, and automated blood pressure monitor. Make sure that alarm limits are set appropriately for the patient's current condition, and that alarms are turned on, functioning properly, and audible to staff.[23,24,25,26]
■ Obtain the patient's baseline vital signs. Then closely monitor vital signs at an interval determined by your facility and the patient's condition *to detect changes in condition.*
■ Administer supplemental oxygen, as necessary and prescribed.
■ Screen a patient with suspected infection for sepsis using your facility's screening tool *to ensure prompt recognition and treatment of sepsis.*[1,2,3] If the patient displays signs and symptoms of sepsis, notify the practitioner and the rapid response team, as necessary.

Initiate within 1 hour of presentation (time of emergency department triage or from earliest documentation of sepsis)

■ Obtain specimens for routine microbiologic cultures, including blood cultures (at least two sets: anaerobic and anaerobic),[6,27] as well as for a complete blood count, electrolyte and lactate levels, coagulation studies, and other laboratory tests, as ordered, *to identify the causative organism and evaluate for infection-related organ dysfunction.* Collect blood cultures before administering antibiotics.[5] Label the specimen in the presence of the patient *to prevent mislabeling.*[13] Place the samples in a laboratory biohazard transport bag and send them to the laboratory immediately with the appropriate laboratory request forms (if necessary).[22] Notify the practitioner of critical test results within your facility's established time frame *so that the patient can be promptly treated.*[28]
■ Make sure that the patient has adequate IV access. Assist with central venous access catheter insertion if necessary. *Research doesn't support required use of a central venous access catheter to monitor CVP and central venous oxygen saturation (ScvO₂) in all patients with septic shock who have received timely antibiotics and fluid resuscitation or in all patients with a lactate level lower than 36 mg/dL (4 mmol/L).* (See the "Central venous access catheter care" procedure.)

■ Assist the practitioner with removing—or, as ordered, remove—IV access devices that are a possible source of sepsis or septic shock after other vascular access has been established.[6]
■ Administer broad-spectrum antibiotics, as prescribed, following safe medication administration practices.[5,6,29,30,31,32] If the source of infection is known, ensure that the patient receives antibiotics specific to the organism's sensitivity.[5]
■ Administer 30 mL/kg of crystalloid IV fluids, as ordered, for sepsis-induced hypotension or a lactate level greater than or equal to 36 mg/dL (4 mmol/L).[6,33] Note that some patients may need more rapid administration and greater volumes of fluid.[6] Guidelines recommend completing the infusion within 3 hours of sepsis recognition.[5]
■ Assist with arterial catheter insertion, if necessary and ordered, *to monitor blood pressure.*[6]
■ Administer vasopressors, as prescribed, following safe medication administration practices, to treat hypotension during or after fluid resuscitation to maintain a MAP of 65 mm Hg or above.[29,30,31,32] *Urgently restoring adequate perfusion pressure to vital organs is key to successful resuscitation.*[5,6]
■ If required by your facility, before administering a vasopressor, have another nurse perform an independent double-check *to verify the patient's identity and make sure that the correct medication is in the prescribed concentration, the medication's indication corresponds with the patient's diagnosis, the dosage calculations are correct, the dosing formula used to derive the final dose is correct, the prescribed administration route is safe and proper for the patient, the prescribed time and frequency of administration are safe and proper for the patient, the electronic infusion device settings are correct, and the infusion line is attached to the correct port.*[34]

NURSING ALERT Vasopressors, such as norepinephrine, EPINEPHrine, and vasopressin, are considered high-alert medications *because they can cause significant patient harm when used in error.*[35]

■ Compare the results of the independent double-check (if required). If no discrepancies exist, begin infusing the medication. If discrepancies exist, rectify them before beginning the infusion.[34]
■ Make sure that the electronic infusion device's alarm limits are set appropriately, and that alarms are turned on, functioning properly, and audible to staff.[23,24,26]
■ Administer norepinephrine, as prescribed, following safe medication administration practices.[29,30,31,32] *Norepinephrine is the vasopressor of choice for septic shock.*
■ Administer EPINEPHrine, as prescribed, following safe medication administration practices, when an additional agent is necessary to maintain adequate blood pressure.[29,30,31,32] Alternatively, administer vasopressin in addition to norepinephrine *to raise the patient's blood pressure or reduce the norepinephrine requirement.*
■ Administer DOBUTamine, as prescribed, following safe medication administration practices,[29,30,31,32] if the patient shows signs of persistent hypoperfusion despite adequate fluid resuscitation and the use of vasopressors.[6]

Completing the procedure

■ Assist the practitioner with assessing the patient's fluid volume status and tissue perfusion if the patient remains hypotensive despite initial fluid resuscitation. Assess the patient's vital signs (including MAP),[6] cardiac and respiratory status, capillary refill time, pulse pressure variation, and skin condition.[6,33] Measure CVP and ScvO₂, assess fluid responsiveness using the passive leg raise or fluid challenge test, or assist with bedside cardiovascular ultrasonography.[6,33]
■ Administer IV fluids, as ordered and necessary, according to the patient's fluid volume status. Use a fluid challenge technique, continuing fluid administration as long as hemodynamic improvement continues.[6,33] Keep in mind that fluid resuscitation beyond the initial resuscitation requires careful assessment *to make sure that the patient remains responsive to fluids.* Some evidence suggests that a sustained positive fluid balance during the ICU stay may be harmful.[5]
■ If the patient's initial lactate level was elevated (greater than 2 mmol/L), remeasure the lactate level within 4 hours, as ordered, *to guide resuscitation.*[5,6,33]
■ Closely monitor the patient's urine output.[6,33]

- Monitor the procalcitonin level, as ordered, *to assist with the de-escalation of antibiotic therapy.*
- If the patient experiences refractory shock after receiving adequate IV fluid resuscitation and vasopressor therapy, administer an IV corticosteroid, as ordered, following safe medication administration practices.[29,30,31,32]
- Follow the practitioner's order or your facility's protocol for monitoring and managing the patient's glucose level. Guidelines recommend administering insulin when two consecutive blood glucose levels exceed 180 mg/dL (10 mmol/L). If the patient has an arterial catheter, guidelines suggest using the arterial blood instead of capillary blood for point-of-care testing using a glucose meter.[6] (See the "Blood glucose monitoring" procedure.)
- If the patient can't consume nutrition orally, initiate enteral tube feedings, as ordered, within 48 hours *to maintain gut integrity and prevent intestinal permeability, dampen the inflammatory response, and modulate metabolic responses that may reduce insulin resistance.*[6]
- Assess the patient's risk of delirium using a facility-approved delirium assessment tool, such as the Confusion Assessment Method for ICU or the Intensive Care Delirium Screening Checklist.[36]
- Use pharmacologic and mechanical measures to prevent VTE, as prescribed.[6]
- Assess the patient's risk of pressure injury using a facility-approved risk assessment tool. Reposition the patient and use support surfaces, as necessary, *to prevent skin breakdown.*[37]

HOSPITAL-ACQUIRED CONDITION ALERT Keep in mind that the Centers for Medicare and Medicaid Services considers a stage 3 or stage 4 pressure injury to be a hospital-acquired condition, *because use of best practices can reasonably prevent it.* Be sure to follow evidence-based pressure injury prevention practices, such as assessing skin integrity, encouraging early mobility, and repositioning the patient, *to reduce the risk of pressure injuries.*[37,38,39]

- Continue to monitor closely until the patient is stable.
- Return the bed to the lowest position *to prevent falls and maintain patient safety.*[40]
- Discard used supplies in appropriate receptacles.[22]
- Remove and discard your gloves and any other personal protective equipment worn.[22]
- Perform hand hygiene.[7,8,9,10,11,12]
- Clean and disinfect your stethoscope using a disinfectant pad.[21,41]
- Perform hand hygiene.[7,8,9,10,11,12]
- Put on gloves and, as necessary, other personal protective equipment *to comply with standard precautions.*[22]
- Clean and disinfect other reusable equipment according to the manufacturer's instructions *to prevent the spread of infection.*[21,42]
- Remove and discard your gloves and other personal protective equipment worn.[22]
- Perform hand hygiene.[7,8,9,10,11,12]
- Document the procedure.[43,44,45,46]

Special considerations

- *Because sepsis is one of the leading causes of death in hospitalized patients worldwide,* infection prevention is the best strategy for protecting patients from sepsis. *To help prevent infection,* the Centers for Disease Control and Prevention recommends performing hand hygiene before and after contact with a patient or a patient's environment, removing invasive devices as soon as they're no longer necessary, and following other best practices for infection prevention when providing patient care.[9]
- Patient populations most at risk for developing sepsis include older adults and neonates, as well as patients who are immunocompromised, have a chronic illness (such as diabetes, lung disease, kidney disease, or cancer), are receiving immunosuppressive therapy, or are malnourished or debilitated.[47]
- The Joint Commission has issued a sentinel event alert about medical device alarm safety, *because alarm-related events have been associated with permanent loss of function and death.* Among the major contributing factors were improper alarm settings, alarms turned off inappropriately, and alarm signals not audible to staff. Make sure that alarm limits are set appropriately, and that alarms are turned on, functioning properly, and audible to staff. Follow facility guidelines for preventing alarm fatigue.[26]

Complications

Failure to follow appropriate emergency procedures for a patient with sepsis can result in multiple organ dysfunction syndrome and death.[6]

Documentation

Record the patient's vital signs, your assessment findings, and laboratory test results. Document the name of the practitioner notified of the patient's condition, critical laboratory test results, the date and time of notification, and any prescribed interventions and the patient's response. Document the medication strength, dose, route of administration, and date and time of administration. Record any adverse reactions to the prescribed medication, the date and time you notified the practitioner, and prescribed interventions and the patient's response. Record any vascular access devices you inserted; the indication for use; insertion site location; specific site preparation; local anesthetic (if used); infection prevention and safety precautions you took; type, length, size, and lot number of the catheter you inserted; date and time of insertion; number of insertion attempts; device functionality; insertion method, including visualization and guidance technology; confirmation of the anatomic location of the catheter tip; condition of the site; method of catheter stabilization; dressing; and the patient's tolerance of the procedure. Document any enteral feeding tube insertion, the addition of supplemental oxygen, and the patient's tolerance of the procedures. Document teaching you provided to the patient and family (if applicable), their understanding of that teaching, and any need for follow-up teaching.

References

1 Singer, M., et al. (2016). The third international consensus definitions for sepsis and septic shock (sepsis-3). *Journal of the American Medical Association, 315*(8), 801–810. https://www.ncbi.nlm.nih.gov/pmc/articles/PMC4968574/ (Level VII)

2 Society of Critical Care Medicine. (n.d.). Sepsis definitions. https://www.sccm.org/Research/Quality/Sepsis-Definitions

3 Shankar-Hari, M., et al. (2016). Developing a new definition and assessing new clinical criteria for septic shock: For the third international consensus definitions for sepsis and septic shock (sepsis-3). *Journal of the American Medical Association, 315*(8), 775–787. https://www.ncbi.nlm.nih.gov/pmc/articles/PMC4910392/ (Level VII)

4 Rudd, K. E., et al. (2018). Association of the Quick Sequential (sepsis-related) Organ Failure Assessment (qSOFA) score with excess hospital mortality in adults with suspected infection in low- and middle-income countries. *JAMA, 319*(21), 2202–2211. https://www.ncbi.nlm.nih.gov/pmc/articles/PMC6134436/ (Level IV)

5 Levy, M. M., et al. (2018). The Surviving Sepsis Campaign bundle: 2018 Update. *Critical Care Medicine, 46*(6), 997–1000. https://journals.lww.com/ccmjournal/Fulltext/2018/06000/The_Surviving_Sepsis_Campaign_Bundle__2018_Update.21.aspx (Level VII)

6 Rhodes, A., et al. (2017). Surviving Sepsis Campaign: International guidelines for management of sepsis and septic shock, 2016. *Critical Care Medicine, 45*(3), 486–552. https://journals.lww.com/ccmjournal/Fulltext/2017/03000/Surviving_Sepsis_Campaign___International.15.aspx (Level I)

7 The Joint Commission. (2021). Standard NPSG.07.01.01. *Comprehensive accreditation manual for hospitals.* (Level VII)

8 World Health Organization. (2009). WHO guidelines on hand hygiene in health care: First global patient safety challenge, clean care is safer care. https://apps.who.int/iris/bitstream/handle/10665/44102/9789241597906_eng.pdf?sequence=1 (Level IV)

9 Centers for Disease Control and Prevention. (2002). Guideline for hand hygiene in health-care settings: Recommendations of the Healthcare Infection Control Practices Advisory Committee and the HICPAC/SHEA/APIC/IDSA Hand Hygiene Task Force. *MMWR Recommendations and Reports, 51*(RR-16), 1–45. https://www.cdc.gov/mmwr/pdf/rr/rr5116.pdf (Level II)

10 Accreditation Association for Hospitals and Health Systems. (2020). Standard 07.01.21. *Healthcare Facilities Accreditation Program: Accreditation requirements for acute care hospitals.* (Level VII)

11 DNV GL-Healthcare USA, Inc. (2020). IC.1.SR.1. *NIAHO® accreditation requirements, interpretive guidelines and surveyor guidance—revision 20.0.* (Level VII)

12 Centers for Medicare and Medicaid Services, Department of Health and Human Services. (2020). Condition of participation: Infection control. 42 C.F.R. § 482.42.

13 The Joint Commission. (2021). Standard NPSG.01.01.01. *Comprehensive accreditation manual for hospitals.* (Level VII)

14 Centers for Medicare and Medicaid Services, Department of Health and Human Services. (2020). Condition of participation: Patient's rights. 42 C.F.R. § 482.13(c)(1).

15 The Joint Commission. (2021). Standard RI.01.01.01. *Comprehensive accreditation manual for hospitals.* (Level VII)

16 DNV GL-Healthcare USA, Inc. (2020). PR.2.SR.5. *NIAHO® accreditation requirements, interpretive guidelines and surveyor guidance—revision 20.0.* (Level VII)

17 Accreditation Association for Hospitals and Health Systems. (2020). Standard 15.01.16. *Healthcare Facilities Accreditation Program: Accreditation requirements for acute care hospitals.* (Level VII)

18 The Joint Commission. (2021). Standard PC.02.01.21. *Comprehensive accreditation manual for hospitals.* (Level VII)

19 Waters, T. R., et al. (2009). Safe patient handling training for schools of nursing. https://www.cdc.gov/niosh/docs/2009-127/pdfs/2009-127.pdf (Level VII)

20 Siegel, J. D., et al. (2007, revised 2019). 2007 guideline for isolation precautions: Preventing transmission of infectious agents in healthcare settings. https://www.cdc.gov/infectioncontrol/pdf/guidelines/isolation-guidelines-H.pdf (Level II)

21 Accreditation Association for Hospitals and Health Systems. (2020). Standard 07.01.10. *Healthcare Facilities Accreditation Program: Accreditation requirements for acute care hospitals.* (Level VII)

22 Occupational Safety and Health Administration. (2012). Bloodborne pathogens, standard number 1910.1030. https://www.osha.gov/pls/oshaweb/owadisp.show_document?p_id=10051&p_table=STANDARDS (Level VII)

23 The Joint Commission. (2021). Standard NPSG.06.01.01. *Comprehensive accreditation manual for hospitals.* (Level VII)

24 Graham, K. C., & Cvach, M. (2010). Monitor alarm fatigue: Standardizing use of physiological monitors and decreasing nuisance alarms. *American Journal of Critical Care, 19,* 28–37.

25 American Association of Critical-Care Nurses. (2018). AACN practice alert: Managing alarms in acute care across the life span—electrocardiography and pulse oximetry. https://www.aacn.org/clinical-resources/practice-alerts/managing-alarms-in-acute-care-across-the-life-span (Level VII)

26 The Joint Commission. (2013). Sentinel event alert 50: Medical device alarm safety in hospitals. https://www.jointcommission.org/resources/patient-safety-topics/sentinel-event/sentinel-event-alert-newsletters/sentinel-event-alert-issue-50-medical-device-alarm-safety-in-hospitals/ (Level VII)

27 Centers for Medicare and Medicaid Services & the Joint Commission. (2022). Specifications manual for national hospital inpatient quality measures (version 5.11a). https://www.qualitynet.org/inpatient/specifications-manuals#tab1

28 The Joint Commission. (2021). Standard NPSG.02.03.01. *Comprehensive accreditation manual for hospitals.* (Level VII)

29 The Joint Commission. (2021). Standard MM.06.01.01. *Comprehensive accreditation manual for hospitals.* (Level VII)

30 Centers for Medicare and Medicaid Services, Department of Health and Human Services. (2020). Condition of participation: Nursing services. 42 C.F.R. § 482.23(c).

31 Accreditation Association for Hospitals and Health Systems. (2020). Standard 16.01.03. *Healthcare Facilities Accreditation Program: Accreditation requirements for acute care hospitals.* (Level VII)

32 DNV GL-Healthcare USA, Inc. (2020). MM.1.SR.3. *NIAHO® accreditation requirements, interpretive guidelines and surveyor guidance—revision 20.0.* (Level VII)

33 Dellinger, R. P., et al. (2017). A users' guide to the 2016 Surviving Sepsis Guidelines. *Intensive Care Medicine, 43,* 299–303. https://link.springer.com/article/10.1007/s00134-017-4681-8 (Level IV)

34 Institute for Safe Medication Practice. (2019). Independent double checks: Worth the effort if used judiciously and properly. https://www.ismp.org/resources/independent-double-checks-worth-effort-if-used-judiciously-and-properly (Level VII)

35 Institute for Safe Medication Practices. (2018). ISMP list of high-alert medications in acute care settings. https://www.ismp.org/sites/default/files/attachments/2018-08/highAlert2018-Acute-Final.pdf (Level VII)

36 Krewulak, K. D., et al. (2020). The CAM-ICU-7 and ICDSC as measures of delirium severity in critically ill adult patients. *PLoS One, 15*(11), e0242378. https://journals.plos.org/plosone/article?id=10.1371/journal.pone.0242378 (Level IV)

37 European Pressure Ulcer Advisory Panel, et al. (2019). Prevention and treatment of pressure ulcers/injuries: Quick reference guide. http://www.internationalguideline.com/static/pdfs/Quick_Reference_Guide-10Mar2019.pdf (Level VII)

38 Jarrett, N., & Callaham, M. (2016). Evidence-based guidelines for selected hospital-acquired conditions: Final report. https://www.cms.gov/Medicare/Medicare-Fee-for-Service-Payment/HospitalAcqCond/Downloads/2016-HAC-Report.pdf

39 Wound Ostomy and Continence Nurses Society (WOCN). (2016). *Guideline for prevention and management of pressure ulcers (injuries): WOCN clinical practice guideline series 2.* Mt. Laurel, NJ: WOCN.

40 Ganz, D. A., et al. (2013, reviewed 2021). *Preventing falls in hospitals: A toolkit for improving quality of care* (AHRQ publication no. 13-0015-EF). Agency for Healthcare Research and Quality. https://www.ahrq.gov/professionals/systems/hospital/fallpxtoolkit/index.html (Level VII)

41 Rutala, W. A., et al. (2008, revised 2019). Guideline for disinfection and sterilization in healthcare facilities, 2008. https://www.cdc.gov/infection-control/pdf/guidelines/disinfection-guidelines-H.pdf (Level I)

42 Accreditation Association for Hospitals and Health Systems. (2020). Standard 07.02.03. *Healthcare Facilities Accreditation Program: Accreditation requirements for acute care hospitals.* (Level VII)

43 The Joint Commission. (2021). Standard RC.01.03.01. *Comprehensive accreditation manual for hospitals.* (Level VII)

44 DNV GL-Healthcare USA, Inc. (2020). MR.2.SR.1. *NIAHO® accreditation requirements, interpretive guidelines and surveyor guidance—revision 20.0.* (Level VII)

45 Accreditation Association for Hospitals and Health Systems. (2020). Standard 10.00.03. *Healthcare Facilities Accreditation Program: Accreditation requirements for acute care hospitals.* (Level VII)

46 Centers for Medicare and Medicaid Services, Department of Health and Human Services. (2020). Condition of participation: Medical record services. 42 C.F.R. § 482.24(b).

47 Cleveland Clinic. (2019). Sepsis. https://my.clevelandclinic.org/health/diseases/12361-sepsis

SEQUENTIAL COMPRESSION THERAPY

Sequential compression therapy helps prevent venous thromboembolism, which includes deep vein thrombosis (DVT) and pulmonary embolism, in patients at risk for the disorder. This safe, effective, noninvasive therapy massages the legs in a wavelike, milking motion that promotes blood flow in the lower extremities to decrease the risk of thrombosis.

HOSPITAL-ACQUIRED CONDITION ALERT Keep in mind that the Centers for Medicare and Medicaid Services considers venous thromboembolism (VTE) a hospital-acquired condition, in patients who underwent total knee or hip replacement *because it can be reasonably prevented using a variety of best practices.* Make sure to follow evidence-based VTE prevention practices, such as the use of mechanical compression devices (including antiembolism stockings and intermittent pneumatic compression devices), early ambulation, and pharmacologic prophylaxis, *to reduce the risk of VTE.*[1,2,3]

Sequential compression therapy is used in combination with anticoagulant medications to prevent DVT in low- to moderate-risk patients. For patients at high risk for bleeding, however, sequential compression is used without anticoagulants.[4,5] Preventive measures continue for as long as the patient remains at risk.

Both antiembolism stockings and sequential compression sleeves are commonly used preoperatively and postoperatively, *because blood clots tend to form during surgery.* Sequential compression therapy counteracts blood stasis and coagulation changes, two of the three major factors that promote DVT. It reduces stasis by increasing peak blood flow velocity, which helps empty the femoral vein's valve cusps of pooled or static blood. The compressions also have an anticlotting effect by increasing fibrinolytic activity, which stimulates the release of a plasminogen activator.

Studies show that many patients at risk for developing DVT don't comply with sequential compression therapy.[4] Providing education about the therapy to patients, including the importance of adhering to therapy, may promote adherence.

Sequential compression therapy isn't appropriate for patients with acute DVT (or DVT diagnosed within the last 6 months), serious arterial insufficiency, ischemic vascular disease, massive edema of the legs resulting from pulmonary edema or heart failure, or any local condition that the compression sleeves would aggravate, such as dermatitis, recent skin graft, cellulitis, gangrene, or vein ligation (in the immediate postoperative period). It's also unlikely to benefit patients with pronounced leg deformities.

Equipment

Measuring tape and brand-specific sizing chart ■ appropriately sized compression sleeves ■ connecting tubing ■ compression controller ■ facility-approved disinfectant.

Preparation of equipment

Inspect all equipment and supplies. If a product is expired, is defective, or has compromised integrity, remove it from patient use, label it as expired or defective, and report the expiration or defect as directed by your facility.

Implementation

■ Verify the practitioner's order.
■ Gather and prepare the necessary equipment and supplies.
■ Perform hand hygiene.[6,7,8,9,10,11]
■ Confirm the patient's identity using at least two patient identifiers.[12]
■ Provide privacy.[13,14,15,16]
■ Explain the procedure to the patient and family (if appropriate) according to their individual communication and learning needs *to increase their understanding, allay their fears, and enhance cooperation.*[17]
■ Perform hand hygiene.[6,7,8,9,10,11]
■ Determining the proper sleeve size according to the manufacturer's instructions.
■ Remove the compression sleeves from the package and unfold them.
■ Lay the unfolded sleeves on a flat surface with the cotton lining facing up (as shown below).

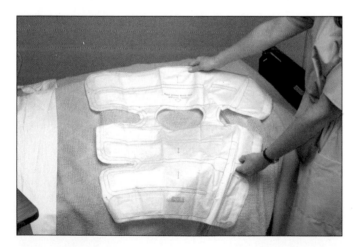

■ Note the markings on the lining denoting the ankle and the area behind the knee at the popliteal pulse point. Use these markings to position the sleeve at the appropriate landmarks.
■ Place the patient's leg on the sleeve lining. Position the back of the knee over the popliteal opening.
■ Make sure that the back of the ankle is over the ankle marking.
■ Starting at the side opposite the clear plastic tubing, wrap the sleeve snugly around the patient's leg.
■ Fasten the sleeve securely with the Velcro fasteners. *For the best fit,* first secure the ankle and calf sections, and then the thigh, if applicable. The sleeve should fit snugly, but not tightly. Check the fit by inserting two fingers between the sleeve and the patient's leg. Loosen or tighten the sleeve by readjusting the Velcro fasteners.
■ Using the same procedure, apply the second sleeve (as shown on top right).

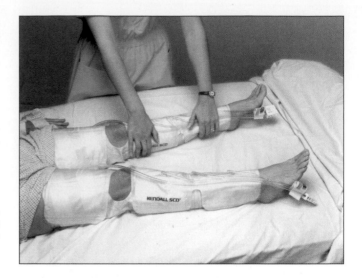

Operating the system

■ Connect each sleeve to the tubing leading to the controller. (Some devices require that both sleeves be attached to the controller for the controller to function, whereas others can operate with one or both attached. Follow your manufacturer's instructions for use.) Line up the blue arrows on the sleeve connector with the arrows on the tubing connectors and push the ends together firmly. Listen for a click, signaling a firm connection. Make sure that the tubing is not kinked.
■ Plug the compression controller into the proper wall outlet. Turn on the power. If your controller can function with one or both sleeves attached, be sure to turn on the sleeves that are needed. The controller automatically sets the compression sleeve pressure at 45 mm Hg, which is the midpoint of the normal range (35 to 55 mm Hg).
■ Observe to see how well the patient tolerates the therapy and to make sure the controller is working properly as the system completes its first cycle.
■ Check the AUDIBLE ALARM key. The green light should be lit, indicating that the alarm is working.
■ Perform hand hygiene.[6,7,8,9,10,11]
■ Document the procedure.[18,19,20,21]

Discontinuing compression therapy

■ Verify the practitioner's order.
■ Perform hand hygiene.[6,7,8,9,10,11]
■ Confirm the patient's identity using at least two patient identifiers.[12,22]
■ Provide privacy.[13,14,15,16]
■ Explain the procedure to the patient and family (if appropriate) according to their individual communication and learning needs *to increase their understanding, allay their fears, and enhance cooperation.*[17]
■ Turn off the power.
■ Open the Velcro fasteners on the sleeves and remove them from the extremities.
■ Discard the sleeves in the appropriate receptacle.
■ Disconnect the tubing from the compressor by depressing the latches on each side of the connector and pull them apart.
■ Clean and disinfect the tubing and compressor using a facility-approved disinfectant.[23,24]
■ Store the tubing and compressor as determined by your facility, *because this equipment isn't disposable.*
■ Perform hand hygiene.[6,7,8,9,10,11]
■ Document the procedure.[18,19,20,21]

Special considerations

■ The compression sleeves should function continuously (24 hours daily) until the patient is fully ambulatory. Check the sleeves at least once each shift to *ensure proper fit and inflation.*
■ Remove the sleeves when the patient is walking, bathing, or leaving the room for tests or other procedures by undoing the Velcro fasteners. Reapply them immediately after any of these activities.

■ Assess the patient's skin under the sleeves at least every 8 hours *for signs of pressure-related injury.*[25]

■ Assess the extremities for peripheral pulses, edema, changes in sensation, and movement at least once each shift.

■ Be aware that the compression controller also has a mechanism to help cool the patient.

■ If a malfunction triggers the instrument's alarm, you'll hear beeping. The system shuts off whenever the alarm is activated. To respond to the alarm, follow the instructions provided by the manufacturer.

Complications

The most common complication of compression therapy is skin irritation, which usually results from sweating or sensitivity to the sleeve material.

Documentation

Document the procedure, the patient's response to and understanding of the procedure, the status of the alarm and cooling settings, and your skin assessment findings. Document teaching provided to the patient and family (if applicable), their understanding of that teaching, and any need for follow-up teaching.

REFERENCES

1 Jarrett, N., & Callaham, M. (2016). Evidence-based guidelines for selected hospital-acquired conditions: Final report. https://www.cms.gov/Medicare/Medicare-Fee-for-Service-Payment/HospitalAcqCond/Downloads/2016-HAC-Report.pdf

2 Falck-Ytter, Y., et al. (2012). Prevention of VTE in orthopedic surgery patients: Antithrombotic therapy and prevention of thrombosis (9th ed.). *Chest, 141*(2 Suppl), e278S–e325S. https://www.ncbi.nlm.nih.gov/pmc/articles/PMC3278063/ (Level VII)

3 Balk, E. M., et al. (2017). *Venous thromboembolism prophylaxis in major orthopedic surgery: Systematic review update* (AHRQ publication no. 17-EHC021-EF). Rockville, MD: Agency for Healthcare Research and Quality. https://effectivehealthcare.ahrq.gov/topics/thromboembolism-update/research-2017 (Level I)

4 American Association of Critical Care Nurses. (2016). AACN practice alert: Preventing venous thromboembolism in adults. https://www.aacn.org/clinical-resources/practice-alerts/venous-thromboembolism-prevention (Level VII)

5 Zareba, P., et al. (2014). Meta-analysis of randomized trials comparing combined compression and anticoagulation with either modality alone for prevention of venous thromboembolism after surgery. *British Journal of Surgery, 101*, 1053–1062. (Level I)

6 The Joint Commission. (2021). Standard NPSG.07.01.01. *Comprehensive accreditation manual for hospitals.* Oakbrook Terrace, IL: The Joint Commission. (Level VII)

7 Centers for Disease Control and Prevention. (2002). Guideline for hand hygiene in health-care settings: Recommendations of the Healthcare Infection Control Practices Advisory Committee and the HICPAC/SHEA/APIC/IDSA Hand Hygiene Task Force. *MMWR Recommendations and Reports, 51*(RR-16), 1–45. https://www.cdc.gov/mmwr/pdf/rr/rr5116.pdf (Level II)

8 World Health Organization. (2009). WHO guidelines on hand hygiene in health care: First global patient safety challenge, clean care is safer care. https://apps.who.int/iris/bitstream/handle/10665/44102/9789241597906_eng.pdf?sequence=1 (Level IV)

9 Accreditation Association for Hospitals and Health Systems. (2020). Standard 07.01.21 *Healthcare Facilities Accreditation Program: Accreditation requirements for acute care hospitals.* Chicago, IL: Accreditation Association for Hospitals and Health Systems. (Level VII)

10 Centers for Medicare and Medicaid Services, Department of Health and Human Services. (2020). Condition of participation: Infection control. 42 C.F.R. § 482.42.

11 DNV GL-Healthcare USA, Inc. (2020). IC.1.SR.1. *NIAHO® accreditation requirements, interpretive guidelines and surveyor guidance—revision 20.0.* Milford, OH: DNV GL-Healthcare USA, Inc. (Level VII)

12 The Joint Commission. (2021). Standard NPSG.01.01.01. *Comprehensive accreditation manual for hospitals.* Oakbrook Terrace, IL: The Joint Commission. (Level VII)

13 Accreditation Association for Hospitals and Health Systems. (2020). Standard 15.01.16. *Healthcare Facilities Accreditation Program: Accreditation requirements for acute care hospitals.* Chicago, IL: Accreditation Association for Hospitals and Health Systems. (Level VII)

14 Centers for Medicare and Medicaid Services, Department of Health and Human Services. (2020). Condition of participation: Patient's rights. 42 C.F.R. § 482.13(c)(1).

15 DNV GL-Healthcare USA, Inc. (2020). PR.2.SR.5. *NIAHO® accreditation requirements, interpretive guidelines and surveyor guidance—revision 20.0.* Milford, OH: DNV GL-Healthcare USA, Inc. (Level VII)

16 The Joint Commission. (2021). Standard RI.01.01.01. *Comprehensive accreditation manual for hospitals.* Oakbrook Terrace, IL: The Joint Commission. (Level VII)

17 The Joint Commission. (2021). Standard PC.02.01.21. *Comprehensive accreditation manual for hospitals.* Oakbrook Terrace, IL: The Joint Commission. (Level VII)

18 The Joint Commission. (2021). Standard RC.01.03.01. *Comprehensive accreditation manual for hospitals.* Oakbrook Terrace, IL: The Joint Commission. (Level VII)

19 Accreditation Association for Hospitals and Health Systems. (2020). Standard 10.00.03. *Healthcare Facilities Accreditation Program: Accreditation requirements for acute care hospitals.* Chicago, IL: Accreditation Association for Hospitals and Health Systems. (Level VII)

20 Centers for Medicare and Medicaid Services, Department of Health and Human Services. (2020). Condition of participation: Medical record services. 42 C.F.R. § 482.24(b).

21 DNV GL-Healthcare USA, Inc. (2020). MR.2.SR.1. *NIAHO® accreditation requirements, interpretive guidelines and surveyor guidance—revision 20.0.* Milford, OH: DNV GL-Healthcare USA, Inc. (Level VII)

22 Accreditation Association for Hospitals and Health Systems. (2020). Standard 30.00.14. *Healthcare Facilities Accreditation Program: Accreditation requirements for acute care hospitals.* Chicago, IL: Accreditation Association for Hospitals and Health Systems. (Level VII)

23 Rutala, W. A., et al. (2008, revised 2019). Guideline for disinfection and sterilization in healthcare facilities, 2008. https://www.cdc.gov/infection-control/pdf/guidelines/disinfection guidelines H.pdf (Level I)

24 Accreditation Association for Hospitals and Health Systems. (2020). Standard 07.02.03. *Healthcare Facilities Accreditation Program: Accreditation requirements for acute care hospitals.* Chicago, IL: Accreditation Association for Hospitals and Health Systems. (Level VII)

25 European Pressure Ulcer Advisory Panel, et al. (2019). Prevention and treatment of pressure ulcers/injuries: Quick reference guide. http://www.internationalguideline.com/static/pdfs/Quick_Reference_Guide-10Mar2019.pdf (Level VII)

SEXUAL ASSAULT EXAMINATION

You should emergently triage a patient who has been the victim of a sexual assault as soon as the patient arrives at the emergency department; place the patient in a treatment room as quickly as possible.[1,2] Providing care for the patient is a multi-step process. Key components including obtaining a medical history and event history, performing a head-to-toe assessment (including an anogenital assessment), and collecting evidence as indicated.[3]

Each facility or agency has a specific protocol for specimen collection in cases of sexual assault. Evidence collection kits may vary by facility; however, all kits should meet or exceed the minimum guidelines for content as determined by the U.S. Department of Justice.[2] Specimens may be collected from various sources, and can include blood, hair, nails, tissues, and such body fluids as urine, semen, saliva, and cervical and vaginal secretions. In addition, evidence can be obtained from the results of diagnostic tests, such as computed tomography and radiography. Regardless of the protocol or specimen source, accurate and precise specimen collection is essential in conjunction with thorough, objective documentation, *because in many cases this information will be used as evidence in legal proceedings.*

Some facilities have a sexual assault forensic examiner (SAFE), also known as a sexual assault nurse examiner, available to care for a patient who has reported sexual assault. The SAFE is a skilled professional nurse trained to provide comprehensive care and collect evidence. The SAFE may also be called upon at a later date to testify in legal proceedings.

If you're responsible for collecting specimens in a sexual assault case, follow these guidelines:

- Know your facility's method for specimen collection in sexual assault cases.
- When obtaining specimens, collect them from the victim and, if possible, from the suspect.
- Except in situations covered by mandatory reporting laws, inform local law enforcement agencies of the suspected assault after consent for release of information has been obtained from the patient.[2,4,5]
- Check with local law enforcement agencies about additional specimens they may need—for example, such trace evidence as soot, grass, gravel, glass, and other debris.
- Wear gloves and change them frequently; use disposable equipment and instruments if possible.[2]
- Avoid coughing, sneezing, or talking over specimens or touching your face, nose, or mouth when collecting specimens.
- Treat the patient's clothing as specimens.
- Place each item collected in a separate paper bag.[2]

NURSING ALERT Never allow a specimen or item considered as evidence to be left unattended.

- Document each item or specimen collected.
- Label each specimen in the presence of the patient *to prevent mislabeling.*[6]
- Obtain photographs of all injuries for documentation before collecting physical evidence.[2]
- Include written documentation of the patient's physical and psychological condition on the first encounter, throughout specimen collection, and afterward.

Equipment

Nonlubricated, powder-free gloves ▪ alternate light source (Ensure alternate light source fluoresces at an appropriate wavelength to detect the intended secretion, stain, or fiber, and that you are aware of the limitation with the specific equipment.)[2] ▪ sexual assault evidence collection kit, including:[2] checklist to guide proper collection of evidence, kit container, forms (such as authorization forms, anatomical diagrams, medical forensic history, and release of evidence), examination paper, tweezers, tape, nail clippers and scrapers, saline solution or distilled water, clean paper bag(s) (one for each article of clothing), envelopes, scissors, sterile containers, pencil or pen, swabs for specimen collection, comb, ethylenediaminetetraacetic acid (EDTA) blood collection tube or blood collection filter paper, slides, and deoxyribonucleic acid (DNA) stain card (Note: Contents vary; some jurisdictions have a customized kit.) ▪ speculum ▪ supplies for venipuncture (see the "Venipuncture" procedure) ▪ supplies for urine specimen collection ▪ patient labels ▪ image capturing device (such as cameras with batteries or other facility-approved image capturing device) ▪ cup of water ▪ forensic scale or ruler ▪ Optional: gown, mask, goggles, face shield, colposcope, anoscope,[2] toluidine blue dye, tetanus toxoid, hepatitis B vaccination, antibiotics, sexually transmitted infection (STI) prophylaxis, human immunodeficiency virus (HIV) prophylaxis, emergency contraception.[7]

Preparation of equipment

Make sure that the sexual assault collection kit contains the necessary items for specimen collection, based on the evidence required by the local crime laboratory. The kit contains a form that must be completed, signed, and dated by the examiner.

Inspect all equipment and supplies. If a product is expired, is defective, or has compromised integrity, remove it from patient use, label it as expired or defective, and report the expiration or defect as directed by your facility.

Implementation

- Confirm that patient authorization for specimen collection has been obtained as required.[2]
- Gather and prepare the necessary equipment and supplies,
- Perform hand hygiene.[8,9,10,11,12,13]
- Confirm the patient's identity using at least two patient identifiers.[6]
- Provide privacy.[2,14,15,16,17]

- Assess the patient's ability to undergo the specimen collection procedure.
- Explain the procedure to the patient and family (if appropriate) according to their individual communication and learning needs *to increase their understanding, allay their fears, and enhance cooperation.*[18]
- Provide emotional support throughout the procedure. Obtain the assistance of a social worker, patient advocate, or sexual assault victim advocate *to advocate and support the patient during the examination,* as indicated.[2]
- Inform the patient that the presence of family, friends, and others offering personal support during the examination may influence or be perceived as influencing the patient's statements. If the patient chooses to have anyone else present despite this knowledge, those present should not actively participate in the process.[2]
- Obtain a detailed forensic history from the patient, which is intended to guide the forensic examination, evidence collection, and medical treatment. If able, coordinate your forensic history taking with a law enforcement investigator.[2]
- Perform hand hygiene.[8,9,10,11,12,13]
- Put on nonlubricated powder-free gloves and, as needed, other personal protective equipment *to comply with standard precautions.*[19,20]
- Ask the patient to stand on a clean piece of examination paper, if possible. If the patient can't stand, then have the patient remain on the examination table or bed.
- Ask the patient to remove each article of clothing, one at a time. Place each article in a separate, clean paper bag.[2]
- If the clothing is wet, allow it to dry first before placing the item into the paper bag, if possible. Notify law enforcement if clothing isn't dry when bagged.[2]

NURSING ALERT Don't use plastic bags to collect clothing. *Plastic promotes bacterial growth and can destroy DNA.*[2]

- Fold the examination paper onto itself and place it into a clean paper bag.
- Fold over, seal, label, and initial each bag.
- Before obtaining specimens, inspect the body using an alternative light source *to help identify areas of trauma and secretion deposits.* Colposcopes (used in the assessment of the skin, mouth, and perineum) have magnifying lenses and a green filter to enhance visualization. They may also have an imaging device attached *to record findings.*[2]

NURSING ALERT In some jurisdictions, toluidine blue dye may be used to highlight areas of genital and perineal trauma; however, its use is controversial, *because it may be perceived by the court as changing the appearance of the tissue*; therefore, it isn't universally used. When used, toluidine blue dye should be applied using a cotton swab before an internal or digital speculum examination is performed.[2]

Collecting oral specimens

- Using two swabs at the same time, swab the patient's mouth and gum area.
- Roll one swab over a slide, if required by your local jurisdiction, and let the slide and swabs air-dry.[2]
- Place the oral swabs in the swab container and close it; place the slide in the cardboard sleeve, close it, and tape it shut.
- Place the swab container and cardboard sleeve in an envelope.
- Seal and label the envelope appropriately.[2,21]

Collecting buccal specimens

- Instruct the patient to rinse the mouth with water.
- Using a swab, swab the patient's buccal area for 15 to 20 times *to provide a DNA control sample.*
- Allow the swab to air-dry.
- Place the buccal swab in the swab container and close it.
- Place the swab container in an envelope.
- Seal and label the envelope appropriately.[2,21]

Collecting vaginal or cervical secretions

- Keep in mind when collecting specimens that the quality of the swabs collected is specific to the type of specimen. For moist secretions, typically a one-swab technique is used; if secretions are dry, then a two-swab technique is used.

- Swab the vaginal area thoroughly with four swabs, or according to local jurisdiction; swab the cervical area with two swabs, making sure to keep the vaginal swabs separate from the cervical swabs.
- Gently roll each vaginal swab over a slide, if required by your jurisdiction, and let the slides and swabs to air-dry; do the same for the cervical swabs.
- Place the vaginal swabs in the swab container and close it; place the slides in the cardboard sleeve, close it, and tape it shut; repeat this procedure for the cervical swabs.
- Place the swab container and cardboard sleeve into the envelope and seal it securely.
- Complete the information requested on the front of the envelope; if vaginal and cervical swabs are obtained, use a separate envelope for each.

Collecting anal or rectal secretions[2]
- Moisten the provided swab(s) with sterile water.
- Insert each swab(s) gently, approximately 1¼" (3.2 cm) into the patient's rectum. An anoscope may be used *to aid visualization and avoid contamination of the specimen*; be aware of the need to obtain an informed consent in some jurisdictions and the potential to further traumatize the patient with its use.[2]
- Rotate the swab(s) gently and then remove the swab(s).
- Allow the swab(s) to air-dry and then place the swab(s) in an envelope.
- Seal and label the envelope appropriately.

Collecting penile secretions
- Moisten the provided swabs with sterile water.
- Swab the entire external surface of the penis.
- Repeat this at least one more time (so that you obtain at least two swabs).
- Allow the swabs to air-dry and then place them in an envelope.
- Seal and label the envelope appropriately.

Collecting pubic hair
- Place the provided collection paper under the patient's buttocks and, using the comb provided in the kit, comb through the pubic hair[2] *to collect any debris, trace evidence, or hair from the suspect that may be present.*
- Fold the collection paper containing the comb, hair, and other debris, and place it in an envelope. Seal and label the envelope appropriately.
- Alternatively, if requested in your local jurisdiction, obtain 20 to 30 plucked hairs from the patient as reference samples; allow the patient the option of plucking the pubic hair.
- Place the plucked hair in the envelope; seal and label it appropriately.

Collecting blood samples
- After performing a venipuncture, obtain at least 5 mL of blood in an EDTA tube.
- Write the patient's name and date on the label of the tube.
- Remove the DNA stain card from the kit and label it with the patient's name.
- Withdraw 1 mL of blood from the EDTA blood collection tube and apply blood to each of the four circles on the card, completely filling each circle if possible.
- Let the card air-dry and then place the card in the envelope.
- Seal and label the envelope appropriately.
- Place the blood tube into the tube holder supplied in the kit and seal the holder with the tape supplied in the kit (it may be referred to as evidence tape).
- Place the tube and holder in the zippered bag provided.
- Collect additional blood samples to test for pregnancy, such STIs as HIV and syphilis, or toxicology, as appropriate, and send them to the laboratory immediately.

Collecting urine specimens
- Obtain a random urine specimen from the patient. Remind the patient not to use cleaning wipes *to avoid destroying possible evidence.*
- Obtain a urine specimen for drug screening immediately if it's suspected that the patient was given drugs to facilitate the sexual assault, and if the examination takes place within 96 hours of the assault.[2]

Taking photographs
- Using an appropriate camera, obtain photographs of each separate injury, such as bruises, lacerations, abrasions, and cuts, as directed by the local jurisdiction. Use a forensic scale or ruler to provide size reference in photographs. Take two photographs of each separate injury, one with the scale and one without it. Also, take photographs at medium range *to show injury in the context of the body area* and take close-ups *to show injuries using a forensic scale.*[2]
- Female victims should have another female in the room if the photographer is a male.[2]
- Shield any uninvolved breast or genital area from photographs, *because graphic photographs may be deemed inadmissible in court.*[2] Respect the patient's privacy and drape the patient appropriately while taking photographs.[2]
- Print and label all photographs and place them in the patient's medical forensic record. Don't place photographs in the kit container with specimens.[2]

Storing specimens
- Place blood samples inside the evidence collection envelope, which must be refrigerated while maintaining the chain of custody.[2]
- Place other specimens (except clothing) in the kit container. These specimens may be stored at room temperature while maintaining the proper chain of custody.[2]

Completing the procedure
- Remove and discard your gloves and, if worn, other personal protective equipment.[19,20]
- Perform hand hygiene.[8,9,10,11,12,13]
- Release all the specimens to the law enforcement officer.
- Carefully document the hand-off of the specimens *to ensure proper chain of custody.*[2]
- Document the procedure.[22,23,74,75]

Special considerations
- Follow the directions in the sexual assault evidence collection kit precisely, *to ensure the proper chain of custody.*[21]
- If a female or transgender male patient is menstruating, collect tampons and sanitary napkins. Air-dry them as much as possible, and then place them in a separate paper collection bag.[2]
- Injuries should be marked on an anatomical diagram as well as photographed.[2]
- Provide culturally sensitive follow-up counseling and support to the patient. Provide referrals as needed.[2]
- If needed, administer ordered medications, such as tetanus toxoid, antibiotics for STI prophylaxis, emergency contraceptives, and HIV prophylaxis following safe medication administration practices.[7,26,27,28]
- Assess the patient's hepatitis B immunization status; vaccinate the patient, as needed and prescribed, following safe medication administration practices.[7,26,27,28]
- If possible, arrange for a support person to accompany the patient home.[2]
- Arrange for a referral to a local support group or a trained sexual assault counselor for follow-up.[2]
- Report cases of suspected child abuse in accordance with state guidelines.[7]

Documentation
For each specimen collected, document the type, location from where the specimen was collected, time, patient's name and identification number, and other relevant information. Include photographs, as appropriate, and include relevant information about each photo.[2] Regardless of the protocol or specimen source, accurate and precise specimen collection is essential, along with thorough and objective documentation, *because this information may serve as evidence in legal proceedings.* Record the name of the sexual assault counselor, if present, and any referrals. Document teaching provided to the patient and family (if appropriate), their understanding of that teaching, and any need for follow-up teaching.

REFERENCES

1 Emergency Nurses Association. (2020). Emergency severity index (ESI): A triage tool for emergency department (version 4). https://www.ena.org/docs/default-source/education-document-library/esi-implementation-handbook-2020.pdf?sfvrsn=fdc327df_2 (Level VII)

2 U.S. Department of Justice, Office on Violence Against Women. (2013). A national protocol for sexual assault medical forensic examinations: Adults/adolescents. https://www.ncjrs.gov/pdffiles1/ovw/241903.pdf (Level VII)

3 International Association of Forensic Nurses. (2018). Sexual assault nurse examiner (SANE) education guidelines. https://cdn.ymaws.com/www.forensicnurses.org/resource/resmgr/education/2018_sane_edguidelines.pdf

4 The Joint Commission. (2021). Standard RI.01.06.03. *Comprehensive accreditation manual for hospitals.* (Level VII)

5 The Joint Commission. (2021). Standard PC.01.02.09. *Comprehensive accreditation manual for hospitals.* (Level VII)

6 The Joint Commission. (2021). Standard NPSG.01.01.01. *Comprehensive accreditation manual for hospitals.* (Level VII)

7 Centers for Disease Control and Prevention. (2021). Sexually transmitted infections treatment guidelines, 2021. *MMWR Recommendations and Reports, 70*(RR-4), 1–192. https://www.cdc.gov/std/treatment-guidelines/STI-Guidelines-2021.pdf (Level II)

8 The Joint Commission. (2021). Standard NPSG.07.01.01. *Comprehensive accreditation manual for hospitals.* (Level VII)

9 Centers for Disease Control and Prevention. (2002). Guideline for hand hygiene in health-care settings: Recommendations of the Healthcare Infection Control Practices Advisory Committee and the HICPAC/SHEA/APIC/IDSA Hand Hygiene Task Force. *MMWR Recommendations and Reports, 51*(RR-16), 1–45. https://www.cdc.gov/mmwr/pdf/rr/rr5116.pdf (Level II)

10 World Health Organization. (2009). WHO guidelines on hand hygiene in health care: First global patient safety challenge, clean care is safer care. https://apps.who.int/iris/bitstream/handle/10665/44102/9789241597906_eng.pdf?sequence=1 (Level IV)

11 Accreditation Association for Hospitals and Health Systems. (2020). Standard 07.01.21. *Healthcare Facilities Accreditation Program: Accreditation standards for acute care hospitals.* (Level VII)

12 Centers for Medicare and Medicaid Services, Department of Health and Human Services. (2020). Condition of participation: Infection control. 42 C.F.R. § 482.42.

13 DNV GL-Healthcare USA, Inc. (2020). IC.1.SR.1. *NIAHO® accreditation requirements, interpretive guidelines and surveyor guidance—revision 20.0.* (Level VII)

14 The Joint Commission. (2021). Standard RI.01.01.01. *Comprehensive accreditation manual for hospitals.* (Level VII)

15 Centers for Medicare and Medicaid Services, Department of Health and Human Services. (2020). Condition of participation: Patient's rights. 42 C.F.R. § 482.13(c)(1).

16 Accreditation Association for Hospitals and Health Systems. (2020). Standard 15.01.16. *Healthcare Facilities Accreditation Program: Accreditation requirements for acute care hospitals.* (Level VII)

17 DNV GL-Healthcare USA, Inc. (2020). PR.2.SR.5. *NIAHO® accreditation requirements, interpretive guidelines and surveyor guidance—revision 20.0.* (Level VII)

18 The Joint Commission. (2021). Standard PC.02.01.21. *Comprehensive accreditation manual for hospitals.* (Level VII)

19 Siegel, J. D., et al. (2007, revised 2019). 2007 guideline for isolation precautions: Preventing transmission of infectious agents in healthcare settings. https://www.cdc.gov/infectioncontrol/pdf/guidelines/isolation-guidelines-H.pdf (Level II)

20 Accreditation Association for Hospitals and Health Systems. (2020). Standard 07.01.10. *Healthcare Facilities Accreditation Program: Accreditation requirements for acute care hospitals.* (Level VII)

21 NYS Division of Criminal Justice Services. (2018). Sexual offense evidence collection kit: Instruction sheet. https://www.health.ny.gov/professionals/safe/docs/evidence_collection_kit_instructions.pdf

22 The Joint Commission. (2021). Standard RC.01.03.01. *Comprehensive accreditation manual for hospitals.* (Level VII)

23 Accreditation Association for Hospitals and Health Systems. (2020). Standard 10.00.03. *Healthcare Facilities Accreditation Program: Accreditation requirements for acute care hospitals.* (Level VII)

24 Centers for Medicare and Medicaid Services, Department of Health and Human Services. (2020). Condition of participation: Medical record services. 42 C.F.R. § 482.24(b).

25 DNV GL-Healthcare USA, Inc. (2020). MR.2.SR.1. *NIAHO® accreditation requirements, interpretive guidelines and surveyor guidance—revision 20.0.* (Level VII)

26 Centers for Medicare and Medicaid Services, Department of Health and Human Services. (2020). Condition of participation: Nursing services. 42 C.F.R. § 482.23(c).

27 Accreditation Association for Hospitals and Health Systems. (2020). Standard 16.01.03. *Healthcare Facilities Accreditation Program: Accreditation requirements for acute care hospitals.* (Level VII)

28 DNV GL-Healthcare USA, Inc. (2020). MM.1.SR.3. *NIAHO® accreditation requirements, interpretive guidelines and surveyor guidance—revision 20.0.* (Level VII)

Sharp debridement

Debridement involves removing necrotic tissue or contaminated foreign debris from a wound. As necrotic tissue develops, it becomes a barrier to wound healing and a medium for bacterial growth.[1] Removing this tissue decreases the risk of infection, accelerates wound healing, and prevents further complications associated with tissue destruction. Surgical debridement is recommended for large or deep wounds. However, when surgical debridement isn't appropriate for the patient's condition, sharp, chemical (or enzymatic), mechanical, autolytic, or biosurgical debridement is an acceptable alternative.[2]

Sharp debridement involves using a scalpel, scissors, or other sharp instrument to excise a wound's necrotic material and accumulated debris (biofilm) up to the viable tissue.[3] It's the most rapid form of debridement and can be used with other forms of debridement as needed. A practitioner, physical therapist, or specially trained nurse may perform sharp debridement as permitted by the facility and state practice acts.[1,4,5]

Sharp debridement should be used cautiously in patients with a compromised immune system, compromised vascular supply to the limb, or sepsis. Relative contraindications for sharp debridement include anticoagulant therapy and bleeding disorders.[5]

Equipment

Prescribed analgesic ▪ labels ▪ gloves ▪ sterile drape or towel ▪ wound measuring device ▪ sterile scalpel or scissors ▪ sterile forceps ▪ prescribed cleaning solutions and medications ▪ dressings ▪ impervious plastic trash bag ▪ Optional: gown, sterile gloves, sterile gown, mask and goggles or mask with a face shield, cap, camera, vital signs monitoring equipment, irrigation container, wound irrigation device.

Preparation of equipment

Inspect all equipment and supplies. If a product is expired or defective, or has compromised integrity, remove it from patient use, label it as expired or defective, and report the expiration or defect as directed by your facility.

Implementation

▪ Review the patient's medical record for a history of allergies to latex or analgesics or contraindications to the procedure.
▪ If required by your facility, confirm that written informed consent has been obtained and that the signed consent form is in the patient's medical record.[6,7,8,9]
▪ Conduct a preprocedure verification *to make sure that all relevant documentation, related information, and equipment are available and correctly identified to the patient identifiers.*[10,11]
▪ Verify that ordered laboratory tests are complete and that the results are in the patient's medical record. Notify the practitioner of any unexpected results.[10,11]
▪ Perform hand hygiene.[12,13,14,15,16,17]
▪ Confirm the patient's identity using at least two patient identifiers.[18]
▪ Provide privacy.[19,20,21,22]
▪ Explain the procedure to the patient and family (if appropriate) according to their individual communication and learning needs *to increase their understanding, allay their fears, and enhance cooperation.*[23] Answer any questions.

- Screen and assess the patient's pain using facility-defined criteria that are consistent with the patient's age, condition, and ability to understand.[24]
- Treat the patient's pain, as needed and ordered, using nonpharmacologic or pharmacologic approaches, or a combination of approaches. Base the treatment plan on evidence-based practices and the patient's clinical condition, past medical history, and pain management goals.[24]
- Teach the patient distraction and relaxation techniques, if possible, *to minimize discomfort.*
- Administer an oral analgesic, following safe medication administration practices, at an appropriate time before debridement begins based on the onset and peak of the medication prescribed, or give an IV analgesic immediately before the procedure, as ordered.[1,5,25,26,27,28,29]
- If the patient is receiving IV opioids, frequently monitor vital signs and the respiratory status and sedation level *to promptly recognize and treat oversedation and respiratory depression related to IV opioid use.* Explain the monitoring process to the patient and family (including that it may be necessary to awaken the patient to assess the medication's effects). Advise the patient and family to alert staff immediately if breathing problems or other changes occur that may be a reaction to the medication.[30]
- Raise the patient's bed to waist level before providing patient care *to prevent caregiver back strain.*[31]
- Perform hand hygiene.[12,13,14,15,16,17]
- Keep the patient warm. Expose only the area to be debrided *to prevent vasoconstriction that reduces wound healing.*[1]
- If the wound to be debrided is on a lower extremity, perform a neurovascular assessment before beginning the procedure *to obtain a baseline for comparison.*[5] *Inadequate perfusion can result in wound extension.*[1]
- Perform hand hygiene.[12,13,14,15,16,17]
- Prepare a sterile field using a sterile drape or towel.[1] Then, using sterile no-touch technique, set up the necessary supplies on the sterile field.[32]
- Label all medications, medication containers, and solutions on and off the sterile field.[33,34]
- Conduct a time-out immediately before starting the procedure *to perform a final assessment that the correct patient, site, positioning, and procedure are identified and, as applicable, that all relevant information and necessary equipment are available.*[35]
- Put on a cap and mask and goggles or a mask and face shield and a gown, as needed, *to comply with standard procedures.*[36,37,38]
- Perform hand hygiene.[12,13,14,15,16,17]
- Put on gloves *to comply with standard precautions.*[32,36,37,38]
- Gently remove the dressings and discard them carefully in an impervious plastic trash bag, *because soiled dressings harbor infectious microorganisms.*[38]
- Remove and discard your gloves.[36,37,38]
- Perform hand hygiene.[12,13,14,15,16,17]
- Put on gloves.[36,37,38,39]
- Clean the wound *to remove debris and bacterial load.*[1,3,25] (See the "Wound irrigation" procedure.)
- Measure the wound *to determine how wound healing is progressing.* If applicable, photograph the wound *for additional documentation.*[5]
- Lift the necrotic tissue with forceps. Use the scalpel or scissors to cut the tissue. Keep the scalpel or scissors parallel to or angled away from the wound bed.
- Replace the dressing over the wound.[1]
- Return the bed to the lowest position *to prevent falls and maintain patient safety.*[40]
- Discard used supplies and debrided tissue in appropriate receptacles.[38]
- Remove and discard your gloves and remove your personal protective equipment.[38]
- Perform hand hygiene.[12,13,14,15,16,17]
- Reassess and respond to the patient's pain by evaluating the response to treatment and progress toward pain management goals. Assess for adverse reactions and risk factors for adverse events that may result from treatment.[24]
- Perform hand hygiene.[12,13,14,15,16,17]
- Document the procedure.[41,42,43,44]

Special considerations

- *Because debridement removes dead tissue*, bleeding should be minimal. If bleeding occurs, apply gentle pressure on the wound with sterile 4"× 4" (10-cm × 10-cm) gauze pads.[1] Then apply a hemostatic agent or calcium alginate dressing, as ordered.[25] If bleeding persists, notify the practitioner, and maintain pressure on the wound until the practitioner arrives. Note that excessive bleeding or spurting vessels may require ligation or cauterization.

Complications

Infection can develop despite the use of sterile technique and equipment. Bleeding, the most common complication, can occur if debridement exposes an eroded blood vessel or if you inadvertently cut a vessel. Fluid and electrolyte imbalances may result from exudate lost during the procedure.

Documentation

Record the date and time of wound debridement, the area debrided, and solutions and medications used. Describe the wound's condition, noting signs of infection or skin breakdown. Document the wound's measurement and whether the wound was photographed. Record the patient's tolerance of and reaction to the procedure. Note indications for additional therapy. Record the administration of preprocedure pain medication and pain assessment findings before, during, and after the procedure. Document teaching provided to the patient and family (if applicable), their understanding of that teaching, and any need for follow-up teaching.

REFERENCES

1 Wiegand, D. (2017). *AACN procedure manual for high acuity, progressive, and critical care* (7th ed.). St. Louis, MO: Elsevier.
2 Harris, C., et al. (2018). Sharp wound debridement: Patient selection and perspectives. *Chronic Wound Care Management and Research, 5*, 29–36. https://dovepress.com/sharp-wound-debridement-patient-selection-and-perspectives-peer-reviewed-fulltext-article-CWCMR
3 Armstrong, D. G., & Meyr, A. J. (2021). Basic principles of wound management. In: *UpToDate,* Eidt, J. F., et al. (Eds.).
4 National Alliance of Wound Care and Ostomy. (n.d.). Scope of practice. https://www.nawccb.org/scope-of-practice
5 European Pressure Ulcer Advisory Panel, et al. (2019). Prevention and treatment of pressure ulcers/injuries: Quick reference guide. http://www.internationalguideline.com/static/pdfs/Quick_Reference_Guide-10Mar2019.pdf (Level VII)
6 Centers for Medicare and Medicaid Services, Department of Health and Human Services. (2020). Condition of participation: Patient's rights. 42 C.F.R. § 482.13(b)(2).
7 The Joint Commission. (2021). Standard RI.01.03.01. *Comprehensive accreditation manual for hospitals.* Oakbrook Terrace, IL: The Joint Commission. (Level VII)
8 Accreditation Association for Hospitals and Health Systems. (2020). Standard 15.01.11. *Healthcare Facilities Accreditation Program: Accreditation requirements for acute care hospitals.* Chicago, IL: Accreditation Association for Hospitals and Health Systems. (Level VII)
9 DNV GL-Healthcare USA, Inc. (2020). PR.2.SR.3. *NIAHO® accreditation requirements, interpretive guidelines and surveyor guidance—revision 20.0.* Milford, OH: DNV GL-Healthcare USA, Inc. (Level VII)
10 The Joint Commission. (2021). Standard UP.01.01.01. *Comprehensive accreditation manual for hospitals.* Oakbrook Terrace, IL: The Joint Commission. (Level VII)
11 Accreditation Association for Hospitals and Health Systems. (2020). Standard 30.00.14. *Healthcare Facilities Accreditation Program: Accreditation requirements for acute care hospitals.* Chicago, IL: Accreditation Association for Hospitals and Health Systems. (Level VII)
12 Centers for Disease Control and Prevention. (2002). Guideline for hand hygiene in health-care settings: Recommendations of the Healthcare Infection Control Practices Advisory Committee and the HICPAC/SHEA/APIC/IDSA Hand Hygiene Task Force. *MMWR Recommendations and Reports, 51*(RR-16), 1–45. https://www.cdc.gov/mmwr/pdf/rr/rr5116.pdf (Level II)

13 World Health Organization. (2009). WHO guidelines on hand hygiene in health care: First global patient safety challenge, clean care is safer care. https://apps.who.int/iris/bitstream/handle/10665/44102/9789241597906_eng.pdf?sequence=1 (Level IV)

14 The Joint Commission. (2021). Standard NPSG.07.01.01. *Comprehensive accreditation manual for hospitals.* Oakbrook Terrace, IL: The Joint Commission. (Level VII)

15 Centers for Medicare and Medicaid Services, Department of Health and Human Services. (2020). Condition of participation: Infection control. 42 C.F.R. § 482.42.

16 Accreditation Association for Hospitals and Health Systems. (2020). Standard 07.01.21. *Healthcare Facilities Accreditation Program: Accreditation requirements for acute care hospitals.* Chicago, IL: Accreditation Association for Hospitals and Health Systems. (Level VII)

17 DNV GL-Healthcare USA, Inc. (2020). IC.1.SR.1. *NIAHO® accreditation requirements, interpretive guidelines and surveyor guidance—revision 20.0.* Milford, OH: DNV GL-Healthcare USA, Inc. (Level VII)

18 The Joint Commission. (2021). Standard NPSG.01.01.01. *Comprehensive accreditation manual for hospitals.* Oakbrook Terrace, IL: The Joint Commission. (Level VII)

19 Accreditation Association for Hospitals and Health Systems. (2020). Standard 15.01.16. *Healthcare Facilities Accreditation Program: Accreditation requirements for acute care hospitals.* Chicago, IL: Accreditation Association for Hospitals and Health Systems. (Level VII)

20 Centers for Medicare and Medicaid Services, Department of Health and Human Services. (2020). Condition of participation: Patient's rights. 42 C.F.R. § 482.13(c)(1).

21 DNV GL-Healthcare USA, Inc. (2020). PR.2.SR.5. *NIAHO® accreditation requirements, interpretive guidelines and surveyor guidance—revision 20.0.* Milford, OH: DNV GL-Healthcare USA, Inc. (Level VII)

22 The Joint Commission. (2021). Standard RI.01.01.01. *Comprehensive accreditation manual for hospitals.* Oakbrook Terrace, IL: The Joint Commission. (Level VII)

23 The Joint Commission. (2021). Standard PC.02.01.21. *Comprehensive accreditation manual for hospitals.* Oakbrook Terrace, IL: The Joint Commission. (Level VII)

24 The Joint Commission. (2021). Standard PC.01.02.07. *Comprehensive accreditation manual for hospitals.* Oakbrook Terrace, IL: The Joint Commission. (Level VII)

25 Woo, K. Y., & Sibbald, R. G. (2010). Local wound care for malignant and palliative wounds. *Advances in Skin and Wound Care, 23,* 417–428. (Level VII)

26 Centers for Medicare and Medicaid Services, Department of Health and Human Services. (2020). Condition of participation: Nursing services. 42 C.F.R. § 482.23(c).

27 Accreditation Association for Hospitals and Health Systems. (2020). Standard 16.01.03. *Healthcare Facilities Accreditation Program: Accreditation requirements for acute care hospitals.* Chicago, IL: Accreditation Association for Hospitals and Health Systems. (Level VII)

28 DNV GL-Healthcare USA, Inc. (2020). MM.1.SR.3. *NIAHO® accreditation requirements, interpretive guidelines and surveyor guidance—revision 20.0.* Milford, OH: DNV GL-Healthcare USA, Inc. (Level VII)

29 The Joint Commission. (2021). Standard MM.06.01.01. *Comprehensive accreditation manual for hospitals.* Oakbrook Terrace, IL: The Joint Commission. (Level VII)

30 Centers for Medicare and Medicaid Services. (2014). Requirements for hospital medication administration, particularly intravenous (IV) medications and post-operative care of patients receiving IV opioids. http://www.cms.gov/Medicare/Provider-Enrollment-and-Certification/SurveyCertificationGenInfo/Downloads/Survey-and-Cert-Letter-14-15.pdf

31 Waters, T. R., et al. (2009). Safe patient handling training for schools of nursing. https://www.cdc.gov/niosh/docs/2009-127/pdfs/2009-127.pdf (Level VII)

32 Wound, Ostomy and Continence Nurses Society Wound Committee & Association for Professionals in Infection Control and Epidemiology. (2012). Clean vs. sterile dressing techniques for management of chronic wounds: A fact sheet. *Journal of Wound, Ostomy and Continence Nursing, 39*(Suppl. 2), S30–S34. https://journals.lww.com/jwocnonline/Fulltext/2012/03001/Clean_vs_Sterile_Dressing_Techniques_for.7.aspx

33 The Joint Commission. (2021). Standard NPSG.03.04.01. *Comprehensive accreditation manual for hospitals.* Oakbrook Terrace, IL: The Joint Commission. (Level VII)

34 Accreditation Association for Hospitals and Health Systems. (2020). Standard 25.01.27. *Healthcare Facilities Accreditation Program: Accreditation requirements for acute care hospitals.* Chicago, IL: Accreditation Association for Hospitals and Health Systems. (Level VII)

35 The Joint Commission. (2021). Standard UP.01.03.01. *Comprehensive accreditation manual for hospital.* Oakbrook Terrace, IL: The Joint Commission. (Level VII)

36 Siegel, J. D., et al. (2007, revised 2019). 2007 guideline for isolation precautions: Preventing transmission of infectious agents in healthcare settings. https://www.cdc.gov/infectioncontrol/pdf/guidelines/isolation-guidelines-H.pdf (Level II)

37 Accreditation Association for Hospitals and Health Systems. (2020). Standard 07.01.10. *Healthcare Facilities Accreditation Program: Accreditation requirements for acute care hospitals.* Chicago, IL: Accreditation Association for Hospitals and Health Systems. (Level VII)

38 Occupational Safety and Health Administration. (2012). Bloodborne pathogens, standard number 1910.1030. https://www.osha.gov/pls/oshaweb/owadisp.show_document?p_id=10051&p_table=STANDARDS (Level VII)

39 Wound, Ostomy, and Continence Nurses Society. (2015). *Methods of wound debridement: Best practices for clinicians.* Mt. Laurel, NJ: Wound, Ostomy, and Continence Nurses Society.

40 Ganz, D. A., et al. (2013, reviewed 2021). *Preventing falls in hospitals: A toolkit for improving quality of care* (AHRQ Publication No. 13-0015-EF). Rockville, MD: Agency for Healthcare Research and Quality. https://www.ahrq.gov/professionals/systems/hospital/fallpxtoolkit/index.html (Level VII)

41 The Joint Commission. (2021). Standard RC.01.03.01. *Comprehensive accreditation manual for hospitals.* Oakbrook Terrace, IL: The Joint Commission. (Level VII)

42 Centers for Medicare and Medicaid Services, Department of Health and Human Services. (2020). Condition of participation: Medical record services. 42 C.F.R. § 482.24(b).

43 Accreditation Association for Hospitals and Health Systems. (2020). Standard 10.00.03. *Healthcare Facilities Accreditation Program: Accreditation requirements for acute care hospitals.* Chicago, IL: Accreditation Association for Hospitals and Health Systems. (Level VII)

44 DNV GL-Healthcare USA, Inc. (2020). MR.2.SR.1. *NIAHO® accreditation requirements, interpretive guidelines and surveyor guidance—revision 20.0.* Milford, OH: DNV GL-Healthcare USA, Inc. (Level VII)

SHAVING

Performed with a safety or electric razor, shaving may be part of a patient's usual daily care.[1] Shaving promotes patient comfort by removing facial hair that can itch and irritate the skin and produce an unkempt appearance. Because nicks and cuts occur more frequently with a safety razor, shaving with an electric razor is indicated for a patient with a clotting disorder or a patient undergoing anticoagulant therapy.[1] Shaving may be contraindicated in the patient with a facial skin disorder or wound.

Equipment

Gloves ■ light source ■ Optional: personal protective equipment (gown, mask and goggles or mask with face shield).

For shaving with a disposable safety razor
Soap or shaving cream ■ bath towel ■ washcloth ■ basin ■ facility-approved disinfectant ■ Optional: aftershave lotion, bedside stand or overbed table.

For shaving with an electric or battery-operated razor
Bath towel ■ disinfectant wipes ■ Optional: preshave and aftershave lotions, grounded three-pronged plug.

Preparation of equipment

For a safety razor, make sure the blade is sharp, clean, even, and rust-free. A razor may be used more than once, but only for the same patient. If the patient is bedridden, gather the equipment on the bedside stand or overbed table; if the patient is ambulatory, gather it at the sink.

For an electric razor, check its cord for fraying or other damage that could create an electrical hazard. If the razor isn't double-insulated or battery operated, use a grounded three-pronged plug. Examine the razor head for sharp edges and dirt. Read the manufacturer's instructions, if available.

Implementation

- Gather and prepare the necessary equipment and supplies.
- Perform hand hygiene.[2,3,4,5,6,7]
- Confirm the patient's identity using at least two patient identifiers.[8]
- Provide privacy.[9,10,11,12]
- Tell the patient that you're going to provide a shave. Ask the patient to assist you as much as possible *to promote independence.*
- Unless contraindicated, place the conscious patient in the high Fowler or semi-Fowler position. If the patient is unconscious, elevate the head *to prevent soap and water from running behind it.*
- If the patient is unable to be placed in the high-Fowler position, raise the bed to waist level before providing care *to prevent caregiver back strain.*[13]
- Make sure there is adequate lighting.
- Perform hand hygiene.[2,3,4,5,6,7]
- Put on gloves and, as necessary, other personal protective equipment *to comply with standard precautions.*[14,15,16]

Using a safety razor

- Drape a bath towel around the patient's shoulders and tuck it under the chin *to protect the bed from moisture and to catch falling facial hair.*
- Fill the basin with warm water. Using the washcloth, wet the patient's entire beard with warm water. Let the warm cloth soak the beard for at least 1 minute *to soften facial hair.*
- Apply shaving cream to the beard; if you're using soap, rub it *to form a lather.*
- Gently stretch the patient's skin taut with one hand and shave with the other, holding the razor firmly. Ask the patient to puff the cheeks or turn the head, as necessary, *to shave hard-to-reach areas.*
- Begin at the patient's sideburns and work toward the chin using short, firm, downward strokes in the direction of hair growth (as shown below). *This method reduces skin irritation and helps prevent nicks and cuts.*

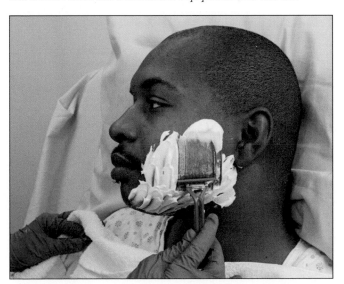

- Rinse the razor often *to remove facial hair and shaving cream.* Apply more warm water or shaving cream to the patient's face, as needed, *to maintain adequate lather.*
- Shave across the patient's chin and up the neck and throat. Use short, gentle strokes for the neck and the area around the nose and mouth *to avoid skin irritation.*
- Change the water, and rinse any remaining lather and facial hair from the patient's face. Then dry the face with a bath towel and, if the patient desires, apply aftershave lotion.

- Rinse the razor and then return the razor to its storage area or dispose of it in a sharps container.[14]
- Remove and discard your gloves.[14]
- Perform hand hygiene.[2,3,4,5,6,7]
- Put on gloves.[14,16]
- Clean and disinfect the basin using a facility-approved disinfectant.[17,18]
- Allow the basin to dry thoroughly and then store it as directed by your facility.

Using an electric or battery-operated razor

- Drape a bath towel around the patient's shoulders and tuck it under the chin *to catch falling facial hair.*
- Plug in the razor, if applicable, and apply preshave lotion, if available, *to remove skin oils.*
- If the razor head is adjustable, select the appropriate setting.
- Using a circular motion and pressing the razor firmly against the patient's skin, shave each area of the patient's face until smooth.
- If the patient desires, apply aftershave lotion.
- Clean and disinfect the razor head as directed by your facility, and return the razor to its storage area.[17,18]

Completing the procedure

- If necessary, return the bed to the lowest position *to prevent falls and maintain the patient's safety.*[19]
- Remove and discard your gloves and, if worn, other personal protective equipment.[14]
- Perform hand hygiene.[2,3,4,5,6,7]
- Document the procedure.[20,21,22,23]

Special considerations

- Don't interchange patients' shaving equipment *to prevent the spread of infections, such as methicillin-resistant* Staphylococcus aureus.[24]
- Be aware of cultural or religious beliefs[1] that may affect the patient's desire for routine shaving to be performed.
- A safety inspection by medical maintenance may need to be performed before using an electric razor brought from the patient's home.[25]

Complications

Cuts and abrasions are the most common complications of shaving. Skin irritation and folliculitis can also occur.[26,27]

Documentation

Document the procedure in the patient's medical record. If applicable, record nicks and cuts resulting from shaving as well as alterations in the condition of the patient's skin. Document teaching provided to the patient and family (if appropriate), their understanding of that teaching, and any need for follow-up teaching.

REFERENCES

1 Craven, R. F., et al. (2021). *Fundamentals of nursing: Concepts and competencies for practice* (9th ed.). Philadelphia, PA: Wolters Kluwer.
2 The Joint Commission. (2021). Standard NPSG.07.01.01. *Comprehensive accreditation manual for hospitals.* Oakbrook Terrace, IL: The Joint Commission. (Level VII)
3 Centers for Disease Control and Prevention. (2002). Guideline for hand hygiene in health-care settings: Recommendations of the Healthcare Infection Control Practices Advisory Committee and the HICPAC/SHEA/APIC/IDSA Hand Hygiene Task Force. *MMWR Recommendations and Reports, 51*(RR-16), 1–45. https://www.cdc.gov/mmwr/pdf/rr/rr5116.pdf (Level II)
4 World Health Organization. (2009). WHO guidelines on hand hygiene in health care: First global patient safety challenge, clean care is safer care. https://apps.who.int/iris/bitstream/handle/10665/44102/9789241597906_eng.pdf?sequence=1 (Level IV)
5 Accreditation Association for Hospitals and Health Systems. (2020). Standard 07.01.21. *Healthcare Facilities Accreditation Program: Accreditation requirements for acute care hospitals.* Chicago, IL: Accreditation Association for Hospitals and Health Systems. (Level VII)

6 Centers for Medicare and Medicaid Services, Department of Health and Human Services. (2020). Condition of participation: Infection control. 42 C.F.R. § 482.42.

7 DNV GL-Healthcare USA, Inc. (2020). IC.1.SR.1. *NIAHO® accreditation requirements, interpretive guidelines and surveyor guidance—revision 20.0.* Milford, OH: DNV GL-Healthcare USA, Inc. (Level VII)

8 The Joint Commission. (2021). Standard NPSG.01.01.01. *Comprehensive accreditation manual for hospitals.* Oakbrook Terrace, IL: The Joint Commission. (Level VII)

9 Accreditation Association for Hospitals and Health Systems. (2020). Standard 15.01.16. *Healthcare Facilities Accreditation Program: Accreditation requirements for acute care hospitals.* Chicago, IL: Accreditation Association for Hospitals and Health Systems. (Level VII)

10 Centers for Medicare and Medicaid Services, Department of Health and Human Services. (2020). Condition of participation: Patient's rights. 42 C.F.R. § 482.13(c)(1).

11 DNV GL-Healthcare USA, Inc. (2020). PR.2.SR.5. *NIAHO® accreditation requirements, interpretive guidelines and surveyor guidance—revision 20.0.* Milford, OH: DNV GL-Healthcare USA, Inc. (Level VII)

12 The Joint Commission. (2021). Standard RI.01.01.01. *Comprehensive accreditation manual for hospitals.* Oakbrook Terrace, IL: The Joint Commission. (Level VII)

13 Waters, T. R., et al. (2009). Safe patient handling training for schools of nursing. https://www.cdc.gov/niosh/docs/2009-127/pdfs/2009-127.pdf (Level VII)

14 Occupational Safety and Health Administration. (2012). Bloodborne pathogens, standard number 1910.1030. https://www.osha.gov/pls/oshaweb/owadisp.show_document?p_id=10051&p_table=STANDARDS (Level VII)

15 Accreditation Association for Hospitals and Health Systems. (2020). Standard 07.01.10. *Healthcare Facilities Accreditation Program: Accreditation requirements for acute care hospitals.* Chicago, IL: Accreditation Association for Hospitals and Health Systems. (Level VII)

16 Siegel, J. D., et al. (2007, revised 2019). 2007 guideline for isolation precautions: Preventing transmission of infectious agents in healthcare settings. https://www.cdc.gov/infectioncontrol/pdf/guidelines/isolation-guidelines-H.pdf (Level II)

17 Rutala, W. A., et al. (2008, revised 2019). Guideline for disinfection and sterilization in healthcare facilities, 2008. https://www.cdc.gov/infectioncontrol/pdf/guidelines/disinfection-guidelines-H.pdf (Level I)

18 Accreditation Association for Hospitals and Health Systems. (2020). Standard 07.02.03. *Healthcare Facilities Accreditation Program: Accreditation requirements for acute care hospitals.* Chicago, IL: Accreditation Association for Hospitals and Health Systems. (Level VII)

19 Ganz, D. A., et al. (2013, reviewed 2021). *Preventing falls in hospitals: A toolkit for improving quality of care* (AHRQ Publication No. 13-0015-EF). Rockville, MD: Agency for Healthcare Research and Quality. https://www.ahrq.gov/professionals/systems/hospital/fallpxtoolkit/index.html (Level VII)

20 Centers for Medicare and Medicaid Services, Department of Health and Human Services. (2020). Condition of participation: Medical record services. 42 C.F.R. § 482.24(b).

21 Accreditation Association for Hospitals and Health Systems. (2020). Standard 10.00.03. *Healthcare Facilities Accreditation Program: Accreditation requirements for acute care hospitals.* Chicago, IL: Accreditation Association for Hospitals and Health Systems. (Level VII)

22 The Joint Commission. (2021). Standard RC.01.03.01. *Comprehensive accreditation manual for hospitals.* Oakbrook Terrace, IL: The Joint Commission. (Level VII)

23 DNV GL-Healthcare USA, Inc. (2020). MR.2.SR.1. *NIAHO® accreditation requirements, interpretive guidelines and surveyor guidance—revision 20.0.* Milford, OH: DNV GL-Healthcare USA, Inc. (Level VII)

24 Centers for Disease Control and Prevention. (2019). Methicillin-resistant *Staphylococcus aureus* (MRSA): General information. https://www.cdc.gov/mrsa/community/index.html

25 The Joint Commission. (2021). Standard EC.02.04.03. *Comprehensive accreditation manual for hospitals.* Oakbrook Terrace, IL: The Joint Commission. (Level VII)

26 Goldstein, B. G., & Goldstein, A. O. (2019). Pseudofolliculitis barbae. In: *UpToDate,* Dellavalle, R. P., & Owen, C. (Eds.).

27 Shenenberger, D. W. (2021). Removal of unwanted hair. In: *UpToDate,* Dellavalle, R. P., & Dover, J. S. (Eds.).

Sitz bath

A sitz bath involves immersion of the pelvic area in warm or hot water. It is used to relieve discomfort, especially after perineal or rectal surgery or childbirth.[1,2,3,4] The bath promotes wound healing by cleaning the perineum and anus, increasing circulation, and reducing inflammation. It also helps relax local muscles.[1]

To be performed correctly, the sitz bath requires frequent checks of water temperature to ensure safety, comfort, and therapeutic effects. Correct draping of the patient during and prompt dressing after the bath help prevent vasoconstriction.

Equipment

Sitz tub, portable sitz bath, or regular bathtub ▪ bath mat ▪ bath (utility) thermometer ▪ two bath blankets ▪ towels ▪ patient gown ▪ facility-approved disinfectant ▪ gloves ▪ Optional: rubber mat, rubber ring, footstool, overbed table, IV pole (to hold irrigation bag), wheelchair or stretcher, wound dressings, personal protective equipment, blood pressure monitoring device, watch or clock with a second hand.

A portable sitz bath kit is available in a commercial disposable kit for single-patient use. The kit includes a plastic basin that fits over a commode and an irrigation bag with tubing and clamp.

Preparation of equipment

Inspect all equipment and supplies. If a product is expired, is defective, or has compromised integrity, remove it from patient use, label it as defective, and report the defect as directed by your facility. Make sure the sitz tub, portable sitz bath, or regular bathtub is clean and disinfected. As an alternative, obtain a disposable sitz bath kit from the central supply department.

Sitz bath and regular bathtub

Position the bath mat next to the bathtub, sitz tub, or commode. If you're using a tub, place the rubber mat on its surface *to prevent falls.* Place the rubber ring on the bottom of the tub *to serve as a seat for the patient,* and cover the ring with a towel *for comfort.* Keep the patient elevated *to improve water flow over the wound site and to avoid unnecessary pressure on tender tissues.*

Fill the sitz tub or bathtub one-third to one-half full *so that the water will reach the seated patient's umbilicus.* Use warm water (94° to 98° F [34.4° to 36.7° C]) for relaxation or wound cleaning and healing, and hot water (110° to 115° F [43.3° to 46.1° C]) for heat application. Run the water slightly warmer than desired, *because it will cool while the patient prepares for the bath.* Measure the water temperature using the bath thermometer.

Commercial sitz bath kit

Open the package and familiarize yourself with the equipment. Fill the basin to the specified line with water at the prescribed temperature. Place the basin under the commode seat, clamp the irrigation tubing to block water flow, and fill the irrigation bag with water of the same temperature as that in the basin. *To create flow pressure,* hang the bag above the patient's head on a hook, towel rack, or IV pole.

Implementation

- Verify the practitioner's order.
- Gather and prepare the necessary equipment and supplies.
- Perform hand hygiene.[5,6,7,8,9,10]
- Confirm the patient's identity using at least two patient identifiers.[11]
- Explain the procedure the patient and family (if appropriate) according to their individual communication and learning needs *to increase their understanding, allay their fears, and enhance cooperation.*[12] Answer any questions.
- Provide privacy.[13,14,15,16]
- Assess the patient's condition.
- Instruct the patient to void.
- Assist the patient to the bath area.

- Make sure that the area is warm and free from drafts.
- Help the patient undress, as needed.
- Perform hand hygiene.[5,6,7,8,9,10]
- Put on gloves and, as needed, other personal protective equipment *to comply with standard precautions.*[8,17,18]
- If the patient has soiled dressings, remove and discard them in the appropriate receptacle, remove and discard your gloves, perform hand hygiene, and put on new gloves.[5,6,7,8,9,10,17,18]
- If a dressing adheres to a wound, allow it to soak off in the water.
- Assist the patient into the tub or onto the commode, as needed. Instruct the patient to use the safety rail *for balance.*
- Explain that the sensation may be unpleasant initially *because the wound area is tender.* Assure the patient that this discomfort will soon be relieved by the warm water.
- For any apparatus except a regular bathtub: if the patient's feet don't reach the floor and the weight of the legs presses against the edge of the equipment, place a small stool under the patient's feet *to decrease pressure on local blood vessels.* Also place a folded towel against the patient's lower back *to prevent discomfort and promote correct body alignment.*
- Drape the patient's shoulders and knees with bath blankets *to avoid chills that may cause vasoconstriction.*
- If you're using a sitz tub or bathtub, check the water temperature frequently with the bath thermometer. If the temperature drops significantly, add warm water. For maximum safety, first help the patient stand up slowly *to prevent dizziness and loss of balance.* Then, with the patient holding the safety rail *for support,* run warm water into the tub. Check the water temperature. When the water reaches the correct temperature, help the patient sit down again to resume the bath.
- If you're using a commercial sitz bath kit, open the clamp on the irrigation tubing *to allow a stream of water to flow continuously over the wound site.* Refill the bag with water of the correct temperature as needed, and encourage the patient to regulate the flow. Place the patient's overbed table in front of the patient *to provide support and comfort.*
- If necessary, stay with the patient during the bath. If you must leave, place the call light within the patient's reach, show the patient how to use it, and ensure privacy.
- Assess the patient's color and general condition frequently. If the patient complains of feeling weak, faint, or nauseated or shows signs of cardiovascular distress, discontinue the bath, check the patient's pulse and blood pressure, and assist the patient back to bed. Use a wheelchair or stretcher for transport to the patient's room, if necessary, and notify the practitioner.
- When the prescribed sitz bath time has elapsed—usually 15 to 20 minutes—tell the patient to use the safety rail *for balance,* and help the patient to a standing position, moving slowly *to prevent dizziness and to allow the patient to regain equilibrium.*
- If necessary, assist the patient to dry.
- Remove and discard your gloves.[17,18]
- Perform hand hygiene[5,6,7,8,9,10] and put on a new pair of gloves.[17,18]
- Redress the wound as needed.
- Provide the patient with a clean gown, and help the patient dress and return to bed or back to the room.
- Dispose of soiled materials properly.[18]
- Empty, clean, and disinfect the sitz tub, bathtub, or portable sitz bath using a facility-approved disinfectant.[19,20] Return the commercial sitz bath kit to the patient's bedside for later use.
- Remove and discard your gloves and other personal protective equipment, if worn,[17,18] and perform hand hygiene.[5,6,7,8,9,10]
- Document the procedure.[21,22,23,24]

Special considerations

- Use a regular bathtub only if a sitz tub, portable sitz bath, or commercial sitz bath kit is unavailable. A regular bathtub is less effective for local treatment than a sitz device, and should be avoided, *because the application of heat to the extremities causes vasodilation and draws blood away from the perineal area,*
- If the patient will be sitting in a bathtub with the extremities immersed in the hot water, check the patient's pulse before, during, and after the bath *to help detect vasodilation that could make the patient feel faint when standing up.*
- Tell the patient never to touch an open wound *to avoid the risk of infection.*

Complications

Weakness or faintness can result from heat or the exertion of changing position during a sitz bath. An irregular or accelerated pulse may indicate cardiovascular distress.

Documentation

Record the date, time, duration, and temperature of the bath; wound condition before and after treatment, including color, odor, and amount of drainage; any complications, your interventions, and the patient's response to your interventions; and the patient's response to treatment. Document teaching you provided to the patient and family (if applicable), their understanding of that teaching, and any need for follow-up teaching.

REFERENCES

1 Bleday, R. (2020). Anal fissure: Medical management. In: *UpToDate*, Weiser, M., & Friedman, L. S. (Eds.).
2 Berkowitz, L. R., & Foust-Wright, C. E. (2020). Postpartum perineal care and management of complications. In: *UpToDate*, Brubaker, L., & Lockwood, C. J. (Eds.).
3 Silbert-Flagg, J., & Pillitteri, A. (2018). *Maternal and child health nursing: Care of the childbearing and childrearing family* (8th ed.). Philadelphia, PA: Wolters Kluwer.
4 Ellis, C. N. (2021). Anal fissure: Surgical management. In: *UpToDate*, Weiser, M. (Ed.)
5 The Joint Commission. (2021). Standard NPSG.07.01.01. *Comprehensive accreditation manual for hospitals.* Oakbrook Terrace, IL: The Joint Commission. (Level VII)
6 Centers for Disease Control and Prevention. (2002). Guideline for hand hygiene in health-care settings: Recommendations of the Healthcare Infection Control Practices Advisory Committee and the HICPAC/SHEA/APIC/IDSA Hand Hygiene Task Force. *MMWR Recommendations and Reports, 51*(RR-16), 1–45. https://www.cdc.gov/mmwr/pdf/rr/rr5116.pdf (Level II)
7 World Health Organization. (2009). WHO guidelines on hand hygiene in health care: First global patient safety challenge, clean care is safer care. https://apps.who.int/iris/bitstream/handle/10665/44102/9789241597906_eng.pdf?sequence=1 (Level IV)
8 Accreditation Association for Hospitals and Health Systems. (2020). Standard 07.01.21. *Healthcare Facilities Accreditation Program: Accreditation requirements for acute care hospitals.* Chicago, IL: Accreditation Association for Hospitals and Health Systems. (Level VII)
9 Centers for Medicare and Medicaid Services, Department of Health and Human Services. (2020). Condition of participation: Infection control. 42 C.F.R. § 482.42.
10 DNV GL-Healthcare USA, Inc. (2020). IC.1.SR.1. *NIAHO® accreditation requirements, interpretive guidelines and surveyor guidance—revision 20.0.* Milford, OH: DNV GL-Healthcare USA, Inc. (Level VII)
11 The Joint Commission. (2021). Standard NPSG.01.01.01. *Comprehensive accreditation manual for hospitals.* Oakbrook Terrace, IL: The Joint Commission. (Level VII)
12 The Joint Commission. (2021). Standard PC.02.01.21. *Comprehensive accreditation manual for hospitals.* Oakbrook Terrace, IL: The Joint Commission. (Level VII)
13 Centers for Medicare and Medicaid Services, Department of Health and Human Services. (2020). Condition of participation: Patient's rights. 42 C.F.R. § 482.13(c)(1).
14 Accreditation Association for Hospitals and Health Systems. (2020). Standard 15.01.16. *Healthcare Facilities Accreditation Program: Accreditation requirements for acute care hospitals.* Chicago, IL: Accreditation Association for Hospitals and Health Systems. (Level VII)
15 DNV GL-Healthcare USA, Inc. (2020). PR.2.SR.5. *NIAHO® accreditation requirements, interpretive guidelines and surveyor guidance—revision 20.0.* Milford, OH: DNV GL-Healthcare USA, Inc. (Level VII)
16 The Joint Commission. (2021). Standard RI.01.01.01. *Comprehensive accreditation manual for hospitals.* Oakbrook Terrace, IL: The Joint Commission. (Level VII)
17 Siegel, J. D., et al. (2007, revised 2019). 2007 guideline for isolation precautions: Preventing transmission of infectious agents in healthcare settings. https://www.cdc.gov/infectioncontrol/pdf/guidelines/isolation-guidelines-H.pdf (Level II)

18 Occupational Safety and Health Administration. (2012). Bloodborne pathogens, standard number 1910.1030. https://www.osha.gov/pls/oshaweb/owadisp.show_document?p_id=10051&p_table=STANDARDS (Level VII)

19 Rutala, W. A., et al. (2008, revised 2019). Guideline for disinfection and sterilization in healthcare facilities, 2008. https://www.cdc.gov/infection-control/pdf/guidelines/disinfection-guidelines-H.pdf (Level I)

20 Accreditation Association for Hospitals and Health Systems. (2020). Standard 07.02.03. *Healthcare Facilities Accreditation Program: Accreditation requirements for acute care hospitals.* Chicago, IL: Accreditation Association for Hospitals and Health Systems. (Level VII)

21 The Joint Commission. (2021). Standard RC.01.03.01. *Comprehensive accreditation manual for hospitals.* Oakbrook Terrace, IL: The Joint Commission. (Level VII)

22 Accreditation Association for Hospitals and Health Systems. (2020). Standard 10.00.03. *Healthcare Facilities Accreditation Program: Accreditation requirements for acute care hospitals.* Chicago, IL: Accreditation Association for Hospitals and Health Systems. (Level VII)

23 Centers for Medicare and Medicaid Services, Department of Health and Human Services. (2020). Condition of participation: Medical record services. 42 C.F.R. § 482.24(b).

24 DNV GL-Healthcare USA, Inc. (2020). MR.2.SR.1. *NIAHO® accreditation requirements, interpretive guidelines and surveyor guidance—revision 20.0.* Milford, OH: DNV GL-Healthcare USA, Inc. (Level VII)

SKIN BIOPSY, ASSISTING

Skin biopsy is a diagnostic test in which a small piece of tissue is removed, under local anesthesia, from a lesion that's suspected of being malignant, or related to another dermatosis. There are no absolute contraindications to skin biopsy. Infection at the biopsy site is a relative contraindication unless infection is the indication for the biopsy. Caution should be used for patient with bleeding diatheses and those who are on anticoagulant therapy.[1,2]

One of three techniques may be used: shave biopsy, punch biopsy, or excisional biopsy. *Shave biopsy* cuts the lesion above the skin line, which allows further biopsy of the site. *Punch biopsy* removes an oval or round core plug from the center of the lesion. *Excisional biopsy* removes the entire lesion and is indicated for subcutaneous or deep dermal lesions; rapidly expanding lesions; malignant or dysplastic tissue; cases in which the margins of the skin surrounding the lesion need to be clear; examining the border of a lesion surrounding normal skin; and sclerotic, bullous, or atrophic lesions.[3]

Lesions suspected of being malignant usually have changed in color, size, or appearance or have failed to heal properly. (See *The ABCDEs of malignant melanoma*.) Fully developed lesions should be selected for biopsy whenever possible, *because they provide more diagnostic information than lesions that are resolving or in early stages of development.* For example, if the skin shows blisters, the biopsy should include the most mature blisters.

Normal skin consists of squamous epithelium (epidermis) and fibrous connective tissue (dermis). Benign growths include cysts, seborrheic keratoses, warts, pigmented nevi (moles), keloids, dermatofibromas, and neurofibromas.[4] Malignant tumors include dysplastic nevi, basal cell carcinoma, squamous cell carcinoma, and malignant melanoma.

Equipment

Gloves ▪ sterile gloves ▪ #15 scalpel for shave or excisional biopsy ▪ antiseptic agent (isopropyl alcohol, povidone-iodine solution, or chlorhexidine) ▪ punch instrument for punch biopsy ▪ local anesthetic ▪ sterile specimen bottle containing 10% formaldehyde solution or other preservative or other sterile container[3] ▪ sterile gauze pads ▪ prescribed topical ointment (petrolatum or antibiotic ointment)[1] ▪ adhesive bandage ▪ sterile forceps ▪ adhesive strips ▪ labels ▪ laboratory biohazard transport bag ▪ Optional: laboratory request form; gown, mask, mask with face shield, goggles, topical hemostatic agent, 3-0, 4-0, or 5-0 sutures, prescribed analgesics, light source.

Preparation of equipment

Some biopsy specimens require special fixation techniques and may need to be delivered to the laboratory in different preservative fluids. Consult your facility's pathologist if you are unsure of any required techniques.[3]

The ABCDEs of malignant melanoma

A simple ABCDE rule outlines the warning signs of malignant melanoma.[5]

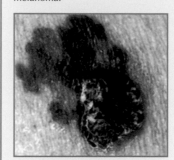

ASYMMETRY: One half of a mole or birthmark doesn't match the other half.

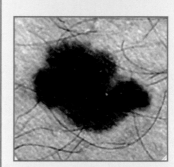

BORDER: The edges are irregular, ragged, notched, or blurred.

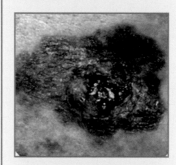

COLOR: The pigmentation isn't uniform; it may have varying degrees of brown, black, or sometimes red.

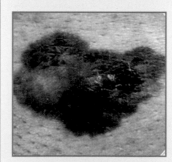

DIAMETER: The diameter is greater than ¼" (0.6 mm), about the size of a pencil eraser. There's a sudden or progressive increase in size.

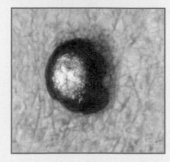

EVOLVING: The size, shape, color, elevation, or another trait has changed, or a new sign or symptom, such as bleeding, itching, or crusting, has developed.

Inspect all equipment and supplies. If a product is expired, is defective, or has compromised integrity, remove it from patient use, label it as expired or defective, and report the expiration or defect as directed by your facility.

Implementation

- Verify the practitioner's order.
- Review the patient's medical record for a history of allergies to latex or to the local anesthetic.
- Conduct a preprocedure verification *to make sure that all relevant documentation, related information, and equipment are available and correctly matched to the patient's identifiers.*[6,7]
- Confirm that informed consent has been obtained and that the signed consent form is in the patient's medical record.[8,9,10,11]
- Gather and prepare the necessary equipment and supplies.
- Perform hand hygiene.[12,13,14,15,16,17]
- Confirm the patient's identity using at least two patient identifiers.[18]
- Provide privacy.[19,20,21,22]
- Reinforce the practitioner's explanation of the procedure to the patient and family (if appropriate) according to their individual communication and learning needs *to increase their understanding, allay their fears, and enhance cooperation.*[23] Answer questions.
- Inform the patient that it's not necessary to restrict food or fluids.
- Tell the patient that a practitioner will administer a local anesthetic for pain.
- Inform the patient that the biopsy will take about 15 minutes and that the test results are usually available within 7 days, depending on the facility.
- Raise the bed to waist level before providing care *to prevent caregiver back strain.*[24]
- Ensure adequate lighting *to visualize the lesion.*
- Perform hand hygiene.[12,13,14,15,16,17]
- Put on gloves and, as needed, other personal protective equipment *to comply with standard precautions.*[25,26,27]
- If appropriate, make sure the surgical site is marked as directed by your facility.[28]
- Label all medications, medication containers, and other solutions on and off the sterile field.[29]
- Position the patient comfortably and clean the skin with an antiseptic agent, such as isopropyl alcohol, povidone-iodine solution, or chlorhexidine, before the practitioner administers the local anesthetic.[3]
- Conduct a time-out immediately before starting the procedure *to perform a final assessment that the correct patient, site, positioning, and procedures are identified and, as applicable, all relevant information and necessary equipment are available.*[30]
- Assist with the biopsy procedure, as needed.
- The practitioner performs hand hygiene and puts on sterile gloves and, as needed, other personal protective equipment.
- For a shave biopsy, the practitioner cuts the growth off at the skin line with a #15 scalpel and immediately places the tissue in a properly labeled specimen bottle containing 10% formaldehyde solution. Apply pressure to the biopsy area *to stop bleeding.* Apply an adhesive bandage. The practitioner may apply a topical hemostatic agent as needed. Apply a thin layer of prescribed topical ointment and an adhesive bandage.[1]
- For a punch biopsy, the practitioner pulls the skin surrounding the lesion taut, introduces the punch into the lesion firmly, and rotates the punch *to obtain a tissue specimen.* The practitioner lifts the plug with forceps and severs as deeply into the fat layer as possible. The practitioner then places the specimen in a properly labeled specimen bottle containing 10% formaldehyde solution or a sterile container, if indicated. After the procedure, the practitioner closes the wound according to the size of the punch; the wound may require an adhesive bandage alone or sutures. Apply a thin layer of prescribed topical ointment to the suture area or before applying an adhesive bandage.[1]
- For an excisional biopsy, the practitioner uses a #15 scalpel *to excise the lesion;* the practitioner makes the incision as wide and as deep as necessary. The practitioner removes the tissue specimen and places it immediately in a properly labeled specimen bottle containing 10% formaldehyde solution. The practitioner applies pressure to the site *to stop bleeding* and then closes the wound according to the location of the biopsy. If the

incision is large, it may need skin grafting; if it's small, adhesive strips may be sufficient.

NURSING ALERT Handle biopsy specimens carefully *to minimize injury and excess tissue drying that may interfere with histopathologic evaluation.*[3]
- Check the biopsy site for bleeding. Apply a topical hemostatic agent, as ordered, following safe medication administration procedures.[3,31,32,33,34]
- Return the bed to the lowest position *to prevent falls and maintain patient safety.*[35]
- Discard used supplies in appropriate receptacles.[27]
- Remove and discard your gloves and other personal protective equipment, if worn.[27]
- Perform hand hygiene.[12,13,14,15,16,17]
- Label the specimen container in the presence of the patient *to prevent mislabeling.*
- Complete the laboratory request form (if required by your facility), place the specimen in a laboratory biohazard transport bag, and send it to the laboratory immediately.[18,27]
- If the patient experiences pain, administer analgesics, as prescribed, following safe medication administration practices.[31,32,33,34]
- Perform hand hygiene.[12,13,14,15,16,17]
- Document the procedure.[36,37,38,39]

Special considerations

- Shave biopsies aren't recommended for suspected melanomas. Biopsy of a suspected melanoma should include a margin of 1 to 3 mm.[40]
- Some facilities may require marking the biopsy site with a skin marking pen or photographing the biopsy site, including body landmarks, as part of their preprocedure process *to reduce processing errors.*[41]
- Placing an ice pack on the biopsy site for 3 to 5 minutes several times during the first 24 hours may help decrease bleeding, hematoma, pain, and edema.[1]

Complications

Possible complications include hematoma, bleeding, pain, edema, and infection of the surrounding tissue as well as subsequent scar formation. Less common complications include vasovagal response during the procedure, and failure of the wound to close properly and wound dehiscence after the procedure.[1,2]

Documentation

Document the date and time of the biopsy, the biopsy site, the appearance of the specimen and site, whether bleeding occurred at the biopsy site, and the patient's tolerance of the procedure. Record the administration of anesthetic or analgesic medication, the patient's response to the medication, any adverse effects, interventions you provided, and the patient's response to those interventions. Document teaching provided to the patient and family (if appropriate), their understanding of that teaching, and any need for follow-up teaching.

REFERENCES

1 Alguire, P. C., & Mathes, B. M. (2021). Skin biopsy techniques. In: *UpToDate,* Berman, R. S., & Miller, S. J. (Eds.).
2 Prather, C. L. (2018). Skin biopsy. https://emedicine.medscape.com/article/1997709-overview
3 Zuber, T. J. (2012). Skin biopsy techniques: When and how to perform shave and excisional biopsy. *Consultant, 52*(7), 522–526.
4 Goldstein, B. G., & Goldstein, A. O. (2021). Overview of benign lesions of the skin. In: *UpToDate,* Dellavalle, R. P. (Ed.).
5 Skin Cancer Foundation. (2021). Melanoma warning signs. https://www.skincancer.org/skin-cancer-information/melanoma/melanoma-warning-signs-and-images/
6 The Joint Commission. (2021). Standard UP.01.01.01. *Comprehensive accreditation manual for hospitals.* Oakbrook Terrace, IL: The Joint Commission. (Level VII)
7 Accreditation Association for Hospitals and Health Systems. (2020). Standard 30.00.14. *Healthcare Facilities Accreditation Program: Accreditation requirements for acute care hospitals.* Chicago, IL: Accreditation Association for Hospitals and Health Systems. (Level VII)

8 Accreditation Association for Hospitals and Health Systems. (2020). Standard 30.01.11. *Healthcare Facilities Accreditation Program: Accreditation requirements for acute care hospitals.* Chicago, IL: Accreditation Association for Hospitals and Health Systems. (Level VII)

9 Centers for Medicare and Medicaid Services, Department of Health and Human Services. (2020). Condition of participation: Patient's rights. 42 C.F.R. § 482.13(b)(2).

10 The Joint Commission. (2021). Standard RI.01.03.01. *Comprehensive accreditation manual for hospitals.* Oakbrook Terrace, IL: The Joint Commission. (Level VII)

11 DNV GL-Healthcare USA, Inc. (2020). PR.2.SR.3. *NIAHO® accreditation requirements, interpretive guidelines and surveyor guidance—revision 20.0.* Milford, OH: DNV GL-Healthcare USA, Inc. (Level VII)

12 The Joint Commission. (2021). Standard NPSG.07.01.01. *Comprehensive accreditation manual for hospitals.* Oakbrook Terrace, IL: The Joint Commission. (Level VII)

13 Centers for Disease Control and Prevention. (2002). Guideline for hand hygiene in health-care settings: Recommendations of the Healthcare Infection Control Practices Advisory Committee and the HICPAC/SHEA/APIC/IDSA Hand Hygiene Task Force. *MMWR Recommendations and Reports, 51*(RR-16), 1–45. https://www.cdc.gov/mmwr/pdf/rr/rr5116.pdf (Level II)

14 World Health Organization. (2009). WHO guidelines on hand hygiene in health care: First global patient safety challenge, clean care is safer care. https://apps.who.int/iris/bitstream/handle/10665/44102/9789241597906_eng.pdf?sequence=1 (Level IV)

15 Accreditation Association for Hospitals and Health Systems. (2020). Standard 07.01.21. *Healthcare Facilities Accreditation Program: Accreditation requirements for acute care hospitals.* Chicago, IL: Accreditation Association for Hospitals and Health Systems. (Level VII)

16 Centers for Medicare and Medicaid Services, Department of Health and Human Services. (2020). Condition of participation: Infection control. 42 C.F.R. § 482.42.

17 DNV GL-Healthcare USA, Inc. (2020). IC.1.SR.1. *NIAHO® accreditation requirements, interpretive guidelines and surveyor guidance—revision 20.0.* Milford, OH: DNV GL-Healthcare USA, Inc. (Level VII)

18 The Joint Commission. (2021). Standard NPSG.01.01.01. *Comprehensive accreditation manual for hospitals.* Oakbrook Terrace, IL: The Joint Commission. (Level VII)

19 DNV GL-Healthcare USA, Inc. (2020). PR.2.SR.5. *NIAHO® accreditation requirements, interpretive guidelines and surveyor guidance—revision 20.0.* Milford, OH: DNV GL-Healthcare USA, Inc. (Level VII)

20 Centers for Medicare and Medicaid Services, Department of Health and Human Services. (2020). Condition of participation: Patient's rights. 42 C.F.R. § 482.13(c)(1).

21 Accreditation Association for Hospitals and Health Systems. (2020). Standard 15.01.16. *Healthcare Facilities Accreditation Program: Accreditation requirements for acute care hospitals.* Chicago, IL: Accreditation Association for Hospitals and Health Systems. (Level VII)

22 The Joint Commission. (2021). Standard RI.01.01.01. *Comprehensive accreditation manual for hospitals.* Oakbrook Terrace, IL: The Joint Commission. (Level VII)

23 The Joint Commission. (2021). Standard PC.02.01.21. *Comprehensive accreditation manual for hospitals.* Oakbrook Terrace, IL: The Joint Commission. (Level VII)

24 Waters, T. R., et al. (2009). Safe patient handling training for schools of nursing. https://www.cdc.gov/niosh/docs/2009-127/pdfs/2009-127.pdf (Level VII)

25 Accreditation Association for Hospitals and Health Systems. (2020). Standard 07.01.10. *Healthcare Facilities Accreditation Program: Accreditation requirements for acute care hospitals.* Chicago, IL: Accreditation Association for Hospitals and Health Systems. (Level VII)

26 Siegel, J. D., et al. (2007, revised 2019). 2007 guideline for isolation precautions: Preventing transmission of infectious agents in healthcare settings. https://www.cdc.gov/infectioncontrol/pdf/guidelines/isolation-guidelines-H.pdf (Level II)

27 Occupational Safety and Health Administration. (2012). Bloodborne pathogens, standard number 1910.1030 https://www.osha.gov/pls/oshaweb/owadisp.show_document?p_id=10051&p_table=STANDARDS (Level VII)

28 The Joint Commission. (2021). Standard UP.01.02.01. *Comprehensive accreditation manual for hospitals.* Oakbrook Terrace, IL: The Joint Commission. (Level VII)

29 The Joint Commission. (2021). Standard NPSG.03.04.01. *Comprehensive accreditation manual for hospitals.* Oakbrook Terrace, IL: The Joint Commission. (Level VII)

30 The Joint Commission. (2021). Standard UP.01.03.01. *Comprehensive accreditation manual for hospitals.* Oakbrook Terrace, IL: The Joint Commission. (Level VII)

31 Accreditation Association for Hospitals and Health Systems. (2020). Standard 16.01.03. *Healthcare Facilities Accreditation Program: Accreditation requirements for acute care hospitals.* Chicago, IL: Accreditation Association for Hospitals and Health Systems. (Level VII)

32 DNV GL-Healthcare USA, Inc. (2020). MM.1.SR.3. *NIAHO® accreditation requirements, interpretive guidelines and surveyor guidance—revision 20.0.* Milford, OH: DNV GL-Healthcare USA, Inc. (Level VII)

33 The Joint Commission. (2021). Standard MM.06.01.01. *Comprehensive accreditation manual for hospitals.* Oakbrook Terrace, IL: The Joint Commission. (Level VII)

34 Centers for Medicare and Medicaid Services, Department of Health and Human Services. (2020). Condition of participation: Nursing services. 42 C.F.R. § 482.23(c).

35 Ganz, D. A., et al. (2013, reviewed 2021). *Preventing falls in hospitals: A toolkit for improving quality of care* (AHRQ Publication No. 13-0015-EF). Rockville, MD: Agency for Healthcare Research and Quality. https://www.ahrq.gov/professionals/systems/hospital/fallpxtoolkit/index.html (Level VII)

36 Centers for Medicare and Medicaid Services, Department of Health and Human Services. (2020). Condition of participation: Medical record services. 42 C.F.R. § 482.24(b).

37 Accreditation Association for Hospitals and Health Systems. (2020). Standard 10.00.03. *Healthcare Facilities Accreditation Program: Accreditation requirements for acute care hospitals.* Chicago, IL: Accreditation Association for Hospitals and Health Systems. (Level VII)

38 The Joint Commission. (2021). Standard RC.01.03.01. *Comprehensive accreditation manual for hospitals.* Oakbrook Terrace, IL: The Joint Commission. (Level VII)

39 DNV GL-Healthcare USA, Inc. (2020). MR.2.SR.1. *NIAHO® accreditation requirements, interpretive guidelines and surveyor guidance—revision 20.0.* Milford, OH: DNV GL-Healthcare USA, Inc. (Level VII)

40 Seiverling, E. V., et al. (2018). Biopsies for skin cancer detection: Dispelling the myths. *The Journal of Family Practice, 67*(5), 270–274. https://www.mdedge.com/clinicianreviews/article/164358/oncology/biopsies-skin-cancer-detection-dispelling-myths (Level V)

41 Stratman, E. J., et al. (2016). Skin biopsy: Identifying and overcoming errors in the skin biopsy pathway. *Journal of the American Academy of Dermatology, 74*(1), 19–25. https://www.jaad.org/article/S0190-9622(15)01813-7/fulltext (Level VII)

SKIN GRAFT CARE

A skin graft is a procedure in which healthy skin is removed either from the patient (autograft) or a donor (allograft) and transplanted to a part of the patient's body to resurface an area damaged by burns, traumatic injury, chronic nonhealing cutaneous ulcers, or surgery (for example removal of cutaneous malignancies).[1] The procedures for caring for an autograft requires care for two sites: the graft site and the donor site.

The graft itself may be one of several types: split-thickness, full-thickness, or pedicle-flap.[2,3] (See *Understanding types of grafts.*) Successful grafting depends on various factors, including clean wound granulation with adequate vascularization, complete contact of the graft with the wound bed, sterile technique to prevent infection, adequate graft immobilization, and skilled care.[4]

The size and depth of a wound determine whether it requires grafting.[2] Grafting usually occurs at the completion of wound debridement. The goal is to cover all wounds with an autograft or allograft within 2 weeks. With enzymatic debridement, grafting may be performed 5 to 7 days after debridement is complete; with surgical debridement, grafting can occur the same day as surgery.

Various dressings are available to cover skin graft and donor sites. Newly grafted tissues needs to be well protected from friction to ensure optimal healing, adherence to the wound bed, and vascularization to the site. Dressings act as protective barriers from shearing forces and infection

Understanding types of grafts

A patient may receive one or more of the graft types described below, based on the location, thickness, extent, and aesthetic concerns of the area that requires grafting.

Split-thickness graft

A split-thickness graft includes the epidermis and part of the dermis.[2] It may be applied as a sheet (usually on the face or neck *to preserve the cosmetic result*) or as a mesh. A mesh graft has tiny slits cut in it, which allow the graft to expand up to nine times its original size. Mesh grafts prevent fluids from collecting under the graft and typically are used over extensive full-thickness burns. A split-thickness graft is used most commonly for covering open burns or areas of extensive skin loss (other than the face).[5]

Full-thickness graft

A full-thickness graft includes the epidermis and the entire dermis.[2] Consequently, the graft contains hair follicles, sweat glands, and sebaceous glands, which typically aren't included in split-thickness grafts. Full-thickness grafts usually are used for small burns that cause deep wounds and for visible areas of the face, hands, and joints, *because they undergo less contraction while healing.*[5]

Pedicle-flap graft

A pedicle-flap graft includes not only skin and subcutaneous tissue but also subcutaneous blood vessels *to ensure a continued blood supply to the graft*. Pedicle-flap grafts may be used during reconstructive surgery *to cover previous defects.*[3]

---

as well as help to prevent the wound from drying out.[2] Examples of materials used include paraffin gauze-based, hydrocolloid, alginate, semipermeable film, silicone, foam, and hydrofiber dressings.[4,6,7,8] Initial skin graft dressings are applied in the operating room and covered with elastic gauze or a compression bandage to promote hemostasis and minimize exudate. Splints may also be applied, if needed, to immobilize and protect the grafted area.[4]

How to care for a donor graft site

Autografts are usually taken from another area of the patient's body with a dermatome, an instrument that cuts uniform, split-thickness skin portions—typically, about 0.013 to 0.05 cm thick. Autografting makes the donor site a partial-thickness wound, which may bleed, drain, and cause pain.

The donor site needs scrupulous care *to prevent infection, which could convert the site to a full-thickness wound.* Depending on the graft's thickness, tissue may be obtained from the donor site again in as little as 10 days.

A donor site dressing is applied intraoperatively and helps protect new epithelial proliferation. In addition to the inner dressing, the donor site may be dressed in antibiotic-impregnated gauze or a synthetic skin substitute. This outer gauze dressing can be taken off on the first postoperative day.

The donor site should receive the same care as the autograft does, using dressing changes at the initial stages *to prevent infection and promote healing.* To dressing the wound, follow these steps:
- Perform hand hygiene[9,10,11,12,13,14] and put on sterile gloves.[15,16,17]
- Remove the outer gauze dressings within 24 hours.
- Inspect the inner dressing for signs of infection, and then leave it open to the air *to speed drying and healing.*
- Leave small amounts of fluid accumulation alone. Using sterile technique, aspirate larger amounts through the dressing with a small-gauge needle and syringe.
- Don't apply any creams to the donor site until it's dry. When dry, you may apply a thin layer of cream daily, according to the practitioner's order, *to keep the skin tissue pliable.*
- As the donor site heals, different types of dressings may be required based on the amount of exudate and level of re-epithelialization.

A practitioner or a specially trained nurse may change graft dressings. The dressings usually stay in place for 3 to 5 days after surgery *to avoid disturbing the graft site.*[2]

The skin graft donor site also requires diligent care. (See *How to care for a donor graft site.*)

Equipment

Prescribed analgesic ▪ gloves ▪ sterile gloves ▪ sterile gown or clean gown ▪ cap ▪ mask ▪ sterile forceps ▪ sterile scissors ▪ sterile 4" × 4" (10-cm × 10-cm) gauze pads ▪ prescribed skin graft dressing ▪ elastic gauze or compression dressing ▪ warm normal saline solution ▪ moisturizing cream ▪ sterile drapes or towels ▪ labels ▪ vital signs monitoring equipment ▪ Optional: facility-approved sedation assessment tool, sterile cotton-tipped applicators, sterile scalpel, supplies for wound specimen collection, prescribed sedative or anxiolytic medication, prescribed topical medication.

Preparation of equipment

Inspect all equipment and supplies. If a product is expired, is defective, or has compromised integrity, remove it from patient use, label it as expired or defective, and report the expiration or defect as directed by your facility.

Implementation

- Verify the practitioner's order.
- Gather and prepare the necessary equipment and supplies.
- Perform hand hygiene.[9,10,11,12,13,14]
- Prepare a sterile field and, using sterile technique, set up the supplies on the sterile field.
- Label all medications, medication containers, and solutions on and off the sterile field.[18,19]
- Perform hand hygiene.[9,10,11,12,13,14]
- Confirm the patient's identity using at least two patient identifiers.[20]
- Provide privacy.[21,22,23,24]
- Explain the procedure to the patient and family (if appropriate) according to their individual communication and learning needs *to increase their understanding, allay their fears, and enhance cooperation.*[25]
- Screen for and assess the patient's pain using facility-defined criteria that are consistent with the patient's age, condition, and ability to understand.[26]
- Treat the patient's pain as needed and ordered using nonpharmacologic or pharmacologic approaches, or a combination of approaches. Base the treatment plan on evidence-based practices and the patient's clinical condition, past medical history, and pain management goals.[26]
- Administer a prescribed sedation or anxiolytic medication, as ordered, following safe medication administration practices, *to reduce anxiety and increase compliance with the procedure.*[2,27,28,29,30]
- Administer an oral analgesic, as ordered, at an appropriate time (depending on the medication's peak and onset of action) before beginning the procedure. Alternatively, give an IV analgesic immediately before the procedure. Follow safe medication administration practices when administering these medications.[27,28,29,30]
- Monitor the patient's vital signs throughout the procedure, *because changes in vital signs may indicate the patient is experiencing pain or anxiety.*[2]
- If the patient is receiving IV opioid medication, frequently monitor vital signs, respiratory status, and sedation level *to promptly recognize and treat oversedation and respiratory depression related to IV opioid use.* Explain the monitoring process to the patient and family (including that it may be necessary to awaken the patient to assess the effects of medication). Advise the patient and family to alert a staff member immediately if breathing problems or other changes occur that might be a reaction to the medication.[29,30,31]
- Raise the bed to waist level before providing care *to prevent caregiver back strain.*[32]
- Remove the patient's splint, if worn.
- Put on a cap and mask.[15,16,17]
- Perform hand hygiene.[9,10,11,12,13,14]
- Put on a sterile or clean gown (based upon the severity of the patient's injuries) and gloves *to comply with standard precautions.* Most facilities use

Evacuating fluid from a sheet graft

When a small pocket of fluid (called a *bleb*) accumulates beneath a sheet graft, the practitioner or specially trained nurse will need to evacuate the fluid using a sterile scalpel and sterile cotton-tipped applicators. First, using the scalpel, carefully make a small nick in the sheet graft directly over the area of the bleb (as shown below). Express the fluid by rolling sterile cotton-tipped applicators gently over the graft toward the nick. Then gently dab away the expressed fluid using a sterile gauze pad moistened with normal saline solution.[2]

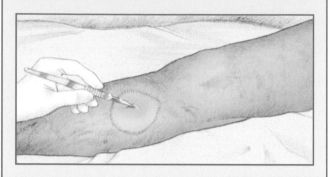

sterile no-touch technique for application of dressings and clean technique for removal of the dressings and cleansing.[2,15,16,17]

- Gently lift off all outer dressings.[2]
- Soak the middle dressings with warm saline solution *to make their removal easier* and then remove them carefully and slowly *to avoid disturbing the graft site*.[2]
- Remove and discard your gloves.[17]
- Perform hand hygiene.[9,10,11,12,13,14]
- Put on the sterile gloves.[15,16,17]
- Assess the condition of the graft site. Estimate the percentage of skin graft that has adhered successfully to the wound bed *to assess the progression of healing*.[2] Assess for signs of infection, such as fever or purulent drainage.[2] Notify the practitioner if you note purulent drainage. Obtain a wound culture, if ordered. (See the "Swab specimen collection" procedure.)
- If ordered, remove the inner graft dressing with sterile forceps, and clean the area gently. If necessary, soak the dressing with warm normal saline solution *to ease removal*.[2]
- Inspect an allograft for signs of rejection, such as infection and delayed healing.
- Inspect a sheet graft frequently for blebs; if ordered and trained to do so, evacuate them carefully with a sterile scalpel.[2] If the sheet graft has been in place for less than 48 hours and the fluid is near the edge of the graft, gently roll the fluid to the edge and out from under the graft using sterile cotton-tipped swabs.[2] (See *Evacuating fluid from a sheet graft*.)
- Apply topical medication, if ordered, following safe medication administration practices.[27,28,29,30]
- If you removed the graft dressing, place a new prescribed graft dressing over the site *to promote wound healing and prevent infection*.[2] Use sterile scissors to cut the new dressing to the appropriate size.
- Cover the inner dressing with sterile 4" × 4" (10-cm × 10-cm) gauze and elastic gauze dressing or a compression bandage.
- Clean the splint and reapply it, if indicated.[2]
- Assess the donor site if the patient received an autograft.
- Clean completely healed areas and apply prescribed moisturizing cream to them *to keep the skin pliable and to retard scarring*.[2]
- Discard used supplies in appropriate receptacles.[17]
- Remove and discard your gloves, gown, mask, and cap.[17]
- Perform hand hygiene.[9,10,11,12,13,14]
- Return the bed to the lowest position *to prevent falls and maintain patient safety*.[33]
- Reassess and respond to the patient's pain by evaluating the response to treatment and progress toward pain management goals. Assess for

adverse reactions and risk factors for adverse events that may result from treatment.[26]

- Perform hand hygiene.[9,10,11,12,13,14]
- Document the procedure.[34,35,36,37]

Special considerations

- *To avoid dislodging the graft,* discontinue hydrotherapy 3 to 4 days after grafting, as ordered by the practitioner; avoid using a blood pressure cuff over the graft; don't tug or pull dressings during dressing changes; and keep the patient from lying on the graft.[2]
- If the graft dislodges, apply sterile skin compresses *to keep the area moist until the surgeon reapplies the graft.* If the graft affects an arm or a leg, elevate the affected extremity *to reduce postoperative edema.* Check for bleeding and signs and symptoms of neurovascular impairment, such as increasing pain, numbness or tingling, coolness, and pallor.[2]
- Apply negative pressure to the graft site, if ordered, *because research indicates that applying topical negative pressure may increase the quantity and quality of split-thickness skin graft success when compared with the application of traditional dressings.*[4,38,39] (See the "Negative-pressure wound therapy" procedure.)

Complications

Graft failure can result from traumatic injury, hematoma or seroma formation, infection, an inadequate graft bed, rejection, mechanical shearing force, or compromised nutritional status.[4]

Documentation

Record the time and date of all dressing changes and any additional treatments provided. Document all medications administered and the patient's response to those medications, including pain assessment findings. Describe the condition of the graft, and note any signs and symptoms of infection or rejection. Also note the patient's reaction to graft care. Document teaching provided to the patient and family (if applicable), their understanding of that teaching, and any need for follow-up teaching.

References

1 Grande, D. J. (2021). Skin grafting. https://emedicine.medscape.com/article/1129479-overview
2 Wiegand, D. (2017). *AACN procedure manual for high acuity, progressive, and critical care* (7th ed.). St. Louis, MO: Elsevier.
3 Morris, D. (2021). Overview of flaps for soft tissue reconstruction. In: *UpToDate,* Butler, C. E. (Ed.).
4 Leon-Villapalos, J., & Dziewulski, P. (2021). Skin autografting. In: *UpToDate,* Butler, C. E., & Jeschke, M. G. (Eds.).
5 Khosh, M. M. (2021). Full-thickness skin grafts. https://emedicine.medscape.com/article/876379-overview
6 Canadian Agency for Drugs and Technologies in Health. (2013). *Dressings and care of skin grafts sites: A review of clinical evidence and guidelines.* https://www.ncbi.nlm.nih.gov/books/NBK195744/
7 Jeong, H. S., et al. (2011). Hydrocolloid dressings in skin grafting for immobilization and compression. *Dermatologic Surgery, 37,* 320–324. (Level IV)
8 Kaiser, D., et al. (2013). Alginate dressing and polyurethane film versus paraffin gauze in the treatment of split-thickness skin graft donor sites: A randomized controlled pilot study. *Advances in Skin & Wound Care, 26,* 67–73. (Level II)
9 Centers for Disease Control and Prevention. (2002). Guideline for hand hygiene in health-care settings: Recommendations of the Healthcare Infection Control Practices Advisory Committee and the HICPAC/SHEA/APIC/IDSA Hand Hygiene Task Force. *MMWR Recommendations and Reports, 51*(RR-16), 1–45. https://www.cdc.gov/mmwr/pdf/rr/rr5116.pdf (Level II)
10 World Health Organization. (2009). WHO guidelines on hand hygiene in health care: First global patient safety challenge, clean care is safer care. https://apps.who.int/iris/bitstream/handle/10665/44102/9789241597906_eng.pdf (Level IV)
11 The Joint Commission. (2021). Standard NPSG.07.01.01. *Comprehensive accreditation manual for hospitals.* Oakbrook Terrace, IL: The Joint Commission. (Level VII)

12 Accreditation Association for Hospitals and Health Systems. (2020). Standard 07.01.21. *Healthcare Facilities Accreditation Program: Accreditation requirements for acute care hospitals.* Chicago, IL: Accreditation Association for Hospitals and Health Systems. (Level VII)

13 Centers for Medicare and Medicaid Services, Department of Health and Human Services. (2020). Condition of participation: Infection control. 42 C.F.R. § 482.42.

14 DNV GL-Healthcare USA, Inc. (2020). IC.1.SR.1. *NIAHO® accreditation requirements, interpretive guidelines and surveyor guidance—revision 20.0.* Milford, OH: DNV GL-Healthcare USA, Inc. (Level VII)

15 Siegel, J. D., et al. (2007, revised 2019). 2007 guideline for isolation precautions: Preventing transmission of infectious agents in healthcare settings. https://www.cdc.gov/infectioncontrol/pdf/guidelines/isolation-guidelines-H.pdf (Level II)

16 Accreditation Association for Hospitals and Health Systems. (2020). Standard 07.01.10. *Healthcare Facilities Accreditation Program: Accreditation requirements for acute care hospitals.* Chicago, IL: Accreditation Association for Hospitals and Health Systems. (Level VII)

17 Occupational Safety and Health Administration. (2012). Bloodborne pathogens, standard number 1910.1030. https://www.osha.gov/pls/oshaweb/owadisp.show_document?p_id=10051&p_table=STANDARDS (Level VII)

18 The Joint Commission. (2021). Standard NPSG.03.04.01. *Comprehensive accreditation manual for hospitals.* Oakbrook Terrace, IL: The Joint Commission. (Level VII)

19 Accreditation Association for Hospitals and Health Systems. (2020). Standard 25.01.27. *Healthcare Facilities Accreditation Program: Accreditation requirements for acute care hospitals.* Chicago, IL: Accreditation Association for Hospitals and Health Systems. (Level VII)

20 The Joint Commission. (2021). Standard NPSG.01.01.01. *Comprehensive accreditation manual for hospitals.* Oakbrook Terrace, IL: The Joint Commission. (Level VII)

21 Accreditation Association for Hospitals and Health Systems. (2020). Standard 15.01.16. *Healthcare Facilities Accreditation Program: Accreditation requirements for acute care hospitals.* Chicago, IL: Accreditation Association for Hospitals and Health Systems. (Level VII)

22 Centers for Medicare and Medicaid Services, Department of Health and Human Services. (2020). Condition of participation: Patient's rights. 42 C.F.R. § 482.13(c)(1).

23 DNV GL-Healthcare USA, Inc. (2020). PR.2.SR.5. *NIAHO® accreditation requirements, interpretive guidelines and surveyor guidance—revision 20.0.* Milford, OH: DNV GL-Healthcare USA, Inc. (Level VII)

24 The Joint Commission. (2021). Standard RI.01.01.01. *Comprehensive accreditation manual for hospitals.* Oakbrook Terrace, IL: The Joint Commission. (Level VII)

25 The Joint Commission. (2021). Standard PC.01.21. *Comprehensive accreditation manual for hospitals.* Oakbrook Terrace, IL: The Joint Commission. (Level VII)

26 The Joint Commission. (2021). Standard PC.01.02.07. *Comprehensive accreditation manual for hospitals.* Oakbrook Terrace, IL: The Joint Commission. (Level VII)

27 The Joint Commission. (2021). Standard MM.06.01.01. *Comprehensive accreditation manual for hospitals.* Oakbrook Terrace, IL: The Joint Commission. (Level VII)

28 Accreditation Association for Hospitals and Health Systems. (2020). Standard 16.01.03. *Healthcare Facilities Accreditation Program: Accreditation requirements for acute care hospitals.* Chicago, IL: Accreditation Association for Hospitals and Health Systems. (Level VII)

29 Centers for Medicare and Medicaid Services, Department of Health and Human Services. (2020). Condition of participation: Nursing services. 42 C.F.R. § 482.23(c).

30 DNV GL-Healthcare USA, Inc. (2020). MM.1.SR.3. *NIAHO® accreditation requirements, interpretive guidelines and surveyor guidance—revision 20.0.* Milford, OH: DNV GL-Healthcare USA, Inc. (Level VII)

31 Centers for Medicare and Medicaid Services. (2014). Requirements for hospital medication administration, particularly intravenous (IV) medications and post-operative care of patients receiving IV opioids. https://www.cms.gov/Medicare/Provider-Enrollment-and-Certification/SurveyCertificationGenInfo/Downloads/Survey-and-Cert-Letter-14-15.pdf

32 Waters, T. R., et al. (2009). Safe patient handling training for schools of nursing. https://www.cdc.gov/niosh/docs/2009-127/pdfs/2009-127.pdf (Level VII)

33 Ganz, D. A., et al. (2013, reviewed 2021). *Preventing falls in hospitals: A toolkit for improving quality of care* (AHRQ Publication No. 13-0015-EF). Rockville, MD: Agency for Healthcare Research and Quality. https://www.ahrq.gov/professionals/systems/hospital/fallpxtoolkit/index.html (Level VII)

34 The Joint Commission. (2021). Standard RC.01.03.01. *Comprehensive accreditation manual for hospitals.* Oakbrook Terrace, IL: The Joint Commission. (Level VII)

35 Centers for Medicare and Medicaid Services, Department of Health and Human Services. (2020). Condition of participation: Medical record services. 42 C.F.R. § 482.24(b).

36 Accreditation Association for Hospitals and Health Systems. (2020). Standard 10.00.03. *Healthcare Facilities Accreditation Program: Accreditation requirements for acute care hospitals.* Chicago, IL: Accreditation Association for Hospitals and Health Systems. (Level VII)

37 DNV GL-Healthcare USA, Inc. (2020). MR.2.SR.1. *NIAHO® accreditation requirements, interpretive guidelines and surveyor guidance—revision 20.0.* Milford, OH: DNV GL-Healthcare USA, Inc. (Level VII)

38 Azzopardi, E. A., et al. (2013). Application of topical negative pressure (vacuum-assisted closure) to split-thickness skin grafts: A structured evidence-based review. *Annals of Plastic Surgery, 70,* 23–29. (Level V)

39 Petkar, K. S., et al. (2011). A prospective randomized controlled trial comparing negative pressure dressing and conventional dressing methods on split-thickness skin grafts in burned patients. *Burns, 37,* 925–929. (Level II)

Skin staple and clip removal

A practitioner may use skin staples or clips instead of standard sutures to close lacerations and surgical wounds. Because they can secure a wound more quickly than sutures, skin staples and clips can substitute for surface sutures where cosmetic results aren't a prime consideration, such as in abdominal closure. When properly placed, staples and clips distribute tension evenly along the suture line with minimal tissue trauma and compression, promoting healing and minimizing scarring. Because staples and clips are made from surgical stainless steel, tissue reaction to them is minimal.[1]

Practitioners typically remove skin staples and clips, but some facilities permit qualified nurses to perform this procedure. The timing of skin staple or clip removal depends on the location of the wound, the condition of the wound (absence of inflammation, drainage, and infection), and the patient's general condition.[2] Sterile technique typically isn't required for removal unless the patient's condition warrants it; a sterile no-touch technique can usually be used.[3]

Equipment

Gloves ▪ sterile staple or clip extractor ▪ 4" × 4" (10-cm × 10-cm) gauze pads ▪ Optional: adhesive remover, adhesive strips or butterfly adhesive strips, sterile drape, antiseptic cleaning agent, sterile normal saline solution, tape, sterile gauze dressing, alcohol-free skin protectant.

Preparation of equipment

Inspect all equipment and supplies. If a product is expired, is defective, or has compromised integrity, remove it from patient use, label it as expired or defective, and report the expiration or defect as directed by your facility.

Implementation

▪ If your facility allows you to remove skin staples and clips, verify the practitioner's order *to confirm the exact timing and details for this procedure.*[4] The practitioner may want you to remove only alternate staples or clips initially[1] and to leave others in place for an additional day or two *to support the incision site.*

▪ Review the patient's medical record for any history of allergies, especially to adhesive tape and topical solutions or medications.

▪ Gather and prepare the necessary equipment and supplies.

▪ Perform hand hygiene.[5,6,7,8,9,10]

▪ Confirm the patient's identity using at least two patient identifiers.[11]

▪ Provide privacy.[12,13,14,15]

■ Explain the procedure to the patient and family (if appropriate) according to their individual communication and learning needs *to increase their understanding, allay their fears, and enhance cooperation.*[16] Tell the patient to expect to feel a slight pulling or tickling sensation—but little discomfort—during staple or clip removal. Reassure the patient that, because the incision is healing properly, removing the supporting staples or clips won't weaken the incision line.

■ Screen and assess the patient's pain using facility-defined criteria that are consistent with the patient's age, condition, and ability to understand.[17]

■ Treat the patient's pain, as needed and ordered, using nonpharmacologic or pharmacologic methods, or a combination of approaches. Base the treatment plan on evidence-based practices and the patient's clinical condition, past medical history, and pain management goals.[17]

■ Raise the patient's bed to waist level before providing care *to prevent caregiver back strain.*[18]

■ Perform hand hygiene.[5,6,7,8,9,10]

■ Assist the patient into a comfortable position for the procedure. Be sure the patient's position doesn't create tension on the incision.

■ Ensure adequate lighting.

■ Drape the patient so that only the incisional area is exposed *to provide privacy.*

■ Perform hand hygiene.[5,6,7,8,9,10]

■ Put on gloves *to comply with standard precautions.*[19,20,21]

■ If the patient's wound has a dressing, carefully remove the dressing *to prevent skin stripping and tearing.* Discard the dressing in a waterproof trash container.[21] Use adhesive remover, if needed, to remove old adhesive from the skin.

■ Assess the incision site. Note redness, warmth, swelling, and drainage, *which may indicate infection.* Be aware that a localized reaction to the staples or clips may cause some faint erythema; this finding is normal, but you must differentiate it from pathologic erythema. Note whether the wound margins are well approximated. Report abnormal findings to the practitioner. *If the wound isn't adequately healed, the staples or clips may need to remain in place longer. Evidence of infection may necessitate pharmacologic intervention.*

■ Remove and discard your gloves.[19,20,21]

■ Perform hand hygiene.[5,6,7,8,9,10]

■ Put on a new pair of gloves.[3,20,21]

■ Open the package containing the sterile staple or clip extractor, maintaining asepsis.

■ Gently clean the incision using an antiseptic agent, if directed, working from the inner aspect to the outer aspects of the wound, *to decrease the number of microorganisms present, thereby reducing the risk of infection.* Alternatively, moisten dried crusts with sterile normal saline solution, if directed, *to ease staple or clip removal.*

■ Pick up the sterile staple or clip extractor.

■ Place the bottom of the staple or clip extractor under the center of the first staple.

■ Keeping the lower jaw of the instrument against the patient's skin, squeeze the handles of the staple or clip extractor together to close it (as shown below). Don't lift the staple or clip extractor while squeezing it *to avoid causing tension on the skin.*

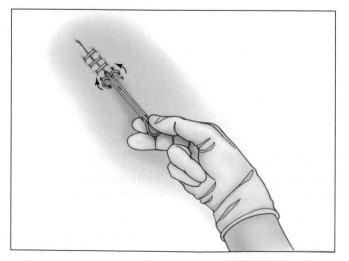

Applying adhesive strips

Adhesive strips made of thin strips of sterile, nonwoven, porous fabric tape are a primary means of keeping a wound closed after staple or clip removal. Use these steps to apply adhesive strips:

■ Apply alcohol-free skin protectant to the outside of the incision, if ordered and according to the manufacturer's instructions.

■ Allow the skin protectant to become tacky before applying the adhesive strips *to help the strips stick to the skin.*

■ Attach one end of an adhesive strip to one side of the incision line, and then pull the strip gently across the incision line and attach it on the opposite side.

■ Continue to place adhesive strips about ½" (1.3 cm) apart or closer, depending on the size and location of the incision line.

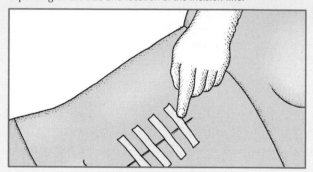

Butterfly adhesive strips are sterile, waterproof adhesive strips that have a narrow, nonadhesive bridge connecting the two expanded adhesive portions. These strips help close small wounds and assist with healing after staple or clip removal.

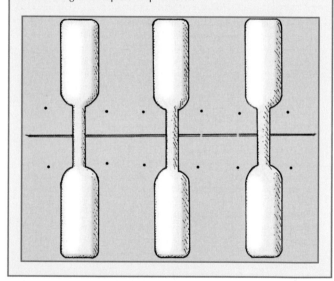

■ Lift the staple or clip out of the skin in a swift, smooth motion *to minimize pain.*

■ Discard the staple or clip onto a gauze pad.

■ Remove every other staple or clip until you reach the end of the incisional area, and then return to the start and remove the rest, as ordered. *This approach facilitates detection of wound dehiscence, and allows for every other staple or clip to be left in place if needed as the wound continues to heal.*[4] Alternatively, remove the staples or clips in succession, as ordered by the practitioner.

■ If an incision is gaping and incompletely healed upon staple or clip removal, apply adhesive strips and notify the practitioner.

■ If desired, apply adhesive strips or butterfly adhesive strips even if the wound is healing normally *to give added support to the incision and to prevent lateral tension from resulting in a wide scar.* Leave the strips in place for 3 to 5 days.[4] (See *Applying adhesive strips.*)

■ Assess the need for a dressing or covering. Apply a sterile gauze dressing, if needed, *to reduce the risk of infection and irritation from clothing.*

- Return the patient's bed to the lowest position *to prevent falls and maintain patient safety.*[22]
- Discard used supplies in appropriate receptacles.[21] If you used a reusable staple or clip extractor, prepare it for reprocessing.[23,24]
- Remove and discard your gloves.[21]
- Perform hand hygiene.[5,6,7,8,9,10]
- Report abnormal findings to the practitioner.
- Reassess and respond to the patient's pain by evaluating the response to treatment and progress toward pain management goals. Assess for adverse reactions and risk factors for adverse events that may result from treatment.[17]
- Perform hand hygiene.[5,6,7,8,9,10]
- Document the procedure.[25,26,27,28]

Special considerations

If skin staple or slip removal is difficult, notify the practitioner; *staples or clips placed too deeply within the skin or left in place too long may resist removal.*

Complications

Potential complications of staple or clip removal include infection, failure to remove a staple or clip, and incomplete healing on removal, which may require application of adhesive strips or wound repair.

Documentation

Record the date and time of staple or clip removal, the number of staples or clips removed, the number of staples or clips remaining, the appearance of the wound (redness, warmth, drainage), the approximation of wound margins, the application of a dressing or adhesive strips, and any signs of wound complications. Note the patient's tolerance of the procedure, any administered pain medication, and pain assessment findings. Document any teaching you provided to the patient and family (if applicable), their understanding of that teaching, and any need for follow-up teaching.

REFERENCES

1 Craven, R. F., et al. (2020). *Fundamentals of nursing: Concepts and competencies for practice.* (9th ed.). Wolters Kluwer.
2 Forsch, R. T., et al. (2017). Laceration repair: A practical approach. *American Family Physician, 95*(10), 628–636. https://www.aafp.org/afp/2017/0515/p628.html (Level VII)
3 World Health Organization. (2009). Glove use information leaflet. https://www.who.int/gpsc/5may/Glove_Use_Information_Leaflet.pdf (Level VII)
4 Wiegand, D. L. (2017). *AACN procedure manual for high acuity, progressive, and critical care* (7th ed.). St. Louis, MO: Elsevier.
5 Centers for Disease Control and Prevention. (2002). Guideline for hand hygiene in health-care settings: Recommendations of the Healthcare Infection Control Practices Advisory Committee and the HICPAC/SHEA/APIC/IDSA Hand Hygiene Task Force. *MMWR Recommendations and Reports, 51*(RR-16), 1–45. https://www.cdc.gov/mmwr/pdf/rr/rr5116.pdf (Level II)
6 World Health Organization. (2009). WHO guidelines on hand hygiene in health care: First global patient safety challenge, clean care is safer care. https://apps.who.int/iris/bitstream/handle/10665/44102/9789241597906_eng.pdf (Level IV)
7 The Joint Commission. (2021). Standard NPSG.07.01.01. *Comprehensive accreditation manual for hospitals.* Oakbrook Terrace, IL: The Joint Commission. (Level VII)
8 Centers for Medicare and Medicaid Services, Department of Health and Human Services. (2020). Condition of participation: Infection control. 42 C.F.R. § 482.42.
9 Accreditation Association for Hospitals and Health Systems. (2020). Standard 07.01.21. *Healthcare Facilities Accreditation Program: Accreditation requirements for acute care hospitals.* Chicago, IL: Accreditation Association for Hospitals and Health Systems. (Level VII)
10 DNV GL-Healthcare USA, Inc. (2020). IC.1.SR.1. *NIAHO® accreditation requirements, interpretive guidelines and surveyor guidance—revision 20.0.* Milford, OH: DNV GL-Healthcare USA, Inc. (Level VII)
11 The Joint Commission. (2021). Standard NPSG.01.01.01. *Comprehensive accreditation manual for hospitals.* Oakbrook Terrace, IL: The Joint Commission. (Level VII)
12 Centers for Medicare and Medicaid Services, Department of Health and Human Services. (2020). Condition of participation: Patient's rights. 42 C.F.R. § 482.13(c)(1).
13 The Joint Commission. (2021). Standard RI.01.01.01. *Comprehensive accreditation manual for hospitals.* Oakbrook Terrace, IL: The Joint Commission. (Level VII)
14 Accreditation Association for Hospitals and Health Systems. (2020). Standard 15.01.16. *Healthcare Facilities Accreditation Program: Accreditation requirements for acute care hospitals.* Chicago, IL: Accreditation Association for Hospitals and Health Systems. (Level VII)
15 DNV GL-Healthcare USA, Inc. (2020). PR.2.SR.5. *NIAHO® accreditation requirements, interpretive guidelines and surveyor guidance—revision 20.0.* Milford, OH: DNV GL-Healthcare USA, Inc. (Level VII)
16 The Joint Commission. (2021). Standard PC.02.01.21. *Comprehensive accreditation manual for hospitals.* Oakbrook Terrace, IL: The Joint Commission. (Level VII)
17 The Joint Commission. (2021). Standard PC.01.02.07. *Comprehensive accreditation manual for hospitals.* Oakbrook Terrace, IL: The Joint Commission. (Level VII)
18 Waters, T. R., et al. (2009). Safe patient handling training for schools of nursing. https://www.cdc.gov/niosh/docs/2009-127/pdfs/2009-127.pdf (Level VII)
19 Siegel, J. D., et al. (2007, revised 2019). 2007 guideline for isolation precautions: Preventing transmission of infectious agents in healthcare settings. https://www.cdc.gov/infectioncontrol/pdf/guidelines/isolation-guidelines-H.pdf (Level II)
20 Accreditation Association for Hospitals and Health Systems. (2020). Standard 07.01.10. *Healthcare Facilities Accreditation Program: Accreditation requirements for acute care hospitals.* Chicago, IL: Accreditation Association for Hospitals and Health Systems. (Level VII)
21 Occupational Safety and Health Administration. (2012). Bloodborne pathogens, standard number 1910.1030. https://www.osha.gov/pls/oshaweb/owadisp.show_document?p_id=10051&p_table=STANDARDS (Level VII)
22 Ganz, D. A., et al. (2013, reviewed 2021). *Preventing falls in hospitals: A toolkit for improving quality of care* (AHRQ Publication No. 13-0015-EF). Rockville, MD: Agency for Healthcare Research and Quality. https://www.ahrq.gov/professionals/systems/hospital/fallpxtoolkit/index.html (Level VII)
23 Rutala, W. A., et al. (2008, revised 2019). Guideline for disinfection and sterilization in healthcare facilities, 2008. https://www.cdc.gov/infection-control/pdf/guidelines/disinfection-guidelines-H.pdf (Level I)
24 Accreditation Association for Hospitals and Health Systems. (2020). Standard 07.02.03. *Healthcare Facilities Accreditation Program: Accreditation requirements for acute care hospitals.* Chicago, IL: Accreditation Association for Hospitals and Health Systems. (Level VII)
25 The Joint Commission. (2021). Standard RC.01.03.01. *Comprehensive accreditation manual for hospitals.* Oakbrook Terrace, IL: The Joint Commission. (Level VII)
26 Centers for Medicare and Medicaid Services, Department of Health and Human Services. (2020). Condition of participation: Medical record services. 42 C.F.R. § 482.24(b).
27 Accreditation Association for Hospitals and Health Systems. (2020). Standard 10.00.03. *Healthcare Facilities Accreditation Program: Accreditation requirements for acute care hospitals.* Chicago, IL: Accreditation Association for Hospitals and Health Systems. (Level VII)
28 DNV GL-Healthcare USA, Inc. (2020). MR.2.SR.1. *NIAHO® accreditation requirements, interpretive guidelines and surveyor guidance—revision 20.0.* Milford, OH: DNV GL-Healthcare USA, Inc. (Level VII)

SOAKS

A soak involves immersion of a body part in warm water or a medicated solution. This treatment is used to soften exudates, facilitate debridement, enhance suppuration, clean wounds or burns, rehydrate wounds, apply medication to infected areas, and increase local blood supply and circulation.

Most soaks are applied with clean tap water and clean technique. Sterile solution and sterile equipment are required for treating wounds, burns, and other breaks in the skin.

Equipment

Soak basin or tub ■ bath (utility) thermometer ■ warm tap water or prescribed solution ■ cup ■ pitcher ■ fluid-impermeable pad ■ pillows ■ towels ■ gloves ■ facility-approved disinfectant ■ Optional: gauze pads, sterile gloves, sterile dressing materials, overbed table, footstool, personal protective equipment.

Preparation of equipment

Inspect all equipment and supplies. If a product is expired, is defective, or has compromised integrity, remove it from patient use, label it as expired or defective, and report the expiration or defect as directed by your facility.

Perform hand hygiene.[1,2,3,4,5,6] Clean and disinfect the basin or tub using a facility-approved disinfectant.[7,8] Alternatively, obtain a new soak basin, if directed by your facility. Run warm tap water into a pitcher or heat the prescribed solution, as applicable. Measure the water or solution temperature with a bath thermometer. If the temperature isn't within the prescribed range (usually 105° to 110° F [40.6° to 43.3° C]), add hot or cold water, or reheat or cool the solution, as needed. If you're preparing the soak outside the patient's room, heat the liquid slightly above the correct temperature *to allow for cooling during transport*. If the solution for a medicated soak isn't premixed, prepare the solution and heat it to the prescribed temperature.

Implementation

- Verify the practitioner's order.
- Gather and prepare the necessary equipment and supplies.
- Review the patient's medical record for a history of an allergy to the prescribed solution, as appropriate. If an allergy exists, notify the practitioner.
- Perform hand hygiene.[1,2,3,4,5,6]
- Confirm the patient's identity using at least two patient identifiers.[9]
- Provide privacy.[10,11,12,13]
- Explain the procedure to the patient and family (if appropriate) according to their individual communication and learning needs *to increase their understanding, allay their fears, and enhance cooperation.*[14]
- Perform hand hygiene.[1,2,3,4,5,6]
- Put on gloves as necessary *to comply with standard precautions.*[15,16,17]
- Position the patient appropriately, according to the area of the body for which the soak is intended. For an arm soak, instruct the patient to sit erect. For a leg or foot soak, instruct the patient to lie down and bend the appropriate knee. For a foot soak in the sitting position, have the patient sit on the edge of the bed or transfer to a chair.
- Place a fluid-impermeable pad under the treatment site and, if necessary, cover the pad with a towel *to absorb spillage.*
- Expose the treatment site and perform a skin assessment. Assess skin temperature, color, moisture balance (assess for dryness or itching), turgor, and integrity. Also assess for edema and any skin lesions.[18]
- Remove and properly discard any dressing and assess the wound.[18] If the dressing is stuck to the wound, leave it in place and proceed with the soak. Remove the dressing several minutes later, when it has begun to soak free. After you've removed and discarded the dressing, remove and discard your gloves, perform hand hygiene, and put on new gloves.[1,2,3,4,5,6,15,17]
- Position the soak basin or tub under the treatment site on the bed, overbed table, footstool, or floor, as appropriate. If the soak basin or tub will be placed in the bed, make sure that the bed is flat beneath it *to prevent spills.*
- Pour the heated liquid into the soak basin or tub.
- Lower the patient's affected area into the basin or tub gradually *to allow adjustment to the temperature change.* Make sure the soak solution covers the treatment site.
- Make the patient comfortable, and ensure proper body alignment. Support other body parts with pillows or towels as needed *to prevent discomfort and muscle strain.*
- Remove and discard your gloves.[15,17]
- Perform hand hygiene.[1,2,3,4,5,6]
- Check the temperature of the soak solution with the bath thermometer every 5 minutes. If the temperature drops below the prescribed range, remove some of the cooled solution with a cup, lift the patient's arm or

leg from the basin *to avoid burns*, and add hot water or solution to the basin. Mix the liquid thoroughly and then recheck the temperature. If the temperature is within the prescribed range, lower the affected area back into the basin.

- Observe the patient for signs of tissue intolerance, including extreme redness at the treatment site, excessive drainage, bleeding, and maceration. If such signs develop, or if the patient complains of pain, discontinue the treatment and notify the practitioner.
- Perform hand hygiene[1,2,3,4,5,6] and put on a new pair of gloves.[15,17]
- After 15 to 20 minutes, or the ordered duration, lift the patient's treatment area from the basin or tub and remove the basin or tub.
- Dry the area thoroughly with a towel. If the patient has a wound, dry the skin around it without touching the wound.
- While the skin is hydrated from the soak, use gauze pads to remove loose scales or crusts, as appropriate.
- Observe the treatment area for general appearance, degree of swelling, debridement, suppuration, and healing.
- If the patient's wound requires redressing, remove and discard your gloves,[15,17] perform hand hygiene,[1,2,3,4,5,6] put on new gloves,[15,17] and then redress the wound.
- Remove the towel and fluid-impermeable pad, and make the patient comfortable in bed.
- Discard the soak solution and discard soiled materials in the appropriate receptacle.[15,17]
- Remove and discard your gloves.[15,17]
- Perform hand hygiene.[1,2,3,4,5,6]
- Put on new gloves.[15,17]
- Clean and disinfect the basin or tub using a facility-approved disinfectant.[7,8]
- Remove and discard your gloves.[15,17]
- Perform hand hygiene.[1,2,3,4,5,6]
- If the soak treatment is to be repeated, store the equipment in the patient's room, out of the patient's reach; otherwise, return it to the central supply department.
- Document the procedure.[19,20,21,22]

Special considerations

- To treat large areas, particularly burns, a soak may be administered in a whirlpool or Hubbard tank.

Complications

Tissue intolerance may occur; its signs and symptoms include extreme redness, excessive drainage, bleeding, maceration, and pain at the treatment site.

Documentation

Record the date, time, and duration of the soak; the treatment site; the solution used and its temperature; skin and wound appearance before, during, and after treatment; and the patient's tolerance of treatment. Document teaching you provided to the patient and family (if applicable), their understanding of that teaching, and any need for follow-up teaching.

REFERENCES

1 The Joint Commission. (2021). Standard NPSG.07.01.01. *Comprehensive accreditation manual for hospitals.* Oakbrook Terrace, IL: The Joint Commission. (Level VII)

2 Centers for Disease Control and Prevention. (2002). Guideline for hand hygiene in health-care settings: Recommendations of the Healthcare Infection Control Practices Advisory Committee and the HICPAC/SHEA/APIC/IDSA Hand Hygiene Task Force. *MMWR Recommendations and Reports, 51*(RR-16), 1–45. https://www.cdc.gov/mmwr/pdf/rr/rr5116.pdf (Level II)

3 World Health Organization. (2009). WHO guidelines on hand hygiene in health care: First global patient safety challenge, clean care is safer care. https://apps.who.int/iris/bitstream/handle/10665/44102/9789241597906_eng.pdf?sequence=1 (Level IV)

4 Accreditation Association for Hospitals and Health Systems. (2020). Standard 07.01.21. *Healthcare Facilities Accreditation Program: Accreditation requirements for acute care hospitals.* Chicago, IL: Accreditation Association for Hospitals and Health Systems. (Level VII)

5 Centers for Medicare and Medicaid Services, Department of Health and Human Services. (2020). Condition of participation: Infection control. 42 C.F.R. § 482.42.

6 DNV GL-Healthcare USA, Inc. (2020). IC.1.SR.1. *NIAHO® accreditation requirements, interpretive guidelines and surveyor guidance—revision 20.0.* Milford, OH: DNV GL-Healthcare USA, Inc. (Level VII)

7 Rutala, W. A., et al. (2008, revised 2019). Guideline for disinfection and sterilization in healthcare facilities, 2008. https://www.cdc.gov/infection-control/pdf/guidelines/disinfection-guidelines-H.pdf (Level I)

8 Accreditation Association for Hospitals and Health Systems. (2020). Standard 07.02.03. *Healthcare Facilities Accreditation Program: Accreditation requirements for acute care hospitals.* Chicago, IL: Accreditation Association for Hospitals and Health Systems. (Level VII)

9 The Joint Commission. (2021). Standard NPSG.01.01.01. *Comprehensive accreditation manual for hospitals.* Oakbrook Terrace, IL: The Joint Commission. (Level VII)

10 Accreditation Association for Hospitals and Health Systems. (2020). Standard 15.01.16. *Healthcare Facilities Accreditation Program: Accreditation requirements for acute care hospitals.* Chicago, IL: Accreditation Association for Hospitals and Health Systems. (Level VII)

11 Centers for Medicare and Medicaid Services, Department of Health and Human Services. (2020). Condition of participation: Patient's rights. 42 C.F.R. § 482.13(c)(1).

12 DNV GL-Healthcare USA, Inc. (2020). PR.2.SR.5. *NIAHO® accreditation requirements, interpretive guidelines and surveyor guidance—revision 20.0.* Milford, OH: DNV GL-Healthcare USA, Inc. (Level VII)

13 The Joint Commission. (2021). Standard RI.01.01.01. *Comprehensive accreditation manual for hospitals.* Oakbrook Terrace, IL: The Joint Commission. (Level VII)

14 The Joint Commission. (2021). Standard PC.02.01.21. *Comprehensive accreditation manual for hospitals.* Oakbrook Terrace, IL: The Joint Commission. (Level VII)

15 Siegel, J. D., et al. (2007, revised 2019). 2007 guideline for isolation precautions: Preventing transmission of infectious agents in healthcare settings. https://www.cdc.gov/infectioncontrol/pdf/guidelines/isolation-guidelines-H.pdf (Level II)

16 Accreditation Association for Hospitals and Health Systems. (2020). Standard 07.01.10. *Healthcare Facilities Accreditation Program: Accreditation requirements for acute care hospitals.* Chicago, IL: Accreditation Association for Hospitals and Health Systems. (Level VII)

17 Occupational Safety and Health Administration. (2012). Bloodborne pathogens, standard number 1910.1030. https://www.osha.gov/pls/oshaweb/owadisp.show_document?p_id=10051&p_table=STANDARDS (Level VII)

18 Baranoski, S., & Ayello, E. A. (2020). *Wound care essentials: Practice principles* (5th ed.). Wolters Kluwer.

19 The Joint Commission. (2021). Standard RC.01.03.01. *Comprehensive accreditation manual for hospitals.* Oakbrook Terrace, IL: The Joint Commission. (Level VII)

20 Accreditation Association for Hospitals and Health Systems. (2020). Standard 10.00.03. *Healthcare Facilities Accreditation Program: Accreditation requirements for acute care hospitals.* Chicago, IL: Accreditation Association for Hospitals and Health Systems. (Level VII)

21 Centers for Medicare and Medicaid Services, Department of Health and Human Services. (2020). Condition of participation: Medical record services. 42 C.F.R. § 482.24(b).

22 DNV GL-Healthcare USA, Inc. (2020). MR.2.SR.1. *NIAHO® accreditation requirements, interpretive guidelines and surveyor guidance—revision 20.0.* Milford, OH: DNV GL-Healthcare USA, Inc. (Level VII)

SPIRITUAL CARE

Religious beliefs can profoundly influence a patient's recovery rate, attitude toward treatment, and overall response to hospitalization. Therefore, it's important to obtain information about the patient's spiritual and religious practices during assessment.[1] In certain religious groups, beliefs can preclude diagnostic tests and therapeutic treatments, require dietary restrictions, and prohibit organ donation and artificial prolongation of life. (See *Beliefs and practices of selected religions*, page 776.)

Effective patient care requires recognition of and respect for the patient's religious beliefs.[10] Recognizing these beliefs and the need for spiritual care may require close attention to nonverbal cues or to seemingly casual remarks that express spiritual concerns. Respecting the patient's beliefs may require setting aside your own beliefs to help the patient follow personal beliefs. Providing spiritual care may require contacting an appropriate clergy member in the facility or community, gathering equipment needed to help the patient perform rites and administer sacraments, and preparing the patient for a pastoral visit.

Equipment

Supplies specific to the patient's religious affiliation ∎ Optional: clean towels (one or two), container of water (for emergency baptism), teaspoon, medicine cup.

Some facilities, particularly those with a religious affiliation, provide baptismal trays. A clergy member may bring holy water, holy oil, or other religious articles to minister to the patient.

Preparation of equipment

For baptism, cover a small table with a clean towel. Fold a second towel and place it on the table, along with the teaspoon or medicine cup. For communion and anointing, cover the bedside stand with a clean towel.

Implementation

∎ Check the patient's admission record *to determine the patient's religious affiliation.* Remember that some patients may claim no religious beliefs. However, even an agnostic may wish to speak with a clergy member, so watch and listen carefully for subtle expressions of this desire.
∎ Perform hand hygiene.[11,12,13,14,15,16]
∎ Confirm the patient's identity using at least two patient identifiers.[17]
∎ Provide privacy.[10,18,19,20]
∎ Assess the patient's spiritual needs, resources, and preferences.[21]
∎ Evaluate the patient's behavior for signs of loneliness, anxiety, or fear, *emotions that may signal the need for spiritual counsel.* Also consider whether the patient is facing a health crisis, which can occur before childbirth or surgery and with chronic illness or impending death. Remember that a patient may feel acutely distressed because of the inability to participate in religious observances; help such a patient verbalize beliefs *to relieve stress.* Listen to the patient, and let the patient express concerns, but carefully refrain from imposing your beliefs on the patient *to avoid conflict and further stress.*[21]
∎ If the patient requests, arrange a visit by an appropriate clergy member. Consult this clergy member if you need more information about the patient's beliefs.
∎ If your patient faces the possibility of abortion, amputation, transfusion, or other medical procedures with important religious implications, try to discover the patient's spiritual attitude. Also, try to determine your patient's attitude toward the importance of laying on of hands, confession, communion, observance of holy days (such as the Sabbath), and restrictions on diet or physical appearance. *Helping the patient continue normal religious practices during hospitalization can help reduce stress.*
∎ If the patient is pregnant, find out about beliefs concerning infant baptism and circumcision, and comply with them after birth.

PEDIATRIC ALERT If a neonate is in critical condition, call an appropriate clergy member immediately. In an extreme emergency, you can perform a Roman Catholic baptism using a container of any available water. If you do so, be sure to notify the priest *because administration of this sacrament should occur only once.*

∎ If a Jewish woman delivers a male infant prematurely or by cesarean birth, ask whether she plans to observe the rite of circumcision, or a bris, a significant ceremony performed on the 8th day after birth. (*Because a patient who delivers a healthy, full-term baby vaginally is usually discharged quickly,* this ceremony is normally performed outside the facility.) For a bris, ensure privacy and, if requested, sterilize the instruments.
∎ If the patient requests communion, prepare for it before the clergy member arrives. Place the patient in the Fowler or semi-Fowler position if condition permits. Otherwise, allow the patient to remain supine. Tuck a clean towel under the patient's chin and straighten the bed linens. If the patient is on a nothing-by-mouth status, contact the practitioner to clarify whether the patient may receive communion, and alert the clergy member to the patient's situation.[22]

Beliefs and practices of selected religions

Religious beliefs can affect the patient's attitudes toward illness and traditional medicine. By trying to accommodate religious beliefs and practices in your plan of care, you can increase the patient's willingness to learn and comply with treatment regimens. *Because religious beliefs may vary within particular sects,* individual practices may differ from those described here.

Adventist
- *Birth and death rituals*: None (baptism of adults only)
- *Dietary restrictions*: Alcohol, coffee, tea, opioids, stimulants, and meat or animal products (in some groups) prohibited
- *Practices in health crisis*: Communion, baptism, divine healing and anointing with oil, prayer, and Saturday Sabbath (in some groups)

Baptist
- *Birth and death rituals*: At birth, none (baptism of believers only); before death, counseling by clergy member and prayer
- *Dietary restrictions*: Alcohol, coffee, and tea (in some groups) prohibited
- *Practices in health crisis*: Healing by laying on of hands (in some groups) as well as resistance to medical therapy (occasionally approved)

Buddhist
- *Birth and death rituals*: At birth, none; when possible, continuation of life and therefore pursuit of Enlightenment to observe Buddhist respect for life; if prolonged life won't permit continued pursuit of Enlightenment, possible acceptance of euthanasia, withdrawal of care, and organ donation
- *Dietary restrictions*: Vegetarian diet, dietary moderation[2]
- *Practices in health crisis*: No specific restrictions, but moderation possibly encouraged to support pursuit of Enlightenment[2]

Christian Scientist
- *Birth and death rituals*: At birth, none; before death, counseling by a Christian Science practitioner
- *Dietary restrictions*: Alcohol, coffee, and tobacco prohibited
- *Practices in health crisis*: Refusal of all treatments (most groups), including drugs, biopsies, physical examination, and blood transfusions; vaccinations permitted only when required by law; alteration of thoughts believed to cure illness; hypnotism and psychotherapy prohibited (Christian Scientist nurses and nursing homes honor these beliefs)

Church of Christ
- *Birth and death rituals*: None (baptism at age 8 or older)
- *Dietary restrictions*: Alcohol discouraged
- *Practices in health crisis*: Communion, anointing with oil, laying on of hands, and counseling (all performed by a minister)

Eastern Orthodox
- *Birth and death rituals*: At birth, baptism and confirmation; before death, last rites; for members of the Russian Orthodox Church, arms are crossed after death, fingers set in a cross, and unembalmed body clothed in natural fiber
- *Dietary restrictions*: For members of the Russian Orthodox Church and usually the Greek Orthodox Church, no meat or dairy products on Wednesdays and Fridays and during Lent
- *Practices in health crisis*: Anointing of the sick; for members of the Russian Orthodox Church, cross necklace is replaced immediately after surgery, and shaving of male patients is prohibited except in preparation for surgery; for members of the Greek Orthodox Church, communion and Sacrament of Holy Unction

Episcopalian
- *Birth and death rituals*: At birth, baptism; before death, occasional last rites
- *Dietary restrictions*: For some members, abstention from meat on Fridays, fasting before communion (which may be daily)
- *Practices in health crisis*: Communion, prayer, and counseling (all performed by a minister)

Hindu
- *Birth and death rituals*: At birth, importance of noting the exact time of birth; Jatakarma (ceremony that involves putting honey into the child's mouth and whispering the name of God in the child's ear to welcome the baby into the family); possibly, postponement of naming until 10 days after birth; if the patient is dying, possible aromatherapy to assist the dying

patient's soul to rest in peace; at death, proper performance of funeral rites to ensure the cycle of life and reincarnation[3,4]
- *Dietary restrictions*: Beef intake prohibited; possibly vegetarian diet; possibly fasting on special occasions, such as holy days (dietary restrictions may vary during different stages of life)[4]
- *Practices in health crisis*: Preference by women for female health care providers; possible desire to wear personal clothing under hospital gown; possible unwillingness to discuss problems involving the genitourinary system; desire to keep small statue or picture of the family god at the bedside and to start each day with prayer

Jehovah's Witnesses
- *Birth and death rituals*: None
- *Dietary restrictions*: Abstention from foods to which blood has been added
- *Practices in health crisis*: Typically, no blood transfusions permitted; a court order may be required for emergency transfusion.

Judaism
- *Birth and death rituals*: Ritual male circumcision on 8th day after birth; burial of a dead fetus; ritual washing of the dead; burial (including organs and other body tissues) as soon as possible; no autopsy or embalming
- *Dietary restrictions*: For Orthodox and Conservative Jews, kosher dietary laws (for example, pork and shellfish prohibited); for Reform Jews, usually no restrictions
- *Practices in health crisis*: Rabbinical consultation required for donation or transplantation of organs; for Orthodox and Conservative Jews, medical procedures possibly prohibited on the Sabbath (from sundown Friday to sundown Saturday) and on special holidays except where withholding the procedure would be detrimental to the person's health.[5]

Lutheran
- *Birth and death rituals*: Baptism usually performed 6 to 8 weeks after birth
- *Dietary restrictions*: None
- *Practices in health crisis*: Communion, prayer, and counseling (all performed by a minister)

Mormon
- *Birth and death rituals*: At birth, none (baptism at age 8 or older); before death, baptism and gospel preaching
- *Dietary restrictions*: Alcohol, tobacco, tea, and coffee prohibited; meat intake limited
- *Practices in health crisis*: Belief in divine healing through the laying on of hands; communion on Sundays; refusal of medical treatment by some members; special undergarment worn by many

Muslim
- *Birth and death rituals*: Fetus aborted spontaneously before 130 days, treated as discarded tissue; after 130 days, fetus treated as a human being; before death, confession of sins with family present; after death, only relatives or friends may touch the body
- *Dietary restrictions*: Pork prohibited; daylight fasting during 9th month of Islamic calendar
- *Practices in health crisis:* Faith healing (for the patient's morale only); rejection of medical therapy by conservative members; possible preference for same-gender health care provider; possibly many visitors for a hospitalized patient to fulfill the religious obligation of charity; possible request for the bed be turned toward Mecca for prayer (if bedridden); possible use of a prayer rug, if physically able; obtain permission before entering the patient's room, if possible.[6,7]

Orthodox Presbyterian
- *Birth and death rituals*: Infant baptism; scripture reading and prayer before death
- *Dietary restrictions*: None
- *Practices in health crisis*: Communion, prayer, and counseling (all performed by a minister)

Beliefs and practices of selected religions *(continued)*

Pentecostal Assembly of God, Foursquare Church
- *Birth and death rituals*: None (baptism only after age of accountability)
- *Dietary restrictions*: Abstention from alcohol, tobacco, meat slaughtered by strangling, any food to which blood has been added, and sometimes pork
- *Practices in health crisis*: Divine healing through prayer, anointing with oil, laying on of hands

Roman Catholic
- *Birth and death rituals*: Infant baptism, including baptism of aborted fetus without sign of clinical death (tissue necrosis); before death, last rites, which includes confession, anointing of the sick, and final communion[8]

- *Dietary restrictions*: Fasting or abstention from meat on Ash Wednesday and on Fridays during Lent (practice usually waived for the hospitalized)
- *Practices in health crisis*: Burial of major amputated limb (sometimes) in consecrated ground; organ donation or transplantation allowed if the benefit to recipient outweighs the donor's potential harm; Anointing of the Sick sacrament performed just before death as well as when patients are ill and sometimes performed shortly after admission[9]

United Methodist
- *Birth and death rituals*: None (baptism of children and adults only)
- *Dietary restrictions*: None
- *Practices in health crisis*: Communion before surgery or similar crisis; donation of body parts encouraged

---

- If a terminally ill patient requests the Anointing of the Sick sacrament or special treatment of the body after death, call an appropriate clergy member. For the Roman Catholic patient, call a Roman Catholic priest to administer the sacrament, even if the patient is unresponsive or comatose. *To prepare the patient for this sacrament*, uncover the arms and fold back the top linens *to expose the feet*. After the clergy member anoints the patient's forehead, eyes, nose, mouth, hands, and feet, straighten and retuck the bed linens.
- Perform hand hygiene.[11,12,13,14,15,16]
- Document the procedure.[23,24,25,26]

Special considerations
- Handle the patient's religious articles carefully *to avoid damage or loss*. As needed, consult the family or spiritual leader about the handling of religious articles.[1]
- Become familiar with religious resources in your facility. Some facilities employ one or more clergy members who counsel patients and staff members and link patients to other pastoral resources.[1]

Documentation
If the patient underwent baptism, complete a baptismal form and attach it to the patient's record; send a copy of the form to the appropriate clergy member. Record the rites of circumcision and Anointing of the Sick sacrament in the patient's medical record.

REFERENCES
1 Craven, R. F., et al. (2020). *Fundamentals of nursing: Concepts and competencies for practice* (9th ed.). Philadelphia, PA: Wolters Kluwer.
2 ElGindy, G. (2013). Understanding Buddhist patients' dietary needs. https://minoritynurse.com/?s=buddhist+patients
3 Shanmugasundaram, S., et al. (n.d.). Culturally competent care at the end of life: A Hindu perspective. https://sigma.nursingrepository.org/bitstream/handle/10755/313364/Shanmugasundaram_S.pdf?sequence=8&isAllowed=y
4 Minority Nurse. (2013). Hindu dietary practices: Feeding the body, mind, and soul. https://minoritynurse.com/hindu-dietary-practices-feeding-the-body-mind-and-soul/
5 Chabad.org (n.d.) Jewish practice 10: in case of emergency. https://www.chabad.org/library/article_cdo/aid/253230/jewish/10-In-Case-of-Emergency.htm
6 Attum, B., & Shamoon, Z. (2021). Cultural competence in the care of Muslim patients and their families. https://www.ncbi.nlm.nih.gov/books/NBK499933/
7 Boucher, N. A., et al. (2017). Supporting Muslim patients during advanced illness. *Permanente Journal, 21*, 16–190. https://www.ncbi.nlm.nih.gov/pmc/articles/PMC5469433/
8 Catholic Answers. (n.d.) Tract: Anointing of the sick. https://www.catholic.com/tract/anointing-of-the-sick
9 Swihart, D. L., et al. (2021). Cultural religious competence in clinical practice. https://www.ncbi.nlm.nih.gov/books/NBK493216/
10 The Joint Commission. (2021). Standard RI.01.01.01. *Comprehensive accreditation manual for hospitals.* Oakbrook Terrace, IL: The Joint Commission. (Level VII)
11 Centers for Disease Control and Prevention. (2002). Guideline for hand hygiene in health-care settings: Recommendations of the Healthcare Infection Control Practices Advisory Committee and the HICPAC/SHEA/APIC/IDSA Hand Hygiene Task Force. *MMWR Recommendations and Reports, 51*(RR-16), 1–45. https://www.cdc.gov/mmwr/pdf/rr/rr5116.pdf (Level II)
12 World Health Organization. (2009). WHO guidelines on hand hygiene in health care: First global patient safety challenge, clean care is safer care. https://apps.who.int/iris/bitstream/handle/10665/44102/9789241597906_eng.pdf?sequence=1 (Level IV)
13 The Joint Commission. (2021). Standard NPSG.07.01.01. *Comprehensive accreditation manual for hospitals.* Oakbrook Terrace, IL: The Joint Commission. (Level VII)
14 Accreditation Association for Hospitals and Health Systems. (2020). Standard 07.01.21. *Healthcare Facilities Accreditation Program: Accreditation requirements for acute care hospitals.* Chicago, IL: Accreditation Association for Hospitals and Health Systems. (Level VII)
15 Centers for Medicare and Medicaid Services, Department of Health and Human Services. (2020). Condition of participation: Infection control. 42 C.F.R. § 482.42.
16 DNV GL-Healthcare USA, Inc. (2020). IC.1.SR.1. *NIAHO® accreditation requirements, interpretive guidelines and surveyor guidance—revision 20.0.* Milford, OH: DNV GL-Healthcare USA, Inc. (Level VII)
17 The Joint Commission. (2021). Standard NPSG.01.01.01. *Comprehensive accreditation manual for hospitals.* Oakbrook Terrace, IL: The Joint Commission. (Level VII)
18 DNV GL-Healthcare USA, Inc. (2020). PR.2.SR.5. *NIAHO® accreditation requirements, interpretive guidelines and surveyor guidance—revision 20.0.* Milford, OH: DNV GL-Healthcare USA, Inc. (Level VII)
19 Centers for Medicare and Medicaid Services, Department of Health and Human Services. (2020). Condition of participation: Patient's rights. 42 C.F.R. § 482.13(c)(1).
20 Accreditation Association for Hospitals and Health Systems. (2020). Standard 15.01.16. *Healthcare Facilities Accreditation Program: Accreditation requirements for acute care hospitals.* Chicago, IL: Accreditation Association for Hospitals and Health Systems. (Level VII)
21 Taylor, E. J. (2011). Spiritual care: Evangelism at the bedside? *Journal of Christian Nursing, 28*, 194–202.
22 Burke, G. F., & McIlvried, R. (2010). Communion for NPO patients. *Ethics and Medics, 35*(5), 1–2. https://static1.squarespace.com/static/5e3ada1a6a2e8d6a131d1dcd/t/5efa410a7efd041c2a142a9b/1593458954721/NCBC_EM_May2010+%28revised%29.pdf
23 The Joint Commission. (2021). Standard RC.01.03.01. *Comprehensive accreditation manual for hospitals.* Oakbrook Terrace, IL: The Joint Commission. (Level VII)
24 Centers for Medicare and Medicaid Services, Department of Health and Human Services. (2020). Condition of participation: Medical record services. 42 C.F.R. § 482.24(b).
25 Accreditation Association for Hospitals and Health Systems. (2020). Standard 10.00.03. *Healthcare Facilities Accreditation Program: Accreditation requirements for acute care hospitals.* Chicago, IL: Accreditation Association for Hospitals and Health Systems. (Level VII)
26 DNV GL-Healthcare USA, Inc. (2020). MR.2.SR.1. *NIAHO® accreditation requirements, interpretive guidelines and surveyor guidance—revision 20.0.* Milford, OH: DNV GL-Healthcare USA, Inc. (Level VII)

Splint application

By immobilizing the site of an injury, a splint alleviates pain and allows the injury to heal in proper alignment. It also minimizes possible complications, such as excessive bleeding into tissues and restricted blood flow caused by bone pressing against vessels.[1] In cases of multiple serious injuries, a splint allows caretakers to move the patient without risking further damage to bones, muscles, nerves, blood vessels, and skin.

Splints have traditionally been made of plaster of Paris; however, in recent years, many different types of splints and splinting materials have become available, including preformed plaster, fiberglass, padded fiberglass, aluminum, air splints, and vacuum splints. Preformed, rigid commercial splints are available for use on various body parts, come in multiple sizes, and are usually made of hard plastic and Velcro.[1] Commercial splints may be removed to enable skin assessment; however, repeated removal by the patient may delay healing or cause additional injury.[1]

A practitioner may order a splint to immobilize a simple or compound fracture, dislocation, or subluxation. (See *Rigid splint.*)

During an emergency, splint any injury you suspect of being a fracture, dislocation, or subluxation.[1] No contraindications exist for rigid splints.

Equipment

Rigid splint ▪ tape measure ▪ padding ▪ Velcro straps, 2" (5-cm) roller gauze, or 2" (5-cm) cloth strips ▪ tape ▪ pillows ▪ vital signs monitoring equipment ▪ Optional: gloves and other personal protective equipment, ice, prescribed pain medication, and scissors, ring cutter, or other equipment to remove clothing or jewelry.

A practitioner may prefer to use an air splint (an inflatable, semirigid splint) to secure an injured extremity. (See *Using an air splint.*)

Implementation

▪ Gather and prepare the necessary equipment and supplies. Perform hand hygiene.[3,4,5,6,7,8]
▪ Confirm the patient's identity using at least two patient identifiers.[9]
▪ Provide privacy.[10,11,12,13]
▪ Obtain a history of the circumstances surrounding the injury (including the time and mechanism of injury) and significant medical history, including alcohol use, medications, allergies, and tetanus immunization status, if known. Ask the time of the patient's last oral intake, and keep the patient on nothing-by-mouth status if procedural sedation or surgical intervention is possible.[2] (See the "Moderate sedation" procedure.)
▪ Explain the procedure to the patient and family (if appropriate) according to their individual communication and learning needs *to increase their understanding, allay their fears, and enhance cooperation.*[14]
▪ Raise the patient's bed to waist level before providing patient care *to prevent caregiver back strain.*[15]
▪ Perform hand hygiene.[3,4,5,6,7,8]

Rigid splint

A rigid splint, as shown below, can help immobilize a fracture or dislocation in an extremity. Ideally, two people should apply a rigid splint to an extremity.

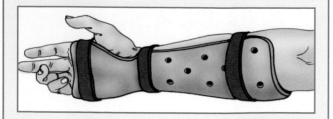

EQUIPMENT

Using an air splint

In an emergency, you can apply an air splint, shown below, *to immobilize a fracture or control bleeding,* especially from a forearm or lower leg. This compact, comfortable splint is made of double-walled plastic and provides gentle, diffuse pressure over an injured area. After choosing the appropriate splint, wrap it around the affected extremity, secure it with Velcro or other strips, and then inflate it. Inflate the splint only to the point where you can slip a finger between the splint and the skin *so that it fits snugly enough to immobilize the extremity without impairing circulation.*[2]

An air splint may actually control bleeding better than a local pressure bandage. Its clear plastic construction simplifies inspection of the affected site for bleeding, pallor, and cyanosis. An air splint also allows the patient to be moved without further damage to the injured limb.

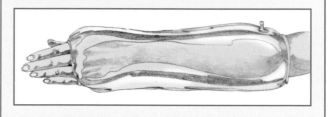

▪ Put on gloves and other personal protective equipment, as needed.[16,17,18]
▪ If necessary, remove or cut away the patient's clothing, and remove jewelry if the injury involves the hand, foot, or toes where jewelry is worn.[2]
▪ Begin a thorough head-to-toe assessment, inspecting for obvious deformities, swelling, or bleeding.
▪ Screen and assess the patient's pain using facility-defined criteria consistent with the patient's age, condition, and ability to understand.[19]
▪ Treat the patient's pain, as needed and ordered, using nonpharmacologic or pharmacologic approaches, or a combination of approaches. Base the treatment plan on evidence-based practices and the patient's clinical condition, past medical history, and pain management goals. If administering pain medications, follow safe medication administration practices.[20,21,22,23] Ensure adequate analgesia during and after splinting, *because splint application may involve painful movement of the injured limb.*
▪ Assess the affected extremity's range of motion (ROM).
▪ Inspect and gently palpate the injured area for evidence of fracture or dislocation.
▪ Assess neurovascular integrity distal to the injury site.[2]
▪ If possible, align the injured extremity in its normal anatomic position.
▪ *To avoid damaging misplaced vessels and nerves,* don't attempt to straighten a dislocation.
▪ Measure the uninjured side *to determine the proper splint size.* Choose a splint that will immobilize the joints above and below the fracture.[1,24]
▪ Pad the splint, as needed, *to protect bony prominences.*[25]
▪ Support the injured extremity above and below the fracture site while applying firm, gentle traction.[24]
▪ Have an assistant place the splint under, beside, or on top of the extremity.
▪ Have the assistant apply the bindings to secure the splint, being careful not to compromise the circulation; the splint should fit snugly but not be constrictive.[26]
▪ Assess the neurovascular status of the extremity. If it's impaired by the bindings, release and reapply them.
▪ Elevate the injured extremity, keeping in mind that excessive elevation may compromise arterial circulation.[2]
▪ Monitor the patient's vital signs frequently *to detect signs of shock. Fractured bones may cause significant bleeding into surrounding tissues.*
▪ Reassess the neurovascular status by assessing skin color, temperature of the extremities, the presence of paresthesia, and pulses, and assess the ability to move and sensation.[1,26] *Numbness or paralysis distal to an injury indicates nerve injury.*

- Reassess and respond to the patient's pain by evaluating the response to treatment and progress toward pain management goals. Assess for adverse reactions and risk factors for adverse events that may result from treatment.[19,27]
- Apply ice to the injury, as needed, *to minimize swelling.*[2]
- Assess the patient for signs of skin breakdown and medical device–related pressure injury on an ongoing basis. *Pressure injury can result from contact between the patient's skin and the splint or from immobility.*[25]
- Return the bed to the lowest position *to prevent falls and maintain patient safety.*[28]
- Remove and discard your gloves and other personal protective equipment, if worn.[16,17]
- Perform hand hygiene.[3,4,5,6,7,8]
- Document the procedure.[29,30,31,32]

Special considerations

- Studies suggest that many splints are applied incorrectly, which can cause unnecessary injuries, such as skin or soft-tissue complications and excessive swelling.[1]
- Prompt identification of impaired nerve or circulatory function is critical to preventing patient harm. Notify the practitioner of any neurovascular changes.[26]

Patient teaching

Teach the patient how to remove and apply the splint properly and the schedule that the patient should follow. Also review permissible activities while wearing the splint. Tell the patient to check the skin beneath the splint several times per day and report numbness, tingling, pain, a change in skin temperature, and skin breakdown in the affected extremity. Instruct the patient never to place foreign objects between the splinting material and the skin.[33]

Complications

Multiple transfers and repeated manipulation of a fracture may cause fat embolism. This complication usually occurs within 36 hours of an injury or manipulation.[34] Symptoms of fat embolism include dyspnea, agitation, hypoxia, changes in mental status, and a petechial rash, most commonly seen on the head, neck, anterior thorax, axillae, and subconjunctiva.[35]

Other possible complications include medical device–associated pressure injuries, contact dermatitis beneath the splint, neurovascular compromise, and decreased ROM.[1,25]

Documentation

Record the circumstances surrounding the injury, including the time and mechanism of injury. Document the patient's complaints, noting whether the symptoms are localized. Document any medication administered; the strength, dose, route, and date and time of administration; and any adverse effects.[36] Record the neurovascular assessment before and after applying the splint. Note the type of wound and the type and amount of any drainage. Note the time of splint and ice application. Be sure to note if the bone end slips into surrounding tissue or if transportation causes a change in the degree of dislocation. Document teaching provided to the patient and family (if applicable), their understanding of that teaching, and any need for follow-up teaching.

REFERENCES

1 Stracciolini, A. (2021). Basic techniques for splinting of musculoskeletal injuries. In: *UpToDate*, Fields, K. B., et al. (Eds.).
2 Emergency Nurses Association. (2020). *Sheehy's emergency nursing: Principles and practice* (7th ed.). St. Louis, MO: Elsevier.
3 Centers for Disease Control and Prevention. (2002). Guideline for hand hygiene in health-care settings: Recommendations of the Healthcare Infection Control Practices Advisory Committee and the HICPAC/SHEA/APIC/IDSA Hand Hygiene Task Force. *MMWR Recommendations and Reports, 51*(RR-16), 1–45. https://www.cdc.gov/mmwr/pdf/rr/rr5116.pdf (Level II)
4 World Health Organization. (2009). WHO guidelines on hand hygiene in health care: First global patient safety challenge, clean care is safer care. https://apps.who.int/iris/bitstream/handle/10665/44102/9789241597906_eng.pdf?sequence=1 (Level IV)
5 The Joint Commission. (2021). Standard NPSG.07.01.01. *Comprehensive accreditation manual for hospitals.* Oakbrook Terrace, IL: The Joint Commission. (Level VII)
6 Centers for Medicare and Medicaid Services, Department of Health and Human Services. (2020). Condition of participation: Infection control. 42 C.F.R. § 482.42.
7 Accreditation Association for Hospitals and Health Systems. (2020). Standard 07.01.21. *Healthcare Facilities Accreditation Program: Accreditation requirements for acute care hospitals.* Chicago, IL: Accreditation Association for Hospitals and Health Systems. (Level VII)
8 DNV GL-Healthcare USA, Inc. (2020). IC.1.SR.1. *NIAHO® accreditation requirements, interpretive guidelines and surveyor guidance—revision 20.0.* Milford, OH: DNV GL-Healthcare USA, Inc. (Level VII)
9 The Joint Commission. (2021). Standard NPSG.01.01.01. *Comprehensive accreditation manual for hospitals.* Oakbrook Terrace, IL: The Joint Commission. (Level VII)
10 Centers for Medicare and Medicaid Services, Department of Health and Human Services. (2020). Condition of participation: Patient's rights. 42 C.F.R. § 482.13(c)(1).
11 Accreditation Association for Hospitals and Health Systems. (2020). Standard 15.01.16. *Healthcare Facilities Accreditation Program: Accreditation requirements for acute care hospitals.* Chicago, IL: Accreditation Association for Hospitals and Health Systems. (Level VII)
12 The Joint Commission. (2021). Standard RI.01.01.01. *Comprehensive accreditation manual for hospitals.* Oakbrook Terrace, IL: The Joint Commission. (Level VII)
13 DNV GL-Healthcare USA, Inc. (2020). PR.2.SR.5. *NIAHO® accreditation requirements, interpretive guidelines and surveyor guidance—revision 20.0.* Milford, OH: DNV GL-Healthcare USA, Inc. (Level VII)
14 The Joint Commission. (2021). Standard PC.02.01.21. *Comprehensive accreditation manual for hospitals.* Oakbrook Terrace, IL: The Joint Commission. (Level VII)
15 Waters, T. R., et al. (2009). Safe patient handling training for schools of nursing. https://www.cdc.gov/niosh/docs/2009-127/pdfs/2009-127.pdf (Level VII)
16 Siegel, J. D., et al. (2007, revised 2019). 2007 guideline for isolation precautions: Preventing transmission of infectious agents in healthcare settings. https://www.cdc.gov/infectioncontrol/pdf/guidelines/isolation-guidelines-H.pdf (Level II)
17 Accreditation Association for Hospitals and Health Systems. (2020). Standard 07.01.10. *Healthcare Facilities Accreditation Program: Accreditation requirements for acute care hospitals.* Chicago, IL: Accreditation Association for Hospitals and Health Systems. (Level VII)
18 Occupational Safety and Health Administration. (2012). Bloodborne pathogens, standard number 1910.1030. https://www.osha.gov/pls/oshaweb/owadisp.show_document?p_id=10051&p_table=STANDARDS (Level VII)
19 The Joint Commission. (2021). Standard PC.01.02.07. *Comprehensive accreditation manual for hospitals.* Oakbrook Terrace, IL: The Joint Commission. (Level VII)
20 Centers for Medicare and Medicaid Services, Department of Health and Human Services. (2020). Condition of participation: Nursing services. 42 C.F.R. § 482.23(c).
21 The Joint Commission. (2021). Standard MM.06.01.01. *Comprehensive accreditation manual for hospitals.* Oakbrook Terrace, IL: The Joint Commission. (Level VII)
22 Accreditation Association for Hospitals and Health Systems. (2020). Standard 16.01.03. *Healthcare Facilities Accreditation Program: Accreditation requirements for acute care hospitals.* Chicago, IL: Accreditation Association for Hospitals and Health Systems. (Level VII)
23 DNV GL-Healthcare USA, Inc. (2020). MM.1.SR.3. *NIAHO® accreditation requirements, interpretive guidelines and surveyor guidance—revision 20.0.* Milford, OH: DNV GL-Healthcare USA, Inc. (Level VII)
24 Bethel, C. A., & Meller, M. M. (2019). Volar splinting. In: *StatPearls.* Treasure Island, FL: StatPearls Publishing.
25 Wound Ostomy and Continence Nurses Society (WOCN). (2016). *Guideline for prevention and management of pressure ulcers (injuries): WOCN clinical practice guideline series 2.* Mount Laurel, NJ: WOCN.
26 Hinkle, J. L., & Cheever, K. H. (2018). *Brunner & Suddarth's textbook of medical-surgical nursing* (14th ed.). Wolters Kluwer.
27 Accreditation Association for Hospitals and Health Systems. (2020). Standard 16.02.05. *Healthcare Facilities Accreditation Program: Accreditation requirements for acute care hospitals.* Chicago, IL: Accreditation Association for Hospitals and Health Systems. (Level VII)

28 Ganz, D. A., et al. (2013, reviewed 2021). *Preventing falls in hospitals: A toolkit for improving quality of care* (AHRQ Publication No. 13-0015-EF). Rockville, MD: Agency for Healthcare Research and Quality. https://www.ahrq.gov/professionals/systems/hospital/fallpxtoolkit/index.html (Level VII)

29 The Joint Commission. (2021). Standard RC.01.03.01. *Comprehensive accreditation manual for hospitals.* Oakbrook Terrace, IL: The Joint Commission. (Level VII)

30 Centers for Medicare and Medicaid Services, Department of Health and Human Services. (2020). Condition of participation: Medical record services. 42 C.F.R. § 482.24(b).

31 Accreditation Association for Hospitals and Health Systems. (2020). Standard 10.00.03. *Healthcare Facilities Accreditation Program: Accreditation requirements for acute care hospitals.* Chicago, IL: Accreditation Association for Hospitals and Health Systems. (Level VII)

32 DNV GL-Healthcare USA, Inc. (2020). MR.2.SR.1. *NIAHO® accreditation requirements, interpretive guidelines and surveyor guidance—revision 20.0.* Milford, OH: DNV GL-Healthcare USA, Inc. (Level VII)

33 Schweich, P. (2021). Patient education: Cast and splint care (Beyond the basics). In: *UpToDate,* Boutis, K. (Ed.).

34 Porpodis, K., et al. (2012). Fat embolism due to bilateral femoral fracture: A case report. *International Journal of General Medicine, 5,* 59–63. (Level VI)

35 Weinhouse, G. L. (2021). Fat embolism syndrome. In: *UpToDate,* Parsons, P. E. (Ed.).

36 The Joint Commission. (2021). Standard RC.02.01.01. *Comprehensive accreditation manual for hospitals.* Oakbrook Terrace, IL: The Joint Commission. (Level VII)

SPONGE BATH

A sponge bath with tepid water involves the use of lukewarm water to reduce fever by dilating superficial blood vessels, which releases heat and lowers body temperature. It may lower systemic temperature when routine fever treatments fail.[1] Guidelines no longer recommend tepid sponge bath use for children, *because it may lead to extreme chilling and shock to an immature nervous system and has little advantage over the use of oral antipyretics.*[2]

Equipment

Basin of tepid water, about 80° to 93° F (26.7° to 33.9° C) ▪ bath (utility) thermometer ▪ bath blanket ▪ fluid-impermeable pad ▪ washcloths ▪ towel ▪ clean hospital gown (for patient) ▪ vital signs monitoring equipment ▪ Optional: gloves, prescribed antipyretic, ice bag and cover, facility-approved disinfectant.

Preparation of equipment

Inspect all equipment and supplies. If a product is expired, is defective, or has compromised integrity, remove it from patient use, label it as expired or defective, and report the expiration or defect as directed by your facility. If needed, prepare an ice bag and cover; *the cover prevents skin irritation and tissue damage.* Then place the bath thermometer in a basin, and run water over it until the temperature reaches the high end of the tepid range (93° F [33.9° C]), *because the water will cool during the sponge bath.* Immerse the washcloths in the tepid solution until saturated.

Implementation

▪ Verify the practitioner's order.
▪ Review the patient's medication record for recent administration of an antipyretic. If not administered recently, administer an antipyretic as ordered 15 to 20 minutes before the sponge bath following safe medication administration practices *to achieve more rapid fever reduction.*[3,4,5,6]
▪ Gather and prepare the necessary equipment and supplies.
▪ Perform hand hygiene.[7,8,9,10,11,12]
▪ Confirm the patient's identity using at least two patient identifiers.[13]
▪ Provide privacy.[14,15,16,17]
▪ Explain the procedure to the patient and family (if appropriate) according to their individual communication and learning needs *to increase their understanding, allay their fears, and enhance cooperation.*[18]

▪ Ensure the room is warm and free from drafts.
▪ Raise the patient's bed to waist level before providing patient care *to prevent caregiver back strain.*[19]
▪ Perform hand hygiene.[7,8,9,10,11,12]
▪ Put on gloves as needed *to comply with standard precautions.*[20,21,22]
▪ Assess the patient's condition.
▪ Obtain and document the patient's vital signs (temperature, pulse, and respirations) *to serve as baseline for comparison.*
▪ Place a fluid-impermeable pad under the patient *to catch any spills,* and a bath blanket on top of the patient *for privacy.* Then remove the patient's gown. Also remove the top bed linen *to avoid wetting it.*
▪ Place a covered ice bag on the patient's head *to prevent headache and nasal congestion from occurring as the rest of the body cools.*
▪ Wring out each washcloth before sponging the patient *so that the water doesn't drip and cause discomfort.*
▪ Place moist washcloths over the major superficial blood vessels in the axillae, groin, and popliteal areas *to accelerate cooling.* Change the washcloths as they warm.
▪ Bathe each extremity separately for about 5 minutes; then sponge the chest and abdomen for 5 minutes. Turn the patient, and bathe the back and buttocks for 5 to 10 minutes. Keep the patient covered except for the body part you're sponging.
▪ Pat each area dry after sponging, but avoid rubbing with the towel, *because rubbing increases cell metabolism and produces heat.*
▪ Add tepid water to the basin as necessary, checking the bath thermometer reading, *to maintain the desired water temperature.*
▪ Monitor the patient's temperature, pulse, respirations, and blood pressure every 10 minutes or as needed. Notify the practitioner if the patient's temperature doesn't fall within 30 minutes.
▪ Observe the patient for chills, shivering, pallor, mottling, cyanosis of the lips or nail beds, and changes in vital signs—especially a rapid, weak, or irregular pulse—*because such signs may indicate an emergency.* If any of these signs occur, discontinue the bath, cover the patient lightly, and notify the practitioner.
▪ If no adverse effects occur, bathe the patient for at least 30 minutes or until the patient's temperature reaches 1° to 2° F (0.6° to 1° C) above the desired level, *because the temperature will continue to fall naturally.* Continue to monitor the temperature until it stabilizes.
▪ After the bath, make sure the patient is dry and comfortable. Dress the patient in a fresh gown and cover lightly.
▪ Return the patient's bed to the lowest position *to prevent falls and maintain patient safety.*[23]
▪ Discard used supplies in the appropriate receptacles.[22]
▪ Remove and discard your gloves, if worn.[20,22]
▪ Perform hand hygiene.[7,8,9,10,11,12]
▪ If the treatment will be repeated, clean and disinfect the reusable equipment according to the manufacturer's instructions *to prevent the spread of infection,*[24,25] and store the equipment in the patient's room.
▪ Perform hand hygiene.[7,8,9,10,11,12]
▪ Obtain the patient's temperature, pulse, respirations, and blood pressure 30 minutes after the bath *to determine the treatment's effectiveness.*
▪ Perform hand hygiene.[7,8,9,10,11,12]
▪ Document the procedure.[26,27,28,29]

Special considerations

▪ Consider covering the patient's trunk with a wet towel for 15 minutes *to speed cooling.* Resaturate the towel as necessary.
▪ Refrain from bathing the breasts of a postpartum patient, *because the nipples could become overly dry or develop fissures.*
▪ *Because temperatures can vary greatly among methods and anatomic sites,* consistently use the same method and site to obtain the patient's temperature throughout the procedures, if possible.[30,31]

Documentation

Record the date, time, and duration of the sponge bath; the temperature of the water; the patient's temperature, pulse, respirations, and blood pressure before, during, and after the procedure; and the patient's tolerance of the procedure. Note any complications that arise, the practitioner you notified, interventions you took, and the patient's response to the intervention. Document teaching you provided to the patient and family (if applicable), their understanding of that teaching, and any need for follow-up teaching.

REFERENCES

1 Dinarello, C. A., & Porat, R. (2021). Pathophysiology and treatment of fever in adults. In: *UpToDate*, Weller, P. F. (Ed.).

2 Silbert-Flagg, J., & Pillitteri, A. (2018). *Maternal and child health nursing: Care of the childbearing and childrearing family* (8th ed.). Philadelphia, PA: Wolters Kluwer.

3 The Joint Commission. (2021). Standard MM.06.01.01. *Comprehensive accreditation manual for hospitals*. Oakbrook Terrace, IL: The Joint Commission. (Level VII)

4 DNV GL-Healthcare USA, Inc. (2020). MM.1.SR.3. *NIAHO® accreditation requirements, interpretive guidelines and surveyor guidance—revision 20.0*. Milford, OH: DNV GL-Healthcare USA, Inc. (Level VII)

5 Centers for Medicare and Medicaid Services, Department of Health and Human Services. (2020). Condition of participation: Nursing services. 42 C.F.R. § 482.23(c).

6 Accreditation Association for Hospitals and Health Systems. (2020). Standard 16.01.03. *Healthcare Facilities Accreditation Program: Accreditation requirements for acute care hospitals*. Chicago, IL: Accreditation Association for Hospitals and Health Systems. (Level VII)

7 The Joint Commission. (2021). Standard NPSG.07.01.01. *Comprehensive accreditation manual for hospitals*. Oakbrook Terrace, IL: The Joint Commission. (Level VII)

8 Centers for Disease Control and Prevention. (2002). Guideline for hand hygiene in health-care settings: Recommendations of the Healthcare Infection Control Practices Advisory Committee and the HICPAC/SHEA/APIC/IDSA Hand Hygiene Task Force. *MMWR Recommendations and Reports, 51*(RR-16), 1–45. https://www.cdc.gov/mmwr/pdf/rr/rr5116.pdf (Level II)

9 World Health Organization. (2009). WHO guidelines on hand hygiene in health care: First global patient safety challenge, clean care is safer care. https://apps.who.int/iris/bitstream/handle/10665/44102/9789241597906_eng.pdf?sequence=1 (Level IV)

10 Accreditation Association for Hospitals and Health Systems. (2020). Standard 07.01.21. *Healthcare Facilities Accreditation Program: Accreditation requirements for acute care hospitals*. Chicago, IL: Accreditation Association for Hospitals and Health Systems. (Level VII)

11 Centers for Medicare and Medicaid Services, Department of Health and Human Services. (2020). Condition of participation: Infection control. 42 C.F.R. § 482.42.

12 DNV GL-Healthcare USA, Inc. (2020). IC.1.SR.1. *NIAHO® accreditation requirements, interpretive guidelines and surveyor guidance—revision 20.0*. Milford, OH: DNV GL-Healthcare USA, Inc. (Level VII)

13 The Joint Commission. (2021). Standard NPSG.01.01.01. *Comprehensive accreditation manual for hospitals*. Oakbrook Terrace, IL: The Joint Commission. (Level VII)

14 Accreditation Association for Hospitals and Health Systems. (2020). Standard 15.01.16. *Healthcare Facilities Accreditation Program: Accreditation requirements for acute care hospitals*. Chicago, IL: Accreditation Association for Hospitals and Health Systems. (Level VII)

15 Centers for Medicare and Medicaid Services, Department of Health and Human Services. (2020). Condition of participation: Patient's rights. 42 C.F.R. § 482.13(c)(1).

16 The Joint Commission. (2021). Standard RI.01.01.01. *Comprehensive accreditation manual for hospitals*. Oakbrook Terrace, IL: The Joint Commission. (Level VII)

17 DNV GL-Healthcare USA, Inc. (2020). PR.2.SR.5. *NIAHO® accreditation requirements, interpretive guidelines and surveyor guidance—revision 20.0*. Milford, OH: DNV GL-Healthcare USA, Inc. (Level VII)

18 The Joint Commission. (2021). Standard PC.02.01.21. *Comprehensive accreditation manual for hospitals*. Oakbrook Terrace, IL: The Joint Commission. (Level VII)

19 Waters, T. R., et al. (2009). Safe patient handling training for schools of nursing. https://www.cdc.gov/niosh/docs/2009-127/pdfs/2009-127.pdf (Level VII)

20 Siegel, J. D., et al. (2007, revised 2019). 2007 guideline for isolation precautions: Preventing transmission of infectious agents in healthcare settings. https://www.cdc.gov/infectioncontrol/pdf/guidelines/isolation-guidelines-H.pdf (Level II)

21 Accreditation Association for Hospitals and Health Systems. (2020). Standard 07.01.10. *Healthcare Facilities Accreditation Program: Accreditation requirements for acute care hospitals*. Chicago, IL: Accreditation Association for Hospitals and Health Systems. (Level VII)

22 Occupational Safety and Health Administration. (2012). Bloodborne pathogens, standard number 1910.1030. https://www.osha.gov/pls/oshaweb/owadisp.show_document?p_id=10051&p_table=STANDARDS (Level VII)

23 Ganz, D. A., et al. (2013, reviewed 2021). *Preventing falls in hospitals: A toolkit for improving quality of care* (AHRQ Publication No. 13-0015-EF). Rockville, MD: Agency for Healthcare Research and Quality. https://www.ahrq.gov/professionals/systems/hospital/fallpxtoolkit/index.html (Level VII)

24 Rutala, W. A., et al. (2008, revised 2019). Guideline for disinfection and sterilization in healthcare facilities, 2008. https://www.cdc.gov/infection-control/pdf/guidelines/disinfection-guidelines-H.pdf (Level I)

25 Accreditation Association for Hospitals and Health Systems. (2020). Standard 07.02.03. *Healthcare Facilities Accreditation Program: Accreditation requirements for acute care hospitals*. Chicago, IL: Accreditation Association for Hospitals and Health Systems. (Level VII)

26 The Joint Commission. (2021). Standard RC.01.03.01. *Comprehensive accreditation manual for hospitals*. Oakbrook Terrace, IL: The Joint Commission. (Level VII)

27 Accreditation Association for Hospitals and Health Systems. (2020). Standard 10.00.03. *Healthcare Facilities Accreditation Program: Accreditation requirements for acute care hospitals*. Chicago, IL: Accreditation Association for Hospitals and Health Systems. (Level VII)

28 Centers for Medicare and Medicaid Services, Department of Health and Human Services. (2020). Condition of participation: Medical record services. 42 C.F.R. § 482.24(b).

29 DNV GL-Healthcare USA, Inc. (2020). MR.2.SR.1. *NIAHO® accreditation requirements, interpretive guidelines and surveyor guidance—revision 20.0*. Milford, OH: DNV GL-Healthcare USA, Inc. (Level VII)

30 McCallum, L., & Higgins, D. (2012). Measuring body temperature. *Nursing Times, 108*(45), 20–22. https://www.nursingtimes.net/clinical-archive/assessment-skills/measuring-body-temperature-06-11-2012/

31 Makic, M. B., et al. (2011). Evidence based practice habits: Putting more sacred cows out to pasture. *Critical Care Nurse, 31*(2), 38–62. (Level V)

SPUTUM COLLECTION

Secreted by mucous membranes lining the bronchioles, bronchi, and trachea, sputum helps protect the respiratory tract from infection. When expelled from the respiratory tract, sputum carries saliva, nasal and sinus secretions, dead cells, and normal oral bacteria from the respiratory tract. Culturing of sputum specimens identifies microorganisms causing infection.[1,2] Laboratory examination of sputum helps in the diagnosis and treatment of such conditions as pneumonia and tuberculosis (TB).[2]

Sputum specimens collected by expectoration are commonly used for cytology, culture and sensitivity, and acid-fast bacilli (AFB) testing.[2] Cytologic examination helps identify abnormal cells. Culture and sensitivity testing identifies specific microorganisms and antibiotic sensitivity. Smear specimens that test positive for AFB must also undergo culture and sensitivity testing to confirm TB.

When a patient is unable to produce an adequate specimen, additional treatments may be needed to help mobilize secretions. These treatments include nebulizer use, chest percussion or vibration, and postural drainage.[2,3,4]

Tracheal suctioning involves secretion removal from the trachea or bronchi via a catheter inserted through the nose. Collection of sputum specimens is easiest early in the morning because secretions usually accumulate overnight. The procedure is absolutely contraindicated in patients with epiglottitis or croup. It is relatively contraindicated in those with occluded nasal passages, epistaxis, acute head, neck, or facial injury, irritable airway, upper respiratory infection, laryngospasm, bronchospasm, tracheal surgery, gastric surgery with high anastomosis, myocardial infarction, or bleeding or clotting problems.[5]

NURSING ALERT For information specific to obtaining specimens for coronavirus disease 2019 (COVID-19) testing, see the Centers for Disease Control and Prevention Web site for the most up-to-date information: https://www.cdc.gov/coronavirus/2019-ncov/lab/guidelines-clinical-specimens.html

Equipment

For expectoration

Sterile specimen container with tight-fitting cap ▪ gloves ▪ glass of water ▪ facial tissues ▪ label ▪ laboratory biohazard transport bag ▪ oral hygiene supplies ▪ Optional: laboratory request form, gown, mask and goggles or mask and face shield, respirator (such as an N95 respirator or a powered air-purifying respirator if TB or other airborne pathogens are suspected), nebulizer treatment equipment, pillow, disinfectant wipes.

For tracheal suctioning

#12 to #14 French sterile suction catheter ▪ sterile gloves ▪ sterile in-line specimen trap ▪ sterile container with sterile normal saline solution ▪ suction source with regulator ▪ suction canister and tubing ▪ oxygen administration equipment ▪ stethoscope ▪ pulse oximeter and probe ▪ label ▪ laboratory biohazard transport bag ▪ supplies for oral care ▪ disinfectant pad ▪ emergency equipment (code cart with emergency medications, defibrillator, handheld resuscitation bag with mask, intubation equipment) ▪ Optional: laboratory request form, respirator (such as an N95 or powered air purifying respirator if TB or other airborne pathogens are suspected), gown, mask with face shield or mask and goggles, sterile water-soluble lubricant.[2]

Commercial suction kits are available, but the content varies. Check the package label when gathering supplies.

Preparation of equipment

Inspect all equipment and supplies. If a product is expired, is defective, or has compromised integrity, remove it from patient use, label it as expired or defective, and report the expiration or defect as directed by your facility.

Implementation

▪ Verify the practitioner's order.
▪ Gather and prepare the necessary equipment and supplies.
▪ Perform hand hygiene.[6,7,8,9,10,11]
▪ Confirm the patient's identity using at least two patient identifiers.[12]
▪ Provide privacy.[13,14,15,16]
▪ Explain the procedure to the patient and family (if appropriate) according to their individual communication and learning needs *to increase their understanding, allay their fears and enhance cooperation.*[17].
▪ Position all supplies within reach.
▪ Instruct the patient to sit in a chair or at the edge of the bed. If the patient can't sit up, place the patient in the high Fowler position. *These positions help the patient exert a greater force when coughing, increasing the likelihood of gathering an adequate sputum sample.*
▪ Perform hand hygiene.[6,7,8,9,10,11]
▪ Put on gloves and, as needed, other personal protective equipment *to comply with standard precautions.*[18,19,20]

NURSING ALERT If the patient requires airborne precautions, wear a powered air-purifying respirator or a fit-tested N95 or higher-level disposable respirator when caring for the patient. Put on the respirator before entering the room and remove it after exiting the room. If you anticipate spraying of respiratory fluids, wear a gown, mask, and face shield or goggles, as well as gloves.[19]

▪ Perform treatment (such as nebulizer use, chest percussion, and postural drainage), as ordered, *to assist in specimen production.*[3] (See the "Chest physiotherapy" and "Nebulizer therapy" procedures.)

Sputum collection by expectoration

▪ Instruct the patient to rinse the mouth with water *to reduce specimen contamination with normal flora.*[2,21] Avoid mouthwash or toothpaste, *because they may affect the mobility of organisms in the sputum sample.*

▪ If the patient has a surgical incision or localized area of discomfort, have the patient place the hands firmly over the affected area or place a pillow over the area *to provide splinting, which reduces tension on the incision during coughing.*
▪ Instruct the patient to take three slow, deep breaths and to then cough deeply from a maximal inspiration while covering the mouth with a tissue.[19,21] Repeat the procedure as necessary until the patient produces sputum. Allow rest periods between each maneuver.
▪ When sputum is mobilized, instruct the patient to expectorate directly into the sterile specimen container[21] without touching the inside or rim of the container. Have the patient continue producing sputum until the amount totals at least 5 mL, if possible.
▪ Assess the sputum to ensure it's actually sputum and not saliva, *because saliva produces inaccurate test results.* Sputum appears thick and opaque, while saliva appears thin, clear, and watery.[1]
▪ Cap the specimen container tightly and, if necessary, clean its exterior with disinfectant wipes.

Sputum collection by tracheal suctioning

▪ Raise the bed to waist level before providing care *to prevent caregiver back strain.*[22]
▪ Position the patient in the high or semi-Fowler position *to promote lung expansion and to facilitate the patient's ability to cough.*
▪ Perform hand hygiene.[6,7,8,9,10,11]
▪ Assess the patient's respiratory status, including respiratory rate, depth, and pattern; breath sounds; oxygen saturation level by pulse oximetry[5]; and the color of the nail beds and mucous membranes *to obtain baseline findings.* Continue to monitor the patient's respiratory status throughout the procedure.
▪ Hyperoxygenate the patient with an appropriate oxygen delivery device, as indicated and ordered, *to prevent hypoxia during tracheal suctioning.*[5]
▪ Perform hand hygiene.[6,7,8,9,10,11]
▪ Put on personal protective equipment, as needed, *to comply with standard precautions.*[18,19,20]
▪ Open equipment packages following sterile no-touch technique.
▪ Put on sterile gloves.[19,20] Consider the suction catheter hand sterile and your other hand clean *to prevent cross-contamination.*[23]
▪ Connect the suction tubing to the male adapter of the in-line specimen trap. Attach the sterile suction catheter to the rubber tubing of the trap. (See *Attaching a specimen trap to a suction catheter.*)
▪ Lubricate the catheter with normal saline solution or water-soluble lubricant.
▪ Gently pass the catheter through the patient's nostril, directing it toward the septum and floor of the nasal cavity, without applying suction.[2,5,23] Gently twist the catheter if you feel resistance in the nostril. If twisting doesn't help, withdraw the catheter and insert it in the other nostril.[2]
▪ When the catheter reaches the larynx, have the patient assume a "sniffing" position *to help align the opening of the larynx with the lower pharynx, easing passage of the catheter through the larynx.* Advance the catheter into the trachea until the patient coughs or you feel resistance.[2] Tell the patient to take several deep breaths through the mouth *to ease insertion.*
▪ To obtain the specimen, apply suction for 5 to 10 seconds, but never for longer than 15 seconds, *to prevent atelectasis and hypoxia.* If the procedure must be repeated, reapply oxygen, monitor the oxygen saturation level by pulse oximetry, and wait at least 1 minute *to allow the patient time to return to preprocedure condition.*[2]
▪ When sputum collection is completed, gently remove the catheter.
▪ Administer oxygen, as ordered, and monitor the patient's response.
▪ Reassess the patient's respiratory status *to verify that the patient is in stable condition.*
▪ Turn off the suction source.
▪ Detach the catheter from the in-line specimen trap, gather it up in your dominant hand, and pull your glove cuff inside out and down around the used catheter. Then discard it appropriately.[20]
▪ Detach the trap from the tubing connected to the suction device. Seal the trap tightly by connecting the rubber tubing to the male adapter of the trap.

EQUIPMENT

Attaching a specimen trap to a suction catheter

Wearing sterile gloves, push the suction tubing onto the male adapter of the in-line specimen trap.

Insert the suction catheter into the rubber tubing of the trap.

After suctioning, disconnect the in-line trap from the suction tubing and catheter. *To seal the container,* connect the rubber tubing to the male adapter of the trap

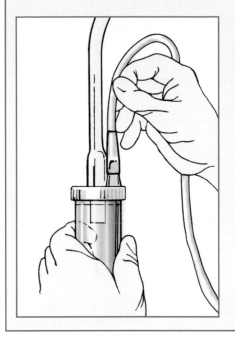 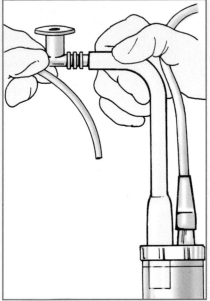 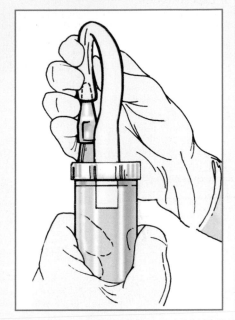

- Clear the suction tubing with normal saline solution.
- Return the bed to the lowest position *to prevent falls and maintain the patient's safety.*[24]

Completing the procedure
- Remove and discard your gloves and any other personal protective equipment worn.[20]
- Perform hand hygiene.[6,7,8,9,10,11]
- Label the specimen container in the presence of the patient *to prevent mislabeling.*[12] Include on the laboratory request form (if required by your facility) whether the patient was febrile or taking antibiotics, and whether sputum was induced, *because such specimens commonly appear watery and may resemble saliva.*[25,26]
- Send the specimen to the laboratory immediately in a laboratory biohazard transport bag.[20] *A delay in transport of the sample to the laboratory could damage the specimen and alter the accuracy of the results.*
- Offer to assist the patient with oral care and hand hygiene.[19]
- Clean and disinfect your stethoscope with a disinfectant pad.[27,28]
- Perform hand hygiene.[6,7,8,9,10,11]
- Document the procedure.[29,30,31,32]

Special considerations
- If possible, collect the specimen early in the morning, before breakfast, *because secretions accumulate overnight, making collection easier, and an empty stomach decreases the risk of vomiting food.*[3,33]
- If normal maximal cough efforts fail to produce a specimen, consider having the patient attempt the forced expiratory technique, also known as huff coughing, which consists of one or two huffs (forced expirations) from mid- to low-lung volumes with the glottis open. Have the patient repeat the process until maximal bronchial clearance occurs; the patient can reinforce the process by compressing the chest wall using a brisk adduction movement of the upper arms.[2,34]
- Ideally, obtain specimens before initiating antibiotic treatment.[35]

- Sputum induction increases TB case detection, is useful for patients who have negative results on spontaneous smear microscopy or who can't expectorate spontaneously, and is well tolerated.[36]
- If TB is suspected, institute airborne precautions (including N95 respirator use) in addition to standard precautions. Also place the patient in an airborne infection isolation room *to reduce the risk of transmission.*[19,37]
- If you can't obtain a sputum specimen, notify the practitioner to see if additional orders are needed. A nebulizer treatment, chest percussion, or postural drainage may be needed *to assist in specimen collection.*[3]

Complications
Patients with cardiac disease may develop arrhythmias or angina during the procedure as a result of coughing.[4] Other potential complications include nasal, pharyngeal and tracheal trauma; infection; discomfort or pain; increased intracranial pressure; increased or decreased blood pressure; vomiting; aspiration; laryngospasm; bronchospasm; hypoxemia and hypoxia; atelectasis; pneumothorax; respiratory arrest;[5] and light-headedness, nausea, and pain after abdominal surgery or chest trauma.

Documentation
Document the sputum collection method used; the time and date of collection; the patient's tolerance of the procedure; the color, volume, and consistency of the specimen; and the specimen's proper disposition. Document your assessment of the patient's respiratory status, including oxygen saturation, before, during, and after the procedure, as well as the patient's tolerance of the procedure. Document teaching provided to the patient and family (if applicable), their understanding of that teaching, and any need for follow-up teaching.

REFERENCES
1 Craven, R. F., et al. (2022). *Fundamentals of nursing: Concepts and competencies for practice* (9th ed.). Philadelphia, PA: Wolters Kluwer.
2 Kacmarek, R. M., et al. (2021). *Egan's fundamentals of respiratory care* (12th ed.). St. Louis, MO: Elsevier.

3   Hinkle, J. L., & Cheever, K. H. (2018). *Brunner & Suddarth's textbook of medical-surgical nursing* (14th ed.). Philadelphia, PA: Wolters Kluwer.

4   NSW Government. (2018). Sputum induction guidelines. https://www.health.nsw.gov.au/Infectious/tuberculosis/Pages/tb-sputum-induction-guidelines.aspx (Level VII)

5   American Association for Respiratory Care (AARC). (2004). AARC clinical practice guideline: Nasotracheal suctioning—2004 revision and update. *Respiratory Care, 49*(9), 1080–1084 http://rc.rcjournal.com/content/respcare/49/9/1080.full.pdf (Level VII)

6   Centers for Disease Control and Prevention. (2002). Guideline for hand hygiene in health-care settings: Recommendations of the Healthcare Infection Control Practices Advisory Committee and the HICPAC/SHEA/APIC/IDSA Hand Hygiene Task Force. *MMWR Recommendations and Reports, 51*(RR-16), 1–45. https://www.cdc.gov/mmwr/pdf/rr/rr5116.pdf (Level II)

7   The Joint Commission. (2021). Standard NPSG.07.01.01. *Comprehensive accreditation manual for hospitals.* Oakbrook Terrace, IL: The Joint Commission. (Level VII)

8   World Health Organization. (2009). WHO guidelines on hand hygiene in health care: First global patient safety challenge, clean care is safer care. https://apps.who.int/iris/bitstream/handle/10665/44102/9789241597906_eng.pdf?sequence=1 (Level IV)

9   Accreditation Association for Hospitals and Health Systems. (2020). Standard 07.01.21. *Healthcare Facilities Accreditation Program: Accreditation requirements for acute care hospitals.* Chicago, IL: Accreditation Association for Hospitals and Health Systems. (Level VII)

10 Centers for Medicare and Medicaid Services, Department of Health and Human Services. (2020). Condition of participation: Infection control. 42 C.F.R. § 482.42.

11 DNV GL-Healthcare USA, Inc. (2020). IC.1.SR.1. *NIAHO® accreditation requirements, interpretive guidelines and surveyor guidance—revision 20.0.* Milford, OH: DNV GL-Healthcare USA, Inc. (Level VII)

12 The Joint Commission. (2021). Standard NPSG.01.01.01. *Comprehensive accreditation manual for hospitals.* Oakbrook Terrace, IL: The Joint Commission. (Level VII)

13 DNV GL-Healthcare USA, Inc. (2020). PR.2.SR.5. *NIAHO® accreditation requirements, interpretive guidelines and surveyor guidance—revision 20.0.* Milford, OH: DNV GL-Healthcare USA, Inc. (Level VII)

14 Centers for Medicare and Medicaid Services, Department of Health and Human Services. (2020). Condition of participation: Patient's rights. 42 C.F.R. § 482.13(c)(1).

15 Accreditation Association for Hospitals and Health Systems. (2020). Standard 15.01.16. *Healthcare Facilities Accreditation Program: Accreditation requirements for acute care hospitals.* Chicago, IL: Accreditation Association for Hospitals and Health Systems. (Level VII)

16 The Joint Commission. (2021). Standard RI.01.01.01. *Comprehensive accreditation manual for hospitals.* Oakbrook Terrace, IL: The Joint Commission. (Level VII)

17 The Joint Commission. (2021). Standard PC.02.01.21. *Comprehensive accreditation manual for hospitals.* Oakbrook Terrace, IL: The Joint Commission. (Level VII)

18 Accreditation Association for Hospitals and Health Systems. (2020). Standard 07.01.10. *Healthcare Facilities Accreditation Program: Accreditation requirements for acute care hospitals.* Chicago, IL: Accreditation Association for Hospitals and Health Systems. (Level VII)

19 Siegel, J. D., et al. (2007, revised 2019). 2007 guideline for isolation precautions: Preventing transmission of infectious agents in healthcare settings. https://www.cdc.gov/infectioncontrol/pdf/guidelines/isolation-guidelines-H.pdf (Level II)

20 Occupational Safety and Health Administration. (2012). Bloodborne pathogens, standard number 1910.1030. https://www.osha.gov/pls/oshaweb/owadisp.show_document?p_id=10051&p_table=STANDARDS (Level VII)

21 Septimus, E. (2019). Collecting cultures: A clinician guide. https://www.cdc.gov/antibiotic-use/core-elements/collecting-cultures.html (Level VII)

22 Waters, T. R., et al. (2009). Safe patient handling training for schools of nursing. https://www.cdc.gov/niosh/docs/2009-127/pdfs/2009-127.pdf (Level VII)

23 Centers for Disease Control and Prevention. (2004). Guidelines for preventing health-care-associated pneumonia, 2003: Recommendations of CDC and the Healthcare Infection Control Practices Advisory Committee. *MMWR Recommendations and Reports, 53*(RR-3), 1–32. https://www.cdc.gov/mmwr/pdf/rr/rr5303.pdf (Level II)

24 Ganz, D. A., et al. (2013, reviewed 2021). *Preventing falls in hospitals: A toolkit for improving quality of care* (AHRQ Publication No. 13-0015-EF). Rockville, MD: Agency for Healthcare Research and Quality. https://www.ahrq.gov/professionals/systems/hospital/fallpxtoolkit/index.html (Level VII)

25 Fischbach, F., & Fischbach, M. A. (2022). *A manual of laboratory and diagnostic tests* (11th ed.). Philadelphia, PA: Wolters Kluwer.

26 Bernardo, J. (2021). Diagnosis of pulmonary tuberculosis in adults. In: *UpToDate,* von Reyn, C. F. (Ed.).

27 Accreditation Association for Hospitals and Health Systems. (2020). Standard 07.02.03. *Healthcare Facilities Accreditation Program: Accreditation requirements for acute care hospitals.* Chicago, IL: Accreditation Association for Hospitals and Health Systems. (Level VII)

28 Rutala, W. A., et al. (2008, revised 2019). Guideline for disinfection and sterilization in healthcare facilities, 2008. https://www.cdc.gov/infection-control/pdf/guidelines/disinfection-guidelines-H.pdf (Level I)

29 The Joint Commission. (2021). Standard RC.01.03.01. *Comprehensive accreditation manual for hospitals.* Oakbrook Terrace, IL: The Joint Commission. (Level VII)

30 Accreditation Association for Hospitals and Health Systems. (2020). Standard 10.00.03. *Healthcare Facilities Accreditation Program: Accreditation requirements for acute care hospitals.* Chicago, IL: Accreditation Association for Hospitals and Health Systems. (Level VII)

31 Centers for Medicare and Medicaid Services, Department of Health and Human Services. (2020). Condition of participation: Medical record services. 42 C.F.R. § 482.24(b).

32 DNV GL-Healthcare USA, Inc. (2020). MR.2.SR.1. *NIAHO® accreditation requirements, interpretive guidelines and surveyor guidance—revision 20.0.* Milford, OH: DNV GL-Healthcare USA, Inc. (Level VII)

33 Boruchoff, S. E., & Weinstein, M. P. (2022). Sputum cultures for the evaluation of bacterial pneumonia. In: *UpToDate,* Ramirez, J. A. (Ed.).

34 Strickland, S. L., et. al. (2013). AARC clinical practice guideline: Effectiveness of nonpharmacologic airway clearance therapies in hospitalized patients. *Respiratory Care, 58*(12), 2187–2193. https://www.aarc.org/wp-content/uploads/2014/08/nonpharmacologic_2013.pdf (Level VII)

35 Centers for Disease Control and Prevention. (n.d.). Specimen collection guidelines. https://www.cdc.gov/urdo/downloads/SpecCollectionGuidelines.pdf (Level VII)

36 Hepple, P., et al. (2012). Microscopy compared to culture for the diagnosis of tuberculosis in induced sputum samples: A systematic review. *International Journal of Tuberculosis and Lung Disease, 16*(6), 579–588. https://www.ingentaconnect.com/content/iuatld/ijtld/2012/00000016/00000005/art00005;jsessionid=9bentob7gq0n.x-ic-live-03 (Level I)

37 Centers for Disease Control and Prevention. (2005). Guidelines for preventing the transmission of *Mycobacterium tuberculosis* in health-care settings, 2005. *MMWR Recommendations and Reports, 54*(RR-17), 1–141. https://www.cdc.gov/mmwr/PDF/rr/rr5417.pdf (Level I)

STANDARD PRECAUTIONS

Standard precautions were developed by the Centers for Disease Control and Prevention (CDC) to protect against the transmission of infection. CDC officials recommend that health care workers assume that all patients are potentially infected or colonized (carriers without signs or symptoms of infection) with an organism that could be transmitted in the health care setting.[1]

Part of routine infection control practices, following standard precautions includes wearing gloves for situations involving known or anticipated contact with blood, body fluids, tissue, mucous membranes, or nonintact skin.[1] If the task or procedure being performed may result in splashing or splattering of blood or body fluids to the face, a mask and goggles or face shield should be worn. If the task or procedure being performed may result in splashing or splattering of blood or body fluids to the body, a fluid-resistant gown or apron should be worn.[1,2] Additional protective clothing such as shoe covers may be appropriate to protect the feet in situations that may expose the health care worker to large amounts of blood or body fluids (or both), such as when caring for a trauma patient in the operating room or emergency department.

Standard precautions should be combined with transmission-based precautions for patients with confirmed or suspected infection with highly transmissible pathogens.[1,3,4] (See *Transmission-based precautions* as

---

Transmission-based precautions[1]

Transmission-based precautions may be necessary in addition to standard precautions, depending on the patient's condition.

PRECAUTION TYPE	INDICATIONS	NURSING ACTIONS
Airborne	To prevent the spread of infection when a patient is suspected of or known to have an infection that's spread by the airborne route	■ Place the patient in an airborne infection isolation room with monitored negative pressure, if available. ■ Caution all people who enter the room to wear a respirator mask (N95).[1] ■ Staff who aren't immune to vaccine-preventable airborne diseases shouldn't care for the patient.[1]
Contact	To prevent the spread of epidemiologically important infectious organisms through direct patient contact or indirect contact with the patient's environment	■ Place the patient in a single-patient room, if possible. ■ Wear a gown and gloves for all interactions with the patient or the patient's environment. ■ Follow your facility's infection-control plan to determine when to initiate contact precautions.[3] ■ Designate patient care equipment if possible.[1]
Droplet	To prevent the spread of infectious organisms through close respiratory or mucous membrane contact with respiratory secretions from an infected patient	■ Place the patient in a single-patient room, if possible. ■ Put on a mask before entering the patient's room if working within 3′ (0.9 m) of the patient. ■ Designate patient care equipment if possible.[1] ■ The patient should wear a mask if transported outside of the room.[1]

---

well as the "Airborne precautions," "Contact precautions," and "Droplet precautions" procedures.)

NURSING ALERT When caring for a patient with known or suspected coronavirus disease 2019 (COVID-19), follow the latest recommendations from the CDC. For details, see https://www.cdc.gov/coronavirus/2019-ncov/hcp/infection-control-recommendations.html

NURSING ALERT When caring for a patient with known or suspected Ebola virus disease, follow the latest recommendations from the CDC. For details, see https://www.cdc.gov/vhf/ebola/clinicians/evd/infection-control.html

Equipment

Gloves ■ mask and goggles, or mask with face shield ■ gown ■ facility-approved disinfectant ■ puncture-resistant sharps disposal container ■ fluid-impervious bags or containers labeled BIOHAZARD ■ paper towels ■ detergent and water ■ laboratory biohazard transport bags ■ labels ■ Optional: shoe covers, apron, alcohol-based hand rub, sterile single-use disposable needles and syringes, safety needles, absorbent material for spills, tools to pick up broken objects, masks, tissues, laboratory requisition forms.

Implementation

■ Gather and prepare the necessary equipment and supplies.
■ Perform hand hygiene before and after patient care and before and after putting on and removing gloves. *Hand hygiene removes microorganisms from your skin.*[5,6,7,8,9,10,11] If your hands aren't visibly soiled, use an alcohol-based hand sanitizer for routine decontamination.[1,6,7,8,9,10,11]
■ Wash your hands immediately if they become contaminated with blood or body fluids, excretions, secretions, or drainage.[3,6,7,8,9,10,11]
■ Wear gloves if you will or could come in contact with blood, specimens, tissue, body fluids, secretions or excretions, mucous membrane, broken skin, or contaminated surfaces or objects.[1,2]
■ Change your gloves and perform hand hygiene when moving from a contaminated to a clean site during patient care and in between patient contacts *to avoid cross-contamination.*[1,5,6,7,8,9,10,11]
■ Wear a fluid-resistant gown as well as a mask and goggles or a mask with face shield during procedures likely to generate splash or splatter of blood or body fluids, such as surgery, endoscopic procedures, dialysis, catheter insertion, intubation, and manipulation of arterial lines.[1,2,5]
■ Wear a mask during lumbar puncture procedures, such as a myelogram and spinal and epidural anesthesia. The practitioner performing the procedure should wear a mask with a face shield.[1]

■ Follow safe injection practices; whenever possible, use single-dose vials instead of multidose vials. Use a sterile, single-use disposable needle and syringe for each injection.[1] Use safety needles if available.[2]
■ Handle used needles and other sharp instruments carefully. Don't bend or break them, reinsert them into their original sheaths, remove needles from syringes, or unnecessarily handle them. Activate any safety mechanisms immediately after use. Discard the instruments intact immediately after use into a puncture-resistant sharps disposal container. Use tools to pick up broken glass or other sharp objects. *These measures reduce the risk of accidental injury and infection.* Use a needleless IV system whenever possible.[1,2]
■ Immediately notify your employee health provider (or the provider's designee) of all needle-stick or other sharp-object injuries, mucosal splashes, or contamination of open wounds or nonintact skin with blood or body fluids, *to allow investigation of the incident and appropriate care and documentation.* Be sure to complete all follow-up screening and care as recommended by your employee health provider.[2]
■ Properly label all specimens collected from patients in the presence of the patient *to prevent mislabeling,* and place them in plastic bags at the collection site.[2,12] Attach requisition slips, if required, to the outside of all bags.[2]
■ Place all items that have come in direct contact with the patient's secretions, excretions, blood, drainage, or body fluids—such as nondisposable utensils or instruments—in a single impervious bag or container labelled BIOHAZARD before removal from the room. Place linens and trash in single bags of sufficient thickness to contain the contents.[1,2]
■ While wearing the appropriate personal protective equipment, promptly clean all blood and body fluid spills. Blot the spill with an absorbent material (such as a paper towel) first, and then clean the area with detergent and water. Notify the environmental services department of the spill *so they can properly clean the area.*[2]
■ If you have an exudative lesion, avoid all direct patient contact until the condition has resolved and you've been cleared by the employee health provider.[13]
■ If you have dermatitis or another condition resulting in broken skin on your hands, avoid situations where you may have contact with blood and body fluids (even if gloves are worn) until the condition has resolved and you've been cleared by the employee health care provider.
■ Perform hand hygiene and put on gloves, if needed, before cleaning and disinfecting reusable equipment. Following the manufacturer's instructions, properly clean and disinfect or sterilize reusable equipment with hospital-grade disinfectant before using it for another patient.[1,14,15] After cleaning and disinfecting reusable equipment, remove and discard your gloves, if worn, and perform hand hygiene.[1,2,5,6,7,8,9,10,11]

■ Teach patients, family members, and visitors about hand hygiene, respiratory hygiene, and cough etiquette. Instruct visitors to perform hand hygiene before and after visiting a patient. Provide a mask for anyone who shows signs or symptoms of a respiratory infection. Tell visitors to cover the mouths and nose with a tissue when coughing or sneezing, dispose of the tissue promptly, and then perform hand hygiene.[1,5,6,7,8,9,10]

Special considerations

■ Keep mouthpieces, resuscitation bags, and other ventilation devices nearby *to eliminate the need for emergency mouth-to-mouth resuscitation, which in turn reduces the risk of exposure to body fluids.*[1]

NURSING ALERT *Because you may not always know which organisms may be present in every clinical situation*, you must use standard precautions for every contact with blood, body fluids, secretions, excretions, drainage, mucous membranes, and nonintact skin.[1] Use your judgment in individual cases about whether to implement additional transmission-based precautions, such as airborne, droplet, or contact precautions or a combination of them. In addition, if your work exposes you to blood, you should receive the hepatitis B virus vaccine series.

Complications

Failure to comply with standard precautions may lead to exposure to bloodborne pathogens or other infectious agents and to all the complications they may cause.

Documentation

Record any transmission-based precautions that may be required in addition to standard precautions.[16,17,18] Document patient, family, and other visitor teaching provided, their understanding of that teaching, and any need for follow-up teaching.

REFERENCES

1 Siegel, J. D., et al. (2007, revised 2019). 2007 guideline for isolation precautions: Preventing transmission of infectious agents in healthcare settings. https://www.cdc.gov/infectioncontrol/pdf/guidelines/isolation-guidelines-H.pdf (Level II)
2 Occupational Safety and Health Administration. (2012). Bloodborne pathogens, standard number 1910.1030. https://www.osha.gov/pls/oshaweb/owadisp.show_document?p_id=10051&p_table=STANDARDS (Level VII)
3 The Joint Commission. (2021). Standard IC.02.01.01. *Comprehensive accreditation manual for hospitals.* (Level VII)
4 Accreditation Association for Hospitals and Health Systems. (2020). Standard 07.01.10. *Healthcare Facilities Accreditation Program: Accreditation requirements for acute care hospitals.* (Level VII)
5 World Health Organization. (2007). Standard precautions in healthcare. https://www.who.int/csr/resources/publications/EPR_AM2_E7.pdf (Level IV)
6 Centers for Disease Control and Prevention. (2002). Guideline for hand hygiene in health care settings: Recommendations of the Healthcare Infection Control Practices Advisory Committee and the HICPAC/SHEA/APIC/IDSA Hand Hygiene Task Force. *MMWR Recommendations and Reports, 51*(RR-16), 1–45. https://www.cdc.gov/mmwr/pdf/rr/rr5116.pdf (Level II)
7 The Joint Commission. (2021). Standard NPSG.07.01.01. *Comprehensive accreditation manual for hospitals.* (Level VII)
8 Centers for Medicare and Medicaid Services, Department of Health and Human Services. (2020). Condition of participation: Infection control. 42 C.F.R. § 482.42.
9 DNV GL-Healthcare USA, Inc. (2020). IC.1.SR.1. *NIAHO® accreditation requirements, interpretive guidelines and surveyor guidance—revision 20.0.* (Level VII)
10 World Health Organization. (2009). WHO guidelines on hand hygiene in health care: First global patient safety challenge, clean care is safer care. https://apps.who.int/iris/bitstream/handle/10665/44102/9789241597906_eng.pdf?sequence=1 (Level IV)
11 Accreditation Association for Hospitals and Health Systems. (2020). Standard 07.01.21. *Healthcare Facilities Accreditation Program: Accreditation requirements for acute care hospitals.* (Level VII)
12 The Joint Commission. (2021). Standard NPSG.01.01.01. *Comprehensive accreditation manual for hospitals.* (Level VII)
13 The Joint Commission. (2021). Standard IC.02.03.01. *Comprehensive accreditation manual for hospitals.* (Level VII)
14 Rutala, W. A., et al. (2008, revised 2019). Guideline for disinfection and sterilization in healthcare facilities, 2008. https://www.cdc.gov/infection-control/pdf/guidelines/disinfection-guidelines-H.pdf (Level I)
15 The Joint Commission. (2021). Standard IC.02.02.01. *Comprehensive accreditation manual for hospitals.* (Level VII)
16 Accreditation Association for Hospitals and Health Systems. (2020). Standard 10.00.03. *Healthcare Facilities Accreditation Program: Accreditation requirements for acute care hospitals.* (Level VII)
17 Centers for Medicare and Medicaid Services, Department of Health and Human Services. (2020). Condition of participation: Medical record services. 42 C.F.R. § 482.24(b).
18 DNV GL-Healthcare USA, Inc. (2020). MR.2.SR.1. *NIAHO® accreditation requirements, interpretive guidelines and surveyor guidance—revision 20.0.* (Level VII)

STERILE TECHNIQUE, BASIC

Sterile technique involves using specific actions and activities to prevent contamination and maintain sterility of specific areas during surgical and other invasive procedure.[1] Sterile technique should be followed whenever a patient's skin is intentionally perforated, during procedures that involve entry into a sterile body cavity,[2] or when contact with nonintact skin resulting from trauma or surgery is possible.

Procedures requiring sterile technique include any surgical procedure, vaginal birth, invasive radiologic procedures, preparation of total parenteral nutrition and chemotherapeutic agents, and vascular access insertion, care, and maintenance.[3] Other procedures, such as urinary catheter insertion, tracheostomy care, and surgical or wound irrigation and dressing changes, may also require sterile technique depending on the patient's condition and facility protocols.

Certain patients with compromised immune systems (such as those with burns or recent organ transplants and those receiving chemotherapy or radiation therapy) may require sterile technique more often, even for some procedures that would normally require only clean technique, *because of their increased susceptibility to infection.*[2]

Equipment

Sterile gloves ■ other personal protective equipment ■ sterile supplies, as required by the procedure to be performed ■ Optional: facility-approved disinfectant, sterile bowl, sterile transfer device, prescribed analgesic, sterile marker, sterile labels (blank or preprinted).[4,5]

Many procedures have commercially prepared kits that provide all of the necessary components.

Preparation of equipment

Inspect all equipment and supplies. If a product is expired, is defective, or has compromised integrity, remove it from patient use, label it as expired or defective, and report the expiration or defect as directed by your facility.

Ensure that the sterilization tape on reusable supplies has turned the appropriate color.[1] (See your facility's guidelines. The color depends on the product used and the sterilization method.) Prepare a clean surface for setting up the equipment for the sterile procedure.

Implementation

■ Verify the practitioner's order *to ensure that the right procedure is being performed on the right patient at the right time.*[6]
■ Review the patient's medical record for history of allergies to latex or medications.
■ If required by your facility, confirm that written informed consent has been obtained and that the signed consent form is in the patient's medical record.[7,8,9,10]
■ Gather and prepare the necessary equipment and supplies.
■ Perform hand hygiene.[11,12,13,14,15,16]
■ Confirm the patient's identity using at least two patient identifiers.[17]
■ Provide privacy.[18,19,20,21]

■ Explain the procedure to the patient and family (if appropriate) according to their individual communication and learning needs *to increase their understanding, allay their fears, and enhance cooperation.*[22]

■ Screen and assess the patient's pain using facility-defined criteria that are consistent with the patient's age, condition, and ability to understand.[23]

■ Treat the patient's pain, as needed and ordered, using nonpharmacologic or pharmacologic methods or a combination of approaches. Base the treatment plan on evidence-based practices and the patient's clinical condition, past medical history, and pain management goals.[23] Consider administering an analgesic 20 to 30 minutes before the procedure, as needed and ordered, following safe medication administration practices, *to promote patient comfort.*[24,25,26,27]

■ Remove you rings, watch, and bracelets.[28]

■ Perform hand hygiene.[11,12,13,14,15,16]

■ Follow standard precautions by putting on the necessary personal protective equipment for the procedure.[29,30,31]

Opening a sterile kit

■ Remove the plastic outer wrapper from the procedure kit, if one is present.

■ Place the inner wrapped kit on a clean, dry, flat surface, *because any moisture on the table could be absorbed through the wrapper and contaminate the sterile supplies.*

■ Position the kit so that the you can open the farthest wrapper first, *because doing so prevents contamination that may occur from moving your unsterile arm over the sterile items.*[1]

■ Grasp the outer portion of the flap and open the flap away from your body, keeping your arm outstretched to the side *so that it doesn't cross over the sterile field* (as shown below).[1]

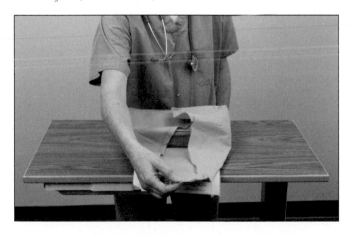

■ Grasp the outer surface of the first side flap with your hand on the same side as the flap (as shown below) *to avoid crossing over the sterile field.* Open the flap fully *to avoid allowing the wrapper to spring back in place.*

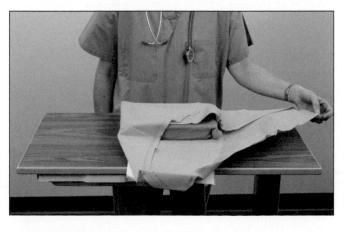

■ Grasp the outer surface of the second side flap and open it with your hand on the same side as the flap (as shown on top right).[1]

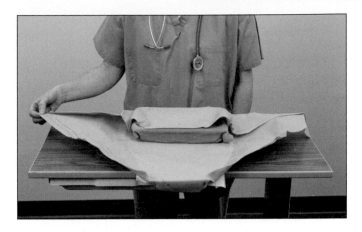

■ Grasp the outer surface of the innermost flap and open it toward your body (as shown below).[1]

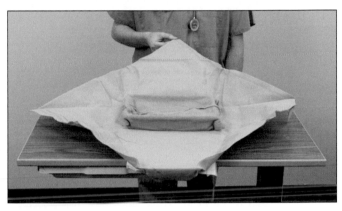

■ Secure the wrapper edges *to prevent them from contaminating sterile areas or items.*[1]

Opening a wrapped sterile item

■ Grasp the sterile item wrapped in paper or linen in your nondominant hand.

■ Break the sterilization tape.

■ Use your dominant hand to grasp the outer surface of the top outermost flap *to avoid touching a sterile surface.*

■ Open the flap away from your body.

■ Grasp the outer surface of the first side flap and open it fully to the side.

■ Repeat with the other side flap.

■ Secure all flaps in your nondominant hand *to avoid dangling and contaminating the sterile field.*

■ Grasp the outer surface of the inner flap and open it toward you.

■ Place the item on the sterile field, ensuring that only sterile surfaces touch other sterile surfaces *to avoid contamination.*[1]

■ Make sure the item is at least 1" (2.5 cm) from the edge of the sterile field.

Opening a peel-pack container or pouch

■ Grasp the unsealed corner of the wrapper and pull it toward you.

■ Open a peel-pack pouch (such as gloves and syringes) by grasping each side of the unsealed edge with the thumb side of each hand parallel to the seal and pulling apart gently.

■ Hold the sides back so the wrap covers your hands and exposes the sterile item.

■ If the item is light, drop it onto the sterile field. Don't allow the item to slide across the package side when dropping the item onto the sterile field. If the item is heavy, give it to a scrubbed person, or open it on a separate surface.[1]

Pouring a sterile solution

■ Open the wrapped package containing the sterile bowl as described above *to avoid contaminating the sterile field.* Label the bowl with the name of the solution to be poured into it.[32]

■ Place the bowl on the edge of the sterile field but inside of the 1" (2.5-cm) safety margin *so that solution can be poured without reaching across the sterile field.*[1]

■ Visually inspect the solution container; don't use the solution if the expiration date has passed or if there is an indication that the solution has been compromised.[1]

■ Unwrap the seal on the sterile solution bottle.

■ Unscrew the cap without touching the edges of the bottle.

■ Pour the solution into the appropriately labeled bowl without reaching over the sterile field.[1] Use a sterile transfer device, if available, *to reduce the risk of contamination of the sterile field from splashing and spilling.*

■ Pour the solution slowly *to avoid splashing onto the drape and contaminating the sterile field.*[1]

■ Discard any unused solution, *because you can't ensure sterility of the contents of the open solution container when replacing the cap.*[1]

Opening and putting on sterile gloves

■ Open the package containing the sterile gloves, touching only the outer side of the glove wrapper. Keep in mind that some commercially prepared kits (such as the kit for inserting an indwelling urinary catheter) include a pair of sterile gloves; if gloves are included they will be the uppermost item in the pack.

■ Perform hand hygiene.[11,12,13,14,15,16]

■ Grasp the paper glove wrapper and place it on a clean, dry, flat surface.

■ Open the inner package, touching only the outer edges of the wrapper (as shown below).

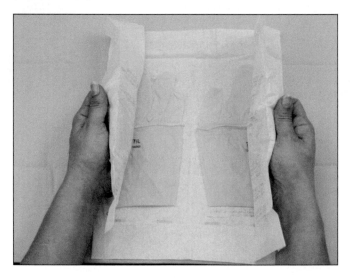

■ Use the thumb and fingers of your nondominant hand to grasp the folded inner surface portion of the glove for the dominant hand, touching only the inner portion of the glove (as shown below) *to avoid contaminating the outer portion of the glove.*

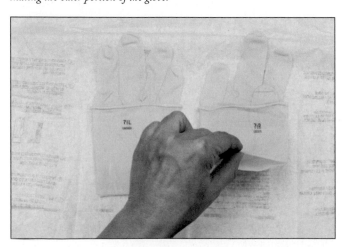

■ Lift up the glove and insert your dominant hand into the glove, palm side up (as shown below).

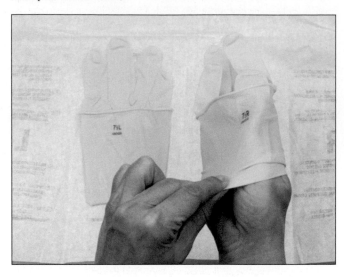

■ Pull down the cuff by touching only the inner surface of the glove. Gently stretch the glove over your hand. Make sure the outside of the glove doesn't touch the nonsterile surface.[33]

■ Insert the four fingers of your dominant gloved hand into the sterile outer cuff of the other glove, keeping your thumb pulled back out of the way (as shown below).

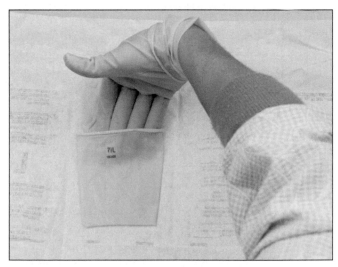

■ Lift up the glove and insert the nondominant hand into the glove. Allow the cuff to come uncuffed as you finish putting it on, but don't touch the skin of the arm with your gloved hand.

■ Adjust the fingers of the gloves after both your hands are gloved.

■ Keep your hands above waist level *to decrease the potential for contamination.*[33]

Special considerations

■ Open supplies away from the already set up sterile field *to avoid contaminating the field.*[28] Present sterile items directly to the sterile team member or place them securely on the sterile field.[1]

■ Be aware that medical asepsis, also called *clean technique*, isn't the same as sterile technique. Medical asepsis is focused on the absence of pathogenic organisms and doesn't require items to be sterile. Sterile technique and surgical asepsis are focused on the elimination of all microorganisms.[2]

Complications

Infection may result from failure to properly follow sterile technique.

Documentation

Document the procedure that you and the health care team performed, using guidelines for that procedure. Within this documentation, note the sterile supplies used and that sterile technique was followed. Note the date and time of the procedure.

REFERENCES

1 Guideline for perioperative practice: Sterile technique. (2021). In Wood, A. (Ed.), *Guidelines for perioperative practice, 2021 edition*. Denver, CO: Association of periOperative Registered Nurses. (Level VII)

2 Craven, R. F., et al. (2021). *Fundamentals of nursing: Concepts and competencies for practice* (9th ed.). Philadelphia, PA: Wolters Kluwer.

3 World Health Organization. (2009). Glove use information leaflet. https://www.who.int/gpsc/5may/Glove_Use_Information_Leaflet.pdf (Level VII)

4 Guideline for perioperative practice: Medication safety. (2021). In Wood, A. (Ed.), *Guidelines for perioperative practice, 2021 edition*. Denver, CO: Association of periOperative Registered Nurses. (Level VII)

5 Sheridan, D. J. (2006). Labeling solution and medications in sterile procedural settings. *Joint Commission Journal on Quality and Patient Safety, 32*, 276–282.

6 The Joint Commission. (2021). Standard UP.01.01.01. *Comprehensive accreditation manual for hospitals*. Oakbrook Terrace, IL: The Joint Commission. (Level VII)

7 The Joint Commission. (2021). Standard RI.01.03.01. *Comprehensive accreditation manual for hospitals*. Oakbrook Terrace, IL: The Joint Commission. (Level VII)

8 Centers for Medicare and Medicaid Services, Department of Health and Human Services. (2020). Condition of participation: Patient's rights. 42 C.F.R. § 482.13(b)(2).

9 Accreditation Association for Hospitals and Health Systems. (2020). Standard 15.01.11. *Healthcare Facilities Accreditation Program: Accreditation requirements for acute care hospitals*. Chicago, IL: Accreditation Association for Hospitals and Health Systems. (Level VII)

10 DNV GL-Healthcare USA, Inc. (2020). PR.2.SR.3. *NIAHO® accreditation requirements, interpretive guidelines and surveyor guidance—revision 20.0*. Milford, OH: DNV GL-Healthcare USA, Inc. (Level VII)

11 The Joint Commission. (2021). Standard NPSG 07.01.01. *Comprehensive accreditation manual for hospitals*. Oakbrook Terrace, IL: The Joint Commission. (Level VII)

12 Centers for Disease Control and Prevention. (2002). Guideline for hand hygiene in health-care settings: Recommendations of the Healthcare Infection Control Practices Advisory Committee and the HICPAC/SHEA/APIC/IDSA Hand Hygiene Task Force. *MMWR Recommendations and Reports, 51*(RR-16), 1–45. https://www.cdc.gov/mmwr/pdf/rr/rr5116.pdf (Level II)

13 World Health Organization. (2009). WHO guidelines on hand hygiene in health care: First global patient safety challenge, clean care is safer care. https://apps.who.int/iris/bitstream/handle/10665/44102/9789241597906_eng.pdf?sequence=1 (Level IV)

14 Accreditation Association for Hospitals and Health Systems. (2020). Standard 07.01.21. *Healthcare Facilities Accreditation Program: Accreditation requirements for acute care hospitals*. Chicago, IL: Accreditation Association for Hospitals and Health Systems. (Level VII)

15 Centers for Medicare and Medicaid Services, Department of Health and Human Services. (2020). Condition of participation: Infection control. 42 C.F.R. § 482.42.

16 DNV GL-Healthcare USA, Inc. (2020). IC.1.SR.1. *NIAHO® accreditation requirements, interpretive guidelines and surveyor guidance—revision 20.0*. Milford, OH: DNV GL-Healthcare USA, Inc. (Level VII)

17 The Joint Commission. (2021). Standard NPSG.01.01.01. *Comprehensive accreditation manual for hospitals*. Oakbrook Terrace, IL: The Joint Commission. (Level VII)

18 DNV GL-Healthcare USA, Inc. (2020). PR.2.SR.5. *NIAHO® accreditation requirements, interpretive guidelines and surveyor guidance—revision 20.0*. Milford, OH: DNV GL-Healthcare USA, Inc. (Level VII)

19 Centers for Medicare and Medicaid Services, Department of Health and Human Services. (2020). Condition of participation: Patient's rights. 42 C.F.R. § 482.13(c)(1).

20 Accreditation Association for Hospitals and Health Systems. (2020). Standard 15.01.16. *Healthcare Facilities Accreditation Program: Accreditation requirements for acute care hospitals*. Chicago, IL: Accreditation Association for Hospitals and Health Systems. (Level VII)

21 The Joint Commission. (2021). Standard RI.01.01.01. *Comprehensive accreditation manual for hospitals*. Oakbrook Terrace, IL: The Joint Commission. (Level VII)

22 The Joint Commission. (2021). Standard PC.02.01.21. *Comprehensive accreditation manual for hospitals*. Oakbrook Terrace, IL: The Joint Commission. (Level VII)

23 The Joint Commission. (2021). Standard PC.01.02.07. *Comprehensive accreditation manual for hospitals*. Oakbrook Terrace, IL: The Joint Commission. (Level VII)

24 Accreditation Association for Hospitals and Health Systems. (2020). Standard 16.01.03. *Healthcare Facilities Accreditation Program: Accreditation requirements for acute care hospitals*. Chicago, IL: Accreditation Association for Hospitals and Health Systems. (Level VII)

25 Centers for Medicare and Medicaid Services, Department of Health and Human Services. (2020). Condition of participation: Nursing services. 42 C.F.R. § 482.23(c).

26 DNV GL-Healthcare USA, Inc. (2020). MM.1.SR.3. *NIAHO® accreditation requirements, interpretive guidelines and surveyor guidance—revision 20.0*. Milford, OH: DNV GL-Healthcare USA, Inc. (Level VII)

27 The Joint Commission. (2021). Standard MM.06.01.01. *Comprehensive accreditation manual for hospitals*. Oakbrook Terrace, IL: The Joint Commission. (Level VII)

28 Guideline for perioperative practice: Hand hygiene. (2021). In Wood, A. (Ed.), *Guidelines for perioperative practice, 2021 edition*. Denver, CO: Association of periOperative Registered Nurses. (Level VII)

29 Accreditation Association for Hospitals and Health Systems. (2020). Standard 07.01.10. *Healthcare Facilities Accreditation Program: Accreditation requirements for acute care hospitals*. Chicago, IL: Accreditation Association for Hospitals and Health Systems. (Level VII)

30 Siegel, J. D., et al. (2007, revised 2019). 2007 guideline for isolation precautions: Preventing transmission of infectious agents in healthcare settings. https://www.cdc.gov/infectioncontrol/pdf/guidelines/isolation-guidelines-H.pdf (Level II)

31 Occupational Safety and Health Administration. (2012). Bloodborne pathogens, standard number 1910.1030. https://www.osha.gov/pls/oshaweb/owadisp.show_document?p_id=10051&p_table=STANDARDS (Level VII)

32 The Joint Commission. (2021). Standard NPSG.03.04.01. *Comprehensive accreditation manual for hospitals*. Oakbrook Terrace, IL: The Joint Commission. (Level VII)

33 Timby, B. K. (2017). *Fundamental nursing skills and concepts* (11th ed.). Philadelphia, PA: Wolters Kluwer.

STOOL SPECIMEN COLLECTION

Stool is collected to determine the presence of blood, ova and parasites, pathogens, leukocytes, and fat. Gross examination of stool characteristics, including color, consistency, and odor, can reveal such conditions as GI bleeding and steatorrhea.[1]

Stool specimens may be collected over a specific time period, such as 24, 48, 72, or 96 hours. Timed specimens are usually collected to test for fat, porphyrins, urobilinogen, nitrogen, and electrolytes.[1] Because stool specimens can't be obtained on demand, proper collection requires careful instructions to the patient to ensure an uncontaminated specimen.

Equipment

Specimen container with lid ■ gloves ■ specimen hat, bedpan or portable commode ■ transfer device (disposable tongue blade, spoon, spatula) ■ laboratory biohazard transport bag ■ specimen label ■ Optional: fluid-impermeable pad, absorbent adult briefs, gown, mask with face shield or mask and goggles, perineal area cleaning supplies, enema equipment (see the "Enema administration" procedure), laboratory request form, ice.

Commercial kits are available for stool specimen collection, preservation, and transport, depending on the specific testing requirements. Follow the manufacturer's instructions for use.

Implementation

- Review the practitioner's order for the stool collection.
- Gather and prepare the necessary equipment and supplies.
- Perform hand hygiene.[2,3,4,5,6,7]
- Confirm the patient's identity using at least two patient identifiers.[8]

- Provide privacy.[9,10,11,12]
- Explain the procedure to the patient and family (if appropriate) according to their individual communication and learning needs *to increase their understanding, allay their fears, and enhance cooperation.*[13]
- Tell the patient to notify you when the urge to defecate occurs. At that time, have the patient defecate into a specimen hat on the toilet, a clean, dry bedpan, or a portable commode. Instruct the patient not to contaminate the sample with urine or toilet tissue, *because urine inhibits fecal bacterial growth, and toilet tissue contains bismuth, which interferes with test results.* Instruct a female patient not to contaminate the sample with menstrual blood, *which may interfere with test results.*[1]
- Perform hand hygiene.[2,3,4,5,6,7]
- Put on gloves and, as needed, other personal protective equipment *to comply with standard precautions.*[14,15,16]

Random stool collection

- If the patient is incontinent, collect a stool sample from a fluid-impermeable pad or absorbent adult briefs.[1]
- Using a transfer device, transfer the entire stool sample from the specimen hat, bedpan, portable commode, or adult briefs to the specimen container, and place the lid on the specimen container.[1]
- If the patient passes blood, mucus, or pus with the stool, include it with the specimen. Notify the practitioner of abnormal findings.
- Discard the transfer device in the appropriate receptacle.[16]

Timed stool collection

- Place a patient care reminder that says SAVE ALL STOOLS over the patient's bed and in the bathroom.[1]
- Begin the timing of collections with the passage of the first stool.
- Perform hand hygiene.[2,3,4,5,6,7]
- Put on gloves and, as needed other personal protective equipment *to comply with standard precautions.*[14,15,16]
- If the patient is incontinent, collect a stool sample from a fluid-impermeable pad or absorbent adult briefs.[1]
- Collect each specimen by using a transfer device to transfer the entire stool from the specimen hat, bedpan, portable commode, or adult briefs to the container, and include all the stool in the total specimen.[9,17]
- Continue to collect stools passed, remembering to transfer all stools to the specimen container. Notify the practitioner of abnormal stools.[1]
- If stool must be obtained with an enema, most tests allow for use of normal saline solution. Contact the laboratory before using an enema *to verify what can be used.*[1]
- Label all specimens in the presence of the patient *to prevent mislabeling.*[8] If you're submitting individual specimens to the laboratory, label each specimen with the day of test (Day 1, Day 2, Day 3, Day 4) and the time of day that it was collected.[1]

Completing the procedure

- Remove and discard your gloves and any other personal protective equipment, if worn.[16]
- Perform hand hygiene.[2,3,4,5,6,7]
- Label all specimens in the presence of the patient *to prevent mislabeling.*[8]
- Provide the patient with the opportunity to thoroughly clean the perianal area and perform hand hygiene. Assist as necessary.
- Place the labeled specimen in the laboratory biohazard bag and immediately send each stool specimen to the laboratory with a laboratory request form (if required in your facility). Depending on the test ordered, the sample may need to be transported on ice. Alternatively, if permitted, refrigerate the specimens collected during the test period and send them to the laboratory when the collection is complete. Contact the laboratory for specific directions.[1,16,17]
- Perform hand hygiene.[2,3,4,5,6,7]
- Document the procedure.[18,19,20,21]

Special considerations

- Never place a stool specimen in a refrigerator that contains food or medication, *to prevent contamination.*[16]

- If testing for *Clostridioides difficile*, collect only diarrheal (unformed) stool unless ileus due to infection is suspected.[22,23]
- Certain drugs and substances render stool specimens unsatisfactory for laboratory testing. These substances include antacids, kaolin, mineral oil and other oily materials, nonabsorbable antidiarrheal preparations, barium or bismuth (which need 7 to 10 days for effects to clear), antimicrobial agents (which need 2 to 3 weeks), and gallbladder dyes (which need 3 weeks). If possible, collect specimens before these substances are administered; otherwise, wait to collect specimens until after the effects have passed.[1,24]

Patient teaching

Instruct the patient who will be obtaining a specimen at home to collect it in a clean container with a tight-fitting lid, wrap the container in a paper bag, and keep it in the refrigerator (separate from food items) until it can be transported.[1]

Documentation

Record the date and time you collected the specimen and sent it to the laboratory. Record the stool's color, odor, and consistency as well as any unusual characteristics; also note whether the patient had difficulty passing the stool and whether you needed to administer an enema to obtain the specimens. Document teaching provided to the patient and family (if appropriate), their understanding of that teaching, and any need for follow-up teaching.

REFERENCES
1 Fischbach, F., & Fischbach, M. A. (2022). *A manual of laboratory and diagnostic tests* (11th ed.). Philadelphia, PA: Wolters Kluwer.
2 The Joint Commission. (2021). Standard NPSG.07.01.01. *Comprehensive accreditation manual for hospitals.* Oakbrook Terrace, IL: The Joint Commission. (Level VII)
3 Centers for Disease Control and Prevention. (2002). Guideline for hand hygiene in health-care settings: Recommendations of the Healthcare Infection Control Practices Advisory Committee and the HICPAC/SHEA/APIC/IDSA Hand Hygiene Task Force. *MMWR Recommendations and Reports, 51*(RR-16), 1–45. https://www.cdc.gov/mmwr/pdf/rr/rr5116.pdf (Level II)
4 World Health Organization. (2009). WHO guidelines on hand hygiene in health care: First global patient safety challenge, clean care is safer care. https://apps.who.int/iris/bitstream/handle/10665/44102/9789241597906_eng.pdf?sequence=1 (Level IV)
5 Accreditation Association for Hospitals and Health Systems. (2020). Standard 07.01.21. *Healthcare Facilities Accreditation Program: Accreditation requirements for acute care hospitals.* Chicago, IL: Accreditation Association for Hospitals and Health Systems. (Level VII)
6 Centers for Medicare and Medicaid Services, Department of Health and Human Services. (2020). Condition of participation: Infection control. 42 C.F.R. § 482.42.
7 DNV GL-Healthcare USA, Inc. (2020). IC.1.SR.1. *NIAHO® accreditation requirements, interpretive guidelines and surveyor guidance—revision 20.0.* Milford, OH: DNV GL-Healthcare USA, Inc. (Level VII)
8 The Joint Commission. (2021). Standard NPSG.01.01.01. *Comprehensive accreditation manual for hospitals.* Oakbrook Terrace, IL: The Joint Commission. (Level VII)
9 The Joint Commission. (2021). Standard RI.01.01.01. *Comprehensive accreditation manual for hospitals.* Oakbrook Terrace, IL: The Joint Commission. (Level VII)
10 Centers for Medicare and Medicaid Services, Department of Health and Human Services. (2020). Condition of participation: Patient's rights. 42 C.F.R. § 482.13(c)(1).
11 Accreditation Association for Hospitals and Health Systems. (2020). Standard 15.01.16. *Healthcare Facilities Accreditation Program: Accreditation requirements for acute care hospitals.* Chicago, IL: Accreditation Association for Hospitals and Health Systems. (Level VII)
12 DNV GL-Healthcare USA, Inc. (2020). PR.2.SR.5. *NIAHO® accreditation requirements, interpretive guidelines and surveyor guidance—revision 20.0.* Milford, OH: DNV GL-Healthcare USA, Inc. (Level VII)
13 The Joint Commission. (2021). Standard PC.02.01.21. *Comprehensive accreditation manual for hospitals.* Oakbrook Terrace, IL: The Joint Commission. (Level VII)

14 Siegel, J. D., et al. (2007, revised 2019). 2007 guideline for isolation precautions: Preventing transmission of infectious agents in healthcare settings. https://www.cdc.gov/infectioncontrol/pdf/guidelines/isolation-guidelines-H.pdf (Level II)

15 Accreditation Association for Hospitals and Health Systems. (2020). Standard 07.01.10. *Healthcare Facilities Accreditation Program: Accreditation requirements for acute care hospitals.* Chicago, IL: Accreditation Association for Hospitals and Health Systems. (Level VII)

16 Occupational Safety and Health Administration. (2012). Bloodborne pathogens, standard number 1910.1030. https://www.osha.gov/pls/oshaweb/owadisp.show_document?p_id=10051&p_table=STANDARDS (Level VII)

17 Sharma, L. (2018). Evidence summary. Fecal specimen: Collection and assessment. *The JBI EBP Database.* AN: JBI211

18 The Joint Commission. (2021). Standard RC.01.03.01. *Comprehensive accreditation manual for hospitals.* Oakbrook Terrace, IL: The Joint Commission. (Level VII)

19 Centers for Medicare and Medicaid Services, Department of Health and Human Services. (2020). Condition of participation: Medical record services. 42 C.F.R. § 482.24(b).

20 Accreditation Association for Hospitals and Health Systems. (2020). Standard 10.00.03. *Healthcare Facilities Accreditation Program: Accreditation requirements for acute care hospitals.* Chicago, IL: Accreditation Association for Hospitals and Health Systems. (Level VII)

21 DNV GL-Healthcare USA, Inc. (2020). MR.2.SR.1. *NIAHO® accreditation requirements, interpretive guidelines and surveyor guidance—revision 20.0.* Milford, OH: DNV GL-Healthcare USA, Inc. (Level VII)

22 Dubberke, E. R., et al. (2014). Strategies to prevent Clostridium difficile infections in acute care hospitals: 2014 update. *Infection Control & Hospital Epidemiology, 35*(6), 628–645. (Level VII)

23 McDonald, L. C., et al. (2018). Clinical practice guidelines for Clostridium difficile infection in adults and children: 2017 update by the Infectious Diseases Society of America (IDSA) and Society for Healthcare Epidemiology of America (SHEA). *Clinical Infectious Diseases, 66*(7), e1–e48. https://www.ncbi.nlm.nih.gov/pmc/articles/PMC6018983/ (Level I)

24 Centers for Disease Control and Prevention. (2016). DPDx—Laboratory identification of parasites of public health concern: Stool specimen—Specimen collection. https://www.cdc.gov/dpdx/diagnosticprocedures/stool/specimencoll.html (Level VII)

ST-SEGMENT MONITORING

A sensitive indicator of myocardial damage, the ST segment is normally flat or isoelectric. A depressed ST segment may result from cardiac glycosides, myocardial ischemia, or a subendocardial infarction. An elevated ST segment suggests myocardial infarction (MI).[1]

Continuous ST-segment monitoring is helpful for patients with acute coronary syndromes and for those who have received thrombolytic therapy or have undergone coronary angioplasty or cardiac surgery.[2] ST-segment monitoring allows early detection of reocclusion. It's also useful for patients who have had previous episodes of cardiac ischemia without chest pain, for those who have difficulty distinguishing cardiac pain from pain associated with other sources, and for those who have difficulty communicating.[3] It enables the practitioner to identify and reverse ischemia by starting early interventions, avoiding myocardial damage.[2] In addition, the American Heart Association recommends ST-segment monitoring for arrhythmias only for suspected ischemia and patients with acute stroke who are at increased risk for cardiac events.[2]

Because ischemia typically occurs in only one portion of the heart muscle, not all electrocardiogram (ECG) leads detect it. Continuous ST-segment monitoring of all 12 leads is preferred if available.[3] If it isn't available, examining ECG tracings obtained during an ischemic episode or identifying an occluded coronary artery that leads to ischemia using angiography allows selection of the most appropriate lead.[2] The leads showing ischemia are the same leads used for ST-segment monitoring; they're referred to as the "ST fingerprint."[2,3]

Because of frequent false alarms, ST-segment monitoring isn't useful for patients who are restless and patients with a ventricular paced rhythm or a rhythm that obscures the ST segment (such as coarse atrial fibrillation or flutter, or intermittent accelerated idioventricular rhythm).[2,4]

Although guidelines typically discourage ST-segment monitoring in patients with existing left bundle-branch block, it may help diagnose MI in these patients.[3]

Equipment

ECG electrodes ∎ ECG monitor cable ∎ lead wires ∎ cardiac monitor programmed for ST-segment monitoring ∎ soap and water or cleaning pads ∎ gauze pad or washcloth ∎ black indelible marker ∎ Optional: gloves, disposable-head clippers, single-patient-use scissors.

Preparation of equipment

Inspect all equipment and supplies. If a product is expired, is defective, or has compromised integrity, remove it from patient use, label it as expired or defective, and report the expiration or defect as directed by your facility.

Bring the equipment to the patient's bedside, plug the cardiac monitor into an electrical outlet, and turn the monitor on.

Implementation

∎ Verify the practitioner's order.
∎ Gather and prepare the necessary equipment and supplies.
∎ Perform hand hygiene.[5,6,7,8,9,10]
∎ Confirm the patient's identity using at least two patient identifiers.[11]
∎ Provide privacy.[12,13,14,15]
∎ Explain the procedure to the patient and family (if appropriate) according to their communication and learning needs *to increase their understanding, allay their fears, and enhance cooperation.*[16]
∎ Raise the patient's bed to waist level when providing patient care *to prevent caregiver back strain.*[17]
∎ Place the patient in the supine position with the head of the bed elevated less than 45 degrees, *because ST-segment changes that mimic ischemia can occur with changes in body position.*[3]
∎ Perform hand hygiene.[5,6,7,8,9,10]
∎ Put on gloves, as necessary, *to comply with standard precautions.*[18,19,20]
∎ Select the sites for electrode placement.[21]
∎ Properly prepare the patient's skin for electrode placement. If necessary, clip excess hair from intended sites with disposable-head clippers or single-patient-use scissors *to ensure good skin contact with the electrodes.*[4,22] Clean the intended sites with soap and water or cleaning pads, and then dry them thoroughly with a washcloth or gauze pad *to enhance electrode contact.* Don't use alcohol for skin preparation *because it dries out the skin.*[22] Gently abrade the skin at the intended sites with a gauze pad or washcloth *to roughen a small area of the skin and promote electrode adherence.*[4]
∎ Mark the intended sites with black indelible ink when electrode placement has been determined *to prevent inaccurate electrode placement and false-positive changes if an electrode needs to be replaced.*[3,4]
∎ Attach the lead wires to the electrodes, check the conductive gel on each electrode placement *to make sure it's sufficiently moist,* and position the electrodes appropriately on the patient's skin.[4]
∎ Activate ST-segment monitoring according to the manufacturer's instruction.
∎ Select the appropriate ECG for each ST channel to be monitored. If continuous 12-lead ST-segment monitoring is unavailable, use the patient's ST fingerprint to determine the leads to monitor. If the ST fingerprint isn't available, choose the leads most likely to show arrhythmias and ST-segment changes:[3] Lead III (or aV_F) is sensitive to inferior wall or right coronary artery ischemia. Lead V_3 (or V_2) is sensitive to anterior wall or left anterior descending artery ischemia. Lead V_5 or V_4 is recommended to identify demand-related ischemia in high-risk patients undergoing noncardiac surgical procedures as well as in those with critical medical illness. Lead V_6 is sensitive to left circumflex artery ischemia. Lead V_4R is recommended to assess for coexisting right ventricular MI in patients with acute ST-segment elevation MI in the inferior wall. Leads III (or aV_F) and V_3 (or V_2) are recommended for patients with suspected acute coronary syndrome who haven't yet shown ECG changes or changes in coronary anatomy.[3]
∎ Identify the ECG complex landmarks, as prompted by the monitor.[4]

■ Adjust the ST point to 60 milliseconds (ms) after the J point (as shown below).[3]

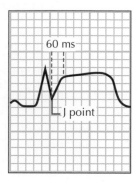

■ Set the alarm limits for each ST-segment parameter by manipulating the high- and low-limit keys. Set the alarm parameter to 1 mm above and below the patient's baseline ST segment in all leads except V_2 and V_3. In those leads, set the upper alarm limit at 1.5 mm from baseline for a female patient and 2 mm from the baseline for a male patient.[3] Make sure the alarms are turned on, functioning properly, and audible to staff members.[22,23,24,25]

■ Press the appropriate key *to return to the display screen.*

■ Assess the waveform shown on the monitor. Print a baseline ECG tracing *to evaluate the quality of the signal.*[4] Evaluate for ST-segment depression or elevation. (See *Changes in the ST segment.*) Measure ST-segment

changes 60 ms beyond the J point of the ECG complex. ST-segment depression or elevation that lasts for at least 1 minute may be clinically significant; assess the patient further and notify the patient's practitioner.[2,3]

■ Return the bed to the lowest position *to prevent falls and maintain patient safety.*[26]

■ Discard supplies in the appropriate receptacles.[20]

■ Remove and discard your gloves, if worn.[20]

■ Perform hand hygiene.[5,6,7,8,9,10]

■ Document the procedure.[27,28,29,30]

Special considerations

■ Check electrode placement every shift, evaluate ST-segment trends when obtaining vital signs, and respond appropriately to all ST-segment alarms. If you note ischemia, obtain a 12-lead ECG and assess the patient for signs and symptoms of acute ischemia (for example, arrhythmias, angina, and hemodynamic changes).[4]

■ Consider changing electrodes daily *to decrease the number of false alarms.*[22]

Complications

Complications include skin irritation at the electrode sites.

Documentation

Document in the patient's medical record the leads you monitored and the ST-segment measurement points. Document the initial ECG strip with the baseline ST-segment monitoring and any strips that suggest ST-segment changes. Document teaching provided to the patient and family (if applicable), their understanding of that teaching, and any need for follow-up teaching.

Changes in the ST segment

Closely monitoring the ST segment on a patient's ECG can help you detect ischemia or injury before the infarction develops.

ST-segment depression

An ST segment is considered depressed when it's 0.5 mm or more below the baseline. A depressed ST segment may indicate myocardial ischemia or digoxin toxicity.

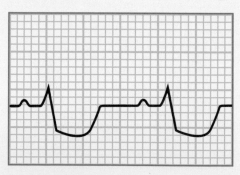

ST-segment elevation

An ST segment is considered elevated when it's 1 mm or more above the baseline. An elevated ST segment may indicate myocardial injury.

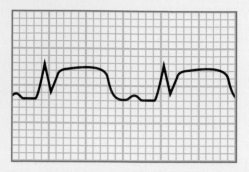

REFERENCES

1 Hinkle, J. L., & Cheever, K. H. (2018). *Brunner & Suddarth's textbook of medical-surgical nursing* (14th ed.). Philadelphia, PA: Wolters Kluwer.

2 Sandau, K. E., et al. (2017). Update to practice standards for electrocardiographic monitoring in hospital settings: A scientific statement from the American Heart Association. *Circulation, 136*(19), e273–e344. https://www.ahajournals.org/doi/pdf/10.1161/CIR.0000000000000527 (Level VII)

3 American Association of Critical-Care Nurses (AACN). (2018). AACN practice alert: Ensuring accurate ST-segment monitoring. https://www.aacn.org/clinical-resources/practice-alerts/st-segment-monitoring (Level VII)

4 Wiegand, D. L. (2017). *AACN procedure manual for high acuity, progressive, and critical care* (7th ed.). St. Louis, MO: Elsevier.

5 World Health Organization (WHO). (2009). WHO guidelines on hand hygiene in health care: First global patient safety challenge, clean care is safer care. https://apps.who.int/iris/bitstream/handle/10665/44102/9789241597906_eng.pdf?sequence=1 (Level IV)

6 Centers for Disease Control and Prevention. (2002). Guideline for hand hygiene in health-care settings: Recommendations of the Healthcare Infection Control Practices Advisory Committee and the HICPAC/SHEA/APIC/IDSA Hand Hygiene Task Force. *MMWR Recommendations and Reports, 51*(RR-16), 1–45. https://www.cdc.gov/mmwr/pdf/rr/rr5116.pdf (Level II)

7 Centers for Medicare and Medicaid Services, Department of Health and Human Services. (2020). Condition of participation: Infection control. 42 C.F.R. § 482.42.

8 The Joint Commission. (2021). Standard NPSG.07.01.01. *Comprehensive accreditation manual for hospitals.* Oakbrook Terrace, IL: The Joint Commission. (Level VII)

9 Accreditation Association for Hospitals and Health Systems. (2020). Standard 07.01.21. *Healthcare Facilities Accreditation Program: Accreditation requirements for acute care hospitals.* Chicago, IL: Accreditation Association for Hospitals and Health Systems. (Level VII)

10 DNV GL-Healthcare USA, Inc. (2020). IC.1.SR.1. *NIAHO® accreditation requirements, interpretive guidelines and surveyor guidance—revision 20.0.* Milford, OH: DNV GL-Healthcare USA, Inc. (Level VII)

11 The Joint Commission. (2021). Standard NPSG.01.01.01. *Comprehensive accreditation manual for hospitals.* Oakbrook Terrace, IL: The Joint Commission. (Level VII)

12 Accreditation Association for Hospitals and Health Systems. (2020). Standard 15.01.16. *Healthcare Facilities Accreditation Program:*

Accreditation requirements for acute care hospitals. Chicago, IL: Accreditation Association for Hospitals and Health Systems. (Level VII)

13 Centers for Medicare and Medicaid Services, Department of Health and Human Services. (2020). Condition of participation: Patient's rights. 42 C.F.R. § 482.13(c)(1).

14 The Joint Commission. (2021). Standard RI.01.01.01. *Comprehensive accreditation manual for hospitals.* Oakbrook Terrace, IL: The Joint Commission. (Level VII)

15 DNV GL-Healthcare USA, Inc. (2020). PR.2.SR.5. *NIAHO® accreditation requirements, interpretive guidelines and surveyor guidance—revision 20.0.* Milford, OH: DNV GL-Healthcare USA, Inc. (Level VII)

16 The Joint Commission. (2021). Standard PC.02.01.21. *Comprehensive accreditation manual for hospitals.* Oakbrook Terrace, IL: The Joint Commission. (Level VII)

17 Waters, T. R., et al. (2009). Safe patient handling training for schools of nursing. https://www.cdc.gov/niosh/docs/2009-127/pdfs/2009-127.pdf (Level VII)

18 Siegel, J. D., et al. (2007, revised 2019). 2007 guideline for isolation precautions: Preventing transmission of infectious agents in healthcare settings. https://www.cdc.gov/infectioncontrol/pdf/guidelines/isolation-guidelines-H.pdf (Level II)

19 Accreditation Association for Hospitals and Health Systems. (2020). Standard 07.01.10. *Healthcare Facilities Accreditation Program: Accreditation requirements for acute care hospitals.* Chicago, IL: Accreditation Association for Hospitals and Health Systems. (Level VII)

20 Occupational Safety and Health Administration. (2012). Bloodborne pathogens, standard number 1910.1030. https://www.osha.gov/pls/oshaweb/owadisp.show_document?p_id=10051&p_table=STANDARDS (Level VII)

21 Kligfield, P., et al. (2007). Recommendations for the standardization and interpretation of the electrocardiogram: Part I—the electrocardiogram and its technology. *Circulation, 115*(10), 1306–1324. https://www.ahajournals.org/doi/pdf/10.1161/circulationaha.106.180200 (Level II)

22 American Association of Critical-Care Nurses (AACN). (2018). AACN practice alert: Managing alarms in acute care across the life span: Electrocardiography and pulse oximetry. https://www.aacn.org/clinical-resources/practice-alerts/managing-alarms-in-acute-care-across-the-life-span (Level VII)

23 The Joint Commission. (2021). Standard NPSG.06.01.01. *Comprehensive accreditation manual for hospitals.* Oakbrook Terrace, IL: The Joint Commission. (Level VII)

24 The Joint Commission. (2013). Sentinel event alert 50: Medical device alarm safety in hospitals. https://www.jointcommission.org/assets/1/6/SEA_50_alarms_4_26_16.pdf (Level VII)

25 Graham, K. C., & Cvach, M. (2010). Monitor alarm fatigue: Standardizing use of physiological monitors and decreasing nuisance alarms. *American Journal of Critical Care, 19*(1), 28–37. https://doi.org/10.4037/ajcc2010651

26 Ganz, D. A., et al. (2013, reviewed 2021). *Preventing falls in hospitals: A toolkit for improving quality of care* (AHRQ Publication No. 13-0015-EF). Agency for Healthcare Research and Quality. https://www.ahrq.gov/professionals/systems/hospital/fallpxtoolkit/index.html (Level VII)

27 The Joint Commission. (2021). Standard RC.01.03.01. *Comprehensive accreditation manual for hospitals.* Oakbrook Terrace, IL: The Joint Commission. (Level VII)

28 Accreditation Association for Hospitals and Health Systems. (2020). Standard 10.00.03. *Healthcare Facilities Accreditation Program: Accreditation requirements for acute care hospitals.* Chicago, IL: Accreditation Association for Hospitals and Health Systems. (Level VII)

29 Centers for Medicare and Medicaid Services, Department of Health and Human Services. (2020). Condition of participation: Medical record services. 42 C.F.R. § 482.24(b).

30 DNV GL-Healthcare USA, Inc. (2020). MR.2.SR.1. *NIAHO® accreditation requirements, interpretive guidelines and surveyor guidance—revision 20.0.* Milford, OH: DNV GL-Healthcare USA, Inc. (Level VII)

SUBCUTANEOUS INJECTION

Subcutaneous injection delivers a drug into the adipose (fatty) tissue beneath the skin.[1] This method allows the drug to move into the bloodstream more rapidly than when given with oral administration, because it's absorbed by the body mainly through capillaries. When compared with intramuscular injection, subcutaneous injection provides slower, more sustained drug delivery, minimizes tissue trauma, and carries little risk of striking large blood vessels and nerves with the syringe needle.

Drugs recommended for subcutaneous injection include nonirritating aqueous solutions and suspensions contained in 0.5 to 2 mL of fluid.[1] Larger volumes may cause discomfort and inadequate medication absorption. Heparin and insulin, for example, are usually administered subcutaneously. (Some diabetic patients may benefit from an insulin infusion pump.) Some vaccines are also administered by subcutaneous injection.

Subcutaneous injections are performed using a relatively short needle. The most common sites are the outer aspect of the upper arm, anterior thigh, loose tissue of the lower abdomen, upper hips, buttocks, and upper back. (See *Locating subcutaneous injection sites.*) Subcutaneous injections are contraindicated in sites that are inflamed, edematous, infected, scarred, or covered by a mole, birthmark, or other lesion. They may also be contraindicated in patients with impaired coagulation mechanisms.

Equipment

Prescribed medication ▪ patient's medication administration record ▪ 25G to 30G ½" (1.3-cm) to ⅝" (1.6-cm) needle ▪ 1- to 3-mL syringe ▪ antiseptic pads ▪ gauze pads ▪ Optional: gloves, other personal protective equipment, filter needle, label.

Implementation

▪ Avoid distractions and interruptions when preparing and administering medication *to prevent medication errors.*[2,3]

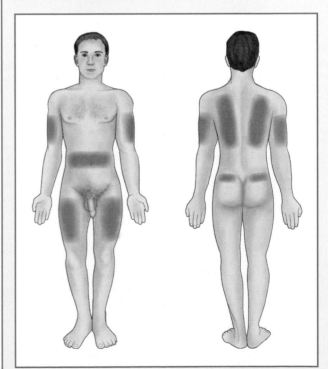

Locating subcutaneous injection sites

Subcutaneous injection sites (highlighted below) include the fat pads on the abdomen, upper hips, and lateral upper arms and thighs. For repeated subcutaneous injections, such as insulin administration, rotate sites. Choose one injection site in one area, move to a corresponding injection site in the next area, and so on. When returning to an area, choose a new site in that area.

Preferred injection sites for insulin are the arms, abdomen, thighs, and buttocks. The preferred injection site for heparin is the lower abdominal fat pad, just below the umbilicus.

- Verify the practitioner's order.[4,5,6,7]
- Reconcile the patient's medications when a new medication is ordered *to reduce the risk of medication errors, including omissions, duplications, dosing errors, and drug interactions.*[8,9]
- Gather the prescribed medication and necessary equipment and supplies.
- Compare the medication label with the order in the patient's medication administration record.[4,5,6,7]
- Review the patient's medical record for allergies or contraindications to the prescribed medication. If an allergy or a contraindication exists, don't administer the medication; instead, notify the practitioner.[4,5,6,7]
- Check the expiration date on the medication. If the medication is expired, return it to the pharmacy and obtain new medication.[4,5,6,7]
- Visually inspect the medication for particles, discoloration, and other signs of loss of integrity; don't administer the medication if its integrity is compromised.[4,5,6,7]
- Discuss any unresolved concerns about the medication with the patient's practitioner.[4,5,6,7]
- Calculate the dosage and have another nurse verify your calculations, if necessary.

NURSING ALERT Insulin and heparin are considered high-alert medications *because they can cause significant patient harm when used in error.*[10] Before administering either medication, have another nurse perform an independent double-check (if required by your facility) *to verify the patient's identity and to make sure that the correct medication is being administered in the prescribed concentration, the medication's indication corresponds with the patient's diagnosis, the dosage calculations are correct and the dosing formula used to derive the final dose is correct, and the route of administration is safe and appropriate for the patient.* Compare your results with the results of the independent double-check and, if no discrepancies exist, administer the medication. If discrepancies exist, rectify them before administering the drug.[11]

- Perform hand hygiene.[12,13,14,15,16,17]

NURSING ALERT If your facility's hazardous drug list contains the drug you're about to administer, put on personal protective equipment, as directed.[18]

- If you need to draw up the medication for injection, read the label again as you draw it up. If you aren't going to administer the medication immediately, label the syringe to help prevent medication administration errors. Immediate administration of a medication includes preparation, direct transport to the patient, and administration without any break in the process.[19,20]

Drawing up medication from a single-dose ampule

- Wrap a gauze pad around the ampule's neck and snap off the top, directing the force away from your body. Alternatively, insert the ampule's head into an ampule breaker. Attach a filter needle to the syringe and withdraw the medication, keeping the needle's bevel tip below the level of the solution. Tap the syringe *to clear air from it.* Cover the needle with the needle sheath.
- Before discarding the ampule, check the medication label against the patient's medication administration record.
- Detach the filter needle, and discard the filter needle and ampule in a puncture-resistant sharps container. Attach the appropriate needle to the syringe.
- Whenever possible, use a single-dose vial instead of a multidose vial. If a single-dose vial isn't available, dedicate a multidose medication vial to one patient whenever possible *to reduce the risk of bloodborne pathogen transmission and infection.* If you must use a multidose vial for more than one patient, keep and access it in a dedicated medication preparation area, away from immediate patient treatment areas, *to prevent inadvertent contamination of the vial through direct or indirect contact with potentially contaminated surfaces or equipment that could lead to infections in subsequent patients.*[21,22,23] Reconstitute powdered medications according to the manufacturer's prescribing information.

Drawing up medication from a single-dose or multidose vial

- Roll the vial between your palms, if necessary, *to ensure the drug is mixed equally throughout.*

- Remove the vial lid and disinfect the vial's rubber stopper with an antiseptic pad using friction, and then allow it to dry.[21,24]
- Pull the syringe plunger back until the volume of air in the syringe equals the volume of drug to be withdrawn from the vial.
- Without inverting the vial, insert the needle into the vial. Inject the air, invert the vial, and keep the needle's bevel tip below the level of the solution as you withdraw the prescribed amount of medication. Tap the syringe *to clear any air from it.*
- Remove the needle from the vial and cover the needle with the needle sheath.
- Check the medication label against the patient's medication record before discarding the single-dose vial or returning the multidose vial to the shelf.

Administering the subcutaneous injection

- Perform hand hygiene.[12,13,14,15,16,17]
- Confirm the patient's identity using at least two patient identifiers.[25]
- Provide privacy.[26,27,28,29]
- Explain the procedure to the patient and family (if appropriate) according to their individual communication and learning needs *to increase their understanding, allay their fears, and enhance cooperation.*[30] Answer any questions the patient has about the procedure.[31,32]
- Teach the patient who is receiving the medication for the first time about potential adverse reactions, and discuss any other concerns related to the medication.[4,5,6,7]
- Verify that the medication is being administered at the proper time, in the prescribed dose, and by the correct route, *to reduce the risk of medication errors.*[4,5,6,7]
- If your facility uses a bar code technology, use it as directed by your facility.
- Assess the patient's condition *to determine the need for the medication.*
- Select an appropriate injection site. Rotate sites according to a schedule for repeated injections, using different areas of the body unless contraindicated.[33] (For example, heparin should be injected only in the abdomen, if possible).
- Position the patient and expose the injection site. If appropriate, raise the bed to waist level before providing care *to prevent caregiver back strain.*[34]
- Perform hand hygiene.[12,13,14,15,16,17]
- Put on gloves if contact with blood or body fluids is likely, or if your skin or the patient's skin isn't intact. (Gloves aren't required for routine subcutaneous injections, *because bleeding is unlikely, and they don't protect against needlestick injury.*)[24,35,36,37]
- Clean the injection site with an antiseptic pad, beginning at the center of the site and moving outward in a circular motion. Allow the skin to dry before injecting the drug *to avoid a stinging sensation from introducing alcohol into subcutaneous tissues.*[36,38]
- Remove the protective needle sheath.
- With your nondominant hand, grasp the skin around the injection site firmly *to elevate the subcutaneous tissue,* forming a 1" (2.5-cm) fat fold.
- While grasping the skin with your nondominant hand, use your dominant hand to position the syringe over the injection site with the needle bevel up. Don't touch the needle.
- Tell the patient to expect to feel a needle prick.
- Insert the needle quickly in one motion at a 45- or 90-degree angle. (See *Technique for subcutaneous injections.*) Release the patient's skin *to avoid injecting the drug into compressed tissue and irritating nerve fibers.*
- Inject the medication.
- Remove the needle gently but quickly at the same angle used for insertion and, if present, activate the safety mechanism *to prevent accidental needle-stick injury.*[35]
- Cover the site with a gauze pad and apply gentle pressure. Don't massage the site.[39]
- Remove and discard the gauze pad.[35]
- Check the injection site for bleeding and bruising.
- Carefully observe the patient for a rash, pruritus, cough, or other signs of an adverse reaction to the medication.
- If appropriate, return the bed to the lowest position *to prevent falls and maintain safety.*[40]

Technique for subcutaneous injections

Before giving the injection, elevate the subcutaneous tissue at the site by grasping it firmly.

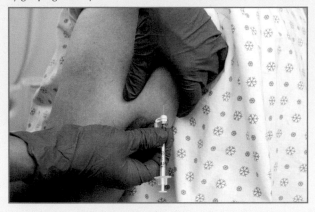

Insert the needle at a 45- or 90-degree angle to the skin surface, depending on needle length and the amount of subcutaneous tissue at the site. Some medications, such as heparin, should always be injected at a 90-degree angle.

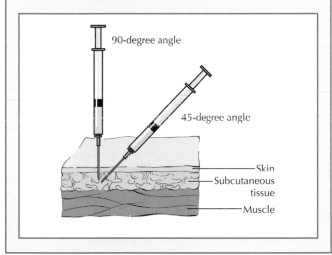

- 90-degree angle
- 45-degree angle
- Skin
- Subcutaneous tissue
- Muscle

- Discard the syringe and needle in a puncture-resistance sharps container. *To avoid needle-stick injuries,* don't resheath the needle.[35]
- Remove and discard your gloves, if worn.[35,37]
- Perform hand hygiene.[12,13,14,15,16,17]
- Document the procedure.[41,42,43,44]

Special considerations

- Best practices no longer recommend aspiration for blood with subcutaneous injections, *because administration into the bloodstream with subcutaneous injections is rare.*[39] Aspiration for blood also isn't recommended by guidelines for the administration of vaccines.[45]
- Vaccine doses shouldn't be drawn up into a syringe until immediately before administration.[36]

For insulin injections

- *To establish more consistent blood insulin levels,* rotate insulin injection sites within anatomic regions. Preferred insulin injection sites are the arms, abdomen, thighs, and buttocks.[33]
- Make sure the type of insulin, unit dosage, and syringe are correct.
- When combining insulins in a syringe, make sure they're compatible. Follow your facility's guidelines regarding which type of insulin to draw up first.

- Before drawing up insulin suspension, gently roll and invert the bottle. Don't shake the bottle, *because shaking can cause foam or bubbles to develop in the syringe.*
- Insulin may be administered through an inserted insulin pump. However, before administering the drug, make sure the patient doesn't already have a pump in place.

For heparin injections

- The preferred site for a heparin injection is the lower abdominal fat pad, 2" (5 cm) beneath the umbilicus, between the right and left iliac crests. *Injecting heparin into this area, which isn't involved in muscle activity, reduces the risk of local capillary bleeding.* Always rotate the sites from one side to the other.
- Inject the drug slowly into the fat pad.
- Remove the needle quickly after injection, and apply an alcohol pad with pressure to the site for 5 to 10 seconds *to prevent loss of heparin.*[46]
- Don't administer any injections within 2" (5 cm) of a scar, a bruise, or the umbilicus.
- Don't rub or massage the site after the injection, *because doing so can cause localized minute hemorrhages and bruises.*
- If the patient bruises easily, apply ice to the site for the first 5 minutes after the injection *to minimize local hemorrhage,* and then apply pressure.

Complications

Complications related to the action of the medication can occur. Concentrated and irritating solutions can cause sterile abscesses to form. Repeated injections in the same site can cause lipodystrophy, a localized reaction that affects adipose tissue.[33]

Documentation

Document the medication name, strength, dose, route of administration, site, and date and time of administration. Record any adverse reactions to the prescribed medication, the date and time you notified the practitioner, prescribed interventions, and the patient's response to those interventions.[47] Document teaching provided to the patient and family (if applicable), their understanding of that teaching, and any need for follow-up teaching.

REFERENCES

1 Ogston-Tuck, S. (2014). Subcutaneous injection technique: An evidence-based approach. *Nursing Standard, 29*(3), 53–58. (Level I)
2 Westbrook, J., et al. (2010). Association of interruptions with an increased risk and severity of medication administration errors. *Archives of Internal Medicine, 170,* 683–690. (Level IV)
3 Institute for Safe Medication Practices. (2012). Side tracks on the safety express: Interruptions lead to errors and unfinished…Wait, what was I doing? *Nurse Advise-ERR, 11*(2), 1–4. https://www.ismp.org/resources/side-tracks-safety-express-interruptions-lead-errors-and-unfinished-wait-what-was-i-doing?id=37
4 Accreditation Association for Hospitals and Health Systems. (2020). Standard 16.01.03. *Healthcare Facilities Accreditation Program: Accreditation requirements for acute care hospitals.* Chicago, IL: Accreditation Association for Hospitals and Health Systems. (Level VII)
5 Centers for Medicare and Medicaid Services, Department of Health and Human Services. (2020). Condition of participation: Nursing services. 42 C.F.R. § 482.23(c).
6 DNV GL-Healthcare USA, Inc. (2020). MM.1.SR.3. *NIAHO® accreditation requirements, interpretive guidelines and surveyor guidance—revision 20.0.* Milford, OH: DNV GL-Healthcare USA, Inc. (Level VII)
7 The Joint Commission. (2021). Standard MM.06.01.01. *Comprehensive accreditation manual for hospitals.* Oakbrook Terrace, IL: The Joint Commission. (Level VII)
8 Accreditation Association for Hospitals and Health Systems. (2020). Standard 25.02.13. *Healthcare Facilities Accreditation Program: Accreditation requirements for acute care hospitals.* Chicago, IL: Accreditation Association for Hospitals and Health Systems. (Level VII)
9 The Joint Commission. (2021). Standard NPSG.03.06.01. *Comprehensive accreditation manual for hospitals.* Oakbrook Terrace, IL: The Joint Commission. (Level VII)
10 Institute for Safe Medication Practices. (2018). ISMP list of high-alert medications in acute care settings. https://www.ismp.org/sites/default/files/attachments/2018-08/highAlert2018-Acute-Final.pdf (Level VII)

11 Institute for Safe Medication Practice. (2019). Independent double checks: Worth the effort if used judiciously and properly. https://www.ismp.org/resources/independent-double-checks-worth-effort-if-used-judiciously-and-properly (Level VII)

12 The Joint Commission. (2021). Standard NPSG.07.01.01. *Comprehensive accreditation manual for hospitals.* Oakbrook Terrace, IL: The Joint Commission. (Level VII)

13 Centers for Disease Control and Prevention. (2002). Guideline for hand hygiene in health-care settings: Recommendations of the Healthcare Infection Control Practices Advisory Committee and the HICPAC/SHEA/APIC/IDSA Hand Hygiene Task Force. *MMWR Recommendations and Reports, 51*(RR-16), 1–45. https://www.cdc.gov/mmwr/pdf/rr/rr5116.pdf (Level II)

14 World Health Organization. (2009). WHO guidelines on hand hygiene in health care: First global patient safety challenge, clean care is safer care. https://apps.who.int/iris/bitstream/handle/10665/44102/9789241597906_eng.pdf?sequence=1 (Level IV)

15 Accreditation Association for Hospitals and Health Systems. (2020). Standard 07.01.21. *Healthcare Facilities Accreditation Program: Accreditation requirements for acute care hospitals.* Chicago, IL: Accreditation Association for Hospitals and Health Systems. (Level VII)

16 Centers for Medicare and Medicaid Services, Department of Health and Human Services. (2020). Condition of participation: Infection control. 42 C.F.R. § 482.42.

17 DNV GL-Healthcare USA, Inc. (2020). IC.1.SR.1. *NIAHO® accreditation requirements, interpretive guidelines and surveyor guidance—revision 20.0.* Milford, OH: DNV GL-Healthcare USA, Inc. (Level VII)

18 United States Pharmacopeial Convention. (2019). USP general chapter <800>: Hazardous drugs—Handling in healthcare settings. https://www.usp.org/compounding/general-chapter-hazardous-drugs-handling-healthcare (Level VII)

19 The Joint Commission. (2021). Standard NPSG.03.04.01. *Comprehensive accreditation manual for hospitals.* Oakbrook Terrace, IL: The Joint Commission. (Level VII)

20 Accreditation Association for Hospitals and Health Systems. (2020). Standard 25.01.18. *Healthcare Facilities Accreditation Program: Accreditation requirements for acute care hospitals.* Chicago, IL: Accreditation Association for Hospitals and Health Systems. (Level VII)

21 Dolan, S., et al. (2016). *APIC position paper: Safe injection, infusion, and medication practices in health care.* Washington, DC: Association for Professionals in Infection Control and Epidemiology. https://www.apic.org/Resource_/TinyMceFileManager/Position_Statements/2016APICSIPPositionPaper.pdf

22 Centers for Disease Control and Prevention. (2019). Injection safety: Questions about multi-dose vials. https://www.cdc.gov/injectionsafety/providers/provider_faqs_multivials.html

23 The Joint Commission. (2014). Sentinel event alert 52: Preventing infection from the misuse of vials. https://www.jointcommission.org/resources/patient-safety-topics/sentinel-event/sentinel-event-alert-newsletters/sentinel-event-alert-issue-52-preventing-infection-from-the-misuse-of-vials/ (Level VII)

24 World Health Organization. (2010). WHO best practices for injections and related procedures toolkit. https://apps.who.int/iris/bitstream/handle/10665/44298/9789241599252_eng.pdf;jsessionid=68518F-C0795633478D5811038B5AAF97?sequence=1 (Level VII)

25 The Joint Commission. (2021). Standard NPSG.01.01.01. *Comprehensive accreditation manual for hospitals.* Oakbrook Terrace, IL: The Joint Commission. (Level VII)

26 Accreditation Association for Hospitals and Health Systems. (2020). Standard 15.01.16. *Healthcare Facilities Accreditation Program: Accreditation requirements for acute care hospitals.* Chicago, IL: Accreditation Association for Hospitals and Health Systems. (Level VII)

27 Centers for Medicare and Medicaid Services, Department of Health and Human Services. (2020). Condition of participation: Patient's rights. 42 C.F.R. § 482.13(c)(1).

28 The Joint Commission. (2021). Standard RI.01.01.01. *Comprehensive accreditation manual for hospitals.* Oakbrook Terrace, IL: The Joint Commission. (Level VII)

29 DNV GL-Healthcare USA, Inc. (2020). PR.2.SR.5. *NIAHO® accreditation requirements, interpretive guidelines and surveyor guidance—revision 20.0.* Milford, OH: DNV GL-Healthcare USA, Inc. (Level VII)

30 The Joint Commission. (2021). Standard PC.02.01.21. *Comprehensive accreditation manual for hospitals.* Oakbrook Terrace, IL: The Joint Commission. (Level VII)

31 The Joint Commission. (2021). Standard RI.01.03.01. *Comprehensive accreditation manual for hospitals.* Oakbrook Terrace, IL: The Joint Commission. (Level VII)

32 Centers for Medicare and Medicaid Services, Department of Health and Human Services. (2020). Condition of participation: Patient's rights. 42 C.F.R. § 482.13(b)(2).

33 Eli Lilly and Company. (2019). Humalog: Prescribing information. https://www.accessdata.fda.gov/drugsatfda_docs/label/2019/020563s196s198s199,205747s022s025s026lbl.pdf

34 Waters, T. R., et al. (2009). Safe patient handling training for schools of nursing. https://www.cdc.gov/niosh/docs/2009-127/pdfs/2009-127.pdf (Level VII)

35 Occupational Safety and Health Administration. (2012). Bloodborne pathogens, standard number 1910.1030. https://www.osha.gov/pls/oshaweb/owadisp.show_document?p_id=10051&p_table=STANDARDS (Level VII)

36 Wolicki, J., & Miller, E. (2021). Vaccine administration. In Hall, E., et al. (Eds.), *Epidemiology and prevention of vaccine-preventable diseases (14th ed.).* National Center for Immunization and Respiratory Diseases, Centers for Disease Control and Prevention. Washington, DC: Public Health Foundation. https://www.cdc.gov/vaccines/pubs/pinkbook/vac-admin.html

37 Siegel, J. D., et al. (2007, revised 2019). 2007 guideline for isolation precautions: Preventing transmission of infectious agents in healthcare settings. https://www.cdc.gov/infectioncontrol/pdf/guidelines/isolation-guidelines-H.pdf (Level II)

38 Injection: Subcutaneous. (2020). *The JBI EBP Database.* AN: JBI24442.

39 Craven, R. F., et al. (2020). *Fundamentals of nursing: Concepts and competencies for practice* (9th ed.). Philadelphia, PA: Wolters Kluwer.

40 Ganz, D. A., et al. (2013, reviewed 2021). *Preventing falls in hospitals: A toolkit for improving quality of care* (AHRQ publication no. 13-0015-EF). https://www.ahrq.gov/professionals/systems/hospital/fallpxtoolkit/index.html (Level VII)

41 The Joint Commission. (2021). Standard RC.01.03.01. *Comprehensive accreditation manual for hospitals.* Oakbrook Terrace, IL: The Joint Commission. (Level VII)

42 Accreditation Association for Hospitals and Health Systems. (2020). Standard 10.00.03. *Healthcare Facilities Accreditation Program: Accreditation requirements for acute care hospitals.* Chicago, IL: Accreditation Association for Hospitals and Health Systems. (Level VII)

43 Centers for Medicare and Medicaid Services, Department of Health and Human Services. (2020). Condition of participation: Medical record services. 42 C.F.R. § 482.24(b).

44 DNV GL-Healthcare USA, Inc. (2020). MR.2.SR.1. *NIAHO® accreditation requirements, interpretive guidelines and surveyor guidance—revision 20.0.* Milford, OH: DNV GL-Healthcare USA, Inc. (Level VII)

45 Kroger, A., et al. (2021). Vaccine recommendations and guidelines of the Advisory Committee on Immunization Practices (ACIP): General best practice guidelines for immunization. https://www.cdc.gov/vaccines/hcp/acip-recs/general-recs/index.html (Level VII)

46 Sandoz Canada, Inc. (2018). Prescribing information: Heparin sodium injection USP. https://www.sandoz.ca/sites/www.sandoz.ca/files/Heparin%20Sodium%20Injection%20Product%20Monograph.pdf

47 The Joint Commission. (2021). Standard RC.02.01.01. *Comprehensive accreditation manual for hospitals.* Oakbrook Terrace, IL: The Joint Commission. (Level VII)

SUBDERMAL DRUG IMPLANT INSERTION, ASSISTING

A method of drug delivery, subdermal implants are flexible capsules or rods that are placed under the skin. This method is used to administer drugs for the palliative treatment of prostate cancer and uterine fibroids, for family planning, for treatment of early puberty in children, and for treatment of opioid addiction. Drugs administered through subdermal implants diffuse slowly and are absorbed into the bloodstream. A subdermal implant is inserted just under the dermis of the skin, typically in the nondominant upper arm about 3" to 4" (8 to 10 cm) above the medial epicondyle of the humerus, avoiding the groove between the biceps and triceps muscles (and the large blood vessels and nerves that lie there in the neurovascular bundle deeper in the subcutaneous tissue) to reduce the risk of neural or vascular injury.[1]

Equipment

Sterile surgical drapes ▪ sterile gloves ▪ antiseptic solution ▪ prescribed implants (commonly including an implantation kit with insertion tool)[1,2] ▪ needles ▪ 5-mL syringe ▪ scalpel ▪ forceps ▪ sterile absorbable sutures, sterile adhesive surgical strips, or liquid skin adhesive ▪ sterile gauze ▪ tape or adhesive bandage ▪ gloves ▪ Optional: surgical marker.

Preparation of equipment

Inspect all equipment and supplies. If a product is expired, is defective, or has compromised integrity, remove it from patient use, label it as expired or defective, and report the expiration or defect as directed by your facility.

Implementation

▪ Avoid distractions and interruptions when preparing and administering medication to prevent medication errors.[3,4]
▪ Verify the practitioner's order.[5,6,7,8]
▪ Reconcile the patient's medications when the practitioner prescribes a new medication *to reduce the risk of medication errors, including omissions, duplications, dosing errors, and drug interactions.*[9,10]
▪ Compare the medication label with the order in the patient's medical record.[5,6,7,8]
▪ If required by your facility, confirm that written informed consent is obtained and that the signed consent form is in the patient's medical record.[11,12,13,14]
▪ Conduct a preprocedure verification *to make sure that all relevant documentation, related information, and equipment are available and correctly identified to the patient's identifiers.*[15,16]
▪ Check the patient's medical record for allergies or contraindications to the prescribed medication. If an allergy or a contraindication exists, don't administer the medication; instead, notify the practitioner.[5,6,7,8]
▪ Check the expiration date on the medication. If the medication has expired, return it to the pharmacy and obtain new medication.[5,6,7,8]
▪ Visually inspect the medication for loss of integrity; don't administer the medication if its integrity is compromised.[5,6,7,8]
▪ Discuss any unresolved concerns about the medication with the patient's practitioner.[5,6,7,8]
▪ Perform hand hygiene.[17,18,19,20,21,22]
▪ Confirm the patient's identity using at least two patient identifiers.[23]
▪ Provide privacy.[24,25,26,27]
▪ Reinforce the practitioner's explanation of the procedure, and answer the patient's questions.
▪ Check the patient's history for hypersensitivity to latex or to the local anesthetic.
▪ If the patient is receiving the medication for the first time, teach the patient and family (if appropriate) about potential adverse reactions, and other concerns related to the medication.[5,6,7,8]
▪ Verify that the medication is being administered at the proper time, in the prescribed dose, and by the correct route *to reduce the risk of medication errors.*[5,6,7,8]
▪ Perform hand hygiene.[17,18,19,20,21,22]
▪ Put on gloves *to comply with standard precautions.*[28,29,30]
▪ Assist the patient into the supine position on the examination table.
▪ If appropriate, make sure that the insertion site is marked as required by your facility.[16,31]
▪ During the procedure, stay and provide support, as necessary, while the practitioner inserts the implants.
▪ The practitioner performs hand hygiene and then puts on sterile gloves.[17,18,19,20,21,22,28,29]
▪ The practitioner cleans the site with antiseptic solution and then drapes the site with sterile drapes.
▪ Conduct a time-out immediately before starting the procedure *to ensure that the correct patient, site, positioning, and procedure are identified and, as applicable, that all relevant information and necessary equipment are available.*[32]
▪ After anesthetizing the upper portion of the nondominant arm, the practitioner inserts the implant(s) following the drug's prescribing information.[1,2,33]

▪ After insertion, the practitioner removes the insertion tool and palpates the area *to verify the placement of the implant.* If the practitioner can't palpate the implant, the insertion tool (if used) should be checked *to see whether it still contains the implant.* Implant placement can also be verified using X-ray, computed tomography (CT), ultrasound, or magnetic resonance imaging. Refer to the drug's prescribing information, *because some implants aren't radiopaque and can't be visualized by X-ray or CT.*[1,2,33]
▪ The practitioner closes the incision with liquid skin adhesive, sterile absorbable sutures, or sterile adhesive surgical strips, and covers it with sterile gauze and tape or an adhesive bandage.
▪ Discard used supplies and sharps in appropriate receptacles.[29]
▪ Remove and discard your gloves.[28,29]
▪ Perform hand hygiene.[17,18,19,20,21,22]
▪ Document the procedure.[34,35,36,37]

Special considerations

▪ If the implant is a contraceptive, confirm that the patient isn't pregnant before implant insertion.[1]

Complications

Potential complications of subdermal drug implant insertion include pain, bleeding, infection, and scarring at the insertion site. Improper insertion can lead to complicated removal if the insert is implanted too deeply, isn't palpable, or migrates.[33] Complications related to the action of the medication can occur.

Documentation

Document the name of the drug, insertion or administration site, date and time of insertion, and patient's response to the procedure. Note the date at which the implant should be removed and a new implant inserted. Document teaching provided to the patient and family (if applicable), their understanding of that teaching, and any need for follow-up teaching.

REFERENCES

1 Merck and Company, Inc. (2020). Nexplanon: Prescribing information. https://www.merck.com/product/usa/pi_circulars/n/nexplanon/nexplanon_pi.pdf
2 Endo Pharmaceuticals Inc. (2019). Vantas-histrelin acetate implant: Prescribing information. https://www.endo.com/File%20Library/Products/Prescribing%20Information/Vantas_prescribing_information.html
3 Institute for Safe Medication Practices. (2012). Side tracks on the safety express: Interruptions lead to errors and unfinished…Wait, what was I doing? *Nurse Advise-ERR, 11*(2), 1–4. https://www.ismp.org/resources/side-tracks-safety-express-interruptions-lead-errors-and-unfinished-wait-what-was-i-doing?id=37
4 Westbrook, J., et al. (2010). Association of interruptions with an increased risk and severity of medication administration errors. *Archives of Internal Medicine, 170,* 683–690. (Level IV)
5 The Joint Commission. (2021). Standard MM.06.01.01. *Comprehensive accreditation manual for hospitals.* Oakbrook Terrace, IL: The Joint Commission. (Level VII)
6 Accreditation Association for Hospitals and Health Systems. (2020). Standard 16.01.03. *Healthcare Facilities Accreditation Program: Accreditation standards for acute care hospitals.* Chicago, IL: Accreditation Association for Hospitals and Health Systems. (Level VII)
7 Centers for Medicare and Medicaid Services, Department of Health and Human Services. (2020). Condition of participation: Nursing services. 42 C.F.R. § 482.23(c).
8 DNV GL-Healthcare USA, Inc. (2020). MM.1.SR.3. *NIAHO® accreditation requirements, interpretive guidelines and surveyor guidance—revision 20.0.* Milford, OH: DNV GL-Healthcare USA, Inc. (Level VII)
9 Accreditation Association for Hospitals and Health Systems. (2020). Standard 25.02.13. *Healthcare Facilities Accreditation Program: Accreditation requirements for acute care hospitals.* Chicago, IL: Accreditation Association for Hospitals and Health Systems. (Level VII)
10 The Joint Commission. (2021). Standard NPSG.03.06.01. *Comprehensive accreditation manual for hospitals.* Oakbrook Terrace, IL: The Joint Commission. (Level VII)

11 The Joint Commission. (2021). Standard RI.01.03.01. *Comprehensive accreditation manual for hospitals.* Oakbrook Terrace, IL: The Joint Commission. (Level VII)

12 Centers for Medicare and Medicaid Services, Department of Health and Human Services. (2020). Condition of participation: Patient's right. 42 C.F.R. § 482.13(b)(2).

13 Accreditation Association for Hospitals and Health Systems. (2020). Standard 15.01.11. *Healthcare Facilities Accreditation Program: Accreditation standards for acute care hospitals.* Chicago, IL: Accreditation Association for Hospitals and Health Systems. (Level VII)

14 DNV GL-Healthcare USA, Inc. (2020). PR.2.SR.3. *NIAHO® accreditation requirements, interpretive guidelines and surveyor guidance—revision 20.0.* Milford, OH: DNV GL-Healthcare USA, Inc. (Level VII)

15 The Joint Commission. (2021). Standard UP.01.01.01. *Comprehensive accreditation manual for hospitals.* Oakbrook Terrace, IL: The Joint Commission. (Level VII)

16 Accreditation Association for Hospitals and Health Systems. (2020). Standard 30.00.14. *Healthcare Facilities Accreditation Program: Accreditation requirements for acute care hospitals.* Chicago, IL: Accreditation Association for Hospitals and Health Systems. (Level VII)

17 The Joint Commission. (2021). Standard NPSG.07.01.01. *Comprehensive accreditation manual for hospitals.* Oakbrook Terrace, IL: The Joint Commission. (Level VII)

18 Centers for Disease Control and Prevention. (2002). Guideline for hand hygiene in health-care settings: Recommendations of the Healthcare Infection Control Practices Advisory Committee and the HICPAC/SHEA/APIC/IDSA Hand Hygiene Task Force. *MMWR Recommendations and Reports, 51*(RR-16), 1–45. https://www.cdc.gov/mmwr/pdf/rr/rr5116.pdf (Level II)

19 World Health Organization. (2009). WHO guidelines on hand hygiene in health care: First global patient safety challenge, clean care is safer care. https://apps.who.int/iris/bitstream/handle/10665/44102/9789241597906_eng.pdf?sequence=1 (Level IV)

20 Accreditation Association for Hospitals and Health Systems. (2020) Standard 07.01.21. *Healthcare Facilities Accreditation Program: Accreditation standards for acute care hospitals.* Chicago, IL: Accreditation Association for Hospitals and Health Systems. (Level VII)

21 Centers for Medicare and Medicaid Services, Department of Health and Human Services. (2020). Condition of participation: Infection control. 42 C.F.R. § 482.42.

22 DNV GL-Healthcare USA, Inc. (2020). IC.1.SR.1. *NIAHO® accreditation requirements, interpretive guidelines and surveyor guidance—revision 20.0.* Milford, OH: DNV GL-Healthcare USA, Inc. (Level VII)

23 The Joint Commission. (2021). Standard NPSG.01.01.01. *Comprehensive accreditation manual for hospitals.* Oakbrook Terrace, IL: The Joint Commission. (Level VII)

24 Accreditation Association for Hospitals and Health Systems. (2020). Standard 15.01.16. *Healthcare Facilities Accreditation Program: Accreditation requirements for acute care hospitals.* Chicago, IL: Accreditation Association for Hospitals and Health Systems. (Level VII)

25 Centers for Medicare and Medicaid Services, Department of Health and Human Services. (2020). Condition of participation: Patient's rights. 42 C.F.R. § 482.13(c)(1).

26 DNV GL-Healthcare USA, Inc. (2020). PR.2.SR.5. *NIAHO® accreditation requirements, interpretive guidelines and surveyor guidance—revision 20.0.* Milford, OH: DNV GL-Healthcare USA, Inc. (Level VII)

27 The Joint Commission. (2021). Standard RI.01.01.01. *Comprehensive accreditation manual for hospitals.* Oakbrook Terrace, IL: The Joint Commission. (Level VII)

28 Siegel, J. D., et al. (2007, revised 2019). 2007 guideline for isolation precautions: Preventing transmission of infectious agents in healthcare settings. https://www.cdc.gov/infectioncontrol/pdf/guidelines/isolation-guidelines-H.pdf (Level II)

29 Occupational Safety and Health Administration. (2012). Bloodborne pathogens, standard number 1910.1030. https://www.osha.gov/pls/oshaweb/owadisp.show_document?p_id=10051&p_table=STANDARDS (Level VII)

30 Accreditation Association for Hospitals and Health Systems. (2020). Standard 07.01.10. *Healthcare Facilities Accreditation Program: Accreditation standards for acute care hospitals.* Chicago, IL: Accreditation Association for Hospitals and Health Systems. (Level VII)

31 The Joint Commission. (2021). Standard UP.01.02.01. *Comprehensive accreditation manual for hospitals.* Oakbrook Terrace, IL: The Joint Commission. (Level VII)

32 The Joint Commission. (2021). Standard UP.01.03.01. *Comprehensive accreditation manual for hospitals.* Oakbrook Terrace, IL: The Joint Commission. (Level VII)

33 Titan Pharmaceuticals, Inc. (2018). Probuphine: Prescribing information. https://s3.amazonaws.com/content.stockpr.com/titanpharm/files/pages/titanpharm/db/339/description/probuphine-PI-Aug2018.pdf

34 The Joint Commission. (2021). Standard RC.01.03.01. *Comprehensive accreditation manual for hospitals.* Oakbrook Terrace, IL: The Joint Commission. (Level VII)

35 Accreditation Association for Hospitals and Health Systems. (2020). Standard 10.00.03. *Healthcare Facilities Accreditation Program: Accreditation standards for acute care hospitals.* Chicago, IL: Accreditation Association for Hospitals and Health Systems. (Level VII)

36 Centers for Medicare and Medicaid Services, Department of Health and Human Services. (2020). Condition of participation: Medical record services. 42 C.F.R. § 482.24(b).

37 DNV GL-Healthcare USA, Inc. (2020). MR.2.SR.1. *NIAHO® accreditation requirements, interpretive guidelines and surveyor guidance—revision 20.0.* Milford, OH: DNV GL-Healthcare USA, Inc. (Level VII)

SURGICAL DRAIN REMOVAL

Surgical drains are important adjuncts to postoperative care: *they promote wound healing by providing an exit site for fluid that accumulates in or near the wound bed.*[1] Drains commonly inserted during surgery include the Hemovac, bulb suction, and Penrose drains. Drains should be removed when they malfunction or when drainage becomes minimal (less than 25 mL in the previous 24 hours).[2,3]

Equipment

Sterile 4" × 4" (10-cm × 10-cm) gauze pads ■ tape (paper or silicone for frail skin)[4] ■ gloves ■ sterile gloves ■ labels ■ Optional: suture removal kit, prescribed pain medication, sterile specimen swabs, sterile scissors, sterile specimen collection containers, laboratory request form, laboratory biohazard transport bag, gown, mask with face shield or mask and goggles, nonadherent contact layers, nonadherent or silicone foam dressing, other topical dressing specifically formulated for fragile skin.

Implementation

- Verify the practitioner's order.
- Review the patient's medical record to determine the type of drain to be removed, its location, and the method used to secure it *to ensure proper removal.*
- Verify whether a surgical drain, drain tip, or drainage needs to be sent for culturing upon drain removal.
- Gather and prepare the necessary equipment and supplies.
- Perform hand hygiene.[5,6,7,8,9,10]
- Confirm the patient's identity using at least two patient identifiers.[11]
- Provide privacy.[12,13,14,15]
- Explain the procedure to the patient and family (if appropriate) according to their individual communication and learning needs *to increase their understanding, allay their fears, and enhance cooperation.*[16]
- Raise the patient's bed to waist level when providing care *to prevent caregiver back strain.*[17]
- Perform hand hygiene.[5,6,7,8,9,10]
- Screen and assess the patient's pain using facility-defined criteria that are consistent with the patient's age, condition, and ability to understand.[18]
- Treat the patient's pain, as needed and ordered, using nonpharmacologic, pharmacologic, or a combination of approaches. Base the treatment plan on evidence-based practices and the patient's clinical condition, past medical history, and pain management goals.[18]
- Perform hand hygiene.[5,6,7,8,9,10]
- Put on gloves and, if necessary, a gown and a mask with a face shield or a mask and goggles *to comply with standard precautions.*[19,20,21]
- Position the patient comfortable and in a manner that provides you with adequate access to the surgical site.
- If the drain contains suction from its initial closure, release the suction from the drain.[3,22,23]
- Empty any remaining drainage; note the volume, color, consistency, and odor of any drainage within the drain.[23]

- Remove the drain dressing *to gain access to the exit site.* Remove the dressing and tape carefully *to prevent skin stripping and tearing.* Discard them in an appropriate receptacle.[20]
- Remove and discard your gloves.[20]
- Perform hand hygiene.[5,6,7,8,9,10]
- Put on sterile gloves.[19,20]
- Using the suture removal kit, cut and remove any sutures present.[23]
- Place a sterile gauze pad close to the drain exit site *to absorb any remaining drainage that escapes while you remove the drain.*[1]
- Have the patient breathe deeply and smoothly. Grasp the drain close to the skin with a sterile-gloved hand.[2]
- Gently withdraw the drain using smooth, steady traction. If you feel resistance, stop the procedure and notify the practitioner.[1,22]
- Maintain pressure over the drain site with the sterile gauze pad for a few minutes until drainage or bleeding is minimal.[3]
- Check that you've removed the entire drain. Examine the drain tip for irregularities or other signs of breakage. The drain should have a clean-cut edge and not appear jagged or torn.[2,23]
- If the drain tip is required for culture, cut it with sterile scissors and place it in a sterile specimen container. Label the specimen container in the presence of the patient *to prevent mislabeling.*[11] Place the specimen container in a laboratory biohazard transport bag[20] and send it to the laboratory with a completed laboratory request form (if required).
- Discard the drain in an appropriate receptacle.[20]
- Assess the patient's skin integrity at the exit site for signs of infection, such as redness, swelling, a foul odor, or purulent drainage, and for signs of fluid accumulation.[1]
- If purulent drainage and inflammation are present at the drain exit site, obtain a specimen using a sterile specimen swab, if ordered. Place the swab in its container and then label the container in the presence of the patient *to prevent mislabeling.*[11] Place the specimen container in a laboratory biohazard transport bag[20] and send it to the laboratory with a completed laboratory request form (if required).
- Remove and discard your gloves,[20] perform hand hygiene,[5,6,7,8,9,10] and put on gloves.[19,20]
- Place a sterile gauze pad over the drain exit site and secure it with tape.[1,23] Alternatively, if the patient has fragile skin, cover the site with nonadherent contact layers, a nonadherent or silicone foam dressing, or other topical dressing specifically formulated for fragile skin, and secure the dressing with paper or silicone tape *to prevent skin stripping or tearing.*[4] Label the dressing as directed by your facility.
- Return the bed to the lowest position *to prevent falls and maintain patient safety.*[24]
- Discard used materials in appropriate receptacles.[20]
- Remove and discard your gloves and, if worn, other personal protective equipment.[20]
- Perform hand hygiene.[5,6,7,8,9,10]
- Reassess and respond to the patient's pain by evaluating the response to treatment and progress toward pain management goals. Assess for adverse reactions and risk factors for adverse events that may result from treatment.[18]
- Perform hand hygiene.[5,6,7,8,9,10]
- Document the procedure.[25,26,27]

Special considerations

- Drainage from the drain exit site should be minimal and should cease within 24 hours of drain removal. If drainage continues, notify the practitioner, *because fluid may be accumulating beneath the skin and require evacuation.*[1]

Complications

Pain may accompany drain removal and persist after removal. Infection and continued drainage with accumulation of fluid underneath the skin may also occur.[1]

Documentation

Document the date and time of drain removal, the type of drain removed, the condition of the drain exit site, and the presence and characteristics of the drainage present. Document pain assessment findings, any interventions taken, and the patient's response to those interventions. Note any specimens collected and sent for microbiologic examination. Document the patient's tolerance of the procedure. Document teaching provided to the patient and family (if applicable), their understanding of that teaching, and any need for follow-up teaching.

REFERENCES

1 Wiegand, D. L. (2017). *AACN procedure manual for high acuity, progressive, and critical care* (7th ed.). St. Louis, MO: Elsevier.
2 Walker, J. (2007). Patient preparation for safe removal of surgical drains. *Nursing Standard, 21*(49), 39–41.
3 Fong, E. (2019). Vacuum drain (surgical): Removal. *JBI EBP Database.* AN: JBI551
4 LeBlanc, K., et al. (2013). International skin tear advisory panel: A tool kit to aid in the prevention, assessment, and treatment of skin tears using a simplified classification system. *Advances in Skin & Wound Care, 26,* 459–476. (Level IV)
5 Centers for Disease Control and Prevention. (2002). Guideline for hand hygiene in health-care settings: Recommendations of the Healthcare Infection Control Practices Advisory Committee and the HICPAC/SHEA/APIC/IDSA Hand Hygiene Task Force. *MMWR Recommendations and Reports, 51*(RR-16), 1–45. https://www.cdc.gov/mmwr/pdf/rr/rr5116.pdf (Level II)
6 The Joint Commission. (2021). Standard NPSG.07.01.01. *Comprehensive accreditation manual for hospitals.* Oakbrook Terrace, IL: The Joint Commission. (Level VII)
7 World Health Organization. (2009). WHO guidelines on hand hygiene in health care: First global patient safety challenge, clean care is safer care. https://apps.who.int/iris/bitstream/handle/10665/44102/9789241597906_eng.pdf?sequence=1 (Level IV)
8 Centers for Medicare and Medicaid Services, Department of Health and Human Services. (2020). Condition of participation: Infection control. 42 C.F.R. § 482.42.
9 Accreditation Association for Hospitals and Health Systems. (2020). Standard 07.01.21. *Healthcare Facilities Accreditation Program: Accreditation requirements for acute care hospitals.* Chicago, IL: Accreditation Association for Hospitals and Health Systems. (Level VII)
10 DNV GL-Healthcare USA, Inc. (2020). IC.1.SR.1. *NIAHO® accreditation requirements, interpretive guidelines and surveyor guidance—revision 20.0.* Milford, OH: DNV GL-Healthcare USA, Inc. (Level VII)
11 The Joint Commission. (2021). Standard NPSG.01.01.01. *Comprehensive accreditation manual for hospitals.* Oakbrook Terrace, IL: The Joint Commission. (Level VII)
12 Centers for Medicare and Medicaid Services, Department of Health and Human Services. (2020). Condition of participation: Patient's rights. 42 C.F.R. § 482.13(c)(1).
13 Accreditation Association for Hospitals and Health Systems. (2020). Standard 15.01.16. *Healthcare Facilities Accreditation Program: Accreditation requirements for acute care hospitals.* Chicago, IL: Accreditation Association for Hospitals and Health Systems. (Level VII)
14 The Joint Commission. (2021). Standard RI.01.01.01. *Comprehensive accreditation manual for hospitals.* Oakbrook Terrace, IL: The Joint Commission. (Level VII)
15 DNV GL-Healthcare USA, Inc. (2020). PR.2.SR.5. *NIAHO® accreditation requirements, interpretive guidelines and surveyor guidance—revision 20.0.* Milford, OH: DNV GL-Healthcare USA, Inc. (Level VII)
16 The Joint Commission. (2021). Standard PC.02.01.21. *Comprehensive accreditation manual for hospitals.* Oakbrook Terrace, IL: The Joint Commission. (Level VII)
17 Waters, T. R., et al. (2009). Safe patient handling training for schools of nursing. https://www.cdc.gov/niosh/docs/2009-127/pdfs/2009-127.pdf (Level VII)
18 The Joint Commission. (2021). Standard PC.01.02.07. *Comprehensive accreditation manual for hospitals.* Oakbrook Terrace, IL: The Joint Commission. (Level VII)
19 Siegel, J. D., et al. (2007, revised 2019). 2007 guideline for isolation precautions: Preventing transmission of infectious agents in healthcare settings. https://www.cdc.gov/infectioncontrol/pdf/guidelines/isolation-guidelines-H.pdf (Level II)
20 Occupational Safety and Health Administration. (2012). Bloodborne pathogens, standard number 1910.1030. https://www.osha.gov/pls/oshaweb/owadisp.show_document?p_id=10051&p_table=STANDARDS (Level VII)
21 Accreditation Association for Hospitals and Health Systems. (2020). Standard 07.01.10. *Healthcare Facilities Accreditation Program: Accreditation requirements for acute care hospitals.* Chicago, IL: Accreditation Association for Hospitals and Health Systems. (Level VII)

22 Durai, R., & Ng, P. C. H. (2010). Surgical vacuum drains: Types, uses, and complications. *AORN Journal, 91*, 266–271.

23 Knowlton, M. C. (2015). Nurse's guide to surgical drain removal. *Nursing, 45*(9), 59–61.

24 Ganz, D. A., et al. (2013, reviewed 2021). *Preventing falls in hospitals: A toolkit for improving quality of care* (AHRQ Publication No. 13-0015-EF). Rockville, MD: Agency for Healthcare Research and Quality. https://www.ahrq.gov/professionals/systems/hospital/fallpxtoolkit/index.html (Level VII)

25 The Joint Commission. (2021). Standard RC.01.03.01. *Comprehensive accreditation manual for hospitals.* Oakbrook Terrace, IL: The Joint Commission. (Level VII)

26 Centers for Medicare and Medicaid Services, Department of Health and Human Services. (2020). Condition of participation: Medical record services. 42 C.F.R. § 482.24(b).

27 Accreditation Association for Hospitals and Health Systems. (2020). Standard 10.00.03. *Healthcare Facilities Accreditation Program: Accreditation requirements for acute care hospitals.* Chicago, IL: Accreditation Association for Hospitals and Health Systems. (Level VII)

SURGICAL WOUND MANAGEMENT

Adhering to certain procedures when caring for a patient with a surgical wound can help prevent infection by preventing pathogens from entering the wound. In addition to promoting patient comfort, performing such procedures protects the skin surface from maceration and excoriation caused by contact with irritating drainage and also enables measurement of wound drainage to monitor fluid balance.[1]

The two primary methods used to manage a draining surgical wound are dressing and pouching. Dressing is preferred, unless caustic or excessive drainage is compromising the patient's skin integrity. Usually, lightly seeping wounds with drains and wounds with minimal purulent drainage can be managed with packing and gauze dressings. Some wounds, such as those that become chronic, may require occlusive dressings. Dressing changes must occur often enough to keep the skin dry. In addition to an appropriate dressing, a patient with a surgical wound requires close monitoring.

When dressing a wound, use sterile no-touch technique and sterile supplies to prevent contamination. Observe the color of the wound; this will help you determine which type of dressing to apply. (See *Tailoring wound care to wound color*.) Change the dressing often enough to keep the skin dry, and always follow standard precautions set by the Centers for Disease Control and Prevention.

Equipment

Gloves ▪ sterile gloves ▪ sterile 4" × 4" (10-cm × 10-cm) gauze pads ▪ prescribed antiseptic cleaning agent ▪ adhesive or other tape ▪ soap and water ▪ sterile drape ▪ Optional: prescribed pain medication, gown, mask, goggles, mask with face shield, acetone-free adhesive remover, sterile normal saline solution, prescribed topical medication, sterile container, wound irrigant and irrigation supplies, sterile cotton-tipped applicators, wound culture collection equipment, protective skin barrier, 2" × 2" (5-cm × 5-cm) gauze pads, sterile 4" × 4" (10-cm × 10-cm) precut gauze drain dressings, forceps, large absorbent dressings, and Montgomery straps, a fishnet tube elasticized dressing support, or a T-binder.

Preparation of equipment

Inspect all equipment and supplies. If a product is expired, is defective, or has compromised integrity, remove it from patient use, label it as expired or defective, and report the expiration or defect as directed by your facility.

Implementation

▪ Verify the practitioner's order for specific wound care and medication instructions.
▪ Review the patient's medical record for history of allergies to tape, topical solutions, latex, and medications.
▪ Gather and prepare the necessary equipment and supplies.
▪ Perform hand hygiene.[2,3,4,5,6,7]
▪ Confirm the patient's identity using at least two patient identifiers.[8]
▪ Provide privacy.[9,10,11,12]
▪ Explain the procedure to the patient and family (if appropriate) according to their individual communication and learning needs *to increase their understanding, allay their fears, and enhance cooperation.*[13]

Tailoring wound care to wound color

To promote healing in any wound, keep it moist, clean, and free of debris. For an open wound, use wound color to guide the specific management approach and to assess how well the wound is healing.

Red wounds
Red, the color of healthy granulation tissue, indicates normal healing. When a wound begins to heal, a layer of pale pink granulation tissue covers the wound bed. As this layer thickens, it becomes beefy red. Cover a red wound, keep it moist and clean, and protect it from trauma. Use a transparent dressing, hydrocolloid dressing, or gauze dressing moistened with sterile normal saline solution or impregnated with petroleum jelly or an antibiotic.

Yellow wounds
Yellow is the color of exudate produced by microorganisms in an open wound. When a wound heals without complications, the immune system removes microorganisms. However, if there are too many microorganisms to remove, exudate accumulates and becomes visible. Exudate usually appears whitish yellow, creamy yellow, yellowish green, or beige. Dry exudate appears darker.

If the patient has a yellow wound, clean it and remove exudate using irrigation; then cover it with a moist dressing. Use absorptive products or a moist gauze dressing with or without an antibiotic. You may also use hydrotherapy with whirlpool or high-pressure irrigation.

Black wounds
Black, the least healthy color, signals necrosis, with dead, avascular tissue that slows healing and provides a site for microorganisms to proliferate.

A black wound should be debrided. As ordered, use enzyme products, surgical debridement, hydrotherapy with whirlpool or irrigation, or a moist gauze dressing. After removing dead tissue, apply a dressing to keep the wound moist and guard against external contamination.

Multicolored wounds
You may note two or even all three colors in a wound. In this case, classify the wound according to the least healthy color present. For example, if your patient's wound is both red and yellow, classify it as a yellow wound.

▪ Raise the patient's bed to waist level when providing patient care *to prevent caregiver back strain.*[14]
▪ Perform hand hygiene.[2,3,4,5,6,7]
▪ Screen for and assess the patient's pain using facility-defined criteria that are consistent with the patient's age, condition, and ability to understand.[15]
▪ Treat the patient's pain, as needed and ordered, using nonpharmacologic, pharmacologic, or a combination of approaches. Base the treatment plan on evidence-based practices and the patient's clinical condition, past medical history, and pain management goals.[15]

Removing the old dressing

▪ Position the patient as necessary to gain access to the wound. *To avoid chilling the patient,* expose only the wound site.
▪ Perform hand hygiene.[2,3,4,5,6,7]
▪ Put on a gown and a face shield or goggles, if necessary, *to comply with standard precautions.*[16,17,18]
▪ Put on gloves.[16,17,18]
▪ Assess the patient's condition.
▪ Loosen the soiled dressing by holding the patient's skin and pulling the tape or dressing toward the wound. *This technique protects the newly formed tissue and prevents stress on the incision.* Moisten the tape with acetone-free adhesive remover, if necessary, *to make the removal less painful (particularly if the skin is hairy).* Don't apply solvents to the incision, *because they could contaminate the wound.*

ELDER ALERT Remove adhesive tape carefully *to prevent skin tears in older adult patients.*

▪ Slowly remove the soiled dressing.[1] If the gauze adheres to the wound, loosen the gauze by moistening it with sterile normal saline solution.
▪ Observe the dressing for the amount, type, color, and odor of drainage.[1]
▪ Discard the dressing and your gloves in the appropriate receptacle.[1,18]
▪ Remove and discard your gloves.[16,18]

Caring for the wound

- Perform hand hygiene.[2,3,4,5,6,7]
- Establish a sterile field with all of the needed equipment and supplies.[1]
- Open and prepare the supplies you'll need to care for the wound, such as sterile dressings and antiseptic cleaning agent.
- Perform hand hygiene.[2,3,4,5,6,7]
- Put on sterile gloves.[1]
- Saturate the sterile gauze pads with the prescribed cleaning agent.[1] Avoid using cotton balls, *because they may shed fibers in the wound, causing irritation, infection, or adhesion.*
- If ordered, irrigate the wound using the specified solution.[1] (See the "Wound irrigation" procedure.)
- Pick up the moistened gauze pad and squeeze out the excess solution.
- For an open wound, clean the wound in a full or half circle, beginning in the center and working outward (as shown below). Use a new pad for each circle. Clean to at least 1" (2.5 cm) beyond the end of the new dressing or 2" (5 cm) beyond the wound margins if you aren't applying a new dressing.

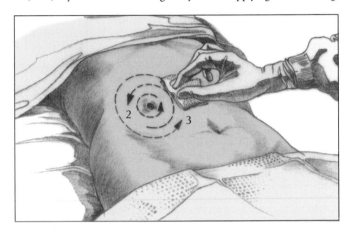

- For a linear incision, work from the top of the incision, wipe once to the bottom, and then discard the gauze pad. With a second moistened pad, wipe from top to bottom in a vertical path next to the incision. Continue to work outward from the incision in lines running parallel to it (as shown below). Always wipe from the clean area toward the less clean area (usually from top to bottom). Use each gauze pad for only one stroke *to avoid tracking wound exudate and normal body flora from surrounding skin to the clean areas.* Remember that the suture line is cleaner than the adjacent skin, and the top of the suture line is usually cleaner than the bottom, *because more drainage collects at the bottom of the wound.*

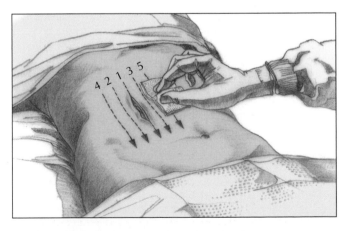

- Use sterile cotton-tipped applicators for efficient cleaning of tight-fitting wire sutures, deep and narrow wounds, and wounds with pockets, if needed. *Because the cotton on the applicator is wrapped tightly, it's less likely to leave fibers in the wound than a cotton ball.* Remember to wipe only once with each applicator.
- Clean all areas of the wound *to wash away debris, pus, blood, and necrotic material.* Try not to disturb sutures or irritate the incision. Clean to at least 1" (2.5 cm) beyond the end of the new dressing.

- Check to make sure the edges of the incision are lined up properly, and check for signs of infection (heat, redness, swelling, induration, and odor), dehiscence, and evisceration.[1] If you observe such signs, or if the patient reports pain at the wound site, notify the practitioner.
- Wash the skin surrounding the wound with soap and water, and pat it dry using a sterile 4" × 4" (10-cm × 10-cm) gauze pad. Avoid oil-based soap, *because it may interfere with tape adherence.*
- If ordered, obtain a wound culture. (See the "Swab specimen collection" procedure.)
- Apply any prescribed topical medication following safe medication administration practices.[19,20,21,22]
- Apply a skin barrier to the skin surrounding the wound that will come in contact with drainage, adhesive tape, dressings, or devices (as needed) following the manufacturer's instructions. Allow it to dry for the length of time specified by the manufacturer.[23,24]
- If ordered, pack the wound with sterile 4" × 4" (10-cm × 10-cm) or 2" × 2" (5-cm × 5-cm) gauze pads or strips folded to fit using a sterile forceps. Avoid using cotton-lined gauze pads, *because cotton fibers can adhere to the wound surface and cause complications.* Pack the wound using the wet-to-damp method. *Soaking the packing material in sterile saline solution and wringing it out so that it's slightly moist provides a moist wound environment that absorbs debris and drainage without disrupting new tissue when the packing is removed.*[1] Don't pack the wound tightly, *because doing so exerts pressure and can damage the wound.*

Applying a fresh gauze dressing

- Gently place sterile 4" × 4" (10-cm × 10-cm) gauze pads at the center of the wound, and move progressively outward to the edges of the wound site. Extend the gauze at least 1" (2.5 cm) beyond the incision in each direction, and cover the wound evenly with enough sterile dressings (usually two or three layers) to absorb all drainage until the next dressing change. Use large absorbent dressings to form outer layers, if needed, *to provide greater absorbency.*[1]
- Secure the dressing's edges to the patient's skin with strips of tape (as shown below) *to maintain the sterility of the wound site.*

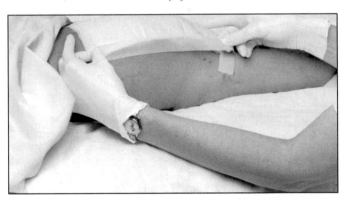

- Alternatively, secure the dressing with a T-binder or Montgomery straps (as shown below) *to prevent skin excoriation,* which can occur with repeated tape removal necessitated by frequent dressing changes.

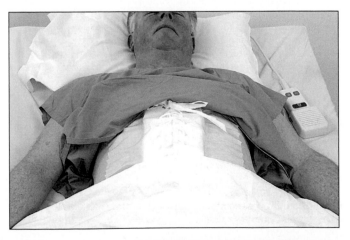

■ If the wound is on a limb, secure the dressing with a fishnet tube elasticized dressing support.

Dressing a wound with a drain
■ Gently press one sterile precut gauze drain dressing close to the skin around the drain so that the tubing fits into the slit.
■ Press a second sterile precut gauze drain dressing around the drain from the opposite direction so that the two dressings encircle the tubing.
■ Layer as many uncut, sterile 4" × 4" (10-cm × 10-cm) gauze pads or large absorbent dressings around the tubing as needed *to absorb expected drainage.*
■ Tape the dressing in place, or use a T-binder or Montgomery straps.

Completing the procedure
■ Make sure the patient is comfortable.
■ Return the bed to the lowest position *to prevent falls and maintain patient safety.*[25]
■ Discard all used supplies in appropriate receptacles.[17,18]
■ Remove and discard your gloves.[16,17,18]
■ Perform hand hygiene.[2,3,4,5,6,7]
■ Reassess and respond to the patient's pain by evaluating the response to treatment and progress toward pain management goals. Assess for adverse reactions and risk factors for adverse events that may result from treatment.[15]
■ Perform hand hygiene.[2,3,4,5,6,7]
■ Document the procedure.[26,27,28,29]

Special considerations
■ If the patient has fragile skin, use dressings and tape specially formulated for fragile skin *to prevent skin stripping and tearing during removal.*[23]
■ *Because many practitioners prefer to change the first postoperative dressing themselves to check the incision,* don't change the first dressing unless you have specific instructions to do so. If you have no such order and drainage comes through the dressings, reinforce the dressing with fresh sterile gauze. Request an order to change the dressing, or ask the practitioner to change it as soon as possible. A reinforced dressing shouldn't remain in place longer than 24 hours, *because it's an excellent medium for bacterial growth.*
■ If the dressing becomes wet from the outside (for example, from spilled drinking water), replace it as soon as possible to prevent wound contamination.

Complications
A complication of surgical wound dressing application is an allergic reaction to an antiseptic cleaning agent, prescribed topical medication, or adhesive tape. An allergic reaction can lead to skin redness, rash, excoriation, and infection. Skin tears are also a potential complication.

Documentation
Document the date, time, and type of wound management procedure; amount of soiled dressing and packing removed; wound appearance (size, condition of margins, and presence of necrotic tissue) and odor (if present); type, color, consistency, and amount of drainage (for each wound); presence and location of drains; additional procedures, such as irrigation, packing, or application of a topical medication; type and amount of new dressing or pouch applied; and the patient's tolerance of the procedure. Document teaching provided to the patient and family (if applicable), their understanding of that teaching, and any need for follow-up teaching.

Document special or detailed wound care instructions and pain management steps in the care plan. Record the color and amount of drainage on the intake-and-output sheet.

REFERENCES

1 Nettina, S. M. (2019). *Lippincott manual of nursing practice* (11th ed.). Philadelphia, PA: Wolters Kluwer.

2 The Joint Commission. (2021). Standard NPSG.07.01.01. *Comprehensive accreditation manual for hospitals.* Oakbrook Terrace, IL: The Joint Commission. (Level VII)

3 Centers for Disease Control and Prevention. (2002). Guideline for hand hygiene in health-care settings: Recommendations of the Healthcare Infection Control Practices Advisory Committee and the HICPAC/SHEA/APIC/IDSA Hand Hygiene Task Force. *MMWR Recommendations and Reports, 51*(RR-16), 1–45. https://www.cdc.gov/mmwr/pdf/rr/rr5116.pdf (Level II)

4 World Health Organization. (2009). WHO guidelines on hand hygiene in health care: First global patient safety challenge, clean care is safer care. https://apps.who.int/iris/bitstream/handle/10665/44102/9789241597906_eng.pdf?sequence=1 (Level IV)

5 Accreditation Association for Hospitals and Health Systems. (2020). Standard 07.01.21. *Healthcare Facilities Accreditation Program: Accreditation requirements for acute care hospitals.* Chicago, IL: Accreditation Association for Hospitals and Health Systems. (Level VII)

6 Centers for Medicare and Medicaid Services, Department of Health and Human Services. (2020). Condition of participation: Infection control. 42 C.F.R. § 482.42.

7 DNV GL-Healthcare USA, Inc. (2020). IC.1.SR.1. *NIAHO® accreditation requirements, interpretive guidelines and surveyor guidance—revision 20.0.* Milford, OH: DNV GL-Healthcare USA, Inc. (Level VII)

8 The Joint Commission. (2021). Standard NPSG.01.01.01. *Comprehensive accreditation manual for hospitals.* Oakbrook Terrace, IL: The Joint Commission. (Level VII)

9 Accreditation Association for Hospitals and Health Systems. (2020). Standard 15.01.16. *Healthcare Facilities Accreditation Program: Accreditation requirements for acute care hospitals.* Chicago, IL: Accreditation Association for Hospitals and Health Systems. (Level VII)

10 Centers for Medicare and Medicaid Services, Department of Health and Human Services. (2020). Condition of participation: Patient's rights. 42 C.F.R. § 482.13(c)(1).

11 The Joint Commission. (2021). Standard RI.01.01.01. *Comprehensive accreditation manual for hospitals.* Oakbrook Terrace, IL: The Joint Commission. (Level VII)

12 DNV GL-Healthcare USA, Inc. (2020). PR.2.SR.5. *NIAHO® accreditation requirements, interpretive guidelines and surveyor guidance—revision 20.0.* Milford, OH: DNV GL-Healthcare USA, Inc. (Level VII)

13 The Joint Commission. (2021). Standard PC.02.01.21. *Comprehensive accreditation manual for hospitals.* Oakbrook Terrace, IL: The Joint Commission. (Level VII)

14 Waters, T. R., et al. (2009). Safe patient handling training for schools of nursing. https://www.cdc.gov/niosh/docs/2009-127/pdfs/2009-127.pdf (Level VII)

15 The Joint Commission. (2021). Standard PC.01.02.07. *Comprehensive accreditation manual for hospitals.* Oakbrook Terrace, IL: The Joint Commission. (Level VII)

16 Siegel, J. D., et al. (2007, revised 2019). 2007 guideline for isolation precautions: Preventing transmission of infectious agents in healthcare settings. https://www.cdc.gov/infectioncontrol/pdf/guidelines/isolation-guidelines-H.pdf (Level II)

17 Accreditation Association. for Hospitals and Health Systems (2020). Standard 07.01.10. *Healthcare Facilities Accreditation Program: Accreditation requirements for acute care hospitals.* Chicago, IL: Accreditation Association for Hospitals and Health Systems. (Level VII)

18 Occupational Safety and Health Administration. (2012). Bloodborne pathogens, standard number 1910.1030. https://www.osha.gov/pls/oshaweb/owadisp.show_document?p_id=10051&p_table=STANDARDS (Level VII)

19 Accreditation Association for Hospitals and Health Systems. (2020). Standard 16.01.03. *Healthcare Facilities Accreditation Program: Accreditation requirements for acute care hospitals.* Chicago, IL: Accreditation Association for Hospitals and Health Systems. (Level VII)

20 Centers for Medicare and Medicaid Services, Department of Health and Human Services. (2020). Condition of participation: Nursing services. 42 C.F.R. § 482.23(c).

21 DNV GL-Healthcare USA, Inc. (2020). MM.1.SR.3. *NIAHO® accreditation requirements, interpretive guidelines and surveyor guidance—revision 20.0.* Milford, OH: DNV GL-Healthcare USA, Inc. (Level VII)

22 The Joint Commission. (2021). Standard MM.06.01.01. *Comprehensive accreditation manual for hospitals.* Oakbrook Terrace, IL: The Joint Commission. (Level VII)

23 LeBlanc, K., et al. (2013). International skin tear advisory panel: A tool kit to aid in the prevention, assessment, and treatment of skin tears using a simplified classification system. *Advances in Skin & Wound Care, 26,* 459–476. (Level IV)

24 Baranoski, S., & Ayello, E. A. (2020). *Wound care essentials: Practice principles* (5th ed.). Philadelphia, PA: Wolters Kluwer.

25 Ganz, D. A., et al. (2013, reviewed 2021). *Preventing falls in hospitals: A toolkit for improving quality of care* (AHRQ Publication No. 13-0015-EF). Rockville, MD: Agency for Healthcare Research and Quality. https://www.ahrq.gov/professionals/systems/hospital/fallpxtoolkit/index.html (Level VII)

26 The Joint Commission. (2021). Standard RC.01.03.01. *Comprehensive accreditation manual for hospitals.* Oakbrook Terrace, IL: The Joint Commission. (Level VII)

27 Accreditation Association for Hospitals and Health Systems. (2020). Standard 10.00.03. *Healthcare Facilities Accreditation Program: Accreditation requirements for acute care hospitals.* Chicago, IL: Accreditation Association for Hospitals and Health Systems. (Level VII)

28 Centers for Medicare and Medicaid Services, Department of Health and Human Services. (2020). Condition of participation: Medical record services. 42 C.F.R. § 482.24(b).

29 DNV GL-Healthcare USA, Inc. (2020). MR.2.SR.1. *NIAHO® accreditation requirements, interpretive guidelines and surveyor guidance—revision 20.0.* Milford, OH: DNV GL-Healthcare USA, Inc. (Level VII)

SUTURE REMOVAL

A practitioner may use skin sutures to close a laceration or surgical wound. The timing of suture removal depends on the patient's condition, the location of the sutured incision, and the condition of the wound (absence of inflammation, drainage, and infection).[1] The goal is to remove the sutures from a healed wound without damaging newly formed tissue. A no-touch technique can usually be used for suture removal unless the patient's condition warrants sterile technique.[2] The method used for suture removal depends on the method of suturing. Sutures are usually removed by a practitioner; however, in many facilities a nurse may remove them according to the practitioner's order.

In general, sutures on the face are removed in 3 to 5 days;[1] on the arm, in 7 to 10 days;[1] on the scalp, in 7 to 14 days;[1,3] on the hand, foot, leg, or trunk, in 10 to 14 days;[1] and on the palm or sole, in 14 to 21 days.[1]

Equipment

Gloves ■ sterile suture removal kit (sterile forceps or hemostat, sterile curved-tipped suture scissors) ■ Optional: adhesive remover, normal saline solution, adhesive strips or adhesive butterfly strips, sterile drape, antiseptic cleaning agent, tape, sterile 4" × 4" (10-cm × 10-cm) dressings, alcohol-free skin protectant.

Preparation of equipment

Inspect all equipment and supplies. If a product is expired, is defective, or has compromised integrity, remove it from patient use, label it as expired or defective, and report the expiration or defect as directed by your facility.

Implementation

■ If your facility allows you to remove sutures, check the practitioner's order *to confirm the exact timing and details of the procedure.*[4]
■ Review the patient's medical record for a history of allergies, especially to adhesive tape, topical solutions, and medications.
■ Gather and prepare the necessary equipment and supplies.
■ Perform hand hygiene.[5,6,7,8,9,10]
■ Confirm the patient's identity using at least two patient identifiers.[11]
■ Provide privacy.[12,13,14,15]
■ Explain the procedure to the patient and family (if appropriate) according to their individual communication and learning needs *to increase their understanding, allay their fears, and enhance cooperation.*[16] Tell the patient to expect to feel a slight pulling or tickling sensation as the sutures are removed from the skin. Reassure the patient that, because the wound is healing properly, removing the sutures won't weaken the incision line.[4]
■ Screen and assess the patient's pain using facility-defined criteria that are consistent with the patient's age, condition, and ability to understand.[17,18]

■ Treat the patient's pain, as needed and ordered, using nonpharmacologic or pharmacologic methods, or a combination of approaches. Base the treatment plan on evidence-based practices and the patient's clinical condition, past medical history, and pain management goals.[17]
■ Raise the patient's bed to waist level while providing direct patient care *to prevent caregiver back strain.*[19]
■ Perform hand hygiene.[5,6,7,8,9,10]
■ Assist the patient to a comfortable position. Make sure that the patient's position doesn't create tension on the suture line. *Because some patients experience nausea and dizziness during the procedure,* have the patient recline, if possible.
■ Drape the patient using a sterile drape, if appropriate, so that only the suture area is exposed *to help provide privacy.*
■ Perform hand hygiene.[5,6,7,8,9,10]
■ Put on gloves *to comply with standard precautions.*[20,21,22]
■ If the patient's suture area is covered with a dressing, remove the dressing carefully *to prevent skin stripping and tearing;* discard the used dressing in the appropriate receptacle.[22] Use adhesive remover, if needed and appropriate, *to remove any old adhesive from the patient's skin.*
■ Assess the suture area for redness, warmth, and drainage, *which may indicate infection.*[4] Be aware that a localized reaction to the skin sutures can cause some faint erythema; this finding is normal, but you must differentiate it from pathologic erythema. Note whether the wound margins appear well approximated.[4] Report any abnormal findings to the practitioner. *If the suture area isn't adequately healed, the skin sutures may need to remain in place longer. Evidence of infection may require pharmacologic intervention.*[4]
■ Remove and discard your gloves[22] and perform hand hygiene.[5,6,7,8,9,10]
■ Put on a new pair of gloves.[2,20,22]
■ Open the sterile suture removal kit, maintaining asepsis.
■ Gently clean the suture line with an antiseptic cleaning agent, if directed, *to decrease the number of microorganisms present, thereby reducing the risk of infection.*[4] Alternatively, moisten dried crusts with normal saline solution, if directed, *to allow for visualization of all sutures and to ease skin suture removal.*[4]
■ With your nondominant hand, use the sterile pair of forceps or the hemostat to grasp the skin suture near the knot and then lift the knot gently slightly up off the patient's skin.[4]
■ Grasp and cut each suture at the appropriate place, according to the suture type, and then remove it. Proceed according to the type of sutures you're removing. (See *Methods for removing sutures,* page 804.) *Because the visible part of a suture is exposed to skin bacteria and is considered contaminated,* be sure to cut sutures at the skin surface on one side of the visible part of the suture. Remove the suture by lifting and pulling the visible end off the skin *to avoid drawing this contaminated portion back through subcutaneous tissue.*[4]
■ If ordered, remove every other skin suture *to maintain some support for the incision and ensure that the incision heals adequately.* Then go back to the starting position and remove the remaining sutures as ordered.[4]
■ After removing skin sutures, wipe the incision gently with gauze pads soaked in an antiseptic cleaning agent, if directed.[4]
■ Assess the site for approximation of margins *to determine whether adhesive strips are needed.*[4]
■ Apply adhesive strips as needed.[4]
■ Assess the need for a dressing or covering; apply one, as needed.[4]
■ Return the bed to the lowest position *to prevent falls and to maintain patient safety.*[23]
■ Discard used supplies in appropriate receptacles. If you used reusable skin suture scissors and forceps or hemostat, prepare them for processing.[24,25]
■ Remove and discard your gloves.[22]
■ Perform hand hygiene.[5,6,7,8,9,10]
■ Report any abnormal findings to the practitioner.[4]
■ Reassess and respond to the patient's pain by evaluating the response to treatment and progress toward pain management goals. Assess for adverse reactions and risk factors for adverse events that may result from treatment.[17]
■ Perform hand hygiene.[5,6,7,8,9,10]
■ Document the procedure.[26,27,28,29]

Methods for removing sutures

Removal techniques usually depend on the type of sutures to be removed. The first two illustrations below depict the cutting and grasping of sutures; the remaining four illustrations show removal steps for four common suture types. Keep in mind that, for all suture types, it's important to grasp and cut sutures in the correct place *to avoid pulling the exposed (and thus contaminated) suture material through subcutaneous tissue.*

Cutting the suture

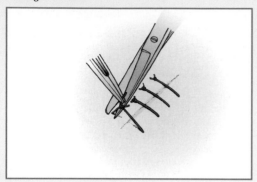

Grasping the suture

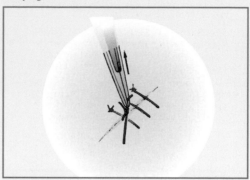

Plain interrupted sutures

Using sterile forceps, grasp the knot of the first suture and raise it off the skin. *Doing so exposes a small portion of the suture that was below skin level.* Place the rounded tips of sterile curved-tip suture scissors against the skin, and cut through the exposed portion of the suture. Then, still holding the knot with the forceps, pull the cut suture up and out of the skin in a smooth, continuous motion to *avoid causing the patient pain.* Discard the suture. Repeat the process for every other suture (alternating sutures) initially; if the wound doesn't gape, you can then remove the remaining sutures as ordered.[4]

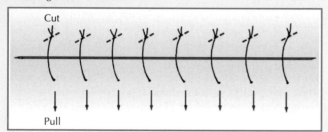

Plain continuous sutures

Cut the first suture on the side opposite the knot. Next, cut the same side of the next suture in line. Then lift the first suture out in the direction of the knot. Proceed along the suture line, grasping each suture where you grasped the knot on the first one.[4]

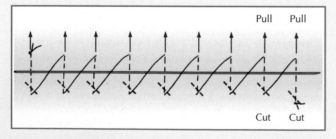

Mattress interrupted sutures

If possible, remove the small, visible portion of the suture opposite the knot by cutting it at each visible end and lifting the small piece away from the skin *to prevent pulling it through and contaminating subcutaneous tissue.* Then remove the rest of the suture by pulling it out in the direction of the knot. If the visible portion is too small to cut twice, cut it once and pull the entire suture out in the opposite direction. Repeat these steps for the remaining sutures.[4]

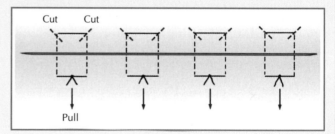

Mattress continuous sutures

Follow the procedure for removing mattress interrupted sutures, first removing the small visible portion of the suture, if possible, *to prevent pulling it through and contaminating subcutaneous tissue.* Then extract the rest of the suture in the direction of the knot.[4]

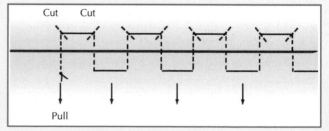

Special considerations

■ If the patient has retention and regular skin sutures in place, check the practitioner's order for the sequence in which they are to be removed. *Because retention sutures link underlying fat and muscle tissue and give added support to the obese patient or one with a slow-healing wound,* they usually remain in place for 14 to 21 days.[4]

■ If the wound dehisces during suture removal, keep the remaining sutures in place, apply adhesive or butterfly adhesive strips *to help support and approximate the wound edges,* and call the practitioner immediately to assess the wound.[4]

■ Adhesive strips generally are left in place for 3 to 5 days, or as ordered.[4,30]

Complications

Potential complications of skin suture removal include infection, missed removal of a suture, and incomplete healing resulting from removing the sutures too soon.[4]

Documentation

Document your assessment findings before and after suture removal, including the appearance of the patient's incision site, the approximation of wound margins, and the presence or absence of redness, warmth, and drainage. Record the date and time of suture removal, the location, type, and number of sutures you removed, number of sutures remaining, and date for assessment for possible removal of the remaining sutures, based on incision site healing. Record the name of the practitioner notified of complications, the date and time of notification, any prescribed interventions, and the patient's response to the interventions. Document the application of a dressing or adhesive strips. Note the patient's tolerance of the procedure, any administered pain medication, and pain assessment findings. Document any teaching you provided to the patient and family (if applicable), their understanding of that teaching, and any need for follow-up teaching.

REFERENCES

1 Forsch, R. T., et al. (2017). Laceration repair: A practical approach. *American Family Physician, 95*(10), 628–636. https://www.aafp.org/afp/2017/0515/p628.html (Level VII)

2 World Health Organization. (2009). Glove use information leaflet. https://www.who.int/gpsc/5may/Glove_Use_Information_Leaflet.pdf (Level VII)

3 Hollander, J. E. (2019). Assessment and management of scalp lacerations. In: *UpToDate*, Stack, A. M., & Wolfson, A. B. (Eds.).

4 Wiegand, D. L. (2017). *AACN procedure manual for high acuity, progressive, and critical care* (7th ed.). St. Louis, MO: Elsevier.

5 Centers for Disease Control and Prevention. (2002). Guideline for hand hygiene in health-care settings: Recommendations of the Healthcare Infection Control Practices Advisory Committee and the HICPAC/SHEA/APIC/IDSA Hand Hygiene Task Force. *MMWR Recommendations and Reports, 51*(RR-16), 1–45. https://www.cdc.gov/mmwr/pdf/rr/rr5116.pdf (Level II)

6 World Health Organization. (2009). WHO guidelines on hand hygiene in health care: First global patient safety challenge, clean care is safer care. https://apps.who.int/iris/bitstream/handle/10665/44102/9789241597906_eng.pdf (Level IV)

7 The Joint Commission. (2021). Standard NPSG.07.01.01. *Comprehensive accreditation manual for hospitals.* Oakbrook Terrace, IL: The Joint Commission. (Level VII)

8 Accreditation Association for Hospitals and Health Systems. (2020). Standard 07.01.21. *Healthcare Facilities Accreditation Program: Accreditation requirements for acute care hospitals.* Chicago, IL: Accreditation Association for Hospitals and Health Systems. (Level VII)

9 Centers for Medicare and Medicaid Services, Department of Health and Human Services. (2020). Condition of participation: Infection control. 42 C.F.R. § 482.42.

10 DNV GL-Healthcare USA, Inc. (2020). IC.1.SR.1. *NIAHO® accreditation requirements, interpretive guidelines and surveyor guidance—revision 20.0.* Milford, OH: DNV GL-Healthcare USA, Inc. (Level VII)

11 The Joint Commission. (2021). Standard NPSG.01.01.01. *Comprehensive accreditation manual for hospitals.* Oakbrook Terrace, IL: The Joint Commission. (Level VII)

12 Accreditation Association for Hospitals and Health Systems. (2020). Standard 15.01.16. *Healthcare Facilities Accreditation Program: Accreditation requirements for acute care hospitals.* Chicago, IL: Accreditation Association for Hospitals and Health Systems. (Level VII)

13 The Joint Commission. (2021). Standard RI.01.01.01. *Comprehensive accreditation manual for hospitals.* Oakbrook Terrace, IL: The Joint Commission. (Level VII)

14 Centers for Medicare and Medicaid Services, Department of Health and Human Services. (2020). Condition of participation: Patient's rights. 42 C.F.R. § 482.13(c)(1).

15 DNV GL-Healthcare USA, Inc. (2020). PR.2.SR.5. *NIAHO® accreditation requirements, interpretive guidelines and surveyor guidance—revision 20.0.* Milford, OH: DNV GL-Healthcare USA, Inc. (Level VII)

16 The Joint Commission. (2021). Standard PC.02.01.21. *Comprehensive accreditation manual for hospitals.* Oakbrook Terrace, IL: The Joint Commission. (Level VII)

17 The Joint Commission. (2021). Standard PC.01.02.07. *Comprehensive accreditation manual for hospitals.* Oakbrook Terrace, IL: The Joint Commission. (Level VII)

18 The Joint Commission. (2010). *Advancing effective communication, cultural competence, and patient- and family-centered care: A roadmap for hospitals.* Oakbrook Terrace, IL: The Joint Commission. https://www.jointcommission.org/assets/1/6/ARoadmapforHospitalsfinalversion727.pdf (Level VII)

19 Waters, T. R., et al. (2009). Safe patient handling training for schools of nursing. https://www.cdc.gov/niosh/docs/2009-127/pdfs/2009-127.pdf (Level VII)

20 Siegel, J. D., et al. (2007, revised 2019). 2007 guideline for isolation precautions: Preventing transmission of infectious agents in healthcare settings. https://www.cdc.gov/infectioncontrol/pdf/guidelines/isolation-guidelines-H.pdf (Level II)

21 Accreditation Association for Hospitals and Health Systems. (2020). Standard 07.01.10. *Healthcare Facilities Accreditation Program: Accreditation requirements for acute care hospitals.* Chicago, IL: Accreditation Association for Hospitals and Health Systems. (Level VII)

22 Occupational Safety and Health Administration. (2012). Bloodborne pathogens, standard number 1910.1030. https://www.osha.gov/pls/oshaweb/owadisp.show_document?p_id=10051&p_table=STANDARDS (Level VII)

23 Ganz, D. A., et al. (2013, reviewed 2021). *Preventing falls in hospitals: A toolkit for improving quality of care* (AHRQ Publication No. 13-0015-EF). Rockville, MD: Agency for Healthcare Research and Quality. https://www.ahrq.gov/professionals/systems/hospital/fallpxtoolkit/index.html (Level VII)

24 Rutala, W. A., et al. (2008, revised 2019). Guideline for disinfection and sterilization in healthcare facilities, 2008. https://www.cdc.gov/infection-control/pdf/guidelines/disinfection-guidelines-H.pdf (Level I)

25 Accreditation Association for Hospitals and Health Systems. (2020). Standard 07.02.03. *Healthcare Facilities Accreditation Program: Accreditation requirements for acute care hospitals.* Chicago, IL: Accreditation Association for Hospitals and Health Systems. (Level VII)

26 The Joint Commission. (2021). Standard RC.01.03.01. *Comprehensive accreditation manual for hospitals.* Oakbrook Terrace, IL: The Joint Commission. (Level VII)

27 Centers for Medicare and Medicaid Services, Department of Health and Human Services. (2020). Condition of participation: Medical record services. 42 C.F.R. § 482.24(b).

28 Accreditation Association for Hospitals and Health Systems. (2020). Standard 10.00.03. *Healthcare Facilities Accreditation Program: Accreditation requirements for acute care hospitals.* Chicago, IL: Accreditation Association for Hospitals and Health Systems. (Level VII)

29 DNV GL-Healthcare USA, Inc. (2020). MR.2.SR.1. *NIAHO® accreditation requirements, interpretive guidelines and surveyor guidance—revision 20.0.* Milford, OH: DNV GL-Healthcare USA, Inc. (Level VII)

30 American Academy of Dermatology Association. (n.d.). Proper wound care: How to minimize a scar. https://www.aad.org/public/skin-hair-nails/injured-skin/wound-care

SWAB SPECIMEN COLLECTION

Correct collection and handling of swab specimens helps laboratory staff members accurately identify pathogens with a minimum of contamination from normal bacterial flora.

Collection methods vary depending on the type of specimen being collected. For instance, collection of throat, nasopharyngeal, external ear, eye, and rectal specimens usually involves sampling inflamed tissues and exudates, typically using sterile swabs of cotton or other absorbent material.[1] Wound specimen collection normally involves sampling wound tissues and exudates expressed from the wound with sterile swabs of cotton or another absorbent material. For antibiotic-resistant wound evaluation and monitoring, quantitative biopsies are preferred over the swab specimen collection technique described in this procedure.[1,2]

Collection of fluid from the middle ear is performed by a practitioner using a needle and syringe to withdraw the fluid through the tympanic membrane; this method is referred to as *tympanocentesis*.[3] Middle ear specimen collection is generally limited to cases where antibiotics have failed to improve the patient's condition, and definitive bacterial identification and susceptibility testing are needed.[4] Middle ear specimen collection is contraindicated if a patient can't cooperate, has tympanostomy tubes in place, or has a history of blood dyscrasia, intratympanic tumor, or vascular anomalies of the middle ear cavity. It's also contraindicated if the tympanic membrane is incompletely or poorly visualized, such as with congenital stenosis of the external auditory canal.[3,5]

Inflammatory eye conditions can result from a number of diseases, and various organisms can cause eye infections. *Streptococcus pneumoniae, Staphylococcus aureus,* and *Haemophilus influenzae* can all be recovered with the use of proper specimen collection technique.[6]

Normal bacterial flora in stool include several potentially pathogenic organisms. Bacteriologic examinations help identify pathogens that cause overt GI disease (such as *Salmonella* and *Shigella* species) and carrier states.[1] A rectal swab may also help identify sexually transmitted disease such as gonorrhea and chlamydia.[7] A sensitivity test may follow isolation of the pathogen. Correctly identifying the causative organism is vital for treating the patient, helping to prevent possible fatal complications (especially in a debilitated patient), and preventing the spread of a severe infectious disease.

After the specimen has been collected, the swab is immediately placed in a sterile tube containing the appropriate transport medium.[1]

NURSING ALERT For information specific to obtaining specimens for coronavirus 2019 (COVID-19) testing, please refer to the Centers for Disease Control and Prevention's website for the most updated information at https://www.cdc.gov/coronavirus/2019-ncov/lab/guidelines-clinical-specimens.html

Equipment

Gloves ■ mask with face shield or mask and goggles ■ penlight ■ sterile swabs (cotton wool or synthetic fiber) ■ sterile culture tube with transport medium or commercial collection kit ■ specimen label ■ laboratory biohazard transport bag ■ Optional: gown, laboratory request form.

Additional equipment for throat and nasopharyngeal specimen collection

Tongue blade ■ Optional: commercially prepared kit with flocked swabs.

Additional equipment for wound specimen collection

Sterile normal saline solution, swab collection and transport system, sterile gauze pads.[8]

Additional equipment for external and middle ear specimen collection

Normal saline solution ■ 2" × 2" (5-cm × 5-cm) gauze pads ■ otoscope ■ ear speculum ■ tympanocentesis aspirator or sterile 3-mL syringe and sterile 21G 3.5" (90-mm) spinal needle[3,5] ■ Optional: wax hook, prescribed local anesthetic.

Additional equipment for rectal specimen collection

Soap and water ■ washcloth ■ normal saline solution or sterile broth medium.

Implementation

■ Verify the practitioner's order.
■ Gather and prepare the necessary equipment and supplies.
■ Perform hand hygiene.[9,10,11,12,13,14]
■ Confirm the patient's identity using at least two patient identifiers.[15]
■ Provide privacy.[16,17,18,19]
■ Explain the procedure to the patient according to individual communication and learning needs *to increase their understanding, allay their fears, and enhance cooperation.*[20]

Throat specimen collection

■ Assist the patient to sit erect at the edge of the bed or in a chair, facing you.
■ Tell the patient that gagging may occur during the swabbing but that the swabbing will take only 10 to 15 seconds.
■ Perform hand hygiene.[9,10,11,12,13,14]
■ Put on gloves and other personal protective equipment as needed *to comply with standard precautions.*[21,22,23]

NURSING ALERT If a patient requires airborne precautions, wear a powered air-purifying respirator or a fit-tested N95 or higher-level disposable respirator when caring for the patient; put on the respirator before entering the room and remove it after exiting the room. If you anticipate spraying of respiratory fluids, wear a gown and a mask and goggles or a mask with face shield as well as gloves.[23]

■ Tell the patient to tilt back the head and open the mouth wide.[6]
■ Depress the back third of the tongue with the tongue blade and illuminate the throat with the penlight.[6,24]
■ Inspect the throat for swelling, pus, and red or white spots.[24]

■ If the patient gags, withdraw the tongue blade and tell the patient to breathe deeply. After the patient is relaxed, reinsert the tongue blade but not as deeply as before. Encourage the patient to close the eyes or stare at the ceiling *to promote cooperation.*
■ Open and remove the swab, taking care not to touch the tip with your hands, *because the swab is sterile.* If you touch the swab, discard it and obtain a new swab.
■ Rub the swab quickly but thoroughly over both tonsils, including inflamed or purulent sites, using light pressure. Don't touch the tongue, cheeks, saliva, or teeth with the swab *to avoid contaminating it with oral bacteria.*[6]
■ Withdraw the swab and immediately place it in the culture tube. If you're using a commercial kit, crush the ampule of culture medium at the bottom of the tube, and then push the swab into the medium *to keep the swab moist.* If you're using a rapid strep test kit, follow the manufacturer's instructions.[6]

Nasopharyngeal specimen collection

■ Tell the patient that gagging or the urge to sneeze may occur during the swabbing but that the procedure takes less than 1 minute.[25]
■ Have the patient sit erect at the edge of the bed or in a chair, facing you.
■ Perform hand hygiene.[9,10,11,12,13,14]
■ Put on gloves, a mask, and other personal protective equipment as necessary.[21,22,23,25,26]
■ Ask the patient to blow the nose into a tissue *to clear the nasal passages.*[26,27]
■ Determine the more patent nostril by having the patient exhale and occlude one nostril at a time, and asking for then patient's assessment of airflow through the nostrils.
■ While it's still in the package, bend the sterile swab in a curve; then open the package without contaminating the swab.
■ Instruct the patient to tilt the head back at a 70-degree angle.[28,29]
■ Gently pass the swab through the more patent nostril into the nasopharynx, keeping the swab near the septum and floor of the nose until you feel resistance or until the swab reaches a distance equivalent to that of the ear to the nostril.[27,30] Rotate the swab gently 2 to 3 times and hold for 5 to 10 seconds *to absorb secretions* and then remove it.[28,29,30] (See *Collecting a nasopharyngeal specimen.*)
■ Alternatively, depress the patient's tongue with a tongue blade, and pass the bent swab up behind the uvula. Rotate the swab and withdraw it.

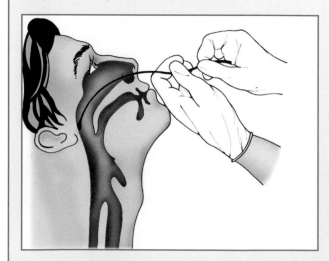

Collecting a nasopharyngeal specimen

After passing the sterile, flexible cotton-tipped swab into the nasopharynx (as shown below), rotate it gently 2 to 3 times and hold for 5 to 10 seconds *to collect a specimen.*[28,29] Then remove the swab, taking care not to injure the nasal mucous membrane.

- Remove the cap from the sterile culture tube, insert the swab into the transport medium, and break off the contaminated end of the swab.[28]
- Close the tube tightly.

Wound specimen collection
- Carefully remove the dressing to expose the wound. Dispose of the soiled dressings properly.[8,21]
- Remove and discard your gloves[22,23] and perform hand hygiene.[9,10,11,12,13,14]
- Put on a new pair of clean or sterile gloves depending on the patient's condition and the type, location, and depth of the wound.[21,22,23,31]
- Irrigate the wound with sterile normal saline solution *to remove surface debris or exudate and to prevent specimen contamination.*[1,8]
- Wipe the surface of the wound with a sterile gauze pad moistened with normal saline solution *to remove surface contaminants.*[8]
- Blot excess normal saline solution gently from the wound bed with a dry sterile gauze pad.
- Assess and measure the wound.[8]
- Assess the wound for malodor after cleaning *to make sure that the odor is from the wound and not the dressing.*[32]
- Remove and discard your gloves.[22,23]
- Perform hand hygiene.[9,10,11,12,13,14]
- Open the swab specimen collection and transport system. Prepare the contents, as needed, following the manufacturer's instructions for use.[8]
- Perform hand hygiene.[9,10,11,12,13,14]
- Put on a new pair of gloves.[21,22]
- To collect an anaerobic specimen, select the culture swab for anaerobic culture collection (if appropriate).[8] *Some swab collection and transport systems contain swabs that are designed for anaerobic and aerobic specimen collection. If your facility's collection system requires only one specimen for both anaerobic and aerobic specimen collection, use the culture swab to collect the specimen.*
- If the wound bed appears dry, moisten the swab with normal saline solution.[8]
- Identify a 1-cm² area of viable wound tissue at or near the center of the wound.[8]
- Rotate the tip of the swab over the identified 1-cm² area of the wound for 5 seconds, applying sufficient pressure to express fluid from the wound.[8,33,34]
- Remove the swab from the wound.[34]
- Insert the swab immediately into the appropriate transport system following the manufacturer's instructions for use. Use caution to avoid contaminating the swab when placing it into the transport system.[8,34]
NURSING ALERT Note that the culture must come from the cleanest tissue possible—not pus, slough, eschar, or necrotic material. Never collect exudate from the skin.[20]

External ear specimen collection
- Gently clean excess debris from the patient's ear with normal saline solution and gauze pads.
- Clean the ear with a disinfectant pad *to prevent contamination of the specimen with skin flora.*[6]
- Insert the sterile swab into the ear canal, and rotate it gently along the walls of the canal *to avoid damaging the eardrum.*
- Withdraw the swab, being careful not to touch other surfaces *to avoid contaminating the specimen.*
- Place the swab in the sterile culture tube with transport medium.

Assisting with middle ear specimen collection
- Clean the patient's outer ear with normal saline solution and gauze pads.
- Assist the practitioner with wax removal, if needed, *to remove any wax that might obscure the view and aid in visualization.*[3]
- If the practitioner prescribes a local anesthetic, assist with administration, as needed.[3] Keep in mind that if eutectic mixture of local anesthetic (EMLA) is used, it requires at least 30 minutes for onset of action.[3]
- The practitioner prepares the syringe and needle, visualizes the affected ear using an otoscope with ear speculum, punctures the eardrum with a sterile needle attached to a syringe, and aspirates fluid into the syringe. The practitioner may also collect a specimen using a sterile culture swab.
- The practitioner places the fluid or swab specimen in a sterile specimen container or culture tube with transport medium.

Eye specimen collection
- Gently clean excess debris around the outside of the patient's eye using warm water. Use a separate sterile gauze pad for each eye, wiping from the inner to the outer canthus.[35]
- Retract the lower eyelid *to expose the conjunctival sac and the inner canthus.* Obtain the specimen gently from the lower conjunctiva or the inner canthus. Hold the sterile swab parallel to the eye, rather than pointed directly at it *to prevent corneal irritation and eye trauma that can result from sudden movement.*
- Immediately place the swab in the sterile culture tube with transport medium.[6]

Rectal swab specimen collection
- Assist the patient into a dorsal lithotomy or lateral recumbent position.[6]
- Clean the area around the patient's anus using a washcloth and soap and water *to minimize contamination of the specimen.*
- Insert a sterile cotton swab, moistened with normal saline solution or sterile broth medium, through the anus and advance it about 1" to 1¼" (2.5 to 3.2 cm).[36] While withdrawing the swab, gently rotate it against the walls of the lower rectum *to sample a large area of the rectal mucosa.*[37] If you push the swab into feces, repeat the procedure with a clean swab.[38]
- Place the swab in a culture tube with transport medium, ensuring that the medium covers the cotton tip.[36,37]

Completing the procedure
- Discard used supplies in appropriate receptacles.[21]
- Remove and discard your gloves and other personal protective equipment, if worn.[21]
- Perform hand hygiene.[9,10,11,12,13,14]
- Label the specimen in the presence of the patient *to prevent mislabeling.*[15]
- Complete a laboratory request form if necessary.
- Place the specimen in a laboratory biohazard transport bag and send it to the laboratory immediately *to prevent growth or deterioration of microbes.*[21]
- Perform hand hygiene.[9,10,11,12,13,14]
- Document the procedure.[39,40,41,42]

Special considerations
- Note recent antibiotic therapy on the laboratory request form (if used in your facility) and indicate whether an organism is strongly suspected—especially *Corynebacterium diphtheriae* (which requires two swabs and special growth medium) or *Neisseria meningitis* (which requires enriched selective media).
- If possible, obtain a specimen before starting antimicrobial therapy.[1]
- Check with the laboratory for special instructions for viral studies.
- *To maximize sensitivity for a large number of viruses,* collection of combined nasopharyngeal and oropharyngeal specimens is the most effective approach.[30]
- *Because throat swabs and anterior nasal swabs have unacceptably low rates of deoxyribonucleic acid recovery,* don't use them for pertussis diagnosis.[43]
- Instruct the patient to avoid antiseptic mouthwash before collecting throat or nasopharyngeal specimens.[44]
- *To avoid stimulating the gag reflex when collecting throat or nasopharyngeal specimens and possibly causing the patient to vomit,* it's advisable to wait 1 hour after a meal before conducting the procedure (if possible).
- Before collecting a throat or nasopharyngeal specimen, notify the practitioner if the patient shows signs or symptoms of a systemic infection or has difficulty breathing because of swelling of the tongue or throat.
- When collecting an eye specimen, don't use an antiseptic before culturing *to avoid irritating the eye and inhibiting growth of organisms in the culture.* If the patient is a child or an uncooperative adult, ask a coworker to restrain the patient's head *to prevent eye trauma resulting from sudden movement.*

■ Collect each eye and ear specimen separately *to avoid cross-contamination*.[6]
■ Don't refrigerate eye specimens.[6]
■ If a corneal scraping is required, this procedure is performed by a practitioner using a wire culture loop.[6]
■ If delivery of the rectal specimen to the laboratory isn't possible within 2 hours of collection, you should refrigerate the specimen at 35.6° to 46.4° F (2° to 8° C) and ensure evaluation within 72 hours. Alternatively, you can store the sample at room temperature (68° to 77° F [20° to 25 °C]) and ensure evaluation within 48 hours. If the rectal specimen is a culture undergoing examination for *Clostridioides difficile*, you should refrigerate the specimen at 35.6° to 46.4° F (2° to 8° C) and ensure evaluation within 48 hours, or store it at room temperature (68° to 77° F [20° to 25 °C]) and ensure evaluation within 24 hours.[36]

Complications

Temporary discomfort may occur during a nasopharyngeal culture.[25] Laryngospasm may occur after the culture is obtained if the patient has epiglottitis or diphtheria. Keep resuscitation equipment nearby.

With ear specimen collection, the patient may experience pain due to sensitivity of the tympanic membrane. Other potential complications include bleeding, risk of permanent perforation, and damage to middle ear structures, including the ossicles and facial nerve.[3]

Improper technique may cause specimen contamination, resulting in inappropriate treatment.

Documentation

Record the time, date, and site of specimen collection, and recent or current antibiotic therapy. Also note whether the specimen has an unusual appearance or odor. Document the patient's tolerance of the procedure. For a wound culture, document the type of dressing that was reapplied to the wound, if applicable.[32] Document teaching provided to the patient and family (if applicable), their understanding of that teaching, and any need for follow-up teaching.

REFERENCES

1 Craven, R. F., et al. (2021). *Fundamentals of nursing: Concepts and competencies for practice* (9th ed.). Philadelphia, PA: Wolters Kluwer.
2 Copeland-Halperin, L. R., et al. (2016). Sample procurement for cultures of infected wounds: A systematic review. *Journal of Wound Care, 25*, S4–S10. (Level I)
3 van Wyk, F. C. (2018). Tympanocentesis. https://emedicine.medscape.com/article/1413525-overview
4 Lieberthal, A. S., et al. (2013). The diagnosis and management of acute otitis media. *Pediatrics, 131*(3), e964–e999. https://pediatrics.aappublications.org/content/131/3/e964 (Level VII)
5 Shaikh, N., et al. (2011). Tympanocentesis in children with acute otitis media. *New England Journal of Medicine, 364*, e4. https://www.nejm.org/doi/full/10.1056/NEJMvcm0706756 (Level VII)
6 Fischbach, F., & Fischbach, M. A. (2022). *A manual of laboratory and diagnostic tests* (11th ed.). Philadelphia, PA: Wolters Kluwer.
7 Ghanem, K. G., & Tuddenham, S. (2020). Screening for sexually transmitted infection. In: *UpToDate*, Marrazzo, J. (Ed.).
8 Wound swab culture using Levine's technique. (2020). *JBI EBP Database*. AN: JBI24743 (Level V)
9 Centers for Disease Control and Prevention. (2002). Guideline for hand hygiene in health care settings: Recommendations of the Healthcare Infection Control Practices Advisory Committee and the HICPAC/SHEA/APIC/IDSA Hand Hygiene Task Force. *MMWR Recommendations and Reports, 51*(RR-16), 1–45. https://www.cdc.gov/mmwr/pdf/rr/rr5116.pdf (Level II)
10 The Joint Commission. (2021). Standard NPSG.07.01.01. *Comprehensive accreditation manual for hospitals*. Oakbrook Terrace, IL: The Joint Commission. (Level VII)
11 World Health Organization. (2009). WHO guidelines on hand hygiene in health care: First global patient safety challenge, clean care is safer care. https://apps.who.int/iris/bitstream/handle/10665/44102/9789241597906_eng.pdf?sequence=1 (Level IV)
12 Accreditation Association for Hospitals and Health Systems. (2020). Standard 07.01.21. *Healthcare Facilities Accreditation Program: Accreditation requirements for acute care hospitals*. Chicago, IL: Accreditation Association for Hospitals and Health Systems. (Level VII)
13 Centers for Medicare and Medicaid Services, Department of Health and Human Services. (2020). Condition of participation: Infection control. 42 C.F.R. § 482.42.
14 DNV GL-Healthcare USA, Inc. (2020). IC.1.SR.1. *NIAHO® accreditation requirements, interpretive guidelines and surveyor guidance—revision 20.0*. Milford, OH: DNV GL-Healthcare USA, Inc. (Level VII)
15 The Joint Commission. (2021). Standard NPSG.01.01.01. *Comprehensive accreditation manual for hospitals*. Oakbrook Terrace, IL: The Joint Commission. (Level VII)
16 DNV GL-Healthcare USA, Inc. (2020). PR.1.SR.5. *NIAHO® accreditation requirements, interpretive guidelines and surveyor guidance—revision 20.0*. Milford, OH: DNV GL-Healthcare USA, Inc. (Level VII)
17 Centers for Medicare and Medicaid Services, Department of Health and Human Services. (2020). Condition of participation: Patient's rights. 42 C.F.R. § 482.13(c)(1).
18 Accreditation Association for Hospitals and Health Systems. (2020). Standard 15.01.16. *Healthcare Facilities Accreditation Program: Accreditation requirements for acute care hospitals*. Chicago, IL: Accreditation Association for Hospitals and Health Systems. (Level VII)
19 The Joint Commission. (2021). Standard RI.01.01.01. *Comprehensive accreditation manual for hospitals*. Oakbrook Terrace, IL: The Joint Commission. (Level VII)
20 The Joint Commission. (2021). Standard PC.02.01.21. *Comprehensive accreditation manual for hospitals*. Oakbrook Terrace, IL: The Joint Commission. (Level VII)
21 Occupational Safety and Health Administration. (2012). Bloodborne pathogens, standard number 1910.1030. https://www.osha.gov/pls/oshaweb/owadisp.show_document?p_id=10051&p_table=STANDARDS (Level VII)
22 Accreditation Association for Hospitals and Health Systems. (2020). Standard 07.01.10. *Healthcare Facilities Accreditation Program: Accreditation requirements for acute care hospitals*. Chicago, IL: Accreditation Association for Hospitals and Health Systems. (Level VII)
23 Siegel, J. D., et al. (2007, revised 2019). 2007 guideline for isolation precautions: Preventing transmission of infectious agents in healthcare settings. https://www.cdc.gov/infectioncontrol/pdf/guidelines/isolation-guidelines-H.pdf (Level II)
24 Association of Public Health Laboratories. (2011). Good laboratory practice: CLIA non-waived tests. https://www.aphl.org/programs/QSA/Documents/CLIA_2011_Non-Waived-Tests.pdf#search=Good%20laboratory%20practice%3A%20%20CLIA%20non%2Dwaived%20tests (Level VII)
25 Yeh, S., & Mink, C. (2020). Pertussis infection in infants and children: Clinical features and diagnosis. In: *UpToDate*, Edwards, M. S. (Ed.).
26 Centers for Disease Control and Prevention. (2019). Pertussis (whooping cough): Specimen collection. https://www.cdc.gov/pertussis/clinical/diagnostic-testing/specimen-collection.html
27 Marty, F. M., et al. (2020). How to obtain a nasopharyngeal swab specimen. *New England Journal of Medicine, 382*, e76. https://www.nejm.org/doi/full/10.1056/NEJMvcm2010260
28 PhysLab. (2017). Nasopharyngeal specimen collection guide. http://www.physlab.com/collect/micronasopharyngeal.pdf
29 Johns Hopkins Medical. (2019). Specimen collection guidelines. https://pathology.jhu.edu/microbiology/files/Specimen_Collection_Guidelines_2019.pdf
30 Centers for Disease Control and Prevention (n.d.) Specimen collection guidelines. https://www.cdc.gov/urdo/downloads/SpecCollectionGuidelines.pdf
31 Wound, Ostomy, and Continence Nurses Society (WOCN). (2012). Clean vs. sterile dressing techniques for management of chronic wounds: A fact sheet. *Journal of Wound, Ostomy and Continence Nursing, 39*, S30–S34. (Level VII)
32 Baranoski, S., & Ayello, E. A. (2020). *Wound care essentials: Practice principles* (5th ed.). Philadelphia, PA: Wolters Kluwer.
33 Stallard, Y. (2018). When and how to perform cultures on chronic wounds? *Journal of Wound Ostomy and Continence Nurses Society, 45*(2), 179–186. https://nursing.ceconnection.com/ovidfiles/00152192-201803000-00013.pdf
34 Bryant, R. A., & Nix, D. P. (2016). *Acute & chronic wounds: Current management concepts* (5th ed.). St. Louis, MO: Mosby.
35 Hearne, B. J., et al. (2018). Eye care in the intensive care unit. *Journal of the Intensive Care Society, 19*, 345–350.

36 Copan Italia Spa. (n.d.). FecalSwab: How to use guide for stool sample collection. https://www.copanusa.com/wp-content/uploads/2019/07/FecalSwab-Instructional-Guide.pdf

37 Centers for Disease Control and Prevention. (2015). Guidelines for specimen collection: Instructions for collecting stool specimens. https://www.cdc.gov/foodsafety/outbreaks/investigating-outbreaks/specimen-collection.html (Level VII)

38 Van Leeuwen, A. M., & Bladh, M. L. (2019). *Davis's comprehensive handbook of laboratory and diagnostic tests with nursing implications* (8th ed.). Philadelphia, PA: F. A. Davis.

39 The Joint Commission. (2021). Standard RC.01.03.01. *Comprehensive accreditation manual for hospitals*. Oakbrook Terrace, IL: The Joint Commission. (Level VII)

40 Accreditation Association for Hospitals and Health Systems. (2020). Standard 10.00.03. *Healthcare Facilities Accreditation Program: Accreditation requirements for acute care hospitals*. Chicago, IL: Accreditation Association for Hospitals and Health Systems. (Level VII)

41 Centers for Medicare and Medicaid Services, Department of Health and Human Services. (2020). Condition of participation: Medical record services. 42 C.F.R. § 482.24(b).

42 DNV GL-Healthcare USA, Inc. (2020). MR.2.SR.1. *NIAHO® accreditation requirements, interpretive guidelines and surveyor guidance—revision 20.0*. Milford, OH: DNV GL-Healthcare USA, Inc. (Level VII)

43 Centers for Disease Control and Prevention. (2015). Chapter 10: Pertussis: Laboratory testing. In *Manual for the surveillance of vaccine-preventable diseases*. https://www.cdc.gov/vaccines/pubs/surv-manual/chpt10-pertussis.html#laboratory (Level VII)

44 U.S. National Library of Medicine. (2021). Throat swab culture. https://medlineplus.gov/ency/article/003746.htm

TEMPERATURE MEASUREMENT

Normal body temperature ranges vary by site, with higher temperatures at the core of the body and lower temperatures at the periphery.[1] Core body temperature can only be measured invasively, commonly with a pulmonary artery catheter; however, even though it's considered the gold standard, pulmonary artery temperature can only be monitored in specialized clinical settings. An esophageal probe or an indwelling urinary catheter with a temperature probe can also be used to measure temperature invasively.[2,3]

The American College of Critical Care and the Infectious Diseases Society of America recommend using the most accurate and reliable method to measure temperature, taking into consideration the clinical circumstances of the patient. They state that temperature is most accurately measured using invasive measures, including rectal, followed (in order) by oral and tympanic membrane measurement. Axillary temperature measurement, temporal artery estimates, and chemical dot thermometers shouldn't be used on the intensive care unit, and rectal temperature measurements should be avoided in neutropenic patients.[2]

Noncontact infrared thermometers (NCITs) provide another method for temperature measurement. These devices are quick, easy to use, and easy to clean and disinfect. Because NCITs don't require patient contact to measure temperature, they reduce the risk of cross-contamination and may subsequently reduce the risk of spreading infection between patients. However, proper use of NCITs requires close distance between the clinician and the patient, which increases the risk of spreading infection between the patient and clinician.[4]

Some research disputes the accuracy of NCITs because they're sensitive to external environmental temperature and the temperature changes associated with head cover use. Improper positioning on the forehead also affects their accuracy.[4]

Normal body temperature is commonly thought to be 98.6° F (37° C).[5] In healthy patients, this temperature may vary by about 0.9° F to 1.8° F (0.5° C to 1° C), according to the patient's circadian rhythm and menstrual cycle. Mean temperature is lower in older adults.[1] With strenuous exercise, temperature can rise about 3.6° F to 5.4° F (2° C to 3° C). In addition to biological process, environmental factors can alter body temperature, including hot lights, specialized mattresses, air conditioning, dialysis, cardiopulmonary bypass, peritoneal lavage, and continuous hemofiltration. Medications and damage to the central or autonomic nervous system can also alter a patient's ability to regulate temperature. With so many factors potentially influencing temperature, it may be difficult to determine whether a change results from a physiologic process, a medication, or an environmental influence.[1,2]

This procedure covers temperature measurement by the rectal, oral, tympanic membrane, and noncontact infrared methods. The best temperature measuring system for the patient is one that provides reliable, reproducible values safely and conveniently. For example, oral temperature measurement is safe, convenient, and familiar for an alert and cooperative patient.[2]

Because temperature can vary greatly among methods and sites, use the same method and site consistently throughout an episode of care, if possible, and document the method, site, and results in the patient's medical record.[6] If a patient develops a new fever, review trends in the patient's temperature data and evaluate other vital signs; don't make clinical decisions based on a single temperature reading.[2,6]

Equipment

Electronic thermometer (standard, tympanic, or noncontact infrared) ▪ disposable thermometer probe cover or sheath ▪ facility-approved disinfectant ▪ Optional: gloves, water-soluble lubricant, wipe, facial tissue, washcloth, toilet paper.

Preparation of equipment

Make sure that any device used to measure temperature is maintained and calibrated appropriately. Follow the manufacturer's instructions for use, and cover the thermometer probe with a cover or sheath, as needed.

Inspect all equipment and supplies. If a product is expired, is defective, or has compromised integrity, remove it from patient use, label it as expired or defective, and report the expiration or defect as directed by your facility.

Implementation

▪ Review the patient's medical record for contraindications to measuring temperature by the chosen method.
▪ Gather and prepare the necessary equipment and supplies.
▪ Perform hand hygiene.[7,8,9,10,11,12]
▪ Confirm the patient's identity using at least two patient identifiers.[13]
▪ Provide privacy.[14,15,16,17]
▪ Explain the procedure to the patient and family (if appropriate) according to their individual communication and learning needs *to increase their understanding, allay their fears, and enhance cooperation.*[18]
▪ Raise the patient's bed to waist level when providing patient care *to prevent caregiver back strain.*[19]

Measuring rectal temperature

▪ Perform hand hygiene.[7,8,9,10,11,12]
▪ Put on gloves *to comply with standard precautions.*[20,21,22]
▪ Assist the patient to a side-lying position with the top leg flexed.
▪ Cover the thermometer probe with a probe cover or sheath.
▪ Lubricate about 1½" (3.8 cm) of the tip of the covered probe *to ease insertion*, or use a prelubricated sheath, if available.
▪ Lift the patient's upper buttock and gently insert the lubricated thermometer probe into the anus about 1½" (3.8 cm).
▪ Hold the thermometer in place for the duration of time indicated by the manufacturer *to ensure that the maximum temperature is displayed.* Read the temperature display.
▪ Carefully remove the thermometer probe.
▪ Remove and dispose of the rectal probe cover or sheath and discard it in an appropriate receptacle.[22]
▪ Clean the lubricant from the patient's anal area, if necessary.
▪ Remove and discard your gloves.[22]
▪ Perform hand hygiene.[7,8,9,10,11,12]
▪ Assist the patient to a comfortable position.

Measuring oral temperature

- If the patient recently ate, drank hot or cold liquids, chewed gum, or smoked, wait at least 30 minutes before taking an oral temperature.[23,24]
- Perform hand hygiene.[7,8,9,10,11,12]
- Cover the thermometer probe with a probe cover or sheath.
- Position the covered tip of the thermometer under the patient's tongue in the posterior sublingual pocket, *because the external carotid artery perfuses the area, reflecting changes in core temperature.*[1]
- Instruct the patient to close the lips around the thermometer but to avoid biting down.
- Leave the thermometer in place for the duration of time indicated by the manufacturer *to ensure that the maximum temperature is displayed.* Read the temperature display.
- Remove the oral probe or sheath and discard it in an appropriate receptacle.[22]

Measuring tympanic membrane temperature

- Make sure the tympanic lens is clean before using the thermometer; *a dirty lens may produce inaccurate temperature measurements.*[2,25]
- If the patient has been lying with the ear on a pillow or has been wearing earplugs or hearing aids, allow 30 minutes to elapse before measuring temperature *to allow the temperature to normalize.*[25]
- Examine the patient's ear, *because cerumen may reduce the accuracy of readings.* Choose the other ear or an alternative method for measuring the patient's temperature if cerumen is present.[25]
- Cover the thermometer probe with a probe cover.
- Gently pull the ear up and back for an adult, as shown below.

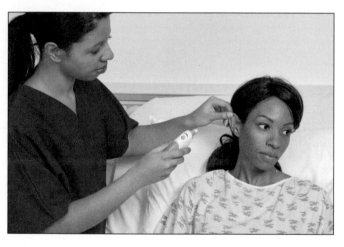

- Insert the thermometer into the patient's ear according to the manufacturer's instructions. *Depending on the thermometer's design, some thermometers require a light seal, whereas others require a full seal and a twist of the thermometer.*[1]
- Press the activation button and hold the thermometer in place for the duration of time indicated by the manufacturer *to ensure that the maximum temperature is displayed.* Read the temperature display.
- Remove the probe cover, and discard it in an appropriate receptacle.[22]

Using an NCIT

- Follow the manufacturer's instructions; *temperature measurement instructions vary by product.* Avoid touching the NCIT sensor, and keep it clean and dry *to help ensure accurate results.*[4]
- Measure temperature in a draft-free location, away from direct light and radiant heat sources. Ensure radiant temperature ranges 60.8° F to 104° F (16° C to 40° C) with relative humidity of 85% or less, if directed by the manufacturer.[4]
- Place the NCIT in the environment where you intend to measure the patient's temperature for 10 to 30 minutes before use, if directed by the manufacturer, *to allow the device to adjust to the environmental conditions.*[4]
- Inspect the patient's forehead to ensure that it's clean, dry, and accessible. *Head coverings or excessive clothing may falsely elevate the temperature reading; moisture, such as from cleansing wipes, may falsely lower the temperature reading.*[4]

- Instruct the patient to remain stationary during temperature measurement.[4]
- Position the thermometer perpendicular to the patient's forehead at the distance specified by the manufacturer's instructions; *distance varies by NCIT.*[4]
- Push the activation button *to measure the patient's temperature.*
- Read the temperature display.

Completing the procedure

- Return the bed to the lowest position *to prevent falls and maintain patient safety.*[26]
- Perform hand hygiene.[7,8,9,10,11,12]
- Clean and disinfect the thermometer following the manufacturer's instructions *to prevent the spread of infection.*[27,28]
- Perform hand hygiene.[7,8,9,10,11,12]
- Document the procedure.[29,30,31,32]

Special considerations

- Rectal temperature measurement has been implicated in the spread of enteric pathogens such as *Clostridioides difficile* and vancomycin-resistant enterococci through the device or health care worker. Make sure the thermometer and probe are properly cleaned and disinfected between use, and that other infection-prevention guidelines are followed *to prevent the spread of infection.*[2]

Complications

Inaccurate results from faulty technique can lead to a delay in treatment or inappropriate treatment. Rectal trauma or perforation can occur with rectal temperature measurement. Oral temperature measurement can cause damage to the oral mucosa, especially in patients with abnormal mucosa due to trauma, thermal injury, infection, surgery, cancer, or cytotoxic medications. Tympanic membrane temperature measurement may cause trauma to the tympanic membrane.[2]

Documentation

Record the time, site, device, and temperature in the patient's medical record. Document prescribed interventions and the patient's response to those interventions. Document teaching provided to the patient and family (if applicable), their understanding of that teaching, and any need for follow-up teaching.

REFERENCES

1 Davie, A., & Amoore, J. (2010). Best practice in the measurement of body temperature. *Nursing Standard, 24*(42), 42–49. (Level VII)
2 O'Grady, N. P., et al. (2008). Guidelines for evaluation of new fever in critically ill adult patients: 2008 update from the American College of Critical Care Medicine and the Infectious Diseases Society of America. *Critical Care Medicine, 36*(4), 1330–1349. https://journals.lww.com/ccmjournal/Fulltext/2008/04000/Guidelines_for_evaluation_of_new_fever_in.40.aspx (Level VII)
3 Munro, N. (2014). Fever in acute and critical care: A diagnostic approach. *AACN Advanced Critical Care, 25*, 237–248. (Level VII)
4 U.S. Food and Drug Administration. (2020). Non-contact infrared thermometers. https://www.fda.gov/medical-devices/general-hospital-devices-and-supplies/non-contact-infrared-thermometers
5 MacLaren, G., & Spelman, D. (2021). Fever in the intensive care unit. In: *UpToDate*, Manaker, S. (Ed.).
6 Makic, M. B., et al. (2011). Evidence-based practice habits: Putting more sacred cows out to pasture. *Critical Care Nurse, 31*(2), 38–62. (Level VII)
7 The Joint Commission. (2021). Standard NPSG.07.01.01. *Comprehensive accreditation manual for hospitals.* Oakbrook Terrace, IL: The Joint Commission. (Level VII)
8 Centers for Disease Control and Prevention. (2002). Guideline for hand hygiene in health-care settings: Recommendations of the Healthcare Infection Control Practices Advisory Committee and the HICPAC/SHEA/APIC/IDSA Hand Hygiene Task Force. *MMWR Recommendations and Reports, 51*(RR-16), 1–45. https://www.cdc.gov/mmwr/pdf/rr/rr5116.pdf (Level II)
9 World Health Organization. (2009). WHO guidelines on hand hygiene in health care: First global patient safety challenge,

clean care is safer care. https://apps.who.int/iris/bitstream/handle/10665/44102/9789241597906_eng.pdf?sequence=1 (Level IV)

10 Centers for Medicare and Medicaid Services, Department of Health and Human Services. (2020). Condition of participation: Infection control. 42 C.F.R. § 482.42.

11 Accreditation Association for Hospitals and Health Systems. (2020). Standard 07.01.21. *Healthcare Facilities Accreditation Program: Accreditation requirements for acute care hospitals.* Chicago, IL: Accreditation Association for Hospitals and Health Systems. (Level VII)

12 DNV GL-Healthcare USA, Inc. (2020). IC.1.SR.1. *NIAHO® accreditation requirements, interpretive guidelines and surveyor guidance—revision 20.0.* Milford, OH: DNV GL-Healthcare USA, Inc. (Level VII)

13 The Joint Commission. (2021). Standard NPSG.01.01.01. *Comprehensive accreditation manual for hospitals.* Oakbrook Terrace, IL: The Joint Commission. (Level VII)

14 Centers for Medicare and Medicaid Services, Department of Health and Human Services. (2020). Condition of participation: Patient's rights. 42 C.F.R. § 482.13(c)(1).

15 Accreditation Association for Hospitals and Health Systems. (2020). Standard 15.01.16. *Healthcare Facilities Accreditation Program: Accreditation requirements for acute care hospitals.* Chicago, IL: Accreditation Association for Hospitals and Health Systems. (Level VII)

16 The Joint Commission. (2021). Standard RI.01.01.01. *Comprehensive accreditation manual for hospitals.* Oakbrook Terrace, IL: The Joint Commission. (Level VII)

17 DNV GL-Healthcare USA, Inc. (2020). PR.2.SR.5. *NIAHO® accreditation requirements, interpretive guidelines and surveyor guidance—revision 20.0.* Milford, OH: DNV GL-Healthcare USA, Inc. (Level VII)

18 The Joint Commission. (2021). Standard PC.02.01.21. *Comprehensive accreditation manual for hospitals.* Oakbrook Terrace, IL: The Joint Commission. (Level VII)

19 Waters, T. R., et al. (2009). Safe patient handling training for schools of nursing. https://www.cdc.gov/niosh/docs/2009-127/pdfs/2009-127.pdf (Level VII)

20 Accreditation Association for Hospitals and Health Systems. (2020). Standard 07.01.10. *Healthcare Facilities Accreditation Program: Accreditation requirements for acute care hospitals.* Chicago, IL: Accreditation Association for Hospitals and Health Systems. (Level VII)

21 Siegel, J. D., et al. (2007, revised 2019). 2007 guideline for isolation precautions: Preventing transmission of infectious agents in healthcare settings. https://www.cdc.gov/infectioncontrol/pdf/guidelines/isolation-guidelines-H.pdf (Level II)

22 Occupational Safety and Health Administration. (2012). Bloodborne pathogens, standard number 1910.1030. https://www.osha.gov/pls/oshaweb/owadisp.show_document?p_id=10051&p_table=STANDARDS (Level VII)

23 Mayo Clinic. (2020). How to take your temperature. https://www.mayoclinic.org/how-to-take-temperature/art-20482578#:~:text=If%20you've%20been%20eating,thermometer%20beep%20indicates%20it's%20done

24 Dinarello, C. A., & Porat, R. (2021). Pathophysiology and treatment of fever in adults. In: *UpToDate*, Weller, P. F. (Ed.)

25 Allyn, Welch (2019). Braun ThermoScan ear thermometer: Directions for use. https://www.hillrom.com/content/dam/hillrom-aem/us/en/sap-documents/LIT/80024/80024839LITPDF.pdf

26 Ganz, D. A., et al. (2013, reviewed 2021). *Preventing falls in hospitals: A toolkit for improving quality of care* (AHRQ Publication No. 13-0015-EF). Rockville, MD: Agency for Healthcare Research and Quality. https://www.ahrq.gov/professionals/systems/hospital/fallpxtoolkit/index.html (Level VII)

27 Rutala, W. A., et al. (2008, revised 2019). Guideline for disinfection and sterilization in healthcare facilities, 2008. https://www.cdc.gov/infection-control/pdf/guidelines/disinfection-guidelines-H.pdf (Level I)

28 Accreditation Association for Hospitals and Health Systems. (2020). Standard 07.02.03. *Healthcare Facilities Accreditation Program: Accreditation requirements for acute care hospitals.* Chicago, IL: Accreditation Association for Hospitals and Health Systems. (Level VII)

29 The Joint Commission. (2021). Standard RC.01.03.01. *Comprehensive accreditation manual for hospitals.* Oakbrook Terrace, IL: The Joint Commission. (Level VII)

30 Centers for Medicare and Medicaid Services, Department of Health and Human Services. (2020). Condition of participation: Medical record services. 42 C.F.R. § 482.24(b).

31 Accreditation Association for Hospitals and Health Systems. (2020). Standard 10.00.03. *Healthcare Facilities Accreditation Program: Accreditation requirements for acute care hospitals.* Chicago, IL: Accreditation Association for Hospitals and Health Systems. (Level VII)

32 DNV GL-Healthcare USA, Inc. (2020). MR.2.SR.1. *NIAHO® accreditation requirements, interpretive guidelines and surveyor guidance—revision 20.0.* Milford, OH: DNV GL-Healthcare USA, Inc. (Level VII)

THERAPEUTIC BATH

Also referred to as *balneotherapy*, the therapeutic bath combines water and additives to soothe and relax the patient, relieve fatigue and sore muscles and joints, clean the skin, relieve inflammation and pruritus, and soften and remove crusts, scales, debris, and old medications. Used primarily for their antipruritic and emollient actions, these baths coat irritated skin with a soothing, protective film. Because they constrict surface blood vessels, they also have an anti-inflammatory effect.

The addition of oatmeal powder, soluble cornstarch, or soybean complex to water creates a colloid bath, which has a soothing effect and is used to treat generalized itching. Oil baths are useful for lubricating dry skin and easing eczematous eruptions. Sodium bicarbonate added to water produces an alkaline bath that has a cooling effect and helps relieve pruritus. A medicated tar bath may help psoriasis; the film of tar left on the skin works in combination with ultraviolet light to inhibit the rapid cell turnover characteristic of psoriasis. (See *Comparing therapeutic baths*.)

A patient confined to bed may benefit from a local soak with the therapeutic additive instead of a therapeutic tub bath. (See the "Soaks" procedure.)

Comparing therapeutic baths

The table below lists the types of therapeutic baths along with their agents and purpose.

TYPE	AGENTS	PURPOSE
Antibacterial	▪ Acetic acid ▪ Potassium permanganate ▪ Povidone-iodine	▪ To treat infected eczema, dirty ulcerations, furunculosis, and pemphigus
Colloidal	▪ Aveeno colloidal oatmeal ▪ Aveeno colloidal oatmeal, oilated ▪ Soybean complex ▪ Starch and baking soda	▪ To relieve pruritus and to soothe and coat irritated skin; indicated for any irritated or oozing condition, such as atopic eczema
Emollient	▪ Bath oils ▪ Chamomile ▪ Mineral oil	▪ To clean and hydrate the skin; indicated for any dry skin condition
Tar	▪ Bath oils with tar ▪ Coal tar concentrate	▪ To treat scaly dermatoses (sometimes in combination with ultraviolet light therapy); loosens scales and relieves pruritus

Equipment

Bathtub ▪ bath mat ▪ rubber mat ▪ bath (utility) thermometer ▪ therapeutic additive ▪ measuring device ▪ washcloths ▪ towels ▪ patient gown or loose-fitting cotton pajamas ▪ gloves ▪ facility-approved disinfectant ▪ Optional: lubricating cream or ointment, plastic apron or protective gown, personal protective equipment, colander, sieve.

Preparation of equipment

Make sure the tub is clean and disinfected,[1] *to reduce the risk for infection.* Place the bath mat next to the tub and the rubber mat on the bottom of the tub *to prevent falls, because the therapeutic additive may make the tub exceptionally slippery.*

Inspect all equipment and supplies. If a product is expired, is defective, or has compromised integrity, remove it from patient use, label it as expired or defective, and report the expiration or defect, as directed by your facility.

If you are giving a tar bath, wear a plastic apron or protective gown, *because tar preparations stain clothing.*[2]

Read the manufacturer's instructions on the therapeutic additive bottle. Look for contraindications, adverse effects, and warnings.

Implementation

- Verify the practitioner's order.
- Gather and prepare the necessary equipment and supplies.
- Review the patient's medical record for a history of allergies or contraindications to the therapeutic additive.
- Draw the bath before bringing the patient to the bath area *to prevent chilling.* Fill the tub with 6" to 8"(15 cm to 20 cm) of water at 95° F to 100° F (35° C to 38° C).
- Measure the correct amount of therapeutic additive, according to the practitioner's order or package instructions. As the tub is filling, thoroughly mix the additive in the water. Add most substances directly to the water, but place oatmeal powder in a sieve or colander under the tub faucet *to help it dissolve.* Begin with 2 tbs (about 30 mL) of oatmeal powder; then add more powder or water as needed *to regulate the thickness of the oatmeal bath.*
- Perform hand hygiene.[3,4,5,6,7,8]
- Confirm the patient's identity using at least two patient identifiers.[9]
- Provide privacy.[10,11,12,13]
- Explain the procedure to the patient and family (if appropriate) according to their individual communication and learning needs *to increase their understanding, allay their fears, and enhance cooperation.*[14]
- Have the patient void, if needed.
- Escort the patient to the bath area.
- Close the door *to maintain privacy and eliminate drafts.*

NURSING ALERT Make sure that the bathroom is well ventilated. Some patients may experience allergic reactions or hypersensitivity to the additive in the water or to its odor. If a reaction occurs, limit the patient's time in the bath and notify the practitioner. If a skin reaction to the additive occurs, gently wash the additive from the skin and notify the practitioner.

- Perform hand hygiene.[3,4,5,6,7,8]
- Put on gloves and other personal protective equipment as needed *to comply with standard precautions.*[15,16,17]
- Check the water temperature using a bath thermometer.
- Help the patient undress, and then help the patient into the tub, if necessary. Advise the patient to use the safety rails *to help prevent falls.*[18]
- Explain that the bath may feel unpleasant at first *because the skin is irritated by the additive*, but assure the patient that the medication will soon coat and soothe the skin.
- Ask the patient to stretch out in the tub and submerge the body up to the chin. Support the head and neck, if needed. If the patient's capable, give the patient a washcloth to apply the bath solution gently to the face and other body areas not immersed if these areas require treatment.

NURSING ALERT Tell the patient taking a tar bath not to get the bath solution in the eyes, *because tar is an eye irritant.* If this occurs, tell the patient to rinse the eyes with water.[2]

- Warn the patient against scrubbing the skin *to prevent further irritation.*

- Add warm water to the bath as needed *to maintain a comfortable temperature.*
- Remove and discard your gloves and other personal equipment, if worn.[15,16,17]
- Perform hand hygiene.[3,4,5,6,7,8]
- Allow the patient to soak for 15 to 30 minutes. *Periods of soaking longer than this may cause skin softening and damage to the skin.* If you stay with the patient, pull the bath curtain *to give the patient some privacy and protect the patient from drafts.* If you must leave the room, show the patient how to use the call light, and ensure the patient's privacy.[18]
- After the bath, assist the patient from the tub. Have the patient use the safety rails *to help prevent falls.*[18]
- Help the patient pat the skin dry with towels. Don't rub the skin, *because rubbing removes some solutes and oils clinging to the skin and produces friction, worsening pruritus.*
- Perform hand hygiene.[3,4,5,6,7,8]
- Put on new gloves and other personal protective equipment as needed.[15,16,17]
- Apply lubricating cream or ointment, if ordered, *to help hold water in the newly hydrated skin.*
- Provide a fresh patient gown or loose-fitting cotton pajamas. *Tight clothing and scratchy or synthetic materials can aggravate skin conditions by causing friction and increasing perspiration.*
- Escort the patient back to the room and make sure the patient is comfortable.
- Drain the bath water, and clean and disinfect the tub using a facility-approved disinfectant.[1,19] If you've given an oatmeal powder bath, drain and rinse the tub immediately; *otherwise the powder will cake, making later removal difficult.*
- Discard soiled materials in the appropriate receptacles.[17]
- Remove and discard your gloves and other personal protective equipment, if worn.[15,17]
- Perform hand hygiene.[3,4,5,6,7,8]
- Document the procedure.[20,21,22,23]

Special considerations

- The treatment's purpose and type of additive used will determine the water temperature. Cool to lukewarm water is used for relieving pruritus and promotes mixing when adding tar or starch. Warm baths soothe, but baths warmer than 100° F (38° C) causes vasodilation, *which could aggravate pruritus.*
- *Because pruritus seems worse at night*, a therapeutic bath is best before bedtime, unless ordered otherwise, *to promote restful sleep.*
- *Because the patient with a skin disorder may be self-conscious*, maintain eye contact during conversation and avoid staring at the skin. Also avoid nonverbal expressions and gestures that show revulsion. Allow the patient who wishes to do so to talk about the condition and how it affects self-esteem.
- Refrain from using soap during a therapeutic bath, *because its drying effect counteracts the bath emollient.*
- *A patient with skin breakdown chills easily*, so protect the patient from drafts. However, avoid covering or dressing the patient too warmly after the bath, *because perspiration aggravates pruritus.* Instruct the patient not to scratch the skin, *to prevent excoriation and infection.*
- If the patient is confined to bed, you can place the therapeutic additive in a basin of water at 95° F to 100° F (35° C to 38°C) and apply it with a washcloth, using light, gentle strokes.

Complications

The patient may experience an allergic reaction or hypersensitivity to the additive.

Documentation

Record the date, time, and duration of the bath. Note the water temperature, type and amount of additive, skin appearance before and after the bath, the patient's tolerance of the treatment, and the bath's effectiveness. Document teaching you provided to the patient and family (if applicable), their understanding of that teaching, and any need for follow-up teaching.

REFERENCES

1 Rutala, W. A., et al. (2008, revised 2019). Guideline for disinfection and sterilization in healthcare facilities, 2008. https://www.cdc.gov/infection-control/pdf/guidelines/disinfection-guidelines-H.pdf (Level I)

2 Multum, C. (2021). Balnetar. https://www.drugs.com/mtm/balnetar.html

3 The Joint Commission. (2021). Standard NPSG.07.01.01. *Comprehensive accreditation manual for hospitals.* Oakbrook Terrace, IL: The Joint Commission. (Level VII)

4 Centers for Disease Control and Prevention. (2002). Guideline for hand hygiene in health-care settings: Recommendations of the Healthcare Infection Control Practices Advisory Committee and the HICPAC/SHEA/APIC/IDSA Hand Hygiene Task Force. *MMWR Recommendations and Reports, 51*(RR-16), 1–45. https://www.cdc.gov/mmwr/pdf/rr/rr5116.pdf (Level II)

5 World Health Organization. (2009). WHO guidelines on hand hygiene in health care: First global patient safety challenge, clean care is safer care. https://apps.who.int/iris/bitstream/handle/10665/44102/9789241597906_eng.pdf?sequence=1 (Level IV)

6 Accreditation Association for Hospitals and Health Systems. (2020). Standard 07.01.21. *Healthcare Facilities Accreditation Program: Accreditation requirements for acute care hospitals.* Chicago, IL: Accreditation Association for Hospitals and Health Systems. (Level VII)

7 Centers for Medicare and Medicaid Services, Department of Health and Human Services. (2020). Condition of participation: Infection control. 42 C.F.R. § 482.42.

8 DNV GL-Healthcare USA, Inc. (2020). IC.1.SR.1. *NIAHO® accreditation requirements, interpretive guidelines and surveyor guidance—revision 20.0.* Milford, OH: DNV GL-Healthcare USA, Inc. (Level VII)

9 The Joint Commission. (2021). Standard NPSG.01.01.01. *Comprehensive accreditation manual for hospitals.* Oakbrook Terrace, IL: The Joint Commission. (Level VII)

10 Accreditation Association for Hospitals and Health Systems. (2020). Standard 15.01.16. *Healthcare Facilities Accreditation Program: Accreditation requirements for acute care hospitals.* Chicago, IL: Accreditation Association for Hospitals and Health Systems. (Level VII)

11 Centers for Medicare and Medicaid Services, Department of Health and Human Services. (2020). Condition of participation: Patient's rights. 42 C.F.R. § 482.13(c)(1).

12 The Joint Commission. (2021). Standard RI.01.01.01. *Comprehensive accreditation manual for hospitals.* Oakbrook Terrace, IL: The Joint Commission. (Level VII)

13 DNV GL-Healthcare USA, Inc. (2020). PR.2.SR.5. *NIAHO® accreditation requirements, interpretive guidelines and surveyor guidance—revision 20.0.* Milford, OH: DNV GL-Healthcare USA, Inc. (Level VII)

14 The Joint Commission. (2021). Standard PC.02.01.21. *Comprehensive accreditation manual for hospitals.* Oakbrook Terrace, IL: The Joint Commission. (Level VII)

15 Siegel, J. D., et al. (2007, revision 2019). 2007 guideline for isolation precautions: Preventing transmission of infectious agents in healthcare settings. https://www.cdc.gov/infectioncontrol/pdf/guidelines/isolation-guidelines-H.pdf (Level II)

16 Accreditation Association for Hospitals and Health Systems. (2020). Standard 07.01.10. *Healthcare Facilities Accreditation Program: Accreditation requirements for acute care hospitals.* Chicago, IL: Accreditation Association for Hospitals and Health Systems. (Level VII)

17 Occupational Safety and Health Administration. (2012). Bloodborne pathogens, standard number 1910.1030. https://www.osha.gov/pls/oshaweb/owadisp.show_document?p_id=10051&p_table=STANDARDS (Level VII)

18 Ganz, D. A., et al. (2013, reviewed 2021). *Preventing falls in hospitals: A toolkit for improving quality of care* (AHRQ Publication No. 13-0015-EF). Rockville, MD: Agency for Healthcare Research and Quality. https://www.ahrq.gov/professionals/systems/hospital/fallpxtoolkit/index.html (Level VII)

19 Accreditation Association for Hospitals and Health Systems. (2020). Standard 07.02.03. *Healthcare Facilities Accreditation Program: Accreditation requirements for acute care hospitals.* Chicago, IL: Accreditation Association for Hospitals and Health Systems. (Level VII)

20 The Joint Commission. (2021). Standard RC.01.03.01. *Comprehensive accreditation manual for hospitals.* Oakbrook Terrace, IL: The Joint Commission. (Level VII)

21 Accreditation Association for Hospitals and Health Systems. (2020). Standard 10.00.03. *Healthcare Facilities Accreditation Program: Accreditation requirements for acute care hospitals.* Chicago, IL: Accreditation Association for Hospitals and Health Systems. (Level VII)

22 Centers for Medicare and Medicaid Services, Department of Health and Human Services. (2020). Condition of participation: Medical record services. 42 C.F.R. § 482.24(b).

23 DNV GL-Healthcare USA, Inc. (2020). MR.2.SR.1. *NIAHO® accreditation requirements, interpretive guidelines and surveyor guidance—revision 20.0.* Milford, OH: DNV GL-Healthcare USA, Inc. (Level VII)

THORACENTESIS, ASSISTING

Thoracentesis involves insertion of a needle into the pleural space to remove a pleural effusion (an accumulation of pleural fluid). The procedure may help diagnose the cause of a pleural effusion of unknown etiology or relieve symptoms caused by pleural effusion.[1]

Pleural effusions develop when there's an overproduction of fluid or fluid fails to reabsorb. They're classified as transudative or exudative. Transudative pleural effusions are commonly associated with systemic conditions (such as heart failure), whereas a local condition (such as an infection or pulmonary embolus) usually causes exudative pleural effusions.[1]

An effusion is classified as exudative when pleural fluid analysis meets one of the following criteria: the protein-to-serum ratio exceeds 0.5 g/dL, the lactate dehydrogenase (LDH)-to-serum ratio exceeds 0.6 international units/mL, or the LDH exceeds more than two-thirds the upper limit of normal.[1] A pleural effusion is classified as transudative if none of the exudative criteria are met.[1]

Relative contraindications for thoracentesis include uncorrectable coagulopathy, current anticoagulation therapy, difficult anatomy, elevated left hemidiaphragm, known pulmonary disease, left-sided pleural effusion, pneumonectomy, current positive end-expiratory pressure therapy, active infection at the needle insertion site, and splenomegaly.[1]

Ultrasound-guided thoracentesis reduces the risk of complications.[1] A practitioner performs the procedure with a nurse assisting, as needed.

Equipment

Most facilities use a prepackaged thoracentesis tray that typically includes the following: sterile fenestrated drape ▪ 1% or 2% lidocaine ▪ 5-mL syringe with 22G and 25G needles for anesthetic injection ▪ 14G thoracentesis needle for aspiration or 16G over-the-needle catheters[1] ▪ 50- or 60-mL syringe ▪ three-way stopcock ▪ drainage tube set ▪ extension set with 16G 1½" (3.8 cm) vacuum needle and vacuum bottle ▪ fluid collection bag[2] ▪ sterile specimen containers ▪ sterile 4"× 4" (10-cm × 10-cm) gauze pads ▪ antiseptic cleaning swabs or applicators (chlorhexidine or povidone iodine) ▪ adhesive bandage.

You'll also need the following: Sterile fine-tip marker ▪ sterile labels ▪ vital signs monitoring equipment ▪ pulse oximeter and probe ▪ sterile gloves ▪ gowns ▪ masks and goggles or masks with face shields ▪ gloves ▪ stethoscope ▪ specimen collection bottles ▪ laboratory biohazard transport bag ▪ prescribed sedative or analgesic ▪ disinfectant pad ▪ facility-approved pain assessment tool ▪ emergency equipment (code cart with cardiac medications, defibrillator, handheld resuscitation bag with mask, intubation equipment) ▪ Optional: preprocedure verification checklist, bedside ultrasound equipment, sterile and clean disposable ultrasound probe covers, sterile ultrasound gel, disposable-head hair clippers, IV catheter insertion equipment, laboratory request forms, sterile hemostat.

Preparation of equipment

Inspect all equipment and supplies. If a product is expired, is defective, or has compromised integrity, remove it from patient use, label it as expired or defective, and report the expiration or defect as directed by your facility. Prepare the necessary laboratory request forms, if applicable. Be sure to list current antibiotic therapy on the laboratory request forms, *because antibiotic therapy affect specimen analysis.* Prepare the ultrasound equipment, if appropriate. Make sure that emergency equipment is functioning properly and readily available.

Implementation

▪ Verify the practitioner's orders.
▪ Check the patient's medical history for any allergies, especially to latex, antiseptic cleaning solution, or the local anesthetic.

Positioning for thoracentesis

The choice of the position may vary. Usually, the patient is sitting upright and leaning forward. If the patient is sitting on the edge of the bed, support the legs and have the patient lean forward and rest the head and arms on a pillow on the overbed table (as shown). If possible, enlist the assistance of another staff member to stand in front of the patient *for additional support*. If the patient can't sit, turn the patient on the unaffected side, positioned at the edge of the bed with the arm of the affected side raised comfortably above the patient's head. Elevate the head of the bed 30 to 45 degrees, unless contraindicated.[1] Recumbent thoracentesis is possible with ultrasound guidance.[37,38] *Proper positioning stretches the chest or back and allows easier access to the intercostal spaces.*

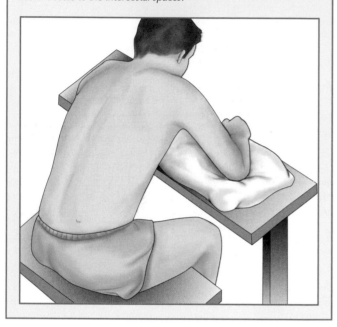

■ Gather and prepare the necessary equipment and supplies at the patient's bedside or in the treatment area.

■ If required by your facility, confirm that an informed consent has been obtained and that the signed consent form is in the patient's medical record.[3,4,5,6]

■ Conduct a preprocedure verification *to make sure that all relevant documentation, related information, and equipment are available and correctly identified to the patient's identifiers.*[7,8,9] If required, complete a preprocedure verification checklist or confirm that one is complete.[7,10,11]

■ Verify that the laboratory and imaging studies have been completed as ordered, and that the results are in the patient's medical record. Notify the practitioner of any unexpected results.[8,9]

■ Perform hand hygiene.[12,13,14,15,16,17]

■ Confirm the patient's identity using at least two patient identifiers.[18]

■ Reinforce the practitioner's explanation of the procedure and answer any questions. Inform the patient that some discomfort and pressure may occur during the needle insertion.[3,4,5,6]

■ Allow the patient's family members to remain throughout the procedure if they wish to do so.[19] Assist them in putting on personal protective equipment, as needed.

■ Provide privacy and emotional support for the patient and family (if appropriate).[20,21,22,23]

■ If required by your facility, make sure that the procedure site is marked.[7,9,10,24]

■ Perform hand hygiene.[12,13,14,15,16,17]

■ Put on gloves, a gown, and a mask with a face shield or a mask and goggles, as needed, *to comply with standard precautions.*[25,26,27]

■ Assess vital signs, pain level, and respiratory function *as a baseline for comparison during and after the procedure.*[1,28]

■ Attach the patient to a continuous pulse oximeter and obtain a baseline oxygen saturation level *for comparison during and after the procedure.*[1]

Make sure that alarm limits are set appropriately for the patient's current condition, and that alarms are turned on, functioning properly, and audible to staff.[29,30,31,32]

■ Auscultate the patient's breath sounds.[1]

■ Ensure that the patient has patent IV access *for administration of procedural and emergency medications.* Initiate IV access, if needed.[1]

■ Administer a sedative or an analgesic as ordered following safe medication administration practices.[33,34,35,36]

■ Position the patient appropriately *to ease the withdrawal of pleural fluid.*[1] Make sure that the patient is firmly supported and comfortable. (See *Positioning for thoracentesis.*)

■ Remind the patient not to cough, breathe deeply, or move suddenly during the procedure *to avoid puncture of the visceral pleura or lung.*[39] If the patient coughs, the practitioner will briefly halt the procedure and withdraw the needle slightly *to prevent puncture.*

■ Expose the patient's entire chest or back as appropriate.[39]

■ Clip hair from the aspiration site using disposable-head hair clippers, if needed.[40,41]

■ Perform hand hygiene.[12,13,14,15,16,17]

■ Put on a gown, a mask and goggles or mask with face shield, and gloves.[25,26,27]

■ Using sterile technique, open the thoracentesis tray. Label all medications, medication containers, and other solutions on and off the sterile field.[42,43]

■ Assist the practitioner as necessary in disinfecting the site and allowing it to dry.

■ Conduct a time-out immediately before starting the procedure *to perform a final assessment to ensure that the correct patient, site, positioning, and procedure are identified, and that, as applicable, all relevant information and necessary equipment are available.*[7,9,44]

■ After draping the patient and injecting the local anesthetic, the practitioner may use ultrasonography to identify landmarks. *Ultrasound guidance reduces the risk of pneumothorax and increases thoracentesis success.*[1,7,37,45]

■ The practitioner attaches a three-way stopcock with tubing to the aspirating needle and opens the stopcock valve between the syringe and the needle, *to enable the aspiration of pleural fluid during needle insertion and to prevent air from entering the pleural space.*[1]

■ Attach the other end of the tubing to the fluid collection bag or vacuum bottle.[2]

■ The practitioner inserts the needle into the pleural space and attaches a 50-mL syringe to the needle's stopcock. A sterile hemostat might be used *to hold the needle in place and prevent a pleural tear or lung puncture.* Alternatively, the practitioner may introduce a catheter into the needle, remove the needle, and attach a stopcock and syringe to the catheter *to reduce the risk of pleural puncture by the needle.*[1]

■ Reassure the patient throughout the procedure, assessing for signs of anxiety. Keep the patient informed of each step.

■ Monitor the patient's vital signs and oxygen saturation level regularly during the procedure.[1] Continually observe the patient for signs of distress such as pallor, vertigo, faintness, weak or rapid pulse, decreased blood pressure, dyspnea, tachypnea, diaphoresis, chest pain, blood-tinged mucus, and excessive coughing. Alert the practitioner if any of these develop, *because they may indicate complications such as hypovolemic shock and tension pneumothorax.*[1]

■ Assist the practitioner as needed with specimen collection, fluid drainage, and site dressing.

■ Label the specimens with the patient's name, identification number, and date and time of collection in the presence of the patient *to prevent mislabeling.* Place the specimens in a laboratory biohazard transport bag and send them to the laboratory immediately with the appropriate laboratory request forms, if necessary.[27]

■ After the practitioner withdraws the needle or catheter, apply pressure to the puncture site using a sterile 4" × 4" (10-cm × 10-cm) gauze pad.[1] Apply an adhesive bandage over the site.[1]

■ Place the patient in a comfortable position.[1]

■ Assess the patient's vital signs, oxygen saturation level, and respiratory status.[1] Continue to monitor vital signs at a frequency determined by the patient's condition and your facility, *because there's no evidence-based research available to indicate best practice for frequency of assessing vital signs after thoracentesis.*[46]

- Screen for and assess the patient's pain using facility-defined criteria that are consistent with the patient's age, condition, and ability to understand.[28]
- Treat the patient's pain, as needed and ordered, using nonpharmacologic or pharmacologic approaches, or a combination. Base the treatment plan on evidence-based practices and the patient's clinical condition, past medical history, and pain management goals.[28]
- Monitor closely if the patient is at high risk for adverse outcomes related to opioid treatment, if prescribed.[28]
- Examine the dressing for drainage.[1]
- Discard used supplies in the appropriate receptacles.[27]
- Obtain a chest X-ray, if ordered, after the procedure. *If not clinically indicated, routine chest X-ray isn't necessary.*[1]
- Reassess and respond to the patient's pain by evaluating the response to treatment and progress toward pain management goals. Assess for adverse reactions and risk factors for adverse events that may result from treatment.[28]
- Remove and discard your gloves and personal protective equipment, if worn.[27]
- Perform hand hygiene.[12,13,14,15,16,17]
- Clean and disinfect your stethoscope with a disinfectant pad.[47,48]
- Perform hand hygiene.[12,13,14,15,16,17]
- Document the procedure.[49,50,51,52]

Special considerations

- The maximum volume of fluid that can be safely removed during therapeutic thoracentesis is unknown; the occurrence of reexpansion pulmonary edema and procedure-related pneumothorax doesn't clearly correlate with the onset of symptoms or the volume of fluid removed. A traditional method to avoid these complications has been to discontinue fluid removal at the onset of chest discomfort or when the total amount of fluid removed reaches 1,000 to 1,500 mL. However, this practice doesn't always prevent adverse effects; in fact, many patients do well with removal of more than 1,500 mL of fluid.[53]
- Some coughing is common as the lung re-expands.[1]
- Pleuritic or shoulder pain may indicate pleural irritation by the needle point.
- The practitioner may decide to place a small-bore (or pigtail) chest tube for continued drainage of a large effusion.[38]

Complications

Potential complications of thoracentesis include shortness of breath or cough, hemorrhage or other bleeding, puncture of the liver or spleen, infection, pain at the insertion site, pneumothorax, empyema, vasovagal events, and reexpansion pulmonary edema.[54]

Documentation

Record the date and time of the procedure and the name of the practitioner who performed it. Include the location of the puncture site; volume and description (color, viscosity, odor) of the fluid withdrawn; specimens sent to the laboratory; vital signs, oxygen saturation level, pain level, and respiratory assessment findings before, during, and after the procedure; any postprocedural tests, such as a chest X-ray; any complications that occurred, the prescribed interventions, and the patient's response to those interventions; and the patient's reaction to the procedure. Document all medications you administered and the patient's response to those medications. Document any complications, the name of the practitioner notified and the date and time of notification, prescribed interventions, and the patient's response to the interventions. Document teaching provided to the patient and family (if applicable), their understanding of that teaching, and any need for follow-up teaching.

REFERENCES

1 Wiegand, D. L. (2017). *AACN procedure manual for high acuity, progressive, and critical care* (7th ed.). St. Louis, MO: Elsevier.
2 Carefusion. (2014). Thora-Para catheter drainage system overview. https://www.bd.com/en-us/offerings/capabilities/interventional-specialties/peritoneal-and-pleural-drainage/thoracentesis-and-paracentesis/thora-para-catheter-drainage-system
3 Centers for Medicare and Medicaid Services. (2020). Condition of participation: Patient's rights. 42 C.F.R. § 482.13(b)(2).
4 The Joint Commission. (2021). Standard RI.01.03.01. *Comprehensive accreditation manual for hospitals.* Oakbrook Terrace, IL: The Joint Commission. (Level VII)
5 Accreditation Association for Hospitals and Health Systems. (2020). Standard 15.01.11. *Healthcare Facilities Accreditation Program: Accreditation requirements for acute care hospitals.* Chicago, IL: Accreditation Association for Hospitals and Health Systems. (Level VII)
6 DNV GL-Healthcare USA, Inc. (2020). PR.2.SR.3. *NIAHO® accreditation requirements, interpretive guidelines and surveyor guidance—revision 20.0.* Milford, OH: DNV GL-Healthcare USA, Inc. (Level VII)
7 DeBiasi, E. M., & Puchalski, J. (2016). Thoracentesis: State-of-the-art in procedural safety, patient outcomes, and physiologic impact. *Pleura, 3,* 1–10. http://journals.sagepub.com/doi/pdf/10.1177/2373997516646554 (Level V)
8 The Joint Commission. (2021). Standard UP.01.01.01. *Comprehensive accreditation manual for hospitals.* Oakbrook Terrace, IL: The Joint Commission. (Level VII)
9 Accreditation Association for Hospitals and Health Systems. (2020). Standard 30.00.14. *Healthcare Facilities Accreditation Program: Accreditation requirements for acute care hospitals.* Chicago, IL: Accreditation Association for Hospitals and Health Systems. (Level VII)
10 Miller, K. E., et al. (2014). Wrong-side thoracentesis: Lessons learned from root cause analysis. *JAMA Surgery, 149*(8), 774–779. https://jamanetwork.com/journals/jamasurgery/fullarticle/1879844 (Level V)
11 World Health Organization. (2009). Implementation manual: WHO surgical safety checklist 2009. https://apps.who.int/iris/bitstream/handle/10665/44186/9789241598590_eng.pdf;sequence=1 (Level IV)
12 The Joint Commission. (2021). Standard NPSG.07.01.01. *Comprehensive accreditation manual for hospitals.* Oakbrook Terrace, IL: The Joint Commission. (Level VII)
13 World Health Organization (WHO). (2009). WHO guidelines on hand hygiene in health care: First global patient safety challenge, clean care is safer care. https://apps.who.int/iris/bitstream/handle/10665/44102/9789241597906_eng.pdf?sequence=1 (Level IV)
14 Centers for Disease Control and Prevention. (2002). Guideline for hand hygiene in health-care settings: Recommendations of the Healthcare Infection Control Practices Advisory Committee and the HICPAC/SHEA/APIC/IDSA Hand Hygiene Task Force. *MMWR Recommendations and Reports, 51*(RR-16), 1–45. https://www.cdc.gov/mmwr/pdf/rr/rr5116.pdf (Level II)
15 Centers for Medicare and Medicaid Services, Department of Health and Human Services. (2020). Condition of participation: Infection control. 42 C.F.R. § 482.42.
16 Accreditation Association for Hospitals and Health Systems. (2020). Standard 07.01.21. *Healthcare Facilities Accreditation Program: Accreditation requirements for acute care hospitals.* Chicago, IL: Accreditation Association for Hospitals and Health Systems. (Level VII)
17 DNV GL-Healthcare USA, Inc. (2020). IC.1.SR.1. *NIAHO® accreditation requirements, interpretive guidelines and surveyor guidance—revision 20.0.* Milford, OH: DNV GL-Healthcare USA, Inc. (Level VII)
18 The Joint Commission. (2021). Standard NPSG.01.01.01. *Comprehensive accreditation manual for hospitals.* Oakbrook Terrace, IL: The Joint Commission. (Level VII)
19 American Association of Critical-Care Nurses (AACN). (2016). AACN practice alert: Family presence during resuscitation and invasive procedures. https://www.aacn.org/clinical-resources/practice-alerts/family-presence-during-resuscitation-and-invasive-procedures (Level VII)
20 Accreditation Association for Hospitals and Health Systems. (2020). Standard 15.01.16. *Healthcare Facilities Accreditation Program: Accreditation requirements for acute care hospitals.* Chicago, IL: Accreditation Association for Hospitals and Health Systems. (Level VII)
21 DNV GL-Healthcare USA, Inc. (2020). PR.2.SR.5. *NIAHO® accreditation requirements, interpretive guidelines and surveyor guidance—revision 20.0.* Milford, OH: DNV GL-Healthcare USA, Inc. (Level VII)
22 The Joint Commission. (2021). Standard RI.01.01.01. *Comprehensive accreditation manual for hospitals.* Oakbrook Terrace, IL: The Joint Commission. (Level VII)
23 Centers for Medicare and Medicaid Services, Department of Health and Human Services. (2020). Condition of participation: Patient's rights. 42 C.F.R. § 482.13(c)(1).

24 The Joint Commission. (2021). Standard UP.01.02.01. *Comprehensive accreditation manual for hospitals*. Oakbrook Terrace, IL: The Joint Commission. (Level VII)

25 Siegel, J. D., et al. (2007, revised 2019). 2007 guideline for isolation precautions: Preventing transmission of infectious agents in healthcare settings. https://www.cdc.gov/infectioncontrol/pdf/guidelines/isolation-guidelines-H.pdf (Level II)

26 Accreditation Association for Hospitals and Health Systems. (2020). Standard 07.01.10. *Healthcare Facilities Accreditation Program: Accreditation requirements for acute care hospitals*. (Level VII)

27 Occupational Safety and Health Administration. (2012). Bloodborne pathogens, standard number 1910.1030. https://www.osha.gov/pls/oshaweb/owadisp.show_document?p_id=10051&p_table=STANDARDS (Level VII)

28 The Joint Commission. (2021). Standard PC.01.02.07. *Comprehensive accreditation manual for hospitals*. Oakbrook Terrace, IL: The Joint Commission. (Level VII)

29 American Association of Critical-Care Nurses (AACN). (2018). AACN practice alert: Managing alarms in acute care across the life span: Electrocardiography and pulse oximetry. https://www.aacn.org/clinical-resources/practice-alerts/managing-alarms-in-acute-care-across-the-life-span (Level VII)

30 The Joint Commission. (2021). Standard NPSG.06.01.01. *Comprehensive accreditation manual for hospitals*. Oakbrook Terrace, IL: The Joint Commission. (Level VII)

31 Graham, K. C., & Cvach, M. (2010). Monitor alarm fatigue: Standardizing use of physiological monitors and decreasing nuisance alarms. *American Journal of Critical Care, 19*(1), 28–37. https://doi.org/10.4037/ajcc2010651

32 The Joint Commission. (2013). Sentinel event alert 50: Medical device alarm safety in hospitals. https://www.jointcommission.org/-/media/tjc/documents/resources/patient-safety-topics/sentinel-event/sea_50_alarms_4_26_16.pdf (Level VII)

33 Centers for Medicare and Medicaid Services, Department of Health and Human Services. (2020). Condition of participation: Nursing services. 42 C.F.R. § 482.23(c).

34 Accreditation Association for Hospitals and Health Systems. (2020). Standard 16.01.03. *Healthcare Facilities Accreditation Program: Accreditation requirements for acute care hospitals*. Chicago, IL: Accreditation Association for Hospitals and Health Systems. (Level VII)

35 DNV GL-Healthcare USA, Inc. (2020). MM.1.SR.3. *NIAHO® accreditation requirements, interpretive guidelines and surveyor guidance – revision 20.0*. Milford, OH: DNV GL-Healthcare USA, Inc. (Level VII)

36 The Joint Commission. (2021). Standard MM.06.01.01. *Comprehensive accreditation manual for hospitals*. Oakbrook Terrace, IL: The Joint Commission. (Level VII)

37 Soldati, G., et al. (2013). Ultrasound-guided pleural puncture in supine or recumbent lateral position—feasibility study. *Multidisciplinary Respiratory Medicine, 8*(1), 18. https://doi.org/10.1186/2049-6958-8-18 (Level IV)

38 Liu, Y. H., et al. (2010). Ultrasound-guided pigtail catheters for drainage of various pleural diseases. *American Journal of Emergency Medicine, 28*(8), 915–921. https://doi.org/10.1016/j.ajem.2009.04.041 (Level IV)

39 Hinkle, J. L., & Cheever, K. H. (2018). *Brunner & Suddarth's textbook of medical-surgical nursing* (14th ed.). Philadelphia, PA: Wolters Kluwer.

40 Guideline for perioperative practice: Patient skin antisepsis. (2021). In Wood, A. (Ed.), *Guidelines for perioperative practice 2021 edition*. Denver CO: Association of periOperative Registered Nurses (AORN). (Level VII)

41 Rothrock, J. C. (2019). *Alexander's care of the surgical patient* (16th ed.). St. Louis, MO: Elsevier.

42 The Joint Commission. (2021). Standard NPSG.03.04.01. *Comprehensive accreditation manual for hospitals*. Oakbrook Terrace, IL: The Joint Commission. (Level VII)

43 Accreditation Association for Hospitals and Health Systems. (2020). Standard 25.01.27. *Healthcare Facilities Accreditation Program: Accreditation requirements for acute care hospitals*. Chicago, IL: Accreditation Association for Hospitals and Health Systems. (Level VII)

44 The Joint Commission. (2021). Standard UP.01.03.01. *Comprehensive accreditation manual for hospitals*. Oakbrook Terrace, IL: The Joint Commission. (Level VII)

45 Perazzo, A., et al. (2014). Can ultrasound guidance reduce the risk of pneumothorax following thoracentesis? *Journal Brasileiro de Pneumologia, 40*(1), 6–12. https://doi.org/10.1590/S1806-37132014000100002 (Level IV)

46 American Society of PeriAnesthesia Nurses (ASPAN). (2020). *2021–2022 Perianesthesia nursing standards, practice recommendations and interpretive statements*. Cherry Hill, NJ: ASPAN. (Level VII)

47 Rutala, W. A., et al. (2008, revised 2019). Guideline for disinfection and sterilization in healthcare facilities, 2008. https://www.cdc.gov/infection-control/pdf/guidelines/disinfection-guidelines-H.pdf (Level I)

48 Accreditation Association for Hospitals and Health Systems. (2020). Standard 07.02.03. *Healthcare Facilities Accreditation Program: Accreditation requirements for acute care hospitals*. Chicago, IL: Accreditation Association for Hospitals and Health Systems. (Level VII)

49 The Joint Commission. (2021). Standard RC.01.03.01. *Comprehensive accreditation manual for hospitals*. Oakbrook Terrace, IL: The Joint Commission. (Level VII)

50 Centers for Medicare and Medicaid Services, Department of Health and Human Services. (2020). Condition of participation: Medical record services. 42 C.F.R. § 482.24(b).

51 Accreditation Association for Hospitals and Health Systems. (2020). Standard 10.00.03. *Healthcare Facilities Accreditation Program: Accreditation requirements for acute care hospitals*. Chicago, IL: Accreditation Association for Hospitals and Health Systems. (Level VII)

52 DNV GL-Healthcare USA, Inc. (2020). MR.2.SR.1. *NIAHO® accreditation requirements, interpretive guidelines and surveyor guidance—revision 20.0*. Milford, OH: DNV GL-Healthcare USA, Inc. (Level VII)

53 Huggins, J. T., & Chopra, A. (2021). Large volume (therapeutic) thoracentesis: Procedure and complications. In: *UpToDate*, Broaddus, V. C. (Ed.).

54 Heffner, J. E., & Mayo, P. (2021). Ultrasound-guided thoracentesis. In: *UpToDate*, Broaddus, V. C. (Ed.).

THORACIC ELECTRICAL BIOIMPEDANCE MONITORING

A noninvasive alternative for tracking hemodynamic status, thoracic electrical bioimpedance monitoring, also known as *impedance cardiography*, provides information about a patient's cardiac index, preload, afterload, contractibility, cardiac output, and blood flow.[1] In this procedure, electrodes placed on the patient's thorax send harmless low-level electricity through the patient's body and detect return electrical signals. These signals, which are interruptions in the electrical flow, come from changes in the volume and velocity of blood as it flows through the aorta. The thoracic electrical bioimpedance monitor interprets the signals as a waveform. Cardiac output is then computed from this waveform and the electrocardiogram (ECG).

Thoracic electrical bioimpedance monitoring eliminates the risk of infection, bleeding, pneumothorax, emboli, and arrhythmias associated with traditional invasive monitoring. It can be used to detect trends in the patient's hemodynamic values to help guide treatment.[2] The accuracy of results obtained by this method is comparable to results obtained by thermodilution; however, the methods aren't considered interchangeable.[3]

Equipment

Thoracic electrical bioimpedance unit ▪ color-coded ECG lead wires ▪ four sets of thoracic electrical bioimpedance electrodes ▪ three ECG electrodes ▪ 3" × 3" (7.6-cm × 7.6-cm) or 4" × 4" (10-cm × 10-cm) gauze pads ▪ warm water ▪ tape measure ▪ Optional: gloves, gown, mask with face shield or mask and goggles, disposable-head hair clippers.

Preparation of equipment

Inspect all equipment and supplies. If a product is expired, is defective, or has compromised integrity, remove it from patient use, label it as expired or defective, and report the expiration or defect as directed by your facility. Follow the manufacturer's instructions for use and care of the thoracic electrical bioimpedance unit.

Implementation

▪ Gather the necessary equipment and supplies.
▪ Perform hand hygiene.[4,5,6,7,8,9]
▪ Confirm the patient's identity using at least two patient identifiers.[10]
▪ Provide privacy.[11,12,13,14]

- Explain the procedure to the patient and family (if appropriate) according to their individual communication and learning needs *to increase their understanding, allay their fears, and enhance cooperation.*[15]
- Plug the thoracic electrical bioimpedance unit into a power supply.
- Press the POWER button.
- Enter the patient's information into the device as prompted by the initial display screen appearing on the unit.
- Raise the patient's bed to waist level when providing patient care *to prevent caregiver back strain.*[16]
- Perform hand hygiene.[4,5,6,7,8,9]
- Put on gloves, a gown, and a mask with a face shield or a mask and goggles, as needed, *to comply with standard precautions.*[17,18,19]
- Assist the patient into a supine position, with the head of the bed elevated no more than 30 degrees.
- Expose the patient's chest.
- Clip the hair at the site to be used for electrode placement, as needed, using disposable-head hair clippers.[20]
- Wet 4" × 4" (10-cm × 10-cm) or 3" × 3" (7.6-cm × 7.6-cm) gauze pads with warm water and using the wet gauze pads clean the skin on each side of the patient's neck from the base of the neck to 2" (5 cm) above the base. Then dry the skin with clean, dry gauze pads. Also clean and dry the skin on both sides of the chest at the midaxillary line directly across the xiphoid process. *To ensure that you've cleaned a large enough area for electrode placement,* clean at least two fingerbreadths above and below the site.
- Place one thoracic bioimpedance electrode set vertically on the side of the neck in line with the ear. Make sure that the bottom of the electrode set isn't lower than the junction of the shoulder at the base of the neck.
- Place the second set of electrodes on the opposite side of the neck in line with the ear and about 180 degrees from the first set.[20]
- Place the remaining two sets of electrodes on either side of the patient's chest. *To determine the correct location,* draw a line with your finger from the xiphoid process to the midaxillary line on one side of the chest and place the first remaining set at this location; ensure that the top electrode is at the level of the xiphoid process. Place the second remaining set on the opposite chest wall.
- Attach the ECG lead wires and try different lead selections until you obtain a consistent QRS signal. Don't remove the patient from the primary monitor, *because the regular system must be maintained to ensure monitoring at the central station and to keep the alarms intact.*
- Attach the lead wires of the bioimpedance harness to the thoracic electrical bioimpedance electrodes and the ECG electrodes.
- Measure the distance between the bottom of an electrode set on one side of the patient's neck and the top of an electrode set on the same side of the chest. This distance, the *thorax length,* is the numeric value required by the thoracic electrical bioimpedance monitor's computer to calculate accurate stroke volume. Enter this value on the patient data screen; then return to the waveform screen.
- Begin monitoring the results provided by the thoracic electrical bioimpedance unit.[1]
- Return the bed to the lowest position *to prevent falls and maintain patient safety.*[21]
- Remove and discard your gloves and other personal protective equipment, if worn.[19]
- Perform hand hygiene.[4,5,6,7,8,8]
- Document the procedure.[22,23,24,25]

Special considerations

- Baseline bioimpedance values may be reduced in patients who have conditions characterized by increased fluid in the chest, such as pulmonary edema and pleural effusion.
- Bioimpedance values may be lower than thermodilution values in patients with tachycardia and other arrhythmias.
- Some bioimpedance devices allow for application of electrodes on an endotracheal tube. Follow the manufacturer's guidelines regarding the proper locations for electrode placement for such devices.[1]
- Electrodes are for single use and should be replaced every 24 hours *to maintain a strong reading.*[1,20]

Complications

Prolonged electrode application can cause skin irritation and tissue breakdown.

Documentation

Document the date and time that you began the monitoring. Note the waveforms and bioimpedance values on the monitor; document these values by pressing PRINT on the waveform screen to print a strip that contains all the values monitored at the ordered interval. Place the strip in the patient's chart. Record the patient's tolerance of the procedure. Document teaching provided to the patient and family (if applicable), their understanding of that teaching, and any need for follow-up teaching.

REFERENCES

1 Wiegand, D. L. (2017). *AACN procedure manual for high acuity, progressive, and critical care* (7th ed.). St. Louis, MO: Elsevier.

2 Kobe, J., et al. (2019). Cardiac output monitoring: Technology and choice. *Annals of Cardiac Anaesthesia, 22*(1), 6–17. https://www.ncbi.nlm. nih.gov/pmc/articles/PMC6350438/ (Level V)

3 Joosten, A., et al. (2017). Accuracy and precision of non-invasive cardiac output monitoring devices in perioperative medicine: A systematic review and meta-analysis. *British Journal of Anaesthesia, 118*(3), 298–310. https:// bjanaesthesia.org/article/S0007-0912(17)30199-X/fulltext (Level I)

4 The Joint Commission. (2021). Standard NPSG.07.01.01. *Comprehensive accreditation manual for hospitals.* Oakbrook Terrace, IL: The Joint Commission. (Level VII)

5 Centers for Disease Control and Prevention. (2002). Guideline for hand hygiene in health-care settings: Recommendations of the Healthcare Infection Control Practices Advisory Committee and the HICPAC/ SHEA/APIC/IDSA Hand Hygiene Task Force. *MMWR Recommendations and Reports, 51*(RR-16), 1–45. https://www.cdc.gov/mmwr/pdf/rr/rr5116. pdf (Level II)

6 World Health Organization (WHO). (2009). WHO guidelines on hand hygiene in health care: First global patient safety challenge, clean care is safer care. https://apps.who.int/iris/bitstream/han- dle/10665/44102/9789241597906_eng.pdf?sequence=1 (Level IV)

7 Accreditation Association for Hospitals and Health Systems. (2020). Standard 07.01.21, *Healthcare Facilities Accreditation Program: Accreditation requirements for acute care hospitals.* Chicago, IL: Accreditation Association for Hospitals and Health Systems. (Level VII)

8 Centers for Medicare and Medicaid Services, Department of Health and Human Services. (2020). Condition of participation: Infection control. 42 C.F.R. § 482.42.

9 DNV GL-Healthcare USA, Inc. (2020). IC.1.SR.1. *NIAHO® accreditation requirements, interpretive guidelines and surveyor guidance—revision 20.0.* Milford, OH: DNV GL-Healthcare USA, Inc. (Level VII)

10 The Joint Commission. (2021). Standard NPSG.01.01.01. *Comprehensive accreditation manual for hospitals.* Oakbrook Terrace, IL: The Joint Commission. (Level VII)

11 Accreditation Association for Hospitals and Health Systems. (2020). Standard 15.01.16. *Healthcare Facilities Accreditation Program: Accreditation requirements for acute care hospitals.* Chicago, IL: Accreditation Association for Hospitals and Health Systems. (Level VII)

12 Centers for Medicare and Medicaid Services, Department of Health and Human Services. (2020). Condition of participation: Patient's rights. 42 C.F.R. § 482.13(c)(1).

13 The Joint Commission. (2021). Standard RI.01.01.01. *Comprehensive accreditation manual for hospitals.* Oakbrook Terrace, IL: The Joint Commission. (Level VII)

14 DNV GL-Healthcare USA, Inc. (2020). PR.2.SR.5. *NIAHO® accreditation requirements, interpretive guidelines and surveyor guidance—revision 20.0.* Milford, OH: DNV GL-Healthcare USA, Inc. (Level VII)

15 The Joint Commission. (2021). Standard PC.02.01.21. *Comprehensive accreditation manual for hospitals.* Oakbrook Terrace, IL: The Joint Commission. (Level VII)

16 Waters, T. R., et al. (2009). Safe patient handling training for schools of nursing. https://www.cdc.gov/niosh/docs/2009-127/pdfs/2009-127.pdf (Level VII)

17 Siegel, J. D., et al. (2007, revised 2019). 2007 guideline for isolation precautions: Preventing transmission of infectious agents in healthcare settings. https://www.cdc.gov/infectioncontrol/pdf/guidelines/isolation- guidelines-H.pdf (Level II)

18 Accreditation Association for Hospitals and Health Systems. (2020). Standard 07.01.10. *Healthcare Facilities Accreditation Program: Accreditation requirements for acute care hospitals.* Chicago, IL: Accreditation Association for Hospitals and Health Systems. (Level VII)

19 Occupational Safety and Health Administration. (2012). Bloodborne pathogens, standard number 1910.1030. https://www.osha.gov/pls/oshaweb/owadisp.show_document?p_id=10051&p_table=STANDARDS (Level VII)

20 CardioDynamics International Corporation. (2009). BioZ Dx ICG Diagnostics operator/service manual. https://www.sonosite.com/sites/default/files/bioz_operator_service_manual.pdf

21 Ganz, D. A., et al. (2013, reviewed 2021). *Preventing falls in hospitals: A toolkit for improving quality of care* (AHRQ Publication No. 13-0015-EF). Agency for Healthcare Research and Quality. https://www.ahrq.gov/professionals/systems/hospital/fallpxtoolkit/index.html (Level VII)

22 The Joint Commission. (2021). Standard RC.01.03.01. *Comprehensive accreditation manual for hospitals.* Oakbrook Terrace, IL: The Joint Commission. (Level VII)

23 Accreditation Association for Hospitals and Health Systems. (2020). Standard 10.00.03. *Healthcare Facilities Accreditation Program: Accreditation requirements for acute care hospitals.* Chicago, IL: Accreditation Association for Hospitals and Health Systems. (Level VII)

24 Centers for Medicare and Medicaid Services, Department of Health and Human Services. (2020). Condition of participation: Medical record services. 42 C.F.R. § 482.24(b).

25 DNV GL-Healthcare USA, Inc. (2020). MR.2.SR.1. *NIAHO® accreditation requirements, interpretive guidelines and surveyor guidance—revision 20.0.* Milford, OH: DNV GL-Healthcare USA, Inc. (Level VII)

TOPICAL SKIN DRUG APPLICATION

Topical drugs are applied directly to the skin surface or mucous membranes, and are absorbed through the epidermal layer into the dermis.[1] The extent of absorption depends on the vascularity of the region. Topical nitroglycerin, fentaNYL, nicotine, and certain supplemental hormone replacements are used for systemic effects. Most other topical medications are used for local effects.

Topical medications may be in the form of lotions, pastes, ointments, creams, powders, shampoos, and aerosol sprays. Ointments have a fatty base, which is an ideal vehicle for such drugs as antimicrobials and antiseptics. Typically, topical medications should be applied two or three times a day to achieve their therapeutic effect.

Equipment

Patient's medication administration record ■ prescribed medication ■ gloves ■ Optional: soap, water, washcloth, towel, white cotton gloves, terry cloth slippers, sterile gauze, transparent semipermeable dressing, adhesive tape, comb or brush, fine-toothed comb (for nits), sterile gloves .

Implementation

■ Avoid distractions and interruptions when preparing and administering the medication *to prevent medication errors.*[2,3]
■ Verify the practitioner's order.[4,5,6,7]
■ Reconcile the patient's medications when the practitioner orders a new medication *to reduce the risk of medication errors, including omissions, duplications, dosing errors, and drug interactions.*[8,9]
■ Compare the medication label with the order in the patient's medical record.[4,5,6,7]
■ Check the patient's medical record for an allergy or a contraindication to the prescribed medication. If an allergy or a contraindication exists, don't administer the medication and notify the practitioner.[4,5,6,7]
■ Check the expiration date on the medication. If the medication is expired, return it to the pharmacy and obtain new medication.[4,5,6,7]
■ Visually inspect the medication for loss of integrity; don't administer the medication if its integrity is compromised.[4,5,6,7]
■ Discuss any unresolved concerns about the medication with the patient's practitioner.[4,5,6,7]
■ Perform hand hygiene.[10,11,12,13,14,15]
■ Confirm the patient's identity using at least two patient identifiers.[16]
■ Provide privacy.[17,18,19,20]

■ Explain the procedure to the patient and family (if appropriate) according to their individual communication and learning needs *to increase their understanding, allay their fears, and enhance cooperation.*[21] Answer any questions.
■ Teach the patient and family (if appropriate) who is receiving the medication for the first time about potential adverse reactions, and discuss any other concerns related to the medication.[4,5,6,7]
■ Verify that the medication is being administered at the proper time, in the prescribed dose, and by the correct route *to reduce the risk of medication errors.*[4,5,6,7]
■ If your facility uses a bar code technology, use it as directed by your facility.
■ Perform hand hygiene.[10,11,12,13,14,15]

NURSING ALERT If your facility's hazardous drug list contains the drug you're about to administer, put on personal protective equipment, as directed.[22]

■ Put on gloves *to comply with standard precautions and prevent absorption of the medication through your skin.*[23,24,25]
■ Help the patient assume a comfortable position that provides access to the area to be treated.
■ Expose the area to be treated. Make sure the skin or mucous membrane is intact (unless the medication has been ordered to treat a skin lesion, such as an ulcer). *Applying medication to broken or abraded skin can cause unwanted systemic absorption and result in further irritation.*
■ If needed, clean the skin of debris, including crusts and epidermal scales, with mild soap and water and a washcloth. Blot gently with a towel.
■ Remove medication from the skin if it remains from a previous dose *to prevent skin irritation from an accumulation of medication.*
■ Change your gloves if they become soiled. Perform hand hygiene before putting on new pair of gloves.[24]

Applying paste, cream, or ointment

■ Open the container. Place the lid or cap upside down *to prevent contamination of the inside surface.*
■ Using your gloved hands, apply the medication to the affected area with long, smooth strokes that follow the direction of hair growth (as shown below). *This technique avoids forcing medication into hair follicles, which can cause irritation and lead to folliculitis.* Avoid excessive pressure when applying the medication, *because excessive pressure could abrade the skin.*

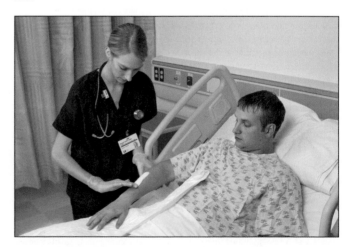

Applying other topical medications

■ To apply shampoos, follow package directions. (See *Using medicated shampoos.*)
■ To apply aerosol sprays, shake the container, if indicated, *to completely mix the medication.* Hold the container 6" to 12" (15 to 30 cm) from the skin, or follow the manufacturer's recommendation. Spray a thin film of medication evenly over the treatment area, away from the patient's face *to prevent direct inhalation of the spray.*

Using medicated shampoos

Medicated shampoos include keratolytic and cytostatic agents, coal tar preparations, and lindane (gamma benzene hexachloride) solutions. They can be used to treat such conditions as dandruff, psoriasis, and head lice.

Because contraindications, adverse effects, warnings, precautions, and application instructions may vary depending on the specific medicated shampoo that you are using, check the label on the shampoo before starting the procedure.[26,27,28]

To apply a medicated shampoo, follow these steps:
- Perform hand hygiene.[10,11,12,13,14,15]
- Put on gloves.[24,25]
- Prepare the patient for shampoo treatment.
- Shake the bottle of shampoo well *to evenly mix the solution.*
- Wet the patient's hair thoroughly and wring out excess water.
- Apply the proper amount of shampoo, as directed on the label.
- Work the shampoo into a lather, adding water as necessary. Part the hair and work the shampoo into the scalp, taking care not to use your fingernails.
- Leave the shampoo on the scalp and hair for as long as instructed (usually 5 to 10 minutes). Then rinse the hair thoroughly.
- Towel-dry the patient's hair.
- After the hair is dry, comb or brush it. Use a fine-tooth comb to remove nits if needed.
- Remove and discard your gloves and perform hand hygiene.[10,11,12,13,14,15]

- To apply powders, dry the skin surface, being sure to spread skin folds where moisture collects. Then apply a thin layer of powder over the treatment area; apply the powder away from the patient's face *to prevent direct inhalation of the powder.*
- *To protect applied medications and prevent them from soiling the patient's clothes,* tape sterile gauze pads or a transparent semipermeable dressing over the treatment area, if appropriate. With certain medications (such as topical steroids), applying a semipermeable dressing may be contraindicated. Check the medication's prescribing information and cautions. If you're applying a topical medication to the patient's hands or feet, cover the hands with white cotton gloves and the feet with terry cloth slippers if appropriate.

Completing the procedure
- Monitor the patient's skin for adverse effects of the medication, such as irritation, an allergic reaction, or skin breakdown.
- Discard used supplies and dressings in the appropriate receptacles.[24,25]
- Remove and discard your gloves,[24,25] and perform hand hygiene.[10,11,12,13,14,15]
- Document the procedure.[29,30,31,32]

Special considerations
- Don't apply ointments to mucous membranes as liberally as you would to skin, *because mucous membranes are usually moist and absorb ointment more quickly than skin does.*
- Never apply ointment to the eyelids or ear canal unless ordered. *The ointment may congeal and occlude the tear duct or ear canal.*

Complications
Skin irritation, a rash, or an allergic reaction may occur.[26,27,28] Complications related to the action of the medication may also occur.[26,27,28]

Documentation
Document the medication strength, dose, route of administration, and the date and time of administration. Record any adverse reactions to the prescribed medication, the date and time that the practitioner was notified, prescribed interventions, and the patient's response to those interventions.[33] Document the patient's response to and tolerance of therapy. Document teaching provided to the patient and family (if applicable), their understanding of that teaching, and any need for follow-up teaching.

REFERENCES
1 Institute for Quality and Efficiency in Health Care. (2020). Using medication: Topical medications. https://www.ncbi.nlm.nih.gov/books/NBK361003/
2 Westbrook, J., et al. (2010). Association of interruptions with an increased risk and severity of medication administration errors. *Archives of Internal Medicine, 170,* 683–690. (Level IV)
3 Institute for Safe Medication Practices. (2012). Side tracks on the safety express: Interruptions lead to errors and unfinished…Wait, what was I doing? *Nurse Advise-ERR, 11*(2), 1–4. https://www.ismp.org/resources/side-tracks-safety-express-interruptions-lead-errors-and-unfinished-wait-what-was-i-doing?id=37
4 Accreditation Association for Hospitals and Health Systems. (2020). Standard 16.01.03. *Healthcare Facilities Accreditation Program: Accreditation requirements for acute care hospitals.* Chicago, IL: Accreditation Association for Hospitals and Health Systems. (Level VII)
5 Centers for Medicare and Medicaid Services, Department of Health and Human Services. (2020). Condition of participation: Nursing services. 42 C.F.R. § 482.23(c).
6 DNV GL-Healthcare USA, Inc. (2020). MM.1.SR.3. *NIAHO® accreditation requirements, interpretive guidelines and surveyor guidance—revision 20.0.* Milford, OH: DNV GL-Healthcare USA, Inc. (Level VII)
7 The Joint Commission. (2021). Standard MM.06.01.01. *Comprehensive accreditation manual for hospitals.* Oakbrook Terrace, IL: The Joint Commission. (Level VII)
8 Accreditation Association for Hospitals and Health Systems. (2020). Standard 25.02.13. *Healthcare Facilities Accreditation Program: Accreditation requirements for acute care hospitals.* Chicago, IL: Accreditation Association for Hospitals and Health Systems. (Level VII)
9 The Joint Commission. (2021). Standard NPSG.03.06.01. *Comprehensive accreditation manual for hospitals.* Oakbrook Terrace, IL: The Joint Commission. (Level VII)
10 The Joint Commission. (2021). Standard NPSG.07.01.01. *Comprehensive accreditation manual for hospitals.* Oakbrook Terrace, IL: The Joint Commission. (Level VII)
11 Centers for Disease Control and Prevention. (2002). Guideline for hand hygiene in health-care settings: Recommendations of the Healthcare Infection Control Practices Advisory Committee and the HICPAC/SHEA/APIC/IDSA Hand Hygiene Task Force. *MMWR Recommendations and Reports, 51*(RR-16), 1–45. https://www.cdc.gov/mmwr/pdf/rr/rr5116.pdf (Level II)
12 World Health Organization. (2009). WHO guidelines on hand hygiene in health care: First global patient safety challenge, clean care is safer care. https://apps.who.int/iris/bitstream/handle/10665/44102/9789241597906_eng.pdf?sequence=1 (Level IV)
13 Accreditation Association for Hospitals and Health Systems. (2020). Standard 07.01.21. *Healthcare Facilities Accreditation Program: Accreditation requirements for acute care hospitals.* Chicago, IL: Accreditation Association for Hospitals and Health Systems. (Level VII)
14 Centers for Medicare and Medicaid Services, Department of Health and Human Services. (2020). Condition of participation: Infection control. 42 C.F.R. § 482.42.
15 DNV GL-Healthcare USA, Inc. (2020). IC.1.SR.1. *NIAHO® accreditation requirements, interpretive guidelines and surveyor guidance—revision 20.0.* Milford, OH: DNV GL-Healthcare USA, Inc. (Level VII)
16 The Joint Commission. (2021). Standard NPSG.01.01.01. *Comprehensive accreditation manual for hospitals.* Oakbrook Terrace, IL: The Joint Commission. (Level VII)
17 Centers for Medicare and Medicaid Services, Department of Health and Human Services. (2020). Condition of participation: Patient's rights. 42 C.F.R. § 482.13(c)(1).
18 Accreditation Association for Hospitals and Health Systems. (2020). Standard 15.01.16. *Healthcare Facilities Accreditation Program: Accreditation requirements for acute care hospitals.* Chicago, IL: Accreditation Association for Hospitals and Health Systems. (Level VII)
19 DNV GL-Healthcare USA, Inc. (2020). PR.2.SR.5. *NIAHO® accreditation requirements, interpretive guidelines and surveyor guidance—revision 20.0.* Milford, OH: DNV GL-Healthcare USA, Inc. (Level VII)
20 The Joint Commission. (2021). Standard RI.01.01.01. *Comprehensive accreditation manual for hospitals.* Oakbrook Terrace, IL: The Joint Commission. (Level VII)

21 The Joint Commission. (2021). Standard PC.02.01.21. *Comprehensive accreditation manual for hospitals.* Oakbrook Terrace, IL: The Joint Commission. (Level VII)

22 The United States Pharmacopeial Convention. (2019). USP general chapter <800> hazardous drugs: Handling in healthcare settings. https://www.usp.org/compounding/general-chapter-hazardous-drugs-handling-healthcare

23 Occupational Safety and Health Administration. (2012). Bloodborne pathogens, standard number 1910.1030. https://www.osha.gov/pls/oshaweb/owadisp.show_document?p_id=10051&p_table=STANDARDS

24 Siegel, J. D., et al. (2007, revised 2019). 2007 guideline for isolation precautions: Preventing transmission of infectious agents in healthcare settings. https://www.cdc.gov/infectioncontrol/pdf/guidelines/isolation-guidelines-H.pdf (Level II)

25 Accreditation Association for Hospitals and Health Systems. (2020). Standard 07.01.10. *Healthcare Facilities Accreditation Program: Accreditation requirements for acute care hospitals.* Chicago, IL: Accreditation Association for Hospitals and Health Systems. (Level VII)

26 Hanes, E. (2021). Medicated shampoos: Why they're used and how they work. https://www.healthgrades.com/right-care/skin-hair-and-nails/medicated-shampoos-why-theyre-used-and-how-they-work

27 RxList. (2017). Lindane shampoo. https://www.rxlist.com/lindane-shampoo-drug.htm#description

28 Cunha, J. P. (2021). Coal tar shampoo. https://www.rxlist.com/consumer_neutrogena_tgel_coal_tar_shampoo/drugs-condition.htm

29 The Joint Commission. (2021). Standard RC.01.03.01. *Comprehensive accreditation manual for hospitals.* Oakbrook Terrace, IL: The Joint Commission. (Level VII)

30 Accreditation Association for Hospitals and Health Systems. (2020). Standard 10.00.03. *Healthcare Facilities Accreditation Program: Accreditation requirements for acute care hospitals.* Chicago, IL: Accreditation Association for Hospitals and Health Systems. (Level VII)

31 Centers for Medicare and Medicaid Services, Department of Health and Human Services. (2020). Condition of participation: Medical record services. 42 C.F.R. § 482.24(b).

32 DNV GL-Healthcare USA, Inc. (2020). MR.2.SR.1. *NIAHO® accreditation requirements, interpretive guidelines and surveyor guidance—revision 20.0.* Milford, OH: DNV GL-Healthcare USA, Inc. (Level VII)

33 The Joint Commission. (2021). Standard RC.02.01.01. *Comprehensive accreditation manual for hospitals.* Oakbrook Terrace, IL: The Joint Commission. (Level VII)

Tracheal cuff pressure measurement

When inflated properly, an endotracheal (ET) or tracheostomy cuff provides a closed system for mechanical ventilation, delivering the desired tidal volume to the patient's lungs. To function properly, the cuff must exert enough pressure on the tracheal wall to seal the airway without compromising the blood supply to the tracheal mucosa. The ideal pressure is the lowest amount needed to seal the airway. Many authorities recommend maintaining a cuff pressure lower than capillary perfusion pressure, which is estimated to be 25 to 30 mm Hg.[1] Therefore, inflating the cuff to 20 to 25 mm Hg is commonly recommended, although some authorities recommend 20 to 30 cm H_2O.[1,2,3] The Intensive Care Society recommends using a cuff pressure that doesn't exceed 25 cm H_2O.[3]

When cuff pressure is inadequate, oropharyngeal secretions can leak around the cuff, increasing the risk of ventilator-associated pneumonia.[4] Cuff leaks can lead to aspiration in ventilator-dependent and spontaneously breathing patients.[2] Overinflation of the cuff can cause tracheal necrosis, tracheomalacia, tracheoinnominate artery fistula, tracheal ulceration, tracheal fibrosis, tracheal stenosis, and tracheoesophageal fistula.[5] Malpositioning the tracheostomy or ET tube or inserting a tube that's too small in diameter can also cause high cuff pressure due to overfilling the cuff to achieve a seal in the trachea.[1] Cuff pressures vary with each patient, the type of tracheostomy tube, and the mode of ventilation.[1] To keep pressure within safe limits, measurement should occur at least once each shift or at an interval determined by the facility.[6] A nurse or respiratory therapist can measure cuff pressure.

Equipment

Cuff pressure manometer ■ suction equipment ■ gloves ■ facility-approved disinfectant ■ handheld resuscitation bag with oxygen source and tubing ■ Optional: communication aids, mechanical ventilator.

Preparation of equipment

Inspect all equipment and supplies. If a product is expired, is defective, or has compromised integrity, remove it from patient use, label it as expired or defective, and report the expiration or defect as directed by your facility.

Assemble all equipment at the patient's bedside. Calibrate the manometer following the manufacturer's instructions. Make sure the oxygen source and handheld resuscitation bag are readily available at the patient's bedside.

Implementation

■ Verify the practitioner's order.
■ Gather and prepare the necessary equipment and supplies.
■ Perform hand hygiene.[7,8,9,10,11,12]
■ Confirm the patient's identity using at least two patient identifiers.[13]
■ Provide privacy.[14,15,16,17]
■ Explain the procedure to the patient and family (if appropriate) according to their individual communication and learning needs *to increase their understanding, allay their fears, and enhance cooperation.*[18]
■ Raise the patient's bed to waist level before providing care *to prevent caregiver back strain.*[19]
■ Perform hand hygiene.[7,8,9,10,11,12]
■ Place the patient in the semi-Fowler position, if appropriate, *to promote oxygenation and reduce the risk of aspiration.*[1,20]
■ Perform hand hygiene.[7,8,9,10,11,12]
■ Put on gloves *to comply with standard precautions.*[21,22,23]
■ Hyperoxygenate the patient, if necessary, by adjusting the fraction of inspired oxygen on the mechanical ventilator or by using the temporary oxygen-rich environment program available on the ventilator, *to prevent hypoxia.*[24]
■ Suction the ET or tracheostomy tube and the patient's oropharynx *to remove accumulated secretions above the cuff.*[1,20,25] (See the "Tracheal suctioning, intubated patient" procedure.)
■ Attach the cuff pressure manometer to the cuff pilot balloon port and then read the measurement.[6]
■ Adjust the pressure, as needed (see the "Tracheostomy care" procedure).
■ If the cuff pressure measures greater than 25 cm H_2O, press the pressure-release button on the device until the pressure reaches 20 to 25 cm H_2O.[1]
■ If the pressure measures less than 20 cm H_2O, add air by squeezing the bulb until the pressure reaches 20 to 25 cm H_2O.[1]
■ If you aren't able to maintain adequate pressure, notify the practitioner.[1]
NURSING ALERT Studies have found that minimal occlusive volume and minimal leak inflation techniques increase the risk of silent aspiration. Guidelines recommend using a measuring device, such as a manometer, to achieve optimal cuff pressure *to decrease the risk of adverse events.*[1,2,26]
■ Disconnect the cuff pressure manometer from the cuff pilot balloon port.
■ Make sure that the ventilator alarms are set appropriately for the patient's current condition, and that alarms are turned on, functioning properly, and audible to staff.[27,28,29]
■ Make sure that the patient is comfortable and can easily reach the call light and communication aids.
■ Return the bed to the lowest position *to prevent falls and maintain patient safety.*[30]
■ Remove and discard your gloves.[23]
■ Perform hand hygiene.[7,8,9,10,11,12]
■ Put on gloves, as needed.[21,23]
■ Clean and disinfect the surface of the manometer according to the manufacturer's instructions *to prevent the spread of infection.*[31,32]
■ Perform hand hygiene.[7,8,9,10,11,12]
■ Document the procedure.[33,34,35,36]

Special considerations

■ Most cuff pressure manometers are designed only for use with air-filled cuffs. Use with a saline-filled cuff can damage the unit.[1]
■ Cuff pressure values vary and decrease over time. Unless you perform continuous monitoring or attach an automatic regulating device,

maintaining a cuff pressure value within the therapeutic range can be difficult *because of changes in body position and head alignment, tube migration, coughing, lung compliance, and airway and intrathoracic pressures.*[37] Guidelines recommend frequent, routine assessment of cuff pressure but don't identify optimal frequency.[37]

Complications

Aspiration of upper airway secretions, underventilation, or coughing spasms can occur if a leak is created during cuff pressure measurement. Overinflation of the cuff can cause tracheal wall injury.[2]

Documentation

Record the date and time of the procedure, cuff pressure, total amount of air in the cuff after the procedure, and the patient's tolerance of the procedure. Document any complications that occurred, the name of the practitioner notified of complications, the date and time of notification, any prescribed interventions, and the patient's response to them. Document teaching provided to the patient and family (if appropriate), their understanding of that teaching, and any need for follow-up teaching.

REFERENCES

1 Wiegand, D. L. (2017). *AACN procedure manual for high acuity, progressive, and critical care* (7th ed.). St. Louis, MO: Elsevier.

2 Kacmarek, R. M. (2021). *Egan's fundamentals of respiratory care* (12th ed.). St. Louis, MO: Mosby.

3 Intensive Care Society. (2014, reviewed 2018). Standards for the care of adult patients with a temporary tracheostomy: Standards and guidelines. https://www.wyccn.org/uploads/6/5/1/9/65199375/ics_tracheostomy_standards__2014_.pdf (Level VII)

4 Morris, L. L., et al. (2013). Tracheostomy care and complications in the intensive care unit. *Critical Care Nurse, 33*(5), 18–30.

5 Morris, L., & Afifi, M. S. (Eds.). (2010). *Tracheostomies: The complete guide.* New York, NY: Springer Publishing Company.

6 Pisano, A., et al. (2019). Assessing the correct inflation of the endotracheal tube cuff: A larger pilot balloon increases the sensitivity of the 'finger-pressure' technique, but it remains poorly reliable in clinical practice. *Journal of Clinical Monitoring and Computing, 33,* 301–305. https://link.springer.com/article/10.1007/s10877-018-0158-8 (Level VI)

7 The Joint Commission. (2021). Standard NPSG.07.01.01. *Comprehensive accreditation manual for hospitals.* Oakbrook Terrace, IL: The Joint Commission. (Level VII)

8 World Health Organization. (2009). WHO guidelines on hand hygiene in health care: First global patient safety challenge, clean care is safer care. https://apps.who.int/iris/bitstream/handle/10665/44102/9789241597906_eng.pdf?sequence=1 (Level IV)

9 Centers for Disease Control and Prevention. (2002). Guideline for hand hygiene in health-care settings: Recommendations of the Healthcare Infection Control Practices Advisory Committee and the HICPAC/SHEA/APIC/IDSA Hand Hygiene Task Force. *MMWR Recommendations and Reports, 51*(RR-16), 1–45. https://www.cdc.gov/mmwr/pdf/rr/rr5116.pdf (Level II)

10 Accreditation Association for Hospitals and Health Systems. (2020). Standard 07.01.21. *Healthcare Facilities Accreditation Program: Accreditation requirements for acute care hospitals.* Chicago, IL: Accreditation Association for Hospitals and Health Systems. (Level VII)

11 Centers for Medicare and Medicaid Services, Department of Health and Human Services. (2020). Condition of participation: Infection control. 42 C.F.R. § 482.42.

12 DNV GL-Healthcare USA, Inc. (2020). IC.1.SR.1. *NIAHO® accreditation requirements, interpretive guidelines and surveyor guidance—revision 20.0.* Milford, OH: DNV GL-Healthcare USA, Inc. (Level VII)

13 The Joint Commission. (2021). Standard NPSG.01.01.01. *Comprehensive accreditation manual for hospitals.* Oakbrook Terrace, IL: The Joint Commission. (Level VII)

14 Accreditation Association for Hospitals and Health Systems. (2020). Standard 15.01.16. *Healthcare Facilities Accreditation Program: Accreditation requirements for acute care hospitals.* Chicago, IL: Accreditation Association for Hospitals and Health Systems. (Level VII)

15 Centers for Medicare and Medicaid Services, Department of Health and Human Services. (2020). Condition of participation: Patient's rights. 42 C.F.R. § 482.13(c)(1).

16 DNV GL-Healthcare USA, Inc. (2020). PR.2.SR.5. *NIAHO® accreditation requirements, interpretive guidelines and surveyor guidance—revision 20.0.* Milford, OH: DNV GL-Healthcare USA, Inc. (Level VII)

17 The Joint Commission. (2021). Standard RI.01.01.01. *Comprehensive accreditation manual for hospitals.* Oakbrook Terrace, IL: The Joint Commission. (Level VII)

18 The Joint Commission. (2021). Standard PC.02.01.21. *Comprehensive accreditation manual for hospitals.* Oakbrook Terrace, IL: The Joint Commission. (Level VII)

19 Waters, T. R., et al. (2009). Safe patient handling training for schools of nursing. https://www.cdc.gov/niosh/docs/2009-127/pdfs/2009-127.pdf (Level VII)

20 American Association of Critical-Care Nurses. (2017). AACN practice alert: Ventilator associated pneumonia. https://www.aacn.org/clinical-resources/practice-alerts/ventilator-associated-pneumonia-vap (Level VII)

21 Siegel, J. D., et al. (2007, revised 2019). 2007 guideline for isolation precautions: Preventing transmission of infectious agents in healthcare settings. https://www.cdc.gov/infectioncontrol/pdf/guidelines/isolation-guidelines-H.pdf (Level II)

22 Accreditation Association for Hospitals and Health Systems. (2020). Standard 07.01.10. *Healthcare Facilities Accreditation Program: Accreditation requirements for acute care hospitals.* Chicago, IL: Accreditation Association for Hospitals and Health Systems. (Level VII)

23 Occupational Safety and Health Administration. (2012). Bloodborne pathogens, standard number 1910.1030. https://www.osha.gov/pls/oshaweb/owadisp.show_document?p_id=10051&p_table=STANDARDS (Level VII)

24 American Association for Respiratory Care. (2010). AARC clinical practice guidelines: Endotracheal suctioning of mechanically ventilated patients with artificial airways 2010. *Respiratory Care, 55*(6), 758–764. https://www.aarc.org/wp-content/uploads/2014/08/06.10.0758.pdf (Level VII)

25 Accreditation Association for Hospitals and Health Systems. (2020). Standard 07.01.02. *Healthcare Facilities Accreditation Program: Accreditation requirements for acute care hospitals.* Chicago, IL: Accreditation Association for Hospitals and Health Systems. (Level VII)

26 Jordan, P., et al. (2012). Endotracheal tube cuff pressure management in adult critical care units. *South African Journal of Critical Care, 28*(1), 15–19. http://www.sajcc.org.za/index.php/SAJCC/article/view/129/148 (Level VI)

27 The Joint Commission. (2021). Standard NPSG.06.01.01. *Comprehensive accreditation manual for hospitals.* Oakbrook Terrace, IL: The Joint Commission. (Level VII)

28 Graham, K. C., & Cvach, M. (2010). Monitor alarm fatigue: Standardizing use of physiological monitors and decreasing nuisance alarms. *American Journal of Critical Care, 19,* 28–37. https://aacnjournals.org/ajcconline/article-abstract/19/1/28/5720/Monitor-Alarm-Fatigue-Standardizing-Use-of?redirectedFrom=fulltext

29 The Joint Commission. (2013). Sentinel event alert: Medical device alarm safety in hospitals. https://www.jointcommission.org/-/media/tjc/documents/resources/patient-safety-topics/sentinel-event/sea_50_alarms_4_26_16.pdf (Level VII)

30 Ganz, D. A., et al. (2013, reviewed 2021). *Preventing falls in hospitals: A toolkit for improving quality of care* (AHRQ Publication No. 13-0015-EF). Rockville, MD: Agency for Healthcare Research and Quality. https://www.ahrq.gov/professionals/systems/hospital/fallpxtoolkit/index.html (Level VII)

31 Rutala, W. A., et al. (2008, revised 2019). Guideline for disinfection and sterilization in healthcare facilities, 2008. https://www.cdc.gov/infection-control/pdf/guidelines/disinfection-guidelines-H.pdf (Level I)

32 Accreditation Association for Hospitals and Health Systems. (2020). Standard 07.02.03. *Healthcare Facilities Accreditation Program: Accreditation requirements for acute care hospitals.* Chicago, IL: Accreditation Association for Hospitals and Health Systems. (Level VII)

33 DNV GL-Healthcare USA, Inc. (2020). MR.2.SR.1. *NIAHO® accreditation requirements, interpretive guidelines and surveyor guidance—revision 20.0.* Milford, OH: DNV GL-Healthcare USA, Inc. (Level VII)

34 The Joint Commission. (2021). Standard RC.01.03.01. *Comprehensive accreditation manual for hospitals.* Oakbrook Terrace, IL: The Joint Commission. (Level VII)

35 Accreditation Association for Hospitals and Health Systems. (2020). Standard 10.00.03. *Healthcare Facilities Accreditation Program: Accreditation requirements for acute care hospitals.* Chicago, IL: Accreditation Association for Hospitals and Health Systems. (Level VII)

36 Centers for Medicare and Medicaid Services, Department of Health and Human Services. (2020). Condition of participation: Medical record services. 42 C.F.R. § 482.24(b).

37 Sole, M. L., et al. (2011). Evaluation of an intervention to maintain endotracheal tube cuff pressure within therapeutic range. *American Journal of Critical Care, 20*(2), 109–118. https://www.ncbi.nlm.nih.gov/pmc/articles/PMC3506174/pdf/nihms419038.pdf (Level II)

TRACHEAL SUCTIONING, INTUBATED PATIENT

Tracheal suction is used to help remove pulmonary secretions from a patient's artificial airway to prevent obstruction. Maintaining a patent airway is essential to promote the optimal exchange of oxygen and carbon dioxide and to prevent pneumonia, which can result from the pooling of secretions.[1,2,3]

There are two methods of tracheal suctioning: open and closed. The open tracheal suction system requires disconnecting the patient from the ventilator for suctioning. The closed tracheal suction system uses a sterile in-line suction catheter attached to the ventilator circuit, which permits suctioning without disconnecting the patient from the ventilator. Closed tracheal suctioning provides continuous mechanical ventilation and oxygenation during the procedure.[3,4] Research doesn't suggest the best practice for a closed or open suctioning technique, nor does it establish that a closed system is better or worse than an open system for reducing bacterial colonization and ventilator-associated pneumonia.[5,6]

Indications for suctioning include presence of secretions in the airway, adventitious breath sounds on auscultation, increased peak airway pressure, an increased respiratory rate, frequent coughing, suspected aspiration of gastric or upper airway secretions, sudden onset of respiratory distress with suspected airway obstruction, a decreased oxygen saturation level, and the need to obtain a sputum specimen to identify infection.[3,4,7]

According to the guidelines from the American Association for Respiratory Care, you should hyperoxygenate the patient with 100% oxygen for 30 to 60 seconds before undertaking tracheal suctioning and before and after each pass of the suction catheter.[1,3,4,7] Each suctioning event, which includes the placement and withdrawal of the suction catheter, should take no longer than 15 seconds.[7] Suction pressure should be set at the lowest level that clears secretions effectively.[8] After suctioning, the patient should be hyperoxygenated again for at least 1 minute using the same technique used for preoxygenating the patient.[3,7]

Equipment

Oxygen source ■ handheld resuscitation bag with tubing ■ suction apparatus ■ collection container ■ connecting tubing ■ suction catheter kit (a sterile suction catheter, one sterile glove, one clean glove, goggles, and a disposable sterile solution container) ■ 1-L bottle of sterile water or normal saline solution ■ label ■ disinfectant pad ■ stethoscope ■ vital signs monitoring equipment ■ pulse oximeter and probe ■ Optional: gown, mask and goggles or mask with face shield, sterile towel, positive end-expiratory pressure (PEEP) valve, extra suction catheter, sterile gloves.

Preparation of equipment

Choose an appropriately sized suction catheter.[4] The catheter diameter should be no larger than half the inside diameter of the tracheostomy or endotracheal (ET) tube *to minimize hypoxia during suctioning.* (A #12 or #14 French catheter may be used for an 8-mm or larger tube.[7,8,9,10]) Place the suction equipment on the patient's overbed table or bedside stand. Position the table or stand on your preferred side of the bed *to facilitate suctioning.*

Inspect all equipment and supplies. If a product is expired, is defective, or has compromised integrity, remove it from patient use, label it as expired or defective, and report the expiration or defect as directed by your facility.

Attach the collection container to the suction apparatus and the connecting tube to the collection container. Label and date the normal saline solution or sterile water bottle. Attach the handheld resuscitation bag to the oxygen source, and make sure it's functioning properly and readily available. Attach the PEEP valve to the handheld resuscitation bag if indicated.

Implementation

- Verify the practitioner's order, if needed.
- Gather and prepare the necessary equipment and supplies.
- Perform hand hygiene.[1,11,12,13,14,15,16]
- Confirm the patient's identity using at least two patient identifiers.[17]
- Provide privacy.[18,19,20,21]
- Explain the procedure to the patient and family (if appropriate) according to their individual communication and learning needs *to increase their understanding, allay their fears, and enhance cooperation.*[22] Provide instruction even if the patient is unresponsive. Explain that tracheal suctioning usually causes transient coughing or gagging but that coughing is helpful for removing secretions. Continue to reassure the patient throughout the procedure *to minimize anxiety, promote relaxation, and decrease oxygen demand.*
- Raise the bed to waist level before providing care *to prevent caregiver back strain.*[23]
- Perform hand hygiene.[1,11,12,13,14,15,16]
- Assess the patient's vital signs, breath sounds, respiratory effort, and general appearance, and whether copious secretions are present, *to establish a baseline for comparison after tracheal suctioning.* Review the patient's arterial blood gas values and oxygen saturation levels if available. Attach the patient to a pulse oximeter to assess oxygen saturation level before, during, and after the procedure.[7] Evaluate the patient's ability to cough and deep-breathe *to help move secretions up the tracheobronchial tree.*[7]
- Unless contraindicated, elevate the head of the bed at a 30- to 45-degree angle *to promote lung expansion and productive coughing and to prevent aspiration and ventilator-associated pneumonia.*[2,5,24]
- Perform hand hygiene.[1,11,12,13,14,15,16]
- Put on a mask and goggles or mask with face shield and other personal protective equipment as needed, *to comply with standard precautions.*[7,25,26,27]
- Open the sterile normal saline or sterile water bottle.
- Open the package containing the disposable sterile solution container.
- Using strict, no-touch technique, open the suction catheter kit and put the sterile glove on your dominant hand and the clean (nonsterile) glove on your nondominant hand. If using individual supplies, open the suction catheter and the gloves, placing the clean (nonsterile) glove on your nondominant hand first and then the sterile glove on your dominant hand.[1,7]
- Using your nondominant (nonsterile) hand, pour the normal saline solution or sterile water into the disposable sterile solution container.
- Place a sterile towel over the patient's chest, if desired, *to provide an additional sterile area.*
- Using your dominant (sterile) hand, remove the catheter from its wrapper. Keep it coiled *to prevent it from touching a nonsterile object.*
- Using your nondominant (nonsterile) hand to manipulate the connecting tubing, attach the suction catheter to the tubing (as shown below).

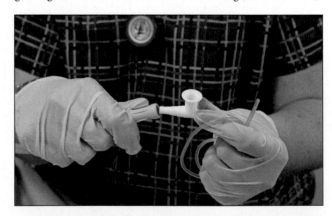

- Using your nondominant (nonsterile) hand, set the suction pressure at the lowest possible level that clears secretions effectively.[3,7,8] *Higher pressures don't enhance secretion removal and may cause traumatic injury.* Occlude the suction port *to assess suction pressure.*[7]

NURSING ALERT Experts recommend using suction pressures of up to 120 mm Hg (15.9 kPa) for open tracheal suction systems and up to 150 mm Hg (20 kPa) for closed systems.[7,10]

■ Dip the catheter tip in the normal saline solution or sterile water (as shown below) *to lubricate the outside of the catheter and reduce tissue trauma during insertion.*

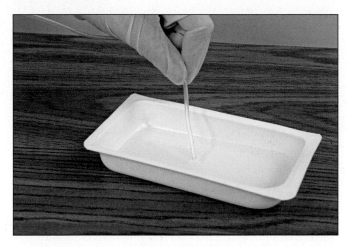

■ With the catheter tip in the sterile normal saline solution or sterile water, occlude the suction control valve with the thumb of your nondominant (nonsterile) hand (as shown below). Suction a small amount of solution or water through the catheter *to lubricate the inside of the catheter, which facilitates passage of secretions through it.* For a closed tracheal suction system, see *Closed tracheal suctioning,* page 824.

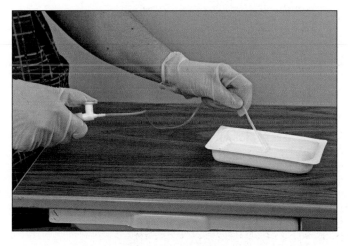

■ Hyperoxygenate the patient with 100% oxygen for 30 to 60 seconds.[2,3,4,7,8] You can do so with a ventilator by pressing the hyperoxygenate button or by increasing the baseline fraction of inspired oxygen level. If these methods aren't available, disconnect the ventilator from the tracheostomy tube, attach the handheld resuscitation bag to the tracheostomy tube, and administer five to six breaths over 30 seconds.[3]

■ Using your nondominant (nonsterile) hand, disconnect the patient from the ventilator.

■ Using your dominant (sterile) hand, advance the suction catheter gently to the premeasured distance needed for insertion (generally, the length of the adapter plus the length of the tracheostomy tube) without applying suction. *Measuring the depth ensures that the suction catheter doesn't extend beyond the end of the tracheostomy or ET tube, which may cause trauma to the tracheal mucosa.*[7,28]

NURSING ALERT Research hasn't shown deep tracheal suctioning to be superior to shallow tracheal suctioning and suggests that it may be associated with more adverse events.[3,7]

■ After inserting the suction catheter, apply suction intermittently by removing and replacing the thumb of your nondominant (nonsterile) hand over the suction control valve. Simultaneously, use your dominant (sterile) hand to withdraw the catheter as you roll it between your thumb and forefinger. *This rotating motion prevents the catheter from pulling tissue into the tube as it exits, avoiding tissue trauma.*

■ Use your nondominant (nonsterile) hand to stabilize the tip of the tracheostomy tube as you withdraw the catheter *to prevent mucous membrane irritation or accidental extubation.* The suctioning event should take no longer than 15 seconds.[4,7]

■ Resume oxygen delivery by reconnecting the source of oxygen or ventilation and hyperoxygenating the patient's lungs with 100% oxygen for 30 to 60 seconds before continuing tracheal suctioning, *to prevent or relieve hypoxia.*[2,3,4,7]

■ Observe and allow the patient to rest for a few minutes before the next tracheal suctioning. The timing of each suctioning and the length of each rest period depend on the patient's tolerance of the procedure and the absence of complications. Encourage the patient to cough between suctioning attempts *to enhance secretion removal.*

■ Observe the secretions. Normal sputum is watery and tends to be sticky. If the secretions are thick, clear the catheter periodically by dipping the tip in the sterile normal saline solution or sterile water and applying suction. Tenacious or thick sputum usually indicates dehydration. Also observe for color variations. Normal sputum is white or translucent; yellow or green may indicate infection, brown usually indicates old blood, and red indicates fresh blood. When sputum contains blood, note whether it's streaked or well mixed. Also, note how often blood appears.

■ If the patient's heart rate and rhythm are being monitored, observe for arrhythmias. If they occur, stop suctioning and ventilate the patient.

■ After tracheal suctioning, hyperoxygenate the patient with 100% oxygen for at least 1 minute using the same technique described earlier.[2,3,4,7]

■ Readjust the FIO₂ and, for a ventilated patient, the parameters and alarms to the ordered settings. Set alarm limits according to the patient's condition, and ensure that the alarms are turned on, functioning properly, and audible to staff.[29,30,31]

■ After suctioning the lower airway, assess the patient's need for upper airway suctioning. (See the "Oronasopharyngeal suctioning" procedure.) Always change the suction catheter and sterile glove before resuctioning the lower airway, if necessary, *to avoid introducing microorganisms into the lower airway.*[1]

■ Clear the connecting tubing by aspirating the remaining sterile normal saline solution or sterile water.[3]

■ Remove and discard your gloves and, if worn, other personal protective equipment

■ Discard used supplies in the appropriate receptacles.[27] Replace supplies as needed.

■ Perform hand hygiene.[1,11,12,13,14,15,16]

■ Maintain the head of the patient's bed at 30 to 45 degrees, if the patient's condition allows, *to prevent ventilator-associated pneumonia.*[5,24]

■ Auscultate the patient's breath sounds bilaterally, obtain vital signs, and monitor oxygen saturation levels, if indicated, *to assess the procedure's effectiveness.*[3]

■ Return the bed to the lowest position *to prevent falls and maintain patient safety.*[32]

■ Perform hand hygiene.[1,11,12,13,14,15,16]

■ Clean and disinfect your stethoscope using a disinfectant pad.[33,34]

■ Perform hand hygiene.[1,11,12,13,14,15,16]

■ Document the procedure.[35,36,37,38]

Special considerations

■ The Joint Commission has issued a sentinel event alert concerning medical device alarm safety, *because alarm-related events have been associated with permanent loss of function or death.* Among the major contributing factors noted were improper alarm settings, alarms inappropriately turned off, and alarm signals that are inaudible to staff. Ensure that alarm limits are set appropriately, and that alarms are turned on, functioning properly, and audible to staff. Follow facility guidelines for preventing alarm fatigue.[31]

■ Although research results are mixed regarding the effects of instilling normal saline into the trachea before suctioning, it isn't a recommended practice.[4,10,39,40] Studies show that instillation of normal saline solution into the trachea before suctioning may stimulate the patient's cough but doesn't liquefy secretions. Keeping the patient adequately hydrated and using bronchial hygiene techniques seem to have a greater effect on mobilizing secretions. In addition, instilling normal

Closed tracheal suctioning

A closed tracheal suction system can ease removal of secretions and reduce patient complications. The system—which consists of a sterile suction catheter in a clear plastic sleeve—allows the patient to remain connected to the ventilator during suctioning, letting the ventilator maintain tidal volume, oxygen concentration, and positive end-expiratory pressure, which reduces the risk of suction-induced hypoxemia.

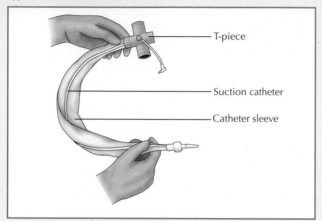

T-piece

Suction catheter

Catheter sleeve

Because the catheter remains in a protective sleeve, you don't need to touch the catheter, and the ventilator circuit remains closed. The closed tracheal suctioning method reduces the risk of spraying of respiratory secretions, especially during suction-induced coughing.[3]

A closed tracheal suction device allows the patient to remain connected to the ventilator during suctioning.[3,4] As a result, the patient may continue to be oxygenated and receive PEEP while undergoing suctioning. In patients receiving intermittent mandatory mechanical ventilation, closed tracheal suctioning may reduce arterial desaturation and eliminate the need for preoxygenation.[7]

On the negative side, closed tracheal suctioning may produce increased negative airway pressure when certain ventilatory modes are used, increasing the risk of atelectasis and hypoxemia.

Implementation

To perform the procedure, gather the equipment for the closed tracheal suction system, which consists of a suction control valve, a T-piece to connect the artificial airway to the ventilator breathing circuit, and a catheter sleeve that encloses the catheter and has connections at each end for the control valve and the T-piece. Then follow these steps:

■ Perform hand hygiene.[1,11,12,13,14,15,16]
■ Put on gloves and, as needed, other personal protective equipment.[25,26,27]
■ Remove the closed tracheal suction system from its wrapping.
■ Attach the control valve to the connecting tubing.

■ Depress the suction control valve, and keep it depressed while setting the suction pressure to the desired level.
■ Connect the T-piece to the ventilator breathing circuit; make sure the irrigation port is closed. Then connect the T-piece to the patient's ET or tracheostomy tube.
■ Hyperoxygenate the patient with 100% oxygen for 30 to 60 seconds.[2,3,4,7,8]
■ Steadying the T-piece, use the thumb and index finger of the other hand to advance the catheter through the ET or tracheostomy tube and into the patient's tracheobronchial tree (as shown). It may be necessary to gently retract the catheter sleeve as you advance the catheter.

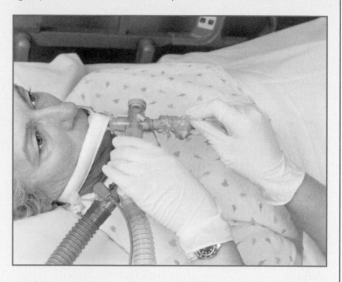

■ While continuing to hold the T-piece and control valve, apply intermittent suction and withdraw the catheter until it reaches its fully extended length in the sleeve for no longer than 10 seconds.[3] Repeat the procedure only if necessary.
■ Hyperoxygenate the patient with 100% oxygen for 30 to 60 seconds.[2,3,4,7,8]
■ After you've completed tracheal suctioning, flush the catheter by maintaining suction while slowly introducing the sterile normal saline solution or sterile water into the irrigation port while applying continuous suction to clear the catheter. Be careful not to lavage the solution down the tube.[3]
■ Turn the suction control valve to the OFF position.
■ Discard used supplies in appropriate receptacles. Replace the suction equipment and supplies, as needed.[27]
■ Remove and discard your gloves and, if worn, other personal protective equipment.[27]
■ Perform hand hygiene.[1,11,12,13,14,15,16]

saline solution may also decrease arterial and mixed venous oxygenation and contribute to lower airway contamination, increasing the risk of ventilator-associated pneumonia.[3,7,8,10] One study showed that instilling normal saline solution into the trachea before suctioning lowered the rate of microbiologically confirmed ventilator-associated pneumonia but had no impact on clinical ventilator-associated pneumonia or patient outcomes.[5]

■ Change the suction catheter and sleeve and ventilator circuit tubing only when visibly soiled *to avoid frequent disruptions in the closed circuit, which increase the risk of ventilator-associated pneumonia.*[5]
■ If the cuff of the ET or tracheostomy tube is inflated and needs to be deflated, suction the lower airway using the above procedure, then suction the upper airway before deflating the cuff using a syringe.[1,2]
■ If appropriate, provide music therapy, as needed, throughout the procedure. *Music therapy has been shown to reduce pain and control sedation levels in patients receiving mechanical ventilation.*[41]

Patient teaching

Teach the patient and family (if applicable) about measures to prevent ventilator-associated pneumonia, and involve them in maintaining the head of the bed at a 30 to 45 degree angle.[24] If the patient will be discharged with an artificial airway, teach the patient and family how to perform tracheal suctioning. Teach about the signs that indicate the need for suctioning and what to expect, *to reduce anxiety.* Encourage the patient to assist in secretion removal by coughing.[3]

Complications

Complications of tracheal suctioning include hypoxemia, dyspnea, atelectasis, tracheal or bronchial mucosal trauma, bacterial colonization of the lower airway, hypotension or hypertension, cardiac arrhythmias, a decreased mixed venous oxygen saturation level, pain, anxiety, pulmonary hemorrhage or bleeding, respiratory arrest, cardiac arrest, laryngospasm or bronchospasm, and increased intracranial pressure.[3,4,7]

Documentation

Record the date and time of the procedure; the technique used; the reason for tracheal suctioning; the amount, color, consistency, and odor (if any) of the secretions; your assessment findings; and the patient's response to the procedure. Document any complications, the name of the practitioner notified, the date and time of notification, prescribed interventions, and the patient's response to them. Document teaching provided to the patient and family (if applicable), their understanding of that teaching, and any need for follow-up teaching.

REFERENCES

1 Centers for Disease Control and Prevention. (2004). Guidelines for preventing health-care-associated pneumonia, 2003: Recommendations of CDC and the Healthcare Infection Control Practices Advisory Committee. *MMWR Recommendations and Reports, 53*(RR-3), 1–32. https://www.cdc.gov/mmwr/preview/mmwrhtml/rr5303a1.htm (Level II)

2 American Association of Critical Care Nurses. (2017). AACN practice alert: Ventilator associated pneumonia. https://www.aacn.org/clinical-resources/practice-alerts/ventilator-associated-pneumonia-vap (Level VII)

3 Wiegand, D. L. (2017). *AACN procedure manual for high acuity, progressive, and critical care* (7th ed.). St. Louis, MO: Elsevier.

4 Kacmarek, R. M., et al. (2021). *Egan's fundamentals of respiratory care* (12th ed.). St. Louis, MO: Mosby.

5 Klompas, M., et al. (2014). Strategies to prevent ventilator-associated pneumonia in acute care hospitals: 2014 update. *Infection Control and Hospital Epidemiology, 35*, 915–936. https://www.jstor.org/stable/10.1086/677144#metadata_info_tab_contents (Level I)

6 Favretto, D. O., et al. (2012). Endotracheal suction in intubated critically ill adult patients undergoing mechanical ventilation: A systematic review. *Revista Latino-Americana de Enfermagem, 20*(5), 997–1007. http://www.scielo.br/pdf/rlae/v20n5/23.pdf (Level I)

7 American Association for Respiratory Care. (2010). AARC clinical practice guidelines: Endotracheal suctioning of mechanically ventilated patients with artificial airways 2010. *Respiratory Care, 55*(6), 758–764. https://www.aarc.org/wp-content/uploads/2014/08/06.10.0758.pdf (Level VII)

8 Bodenham, A., et al. (2014, reviewed 2018). Intensive Care Society standards: Standards for the care of adult patients with a temporary tracheostomy. https://www.wyccn.org/uploads/6/5/1/9/65199375/ics_tracheostomy_standards__2014_.pdf (Level VII)

9 Morris, L., & Afifi, M. S. (Eds.). (2010). *Tracheostomies: The complete guide.* New York, NY: Springer.

10 Nance-Floyd, B. (2011). Tracheostomy care: An evidence-based guide. *American Nurse, 6*(7), 14–16. https://www.americannursetoday.com/tracheostomy-care-an-evidence-based-guide-to-suctioning-and-dressing-changes/

11 Centers for Disease Control and Prevention. (2002). Guideline for hand hygiene in health-care settings: Recommendations of the Healthcare Infection Control Practices Advisory Committee and the HICPAC/SHEA/APIC/IDSA Hand Hygiene Task Force. *MMWR Recommendations and Reports, 51*(RR-16), 1–45. https://www.cdc.gov/mmwr/pdf/rr/rr5116.pdf (Level II)

12 The Joint Commission. (2021). Standard NPSG.07.01.01. *Comprehensive accreditation manual for hospitals.* Oakbrook Terrace, IL: The Joint Commission. (Level VII)

13 World Health Organization. (2009). WHO guidelines on hand hygiene in health care: First global patient safety challenge, clean care is safer care. https://apps.who.int/iris/bitstream/handle/10665/44102/9789241597906_eng.pdf?sequence=1 (Level IV)

14 Centers for Medicare and Medicaid Services, Department of Health and Human Services. (2020). Condition of participation: Infection control. 42 C.F.R. § 482.42.

15 Accreditation Association for Hospitals and Health Systems. (2020). Standard 07.01.21. *Healthcare Facilities Accreditation Program: Accreditation requirements for acute care hospitals.* Chicago, IL: Accreditation Association for Hospitals and Health Systems. (Level VII)

16 DNV GL-Healthcare USA, Inc. (2020). IC.1.SR.1. *NIAHO® accreditation requirements, interpretive guidelines and surveyor guidance—revision 20.0.* Milford, OH: DNV GL-Healthcare USA, Inc. (Level VII)

17 The Joint Commission. (2021). Standard NPSG.01.01.01. *Comprehensive accreditation manual for hospitals.* Oakbrook Terrace, IL: The Joint Commission. (Level VII)

18 The Joint Commission. (2021). Standard RI.01.01.01. *Comprehensive accreditation manual for hospitals.* Oakbrook Terrace, IL: The Joint Commission. (Level VII)

19 DNV GL-Healthcare USA, Inc. (2020). PR.2.SR.5. *NIAHO® accreditation requirements, interpretive guidelines and surveyor guidance—revision 20.0.* Milford, OH: DNV GL-Healthcare USA, Inc. (Level VII)

20 Centers for Medicare and Medicaid Services, Department of Health and Human Services. (2020). Condition of participation: Patient's rights. 42 C.F.R. § 482.13(c)(1).

21 Accreditation Association for Hospitals and Health Systems. (2020). Standard 15.01.16. *Healthcare Facilities Accreditation Program: Accreditation requirements for acute care hospitals.* Chicago, IL: Accreditation Association for Hospitals and Health Systems. (Level VII)

22 The Joint Commission. (2021). Standard PC.02.01.21. *Comprehensive accreditation manual for hospitals.* Oakbrook Terrace, IL: The Joint Commission. (Level VII)

23 Waters, T. R., et al. (2009). Safe patient handling training for schools of nursing. https://www.cdc.gov/niosh/docs/2009-127/pdfs/2009-127.pdf (Level VII)

24 Accreditation Association for Hospitals and Health Systems. (2020). Standard 07.01.02. *Healthcare Facilities Accreditation Program: Accreditation requirements for acute care hospitals.* Chicago, IL: Accreditation Association for Hospitals and Health Systems. (Level VII)

25 Siegel, J. D., et al. (2007, revised 2019). 2007 guideline for isolation precautions: Preventing transmission of infectious agents in healthcare settings. https://www.cdc.gov/infectioncontrol/pdf/guidelines/isolation-guidelines-H.pdf (Level II)

26 Accreditation Association for Hospitals and Health Systems. (2020). Standard 07.01.10. *Healthcare Facilities Accreditation Program: Accreditation requirements for acute care hospitals.* Chicago, IL: Accreditation Association for Hospitals and Health Systems. (Level VII)

27 Occupational Safety and Health Administration. (2012). Bloodborne pathogens, standard number 1910.1030. https://www.osha.gov/pls/oshaweb/owadisp.show_document?p_id=10051&p_table=STANDARDS (Level VII)

28 Pedersen, C. M., et al. (2009). Endotracheal suctioning of the adult intubated patient—What is the evidence? *Intensive and Critical Care Nursing, 25*(1), 21–30. (Level V)

29 Graham, K. C., & Cvach, M. (2010). Monitor alarm fatigue: Standardizing use of physiological monitors and decreasing nuisance alarms. *American Journal of Critical Care, 19*, 28–37.

30 The Joint Commission. (2021). Standard NPSG.06.01.01. *Comprehensive accreditation manual for hospitals.* Oakbrook Terrace, IL: The Joint Commission. (Level VII)

31 The Joint Commission. (2013). Sentinel event alert: Medical device alarm safety in hospitals. https://www.jointcommission.org/-/media/tjc/documents/resources/patient-safety-topics/sentinel-event/sea_50_alarms_4_26_16.pdf (Level VII)

32 Ganz, D. A., et al. (2013, reviewed 2021). *Preventing falls in hospitals: A toolkit for improving quality of care* (AHRQ Publication No. 13-0015-EF). Rockville, MD: Agency for Healthcare Research and Quality. https://www.ahrq.gov/professionals/systems/hospital/fallpxtoolkit/index.html (Level VII)

33 Rutala, W. A., et al. (2008, revised 2019). Guideline for disinfection and sterilization in healthcare facilities, 2008. https://www.cdc.gov/infection-control/pdf/guidelines/disinfection-guidelines-H.pdf (Level I)

34 Accreditation Association for Hospitals and Health Systems. (2020). Standard 07.02.03. *Healthcare Facilities Accreditation Program: Accreditation requirements for acute care hospitals.* Chicago, IL: Accreditation Association for Hospitals and Health Systems. (Level VII)

35 The Joint Commission. (2021). Standard RC.01.03.01. *Comprehensive accreditation manual for hospitals.* Oakbrook Terrace, IL: The Joint Commission. (Level VII)

36 Centers for Medicare and Medicaid Services, Department of Health and Human Services. (2020). Condition of participation: Medical record services. 42 C.F.R. § 482.24(b).

37 Accreditation Association for Hospitals and Health Systems. (2020). Standard 10.00.03. *Healthcare Facilities Accreditation Program: Accreditation requirements for acute care hospitals.* Chicago, IL: Accreditation Association for Hospitals and Health Systems. (Level VII)

38 DNV GL-Healthcare USA, Inc. (2020). MR.2.SR.1. *NIAHO® accreditation requirements, interpretive guidelines and surveyor guidance—revision 20.0.* Milford, OH: DNV GL-Healthcare USA, Inc. (Level VII)

39 Ayhan, H., et al. (2015). Normal saline instillation before endotracheal suctioning: "What does the evidence say? What do the nurses think?": Multimethod study. *Journal of Critical Care, 30*, 762–767. (Level I)

40 Wang, C., et al. (2017). Normal saline instillation before suctioning: A meta-analysis of randomized controlled trials. *Australian Critical Care, 30*, 260–265. (Level I)

41 Aktas, Y. Y., & Karabulut, N. (2016). The effects of music therapy in endotracheal suctioning of mechanically ventilated patients. *Nursing in Critical Care, 21*, 44–52. (Level VI)

TRACHEOSTOMY AND VENTILATOR SPEAKING VALVE USE

Patients with a conventional tracheostomy tube can't speak because the cuffed tracheostomy tube that directs air into the lungs on inspiration expels air through the tracheostomy tube rather than the vocal cords, mouth, and nose. Providing a means of communication for such patients is crucial for their physical and emotional well-being. Nonverbal means of communicating, such as writing, lip-reading, alphabet boards, and gestures, can be frustrating for the patient and family members as well as for health care personnel.

A speaking valve allows a patient with a tracheostomy to speak. Valve brands include Passy-Muir, Montgomery, Shiley, and Shikani. The most common type is the positive-closure-one-way speaking valve, which opens on inspiration to allow the patient to inspire through the tracheostomy tube and then closes after inspiration, redirecting the exhaled air around the tube, through larynx and pharynx, which enables speech when air passes through the vocal cords, and out of the mouth.[1]

Ideally, the tracheostomy tube should be cuffless; however, if the tube is cuffed, it must be *completely* deflated to enable the patient to exhale and to function safely.[1,2] For maximum airflow around the tube, the tube should be no larger than two-thirds the size of the tracheal lumen.[1] Speaking valves fit on the hub of adult, pediatric, and neonatal tracheostomy tubes, and some are also appropriate for placement in ventilator tubing. Generally, valves also include safety ties or lanyards that prevent valve loss if the patient inadvertently coughs the speaking valve out of the tracheostomy tube.

Speaking valve use is contraindicated in patients who are medically unstable or require significant ventilator support (high respiratory rate and minute ventilation requirements, high fraction of inspired oxygen, positive end-expiratory pressure greater than 5 cm H_2O, respiratory distress, frequent bronchospasm, and air-trapping problems). It's also contraindicated in an unconscious or sleeping patient; a patient with pneumothorax with or without air leaks if increased lung pressures are possible; and patients with a larger-diameter tracheostomy tube, a tracheostomy tube with inflated cuff or foam cuff, or an airway obstruction above the tracheostomy, such as bilateral vocal cord paralysis, severe tracheal or laryngeal stenosis, and tumor obstruction. A speaking valve is also contraindicated in patients with copious, excessive, or thick secretions; paralysis of the lips, tongue, and other muscles involved in speech; or laryngectomy.[1,3,4]

Speaking valve use requires a multidisciplinary team approach. A practitioner's order is required for placement and sometimes for cuff deflation. The nurse, speech-language pathologist, and respiratory therapist are responsible for monitoring and assessing the patient while the patient is using the speaking valve.[2] Ventilator adjustments for the ventilator-dependent tracheostomy patient are the respiratory therapist's responsibility. A speech-language pathologist should assess the patient's cognitive, language, and oral motor function, and may also evaluate swallowing status and the risk for aspiration. The patient must also be involved in the decision about whether to use the speaking valve.

An initial trial assesses the patient's tolerance. Make sure that the patient understands how the speaking valve functions and what to expect during the trial. The patient who is anxious, especially during cuff deflation, may be unwilling to use the valve, so provide emotional support. Assess the patient's ability to tolerate cuff deflation before using the speaking valve.[1]

Don't leave the patient unsupervised with the valve in place until you determine tolerance.[1] If the patient can't tolerate the speaking valve initially, the team should troubleshoot to determine the cause. Problem-solving to increase patient tolerance of the one-way speaking valve may include tracheostomy tube downsizing, or continued therapeutic trials with implementation of strengthening programs to address respiration, voice, and swallowing issues.[2] Some patients are only able to wear the speaking valve for a few minutes at a time, building up time gradually as tolerated. If repeated trials fail, the speech-language pathologist should assess the patient for other communication options.

Equipment

Appropriate-sized speaking valve ▪ gloves ▪ stethoscope ▪ pulse oximeter and probe ▪ vital signs monitoring equipment ▪ suction equipment ▪ handheld resuscitation bag ▪ oxygen source ▪ 10-mL Luer-lock syringe ▪ speaking valve manufacturer's instruction booklet ▪ disinfectant pad ▪

cuff-deflation warning sign ▪ label for tracheostomy pilot balloon ▪ Optional: wide-mouth short flex tubing.

Preparation of equipment

Inspect all equipment and supplies. If a product is expired, is defective, or has compromised integrity, remove it from patient use, label it as expired or defective, and report the expiration or defect as directed by your facility.

Make sure that the oxygen source and handheld resuscitation bag are readily available at the patient's bedside.

Implementation

- Verify the practitioner's order.
- Gather and prepare the necessary equipment and supplies.
- Perform hand hygiene.[5,6,7,8,9,10]
- Confirm the patient's identity using at least two patient identifiers.[11]
- Provide privacy.[12,13,14,15]
- Explain the procedure to the patient and family (if appropriate) according to their individual communication and learning needs *to increase their understanding, allay their fears, and enhance cooperation.*[16] Provide the patient and family (if appropriate) with the written instructions included in the speaking valve booklet.
- If this is the patient's first experience, coordinate the trial with the respiratory therapist and speech-language pathologist.[2]
- Raise the bed to waist level before performing patient care *to prevent caregiver back strain.*[17]
- Elevate the head of the patient's bed about 45 degrees *to allow full movement of the respiratory muscles and diaphragm.*[18]
- Perform hand hygiene.[5,6,7,8,9,10]
- Put on gloves *to comply with standard precautions.*[19,20,21]
- Assess the patient's vital signs, color, oxygen saturation level using pulse oximetry, breath sounds, level of consciousness, work of breathing, and tracheal and oral secretions.[3]
- Perform tracheal and oral suctioning *to clear the airway of pooled secretions that could leak past the cuff after the cuff is deflated, increasing the patient's risk of pneumonia.*[3]
- Deflate the cuff slowly *so the patient can become accustomed to using the upper airways again.* Do this by first tracing the tubing from the patient to its point of origin *to make sure that you're connecting the syringe to the pilot balloon.*[22] Then attach a 10-mL syringe to the tracheostomy tube's pilot balloon (as shown below), and remove the air until air can no longer be extracted and a vacuum is created. Suction the trachea and oral cavity as needed. The tracheostomy cuff *must* be completely deflated before the speaking valve is placed *because any air left in the cuff can block airflow in the tracheostomy tube.*[18]

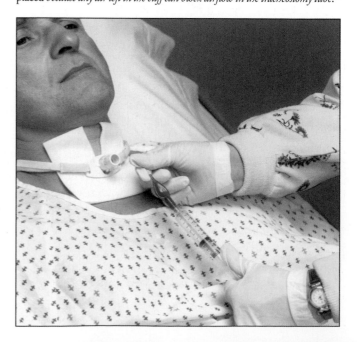

NURSING ALERT Never place a speaking valve on the tracheostomy tube before deflating the cuff, *because the patient won't be able to breathe.*

■ Hold the speaking valve between your fingers. For a patient who isn't ventilator-dependent, attach the speaking valve to the existing tracheostomy hub with a quarter-turn twist (as shown below).

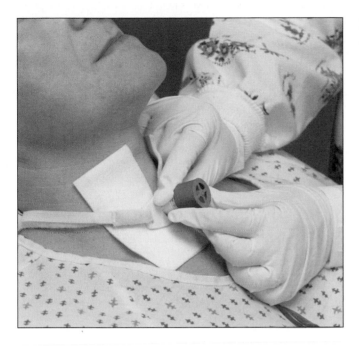

■ For the patient who is ventilator-dependent, insert the speaking valve into the end of the wide-mouth, short-flex tubing (as shown below).

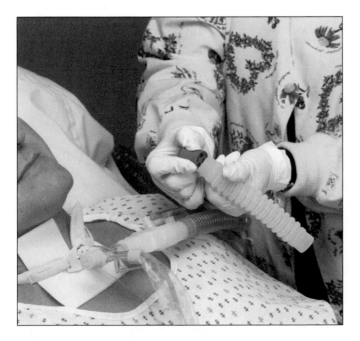

■ Connect the other end of the short-flex tubing to the ventilator tubing.
■ Attach the speaking valve (connected to the short-flex tubing) and the ventilator tubing to the closed-suction system (as shown to the right). Alternatively, attach the speaking valve between the swivel adapter and the short-flex tubing and ventilator tubing.

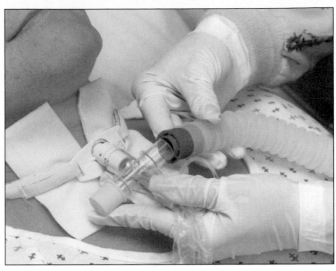

■ Adjust ventilator settings as needed and ordered. You may have to increase the tidal volume if air leaks around the tube.[4] Make sure that the ventilator alarms are set appropriately for the patient's current condition, and that the alarms are turned on, functioning properly, and audible to staff.[23,24,25]
■ After the speaking valve is in place, encourage the patient to relax, and tell the patient to notice how the lungs fill with air when the machine delivers a breath of air. Instruct the patient to breathe out through the nose and mouth.
■ Coach the patient to breathe in first, then speak. Tell the patient to initially try vocalizing simple sounds, such as "Ahhhh," or to count "1, 2, 3, 4."[4]
■ Provide reassurance as needed; the speech-language pathologist can help facilitate voice production and speech as needed.
■ Evaluate the patient's response during speaking valve use. Monitor vital signs, color, breath sounds, level of consciousness, work of breathing, and tracheal and oral secretions.
■ Monitor the patient's oxygen saturation level by pulse oximetry; maintain a level of at least 90% (or as ordered), and be alert for signs of respiratory distress.[4]

NURSING ALERT Remove the speaking valve immediately if the patient shows signs and symptoms of distress, such as a significant change in blood pressure or heart rate, increased respiratory rate, dyspnea, diaphoresis, anxiety, uncontrollable coughing, or arterial oxygen saturation less than 90% (as ordered). Reassess the patient before trying the valve again.[2,3]

■ Remove the valve and suction as needed *to maintain a patent airway.*[4]

NURSING ALERT Secretions can obstruct air passage outside the tube, causing respiratory distress and valve intolerance. Although a one-way speaking valve can improve the strength of the cough, it may be difficult for the patient to cough secretions up to the mouth with the valve in place *because of the small space between the tube and the trachea, thicker secretions, inability to take deep breaths, and weak cough.*[4]

■ Post cuff-deflation warning signs in the room.
■ Label the tracheostomy pilot balloon *to remind health care providers to reinflate the pilot balloon after removing the speaking valve.*[3]
■ Gently twist the speaking valve to remove it. Only when it's removed and the original setup is in place should you return the ventilator settings to their original levels and reinflate the pilot balloon cuff. Always remember to reinflate the tracheostomy cuff *after* removing the speaking valve.
■ Return the bed to the lowest position *to prevent falls and maintain patient safety.*[26]
■ Discard used supplies in appropriate receptacles.[21]
■ Remove and discard your gloves.[21]
■ Perform hand hygiene.[5,6,7,8,9,10]
■ Clean and disinfect your stethoscope using a disinfectant pad *to prevent transmission of microorganisms.*[27,28]
■ Perform hand hygiene.[5,6,7,8,9,10]
■ Document the procedure.[29,30,31,32]

Special considerations

■ Some valves can be used on or off the ventilator, and are convenient to use on patients who are ventilator-dependent *because these valves are tapered to fit into disposable ventilator tubing.* An oxygen port may be available for use with some speaking valves, enabling improved mobility and comfort for patients who require a tracheostomy tube, a speaking valve, and low-flow supplemental oxygen. Be sure to review the instructions for use *to ensure that the valve is appropriate for the patient's needs.*

■ If the patient requiring mechanical ventilation uses a speaking valve, the patient's positive end-expiratory pressure requirement may lessen, *because the speaking valve causes airway pressures to rise.*[3]

■ Remove the speaking valve before administering medicated nebulizer treatments. If the speaking valve is inadvertently used during a nebulizer treatment, remove it immediately and rinse it thoroughly *to remove the medication residue that may affect performance of the diaphragm.*[3,4]

■ Remove the valve when the patient is sleeping.[4]

■ Assess to determine whether the patient's condition permits the use of a cuffless tracheostomy tube *to eliminate the need for cuff deflation during speaking valve use.*[3]

■ A speaking valve may be used 48 to 72 hours after a tracheotomy in a non-ventilator-dependent patient if tracheal edema and secretions from the surgical procedure have decreased.[3]

■ Speaking valve use may need to be delayed for 48 to 72 hours after a tracheostomy tube change if tracheal swelling or bronchospasm occurs as a result of the procedure.[3]

Complications

Complications of ventilator valve use may include aspiration of secretions and respiratory distress.

Documentation

Document the type of speaking valve used and the time the device was placed. Record the patient's response to the procedure, respiratory and hemodynamic status, secretion management, and ability to vocalize. Document teaching provided to the patient and family (if appropriate), their understanding of that teaching, and any need for follow up teaching.

REFERENCES

1 Morris, L., & Afifi, M. S. (Eds.). (2010). *Tracheostomies: The complete guide.* New York, NY: Springer Publishing Company.

2 Windhorst, C., et al. (2009). Patients requiring tracheostomy and mechanical ventilation. A model for interdisciplinary decision-making. *ASHA Leader, 14*(1). https://leader.pubs.asha.org/doi/10.1044/leader. FTR1.14012009.10

3 Passy-Muir, Inc. (n.d.). Passy-Muir tracheostomy and ventilator swallowing and speaking valves instruction booklet. https://www.passy-muir.com/sites/default/files/pdf/instructbklt.pdf

4 Grossbach, I., et al. (2011). Promoting effective communication for patients receiving mechanical ventilation. *Critical Care Nurse, 31*(3), 46–60. http://ccn.aacnjournals.org/content/31/3/46.full.pdf+html (Level VII)

5 World Health Organization. (2009). WHO guidelines on hand hygiene in health care: First global patient safety challenge, clean care is safer care. https://apps.who.int/iris/bitstream/handle/10665/44102/9789241597906_eng.pdf?sequence=1 (Level IV)

6 The Joint Commission. (2021). Standard NPSG.07.01.01. *Comprehensive accreditation manual for hospitals.* Oakbrook Terrace, IL: The Joint Commission. (Level VII)

7 Centers for Disease Control and Prevention. (2002). Guideline for hand hygiene in health-care settings: Recommendations of the Healthcare Infection Control Practices Advisory Committee and the HICPAC/SHEA/APIC/IDSA Hand Hygiene Task Force. *MMWR Recommendations and Reports, 51*(RR-16), 1–45. https://www.cdc.gov/mmwr/pdf/rr/rr5116.pdf (Level II)

8 Centers for Medicare and Medicaid Services, Department of Health and Human Services. (2020). Condition of participation: Infection control. 42 C.F.R. § 482.42.

9 Accreditation Association for Hospitals and Health Systems. (2020). Standard 07.01.21. *Healthcare Facilities Accreditation Program: Accreditation requirements for acute care hospitals.* Chicago, IL: Accreditation Association for Hospitals and Health Systems. (Level VII)

10 DNV GL-Healthcare USA, Inc. (2020). IC.1.SR.1. *NIAHO® accreditation requirements, interpretive guidelines and surveyor guidance—revision 20.0.* Milford, OH: DNV GL-Healthcare USA, Inc. (Level VII)

11 The Joint Commission. (2021). Standard NPSG.01.01.01. *Comprehensive accreditation manual for hospitals.* Oakbrook Terrace, IL: The Joint Commission. (Level VII)

12 The Joint Commission. (2021). Standard RI.01.01.01. *Comprehensive accreditation manual for hospitals.* Oakbrook Terrace, IL: The Joint Commission. (Level VII)

13 DNV GL-Healthcare USA, Inc. (2020). PR.2.SR.5. *NIAHO® accreditation requirements, interpretive guidelines and surveyor guidance—revision 20.0.* Milford, OH: DNV GL-Healthcare USA, Inc. (Level VII)

14 Centers for Medicare and Medicaid Services, Department of Health and Human Services. (2020). Condition of participation: Patient's rights. 42 C.F.R. § 482.13(c)(1).

15 Accreditation Association for Hospitals and Health Systems. (2020). Standard 15.01.16. *Healthcare Facilities Accreditation Program: Accreditation requirements for acute care hospitals.* Chicago, IL: Accreditation Association for Hospitals and Health Systems. (Level VII)

16 The Joint Commission. (2021). Standard PC.02.01.21. *Comprehensive accreditation manual for hospitals.* Oakbrook Terrace, IL: The Joint Commission. (Level VII)

17 Waters, T. R., et al. (2009). Safe patient handling training for schools of nursing. https://www.cdc.gov/niosh/docs/2009-127/pdfs/2009-127.pdf (Level VII)

18 Passy-Muir, Inc. (n.d.). Passy-Muir tracheostomy and ventilator swallowing and speaking valves patient education handbook. https://www.passy-muir.com/sites/default/files/pdf/patienthdbk.pdf

19 Siegel, J. D., et al. (2007, revised 2019). 2007 guideline for isolation precautions: Preventing transmission of infectious agents in healthcare settings. https://www.cdc.gov/infectioncontrol/pdf/guidelines/isolation-guidelines-H.pdf (Level II)

20 Accreditation Association for Hospitals and Health Systems. (2020). Standard 07.01.10. *Healthcare Facilities Accreditation Program: Accreditation requirements for acute care hospitals.* Chicago, IL: Accreditation Association for Hospitals and Health Systems. (Level VII)

21 Occupational Safety and Health Administration. (2012). Bloodborne pathogens, standard number 1910.1030. https://www.osha.gov/pls/oshaweb/owadisp.show_document?p_id=10051&p_table=STANDARDS (Level VII)

22 U.S. Food and Drug Administration. (2021). Examples of medical device misconnections. https://www.fda.gov/medical-devices/medical-device-connectors/examples-medical-device-misconnections

23 The Joint Commission. (2021). Standard NPSG.06.01.01. *Comprehensive accreditation manual for hospitals.* Oakbrook Terrace, IL: The Joint Commission (Level VII)

24 Graham, K. C., & Cvach, M. (2010). Monitor alarm fatigue: Standardizing use of physiological monitors and decreasing nuisance alarms. *American Journal of Critical Care, 19*, 28–37. https://aacnjournals.org/ajcconline/article-abstract/19/1/28/5720/Monitor-Alarm-Fatigue-Standardizing-Use-of?redirectedFrom=fulltext

25 The Joint Commission. (2013). Sentinel event alert 50: Medical device alarm safety in hospitals. https://www.jointcommission.org/-/media/tjc/documents/resources/patient-safety-topics/sentinel-event/sea_50_alarms_4_26_16.pdf (Level VII)

26 Ganz, D. A., et al. (2013, reviewed 2021). *Preventing falls in hospitals: A toolkit for improving quality of care* (AHRQ Publication No. 13-0015-EF). Rockville, MD: Agency for Healthcare Research and Quality. https://www.ahrq.gov/professionals/systems/hospital/fallpxtoolkit/index.html (Level VII)

27 Rutala, W. A., et al. (2008, revised 2019). Guideline for disinfection and sterilization in healthcare facilities, 2008. https://www.cdc.gov/infectioncontrol/pdf/guidelines/disinfection-guidelines-H.pdf (Level I)

28 Accreditation Association for Hospitals and Health Systems. (2020). Standard 07.02.03. *Healthcare Facilities Accreditation Program: Accreditation requirements for acute care hospitals.* Chicago, IL: Accreditation Association for Hospitals and Health Systems. (Level VII)

29 The Joint Commission. (2021). Standard RC.01.03.01. *Comprehensive accreditation manual for hospitals.* Oakbrook Terrace, IL: The Joint Commission. (Level VII)

30 Accreditation Association for Hospitals and Health Systems. (2020). Standard 10.00.03. *Healthcare Facilities Accreditation Program: Accreditation requirements for acute care hospitals.* Chicago, IL: Accreditation Association for Hospitals and Health Systems. (Level VII)

31 Centers for Medicare and Medicaid Services, Department of Health and Human Services. (2020). Condition of participation: Medical record services. 42 C.F.R. § 482.24(b).

32 DNV GL-Healthcare USA, Inc. (2020). MR.2.SR.1. *NIAHO® accreditation requirements, interpretive guidelines and surveyor guidance—revision 20.0.* Milford, OH: DNV GL-Healthcare USA, Inc. (Level VII)

TRACHEOSTOMY CARE

Whether a tracheotomy is performed in an emergency situation or after careful preparation, as a permanent measure or as temporary therapy, tracheostomy care goals remain the same: to ensure airway patency by keeping the tube free of mucus buildup, to maintain mucous membrane and skin integrity, to prevent infection, and to provide psychological support.

The patient may have one of three types of tracheostomy tube: uncuffed, cuffed, or fenestrated.[1] Tube selection depends on the patient's condition and the practitioner's preference. Each type of tube has advantages and disadvantages. An *uncuffed tube*, which may be plastic or metal, allows air to flow freely around the tracheostomy tube and through the larynx, reducing the risk of tracheal damage. A *cuffed tube*, made of plastic, is disposable. The cuff and the tube won't separate accidentally inside the trachea because the cuff is bonded to the tube. A cuffed tube doesn't require periodic deflating to lower pressure, *because cuff pressure is low and evenly distributed against the tracheal wall.* A plastic *fenestrated tube* permits speech through the upper airway when the external opening is capped and the cuff is deflated.[1] It also allows easy removal of the inner cannula for cleaning. However, a fenestrated tube can become occluded. (See *Types of tracheostomy tubes.*)

The maximum acceptable tracheostomy tube cuff pressure shouldn't exceed 25 mm Hg.[1,2] Cuff inflation or deflation may be necessary to maintain this optimal pressure. When cuff pressure is inadequate, oropharyngeal secretions can leak around the cuff, increasing the risk of ventilator-associated pneumonia (VAP).[3] Overinflation of the cuff can cause tracheal necrosis, tracheomalacia, tracheoinnominate artery fistula, tracheal ulceration, fibrosis, tracheoesophageal fistula, and tracheal stenosis.[4] High cuff pressure can also result from malposition of the tracheostomy or insertion of a tube that's too small in diameter, requiring overfilling of the cuff to achieve a seal in the trachea.[1] Actual cuff pressure varies with each patient, however. To keep the pressure within safe limits, measure cuff pressure at least once each shift or at an interval determined by your facility.[5,6] (See the "Tracheal cuff pressure measurement" procedure.) A respiratory therapist or nurse can maintain and measure tracheal cuff pressure.

Tracheostomy cuff deflation is necessary to remove the tube, secure a decannulation cap, attach a speaking valve to the tube, and enable the patient to eat or drink.[2]

To prevent infection, all tracheostomy care should be performed using sterile technique until the stoma has healed. For new tracheotomies, sterile gloves are required for all manipulations at the tracheostomy site. When the stoma has healed, clean gloves can be substituted for sterile ones.

Changing tracheostomy ties helps prevent infection and the skin underneath the ties from becoming excoriated and wet. Two types of tracheostomy ties may be used to secure tracheostomy tubes: twill tape or a commercially prepared tracheostomy tube holder. A commercially prepared tracheostomy tube holder is recommended, *because it protects the patient from pressure on the back of the neck and is easily adjustable.* [7]

Equipment
For cuff inflation and deflation
10-mL syringe ▪ gloves ▪ stethoscope ▪ handheld resuscitation bag ▪ oxygen source and tubing ▪ suction equipment ▪ sterile tracheostomy tubes (same size as the tube currently in place and one a size smaller)[4] ▪ obturator ▪ disinfectant pad ▪ cuff pressure manometer ▪ ventilator or humidified oxygen ▪ Optional: gown, mask, goggles, mask with face shield, communication aids.

EQUIPMENT

Types of tracheostomy tubes

Cuffed and uncuffed tracheostomy tubes each have advantages and disadvantages. Cuffed tubes help seal the area between the tube and trachea, decreasing the patient's risk of aspiration. However, if the cuff pressure isn't regularly monitored, this type of tube can lead to tracheal erosion. Also, when the cuff is inflated, the patient can't talk and needs an alternate means of communication.

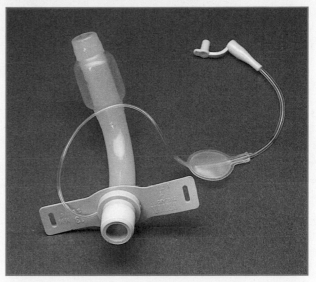

Uncuffed tubes allow the patient to eat and talk. However, this type of tube can't be used in a patient who is receiving mechanical ventilation, *because oxygen may escape from around the tube.*

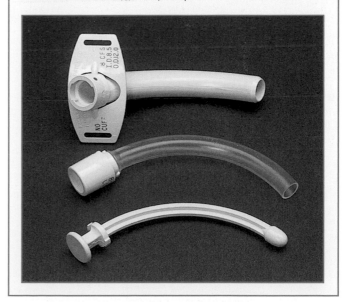

For tracheostomy ties change
Tracheostomy twill tape or a commercially prepared tracheostomy tube holder with Velcro ties ▪ gloves ▪ stethoscope ▪ disinfectant pad ▪ cotton-tipped applicators ▪ normal saline solution ▪ sterile water ▪ sterile container ▪ sterile 4" × 4" (10-cm × 10-cm) gauze pads ▪ oral care supplies ▪ emergency equipment (code cart with emergency medications, defibrillator, handheld resuscitation bag attached to oxygen source and mask, two sterile tracheostomy tubes [one same size as the tube currently in place and one a size smaller],[3] obturator) ▪ bandage scissors ▪ Optional: gown, mask with face shield or mask and goggles, sterile precut tracheostomy dressing, suction equipment, skin barrier.

For tracheostomy tube cannula and stoma care

Disposable inner cannula ▪ two or three sterile solution containers ▪ sterile normal saline solution or sterile water, or other cleaning solution recommended by the manufacturer ▪ sterile cotton-tipped applicators ▪ sterile 4" × 4" (10-cm × 10-cm) gauze pads ▪ sterile gloves ▪ clean gloves ▪ prepackaged sterile tracheostomy dressing ▪ sterile nylon brush ▪ suctioning supplies ▪ stethoscope ▪ disinfectant pad ▪ handheld resuscitation bag connected to an oxygen source ▪ extra tracheostomy tubes and obturator[3] ▪ Optional: skin barrier[8], sterile pipe cleaners, tracheostomy ties, gown, mask and goggles or mask with face shield, extra inner cannula, foam tracheostomy dressing, diluted hydrogen peroxide solution, mechanical ventilator or humidification device.

Note: Commercially prepared tracheostomy care kits are available.

Preparation of equipment
For tracheostomy tube cannula and stoma care

Inspect all equipment and supplies. If a product is expired, is defective, or has compromised integrity, remove it from patient use, label it as expired or defective, and report the expiration or defect as directed by your facility.

Make sure that extra tracheostomy tubes with an obturator are readily available. Also make sure that a handheld resuscitation bag and oxygen source are readily available and functioning.[4]

Place the equipment and supplies on a clean table or stand near the patient's bed. Open the tracheostomy care kit (if available in your facility) using sterile technique. Using sterile technique, pour sterile normal saline solution, sterile water, or other cleaning solution recommended by the manufacturer (such as diluted hydrogen peroxide solution) into one of the sterile solution containers. Then pour sterile normal saline solution or sterile water into the second sterile container for rinsing. For inner cannula care, you may use a third sterile solution container to hold the gauze pads and cotton-tipped applicators saturated with normal saline solution.

If you must replace the disposable inner cannula, open the package containing the new inner cannula while maintaining sterile technique.[1] Obtain or prepare new tracheostomy ties, if indicated. Make sure that the extra tracheostomy tubes and obturator are at the bedside for use in an emergency.

Implementation

▪ Gather and prepare the necessary equipment and supplies.
▪ Read the cuff manufacturer's instructions, *because cuff types and procedures may vary.*
▪ Perform hand hygiene.[9,10,11,12,13,14]
▪ Confirm the patient's identity using at least two patient identifiers.[15]
▪ Provide privacy.[16,17,18,19]
▪ Explain the procedure to the patient and family (if appropriate) according to their individual communication and learning needs *to increase their understanding, allay their fears, and enhance cooperation.*[20]
▪ Raise the patient's bed to waist level before performing patient care *to prevent caregiver back strain.*[21]
▪ Perform hand hygiene.[7,8,9,10,11,12]
▪ Assess the patient's respiratory status *to obtain baseline measurements for comparison.*[1]
▪ Place the patient in a semi-Fowler position, if appropriate, *to prevent aspiration of secretions and promote oxygenation.*[1]
▪ Perform hand hygiene.[9,10,11,12,13,14]
▪ Put on gloves and other personal protective equipment, as needed *to comply with standard precautions.*[22,23,24]
▪ Hyperoxygenate the patient for 30 to 60 seconds, if needed. Then perform oropharyngeal suctioning to remove accumulated secretions from above the cuff, *because these secretions have been implicated in the development of VAP.*[3,25,26]
▪ Remove the ventilation device or humidified oxygen.
▪ Trace the tubing from the patient to its point of origin *to makes sure you're connecting the syringe to the cuff pilot balloon port.*[27]
▪ Insert a 10-mL syringe into the cuff pilot balloon port.

Cuff deflation

▪ To deflate the cuff, ventilate the patient with a handheld resuscitation bag, and slowly withdraw air from the cuff until you hear a small leak with a stethoscope over the larynx during inspiration. *Slow deflation allows positive lung pressure to push secretions upward from the bronchi. Cuff deflation can also stimulate the patient's cough reflex, producing additional secretions.* Remove the syringe if you aren't immediately reinflating the cuff.

Cuff inflation

▪ Inflate the cuff per the manufacturer's recommendation or practitioner's order.
▪ Remove the syringe.
▪ Attach a cuff pressure manometer to the cuff pilot balloon port and read the measurement.
▪ Adjust the pressure as needed. If the cuff pressure measures greater than 25 cm H_2O, press the pressure-release button on the device until the pressure reaches 20 to 25 cm H_2O.[1] If the pressure measures less than 20 cm H_2O, add air by squeezing the bulb until the pressure reaches 20 to 25 cm H_2O.[1]
▪ Note the exact amount of air you used to inflate the cuff *to help detect tracheomalacia if more air becomes consistently necessary.*
▪ If you're not able to maintain adequate pressure, notify the practitioner.[1]

NURSING ALERT Minimal occlusive volume and minimal leak inflation techniques have been found to increase the risk of silent aspiration. Guidelines recommend using a measuring device, such as a manometer, *to achieve optimal cuff pressures and decrease the risk of adverse events.*[1,5,28]

▪ Disconnect the cuff pressure manometer from the cuff pilot balloon port.
▪ Reconnect the ventilation device or humidified oxygen.
▪ If the patient is on a ventilator, make sure that the ventilator alarms are set appropriately for the patient's current condition, and that the alarms are turned on, functioning properly, and audible to staff.[29,30,31]
▪ Reassess the patient's respiratory status and compare the findings to baseline findings.[1]
▪ Note the exact amount of air used to inflate the cuff *to help detect tracheomalacia if more air is consistently needed.*

Tracheostomy ties change

▪ Obtain assistance from another nurse or a respiratory therapist *because of the risk of accidental tube dislodgement.*[8]

NURSING ALERT Research overwhelmingly recommends a two-person technique for changing a tracheostomy tube securing device *to prevent tube dislodgment.* In the two-person technique, one person holds the tracheostomy tube in place while the other person changes the securing device.[8]

▪ Inspect the skin around the stoma and in areas where rubbing may occur, such as the neck and chin. Look for redness, a rash, abrasions, and ulceration.[3,32] If the patient's neck or stoma is excoriated or infected, notify the practitioner. *If not detected early and treated appropriately, skin irritation can lead to breakdown and infection.*
▪ Clean the stomal area with cotton-tipped applicators moistened with normal saline solution *to remove debris at the juncture of the stoma and tracheostomy tube.* Don't use the applicator for more than one pass over the skin. Place sterile gauze pads in a sterile container with normal saline solution or sterile water and use the moistened gauze pads to clean the surrounding skin.[1]
▪ Dry the area thoroughly with additional sterile gauze pads. Apply a skin barrier, as needed.[8]

Ties change using twill tape

▪ Cut a piece of twill tape that's long enough to encircle the patient's neck twice. Cut the ends diagonally.[1]

- Instruct the assistant to hold the tracheostomy tube in place *to prevent its expulsion during replacement of the ties and to minimize irritation and coughing due to tube manipulation.*[1,3,33]
- With the assistant's gloved fingers holding the tracheostomy tube in place, cut the soiled tracheostomy ties with the bandage scissors, or untie them and discard the ties. Be careful not to cut the tube of the pilot balloon.
- Insert one end of the new twill tape through one eye of tracheostomy tube flange and pull the ends of the twill tape even.[1]
- Pass both ends of the twill tape around the patient's neck and insert one end through the second eye of the flange.
- Instruct the patient to flex the neck while you pull snugly on the ties, allowing space for one finger between the tie and the patient's neck.[4]
- Instruct the assistant to place one finger under the twill tape as you tie the ends securely with a double square knot.[1] Make sure that the knot rests on the side of the patient's neck *for easy access.*[1,3,4]

Changing a commercially prepared tracheostomy tube holder

- Instruct the assistant to hold the tracheostomy tube in place *to prevent its dislodgement or expulsion during replacement of the Velcro tabs.*[1,4,8,33]
- Remove the old tracheostomy tube holder by opening the Velcro tabs.
- Thread one Velcro tab through the flange and secure it to the body of the tracheostomy tube holder.
- Bring the loose end of the tracheostomy tube holder around the back of the patient's neck.
- Thread the remaining Velcro tab through the other flange and secure it to the body of the tracheostomy tube holder.
- Adjust the right and left Velcro tabs, as needed, *to ensure that only one finger can slide under the tie at the back of the neck.*[4] *Fastening too tightly can lead to skin breakdown and vascular obstruction; fastening too loosely can lead to tube decannulation.*[3]
- Check tracheostomy tie tension frequently on a patient with traumatic injury, radical neck dissection, or cardiac failure, *because neck diameter can increase from swelling and cause constriction*; also check a restless patient frequently, *because ties can loosen and cause tube dislodgment.*
- If necessary, apply a sterile, precut tracheostomy dressing by sliding the dressing under the flanges of the tracheostomy tube, starting at the bottom and moving to the top.

NURSING ALERT Use a manufactured split dressing; don't cut a gauze pad, *because loose fibers around the stoma or tracheostomy tube can cause irritation and increase the risk of infection.*[8,33]

Tracheostomy tube cannula and stoma care

- Perform hand hygiene.[9,10,11,12,13,14]
- Put on gloves and other personal protective equipment as needed.[22,23,24] Use a mask with face shield or mask and goggles if spraying of respiratory secretions is likely.[26]
- Assess the patient's respiratory status and the need for suctioning.[1]
- Hyperoxygenate the patient for 30 to 60 seconds before suctioning (if needed) by adjusting the fraction of inspired oxygen on the mechanical ventilator or by using the temporary oxygen-enrichment program available on the ventilator *to prevent hypoxemia.*[26]
- If needed, suction the tracheostomy tube by inserting the suction catheter to a premeasured distance[1,8] *to clear the airway of any secretions that may hinder oxygenation.* Determine the volume of secretions, and assess them for color, consistency, and odor. (See the "Tracheal suctioning, intubated patient" procedure.)
- With your nondominant hand, reconnect the patient to the humidifier or ventilator, if necessary. Hyperoxygenate the patient for at least 1 minute following suctioning.[1,26]
- Remove the patient's tracheostomy dressing, inspect it for drainage, and then discard it.[1,24]
- Assess the patient's cardiac and respiratory status *to evaluate response to suctioning.*[26,34]

- Remove and discard your gloves.[24]
- Perform hand hygiene.[9,10,11,12,13,14]

Cleaning a nondisposable inner cannula

- Put on sterile gloves.[1,22,23,24]
- Using your nondominant hand, disconnect the ventilator or humidification device and unlock the tracheostomy tube's inner cannula by rotating it counterclockwise (as shown below).[1]

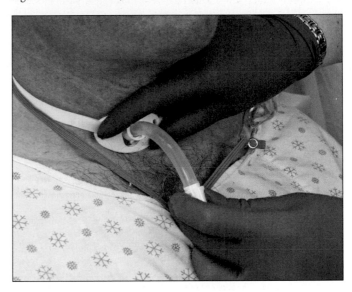

- Remove the inner cannula and place it in the container of sterile normal saline solution or sterile water, or other cleaning solution recommended by the manufacturer—but don't allow it to soak.
- Place the ventilator oxygen device or humidification device over or near the outer cannula *to maintain the oxygen supply.* Alternatively, have another staff member maintain oxygen supply for the patient.
- Working quickly, use your dominant hand to scrub the cannula with the sterile nylon brush (as shown below).[1] You may also use a sterile pipe cleaner (provided in a commercially prepared tracheostomy care kit) if necessary to clean the inner cannula.[34]

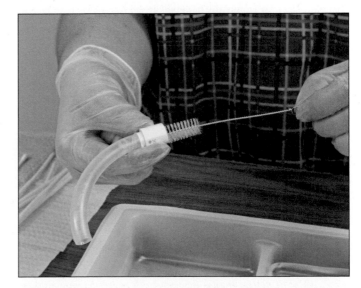

- Immerse the cannula in the container of normal saline solution or sterile water (as shown on the next page), and agitate it for about 10 seconds *to rinse it thoroughly.*

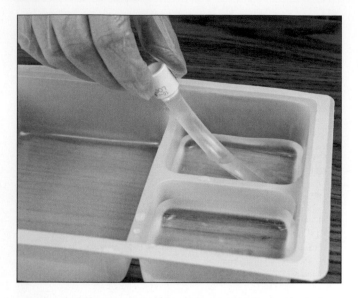

■ Inspect the cannula for cleanliness. Repeat the cleaning process if necessary. When it's clean, tap it gently against the inside edge of the sterile container *to remove excess liquid and prevent aspiration.* Alternatively, you can use a pipe cleaner to dry the inside of the inner cannula.[3] Don't dry the outer surface, *because a thin film of moisture acts as a lubricant during insertion.*

■ Reinsert the inner cannula into the patient's tracheostomy tube. Lock it in place and then gently pull on it *to make sure it's positioned securely.* Reconnect the mechanical ventilator or humidification device.[1]

■ If the patient can't tolerate being disconnected from the ventilator for the time it takes to clean the inner cannula, replace the existing inner cannula with a clean one and reattach the mechanical ventilator. Then clean the cannula that you just removed from the patient and store it in a sterile container for the next time.[1]

Replacing a disposable inner cannula

■ Perform hand hygiene.[9,10,11,12,13,14]
■ Put on clean gloves.[1,22,23,24]
■ Using your dominant hand, remove the patient's inner cannula.[1] After evaluating the secretions in the cannula, discard it properly.
■ Pick up the new inner cannula, touching only the outer locking portion. Insert the cannula into the tracheostomy and, following the manufacturer's instructions, lock it securely.[1]
■ Replace any humidification or ventilation device.[1]
■ Remove and discard your gloves.[24]
■ Perform hand hygiene.[9,10,11,12,13,14]

Cleaning the stoma and outer cannula

■ Perform hand hygiene.[9,10,11,12,13,14]
■ Put on clean gloves.[22,23]
■ With your dominant hand, moisten a sterile gauze pad with sterile normal saline solution or sterile water. Squeeze out the excess liquid *to prevent accidental aspiration.* Then wipe the patient's neck under the tracheostomy tube flanges and tracheostomy ties.
■ Assess the stoma site and surrounding skin for redness, swelling, and drainage, *which may indicate infection.*[1,3]
■ Use a sterile cotton-tipped applicator and a sterile gauze pad to clean the stoma site and the tube's flanges. Wipe only once with each applicator or gauze pad and then discard it, *to prevent contamination of a clean area with a soiled applicator or pad.*[1] Loosen dried secretions with a sterile, cotton-tipped applicator or sterile gauze pad containing diluted hydrogen peroxide solution, if necessary. However, keep in mind that hydrogen peroxide can delay wound healing.[35]
■ Rinse debris with one or more sterile 4" × 4" (10-cm × 10-cm) gauze pads dampened in sterile normal saline solution or sterile water.
■ Dry the area thoroughly with additional sterile gauze pads; apply a skin barrier, as needed.[8]

■ Remove the tracheostomy ties and apply new ties, if needed.
■ Apply a new sterile tracheostomy dressing.[1,3] Sites with excessive moisture may require a foam tracheostomy dressing.[8]
NURSING ALERT Always use a manufactured split dressing; don't cut a gauze pad, *because loose fibers around the stoma or tracheostomy tube can cause irritation and increase the risk of infection.*[8]
■ If the patient is receiving mechanical ventilation, make sure that alarm limits are set appropriately for the patient's current condition, and that alarms are turned on, functioning properly, and audible to staff.[29,30,31]

Completing the procedure

■ Return the bed to the lowest position *to prevent falls and maintain patient safety.*[36]
■ Make sure that the patient is comfortable, the head of the patient's bed is elevated 30 to 45 degrees *to prevent ventilator-associated pneumonia,*[37,38] and the patient can easily reach the call light and communication aids.
■ Discard used supplies in appropriate receptacles.[24]
■ Remove and discard your gloves and any other personal protective equipment worn.[24]
■ Perform hand hygiene.[9,10,11,12,13,14]
■ As needed, clean and disinfect your stethoscope using a disinfectant pad.[39,40]
■ Perform hand hygiene.[9,10,11,12,13,14]
■ Document the procedure.[41,42,43,44]

Special considerations

■ Note that cuff pressure values vary and decrease over time. Unless you perform continuous monitoring or attach an automatic regulating device, maintaining a cuff pressure value within the therapeutic range can be difficult owing to changes in body position and head alignment, tube migration, coughing, lung compliance, and airway and intrathoracic pressures.[45,46] Guidelines recommend frequent, routine assessment of cuff pressure but don't identify the optimal frequency.[5]

■ Follow your facility's guidelines regarding the correct procedure if a tracheostomy tube is expelled or if the outer cannula becomes blocked. If the patient's breathing is obstructed—for example, when the tube is blocked with mucus that can't be removed by suctioning or by withdrawing the inner cannula—call the appropriate code and provide manual resuscitation with a handheld resuscitation bag, or reconnect the patient to the ventilator. Don't remove the tracheostomy tube entirely, *because removal may allow the airway to completely close.* Use extreme caution when attempting to reinsert an expelled tracheostomy tube *because of the risk of tracheal trauma, perforation, compression, and asphyxiation.*

■ Frequently check the ties or tube holder for moisture, tightness, or friction. Inspect the skin under the medical device at least twice daily. Use padding under the ties or holder, as needed.[32]

■ Provide oral care with chlorhexidine routinely at an interval determined by your facility *to prevent VAP and to prevent the oral cavity from becoming dry and malodorous or developing sores from encrusted secretions.*[37,38,47]

■ The optimal frequency for cleaning the inner cannula is undetermined.[3,4] Clean or change the inner cannula when needed, and inspect it regularly, at least two times per day.[3,4]

■ Clean the stoma site every 4 to 8 hours.[3]

■ Change the dressing frequently whenever secretions begin to collect, *because a wet dressing with exudate or secretions predisposes the patient to skin excoriation, breakdown, and infection.*[4]

■ Replace all equipment, including solutions, regularly at an interval determined by your facility *to reduce the risk of health care–acquired infections.*

Patient teaching

Educate the patient and family (if appropriate) in the proper technique for changing tracheostomy ties and performing tracheostomy tube cannula and stoma care. Provide written instructions and observe return demonstrations. Coordinate with the patient and family and the durable medical equipment supplier to ensure that all necessary supplies are available for home use before discharge. Teach the patient and family to always have tracheostomy emergency supplies within reach whenever they leave home.[48]

Instruct the patient and family to contact the practitioner if they observe signs of infection, such as redness, breaks in the skin, odor, drainage, and yellow or green mucus.

Teach the patient and family about measures to prevent VAP, including maintaining the head of the bed at 30 to 45 degrees. Encourage them to alert a staff member when the bed doesn't appear to be positioned correctly.[37,47]

Complications

Hardened mucus or a slipped cuff can occlude the cannula opening and obstruct the airway. Tube displacement can stimulate the cough reflex if the tip rests on the carina, or it can cause blood vessel erosion and hemorrhage. Just the presence of the tube or excessive cuff pressure can produce tracheal erosion and necrosis. The cuff can rupture from overinflation, or the tube can dislodge during deflation. Tracheal wall injury and aspiration are possible with inadequate cuff pressures.[28]

Complications associated with changing tracheostomy ties include dislodgement of the tube. Skin breakdown and vascular obstruction can occur if the ties are too tight. Decannulation can occur if the ties are too loose.

Documentation

Record the date and time of the procedure; the type of procedure; the amount, consistency, color, and odor of secretions; the patient's respiratory status before and after the procedure; changing of the tracheostomy tube by the practitioner; the duration of any cuff deflation; the amount of air used for cuff inflation; and cuff pressure readings, including specific body position. Note complications that occurred, the name of the practitioner notified, the date and time of the notification, the resulting interventions, any prescribed medications, and the patient's tolerance of them. Document teaching provided to the patient and family (if appropriate), their understanding of that teaching, and any need for follow-up teaching.

REFERENCES

1 Wiegand, D. L. (2017). *AACN procedure manual for high acuity, progressive, and critical care* (7th ed.). St. Louis, MO: Elsevier.
2 Intensive Care Society. (2008, reviewed 2011). Standards for the care of adult patients with a temporary tracheostomy: Standards and guidelines. https://nanopdf.com/download/ics-tracheostomy-standards_pdf (Level VII)
3 Morris, L., & Afifi, M. S. (Eds.). (2010). *Tracheostomies: The complete guide*. New York, NY: Springer.
4 Morris, L. L., et al. (2013). Tracheostomy care and complications in the intensive care unit. *Critical Care Nurse, 33*(5), 18–30. (Level VII)
5 Khan, M. U., et al. (2016). Measurement of endotracheal tube cuff pressure: Instrumental versus conventional method. *Saudi Journal of Anaesthesia, 10*(4), 428–431. https://www.ncbi.nlm.nih.gov/pmc/articles/PMC5044728/ (Level VI)
6 Pisano, A., et al. (2019). Assessing the correct inflation of the endotracheal tube cuff: A larger pilot balloon increases the sensitivity of the 'finger-pressure' technique, but it remains poorly reliable in clinical practice. *Journal of Clinical Monitoring and Computing, 33*, 301–305. https://link.springer.com/article/10.1007/s10877-018-0158-8 (Level VI)
7 Bodenham, A., et al. (2014, reviewed 2018). Standards for the care of adult patients with a temporary tracheostomy: Standards and guidelines. https://www.semanticscholar.org/paper/Standards-for-the-care-of-adult-patients-with-a-and-Bodenham-Bell/c8b6a451283360197389b718cd-219b3a14ff3acb (Level VII)
8 Nance-Floyd, B. (2011). Tracheostomy care: An evidence-based guide. https://www.americannursetoday.com/tracheostomy-care-an-evidence-based-guide-to-suctioning-and-dressing-changes/ (Level VII)
9 World Health Organization. (2009). WHO guidelines on hand hygiene in health care: First global patient safety challenge, clean care is safer care. https://apps.who.int/iris/bitstream/handle/10665/44102/9789241597906_eng.pdf?sequence=1 (Level IV)
10 The Joint Commission. (2021). Standard NPSG.07.01.01. *Comprehensive accreditation manual for hospitals*. Oakbrook Terrace, IL: The Joint Commission. (Level VII)
11 Centers for Disease Control and Prevention. (2002). Guideline for hand hygiene in health-care settings: Recommendations of the Healthcare Infection Control Practices Advisory Committee and the HICPAC/SHEA/APIC/IDSA Hand Hygiene Task Force. *MMWR Recommendations and Reports, 51*(RR-16), 1–45. https://www.cdc.gov/mmwr/pdf/rr/rr5116.pdf (Level II)
12 Accreditation Association for Hospitals and Health Systems. (2020). Standard 07.01.21. *Healthcare Facilities Accreditation Program: Accreditation requirements for acute care hospitals*. Chicago, IL: Accreditation Association for Hospitals and Health Systems. (Level VII)
13 Centers for Medicare and Medicaid Services, Department of Health and Human Services. (2020). Condition of participation: Infection control. 42 C.F.R. § 482.42.
14 DNV GL-Healthcare USA, Inc. (2020). IC.1.SR.1. *NIAHO® accreditation requirements, interpretive guidelines and surveyor guidance—revision 20.0.* Milford, OH: DNV GL-Healthcare USA, Inc. (Level VII)
15 The Joint Commission. (2021). Standard NPSG.01.01.01. *Comprehensive accreditation manual for hospitals*. Oakbrook Terrace, IL: The Joint Commission. (Level VII)
16 Accreditation Association for Hospitals and Health Systems. (2020). Standard 15.01.16. *Healthcare Facilities Accreditation Program: Accreditation requirements for acute care hospitals*. Chicago, IL: Accreditation Association for Hospitals and Health Systems. (Level VII)
17 Centers for Medicare and Medicaid Services, Department of Health and Human Services. (2020). Condition of participation: Patient's rights. 42 C.F.R. § 482.13(c)(1).
18 The Joint Commission. (2021). Standard RI.01.01.01. *Comprehensive accreditation manual for hospitals*. Oakbrook Terrace, IL: The Joint Commission. (Level VII)
19 DNV GL-Healthcare USA, Inc. (2020). PR.2.SR.5. *NIAHO® accreditation requirements, interpretive guidelines and surveyor guidance—revision 20.0.* Milford, OH: DNV GL-Healthcare USA, Inc. (Level VII)
20 The Joint Commission. (2021). Standard PC.02.01.21. *Comprehensive accreditation manual for hospitals*. Oakbrook Terrace, IL: The Joint Commission. (Level VII)
21 Waters, T. R., et al. (2009). Safe patient handling training for schools of nursing. https://www.cdc.gov/niosh/docs/2009-127/pdfs/2009-127.pdf (Level VII)
22 Siegel, J. D., et al. (2007, revised 2019). 2007 guideline for isolation precautions: Preventing transmission of infectious agents in healthcare settings. https://www.cdc.gov/infectioncontrol/pdf/guidelines/isolation-guidelines-H.pdf (Level II)
23 Accreditation Association for Hospitals and Health Systems. (2020). Standard 07.01.10. *Healthcare Facilities Accreditation Program: Accreditation requirements for acute care hospitals*. Chicago, IL: Accreditation Association for Hospitals and Health Systems. (Level VII)
24 Occupational Safety and Health Administration. (2012). Bloodborne pathogens, standard number 1910.1030. https://www.osha.gov/pls/oshaweb/owadisp.show_document?p_id=10051&p_table=STANDARDS (Level VII)
25 American Association of Critical-Care Nurses. (2017). AACN practice alert: Ventilator-associated pneumonia. https://www.aacn.org/clinical-resources/practice-alerts/ventilator-associated-pneumonia-vap (Level VII)
26 American Association for Respiratory Care (AARC). (2010). AARC clinical practice guidelines: Endotracheal suctioning of mechanically ventilated patients with artificial airways 2010. *Respiratory Care, 55*(6), 758–764. https://www.aarc.org/wp-content/uploads/2014/08/06.10.0758.pdf (Level VII)
27 U.S. Food and Drug Administration. (2017). Examples of medical device misconnections. https://www.fda.gov/medical-devices/medical-device-connectors/examples-medical-device-misconnections
28 Kacmarek, R. M. (2021). *Egan's fundamentals of respiratory care* (12th ed.). St. Louis, MO: Mosby.
29 The Joint Commission. (2021). Standard NPSG.06.01.01. *Comprehensive accreditation manual for hospitals*. Oakbrook Terrace, IL: The Joint Commission. (Level VII)
30 Graham, K. C., & Cvach, M. (2010). Monitor alarm fatigue: Standardizing use of physiological monitors and decreasing nuisance alarms. *American Journal of Critical Care, 19*, 28–37. https://aacnjournals.org/ajcconline/article-abstract/19/1/28/5720/Monitor-Alarm-Fatigue-Standardizing-Use-of?redirectedFrom=fulltext
31 The Joint Commission. (2013). Sentinel event alert 50: Medical device alarm safety in hospitals. https://www.jointcommission.org/-/media/tjc/documents/resources/patient-safety-topics/sentinel-event/sea_50_alarms_4_26_16.pdf (Level VII)

32 European Pressure Ulcer Advisory Panel, et al. (2019). Prevention and treatment of pressure ulcers/injuries: Quick reference guide. http://www.internationalguideline.com/static/pdfs/Quick_Reference_Guide-10Mar2019.pdf (Level VII)

33 Schreiber, M. L. (2015). Tracheostomy: Site care, suctioning, and readiness. *MedSurg Nursing, 24,* 121–124.

34 Regan, E. N., & Dallachiesa, L. (2009). How to care for a patient with a tracheostomy. *Nursing, 39*(8), 34–39. (Level V)

35 Thomas, G. W., et al. (2009). Mechanisms of delayed wound healing by commonly used antiseptics. *Journal of Trauma, 66,* 82–90. (Level VI)

36 Ganz, D. A., et al. (2013, reviewed 2021). *Preventing falls in hospitals: A toolkit for improving quality of care* (AHRQ Publication No. 13-0015-EF). Rockville, MD: Agency for Healthcare Research and Quality. https://www.ahrq.gov/professionals/systems/hospital/fallpxtoolkit/index.html (Level VII)

37 Accreditation Association for Hospitals and Health Systems. (2020). Standard 07.01.02. *Healthcare Facilities Accreditation Program: Accreditation requirements for acute care hospitals.* Chicago, IL: Accreditation Association for Hospitals and Health Systems. (Level VII)

38 Klompas, M., et al. (2014). Strategies to prevent ventilator-associated pneumonia in acute care hospitals: 2014 update. *Infection Control and Hospital Epidemiology, 35*(8), 915–936. https://www.jstor.org/stable/10.1086/677144#metadata_info_tab_contents (Level I)

39 Rutala, W. A., et al. (2008, revised 2019). Guideline for disinfection and sterilization in healthcare facilities, 2008. https://www.cdc.gov/infection-control/pdf/guidelines/disinfection-guidelines-H.pdf (Level I)

40 Accreditation Association for Hospitals and Health Systems. (2020). Standard 07.02.03. *Healthcare Facilities Accreditation Program: Accreditation requirements for acute care hospitals.* Chicago, IL: Accreditation Association for Hospitals and Health Systems. (Level VII)

41 The Joint Commission. (2021). Standard RC.01.03.01. *Comprehensive accreditation manual for hospitals.* Oakbrook Terrace, IL: The Joint Commission. (Level VII)

42 Centers for Medicare and Medicaid Services, Department of Health and Human Services. (2020). Condition of participation: Medical record services. 42 C.F.R. § 482.24(b).

43 Accreditation Association for Hospitals and Health Systems. (2020). Standard 10.00.03. *Healthcare Facilities Accreditation Program: Accreditation requirements for acute care hospitals.* Chicago, IL: Accreditation Association for Hospitals and Health Systems. (Level VII)

44 DNV GL-Healthcare USA, Inc. (2020). MR.2.SR.1. *NIAHO® accreditation requirements, interpretive guidelines and surveyor guidance—revision 20.0.* Milford, OH: DNV GL-Healthcare USA, Inc. (Level VII)

45 Sole, M. L., et al. (2011). Evaluation of an intervention to maintain endotracheal tube cuff pressure within therapeutic range. *American Journal of Critical Care, 20*(2), 109–118. https://www.ncbi.nlm.nih.gov/pmc/articles/PMC3506174/ (Level IV)

46 Lizy, C., et al. (2014). Cuff pressure of endotracheal tubes after changes in body position in critically ill patients treated with mechanical ventilation. *American Journal of Critical Care, 23,* e1–e8. (Level IV)

47 Institute for Healthcare Improvement. (2012). *How-to guide: Prevent ventilator-associated pneumonia.* Cambridge, MA: Institute for Healthcare Improvement. (Level VII)

48 Miske, L., et al. (2017). Preventing catastrophe: Verification of tracheostomy emergency supplies for patients living at home with an artificial airway. *Chest, 152*(Suppl.), A572. (Level VI)

TRACHEOTOMY, ASSISTING

A tracheotomy involves surgically creating a temporary or permanent external opening, or stoma, in the anterior neck to provide a patent airway. A tracheostomy tube inserted into the stoma after the procedure maintains the patent airway. The practitioner may perform this procedure percutaneously at the bedside or surgically in the operating room.[1]

A tracheotomy is indicated for various conditions, including upper airway obstruction, respiratory failure with the inability to wean from mechanical ventilation, the need for prolonged mechanical ventilation or an artificial airway, copious or retained secretions, a difficult airway, airway protection, and emergency airway securement.[2,3]

Equipment

Appropriate-sized tracheostomy tube with obturator ▪ sterile tracheotomy tray (usually contains tracheal dilator, vein retractor, hemostats, and clamps) ▪ sutures and needles ▪ 4" × 4" (10-cm ×10-cm) gauze pads ▪ sterile drapes ▪ sterile gloves ▪ gloves ▪ gown ▪ mask with face shield or mask and goggles ▪ sterile gown ▪ sterile bowls ▪ stethoscope ▪ disinfectant pad ▪ prepackaged, sterile tracheostomy dressing ▪ blanket or towel ▪ tracheostomy ties or commercially prepared tracheostomy tube holder ▪ suction apparatus and tubing ▪ alcohol pad ▪ antiseptic cleaning solution ▪ sterile water ▪ 5-mL syringe with 22G needle ▪ local anesthetic ▪ prescribed sedative ▪ oxygen therapy device ▪ oxygen source ▪ humidification source or device ▪ syringe for cuff inflation ▪ manometer (or other cuff pressure measurement device) ▪ cardiac monitoring equipment ▪ pulse oximeter and probe ▪ end-tidal carbon dioxide detector ▪ vital signs monitoring equipment ▪ emergency equipment (code cart with emergency medications, defibrillator, handheld resuscitation bag, intubation equipment) ▪ facility-approved disinfectant ▪ Optional: IV catheter insertion kit, mechanical ventilator.

Many facilities use prepackaged, sterile tracheotomy trays.

Preparation of equipment

Inspect all equipment and supplies. If a product is expired, is defective, or has compromised integrity, remove it from patient use, label it as expired or defective, and report the expiration or defect as directed by your facility.

Make sure emergency equipment is functioning properly and readily available.

Perform hand hygiene[4,5,6,7,8,9] and then, maintaining sterile technique, open the tray. Take the tracheostomy tube from its container and place it on the sterile field. If necessary, set up the suction equipment and make sure it works. When the practitioner opens the sterile bowls, pour in the antiseptic cleaning solution.

Implementation

▪ Have one person stay with the patient while another gathers and prepares the necessary equipment and supplies.
▪ Perform hand hygiene.[4,5,6,7,8,9]
▪ Confirm the patient's identity using at least two patient identifiers.[10]
▪ Provide privacy.[11,12,13,14]
▪ Explain the procedure to the patient and family (if appropriate) according to their individual communication and learning needs *to increase their understanding, allay their fears, and enhance cooperation.*[15] Do this even if the patient is unresponsive.
▪ If possible, and required by your facility, confirm that written informed consent has been obtained and that the signed consent form is in the patient's medical record.[16,17,18,19]
▪ Check the patient's medical record for allergies, especially to anesthetics or latex.
▪ Conduct a preprocedure verification *to make sure that all relevant documentation, related information, and equipment are available and correctly identified to the patient's identifiers.*[20,21]
▪ Perform hand hygiene.[4,5,6,7,8,9]
▪ Put on a gown, a mask with face shield or a mask and goggles, and gloves *to comply with standard precautions.*[22,23,24]
▪ Assess the patient's condition.
▪ Maintain ventilation until the tracheotomy is performed.
▪ Make sure the patient has patent IV access; insert an IV catheter if ordered and if necessary.[25]
▪ Administer a sedative for the procedure, as ordered, following safe medication administration practices *to decrease pain and anxiety.*[26,27,28,29]
▪ Monitor the patient's cardiac rhythm, oxygen saturation level using pulse oximetry, blood pressure, and exhaled carbon dioxide level using an end-tidal carbon dioxide detector throughout the procedure.[25]
▪ Make sure that the alarm limits are appropriately set for the patient's current condition, and that the alarms are turned on, functioning properly, and audible to staff.[30,31,32,33]
▪ Raise the patient's bed to waist level before providing care *to allow access to the tracheotomy site and to prevent caregiver back strain.*[34]
▪ Roll a blanket or towel to form a shoulder roll, and place it under the patient's shoulders and neck *to extend the neck.* If the patient is in respiratory distress and optimal neck extension isn't tolerated, place the patient in the semi-Fowler position.[25]

Assisting with a tracheotomy

After preparing the skin with an antiseptic and allowing it to dry, the practitioner will make a horizontal or vertical incision into the skin. (A vertical incision helps avoid arteries, veins, and nerves on the lateral borders of the trachea.) Then the practitioner will dissect subcutaneous fat and muscle and move the muscle aside with vein retractors *to locate the tracheal rings*. The practitioner will make an incision between the second and third tracheal rings, using hemostats *to control bleeding.*[1]

The practitioner will inject a local anesthetic into the tracheal lumen *to suppress the cough reflex* and create a stoma in the trachea. When this is done, carefully apply suction *to remove blood and secretions that may obstruct the airway or be aspirated into the lungs*. The practitioner will then insert the tracheostomy tube and obturator into the stoma (as shown below). After inserting the tube, the practitioner will remove the obturator.

Apply a sterile tracheostomy dressing, and anchor the tube with tracheostomy ties (as shown below). Check for air movement through the tube, and auscultate breath sounds *to ensure proper placement.*

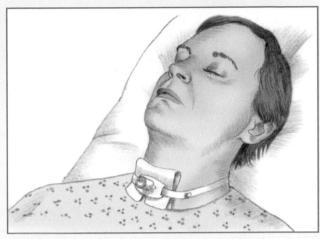

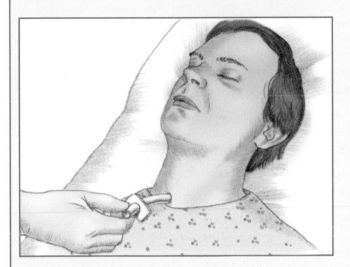

An alternative approach

A minimally invasive percutaneous tracheotomy may also be performed at the bedside. Unlike the surgical technique, this method dilates rather than cuts the tissue structures. During this procedure, the practitioner passes a needle into the trachea and then threads a dilator over a guidewire, which progressively dilates until a tracheostomy tube can be placed. This method has a similar success rate compared with the surgical approach.[37,38]

After the skin is prepared and anesthetized, the practitioner makes a 1-cm midline incision. When the stoma reaches the desired size, the practitioner inserts the tracheostomy tube. After the tube is in place, inflate the cuff, secure the tube, and check the patient's breath sounds. The practitioner will suture the corners of the incision. Then obtain a portable chest X-ray, as ordered.

NURSING ALERT Use caution and don't extend the neck in a patient with a cervical spine injury *to prevent further injury.*[35]

- Conduct a time-out immediately before starting the procedure *to perform a final assessment that the correct patient, site, positioning, and procedure are identified, and that, as applicable, all relevant information and necessary equipment are available during and after the procedure.*[21,36]
- Disinfect the top of the local anesthetic vial with an alcohol pad and allow it to dry. Invert the vial so that the practitioner can withdraw the anesthetic using the 22G needle attached to the 5-mL syringe.
- The practitioner will put on a sterile gown, a mask with face shield or a mask and goggles, and sterile gloves.[22,23,24] Assist with the procedure as needed. (See *Assisting with a tracheotomy.*)
- When the tube is in position, attach it to the appropriate oxygen therapy device connected to an oxygen source.
- Provide adequate humidification of inspired oxygen, *because when a tracheostomy bypasses the upper airway, alternative methods of conditioning inspired air must be used to avoid airway damage and thickening of mucosal secretions.*[1,39]
- Inject air into the distal cuff port *to inflate the cuff*. Measure the tracheal cuff pressure. (See the "Tracheal cuff pressure measurement" procedure.) If the patient is receiving mechanical ventilation, make sure that ventilator alarm limits are set appropriately for the patient's current condition, and that alarms are turned on, functioning properly, and audible to staff.[30,32,33]

NURSING ALERT Limit tracheostomy tube cuff pressure to 25 mm Hg to prevent ischemia and mucosal injury.[37]

- Auscultate the patient's breath sounds using a stethoscope.
- Remove and discard your gloves,[24] perform hand hygiene,[4,5,6,7,8,9] and put on sterile gloves.[22,24]
- Apply the sterile tracheostomy dressing under the tracheostomy tube flange. Place the tracheostomy ties through the openings of the tube flanges and tie them on the side of the patient's neck; alternately, apply commercially prepared tracheostomy tube holder straps through the openings of the tube flanges and fasten the straps on the side of the patient's neck following the manufacturer's instructions. *Doing so allows easy access and prevents pressure necrosis at the back of the neck.*[37]

- Discard used supplies in appropriate receptacles.[24]
- Assess the patient's vital signs and respiratory status at an interval determined by your facility or the patient's condition; *there's no evidence-based research to indicate best practice for frequency of vital signs monitoring, so it should be determined by each facility.*[40]
- Return the bed to the lowest position *to prevent falls and maintain patient safety.*[41]
- Make sure the head of the patient's bed is elevated 30 to 45 degrees (unless contraindicated) *to prevent ventilator-associated pneumonia and to make sure that the patient is comfortable and can easily reach the call light.*[42,43]
- Obtain a chest X-ray as ordered *to confirm tube placement.*
- Remove and discard your gloves and other personal protective equipment.[24]
- Perform hand hygiene.[4,5,6,7,8,9]
- Put on gloves, as necessary.[22,24]
- Clean and disinfect reusable equipment according to the manufacturer's instructions *to prevent the spread of infection.*[44,45] Send surgical equipment for reprocessing, as indicated.
- If you wore gloves, remove and discard them.[24]
- Perform hand hygiene.[4,5,6,7,8,9]
- Clean and disinfect your stethoscope using a disinfectant pad.[44,45]
- Perform hand hygiene.[4,5,6,7,8,9]
- Document the procedure.[46,47,48,49]

Special considerations

■ Monitor the patient carefully for signs of infection. Ideally, the tracheotomy should be performed using sterile technique as described; however, in an emergency, this may not be possible, *increasing the risk of infection.*[50]

■ Make sure the following equipment is always at the patient's bedside: suctioning equipment, *because the patient may need the airway cleared at any time;* the sterile obturator used to insert the tracheostomy tube *in case the tube is expelled;* a sterile tracheostomy tube and obturator (the same size as the one used) *in case the tube must be replaced quickly;* a spare, sterile inner cannula *that can be used if the cannula is expelled;* a sterile tracheostomy tube and obturator one size smaller than the one used, *which may be needed if the tube is expelled and the trachea begins to close;* and a sterile tracheal dilator or sterile hemostats *to maintain an open airway before inserting a new tracheostomy tube.*

Complications

A tracheotomy can cause an airway obstruction (from improper tube placement), hemorrhage, edema, a perforated esophagus, subcutaneous or mediastinal emphysema, aspiration of secretions, tracheal necrosis (from cuff pressure), infection, tracheoinnominate fistula, and lacerations of arteries, veins, and nerves.

Documentation

Record the reason for the procedure, the date and time it took place, the patient's respiratory status before and after the procedure, and the results of the chest X-ray. Note the type and size of tube used. Include any complications that occurred during the procedure, any prescribed interventions for the complications, and the patient's response to those interventions. Document the amount of cuff pressure and the respiratory therapy initiated after the procedure. Also note the patient's response to respiratory therapy. Document teaching provided to the patient and family (if applicable), their understanding of that teaching, and any need for follow-up teaching.

REFERENCES

1 Kacmarek, R. M., et al. (2021). *Egan's fundamentals of respiratory care* (12th ed.). St. Louis, MO: Mosby.

2 Cheung, N. H., & Napolitano, L. M. (2014). Tracheostomy: Epidemiology, indications, timing, technique, and outcomes. *Respiratory Care, 59,* 895–919. (Level VII)

3 De Leyn, P., et al. (2007). Tracheotomy: Clinical review and guidelines. *European Journal of Cardio-thoracic Surgery, 32*(3), 412–421. https://academic.oup.com/ejcts/article/32/3/412/529979

4 The Joint Commission. (2021). Standard NPSG.07.01.01. *Comprehensive accreditation manual for hospitals.* Oakbrook Terrace, IL: The Joint Commission. (Level VII)

5 Centers for Disease Control and Prevention. (2002). Guideline for hand hygiene in health-care settings: Recommendations of the Healthcare Infection Control Practices Advisory Committee and the HICPAC/SHEA/APIC/IDSA Hand Hygiene Task Force. *MMWR Recommendations and Reports, 51*(RR-16), 1–45. https://www.cdc.gov/mmwr/pdf/rr/rr5116.pdf (Level II)

6 World Health Organization. (2009). WHO guidelines on hand hygiene in health care: First global patient safety challenge, clean care is safer care. https://apps.who.int/iris/bitstream/handle/10665/44102/9789241597906_eng.pdf?sequence=1 (Level IV)

7 Centers for Medicare and Medicaid Services, Department of Health and Human Services. (2020). Condition of participation: Infection control. 42 C.F.R. § 482.42.

8 Accreditation Association for Hospitals and Health Systems. (2020). Standard 07.01.21. *Healthcare Facilities Accreditation Program: Accreditation requirements for acute care hospitals.* Chicago, IL: Accreditation Association for Hospitals and Health Systems. (Level VII)

9 DNV GL-Healthcare USA, Inc. (2020). IC.1.SR.1. *NIAHO® accreditation requirements, interpretive guidelines and surveyor guidance—revision 20.0.* Milford, OH: DNV GL-Healthcare USA, Inc. (Level VII)

10 The Joint Commission. (2021). Standard NPSG.01.01.01. *Comprehensive accreditation manual for hospitals.* Oakbrook Terrace, IL: The Joint Commission. (Level VII)

11 Accreditation Association for Hospitals and Health Systems. (2020). Standard 15.01.16. *Healthcare Facilities Accreditation Program: Accreditation requirements for acute care hospitals.* Chicago, IL: Accreditation Association for Hospitals and Health Systems. (Level VII)

12 Centers for Medicare and Medicaid Services, Department of Health and Human Services. (2020). Condition of participation: Patient's rights. 42 C.F.R. § 482.13(c)(1).

13 DNV GL-Healthcare USA, Inc. (2020). PR.2.SR.5. *NIAHO® accreditation requirements, interpretive guidelines and surveyor guidance—revision 20.0.* Milford, OH: DNV GL-Healthcare USA, Inc. (Level VII)

14 The Joint Commission. (2021). Standard RI.01.01.01. *Comprehensive accreditation manual for hospitals.* Oakbrook Terrace, IL: The Joint Commission. (Level VII)

15 The Joint Commission. (2021). Standard PC.02.01.21. *Comprehensive accreditation manual for hospitals.* Oakbrook Terrace, IL: The Joint Commission. (Level VII)

16 The Joint Commission. (2021). Standard RI.01.03.01. *Comprehensive accreditation manual for hospitals.* Oakbrook Terrace, IL: The Joint Commission. (Level VII)

17 Centers for Medicare and Medicaid Services, Department of Health and Human Services. (2020). Condition of participation: Patient's rights. 42 C.F.R. § 482.13(b)(2).

18 Accreditation Association for Hospitals and Health Systems. (2020). Standard 15.01.11. *Healthcare Facilities Accreditation Program: Accreditation requirements for acute care hospitals.* Chicago, IL: Accreditation Association for Hospitals and Health Systems. (Level VII)

19 DNV GL-Healthcare USA, Inc. (2020). PR.2.SR.3. *NIAHO® accreditation requirements, interpretive guidelines and surveyor guidance—revision 20.0.* Milford, OH: DNV GL-Healthcare USA, Inc. (Level VII)

20 The Joint Commission. (2021). Standard UP.01.01.01. *Comprehensive accreditation manual for hospitals.* Oakbrook Terrace, IL: The Joint Commission. (Level VII)

21 Accreditation Association for Hospitals and Health Systems. (2020). Standard 30.00.14. *Healthcare Facilities Accreditation Program: Accreditation requirements for acute care hospitals.* Chicago, IL: Accreditation Association for Hospitals and Health Systems. (Level VII)

22 Siegel, J. D., et al. (2007, revised 2019). 2007 guideline for isolation precautions: Preventing transmission of infectious agents in healthcare settings. https://www.cdc.gov/infectioncontrol/pdf/guidelines/isolation-guidelines-H.pdf (Level II)

23 Accreditation Association for Hospitals and Health Systems. (2020). Standard 07.01.10. *Healthcare Facilities Accreditation Program: Accreditation requirements for acute care hospitals.* Chicago, IL: Accreditation Association for Hospitals and Health Systems. (Level VII)

24 Occupational Safety and Health Administration. (2012). Bloodborne pathogens, standard number 1910.1030. https://www.osha.gov/pls/oshaweb/owadisp.show_document?p_id=10051&p_table=STANDARDS(Level VII)

25 Morris, L., & Afifi, M. S. (Eds.). (2010). *Tracheostomies: The complete guide.* New York, NY: Springer Publishing Company.

26 The Joint Commission. (2021). Standard MM.06.01.01. *Comprehensive accreditation manual for hospitals.* Oakbrook Terrace, IL: The Joint Commission. (Level VII)

27 Accreditation Association for Hospitals and Health Systems. (2020). Standard 16.01.03. *Healthcare Facilities Accreditation Program: Accreditation requirements for acute care hospitals.* Chicago, IL: Accreditation Association for Hospitals and Health Systems. (Level VII)

28 Centers for Medicare and Medicaid Services, Department of Health and Human Services. (2020). Condition of participation: Nursing services. 42 C.F.R. § 482.23(c).

29 DNV GL-Healthcare USA, Inc. (2020). MM.1.SR.3. *NIAHO® accreditation requirements, interpretive guidelines and surveyor guidance—revision 20.0.* Milford, OH: DNV GL-Healthcare USA, Inc. (Level VII)

30 Graham, K. C., & Cvach, M. (2010). Monitor alarm fatigue: Standardizing use of physiological monitors and decreasing nuisance alarms. *American Journal of Critical Care, 19,* 28–37.

31 American Association of Critical-Care Nurses. (2018). AACN practice alert: Managing alarms in acute care across the life span—electrocardiography and pulse oximetry. *Critical Care Nurse, 38*(2), e16–e20. (Level VII)

32 The Joint Commission. (2021). Standard NPSG.06.01.01. *Comprehensive accreditation manual for hospitals.* Oakbrook Terrace, IL: The Joint Commission. (Level VII)

33 The Joint Commission. (2013). Sentinel event alert 50: Medical device alarm safety in hospitals. https://www.jointcommission.org/assets/1/6/SEA_50_alarms_4_26_16.pdf (Level VII)

34 Waters, T. R., et al. (2009). Safe patient handling training for schools of nursing. https://www.cdc.gov/niosh/docs/2009-127/pdfs/2009-127.pdf (Level VII)

35 Roberts, J. R., et al. (Eds.). (2019). *Roberts and Hedges' clinical procedures in emergency medicine and acute care* (7th ed.). St. Louis, MO: Elsevier.

36 The Joint Commission. (2021). Standard UP.01.03.01. *Comprehensive accreditation manual for hospitals*. Oakbrook Terrace, IL: The Joint Commission. (Level VII)

37 Wiegand, D. L. (2017). *AACN procedure manual for high acuity, progressive, and critical care* (7th ed.). St. Louis, MO: Elsevier.

38 Hyzy, R. C., & McSparron, J. I. (2020). Overview of tracheostomy. In: *UpToDate*, Feller-Kopman, D. J. (Ed.).

39 American Association for Respiratory Care. (2002). AARC clinical practice guideline: Oxygen therapy for adults in the acute care facility—2002 revision and update. *Respiratory Care, 47*(6), 717–720. https://www.aarc.org/wp-content/uploads/2014/08/06.02.717.pdf (Level VII)

40 American Society of PeriAnesthesia Nurses. (2019). *2019–2020 perianesthesia nursing standards, practice recommendations and interpretive statements*. Cherry Hill, NJ: American Society of PeriAnesthesia Nurses. (Level VII)

41 Ganz, D. A., et al. (2013, reviewed 2021). Preventing falls in hospitals: A toolkit for improving quality of care (AHRQ publication no. 13-0015-EF). https://www.ahrq.gov/professionals/systems/hospital/fallpxtoolkit/index.html (Level VII)

42 Klompas, M., et al. (2014). Strategies to prevent ventilator-associated pneumonia in acute care hospitals: 2014 update. *Infection Control and Hospital Epidemiology, 35*(8), 915–936. https://www.jstor.org/stable/10.1086/677144#metadata_info_tab_contents (Level I)

43 Accreditation Association for Hospitals and Health Systems. (2020). Standard 07.01.02. *Healthcare Facilities Accreditation Program: Accreditation requirements for acute care hospitals*. Chicago, IL: Accreditation Association for Hospitals and Health Systems. (Level VII)

44 Rutala, W. A., et al. (2008, revised 2019). Guideline for disinfection and sterilization in healthcare facilities, 2008. https://www.cdc.gov/infection-control/pdf/guidelines/disinfection-guidelines-H.pdf (Level I)

45 Accreditation Association for Hospitals and Health Systems. (2020). Standard 07.02.03. *Healthcare Facilities Accreditation Program: Accreditation requirements for acute care hospitals*. Chicago, IL: Accreditation Association for Hospitals and Health Systems. (Level VII)

46 The Joint Commission. (2021). Standard RC.01.03.01. *Comprehensive accreditation manual for hospitals*. Oakbrook Terrace, IL: The Joint Commission. (Level VII)

47 Accreditation Association for Hospitals and Health Systems. (2020). Standard 10.00.03. *Healthcare Facilities Accreditation Program: Accreditation requirements for acute care hospitals*. Chicago, IL: Accreditation Association for Hospitals and Health Systems. (Level VII)

48 Centers for Medicare and Medicaid Services, Department of Health and Human Services. (2020). Condition of participation: Medical record services. 42 C.F.R. § 482.24(b).

49 DNV GL-Healthcare USA, Inc. (2020). MR.2.SR.1. *NIAHO® accreditation requirements, interpretive guidelines and surveyor guidance—revision 20.0*. Milford, OH: DNV GL-Healthcare USA, Inc. (Level VII)

50 Trouillet, J., et al. (2018). Tracheotomy in the intensive care unit: Guidelines from a French expert panel. *Annals of Intensive Care, 8*, 37. https://www.ncbi.nlm.nih.gov/pmc/articles/PMC5854567/pdf/13613_2018_Article_381.pdf (Level VII)

TRANSCRANIAL DOPPLER MONITORING

Transcranial Doppler ultrasonography is a noninvasive method of monitoring blood flow velocity in the intracranial vessels, specifically the internal carotid, middle cerebral, posterior cerebral and the anterior cerebral arteries.[1,2] This procedure is used on the intensive care unit to monitor patients who have experienced cerebrovascular disorders, such as stroke, head trauma, and subarachnoid hemorrhage. It can help detect intracranial stenosis, vasospasm, and arteriovenous malformations as well as assess collateral pathways.[3,4] Because it also allows monitoring of a continuous waveform, it can be used in intraoperative monitoring of cerebral circulation.

Transcranial Doppler ultrasonography is also used to monitor the effect of intracranial pressure changes on the cerebral circulation, to monitor patient response to various medications, and to evaluate carbon dioxide reactivity, which may be impaired or lost from arterial obstruction or trauma. It has also been used to confirm brain death.[4,5]

The transcranial Doppler unit transmits pulses of high-frequency ultrasound, which are then reflected back to the transducer by the red blood cells moving in the vessel being monitored. This information is then processed by the instrument into an audible signal and a velocity waveform, which is displayed on the monitor. The displayed waveform is actually a moving graph of blood flow velocities with *time* displayed along the horizontal axis, *velocity* displayed along the vertical axis, and *amplitude* represented by various colors or intensities within the waveform. The heart's contractions speed up the movement of blood cells during systole and slow it down during diastole, resulting in a waveform that varies in velocity over the cardiac cycle.

The major benefits of transcranial Doppler monitoring are that it provides instantaneous, real-time information about cerebral blood flow and that it's noninvasive and painless for the patient.[6] Also, the unit itself is portable and easy to use. The major disadvantage is that it relies on the ability of the ultrasound waves to penetrate thin areas of the cranium; this is difficult if the patient has thickening of the temporal bone, which increases with age.

Cerebral blood flow velocities are variable and affected by the patient's age, arterial carbon dioxide level, cerebral and systemic perfusion, body temperature, and state of arousal as well as by mechanical ventilation, suctioning, and the presence of systemic shunts, cardiac disease, and anemia.[5,7] Monitoring should optimally occur while the patient is awake and calm but not sedated or anesthetized; however, those considerations don't apply if monitoring is performed to determine brain death or detect intraoperative or postoperative perfusion abnormalities.[5]

This procedure requires specialized training to ensure accurate vessel identification and correct interpretation of the signals. The transcranial Doppler unit should always be used with its power set at the lowest level needed to provide an adequate waveform.

Equipment

Transcranial Doppler unit ▪ transducer with an attachment system ▪ terry cloth headband ▪ ultrasonic coupling gel ▪ marker ▪ Optional: headphones, gloves, gown, mask with face shield or mask and goggles.

Preparation of equipment

Inspect all equipment and supplies. If a product is expired, is defective, or has compromised integrity, remove it from patient use, label it as expired or defective, and report the expiration or defect as directed by your facility. Follow the manufacturer's recommendations for setup, use, and care of the transcranial Doppler unit.

Implementation

▪ Verify the practitioner's order.
▪ Gather and prepare the necessary equipment and supplies,
▪ Perform hand hygiene.[8,9,10,11,12,13]
▪ Confirm the patient's identity using at least two patient identifiers.[14]
▪ Provide privacy.[15,16,17,18]
▪ Explain the procedure to the patient and family (if appropriate) according to their communication and learning needs *to increase understanding, allay fears, and enhance cooperation.*[19] If appropriate, remind the patient to lie quietly without moving or talking.[7]
▪ Raise the bed to waist level before providing care *to prevent caregiver back strain.*[20]
▪ Perform hand hygiene.[8,9,10,11,12,13]
▪ Put on gloves, a gown, and a mask with a face shield or a mask and goggles, as needed, *to comply with standard precautions.*[21,22,23]
▪ Place the patient in the proper position, usually the supine position.[5]
▪ Turn the Doppler unit on and observe as it performs a self-test.
▪ Enter information as prompted by the Doppler unit. Depending on the unit you're using, you may need to enter the patient's name, identification number, and diagnosis, or the practitioner's name.
▪ Indicate the vessel you wish to monitor, typically the right or left middle cerebral artery, and set the approximate depth of the vessel within the skull (50 mm to 56 mm for the middle cerebral artery).
▪ Increase the power level to 100% initially *to locate the signal.*[5] You can later decrease the level as needed, depending on the thickness of the patient's skull.

■ Examine the temporal region of the patient's head, and mentally identify the three windows of the transtemporal access route: posterior, middle, and anterior (as shown below).

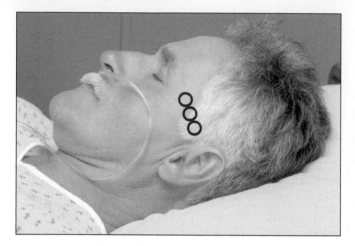

■ Apply a generous amount of ultrasonic gel at the level of the temporal bone between the tragus of the ear and the end of the eyebrow, over the area of the three windows.
■ Place the transducer on the posterior window. Angle the transducer slightly in an anterior direction, and slowly move it in a narrow circle. As you hold the transducer at an angle and perform this technique, also begin to very slowly move the transducer forward across the temporal area. As you do this, listen for the audible signal with the highest pitch. This sound corresponds to the highest velocity signal, which corresponds to the signal of the vessel you are assessing. You can also use headphones *to let you better evaluate the audible signal and provide patient privacy.*
■ After you've located the highest-pitched signal, use a marker to draw a circle around the transducer head on the patient's temple (as shown below). Note the angle of the transducer *so that you can duplicate it after the transducer attachment system is in place.*

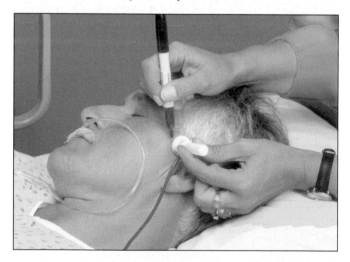

■ Next, place the transducer system on the patient. To do this, first place the plate of the transducer attachment system over the patient's temporal area; match the circular opening in the plate exactly with the circle drawn on the patient's head. Then, holding the plate in place, encircle the patient's head with the straps attached to the system. Finally, tighten the straps *so that the transducer attachment system will stay in place on the patient's head.*
■ Fill the circular opening in the plate with the ultrasonic gel.
■ Place the transducer in the gel-filled opening in the attachment system plate. Using the plastic screws provided, loosely secure the two plates together *to hold the transducer in place while allowing it to rotate for the best angle.*
■ Adjust the position and angle of the transducer until you again hear the highest-pitched audible signal. When you hear this signal, look at the

waveform on the monitor screen. You should see a clear waveform with a bright white line (called an *envelope*) at the upper edge of the waveform. The envelope exactly follows the contours of the waveform itself.
■ If the envelope doesn't follow the waveform's contours, adjust the GAIN setting. If the signal is wrapping around the screen, increase the scale *to drop the baseline.*
■ When you've determined that you have the strongest, highest-pitched signal and the best waveform, lock the transducer in place by tightening the plastic screws (as shown below). The tightened plates will hold the transducer at the angle you've chosen.

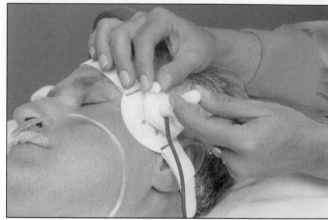

■ Disconnect the transducer handle.
■ Place a wide terry cloth headband over the transducer attachment system, and secure it around the patient's head *to provide additional stability for the transducer.*
■ Look at the monitor screen. You should be able to see a waveform and read the numeric values of the peak, mean velocities, and pulsatility index (PI+) above the displayed waveform. The shape of the waveform reveals more information. (See *Comparing velocity waveforms.*)
■ Return the bed to the lowest position *to prevent falls and maintain patient safety.*[24]
■ Remove and discard your gloves and other personal protective equipment, if worn.[23]
■ Perform hand hygiene.[8,9,10,11,12,13]
■ Document the procedure.[25,26,27,28]

Special considerations

■ Before using the transcranial Doppler system, remove turban head dressings or thick dressings over the test site.
■ Consider behavioral or pharmacologic intervention for a combative or confused patient before beginning the procedure. *The patient must cooperate and lie still to ensure accurate tracings.*[29]
■ Velocity changes in the transcranial Doppler signal correlate with changes in cerebral blood flow. The parameter that most clearly reflects this change is the mean velocity. To determine this, first establish a baseline for the mean velocity. After a baseline for the mean velocity has been established, the value (%) will change negatively or positively from the baseline as the patient's velocity increases or decreases.[4]
■ Emboli appear as high-intensity transients occurring randomly during the cardiac cycle. Emboli make a distinctive clicking, chirping, or plunking sound.[4,5] You can set up an emboli counter to count either the total number of emboli aggregates or the rate of embolic events per minute.
■ Various screens can be stored on the system's hard drive and then recalled or printed.

Documentation

Record the date and the time that the monitoring started and the artery monitored. Document the patient's tolerance of the procedure. Document teaching provided to the patient and family (if applicable), their understanding of that teaching, and any need for follow-up teaching.

Comparing velocity waveforms

A normal transcranial Doppler signal is usually characterized by mean velocities that fall within the normal reported values. Additional information can be gathered by evaluating the shape of the velocity waveform.

Effect of significant proximal vessel obstruction

A delayed systolic upstroke can be seen in a waveform when significant proximal vessel obstruction is present.

Normal

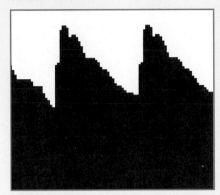

Proximal vessel obstruction

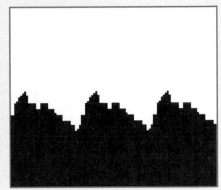

Effect of increased cerebrovascular resistance

Changes in cerebrovascular resistance, such as those that occur with increased intracranial pressure, cause a decrease in diastolic flow.

Normal

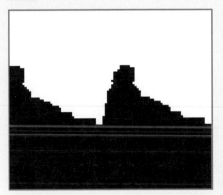

Increased resistance

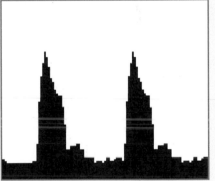

REFERENCES

1 Fillio, J. O., & Lansberg, M. G. (2021). Neuroimaging of acute ischemic stroke. In: *UpToDate*, Kasner, S. E., & Tung, G. A. (Eds.).

2 D'Andrea, A., et al. (2016). Transcranial Doppler ultrasonography: From methodology to major clinical applications. *World Journal of Cardiology, 8*(7), 383–400. https://www.ncbi.nlm.nih.gov/pmc/articles/PMC4958690/

3 Le Roux, P., et al. (2014). Consensus summary statement of the International Multidisciplinary Consensus Conference on Multimodality Monitoring in Neurocritical Care: A statement for healthcare professionals from the Neurocritical Care Society and the European Society of Intensive Care Medicine. *Neurocritical Care, 21*(Suppl. 2), S1–S26. https://link.springer.com/article/10.1007/s12028-014-0041-5 (Level VII)

4 Naqvi, J., et al. (2013). Transcranial Doppler ultrasound: A review of the physical principles and major applications in critical care. *International Journal of Vascular Medicine,* 2013, 629378. https://www.hindawi.com/journals/ijvm/2013/629378/ (Level V)

5 American Institute of Ultrasound in Medicine (AIUM). (2017). AIUM practice parameter for the performance of a transcranial Doppler ultrasound examination for adults and children. https://www.aium.org/resources/guidelines/transcranial.pdf (Level VII)

6 Wiegand, D. L. (2017). *AACN procedure manual for high acuity, progressive, and critical care* (7th ed.). St. Louis, MO: Elsevier.

7 Purkayastha, S., & Sorond, F. (2012). Transcranial Doppler ultrasound: Technique and application. *Seminars in Neurology, 32*(4), 411–420. https://www.ncbi.nlm.nih.gov/pmc/articles/PMC3902805/ (Level V)

8 World Health Organization (WHO). (2009). WHO guidelines on hand hygiene in health care: First global patient safety challenge, clean care is safer care. https://apps.who.int/iris/bitstream/handle/10665/44102/9789241597906_eng.pdf?sequence=1 (Level IV)

9 The Joint Commission. (2021). Standard NPSG.07.01.01. *Comprehensive accreditation manual for hospitals.* Oakbrook Terrace, IL: The Joint Commission. (Level VII)

10 Centers for Disease Control and Prevention. (2002). Guideline for hand hygiene in health-care settings: Recommendations of the Healthcare Infection Control Practices Advisory Committee and the HICPAC/SHEA/APIC/IDSA Hand Hygiene Task Force. *MMWR Recommendations and Reports, 51*(RR-16), 1–45. https://www.cdc.gov/mmwr/pdf/rr/rr5116.pdf (Level II)

11 Centers for Medicare and Medicaid Services, Department of Health and Human Services. (2020). Condition of participation: Infection control. 42 C.F.R. § 482.42.

12 Accreditation Association for Hospitals and Health Systems. (2020). Standard 07.01.21. *Healthcare Facilities Accreditation Program: Accreditation requirements for acute care hospitals.* Chicago, IL: Accreditation Association for Hospitals and Health Systems. (Level VII)

13 DNV GL-Healthcare USA, Inc. (2020). IC.1.SR.1. *NIAHO® accreditation requirements, interpretive guidelines and surveyor guidance—revision 20.0.* Milford, OH: DNV GL-Healthcare USA, Inc. (Level VII)

14 The Joint Commission. (2021). Standard NPSG.01.01.01. *Comprehensive accreditation manual for hospitals.* Oakbrook Terrace, IL: The Joint Commission. (Level VII)

15 The Joint Commission. (2021). Standard RI.01.01.01. *Comprehensive accreditation manual for hospitals.* Oakbrook Terrace, IL: The Joint Commission. (Level VII)

16 DNV GL-Healthcare USA, Inc. (2020). PR.2.SR.5. *NIAHO® accreditation requirements, interpretive guidelines and surveyor guidance—revision 20.0.* Milford, OH: DNV GL-Healthcare USA, Inc. (Level VII)

17 Centers for Medicare and Medicaid Services, Department of Health and Human Services. (2020). Condition of participation: Patient's rights. 42 C.F.R. § 482.13(c)(1).

18 Accreditation Association for Hospitals and Health Systems. (2020). Standard 15.01.16. *Healthcare Facilities Accreditation Program: Accreditation requirements for acute care hospitals.* Chicago, IL: Accreditation Association for Hospitals and Health Systems. (Level VII)

19 The Joint Commission. (2021). Standard PC.02.01.21. *Comprehensive accreditation manual for hospitals.* Oakbrook Terrace, IL: The Joint Commission. (Level VII)

20 Waters, T. R., et al. (2009). Safe patient handling training for schools of nursing. https://www.cdc.gov/niosh/docs/2009-127/pdfs/2009-127.pdf (Level VII)

21 Siegel, J. D., et al. (2007, revised 2019). 2007 guideline for isolation precautions: Preventing transmission of infectious agents in healthcare settings. https://www.cdc.gov/infectioncontrol/pdf/guidelines/isolation-guidelines-H.pdf (Level II)

22 Accreditation Association for Hospitals and Health Systems. (2020). Standard 07.01.10. *Healthcare Facilities Accreditation Program: Accreditation requirements for acute care hospitals.* Chicago, IL: Accreditation Association for Hospitals and Health Systems. (Level VII)

23 Occupational Safety and Health Administration. (2012). Bloodborne pathogens, standard number 1910.1030. https://www.osha.gov/pls/oshaweb/owadisp.show_document?p_id=10051&p_table=STANDARDS (Level VII)

24 Ganz, D. A., et al. (2013, reviewed 2021). *Preventing falls in hospitals: A toolkit for improving quality of care* (AHRQ Publication No. 13-0015-EF). Agency for Healthcare Research and Quality. https://www.ahrq.gov/professionals/systems/hospital/fallpxtoolkit/index.html (Level VII)

25 The Joint Commission. (2021). Standard RC.01.03.01. *Comprehensive accreditation manual for hospitals.* Oakbrook Terrace, IL: The Joint Commission. (Level VII)

26 Accreditation Association for Hospitals and Health Systems. (2020). Standard 10.00.03. *Healthcare Facilities Accreditation Program: Accreditation requirements for acute care hospitals.* Chicago, IL: Accreditation Association for Hospitals and Health Systems. (Level VII)

27 Centers for Medicare and Medicaid Services, Department of Health and Human Services. (2020). Condition of participation: Medical record services. 42 C.F.R. § 482.24(b).

28 DNV GL-Healthcare USA, Inc. (2020). MR.2.SR.1. *NIAHO® accreditation requirements, interpretive guidelines and surveyor guidance—revision 20.0.* Milford, OH: DNV GL-Healthcare USA, Inc. (Level VII)

29 Harris, C. (2014). Neuromonitoring indications and utility in the intensive care unit. *Critical Care Nurse, 34*(3), 30–39. https://doi.org/10.4037/ccn2014506

Transcutaneous electrical nerve stimulation

Transcutaneous electrical nerve stimulation (TENS) is the application of electrical stimulation to the skin for pain relief. It's based on the gate-control theory of pain, which proposes that painful impulses pass through a "gate" in the brain. TENS is performed with a portable, battery-powered device that transmits painless electrical current to peripheral nerves or directly to a painful area over relatively large nerve fibers. This treatment effectively alters the patient's perception of pain by blocking painful stimuli traveling over smaller fibers. In addition, with repeated applications, the secretion of endogenous endorphins increases over time, resulting in pain reduction.[1]

TENS is used for postoperative patients and those with acute and chronic pain as part of a multimodal therapy, and may have the additive effects of reducing the need for analgesic drugs and allowing the patient to resume normal activities.[2] Typically, a course of TENS treatments lasts 3 to 5 days. Some conditions, such as phantom limb pain, may require continuous stimulation; other conditions, such as a painful arthritic joint, require shorter periods (3 to 4 hours). TENS has also been found to decrease knee pain associated with osteoarthritis. However, recent studies have shown TENS isn't helpful in patients with chronic lower back pain.[3,4] (See *Current uses of TENS.*)[5]

TENS is contraindicated for patients with cardiac pacemakers, *because it can interfere with pacemaker function.*[2,7] The procedure should be used with caution in pregnant patients not in labor and in patients with cardiac disease (*because it may cause arrhythmias*), lymphedema, a spinal cord stimulator, or an intrathecal pump.[8] You should avoid electrode placement on the anterior neck, *because the electrodes may cause laryngospasm.*

Current uses of TENS

Transcutaneous electrical nerve stimulation (TENS) has been helpful in temporary relief of acute pain, such as postoperative pain, and in ongoing relief of chronic pain, such as sciatica. It can also be used to prevent migraine headache pain.[5] Additionally, randomized control trials have shown successful use of TENS in patients experiencing labor pain.[6]

Other the types of pain that may respond to TENS are arthritis, bone fracture pain, bursitis, cancer-related pain, diabetic neuropathy pain, dysmenorrhea, musculoskeletal pain, myofascial pain, neuralgias and neuropathies, phantom limb pain, and whiplash.

A practitioner must prescribe TENS when used in the facility setting. Use of the device is most successful if administered and taught to the patient by a therapist skilled in its use.

You should also avoid placement over an area with sensory impairment, *because the device may cause burns.*[2,8]

Equipment

TENS device ■ pregelled, self-stick electrodes ■ warm water and soap ■ washcloth ■ towel ■ lead wires ■ charged battery pack ■ battery recharger ■ Optional: facility-approved pain scale, alcohol pads, hypoallergenic tape.

Commercial TENS kits are available. They include the stimulator, lead wires, electrodes, spare battery pack, battery recharger, and sometimes the adhesive patch.

Preparation of equipment

Inspect all equipment and supplies. If a product is expired, is defective, or has compromised integrity, remove it from patient use, label it as expired or defective, and report the expiration or defect as directed by your facility.

Before beginning the procedure, always test the battery pack *to make sure it's fully charged.* Follow the manufacturer's instructions for use and care of the TENS device.

Implementation

■ Verify the practitioner's order.
■ Review the patient's medical record for history of any contraindications to the procedure or allergies to adhesives in the pregelled, self-stick electrodes.
■ Gather and prepare the necessary equipment and supplies.
■ Perform hand hygiene.[9,10,11,12,13,14]
■ Confirm the patient's identity using at least two patient identifiers.[15]
■ Provide privacy.[16,17,18,19]
■ If the patient has never used a TENS unit, show the patient the device and explain the procedure to the patient and family (if appropriate) according to their individual communication and learning needs *to increase their understanding, allay their fears, and enhance cooperation.*[20]

Before TENS treatment

■ Using soap and water, thoroughly clean the skin where you'll apply the electrodes. Dry the skin before application. Use an alcohol pad, if necessary, *to remove excess oil or lotion.*
■ Apply the ordered number of electrodes on the proper skin area, leaving at least 2″ (5 cm) between them. (See *Positioning TENS electrodes.*) If necessary, secure them with hypoallergenic tape. Tape all sides evenly *so that the electrodes are firmly attached to the skin.*
■ Plug the pin connectors into the electrode sockets. *To protect the cords,* hold the connectors—not the cords themselves—during insertion.
■ Turn the channel controls to the OFF position or as recommended in the operator's manual.
■ Plug the lead wires into the jacks in the control box.
■ Turn the AMPLITUDE and RATE dials slowly as the manual directs. (The patient should feel a tingling sensation.) Then adjust the controls on this device to the prescribed settings or to settings that are most

EQUIPMENT

Positioning TENS electrodes

In transcutaneous electrical nerve stimulation (TENS), electrodes placed around peripheral nerves (or an incisional site) transmit mild electrical pulses to the brain. The current is thought to block pain impulses. The patient can influence the level and frequency of pain relief by adjusting the controls on the device.

Typically, electrode placement varies, even in patients who have similar complaints. You can place electrodes in several ways:
- to cover the painful area or surround it, as with painful joints or muscle tenderness or spasm
- to "capture" the painful area between electrodes, as with incisional pain
- to evoke "sensory analgesia" at trigger points.[8]

In peripheral nerve injury, place electrodes proximal to the injury (between the brain and the injury site) *to avoid increasing pain.* Placing electrodes in a hypersensitive area also increases pain. In an area lacking sensation, you should place electrodes on adjacent dermatomes.

In labor pain, one pair of electrodes is usually placed paravertebrally at the level of T10 to L1, and another at the level of S2 to S4. This produces a buzzing or prickling sensation, reducing the awareness of contraction pain. The patient controls the intensity of the current and stimulation pattern.[6]

The illustrations show combinations of electrode placement (red squares) and areas of nerve stimulation (shaded red) for lower back and leg pain.

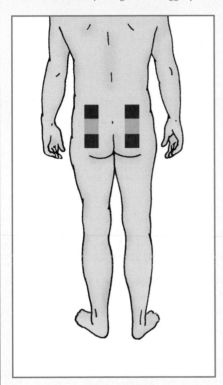
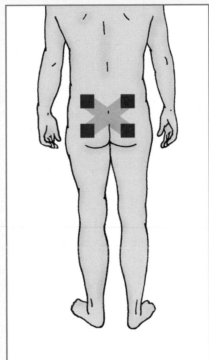
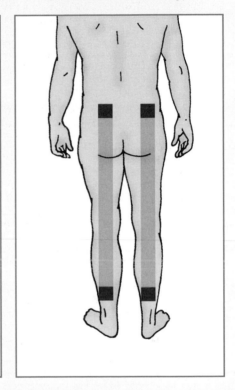

---

comfortable for the patient. Most patients select stimulation frequencies of 60 to 100 Hz.
- Attach the TENS control box to part of the patient's clothing, such as a belt, pocket, or bra.
- *To make sure the device is working effectively,* monitor the patient for signs of excessive stimulation, such as muscle twitches, and for signs of inadequate stimulation, signaled by the patient's inability to feel a mild tingling sensation.
- Perform hand hygiene hygiene.[9,10,11,12,13,14]

To remove the device
- Perform hand hygiene hygiene.[9,10,11,12,13,14]
- Turn off the controls and unplug the electrode lead wires from the control box. If removing the TENS device, lift the central part of the device off the pin on the electrode and take off the device.
- If another treatment will be given soon, leave the electrodes in place; if not, remove them by lifting the edge of each electrode and pulling each one off the skin gently.
- Clean the patient's skin with soap and water, and dry it with a towel.
- Screen for and assess the patient's pain using facility-defined criteria that are consistent with the patient's age, condition, and ability to understand.[21]
- Treat the patient's pain, as needed and ordered, using nonpharmacologic or pharmacologic approached, or a combination. Base the treatment plan on evidence-based practices and on the patient's

clinical condition, past medical history, and pain management goals.[21]
- Recharge the used battery pack *so that it's always ready for use.*
- Reassess and respond to the patient's pain by evaluating the response to treatment and progress toward pain management goals. Assess for adverse reactions and risk factors for adverse events that my result from treatment.[21]

Completing the procedure
- Perform hand hygiene hygiene.[9,10,11,12,13,14]
- Document the procedure.[22,23,24,25]

Special considerations
- If you must move the electrodes during the procedure, turn off the controls first. Follow the practitioner's orders regarding electrode placement and control settings. *Incorrect placement of the electrodes will result in inappropriate pain control.*
- Keep in mind that setting the controls too high can cause pain, and setting them too low will fail to relieve pain.

NURSING ALERT Never place the electrodes near the patient's eyes or over the nerves that innervate the carotid sinus or laryngeal or pharyngeal muscles *to avoid interference with critical nerve function.*[8]
- If TENS is used continuously for pain, remove the electrodes at least daily *to check for skin irritation, provide skin care, and rotate sites of electrode placement.*[26]

■ Patients using TENS therapy at home have reported problems with electrode connectivity, difficulty with correct electrode placement, and unpleasant sensations.[22]

Documentation

Record on the patient's medical record and the nursing care plan the TENS electrode placement sites and control settings you used. Document the patient's tolerance of the treatment and the time of device removal. Also evaluate pain control; record the location of the pain and the patient's rating of it using a facility-approved pain scale. Note the condition of the patient's skin at the sites of removed electrodes. Document teaching provided to the patient and family (if appropriate), their understanding of that teaching, and any need for follow-up teaching.

REFERENCES

1 Grover, C. A., et al. (2018). Transcutaneous electrical nerve stimulation in the ED for pain relief: A preliminary study of feasibility and efficacy. *Western Journal of Emergency Medicine, 19*(5), 72–76. https://westjem.com/original-research/transcutaneous-electrical-nerve-stimulation-tens-in-the-emergency-department-for-pain-relief-a-preliminary-study-of-feasibility-and-efficacy.html (Level VI)

2 Chou, R., et al. (2016). Management of postoperative pain: A clinical practice guideline from the American Pain Society, the American Society of Regional Anesthesia and Pain Medicine, and the American Society of Anesthesiologists' Council on Regional Anesthesia, Executive Committee and Administration Council. *The Journal of Pain, 17*(2), 131–157. https://www.jpain.org/article/S1526-5900(15)00995-5/pdf (Level VII)

3 Chou, R. (2021). Subacute and chronic low back pain: Nonpharmacologic and pharmacologic treatment. In: *UpToDate*, Atlas, S. J. (Ed.).

4 Wu, L. C., et al. (2018). Literature review and meta-analysis of transcutaneous electrical nerve stimulation in treating chronic back pain. *Regional Anesthesia and Pain Medicine, 43*(4), 425–433. https://www.ncbi.nlm.nih.gov/pmc/articles/PMC5916478/ (Level I)

5 U.S. Food and Drug Administration. (2017). Treating migraines: More ways to fight the pain. https://www.fda.gov/consumers/consumer-updates/treating-migraines-more-ways-fight-pain

6 Caughey, A. B., & Tilden, E. (2021). Nonpharmacologic approaches to management of labor pain. In: *UpToDate*, Lockwood, C. (Ed.).

7 Portugal, S. E. (2021). Rehabilitative measures for treatment of pain and inflammation. https://www.merckmanuals.com/professional/special-subjects/rehabilitation/rehabilitative-measures-for-treatment-of-pain-and-inflammation

8 Kaye, V., & Brandstater, M. E. (2019). Transcutaneous electrical nerve stimulation. https://emedicine.medscape.com/article/325107-overview#a1

9 World Health Organization. (2009). WHO guidelines on hand hygiene in health care: First global patient safety challenge, clean care is safer care. https://apps.who.int/iris/bitstream/handle/10665/44102/9789241597906_eng.pdf?sequence=1 (Level IV)

10 The Joint Commission. (2021). Standard NPSG.07.01.01. *Comprehensive accreditation manual for hospitals*. Oakbrook Terrace, IL: The Joint Commission. (Level VII)

11 Centers for Disease Control and Prevention. (2002). Guideline for hand hygiene in health-care settings: Recommendations of the Healthcare Infection Control Practices Advisory Committee and the HICPAC/SHEA/APIC/IDSA Hand Hygiene Task Force. *MMWR Recommendations and Reports, 51*(RR-16), 1–45. https://www.cdc.gov/mmwr/pdf/rr/rr5116.pdf (Level II)

12 Centers for Medicare and Medicaid Services, Department of Health and Human Services. (2020). Condition of participation: Infection control. 42 C.F.R. § 482.42.

13 Accreditation Association for Hospitals and Health Systems. (2020). Standard 07.01.21. *Healthcare Facilities Accreditation Program: Accreditation requirements for acute care hospitals*. Chicago, IL: Accreditation Association for Hospitals and Health Systems. (Level VII)

14 DNV GL-Healthcare USA, Inc. (2020). IC.1.SR.1. *NIAHO® accreditation requirements, interpretive guidelines and surveyor guidance—revision 20.0*. Milford, OH: DNV GL-Healthcare USA, Inc. (Level VII)

15 The Joint Commission. (2021). Standard NPSG.01.01.01. *Comprehensive accreditation manual for hospitals*. Oakbrook Terrace, IL: The Joint Commission. (Level VII)

16 Centers for Medicare and Medicaid Services, Department of Health and Human Services. (2020). Condition of participation: Patient's rights. 42 C.F.R. § 482.13(c)(1).

17 Accreditation Association for Hospitals and Health Systems. (2020). Standard 15.01.16. *Healthcare Facilities Accreditation Program: Accreditation requirements for acute care hospitals*. Chicago, IL: Accreditation Association for Hospitals and Health Systems. (Level VII)

18 DNV GL-Healthcare USA, Inc. (2020). PR.2.SR.5. *NIAHO® accreditation requirements, interpretive guidelines and surveyor guidance—revision 20*. Milford, OH: DNV GL-Healthcare USA, Inc. (Level VII)

19 The Joint Commission. (2021). Standard RI.01.01.01. *Comprehensive accreditation manual for hospitals*. Oakbrook Terrace, IL: The Joint Commission. (Level VII)

20 The Joint Commission. (2021). Standard PC.02.01.21. *Comprehensive accreditation manual for hospitals*. Oakbrook Terrace, IL: The Joint Commission. (Level VII)

21 The Joint Commission. (2021). Standard PC.01.02.07. *Comprehensive accreditation manual for hospitals*. Oakbrook Terrace, IL: The Joint Commission. (Level VII)

22 The Joint Commission. (2021). Standard RC.01.03.01. *Comprehensive accreditation manual for hospital*. Oakbrook Terrace, IL: The Joint Commission. (Level VII)

23 Accreditation Association for Hospitals and Health Systems. (2020). Standard 10.00.03. *Healthcare Facilities Accreditation Program: Accreditation requirements for acute care hospitals*. Chicago, IL: Accreditation Association for Hospitals and Health Systems. (Level VII)

24 Centers for Medicare and Medicaid Services, Department of Health and Human Services. (2020). Condition of participation: Medical record services. 42 C.F.R. § 482.24(b).

25 DNV GL-Healthcare USA, Inc. (2020). MR.2.SR.1. *NIAHO® accreditation requirements, interpretive guidelines and surveyor guidance—revision 20.0*. Milford, OH: DNV GL-Healthcare USA, Inc. (Level VII)

26 Craven, R. F., et al. (2017). *Fundamentals of nursing: Human health and function* (8th ed.). Philadelphia, PA: Wolters Kluwer.

TRANSCUTANEOUS PACING

Transcutaneous pacing is a method of external electrical stimulation of the heart through a set of electrode pads. It is used to temporarily restore electrical activity when the cardiac condition is abnormal and the patient is hemodynamically unstable.[1] The device works by monitoring cardiac rate and rhythm continuously and delivering pacing impulses through the skin and chest wall muscles when needed, causing electrical depolarization and subsequent cardiac contraction to maintain cardiac output.

A transcutaneous pacing device may be used as a temporary intervention, *because it can be easily applied and managed until the patient can receive more-definitive treatment, such as temporary transvenous pacing or the insertion of a permanent cardiac pacemaker.*[2] The use of a transcutaneous pacing device is the best choice in a life-threatening situation in which time is critical. (See *Indications for transcutaneous pacing*.)

Transcutaneous pacing works by sending an electrical impulse from the pulse generator to the patient's heart by way of two electrodes, which are placed on the front and back of the patient's chest.[2]

Transcutaneous pacing is recommended by the American Heart Association Guidelines for cardiopulmonary resuscitation and emergency cardiovascular care for symptomatic bradycardia when a pulse is present. It isn't recommended for cardiac arrest, because research shows that it's ineffective in that situation.[3]

Indications for transcutaneous pacing

The American Heart Association recommends transcutaneous pacing for these Class IIa indications:

■ bradycardia with hemodynamic instability unresponsive to atropine while preparing for emergent transvenous pacing
■ high-degree block (Mobitz type II second-degree block or third-degree atrioventricular block)
■ symptomatic bradycardia
■ sinus arrest.[3]

Equipment

Transcutaneous pacing pulse generator with pacemaker cable ▪ transcutaneous pacing electrodes ▪ monitoring electrodes ▪ 12-lead electrocardiogram (ECG) machine ▪ ECG cables and monitor ▪ washcloth ▪ towel ▪ nonemollient soap ▪ tap water ▪ vital signs monitoring equipment ▪ emergency equipment (code cart with emergency medications, defibrillator, handheld resuscitation bag with mask, intubation equipment) ▪ Optional: disposable-head clippers, prescribed analgesic or sedative.

Preparation of equipment

Inspect all equipment and supplies. If a product is expired, is defective, or has compromised integrity, remove it from patient use, label it as expired or defective, and report the expiration or defect as directed by your facility. Make sure emergency equipment is functioning properly and readily available.

Follow the manufacturer's recommendations for use and care of the transcutaneous pacemaker.

Implementation

- Gather and prepare the necessary equipment and supplies.
- Perform hand hygiene[4,5,6,7,8,9]
- Confirm the patient's identity using at least two patient identifiers.[10]
- Provide privacy[11,12,13,14]
- Explain the procedure to the patient and family (if appropriate) according to their individual communication and learning needs *to increase their understanding, allay their fears, and enhance cooperation.*[15]
- Assist the patient to the supine position and expose the torso.[1]
- If needed, clip the patient's hair over the areas of electrode placement. However, don't shave the area, *because if you nick the skin, the current from the pulse generator could cause discomfort,*[1] *and the nicks could become irritated or infected after the electrodes are applied.*
- Prepare the skin on the patient's chest and back by washing it with a washcloth, nonemollient soap, and tap water; dry the skin thoroughly *to improve electrode adherence.*[1] Remove any transdermal patches or skin preparation products (such as ointments, alcohol, and povidone iodine).[1]
- Plug the ECG cable into the ECG input connection on the front of the transcutaneous pacing pulse generator. Turn on the monitor.
- Attach the monitoring electrodes to the patient in lead I, II, or III position *to monitor the rhythm.* Do this even if the patient is already on telemetry monitoring, *to allow the monitoring electrodes connected to the transcutaneous pacemaker.* If you select the lead II position, adjust the left leg (LL) monitoring electrode placement *to accommodate the anterior transcutaneous pacing electrode and the patient's anatomy.* You should see the ECG waveform on the monitor.
- Adjust the ECG size to the maximum R-wave size, and look for the device indicator signaling that the device senses the QRS complex of the patient's intrinsic rhythm.[1] Adjust the audible R-wave signal to a suitable volume level, and activate the alarm by pressing the appropriate button. Make sure the alarm limits are set properly for the patient's current condition, and that the alarms are turned on, functioning properly, and audible to staff.[16,17,18]
- Press the appropriate button for a printout of the waveform.
- Apply the posterior transcutaneous pacing electrode (marked BACK), to the skin on the left side of the patient's back, just below the scapula and to the left of the spine. Alternatively, if anterolateral pacing electrode placement is indicated (such as with hemodynamic instability or if the patient's back is difficult to access), place the back (posterior) electrode over the patient's right sternal area at the third intercostal space.[1] Follow the manufacturer's instructions for electrode application. Avoid placing the pacing electrodes directly over lesions, injuries, large bone structures (such as the sternum, spine, and scapula), implanted devices, dressings, tubes, drains, or fresh incisions.[19]
- Apply the anterior transcutaneous pacing electrode (marked FRONT) to the left side of the precordium in the usual lead V_2 to V_5 position. With female patients, place the anterior electrode under and lateral to the patient's breast tissue, but avoid placing it over the diaphragm.[1] Follow the manufacturer's instructions for electrode application. (See *Transcutaneous electrode placement.*)
- After ensuring the energy output in milliamperes (mA) is set to 0, connect the transcutaneous pacing electrodes to the pacemaker cable, which is connected to the pulse generator.

Transcutaneous electrode placement

For a noninvasive temporary pacemaker, the two pacing electrodes are placed at heart level on the patient's chest (anterior) and back (posterior), as shown below.

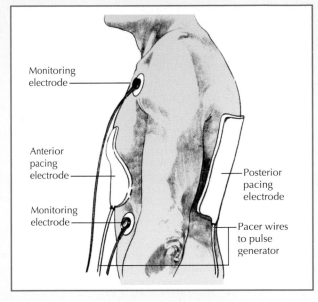

Monitoring electrode
Anterior pacing electrode
Monitoring electrode
Posterior pacing electrode
Pacer wires to pulse generator

Alternatively, place the back (posterior electrode over the patient's right sternal area at the second or third intercostal space (as shown below).[1]

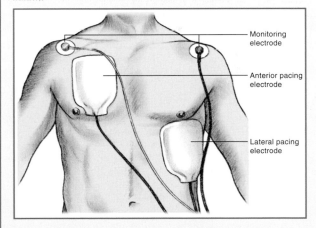

Monitoring electrode
Anterior pacing electrode
Lateral pacing electrode

You can initiate this type of pacing quickly in an emergency.

- Check the waveform, looking for a tall QRS complex in lead II.
- Turn on the pulse generator. Inform the patient that a thumping or twitching sensation may occur. Reassure the patient that you'll provide medication if the discomfort is intolerable.
- Set the pulse generator mode (demand or asynchronous) as ordered. The demand mode senses intrinsic myocardial activity and only paces when the patient's intrinsic rate falls below the set rate. In the asynchronous mode, pacing occurs at a set rate regardless of the patient's intrinsic rate.
- Set the pacemaker rate to maintain an adequate cardiac output. Some pacemakers have a default setting (for example, 80 beats/minute) that can be adjusted as needed.[1]
- Set the energy output. Slowly increase the amount of energy delivered to the heart by adjusting the mA setting. Do this until capture is achieved; you'll see a pacing spike followed by a widened QRS complex that resembles a premature ventricular contraction. This is the pacing threshold.

To ensure consistent capture, increase output by 10%. Don't increase output any higher; *doing so may cause the patient needless discomfort.*

■ With full capture, the patient's heart rate should be approximately the same as the pacing rate set on the machine (pacemaker). The usual pacing threshold is between 40 and 70 mA. Assess the patient's pulse *to ensure adequate blood flow with paced complexes;*[1] don't rely on the monitor alone to determine the patient's heart rate.

■ Assess the patient's vital signs, skin color, level of consciousness, and peripheral pulses *to determine the effectiveness of the paced rhythm.*[1]

■ Obtain a 12-lead ECG tracing *to serve as a baseline for comparison,* and then obtain additional ECGs as required by your facility or when clinical changes occur.

■ Screen for and assess the patient's pain using facility-defined criteria that are consistent with the patient's age, condition, and ability to understand.[20,21]

■ Treat the patient's pain, as needed and ordered, using nonpharmacologic or pharmacologic approaches, or a combination. Base the treatment plan on evidence-based practices and the patient's clinical condition, past medical history, and pain management goals.[20]

■ Administer an analgesic or sedative as ordered and indicated following safe medication administration practices.[1,22,23,24]

■ Monitor closely if the patient is at high risk for adverse outcomes related to opioid treatment, if prescribed.[20]

■ Perform hand hygiene.[4,5,6,7,8,9]

■ Document the procedure.[25,26,27,28]

Special considerations

■ Obtain a rhythm strip before, during, and after pacemaker placement; any time that pacemaker settings are changed; and whenever the patient receives treatment for a complication due to the pacemaker.

■ Monitor the ECG reading continuously, noting capture, sensing, rate, intrinsic beats, and competition of paced and intrinsic heart rhythms. If the pacemaker is sensing correctly, the sense indicator on the pulse generator should flash with each beat.

Complications

Complications of transcutaneous pacemaker therapy include inability to achieve capture and successfully pace the heart, as well as patient discomfort.[2] Arrhythmias and skin breakdown can also occur.[1]

Documentation

Record the reason for transcutaneous pacing, the date and time it was initiated, the type of pacemaker used, and the locations of the electrodes. Also record the pacemaker settings. Note the patient's response to the procedure, along with any complications and interventions implemented. If possible, obtain ECG tracings before, during, and after pacemaker placement; whenever pacemaker settings are changed; and when the patient receives treatment for a complication caused by the pacemaker. Document teaching provided to the patient and family (if applicable), their understanding of that teaching, and any need for follow-up teaching.

REFERENCES

1 Wiegand, D. L. (2017). *AACN procedure manual for high acuity, progressive, and critical care* (7th ed.). St. Louis, MO: Elsevier.

2 Ganz, L. I. (2019). Temporary cardiac pacing. In: *UpToDate,* Estes, N. A, (Ed.).

3 American Heart Association. (2020). 2020 American Heart Association Guidelines for CPR and ECC—Part 3: Adult Basic and Advanced Life Support. https://cpr.heart.org/en/resuscitation-science/cpr-and-ecc-guidelines/adult-basic-and-advanced-life-support (Level II)

4 The Joint Commission. (2021). Standard NPSG.07.01.01. *Comprehensive accreditation manual for hospitals.* Oakbrook Terrace, IL: The Joint Commission. (Level VII)

5 Centers for Disease Control and Prevention. (2002). Guideline for hand hygiene in health-care settings: Recommendations of the Healthcare Infection Control Practices Advisory Committee and the HICPAC/SHEA/APIC/IDSA Hand Hygiene Task Force. *MMWR Recommendations and Reports, 51*(RR–16), 1–45. https://www.cdc.gov/mmwr/pdf/rr/rr5116.pdf (Level II)

6 World Health Organization (WHO). (2009). WHO guidelines on hand hygiene in health care: First global patient safety challenge, clean care is safer care. https://apps.who.int/iris/bitstream/handle/10665/44102/9789241597906_eng.pdf?sequence=1 (Level IV)

7 Accreditation Association for Hospitals and Health Systems. (2020). Standard 07.01.21. *Healthcare Facilities Accreditation Program: Accreditation requirements for acute care hospitals.* Chicago, IL: Accreditation Association for Hospitals and Health Systems. (Level VII)

8 Centers for Medicare and Medicaid Services, Department of Health and Human Services. (2020). Condition of participation: Infection control. 42 C.F.R. § 482.42.

9 DNV GL-Healthcare USA, Inc. (2020). IC.1.SR.1. *NIAHO® accreditation requirements, interpretive guidelines and surveyor guidance—revision 20.0.* Milford, OH: DNV GL-Healthcare USA, Inc. (Level VII)

10 The Joint Commission. (2021). Standard NPSG.01.01.01. *Comprehensive accreditation manual for hospitals.* Oakbrook Terrace, IL: The Joint Commission. (Level VII)

11 DNV GL-Healthcare USA, Inc. (2020). PR.2.SR.5. *NIAHO® accreditation requirements, interpretive guidelines and surveyor guidance—revision 20.0.* Milford, OH: DNV GL-Healthcare USA, Inc. (Level VII)

12 The Joint Commission. (2021). Standard RI.01.01.01. *Comprehensive accreditation manual for hospitals.* Oakbrook Terrace, IL: The Joint Commission. (Level VII)

13 Centers for Medicare and Medicaid Services, Department of Health and Human Services. (2020). Condition of participation: Patient's rights. 42 C.F.R. § 482.13(c)(1).

14 Accreditation Association for Hospitals and Health Systems. (2020). Standard 15.01.16. *Healthcare Facilities Accreditation Program: Accreditation requirements for acute care hospitals.* Chicago, IL: Accreditation Association for Hospitals and Health Systems. (Level VII)

15 The Joint Commission. (2021). Standard PC.02.01.21. *Comprehensive accreditation manual for hospitals.* Oakbrook Terrace, IL: The Joint Commission. (Level VII)

16 The Joint Commission. (2013). Sentinel event alert 50: Medical device alarm safety in hospitals. https://www.jointcommission.org/-/media/tjc/documents/resources/patient-safety-topics/sentinel-event/sea_50_alarms_4_26_16.pdf (Level VII)

17 Graham, K. C., & Cvach, M. (2010). Monitor alarm fatigue: Standardizing use of physiological monitors and decreasing nuisance alarms. *American Journal of Critical Care, 19*(1), 28–37. https://doi.org/10.4037/ajcc2010651

18 American Association of Critical-Care Nurses (AACN). (2018). *AACN practice alert: Managing alarms in acute care across the life span: Electrocardiography and pulse oximetry.* https://www.aacn.org/clinical-resources/practice-alerts/managing-alarms-in-acute-care-across-the-life-span (Level VII)

19 Philips Healthcare. (2013). Non-invasive transcutaneous pacing: Application note. http://incenter.medical.philips.com/doclib/enc/fetch/577817/577869/Non-Invasive_Transcutaneous_Pacing.pdf%3Fnodeid%3D8615795%26vernum%3D2

20 The Joint Commission. (2021). Standard PC.01.02.07. *Comprehensive accreditation manual for hospitals.* Oakbrook Terrace, IL: The Joint Commission. (Level VII)

21 Institute for Safe Medication Practices. (2012). Side tracks on the safety express: Interruptions lead to errors and unfinished…Wait, what was I doing? *Nurse Advise-ERR, 11*(2), 1–4. https://www.ismp.org/resources/side-tracks-safety-express-interruptions-lead-errors-and-unfinished-wait-what-was-i-doing?id=37

22 DNV GL-Healthcare USA, Inc. (2020). MM.1.SR.3. *NIAHO® accreditation requirements, interpretive guidelines and surveyor guidance—revision 20.0.* Milford, OH: DNV GL-Healthcare USA, Inc. (Level VII)

23 Accreditation Association for Hospitals and Health Systems. (2020). Standard 16.01.03. *Healthcare Facilities Accreditation Program: Accreditation requirements for acute care hospitals.* Chicago, IL: Accreditation Association for Hospitals and Health Systems. (Level VII)

24 Centers for Medicare and Medicaid Services, Department of Health and Human Services. (2020). Condition of participation: Nursing services. 42 C.F.R. § 482.23(c).

25 The Joint Commission. (2021). Standard RC.01.03.01. *Comprehensive accreditation manual for hospitals.* Oakbrook Terrace, IL: The Joint Commission. (Level VII)

26 Accreditation Association for Hospitals and Health Systems. (2020). Standard 10.00.03. *Healthcare Facilities Accreditation Program: Accreditation requirements for acute care hospitals.* Chicago, IL: Accreditation Association for Hospitals and Health Systems. (Level VII)

27 Centers for Medicare and Medicaid Services, Department of Health and Human Services. (2020). Condition of participation: Medical record services. 42 C.F.R. § 482.24(b).

28 DNV GL-Healthcare USA, Inc. (2020). MR.2.SR.1. *NIAHO® accreditation requirements, interpretive guidelines and surveyor guidance—revision 20.0.* Milford, OH: DNV GL-Healthcare USA, Inc. (Level VII)

TRANSDERMAL DRUG APPLICATION

Through a measured dose of ointment or an adhesive patch applied to the skin, transdermal drugs deliver constant, controlled medication directly into the bloodstream for a prolonged systemic effect.

Nitroglycerin is a commonly administered transdermal medication. It's indicated for the treatment of angina in patients with coronary artery disease. Nitroglycerin ointment dilates coronary vessels for up to 7 hours.[1] (See *Applying nitroglycerin ointment.*)

Medications available as transdermal patches include scopolamine, which treats motion sickness; granisetron for chemotherapy-induced nausea and vomiting; estradiol for postmenopausal hormone replacement; estrogen and progesterone for hormonal contraception; cloNIDine for hypertension; nicotine for smoking cessation; and fentaNYL, an opioid analgesic for controlling chronic pain.[3]

Contraindications for transdermal drug application include skin allergies or skin reactions to the medication. Transdermal drugs shouldn't be applied to broken or irritated skin, which would increase irritation, or to scarred or callused skin, which might impair absorption.

NURSING ALERT Don't apply heat over a fentaNYL transdermal system or its surrounding area, *because an increase in temperature increases fentaNYL release, which can result in overdose and death.*[4,5]

Equipment

Patient's medication administration record ▪ prescribed medication ▪ application strip or ruled measuring paper (for nitroglycerin ointment) ▪ adhesive tape ▪ pen or marker ▪ Optional: gloves, other personal protective equipment, transparent semipermeable dressing, disposable-head clippers, blood pressure equipment, supplies to remove previously applied medication (tissue or soap, water, and a washcloth).

Implementation

▪ Avoid distractions and interruptions when preparing and administering the medication *to prevent medication errors.*[6,7]

▪ Verify the practitioner's order.[8]

▪ Reconcile the patient's medications when the practitioner orders a new medication *to reduce the risk of medication errors, including omissions, duplications, dosing errors, and drug interactions.*[9,10]

▪ Compare the medication label with the order in the patient's medical record and verify that the medication is correct.[8,11,12,13]

▪ Check the patient's medical record for allergies or contraindications to the prescribed medication. If an allergy or a contraindication exists, don't administer the medication; notify the practitioner.[8,11,12,13]

▪ Check the expiration date on the medication. If the medication has expired, return it to the pharmacy and obtain new medication.[8,11,12,13]

▪ Visually inspect the medication for loss of integrity; don't administer the medication if its integrity has been compromised.[8,11,12,13]

▪ Discuss any unresolved concerns about the medication with the practitioner.[8,11,12,13]

▪ Perform hand hygiene.[14,15,16,17,18,19]

▪ Confirm the patient's identity using at least two patient identifiers.[20]

▪ Provide privacy.[21,22,23,24]

▪ Explain the procedure to the patient and family (if appropriate) according to their individual communication and learning needs *to increase their understanding, allay their fears, and enhance cooperation.*[25] Answer any questions.

▪ Teach the patient who is receiving the medication for the first time about potential adverse reactions, and discuss any other concerns related to the medication.[8,11,12,13]

▪ Verify that the medication is being administered at the correct time, in the prescribed dose, and by the correct route *to reduce the risk of medication errors.*[8,11,12,13]

Applying nitroglycerin ointment

Unlike many topical medications, nitroglycerin ointment is used for its transdermal systemic effects. It's used to dilate the veins and arteries, improving cardiac perfusion in a patient with cardiac ischemia or angina pectoris.

To apply nitroglycerin ointment transdermally, start by taking the patient's baseline blood pressure *so that you can compare it with later readings.* Remove any previously applied nitroglycerin ointment. Nitroglycerin ointment, which is prescribed by the inch, comes with a rectangular piece of ruled paper to be used in applying the medication. Put on gloves if needed. Squeeze the prescribed amount of ointment onto the ruled measuring paper (as shown below).

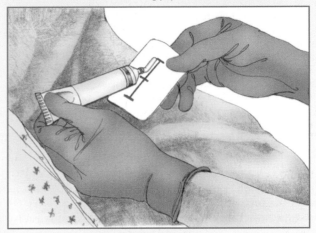

After measuring the correct amount of ointment, tape the ruled measuring paper, drug side down, directly to the skin, usually on the chest or arm. Do so by spreading a thin layer of the ointment over an area of 3" [7.5 cm].) For increased absorption, the practitioner may request that you cover the site with a transparent semipermeable dressing (as shown below).

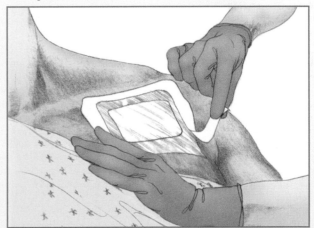

Monitor closely and document the patient's blood pressure throughout treatment, as ordered.[1,2] If the blood pressure has dropped significantly and the patient has a headache (from vasodilation of blood vessels in the head), notify the practitioner immediately; the practitioner may reduce the medication dose. If the patient's blood pressure has dropped but the patient has no symptoms, instruct the patient to lie still until the blood pressure returns to normal.

▪ If your facility uses a bar code technology, use it as directed by your facility.

▪ Perform hand hygiene.[14,15,16,17,18,19]

NURSING ALERT If your facility's hazardous drug list contains the drug that you're about to administer, put on personal protective equipment, as directed.[26]

- Put on gloves if needed *to comply with standard precautions*.[27,28,29]
- Remove any previously applied medication.
- To apply ointment, place the prescribed amount of transdermal ointment on the applicator strip or ruled measuring paper, taking care not to get any on your skin.
- To apply a transdermal patch, open the package and remove the patch. Without touching the adhesive surface, remove the clear plastic backing.
- Apply the application strip, ruled measuring tape, or transdermal patch to any dry, hairless area of the body.
- Alternatively, cover an ointment application site with a transparent semipermeable dressing.
- If needed, use disposable-head clippers to remove excess hair before application, but avoid shaving an area to apply ointment, *because shaving removes the top layer of skin, which can cause the medication to absorb faster that it would with unshaved skin.*
- Follow the medications' prescribing information for specific application instructions.
- Don't rub the ointment into the skin.[1]
- Write the date, the time, and your initials on the new application strip, ruled measuring tape, transparent semipermeable dressing, or patch, as directed by your facility.
- Instruct the patient to keep the area around the ointment or patch as dry as possible.
- Remove and discard your gloves and other personal protective equipment, if worn,[28,29] and perform hand hygiene.[14,15,16,17,18,19]
- Document the procedure.[30,31,32,33]

Special considerations

- Reapply transdermal medications at the same time every day *to ensure a continuous effect*, but alternate the application sites *to avoid skin irritation*.
- Store the transdermal medication at room temperature with the cap closed tightly.
- When applying a scopolamine or fentaNYL patch, instruct the patient not to drive or operate machinery until the response to the drug has been determined.[4,34]
- Warn a patient using a cloNIDine patch to check with the practitioner before taking an over-the-counter cough preparation, *because such drugs may counteract cloNIDine's effects*.[35]
- If a fentaNYL patch won't adhere, tape the edges of the patch with adhesive tape; if problems with adhesion persist, apply a transparent semipermeable dressing over the patch.[4]
- Some transdermal patches aren't compatible with magnetic resonance imaging (MRI) and may cause skin burns if not removed before testing. Consult with the practitioner about removing a transdermal patch prior to MRI, as applicable.[35]
- Remove transdermal patches from the chest before applying defibrillator pads or paddles, *because these patches may block the transfer of energy from the pad or paddles to the patient and cause burns when the pad or paddle is placed over the patch*. Alternatively, ensure that the paddle or pad does not touch the transdermal patch.[36]

Patient teaching

Teach the patient how to apply the patch. (See *Applying a transdermal medication patch*.)

Complications

Transdermal medications can cause skin irritation, such as pruritus and a rash. The patient may also suffer adverse effects of the specific drug administered. For example, transdermal nitroglycerin may cause headaches and orthostatic hypotension.[1] Adverse effects of scopolamine include dry mouth and drowsiness (most common); for estradiol, increased risk of endometrial cancer and thromboembolic disease; and for clonidine, possible severe rebound hypertension, especially if withdrawn suddenly.[34,35,39] An anaphylactic reaction to

APPLYING A TRANSDERMAL MEDICATION PATCH

Instruct the patient who will be receiving medication by transdermal patch in its proper use. Explain to the patient that the patch consists of several layers. The layer closest to the skin contains a small amount of the drug and allows prompt introduction of the drug into the bloodstream. The next layer controls release of the drug from the main portion of the patch. The third layer contains the main dose of the drug. The outermost layer consists of an aluminized polyester barrier.

Teach the patient to apply the patch to appropriate skin areas, such as the upper arm or chest or behind the ear, and to use a different site for each application *to avoid skin irritation*. If necessary, you can clip the hair at the site. Caution the patient to avoid any area that may cause uneven absorption, such as skin folds, scars, and calluses, or any irritated or damaged skin areas. Also, tell the patient not to apply the patch below the elbow or knee.

Warn the patient to avoid touching the gel or surrounding tape during application. Instruct the patient to wash the skin where the old patch was removed and to wash the hands after application *to remove any medication that may have rubbed off*.

Warn the patient not to get the patch wet, and to discard it if it leaks or falls off, and then to clean the site and apply a new patch at a different site. If the transdermal patch contains fentaNYL or granisetron, warn the patient to avoid applying heat over the fentaNYL or granisetron transdermal system or its surrounding area, *because an increase in temperature increases drug release from the system, which can result in overdose*.[4,37]

Instruct the patient to apply the patch at the same time at the prescribed interval *to ensure continuous drug delivery*. Bedtime application is ideal *because body movement is reduced during the night*. Lastly, tell the patient not to forget to remove the old patch, and to dispose of it properly.

Caution the patient that accidental exposure to a fentaNYL patch, especially by a child, can be fatal. Exposure can occur when a child or caregiver touches skin that hasn't been cleansed after removal of an old patch or by contact with a removed patch. The patient should fold the old patch in half and then flush it down the toilet to prevent inadvertent contact.[4,38]

the medication can also occur; monitor for signs and symptoms of this complication.

Documentation

Document the medication's name, dose, strength, route, and administration site as well as the date and time of administration in the patient's medication administration record. Document the skin's appearance and integrity before administration. Record whether adverse effects were present or absent and, if present, the date and time that you notified the practitioner, prescribed interventions, and the patient's response to those interventions.[40] Document the patient's response to and tolerance of therapy. Document teaching provided to the patient and family (if applicable), their understanding of that teaching, and any need for follow-up teaching. Include whether you provided the patient with written information about the prescribed medication.

REFERENCES

1 Fougera, E. & Company. (2019). Nitro-Bid nitroglycerin ointment. https://dailymed.nlm.nih.gov/dailymed/drugInfo. cfm?setid=30934ddc-0823-4097-8699-d10988011d7c

2 Kannam, J. P., & Gersh, B. J. (2021). Nitrates in the management of chronic coronary syndrome. In: *UpToDate*, Kaski, J. C. (Ed.).

3 Al Hanbali, O. A., et al. (2019). Transdermal patches: Design and current approaches to painless drug delivery. *Acta Pharmaceutica, 69*, 197–215.

4 Janssen Pharmaceuticals, Inc. (2016). Duragesic (fentanyl transdermal system) for transdermal administration. At https://www.accessdata.fda.gov/drugsatfda_docs/label/2016/019813s069lbl.pdf

5 Institute for Safe Medication Practices. (2015). Transdermal patches and heat sources. *Nurse Advise ERR, 13*(4), 1–5. https://www.ismp.org/sites/default/files/attachments/2018-04/NurseAdviseERR201504.pdf

6 Westbrook, J., et al. (2010). Association of interruptions with an increased risk and severity of medication administration errors. *Archives of Internal Medicine, 170*, 683–690. (Level IV)

7 Institute for Safe Medication Practices. (2012). Side tracks on the safety express: Interruptions lead to errors and unfinished…Wait, what was I doing? *Nurse Advise-ERR, 11*(2), 1–4. https://www.ismp.org/resources/side-tracks-safety-express-interruptions-lead-errors-and-unfinished-wait-what-was-i-doing?id=37

8 Accreditation Association for Hospitals and Health Systems. (2020). Standard 16.01.03. *Healthcare Facilities Accreditation Program: Accreditation requirements for acute care hospitals.* Chicago, IL: Accreditation Association for Hospitals and Health Systems. (Level VII)

9 The Joint Commission. (2021). Standard NPSG.03.06.01. *Comprehensive accreditation manual for hospitals.* Oakbrook Terrace, IL: The Joint Commission. (Level VII)

10 Accreditation Association for Hospitals and Health Systems. (2020). Standard 25.02.13. *Healthcare Facilities Accreditation Program: Accreditation requirements for acute care hospitals.* Chicago, IL: Accreditation Association for Hospitals and Health Systems. (Level VII)

11 Centers for Medicare and Medicaid Services, Department of Health and Human Services. (2020). Condition of participation: Nursing services. 42 C.F.R. § 482.23(c).

12 DNV GL-Healthcare USA, Inc. (2020). MM.1.SR.3. *NIAHO® accreditation requirements, interpretive guidelines and surveyor guidance—revision 20.0.* Milford, OH: DNV GL-Healthcare USA, Inc. (Level VII)

13 The Joint Commission. (2021). Standard MM.06.01.01. *Comprehensive accreditation manual for hospitals.* Oakbrook Terrace, IL: The Joint Commission. (Level VII)

14 Centers for Disease Control and Prevention. (2002). Guideline for hand hygiene in health-care settings: Recommendations of the Healthcare Infection Control Practices Advisory Committee and the HICPAC/SHEA/APIC/IDSA Hand Hygiene Task Force. *MMWR Recommendations and Reports, 51*(RR-16), 1–45. https://www.cdc.gov/mmwr/pdf/rr/rr5116.pdf (Level II)

15 The Joint Commission. (2021). Standard NPSG.07.01.01. *Comprehensive accreditation manual for hospitals.* Oakbrook Terrace, IL: The Joint Commission. (Level VII)

16 World Health Organization. (2009). WHO guidelines on hand hygiene in health care: First global patient safety challenge, clean care is safer care. https://apps.who.int/iris/bitstream/handle/10665/44102/9789241597906_eng.pdf?sequence=1 (Level IV)

17 Accreditation Association for Hospitals and Health Systems. (2020). Standard 07.01.21. *Healthcare Facilities Accreditation Program: Accreditation requirements for acute care hospitals.* Chicago, IL: Accreditation Association for Hospitals and Health Systems. (Level VII)

18 Centers for Medicare and Medicaid Services, Department of Health and Human Services. (2020). Condition of participation: Infection control. 42 C.F.R. § 482.42.

19 DNV GL-Healthcare USA, Inc. (2020). IC.1.SR.1. *NIAHO® accreditation requirements, interpretive guidelines and surveyor guidance—revision 20.0.* Milford, OH: DNV GL-Healthcare USA, Inc. (Level VII)

20 The Joint Commission. (2021). Standard NPSG.01.01.01. *Comprehensive accreditation manual for hospitals.* Oakbrook Terrace, IL: The Joint Commission. (Level VII)

21 Accreditation Association for Hospitals and Health Systems. (2020). Standard 15.01.16. *Healthcare Facilities Accreditation Program: Accreditation requirements for acute care hospitals.* Chicago, IL: Accreditation Association for Hospitals and Health Systems. (Level VII)

22 Centers for Medicare and Medicaid Services, Department of Health and Human Services. (2020). Condition of participation: Patient's rights. 42 C.F.R. § 482.13(c)(1).

23 DNV GL-Healthcare USA, Inc. (2020). PR.2.SR.5. *NIAHO® accreditation requirements, interpretive guidelines and surveyor guidance—revision 20.0.* Milford, OH: DNV GL-Healthcare USA, Inc. (Level VII)

24 The Joint Commission. (2021). Standard RI.01.01.01. *Comprehensive accreditation manual for hospitals.* Oakbrook Terrace, IL: The Joint Commission. (Level VII)

25 The Joint Commission. (2021). Standard PC.02.01.21. *Comprehensive accreditation manual for hospitals.* Oakbrook Terrace, IL: The Joint Commission. (Level VII)

26 The United States Pharmacopeial Convention. (2019). USP general chapter <800> Hazardous drugs—Handling in healthcare settings. https://www.usp.org/compounding/general-chapter-hazardous-drugs-handling-healthcare

27 Occupational Safety and Health Administration. (2012). Bloodborne pathogens, standard number 1910.1030. https://www.osha.gov/pls/oshaweb/owadisp.show_document?p_id=10051&p_table=STANDARDS (Level VII)

28 Siegel, J. D., et al. (2007, revised 2019). 2007 guideline for isolation precautions: Preventing transmission of infectious agents in healthcare settings. https://www.cdc.gov/infectioncontrol/pdf/guidelines/isolation-guidelines-H.pdf (Level II)

29 Accreditation Association for Hospitals and Health Systems. (2020). Standard 07.01.10. *Healthcare Facilities Accreditation Program: Accreditation requirements for acute care hospitals.* Chicago, IL: Accreditation Association for Hospitals and Health Systems. (Level VII)

30 The Joint Commission. (2021). Standard RC.01.03.01. *Comprehensive accreditation manual for hospitals.* Oakbrook Terrace, IL: The Joint Commission. (Level VII)

31 Accreditation Association for Hospitals and Health Systems. (2020). Standard 10.00.03. *Healthcare Facilities Accreditation Program: Accreditation requirements for acute care hospitals.* Chicago, IL: Accreditation Association for Hospitals and Health Systems. (Level VII)

32 Centers for Medicare and Medicaid Services, Department of Health and Human Services. (2020). Condition of participation: Medical record services. 42 C.F.R. § 482.24(b).

33 DNV GL-Healthcare USA, Inc. (2020). MR.2.SR.1. *NIAHO® accreditation requirements, interpretive guidelines and surveyor guidance—revision 20.0.* Milford, OH: DNV GL-Healthcare USA, Inc. (Level VII)

34 Perrigo. (2014). Scopolamine transdermal system: Prescribing information. https://www.accessdata.fda.gov/drugsatfda_docs/label/2015/078830Orig1s000lbl.pdf

35 Boehringer Ingelheim. (2011). Catapres-TTS® (clonidine): Prescribing information. https://www.accessdata.fda.gov/drugsatfda_docs/label/2012/018891s028lbl.pdf

36 Wiegand, D. L. (2017). *AACN procedure manual for high acuity, progressive, and critical care* (7th ed.). St. Louis, MO: Elsevier.

37 Kyowa Kirin, Inc. (2017). Sancuso (granisetron transdermal system): Prescribing information. https://www.accessdata.fda.gov/drugsatfda_docs/label/2017/022198s016lbl.pdf

38 U.S. Food and Drug Administration. (2018). FDA drug safety communication: FDA requiring color changes to Duragesic (fentanyl) pain patches to aid safety—emphasizing that accidental exposure to used patches can cause death. https://www.fda.gov/drugs/drug-safety-and-availability/fda-drug-safety-communication-fda-requiring-color-changes-duragesic-fentanyl-pain-patches-aid-safety

39 Burkman, R. T. (2021). Contraception: Transdermal contraceptive patch. In: *UpToDate*, Schreiber, C. A. (Ed.).

40 The Joint Commission. (2021). Standard RC.02.01.01. *Comprehensive accreditation manual for hospitals.* Oakbrook Terrace, IL: The Joint Commission. (Level VII)

TRANSDUCER SYSTEM SETUP

Transducer systems detect intravascular and intracardiac pressures and convert them to an electrical signal that's transmitted to a monitor. The exact type of transducer system used depends on the type of monitoring system, the patient's needs, and the practitioner's preference. Some systems monitor pressure continuously, others intermittently. Single-pressure transducers monitor only one type of pressure—for example, pulmonary artery pressure (PAP). Multiple-pressure transducers can monitor two or more types of pressure, such as PAP and central venous pressure.

Use sterile no-touch technique when setting up a transducer system to reduce the risk of vascular catheter–associated infection.

Keep in mind that the Centers for Medicare and Medicaid Services considers vascular catheter–associated infection a hospital-acquired condition, *because it can be reasonably prevented using a variety of best practices.* Make sure to follow evidence-based infection-prevention practices (such as performing hand hygiene, using sterile no-touch technique, and changing the transducer system setup when indicated) *to reduce the risk of vascular catheter–associated infection.*[1,2,3,4,5,6]

Equipment

Bag of flush solution (usually 500 mL of normal saline solution) ■ pressure infuser bag ■ preassembled disposable pressure tubing with flush device and disposable transducer ■ monitor, pressure module, and pressure cable ■ IV pole with transducer mount ■ leveling device (carpenter's level or laser) ■ sterile, nonvented stopcock caps ■ labels ■ gloves ■ Optional: 500 to 1,000 units of heparin, syringe, gown, mask and goggles or mask with face shield.

Preparation of equipment

Inspect all equipment and supplies. If a product is expired, is defective, or has compromised integrity, remove it from patient use, label it as expired or defective, and report the expiration or defect as directed by your facility.

For initial setup, turn on the monitor and insert the correct pressure module. Plug the pressure cable into the appropriate pressure module. Turn on the correct parameters (for example, pulmonary artery, right atrial, or arterial pressure) *to visualize the correct waveforms.* Set the appropriate scale for the pressure monitored *to obtain accurate pressure readings.*[7]

Implementation

Setting up the system

■ Verify the practitioner's orders.
■ Gather and prepare the necessary equipment and supplies.
■ Perform hand hygiene.[8,9,10,11,12,13]
■ Confirm the patient's identity using at least two patient identifiers.[14]
■ Explain the procedure to the patient and family (if appropriate) according to their individual communication and learning needs *to increase their understanding, allay their fears, and enhance cooperation.*[15]
■ If used in your facility, add the heparin to the flush solution—usually, 1 to 2 units of heparin per milliliter of solution drawn up in a syringe.
NURSING ALERT Although heparin may prevent thrombosis, its use has been associated with thrombocytopenia and other hematologic risks. Because the risks outweigh the benefits, many facilities no longer use it in flush solutions.[7,16]
■ Label the IV flush solution bag with the date and time the solution was prepared, the dose of heparin (if added), and your initials.[7]
■ Remove the preassembled pressure tubing from the package. If necessary, connect the pressure tubing to the transducer. Tighten all tubing connections *to prevent dangerous disconnections.*[17]
■ Spike the outlet port of the IV flush solution bag with the pressure tubing spike, invert the bag, and open the tubing's roller clamp. Then compress the tubing's drip chamber, filling it halfway with the flush solution *to help prevent air bubbles from entering the tubing.*[7] Roll the roller clamp to the closed position.
NURSING ALERT Air in the tubing may dampen the waveform and cause an air embolism.[7]
■ Place the IV flush solution bag into the pressure infuser bag. To do this, hang the pressure infuser bag on the IV pole, and then position the IV flush solution bag inside the pressure infuser bag. Don't inflate the pressure bag, *because priming the tubing under pressure can cause air bubbles to enter the system.*[7]
■ Open the tubing's roller clamp, uncoil the tube if you haven't already done so, and remove the protective cap at the end of the pressure tubing. Slowly activate the continuous flush device *to prime the entire system,* including the stopcock ports, with the IV flush solution *to eliminate air from the transducer system.*
■ As the IV flush solution nears the disposable transducer, hold the transducer at a 45-degree angle (as shown to the right) *to force any air out of the transducer system.*

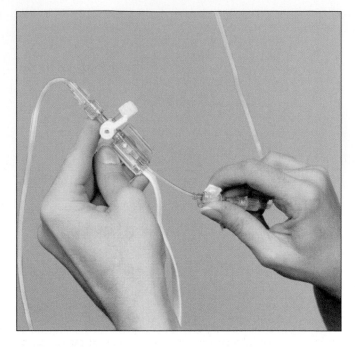

■ When the IV flush solution nears the stopcock, open the stopcock to air, allowing the solution to flow into the stopcock (as shown below). When the stopcock fills, close it to air and turn it open to the remainder of the tubing.

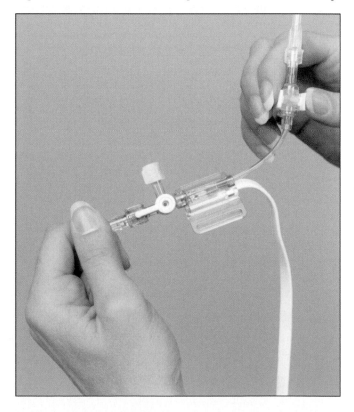

■ After removing the air from the stopcock, replace the vented cap with a sterile, nonvented cap *to prevent bacteria and air from entering the transducer system.*[7]
■ After you've completely primed the system, replace the protective cap at the end of the pressure tubing.
■ Inflate the pressure infuser bag to 300 mm Hg *to allow delivery of 1 to 3 mL/hour of IV flush solution through the access catheter, minimizing clot formation and maintaining access catheter patency.*[7] Ensure that the pressure tubing's drip chamber doesn't completely fill with fluid as you inflate the pressure bag.
■ Insert the transducer device into the IV pole mount holder *to secure the transducer,* if used.[7]

■ Label the pressure tubing with the date of initiation or the date of change as directed by your facility.[18]

■ Before connecting the pressure monitoring system to the patient's access catheter, level and zero the transducer. Zero the system during initial setup, if the transducer system is disconnected from the monitoring cable, if the monitoring cable is disconnected from the monitor, and when blood pressure values don't correspond with the patient's clinical status *to minimize the number of entries into the pressure monitoring system, which reduces the risk of vascular catheter-associated infection.*[7]

Leveling and zeroing the system

■ Perform hand hygiene.[8,9,10,11,12,13]

■ Put on gloves and, as needed, other personal protective equipment *to comply with standard precautions.*[19,20,21]

■ Position the patient supine, with the head of the bed elevated up to 60 degrees.[22] If the patient can't tolerate such positioning, use a prone or a 20-, 30-, or 90-degree lateral position, as appropriate.[7,22]

■ If the patient is in the supine or prone position, use a leveling device to position the air-reference stopcock or the air–fluid interface of the transducer level with the phlebostatic axis (midway between the posterior chest and the sternum at the fourth intercostal space, midaxillary line).[7,22] If the patient is in a lateral position, level the air-reference stopcock or the air–fluid interface of the transducer at the lateral angle–specific reference.[22]

■ After leveling the transducer, turn the stopcock located next to the transducer off to the patient and open to air. Remove the cap to the stopcock port.

■ Zero the transducer following the manufacturer's directions for zeroing.

■ When you've finished zeroing the transducer, turn the stopcock so that it's in a monitoring position with the stopcock closed to air and open to the side of the pressure tubing that leads to the patient. Place a new, sterile, nonvented cap on the stopcock *to maintain sterility.* Now you've assembled a single-pressure transducer system (as shown below).

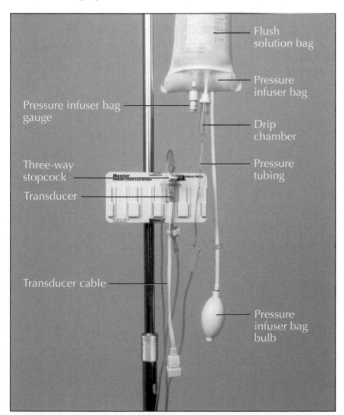

Pressure infuser bag gauge

Three-way stopcock

Transducer

Transducer cable

Flush solution bag

Pressure infuser bag

Drip chamber

Pressure tubing

Pressure infuser bag bulb

Connecting the pressure tubing to the appropriate IV catheter port

■ Using sterile no-touch technique, remove the cap at the end of the pressure tubing and then connect the end of the pressure tubing to the

appropriate catheter port (pulmonary artery, right atrial, or arterial) *to enable pressure monitoring.*[7]

■ Trace the tubing from the patient to its point of origin *to make sure that you've connected it to the proper port.*[17,23]

■ Assess the pressure waveforms *to ensure that the transducer system is functioning properly.* Perform a square wave test *to ensure that the pressure waveform components are clearly defined to aid in accurate pressure measurement.*[7]

■ Ensure that the hemodynamic monitoring system alarms are turned on, alarm limits are appropriate for the patient's present condition, and alarms are audible and functioning properly.[24,25,26]

■ Remove and discard your gloves, and other personal protective equipment if worn.[19]

Completing the procedure

■ Perform hand hygiene.[8,9,10,11,12,13]

■ Document the procedure.[27,28,29,30]

Special considerations

■ The Joint Commission has issued a sentinel event alert concerning medical device alarm safety, *because alarm-related events have been associated with permanent loss of function or death.* Among the major contributing factors were improper alarm settings, alarms turned off improperly, and alarm signals that were inaudible to staff. Ensure that alarm limits are set appropriately, and that alarms are turned on, functioning properly, and audible to staff. Follow facility guidelines for preventing alarm fatigue.[24]

■ Regularly assess the transducer system *to make sure that the IV flush solution bag contains fluid, the system is free of air bubbles, the pressure infuser bag pressure is maintained at 300 mm Hg, and all connections are secured tightly.*[7]

■ Change disposable or reusable transducer systems, including administration set, continuous flush device, and flush solution used for invasive hemodynamic pressure monitoring, every 96 hours; change immediately when contamination is suspected or when the integrity of the product or system is compromised. Limit the number of manipulations and entries to the system.[18]

Complications

Infection may result if sterility of the transducer system isn't maintained.

Documentation

Document the patient's position for leveling and zeroing so that other health care team members can replicate the positioning for subsequent assessments. Document the type of IV flush solution used and the date and time of pressure tubing changes. Record any unexpected outcomes and your interventions. Document teaching provided to the patient and family (if applicable), their understanding of that teaching, and any need for follow-up teaching.

REFERENCES

1 Centers for Disease Control and Prevention. (2011, revised 2017). Guidelines for the prevention of intravascular catheter-related infections. https://www.cdc.gov/infectioncontrol/guidelines/bsi/recommendations. html (Level I)

2 Jarrett, N., & Callaham, M. (2016). Evidence-based guidelines for selected hospital-acquired conditions: Final report. https://www.cms.gov/Medicare/ Medicare-Fee-for-Service-Payment/HospitalAcqCond/Downloads/2016-HAC-Report.pdf

3 Association of Professionals in Infection Control and Epidemiology. (2015). Guide to preventing central line-associated bloodstream infections. http://apic.org/Resource_/TinyMceFileManager/2015/APIC_CLABSI_ WEB.pdf (Level IV)

4 Marschall, J., et al. (2014). SHEA/IDSA practice recommendation: Strategies to prevent central line-associated bloodstream infections in acute care hospitals. *Infection Control and Hospital Epidemiology, 35*(7), 753–771. https://www.jstor.org/stable/10.1086/676533#metadata_info_ tab_contents (Level I)

5 Standard 50. Infection. Infusion therapy standards of practice (8th ed.). (2021). *Journal of Infusion Nursing, 44*(Suppl. 1), S153–S157. (Level VII)

6 The Joint Commission. (2021). Standard NPSG.07.04.01. *Comprehensive accreditation manual for hospitals*. Oakbrook Terrace, IL: The Joint Commission. (Level VII)

7 Wiegand, D. L. (2017). *AACN procedure manual for high acuity, progressive, and critical care* (7th ed.). St. Louis, MO: Elsevier.

8 The Joint Commission. (2021). Standard NPSG.07.01.01. *Comprehensive accreditation manual for hospitals*. Oakbrook Terrace, IL: The Joint Commission. (Level VII)

9 Centers for Disease Control and Prevention. (2002). Guideline for hand hygiene in health-care settings: Recommendations of the Healthcare Infection Control Practices Advisory Committee and the HICPAC/SHEA/APIC/IDSA Hand Hygiene Task Force. *MMWR Recommendations and Reports, 51*(RR-16), 1–45. https://www.cdc.gov/mmwr/pdf/rr/rr5116.pdf (Level II)

10 World Health Organization (WHO). (2009). WHO guidelines on hand hygiene in health care: First global patient safety challenge, clean care is safer care. https://apps.who.int/iris/bitstream/handle/10665/44102/9789241597906_eng.pdf?sequence=1 (Level IV)

11 Accreditation Association for Hospitals and Health Systems. (2020). Standard 07.01.21. *Healthcare Facilities Accreditation Program: Accreditation requirements for acute care hospitals*. Chicago, IL: Accreditation Association for Hospitals and Health Systems. (Level VII)

12 Centers for Medicare and Medicaid Services. (2020). Condition of participation: Infection control. 42 C.F.R. § 482.42.

13 DNV GL-Healthcare USA, Inc. (2020). IC.1.SR.1. *NIAHO® accreditation requirements, interpretive guidelines and surveyor guidance—revision 20.0*. Milford, OH: DNV GL-Healthcare USA, Inc. (Level VII)

14 The Joint Commission. (2021). Standard NPSG.01.01.01. *Comprehensive accreditation manual for hospitals*. Oakbrook Terrace, IL: The Joint Commission. (Level VII)

15 The Joint Commission. (2021). Standard PC.02.01.21. *Comprehensive accreditation manual for hospitals*. Oakbrook Terrace, IL: The Joint Commission. (Level VII)

16 Coutre, S., & Crowther, M. (2021). Clinical presentation and diagnosis of heparin-induced thrombocytopenia. In: *UpToDate*, Leung, L. L. K. (Ed.).

17 U.S. Food and Drug Administration. (2017). Examples of medical device misconnections. https://www.fda.gov/medical-devices/medical-device-connectors/examples-medical-device-misconnections

18 Standard 43. Administration set management. Infusion therapy standards of practice (8th ed.). (2021). *Journal of Infusion Nursing, 44*(Suppl. 1), S123–S125. (Level VII)

19 Occupational Safety and Health Administration. (2012). Bloodborne pathogens, standard number 1910.1030. https://www.osha.gov/pls/oshaweb/owadisp.show_document?p_id=10051&p_table=STANDARDS (Level VII)

20 Accreditation Association for Hospitals and Health Systems. (2020). Standard 07.01.10. *Healthcare Facilities Accreditation Program: Accreditation requirements for acute care hospitals*. Chicago, IL: Accreditation Association for Hospitals and Health Systems. (Level VII)

21 Siegel, J. D., et al. (2007, revised 2019). 2007 guideline for isolation precautions: Preventing transmission of infectious agents in healthcare settings. https://www.cdc.gov/infectioncontrol/pdf/guidelines/isolation-guidelines-H.pdf (Level II)

22 American Association of Critical-Care Nurses (AACN). (2017). AACN practice alert: Pulmonary artery/central venous pressure monitoring in adults. https://www.aacn.org/-/media/aacn-website/linical-resources/practice-alerts/pap2017practicealert.pdf (Level VII)

23 The Joint Commission. (2014). Sentinel event alert 53: Managing risk during transition to new ISO tubing connector standards. https://www.jointcommission.org/-/media/tjc/documents/resources/patient-safety-topics/sentinel-event/sea_53_connectors_8_19_14_final.pdf (Level VII)

24 The Joint Commission. (2013). Sentinel event alert 50: Medical device alarm safety in hospitals. https://www.jointcommission.org/-/media/tjc/documents/resources/patient-safety-topics/sentinel-event/sea_50_alarms_4_26_16.pdf (Level VII)

25 Graham, K. C., & Cvach, M. (2010). Monitor alarm fatigue: Standardizing use of physiological monitors and decreasing nuisance alarms. *American Journal of Critical Care, 19*(1), 28–37. https://doi.org/10.4037/ajcc2010651

26 The Joint Commission. (2021). Standard NPSG.06.01.01. *Comprehensive accreditation manual for hospitals*. Oakbrook Terrace, IL: The Joint Commission. (Level VII)

27 The Joint Commission. (2021). Standard RC.01.03.01. *Comprehensive accreditation manual for hospitals*. Oakbrook Terrace, IL: The Joint Commission. (Level VII)

28 Accreditation Association for Hospitals and Health Systems. (2020). Standard 10.00.03. *Healthcare Facilities Accreditation Program: Accreditation requirements for acute care hospitals*. Chicago, IL: Accreditation Association for Hospitals and Health Systems. (Level VII)

29 Centers for Medicare and Medicaid Services, Department of Health and Human Services. (2020). Condition of participation: Medical record services. 42 C.F.R. § 482.24(b).

30 DNV GL-Healthcare USA, Inc. (2020). MR.2.SR.1. *NIAHO® accreditation requirements, interpretive guidelines and surveyor guidance—revision 20.0*. Milford, OH: DNV GL-Healthcare USA, Inc. (Level VII)

TRANSFER WITHIN A FACILITY

Patient transfer requires thorough preparation and documentation. Preparation includes an explanation of the transfer to the patient and family and discussion of the patient's condition and care plan with staff members on the receiving unit.[1] Documentation of the patient's condition before and during transfer and adequate communication between the nursing staff members ensures continuity of nursing care, and provides legal protection for the transferring unit and its staff.[2]

Equipment

Admission inventory of belongings ▪ patient's medical and medication record ▪ prescribed medications ▪ patient belongings ▪ bag ▪ transfer vehicle (wheelchair, bed, or stretcher) ▪ Optional: oxygen tank, oxygen administration tubing, blankets, pulse oximeter, cardiac monitor and defibrillator, handheld resuscitation bag and mask, equipment specific to the patient's condition, reusable supplies, wheeled poles for equipment.

Implementation

▪ Verify the practitioner's order for transfer.

▪ If the patient is being transferred from or to an intensive care unit, your facility may require new care orders from the patient's practitioner. If so, review the new orders with the nursing staff at the receiving unit during hand-off communication.[2,3]

▪ Perform hand hygiene.[4,5,6,7,8,9]

▪ Confirm the patient's identity using at least two patient identifiers.[10]

▪ Provide privacy.[11,12,13,14]

▪ Explain the transfer to the patient and family (if appropriate) according to their individual communication and learning needs *to increase their understanding, allay their fears, and enhance cooperation*.[15] If the patient is anxious about the transfer or the patient's condition precludes patient teaching, be sure to explain the reason for the transfer to family, especially if the transfer is the result of a serious change in the patient's condition.[1]

▪ Assess the patient's physical condition *to determine the means of transfer, such as a wheelchair, bed, or stretcher*.[16]

▪ If the patient requires continuous oxygen or mechanical ventilation, arrange for the respiratory therapy department to provide support during the transfer.[3]

▪ Provide hand-off communication to the nurse who will assume responsibility for the patient's care in the receiving unit. Make sure to cover everything needed to safely care for the patient in a timely fashion, including the patient's medication regimen and the nursing care plan, *to ensure continuity of care*.[3,17,18] Provide face-to-face hand-off communication when possible. If not possible, communicate in real time by telephone or video conference.[18] Provide ample time and opportunity for questions *to avoid miscommunications that can cause patient care errors*.[3,17,18] Use a hand-off communication technique, such as the Situation-Background-Assessment-Recommendation (SBAR) or other facility-approved communication technique, *to improve communication and reduce errors*.[18,19]

▪ Ensure that the reconciled list of the patient's medications has been communicated to the next practitioner who will be caring for the patient, and that the communication is documented in the patient's medical record, *to reduce the risk of transition-related adverse medication events*.[20,21]

▪ Verify that the new room in the receiving unit is ready for the patient's arrival.

■ Use the admissions inventory of patient property from the patient's medical record as a checklist to collect the patient's belongings and place them in a patient's belongings bag. Be sure to check the entire room, including the closet, bedside stand, overbed table, and bathroom.

■ Gather the patient's medications that are stored outside of the automated dispensing machine and send them to the receiving unit upon transfer. Send any special equipment and other required materials to the receiving unit.[3] *Moving such articles with the patient helps prevent loss and duplicate charges for equipment and supplies.*

■ Obtain assistance as needed. *Additional personnel may be needed based on the patient's condition and the amount of support equipment being transferred.*

■ Secure all IV lines, feeding tubes, monitoring leads, and other equipment, as needed, *to help prevent lines from becoming dislodged during the transfer.* If possible, attach electronic infusion devices and other equipment to the transfer vehicle. If equipment can't be attached to the transfer vehicle, have someone assist with wheeling the poles.

■ Use a wheelchair to transport the ambulatory patient to the newly assigned room unless it's on the same unit as the present room, in which case you may allow the patient to walk. Use a stretcher or bed to transport a patient whose condition doesn't permit transfer in a wheelchair.

■ Cover the patient with blankets, as needed, *to prevent the patient from becoming hypothermic.*

■ Raise the patient's bed to waist level before transferring the patient in a bed or stretcher *to prevent caregiver back strain.*[22] Then take the patient to the assigned room and, depending on the patient's condition, place the patient in the bed or seat the patient in a chair.

■ Notify the receiving unit's nursing staff of the patient's arrival.

■ Set up electronic infusion devices and monitors, as appropriate. If medical devices are necessary, make sure that that alarm limits are set appropriately for the patient's condition, and that the alarms are turned on, functioning properly, and audible to staff.[23,24,25,26,27]

■ If present, trace IV tubing from the patient to the point of origin *to make sure it's connected to the proper port.* Route the tubing in a standardized direction if the patient has other tubing and catheters that have different purposes. If the patient requires multiple IV lines, label the tubing at the distal end (near the patient) and proximal end (near the source container) *to reduce the risk of misconnection.*[28,29]

■ Return the bed to the lowest position *to prevent falls and maintain patient safety.*[30]

■ Introduce the patient and family to the receiving nurse on the new unit. Tell the patient about any unfamiliar equipment, such as the call light. Make sure the call light is within the patient's reach *to ensure patient safety.*

■ Provide additional hand-off communication to the patient's new nurse, as needed. Answer any questions the nurse on the receiving unit may have regarding the patient's condition or care, *to avoid miscommunication that can cause patient care errors during transition of care.*[3,17,18] As part of the hand-off process, allow time for the receiving staff member to trace each tubing and catheter from the patient to its point of origin using a standardized line reconciliation process.[29]

■ Perform hand hygiene.[4,5,6,7,8,9]

■ Document the procedure.[31,32,33,34]

Special considerations

■ Before transferring the patient, make sure that, as appropriate, you have suctioned the patient's airway, administered prescribed medications, completed scheduled procedures, changed soiled dressings, bathed the incontinent patient, and emptied drainage collection devices.

Complications

A change in the patient's condition may occur or go unnoticed if the equipment is dislodged or disconnected during transfer.

Documentation

Record the time and date of transfer, the patient's condition during transfer, the name of the receiving unit, and the mode of transfer. Document equipment accompanying the patient, such as IV lines and electronic infusion devices, surgical drains, and oxygen therapy equipment. Note the name and title of the person to whom you provided hand-off communication in the receiving unit; also, include the names of staff or family accompanying the patient. Document teaching provided to the patient and family (if applicable), their understanding of that teaching, and any need for follow-up teaching.

REFERENCES

1 The Joint Commission. (2021). Standard PC.04.01.05. *Comprehensive accreditation manual for hospitals.* Oakbrook Terrace, IL: The Joint Commission. (Level VII)

2 The Joint Commission. (2021). Standard PC.04.01.01. *Comprehensive accreditation manual for hospitals.* Oakbrook Terrace, IL: The Joint Commission. (Level VII)

3 The Joint Commission. (2021). Standard PC.04.02.01. *Comprehensive accreditation manual for hospitals.* Oakbrook Terrace, IL: The Joint Commission. (Level VII)

4 Centers for Disease Control and Prevention. (2002). Guideline for hand hygiene in health-care settings: Recommendations of the Healthcare Infection Control Practices Advisory Committee and the HICPAC/SHEA/APIC/IDSA Hand Hygiene Task Force. *MMWR Recommendations and Reports, 51*(RR-16), 1–45. https://www.cdc.gov/mmwr/pdf/rr/rr5116.pdf (Level II)

5 World Health Organization. (2009). WHO guidelines on hand hygiene in health care: First global patient safety challenge, clean care is safer care. https://apps.who.int/iris/bitstream/handle/10665/44102/9789241597906_eng.pdf?sequence=1 (Level IV)

6 The Joint Commission. (2021). Standard NPSG.07.01.01. *Comprehensive accreditation manual for hospitals.* Oakbrook Terrace, IL: The Joint Commission. (Level VII)

7 Accreditation Association for Hospitals and Health Systems. (2020). Standard 07.01.21. *Healthcare Facilities Accreditation Program: Accreditation requirements for acute care hospitals.* Chicago, IL: Accreditation Association for Hospitals and Health Systems. (Level VII)

8 Centers for Medicare and Medicaid Services, Department of Health and Human Services. (2020). Condition of participation: Infection control. 42 C.F.R. § 482.42

9 DNV GL-Healthcare USA, Inc. (2020). IC.1.SR.1. *NIAHO® accreditation requirements, interpretive guidelines and surveyor guidance—revision 20.0.* Milford, OH: DNV GL-Healthcare USA, Inc. (Level VII)

10 The Joint Commission. (2021). Standard NPSG.01.01.01. *Comprehensive accreditation manual for hospitals.* Oakbrook Terrace, IL: The Joint Commission. (Level VII)

11 Accreditation Association for Hospitals and Health Systems. (2020). Standard 15.01.16. *Healthcare Facilities Accreditation Program: Accreditation requirements for acute care hospitals.* Chicago, IL: Accreditation Association for Hospitals and Health Systems. (Level VII)

12 The Joint Commission. (2021). Standard RI.01.01.01. *Comprehensive accreditation manual for hospitals.* Oakbrook Terrace, IL: The Joint Commission. (Level VII)

13 DNV GL-Healthcare USA, Inc. (2020). PR.2.SR.5. *NIAHO® accreditation requirements, interpretive guidelines and surveyor guidance—revision 20.0.* Milford, OH: DNV GL-Healthcare USA, Inc (Level VII)

14 Centers for Medicare and Medicaid Services, Department of Health and Human Services. (2020). Condition of participation: Patient's rights. 42 C.F.R. § 482.13(c)(1).

15 The Joint Commission. (2021). Standard PC.02.01.21. *Comprehensive accreditation manual for hospitals.* Oakbrook Terrace, IL: The Joint Commission. (Level VII)

16 The Joint Commission. (2021). Standard PC.04.01.03. *Comprehensive accreditation manual for hospitals.* Oakbrook Terrace, IL: The Joint Commission. (Level VII)

17 The Joint Commission. (2021). Standard PC.02.02.01. *Comprehensive accreditation manual for hospitals.* Oakbrook Terrace, IL: The Joint Commission. (Level VII)

18 The Joint Commission. (2017). Sentinel event alert 58: Inadequate hand-off communication" https://www.jointcommission.org/-/media/tjc/documents/resources/patient-safety-topics/sentinel-event/sea_58_hand_off_comms_9_6_17_final_(1).pdf (Level VII)

19 Institute for Healthcare Improvement. (n.d.). SBAR tool: Situation-Background-Assessment-Recommendation. http://www.ihi.org/resources/Pages/Tools/SBARToolkit.aspx (Level V)

20 The Joint Commission. (2021). Standard NPSG.03.06.01. *Comprehensive accreditation manual for hospitals.* Oakbrook Terrace, IL: The Joint Commission. (Level VII)

21 Accreditation Association for Hospitals and Health Systems. (2020). Standard 25.02.13. *Healthcare Facilities Accreditation Program: Accreditation requirements for acute care hospitals.* Chicago, IL: Accreditation Association for Hospitals and Health Systems. (Level VII)

22 Waters, T. R., et al. (2009). Safe patient handling training for schools of nursing. https://www.cdc.gov/niosh/docs/2009-127/pdfs/2009-127.pdf (Level VII)

23 The Joint Commission. (2013). Sentinel event alert 50: Medical device alarm safety in hospitals. https://www.jointcommission.org/assets/1/6/ SEA_50_alarms_4_26_16.pdf (Level VII)

24 The Joint Commission. (2021). Standard NPSG.06.01.01. *Comprehensive accreditation manual for hospitals.* Oakbrook Terrace, IL: The Joint Commission. (Level VII)

25 American Association of Critical-Care Nurses. (2018). AACN practice alert: Managing alarms in acute care across the life span: Electrocardiography and pulse oximetry. https://www.aacn.org/clinical-resources/practice-alerts/managing-alarms-in-acute-care-across-the-life-span (Level VII)

26 Graham, K. C., & Cvach, M. (2010). Monitor alarm fatigue: Standardizing use of physiological monitors and decreasing nuisance alarms. *American Journal of Critical Care, 19,* 28–37.

27 Jacques, S., & Williams, E. (2016). Reducing the safety hazards of monitor alert and alarm fatigue. https://psnet.ahrq.gov/perspective/reducing-safety-hazards-monitor-alert-and-alarm-fatigue (Level VII)

28 U.S. Food and Drug Administration. (2017). Examples of medical device misconnections. https://www.fda.gov/medical-devices/ medical-device-connectors/examples-medical-device-misconnections

29 The Joint Commission. (2014). Sentinel event alert 53: Managing risk during transition to new ISO tubing connector standards. https://www. jointcommission.org/-/media/tjc/documents/resources/patient-safety-topics/sentinel-event/sea_53_connectors_8_19_14_final.pdf (Level VII)

30 Ganz, D. A., et al. (2013, reviewed 2021). *Preventing falls in hospitals: A toolkit for improving quality of care* (AHRQ Publication No. 13-0015-EF). Rockville, MD: Agency for Healthcare Research and Quality. https://www. ahrq.gov/professionals/systems/hospital/fallpxtoolkit/index.html (Level VII)

31 The Joint Commission. (2021). Standard RC.01.03.01. *Comprehensive accreditation manual for hospitals.* Oakbrook Terrace, IL: The Joint Commission. (Level VII)

32 Centers for Medicare and Medicaid Services, Department of Health and Human Services. (2020). Condition of participation: Medical record services. 42 C.F.R. § 482.24(b).

33 Accreditation Association for Hospitals and Health Systems. (2020). Standard 10.00.03. *Healthcare Facilities Accreditation Program: Accreditation requirements for acute care hospitals.* Chicago, IL: Accreditation Association for Hospitals and Health Systems. (Level VII)

34 DNV GL-Healthcare USA, Inc. (2020). MR.2.SR.1. *NIAHO® accreditation requirements, interpretive guidelines and surveyor guidance—revision 20.0.* Milford, OH: DNV GL-Healthcare USA, Inc. (Level VII)

Transfusion of blood and blood products

The transfusion of blood and blood products can be a lifesaving procedure, but it does have its risks. Errors, such as the administration of the wrong blood to the wrong patient, can lead to long-term health problems and even death. Use extreme caution when preparing a patient to receive a blood transfusion. Following procedures that ensure accurate identification of the patient and verifying blood transfusion components can help prevent potentially fatal errors.[1]

HOSPITAL-ACQUIRED CONDITION ALERT Keep in mind that the Centers for Medicare and Medicaid Services considers a blood incompatibility errors a hospital-acquired condition, *because it can be reasonably prevented using a variety of best practices.* Make sure to follow evidence-based prevention practices, such as carefully identifying the patient and blood sample for compatibility testing, and participating in a two-person verification process before blood or blood product administration, *to reduce the risk of incompatibility errors.*[2,3]

When implementing your facility's identification and verification process, don't transfuse any blood product that doesn't match the patient's assigned identification number. Keep in mind that plasma, platelets, and blood derivatives can also cause serious transfusion reactions, so administer them with care.[1]

Before administering blood or a blood product, health care professionals should be familiar with the different types of blood and blood products. (See *Transfusing blood and selected blood products.*)

Equipment

Blood or blood component administration set ▪ IV pole ▪ gloves ▪ blood or blood product ▪ preservative-free normal saline solution ▪ 3-mL syringe ▪ antiseptic pad (chlorhexidine-based, povidone-iodine, or alcohol) ▪ disinfectant pad ▪ stethoscope ▪ vital signs monitoring equipment ▪ blood request form ▪ Optional: prescribed premedications, 250 mL of normal saline solution, IV catheter equipment (should include 18G to 24G catheters),[6] electronic infusion device indicated for blood transfusion use,[6] blood warming device and administration set, mask, protective eyewear, gown, pulse oximeter and probe, venipuncture equipment, labels.

Straight line and Y-type blood administration sets contain a standard 170- to 260-micron blood filter designed to eliminate blood clots and cellular debris that occur during blood storage.[6] Sometimes, however, a specialized blood filter may be required.[1] (See *Specialized blood filters,* page 854.)

Preparation of equipment

Inspect all equipment and supplies. If a product is expired, is defective, or has compromised integrity, remove it from patient use, label it as expired or defective, and report the expiration or defect as directed by your facility.

Avoid obtaining the blood or blood product until you're ready to begin the transfusion. Prepare the equipment when you're ready to start the infusion. If the patient has a history of adverse reactions, administer premedication, as prescribed, following safe medication administration practices.[8,9,10,11] *To ensure effectiveness,* administer oral medication 30 minutes before starting the transfusion. If IV medication is prescribed, administer it immediately before starting the transfusion.[1]

Implementation

▪ Verify the practitioner's order. Confirm that the order addresses the indication for transfusion, the preparation of the product, and administration (including the start time and rate of infusion).[1,12] Confirm that the order and the medical record are labeled with the patient's first and last name and unique identification number.[6]

▪ Unless the transfusion is an emergency, confirm that informed consent has been obtained before initiating transfusion therapy, and that the signed consent form is in the patient's medical record.[13,14,15,16,17]

▪ Review the patient's medication regimen; *certain medications, such as antifungal agents and chemotherapy, might not be recommended for infusion during blood transfusion.*[1] Consult with the patient's practitioner if necessary.

▪ Ensure that a blood sample was obtained for compatibility testing; collect a blood sample if one hasn't been collected. (See the "Venipuncture" procedure.) Blood samples must be collected within 3 days of red blood cell (RBC) transfusion if the patient has been pregnant within the preceding 3 months or has been transfused within the preceding 3 months, or if the patient's history is uncertain or unavailable.[1]

▪ Make sure that transfusion services receives a blood request form that contains the patient's first and last name, an identification number unique to the patient, the prescribed blood component and amount ordered, and the name of the responsible practitioner. (A computer-transmitted request is acceptable if it contains the required information.) Additional information, such as the patient's age, sex, diagnosis, transfusion history, pregnancy history, and special blood component or service needs, as well as the date and time of blood sample collection for compatibility testing, may be helpful in resolving any problems that may occur.[1]

▪ Gather and prepare the necessary equipment and supplies.

▪ Perform hand hygiene.[18,19,20,21,22,23,24,25]

▪ Confirm the patient's identity using at least two patient identifiers.[1,26]

▪ Provide privacy.[27,28,29,30]

▪ Verify that the patient's religious beliefs don't prohibit blood transfusion therapy.[1]

Transfusing blood and selected blood products

BLOOD COMPONENT	INDICATIONS	COMPATIBILITY	NURSING CONSIDERATIONS
Red blood cells (RBCs) Concentrate of RBCs from whole blood[4]	■ To restore or maintain oxygen-carrying capacity in symptomatic anemia ■ To increase RBC mass in acute anemia caused by trauma, surgical blood loss, or chemotherapy[1] ■ To increase RBC mass in chronic anemia with associated cardiovascular decompensation[1]	■ Group A receives A or O.[1] ■ Group B receives B or O.[1] ■ Group AB receives AB, A, B, or O.[1] ■ Group O receives O.[1] ■ Rh-negative recipients can only receive Rh-negative RBCs.[1] ■ Rh-positive recipients can receive Rh-positive or Rh-negative RBCs.	■ Transfuse RBCs through a sterile, pyrogen-free transfusion set with an appropriate filter. ■ Prime the administration set with normal saline solution if using a Y-type administration set. ■ Ensure that the transfusion is started within the facility-designated time of removal from transfusion services (for example, 30 minutes).[1,5] ■ Start the transfusion at a slow rate, as prescribed, and increase the rate as prescribed if no signs of a reaction occur to ensure completion of the transfusion within 4 hours.[1,6,7] ■ Avoid administration for anemia that's correctable with nutrition or drug therapy.[1]
Leukocyte-reduced RBCs Concentrate of RBCs from whole blood with white blood cells removed from the blood component during apheresis collection or by filtration of the blood product.[4]	■ To restore or maintain oxygen-carrying capacity in symptomatic anemia in patients at risk for reactions caused by leukocyte antibodies[1] ■ To treat symptomatic anemia in immunocompromised patients ■ To increase RBC mass in acute anemia caused by trauma, surgical blood loss, or chemotherapy in patients at risk for reactions caused by leukocyte antibodies ■ To increase RBC mass in chronic anemia with associated cardiovascular decompensation in patients at risk for reactions caused by leukocyte antibodies	■ Group A receives A or O.[1] ■ Group B receives B or O.[1] ■ Group AB receives AB, A, B, or O.[1] ■ Group O receives O.[1] ■ Rh-positive recipients receive Rh-positive or Rh-negative RBCs.[1] ■ Rh-negative recipients receive only Rh-negative RBCs.[1]	■ Transfuse the RBCs through a sterile, pyrogen-free transfusion set with an appropriate filter. ■ Prime the administration set with normal saline solution if using a Y-type administration set. ■ Ensure that the transfusion is started within the facility-designated time of removal from transfusion services (for example, 30 minutes).[5] ■ Start the transfusion at a slow rate, as prescribed, and increase the rate as prescribed if no signs of a reaction occur to ensure completion of the transfusion within 4 hours.[1,7] ■ RBCs can be collected in special multiple-bag units so that the patient can receive a small volume of blood multiple times from the same donor. ■ Avoid administration for anemia that's correctable with nutrition or drug therapy.[1]
Platelets Concentrate of platelets separated from whole blood obtained by apheresis or pooled from multiple donors	■ To control bleeding that results from decreased circulating platelets or malfunctioning platelets.[1] ■ To increase platelet count in a patient who requires an invasive procedure ■ To prevent bleeding in a patient with a low platelet count	■ Donor plasma should be ABO-compatible with the recipient's RBCs when large volumes are given to adults ■ Rh-negative recipients receive Rh-negative platelets when possible, especially in women going through childbirth	■ Transfuse through a sterile, pyrogen-free transfusion set with an appropriate filter. (Don't use a microaggregate filter.)[1] A leukocyte-reduction filter may be necessary if leukocyte-reduced platelets aren't available. ■ Transfusion may proceed as quickly as tolerated, but must take less than 4 hours. ■ Patients who don't benefit from transfusion with non-human leukocyte antigen (HLA) platelets may benefit from HLA platelets.
Plasma Noncellular portion of blood that's separated and frozen after donation and contains coagulation factors and other proteins	■ To temporarily reverse the effects of warfarin[1] ■ For plasma exchange (especially for thrombotic thrombocytopenia)[1] ■ To treat factor deficiency if concentrate is unavailable[1] ■ To correct abnormal coagulation test results before invasive procedures[1] ■ To treat liver disease with protein synthetic defect[1] ■ To treat dilutional coagulopathy[1] ■ To treat consumptive coagulopathy[1]	■ Group A receives A or AB ■ Group B receives B or AB ■ Group AB receives AB ■ Group O receives O, A, B, or AB ■ Rh matching not required	■ Transfuse through a sterile, pyrogen-free transfusion set with an appropriate filter. ■ Infuse immediately after thawing. ■ Administration is usually over 30 to 60 minutes.[1]
Cryoprecipitate Also known as *cryoprecipitated antihemophilic factor*; noncellular blood component that's prepared by thawing fresh frozen plasma, recovering the insoluble precipitate, and then refreezing the precipitate within 1 hour of collection; contains concentrated levels of fibrinogen, Factor VIII, von Willebrand factor, Factor XIII, and fibronectin[4]	■ To treat factor deficiency when factor-specific concentrate is unavailable[1] ■ To treat hypofibrinogenemia[1] ■ To treat dysfibrinogenemia[1] ■ To treat von Willebrand disease[1] ■ To correct fibronectin deficiency[1]	■ ABO compatibility not required but preferred[1] ■ Rh matching not required	■ Transfuse through a sterile, pyrogen-free transfusion set with an appropriate filter. ■ Infuse immediately after thawing. ■ May be administered through a small-gauge IV catheter. ■ Administration is usually over 15 to 30 minutes.[1]

EQUIPMENT

Specialized blood filters

When determined to be medically necessary, specialized filters are used to transfuse blood and blood products.[6]

FILTER TYPE	CONSIDERATIONS
Microaggregate filter	■ Eliminates debris as small as 20 microns ■ Use isn't warranted in routine transfusion therapy[1,6] ■ Not appropriate for granulocyte infusions[1] ■ May be indicated for use with extracorporeal membrane oxygenation circuits, preparation of intraoperative blood recovery collections, or infusion of wound drainage collections[1]
Leucocyte reduction filter	■ Reduces the number of leukocytes by 99.9% in red blood cell and platelet units ■ May be used to reduce the risk of transfusion complications if a prestorage leukocyte-reduced blood unit isn't available[1,6] ■ Requires close following of the manufacturer's instructions for use[1]

■ Explain the procedure to the patient and family (if appropriate) according to their individual communication and learning needs *to increase their understanding, allay their fears, and enhance cooperation.*[31]
■ Perform hand hygiene.[18,19,20,21,22,23,24,25]
■ Put on gloves *to comply with standard precautions.*[22,32,33,34,35,36]
■ Ensure that the patient has adequate venous access with an appropriate-sized catheter (for short peripheral catheters, 20G to 24G based on vein size and patient preference; 18G to 20G if rapid infusion is required).[6] Verify patency by aspirating for blood return.[6,37] Insert an IV catheter if necessary. (See the "IV catheter insertion and removal" procedure.) A central venous catheter is also an acceptable option for blood transfusion.[1,6]
■ Remove and discard your gloves.[32,34,38]
■ Perform hand hygiene.[18,19,20,21,22,23,24,25]
■ Obtain and record the patient's vital signs immediately before initiating the transfusion *to serve as a baseline for comparison.*[1,6]
■ Assess the patient's breath and heart sounds, skin color, and current laboratory test results, such as hemoglobin and hematocrit. Identify any conditions that may increase the risk of a transfusion reaction, such as fever, heart failure, kidney disease, or the risk of fluid volume excess.[5,6]
■ Question the patient about the presence of signs and symptoms that may later be mistaken for a transfusion reaction, such as chills, itching, rash, hematuria, muscle aches, and difficulty breathing.[1]
■ Assist the patient to the bathroom if necessary before beginning the transfusion.[1]
■ Help the patient assume a comfortable position either in a chair or bed; *providing patient comfort before the transfusion helps to reduce the number of manipulations of the blood and tubing during the course of the procedure.*[1]
■ If the patient is in bed, raise the bed to waist level before providing care *to prevent caregiver back strain.*[39]
■ Offer the patient diversional activities, such as reading materials, television, radio, and games, *to allay anxiety during the transfusion.*[1]
■ Perform hand hygiene.[18,19,20,21,22,23,24,25]
■ Obtain the blood or blood product from transfusion services. When receiving the blood or blood product from the transfusion services representative, verify the patient's two independent identifiers; ABO group and Rh type; the donor identification number, ABO group, and (if required) Rh type; interpretation of crossmatch tests (if required); special transfusion requirements (if applicable); the expiration date and time (if applicable); and the date and time of blood issue. Wear gloves, or transport the blood component units in a container that prevents direct contact with the blood unit bag.[1,34]
■ If not already wearing gloves, perform hand hygiene.[18,19,20,21,22,23,24,25]

■ Put on gloves and other personal protective equipment as needed *to comply with standard precautions.*[22,32,33,34,35,36]
■ Use a two-person verification process in the presence of the patient *to match the blood or blood component with the practitioner's order and the patient with the blood component.*[6,40] One of the individuals conducting the verification must be qualified to administer the blood or blood product, and is usually a registered nurse. The second individual conducting the verification must be qualified to participate in the process as determined by your facility.[40] Each employee must independently compare the information as follows:[1] compare the name and identification number on the patient's identification bracelet with those on the blood bag label; check the blood bag identification number, ABO blood group, Rh compatibility, and interpretation of compatibility testing; compare the patient's blood bank identification number with the number on the blood bag.[1]
■ Check the expiration date on the blood bag, and observe for leaks, abnormal color, clots, excessive air or bubbling, and unusual odor.[1,6] Return expired or abnormal blood to transfusion services.[1]
■ After checking all of the identifying information, sign the transfusion form *to indicate that the identification was correct and that you're the person starting the transfusion*; other items that may be included on the transfusion form include the name and volume of the blood product, the blood product's identification number, and the date and time of the transfusion.[1]

NURSING ALERT All identification attached to the blood or blood product bag should remain attached until you've terminated the transfusion.[1]

■ If your facility uses a bar code technology, use it as directed by your facility.
■ Prime the blood administration set according to the manufacturer's instructions. When using a Y-type set, use normal saline solution to prime the tubing; when using a straight set, use the prescribed blood product.[1]

NURSING ALERT Medications should never be mixed with blood components.[6] If the patient requires IV medications during transfusion, start a separate IV line for the administration of medications *so that the patient can receive the therapeutic benefits of the blood component and the medication simultaneously.* Other IV solutions (with the exception of Plasma-Lyte 148) aren't compatible with blood products and should not be administered through the same IV line.[1]

■ If you're using a blood warmer or an electronic infusion device, insert the tubing into the device and operate the device following the manufacturer's instructions for use.[1,6] (See *Blood warmers.*)
■ Perform a vigorous mechanical scrub of the vascular access device hub for at least 5 seconds using an antiseptic pad. Allow it to dry completely.[42,43]
■ Trace the blood administration set tubing from the patient to its point of origin before beginning the transfusion *to make sure that you're connecting the tubing to the correct port,* and then attach it to the venous access device.[37,44] Route the tubing in a standardized direction if the patient has other tubing and catheters that have different purposes. Label the tubing

EQUIPMENT

Blood warmers

Blood warmers may be used to prevent hypothermia, which can result from rapid infusion of large volumes of refrigerated blood.[1] Various types of blood and fluid warmers are available.

The ideal blood and fluid warmer should be capable of safely delivering fluids and blood products at normothermia at both high and low flow rates and must be tested and approved for use with blood components.[1] The blood and fluid warmer should be equipped with a visible temperature gauge and an audible alarm system.[41] No matter what type of device is available at your facility, be sure to follow the manufacturer's instructions for use.

A blood warmer may be indicated for use:
■ in a plasma exchange transfusion
■ during surgery
■ in a trauma patient
■ in a patient with cold agglutinin disease.[1,41]

at both the distal end (near the patient connection) and proximal end (near the source container) *to reduce the risk of misconnections* if multiple IV lines will be used.[44,45]

■ Start the blood transfusion at a slow rate for the first 15 minutes, and increase the rate as prescribed if there are no signs of a reaction *to ensure completion of the transfusion within 4 hours.*[1,6,7]

■ Remain near the patient during the first 15 minutes to monitor for signs and symptoms of a transfusion reaction, *because if a major incompatibility exists, or a severe allergic reaction such as anaphylaxis occurs, signs and symptoms usually appear before the first 50 mL of the unit have been transfused.*[6]

■ If a reaction occurs, immediately stop the transfusion and notify transfusion services and the patient's practitioner.[1,6] (See the "Transfusion reaction management" procedure.)

■ Assess the patient's respiratory status (including breath sounds and, if indicated, oxygen saturation level), skin appearance, and urine output.[46]

■ If no evidence of a transfusion reaction occurs within the first 15 minutes of the transfusion, increase the infusion rate to the prescribed rate.[6]

■ Before leaving the patient's room, instruct the patient and family (if applicable) to immediately report anything unusual.[1]

■ Observe the patient periodically during the transfusion *to identify early signs and symptoms of a possible transfusion reaction.*[1] Monitor vital signs during the transfusion if directed by your facility or if the patient's condition warrants.[33]

■ Closely monitor the flow rate and inspect the IV insertion site for signs of infiltration. If signs of infiltration are present, stop the transfusion immediately, disconnect the administration set, and aspirate fluid from the catheter using a small syringe. Remove the catheter and estimate the volume of fluid infiltrated. Notify the practitioner, and insert a new IV catheter in a different location *to prevent an interruption in transfusion therapy.*[47]

■ Remove and discard your gloves and, if worn, other personal protective equipment.[32,34,38]

■ Perform hand hygiene.[18,19,20,21,22,23,24,25]

■ At the completion of blood product administration, obtain the patient's vital signs *to compare with baseline measurements to detect signs of a possible transfusion reaction.*[1]

■ If you must administer additional units, repeat the procedure. Follow manufacturer's instructions regarding changing of transfusion administration sets and filters.[1,6,48]

■ If no additional units are prescribed, perform hand hygiene,[18,19,20,21,22,23,24,25] put on gloves,[32,33,34] and reconnect the original IV fluid, saline-lock the catheter, or discontinue the IV infusion, as prescribed.[5,49]

■ Return the bed to the lowest position, if applicable, *to prevent falls and maintain the patient's safety.*[50]

■ Discard used infusion supplies in an appropriate container, and discard the blood bag, tubing, and filter in an appropriate hazardous waste container.[32,34,38]

■ Clean and disinfect your stethoscope using a disinfectant pad.[51,52]

■ Remove and discard your gloves.[32,34,38]

■ Perform hand hygiene.[18,19,20,21,22,23,24,25]

■ Continue to assess and monitor the patient for signs and symptoms of a delayed transfusion reaction for 4 to 6 hours after the transfusion.[6] If the patient isn't under direct observation after the transfusion (for example, if the patient receives a transfusion as an outpatient), provide patient teaching about signs and symptoms of a delayed transfusion reaction and the importance of reporting them.[1,6]

■ Document the procedure.[53,54,55,56]

Special considerations

■ Use of automated identification technology, such as bar code technology, radio-frequency identification devices, and biometric scanning, is acceptable if permitted by your facility *to improve the identification system.*[6,40]

■ If necessary, using sterile technique, change the blood or blood component administration set and filter according to the manufacturer's instructions. Change it immediately if you suspect contamination, or if the integrity of the product or system has been compromised.[48]

■ Be aware that a donor unit of blood can be split if a patient might not be able to tolerate the fluid volume of an entire unit at one time. Individual portions of the unit can be released for administration while the remainder is safely stored.[1,6] Consult with transfusion services if unit splitting is necessary.

■ Note that the U.S. Food and Drug Administration has approved the compatibility of Plasma-Lyte 148 with blood components; it may be administered before or after the infusion of blood through the same administration set (for example, as priming solution), added to or infused concurrently with blood components, and used as a diluent in the transfusion of RBCs.[1]

■ If the blood bag empties before the next one arrives, administer normal saline solution slowly *to keep the vein patent.* If you're using a Y-type set, close the blood-line clamp, open the clamp to the normal saline solution, and let it infuse slowly until the new unit of blood arrives. Decrease the flow rate or clamp the line before attaching the new unit of blood.

■ Blood products must be infused within 4 hours of removal from the transfusion services refrigerator.[1,6,7] If any blood product remains after 4 hours, discontinue the infusion and discard the remaining product, as directed.

■ Many organized religions don't prohibit the use of blood products by their members when a medical need arises. However, Jehovah's Witnesses and Christian Scientists include teachings that prohibit transfusion therapy (although some believers of these and other faiths accept some blood components). Provide the opportunity for all patients to discuss their beliefs regarding blood transfusion.[1]

■ Be aware that whole blood is rarely used. It may be used on rare occasions to restore blood volume from hemorrhage or in an exchange transfusion.

■ The Joint Commission considers a blood incompatibility error a sentinel event. A sentinel event is an unexpected occurrence involving death or serious physical or psychological injury or the risk thereof. Sentinel events require immediate investigation and response. Follow your facility's process for reporting a suspected blood incompatibility error.[57]

Patient teaching

Because blood transfusion reactions can occur after a transfusion is complete, teach the patient and family (if applicable) about signs and symptoms of a transfusion reaction. Tell them to be alert to the possibility of a delayed reaction, and advise them to report signs and symptoms promptly to the practitioner. (See *Teaching about blood and blood product transfusion,* page 856.)

Complications

Despite improvements in crossmatching precautions, transfusion reactions can still occur during a transfusion or within 96 hours after a transfusion. Transfusion reactions typically stem from a major antigen-antibody reaction. Monitor the patient closely for signs and symptoms, especially if the patient can't report the symptoms. A transfusion reaction requires prompt action *to prevent further complications and, possibly, death.*

Unlike a transfusion reaction, an infectious disease transmitted during a transfusion may go undetected until days, weeks, or even months later, when it produces signs and symptoms. Measures to prevent disease transmission include laboratory testing of blood products and careful screening of potential donors, neither of which is guaranteed. Hepatitis C accounts for most posttransfusion hepatitis cases. The tests that detect hepatitis B and hepatitis C can produce false-negative results and may allow some hepatitis cases to go undetected. The risk of transmitting human immunodeficiency virus during transfusion is very low. Blood products are tested rigorously using highly sensitive testing methods.[58,59] Many transfusion services screen blood for cytomegalovirus (CMV); blood with CMV is especially dangerous for an immunosuppressed, seronegative patient. Transfusion services also test blood for syphilis, but refrigerating blood virtually eliminates the risk of transfusion-related syphilis. Transfusion services also screen for human T-lymphotropic viruses I and II and for the mosquito-borne diseases West Nile virus and Zika virus, which can be transmitted through blood transfusion; however, cases are rare.[58]

PATIENT TEACHING

TEACHING ABOUT BLOOD AND BLOOD PRODUCT TRANSFUSION

When developing a teaching plan, set objectives based on the information you gathered during your assessment. Set criteria for evaluating whether your objectives were met. Make sure that your teaching plan contains content that's directly related to your objectives and covers the following information.[1]

Sequence of events
- Reasons for the transfusion
- Performance of compatibility testing
- IV catheter insertion, if an appropriately sized catheter isn't already in place
- Premedication administration, as needed and prescribed
- Monitoring of vital signs and other parameters before, during, and after the transfusion
- Activity limitations during the transfusion
- Expectations after the transfusion

Benefits of the transfusion
- Improved oxygen-carrying capacity of red blood cells (RBCs), for example, if RBCs are prescribed for treatment of symptomatic anemia
- Provision of coagulation factors to prevent or control bleeding

Risks associated with the transfusion
- Immunologic complications, such as hemolytic and nonhemolytic reactions
- Transmission of infectious disease
- Fluid overload and subsequent pulmonary edema
- Sepsis

Signs and symptoms of complications associated with the transfusion
- Vague, uneasy feeling
- Onset of pain (especially at the IV site, back, or chest)
- Chills
- Flushing
- Fever
- Nausea
- Dizziness
- Rash
- Itching
- Dark or red urine

Documenting blood transfusions

After matching the patient's name, medical record number, blood group (or type) and Rh factor (the patient's and the donor's); the crossmatch data; and the transfusion services identification number with the label on the blood bag, you'll need to clearly document that you did so. The blood or blood product must be identified and documented properly by two health care professionals as well unless one-person verification accompanied by automated identification technology is permitted in your facility.

On the transfusion record, document
- the date and time the transfusion was started and completed
- the name of the health care professional who verified the information
- the type and gauge of the catheter
- the total amount of the transfusion
- the patient's vital signs before, during, and after the transfusion
- any infusion device used
- the flow rate
- any blood warming unit used.

If the patient receives autologous blood, document on the intake and output record
- the amount of autologous blood retrieved
- the amount reinfused
- laboratory data during and after the autotransfusion
- the patient's pretransfusion and posttransfusion vital signs.

Pay particular attention to the patient's:
- coagulation profile
- hemoglobin level, hematocrit, arterial blood gas values, and calcium level
- tolerance of the procedure, especially fluid status.

Transfusion-associated circulatory overload, transfusion-related acute lung injury, and hemolytic, allergic, febrile, and pyogenic reactions can result from any transfusion. Coagulation disturbances, citrate intoxication, hyperkalemia, acid-base imbalance, ammonia intoxication, hypothermia, and loss of 2,3-diphosphoglycerate can result from massive transfusion.

Documentation

Record the date and time of the transfusion; confirmation that informed consent was obtained; the indications for the transfusion; any premedications administered; the donor identification number; the type and amount of transfusion product transfused; the amount of normal saline solution infused; the patient's vital signs before, during (if required), and after the transfusion; your check of all identification data; and the patient's response. Document any transfusion reaction, the name of the practitioner notified, time of notification, interventions performed, and the patient's response to those interventions. Document teaching provided to the patient and family (if applicable), their understanding of that teaching, and any need for follow-up teaching.[1] (See *Documenting blood transfusions*.)

REFERENCES

1 Association for the Advancement of Blood & Biotherapies (AABB). (2018). *Primer of blood administration*. Bethesda, MD: AABB.(Level VII)

2 Jarrett, N., & Callaham, M. (2016). Evidence-based guidelines for selected hospital-acquired conditions: Final report. https://www.cms.gov/Medicare/Medicare-Fee-for-Service-Payment/HospitalAcqCond/Downloads/2016-HAC-Report.pdf

3 Centers for Medicare and Medicaid Services, Department of Health and Human Services. (2021). Appendix I: Hospital-acquired conditions (HACS) list. https://www.cms.gov/Medicare/Medicare-Fee-for-Service-Payment/HospitalAcqCond/icd10_hacs

4 American Red Cross. (2021). A compendium of transfusion practice guidelines (edition 4.0). https://www.redcrossblood.org/content/dam/redcrossblood/hospital-page-documents/334401_compendium_v04jan2021_bookmarkedworking_rwv01.pdf (Level VII)

5 Infusion Nurses Society. (2016). *Policies and procedures for infusion therapy* (5th ed.). Boston, MA: Infusion Nurses Society.

6 Standard 64. Blood administration. Infusion therapy standards of practice (8th ed.). (2021). *Journal of Infusion Nursing, 44*(Suppl. 1), S191–S194. (Level VII)

7 Association for the Advancement of Blood & Biotherapies (AABB), et al. (2017). *Circular of information for use of human blood and blood components*. https://www.aabb.org/news-resources/resources/circular-of-information (Level VII)

8 The Joint Commission. (2021). Standard MM.06.01.01. *Comprehensive accreditation manual for hospitals*. Oakbrook Terrace, IL: The Joint Commission. (Level VII)

9 Centers for Medicare and Medicaid Services, Department of Health and Human Services. (2020). Condition of participation: Nursing services. 42 C.F.R. § 23(c).

10 Accreditation Association for Hospitals and Health Systems. (2020). Standard 16.01.03. *Healthcare Facilities Accreditation Program: Accreditation requirements for acute care hospitals*. Chicago, IL: Accreditation Association for Hospitals and Health Systems. (Level VII)

11 DNV GL-Healthcare USA, Inc. (2020). MM.1.SR.3. *NIAHO® accreditation requirements, interpretive guidelines and surveyor guidance—revision 20.0*. Milford, OH: DNV GL-Healthcare USA, Inc. (Level VII)

12 The Joint Commission. (2017). Patient blood management certification review process guide for health care organizations. https://www.jointcommission.org/-/media/enterprise/tjc/imported-resource-assets/

documents/2017_pbm_org_rpgpdf.pdf?db=web&hash=BC1A07CF-934CA30555312ECC65DBD522&hash=BC1A07CF934CA30555312E-CC65DBD522

13 The Joint Commission. (2021). Standard RI.01.03.01. *Comprehensive accreditation manual for hospitals.* Oakbrook Terrace, IL: The Joint Commission. (Level VII)

14 Centers for Medicare and Medicaid Services, Department of Health and Human Services. (2020). Condition of participation: Patient's rights. 42 C.F.R. § 482.13(b)(2).

15 Standard 9. Informed consent. Infusion therapy standards of practice (8th ed.). (2021). *Journal of Infusion Nursing, 44*(Suppl. 1), S37–S39. (Level VII)

16 Accreditation Association for Hospitals and Health Systems. (2020). Standard 15.01.11. *Healthcare Facilities Accreditation Program: Accreditation requirements for acute care hospitals.* Chicago, IL: Accreditation Association for Hospitals and Health Systems. (Level VII)

17 DNV GL-Healthcare USA, Inc. (2020). PR.2.SR.3. *NIAHO® accreditation requirements, interpretive guidelines and surveyor guidance—revision 20.0.* Milford, OH: DNV GL-Healthcare USA, Inc. (Level VII)

18 The Joint Commission. (2021). Standard NPSG.07.01.01. *Comprehensive accreditation manual for hospitals.* Oakbrook Terrace, IL: The Joint Commission. (Level VII)

19 Centers for Disease Control and Prevention. (2002). Guideline for hand hygiene in health-care settings: Recommendations of the Healthcare Infection Control Practices Advisory Committee and the HICPAC/SHEA/APIC/IDSA Hand Hygiene Task Force. *MMWR Recommendations and Reports, 51*(RR-16), 1–45. https://www.cdc.gov/mmwr/pdf/rr/rr5116.pdf (Level II)

20 World Health Organization. (2009). WHO guidelines on hand hygiene in health care: First global patient safety challenge, clean care is safer care. https://apps.who.int/iris/bitstream/handle/10665/44102/9789241597906_eng.pdf?sequence=1 (Level IV)

21 Standard 16. Hand hygiene. Infusion therapy standards of practice (8th ed.). (2021). *Journal of Infusion Nursing, 44*(Suppl. 1), S53–S54. (Level VII)

22 Centers for Disease Control and Prevention. (2011, revised 2017). Guidelines for the prevention of intravascular catheter–related infections. https://www.cdc.gov/infectioncontrol/guidelines/bsi/recommendations.html (Level I)

23 Centers for Medicare and Medicaid Services, Department of Health and Human Services. (2020). Condition of participation: Infection control. 42 C.F.R. § 482.42.

24 Accreditation Association for Hospitals and Health Systems. (2020). Standard 07.01.21. *Healthcare Facilities Accreditation Program: Accreditation requirements for acute care hospitals.* Chicago, IL: Accreditation Association for Hospitals and Health Systems. (Level VII)

25 DNV GL-Healthcare USA, Inc. (2020). IC.1.SR.1. *NIAHO® accreditation requirements, interpretive guidelines and surveyor guidance—revision 20.0.* Milford, OH: DNV GL-Healthcare USA, Inc. (Level VII)

26 The Joint Commission. (2021). Standard NPSG.01.01.01. *Comprehensive accreditation manual for hospitals.* Oakbrook Terrace, IL: The Joint Commission. (Level VII)

27 Accreditation Association for Hospitals and Health Systems. (2020). Standard 15.01.16. *Healthcare Facilities Accreditation Program: Accreditation requirements for acute care hospitals.* Chicago, IL: Accreditation Association for Hospitals and Health Systems. (Level VII)

28 Centers for Medicare and Medicaid Services, Department of Health and Human Services. (2020). Condition of participation: Patient's rights. 42 C.F.R. § 482.13(c)(1).

29 DNV GL-Healthcare USA, Inc. (2020). PR.2.SR.5. *NIAHO® accreditation requirements, interpretive guidelines and surveyor guidance—revision 20.0.* Milford, OH: DNV GL-Healthcare USA, Inc. (Level VII)

30 The Joint Commission. (2021). Standard RI.01.01.01. *Comprehensive accreditation manual for hospitals.* Oakbrook Terrace, IL: The Joint Commission. (Level VII)

31 The Joint Commission. (2021). Standard PC.02.01.21. *Comprehensive accreditation manual for hospitals.* Oakbrook Terrace, IL: The Joint Commission. (Level VII)

32 Siegel, J. D., et al. (2007, revised 2019). 2007 guideline for isolation precautions: Preventing transmission of infectious agents in healthcare settings. https://www.cdc.gov/infectioncontrol/pdf/guidelines/isolation-guidelines-H.pdf (Level II)

33 Standard 17. Standard precautions. Infusion therapy standards of practice (8th ed.). (2021). *Journal of Infusion Nursing, 44*(Suppl. 1), S54–S55. (Level VII)

34 Occupational Safety and Health Administration. (2012). Bloodborne pathogens, standard number 1910.1030. https://www.osha.gov/pls/oshaweb/owadisp.show_document?p_id=10051&p_table=STANDARDS (Level VII)

35 DNV GL-Healthcare USA, Inc. (2020). IC.1.SR.2. *NIAHO® accreditation requirements, interpretive guidelines and surveyor guidance—revision 20.0.* Milford, OH: DNV GL-Healthcare USA, Inc. (Level VII)

36 Accreditation Association for Hospitals and Health Systems. (2020). Standard 07.01.10. *Healthcare Facilities Accreditation Program: Accreditation requirements for acute care hospitals.* Chicago, IL: Accreditation Association for Hospitals and Health Systems. (Level VII)

37 Standard 59. Infusion medication and solution administration. Infusion therapy standards of practice (8th ed.). (2021). *Journal of Infusion Nursing, 44*(Suppl. 1), S180–S183. (Level VII)

38 Standard 21. Medical waste and sharps safety. Infusion therapy standards of practice (8th ed.). (2021). *Journal of Infusion Nursing, 44*(Suppl. 1), S60–S62. (Level VII)

39 Waters, T. R., et al. (2009). Safe patient handling training for schools of nursing. https://www.cdc.gov/niosh/docs/2009-127/pdfs/2009-127.pdf (Level VII)

40 The Joint Commission. (2021). Standard NPSG.01.03.01. *Comprehensive accreditation manual for hospitals.* Oakbrook Terrace, IL: The Joint Commission. (Level VII)

41 Standard 25. Blood and fluid warming. Infusion therapy standards of practice (8th ed.). (2021). *Journal of Infusion Nursing, 44*(Suppl. 1), S72–S73. (Level VII)

42 Marschall, J., et al. (2014). SHEA/IDSA practice recommendation: Strategies to prevent central line–associated bloodstream infections in acute care hospitals. *Infection Control and Hospital Epidemiology, 35*(7), 753–771. https://www.jstor.org/stable/10.1086/676533#metadata_info_tab_contents (Level I)

43 Standard 36. Needleless connectors. Infusion therapy standards of practice (8th ed.). (2021). *Journal of Infusion Nursing, 44*(Suppl. 1), S104–S107. (Level VII)

44 U.S. Food and Drug Administration. (2017). Examples of medical device misconnections. https://www.fda.gov/medical-devices/medical-device-connectors/examples-medical-device-misconnections

45 The Joint Commission. (2014). Sentinel event alert 53: Managing risk during transition to new ISO tubing connector standards. https://www.jointcommission.org/-/media/tjc/documents/resources/patient-safety-topics/sentinel-event/sea_53_connectors_8_19_14_final.pdf (Level VII)

46 Fredrich, N. L. (2016). Evidence-based practice for red blood cell transfusions. *Nursing2016 Critical Care, 11*(1), 31–37. (Level VII)

47 Standard 47. Infiltration and extravasation. Infusion therapy standards of practice (8th ed.). (2021). *Journal of Infusion Nursing, 44*(Suppl. 1), S142–S1147. (Level VII)

48 Standard 43. Administration set management. Infusion therapy standards of practice (8th ed.). (2021). *Journal of Infusion Nursing, 44*(Suppl. 1), S123–S125. (Level VII)

49 Infusion Nurses Society. (2016). *Policies and procedures for infusion nursing of the older adult* (3rd ed.). Boston, MA: Infusion Nurses Society.

50 Ganz, D. A., et al. (2013, reviewed 2021). *Preventing falls in hospitals: A toolkit for improving quality of care* (AHRQ Publication No. 13-0015-EF). Agency for Healthcare Research and Quality. https://www.ahrq.gov/professionals/systems/hospital/fallpxtoolkit/index.html (Level VII)

51 Rutala, W. A., et al. (2008, revised 2019). Guideline for disinfection and sterilization in healthcare facilities, 2008. https://www.cdc.gov/infection-control/pdf/guidelines/disinfection-guidelines-H.pdf (Level I)

52 Accreditation Association for Hospitals and Health Systems. (2020). Standard 07.02.03. *Healthcare Facilities Accreditation Program: Accreditation requirements for acute care hospitals.* Chicago, IL: Accreditation Association for Hospitals and Health Systems. (Level VII)

53 The Joint Commission. (2021). Standard RC.01.03.01. *Comprehensive accreditation manual for hospitals.* Oakbrook Terrace, IL: The Joint Commission. (Level VII)

54 Centers for Medicare and Medicaid Services, Department of Health and Human Services. (2020). Condition of participation: Medical record services. 42 C.F.R. § 482.24(b).

55 Accreditation Association for Hospitals and Health Systems. (2020). Standard 10.00.03. *Healthcare Facilities Accreditation Program:*

Accreditation requirements for acute care hospitals. Chicago, IL: Accreditation Association for Hospitals and Health Systems. (Level VII)

56 DNV GL-Healthcare USA, Inc. (2020). MR.2.SR.1. *NIAHO® accreditation requirements, interpretive guidelines and surveyor guidance—revision 20.0.* Milford, OH: DNV GL-Healthcare USA, Inc. (Level VII)

57 The Joint Commission. (1999). Sentinel event alert 10: Blood Transfusion Errors: Preventing Future Occurrences. https://www.jointcommission.org/-/media/tjc/documents/resources/patient-safety-topics/sentinel-event/sea_10.pdf (Level VII)

58 American Red Cross. (n.d.). Infectious disease, HLA, and ABO donor qualification testing. https://www.redcrossblood.org/biomedical-services/blood-diagnostic-testing/blood-testing.html (Level VII)

59 Centers for Disease Control and Prevention. (2019). Blood safety: Diseases and organisms. http://www.cdc.gov/bloodsafety/bbp/diseases-organisms.html (Level VII)

TRANSFUSION REACTION MANAGEMENT

A transfusion reaction is any unfavorable event that occurs in a patient during or after transfusion of blood or a blood component that can be related to the transfusion.[1] When caring for a patient who has received a blood or blood component transfusion, health care providers should consider any adverse change in the patient's condition a possible symptom of a transfusion reaction and evaluate the patient promptly to prevent further complications.[1] (See *A guide to transfusion reactions.*)

Equipment

Gloves ■ sterile cap ■ normal saline solution ■ IV administration set ■ supplies for blood collection (see the "Venipuncture" procedure) ■ transfusion reaction report form ■ stethoscope ■ pulse oximeter and probe ■ vital signs monitoring equipment ■ laboratory specimen labels ■ laboratory biohazard transport bags ■ disinfectant pad ■ Optional: oxygen, EPINEPHrine, hypothermia blanket, indwelling urinary catheter and insertion kit, prescribed medications, prescribed IV fluid, emergency equipment (code cart with emergency medications, defibrillator, hand-held resuscitation bag with mask, intubation equipment.

Preparation of equipment

Inspect all IV equipment and supplies. If a product is expired, is defective, or has compromised integrity, remove it from patient use, label it as expired or defective, and report the expiration or defect as directed by your facility.[7]

Implementation

■ Gather and prepare the necessary equipment and supplies.
■ Perform hand hygiene.[8,9,10,11,12,13,14,15]
■ Confirm the patient's identity using at least two patient identifiers.[16]
■ Provide privacy.[17,18,19,20]
■ Explain the procedure, as time allows, to the patient and family (if appropriate) according to their individual communication and learning needs *to increase their understanding, allay their fears, and enhance cooperation.*[21]
■ Raise the bed to waist level before performing care *to prevent caregiver back strain.*[22]
■ Put on gloves *to comply with standard precautions.*[23,24,25,26,27]
■ If you suspect a transfusion reaction, stop the transfusion immediately; don't allow the blood remaining in the filter and tubing to infuse.[1,28]
■ Trace the blood administration tubing from the patient to its point of origin, disconnect it from the IV catheter, and cover the hub with a sterile cap; don't discard the administration set or the blood product.[1,29]
■ Prime a new administration set with normal saline solution, attach the administration set to the IV catheter, and infuse normal saline solution at a keep-vein-open rate.[1] Trace the tubing from the patient to its point of origin *to make sure that you've connected the tubing to the correct port.*[29]
■ Remain with the patient and notify the patient's practitioner and transfusion services personnel immediately.[1]
■ Verify that the patient received the correct blood by comparing the patient's identifying information on the blood bag, attached tag, and the patient's wrist band. If the information doesn't match, notify transfusion services *to help prevent further mismatching.*[1]
■ Closely monitor the patient's vital signs for indications of shock.[1] Monitor oxygen saturation level using pulse oximetry and assess cardiac and respiratory status frequently, as indicated by the patient's condition and the type of reaction suspected.
■ Administer treatment as prescribed *to provide symptomatic relief.*[1,28]
■ Place the blood bag (even if it's empty), attached IV fluids, and administration set with the related forms and labels in a laboratory biohazard transport bag[23] and return them to transfusion services, *because transfusion services will test these materials to further evaluate the reaction.*[1]
■ Perform a venipuncture in a different vein and obtain blood samples for laboratory testing for hemolysis; obtain a blood sample for repeat ABO group determination and direct antiglobulin testing, as ordered.[1] The practitioner may order additional laboratory testing such as blood cultures *if bacterial contamination is suspected.* The practitioner may also order blood urea nitrogen and creatinine levels *to monitor renal function* as well as coagulation studies, such as prothrombin time, partial thromboplastin time, fibrinogen level, and D-dimer, *to identify red blood cell destruction and to monitor for disseminated intravascular coagulation.* Report critical test results to the practitioner within the time frame determined by your facility *to ensure prompt treatment.*

NURSING ALERT Limit phlebotomy and blood loss from laboratory testing *to reduce the risk of iatrogenic anemia.*[30]

■ Label all samples in the presence of the patient *to prevent mislabeling.*[16]
■ Complete and send the appropriate documentation—usually a transfusion reaction form—to the laboratory along with the samples in a laboratory biohazard transport bag.[23]
■ Discard used supplies in the appropriate receptacles.[23,24,31]
■ Return the bed to the lowest position *to prevent falls and maintain patient safety.*[32]
■ Remove and discard your gloves, if worn.[23,24,31]
■ Perform hand hygiene.[8,9,10,11,12,13,14,15]
■ Closely monitor intake and output; insert an indwelling urinary catheter, if ordered, *to monitor urine output in a critically ill patient.* (See the "Indwelling urinary catheter insertion" procedure.)[1,33] Note evidence of oliguria or anuria, *because hemoglobin deposition in the renal tubes can cause renal damage.*
■ Make sure the patient is comfortable, and provide reassurance to the patient and family as needed.
■ Clean and disinfect your stethoscope using a disinfectant pad.[34,35]
■ Perform hand hygiene.[8,9,10,11,12,13,14,15]
■ Put on gloves, as needed.[23,24,25,26,27]
■ Clean and disinfect other reusable equipment according to the manufacturer's instructions *to prevent the spread of infection.*[34,35]
■ Remove and discard your gloves, if worn.[23,24,31]
■ Perform hand hygiene.[8,9,10,11,12,13,14,15]
■ Document the procedure.[36,37,38,39,40]

Special considerations

HOSPITAL-ACQUIRED CONDITION ALERT Keep in mind that the Centers for Medicare and Medicaid Services considers a blood incompatibility error a hospital-acquired condition *because it can reasonably be prevented using a variety of best practices.* Make sure to follow evidence-based prevention practices, such as carefully identifying the patient and blood sample for compatibility testing and participating in a two-person verification process before blood or blood product administration, *to reduce the risk of incompatibility errors.*[41,42,43]

■ The Joint Commission considers a blood incompatibility error a sentinel event. A *sentinel event* is an unexpected occurrence involving death or serious physical or psychological injury or the risk thereof. Sentinel events require immediate investigation and response. Follow your facility's process for reporting a blood incompatibility error if you suspect one.[44]
■ Be aware that the compatibility testing facility must report recipient fatalities from transfusion of blood or a blood product to the U.S. Food and Drug Administration (FDA) as soon as possible after the event by phone (240-402-9160), e-mail (fatalities2@fda.hhs.gov), or fax (301-827-0333). The reporting facility must also send a written report within 7 days after the fatality addressed to the FDA Center for Biologics

A guide to transfusion reactions

Any patient receiving a transfusion of blood or blood products is at risk for a transfusion reaction. A transfusion reaction may be immediate (occurring during the transfusion or within several hours of transfusion completion) or delayed. The chart below describes immediate and delayed reactions.[1]

REACTIONS (AND CAUSES)	SIGNS AND SYMPTOMS	PREVENTIVE MEASURES AND NURSING INTERVENTIONS
IMMEDIATE REACTIONS		
Acute hemolytic reaction (caused by administration of incompatible blood)	■ Chills ■ Shaking ■ Fever (temperature increase of 2° F [1° C] or more) ■ Increased pulse rate ■ Pain at the IV insertion site ■ Nausea and vomiting ■ Chest tightness ■ Headache ■ Flank pain ■ Hypotension ■ Renal failure or shock (if allowed to progress)	■ Properly label all blood samples in the presence of the patient. ■ Positively identify the patient and donor blood types and groups before the transfusion.[1] ■ Use a two-person verification process *to verify the patient and blood component.*[2] ■ Transfuse the blood slowly for the first 15 minutes and remain with the patient.[2] ■ Save the donor blood *to reattempt crossmatching with the patient's blood.*[1] ■ If an acute hemolytic reaction occurs, stop the transfusion immediately and notify transfusion services personnel and the patient's practitioner.[2] ■ Maintain patent IV access. ■ Monitor vital signs for signs of shock. ■ Insert an indwelling urinary catheter, if ordered, *to monitor urine output.*[1] ■ Send a blood sample *to check for intravascular hemolysis.* ■ Assess for signs of disseminated intravascular coagulation.[1] ■ Provide supportive medical therapies, as ordered, *to reverse shock.*[1]
Bacterial sepsis (blood product contamination)	■ Rigors ■ Chills ■ High fever (temperature increase of 3.5° F [2° C] or more) ■ Shock	■ Use sterile technique when collecting and administering blood products. ■ Ensure that the transfusion is started within the facility's designated time of removal from transfusion services (for example, 30 minutes).[3] ■ Complete the transfusion in 4 hours or less.[1,4] ■ Don't reuse the filter or tubing if the first unit of blood takes 4 hours or longer to infuse. ■ If signs or symptoms of bacterial sepsis occur, immediately stop the transfusion and notify the practitioner and transfusion services personnel.[1] ■ Treat the patient's fever as prescribed.[1] ■ Send blood samples from the patient and blood component for culture and sensitivity testing.[1] ■ Administer antibiotics as prescribed.[1]
Febrile nonhemolytic reactions (caused by leukocyte or platelet antibodies, plasma protein antibodies, or cytokines from donor leukocytes)	■ Fever (temperature increase of 2° F [1° C] or more occurring during or shortly after a transfusion in the absence of any other stimulus for fever) ■ Chills	■ Administer acetaminophen or an antihistamine before the transfusion, as prescribed.[1] ■ Administer leukocyte-reduced red blood cells (RBCs), as prescribed, *because they're less likely to cause a reaction.* ■ If signs or symptoms occur, stop the transfusion immediately and notify the practitioner and transfusion services personnel.[1]
Transfusion-related acute lung injury (TRALI) (caused by complement and histamine release caused by granulocyte antibodies in donor or recipient)	■ Dyspnea ■ Pulmonary edema ■ Normal pulmonary artery wedge pressure	■ Stop the transfusion immediately.[5] ■ Administer treatment to support blood pressure, as prescribed. ■ Administer supplemental oxygen, as prescribed. ■ Prepare for endotracheal intubation and mechanical ventilation, if necessary.
Allergic reaction (caused by allergen in donor's plasma)	■ Urticaria ■ Flushing ■ Wheezing ■ Dyspnea ■ Laryngeal edema	■ Administer antihistamines before the transfusion, as prescribed, if the patient tends to experience allergic reactions.[1] ■ If the patient develops mild itching, reduce the transfusion rate.[1] ■ If signs and symptoms are more severe than mild itching, stop the transfusion immediately and notify the patient's practitioner and transfusion services personnel.[1] ■ Administer EPINEPHrine as prescribed *to treat wheezing and anaphylactic reactions.*[1] ■ Restart the transfusion, as ordered, if no other cause or signs and symptoms are found, or if an antihistamine provides relief from itching.[1] ■ Don't restart the transfusion if the patient has a fever, pulmonary or airway signs and symptoms, or anaphylaxis.[1]

(Continued)

A guide to transfusion reactions *(continued)*

REACTIONS (AND CAUSES)	SIGNS AND SYMPTOMS	PREVENTIVE MEASURES AND NURSING INTERVENTIONS
Transfusion-associated circulatory overload (TACO) (caused by rapid infusion or excessive volume of blood)	■ Precordial pain ■ Dyspnea ■ Crackles[6] ■ Wheezing[6] ■ Cyanosis ■ Dry cough ■ Jugular vein distention[6] ■ Hypertension[6] ■ Tachycardia[6] ■ Wide pulse pressure[6]	■ Administer blood components slowly.[1] ■ Use volume-reduced platelets *to prevent fluid overload.*[1] ■ Administer the component using an electronic infusion device *to maintain flow rate.* ■ Position the patient in a semi-Fowler or upright position *to increase venous resistance.*[1] ■ If the patient develops signs and symptoms of TACO, stop the transfusion immediately and notify the practitioner and transfusion services personnel.[1]

DELAYED REACTIONS

Delayed hemolytic reaction (caused by production of antibodies by recipient's RBCs to antigen on transfused cells)	Occurring 5 to 10 days after transfusion: ■ Fever ■ RBC destruction	■ Monitor laboratory test results for anemia and reduced benefit from successive transfusions.[1] ■ If the patient develops signs and symptoms of delayed hemolytic reaction, notify the practitioner and transfusion services personnel.[1]
Alloimmunization—unpredictable development of antibodies to RBCs, white blood cells, platelets, or plasma proteins	■ Increases risk of hemolytic, febrile, and allergic reactions.	■ Keep in mind that patients who receive multiple transfusions are at risk.[1] ■ If signs or symptoms of a reaction occur, notify the practitioner and transfusion services personnel.[1]
Posttransfusion purpura (due to sensitization caused by pregnancy or previous transfusion)	Occurring 7 to 10 days after transfusion: ■ Sudden, dramatic thrombocytopenia	■ Administer high-dose immune globulin IV, as prescribed. ■ Monitor the patient's platelet count.
Transfusion-associated graft-versus-host disease (caused by engrafting of the T lymphocytes from the donor's component in the recipient that then react against the recipient's tissue antigens)	Typically developing 10 to 12 days after transfusion: ■ Fever ■ Rash ■ Diarrhea ■ Desquamation ■ Pancytopenia	■ Provide supportive care as ordered.

Evaluation and Research Document Control Center, 10903 New Hampshire Avenue, WO71, G112, Silver Spring, MD 20993-0002.[45]

Documentation

Record the time and date that the transfusion was started, the type of blood component transfused, the unit identification number, the patient's condition at the start of the transfusion, the patient's vital signs, and your other assessment findings. Record the time the transfusion was stopped, the volume infused, the patient's condition, the identity of the person who stopped the transfusion and observed the patient, the date and time the practitioner was notified, prescribed interventions, and the patient's response to those interventions. Record any samples sent to the laboratory for analysis, any nursing interventions performed, and the patient's response to those interventions. If required by your facility, complete a transfusion reaction report form. Document teaching provided to the patient and family (if applicable), their understanding of that teaching, and any need for follow-up teaching.

REFERENCES

1 Association for the Advancement of Blood & Biotherapies (AABB). (2018). *Primer of blood administration.* Bethesda, MD: AABB. (Level VII)
2 Standard 12. Product evaluation, integrity, and defect reporting. Infusion therapy standards of practice (8th ed.). (2021). *Journal of Infusion Nursing, 44*(Suppl. 1), S45–S146. (Level VII)
3 Infusion Nurses Society. (2016). *Policies and procedures for infusion therapy* (5th ed.). Boston, MA: Infusion Nurses Society.
4 Association for the Advancement of Blood & Biotherapies (AABB), et al. (2017). *Circular of information for use of human blood and blood components.* Bethesda, MD: AABB. https://www.aabb.org/tm/coi/Documents/coi1017.pdf

5 Kleinman, S., & Kor, D. J. (2020). Transfusion-related acute lung injury (TRALI). In: *UpToDate*, Silvergleid, A. J., & Manaker, S. (Eds.).
6 Silvergleid, A. J. (2021). Transfusion-associated circulatory overload (TACO). In *UpToDate*, Kleinman, S. (Ed.)
7 Standard 12. Product evaluation, integrity, and defect reporting. Infusion therapy standards of practice (8th ed.). (2021). *Journal of Infusion Nursing, 44*(Suppl. 1), S45–S46. (Level VII)
8 Centers for Disease Control and Prevention. (2002). Guideline for hand hygiene in health-care settings: Recommendations of the Healthcare Infection Control Practices Advisory Committee and the HICPAC/SHEA/APIC/IDSA Hand Hygiene Task Force. *MMWR Recommendations and Reports, 51*(RR-16), 1–45. https://www.cdc.gov/mmwr/pdf/rr/rr5116.pdf (Level II)
9 World Health Organization (WHO). (2009). WHO guidelines on hand hygiene in health care: First global patient safety challenge, clean care is safer care. https://apps.who.int/iris/bitstream/handle/10665/44102/9789241597906_eng.pdf?sequence=1 (Level IV)
10 Centers for Disease Control and Prevention. (2011, revised 2017). Guidelines for the prevention of intravascular catheter-related infections. https://www.cdc.gov/infectioncontrol/guidelines/bsi/recommendations.html (Level I)
11 Standard 16. Hand hygiene. Infusion therapy standards of practice (8th ed.). (2021). *Journal of Infusion Nursing, 44*(Suppl. 1), S53–S54. (Level VII)
12 The Joint Commission. (2021). Standard NPSG.07.01.01. *Comprehensive accreditation manual for hospitals.* Oakbrook Terrace, IL: The Joint Commission. (Level VII)
13 Centers for Medicare and Medicaid Services, Department of Health and Human Services. (2020). Condition of participation: Infection control. 42 C.F.R. § 482.42.
14 Accreditation Association for Hospitals and Health Systems. (2020). Standard 07.01.21. *Healthcare Facilities Accreditation Program:*

15 DNV GL-Healthcare USA, Inc. (2020). IC.1.SR.1. *NIAHO® accreditation requirements, interpretive guidelines and surveyor guidance—revision 20.0.* Milford, OH: DNV GL-Healthcare USA, Inc. (Level VII)

16 The Joint Commission. (2021). Standard NPSG.01.01.01. *Comprehensive accreditation manual for hospitals.* Oakbrook Terrace, IL: The Joint Commission. (Level VII)

17 Accreditation Association for Hospitals and Health Systems. (2020). Standard 15.01.16. *Healthcare Facilities Accreditation Program: Accreditation requirements for acute care hospitals.* Chicago, IL: Accreditation Association for Hospitals and Health Systems. (Level VII)

18 Centers for Medicare and Medicaid Services. (2020). Condition of participation: Patient's rights. 42 C.F.R. § 482.13(c)(1).

19 DNV GL-Healthcare USA, Inc. (2020). PR.2.SR.5. *NIAHO® accreditation requirements, interpretive guidelines and surveyor guidance—revision 20.0.* Milford, OH: DNV GL-Healthcare USA, Inc. (Level VII)

20 The Joint Commission. (2021). Standard RI.01.01.01. *Comprehensive accreditation manual for hospitals.* Oakbrook Terrace, IL: The Joint Commission. (Level VII)

21 The Joint Commission. (2021). Standard PC.02.01.21. *Comprehensive accreditation manual for hospitals.* Oakbrook Terrace, IL: The Joint Commission. (Level VII)

22 Waters, T. R., et al. (2009). Safe patient handling training for schools of nursing. https://www.cdc.gov/niosh/docs/2009-127/pdfs/2009-127.pdf (Level VII)

23 Occupational Safety and Health Administration. (2012). Bloodborne pathogens, standard number 1910.1030. https://www.osha.gov/pls/oshaweb/owadisp.show_document?p_id=10051&p_table=STANDARDS (Level VII)

24 Siegel, J. D., et al. (2007, revised 2019). 2007 guideline for isolation precautions: Preventing transmission of infectious agents in healthcare settings. https://www.cdc.gov/infectioncontrol/pdf/guidelines/isolation-guidelines-H.pdf (Level II)

25 Standard 17. Standard precautions. Infusion therapy standards of practice (8th ed.). (2021). *Journal of Infusion Nursing, 44*(Suppl. 1), S54–S55. (Level VII)

26 Accreditation Association for Hospitals and Health Systems. (2020). Standard 07.01.10. *Healthcare Facilities Accreditation Program: Accreditation requirements for acute care hospitals.* Chicago, IL: Accreditation Association for Hospitals and Health Systems. (Level VII)

27 DNV GL-Healthcare USA, Inc. (2020). IC.1.SR.2. *NIAHO® accreditation requirements, interpretive guidelines and surveyor guidance—revision 20.0.* Milford, OH: DNV GL-Healthcare USA, Inc. (Level VII)

28 Standard 64. Blood administration. Infusion therapy standards of practice (8th ed.). (2021). *Journal of Infusion Nursing, 44*(Suppl. 1), S191–S194. (Level VII)

29 U.S. Food and Drug Administration. (2017). Examples of medical device misconnections. https://www.fda.gov/medical-devices/medical-device-connectors/examples-of-medical-device-misconnections

30 Tolich, D. J., et al. (2013). Blood management: Best-practice transfusion strategies. *Nursing, 43*(1), 40–47. https://journals.lww.com/nursing/Fulltext/2013/01000/Blood_management_Best_practice_transfusion.13.aspx (Level V)

31 Standard 21. Medical waste and sharps safety. Infusion therapy standards of practice (8th ed.). (2021). *Journal of Infusion Nursing, 44*(Suppl. 1), S60–S62. (Level VII)

32 Ganz, D. A., et al. (2013, reviewed 2021). *Preventing falls in hospitals: A toolkit for improving quality of care* (AHRQ Publication No. 13-0015-EF). Rockville, MD: Agency for Healthcare Research and Quality. https://www.ahrq.gov/professionals/systems/hospital/fallpxtoolkit/index.html (Level VII)

33 Healthcare Infection Control Practices Advisory Committee. (2010, revised 2019). Guideline for prevention of catheter-associated urinary tract infections 2009. https://www.cdc.gov/infectioncontrol/pdf/guidelines/cauti-guidelines-H.pdf (Level I)

34 Rutala, W. A., et al. (2008, revised 2019). Guideline for disinfection and sterilization in healthcare facilities, 2008. https://www.cdc.gov/infection-control/pdf/guidelines/disinfection-guidelines-H.pdf (Level I)

35 Accreditation Association for Hospitals and Health Systems. (2020). Standard 07.02.03. *Healthcare Facilities Accreditation Program: Accreditation requirements for acute care hospitals.* (Level VII)

36 The Joint Commission. (2021). Standard RC.01.03.01. *Comprehensive accreditation manual for hospitals.* Oakbrook Terrace, IL: The Joint Commission. (Level VII)

37 Centers for Medicare and Medicaid Services. (2020). Condition of participation: Medical record services. 42 C.F.R. § 482.24(b).

38 Accreditation Association for Hospitals and Health Systems. (2020). Standard 10.00.03. *Healthcare Facilities Accreditation Program: Accreditation requirements for acute care hospitals.* Chicago, IL: Accreditation Association for Hospitals and Health Systems. (Level VII)

39 DNV GL-Healthcare USA, Inc. (2020). MR.2.SR.1. *NIAHO® accreditation requirements, interpretive guidelines and surveyor guidance—revision 20.0.* Milford, OH: DNV GL-Healthcare USA, Inc. (Level VII)

40 Standard 10. Documentation in the medical record. Infusion therapy standards of practice (8th ed.). (2021). *Journal of Infusion Nursing, 44*(Suppl. 1), S39–S42. (Level VII)

41 The Joint Commission. (2021). Standard NPSG.01.03.01. *Comprehensive accreditation manual for hospitals.* Oakbrook Terrace, IL: The Joint Commission. (Level VII)

42 Jarrett, N., & Callaham, M. (2016). Evidence-based guidelines for selected hospital-acquired conditions: Final report. https://www.cms.gov/Medicare/Medicare-Fee-for-Service-Payment/HospitalAcqCond/Downloads/2016-HAC-Report.pdf (Level VII)

43 Centers for Medicare and Medicaid Services. (2021). Appendix I: Hospital-acquired conditions (HACS) list. https://www.cms.gov/Medicare/Medicare-Fee-for-Service-Payment/HospitalAcqCond/icd10_hacs

44 The Joint Commission. (2021). Most commonly reviewed sentinel event types. https://www.jointcommission.org/-/media/tjc/documents/resources/patient-safety-topics/sentinel-event/most-frequently-reviewed-event-types-2020.pdf (Level VII)

45 U.S. Food and Drug Administration. (2021). Transfusion/donation fatalities: Notification process for transfusion related fatalities and donation related deaths. https://www.fda.gov/vaccines-blood-biologics/report-problem-center-biologics-evaluation-research/transfusiondonation-fatalities

TRANSVENOUS PACING

The insertion of a temporary pacemaker for use in transvenous pacing may be done in an emergency or as an elective procedure. The pacemaker system consists of an external, battery-powered pulse generator and a lead or electrode system. The purpose of a transvenous pacemaker (the most common type of temporary pacemaker) is to maintain circulatory integrity by providing for standby pacing if sudden complete heart block occurs, to increase the heart rate during periods of symptomatic bradycardia, and, occasionally, to control sustained supraventricular or ventricular tachycardia.[1] In addition to being more comfortable for the patient, a transvenous pacemaker is more reliable than a transcutaneous pacemaker.

Transvenous pacing involves threading an electrode catheter through a vein into the patient's right atrium or right ventricle; single-chamber pacing is most appropriate in an emergency, because the goal is to establish the patient's heart rate as quickly as possible.[1] Dual-chamber pacing can be used if the patient requires atrial contraction for improved hemodynamics.[1] Veins used for insertion include the subclavian, brachial, internal jugular, and femoral.[1] The femoral site should be used as a last resort because it's associated with an increased risk of infection. The electrode then attaches to an external pulse generator, which can provide an electrical stimulus directly to the endocardium. Transvenous pacemaker insertion is performed by a practitioner with a nurse assisting.[1]

Indications for transvenous pacing include management of symptomatic bradycardia, tachyarrhythmias, and other conduction system disturbances as well as persistent hemodynamically unstable sinus node dysfunction refractory to medical therapy.[1,2] It may also help diagnose conduction abnormalities. According to the American Heart Association, pacing isn't recommended in cardiac arrest.[3]

Equipment

Temporary pacemaker generator with new battery ■ guidewire or introducer ■ pacing electrode catheter ■ gloves ■ sterile gloves ■ sterile occlusive dressing supplies ■ antiseptic solution (2% chlorhexidine-based solution) ■ emergency equipment (code cart with emergency medications, defibrillator, handheld resuscitation bag with mask, intubation equipment) ■ vital signs monitoring equipment ■ prescribed analgesic or sedative ■ cardiac monitor with strip-chart recorder ■ prescribed local anesthetic ■ sterile syringe and 25G needle (for local anesthetic administration) ■ bridging cable ▪ percutaneous introducer tray or venous cutdown tray ▪ sterile gowns ▪ head covers ▪ masks and goggles or masks with face shield ▪ sterile fenestrated drape ▪ suturing equipment ▪ Optional: alligator clip, fluoroscopy equipment and protective aprons, ultrasound equipment, disposable-head clippers, peripheral IV insertion equipment, prescribed IV fluids, gown.

Preparation of equipment

Inspect all equipment and supplies. If a product is expired, is defective, or has compromised integrity, remove it from patient use, label it as expired or defective, and report the expiration or defect as directed by your facility. Connect the patient to a cardiac monitor. Make sure that emergency equipment is functioning properly and readily available.

Implementation

- Verify the practitioner's order.
- Gather and prepare the necessary equipment and supplies.
- If required by your facility, confirm that written informed consent has been obtained and that the signed consent form is in the patient's medical record.[4,5,6,7]
- Conduct a preprocedure verification *to make sure that all relevant documentation, related information, and equipment are available and correctly identified to the patient's identifiers.*[8,9]
- Perform hand hygiene.[10,11,12,13,14,15]
- Confirm the patient's identity using at least two patient identifiers.[9,16]
- Provide privacy.[17,18,19,20]
- Explain the procedure to the patient and family (if appropriate) according to their individual communication and learning needs *to increase their understanding, allay their fears, and enhance cooperation.*[21]
- Review the patient's medical record for a history of allergies to local anesthetics or latex.
- Raise the patient's bed to waist level before providing patient care *to prevent caregiver back strain.*[22]
- Perform hand hygiene[10,11,12,13,14,15] and put on gloves and, as needed, other personal protective equipment *to comply with standard precautions.*[23,24,25]
- Assess the patient's vital signs, skin color, level of consciousness (LOC), heart rate and rhythm, peripheral pulses, and emotional state *to serve as a baseline for comparison during and after the procedure.*
- If ordered, insert a peripheral IV catheter and initiate the ordered IV infusion at the ordered rate. (See the "IV catheter insertion and removal" procedure.)
- Insert a new battery into the external pacemaker generator, and test it *to make sure it has a strong charge.* Connect the bridging cable to the generator, and align the positive and negative poles. *This cable allows slack between the electrode catheter and the generator, reducing the risk of accidental catheter displacement.*
- Connect the patient to the bedside monitoring system and monitor the electrocardiogram (ECG) continuously.[1] Make sure that alarm limits are set appropriately for the patient's current condition, and that alarms are turned on, functioning properly, and audible to staff.[26,27,28,29]
- Place the patient in the supine position.
- Place a fluid-impermeable pad under the patient *to prevent the bed from becoming soiled.*
- If necessary, clip the hair around the insertion site using disposable-head hair clippers.[30]
- Screen for and assess the patient's pain using facility-defined criteria that are consistent with the patient's age, condition, and ability to understand.[31]
- Treat the patient's pain, as needed and ordered, using nonpharmacologic, pharmacologic, or a combination of approaches. Base the treatment plan on evidence-based practices and the patient's clinical condition, past medical history, and pain management goals.[31]
- Administer an analgesic or a sedative, as ordered, following safe medication administration practices.[1,32,33,34,35] Alternatively, ensure that a second person administers an analgesic or a sedative as ordered.
- Remove and discard your gloves and other personal protective equipment, if worn,[24] and perform hand hygiene.[10,11,12,13,14,15]
- Open the appropriate supply tray while maintaining a sterile field. Label all medications, medication containers, and other solutions on and off the sterile field.[36]

- Assist the practitioner in putting on a sterile gown, a mask and goggles or a mask with face shield, a head cover, and sterile gloves. If assisting, put on the same personal protective equipment.[23,24]
- Assist the practitioner with insertion as necessary. The practitioner may use fluoroscopy-guided technique, ultrasound-guided technique, or ECG-guided technique. If the practitioner is using fluoroscopy-guided technique, place a protective apron on the patient below the waist; ensure all staff members also put on protective aprons. If the practitioner is using ultrasound-guided technique for placement, prepare the ultrasound equipment. If the practitioner is using ECG-guided technique, connect an alligator clip to the V lead of the cardiac monitor and the distal end of the electrode catheter. Set the cardiac monitor to display the V lead continuously.[1]
- The practitioner disinfects the insertion site with an antiseptic solution and allows it to dry completely. Assist as needed.
- Following maximal barrier precautions, the practitioner covers the patient from head to toe with a sterile fenestrated drape, leaving a small opening for the insertion site.
- Conduct a time-out immediately before starting the procedure *to perform a final assessment that the correct patient, site, positioning, and procedure are identified, and that, as applicable, all relevant information and necessary equipment are available.*[9,37]
- After anesthetizing the insertion site, the practitioner will puncture the brachial, femoral, subclavian, or jugular vein. The practitioner will insert a guidewire or an introducer and advance the electrode catheter.
- As the catheter advances, watch the cardiac monitor.[1] If the practitioner is using ECG-guided technique, when the electrode catheter reaches the right atrium, you'll notice large P waves and small QRS complexes. Then, as the catheter reaches the right ventricle, the P waves will become smaller while the QRS complexes enlarge. When the catheter touches the right ventricular endocardium, expect to see elevated ST segments, premature ventricular contractions, or both.[1] When the electrode catheter reaches the right ventricle, it will send an impulse to the myocardium, causing depolarization. If the patient needs atrial pacing, either alone or with ventricular pacing, the practitioner may place an electrode in the right atrium.

Sensitivity and stimulation threshold testing

Sensitivity and stimulation threshold testing helps determine the appropriate pacemaker rate and amount of electrical current needed to initiate depolarization of the myocardium. Testing should occur on both chambers, as appropriate. Sensitivity threshold testing isn't necessary if the patient has no intrinsic rhythm. In some facilities, critical care nurses are permitted to perform sensitivity and stimulation threshold testing; in other facilities, the practitioner must perform the testing. Frequency of testing also varies by facility. Testing typically occurs at least every 24 hours *to make sure that the pacemaker is functioning properly and that it isn't delivering high levels of energy to the myocardium.*[1]

Performing sensitivity threshold testing

- Slowly turn the sensitivity dial to a higher numeric setting until the sensing indicator light stops flashing; this occurs when the device no longer senses the patient's intrinsic rhythm.[1,38]
- Gradually turn the sensitivity dial to a lower numeric setting until the sensing light begins flashing with each complex and the pacing light stops flashing; this setting is the sensing threshold.[1,38]
- Set the sensitivity dial to the setting that's one-half the value of the sensing threshold.[1,38]

Performing stimulation threshold testing

- Set the pacing rate about 10 beats/minute above the patient's intrinsic rate.[1]
- Beginning at 20 milliamperes (mA), slowly decrease the output until capture is lost.[1]
- Gradually increase the mA until you see a 1:1 capture and the pacing light flashes; this is the stimulation threshold.[1]
- Set the mA at least two times higher than the stimulation threshold.[1]

■ Meanwhile, continuously monitor the patient's cardiac status and treat arrhythmias, as appropriate.[1] Also assess the patient for jaw pain and earache; *these symptoms indicate that the electrode catheter has missed the superior vena cava and has moved into the neck instead.*

■ When the electrode catheter is in place, attach the catheter leads to the bridging cable, lining up the positive and negative poles. Make sure all connections are secure.[1]

■ Turn the pacemaker on and obtain settings (mode, rate, and energy level) from the practitioner. Set the pacing mode, rate, and energy level (output and milliamperes) according to the practitioner's order or as determined by sensitivity testing (the level of intrinsic cardiac activity as sensed by electrodes) and stimulation threshold testing (the minimum amount of voltage necessary to initiate depolarization).[1] (See *Sensitivity and stimulation threshold testing.*) Ensure that the settings are correct.

■ The practitioner will then secure the catheter to the insertion site, usually by suturing.

■ Apply a sterile occlusive dressing to the site.[1] Label the dressing with the date, the time, and your initials. Secure the pulse generator and pacemaker wires, as necessary.

■ Assess the patient's vital signs, skin color, LOC, heart rate and rhythm, peripheral pulses, and emotional state *to determine the effectiveness of the paced rhythm.*[1]

TROUBLESHOOTING

HANDLING PACEMAKER MALFUNCTIONS

Occasionally, a temporary pacemaker may fail to function properly. When failure occurs, you need to take immediate action to correct the problem. Follow these guidelines when your patient's pacemaker fails to pace, capture, or sense intrinsic beats.

Failure to pace
Failure to pace happens when the pacemaker either doesn't fire or fires too often. The pulse generator may not be working properly, or it may not be conducting the impulse to the patient.

Nursing interventions
■ If the pacing or sensing indicator flashes, check the patient, all connections, and the battery. Check the position of the pacing electrode in the patient by X-ray, as ordered.
■ If the pulse generator is turned on but the indicators still aren't flashing, change the battery. If that doesn't help, use a different pulse generator.
■ Check the settings if the pacemaker is firing too rapidly. If the rate is correct or if increasing the sensitivity (according to the practitioner's order) doesn't help, change the pulse generator.
■ Have a transcutaneous pacemaker on standby in case the pacemaker continues to malfunction and the patient becomes symptomatic.
■ Notify the practitioner.

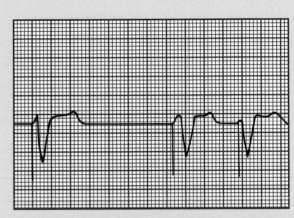

Failure to capture
In failure to capture, pacemaker spikes appear on the rhythm strip but the heart isn't responding. This malfunction can be caused by changes in the pacing threshold due to ischemia, an electrolyte imbalance (high or low potassium or magnesium levels), acidosis, an adverse reaction to a medication, a perforated ventricle, fibrosis, or the electrode position.

Nursing interventions
■ Verify that the settings are correct according to the practitioner's order.
■ If the heart isn't responding, carefully check all connections, increase the milliamperes slowly as determined by your facility, and notify the practitioner of the failure to capture.
■ Have a transcutaneous pacemaker on standby in case the pacemaker continues to malfunction and the patient become symptomatic.
■ Notify the practitioner.

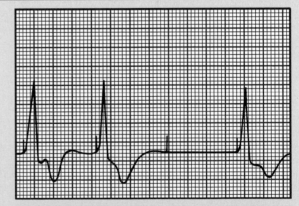

Failure to sense intrinsic beats
Failure to sense intrinsic beats could cause ventricular tachycardia or ventricular fibrillation if the pacemaker fires on the vulnerable T wave. Possible causes include the pacemaker sensing an external stimulus such as a QRS complex, which could lead to asystole, or the pacemaker not being sensitive enough, which means it could fire anywhere within the cardiac cycle.

Nursing interventions
■ If the pacemaker is undersensing, increase the sensitivity by turning down the voltage, usually to 2 to 5 millivolts (mV). If it's oversensing, decrease the sensitivity by turning the voltage to 5 mV or higher.
■ Change the battery and then the pulse generator.
■ Remove items in the room that could be causing electromechanical interference (such as razors, radios, and cautery devices). Check the ground wires on the bed and other equipment for obvious damage. Unplug each piece and see if the interference stops. When you locate the cause, notify the staff engineer and ask for it to be checked.
■ If the pacemaker is still firing on the T wave and all other efforts to correct it have failed, attach the patient to a transcutaneous pacemaker, turn off the epicardial pacemaker, and notify the practitioner.

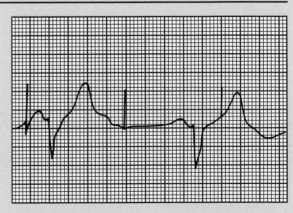
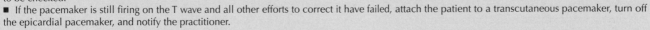

- Reassess and respond to the patient's pain by evaluating the response to treatment and progress toward pain management goals. Assess for adverse reactions and risk factors for adverse events that may result from treatment.[31]
- Return the bed to the lowest position *to prevent falls and maintain patient safety.*[39]
- Obtain a chest X-ray, as ordered, *to detect complications associated with insertion, such as pneumothorax.*[1]
- Discard supplies in the appropriate receptacles.[24]
- Remove and discard your personal protective equipment.[24]
- Perform hand hygiene.[10,11,12,13,14,15]
- Document the procedure.[40,41,42,43]

Special considerations

- Confirm positioning of the lead wire by ultrasonography, fluoroscopy, or chest X-ray, as ordered.[1]
- Take safety measures, including placing a plastic cover supplied by the manufacturer over the pacemaker controls and using the setting lock feature, if available, *to avoid an accidental setting change.*[38]
- Disconnect the temporary pacemaker from the lead system before defibrillation or cardioversion whenever possible *to ensure patient safety and to avoid damage to the pacemaker.*[38]
- Perform a 12-lead ECG before the procedure *to serve as a baseline*, and then perform additional ECGs daily or as needed with clinical changes. Also, if possible, obtain a rhythm strip before, during, and after pacemaker placement; any time that pacemaker settings change; and whenever the patient receives treatment for a complication caused by the pacemaker.
- Continuously monitor the ECG reading, noting capture, sensing, rate, intrinsic beats, and competition of paced and intrinsic rhythms.[44] If the pacemaker is sensing correctly, the sense indicator on the pulse generator should flash with each beat. (See *Handling pacemaker malfunctions*, page 863.)

Complications

Complications associated with pacemaker therapy include microshock, equipment failure, and competitive or fatal arrhythmias. Transvenous pacemakers can cause such complications as pneumothorax or hemothorax, cardiac perforation and tamponade, diaphragmatic stimulation, pulmonary embolism, thrombophlebitis, infection, air embolism, and bleeding.[45] Also, if the practitioner threads the electrode through the antecubital or femoral vein, venous spasm, thrombophlebitis, or lead displacement can result.

Documentation

Record the reason for the temporary pacing, the date and time of pacemaker insertion, the time pacing started, pacemaker settings, and the locations of the electrodes. Document the patient's vital signs, heart rate and rhythm, skin color, LOC, peripheral pulse, and emotional state before and after the procedure. Note the patient's pain assessment, any interventions provided, and the patient's response to the interventions. Note the patient's response to the procedure along with any complications that occurred and interventions performed in response. Document confirmation of electrode placement. If possible, obtain rhythm strips before, during, and after pacemaker placement; whenever pacemaker settings change; and when the patient receives treatment for a complication caused by the pacemaker. As you monitor the patient, record responses to temporary pacing and note changes in the patient's condition. Document teaching provided to the patient and family (if applicable), their understanding of that teaching, and any need for follow-up teaching.

REFERENCES

1 Wiegand, D. L. (2017). *AACN procedure manual for high acuity, progressive, and critical care* (7th ed.). St. Louis, MO: Elsevier.

2 Kusumoto, F. M., et al. (2018). 2018 ACC/AHA/HRS guideline on the evaluation and management of patients with bradycardia and cardiac conduction delay. *Journal of the American College of Cardiology, 74*(7), e51–e156. https://www.sciencedirect.com/science/article/pii/S073510971838985X?viaDihub (Level VII)

3 American Heart Association. (2020). 2020 American Heart Association Guidelines for CPR and ECC—Part 3: Adult basic and advanced life support. https://cpr.heart.org/en/resuscitation-science/cpr-and-ecc-guidelines (Level II)

4 The Joint Commission. (2021). Standard RI.01.03.01. *Comprehensive accreditation manual for hospitals.* Oakbrook Terrace, IL: The Joint Commission. (Level VII)

5 Centers for Medicare and Medicaid Services, Department of Health and Human Services. (2020). Condition of participation: Patient's rights. 42 C.F.R. § 482.13(b)(2).

6 Accreditation Association for Hospitals and Health Systems. (2020). Standard 30.01.11. *Healthcare Facilities Accreditation Program: Accreditation requirements for acute care hospitals.* Chicago, IL: Accreditation Association for Hospitals and Health Systems. (Level VII)

7 DNV GL-Healthcare USA, Inc. (2020). PR.2.SR.3. *NIAHO® accreditation requirements, interpretive guidelines and surveyor guidance—revision 20.0.* Milford, OH: DNV GL-Healthcare USA, Inc. (Level VII)

8 The Joint Commission. (2021). Standard UP.01.01.01. *Comprehensive accreditation manual for hospitals.* Oakbrook Terrace, IL: The Joint Commission. (Level VII)

9 Accreditation Association for Hospitals and Health Systems. (2020). Standard 30.00.14. *Healthcare Facilities Accreditation Program: Accreditation requirements for acute care hospitals.* Chicago, IL: Accreditation Association for Hospitals and Health Systems. (Level VII)

10 Centers for Disease Control and Prevention. (2002). Guideline for hand hygiene in health-care settings: Recommendations of the Healthcare Infection Control Practices Advisory Committee and the HICPAC/SHEA/APIC/IDSA Hand Hygiene Task Force. *MMWR Recommendations and Reports, 51*(RR-16), 1–45. https://www.cdc.gov/mmwr/pdf/rr/rr5116.pdf (Level II)

11 The Joint Commission. (2021). Standard NPSG.07.01.01. *Comprehensive accreditation manual for hospitals.* Oakbrook Terrace, IL: The Joint Commission. (Level VII)

12 World Health Organization (WHO). (2009). WHO guidelines on hand hygiene in health care: First global patient safety challenge, clean care is safer care. https://apps.who.int/iris/bitstream/handle/10665/44102/9789241597906_eng.pdf?sequence=1 (Level IV)

13 Accreditation Association for Hospitals and Health Systems. (2020). Standard 07.01.21. *Healthcare Facilities Accreditation Program: Accreditation requirements for acute care hospitals.* Chicago, IL: Accreditation Association for Hospitals and Health Systems. (Level VII)

14 Centers for Medicare and Medicaid Services, Department of Health and Human Services. (2020). Condition of participation: Infection control. 42 C.F.R. § 482.42.

15 DNV GL-Healthcare USA, Inc. (2020). IC.1.SR.1. *NIAHO® accreditation requirements, interpretive guidelines and surveyor guidance—revision 20.0.* Milford, OH: DNV GL-Healthcare USA, Inc. (Level VII)

16 The Joint Commission. (2021). Standard NPSG.01.01.01. *Comprehensive accreditation manual for hospitals.* Oakbrook Terrace, IL: The Joint Commission. (Level VII)

17 Accreditation Association for Hospitals and Health Systems. (2020). Standard 15.01.16. *Healthcare Facilities Accreditation Program: Accreditation requirements for acute care hospitals.* Chicago, IL: Accreditation Association for Hospitals and Health Systems. (Level VII)

18 Centers for Medicare and Medicaid Services, Department of Health and Human Services. (2020). Condition of participation: Patient's rights. 42 C.F.R. § 482.13(c)(1).

19 DNV GL-Healthcare USA, Inc. (2020). PR.2.SR.5. *NIAHO® accreditation requirements, interpretive guidelines and surveyor guidance—revision 20.0.* Milford, OH: DNV GL-Healthcare USA, Inc. (Level VII)

20 The Joint Commission. (2021). Standard RI.01.01.01. *Comprehensive accreditation manual for hospitals.* Oakbrook Terrace, IL: The Joint Commission. (Level VII)

21 The Joint Commission. (2021). Standard PC.02.01.21. *Comprehensive accreditation manual for hospitals.* Oakbrook Terrace, IL: The Joint Commission. (Level VII)

22 Waters, T. R., et al. (2009). Safe patient handling training for schools of nursing. https://www.cdc.gov/niosh/docs/2009-127/pdfs/2009-127.pdf (Level VII)

23 Siegel, J. D., et al. (2007, revision 2019). 2007 guideline for isolation precautions: Preventing transmission of infectious agents in healthcare settings. https://www.cdc.gov/infectioncontrol/pdf/guidelines/isolation-guidelines-H.pdf (Level II)

24 Occupational Safety and Health Administration. (2012). Bloodborne pathogens, standard number 1910.1030. https://www.osha.gov/pls/oshaweb/owadisp.show_document?p_id=10051&p_table=STANDARDS (Level VII)

25 Accreditation Association for Hospitals and Health Systems. (2020). Standard 07.01.10. *Healthcare Facilities Accreditation Program: Accreditation requirements for acute care hospitals.* Chicago, IL: Accreditation Association for Hospitals and Health Systems. (Level VII)

26 The Joint Commission. (2021). Standard NPSG.06.01.01. *Comprehensive accreditation manual for hospitals.* Oakbrook Terrace, IL: The Joint Commission. (Level VII)

27 American Association of Critical-Care Nurses (AACN). (2018). AACN practice alert: Managing alarms in acute care across the life span: Electrocardiography and pulse oximetry. https://www.aacn.org/clinical-resources/practice-alerts/managing-alarms-in-acute-care-across-the-life-span (Level VII)

28 Graham, K. C., & Cvach, M. (2010). Monitor alarm fatigue: Standardizing use of physiological monitors and decreasing nuisance alarms. *American Journal of Critical Care, 19*(1), 28–37. https://doi.org/10.4037/ajcc2010651

29 The Joint Commission. (2013). Sentinel event alert 50: Medical device alarm safety in hospitals. https://www.jointcommission.org/-/media/tjc/documents/resources/patient-safety-topics/sentinel-event/sea_50_alarms_4_26_16.pdf (Level VII)

30 The Joint Commission. (2021). Standard NPSG.07.05.01. *Comprehensive accreditation manual for hospitals.* Oakbrook Terrace, IL: The Joint Commission. (Level VII)

31 The Joint Commission. (2021). Standard PC.01.02.07. *Comprehensive accreditation manual for hospitals.* Oakbrook Terrace, IL: The Joint Commission. (Level VII)

32 Accreditation Association for Hospitals and Health Systems. (2020). Standard 16.01.03. *Healthcare Facilities Accreditation Program: Accreditation requirements for acute care hospitals.* Chicago, IL: Accreditation Association for Hospitals and Health Systems. (Level VII)

33 Centers for Medicare and Medicaid Services, Department of Health and Human Services. (2020). Condition of participation: Nursing services. 42 C.F.R. § 482.23(c).

34 DNV GL Healthcare USA, Inc. (2020). MM.1.SR.3. *NIAHO® accreditation requirements, interpretive guidelines and surveyor guidance—revision 20.0.* Milford, OH: DNV GL-Healthcare USA, Inc. (Level VII)

35 The Joint Commission. Oakbrook Terrace, IL: The Joint Commission. (2021). Standard MM.06.01.01. *Comprehensive accreditation manual for hospitals.* (Level VII)

36 The Joint Commission. (2021). Standard NPSG.03.04.01. *Comprehensive accreditation manual for hospitals.* Oakbrook Terrace, IL: The Joint Commission. (Level VII)

37 The Joint Commission. (2021). Standard UP.01.03.01. *Comprehensive accreditation manual for hospitals.* Oakbrook Terrace, IL: The Joint Commission. (Level VII)

38 Medtronic. (2020). 5392: Dual chamber temporary external pacemaker: Technical manual. https://manuals.medtronic.com/content/dam/emanuals/crdm/M811268A001A_view.pdf

39 Ganz, D. A., et al. (2013, reviewed 2021). *Preventing falls in hospitals: A toolkit for improving quality of care* (AHRQ Publication No. 13-0015-EF). Agency for Healthcare Research and Quality. https://www.ahrq.gov/professionals/systems/hospital/fallpxtoolkit/index.html (Level VII)

40 The Joint Commission. (2021). Standard RC.01.03.01. *Comprehensive accreditation manual for hospitals.* Oakbrook Terrace, IL: The Joint Commission. (Level VII)

41 Centers for Medicare and Medicaid Services, Department of Health and Human Services. (2020). Condition of participation: Medical record services. 42 C.F.R. § 482.24(b).

42 Accreditation Association for Hospitals and Health Systems. (2020). Standard 10.00.03. *Healthcare Facilities Accreditation Program: Accreditation requirements for acute care hospitals.* Chicago, IL: Accreditation Association for Hospitals and Health Systems. (Level VII)

43 DNV GL-Healthcare USA, Inc. (2020). MR.2.SR.1. *NIAHO® accreditation requirements, interpretive guidelines and surveyor guidance—revision 20.0.* Milford, OH: DNV GL-Healthcare USA, Inc. (Level VII)

44 Sandau, K. E., et al. (2017). Update to practice standards for electrocardiographic monitoring in hospital settings: A scientific statement from the American Heart Association. *Circulation, 136*(9), e273–e344. https://www.ahajournals.org/doi/full/10.1161/CIR.0000000000000527 (Level I)

45 Ganz, L. I. (2019). Temporary cardiac pacing. In: *UpToDate,* Estes, N. A. M. (Ed.).

TRAUMATIC WOUND MANAGEMENT

Traumatic wounds include puncture wounds, abrasions, lacerations, and amputations.

A *puncture wound* occurs when a pointed object, such as a knife, glass fragment, or nail, pierces or penetrates the skin. It can also result from a human or animal bite. A puncture wound typically doesn't cause excessive bleeding, and may appear to close almost immediately; however, puncture wounds can be dangerous because of the risk of infection. Puncture wounds caused by human or animal bites are particularly prone to infection.[1,2]

In a *traumatic abrasion*, contact with a hard object, such as the road, floor, or carpet, scrapes the skin,[3] resulting in loss of the epidermis and partial loss of the dermis. These partial-thickness wounds are typically shallow, red, painful, and highly exudative, and may contain debris from the surface that caused the abrasion-producing event.[4] Abrasions are sometimes full-thickness, involving the complete epidermis and dermis; these wounds may require debridement and skin grafting or flap coverage. Abrasions can occur on any part of the body, but usually affect bony areas (such as the hands, forearms, elbows, knees, and chin). They're typically more painful than lacerations because they involve a larger area of skin and expose more nerve endings. If they involve the head or neck, they may appear worse than they are because of the increased blood supply in these areas. A patient doesn't typically seek medical treatment for an isolated traumatic abrasion; in most cases, this type of wound is treated with other traumatic injuries. Abrasions in nonexposed areas, such as the neck or genitalia, require additional questioning to determine the cause.[4]

A *traumatic laceration* is a tear in the skin that occurs from an injury. Most wounds of this type are located on the head, the neck, or an upper extremity. The most common mechanism of injury is the application of blunt force that crushes the skin against underlying bone, causing the skin to split. Other causes of lacerations include sharp instruments, glass, and wooden objects.[5]

A *traumatic amputation* is the severing of part of the body, such as a limb or part of a limb.

When caring for a patient with a traumatic wound, your first priority is to assess the patient's circulation, airway, and breathing.[6] Once these are stabilized, you can address the traumatic wound. Initial management focuses on controlling bleeding, usually by applying firm, direct pressure and elevating the extremity. If bleeding continues, you may need to compress a pressure point. You must also assess the condition of the wound; puncture wounds may contain foreign bodies, such as fragments from the object that caused the wound or from clothing driven into the wound by the object.[7] You would then clean and manage the wound according to the extent of the injury.

Equipment

Soap and water ■ washcloth ■ sterile basin ■ normal saline solution or potable tap water ■ wound irrigation device (a commercial wound irrigation device or a 35-mL or 65-mL catheter-tip syringe with a 19G needle or angiocatheter ■ sterile 4″ × 4″ (10-cm × 10-cm) gauze pads ■ gloves (clean or sterile) ■ sterile dressing ■ fluid-impermeable pad ■ wound measuring device ■ facility-approved pain assessment tool ■ light source ■ vital signs monitoring equipment ■ sutures and suture kit or skin-closure strips ■ cardiac monitor ■ pulse oximeter and probe ■ prescribed IV fluid ■ two watertight containers or bags and labels ■ ice ■ Optional: mask and goggles or mask with face shield, gown, single-patient-use scissors, disposable-head clippers, tetanus toxoid vaccine or tetanus immune globulin, rabies prophylaxis vaccine, appropriately-sized syringe and needle, anesthetic agent, prescribed pain medication, camera, prescribed antibacterial ointment, prescribed systemic antibiotics, splint, blood collection equipment (test tubes, labels, laboratory biohazard transport bag), oxygen and oxygen delivery system.

Preparation of equipment

Inspect all equipment and supplies. If a product is expired, is defective, or has compromised integrity, remove it from patient use, label it as expired or defective, and report the expiration or defect as directed by your facility.

Fill a sterile basin with normal saline solution or potable tap water. Make sure the treatment area has enough light *to allow close observation of the wound.*

Implementation

■ Gather and prepare the necessary equipment and supplies.
■ Perform hand hygiene.[8,9,10,11,12,13]
■ Put on gloves and, as needed, other personal protective equipment *to comply with standard precautions.*[14,15,16]
■ Confirm the patient's identity using at least two patient identifiers.[17]
■ Assess the patient's circulation, airway, and breathing. If necessary, begin cardiopulmonary resuscitation, *because a wound may be associated with a more serious, life-threatening injury.*[6] (See the "Cardiopulmonary resuscitation" procedures.)
■ Provide privacy.[18,19,20,21]
■ Explain the procedure to the patient and family (if appropriate) according to their individual communication and learning needs *to increase their understanding, allay their fears, and enhance cooperation.*[22]
■ Raise the patient's bed to waist level before providing patient care *to prevent caregiver back strain.*[23]
■ Remove the patient's clothing *to expose the wound,* if necessary.
■ Control bleeding by applying gentle pressure using a sterile gauze pad, elevating the injured area (if applicable), or, if necessary, applying compression to pressure points.[24]
■ Obtain a history from the patient, if possible, or from an eye witnesses to the injury or a family member. The history should include the date, time, and mechanism of injury; whether any contaminants were present; the type, size, or weight of the object involved and details about the object, including whether the object was sharp or dull; the angle and speed of penetration; the environment in which the injury occurred; and the patient's tetanus immunization history.[25]
■ Ask about risk factors that may complicate wound healing, such as diabetes mellitus, peripheral vascular disease, chronic renal failure, human immunodeficiency virus infection, immunosuppressive medication or anticoagulant use, and bleeding disorders. Inquire about allergies to latex, medications, and dressing materials.
■ Obtain the patient's vital signs, and assess for other injuries, *because traumatic wounds are commonly associated with other injuries.*[24]
■ Screen for and assess the patient's pain using facility-defined criteria that are consistent with the patient's age, condition, and ability to understand.[26]
■ Treat the patient's pain, as needed and ordered, using nonpharmacologic or pharmacologic approaches, or a combination. Base the treatment plan on evidence-based practices and the patient's clinical condition, past medical history, and pain management goals.[26]
■ Remove jewelry near and distal to the wound *to prevent neurovascular compromise as swelling occurs in response to the injury.*
■ Place a fluid-impermeable pad under the injured area.

For a traumatic puncture wound

■ Clean the skin surrounding the puncture wound with soap and water and a washcloth *to prevent skin contaminants from entering the wound.*
■ Inspect the wound; estimate its depth, and determine the degree of contamination and the likelihood of injury to internal tissues.[25]
■ If a penetrating object remains in the wound, support the object until removal is possible. If the foreign body is in a joint or a highly mobile area, splint the joint or area *to prevent further damage.*
■ Assist the practitioner during inspection of the wound and assessment of the injured area and the area distal to the injury for sensation, muscle movement, and adequate circulation *to determine whether significant nerve or vessel damage has occurred.*[25]
■ Screen for and assess the patient's pain using facility-defined criteria that are appropriate for the patient's age, condition, and ability to understand.[26]
■ Monitor closely if the patient is at high risk for adverse outcomes related to opioid treatment, if prescribed.[26]
■ If the wound is deep, assist the practitioner with the administration of a local or regional anesthetic, as needed, following safe medication practices, *to further inspect the wound.*

■ Irrigate the wound with sterile normal saline solution or potable tap water using an irrigation device *to remove debris and bacteria from the wound.*[5,24] Flush the wound gently with solution until the solution runs clear, being sure to hold the syringe 1" (2.54 cm) above the wound and rinsing from the least to the most contaminated area (See the "Wound irrigation" procedure).
■ Arrange for an X-ray, ultrasonography, or computed tomography scan, as ordered, *to locate or assess for a retained foreign body.*[25]
■ Obtain consent and photograph the wound, if indicated. (See the "Wound photography" procedure.)
■ Clip local hair using single-patient-use scissors or disposable-head clippers, as needed, *to prevent wound contamination;* don't clip eyebrows, *because regrowth is unpredictable.*[5,24]
■ Remove and discard your gloves.[15]
■ Perform hand hygiene.[8,9,10,11,12,13]
■ Put on new gloves (clean or sterile, depending on the nature and location of the wound).[14,15]
■ Assist the practitioner with foreign body removal and wound closure using sutures or skin-closure strips, as indicated. You'll usually allow puncture wounds to heal by secondary intentions without sutures or staples *to allow wound drainage and decrease the risk of infection.*[25]
■ Apply antibacterial ointment, if prescribed, following safe medication administration practices *to help prevent infection.*[5,24,27,28,29,30]
■ Apply a dry, sterile dressing over the wound *to absorb drainage and help prevent bacterial contamination.*[5]
■ Administer the tetanus toxoid vaccine or tetanus immune globulin, as needed and ordered, following safe medication administration practices.[24,27,28,29,30]
■ If the puncture wound was caused by an animal and the immunization status of the animal is unknown or not current, administer rabies prophylaxis vaccine, as needed and as ordered, following safe medication administration practices.[24,27,28,29,30]
■ Reassess and respond to the patient's pain by evaluating the response to treatment and progress toward pain management goals. Assess for adverse reactions and risk factors for adverse events that may result from treatment.[26]
■ Administer systemic antibiotics, if ordered, following safe medication administration practices.[27,28,29,30]
■ Discard used supplies in appropriate receptacles.[15]
■ Return the bed to the lowest position *to prevent falls and maintain the patient's safety.*[31]
■ Remove and discard your gloves and other personal protective equipment, if worn.[15]
■ Perform hand hygiene.[8,9,10,11,12,13]
■ Document the procedure.[32,33,34,35]

For a traumatic abrasion

■ Irrigate the wound with normal saline solution or tap water (as directed) using a wound irrigation device *to remove wound debris and bacteria.*[3,24,36] Alternatively, if the patient is able, have the patient shower and clean the wound with a surgical scrub brush or sponge containing chlorhexidine (or another prescribed antiseptic solution) or, if the wound is small and the patient is able, use a shower attachment at a faucet to clean the wound with tap water.
■ Obtain consent and then photograph the wound, if indicated.
■ Assess the wound, measure the wound size, and remove any remaining debris using a surgical scrub sponge or brush containing chlorhexidine or another prescribed antiseptic solution, *to reduce the risk of infection,* if needed.[24]
■ If debris continues to remain in the wound, notify the patient's practitioner, *because the site may need to be anesthetized before further cleaning. Be sure to remove all debris from the wound to prevent tattooing, which occurs when debris becomes embedded in the dermal layer.*
■ Arrange for an X-ray, if ordered, *to rule out the presence of a foreign body, especially if gravel or other material is present in the wound.*
■ If surgical intervention is necessary to clean the wound, prepare the patient for transfer to an operating room.
■ Apply antibacterial ointment, if ordered, following safe medication administration practices.[27,28,29,30]

- Cover the wound with a sterile, occlusive, low-adherent dressing, *because occlusive dressings promote wound healing.*[37]
- Administer a tetanus toxoid vaccine, if needed and prescribed, following safe medication administration practices.[27,28,29,30]

For a traumatic laceration

- Irrigate the wound with normal saline solution or tap water (as directed) using an irrigation device *to remove wound debris and bacteria.*[5]
- Assess the wound to determine its severity as well as the involvement of underlying muscle, tendons, nerves, blood vessels, and bones. Determine whether your clinical findings are consistent with the patient's history.[5]
- Arrange for an X-ray or ultrasound, if ordered, *to assess the extent of injury and detect the presence of any foreign body.*[5]
- Obtain consent and photograph the wound, if indicated.
- Clip local hair using single-patient-use scissors or disposable-head clippers, as needed, *to prevent wound contamination;* don't clip eyebrows, *because regrowth is unpredictable.*[5]
- Remove and discard your gloves.[15]
- Perform hand hygiene.[8,9,10,11,12,13]
- Put on gloves.[14,15,38]
- Assist as the practitioner administers a local anesthetic (for a small wound) or a regional block (for a large extremity wound) and provides wound care; the practitioner will remove any visible foreign matter with forceps and devitalized tissue with sharp debridement *to reduce the risk of infection.*
- If indicated, prepare the patient for surgical intervention *to control bleeding and treat underlying injuries immediately.* Surgical intervention may be needed to repair deep wounds of the hand or foot; full-thickness lacerations of the eyelid, lip, or ear; lacerations involving nerves, arteries, bones, or joints; penetrating wounds of unknown depth; severe crush injuries; severely contaminated wounds that require drainage; and wounds for which the cosmetic outcome is a strong concern.[5]
- Assist the practitioner with wound closure (if appropriate) using sutures, tissue adhesive, staples, or skin-closure strips. If closure must be delayed, assist the practitioner with packing the wound.
- Apply antibacterial ointment or petrolatum jelly, if ordered, following safe medication administration practices,[5,27,28,29,30] *to help prevent infection.* Don't apply a topical ointment if the wound was closed with a tissue adhesive, *because topical ointments loosen the adhesive and can cause wound dehiscence.*
- Apply a dry, sterile dressing over the wound, if ordered; cover sutured or stapled wounds with a protective nonadherent dressing for 24 to 48 hours until adequate epithelization takes place *to protect the wound from gross contamination.*[5] An occlusive or semi-occlusive dressing may be applied, if appropriate, *because wounds may heal faster in a moist environment.*[38,39]
- Administer tetanus toxoid vaccine or tetanus immune globulin, as needed and prescribed, following safe medication administration practices.[27,28,29,30]

For a traumatic amputation

- Control bleeding by applying direct pressure to the wound using sterile gauze, elevating the injured area, or, if necessary, applying compression to pressure points. If bleeding continues, apply a tourniquet as close to the amputation site as possible.[40,41]

NURSING ALERT Keep in mind that prolonged tourniquet use can cause complications, including compartment syndrome, nerve palsy, damage to blood vessels, thrombosis, pressure injuries, and further amputation related to tourniquet pressure and duration of occlusion. A time beyond which irreversible complications may occur has not been determined; however, a recent study found that tourniquet use for longer than 2 hours was associated with amputation and fasciotomy but not other morbidities. It's essential to communicate the time a tourniquet is first applied to emergency medical service providers and emergency department staff.[42,43]

- Obtain a history from the patient (or from an eyewitnesses to the injury or a family member), if able, that includes the date, time, and mechanism of injury; information about any contaminants present; the type, size, or weight of any instrument or machinery involved; details about the instrument, including whether it was dull or sharp; the angle and speed of penetration; the environment in which the injury occurred; and the date of the patient's last tetanus immunization. Also inquire about any allergies to latex, medications, or dressing materials.

- Ask about risk factors that may complicate wound healing, such as diabetes mellitus, stage 5 kidney disease, peripheral vascular disease, human immunodeficiency virus infection, immunosuppressive drug or anticoagulant use, and bleeding disorders.[44]
- Attach the patient to a continuous cardiac monitor, pulse oximeter, and automated blood pressure device, as indicated. Make sure that the alarm limits are set appropriately for the patient's current condition, and that the alarms are turned on, functioning properly, and audible to staff.[45,46,47,48]
- Obtain the patient's vital signs and assess for signs of shock, such as hypotension, tachycardia, diminished pulses, altered level of consciousness, and pallor. Assess for other injuries.
- Administer supplemental oxygen, as prescribed.[37]
- Insert an IV catheter, as ordered, if the patient doesn't already have one in place. (See the "IV catheter insertion and removal" procedure.) Administer IV fluids as prescribed.
- Screen for and assess the patient's pain using facility-defined criteria that are appropriate for the patient's age, condition, and ability to understand.[26]
- Treat the patient's pain, as needed and ordered, using nonpharmacologic or pharmacologic approaches, or a combination. Base the treatment plan on evidence-based practices and the patient's clinical condition, past medical history, and pain management goals.[26] Administer pain medication, as needed and as ordered, following safe medication administration practices; *administering pain medication as soon as possible after injury controls acute pain and reduces the risk of chronic pain.*[27,28,29,30,40]
- Monitor closely if the patient is at high risk for adverse outcomes related to opioid treatment, if prescribed.[26]
- If directed by your facility, obtain consent and photograph the wound.
- For a complete amputation, irrigate the residual limb with sterile normal saline solution *to remove gross contamination.*[37]
- For a partial amputation, support the limb and splint it in a position of anatomic function.[37]
- Remove jewelry near the amputation site *to prevent neurovascular compromise because swelling occurs in response to the injury.*[24]

Caring for a severed body part

After traumatic amputation, a surgeon may be able to reimplant the severed body part through microsurgery. The chance of successful reimplantation is much greater if the amputated part has received proper care.

If a patient arrives at the hospital with a severed body part, first make sure that bleeding at the amputation site has been controlled. Then follow these guidelines for preserving the body part:
- Perform hand hygiene[8,9,10,11,12,13] and put on sterile gloves.[14,15]
- Place several sterile gauze pads and an appropriate amount of sterile roller gauze in a sterile basin, and pour sterile normal saline or sterile lactated Ringer solution over them. *Never use any other solution,* and don't try to scrub or debride the part.
- Holding the body part in one gloved hand, carefully pat it dry with sterile gauze. Place saline-moistened gauze pads over the severed end; then wrap the whole body part with saline-moistened roller gauze. Wrap the gauze with a sterile towel, if available. Then put this package in a watertight bag or container and seal it.[24]
- Fill another plastic bag with ice and water *to make an ice-water slurry* and place the part (still in its watertight container) inside the outer bag. Seal the outer bag. (Always protect the part from direct contact with ice—and never use dry ice—*to prevent irreversible tissue damage, which would make the part unsuitable for reimplantation.*) Keep this bag ice-cold until the surgeon is ready to do the reimplantation surgery.[24]
- Label the bag with the patient's name and identification number, identification of the amputated part, the health care facility's identification number, and the date and time when cooling began.[24]

Note: The body part must be wrapped and cooled quickly. *Irreversible tissue damage occurs after only 6 hours at ambient temperature.* However, hypothermic management seldom preserves tissues for more than 24 hours.

■ Cover the wound with sterile gauze soaked in normal saline solution and then cover the gauze with an adhesive film dressing *to prevent evaporation*. Avoid repeated wound inspection and dressing changes, *because they increase the risk of infection*.

■ Administer antibiotics, as ordered, *to prevent infection* following safe medication administration practices.[27,28,29,30]

■ As ordered, obtain blood samples for coagulation studies; hemoglobin level, hematocrit, electrolyte levels, and typing and crossmatching *in the event blood transfusion is needed*.

■ Administer tetanus toxoid vaccine or tetanus immune globulin, as needed and prescribed, following safe medication administration practices.[27,28,29,30]

■ Preserve the severed body part, if possible. (See *Caring for a severed body part*, page 867.)

■ Arrange for an X-ray of the extremity, if ordered.

■ Prepare the patient for surgery, as indicated.

Completing the procedure

■ Return the bed to the lowest position *to prevent falls and maintain the patient's safety*.[31]

■ Discard used supplies in appropriate receptacles.[15]

■ Reassess and respond to the patient's pain by evaluating the response to treatment and progress toward pain management goals. Assess for adverse reactions and risk factors for adverse events that may result from treatment.[26]

■ Remove and discard your gloves and any other personal protective equipment worn.[15]

■ Perform hand hygiene.[8,9,10,11,12,13]

■ Document the procedure.[32,33,34,35]

Special considerations

■ When irrigating a traumatic wound, avoid using more than 8 psi of pressure. *High-pressure irrigation can seriously interfere with healing, kill cells, and allow bacteria to infiltrate the tissue*.[38,49]

■ Observe for signs of infection, such as warm, red skin at the site and purulent discharge.[3] Be aware that infection of a traumatic wound can delay healing, increase scar formation, and trigger systemic infection such as septicemia.[4]

■ Observe all dressings for tightness, *which may be a sign of edema*. If edema is present, adjust the dressing *to avoid impairing circulation to the area*.

■ Note that cyanoacrylate topical bandage (skin glue), lipidocolloid-based mesh dressings, soft silicone foam dressings, and clear acrylic dressings may promote healing and lower infection rates. Use these products as ordered or as directed by your facility.[50,51]

Complications

Cleaning and care of traumatic wounds may temporarily increase the patient's pain. Excessive, vigorous cleaning may further disrupt tissue integrity.[24] Localized or systemic infection can result from a traumatic puncture wound. Significant blood loss and local and systemic infection are other potential complications of traumatic amputation.[40] Complications from an infected animal or human bite may include septic arthritis, osteomyelitis, abscess, tendinitis, and bacteremia.[3]

Documentation

Document the date and time of the procedure, wound size and condition, assessment findings (including vital signs), medication administration, pain assessment, and specific wound care measures you performed. Document the location and type of injury, evidence that you collected (if appropriate), and a brief description on a body diagram (if used in your facility), as indicated.[37] Document teaching provided to the patient and family (if applicable), their understanding of that teaching, and any need for follow-up teaching.

REFERENCES

1 Baddour, L. M., & Harper, M. (2021). Animal bites (dogs, cats, and other animals): Evaluation and management. In: *UpToDate*, Wolfson, A. B. (Ed.).

2 Baddour, L. M., & Harper, M. (2021). Human bites: Evaluation and management. In: *UpToDate*, Wolfson, A. B. (Ed.).

3 Worster, B., et al. (2015). Common questions about wound care. *American Family Physician, 91*(2), 86–92. https://www.aafp.org/afp/2015/0115/p86.html

4 Shrestha, R., et al. (2020). Abrasions. https://www.ncbi.nlm.nih.gov/books/NBK554465/

5 deLemos, D. (2021). Skin laceration repair with sutures. In: *UpToDate*, Stack, A. M., & Wolfson, A. B. (Eds.).

6 American Heart Association. (2020). 2020 American Heart Association Guidelines for CPR and ECC—Part 3: Adult basic and advanced life support. https://cpr.heart.org/en/resuscitation-science/cpr-and-ecc-guidelines (Level II)

7 American College of Foot and Ankle Surgeons. (n.d.). Puncture wounds. https://www.acfas.org/footankleinfo/puncture-wounds.htm

8 The Joint Commission. (2021). Standard NPSG.07.01.01. *Comprehensive accreditation manual for hospitals*. Oakbrook Terrace, IL: The Joint Commission. (Level VII)

9 Centers for Disease Control and Prevention. (2002). Guideline for hand hygiene in health-care settings: Recommendations of the Healthcare Infection Control Practices Advisory Committee and the HICPAC/SHEA/APIC/IDSA Hand Hygiene Task Force. *MMWR Recommendations and Reports, 51*(RR-16), 1–45. https://www.cdc.gov/mmwr/pdf/rr/rr5116.pdf (Level II)

10 World Health Organization (WHO). (2009). WHO guidelines on hand hygiene in health care: First global patient safety challenge, clean care is safer care. https://apps.who.int/iris/bitstream/handle/10665/44102/9789241597906_eng.pdf?sequence=1 (Level IV)

11 Accreditation Association for Hospitals and Health Systems. (2020). Standard 07.01.21. *Healthcare Facilities Accreditation Program: Accreditation requirements for acute care hospitals*. Chicago, IL: Accreditation Association for Hospitals and Health Systems. (Level VII)

12 Centers for Medicare and Medicaid Services, Department of Health and Human Services. (2020). Condition of participation: Infection control. 42 C.F.R. § 482.42.

13 DNV GL-Healthcare USA, Inc. (2020). IC.1.SR.1. *NIAHO® accreditation requirements: Interpretive guidelines and surveyor guidance—revision 20.0*. Milford, OH: DNV GL-Healthcare USA, Inc. (Level VII)

14 Siegel, J. D., et al. (2007, revised 2019). 2007 guideline for isolation precautions: Preventing transmission of infectious agents in healthcare settings. https://www.cdc.gov/infectioncontrol/pdf/guidelines/isolation-guidelines-H.pdf (Level II)

15 Occupational Safety and Health Administration. (2012). Bloodborne pathogens, standard number 1910.1030. fromhttps://www.osha.gov/pls/oshaweb/owadisp.show_document?p_id=10051&p_table=STANDARDS (Level VII)

16 Accreditation Association for Hospitals and Health Systems. (2020). Standard 07.01.10. *Healthcare Facilities Accreditation Program: Accreditation requirements for acute care hospitals*. Chicago, IL: Accreditation Association for Hospitals and Health Systems. (Level VII)

17 The Joint Commission. (2021). Standard NPSG.01.01.01. *Comprehensive accreditation manual for hospitals*. Oakbrook Terrace, IL: The Joint Commission. (Level VII)

18 DNV GL-Healthcare USA, Inc. (2020). PR.2.SR.5. *NIAHO® accreditation requirements: Interpretive guidelines and surveyor guidance—revision 20.0*. Milford, OH: DNV GL-Healthcare USA, Inc. (Level VII)

19 Accreditation Association for Hospitals and Health Systems. (2020). Standard 15.01.16. *Healthcare Facilities Accreditation Program: Accreditation requirements for acute care hospitals*. Chicago, IL: Accreditation Association for Hospitals and Health Systems. (Level VII)

20 Centers for Medicare and Medicaid Services, Department of Health and Human Services. (2020). Condition of participation: Patient's rights. 42 C.F.R. § 482.13(c)(1).

21 The Joint Commission. (2021). Standard RI.01.01.01. *Comprehensive accreditation manual for hospitals*. Oakbrook Terrace, IL: The Joint Commission. (Level VII)

22 The Joint Commission. (2021). Standard PC.02.01.21. *Comprehensive accreditation manual for hospitals*. Oakbrook Terrace, IL: The Joint Commission. (Level VII)

23 Waters, T. R., et al. (2009). Safe patient handling training for schools of nursing. https://www.cdc.gov/niosh/docs/2009-127/pdfs/2009-127.pdf (Level VII)

24 Roberts, J. R., et al. (2019). *Roberts and Hedges' clinical procedures in emergency medicine and acute care* (7th ed.). St. Louis, MO: Elsevier.

25 Baddour, L. M., & Brown, A. M. (2020). Infectious complications of puncture wounds. In: *UpToDate*, Sexton, D. J. (Ed.).

26 The Joint Commission. (2021). Standard PC.01.02.07. *Comprehensive accreditation manual for hospitals*. Oakbrook Terrace, IL: The Joint Commission. (Level VII)

27 DNV GL-Healthcare USA, Inc. (2020). MM.1.SR.3. *NIAHO® accreditation requirements: Interpretive guidelines and surveyor guidance—revision 20.0*. Milford, OH: DNV GL-Healthcare USA, Inc. (Level VII)

28 Centers for Medicare and Medicaid Services, Department of Health and Human Services. (2020). Condition of participation: Nursing services. 42 C.F.R. § 482.23(c).

29 Accreditation Association for Hospitals and Health Systems. (2020). Standard 16.01.03. *Healthcare Facilities Accreditation Program: Accreditation requirements for acute care hospitals*. Chicago, IL: Accreditation Association for Hospitals and Health Systems. (Level VII)

30 The Joint Commission. (2021). Standard MM.06.01.01. *Comprehensive accreditation manual for hospitals*. Oakbrook Terrace, IL: The Joint Commission. (Level VII)

31 Ganz, D. A., et al. (2013). *Preventing falls in hospitals: A toolkit for improving quality of care* (AHRQ Publication No. 13-0015-EF). Agency for Healthcare Research and Quality. https://www.ahrq.gov/professionals/systems/hospital/fallpxtoolkit/index.html (Level VII)

32 The Joint Commission. (2021). Standard RC.01.03.01. *Comprehensive accreditation manual for hospitals*. Oakbrook Terrace, IL: The Joint Commission. (Level VII)

33 Accreditation Association for Hospitals and Health Systems. (2020). Standard 10.00.03. *Healthcare Facilities Accreditation Program: Accreditation requirements for acute care hospitals*. Chicago, IL: Accreditation Association for Hospitals and Health Systems. (Level VII)

34 Centers for Medicare and Medicaid Services, Department of Health and Human Services. (2020). Condition of participation: Medical record services. 42 C.F.R. § 482.24(b).

35 DNV GL-Healthcare USA, Inc. (2020). MR.2.SR.1. *NIAHO® accreditation requirements: Interpretive guidelines and surveyor guidance—revision 20.0*. Milford, OH: DNV GL-Healthcare USA, Inc. (Level VII)

36 Butcher, H. K., et al. (2018). *Nursing interventions classification (NIC)* (7th ed.). St. Louis, MO: Elsevier.

37 Emergency Nurses Association. (2013). *Sheehy's manual of emergency care* (7th ed.). St. Louis, MO: Elsevier.

38 Forsch, R. T., et al. (2017). Laceration repair: A practical approach. *American Family Physician* 95(10), 628–636. https://www.aafp.org/afp/2017/0515/p628.html (Level V)

39 Mankowitz, S. L. (2017). Laceration management. *Journal of Emergency Medicine, 53*(3), 369–382. https://doi.org/10.1016/j.jemermed.2017.05.026

40 Kalapatapu, V. (2021). Lower extremity amputation. In: *UpToDate*, Mills, J. L., & Eidt, J. F. (Eds.).

41 Drew, B., et al. (2015). Tourniquet conversion: A recommended approach in the prolonged field care setting. *Journal of Special Operations Medicine, 15*(3), 81–85. http://www.specialoperationsmedicine.org/Documents/PFC%20WG/Drew%20JSOM%20Fall%202015%20Edition-2.pdf (Level V)

42 American Heart Association. (2020). 2020 American Heart Association Guidelines for CPR and ECC—Part 8: First aid. https://cpr.heart.org/en/resuscitation-science/cpr-and-ecc-guidelines (Level II)

43 Kragh, J. F., et al. (2009). Survival with emergency tourniquet use to stop bleeding in major limb trauma. *Annals of Surgery, 249*(1), 1–7. https://journals.lww.com/annalsofsurgery/Fulltext/2009/01000/Survival_With_Emergency_Tourniquet_Use_to_Stop.1.aspx (Level IV)

44 Trott, A. T. (2012). *Wounds and lacerations: Emergency care and closure* (4th ed.). Philadelphia, PA: Saunders.

45 Graham, K. C., & Cvach, M. (2010). Monitor alarm fatigue: Standardizing use of physiological monitors and decreasing nuisance alarms. *American Journal of Critical Care, 19*(1), 28–37. https://doi.org/10.4037/ajcc2010651

46 The Joint Commission. (2021). Standard NPSG.06.01.01. *Comprehensive accreditation manual for hospitals*. Oakbrook Terrace, IL: The Joint Commission. (Level VII)

47 The Joint Commission. (2013). Sentinel event alert 50: Medical device alarm safety in hospitals. https://www.jointcommission.org/-/media/tjc/documents/resources/patient-safety-topics/sentinel-event/sea_50_alarms_4_26_16.pdf (Level VII)

48 American Association of Critical-Care Nurses (AACN). (2018). *AACN practice alert: Managing alarms in acute care across the life span: Electrocardiography and pulse oximetry*. https://www.aacn.org/clinical-resources/practice-alerts/managing-alarms-in-acute-care-across-the-life-span (Level VII)

49 Baranoski, S., & Ayello, E. A. (2020). *Wound care essentials: Practice principles* (5th ed.). Philadelphia, PA: Wolters Kluwer.

50 Singer, A. J., et al. (2015). Evaluation of a liquid dressing for minor nonbleeding abrasions and class I and II skin tears in the emergency department. *Journal of Emergency Medicine, 48*(2), 178–185. https://doi.org/10.1016/j.jemermed.2014.10.008 (Level IV)

51 Eberlein, T., et al. (2016). Advantages in wound healing by a topical easy to use wound healing lipo-gel for abrasive wounds—evidence from a randomized, controlled experimental clinical study. *Wound Medicine, 15,* 11–19. https://doi.org/10.1016/j.wndm.2016.09.003 (Level II)

Tub baths and showers

Tub baths and showers provide personal hygiene, stimulate circulation, and reduce tension for the patient. They also allow you to observe skin conditions and assess joint mobility and muscle strength.[1] If not precluded by the patient's condition or safety considerations, privacy during bathing promotes the patient's sense of well-being by allowing the patient to assume responsibility for personal care.

Patients who are recovering from recent surgery, who are emotionally unstable, or who have casted extremities or dressings in place usually require the practitioner's permission for a tub bath or shower.

Equipment

Washcloths ▪ bath towels ▪ bath blanket ▪ skin cleanser ▪ towel mat ▪ OCCUPIED sign ▪ clean clothing or hospital gown ▪ facility-approved disinfectant ▪ Optional: gloves, chair, shower cap, shampoo, plastic bag, nonskid shower chair, nonskid bath mat.

Preparation of equipment

Inspect all equipment and supplies. If a product is expired, is defective, or has compromised integrity, remove it from patient use, label it as expired or defective, and report the expiration or defect as directed by your facility.

Prepare the bathing area before the patient arrives. Close all doors and windows and adjust the room temperature *to avoid chilling the patient*. Check that the bathtub or shower is clean and disinfected.[1,2] Then gather bathing articles and observe appropriate safety measures. Remove electrical appliances, such as hair dryers and heaters, from the patient's reach, *to prevent electrical shock*.[1]

For a bath

Position a chair next to the tub *to help the patient get in and out of the tub and to provide a seat if the patient becomes weak*. Place a bath blanket over the chair *to cover the patient if the patient becomes chilled*. If the tub doesn't have nonskid strips, place a rubber mat or other nonskid mat in the tub. Then, fill the tub halfway with warm water and test the temperature;[1] it should feel comfortable to the touch. Adjust water flow and temperature just before the patient gets into the tub. Place a towel mat on the floor in front of the tub *to avoid contact with the cold flooring and prevent slipping*.[1]

For a shower

Cover the floor of the shower with a nonskid mat unless it already has nonskid strips. Place a nonskid shower chair in the locked position in the shower, if needed, *to provide support and a place where the patient can sit down to wash the legs and feet, to reduce the risk of falling*. Next, place a towel mat next to the bathing area *to avoid contact with cold flooring and to prevent slipping*.[1] Adjust water flow and temperature just before the patient gets into the shower.[1]

Implementation

- Verify the practitioner's order, if required.
- Gather and prepare the necessary equipment and supplies.
- Perform hand hygiene.[3,4,5,6,7,8]
- Confirm the patient's identity using at least two patient identifiers.[9]
- Explain the procedure to the patient and family (if appropriate) according to their individual communication and learning needs *to increase their understanding, ally their fears, and enhance cooperation*.[10]
- Escort the patient to the bathing area.[1]

- Provide privacy.[11,12,13,14]
- Perform hand hygiene.[3,4,5,6,7,8]
- Put on gloves, as necessary, *to comply with standard precautions.*[15,16,17]
- Help the patient undress, as necessary.
- Offer the patient a shower cap if the patient wants to keep the hair dry. Otherwise, provide shampoo. Place all items within easy reach of the patient *to prevent reaching and maintain patient safety.*
- Help the patient into the tub or shower.[1] Encourage the patient to use the handrails *to prevent falling.* Alternatively, assist the patient into the tub using a hydraulic bath lift.
- Place a towel on the shower chair, if necessary, *to increase patient comfort and warmth.*[18]
- Provide washcloths and skin cleaner. Avoid adding bath oil to the water, *because oil makes the tub slick and increases the risk of falling.*[1]
- Taking care to respect privacy, help the patient bathe, as needed. Be aware of signs of discomfort with bathing.[18]
- Allow family members to assist the patient with bathing, as desired, *to minimize fear.* Allow the patient to schedule bathing according to the patient's energy level and other preferences.[18]
- If you can safely leave the patient alone, place the call light within reach and show the patient how to use it. If the patient is confused, don't leave the patient alone.
- Tell the patient to leave the door unlocked *for safety,* but assure the patient that you'll post an OCCUPIED sign on the door.[1] Stay nearby in case of emergency, and check on the patient every 5 to 10 minutes.
- When the patient finishes bathing, drain the tub or turn off the shower (if necessary).[1]
- Assist the patient onto the towel mat *to prevent falling.*[1] Help the patient dry off and put on a clean gown or other clothing, as appropriate.[1]
- Escort the patient to the room or bed.[1]
- Dry the floor of the bathing area well *to prevent slipping.*
- Clean and disinfect the tub or shower and shower chair, if used, with facility-approved disinfectant.[2,19]
- Discard used washcloths and towels in the appropriate receptacle.[17]
- Remove and discard your gloves, if worn.[17]
- Perform hand hygiene.[3,4,5,6,7,8]
- Return the patient's personal belongings to the bedside.
- Perform hand hygiene.[3,4,5,6,7,8]
- Document the procedure.[20,21,22,23]

Special considerations

- Separate hair washing from body washing if either is distressing or overwhelming for the patient.[18]
- Encourage the patient to use safety devices, bars, and rails when bathing.[1]
- If the patient has dry skin, have the patient apply or assist with applying lotion or oil after the tub bath or shower.[1]
- *Because bathing in water that is too warm may cause vasodilation,* be alert for orthostatic hypotension.[1]
- If a walk-in tub is available at your facility, follow the manufacturer's instructions for use and cleaning.

Complications

A patient fall or burns may occur if safety precautions aren't followed.

Documentation

Describe the patient's skin condition and record any discoloration or redness in your notes. Document the patient's tolerance of the procedure. Document teaching provided to the patient and family (if applicable), their understanding of that teaching, and any need for follow-up teaching.

REFERENCES

1 Craven, R. F., et al. (2021). *Fundamentals of nursing: Concepts and competencies for practice.* (9th ed.). Philadelphia, PA: Wolters Kluwer.

2 Rutala, W. A., et al. (2008, revised 2019). Guideline for disinfection and sterilization in healthcare facilities, 2008. https://www.cdc.gov/infection-control/pdf/guidelines/disinfection-guidelines-H.pdf (Level I)

3 The Joint Commission. (2021). Standard NPSG.07.01.01. *Comprehensive accreditation manual for hospitals.* Oakbrook Terrace, IL: The Joint Commission. (Level VII)

4 Centers for Disease Control and Prevention. (2002). Guideline for hand hygiene in health-care settings: Recommendations of the Healthcare Infection Control Practices Advisory Committee and the HICPAC/SHEA/APIC/IDSA Hand Hygiene Task Force. *MMWR Recommendations and Reports, 51*(RR-16), 1–45. https://www.cdc.gov/mmwr/pdf/rr/rr5116.pdf (Level II)

5 World Health Organization. (2009). WHO guidelines on hand hygiene in health care: First global patient safety challenge, clean care is safer care. https://apps.who.int/iris/bitstream/handle/10665/44102/9789241597906_eng.pdf?sequence=1 (Level IV)

6 Centers for Medicare and Medicaid Services, Department of Health and Human Services. (2020). Condition of participation: Infection control. 42 C.F.R. § 482.42.

7 Accreditation Association for Hospitals and Health Systems. (2020). Standard 07.01.21. *Healthcare Facilities Accreditation Program: Accreditation requirements for acute care hospitals.* Chicago, IL: Accreditation Association for Hospitals and Health Systems. (Level VII)

8 DNV GL-Healthcare USA, Inc. (2020). IC.1.SR.1. *NIAHO® accreditation requirements, interpretive guidelines and surveyor guidance—revision 20.0.* Milford, OH: DNV GL-Healthcare USA, Inc. (Level VII)

9 The Joint Commission. (2021). Standard NPSG.01.01.01. *Comprehensive accreditation manual for hospitals.* Oakbrook Terrace, IL: The Joint Commission. (Level VII)

10 The Joint Commission. (2021). Standard PC.02.01.21. *Comprehensive accreditation manual for hospitals.* Oakbrook Terrace, IL: The Joint Commission. (Level VII)

11 DNV GL-Healthcare USA, Inc. (2020). PR.2.SR.5. *NIAHO® accreditation requirements, interpretive guidelines and surveyor guidance—revision 20.0.* Milford, OH: DNV GL-Healthcare USA, Inc. (Level VII)

12 Centers for Medicare and Medicaid Services, Department of Health and Human Services. (2020). Condition of participation: Patient's rights. 42 C.F.R. § 482.13(c)(1).

13 Accreditation Association for Hospitals and Health Systems. (2020). Standard 15.01.16. *Healthcare Facilities Accreditation Program: Accreditation requirements for acute care hospitals.* Chicago, IL: Accreditation Association for Hospitals and Health Systems. (Level VII)

14 The Joint Commission. (2021). Standard RI.01.01.01. *Comprehensive accreditation manual for hospitals.* Oakbrook Terrace, IL: The Joint Commission. (Level VII)

15 Siegel, J. D., et al. (2007, revised 2019). 2007 guideline for isolation precautions: Preventing transmission of infectious agents in healthcare settings. https://www.cdc.gov/infectioncontrol/pdf/guidelines/isolation-guidelines-H.pdf (Level II)

16 Accreditation Association for Hospitals and Health Systems. (2020). Standard 07.01.10. *Healthcare Facilities Accreditation Program: Accreditation requirements for acute care hospitals.* Chicago, IL: Accreditation Association for Hospitals and Health Systems. (Level VII)

17 Occupational Safety and Health Administration. (2012). Bloodborne pathogens, standard number 1910.1030. https://www.osha.gov/pls/oshaweb/owadisp.show_document?p_id=10051&p_table=STANDARDS (Level VII)

18 Rader, J., et al. (2006). The bathing of older adults with dementia: Easing the unnecessarily unpleasant aspects of assisted bathing. *American Journal of Nursing, 106*(4), 40–48. https://journals.lww.com/ajnonline/pages/articleviewer.aspx?year=2006&issue=04000&article=00026&type=fulltext (Level VII)

19 Accreditation Association for Hospitals and Health Systems. (2020). Standard 07.02.03. *Healthcare Facilities Accreditation Program: Accreditation requirements for acute care hospitals.* Chicago, IL: Accreditation Association for Hospitals and Health Systems. (Level VII)

20 The Joint Commission. (2021). Standard RC.01.03.01. *Comprehensive accreditation manual for hospitals.* Oakbrook Terrace, IL: The Joint Commission. (Level VII)

21 Accreditation Association for Hospitals and Health Systems. (2020). Standard 10.00.03. *Healthcare Facilities Accreditation Program: Accreditation requirements for acute care hospitals.* Chicago, IL: Accreditation Association for Hospitals and Health Systems. (Level VII)

22 Centers for Medicare and Medicaid Services, Department of Health and Human Services. (2020). Condition of participation: Medical record services. 42 C.F.R. § 482.24(b).

23 DNV GL-Healthcare USA, Inc. (2020). MR.2.SR.1. *NIAHO® accreditation requirements, interpretive guidelines and surveyor guidance—revision 20.0.* Milford, OH: DNV GL-Healthcare USA, Inc. (Level VII)

Ultraviolet light therapy

Ultraviolet (UV) light exposure causes profound biological changes, including UV light–induced immune suppression, inhibition of skin cell proliferation, and stimulation of melanocyte proliferation.[1,2] Some skin conditions, including psoriasis, eczema, vitiligo, mycosis fungoides, atopic dermatitis, uremic pruritus, and graft-versus-host disease, may respond to therapy that uses timed exposure to UV light rays.[1,2]

Emitted by the sun, the UV spectrum is subdivided into three bands—A, B, and C—each of which affects the skin differently. Ultraviolet A (UVA) radiation (with a relatively long wavelength of 320 to 400 nanometers [nm]) rapidly darkens preformed melanin pigment, may augment ultraviolet B (UVB) in causing sunburn and skin aging, and may induce phototoxicity in the presence of some drugs. UVB radiation (with a wavelength of 280 to 320 nm) causes sunburn and erythema. Ultraviolet C (UVC) radiation (with a wavelength of 200 to 280 nm) normally is absorbed by the earth's ozone layer and doesn't reach the ground; it's used in operating-room germicidal lamps because it kills bacteria.[1,2,3]

Treating skin with the administration of a photosensitizing psoralen plus exposure to UVA is called *psoralen-plus-ultraviolet A (PUVA) therapy,* or *photochemotherapy.* The psoralen agent, such as methoxsalen, creates artificial sensitivity to UVA by binding with the deoxyribonucleic acid in epidermal basal cells. Administered before UV light therapy, the agent photosensitizes the skin to enhance therapeutic effects. Other drugs used in PUVA therapy include acitretin (an oral vitamin A derivative) and methotrexate. Psoralen agents are commonly prescribed in pill form, but may be prescribed in topical form for localized therapy or when a patient can't tolerate adverse effects associated with systemic therapy.[1]

For PUVA therapy, the initial dose is based on the patient's skin type, and subsequent doses are increased according to the treatment protocol and as tolerated.[4] The practitioner calculates the UVB dose based on skin type estimation or by determining a minimal erythema dose—the smallest amount of UV light needed to produce mild erythema.[4] Targeted UVB therapy delivered by a high-energy laser is available and allows for targeted therapy of higher doses of UVB, which may have a more rapid response time and therefore a shorter therapy period, protect unaffected skin, and have fewer complications.[2,4] Treatment is generally continued until complete remission or until no further improvement is seen. Maintenance therapy may then be ordered to prolong remission, or the patient may be tapered off of treatment.[2,4] (See *Comparing skin types.*)

Comparing skin types

The table below compares different skin types based on their susceptibility to ultraviolet light and their subsequent sunburn and tanning history.[1,2,4]

Skin type	Sunburn and tanning history
I	Always burns; never tans; sensitive ("Celtic" skin)
II	Burns easily; tans minimally
III	Burns moderately; tans gradually to light brown (average Caucasian skin)
IV	Burns minimally; always tans well to moderately brown (olive skin)
V	Rarely burns; tans profusely to dark (brown skin)
VI	Never burns; deeply pigmented; not sensitive (black skin)

Contraindications to PUVA therapy include lupus erythematosus in patients with a history of photosensitivity or a positive Ro antibody, porphyria, xeroderma pigmentosa, or a personal history of melanoma; PUVA therapy is also contraindicated for children younger than age 10.[1,4,5] Caution should be used in patients with skin types I and II; patients with a history of liver, renal, or cardiac disease, photosensitivity disease, skin cancer, extensive sun-damaged skin, or arsenic ingestion; patients currently using photosensitivity-inducing drugs other than a psoralen agent; children between 10 and 18 years of age; patient's with a family history of melanoma; and patients with previous skin irradiation (which can induce skin cancer).[1,4,6] PUVA therapy is contraindicated in lactating women, and in pregnant women *because of increased risk of birth defects from psoralen agents.*[4] Women of childbearing age who undergo PUVA therapy should have a pregnancy test before beginning therapy, and both men and women of childbearing age and men with partners of childbearing age should use a reliable form of birth control as recommended by the prescribing information for the psoralen agent.[7,8,9]

Contraindications to UVB therapy include lupus erythematosus and xeroderma pigmentosum.[2] Caution should be used in patients with skin types I and II; patients with a history of photosensitivity disease, skin cancer, or arsenic ingestion; patients currently using photosensitivity-inducing drugs or immunosuppression for organ transplantation; and patients with previous skin irradiation.[2,4] According to established guidelines, UVB therapy is considered safe during pregnancy.[4]

A patient can undergo UV light therapy in a hospital, in practitioner's office, or at home. Typically set into a reflective cabinet, the light source consists of a bank of high-intensity fluorescent bulbs. The patient can stand or lie down for the therapy. At home, the patient may use a home phototherapy unit prescribed by the practitioner.[10] Treatment schedules vary according to the patient's diagnosis and the UV therapy prescribed.[4]

Equipment
For UVA radiation
Fluorescent black-light lamp ■ high-intensity UVA fluorescent bulbs ■ UV-opaque sunglasses.

For UVB radiation
UVB fluorescent lamp ■ UVB florescent bulbs ■ goggles with gray or green polarized lenses.

For all UV treatments
Phototherapy unit ■ hospital gown ■ Optional: prescribed oral or topical phototherapeutic medications, sunscreen, towels, underwear or athletic supporter for male patient.

Preparation of equipment
Inspect all equipment and supplies. If a product is expired, is defective, or has compromised integrity, remove it from patient use, label it as expired or defective, and report the expiration or defect as directed by your facility. Make sure that the equipment functions properly before use. Replace the UVB fluorescent bulbs, if needed.

Implementation
■ Review the patient's health history for contraindications to UV light therapy.
■ Verify the practitioner's orders *to confirm the UV light treatment type and dose.*
■ Perform hand hygiene.[11,12,13,14,15,16]
■ Confirm the patient's identity using at least two patient identifiers.[17]
■ Provide privacy.[18,19,20,21]
■ Review the patient's current medications, herbs, and supplements. Ask the patient about the use of photosensitizing drugs, such as anticonvulsants, certain antihypertensives, fluoroquinolones, phenothiazines, salicylates, sulfonamides, tetracyclines, thiazides, tretinoin, and various cancer drugs, *which may increase the risk of acute phototoxic erythema.*[1,22]
■ Explain the procedure to the patient and family (if appropriate) according to their individual communication and learning needs *to*

increase their understanding, allay their fears, and enhance cooperation.[23] Inform the patient that UV light treatments produce a mild sunburn that will help reduce or resolve skin lesions.

For PUVA therapy

- Confirm that the patient took the prescribed psoralen agent before therapy, as directed. Methoxsalen should be taken 1 to 2 hours before treatment. In patients who experience nausea, it may be taken with milk or a small amount of high-fat-content food (such as cheese) or in two divided portions about 30 minutes apart.[1,7]
- Instruct the patient to disrobe and put on a hospital gown.
- Ensure that the patient uses sunscreen with a sun protection factor (SPF) of 50+, towels, or a hospital gown *to protect vulnerable skin areas.* All male patients receiving PUVA must wear protection (underwear or athletic supporter) over the groin area.[1]
- Have the patient enter or assume an appropriate position in the phototherapy unit.
- Instruct the patient to remove the gown or expose only the area to undergo therapy.
- Instruct the patient to put on UV-opaque sunglasses, and ensure that the patient wears them throughout UV light therapy *to protect the eyes from harmful UV light.* Tell the patient to wear these glasses after treatment until sunset the same day, *because the prescribed psoralen agent can cause photosensitivity.* Advise the patient that photoprotection isn't necessary from common florescent lights.[1]

For local UVB therapy

- Instruct the patient to disrobe and put on a hospital gown, if necessary.
- Position the patient at the correct distance from the light source, as prescribed or per the manufacturer's instructions.[24]
- If the patient must stand during UVB therapy, ask the patient to report any dizziness *to ensure safety.*
- If the face isn't involved in the disease process, ensure that the patient applies sunscreen with an SPF of 50+ or uses a cloth barrier for protection. Instruct a male patient undergoing UVB therapy to protect the genitalia, if not involved in the disease process, by wearing underwear.[2]
- Instruct the patient to put on dark, polarized goggles, and ensure that the patient wears them throughout UV light therapy *to protect the eyes from harmful UV light.*[2]
- Instruct the patient to remove the gown or expose only the area that will undergo therapy.
- If you're observing the patient through light-chamber windows, put on goggles.

Completing the procedure

- After delivering the prescribed UV dose, allow the patient to dress and then help the patient out of the phototherapy unit.
- Instruct the patient to avoid sun exposure to treated areas after therapy.[10]
- Perform hand hygiene.[11,12,13,14,15,16]
- Document the procedure.[25,26,27,28]

Special considerations

- If the patient is prescribed methoxsalen, ensure that baseline liver function studies have been completed before administration *to evaluate for hepatic involvement.*[7,29]
- If the patient is prescribed acitretin, confirm completion of liver function and blood lipid studies before administration and at regular intervals during therapy. Refer to prescribing information for rigid informed consent, pregnancy prevention requirements, and blood donation prohibition guidelines.[9,29]
- If the patient is prescribed methotrexate, confirm completion of liver function studies and a complete blood count before administration, and at regular intervals during therapy (as ordered) according to dosage adjustments, the patient's condition, and previous test results.[29,30]
- Tar and carbonis detergens (a tar distillate) applied before UVB therapy *decrease effectiveness of treatment* and should be avoided.[4]

- A thin layer of emollient, such as petroleum jelly, may be applied before UVB treatment *to increase the effectiveness of treatment and reduce erythema.*[4]
- Note that a patient with psoriasis may benefit from bathing or a hand and foot soak before UV exposure *to remove plaques gently.*[5,10,22] The patient will soak in water with dissolved methoxsalen for 30 minutes before UV exposure, dry off without rinsing, and then begin UV exposure.[22]
- Treatment duration should be individualized. Treatment is commonly continued until the patient's response plateaus or remission occurs. Maintenance therapy may be necessary once a month *to increase remission time*; however, maintenance therapy may increase the risk of cumulative effects. Therapy may resume or the frequency of maintenance therapy may increase if relapse occurs.[1]

Patient teaching

Instruct the patient and family (if applicable) to look for marked erythema, blistering, peeling, or other signs of UV light overexposure 4 to 6 hours after UVB therapy and 24 to 48 hours after UVA/PUVA therapy. In either case, the erythema should disappear within another 24 hours of therapy. Explain to the patient that mild dryness and desquamation (skin peeling) will occur in 1 to 2 days after therapy. Teach the patient appropriate skin care measures. (See *Skin care guidelines.*) Advise the patient to notify the practitioner if UV light overexposure occurs. Typically, the practitioner recommends stopping UV light treatment for a few days and then starting over at a lower exposure level. The practitioner may also prescribe a topical corticosteroid, a nonsteroidal anti-inflammatory drug, or a systemic corticosteroid for severe exposure.

PATIENT TEACHING

SKIN CARE GUIDELINES

A patient who's receiving ultraviolet light therapy must know how to protect the skin from injury. Provide your patient with the following skin care tips:

- Encourage the patient to use sunscreen and fragrance-free moisturizers and drink plenty of fluids *to protect the skin, combat dry skin and maintain adequate hydration.* Warn the patient to avoid hot baths or showers and to use soap sparingly, *because heat and soap promote dry skin.*[31]
- Instruct the patient to notify the practitioner before taking any medication, including aspirin, *to prevent heightened photosensitivity.*[5]
- If the patient is receiving psoralen plus UVA therapy, review the psoralen agent dosage schedule. Explain that deviating from it could result in burns or ineffective treatment. Urge the patient to wear appropriate sunglasses outdoors for at least 24 hours after taking the psoralen agent. Recommend annual eye examinations *to detect cataract formation.*[1,4]
- If the patient uses a UVB lamp at home, advise the patient to follow the manufacturer's instructions. Stress the importance of exposing the skin to the light for the exact amount of time prescribed by the practitioner. Instruct the patient to protect the eyes with goggles and to use a dependable timer or have someone else time the therapy. Above all, urge the patient never to use the UVB lamp when tired, *to avoid falling asleep under the lamp and sustaining a burn.*
- Teach the patient first aid procedures for localized burning. Tell the patient to apply cool water soaks for 20 minutes or until skin temperature cools. For more extensive burns, recommend tepid tap water baths after notifying the practitioner about the burn. After the patient bathes, suggest using an oil-in-water moisturizing lotion (not a petroleum jelly–based product, which can trap radiant heat).
- Instruct the patient to limit natural-light exposure (not only to outside light but also to light through windows), to use a sunscreen when outdoors, and to notify the practitioner immediately if the patient discovers any unusual skin lesions.
- Advise the patient to avoid harsh soaps and chemicals, such as paints and solvents, and to discuss ways to manage physical and psychological stress, *which may exacerbate skin disorders.*[31]

Complications

Overexposure to UV light (sunburn) can result from prolonged therapy or an inadequate distance between the patient and the light source. Sunburn can also result from the use of photosensitizing drugs and from overly sensitive skin.[1]

Erythema, nausea, and pruritus are the three major short-term adverse effects of PUVA therapy. Long-term adverse effects are similar to those caused by excessive exposure to sunlight, including premature aging (xerosis, wrinkles, and mottled skin), folliculitis, telangiectasia, increased risk of skin cancer, and cataracts (if eye protection isn't used). Photo-onycholysis (lifting of the nail bed) and melanonychia (darkening of the nail plate) can also occur. Less commonly, neuropathic pain due to phototoxic damage of the dermal nerve endings can occur.[1]

Erythema is the major adverse effect of UVB therapy. Although minimal erythema without discomfort is acceptable, UVB therapy is suspended if marked edema, swelling, or blistering occurs. Skin dryness, pruritus, and increased frequency of recurrent herpes simplex can also occur.[2]

Documentation

Record the date and time of initial and subsequent UV light therapy treatments, the UV light wavelength used, and the name, route, time, and dose of any oral or topical medications administered. Record the exact location on the patient's body where a topical medication was applied. Record the exact duration of UV light therapy, the distance between the light source and the patient's skin, and the patient's tolerance of the procedure. Note any safety measures used, including eye protection. Also describe the condition of the patient's skin before and after UV light therapy. Note improvements and adverse reactions, such as increased pruritus, oozing, and scaling, experienced by the patient. Document teaching provided to the patient and family (if applicable), their understanding of that teaching, and any need for follow-up teaching.

REFERENCES

1 Richard, E. G. (2021). Psoralen plus ultraviolet A (PUVA) photochemotherapy. In: *UpToDate*, Elmets, C. A. (Ed.).

2 Hönigsmann, H. (2020). UVB therapy (broadband and narrowband). In: *UpToDate*, Elmets, C. A. (Ed.).

3 American Osteopathic College of Dermatology (n.d.) Phototherapy: UVB. https://www.aocd.org/page/PhototherapyUVB

4 Elmets, C. A., et al. (2019). Joint American Academy of Dermatology—National Psoriasis Foundation guidelines of care for the management and treatment of psoriasis with phototherapy. *Journal of the American Academy of Dermatology, 81*(3), 775–804. https://www.jaad.org/article/S0190-9622(19)30637-1/pdf (Level VII)

5 National Psoriasis Foundation. (2018). Phototherapy. https://www.psoriasis.org/phototherapy/

6 Menter, A., et al. (2010). Guidelines of care for the management of psoriasis and psoriatic arthritis: Section 5. Guidelines of care for the treatment of psoriasis with phototherapy and photochemotherapy. *Journal of the American Academy of Dermatology, 62*(1), 114–135. https://www.psoriasis.org/phototherapy/

7 Drugs.com. (2021). Methoxsalen. https://www.drugs.com/mtm/methoxsalen.html

8 American Academy of Dermatology Association. (n.d.). Psoriasis treatment: Methotrexate. https://www.aad.org/public/diseases/scaly-skin/psoriasis/diagnosis-and-treatment-of-psoriasis/methotrexate

9 Stiefel Laboratories, Inc. (2017). Soriatane (acitretin) capsules" https://www.accessdata.fda.gov/drugsatfda_docs/label/2017/019821s028lbl.pdf

10 Feldman, S. R. (2021). Treatment of psoriasis in adults. In: *UpToDate*, Dellavale, R. P. & Duffin, K. C. (Eds.).

11 Centers for Disease Control and Prevention. (2002). Guideline for hand hygiene in health-care settings: Recommendations of the Healthcare Infection Control Practices Advisory Committee and the HICPAC/SHEA/APIC/IDSA Hand Hygiene Task Force. *MMWR Recommendations and Reports, 51*(RR-16), 1–45. https://www.cdc.gov/mmwr/pdf/rr/rr5116.pdf (Level II)

12 World Health Organization. (2009). WHO guidelines on hand hygiene in health care: First global patient safety challenge, clean care is safer care. https://apps.who.int/iris/bitstream/handle/10665/44102/9789241597906_eng.pdf?sequence=1 (Level IV)

13 The Joint Commission. (2021). Standard NPSG.07.01.01. *Comprehensive accreditation manual for hospitals.* Oakbrook Terrace, IL: The Joint Commission. (Level VII)

14 Accreditation Association for Hospitals and Health Systems. (2020). Standard 07.01.21. *Healthcare Facilities Accreditation Program: Accreditation requirements for acute care hospitals.* Chicago, IL: Accreditation Association for Hospitals and Health Systems. (Level VII)

15 Centers for Medicare and Medicaid Services, Department of Health and Human Services. (2020). Condition of participation: Infection control. 42 C.F.R. § 482.42.

16 DNV GL-Healthcare USA, Inc. (2020). IC.1.SR.1. *NIAHO® accreditation requirements, interpretive guidelines and surveyor guidance – revision 20.0.* Milford, OH: DNV GL-Healthcare USA, Inc. (Level VII)

17 The Joint Commission. (2021). Standard NPSG.01.01.01. *Comprehensive accreditation manual for hospitals.* Oakbrook Terrace, IL: The Joint Commission. (Level VII)

18 Accreditation Association for Hospitals and Health Systems. (2020). Standard 15.01.16. *Healthcare Facilities Accreditation Program: Accreditation requirements for acute care hospitals.* Chicago, IL: Accreditation Association for Hospitals and Health Systems. (Level VII)

19 Centers for Medicare and Medicaid Services, Department of Health and Human Services. (2020). Condition of participation: Patient's rights. 42 C.F.R. § 482.13(c)(1).

20 DNV GL-Healthcare USA, Inc. (2020). PR.2.SR.5. *NIAHO® accreditation requirements, interpretive guidelines and surveyor guidance – revision 20.0.* Milford, OH: DNV GL-Healthcare USA, Inc. (Level VII)

21 The Joint Commission. (2021). Standard RI.01.01.01. *Comprehensive accreditation manual for hospitals.* Oakbrook Terrace, IL: The Joint Commission. (Level VII)

22 Farahnik, B., et al. (2016). The patient's guide to psoriasis treatment. Part 2: PUVA phototherapy. *Dermatology and Therapy, 6*(3), 315–324. https://www.ncbi.nlm.nih.gov/pmc/articles/PMC4972736/ (Level VII)

23 The Joint Commission. (2021). Standard PC.02.01.21. *Comprehensive accreditation manual for hospitals.* Oakbrook Terrace, IL: The Joint Commission. (Level VII)

24 National Psoriasis Foundation. (2021). Expanding phototherapy research and access through self-advocacy. https://www.psoriasis.org/advance/expanding-litestudy-patient-psoriasis-uvb-phototherapy/

25 The Joint Commission. (2021). Standard RC.01.03.01. *Comprehensive accreditation manual for hospitals.* Oakbrook Terrace, IL: The Joint Commission.(Level VII)

26 Centers for Medicare and Medicaid Services, Department of Health and Human Services. (2020). Condition of participation: Medical record services. 42 C.F.R. § 482.24(b).

27 Accreditation Association for Hospitals and Health Systems. (2020). Standard 10.00.03. *Healthcare Facilities Accreditation Program: Accreditation requirements for acute care hospitals.* Chicago, IL: Accreditation Association for Hospitals and Health Systems. (Level VII)

28 DNV GL-Healthcare USA, Inc. (2020). MR.2.SR.1. *NIAHO® accreditation requirements, interpretive guidelines and surveyor guidance – revision 20.0.* Milford, OH: DNV GL-Healthcare USA, Inc. (Level VII)

29 Menter, A., et al. (2020). Joint American Academy of Dermatology–National Psoriasis Foundation guidelines of care for the management of psoriasis with systemic nonbiologic therapies. *Journal of the American Academy of Dermatology, 82*(6), 1445–1486. https://www.sciencedirect.com/science/article/pii/S019096222030284X (Level VII)

30 American Academy of Dermatology. (2010). *Psoriasis: Treatment guide for methotrexate.* Schaumburg, IL: American Academy of Dermatology.

31 American Academy of Dermatology Association. (n.d.). Psoriasis resource center. https://www.aad.org/public/diseases/scaly-skin/psoriasis#tips

UNNA BOOT APPLICATION

Named for dermatologist Paul Gerson Unna, the nonelastic paste bandage Unna boot can be used to treat uninfected, nonnecrotic leg and foot ulcers that result from such conditions as venous insufficiency and stasis dermatitis.[1] A commercially prepared Unna boot is a gauze compression dressing that's impregnated with a preparation known as *Unna paste* (gelatin, zinc oxide, calamine lotion, and glycerin). The dressing wraps around the affected foot and leg. The boot's effectiveness results from compression applied by the bandage, which decreases edema, combined with moisture supplied by the paste.[1,2]

The Unna boot is contraindicated in patients allergic to any ingredient used in the paste and in patients with arterial ulcers, mixed venous and arterial ulcers, suspected or known lower extremity venous thrombosis, weeping eczema, necrotic tissue, or cellulitis.[3,4] Unna boots should be used cautiously in patients with heart failure, *because fluid volume shifts can affect cardiac function.*[3]

Equipment

Gauze sponges ▪ prescribed cleaning agent ▪ normal saline solution ▪ commercially prepared paste bandage impregnated with zinc oxide, glycerin, gelatin, and calamine ▪ gloves ▪ elastic bandage or self-adherent wrap to cover the Unna boot ▪ tape or clip ▪ pillow ▪ disposable wound measuring device ▪ Optional: roller gauze for excessive drainage, bandage scissors, Doppler ultrasound equipment.

Implementation

▪ Gather and prepare the necessary equipment and supplies.
▪ Perform hand hygiene.[5,6,7,8,9,10]
▪ Confirm the patient's identity using at least two patient identifiers.[11]
▪ Provide privacy.[12,13,14,15]
▪ Explain the procedure to the patient and family (if appropriate) according to their individual communication and learning needs *to increase their understanding, allay their fears, and enhance cooperation.*[16]
▪ Raise the patient's bed to waist level before providing patient care *to prevent caregiver back strain.*[17]
▪ Perform hand hygiene.[5,6,7,8,9,10]
▪ Put on gloves.[18,19,20]
▪ Assess the ulcer and the surrounding skin. Measure ulcer size with the disposable wound-measuring device, and evaluate the ulcer's drainage, and appearance.[1,2]
▪ Perform a neurovascular assessment of the affected foot *to ensure adequate circulation.*[1] If you don't detect a dorsalis pedis or posterior tibial pulse in the foot by palpation, Doppler ultrasound, or ankle-brachial index, report the finding before applying the Unna boot.
▪ Place the patient in the supine position, elevating the leg on which you're going to place the Unna boot.
▪ Open all the bandage wrappers. Make sure that you have enough supplies to cover the extremity.
▪ Have the patient dorsiflex the foot 90 degrees.[21]
▪ Clean the affected area gently with the gauze sponge and prescribed cleaning agent[1] *to slow bacterial growth and to remove dirt and wound debris, which can create pressure points after you apply the bandage.*
▪ Rinse the affected area with normal saline solution and dry it thoroughly with a gauze sponge.
▪ Remove and discard your gloves.[20]
▪ Perform hand hygiene.[5,6,7,8,9,10]
▪ Put on new gloves.[18,19,20]
▪ Have the patient flex the knee.
▪ Starting with the foot positioned at a right angle to the leg, wrap the impregnated gauze bandage firmly in a spiral motion, beginning just above the toes. Wrap the bandage twice around, just above the toes, without tension. Continue wrapping upward, overlapping the dressing 50% or more with each turn.[21] Make sure the dressing covers the heel. Smooth the boot with your free hand as you go (as shown below).

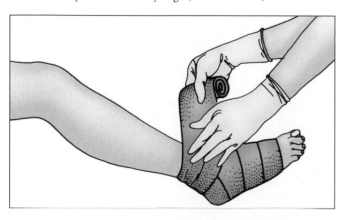

▪ Stop wrapping about 1" (2.5 cm) below the knee and popliteal fossa, as shown below, *to prevent irritation when the knee is bent.* The wrap should be snug but not tight. Mold the boot with your free hand as you apply the bandage *to make it smooth and even.* If necessary, make a 2" (5-cm) slit in the boot just below the knee *to relieve constriction that may develop as the dressing hardens.*

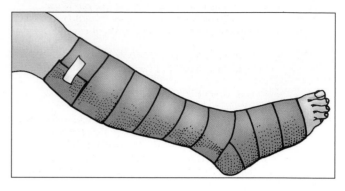

▪ If drainage is excessive, you may wrap a roller gauze dressing over the Unna boot.
▪ As the final layer, wrap an elastic bandage in a figure-eight pattern *to provide external compression,* and secure it in place using a clip or tape.
▪ Instruct the patient to remain in bed with the leg outstretched and elevated on a pillow until the paste dries (approximately 30 minutes).
▪ Observe the patient's foot for signs and symptoms of neurovascular impairment, such as cyanosis, loss of sensation, and swelling. *These findings indicate that the bandage is too tight and must be removed.*[1]
▪ Remove and discard your gloves.[20]
▪ Return the bed to the lowest position *to prevent falls and maintain patient safety.*[22]
▪ Perform hand hygiene.[5,6,7,8,9,10]
▪ Document the procedure.[23,24,25,26]

Special considerations

▪ Change the boot as ordered *to assess the underlying skin and ulcer healing;* also change the boot when the patient detects a loosening of the boot, or anytime the wrap becomes saturated with drainage. Remove the boot by unwrapping the bandage from the knee down to the foot.
▪ If the boot is applied over a swollen leg, change the boot as the edema subsides—if necessary, more frequently than every 3 days.[27]
▪ Don't make reverse turns while wrapping the bandage. *This could create excessive pressure areas that may cause discomfort as the bandage hardens.*
▪ Other two- or four-layer wraps are available that follow the same principles as an Unna boot. Some products can be removed daily, such as compression stockings, which require measurement for accurate fit after any edema has subsided.[21]

Complications

Contact dermatitis may result from hypersensitivity to Unna paste. Neurovascular impairment (cyanosis, loss of sensation, swelling, and necrosis) may also occur if the boot is too tight. Fungal infections may occur with exudate moisture collection beneath the dressing. An improperly applied boot may worsen the existing or create new venous ulcers.[3]

Documentation

Record the date and time of application and the presence of a pulse in the affected foot. Specify which leg you bandaged. Describe the appearance of the patient's skin before and after boot application. Name the equipment used (a commercially prepared bandage or Unna paste and lightweight gauze). Describe any allergic reaction. Document teaching you provided to the patient and family (if applicable), their understanding of that teaching, and any need for follow-up teaching.

REFERENCES

1 Kelechi, T. J., et al. (2020). 2019 guideline for management of wounds in patients with lower-extremity venous disease (LEVD): An executive summary. *Journal of Wound, Ostomy, and Continence Nursing, 47*, 97–110. (Level VII)

2 Bolton, L. L., et al. (2014). Association for the Advancement of Wound Care (AAWC) venous and pressure ulcer guidelines. *Ostomy Wound Management, 60*(11), 24–66. https://www.o-wm.com/article/association-advancement-wound-care-aawc-venous-and-pressure-ulcer-guidelines (Level I)

3 Armstrong, D. G., & Meyr, A. J. (2021). Compression therapy for the treatment of chronic venous insufficiency. In: *UpToDate*, Mills, J. L., & Eidt, J. F. (Eds.).

4 WoundSource. (n.d.). Unna-FLEX elastic Unna boot. https://www.woundsource.com/product/unna-flex-elastic-unna-boot

5 Centers for Disease Control and Prevention. (2002). Guideline for hand hygiene in health-care settings: Recommendations of the Healthcare Infection Control Practices Advisory Committee and the HICPAC/SHEA/APIC/IDSA Hand Hygiene Task Force. *MMWR Recommendations and Reports, 51*(RR-16), 1–45. https://www.cdc.gov/mmwr/pdf/rr/rr5116.pdf (Level II)

6 World Health Organization. (2009). WHO guidelines on hand hygiene in health care: First global patient safety challenge, clean care is safer care. http://apps.who.int/iris/bitstream/10665/44102/1/9789241597906_eng.pdf (Level IV)

7 The Joint Commission. (2021). Standard NPSG.07.01.01. *Comprehensive accreditation manual for hospitals*. Oakbrook Terrace, IL: The Joint Commission. (Level VII)

8 Accreditation Association for Hospitals and Health Systems. (2020). Standard 07.01.21. *Healthcare Facilities Accreditation Program: Accreditation requirements for acute care hospitals*. Chicago, IL: Accreditation Association for Hospitals and Health Systems. (Level VII)

9 Centers for Medicare and Medicaid Services, Department of Health and Human Services. (2020). Condition of participation: Infection control. 42 C.F.R. § 482.42.

10 DNV GL-Healthcare USA, Inc. (2020). IC.1.SR.1. *NIAHO® accreditation requirements, interpretive guidelines and surveyor guidance – revision 20*. Milford, OH: DNV GL-Healthcare USA, Inc. (Level VII)

11 The Joint Commission. (2021). Standard NPSG.01.01.01. *Comprehensive accreditation manual for hospitals*. Oakbrook Terrace, IL: The Joint Commission. (Level VII)

12 Accreditation Association for Hospitals and Health Systems. (2020). Standard 15.01.16. *Healthcare Facilities Accreditation Program: Accreditation requirements for acute care hospitals*. Chicago, IL: Accreditation Association for Hospitals and Health Systems. (Level VII)

13 Centers for Medicare and Medicaid Services, Department of Health and Human Services. (2020). Condition of participation: Patient's rights. 42 C.F.R. § 482.13(c)(1).

14 DNV GL-Healthcare USA, Inc. (2020). PR.2.SR.5. *NIAHO® accreditation requirements, interpretive guidelines and surveyor guidance – revision 20.0*. Milford, OH: DNV GL-Healthcare USA, Inc. (Level VII)

15 The Joint Commission. (2021). Standard RI.01.01.01. *Comprehensive accreditation manual for hospitals*. Oakbrook Terrace, IL: The Joint Commission. (Level VII)

16 The Joint Commission. (2021). Standard PC.02.01.21. *Comprehensive accreditation manual for hospitals*. Oakbrook Terrace, IL: The Joint Commission. (Level VII)

17 Waters, T. R., et al. (2009). Safe patient handling training for schools of nursing. https://www.cdc.gov/niosh/docs/2009-127/pdfs/2009-127.pdf (Level VII)

18 Siegel, J. D., et al. (2007, revised 2019). 2007 guideline for isolation precautions: Preventing transmission of infectious agents in healthcare settings. https://www.cdc.gov/infectioncontrol/pdf/guidelines/isolation-guidelines-H.pdf (Level II)

19 Accreditation Association for Hospitals and Health Systems. (2020). Standard 07.01.10. *Healthcare Facilities Accreditation Program: Accreditation requirements for acute care hospitals*. Chicago, IL: Accreditation Association for Hospitals and Health Systems. (Level VII)

20 Occupational Safety and Health Administration. (2012). Bloodborne pathogens, standard number 1910.1030. https://www.osha.gov/pls/oshaweb/owadisp.show_document?p_id=10051&p_table=STANDARDS (Level VII)

21 Hinkle, J. L., & Cheever, K. H. (2017). *Brunner & Suddarth's textbook of medical-surgical nursing* (14th ed.). Philadelphia, PA: Wolters Kluwer.

22 Ganz, D. A., et al. (2013, reviewed 2021). *Preventing falls in hospitals: A toolkit for improving quality of care* (AHRQ Publication No. 13-0015-EF). Rockville, MD: Agency for Healthcare Research and Quality. https://www.ahrq.gov/professionals/systems/hospital/fallpxtoolkit/index.html (Level VII)

23 The Joint Commission. (2021). Standard RC.01.03.01. *Comprehensive accreditation manual for hospitals*. Oakbrook Terrace, IL: The Joint Commission. (Level VII)

24 Centers for Medicare and Medicaid Services, Department of Health and Human Services. (2020). Condition of participation: Medical record services. 42 C.F.R. § 482.24(b).

25 Accreditation Association for Hospitals and Health Systems. (2020). Standard 10.00.03. *Healthcare Facilities Accreditation Program: Accreditation requirements for acute care hospitals*. Chicago, IL: Accreditation Association for Hospitals and Health Systems. (Level VII)

26 DNV GL-Healthcare USA, Inc. (2020). MR.2.SR.1. *NIAHO® accreditation requirements, interpretive guidelines and surveyor guidance – revision 20*. Milford, OH: DNV GL-Healthcare USA, Inc. (Level VII)

27 Dissemond, J., et al. (2016). Compression therapy in patients with venous leg ulcers. *Journal of the German Society of Dermatology, 14*(11), 1072–1087. https://onlinelibrary.wiley.com/doi/full/10.1111/ddg.13091

URINARY DIVERSION STOMA CARE

Urinary diversions provide an alternative route for urine flow when a disorder impedes normal drainage, as in the case of an invasive bladder tumor.[1] A permanent urinary diversion is indicated in any condition that requires a total cystectomy. In conditions requiring temporary urinary drainage or diversion, a suprapubic or urethral catheter is usually inserted to divert the flow of urine temporarily. The catheter remains in place until the incision heals. Urinary diversions may also be indicated for patients with neurogenic bladder, congenital anomaly, traumatic injury to the lower urinary tract, strictures, pelvic malignancy, or severe chronic urinary tract infection causing severe ureteral and renal damage.[1]

Ileal conduit and continent urinary diversion are the two types of permanent urinary diversions with stomas.[1] (See *Types of permanent urinary diversion*, page 876.) These procedures usually require the patient to wear a urine-collection appliance and to care for a newly created stoma. Evaluation by a wound, ostomy, and continence nurse (WOCN) will facilitate site selection and postoperative stoma care.

Equipment

Gloves ▪ fluid-impermeable pad ▪ graduated cylinder ▪ washcloth ▪ warm water ▪ absorbent, lint-free material for wicking (rolled gauze pad or tampon) ▪ gauze pads ▪ pouching system (one-piece or two-piece, disposable or reusable, with a spout for ease of emptying; see *Urinary diversion pouching systems*, page 876) ▪ stoma measuring guide ▪ Optional: scissors, gown, goggles and mask or mask with face shield, marker or pen, disposable-head clippers, electric razor, safety razor and ostomy barrier powder, shaving foam (no moisturizers or perfumes), mild soap (oil-, perfume-, and deodorant-free).[2]

Implementation

▪ Gather and prepare the necessary equipment and supplies.
▪ Perform hand hygiene.[3,4,5,6,7,8]
▪ Confirm the patient's identity using at least two patient identifiers.[9]
▪ Provide privacy.[10,11,12,13]
▪ Explain the procedure to the patient and family (if appropriate) according to their individual communication and learning needs *to increase their understanding, allay their fears, and enhance cooperation.*[14] Offer constant reinforcement and reassurance *to counteract negative reactions that stoma care may elicit. The patient or a family member will eventually need to perform the procedure.*
▪ Raise the patient's bed to waist level before providing care *to prevent caregiver back strain.*[15]
▪ Position the patient in a low Fowler position *so the patient's abdomen is flat. This position eliminates skin folds that could cause the appliance to slip or irritate the skin, and allows the patient to observe or participate.*

Types of permanent urinary diversion

The two types of permanent urinary diversion are the ileal conduit and the continent urinary diversion, or Indiana pouch,[1] both described below. Other types of catheterizable continent pouches include the Kock, Mainz, and Florida pouches. Another type of continent urinary diversion, the orthotopic neobladder, hooks back to the urethra, making a stoma unnecessary.

Ileal conduit
A segment of the ileum is excised, and the two ends of the ileum that result from excision of the segment are sutured closed. Then the ureters are dissected from the bladder and anastomosed to the ileal segment. One end of the ileal segment is closed with sutures; the opposite end is brought through the abdominal wall, forming a stoma.

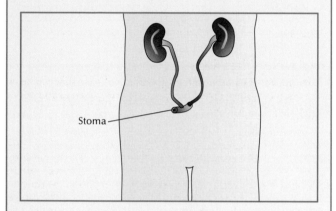

Continent urinary diversion (Indiana pouch)
The surgeon introduces the ureters into a segment of ileum and cecum. Urine is drained periodically by inserting a catheter into the stoma.

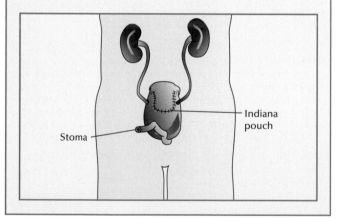

- Perform hand hygiene.[3,4,5,6,7,8]
- Put on gloves and, as needed, other personal protective equipment *to comply with standard precautions.*[16,17,18]
- Place a fluid-impermeable pad under the patient's side, near the stoma.
- Open the drain valve of the appliance you're replacing and empty the urine in the pouch into a graduated cylinder.
- Remove the appliance by loosening and lifting the edges of the pouch while pushing the skin back from the pouch, starting at the top of the pouch and working down to the bottom.[2]
- If the appliance is disposable, discard it into the waste receptacle.[18] If it's reusable, follow the manufacturer's cleaning instructions.
- *To prevent a constant flow of urine onto the skin while you're changing the appliance,* wick the urine with an absorbent, lint-free material,[1] as shown to the right.

 ## Urinary diversion pouching systems

Disposable pouching systems
Options for disposable pouching systems include a one-piece disposable system with spout closure and a two-piece drainable, disposable pouch with a skin barrier. The one-piece system consists of a transparent or opaque, odor-proof plastic pouch with attached adhesive backing. Some pouches have microporous tape edges or belt tabs. The spout opening enables easy draining.

The two-piece drainable, disposable pouch with a separate skin barrier permits more frequent pouch changes. Also made of transparent or opaque, odor-proof plastic, this style comes with belt tabs and usually snaps to the skin barrier with a flange mechanism. Newer two-piece pouches have an adhesive coupling. The pouch sticks to the wafer, allowing greater flexibility and comfort.

Reusable pouching system
Typically manufactured from sturdy, opaque, hypoallergenic plastic, the reusable pouch comes with a separate, custom-made faceplate and O-ring. The device has a 1- to 3-month life span, depending on how frequently the patient empties the pouch. Reusable equipment may benefit a patient who needs a firm faceplate, has sensitivity to any type of adhesive, or wishes to minimize cost.

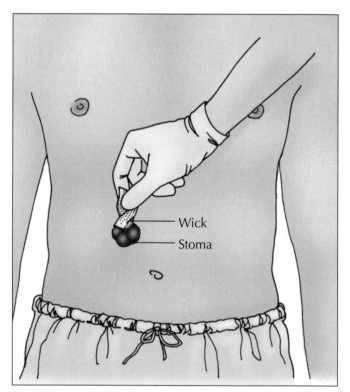

- Using warm water and a washcloth, carefully wash around the stoma.[2] Note that you need not use soap and water around the stoma; however, if the patient prefers that you use soap, use a very mild soap without oils, perfumes, or deodorants.[2] Be sure to rinse the soap off the skin around the stoma very well, *because soap residue can cause skin irritation and prevent adherence of the skin barrier.*[2]
- Dry the peristomal area thoroughly with a gauze pad, *because moisture will keep the appliance from sticking.*[2]

NURSING ALERT Don't use alcohol or other harsh chemicals to clean the skin around the stoma, *because they can irritate the skin.* Don't apply any powders or creams to the skin around the stoma unless recommended by the wound ostomy continence nurse or practitioner, *because they can prevent the pouching system from sticking properly.*[2]

- If necessary, remove any hair from the area with clippers or by shaving with an electric razor or a safety razor and an ostomy skin barrier powder or mild soap and water. Always shave in the direction of the hair growth and away from the stoma *to limit skin irritation and avoid injury to the stoma.* If using shaving foam, avoid moisturizers or perfumed foam *because they can irritate the skin as well as keep the pouching system from sticking properly.* Rinse the skin thoroughly with water after shaving.[2]
- Inspect the stoma *for proper healing and to detect complications.* Check the color and the appearance of the suture line, and examine any moisture or drainage. Inspect the peristomal skin for redness, irritation, and intactness.
- Consult with a WOCN, if needed, when skin problems arise.
- For a pouch with an attached skin barrier (one-piece system), measure the stoma with the measuring guide. Select an opening size that matches the stoma.
- For an adhesive-backed pouch with a separate skin barrier (two-piece), measure the stoma with the measuring guide and select the opening that matches the stoma. Trace the selected size opening onto the paper back of the skin barrier's adhesive side. Cut out the opening. (If the pouch has precut openings, which can be handy for a round stoma, select an opening no more than ⅛" [3.2 mm] larger than the stoma. If the pouch comes without an opening, cut a hole ⅛" [3.2 mm] wider than the measured tracing.) Many pouching systems can be fit up to the stoma edge

without risk of trauma to the stoma. The cut-to-fit system works best for an irregularly shaped stoma.

- Remove the material used for wicking urine and place it in the appropriate receptacle.[18]
- When using a one-piece system, center it over the stoma, adhesive side down, and gently press it to the skin.
- When using a two-piece system with a wafer, apply the wafer, then gently press the pouch opening onto the ring until it snaps into place.
- When using a two-piece adhesive system with a coupling device, line up the adhesive portion of the pouch to the "landing zone" of the wafer. Press together *for adhesion.* You can attach the pouches used in a two-piece system to the wafer before application if the patient is still experiencing incisional discomfort.
- Return the bed to the lowest position *to prevent falls and maintain patient safety.*[19]
- Discard used materials in appropriate receptacles.[18]
- Remove and discard your gloves and other personal protective equipment if worn.[18]
- Perform hand hygiene.[3,4,5,6,7,8]
- Document the procedure.[20,21,22,23]

Special considerations

- If the patient has a continent urinary diversion, make sure you know how to meet the patient's special needs. (See *Caring for the patient with a continent urinary diversion.*)

Patient teaching

The patient or a family member can learn to care for a urinary diversion stoma at home (see *Home care for the patient with a continent urinary diversion*). However, you must give special consideration to the patient's emotional adjustment to the stoma before you can expect the patient to maintain it properly. *To encourage a positive attitude,* help the patient get used to the idea of caring for the stoma and the appliance as though

---

Caring for the patient with a continent urinary diversion

With a continent urinary diversion, an alternative to the traditional ileal conduit, a pouch created from the ascending colon and terminal ileum serves as a new bladder, which empties through a stoma. To drain urine continuously, several drains are inserted into this reconstructed bladder by the practitioner and left in place for 3 to 6 weeks until the new stoma heals. The patient is discharged from the health care facility with the drains in place and must return to have them removed and to learn to catheterize the stoma.

First hospitalization care
- Immediately after surgery, monitor intake and output from each drain.[1] Be alert for decreased output, *which may indicate that urine flow is obstructed.*
- Watch for common postoperative complications, such as infection or bleeding. Also watch for signs of urinary leakage, which include increased abdominal distention and urine appearing around the drains or midline incision.
- Irrigate the drains as ordered.
- Perform hand hygiene[3,4,5,6,7,8] and put on gloves.[16,17,18] Clean the area around the drains daily, first with an antiseptic swab and then with sterile water. Apply a dry, sterile dressing to the area. Use precut 4" × 4" (10-cm × 10-cm) drain dressings around the drains *to absorb leakage.*
- *To increase the patient's mobility and comfort,* connect the drains to a leg bag.

Second hospitalization or outpatient care
- After the patient's drains are removed by the practitioner, teach the patient how to catheterize the stoma. Begin by gathering the following equipment on a clean towel: latex-free catheter (usually #14 or #16 French), water-soluble lubricant, washcloth, towel, urine-collection container, and an irrigating solution (optional).
- Apply water-soluble lubricant to the catheter tip *to facilitate insertion.*
- Remove and discard the stoma cover.[18] Using the washcloth and water, clean the stoma and the area around it, starting at the stoma and working outward in a circular motion. Dry the area thoroughly with a towel.
- Hold the urine-collection container under the catheter, then slowly insert the catheter into the stoma. Urine should begin to flow into the container. If it doesn't, gently rotate the catheter or redirect its angle. If the catheter drains slowly, it may be plugged with mucus. Irrigate it with sterile saline solution or sterile water to clear it. When the flow stops, pinch the catheter closed and remove it.

PATIENT TEACHING

HOME CARE FOR THE PATIENT WITH A CONTINENT URINARY DIVERSION

- Explain that the stoma is commonly edematous (swollen) in the initial postoperative period, and that its size will gradually reduce over 6 to 8 weeks.
- Teach the patient how to care for the drains and their insertion sites during the 3 to 6 weeks the patient will be at home before their removal, and teach the patient how to attach them to a leg bag. Also teach the patient how to recognize the signs and symptoms of infection and obstruction.
- After the drains are removed, teach the patient how to empty the pouch, and establish a schedule. Initially, the patient should catheterize the stoma and empty the pouch every 2 to 3 hours. Later, the patient should catheterize every 4 hours while awake and also irrigate the pouch each morning and evening, if ordered. Instruct the patient to empty the pouch whenever the patient feels a sensation of fullness.
- Tell the patient that the catheters are reusable, but only after they've been cleaned. The patient should clean the catheter thoroughly with warm, soapy water; rinse it thoroughly; and hang it to dry over a clean towel. The patient should store cleaned and dried catheters in plastic bags. Tell that patient to reuse catheters for up to 1 month before discarding them. However, the patient should immediately discard any catheter that becomes discolored or cracked.
- Provide a contact telephone number for acute problems or questions.
- Provide the patient with information on what to do when such problems as odor, urinary tract infection, and leakage occur.
- Explain that mucus is a normal finding, and tell the patient what to do when there is more mucus than is normally observed.
- Explain that the stoma can bleed easily on contact.
- Discuss with the patient how to manage the stoma while performing activities of daily living, such as bathing, dressing, traveling, working, engaging in hobbies, and sexual activity.[24]

they're natural extensions of the patient. When teaching the patient how to perform the procedure, give the patient written instructions and provide positive reinforcement after the patient completes each step.[1] Suggest that the patient perform the procedure in the morning when urine flows most slowly.

Arrange for a visiting nurse or a wound ostomy continence nurse to assist the patient at home. Tell the patient about ostomy support groups, the United Ostomy Associations of America, and the American Cancer Society. Members of these organizations routinely visit health care facilities to explain ostomy care and the types of appliances available, and to help patients learn to function normally with a stoma.

Help the patient choose between disposable and reusable appliances by telling the patient the advantages and disadvantages of each. Emphasize the importance of correct placement and of a well-fitted appliance *to prevent seepage of urine onto the skin.* When positioned correctly, most appliances remain in place for at least 3 days and for as long as 7 days if no leakage occurs.[2] With the improved adhesives and pouches available, belts aren't always necessary.

Because urine flows constantly, it accumulates quickly, becoming even heavier than stools. *To prevent the weight of the urine from loosening the seal around the stoma and separating the appliance from the skin,* tell the patient to empty the appliance through the drain valve when it's one-third to one-half full.[2] Teach the patient sanitary and dietary measures that can protect the peristomal skin and control the odor that commonly results from alkaline urine, infection, and poor hygiene. Explain that generous fluid intake also helps to reduce odor by diluting the urine. Instruct the patient to connect the appliance to a urine-collection container before going to sleep. *The continuous flow of urine into the container during the night prevents the urine from accumulating and stagnating in the appliance.*

Advise the patient to wash reusable appliances with soap and lukewarm water and then air-dry them thoroughly *to prevent brittleness.*

Complications

Complications may include bleeding, which is especially likely with an ileal conduit, or reddened or excoriated peristomal skin. Other complications include mechanical injury, pressure injuries, skin-stripping injuries, mucocutaneous separation, hyperplastic skin around the stoma, folliculitis, and infection.[25,26]

Documentation

Record the appearance and color of the stoma and whether it's inverted, flush with the skin, or protruding. If it protrudes, note the amount it protrudes above the skin (the normal range is ½" to ¾"[1.3 to 2 cm].) Record the appearance and condition of the peristomal skin, noting any redness or irritation; complaints by the patient of itching or burning; and any nursing interventions performed, including consultation with the WOCN. Document teaching provided to the patient and family (if appropriate), their understanding of that teaching, and any need for follow-up teaching.

References

1 Hinkle, J. L., & Cheever, K. H. (2018). *Brunner & Suddarth's textbook of medical-surgical nursing* (14th ed.). Philadelphia, PA: Wolters Kluwer.

2 Wound, Ostomy and Continence Nurses Society (WOCN). (2018). *Basic ostomy skin care: A guide for patients and health care providers.* Mt. Laurel, NJ: WOCN. https://www.ostomy.org/wp-content/uploads/2018/11/wocn_basic_ostomy_skin_care_2018.pdf

3 The Joint Commission. (2021). Standard NPSG.07.01.01. *Comprehensive accreditation manual for hospitals.* Oakbrook Terrace, IL: The Joint Commission. (Level VII)

4 Centers for Disease Control and Prevention. (2002). Guideline for hand hygiene in health-care settings: Recommendations of the Healthcare Infection Control Practices Advisory Committee and the HICPAC/SHEA/APIC/IDSA Hand Hygiene Task Force. *MMWR Recommendations and Reports, 51*(RR-16), 1–45. https://www.cdc.gov/mmwr/pdf/rr/rr5116.pdf (Level II)

5 World Health Organization. (2009). WHO guidelines on hand hygiene in health care: First global patient safety challenge, clean care is safer care. https://apps.who.int/iris/bitstream/handle/10665/44102/9789241597906_eng.pdf?sequence–1 (Level IV)

6 Accreditation Association for Hospitals and Health Systems. (2020). Standard 07.01.21. *Healthcare Facilities Accreditation Program: Accreditation requirements for acute care hospitals.* Chicago, IL: Accreditation Association for Hospitals and Health Systems. (Level VII)

7 Centers for Medicare and Medicaid Services, Department of Health and Human Services. (2020). Condition of participation: Infection control. 42 C.F.R. § 482.42.

8 DNV GL-Healthcare USA, Inc. (2020). IC.1.SR.1. *NIAHO® accreditation requirements, interpretive guidelines and surveyor guidance – revision 20.0.* Milford, OH: DNV GL-Healthcare USA, Inc. (Level VII)

9 The Joint Commission. (2021). Standard NPSG.01.01.01. *Comprehensive accreditation manual for hospitals.* Oakbrook Terrace, IL: The Joint Commission. (Level VII)

10 The Joint Commission. (2021). Standard RI.01.01.01. *Comprehensive accreditation manual for hospitals.* Oakbrook Terrace, IL: The Joint Commission. (Level VII)

11 DNV GL-Healthcare USA, Inc. (2020). PR.2.SR.5. *NIAHO® accreditation requirements, interpretive guidelines and surveyor guidance – revision 20.0.* Milford, OH: DNV GL-Healthcare USA, Inc. (Level VII)

12 Centers for Medicare and Medicaid Services, Department of Health and Human Services. (2020). Condition of participation: Patient's rights. 42 C.F.R. § 482.13(c)(1).

13 Accreditation Association for Hospitals and Health Systems. (2020). Standard 15.01.16. *Healthcare Facilities Accreditation Program: Accreditation requirements for acute care hospitals.* Chicago, IL: Accreditation Association for Hospitals and Health Systems. (Level VII)

14 The Joint Commission. (2021). Standard PC.02.01.21. *Comprehensive accreditation manual for hospitals.* Oakbrook Terrace, IL: The Joint Commission. (Level VII)

15 Waters, T. R., et al. (2009). Safe patient handling training for schools of nursing. https://www.cdc.gov/niosh/docs/2009-127/pdfs/2009-127.pdf (Level VII)

16 Siegel, J. D., et al. (2007, revised 2019). 2007 guideline for isolation precautions: Preventing transmission of infectious agents in healthcare settings. https://www.cdc.gov/infectioncontrol/pdf/guidelines/isolation-guidelines-H.pdf (Level II)

17 Accreditation Association for Hospitals and Health Systems. (2020). Standard 07.01.10. *Healthcare Facilities Accreditation Program: Accreditation requirements for acute care hospitals.* Chicago, IL: Accreditation Association for Hospitals and Health Systems. (Level VII)

18 Occupational Safety and Health Administration. (2012). Bloodborne pathogens, standard number 1910.1030. https://www.osha.gov/pls/oshaweb/owadisp.show_document?p_id=10051&p_table=STANDARDS (Level VII)

19 Ganz, D. A., et al. (2013, reviewed 2021). *Preventing falls in hospitals: A toolkit for improving quality of care*(AHRQ Publication No. 13-0015-EF). Rockville, MD: Agency for Healthcare Research and Quality. https://www.ahrq.gov/professionals/systems/hospital/fallpxtoolkit/index.html (Level VII)

20 The Joint Commission. (2021). Standard RC.01.03.01. *Comprehensive accreditation manual for hospitals.* Oakbrook Terrace, IL: The Joint Commission. (Level VII)

21 Accreditation Association for Hospitals and Health Systems. (2020). Standard 10.00.03. *Healthcare Facilities Accreditation Program: Accreditation requirements for acute care hospitals.* Chicago, IL: Accreditation Association for Hospitals and Health Systems. (Level VII)

22 Centers for Medicare and Medicaid Services, Department of Health and Human Services. (2020). Condition of participation: Medical record services. 42 C.F.R. § 482.24(b).

23 DNV GL-Healthcare USA, Inc. (2020). MR.2.SR.1. *NIAHO® accreditation requirements, interpretive guidelines and surveyor guidance – revision 20.0.* Milford, OH: DNV GL-Healthcare USA, Inc. (Level VII)

24 National Institute of Diabetes and Digestive and Kidney Diseases. (2020). Urinary diversion. https://www.niddk.nih.gov/health-information/urologic-diseases/urinary-diversion

25 Szymanski, K. M., et al. (2010). External stoma and peristomal complications following radical cystectomy and ileal conduit diversion: A systematic review. *Ostomy Wound Management, 56,* 28–35. https://pubmed.ncbi.nlm.nih.gov/20093715/ (Level I)

26 Northwestern Memorial HealthCare. (2019). A patient guide to urinary diversions. https://www.nm.org/-/media/northwestern/resources/patients-and-visitors/patient-education-care-and-treatment/northwestern-medicine-a-patients-guide-to-urinary-diversions.pdf

URINE COLLECTION, 12- OR 24-HOUR TIMED

Because hormones, proteins, and electrolytes are excreted in small, variable amounts in urine, specimens for measuring these substances must typically be collected over an extended period to yield quantities of diagnostic value. A 24-hour specimen is used most commonly because it provides an average excretion rate for substances. Timed specimens may also be collected for shorter periods, such as 12 hours, depending on the specific information needed.

All urine voided within the prescribed time period is collected in a suitable collection container. Depending on the intended test, a preservative may be added to the specimen collection container, and the specimen may need to be kept refrigerated or on ice.[1]

Equipment

24-hour urine specimen collection container ▪ gloves ▪ specimen label ▪ laboratory biohazard transport bag ▪ patient-care reminders ▪ facility-approved disinfectant ▪ Optional: specimen preservative, specimen collection hat, refrigerator or ice-filled basin(s), graduated container, bedpan, urinal, bedside commode, laboratory request form, gown.

Preparation of equipment

Inspect all equipment and supplies. If a product is expired, is defective, or has compromised integrity, remove it from patient use, label it as expired or defective, and report the expiration or defect as directed by your facility.

If a preservative is needed, check the expiration date on the preservative container and add the preservative to the specimen collection container.

Implementation

▪ Verify the practitioner's order.
▪ Check with the laboratory *to determine the proper container and preservative (if needed) for the ordered test and whether the specimen requires refrigeration during the collection period.*
▪ Gather and prepare the necessary equipment and supplies.
▪ Perform hand hygiene.[2,3,4,5,6,7]
▪ Confirm the patient's identity using at least two patient identifiers.[8]
▪ Label the specimen container in the presence of the patient *to help prevent mislabeling.*[8] The label should include the patient's name and identification number, the date, the start time of the collection, the time the collection should end, the test ordered, any other pertinent information, and your initials.[1]
▪ Provide privacy.[9,10,11,12]
▪ Explain the procedure to the patient and family members (if appropriate) according to their individual communication and learning needs *to help increase their understanding, allay their fears, enhance cooperation, and prevent accidental disposal of urine during the collection period.*[13] Emphasize that failure to collect even one specimen during the collection period invalidates the test and requires that it be started over.[1]
▪ If you are collecting a voided specimen, explain that the patient should empty the bladder just before the 12- or 24-hour collection period begins, and that this specimen will be discarded.[1] Explain that the patient should save and store all urine voided during the 12- or 24-hour collection period in one specimen collection container.[1] Instruct the patient to notify you after each void and to avoid contaminating the urine with stool or toilet tissue.[1]
▪ Instruct the patient to avoid exercise and ingestion of coffee, tea, and certain drugs (unless directed otherwise by the practitioner) right before and during the test *to avoid altering test results.* Make sure that the patient understands the instructions and is willing to adhere to the restrictions.
▪ Place patient-care reminders over the patient's bed, in the bathroom, and on the urinal, bedpan, bedside commode, or indwelling catheter collection bag. Include the date and the collection interval.

Collecting a voided specimen

▪ If the patient is using the bathroom toilet, place a specimen collection hat in the toilet bowl *to collect and measure urine.*[1] If the patient can't use the bathroom toilet, use a urinal, bedpan, or bedside commode, as appropriate, *to collect urine as the patient voids.*

▪ At the beginning of the collection period, ask the patient to void.[1]
▪ Perform hand hygiene[2,3,4,5,6,7] and then put on gloves *to comply with standard precautions.*[14,15]
▪ Measure the amount of urine using a graduated collection container, if output is being recorded.[1]
▪ Discard the urine specimen *so that the patient starts the collection period with an empty bladder.*[1]
▪ Note the time as the beginning time for the collection period.[1]
▪ Remove and discard your gloves.[14,15]
▪ Perform hand hygiene.[2,3,4,5,6,7]
▪ After each time the patient voids during the collection period, perform hand hygiene[2,3,4,5,6,7] and put on gloves *to comply with standard precautions.*[14,15] Measure the amount of urine using a graduated container, if output is to be recorded.[1] Pour the urine specimen to be saved into the specimen collection container.[1] Then remove and discard your gloves,[14,15] and perform hand hygiene.[2,3,4,5,6,7]
▪ Keep the specimen collection container refrigerated or on ice *to preserve the specimen,* as appropriate.[1]
▪ At the end of the collection period, perform hand hygiene[2,3,4,5,6,7] and put on gloves *to comply with standard precautions.*[14,15] Instruct the patient to void again, if possible. Measure the amount of urine (if output is being recorded), and add this final specimen to the collection container.[1] Note the ending time on the specimen label.[1]

Collecting an indwelling urinary catheter specimen

▪ Perform hand hygiene[2,3,4,5,6,7] at the beginning of the collection period and put on gloves *to comply with standard precautions.*[14,15]
▪ Empty the urine collection bag. During emptying, avoid splashing, and don't allow the drainage spigot to come in contact with the nonsterile container *to help reduce the risk of catheter-associated urinary tract infections.*[16,17,18,19]

HOSPITAL-ACQUIRED CONDITION ALERT Keep in mind that the Centers for Medicare and Medicaid Services considers catheter-associated urinary tract infection (CAUTI) a hospital-acquired condition, *because it can be reasonably prevented using a variety of best practices.* Make sure to follow evidence-based CAUTI prevention practices—such as performing hand hygiene before and after any catheter manipulation; maintaining a sterile, continuously closed drainage system; maintaining unobstructed urine flow; emptying the urine collection bag regularly; replacing the catheter and urine collection system using sterile technique when a break in sterile technique, disconnection, or leakage occurs; and discontinuing the catheter as soon as it's no longer indicated clinically—when caring for a patient with an indwelling urinary catheter *to help reduce the risk of CAUTI.*[16,17,18,19,20,21]

▪ Measure the amount of urine if output is being recorded.
▪ Discard the urine.[1]
▪ Note the time as the beginning time for the collection period.[1]
▪ Put the urine drainage bag in an ice-filled basin at the bedside.[1]
▪ Remove and discard your gloves.[14,15]
▪ At regular intervals during the collection period, perform hand hygiene[2,3,4,5,6,7] and put on gloves *to comply with standard precautions.*[14,15] Empty the urine drainage bag. Measure the amount of urine, if output is being recorded.[1] Pour the urine specimen to be saved into the specimen collection container.[1] Remove and discard your gloves,[14,15] and perform hand hygiene.[2,3,4,5,6,7]
▪ Keep the collection container refrigerated or on ice *to preserve the specimen,* as appropriate.[1]
▪ At the end of the collection period, perform hand hygiene[2,3,4,5,6,7] and put on gloves *to comply with standard precautions.*[14,15] Collect the remaining urine from the indwelling urinary catheter collection bag. If recording output, measure the volume of urine, and then add this final specimen to the collection container.[1] Note the ending time on the specimen label.[1]

Completing the procedure

▪ Place the specimen collection container in an approved laboratory biohazard transport container.[22]
▪ Discard used supplies in appropriate receptacles.[22]
▪ Remove and discard your gloves.[14,15]
▪ Perform hand hygiene.[2,3,4,5,6,7]

■ Immediately send the container to the laboratory with a properly completed laboratory request form, if required by your facility.[22]

■ Remove the patient-care reminders, and inform the patient and family that the specimen collection period is complete.

■ Perform hand hygiene.[2,3,4,5,6,7]

■ Put on gloves and, as needed, a gown *to comply with standard precautions.*[22]

■ Clean and disinfect reusable equipment according to the manufacturer's instructions *to prevent the spread of infection.*[23,24]

■ Remove and discard your gloves and, if worn, your gown.[22]

■ Perform hand hygiene.[2,3,4,5,6,7]

■ Document the procedure.[25,26,27,28]

Special considerations

■ If appropriate, keep the patient well hydrated before and during the test *to ensure adequate urine flow.*

■ Never store a specimen in a refrigerator that contains food or medication *to avoid contamination.*[1]

■ If a urine specimen is accidentally discarded during the collection period, restart the procedure.[1] Emphasize the need to save all of the patient's urine during the collection period to everyone involved in the patient's care as well as to the patient, family, and other visitors.

■ Notify the practitioner if the patient is menstruating, *because the test may need to be postponed to avoid specimen contamination.*[1]

Patient teaching

If the patient must collect urine at home, provide written instructions for the appropriate method. Instruct the patient to keep the collection container in a brown bag in a refrigerator at home, separate from other refrigerator contents.

Documentation

Record the dates, starting and ending times, and method of urine specimen collection. Also record the name of the test, the amount of urine collected (if needed), any preservative or refrigeration used, and the time of specimen transport to the laboratory. Document teaching provided to the patient and family (if applicable), their understanding of that teaching, and any need for follow-up teaching.

REFERENCES

1 Fischbach, F., & Fischbach, M. A. (2022). *A manual of laboratory and diagnostic tests* (11th ed.). Philadelphia, PA: Wolters Kluwer.

2 The Joint Commission. (2021). Standard NPSG.07.01.01. *Comprehensive accreditation manual for hospitals.* Oakbrook Terrace, IL: The Joint Commission. (Level VII)

3 World Health Organization. (2009). WHO guidelines on hand hygiene in health care: First global patient safety challenge, clean care is safer care. https://apps.who.int/iris/bitstream/handle/10665/44102/9789241597906_eng.pdf?sequence=1 (Level IV)

4 Centers for Disease Control and Prevention. (2002). Guideline for hand hygiene in health-care settings: Recommendations of the Healthcare Infection Control Practices Advisory Committee and the HICPAC/SHEA/APIC/IDSA Hand Hygiene Task Force. *MMWR Recommendations and Reports, 51*(RR-16), 1–45. https://www.cdc.gov/mmwr/pdf/rr/rr5116.pdf (Level II)

5 Centers for Medicare and Medicaid Services, Department of Health and Human Services. (2020). Condition of participation: Infection control. 42 C.F.R. § 482.42.

6 Accreditation Association for Hospitals and Health Systems. (2020). Standard 07.01.21. *Healthcare Facilities Accreditation Program: Accreditation requirements for acute care hospitals.* Chicago, IL: Accreditation Association for Hospitals and Health Systems. (Level VII)

7 DNV GL-Healthcare USA, Inc. (2020). IC.1.SR.1. *NIAHO® accreditation requirements, interpretive guidelines and surveyor guidance – revision 20.0.* Milford, OH: DNV GL-Healthcare USA, Inc. (Level VII)

8 The Joint Commission. (2021). Standard NPSG.01.01.01. *Comprehensive accreditation manual for hospitals.* Oakbrook Terrace, IL: The Joint Commission. (Level VII)

9 Centers for Medicare and Medicaid Services, Department of Health and Human Services. (2020). Condition of participation: Patient's rights. 42 C.F.R. § 482.13(c)(1).

10 Accreditation Association for Hospitals and Health Systems. (2020). Standard 15.01.16. *Healthcare Facilities Accreditation Program: Accreditation requirements for acute care hospitals.* Chicago, IL: Accreditation Association for Hospitals and Health Systems. (Level VII)

11 The Joint Commission. (2021). Standard RI.01.01.01. *Comprehensive accreditation manual for hospitals.* Oakbrook Terrace, IL: The Joint Commission. (Level VII)

12 DNV GL-Healthcare USA, Inc. (2020). PR.2.SR.5. *NIAHO® accreditation requirements, interpretive guidelines and surveyor guidance – revision 20.0.* Milford, OH: DNV GL-Healthcare USA, Inc. (Level VII)

13 The Joint Commission. (2021). Standard PC.02.01.21. *Comprehensive accreditation manual for hospitals.* Oakbrook Terrace, IL: The Joint Commission. (Level VII)

14 Siegel, J. D., et al. (2007, revised 2019). 2007 guideline for isolation precautions: Preventing transmission of infectious agents in healthcare settings. https://www.cdc.gov/infectioncontrol/pdf/guidelines/isolation-guidelines-H.pdf (Level II)

15 Accreditation Association for Hospitals and Health Systems. (2020). Standard 07.01.10. *Healthcare Facilities Accreditation Program: Accreditation requirements for acute care hospitals.* Chicago, IL: Accreditation Association for Hospitals and Health Systems. (Level VII)

16 Lo, E., et al. (2014). SHEA/IDSA practice recommendation: Strategies to prevent catheter-associated urinary tract infections in acute care hospitals: 2014 update. *Infection Control and Hospital Epidemiology, 35,* 464–479. https://www.jstor.org/stable/10.1086/675718#metadata_info_tab_content (Level I)

17 Accreditation Association for Hospitals and Health Systems. (2020). Standard 07.01.02. *Healthcare Facilities Accreditation Program: Accreditation requirements for acute care hospitals.* Chicago, IL: Accreditation Association for Hospitals and Health Systems. (Level VII)

18 The Joint Commission. (2021). Standard NPSG.07.06.01. *Comprehensive accreditation manual for hospitals.* Oakbrook Terrace, IL: The Joint Commission. (Level VII)

19 Healthcare Infection Control Practices Advisory Committee. (2010, revised 2019). Guideline for prevention of catheter-associated urinary tract infections 2009. https://www.cdc.gov/infectioncontrol/pdf/guidelines/cauti-guidelines-H.pdf (Level I)

20 Association of Professionals in Infection Control and Epidemiology (APIC). (2014). APIC Implementation Guide: Guide to preventing catheter-associated urinary tract infections. https://apic.org/wp-content/uploads/2019/02/APIC_CAUTI_IG_FIN_REVD0815.pdf (Level IV)

21 Jarrett, N., & Callaham, M. (2016). Evidence-based guidelines for selected hospital-acquired conditions: Final report. https://www.cms.gov/Medicare/Medicare-Fee-for-Service-Payment/HospitalAcqCond/Downloads/2016-HAC-Report.pdf

22 Occupational Safety and Health Administration. (2012). Bloodborne pathogens, standard number 1910.1030. https://www.osha.gov/pls/oshaweb/owadisp.show_document?p_id=10051&p_table=STANDARDS (Level VII)

23 Accreditation Association for Hospitals and Health Systems. (2020). Standard 07.02.03. *Healthcare Facilities Accreditation Program: Accreditation requirements for acute care hospitals.* Chicago, IL: Accreditation Association for Hospitals and Health Systems. (Level VII)

24 Rutala, W. A., et al. (2008, revised 2019). Guideline for disinfection and sterilization in healthcare facilities, 2008. https://www.cdc.gov/infectioncontrol/pdf/guidelines/disinfection-guidelines-H.pdf (Level I)

25 The Joint Commission. (2021). Standard RC.01.03.01. *Comprehensive accreditation manual for hospitals.* Oakbrook Terrace, IL: The Joint Commission. (Level VII)

26 Centers for Medicare and Medicaid Services, Department of Health and Human Services. (2020). Condition of participation: Medical record services. 42 C.F.R. § 482.24(b).

27 Accreditation Association for Hospitals and Health Systems. (2020). Standard 10.00.03. *Healthcare Facilities Accreditation Program: Accreditation requirements for acute care hospitals.* Chicago, IL: Accreditation Association for Hospitals and Health Systems. (Level VII)

28 DNV GL-Healthcare USA, Inc. (2020). MR.2.SR.1. *NIAHO® accreditation requirements, interpretive guidelines and surveyor guidance – revision 20.0.* Milford, OH: DNV GL-Healthcare USA, Inc. (Level VII)

URINE GLUCOSE AND KETONE TESTS

Glucose and ketones aren't normally found in urine,[1] so their presence signifies an underlying condition. Reagent strip tests help monitor urine glucose and ketone levels and screen for diabetes. Urine ketone tests monitor fat metabolism, help diagnose carbohydrate deprivation and diabetic ketoacidosis, and help distinguish between diabetic and nondiabetic coma. Urine glucose testing isn't as accurate as blood glucose testing,[2] and should be used only when blood glucose testing isn't available.[3,4]

Glucose oxidase tests (such as Diastix and Clinistix strips) produce color changes when patches of reagents implanted in handheld plastic strips react with glucose in the patient's urine. Urine ketone strip tests (such as Keto-Diastix and Ketostix) work similarly. Test results are read by comparing color changes with a standardized reference chart.[5] In some facilities, the nurse collects the urine specimen, performs the test, and then interprets the results using one of the described methods; in others, the nurse collects the urine specimen and sends it to the laboratory for interpretation. Nursing staff members should follow their facility's process for urine glucose and ketone testing.

Equipment

Urine specimen container ▪ gloves ▪ Optional: glucose oxidase or ketone test strips, timer (or watch or clock with second hand), appropriate equipment for the specific type of urine collection method, label, laboratory biohazard transport bag.

Preparation of equipment

Check the expiration date on the reagent strips and discard them if they're expired. Allow time for refrigerated items, including reagents and patient specimens, to reach room temperature before testing, if specified in the product insert.[5] Check and record lot numbers for test kits, test devices, and controls. (Don't mix reagents from different products or lot numbers. If you're using a new lot, set up quality control, as needed, and refer to the product insert for changes in control ranges.) Visually inspect reagent vials and the strips within them for damage, discoloration, and contamination. Prepare and store reagents according to the manufacturer's instructions. If opening a new reagent strip vial or kit, write the date opened on the outside of the vial or test kit *to record when it was opened*.[6]

Implementation

▪ Verify the practitioner's order.
▪ Gather and prepare the necessary equipment and supplies.
▪ Check the patient's history for medications that may interfere with test results.
▪ Perform hand hygiene.[7,8,9,10,11,12]
▪ Confirm the patient's identity using at least two patient identifiers.[13]
▪ Provide privacy.[14,15,16,17]
▪ Explain the procedure to the patient and family (if appropriate) according to their individual communication and learning need *to increase their understanding, allay fears and enhance cooperation*.[18]
▪ Obtain a random or clean-catch urine specimen.[19] (See the section titled "Collecting a random specimen," "Collecting a clean-catch midstream specimen, female," "Collecting a clean-catch midstream specimen, male," or "Collecting an indwelling catheter specimen" in the "Urine specimen collection" procedure.)
▪ Perform hand hygiene.[7,8,9,10,11,12]
▪ Put on gloves *to comply with standard precautions*.[20,21,22]
▪ Test the urine specimen immediately after the patient voids. Alternatively, if directed by your facility, label the specimen in the presence of the patient *to prevent mislabeling*,[13] place the specimen in a laboratory biohazard transport bag, and send the specimen to the laboratory for urine glucose and ketone testing.[22]

Glucose oxidase strip tests

▪ If you're using a Clinistix strip, dip the reagent end of the strip into the urine specimen for 2 seconds. Remove excess urine by tapping the strip against the container's rim, wait for exactly 10 seconds, and then compare its color with the standardized color chart on the test strip container. Ignore color changes that occur after 10 seconds. Record the result.

▪ If you're using a Diastix strip, dip the reagent end of the strip into the urine specimen for 2 seconds. Remove excess urine by tapping the strip against the container's rim, wait for exactly 30 seconds, and then compare the strip's color with the standardized color chart on the test strip container. Ignore color changes that occur after 30 seconds. Record the result.

Ketone strip tests

▪ If you're using a Ketostix strip, dip the reagent end of the strip into the urine specimen and remove it immediately. Wait exactly 15 seconds, and then compare the color of the strip with the standardized color chart on the test strip container. Ignore color changes that occur after 15 seconds. Record the result.
▪ If you're using a Keto-Diastix strip, dip the reagent end of the strip into the urine specimen and remove it immediately. Remove excess urine by tapping the strip against the container's rim, and hold the strip horizontally *to prevent mixing of chemicals between the two reagent squares*. Wait exactly 15 seconds, and then compare the color of the ketone part of the strip with the standardized color chart on the test strip container. After 30 seconds, compare the color of the glucose part of the strip with the color chart. Record the result.

NURSING ALERT Always be sure to read results during the correct timeframe, especially if you're conducting more than one test at a time.[5] *Time intervals longer than those specified in the product insert can result in false-positive, false-negative, or invalid results because of exaggerated color development, fading of reaction products, and migration beyond a visible range.*[6]

Completing the procedure

▪ Measure and record the amount of urine collected if the patient's intake and output is being monitored.
▪ Discard the urine specimen, specimen container, and reagent strips in appropriate receptacles.[22]
▪ Remove and discard your gloves.[22]
▪ Perform hand hygiene.[7,8,9,10,11,12]
▪ Notify the practitioner of critical test results within your facility's established time frame *so the patient can be promptly treated*.[23]
▪ Document the procedure and the test results.[19,24,25,26]

Special considerations

▪ If you're testing a refrigerated urine specimen, allow it to warm to room temperature and mix the specimen before testing.[27]
▪ Agents containing free sulfhydryl groups can cause interference with ketone detection.[1]
▪ Highly pigmented urine can result in false-positive results.[1]
▪ Improper specimen or test strip storage may result in false-negative results.[1]

Complications

Improper collection technique or testing procedure may affect the accuracy of the results.[5]

Documentation

Record the test results according to the information on the reagent containers, or use a flowchart designed to record this information. Indicate whether the practitioner was notified of the test results and the time of the notification. Also, record any treatment given as a result of the testing. Document teaching provided to the patient and family (if applicable), their understanding of the teaching, and any need for follow-up teaching.

REFERENCES

1 Dumonceaux, M. (2016). Rediscovering urine chemistry—and understanding its limitations. *Medical Laboratory Observer, 48*(12), 12–14. https://www.mlo-online.com/continuing-education/article/13008884/rediscovering-urine-chemistryand-understanding-its-limitations

2 Kuru, B., et al. (2014). Comparing finger-stick beta-hydroxybutyrate with dipstick urine tests in the detection of ketone bodies. *Turkish Journal of Emergency Medicine, 14*(2), 47–52. https://www.ncbi.nlm.nih.gov/pmc/articles/PMC4909883/ (Level IV)

3 Klocker, A. A., et al. (2013). Blood β-hydroxybutyrate vs. urine acetoacetate testing for the prevention and management of ketoacidosis in type 1 diabetes: A systematic review. *Diabetic Medicine, 30,* 818–824. (Level I)

4 National Collaborating Centre for Women's and Children's Health. (2015, updated 2020). *Diabetes (type 1 and type 2) in children and young people: Diagnosis and management.* London, UK: National Institute for Health and Care Excellence. https://www.nice.org.uk/guidance/ng18 (Level VII)

5 Yates, A. (2016). Urinalysis: How to interpret results. *Nursing Times, 2,* 1–3. https://www.nursingtimes.net/clinical-archive/continence/urinalysis-how-to-interpret-results-07-06-2016/

6 Centers for Disease Control and Prevention. (2005). Good laboratory practices for waived testing sites: Survey findings from testing sites holding a certificate of waiver under the Clinical Laboratory Improvement Amendments of 1988 and recommendations for promoting quality testing. *MMWR Recommendations and Reports, 54*(RR-13), 1–25. https://www.cdc.gov/mmwr/PDF/rr/rr5413.pdf (Level II)

7 The Joint Commission. (2021). Standard NPSG.07.01.01. *Comprehensive accreditation manual for hospitals.* Oakbrook Terrace, IL: The Joint Commission. (Level VII)

8 Centers for Disease Control and Prevention. (2002). Guideline for hand hygiene in health-care settings: Recommendations of the Healthcare Infection Control Practices Advisory Committee and the HICPAC/SHEA/APIC/IDSA Hand Hygiene Task Force. *MMWR Recommendations and Reports, 51*(RR-16), 1–45. https://www.cdc.gov/mmwr/pdf/rr/rr5116.pdf (Level II)

9 World Health Organization. (2009). WHO guidelines on hand hygiene in health care: First global patient safety challenge, clean care is safer care. https://apps.who.int/iris/bitstream/handle/10665/44102/9789241597906_eng.pdf?sequence=1 (Level IV)

10 Centers for Medicare and Medicaid Services, Department of Health and Human Services. (2020). Condition of participation: Infection control. 42 C.F.R. § 482.42.

11 Accreditation Association for Hospitals and Health Systems. (2020). Standard 07.01.21. *Healthcare Facilities Accreditation Program: Accreditation requirements for acute care hospitals.* Chicago, IL: Accreditation Association for Hospitals and Health Systems. (Level VII)

12 DNV GL-Healthcare USA, Inc. (2020). IC.1.SR.1. *NIAHO® accreditation requirements, interpretive guidelines and surveyor guidance – revision 20.0.* Milford, OH: DNV GL-Healthcare USA, Inc. (Level VII)

13 The Joint Commission. (2021). Standard NPSG.01.01.01. *Comprehensive accreditation manual for hospitals.* Oakbrook Terrace, IL: The Joint Commission. (Level VII)

14 DNV GL-Healthcare USA, Inc. (2020). PR.2.SR.5. *NIAHO® accreditation requirements, interpretive guidelines and surveyor guidance – revision 20.0.* Milford, OH: DNV GL-Healthcare USA, Inc. (Level VII)

15 Centers for Medicare and Medicaid Services, Department of Health and Human Services. (2020). Condition of participation: Patient's rights. 42 C.F.R. § 482.13(c)(1).

16 Accreditation Association for Hospitals and Health Systems. (2020). Standard 15.01.16. *Healthcare Facilities Accreditation Program: Accreditation requirements for acute care hospitals.* Chicago, IL: Accreditation Association for Hospitals and Health Systems. (Level VII)

17 The Joint Commission. (2021). Standard RI.01.01.01. *Comprehensive accreditation manual for hospitals.* Oakbrook Terrace, IL: The Joint Commission. (Level VII)

18 The Joint Commission. (2021). Standard PC.02.01.21. *Comprehensive accreditation manual for hospitals.* Oakbrook Terrace, IL: The Joint Commission. (Level VII)

19 DNV GL-Healthcare USA, Inc. (2020). MR.2.SR.1. *NIAHO® accreditation requirements, interpretive guidelines and surveyor guidance – revision 20.0.* Milford, OH: DNV GL-Healthcare USA, Inc. (Level VII)

20 Accreditation Association for Hospitals and Health Systems. (2020). Standard 07.01.10. *Healthcare Facilities Accreditation Program: Accreditation requirements for acute care hospitals.* Chicago, IL: Accreditation Association for Hospitals and Health Systems. (Level VII)

21 Siegel, J. D., et al. (2007, revised 2019). 2007 guideline for isolation precautions: Preventing transmission of infectious agents in healthcare settings. https://www.cdc.gov/infectioncontrol/pdf/guidelines/isolation-guidelines-H.pdf (Level II)

22 Occupational Safety and Health Administration. (2012). Bloodborne pathogens, standard number 1910.1030. https://www.osha.gov/pls/oshaweb/owadisp.show_document?p_id=10051&p_table=STANDARDS (Level VI)

23 The Joint Commission. (2021). Standard NPSG.02.03.01. *Comprehensive accreditation manual for hospitals.* Oakbrook Terrace, IL: The Joint Commission. (Level VII)

24 The Joint Commission. (2021). Standard RC.01.03.01. *Comprehensive accreditation manual for hospitals.* Oakbrook Terrace, IL: The Joint Commission. (Level VII)

25 Centers for Medicare and Medicaid Services, Department of Health and Human Services. (2020). Condition of participation: Medical record services. 42 C.F.R. § 482.24(b).

26 Accreditation Association for Hospitals and Health Systems. (2020). Standard 10.00.03. *Healthcare Facilities Accreditation Program: Accreditation requirements for acute care hospitals.* Chicago, IL: Accreditation Association for Hospitals and Health Systems. (Level VII)

27 Fischbach, F., & Fischbach, M. A. (2022). *A manual of laboratory and diagnostic tests* (11th ed.). Philadelphia, PA: Wolters Kluwer.

Urine pH measurement

The pH of urine—its alkalinity or acidity—reflects the kidneys' ability to maintain a normal hydrogen ion concentration in plasma and extracellular fluids. The normal hydrogen ion concentration in urine varies, ranging from 4.6 to 8, but it usually averages around a pH of 6.[1,2]

The simplest procedure for testing the pH of urine consists of dipping a reagent strip (such as Combistix) into a fresh specimen of the patient's urine and comparing the resulting color change with a standardized color chart.[3] In some facilities, the nurse collects the urine specimen and measures urine pH. In others, the nurse collects the specimen and sends it to the laboratory for interpretation. Nursing staff members should follow the facility's process for urine pH measurement.

An alkaline pH (above 7) may result from a diet low in meat and carbohydrates but high in vegetables, dairy products, and citrus fruits.[4] Alkaline urine causes turbidity and the formation of phosphate, carbonate, and amorphous crystals. Alkaline urine may also result from urinary tract infection (UTI) with urease-producing bacteria, gastric suctioning, vomiting, hyperventilation, and metabolic or respiratory alkalosis.[1,4]

An acidic pH (below 7), which may result from a high-protein diet and a diet high in cranberries, also causes turbidity as well as the formation of oxalate, cystine, amorphous urate, and uric acid crystals. Acidic urine may also result from renal tuberculosis, phenylketonuria, alkaptonuria, pyrexia, diarrhea, starvation, diabetic ketoacidosis, kidney failure, chronic lung disease, UTI caused by acid-producing bacteria (such as *Escherichia coli*), and all forms of acidosis.[1,4] Low urine pH is also associated with insulin resistance and metabolic syndrome.[5,6]

Measuring urine pH can also help monitor some medications—including methenamine, ammonium chloride, and such diuretics as thiazides—that are active only at certain pH levels.[2,7]

Equipment

Urine specimen container ▪ gloves ▪ Optional: reagent strips that include pH indicators, appropriate equipment for the specific type of urine collection method, label and laboratory biohazard transport bag.

Preparation of equipment

Check the expiration dates on the reagent strips and discard them if they're expired. Allow time for refrigerated items to reach room temperature before testing, if specified in the product insert.[3] Check and record lot numbers for test kits, test devices, and controls. (Don't mix reagents from different products or lot numbers. If you're using a new lot, set up quality control, as needed, and refer to the product insert for changes in control ranges.) Visually inspect the reagent vials and the strips within them for damage, discoloration, and contamination. Prepare and store reagents strips according to the manufacturer's instructions. If opening a new reagent strip vial or kit, write the date opened on the outside of the vial or test kit.[8]

Implementation

- Verify the practitioner's order, if required.
- Gather and prepare the necessary equipment and supplies.
- Perform hand hygiene.[9,10,11,12,13,14]
- Confirm the patient's identity using at least two patient identifiers.[15]
- Provide privacy.[16,17,18,19]
- Explain the procedure to the patient and family (if appropriate) according to their individual communication and learning needs *to increase their understanding, allay their fears and enhance cooperation.*[20]
- Perform hand hygiene.[9,10,11,12,13,14]
- Put on gloves *to comply with standard precautions.*[21,22,23]
- Obtain a random or clean-catch urine specimen.[2] (See the section titled "Collecting a random specimen," "Collecting a clean-catch midstream specimen, female," "Collecting a clean-catch midstream specimen, male," or "Collecting an indwelling catheter specimen" in the "Urine specimen collection" procedure.)
- Measure urine pH as permitted by your facility. Alternatively, label the specimen in the presence of the patient *to prevent mislabeling,*[15] place the specimen in a laboratory biohazard transport bag, and send the specimen to the laboratory for urine pH measurement.[23]
- To measure urine pH yourself, dip a reagent strip into the urine, remove it, and tap the reagent strip against the container's rim *to remove excess urine.*[3]
- While holding the strip horizontally *to avoid mixing reagents from adjacent test areas on the strip,* compare the color on the strip with the standardized color chart on the strip package.[3] This comparison can be made up to 60 seconds after immersing the strip.

NURSING ALERT Always be sure to read results during the correct time frame, especially if conducting more than one test at a time.[3] *Reading test results during time intervals longer than those specified in the product insert may result in false-positive, false-negative, or invalid results because of exaggerated color development, fading reaction products, and migration beyond a visible range.*[8]

- If you're monitoring the patient's urinary intake and output, measure and record the amount of urine collected.
- Discard the urine specimen, specimen container, and reagent strip in appropriate receptacles.[23]
- Remove and discard your gloves.[23]
- Perform hand hygiene.[9,10,11,12,13,14]
- If you performed the test, record the urine pH measurement test results in the patient's medical record.[3]
- Notify the practitioner of critical test results within your facility's established time frame *so the patient can be promptly treated.*[24]
- Document the procedure.[25,26,27,28]

Special considerations

- Use only a fresh urine specimen to measure urine pH, *because bacterial growth at room temperature for a prolonged time may change urine pH.* If you are unable to test a urine specimen immediately, store the specimen according to the reagent strip manufacturer's instructions (usually 35.6° F to 39.2° F [2° C to 4° C]) and then bring the specimen to room temperature before testing.[3]
- Avoid letting a drop of urine run onto adjacent reagent spots on the strip, *because the other reagents can change the pH result.*[2]
- Urine pH may be lowest in the morning and after an overnight fasting, and higher after meals.[3]

Complications

Improper collection technique or testing procedure may affect the accuracy of the results.[3]

Documentation

Record the urine pH measurement test results, the date and time of voiding, and the amount of urine voided, if applicable. Document the name of the practitioner notified of test results, the date and time of notification, prescribed interventions, and the patient's response to those interventions, if applicable. Document teaching you provided to the patient and family (if applicable), their understanding of that teaching, and any need for follow-up teaching.

REFERENCES

1 Wald, R. (2021). Urinalysis in the diagnosis of kidney disease. In: *UpToDate*, Curhan, G. C. (Ed.).

2 Fischbach, F., & Fischbach, M. A. (2022). *A manual of laboratory and diagnostic tests* (11th ed.). Philadelphia, PA: Wolters Kluwer.

3 Yates, A. (2016). Urinalysis: How to interpret results. *Nursing Times, 2,* 1–3. https://www.nursingtimes.net/clinical-archive/continence/urinalysis-how-to-interpret-results-07-06-2016/

4 Dumonceaux, M. (2016). Rediscovering urine chemistry—and understanding its limitations. *Medical Laboratory Observer, 48*(12), 12–14. https://www.mlo-online.com/continuing-education/article/13008884/rediscovering-urine-chemistryand-understanding-its-limitations

5 Shimodaira, M., et al. (2018). Association of low urine pH with insulin resistance in non-diabetic Japanese subjects. *Experimental and Clinical Endocrinology & Diabetes, 126,* 357–361. (Level IV)

6 Chung, S. M., et al. (2018). Low urine pH affects the development of metabolic syndrome, associative with the increase of dyslipidemia and dysglycemia: Nationwide cross-sectional study (KNHANES 2013-2015) and a single-center retrospective cohort study. *PLoS One, 13*(8), e0202757. (Level IV)

7 Edenbridge Pharmaceuticals, LLC. (n.d.). Methenamine mandelate tablets, USP. http://www.edenbridgepharma.com/products-methenamine.php

8 Centers for Disease Control and Prevention. (2005). Good laboratory practices for waived testing sites: Survey findings from testing sites holding a certificate of waiver under the Clinical Laboratory Improvement Amendments of 1988 and recommendations for promoting quality testing. *MMWR Recommendations and Reports, 54*(RR-13), 1–25. http://www.cdc.gov/mmwr/PDF/rr/rr5413.pdf (Level II)

9 The Joint Commission. (2021). Standard NPSG.07.01.01. *Comprehensive accreditation manual for hospitals.* Oakbrook Terrace, IL: The Joint Commission. (Level VII)

10 Centers for Disease Control and Prevention. (2002). Guideline for hand hygiene in health-care settings: Recommendations of the Healthcare Infection Control Practices Advisory Committee and the HICPAC/SHEA/APIC/IDSA Hand Hygiene Task Force. *MMWR Recommendations and Reports, 51*(RR-16), 1–45. https://www.cdc.gov/mmwr/pdf/rr/rr5116.pdf (Level II)

11 World Health Organization. (2009). WHO guidelines on hand hygiene in health care: First global patient safety challenge, clean care is safer care. https://apps.who.int/iris/bitstream/handle/10665/44102/9789241597906_eng.pdf?sequence=1 (Level IV)

12 Accreditation Association for Hospitals and Health Systems. (2020). Standard 07.01.21. *Healthcare Facilities Accreditation Program: Accreditation requirements for acute care hospitals.* Chicago, IL: Accreditation Association for Hospitals and Health Systems. (Level VII)

13 Centers for Medicare and Medicaid Services, Department of Health and Human Services. (2020). Condition of participation: Infection control. 42 C.F.R. § 482.42.

14 DNV GL-Healthcare USA, Inc. (2020). IC.1.SR.1. *NIAHO® accreditation requirements, interpretive guidelines and surveyor guidance – revision 20.0.* Milford, OH: DNV GL-Healthcare USA, Inc. (Level VII)

15 The Joint Commission. (2021). Standard NPSG.01.01.01. *Comprehensive accreditation manual for hospitals.* Oakbrook Terrace, IL: The Joint Commission. (Level VII)

16 DNV GL-Healthcare USA, Inc. (2020). PR.2.SR.5. *NIAHO® accreditation requirements, interpretive guidelines and surveyor guidance – revision 20.0.* Milford, OH: DNV GL-Healthcare USA, Inc. (Level VII)

17 Centers for Medicare and Medicaid Services, Department of Health and Human Services. (2020). Condition of participation: Patient's rights. 42 C.F.R. § 482.13(c)(1).

18 Accreditation Association for Hospitals and Health Systems. (2020). Standard 15.01.16. *Healthcare Facilities Accreditation Program: Accreditation requirements for acute care hospitals.* Chicago, IL: Accreditation Association for Hospitals and Health Systems. (Level VII)

19 The Joint Commission. (2021). Standard RI.01.01.01. *Comprehensive accreditation manual for hospitals.* Oakbrook Terrace, IL: The Joint Commission. (Level VII)

20 The Joint Commission. (2021). Standard PC.02.01.21. *Comprehensive accreditation manual for hospitals.* Oakbrook Terrace, IL: The Joint Commission. (Level VII)

21 Accreditation Association for Hospitals and Health Systems. (2020). Standard 07.01.10. *Healthcare Facilities Accreditation Program: Accreditation requirements for acute care hospitals.* Chicago, IL: Accreditation Association for Hospitals and Health Systems. (Level VII)

22 Siegel, J. D., et al. (2007, revised 2019). 2007 guideline for isolation precautions: Preventing transmission of infectious agents in healthcare settings. https://www.cdc.gov/infectioncontrol/pdf/guidelines/isolation-guidelines-H.pdf (Level II)

23 Occupational Safety and Health Administration. (2012). Bloodborne pathogens, standard number 1910.1030. (Level VII)

24 The Joint Commission. (2021). Standard NPSG.02.03.01. *Comprehensive accreditation manual for hospitals*. Oakbrook Terrace, IL: The Joint Commission.

25 The Joint Commission. (2021). Standard RC.01.03.01. *Comprehensive accreditation manual for hospitals*. Oakbrook Terrace, IL: The Joint Commission. (Level VII)

26 Accreditation Association for Hospitals and Health Systems. (2020). Standard 10.00.03. *Healthcare Facilities Accreditation Program: Accreditation requirements for acute care hospitals*. Chicago, IL: Accreditation Association for Hospitals and Health Systems. (Level VII)

27 Centers for Medicare and Medicaid Services, Department of Health and Human Services. (2020). Condition of participation: Medical record services. 42 C.F.R. § 482.24(b).

28 DNV GL-Healthcare USA, Inc. (2020). MR.2.SR.1. *NIAHO® accreditation requirements, interpretive guidelines and surveyor guidance – revision 20.0*. Milford, OH: DNV GL-Healthcare USA, Inc. (Level VII)

URINE SPECIMEN COLLECTION

A *random urine specimen* is usually collected as part of the physical examination or at various times during hospitalization. A random urine specimen may be used when a sterile specimen is not required.[1] This specimen permits laboratory screening for urinary and systemic disorders; it's also used for drug screening. For a random collection, a first-void morning specimen should be used, if possible.[2]

A clean-catch urine specimen collection, also called the *clean-catch midstream urine specimen collection*, is a method performed to detect bladder bacteriuria.[3,4] Because urine is most concentrated on the first void in the morning, a clean-catch midstream urine specimen should be collected on the first void of the day, if possible.[3] The optimal clean-catch urine sample is collected after cleaning the urinary meatus to decrease the likelihood of contamination of the specimen with bacteria from the urethra. However, clinical studies do not show that cleaning the urinary meatus is associated with lower rates of contamination.[3,4]

An *indwelling urinary catheter specimen*—obtained by aspiration with a syringe—requires maintaining a closed urinary drainage system and using sterile collection technique to prevent catheter-associated urinary tract infections.[4,5,6]

Collection of a urine specimen from a urostomy, an ileal conduit, or a colon conduit may be necessary to confirm a suspected urinary tract infection. Collection of a urine specimen through these devices can occur by sterile catheterization or by collecting urine into a specimen collection container as it flows from the stoma using the clean-catch method. To avoid specimen contamination, collection of a urine specimen for culture should never occur directly from an ostomy pouch or a bedside drainage bag. Improper specimen collection can lead to inaccurate culture results, causing inappropriate diagnosis and treatment.[7]

Urine specimens for culture should be processed as soon as possible, preferably within 2 hours. If urine specimens can't be processed within 30 minutes of collection, they should be refrigerated. Refrigerated specimens should be cultured within 24 hours.[8] If adhering to this guideline isn't possible, a culture tube that contains preservative should be used to prevent bacterial growth.[9]

Equipment
For a random specimen
Bedpan, bedside commode, urinal with cover, or specimen collection hat ■ gloves ■ specimen container with lid ■ label ■ laboratory biohazard transport bag ■ soap ■ water ■ washcloth ■ Optional: graduated container, perineal care supplies, ice, laboratory request form, gown, mask and goggles or mask with face shield.

For a clean-catch midstream specimen
Gloves ■ cleansing towelettes ■ sterile specimen container with lid ■ label ■ laboratory biohazard transport bag ■ Optional: laboratory request form, graduated container, specimen collection hat (if using a bathroom toilet), bedside commode, illustrations, ice, preservative-filled urine specimen tube.

Commercial clean-catch kits are available that contain the necessary equipment.

For an indwelling catheter specimen
Gloves ■ antiseptic pad ■ syringe (3-mL to 30-mL, depending on the volume of urine required for the ordered test) or Luer-lock access device ■ sterile or nonsterile specimen container with lid (depending on the ordered test) or urine collection tube (with preservative) ■ label ■ laboratory biohazard transport bag ■ Optional: ice, laboratory request form.

For a specimen from a urostomy, ileal conduit, or colon conduit
Gloves ■ sterile gloves ■ cleaning solution (chlorhexidine, povidone-iodine, or soap and water)[5,7] ■ sterile 4" × 4" (10-cm × 10-cm) gauze pads ■ straight catheter (#16 French catheter is preferred for mucus drainage)[7] ■ sterile water-soluble lubricant ■ sterile specimen container with lid ■ label ■ laboratory biohazard transport bag ■ washcloth or soft paper towels ■ towel or absorbent pad ■ Optional: other personal protective equipment, laboratory request form, pouching system, towel, nonsterile gauze pads.

Preparation of equipment
Inspect all equipment and supplies. If a product is expired, is defective, or has compromised integrity, remove it from patient use, label it as expired or defective, and report the expiration or defect as directed by your facility. Set up a sterile field, and then open and place sterile items on the field, as necessary.

Implementation
■ Gather and prepare the necessary equipment and supplies.
■ Verify the practitioner's order for the urine specimen.
■ Perform hand hygiene.[10,11,12,13,14,15]
■ Confirm the patient's identity using at least two patient identifiers.[16]
■ Provide privacy.[17,18,19,20]
■ Explain the procedure and its purpose to the patient and family (if appropriate) according to their individual communication and learning needs *to increase their understanding, allay their fears, and enhance cooperation.*[21]

Collecting a random specimen
■ Instruct the patient on bed rest to void into a clean bedpan or urinal; instruct the ambulatory patient to void into a clean bedpan or urinal or into a specimen collection hat placed in the bedside commode or in the toilet in the bathroom. The urine specimen shouldn't be contaminated with feces or toilet paper. Note on the specimen if the patient is menstruating.[1]
■ Perform hand hygiene.[10,11,12,13,14,15]
■ Put on gloves and, as needed, other personal protective equipment *to comply with standard precautions.*[22,23,24] Then pour 30 to 60 mL of urine into the specimen container and place the lid on the container securely.
■ If the patient's urine output must be measured and recorded, pour the remaining urine into the graduated container. Otherwise, discard the remaining urine. If you inadvertently spill urine on the outside of the container, clean and dry it *to prevent cross-contamination.*

Collecting a clean-catch midstream specimen, female
■ Instruct the patient perform hand hygiene, and then to sit far back on the bedside commode or facing the back of the toilet *to promote better positioning of the thighs,* with her legs spread apart.
■ If you're using a commercial clean-catch kit, open it.
■ Perform hand hygiene.[10,11,12,13,14,15]

- Put on gloves *to comply with standard precautions.*[22,23,24]
- Open the sterile specimen container and place the cap down with the sterile inside surface facing up. *To prevent contamination of the specimen,* avoid touching the inside of the container and lid, and instruct the patient to avoid touching them.[25]
- Instruct the patient to separate the folds of skin around the urinary opening.[25] Instruct her to clean the urinary opening and surrounding area from front to back using a towelette and then discard the towelette in a waste receptacle, and to repeat this step with a second towelette.[25] Assist the patient, as needed.
- Instruct the patient to straddle the bedside commode sitting as far back on the commode as possible, or face the back of the toilet *to allow labial spreading* and to keep her skin folds separated while voiding. Assist as needed.[4]
- Instruct the patient to begin voiding into the bedside commode or toilet, *because the first urine voided washes microorganisms and cellular debris out of the meatus.*[1,25] Then, without stopping the urine stream, the patient (or you, if assisting) should move the collection container into the stream, collecting 30 to 50 mL at the midstream portion of the voiding.[9]
- Tell the patient to move the container out of the continuing urine stream after she has collected the specimen, and to finish voiding into the bedside commode or toilet.
- Take the sterile container from the patient and cap it securely. Avoid touching the inside of the container and lid *to prevent contamination.* If the outside of the container is soiled, clean it and wipe it dry.
- If intake and output are being recorded, measure the remaining urine (from the first and last portions of the voiding) in a graduated container. Include the amount in the specimen container when recording the total amount voided.

Collecting a clean-catch midstream specimen, male
- If you're using a commercial clean-catch kit, open it.
- Perform hand hygiene.[10,11,12,13,14,15]
- Put on gloves *to comply with standard precautions.*[22,23,24]
- Open the sterile specimen container and place the cap down with the sterile inside surface facing up. Avoid touching the inside of the container and lid, and instruct the patient to avoid touching them *to prevent contamination of the specimen.*[25]
- Instruct the patient to perform hand hygiene, and then hold his penis with one hand and use the other hand to clean the end of the penis with a towelette, beginning with the urethral opening and working away from it. (The foreskin of an uncircumcised male must first be retracted). Instruct the patient to discard the towelette in a waste receptacle. Then instruct the patient to repeat using a second clean towelette.[25] Assist patient as needed.
- Instruct the patient to begin voiding into the bedside commode or toilet, *because the first urine washes microorganisms and cellular debris from the urethra.*[1] Then, without stopping the urine stream, the patient (or you, if assisting) should move the collection container into the stream, collecting 30 to 50 mL at the midstream portion of the voiding.[9]
- Tell the patient to move the container out of the stream after he has collected the specimen, and to finish voiding into the bedside commode or toilet.
- Take the sterile container from the patient and cap it securely. Avoid touching the inside of the container and lid *to prevent contamination.* If the outside of the container is soiled, clean it and wipe it dry.
- If intake and output are being recorded, measure the remaining urine (from the first and last portions of the voiding) in a graduated container. Include the amount in the specimen container when recording the total amount voided.

Collecting an indwelling catheter specimen
- Perform hand hygiene[10,11,12,13,14,15] and put on gloves *to comply with standard precautions.*[22,23,24]
- Drain urine from the drainage tube into the collection bag.
- Disinfect the sampling port with an antiseptic pad and allow it to dry.[5]
- If using a syringe, attach the syringe to the sampling port. When fresh urine appears in the tubing, aspirate the specimen into the syringe.

Remove the syringe from the sampling port. Slowly transfer the specimen to the appropriate container. Dispose of the syringe in an appropriate receptacle.[24]
- If using a Luer-lock access device, attach the device to the sampling port. When fresh urine appears in the tubing, grasp the access device securely and push the collection tube into the device. Allow the natural vacuum of the tube to draw the specimen into the tube until the vacuum no longer continues to draw, *which indicates complete filling.*[26] Remove the Luer-lock access device from the sampling port. Discard the Luer-lock access device in an appropriate receptacle.[24]

Collecting a specimen from a urostomy, ileal conduit, or colon conduit
- Put on gloves and, as needed, other personal protective equipment *to comply with standard precautions.*[22,23,24]
- Drape a towel or an absorbent pad under the stoma *to promote privacy and provide absorption, if needed.*[7]
- If the patient is using a one-piece pouch system, remove the pouch system. If the patient is using a two-piece pouch system, remove the pouch from the skin barrier flange or completely remove the pouch system.[7]
- Remove and discard your gloves.[22,23,24]
- Perform hand hygiene.[10,11,12,13,14,15]
- Put on sterile gloves.[22,23,24]
- Clean the stoma with cleaning solution using a circular motion from the stoma opening outward.[7]
- Blot the stoma using a sterile gauze pad.[7]
- If using a catheter, while maintaining the sterility of the catheter, place the open end of the catheter into the specimen container.[7] Lubricate the catheter with water-soluble lubricant *to facilitate insertion.*[7] Gently insert the catheter tip into the stoma, but be sure to insert it no more than 3" (7.5 cm). If you meet resistance, rotate the catheter until it slides into place; don't force it.[7] Hold the catheter in place until urine begins to flow; collect 5 to 10 mL of urine. Note that collecting a sufficient specimen may take 5 to 15 minutes.[7] After obtaining a sufficient urine specimen, remove the catheter.[7]

NURSING ALERT Don't insert a catheter to obtain a specimen when stents are present in a urinary stoma.[7]
- If using the clean-catch method, allow a few drops of urine to flow from the stoma onto a sterile gauze pad.[7] Maintaining the sterility of the specimen container, hold the container under the stoma and collect 5 to 10 mL of urine. Note that collecting a sufficient specimen may take 5 to 15 minutes.[7] After obtaining a sufficient specimen, remove the specimen container from under the stoma.[7]
- If stents are present in a urostomy stoma, clean the outside ends of the stents with cleaning solution.[7] Blot the stents with sterile gauze.[7] Allow a few drops of urine to flow from the stents onto a sterile gauze pad.[7] Maintaining the sterility of the specimen container, hold the container under the stents and collect 5 to 10 mL of urine. Note that collecting a sufficient specimen may take 5 to 15 minutes.[7] After obtaining a sufficient specimen, remove the specimen container from under the stents.[7]

Completing the procedure
- Label the specimen container in the presence of the patient *to prevent mislabeling.*[16]
- Place the specimen container in the laboratory biohazard transport bag with a laboratory request form (if required in your facility), and send it to the laboratory immediately, or refrigerate it if transport may be delayed.[2,24,27] *Delayed transport of the specimen at room temperature may alter test results.*
- Assist the patient with perineal care, as needed.
- Offer the patient a washcloth and soap and water to wash the hands.
- Clean the graduated container. Also clean the urinal, bedside commode, or bedpan and return it to its proper storage area.[28]
- Discard disposable items in appropriate receptacles.[24]
- Remove and discard your gloves, and other personal protective equipment if worn.[24]
- Perform hand hygiene.[10,11,12,13,14,15]
- Document the procedure.[29,30,31,32]

Special considerations

■ Contact the laboratory if specialized urine testing is ordered to determine whether there are unique instructions for storage or transport.[33]

■ Never store a urine specimen in a refrigerator that contains food or medication *to reduce the risk of contamination from potentially infectious material.*[24]

■ Collecting urine with a syringe increases the potential for contamination. Using a Luer-lock access device is the preferred method.[9]

■ If a large volume of urine is needed for special analyses (not culture), obtain the urine specimen directly from the indwelling urinary catheter drainage bag, not the sampling port.[2]

Complications

Contamination of the specimen (such as with stool) may alter results. Catheter-associated urinary tract infection may result from improper technique.[8] Improper specimen collection can cause inaccurate culture results, leading to inappropriate diagnosis and treatment. Trauma to the stoma can occur with specimen collection using a catheter.

Documentation

Record the date and time of specimen collection and when the specimen was transported to the laboratory. Specify the test as well as the appearance, odor, color, and any unusual characteristics of the specimen. If necessary, record the urine volume on the intake and output record. Document your preparation of the stoma for collection, the date and time of specimen collection, the volume of urine you collected, and the collection method you used. Document teaching provided to the patient and family (if applicable), their understanding of that teaching, and any need for follow-up teaching.

REFERENCES

1 Craven, R. F., et al. (2017). *Fundamentals of nursing: Human health and function.* (8th ed.). Philadelphia, PA: Wolters Kluwer.

2 Health Network Laboratories. (2021). Urinalysis with reflex microscopic. https://www.testmenu.com/healthnetworklaboratories/Tests/511443

3 Meyrier, A. (2021). Sampling and evaluation of voided urine in the diagnosis of urinary tract infection in adults. In: *UpToDate,* Calderwood, S. B. (Ed.).

4 Brusch, J. L., et al. (2020). What is the recommended method and procedure for urine specimen collection in evaluation for urinary tract infection (UTI)? https://www.medscape.com/answers/233101-3241/what-is-the-recommended-method-and-procedure-for-urine-specimen-collection-in-evaluation-for-urinary-tract-infection-uti

5 Healthcare Infection Control Practices Advisory Committee. (2010, revised 2019). Guideline for prevention of catheter-associated urinary tract infections 2009. https://www.cdc.gov/infectioncontrol/pdf/guidelines/cauti-guidelines-H.pdf (Level I)

6 The Joint Commission. (2021). Standard NPSG.07.06.01. *Comprehensive accreditation manual for hospitals.* Oakbrook Terrace, IL: The Joint Commission. (Level VII)

7 Wound, Ostomy and Continence Nurses Society (WOCN). (2018). *Catheterization of an ileal or colon conduit stoma: Best practice for clinicians.* Mount Laurel, NJ: WOCN. https://www.ostomy.org/wp-content/uploads/2018/11/Catheterization-of-Urinary-Stoma-2018.pdf (Level VII)

8 Association of Professionals in Infection Control and Epidemiology (APIC). (2014). APIC implementation guide: Guide to preventing catheter-associated urinary tract infections. https://apic.org/wp-content/uploads/2019/02/APIC_CAUTI_IG_FIN_REVD0815.pdf (Level IV)

9 Garcia, R., & Spitzer, E. D. (2017). Promoting appropriate urine culture management to improve health care outcomes and the accuracy of catheter-associated urinary tract infections. *American Journal of Infection Control, 45,* 1143–1153.

10 Centers for Disease Control and Prevention. (2002). Guideline for hand hygiene in health-care settings: Recommendations of the Healthcare Infection Control Practices Advisory Committee and the HICPAC/SHEA/APIC/IDSA Hand Hygiene Task Force. *MMWR Recommendations and Reports, 51*(RR-16), 1–45. https://www.cdc.gov/mmwr/pdf/rr/rr5116.pdf (Level II)

11 World Health Organization. (2009). WHO guidelines on hand hygiene in health care: First global patient safety challenge, clean care is safer care. https://apps.who.int/iris/bitstream/handle/10665/44102/9789241597906_eng.pdf?sequence=1 (Level IV)

12 The Joint Commission. (2021). Standard NPSG.07.01.01. *Comprehensive accreditation manual for hospitals.* Oakbrook Terrace, IL: The Joint Commission. (Level VII)

13 Accreditation Association for Hospitals and Health Systems. (2020). Standard 07.01.21. *Healthcare Facilities Accreditation Program: Accreditation requirements for acute care hospitals.* Chicago, IL: Accreditation Association for Hospitals and Health Systems. (Level VII)

14 Centers for Medicare and Medicaid Services, Department of Health and Human Services. (2020). Condition of participation: Infection control. 42 C.F.R. § 482.42.

15 DNV GL-Healthcare USA, Inc. (2020). IC.1.SR.1. *NIAHO® accreditation requirements, interpretive guidelines and surveyor guidance – revision 20.0.* Milford, OH: DNV GL-Healthcare USA, Inc. (Level VII)

16 The Joint Commission. (2021). Standard NPSG.01.01.01. *Comprehensive accreditation manual for hospitals.* Oakbrook Terrace, IL: The Joint Commission. (Level VII)

17 Accreditation Association for Hospitals and Health Systems. (2020). Standard 15.01.16. *Healthcare Facilities Accreditation Program: Accreditation requirements for acute care hospitals.* Chicago, IL: Accreditation Association for Hospitals and Health Systems. (Level VII)

18 Centers for Medicare and Medicaid Services, Department of Health and Human Services. (2020). Condition of participation: Patient's rights. 42 C.F.R. § 482.13(c)(1).

19 The Joint Commission. (2021). Standard RI.01.01.01. *Comprehensive accreditation manual for hospitals.* Oakbrook Terrace, IL: The Joint Commission. (Level VII)

20 DNV GL-Healthcare USA, Inc. (2020). PR.2.SR.5. *NIAHO® accreditation requirements, interpretive guidelines and surveyor guidance – revision 20.0.* Milford, OH: DNV GL-Healthcare USA, Inc. (Level VII)

21 The Joint Commission. (2021). Standard PC.02.01.21. *Comprehensive accreditation manual for hospitals.* Oakbrook Terrace, IL: The Joint Commission. (Level VII)

22 Siegel, J. D., et al. (2007, revised 2019). 2007 guideline for isolation precautions: Preventing transmission of infectious agents in healthcare settings. https://www.cdc.gov/infectioncontrol/pdf/guidelines/isolation-guidelines-H.pdf (Level II)

23 Accreditation Association for Hospitals and Health Systems. (2020). Standard 07.01.10. *Healthcare Facilities Accreditation Program: Accreditation requirements for acute care hospitals.* Chicago, IL: Accreditation Association for Hospitals and Health Systems. (Level VII)

24 Occupational Safety and Health Administration. (2012). Bloodborne pathogens, standard number 1910.1030. https://www.osha.gov/pls/oshaweb/owadisp.show_document?p_id=10051&p_table=STANDARDS (Level VII)

25 Becton, Dickinson and Company. (2004). Midstream clean catch urine procedure. http://legacy.bd.com/resource.aspx?IDX=11181

26 Becton, Dickinson and Company. (n.d.). BD Vacutainer complete urine collection kits. https://www.bd.com/en-us/offerings/capabilities/specimen-collection/urine-specimen-collection/bd-vacutainer-collection-and-transfer-products/bd-vacutainer-complete-urine-collection-kits

27 Skobe, C. (n.d.). The basics of specimen collection and handling of urine testing. https://www.bd.com/en-us/offerings/capabilities/specimen-collection/vacutainer-educational-services-and-materials/labnotes/labnotes-14-2-2004

28 Accreditation Association for Hospitals and Health Systems. (2020). Standard 07.02.03. *Healthcare Facilities Accreditation Program: Accreditation requirements for acute care hospitals.* Chicago, IL: Accreditation Association for Hospitals and Health Systems. (Level VII)

29 The Joint Commission. (2021). Standard RC.01.03.01. *Comprehensive accreditation manual for hospitals.* Oakbrook Terrace, IL: The Joint Commission. (Level VII)

30 Centers for Medicare and Medicaid Services, Department of Health and Human Services. (2020). Condition of participation: Medical record services. 42 C.F.R. § 482.24(b).

31 Accreditation Association for Hospitals and Health Systems. (2020). Standard 10.00.03. *Healthcare Facilities Accreditation Program: Accreditation requirements for acute care hospitals.* Chicago, IL: Accreditation Association for Hospitals and Health Systems. (Level VII)

32 DNV GL-Healthcare USA, Inc. (2020). MR.2.SR.1. *NIAHO® accreditation requirements, interpretive guidelines and surveyor guidance – revision 20.0.* Milford, OH: DNV GL-Healthcare USA, Inc. (Level VII)

33 Quest Diagnostics. (n.d.). Urine collection. https://www.questdiagnostics.com/healthcare-professionals/test-directory/specimen-handling/urine-collection

Urine straining, for calculi

Renal calculi, commonly called kidney stones, are abnormal clusters or crystals of mineral and acid salts that may develop in one or both kidneys. They can be excreted with urine or become lodged in the urinary tract, causing pain, hematuria, urine retention, renal colic, and possibly hydronephrosis.[1]

Ranging in size from microscopic to several centimeters, calculi form in the kidneys when mineral salts—principally calcium oxalate or calcium phosphate—collect around a nucleus of bacterial cells, blood clots, or other particles. Other substances involved in calculus formation include uric acid, struvite (magnesium ammonium phosphate), and cystine.[2] To prevent recurrence, the practitioner can order laboratory tests to determine the components of the calculi and use this information to help in planning therapy.[1]

Renal calculi result from many causes, including hypercalcemia (which may occur with hyperparathyroidism, excessive dietary intake of calcium, and prolonged immobility), abnormal urine pH levels, dehydration, hyperuricemia associated with gout, and some hereditary disorders. Most commonly, calculi form as a result of urine stasis stemming from dehydration (which concentrates urine), benign prostatic hyperplasia, neurologic disorders, or urethral strictures. Anatomic abnormalities, such as ureteropelvic junction obstruction or horseshoe kidney, may worsen calculi formation.[3]

Testing to determine the presence of calculi requires careful straining of all of the patient's urine through a gauze pad or fine-mesh sieve and, at times, quantitative laboratory analysis of questionable specimens. Such testing typically continues until the patient passes the calculi or until surgery, as ordered.

Equipment

Commercial strainer ■ graduated collection container ■ bedpan, urinal or specimen collection hat ■ gloves ■ three patient-care reminder signs stating STRAIN ALL URINE ■ specimen container ■ specimen label ■ biohazard laboratory transport bag ■ Optional: rubber band, 4" × 4" (10-cm × 10-cm) gauze pad, laboratory request form.

Implementation

- Verify the practitioner's order, if needed.
- Gather and prepare all necessary equipment and supplies.
- Perform hand hygiene.[4,5,6,7,8,9]
- Confirm the patient's identity using at least two patient identifiers.[10]
- Provide privacy.[11,12,13,14]
- Explain the procedure to the patient and family (if appropriate) according to their individual communication and learning needs *to increase their understanding, allay their fears, and enhance cooperation.*[15]
- Post patient-care reminder signs stating STRAIN ALL URINE over the patient's bed, in the bathroom, and on the graduated collection container.
- Tell the patient to notify you after each voiding.
- Leave the urinal or bedpan within the patient's reach, or ensure that a specimen collection hat is in place for an ambulatory patient.
- After the patient voids, perform hand hygiene.[4,5,6,7,8,9]
- Put on gloves *to comply with standard precautions.*[16,17,18]
- Secure a commercial strainer over the mouth of a graduated collection container. If a commercial strainer isn't available, unfold a 4" × 4" (10-cm × 10-cm) gauze pad, place it over the top of a graduated collection container, and secure it with a rubber band.
- Pour the specimen from the urinal, bedpan, or specimen collection hat into the graduated collection container. If the patient has an indwelling urinary catheter in place, strain all urine from the collection bag before discarding it.
- Examine the strainer (or gauze pad) for calculi. If you detect calculi, place them in a specimen container. If you aren't sure whether calculi are present, notify the practitioner and place the filtrate (the urine that has passed through the strainer) in a specimen container.
- Label the specimen in the presence of the patient *to help prevent mislabeling.*[10]
- Place the specimen in a biohazard laboratory transport bag and send it to the laboratory immediately with the appropriate laboratory request form, if needed.[18]

- If the strainer is intact, rinse it carefully for reuse.[19] If it has become damaged, discard it and replace it with a new strainer. If a gauze pad was used, replace it with a new gauze pad.[17,18]
- Remove and discard your gloves.[17,18]
- Perform hand hygiene.[4,5,6,7,8,9]
- Put on gloves.[17,18]
- Clean and disinfect other reusable equipment (such as the bedpan, urinal, or specimen collection hat and graduated collection container) according to the manufacturer's instructions *to prevent the spread of infection.*[19,20]
- Remove and discard your gloves.[17,18]
- Perform hand hygiene.[4,5,6,7,8,9]
- Document the procedure.[21,22,23,24]

Special considerations

- Don't leave calculi in contact with urine or other fluids, *because this contact may alter the results of the analysis.*[25]
- Be aware that calculi may appear in various colors, each of which has diagnostic value.[26]

Documentation

Document the date and time of specimen collection as well as specimen transport to the laboratory. Note the characteristics of the urine and describe any calculi passed, including the size and number of calculi. Also note pain or hematuria that occurred during voiding. Document teaching provided to the patient and family (if applicable), their understanding of that teaching, and any need for follow-up teaching.

REFERENCES

1 Curhan, G. C., et al. (2021). Kidney stones in adults: Diagnosis and acute management of suspected nephrolithiasis. In: *UpToDate*, Goldfarb, S., & O'Leary, M. P. (Eds.).

2 Alelign, T., & Petros, B. (2018). Kidney stone disease: An update on current concepts. *Advances in Urology*, 2018, 3068365. https://www.hindawi.com/journals/au/2018/3068365/ (Level V)

3 Cunningham, P., et al. (2016). Kidney stones: Pathophysiology, diagnosis and management. *British Journal of Nursing, 25,* 1112–1116.

4 Centers for Disease Control and Prevention. (2002). Guideline for hand hygiene in health-care settings: Recommendations of the Healthcare Infection Control Practices Advisory Committee and the HICPAC/SHEA/APIC/IDSA Hand Hygiene Task Force. *MMWR Recommendations and Reports, 51*(RR-16), 1–45. https://www.cdc.gov/mmwr/pdf/rr/rr5116.pdf (Level II)

5 The Joint Commission. (2021). Standard NPSG.07.01.01. *Comprehensive accreditation manual for hospitals.* Oakbrook Terrace, IL: The Joint Commission. (Level VII)

6 World Health Organization. (2009). WHO guidelines on hand hygiene in health care: First global patient safety challenge, clean care is safer care. https://apps.who.int/iris/bitstream/handle/10665/44102/9789241597906_eng.pdf?sequence=1 (Level IV)

7 Accreditation Association for Hospitals and Health Systems. (2020). Standard 07.01.21. *Healthcare Facilities Accreditation Program: Accreditation requirements for acute care hospitals.* Chicago, IL: Accreditation Association for Hospitals and Health Systems. (Level VII)

8 Centers for Medicare and Medicaid Services, Department of Health and Human Services. (2020). Condition of participation: Infection control. 42 C.F.R. § 482.42.

9 DNV GL-Healthcare USA, Inc. (2020). IC.1.SR.1. *NIAHO® accreditation requirements, interpretive guidelines and surveyor guidance – revision 20.0.* Milford, OH: DNV GL-Healthcare USA, Inc. (Level VII)

10 The Joint Commission. (2021). Standard NPSG.01.01.01. *Comprehensive accreditation manual for hospitals.* Oakbrook Terrace, IL: The Joint Commission. (Level VII)

11 DNV GL-Healthcare USA, Inc. (2020). PR.2.SR.5. *NIAHO® accreditation requirements, interpretive guidelines and surveyor guidance – revision 20.0.* Milford, OH: DNV GL-Healthcare USA, Inc. (Level VII)

12 Centers for Medicare and Medicaid Services, Department of Health and Human Services. (2020). Condition of participation: Patient's rights. 42 C.F.R. § 482.13(c)(1).

13 Accreditation Association for Hospitals and Health Systems. (2020). Standard 15.01.16. *Healthcare Facilities Accreditation Program: Accreditation requirements for acute care hospitals.* Chicago, IL: Accreditation Association for Hospitals and Health Systems. (Level VII)

14 The Joint Commission. (2021). Standard RI.01.01.01. *Comprehensive accreditation manual for hospitals.* Oakbrook Terrace, IL: The Joint Commission. (Level VII)

15 The Joint Commission. (2021). Standard PC.02.01.21. *Comprehensive accreditation manual for hospitals.* Oakbrook Terrace, IL: The Joint Commission. (Level VII)

16 Accreditation Association for Hospitals and Health Systems. (2020). Standard 07.01.10. *Healthcare Facilities Accreditation Program: Accreditation requirements for acute care hospitals.* Chicago, IL: Accreditation Association for Hospitals and Health Systems. (Level VII)

17 Siegel, J. D., et al. (2007, revised 2019). 2007 guideline for isolation precautions: Preventing transmission of infectious agents in healthcare settings. https://www.cdc.gov/infectioncontrol/pdf/guidelines/isolation-guidelines-H.pdf (Level II)

18 Occupational Safety and Health Administration. (2012). Bloodborne pathogens, standard number 1910.1030. https://www.osha.gov/pls/oshaweb/owadisp.show_document?p_id=10051&p_table=STANDARDS (Level VII)

19 Accreditation Association for Hospitals and Health Systems. (2020). Standard 07.02.03. *Healthcare Facilities Accreditation Program: Accreditation requirements for acute care hospitals.* Chicago, IL: Accreditation Association for Hospitals and Health Systems. (Level VII)

20 Rutala, W. A., et al. (2008, revised 2019). Guideline for disinfection and sterilization in healthcare facilities, 2008. https://www.cdc.gov/infection-control/pdf/guidelines/disinfection-guidelines-H.pdf (Level I)

21 The Joint Commission. (2021). Standard RC.01.03.01. *Comprehensive accreditation manual for hospitals.* Oakbrook Terrace, IL: The Joint Commission. (Level VII)

22 Accreditation Association for Hospitals and Health Systems. (2020). Standard 10.00.03. *Healthcare Facilities Accreditation Program: Accreditation requirements for acute care hospitals.* Chicago, IL: Accreditation Association for Hospitals and Health Systems. (Level VII)

23 Centers for Medicare and Medicaid Services, Department of Health and Human Services. (2020). Condition of participation: Medical record services. 42 C.F.R. § 482.24(b).

24 DNV GL-Healthcare USA, Inc. (2020). MR.2.SR.1. *NIAHO® accreditation requirements, interpretive guidelines and surveyor guidance – revision 20.0.* Milford, OH: DNV GL-Healthcare USA, Inc. (Level VII)

25 Mayo Foundation for Medical Education and Research. (2018). Patient collection instructions for kidney stones. https://www.mayocliniclabs.com/it-mmfiles/StoneCollect0809.pdf

26 Fischbach, F., & Fischbach, M. A. (2022). *A manual of laboratory and diagnostic tests* (11th ed.). Philadelphia, PA: Wolters Kluwer.

VAGINAL MEDICATION ADMINISTRATION

Vaginal medications include creams, gels, ointments, and suppositories. The medications may be contraceptives, topical treatments for inflammation or infection (caused by bacterial vaginosis or *Candida*), lubricants, moisturizers, or hormone replacement therapy for menopausal women.[1,2]

Vaginal suppositories can also be used as a method to introduce probiotics to restore vaginal flora.[2] Low-dose vaginal estrogen by vaginal suppository is an effective treatment for symptoms of vaginal atrophy not responsive to nonhormonal intervention.[3] Progesterone administered vaginally has also been effective in decreasing the risk of preterm birth and improving perinatal outcomes.[4] Suppositories melt when they come into contact with the vaginal mucosa, allowing the medication to diffuse topically as effectively as creams, gels, and ointments.

Vaginal medications usually come with a disposable applicator that enables placement of medication in the anterior and posterior fornices. Administration is most effective when the patient can remain lying down afterward to retain the medication.

Equipment

Medication administration record ■ prescribed medication ■ applicator ■ water-soluble lubricant ■ gloves ■ small sanitary pad ■ fluid-impermeable pad ■ washcloth and warm water ■ towel ■ Optional: label.

Implementation

■ Avoid distractions and interruptions when preparing and administering medications *to prevent medication administration errors.*[5,6]
■ Verify the practitioner's order.[7,8,9,10]
■ Reconcile the patient's medications when the practitioner orders a new medication *to reduce the risk of medication errors, including omissions, duplications, dosing errors, and drug interactions.*[11]
■ Gather and prepare the necessary equipment and supplies.
■ Compare the medication label with the order in the patient's medical record.[7,8,9,10]
■ Check the patient's medical record for an allergy or a contraindication to the prescribed medication. If an allergy or a contraindication exists, don't administer the medication; notify the practitioner.[7,8,9,10]
■ Check the expiration date on the medication. If the medication is expired, return it to the pharmacy and obtain new medication.[7,8,9,10]
■ Visually inspect the medication for signs of loss of integrity; if its integrity is compromised, return it to the pharmacy.[7,8,9,10]
■ Discuss any unresolved concerns about the medication with the patient's practitioner.[7,8,9,10]
■ Perform hand hygiene.[12,13,14,15,16,17]
■ Confirm the patient's identity using at least two patient identifiers.[7,18]
■ Provide privacy.[19,20,21,22]
■ Explain the procedure to the patient and family (if appropriate) according to their individual communication and learning needs *to increase their understanding, allay their fears, and enhance cooperation.*[23]
■ If the patient is receiving the medication for the first time, teach the patient and family (if appropriate) about potential adverse effects, and discuss any other concerns related to the medication.[7,8,9,10]
■ Verify that the medication is being administered to the correct patient, at the proper time, in the prescribed dose, and by the correct route, and that its indication is appropriate for the patient's condition, *to prevent medication administration errors.*[7,8,9,10]
■ Ask the patient to void.
■ If your facility uses a bar code technology, use it as directed by your facility.
■ Ask whether the patient would prefer to insert the medication. If so, provide appropriate instructions.
■ If you're inserting the medication, proceed with the following steps.
■ If applicable, raise the patient's bed to waist level before providing patient care to prevent caregiver back strain.[24]
■ Perform hand hygiene.[12,13,14,15,16,17]
■ Put on gloves *to comply with standard precautions.*[25,26]
■ Help the patient into the lithotomy position or the supine position with the knees bent, and expose the perineum.
■ Place a fluid-impermeable pad underneath the patient.
■ Wash the vaginal orifice using a washcloth and warm water. Dry the area with a towel, wiping from front to back

Administration of vaginal creams, gels, and ointments

■ Insert the plunger into the applicator. Then attach the applicator to the tube of medication.
■ Gently squeeze the tube to fill the applicator with the prescribed amount of medication. Detach the applicator from the tube, and lubricate the applicator or apply a small amount of ointment to the outside of the applicator.
■ Expose the vagina by spreading the labia with your fingers.
■ Insert the applicator following the manufacturer's instructions.
■ Administer the medication by depressing the plunger on the applicator.
■ Remove the applicator.
■ Provide the patient with a sanitary pad *to prevent the medication from soiling the patient's clothing and bedding.*
■ Cover the patient *to promote dignity and comfort.*
■ Remove and discard your gloves[25,26] and perform hand hygiene.[12,13,14,15,16,17]
■ Help the patient into a comfortable position and advise the patient to remain recumbent in bed as much as possible for the next several hours.
■ If applicable, return the bed to the lowest position *to prevent falls and maintain patient safety.*[27]
■ Perform hand hygiene.[12,13,14,15,16,17]

- Put on gloves[25,26]
- If the applicator can be used again, wash it with soap and warm water, label it, and store it. If the applicator is disposable, discard it in the appropriate receptacle.

Administration of a vaginal suppository
- Remove the suppository from the wrapper and lubricate it with water-soluble lubricant.
- Expose the vagina by spreading the labia with your fingers.
- With an applicator or the forefinger of your free hand, insert the suppository about 2″ (5 cm) into the vagina.

Completing the procedure
- Remove and discard your gloves.[25,26]
- Perform hand hygiene.[12,13,14,15,16,17]
- *To prevent the medication from soiling the patient's clothing and bedding,* provide a sanitary pad.
- Document the procedure.[28,29,30,31]

Special considerations
- If possible, plan to insert vaginal medications at bedtime, *when the patient is most likely to be recumbent for several hours after administration.*
- Refrigerate vaginal suppositories that melt at room temperature.

Patient teaching
If the patient will have to administer the medication after discharge, teach the patient how to insert it, and provide a patient teaching aid if available. Instruct the patient not to wear a tampon after inserting vaginal medication, *because it would absorb the medication and decrease its effectiveness.* Also instruct the patient to avoid sexual intercourse during treatment unless the product is prescribed for lubrication or moisturizing. The patient should not douche during treatment. Instruct the patient to monitor the response to the medication and to inform the practitioner of unusual discharges, bleeding, pain, fever, or other adverse effects.

Complications
Vaginal medications may cause local irritation. Medications contained in the ointment, cream, or gel may have local and systemic adverse effects.

Documentation
Record the name and dose of the medication administered as well as the date and time of administration. Note any adverse reactions that occur, the name of the practitioner you notified of those adverse reactions, the date and time of notification, prescribed interventions, and the patient's response to those interventions. Document the patient's response to and tolerance of the treatment. Also document teaching provided to the patient and family (if applicable), their understanding of that teaching, and any need for follow-up teaching.

REFERENCES

1 North American Menopause Society (NAMS). (2018). MenoNote: Vaginal dryness. http://www.menopause.org/docs/default-source/for-women/mn-vaginal-dryness.pdf

2 Recine, N., et al. (2015). Restoring vaginal microbiota: Biological control of bacterial vaginosis. A prospective case-control study using *Lactobacillus rhamnosus* BMX 54 as adjuvant treatment against bacterial vaginosis. *Archives of Gynecology and Obstetrics, 293*(1), 101–107. https://www.researchgate.net/publication/279754341_Restoring_vaginal_microbiota_biological_control_of_bacterial_vaginosis_A_prospective_case-control_study_using_Lactobacillus_rhamnosus_BMX_54_as_adjuvant_treatment_against_bacterial_vaginosis (Level IV)

3 Bachmann, G., & Santen, R. J. (2021). Genitourinary syndrome of menopause (vulvovaginal atrophy): Treatment. In *UpToDate*, Barbieri, R. L., & Burstein, H. J. (Eds.).

4 Romero, R., et al. (2018). Vaginal progesterone for preventing preterm birth and adverse perinatal outcomes in singleton gestations with a short cervix: A meta-analysis of individual patient data. *American Journal of Obstetrics & Gynecology, 218*(2), 161–180. https://www.ncbi.nlm.nih.gov/pmc/articles/PMC5987201/ (Level I)

5 Westbrook, J., et al. (2010). Association of interruptions with an increased risk and severity of medication administration errors. *Archives of Internal Medicine, 170*, 683–690. (Level IV)

6 Institute for Safe Medication Practices. (2012). Side tracks on the safety express: Interruptions lead to errors and unfinished…Wait, what was I doing? *Nurse Advise-ERR, 11*(2), 1–4. https://www.ismp.org/resources/side-tracks-safety-express-interruptions-lead-errors-and-unfinished-wait-what-was-i-doing?id=37

7 Accreditation Association for Hospitals and Health Systems. (2020). Standard 16.01.03. *Healthcare Facilities Accreditation Program: Accreditation requirements for acute care hospitals.* Chicago, IL: Accreditation Association for Hospitals and Health Systems. (Level VII)

8 Centers for Medicare and Medicaid Services, Department of Health and Human Services. (2020). Condition of participation: Nursing services. 42 C.F.R. § 482.23(c).

9 DNV GL-Healthcare USA, Inc. (2020). MM.1.SR.3. *NIAHO® accreditation requirements: Interpretive guidelines and surveyor guidance—revision 20.0.* Milford, OH: DNV GL-Healthcare USA, Inc. (Level VII)

10 The Joint Commission. (2021). Standard MM.06.01.01. *Comprehensive accreditation manual for hospitals.* Oakbrook Terrace, IL: The Joint Commission. (Level VII)

11 Accreditation Association for Hospitals and Health Systems. (2020). Standard 25.02.13. *Healthcare Facilities Accreditation Program: Accreditation requirements for acute care hospitals.* Chicago, IL: Accreditation Association for Hospitals and Health Systems. (Level VII)

12 The Joint Commission. (2021). Standard NPSG.07.01.01. *Comprehensive accreditation manual for hospitals.* Oakbrook Terrace, IL: The Joint Commission. (Level VII)

13 Centers for Disease Control and Prevention. (2002). Guideline for hand hygiene in health-care settings: Recommendations of the Healthcare Infection Control Practices Advisory Committee and the HICPAC/SHEA/APIC/IDSA Hand Hygiene Task Force. *MMWR Recommendations and Reports, 51*(RR-16), 1–45. https://www.cdc.gov/mmwr/pdf/rr/rr5116.pdf (Level II)

14 World Health Organization. (2009). WHO guidelines on hand hygiene in health care: First global patient safety challenge, clean care is safer care. https://apps.who.int/iris/bitstream/handle/10665/44102/9789241597906_cng.pdf?sequence=1 (Level IV)

15 Accreditation Association for Hospitals and Health Systems. (2020). Standard 07.01.21. *Healthcare Facilities Accreditation Program: Accreditation requirements for acute care hospitals.* Chicago, IL: Accreditation Association for Hospitals and Health Systems. (Level VII)

16 Centers for Medicare and Medicaid Services, Department of Health and Human Services. (2020). Condition of participation: Infection control. 42 C.F.R. § 482.42.

17 DNV GL-Healthcare USA, Inc. (2020). IC.1.SR.1. *NIAHO® accreditation requirements: Interpretive guidelines and surveyor guidance—revision 20.0.* Milford, OH: DNV GL-Healthcare USA, Inc. (Level VII)

18 The Joint Commission. (2021). Standard NPSG.01.01.01. *Comprehensive accreditation manual for hospitals.* Oakbrook Terrace, IL: The Joint Commission. (Level VII)

19 Accreditation Association for Hospitals and Health Systems. (2020). Standard 15.01.16. *Healthcare Facilities Accreditation Program: Accreditation requirements for acute care hospitals.* Chicago, IL: Accreditation Association for Hospitals and Health Systems. (Level VII)

20 Centers for Medicare and Medicaid Services, Department of Health and Human Services. (2020). Condition of participation: Patient's rights. 42 C.F.R. § 482.13(c)(1).

21 The Joint Commission. (2021). Standard RI.01.01.01. *Comprehensive accreditation manual for hospitals.* Oakbrook Terrace, IL: The Joint Commission. (Level VII)

22 DNV GL-Healthcare USA, Inc. (2020). PR.2.SR.5. *NIAHO® accreditation requirements: Interpretive guidelines and surveyor guidance—revision 20.0.* Milford, OH: DNV GL-Healthcare USA, Inc. (Level VII)

23 The Joint Commission. (2021). Standard PC.02.01.21. *Comprehensive accreditation manual for hospitals.* Oakbrook Terrace, IL: The Joint Commission. (Level VII)

24 Waters, T. R., et al. (2009). Safe patient handling training for schools of nursing. https://www.cdc.gov/niosh/docs/2009-127/pdfs/2009-127.pdf (Level VII)

25 Siegel, J. D., et al. (2007, revised 2019). 2007 guideline for isolation precautions: Preventing transmission of infectious agents in healthcare

settings. https://www.cdc.gov/infectioncontrol/pdf/guidelines/isolation-guidelines-H.pdf (Level II)

26 Accreditation Association for Hospitals and Health Systems. (2020). Standard 07.01.10. *Healthcare Facilities Accreditation Program: Accreditation requirements for acute care hospitals.* Chicago, IL: Accreditation Association for Hospitals and Health Systems. (Level VII)

27 Ganz, D. A., et al. (2013). *Preventing falls in hospitals: A toolkit for improving quality of care* (AHRQ Publication No. 13-0015-EF). https://www.ahrq.gov/professionals/systems/hospital/fallpxtoolkit/index.html (Level VII)

28 The Joint Commission. (2021). Standard RC.01.03.01. *Comprehensive accreditation manual for hospitals.* Oakbrook Terrace, IL: The Joint Commission. (Level VII)

29 Accreditation Association for Hospitals and Health Systems. (2020). Standard 10.00.03. *Healthcare Facilities Accreditation Program: Accreditation requirements for acute care hospitals.* Chicago, IL: Accreditation Association for Hospitals and Health Systems. (Level VII)

30 Centers for Medicare and Medicaid Services, Department of Health and Human Services. (2020). Condition of participation: Medical record services. 42 C.F.R. § 482.24(b).

31 DNV GL-Healthcare USA, Inc. (2020). MR.2.SR.1. *NIAHO® accreditation requirements: Interpretive guidelines and surveyor guidance—revision 20.0.* Milford, OH: DNV GL-Healthcare USA, Inc. (Level VII)

VENIPUNCTURE

Venipuncture involves puncturing a vein with a needle or winged collection device to collect a venous blood sample in an evacuated tube or syringe.

Blood collected using a syringe should be transferred cautiously to the appropriate tubes using a needleless device *to prevent needlestick injury.* Depressing the syringe plunger during transfer can create positive pressure, displacing the stopper and potentially resulting in exposure to the patient's blood. Using a syringe may also result in overfilling or underfilling of tubes with blood, leading to inaccurate test results.[1]

When performing venipuncture for phlebotomy, use the extremity opposite an IV infusion. If you must perform venipuncture in the extremity with a vascular access device infusion, use a vein below the device or infusion. Avoid venipuncture on the side of the body where a patient has had lymphedema or has undergone radiation therapy or breast surgery with axillary node dissection. It also shouldn't be performed in an extremity where there is altered blood flow, such as an extremity that has been affected by stroke, injury, or deformity.[2,3,4] Restrict venipuncture to the hands in patients with actual or planned dialysis graft or fistula.[2]

The most commonly used veins for venipuncture for phlebotomy include the median cubital, the cephalic, and the basilic veins in the antecubital area. Only the volume of blood needed for accurate testing should be obtained, *because phlebotomy contributes to iron deficiency and blood loss in critically ill patients, making the patient susceptible to other complications.* Measures to conserve the patient's blood include using low-volume blood collection tubes when possible, recording the volume of blood obtained for laboratory testing, avoiding routine testing, consolidating daily tests into one blood draw, and using point-of-care testing methods when possible.[2,3,4]

Although phlebotomy personnel commonly perform this procedure in health care facilities, nurses and other trained personnel may also perform venipuncture. *To reduce the risk of culture contamination,* a dedicated phlebotomy team is recommended for obtaining blood cultures.[2]

Before performing venipuncture, assess the patient for possible risks factors, such as anticoagulant therapy, low platelet count, bleeding disorders, and other abnormalities that increase the risk of bleeding and hematoma formation.

Equipment

Gloves ▪ syringe or needle holder (Vacutainer) ▪ antiseptic agent (alcohol-based chlorhexidine preferred; if contraindicated, use an iodophor such as povidone-iodine or 70% alcohol) ▪ evacuated blood collection tubes ▪ venipuncture needle (21G to 23G) or winged collection device (21G, 23G, or 25G) ▪ single-patient-use tourniquet ▪ labels ▪ laboratory transport bag ▪ 2″ × 2″ (5-cm × 5-cm) gauze pads ▪ adhesive bandage

▪ Optional: needleless device, ice or cold pack, tape, laboratory request form, sterile gloves, gown, mask with face shield or mask and goggles.

Preparation of equipment

If you're using evacuated tubes, open the needle packet or winged collection device and attach the needle or winged device to the needle holder. If you're using a syringe, attach the appropriate needle to it. Be sure to choose a syringe large enough to hold all the blood required for the test. Gather the appropriate collection tubes for the ordered laboratory tests. (See *Collection tube guide.*) Check the expiration date on the blood collection tubes; obtain a new tube if any are expired. Inspect the collection tube additives; don't use the collection tubes if additives are discolored. Gently tap collection tubes containing additives *to dislodge any material that may be adhering to the stopper.* Inspect the needle *to make sure its integrity is intact.*[1]

Implementation

▪ Verify the practitioner's order.
▪ Review the patient's medical record for allergies to antiseptic, adhesive, and latex (if used in your facility). Use an alternative product if necessary *to avoid adverse reactions.*[5] Also review the patient's medical record for factors that may affect peripheral vasculature, such as conditions that result in structural vessel changes, history of frequent venipuncture or lengthy infusion therapy, skin variations, skin alterations, patient age, obesity, or fluid volume deficit, *to determine the need for vascular visualization technology.*[6]
▪ Check the laboratory labels *to verify the patient and testing information.* If a requisition form is also needed by your facility, verify the information.
▪ Determine whether fasting requirements, dietary and medication restrictions, or scheduling and medical treatment considerations are associated with the ordered test. Note these factors on the laboratory request form, as applicable, *to ensure accuracy of the test results.*[7]
▪ Gather and prepare the appropriate equipment and supplies.
▪ Perform hand hygiene.[1,8,9,10,11,12,13,14,15]
▪ Confirm the patient's identity using at least two patient identifiers.[16]
▪ Provide privacy.[17,18,19,20]
▪ Explain the procedure to the patient and family (if appropriate) according to their individual communication and learning needs *to increase their understanding, allay their fears, and enhance cooperation.*[21]
▪ Ask whether the patient has ever felt faint, sweaty, or nauseated when having blood drawn, *to prepare to manage a vasovagal reaction in the patient at risk.*
▪ If fasting or other dietary restrictions were required for an ordered test, confirm that the patient has implemented these restrictions.[2]
▪ If the patient is in bed, raise the bed to waist level before performing patient care *to prevent caregiver back strain.*[22]
▪ Put on gloves and, if needed, other personal protective equipment *to comply with standard precautions.*[8,23,24]
▪ Ask the patient in bed to lie in the supine position, with the head slightly elevated and arms at the sides. Ask the ambulatory patient to sit in a chair and support the arm securely on an armrest or table.[1] Position the patient's arm horizontally or slanting downward.[1]

NURSING ALERT Don't collect a blood specimen while the patient is sitting upright on any surface without armrests or other barriers designed to prevent a fall.[1]

▪ Assess the patient's veins *to determine the best puncture site and needle size.* (See *Common venipuncture sites.*) The preferred venipuncture site is the antecubital fossa, *because a number of large veins lie relatively near the skin's surface.* When the antecubital veins aren't acceptable or unavailable, use veins on the back of the hand.[1] Limit 25G needles to situations in which veins are too fragile to use a larger-size needle; however, keep in mind that improper technique may cause hemolysis.
▪ Assess the patient for such factors as easy bruising, increased risk of bleeding, compromised circulation, and fragile veins or skin, *which indicate that you should either not apply a tourniquet or apply it loosely.*
▪ Apply a tourniquet about 2″(5 cm) above the intended venipuncture site *to accurately identify and prioritize the veins for use to minimize the potential for injury and complications.*[1] Make sure you can palpate an

EQUIPMENT

Collection tube guide

The table below shows the recommended order of draw for commonly used collection tubes, the stopper or closure color, the typical laboratory studies performed, and the number of tube inversions needed to mix the sample. Consult with laboratory personnel for information about less commonly ordered testing.[1,5]

ORDER OF DRAW	COLLECTION TUBE TYPE	STOPPER OR CLOSURE COLOR	COMMON LABORATORY USE	NUMBER OF INVERSIONS
1	Blood culture or other sterile test	▪ Blood culture bottles	▪ Blood culture (ideally, samples should be from two to three blood draws from separate venipuncture sites and not collected through a vascular catheter)[2]	8 to 10
2	Citrate	▪ Blue stopper (tube must be filled completely)	▪ Coagulation studies	3 to 4
3	Gel, serum	▪ Red and black stopper ▪ Gold closure	▪ Serum chemistry ▪ Routine blood donor screening	5
4	No gel, serum	▪ Red stopper or closure	▪ Serum chemistry ▪ Routine blood donor screening	5 (plastic) 0 (glass)
5	Heparin	▪ Green stopper or closure ▪ Green and gray stopper or light green closure	▪ Plasma chemistry	8 to 10
6	EDTA	▪ Lavender stopper or closure ▪ Pink stopper or closure	▪ Whole blood hematology ▪ Routine immunohematology and blood donor screening ▪ Cross-matching (pink stopper or closure; tube contains special label for required blood bank information)	8 to 10
7	Potassium EDTA	▪ White closure	▪ Molecular diagnostic testing	8 to 10
8	Sodium fluoride	▪ Gray stopper or closure	▪ Glucose testing	8 to 10

EDTA, ethylenediaminetetraacetic acid

Common venipuncture sites

The illustrations below show the anatomic locations of veins commonly used for venipuncture. The most commonly used veins include the median cubital, cephalic, and basilic veins in the antecubital area. You may also use veins in the hand if necessary. *Because of the risk of nerve, tendon, and arterial involvement,* don't use veins on the palmar surface of the wrist or the lateral wrist above the thumb to mid-forearm.[1]

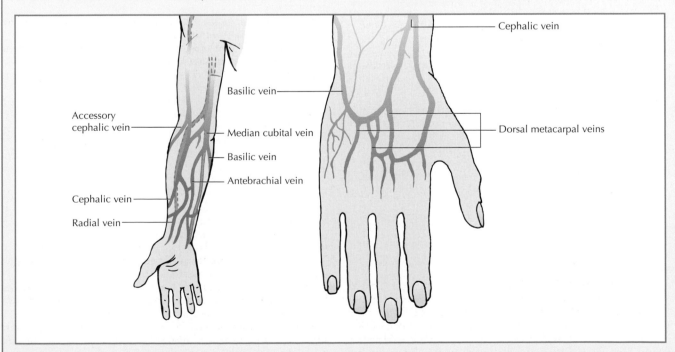

arterial pulse distal to the tourniquet *to prevent circulatory impairment. To prevent venous stasis and other causes of collection-related abnormal test results,* don't ask the patient to tightly clench or repetitively open and close the fist, and limit tourniquet application time to less than 1 minute.[2] If a tourniquet has been in place for more than 1 minute before accessing the vein, release it and reply after 2 minutes before performing the venipuncture.[1]

■ Prepare the venipuncture site using an antiseptic agent. (Alcohol-based chlorhexidine is preferred; if contraindicated, use an iodophor such as povidone-iodine or 70% alcohol.) Apply the agent using a single-use sterile applicator. Allow the agent to dry completely without fanning, wiping, or blowing on it.[25] Don't touch the intended venipuncture site after preparation; if you need to, put on sterile gloves *to prevent contamination.*[2,25] For alcohol-based chlorhexidine, apply with an applicator using a vigorous side-to-side motion for 30 seconds. Allow the area to dry completely.[25,26] For povidone-iodine solution, apply using a swab. Begin at the intended insertion site and move outward in concentric circles. Allow the solution to dry completely (typically at least 2 minutes).[25,27]

NURSING ALERT Don't use an alcohol-based antiseptic to clean the venipuncture site if you're collecting samples for blood alcohol testing *to avoid any question of cross-contamination.*[1]

■ Firmly hold the patient's arm distal to the intended venipuncture site. Immobilize the vein by pressing 1" to 2" (2.5 to 5 cm) below the venipuncture site with your thumb and drawing the skin taut.[1]

■ Position the needle holder or syringe with the needle bevel up and the shaft parallel to the path of the vein and at a 30-degree angle to the arm. If you're using a winged collection device attached to a needle holder, grasp the wings and position the bevel up.

■ Tell the patient that you're about to perform the venipuncture *to prepare the patient.*[1]

■ Insert the needle into the vein. If you're using a syringe, venous blood will appear in the hub; withdraw the blood slowly, pulling the plunger of the syringe gently *to create steady suction* until you obtain the required sample. *Pulling the plunger too forcibly may collapse the vein.* If you're using a needle holder and an evacuated tube, grasp the holder securely *to stabilize it in the vein,* and push down on the collection tube until the needle punctures the rubber stopper. Blood will flow into the tube automatically.[1]

■ For coagulation studies, don't discard the initial sample unless you're using a winged needle with an attached extension set, *because air in the extension set prevents the correct ratio of blood to anticoagulant additive in the tube.*[2]

■ Immediately release the tourniquet (if used) when blood begins to flow into the collection container.[2]

■ When the first tube has filled to its correct volume and blood flow ceases, remove it from the holder. Continue to fill the required tubes using the correct order of draw, removing one and inserting another. Gently invert each tube and then return it to an upright position as you remove it *to help mix the additive with the sample;*[1] this counts as one complete inversion for each tube.

■ After you've drawn the sample, place a gauze pad over the puncture site, and slowly and gently remove the needle from the vein. When you're using an evacuated tube, remove it from the needle holder *to release the vacuum* before withdrawing the needle from the vein.

■ Activate the needle protector safety device if necessary.[1]

■ Apply gentle pressure to the puncture site for as long as necessary until bleeding stops *to prevent extravasation into the surrounding tissue, which can cause a hematoma.*[1]

■ After bleeding stops, apply an adhesive bandage or tape a gauze bandage in place.[1]

■ If you've used a syringe, transfer the sample to a collection tube immediately using a needleless device. Be careful to avoid foaming, *which can cause hemolysis.*[1]

■ *To make sure that tube additives are properly mixed with the blood sample,* carefully invert each tube the appropriate number of times indicated by the tube's additive. Don't shake the collection tubes; *vigorous mixing may causing foaming and hemolysis.*[1]

■ Label all specimens in the presence of the patient *to help prevent mislabeling.*[16] At a minimum, the label should contain the patient's first and last name and identification number, the date and time of collection, and your initials or name, if required.[1,16] If you're obtaining a blood bank sample, sign the collection tube label if required by your facility.

■ Discard syringes and needles in a puncture-resistant sharps disposal container.[24,28]

■ Check the venipuncture site *to see if a hematoma has developed.* If it has, apply pressure until you're sure the bleeding has stopped.[1]

■ If the patient is in bed, return the bed to the lowest position *to prevent falls and maintain patient safety.*[29]

■ Remove and discard your gloves and any other personal protective equipment worn.[24]

■ Perform hand hygiene.[8,9,10,11,12,13,14,15]

■ Place the samples in a laboratory biohazard transport bag and send them immediately to the laboratory with the appropriate laboratory request forms (if necessary).[24]

■ Provide ice or a cold pack for transport, if required; *coagulation studies may require ice or a cold pack for transport.*

■ Document the procedure.[30,31,32,33]

Special considerations

■ Don't collect a venous sample from an infection site, *because pathogens may be introduced into the vascular system.*[1] Likewise, avoid drawing blood from edematous areas or sites of previous hematoma or vascular injury.[2]

■ Limit your attempts at venipuncture to two; after two attempts, notify a specially trained phlebotomist or the practitioner to obtain the sample.[1,7]

Complications

Potential complications of venipuncture include accidental arterial puncture, nerve injury, hematoma at the needle insertion site, and hemolysis of the sample. The patient may also experience dizziness, syncope, fainting, nausea, vomiting, and seizures.[1]

Documentation

Record the date, time, and site of venipuncture; name of the test; time you sent the sample to the laboratory; and amount of blood you collected. Note any adverse reactions and how the patient tolerated the procedure. Document teaching provided to the patient and family (if applicable), their understanding of that teaching, and any need for follow-up teaching.

REFERENCES

1 Clinical and Laboratory Standards Institute (CLSI). (2017). *CLSI Standard GP41: Collection of diagnostic venous blood specimens* (7th edition). Wayne, PA: CLSI. (Level VII)

2 Standard 44. Blood sampling. Infusion therapy standards of practice (8th ed.). (2021). *Journal of Infusion Nursing, 44*(Suppl. 1), S125–S133. (Level VII)

3 Infusion Nurses Society. (2016). *Policies and procedures for infusion therapy* (5th ed.). Boston, MA: Infusion Nurses Society.

4 Infusion Nurses Society. (2016). *Policies and procedures for infusion therapy of the older adult* (3rd ed.). Boston, MA: Infusion Nurses Society.

5 Standard 14. Latex sensitivity or allergy. Infusion therapy standards of practice (8th ed.). (2021). *Journal of Infusion Nursing, 44*(Suppl. 1), S49–S50. (Level VII)

6 Standard 22. Vascular visualization. Infusion therapy standards of practice (8th ed.). (2021). *Journal of Infusion Nursing, 44*(Suppl. 1), S63–S65. (Level VII)

7 Fischbach, F., & Fischbach, M. A. (2022). *A manual of laboratory and diagnostic tests* (11th ed.). Philadelphia, PA: Wolters Kluwer.

8 Accreditation Association for Hospitals and Health Systems. (2020). Standard 07.01.10. *Healthcare Facilities Accreditation Program: Accreditation requirements for acute care hospitals.* Chicago, IL: Accreditation Association for Hospitals and Health Systems. (Level VII)

9 The Joint Commission. (2021). Standard NPSG.07.01.01. *Comprehensive accreditation manual for hospitals.* Oakbrook Terrace, IL: The Joint Commission. (Level VII)

10 Centers for Disease Control and Prevention. (2002). Guideline for hand hygiene in health-care settings: Recommendations of the Healthcare Infection Control Practices Advisory Committee and the HICPAC/SHEA/APIC/IDSA Hand Hygiene Task Force. *MMWR Recommendations*

and Reports, *51*(RR-16), 1–45. https://www.cdc.gov/mmwr/pdf/rr/rr5116.pdf (Level II)

11 World Health Organization. (2009). *WHO guidelines on hand hygiene in health care: First global patient safety challenge, clean care is safer care.* https://apps.who.int/iris/bitstream/handle/10665/44102/9789241597906_eng.pdf?sequence=1 (Level IV)

12 Standard 16. Hand hygiene. Infusion therapy standards of practice (8th ed.). (2021). *Journal of Infusion Nursing, 44*(Suppl. 1), S53–S54. (Level VII)

13 Centers for Medicare and Medicaid Services, Department of Health and Human Services. (2020). Condition of participation: Infection control. 42 C.F.R. § 482.42.

14 Accreditation Association for Hospitals and Health Systems. (2020). Standard 07.01.21. *Healthcare Facilities Accreditation Program: Accreditation requirements for acute care hospitals.* Chicago, IL: Accreditation Association for Hospitals and Health Systems. (Level VII)

15 DNV GL-Healthcare USA, Inc. (2020). IC.1.SR.1. *NIAHO® accreditation requirements, interpretive guidelines and surveyor guidance—revision 20.0.* Milford, OH: DNV GL-Healthcare USA, Inc. (Level VII)

16 The Joint Commission. (2021). Standard NPSG.01.01.01. *Comprehensive accreditation manual for hospitals.* Oakbrook Terrace, IL: The Joint Commission. (Level VII)

17 DNV GL-Healthcare USA, Inc. (2020). PR.2.SR.5. *NIAHO® accreditation requirements, interpretive guidelines and surveyor guidance—revision 20.0.* Milford, OH: DNV GL-Healthcare USA, Inc. (Level VII)

18 Centers for Medicare and Medicaid Services, Department of Health and Human Services. (2020). Condition of participation: Patient's rights. 42 C.F.R. § 482.13(c)(1).

19 Accreditation Association for Hospitals and Health Systems. (2020). Standard 15.01.16. *Healthcare Facilities Accreditation Program: Accreditation requirements for acute care hospitals.* Chicago, IL: Accreditation Association for Hospitals and Health Systems. (Level VII)

20 The Joint Commission. (2021). Standard RI.01.01.01. *Comprehensive accreditation manual for hospitals.* Oakbrook Terrace, IL: The Joint Commission. (Level VII)

21 The Joint Commission. (2021). Standard PC.02.01.21. *Comprehensive accreditation manual for hospitals.* Oakbrook Terrace, IL: The Joint Commission. (Level VII)

22 Waters, T. R., et al. (2009). *Safe patient handling training for schools of nursing.* https://www.cdc.gov/niosh/docs/2009-127/pdfs/2009-127.pdf (Level VII)

23 Siegel, J. D., et al. (2007, revised 2019). 2007 guideline for isolation precautions: Preventing transmission of infectious agents in healthcare settings. https://www.cdc.gov/infectioncontrol/pdf/guidelines/isolation-guidelines-H.pdf (Level II)

24 Occupational Safety and Health Administration. (2012). Bloodborne pathogens, standard number 1910.1030. https://www.osha.gov/pls/oshaweb/owadisp.show_document?p_id=10051&p_table=STANDARDS (Level VII)

25 Standard 33. Vascular access site preparation and skin antisepsis. Infusion therapy standards of practice (8th ed.). (2021). *Journal of Infusion Nursing, 44*(Suppl. 1), S96. (Level VII)

26 CareFusion. (2015). ChloraPrep Single Swabstick/ChloraPrep Triple swabstick. CareFusion. https://go.bd.com/ChloraPrep-PurPrep-Portfolio.html?utm_source=google&utm_medium=cpc&utm_content=su-purprep-portf-google-ads-fy21&utm_campaign=7014W000001B0Ts&gclid=Cj0KCQjwg7KJBhDyARIsAHrAXaGkNuStaonLeNUxW8O8Uvb2A-9OnPm-LAbnGS9J0L4Jluu6MUQS6gAaAkiMEALw_wcB.

27 CareFusion. (n.d.). Scrub Care 10% povidone-iodine, paint. CareFusion. https://www.bd.com/documents/labels/IP_PVP-I-Topical-Solution-10-Percent-2-oz-29906-002_PL_EN.pdf.

28 Standard 21. Medical waste and sharps safety. Infusion therapy standards of practice (8th ed.). (2021). *Journal of Infusion Nursing, 44*(Suppl. 1), S60–S62. (Level VII)

29 Ganz, D. A., et al. (2013). *Preventing falls in hospitals: A toolkit for improving quality of care* (AHRQ Publication No. 13-0015-EF). Agency for Healthcare Research and Quality. https://www.ahrq.gov/professionals/systems/hospital/fallpxtoolkit/index.html (Level VII)

30 The Joint Commission. (2021). Standard RC.01.03.01. *Comprehensive accreditation manual for hospitals.* Oakbrook Terrace, IL: The Joint Commission. (Level VII)

31 Accreditation Association for Hospitals and Health Systems. (2020). Standard 10.00.03. *Healthcare Facilities Accreditation Program: Accreditation requirements for acute care hospitals.* Chicago, IL: Accreditation Association for Hospitals and Health Systems. (Level VII)

32 Centers for Medicare and Medicaid Services, Department of Health and Human Services. (2020). Condition of participation: Medical record services. 42 C.F.R. § 482.24(b).

33 DNV GL-Healthcare USA, Inc. (2020). MR.2.SR.1. *NIAHO® accreditation requirements, interpretive guidelines and surveyor guidance—revision 20.0.* Milford, OH: DNV GL-Healthcare USA, Inc. (Level VII)

VENTRICULAR ASSIST DEVICE CARE

A ventricular assist device (VAD) is implanted to provide support to a failing heart by assisting with the pumping function. VADs are designed to decrease the heart's workload and increase cardiac output in patients with ventricular failure. They're commonly used as a bridge to cardiac transplantation in patients who are at risk for death from refractory end-stage left ventricular heart failure, as a bridge to recovery from cardiogenic shock, or as destination therapy for patients who don't qualify for or desire cardiac transplantation.[1,2] Other indications for VAD therapy include an inability to be weaned from cardiopulmonary bypass and heart failure that doesn't respond to optimal medical therapy.[1,2] VADs are associated with improved secondary organ function, reduced pulmonary hypertension, and improved nutritional status. These benefits may also give time for improvement to patients who previously received a VAD as destination therapy so that they can become eligible for cardiac transplantation.[3,4]

Inserting a VAD involves a specific surgical procedure in which blood flow is diverted from a ventricle to an artificial pump. Commonly used devices include the HeartWare and HeartMate VADs. The HeartWare and HeartMate 3 VADs use a centrifugal blood pump that's implanted in the pericardial space with left ventricular apex to ascending aortic cannulation to provide left ventricular support.[5] The inflow conduit is integrated with the pump, and an outflow graft with a strain relief is attached to the pump. A percutaneous driveline connects the pump to an external controller, powered by batteries or electricity from an outlet. The monitor is used to display system performance and to change controller operating parameters.[1] The HeartMate II VAD, an axial-flow, rotary ventricular assist system, generates blood flow at a rate of up to 10 L/minute. One end of the VAD is attached to the apex of the left ventricle; the other end connects to the ascending aorta. The VAD diverts blood from the weakened left ventricle and propels it into the aorta. A small external computer monitors the system's operation. A drive line, which passes through the patient's abdomen, connects the implanted pump to the system controller. The system is powered by two lithium batteries or a power module that connects to an electrical outlet.[6]

VAD use is contraindicated in patients who are allergic to or can't tolerate anticoagulation therapy, as well as in pregnant patients (because of the need for anticoagulation). Because VADs have limited use in patients with artificial mitral or aortic valves, the risks are currently unknown.[1] Other relative contraindications include body surface area of less than 1.2 m², irreversible end-stage organ damage, unrepairable ventricular septal defect, comorbidities that limit life expectancy to less than 3 years, active neuropathy, active infection, diabetes-related retinopathy, poor glycemic control, severe neuropathy, peripheral neuropathy, active long-term institutionalized psychiatric illness, and conditions that limit the patient's ability to care for the device (such as neuromuscular disease, psychosocial or cognitive conditions, lack of a caregiver or increased caregiver burden, active substance abuser, or medical nonadherence).[2]

Equipment

VAD ▪ VAD batteries ▪ AC or DC adapter ▪ battery charger ▪ system monitor ▪ system controller ▪ mild antiseptic soap or cleaning agent (preferably chlorhexidine) ▪ sterile normal saline solution ▪ sterile gauze pad ▪ prescribed analgesics ▪ other prescribed medications ▪ vital signs monitoring equipment ▪ dressing supplies ▪ gloves ▪ sterile gloves ▪ mask ▪ cap ▪ stethoscope ▪ disinfectant pad ▪ prescribed IV fluid ▪ IV administration set ▪ electronic infusion device (preferably a smart pump with dose-error software and interoperability with electronic health records) ▪ suction equipment ▪ oral care supplies ▪ cardiac monitor ▪ hemodynamic monitoring equipment ■ emergency equipment (code cart with emergency medications, defibrillator, handheld resuscitation bag with mask, intubation equipment) ■ Optional: sterile gown, specialized clip, Montgomery strap, customized percutaneous lead immobilization binder or belt, gown, mask and goggles or mask with face shield, antiembolism stockings or sequential compression device, Doppler ultrasound device, ultrasound gel, 12-lead electrocardiograph (ECG) machine, IV dextran, arterial catheter monitoring supplies, scale.

Preparation of equipment

Inspect all equipment and supplies. If a product is expired, is defective, or has compromised integrity, remove it from patient use, label it as expired or defective, and report the expiration or defect as directed by your facility.

Make sure emergency equipment is functioning properly and readily available. Have a backup controller available and programmed identically to the primary controller *in case the primary controller fails or malfunctions; using a backup controller with settings different from the patient's current system may result in diminished support and patient harm.* Ensure that fully charged batteries are available at all times.[1]

Implementation

■ Review the patient's medical record for medical and surgical history, allergies, and current medications.
■ Verify the practitioner's orders.
■ Perform hand hygiene.[7,8,9,10,11,12]
■ Confirm the patient's identity using at least two patient identifiers.[13]
■ Provide privacy.[14,15,16,17]
■ Explain the procedure to the patient and family (if appropriate) according to their communication and learning needs *to increase their understanding, allay their fears, and enhance cooperation.*[18]
■ Provide emotional support to the patient and family.
■ Raise the patient's bed to waist level when providing patient care *to prevent caregiver back strain.*[19]
■ Perform hand hygiene.[7,8,9,10,11,12]
■ Put on gloves and, as needed, other personal protective equipment *to comply with standard precautions.*[20,21,22]
■ Receive hand-off communication from the person who was responsible for the patient's care. Ask questions as necessary *to avoid miscommunications that could lead to patient care errors during transitions of care.*[23,24,25] As part of the hand-off process, trace each tubing and catheter from the patient to its point of origin; use a standardized reconciliation process.[25]
■ Make sure that the VAD, controller, monitor, and power sources are set up according to the device manufacturer's instructions for use.
■ Attach the patient to a continuous cardiac monitor, and attach hemodynamic monitoring equipment to the monitor modules if present. Make sure that alarm limits are set appropriately for the patient's current condition, and that the alarms are turned on, functioning properly, and audible to staff members.[26,27]
■ Closely monitor the patient's vital signs at an interval determined by your facility and the patient's condition. Manually auscultate the patient's blood pressure *to ensure accurate results.* If you can't manually auscultate blood pressure, use a Doppler ultrasound device.[1] Blood pressure monitoring using an arterial catheter should be considered if blood flow is pulseless or hypotension precludes use of the manual or Doppler methods.[5,6] To measure blood pressure using a Doppler ultrasound device, place an appropriately sized blood pressure cuff around the patient's upper arm so that the end of the cuff is ¾" to 1" (2 to 2.5 cm) above the antecubital fossa. Align the cuff so that the mark on the cuff for "artery" is positioned over the artery.[28] Alternatively, place the cuff on the patient's forearm for radial artery measurement or the ankle for tibial artery measurement.[29] Apply ultrasound gel to the general location of the artery intended for blood pressure measurement.[29] Locate the vessel by turning on the Doppler ultrasound device and placing the probe over the area until you locate the audible blood flow.[29] Hold the probe still over the artery; don't press down too hard or you'll compress the vessel and be unable to hear blood flow.[29] Inflate the blood pressure cuff until the flow sounds disappear, and then add an additional 30 mm Hg.[29] Release the

bulb and slowly deflate the cuff while watching the pressure manometer.[29] Note the pressure at the point where flow returns to the artery, as indicated by continuous flow or a mildly pulsatile sound.[29] Document this pressure as XX/Doppler or XX/D (for example, 88/Doppler or 88/D); note the location where you measured the pressure.[29]
■ Monitor the patient's cardiovascular, respiratory, and neurologic status *to enable prompt recognition of changes in the patient's condition.* Assess the exit site, and monitor the mediastinal and chest tube sites and drainage.[6] Report immediately bleeding from the exit site, a sudden increase or cessation of chest or mediastinal tube drainage, and other associated complications.
■ Screen for and assess the patient's pain using facility-defined criteria that are consistent with the patient's age, condition, and ability to understand.[30]
■ Treat the patient's pain, as needed and ordered, using nonpharmacologic or pharmacologic approaches, or a combination. Base the treatment plan on evidence-based practices and the patient's clinical condition, past medical history, and pain management goals.[30] Administer analgesics, as needed and ordered, following safe medication administration practices.[31,32,33,34]
■ Monitor closely if the patient is at high risk for adverse outcomes related to opioid treatment, if prescribed.[30]
■ If the patient requires endotracheal intubation and mechanical ventilation during the immediate postoperative period, confirm the ventilator settings and keep the head of the bed elevated at least 30 degrees, if tolerated. Assess the patient's readiness for extubation; extubate the patient as soon as clinically indicated *to reduce the risk of ventilator-associated pneumonia.*[1]
■ Weigh the patient and record the weight in kilograms *to ensure accurate medication dosing.*[35]

For the patient with a HeartWare VAD

■ Confirm the controller settings on the monitor, including the pump speed, hematocrit setting, VAD identification, pump serial number, suction response setting, controller date and time, low-flow alarm limit, high-power alarm limit, and patient identification.[1] Make sure the connections to the power, monitor, and driveline are secure.[1] Make sure that alarms are turned on, functioning properly, and audible to staff members.[26,27]
■ Closely monitor the VAD parameters *to enable prompt recognition of changes in the patient's condition.*
■ Monitor the patient's cardiac index, *because pump speeds are adjusted according to a calculated cardiac index; pump speeds of 2,400 to 3,200 revolutions per minute (RPM) are recommended by guidelines.* Unless there's a clear clinical need for higher flows, the cardiac index should be set at or above 2.2 L/minute/m².[1]
■ Administer IV fluid, as prescribed, to maintain a pump flow index (pump flow ÷ body surface area) greater than 2 L/minute/m², with central venous pressure and left atrial pressure less than 20 mm Hg. Maintain mean arterial pressure at less than 85 mm Hg as tolerated; *the VAD pump is sensitive to preload and afterload.*[1]
■ Administer a vasopressor or vasodilator as prescribed, following safe medication administration practices, *to adjust vasomotor tone as needed.*[1,31,32,33,34]
■ Administer an inotropic agent, as ordered and needed, *to improve right ventricular function.*[1,31,32,33,34]
■ Administer anticoagulant therapy as prescribed, following safe medication administration practices, *to reduce the risk of stroke.*[1,31,32,33,34] Anticoagulation therapy should be individualized for each patient. Before starting anticoagulation, make sure chest tube drainage is less than 40 mL/hour for about 3 hours, hematocrit is stable without the need for blood transfusion, and coagulation factors are approaching normal.[1] Administer low-dose heparin at 10 units/kg/hour on postoperative day 1 to a target partial thromboplastin time (PTT) of 40 to 50 seconds as ordered.[1] Gradually increase the heparin dosage as prescribed to maintain the PTT between 50 and 60 seconds.[1] Monitor platelet reactivity as ordered *to assess for aspirin resistance*; administer aspirin monotherapy or combination therapy with dipyridamole or clopidogrel as prescribed within 24 hours after implantation if there are no postoperative bleeding complications, *to reduce the risk of stroke.*[1] For patients who are aspirin sensitive or otherwise intolerant, administer clopidogrel as ordered.[1]

Begin warfarin within 4 days postoperatively and titrate to maintain the patient's International Normalized Ratio (INR) at 2 to 3 for long-term therapy as ordered.[1]

NURSING ALERT Anticoagulant medications are considered high-alert medications *because they can cause significant patient harm when used in error.*[36] If required by your facility, before administering an anticoagulant, have another nurse perform an independent double-check *to verify the patient's identity and make sure that you have the correct medication in the prescribed strength or concentration; the medication's indication corresponds with the patient's diagnosis; the dosage calculations are correct and the dosing formula used to derive the final dose is correct; the prescribed route of administration is safe and proper for the patient; the prescribed time and frequency of administration are safe and proper for the patient; and, if an infusion, the pump settings are correct, and the infusion line is attached to the correct port.*[37]

■ Administer systemic antibiotics as ordered for 48 to 72 hours following safe medication administration practices *to reduce the risk of infection.*[1,31,32,33,34]

■ Turn the patient from side to side at least every 2 hours as soon as the patient is clinically stable; begin physical therapy and range-of-motion (ROM) exercises on the first postoperative day if possible *to reduce the risk of pressure injuries and other complications of immobility.*[1,2] As soon as the patient is able, assist the patient to a chair; progress to ambulation in the hallways within a few days of VAD implantation.[1]

■ Perform driveline (the line connecting the pump to the external controller and power source) exit site care routinely (every 24 to 48 hours) as ordered, following strict sterile technique. Perform hand hygiene.[7,8,9,10,11,12] Put on a cap, a mask, and sterile gloves.[1,2] Put on a sterile gown and use maximal barrier precautions if required in your facility.[29] Remove and discard the dressing in an appropriate receptacle.[20] Remove and discard your gloves.[20] Perform hand hygiene.[7,8,9,10,11,12] Put on a new pair of sterile gloves.[2,20,21] Inspect the driveline for kinks, tears, punctures, breakdown of material, and other damage. Notify the practitioner if you see blood within the driveline lumen or if the driveline is damaged.[1] Clean the exit site with an antiseptic cleaning agent (diluted chlorhexidine scrub solution is preferred), and dry the site with a sterile gauze pad *to avoid tissue injury.*[1,7] Immobilize the percutaneous lead with a sterile occlusive dressing and, if necessary, a specialized clip, Montgomery strap, or customized percutaneous lead immobilization binder or belt. Keep the extra external length of the driveline under a binder or clothing.[1]

■ If the patient requires defibrillation, use an external defibrillator to deliver shocks as indicated, following Advanced Cardiac Life Support (ACLS) protocol; the VAD can be left intact and doesn't need to be turned off.[1] If internal defibrillation is required, the VAD can also be left intact and doesn't need to be turned off as the practitioner delivers the shock.[1]

■ Respond to alarms promptly, and troubleshoot the device as permitted and necessary. Always refer to the manufacturer's instructions for use.

For the patient with a HeartMate II or HeartMate 3 VAD

■ Assess the system settings and parameters, including pump flow (estimate of blood flow out of the pump, which is based on pump speed and the amount of power provided to the pump motor); pump speed (speed of the pump in RPM); pulsatility index (displayed as pulse index, a calculation related to the amount of assistance that's provided by the pump, which typically ranges from 1 to 10; higher values indicate higher pulsatility, which means the pump is providing less support and the heart is providing more support); and pump power (amount of power provided by the pump motor, which ranges from 0 to 25.5 watts).[6] Make sure that alarm limits are set appropriately for the patient's current condition, and that alarms are turn on, functioning properly, and audible to staff members.[26,27]

■ Suspect thrombus formation if you note an increase in the VAD system power requirement and a reduction in the pulse index. Notify the practitioner of your findings, *because pump replacement may be necessary.*[6]

■ Monitor the patient for signs and symptoms of blood leak from any system component (unexplained internal bleeding, possibly with painful abdominal distention; blood draining from the driveline exit site; or decreased hemoglobin and hematocrit).[5,6]

■ Closely monitor the patient's hemodynamic status; small increases in afterload (systemic vascular resistance) and small decreases in preload (left ventricular filling) may result in diminished pump flow, a reduction that may result in a clinically significant decrease in perfusion.[6] Assess the patient for signs and symptoms of decreased perfusion with changes in preload and afterload. Monitor mixed venous oxygen saturation levels as ordered.[6]

■ If the patient exhibits condition changes, auscultate over the pump pocket *to verify that the pump is running.*[6]

■ Administer IV fluid as prescribed.

■ Administer medications as prescribed, following safe medication administration practices, *to maintain mean arterial pressure at less than 90 mm Hg.*[6,31,32,33,34]

■ Administer 10% low-molecular-weight dextran at 25 mL/hour if prescribed, following safe medication administration practices.[5,31,32,33,34]

■ Administer anticoagulant therapy as prescribed *to reduce the risk of stroke,* following safe medication administration practices.[6,31,32,33,34] Anticoagulation therapy should be individualized for each patient. Begin IV heparin therapy 12 to 24 hours after surgery or when chest tube drainage is less than 50 mL/hour for a period of 2 to 3 hours, as ordered.[5] Initially, titrate the heparin dose to maintain a PTT of 45 to 50 seconds for 24 hours, as ordered.[5] After 24 hours, increase the heparin dose and titrate to a PTT of 50 to 60 seconds, as ordered.[5] After another 24 hours, increase the heparin dose and titrate to a PTT 55 to 65 seconds, as ordered.[5] Day 2 to 3 postoperatively, administer aspirin and dipyridamole, as prescribed.[5] Day 3 to 5 postoperatively, after chest tubes have been removed and there's no evidence of bleeding, begin warfarin (overlapping with heparin), as ordered.[5] Discontinue heparin as ordered after the patient's INR stabilizes to a range of 2 to 3 on warfarin therapy.[5]

■ If the patient requires defibrillation, use an external defibrillator to deliver shocks, as indicated, following ACLS protocol; leave the pump running, and don't disconnect the system controller from the percutaneous lead before delivering the shock. If internal defibrillation is required, disconnect the VAD from the controller, *because the paddles will be in close proximity to the device. Because retrograde flow may occur through the pump when it's off,* it may be necessary to clamp the outflow graft while the device is stopped.[5,6]

■ Administer prophylactic antibiotics postoperatively, as prescribed, *to reduce the risk of infection.*[5,6,31,32,33,34]

■ If the patient reports dizziness, immediately assess the patient and evaluate the system.[6]

■ Turn the patient from side to side at least every 2 hours as soon as the patient is clinically stable; begin physical therapy and ROM exercises on the first postoperative day, if possible, *to reduce the risk of pressure injuries and other complications of immobility.*[1,2,6] As soon as the patient is able, assist the patient to a chair; progress to ambulation in the hallways within a few days of VAD implantation.[1,6]

■ Respond to alarms promptly, and troubleshoot the device as permitted and necessary. Always refer to the manufacturer's instructions for use.

■ If an alarm signals controller failure, change the controller per manufacturer's instructions.

■ Perform percutaneous lead exit site care daily, using strict sterile technique. Perform hand hygiene.[7,8,9,10,11,12] Put on a cap, a mask, and sterile gloves.[5,6] Put on a sterile gown and use maximal barrier precautions if required in your facility.[29] Remove and discard the dressing in an appropriate receptacle.[20] Remove and discard your gloves, perform hand hygiene, and put on sterile gloves.[5,6,7,8,9,10,11,12,20,21] Gently clean the site with a mild antiseptic soap (preferably chlorhexidine solution), and then dry the clean site with a sterile gauze pad.[6] Inspect the percutaneous lead *to make sure it's free from bending or kinking.* Cover the site with a dry sterile dressing.[5,6] Immobilize the percutaneous lead with a stabilization belt or abdominal binder *to reduce trauma to the exit site.* Keep the stabilization belt or abdominal binder in place at all times except when the patient showers (if permitted), or when the belt or binder is being replaced with a newly cleaned belt or binder.[6]

■ Arrange for echocardiography, if ordered, to perform a ramped speed study *to determine the patient's appropriate fixed-speed setting.* A ramped speed study is intended for hemodynamically stable, euvolemic patients in the postoperative period or later.[6]

Completing the procedure

■ Monitor the patient's intake and output closely *to promptly detect changes in the patient's condition.*[2]

■ Monitor the patient for signs of cardiac tamponade, such as unexplained low VAD flow or cardiac output despite adequate intravascular fluid volume (right atrial pressure [RAP] or pulmonary artery occlusion pressure [PAOP] 10 to 15 mm Hg), narrowed pulse pressure beyond what's expected from a device recipient, elevated RAP or PAOP despite inadequate pump or cardiac output, reduced mixed venous oxygen saturation, tachycardia, reduced urine output, sudden cessation of chest tube drainage, decreased electrical voltage on the ECG, and enlargement of the cardiac silhouette or widened mediastinum on chest X-ray. Notify the practitioner immediately if such signs occur.[29]

■ If the patient suffers cardiac arrest and needs cardiopulmonary resuscitation, compressions may pose a risk because of the pump location and position of the outflow graft on the aorta. Collaborate with the patient's practitioner in advance, and be familiar with your facility's guidelines for which ACLS measure to follow in the event of cardiac arrest. If compressions are performed, make sure function and positioning of the VAD are confirmed after the patient's condition stabilizes. Cardiac massage under direct vision performed by a skilled surgeon may be effective for a patient who has had recent device implantation (before mediastinal healing).[1,29,38]

■ Obtain a 12-lead ECG as ordered if the patient complains of "feeling different" *to determine an underlying cause.*[6]

■ Provide oral nutrition as ordered as soon as the patient's condition warrants *to correct nutritional deficiencies and reduce the risk of infection.* Alternatively, if the patient remains intubated, begin an enteral tube feeding, as ordered.[1,6]

■ Remove invasive monitoring lines and catheters, as ordered, as soon as the patient's condition allows, *to reduce the risk of infection.*[1,6]

■ Monitor laboratory test results (electrolyte and lactate levels, complete blood count, prothrombin time, INR, and PTT) as ordered.[1,6] Notify the practitioner of critical test results within your facility's established time frame *so the patient can be treated promptly.*[39]

■ Monitor the patient's blood glucose levels, and administer antidiabetic agents as prescribed following safe medication administration practices *to maintain strict blood glucose control, which helps to reduce the risk of infection.*[6,31,32,33,34]

■ Avoid situations and use of devices that can cause strong electrostatic discharges, *because electrostatic discharges can damage the electrical parts of the VAD system and cause the VAD to stop or perform improperly.*[1,6]

■ Provide oral care *to reduce oral bacterial colonization, which helps reduce the risk of health care–associated pneumonia.* Gently brush the patient's teeth, gums, and tongue at least twice daily using a soft-bristle toothbrush, toothpaste, and sterile water.[40] Moisturized the oral mucosa and lips every 2 to 4 hours *to reduce oral inflammation and improve oral health.*[40] Use a chlorhexidine mouth rinse twice daily during the perioperative period, as prescribed, *to prevent ventilator-associated pneumonia.*[40]

■ Use antiembolism prevention strategies, such as applying antiembolism stockings or a sequential compression device, as ordered, *to promote venous return and prevent venous thromboembolism.*

■ If the patient was receiving a beta-adrenergic blocker before surgery, collaborate with the patient's practitioner to make sure the patient receives it during the perioperative period, as appropriate.[41]

■ If the patient has an indwelling urinary catheter inserted for surgery, remove the catheter on postoperative day 1 or 2 (with the day of surgery considered day 0) or as soon as the patient no longer needs it, *to reduce the risk of catheter-associated urinary tract infection.*[41,42,43] (See the "Indwelling urinary catheter care and removal" procedure.)

HOSPITAL-ACQUIRED CONDITION ALERT Keep in mind that the Centers for Medicare and Medicaid Services considers catheter-associated urinary tract infection (CAUTI) a hospital-acquired condition, *because it can be reasonably prevented using a variety of best practices. To reduce the risk of CAUTI when caring for a patient with an indwelling urinary catheter*, make sure to follow evidence-based CAUTI prevention practices, such as performing hand hygiene before and after any catheter manipulation; maintaining a sterile, continuously closed drainage system; maintaining unobstructed urine flow; emptying the collection bag regularly; replacing the catheter and drainage system using sterile technique when breaks in sterile technique, disconnection, or leakage occurs; and discontinuing the catheter as soon as it's no longer clinically indicated.[42,43,44,45,46]

■ Return the bed to the lowest position *to prevent falls and maintain patient safety.*[47]

■ Maintain the device following the manufacturer's instructions for use.

■ Remove and discard your gloves and other personal protective equipment.[20]

■ Perform hand hygiene.[7,8,9,10,11,12]

■ Clean and disinfect your stethoscope using a disinfectant pad.[48]

■ Perform hand hygiene.[7,8,9,10,11,12]

■ Reassess and respond to the patient's pain by evaluating the response to the treatment and progress toward pain management goals. Assess for adverse reactions and risk factors for adverse events that may result from treatment.[30]

■ Perform hand hygiene.[7,8,9,10,11,12]

■ Document the procedure.[49,50,51,52]

Special considerations

■ Don't subject the patient to magnetic resonance imaging (MRI), *because the VAD contains magnetic components; MRI can cause device failure or patient injury.*[1,5,6]

■ Keep cell phones at least 20" (50 cm) from the controller, *because phones may interfere with the device function.*[1,6]

■ Don't expose the patient to therapeutic levels of ultrasound energy, *because lithotripsy and other procedures that use high-intensity ultrasound may cause harm if the implanted device inadvertently concentrates the ultrasound field.*[1,6]

■ Don't expose the patient to high-power electrical treatments such as diathermy.[1,6]

■ Keep in mind that therapeutic ionizing radiation may damage the device, although the damage may not be immediately detectable.[1,6]

NURSING ALERT Electrostatic discharge, such as from walking across carpet or when taking clothes out of a dryer, can interfere with electrical parts of the HeartMate 3 and cause it to stop functioning. In addition, the device can interfere with implantable cardiac defibrillators, requiring adjustment of device sensitivity or repositioning of the lead.[5]

■ The Joint Commission issued a sentinel event alert concerning medical device alarm safety, *because alarm-related events have been associated with permanent loss of function or death.* Among the major contributing factors were improper alarm settings, alarm settings inappropriately turned off, and alarm signals that were inaudible to staff. Make sure that alarm limits are set appropriately for the patient's current condition, and that alarms are turned on, functioning properly, and audible to staff. Follow facility guidelines for preventing alarm fatigue.[25]

Complications

Complications associated with the HeartWare and HeartMate devices include death, bleeding (perioperative or late), cardiac arrhythmias, local infection, respiratory failure, device malfunction, sepsis, right-sided heart failure, driveline infection, kidney failure, stroke, neurologic dysfunction, psychiatric episodes, peripheral thromboembolism, hemolysis, hepatic dysfunction, device thrombosis, and myocardial infarction.[1,6] Other potential complications associated with the HeartWare device include air embolism, aortic insufficiency, driveline perforation, erosions and other tissue damage, GI bleeding, arteriovenous malformations, hypertension, multiorgan failure, pericardial effusion or tamponade, platelet dysfunction, worsening heart failure, and wound dehiscence.[1]

Documentation

Document the patient's vital signs, hemodynamic parameters, your assessment findings, system parameters, any pump adjustments, and medications you administered. Document complications, the date and time, the name of the practitioner you notified, prescribed interventions, and the patient's response to those interventions. Record dressing changes and the condition of the insertion site. Document teaching provided to the patient and family (if applicable), their understanding of that teaching, and any need for follow-up teaching.

REFERENCES

1 HeartWare, Inc. (2018). HeartWare HVAD system: Instructions for use. https://bchcicu.org/wp-content/uploads/2018/07/ifu00375_rev05_hvad_ifu_en-english_electronic.pdf

2 Wiegand, D. L. (2017). *AACN procedure manual for high acuity, progressive, and critical care* (7th ed.). St. Louis, MO: Elsevier.

3 Birks, E. J. (2020). Intermediate- and long-term mechanical circulatory support. In: *UpToDate*, Mancini, D., & Hunt, S. A. (Eds.).

4 Feldman, D., et al. (2013). The 2013 International Society for Heart and Lung Transplantation guidelines for mechanical circulatory support: Executive summary. *Journal of Heart and Lung Transplantation, 32*(2), 157–187. https://doi.org/10.1016/j.healun.2012.09.013 (Level VII)

5 Thoratec Corporation. (2018). HeartMate3 left ventricular assist system: Instructions for use. https://fda.report/PMA/P160054/16/P160054S008D.pdf

6 Thoratec Corporation. (2017). HeartMate II left ventricular assist system: Instructions for use. https://www.cardiovascular.abbott/us/en/hcp/products/heart-failure/left-ventricular-assist-devices/heartmate-2/manuals-resources.html

7 Centers for Disease Control and Prevention. (2002). Guideline for hand hygiene in health-care settings: Recommendations of the Healthcare Infection Control Practices Advisory Committee and the HICPAC/SHEA/APIC/IDSA Hand Hygiene Task Force. *MMWR Recommendations and Reports, 51*(RR-16), 1–45. https://www.cdc.gov/mmwr/pdf/rr/rr5116.pdf (Level VII)

8 World Health Organization (WHO). (2009). WHO guidelines on hand hygiene in health care: First global patient safety challenge, clean care is safer care. https://apps.who.int/iris/bitstream/handle/10665/44102/9789241597906_eng.pdf?sequence=1 (Level IV)

9 The Joint Commission. (2021). Standard NPSG.07.01.01. *Comprehensive accreditation manual for hospitals*. Oakbrook Terrace, IL: The Joint Commission. (Level VII)

10 Accreditation Association for Hospitals and Health Systems. (2020). Standard 07.01.21. *Healthcare Facilities Accreditation Program: Accreditation requirements for acute care hospitals*. Chicago, IL: Accreditation Association for Hospitals and Health Systems. (Level VII)

11 Centers for Medicare and Medicaid Services, Department of Health and Human Services. (2020). Condition of participation: Infection control. 42 C.F.R. § 482.42.

12 DNV GL-Healthcare USA, Inc. (2020). IC.1.SR.1. *NIAHO® accreditation requirements, interpretive guidelines and surveyor guidance—revision 20.0*. Milford, OH: DNV GL-Healthcare USA, Inc. (Level VII)

13 The Joint Commission. (2021). Standard NPSG.01.01.01. *Comprehensive accreditation manual for hospitals*. Oakbrook Terrace, IL: The Joint Commission. (Level VII)

14 Accreditation Association for Hospitals and Health Systems. (2020). Standard 15.01.16. *Healthcare Facilities Accreditation Program: Accreditation requirements for acute care hospitals*. Chicago, IL: Accreditation Association for Hospitals and Health Systems. (Level VII)

15 Centers for Medicare and Medicaid Services, Department of Health and Human Services. (2020). Condition of participation: Patient's rights. 42 C.F.R. § 482.13(c)(1).

16 DNV GL-Healthcare USA, Inc. (2020). PR.2.SR.5. *NIAHO® accreditation requirements, interpretive guidelines and surveyor guidance—revision 20.0*. Milford, OH: DNV GL-Healthcare USA, Inc. (Level VII)

17 The Joint Commission. (2021). Standard RI.01.01.01. *Comprehensive accreditation manual for hospitals*. Oakbrook Terrace, IL: The Joint Commission. (Level VII)

18 The Joint Commission. (2021). Standard PC.02.01.21. *Comprehensive accreditation manual for hospitals*. Oakbrook Terrace, IL: The Joint Commission. (Level VII)

19 Waters, T. R., et al. (2009). Safe patient handling training for schools of nursing. https://www.cdc.gov/niosh/docs/2009-127/pdfs/2009-127.pdf (Level VII)

20 Occupational Safety and Health Administration. (2012). Bloodborne pathogens, standard number 1910.1030. https://www.osha.gov/pls/oshaweb/owadisp.show_document?p_id=10051&p_table=STANDARDS (Level VII)

21 Siegel, J. D., et al. (2007, revised 2019). 2007 guideline for isolation precautions: Preventing transmission of infectious agents in healthcare settings. https://www.cdc.gov/infectioncontrol/pdf/guidelines/isolation-guidelines-H.pdf (Level II)

22 Accreditation Association for Hospitals and Health Systems. (2020). Standard 07.01.10. *Healthcare Facilities Accreditation Program: Accreditation requirements for acute care hospitals*. Chicago, IL: Accreditation Association for Hospitals and Health Systems. (Level VII)

23 The Joint Commission. (2021). Standard PC.02.02.01. *Comprehensive accreditation manual for hospitals*. Oakbrook Terrace, IL: The Joint Commission. (Level VII)

24 The Joint Commission. (2012). Hot topics in health care: Transitions of care: The need for a more effective approach to continuing patient care. https://flbog.sip.ufl.edu/risk-rx-article/transitions-of-care-the-need-for-a-more-effective-approach-to-continuing-patient-care/

25 The Joint Commission. (2013). Sentinel event alert 50: Medical device alarm safety in hospitals. https://www.jointcommission.org/-/media/tjc/documents/resources/patient-safety-topics/sentinel-event/sea_50_alarms_4_26_16.pdf (Level VII)

26 Graham, K. C., & Cvach, M. (2010). Monitor alarm fatigue: Standardizing use of physiological monitors and decreasing nuisance alarms. *American Journal of Critical Care, 19*(1), 28–37. https://doi.org/10.4037/ajcc2010651

27 American Association of Critical-Care Nurses (AACN). (2016). *AACN practice alert: Obtaining accurate noninvasive blood pressure measurements in adults*. https://www.aacn.org/clinical-resources/practice-alerts/obtaining-accurate-noninvasive-blood-pressure-measurements-in-adults (Level VII)

28 O'Shea, G. (2012). Ventricular assist devices: What intensive care unit nurses need to know about postoperative management. *AACN Advanced Critical Care, 23*(1), 69–83. https://doi.org/10.1097/nci.0b013e318240aaa9 (Level V)

29 The Joint Commission. (2021). Standard PC.01.02.07. *Comprehensive accreditation manual for hospitals*. Oakbrook Terrace, IL: The Joint Commission. (Level VII)

30 DNV GL-Healthcare USA, Inc. (2020). MM.1.SR.2. *NIAHO® accreditation requirements, interpretive guidelines and surveyor guidance—revision 20.0*. Milford, OH: DNV GL-Healthcare USA, Inc. (Level VII)

31 Accreditation Association for Hospitals and Health Systems. (2020). Standard 16.01.03. *Healthcare Facilities Accreditation Program: Accreditation requirements for acute care hospitals*. Chicago, IL: Accreditation Association for Hospitals and Health Systems. (Level VII)

32 Centers for Medicare and Medicaid Services, Department of Health and Human Services. (2020). Condition of participation: Nursing services. 42 C.F.R. § 482.23(c).

33 The Joint Commission. (2021). Standard MM.06.01.01. *Comprehensive accreditation manual for hospitals*. Oakbrook Terrace, IL: The Joint Commission. (Level VII)

34 Institute for Safe Medication Practices. (2020). 2020–2021 targeted medication safety best practices for hospitals. https://www.ismp.org/sites/default/files/attachments/2020-02/2020-2021%20TMSBP-%20FINAL_1.pdf

35 Institute for Safe Medication Practices. (2018). ISMP list of high-alert medications in acute care settings. https://www.ismp.org/sites/default/files/attachments/2018-08/highAlert2018-Acute-Final.pdf

36 Thoratec Corporation. (2017). HeartMate 3 left ventricular assist system: Alarms for clinicians. https://www.accessdata.fda.gov/cdrh_docs/pdf16/P160054C.pdf

37 Peberdy, M. A., et al. (2017). Cardiopulmonary resuscitation in adults and children with mechanical circulatory support: A scientific statement from the American Heart Association. *Circulation, 135*(24), e1115–e1134. https://www.ahajournals.org/doi/full/10.1161/CIR.0000000000000504 (Level VII)

38 The Joint Commission. (2021). Standard NPSG.02.03.01. *Comprehensive accreditation manual for hospitals*. Oakbrook Terrace, IL: The Joint Commission. (Level VII)

39 American Association of Critical-Care Nurses (AACN). (2017). *AACN practice alert: Oral care for acutely and critically ill patients*. https://www.aacn.org/clinical-resources/practice-alerts/oral-care-for-acutely-and-critically-ill-patients (Level VII)

40 Centers for Medicare and Medicaid Services & The Joint Commission. (2022). The specifications manual for national hospital inpatient quality measures (version 5.11a) https://www.qualitynet.org/inpatient/specifications-manuals#tab1

41 Healthcare Infection Control Practices Advisory Committee. (2010, revised 2019). Guideline for prevention of catheter-associated urinary tract infections 2009. https://www.cdc.gov/infectioncontrol/pdf/guidelines/cauti-guidelines-H.pdf (Level I)

42 The Joint Commission. (2021). Standard NPSG.07.06.01. *Comprehensive accreditation manual for hospitals*. Oakbrook Terrace, IL: The Joint Commission. (Level VII)

43 Jarrett, N., & Callaham, M. (2016). Evidence-based guidelines for selected hospital-acquired conditions: Final report. https://www.cms.gov/Medicare/Medicare-Fee-for-Service-Payment/HospitalAcqCond/Downloads/2016-HAC-Report.pdf

44 Agency for Healthcare Research and Quality & U.S. Department of Health and Human Services. (2015). Toolkit for reducing catheter-associated

urinary tract infections in hospital units: Implementation guide. http://www.ahrq.gov/professionals/quality-patient-safety/hais/cauti-tools/impl-guide/index.html

45 Lo, E., et al. (2014). SHEA/IDSA practice recommendation: Strategies to prevent catheter-associated urinary tract infections in acute care hospitals: 2014 update. *Infection Control and Hospital Epidemiology, 35*(5), 464–479. https://www.jstor.org/stable/10.1086/675718#metadata_info_tab_contents (Level I)

46 Ganz, D. A., et al. (2013, reviewee 2021). *Preventing falls in hospitals: A toolkit for improving quality of care* (AHRQ Publication No. 13-0015-EF). Agency for Healthcare Research and Quality. https://www.ahrq.gov/professionals/systems/hospital/fallpxtoolkit/index.html (Level VII)

47 Accreditation Association for Hospitals and Health Systems. (2020). Standard 07.02.03. *Healthcare Facilities Accreditation Program: Accreditation requirements for acute care hospitals.* Chicago, IL: Accreditation Association for Hospitals and Health Systems. (Level VII)

48 Rutala, W. A., et al. (2008, revised 2019). Guideline for disinfection and sterilization in healthcare facilities, 2008. https://www.cdc.gov/infection-control/pdf/guidelines/disinfection-guidelines-H.pdf (Level I)

49 The Joint Commission. (2021). Standard RC.01.03.01. *Comprehensive accreditation manual for hospitals.* Oakbrook Terrace, IL: The Joint Commission. (Level VII)

50 Accreditation Association for Hospitals and Health Systems. (2020). Standard 10.00.03. *Healthcare Facilities Accreditation Program: Accreditation requirements for acute care hospitals.* Chicago, IL: Accreditation Association for Hospitals and Health Systems. (Level VII)

51 Centers for Medicare and Medicaid Services, Department of Health and Human Services. (2020). Condition of participation: Medical record services. 42 C.F.R. § 482.24(b).

52 DNV GL-Healthcare USA, Inc. (2020). MR.2.SR.1. *NIAHO® accreditation requirements, interpretive guidelines and surveyor guidance—revision 20.0.* Milford, OH: DNV GL-Healthcare USA, Inc. (Level VII)

VOLUME-CONTROL SET PREPARATION

A volume-control set, also referred to as a *burette set*, is similar to a standard IV administration set, with the addition of a graduated chamber immediately above the drip chamber of the tubing. This chamber, which includes a separate medication port and air filter, allows administration of medications or a precise volume of fluid.

Accurate control of the flow rate permits optimal patient management and prevents IV dosing errors. Controlling the dose and flow rate is particularly important when administering highly potent, irritating, or potentially toxic IV medications to children or older adults. The volume-control set design also prevents free flow of fluid and shuts off when the fluid is exhausted, preventing air from entering the IV catheter.

Despite the potential advantages, there's little evidence to support the use of volume-control sets, and research has identified medication and flushing errors associated with their use.[1] Volume-control sets haven't been used frequently since the advent of volumetric and smart pumps for IV infusion. Some IV pump systems can accommodate a volume-control set. Refer to the pump manufacturer's instructions for safe use together.[2]

HOSPITAL-ACQUIRED CONDITION ALERT Keep in mind that the Centers for Medicare and Medicaid Services considers vascular catheter–associated infection a hospital-acquired condition *because it can be reasonable prevented using a variety of best practices.* Make sure to follow evidence-based infection prevention practices, such as performing hand hygiene and following sterile, no-touch technique, *to reduce the risk of vascular catheter–associated infections.*[3,4,5,6,7]

Equipment

Volume-control set ■ IV pole ■ prescribed IV solution ■ antiseptic pads (alcohol, tincture of iodine, or chlorhexidine-based) ■ medication in labeled syringe ■ label.

Although various models of volume-control sets are available, each one consists of a graduated fluid chamber (120 to 250 mL) with a spike and a filtered air line on the top and administration tubing underneath. Floating valve sets have a valve at the bottom that closes when the chamber empties; membrane filter sets have a rigid filter at the bottom that, when wet, prevents the passage of air.

NURSING ALERT Make sure the volume-control set is labeled clearly when medications are added to the system. Check with the pharmacy for incompatibilities before adding the drug, and always use sterile technique. Keep in mind that chemical inactivation or precipitation can occur when multiple medications are administered using the same volume-control set.[1,8]

Preparation of equipment

Prepare any ordered medication and verify compatibility of the medication and diluent before administration. Whenever possible, administer pharmacy-prepared or commercially available products.[9]

Inspect all IV equipment and supplies. If a product is expired, is defective, or has compromised integrity, remove it from patient use, label it as expired or defective, and report the expiration or defect as directed by your facility.[10]

Implementation

■ Avoid distractions and interruptions when preparing and administering IV solutions and medication *to prevent administration errors.*[11,12]

■ Review the practitioner's order to make sure that the prescribed infusion solution or medication, dose, rate, and route of administration are appropriate for the patient's age, condition, and access device, and that the infusion or medication is compatible with other solutions or medications. Make sure the order includes any test results that require monitoring. Address concerns about the order with the practitioner, pharmacist, or your supervisor, the risk management department, or as directed by your facility.[13]

■ Gather and prepare the necessary equipment and supplies.

■ Compare the label on the solution container and prescribed medication with the order in the patient's medical record. Verify the practitioner's order, patient's name, dosage, concentration, administration route, frequency, and infusion rate.[13,14]

■ Check the patient's medical record for an allergy or contraindication to the prescribed medication or solution. If an allergy or contraindication exists, don't administer the medication; notify the practitioner.[15,16,17,18]

■ Check the expiration date on the prescribed medication or solution. If the medication or solution is expired, return it to the pharmacy and obtain new medication or solution.[15,16,17,18]

■ Visually inspect the solution for particles, discoloration, or other loss of integrity; don't administer the medication or solution if its integrity is compromised.[15,16,17,18]

■ Discuss any unresolved concerns about the IV solution or medication with the patient's practitioner.[15,16,17,18]

■ Perform hand hygiene.[3,19,20,21,22,23,24]

■ Confirm the patient's identity using at least two patient identifiers.[25]

■ Provide privacy.[26,27,28,29]

■ Explain the procedure to the patient and family (if appropriate) according to their individual communication and learning needs *to increase their understanding, allay their fears, and enhance cooperation.*[30,31]

■ If the patient is receiving the mediation for the first time, teach the patient and family (if appropriate) about the potential adverse reactions and other concerns related to the medications.[15,16,17,18,31]

■ If an IV catheter is already in place, assess the insertion site for signs of infiltration and infection.[32,33]

■ Remove the volume-control set from its box and close all the clamps.

■ Remove the protective cap from the volume-control set spike, insert the spike into the prescribed IV solution container, and hang the container on the IV pole.

■ Open the air vent clamp and close the upper slide clamp.

■ Open the lower clamp on the IV tubing, slide it upward until it's slightly below the drip chamber, and close the clamp.

■ Open the upper clamp until the fluid chamber fills with about 30 mL of solution. Then close the clamp.

■ Gently squeeze the drip chamber.

■ Release the drip chamber and let it fill to the level recommended by the manufacturer.

■ Open the lower clamp, prime the tubing, and close the clamp.

■ To use the set as a primary line, perform a vigorous mechanical scrub of the catheter hub or needleless connector for at least 5 seconds[5] using an antiseptic pad. Allow it to dry completely.[6,34] Then, attach the distal end of the tubing directly to the catheter hub or needleless access device.

■ To use the set as a secondary line, perform a vigorous mechanical scrub of the Y-port of the primary tubing for at least 5 seconds using an antiseptic pad. Allow it to dry completely.[6,34] Then attach the distal end of the tubing to the Y-port of the primary tubing, following the manufacturer's instructions.

■ To add medication, perform a vigorous mechanical scrub of the injection port on the volume-control set for at least 5 seconds using an antiseptic pad. Allow it to dry completely.[6,34] Inject the medication (as shown below). Follow safe medication administration practices.[6,16,17,18]

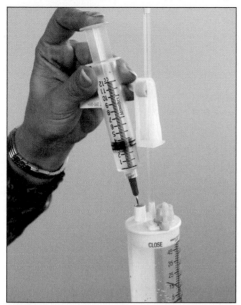

NURSING ALERT Don't administer continuous high-alert medications as secondary infusions or connect a secondary medication to a high-alert primary continuous infusion, *to avoid patient harm caused by inadvertent medication administration at incorrect or indeterminate rates.*[35]

■ Place a label on the chamber indicating the drug, dose, date, and your initials. Don't write directly on the chamber, *because the plastic absorbs ink.*[36]

■ Open the upper clamp (as shown below), fill the fluid chamber with the prescribed amount of solution, and close the clamp. Gently rotate the chamber *to mix the medication.*

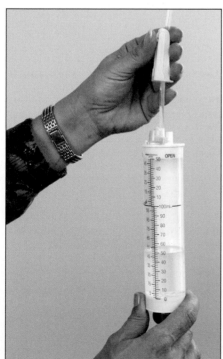

■ If using the volume-control set to deliver a secondary infusion, turn off the primary solution or lower the drip rate *to maintain an open line.* Verify that the secondary infusion is active and the primary infusion is inactive by viewing the drip chambers, as indicated.

■ Trace the IV tubing from the patient to the point of origin *to make sure that the set is connected to the proper port.* Route the tubing in a standardized direction if the patient has other tubing and catheters that have different purposes. If you're using multiple IV lines, label the tubing at the distal end (near the patient connection) and the proximal end (near the source container) *to reduce the risk of misconnection.*[14,37,38]

■ Open the lower clamp on the volume-control set and adjust the drip rate as ordered.

■ After completion of the infusion, open the upper clamp and let 10 mL of IV solution flow into the chamber. Infuse the fluid at the same rate as the initial infusion *to flush the tubing.*

■ If you're using the volume-control set as a secondary IV line, close the lower clamp and reset the flow rate of the primary line. If you're using the set as a primary IV line, close the lower clamp, refill the chamber to the prescribed amount, and begin the infusion again.

■ Monitor the IV volume-control set regularly, inspect the IV insertion site for complications, and evaluate the patient's response to therapy.[14]

■ Perform hand hygiene.[3,19,20,21,22,23,24]

■ Document the procedure.[39,40,41,42,43]

Special considerations

■ Administration sets for primary and secondary continuous infusion of fluids other than lipids, blood, or blood products should be changed no more frequently than every 96 hours, but at least every 7 days (unless otherwise directed by manufacturer's instructions) and immediately upon suspected contamination or when the integrity of the product or system has been compromised. In addition to routine changes, change the administration set whenever the vascular access device is changed or when a new vascular access device is inserted. Change a secondary administration set that is detached from the primary administration set every 24 hours. Change a primary intermittent administration set every 24 hours.[38]

■ Label any medication added to volume-control sets *to avoid the inadvertent addition of multiple, potentially incompatible medications.*

Complications

Complications of IV infusion therapy include local or systemic infection, infiltration, extravasation, air embolism, catheter occlusion or dislodgment, and circulatory overload. Improper labeling and flushing may result in drug incompatibilities or medication administration errors.[14,33,44,45]

Documentation

Document the type of fluid administered; the rate, time, route, and method of administration; and the condition of the venipuncture or access site before and after infusion therapy. If you add a drug to the volume-control set, record the name, strength, and dosage of the medication, the amount of fluid used to dilute it, and the date and time of the infusion. Document the patient's response to the medication. Record any adverse reactions to the prescribed medication, the date and time that the practitioner was notified, prescribed interventions, and the patient's response to those interventions.[14] Document teaching provided to the patient and family (if applicable), their understanding of that teaching, and any need for follow-up teaching.[3]

REFERENCES

1 Institute for Safe Medication Practices. (2009). Volume control set safety. *ISMP Medication Safety Alert!, 14*(11), 2. (Level VII)

2 BD. (2014). Burette set tip sheet: Burette set use: Alaris System. https://www.bd.com/assets/documents/guides/tip-sheets/IF_Using-Burette-Set-With-Alaris-System_TS_EN.pdf

3 Centers for Disease Control and Prevention. (2002). Guideline for hand hygiene in health-care settings: Recommendations of the Healthcare Infection Control Practices Advisory Committee and the HICPAC/SHEA/APIC/IDSA Hand Hygiene Task Force. *MMWR Recommendations and Reports, 51*(RR-16), 1–45. https://www.cdc.gov/mmwr/pdf/rr/rr5116.pdf (Level II)

4 The Joint Commission. (2021). Standard NPSG.07.04.01. *Comprehensive accreditation manual for hospitals.* (Level VII)

5 Infusion Nurses Society. (2016). *Policies and procedures for infusion therapy* (5th ed.). Infusion Nurses Society.

6 Marschall, J., et al. (2014). SHEA/IDSA practice recommendation: Strategies to prevent central line–associated bloodstream infections in

acute care hospitals. *Infection Control and Hospital Epidemiology, 35*(7), 753–771. https://www.jstor.org/stable/10.1086/676533#metadata_info_tab_contents (Level I)

7 Jarrett, N., & Callaham, M. (2016). Evidence-based guidelines for selected hospital-acquired conditions: Final report. https://www.cms.gov/Medicare/Medicare-Fee-for-Service-Payment/HospitalAcqCond/Downloads/2016-HAC-Report.pdf

8 Foinard, A., et al. (2012). Impact of physical incompatibility on drug mass flow rates: Example of furosemide-midazolam incompatibility. *Annals of Intensive Care, 2*, Article 28. https://annalsofintensivecare.springeropen.com/track/pdf/10.1186/2110-5820-2-28 (Level IV)

9 Standard 20. Compounding and preparation of parenteral solutions and medications. Infusion therapy standards of practice (8th ed.). (2021). *Journal of Infusion Nursing, 44*(Suppl. 1), S59–S60. (Level VII)

10 Standard 12. Product evaluation, integrity, and defect reporting. Infusion therapy standards of practice (8th ed.). (2021). *Journal of Infusion Nursing, 44*(Suppl. 1), S45–S46. (Level VII)

11 Institute for Safe Medication Practices. (2012). Side tracks on the safety express: Interruptions lead to errors and unfinished...Wait, what was I doing? *Nurse Advise-ERR, 11*(2), 1–4. https://www.ismp.org/resources/side-tracks-safety-express-interruptions-lead-errors-and-unfinished-wait-what-was-i-doing?id=37

12 Westbrook, J., et al. (2010). Association of interruptions with an increased risk and severity of medication administration errors. *Archives of Internal Medicine, 170*(8), 683–690. https://doi.org/10.1001/archinternmed.2010.65 (Level IV)

13 Standard 13. Medication verification. Infusion therapy standards of practice (8th ed.). (2021). *Journal of Infusion Nursing, 44*(Suppl. 1), S46–S49. (Level VII)

14 Standard 59. Infusion medication and solution administration. Infusion therapy standards of practice (8th ed.). (2021). *Journal of Infusion Nursing, 44*(Suppl. 1), S180–S183. (Level VII)

15 The Joint Commission. (2021). Standard MM.06.01.01. *Comprehensive accreditation manual for hospitals.* Oakbrook Terrace, IL: The Joint Commission. (Level VII)

16 DNV GL-Healthcare USA, Inc. (2020). MM.1.SR.3. *NIAHO® accreditation requirements, interpretive guidelines and surveyor guidance—revision 20.0.* Milford, OH: DNV GL-Healthcare USA, Inc. (Level VII)

17 Centers for Medicare and Medicaid Services, Department of Health and Human Services. (2020). Condition of participation: Nursing services. 42 C.F.R. § 482.23(c).

18 Accreditation Association for Hospitals and Health Systems. (2020). Standard 16.01.03. *Healthcare Facilities Accreditation Program: Accreditation requirements for acute care hospitals.* Chicago, IL: Accreditation Association for Hospitals and Health Systems. (Level VII)

19 The Joint Commission. (2021). Standard NPSG.07.01.01. *Comprehensive accreditation manual for hospitals.* Oakbrook Terrace, IL: The Joint Commission. (Level VII)

20 Standard 16. Hand hygiene. Infusion therapy standards of practice (8th ed.). (2021). *Journal of Infusion Nursing, 44*(Suppl. 1), S53–S54. (Level VII)

21 World Health Organization. (2009). WHO guidelines on hand hygiene in health care: First global patient safety challenge, clean care is safer care. https://apps.who.int/iris/bitstream/handle/10665/44102/9789241597906_eng.pdf?sequence=1 (Level IV)

22 Centers for Medicare and Medicaid Services, Department of Health and Human Services. (2020). Condition of participation: Infection control. 42 C.F.R. § 482.42.

23 Accreditation Association for Hospitals and Health Systems. (2020). Standard 07.01.21. *Healthcare Facilities Accreditation Program: Accreditation requirements for acute care hospitals.* Chicago, IL: Accreditation Association for Hospitals and Health Systems. (Level VII)

24 DNV GL-Healthcare USA, Inc. (2020). IC.1.SR.1. *NIAHO® accreditation requirements, interpretive guidelines and surveyor guidance—revision 20.0.* Milford, OH: DNV GL-Healthcare USA, Inc. (Level VII)

25 The Joint Commission. (2021). Standard NPSG.01.01.01. *Comprehensive accreditation manual for hospitals.* Oakbrook Terrace, IL: The Joint Commission. (Level VII)

26 The Joint Commission. (2021). Standard RI.01.01.01. *Comprehensive accreditation manual for hospitals.* Oakbrook Terrace, IL: The Joint Commission. (Level VII)

27 DNV GL-Healthcare USA, Inc. (2020). PR.2.SR.5. *NIAHO® accreditation requirements, interpretive guidelines and surveyor guidance—revision 20.0.* Milford, OH: DNV GL-Healthcare USA, Inc. (Level VII)

28 Centers for Medicare and Medicaid Services, Department of Health and Human Services. (2020). Condition of participation: Patient's rights. 42 C.F.R. § 482.13(c)(1).

29 Accreditation Association for Hospitals and Health Systems. (2020). Standard 15.01.16. *Healthcare Facilities Accreditation Program: Accreditation requirements for acute care hospitals.* Chicago, IL: Accreditation Association for Hospitals and Health Systems. (Level VII)

30 The Joint Commission. (2021). Standard PC.02.01.21. *Comprehensive accreditation manual for hospitals.* Oakbrook Terrace, IL: The Joint Commission. (Level VII)

31 Standard 8. Patient education. Infusion therapy standards of practice (8th ed.). (2021). *Journal of Infusion Nursing, 44*(Suppl. 1), S35–S37. (Level VII)

32 Standard 42. Vascular access device assessment, care and dressing changes. Infusion therapy standards of practice (8th ed.). (2021). *Journal of Infusion Nursing, 44*(Suppl. 1), S119–S123. (Level VII)

33 Standard 47. Infiltration and extravasation. Infusion therapy standards of practice (8th ed.). (2021). *Journal of Infusion Nursing, 44*(Suppl. 1), S142–S147. (Level VII)

34 Standard 36. Needleless connectors. Infusion therapy standards of practice (8th ed.). (2021). *Journal of Infusion Nursing, 44*(Suppl. 1), S104–S107. (Level VII)

35 Wollitz, A., & Grissinger, M. (2014). Aligning the lines: An analysis of IV line errors. *Pennsylvania Patient Safety Advisory, 11*(1),1–8. http://patientsafety.pa.gov/ADVISORIES/documents/201403_01.pdf

36 Accreditation Association for Hospitals and Health Systems. (2020). Standard 25.01.18. *Healthcare Facilities Accreditation Program: Accreditation requirements for acute care hospitals.* Chicago, IL: Accreditation Association for Hospitals and Health Systems. (Level VII)

37 The Joint Commission. (2014). Sentinel event alert 53: Managing risk during transition to new ISO tubing connector standards. https://www.jointcommission.org/-/media/tjc/documents/resources/patient-safety-topics/sentinel-event/sea_53_connectors_8_19_14_final.pdf (Level VII)

38 Standard 43. Administration set management. Infusion therapy standards of practice (8th ed.). (2021). *Journal of Infusion Nursing, 44*(Suppl. 1), S123–S125. (Level VII)

39 The Joint Commission. (2021). Standard RC.01.03.01. *Comprehensive accreditation manual for hospitals.* Oakbrook Terrace, IL: The Joint Commission. (Level VII)

40 Centers for Medicare and Medicaid Services, Department of Health and Human Services. (2020). Condition of participation: Medical record services. 42 C.F.R. § 482.24(b).

41 Accreditation Association for Hospitals and Health Systems. (2020). Standard 10.00.03. *Healthcare Facilities Accreditation Program: Accreditation requirements for acute care hospitals.* Chicago, IL: Accreditation Association for Hospitals and Health Systems. (Level VII)

42 DNV GL-Healthcare USA, Inc. (2020). MR.2.SR.1. *NIAHO® accreditation requirements, interpretive guidelines and surveyor guidance—revision 20.0.* Milford, OH: DNV GL-Healthcare USA, Inc. (Level VII)

43 Standard 10. Documentation in the health record. Infusion therapy standards of practice (8th ed.). (2021). *Journal of Infusion Nursing, 44*(Suppl. 1), S39–S42. (Level VII)

44 Standard 50. Infection. Infusion therapy standards of practice (8th ed.). (2021). *Journal of Infusion Nursing, 44*(Suppl. 1), S153–S157. (Level VII)

45 Standard 52. Air embolism. Infusion therapy standards of practice (8th ed.). (2021). *Journal of Infusion Nursing, 44*(Suppl. 1), S160–S161. (Level VII)

WALKER USE TRAINING

A walker—an assistive device that consists of a metal frame with handgrips and four legs— supports the patient on three sides, with the fourth side remaining open. Because this device provides greater stability and security than other ambulatory aids, it's recommended for the patient who has insufficient strength and balance to use crutches or a cane, or who is weak and requires frequent rest periods. A walker may help improve balance, increase mobility, reduce pain, and increase confidence.[1]

Attachments for standard walkers and modified walkers help meet special needs. For example, a walker may have a platform added to support an injured arm, brakes to assist in controlling descents, or a seat to allow for rest breaks.

Various types of walkers are available. A standard walker requires arm strength and balance, *because it must be lifted off the ground to advance forward.* This type of walker is the most stable and promotes a slow gait pattern. A bariatric or heavy-duty walker has extra strength and width to accommodate patients weighing more than 300 lb (136 kg) and up to 1,000 lb (453.5 kg). It's available as a rolling walker and with a support for a large abdominal pannus that would otherwise shift the patient's center of gravity and increase the risk of falls.[2,3] A rolling walker may have two or four wheels and may have a seat; it offers the patient a more fluid gait pattern as well as enhanced maneuverability with turns. This type of walker is appropriate only for patients with intact cognition *because of the increased risk of falls.* A walker with a seat offers instantly available seating for patients with poor endurance or cardiopulmonary disease. A platform walker has one or two platforms attached to the frame of the walker for a patient who can't bear weight directly on hand, wrist, or forearm because of pain, upper extremity weight-bearing limitations, or both. This type of walker is also a rolling walker, *because a patient with concurrent upper extremity limitations is typically unable to lift and advance a standard walker.* A reciprocal walker is used by a patient with very weak arms or impaired balance; it allows one side to be advanced ahead of the other. A stair walker has an extra set of handles extending toward the patient on the open side to allow for use on stairs.

Because research shows that 30% to 50% of patients stop using their assistive device soon after receiving it, selection of the appropriate device and thorough instruction on its benefits and use become even more important to effectively increase mobility and reduce disability.[1]

Equipment

Walker ■ nonskid shoes or slippers ■ Optional: platform, wheel attachments.

Preparation of equipment

Obtain the appropriate walker with the advice of a physical therapist, and ensure that it has been cleaned and disinfected before patient use.[4] Adjust the walker to the patient's height. The top of the walker should align with the inside crease of the patient's wrist; elbows should be flexed at a 15- to 30-degree angle when standing comfortably within the walker with hands on the grips. To adjust the walker height, turn the walker upside down and change the leg length by pushing in the button on each shaft, and release it when the leg is in the desired position. Make sure the walker is level before the patient attempts to use it.

Inspect the walker for defects. If the walker is defective, remove it from patient use, label it as defective, and report the defect as directed by your facility.

Implementation

■ Gather and prepare the necessary equipment and supplies.
■ Review the patient's medical record for appropriateness of treatment, including history of falls and current fall risk.[5,6,7]
■ Verify the practitioner's order, if needed.[5]
■ Perform hand hygiene.[8,9,10,11,12,13]
■ Confirm the patient's identity using at least two patient identifiers.[14]
■ Provide privacy.[15,16,17,18]
■ Explain the procedure to the patient and family (if appropriate) according to their individual communication and learning needs *to increase their understanding, allay their fears, and enhance cooperation.*[19]
■ Make sure the patient is wearing nonskid shoes or slippers.
■ Help the patient stand within the walker, and instruct the patient to hold the hand grips firmly and equally *to help stabilize the walker and promote safety.* Make sure that the patient is standing as upright as possible. Stand behind the patient, closer to the involved leg.
■ If the patient has equal strength in both legs, instruct the patient to advance the walker 6" to 8" (15 to 20 cm) and to step forward with either leg.

■ If the patient has one-sided leg weakness, tell the patient to advance the walker 6" to 8" (15 to 20 cm), and to step forward with the involved leg and follow with the uninvolved leg, supporting the weight on the arms. Encourage the patient to take equal strides.
■ If the patient is using a reciprocal walker, teach the two-point or four-point gait. For a two-point gate, instruct the patient to stand with the weight evenly distributed between the legs and the walker. Stand behind the patient, slightly to one side. Tell the patient to simultaneously advance the walker's right side and the left foot. Then have the patient advance the walker's left side and the right foot.
■ For a four-point gait, instruct the patient to evenly distribute the weight between the legs and the walker. Stand behind the patient and slightly to one side. Have the patient move the right side of the walker forward; then have the patient move the left foot forward. Next, instruct the patient to move the left side of the walker forward; then have the patient move the right foot forward.
■ Instruct the patient to step into the walker with each step, and not to walk behind it.
■ If the patient is using a wheeled or stair walker, reinforce the physical therapist's instructions. Stress the need for caution when using a stair walker.
■ Teach the patient how to use a walker safely to sit and stand. (See *Teaching safe use of a walker,* page 902.)
■ Observe as the patient returns the demonstration, assisting as necessary.
■ Perform hand hygiene.[8,9,10,11,12,13]
■ Document the procedure.[20,21,22,23]

Special considerations

■ If the patient starts to fall, support the hips and shoulders *to help maintain an upright position if possible.* If unsuccessful, ease the patient slowly to the closest surface—bed, floor, or chair—*to prevent injury.*[24]
■ Routinely observe a patient using the walker, and regularly assess the walker for appropriateness and maintenance, including checking proper height and the condition of the walker's legs, wheels, tips, and hand grips.[1] *The frequency of fall injuries in people using walkers suggests that they may not use these walking aids correctly.*[6]
■ Refer the patient to a home health agency for a home environment assessment, if needed, *because extrinsic (environmental) factors may increase the risk of falling.*[6,7]

Patient teaching

Focus patient teaching on the practitioner's and physical therapist's treatment plans, and include these safety instructions:[25]
■ Maintain an erect posture, and avoid looking down while using the walker.
■ Maintain the rubber tips of the walker, and replace them when they become worn.
■ Use firm chairs with armrests if possible.
■ Avoid pulling on the walker to stand.
■ Avoid stepping too far into the walker while walking.
■ Avoid leaning on the walker when getting up or attempting to sit down.
■ Feel for chair arms to redistribute weight when sitting down or standing up.
■ Avoid wet surfaces. If you're unable to avoid ambulating on a wet or slippery surface, take small steps.
■ Remove throw rugs, cords, furniture, or anything that may interfere with walking.
■ Avoid hurrying and taking large steps with turns.
■ Change direction slowly and carefully.

Complications

An improperly fitted walker can lead to falls and injury.[26]

Documentation

Record the type of walker and attachments used, the degree of guarding required, the distance walked, and the patient's tolerance of and proficiency with safe ambulation.[1] Document teaching provided to the patient and family (if applicable), their understanding of that teaching, and any need for follow-up teaching.

PATIENT TEACHING

TEACHING SAFE USE OF A WALKER

Sitting down

■ First, tell the patient to stand with the back of the stronger leg against the front of the chair, the weaker leg slightly off the floor, and the walker directly in front.

■ Then tell the patient to grasp the armrests on the chair, one arm at a time, while supporting most of the weight on the stronger leg. (In the illustrations below, the patient has left leg weakness.)

■ Finally, tell the patient to lower into the chair and slide backward. Once seated, have the patient place the walker beside the chair.

Getting up

■ After bringing the walker to the front of the chair, tell the patient to slide forward in the chair. Have the patient place the back of the stronger leg against the seat and then advance the weaker leg.

■ Next, instruct the patient to place both hands on the chair's armrests and push to a standing position. Have the patient use the stronger leg and the opposite hand for support while grasping the walker's handgrip with the free hand.

■ Then have the patient grasp the free handgrip with the other hand.

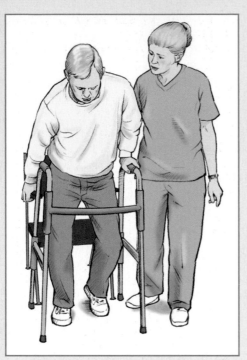

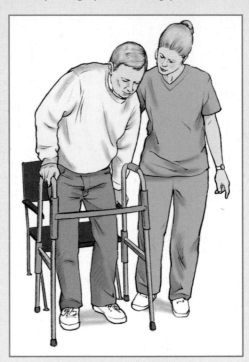

REFERENCES

1 Bradley, S. M., & Hernandez, C. R. (2011). Geriatric assistive devices. *American Family Physician, 84*(4), 405–411. https://www.aafp.org/afp/2011/0815/p405.html (Level VII)

2 VHA Center for Engineering & Occupational Safety and Health (CEOSH). (2015). Bariatric safe patient handling and mobility guidebook: A resource guide for care of persons of size. https://www.asphp.org/wp-content/uploads/2011/05/Baraiatrice-SPHM-guidebook-care-of-Person-of-Size.pdf

3 Lim, R. B. (2020). Hospital accreditation, accommodations, and staffing for care of the bariatric surgical patient. In: *UpToDate*, Jones, D. (Ed.).

4 Rutala, W. A., et al. (2008, revised 2019). Guideline for disinfection and sterilization in healthcare facilities, 2008. https://www.cdc.gov/infection-control/pdf/guidelines/disinfection-guidelines-H.pdf

5 The Joint Commission. (2021). Standard NPSG.09.02.01. *Comprehensive accreditation manual for hospitals.* Oakbrook Terrace, IL: The Joint Commission. (Level VII)

6 Stevens, J. A., et al. (2009). Unintentional fall injuries associated with walkers and canes in older adults treated in U.S. emergency departments. *Journal of the American Geriatrics Society, 57*, 1464–1469. (Level IV)

7 Panel on Prevention of Falls in Older Persons, American Geriatrics Society and British Geriatrics Society. (2011). Summary of the updated American Geriatrics Society/British Geriatrics Society clinical practice guideline for prevention of falls in older persons. *Journal of the American Geriatrics Society, 59*, 148–157. (Level VII)

8 The Joint Commission. (2021). Standard NPSG.07.01.01. *Comprehensive accreditation manual for hospitals.* Oakbrook Terrace, IL: The Joint Commission. (Level VII)

9 Centers for Disease Control and Prevention. (2002). Guideline for hand hygiene in health-care settings: Recommendations of the Healthcare Infection Control Practices Advisory Committee and the HICPAC/SHEA/APIC/IDSA Hand Hygiene Task Force. *MMWR Recommendations and Reports, 51*(RR-16), 1–45. https://www.cdc.gov/mmwr/pdf/rr/rr5116.pdf (Level II)

10 World Health Organization. (2009). WHO guidelines on hand hygiene in health care: First global patient safety challenge, clean care is safer care. https://apps.who.int/iris/bitstream/handle/10665/44102/9789241597906_eng.pdf?sequence=1 (Level IV)

11 Accreditation Association for Hospitals and Health Systems. (2020). Standard 07.01.21. *Healthcare Facilities Accreditation Program: Accreditation requirements for acute care hospitals.* Chicago, IL: Accreditation Association for Hospitals and Health Systems. (Level VII)

12 Centers for Medicare and Medicaid Services, Department of Health and Human Services. (2020). Condition of participation: Infection control. 42 C.F.R. § 482.42.

13 DNV GL-Healthcare USA, Inc. (2020). IC.1.SR.1. *NIAHO® accreditation requirements, interpretive guidelines and surveyor guidance—revision 20.0.* Milford, OH: DNV GL-Healthcare USA, Inc. (Level VII)

14 The Joint Commission. (2021). Standard NPSG.01.01.01. *Comprehensive accreditation manual for hospitals.* Oakbrook Terrace, IL: The Joint Commission. (Level VII)

15 DNV GL-Healthcare USA, Inc. (2020). PR.1.SR.5. *NIAHO® accreditation requirements, interpretive guidelines and surveyor guidance—revision 20.0.* Milford, OH: DNV GL-Healthcare USA, Inc. (Level VII)

16 Centers for Medicare and Medicaid Services, Department of Health and Human Services. (2020). Condition of participation: Patient's rights. 42 C.F.R. § 482.13(c)(1).

17 Accreditation Association for Hospitals and Health Systems. (2020). Standard 15.01.16. *Healthcare Facilities Accreditation Program: Accreditation requirements for acute care hospitals.* Chicago, IL: Accreditation Association for Hospitals and Health Systems. (Level VII)

18 The Joint Commission. (2021). Standard RI.01.01.01. *Comprehensive accreditation manual for hospitals.* Oakbrook Terrace, IL: The Joint Commission. (Level VII)

19 The Joint Commission. (2021). Standard PC.02.01.21. *Comprehensive accreditation manual for hospitals.* Oakbrook Terrace, IL: The Joint Commission. (Level VII)

20 The Joint Commission. (2021). Standard RC.01.03.01. *Comprehensive accreditation manual for hospitals.* Oakbrook Terrace, IL: The Joint Commission. (Level VII)

21 Accreditation Association for Hospitals and Health Systems. (2020). Standard 10.00.03. *Healthcare Facilities Accreditation Program: Accreditation requirements for acute care hospitals.* Chicago, IL: Accreditation Association for Hospitals and Health Systems. (Level VII)

22 Centers for Medicare and Medicaid Services, Department of Health and Human Services. (2020). Condition of participation: Medical record services. 42 C.F.R. § 482.24(b).

23 DNV GL-Healthcare USA, Inc. (2020). MR.2.SR.1. *NIAHO® accreditation requirements, interpretive guidelines and surveyor guidance—revision 20.0.* Milford, OH: DNV GL-Healthcare USA, Inc. (Level VII)

24 Craven, R. F., et al. (2021). *Fundamentals of nursing: Concepts and competencies for practice.* (9th ed.). Philadelphia, PA: Wolters Kluwer.

25 American Academy of Orthopaedic Surgeons. (2015). How to use crutches, canes, and walkers. https://orthoinfo.aaos.org/en/recovery/how-to-use-crutches-canes-and-walkers (Level VII)

26 Luz, C., et al. (2017). Do canes or walkers make any difference? Nonuse and fall injuries. *The Gerontologist, 57*(2), 211–218. https://academic.oup.com/gerontologist/article/57/2/211/2631943 (Level IV)

WATER INTOXICATION ASSESSMENT

Water intoxication occurs when the body's water and sodium levels become imbalanced as a result of excessive water intake that's accompanied by inadequate sodium intake.[1] Resulting in severe hyponatremia, this imbalance allows more water to enter the cells, causing them to swell and place excess pressure on the body's organs, especially the brain.

Excess water intake leading to water intoxication may be seen in competitive athletes, especially runners, and in users of 3,4-methylenedioxymethamphetamine (also known as ecstasy).[1,2,3] In patients with chronic psychiatric disorders, water intoxication may result from compulsive water drinking, also known as *psychogenic polydipsia* or *primary polydipsia*.[2,4] Although the cause of psychogenic polydipsia is unknown, it is thought that a central defect in thirst regulation may be a significant component.[2] The condition may be related to the interaction of several factors, including delusions about fluid intake, adverse effects of medications (such as dry mouth), and hyperactivity of the hypothalamic thirst centers.[2,4]

Water intoxication typically produces no signs and symptoms in its early stages; however, over time, it causes neurologic, GI, cardiac, behavioral, and cognitive changes.[1] The signs and symptoms of water intoxication are commonly mistaken for those of alcohol intoxication, and behavioral changes are commonly attributed to the patient's psychiatric diagnosis. (See *Signs and symptoms of water intoxication.*)

Early detection of water intoxication is crucial to prevent seizures, coma, and death, which may occur with severe hyponatremia when serum sodium concentration drops below 120 mmol/L.[5]

Equipment

Vital signs monitoring equipment ▪ scale ▪ graduated urine collection container ▪ venipuncture supplies ▪ Optional: gloves, IV infusion equipment and prescribed fluids, prescribed medications.

Implementation

▪ Review the patient's medical history, psychiatric diagnosis, and therapeutic regimen.
▪ Perform hand hygiene.[6,7,8,9,10,11]
▪ Confirm the patient's identity using at least two patient identifiers.[12]
▪ Provide privacy.[13,14,15,16]

Signs and symptoms of water intoxication

These signs and symptoms of water intoxication may occur over time.

Neurologic
▪ Headache
▪ Vertigo
▪ Drowsiness
▪ Blurred vision
▪ Weakness
▪ Tremors
▪ Lethargy
▪ Seizures

GI
▪ Nausea
▪ Repeated vomiting

Cardiac
▪ Hypotension
▪ Tachycardia
▪ Cardiac arrhythmias
▪ Heart failure

Behavioral and cognitive
▪ Restlessness
▪ Agitation
▪ Disorientation
▪ Confusion
▪ Delirium

Other
▪ Rapid breathing
▪ Decreased urination
▪ Sudden weight gain
▪ Metabolic abnormalities
▪ Muscle cramps[1]

Calculating maintenance fluid requirements

The formula below helps you calculate the maintenance fluid requirements for your patient:

(1,500 mL for the first 20 kg) + (20 mL for each kg over 20 kg)

For example, if you have a patient who weighs 75 kg, use the formula as follows:

1,500 mL + (20 mL × 55) = 1,500 + 1,100 = 2,600 mL of fluid per day.

▪ Explain the procedure to the patient and family (if appropriate) according to their individual communication and learning needs *to increase their understanding, allay their fears, and enhance cooperation.*[17]
▪ Ask the patient and family (if appropriate) to describe any signs or symptoms the patient has experienced *to help identify signs and symptoms that would indicate water intoxication.* Ask them to quantify the patient's water intake, if able.
NURSING ALERT Be aware that patients with psychiatric disorders may not recognize the signs and symptoms of water intoxication or may not admit to having them.
▪ Assess the patient for signs and symptoms of water intoxication.
▪ Obtain the patient's vital signs.
▪ Weigh the patient in kilograms on the appropriate scale.[18]
▪ Calculate the patient's estimated total daily fluid requirement based on the patient's body weight *to assess for excess water intake.* (See *Calculating maintenance fluid requirements.*)
▪ Perform hand hygiene.[6,7,8,9,10,11]
▪ Put on gloves *to comply with standard precautions.*[19,20,21]
▪ Perform a venipuncture *to obtain baseline and serial serum sodium levels,* as ordered. Notify the practitioner of critical test results within your facility's established time frame *so that the patient can be treated promptly.*
▪ Verify the practitioner's treatment orders based on your assessment findings.
▪ Provide interventions (which may include IV administration of a hypertonic saline solution) and administer medications (such as cloZAPine or an oral vasopressin antagonist), as ordered, following safe medication administration practices. Treatment may also include discontinuing contributing medications.
▪ Monitor the patient's water intake *to prevent self-induced water intoxication.*
▪ Measure the patient's urine output hourly or as ordered. Immediately report an output of less than 30 mL/hour to the patient's practitioner.

■ Monitor the patient, using one-to-one safety precautions as necessary, *to decrease excessive water intake.*

■ Provide alternative activities *to redirect the patient from drinking excessive amounts of water while awake.*

■ Continue to monitor the patient's mental status, behavior, level of consciousness, weight, vital signs, and serum sodium levels.

■ Remove and discard your gloves, if worn.[19]

■ Perform hand hygiene.[6,7,8,9,10,11]

■ Document the procedure.[22,23,24,25]

Special considerations

■ If the patient has severe water intoxication, the practitioner may order IV furosemide *to promote diuresis.*[1]

Patient teaching

Teach the patient and family about the dangers related to excess water intake. Provide suggestions on ways for the family to redirect the patient during waking hours. If the patient demonstrates a willingness to cooperate with restrictions, suggest alternative behaviors when the patient has the urge to drink excessively.

Provide the patient and family with the patient's estimated total daily fluid requirement based on body weight *to ensure that the patient is adequately hydrated.* Review the signs and symptoms of water intoxication with family members, and instruct them to call the practitioner or seek medical attention immediately if the patient develops them.

Complications

Untreated or undiagnosed water intoxication can lead to rhabdomyolysis, seizures, coma, and death.[4] Too-rapid correction of hyponatremia may lead to osmotic demyelination syndrome, a severe and sometimes irreversible neurologic disorder.[1]

Documentation

Record your assessment findings and the patient's vital signs, serum sodium levels, and weight in the patient's medical record. Also record all signs and symptoms of water intoxication, prescribed interventions, and the patient's response to those interventions. Document the patient's estimated total daily fluid requirements and the efforts made to maintain this amount. Record intake and output. Document teaching provided to the patient and family (if applicable), their understanding of that teaching, and any need for follow-up teaching.

REFERENCES

1 Sterns, R. H. (2020). Diagnostic evaluation of adults with hyponatremia. In: *UpToDate*, Emmett, M. (Ed.).

2 Sterns, R. H. (2020). Causes of hypotonic hyponatremia in adults. In: *UpToDate*, Emmett, M. (Ed.).

3 Siegel, A. J. (2015). Fatal water intoxication and cardiac arrest in runners during marathons: Prevention and treatment based on validated clinical paradigms. *American Journal of Medicine, 128*(10), 1070–1075.https://www.amjmed.com/article/S0002-9343(15)00353-8/fulltext (Level VII)

4 Fernando, S., et al. (2019). A compulsive act of excess water intake leading to hyponatremia and rhabdomyolysis: A case report. *International Journal of Emergency Medicine, 12,* 34. https://intjem.biomedcentral.com/articles/10.1186/s12245-019-0255-6

5 Braun, M. M., et al. (2015). Diagnosis and management of sodium disorders: Hyponatremia and hypernatremia. *American Family Physician, 91*(5), 299–307 https://www.aafp.org/afp/2015/0301/p299.html (Level VII)

6 The Joint Commission. (2021). Standard NPSG.07.01.01. *Comprehensive accreditation manual for hospitals.* Oakbrook Terrace, IL: The Joint Commission. (Level VII)

7 Centers for Disease Control and Prevention. (2002). Guideline for hand hygiene in health-care settings: Recommendations of the Healthcare Infection Control Practices Advisory Committee and the HICPAC/SHEA/APIC/IDSA Hand Hygiene Task Force. *MMWR Recommendations and Reports, 51*(RR-16), 1–45. https://www.cdc.gov/mmwr/pdf/rr/rr5116.pdf (Level II)

8 World Health Organization. (2009). WHO guidelines on hand hygiene in health care: First global patient safety challenge,

clean care is safer care. https://apps.who.int/iris/bitstream/handle/10665/44102/9789241597906_eng.pdf?sequence=1 (Level IV)

9 Centers for Medicare and Medicaid Services, Department of Health and Human Services. (2020). Condition of participation: Infection control. 42 C.F.R. § 482.42.

10 Accreditation Association for Hospitals and Health Systems. (2020). Standard 07.01.21. *Healthcare Facilities Accreditation Program: Accreditation requirements for acute care hospitals.* Chicago, IL: Accreditation Association for Hospitals and Health Systems. (Level VII)

11 DNV GL-Healthcare USA, Inc. (2020). IC.1.SR.1. *NIAHO® accreditation requirements, interpretive guidelines and surveyor guidance—revision 20.0.* Milford, OH: DNV GL-Healthcare USA, Inc. (Level VII)

12 The Joint Commission. (2021). Standard NPSG.01.01.01. *Comprehensive accreditation manual for hospitals.* Oakbrook Terrace, IL: The Joint Commission. (Level VII)

13 DNV GL-Healthcare USA, Inc. (2020). PR.2.SR.5. *NIAHO® accreditation requirements, interpretive guidelines and surveyor guidance—revision 20.0.* Milford, OH: DNV GL-Healthcare USA, Inc. (Level VII)

14 Centers for Medicare and Medicaid Services, Department of Health and Human Services. (2020). Condition of participation: Patient's rights. 42 C.F.R. § 482.13(c)(1).

15 Accreditation Association for Hospitals and Health Systems. (2020). Standard 15.01.16. *Healthcare Facilities Accreditation Program: Accreditation requirements for acute care hospitals.* Chicago, IL: Accreditation Association for Hospitals and Health Systems. (Level VII)

16 The Joint Commission. (2021). Standard RI.01.01.01. *Comprehensive accreditation manual for hospitals.* Oakbrook Terrace, IL: The Joint Commission. (Level VII)

17 The Joint Commission. (2021). Standard PC.02.01.21. *Comprehensive accreditation manual for hospitals.* Oakbrook Terrace, IL: The Joint Commission. (Level VII)

18 Institute for Safe Medication Practices. (2020). 2020-2021 targeted medication safety best practices for hospitals. https://www.ismp.org/sites/default/files/attachments/2020-02/2020-2021%20TMSBP-%20FINAL_1.pdf

19 Occupational Safety and Health Administration. (2012). Bloodborne pathogens, standard number 1910.1030. https://www.osha.gov/pls/oshaweb/owadisp.show_document?p_id=10051&p_table=STANDARDS (Level VII)

20 Siegel, J. D., et al. (2007, revised 2019). 2007 guideline for isolation precautions: Preventing transmission of infectious agents in healthcare settings. https://www.cdc.gov/infectioncontrol/pdf/guidelines/isolation-guidelines-H.pdf (Level II)

21 Accreditation Association for Hospitals and Health Systems. (2020). Standard 07.01.10. *Healthcare Facilities Accreditation Program: Accreditation requirements for acute care hospitals.* Chicago, IL: Accreditation Association for Hospitals and Health Systems. (Level VII)

22 Accreditation Association for Hospitals and Health Systems. (2020). Standard 10.00.03. *Healthcare Facilities Accreditation Program: Accreditation requirements for acute care hospitals.* Chicago, IL: Accreditation Association for Hospitals and Health Systems. (Level VII)

23 Centers for Medicare and Medicaid Services, Department of Health and Human Services. (2020). Condition of participation: Medical record services. 42 C.F.R. § 482.24(b).

24 DNV GL-Healthcare USA, Inc. (2020). MR.2.SR.1. *NIAHO® accreditation requirements, interpretive guidelines and surveyor guidance—revision 20.0.* Milford, OH: DNV GL-Healthcare USA, Inc. (Level VII)

25 The Joint Commission. (2021). Standard RC.01.03.01. *Comprehensive accreditation manual for hospitals.* Oakbrook Terrace, IL: The Joint Commission. (Level VII)

WEANING A PATIENT FROM A VENTILATOR

Successful weaning from a ventilator depends on the patient's ability to breathe independently, which means that the patient must have a spontaneous respiratory effort for effective gas exchange, a stable cardiovascular system, and sufficient respiratory muscle strength and level of consciousness for weaning.

Weaning entails gradually reducing ventilator support until the patient can be removed from mechanical ventilation and successfully extubated. As soon as the patient's condition allows, sedation should be reduced so that the multidisciplinary team can adequately assess the patient's readiness to wean. The team should then plan to use either a facility-approved weaning protocol or an individualized weaning plan.[1]

Weaning should be initiated as soon as possible, because ventilator use exceeding 24 hours increases the patient's risk of developing such complications as ventilator-associated pneumonia, ventilator induced lung injury, pulmonary barotrauma, airway injury, GI bleeding, venous thromboembolism, sinusitis, and increased mortality.[1,2] Common methods for weaning a patient from ventilatory support include:
- spontaneous breathing trials using the ventilator's continuous positive airway pressure mode or a T-tube (alternating with mechanical ventilation)
- synchronized intermittent mandatory ventilation
- pressure support ventilation (PSV).[3]

Regardless of the approach used, all multidisciplinary team members who are involved with weaning the patient from the ventilator must understand the process and the schedule, and be aware of the measures of success or failure appropriate to that approach. Before weaning, you should assess the patient's readiness to wean, which is usually determined by spontaneous breathing trials—the most widely accepted tool for such assessments.[4,5] Weaning is indicated for all patients who are determined to be ready to wean. It's contraindicated for those who are determined to be unready to wean, as well as those for whom weaning would be considered futile, such as in the presence of irreversible disease.[6]

Equipment

Ventilator ■ alternative oxygen delivery system ■ weaning protocol (practitioner-ordered or facility-approved) ■ pulse oximeter and probe ■ stethoscope ■ vital signs monitoring equipment ■ cardiac monitor ■ disinfectant pad ■ gloves ■ suction equipment ■ emergency equipment (code cart with emergency medication, defibrillator, handheld resuscitation bag with mask, intubation equipment) ■ Optional: gown, mask and goggles or mask with face shield, capnography equipment, arterial blood gas sampling equipment.

Preparation of equipment

Inspect all equipment and supplies. If a product is expired, is defective, or has compromised integrity, remove it from patient use, label it as expired or defective, and report the expiration or defect as directed by your facility. Make sure that the alternative oxygen delivery system, suction equipment, and emergency equipment are readily available and functioning properly.

Implementation

- Verify the practitioner's order.
- Gather and prepare the necessary equipment and supplies.
- Perform hand hygiene.[7,8,9,10,11,12]
- Put on gloves and other personal protective equipment as needed.[13,14,15]
- Confirm the patient's identity using at least two patient identifiers.[16]
- Provide privacy.[17,18,19,20]
- In collaboration with the respiratory therapist, initiate a spontaneous awakening trial. Interrupt the patient's sedative infusion according to the practitioner's order or your facility-approved weaning protocol.[21,22]
- Explain the procedure to the patient and family (if appropriate) according to their individual communication and learning needs *to increase their understanding, allay their fears, and enhance cooperation.*[23]
- Assure the patient that you'll provide coaching through the weaning process.
- Raise the patient's bed to waist level before providing care *to prevent caregiver back strain.*[24]
- Perform hand hygiene.[7,8,9,10,11,12]
- Make sure that the patient is attached to a cardiac monitor, as ordered. Make sure that the alarm limits are set appropriately for the patient's current condition, and that the alarms are turned on, functioning properly, and audible to staff.[25,26,27,28]
- Perform a complete physical assessment *to evaluate patient readiness*, and discuss your results during multidisciplinary rounds.[6] (See *Weaning readiness criteria.*)
- In collaboration with a respiratory therapist, if the patient passes the awakening trial, institute a spontaneous breathing trial (SBT), as ordered

or according to your facility's protocol (usually 5 to 10 minutes). *After a patient is deemed ready to wean, the best method to assess whether the patient can breathe independently is to perform an SBT.*[6] The evidence suggests that AN SBT with pressure augmentation of 5 to 8 cm H_2O is more likely to be successful than an SBT performed without pressure augmentation.[29]
- Instruct the patient to breath normally.[1]
- Assess the patient's vital signs, oxygenation, and mental status.[1]
- Monitor for findings associated with weaning intolerance: respiratory rate greater than 35 breaths/minute; arterial pH less than 7.32; oxygen saturation level by pulse oximetry less than 90%; end-tidal carbon dioxide increased by more than 10 mm Hg; heart rate greater than 140 beats/minute or a 20% increase over baseline; increased respiratory effort; systolic blood pressure greater than 180 mm Hg, diastolic blood pressure greater than 90 mm Hg, or hypotension; anxiety; and marked diaphoresis.[30,31]
- If the patient doesn't tolerate the SBT, if the cardiac monitor reveals a cardiac arrhythmia, or if the patient develops chest pain, immediately return the patient to resting ventilator settings; then monitor the patient's vital signs *to make sure that they return to baseline*, and notify the practitioner.
- Reassure the patient that setbacks are common, and encourage the patient to rest. Explain that the patient will have another SBT the next day if the patient meets the readiness criteria.[1]
- If the patient tolerates the SBT, follow your facility's weaning protocol (or the practitioner's order), or continue the SBT for up to 2 hours[6] (1 hour is usually sufficient)[1] and then return to resting ventilator settings.[1] (See *After weaning.*)

Weaning readiness criteria

Criteria to consider when evaluating the patient's readiness to wean:
- Resolved or improved condition that no longer requires ventilation
- Adequate natural airway or a functioning tracheostomy
- Ability to cough and mobilize secretions
- Successful withdrawal of sedation
- Clear or clearing chest x-ray
- Arterial oxygen saturation greater than 92% or partial pressure of oxygen/fraction of inspired oxygen (PaO_2/FIO_2) ratio greater than or equal to 150 mm Hg (19.75 kPa) on FIO_2 less than or equal to 40% with positive end-expiratory pressure less than or equal to 5 cm H_2O (0.49 kPa)[2] (PaO_2/FIO_2 ratio of greater than or equal to 120 mm Hg for patients with chronic hypoxemia)[2]
- Arterial blood gas values within normal limits or at patient's baseline with pH greater than 7.25[2]
- Hemoglobin greater than or equal to 7 g/dL (70g/L)[2]
- Hemodynamic stability, without myocardial ischemia, adequate resuscitation, and no need for vasoactive support, or requires low-dose vasoactive support[2]
- Core body temperature greater than 96.8° F (36° C) and less than 102.2° F (39° C)
- Absence of infection, acid-base or electrolyte imbalance, hyperglycemia, arrhythmias, kidney failure, anemia, or excessive fatigue
- Adequate pain management with minimal use of pain medication
- Awake and alert or easily arousable[2]

After weaning

After being weaned, the patient should demonstrate:
- respiratory rate less than 24 breaths/minute
- heart rate and blood pressure within 15% of personal baseline
- tidal volume of 3 to 5 mL/kg
- arterial pH greater than 7.35
- partial pressure of arterial oxygen maintained at greater than 60 mm Hg (7.9 kPa)
- partial pressure of arterial carbon dioxide maintained at less than 45 mm Hg (5.9 kPa)
- oxygen saturation level maintained at greater than 90%
- absence of cardiac arrhythmias
- absence of accessory muscle use.[1]

The patient may require supplemental oxygen to achieve these goals.

- Assess the patient's vital signs, cardiac status, breath sounds, and oxygen saturation level by pulse oximetry frequently throughout the weaning process.[1] Notify the practitioner if you note signs of weaning intolerance.[6]
- Return the bed to the lowest level *to prevent falls and maintain patient safety*.[32]
- Remove and discard your gloves and other personal protective equipment.[15]
- Perform hand hygiene.[7,8,9,10,11,12]
- Clean and disinfect your stethoscope using a disinfectant pad.[33,34]
- Perform hand hygiene.[7,8,9,10,11,12]
- Document the procedure.[35,36,37,38]

Special considerations

- Be aware that capnography may be useful during ventilator management and weaning.[39]
- Make sure the patient gets adequate rest and sleep, *because altered sleep may prolong weaning from the ventilator*. Provide subdued lighting, safely muffle equipment noises, and restrict staff access to the area *to promote quiet during rest periods*.

Complications

Hypoxia may occur if the patient isn't ready to breathe independently or tolerate decreased ventilator settings.

Documentation

Record your assessment findings that determined the patient's readiness to wean. Record the results after each weaning episode, including specific parameters and the patient's tolerance of the weaning trial. List all complications, unexpected outcomes, the practitioner notified of complications and the date and time of notification, the prescribed interventions, and the patient's response to those interventions. If the patient was receiving PSV or using a T-piece or tracheostomy collar, note the duration of spontaneous breathing and the patient's ability to maintain the weaning schedule. If intermittent mandatory ventilation was used, with or without PSV, record the control breath rate, the time of each breath reduction, and the rate of spontaneous respirations. Also document any teaching provided to the patient and family (if appropriate), their understanding of that teaching, and any need for follow-up teaching.

REFERENCES

1 Wiegand, D. L. (Ed.). (2017). *AACN procedure manual for high acuity, progressive, and critical care* (7th ed.). St. Louis, MO: Elsevier.

2 Epstein, S. K. (2021). Weaning from mechanical ventilation: Readiness testing. In: *UpToDate*, Parsons, P. E. (Ed.).

3 Hetland, B., et al. (2018). Mechanical ventilation weaning: An evidence-based review. *Nursing Critical Care, 13*(6), 5–16. https://journals.lww.com/nursingcriticalcare/Fulltext/2018/11000/Mechanical_ventilation_weaning__An_evidence_based.2.aspx

4 Haas, C. F., & Loik, P. S. (2012). Ventilator discontinuation protocols. *Respiratory Care, 57*(10), 1649–1662. http://rc.rcjournal.com/content/57/10/1649

5 MacIntyre, N. R. (2013). The ventilator discontinuation process: An expanding evidence base. *Respiratory Care, 58*(6), 1074–1086. http://rc.rcjournal.com/content/58/6/1074

6 American College of Chest Physicians, et al. (2002). Evidence-based guidelines for weaning and discontinuing ventilatory support. *Respiratory Care, 47*(1), 69–90. https://www.aarc.org/wp-content/uploads/2014/08/ebgwdvscpg.pdf (Level VII)

7 Centers for Disease Control and Prevention. (2002). Guideline for hand hygiene in health-care settings: Recommendations of the Healthcare Infection Control Practices Advisory Committee and the HICPAC/SHEA/APIC/IDSA Hand Hygiene Task Force. *MMWR Recommendations and Reports, 51*(RR-16), 1–45. https://www.cdc.gov/mmwr/pdf/rr/rr5116.pdf (Level II)

8 The Joint Commission. (2021). Standard NPSG.07.01.01. *Comprehensive accreditation manual for hospitals*. Oakbrook Terrace, IL: The Joint Commission. (Level VII)

9 World Health Organization. (2009). WHO guidelines on hand hygiene in health care: First global patient safety challenge, clean care is safer care. https://apps.who.int/iris/bitstream/handle/10665/44102/9789241597906_eng.pdf (Level IV)

10 Accreditation Association for Hospitals and Health Systems. (2020). Standard 07.01.21. *Healthcare Facilities Accreditation Program: Accreditation requirements for acute care hospitals*. Chicago, IL: Accreditation Association for Hospitals and Health Systems. (Level VII)

11 Centers for Medicare and Medicaid Services, Department of Health and Human Services. (2020). Condition of participation: Infection control. 42 C.F.R. § 482.42.

12 DNV GL-Healthcare USA, Inc. (2020). IC.1.SR.1. *NIAHO® accreditation requirements, interpretive guidelines and surveyor guidance—revision 20.0*. Milford, OH: DNV GL-Healthcare USA, Inc. (Level VII)

13 Siegel, J. D., et al. (2007, revised 2019). 2007 guideline for isolation precautions: Preventing transmission of infectious agents in healthcare settings. https://www.cdc.gov/infectioncontrol/pdf/guidelines/isolation-guidelines-H.pdf (Level II)

14 Accreditation Association for Hospitals and Health Systems. (2020). Standard 07.01.10. *Healthcare Facilities Accreditation Program: Accreditation requirements for acute care hospitals*. Chicago, IL: Accreditation Association for Hospitals and Health Systems. (Level VII)

15 Occupational Safety and Health Administration. (2012). Bloodborne pathogens, standard number 1910.1030. https://www.osha.gov/pls/oshaweb/owadisp.show_document?p_id=10051&p_table=STANDARDS (Level VII)

16 The Joint Commission. (2021). Standard NPSG.01.01.01. *Comprehensive accreditation manual for hospitals*. Oakbrook Terrace, IL: The Joint Commission. (Level VII)

17 DNV GL-Healthcare USA, Inc. (2020). PR.2.SR.5. *NIAHO® accreditation requirements, interpretive guidelines and surveyor guidance—revision 20.0*. Milford, OH: DNV GL-Healthcare USA, Inc. (Level VII)

18 The Joint Commission. (2021). Standard RI.01.01.01. *Comprehensive accreditation manual for hospitals*. Oakbrook Terrace, IL: The Joint Commission. (Level VII)

19 Centers for Medicare and Medicaid Services, Department of Health and Human Services. (2020). Condition of participation: Patient's rights. 42 C.F.R. § 482.13(c)(1).

20 Accreditation Association for Hospitals and Health Systems. (2020). Standard 15.01.16. *Healthcare Facilities Accreditation Program: Accreditation requirements for acute care hospitals*. Chicago, IL: Accreditation Association for Hospitals and Health Systems. (Level VII)

21 Klompas, M., et al. (2014). Strategies to prevent ventilator-associated pneumonia in acute care hospitals: 2014 update. *Infection Control and Hospital Epidemiology, 35*(8), 915–936. https://www.jstor.org/stable/10.1086/677144#metadata_info_tab_contents (Level I)

22 Vanderbilt University. (2008). "Wake up and breathe" protocol: Spontaneous awakening trials (SATS) + spontaneous breathing trials (SBTs). https://www.mnhospitals.org/Portals/0/Documents/ptsafety/LEAPT%20Delirium/Vanderbilt%20Wake%20Up%20and%20Breath%20Protocol%20Flowsheet.pdf

23 The Joint Commission. (2021). Standard PC.02.01.21. *Comprehensive accreditation manual for hospitals*. Oakbrook Terrace, IL: The Joint Commission. (Level VII)

24 Waters, T. R., et al. (2009). Safe patient handling training for schools of nursing. [https://www.cdc.gov/niosh/docs/2009-127/pdfs/2009-127.pdf (Level VII)

25 American Association of Critical-Care Nurses. (2018). AACN practice alert: Managing alarms in acute care across the life span: Electrocardiography and pulse oximetry. https://www.aacn.org/clinical-resources/practice-alerts/managing-alarms-in-acute-care-across-the-life-span (Level VII)

26 Graham, K. C., & Cvach, M. (2010). Monitor alarm fatigue: Standardizing use of physiological monitors and decreasing nuisance alarms. *American Journal of Critical Care, 19*, 28–37.

27 The Joint Commission. (2021). Standard NPSG.06.01.01. *Comprehensive accreditation manual for hospitals*. Oakbrook Terrace, IL: The Joint Commission. (Level VII)

28 The Joint Commission. (2013). Sentinel event alert 50: Medical device alarm safety in hospitals. https://www.jointcommission.org/-/media/tjc/documents/resources/patient-safety-topics/sentinel-event/sea_50_alarms_4_26_16.pdf (Level VII)

29 Schmidt, G. A., et al. (2017). Official executive summary of the American Thoracic Society/American College of Chest Physicians clinical practice

guideline: Liberation from mechanical ventilation in critically ill adults. *American Journal of Respiratory Critical Care Medicine, 195*(1), 115–119. https://www.atsjournals.org/doi/full/10.1164/rccm.201610-2076ST#read cube-epdf (Level VII)

30 Amri, P., et al. (2016). Weaning the patient from the mechanical ventilator: A review article. *Archives of Critical Care Medicine, 1*(4), e8363.

31 Abdo, M., et al. (2014). Difficult weaning from mechanical ventilation in the pediatric ICU. *Ain-Shams Journal of Anaesthesiology, 7*(1), 76–79. http://www.asja.eg.net/article.asp?issn=1687-7934;year=2014;volume=7;issue=1;spage=76;epage=79;aulast=Abdo (Level IV)

32 Ganz, D. A., et al. (2013, reviewed 2021). *Preventing falls in hospitals: A toolkit for improving quality of care* (AHRQ Publication No. 13-0015-EF). Rockville, MD: Agency for Healthcare Research and Quality. https://www.ahrq.gov/professionals/systems/hospital/fallpxtoolkit/index.html (Level VII)

33 Rutala, W. A., et al. (2008, revised 2019). Guideline for disinfection and sterilization in healthcare facilities, 2008. https://www.cdc.gov/infection-control/pdf/guidelines/disinfection-guidelines-H.pdf (Level I)

34 Accreditation Association for Hospitals and Health Systems. (2020). Standard 07.02.03. *Healthcare Facilities Accreditation Program: Accreditation requirements for acute care hospitals.* Chicago, IL: Accreditation Association for Hospitals and Health Systems. (Level VII)

35 The Joint Commission. (2021). Standard RC.01.03.01. *Comprehensive accreditation manual for hospitals.* Oakbrook Terrace, IL: The Joint Commission. (Level VII)

36 Accreditation Association for Hospitals and Health Systems. (2020). Standard 10.00.03. *Healthcare Facilities Accreditation Program: Accreditation requirements for acute care hospitals.* Chicago, IL: Accreditation Association for Hospitals and Health Systems. (Level VII)

37 Centers for Medicare and Medicaid Services, Department of Health and Human Services. (2020). Condition of participation: Medical record services. 42 C.F.R. § 482.24(b).

38 DNV GL-Healthcare USA, Inc. (2020). MR.2.SR.1. *NIAHO® accreditation requirements, interpretive guidelines and surveyor guidance—revision 20.0.* Milford, OH: DNV GL-Healthcare USA, Inc. (Level VII)

39 Walsh, B. K., et al. (2011). AARC clinical practice guideline: Capnography/capnometry during mechanical ventilation: 2011. *Respiratory Care, 56*(4), 503–509. https://www.aarc.org/wp-content/uploads/2014/08/04.11.0503.pdf (Level VII)

WOUND DEHISCENCE AND EVISCERATION MANAGEMENT

Wound dehiscence and evisceration are most likely to occur 4 or 14 days after surgery, with a mean of 8 days.[1,2] This can be a surgical emergency and a potentially life-threatening event.[1] (See *Recognizing dehiscence and evisceration*.)

The World Union of Wound Healing Societies identifies three categories of factors that cause surgical wound dehiscence: technical issues, mechanical stress, and disrupted healing. Technical issues occur when the method of closure isn't strong enough to hold the edges of the wound together. This includes unravelling or slipping of suture knots, sutures placed too close to the edge of the incision, and sutures placed too far apart or under too much tension. Mechanical stress may include a sudden increase in intra-abdominal or intra-thoracic pressure from retching, vomiting, coughing, sneezing, or lifting heavy weights. It can also be caused by swelling of the tissue around the incision from a hematoma, a seroma, or an abscess. Disrupted healing can occur for many reasons and in any phase of healing. It may be related to wound infection, large initial wound size, or patient-related comorbidities. Major patient risk factors include obesity, diabetes, smoking, emergency or unusually long surgery, perioperative hypothermia, and age greater than 65. Additional risk factors are numerous, and include alcohol abuse, chronic obstructive pulmonary disease, male gender, peripheral vascular disease, long-term steroid use, and malnutrition.[2]

Equipment

Sterile towels ▪ sterile normal saline solution ▪ sterile irrigation set (including a basin, a solution container, and a 50- or 60-mL catheter-tip syringe) ▪ labels ▪ sterile abdominal dressings ▪ sterile, waterproof drape ▪ sterile gloves.

Recognizing dehiscence and evisceration

Although surgical wounds typically heal without incident, occasionally they don't heal, leading to wound dehiscence and possibly evisceration.

Wound dehiscence
In wound dehiscence, the edges of a wound fail to join, or they separate even after they seem to be healing normally (as shown below). Wound dehiscence can lead to evisceration.

Evisceration
With wound evisceration—an even more serious complication than dehiscence—a portion of the viscera (usually a bowel loop) protrudes through the surgical incision (as shown below). Evisceration can lead to peritonitis and septic shock.

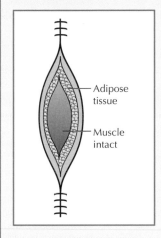

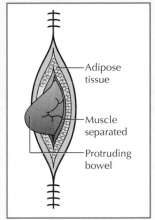

If the patient will return to the operating room (OR), be sure you also gather the following equipment: Prescribed preoperative medications ▪ preoperative checklist ▪ Optional: IV administration set, prescribed IV fluids, IV catheter insertion equipment, equipment for nasogastric (NG) tube intubation equipment, NG tube suction equipment.

Implementation

▪ Perform hand hygiene.[3,4,5,6,7,8]
▪ Confirm the patient's identity using at least two patient identifiers.[9]
▪ Provide privacy.[10,11,12,13]
▪ Reassure and support the patient *to ease the patient's anxiety*.[2] Instruct the patient to stay in bed. If possible, remain with the patient while someone else notifies the practitioner and collects the necessary equipment.
▪ Explain the procedure to the patient and family (if appropriate) according to their individual communication and learning needs *to increase their understanding, allay their fears, and enhance cooperation.*[14]
▪ Raise the bed to waist level before providing care *to prevent caregiver back strain.*[15]
▪ Perform hand hygiene.[3,4,5,6,7,8]
▪ Using sterile technique (see the "Sterile technique, basic" procedure), unfold a sterile towel *to create a sterile field.*
▪ Open the package containing the irrigation set, and place the basin, solution container, and 50- or 60-mL syringe on the sterile field.
▪ Pour sterile normal saline solution into the sterile basin.
▪ Label all solutions on and off the sterile field while maintaining the sterility of the sterile field *to provide information regarding the solutions they contain.*[16,17]
▪ Open the sterile abdominal dressings and place them on the sterile field.
▪ Perform hand hygiene.[3,4,5,6,7,8]
▪ Put on sterile gloves *to comply with standard precautions.*[18,19,20]
▪ Place the sterile abdominal dressings in the sterile basin *to saturate them with sterile normal saline solution.*
▪ Place the moistened sterile abdominal dressings over the exposed viscera and then cover the dressings with a sterile, waterproof drape *to retain the moisture.*[1]

- Remove and discard your gloves.[20]
- Perform hand hygiene.[3,4,5,6,7,8]
- Return the bed to the lowest position *to prevent falls and maintain the patient's safety.*[21]
- Monitor the patient's wound regularly, and moisten the dressings as needed to maintain moisture. To moisten the dressings, pour sterile normal saline solution into the irrigation solution container. Use the syringe to withdraw normal saline solution from the container; remove the waterproof drape from the dressings, and then irrigate the abdominal dressings gently using the syringe. Inspect the color of the viscera; if they appear dusky or black, notify the practitioner immediately. *With their blood supply interrupted, protruding viscera may become ischemic and necrotic.* Cover the dressings with the waterproof drape.
- Maintain the patient on bed rest in a semi-Fowler position with the knees flexed *to prevent injury and reduce stress on an abdominal incision.*
- Don't allow the patient to have anything by mouth, *to decrease the risk of aspiration during surgery.*
- Monitor the patient's vital signs frequently *to help in recognizing a change in the patient's condition promptly.*

Preparing the patient for return to the OR
- If required by your facility, confirm that written informed consent has been obtained and that the signed consent form is in the patient's medical record.[22,23,24,25]
- Conduct a preprocedure verification *to make sure that all relevant documentation, related information, and equipment are available and correctly identified to the patient's identifiers.*[26,27]
- Gather and prepare the necessary equipment and supplies.
- Perform hand hygiene.[3,4,5,6,7,8]
- Confirm the patient's identity using at least two patient identifiers.[9]
- Provide privacy.[10,11,12,13]
- Confirm that the patient has adequate IV access. Insert an IV catheter, if needed and ordered. Administer IV fluids if prescribed.
- Insert an NG tube if ordered. Connect the NG tube to continuous or low intermittent suction, as ordered.
- Administer preoperative medications, as ordered, following safe medication administration practices.[28,29,30,31]
- Complete a preoperative checklist as required by your facility.
- Continue to reassure the patient while you prepare the patient for surgery.[2]
- Ensure that the OR staff has been informed about the surgical procedure. Provide hand-off communication for the person who'll assume responsibility for care of the patient during surgery. Allow time for questions, as necessary, *to avoid miscommunications that may cause patient care errors during transitions of care.* As part of the hand-off process, allow time for the receiving staff member to trace each tubing and catheter from the patient to its point of origin; a standardized line reconciliation process should be used.[32,33]
- Perform hand hygiene.[3,4,5,6,7,8]
- Document the procedure.[34,35,36,37]

Special considerations
- Depending on the patient's condition, you may not perform some of these procedures at the bedside. For instance, NG intubation may make the patient gag or vomit, causing further evisceration. For this reason, the practitioner may choose to have the NG tube inserted in the OR with the patient under anesthesia.

Complications
The most common complication of wound dehiscence and evisceration management is infection, which can lead to septic shock. Additional complications are pain, organ injury (protruding viscera may become ischemic and necrotic), hypovolemic shock, and complications related to the surgical repair procedure.[1,2]

Documentation
Note the date and time that the wound problem occurred, the patient's activity preceding the wound problem, the patient's condition, the time when you notified the practitioner, and the name of the practitioner notified. Describe the appearance of the wound or eviscerated organ; the amount, color, consistency, and odor of any drainage; and any nursing actions taken. Record the patient's vital signs, the patient's response to the wound problem, and the practitioner's actions. If the patient returns to the operating room, complete the preoperative checklist used by your facility. Note the name and title of the person who received your hand-off communication. Document teaching provided to the patient and family (if applicable), their understanding of that teaching, and any need for follow-up teaching.

REFERENCES

1 Mizell, J. S. (2020). Complications of abdominal surgical incisions. In: *UpToDate*, Rosen, M. (Ed.).
2 Wounds International. (2018). World Union of Wound Healing Societies (WUWHS) Consensus Document: Surgical wound dehiscence: Improving prevention and outcomes. https://www.woundsinternational.com/resources/details/consensus-document-surgical-wound-dehiscence-improving-prevention-and-outcomes (Level VII)
3 Centers for Disease Control and Prevention. (2002). Guideline for hand hygiene in health-care settings: Recommendations of the Healthcare Infection Control Practices Advisory Committee and the HICPAC/SHEA/APIC/IDSA Hand Hygiene Task Force. *MMWR Recommendations and Reports, 51*(RR-16), 1–45. https://www.cdc.gov/mmwr/pdf/rr/rr5116.pdf (Level II)
4 World Health Organization. (2009). WHO guidelines on hand hygiene in health care: First global patient safety challenge, clean care is safer care. t https://apps.who.int/iris/bitstream/handle/10665/44102/9789241597906_eng.pdf?sequence=1 (Level IV)
5 The Joint Commission. (2021). Standard NPSG.07.01.01. *Comprehensive accreditation manual for hospitals*. Oakbrook Terrace, IL: The Joint Commission. (Level VII)
6 Accreditation Association for Hospitals and Health Systems. (2020). Standard 07.01.21. *Healthcare Facilities Accreditation Program: Accreditation requirements for acute care hospitals*. Chicago, IL: Accreditation Association for Hospitals and Health Systems. (Level VII)
7 Centers for Medicare and Medicaid Services, Department of Health and Human Services. (2020). Condition of participation: Infection control. 42 C.F.R. § 482.42.
8 DNV GL-Healthcare USA, Inc. (2020). IC.1.SR.1. *NIAHO® accreditation requirements, interpretive guidelines and surveyor guidance—revision 20.0.* Milford, OH: DNV GL-Healthcare USA, Inc. (Level VII)
9 The Joint Commission. (2021). Standard NPSG.01.01.01. *Comprehensive accreditation manual for hospitals*. Oakbrook Terrace, IL: The Joint Commission. (Level VII)
10 DNV GL-Healthcare USA, Inc. (2020). PR.2.SR.5. *NIAHO® accreditation requirements, interpretive guidelines and surveyor guidance—revision 20.0.* Milford, OH: DNV GL-Healthcare USA, Inc. (Level VII)
11 Centers for Medicare and Medicaid Services, Department of Health and Human Services. (2020). Condition of participation: Patient's rights. 42 C.F.R. § 482.13(c)(1).
12 Accreditation Association for Hospitals and Health Systems. (2020). Standard 15.01.16. *Healthcare Facilities Accreditation Program: Accreditation requirements for acute care hospitals*. Chicago, IL: Accreditation Association for Hospitals and Health Systems. (Level VII)
13 The Joint Commission. (2021). Standard RI.01.01.01. *Comprehensive accreditation manual for hospitals*. Oakbrook Terrace, IL: The Joint Commission. (Level VII)
14 The Joint Commission. (2021). Standard PC.02.01.21. *Comprehensive accreditation manual for hospitals*. Oakbrook Terrace, IL: The Joint Commission.
15 Waters, T. R., et al. (2009). Safe patient handling training for schools of nursing. https://www.cdc.gov/niosh/docs/2009-127/pdfs/2009-127.pdf (Level VII)
16 Accreditation Association for Hospitals and Health Systems. (2020). Standard 25.01.27. *Healthcare Facilities Accreditation Program: Accreditation requirements for acute care hospitals*. Chicago, IL: Accreditation Association for Hospitals and Health Systems. (Level VII)
17 The Joint Commission. (2021). Standard NPSG.03.04.01. *Comprehensive accreditation manual for hospitals*. Oakbrook Terrace, IL: The Joint Commission. (Level VII)
18 Siegel, J. D., et al. (2007, revised 2019). 2007 guideline for isolation precautions: Preventing transmission of infectious agents in healthcare

settings. https://www.cdc.gov/infectioncontrol/pdf/guidelines/isolation-guidelines-H.pdf (Level II)

19 Accreditation Association for Hospitals and Health Systems. (2020). Standard 07.01.10. *Healthcare Facilities Accreditation Program: Accreditation requirements for acute care hospitals.* Chicago, IL: Accreditation Association for Hospitals and Health Systems. (Level VII)

20 Occupational Safety and Health Administration. (2012). Bloodborne pathogens, standard number 1910.1030. https://www.osha.gov/pls/oshaweb/owadisp.show_document?p_id=10051&p_table=STANDARDS (Level VII)

21 Ganz, D. A., et al. (2013, reviewed 2021). *Preventing falls in hospitals: A toolkit for improving quality of care* (AHRQ Publication No. 13-0015-EF). Rockville, MD: Agency for Healthcare Research and Quality. https://www.ahrq.gov/professionals/systems/hospital/fallpxtoolkit/index.html (Level VII)

22 The Joint Commission. (2021). Standard RI.01.03.01. *Comprehensive accreditation manual for hospitals.* Oakbrook Terrace, IL: The Joint Commission. (Level VII)

23 Centers for Medicare and Medicaid Services, Department of Health and Human Services. (2020). Condition of participation: Patient's rights. 42 C.F.R. § 482.13(b)(2).

24 Accreditation Association for Hospitals and Health Systems. (2020). Standard 30.01.11. *Healthcare Facilities Accreditation Program: Accreditation requirements for acute care hospitals.* Chicago, IL: Accreditation Association for Hospitals and Health Systems. (Level VII)

25 DNV GL-Healthcare USA, Inc. (2020). PR.2.SR.3. *NIAHO® accreditation requirements, interpretive guidelines and surveyor guidance—revision 20.0.* Milford, OH: DNV GL-Healthcare USA, Inc. (Level VII)

26 The Joint Commission. (2021). Standard UP.01.01.01. *Comprehensive accreditation manual for hospitals.* Oakbrook Terrace, IL: The Joint Commission. (Level VII)

27 Accreditation Association for Hospitals and Health Systems. (2020). Standard 30.00.14. *Healthcare Facilities Accreditation Program: Accreditation requirements for acute care hospitals.* Chicago, IL: Accreditation Association for Hospitals and Health Systems. (Level VII)

28 Accreditation Association for Hospitals and Health Systems. (2020). Standard 16.01.03. *Healthcare Facilities Accreditation Program: Accreditation requirements for acute care hospitals.* Chicago, IL: Accreditation Association for Hospitals and Health Systems. (Level VII)

29 Centers for Medicare and Medicaid Services, Department of Health and Human Services. (2020). Condition of participation: Nursing services. 42 C.F.R. § 482.23(c).

30 The Joint Commission. (2021). Standard MM.06.01.01. *Comprehensive accreditation manual for hospitals.* Oakbrook Terrace, IL: The Joint Commission. (Level VII)

31 DNV GL-Healthcare USA, Inc. (2020). MM.1.SR.3. *NIAHO® accreditation requirements, interpretive guidelines and surveyor guidance—revision 20.0.* Milford, OH: DNV GL-Healthcare USA, Inc. (Level VII)

32 The Joint Commission. (2021). Standard PC.02.02.01. *Comprehensive accreditation manual for hospitals.* Oakbrook Terrace, IL: The Joint Commission. (Level VII)

33 The Joint Commission. (2014). Sentinel event alert 53: Managing risk during transition to new ISO tubing connector standards. https://www.jointcommission.org/-/media/tjc/documents/resources/patient-safety-topics/sentinel-event/sea_53_connectors_8_19_14_final.pdf (Level VII)

34 Accreditation Association for Hospitals and Health Systems. (2020). Standard 10.00.03. *Healthcare Facilities Accreditation Program: Accreditation requirements for acute care hospitals.* Chicago, IL: Accreditation Association for Hospitals and Health Systems. (Level VII)

35 Centers for Medicare and Medicaid Services, Department of Health and Human Services. (2020). Condition of participation: Medical record services. 42 C.F.R. § 482.24 (b).

36 DNV GL-Healthcare USA, Inc. (2020). MR.2.SR.1. *NIAHO® accreditation requirements: Interpretive guidelines & surveyor guidance—revision 20.0.* Milford, OH: DNV GL-Healthcare USA, Inc. (Level VII)

37 The Joint Commission. (2021). Standard RC.01.03.01. *Comprehensive accreditation manual for hospitals.* Oakbrook Terrace, IL: The Joint Commission. (Level VII)

WOUND IRRIGATION

Wound irrigation involves directing a steady flow of an irrigation solution across an open wound to remove debris and drainage from the wound. Wound irrigation can be performed using a catheter-tip syringe with a 19G angiocatheter or a commercial wound irrigation device. Irrigation pressure should be adequate to clean the surface of the wound without causing trauma to the wound bed; 5 to 15 psi (0.35 to 1.05 kg/cm²) generally is considered safe and sufficient for cleaning an open wound.[1,2]

After irrigation, open wounds usually are packed to absorb additional drainage. Follow standard precautions when irrigating a wound to prevent exposure to blood or body fluids.[3]

Equipment

Waterproof trash container ▪ emesis basin ▪ gloves ▪ goggles and mask or mask with face shield ▪ gown ▪ irrigation solution (normal saline solution or other prescribed wound cleanser) ▪ irrigation container (sterile or clean) ▪ sterile gauze pad ▪ sterile dressing ▪ wound irrigation device (35-mL catheter-tip syringe with 19G angiocatheter or commercial wound irrigation device)[2] ▪ skin-protectant wipe ▪ Optional: prescribed pain medication, wound packing material, fluid-impermeable pad.

Preparation of equipment

Inspect all equipment and supplies. If a product is expired, is defective, or has compromised integrity, remove it from patient use, label it as expired or defective, and report the expiration or defect as directed by your facility. Check the expiration date on each sterile package and inspect the packages for tears. Follow the manufacturer's recommendations and your facility's guidelines regarding the shelf life of solutions once they have been opened. Ensure that the irrigation solution is at room temperature.

Implementation

- Verify the practitioner's order.
- Gather and prepare the necessary equipment and supplies.
- Perform hand hygiene.[4,5,6,7,8,9]
- Confirm the patient's identity using at least two patient identifiers.[10]
- Provide privacy.[11,12,13,14]
- Explain the procedure to the patient and family (if appropriate) according to their individual communication and learning needs *to increase their understanding, allay their fears, and enhance cooperation.*[15]
- Screen and assess the patient's pain using facility-defined criteria that are consistent with the patient's age, condition, and ability to understand.[16]
- Treat the patient's pain as needed and ordered using nonpharmacologic or pharmacologic methods, or a combination of approaches.[16] Administer prescribed pain medication to the patient at least 20 minutes before wound irrigation, as needed and ordered, following safe medication administration practices, *because dressing changes may be painful.*[17,18,19,20] Base the treatment plan on evidence-based practices and the patient's clinical condition, medical history, and pain management goals.[16]
- Encourage the patient to request a time-out during the procedure if the patient experiences pain.
- Raise the bed to waist level before providing care *to prevent caregiver back strain.*[21]
- Perform hand hygiene.[4,5,6,7,8,9]
- Position the patient in a way that maximizes comfort while allowing easy access to the wound site.
- Depending on the location of the wound, cover the bed linens with a fluid-impermeable pad *to help prevent soiling.*
- Place an emesis basin below the wound *so that the irrigation solution flows from the wound into the basin and drains from the clean to the dirty end of the wound.*
- Perform hand hygiene.[4,5,6,7,8,9]
- Put on a gown, a mask with a face shield or goggles and a mask, and gloves *to comply with standard precautions, because splashing may occur during pressurized irrigation.*[1,3,22,23]
- Remove the existing dressing gently, irrigating it with normal saline if necessary *to help ease removal.*
- Discard the soiled dressing in a waterproof trash container.[23]
- Remove and discard your gloves.[23]
- Perform hand hygiene.[4,5,6,7,8,9]
- Inspect the wound and surrounding tissue *to gauge the healing process and to assess for the presence of infection.*

- Establish a clean field that contains all of the equipment and supplies you'll need for irrigation and wound care.
- Pour the prescribed amount of irrigating solution into a clean or sterile irrigation container.
- Perform hand hygiene.[4,5,6,7,8,9]
- Put on gloves.[3,22,23]
- If you're using a 35-mL catheter-tip syringe and 19G angiocatheter, attach the angiocatheter to the syringe and then irrigate the wound using normal saline solution or another prescribed wound cleanser. Alternatively, irrigate the wound using a commercial wound irrigation device.[2] Apply sufficient irrigation pressure to clean the wound without damaging tissue. Also irrigate the surrounding skin. Ensure that the solution flows from the clean to the dirty area of the wound *to help prevent contamination of clean tissue by the exudate.* Also, ensure that the solution reaches all areas of the wound.
- Continue to irrigate the wound until you've administered the prescribed amount of irrigation solution or until the solution returns clear.[24] Note the amount of solution administered.
- Discard the syringe (if used) in a puncture-resistant sharps container.[23]
- Keep the patient positioned *to allow further wound drainage into the basin.*
- Dry the patient's intact skin with a sterile gauze pad.
- Apply a skin-protectant wipe and allow it to dry completely *to help prevent skin breakdown and infection.*
- Pack the wound loosely, if ordered, *to stimulate granulation.*[2]
- Apply the prescribed dressing.[2]
- Dispose of drainage and solutions properly, and clean or discard soiled equipment and supplies.[23] *To prevent contamination of other equipment,* don't return unopened sterile supplies to the sterile supply cabinet. Store them in an appropriate location in the patient's room or as directed by your facility.
- Return the patient's bed to the lowest position *to help prevent falls and maintain patient safety.*[25]
- Remove and discard your gloves and other personal protective equipment in the appropriate receptacles.[25]
- Perform hand hygiene.[4,5,6,7,8,9]
- Reassess and respond to the patient's pain by evaluating the response to treatment and progress toward pain management goals. Assess the patient for any adverse reactions and risk factors for adverse events that may result from treatment.[16]
- Perform hand hygiene.[4,5,6,7,8,9]
- Document the procedure.[26,27,28,29]

Special considerations

- Try to coordinate wound irrigation with the practitioner's visit *so the practitioner can inspect the patient's wound.*
- Use only the irrigation solution specified by the practitioner, *because other irrigants may be erosive or otherwise harmful.*
- Note that some facilities may use a splash guard for wound irrigation *to help prevent exposure to contaminated returned irrigation solution.*

Patient teaching

If the wound must be irrigated at home, teach the patient and family (if appropriate) how to perform the procedure. Ask for a return demonstration of the proper technique. Provide written instructions. Arrange for home health supplies and nursing visits, as appropriate. Urge the patient to call the practitioner if there are signs of infection.

Complications

Wound irrigation may cause excoriation and increased pain. Poor technique may increase the risk of infection. Pressure over 15 psi causes trauma to the wound and directs bacteria back into the tissue.[2]

Documentation

Record the date and time of wound irrigation, the amount and type of irrigation solution used, the appearance of the wound, the presence of any sloughing tissue or exudate, the amount of solution returned, any skin care performed around the wound, the dressings applied, and the patient's tolerance of the treatment. Document teaching provided to the patient and family (if applicable), their understanding of that teaching, and any need for follow-up teaching.

REFERENCES

1 European Pressure Ulcer Advisory Panel, et al. (2019). Prevention and treatment of pressure ulcers/injuries: Quick reference guide. http://www.internationalguideline.com/static/pdfs/Quick_Reference_Guide-10Mar2019.pdf (Level VII)
2 Baranoski, S., & Ayello, E. A. (2020). *Wound care essentials: Practice principles* (5th ed.). Philadelphia, PA: Wolters Kluwer.
3 Siegel, J. D., et al. (2007, revised 2019). 2007 guideline for isolation precautions: Preventing transmission of infectious agents in healthcare settings. https://www.cdc.gov/infectioncontrol/pdf/guidelines/isolation-guidelines-H.pdf (Level II)
4 The Joint Commission. (2021). Standard NPSG.07.01.01. *Comprehensive accreditation manual for hospitals.* Oakbrook Terrace, IL: The Joint Commission. (Level VII)
5 Centers for Disease Control and Prevention. (2002). Guideline for hand hygiene in health-care settings: Recommendations of the Healthcare Infection Control Practices Advisory Committee and the HICPAC/SHEA/APIC/IDSA Hand Hygiene Task Force. *MMWR Recommendations and Reports, 51*(RR-16), 1–45. https://www.cdc.gov/mmwr/pdf/rr/rr5116.pdf (Level II)
6 World Health Organization. (2009). WHO guidelines on hand hygiene in health care: First global patient safety challenge, clean care is safer care. https://apps.who.int/iris/bitstream/handle/10665/44102/9789241597906_eng.pdf?sequence=1 (Level IV)
7 Accreditation Association for Hospitals and Health Systems. (2020). Standard 07.01.21. *Healthcare Facilities Accreditation Program: Accreditation requirements for acute care hospitals.* Chicago, IL: Accreditation Association for Hospitals and Health Systems. (Level VII)
8 Centers for Medicare and Medicaid Services, Department of Health and Human Services. (2020). Condition of participation: Infection control. 42 C.F.R. § 482.42.
9 DNV GL-Healthcare USA, Inc. (2020). IC.1.SR.1. *NIAHO® accreditation requirements, interpretive guidelines and surveyor guidance—revision 20.0.* Milford, OH: DNV GL-Healthcare USA, Inc. (Level VII)
10 The Joint Commission. (2021). Standard NPSG.01.01.01. *Comprehensive accreditation manual for hospitals.* Oakbrook Terrace, IL: The Joint Commission. (Level VII)
11 Accreditation Association for Hospitals and Health Systems. (2020). Standard 15.01.16. *Healthcare Facilities Accreditation Program: Accreditation requirements for acute care hospitals.* Chicago, IL: Accreditation Association for Hospitals and Health Systems. (Level VII)
12 Centers for Medicare and Medicaid Services, Department of Health and Human Services. (2020). Condition of participation: Patient's rights. 42 C.F.R. § 482.13(c)(1).
13 DNV GL-Healthcare USA, Inc. (2020). PR.2.SR.5. *NIAHO® accreditation requirements, interpretive guidelines and surveyor guidance—revision 20.0.* Milford, OH: DNV GL-Healthcare USA, Inc. (Level VII)
14 The Joint Commission. (2021). Standard RI.01.01.01. *Comprehensive accreditation manual for hospitals.* Oakbrook Terrace, IL: The Joint Commission. (Level VII)
15 The Joint Commission. (2021). Standard PC.02.01.21. *Comprehensive accreditation manual for hospitals.* Oakbrook Terrace, IL: The Joint Commission. (Level VII)
16 The Joint Commission. (2021). Standard PC.01.02.07. *Comprehensive accreditation manual for hospitals.* Oakbrook Terrace, IL: The Joint Commission. (Level VII)
17 Accreditation Association for Hospitals and Health Systems. (2020). Standard 16.01.03. *Healthcare Facilities Accreditation Program: Accreditation requirements for acute care hospitals.* Chicago, IL: Accreditation Association for Hospitals and Health Systems. (Level VII)
18 Centers for Medicare and Medicaid Services, Department of Health and Human Services. (2020). Condition of participation: Nursing services. 42 C.F.R. § 482.23(c).
19 The Joint Commission. (2021). Standard MM.06.01.01. *Comprehensive accreditation manual for hospitals.* Oakbrook Terrace, IL: The Joint Commission. (Level VII)
20 DNV GL-Healthcare USA, Inc. (2020). MM.1.SR.3. *NIAHO® accreditation requirements, interpretive guidelines and surveyor guidance—revision 20.0.* Milford, OH: DNV GL-Healthcare USA, Inc. (Level VII)

21 Waters, T. R., et al. (2009). Safe patient handling training for schools of nursing. https://www.cdc.gov/niosh/docs/2009-127/pdfs/2009-127.pdf (Level VII)

22 Accreditation Association for Hospitals and Health Systems. (2020). Standard 07.01.10. *Healthcare Facilities Accreditation Program: Accreditation requirements for acute care hospitals.* Chicago, IL: Accreditation Association for Hospitals and Health Systems. (Level VII)

23 Occupational Safety and Health Administration. (2012). Bloodborne pathogens, standard number 1910.1030. https://www.osha.gov/pls/oshaweb/owadisp.show_document?p_id=10051&p_table=STANDARDS (Level VII)

24 Mak, S. S., et al. (2015). Pressurised irrigation versus swabbing method in cleansing wounds healed be secondary intention: A randomised controlled trial with cost-effectiveness analysis. *International Journal of Nursing Studies, 52,* 88–101. (Level II)

25 Ganz, D. A., et al. (2013, reviewed 2021). *Preventing falls in hospitals: A toolkit for improving quality of care* (AHRQ Publication No. 13-0015-EF). Rockville, MD: Agency for Healthcare Research and Quality. https://www.ahrq.gov/professionals/systems/hospital/fallpxtoolkit/index.html (Level VII)

26 The Joint Commission. (2021). Standard RC.01.03.01. *Comprehensive accreditation manual for hospitals.* Oakbrook Terrace, IL: The Joint Commission. (Level VII)

27 Centers for Medicare and Medicaid Services, Department of Health and Human Services. (2020). Condition of participation: Medical record services. 42 C.F.R. § 482.24(b).

28 Accreditation Association for Hospitals and Health Systems. (2020). Standard 10.00.03. *Healthcare Facilities Accreditation Program: Accreditation requirements for acute care hospitals.* Chicago, IL: Accreditation Association for Hospitals and Health Systems. (Level VII)

29 DNV GL-Healthcare USA, Inc. (2020). MR.2.SR.1. *NIAHO® accreditation requirements, interpretive guidelines and surveyor guidance—revision 20.0.* Milford, OH: DNV GL-Healthcare USA, Inc. (Level VII)

Wound photography

Wound photography may be used in conjunction with traditional wound assessment and documentation to help monitor, communicate, and record wound healing progression, complications, or failure to heal, *to better manage chronic wounds.* Wound photography isn't intended to replace traditional written documentation; instead, it's an adjunct method to support detailed, written documentation through the use of a visual record of the wound.[1,2] When obtained with a digital camera, digital wound images may be uploaded via a universal serial bus (USB) connection or a secure wireless connection to a secure server, where the image may be viewed, evaluated, and stored in the electronic medical record.[3]

Equipment

Digital camera (high resolution, preferably with automatic light and focus adjustment and a zoom feature) ▪ fluid-impermeable pad ▪ gloves ▪ sterile normal saline solution ▪ sterile gauze pads ▪ disposable ruler with metric demarcation ▪ sterile dressing supplies ▪ secure connection equipment and software (USB or wireless) ▪ Optional: prescribed pain medication, personal protective equipment (gown, mask and goggles or mask with face shield), prescribed wound cleanser, wound irrigation device, prescribed topical wound treatments and applicators.

Preparation of equipment

Inspect all equipment and supplies. If a product is expired, is defective, or has compromised integrity, remove it from patient use, label it as expired or defective, and report the expiration or defect as directed by your facility. Ensure that the camera batteries are charged and that the camera is maintained according to the manufacturer's instructions *to ensure its functionality.* Set the camera's light and focus settings to automatic if this feature is available.

Implementation

▪ Review the patient's medical record for pertinent history, the type of wound, previous assessment findings, and the treatment plan. Review prior wound images, if available.

▪ Gather and prepare the necessary equipment and supplies. Place the camera on a clean surface away from patient care items *to prevent cross-contamination.*[4]

▪ Perform hand hygiene.[5,6,7,8,9,10]

▪ Confirm the patient's identity using at least two patient identifiers.[11]

▪ Provide privacy.[12,13,14,15]

▪ Explain the procedure to the patient and family (if appropriate) according to their individual communication and learning needs *to increase their understanding, allay their fears, and enhance cooperation.*[16]

▪ If required by your facility, confirm that informed consent has been obtained and that the signed consent form is in the patient's medical record.[1,17]

▪ Screen for and assess the patient's pain using facility-defined criteria that are consistent with the patient's age, condition, and ability to understand.[18]

▪ Treat the patient's pain, as needed and ordered, using nonpharmacologic or pharmacologic approaches, or a combination. Base the treatment plan on evidence-based practices and the patient's clinical condition, past medical history, and pain management goals. Administer pain medication, as needed and ordered, following safe medication administration practices, *because wound care can be painful.* Allow adequate time for the medication to take effect.[2,18,19,20,21,22]

▪ Ensure that ambient lighting is adequate *to visualize the wound and optimize wound photography.*[23,24]

▪ Raise the bed to waist level before providing care *to prevent caregiver back strain.*[25]

▪ Perform hand hygiene.[5,6,7,8,9,10]

▪ Assist the patient to a position that maximizes comfort while allowing easy access to the wound. Expose only the wound and surrounding area *to maintain warmth and modesty.*[4,24]

▪ Place a fluid-impermeable pad under the wound *to prevent soiling.*

▪ Perform hand hygiene.[5,6,7,8,9,10]

▪ Put on gloves and, as needed, other personal protective equipment *to comply with standard precautions.*[26,27,28]

▪ Remove the existing dressing gently, irrigating it with normal saline solution (if needed) *to ease removal.*[3]

▪ Inspect the soiled dressing, note the type and amount of drainage, and discard it in an appropriate receptacle.[27]

▪ Assess the wound, wound edges, and surrounding tissue.

▪ Clean the wound with gauze pads moistened with normal saline solution or other prescribed wound cleanser, removing as much devitalized tissue and debris as possible. If adherent material is present in the wound, irrigate the wound using a wound irrigation device.[23,24]

▪ Place the disposable ruler flat against the most distal edge of the wound and outside any areas of callus or cellulitis *to allow for accurate wound size assessment upon image review.*[2,3,23,24]

▪ Remove and discard your gloves.[27]

▪ Perform hand hygiene.[5,6,7,8,9,10]

▪ Position the camera parallel to the plane of the wound or as directed by your facility, *because using the wrong camera angle can cause the wound to appear larger than it actually is.*[4]

▪ When photographing a wound, ensure that you use proper technique. Improper technique (below left), which entails positioning the camera at an angle that isn't parallel to the wound, produces a distorted photo. For proper technique (below right), position the camera parallel to the plane of the wound to produce a photo that accurately portrays the wound.

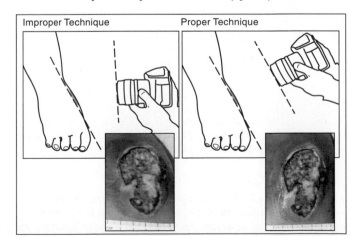

■ Adjust the distance between the camera and wound (or use the zoom feature, if present) so that the image obtained includes the entire wound, a sample of the surrounding skin, and the disposable ruler in the image frame but excludes the rest of the patient (especially the face or any other identifying characteristics) and surrounding objects.[3,4,23,24]

■ If an automatic focus feature isn't present on the camera, focus the image so that the lines on the ruler are well-defined, *to capture a clear image.*[3,24]

■ Review the image on the digital display screen *to ensure that the image is high quality.* Repeat the process, as needed, *to capture a high-quality image.* Distance from the wound should be as directed by your facility protocol, but serial photographs of the same wound should be at a consistent distance.[3,24]

■ Perform hand hygiene.[5,6,7,8,9,10]

■ Put on gloves *to comply with standard precautions.*[26,27,28]

■ Apply topical wound treatments, if prescribed, following safe medication administration practices.[19,20,21,22]

■ Apply the appropriate type of sterile dressing based on the type of wound and degree of drainage and according to practitioner orders.[29,30]

■ Return the bed to the lowest position *to prevent falls and maintain the patient's safety.*[31]

■ Discard used supplies in appropriate receptacles.[27]

■ Remove and discard your gloves and, if worn, any other personal protective equipment.[27]

■ Perform hand hygiene.[5,6,7,8,9,10]

■ Reassess and respond to the patient's pain by evaluating the response to treatment and progress toward pain management goals. Assess for adverse reactions and risk factors for adverse events that may result from treatment.[18]

■ Perform hand hygiene.[5,6,7,8,9,10]

■ Upload the images and required associated information (patient identifying information, anatomic location, and date and time the images were taken, if not automatically recorded) via a USB connection or a secure wireless connection to the patient's electronic medical record on your facility's secure server.[1,2,3,17]

■ Delete the images from the digital camera's storage.[32]

■ Document the procedure.[33,34,35,36]

Special considerations

■ Avoid using flash photography and flashlights during wound photography, *because they can cause shadows and glare, especially on moist wound surfaces.*[4,24]

■ When photographing wounds undergoing debridement, photograph the wound before and after debridement.[3]

Documentation

Record the date and time of wound photography, the anatomic location of the wound, and the number of images captured. Note the angle of the camera from the wound. Document your assessment of the wound as well as the patient's pain assessments. Document wound care provided, the patient's tolerance of the procedure, and any interventions implemented, including medications administered. Document teaching provided to the patient and family (if applicable), their understanding of that teaching, and any need for follow-up teaching.

REFERENCES

1   Wound, Ostomy, and Continence Nurses Society (WOCN). (2012). Photography in wound documentation: Fact sheet. https://pdf4pro.com/fullscreen/photography-in-wound-documentation-fact-sheet-167a11.html (Level VII)

2   Baranoski, S., & Ayello, E. A. (2020). *Wound care essentials: Practice principles* (5th ed.). Philadelphia, PA: Wolters Kluwer.

3   Rennert, R., et al. (2009). Standardization of wound photography using the wound electronic medical record. *Advances in Skin & Wound Care, 22,* 32–38.

4   Bradshaw, L. M., et al. (2011). Collaboration in wound photography competency development: A unique approach. *Advances in Skin & Wound Care, 24,* 85–92.

5   Accreditation Association for Hospitals and Health Systems. (2020). Standard 07.01.21. *Healthcare Facilities Accreditation Program: Accreditation requirements for acute care hospitals.* Chicago, IL: Accreditation Association for Hospitals and Health Systems. (Level VII)

6   Centers for Disease Control and Prevention. (2002). Guideline for hand hygiene in health-care settings: Recommendations of the Healthcare Infection Control Practices Advisory Committee and the HICPAC/SHEA/APIC/IDSA Hand Hygiene Task Force. *MMWR Recommendations and Reports, 51*(RR-16), 1–45. https://www.cdc.gov/mmwr/pdf/rr/rr5116.pdf (Level II)

7   Centers for Medicare and Medicaid Services, Department of Health and Human Services. (2020). Condition of participation: Infection control. 42 C.F.R. § 482.42.

8   DNV GL-Healthcare USA, Inc. (2020). IC.1.SR.1. *NIAHO® accreditation requirements, interpretive guidelines and surveyor guidance—revision 20.0.* Milford, OH: DNV GL-Healthcare USA, Inc. (Level VII)

9   The Joint Commission. (2021). Standard NPSG.07.01.01. *Comprehensive accreditation manual for hospitals.* Oakbrook Terrace, IL: The Joint Commission. (Level VII)

10 World Health Organization. (2009). WHO guidelines on hand hygiene in health care: First global patient safety challenge, clean care is safer care. https://apps.who.int/iris/bitstream/handle/10665/44102/9789241597906_eng.pdf?sequence=1 (Level IV)

11 The Joint Commission. (2021). Standard NPSG.01.01.01. *Comprehensive accreditation manual for hospitals.* Oakbrook Terrace, IL: The Joint Commission. (Level VII)

12 Accreditation Association for Hospitals and Health Systems. (2020). Standard 15.01.16. *Healthcare Facilities Accreditation Program: Accreditation requirements for acute care hospitals.* Chicago, IL: Accreditation Association for Hospitals and Health Systems. (Level VII)

13 Centers for Medicare and Medicaid Services, Department of Health and Human Services. (2020). Condition of participation: Patient's rights. 42 C.F.R. § 482.13(c)(1).

14 DNV GL-Healthcare USA, Inc. (2020). PR.2.SR.5. *NIAHO® accreditation requirements, interpretive guidelines and surveyor guidance– revision 20.0.* Milford, OH: DNV GL-Healthcare USA, Inc. (Level VII)

15 The Joint Commission. (2021). Standard RI.01.01.01. *Comprehensive accreditation manual for hospitals.* Oakbrook Terrace, IL: The Joint Commission. (Level VII)

16 The Joint Commission. (2021). Standard PC.02.01.21. *Comprehensive accreditation manual for hospitals.* Oakbrook Terrace, IL: The Joint Commission. (Level VII)

17 Wiedemann, L. A. (2010). Using clinical photos in EHRs. *Journal of the American Health Information Management Association, 81*(4), 44–45.

18 The Joint Commission. (2021). Standard PC.01.02.07. *Comprehensive accreditation manual for hospitals.* Oakbrook Terrace, IL: The Joint Commission. (Level VII)

19 Accreditation Association for Hospitals and Health Systems. (2020). Standard 16.01.03. *Healthcare Facilities Accreditation Program: Accreditation requirements for acute care hospitals.* Chicago, IL: Accreditation Association for Hospitals and Health Systems. (Level VII)

20 Centers for Medicare and Medicaid Services, Department of Health and Human Services. (2020). Condition of participation: Nursing services. 42 C.F.R. § 482.23(c).

21 DNV GL-Healthcare USA, Inc. (2020). MM.1.SR.3. *NIAHO® accreditation requirements, interpretive guidelines and surveyor guidance—revision 20.0.* Milford, OH: DNV GL-Healthcare USA, Inc. (Level VII)

22 The Joint Commission. (2021). Standard MM.06.01.01. *Comprehensive accreditation manual for hospitals.* Oakbrook Terrace, IL: The Joint Commission. (Level VII)

23 Li, D., et al. (2018). The characteristics of pressure injury photographs from the electronic health record in clinical settings. *Journal of Clinical Nursing, 27,* 819–828. (Level VI)

24 Thompson, N., et al. (2013). Reliability and validity of the revised photographic wound assessment tool on digital images taken of various types of chronic wounds. *Advances in Skin & Wound Care, 26,* 360–373. (Level VI)

25 Waters, T. R., et al. (2009). Safe patient handling training for schools of nursing. http://www.cdc.gov/niosh/docs/2009-127/pdfs/2009-127.pdf (Level VII)

26 Accreditation Association for Hospitals and Health Systems. (2020). Standard 07.01.10. *Healthcare Facilities Accreditation Program: Accreditation requirements for acute care hospitals.* Chicago, IL: Accreditation Association for Hospitals and Health Systems. (Level VII)

27 Occupational Safety and Health Administration. (2012). Bloodborne pathogens, standard number 1910.1030. https://www.osha.gov/pls/oshaweb/owadisp.show_document?p_id=10051&p_table=STANDARDS (Level VII)

28 Siegel, J. D., et al. (2007, revised 2019). *2007 guideline for isolation precautions: Preventing transmission of infectious agents in healthcare settings.* https://www.cdc.gov/infectioncontrol/pdf/guidelines/isolation-guidelines-H.pdf (Level II)

29 Dhivya, S., et al. (2015). Wound dressings—A review. *BioMedicine, 5*(4), 24–28. https://biomedicine.cmu.edu.tw/doc/17-4.pdf

30 Skórkowska-Telichowska, K., et al. (2013). The local treatment and available dressings designed for chronic wounds. *Journal of the American Academy of Dermatology, 68,* e117–e126.

31 Ganz, D. A., et al. (2013, reviewed 2021). *Preventing falls in hospitals: A toolkit for improving quality of care* (AHRQ Publication No. 13-0015-EF). Rockville, MD: Agency for Healthcare Research and Quality. https://www.ahrq.gov/sites/default/files/publications/files/fallpxtoolkit_0.pdf (Level VII)

32 Spear, M. (2011). Wound photography: Considerations and recommendations. *Plastic Surgical Nursing, 31,* 82–83.

33 Accreditation Association for Hospitals and Health Systems. (2020). Standard 10.00.03. *Healthcare Facilities Accreditation Program: Accreditation requirements for acute care hospitals.* Chicago, IL: Accreditation Association for Hospitals and Health Systems. (Level VII)

34 Centers for Medicare and Medicaid Services, Department of Health and Human Services. (2020). Condition of participation: Medical record services. 42 C.F.R. § 482.24(b).

35 DNV GL-Healthcare USA, Inc. (2020). MR.2.SR.1. *NIAHO® accreditation requirements, interpretive guidelines and surveyor guidance– revision 20.0.* Milford, OH: DNV GL-Healthcare USA, Inc. (Level VII)

36 The Joint Commission. (2021). Standard RC.01.03.01. *Comprehensive accreditation manual for hospitals.* Oakbrook Terrace, IL: The Joint Commission. (Level VII)

Z-TRACK INJECTION

The Z-track method is the preferred method for administering IM injections *because it prevents leakage, or tracking, of medication into the subcutaneous tissue (which can cause patient discomfort and may permanently stain some tissue).* Lateral displacement of the skin during the injection helps to seal the drug in the muscle.[1] This procedure requires careful attention to technique.

Equipment

Patient's medication record ▪ single-use sterile syringe with a needle of appropriate size (at least 1½" [3.8 cm] recommended)[1] and gauge (self-sheathing needle recommended)[2] ▪ prescribed medication ▪ alcohol pads ▪ puncture-resistant sharps container ▪ Optional: labels, gloves, 1" (2.5-cm) filter needle, ampule breaker.

Implementation

▪ Avoid distractions and interruptions when preparing and administering medication *to prevent medication errors.*[3,4]

▪ Verify the practitioner's order for medication.[5,6,7,8]

▪ Reconcile the patient's medications when a new medication is prescribed by the practitioner *to reduce the risk of medication administration errors, including omissions, duplications, dosing errors, and drug interactions.*[9,10]

▪ Gather and prepare the necessary equipment and supplies.

▪ Compare the medication label to the practitioner's order in the patient's medical record.[5,6,7,8]

▪ Check the patient's medical record for an allergy or a contraindication to the prescribed medication. If an allergy or a contraindication exists, don't administer the medication; instead, notify the practitioner.[5,6,7,8]

▪ Check the expiration date on the prescribed medication. If the medication is expired, return it to the pharmacy and obtain new medication.[5,6,7,8]

▪ Visually inspect the solution for particles, discoloration, or other loss of integrity; don't administer the medication if its integrity is compromised.[5,6,7,8] Keep in mind that for some drugs (such as suspensions), the presence of drug particles is normal. If in doubt, check with the pharmacist and the manufacturer's instructions.

▪ Discuss any unresolved concerns about the prescribed medication with the patient's practitioner.[5,6,7,8]

▪ Perform hand hygiene.[11,12,13,14,15,16]

▪ Carefully calculate the prescribed medication dose. If you're administering a high-alert medication that may cause significant patient harm when used in error, perform an independent double-check with another nurse if required by your facility.[17,18,19]

▪ Read the prescribed medication label again as you draw up the medication for injection, if needed.

▪ Perform hand hygiene.[11,12,13,14,15,16]

▪ Confirm the patient's identity using at least two patient identifiers.[5,20]

▪ Provide privacy.[21,22,23,24]

▪ If the patient is receiving the medication for the first time, teach the patient about potential adverse reactions and discuss any other concerns related to the medication.[5,6,7,8]

▪ Verify that the medication is being administered at the proper time, in the prescribed dose, and by the correct route *to reduce the risk of medication administration errors.*[5,6,7,8]

▪ Explain the procedure to the patient and family (if appropriate) according to their individual communication and learning needs *to increase their understanding, allay their fears, and enhance cooperation.*[25]

▪ If your facility uses a bar code technology, use it as directed by your facility.

▪ Raise the bed to waist level before providing care *to prevent caregiver back strain.*[26]

▪ Perform hand hygiene.[11,12,13,14,15,16]

NURSING ALERT If your facility's hazardous drug list contains the medication you are about to administer, put on personal protective equipment, as directed.[27]

▪ Put on gloves if contact with blood or body fluids is likely, or if your skin or the patient's skin isn't intact; glove use isn't necessary for routine IM injection.[28,29]

▪ Select an appropriate injection site. The ventrogluteal site is used most commonly for healthy adults, although the deltoid muscle may be used for a small-volume injection (2 mL or less). Remember to always rotate injection sites for patients who require repeated injections.

▪ Position and drape the patient appropriately using the bed linens, making sure the site is well exposed and that lighting is adequate.

▪ Clean the patient's skin at the injection site with an alcohol pad, moving the pad outward in a circular motion to a circumference of about 2" (5 cm) from the injection site. Then allow the skin to dry.[28]

▪ Remove the needle sheath.

▪ With your nondominant hand, displace the patient's skin laterally by pulling or pushing it ¾" to 1¼" (2 to 3 cm) away from the injection site.[1]

▪ Position the syringe at a 90-degree angle to the patient's skin surface, with the needle about 2" (5 cm) from the skin. Tell the patient to expect to feel a prick as you insert the needle. Insert the needle quickly and smoothly through the skin and subcutaneous tissue and deep into the muscle at a 90-degree angle.[1]

▪ Inject the medication slowly according to the manufacturer's prescribing information.

▪ Wait 10 seconds *to ensure dispersion of the medication,* and then withdraw the needle slowly at a 90-degree angle.[30]

▪ Remove your thumb and index finger from the surface of the patient's skin, allowing the displaced skin and subcutaneous tissue to return to their normal positions *to seal the needle track,* trapping the medication in the muscle. Don't massage the injection site or allow the patient to wear a tight-fitting garment over the site, *because doing so may force the medication into subcutaneous tissue.*

- Activate the needle safety device, if available, and discard the needle and syringe in a puncture-resistant sharps container. *To avoid needle-stick injuries,* don't recap needles.[2]
- Return the bed to the lowest position *to prevent falls and maintain patient safety.*[31]
- Remove and discard your gloves, if worn.[2,29]
- Perform hand hygiene.[11,12,13,14,15,16]
- Document the procedure.[32,33,34,35]

Special considerations

- The Joint Commission issued a sentinel event alert concerning the transmission of pathogens related to the misuse of vials that have caused viral and bacterial infections, including hepatitis B, hepatitis C, meningitis, and epidural abscesses. These infections have been attributed to the reuse of single-dose vials that don't typically contain preservatives, re-entering multidose vials with used syringes and needles, and using multidose vials for multiple patients. To prevent these infections, follow evidence-based best practices, such as disinfecting the vial's rubber stopper before piercing, using single-dose vials only once and then discarding the vial, dedicating multidose vials to a single patient, and using a new syringe and needle when re-entering a multidose vial. Assign the appropriate "beyond-use" date when first entering a multidose vial, and store multidose vials as directed by your facility and according to the manufacturer's instructions.[36]
- If the patient is receiving multiple injections or an injection daily, rotate IM injection sites.

Complications

Discomfort and tissue irritation may result from drug leakage into subcutaneous tissue. Failure to rotate IM injection sites in patients who require repeated injections can interfere with the absorption of medication. Unabsorbed medications may build up in deposits that may reduce the desired pharmacologic effect and may lead to abscess formation or tissue fibrosis. Improper technique can result in injury to blood vessels, bone, and peripheral nerves.[1] Other complications may occur depending on the medication administered.

Documentation

Record the prescribed medication, dosage, date and time of administration, and IM injection site on the patient's medication record. Include the patient's response to the injected medication. Document teaching provided to the patient and family (if applicable), their understanding of that teaching, and any need for follow-up teaching.

REFERENCES

1 Hopkins, U., & Arias, C. Y. (2013). Large-volume IM injections: A review of best practices. *Oncology Nurse Advisor*, 2013, 32–37. (Level V)
2 Occupational Safety and Health Administration. (2012). Bloodborne pathogens, standard number 1910.1030. https://www.osha.gov/pls/oshaweb/owadisp.show_document?p_id=10051&p_table=STANDARDS (Level VII)
3 Westbrook, J., et al. (2010). Association of interruptions with an increased risk and severity of medication administration errors. *Archives of Internal Medicine, 170*, 683–690. (Level IV)
4 Institute for Safe Medication Practices. (2012). Side tracks on the safety express: Interruptions lead to errors and unfinished…Wait, what was I doing? *Nurse Advise-ERR, 11*(2), 1–4. https://www.ismp.org/resources/side-tracks-safety-express-interruptions-lead-errors-and-unfinished-wait-what-was-i-doing?id=37
5 Accreditation Association for Hospitals and Health Systems. (2020). Standard 16.01.03. *Healthcare Facilities Accreditation Program: Accreditation requirements for acute care hospitals.* Chicago, IL: Accreditation Association for Hospitals and Health Systems. (Level VII)
6 Centers for Medicare and Medicaid Services, Department of Health and Human Services. (2020). Condition of participation: Nursing services. 42 C.F.R. § 482.23(c).
7 DNV GL-Healthcare USA, Inc. (2020). MM.1.SR.3. *NIAHO accreditation requirements, interpretive guidelines and surveyor guidance—revision 20.0.* Milford, OH: DNV GL-Healthcare USA, Inc. (Level VII)
8 The Joint Commission. (2021). Standard MM.06.01.01. *Comprehensive accreditation manual for hospitals.* Oakbrook Terrace, IL: The Joint Commission. (Level VII)
9 Accreditation Association for Hospitals and Health Systems. (2020). Standard 25.02.13. *Healthcare Facilities Accreditation Program: Accreditation requirements for acute care hospitals.* Chicago, IL: Accreditation Association for Hospitals and Health Systems. (Level VII)
10 The Joint Commission. (2021). Standard NPSG.03.06.01. *Comprehensive accreditation manual for hospitals.* Oakbrook Terrace, IL: The Joint Commission. (Level VII)
11 The Joint Commission. (2021). Standard NPSG.07.01.01. *Comprehensive accreditation manual for hospitals.* Oakbrook Terrace, IL: The Joint Commission. (Level VII)
12 Centers for Disease Control and Prevention. (2002). Guideline for hand hygiene in health-care settings: Recommendations of the Healthcare Infection Control Practices Advisory Committee and the HICPAC/SHEA/APIC/IDSA Hand Hygiene Task Force. *MMWR Recommendations and Reports, 51*(RR-16), 1–45. https://www.cdc.gov/mmwr/pdf/rr/rr5116.pdf (Level II)
13 World Health Organization. (2009). WHO guidelines on hand hygiene in health care: First global patient safety challenge, clean care is safer care. https://apps.who.int/iris/bitstream/handle/10665/44102/9789241597906_eng.pdf?sequence=1 (Level IV)
14 Accreditation Association for Hospitals and Health Systems. (2020). Standard 07.01.21. *Healthcare Facilities Accreditation Program: Accreditation requirements for acute care hospitals.* Chicago, IL: Accreditation Association for Hospitals and Health Systems. (Level VII)
15 Centers for Medicare and Medicaid Services, Department of Health and Human Services. (2020). Condition of participation: Infection control. 42 C.F.R. § 482.42.
16 DNV GL-Healthcare USA, Inc. (2020). IC.1.SR.1. *NIAHO® accreditation requirements, interpretive guidelines and surveyor guidance—revision 20.0.* Milford, OH: DNV GL-Healthcare USA, Inc. (Level VII)
17 Institute for Safe Medication Practices. (2018). ISMP list of high-alert medications in acute care settings. https://www.ismp.org/sites/default/files/attachments/2018-08/highAlert2018-Acute-Final.pdf
18 Institute for Safe Medication Practice. (2019). Independent double checks: Worth the effort if used judiciously and properly. https://www.ismp.org/resources/independent-double-checks-worth-effort-if-used-judiciously-and-properly (Level VII)
19 Institute for Safe Medication Practices ISMP). (2020). 2020-2021 targeted medication safety best practices for hospitals. https://www.ismp.org/sites/default/files/attachments/2020-02/2020-2021%20TMSBP-%20FINAL_1.pdf
20 The Joint Commission. (2021). Standard NPSG.01.01.01. *Comprehensive accreditation manual for hospitals.* Oakbrook Terrace, IL: The Joint Commission. (Level VII)
21 Centers for Medicare and Medicaid Services, Department of Health and Human Services. (2020). Condition of participation: Patient's rights. 42 C.F.R. § 482.13(c)(1).
22 Accreditation Association for Hospitals and Health Systems. (2020). Standard 15.01.16. *Healthcare Facilities Accreditation Program: Accreditation requirements for acute care hospitals.* Chicago, IL: Accreditation Association for Hospitals and Health Systems. (Level VII)
23 DNV GL-Healthcare USA, Inc. (2020). PR.2.SR.5. *NIAHO® accreditation requirements, interpretive guidelines and surveyor guidance – revision 20.0.* Milford, OH: DNV GL-Healthcare USA, Inc. (Level VII)
24 The Joint Commission. (2021). Standard RI.01.01.01. *Comprehensive accreditation manual for hospitals.* Oakbrook Terrace, IL: The Joint Commission. (Level VII)
25 The Joint Commission. (2021). Standard PC.02.01.21. *Comprehensive accreditation manual for hospitals.* Oakbrook Terrace, IL: The Joint Commission. (Level VII)
26 Waters, T. R., et al. (2009). Safe patient handling training for schools of nursing. https://www.cdc.gov/niosh/docs/2009-127/pdfs/2009-127.pdf (Level VII)
27 The United States Pharmacopeial Convention. (2019). USP general chapter <800> Hazardous drugs—Handling in healthcare settings. https://www.usp.org/compounding/general-chapter-hazardous-drugs-handling-healthcare (Level VII)
28 World Health Organization. (2010). WHO best practices for injections and related procedures toolkit. https://apps.who.int/iris/bitstream/handle/10665/44298/9789241599252_eng.pdf;jsessionid=3DA960E-1CD99D06B06264613DE77A19F?sequence=1 (Level IV)

29 Accreditation Association for Hospitals and Health Systems. (2020). Standard 07.01.10. *Healthcare Facilities Accreditation Program: Accreditation requirements for acute care hospitals.* Chicago, IL: Accreditation Association for Hospitals and Health Systems. (Level VII)

30 Ogston-Tuck, S. (2014). Intramuscular injection technique: An evidence-based approach. *Nursing Standard.* 29(4), 52–59.

31 Ganz, D. A., et al. (2013, reviewed 2021). *Preventing falls in hospitals: A toolkit for improving quality of care* (AHRQ Publication No. 13-0015-EF). Rockville, MD: Agency for Healthcare Research and Quality. https://www.ahrq.gov/professionals/systems/hospital/fallpxtoolkit/index.html (Level VII)

32 The Joint Commission. (2021). Standard RC.01.03.01. *Comprehensive accreditation manual for hospitals.* Oakbrook Terrace, IL: The Joint Commission. (Level VII)

33 Accreditation Association for Hospitals and Health Systems. (2020). Standard 10.00.03. *Healthcare Facilities Accreditation Program: Accreditation requirements for acute care hospitals.* Chicago, IL: Accreditation Association for Hospitals and Health Systems. (Level VII)

34 Centers for Medicare and Medicaid Services, Department of Health and Human Services. (2020). Condition of participation: Medical record services. 42 C.F.R. § 482.24(b).

35 DNV GL-Healthcare USA, Inc. (2020). MR.2.SR.1. *NIAHO® accreditation requirements, interpretive guidelines and surveyor guidance—revision 20.0.* Milford, OH: DNV GL-Healthcare USA, Inc. (Level VII)

36 The Joint Commission. (2014). Sentinel event alert 52: Preventing infection from the misuse of vials. https://www.jointcommission.org/-/media/tjc/documents/resources/patient-safety-topics/sentinel-event/sea_52.pdf (Level VII)

Index

Note: The letter i following a page number indicates an illustration; t indicates a table